GASTROENTEROLOGY

GYNECOLOGY AND OBSTETRICS

HEMATOLOGY/ONCOLOGY

Expert CONSULT

Activate your access at expertconsult.com

1 REGISTER

- Visit **expertconsult.com.**
- Click **"Register Now."**
- Fill in your **user information.**
- Click **"Create Account."**

2 ACTIVATE YOUR BOOK

- Scratch off your **Activation Code** below and enter it into the **"Add a title"** box.
- **You're done!** Click on the book's title under **"My Titles."**

For technical assistance, email **online.help@elsevier.com** or call **800-401-9962** (inside the US) or **+1-314-995-3200** (outside the US).

Scratch off Below
Ferri

Activation Code MKF[illegible]

MISCELLANEOUS

NEPHROLOGY

NEUROLOGY

2011 Ferri's CLINICAL ADVISOR

5 Books in 1

FRED F. FERRI, M.D., F.A.C.P.
Clinical Professor
Alpert Medical School
Brown University
Providence, Rhode Island

ELSEVIER
MOSBY

ELSEVIER
MOSBY

1600 John F. Kennedy Blvd.
Ste 1800
Philadelphia, PA 19103-2899

FERRI'S CLINICAL ADVISOR 2011: INSTANT DIAGNOSIS AND TREATMENT ISSN: 1541-4515

Notice

Knowledge and best practice in this field are constantly changing. As new research and experience broaden our knowledge, changes in practice, treatment, and drug therapy may become necessary or appropriate. Readers are advised to check the most current information provided (i) on procedures featured or (ii) by the manufacturer of each product to be administered, to verify the recommended dose or formula, the method and duration of administration, and contraindications. It is the responsibility of the practitioner, relying on their own experience and knowledge of the patient, to make diagnoses, to determine dosages and the best treatment for each individual patient, and to take all appropriate safety precautions. To the fullest extent of the law, neither the Publisher nor the Editors assume any liability for any injury and/or damage to persons or property arising out of or related to any use of the material contained in this book.

The Publisher

ISSN: 1541-4515

Acquisitions Editor: Druanne Martin
Developmental Editor: Lucia Gunzel
Editorial Assistant: John Ingram
Design Direction: Ellen Zanolle
Marketing Manager: Helena Mutak

Printed in the United States of America

Last digit is the print number: 9 8 7 6 5 4 3 2 1

Section Editors

RUBEN ALVERO, M.D.
Associate Professor
Obstetrics and Gynecology
University of Colorado Health Sciences Center
Aurora, Colorado
SECTION I

JEFFREY M. BORKAN, M.D., PH.D.
Professor and Chair
Department of Family Medicine
Physician-in-Chief
Alpert Medical School
Brown University
Providence, Rhode Island
Memorial Hospital of Rhode Island
Pawtucket, Rhode Island
SECTION I

MICHAEL R. DOBBS, M.D.
Assistant Professor
Neurology and Preventative Medicine
Neurology Residency Program Director
Medical Director
Stroke Care
Chandler Medical Center
University of Kentucky
Lexington, Kentucky
SECTION I

MITCHELL D. FELDMAN, M.D., M.PHIL.
Professor of Medicine
Director of Faculty Mentoring
University of California, San Francisco
Division of General Internal Medicine
San Francisco, California
SECTION I

FRED F. FERRI, M.D., F.A.C.P.
Clinical Professor
Alpert Medical School
Brown University
Providence, Rhode Island
SECTIONS I-V

GLENN G. FORT, M.D., M.P.H., F.A.C.P., F.I.D.S.A.
Clinical Associate Professor of Medicine
Alpert Medical School
Brown University
Chief
Infectious Diseases
Our Lady of Fatima Hospital
North Providence, Rhode Island
SECTION I

LONNIE R. MERCIER, M.D.
Clinical Instructor
Department of Orthopedic Surgery
Creighton University School of Medicine
Omaha, Nebraska
SECTION I

DENNIS J. MIKOLICH, M.D., F.A.C.P., F.C.C.P.
Chief
Division of Infectious Diseases
VA Medical Center
Clinical Associate Professor of Medicine
Alpert Medical School
Brown University
Providence, Rhode Island
SECTION I

IRIS TONG, M.D.
Assistant Professor (Clinical)
Alpert Medical School
Brown University
Division of Ambulatory General Internal Medicine
Rhode Island Hospital
Providence, Rhode Island
SECTION I

WEN-CHIH WU, M.D.
Assistant Professor of Medicine
Alpert Medical School
Brown University
Cardiologist
Providence VA Medical Center
Providence, Rhode Island
SECTION I

Contributors

SONYA S. ABDEL-RAZEQ, M.D.
Clinical Assistant Instructor
Department of Obstetrics and Gynecology/Resident Education
State University of New York at Buffalo
Women's and Children's Hospital
Buffalo, New York

ABDULRAHMAN ABDULBAKI, M.D.
Assistant Instructor of Medicine
Department of Internal Medicine
Memorial Hospital of Rhode Island
Alpert Medical School
Brown University
Providence, Rhode Island

TANYA ALI, M.D.
Clinical Assistant Professor of Medicine
Department of Medicine
Alpert Medical School
Brown University
Providence, Rhode Island

PHILIP J. ALIOTTA, M.D., M.S.H.A., F.A.C.S.
Clinical Instructor
Department of Urology
School of Medicine and Biomedical Sciences
State University of New York at Buffalo
Buffalo, New York
Medical Director
Center for Urologic Research of Western New York
Williamsville, New York

RUBEN ALVERO, M.D.
Associate Professor
Obstetrics and Gynecology
University of Colorado Health Sciences Center
Aurora, Colorado

SRIVIDYA ANANDAN, M.D.
Attending Physician
Internal Medicine
Harvard Vanguard Medical Associates
Quincy, Massachusetts

GOWRI ANANDARAJAH, M.D.
Clinical Associate Professor
Department of Family Medicine
Alpert Medical School
Brown University
Providence, Rhode Island

MEL L. ANDERSON, M.D., F.A.C.P.
Assistant Professor of Medicine
University of Colorado School of Medicine
Denver Veterans Affairs Medical Center
Denver, Colorado

MICHELLE STOZEK ANVAR, M.D.
Clinical Instructor
Division of General Internal Medicine
Rhode Island Hospital
Clinical Instructor
Alpert Medical School
Brown University
Providence, Rhode Island

ETSUKO AOKI, M.D., PH.D.
Attending Physician
Department of Hematology
Nagoya Medical Center
Nagoya, Japan

NICOLE APPELLE, M.D., M.P.H.
Department of Medicine
University of San Francisco
San Francisco, California

WISSAM S.Z. ASFAHANI, M.D.
Department of Neurosurgery
University of Kentucky
Lexington, Kentucky

SUDEEP KAUR AULAKH, M.D., C.M., F.R.C.P.C.
Director of Ambulatory Education
High Street Health Center
Assistant Professor of Medicine
Tufts University School of Medicine
Baystate Medical Center
Springfield, Massachusetts

OMRI BERGER, M.D.
Department of Psychiatry
University of California, San Francisco
San Francisco, California

SETH BERKOWITZ, M.D.
Department of Medicine
University of California, San Francisco
San Francisco, California

AGNIESZKA K. BIALIKIEWICZ, M.D.
Assistant Clinical Instructor
Department of Family Medicine
Alpert Medical School
Brown University
Providence, Rhode Island

MICHAEL BLUNDIN, M.D.
Pulmonary and Critical Care
Rhode Island Hospital

SHEENAGH M. BODKIN, M.D.
Internal Medicine
The Center for Women's Health
Providence, Rhode Island

NIRALI BORA, M.D.
Family Medicine Resident
Department of Family Medicine
Memorial Hospital of Rhode Island
Alpert Medical School
Brown University
Pawtucket, Rhode Island

JEFFREY M. BORKAN, M.D., PH.D.
Professor and Chair
Department of Family Medicine
Physician-in-Chief
Alpert Medical School
Brown University
Providence, Rhode Island
Memorial Hospital of Rhode Island
Pawtucket, Rhode Island

LYNN BOWLBY, M.D.
Attending Physician
Division of General Internal Medicine
Rhode Island Hospital
Clinical Instructor of Medicine
Alpert Medical School
Brown University
Providence, Rhode Island

MARK BRADY, M.D., M.P.H., M.M.S.
Yale-New Haven Hospital
Department of Emergency Medicine
New Haven, Connecticut

SCOTT BRANCATO, M.D.
Fellow in Cardiology
Alpert Medical School
Brown University
Providence, Rhode Island

MANDEEP K. BRAR, M.D., M.P.H.
Clinical Assistant Professor
Department of Obstetrics and Gynecology
State University of New York at Buffalo
Buffalo, New York

GAVIN BROWN, M.D.
Neuromuscular Fellow
Emory University
Atlanta, Georgia

JENNIFER BUCKLEY, M.D.
Family Medicine Resident
Memorial Hospital of Rhode Island
Alpert Medical School
Brown University
Providence, Rhode Island

JONATHAN BURNS, M.A., M.D.
Assistant Clinical Instructor
Department of Family Medicine
Alpert Medical School
Brown University
Providence, Rhode Island

DOUGLAS BURTT, M.D.
Clinical Assistant Professor of Medicine
Division of Cardiology
Alpert Medical School
Brown University
Providence, Rhode Island

STEVEN BUSSELEN, M.D.
Medical Director
Tri-Town Health Center
Johnston, Rhode Island

CLAUDIA RODRIGUEZ CABRERA, M.D.
Internal Medicine Residency Program Director
Hospital Regional Universitario de Jose Maria
Cabral y Baez
Santiago, Dominican Republic

GAURAV CHOUDHARY, M.D.
Assistant Professor of Medicine
Alpert Medical School
Brown University
Providence, Rhode Island

STEPHANIE W. CHOW, M.D.
Assistant Instructor
Department of Family Medicine
Alpert Medical School
Brown University
Providence, Rhode Island

SCOTT COHEN, M.D.
Fellow in Cardiology
Alpert Medical School
Brown University
Providence, Rhode Island

KAILA COMPTON, M.D., PH.D.
Department of Psychiatry
Residency Training Program
University of California, San Francisco
San Francisco, California

MARIA A. CORIGLIANO, M.D., F.A.C.O.G.
Clinical Assistant Professor
Department of Obstetrics and Gynecology
State University of New York at Buffalo
Buffalo, New York

BRIAN J. COWLES, PHARM.D.
Assistant Professor of Pharmacy
Department of Pharmacy Practice
Albany College of Pharmacy and Health Sciences, Vermont Campus
Colchester, Vermont

PATRICIA CRISTOFARO, M.D.
Assistant Professor of Medicine
Alpert Medical School
Brown University
Physician
Veteran's Hospital
Providence, Rhode Island

JOHN E. CROOM, M.D., PH.D.
Co-Director
Comprehensive Epilepsy Center
Saint Luke's Mid America Brain and Stroke Institute
Neurological Consultants of Kansas City, Inc.
Kansas City, Missouri

ALICIA J. CURTIN, Ph.D., G.N.P.
Assistant Professor
Division of Geriatrics
Alpert Medical School
Brown University
Providence, Rhode Island

CLAUDIA L. DADE, M.D.
Attending Physician
Division of Infectious Diseases
Elmhurst Hospital Center
Elmhurst, New York
Instructor in Medicine
Mount Sinai School of Medicine
New York, New York

GEORGE T. DANAKAS, M.D., F.A.C.O.G.
Clinical Assistant Professor
Department of Obstetrics and Gynecology
State University of New York at Buffalo
Buffalo, New York

ALEXANDRA DEGENHARDT, M.D.
Director
Multiple Sclerosis Center
New York Methodist Hospital
Brooklyn, New York

JOSEPH A. DIAZ, M.D.
Assistant Professor of Medicine
Division of General Internal Medicine
Memorial Hospital of Rhode Island
Alpert Medical School
Brown University
Providence, Rhode Island

MICHAEL R. DOBBS, M.D.
Assistant Professor
Neurology and Preventative Medicine
Neurology Residency Program Director
Medical Director
Stroke Care
Chandler Medical Center
University of Kentucky
Lexington, Kentucky

CHRISTINE M. DUFFY, M.D., M.P.H.
Fellow
Center for Gerontology and Health Care Research
Alpert Medical School
Brown University
Providence, Rhode Island

ANDREW DUKER, M.D.
Assistant Professor of Neurology
James J. and Joan A. Gardner Family Center for Parkinson's Disease and Movement Disorders
University of Cincinnati
Cincinnati, Ohio

JEFFREY S. DURMER, M.D., Ph.D., D.ABSM.
Chief Medical Officer
Fusion Sleep Center
Johns Creek, Georgia

THOMAS J. EARL, M.D.
Fellow in Cardiovascular Disease
Department of Medicine
Division of Cardiology
Alpert Medical School
Brown University
Providence, Rhode Island

STUART J. EISENDRATH, M.D.
Professor of Clinical Psychiatry
University of California, San Francisco
San Francisco, California

CHRISTINE EISENHOWER, Pharm.D
Doctor of Pharmacy Candidate
University of Rhode Island

PAMELA ELLSWORTH, M.D.
Associate Professor of Urology
Alpert Medical School
Brown University
Providence, Rhode Island

HODA ELTOMI, M.D.
Assistant Instructor
Department of Family Medicine
Memorial Hospital of Rhode Island
Alpert Medical School
Brown University
Pawtucket, Rhode Island

GREGORY J. ESPER, M.D.
Director
General Neurology
Emory University
Atlanta, Georgia

VALERIA FABRE, M.D.
Resident
Internal Medicine
Memorial Hospital of Rhode Island
Alpert Medical School
Brown University
Providence, Rhode Island

MARK J. FAGAN, M.D.
Director
Medical Primary Care Unit
Rhode Island Hospital
Associate Professor of Medicine
Alpert Medical School
Brown University
Providence, Rhode Island

GIL M. FARKASH, M.D.
Assistant Clinical Professor
State University of New York at Buffalo
School of Medicine
Buffalo, New York

TIMOTHY W. FARRELL, M.D.
Assistant Professor of Medicine (Clinical)
Adjunct Assistant Professor of Family Medicine
Division of Geriatrics
University of Utah School of Medicine
Salt Lake City, Utah

KELLY BOSSENBROK FEDORIW, M.D.
Assistant Clinical Instructor
Alpert Medical School
Brown University
Providence, Rhode Island

MITCHELL D. FELDMAN, M.D., M.PHIL.
Professor of Medicine
Director of Faculty Mentoring
University of California, San Francisco
Division of General Internal Medicine
San Francisco, California

FRED F. FERRI, M.D., F.A.C.P.
Clinical Professor
Alpert Medical School
Brown University
Providence, Rhode Island

STACI A. FISCHER, M.D., F.A.C.P.
Assistant Professor of Medicine
Division of Infectious Diseases
Alpert Medical School
Brown University
Rhode Island Hospital
Providence, Rhode Island

MARLENE FISHMAN, M.P.H., C.I.C.
Director
Nosocomial Infection
St. Joseph Health Services of Rhode Island

ILJIE KIM FITZGERALD, M.D., M.S.
Department of Psychiatry
University of California, San Francisco
San Francisco, California

TAMARA G. FONG, M.D., PH.D.
Instructor in Neurology
Beth Israel Deaconess Medical Center
Harvard Medical School
Boston, Massachusetts

GLENN G. FORT, M.D., M.P.H., F.A.C.P., F.I.D.S.A.
Clinical Associate Professor of Medicine
Alpert Medical School
Brown University
Chief
Infectious Diseases
Our Lady of Fatima Hospital
North Providence, Rhode Island

GENNA GEKHT, M.D.
Chief Resident in Neurology
Department of Neurology
Emory University
Atlanta, Georgia

ANTHONY S. GEMINIAGNI, M.D.
Fellow in Cardiology
Alpert Medical School
Brown University
Providence, Rhode Island

PAUL F. GEORGE, M.D.
Assistant Clinical Instructor
Department of Family Medicine
Alpert Medical School
Brown University
Pawtucket, Rhode Island

DAVID R. GIFFORD, M.D., M.P.H.
Director
Rhode Island Department of Health
Assistant Professor of Community Health and Medicine
Alpert Medical School
Brown University
Providence, Rhode Island

ANNGENE A. GIUSTOZZI, M.D., M.P.H.
Assistant Professor
Department of Family Medicine
Alpert Medical School
Brown University
Providence, Rhode Island

CINDY GLEIT, M.D.
Assistant Clinical Instructor
Department of Family Medicine
Alpert Medical School
Brown University
Providence, Rhode Island

GEETHA GOPALAKRISHNAN, M.D.
Assistant Professor of Medicine
Alpert Medical School
Brown University
Providence, Rhode Island

PAUL GORDON, M.D.
Clinical Assistant Professor of Medicine
Division of Cardiology
Alpert Medical School
Brown University
Providence, Rhode Island

NANCY R. GRAFF, M.D.
Associate Clinical Professor
Department of Pediatrics
University of California, San Diego
San Diego, California

JOHN A. GRAY, M.D., PH.D.
Department of Psychiatry
Postdoctoral Fellow
Department of Cellular and Molecular Pharmacology
University of California, San Francisco
San Francisco, California

ALLISON D. GRAZIADEI, M.D.
Endocrinology Fellow
Division of Endocrinology
Alpert Medical School
Brown University
Providence, Rhode Island

REBECCA A. GRIFFITH, M.D.
Attending Physician
Department of Medicine
Morristown Memorial Hospital
Morristown, New Jersey

NAWAZ HACK, M.D.
Department of Neurology
Chandler Medical Center
University of Kentucky
Lexington, Kentucky

MUSTAFA A. HAMMAD, M.D.
Clinical Neurophysiology Fellow
Department of Neurology
Emory University
Atlanta, Georgia

SAJEEV HANDA, M.D.
Director
Division of Hospitalist Medicine
Rhode Island Hospital
Clinical Instructor of Medicine
Alpert Medical School
Brown University
Providence, Rhode Island

TAYLOR HARRISON, M.D.
Assistant Professor of Neurology
Department of Neurology
Emory University
Atlanta, Georgia

CHRISTINE HARTLEY, M.D.
Assistant Clinical Instructor
Department of Family Medicine
Memorial Hospital of Rhode Island
Alpert Medical School
Brown University
Providence, Rhode Island

DON HAYES, JR., M.D.
Assistant Professor of Pediatrics and Internal Medicine
University of Kentucky College of Medicine
Director
University of Kentucky Pediatric Sleep Program
Kentucky Children's Hospital
Associate Director
University of Kentucky Healthcare Sleep Disorders Center
Lexington, Kentucky

CHRISTINE HEALY, D.O.
Assistant Clinical Instructor
Department of Family Medicine
Alpert Medical School
Brown University
Providence, Rhode Island

WILLIAM H. HEWITT, M.D.
Clinical Neurophysiology Fellow
Emory University School of Medicine
Atlanta, Georgia

KHIET C. HOANG, M.D.
Fellow in Cardiology
Irvine Medical School
University of California, Irvine
Orange, California

N. WILSON HOLLAND, M.D., F.A.C.P.
Assistant Professor of Medicine
Fellowship Director
Department of Medicine
Division of Geriatrics and Gerontology
Emory University School of Medicine
Atlanta Veterans Administration Medical Center
Atlanta, Georgia

ANNE L. HUME, PHARM.D.
Professor of Pharmacy
Department of Pharmacy Practice
University of Rhode Island
Kingston, Rhode Island
Adjunct Professor of Family Medicine
Memorial Hospital of Rhode Island
Pawtucket, Rhode Island

JENNIFER ROH HUR, M.D.
Assistant Professor of Clinical Medicine
Indiana University School of Medicine
Indianapolis, Indiana

RICHARD S. ISAACSON, M.D.
Resident in Neurology
Beth Israel Deaconess Medical Center
Harvard Medical School
Boston, Massachusetts

JENNIFER JEREMIAH, M.D.
Clinical Associate Professor of Medicine
Alpert Medical School
Brown University
Providence, Rhode Island

MICHAEL P. JOHNSON, M.D.
Staff Physician
Division of General Internal Medicine
Rhode Island Hospital
Assistant Professor of Medicine
Alpert Medical School
Brown University
Providence, Rhode Island

BREE JOHNSTON, M.D., M.P.H.
Associate Professor of Medicine
Division of Geriatrics
Department of Medicine
Veterans Affairs Medical Center
University of California, San Diego
San Diego, California

KIMBERLY JONES, M.D.
Resident Physician
Department of Child Neurology
University of Kentucky
Lexington, Kentucky

KOHAR JONES, M.D.
Clinical Assistant Professor
Department of Family Medicine
University of Chicago
Family Physician Chicago Family Health Center
Chicago, Illinois

LUCY KALANITHI, M.D.
Internal Medicine/Primary
University of California, San Francisco
San Francisco, California

KARA A. KENNEDY, D.O.
Department of Neurology
KY Clinic L-445
University of Kentucky
Lexington, Kentucky

BEVIN KENNEY, M.D.
Chief Medical Resident
Alpert Medical School
Brown University
Providence, Rhode Island

WAN J. KIM, M.D.
Clinical Instructor
Department of Obstetrics and Gynecology
State University of New York at Buffalo
Buffalo, New York

ROBERT M. KIRCHNER, M.D.
Cardiology Fellow
Division of Cardiology
Alpert Medical School
Brown University
Providence, Rhode Island

MICHAEL KLEIN, M.D.
Clinical Assistant Professor
Department of Family Medicine
Alpert Medical School
Brown University
Providence, Rhode Island

MELVYN KOBY, M.D.
Associate Clinical Professor of Medicine
Department of Ophthalmology
University of Louisville School of Medicine
Louisville, Kentucky

KENNETH KORR, M.D.
Associate Professor of Medicine
Division of Cardiology
Alpert Medical School
Brown University
Providence, Rhode Island

KRISTINA KRAMER, M.D.
Medical Director
Intensive Care Unit
John Muir Medical Center
Walnut Creek, California

DAVID I. KURSS, M.D., F.A.C.O.G.
Clinical Assistant Professor
Department of Obstetrics and Gynecology
State University of New York at Buffalo
Buffalo, New York

CINDY LAI, M.D.
Department of Medicine
University of California, San Francisco
San Francisco, California

QUANG P. LE, M.D., M.P.H.
Assistant Instructor
Department of Family Medicine
Memorial Hospital of Rhode Island
Alpert Medical School
Brown University
Providence, Rhode Island

KACHIU LEE, B.A.
Medical Student
Department of Dermatology
Feinberg School of Medicine
Northwestern University
Chicago, Illinois

MARGARET LEKANDER, M.D.
Clinical Instructor
Department of Family Medicine
Memorial Hospital of Rhode Island
Alpert Medical School
Brown University
Pawtucket, Rhode Island

DONITA DILLON LIGHTNER, M.D.
Pediatric Neurology
Department of Neurology
University of Kentucky
Lexington, Kentucky

CHUN LIM, M.D., PH.D.
Department of Neurology
Beth Israel Deaconess Medical Center
Boston, Massachusetts

RICHARD LONG, M.D.
Clinical Associate Professor
Department of Family Medicine
Alpert Medical School
Brown University
Providence, Rhode Island
Clinical Associate Professor of Family Medicine
Department of Family Medicine
Boston University School of Medicine
Boston, Massachusetts

SUSANNA R. MAGEE, M.D., M.P.H.
Assistant Professor of Family Medicine
Department of Family Medicine
Alpert Medical School
Brown University
Director of Maternal and Child Health
Memorial Hospital of Rhode Island
Pawtucket, Rhode Island

MICHAEL MAHER, M.D.
Assistant Professor of Internal Medicine
Alpert Medical School
Brown University
Rhode Island Hospital
Providence, Rhode Island

GARY S. MAK, M.D.
Cardiology Fellow
University of California, Irvine
Orange, California

ACHRAF A. MAKKI, M.D., M.Sc.
Resident
Department of Neurology
Emory University
Atlanta, Georgia

MONZR M. AL MALKI, M.D.
Biotherapeutics Development Lab
Division of Surgical Research
Boston University School of Medicine
Roger Williams Medical Center
Providence, Rhode Island

DOUGLAS W. MARTIN, M.D.
Fellow in Pulmonary Diseases and Critical Care
Alpert Medical School
Brown University
Providence, Rhode Island

DANIEL T. MATTSON, M.D., M.Sc. (MED.)
St. Louis Neurological Institute
St. Louis, Missouri

KATE MAVRICH, M.D.
Medical Resident
Alpert Medical School
Brown University
Providence, Rhode Island

ALISON MAY, M.D.
Department of Psychiatry
VA Medical Center
University of California, San Francisco
Clinical Instructor
Lyon-Martin Health Services
San Francisco, California

MAITREYI MAZUMDAR, M.D., M.P.H., M.Sc.
Instructor in Neurology
Harvard Medical School
Children's Hospital Boston
Department of Neurology
Boston, Massachusetts

KELLY A. McGARRY, M.D.
Associate Program Director
General Internal Medicine Residency Program
Rhode Island Hospital
Assistant Professor of Medicine
Alpert Medical School
Brown University
Providence, Rhode Island

LYNN McNICOLL, M.D.
Assistant Professor of Medicine
Alpert Medical School
Brown University
Geriatrician
Division of Geriatrics
Rhode Island Hospital
Providence, Rhode Island

AKANKSHA MEHTA, M.D.
Surgical Resident
Department of Urology
Brown University
Providence, Rhode Island

SHALIN B. MEHTA, M.D.
Brown Medical School
Providence, Rhode Island

LONNIE R. MERCIER, M.D.
Clinical Instructor
Department of Orthopedic Surgery
Creighton University School of Medicine
Omaha, Nebraska

DENNIS J. MIKOLICH, M.D., F.A.C.P., F.C.C.P.
Chief
Division of Infectious Diseases
VA Medical Center
Clinical Associate Professor of Medicine
Alpert Medical School
Brown University
Providence, Rhode Island

JENNIFER MIRANDA, M.D.
Endocrinology Fellow
Rhode Island Hospital
Alpert Medical School
Brown University
Providence, Rhode Island

NADIA MUJAHID, M.D.
Assistant Instructor
Department of Family Medicine
Memorial Hospital of Rhode Island
Alpert Medical School
Brown University
Pawtucket, Rhode Island

BILAL H. NAQVI, M.D.
Hematologist/Oncologist
Marshfield Clinic Regional Cancer Center
Eau Claire, Wisconsin

TAKUMA NEMOTO, M.D.
Research Associate Professor of Surgery
State University of New York at Buffalo
Buffalo, New York

JAMES J. NG, M.D.
Staff Physician
The Vancouver Clinic
Vancouver, Washington

MELISSA NOTHNAGLE, M.D.
Assistant Professor of Family Medicine
Alpert Medical School
Brown University
Providence, Rhode Island

BETH NOWAK, M.D.
Fellow
Geriatric Medicine
Boston Medical Center
Boston, Massachusetts

JUDITH NUDELMAN, M.D.
Clinical Assistant Professor
Department of Family Medicine
Alpert Medical School
Brown University
Providence, Rhode Island

GAIL M. O'BRIEN, M.D.
Medical Director
Adult Ambulatory Services
Rhode Island Hospital
Clinical Associate Professor of Medicine
Alpert Medical School
Brown University
Providence, Rhode Island

CAROLYN J. O'CONNOR, M.D.
Assistant Clinical Professor
Yale University School of Medicine
Department of Medicine
St. Mary's Hospital
Waterbury, Connecticut

ALEXANDER B. OLAWAIYE, M.D.
Fellow
Division of Gynecologic Oncology
Vincent Department of Obstetrics, Gynecology and Reproductive Biology
Massachusetts General Hospital
Harvard Medical School
Boston, Massachusetts

MICHAEL K. ONG, M.D., PH.D.
Assistant Professor
UCLA Division of General Internal Medicine/Health Services Research
UCLA School of Medicine
Los Angeles, California

STEVEN M. OPAL, M.D.
Professor of Medicine
Infectious Disease Division
Alpert Medical School
Brown University
Providence, Rhode Island

JOSEPH R. OWENS, M.D.
Department of Neurology
KY Clinic L-445
University of Kentucky
Lexington, Kentucky

CHRISTINA A. PACHECO, M.D.
Clinical Assistant Professor
Department of Family Medicine
Alpert Medical School
Brown University
Providence, Rhode Island

ROBERTO PACHECO, M.D.
Fellow in Interventional Cardiology
Alpert Medical School
Brown University
Providence, Rhode Island

JANICE PATACSIL-TRULL, M.D.
Family Practitioner
Family Medicine Associates of South Attleboro
South Attleboro, Massachusetts

BIRJU B. PATEL, M.D., F.A.C.P.
Assistant Professor of Medicine
Department of Medicine
Division of Geriatrics and Gerontology
Emory University School of Medicine
Atlanta Veterans Administration Medical Center
Atlanta, Georgia

PRANAV M. PATEL, M.D., F.A.C.C., F.S.C.A.I.
Assistant Professor of Medicine
Director
Cardiac Catheterization Laboratory
Division of Cardiology
University of California, Irvine
UCI Medical Center
Orange, California

ELENI PATROZOU, M.D.
Division of Infectious Diseases
Alpert Medical School
Brown University
Rhode Island Hospital
Providence, Rhode Island

STEVEN PELIGIAN, D.O.
Medical Director
CODAC Behavioral Healthcare
Providence, Rhode Island

HEIDI H. PETERSON, M.D.
Clinical Assistant Professor
Department of Family Medicine
Alpert Medical School
Brown University
Memorial Hospital of Rhode Island
Pawtucket, Rhode Island

PAUL A. PIRRAGLIA, M.D., M.P.H.
Assistant Professor of Medicine
Alpert Medical School
Brown University
Rhode Island Hospital
Providence, Rhode Island

SHARON S. HARTMAN POLENSEK, M.D., PH.D.
Clinical Associate
Department of Neurology
Emory University
Atlanta, Georgia

MAURICE POLICAR, M.D.
Chief of Infectious Diseases
Elmhurst Hospital Center
Elmhurst, New York
Assistant Professor of Medicine
Mount Sinai School of Medicine
New York, New York

ARUNDATHI G. PRASAD, M.D.
Clinical Instructor
Department of Obstetrics and Gynecology/Resident Education
State University of New York at Buffalo
Women's and Children's Hospital
Buffalo, New York

KITTICHAI PROMRAT, M.D.
Assistant Professor
Division of Gastroenterology
Department of Medicine
Alpert Medical School
Brown University
Chief
Gastroenterology Section
Providence Veterans Affairs Medical Center
Providence, Rhode Island

SHAHNAZ PUNJANI, M.D.
Fellow
Preventive Cardiology
Providence VA Medical Center
Alpert Medical School
Brown University
Providence, Rhode Island

JOHN RAGSDALE, M.D.
Clinical Assistant Professor of Family Medicine
Duke University Medical Center

RADHIKA RAMANAN, M.D., M.P.H.
Department of Medicine
Division of General Internal Medicine
University of California, San Francisco
San Francisco, California

CHRISTIAN N. RAMSEY III, M.D.
Assistant Professor
Department of Neurosurgery
University of Kentucky
Lexington, Kentucky

CHAITANYA V. REDDY, D.O.
Assistant Clinical Instructor
Department of Family Medicine
Alpert Medical School
Brown University
Providence, Rhode Island

RICHARD REGNANTE, M.D.
Fellow in Cardiovascular Disease
Division of Cardiovascular Medicine
Alpert Medical School
Brown University
Providence, Rhode Island

VICTOR I. REUS, M.D.
Professor of Psychiatry
Department of Psychiatry
Langley Porter Psychiatric Institute
University of California, San Francisco
San Francisco, California

HARLAN G. RICH, M.D.
Director of Endoscopy
Rhode Island Hospital
Associate Professor of Medicine
Alpert Medical School
Brown University
Providence, Rhode Island

JESSICA RISSER, M.D., M.P.H.
Third Year Dermatology Resident
Department of Dermatology
Alpert Medical School
Brown University
Providence, Rhode Island

LUTHER K. ROBINSON, M.D.
Associate Professor of Pediatrics
Director
Dysmorphology and Clinical Genetics
State University of New York at Buffalo
Buffalo, New York

AMITY RUBEOR, D.O.
Assistant Professor (Clinical) of Family Medicine
Memorial Hospital of Rhode Island
Alpert Medical School
Brown University
Pawtucket, Rhode Island

IMMAD SADIQ, M.D.
Clinical Assistant Professor of Medicine
Division of Cardiology
Alpert Medical School
Brown University
Providence, Rhode Island

HEMANT K. SATPATHY, M.D.
Fellow
Division of Maternal-Fetal Medicine
Department of Obstetrics and Gynecology
Emory University
Atlanta, Georgia

RUBY SATPATHY, M.D.
Fellow, Cardiology
Department of Internal Medicine
Creighton University
Omaha, Nebraska

JASON M. SATTERFIELD, PH.D.
Director
Behavioral Medicine
Associate Professor of Clinical Medicine
University of California, San Francisco
San Francisco, California

SEAN I. SAVITZ, M.D.
Assistant Professor of Neurology
University of Texas
Houston, Texas

SYEDA M. SAYEED, M.D.
Internal Medicine Department
Memorial Hospital of Rhode Island
Alpert Medical School
Brown University
Providence, Rhode Island

MICHAEL SCHAEFER, M.D.
Endocrinology Fellow
Rhode Island Hospital
Alpert Medical School
Brown University
Providence, Rhode Island

JACK L. SCHWARTZWALD, M.D.
Clinical Assistant Professor of Medicine
Rhode Island Hospital
Providence, Rhode Island

CATHERINE SHAFTS, D.O.
Assistant Clinical Instructor
Alpert Medical School
Brown University
Providence, Rhode Island

MADHAVI SHAH, M.D.
Assistant Clinical Instructor
Department of Family Medicine
Alpert Medical School
Brown University
Providence, Rhode Island

GRACE SHIH, M.D.
Assistant Clinical Instructor
Department of Family Medicine
Alpert Medical School
Brown University
Providence, Rhode Island

VICTOR SHIN, M.D.
Staff Cardiologist
Providence VA Medical Center
Instructor of Medicine
Alpert Medical School
Brown University
Providence, Rhode Island

MARK SIGMAN, M.D.
Associate Professor of Surgery (Urology)
Division of Urology
Alpert Medical School
Brown University
Providence, Rhode Island

JOANNE M. SILVIA, M.D.
Assistant Clinical Instructor
Department of Family Medicine
Alpert Medical School
Brown University
Providence, Rhode Island

U. SHIVRAJ SOHUR, M.D., PH.D.
Assistant Professor of Neurology
Harvard Medical School
Boston, Massachusetts

DIVJOT SOOCH, M.D.
Assistant Instructor of Family Medicine
Department of Family Medicine
Memorial Hospital of Rhode Island
Alpert Medical School
Brown University
Pawtucket, Rhode Island

JENNIFER R. SOUTHER, M.D.
Attending Physician
Department of Family Practice
Memorial Hospital of Rhode Island
Pawtucket, Rhode Island

JULIE ANNE SZUMIGALA, M.D.
Clinical Instructor
Department of Obstetrics and Gynecology
State University of New York at Buffalo
Buffalo, New York

DOMINICK TAMMARO, M.D.
Associate Director
Categorical Internal Medicine Residency
Co-Director
Medicine-Pediatrics Residency
Division of General Internal Medicine
Rhode Island Hospital
Associate Professor of Medicine
Alpert Medical School
Brown University
Providence, Rhode Island

SARAH TAPYRIK, M.D.
Pulmonary Fellow
NYU Department of Pulmonary and Critical Care
New York, New York

GLADYS TELANG, M.D.
Associate Professor of Dermatology
Alpert Medical School
Brown University
Providence, Rhode Island

IRIS TONG, M.D.
Assistant Professor (Clinical)
Alpert Medical School
Brown University
Division of Ambulatory General Internal Medicine
Rhode Island Hospital
Providence, Rhode Island

FREDERICK D. TRONCALES, M.D.
Fellow in Pulmonary Diseases and Critical Care
Alpert Medical School
Brown University
Providence, Rhode Island

MARGARET TRYFOROS, M.D.
Clinical Assistant Professor
Department of Family Medicine
Alpert Medical School
Brown University
Memorial Hospital of Rhode Island
Providence, Rhode Island

EROBOGHENE E. UBOGU, M.B.B.S. (HONS.)
Assistant Professor of Neurology
Case Western Reserve University School of Medicine
Staff Neurologist
Louis Stokes Cleveland Veterans Affairs Medical Center
Cleveland, Ohio

SEAN H. UITERWYK, M.D.
Clinical Assistant Professor
Department of Family Medicine
Alpert Medical School
Brown University
Providence, Rhode Island

NICOLE J. ULLRICH, M.D., PH.D.
Assistant Professor
Harvard Medical School
Department of Neurology
Children's Hospital Boston
Boston, Massachusetts

MARISA E. VAN POZNAK, M.D.
Attending Physician
Internal Medicine
Women and Infants Hospital
Alpert Medical School
Brown University
Providence, Rhode Island

JORGE A. VILLAFUERTE, M.D.
Attending Orthopedic Surgeon
VA Medical Center
West Roxbury, Massachusetts

HANNAH VU, D.O.
Assistant Clinical Instructor
Department of Family Medicine
Alpert Medical School
Brown University
Providence, Rhode Island

TOM J. WACHTEL, M.D.
Physician-in-Charge
Division of Geriatrics
Rhode Island Hospital
Professor of Community Health and Medicine
Alpert Medical School
Brown University
Providence, Rhode Island

TARA M. WAYT, D.O.
Resident Physician
University of Connecticut
Department of Emergency Medicine

DENNIS M. WEPPNER, M.D., F.A.C.O.G.
Associate Professor of Clinical Gynecology/Obstetrics
State University of New York at Buffalo
Clinical Chief
Department of Gynecology/Obstetrics
Millard Fillmore Hospital
Buffalo, New York

JORDAN WHITE, M.D.
Assistant Instructor
Department of Family Medicine
Alpert Medical School
Brown University
Memorial Hospital of Rhode Island
Pawtucket, Rhode Island

LAUREL M. WHITE, M.D.
Clinical Assistant Professor
Department of Obstetrics and Gynecology
Division of Maternal Fetal Medicine
State University of New York at Buffalo
Buffalo, New York

MATTHEW P. WICKLUND, M.D., F.A.A.N.
Chairman
Department of Neurology
San Antonio Military Medical Center
San Antonio, Texas

DAVID P. WILLIAMS, M.D.
Neurologist
Peachtree Neurological Clinics, PC
Atlanta, Georgia

CHARLES WOLFF, M.D.
Board Certified Family Medicine
Board Certified Hospice and Palliative Care Medicine
Interim Chief of Geriatrics and Assistant Professor of Clinical Medicine
Department of Family Medicine
Alpert Medical School
Brown University
Pawtucket, Rhode Island

MARIE ELIZABETH WONG, M.D.
Physician
Family Medicine
Baystate Brightwood Health Center
Springfield, Massachusetts

WEN-CHIH WU, M.D.
Assistant Professor of Medicine
Alpert Medical School
Brown University
Cardiologist
Providence VA Medical Center
Providence, Rhode Island

WEN Y. (HELENA) WU-CHEN, M.D.
Department of Neurology
Temple University Hospital
Philadelphia, Pennsylvania

BETH J. WUTZ, M.D.
Clinical Assistant Professor of Medicine
Division of Internal Medicine/Pediatrics
Kajeida Health–Buffalo General Hospital
State University of New York at Buffalo
Buffalo, New York

JOHN Q. YOUNG, M.D., M.P.P.
Clinic
Associate Program Director
Residency Training Program
Department of Psychiatry
UCSF School of Medicine
University of California, San Francisco
San Francisco, California

CINDY ZADIKOFF, M.D., F.R.C.P.C.
Assistant Professor of Neurology
Parkinson's Disease and Movement Disorders Center
Davee Department of Neurology and Clinical Neurological Sciences
Feinberg School of Medicine
Northwestern University
Chicago, Illinois

FARIHA ZAHEER, M.D.
Department of Neurology
University of Kentucky
Lexington, Kentucky

SCOTT J. ZUCCALA, D.O., F.A.C.O.G.
Staff Physician
Mercy Hospital of Buffalo
Buffalo, New York

RYAN W. ZUZEK, M.D.
Clinical Cardiology Fellow
Division of Cardiology
Alpert Medical School
Brown University
Providence, Rhode Island

To our families.
Their constant support and encouragement made this book a reality.

Preface

This book is intended to be a clear and concise reference for physicians and allied health professionals. Its user-friendly format was designed to provide a fast and efficient way to identify important clinical information and to offer practical guidance in patient management. The book is divided into five sections and an appendix, each with emphasis on clinical information.

The tremendous success of the previous editions and the enthusiastic comments from numerous colleagues have brought about several positive changes. Each section has also been significantly expanded from prior editions, bringing the total number of medical topics covered in this book to more than 1000. Illustrations have been added to several topics to enhance recollection of clinically important facts. The use of ICD-9CM codes in all the topics will expedite claims submission and reimbursement.

Section I describes in detail well over 700 medical disorders. Several new topics have been added to the 2011 edition. Each medical topic in this section is arranged alphabetically, and the material in each topic is presented in outline format for ease of retrieval. Topics with an accompanying algorithm in Section III are identified with an algorithm symbol (ALG). Similarly, if topics also have a Patient Teaching Guide (PTG) available online, this has been noted. All the PTGs have been completely revised for the 2011 edition. Throughout the text, key, quick-access information is consistently highlighted; clinical photographs are used to further illustrate selected medical conditions; and relevant ICD-9CM codes are listed. Most references focus on current peer-reviewed journal articles rather than outdated textbooks and old review articles. Evidence-based medicine data have been added to relevant topics.

Topics in this section use the following structured approach:

1. Basic Information (Definition, Synonyms, ICD-9CM Codes, Epidemiology & Demographics, Physical Findings & Clinical Presentation, Etiology)
2. Diagnosis (Differential Diagnosis, Workup, Laboratory Tests, Imaging Studies)
3. Treatment (Nonpharmacologic Therapy, Acute General Rx, Chronic Rx, Disposition, Referral)
4. Pearls & Considerations (Comments, Suggested Readings)
5. Evidence-Based Data and References

Section II includes the differential diagnosis, etiology, and classification of signs and symptoms. This section has been significantly expanded for the 2011 edition. It is a practical section that allows the user investigating a physical complaint or abnormal laboratory value to follow a "workup" leading to a diagnosis. The physician can then easily look up the presumptive diagnosis in Section I for the information specific to that illness.

Section III includes clinical algorithms to guide and expedite the patient's workup and therapy. For the 2011 edition, several new algorithms have been added and many others have been revised. To limit the size of the book, several algorithms have been moved to online-only format. Many physicians describe this section as particularly valuable in today's managed-care environment.

Section IV includes normal laboratory values and interpretation of results of commonly ordered laboratory tests. By providing interpretation of abnormal results, this section facilitates the diagnosis of medical disorders and further adds to the comprehensive, "one-stop" nature of our text. This section has also expanded for the 2011 edition.

Section V focuses on preventive medicine and offers essential guidelines from the U.S. Preventive Services Task Force. Information in this section includes recommendations for the periodic health examination, screening for major diseases and disorders, patient counseling, and immunization and chemoprophylaxis recommendations. A portion of this section has been moved to the electronic-only format to limit the total page count for the 2011 edition.

The **Appendix** has been divided into two major sections. Section I contains extensive information on complementary and alternative medicine (CAM). With the material in this appendix, we hope to lessen the current scarcity of exposure of allopathic and osteopathic physicians to the diversity of CAM therapies. Section II of the Appendix, available online, contains an extensive section on primary care procedures.

As clinicians, we all realize the importance of patient education and the need for clear communication with our patients. Toward that end, practical patient instruction sheets, organized alphabetically and covering the majority of the topics in this book, are available online and can be easily customized and printed from any computer. All of them have been updated, and over 100 new ones have been added to the 2011 edition. They represent a valuable addition to patient care and are useful to improve physician-patient communication, patient satisfaction, and quality of care.

I believe that we have produced a state-of-the-art information system with significant differences from existing texts. It contains five sections and patient education guides that could be sold separately based on their content, yet are available under a single cover, offering the reader a tremendous value. I hope that the *Clinical Advisor*'s user-friendly approach, numerous unique features, and yearly updates will make this book a valuable medical reference, not only to primary care physicians but also to physicians in other specialties, medical students, and allied health professionals.

Fred F. Ferri, M.D., F.A.C.P.

Note: Comments from readers are always appreciated and can be forwarded directly to Dr. Ferri at fred_ferri@brown.edu.

EVALUATION OF EVIDENCE

Ferri's Clinical Advisor evaluates all evidence based on a rating system published by the American Academy of Family Physicians. In order to indicate the strength of the supporting evidence, each summary statement is accorded one of three levels:

LEVEL A

- Systematic reviews of randomized controlled trials, including meta-analyses
- Good-quality randomized controlled trials

LEVEL B

- Good-quality nonrandomized clinical trials
- Systematic reviews not in Level A
- Lower-quality randomized controlled trials not in Level A
- Other types of study: case-control studies, clinical cohort studies, cross-sectional studies, retrospective studies, and uncontrolled studies

LEVEL C

- Evidence-based consensus statements and expert guidelines

SOURCES OF EVIDENCE

Evidence is summarized principally from three critically evaluated, very highly regarded sources:

- **Cochrane Systematic Reviews** are respected throughout the world as one of the most rigorous searches of medical journals for randomized controlled trials. They provide highly structured systematic reviews, with evidence included or excluded on the basis of explicit quality-related criteria, and they often use meta-analyses to increase the power of the findings of numerous studies.
- ***Clinical Evidence*** is produced by the BMJ Publishing Group. It provides synopses of the best currently available evidence on the treatment and prevention of many clinical conditions, based on searches and appraisals of the available literature.
- **The National Guideline Clearinghouse™** is a comprehensive database of evidence-based clinical practice guidelines and related documents produced by the Agency for Healthcare Research and Quality in partnership with the American Medical Association and the American Association of Health Plans.

In addition, where evidence exists that has not yet been critically reviewed in one of the three sites above, the evidence is summarized briefly, categorized, and fully referenced. Guidelines are also sourced from government and professional bodies.

Contents

Detailed Contents

SECTION I Diseases and Disorders

PTG indicates that a Patient Teaching Guide is available at www.expertconsult.com.

SECTION II **Differential Diagnosis**

SECTION III **Clinical Algorithms**

SECTION IV Laboratory Tests and Interpretation of Results

SECTION V **Clinical Practice Guidelines**

PART A • THE PERIODIC HEALTH EXAMINATION

PART B • IMMUNIZATIONS AND CHEMOPROPHYLAXIS

APPENDIX I **Complementary and Alternative Medicine**

APPENDIX II **Primary Care Procedures, available at www.expertconsult.com**

Additional PTGs Available at www.expertconsult.com Not Linked to Topics in Section I

Additional Algorithms Available at www.expertconsult.com

SECTION I

Diseases and Disorders

BASIC INFORMATION

DEFINITION

Abruptio placentae is the separation of placenta from the uterine wall before delivery of the fetus. There are three classes of abruption based on maternal and fetal status, including an assessment of uterine contractions, quantity of bleeding, fetal heart rate monitoring, and abnormal coagulation studies (fibrinogen, prothrombin time, partial thromboplastin time).

- Grade I: mild vaginal bleeding, uterine irritability, stable vital signs, reassuring fetal heart rate, normal coagulation profile (fibrinogen 450 mg%)
- Grade II: moderate vaginal bleeding, hypertonic uterine contractions, orthostatic blood pressure measurements, unfavorable fetal status, fibrinogen 150 to 250 mg%
- Grade III: severe bleeding (may be concealed), hypertonic uterine contractions, overt signs of hypovolemic shock, fetal death, thrombocytopenia, fibrinogen <150 mg%

SYNONYMS

Premature separation of placenta

ICD-9CM CODES

641.2 Premature separation of placenta

EPIDEMIOLOGY & DEMOGRAPHICS

INCIDENCE (IN U.S.): One in 86 to 206 births; incidence by grade: I = 40%, II = 45%, III = 15%; 80% occur before the onset of labor

RISK FACTORS: Hypertension (greatest association), trauma, polyhydramnios, multifetal gestation, smoking, use of crack cocaine, chorioamnionitis, preterm premature rupture of membranes

RECURRENCE RATE: 5% to 17%; with two prior episodes, 25%

PHYSICAL FINDINGS & CLINICAL PRESENTATION

- Triad of uterine bleeding (concealed or per vagina), hypertonic uterine contractions or signs of preterm labor, and evidence of fetal compromise exists.
- More than 80% of cases have external bleeding; 20% of cases have no bleeding but have indirect evidence of abruption, such as failed tocolysis for preterm labor.
- Tetanic uterine contractions are found in only 17% of cases unless grade II or III abruption.

ETIOLOGY

- Primary etiology: unknown
- Hypertension: found in 40% to 50% of grade III abruptions
- Rapid decompression of uterine cavity, as can occur in polyhydramnios or multifetal gestation
- Blunt external trauma (motor vehicle accident, spousal abuse)

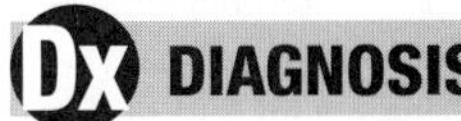

DIAGNOSIS

DIFFERENTIAL DIAGNOSIS

- Placenta previa
- Cervical or vaginal trauma
- Labor
- Cervical cancer
- Rupture of membranes
- The differential diagnosis of vaginal bleeding in pregnancy is described in Section II

WORKUP

- Initial assessment should evaluate for the source of bleeding, ruling out placenta previa and associated conditions that contraindicate any type of vaginal examination (e.g., pelvic speculum examination).
- Continuous fetal heart monitoring is indicated for all viable gestations (60% incidence of fetal distress in labor); may show early signs of maternal hypovolemia (late decelerations or fetal tachycardia) before overt maternal vital sign changes.
- Actual amount of blood loss is often greater than initially perceived because of the possibility of concealed retroplacental bleeding and apparent "normal" vital signs. The relative hypervolemia of pregnancy initially protects the patient until late in the course of bleeding, when abrupt and sudden cardiovascular collapse can occur.

LABORATORY TESTS

- Baseline hemoglobin and hematocrit help quantify blood loss and establish baseline values for serial comparisons during expectant management.
- Coagulation profile: platelets, fibrinogen, prothrombin, and partial thromboplastin time. Diffuse intravascular coagulation can develop with severe abruption. If fibrinogen is <150 mg%, estimated blood loss is approximately 2000 ml; if fibrinogen is <100 mg%, consider fresh frozen plasma to prevent further bleeding.
- Type and antibody screen is important to identify Rh-negative patients who may need Rh immune globulin.

IMAGING STUDIES

Ultrasound should include fetal presentation and status, amniotic fluid volume, placental location, as well as any evidence of hematoma (retroplacental, subchorionic, or preplacental).

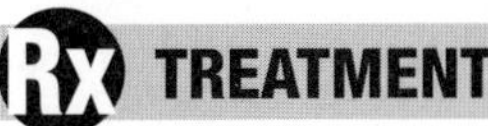

TREATMENT

ACUTE GENERAL Rx

- Stabilization of the mother is the first priority.
- Treatment depends on gestational age of the fetus, severity of the abruption, and maternal status.
- Initial assessment for signs of maternal hemodynamic compromise or hemorrhagic shock; large-bore intravenous access, with crystalloid fluid resuscitation using a replacement of 3 ml lactated Ringer's solution for every 1 ml estimated blood loss.
- Indwelling Foley catheter to monitor urine output and maternal volume status, with a goal of 30 ml/hr urine output.
- Assess fetal status and gestational age by sonogram and continuous fetal heart rate monitoring.
- Because of the unpredictable nature of abruptions, cross-matched blood should be made available during the initial resuscitation period.

CHRONIC Rx

- In the term fetus or when lung maturity has been documented, delivery is indicated.
- In the preterm fetus or a fetus with an immature lung profile, consider betamethasone 12.5 mg IM q24h for two doses and then delivery, depending on the severity of the abruption and the likelihood of fetal complications from preterm birth.
- Cesarean section should be reserved for cases of fetal distress or for standard obstetric indications.
- In select cases, such as severe prematurity with a stable mother and mild contractions, magnesium sulfate can be used for tocolysis, 6 g IV loading dose then 3 g/hr maintenance, to allow for course of steroids.

DISPOSITION

Because of the unpredictable nature of abruptions, expectant management should occur only under controlled circumstances.

REFERRAL

Abruptio placentae places mother and fetus in a high-risk situation and should be managed by a qualified obstetrician in a facility with capability for neonatal and maternal resuscitation and ability to perform emergency cesarean sections.

AUTHOR: **SCOTT J. ZUCCALA, D.O.**

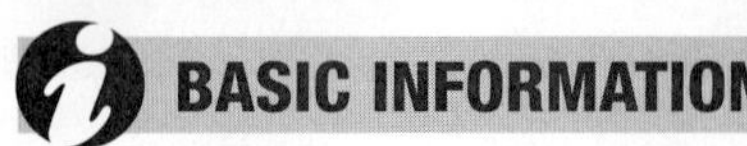

BASIC INFORMATION

DEFINITION

A brain abscess is a focal, intracerebral infection that begins as a localized area of cerebritis and develops into a collection of pus surrounded by a well-vascularized capsule.

ICD-9CM CODES
324.0 Brain abscess

EPIDEMIOLOGY & DEMOGRAPHICS

INCIDENCE: Quite uncommon (occurs about 2% as commonly as brain tumors)
PEAK INCIDENCE: Preadolescence and middle age
PREDOMINANT AGE: Occurs at any age
PREDOMINANT SEX:
- Men affected more than women
- Most common source of underlying infection: contiguous spread from the paranasal sinuses, middle ear, or teeth

PHYSICAL FINDINGS & CLINICAL PRESENTATION

- Classic triad: fever, headache, and focal neurologic deficit are present in 50% of cases.
- Fever is present in only 50% of patients.
- Headache is usually localized to the side of the abscess; onset can be gradual or severe; present in 70% of cases.
- Focal neurologic findings (e.g., seizures, hemiparesis, aphasia, ataxia) depend on the location of the abscess and are seen in 30% to 50% of cases.
- Papilledema is present in 25% of cases.
- Presence of adjacent infections (dental abscess, otitis media, and sinusitis) may be a clue to the underlying diagnosis and should be sought in any suspected case.
- Time course from symptom onset to presentation ranges from hours in fulminant cases to more than 1 mo; 75% present in the first 2 wk.
- The nonspecific presentation of a brain abscess warrants that clinicians maintain a high index of suspicion.

ETIOLOGY

- Brain abscesses arise from:
  Contiguous infection
  Hematogenous spread from a remote site
- They are classified based on the likely portal of entry.

Likely source of abscess:

A. Contiguous focus or primary infection (55% of all brain abscesses):
   1. Paranasal sinus: occur in frontal lobe; streptococci, *Bacteroides, Haemophilus,* and *Fusobacterium* spp.
   2. Otitis media/mastoiditis: occur in temporal lobe and cerebellum; streptococci, Enterobacteriaceae, *Bacteroides,* and *Pseudomonas* spp.
   3. Dental sepsis: occur in frontal lobe; mixed *Fusobacterium, Bacteroides,* and *Streptococcus* spp.
   4. Penetrating head injury: site of abscess depends on site of wound; *Staphylococcus aureus, Clostridium* spp., Enterobacteriaceae
   5. Postoperative: *Staphylococcus epidermidis* and *S. aureus,* Enterobacteriaceae, and Pseudomonadaceae

B. Hematogenous spread/distant site of infection (25% of all brain abscesses): abscesses most commonly multiple, especially in middle cerebral artery distribution; infecting organisms depend on source.
   1. Congenital heart disease: streptococci, *Haemophilus* spp.
   2. Endocarditis: *S. aureus,* viridans streptococci
   3. Urinary tract: Enterobacteriaceae, Pseudomonadaceae
   4. Intraabdominal: streptococci, Enterobacteriaceae, anaerobes
   5. Lung: streptococci, *Actinomyces* species, *Fusobacterium* spp.
   6. Immunocompromised host: *Toxoplasma* species, fungi, Enterobacteriaceae, *Nocardia* spp., tuberculosis, listeriosis

C. Cryptogenic (unknown source): 20% of all brain abscesses

Dx DIAGNOSIS

DIFFERENTIAL DIAGNOSIS

- Other parameningeal infections: subdural empyema, epidural abscess, thrombophlebitis of the major dural venous sinuses and cortical veins
- Embolic strokes in patients with bacterial endocarditis
- Mycotic aneurysms with leakage
- Viral encephalitis (usually resulting from herpes simplex)
- Acute hemorrhagic leukoencephalitis
- Parasitic infections: toxoplasmosis, echinococcosis, cysticercosis
- Metastatic or primary brain tumors
- Cerebral infarction
- CNS vasculitis
- Chronic subdural hematoma

WORKUP

Physical examination, laboratory tests, and imaging studies

LABORATORY TESTS

- White blood cell counts are elevated in 60% of patients.
- Erythrocyte sedimentation rate is usually elevated but may be normal.
- Blood cultures are most often negative (10% positive).
- Lumbar puncture is contraindicated in patients with suspected abscess (20% die or experience neurologic decline).
- The yield of Gram stain and culture of material aspirated at time of surgical drainage approaches 100%.

IMAGING STUDIES

- MRI with and without gadolinium is the diagnostic procedure of choice; provides superior detail compared with CT scan (higher sensitivity and specificity than CT scan, but not always immediately available).
- CT scan (Fig. 1-1) with intravenous contrast is still an excellent test (sensitivity 95%-99%).
- Serial CT or MRI scanning is recommended to follow the response to therapy.

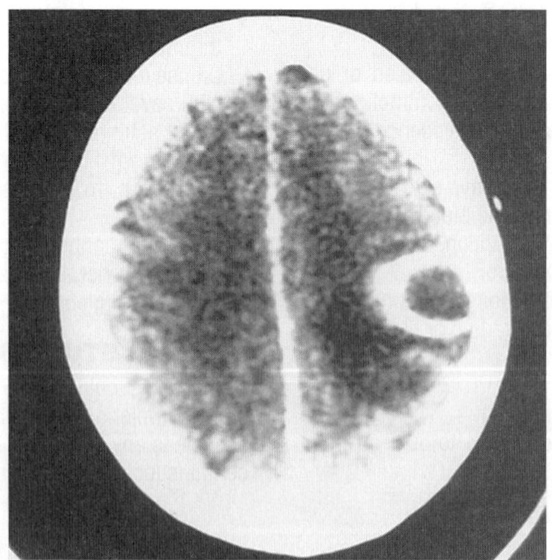

FIGURE 1-1 Computed tomographic (CT) scan showing a brain abscess. A woman presented to physicians after a focal seizure followed by headache and weakness of the arm. Dental work had been performed several weeks before. CT scan revealed a contrast-enhanced, ringlike mass surrounded by edema. It is not possible on this scan to differentiate tumor from abscess. At surgery a well-encapsulated abscess was encountered. (From Andreoli TE [ed]: *Cecil essentials of medicine,* ed 4, Philadelphia, 1997, WB Saunders.)

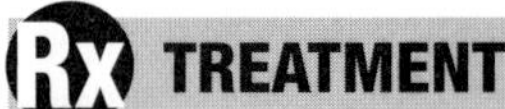

TREATMENT

ACUTE GENERAL Rx

- Effective treatment involves a combination of empiric antibiotic therapy and timely excision or aspiration of the abscess.
- If evidence of edema or mass effect, treatment of elevated intracranial pressure is paramount.
  - Hyperventilation of mechanically ventilated patient.
  - Dexamethasone initially in a dosage of 10 mg IV followed by 4 mg IV q6h until symptoms of cerebral edema subside. Dosage may be reduced after 2 to 4 days and gradually discontinued over a period of 5 to 7 days.
  - Mannitol 0.25 to 1 g/kg IV over 20 to 30 min q6-8h; maximum of 6 g/kg in 24 hr.
- Medical therapy is never a substitute for surgical intervention to relieve increased intracranial pressure. Neurologic deterioration usually mandates surgery.
- Steroids should be limited to patients with severe cerebral edema or midline shift.

MEDICAL Rx

If abscess <2.5 cm and patient is neurologically stable and conscious, may start antibiotics and observe. Empiric antibiotic therapy guided by:

- Abscess location
- Suspicion of primary source
- Presence of single or multiple abscesses
- Patient's underlying medical conditions (e.g., HIV, immunocompromised)

Selection of empiric antibiotic therapy:

- Primary infection or contiguous source:
  1. Otitis media/mastoiditis, sinusitis, dental infection: third-generation cephalosporin (cefotaxime 2 g q6h IV or ceftriaxone 2 g q12h IV) plus metronidazole 15 mg/kg IV as a loading dose, then 7.5 mg/kg q6h IV or 15 mg/kg q12h IV
  2. Dental infection: penicillin G 6 million units q6h plus metronidazole 15 mg/kg IV as a loading dose, then 7.5 mg/kg IV q6h or 15 mg/kg IV q12h
  3. Head trauma: third-generation cephalosporin (cefotaxime 2 g IV q6h or ceftriaxone 2 g IV q12h) plus nafcillin 2 g IV q4h or vancomycin (30 mg/kg IV in two divided doses adjusted for renal function)
  4. Postoperative neurosurgery: vancomycin (dose as above) plus ceftazidime (2g IV q8h)
- Hematogenous spread (congenital heart disease, endocarditis, urinary tract, lung, intraabdominal): nafcillin or vancomycin plus metronidazole plus third-generation cephalosporin (cefotaxime 2 g IV q6h or ceftriaxone 2 g IV q12h)

Duration of antibiotic therapy is unclear. Most recommend parenteral treatment for 4 to 8 wk, with repeated neuroimaging to ensure adequate treatment. (Imaging suggested every week for first 2 wk of therapy, then every 2 wk until antibiotics finished, and then every 2 to 4 mo for 1 yr to monitor for disease recurrence.)

SURGICAL Rx

- Two indications for surgical intervention:
  1. Collect specimens for culture and sensitivity
  2. Reduce mass effect
- Stereotactic biopsy or aspirate of the abscess if surgically feasible
- Essential to selection of targeted antimicrobial coverage
- Timing and choice of surgery depends on:
  - Primary infection source
  - Number and location of the abscesses
  - Whether the procedure is diagnostic or therapeutic
  - Neurologic status of the patient

DISPOSITION

- Prompt diagnostic consideration, early institution of appropriate antimicrobial therapy, and advanced neuroradiologic imaging have reduced the mortality rate from brain abscesses from 40% to 80% in the preantibiotic era to 10% to 20% at present.
- Morbidity is usually manifest as persistent neurologic sequelae (seizures, intellectual or behavioral impairment, motor deficits) seen in 20% to 60% of patients.

REFERRAL

Consultation with a neurosurgeon is mandatory.

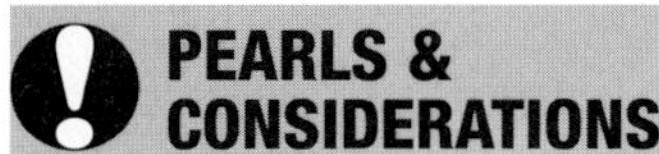

PEARLS & CONSIDERATIONS

COMMENTS

- It is important to maintain a high index of suspicion because a brain abscess often presents with nonspecific symptoms.
- Rapid imaging and early institution of appropriate antimicrobial therapy improve patient morbidity and mortality.
- Neurosurgical consultation is mandatory.

PREVENTION

Because brain abscesses arise from either contiguous infections or hematogenously from a remote site, early and appropriate treatment of inciting infections is paramount to prevent brain abscess.

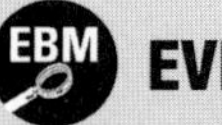

EVIDENCE

Although antimicrobial therapy and surgical drainage are the mainstays of the clinical management of brain abscess, evidence for these therapies is limited.

SUGGESTED READINGS

Bhand AA: Brain abscess—diagnosis and management, *J Coll Physicians Surg Pak* 14:7, 2004.

Carpenter J et al: Retrospective analysis of 49 cases of brain abscess and review of the literature, *Eur J Clin Microbiol Infect Dis* 26:1, 2007.

Gomes JA et al: Glucocorticoid therapy in neurologic critical care, *Crit Care Med* 33(6):1214, 2005.

Kao PT et al: Brain abscess: clinical analysis of 53 cases, *J Microbiol Immunol Infect* 36:2, 2003.

McClelland S 3rd et al: Postoperative central nervous system infections: incidence and associated factors in 2111 neurosurgical procedures, *Clin Infect Dis* 45:1, 2007.

Tattevin P et al: Bacterial brain abscesses: a retrospective study of 94 patients admitted to an intensive care unit (1980–1999), *Am J Med* 115:143, 2003.

The rational use of antibiotics in the treatment of brain abscess: Report by the "Infection in Neurosurgery" Working Party of the British Society for Antimicrobial Chemotherapy, *Br J Neurosurg* 14(6):525, 2000.

AUTHOR: **KELLY A. MCGARRY, M.D.**

Abscess, Breast (PTG)

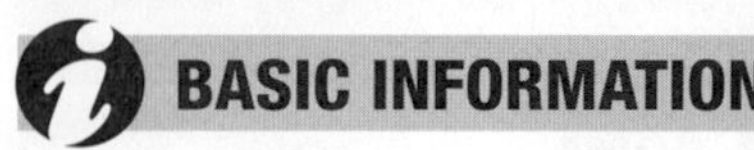

BASIC INFORMATION

DEFINITION

Breast abscess is an acute inflammatory process resulting in the formation of a collection of pus. Typically there is painful erythematous mass formation in the breast, occasionally draining through the overlying skin or nipple duct.

SYNONYMS

Subareolar abscess
Lactational or puerperal abscess

ICD-9CM CODES

6.110	Abscess of the breast
675.0	Abscess of the nipple related to childbirth
675.1	Abscess of the breast related to childbirth

EPIDEMIOLOGY & DEMOGRAPHICS

INCIDENCE: 10% to 30% of all breast abscesses are lactational; acute mastitis occurs in 2.5% of nursing mothers, with one in 15 of these women developing abscess.

PHYSICAL FINDINGS & CLINICAL PRESENTATION

Painful erythematous induration involving breast and leading to fluctuant abscess

ETIOLOGY

- Lactational abscess: milk stasis and bacterial infection leading to mastitis and then abscess, with *Staphylococcus aureus* the most common causative agent
- Subareolar abscess:
  1. Central ducts involved, with obstructive nipple duct changes leading to bacterial infection
  2. Cultured organisms mixed, including anaerobes, staphylococci, streptococci, and others

Dx DIAGNOSIS

DIFFERENTIAL DIAGNOSIS

- Inflammatory carcinoma
- Advanced carcinoma with erythema, edema, and/or ulceration
- Tuberculous abscess (rare in the United States)
- Hydradenitis of breast skin
- Sebaceous cyst with infection

WORKUP

- Clinical examination sufficient
- If abscess suspected, referral to surgeon for incision, drainage, and biopsy
- If possible abscess or advanced carcinoma, referral for workup required

LABORATORY TESTS

- Perform culture and sensitivity test of abscess contents.
- If mammogram or ultrasound is required but prevented by discomfort, perform after resolution of abscess.

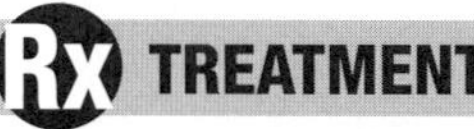

TREATMENT

NONPHARMACOLOGIC THERAPY

- Established abscess: incision and drainage, preferably with general anesthesia
- Biopsy of abscess cavity wall to exclude carcinoma

ACUTE GENERAL Rx

- Antibiotics: generally staphylococci in lactational abscess. Recommended initial antibiotic therapy is nafcillin or oxacillin 2 g q4h IV or cefazolin 1 g q8h IV for 10 to 14 days. Alternative includes vancomycin 1 g IV q12h.
- If acute mastitis is treated early, resolution without drainage is possible.
- Subareolar abscess: broad-spectrum antibiotic treatment (e.g., cephalexin 500 mg PO qid or cefazolin 1 g q8h IV for 10 to 14 days for more severe infection) and drainage are needed to control acute phase.

CHRONIC Rx

Further surgical treatment for recurrences or fistula

DISPOSITION

- Lactational abscess: possible to continue breastfeeding without apparent risk of infection to the infant
- Subareolar abscess:
  1. Notorious for recurrence or complication of fistula formation
  2. Patient informed and referred for subsequent care

REFERRAL

- If abscess drainage required
- For surgical consultation if subareolar abscess involved

SUGGESTED READINGS

Schwarz RJ, Shrestha R: Needle aspiration of breast abscesses, *Am J Surg* 182(2):117, 2001.

Tan YM et al: Breast abscess as the initial presentation of squamous cell of the breast, *Eur J Surg Oncol* 28(1):91, 2002.

AUTHORS: **TAKUMA NEMOTO, M.D.,** and **RUBEN ALVERO, M.D.**

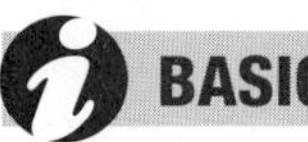

BASIC INFORMATION

DEFINITION

Liver abscess is a necrotic infection of the liver usually classified as pyogenic or amebic.

SYNONYMS

Pyogenic hepatic abscess
Amebic hepatic abscess

ICD-9CM CODES
572.0 Abscess of liver

EPIDEMIOLOGY & DEMOGRAPHICS

INCIDENCE: Incidence of pyogenic liver abscess is 2.3 cases per 100,000 population.
PREVALANCE (WORLDWIDE): Amebic liver abscess is more common than pyogenic liver abscess.
PREVALENCE (IN U.S.): Pyogenic liver abscess is more common than amebic liver abscess.
PREDOMINANT SEX AND AGE: More common in men than women; male/female ratio of 2:1; most common in fourth to sixth decades of life.

PHYSICAL FINDINGS & CLINICAL PRESENTATION

- Fever, chills, and sweats
- Weakness/malaise
- Anorexia with weight loss
- Nausea, vomiting, and diarrhea
- Cough with pleuritic chest pain
- Right upper quadrant abdominal pain
- Hepatomegaly
- Splenomegaly
- Jaundice
- Pleural effusions, rales, and friction rubs may be present
- Most abscesses occur on the right lobe of the liver

ETIOLOGY

- Pyogenic liver abscess is usually polymicrobial (*Klebsiella pneumoniae* [43%], *Escherichia coli* [33%], *Streptococcus* spp. [37%], *Pseudomonas aeruginosa, Proteus* spp., *Bacteroides* spp. [24%], *Fusobacterium* spp., *Actinomyces* spp., gram-positive anaerobes, and *Staphylococcus aureus*).
- Pyogenic liver abscess occurs from:
  1. Biliary disease with cholangitis (accounts for approximately 40% to 60%).
  2. Gallbladder disease with contiguous spread to the liver.
  3. Diverticulitis or appendicitis with spread via the portal circulation.
  4. Hematogenous spread via the hepatic artery, though uncommon; if a solitary organism is isolated, a distant source of hematogenous seeding should be sought.
  5. Penetrating wounds.
  6. Cryptogenic.
  7. Infection by way of portal system (portal pyemia).
  8. No causes found in approximately half of cases.
  9. Incidence increased in patients with diabetes and metastatic cancer.
- Amebic hepatic abscess is caused by the parasite *Entamoeba histolytica.* Amebiasis is usually due to fecal-oral contamination and invades the intestinal mucosa, gaining entry into the portal system to reach the liver.

Dx DIAGNOSIS

The diagnosis of liver abscess requires a high index of suspicion after a detailed history and physical examination. Imaging studies and microbiologic, serologic, and percutaneous techniques (e.g., aspiration) confirm the presence of a liver abscess.

DIFFERENTIAL DIAGNOSIS

- Cholangitis
- Cholecystitis
- Diverticulitis
- Appendicitis
- Perforated viscus
- Mesentery ischemia
- Pulmonary embolism
- Pancreatitis

WORKUP

- The workup of a liver abscess should focus on differentiating between amebic and pyogenic causes.
- Features suggesting an amebic cause include travel to an endemic area, single abscess rather than multiple abscesses, subacute onset of symptoms, and absence of conditions predisposing to pyogenic liver abscess, as highlighted under "Etiology."
- Laboratory studies are not specific but are useful as adjunctive tests.
- Imaging studies cannot differentiate between the two, and bacteriologic cultures may be sterile in 50% of the cases.

LABORATORY TESTS

- Complete blood count showing leukocytosis
- Liver function tests: alkaline phosphatase is most commonly elevated (95% to 100%); aspartate transaminase (AST) and alanine transaminase (ALT) elevated in 50% of cases; elevated bilirubin (28% to 30%); decreased albumin
- Prothrombin time (INR) prolonged (70%)
- Blood cultures positive in 50% of cases
- Aspiration (50% sterile)
- Stool samples for *E. histolytica* trophozoites (positive in 10% to 15% of amebic liver abscess cases)
- Serologic testing for *E. histolytica* does not differentiate acute from old infections

IMAGING STUDIES

- Ultrasound (80% to 100% sensitivity in detecting abscesses) shows round or oval hypoechogenic mass.
- CT scan is more sensitive in detecting hepatic abscesses and contiguous organ extension and is the imaging study of choice (Fig. 1-2).
- Chest x-ray examination abnormal in 50% of the cases, showing elevated right hemidiaphragm, subdiaphragmatic air-fluid levels, pleural effusions, and consolidating infiltrates.
- Most liver abscesses are single; however, multiple liver abscesses are seen with systemic bacteremia.

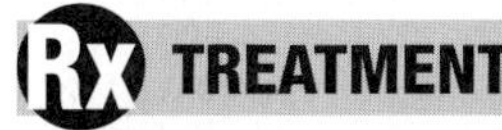

TREATMENT

NONPHARMACOLOGIC THERAPY

- The management of pyogenic liver abscess differs from that of amebic liver abscess.
- Medical management is the cornerstone of therapy in amebic liver abscess, whereas early intervention in the form of surgical

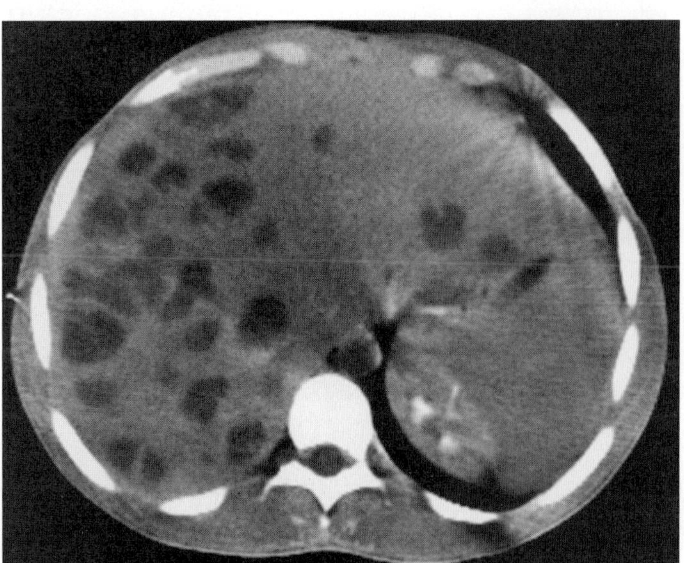

FIGURE 1-2 CT scan demonstrating multiple pyogenic liver abscesses in a 25-year-old man. (From Goldman L, Bennett JC [ed]: *Cecil textbook of medicine,* ed 21, Philadelphia, 2000, WB Saunders.)

therapy or catheter drainage and parenteral antibiotics is the rule in pyogenic liver abscess.

ACUTE GENERAL Rx

- Percutaneous drainage under CT or ultrasound guidance is essential in the treatment of pyogenic liver abscesses.
- Aspiration of hepatic amebic abscesses is not required unless there is no response to treatment or a pyogenic cause is being considered.
- Empiric broad spectrum antibiotics are recommended initially until culture results are available. Common choices include:
  1. Metronidazole (500 mg IV q8h) plus a fluoroquinolone (ciprofloxacin 400 mg IV q12h or levofloxacin 500 mg IV daily).
  2. Monotherapy with a beta-lactam/beta-lactamase inhibitor, such as piperacillin/tazobactam (4.5 g q6h), ticarcillin-clavulanate (3.1 g q4h), or ampicillin-sulbactam (3 g q6h).
  3. Monotherapy with a carbapenem, such as imipenem (500 mg IV q6h), meropenem (1 g q8h), or ertapenem (1 g daily).
  4. In patients with penicillin allergy, clindamycin 600 to 900 mg IV q8h with an aminoglycoside can be considered.
  5. Duration of antibiotic treatment is usually 4 to 6 wk with IV antibiotics used for the first 1 to 2 wk or until a favorable clinical response, followed thereafter with oral antibiotics (e.g., metronidazole 500 mg PO q8h plus ciprofloxacin 500 mg PO q12h).
  6. Third-generation cephalosporins should not be used for empiric therapy because of risk of the emergence of beta-lactamase-producing bacteria.
- Antibiotic coverage for amebic liver abscesses includes:
  1. Tissue agent: metronidazole 750 mg PO tid for 10 days
  2. Luminal agent: after therapy with tissue agent treatment with any luminal agent is required even if the stool is negative, such as paromomycin for 10 days or diiodohydroxyquin for 20 days.

CHRONIC Rx

- If fever persists for 2 wk despite percutaneous drainage and antibiotic therapy as outlined under "Acute General Rx," or if there is failure of aspiration or failure of percutaneous drainage, surgery is indicated.
- In patients not responding to intravenous antibiotics and percutaneous drainage, hepatic artery antibiotic infusion can be considered.
- In patients with evidence of metastatic disease that is causing biliary obstruction, a gastroenterology consultation for endoscopic retrograde cholangiopancreatography and stenting should be considered.

DISPOSITION

- Most patients with pyogenic liver abscesses defervesce within 2 wk of treatment with antibiotics and drainage.
- No randomized controlled studies have evaluated the optimal duration of antibiotic therapy for pyogenic liver abscess. Typical duration of antibiotic therapy is at least 4 to 6 wk.
- Pyogenic liver abscess cure rates using percutaneous drainage and antibiotics have been reported to be between 88% and 100%.
- Mortality rate of untreated pyogenic liver abscess is nearly 100%.
- Most patients with amebic liver abscesses defervesce within 4 to 5 days of treatment.
- Amebic liver abscess mortality rate is <1% unless complications occur (see "Comments").
- Follow-up imaging should be used to monitor response to therapy; continue treatment until CT scan shows complete or near complete resolution of cavity.

REFERRAL

Infectious disease, gastroenterology, interventional radiology, and general surgical consultations are recommended in any patient with hepatic abscess.

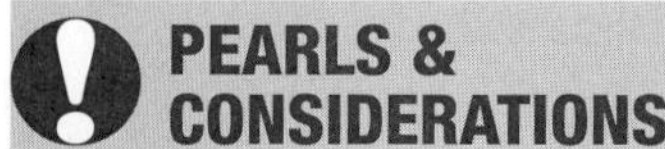

PEARLS & CONSIDERATIONS

COMMENTS

- Complications of pyogenic and amebic liver abscesses include:
  1. Pleuropulmonary extension, resulting in empyema, abscess, and fistula formation
  2. Peritonitis
  3. Purulent pericarditis
  4. Sepsis
- Amebic liver abscesses complicate amebic colitis in nearly 10% of cases.

SUGGESTED READINGS

Blessman J et al: Treatment of amoebic liver abscess with metronidazole alone or in combination with ultrasound guided needle aspiration: a comparative, prospective and randomized study, *Trop Med Int Health* 8(11):1030, 2003.

Kaplan GG et al: Population-based study of the epidemiology of and the risk factors for pyogenic liver abscess, *Clin Gastroenterol Hepatol* 2(11):1032, 2004.

Kurland JE et al: Pyogenic and amebic liver abscess, *Curr Gastroenterol Rep* 6(4):273, 2004.

Lodhi S et al: Features distinguishing amebic from pyogenic liver abscess: a review of 577 adult cases, *Trop Med Int Health* 9(6):718, 2004.

Yu SC et al: Treatment of pyogenic liver abscess: prospective randomized comparison of catheter drainage and needle aspiration, *Hepatology* 39(9):932, 2004.

AUTHOR: **TANYA ALI, M.D.**

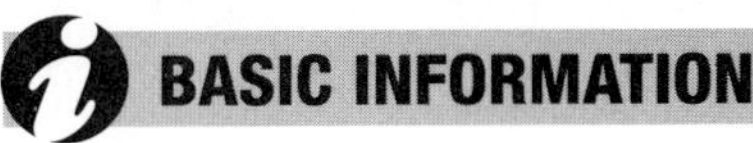

BASIC INFORMATION

DEFINITION

A lung abscess is an infection of the lung parenchyma resulting in a necrotic cavity containing pus.

SYNONYMS

Pulmonary abscess

ICD-9CM CODES

513.0 Abscess of lung

EPIDEMIOLOGY & DEMOGRAPHICS

INCIDENCE: Has decreased over the last 30 years as a result of antibiotic therapy.

- Lung abscess in patients age 50 and over is associated with primary lung neoplasia in 30% of the cases.
- Lung abscesses commonly coexist with empyemas.

RISK FACTORS:

1. Alcohol-related problems
2. Seizure disorders
3. Cerebrovascular disorders with dysphagia
4. Drug abuse
5. Esophageal disorders (e.g., scleroderma, esophageal carcinoma, etc.)
6. Poor oral hygiene
7. Obstructive malignant lung disease
8. Bronchiectasis

PHYSICAL FINDINGS & CLINICAL PRESENTATION

- Symptoms are generally insidious and prolonged, occurring for weeks to months
- Fever, chills, and sweats
- Cough
- Sputum production (purulent with foul odor)
- Pleuritic chest pain
- Hemoptysis
- Dyspnea
- Malaise, fatigue, and weakness
- Tachycardia and tachypnea
- Dullness to percussion, whispered pectoriloquy, and bronchophony
- Amphoric breath sounds (low pitched sound of air moving across a large open cavity)

ETIOLOGY

- The most important factor predisposing to lung abscess is aspiration.
- Following aspiration as a major predisposing factor is periodontal disease.
- Lung abscess is rare in an edentulous person.
- Approximately 90% of lung abscesses are caused by anaerobic microorganisms (*Bacteroides fragilis, Fusobacterium nucleatum,* peptostreptococci, microaerophilic streptococci). Pulmonary actinomycosis will also generate lung abscess.
- In most cases anaerobic infection is mixed with aerobic or facultative anaerobic organisms *(S. aureus, E. coli, K. pneumoniae, P. aeruginosa).*
- Parasitic organisms including Paragonimus westermani and Entamoeba histolytica.
- Fungi including *Aspergillus, Cryptococcus, Histoplasma, Blastomyces,* and *Coccidioides* spp.
- Immunocompromised hosts may become infected with *Aspergillus,* mycobacteria, *Nocardia, Legionella micdadei,* and *Rhodococcus equi.*

Dx DIAGNOSIS

Lung abscess may be primary or secondary.

- Primary lung abscess refers to infection from normal host organisms within the lung (e.g., aspiration, pneumonia).
- Secondary lung abscess results from other preexisting conditions (e.g., endocarditis, underlying lung cancer, pulmonary emboli).

Lung abscess may be acute or chronic.

- Acute lung abscess is present if symptoms are of less than 4 to 6 wk.
- Chronic lung abscess is present if symptoms last longer than 6 wk.

DIFFERENTIAL DIAGNOSIS

The differential diagnosis is similar to that for cavitary lung lesions:

- Bacterial (anaerobic, aerobic, infected bulla, empyema, actinomycosis, tuberculosis)
- Fungal (histoplasmosis, coccidioidomycosis, blastomycosis, aspergillosis, cryptococcosis)
- Parasitic (amebiasis, echinococcosis)
- Malignancy (primary lung carcinoma, metastatic lung disease, lymphoma, Hodgkin's disease)
- Wegener's granulomatosis, sarcoidosis, endocarditis, and septic pulmonary emboli

WORKUP

- The workup of a patient with lung abscess attempts to elicit a primary or a secondary cause.
- Blood tests are not specific in diagnosing lung abscesses.
- Most diagnoses are made from imaging studies; however, to diagnose a specific cause bacteriologic studies are needed.

LABORATORY TESTS

- CBC with leukocytosis
- Bacteriologic studies
  1. Sputum Gram stain and culture (commonly contaminated by oral flora)
  2. Percutaneous transtracheal aspiration
  3. Percutaneous transthoracic aspiration
  4. Fiberoptic bronchoscopy using bronchial brushings or bronchoalveolar lavage is the most widely used intervention when trying to obtain diagnostic bacteriologic cultures
- Blood cultures on some occasions may be positive
- If an empyema is present, obtaining empyema fluid via thoracentesis may isolate the organism

IMAGING STUDIES

- Chest x-ray examination makes the diagnosis of lung abscess showing the cavitary lesion with an air fluid level.
- Lung abscesses are most commonly found in the posterior segment of the right upper lobe.
- Chest CT scan can localize and size the lesion and assist in differentiating lung abscesses from other pathologic processes (e.g., tumor, empyema, infected bulla, etc.) (Fig. 1-3).

Rx TREATMENT

NONPHARMACOLOGIC THERAPY

- Oxygen therapy
- Postural drainage
- Respiratory therapy maneuvers

ACUTE GENERAL Rx

- Penicillin 1 to 2 million units IV q4h until improvement (e.g., afebrile, decrease in sputum production, etc.) followed by penicillin VK 500 mg PO qid for the next 2 to 3 wk but usually requiring longer 6- to 8-wk courses.
- Metronidazole is given with penicillin at doses of 7.5 mg/kg IV q6h followed by PO 500 mg bid to qid dosing.
- Clindamycin is an alternative choice if concerned about penicillin-resistant organisms. The dose is 600 mg IV q8h until improvement followed by 300 mg to 600 mg PO q6h.

CHRONIC Rx

- Bronchoscopy to assist with drainage and/or diagnosis is indicated in patients who fail to respond to antibiotics or if there is suspected underlying malignancy.
- Surgery is indicated on rare occasions (<10%) in patients with complications of lung abscess (see "Comments").

DISPOSITION

- More than 95% of patients are cured with the use of antibiotics alone.
- Complications of lung abscesses include:
  1. Empyema
  2. Massive hemoptysis
  3. Pneumothorax
  4. Bronchopleural fistula
- Mortality is low in community-acquired lung abscess (2.5%).
- Hospital-acquired lung abscess carries a high mortality rate (65%).

REFERRAL

If lung abscess is present, consultation with pulmonary and infectious disease specialist is recommended.

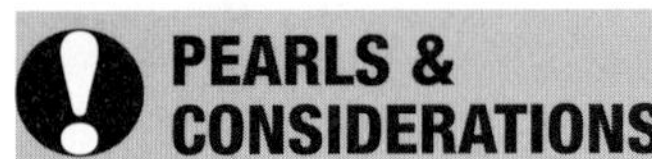

PEARLS & CONSIDERATIONS

COMMENTS

- Complications of lung abscesses include:
  1. Empyema
  2. Bronchopleural fistula
  3. Hepatobronchial fistula
  4. Brain abscess
  5. Bronchiectasis

- Refractory cases are usually the result of:
  1. Large cavity size (>6 cm)
  2. Recurrent aspiration
  3. Thick-walled cavities
  4. Underlying lung carcinoma
  5. Empyema formation
- Necrotizing pneumonia is similar to a lung abscess but differs in size (<2 cm in diameter) and number (usually multiple suppurative cavitary lesions).

SUGGESTED READINGS

Herth F et al: Endoscopic drainage of lung abscesses: technique and outcome, *Chest* 127(4):1378, 2005.

Lorber B: Lung abscess. In *Mandell, Douglas, and Bennett's principles and practice of infectious diseases,* ed 6, New York, 2005, Churchill Livingstone.

Levison J et al: The value of a CT-guided fine needle aspirate in infants with lung abscess, *J Paediatr Child Health* 40(8):474, 2004.

Mansharamani NG, Koziel H: Chronic lung sepsis: lung abscess, bronchiectasis, and empyema, *Curr Opin Pulm Med* 9(3):181, 2003.

Mansharamani N et al: Lung abscess in adults: clinical comparison of immunocompromised to non-immunocompromised patients, *Respir Med* 96(3): 178, 2002.

Schiza S, Siafakas NM: Clinical presentation and management of empyema, lung abscess and pleural effusion, *Curr Opin Pulm Med* 12(3):205, 2006.

AUTHORS: **GLENN G. FORT, M.D., M.P.H.,** and **DENNIS J. MIKOLICH, M.D.**

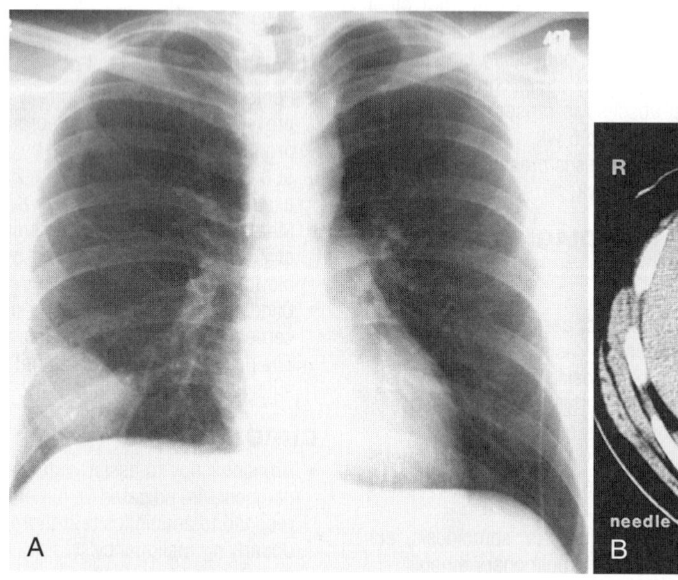

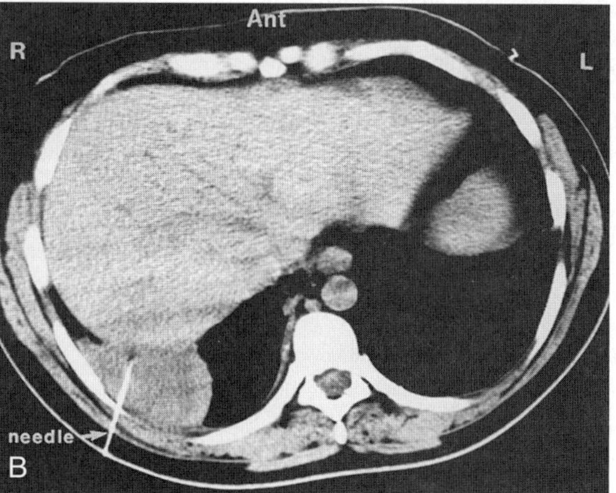

FIGURE 1-3 Lung abscess. On a chest radiograph, a lung abscess may look to be a solid rounded lesion **(A),** or, if it has a connection with the bronchus, there may be an air fluid level in a thick-walled cavitary lesion. CT scanning **(B)** can be used to localize the lesion and to place a needle for drainage and aspiration of contents for culture. (From Mettler FA [ed]: *Primary care radiology,* Philadelphia, 2000, WB Saunders.)

BASIC INFORMATION

DEFINITION

Pelvic abscess is an acute or chronic infection, most commonly involving the pelvic viscera, initially localized and creating its own unique environment so that treatment and possible cure require directed therapy. There are four categories based on etiologic factors:

- Ascending infection, spreading from cervix through endometrial cavity to adnexa, forming a tuboovarian complex
- Infection occurring in the puerperium, which spreads to the adnexa from the endometrium or myometrium by a hematogenous or lymphatic route
- Abscess complicating pelvic surgery
- Involvement of the pelvic viscera as a result of spread from contiguous organs, such as appendicitis or diverticulitis

SYNONYMS

Tuboovarian abscess (TOA)
Vaginal cuff abscess

ICD-9CM CODES
614.2 Salpingitis and oophoritis not specified as acute, subacute, or chronic

EPIDEMIOLOGY & DEMOGRAPHICS

INCIDENCE:

- 34% of hospitalized patients with pelvic inflammatory disease
- 1% to 2% of patients undergoing hysterectomy, most with vaginal approach
- Peak incidence third to fourth decade
- 25% to 50% are nulliparous

RISK FACTORS: Same risk factors as for pelvic inflammatory disease, although in 30% to 50% of patients there is no prior history of salpingitis before abscess forms.

PHYSICAL FINDINGS & CLINICAL PRESENTATION

- Abdominal or pelvic pain (90%)
- Fever or chills (50%)
- Abnormal bleeding (21%)
- Vaginal discharge (28%)
- Nausea (26%)
- Up to 60% to 80% present in the absence of fever or leukocytosis; absence of these findings should not rule out diagnosis

ETIOLOGY

- Mixed flora of anaerobes, aerobes, and facultative anaerobes, such as *Escherichia coli, Bacteroides fragilis, Prevotella* spp., aerobic streptococci, and *Peptococcus* and *Peptostreptococcus* spp.
- *Nesseria gonorrhoeae* and *Chlamydia* are the major etiologic bacteria in cervicitis and salpingitis but are rarely found in abscess cavity cultures.
- In elderly patients consider diverticular disease.

Dx DIAGNOSIS

DIFFERENTIAL DIAGNOSIS

- Pelvic neoplasms, such as ovarian tumors and leiomyomas.
- Inflammatory masses involving adjacent bowel or omentum, such as ruptured appendicitis or diverticulitis.
- Pelvic hematomas, as may occur after cesarean section or hysterectomy.
- Section III describes the diagnostic approach to patients with a pelvic mass; the differential diagnosis of pelvic mass is described in Section II.
- The differential diagnosis of pelvic pain is described in Section II.
- Sonogram or CT scan: commonly used because, owing to associated pain and guarding, a suboptimal abdominal or pelvic examination is the rule rather than the exception.
- Most common cause of preventable death: physician delay in diagnosis.

LABORATORY TESTS

- Complete blood count, including white blood count with differential, hemoglobin, and hematocrit
- Aerobic as well as anaerobic cultures of cervix, blood, urine, sputum, peritoneal cavity (if entered), and abscess cavity before starting antibiotics
- Pregnancy test in patients of reproductive age

IMAGING STUDIES

- Sonogram: noninvasive, inexpensive study to confirm diagnosis, estimate size of abscess, and monitor response to therapy; sensitivity >90%
- CT scan: used for both diagnosis and therapy (CT-guided drainage)
  1. Useful where sonogram provides insufficient information, as with intraabdominal abscesses
  2. Success rate with CT-guided abscess drainage: unilocular, 90%; multilocular, 40%

Rx TREATMENT

Major concerns:

1. Desire for future fertility
2. Likelihood of rupture of abscess, with resulting peritonitis, septic shock, and morbid sequelae

ACUTE GENERAL Rx

- Clinical quandary is whether patient requires immediate surgery (uncertain diagnosis or suspicion of rupture) or management with IV antibiotics, reserving surgery for those with inadequate clinical response (e.g., 48 to 72 hr of therapy, with persistent fever or leukocytosis, increasing size of mass, or suspicion of rupture)
- Surgery indicated in poor response to medical therapy, in those with large adnexal masses (>8 cm), or immunocompromised patients
- Antibiotic combinations:
  1. Clindamycin 900 mg IV q8h or metronidazole 500 mg IV q6-8h plus gentamicin either 5 to 7 mg/kg q24h or 1.5 mg/kg q8h
  2. Alternatives: ampicillin sulbactam 3 g IV q6h or cefoxitin 2 g IV q6h or cefotetan 2 g IV q12h plus doxycycline 100 mg IV q12h
- During medical management, high index of suspicion for acute rupture, such as acute worsening of abdominal pain or new-onset tachycardia and hypotension, mandating immediate surgical intervention after patient stabilization
- Surgical options:
  1. Laparoscopy with drainage and irrigation
  2. Transvaginal colpotomy (abscess must be midline, dissect rectovaginal septum, and be adherent to vaginal fornix)
  3. Laparotomy, including total abdominal hysterectomy with bilateral salpingo-oophorectomy or unilateral salpingo-oophorectomy
  4. Evidence of ruptured tuboovarian abscess is a surgical emergency

DISPOSITION

- Of patients treated with medical therapy, response in 75%, with a 50% pregnancy rate
- No response in 30% to 40%; can be treated with either CT-guided drainage or surgical intervention, keeping in mind that unilateral adnexectomy may give equal chance of cure versus hysterectomy, yet preserve reproductive potential

REFERRAL

If patient has a tuboovarian abscess, refer to gynecologist.

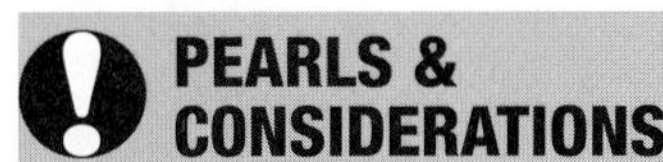

PEARLS & CONSIDERATIONS

COMMENTS

If *Actinomyces* species is isolated from culture, treatment with penicillin is required for an extended period (6 wk to 3 mo).

SUGGESTED READINGS

Aimakhu CO et al: Surgical management of pelvic abscess: laparotomy versus colpotomy, *J Obstet Gynaecol* 23(1):71, 2003.

Sudakoff GS et al: Transrectal and transvaginal sonographic intervention of infected pelvic fluid collections: a complete approach, *Ultrasound Q* 21(3):175, 2005.

AUTHORS: **SCOTT J. ZUCCALA, D.O.,** and **RUBEN ALVERO, M.D.**

Abscess, Perirectal (PTG)

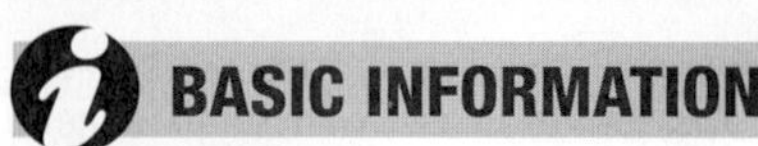

BASIC INFORMATION

DEFINITION

A perirectal abscess is a localized inflammatory process that can be associated with infections of soft tissue and anal glands based on anatomic location. Perianal and perirectal abscesses may be simple or complex, causing suppuration. Infections in these spaces may be classified as superficial perianal or perirectal with involvement in the following anatomic spaces: ischiorectal, intersphincteric, perianal, and supralevator (Fig. 1-4).

SYNONYMS

Rectal abscess
Perianal abscess
Anorectal abscess

ICD-9CM CODES
566 Perirectal abscess

EPIDEMIOLOGY & DEMOGRAPHICS

INCIDENCE (IN U.S.): Commonly encountered
PREDOMINANT SEX: Male > female
PREDOMINANT AGE: All ages
PEAK INCIDENCE: Not seasonal; common
GENETICS: None known

PHYSICAL FINDINGS & CLINICAL PRESENTATION

- Localized perirectal or anal pain—often worsened with movement or straining
- Perirectal erythema or cellulitis
- Perirectal mass by inspection or palpation
- Fever and signs of sepsis with deep abscess
- Urinary retention

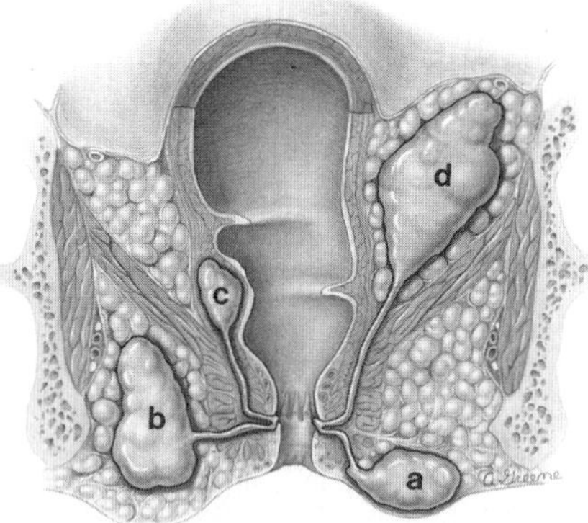

FIGURE 1-4 Common sites of anorectal abscesses: perianal **(a)**, ischiorectal **(b)**, intersphincteric **(c)**, and supralevator **(d)**. (From Noble J [ed]: *Textbook of primary care medicine,* ed 2, St Louis, 1996, Mosby.)

ETIOLOGY

- Polymicrobial aerobic and anaerobic bacteria involving one of the anatomic spaces (see "Definition"), often associated with localized trauma
- Microbiology: most bacteria are polymicrobial, mixed enteric and skin flora
- Predominant anaerobic bacteria:
  1. *Bacteroides fragilis*
  2. *Peptostreptococcus* spp.
  3. *Prevotella* spp.
  4. *Porphyromonas* spp.
  5. *Clostridium* spp.
  6. *Fusobacterium* spp.
- Predominant aerobic bacteria:
  1. *Staphylococcus aureus*
  2. *Streptococcus* spp.
  3. *Escherichia coli*
  4. *Enterococcus* spp.

DIAGNOSIS

Many patients will have predisposing underlying conditions including:

- Malignancy or leukemia
- Immune deficiency
- Diabetes mellitus
- Recent surgery
- Steroid therapy

DIFFERENTIAL DIAGNOSIS

- Neutropenic enterocolitis
- Crohn's disease (inflammatory bowel disease)
- Pilonidal disease
- Hidradenitis suppurativa
- Tuberculosis or actinomycosis; Chagas' disease
- Cancerous lesions
- Chronic anal fistula
- Rectovaginal fistula
- Proctitis—often STD-associated, including: syphilis, gonococcal, chlamydia, chancroid, condylomata acuminata
- AIDS-associated: Kaposi's sarcoma, lymphoma, CMV

WORKUP

- Examination of rectal, perirectal/perineal areas
- Rule out necrotic process and crepitance suggesting deep tissue involvement
- Local aerobic and anaerobic culture
- Blood cultures if toxic, febrile, or compromised
- Possible sigmoidoscopy

IMAGING STUDIES

Usually not indicated unless extensive disease abscess but can include CT

TREATMENT

ACUTE GENERAL Rx

- Incision and drainage of abscess
- Debridement if necrotic tissue
- Rule out need for fistulectomy
- Local wound care—packing
- Sitz baths

Antibiotic treatment: Directed toward coverage for mixed skins and enteric flora
Outpatient—oral:
Amoxicillin/clavulanic acid 875 to 1000 mg bid
Ciprofloxacin 750 mg by mouth every 12 hr plus metronidazole 500 to 750 mg by mouth every 8 hr
Clindamycin 150 to 300 mg by mouth every 8 hr
Inpatient—intravenous:
Ampicillin/sulbactam (Unasyn) 1.5 to 3 gm IV every 6 hr
Cefotetan 1 to 2 gm IV every 8 hr
Piperacillin/Tazobactam 3.375 gm IV every 6 to 8 hr
Imipenem 500 to 1000 mg IV every 8 hr

DISPOSITION

Follow-up with a general surgeon or infectious disease physician is often warranted.

REFERRAL

- General surgeon or colorectal surgeon for drainage.
- AIDS specialist may be needed for perirectal complications of HIV infection.
- Gastroenterologist follow-up may be warranted in Crohn's disease with perirectal fistula and other complications.

PEARLS & CONSIDERATIONS

Perirectal abscess may be a presenting manifestation of type 2 diabetes mellitus in older adults. Check the blood sugar in patients to exclude the possibility of unrecognized diabetes mellitus.

SUGGESTED READING

Marcus RH et al: Perirectal abscess, *Ann Emerg Med* 25(5):597-603, 1995.

AUTHORS: **GLENN G. FORT, M.D., M.P.H.,** and **DENNIS J. MIKOLICH, M.D.**

BASIC INFORMATION

DEFINITION

Definition from the Federal Child Abuse Prevention and Treatment Act (CAPTA): any recent act or failure to act on the part of a parent or caretaker which results in death, serious physical or emotional harm, sexual abuse or exploitation of a child; or an act or failure to act which presents an imminent risk of serious harm to a child.

- Neglect: failure to provide for the basic needs of a child (e.g., food, shelter, supervision)
  1. Medical neglect: failure to provide necessary medical or mental health care
  2. Educational neglect: failure to meet educational needs
  3. Emotional neglect: failure to attend to emotional needs, exposure to domestic violence
- Physical abuse: injury inflicted by an adult intentionally or in the course of excessive discipline
- Sexual abuse: sexual act inflicted by parent or caretaker; includes exploitation and pornography
- Emotional abuse: pattern of behavior of caretaker toward a child that impairs emotional development, such as verbal abuse or cruelty

SYNONYMS

Child maltreatment syndrome
Physical abuse
Sexual abuse
Battered child syndrome
Shaken baby syndrome
Shaken impact syndrome
Abusive head trauma

ICD-9CM CODES

995.5 Child maltreatment
995.50 Child abuse, unspecified
995.51 Child abuse, emotional or psychological
995.52 Child neglect
995.53 Child abuse, sexual
995.54 Child abuse, physical
995.55 Shaken infant syndrome
995.59 Multiple forms of child abuse

EPIDEMIOLOGY & DEMOGRAPHICS

INCIDENCE (IN U.S.): Any reports of incidence are underestimates because many cases are never recognized or reported. These are collected based on Child Protective Services (CPS) state aggregates. In 2007, roughly 735,000 children were determined to be victims of abuse or neglect.

- Types of abuse by percentage.
  1. Neglect: 59%
  2. Physical abuse: 10.8%
  3. Sexual abuse: 7.6%
  4. Emotional abuse: 4.2%
  5. Medical neglect: 1%
  6. Other: 4.2% (e.g., abandonment, threats of harm, congenital drug addiction)
  7. Multiple types: 13%
- For 2007, an estimated 1760 child deaths were caused by abuse or neglect.
  - Overall annual death rate resulting from abuse or neglect is estimated to be 2.35 deaths/100,000 children.
  - More than 30% of these deaths are due to neglect; 26% are due to physical abuse.
  - 75% of these children are <4 yr of age.
  - Most fatalities are directly caused by one or both parents (70%).
  - Many child abuse fatalities are underreported because of misdiagnosis or variations in state definitions and coding.
- More than 73% of abused children were victimized by one or both of their parents.
- One fifth of adult women report history of molestation or sexual assault as a child or adolescent.

PREDOMINANT SEX:

- There is a slight predominance of girls as victims.
- Infant boys (<1 yr) have the highest death rate: 18.8 per 100,000 boys of the same age versus 15.4 per 100,000 infant girls of the same age.

PREDOMINANT AGE: Youngest children (0 to 3 years old) have the highest rates of victimization.

GENETICS: No known genetic factors.

ETIOLOGY

Multiple factors contribute to the incidence. No factor or combination of factors can definitively predict which children will be victimized. Factors contributing to risk of abuse or neglect include the following:

- Parent
  1. Substance abuse
  2. Mental illness
  3. Intellectual impairment
  4. Parental history of being abused as a child
- Child
  1. Low birth weight or prematurity
  2. Chronic physical disability
- Family
  1. Social isolation
  2. Poor parent-child bonding
  3. Stress: unemployment, chronic illness, eviction, arrest, poverty
  4. Domestic violence
- Community/society
  1. Limited transportation
  2. Limited day care
  3. Unsafe neighborhoods
  4. Poverty

Dx DIAGNOSIS

Careful history and physical examination are the most important aspects of the evaluation. Careful documentation of any statements regarding origin of injuries or history of abuse is crucial. Chart and photographic documentation of injuries is also essential. The following are keys to the final diagnosis:

- Patterned bruising (e.g., loop-shaped, square, oval) is indicative of being struck with an object.
- Injury observed is incompatible with the history provided.
- History of injury provided is incompatible with the developmental capabilities of the child.
- Delay in seeking care for a significant injury (e.g., callus formation on a fracture, eschar formation on a burn).
- Bruising is rare in healthy precruising infants and warrants further investigation.
- Multiple significant injuries of different ages.
- Infant with clinically significant head trauma attributed to a trivial cause (e.g., a short fall). Often associated with retinal hemorrhages and skeletal fractures, which are indicative of shaken baby syndrome or abusive head trauma.
- Certain fractures in infants without a history of significant trauma (e.g., motor vehicle accident) are characteristic of abuse: metaphyseal, rib, sternum, scapula, vertebral body.
- Inflicted contact burns are indicated by an impression of the burning object: lighter, iron, cigarette.
- Inflicted immersion burns are indicated by "stocking" burns of the feet or "glove" burns of the hands. Stocking burns are often associated with buttocks/perineal burns from immersion of a minor in a flexed position.
- Most sexual abuse victims will have a normal or nonspecific genital examination. A normal genital examination does not mean the child was not abused. History is the most important part of the diagnosis. Forensic interview by a trained professional is recommended, as is an examination by an experienced health care provider for child and adolescent victims of sexual abuse.
- The identification of a sexually transmitted disease in a prepubertal child who is beyond the neonatal period is suggestive of sexual abuse. Reporting and further careful investigation are warranted. Consult current CDC guidelines and a child sexual abuse expert for further guidance.

DIFFERENTIAL DIAGNOSIS

In all categories, accidental injury is the most common entity to be distinguished from abuse. Accidental injuries are most common over bony prominences: forehead, elbows, knees, shins; soft, fleshy areas are more common for inflicted injury: buttocks, thighs, upper arms.

BRUISING

- Bleeding disorder (idiopathic thrombocytopenic purpura, hemophilia, leukemia, hemorrhagic disease of the newborn, von Willebrand disease)
- Connective tissue disorder (Ehlers-Danlos syndrome, vasculitis)
- Pigments (Mongolian spots)
- Dermatitis (phytophotodermatitis, nickel allergy)
- Folk treatment (coining, cupping)

BURNS

- Chemical burn
- Impetigo
- Folk treatment (moxibustion)
- Dermatitis (phytophotodermatitis)

INTRACRANIAL HEMORRHAGE
- Bleeding disorder
- Perinatal trauma (should resolve by 4 wk)
- Arteriovenous malformation rupture
- Glutaric aciduria

FRACTURES
- Osteogenesis imperfecta
- Rickets
- Congenital syphilis
- Very low birth weight (osteopenia of prematurity)

SEXUAL ABUSE
- Normal variants
- Lichen sclerosis et atrophicus
- Congenital abnormalities
- Urethral prolapse
- Hemangioma
- Nonsexually acquired infection (group A *Streptococcus, Shigella*)

WORKUP

History and physical examination:
- Careful history from all caretakers and child.
- Scene investigation may be necessary.
- Complete physical examination.
- Sexual abuse: forensic interview and magnified examinations by trained professionals are the standard for evaluation and evidence collection.

Laboratory tests for physical abuse:
- Tests performed may vary depending on the severity of abuse and clinical presentation of the child.
- CBC with differential and platelets.
- Prothrombin time, activated partial thromboplastin time.
- Consider closure time (PFA-100), von Willebrand panel.
- Alanine aminotransferase, amylase, urinalysis.

Laboratory tests for sexual abuse:
- If within 72 hr of acute sexual assault/abuse, swabs are obtained for sperm, acid phosphatase, P30, MHS-5 antigen, blood group typing, DNA testing. Also collect samples of foreign hair, blood, saliva, or other tissue if present.
- Per current CDC recommendations, adolescent victims of acute assault should have appropriate specimens collected from sites of penetration for *Neisseria gonorrhea* and *Chlamydia.* Nucleic acid amplification tests (NAATs) may be used and are preferred. In females, wet mount for bacterial vaginosis and trichomonas should also be done. Serum should be obtained for HIV, hepatitis B, and syphilis testing acutely. If negative, HIV and syphilis testing should be repeated 6, 12, and 24 wk after the assault.
- Child victims (i.e., prepubertal) should have specimens collected if considered high risk for a sexually transmitted disease (STD) per current CDC recommendations. Cervical specimens are not collected and vaginal specimens must be collected with care by an experienced provider to avoid further trauma to the child. *Gonorrhea* and *Chlamydia* culture is the gold standard for diagnosis and legal purposes. However, some providers analyze specimens with NAAT followed by culture confirmation if any positive results are obtained. Any culture testing positive for *N. gonorrhea* should be confirmed by at least two laboratory tests that are based on different principles. Specimens should be collected for *Gonorrhea* and *Chlamydia,* wet mount, and blood for serologic testing (HIV, hepatitis B, syphilis) in the following cases:
  1. Presence of vaginal discharge or genital ulcer
  2. Alleged assailant is known to have an STD or be at high risk for an STD
  3. A sibling or adult in the same household has a known STD
  4. High prevalence of STDs in the community
  5. Evidence of ejaculation or penetration is present on the examination
  6. Child or parent requests testing

IMAGING STUDIES

Physical abuse:
- Radiographic skeletal survey for all children <2 yr; for 2- to 5-yr-olds, done only for severe abuse. Consider repeat skeletal survey in 2 wk if severe physical injury is present.
- Noncontrast head CT scan or MRI for all children <1 yr; for children >1 yr, clinical judgment should be used.
- Head MRI for children with significant abusive head trauma. This is used as an adjunct a few days after initial head CT.
- Abdominal CT scan if indicated by clinical examination or laboratory evaluation.

Rx TREATMENT

ACUTE GENERAL Rx

- Stabilize and treat acute medical injuries.
- Report to Child Protective Services. HIPAA allows reports for suspected child abuse without parental authorization.
- Early report to law enforcement for suspected physical abuse or sexual abuse to allow scene investigation.
- Disposition, once medically stable, is dependent on CPS. The child cannot be returned home if the environment is not safe.
- Physician should remain available to discuss with investigators. This is often critical to determining the outcome of the case and placement of the child.
- Because follow-up of adolescent sexual assault victims can be difficult, many experts recommend empiric treatment for *Gonorrhea, Chlamydia,* trichomonas, and bacterial vaginosis. Pregnancy prophylaxis should also be offered. Hepatitis B immunization should be offered if not previously given. HIV prophylaxis is offered in certain situations depending on local epidemiology and type of assault. Consult local infectious disease experts for current recommendations. Repeat examination should be done in 2 wk for all victims of sexual assault, especially if they declined empiric treatment.
- Empiric treatment of child victims of sexual abuse is generally not recommended. This is especially important if NAATs are used for screening for STDs because culture confirmation is necessary for any positive results. Careful follow-up within 2 wk and treatment based on culture results are indicated. HIV prophylaxis is offered in certain circumstances according to local epidemiology and risk. Consult with a local infectious disease expert for further recommendations.

CHRONIC Rx

- Often depends on CPS and court-ordered interventions
- Treatment of parental mental illness
- Treatment of parental substance abuse, including requirements for random drug testing
- Instruction for parents in behavior management skills, including appropriate limit setting and discipline
- Anger management classes for parents
- Trauma-focused cognitive-behavioral therapy for victims of sexual abuse and exposure to domestic violence; useful to include nonoffending parent/caregiver
- Ongoing individual and family therapy
- May need long-term placement in foster care before it is safe to return home

DISPOSITION

- Victims of chronic abuse and neglect have higher rates of mental illness (depression, suicide, posttraumatic stress disorder, eating disorders)
- Victims have more cognitive difficulties and often have impaired academic performance
- Victims are more likely to become aggressive
- Victims, as adults, are more likely to have adverse physical health outcomes (cardiovascular disease, cancer, STDs)
- Victims of abusive head trauma:
  1. One third die.
  2. One third have severe disability.
  3. One third appear normal in the short term.

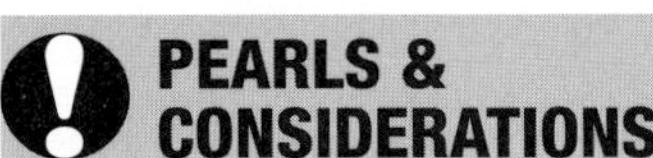

PEARLS & CONSIDERATIONS

PREVENTION

- Home visitation to high-risk families during pregnancy and infancy has shown positive outcomes.
- Anticipatory guidance at health visits to teach normal developmental expectations and appropriate discipline.
- Screening to identify at-risk or abused children.
- Targeted education in the newborn nursery for shaken baby prevention has been shown to be effective.
- Substance abuse prevention and treatment.
- Identification and intervention for domestic violence before children are born.

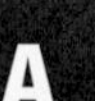

A

Diseases and Disorders

EVIDENCE

Please note: Complete text of EBM for this topic is available online.

Key trials and commentary:

This study analyzed the interaction of four SNPs of the *FKBP5* gene with severity of child abuse as a predictor of adult PTSD symptoms. There were no main effects of the SNPs on PTSD symptoms and no significant genetic interactions with level of non-child abuse trauma as predictor of adult PTSD symptoms, suggesting a potential gene-childhood environment interaction for adult PTSD.

This is an important study illustrating the powerful effects of gene–environment interactions in childhood upon adult psychopathology. The study was meticulous in its design. Gene effects on PTSD risk do not appear to be confounded by the usual suspect, that is, comorbid depression and familial risk for PTSD. What is perhaps most powerful in this study is the extent of the "signal" from the trauma of childhood abuse. The effect is distinct and independent from other trauma experienced in this sample of patients with PTSD. This is an extremely important article in that it illustrates gene–early environment interactions for psychiatric illness in genes. It is also important because of the strength of the "signal" from childhood abuse as a risk factor for the later development of PTSD in adult life.[1] Ⓐ

Evidence-Based Reference

1. Binder EB et al: Association of Fkbp5 polymorphisms and childhood abuse with risk of posttraumatic stress disorder symptoms in adults, *J Am Med Assoc* 299:1291-1305, 2008. Commentary by P. Buckley, M.D. Ⓐ

SUGGESTED READINGS

Adams JA et al: Guidelines for medical care of children who may have been sexually abused, *J Pediatric Adolesc Gynecol* 10:163, 2007.

Dubowitz H: Tackling child neglect: a role for pediatricians, *Pediatr Clin North Am* 56(2):363-378, 2009.

Gilbert R et al: Burden and consequences of child maltreatment in high-income countries, *Lancet* 373(9657):68-81, 2009.

Girardet RG et al: Epidemiology of sexually transmitted infections in suspected child victims of sexual assault, *Pediatrics* 124(1):79-86, 2009.

Saperia J et al: Guideline Development Group and Technical Team: When to suspect child maltreatment: summary of NICE guidelines, *BMJ* 339:b2689, 2009.

United States Department of Health and Human Services: Child Maltreatment 2007. Available at http://www.acf.hhs.gov/programs/cb/pubs/cm07/.

AUTHOR: **NANCY R. GRAFF, M.D.**

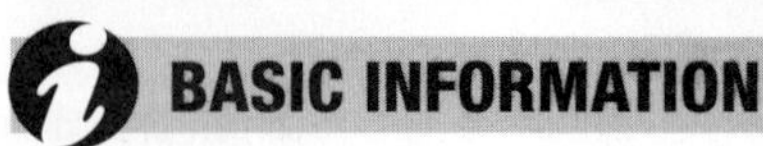

BASIC INFORMATION

DEFINITION

Drug abuse is a recurring pattern of harmful use of a substance despite adverse consequences to work, school, relationships, the legal system, and personal health. This may occur concurrently with or independently from *substance dependence,* in which the impairment or distress is more pervasive and that often (though not necessarily) includes physical dependence and withdrawal symptoms (Table 1-1).

SYNONYMS

Substance use disorder
Substance abuse
Addiction

ICD-9CM CODES

Defined by specific substance F10-F19 (DSM-IV code is also defined by specific substance 291-292, 303-305)

EPIDEMIOLOGY & DEMOGRAPHICS

INCIDENCE (IN U.S.): Alcohol or drug dependence: 5% to 10% of population

PREVALENCE (IN U.S.): Approximately 15% of patients in primary care practice have an at-risk pattern of drug and/or alcohol use; lifetime prevalence of any alcohol use disorder: 30%; prescription drug misuse is on the rise with 5% past-year prevalence.

PREDOMINANT SEX: Males > females

PREDOMINANT AGE:
- Problematic use of substances may begin in early life (8 to 10 yr).
- Mean age of onset of problem drinking is approximately 25 yr for men and 30 yr for women.

PEAK INCIDENCE: For most substances: age 15 to 30 yr

DURATION OF CONDITION:
- Men: average >20 yr of heavy drinking
- Women: average 15 yr of heavy drinking

GENETICS: There is evidence of nonspecific genetic factors.

PHYSICAL FINDINGS & CLINICAL PRESENTATION

- Polysubstance use and comorbidity with psychiatric disorders is common.
- History often reveals recurring behavioral problems, such as relationship, work, or legal problems; violence and traumatic injuries; and anxiety, depression, insomnia, and cognitive and memory dysfunction. Repeated requests for early refills of controlled substances and obtaining prescriptions from multiple providers should raise concern for prescription drug abuse.
- Physical findings are limited but may include injection marks, nasal lesions or recurrent epistaxis, poor dentition, or poor nutritional status; signs/symptoms of intoxication or withdrawal are highly suggestive of substance use disorder.

ETIOLOGY

Two models of addiction:
1. Conditioning (reward driven): Substance use is paired with enforcing and triggering stimuli.
2. Homeostatic (self-medicating): Either preexisting abnormalities or drug-induced abnormalities lead to initial or continued use of the drug.

Dx DIAGNOSIS

DIFFERENTIAL DIAGNOSIS

- Psychiatric disorders such as depression, mania, social phobia, or other anxiety disorders may coexist or occur as a consequence of substance abuse.
- Rule out seizure disorder and underlying illness in persons presenting with substance use.

WORKUP

- A thorough history is crucial for diagnosis of any substance abuse disorder.
- The physician's history-taking style and techniques strongly affect patient's willingness to report use and participate in future treatment activities.
- A structured, nonjudgmental approach is generally preferable. Possibilities include the following:
  1. Ask about alcohol or drug use in the past year.
  2. Use a short screening instrument such as the two-item screen ("In the last year, have you ever consumed alcohol or used drugs more than you meant to? Have you felt you wanted or needed to cut down on your drinking or drug use in the last year?").
  3. Ask about quantity and frequency. For example, the National Institute on Alcohol and Alcoholism declares that problem drinking for men is defined as more than 14 drinks/wk or more than 4 drinks on any one occasion; for women and anyone older than 65 yr, the limits are 7 drinks and no more than 3 on any one occasion.
- Problematic behavior during intoxication or withdrawal is diagnostic.

LABORATORY TESTS

- Consider toxicology screen or blood alcohol level.
- Elevated mean corpuscular volume and γ-glutamyltransferase are most sensitive indicators of alcohol intake.

IMAGING STUDIES

Not helpful in routine diagnosis and management of substance abuse, but possibly useful in the management of sequelae of substance abuse (e.g., brain imaging to evaluate the alcohol abuse–associated increased risk of subdural hematomas or increased evidence of cerebral atrophy).

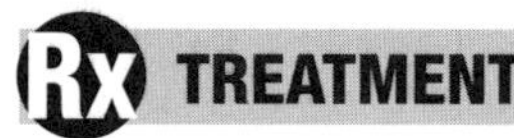

Rx TREATMENT

NONPHARMACOLOGIC THERAPY

- First assess readiness for change; if precontemplative or contemplative, counsel about risks of use and benefits of abstinence; a

TABLE 1-1 Diagnostic Criteria for Dependence and Drug Abuse

Dependence (>3 Needed)	Abuse (>1 for 12 mo)
1. Tolerance	1. Recurrent substance use resulting in failure to fulfill major role obligations at work, school, or home
2. Withdrawal	2. Recurrent substance use in situations in which it is physically hazardous
3. The substance is often taken in larger amounts over a longer period than intended	3. Recurrent substance-related legal problems
4. Any unsuccessful effort or a persistent desire to cut down or control substance use	4. Continued substance use despite having persistent or recurrent social or interpersonal problems caused or exacerbated by the effects of the substance
5. A great deal of time is spent in activities necessary to obtain the substance or recover from its effects	5. Never met criteria for dependence
6. Important social, occupational, or recreational activities given up or reduced because of substance use	
7. Continued substance use despite knowledge of having had persistent or recurrent physical or psychological problems that are likely to be caused or exacerbated by the substance	

Reprinted from Goldman L, Bennett JC (eds): *Cecil textbook of medicine,* ed 21, Philadelphia, 2000, WB Saunders.

motivational interviewing approach has been shown to be effective.

- Nonpharmacologic strategies have the greatest documented efficacy. Effective nonpharmacologic interventions generally include advice, feedback, goal setting, problem solving, and additional contacts for further assistance and support.
- Relapse prevention by avoidance of trigger stimuli or by uncoupling trigger stimuli from substance ingestion.
- Self-help and support groups such as Alcoholics Anonymous, Narcotics Anonymous, and Al-Anon.

ACUTE GENERAL Rx

- Detoxification is an important first step in substance abuse treatment. Its goals are to facilitate withdrawal and reduce symptoms, initiate abstinence, and refer the patient to ongoing treatment.
- Benzodiazepines, particularly long-acting ones, are safe and effective in acute alcohol withdrawal. One strategy is to give the patient a loading dose of a long-acting benzodiazepine (e.g., 20 mg of diazepam) and then follow the patient clinically. An alternative "symptom driven" strategy is to follow the patient closely with serial assessments, such as the Clinical Institute Withdrawal Assessment for Alcohol scale, and to dose with 5 to 10 mg of diazepam as needed to treat withdrawal symptoms.
- Beta-blockers and clonidine generally should be avoided in alcohol withdrawal; they may mask markers of the severity of the withdrawal (blood pressure and pulse rate).
- Clonidine alleviates the discomfort of opiate withdrawal. For treatment of opiate withdrawal, prescribe 0.2 mg q8h for 10 to 14 days. Antidiarrheals, ibuprofen, and baclofen can be used as adjuncts to treat opiate withdrawal symptoms.
- Methadone taper is an effective approach for detoxification in opioid dependence.
- Buprenorphine is a partial μ-opioid receptor agonist that may be used for both detoxification and maintenance in treatment of opioid dependence (see dosing in next section).

CHRONIC Rx

- Naltrexone helps reduce craving for alcohol. Naltrexone 50 mg once daily for 12 wk can be a useful adjunct to substance abuse counseling or rehabilitation programs. Randomized treatment studies are equivocal for long-term outcomes. Naltrexone reduces relapse and the intensity or frequency of any drinking that does occur. It can be hepatotoxic and is contraindicated in opiate users. Intramuscular naltrexone (380 mg monthly) may be considered if adherence to treatment is an issue.
- Acamprosate also helps reduce craving for alcohol. Acamprosate 666 mg three times daily may be an effective adjunct to counseling. A recent meta-analysis showed overall benefit with increase in the number of abstinent days.
- Disulfiram (Antabuse) provokes acetaldehyde accumulation after alcohol ingestion, producing a toxic state manifested by nausea, headache, flushing, and respiratory distress. Studies have shown limited efficacy.
- Topiramate may be an alternative treatment for alcoholism. In a recent 14-wk randomized trial topiramate up to 300 mg daily significantly reduced the number of heavy drinking days.
- Methadone maintenance for opiate addiction is effective and involves once-daily dosing of methadone in a controlled setting.
- Buprenorphine is as effective as low-dose methadone and may be prescribed by physicians who have completed approved training. For induction, initiate 12 to 24 hr after short-acting opioid use and 24 to 48 hr after long-acting opioid use. Use buprenorphine/naloxone tablets in most patients; buprenorphine only on day 1 for patients with dependence on long-acting opioids. Maximum first-day dosage is 8 to 12 mg of buprenorphine (2 mg buprenorphine q2h for signs of withdrawal). Titrate buprenorphine dose up to 16 mg on day 2 for signs of withdrawal and up to 32 mg daily by end of week 1. Then adjust dosage to minimum needed for maintenance. Naltrexone (oral) may also be used for maintenance in opioid dependence treatment, though evidence of effectiveness is limited.
- Always combine pharmacotherapy with counseling.
- Treatment of comorbid psychiatric disorders improves outcomes.
- The effect of any intervention wanes after discontinuation of the intervention.

DISPOSITION

- Substance abuse is a chronic relapsing illness.
- The goal of treatment is always abstinence, but success of treatment is measured by return of function, increasing duration between relapses, and prevention of sequelae of use.

REFERRAL

Physicians should refer any patients who do not make good progress on changing substance use patterns.

PEARLS & CONSIDERATIONS

- Withdrawal from opioids can resemble a severe case of the flu.
- A brief intervention (providing information and advising the patient to reduce consumption of alcohol) by the primary care doctor has been demonstrated in randomized trials to reduce drinking in at-risk patients.
- Treatment rates for alcohol use disorders remain low despite available effective treatments.

EBM EVIDENCE

Please note: Complete text of EBM for this topic is available online.

Key trials and commentary:

This study revealed that cannabis withdrawal was prevalent and clinically significant among a representative sample of frequent cannabis users. Similar results in the subset without polysubstance abuse confirmed the specificity of symptoms to cannabis. Cannabis withdrawal should be added to DSM-V, and the etiology and treatment implications of cannabis withdrawal symptoms should be investigated.

The authors make a good argument for including cannabis withdrawal in the DSM-V as a true withdrawal syndrome. Clinicians familiar with the symptoms reported as withdrawal might wonder whether this has any implications for their actual practice, because they are certainly not going to prescribe cannabinoid therapy. In fact, a defined withdrawal syndrome may result in the all-important recognitions by insurers and other payers, and that would pave the way for further treatment other than supportive care.[1] Ⓐ

Another study examined the association between stimulant treatment in childhood and adolescence and subsequent substance use disorders (alcohol, drug, and nicotine) into the young adult years. The findings revealed no evidence that stimulant treatment increases or decreases the risk for subsequent substance use disorders in children and adolescents with ADHD when they reach young adulthood.

Despite several previous studies to the contrary, the concern that stimulant use in ADHD promotes risk for substance use disorders is a persistent worry. The basic understanding has been that properly treating ADHD mitigates the risk for substance use that is naturally higher among those with ADHD. This study is further evidence of this tenet. The authors gathered data on a large number of males with ADHD and reviewed previous exposure to stimulants. Figure 1 in the original article includes the Kaplan-Meier curves for substance use as an outcome stratified by previous exposure to stimulant medications, which leads to no significant differences. In general, the risks of abuse do seem to be mitigated by proper ADHD treatment, even if at a young age. The authors had, in past years, promoted that stimulant treatment imparted a reduced risk; there is a need to find further data coordinating these two perspectives.

It should be remembered that this study is focused on males only.[2] Ⓑ

There is no approved pharmacotherapy for cocaine dependence. Risperidone is an atypical antipsychotic drug with combined dopamine-2/serotonin-2 (D_2/5-HT_2) antagonist activity that has been effective in reducing cocaine use in some animal studies. This study analyzed the efficacy of a long-acting, injectable preparation of risperidone on cocaine use in active cocaine users.

It revealed that treatment with long-acting injectable risperidone in active cocaine users was not associated with reduction in cocaine use or craving and was associated with worsening of depressive symptoms and weight gain.

Although this study found negative results for the antipsychotic depot medication risperidone in the treatment of cocaine addiction, it is important for clinicians to be aware of this finding. Many clinicians are tempted to try off-label uses of antipsychotics such as risperidone for cocaine addiction because it intuitively makes sense. The paranoia and psychotogenic aspects of cocaine intoxication make these medications likely candidates for trying as treatments. In addition, depot medications are promising for this population because this population is likely to be noncompliant in taking their medications. However, this study found that not only was the risperidone ineffective—it led to increased depression and to increased weight gain, both undesirable side effects. The search for effective agents in the treatment of stimulant abuse should be one of high priority, even though previous efforts have not borne much fruit. Another value of this study is that it reminds us that clinicians should also be cautious about their off-label uses of medications.[3] Ⓐ

Evidence-Based References

1. Hasin DS et al: Cannabis withdrawal in the United States: results from NESARC, *J Clin Psychiatry* 69:1354-1363, 2008. Commentary by R.J. Hamilton, M.D. Ⓐ
2. Biederman J et al: Stimulant therapy and risk for subsequent substance use disorders in male adults with ADHD: a naturalistic controlled 10-year follow-up study, *Am J Psychiatry* 165:597-603, 2008. Commentary by A. Mack, M.D. Ⓐ
3. Loebl T et al: A randomized, double-blind, placebo-controlled trial of long-acting risperidone in cocaine-dependent men, *J Clin Psychiatry* 69:480-486, 2008. Commentary by R. Frances, M.D. Ⓐ

SUGGESTED READINGS

Center for Substance Abuse Treatment, U.S. Department of Health and Human Services: www.csat.samhsa.gov.

Kleber HD et al: Treatment of patients with substance use disorders, second edition, *Am J Psychiatry* 164(4 suppl):5-123, 2007.

Lucey MR et al: Alcoholic hepatitis, *N Engl J Med* 360(26):2758-2759, 2009.

Willenbring ML et al: Helping patients who drink too much: an evidence-based guide for primary care physicians, *Am Fam Phys* 80(1):44-50, 2009.

AUTHORS: **OMRI BERGER, M.D.,** and **RADHIKA RAMANAN, M.D., M.P.H.**

BASIC INFORMATION

DEFINITION

Elder abuse includes domestic elder abuse, institutional elder abuse, and self-neglect.

- Physical abuse: inflicting physical pain or injury
- Sexual abuse: inflicting nonconsensual sexual activity
- Psychological abuse: inflicting mental anguish, including intimidation, humiliation, or threats
- Financial abuse: improper use of the resources without the person's consent
- Abandonment: desertion by the responsible caregiver
- Neglect: failure to fulfill a care-taking obligation, including provision of food, safe shelter, health care, or basic custodial care
- Self-neglect: behavior that threatens the elder's health or safety

SYNONYMS

Battered elder syndrome
Elder mistreatment
Domestic violence in the elderly
Diogenes syndrome

ICD-9CM CODES

995.80 Adult maltreatment, unspecified
995.81 Adult physical abuse
995.82 Adult emotional/psychological abuse
995.83 Adult sexual abuse
995.84 Adult neglect, nutritional
995.85 Other adult abuse and neglect

EPIDEMIOLOGY & DEMOGRAPHICS

INCIDENCE: According to the National Center on Elder Abuse, between 1-2 million Americans aged 65 and older have been injured, exploited, or mistreated by someone whom they depend on for care.

PEAK INCIDENCE: >80 yr of age.

PREVALENCE:

- Most studies estimate a prevalence rate of 2% to 5% in those older than 65 yr.
- Neglect is the most common form of elder mistreatment, representing approximately 27% of all cases.
- In a study of caregivers of patients with dementia in the U.K., one half reported behaving abusively at least some of the time, and one third reported "important" levels of abuse. Verbal abuse was most common and physical abuse was rare.
- Elder self-neglect and abuse are associated with increased risk of mortality.

RISK FACTORS (VICTIM):

- Impaired cognition
- Shared living situation
- Social isolation

RISK FACTORS (PERPETRATOR):

- Substance abuse
- Mental illness, particularly depression
- Dependence on the victim
- Being an involuntary caregiver
- History of violence

PHYSICAL FINDINGS & CLINICAL PRESENTATION

- Physical abuse with multiple injuries at various stages with implausible descriptions of their origins.
- Fear, hypervigilance, or withdrawal.
- Evidence of poor nutrition, poor hygiene, multiple or neglected pressure ulcers, neglected medical conditions, or evidence of restraint use (bruises around wrists or ankles).
- Toxicologic evidence of unprescribed medications.
- Poor adherence, frequent no-shows, or little contact with health care system.

DIAGNOSIS

DIFFERENTIAL DIAGNOSIS

- Advancing dementia
- Depression or other psychiatric disorder
- Malnutrition from intrinsic causes
- Conscious nonadherence
- Financial hardship
- Falling

WORKUP

1. Ask direct specific questions such as*:
   - "Has anyone close to you called you names or put you down recently?"
   - "Are you afraid of anyone in your life?"
   - "Are you able to use the telephone anytime you want to?"
   - "Has anyone forced you to do things you didn't want to do?"
   - "Has anyone taken things or money that belong to you without your OK?"
   - "Has anyone close to you tried to hurt you or harm you recently?"
2. Interview patient separately from the suspected abuser.
3. Pelvic examination if sexual abuse suspected.
4. Take photographs of physical injuries as legal evidence.

LABORATORY TESTS & IMAGING STUDIES

- Toxicology screens and therapeutic drug monitoring are sometimes helpful.
- Other laboratory tests and radiology studies should be ordered according to presentation.

TREATMENT

NONPHARMACOLOGIC THERAPY

- Separate patient and abuser.
- Patient and caregiver may benefit from screening and treatment for substance abuse, mental illness, or cognitive impairment.

*University of Maine Center on Aging: Elder abuse screening protocol for physicians: lessons learned from the Maine partners for elder protection pilot project, http://www.umaine.edu/mainecenteronaging/documents/elderabusescreeningmanual.pdf)

ACUTE GENERAL Rx

As indicated for injury or pain relief

DISPOSITION

If the patient's level of disability does not allow independent living, institutionalization may be required. Guidelines vary at the state and county levels regarding guardianship and conservatorship requirements.

REFERRAL

- For outpatients, report to local adult protective services agency. Reporting is mandatory in most states.
- For nursing home patients, report to regional long-term care ombudsman. Reporting is mandatory under federal law.
- In the U.S., the elder care help line is 1-800-677-1116.
- National Center on Elder Abuse: http://www.ncea.aoa.gov.

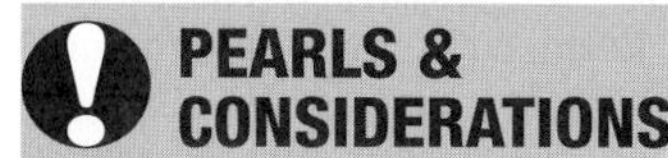

PEARLS & CONSIDERATIONS

COMMENTS

Care should be taken in interacting with the alleged abuser so that access to the victim is not lost.

PREVENTION

- Offer social services (e.g., respite care) for stressed caregivers.
- Make financial arrangements and arrange durable power of attorney for health care and finances while patient is still cognitively intact.

PATIENT & FAMILY EDUCATION

National Center on Elder Abuse: http://www.ncea.aoa.gov

JAMA Patient Page: Hildreth CJ et al: JAMA patient page. Elder abuse, *JAMA* 302(5):588, 2009

SUGGESTED READINGS

Cohen M et al: Elder abuse: disparities between older people's disclosure of abuse, evident signs of abuse, and high risk of abuse, *J Am Geriatr Soc* 55: 1224, 2007.

Cooper C et al: Abuse of people with dementia by family carers: representative cross sectional survey, *BMJ* 338:b155, 2009.

Dong X et al: Elder self-neglect and abuse and mortality risk in a community-dwelling population, *JAMA* 302(5):517-526, 2009.

Dyer CB et al: Vulnerable elders: when it is no longer safe to live alone, *JAMA* 298(12):1448, 2007.

Gill TM: Elder self-neglect: medical emergency or marker of extreme vulnerability, *JAMA* 302(5):570-571, 2009.

AUTHOR: **BREE JOHNSTON, M.D., M.P.H.**

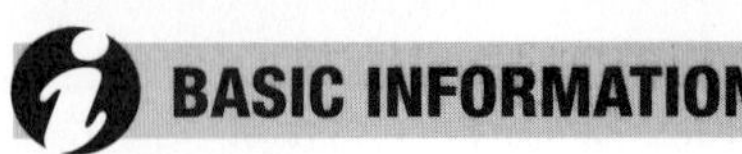

BASIC INFORMATION

DEFINITION

Acetaminophen (APAP) poisoning is a disorder manifested by jaundice, somnolence, diaphoresis, and potential death if not treated appropriately. Pathologically there is hepatic necrosis.

SYNONYMS

Paracetamol poisoning

ICD-9CM CODES

965.4 Acetaminophen poisoning

EPIDEMIOLOGY & DEMOGRAPHICS

- Potentially toxic ingestions of acetaminophen-containing medications exceed 100,000 cases annually in the U.S.
- APAP toxicity is the number one cause of acute liver failure in the U.S.
- Death rate is approximately one in 1000 persons. Nearly 50% of exposures occur in children <6 yr.
- Hepatic necrosis is most likely to occur in people who are chronically malnourished, who regularly abuse alcohol, and who are using other potentially hepatotoxic medications.

PHYSICAL FINDINGS & CLINICAL PRESENTATION

- The physical examination may vary depending on the number of hours lapsed from the ingestion of acetaminophen.
- Symptoms initially may be mild or absent and may consist of diaphoresis, malaise, nausea, and vomiting.
- After 12 to 24 hr, patients may report right upper quadrant pain with associated vomiting, diaphoresis, and subsequent somnolence in concurrence with an increase in lab values.
- In massive overdoses, jaundice may occur within the initial 72 hr.
- Subsequent coma, somnolence, and confusion follow and can ultimately lead to death or need for liver transplant if not treated appropriately.

ETIOLOGY

- The amount of acetaminophen necessary for hepatic toxicity varies with the patient's body size and hepatic function. It is recommended that APAP intake should not exceed 4 g within a 24-hr period.
- Using standardized nomograms calculating the acetaminophen plasma level and the number of hours after ingestion, the clinician can determine potential hepatic toxicity. See the acetaminophen ingestion algorithm in Section III.

Dx DIAGNOSIS

DIFFERENTIAL DIAGNOSIS

- Liver disease from alcohol abuse or hepatitis
- Ingestion of other hepatotoxic substances

WORKUP

Initial workup is aimed at confirming acetaminophen overdose with plasma acetaminophen level and assessment of hepatic damage and potential damage to other organ systems, such as kidneys, pancreas, and heart (see "Laboratory Tests").

LABORATORY TESTS

- Initial laboratory evaluation should include a STAT plasma acetaminophen level with a second level drawn approximately 4 to 6 hr after the initial level. Subsequent levels can be obtained every 2 to 4 hr until the levels stabilize or decline. These levels can be plotted by using the Rumack-Matthew nomogram (see acetaminophen ingestion algorithm [Fig. 3-3] in Section III) to calculate potential hepatic toxicity and for initiation of antidote therapy. The nomogram cannot be used when patients present >24 h after ingestion, for those who ingested an extended-release preparation, in patients who had a repeated supratherapeutic ingestion, or when the time of ingestion is unknown.
- Transaminases (AST, ALT), bilirubin level, prothrombin time (INR), blood urea nitrogen, and creatinine should be initially obtained on all patients.
- Serum and urine toxicology screen for other potential toxic substances is also recommended on admission. Screening for infectious hepatitis should also be considered.

Rx TREATMENT

NONPHARMACOLOGIC THERAPY

Consultation with a Poison Control Center is recommended for patients who have ingested a large amount of acetaminophen and/or other toxic substances. A toxic dose of acetaminophen usually exceeds 7.5 g in the adult or 140 mg/kg.

ACUTE GENERAL Rx

- Hepatotoxicity is defined as any increase in alanine aminotransferase (ALT), severe hepatotoxicity is aspartate aminotransferase (AST) >1000 IU/L, and hepatic failure is hepatotoxicity with hepatic encephalopathy. For those who cannot be risk stratified using the nomogram, the American College of Emergency Physicians recommends that *N*-acetylcysteine be administered to those older than 12 yr with hepatic failure thought to be caused by acetaminophen. It should also be administered to patients >12 yr who have hepatotoxicity thought to be caused by acetaminophen and a suspected or known acetaminophen overdose.
- Perform gastric lavage and administer activated charcoal if the patient is seen within 1 hr of ingestion or the clinician suspects polydrug ingestion.
- Determine blood levels 4 hr after ingestion; if the 4° level is >150 mg/dl, start *N*-acetylcysteine either IV (Acetadote) or PO (Mucomyst). Acetylcysteine IV loading dose is 150 mg/kg over 15 to 60 min ×1. Maintenance dose is 50 mg/kg over 4 hr, followed by 100 mg/kg over 16 hr. The dose does not require adjustment for renal or hepatic impairment or for dialysis. Oral administration consists of 140 mg/kg PO as a loading dose, followed by 70 mg/kg PO q4h for a total of 17 doses. *N*-acetylcysteine therapy should be started within 24 hr of acetaminophen overdose. If charcoal therapy was initially instituted, lavage the stomach and recover as much charcoal as possible; then instill *N*-acetylcysteine, increasing the loading dose by 40%. Advantages of IV administration include more reliable absorption, fewer doses, and shorter duration of treatment (1 day vs. 3 days).
- Monitor acetaminophen level; use graph to plot possible hepatic toxicity. Some toxicologists recommend repeating ALT and acetaminophen levels after 12 to 14 hr of IV acetylcysteine infusion and continuing infusion longer than 16 hr if AST levels are elevated or if the serum acetaminophen concentration is measurable.
- Provide adequate IV hydration (e.g., D_5½NS at 150 ml/hr).
- In patients on IV *N*-acetylcysteine with liver failure, frequent monitoring of vital signs, oxygen saturation by pulse oximetry, AST and serum creatinine as well as signs of hypoglycemia and infection is essential.
- If acetaminophen level is nontoxic, *N*-acetylcysteine therapy may be discontinued.
- If evidence of liver injury is present, continue treatment for 72 hr.

DISPOSITION

Most patients will recover fully without persisting hepatic abnormalities. Hepatic failure is particularly unusual in children <6 yr.

REFERRAL

Psychiatric referral is recommended after intentional ingestions.

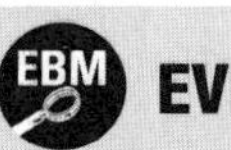

EVIDENCE

A systematic review found that activated charcoal is able to reduce absorption of acetaminophen if taken within 2 hours of ingestion but the clinical benefits are unclear.[1] Ⓐ

IV acetylcysteine may reduce mortality rate in patients with established acetaminophen-induced liver failure.[1-3] Ⓐ

Evidence-Based References

1. Brok J et al: Interventions for paracetamol (acetaminophen) overdoses, *Cochrane Rev* 3:CD00328, 2002. Ⓐ
2. Keays R et al: Intravenous acetylcysteine in paracetamol induced fulminant hepatic failure: a prospective controlled trial, *BMJ* 303:1026, 1991. Ⓐ
3. Brok J et al: Interventions for paracetamol (acetaminophen) overdoses, *Cochrane Database Rev* 12:IP54, 2004.

SUGGESTED READING

Heard KJ: Acetylcysteine for acetaminophen poisoning, *N Engl J Med* 359:285-292, 2008.

AUTHOR: **TARA M. WAYT, D.O.**

BASIC INFORMATION

DEFINITION

Achalasia is a motility disorder of the esophagus characterized by incomplete relaxation of the lower esophageal sphincter (LES) and aperistalsis of esophageal smooth muscle. The result is functional obstruction of the esophagus.

SYNONYMS

Achalasia and cardiospasm
Achalasia (of cardia)
Aperistalsis of esophagus
Megaesophagus
Esophageal achalasia
Esophageal cardiospasm

ICD-9CM CODES

530.0 Achalasia

EPIDEMIOLOGY & DEMOGRAPHICS

- Annual incidence is approximately 0.5 in 100,000 persons.
- Prevalence is <10 per 100,000 persons.
- Although the onset of symptoms may occur at any age, incidence is typically bimodal, 20 to 40 yr, then after 60 yr, with greater incidence in the older group.
- Men and women are affected equally.

PHYSICAL FINDINGS & CLINICAL PRESENTATION

Symptoms:
- Dysphagia with both solids and liquids
- Difficulty belching
- Regurgitation
- Chest pain and/or heartburn
- Globus
- Frequent hiccups
- Vomiting of undigested food
- Symptoms of aspiration such as nocturnal cough; possible dyspnea and pneumonia

Physical findings:
- Focal lung examination abnormalities and wheezing also possible

ETIOLOGY

- Etiology is poorly understood.
- Loss of myenteric nerve fibers in the lower esophageal sphincter and smooth muscle portion of the esophagus. This has been associated with lymphocytic and eosinophilic infiltrates and fibrosis in later stages of disease.
- Loss of intrinsic inhibitory neurons in the myenteric plexus, producing nitric oxide synthase, as well as depletion of networks of interstitial cells of Cajal of the LES, leads to incomplete relaxation.
- This motility disorder may be caused by autoimmune degeneration of the esophageal myenteric plexus because association with the HLA class II antigen DQw1 has been noted. Antimyenteric plexus antibodies have also been described.
- Abnormal immune reactions to neurotropic viruses such as varicella zoster, herpes simplex type 1, and measles viruses have been implicated, but the association has not been confirmed.
- Achalasia is also seen in the rare autosomal recessive disorder Allgrove syndrome (achalasia, alacrima, autonomic disturbance, and acetylcholine insensitivity), which has been linked to a gene mutation on chromosome 12q13.

Dx DIAGNOSIS

DIFFERENTIAL DIAGNOSIS

- Primary achalasia:
  - Idiopathic
- Secondary achalasia:
  - Chagas disease
  - Vagal injury or surgery, including fundoplication
- Pseudoachalasia:
  - Esophageal cancer
  - Infiltrating gastric cancer
  - Oat cell and bronchogenic lung cancer
  - Lymphoma
  - Amyloidosis
  - Paraneoplastic syndrome
- Angina
- Bulimia
- Anorexia nervosa
- Gastric bezoar
- Gastritis
- Peptic ulcer disease
- Postvagotomy dysmotility
- Esophageal disease:
  - Gastroesophageal reflux disease
  - Sarcoidosis
  - Amyloidosis
  - Esophageal stricture
  - Esophageal webs and rings
  - Scleroderma
  - Barrett's esophagus
  - Esophagitis
  - Diffuse esophageal spasm

WORKUP

- Physical examination and laboratory analyses to rule out other causes and assess complications
- Imaging studies, manometry, and endoscopy

LABORATORY TESTS

- Assessment of nutritional status
- Complete blood count, ECG, stress test if diagnosis is in doubt
- Serologic assays for trypanosoma cruzi (Chagas disease) in appropriate individuals

IMAGING STUDIES

Barium swallow with fluoroscopy may demonstrate:
- Uncoordinated or absent esophageal contractions
- An acutely tapered contrast column ("bird's beak"; Fig. 1-5)
- Dilation of the distal (smooth muscle portion) esophagus
- Esophageal air fluid level

Manometry is generally required to confirm the diagnosis. Characteristic abnormalities are as follows:
- Low-amplitude disorganized contractions/aperistalsis
- Incomplete or absent LES relaxation after swallow
- High LES pressure
- A subset of patients with vigorous achalasia may have high-amplitude, long-duration, simultaneous esophageal contractions
- High resolution manometry is being used to define subsets of patients with achalasia who may have different responses to medical or surgical therapies
- Direct visualization by endoscopy should be performed to exclude other causes of dysphagia, including secondary causes of achalasia

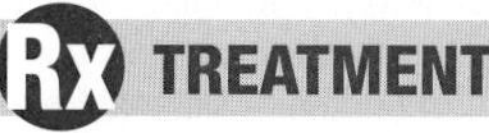

TREATMENT

NONPHARMACOLOGIC THERAPY

- The goals of therapy are to decrease LES pressure, relieve symptoms, and prevent progression to a dilated or megaesophagus.
- Pneumatic dilation may benefit 65% to 90% of patients. Esophageal rupture or perforation is a rare complication (2% to 3%) that can be managed conservatively in some stable patients. Multiple sessions may be required.
- Surgical: laparoscopic or, now less commonly, open esophagomyotomy is effective (90%). This approach currently offers the

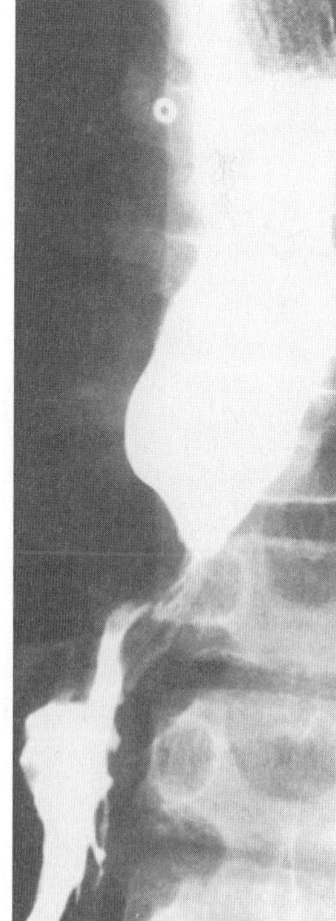

FIGURE 1-5 Classic appearance of achalasia of the esophagus. The dilated esophagus ends in a narrow segment. (From Hoekelman R [ed]: *Primary pediatric care,* ed 3, St Louis, 1997, Mosby.)

A

Diseases and Disorders

most durable symptom relief. Approximately 35% of patients undergoing surgery will develop reflux disease. As a result, some surgeons will perform a "loose" antireflux repair as part of the surgical procedure. An observational study has suggested that those who have had prior endoscopic treatment before myotomy may not do as well as those who have a primary myotomy.

GENERAL Rx

- Medications may be useful for short-term symptom relief and in patients with refractory chest pain. They should only be considered in patients unable to receive, or who are scheduled for, more definitive procedures. LES pressure may be lowered by 50% through sublingual use of long-acting nitrates (e.g., isosorbide dinitrate 5 to 20 mg) or calcium channel blockers (e.g., nifedipine 10 to 30 mg). Side effects are common and duration of relief tends to be short. Sildenafil was shown to be effective in a few small, short-term studies, but it is generally not recommended.
- Botulinum toxin injection will benefit up to 85% of patients by inhibiting acetylcholine release from cholinergic nerve endings, but up to half of these patients will require repeat injections by 6 months. A few studies have suggested that repeated injections can lead to fibrosis, which may complicate subsequent attempts at surgical therapy.

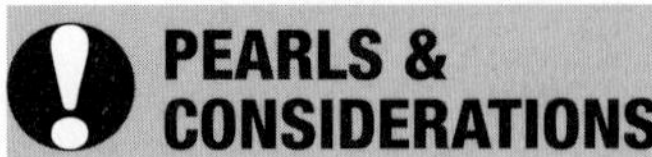

PEARLS & CONSIDERATIONS

COMMENTS

- Medication has a limited role in treatment.
- Botulinum toxin is transiently effective in improving symptoms. Pneumatic dilation and surgical myotomy provide more durable long-term responses. Botulinum toxin should be considered primarily in patients too elderly or ill to be considered for these other therapies.
- Surgical myotomy and mechanical dilation are treatments of choice.
- Patients with achalasia may be at long-term risk of squamous cell carcinoma of the esophagus and non–reflux-associated esophagitis. Treated patients may be at long-term risk for reflux esophagitis, Barrett's esophagus, and adenocarcinoma.

SUGGESTED READINGS

Campos et al: Endoscopic and surgical treatments for achalasia: a systematic review and meta-analysis, *Ann Surg* 249:45-57, 2009.

Di Nardo G et al: Review article: molecular, pathological and therpeutic features of human enteric neuropathies, *Aliment Pharmacol Ther* 28:25, 2008.

Kraichely RE et al: Achalasia: physiology and etiopathogenesis, *Dis Esophagus* 19:213, 2006.

Leyden JE et al: Endoscopic pneumatic dilation versus botulinum toxin injection in the management of primary achalasia, *Cochrane Database Syst Rev* 4:CD005046, 2006.

Smith CD et al: Endoscopic therapy for achalasia before Heller myotomy results in worse outcomes than Heller myotomy alone, *Ann Surg* 243(5):579, 2006.

AUTHOR: **HARLAN G. RICH, M.D.**

BASIC INFORMATION

DEFINITION

Achilles tendon rupture refers to the loss of continuity of the *tendo Achillis,* usually from attrition.

ICD-9CM CODES
845.09 Achilles tendon rupture

EPIDEMIOLOGY & DEMOGRAPHICS

PREDOMINANT AGE: 30 to 55 yr

PHYSICAL FINDINGS & CLINICAL PRESENTATION

Injury often occurs during an activity that puts great stress on the tendon. Sudden "pop" is often felt followed by weakness and swelling. Sometimes the patient feels like he or she has been shot in the calf.

- Patient walks flat footed and is unable to stand on the ball of the foot.
- Tenderness and hemorrhage are present at the site of injury, and a sulcus is usually palpable but may be obscured by an organizing clot if the examination is delayed.
- Although active plantar flexion is usually lost, some plantar flexion occasionally remains because of the activity of the other posterior compartment muscles.
- Thompson's test is usually positive. Test measures plantar flexion of the foot when the calf is squeezed with the patient kneeling on a chair; normal foot plantar flexes with calf compression, but movement is absent when *tendo Achillis* is ruptured.
- Excessive passive dorsiflexion of the foot is also present on the injured side (Fig. 1-6).

ETIOLOGY

- Relative hypovascularity predisposing to tendon rupture in several tendons (Achilles, biceps, and supraspinatus)
- With advancing age, vascular supply to the tendon further compromised
- Repetitive trauma leading to degeneration of this critical area and weakness
- Rupture of *tendo Achillis* usually 2.5 to 5 cm from the insertion of the tendon into the os calcis
- Most common causative event leading to rupture: sudden dorsiflexion of the plantar flexed foot (landing from a height) or sudden pushing off with the weight on the forefoot
- The tendon may be adversely affected by the use of fluoroquinolone antibiotics

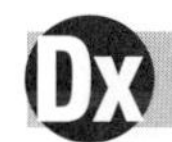

DIAGNOSIS

DIFFERENTIAL DIAGNOSIS

- Incomplete (partial) *tendo Achillis* rupture
- Partial rupture of gastrocnemius muscle, often medial head (previously thought to be "plantaris tendon rupture")

WORKUP

- Clinical diagnosis of complete *tendo Achillis* rupture is usually obvious.
- MRI helpful in partial ruptures.

Rx TREATMENT

- Early referral is necessary for open, end-to-end surgical repair.
- If surgery is contraindicated, a short leg cast applied with the foot in equinus may allow healing.
- In cases of neglected rupture, reconstruction is usually indicated.
- Physical therapy is helpful after repair to restore strength and flexibility.
- Bracing is required for partial rupture.

DISPOSITION

- Prognosis for recovery after surgical repair of the acute rupture is good, but recurrence is not uncommon regardless of treatment.
- *Tendo Achillis* must be protected from excessive activity for up to 1 yr.
- Results of reconstruction for neglected cases are worse than with primary repair.
- Return to work with limited weight-bearing is possible in 2 to 4 wk.

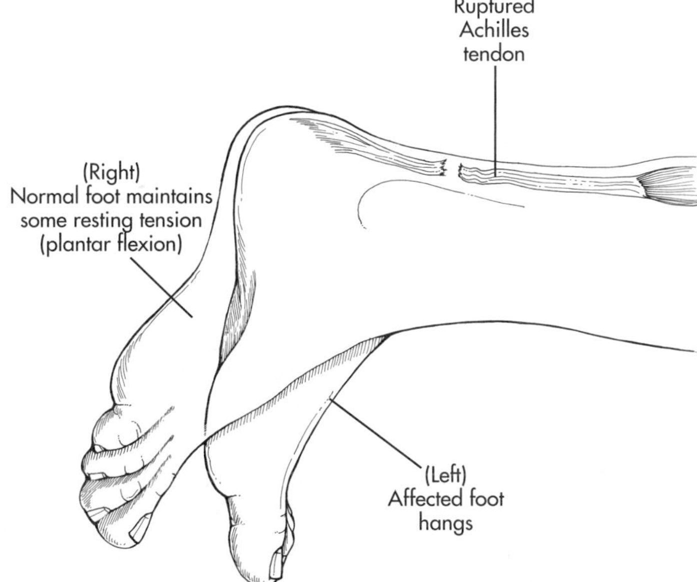

FIGURE 1-6 Observation of Achilles tendon rupture. The patient is asked to lie prone on the examining table with feet hanging off the end. The intact leg retains inherent plantar flexion, whereas on the injured side the foot hangs straight down with gravity. (From Scudieri G [ed]: *Sports medicine: principles of primary care,* St Louis, 1997, Mosby.)

SUGGESTED READINGS

Bhandari M et al: Treatment of acute Achilles tendon rupture: a systematic overview and metaanalysis, *Clin Orthop* (400):190, 2002.

Khan RJ et al: Treatment of acute Achilles tendon ruptures: a meta-analysis of randomized controlled trials, *J Bone Joint Surg Am* 87A:2202, 2005.

Lawrence SJ, Grau GF: Management of acute Achilles tendon ruptures, *Orthopedics* 27:579, 2004.

Maffulli N et al: Chronic rupture of tendo Achilles, *Foot Ankle Clin* 12:583, 2007.

Reddy SS et al: Surgical treatment for chronic disease and disorders of the Achilles tendon, *J Am Acad Orthop Surg* 17:3, 2009.

Rettig AC et al: Potential risk of rerupture in primary Achilles tendon repair in athletes younger than 30 years of age, *Am J Sports Med* 33:119, 2005.

Roberts C, Deliss L: Acute rupture of tendo Achillis, *J Bone Joint Surg Br* 84(4):620, 2002.

Smigielski R: Management of partial tears of the gastro-soleus complex, *Clin Sports Med* 27:219, 2008.

Wallace RG et al: Combined conservative and orthotic management of acute ruptures of the Achilles tendon, *J Bone Joint Surg Am* 86A:1198, 2004.

Wick MC, Reiger M: Images in clinical medicine. Rupture of a calcified Achilles' tendon, *N Engl J Med* 358:2618, 2008.

Worth N et al: Management of acute Achilles tendon ruptures in the United Kingdom, *J Orthop Surg (Hong Kong)* 15:311, 2007.

AUTHOR: **LONNIE R. MERCIER, M.D.**

Acne Vulgaris (PTG)

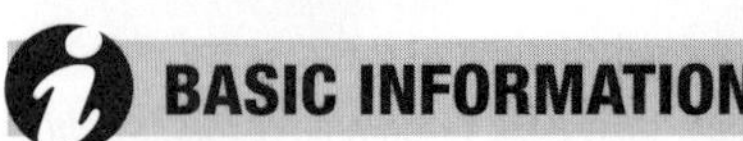

BASIC INFORMATION

DEFINITION

Acne vulgaris is a chronic disorder of the pilosebaceous apparatus caused by abnormal desquamation of follicular epithelium leading to obstruction of the pilosebaceous canal, resulting in inflammation and subsequent formation of papules, pustules, nodules, comedones, and scarring. Acne can be classified by the type of lesion (comedonal, papulopustular, and nodulocystic). The American Academy of Dermatology classification scheme for acne denotes the following three levels:

1. Mild acne: characterized by the presence of comedones (noninflammatory lesions), few papules and pustules (generally <10), but no nodules.
2. Moderate acne: presence of several to many papules and pustules (10 to 40) along with comedones (10 to 40). The presence of >40 papules and pustules along with larger, deeper nodular inflamed lesions (up to five) denotes moderately severe acne (Fig. 1-7).
3. Severe acne: presence of numerous or extensive papules and pustules as well as many nodular lesions.

SYNONYMS

Acne

ICD-9CM CODES
706.1 Acne vulgaris

EPIDEMIOLOGY & DEMOGRAPHICS

- Acne is the most common skin disease in the U.S.
- It is most common in teenagers (highest incidence between ages of 16 and 18 yr).

PHYSICAL FINDINGS & CLINICAL PRESENTATION

- Open comedones (blackheads), closed comedones (whiteheads)
- Greasiness (oily skin)
- Presence of scars from prior acne cysts
- Various stages of development and severity may be present concomitantly
- Common distribution of acne: face, back, and upper chest
- Inflammatory papules, pustules, and ectatic pores

ETIOLOGY

- Overactivity of the sebaceous glands and blockage in the ducts. The obstruction leads to the formation of comedones, which can become inflamed because of overgrowth of *Propionibacterium acnes.*
- Exacerbated by environmental factors (hot, humid, tropical climate), medications (e.g., iodine in cough mixtures, hair greases), industrial exposure to halogenated hydrocarbons.

Dx DIAGNOSIS

DIFFERENTIAL DIAGNOSIS

- Gram-negative folliculitis
- Staphylococcal pyoderma
- Acne rosacea
- Drug eruption
- Sebaceous hyperplasia
- Angiofibromas, basal cell carcinomas, osteoma cutis
- Occupational exposures to oils or grease
- Steroid acne

WORKUP

History and physical examination:

- Inquire about previous treatment
- Careful drug history
- Family history, history of cyclic menstrual flares
- History of use of cosmetics and cleansers
- Oral contraceptive use

LABORATORY TESTS

- Laboratory evaluation is generally not helpful.
- Patients who are candidates for therapy with isotretinoin (Accutane) should have baseline liver enzymes, cholesterol, and triglycerides checked because this medication may result in elevation of lipids and liver enzymes.
- A negative serum pregnancy test or two negative urine pregnancy tests should also be obtained in females 1 wk before initiation of isotretinoin; it is also imperative to maintain effective contraception during and 1 mo after therapy with isotretinoin ends because of its teratogenic effects. Pregnancy status should be rechecked at monthly visits.
- If hyperandrogenism is suspected in female patients, levels of dehydroepiandrosterone sulfate, testosterone (total and free), and androstenedione should be measured. For women with regular menstrual cycles, serum androgen measurements generally are not necessary.

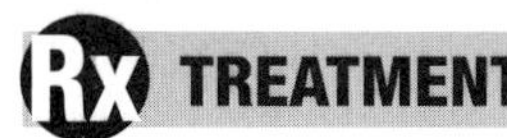

TREATMENT

NONPHARMACOLOGIC THERAPY

- Blue light (ClearLight therapy system) can be used for treatment of moderate inflammatory acne vulgaris. Light in the violet/blue range can cause bacterial death by a photoreaction in which porphyrins react with oxygen to generate reactive oxygen species, which damage the cell membranes of *P. acnes.* Treatment usually consists of 15-min exposures twice weekly for 4 wk.

ACUTE GENERAL Rx

Treatment generally varies with the type of lesions (comedones, papules, pustules, cystic lesions) and the severity of acne.

- Comedones (noninflammatory acne) can be treated with retinoids or retinoid analogs. Topical retinoids are comedolytic and work by normalizing follicular keratinization. Commonly available agents are Adapalene (Differin, 0.1% gel or cream, applied once or twice daily), tazarotene (Tazorac 0.1% cream or gel applied daily), tretinoin (Retin-A 0.1% cream or 0.025 gel applied once daily), tretinoin microsphere (Retin-A Micro, 0.1% gel, applied at bedtime). Tretinoin is inactivated by ultraviolet light and oxidized by benzoyl peroxide; therefore it should only be applied at night and not used concomitantly with benzoyl peroxide.
- Tretinoin is pregnancy category C and tazarotene is pregnancy category X. Salicylic acid preparations (e.g., Neutrogena 2% wash) have keratolytic and antiinflammatory properties and are also useful in the treatment of comedones. Large, open comedones (blackheads) should be expressed.

FIGURE 1-7 Acne on back and shoulders. This acne is typically inflammatory and usually needs oral antibiotics or possibly isotretinoin, but the patient may apply topical medication as well. Heat and sweat may aggravate the condition. (From White GM, Cox NH [eds]: *Diseases of the skin*, ed 2, St Louis, 2006, Mosby.)

- Patients should be reevaluated after 4 to 6 wk. Benzoyl peroxide gel (2.5% or 5%) may be added if the comedones become inflamed or form pustules. The most common adverse effects are dryness, erythema, and peeling. Topical antibiotics (erythromycin, clindamycin lotions or pads) can also be used in patients with significant inflammation. They reduce *P. acnes* in the pilosebaceous follicle and have some antiinflammatory effects. The combination of 5% benzoyl peroxide and 3% erythromycin (Benzamycin) or 1% clindamycin with 5% benzoyl peroxide (BenzaClin) is highly effective in patients who have a mixture of comedonal and inflammatory acne lesions.
- Pustular acne can be treated with tretinoin and benzoyl peroxide gel applied on alternate evenings; drying agents (sulfacetamide-sulfa lotions [Novacet, Sulfacet]) are also effective when used in combination with benzoyl peroxide; oral antibiotics (doxycycline 100 mg qd or erythromycin 1 g qd given in 2 to 3 divided doses) are effective in patients with moderate to severe pustular acne. Patients not responding well to these antibiotics can be switched to minocycline 50 to 100 mg bid; however, this medication is more expensive.
- Patients with nodular cystic acne can be treated with systemic agents: antibiotics (erythromycin, tetracycline, doxycycline, minocycline), isotretinoin (Accutane), or oral contraceptives. Periodic intralesional triamcinolone (Kenalog) injections by a dermatologist are also effective. The possibility of endocrinopathy should be considered in patients responding poorly to therapy.
- Isotretinoin is indicated for acne resistant to antibiotic therapy and severe acne; dosage is 0.5 to 1 mg/kg/day in 2 divided doses (maximum of 2 mg/kg/day); duration of therapy is generally 20 wk for a cumulative dose ≥120 mg/kg for severe cystic acne. Before using this medication patients should undergo baseline laboratory evaluation (see "Laboratory Tests"). This drug is absolutely contraindicated during pregnancy because of its teratogenicity. It should be used with caution in patients with history of depression. To prescribe this drug, physicians must be registered members of the manufacturer's System to Manage Accutane-Related Teratogenicity (SMART) program.
- Azelaic acid is a bacteriostatic dicarboxylic acid used to normalize keratinization and reduce inflammation.
- Oral contraceptives reduce androgen levels and therefore sebum production. They represent a useful adjunctive therapy for all types of acne in women and adolescent girls. Commonly used agents are norgestimate/ethinyl estradiol (Ortho Tri-Cyclen) and drosperinone/ethinyl estradiol (Yasmin).

REFERRAL

Referral for intralesional injection and dermabrasion should be considered in patients with severe acne unresponsive to conventional therapy.

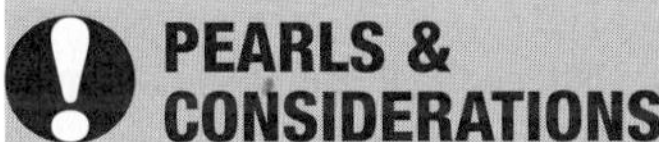

PEARLS & CONSIDERATIONS

- Gram-negative folliculitis should be suspected if inflammatory acne worsens after several months of oral antibiotic therapy.
- Acne may worsen during the first 3 to 4 wk of retinoid therapy before improving.

COMMENTS

Indications for systemic therapy of acne are:

- Painful deep papules or nodules
- Extensive lesions
- Active acne with severe scarring or hyperpigmentation
- Patient's morale

Patients should be educated that in most cases acne can be controlled but not cured and that at least 4 to 6 wk of initial therapy should be required before significant improvement is noted.

EBM EVIDENCE

A systematic review compared different types of combined oral contraceptive pill with placebo or other active treatments for women with acne vulgaris. It found that combined oral contraceptive pills reduced acne lesion counts, severity grades, and self-assessed acne compared with placebo. It was less clear how the effect varied according to type of progestagen used.[1] Ⓐ

A systematic review found that topical retinoids were the mainstay of therapy in patients with comedones only, although good results were also achieved with topical antimicrobials, oral antibiotics, hormonal therapy (in women), and isotretinoin. Researchers concluded that mild to moderately severe inflammatory acne with papules and pustules should be treated with topical antibiotics combined with retinoids. They suggest oral isotretinoin is indicated for severe nodular acne, treatment failures, scarring, frequent relapses, or in cases of severe psychological distress.[2] Ⓑ

Evidence-Based References

1. Arowojolu AO et al: Combined oral contraceptive pills for treatment of acne, *Cochrane Rev* 3, 2004. Ⓐ
2. Haider A, Shaw JC: Treatment of acne vulgaris, *JAMA* 292:726, 2004. Ⓑ

SUGGESTED READINGS

Feldman S et al: Diagnosis and treatment of acne, *Am Fam Physician* 69:2123, 2004.

Haider A, Shaw JC: Treatment of acne vulgaris, *JAMA* 292:726, 2004.

James WD: Acne, *N Engl J Med* 352:1463, 2005.

AUTHOR: **FRED F. FERRI, M.D.**

BASIC INFORMATION

DEFINITION

Acoustic neuroma is a benign proliferation of the Schwann cells that cover the vestibular branch of the eighth cranial nerve (CN VIII). Symptoms are commonly a result of compression of the acoustic branch of CN VIII, the facial nerve (CN VII), and the trigeminal nerve (CN V). The glossopharyngeal nerve (CN IX) and vagus nerve (CN X) are less commonly involved. In extreme cases compression of the brain stem may lead to obstruction of cerebrospinal fluid (CSF) outflow and elevated intracranial pressure (ICP).

SYNONYMS

Vestibular schwannoma

ICD-9CM CODES
225.1 Acoustic neuroma

EPIDEMIOLOGY & DEMOGRAPHICS

Annual incidence is approximately one in 100,000 patients per year. There may be a slight female predominance. The tumor most commonly presents in the fifth and sixth decades.

PHYSICAL FINDINGS & CLINICAL PRESENTATION

- Most frequently unilateral hearing loss and/or tinnitus. Also balance problems, vertigo, facial pain (trigeminal neuralgia) and weakness, difficulty swallowing, fullness or pain of the involved ear. Headache may occur.
- With elevated ICP, patients may also have vomiting, fever, and visual changes.
- Hearing loss is the most common presenting complaint and is usually high frequency.

ETIOLOGY

The etiology is incompletely understood, but long-term exposure to acoustic trauma has been implicated. Bilateral acoustic neuromas may be inherited in an autosomal-dominant manner as part of neurofibromatosis type 2. This disease is associated with a defect on chromosome 22q1.

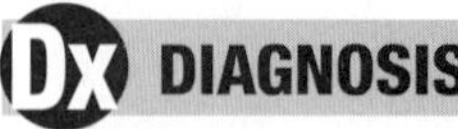

DIAGNOSIS

DIFFERENTIAL DIAGNOSIS

- Benign positional vertigo
- Menière's disease
- Trigeminal neuralgia
- Cerebellar disease
- Normal-pressure hydrocephalus
- Presbycusis
- Glomus tumors
- Vertebrobasilar insufficiency
- Ototoxicity from medications
- Other tumors:
    - Meningioma, glioma
    - Facial nerve schwannoma
    - Cavernous hemangioma
    - Metastatic tumors

WORKUP

- A detailed neurologic examination with special attention to the cranial nerves is crucial.
- Otoscopic evaluation may help rule out other causes of hearing loss.

LABORATORY TESTS

- Audiometry is useful, often showing asymmetric, sensorineural, high-frequency hearing loss.
- CSF protein may be elevated.

IMAGING STUDIES

- MRI with gadolinium is the preferred test. It can detect tumors as small as 2 mm in diameter.
- CT scan with contrast can detect tumors 1 cm in diameter or larger.
- Treatment decisions should be based on the size of the tumor, rate of growth (older patients tend to have slower growing tumors), degree of neurologic deficit, desire to preserve hearing, life expectancy, age of the patient, and surgical risk. A combination of treatments can also be used.

Rx TREATMENT

NONPHARMACOLOGIC THERAPY

- Surgery is the definitive treatment. Choice of approach (middle cranial fossa, translabyrinthine, or retromastoid suboccipital) may vary depending on the size of the tumor, amount of residual hearing desired, and degree of surgical risk that can be tolerated. Partial resection is sometimes undertaken to minimize the risk of injury to nearby structures. Intraoperative facial nerve monitoring is recommended.
- Radiation therapy (stereotactic radiotherapy, stereotactic radiosurgery, or proton beam radiotherapy) is useful for tumors <3 cm in diameter or for those in whom surgery is not an option. Radiotherapy after partial resection has also been used to minimize complications.
- Age alone is not a contraindication to surgery.

ACUTE GENERAL Rx

Not applicable

CHRONIC Rx

Observation with MRI every 6 to 12 mo may be appropriate for frail patients with small tumors, but risk of unrecoverable hearing loss may increase if surgery is delayed.

DISPOSITION

Hearing can be preserved at near-preoperative levels in more than two thirds of patients with small- to medium-sized tumors.

REFERRAL

Prompt referral to an ear-nose-throat specialist or neurosurgeon who is facile with all three surgical approaches is recommended.

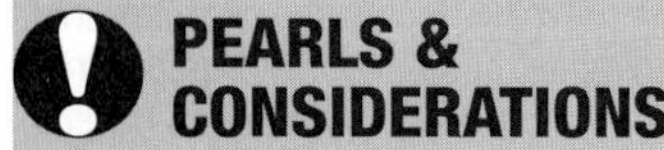

PEARLS & CONSIDERATIONS

COMMENTS

- Presents most commonly as unilateral, sensorineural hearing loss.
- Treatment outcomes are generally good, with cure rates approaching 90% at 5 years.
- Of those who are managed with observation only, approximately half have continued enlargement and approximately one fifth eventually have a surgical intervention.

PATIENT/FAMILY EDUCATION

Acoustic Neuroma Association: http://anausa.org.

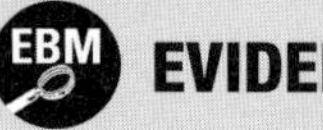

EVIDENCE

A systematic review found no evidence to support the use of *Ginkgo biloba* in the treatment of tinnitus.[1] Ⓐ

Evidence-Based Reference

1. Hilton M, Stuart E: Ginkgo biloba for tinnitus, Cochrane Database of Syst Rev (2):CD003852, 2004. Ⓐ

SUGGESTED READINGS

Kondziolka D et al: Long-term outcomes after radiosurgery for acoustic neuromas, *N Engl J Med* 339: 1426, 1999.

Mendenhall WM et al: Management of acoustic schwannoma, *Am J Otolaryngol* 25(1):38, 2004.

Pitts LH, Jackler RK: Treatment of acoustic neuromas, *N Engl J Med* 339:1471, 1998.

Yoshimoto Y: Systematic review of the natural history of vestibular schwannoma, *J Neurosurg* 103(1):59, 2005.

AUTHORS: **SRIVIDYA ANANDAN, M.D.,** and **PAUL A. PIRRAGLIA, M.D., M.P.H.**

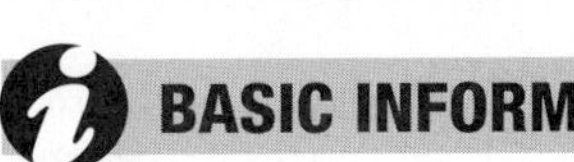

BASIC INFORMATION

DEFINITION

Acquired immunodeficiency syndrome (AIDS) is a disorder caused by infection with the human immunodeficiency virus, type 1 (HIV-1), and marked by progressive deterioration of the cellular immune system, leading to secondary infections or malignancies.

SYNONYMS

AIDS

ICD-9CM CODES
042.9 AIDS, unspecified

EPIDEMIOLOGY & DEMOGRAPHICS

INCIDENCE (IN U.S.):
- 27.1 cases/100,000 persons
- Varies widely by location
- 85% of cases in large cities

PREVALENCE (IN U.S.): 62 cases/100,000 persons

PREDOMINANT SEX: Males 84%, females 16% (through 1998); 40% of newly reported U.S. cases in 1999 were in females

PREDOMINANT AGE: 80% between ages 20 and 40 yr

PEAK INCIDENCE: See "Incidence"

GENETICS:
- Familial disposition: Although there is no proven genetic predisposition, individuals with deletions in the CCR5 gene are immune from infection with macrophage tropic virus (the predominant virus in sexual transmission).
- Congenital infection:
  1. Transmittable from an infected mother to the fetus in utero in as many as 30% of pregnancies.
  2. No specific congenital malformations associated with infection; low birth weight and spontaneous abortion are possible.
- Neonatal infection: transmission possible to the neonate intrapartum or postpartum through breastfeeding.

PHYSICAL FINDINGS & CLINICAL PRESENTATION

- Nonspecific findings: fever, weight loss, anorexia
- Specific syndromes:
  1. Seen in association with opportunistic infection and malignancies, so-called indicator diseases; these include:
     a. Opportunistic infections:
        Disseminated strongyloidiasis
        Disseminated toxoplasmosis, cryptococcosis, histoplasmosis, CMV, herpes simplex, or mycobacterial disease
        Candida esophagitis or bronchopulmonary disease
        Chronic *Cryptosporidia* spp. diarrhea
        Pneumocystis jiroveci pneumonia
        Extensive pulmonary and extrapulmonary tuberculosis
        Recurrent bacterial pneumonia
        Progressive multifocal leukoencephalopathy
     b. AIDS-related neoplasms:
        Kaposi's sarcoma in a person <60 yr of age
        Primary brain lymphoma
        Invasive cervical carcinoma
        High grade B cell non-Hodgkin's lymphoma, Burkitt's lymphoma, undifferentiated non-Hodgkin's lymphoma, or immunoblastic lymphoma
  2. Most common:
     Respiratory infections (*Pneumocystis jiroveci* [formerly known as *Pneumocystis carinii*] pneumonia, TB, bacterial pneumonia, fungal infection)
     CNS infections (toxoplasmosis, cryptococcal meningitis, TB)
     GI (cryptosporidiosis, isosporiasis, cytomegalovirus); Sections II and III describe organisms associated with diarrhea in patients with AIDS
     Eye infections (cytomegalovirus, toxoplasmosis)
     Kaposi's sarcoma (cutaneous or visceral) or lymphoma (nodal or extranodal)
- Possibly asymptomatic
- Diagnosis of AIDS if T-lymphocyte subset analysis demonstrating CD4 cell count <200 or <14% of total lymphocyte in the presence of proven HIV infection even in the absence of other infections
- The various manifestations of HIV infection are described in Section II

ETIOLOGY

- Caused by infection with HIV-1
- Transmitted by heterosexual or male homosexual contact, needle-sharing (during IV drug use), transfusion of contaminated blood or blood products, and from infected mother to fetus or neonate as described previously

DIAGNOSIS

DIFFERENTIAL DIAGNOSIS

- Other wasting illnesses mimicking the nonspecific features of AIDS:
  1. TB
  2. Neoplasms
  3. Disseminated fungal infection
  4. Malabsorption syndromes
  5. Depression
- Other disorders associated with dementia or demyelination producing encephalopathy, myelopathy, or neuropathy

WORKUP

Prompt evaluation of respiratory, CNS, and GI complaints

LABORATORY TESTS

- HIV antibody testing
- T-lymphocyte subset analysis: performed to determine the degree of immunodeficiency
- Viral load assay: to plan long-term antiviral therapy consider genotype or phenotype sensitivity testing for patients failing therapy
- CSF examination: for meningitis
- Serologic tests for syphilis, hepatitis B, hepatitis C, and toxoplasmosis
- Genotypic resistance testing: used to assess for primary resistance in naïve patients and secondary resistance in patients failing a regimen
- Eye exam: to evaluate for CMV retinitis in patients with CD4 counts <50 cells/mm^3
- Cryptococcal antigen: part of the evaluation in AIDS patients with CD4 <100 cells/mm^3 who have fever, diffuse pneumonia, or symptoms of meningitis

IMAGING STUDIES

- Cerebral CT for encephalopathy or focal CNS complications (e.g., toxoplasmosis, lymphoma)
- Pulmonary gallium scanning to aid in the diagnosis of *Pneumocystis jiroveci* (*P. carinii*) pneumonia
- Baseline chest x-ray

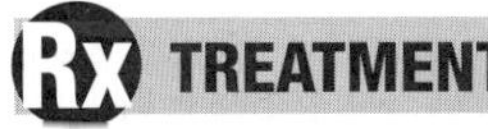

TREATMENT

NONPHARMACOLOGIC THERAPY

- Maintain adequate caloric intake.
- Encourage good oral hygiene, regular dental care.
- Avoid high risk behaviors that increase the risk of repeated exposure to HIV and other potential pathogens—safer sexual practices, avoid sharing needles, etc.
- Update vaccines—particularly the pneumococcal and hepatitis B vaccine along with annual influenza vaccines.
- Avoid administration of any live attenuated vaccines that may be a risk to these immunocompromised patients.
- When feasible, avoid activities that might increase risk of exposure to opportunistic infections (i.e., cleaning out a cat litter box [toxoplasmosis], getting scratched by a cat [*Bartonella* infections], exposure to pet reptiles [salmonellosis], traveling to developing countries [cryptosporidiosis, tuberculosis], eating undercooked foods and drinking from unsafe water supplies, etc.).

ACUTE GENERAL Rx

Acute management of opportunistic infections and malignancies is reviewed elsewhere in this text under specific AIDS-related disorders.

CHRONIC Rx

For all HIV-infected patients, particularly those meeting the case definition of AIDS:
- Preventive therapy for *Pneumocystis jiroveci* pneumonia and TB (see specific chapters elsewhere in this text). With the advent of modern antiretroviral therapy many patients have experienced substantial restoration of cellular immune function. It has become clear that preventive therapy for *Pneumocystis jiroveci* and *Mycobacterium avium* complex as

well as suppressive therapy for cytomegalo-viral and cryptococcal infection can often be safely withdrawn if the CD4 cell count rises above 200 for at least 6 mo.

- Begin HAART (highly active antiretroviral therapy) when any of the following are present:
  1. Symptomatic HIV infection is associated with any opportunistic infection
  2. CD4 count <200 cells/mm^3
  3. CD4 count <350 cells/mm^3 and before it reaches 200 cells/mm^3, especially if the viral load >30,000 copies/ml
  4. Consider therapy if CD4 count is rapidly decreasing and viral load >100,000 copies/ml
- Antiretroviral therapy employing combinations of nucleoside reverse transcriptase inhibitor (NRTI) agents: zidovudine (AZT), didanosine (DDI), zalcitabine (DDC), lamivudine (3TC), Emtricitabine (FTC), stavudine (D4T), abacavir in addition to protease inhibitors (PI) (saquinavir, indinavir, nelfinavir, agenerase, ritonavir/lopinavir, atazanavir), nonnucleoside reverse transcriptase inhibitors (NNRTI) (nevirapine, delavirdine, efavirenz), or the nucleotide agent tenofovir according to current recommendations based on clinical stage and viral load studies. The protease inhibitor ritonavir should be used, in low dose, in combination with other protease inhibitors to obtain more sustained drug levels. Usual initial dosing regimen consists of two NRTIs and an NNRTI (or a PI). Common regimens include:
  1. Combivir (AZT and 3TC) one tablet by mouth twice a day and efavirenz 600 mg by mouth once daily
  2. Combivir (AZT and 3TC) one tablet by mouth twice a day and ritonavir/lopinavir 3 tablets by mouth twice daily with food
  3. Truvada (tenofovir plus Emtricitabine [FTC]) one tablet once daily and efavirenz 600 mg by mouth once daily

  All these drugs have unique and class-specific side effects and require careful and expert follow-up to achieve optimal antiviral effects, ensure compliance, and maintain efficacy. Antiviral response should be monitored by baseline HIV viral load and CD4 count and repeat measurement at 2 wk and 4 wk into treatment and then periodically (every 3 mo) to ensure viral suppression.
- An approach to evaluating chronic diarrhea in patients with HIV infection, the approach to the acutely ill HIV-infected patient, and the evaluation of respiratory complaints are described in Section III. Approach to a patient with a suspected CNS lesion is also described in Section III.
- Genotypic resistance testing should be strongly considered for any patient failing antiretroviral therapy. Poor adherence to therapy, however, often underlies virologic failure.

DISPOSITION

The outlook for AIDS has changed radically since the advent of HAART therapy from an essentially uniformly fatal disease to a chronic medical illness compatible with long-term survival and remarkably good quality of life. Patients should be aggressively supported in the presence of severe illness as outcomes following ICU admissions remain good. This is accomplished through expert and continuous follow-up, use of highly active antiretroviral drugs, and careful detail to compliance to medications and lifestyle modification.

REFERRAL

All patients with AIDS: to a physician knowledgeable and experienced in the management of the disease and its complications

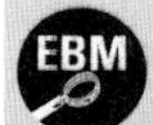

EVIDENCE

Please note: Complete text of EBM for this topic is available online.

Key trials and commentary:

The benefits of continuing antiretroviral therapy are questionable in human immunodeficiency virus (HIV) type 1–infected patients with profound immunodeficiency and multiple treatment failure caused by viral resistance. This study revealed that even when effective virological control is no longer achievable, cART still reduces the risk of ADEs in profoundly immunodeficient HIV-infected patients.

The goal of cART in HIV disease is to improve immune status by suppressing viral replication. Incomplete virologic response is associated with antiretroviral-resistant mutations. Regimens containing five or six drugs or "gigatherapy" are recommended for patients with multiple treatment failures and a highly resistant HIV quasispecies. Gigatherapy has been partially effective. The intervention of treatment interruption to allow wild-type (susceptible to ART) virus to become predominant has not been found to be beneficial in most studies. Immunological, rather than virological factors, may determine progression, particularly in patients with very advanced HIV disease. This study has evaluated the option of continued ART in the most immunosuppressed patients with HIV disease. Compared with patients with virological failure who interrupted cART at least once, profoundly immunodeficient HIV-infected patients who continued cART experienced reduced risk of ADEs. Continued treatment with cART, even with effective virological control, is no longer achievable; however, it may still be beneficial, unless the drug-related adverse events become unmanageable.[1] Ⓐ

Evidence-Based Reference

1. Kousignian I et al: Maintaining antiretroviral therapy reduces the risk of aids-defining events in patients with uncontrolled viral replication and profound immunodeficiency, *Clin Infect Dis* 46:296-304, 2008. Commentary by N. Khardori, M.D. Ⓐ

SUGGESTED READINGS

d'Arminio Monforte A et al: The changing incidence of AIDS events in patients receiving highly active antiretroviral therapy, *Arch Intern Med* 165(4):416, 2005.

Hammer SM et al: Treatment for adult HIV infection: 2006 recommendations of the International AIDS Society—USA panel, *JAMA* 296(7):827, 2006.

Hermsen ED, Wynn HE, McNabb J: Discontinuation of prophylaxis for HIV-associated opportunistic infections in the era of highly active antiretroviral therapy, *Am J Health Syst Pharm* 61(3):245, 2004.

Huang L et al: Intensive care of patients with HIV infection, *N Engl J Med* 355(2):173, 2006.

Kantor R et al: Evolution of resistance to drugs in HIV-1-infected patients failing antiretroviral therapy, *AIDS* 18(11):1503, 2004.

Monier PL, Wilcox R: Metabolic complications associated with the use of highly active antiretroviral therapy in HIV-1-infected adults, *Am J Med Sci* 328(1):48, 2004.

Olsen CH et al: Risk of AIDS and death at given HIV-RNA and CD4 cell count, in relation to specific antiretroviral drugs in regimen, *AIDS* 19(3):319, 2005.

AUTHORS: **GLEN G. FORT, M.D., M.P.H.,** and **DENNIS J. MIKOLICH, M.D.**

BASIC INFORMATION

DEFINITION

Acromegaly is a chronic debilitating disease with an insidious onset, resulting from the effects of either hypersecretion of growth hormone (GH) or increased amounts of an insulin-like growth factor I (IGF-I).

SYNONYMS Marie's disease

ICD-9CM CODES
253.0 Acromegaly

EPIDEMIOLOGY & DEMOGRAPHICS

INCIDENCE: Three to four new cases per 1 million persons annually

PREVALENCE: 50 to 60 cases/1 million persons, with some estimates as high as 90 cases/1 million persons

PREDOMINANT SEX: No sexual predominance

MEAN AGE AT DIAGNOSIS: Males: 40 yr; females: 45 yr

RISK FACTORS

- Increased mortality rate, primarily from cardiovascular and respiratory causes
- Death in 50% of untreated patients by age 50 yr
- Increased prevalence of colon carcinoma and other malignancies

PHYSICAL FINDINGS & CLINICAL PRESENTATION

- Coarse features resulting from growth of soft tissue
- Coarse, oily skin
- Hands and feet that are spadelike, fleshy, and moist
- Prognathism, which can give an underbite
- Carpal tunnel syndrome
- Excessive sweating
- Arthralgias and severe osteoarthritis
- History of increased hat, glove, and/or shoe size
- Hypertension
- Skin tags
- Muscle weakness and decreased exercise capacity
- Headache, often severe
- Diabetes mellitus
- Visual field defects

ETIOLOGY

Cause is usually a pituitary adenoma affecting the anterior lobe.

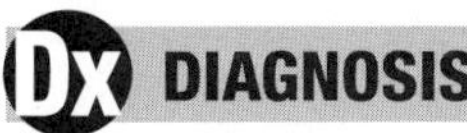

DIAGNOSIS

DIFFERENTIAL DIAGNOSIS

Ectopic production of GH-releasing hormone (GHRH) from a carcinoid or other neuroendocrine tumor

WORKUP

1. First screening test: measure serum IGF-I level.
   a. Direct measurement of the GH level is not as useful because it is secreted in a pulsatile fashion and a random level may be falsely normal.
   b. Upper limits of a normal IGF-I level, depending on the assay: >380 ng/ml or 2.5 U/ml.
2. Failure to suppress serum GH to less than 2 ng/ml after 100 g oral glucose is considered conclusive.
   a. Patients may show suppression of GH (paradoxic response).
   b. Patients will not suppress GH to 2 ng/ml or less (typical response in patients with acromegaly).
   c. GHRH level >300 ng/ml is indicative of an ectopic source of GH.

LABORATORY TESTS

- Elevated serum phosphate
- Elevated urine calcium

IMAGING STUDIES

- Imaging studies of choice: MRI of the pituitary and hypothalamus
- CT of the pituitary and hypothalamus used initially

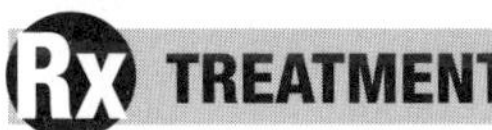

TREATMENT

SURGERY

Treatment of choice: transsphenoidal microsurgical adenomectomy

- Surgical failure rate: approximately 13.3% for microadenomas (tumors <10 mm) and 11.1% for macroadenomas (tumors >10 mm confined to the sella)
- Preoperative IGF-I level: indicator of surgical outcome with higher levels associated with surgical failure

RADIOTHERAPY

- Radiotherapy is usually reserved for tumor recurrence or persistence after surgery in patients with resistance to or intolerance of medical treatment
- Major complication: hypopituitarism, which may occur in up to 50% of patients; this complication is more likely in patients who had surgery irradiation

MEDICAL THERAPY

- Indicated when patients have not responded to surgical therapy, when surgery is contraindicated, and in patients waiting for the effects of radiotherapy to begin
- Somastatin receptor ligands: octreotide, lanreotide:
  - Important in the preoperative shrinkage of pituitary tumors and softening of adenomatous tissue.
  - Pegvisomant is a growth hormone receptor antagonist that has shown promising results in the treatment of acromegaly. It is generally used in patients with resistance to or intolerance of somastatin analogues. It should be used in patients who do not have central compressive symptoms and those with resistant diabetes.
  - Dopamine receptor agonists: Bromocriptine, cabergoline: can be used in addition to somastatin receptor ligands.

CHRONIC Rx

Combination of bromocriptine and octreotide may be synergistic, allowing a lower combination dosage than either alone.

DISPOSITION

- Patients receiving radiotherapy need long-term follow-up to monitor the potential development of hypopituitarism.
- Continuation of medical therapy should be based on the normalization of IGF-I levels.

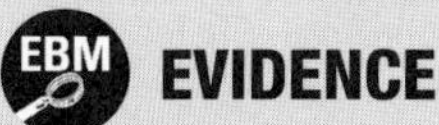

EVIDENCE

Please note: Complete text of EBM for this topic is available online.

Key trials and commentary:

The objective of this study was to address the all-cause mortality risk in patients with acromegaly. This meta-analysis showed increased all-cause mortality in patients with acromegaly, compared with the general population, even after transsphenoidal surgery.

Acromegaly is a relatively rare disorder that is accompanied by a host of potentially life-shortening diseases and complications including hypertension, diabetes mellitus, sleep apnea (with potential cor pulmonale), cardiomyopathy, cardiovascular disease, and colon polyps (with concern for increased risk of colon cancer). Furthermore, the presence of pituitary adenomas or the need for irradiation can lead to pituitary dysfunction. However, although most studies looking at mortality have suggested an increased mortality associated with untreated acromegaly, most of these studies were small and did not reach statistical significance. The aim of this study was to assess the all-cause risk of mortality in acromegaly through a meta-analysis. Sixteen studies were reviewed. The weighted mean of the standardized mortality ratio (SMR) was 1.72, which reflects a 72% increase in mortality in patients with acromegaly compared with the general population. In those studies where more than 80% of the patients were treated with transsphenoidal surgery (i.e., the more recent studies), the SMR was 1.32, which reflects a 32% increase in mortality in patients with acromegaly compared with the general population. This meta-analysis effectively supports earlier conclusions that acromegaly increases risk of mortality from all causes despite the current wide use of the transsphenoidal approach to pituitary adenectomy.[1] Ⓐ

The objective of a separate study was to assess whether weekly administration of 40 mg pegvisomant (PEG-V) improves quality of life (QoL) and metabolic parameters in patients with acromegaly who have normal age-adjusted IGF-1 concentrations during long-acting somatostatin analogue (SSA) treatment. Improvement in quality of life was observed without significant change in IGF-1 after the addition of 40 mg pegvisomant weekly to monthly SSA therapy in acromegalic patients who had normalized IGF-1 on

SSA monotherapy. These data question the current recommendations in how to assess disease activity in acromegaly. Moreover, the findings question the validity of the current approach of medical treatment in which pegvisomant is used only when SSA therapy has failed to normalize IGF-1.

Quality of life is often suboptimal in acromegaly patients effectively treated biochemically. This issue poses a significant challenge for the treating physician. One possible explanation for the discordance between the normalization of growth hormone (GH) levels and persistent symptoms is that achieving traditionally accepted biochemical treatment goals may not truly normalize the effects of GH overproduction. To address this question, these authors performed a double-blind, placebo-controlled, crossover study in which patients who were already "well controlled" on long-term somatostatin analogue (SA) treatment (i.e., had normal IGF-1 levels) were additionally treated with 40 mg PEG-V per week. They found that quality of life in patients treated with both SA and PEG-V had significant improvement in quality of life as measured by both the AcroQoL and the PASQ. These authors believe that their data (1) challenge the biochemical parameters that are considered acceptable in assessing effective treatment of acromegaly, and (2) the algorithm that PEG-V should be used only when SA monotherapy is inadequate to normalize IGF-1.[2] Ⓐ

A separate prospective randomized study evaluated the efficacy and safety of octreotide LAR vs. surgery in newly diagnosed acromegalic patients. This first randomized study in unselected patients indicates that the 48-week treatment outcome of octreotide LAR as first-line treatment of acromegaly does not significantly differ from surgery. Because a complete response to surgery in GH-secreting macroadenomas can be difficult to achieve, first-line therapy with octreotide LAR can be considered as a viable alternative for most patients with acromegaly, owing to its low complication rate.

Pituitary surgery is used as the first-line treatment for acromegaly in most treatment algorithms. However, when surgery is not likely to cure the patient (e.g., when the tumor invades the cavernous sinus), or when surgery is contraindicated, there are few data as to whether medical treatment as opposed to surgical treatment of such tumors produces acceptable efficacy. The goal of this study was to evaluate the safety and efficacy of octreotide LAR (oLAR) vs. surgery in patients newly diagnosed with acromegaly. 104 patients were enrolled in this prospective study and were randomized to either oLAR or surgery over a 48-week period. These authors found that surgically debulking tumors had modest biochemical improvement at 24 weeks, but that the difference was no longer statistically significant by 48-weeks post treatment. Tumor shrinkage and safety parameters were acceptable in both treatment groups. These authors, therefore, conclude that medical treatment of GH-producing pituitary tumors may be an acceptable first-line treatment option in some circumstances.[3] Ⓐ

Evidence-Based References

1. Dekkers OM et al: Mortality in acromegaly: a metaanalysis, *J Clin Endocrinol Metab* 93:61-67, 2008. Commentary by W.H. Ludlam, M.D., Ph.D. Ⓐ

2. Neggers SJCMM et al: Quality of life in acromegalic patients during long-term somatostatin analog treatment with and without pegvisomant, *J Clin Endocrinol Metab* 93:3853-3859, 2008. Commentary by W.H. Ludlam, M.D., Ph.D. Ⓐ

3. Colao A et al: Octreotide LAR vs. surgery in newly diagnosed patients with acromegaly: a randomized, open-label, multicentre study, *Clin Endocrinol* 70:757-768, 2009. Commentary by W.H. Ludlam, M.D., Ph.D. Ⓐ

SUGGESTED READINGS

Doga M et al: Diagnostic and therapeutic consensus on acromegaly, *J Endocrinol Invest* 28(5 suppl):56, 2005.

Ezzat S: Pharmacological options in the treatment of acromegaly, *Cur Opin Invest Drugs* 6(10):1023, 2005.

Ketznelson L: Diagnosis and treatment of acromegaly, *Growth Horm IGF Res* 15(suppl A):S31, 2005.

Melmed S: Acromegaly, *N Engl J Med* 355:2558-2573, 2006.

AUTHORS: **BETH J. WUTZ, M.D.,** and **RUBEN ALVERO, M.D.**

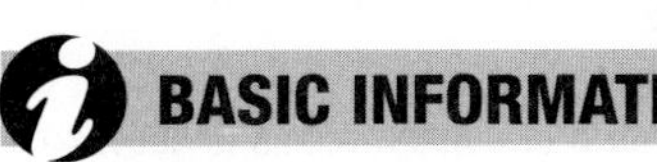

BASIC INFORMATION

DEFINITION

Actinomycosis is an indolent, slowly progressive infection caused by both anaerobic or microaerophilic bacteria that normally colonize the mouth, vagina, and colon. Actinomycosis is characterized by the formation of painful abscesses, soft tissue infiltration, and draining sinuses.

SYNONYMS

Actinomyces infection
Lumpy jaw

ICD-9CM CODES
039.9 Actinomycosis

EPIDEMIOLOGY & DEMOGRAPHICS

Geographic distribution:

- Actinomycosis is worldwide in distribution.
- Commonly found as normal flora of the oral cavity (within gingival crevices, tonsillar crypts, periodontal pockets, dental plaques, and carious teeth), pharynx, tracheobronchial tree, gastrointestinal tract, and female urogenital tract.

Incidence and prevalence:

- Incidence 1:300,000.
- Males infected more often than females 3:1.
- Can occur at any age but commonly seen in midlife.
- Incidence has decreased since the 1950s and is attributed to better oral hygiene and antibiotics.

PHYSICAL FINDINGS & CLINICAL PRESENTATION

Actinomycosis can affect any organ. Although not typically considered as opportunistic pathogens, *Actinomyces* species capitalize on tissue injury or mucosal breach to invade adjacent structures in the head and neck regions. As a result, dental infections and oromaxillofacial trauma are common antecedent events. Characteristic manifestations include:

- Cervicofacial disease (most common site):
  1. Occurs in the setting of poor dental hygiene, recent dental surgery, or minor oral trauma
  2. Painful soft tissue swelling commonly seen at the angle of the mandible
  3. Fever, chills, and weight loss
  4. Trismus
  5. Soft tissue facial infection with sinus tract or fistula formation
- Thoracic disease:
  1. Can involve the lungs, pleura, mediastinum, or chest wall.
  2. Presumed secondary to aspiration of *Actinomyces* organisms in patients with poor oral hygiene.
  3. Fever, cough, weight loss, and pleuritic chest pains are common symptoms.
  4. Signs of pneumonia or pleural effusion may be present.
  5. With extension beyond the lungs to mediastinal structures and the chest wall, signs and symptoms of pericarditis, empyema, chest wall sinus drainage, and tracheoesophageal fistula can all occur (Fig. 1-8).
- Abdominal disease:
  1. Occurs most commonly after appendectomy, perforated bowel, diverticulitis, or surgery to the gastrointestinal tract.
  2. Lesions develop most commonly in the ileocecal valve, causing abdominal pain, fever, weight loss, and a palpable mass.
  3. Extension may occur to the liver, causing jaundice and abscess formation.
  4. Sinus tracts to the abdominal wall can occur.
- Pelvic disease:
  1. Commonly occurs by extension from abdominal disease of the ileocecal valve to the right adnexa (80% of cases).
  2. Endometritis.

ETIOLOGY

- Actinomycosis is most commonly caused by *Actinomyces israelii.* Other causes are *A. naeslundii, A. odontolyticus, A. viscosus,* and *A. meyeri.*
- *Actinomyces* are gram-positive, non–spore-forming, filamentous, anaerobic or microaerophilic rods.
- Actinomycosis infections are polymicrobial, usually associated with *Streptococcus, Bacteroides, Eikenella corrodens, Enterococcus,* and *Fusobacterium* spp.
- Infects individuals only after entry into disrupted mucosa or tissue injury.

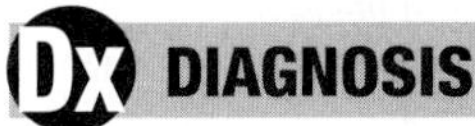

DIAGNOSIS

Isolating the bacteria in the proper clinical setting makes the diagnosis of actinomycosis.

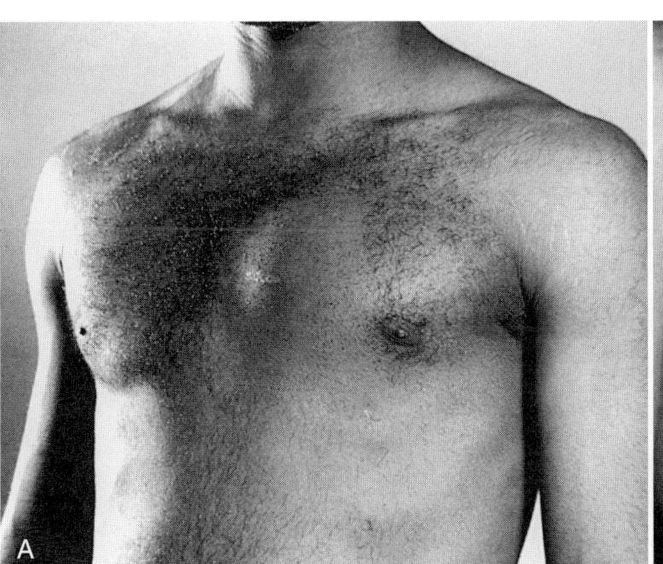

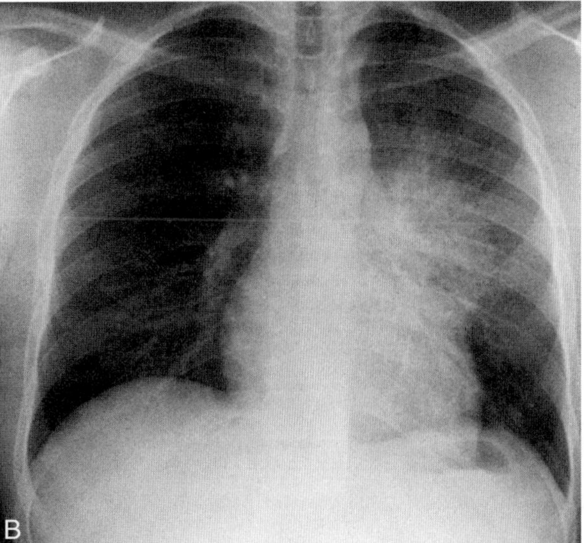

FIGURE 1-8 Thoracic actinomycosis. A, Initial presentation with a bulging mass lesion in the chest wall with a central sinus tract. **B,** The chest radiograph with the associated pulmonary infiltrate. (From Gorbach SL: *Infectious diseases,* ed 2, Philadelphia, 1998, WB Saunders.)

DIFFERENTIAL DIAGNOSIS

- Cervicofacial disease: odontogenic abscesses, brachial cleft cyst
- Pulmonary disease: nocardiosis, botryomycosis, chromomycosis, fungal disease of the lung, tuberculosis
- Intestinal disease: intestinal tuberculosis, ameboma, Crohn's disease, colon cancer
- Pelvic disease: chronic pelvic inflammatory disease, Crohn's disease
- CNS disease: other forms of brain abscess, brain tumors, toxoplasmosis, intracranial hematoma

WORKUP

The workup includes obtaining specimens either by aspirating abscesses, excising sinus tracts, or tissue biopsies. All specimens should be set up to culture anaerobic bacteria and held at least 5 to 7 days.

LABORATORY TESTS

- Isolating "sulfur granules" from tissue specimens or draining sinuses confirms the diagnosis of actinomycosis. *Actinomyces* are noted for forming characteristic sulfur granules in infected tissue but not in vitro. The term *sulfur granule* is a misnomer, reflecting only the yellow color of the granule in pus, because the granules are not composed of any sulfur at all.
  1. Sulfur granules are nests of *Actinomyces* species. Sulfur granules may be macroscopic or microscopic (Fig. 1-9).
  2. Sulfur granules are crushed and stained for identification of *Actinomyces* organisms and may take up to 3 wk to grow in culture media.

IMAGING STUDIES

Imaging studies are useful adjunctive tests in localizing the site and spread of infection.

1. Chest x-ray examination
2. CT scan of the head, chest, abdomen, and pelvic areas is useful

Rx TREATMENT

NONPHARMACOLOGIC THERAPY

- Incision and drainage of abscesses
- Excision of sinus tract

ACUTE GENERAL Rx

- Penicillin 10 to 20 million units per day in 4 divided doses for 4 to 6 wk.
- In penicillin-allergic patients, erythromycin, tetracycline, clindamycin, or cephalosporins (depending on the type of penicillin allergy) are reasonable alternatives.
- Chloramphenicol 50 to 60 mg/kg/day can be used for CNS actinomycosis.

CHRONIC Rx

- Following 4 to 6 wk IV penicillin, oral penicillin V 500 mg PO qid for 6 to 12 mo.
- Treatment of associated microorganisms is not needed.

DISPOSITION

- Clinical actinomycosis, if not treated, spreads to contiguous tissues and structures ignoring tissue planes. Hematogenous spread, although possible, is rare.
- Actinomycosis is very sensitive to antibiotics but requires chronic long-term treatment to prevent relapse.

REFERRAL

If the diagnosis of actinomycosis is suspected, consultation with an infectious disease specialist is suggested. General surgical consultation for excision of sinus tracts and abscess incision and drainage is recommended.

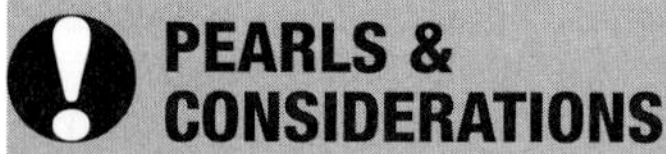

PEARLS & CONSIDERATIONS

COMMENTS

- There is no person-to-person transmission of *Actinomyces.*
- Isolation of the organism in an asymptomatic individual does not mean the person has actinomycosis. Active symptoms must be present to make the diagnosis.
- Pelvic actinomycosis has been associated with use of an intrauterine device (IUD).
- Actinomycosis can also involve the CNS, causing multiple brain abscesses.

SUGGESTED READINGS

Choi J: Optimal duration of IV and oral antibiotics in the treatment of thoracic actinomycosis, *Chest* 128(4):2211, 2005.

Russo TA: Agents of actinomycosis. In *Mandell, Douglas, and Bennett's principles and practice of infectious diseases,* ed 5, New York, 2000, Churchill Livingstone.

Sharkawy AA: Cervicofacial actinomycosis and mandibular osteomyelitis, *Infect Dis Clin North Am* 21, 543-556, 2007.

AUTHORS: **GLENN G. FORT, M.D., M.P.H.,** and **DENNIS J. MIKOLICH, M.D.**

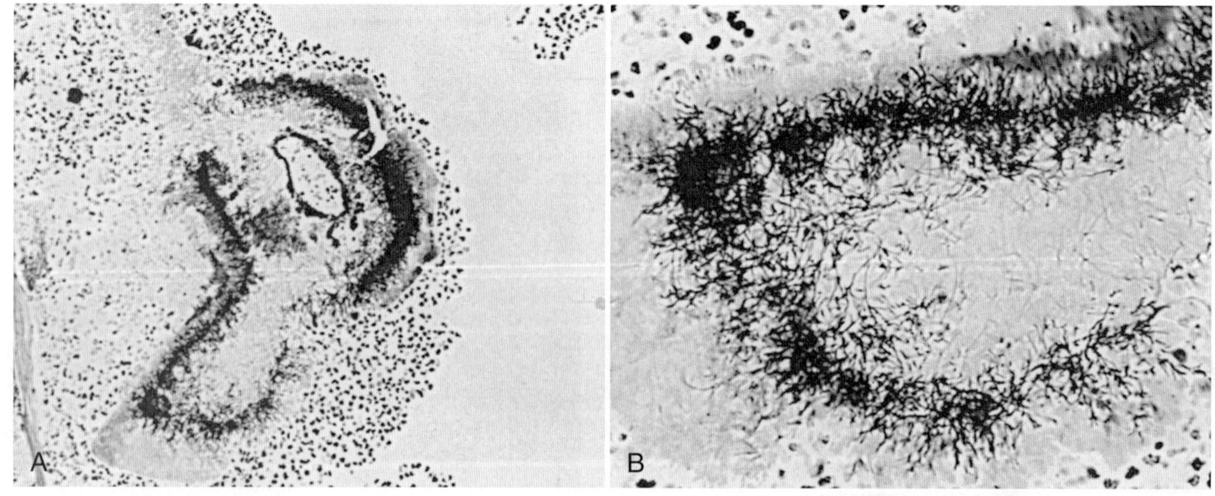

FIGURE 1-9 A, Actinomycotic sulfur granule surrounded by inflammatory cells (Brown-Brenn stain, ×250). **B,** Increased magnification (×1000) demonstrates the delicate, branched filaments of *Actinomyces.* (From Mandell GL [ed]: *Mandell, Douglas, and Bennett's principles and practice of infectious diseases,* ed 5, New York, 2000, Churchill Livingstone.)

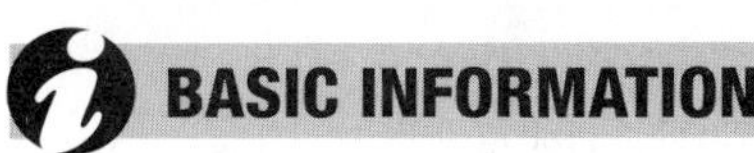

BASIC INFORMATION

DEFINITION

Acute bronchitis is the inflammation of trachea and bronchi.

SYNONYMS Chest cold

ICD-9CM CODES
466.0 Acute bronchitis

EPIDEMIOLOGY & DEMOGRAPHICS

- Highest incidence in smokers, older adults, and young children and during winter months.
- In the U.S. there are nearly 30 million ambulatory visits annually for cough, leading to more than 12 million diagnoses of "bronchitis."
- Acute lower respiratory tract infection is the most common condition treated in primary care.

PHYSICAL FINDINGS & CLINICAL PRESENTATION

- Cough, usually worse in the morning, often productive; mainly caused by transient bronchial hyperresponsiveness
- Low-grade fever
- Substernal discomfort worsened by coughing
- Postnasal drip, pharyngeal injection
- Rhonchi that may clear after cough, occasional wheezing

ETIOLOGY

- Viral infections are the leading cause of bronchitis (rhinovirus, influenza virus, adenovirus, respiratory syncytial virus)
- Atypical organisms *(Mycoplasma, Chlamydia pneumoniae)*
- Bacterial infections *(Haemophilus influenzae, Moraxella, Streptococcus pneumoniae)*

Dx DIAGNOSIS

DIFFERENTIAL DIAGNOSIS

- Pneumonia
- Asthma
- Sinusitis
- Bronchiolitis
- Aspiration
- Cystic fibrosis
- Pharyngitis
- Cough secondary to medications
- Neoplasm (elderly patients)
- Influenza
- Allergic aspergillosis
- Gastroesophageal reflux disease
- Congestive heart failure (in elderly patients)
- Bronchogenic neoplasm

WORKUP

Seldom necessary (e.g., to rule out pneumonia, neoplasm)

LABORATORY TESTS

Laboratory tests are generally not necessary.

IMAGING STUDIES

Chest x-ray examination is usually reserved for patients with suspected pneumonia, influenza, or underlying chronic obstructive pulmonary disease (COPD) and no improvement with therapy.

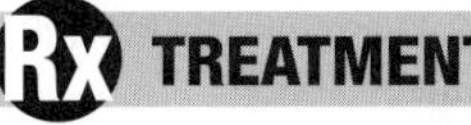

Rx TREATMENT

NONPHARMACOLOGIC THERAPY

- Avoidance of tobacco and other pulmonary irritants
- Increased fluid intake
- Use of vaporizer to increase room humidity

ACUTE GENERAL Rx

- Inhaled bronchodilators (e.g., albuterol, metaproterenol) prn for 1 to 2 wk in patients with wheezing or troublesome cough. Inhaled albuterol has been proven effective in reducing the duration of cough in adults with uncomplicated acute bronchitis.
- Cough suppression with dextromethorphan and guaifenesin is commonly recommended; addition of codeine for cough suppression if cough is severe and is significantly interrupting patient's sleep pattern.
- Use of antibiotics (TMP-SMX, amoxicillin, doxycycline, cefuroxime) for acute bronchitis is generally not indicated; should be considered only in patients with concomitant COPD and purulent sputum or in patients unresponsive to prolonged conservative treatment.
- Antibiotics are overused in patients with acute bronchitis (70% to 90% of office visits for acute bronchitis result in treatment with antibiotics); this practice pattern is contributing to increases in resistant organisms.

CHRONIC Rx

Avoidance of tobacco and other pulmonary irritants

DISPOSITION

- Complete recovery within 7 to 10 days in most patients.
- Patients should be informed to expect to have a cough for 10 to 14 days after the visit.

REFERRAL

For pulmonary function testing only in patients with recurrent bronchitis and suspected underlying asthma

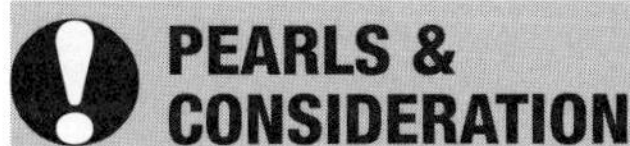

PEARLS & CONSIDERATIONS

COMMENTS

- Intervention studies reveal that patient and physician education are effective in reducing the use of antibiotic therapy. No offer or delayed offer of antibiotics for acute uncomplicated lower respiratory tract infection is acceptable, is associated with little difference in symptom resolution, and is likely to reduce antibiotic use and beliefs in the effectiveness of antibiotics.
- It is helpful to refer to acute bronchitis as a "chest cold." Patients should be informed that antibiotics are probably not going to be beneficial and may result in significant side effects.

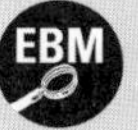

EVIDENCE

Overall, the evidence for the use of beta-2 agonists in acute bronchitis is not strong, especially for those with no evidence of airflow obstruction.[1] Ⓐ

Adults suffering acute infective exacerbations of COPD may find that beta-2 agonists reduce symptoms, but the benefit should be weighed against the possible adverse effects.[1] Ⓐ

Further evidence concerning inhaled short- and long-acting beta-2 agonists and ipratropium for the management of exacerbations in people with existing COPD can be found in the medical topic Chronic Obstructive Pulmonary Disease.

Antibiotics for the treatment of acute bronchitis in people with no underlying lung condition may produce modest benefits, but these must be weighed against the increased risk of adverse effects.[2] Ⓐ

There is little evidence that one antibiotic is preferred over any other.[3] Ⓐ

Even though physicians may be more likely to prescribe antibiotics for smokers with acute bronchitis rather than nonsmokers, seven trials in a systematic review found no difference between the two groups in their response to treatment.[2] Ⓐ

A randomized, controlled trial concluded that people with uncomplicated acute lower respiratory infections given no offer of antibiotics or a delayed prescription of antibiotics demonstrated little difference in the duration of symptoms compared with those treated with antibiotics.[4] Ⓑ

There is no good evidence that dextromethorphan is effective in acute bronchitis.[5] Ⓑ

Evidence-Based References

1. Smucny J et al: β2 agonists for acute bronchitis, *Cochrane Rev* 4, 2006. Ⓐ
2. Smucny J et al: Antibiotics for acute bronchitis, *Cochrane Rev* 4, 2004. Ⓐ
3. Wark P: Bronchitis (acute). In *Clinical evidence,* London, 2007, BMJ Publishing. Ⓐ
4. Little P et al: Information leaflet and antibiotic prescribing strategies for acute lower respiratory tract infection: a randomized controlled trial, *JAMA* 293:3029, 2005. Ⓑ
5. Schroeder K, Fahey T: Over-the-counter medications for acute cough in children and adults in ambulatory settings, *Cochrane Rev* 4, 2004. Ⓑ

SUGGESTED READING

Wenzel R, Fowler A: Acute bronchitis, *N Engl J Med* 355:2125, 2006.

AUTHOR: **FRED F. FERRI, M.D.**

Acute Respiratory Distress Syndrome 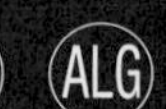

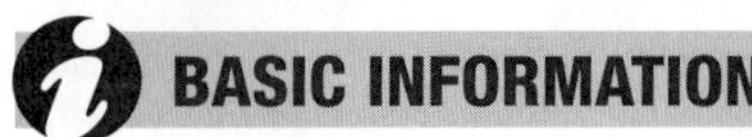

BASIC INFORMATION

DEFINITION

Acute respiratory distress syndrome (ARDS) is a form of noncardiogenic pulmonary edema that results from acute damage to the alveoli. It is characterized by acute diffuse infiltrative lung lesions with resulting interstitial and alveolar edema, severe hypoxemia, and respiratory failure. The definition of ARDS includes the following three components:

1. A ratio of Pa_{O_2} to Fi_{O_2} $\leq$200 regardless of the level of positive end expiratory pressure (PEEP)
2. The detection of bilateral pulmonary infiltrates on frontal chest radiograph
3. Absence of congestive heart failure (pulmonary artery wedge pressure [PAWP] $\leq$18 mm Hg or no clinical evidence of elevated left atrial pressure on the basis of chest radiograph or other clinical data)

The cardinal feature of ARDS, refractory hypoxemia, is caused by formation of protein-rich alveolar edema after damage to the integrity of the lung's alveolar-capillary barrier.

SYNONYMS

ARDS

Adult respiratory distress syndrome

ICD-9CM CODES

518.82 Acute respiratory distress syndrome

EPIDEMIOLOGY & DEMOGRAPHICS

- More than 150,000 ARDS cases per year in the U.S.
- Incidence is 1.5 to 8.3 cases per 100,000 per year.
- Approximately 50% of patients who develop ARDS do so within 24 hours of the inciting event. Mortality rate is 40% to 50%.

PHYSICAL FINDINGS & CLINICAL PRESENTATION

- Signs and symptoms
  1. Dyspnea
  2. Chest discomfort
  3. Cough
  4. Anxiety
- Physical examination
  1. Tachypnea
  2. Tachycardia
  3. Hypertension
  4. Coarse crepitations of both lungs
  5. Fever may be present if infection is the underlying etiology

ETIOLOGY

- Sepsis (>40% of cases)
- Aspiration: near drowning, aspiration of gastric contents (>30% of cases)
- Trauma (>20% of cases)
- Multiple transfusions, blood products
- Drugs (e.g., overdose of morphine, methadone, heroin; reaction to nitrofurantoin)
- Noxious inhalation (e.g., chlorine gas, high O_2 concentration)
- Postresuscitation
- Cardiopulmonary bypass
- Pneumonia
- Burns
- Pancreatitis
- A history of chronic alcohol abuse significantly increases the risk of developing ARDS in critically ill patients

DIAGNOSIS

DIFFERENTIAL DIAGNOSIS

- Cardiogenic pulmonary edema
- Viral pneumonitis
- Lymphangitic carcinomatosis

WORKUP

The search for an underlying cause should focus on treatable causes (e.g., infections such as sepsis or pneumonia)

- Arterial blood gases (ABGs)
- Hemodynamic monitoring
- Bronchoalveolar lavage (selected patients)

LABORATORY TESTS

- ABGs:
  1. Initially: varying degrees of hypoxemia, generally resistant to supplemental oxygen
  2. Respiratory alkalosis, decreased P_{CO_2}
  3. Widened alveolar-arterial gradient
  4. Hypercapnia as the disease progresses
- Bronchoalveolar lavage:
  1. The most prominent finding is an increased number of polymorphonucleocytes.
  2. The presence of eosinophilia has therapeutic implications because these patients respond to corticosteroids.
- Blood and urine cultures

IMAGING STUDIES

Chest radiograph (Fig. 1-10).

- The initial chest radiograph might be normal in the initial hours after the precipitating event.
- Bilateral interstitial infiltrates are usually seen within 24 hr; they often are more prominent in the bases and periphery.
- "White out" of both lung fields can be seen in advanced stages.
- CT scan of chest: diffuse consolidation with air bronchograms, bullae, pleural effusions. Pneumomediastinum and pneumothoraces may also be present.

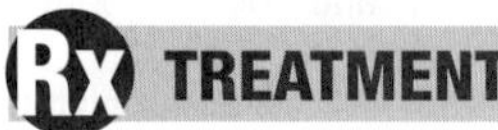

TREATMENT

NONPHARMACOLOGIC THERAPY

Hemodynamic monitoring:

- Can be used for the initial evaluation of ARDS (in ruling out cardiogenic pulmonary edema) and its subsequent management. Recent studies, however, have shown that clinical management involving the early use of pulmonary artery catheters in patients with ARDS did not significantly affect mortality and morbidity rates.
- Although no dynamic profile is diagnostic of ARDS, the presence of pulmonary edema, a high cardiac output, and a low pulmonary capillary wedge pressure (PCWP) is characteristic of ARDS.
- It is important to remember that partially treated intravascular volume overload and flash pulmonary edema can have the hemodynamic features of ARDS; filling pressures can also be elevated by increased intrathoracic pressures or with fluid administration; cardiac function can be depressed by acidosis, hypoxemia, or other factors associated with sepsis.

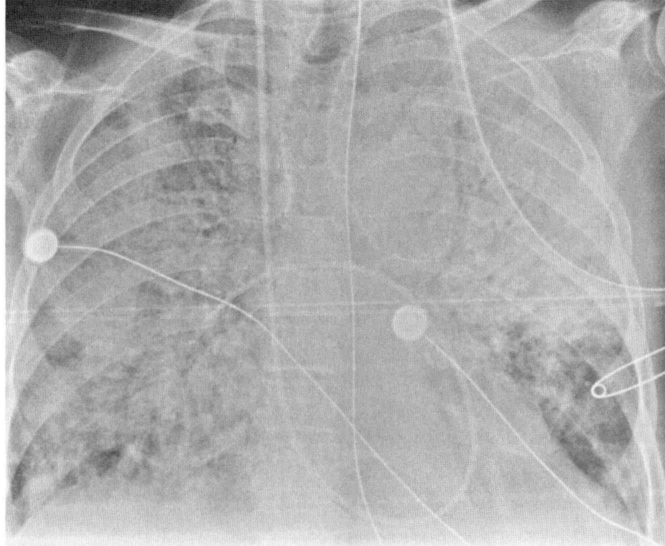

FIGURE 1-10 ARDS. Anteroposterior radiograph in an elderly woman reveals widespread consolidation with air bronchograms. The heart size is normal. There are no pleural effusions. (From McLoud TC: *Thoracic radiology: the requisites,* St Louis, 1998, Mosby.)

Ventilatory support: mechanical ventilation is generally necessary to maintain adequate gas exchange (see Section III). A low tidal volume and low plateau pressure ventilator strategy are recommended to avoid ventilator-induced injury. Assist-control is generally preferred initially with the following ventilator settings:

- FiO_2 1.0 (until a lower value can be used to achieve adequate oxygenation). When possible, minimize oxygen toxicity by maintaining FiO_2 at <60%.
- Tidal volume: Set initial tidal volume at 6 ml/kg of predicted body weight (PBW = 50.0 + 0.91 [height: 152.4 cm] for men, PBW = 45.5 + 0.91 [height: 152.4 cm] for women). The concept of using PBW is based on the fact that lung size depends most strongly on height and sex; PBW normalizes the tidal volume to lung size. Aim to maintain plateau pressure (Pplat) at <30 mm Hg.
- PEEP 5 cm H_2O or greater (to increase lung volume and keep alveoli open). PEEP should be applied in small increments of 3 to 5 cm H_2O (up to a maximum of 15 cm H_2O) to achieve acceptable arterial saturation (>0.9) with nontoxic FiO_2 values (<0.6) and acceptable airway plateau pressures (>30 to 35 cm H_2O). It is important to remember that an increase in PEEP may lower cardiac output and, despite improvement in PaO_2, may actually have a negative effect on tissue oxygenation (the major determinants of tissue oxygenation are hemoglobin, percent saturation, and cardiac output).
- Inspiratory flow: 60 L/min.
- Ventilatory rate: high ventilatory rates of 18 to 24 breaths/min are often necessary in patients with ARDS because of their increased physiologic dead space and smaller lung volumes. Patients must be monitored for excessive intrathoracic gas trapping (auto-PEEP or intrinsic PEEP) that can depress cardiac output.
- Sedation: GABA receptor agonists (including propofol and benzodiazepines such as midazolam) have traditionally been the most commonly administered sedative drugs for ICU patients. Recent trials indicate that the alpha-2 agonist dexmedetomidine may have distinct advantages. At comparable sedation levels, dexmedetomidine-treated patients spent less time on ventilator, experienced less delirium, and developed less tachycardia and hypertension. The most notable adverse effect of dexmedetomidine was bradycardia.

ACUTE GENERAL Rx

Identify and treat precipitating conditions:

- Blood and urine cultures and trial of antibiotics in presumed sepsis (routine administration of antibiotics in all cases of ARDS is not recommended).
- Prompt repair of bone fractures in patients with major trauma.
- Bowel rest and crystalloid resuscitation in pancreatitis.
- Fluid management: optimal fluid and hemodynamic management of patients with ARDS is patient specific; in general, administration of crystalloids is recommended if a downward trend in PCWP is associated with diminished cardiac index, resulting in prerenal azotemia, oliguria, and relative tachycardia. On the other hand, if PCWP increases with little or no change in cardiac index, one should begin diuretic therapy and use low-dose dopamine (2 to 4 μg/kg/min) to maintain natriuresis and support adequate renal flow.
- Positioning the patient: changes in position can improve oxygenation by improving the distribution of perfusion to ventilated lung regions; repositioning (lateral decubitus positioning) should be attempted in patients with hypoxemia that is not responsive to other medical interventions. Placing patients with acute respiratory failure in a prone position improves their oxygenation but does not improve their survival.
- Corticosteroids: routine use of corticosteroids in ARDS is not recommended; corticosteroids may be beneficial in patients with many eosinophils in the bronchoalveolar lavage fluid. Systemic infections should be ruled out or adequately treated before administration of corticosteroids. Use of methylprednisolone has not been shown to increase the rate of infectious complications but is associated with a higher rate of neuromuscular weakness. In addition, starting methylprednisolone therapy more than 2 wk after the onset of ARDS may increase the risk of death.
- Nutritional support: nutritional support, preferably administered by the enteral route, is necessary to maintain adequate colloid oncotic pressure and intravascular volume. The inclusion of eicosapentaenoic acid from fish oil may be beneficial in improving ventilation requirements and length of stay in patients with ARDS.
- Tracheostomy: tracheostomy is warranted in patients requiring >2 wk of mechanical ventilation; discussion regarding tracheostomy should begin with patient (if alert and oriented) and family members/legal guardian after 5 to 7 days of ventilatory support.
- Some form of deep vein thrombosis prophylaxis is indicated in all patients with ARDS.
- Stress ulcer prophylaxis with sucralfate suspension (by nasogastric tube), or IV proton pump inhibitors or H_2 blockers.
- The use of surfactant remains controversial. Patients who receive surfactant have a greater improvement in gas exchange in the initial 24-hour period than patients who receive standard therapy alone; however, the use of exogenous surfactant does not improve survival.

DISPOSITION

- Prognosis for ARDS varies with the underlying cause. Prognosis is worse in patients with chronic liver disease, nonpulmonary organ dysfunction, sepsis, and advanced age.
- Elevated values of dead space fraction ($[PaCO_2 - PeCO_2]/PaCO_2$; normal is <0.3) is associated with an increased risk of death.
- In ARDS, the percentage of potentially recruitable lung is variable and associated with the response to PEEP.
- Overall mortality rate varies between 32% and 45%. Most deaths are attributable to sepsis or multiorgan dysfunction rather than primary respiratory causes.
- Recent trials have shown that as compared with the current standard of care, a ventilator strategy using esophageal measures to estimate the transpulmonary pressure significantly improves oxygenation and compliance. Further trials will determine if this approach should be widely adapted.

REFERRAL

Surgical referral for tracheostomy (see "Acute General Rx").

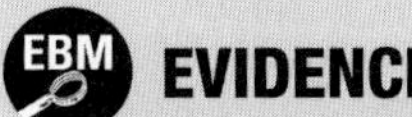

Please note: Complete text of EBM for this topic is available online.

SUGGESTED READINGS

Malhotra A: Low tidal volume ventilation in the acute respiratory distress syndrome, *N Engl J Med* 357: 1113, 2007.

Mercat A et al: Positive end-respiratory pressure setting in adults with acute lung injury and acute respiratory distress syndrome, *JAMA* 299(6):646-655, 2008.

Riker RR et al: Dexmedetomidine vs. midazolam for sedation of critically ill patients, *JAMA* 301(5):489-499, 2009.

Talmor D et al: Mechanical ventilation by esophageal pressure in acute lung injury, *N Engl J Med* 359: 2095-2104, 2008.

Wheeler AP: Acute lung injury and the acute respiratory distress syndrome, *Lancet* 369:1553, 2007.

AUTHOR: **FRED F. FERRI, M.D.**

Addison's Disease (PTG)

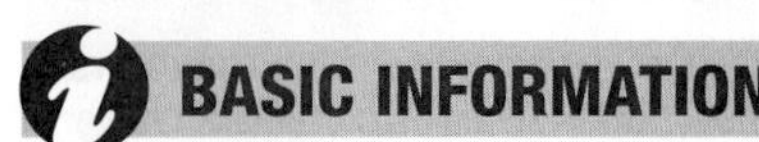

BASIC INFORMATION

DEFINITION

Addison's disease is characterized by inadequate secretion of corticosteroids resulting from partial or complete destruction of the adrenal glands.

SYNONYMS

Primary adrenocortical insufficiency
Adrenal insufficiency

ICD-9CM CODES
255.4 Addison's disease

EPIDEMIOLOGY & DEMOGRAPHICS

PREVALENCE: Five cases/100,000 persons
PREDOMINANT SEX: Female/male ratio of 2:1

PHYSICAL FINDINGS & CLINICAL PRESENTATION

- Hyperpigmentation: more prominent in palmar creases, buccal mucosa, pressure points (elbows, knees, knuckles), perianal mucosa, and around areolas of nipples
- Hypotension
- Generalized weakness
- Amenorrhea and loss of axillary hair in females

ETIOLOGY

- Autoimmune destruction of the adrenal glands (80% of cases)
- Tuberculosis (TB) (15% of cases)
- Carcinomatous destruction of the adrenal glands
- Adrenal hemorrhage (anticoagulants, trauma, coagulopathies, pregnancy, sepsis)
- Adrenal infarction (arteritis, thrombosis)
- AIDS (adrenal insufficiency develops in 30% of patients with AIDS)
- Other: sarcoidosis, amyloidosis, hemochromatosis, Wegener's granulomatosis, postoperative, fungal infections (candidiasis, histoplasmosis)

Dx DIAGNOSIS

DIFFERENTIAL DIAGNOSIS

Sepsis, hypovolemic shock, acute abdomen, apathetic hyperthyroidism in the elderly, myopathies, gastrointestinal malignancy, major depression, anorexia nervosa, hemochromatosis, salt-losing nephritis, chronic infection

WORKUP

- If the clinical picture is highly suggestive of adrenocortical insufficiency, the diagnosis can be made with the rapid adrenocorticotropic hormone (ACTH) test (Corticotropin test):
  1. Give 250 mcg ACTH (Corticotropin) by IV push and measure cortisol levels at 0 and 30 min.
  2. An increase in serum cortisol level to peak concentration >500 nmol/L (18 mcg/dl) indicates a normal response. Cortisol level <18 mcg/dl at 30 or 60 min is suggestive of adrenal insufficiency.
  3. Measure plasma ACTH. A high ACTH level confirms primary adrenal insufficiency.
- Critical illness-related corticosteroid insufficiency (e.g., in sepsis) is best established with the 1 mcg Corticotropin stimulation test in which cortisol levels are measured at baseline and 30 min after administration of corticotropin. A level <25 mcg/dl (690 nmol/L) or an increment over baseline of <9 mcg (250 nmol/L) represents an inadequate adrenal response.
- Secondary adrenocortical insufficiency (caused by pituitary dysfunction) can be distinguished from primary adrenal insufficiency by the following:
  1. Normal or low plasma ACTH level after rapid ACTH (Corticotropin test)
  2. Absence of hyperpigmentation
  3. No significant impairment of aldosterone secretion (because aldosterone secretion is under control of the renin-angiotensin system)
  4. Additional evidence of hypopituitarism (e.g., hypogonadism, hypothyroidism)

LABORATORY TESTS

- Increased potassium, decreased sodium and chloride
- Decreased glucose
- Increased blood urea nitrogen/creatinine ratio (prerenal azotemia)
- Mild normocytic, normochromic anemia, neutropenia, lymphocytosis, eosinophilia (significant dehydration may mask hyponatremia and anemia)
- Purified protein derivative (PPD) and antiadrenal antibodies

IMAGING STUDIES

- Chest x-ray may reveal a small heart.
- Abdominal x-ray film: adrenal calcifications may be noted if the adrenocortical insufficiency is secondary to TB or fungus.
- Abdominal CT scan: small adrenal glands generally indicate either idiopathic atrophy or longstanding TB, whereas enlarged glands are suggestive of early TB or potentially treatable diseases.

Rx TREATMENT

NONPHARMACOLOGIC THERAPY

- Perform periodic monitoring of serum electrolytes, vital signs, and body weight; liberal sodium intake is suggested.
- Periodic measurement of bone density may be helpful in identifying patients at risk for the development of osteoporosis.
- Patients should carry a MedicAlert bracelet and an emergency pack containing hydrocortisone 100 mg ampule, syringe, and needle.
- Patients and partners should be educated on how to give IM injection in case of vomiting or coma.

ACUTE GENERAL Rx

- Addisonian crisis is an acute complication of adrenal insufficiency characterized by circulatory collapse, dehydration, nausea, vomiting, hypoglycemia, and hyperkalemia.
  1. Draw plasma cortisol level; do not delay therapy while waiting for confirming laboratory results.
  2. Administer hydrocortisone 100 mg IV immediately, followed by 100 to 200 mg of hydrocortisone every 24 hours; if patient shows good clinical response, gradually taper dosage and change to oral maintenance dose (usually prednisone 7.5 mg/day).
  3. Provide adequate volume replacement with D_5NS solution until hypotension, dehydration, and hypoglycemia are completely corrected. Large volumes (2 to 3 L) under continuous cardiac monitoring may be necessary in the first 2 to 3 hr to correct the volume deficit and hypoglycemia and to avoid further hyponatremia.
- Identify and correct any precipitating factor (e.g., sepsis, hemorrhage).

CHRONIC Rx

- Give hydrocortisone 15 to 20 mg PO every morning and 5 to 10 mg in late afternoon or prednisone 5 mg in morning and 2.5 mg hs.
- Give oral fludrocortisone 0.05 mg/day to 0.20 mg/day: this mineralocorticoid is necessary if the patient has primary adrenocortical insufficiency. The dose is adjusted based on the serum sodium level and the presence of postural hypotension or marked orthostasis.
- Instruct patients to increase glucocorticoid replacement in times of stress and to receive parenteral glucocorticoids if diarrhea or vomiting occurs. Typical supplementation varies from 25 mg PO qd of hydrocortisone for minor medical and surgical stress to 50 to 100 mg IV hydrocortisone q8h for sepsis-induced hypotension or shock.
- The administration of dehydroepiandrosterone 50 mg PO qd improves well-being and sexuality in women with adrenal insufficiency.

SUGGESTED READING

Bornstein SR: Predisposing factors for adrenal insufficiency, *N Engl J Med* 360:2328-2339, 2009.

AUTHOR: **FRED F. FERRI, M.D.**

BASIC INFORMATION

DEFINITION

Although defining alcoholism precisely is impossible, among the commonly used screening instruments for this disorder are the CAGE questionnaire, short Michigan Alcoholism Screening Test (SMAST), National Council on Alcoholism criteria, and DSM-IV-R criteria. Moderate drinking has been defined as two standard drinks (e.g., 12 oz of beer) per day and one drink per day for women and persons older than 65 yr. Although not generally included under the alcoholism topic, hazardous or at-risk drinking should also be considered. For men, *at-risk drinking* is defined as more than 14 drinks/wk or more than 4 drinks/occasion. For women, at-risk drinking is defined as approximately half that given for men.

The American Psychiatric Association defines diagnostic criteria for *alcohol withdrawal* as follows:

A. Cessation of (or reduction in) alcohol use that has been heavy and prolonged.
B. Two (or more) of the following, developing within several hours to a few days after criterion A:
   1. Autonomic hyperactivity (e.g., sweating or pulse rate >100 beats/min)
   2. Increased hand tremor
   3. Insomnia
   4. Nausea and vomiting
   5. Transient visual, tactile, or auditory hallucinations or illusions
   6. Psychomotor agitation
   7. Anxiety
   8. Grand mal seizures
C. The symptoms in criterion B cause clinically significant distress or impairment in social, occupational, or other important areas of functioning.

The symptoms are not attributable to a general medical condition and are not better accounted for by another mental disorder.

SYNONYMS

Alcohol abuse
Substance abuse

ICD-9CM CODES
303.9 Alcoholism

EPIDEMIOLOGY & DEMOGRAPHICS

INCIDENCE (IN U.S.):

- The clinical history suggests alcohol problems in 15% to 20% of patients in primary care and hospitalized patients. In the U.S. alcohol abuse generates nearly $185 billion in annual economic costs. An estimated 8 million adults in the U.S. have alcohol dependence.
- 20% achieve abstinence without help; 70% achieve sobriety for 1 yr.

PREVALENCE (IN U.S.): 7% of population ≥18 yr

PREDOMINANT SEX:

- Lifetime risk for males 8% to 10%
- Lifetime risk for females 3% to 5%

PEAK INCIDENCE: 20 to 40 yr. The most common age range for initial treatment of alcohol dependence is 35 to 45 yr. However, the peak period for meeting alcohol dependence criteria is ≥10 years earlier.

GENETICS: More common with a family history of alcoholism and in patients of Irish, Scandinavian, and Native American descent

PHYSICAL FINDINGS & CLINICAL PRESENTATION

- Recurring minor trauma
- Gastrointestinal bleeding from gastritis and/or varices
- Pancreatitis (acute and chronic)
- Liver disease
- Odor of alcohol on breath
- Tremulousness
- Tachycardia
- Peripheral neuropathy
- Recent memory loss

ETIOLOGY

- Social and genetic factors important
- Risk factors:
  1. Broken homes
  2. Unemployment
  3. Divorce
  4. Recurrent depression
  5. Addiction to another substance, including tobacco

DIAGNOSIS

WORKUP

- Several screening tests (CAGE, AUDIT, TWEAK, CRAFFT, SMAST) are available. The four-item CAGE (feeling need to Cut down, Annoyed by criticism, Guilty about drinking, and need for an Eye-opener in the morning) is the most popular screening test in primary care. A positive response should lead to further questioning. The sensitivity of the CAGE ranges from 43% to 94% and its specificity ranges from 70% to 97%. The five-item TWEAK scale (Tolerance, Worry, Eye-openers, Amnesia, [K] cut down) and the T-ACE questionnaire (Tolerance, Annoyance, Cut down, Eye-opener) are designed to screen pregnant women for alcohol misuse. They detect lower levels of alcohol consumption that may pose risks during pregnancy. The CRAFFT questionnaire (riding in Car with someone who was drinking, using alcohol to Relax, using alcohol while Alone, Forgetfulness, criticism from Friends and Family, Trouble) is useful as a screening tool for adolescents. Its sensitivity is 92% and specificity 64% for alcohol abuse. Single-question screening about alcohol consumption in a day ("When was the last time you had more than X drinks in a day?" [where X = 5 for men and 4 for women]) with the threshold set at "in the past 3 months" is 85% sensitive and 70% specific in men and 82% and 70% in women for unhealthy alcohol use.
- Blood studies (see later section).

LABORATORY TESTS

- Lab tests alone do not accurately detect alcohol problems but can help identify medical complications related to alcohol use, such as pancreatitis or cirrhosis.
- Gamma-glutamyltransferase (GGTP), generally elevated
- Liver transaminases (alanine aminotransferase [ALT], aspartate aminotransferase [AST]), often elevated, may be normal or low in advanced liver disease
- Low albumin level, hypophosphatemia, hypomagnesemia from malnutrition
- Complete blood count (CBC) reveals elevated mean corpuscular volume from toxic effect of alcohol on erythrocyte development in nutritional deficiencies
- Stool for occult blood may be positive as a result of gastritis or variceal bleeding

IMAGING STUDIES

Indicated only with a history of trauma. CT or ultrasound of abdomen may reveal fatty liver or cirrhosis in advanced stages.

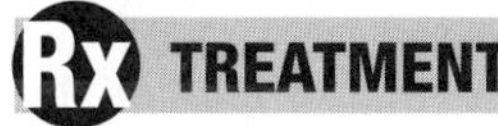

TREATMENT

NONPHARMACOLOGIC THERAPY

- Twelve-step facilitation, cognitive behavioral therapy, and motivational enhancement therapy improve the chances of recovery in patients with alcohol abuse and dependence.
- Depression, if present, should be treated at same time alcohol is withdrawn.

ACUTE GENERAL Rx

Alcohol withdrawal syndrome occurs when a person stops ingesting alcohol after prolonged consumption. It can result in four possible clinical patterns depending on the severity of the patient's alcohol abuse and the time from the patient's previous alcohol ingestion. Blood ethanol level decreases by 20 mg/dl/hr in a normal person. Although discussed separately, these withdrawal states blend together in real life.

1. **Tremulous state** (early alcohol withdrawal, "impending DTs," "shakes," "jitters").
   a. Time interval: usually occurs 6 to 8 hr after the last drink or 12 to 48 hr after reduction of alcohol intake; becomes most pronounced at 24 to 36 hr.
   b. Manifestation: tremors, mild agitation, insomnia, tachycardia; symptoms are relieved by alcohol.
   c. Detoxification can be in the outpatient (ambulatory) or inpatient setting. Candidates for outpatient detoxification should have a reasonable support system (e.g., reliable contact person) who can monitor progress and lack of any significant comorbid conditions (e.g., suicide risk, seizure disorder, coexisting benzodiazepine dependence, prior unsuccessful outpatient detoxification, pregnancy, cirrhosis) or risk factors for severe withdrawal (age >40 yr, drinking >100 g of ethanol daily

[e.g., 1 pint of liquor or eight 12-oz cans of beer, random blood alcohol concentration >200 mg/dl]).

d. Inpatient treatment:
   (1) Admit to medical floor (private room); monitor vital signs q4h; institute seizure precautions; maintain adequate sedation.
   (2) Administer lorazepam as follows:
      (a) Day 1: 2 mg PO q4h while awake and not lethargic.
      (b) Day 2: 1 mg PO q4h while awake and not lethargic.
      (c) Day 3: 0.5 mg PO q4h while awake and not lethargic.
      (d) NOTE: Hold sedation for lethargy or abnormal vital or neurologic signs. The preceding doses are only guidelines; it is best to titrate the dose case by case.
   (3) In patients with mild to moderate withdrawal and without history of seizures, individualized benzodiazepine administration (rather than a fixed-dose regimen) results in lower benzodiazepine administration and avoids unnecessary sedation. The Clinical Institute Withdrawal Assessment-Alcohol (CIWA-A) scale can be used to measure the severity of alcohol withdrawal. It consists of 10 items: nausea; tremor; autonomic hyperactivity; anxiety; agitation; tactile, visual, and auditory disturbances; headache; and disorientation. Each item is assigned a score from 0 to 7. For example, in the "agitation" category 0 indicates normal activity, and 7 indicates that the patient constantly thrashes about. For the category of "tremor," 0 indicates that tremor is not present and 7 tremor is severe, even with arms not extended. The maximum total score is 67. Benzodiazepines are recommended in patients with substantial withdrawal symptoms (CIWA-Ar score >12).
   (4) Beta-adrenergic blockers: beta-blockers are useful for controlling blood pressure and tachyarrhythmias. However, they do not prevent progression to more serious symptoms of withdrawal and, if used, should not be administered alone but in conjunction with benzodiazepines. Beta-blockers should be avoided in patients with contraindications to their use (e.g., bronchospasm, bradycardia, or severe congestive heart failure). Centrally acting alpha-adrenergic agonists such as clonidine ameliorate symptoms in patients with mild to moderate withdrawal but do not reduce delirium or seizures.
   (5) Vitamin replacement: thiamine 100 mg IV or IM for at least 5 days plus oral multivitamins. The IV administration of glucose can precipitate Wernicke's encephalopathy in alcoholics with thiamine deficiency; therefore thiamine administration should precede IV dextrose.
   (6) Hydration PO or IV (high-caloric solution): if IV, glucose with Na^+, K^+, Mg^{2+}, and phosphate replacement prn.
   (7) Laboratory studies.
      (a) CBC, platelet count, INR.
      (b) Electrolytes, glucose, blood urea nitrogen, creatinine.
      (c) GGTP, ALT, AST.
      (d) Phosphorus and magnesium.
      (e) Serum vitamin B_{12} and folic acid (if megaloblastic features in blood smear).
   (8) Diagnostic imaging: generally not necessary; if subdural hematoma is suspected (evidence of trauma, persistent lethargy), a CT scan should be ordered.
   (9) Social rehabilitation: group therapy such as Alcoholics Anonymous; identification and treatment of social and family problems should be initiated during the patient's hospital stay.

2. Alcoholic hallucinosis:
   a. Manifestations: hallucinations usually are auditory, but hallucinations occasionally are visual, tactile, or olfactory; usually there is no clouding of sensorium as in delirium (clinical presentation may be mistaken for an acute schizophrenic episode). Disordered perceptions become most pronounced after 24 to 36 hr of abstinence.
   b. Treatment: same as for DTs (see "withdrawal seizures").
3. Withdrawal seizures ("rum fits"):
   a. Time interval: usually occurs 7 to 30 hr after cessation of drinking, with a peak incidence between 13 and 24 hr.
   b. Manifestations: generalized convulsions with loss of consciousness; focal signs are usually absent; consider further investigation with CT scan of head and electroencephalography if clearly indicated (e.g., presence of focal neurologic deficits, prolonged postictal confusion state). In addition, in a febrile patient who is having a seizure or altered mental state, a lumbar puncture is necessary.
   c. Treatment:
      (1) Diazepam 2.5 mg/min IV until seizure is controlled (check for respiratory depression or hypotension) may be beneficial for prolonged seizure activity; IV lorazepam 1 to 2 mg q2h can be used in place of diazepam. Withdrawal seizures generally are self-limited and treatment is not required; the use of phenytoin or other anticonvulsants for short-term treatment of alcohol withdrawal seizures is not recommended.
      (2) Thiamine 100 mg IV, followed by IV dextrose, should also be administered.
      (3) Electrolyte imbalances (increased Mg^{2+}, decreased K^+, increased or decreased Na^+, decreased PO_4^{-3}) that may exacerbate seizures should be corrected.
4. DTs:
   a. Time interval: variable; usually occurs within 1 wk after reduction or cessation of heavy alcohol intake and persists for 1 to 3 days. Peak incidence is 72 hr and 96 hr after the cessation of alcohol consumption.
   b. Manifestations: profound confusion, tremors, vivid visual and tactile hallucinations, autonomic hyperactivity; this is the most serious clinical presentation of alcohol withdrawal (mortality rate is approximately 15% in untreated patients).
   c. Treatment
      (1) Admission to a detoxification unit where patient can be observed closely.
      (2) Vital signs q30min (neurologic signs, if necessary).
      (3) Use of lateral decubitus or prone position if restraints are necessary
      (4) NPO: nasogastric tube for abdominal distention may be necessary but should not be routinely used.
      (5) Laboratory studies: same as for early alcohol withdrawal.
      (6) Vigorous hydration (4 to 6 L/day): IV with glucose (Na^+, K^+, PO_4^{-3} and Mg^{2+} replacement).
      (7) Vitamins: thiamine 100 mg IV qd. The initial dose of thiamine should precede the administration of IV dextrose; multivitamins (may be added to the hydrating solution).
      (8) Sedation: control of agitation should be achieved with rapid-acting sedative-hypnotic agents in adequate doses to maintain light somnolence for the duration of delirium.
         (a) Initially: lorazepam 2 to 5 mg IM/IV repeated prn.
         (b) Maintenance (individualized dosage): chlordiazepoxide, 50 to 100 mg PO q4-6h, lorazepam 2 mg PO q4h, or diazepam 5 to 10 mg PO tid; withhold doses or decrease subsequent doses if signs of oversedation are apparent.
         (c) Midazolam is also effective for managing DTs. Its rapid onset (sedation within 2 to 4 min of IV injection) and short duration of action (approximately 30 min) make it an ideal agent for titration in continuous infusion.
      (9) Treatment of seizures (as previously described).
      (10) Diagnosis and treatment of concomitant medical, surgical, or psychiatric conditions.

CHRONIC Rx

- See "Referral."
- Pharmacotherapies for alcoholism include:
    - Acamprosate is a synthetic compound with a chemical structure similar to the neurotransmitter gamma-aminobutyric acid and the amino acid neuromodulator taurine. Its mechanism of action is not completely understood. It is indicated for the maintenance of abstinence from alcohol in patients with alcohol dependence who are abstinent at treatment initiation. It should be used only as part of a comprehensive psychosocial treatment program. It does not cause a disulfiram-like reaction as a result of ethanol ingestion. Dose is two 333-mg tablets tid. Treatment should be initiated as soon as possible after the period of alcohol withdrawal, when the patient has achieved abstinence, and should be maintained if the patient relapses.
    - The long-acting opiate antagonist naltrexone inhibits the rewarding effects of alcohol. The starting dose is 25 mg/day, increased to 50 mg PO qd after 1 wk. An extended-release, once-monthly injection of naltrexone is also available and can be used along with psychosocial support to maintain alcohol abstinence. In patients with opioid dependence, naltrexone can precipitate acute withdrawal syndrome and should not be used at least 7 days from last opioid use.
    - Disulfiram (Antabuse). Dosage is 500 mg max qd for 1 to 2 wk, then 125 to 500 mg qd. It interferes with the metabolism of alcohol by inhibiting aldehyde dehydrogenase, causing an accumulation of acetaldehyde. It produces unpleasant symptoms (nausea, flushing, elevated blood pressure, headache, weakness) when alcohol is ingested. It is an older drug that is now rarely used.

DISPOSITION

See "Referral."

REFERRAL

- To Alcoholics Anonymous or Adult Children of Alcoholics
- Family members to Al-Anon or Al-A-Teen
- Many cities have Salvation Army Adult Rehabilitation centers; all patients accepted, regardless of ability to pay

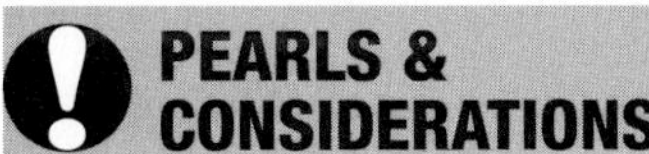

PEARLS & CONSIDERATIONS

COMMENTS

- Relative indications for inpatient alcohol detoxification are as follows: history of DTs or withdrawal seizures, severe withdrawal symptoms, concomitant psychiatric or medical illness, pregnancy, multiple previous detoxifications, recent high levels of alcohol consumption, and lack of reliable support network.
- Detoxification is not a stand-alone treatment but should serve as a bridge to a formal treatment program for alcohol dependence.
- The cure rate for alcoholism is highly disappointing, regardless of the modality. Only those who want to be helped will be helped. An effective strategy for the primary care physician is a prominently displayed sign in the office that states, "If you think you consume too many alcoholic beverages, please discuss it with me." Those who do open up the discussion can be given the facts in a nonjudgmental way and often can be helped. All too often problem drinkers lie on the questionnaire until they face a life-threatening health issue—and even then denial often reigns supreme.
- In a recent clinical trial, patients receiving medical management with naltrexone (100 mg/day), combined behavioral intervention (CBI), or both fared better on drinking outcomes, whereas acamprosate showed no evidence of efficacy, with or without CBI. No combination produced better efficacy than naltrexone or CBI alone in the presence of medical management.

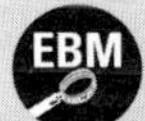

EVIDENCE

Please note: Complete text of EBM for this topic is available online.

Key trials and commentary:

One evidence-based trial sought to determine the time course for onset of effect of intramuscular injectable extended-release naltrexone (XR-NTX), which has demonstrated efficacy for alcohol. XR-NTX 380 mg provided a rapid onset of therapeutic effect in the first 2 days after the first injection that was sustained throughout the 24-week trial. Potential clinical implications of the rapid, early onset of effect of this medication's delivery system for patients who are dependent on alcohol include facilitation of early engagement in treatment, motivation to continue treatment, and focus on the goals established in counseling.

This study finds a rapid onset of effectiveness for depot XR-NTX in reducing heavy drinking, and points to the need for clinicians to use the advances in the pharmacologic treatment of alcoholism and addictions. The National Institute on Alcohol Abuse and Alcoholism recommends that patients with alcoholism be treated with the three FDA-approved medications; yet, only 1% of alcoholics are receiving this treatment. Of the available treatments, XR-NTX has had the best results in studies. Although none of the medications are a panacea in solving the complex psychosocial problem of addiction, they add enough to recovery rates to make their use very worthwhile. The introduction of depot XR-NTX has been a significant advance because of the compliance problem of getting patients motivated to take their medications as prescribed, a major problem for all patients, but especially for the chemically dependent patient. Continued research and drug development in the addiction field is much needed and the pharmaceutical industry, unfortunately, has been reluctant to invest in this area because so far the profits have been meager.[1] Ⓐ

Another study analyzed the effect of naltrexone, ondansetron hydrochloride, or the combination of these medications on cue-induced craving and ventral striatum activation. Consistent with animal data that suggest that both naltrexone and ondansetron reduce alcohol-stimulated dopamine output in the ventral striatum, the current study found evidence that these medications, alone or in combination, could decrease alcohol cue-induced activation of the ventral striatum, consistent with their putative treatment efficacy.

This South Carolina research group has been involved with many of the best treatment outcome studies for pharmacologic treatments of alcoholism. They were also involved with Project Combine, which found better efficacy for naltrexone than acamprosate. Here they find both naltrexone and ondansetron alone or in combination effective in the treatment of alcoholism. Moreover, they are able to measure brain activation effects in the ventral striatum and of cue-induced craving of both drugs and in combination using magnetic resonance imaging. Naltrexone is approved by the Food and Drug Administration (FDA) and is generally available in a generic form, and also in a depot product, whereas ondansetron is experimental, though animal and human studies have been promising, having positive results. Although both drugs have had dramatic results and there have been some negative treatment outcome studies for naltrexone, incremental improvement is of great value to the patient and clinician in helping to treat what is a highly prevalent illness that has enormous social costs. New medications also add to hope and a sense of self-efficacy that can enhance psychotherapy results.[2] Ⓐ

Although disulfiram and naltrexone have been approved by the FDA for the treatment of alcoholism, no medications have been approved for individuals with alcohol dependence and comorbid psychiatric disorders. In particular, the effect of these medications on alcohol use outcomes and on specific psychiatric symptoms is still unknown in patients with the most common co-occurring disorder, major depression. The results of this study suggest that disulfiram and naltrexone are safe pharmacotherapeutic agents for dually diagnosed individuals with depression for the treatment of alcohol use disorders.

Disulfiram and naltrexone have been two of the very few drugs approved by the FDA for the treatment of alcoholism. Currently, there are no medications with FDA approval for patients with alcohol dependence and comorbid psychiatric disorders, despite how frequently they occur.

In this trial, the researchers studied the use of both disulfiram and naltrexone in 139 depressed alcoholic subjects. Of the 254 alcoholic subjects, 54.7% (139) met DSM-IV criteria for major depression. Fascinatingly, they found no relationship between the diagnosis of depression and medication effects on alcohol use outcomes, psychiatric symptoms, or side effects. However, there was a significant interaction between diagnosis and medication and craving. Subjects with depression on disulfiram had lower craving over time than depressed subjects on naltrexone. All these findings are largely new and good news for those of us trying to treat these very difficult patients.[3] Ⓐ

Evidence-Based References

1. Ciraulo DA et al: Early treatment response in alcohol dependence with extended-release naltrexone, *J Clin Psychiatry* 69:190-195, 2008. Commentary by R. Frances, M.D. Ⓐ

2. Myrick H et al: Effect of naltrexone and ondansetron on alcohol cue–induced activation of the ventral striatum in alcohol-dependent people, *Arch Gen Psychiatry* 65:466-475, 2008. Commentary by R. Frances, M.D. Ⓐ

3. Petrakis I, the VA VISN I MIRECC Study Group: Naltrexone and disulfiram in patients with alcohol dependence and current depression, *J Clin Psychopharmacol* 27:160-165, 2007. Commentary by J.C. Ballenger, M.D. Ⓐ

SUGGESTED READINGS

American College of Physicians: Alcohol-use, *Annals of Internal Med: In the Clinic* 3-11, 2009.

Anton RF: Naltrexone for the management of alcohol dependence, *N Engl J Med* 359:715, 2008.

Anton RF et al: Combined pharmacotherapies and behavioral interventions for alcohol dependence, the COMBINE study: a randomized clinical trial, *JAMA* 295:2003, 2006.

Johnson B et al: Topiramate for treating alcohol dependence, a randomized controlled trial, *JAMA* 298(14):1641-1651, 2007.

Moss M, Burnham EL: Alcohol abuse in the critically ill patient, *Lancet* 368:2231, 2006.

Willenbring ML et al: Helping patients who drink too much: an evidence-based guide for primary care physicians, *Am Fam Physician* 80(1):44-50, 2009.

AUTHOR: **FRED F. FERRI, M.D.**

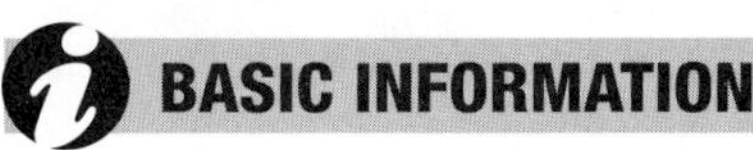

DEFINITION

Alopecia is the term used to describe involuntary hair loss, typically on the scalp or beard, but possibly over the entire body. *Nonscarring alopecia* is hair loss without clinically apparent scarring, inflammation, or skin atrophy. *Scarring alopecia* is characterized by hair loss accompanied by tissue destruction in the form of scarring, inflammation, and/or skin atrophy.

SYNONYMS

Hair loss
Balding

ICD-9CM CODES
704.0 Alopecia
704.01 Alopecia areata
704.02 Telogen effluvium

EPIDEMIOLOGY & DEMOGRAPHICS

INCIDENCE: Depends on etiology, for example:

- Alopecia areata affects 1% of the U.S. population by age 50 yr.
- Androgenetic alopecia affects females less than the male sex but affects up to 40% of women by age 60, increasing after menopause.

GENETICS: Depends on etiology, for example:

- Androgenetic alopecia is autosomal dominant +/− polygenic and can be inherited from one or both parents.
- Certain scarring alopecias are more predominant in people with more coarse hair.

PHYSICAL FINDINGS & CLINICAL PRESENTATION

HISTORY: A careful history must be taken and should include time course for hair loss, the pattern of hair loss, any recent change in life situation/stresses, any associated medical conditions, new medications, any family history of hair loss, and other skin/nail symptoms.

PHYSICAL EXAMINATION:

- General: patient's emotional response to hair loss
- Hair/skin:
  - Hair thinning/loss
  - May have fine, downy hairs also referred to as vellus hairs
  - Skin may show changes consistent with inflammation, infection, and/or atrophy
  - Women may show virilization
  - Exclamation point hairs can be seen in alopecia areata
  - Broken hairs of different length may be seen in traumatic alopecia
  - Hairs that crack or crumble with palpation most often signify shaft damage because of overprocessing

ETIOLOGY

NONSCARRING

- Failure of follicle production
- Hair shaft abnormality
- Pattern hair loss: androgenetic alopecia
- Hair breakage: trichotillomania, traction alopecia, cosmetic overprocessing
- Problem with cycling (excess shedding): telogen effluvium, anagen effluvium, loose anagen syndrome, alopecia areata, syphilis

SCARRING

- Infectious: tinea capitis with inflammation (kerion), bacterial folliculitis as in dissecting folliculitis and folliculitis decalvans
- Neoplasm: alopecia mucinosa in cutaneous T cell lymphoma or alopecia neoplastica caused by metastatic carcinoma (breast cancer)
- Autoimmune: chronic cutaneous lupus erythematosus
- Congenital

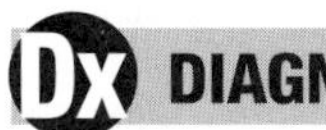

DIFFERENTIAL DIAGNOSIS

1. Nonscarring

- *Telogen effluvium:* This type of alopecia is usually diffuse thinning that follows significant life stress (death of loved one, high fever, severe infection, crash dieting) or change in hormones (postpartum, change or cessation of oral contraceptive pill). Patient often presents with a bag of hair that has fallen out. This is caused by a large number of anagen (growing) hairs entering telogen (dying phase) simultaneously. Telogen effluvium is more common in women.
- *Androgenetic alopecia:* Gradual thinning of hair and a trend toward finer hair, which in men has a typical pattern of receding anterior bitemporal hairline resulting in an M-shaped pattern and in women has a typical pattern of thinning along crown with or without frontotemporal thinning. This type of thinning is due to a combination of genetic predisposition and androgenic conversion of hair follicles into vellus-like follicles.
- *Alopecia areata:* This type of hair loss results in patches of hair loss, typically 2 to 5 cm in diameter, with normal-appearing skin (including presence of follicular openings) at the base, as well as occasional "exclamation point hairs," which are evidence of hair breaking off. Fingernails may show fine pitting. On biopsy, lymphocytes surround the hair bulb "like a swarm of bees," evidence of the autoimmune etiology.

  Alopecia areata universalis (AAU): generalized loss of body hair

  Alopecia areata totalis (AAT): complete loss of scalp hair
- *Tinea:* This type of hair loss is evident in round patches, possibly with scarring, erythema, and lymphadenopathy. This is the more common type of hair loss in children. Diagnosis can be made by scraping the erythematous edge and placing the scraping with KOH under a microscope to check for hyphae. Woods lamp only fluoresces if tinea is caused by *Microsporum* spp.; however, the more common (in the United States) *Trichophyton* spp. does not fluoresce. If a kerion (severe alopecia associated with bogginess) is present, it may cause scarring.
- *Traumatic alopecia:* This type of hair loss is in a pattern consistent with breaking off of hairs because of traction (hair pulling) or chemical agents (hair straightening or permanent). Etiology usually becomes apparent with careful history taking and visualizing the pattern of hair loss.

2. Scarring

- *Lichen planus:* The hair loss associated with lichen planus is typically associated with scaling and atrophy of pruritic, painful skin underlying the hair loss. This hair loss is more common in middle-aged women. Although there are numerous variations in clinical presentation, the general clinical picture is one of a chronic inflammatory condition of the skin, nails, mucous membranes, and/or hair. A classic finding on the scalp is a perifollicular erythema with small keratinous plugs, referred to as hyperkeratosis. The typical skin lesions are flat-topped, violaceous lesions with white lines (Wickham's striae), whereas the typical oral lesions are milky white.
- *Chronic cutaneous (discoid) lupus erythematosus:* This type of hair loss frequently is evident in well-demarcated, erythematous plaques in chronically sun-exposed areas of skin. Lesions exhibit hypopigmentations or hyperpigmentations, atrophy, erythema, and scaling. It may be present concurrently with systemic lupus erythematosus or be the first presenting symptom of systemic lupus erythematosus, but in most cases is a purely cutaneous condition.
- *Tinea with kerion:* A kerion represents an exuberant delayed type hypersensitivity reaction to the tinea capitus, resulting in one (or many) inflamed boggy plaque(s) on the scalp depending on the severity of the infection.

WORKUP

- Hair pull: no shower for 24 hr, scalp with ~60 hairs is gently pulled, <6 hairs pulled is normal and more is suggestive of telogen effluvium, look for telogen bulbs on recovered hairs
- Punch biopsy: send two punches—one for vertical and one for horizontal sectioning—for histopathological analysis preferably by a dermatopathologist

LABORATORY TESTS

Initiate laboratory studies if not clear based on clinical presentation:

- CBC: rule out Fe deficiency
- Total Fe/ferritin: rule out subclinical Fe deficiency
- Thyroid-stimulating hormone (TSH): rule out underlying thyroid disease
- Antinuclear antibody (ANA): screen for autoimmune disease
- Rapid plasma reagin (RPR): rule out cutaneous syphilis if history suggestive of increased risk

Rx TREATMENT

- *Telogen effluvium:* Stop insulting stress/medication and in 3 to 4 mo anagen recurs, and hair density should be normalized by 12 mo. Multiple medications have been shown to be an inciting factor and one should consider stopping them (these include but are not limited to enalapril, colchicine, levodopa, metoprolol, propranolol, oral contraceptives, and lithium). Full regrowth is expected in most cases.
- *Androgenetic alopecia:* For men, the most likely first-line treatment is oral finesteride (type II 5a-reductase inhibitor), which leads to lower levels of dihydrotestosterone. This leads to hair regrowth in about 6 mo, but with cessation, hair returns to pattern of loss within 12 mo. Topical minoxidil can be useful in partially restoring lost hair in both men and women. In women with elevated androgens, antiandrogens such as spironolactone, flutamide, and cimetidine may be considered. Other options include surgical intervention with hair transplantation or hair flaps, or the use of a hairpiece.
- *Alopecia areata:* Spontaneous remission occurs in patchy alopecia areata, but less commonly in AAT or AAU. Glucocorticoids (GCs) are the mainstay of treatment but have little effect on the long-term outcome of hair loss—topical GCs for small patches, intralesional injection of high-potency GCs, and even systemic steroids can all be temporarily effective but at the cost of GC exposure. Under the care of a dermatologist, induction of allergic contact dermatitis using short contact anthralin therapy or squaris acid sensitization can be effective but tends to have significant local discomfort, limiting its use. Topical photochemotherapy has shown some beneficial outcomes with alopecia areata. Photochemotherapy to the entire body is effective ~30% of the time.
- *Tinea capitis:* Oral antifungal agents must be used to effectively treat tinea capitis. Griseofulvin is considered the drug of choice in the United States, and the recommended time course is 6 wk to several months. Other oral agents to consider include terbinafine, itraconazole, fluconazole, or ketoconazole. If there is a kerion (area of boggy, purulent inflammation underlying the area of hair loss), the patient is at increased risk for scarring alopecia because of likely bacterial super infection, and a short course of oral steroids and treatment with an oral antibiotic must be considered.
- *Traumatic alopecia:* First priority is stopping inciting activity/agent, which ideally will lead to gradual resolution of hair loss and hair regrowth.
- *Lichen planus:* Associated hair loss is often permanent; however, for symptomatic control of itching and pain, topical or oral GCs may be considered.
- *Chronic cutaneous discoid erythematosus:* The best prevention is sun protection, with SPF lotion. Treatment options center around the cautious use of topical or intralesional GCs. Hydroxychloroquine and retinoids are also used with caution.

REFERRAL

Dermatology

PATIENT/FAMILY EDUCATION

National Alopecia Areata Foundation: www.naaf.org

SUGGESTED READING

Mounse A, Reed S: Diagnosing and treating hair loss, *Am Fam Phys* 80(4):356, 2009.

AUTHORS: **MARGARET LEKANDER, M.D., AMITY RUBEOR, D.O.,** and **GLADYS TELANG, M.D.**

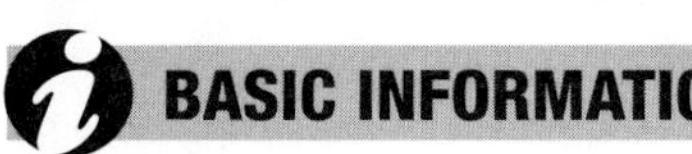

BASIC INFORMATION

DEFINITION

Alpha-1-antitrypsin deficiency is a genetic deficiency of the protease inhibitor alpha-1-antitrypsin that results in a predisposition to pulmonary emphysema and hepatic cirrhosis.

SYNONYMS

AAT

ICD-9CM CODES

277.6 Alpha-1-antitrypsin deficiency

EPIDEMIOLOGY & DEMOGRAPHICS

- Accounts for approximately 2% of chronic obstructive pulmonary disease (COPD) cases in Americans
- Inherited as an autosomal codominant disorder
- Most frequent mutation is in the *SERPINA 1* gene (previously known as *PI* gene)
- Most common alleles are:
  - normal "M" allele (95% frequency in the U.S.)
  - deficient variant "Z" allele (1% to 2%)
  - deficient variant "S" allele (2% to 3%)
- Severe deficiency is most commonly due to homozygotes ZZ
- Risk of COPD is increased with SZ genotype, especially in those who smoke
- Risk of lung disease in heterozygotes (MZ) is uncertain
- One in 10 individuals of European descent carries one of two mutations that may result in partial alpha-1-antitrypsin deficiency

PHYSICAL FINDINGS & CLINICAL PRESENTATION

- Physical findings and clinical presentation are varied and depend on phenotype (see "Etiology")
- Most often affects the lungs but can also involve liver and skin
- Classically associated with early-onset, severe, lower-lobe predominant panacinar emphysema; bronchiectasis may also be seen
- Symptoms are similar to "typical" COPD presentation (dyspnea, cough, sputum production)
- Liver involvement includes neonatal cholestasis, cirrhosis in children and adults, and primary carcinoma of the liver
- Panniculitis is the major dermatologic manifestation

ETIOLOGY

- Degree of alpha-1-antitrypsin deficiency depends on phenotype.
- "MM" represents the normal genotype and is associated with alpha-1-antitrypsin levels in the normal range.
- Mutation most commonly associated with emphysema is Z, with homozygote (ZZ) resulting in approximately 85% deficit in plasma alpha-1-antitrypsin concentrations.
- Development of emphysema is believed to result from an imbalance between the proteolytic enzyme elastase, produced by neutrophils, and alpha-1-antitrypsin, which normally protects lung elastin by inhibiting elastase.
- Deficiency of alpha-1-antitrypsin increases risk of early-onset emphysema, but not all alpha-1-antitrypsin deficient individuals will develop lung disease.
- Smoking increases risk and accelerates onset of COPD.
- Liver disease is caused by pathologic accumulation of alpha-1-antitrypsin in hepatocytes.
- Similar to lung disease, skin involvement is thought to be attributable to unopposed proteolysis in skin.

Dx DIAGNOSIS

DIFFERENTIAL DIAGNOSIS

See "COPD."
See "Cirrhosis."

WORKUP

- Suspicion for alpha-1-antitrypsin deficiency usually results from emphysema developing at an early age and with basilar predominance of disease.
- Suspicion for alpha-1-antitrypsin deficiency resulting in liver disease or skin involvement may arise when other more common etiologies are excluded.

LABORATORY TESTS

- Serum level of alpha-1-antitrypsin can confirm or reject suspicion of deficiency.
- Investigate possibility of abnormal alleles with genotyping.
- Pulmonary function testing is generally consistent with "typical" COPD.

IMAGING STUDIES

- Chest x-ray examination shows characteristic emphysematous changes at lung bases.
- High-resolution chest CT usually confirms the lower-lobe predominant emphysema and may also show significant bronchiectasis.

Rx TREATMENT

NONPHARMACOLOGIC THERAPY

- Avoidance of smoking is paramount.
- Avoidance of other environmental and occupational exposures that may increase risk of COPD.

ACUTE GENERAL Rx

Acute exacerbations of COPD from alpha-1-antitrypsin deficiency are treated in a similar fashion to "typical" COPD exacerbations.

CHRONIC Rx

- The goal of treatment in alpha-1-antitrypsin deficiency is to increase serum alpha-1-antitrypsin levels above a minimum, "protective" threshold.
- Although several therapeutic options are under investigation, IV administration of pooled human alpha-1-antitrypsin is currently the only approved method to raise serum alpha-1-antitrypsin levels. AAT augmentation therapy has been approved by the FDA for patients with AAT deficiency (defined as a protein level <11 micromol/L) who have COPD. Augmentation therapy is expensive ($60,000 to $150,000/year) and requires lifelong treatment.
- Organ transplantation for patients with end-stage lung or liver disease is also an option.

DISPOSITION

- Prognosis of patients with alpha-1-antitrypsin deficiency will depend on phenotype and level of deficiency.
- Among patients with severe alpha-1-antitrypsin deficiency, the most common underlying causes of death are emphysema (72%) and cirrhosis (10%).

REFERRAL

- Referral to specialists with experience in AAT deficiency is preferred
- Pulmonary and hepatology referrals for advanced lung and liver disease, or if replacement therapy is contemplated (e.g., moderate-severe lung disease)
- Lung and liver transplantation in suitable cases

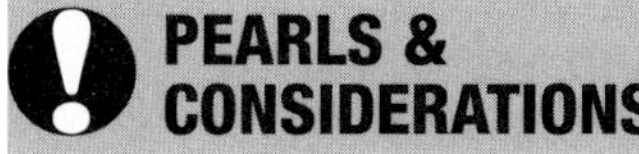

PEARLS & CONSIDERATIONS

- The liver damage arising from the mutation is not from a deficiency in alpha-1-antitrypsin but from a pathologic accumulation of alpha-1-antitrypsin in hepatocytes.
- Consider alpha-1-antitrypsin deficiency in patients presenting with lower-lobe predominant emphysema; in most smokers without alpha-1-antitrypsin deficiency, emphysema predominates in the upper lobes.
- Alpha-1-antitrypsin deficiency is believed to be under-recognized.
- The American Thoracic Society and the European Respiratory Society recommend testing for AAT deficiency in all patients with COPD, emphysema, or asthma with irreversible obstruction, whereas the Global Initiative for Chronic Obstructive Lung Disease only recommends testing for those with early-onset COPD (age <45 years) or a strong family history of COPD.

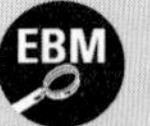

EVIDENCE

There is a lack of randomized trials that have evaluated the use of specific therapies in patients with alpha-1-antitrypsin (AAT) deficiency. The rationale for the use of general measures including management of associated chronic obstructive pulmonary disease (COPD) is based upon their use in those patients with COPD with normal levels of AAT.

However, some statements may be made about therapies specific to those patients with AAT deficiency.

The use of liver transplantation in the treatment of AAT deficiency is supported by expert opinion and by limited data from clinical studies.

Evidence-based professional guidelines from the American Association for the Study of Liver Diseases recommend that liver transplantation is the only effective treatment for decompensated cirrhosis secondary to AAT deficiency. In addition they state that careful assessment for lung disease should be performed before transplantation in patients with cirrhosis secondary to AAT deficiency, although coexistent disease is uncommon.[1] Ⓒ

Follow-up data from patient series of liver transplantation in patients with AAT deficiency has shown that survival is comparable to that found for other liver disease requiring transplantation. In addition, comparison with patients with AAT deficiency and end-stage liver disease prior to the availability of liver transplant shows a significant improvement in survival.[2] Ⓑ

Evidence-Based References

1. Murray KF, Carithers RL Jr: AASLD practice guidelines: evaluation of the patient for liver transplantation, *Hepatology* 41:1407-1432, 2005. Ⓒ

2. Roberts MS et al: Survival after liver transplantation in the United States: a disease-specific analysis of the UNOS database, *Liver Transpl* 10: 886-897, 2004. Ⓑ

SUGGESTED READINGS

American Thoracic Society/European Respiratory Society Statement: Standards for the diagnosis and management of individuals with alpha-1 antitrypsin deficiency, *Am J Respir Crit Care Med* 168:818, 2003.

Hersh CP et al: Chronic obstructive pulmonary disease in alpha1-antitrypsin PI MZ heterozygotes: a meta-analysis, *Thorax* 59(10):843, 2004.

Kohnlgin T, Welte T: Alpha-1-antitrypsin deficiency: pathogenesis, clinical presentation, diagnosis, and treatment, *Am J Med* 121:3-9, 2008.

Silverman EK, Sandhaus RA: Clinical practice: alpha-1-antitrypsin deficiency, *N Engl J Med* 360(26): 2749-2757, 2009.

AUTHOR: **JOSEPH A. DIAZ, M.D.**

BASIC INFORMATION

DEFINITION

Altitude sickness refers to a spectrum of illnesses related to hypoxemia occurring during rapid ascension to high altitudes. Common acute syndromes occurring at high altitudes include acute mountain sickness (AMS), high-altitude pulmonary edema (HAPE), and high-altitude cerebral edema (HACE).

SYNONYMS

Acute mountain sickness
High-altitude pulmonary edema
High-altitude cerebral edema

ICD-9CM CODES
289 Mountain sickness, acute
993.2 High altitude, effects

EPIDEMIOLOGY & DEMOGRAPHICS

- More than 30 million people are at risk of developing altitude sickness.
- AMS is the most common of the altitude diseases.
  - Approximately 40% to 50% of people ascending to 14,000 feet (4200 m) from lowland living develop AMS.
- HAPE generally arises in people who rapidly ascend to 12,000 to 13,000 feet (3600 to 3900 m); however, it has been reported at altitudes as low as 8000 feet.
- Men are five times more likely to develop HAPE than are women.
- AMS and HACE affect men and women equally.

PHYSICAL FINDINGS & CLINICAL PRESENTATION

AMS
- Occurs within hours to a few days after rapid ascent over 8000 ft (2500 m)
- Headache is the most common symptom
- Dizziness and lightheadedness
- Nausea, vomiting, and loss of appetite
- Fatigue
- Sleep disturbance from an exaggerated hyperventilatory phase of Cheyne-Stokes respiration in response to hypoxemia and alkalosis
- AMS can evolve into HAPE and HACE

HAPE (Fig. 1-11)
- Typically occurs 2 to 4 days after ascent over 8000 ft (2500 m).
- Dyspnea
- Dry cough or cough with frothy rust- or pink-tinged sputum
- Chest tightness
- Tachycardia, tachypnea, rales, cyanosis

HACE
- Usually presents several days after AMS
- Confusion, irritability, drowsiness, stupor, hallucinations
- Headache, nausea, vomiting
- Ataxia, paralysis, and seizures
- Coma and death may develop within hours of the first symptoms

ETIOLOGY

- During ascension to altitudes above sea level, the atmospheric pressure decreases. Although the percentage of oxygen in the air remains the same, the partial pressure of oxygen decreases with increased altitude. This can cause hypoxemia.
- The body responds to low oxygen partial pressures through a process of acclimatization (see "Comments").

Dx DIAGNOSIS

Made by clinical presentation and physical findings.

DIFFERENTIAL DIAGNOSIS

- Dehydration
- Carbon monoxide poisoning
- Hypothermia
- Infection
- Substance abuse
- Congestive heart failure
- Pulmonary embolism
- Cerebrovascular accident

WORKUP

Typically the diagnosis is self-evident after history and physical examination. Laboratory tests and imaging studies help monitor cardiopulmonary and central nervous system status in patients admitted to the intensive care unit for pulmonary and/or cerebral edema. In patients with HAPE occurring at lower altitudes (<8000 feet), an evaluation of preexisting pulmonary hypertension or a left-to-right shunt should be considered.

LABORATORY TESTS

Not useful

IMAGING STUDIES

- Chest x-ray examination showing Kerley B-lines and patchy edema (see Fig. 1-11)
- CT scan of the head showing diffuse or patchy edema

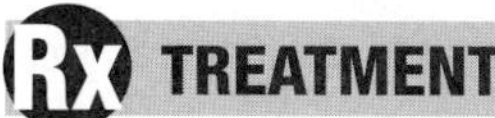

TREATMENT

NONPHARMACOLOGIC THERAPY

- Stop the ascent to allow acclimatization or start to descend until symptoms have resolved.
- Oxygen 4 to 6 L/min is used for severe AMS, HAPE, and HACE.
- Portable hyperbaric bags are useful if available at the site.
- Altitude can cause diuresis that may be mediated by enhanced release of atrial natriuretic peptide. When coupled with the increased fluid loss through increased ventilation, there is a higher risk for dehydration, and adequate hydration should be maintained.

ACUTE PHARMACOLOGIC Rx

- Nonsteroidal antiinflammatory drugs or aspirin is effective in treating headaches in AMS.

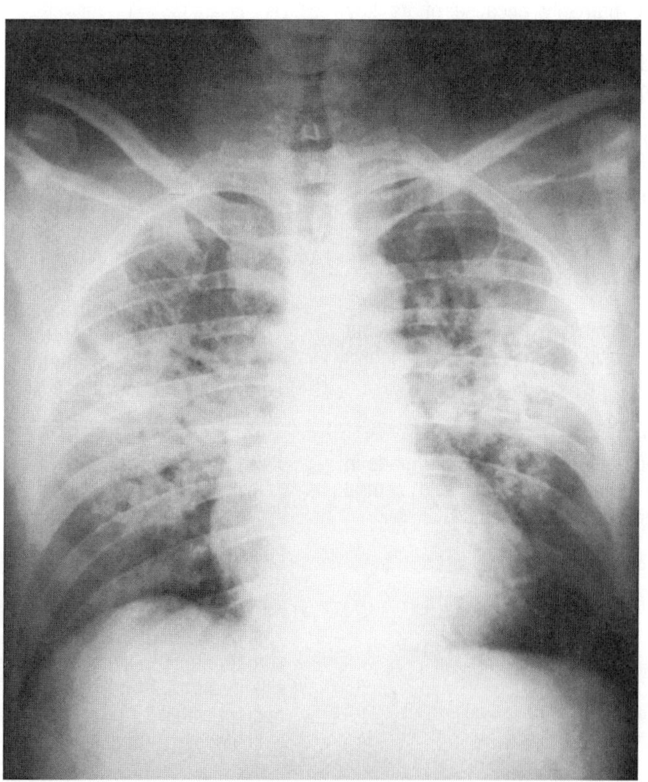

FIGURE 1-11 Chest radiograph showing high-altitude pulmonary edema. (From Strauss RH [ed]: *Sports medicine,* ed 2, Philadelphia, 1991, WB Saunders.)

- Acetazolamide 125 to 250 mg PO bid has been effective for both prevention and acute therapy in patients with AMS and HAPE.
- Nifedipine 10 mg sublingual followed by long-acting nifedipine 30 mg bid is used for patients with HAPE who cannot descend immediately.
- Dexamethasone 4 mg PO every 6 hr is used in patients with severe AMS, HAPE, or HACE.

CHRONIC Rx

Prevention is the most prudent therapy.

1. Slow, staged ascent to avoid altitude sickness.
2. Start the ascent below 8000 feet.
3. Ascend 1000 feet/day (300 m/day).
4. Spend two nights at the same altitude every 3 days.
5. Sleep at lower heights than the altitude climbed ("climb high, sleep low").
6. Prophylactic therapy with acetazolamide up to 750 mg daily and/or dexamethasone 8 to 16 mg daily decreases the risk of developing AMS (combination may have additive benefit). The drugs should be used until acclimatization occurs.
7. Prophylactic inhalation of a β-adrenergic agonist, salmeterol 125 mcg q12h, or the use of slow-release nifedipine 20 mg bid have both been shown to reduce the risk of HAPE in susceptible individuals.
8. Tadalafil, a long-acting phosphodiesterase inhibitor, has recently been shown to decrease the incidence of HAPE in susceptible individuals.
9. The over-the-counter herbal supplement Ginkgo biloba has gained interest in AMS prophylaxis, primarily because of its low adverse effect profile. However, recent randomized clinical trials have failed to show benefit compared with placebo.

DISPOSITION

- AMS improves over a period of 2 to 3 days.
- HAPE is the most common cause of death among patients with altitude illnesses.
- More than 60% of patients with HAPE will have recurrence of symptoms on subsequent climbs.
- Neurologic deficits may persist for weeks but eventually resolve. If coma occurs, prognosis is poor.

REFERRAL

Cardiology and neurology referrals are made in patients with pulmonary edema and central nervous system findings, respectively.

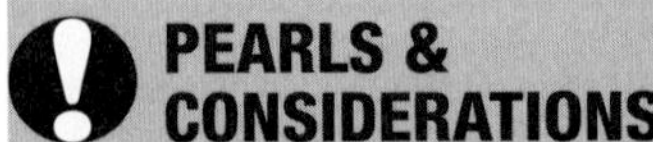

PEARLS & CONSIDERATIONS

COMMENTS

- Acclimatization is the process in which an individual who normally resides at low altitude adapts to hypobaric hypoxia to improve tolerance and performance at higher altitude. These mechanisms include:
  1. An increase in respiratory rates and tidal volume. This hyperventilation allows lowering of arterial carbon dioxide to preserve oxygen delivery, even at extreme altitudes.
  2. An early increase in heart rate and stroke volume to improve oxygen delivery. After 1 wk, both parameters decrease because of diuresis and lower catecholamine levels.
  3. Pulmonary hypertension develops in response to hypoxemia, resulting in improvement of the ventilation-perfusion mismatch but may be maladaptive and lead to the development of HAPE.
  4. Cerebral vasodilation to increase blood flow to the brain.
  5. Rise in hemoglobin and hematocrit. This is a long-term process that takes up to 1 wk to occur in response to the need for improved oxygen delivery.
- Adaptation to altitude is different from acclimatization and refers to physiologic differences in permanent residents at high altitude (e.g., an increased oxygen diffusion capacity).
- Risk factors for the development of altitude sicknesses are:
  1. Rapid ascent
  2. Previous history of altitude sickness
  3. Strenuous exertion on arrival
  4. Obesity
  5. Male gender
- Physical fitness is not protective against high-altitude illness.
- HAPE is characterized by elevated pulmonary pressures, resulting in protein-rich, hemorrhagic exudates into the lung alveoli.
- Both dexamethasone and tadalafil decrease systolic pulmonary artery pressure and may reduce the incidence of HAPE in adults with a history of HAPE. Dexamethasone prophylaxis may also reduce the incidence of AMS in these adults.

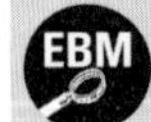

EVIDENCE

Please note: Complete text of EBM for this topic is available online.

Key trials and commentary:

This study sought to determine the impact of sumatriptan prophylaxis on acute mountain sickness (AMS) and altitude headache development within 24 hours of ascent. The results indicate that sumatriptan prophylaxis is effective to prevent AMS development. Furthermore, the findings confirm cerebral vasodilative and edematous mechanisms of AMS progression, whereas sumatriptan is a selective 5-hydroxytryptamine$_1$ receptor subtype agonist and a selective cerebral vasoconstrictor as a result (http://www.controlled-trials.com/ISRCTN87201238/).

Substantial doses of acetazolamide are generally an effective remedy for AMS, but in some patients undesirable side effects develop so that alternative remedies are welcome. This article reports a small, double-blind, controlled trial of sumatriptan, a selective 5-hydroxytryptamine agonist originally developed for the control of migraine. The basis of action is thought to be a vasoconstriction of carotid and middle cerebral vessels.

Several previous authors have found either no benefit or only a transient benefit from this drug when treating an established high-altitude headache. One possible reason why Jafarian and associates were more successful was that they administered the sumatriptan prophylactically, at the time of ascent to an altitude of 3500 m.

The headaches tend to disappear with time at altitude, and if they are prevented from occurring, the transient action of sumatriptan may be a less important criticism. Certainly, further trials comparing sumatriptan prophylaxis with acetazolamide and dexamethasone are warranted. It may also be worth examining the actions of longer-acting triptans. In all of these comparisons, due account needs to be taken of potential cardiovascular side effects from the triptans.[1] Ⓐ

Evidence-Based Reference

1. Jafarian S et al: Sumatriptan for prevention of acute mountain sickness: randomized clinical trial, *Ann Neurol* 62:273-277, 2007. Commentary by R.J. Shephard, M.D., Ph.D., D.P.E. Ⓐ

SUGGESTED READINGS

Basnyat B, Murcoch DR: High-altitude illness, *Lancet* 361:1967, 2003.

Gallagher SA, Hackett PH: High-altitude illness, *Emerg Med Clin North Am* 22:329, 2004.

Hackett P, Rennie D: High altitude pulmonary edema, *JAMA* 287:2275, 2002.

Hachett PH, Roach RC: High-altitude illness, *N Engl J Med* 345:107, 2001.

Maggiorini M et al: Both tadalafil and dexamethasone may reduce the incidence of high-altitude pulmonary edema, *Ann Intern Med* 145:497-506, 2006.

Rodway GW et al: High-altitude related disorders. Part 1. Pathophysiology, differential diagnosis and treatment, *Heart Lung* 32:353, 2003.

West JB: The physiologic basis of high-altitude diseases, *Ann Intern Med* 141:789, 2004.

AUTHORS: **RICHARD REGNANTE, M.D.,** and **PAUL GORDON, M.D.**

BASIC INFORMATION

DEFINITION

Dementia is a syndrome characterized by progressive loss of previously acquired cognitive skills including memory, language, insight, and judgment. Alzheimer's disease (AD) is believed to account for the majority (50% to 75%) of all cases of dementia.

ICD-9CM CODES
331.0 Alzheimer's disease
290.0 Senile dementia, uncomplicated

EPIDEMIOLOGY & DEMOGRAPHICS

INCIDENCE: Risk doubles every 5 yr after the age of 65; above the age of 85 the incidence is about 8%.
PREVALENCE: Currently an estimated 4 million Americans have AD; 7% between the ages of 65 and 74, 53% between 75 and 84, and 40% 85 years and older.
PREDOMINANT SEX: Female

PHYSICAL FINDINGS & CLINICAL PRESENTATION

- Spouse or other family member, usually not the patient, notes insidious memory impairment.
- Patients have difficulties learning and retaining new information and handling complex tasks (e.g., balancing the checkbook), and have impairments in reasoning, judgment, spatial ability, and orientation (e.g., difficulty driving, getting lost away from home).
- Behavioral changes, such as mood changes and apathy, may accompany memory impairment. In later stages patients may develop agitation and psychosis.
- Atypical presentations include early and severe behavioral changes, focal findings on examination, parkinsonism, hallucinations, falls, or onset of symptoms younger than the age of 65.

Dx DIAGNOSIS

There is no definitive imaging or laboratory test for the diagnosis of Alzheimer's disease; rather, diagnosis is dependent on clinical history, a thorough physical and neurologic examination, and use of reliable and valid diagnostic criteria (i.e., DSM-IV or NINDCS-ADRDA) such as the following:

- Loss of memory and one or more additional cognitive abilities (aphasia, apraxia, agnosia, or other disturbance in executive functioning)
- Impairment in social or occupational functioning that represents a decline from a previous level of functioning and results in significant disability
- Deficits that do not occur exclusively during the course of delirium
- Insidious onset and gradual progression of symptoms
- Cognitive loss documented by neuropsychologic tests
- No physical signs, neuroimaging, or laboratory evidence of other diseases that can cause dementia (i.e., metabolic abnormalities, medication or toxin effects, infection, stroke, Parkinson's disease, subdural hematoma, or tumors)

Patients with isolated memory loss who lack functional impairment at home or work do not meet criteria for dementia but may have a mild cognitive impairment (MCI). Identifying patients with MCI is important because patients with MCI may have a slightly higher rate of progression to dementia.

DIFFERENTIAL DIAGNOSIS

- Cancer (brain tumor, meningeal neoplasia)
- Infection (AIDS, neurosyphilis, PML)
- Toxic/metabolic (EtOH, hypothyroidism, B_{12} deficiency, mercury exposure, drug effects)
- Organ failure (dialysis dementia, Wilson's disease)
- Vascular disorder (multiple strokes, severe small vessel changes, chronic vasculitides, or chronic subdural hematoma)
- Depression (pseudodementia)

WORKUP

HISTORY & GENERAL PHYSICAL EXAMINATION:

- Medication lists should always be reviewed for drugs or home remedies that may cause mental status changes.
- Patients should be screened for depression, because it can sometimes mimic dementia but also often occurs as a coexisting condition and should be treated.
- On examination, look for signs of metabolic disturbance, presence of psychiatric features, or focal neurologic deficits.

MENTAL STATUS TESTING:
Brief mental status testing can be done easily and quickly in the office. Most commonly used is the Folstein Mini-Mental Status Examination (MMSE). The MMSE is widely available in many reference books and on the Internet. An MMSE score <24 (scores range from 0 to 30, with lower scores reflecting poorer performance) suggests cognitive impairment; however, the MMSE is not sensitive enough to detect mild dementia or dementia in patients with high baseline IQ. Scores may be spuriously low in patients with limited education, poor motor function, African American or Hispanic ethnicity, poor language skills, or impaired vision. The MMSE is perhaps most useful to follow AD patients for long-term outcomes.

Mental status testing should include tests that assess the following cognitive functions:

- *Orientation:* ask the patient to give the day, date, month, year, and place, and to name the current president.
- *Attention:* ask the patient to recite the months of the year forward and in reverse.
- *Verbal recall:* ask the patient to remember four items; test for recall after a 1- and 5-min delay.
- *Language:* ask the patient to write and then read a sentence; have the patient name both common and less common objects.
- *Visual-spatial:* ask the patient to draw a clock and to set the hands of the clock at 11:10.

Patients with AD typically have trouble with verbal recall, plus visual-spatial or language deficits. Attention is usually preserved until the late stages of AD, so consider alternate diagnoses in patients who perform poorly on tests of attention.

LABORATORY TESTS

- CBC
- Serum electrolytes
- Glucose
- BUN/creatinine
- Liver and thyroid function tests
- Serum vitamin B_{12}
- Syphilis serology (RPR)
- HIV screening as appropriate
- Lumbar puncture if history or signs of cancer, infectious process, or when the clinical presentation is unusual (i.e., rapid progression of symptoms)
- EEG if there is history of seizures, episodic confusion, rapid clinical decline, or suspicion of Creutzfeldt-Jakob disease
- Measurement of apolipoprotein E genotyping, CSF tau and amyloid, and functional imaging including positron emission tomography (PET) or scanning proton emission computed tomography (SPECT) are not routinely indicated
- Brain biopsy (usually reserved for diagnoses such as prion disease, certain vasculitides)

IMAGING STUDIES

CT scan or MRI to rule out hydrocephalus and mass lesions, including subdural hematoma

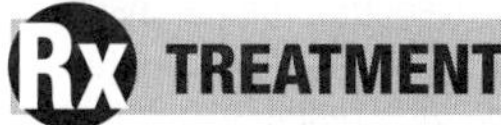

Rx TREATMENT

NONPHARMACOLOGIC THERAPY

- Patient safety, including risks associated with impaired driving, wandering behavior, leaving stoves unattended, and accidents, must be addressed with the patient and family early and appropriate measures implemented.
- Wandering, hoarding or hiding objects, repetitive questioning, withdrawal, and social inappropriateness often respond to behavioral therapies.

ACUTE GENERAL Rx

None

CHRONIC Rx

1. Symptomatic treatment of memory disturbance (Table 1-2):
   a. Cholinesterase inhibitors (ChEI):
      FDA approved for the treatment of mild to moderate AD. Common side effects include nausea, diarrhea, and anorexia and may be bothersome enough to require a slower escalation of dosage, or switching to another agent.
   b. NMDA receptor antagonist: Memantine (Namenda)
      FDA approved for the treatment of moderate to severe AD. Common side effects include constipation, dizziness, or headache. Memantine is contraindicated in patients with renal insufficiency or history of seizures.

2. Symptomatic treatment of neuropsychiatric and behavioral disturbances (Table 1-3): Depression, agitation, delusions, or hallucinations may respond to medications.

DISPOSITION & REFERRAL

- Patients with complex or atypical presentations or challenging management issues should be referred to a neurologist or another specialist with expertise in dementia.
- Family education and support may help reduce need for skilled nursing facility, and reduce caregiver stress, depression, and burnout.

PEARLS & CONSIDERATIONS

The physician should make a thorough search for the treatable causes of dementia. Current American Academy of Neurology practice parameters recommend:

- Treat cognitive symptoms of AD with cholinesterase inhibitors.
- Treat agitation, psychosis, and depression.
- Encourage caregivers to participate in educational programs and support groups.

COMMENTS

The APOE genotype provides information on the risk for AD, but the genotyping of patients raises ethical and emotional concerns. Because the benefits of genetic testing are often modest, and the tests themselves often imprecise in identifying risk, the test is generally discouraged. Recent trials, however, reveal that the disclosure of APOE genotyping results to adult children of patients with AD did not result in significant short-term psychological risks. Test-related distress was reduced among those who learned that they were APOE4 negative. Persons with high levels of emotional distress before undergoing genetic testing are more likely to have emotional difficulties after disclosure.

For additional information for patients, families, and clinicians, contact the following organizations:

- Alzheimer's Association (www.alz.org; 800-272-3900)
- Alzheimer's Disease Education and Referral Center (http://www.nia.nih.gov/Alzheimers; 800-438-4380)

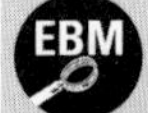

EVIDENCE

Please note: Complete text of EBM for this topic is available online.

Key trials and commentary:

One randomized trial attempted to identify putative genetic loci related to the risk of late-onset Alzheimer's disease (LOAD). It revealed that several additional loci may harbor genetic variants associated with LOAD. This data set provides a wealth of phenotypic and genotypic information for use as a resource in discovery and confirmatory research.

This is a very important study that highlights the complexity of genetics in Alzheimer's disease. It is highly likely that additional loci will be identified in the future.[1] Ⓐ

Evidence of a relation between use of lipid-lowering drugs and cognitive outcomes is mixed. Another study aimed to test the association between use of statins and incidence of dementia and cognitive impairment without dementia (CIND) over 5 years of follow-up. It revealed that statin users were less likely to have incident dementia/cognitive impairment without dementia during a 5-year follow-up. These results add to the emerging evidence suggesting a protective effect of statin use on cognitive outcomes.

There is real concern now about metabolic-related side effects during the long-term pharmacotherapy in schizophrenia. As a result, clinicians are now increasingly prescribing statins. Therefore, this may be a particularly interesting reanalysis study, which suggests that people at high risk for dementia who were prescribed cholesterol-lowering statin agents were half as likely to go on to develop dementia as those people who did not receive statins. The original longitudinal study was funded in 1997 to look at metabolic and vascular conditions such as hypertension and diabetes and their effect on the risk of dementia and Alzheimer's disease. For instance, they found that people with type 2 diabetes are up to 3 times more likely to develop Alzheimer's disease. In this study of 1674 participants who were free of dementia at the start of the study, 27% (452 people) took statins at some point in the study. Over the 5-year follow-up period, 130 participants developed dementia or cognitive impairment. The study is provocative because it suggests that if a patient takes statins over a course of about 5 to 7 years, the risk of dementia might be reduced to half. Also, while statins lowered the dementia risk in the study population, this effect was most pronounced in the patient group at high risk due to metabolic syndrome. The study also took into account potentially confounding variables such as education, smoking status, the presence of an APOE allele, and history of stroke or diabetes. How this effect might occur is unclear. Nevertheless, this is a provocative study.[2] Ⓐ

Evidence-Based References

1. Lee JH et al: Analyses of the National Institute on Aging Late-Onset Alzheimer's Disease Family Study: implication of additional loci, *Arch Neur* 65:1518-1526, 2008. Commentary by D. Drubach, M.D. Ⓐ
2. Cramer C et al: Use of statins and incidence of dementia and cognitive impairment without dementia in a cohort study, *Neurology* 71:344-350, 2008. Commentary by P. Buckley, M.D. Ⓐ

TABLE 1-2 Symptomatic Treatment of Memory Disturbance

	Initial Dose	Target Dose
Donepezil (Aricept)	5 mg qd for 4-6 weeks	10 mg qd
Rivastigmine (Exelon)	1.5 mg bid with food, increase by 1.5 mg bid weekly	3 to 6 mg bid
Galantamine (Reminyl)	4 mg bid with food, increase by 4 mg bid every 4 weeks	8 to 12 mg bid
Memantine (Namenda)	5 mg qd, increase by 5 mg weekly	10 mg bid

TABLE 1-3 Treatment of Behavioral and Neuropsychiatric Symptoms

	Initial Dose	Maximum Dose
Atypical antipsychotics		
Olanzapine (Zyprexa)	2.5 mg qd to bid, may increase by 2.5 mg as needed	7.5 mg bid
Quetiapine (Seroquel)	25 mg bid, may increase by 25 mg every 2 days	250 mg tid
Antidepressants		
Sertraline (Zoloft)	25-50 mg qd, may increase by 25 mg every week	200 mg qd
Citalopram (Celexa)	10 mg qd, may increase after 1 week	20 mg qd

SUGGESTED READINGS

Cummings, JL: Alzheimer's disease, *N Engl J Med* 351:56, 2004.

DeKosky ST et al: Ginkgo-biloba for prevention of dementia, *JAMA* 300(19):2253-2262, 2009.

Doody RS et al: Management of dementia (an evidence-based review): report of the Quality Standards Subcommittee of the American Academy of Neurology, *Neurology* 56:1154, 2001.

DSM-IV: Diagnostic and Statistical Manual of Mental Disorders, ed 4, Washington, DC, 1994, American Psychiatric Association.

Folstein MF et al: "Mini-mental state": a practical method for grading the cognitive state of patients for the clinician, *J Psychiatr Res* 12:189, 1975.

Green RC et al: Disclosure of APOE genotype for risk of Alzheimer's disease, *N Engl J Med* 361:245-254, 2009.

Kawas CH: Early Alzheimer's disease, *N Engl J Med* 349(11):1056, 2003.

Mattsson N et al: CSF biomarkers and insipient Alzheimer's disease in patients with mild cognitive impairment, *JAMA* 302(4):385-393, 2009.

AUTHOR: **TAMARA G. FONG, M.D., PH.D.**

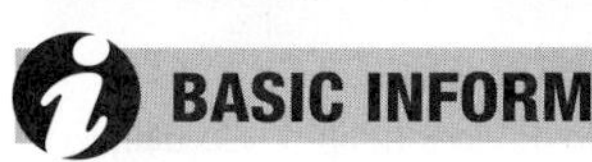

BASIC INFORMATION

DEFINITION

Amaurosis fugax (AF) is a temporary loss of monocular vision caused by transient retinal ischemia.

ICD-9CM CODES
362.34 Amaurosis fugax

EPIDEMIOLOGY & DEMOGRAPHICS

INCIDENCE (IN U.S.): An uncommon but important presentation of carotid artery disease
PEAK INCIDENCE: ≥55 yr

PHYSICAL FINDINGS & CLINICAL PRESENTATION

- Onset is sudden, typically lasting seconds to minutes, and often accompanied by scotomas such as a shade or curtain being pulled over the front of the eye (usually downward).
- Vision loss can be complete or quadrantic.
- Acute stage: cholesterol emboli may be seen in retinal artery (Hollenhorst plaque): carotid bruits or other evidence of generalized atherosclerosis.
- If embolus is cardiac in origin, atrial fibrillation is often present.

ETIOLOGY

- Usually embolic from the internal carotid artery or the heart
- May also be caused by vasculitis, such as giant cell arteritis (GCA), or hyperviscosity syndromes, such as sickle cell disease, that cause ischemia in the vascular territory of the ophthalmic artery

Dx DIAGNOSIS

DIFFERENTIAL DIAGNOSIS

- Retinal migraine: in contrast to amaurosis, the onset of visual loss develops more slowly, usually over 15 to 20 min.
- Transient visual obscurations occur in the setting of papilledema; intermittent rises in intracranial pressure briefly compromise optic disc perfusion and cause transient visual loss lasting 1 to 2 seconds. The episodes may be binocular. If the visual loss persists at the time of evaluation (i.e., vision has not yet recovered), then the differential diagnosis should be broadened to include:
  - Anterior ischemic optic neuropathy: arteritic (classically GCA) or nonarteritic
  - Central retinal vein occlusion

WORKUP

- Workup should focus on embolic sources, but GCA should always be considered.
- Careful examination of retina; embolus may be visible and confirm the diagnosis (Fig. 1-12).
- Auscultation of arteries for carotid bruits.
- Examination of all pulses and for temporal artery tenderness.
- Inquire about symptoms of GCA (scalp tenderness, jaw claudication).
- Examine for signs of hemispheric stroke resulting from intracranial aneurysm (contralateral limb and facial weakness or sensory loss, aphasia, etc.).

LABORATORY TESTS

- Complete blood count with erythrocyte sedimentation rate and C-reactive protein.
- Serum chemistries, including lipid profile.
- ECG and possibly cycling cardiac enzymes.
- Hypercoagulable workup is discretionary based on younger age and history.

IMAGING STUDIES

- Carotid Doppler imaging followed by MR or CT angiography as indicated.
- Transthoracic echocardiography is indicated to screen for embolization in patients with evidence of heart disease and in patients without an evident source for transient neurologic deficit. Transesophageal echocardiography is more sensitive for detecting cardiac sources of embolization (ventricular mural thrombus, atrial appendage, patent foramen ovale, aortic arch).
- Consider MRI of the brain with diffusion-weighted imaging to look for infarcts.

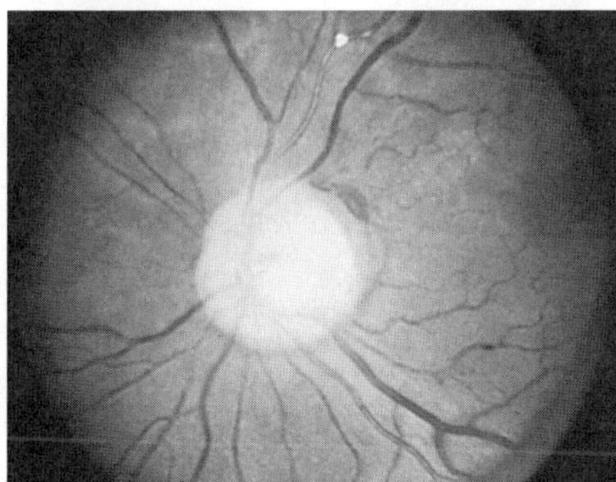

FIGURE 1-12 A cholesterol crystal embolus lodged at an arterial bifurcation. (From Stein JH [ed]: *Internal medicine,* ed 5, St Louis, 1998, Mosby.)

Rx TREATMENT

NONPHARMACOLOGIC THERAPY

- Diet (decrease saturated fatty acids and high-cholesterol foods)
- Exercise
- Cessation of tobacco use

ACUTE GENERAL Rx

- Investigate as an emergency.
- Give aspirin if etiology is presumed embolic.
- If GCA is suspected, start prednisone and refer for temporal artery biopsy within 48 hr (see Giant Cell Arteritis in Section I).

CHRONIC Rx

- Reduce risks by carotid endarterectomy if stenosis >70%. Stenting may be performed in high-risk surgical candidates.
- Control hypertension and manage vascular risk factors.
- Antiplatelet therapy.
- Consider starting an HMG-CoA reductase inhibitor.

DISPOSITION

Among patients with >50% carotid stenosis who do not undergo carotid endarterectomy, those who present with transient monocular blindness have an approximate 10% risk of stroke in 3 yr compared with an approximate 20% risk in patients who present with a hemispheric transient ischemic attack (TIA).

REFERRAL

- Recommend referral to a neurologist for an evaluation and workup.
- If significant carotid stenosis, consider carotid endarterectomy or carotid stenting for the following:
  1. High-grade (≥70%) stenosis
  2. Multiple TIAs despite medical therapy in the setting of high-grade or ulcerative disease

PEARLS & CONSIDERATIONS

- Cholesterol emboli in retinal arteries on funduscopy confirm the diagnosis.
- Recognize that transient visual loss has multiple other causes.

SUGGESTED READING

Murtha T, Stasheff SF: Visual dysfunction in retinal and optic nerve disease, *Neurol Clin* 21:445, 2003.

AUTHOR: **SEAN I. SAVITZ, M.D.**

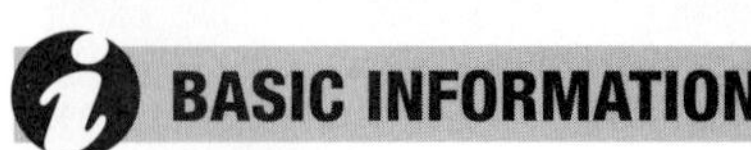

BASIC INFORMATION

DEFINITION

Amblyopia refers to a decrease in vision in one or both eyes in the presence of an otherwise normal ophthalmologic examination.

SYNONYMS

Deprivation amblyopia
Occlusion amblyopia
Strabismus amblyopia
Refractive amblyopia
Organic or toxic amblyopias
Lazy eye

ICD-9CM CODES

368.00 Amblyopia

EPIDEMIOLOGY & DEMOGRAPHICS

INCIDENCE (IN U.S.): 1% to 4% of the general population
PREVALENCE (IN U.S.): High incidence in premature infants with drug-dependent mothers and in neurologically impaired children
PREDOMINANT SEX: None
PREDOMINANT AGE: Childhood
PEAK INCIDENCE: Childhood

PHYSICAL FINDINGS & CLINICAL PRESENTATION

Decreased vision using best refraction in the presence of normal corneal, lens, retinal, and optic nerve appearance (Fig. 1-13)

ETIOLOGY

- Visual deprivation
- Strabismus
- Occlusion with patching
- Refractive error organic lesions in the nervous system
- Toxins

Dx DIAGNOSIS

DIFFERENTIAL DIAGNOSIS

- Central nervous system (CNS) disease (brainstem)
- Optic nerve disorders
- Corneal or other eye diseases
- Retinal disorders

WORKUP

- Complete eye examination to find cause of amblyopia or deprivation of vision. Referral to an ophthalmologist is recommended for any child with a visual acuity in either eye of ≤20/40 at age 3 to 5 yr or worse at age ≥6 yr or a two-line difference in acuity between eyes.
- Motility evaluation.

LABORATORY TESTS

Usually none

IMAGING STUDIES

Usually not necessary unless central nervous system (CNS) lesion suspected

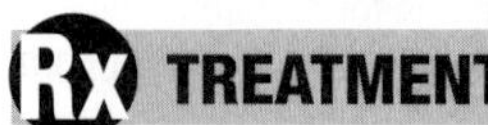

Rx TREATMENT

NONPHARMACOLOGIC THERAPY

- Glasses or prisms to align eyes with minor deviations and improve vision.
- Patches, mechanical versus atropine: patching and atropine both work. Atropine 1% is used daily for 6 mo; patching is used 6 hr/day for 6 mo. Patching may be more effective; 50% get best vision improvement by 16 wk.
- Removal of the cause of the amblyopia if possible.
- Surgery to align the eyes or remove obstruction to vision.

CHRONIC Rx

Patching or optics, including prisms and atropine, most effective in 3- to 7-yr-olds only; minimal or no help after 7 yr

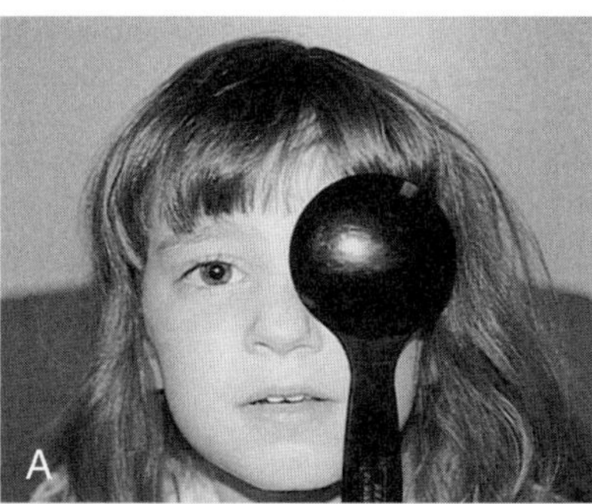

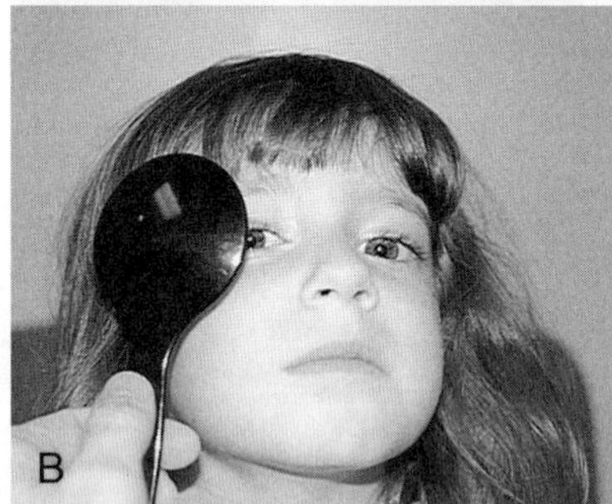

FIGURE 1-13 **A,** This child happily fixes with her right eye and does not object if the left eye is covered. **B,** When the right eye is covered she moves her head away and tries to remove the cover, demonstrating a fixation preference for the right eye and amblyopia of the left eye. (From Hoekelman R [ed]: *Primary pediatric care,* ed 3, St Louis, 1997, Mosby.)

DISPOSITION

Immediate patching, alternating eyes daily

REFERRAL

To ophthalmologist if vision is compromised

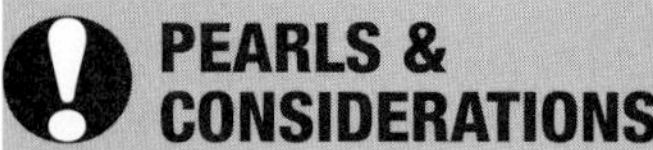

PEARLS & CONSIDERATIONS

COMMENTS

- The earlier the referral, the better the outcome.
- The success of therapy is highly dependent on treatment compliance.
- Amblyopia causes unilateral vision loss in 2% to 4% of the population.

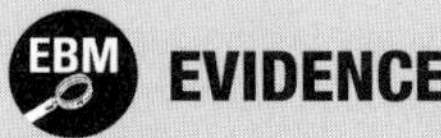

EVIDENCE

A randomized, controlled trial assessed whether full treatment with glasses and patching, compared with glasses only or no treatment, was effective in 177 children aged 3 to 5 yr with mild to moderate unilateral impairment of acuity (6/9 to 6/36) detected by screening. Effects of treatment depended on initial acuity: full treatment showed a substantial effect in moderate acuity (6/36 to 6/18 at recruitment) and no significant effect in mild acuity (6/9 to 6/12 at recruitment). Children in the treatment groups had better visual acuity at follow-up than those in the no treatment group.[1] Ⓑ

A randomized, controlled trial compared atropine sulfate eye drops with patching in the treatment of moderate amblyopia in children younger than 7 yr. Both therapies were equally effective in improving visual acuity after 6 mo of treatment.[2] Ⓑ

Evidence-Based References

1. Clarke MP et al: Randomized controlled trial of treatment of unilateral visual impairment detected at preschool vision screening, *BMJ* 327:1251, 2003. Ⓑ
2. Pediatric Eye Disease Investigator Group: A randomized trial of atropine vs. patching for treatment of moderate amblyopia in children, *Arch Ophthalmol* 120:268, 2002. Ⓑ

SUGGESTED READING

Doshi NR, Rodriguez ML: Amblyopia, *Am Fam Physician* 75:361, 2007.

AUTHOR: **MELVYN KOBY, M.D.**

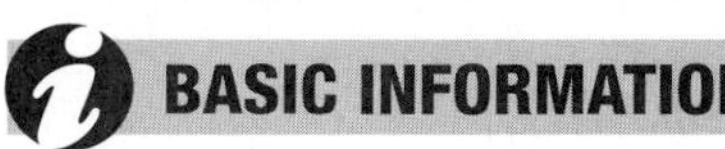

BASIC INFORMATION

DEFINITION

Amebiasis is an infection caused by the protozoal parasite *Entamoeba histolytica.* Although primarily an infection of the colon, amebiasis may cause extraintestinal disease, particularly liver abscess.

SYNONYMS

Amebic dysentery (when severe intestinal infection)

ICD-9CM CODES
006.9 Amebiasis

EPIDEMIOLOGY & DEMOGRAPHICS

INCIDENCE (IN U.S.): Highest in institutionalized patients, sexually active homosexual men

PREVALENCE (IN U.S.): 4% (80% of infections asymptomatic)

PREDOMINANT SEX:
- Equal sex distribution in general
- Striking male predominance of liver abscess

PREDOMINANT AGE: Second through sixth decades

PEAK INCIDENCE: Peaks at age 2 to 3 yr and >40 yr

GENETICS: Infection more likely to be fulminant in young infants

PHYSICAL FINDINGS & CLINICAL PRESENTATION

- Often nonspecific
- Approximately 20% of cases symptomatic
  1. Diarrhea, which may be bloody
  2. Abdominal and back pain
- Abdominal tenderness in 83% of severe cases
- Fever in 38% of severe cases
- Hepatomegaly, RUQ tenderness, and fever in almost all patients with liver abscess (may be absent in fulminant cases)

ETIOLOGY

- Caused by the protozoal parasite *E. histolytica* (Fig. 1-14)
- Transmission by the fecal-oral route
- Infection usually localized to the large bowel, particularly the cecum where a localized mass lesion (ameboma) may form
- Extraintestinal infection in which the organism invades the bowel mucosa and gains access to the portal circulation

Dx DIAGNOSIS

DIFFERENTIAL DIAGNOSIS

- Severe intestinal infection possibly confused with ulcerative colitis or other infectious enterocolitis syndromes, such as those caused by *Shigella, Salmonella, Campylobacter,* or invasive *Escherichia coli*
- In elderly patients: ischemic bowel possibly producing a similar picture

WORKUP

- Three stool specimens over a period of 7 to 10 days to exclude the diagnosis (sensitivity 50% to 80%)
- Concentration and staining the specimen with Lugol's iodine or methylene blue to increase the diagnostic yield
- Available culture (rarely necessary in routine cases)

LABORATORY TESTS

- Stool examination is generally reliable.
- Mucosal biopsy is occasionally necessary.
- Serum antibody may be detected and is particularly sensitive and specific for extraintestinal infection or severe intestinal disease.
- Aspiration of abscess fluid is used to distinguish amebic from bacterial abscesses.

IMAGING STUDIES

Abdominal imaging studies (sonography or CT scan) to diagnose liver abscess

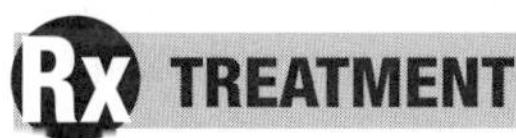

TREATMENT

ACUTE GENERAL Rx

- Metronidazole (750 mg PO tid for 10 days) is used in the treatment of mild to severe intestinal infection and amebic liver abscess; it may be administered intravenously when necessary.
- Follow with iodoquinol (650 mg PO tid for 20 days) to eradicate persistent cysts.
- For asymptomatic patients with amebic cysts on stool examination, use iodoquinol or paromomycin (500 mg PO tid for 7 days).
- Avoid antiperistaltic agents in severe intestinal infections to avoid risk of toxic megacolon.
- Liver abscess is generally responsive to medical management but surgical intervention indicated for extension of liver abscess into pericardium or for toxic megacolon.

DISPOSITION

Host immunity incomplete and reinfection rate high for patients remaining at risk

REFERRAL

- For consultation with infectious diseases specialist for extraintestinal infection or persistent or relapsing intestinal infection
- For surgical consultation:
  1. For toxic megacolon
  2. For impending rupture of or extension of liver abscess into adjacent structures

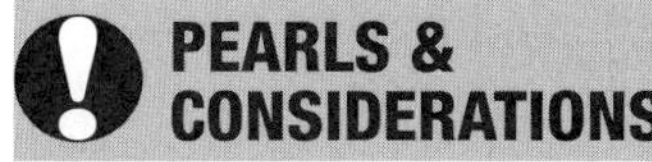

PEARLS & CONSIDERATIONS

COMMENTS

Infection with other intestinal parasites, particularly *Giardia lamblia,* may coexist with amebiasis.

SUGGESTED READINGS

Haque R et al: Entamoeba histolytica infection in children and protection from subsequent amebiasis, *Infect Immun* 74(2):904, 2006.

Pritt BS, Clark CG: Amebiasis, *Mayo Clinic Proc* 83(10): 1159-1160, 2008.

AUTHORS: **GLENN G. FORT, M.D., M.P.H.,** and **DENNIS J. MIKOLICH, M.D.**

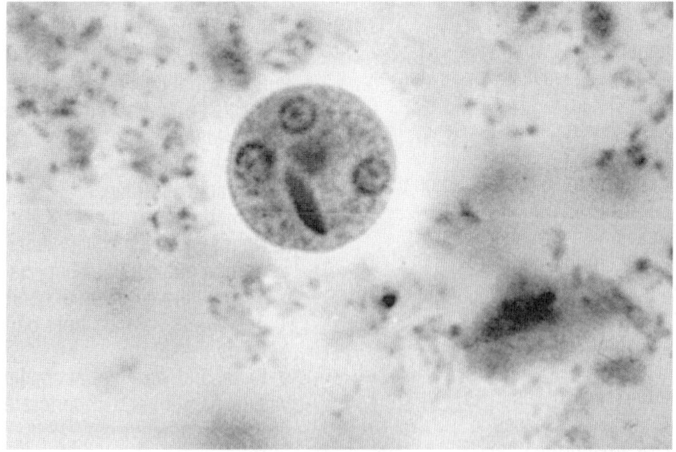

FIGURE 1-14 Mature cyst of *Entamoeba histolytica.* Three of the four nuclei are seen in the plane of focus of this photomicrograph. (From Mandell GL [ed]: *Mandell, Douglas, and Bennett's principles and practice of infectious diseases,* ed 5, New York, 2000, Churchill Livingstone.)

Amenorrhea

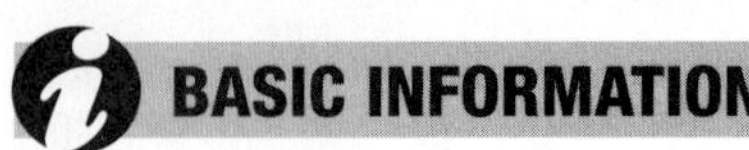

BASIC INFORMATION

DESCRIPTION

Amenorrhea means absence of menstruation. It is classified as either primary or secondary depending on its occurrence before and after menarche, respectively.

- Primary amenorrhea is defined as the absence of menses by age 16 in the presence of secondary sexual characteristics. However, in the absence of these secondary sexual features by the age of 13 to 14 years, one should begin the workup for primary amenorrhea.
- Secondary amenorrhea is the absence of menses for more than three cycles or six months.

ICD-9CM CODES
626.0 Absence of menstruation

EPIDEMIOLOGY & DEMOGRAPHICS

- Incidence of primary amenorrhea and secondary amenorrhea in the U.S. is $<1\%$ and 5% to 7%, respectively.
- It has no racial or ethnic predilection.

ETIOLOGY

- Physiologic amenorrhea
  1. Pregnancy
  2. Lactation
  3. Menopause
- Pathologic amenorrhea
  A. Primary amenorrhea
    1. Hypergonadotropic hypogonadism (frequency: 43%)
      a. Turner syndrome (27%)
      b. Pure gonadal dysgenesis
      c. Autoimmune oophoritis
      d. 17, 20-desmolase deficiency or 17-hydroxylase deficiency
      e. Galactosemia
    2. Eugonadism (30%)
      a. Müllerian agnesis (15%)
      b. Vaginal septum (3%)
      c. Imperforate hymen (1%)
      d. Androgen insensitivity syndrome (AIS) (1%)
      e. 5-alpha reductase deficiency
      f. PCOS (7%)
      g. Adult-onset congenital adrenal hyperplasia (CAH) (1%)
      h. Cushing syndrome
      i. Hypothyroidism
    3. Hypogonadotrophic hypogonadism (27%)
      a. Constitutional delay (14%)
      b. Hypothalamic disorders
      c. Pituitary diseases (5%)
      d. Other CNS diseases
  B. Secondary amenorrhea
    1. Ovarian diseases (40%)
      a. PCOS (20%)
      b. Iatrogenic (oophorectomy, S/P radiation)
      c. Premature ovarian failure (POF)
      d. Ovarian tumors
    2. Hypothalamic dysfunction (35%)
      a. Functional (eating disorders, exercise, stress)
      b. Congenital GNRH deficiency
      c. Infiltrative diseases (sarcoidosis, histiocytosis, lymphoma)
    3. Pituitary diseases (19%)
      a. Hyperprolactinemia (drug induced, hypothyroidism, prolactinoma)
      b. Craniopharyngiomas
      c. Empty sella syndrome
      d. Sheehan's syndrome
      e. S/P radiation
      f. Infiltrative diseases
    4. Uterine diseases (5%)
      Asherman's syndrome
    5. Others
      Hypothyroidism, Cushing's syndrome, adult-onset congenital adrenal hyperplasia, drug induced (Lupron Depot, Depo-Provera, progesterone IUD, danazol, etc.), chronic illnesses

PHYSICAL FINDINGS & CLINICAL PRESENTATION

- Turner's syndrome
  - Mostly present with primary amenorrhea
  - Short stature
  - Epicanthic folds
  - Low set ears
  - High arched palate
  - Micrognathia
  - Sensorineural hearing loss
  - Otitis media
  - Webbing of the neck
  - Pigmented nevi
  - Square/shield chest
  - Widely spaced nipples
  - Absent breast development
  - Bicuspid aortic valve
  - Coarctation of aorta
  - Cubit valgus
  - Short fourth metacarpal
  - Hyperconvex nails
  - Leg edema
  - Renal abnormalities
  - Autoimmune disorders including thyroiditis
  - Diabetes mellitus
- Pure gonadal dysgenesis
  - Unlike Turner's syndrome has no dysmorphic features
- Müllerian agnesis
  - Sporadic inheritance
  - Primary amenorrhea
  - Normal breast development
  - Normal pubic and axillary hair
  - Normal female external genitalia
  - Absent uterus and upper part of vagina
  - Ovary present
  - Renal and vertebral anomalies
- Vaginal septum and imperforate hymen
  - Primary amenorrhea
  - Cyclic lower abdominal pain
  - Imperforate hymen or vaginal septum on pelvic examination
  - Perirectal fullness from hematocolpos
- Androgen insensitivity syndrome
  - Primary amenorrhea
  - X-linked recessive inheritance
  - Normal breast development
  - Absent pubic and axillary hair
  - Testis may be present in the groin or inguinal canal
  - Uterus and vagina absent
  - No associated renal or vertebral anomalies
- Adult-onset congenital adrenal hyperplasia
  - Commonly seen in Ashkenazi Jewish population
  - Mimics the presentation of PCOS
  - Features of hyperandrogenism (virilization, hirsutism, acne)
  - Hypertension
- 5-alpha reductase deficiency
  - Primary amenorrhea
  - Undergo striking virilization at puberty
- PCOS
  - Usually present with secondary amenorrhea and oligomenorrhea
  - Features of hyperandrogenism
  - Obesity
  - Infertility
- Cushing's syndrome
  - Secondary amenorrhea
  - Features of hyperandrogenism
  - Abnormal fat distribution (buffalo hump, spider legs, significant central obesity)
  - Abdominal striae
  - Easy bruising
  - Hypertension
  - Proximal muscle weakness
- Hypothyroidism
  - Secondary amenorrhea
  - Lethargy
  - Constipation
  - Decreased appetite
  - Weight gain
  - Cold intolerance
  - Hair loss
  - Dry skin
  - Hypotension
  - Bradycardia
- Premature ovarian failure
  - Secondary amenorrhea prior to the age of 40
  - History of oophorectomy or pelvic radiation or chemotherapy
  - Vasomotor symptoms
  - Dry, thin vaginal mucosa without rugosity
- Hyperprolactinemia
  - Usually present with secondary amenorrhea
  - History of use of drugs such as antipsychotics, OC pills, antidepressants, antihypertensives, H_2 blockers, opioids, etc.
  - Pituitary adenomas may be associated with headache, vomiting, vision changes
  - Galactorrhea
- Sheehan syndrome
  - History of secondary amenorrhea following postpartum hemorrhagia
  - Failure of lactation
  - Other features of hypopituitarism
- Asherman's syndrome
  - History of D&C
  - Secondary amenorrhea
  - Recurrent miscarriage/infertility

- Functional hypothalamic disorders
  - Usually present with secondary amenorrhea
  - History of eating disorders, severe exercise or stress
  - Use of street drugs
- Kallmann's syndrome
  - Usually present with anosmia

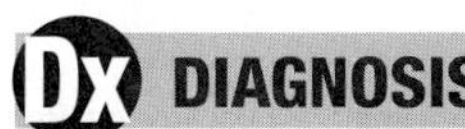

DIAGNOSIS

- First step in the workup of amenorrhea is to rule out pregnancy by serum/urine pregnancy test.
- Diagnostic workup depends on history and physical.
- Primary amenorrhea:
  - Pelvic ultrasonography or MRI to detect any anatomic abnormalities of uterus, cervix, ovaries, or vagina. At times examination under anesthesia is needed to assess the pelvic organs.
  - Karyotyping (46,XX in Müllerian agenesis; 46,XY in AIS; 45,XO in Turner's syndrome) is done when uterus is absent or Turner's syndrome is suspected.
  - Serum FSH, TSH/FT4, prolactin, estradiol:
    FSH>40 mIU/ml along with estradiol <20 pg/ml is indicative of ovarian insufficiency.
    Prolactin >200 ng/ml is suggestive of prolactinoma.
  - Check serum testosterone (male range in AIS; female range in Müllerian agenesis) when uterus is absent or in presence of features of hyperandrogenism.
  - 17 alpha hydroxyprogesterone level in presence of features of hyperandrogenism to rule out CAH. In addition to low level of 17 alpha hydroxyprogesterone, these patients have elevated level of serum progesterone and deoxycorticosterone, hypernatremia, and hypokalemia.
  - MRI of head in presence of:
    Primary hypogonadotrophic hypogonadism.
    Hyperprolactinemia.
    Visual field defects.
    Headaches.
    Signs of hypothalamic-pituitary dysfunction.
- Secondary amenorrhea:
  - Serum FSH, TSH/FT4, prolactin, estradiol:
    Low serum FSH with low estradiol indicates secondary (hypogondotrophic) hypogonadism.
    High serum FSH with low estradiol suggests primary (hypergonadotrophic) hypogonadism.
    Progesterone withdrawal bleeding.
    10 mg medroxyprogesterone is given for 10 days.
    Withdrawal bleeding suggests anovulation in presence of normal endorgan (outflow tract) and ovarian function.
  - Estrogen-progesterone withdrawal bleeding:
    In the absence of progesterone withdrawal bleeding, the patients are exposed to 25 to 35 days of estrogen (0.625-2.5 mg Premarin daily) followed by 10 days of medroxyprogesterone.
    Withdrawal bleeding indicates hypogonadism.
    Absence of bleeding indicates defects with endorgan (e.g., Asherman's syndrome).
  - Serum LH, testosterone and DHEA-S:
    When features of hyperandrogenism seen these tests are ordered.
    Serum testosterone > 200 ng/ml suggests androgen-producing adrenal or ovarian tumors. This level may be mildly elevated in patients with PCOS.
    DHEA-S >700 mcg/dl suggest adrenal origin over ovarian.
    LH/FSH ratio >2 in patient with PCOS.
  - Pelvic ultrasound when PCOS or ovarian tumor suspected.
  - Abdominal CT when adrenal tumor suspected.
  - MRI of head when indicated.
  - HSG, sonohysterography, or diagnostic hysteroscopy in patients with suspected Asherman's syndrome.
  - Karyotyping is indicated when POF occurs before the age of 30.
  - Other tests which are rarely needed:
    Serum transferrin when hemochromatosis is suspected.
    Serum ACE when sarcoidosis is suspected.

TREATMENT

- The treatment of amenorrhea depends on the etiology, as well as the aims of the patient, such as a desire to treat hirsutism or to become pregnant.
- In the absence of pregnancy, withdrawal bleeding may be induced in the majority of patients with amenorrhea using 5 to 10 mg of medroxyprogesterone for 10 days.
- Estrogen replacement along with calcium and vitamin D should be instituted in essentially every patient with hypogonadism to avoid osteoporosis. Women with a uterus require continuous or intermittent progesterone administration to protect against endometrial hyperplasia or cancer. Frequently, it is easiest to prescribe combination oral contraceptive pills. For most patients, continuation until ~50 years, the usual age of menopause, seems reasonable. Young women in whom secondary sex characteristics have failed to develop fully should be exposed initially to very low dose estrogen (0.3 mg of conjugated equine estrogen) given unopposed daily for 6 months with incremental dose increases at 6-month intervals until the required maintenance dose is achieved. Cyclic progesterone therapy, 12 to 14 days per month, should be instituted once vaginal bleeding ensues.
- If possible, patients with anatomic abnormalities will require surgical correction. Creation of a new vagina for patients with Müllerian failure is usually delayed until the woman is emotionally mature and ready to participate in the postoperative care required to maintain vaginal patency. However, if adequate correction is impossible, pregnancy will often require a surrogate to carry a gestation. One should not forget to look for the associated urogenital anomalies in these patients and, when present, treat them appropriately.
- In patients with androgen insensitivity syndrome, the incidence of gonadal malignancy is 22%. However, it rarely occurs before the age of 20. So one should remove the gonads following breast development and the attainment of adult stature. In the absence of a uterus these individuals only need estrogen replacement without progesterone.
- Women with adult-onset CAH may be treated with low-dose corticosteroids in addition to sex steroids to partially block ACTH stimulation of adrenal function and thereby decrease overproduction of adrenal androgens.
- Patients with POF will need estrogen and progesterone replacement. If POF cannot be corrected, these patients will require in vitro fertilization using donor oocytes to conceive. These patients have an increased risk of osteoporosis and heart disease. It can also be associated with autoimmune disorders such as hypothyroidism, Addison's disease, and diabetes mellitus. Therefore, fasting blood glucose, TSH, and, if clinically appropriate, morning cortisol should be measured. In the presence of a Y chromosome, removal of gonadal tissue is recommended at the time of diagnosis to avoid gonadal tumors.
- Hypothyroidism should be treated with thyroid replacement.
- Hyperprolactinemia is treated by avoiding the culprit drugs or by giving dopamine agonists, such as bromocriptine or cabergoline. Pituitary adenomas may require surgery if secondary deficits such as visual changes are observed or when it is resistant to medical therapy or the lesion is rapidly growing.
- Treatment of hypothalamic amenorrhea depends on the etiology. Patients with eating disorders or who exercise excessively will require behavioral modification and nutritional counseling. Elite athletes may choose not to alter their exercise regimens and will therefore require estrogen treatment and prevention of osteoporosis. When associated with infertility, ovulation induction with clomiphene citrate, exogenous gonadotropins, or pulsatile GNRH therapy should be offered.
- The primary treatment of PCOS is weight loss through diet and exercise. Other treatment options include:
  1. Use of OC pills or cyclic progestational agents to help maintain a normal endometrium.
  2. Insulin-sensitizing agents such as metformin to reduce insulin resistance and improve ovulatory function.
  3. Oral contraceptives and/or spironolactone to treat hyperandrogenism.
  4. Clomiphene citrate to induce ovulation.
- In patients with Asherman's syndrome, hysteroscopic lysis of intrauterine adhesions is

followed by administration of long-term exogenous estrogen to stimulate regrowth of endometrial tissue.
- Geneticist consult is given in patients with hereditary causes of amenorrhea.
- Psychiatrist consult is needed in patients with major depression, anorexia nervosa, bulimia nervosa, or other major psychiatric disorders.

COMPLICATIONS

- Osteoporosis
- Endometrial hyperplasia and uterine cancer
- Infertility

PROGNOSIS

Depends on the primary cause of amenorrhea

PATIENT EDUCATION

- Patients with amenorrhea should be reassured that this is, in and of itself, not a concern.
- All women with an intact endometrium should understand the risks of unopposed estrogen action, whether the estrogen is exogenous such as through hormone therapy, or endogenous such as PCOS.
- Hypoestrogenic women should be counseled about the importance of estrogen replacement to protect against bone loss.
- Potential for future child bearing should be discussed.

SUGGESTED READINGS

Master-Hunter T, Heiman DL: Amenorrhea: evaluation and treatment, *Am Fam Physician* 73(8):1374-1382, 2006.

Practice Committee of the American Society for Reproductive Medicine: Current evaluation of amenorrhea, *Fertil Steril* 82(suppl 1):S33-39, 2004.

AUTHOR: **HEMANT K. SATPATHY, M.D.**

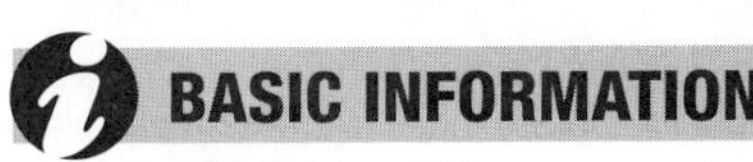

BASIC INFORMATION

DEFINITION

The acquired inability to learn new information or recall new information. The impairment compromises personal, social, and occupational functioning. Disorder is not caused by delirium or dementia.

SYNONYMS

Korsakoff's syndrome
Amnesia

ICD-9CM CODES

780.9 Amnesia (retrograde); memory disturbance, loss or lack

DSM-IV-TR CODES

294 Amnestic disorder due to . . . [indicate the general medical condition]
294.8 Amnestic disorder NOS

EPIDEMIOLOGY & DEMOGRAPHICS

INCIDENCE: Data not available on true incidence or lifetime risk.
PREDOMINANT AGE: Transient global amnesia onset usually after age 50 yr.
GENETICS: Genetic defect for thiamine metabolism has been described in some patients.

PHYSICAL FINDINGS & CLINICAL PRESENTATION

HISTORY

- Diagnosis depends on history.
- The inability to learn or recall new information is the key feature of this disorder.
- The Mini-Mental Status Examination is useful. Patients unable to recall events that transpire during the interview but may have a normal digit span and be able to attend to the conversation.
- Patients are unable to recall events subsequent to the onset of the amnesia.
- Individuals may learn new motor tasks but are unable to recall those learning experiences.
- Amnesia generally is both anterograde and retrograde.

ETIOLOGY

- Traumatic brain injury
- Focal tumors or infarction
- Herpes simplex encephalitis
- Cerebral anoxia
- Korsakoff syndrome (thiamine deficiency)
- Carbon monoxide poisoning
- Transient amnesia may arise from concussion, acute intoxication, anesthesia, medications, seizures, transient global amnesia, and electroconvulsant therapy

Dx DIAGNOSIS

DIFFERENTIAL DIAGNOSIS

- Dementia
- Delirium
- Major depression
- Benign senescent forgetfulness

WORKUP

- Complete medical history and mental status testing
- Neuropsychological testing

LABORATORY TESTS

No current role in diagnosis of amnestic disorders

IMAGING STUDIES

- No specific or diagnostic features of amnestic disorder are detectable on imaging.
- Brain MRI indicates specific atrophy in diencephalic structures in Korsakoff syndrome and in the hippocampus in hypoxic amnesia.
- Neuroradiological examination with MRI is valuable in the diagnosis of acute Wernicke's encephalopathy.
- Brain MR diffusion-weighted imaging may show hippocampal lesions in transient global amnesia.

Rx TREATMENT

NONPHARMACOLOGIC THERAPY

- Cognitive rehabilitation to promote recovery from brain injury may be helpful.
- Supervised living to ensure appropriate long-term care.

ACUTE GENERAL Rx

Initial treatment directed to the underlying etiology

CHRONIC Rx

No known effective treatments to reverse or ameliorate memory deficits.

DISPOSITION

Amnesias may be chronic or transient depending upon etiology.

REFERRAL

Refer for neuropsychological testing.

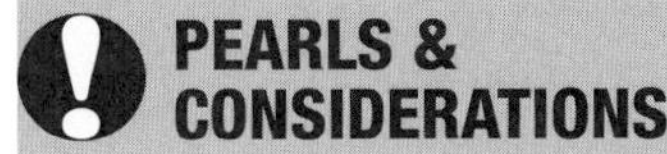

PEARLS & CONSIDERATIONS

COMMENTS

In Korsakoff syndrome, anterograde amnesia (disturbance in acquisition of new information) is more prominent than retrograde amnesia (problems remembering old information).

PREVENTION

High-dose thiamine for prevention of Korsakoff syndrome

PATIENT & FAMILY EDUCATION

Respite care and in-home services for family caregivers

SUGGESTED READINGS

Butler CR et al: Recent insights into the impairment of memory in epilepsy: transient epileptic amnesia, accelerated long-term forgetting and remote memory impairment, *Brain* 131(9):2243-2263, 2008.

Kopelman MD, Thomson AD, Guerrini I, Marshall EJ: The Korsakoff syndrome: clinical aspects, psychology and treatment, *Alcohol Alcohol* 44(2):148-154, 2009.

AUTHOR: **MITCHELL D. FELDMAN, M.D., M.PHIL.**

Amyloidosis

BASIC INFORMATION

DEFINITION

The term *amyloidosis* refers to a heterogenous group of disorders that are all characterized by the deposition of an amorphous, extracellular fibrillar protein in various organs and tissues of the body. It has the following subtypes:
- Primary amyloidosis (AL)
- Secondary amyloidosis (AA)
- Hereditary amyloidosis
- Localized amyloidosis

ICD-9CM CODES
277.3 Amyloidosis

EPIDEMIOLOGY & DEMOGRAPHICS

INCIDENCE (IN U.S.): Between 1500 and 3500 new cases are diagnosed annually. The most common type is AL.

PREVALENCE: Amyloidosis primarily affects men between the ages of 60 and 70 yr.

PHYSICAL FINDINGS & CLINICAL PRESENTATION

- The most common presenting symptoms of amyloidosis are fatigue, dyspnea, edema, paresthesias, and weight loss. Other findings depend on organ system involvement.
- Signs and symptoms of nephrotic syndrome may be present with renal involvement.
- Fatigue and dyspnea may occur with pulmonary involvement.
- GI involvement is uncommon but presents with diarrhea, nausea, abdominal pain, and macroglossia.
- Patients with cardiac involvement have an infiltrative cardiomyopathy and present with a preserved ejection fraction (EF) and diastolic dysfunction.
- Patients may present with bleeding problems caused by either Factor X deficiency or fragile bood vessels caused by infiltration by amyloid. Bleeding around the eyes (raccoon eyes) is a characteristic finding.
- Involvement of the nervous system presents with peripheral neuropathy, muscle weakness, numbness, syncope, or dizziness. Associated autonomic neuropathy can also cause severe disabling symptoms.

ETIOLOGY

The deposition of an amorphous, extracellular fibrillar protein in various tissues that stains with Congo red is the common underlying mechanism, but there are important differences among various subtypes:
- AL is associated with an underlying clonal plasma cell disorder making an abnormal light chain protein with possible deposition in multiple organ system.
- AA has no underlying plasma cell disorder and is a consequence of longstanding systemic inflammation (e.g., tuberculosis, leprosy, malaria, untreated syphilis).
- Localized amyloidosis results from localized synthesis of fibrillar material with no underlying plasma cell disorder.
- Familial amyloidosis is another subtype, with the most common form resulting from mutation of transthretin gene *(TTR)*.

Dx DIAGNOSIS

DIFFERENTIAL DIAGNOSIS

Differential diagnosis varies depending on the organ involvement:
- Renal involvement (toxin- or drug-induced necrosis, glomerulonephritis, renal vein thrombosis)
- Interstitial lung disease (sarcoidosis, connective tissue disease, infectious causative factors)
- Restrictive cardiomyopathy (endomyocardial fibrosis, viral myocarditis)
- Carpal tunnel (rheumatoid arthritis, hypothyroidism, overuse)
- Peripheral neuropathy (alcohol abuse, vitamin deficiencies, diabetes mellitus)

WORKUP

Workup consists of performing blood and urine tests to look for abnormal light chain in urine or blood, performing various tests to look for target organ damage, and getting histologic confirmation by doing a fat pad and bone marrow biopsy and then performing Congo red staining on that.

LABORATORY TESTS

- Immunofixation of serum and urine to look for immunoglobulin light chain is a sensitive screening test
- CBC, blood urea nitrogen (BUN)/creatinine, liver function tests, thyroid functions, and urine for albumin
- Histologic confirmation is necessary with a fat pad and bone marrow biopsy with Congo red staining to establish a diagnosis
- If a noninvasive fat pad biopsy does not establish a diagnosis, then a biopsy of the affected organ may be needed

IMAGING STUDIES

- Two-dimensional Doppler echocardiography to study diagnostic filling is useful to evaluate for cardiac involvement.
- Nuclear imaging with technetium-labeled aprotinin may detect cardiac amyloidosis. Serum amyloid P component (SAP) scintigraphy has high sensitivity for the detection of amyloid deposits in liver, spleen, kidneys, adrenal glands, and bones.

Rx TREATMENT

ACUTE GENERAL Rx

- The goal of therapy is to decrease the production of the amyloidogenic light chain with therapy directed at the clonal plasma cells.
- All agents used to treat multiple myeloma are effective against AL including melphalan, prednisone, oral dexamethasone, systemic chemotherapy like cyclophosphamide, doxorubicin (Adriamycin), and more recently immunomodulatory compounds (IMiDs) molecules like thalidomide or lenalidomide, but none has shown to be superior to melphalan and prednisone, which remain the treatment of choice.
- In highly selected patients with preserved organ function, autologous bone marrow transplant can have good results.
- Patients who experience development of renal failure can be supported with hemodialysis or renal transplant.
- Liver transplantation has been used successfully in patients with familial amyloidosis.
- Recognition and treatment of the underlying disorder is needed for secondary amyloidosis.

DISPOSITION

Prognosis is determined primarily by the presence or absence of cardiac involvement and the form of amyloidosis:
- In AA, eradication of the predisposing disease slows and can occasionally reverse the progression of amyloid disease. Median survival after diagnosis is 133 mo.
- Patients with familial amyloidotic polyneuropathy generally have a prolonged course lasting 10 to 15 yr.
- Amyloidosis associated with immunocytic processes carries the worst prognosis (life expectancy $<$1 yr).
- The progression of amyloidosis associated with renal hemodialysis can be improved with newer dialysis membranes that can pass beta 2-microglobulin.
- Median survival in patients with overt CHF is ~6 mo; it is 30 mo without CHF.
- Serum uric acid has a prognostic value in primary systemic amyloidosis. Patients with uric acid levels $>$8 mg/dl have a median overall survival of 9 mo from diagnosis compared with 20.3 mo for those with lower levels.

EBM EVIDENCE

Please note: Complete text of EBM for this topic is available online.

SUGGESTED READINGS

Kyle RA et al: A trial of three regimen for primary amyloidosis: colchicine, melphalan, prednisone and melphalan prednisone and colchicine, *N Engl J Med* 336(17):1202-1207, 1997.

Sideras K et al: Amyloidosis, *Adv Clin Chem* 47:1-44, 2009.

Wang AK et al: Patterns of neuropathy and autonomic failure in patients with amyloidosis, *Mayo Clin Proc* 83(11):1226-1230, 2008.

AUTHORS: **BILAL H. NAQVI, M.D.,** and **FRED F. FERRI, M.D.**

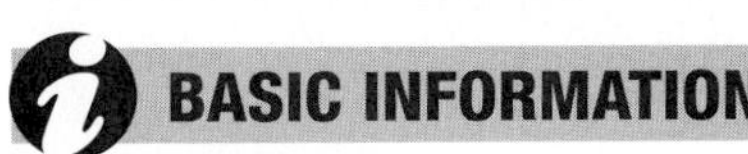

BASIC INFORMATION

DEFINITION

Amyotrophic lateral sclerosis (ALS) is a progressive, degenerative neuromuscular condition of undetermined etiology affecting corticospinal tracts and anterior horn cells, resulting in dysfunction of both upper motor neurons (UMN) and lower motor neurons (LMN), respectively.

SYNONYMS

Lou Gehrig's Disease

ICD-9CM CODES

335.20 Amyotrophic lateral sclerosis

EPIDEMIOLOGY & DEMOGRAPHICS

INCIDENCE: 0.5 to 2 cases per 100,000 persons. Onset is usually between the ages of 50 and 70 yr. Male/female ratio is 2:1.
PREVALENCE: Five in 100,000 persons

PHYSICAL FINDINGS & CLINICAL PRESENTATION

- LMN signs (weakness, hypotonia, wasting, fasciculations, hyporeflexia or areflexia).
- UMN signs (loss of fine motor dexterity, spasticity, extensor plantar responses, hyperreflexia, clonus).
- Preservation of extraocular movements, sensation, bowel and bladder function.
- Dysarthria, dysphagia, pseudobulbar affect, frontal lobe dysfunction.
- Respiratory insufficiency typically occurs late in the disease.
- ALS comprises approximately 90% of adult-onset motor neuron diseases. Other presentations of motor neuron disease include progressive muscular atrophy, primary lateral sclerosis, progressive bulbar palsy, progressive pseudobulbar palsy, and ALS-parkinsonism-dementia complex.

ETIOLOGY

- 90% to 95% of all cases are sporadic; of the familial cases, 10% to 20% are associated with a genetic defect in the copper-zinc superoxide dismutase enzyme.

Dx DIAGNOSIS

DIFFERENTIAL DIAGNOSIS

- Multifocal motor neuropathy with conduction block
- Cervical spondylotic myelopathy with polyradiculopathy
- Spinal stenosis with compression of lumbosacral nerve roots
- Chronic inflammatory demyelinating polyneuropathy with central nervous system lesions
- Syringomyelia
- Syringobulbia
- Foramen magnum tumor
- Meningeal carcinomatosis
- Spinal muscular atrophy
- Polyglucosan body disease
- Bulbospinal muscular atrophy (Kennedy disease)
- Monomyelic amyotrophy
- ALS-like syndromes have been reported in the setting of lead intoxication, HIV, hyperparathyroidism, hyperthyroidism, lymphoma, and B_{12} deficiency.

WORKUP

- Electromyography and nerve conduction studies (El Escorial criteria)
- Assessment of respiratory function (forced vital capacity [FVC], negative inspiratory force)

LABORATORY TESTS

- Vitamin B_{12}, thyroid function, parathyroid hormone, HIV may be considered.
- Serum protein and immunofixation electrophoresis.
- DNA studies for SMA or bulbospinal atrophy, hexosaminidase levels in pure LMN syndrome.
- 24-hour urine for heavy metals if indicated.

IMAGING STUDIES

- Craniospinal neuroimaging contingent on clinical scenario
- Modified barium swallow to evaluate aspiration risk

Rx TREATMENT

NONPHARMACOLOGIC THERAPY

- Noninvasive positive-pressure ventilation may improve quality of life and may increase tracheostomy-free survival in patients with respiratory difficulty (defined by orthopnea or FVC 50% of predicted).
- Percutaneous endoscopic gastrostomy (PEG) tube placement improves nutritional intake, promotes weight stabilization, and eases medication administration. Some studies suggest PEG placement may prolong life 1 to 4 mo, particularly when placed before FVC falls to ≤50% of predicted value.
- Nutrition, speech therapy, physical and occupational therapy services.
- Suction device for sialorrhea.
- Communication may be eased with computerized assistive devices.
- Early discussion of living will, resuscitation orders, desire for PEG and tracheostomy, potential long-term care options.
- Encourage contact with local support groups.

ACUTE GENERAL Rx

Riluzole (Rilutek), a glutamate antagonist, is the only FDA-approved medication known to extend tracheostomy-free survival in patients with ALS. Dosage is 50 mg q12h, at least 1 hr before or 2 hr after meals. It is shown to prolong survival by 2 to 3 months. Manufacturer recommends checking alanine aminotransferase (ALT) once a month for 3 months initially, followed by once every 3 months until the first year of therapy is completed. ALT should be checked periodically thereafter.

CHRONIC Rx

- Sialorrhea may respond to either glycopyrrolate or amitriptyline (consider either propranolol or metoprolol if secretions are thick). Botulinum toxin may be effective in medically refractory cases.
- Spasticity may be treated pharmacologically with baclofen, tizanidine, clonazepam.
- Pseudobulbar affect may improve with amitriptyline, sertraline (Zoloft), or dextromethorphan/quinine.

DISPOSITION

- Mean duration of symptoms is 3 to 5 yr.
- Approximately 20% of patients survive >5 yr.

REFERRAL

- Referral to a neurologist experienced in neuromuscular disease is recommended to confirm the diagnosis. One prospective, population-based study suggested improved survival in subjects treated in a multidisciplinary clinic.
- Gastrointestinal referral for PEG placement is recommended while FVC remains >50% to minimize morbidity attributable to risks inherent to the procedure.

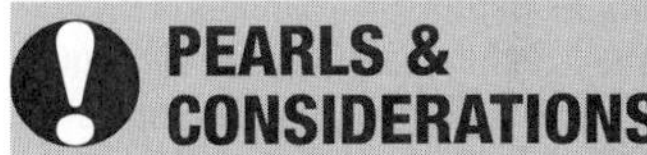

PEARLS & CONSIDERATIONS

- Patient-physician communication is an integral and essential part in both the initial diagnosis and subsequent treatment of ALS.
- A multidisciplinary approach to supportive care may lead to an improved level of daily functioning and foster an increased sense of independence.

SUGGESTED READINGS

Dunkley T et al: Whole-genome analysis of sporadic amyotrophic lateral sclerosis, *N Engl J Med* 357:775-788, 2007.

Miller RG et al: Practice parameter update: The care of the patient with amyotrophic lateral stenosis: Drug, nutritional, and respiratory therapies (an evidence-based review): Report of the Quality Standards Subcommittee of the American Academy of Neurology, *Neurology* 73:1218-1226, 2009.

Mitchell JD, Borasio GD: Amyotrophic lateral sclerosis, *Lancet* 369:2031-2041, 2007.

AUTHOR: **TAYLOR HARRISON, M.D.**

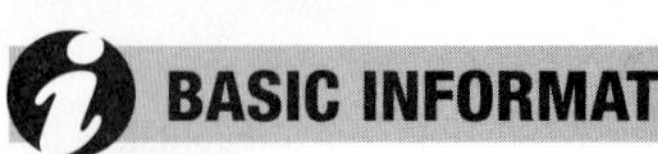

BASIC INFORMATION

DEFINITION

An anaerobic infection is caused by one of a group of bacteria that requires a reduced oxygen tension for growth.

ICD-9CM CODES

See specific condition.

PHYSICAL FINDINGS & CLINICAL PRESENTATION

- May occur at any site, but most are anatomically related to mucosal surfaces
- Should be suspected when there is foul-smelling tissue, soft tissue gas, necrotic tissue, or abscesses
- Head and neck
    1. Odontogenic infections from dental or soft tissue possibly progressing to periapical abscesses, at times extending to bone
    2. Both anaerobic and aerobic pathogens in chronic sinusitis, chronic mastoiditis, peritonsillar abscess, and chronic otitis media
    3. Complications: deep neck space infections, brain abscesses, mediastinitis
- Pleuropulmonary
    1. May involve anaerobes present in the oropharynx
    2. Aspiration more common in persons with altered mental status or seizures
    3. Anaerobic bacteria more likely in those with gingivitis or periodontitis
    4. Manifestations: necrotizing pneumonia, empyema, lung abscess
- Intraabdominal
    1. Disruption of intestinal integrity leading to infection involving anaerobic bacteria
    2. Bacteria from colonic neoplasm, perforated appendicitis, diverticulitis, or bowel surgery, causing bacteremia, peritonitis, at times intraabdominal abscesses
    3. Resulting infections usually mixed, containing both anaerobes and aerobes
- Female genital tract
    1. Anaerobes in bacterial vaginosis, salpingitis, endometritis, pelvic abscesses, septic abortion; infections tend to be mixed
    2. Possible pelvic thrombophlebitis when resolving pelvic infection is accompanied by new or persistent fever
- Other anaerobic infections
    1. Skin and soft tissue infection at any site
    2. More commonly associated infections: synergistic gangrene, bite wound infections, infected decubitus ulcers
    3. Clinical significance of anaerobes in diabetic foot infections unclear
    4. Anaerobic bacteremia uncommon with source usually intraabdominal, followed by female genital tract, pleuropulmonary, and head and neck infections
    5. Osteomyelitis especially when associated with decubitus ulcers or vascular insufficiency
    6. Facial bone osteomyelitis from adjacent infections of the teeth or sinuses

ETIOLOGY

- Most commonly endogenous, arising from bacteria that normally line mucosal surfaces
- Disruption of mucosal barriers resulting from various conditions (trauma, ischemia, surgery, perforation), with infection occurring when organisms gain access to normally sterile sites, causing tissue destruction and abscess formation
- Synergy between different anaerobes or between anaerobes and aerobes important

Dx DIAGNOSIS

DIFFERENTIAL DIAGNOSIS

- Primary differential possibility is an aerobic bacterial infection without the presence of anaerobic bacteria.
- Ischemic necrosis without accompanying anaerobic infection (or "dry" gangrene [noninfected necrosis] vs. "wet" gangrene [infected tissue with anaerobic infection]).

WORKUP

- Specimens submitted for anaerobic culture should be processed within 30 min and may take up to 5 to 7 days to grow
- Large volume of material more likely to have significant growth; swabs less efficient for transporting infected material
- Blood cultures—preferably before antibiotic administration

LABORATORY TESTS

- Elevated WBC count, with extremely high WBC counts sometimes seen with pseudomembranous colitis
- Positive stool *C. difficile* toxin A and B assay
- Increased lactate levels in ischemia or perforation
- Possible positive blood or wound cultures, but failure to grow anaerobes in culture may be common, attributed to inadequate culturing techniques or fastidious organisms

IMAGING STUDIES

- Plain film of an affected area to show gas in tissues, free air resulting from a perforated viscus, or an air/fluid level inside an abscess
- Ultrasound, CT scan, or MRI to reveal abscesses or tissue destruction

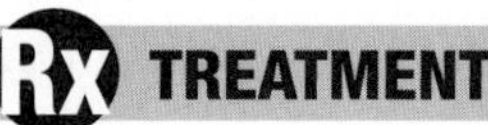

TREATMENT

NONPHARMACOLOGIC THERAPY

- Removal of necrotic tissue
- Drainage of abscesses (accomplished by CT scan–guided percutaneous drainage)

ACUTE GENERAL Rx

Oral antibiotics with anaerobic activity: clindamycin, metronidazole, and chloramphenicol

- Broader spectrum of activity with amoxicillin/clavulanate
- Penicillin VK in odontogenic infections
- Oral metronidazole for *C. difficile*–associated diarrhea, with oral vancomycin used for severe, recurrent, or recalcitrant infections

Parenteral antibiotics for more serious illness

- IV clindamycin, metronidazole, and chloramphenicol
- Cephalosporins (anaerobic or mixed infections): cefoxitin and cefotetan
- Extended-spectrum penicillins (e.g., piperacillin) and combination beta-lactamase plus beta-lactamase inhibitor drugs (e.g., clavulanic acid, sulbactam, tazobactam)
    1. Significant anaerobic activity, plus various degrees of broad-spectrum coverage
    2. Include ampicillin/sulbactam, ticarcillin/clavulanate, and piperacillin/tazobactam
- Imipenem or other carbapenems, such as meropenem or ertapenem, which are broad-spectrum agents with extensive anaerobic activity
- Actinomycosis treated with penicillin for 6 to 12 mo
- SMX/TMP and fluoroquinolones are generally ineffective, but some newer quinolones (e.g., moxifloxacin) have inhibitory activity against anaerobes

DISPOSITION

It is essential that all necrotic debris be removed when treating an anaerobic infection or it will recur; follow-up is critically important to ensure resolution of the process.

REFERRAL

Refer to a surgeon if drainage is required; infectious disease consultation may be useful in complicated patients or if treatment regimen is failing or slow to respond.

SUGGESTED READING

Stein GE, Goldstein EJ: Fluoroquinolones and anaerobes, *Clin Infect Dis* 42(11):1598, 2006.

AUTHORS: **GLENN G. FORT, M.D., M.P.H.,** and **DENNIS J. MIKOLICH, M.D.**

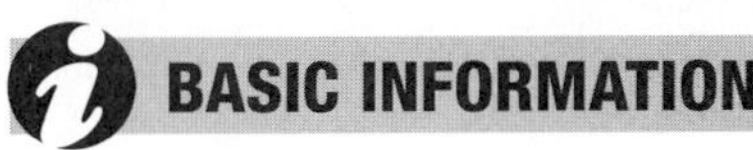

BASIC INFORMATION

DEFINITION

A fissure is a tear in the epithelial lining of the anal canal (i.e., from the dentate line to the anal verge).

SYNONYMS

Anorectal fissure
Anal ulcer

ICD-9CM CODES
565.0 Anal fissure

EPIDEMIOLOGY & DEMOGRAPHICS

PREDOMINANT SEX: Occurs in men more than women. Women are more likely to have anterior fissure than men (10% vs. 1%, respectively). Common in women before and after childbirth.

PREDOMINANT AGE: Can occur at any age. Most common in young and middle-aged adults. Most common cause of rectal bleeding in infants.

PHYSICAL FINDINGS & CLINICAL PRESENTATION

With separation of the buttocks will see a tear in the posterior midline or, less frequently, in the anterior midline (Fig. 1-15)

- Acute anal fissure:
  1. Sharp burning or tearing pain exacerbated by bowel movements
  2. Bright-red blood on toilet paper, a streak of blood on the stool or in the water

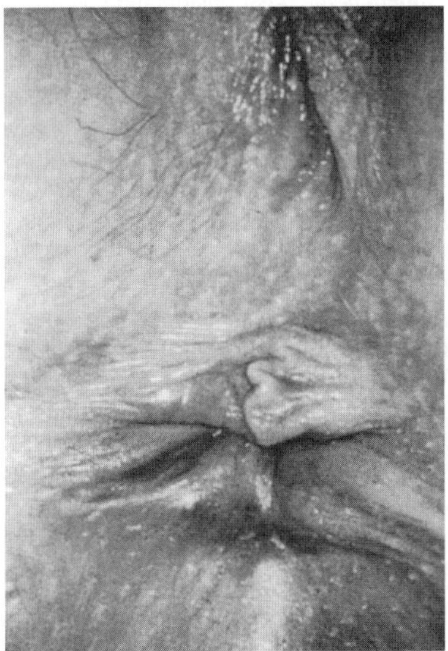

FIGURE 1-15 Lateral anal fissure. (In Seidel HM et al: *Mosby's guide to physical examination,* ed 3, St Louis, 1995, Mosby. Courtesy Gershon Efron, MD, Sinai Hospital of Baltimore.)

- Chronic anal fissure:
  1. Pruritus ani
  2. Pain seldom present
  3. Intermittent bleeding
  4. Sentinel tag at the caudal aspect of the fissure, hypertrophied anal papilla at the proximal end
- Underlying disease possible if the fissure:
  1. Is ectopically located
  2. Extends proximal to the dentate line
  3. Is broad-based or deep
  4. Is especially purulent

ETIOLOGY

- Most initiated after passage of a large, hard stool
- May result from frequent defecation and diarrhea
- Bacterial infections: tuberculosis (TB), syphilis, gonorrhea, chancroid, lymphogranuloma venereum
- Viral infections: herpes simplex virus, cytomegalovirus, human immunodeficiency virus
- Inflammatory bowel disease (IBD): Crohn's disease, ulcerative colitis
- Trauma: surgery (hemorrhoidectomy), foreign bodies, anal intercourse
- Malignancy: carcinoma, lymphoma, Kaposi sarcoma

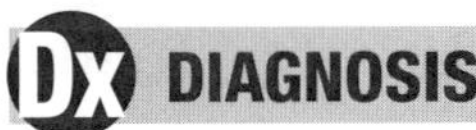

DIAGNOSIS

DIFFERENTIAL DIAGNOSIS

- Proctalgia fugax
- Thrombosed hemorrhoid

WORKUP

- Digital rectal examination after lubricating the entire anus with anesthetic jelly (i.e., 2% lidocaine) and waiting 5 to 10 min
- Anoscopy
- Proctosigmoidoscopy to exclude inflammatory or neoplastic disease
- Biopsy if doubt exists about the etiology of the condition
- All studies done under adequate anesthesia

IMAGING STUDIES

- Colonoscopy or barium enema if diagnosis of IBD or malignancy is suspected
- Small-bowel series occasionally obtained for similar reasons
- Biopsy to reveal caseating granuloma if TB is suspected
- Wet prep with darkfield examination to demonstrate treponemes if syphilis is suspected

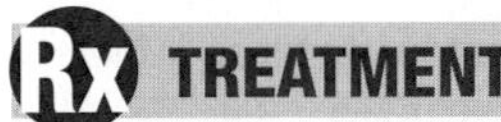

TREATMENT

NONPHARMACOLOGIC THERAPY

- Sitz baths
- High-fiber diet
- Increased oral fluid intake

ACUTE GENERAL Rx

- Bulk-producing agent (e.g., Metamucil) or stool softener
- Local anesthetic jelly (may exacerbate pruritus ani)
- Nitroglycerin ointment
- Suppositories *not* recommended
- Surgery

CHRONIC Rx

- Surgery: lateral internal anal sphincterotomy
- Topical glyceryl trinitrate ointment
- Injection of botulinum toxin (an injection into each side of the internal anal sphincter) is effective in healing chronic anal fissures in more than 90% of patients

DISPOSITION

Outpatient surgery

REFERRAL

- If fissure does not resolve with conservative therapy in 4 to 6 wk
- If patient prefers surgery for acute fissure
- If patient has chronic fissure

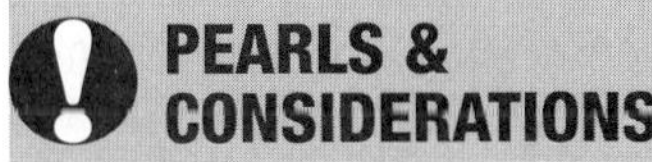

PEARLS & CONSIDERATIONS

COMMENTS

HIV-positive patients should be referred to clinicians who are well versed in the myriad infectious and neoplastic conditions that masquerade as anal ulcers in these patients.

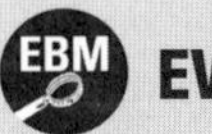

EVIDENCE

Please note: Complete text of EBM for this topic is available online.

SUGGESTED READINGS

Brisinda G et al: A comparison of injection of botulinum toxin and topical nitroglycerin ointment for the treatment of chronic anal fissure, *N Engl J Med* 341:65, 1999.

Brisinda G et al: Treating chronic anal fissure with botulinum neurotoxin, *Nat Clin Pract Gastroenterol Hepatol* 1(2):82, 2004.

Dwarkasing S et al: Magnetic resonance imaging of perianal fistulas, *Semin Ultrasound CT MR* 26(4):247, 2005.

Pfenninger JL, Zainea GG: Common anorectal conditions, *Am Fam Physician* 64:77, 2001.

AUTHORS: **GEORGE T. DANAKAS, M.D.,** and **RUBEN ALVERO, M.D.**

Anaphylaxis

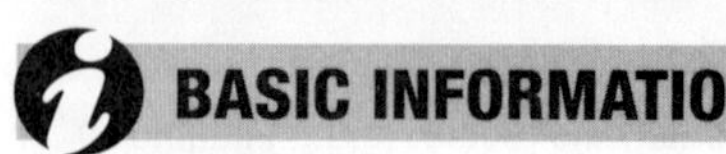

BASIC INFORMATION

DEFINITION

Anaphylaxis is a sudden-onset, life-threatening type I hypersensitivity reaction characterized by bronchial contractions in conjunction with hemodynamic changes. Its clinical presentation may include respiratory, cardiovascular, cutaneous, or gastrointestinal manifestations.

SYNONYMS

Anaphylactoid reaction is closely related to anaphylaxis. It is caused by release of mast cells and basophil mediators triggered by non–IgE–mediated events.

ICD-9CM CODES	
995.0	Anaphylactic shock
995.60	Anaphylaxis due to food
999.4	Anaphylaxis due to immunization
977.9	Anaphylaxis due to drugs
989.5	Anaphylaxis following stings

EPIDEMIOLOGY & DEMOGRAPHICS

INCIDENCE: 20,000 to 50,000 persons each year in the U.S. Anaphylaxis rates are 0.0004% for food, 0.7% to 10% for penicillin, 0.22% to 1% for radiocontrast media, and 0.5% to 5% after insect stings. An estimated one in every 3000 inpatients in U.S. hospitals develops an anaphylactic reaction.

PHYSICAL FINDINGS & CLINICAL PRESENTATION

- Urticaria, pruritus, skin flushing, angioedema, weakness, dizziness
- Dyspnea, cough, malaise, difficulty swallowing
- Wheezing, tachycardia, diarrhea
- Hypotension, vascular collapse

ETIOLOGY

Anaphylaxis results from sudden release into the systemic circulation of histamine, tryptase, and other inflammatory mediators from basophils and mast cells. Virtually any substance may induce anaphylaxis in a given individual.

- Commonly implicated medications are antibiotics, insulin, allergen extracts, opiates, vaccines, nonsteroidal antiinflammatory drugs (NSAIDs), contrast media, and streptokinase
- Foods and food additives, nuts, egg whites, shellfish, fish, milk, fruits, and berries
- Blood products, plasma, immunoglobulin, cryoprecipitate, whole blood
- Venoms such as snake venom, fire ant venom, bee sting (*Hymenoptera* stings)
- Latex

Dx DIAGNOSIS

DIFFERENTIAL DIAGNOSIS

- Endocrine disorders (carcinoid, pheochromocytoma)
- Globus hystericus, anxiety disorder
- Systemic mastocytosis
- Pulmonary embolism, serum sickness, vasovagal reactions
- Severe asthma (the key clinical difference is the abrupt onset of symptoms in anaphylaxis without a history of progressive worsening of symptoms)
- Septic shock or other form of shock
- Airway foreign body

WORKUP

Workup is aimed mainly at eliminating other conditions that may mimic anaphylaxis (e.g., vasovagal syncope may be differentiated by the presence of bradycardia as opposed to the tachycardia seen in anaphylaxis; the absence of hypoxemia in arterial blood gas [ABG] analysis may be useful to exclude pulmonary embolism or foreign body aspiration).

LABORATORY TESTS

- Laboratory evaluation is generally not helpful because the diagnosis of anaphylaxis is a clinical one.
- ABG analysis may be useful to exclude pulmonary embolism, status asthmaticus, and foreign body aspiration.
- Elevated serum and urine histamine levels can be useful for diagnosis of anaphylaxis, but these tests are not commonly available.

IMAGING STUDIES

Generally not helpful.

- Chest radiograph is indicated in patients with acute respiratory compromise.
- ECG should be considered in all patients with sudden loss of consciousness or reports of chest pains or dyspnea and in any elderly patient.

Rx TREATMENT

NONPHARMACOLOGIC THERAPY

- Establish and protect airway.
- IV access should be rapidly established, and IV fluids (i.e., saline) should be administered. The patient should be placed supine or in Trendelenburg position.
- Supplemental oxygen and cardiac monitoring are also recommended.

ACUTE GENERAL Rx

- Epinephrine should be rapidly administered as an SC or IM injection at a dose of 0.01 ml/kg of aqueous epinephrine 1:1000 (maximum adult dose, 0.3 to 0.5 ml). The dose may be repeated approximately q5-10min if there is persistence or recurrence of symptoms. Endotracheal epinephrine should be considered if IV access is not possible during life-threatening reactions.
- Administration of H_1 and H_2 receptor antagonists is also recommended in the initial treatment of anaphylaxis.
  1. Administer diphenhydramine 50 to 75 mg IV or IM.
  2. Cimetidine 300 mg IV over 3 to 5 min, or ranitidine 50 mg IV, should be given initially; subsequent doses of H_1 and H_2 blockers can be given orally q6h for 48 hr.
- Corticosteroids are not useful in the acute episode because of their slow onset of action; however, they should be administered in most cases to prevent prolonged or recurrent anaphylaxis. Commonly used agents are hydrocortisone sodium succinate 250 to 500 mg IV q4-6h in adults (4 to 8 mg/kg for children) or methylprednisolone 60 to 125 mg IV in adults (1 to 2 mg/kg in children).
- Aerosolized β-agonists (e.g., albuterol, 2.5 mg, repeat prn 20 min) are useful to control bronchospasm.
- Additional useful agents in specific circumstances: atropine for refractory bradycardia, dopamine for refractory hypotension (despite volume expansion), and glucagon in patients on β-blocking drugs.

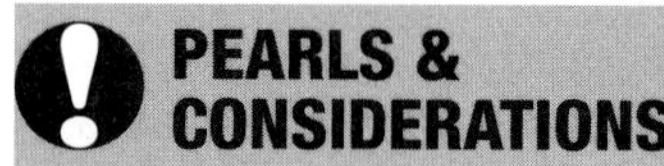

PEARLS & CONSIDERATIONS

COMMENTS

- Patient education regarding the nature of the illness and preventive measures is recommended. A documented history of previous anaphylactic episodes or known anaphylaxis triggers is the most reliable method of identifying individuals at risk.
- Prescription for prefilled epinephrine syringe (EpiPen) should be given, and the patient should be instructed on the use of this emergency kit in case of recurrent anaphylactic episodes.
- Patients should also be advised to carry or wear a MedicAlert ID describing substances that have caused anaphylaxis.
- Avoidance of radiologic contrast is also recommended.
- Venom immunotherapy immediately after a sting is effective and recommended for up to 5 yr after the anaphylactic incident.

SUGGESTED READING

Kemp SF: Office approach to anaphylaxis: sooner better than later, *Am J Med* 120:664-668, 2007.

AUTHOR: **TARA M. WAYT, D.O.**

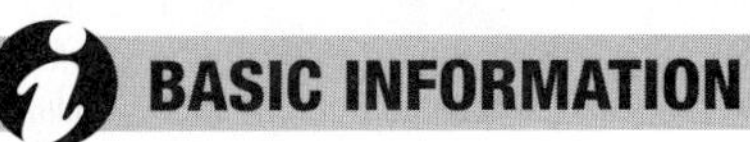

DEFINITION

The anemia of chronic disease refers to mild to moderately severe anemias (with hemoglobin [Hb] ranging from 7-12 g/dl), associated with chronic infections and inflammatory disorders, and some malignancies. Anemia of chronic disease may also refer to normal total body iron stores with low circulating iron (<60 mcg/dl).

SYNONYMS

Anemia of inflammation

ICD-9CM CODES	
285.21	Anemia in chronic kidney disease
285.22	Anemia in neoplastic disease
285.29	Anemia of other chronic illness
285.3	Antineoplastic chemotherapy induced anemia (effective October 1, 2009)
281.9	Unspecified deficiency anemia

EPIDEMIOLOGY & DEMOGRAPHICS

PREVALENCE: The prevalence rate in the elderly ranges from 8% to 44%, with the greatest prevalence in men 85 yr and older.

- Second-most prevalent anemia after iron deficiency anemia
- Perhaps one third of elderly adults with anemia suffer from anemia of chronic disease, anemia of chronic renal failure, or both
  - 11% of men and 10.2% of women age 65 to 85 yr
  - >20% of adults older than 85 yr

PREDOMINANT SEX AND AGE: Male sex >85 yr of age

RISK FACTORS:

- Chronic inflammatory conditions like autoimmune disorders (e.g., rheumatoid arthritis, systemic lupus erythematosus, vasculitis and sarcoidosis, inflammatory bowel disease [Crohn's disease/ulcerative colitis])
- Neoplasia (both hematologic cancer and solid tumors)
- Renal insufficiency/chronic kidney disease
- Infection (acute/chronic—viral, bacterial, parasitic, and fungal)
- Chronic rejection (graft vs. host disease) after solid-organ transplantation

PHYSICAL FINDINGS & CLINICAL PRESENTATION

Most patients are asymptomatic but may have general findings like skin pallor and conjunctival pallor.

ETIOLOGY

It is caused by several mechanisms (e.g., erythrocyte survival, increased uptake and retention of iron within cells of the reticuloendothelial system, inadequate transfer of iron from the reticuloendothelial system, limited availability of iron from erythroid progenitor cells, iron-restricted erythropoiesis.

Dx DIAGNOSIS

DIFFERENTIAL DIAGNOSIS

Iron deficiency anemia
Other causes of normocytic anemia
- Red blood cell loss or destruction
  - Acute blood loss
  - Hypersplenism
  - Hemolysis
- Decreased red blood cell production
  - Primary causes
    - Marrow hypoplasia or aplasia
    - Myelopathies
    - Myeloproliferative disease
    - Pure red blood cell aplasia
  - Secondary causes
    - Chronic renal failure
    - Liver disease
    - Endocrine deficiencies states
    - Sideroblastic anemia

WORKUP

Detailed history and physical examination

LABORATORY TESTS

CBC, reticulocyte count, reticulocyte index and pheripheral smear, serum iron levels, total iron-binding capacity, percentage saturation, and ferritin and erythropoietin level, and sometimes even bone marrow biopsy. Usual findings are as follows:

- Hb levels (typically): 8 to 9.5 g/dl
- Low reticulocyte count (reflecting ineffective erythropoiesis)
- Low serum iron concentration (also low in iron deficiency anemia)
- Low transferrin saturation (also low in iron deficiency anemia)
- Serum ferritin (marker of iron storage) normal or increased[1]
  - Acute inflammatory states may mimic the hematologic profile of anemia of chronic disease
- Soluble transferrin receptor levels remain within normal limits (decreased in and deficiency anemia)
  - Transferrin receptor assay can distinguish iron deficiency anemia from anemia of chronic disease, even in patients with rheumatologic or other inflammatory disorders; number of transferrin receptors increased in iron deficiency anemia and normal in anemia of chronic disease; enzyme-linked immunosorbent assay (ELISA) testing seems as reliable as bone marrow aspiration
- Erythropoietin level
  - Levels become increased only when Hb <10 g/dl
- Mean corpuscular volume (MCV): 81 to 99 femtoliter (fl)

Rx TREATMENT

Treat the underlying disorder/disease.

ACUTE GENERAL Rx

Blood transfusion usually reserved for severe anemia (Hb level <8.0 g/dl) or life-threatening anemia (Hb level <6.5 g/dl), particularly if complicated with ongoing bleeding. Increases survival rates in patients with anemia with myocardial infarction.

CHRONIC Rx

FDA-approved uses of erythropoiesis-stimulating agents epoetin alfa (Epogen, Procrit) and darbepoetin alfa (Aranesp):

- Treatment of anemia with target Hb level ≤12 g/dl in the following patients:
  - Patients with chronic kidney failure
  - Cancer patients receiving chemotherapy
  - Patients with HIV infection who are taking zidovudine

REFERRAL

Hematology and oncology

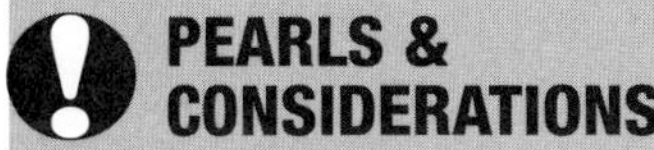

COMMENTS

The anemia of inflammation, which also includes anemia of critical illness, is a condition that presents similarly to anemia of chronic disease but develops within days of the onset of illness. An anemia similar to anemia of inflammation is seen in some elderly patients in the absence of identifiable chronic disease.

PREVENTION

Consider checking Hb levels or CBC in patients with renal failure, cancer, or other chronic disease for screening purposes.

PATIENT/FAMILY EDUCATION

Am Fam Physician 2000 Nov 15;62(10):2264
http://www.mdconsult.com/das/patient/view/0/10041/32120.html/top (English version)
http://www.mdconsult.com/das/patient/view/0/10041/32121.html/top (Spanish version)

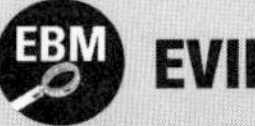

EVIDENCE

Erythropoietin-stimulating agents (ESAs) may cause or worsen hypertension. Excessive dose or duration can lead to polycythemia and dangerous thrombotic events, including myocardial infarction and stroke. Patients with uncontrolled hypertension should not receive ESAs.[1]

Erythropoietin receptor agonists are NOT recommended for routine use in critically ill patients. B

- Epoetin alfa once every 2 weeks is effective for initiation of treatment of anemia of chronic kidney disease.[2]
- There is a concern for severe red cell aplasia (caused by suppression of erythropoi-

esis) and risk for thrombosis secondary to treatment with recombinant human erythropoietin therapy.[3]

Evidence-Based References

1. American Medical Directors Association (AMDA): *Anemia in the long-term care setting*. Columbia, MD, 2007, American Medical Directors Association (AMDA).

2. Benz R et al: Epoetin alfa once every 2 weeks is effective for initiation of treatment of anemia of chronic kidney disease, *Clin J Am Soc Nephrol* 2(2):215-221, 2007.

3. Bunn HF: End run around Epo, *N Engl J Med* 361:1901-1903, 2009.

SUGGESTED READINGS

American Medical Directors Association (AMDA): *Anemia in the long-term care setting*. Columbia, MD, 2007, American Medical Directors Association (AMDA).

Artz AS, Ershler WB: Anemia in elderly persons, *eMedicine Journal,* last updated Sep 29, 2009. Available at www.emedicine.com.

Bunn HF: End run around Epo, *N Engl J Med* 361:1901-1903, 2009.

Chiari MM: Influence of acute inflammation on iron and nutritional status indexes in older inpatients, *J Am Geriatr Soc* 43(7):767-771, 1995.

AUTHOR: **NADIA MUJAHID, M.D.**

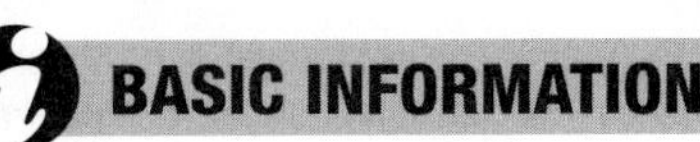

BASIC INFORMATION

DEFINITION

Aplastic anemia is a bone marrow failure syndrome defined by peripheral blood pancytopenia and hypocellular bone marrow.

SYNONYMS

Refractory anemia
Hypoplastic anemia

ICD-9CM CODES
284.9 Aplastic anemia
284.8 Acquired aplastic anemia
284.0 Congenital aplastic anemia

EPIDEMIOLOGY & DEMOGRAPHICS

INCIDENCE: The annual incidence of aplastic anemia is 2 cases per million.

PREDOMINANT SEX AND AGE: The incidence has two peaks, with most patients presenting between age 15 and 25 or after 60 yr.

PHYSICAL FINDINGS & CLINICAL PRESENTATION

- Mucosal bleeding, easy bruising, petechiae or heavy menstrual bleeding is seen secondary to thrombocytopenia.
- Fatigue, lassitude, skin pallor, exertional dyspnea, or palpitations are seen secondary to anemia.
- Infection is an uncommon presentation, but neutropenia may lead to fever and sore throat.
- Various physical manifestations like short stature, skeletal or nail changes may be seen in congenital forms of aplastic anemia.

ETIOLOGY

- In most patients with idiopathic aplastic anemia, bone marrow failure results from immunologically mediated, active destruction of blood-forming cells by lymphocytes. Section II describes the various disorders associated with aplastic anemia.
- Mutations in *TERT,* the gene for the RNA component of telomerase, cause short telomerases in congenital aplastic anemia and in some cases of apparently acquired hematopoietic failure.
- Common etiologic factors in acquired aplastic anemia include:
    - Toxins (e.g., benzene, insecticides)
    - Drugs (e.g., felbamate [Felbatol], cimetidine, NSAIDS, antiepileptics, gold salts, chloramphenicol, sulfonamides, trimethadione, quinacrine, phenylbutazone)
    - Ionizing irradiation
    - Infections (e.g., hepatitis C, HIV, Epstein-Barr virus, parvovirus B_{19})
- Inherited aplastic anemia
    - Fanconi's anemia
    - Reticular dysgenesis
    - Dyskeratosis congenita
    - Nonhematologic syndromes (Down syndrome, etc.)
    - Shwachman-Diamond syndrome
- Pregnancy
- Idiopathic

Dx DIAGNOSIS

DIFFERENTIAL DIAGNOSIS

- Bone marrow infiltration from lymphoma, carcinoma, myelofibrosis
- Severe infection
- Hypoplastic myelodysplastic syndrome or hypoplastic acute myeloid leukemia in adults
- Hypersplenism
- Hairy cell leukemia

WORKUP

- Diagnostic workup consists primarily of bone marrow aspiration and biopsy, and laboratory evaluation (CBC and examination of blood film).
- Bone marrow examination generally shows paucity or absence of erythropoietic and myelopoietic precursor cells; patients with pure red cell aplasia demonstrate only absence of red blood cell (RBC) precursors in the marrow.

LABORATORY TESTS

- CBC reveals pancytopenia. Macrocytosis and toxic granulation of neutrophils may also be present. Isolated cytopenias may occur in the early stages.
- Reticulocyte count reveals reticulocytopenia.
- Additional initial laboratory evaluation should include Ham test to exclude paroxysmal nocturnal hemoglobinuria and testing for hepatitis C.

IMAGING STUDIES

MRI with spin-echo sequence is helpful in the study of bone marrow disease, and the high fat content of an aplastic marrow can be easily seen on MRI.

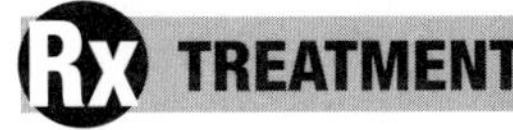

TREATMENT

NONPHARMACOLOGIC THERAPY

Discontinue any offending drugs or agents.

ACUTE GENERAL Rx

- Aggressive treatment of neutropenic fevers with parenteral broad-spectrum antibiotics.
- Administer platelet and RBC transfusions as needed; however, it is important to avoid transfusions in patients who are candidates for bone marrow transplantation.
- A treatment algorithm for aplastic anemia is described in Section III.

CHRONIC Rx

- Allogenic bone marrow transplantation (ABMT) from a human leukocyte antigen (HLA)–matched sibling donor is curative.
- Patients who do not have a matched sibling can be treated with a matched unrelated transplant, but the mortality rate is higher.
- Immunosuppressive therapy with anti-thymocyte globulin (ATG) is an effective alternate treatment for patients who are not candidates for ABMT.
- Other immunosuppressive agents such as cyclosporin, cyclophosphamide, or corticosteroids also have a role in the treatment of aplastic anemia.
- Androgens such as danazol are effective second-line agents.

DISPOSITION

- The most recent update of the European Group for Bone Marrow Translantation long-term survival rate has been reported to be 80%.
- Graft rejection and graft-versus-host disease are the major complications of ABMT.

REFERRAL

Hematology referral is indicated in all patients with aplastic anemia.

SUGGESTED READINGS

Bacigalupo A: Diagnosis and treatment of aplastic anemia, *Hematol Oncol Clin North Am* 23(2):159-170, 2009.

Gafter-Gavili A et al: ATG plus cyclosporine reduces all cause mortality in patients with aplastic anemia. Systemic review and meta analysis, *Acta Hematol* 120(4):237-243, 2008.

Sloand EM et al: Successful treatment of pure red-cell aplasia with an anti-interleukin-2 receptor antibody (Daclizumab), *Ann Intern Med* 144:181, 2006.

AUTHORS: **BILAL H. NAQVI, M.D.,** and **FRED F. FERRI, M.D.**

Anemia, Autoimmune Hemolytic

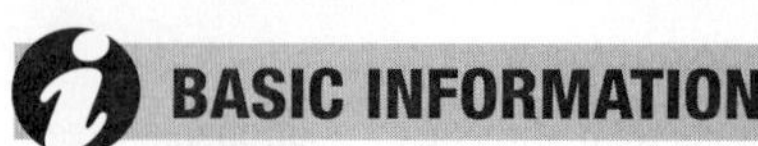

DEFINITION

Autoimmune hemolytic anemia (AIHA) is anemia secondary to premature destruction of red blood cells (RBCs) caused by the binding of autoantibodies and/or complement to RBCs.

ICD-9CM CODES
283.0 Autoimmune hemolytic anemia

EPIDEMIOLOGY & DEMOGRAPHICS

Predominant sex and age: most common in women <50 yr.

PHYSICAL FINDINGS & CLINICAL PRESENTATION

- Pallor, jaundice.
- Tachycardia with a flow murmur may be present if anemia is pronounced.
- Most common presentation is dyspnea and fatigue.
- Patients with intravascular hemolysis may present with dark urine and back pain.
- The presence of hepatomegaly and/or lymphadenopathy suggests an underlying lymphoproliferative disorder or malignancy; splenomegaly may indicate hypersplenism as a cause of hemolysis.

ETIOLOGY

- Warm antibody mediated: immunoglobulin (Ig) G (often idiopathic or associated with leukemia, lymphoma, thymoma, myeloma, viral infections, and collagen-vascular disease)
- Cold antibody mediated: IgM and complement in majority of cases (often idiopathic; at times associated with infections, lymphoma, or cold agglutinin disease)
- Drug induced: three major mechanisms:
  1. Antibody directed against Rh complex (e.g., methyldopa)
  2. Antibody directed against RBC-drug complex (hapten induced; e.g., penicillin)
  3. Antibody directed against complex formed by drug and plasma proteins; the drug-plasma protein-antibody complex causes destruction of RBCs (innocent bystander; e.g., quinidine)

Dx DIAGNOSIS

DIFFERENTIAL DIAGNOSIS

- Hemolytic anemia caused by membrane defects (paroxysmal nocturnal hemoglobinuria, spur cell anemia, Wilson disease)
- Non–immune mediated (microangiopathic hemolytic anemia, hypersplenism, cardiac valve prosthesis, giant cavernous hemangiomas, march hemoglobinuria, physical agents, infections, heavy metals, certain drugs [nitrofurantoin, sulfonamides])

WORKUP

Evaluation consists primarily of laboratory evaluation to confirm hemolysis and exclude other causes of the anemia. Although most cases of AIHA are idiopathic, potential causes should always be sought. Section III describes an algorithm for evaluation of suspected hemolytic anemia.

LABORATORY TESTS

- Initial laboratory tests: complete blood count (anemia), reticulocyte count (elevated), liver function studies (elevated indirect bilirubin, lactate dehydrogenase), evaluation of peripheral smear, Coombs test (positive direct Coombs test indicates presence of antibodies or complement on the surface of RBCs; positive indirect Coombs test implies presence of anti-RBC antibodies freely circulating in the patient's serum), haptoglobin level (decreased)
- IgG antibody and IgM antibody
- Hepatitis serology, antinuclear antibody
- Urinary tests may reveal hemosiderinuria or hemoglobinuria

IMAGING STUDIES

- Chest radiograph
- CT scan of chest and abdomen to rule out lymphoma should be considered

Rx TREATMENT

NONPHARMACOLOGIC THERAPY

- Discontinuation of any potentially offensive drugs
- Plasmapheresis exchange transfusion for severe life-threatening cases only
- Avoid cold exposure in patients with cold antibody

ACUTE GENERAL Rx

- Prednisone 1 to 2 mg/kg/day in divided doses initially in warm antibody autoimmune hemolytic anemia. Corticosteroids are generally ineffective in cold antibody autoimmune hemolytic anemia.
- Splenectomy in patients responding inadequately to corticosteroids when RBC sequestration studies indicate splenic sequestration.
- Immunosuppressive drugs and/or immunoglobulins only after both corticosteroids and splenectomy (unless surgery is contraindicated) have failed to produce an adequate remission.
- Danazol, typically used in conjunction with corticosteroids (may be useful in warm antibody autoimmune hemolytic anemia).
- Immunosuppressive drugs (azathioprine, cyclophosphamide) may be useful in warm antibody autoimmune hemolytic anemia but are indicated only after both corticosteroids and splenectomy (unless surgery is contraindicated) have failed to produce an adequate remission.

DISPOSITION

Prognosis is generally good unless anemia is associated with underlying disorder with a poor prognosis (e.g., leukemia, myeloma).

REFERRAL

- Hematology referral in all cases of AIHA
- Surgical referral for splenectomy in refractory cases

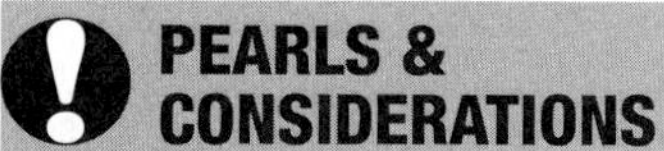

COMMENTS

- The direct Coombs test (also known as the direct antiglobulin test) demonstrates the presence of antibodies or complement on the surface of RBCs and is the hallmark of autoimmune hemolysis.
- Warm AIHA is often associated with autoimmune diseases, whereas cold AIHA often follows viral infections (e.g., mononucleosis) and *Mycoplasma pneumoniae* infections.
- HIV can induce both warm and cold AIHA.

SUGGESTED READINGS

Dhaliwal G et al: Hemolytic anemia, *Am Fam Physician* 69:2599, 2004.

Gehrs BC, Friedberg RC: Autoimmune hemolytic anemia, *Am J Hematol* 69:258, 2002.

AUTHOR: **FRED F. FERRI, M.D.**

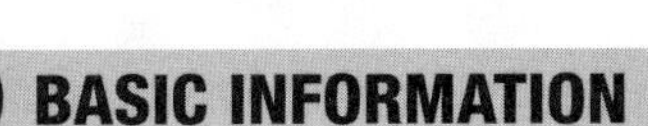

BASIC INFORMATION

DEFINITION

Iron deficiency anemia is anemia resulting from inadequate iron supplementation or excessive blood loss.

ICD-9CM CODES
280.9 Iron deficiency anemia
648.2 Iron deficiency anemia complicating pregnancy

EPIDEMIOLOGY & DEMOGRAPHICS

- Dietary iron deficiency occurs often in infants as a result of unsupplemented milk diets. It is also commonly seen in women during their reproductive years, as a result of heavy menstrual periods, and during pregnancy (increased demand).
- Iron deficiency is the most common nutritional deficiency worldwide.
- The prevalence of iron deficiency is greatest among toddlers ages 1 to 2 yr (7%) from inadequate intake and female individuals ages 12 to 49 yr (9% to 16%) from menstrual losses.
- The prevalence of iron deficiency is 2% in adult men, 9% to 12% in non-Hispanic white women, and 20% in black and Mexican American women.
- GI cancer is diagnosed in 10% of elderly patients with iron deficiency anemia.

PHYSICAL FINDINGS & CLINICAL PRESENTATION

- Most patients have normal examination results.
- Skin pallor and conjunctival pallor may be present.
- Signs and symptoms specific for iron deficiency are koilonychias, pica, pagophagia, and blue sclera.
- Patients with severe anemia can have palpitations, headache, weakness, dizziness, and easy fatigability.

ETIOLOGY

- Blood loss from GI or menstrual bleeding (genitourinary blood loss less often the cause)
- Dietary iron deficiency (rare in adults)
- Poor iron absorption in patients with gastric or small-bowel surgery
- Repeated phlebotomy
- Increased requirements (e.g., during pregnancy)
- Other: traumatic hemolysis (abnormally functioning cardiac valves), idiopathic pulmonary hemosiderosis (iron sequestration in pulmonary macrophages), paroxysmal nocturnal hemoglobinuria (intravascular hemolysis)
- The most common cause worldwide is hookworm infection

Dx DIAGNOSIS

DIFFERENTIAL DIAGNOSIS

- Anemia of chronic disease
- Sideroblastic anemia
- Thalassemia trait
- Lead poisoning

WORKUP

Diagnostic workup consists primarily of laboratory evaluation. Most patients with iron deficiency anemia are asymptomatic in the early stages. With progressive anemia, the major symptoms are fatigue, dizziness, exertional dyspnea, pagophagia (ice eating), and pica. Patient history may also suggest GI blood loss (melena, hematochezia, hemoptysis).

LABORATORY TESTS

- Laboratory results vary with the stage of deficiency.
- Absent iron marrow stores and decreased serum ferritin are the initial abnormalities.
- Decreased serum iron and increased total iron-binding capacity (TIBC) are the next abnormalities.
- Hypochromic microcytic anemia is present with significant iron deficiency.
- Peripheral smear in patients with iron deficiency generally reveals microcytic hypochromic red blood cells (RBCs) with a wide area of central pallor, anisocytosis, and poikilocytosis when severe.
- Laboratory abnormalities consistent with iron deficiency are low serum ferritin level, increased RBC distribution width with values generally >15, low mean corpuscular volume, low mean corpuscular hemoglobin, increased TIBC, and low serum iron.
- In patients diagnosed with iron deficiency anemia, a GI workup including an upper endoscopy and colonoscopy is necessary to look for source of iron loss.

Rx TREATMENT

The goal of therapy is to supply sufficient iron to correct the low hemoglobin and replenish iron stores.

NONPHARMACOLOGIC THERAPY

Patients should be instructed to consume foods that contain large amounts of iron, such as liver, red meat, and legumes.

ACUTE GENERAL Rx

- Treatment consists of ferrous sulfate 325 mg PO daily for at least 6 mo. Calcium supplements can decrease iron absorption; therefore, these two medications should be staggered.
- Parenteral iron therapy is reserved for patients with poor tolerance, noncompliance with oral preparations, or malabsorption.
- Transfusion of packed RBCs is indicated in patients with severe symptomatic anemia (e.g., angina) or life-threatening anemia.

CHRONIC Rx

Patients should be instructed to continue their iron supplements for at least 6 mo or longer to correct depleted body iron stores.

DISPOSITION

Most patients respond rapidly to iron supplementation with improvement in CBC and general well-being. GI side effects from oral iron therapy are common and may require decreased dosage to once every other day or to change to parenteral iron.

REFERRAL

GI referral for evaluation of GI malignancy is recommended in all patients with iron deficiency and suspected GI blood loss.

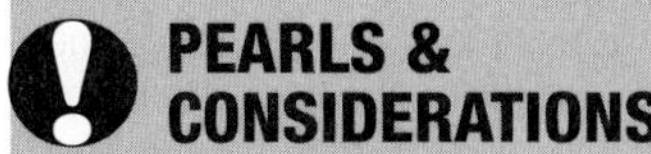

PEARLS & CONSIDERATIONS

COMMENTS

If the diagnosis of iron deficiency anemia is made, locating the suspected site of iron loss is mandatory.

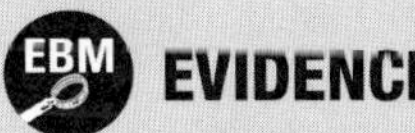

EVIDENCE

Please note: Complete text of EBM for this topic is available online.

Key trials and commentary:

One study assessed whether recombinant human erythropoietin (rhEPO) enhances a rise in hemoglobin concentration in postpartum anemia compared to intravenous iron alone. It revealed that in comparison to intravenous iron alone, the addition of rhEPO did not further increase haemoglobin concentration in women with postpartum anemia.

The authors of this study assessed 60 women postpartum who had a hemoglobin value of <80 g/L. They evaluated the impact of iron and iron plus rhEPO on recovery of the hemoglobin level postpartum. Three groups of patients were treated. All patients were given a single IV dose of 450 mg iron sucrose, and two groups were given either 20,000 or 40,000 U of rhEPO.

For the patients receiving rhEPO and iron, the doses were given on days 0 and 3. The end point of the study was the incremental improvement in hemoglobin level after 1 and 2 weeks. The trial was small, but no significant or dramatic difference was seen with regard to the administration of rhEPO in conjunction with IV iron. The mean increments in hemoglobin levels were 1.8 g/L after 1 week and 2.8 g/L after 2 weeks, regardless of the administration of rhEPO; hence, it remains clear that the administration of iron sucrose in this setting has the potential to significantly improve hemoglobin levels and that the addition of rhEPO does not seem to improve this. What is not clear is whether oral iron supplementation or simple observation would have a similar impact. However, because it is known that women in their third trimester of pregnancy develop iron deficiency anemia and that blood loss associated with parturition can be associated with iron deficiency anemia, it would seem logical that iron repletion would be appropriate in this setting.[1] Ⓐ

Another trial analyzed the effect of IV ferrous sucrose compared with oral ferrous sulphate on hematological parameters and quality of life in women with postpartum anemia. It revealed that women who received 600 mg IV iron sucrose followed by standard oral iron after four weeks, replenished their iron stores more rapidly and had a more favorable development of the fatigue score indicating improved quality of life.

This study addresses an important consideration for patients with iron deficiency anemia. That is, whether induction with IV iron sucrose therapy accelerates the recovery from anemia in patients with an uncomplicated anemia due to blood loss. Unlike patients with chronic illnesses such as autoimmune disorders or inflammatory conditions where mobilization of iron stores may be a problem, postpartum anemia is related to iron deficiency in a normal host. In this study, subjects received 3 doses of iron sucrose followed by oral maintenance therapy compared with oral replacement from day 1 in the standard-of-care group. Compliance was monitored by pill count, and both groups were equally compliant. Not surprisingly, the IV experimental arm was found to have a faster recovery of iron stores compared with oral replacement. In addition, this group had less fatigue, although no differences in the SF-36 quality of life scores were noted. Objectively, the IV group did not recover their hemoglobin any faster than the oral group, and there was no difference at longer time points. Hence, initial IV iron induction was not associated with any objective benefit in terms of the major endpoint, which was hemoglobin recovery. Explanation for the improvement in fatigue may well lie with the fact that the two arms of the study were not double blinded, and, hence, patients receiving IV iron may have experienced an improvement in their fatigue due to the impression that the experimental arm would be superior. This trial is an excellent example of the need for double blinding. One cannot conclude that IV iron, clearly more expensive, provides any objective evidence of benefit in this patient population with normal bone marrow function.[2] Ⓐ

Evidence-Based References

1. Wågström E, Åkesson A, van Rooijen M: Erythropoietin and intravenous iron therapy in postpartum anaemia, *Acta Obstet Gynecol Scand* 86:957-962, 2007. Commentary by M.S. Gordon, M.D. Ⓐ

2. Westad S, Backe B, Salvesen KÅ: A 12-week randomised study comparing intravenous iron sucrose versus oral ferrous sulphate for treatment of postpartum anemia, *Acta Obstet Gynecol Scand* 87:916-923, 2008. Commentary by M.S. Gordon, M.D. Ⓐ

SUGGESTED READINGS

Alleyne A et al: Individualized treatment for iron-deficiency anemia in adults, *Am J Med* 121:943-948, 2008.

Clark SF: Iron deficiency anemia diagnosis and management, *Curr Opin Gastroenterol* 25(2):122-128, 2009. Review.

Killip S et al: Iron deficiency anemia, *Am Fam Physician* 75:671, 2007.

AUTHORS: **BILAL H. NAQVI, M.D.,** and **FRED F. FERRI, M.D.**

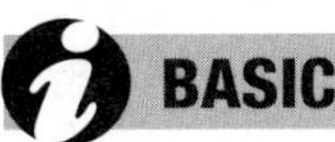

BASIC INFORMATION

DEFINITION

Pernicious anemia (PA) is an autoimmune disease resulting from antibodies against intrinsic factor and gastric parietal cells.

SYNONYMS

Megaloblastic anemia resulting from vitamin B_{12} deficiency

ICD-9CM CODES
281.0 Pernicious anemia

EPIDEMIOLOGY & DEMOGRAPHICS

- Increased incidence in females and older adults (diagnosis is unusual before age 35 yr)
- The overall prevalence of undiagnosed PA after age 60 yr is 1.9%
- Prevalence is highest in women (2.7%), particularly in black women (4.3%)
- Increased incidence of autoimmune disease (e.g., type 1 diabetes mellitus, Graves disease, Addison disease), *Helicobacter pylori* infection

PHYSICAL FINDINGS & CLINICAL PRESENTATION

- Mucosal pallor, glossitis
- Peripheral sensory neuropathy with paresthesias initially and absent reflexes in advanced cases
- Loss of joint position sense, pyramidal or long track signs
- Possible splenomegaly and mild hepatomegaly
- Generalized weakness and delirium/dementia

ETIOLOGY

- Gastric/antiparietal cell antibodies in >70% of patients; antiintrinsic factor antibodies in >50% of patients
- Atrophic gastric mucosa
- Inborn errors of cobalamin-cofactor synthesis are rare. The cobalamin gene *(cblD)* is localized to human chromosome 2q23.2. Mutations in the gene designated MMADHC (methylmalonic aciduria, cblD type, and homocystinuria) are responsible for the cblD defect in vitamin B_{12} metabolism.
- An etiopathophysiologic classification of cobalamin deficiency is described in Section II.

DIAGNOSIS

DIFFERENTIAL DIAGNOSIS

- Nutritional vitamin B_{12} deficiency
- Malabsorption
- Chronic alcoholism (multifactorial)
- Chronic gastritis related to *H. pylori* infection
- Folic acid deficiency
- Myelodysplasia

WORKUP

- The clinical presentation of pernicious anemia varies with the stage. Initially, patients may be asymptomatic. In advanced stages patients may have impaired memory, depression, gait disturbances, paresthesias, and reports of generalized weakness.
- Investigation consists primarily of laboratory evaluation.
- Endoscopy and biopsy for atrophic gastritis may be performed in selected cases.
- Diagnosis is crucial because failure to treat may result in irreversible neurologic deficits.

LABORATORY TESTS

- Complete blood count generally reveals macrocytic anemia and leukopenia with hypersegmented neutrophils.
- Mean corpuscular volume (MCV) is generally significantly elevated in the advanced stages.
- Reticulocyte count is low to normal.
- Falsely low serum cobalamin levels can occur in patients with severe folate deficiency, in patients using high doses of ascorbic acid, and when cobalamin levels are measured after nuclear medicine studies (radioactivity interferes with cobalamin radioimmunoassay measurement).
- Falsely high normal levels in patients with cobalamin deficiency can occur in severe liver disease or chronic granulocytic leukemia.
- The absence of anemia or macrocytosis does not exclude the diagnosis of cobalamin deficiency. Anemia is absent in 20% of patients with cobalamin deficiency, and macrocytosis is absent in >30% of patients at the time of diagnosis. It can be blocked by concurrent iron deficiency or anemia of chronic disease and may be masked by thalassemia trait.
- Schilling test is abnormal in part I; part II corrects to normal after administration of intrinsic factor.
- Laboratory tests used for detecting cobalamin deficiency in patients with normal vitamin B_{12} levels include serum and urinary methylmalonic acid level (elevated), total homocysteine level (elevated), intrinsic factor antibody (positive).
- An increased concentration of plasma methylmalonic acid does not predict clinical manifestations of vitamin B_{12} deficiency and should not be used as the only marker for diagnosis of B_{12} deficiency.
- Additional laboratory abnormalities can include elevated lactate dehydrogenase, direct hyperbilirubinemia, and decreased haptoglobin.

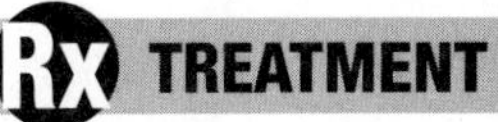

TREATMENT

NONPHARMACOLOGIC THERAPY

Avoid folic acid supplementation without proper vitamin B_{12} supplementation.

ACUTE GENERAL Rx

Traditional therapy of a cobalamin deficiency consists of IM injections of vitamin B_{12} 1000 μg/wk for the initial 4 to 6 wk followed by 1000 μg/mo IM indefinitely. When hematologic parameters have returned to normal range, intranasal cyanocobalamin may be used in place of IM cyanocobalamin. The initial dose of intranasal cyanocobalamin (Nascobal) is 1 spray (500 μg) in one nostril once per week. Cost generally exceeds $120/mo. Monitor response and increase dose if serum B_{12} levels decline. Consider return to intramuscular vitamin B_{12} supplementation if decline persists.

CHRONIC Rx

Parenteral vitamin B_{12} 1000 μg/mo or intranasal cyanocobalamin 500 μg/wk (see "Acute General Rx") for the remainder of life

DISPOSITION

Anemia generally resolves with appropriate treatment. Neurologic deficits, if present at diagnosis, may be permanent.

REFERRAL

Gastrointestinal referral for endoscopy on diagnosis of pernicious anemia and surveillance endoscopy every 5 yr to rule out gastric carcinoma

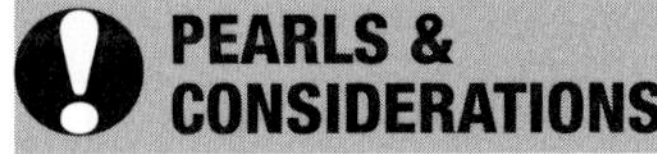

PEARLS & CONSIDERATIONS

COMMENTS

- Patients must understand that therapy is lifelong.
- Self-injection of vitamin B_{12} may be taught in selected patients. Cost of monthly injection is less than $5.
- Oral cobalamin (1000 to 2000 μg/day) has been reported as also being effective in mild cases of pernicious anemia because approximately 1% of an oral dose is absorbed by passive diffusion, a pathway that does not require intrinsic factor. Cost for 1 mo of therapy is approximately $5.

SUGGESTED READING

Coelho D et al: Gene identification for the cblD defect of vitamin B_{12} metabolism, *N Engl J Med* 358:1454-1464, 2008.

AUTHOR: **FRED F. FERRI, M.D.**

Anemia, Sideroblastic (ALG)

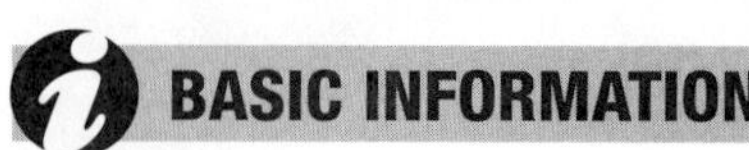

BASIC INFORMATION

DEFINITION

Sideroblastic anemia is a heterogenous group of blood disorders whose two distinctive features are ring sideroblasts in the bone marrow (abnormal erythroblasts with excessive iron accumulation in the mitochondria) and impaired heme biosynthesis. They are classified as hereditary, acquired, and reversible.

SYNONYMS

Hereditary sideroblastic anemias
Acquired idiopathic sideroblastic anemia (AISA)
Reversible sideroblastic anemias

ICD-9CM CODES
285.0 Sideroblastic anemia

EPIDEMIOLOGY & DEMOGRAPHICS

- Sex-linked; primarily affects males.
- AISA affects middle-aged and older adults.

PHYSICAL FINDINGS & CLINICAL PRESENTATION

The symptoms for sideroblastic anemia are the same for any anemia and iron overload:

- Fatigue, weakness, palpitations, shortness of breath, headaches, irritability, and chest pain.
- Physical findings may include pallor, tachycardia, hepatosplenomegaly, S3 gallop, jugular vein distension, and rales.

ETIOLOGY

- The hereditary forms can be X-linked, autosomal dominant or autosomal recessive.
- Acquired forms may be associated with chemotherapy or irradiation.
- Refractory anemia with ringed sideroblast develops as a subtype of myelodysplacia.
- Reversible sideroblastic anemia can be caused by alcohol, isoniazid, pyrazinamide, cycloserine, chloramphenicol, or copper deficiency.

Dx DIAGNOSIS

The principle feature is indolent and progressive, mild, lifelong anemia that goes unnoticed. Symptoms of iron overload may lead to discovery of the underlying disorder. The history and clinical findings, together with typical laboratory findings, usually permit accurate diagnosis of each type of sideroblastic anemia. The molecular defects can be identified in several hereditary forms and in some patients with AISA.

DIFFERENTIAL DIAGNOSIS

- Sideroblastic anemia must be differentiated from other causes of microcytic hypochromic anemia: iron deficiency anemia, thalassemia, anemia of chronic disease, and lead poisoning.
- Tissue iron overload from sideroblastic anemia may act similar to hereditary hemochromatosis with liver cirrhosis, diabetes, congestive heart failure, or cardiac arrhythmias.

WORKUP

Laboratory evaluation: complete blood count, iron studies, free erythrocyte protoporphyrin level (FEP); MRI, bone marrow aspiration, and liver biopsy.

LABORATORY TESTS

- Hypochromic microcytic anemia for the hereditary type and normo or macrocytic anemia for AISA.
- High serum iron levels, low transferrin along with increased transferrin saturation and high serum ferritin.
- Peripheral smear: dimorphic large and small cells revealing Pappenheimer bodies or siderocytes when stained for iron.
- Bone marrow shows the classic ringed sideroblasts not seen in normal bone marrow tissue (Fig. 1-16). The ringed sideroblasts represent iron storage in the mitochondria of normoblasts.
- In transfusion-dependent anemias, monitoring of ferritin and transferrin saturation levels is recommended despite minimal transfusion needs to avoid iron overload.
- Features of infective erethropoeisis like increase in bilirubin concentration, decrease in hepatoglobin, increase in LDH, and normal or increase in reticulocyte no is seen.

Rx TREATMENT

Treatment is directed at controlling symptoms of anemia and preventing organ damage from iron overload.

NONPHARMACOLOGIC THERAPY

Avoid alcohol

ACUTE GENERAL Rx

- A trial of pyridoxine (100-200 mg) is indicated for all patients with hereditary sideroblastic anemia.
- 25% to 50% may show full or partial response to pyridoxine.
- Patients who do not respond will need to be treated with blood transfusion.
- Chelation therapy is needed for patients with transfusion-dependant anemia to prevent complications of iron overload.
- Erythropoietin and granulocyte colony-stimulating factor may show some success in treating MDS-associated refractory anemia with ringed sideroblast.
- Secondary sideroblastic anemia caused by medication can be reversed by withdrawing the medication and administering vitamin B_6 (50 to 200 mg/day).

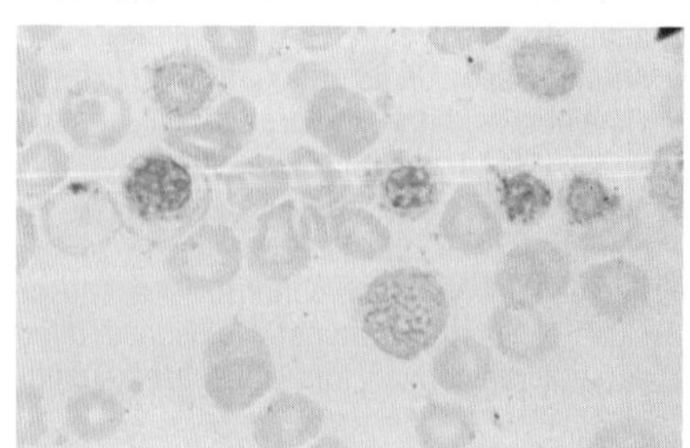

FIGURE 1-16 Prussian blue iron stain of the bone marrow shows ringed sideroblasts. (From Goldman L, Ausiello D [eds]: *Cecil textbook of medicine,* ed 22, Philadelphia, 2004, WB Saunders.)

CHRONIC Rx

- Organ dysfunction resulting from iron overload will require periodic phlebotomy to keep serum ferritin level <500 mcg/L.
- Iron chelating therapy for patients with moderately severe anemia in those who require regular red cell transfusion: deferoxamine continuous infusion or the oral agent deferasirox (EXJADE)
- Splenectomy should be avoided at all costs.

DISPOSITION

In patients with anemia alone, life expectancy is normal. In patients dependent on blood transfusions, morbidity from iron overload can be expected. Some patients with acquired sideroblastic anemia develop leukemia. There are two types of AISA:

1. Pure sideroblastic anemia: with dysplasia confined to the erythroid cell lineage; survival similar to age-matched controls; no incidence of leukemic transformation.
2. Refractory anemia with ringed sideroblasts: dysplastic features involving the red cell lineage, granulopoeisis and/or megakaryopoiesis; approximately 5% will develop acute leukemia. Erythropoietin and granulocyte colony-stimulating factor therapy do not change survival.

REFERRAL

- Hematology.
- Families with severe forms of hereditary sideroblastic anemia should receive genetic counseling.

PEARLS & CONSIDERATIONS

- Sideroblastic anemia can be thought of as an iron-loading anemia secondary to defective heme synthesis.
- A predisposition to leukemia evolution has not been observed in patients with hereditary forms.
- Symptoms rather than an absolute hemoglobin level or hematocrit should guide transfusion therapy.

COMMENTS

Vitamin B_6, or pyridoxal phosphate, is a required cofactor in heme synthesis, and drugs such as isoniazid, cycloserine, and pyrazinamide can inhibit its function.

SUGGESTED READINGS

Alcindor T, Bridges KR: Sideroblastic anemias, *Br J Hematol* 116(4):733, 2002.
Bottomley SS: Congenital sideroblastic anemias, *Current Hematol Rep* 5(1):41, 2006.

AUTHOR: **BILAL H. NAQVI, M.D.**

BASIC INFORMATION

DEFINITION

An abdominal aortic aneurysm (AAA) is a permanent localized dilation of the abdominal aortic artery to at least 1.5 times the diameter measured at the level of the renal arteries. The normal diameter at the renal arteries is 2.0 cm (range, 1.4 to 3.0 cm), and a diameter >3.0 cm is generally considered aneurysmal.

SYNONYMS

AAA

ICD-9CM CODES

441.4 Aneurysm, abdominal (aorta)
441.3 Ruptured abdominal aortic aneurysm

EPIDEMIOLOGY & DEMOGRAPHICS

- AAA is predominantly a disease of older adults, affecting men more than women (4:1).
- The prevalence rate ranges from 4% to 9% in men >60 yr.
- Clinically important AAAs >4.0 cm are present in 1% of men ages 55 to 64 yr, and the prevalence rate increases by 2% to 4% per decade thereafter.
- Approximately 15,000 deaths/yr in the U.S. are attributed to AAA.
- Rupture of an AAA is the tenth leading cause of death in men >55 yr.
- Risk factors for AAA are similar to other atherosclerotic cardiovascular diseases, including smoking, hypertension, hyperlipidemia, male sex, peripheral vascular disease, and family history of AAA.

PHYSICAL FINDINGS & CLINICAL PRESENTATION

- Most aneurysms are asymptomatic and incidentally discovered on imaging studies; however, symptomatic aneurysms are at an increased risk for rupture
- Physical examination has a sensitivity of 76% for detecting AAAs >5 cm and only 29% for AAAs 3.0 to 3.9 cm
- Pulsatile epigastric mass that may or may not be tender
- Abdominal pain radiating to the back, flank, and groin
- Early satiety, nausea, and vomiting caused by compression of adjacent bowel
- Venous thrombosis from iliocaval venous compression
- Discoloration and pain of the feet from distal embolization of the thrombus within the aneurysm
- Flank and groin pain from ureteral obstruction and hydronephrosis
- Rupture presents as shock, organ hypoperfusion, and abdominal distention
- Rare presentations include hematemesis or melena associated with abdominal and back pain in patients with aortoenteric fistulas
- Aortocaval fistulas may also form and produce loud abdominal bruits

ETIOLOGY

- Atherosclerotic (degenerative or nonspecific)
- Genetic (e.g., Ehlers-Danlos syndrome)
- Traumatic
- Cystic medial necrosis (Marfan's syndrome)
- Arteritis, inflammatory
- Mycotic, infected (syphilis)
- Familial clusters (genetic defects in elastin and collagen degradation by proteases such as plasmin, matrix metalloproteinases, and cathepsin S and K)

NATURAL HISTORY

- Understanding the natural history of AAA is important in its management. The likelihood that an aneurysm will rupture is largely influenced by aneurysm diameter, rate of expansion, and sex. Other factors associated with increased risk for rupture include continued smoking, uncontrolled hypertension, and increased wall stress.
- The 5-yr rupture rate of asymptomatic AAAs is 25% to 40% for aneurysms >5.0 cm, 1% to 7% for AAAs of 4.0 to 5.0 cm, and nearly 0% for AAAs <4.0 cm.
- One study showed that the mean expansion rate for ruptured aneurysms was 0.82 vs. 0.42 cm/yr for nonruptured aneurysms.
- The rate of rupture of aneurysms that were 4.0 to 5.5 cm in diameter is four times greater in women compared with men.
- Mortality rate after rupture is >90% because most patients do not reach the hospital in time for surgical repair. Of those who reach the hospital, the mortality rate is still 50% compared with the 1% to 4% mortality rate for elective repair of a nonruptured AAA.

DIAGNOSIS

DIFFERENTIAL DIAGNOSIS

Almost 75% of AAAs are asymptomatic and are discovered on routine examination or serendipitously when ordering studies for other symptoms. Diagnosis of AAA should be considered in the differential of the following conditions:

- Abdominal pain
- Back pain
- Pulsatile abdominal mass

IMAGING STUDIES

- Abdominal ultrasound is nearly 100% accurate in identifying an aneurysm and estimating the size to within 0.3 to 0.4 cm. It is not accurate in estimating the extension to the renal arteries or the iliac arteries.
- CT scan is recommended for preoperative aneurysm imaging and estimates the size of the AAA to within 0.3 mm. There are no false-negative results, and the scan can localize the extent to renal vessels with more precision than ultrasound. CT can also detect the integrity of the wall and exclude rupture.
- Angiography gives detailed arterial anatomy, localizing the aneurysm relative to the renal and visceral arteries. This is the definitive preoperative study before surgery.
- Magnetic resonance angiography may also be used and is at least as accurate as CT, but it is more expensive and not as readily available.

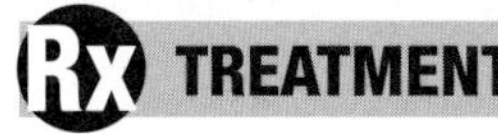

TREATMENT

NONPHARMACOLOGIC THERAPY

- Despite lack of data substantiating reduction in expansion rate through treatment of cardiac risk factors, nonpharmacologic treatment continues to focus on risk factor modification (most importantly smoking cessation, diet, and exercise).
- Serial studies have shown that expansion rates are faster in current smokers than in former smokers.
- Definitive treatment depends on the size of the aneurysm (see "Chronic Rx").

ACUTE GENERAL Rx

- AAA rupture is an emergency.
- Emergent open repair is the traditional method of treatment. However, more centers are increasingly using endovascular repair for patients who fit certain anatomic and physiologic criteria.

CHRONIC Rx

- Blood pressure and fasting lipids should be monitored and controlled as recommended for patients with atherosclerotic disease. Antihyperlipidemic agents such as the statin family of drugs should be prescribed unless contraindications are present.
- The most commonly used predictor of rupture is the maximum diameter of the AAA.
- Monitoring by ultrasound or CT scan should be performed every 6 to 12 months for AAAs measuring 4.0 to 5.4 cm. In patients with AAAs smaller than 4.0 cm, every 2 to 3 yr is reasonable.
- Beta-blocker therapy may have a role in slowing AAA expansion rates, but conclusive evidence is still lacking.
- Antibiotics such as doxycycline and roxithromycin have potential to limit the growth of AAAs, as shown in small human studies with promising results.
- Surgical repair to eliminate the risk for rupture should be performed for patients with infrarenal or juxtarenal AAA of approximately 5.5 cm. Repair is possibly beneficial for AAAs of 5.0 to 5.4 cm.
- Intervention is not recommended for asymptomatic infrarenal or juxtarenal AAAs <5.0 cm in men or 4.5 cm in women.
- For the high-risk patient, percutaneous, endovascular, stent-anchored grafts placed with the patient under local anesthesia have provided an alternative approach (Fig. 1-17).
- Research is ongoing to determine the appropriate low or average surgical risk patients for which the endovascular approach may be an elective option. Short-term outcomes are comparable, if not better than open repair, and long-term outcome data are accumulating and promising.

REFERRAL

Vascular surgical referral should be made in asymptomatic patients with AAAs that are approximately 4.0 cm or in rapidly expanding aneurysms of 0.6 to 0.8 cm/yr, especially if symptoms are present.

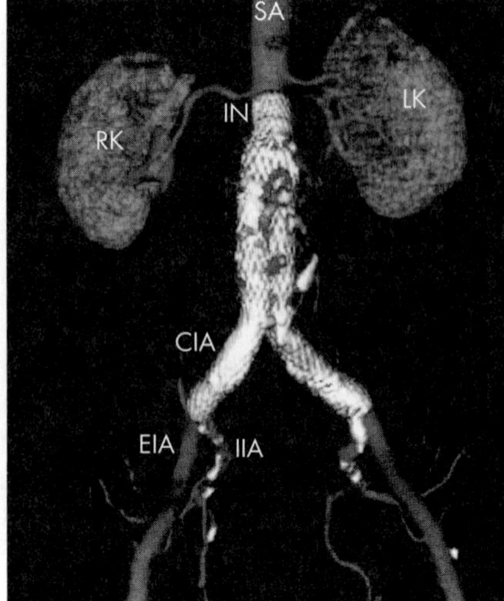

FIGURE 1-17 Endovascular abdominal aortic aneurysm repair involves aneurysm exclusion with an endoluminal aortic stent-graft introduced remotely, usually through the femoral artery. An endovascular graft extends from the infrarenal aorta to both common iliac arteries, preserving the flow to the internal iliac arteries. *SA,* Suprarenal aorta; *IN,* infrarenal aortic neck; *CIA,* common iliac artery; *IIA,* internal iliac artery; *RK,* right kidney; *LK,* left kidney. (From Townsend CM et al [eds]: *Sabiston textbook of surgery,* ed 17, Philadelphia, 2004, Saunders.)

PEARLS & CONSIDERATIONS

- Screening by physical examination and ultrasound should be performed for men age 60 yr who are either the siblings or offspring of patients with AAA and for men ages 65 to 75 yr who have ever smoked.
- Repairing AAAs smaller than 5.5 cm has not been shown to improve survival.
- Endovascular repair is associated with lower operative mortality than open repair, similar mid-term mortality and unknown long-term mortality, and it has not been shown to improve survival in patients unfit for open repair.

COMMENTS

- Most AAAs are infrarenal.
- Surgical risk is increased in patients with coexisting coronary artery disease, pulmonary disease, liver cirrhosis, or chronic renal failure. Evaluation for ischemia and aggressive perioperative hemodynamic monitoring help identify high-risk patients and decrease postoperative complications.
- It is estimated that AAAs <5 cm expand at a rate of 0.4 cm/yr.

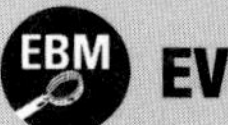

EVIDENCE

Although one multicenter randomized controlled trial (RCT) documented improved perioperative mortality and lower complication rates up to 30 days after surgery in patients randomized to endovascular repair of aneurysms >5 cm vs. open repair, another large RCT found no difference in all-cause mortality between these two treatments at 4-yr follow-up in patients >60 yr old with aneurysms of at least 5.5 cm in diameter.[1,2] Ⓐ

A further RCT in patients >60 yr old, unfit for open repair, with aneurysms >5.5 cm in diameter, found no difference in all-cause mortality at 4 yr between those treated with endovascular repair and those receiving no intervention.[3] Ⓐ

Evidence-Based References

1. Prinssen M et al: Dutch Randomized Endovascular Aneurysm Management (DREAM) trial group. A randomized trial comparing conventional and endovascular repair of abdominal aortic aneurysms, *N Engl J Med* 351:1607-1618, 2004. Ⓐ

2. EVAR trial participants: Endovascular aneurysm repair versus open repair in patients with abdominal aortic aneurysm (EVAR trial 1), *Lancet* 365:2179-2186, 2005. Ⓐ

3. EVAR trial participants: Endovascular aneurysm repair and outcome in patients unfit for open repair of abdominal aortic aneurysm (EVAR trial 2), *Lancet* 365:2187-2192, 2005. Ⓐ

SUGGESTED READINGS

Fleming C et al: Screening for abdominal aortic aneurysm: a best-evidence systematic review for the U.S. Preventive Services Task Force, *Ann Intern Med* 142(3):203, 2005.

Hirsch AT et al: ACC/AHA 2005. Practice guidelines for the management of patients with peripheral arterial disease (lower extremity, renal, mesenteric, and abdominal aortic): a collaborative report, *Circulation* 113(11):e463-e465, 2006.

Lederle FA et al: Systematic review: repair of unruptured abdominal aortic aneurysm, *Ann Intern Med* 146(10):735, 2007.

Upchurch GR, Schaub TA: Abdominal aortic aneurysm, *Am Fam Physician* 73:1198, 2006.

AUTHORS: **KHIET C. HOANG, M.D.,**
and **PRANAV M. PATEL, M.D.**

BASIC INFORMATION

DEFINITION

Angina pectoris is characterized by discomfort that occurs when myocardial oxygen demand exceeds supply. Myocardial ischemia can be asymptomatic (silent ischemia), particularly in diabetics. Angina can be classified as follows:

1. Chronic (stable):
   - Usually follows a precipitating event (e.g., climbing stairs, sexual intercourse, a heavy meal, emotional stress, cold weather).
   - Generally same severity as previous attacks; relieved by rest or by the customary dose of nitroglycerin.
   - Caused by a fixed coronary artery obstruction secondary to atherosclerosis. The presence of one or more obstructions in major coronary arteries is likely; the severity of stenosis is usually >70%.
2. Unstable (rest or crescendo, coronary syndrome):
   - Recent onset
   - Increasing severity, duration, or frequency of chronic angina
   - Occurs at rest or with minimal exertion
3. Prinzmetal's variant:
   - Occurs at rest
   - Manifests electrocardiographically as episodic ST-segment elevations
   - Caused by coronary artery spasms with or without superimposed coronary artery disease (CAD)
   - Patients also more likely to develop ventricular arrhythmias
4. Microvascular angina (syndrome X):
   - Refers to patients with normal coronary angiograms and no coronary spasm but chest pain resembling angina and positive exercise test.
   - Defective endothelium-dependent dilation in the coronary microcirculation contributing to the altered regulation of myocardial perfusion and the ischemic manifestations in these patients.
   - Patients with chest pain and normal or nonobstructive coronary angiograms are predominantly women, and many have a prognosis that is not as benign as commonly thought (2% risk of death or myocardial infarction [MI] at 30 days of follow-up).
   - Useful therapeutic agents for symptom relief are beta-blockers, angiotensin-converting enzyme (ACE) inhibitors, and tricyclic agents. Aggressive antiatherosclerotic therapy with statins should also be undertaken.
5. Other:
   - Angina due to aortic stenosis and idiopathic hypertrophic subaortic stenosis, cocaine-induced coronary vasoconstriction.
6. Refractory angina:
   - Refers to patients who, despite optimal medical therapy, have both angina and objective evidence of ischemia and are not considered candidates for revascularization.
   - Current FDA-approved therapies consist of enhanced external counterpulsation; transcutaneous electrical nerve stimulation; and invasive therapies such as spinal cord stimulation, transmyocardial revascularization, and percutaneous myocardial revascularization. Although some of these therapies may improve symptoms and quality of life, they have not been shown to improve mortality rate.

FUNCTIONAL CLASSIFICATION

- New York Heart Association Functional Classification of angina:
  - Class I: angina only with unusually strenuous activity.
  - Class II: angina with slightly more prolonged or rigorous activity than usual.
  - Class III: angina with usual daily activity.
  - Class IV: angina at rest.
- Grading of angina by the Canadian Cardiovascular Society Classification System:
  - Class I: ordinary physical activity does not cause angina, such as walking, climbing stairs. Angina occurs with strenuous, rapid, or prolonged exertion at work or recreation.
  - Class II: Slight limitation of ordinary activity. Angina occurs on walking or climbing stairs rapidly; walking uphill; walking or stair climbing after meals, in cold, in wind, or under emotional stress; or only during the few hours after awakening. Angina occurs on walking more than two level blocks and climbing more than one flight of ordinary stairs at a normal pace and in normal condition.
  - Class III: Marked limitations of ordinary physical activity. Angina occurs on walking one to two level blocks and climbing one flight of stairs in normal conditions and at a normal pace.
  - Class IV: Inability to carry on any physical activity without discomfort; anginal symptoms may be present at rest.

ICD-9CM CODES

411.1 Angina, stable
413 Angina pectoris
413.1 Prinzmetal's angina
413.9 Angina, unspecified

EPIDEMIOLOGY & DEMOGRAPHICS

- Angina is most common in middle-aged and elderly men.
- Women are usually affected after menopause.
- Prevalence of angina pectoris in people older than 30 yr is >3%.
- Within 12 mo of initial diagnosis, 10% to 20% of patients with diagnosis of stable angina progress to MI or unstable angina.

PHYSICAL FINDINGS & CLINICAL PRESENTATION

- Although there is significant individual variation, most patients report substernal chest pain (pressure, tightness, heaviness, sharp pain, sensation similar to intestinal gas or dysphagia).
- The pain is of short duration (30 sec to 30 min); nonpleuritic; and often accompanied by shortness of breath, nausea, diaphoresis, and numbness or pain in the left arm, jaw, or shoulder.
- Women are significantly less likely to report chest pain or discomfort compared with men.

ETIOLOGY

UNCONTROLLABLE RISK FACTORS FOR ANGINA:

- Advanced age
- Male sex
- Genetic predisposition

MODIFIABLE RISK FACTORS FOR ANGINA:

- Smoking (risk is almost double).
- Hypertension (risk is double if systolic blood pressure is >180 mm Hg).
- Hyperlipidemia.
- Impaired glucose tolerance or diabetes mellitus.
- Obesity (weight >30% over ideal). A higher body mass index during childhood is also associated with an increased risk of coronary heart disease (CHD) in adulthood.
- Hypothyroidism.
- Left ventricular hypertrophy (LVH).
- Sedentary lifestyle.
- Oral contraceptive use.
- Cocaine use (cocaine is used by >5 million Americans regularly and is responsible for >64,000 emergency department [ED] evaluations yearly to rule out myocardial ischemia).
- Metabolic syndrome.
- The development of coronary artery calcium is associated with an increased risk of MI.
- Long-term use of nonsteroidal antiinflammatory drugs is associated with increased cardiovascular risk.
- Exposure to air pollution from traffic (dilute diesel exhaust) promotes myocardial ischemia and is associated with adverse cardiovascular events.
- Low serum folate levels. (Folate is required for conversion of homocysteine to methionine. Hyperhomocysteinemia has a toxic effect on vascular endothelium and interferes with proliferation of arterial wall smooth muscle cells. Folate deficiencies are associated with an increased risk of fatal CHD.)
- Elevated homocysteine levels. Elevated plasma homocysteine level is a strong and independent risk factor for CHD events, especially in patients with type 2 diabetes mellitus. Trials lowering homocysteine levels have, however, been disappointing because lowering therapy with folate did not prevent cardiovascular events among patients with coronary disease.
- Elevated levels of highly sensitive C-reactive protein (hs-CRP, cardio CRP).
- Depression.
- Vasculitis.
- Elevated levels of lipoprotein-associated phospholipase A2.
- Elevated fibrinogen levels.

- Low level of red blood cell glutathione peroxidase-1 activity.

Dx DIAGNOSIS

DIFFERENTIAL DIAGNOSIS

Noncardiac pain mimicking angina may be caused by:

- Pulmonary diseases (pulmonary hypertension, pulmonary embolism, pleurisy, pneumothorax, pneumonia)
- Gastrointestinal disorders (peptic ulcer disease, pancreatitis, esophageal spasm or spontaneous esophageal muscle contraction, esophageal reflux, cholecystitis, cholelithiasis)
- Musculoskeletal conditions (costochondritis, chest wall trauma, cervical arthritis with radiculopathy, muscle strain, myositis)
- Acute aortic dissection
- Herpes zoster
- Anxiety disorder

WORKUP

- In patients with chest pain, the probability of CAD should be estimated on the basis of patient age, sex, cardiovascular risk factors, and pain characteristics.
- The most important diagnostic factor is the history. Chest pain or left arm pain or discomfort reproducing previously documented angina and a known history of CAD or MI are indicative of high likelihood of acute coronary syndrome.
- The physical examination is of little diagnostic help and may be completely normal in many patients, although the presence of an S_4 gallop is suggestive of ischemic chest pain. Transient mitral regurgitation, hypotension, diaphoresis, and rales indicate a high likelihood of acute coronary syndrome.
- An ECG taken during the acute episode may show transient T-wave inversion or ST-segment depression or elevation, but more than 50% of patients with chronic stable angina have normal results on resting ECG.
- Patients with intermediate or high probability should undergo risk stratification through further testing. Treadmill exercise tolerance test is useful to identify patients with CAD who would benefit from cardiac catheterization. Stress echocardiogram or radionuclide testing (e.g., thallium, Persantine, dobutamine) is useful and sensitive in the detection of myocardial ischemia.
- Although invasive, coronary angiography remains the gold standard for the identification of clinically significant CAD. Coronary magnetic resonance angiography can also detect CAD of the proximal and middle segments. This noninvasive approach, where available, can be used to reliably identify (or rule out) left main coronary artery or three-vessel disease.
- Multidetector computed tomography (MDCT) is a newer screening modality for CAD. Its advantages are its speed, safety, and low cost compared with angiography. It has high sensitivity and negative predictive value. Its limitations are as follows: limited to patients with a regular rhythm and slow rates, poor image in morbidly obese patients, inaccurate visualization of the coronary artery within a stent, and decreased diagnostic accuracy in older patients from the prevalence and severity of coronary calcifications with increasing age. Its routine use in clinical practice is not justified. However, it may be useful in excluding coronary disease in selected patients in whom a false-positive result or inconclusive stress test is suspected.

LABORATORY TESTS

- Initial laboratory tests in patients with chronic stable angina should include hemoglobin, fasting glucose, and fasting lipid panel.
- Cardiac isoenzymes (CK-MB q8h $\times$ 2) should be obtained to rule out MI in patients with acute chest pain.
- Cardiac troponins I and T are specific markers of myocardial necrosis and are useful in evaluating patients with acute chest pain. Elevation of either of these proteins in the setting of an acute coronary syndrome identifies patients with a several-fold increased risk of death in subsequent weeks. Patients with negative troponin assays on arrival in the ED and repeated 4 hr later are at a low level of risk for cardiac events within the following 30 days, and most of these patients can be safely discharged. Troponin T tests can be false-positive in patients with renal failure, sepsis, rhabdomyolysis, fibrin clots, and heterophile antibodies. The presence of jaundice or the concurrent use of heparin can result in underestimation of troponin.
- Cardio-CRP (hs-CRP): elevation of cardio-CRP is a relatively moderate predictor of CHD, and it adds prognostic information to that conveyed by the Framingham risk score. However, based on current data, it may be premature to adapt widespread assessment of cardio-CRP.
- Measurement of total cholesterol, low-density lipoprotein cholesterol (LDL-C), high-density lipoprotein cholesterol (HDL-C), and fasting serum triglycerides is recommended for cardiovascular screening. Non-HDL-C and the ratio of total cholesterol to HDL-C and measurements of apolipoprotein fractions (e.g., apolipoprotein B100, apolipoprotein A1) can also be used to estimate cardiovascular risk.
- A single measurement of B-type natriuretic peptide (BNP), a natriuretic and vasodilative peptide regulated by ventricular wall tension and stored mainly in the ventricular myocardium, obtained in the first few days after the onset of ischemic symptoms provides predictive information for risk stratification in acute coronary syndromes. NT-pro-BNP is also a marker of long-term mortality in patients with stable coronary disease and provides prognostic information beyond that provided by conventional cardiovascular risk factors and the degree of left ventricular systolic dysfunction.

IMAGING STUDIES

- Echocardiography is indicated in patients with systolic murmur suggestive of aortic stenosis, mitral valve prolapse, or hypertrophic cardiomyopathy. It is also useful in the detection of ischemia-induced regional wall motion abnormalities or mitral regurgitation. Echocardiography combined with treadmill exercise (stress echo) or pharmacologic stress with dobutamine can be used to detect regional wall abnormalities that occur during myocardial ischemia associated with CAD.
- Coronary angiography is performed to define the location and extent of coronary disease; this is indicated in selected patients who are candidates for coronary artery bypass graft (CABG) surgery or angioplasty.
- Noninvasive methods for assessing myocardial viability to predict which patients will have increased left ventricular ejection fraction and improved survival after revascularization include positron-emission tomography, dobutamine echocardiography, multidetector CT, and contrast-enhanced MRI. Cardiac CT is useful for the detection of subclinical CAD in asymptomatic patients with an intermediate Framingham 10-year risk estimate of 10% to 20%. It detects and quantifies coronary calcium and evaluates the lumen and wall of the coronary artery. The calcium score is a strong predictor of incident CHD and provides predictive information beyond that provided by standard risk factors. Cardiac MRI, in addition to its use for diagnosis of arrhythmogenic right ventricular dysplasia, can also be used to assess myocardial perfusion and viability as well as function. Additional studies are needed to determine the cost effectiveness of these studies in patients with ischemic cardiomyopathy.

Rx TREATMENT

NONPHARMACOLOGIC THERAPY

- Aggressive modification of preventable risk factors (weight reduction in obese patients, regular aerobic exercise program, correction of folate deficiency, low-cholesterol and low-sodium diet, cessation of tobacco use).
- Diets using nonhydrogenated unsaturated fats as the predominant form of dietary fat, whole grains as the main form of carbohydrates, an abundance of fruits and vegetables, and adequate omega-3 fatty acids are optimal for prevention of CHD.
- Correction of possible aggravating factors (e.g., anemia, hypertension, diabetes mellitus, hyperlipidemia, thyrotoxicosis, hypothyroidism). Blood transfusion in the setting of acute coronary syndromes is associated with higher mortality rates. Use caution regarding the routine use of blood transfusions to maintain arbitrary hematocrit levels in stable patients with ischemic heart disease.

ACUTE GENERAL Rx

The major classes of antiischemic agents are nitrates, beta-adrenergic blockers, calcium channel blockers, aspirin, and heparin; they can be used alone or in combination.

- Nitrates cause venodilation and relaxation of vascular smooth muscle; the decreased venous return from venodilation decreases diastolic ventricular wall tension (preload) and thereby reduces mechanical activity (and myocardial oxygen consumption) during systole. Relaxation of vascular smooth muscle increases coronary blood flow and reduces systemic pressure. Tolerance to nitrates can be minimized by avoiding sustained blood levels with a daily nitrate-free period (e.g., omission of bedtime dose of oral isosorbide dinitrate or 12 hr on/12 hr off transdermal nitroglycerin therapy). Nitrates are relatively contraindicated in patients with hypertrophic obstructive cardiomyopathy, and should also be avoided in patients with severe aortic stenosis. Nitrates should not be used within 24 hr of sildenafil (Viagra) or vardenafil (Levitra) or within 48 hr of tadalafil (Cialis) because of the potential for hypotension.
- Beta-adrenergic blockers achieve their major antianginal effect by decreasing myocardial oxygen consumption by reducing heart rate and systolic blood pressure. Absent contraindications, they should be regarded as initial therapy for stable angina for all patients. Their dose should generally be adjusted to reduce the resting heart rate to 50 to 60 beats/min.
- Calcium channel blockers dilate coronary and systemic arteries, increase coronary blood flow, and decrease myocardial oxygen consumption. They play a major role in preventing and terminating myocardial ischemia induced by coronary artery spasm. They are particularly effective in treating microvascular angina. Short-acting calcium channel blockers should be avoided. Calcium channel blockers should generally also be avoided after complicated MI (congestive heart failure [CHF]) and in patients with CHF secondary to systolic dysfunction (unless necessary to control heart rate).
- Aspirin: use of aspirin reduces cardiovascular mortality and morbidity rates by 20% to 25% among patients with CAD. Initial dose is at least 160 mg/day followed by 81 to 325 mg/day. Aspirin inhibits cyclooxygenics and synthesis of thromboxane A_2 and reduces the risk of adverse cardiovascular events by 33% in patients with unstable angina. Patients intolerant to aspirin can be treated with the antiplatelet agent clopidogrel.
- Anticoagulant therapy is useful in patients with unstable angina and reduces the frequency of MI and refractory angina. Patients with unstable angina treated with aspirin plus heparin have a 32% reduction in the risk of MI and death compared with those treated with aspirin alone. Enoxaparin (low molecular weight heparin) and Fondaparinux (selective Factor Xa inhibitor) are as effective as unfractionated heparin in the treatment of unstable angina. Bivalirudin (direct thrombin inhibitor) is another choice if angiography is planned.
- Clopidogrel is a thienopyridine, which acts by irreversibly blocking the P2Y12 adenosine diphosphate receptor on the platelet surface, thereby interrupting platelet activation and aggregation. Initiation is recommended for patients undergoing conservative management of unstable angina along with aspirin and anticoagulant therapy or as an alternative to IIb/IIIa receptor antagonists for patients undergoing angiography.
- Addition of platelet glycoprotein (GP) IIb/IIIa receptor antagonists (eptifibatide or tirofiban) can be considered as an adjunctive therapy in conservative treatment of unstable angina. If a more invasive strategy is planned with angiography, then either clopidogrel or a IIb/IIIa receptor antagonist is given. However, administration of both may be considered in high-risk patients with positive troponin tests, refractory angina, or if delay to percutaneous revascularization is anticipated. Abciximab, the first GP IIb/IIa inhibitor, is an important component of percutaneous revascularization. Started in the catheterization lab, it reduces the incidence of ischemic events. Abciximab is contraindicated in patients for whom an early invasive strategy is not planned. Contraindications to the use of GP IIb/IIa inhibitors are severe hypertension (>180/110 mm Hg), internal bleeding within 30 days, history of intracranial hemorrhage, neoplasm, NVM, aneurysm, cerebrovascular accident (CVA) within 30 days or history of hemorrhagic CVA, thrombocytopenia (<100 k), acute pericarditis, history or symptoms suggestive of aortic dissection, and major surgical procedures or severe physical trauma within previous month.

CHRONIC Rx

- Use of lipid-lowering drugs is recommended in patients with CAD and in patients with hyperlipidemia refractory to diet and exercise. Among patients who have recently had an acute coronary syndrome, an intensive lipid-lowering statin regimen to reduce LDL cholesterol to <70 mg/dL is a reasonable treatment objective. Statins also decrease the level of the inflammatory marker hs-CRP independently of the magnitude of change in lipid parameters.
- ACE inhibition (e.g., ramipril 10 mg/day) has been shown to be effective in reducing cardiovascular death, MI, and stroke in patients who are at risk for or who had vascular disease (without heart failure). Currently evidence for routine use of ACEs in chronic stable angina is insufficient.
- Ranolazine is a newer agent indicated for treatment of chronic angina that is inadequately controlled with other antianginals. It represents a new class of drugs known as *metabolic modulators.* Its exact mechanism of action is unknown. It seems to increase the efficiency of energy production in the heart, maintaining cardiac function. Its antianginal and antiischemic effects do not depend on reductions in heart rate or blood pressure. It is labeled for use in combination with beta-blockers, amlodipine, or nitrates in patients without an adequate antianginal response to those agents. Side effects include prolongation of QT interval.

REFERRAL

Revascularization:

- Revascularization includes either percutaneous coronary intervention (balloon angioplasty and stenting) or CABG.
- CABG surgery is recommended for patients with left main coronary disease, for those with symptomatic three-vessel disease, and for those with LVEF <40% and critical (>70% stenosis) in all three major coronary arteries. Surgical therapy improves prognosis, particularly in diabetic patients with multivessel disease. Compared with percutaneous coronary intervention (PCI), CABG is more effective in relieving angina and leads to fewer repeated revascularizations but has a higher risk for procedural stroke. Survival to 10 years is similar for both procedures.

Angioplasty and coronary stents:

- PCI should be considered for patients with one- or two-vessel disease that does not involve the main left coronary artery and in whom ventricular function is normal or near normal. PCI has an established place in treating angina but is not superior to intensive medical therapy to prevent MI and death in symptomatic or asymptomatic patients. Patients selected for PCI should also be candidates for CABG. In patients with unstable angina who are candidates for PCI, a door-to-balloon time of 90 min or less has been defined as the optimal time from first presentation to treatment to attain the lowest in-hospital mortality rate. The types of lesions best suited for angioplasty are proximal lesions, noncalcified, concentric, and preferably less than 5 mm (should not exceed 10 mm). Approximately 80% of patients show immediate benefit after PCI. The frequency of abrupt closure postangioplasty can be reduced by pretreatment with IV GP IIb/IIIa receptor inhibitors, which block the final common pathway of platelet aggregation. In patients with clinically documented acute coronary syndrome who are treated with GP IIb/IIa inhibitors, even small elevations in troponins I and T identify high-risk patients who derive a large clinical benefit from an early invasive strategy. Abciximab (ReoPro) and eptifibatide (Integrilin) are approved for use before and during PCIs. They are expensive and can cause thrombocytopenia in 0.5% to 1% of patients. Platelet counts should be monitored for 24 hr after starting GP IIb/IIIa inhibitors. Reversal of thrombocytopenia (e.g., patients undergoing emergency CABG) can be achieved with platelet transfusions. Optimal long-term care after PCI requires aggressive systemic pharmacotherapy (antiplatelet agents [aspirin + clopidogrel], statins, beta-blockers, and ACE inhibitors) and therapeutic lifestyle to minimize the risk of future atherothrombotic events.

- The development of coronary stents has increased the number of patients who can be treated in the cardiac laboratory. Cardiac stents are currently used in nearly 95% of all PCI lesions. The rate of restenosis may be reduced by placing a stent electively in primary atheromatous lesions. In patients with symptomatic isolated stenosis of the proximal left anterior descending artery, stenting has advantages over standard coronary angioplasty in that it is associated with both a lower rate of restenosis and a better clinical outcome. The major limitations of stenting are subacute thrombosis, restenosis within the stent, bleeding complications when anticoagulants are used after stenting, and higher cost. The combination of aspirin and clopidogrel is effective in preventing coronary stent thrombosis. Vitamin therapy to lower homocysteine levels has been recommended by some for the prevention of restenosis after coronary angioplasty; however, recent reports indicate that the administration of folate, vitamin B_6, and vitamin B_{12} after coronary stenting may increase the risk of in-stent restenosis and the need for target-vessel revascularization. Regarding the use of various drug-eluting coronary stents, there are no significant differences in clinical outcomes between patients receiving sirolimus- and paclitaxel-eluting stents.

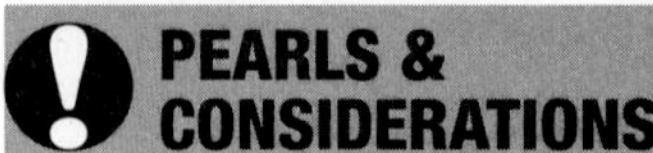

PEARLS & CONSIDERATIONS

COMMENTS

- Although nitrate responsiveness is usually an integral part of a diagnostic strategy for chronic stable chest pain, recent reports question its value and conclude that in a general population admitted for chest pain, relief of pain after nitroglycerin treatment does not predict active CAD and should not be used to guide diagnosis in the acute care setting.
- CABG is associated with higher long-term survival rates and lower rates of repeat revascularization than PCI and stenting; however, patients often prefer stenting because it is less invasive, involves a shorter hospital stay, and has a lower in-hospital mortality rate.
- Section III describes an algorithm for the surgical management of ischemic cardiomyopathy.

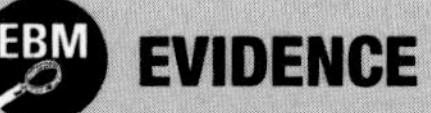

EVIDENCE

Please note: Complete text of EBM for this topic is available online.

SUGGESTED READINGS

Anderson JL et al: ACC/AHA 2007 guidelines for the management of patients with unstable angina/non ST elevation myocardial infarction, *J Am Coll Cariol* 50:1-157, 2007.

Hilas O: Ranolazine for chronic angina, *Am Fam Physician* 75:544, 2007.

Serruys PW et al: Percutaneous coronary interventions versus coronary-artery bypass for severe coronary artery disease, *N Engl J Med* 360:961-972, 2009.

Smith SC et al: AHA/ACC guidelines for secondary prevention for patients with coronary and other atherosclerotic vascular disease: 2006 update, *Circulation* 113:2363, 2006.

Snow V et al: Evaluation of primary care patients with chronic stable angina: guidelines from the American College of Physicians, *Ann Intern Med* 141:57, 562, 2004.

Stone GW, Aronow HD: Long-term care after percutaneous coronary intervention: focus on the role of antiplatelet therapy, *Mayo Clin Proc* 81(5):641, 2006.

AUTHORS: **VICTOR SHIN, M.D.,**
and **FRED F. FERRI, M.D.**

BASIC INFORMATION

DEFINITION

- The mucocutaneous swelling caused by the release of vasoactive mediators is called urticaria and angioedema.
- Urticaria causes edema of the superficial dermis.
- Angioedema involves the deep layers of the dermis and the subcutaneous tissue.

SYNONYMS

Angioneurotic edema

ICD-9CM CODES
995.1 Angioedema (allergic)
277.6 Angioedema (hereditary)

EPIDEMIOLOGY & DEMOGRAPHICS

INCIDENCE: 100 to 3000/100,000 persons (for urticaria and angioedema)

LIFETIME PREVALENCE: Approximately 20% of the population experiences urticaria and/or angioedema at some time during life. The prevalence of hereditary angioedema is 1 case per 50,000 persons.

DEMOGRAPHICS: Race: Slightly more common among African Americans. Sex: More occurrences in women than men. Angioedema commonly occurs after adolescence in the third decade of life.

Angioedema can occur together with urticaria (40%) or alone (20%); the remaining 40% have urticaria alone.

PHYSICAL FINDINGS & CLINICAL PRESENTATION

- Angioedema may be acute or chronic.
  1. Acute angioedema is defined as symptoms lasting 6 wk.
  2. Chronic angioedema is defined as symptoms lasting >6 wk.
- Urticaria is commonly known as "hives" and is:
  1. Pruritic
  2. Palpable and well demarcated
  3. Erythematous
  4. Millimeters to centimeters in size
  5. Multiple in number
  6. Fades within 12 to 24 hr
  7. Reappears at other sites
- Angioedema is characterized by the following:
  1. Nonpruritic
  2. Burning
  3. Not well demarcated
  4. Involves eyelids (Fig. 1-18), lips, tongue, and extremities
  5. Can involve the upper airway, causing respiratory distress
  6. Can involve the gastrointestinal tract, leading to cyclic abdominal pain
  7. Resolves slowly

ETIOLOGY

- Angioedema, with or without urticaria, is classified as acquired (allergic or idiopathic) or hereditary.
- Angioedema is primarily caused by mast cell activation and degranulation with release of vasoactive mediators (e.g., histamine, serotonin, bradykinins), resulting in postcapillary venule inflammation, vascular leakage, and edema in the deep layers of the dermis and subcutaneous tissue.
- Pathologically, angioedema has both immunologic- and nonimmunologic-mediated mechanisms.
  1. Immunoglobulin E–mediated angioedema may result from antigen exposure (e.g., foods [milk, eggs, peanuts, shellfish, tomatoes, chocolate, sulfites] or drugs [penicillin, aspirin, nonsteroidal antiinflammatory drugs, phenytoin, sulfonamides, recombinant tissue plasminogen activator]).
  2. Complement-mediated angioedema involving immune complex mechanisms can also lead to mast cell activation that manifests as serum sickness.
  3. Hereditary angioedema is an autosomal-dominant disease caused by a deficiency of or mutation in C1 esterase inhibitor (C1-INH). C1-INH is a protease inhibitor normally present in high concentrations in the plasma. C1-INH serves many functions, one of which is to inhibit plasma kallikrein, a protease that cleaves kininogen and releases bradykinin. Deficient C1-INH activity results in excess concentration of kininogen and the subsequent release of kinin mediators.
  4. Acquired angioedema is usually associated with other diseases, most commonly B-cell lymphoproliferative disorders, but may also result from the formation of autoantibodies directed against C1 inhibitor protein.
  5. Other causes of angioedema include infection (e.g., herpes simplex, hepatitis B, Coxsackie A and B, *Streptococcus, Candida, Ascaris,* and *Strongyloides*), insect bites and stings, stress, physical factors (e.g., cold, exercise, pressure, and vibration), connective tissue diseases (e.g., systemic lupus erythematosus, Henoch-Schönlein purpura), and idiopathic causes. Angiotensin-converting enzyme (ACE) inhibitors can increase kinin activity and lead to angioedema.

Dx DIAGNOSIS

A detailed history and physical examination usually establish the diagnosis of angioedema. Extensive laboratory testing is of limited value.

DIFFERENTIAL DIAGNOSIS

- Cellulitis
- Arthropod bite
- Hypothyroidism
- Contact dermatitis
- Atopic dermatitis
- Mastocytosis
- Granulomatous cheilitis
- Bullous pemphigoid
- Urticaria pigmentosa
- Anaphylaxis
- Erythema multiforme
- Epiglottitis
- Peritonsillar abscess

WORKUP

- An extensive workup searching for the cause of angioedema is often unrevealing (90%).
- Workup, including diagnostic blood tests and allergy testing, is performed according to results of the history and physical examination.

LABORATORY TESTS

- Complete blood count, erythrocyte sedimentation rate, and urinalysis are sometimes helpful as part of the initial evaluation.
- Stools for ova and parasites.
- Serology testing.
- C4 levels are usually reduced in acquired and hereditary angioedema (occurring without urticaria). If C4 levels are low, C1-INH levels and activity should be obtained. There are isolated reports of hereditary angioedema with normal C4 levels but reduced C1-INH levels.
- Skin and radioallergosorbent testing may be done if food allergies are suspected.
- Skin biopsy is usually done in patients with chronic angioedema refractory to corticosteroid treatment.

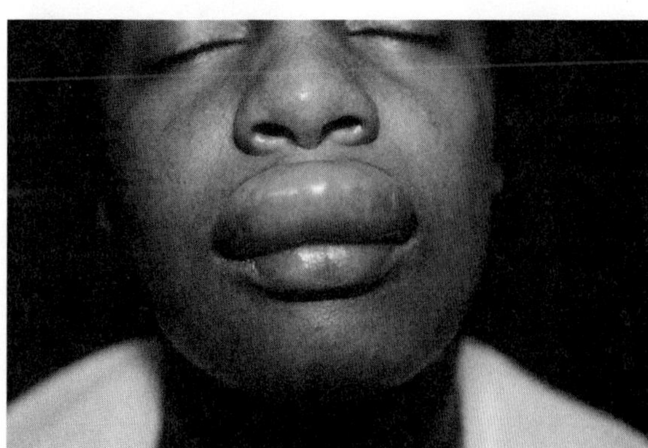

FIGURE 1-18 Angioedema of the upper lip, with severe swelling of deeper tissues. (From Goldstein BG, Goldstein AO: *Practical dermatology,* ed 2, St Louis, 1997, Mosby.)

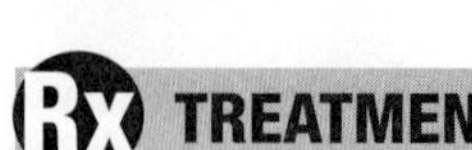

NONPHARMACOLOGIC THERAPY

- Eliminate the offending agent
- Avoid triggering factors (e.g., cold, stress)
- Cold compresses to affected areas

ACUTE GENERAL Rx

- Acute life-threatening angioedema involving the larynx is treated with:
  1. Epinephrine 0.3 mg in a solution of 1:1000 given SC
  2. Diphenhydramine 25 to 50 mg IV or IM
  3. Cimetidine 300 mg IV or ranitidine 50 mg IV
  4. Methylprednisolone 125 mg IV
- Mainstay therapy in nonhereditary angioedema is H_1 antihistamines
  1. Diphenhydramine 25 to 50 mg q6h
  2. Chlorpheniramine 4 mg q6h
  3. Hydroxyzine 10 to 25 mg q6h
  4. Cetirizine 5 to 10 mg qd
  5. Loratadine 10 mg qd
  6. Fexofenadine 60 mg qd
- H_2 antihistamines can be added to H_1 antihistamines
  1. Ranitidine 150 mg bid
  2. Cimetidine 400 mg bid
  3. Famotidine 20 mg bid
- Tricyclic antidepressants
  1. Doxepin 25 to 50 mg qd
- Corticosteroids are rarely required for symptomatic relief of acute angioedema.
- Antihistamines are probably ineffective in acute hereditary angioedema.
- Purified plasma-derived C1-INH replacement therapy is highly effective but is presently unavailable in the U.S.

CHRONIC Rx

- Chronic angioedema is treated as described under "Acute General Rx."
- Corticosteroids are used more often in chronic nonhereditary angioedema.
- Prednisone 1 mg/kg/day for 5 days and then tapered over a period of weeks.
- Androgens (danazol, stanozolol, oxandrolone, methyltestosterone) and antifibrinolytic agents are used for the treatment of chronic hereditary angioedema, which does not respond to antihistamines or corticosteroids. C1-INH replacement therapy is available in some countries.

DISPOSITION

- Antihistamines achieve symptomatic relief in more than 80% of patients with nonhereditary acute angioedema.
- In chronic nonhereditary angioedema, corticosteroids are given in addition to antihistamines.
- A small percentage of people will have recurrence of symptoms after steroid treatment.
- Chronic angioedema can last for months and even years.

REFERRAL

Dermatology consultation is recommended in patients with chronic angioedema, hereditary angioedema, and recurring angioedema.

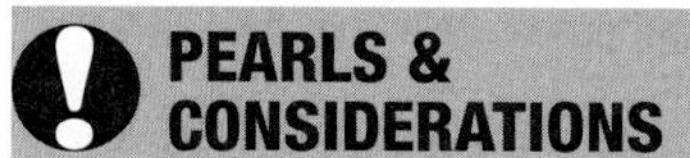

ACE inhibitors can cause angioedema up to many months after initiation. There are multiple case reports and case series of angiotensin receptor blocker–induced angioedema, although the risk is substantially less than that of ACE inhibitors.

COMMENTS

- Identifying a cause for angioedema in patients is often difficult and met with frustration.
- Chronic angioedema, unlike acute angioedema, is rarely caused by an allergic reaction.

SUGGESTED READINGS

Baxi S, Dinakar C: Urticaria and angioedema, *Immunol Allergy Clin North Am* 25(2):353, 2005.

Bork K, Hardt J: Hereditary angioedema: Increased number of attacks after frequent treatments with C1 inhibitor concentrate, *Am J Med* 122:780-783, 2009.

Bowen T et al: Hereditary angioedema: a current state-of-the-art review, VII: Canadian Hungarian 2007 International Consensus Algorithm for the Diagnosis, Therapy, and Management of Hereditary Angioedema, *Ann Allergy Asthma Immunol* 100(1 suppl 2):S30-40, 2008.

Frigas E, Park M: Idiopathic recurrent angioedema, *Immunol Allergy Clin North Am* 26(4):739, 2006.

Temino VM: The spectrum and treatment of angioedema, *Am J Med* 121(4):282, 2008.

Temino VM, Peebles S: The spectrum and treatment of angioedema, *Am J Med* 121:282-286, 2008.

Zuraw BL et al: Hereditary angioedema, *N Engl J Med* 359:1027-1036, 2008.

AUTHOR: **MEL L. ANDERSON, M.D.**

BASIC INFORMATION

DEFINITION

Ankle fractures involve the lateral, medial, or posterior malleolus of the ankle and may occur either alone or in some combination. Associated ligamentous injuries are included.

ICD-9CM CODES
824.8 Ankle fracture (malleolus) (closed)
824.2 Lateral malleolus fracture (fibular)
824.0 Medial malleolus fracture (tibial)

PHYSICAL FINDINGS & CLINICAL PRESENTATION

- Deformity usually depends on extent of displacement
- Pain, tenderness, and hemorrhage at the site of injury
- Gentle palpation of ligamentous structures (especially deltoid ligament) to determine the extent of soft tissue injury
- Evaluation of distal neurovascular status; results recorded

ETIOLOGY

- The ankle depends on its ligamentous and bony support for stability. The joint, or *mortise,* is an inverted U with the dome of the talus fitting into the medial and lateral malleoli. The posterior margin of the tibia is often called the *third* or *posterior malleolus.*
- Most common ankle fractures are the result of eversion or lateral rotation forces on the talus (in contrast with common sprains, which are usually caused by inversion).

Dx DIAGNOSIS

The diagnosis is usually established on the basis of the nature of the injury, the presence of typical findings of bony tenderness with swelling, and abnormal imaging studies.

DIFFERENTIAL DIAGNOSIS

- Ankle sprain
- Avulsion fracture of hindfoot or metatarsal

IMAGING STUDIES

Standard AP and lateral views accompanied by an AP taken 15° internally rotated. The last view is taken to properly visualize the mortise.

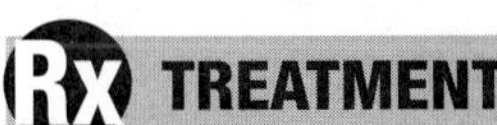

TREATMENT

All fractures: elevation and ice to control swelling for 48 to 72 hr.

ACUTE GENERAL Rx

- Clinical and roentgenographic assessment of the status of the ankle mortise and stability of the injury is mandatory to determine treatment.
- There is potential for displacement if both sides of the joint are significantly injured (e.g., fracture of the lateral malleolus with deltoid ligament injury).
- Deviation of the position of the talus in the mortise could lead to traumatic arthritis.
- If there is no widening of the ankle mortise, many injuries can be safely treated with simple casting without reduction:
  1. Undisplaced or avulsion fractures of either malleolus below the ankle joint line:
     a. Stability of the joint is not compromised and a short leg walking cast or ankle support is sufficient.
     b. Weight bearing is allowed as tolerated.
     c. In 4 to 6 wk, protection may be discontinued.
  2. Isolated undisplaced fractures of the medial, lateral, or posterior malleolus:
     a. Usually stable and require only the application of a short leg walking cast with the ankle in the neutral position or fracture cast boot.
     b. Immobilization should be continued for 8 wk.
     c. Fracture line of lateral malleolus may persist roentgenographically for several months, but immobilization beyond 8 wk is usually unnecessary.
     d. Undisplaced bimalleolar fractures are treated with a long leg cast flexed 30 degrees at the knee to prevent motion and displacement of the fracture fragments. In 4 wk, a short leg walking cast may be applied for an additional 4 wk.
  3. Isolated fractures of the lateral malleolus that are slightly displaced:
     a. May be treated with casting if no medial injury is present.
     b. A below-knee walking cast is applied with ankle in the neutral position; weight bearing is allowed as tolerated.
     c. Six wk of immobilization is sufficient.
     d. If medial tenderness is present, suggesting deltoid ligament rupture, a carefully molded cast may suffice if weight bearing is not allowed and the patient is followed up closely for signs of instability, especially after swelling recedes. If significant widening of the medial ankle mortise (increase in the "medial clear space") develops as a result of lateral displacement of the talus, referral for possible reduction is indicated.
     e. If signs of instability are already present at initial examination (widening of the medial clear space with medial tenderness), referral is indicated.
  4. Undisplaced fracture of the distal fibular epiphysis:
     a. Often diagnosed clinically.
     b. There is tenderness over the epiphyseal plate.
     c. Roentgenographic findings are often negative.
     d. A short leg walking cast or fracture boot is applied for 4 wk.
     e. Growth disturbance is rare.
  5. Isolated posterior malleolar fractures involving less than 25% of the joint surface on the lateral roentgenogram:
     Safely treated by applying a short leg walking cast or fracture brace. (Fractures involving >25% of the weight-bearing surface should be referred because of the potential for instability and subsequent traumatic arthritis.)

CHRONIC Rx

- Early motion is encouraged through a home exercise program.
- Protection from reinjury is appropriate for 4 to 6 wk after cast or brace removal.
- Temporary increase in lower extremity swelling that frequently occurs after short leg cast removal may benefit from the use of support hose.

DISPOSITION

Significant factors involved in the development of traumatic arthritis:
- Amount of joint trauma at the time of injury
- Eventual position of the talus in the mortise

Fracture nonunion is uncommon unless displacement is significant.

REFERRAL

Orthopedic consultation for:
- Unstable ankle joint
- Widened ankle mortise
- Posterior malleolar fracture over 25% of joint with incongruity
- Marked displacement of fracture fragment

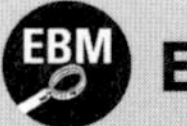

EVIDENCE

Please note: Complete text of EBM for this topic is available online.

SUGGESTED READINGS

Chaudhary SB et al: Complications of ankle fracture in patients with diabetes, *J Am Acad Orthop Surg* 16:159, 2008.

Egol KA et al: Predictors of short-term functional outcome following ankle fracture surgery, *J Bone Joint Surg Am* 88A:974, 2006.

Haraguchi N et al: Pathoanatomy of posterior malleolar fractures of the ankle, *J Bone Joint Surg Am* 88A:1085, 2006.

Leontaritis N et al: Arthroscopically deleted intraarticular lesions associated with acute ankle fractures, *J Bone Joint Surg* 9:333, 2009.

Park JC, Laurin TM: Acute syndesmosis injuries associated with ankle fractures: current perspectives in management, *Bull NYU Hosp Jt Dis* 67:39, 2009.

Schnetzler KA, Hoernschemeyer D: The pediatric triplane fracture, *J Am Acad Orthop Surg* 15:738, 2007.

Tejwani NC et al: Are outcomes of bimalleolar fractures poorer than those of lateral malleolar fractures with medial ligamentous injury? *J Bone Joint Surg Am* 89:1438, 2007.

AUTHOR: **LONNIE R. MERCIER, M.D.**

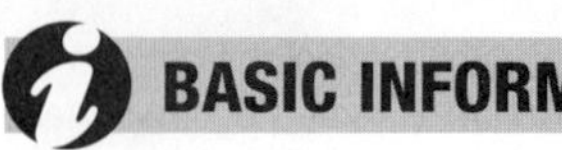

BASIC INFORMATION

DEFINITION

An ankle sprain is an injury to the ligamentous support of the ankle. Most (85%) involve the lateral ligament complex (Fig. 1-19). The anterior inferior tibiofibular (AITF) ligament, deltoid ligament, and interosseous membrane may also be injured. Damage to the tibiofibular syndesmosis is sometimes called a *high sprain* because of pain above the ankle.

ICD-9CM CODES
845.00 Sprain, ankle or foot

EPIDEMIOLOGY & DEMOGRAPHICS

PREVALENCE: One case/10,000 people each day

PREDOMINANT SEX: Varies according to age and level of physical activity

PHYSICAL FINDINGS & CLINICAL PRESENTATION

- Often a history of a "pop"
- Variable amounts of tenderness and hemorrhage
- Possible abnormal anterior drawer test (pulling the plantar flexed foot forward to determine if there is any abnormal increase in forward movement of the talus in the ankle mortise) (Fig. 1-20)
- Inversion sprains: tender laterally; syndesmotic injuries: area of tenderness is more anterior and proximal
- Evaluation of motor function (Fig. 1-21)

ETIOLOGY

- Lateral injuries usually result from inversion and plantar flexion injuries.
- Eversion and rotational forces may injure the deltoid or AITF ligament or the interosseous membrane.

Dx DIAGNOSIS

DIFFERENTIAL DIAGNOSIS

- Fracture of the ankle or foot, particularly involving the distal fibular growth plate in the immature patient
- Avulsion fracture of the fifth metatarsal base

WORKUP

- History and clinical examination are usually sufficient to establish the diagnosis.
- Plain radiographs are always needed.

IMAGING STUDIES

Roentgenographic evaluation:

1. Usually normal but always performed
2. Should include the fifth metatarsal base
3. All minor avulsion fractures noted

Varying opinions on the usefulness of arthrograms, tenograms, and stress films

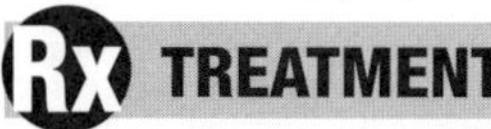

TREATMENT

ACUTE GENERAL Rx

- Ankle sprains are often graded I, II, or III, according to severity, with grade III injury implying complete rupture. The first line of treatment is described by the mnemonic *RICE:*
  - ***R**est*
  - ***I**ce*
  - ***C**ompression*
  - ***E**levation*
- Varying opinions regarding the initial use of NSAIDs
- In 48 to 72 hr, active range of motion and weight bearing as tolerated
- In 4 to 5 days, exercise against resistance added
- Possible cast immobilization for some patients who require early independent walking; short leg orthoses also available for the same purpose

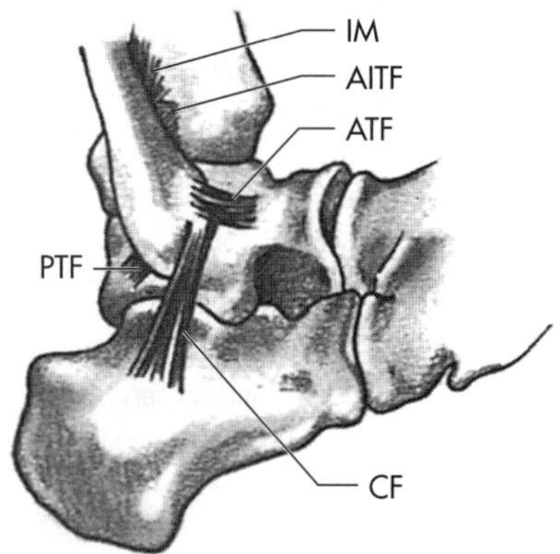

FIGURE 1-19 The lateral ankle ligaments, anterior and posterior talofibular *(ATF, PTF)* and calcaneofibular *(CF)*. Also shown are the anterior inferior tibiofibular ligament *(AITF)* and the beginning of the interosseous membrane *(IM)*. (From Mercier LR [ed]: *Practical orthopaedics,* ed 4, St Louis, 1995, Mosby.)

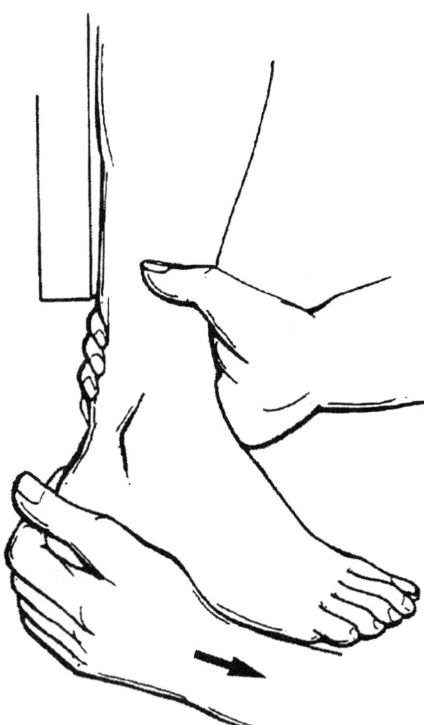

FIGURE 1-20 Anterior drawer test of the ankle (tests the integrity of the anterior talofibular ligament). (From Brinker MR, Miller MD: *Fundamentals of orthopaedics,* Philadelphia, 1999, WB Saunders.)

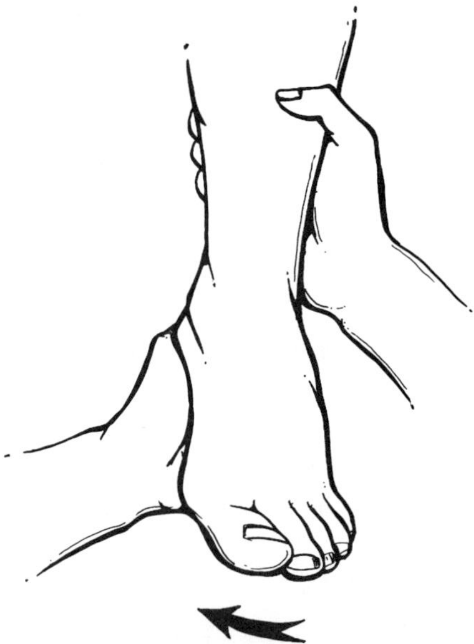

FIGURE 1-21 Talar tilt test (inversion stress) of the ankle (tests the integrity of the anterior talofibular ligament and the calcaneofibular ligament). (From Brinker MR, Miller MD: *Fundamentals of orthopaedics,* Philadelphia, 1999, WB Saunders.)

- Surgery is rarely recommended, even for grade III sprains; reports of equally satisfactory outcomes with nonsurgical treatment

CHRONIC Rx

- Lateral heel and sole wedge to prevent inversion
- Protective taping or bracing during vigorous activities (Fig. 1-22)
- Strengthening exercises

DISPOSITION

- Lateral sprains of any severity may cause lingering symptoms for weeks and months.
    1. Some syndesmotic sprains take even longer to heal.
    2. Heterotopic ossification may even develop in the interosseous membrane, but long-term results do not seem to be affected by such ossification.
- Continuing lateral symptoms may require surgical reconstruction, although late traumatic arthritis or long-term instability is rare regardless of treatment.

REFERRAL

For orthopedic consultation for patients who do not respond to conservative treatment

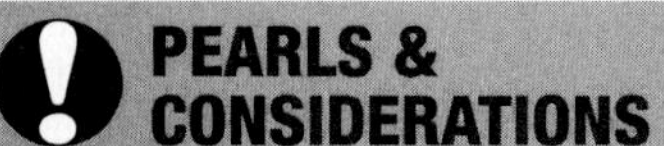

PEARLS & CONSIDERATIONS

COMMENTS

If healing seems delayed (more than 6 wk), the following conditions should be considered:

1. Talar dome fracture
2. Reflex sympathetic dystrophy
3. Chronic tendinitis
4. Peroneal tendon subluxation
5. Other occult fracture
6. Peroneal weakness (poor rehabilitation)
7. A "high" (syndesmotic) sprain

Repeat plain roentgenograms, bone scan, or MRI may be indicated.

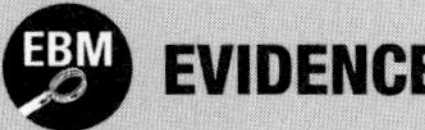

EVIDENCE

Please note: Complete text of EBM for this topic is available online.

SUGGESTED READINGS

Dahners LE, Mullis BH: Effects of nonsteroidal anti-inflammatory drugs on bone formation and soft tissue healing, *J Am Acad Orthop Surg* 12:139, 2004.

Hale SA et al: The effect of a 4-week comprehensive rehabilitation program on postural control and lower extremity function in individuals with chronic ankle instability, *J Orthop Sports Phys Ther* 37:303, 2007.

Ivins D: Acute ankle sprain: an update, *Am Fam Physician* 74:1714, 2006.

Le Gall F et al: Injuries in young elite female soccer players: an 8-season prospective study, *Am J Sports Med* 36:276, 2008.

Maffulli N, Ferran N: Management of acute and chronic ankle instability, *J Am Acad Orthop Surg* 16:608, 2008.

Mizel MS et al: Evaluation and treatment of chronic ankle pain, *J Bone Joint Surg Am* 86A:622, 2004.

O'Neill PJ et al: Excursion and strain of the superficial peroneal nerve during inversion ankle sprain, *J Bone Joint Surg Am* 89A:979, 2007.

Pedowtiz DI et al: Prophylactic bracing decreases ankle injuries in collegiate female volleyball players, *Am J Sports Med* 36:324, 2008.

Van Rijin RG et al: What is the clinical course of acute ankle sprains? A systematic literature review, *Am J Med* 121:324, 2008.

Zalavras C, Thordarson D: Ankle syndesmotic injury, *J Am Acad Orthop Surg* 15:330, 2007.

AUTHOR: **LONNIE R. MERCIER, M.D.**

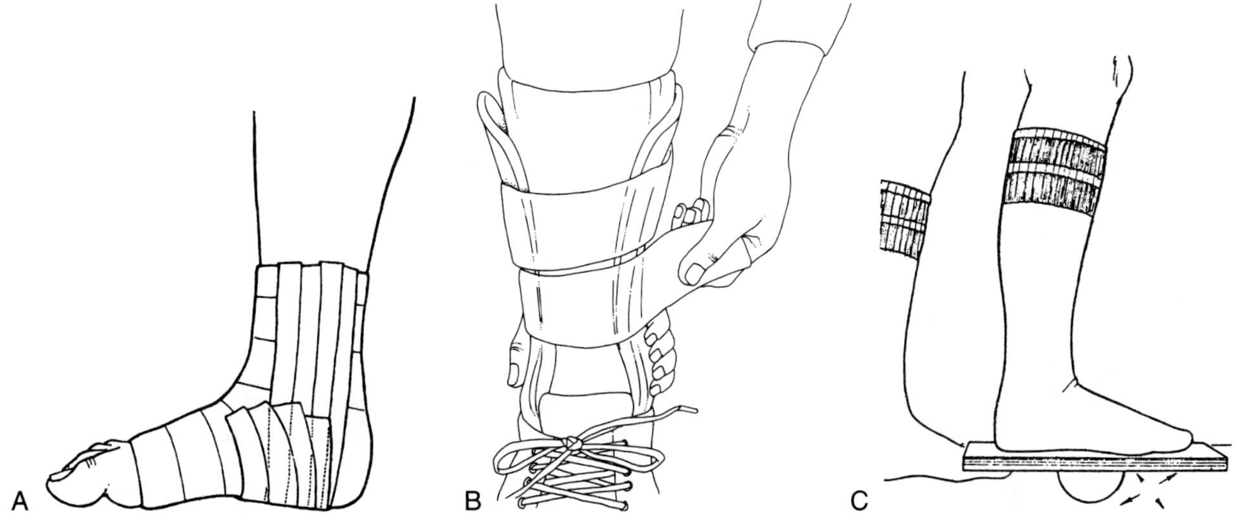

FIGURE 1-22 A, The most effective method of supporting most acute ankle sprains is by using an ACE wrap (BD, Franklin Lakes, NJ) reinforced with 1-inch medial and lateral tape strips. The anterior and posterior aspects of the ankle are left free to allow the patient to flex and extend the ankle. The patient is encouraged to bear weight with crutches. **B,** Diagram of an air splint. Straps are adjusted to heel size, the lower straps are wrapped about the ankle, and the side extensions are centered. The splint is then pressurized and straps adjusted until comfortable support and pressure are attained. **C,** As the ankle pain subsides, about the third to fifth day, balancing exercises can begin to allow the patient to regain ankle proprioception and avoid recurrent instability problems. (From Jardon OM, Mathews MS: Orthopedics. In Rakel RE [ed]: *Textbook of family practice,* ed 5, Philadelphia, 1995, WB Saunders.)

BASIC INFORMATION

DEFINITION

Ankylosing spondylitis is a chronic inflammatory condition involving the sacroiliac joints and axial skeleton characterized by ankylosis and enthesitis (inflammation at tendon insertions). It is one of a group of several overlapping syndromes, including spondylitis associated with Reiter's syndrome, psoriasis, and inflammatory bowel disease. Patients are typically seronegative for the rheumatoid factor. These disorders are now commonly called *rheumatoid variants* or *seronegative spondyloarthropathies.*

SYNONYMS

Marie-Strümpell disease

ICD-9CM CODES

720.0 Ankylosing spondylitis

EPIDEMIOLOGY & DEMOGRAPHICS

PREVALENCE: 0.15% of male population (rare in blacks)
PREDOMINANT AGE AT ONSET: 15 to 35 yr
PREDOMINANT SEX: Male/female ratio of 10:1

PHYSICAL FINDINGS & CLINICAL PRESENTATION

- Morning stiffness
- Fatigue, weight loss, anorexia, and other systemic symptoms in more severe forms
- Bilateral sacroiliac tenderness (sacroiliitis)
- Limited lumbar spine motion (Fig. 1-23)
- Loss of chest expansion measured at the nipple line <2.5 cm, reflecting rib cage involvement

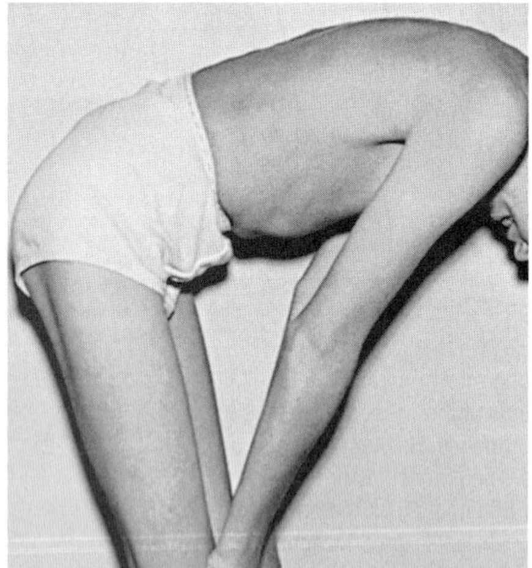

FIGURE 1-23 Loss of lumbodorsal spine mobility in a boy with ankylosing spondylitis. The lower spine remains straight when the patient bends forward. (From Behrman RE: *Nelson textbook of pediatrics,* 17th ed, Philadelphia, 2005, WB Saunders.)

- Occasionally, peripheral joint involvement (large joints are more commonly affected)
- Possible extraskeletal manifestations affecting the cardiovascular system (aortic insufficiency, heart block, cardiomegaly), lungs (pulmonary fibrosis), and eye (uveitis)
- Tenderness at tendon insertion sites, especially the Achilles tendons, plantar fascia
- Radiation below the knee is rare

ETIOLOGY

Unknown. Genetic factors play an important role. Destructive changes probably from release of cytokines and tumor necrosis factor.

DIAGNOSIS

DIFFERENTIAL DIAGNOSIS

- Diffuse idiopathic skeletal hyperostosis (Forestier disease)
- Other spondyloarthropathies
- A clinical algorithm for the evaluation of back pain is described in Section III

WORKUP

The modified New York criteria are often used for diagnosis:

- Low back pain of at least 3 mo duration improved by exercise and not relieved by rest
- Limitation of lumbar spine movement in sagittal and frontal planes
- Decreased chest expansion below normal values for age and sex
- Bilateral sacroiliitis of minimal grade or greater
- Unilateral sacroiliitis of moderate grade or greater

LABORATORY TESTS

- Elevated sedimentation rate, C-reactive protein
- Absence of rheumatoid factor and antinuclear antibody
- Possible mild hyperchromic anemia
- Presence of HLA/B27 antigen in >90% of patients (although this antigen is often present in the general population)

IMAGING STUDIES

- Early roentgenographic features are those of bilateral sacroiliitis on plain films.
- Vertebral bodies may become demineralized and a typical "squaring off" occurs.
- With progression, calcification of the annulus fibrosus and paravertebral ligaments develop, giving rise to the so-called bamboo spine appearance.
- End result may be a forward protruding cervical spine and fixed dorsal kyphosis.
- MRI may be helpful in detecting early inflammatory lesions and is especially helpful when the history is suggestive but plain films are normal.

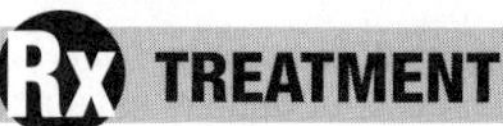

TREATMENT

NONPHARMACOLOGIC THERAPY

- Exercises primarily to maintain flexibility; general aerobic activity also important
- Postural training
  1. Patients must be instructed to sit in the erect position and to avoid stooping; otherwise, a flexion contracture of the spine may develop, which can become so severe that the patient cannot see forward.
  2. Sleeping should be in the supine position on a firm mattress; pillows should not be placed under the head or knees.

CHRONIC Rx

- NSAIDs: indomethacin is often successful in relieving symptoms; newer nonsteroidal agents may be tried as well.
- New research into the use of tumor necrosis factor antagonists such as etanercept appears promising.

DISPOSITION

- Most patients have a normal life span.
- The usual course of the disease is not life threatening, but death may occur as a result of aortic insufficiency or secondary amyloidosis with renal disease.

REFERRAL

- Orthopedic consultation for pain or deformity
- Ophthalmologic consultation for ocular complications
- Rheumatology consultation for uncontrolled symptoms

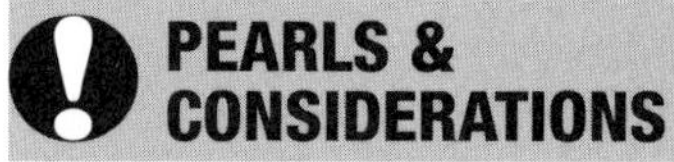

PEARLS & CONSIDERATIONS

COMMENTS

Years may pass between the onset of symptoms and the ultimate diagnosis because of the frequency of nonspecific low back pain.

SUGGESTED READINGS

Brown J: Ankylosing spondylitis, *Lancet* 369:1379-1390, 2007.

Davis JC Jr et al: Health-related quality of life outcomes in patients with active ankylosing spondylitis treated with adalimumab: results from a randomized controlled study, *Arthritis Rheum* 57(6): 1050, 2007.

Heiberg MS et al: The comparative one-year performance of anti-tumor necrosis factor alpha drugs in patients with rheumatoid arthritis, psoriatic arthritis, and ankylosing spondylitis: results from a longitudinal, observational, multicenter study, *Arthritis Rheum* 59:234, 2008.

AUTHOR: **LONNIE R. MERCIER, M.D.**

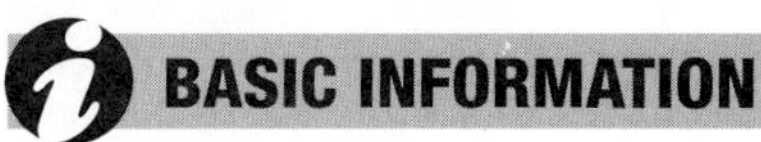

BASIC INFORMATION

DEFINITION

A fistula is an inflammatory tract with a secondary (external) opening in the perianal skin and a primary (internal) opening in the anal canal at the dentate line. It originates in an abscess in the intersphincteric space of the anal canal. Fistulas can be classified as follows:

1. Intersphincteric: fistula track passes within the intersphincteric plane to the perianal skin (most common)
2. Transsphincteric: fistula track passes from the internal opening, through the internal and external sphincter, and into the ischiorectal fossa to the perianal skin (frequent)
3. Suprasphincteric: after passing through the internal sphincter, fistula tract passes above the puborectalis and then tracts downward, lateral to the external sphincter, into the ischiorectal space to the perianal skin (uncommon); if abscess cavity extends cephalad, a supralevator abscess possibly palpable on rectal examination
4. Extrasphincteric: fistula tract passes from the rectum, above the levators, through the levator muscles to the ischiorectal space and perianal skin (rare)

With a horseshoe fistula, the tract passes from one ischiorectal fossa to the other behind the rectum.

SYNONYMS

Fistula-in-ano

ICD-9CM CODES

565.1 Anal fistula

EPIDEMIOLOGY & DEMOGRAPHICS

- Common in all ages
- Occurs equally in men and women
- Associated with constipation
- Pediatric age group: more common in infants; boys more than girls

PHYSICAL FINDINGS & CLINICAL PRESENTATION

- Acute stage: perianal swelling, pain, and fever
- Chronic stage: history of rectal drainage or bleeding; previous abscess with drainage
- Tender external fistulous opening, within 2 to 3 cm of the anal verge, with purulent or serosanguineous drainage on compression; the greater the distance from the anal margin, the greater the probability of a complicated upward extension
- Goodsall's rule:
  1. Location of the internal opening related to the location of the external opening.
  2. With external opening anterior to an imaginary line drawn horizontally across the midpoint of the anus: fistulous tract runs radially into the anal canal.
  3. With opening posterior to the transanal line: tract is usually curvilinear, entering the anal canal in the posterior midline.
  4. Exception to this rule: an external, anterior opening that is >3 cm from the anus. In this case the tract may curve posteriorly and end in the posterior midline.
- If perianal abscess recurs, presence of a fistula is suggested

ETIOLOGY

- Most common: nonspecific cryptoglandular infection (skin or intestinal flora)
- Fistulas more common when intestinal microorganisms are cultured from the anorectal abscess
- Tuberculosis
- Lymphogranuloma venereum
- Actinomycosis
- Inflammatory bowel disease (IBD): Crohn's disease, ulcerative colitis
- Trauma: surgery (episiotomy, prostatectomy), foreign bodies, anal intercourse
- Malignancy: carcinoma, leukemia, lymphoma
- Treatment of malignancy: surgery, radiation

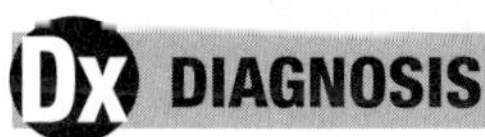

DIAGNOSIS

DIFFERENTIAL DIAGNOSIS

- Hidradenitis suppurativa
- Pilonidal sinus
- Bartholin's gland abscess or sinus
- Infected perianal sebaceous cysts

WORKUP

- Digital rectal examination:
  1. Assess sphincter tone and voluntary squeeze pressure
  2. Determine the presence of an extraluminal mass
  3. Identify an indurated track
  4. Palpate an internal opening or pit
- Gentle probing of external orifice to avoid creating a false tract; 50% do not have clinically detectable opening
- Anoscopy
- Proctosigmoidoscopy to exclude inflammatory or neoplastic disease
- All studies done under adequate anesthesia

LABORATORY TESTS

- Complete blood count
- Rectal biopsy if diagnosis of IBD or malignancy suspected; biopsy of external orifice is useless

IMAGING STUDIES

- Colonoscopy or barium enema if:
  1. Diagnosis of IBD or malignancy is suspected
  2. History of recurrent or multiple fistulas
  3. Patient <25 yr
- Small bowel series: occasionally obtained for reasons similar to above
- Fistulography: unreliable but may be helpful in complicated fistulas

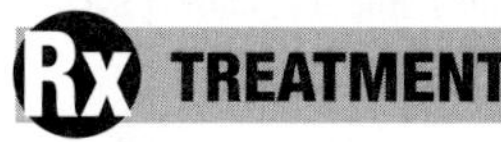

TREATMENT

NONPHARMACOLOGIC THERAPY

Sitz baths

ACUTE GENERAL Rx

- Treatment of choice: surgery
- Broad-spectrum antibiotic given if:
  1. Cellulitis present
  2. Patient is immunocompromised
  3. Valvular heart disease present
  4. Prosthetic devices present
- Stool softener/laxative

CHRONIC Rx

- Surgery
- Surgical goals are as follows:
  1. Cure the fistula
  2. Prevent recurrence
  3. Preserve sphincter function
  4. Minimize healing time
- Methods for the management of anal fistulas: fistulotomy, setons, rectal advancement flaps, colostomy

DISPOSITION

Outpatient surgery

REFERRAL

Refer to a surgeon with expertise in this area

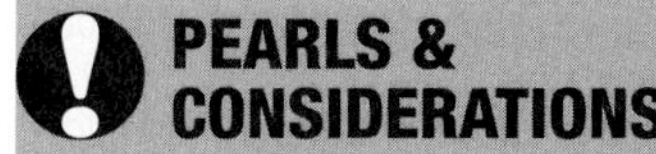

PEARLS & CONSIDERATIONS

COMMENTS

- HIV-positive and diabetic patients with perirectal abscesses/fistulas are true surgical emergencies.
- Risk of septicemia, Fournier's gangrene, and other septic complications make immediate drainage imperative.

SUGGESTED READINGS

Pfenninger JL, Zainea GG: Common anorectal condition, *Am Fam Physician* 64:22, 2001.

Rickard MJ: Anal abscesses and fistulas, *ANZ J Surg* 75(1-2):64, 2005.

Schwartz DA, Herdman CR: The medical treatment of Crohn's perianal fistulas, *Aliment Pharmacol Ther* 19(9):953, 2004.

AUTHORS: **GEORGE T. DANAKAS, M.D.,** and **RUBEN ALVERO, M.D.**

BASIC INFORMATION

DEFINITION

Anorexia nervosa is a psychiatric disorder characterized by abnormal eating behavior, severe self-induced weight loss, and a specific psychopathology (see "Workup").

ICD-9CM CODES
307.1 Anorexia nervosa

EPIDEMIOLOGY & DEMOGRAPHICS

INCIDENCE/PREVALENCE (IN U.S.):

- Anorexia nervosa occurs in 0.2% to 1.3% of the general population, with an annual incidence of five to 10 cases per 100,000 persons.
- Participation in activities that promote thinness (athletics, modeling) is associated with a higher incidence of anorexia nervosa.

PREDOMINANT SEX: Female/male ratio is 9:1. Approximately 0.5% to 1% of women between the ages of 15 and 30 yr have anorexia nervosa.
PREDOMINANT AGE: Adolescence to young adulthood is the predominant age. Mean age of onset is 17 yr. Approximately 0.5% to 1% of college-aged women have anorexia nervosa.

PHYSICAL FINDINGS & CLINICAL PRESENTATION

Primary care physicians must be skilled at recognizing this disorder because patients with mild cases usually present with nonspecific symptoms such as asthenia, cold intolerance, lack of energy, or dizziness. The physical examination may be normal in the early stages or in mild cases. Patients with moderate to severe anorexia have the following physical characteristics:

- Patient is emaciated and bundled in clothing.
- Skin is dry and has excessive growth of lanugo. Skin may also be yellow-tinged from carotenodermia.
- Brittle nails, thinning scalp hair are present.
- Bradycardia, hypotension, hypothermia, and bradypnea are common.
- Female fat distribution pattern is no longer evident.
- Axillary and pubic hair is preserved.
- Peripheral edema may be present.

ETIOLOGY

- Etiology is unknown, but probably multifactorial (sociocultural, psychologic, familial, and genetic factors).
- A history of sexual abuse has been reported in as many as 50% of patients with anorexia nervosa.
- Psychologic factors: anorexics often have an incompletely developed personal identity. They struggle to maintain a sense of control over their environment, they usually have a low self-esteem, and they lack the sense that they are valued and loved for themselves.

Dx DIAGNOSIS

DIFFERENTIAL DIAGNOSIS

- Depression with loss of appetite
- Schizophrenia
- Conversion disorder
- Occult carcinoma, lymphoma
- Endocrine disorders: Addison disease, diabetes mellitus, hypothyroidism or hyperthyroidism, panhypopituitarism
- Gastrointestinal disorders: celiac disease, Crohn disease, intestinal parasitosis
- Infectious disorders: AIDS, tuberculosis
- A clinical algorithm for the evaluation of anorexia is described in Section III

WORKUP

- A diagnosis can be made by using the following DSM-IV diagnostic criteria for anorexia nervosa:
  1. Refusal to maintain body weight (BW) at or above a minimally normal weight for age and height (e.g., weight loss leading to maintenance of BW <85% of that expected or failure to make expected weight gain during a period of growth, leading to BW <85% of that expected)
  2. Intense fear of gaining weight or becoming fat, even though underweight
  3. Disturbance in the way in which BW or shape is experienced, undue influence of BW or shape on self-evaluation, or denial of the seriousness of the current low BW
  4. In postmenarchal females, amenorrhea—that is, the absence of at least three consecutive menstrual cycles (A woman is considered to have amenorrhea if her periods occur only after hormone administration, such as estrogen.)

Specify type:
Restricting type: During the current episode of anorexia nervosa, the person has not regularly engaged in binge eating or purging behavior (i.e., self-induced vomiting or the misuse of laxatives, diuretics, or enemas).
Binge-eating/purging type: During the current episode of anorexia nervosa, the person has regularly engaged in binge eating or purging behavior (i.e., self-induced vomiting or the misuse of laxatives, diuretics, or enemas).

- The SCOFF questionnaire is a screening tool for eating disorders used in England. It consists of the following five questions:
  1. Do you make yourself ***s***ick because you feel full?
  2. Have you lost ***c***ontrol over how much you eat?
  3. Have you lost more than ***o***ne stone (approximately 6 kg) recently?
  4. Do you believe yourself to be ***f***at when others say you are thin?
  5. Does ***f***ood dominate your life?
- A positive response to two or more questions has a reported sensitivity of 100% for anorexia and bulimia and an overall specificity of 87.5%.
- In college-aged women a positive response to any of the following screening questions also warrants further evaluation:
  1. How many diets have you been on in the past year?
  2. Do you think you should be dieting?
  3. Are you dissatisfied with your body size?
  4. Does your weight affect the way you think about yourself?
- Baseline ECG should be performed on all patients with anorexia nervosa. Routine monitoring of patients with prolonged QT interval is necessary; sudden death in these patients is often caused by ventricular arrhythmias related to QT interval prolongation.
- A dual-energy x-ray absorptiometry (DEXA) scan to screen for osteopenia should be considered after 6 mo of amenorrhea in patients suspected of anorexia nervosa.

LABORATORY TESTS

- In mild cases, laboratory findings may be completely normal.
- Endocrine abnormalities:
  1. Decreased follicle-stimulating hormone, luteinizing hormone, T_4, T_3, estrogens, urinary 17-OH steroids, estrone, and estradiol
  2. Normal free T_4, thyroid-stimulating hormone
  3. Increased cortisol, growth hormone, rT_3, T_3RU
  4. Absence of cyclic surge of luteinizing hormone
- Leukopenia, thrombocytopenia, anemia, reduced erythrocyte sedimentation rate, reduced complement levels, and reduced CD4 and CD8 cells may be present.
- Metabolic alkalosis, hypocalcemia, hypokalemia, hypomagnesemia, hypercholesterolemia, and hypophosphatemia may be present.
- Increased plasma β-carotene levels are useful to distinguish these patients from others on starvation diets.

Rx TREATMENT

NONPHARMACOLOGIC THERAPY

- A multidisciplinary approach with psychologic, medical, and nutritional support is necessary.
- A goal weight should be set and the patient should be initially monitored at least once a week in the office setting. The target weight is 100% of ideal BW for teenagers and 90% to 100% for older patients.
- Weight gain should be gradual (1 to 3 lb/wk) to prevent gastric dilation. Begin with 800 to 1200 kcal in frequent small meals (to avoid bloating sensation), then increase calories to 1500 to 3000 depending on height and age.
- Add, as necessary, vitamin and mineral supplements.
- In severe cases, total parenteral nutrition must be used (starting at 800 to 1200 kcal/day).
- Electrolyte levels should be strictly monitored.
- Mealtime should be a time for social interaction, not confrontation.
- Postprandially, sedentary activities are recommended. The patient's access to a bathroom should be monitored to prevent purging.

ACUTE GENERAL Rx

- Criteria to decide on the appropriate initial course of treatment for patients with anorexia nervosa are usually based on the presence of complications, percentage of ideal BW, and severity of body image distortion.
- Outpatient treatment is adequate for most patients.
- Indications for hospitalization are described under "Referral" section.
- Medically stable patients who are within 85% of ideal BW can be followed up by the primary care physician at 3- or 4-wk intervals, which can be lengthened as the patient improves.
- Pharmacologic treatment generally has no role in anorexia nervosa unless major depression or another psychiatric disorder is present. SSRIs can be used to alleviate the depressed mood and moderate obsessive-compulsive behavior in some individuals.

CHRONIC Rx

- Psychotherapy continued for years and focused specifically on self-image, family and peer interactions, and relapse prevention is an integral part of a successful recovery.
- Family therapy is also recommended, especially in younger patients.

DISPOSITION

- The long-term prognosis is generally poor and marked by recurrent exacerbations. The percentage of patients with anorexia nervosa who fully recover is modest. Most patients continue to have a distorted body image, disordered eating habits, and psychic difficulties.
- Most patients with anorexia nervosa will recover menses within 6 mo of reaching 90% of their ideal BW. It is important to note that patients with anorexia nervosa can become pregnant despite amenorrhea.
- Mortality rates vary from 5% to 20% and are six times that of peers without anorexia. Frequent causes of death are electrolyte abnormalities, starvation, or suicide.
- Factors that predict improved outcome in patients with eating disorders include early age at diagnosis, brief interval before initiation of treatment, good parent-child relationships, and having other healthy relationships with friends or therapists.
- A prolonged QT interval is a marker for risk of sudden death.

REFERRAL

Hospitalization should be considered in the following situations:

1. Severe dehydration or electrolyte imbalance
2. ECG abnormalities (prolonged QT interval, arrhythmias)
3. Significant physiologic instability (hypotension, orthostatic changes)
4. Intractable vomiting, purging, or bingeing
5. Suicidal thoughts
6. Weight loss exceeding 30% of ideal BW and unresponsiveness to outpatient treatment
7. Rapidly progressing weight loss (>2 lb in a week)
8. Failure to progress in nutritional rehabilitation in outpatient treatment

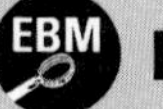

EVIDENCE

Please note: Complete text of EBM for this topic is available online.

Key trials and commentary:

This article provides a succinct summary of state-of-the-art treatment for anorexia nervosa, a difficult-to-treat and persistent illness. There appears to be widespread agreement that refeeding is an essential part of the treatment program, with behavioral treatments likely to be helpful. What distinguishes anorexia nervosa from most psychiatric illnesses is the need for a multidisciplinary approach, with mental health professionals, internists, and nutritionists all playing important parts. This is a disorder that is expensive to treat, with hospitalization often required. Although treatment is often successful in the short-term (e.g., while the patient remains under the watchful eye of the treatment team in the hospital), relapse is common, and the risk of death, either through cardiac arrhythmias or suicide, is high. This disorder affects a relatively small number of patients, but the risk of potentially lethal consequences is high. The article is helpful in condensing a good deal of information about this eating disorder into a concise summary, with useful headings to direct the readers' attention. Although one might wish that there was more empirical evidence about psychological treatments to share, the authors clearly lay out what is known and what interventions have been found effective.[1] Ⓐ

The aim of another study was to compare two cognitive-behavioral treatments for outpatients with eating disorders, one focusing solely on eating disorder features and the other a more complex treatment that also addresses mood intolerance, clinical perfectionism, low self-esteem, or interpersonal difficulties. It revealed that these two transdiagnostic treatments appear to be suitable for the majority of outpatients with an eating disorder. The simpler treatment may best be viewed as the default version, with the more complex treatment reserved for patients with marked additional psychopathology of the type targeted by the treatment.

This is a nicely conducted study that addresses highly prevalent disorders. What makes it particularly clinically relevant is that it extends Fairburn et al's work with patients with bulimia nervosa to eating disorders NOS, the big "catch-all" category for the many patients who do not fit criteria for anorexia or bulimia. There is already a good deal of evidence for Fairburn's cognitive-behavioral therapy (CBT) approach for bulimia, so the finding that two variants of this approach also work well for the more expanded group adds to the evidence base.

It was interesting to learn that although the simpler version and the more complex version of the treatment were not significantly different in their outcomes, patients with mood intolerance, clinical perfectionism, low self-esteem, or interpersonal difficulties did better with the variant that addressed those issues rather than simply focusing on issues specific to eating, for example, over concern with shape and weight. It seems likely that the vast majority of patients with eating disorders would suffer from at least one of those issues, however. It would have been helpful to know a bit more about the prevalence of eating disorder patients who do not suffer from comorbid mood disorders or interpersonal problems.

A major concern about this study is that 40% of potentially eligible patients refused to take part, mainly because they would not be available for the 28 weeks required for participation in the study or because they did not wish to participate in research. This is an extremely high number, and the authors should have determined if there were significant demographic or other types of relevant differences between the group that agreed to participate and the group that did not. If the nonparticipants had more severe disorders, would their outcomes have been as good?

Overall, the specific adaptations that have been made to make CBT specifically relevant to eating disorders (with the exception of anorexia nervosa, which requires a different type of approach) appear to be quite effective. The follow-up of 60 weeks is also a strength given the high rate of relapse with this type of problem.[2] Ⓐ

Evidence-Based References

1. Attia E, Walsh BT: Behavioral management for anorexia nervosa, *N Engl J Med* 360:500-506, 2009. Commentary by J.L. Krupnick, Ph.D. Ⓐ

2. Fairburn CG et al: Transdiagnostic cognitive-behavioral therapy for patients with eating disorders: a two-site trial with 60-week follow-up, *Am J Psychiatry* 166:311-319, 2009. Commentary by J.L. Krupnick, Ph.D. Ⓐ

SUGGESTED READINGS

American Psychiatric Association: Practice guideline for the treatment of patients with eating disorders, *Am J Psychiatry* 157(suppl):4, 2000.

Anstine D, Grinenko D: Rapid screening for disordered eating in college-aged females in the primary care setting, *J Adolesc Health* 26:338, 2000.

Attia E, Walsh BT: Behavioral management for anorexia nervosa, *N Engl J Med* 360:500-506, 2009.

Mehler PS: Diagnosis and care of patients with anorexia nervosa in primary care setting, *Ann Intern Med* 134:1048, 2001.

Miller KK et al: Medical findings in outpatients with anorexia nervosa, *Arch Intern Med* 165:561, 2005.

Morgan JF et al: The SCOFF questionnaire: assessment of a new screening tool for eating disorders, *BMJ* 319:1467, 1999.

Pritts SD, Susman J: Diagnosis of eating disorders in primary care, *Am Fam Physician* 67:297, 2003.

Williams PM et al: Treating eating disorders in primary care, *Am Fam Physician* 77(2):187-195, 2008.

Yager J, Andersen AE: Anorexia nervosa, *N Engl J Med* 353:1481, 2005.

AUTHOR: **FRED F. FERRI, M.D.**

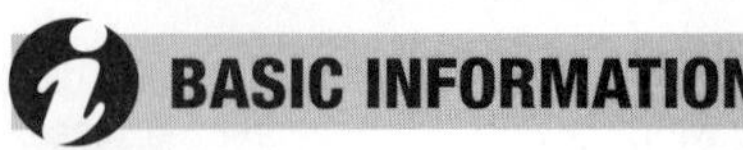

BASIC INFORMATION

DEFINITION

Anthrax is an acute infectious disease caused by the spore-forming bacterium *Bacillus anthracis.*

ICD-9CM CODES
022.0 Cutaneous anthrax
022.1 Inhalation anthrax
022.2 Gastrointestinal anthrax
022.3 Sepsis from anthrax

EPIDEMIOLOGY & DEMOGRAPHICS

- Anthrax most commonly occurs in hoofed animals and can only incidentally infect human beings who come in contact with infected animals or animal products. Between 20,000 and 100,000 cases of cutaneous anthrax occur worldwide annually. In the U.S. the annual incidence was about 130 cases before 2001.
- Until the recent bioterrorism attack in 2001, most cases of anthrax occurred in industrial environments (contaminated raw materials used in manufacturing process) or in agriculture.
- In 2001 there were more than 20 confirmed cases of anthrax resulting from bioterrorism, most of which were associated with handling of contaminated mail. Inhalation anthrax is the most lethal form of anthrax and results from inspiration of 8000 to 50,000 spores of *B. anthracis.* Before 2001 there had not been a case of inhalation anthrax in the U.S. for 20 years.
- Direct person-to-person spread of anthrax is extremely unlikely, if it occurs at all; therefore there is no need to immunize or treat contacts of persons ill with anthrax, such as household contacts, friends, or co-workers, unless they also were exposed to the same source of infection.

PHYSICAL FINDINGS & CLINICAL PRESENTATION

Symptoms of disease vary depending on how the disease was contracted but usually occur within 7 days after exposure. The serious forms of human anthrax are inhalation anthrax, cutaneous anthrax, and gastrointestinal anthrax.

- **Inhalation anthrax** begins with a brief prodrome resembling a viral respiratory illness followed by development of hypoxia and dyspnea, with radiographic evidence of mediastinal widening. Host factors, dose of exposure, and chemoprophylaxis may affect the duration of the incubation period. Initial symptoms include mild fever, muscle aches, and malaise and may progress to respiratory failure and shock; meningitis often develops.
- **Cutaneous anthrax** is characterized by a skin lesion evolving from a papule, through a vesicular stage, to a depressed black eschar. The incubation period ranges from 1 to 12 days. The lesion is usually painless, but patients also may have fever, malaise, headache, and regional lymphadenopathy. The eschar dries and falls off in 1 to 2 wk with little scarring.
- **Gastrointestinal anthrax** is characterized by severe abdominal pain followed by fever and signs of septicemia. Bloody diarrhea and signs of acute abdomen may occur. This form of anthrax usually follows after eating raw or undercooked contaminated meat and can have an incubation period of 1 to 7 days. Gastric ulcers may occur and may be associated with hematemesis. Oropharyngeal and abdominal forms of the disease have been described. Involvement of the pharynx is usually characterized by lesions at the base of the tongue, dysphagia, fever, and regional lymphadenopathy. Lower bowel inflammation typically causes nausea, loss of appetite, and fever followed by abdominal pain, hematemesis, and bloody diarrhea.

ETIOLOGY

The disease is caused by *B. anthracis,* a gram-positive, spore-forming bacillus. It is aerobic, nonmotile, nonhemolytic on sheep's blood agar and grows readily at temperature of 37° C, forming large colonies with irregularly tapered outgrowths (a Medusa's head appearance). In the host it appears as single organisms or chains of two or three bacilli.

DIAGNOSIS

DIFFERENTIAL DIAGNOSIS

- Inhalation anthrax must be distinguished from influenza-like illness (ILI) and tularemia. Most cases of ILI are associated with nasal congestion and rhinorrhea, which are unusual in inhalation anthrax. Additional distinguishing factors are the usual absence of abnormal chest radiograph in ILI (see below).
- Cutaneous anthrax should be distinguished from staphylococcal disease, ecthyma, ecthyma gangrenosum, plague, brown recluse spider bite, and tularemia.
- The differential diagnosis of gastrointestinal anthrax includes viral gastroenteritis, shigellosis, and yersiniosis.

LABORATORY TESTS

- Presumptive identification is based on Gram stain of material from skin lesion, CSF, or blood showing encapsulated gram-positive bacilli.
- Confirmatory tests are performed at specialized laboratories. Virulent strains grow on nutrient agar in the presence of 5% CO_2. Susceptibility to lysis by gamma phage and DFA staining of cell-wall polysaccharide antigen are also useful confirmatory tests.
- Nasal swab culture to determine inhalation exposure is of limited diagnostic value. A negative result does not exclude the possibility of exposure. It may be used by public health officials to assist in epidemiologic investigations of exposed persons to evaluate the dispersion of spores.
- Serologic testing by enzyme-linked immunosorbent assay (ELISA) can confirm the diagnosis.
- A skin test (Anthracin test) that detects anthrax cell-mediated immunity is also available in specialized laboratories.

IMAGING STUDIES

Chest radiographs usually reveal mediastinal widening. Additional findings include infiltrates and pleural effusion.

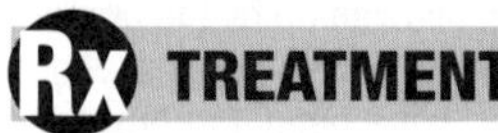

TREATMENT

NONPHARMACOLOGIC Rx

IV hydration and ventilator support may be necessary with inhalation anthrax.

ACUTE GENERAL Rx

- Most naturally occurring *B. anthracis* strains are sensitive to penicillin. The FDA has approved penicillin, doxycycline, and ciprofloxacin for the treatment of inhalational anthrax infection.
- Table 1-4 describes a treatment protocol for inhalation anthrax.
- Initial postexposure prophylaxis therapy in adults is with ciprofloxacin, 500 mg PO bid, or doxycycline 100 mg bid. The total duration of treatment is 60 days.
- A single dose of raxibacumab, a human monoclonal antibody directed against protective antigen, a component of the anthrax toxin, has been reported effective in improving survival in rabbits and monkeys with symptomatic inhalational anthrax.

DISPOSITION

- Case fatality estimates for inhalation anthrax are extremely high (>90%).
- The case fatality rate for cutaneous anthrax is 20% without and <1% with antibiotic treatment.
- The case fatality rate for gastrointestinal anthrax is estimated to be 25% to 60%.

REFERRAL

Consultation with an infectious disease specialist is recommended in all cases of anthrax. Local and state authorities should also be notified of suspected cases of anthrax.

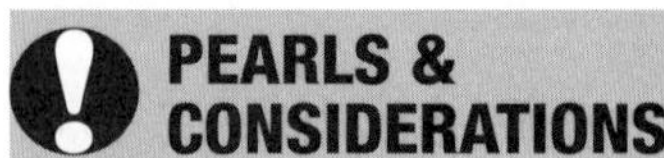

PEARLS & CONSIDERATIONS

COMMENTS

- Postexposure prophylaxis: If the exposure to *B. anthracis* is confirmed and anthrax vaccine is available, 3 doses of the vaccine should be given at 0, 2, and 4 wk, and antibiotics should be continued throughout the 4-wk period. If vaccine is not available, antibiotics should be continued for 60 days.
- Preexposure vaccination is limited to groups at risk for repeated exposures to *B. anthracis* spores, such as bioterrorism level-B laboratories and workers who will be making re-

peated entries into known *B. anthracis* spore-contaminated areas.

- The U.S. anthrax vaccine is an inactivated cell-free product licensed to be given in a 6-dose series.

SUGGESTED READINGS

Holty JE et al: Systematic review: a century of inhalational anthrax cases from 1900 to 2005, *Ann Intern Med* 144:270, 2006.

Hupert N et al: Accuracy of screening for inhalational anthrax after a bioterrorist attack, *Ann Intern Med* 139:337, 2003.

Inglesby TV et al: Anthrax as a biological weapon, 2002, *JAMA* 287:2236, 2002.

Interim guidelines for investigation of and response to *Bacillus anthracis* exposures, *MMWR Morb Mortal Wkly Rep* 50:987, 2001.

Migone TS et al: Raxibacumab for the treatment of inhalational anthrax, *N Engl J Med* 361:135-144, 2009.

Post-exposure anthrax prophylaxis, *Med Lett Drugs Ther* 43:91, 2001.

Swartz MN: Recognition and management of anthrax: an update, *N Engl J Med* 345:1621, 2001.

Use of anthrax vaccine for pre-exposure vaccination, *MMWR Morb Mortal Wkly Rep* 51:1024, 2002.

AUTHOR: **FRED F. FERRI, M.D.**

TABLE 1-4 Inhalation Anthrax Treatment Protocol[a,b]

Category	Initial Therapy (IV)[c,d]	Duration
Adults	Ciprofloxacin 400 mg q12h[a] **or** Doxycycline 100 mg q12h[f] **and** One or two additional antimicrobials[d]	IV treatment initially.[e] Switch to oral antimicrobial therapy when clinically appropriate: Ciprofloxacin 500 mg PO bid **or** Doxycycline 100 mg PO bid Continue for 60 days (IV and PO combined)[g]
Children	Ciprofloxacin 10-15 mg/kg q12h[h,i] **or** Doxycycline[f,j]: >8 yr and >45 kg: 100 mg q12h >8 yr and ≤45 kg: 2.2 mg/kg q12h ≤8 yr: 2.2 mg/kg q12h **and** One or two additional antimicrobials[d]	IV treatment initially.[e] Switch to oral antimicrobial therapy when clinically appropriate: Ciprofloxacin 10-15 mg/kg PO q12h[i] **or** Doxycycline[j]: >8 yr and >45 kg: 100 mg PO bid >8 yr and ≤45 kg: 2.2 mg/kg PO bid ≤8 yr: 2.2 mg/kg PO bid Continue for 60 days (IV and PO combined)[g]
Pregnant women[k]	Same for nonpregnant adults (the high death rate from the infection outweighs the risk posed by the antimicrobial agent)	IV treatment initially. Switch to oral antimicrobial therapy when clinically appropriate.[b] Oral therapy regimens same for nonpregnant adults.
Immunocompromised persons	Same for nonimmunocompromised persons and children	Same for nonimmunocompromised persons and children

From *MMWR Morb Mortal Wkly Rep* 5:987, 2001.

[a]For gastrointestinal and oropharyngeal anthrax, use regimens recommended for inhalational anthrax.

[b]Ciprofloxacin or doxycycline should be considered an essential part of first-line therapy for inhalational anthrax.

[c]Steroids may be considered as an adjunct therapy for patients with severe edema and for meningitis based on experience with bacterial meningitis of other etiologies.

[d]Other agents with in vitro activity include rifampin, vancomycin, penicillin, ampicillin, chloramphenicol, imipenem, clindamycin, and clarithromycin. Because of concerns of constitutive and inducible beta-lactamases in *Bacillus anthracis,* penicillin and ampicillin should not be used alone. Consultation with an infectious disease specialist is advised.

[e]Initial therapy may be altered based on clinical course of the patient; one or two antimicrobial agents (e.g., ciprofloxacin or doxycycline) may be adequate as the patient improves.

[f]If meningitis is suspected, doxycycline may be less optimal because of poor central nervous system penetration.

[g]Because of the potential persistence of spores after an aerosol exposure, antimicrobial therapy should be continued for 60 days.

[h]If IV ciprofloxacin is not available, oral ciprofloxacin may be acceptable because it is rapidly and well absorbed from the gastrointestinal tract with no substantial loss by first-pass metabolism. Maximum serum concentrations are attained 1 to 2 hr after oral dosing but may not be achieved if vomiting or ileus is present.

[i]In children, ciprofloxacin dosage should not exceed 1 g/day.

[j]The American Academy of Pediatrics recommends treatment of young children with tetracyclines for serious infections (e.g., Rocky Mountain spotted fever).

[k]Although tetracyclines are not recommended during pregnancy, their use may be indicated for life-threatening illness. Adverse effects on developing teeth and bones are dose related; therefore doxycycline might be used for a short time (7 to 14 days) before 6 mo of gestation.

BASIC INFORMATION

DEFINITION

The antiphospholipid antibody syndrome (APS) is characterized by arterial or venous thrombosis and/or pregnancy loss *and* the presence of antiphospholipid antibodies (aPL). aPL are antibodies directed against either phospholipids or proteins bound to anionic phospholipids. Three types of aPL have been characterized:
- Lupus anticoagulants
- Anticardiolipin antibodies
- Anti-β_2 glycoprotein-1 antibodies

The syndrome is referred to as primary APS when it occurs alone and as secondary APS when in association with systemic lupus erythematosus (SLE), other rheumatic disorders, or certain infections or medications. APS can affect all organ systems and includes venous and arterial thrombosis, recurrent fetal losses, and thrombocytopenia.

ICD-9CM CODES

795.79 Antiphospholipid antibody syndrome

EPIDEMIOLOGY & DEMOGRAPHICS

PREVALENCE:
- 1% to 5% of healthy individuals have anticardiolipin (ACL) and lupus anticoagulant (LA) antibodies.
- 12% to 30% of patients with SLE have ACL antibodies and 15% to 34% have LA antibodies.

PREDOMINANT AGE: Young to middle-age adults.

RISK FACTORS:
- Underlying SLE and collagen-vascular diseases; other autoimmune disorders including rheumatoid arthritis, Sjögren's syndrome, Behçet's syndrome, and idiopathic thrombocytopenic purpura; AIDS.
- Most individuals are otherwise healthy and have no underlying medical condition.
- Several studies assessing presence of aPL in patients with cardiovascular and cerebrovascular disease have found a higher than expected prevalence of antibody.

GENETICS: Some APS-positive families exist, and human leukocyte antigen (HLA) studies have suggested associations with HLA DR7, DR4, and Dqw7 plus Drw53.

PHYSICAL FINDINGS & CLINICAL PRESENTATION

- **Thrombosis:** Patients with APS are at risk for both venous and arterial thromboses. Venous thromboses are more common, occurring as the initial manifestation of APS in approximately 30% of APS patients. Of all patients with venous thrombosis, 5% to 20% have aPL. The most common site for deep vein thrombosis is the calf, but thromboses may also occur in the renal, hepatic, axillary, subclavian, vena cava, and retinal veins. The most common site of arterial thrombosis is the cerebral vessels. Other common sites are the coronary, renal, mesenteric, and bypass arteries. Recurrent thrombosis is common with APS.
- **Central nervous system:** stroke, transient ischemic attack, migraine, multiinfarct dementia, epilepsy, movement disorders, transverse myelopathy, depression, and Guillain-Barré syndrome.
- **Pulmonary:** pulmonary embolism and infarction, pulmonary hypertension, acute respiratory distress syndrome, intraalveolar pulmonary hemorrhage, a postpartum syndrome characterized by fever, pleuritic chest pain, dyspnea, and patchy infiltrates with pleural effusion on chest radiograph.
- **Cardiology:** Libman-Sacks endocarditis, intracardiac thrombosis, coronary artery disease, myocardial infarction.
- **Gastrointestinal:** abdominal pain, gastrointestinal bleed secondary to ischemia, splenic or pancreatic infarction, hepatic vein thrombosis, Budd-Chiari syndrome (second most common cause of syndrome).
- **Renal:** proteinuria, acute renal failure, hypertension, renal infarct, renal artery or vein thrombosis, postpartum hemolytic-uremic syndrome.
- **Hematology:** thrombocytopenia, hemolytic anemia.
- **Endocrine:** Addison's disease secondary to adrenal hemorrhage and, less frequently, thrombosis.
- **Cutaneous:** livedo reticularis, cutaneous necrosis, skin ulcerations, gangrene of digits.
- **Obstetrics:** recurrent spontaneous abortion (secondary to placental vessel thrombosis and ischemia).
- **Catastrophic APS:** widespread thrombotic disease with visceral damage. To make the diagnosis of catastrophic APS, four criteria must be satisfied:
  1. Evidence of involvement of ≥3 organs, systems, and/or tissues
  2. Development of manifestations simultaneously or in ≤1 week
  3. Confirmation by histopathology of small-vessel occlusion in at least one organ or tissue
  4. Laboratory confirmation of the presence of aPL

ETIOLOGY

- aPL react with negatively charged phospholipids.
- Possible mechanisms of thrombosis include effects of aPL on platelet membranes, endothelial cells, and clotting components such as prothrombin, protein C or S.
- Recently shown that prephospholipids are not immunogenic and that a binding protein (β_2-glycoprotein I) may be the key immunogen in the APS.

DIAGNOSIS

DIFFERENTIAL DIAGNOSIS

Other hypercoagulable states (inherited or acquired)
- Inherited: ATIII, protein C, S deficiencies, factor V Leiden, prothrombin gene mutation
- Acquired: heparin-induced thrombocytopenia, myeloproliferative syndromes, cancer, hyperviscosity
- Hyperhomocysteinemia
- Nephrotic syndrome

WORKUP

Diagnostic criteria of APS include at least one clinical criterion and at least one laboratory criterion.
- Clinical:
  1. Venous, arterial, or small vessel thrombosis *or*
  2. Morbidity with pregnancy defined as
     - Fetal death at ≥10 wk gestation *or*
     - ≥1 premature births before 34 wk gestation secondary to eclampsia, preeclampsia, or severe placental insufficiency *or*
     - ≥3 unexplained consecutive spontaneous abortions at <10 wk gestation
- Laboratory:
  1. IgG and/or IgM anticardiolipin antibody in medium or high titers *or*
  2. Lupus anticoagulant activity found *or*
  3. Anti-β_2 glycoprotein-1 IgM or IgG antibodies found on ≥2 occasions, at least 12 wk apart

LABORATORY TESTS

Laboratory testing of ACL and LA antibodies indicated in:
- Patient with underlying SLE or collagen-vascular disease with thrombosis
- Patient with recurrent, familial, or juvenile deep vein thrombosis (DVT) or thrombosis in an unusual location (mesenteric or cerebral)
- Possibly in patients with lupus or lupuslike disorders in high-risk situations (e.g., surgery, prolonged immobilization, pregnancy)

Abnormal tests include:
- False-positive test for syphilis (RPR/VDRL)
- Lupus anticoagulant activity, demonstrated by prolongation of activated partial thromboplastin time that does not correct with 1:1 mixing study
- Presence of anticardiolipin antibodies (ELISA for anticardiolipin is most sensitive and specific test [>80%])
- Presence of anti β_2-glycoprotein I antibody

TREATMENT

ACUTE GENERAL Rx

- For positive aPL and venous thrombosis:
  - Initial anticoagulation with heparin, then lifelong warfarin treatment, INR 2.0 to 3.0
- For positive aPL with arterial thrombosis:
  - Cerebral arterial thrombosis: aspirin (ASA) 325 mg daily or warfarin therapy (INR 1.4 to 2.8)
  - Noncerebral arterial thrombosis: warfarin therapy (INR 2.0 to 3.0)
- For pregnant women with previously diagnosed APS:
  - Warfarin should be discontinued secondary to its teratogenic effects.

- ASA, 81 mg, and unfractionated heparin (UFH) SC to partial thromboplastin time (PTT) of 1.5 to 2 times control value.
- Intravenous immunoglobulin (IVIG) and prednisone have also been used with success if aspirin and heparin fail.
- Low-molecular-weight (LMW) heparin can be used in place of unfractionated heparin and should be titrated to factor Xa levels in the recommended therapeutic range.
- Pregnant patients on LMW heparin should be transitioned to unfractionated heparin prior to delivery as unfractionated heparin is more easily managed in patients who wish to have epidural anesthesia for childbirth as it has a shorter half-life and is more easily reversed.

- For pregnant women with (+) aPL antibodies and a history of <3 spontaneous abortions:
    - ASA 81 mg daily at conception and UFH 5000 to 10,000 IU SC q12h at time of documented viable intrauterine pregnancy (approximately 7 wk gestation) until 6 wk postpartum.
    - A mid-interval PTT should be checked and should be normal or similar to baseline before therapy.
    - LMW heparin can be used in place of unfractionated heparin and should be titrated to factor Xa levels in the recommended prophylactic range. The combination of ASA 75 mg daily + LMW heparin has been associated with a higher live birth rate when compared to IVIG.
- For pregnant women with (+) aPL antibodies without a history of DVT or pregnancy loss:
    - Consider low-dose UFH or LMW heparin SC, ASA 81 mg, or surveillance.
- For catastrophic APS:
    - Highest survival rate achieved with the combination of anticoagulation, corticosteroids, and IVIG or plasma exchange.
    - Case reports of Rituximab as successful therapy for patients with life-threatening thrombosis refractory to anticoagulation.

CHRONIC Rx

- Anticoagulation with warfarin therapy.
- Immunosuppressive agents such as corticosteroids and cyclophosphamide not effective.
- Limited data suggest that hydroxychloroquine may be effective.

DISPOSITION

- APS patients have a 20% to 70% risk for recurrent thrombosis.
- Initial arterial thrombosis tends to be followed by arterial events, and initial venous thrombosis tends to be followed by venous events.
- Catastrophic APS is associated with a high mortality rate, approaching 50%.
- Incidence of developing catastrophic APS is approximately 0.8% among APS patients.

REFERRAL

To hematology and/or obstetric medicine when diagnosis is made

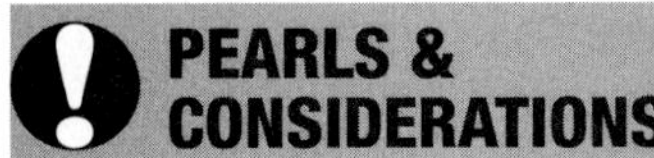

PEARLS & CONSIDERATIONS

COMMENTS

Cerebral features of SLE may be more related to thrombosis than inflammation and may respond better to anticoagulants than immunosuppression.

PREVENTION

Prophylaxis for asymptomatic patients with (+) aPL without previous thrombosis:

- No routine prophylaxis is recommended.
- Questionable whether ASA 81 mg daily is effective.
- Antithrombotic prophylaxis for major surgery, prolonged immobilization, and pregnancy.
- Avoid oral contraceptive pills in women with (+) aPL.

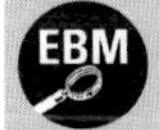

EVIDENCE

Prevention of thrombosis in APLAS.

There is evidence that anticoagulation is effective in the prevention of thrombosis in patients with APLAS.

- An RCT found that aspirin was equally effective to warfarin in preventing recurrent ischemic stroke in patients with APLAS.[1] Ⓑ

Management of APLAS in pregnancy.

- Systematic reviews have found that there is a lack of quality trials that evaluated the therapeutic options for APLAS in pregnancy.[2,3] Ⓐ

As such, the evidence for the use of therapies in this setting is limited. The use of some treatment options are supported by expert opinion:

For patients with antiphospholipid antibodies without previous thrombosis or pregnancy loss, the use of alternatives to warfarin as prophylactic anticoagulation is supported by expert opinion.

- Patients with antiphospholipid antibodies and no prior VTE or pregnancy loss should be considered to have an increased risk for the development of venous thrombosis and, perhaps, pregnancy loss. Suggested approaches for these women include: surveillance, minidose heparin, prophylactic LMWH, and/or low-dose aspirin, 75-162 mg/d.[4] Ⓒ

For patients with APLAS, with a history of prior thrombosis and/or pregnancy loss, the use of alternatives to warfarin as prophylactic anticoagulation is supported by expert opinion.

- For pregnant patients with APLAS and a history of multiple (two or more) early pregnancy losses or one or more late pregnancy losses, preeclampsia, IUGR, or abruption, we suggest administration of antepartum aspirin plus minidose or moderate-dose UFH or prophylactic LMWH.[4] Ⓒ
- Patients with APLAS and a history of venous thrombosis are usually receiving long-term oral anticoagulation therapy because of the high risk of recurrence. During pregnancy, we recommend adjusted-dose LMWH or UFH therapy plus low-dose aspirin and resumption of long-term oral anticoagulation therapy postpartum.[4] Ⓒ

Evidence-Based References

1. Levine SR et al: APASS Investigators. Antiphospholipid antibodies and subsequent thrombo-occlusive events in patients with ischemic stroke, *JAMA* 291:576-584, 2004. Ⓑ

2. Empson M et al: Prevention of recurrent miscarriage for women with antiphospholipid antibody or lupus anticoagulant, *Cochrane Database Rev* (2), 2005. Ⓐ

3. Wisloff F, Crowther M: Evidence-based treatment of the antiphospholipid syndrome: I. Pregnancy failure, *Thromb Res* 114:75-81, 2004. Ⓐ

4. Bates SM et al: Use of antithrombotic agents during pregnancy: the Seventh ACCP Conference on Antithrombotic and Thrombolytic Therapy, *Chest* 126:627S-44S, 2004. Ⓒ

SUGGESTED READINGS

Ahn ER et al: Long-term remission from life-threatening hypercoagulable state associated with lupus anticoagulant (LA) following rituximab therapy, *Am J Hematol* 78(2):127, 2005.

Asherson RA et al: Catastrophic antiphospholipid syndrome: international consensus statement on classification criteria and treatment guidelines, *Lupus* 12:530, 2003.

Charakida M et al: Vascular abnormalities, paraoxonase activity, and dysfunctional HDL in primary antiphospholipid syndrome, *JAMA* 302(11):1210-1217, 2006.

Erkan D, Lockshin MD: New treatments for antiphospholipid syndrome, *Rheum Dis Clin North Am* 32: 129, 2006.

Espinosa G, Cervera R: Thromboprophylaxis and obstetric management of the antiphospholipid syndrome, *Expert Opin Pharmacother* 10(4):601, 2009.

Lim W et al: Management of antiphospholipid antibody syndrome: a systematic review, *JAMA* 295(9):1050, 2006.

Miyakis S et al: International consensus statement on an update of the classification criteria for definite antiphospholipid syndrome, *J Thromb Haemost* 4: 295, 2006.

Rubenstein E et al: Rituximab treatment for resistant antiphospholipid syndrome, *J Rheumatol* 33(2):355, 2006.

AUTHOR: **IRIS TONG, M.D.**

Anxiety (Generalized Anxiety Disorder) 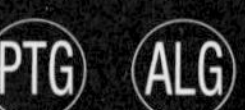

BASIC INFORMATION

DEFINITION

Generalized anxiety disorder (GAD) is most likely to present in combination with other psychiatric and medical conditions. GAD commonly presents with excessive anxiety, fear, and worry for most days over at least a 6-mo period. The subjective anxiety must be accompanied by at least three somatic symptoms (e.g., restlessness, irritability, sleep disturbance, muscle tension, difficulty concentrating, or fatigability). GAD cannot be diagnosed if it occurs only in the setting of an active mood disorder, such as depression.

SYNONYMS

Anxiety neurosis (former name for a subset of anxiety disorders)
Chronic anxiety
GAD

ICD-9CM CODES

F41.1 (DSM-IV Code 300.02)

EPIDEMIOLOGY & DEMOGRAPHICS

INCIDENCE (IN U.S.): 6% to 9% per year in adult primary care clinics

PEAK INCIDENCE: Chronic condition with onset early in life

PREVALENCE (IN U.S.):

- In general population: prevalence of 5% lifetime
- In primary care setting: 3% (the most common anxiety disorder in this setting)

PREDOMINANT SEX: Women are more frequently affected (2:1 ratio) but may present for treatment less often (3:2 female/male).

PREDOMINANT AGE:

- 30% of patients report onset of symptoms before age 11 yr
- 50% of patients have onset before age 18 yr

GENETICS: Concordance rates in dizygotic twins and monozygotic twins are not different (0% to 5%)

PHYSICAL FINDINGS & CLINICAL PRESENTATION

- Report of being "anxious" all of their lives.
- Excessive worry, usually regarding family, finances, work, or health.
- Sleep disturbance, particularly early insomnia.
- Muscle tension (typically in the muscles of neck and shoulders) or headache.
- Difficulty concentrating.
- Daytime fatigue.
- Gastrointestinal symptoms compatible with IBS (one third of patients).
- Physical consequences of anxiety are often the driving force for patients seeking medical attention.
- Comorbid psychiatric illness (e.g., dysthymia or major depression) and substance abuse (e.g., alcohol abuse) are frequent.

ETIOLOGY

- There is no clear etiology.
- Hypotheses centering on neurotransmitters (catecholamines, indolamines) and developmental psychology have been used as an explanatory framework to guide treatment recommendations.
- Prevalence may be increased in the setting of a family history, increase in stress, history of physical or emotional trauma, and medical illness.

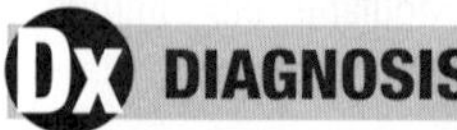

DIAGNOSIS

DIFFERENTIAL DIAGNOSIS

- Wide range of psychiatric and medical conditions; however, for a diagnosis of GAD to be made a person must experience anxiety with coexisting physical symptoms for the majority of the time for at least 6 mo.
- Cardiovascular and pulmonary disease, such as cardiac arrhythmias or COPD.
- Hyperthyroidism.
- Consequence of substance abuse (e.g., cocaine, amphetamines, and PCP) or withdrawal (e.g., alcohol or benzodiazepines).

WORKUP

- History: required for diagnosis. Anxiety disorders are prevalent, disabling, and often untreated in primary care. Screening tests may enhance detection. A simple 7 item in-office case finding instrument, the GAD-7, can detect GAD with sensitivity of 89% and specificity of 82%.
- Physical examination: useful in evaluation for other explanations of complaints.
- Exclusion of other basis for the complaints may require additional laboratory and radiologic workup depending on the presenting symptoms.
- Iatrogenic cause should be suspected if anxiety follows recent changes in medication.

Rx TREATMENT

NONPHARMACOLOGIC THERAPY

- Cognitive-behavioral therapy
- Relaxation training
- Biofeedback
- Psychodynamic psychotherapy

PHARMACOLOGIC THERAPY

- SSRIs/SNRIs
- Azapirones (e.g., buspirone)
- Benzodiazepines (less favored)

ACUTE GENERAL Rx

- Acute treatment is rarely indicated because GAD is a chronic condition.
- If patients are in acute distress, the possibility of another cause, including another anxiety disorder such as panic disorder, should be considered. Benzodiazepine-sparing therapy may preserve future therapeutic options such as azapirones. In addition, caution should be taken in prescribing benzodiazepines because of the propensity for misuse and dependence. If provided, the patient should be educated about the use of other medications and the risks in using benzodiazepines.

CHRONIC Rx

- SSRIs and SNRIs (e.g., venlafaxine and duloxetine) are effective in GAD and are typically given as a first-line treatment. These are particularly useful if comorbid depression is present.
- Buspirone can be effective with minimal potential for tolerance or abuse but may be less effective in patients with previous benzodiazepine exposure and may also require a titration to high doses to be effective.
- Benzodiazepines can be effective if prescribed under good supervision; however, tolerance to benzodiazepines is common, and for this reason they have fallen from a first-line treatment to second-line treatment for GAD. In addition, benzodiazepines can create significant functional impairment at work or while operating motor vehicles.
- Sedating antidepressants may also be useful in ameliorating initial insomnia secondary to anxious ruminations.

DISPOSITION

- This condition is chronic with periodic exacerbations.
- Treatment is given to provide a significant degree of improvement, but symptoms and dysfunction may persist.
- The risk for suicide is higher than in the general population.

REFERRAL

- If the symptoms are refractory to treatment
- If the case is complicated with a comorbid psychiatric condition
- If treatment response is suboptimal with residual dysfunction

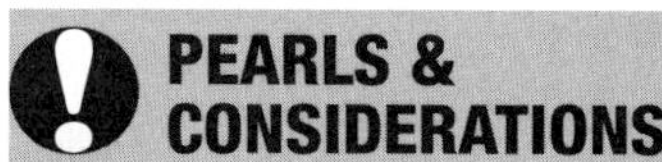

PEARLS & CONSIDERATIONS

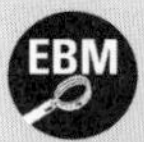

EVIDENCE

Please note: Complete text of EBM for this topic is available online.

Key trials and commentary:

The close association between generalized anxiety disorder (GAD) and major depressive disorder (MDD) prompts questions about how to characterize this association in future diagnostic systems. Most information about GAD-MDD comorbidity comes from patient samples and retrospective surveys. This study analyzed the sequential and cumulative comorbidity between GAD and MDD using data from a prospective longitudinal cohort. Challenging the prevailing notion that generalized anxiety usually precedes depression and eventually develops into depression, these findings show that the reverse pattern occurs almost as often. The GAD-MDD relation is strong, suggesting that the disorders could be classified in one category of distress disorders. Their developmental relation seems more symmetrical than heretofore presumed, suggesting that MDD is not necessarily primary over GAD in diagnostic hierarchy. This prospective study suggests that the lifetime prevalence of GAD and MDD may be underestimated by retrospective surveys and that comorbid GAD+MDD constitutes a greater mental health burden than previously thought.

There has been a great deal of discussion about the relationship between anxiety and depression, and this has become increasingly important as we are trying to develop the database for DSM-V. As previous readers remember, we have followed the studies, which have generally suggested that anxiety comes first with an eventual development into depression in a high percentage of cases. This large cohort study of 1037 individuals followed prospectively to age 32 years actually provides data reversing these general understandings. Although anxiety did precede depression in a third of the cases, it was equally common for depression to occur first and also in an equal number to begin concurrently. Like so many phenomena this occurs one third, one third, and one third. These data do turn the discussion about diagnosis of depression vs. anxiety on its ear. These data certainly argue against using the idea that MDD is hierarchically superior to GAD. It is also clear that GAD-MDD is a greater issue than we have recognized.[1] Ⓐ

Affective and anxiety disorders in early adulthood are associated with internalizing and externalizing disorders in childhood. Previous studies have not examined whether the risk associated with childhood psychological ill health persists for midlife psychological health. Another study analyzed whether childhood and adulthood psychological health are associated with midlife affective and anxiety disorders and to examine sex differences in these associations. This study revealed that childhood psychological health is an important independent distal factor in adulthood psychological health. Adulthood psychological health shows stronger associations with midlife disorders, indicating a poorer prognosis for adulthood than childhood psychological ill health. Men may be more susceptible than women to the effects of psychological ill health in early adulthood on midlife disorders. Targeting prevention, recognition, and treatment efforts in early adulthood, as well as in childhood and adolescence, may significantly reduce the burden of disease.

We increasingly have better data on psychiatric or psychological problems in childhood, and what the sequelae are psychiatrically in adulthood is an issue we have followed in previous editions. This study followed 9297 participants in a 45-year longitudinal study of a cohort born in 1958. They were able to follow children who had internalizing disorders as children ("worries, solitary, miserable, fearful, and fussy") and externalizing disorders ("destructive, fights, not liked, irritable, disobedient, lies, steals, and aggressive") to adulthood and did find a 1.5- to 2-fold increase in midlife anxiety and affective disorders. If they were psychologically ill at ages 23, 33, and 42, there was a 2- to 7-fold increase in midlife disorders, an even stronger association. This and other studies make it clear that when children are "ill" psychologically, these are not trivial disorders and are associated with greater increases in lifelong psychiatric problems. It makes a strong argument that we should pay more attention to treatment and preventive efforts in children. Whether we do this or not is a societal issue, and we are far from consensus on what to do about that.[2] Ⓐ

Evidence-Based References

1. Moffitt TE, Harrington HL, Caspi A: Depression and generalized anxiety disorder: cumulative and sequential comorbidity in a birth cohort followed prospectively to age 32 years, *Arch Gen Psychiatry* 64:651-660, 2007. Commentary by J.C. Ballenger, M.D. Ⓐ

2. Clark C, Rodgers B, Caldwell T: Childhood and adulthood psychological ill health as predictors of midlife affective and anxiety disorders: the 1958 British Birth Cohort, *Arch Gen Psychiatry* 64:668-678, 2007. Commentary by J.C. Ballenger, M.D. Ⓐ

SUGGESTED READINGS

Davidson JR: First-line pharmacotherapy approaches for generalized anxiety disorder, *J Clin Psychiatry* 70(suppl 2):25-31, 2009.

Fricchione G: Clinical practice. Generalized anxiety disorder, *N Engl J Med* 351(7):675, 2004.

Kroenke K et al: Anxiety disorders in primary care: prevalence, impairment, comorbidity, and detection, *Ann Intern Med* 146(5):317-325, 2007.

Stanley MA et al: Cognitive behavior therapy for generalized anxiety disorder among older adults in primary care, *JAMA* 301(14):1460-1467, 2009.

Stewart RE, Chambless DL: Cognitive-behavioral therapy for adult anxiety disorders in clinical practice: a meta-analysis of effectiveness studies, *J Consult Clin Psychol* 77(4):595-606, 2009.

Weisberg RB: Overview of generalized anxiety disorder: epidemiology, presentation, and course, *J Clin Psychiatry* 70(suppl 2):4-9, 2009.

AUTHORS: **SETH A. BERKOWITZ, M.D.,** and **ILJIE KIM FITZGERALD M.D., M.S.**

Aortic Dissection (ALG)

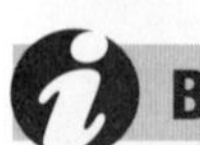

BASIC INFORMATION

DEFINITION

Aortic dissection occurs when blood passes through an intimal tear, separating the intima from the medial layers and creating a false lumen.

SYNONYMS

Dissecting aortic aneurysm

ICD-9CM CODES
441.00 Aortic dissection
444.01 Aortic dissection, thoracic

EPIDEMIOLOGY & DEMOGRAPHICS

PREDOMINANT SEX AND AGE: Males > females (ratio 3:1), ages 60 to 80 yr; mean, 63 yr

INCIDENCE: Approximately 2000 cases per year; thirteenth leading cause of death in U.S.

RISK FACTORS:

- Hypertension
- Atherosclerosis
- Family history of aortic aneurysms/dissection
- History of cardiac surgery, intraaortic catheterization
- Disorders of collagen (Marfan syndrome, Ehlers-Danlos syndrome)
- Vascular inflammation (giant cell arteritis, Takayasu arteritis, rheumatoid arthritis, syphilitic aortitis)
- Aortic coarctation, bicuspid aortic valve
- Turner's syndrome
- Cocaine abuse
- Trauma

CLASSIFICATION

Two main classification schemes based on the location of dissection (Fig. 1-24):

- DeBakey: type I ascending and descending aorta, type II ascending aorta, type III descending aorta
- Stanford: type A ascending aorta (proximal), type B descending aorta (distal)

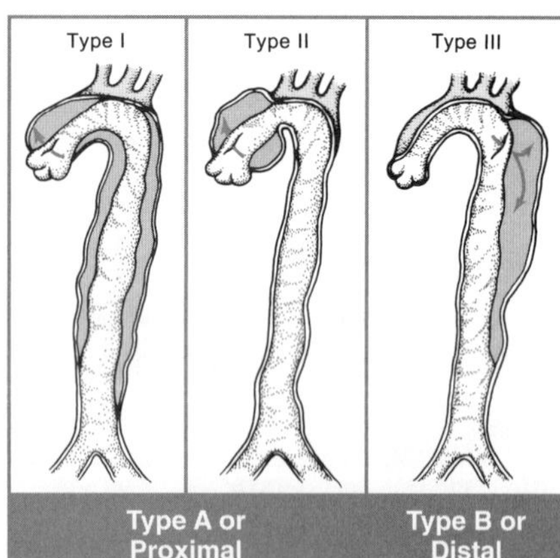

FIGURE 1-24 Classification systems for aortic dissection. (From Isselbacher EM et al: Disease of the aorta. In Braunwald E [ed]: *Heart disease: a textbook of cardiovascular medicine,* ed 5, Philadelphia, 1997, WB Saunders.)

PHYSICAL FINDINGS & CLINICAL PRESENTATION

- Sudden onset of severe sharp, tearing, or ripping chest pain
- Anterior chest pain (ascending dissection)
- Back pain, abdominal pain (descending dissection)
- Syncope, congestive heart failure (CHF), malperfusion may occur
- Most present with severe hypertension, 25% with hypotension (systolic blood pressure <100 mm Hg), which can indicate bleeding, cardiac tamponade, or severe aortic regurgitation
- Pulse and blood pressure differentials (>20 mm Hg between arms) in 9% to 30% of cases, caused by partial compression of subclavian arteries
- Aortic regurgitation in 18% to 50% of cases of proximal dissection, often with diastolic decrescendo murmur
- Myocardial ischemia caused by coronary artery occlusion
- Stroke in 5% to 10% of patients
- Horner syndrome
- Vocal cord paralysis/hoarse voice

ETIOLOGY

- Degeneration or alteration of the intimal and medial layers seems to be the common pathology involved with acquired (e.g., hypertension, vascular inflammation) and genetic (e.g., collagen vascular disease) risk factors for dissection.
- Aortic dissection reflects systemic illness of vasculature.

Dx DIAGNOSIS

DIFFERENTIAL DIAGNOSIS

- Known as the great imitator: PE, ACS, aortic stenosis/insufficiency, nondissecting aneurysm, pericarditis, cholecystitis, peptic ulcer disease, pancreatitis, musculoskeletal pain
- Acute MI needs to be ruled out.
- Consider aortic dissection in patients with unexplained stroke, chest pain, syncope, acute onset CHF, abdominal pain, back pain, and malperfusion of extremities or internal organs.

LABORATORY TESTS

- ECG: helpful to rule out MI, although dissection can lead to coronary ischemia
- Currently no readily available, reliable serum biomarker
- Use of D-dimer dissection is controversial.
- Smooth muscle myosin heavy chain protein (released from damaged medial smooth muscle), C-reactive protein, fibrinogen, and elastin fragments under investigation

IMAGING STUDIES

- Chest radiograph may show widened mediastinum (62%) and displacement of aortic intimal calcium.
- Although the diagnostic sensitivity of transthoracic echocardiography is suboptimal, it is useful in assessing potential high risk features or complications, such as pericardial effusion, and making other potential diagnoses. A negative transthoracic echocardiography, however, does not exclude aortic dissection.
- Transesophageal echocardiography (TEE) is study of choice in unstable patients but is operator dependent.
- MRI has the highest sensitivity and specificity but limited availability; not suitable for unstable patients; contraindicated with pacemakers, metal devices.
- Helical CT is least operator dependent but involves intravenous contrast.
- TEE, MRI, helical CT are imaging modalities of choice. Sensitivities (98% to 100%) and specificities (95% to 98%) nearly equal in skilled hands. Test of choice depends on clinical circumstances and availability.
- With medium or high pretest probability, a second diagnostic test should be done if the first is negative.
- Coronary computed tomographic angiography (CTA) may be an alternative and useful diagnostic study when evaluating for pulmonary embolism, acute coronary syndrome, and aortic dissection.
- Aortography rarely done now.

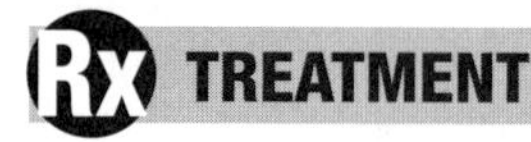

Rx TREATMENT

ACUTE GENERAL Rx

- Admit to ICU for monitoring.
- Target SBP 100 to 120 mm Hg or as low as tolerated; heart rate <60 beats/min to reduce aortic wall stress.
- IV beta-blockers are cornerstones of treatment.
- Propanolol 1 mg every 3 to 5 min; metoprolol 5 mg IV every 5 min; or labetalol 20 mg IV, then 20 to 80 mg every 10 min, followed by nitroprusside 0.3 to 10 mg/kg/min.
- Nitroprusside should not be used without beta-blockade because vasodilation can induce reflex sympathetic stimulation and increased aortic sheer stress.
- IV calcium channel blockers with negative inotropy may be used.
- Pain control, often with morphine.
- Multiple medications may be needed.
- Proximal dissections require emergent surgery to prevent rupture or pericardial effusion.
- Distal dissections are usually treated medically unless distal organ involvement or impending rupture occurs.
- Endovascular repair is feasible for both acute aortic dissection and coronary artery disease.

Literature has shown favorable short- and mid-term outcomes. However, long-term outcome data are still under investigation.

CHRONIC Rx

- Chronic aortic dissection (>2 wk) managed with aggressive blood pressure control: target <120/80 mm Hg in most patients.
- Target low-density lipoprotein <70 mg/dl.
- Minimize strenuous physical activity.
- Serial imaging of the aorta, usually with contrast CT.
- Endovascular repair in chronic type B dissection should be considered when the aortic diameter exceeds 5.5-6.0 cm, when there is uncontrolled pain or blood pressure, or when there is rapid growth of the dissecting aneurysm (>1 cm per year). Long-term outcome data are still under investigation.

DISPOSITION

- 85% mortality rate within 2 wk if untreated.
- Proximal dissection is a surgical emergency. Time is critical; mortality rate is 1% to 3% per hour.
- Overall, in-hospital mortality rate is 30% with proximal dissections and 10% with distal dissections.

REFERRAL

For ICU management and surgery

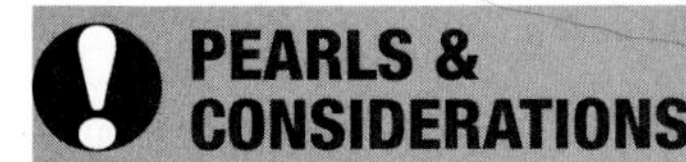

PEARLS & CONSIDERATIONS

- Blood pressure control is essential; beta-blocker is first-line medication.
- Proximal dissection is a surgical emergency.

SUGGESTED READINGS

Akin I, Kische S: Indication, timing, and results of endovascular treatment of type B dissection, *Eur J Vasc Endovasc Surg* 37(3):289-296, 2009.

Golledge J, Eagle KA: Acute aortic dissection, *Lancet* 372(9632):55, 2008.

Himanshu, P, Deeb, M: Ascending and arch aorta pathology, natural history, and treatment, *Circulation* 118:188, 2008.

Kische SE, Ehrlich MP: Endovascular treatment of acute and chronic aortic dissection: midterm results from the Talent Thoracic Retrospective Registry, *J Thorac Cardiovasc Surg* 138(1):115-124, 2009.

Ramanath VS et al: Acute aortic syndromes and thoracic aortic aneurysm, *Mayo Clin Proc* 84(5):465-481, 2009.

Shiga T et al: Diagnostic accuracy of TEE, helical CT, and MRI for suspected thoracic aortic dissection *Arch Intern Med* 166:1350-296, 2006.

AUTHORS: **LYNN BOWLBY, M.D.,** and **ABDULRAHMAN ABDULBAKI, M.D.**

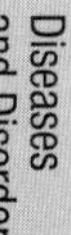

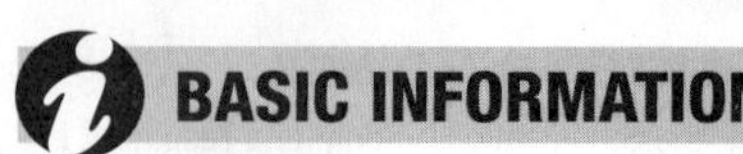

BASIC INFORMATION

DEFINITION

Aortic regurgitation is retrograde blood flow into the left ventricle from the aorta as a result of an incompetent aortic valve.

SYNONYMS

Aortic insufficiency
AI
AR

ICD-9CM CODES
424.1 Aortic valve disorders

EPIDEMIOLOGY & DEMOGRAPHICS

- Prevalence ranges from 4.9% to 10% and increases with age.
- The most common cause of isolated severe aortic regurgitation is aortic root dilation.
- Infectious endocarditis is the most frequent cause of acute aortic regurgitation.

PHYSICAL FINDINGS & CLINICAL PRESENTATION

The clinical presentation varies depending on whether aortic insufficiency is acute or chronic. Chronic aortic insufficiency is well tolerated (except when secondary to infective endocarditis), and the patients remain asymptomatic for years. Common manifestations after significant deterioration of left ventricular function are dyspnea on exertion, syncope, chest pain, and congestive heart failure (CHF). Acute aortic insufficiency manifests primarily with hypotension caused by a sudden fall in cardiac output. A rapid rise in left ventricular diastolic pressure results in a further decrease in coronary blood flow.

Physical findings in chronic aortic insufficiency include the following:

- Widened pulse pressure (markedly increased systolic blood pressure, decreased diastolic blood pressure).
- Bounding pulses, head "bobbing" with each systole (de Musset's sign); "water hammer" or collapsing pulse (Corrigan's pulse) can be palpated at the wrist or on the femoral arteries ("pistol shot" femorals) and is caused by rapid rise and sudden collapse of the arterial pressure during late systole; capillary pulsations (Quincke's pulse) may occur at the base of the nail beds.
- A to-and-fro "double Duroziez" murmur may be heard over femoral arteries with slight compression.
- Popliteal systolic pressure is increased over brachial systolic pressure ≥40 mm Hg (Hill's sign).
- Cardiac auscultation reveals:
  1. Displacement of cardiac impulse downward and to the patient's left
  2. S_3 heard over the apex
  3. Decrescendo, blowing diastolic murmur heard along left sternal border
  4. Low-pitched apical diastolic rumble (Austin-Flint murmur) caused by contrast of the aortic regurgitant jet with the left ventricular wall
  5. Early systolic apical ejection murmur

In patients with acute aortic insufficiency both the wide pulse pressure and the large stroke volume are absent. A short blowing diastolic murmur may be the only finding on physical examination.

ETIOLOGY

- Infective endocarditis
- Rheumatic fibrosis (most common cause in developing countries)
- Trauma with valvular rupture
- Congenital bicuspid aortic valve (most common cause in U.S.)
- Myxomatous degeneration
- Annuloaortic ectasia
- Syphilitic aortitis
- Rheumatic spondylitis
- Systemic lupus erythematosus (SLE)
- Aortic dissection
- Fenfluramine, dexfenfluramine, pergolide, cabergoline
- Takayasu's arteritis, granulomatous arteritis

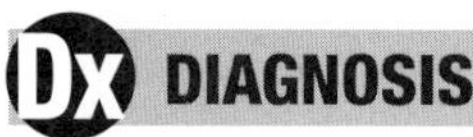

DIAGNOSIS

DIFFERENTIAL DIAGNOSIS

- Patent ductus arteriosus, pulmonary regurgitation, and other valvular abnormalities
- The differential diagnosis of cardiac murmurs is described in Section II

WORKUP

- Echocardiogram, chest radiograph, ECG, and cardiac catheterization (selected patients)
- Medical history and physical examination focused on the following clinical manifestations:
  1. Dyspnea on exertion
  2. Syncope
  3. Chest pain
  4. CHF

IMAGING STUDIES

- Chest radiography:
  1. Left ventricular hypertrophy (chronic aortic regurgitation)
  2. Aortic dilation
  3. Normal cardiac silhouette with pulmonary edema: possible in patients with acute aortic regurgitation
- ECG: left ventricular hypertrophy (LVH).
- Echocardiography is the main imaging modality to diagnose aortic regurgitation and assess left ventricular size and function. Quantification of the severity of regurgitation can be made either qualitatively or quantitatively by effective regurgitant orifice area (severe if >0.30 cm^2) and/or regurgitant volume (severe if >60 ml per beat).
- Cardiac catheterization in selected patients to assess degree of left ventricular dysfunction, to assess the degree of aortic regurgitation when echocardiographic parameters are inclusive, and determine if there is coexistent coronary artery disease.

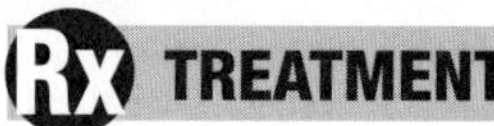

TREATMENT

NONPHARMACOLOGIC THERAPY

- Avoidance of competitive sports and heavy weight lifting if the aortic regurgitation is severe.
- Salt restriction
- Antibiotic prophylaxis is reasonable for high-risk patients who undergo dental procedures. High-risk patients include those with artificial values, previous endocarditis, unrepaired or partially-repaired cyanotic congenital heart disease, or cardiac transplant recipients. Prophylaxis is no longer indicated for intermediate to low-risk patients.

ACUTE GENERAL Rx

MEDICAL:

- Angiotensin-converting enzyme (ACE) inhibitors, diuretics, and sodium restriction for CHF; nitroprusside in patients with acute aortic regurgitation
- Long-term vasodilator therapy with ACE inhibitors who are not candidates for valve replacement in asymptomatic patients with severe aortic regurgitation and normal left ventricular function or asymptomatic patients with severe aortic regurgitation and left ventricular dysfunction.

SURGICAL: Reserved for:

- Symptomatic patients with chronic aortic regurgitation despite optimal medical therapy
- Patients with acute aortic regurgitation (i.e., infective endocarditis) producing left ventricular failure
- Evidence of systolic dysfunction:
  1. Echocardiographic end systolic dimension >55 mm
  2. Echocardiographic end diastolic dimension >75 mm
  3. Left ventricular ejection fraction of 50% or less
- Evidence of heart failure.

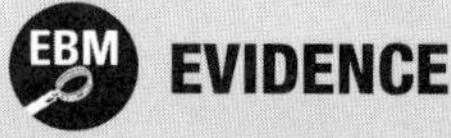

EVIDENCE

Please note: Complete text of EBM for this topic is available online.

SUGGESTED READINGS

Bonow RO et al: ACC/AHA 2006 guidelines for the management of patients with valvular heart disease: a report of the American College of Cardiology/American Heart Association Task Force on Practice Guidelines. Available at http://www.acc.org/clinical/guidelines/valvular/index.pdf.

Bonow RO et al: 2008 focused update incorporated into the ACC/AHA 2006 guidelines for the management of patients with valvular heart disease, *J Am Coll Cardiol* 52:1-142, 2008.

Enriquez-Sarano M, Tajik J: Aortic regurgitation, *N Engl J Med* 351:1539, 2004.

AUTHORS: **WEN-CHIH WU, M.D.,** and **FRED F. FERRI, M.D.**

BASIC INFORMATION

DEFINITION

Aortic stenosis is obstruction to systolic left ventricular outflow across the aortic valve. Symptoms appear when the valve orifice decreases to $<$1 cm^2 (normal orifice is 3 cm^2). The stenosis is considered severe when the orifice is $<$0.5 cm^2/m^2 or the pressure gradient is $\geq$50 mm Hg.

SYNONYMS

Aortic valvular stenosis
AS

ICD-9CM CODES
424.1 Aortic valvular stenosis

EPIDEMIOLOGY & DEMOGRAPHICS

- Aortic stenosis is the most common valve lesion in adults in Western countries.
- Calcific stenosis (most common cause in patients $>$60 yr) occurs in 75% of patients.

PHYSICAL FINDINGS & CLINICAL PRESENTATION

- Rough, loud, systolic, diamond-shaped murmur best heard at base of heart and transmitted into neck vessels; often associated with a thrill or ejection click; may also be heard well at the apex.
- Absence or diminished intensity of sound of aortic valve closure (in severe aortic stenosis).
- Late, slow-rising carotid upstroke with decreased amplitude.
- Strong apical pulse.
- Narrowing of pulse pressure in later stages of aortic stenosis.
- Some patients with aortic stenosis experience bleeding into their GI tract or skin. This is caused by an acquired defect in von Willebrand factor. Aortic valve replacement restores normal hemostasis.

ETIOLOGY

- Rheumatic inflammation of aortic valve
- Progressive stenosis of congenital bicuspid valve (found in 1% to 2% of population)
- Idiopathic calcification of the aortic valve
- Congenital (major cause of aortic stenosis in patients $<$30 yr)

Dx DIAGNOSIS

DIFFERENTIAL DIAGNOSIS

- Hypertrophic cardiomyopathy
- Mitral regurgitation
- Ventricular septal defect
- Aortic sclerosis. Aortic stenosis is distinguished from aortic sclerosis by the degree of valve impairment. In aortic sclerosis, the valve leaflets are abnormally thickened but obstruction to outflow is minimal.

WORKUP

- Echocardiography.
- Chest radiographs, ECG.
- Laboratory: B-type natriuretic peptide or *N*-terminal pro-B-type natriuretic peptide (NT-proBNP) correlates with the mean pressure gradient, aortic valve area, and functional status. It is a useful biochemical marker to evaluate severity of aortic stenosis (AS), monitor disease progression at an early stage, and decide on the optimal time for aortic valve replacement. An increased level of BNP correlates with severity of AS and New York Heart Association functional class.
- Cardiac catheterization in selected patients (see "Imaging Studies")
- Medical history focusing on symptoms and potential complications:
  1. Angina
  2. Syncope (particularly with exertion)
  3. Congestive heart failure (CHF)
  4. GI bleeding: in patients with associated hemorrhagic telangiectasia (AVM)
- Section III describes an algorithm for evaluation of suspected aortic stenosis

IMAGING STUDIES

- Chest x-ray examination:
  1. Poststenotic dilation of the ascending aorta
  2. Calcification of aortic cusps
  3. Pulmonary congestion (in advanced stages of aortic stenosis)
- ECG:
  1. Left ventricular hypertrophy (found in $>$80% of patients)
  2. ST-T wave changes
  3. Atrial fibrillation: frequent
- Doppler echocardiography: thickening of the left ventricular wall; if the patient has valvular calcifications, multiple echoes may be seen from within the aortic root and there is poor separation of the aortic cusps during systole. Gradient across the valve can be estimated but is less precise than with cardiac catheterization. Section III describes an algorithm for the management of patients with aortic stenosis detected by echocardiography.
- Cardiac catheterization: indicated in symptomatic patients; it confirms the diagnosis and estimates the severity of the disease by measuring the gradient across the valve, allowing calculation of the valve area. It also detects coexisting coronary artery stenosis that may need bypass at the same time as aortic valve replacement.

Rx TREATMENT

NONPHARMACOLOGIC THERAPY

- Strenuous activity should be avoided
- Sodium restriction if CHF is present

GENERAL Rx

MEDICAL:

- Diuretics and sodium restriction are needed if CHF is present; digoxin is used only to control rate of atrial fibrillation.
- ACE inhibitors are relatively contraindicated.
- The calcium channel blocker verapamil may be useful only to control rate of atrial fibrillation.
- Antibiotic prophylaxis is reasonable for high-risk patients who undergo dental procedures. High-risk patients include those with artificial valves, previous endocarditis, unrepaired or partially-repaired cyanotic congenital heart disease, or cardiac transplant recipients. Prophylaxis is no longer indicated for intermediate to low-risk patients.

SURGICAL:

- Valve replacement is the treatment of choice in symptomatic patients because the 5-yr mortality rate after onset of symptoms is extremely high, even with optimal medical therapy. Valve replacement is indicated if cardiac catheterization establishes a pressure gradient $>$50 mm Hg and valve area $<$1 cm^2.
- Percutaneous aortic balloon valvuloplasty serves best as palliative therapy in severely symptomatic patients and as a bridge to surgery in hemodynamically unstable adult patients. It is not an option in patients who are good candidates for surgical valve replacement.

DISPOSITION

- 15% to 20% of patients with severe aortic stenosis die before age 20 yr.
- The 5-yr survival rate in adults is 40%.
- The average duration of symptoms before death is angina, 60 mo; syncope, 36 mo; CHF, 24 mo.
- Approximately 75% of patients with symptomatic aortic stenosis will be dead 3 yr after onset of symptoms unless the aortic valve is replaced.

REFERRAL

- Surgical referral for valve replacement in symptomatic patients. However, the presence of moderate or severe valvular calcification, together with a rapid increase in aortic jet velocity and elevated BNP, identify patients with a very poor prognosis who should be considered for early valve replacement rather than have surgery delayed until symptoms develop.
- Surgical mortality rate for valve replacement is 3% to 5%; however, it varies with patient's age ($>$8% in patients $>$75 yr).
- Balloon valvuloplasty is useful in infants and children or poor surgical candidates who do not have calcified valve apparatus; it can be done as an intermediate procedure to stabilize high-risk patients before surgery.
- When performed in adults who have calcified valves, balloon valvuloplasty is useful only for short-term reduction in severity of aortic stenosis when surgery is contraindicated because restenosis occurs rapidly.

 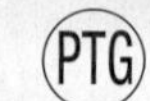

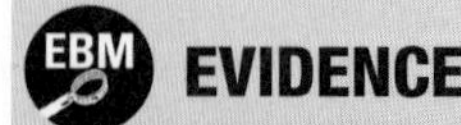

EVIDENCE

Please note: Complete text of EBM for this topic is available online.

SUGGESTED READINGS

Bonow RO et al: ACC/AHA 2006 guidelines for the management of patients with valvular heart disease: a report of the American College of Cardiology/American Heart Association Task Force on practice guidelines. Available at http://www.acc.org/clinical/guidelines/valvular/index.pdf.

Bonow RO et al: 2008 focused update incorporated into the ACC/AHA 2006 guidelines for the management of patients with valvular heart disease, *J Am Coll Cardiol* 52:1-142, 2008.

Kapadia SR et al: Percutaneous treatment of aortic valve stenosis, *Clev Clin J of Med* 75:11, 805-812, 2008.

AUTHORS: **VICTOR SHIN, M.D.,**
and **FRED F. FERRI, M.D.**

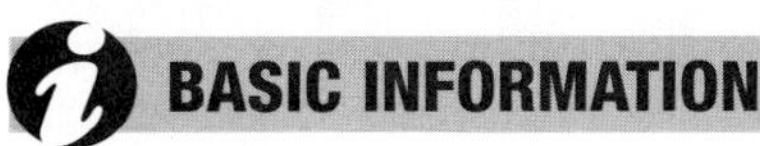

BASIC INFORMATION

DEFINITION

Appendicitis is the acute inflammation of the appendix.

ICD-9CM CODES
540.9 Appendicitis
540.0 Appendicitis with generalized peritonitis

EPIDEMIOLOGY & DEMOGRAPHICS

- Appendicitis occurs in 10% of the population, most commonly between the ages of 10 and 30 yr.
- More than 250,000 appendectomies are performed in the U.S. each year.
- It is the most common abdominal surgical emergency.
- Incidence of appendicitis has declined over the past 30 yr.
- Male/female ratio is 3:2 until mid-20s; it equalizes after age 30 yr.

PHYSICAL FINDINGS & CLINICAL PRESENTATION

- In children with abdominal pain, fever is the single most useful sign associated with appendicitis. Vomiting, rectal tenderness, and rebound tenderness along with fever are more indicative of appendicitis in children than in adults.
- Abdominal pain: initially the pain may be epigastric or periumbilical in nearly 50% of patients; it subsequently localizes to the right lower quadrant within 12 to 18 hr. Pain can be found in back or right flank if appendix is retrocecal or in other abdominal locations if there is malrotation of the appendix.
- Pain with right thigh extension (psoas sign), low-grade fever: temperature may be >38° C if there is appendiceal perforation.
- Pain with internal rotation of the flexed right thigh (obturator sign) is present.
- Right lower quadrant (RLQ) pain on palpation of the left lower quadrant (LLQ) (Rovsing's sign): physical examination may reveal right-sided tenderness in patients with pelvic appendix.
- Point of maximum tenderness is in the RLQ (McBurney's point).
- Nausea, vomiting, tachycardia, cutaneous hyperesthesias at the level of T12 can be present.

ETIOLOGY

Obstruction of the appendiceal lumen with subsequent vascular congestion, inflammation, and edema; common causes of obstruction are:

- Fecaliths: 30% to 35% of cases (most common in adults)
- Foreign body: 4% (fruit seeds, pinworms, tapeworms, roundworms, calculi)
- Inflammation: 50% to 60% of cases (submucosal lymphoid hyperplasia [most common etiology in children, teens])
- Neoplasms: 1% (carcinoids, metastatic disease, carcinoma)

Dx DIAGNOSIS

DIFFERENTIAL DIAGNOSIS

- Intestinal: regional cecal enteritis, incarcerated hernia, cecal diverticulitis, intestinal obstruction, perforated ulcer, perforated cecum, Meckel's diverticulitis
- Reproductive: ectopic pregnancy, ovarian cyst, torsion of ovarian cyst, salpingitis, tubo-ovarian abscess, mittelschmerz, endometriosis, seminal vesiculitis
- Renal: renal and ureteral calculi, neoplasms, pyelonephritis
- Vascular: leaking aortic aneurysm
- Psoas abscess
- Trauma
- Cholecystitis
- Mesenteric adenitis

WORKUP

Patients with RLQ pain, nausea, vomiting, anorexia, and RLQ rebound tenderness should undergo prompt clinical and laboratory evaluation. Imaging studies are generally not necessary in typical appendicitis and generally reserved for patients with an equivocal likelihood of appendicitis. They are useful when the diagnosis is uncertain. Laparoscopy may be useful as both a diagnostic and a therapeutic modality.

LABORATORY TESTS

- Complete blood count with differential reveals leukocytosis with a left shift in 90% of patients with appendicitis. Total white blood cell (WBC) count is generally lower than 20,000/mm^3. Higher counts may be indicative of perforation. Less than 4% have a normal WBC and differential. A WBC count <10,000/mm^3 decreases the likelihood of appendicitis. Low hemoglobin and hematocrit levels in an older patient should raise suspicion for GI tract carcinoma.
- Microscopic hematuria and pyuria may occur in <20% of patients.

IMAGING STUDIES

- CT of the abdomen/pelvis without contrast has a sensitivity of >90% and an accuracy >94% for acute appendicitis. A distended appendix, periappendiceal inflammation, and a thickened appendiceal wall are indicative of appendicitis.
- Ultrasonography has a sensitivity of 75% to 90% for the diagnosis of acute appendicitis, although it is highly operator dependent and difficult in patients with large body habitus. Ultrasound is useful, especially in younger women when diagnosis is unclear. Normal ultrasonographic findings should not deter surgery if the history and physical examination are indicative of appendicitis.

Rx TREATMENT

NONPHARMACOLOGIC THERAPY

- Nothing by mouth
- Do not administer analgesics or antibiotics until the diagnosis is made (may mask signs of peritonitis)

ACUTE GENERAL Rx

- Urgent appendectomy (laparoscopic or open), correction of fluid and electrolyte imbalance with vigorous IV hydration and electrolyte replacement
- IV antibiotic prophylaxis to cover gram-negative bacilli and anaerobes (ampicillin-sulbactam [Unasyn] 3 g IV q6h or piperacillin-tazobactam [Zosyn] 4.5 g IV q8h in adults)

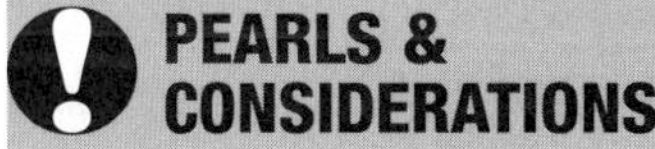

PEARLS & CONSIDERATIONS

COMMENTS

- Perforation is common (20% in adult patients). Indicators of perforation are pain lasting >24 hr, leukocytosis >20,000/mm^3, temperature >102° F, palpable abdominal mass, and peritoneal findings.
- In general, prognosis is excellent. Mortality rate is <1% in young adults without complications; however, it exceeds 10% in elderly patients with ruptured appendix.
- In approximately 20% of patients who undergo exploratory laparotomy because of suspected appendicitis, the appendix is normal.

SUGGESTED READINGS

Bundy DG et al: Does this child have appendicitis? *JAMA* 298(4):438, 2007.

Ebell MH: Diagnosis of appendicitis: laboratory and imaging tests, *Am Fam Physician* 77:1153, 2008

Teresawa T et al: Systematic review: computed tomography and ultrasonography to detect acute appendicitis in adults and adolescents, *Ann Intern Med* 141:537, 2004.

AUTHOR: **FRED F. FERRI, M.D.**

Arrhythmogenic Right Ventricular Dysplasia

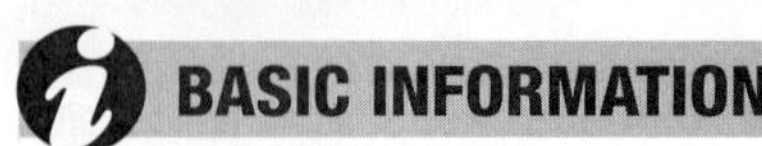

BASIC INFORMATION

DEFINITION

Arrhythmogenic right ventricular dysplasia (ARVD) is a disorder in which normal myocardium is replaced by fibrofatty tissue. It is defined clinically by life-threatening ventricular arrhythmias in apparently healthy young people.

SYNONYMS

Arrhythmogenic right ventricular cardiomyopathy

ICD-9CM CODES:
427.1 Paroxysmal ventricular tachycardia
425.4 Other primary cardiomyopathies
427.89 Other specified cardiac dysrhythmias

ICD-10 CODES:
I47.2 Paroxysmal ventricular tachycardia
I42.8 Other cardiomyopathies
I49.8 Other specified cardiac arrhythmias

EPIDEMIOLOGY & DEMOGRAPHICS

INCIDENCE: Unknown
PREVALENCE: 1/5000 persons
PREDOMINANT SEX AND AGE: Men <35 yr old
RISK FACTORS: Family history of ARVD
GENETICS:
- Autosomal dominant with variable penetrance, and polymorphic phenotypic expression
- Desmosomal dysfunction

PHYSICAL FINDINGS & CLINICAL PRESENTATION

- Suspect when young male individuals have arrhythmia of right heart origin.
- Symptoms vary and range from palpitations, dizziness, and syncope to atypical chest pain, dyspnea, and fatigue.
- Cardiac arrest after physical exertion may be the initial presentation.
- Physical examination will be normal in most patients. Widely split S2 is an important diagnostic clue.

ETIOLOGY

Progressive replacement of the right ventricular myocardium by fibro fatty tissue

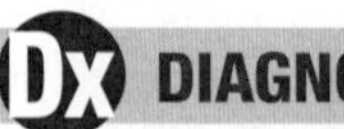

DIAGNOSIS

- Diagnosis is usually made after tachycardia workup in an otherwise healthy adult.
- Diagnosis is made when two major criteria, one major and two minor, or four minor criteria are met.
- See Table 1-5 for diagnostic criteria.

DIFFERENTIAL DIAGNOSIS

- Cardiomyopathy with involvement of the right ventricle
- Uhl's anomaly: rare anomaly characterized by deficiency of the right ventricular (RV) myocardium
- Idiopathic RV tachycardia
- Left dominant arrhythmogenic cardiomyopathy

WORKUP

- Resting ECG will have diagnostic findings in 50% to 90% of patients with ARVD. These changes include T-wave inversions in anterior precordial leads V1-6, epsilon waves (Fig. 1-25), and ventricular tachycardia (VT) with left bundle branch block pattern.
- Endomyocardial biopsy is the preferred method for diagnosis of ARVD. It has specificity of 92%, but it lacks sensitivity (<20%).
- Electrophysiologic study is important to identify delayed potentials that can lead to tachycardiac events.
- Routine immunohistochemical analysis of a conventional endomyocardial-biopsy sample appears to be a highly sensitive and specific diagnostic test for arrhythmogenic right ventricular cardiomyopathy.

TABLE 1-5 Criteria for the Diagnosis of Arrhythmogenic Right Ventricular Dysplasia

Criteria
Global and/or regional dysfunction and structural alterations
Major
Severe dilatation and reduction of right ventricular ejection fraction with no (or only mild) left ventricular impairment Localized right ventricular aneurysms Severe segmental dilatation of the right ventricle
Minor
Mild global right ventricular dilatation and/or ejection fraction with a normal left ventricle Mild segmental dilatation of the right ventricle Regional right ventricular hypokinesis
Tissue characterization of the walls
Major
Fibrofatty replacement of myocardium on endomyocardial biopsy
ECG repolarization abnormalities
Minor
Inverted T waves in the right precordial leads (V2 and V3) in patients older than 12 years and in the absence of right bundle branch block
ECG depolarization/conduction abnormalities
Major
Epsilon waves or localized prolongation (greater than 110 milliseconds) of the QRS complex in right precordial leads (V1 through V3)
Minor
Late potentials visible on signal-averaged ECG
Arrhythmias
Minor
Sustained or nonsustained left bundle branch block type VT documented on ECG, Holter monitoring, or during exercise stress testing Frequent ventricular extrasystoles (more than 1000 per 24 hours on Holter monitoring)
Family history
Major
Familial disease confirmed at autopsy or surgery
Minor
Family history of premature sudden death (younger than 35 years) caused by suspected ARVD/C Family history (clinical diagnosis based on present criteria)

The diagnosis of ARVD is made if one of the following is met: two major criteria, one major and two minor criteria, or four minor criteria.
ARVD, Arrhythmogenic right ventricular dysplasia; *ARVD/C,* arrhythmogenic right ventricular dysplasia/cardiomyopathy; *ECG,* electrocardiography; *VT,* ventricular tachycardia.
(From *Am Fam Physician* 73(8):1391-1398, 2006.)

IMAGING STUDIES

- MRI is a noninvasive method to detect structural changes and regional dysfunction. Cardiac MRI is the most sensitive method to detect ARVD, but has high false-positive rates.
- Echocardiography will show right ventricular dilatation with regional wall motion abnormalities that varied with the severity of the disease.

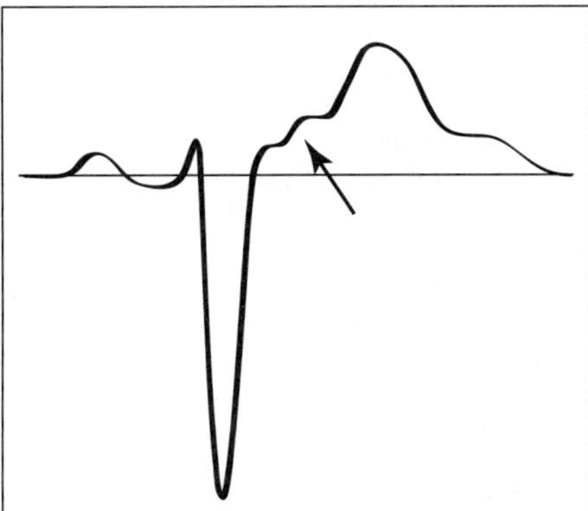

FIGURE 1-25 *Epsilon waves* are small deflection just beyond the QRS complex. Best visualized in leads V1-3. Any potential in leads V1-3 that exceeds the QRS in leads V6 by more than 25 millisecond should be considered epsilon wave. (From Anderson EL: Arrhythmogenic right ventricular dysplasia, *Am Fam Physician* 73(8):1391-1398, 2006.)

- Radionuclide ventriculography can be used to detect wall motion abnormality.

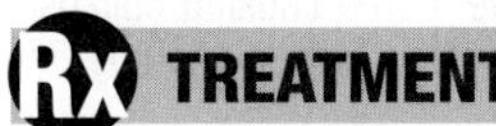

TREATMENT

- Treatment goal is to prevent sudden cardiac death. No definitive therapy is available.

NONPHARMACOLOGIC THERAPY

- Avoidance of activity that may trigger tachycardia
- Right ventriculotomy
- Cardiac transplantation

ACUTE GENERAL Rx

- Intravenous (IV) amiodarone has been proved to be effective in terminating VT.

CHRONIC Rx

- Antiarrhythmic therapy with sotalol, amiodarone, propafenone, beta-blocker alone or in combination can be used
- Radiofrequency ablation is used in cases of refractory VT, frequent tachycardia after defibrillator placement, or localized arrhythmia sites
- Implantable cardioverted defibrillator

REFERRAL

Early cardiology and electrophysiology referral

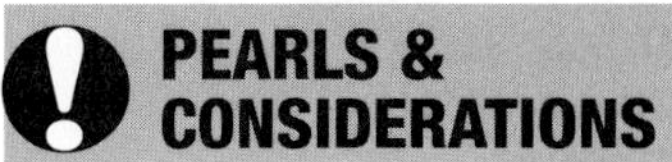

PEARLS & CONSIDERATIONS

PREVENTION

Test first-degree relatives if there is a positive history of sudden cardiac death or death at an early age.

EDUCATION

Patient handout can be found in *American Family Physician* (American Academy of Family Physicians: Information from your family doctor. Arrhythmogenic right ventricular dysplasia: what you should know. *Am Fam Physician* 73(8):1401, 2006).

SUGGESTED READINGS

Anderson EL: Arrhythmogenic right ventricular dysplasia, *Am Fam Physician* 73(8):1391-1398, 2006. Review.

Bomma C et al: Misdiagnosis of arrhythmogenic right ventricular dysplasia/cardiomyopathy, *J Cardiovasc Electrophysiol* 15(3):300-306, 2004.

Calkins H et al: Arrhythmogenic right ventricular cardiomyopathy/dysplasia: an update, *Curr Cardiol Rep* 10(5):367-375, 2008.

Kies P et al: Arrhythmogenic right ventricular dysplasia/cardiomyopathy: screening, diagnosis, and treatment, *Heart Rhythm* 3(2):225-234, 2006.

AUTHORS: **ABDULRAHMAN ABDULBAKI, M.D.,** and **NADIA MUJAHID, M.D.**

Arthritis, Granulomatous

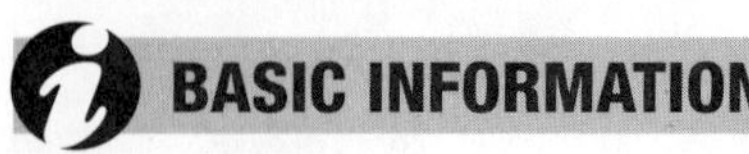

BASIC INFORMATION

DEFINITION

The prototype of granulomatous arthritis is tuberculous arthritis. Atypical mycobacteria, sarcoidosis, and sporotrichosis can cause granulomatous involvement of the synovium, but these entities are much less common.

SYNONYMS

Tuberculous arthritis
Pott's disease

ICD-9CM CODES

711.40 Arthropathy associated with other bacterial disease
730.88 Other infection involving bone

EPIDEMIOLOGY & DEMOGRAPHICS

INCIDENCE (IN U.S.): Unknown
PEAK INCIDENCE: No seasonal predilection
PREVALENCE (IN U.S.): Unknown
PREDOMINANT SEX: Male = female
PREDOMINANT AGE: Rare in childhood

PHYSICAL FINDINGS & CLINICAL PRESENTATION

- Often no constitutional symptoms (fever and weight loss)
- Possibly no clinical or radiographic evidence of pulmonary TB
- Spinal infection most often in the thoracic or upper lumbar area, with back pain as the most common symptom
- Considerable local muscle spasm possible
- Kyphosis and neurologic symptoms resulting from spinal cord compression in advanced disease
- Chronic monoarticular arthritis in the peripheral joints
- Single joint involved in 85% of patients
- Pain, swelling, limitation of motion, and joint stiffness less dramatic than in acute bacterial arthritis; possibly present for months to years
- Seen more often in persons from developing countries, elderly patients, and hemodialysis patients

ETIOLOGY

- Hematogenous spread of organisms from a distant site of infection or by direct spread from bone
- Most commonly affected area: 50% of cases in the spine; next most commonly affected area: large joints (knee and hip)
- Primary infection beginning in the lungs and spreading to the highly vascular synovium
- Tuberculous osteomyelitis commonly involving an adjacent joint
- In peripheral joints, a granulomatous reaction in the synovium causing joint effusion and eventual destruction of underlying bone
- In the spine, infection of the intervertebral disk spreading to adjacent vertebrae
- Osteomyelitis of vertebrae causing collapse, kyphosis, or gibbous deformity, and possibly paraspinal "cold" abscess

Dx DIAGNOSIS

DIFFERENTIAL DIAGNOSIS

- Sarcoidosis
- Fungal arthritis
- Metastatic cancer
- Primary or metastatic synovial tumors

WORKUP

- High index of suspicion needed
- Gold standard: synovial biopsy
- Joint aspiration and culture of the synovial fluid performed while awaiting biopsy
- Positive synovial fluid smear for acid-fast bacilli in 20% of cases; positive culture in 80%
- Elevated synovial fluid protein, low glucose
- Considerable variation in synovial fluid WBC count, but values of 10,000 to 20,000 cells/mm^3 typical; may be predominantly polymorphonuclear leukocytes
- Usually positive tuberculin skin test
- Anergy in elderly patients or in advanced disease
- In spinal infections, percutaneous or open biopsy to obtain accurate C&S data

LABORATORY TESTS

Peripheral WBC count and ESR are elevated but nonspecific.

IMAGING STUDIES

- Plain radiographs of the affected joint
  1. Typically demonstrate bony destruction with little new bone formation
  2. Osteopenia and soft tissue swelling in early infections
  3. Later, erosions at the joint margins
  4. In the spine, disk space narrowing with vertebral collapse (wedging) causing characteristic kyphosis
- CT scan: useful in early diagnosis of infections of the spine and to detect paraspinal abscess
- Technetium and gallium scintigraphic scans: may be positive, but do not permit differentiation from inflammation or osteoarthritis

Rx TREATMENT

NONPHARMACOLOGIC THERAPY

Encourage range-of-motion exercises of the affected joint to prevent contractures.

ACUTE GENERAL Rx

- Combination chemotherapy
  1. If sensitive TB suspected, give isoniazid 5 mg/kg/day (maximum 300 mg/day) plus rifampin 10 mg/kg/day (maximum 600 mg/day) for at least 6 mo and pyrazinamide 15 to 30 mg/kg/day (maximum 2 g/day) for at least the first 2 mo plus ethambutol 15 to 25 mg/kg/day until sensitivity results are available.
  2. Most patients are treated successfully with chemotherapy alone.
  3. Urgent surgical intervention is necessary if spinal cord compression causes neurologic changes.
- Surgical debridement in cases of extensive bone involvement

CHRONIC Rx

In longstanding extensive disease, arthrodesis of weight-bearing joints

DISPOSITION

Loss of cartilage and destruction of underlying bone if treatment is not initiated promptly

REFERRAL

- To a physician experienced in the management of TB
- For consultation with an infectious diseases specialist if drug resistance is suspected or documented
- For neurosurgical and/or orthopedic consultation if neurologic impairment suspected

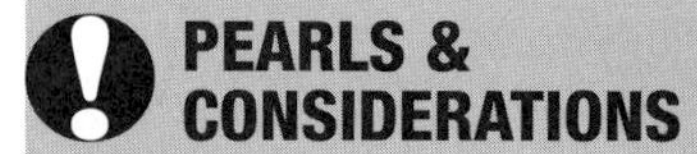

PEARLS & CONSIDERATIONS

COMMENTS

As TB has become less prevalent in the U.S. in the last 10 yr, TB arthritis and osteomyelitis have also become less common.

SUGGESTED READINGS

Crowson AN, Magro C: Interstitial granulomatous dermatitis with arthritis, *Hum Pathol* 35(7):779, 2004.
Gardam M, Lim S: Mycobacterial osteomyelitis and arthritis, *Infect Dis Clin N Am* 19:819-830, 2005.
Rose CD et al: Blau syndrome mutation of CARD15/NOD2 in sporadic early onset granulomatous arthritis, *J Rheumatol* 32(2):373, 2005.
van de Loo FA et al: Deficiency of NADPH oxidase components p47phox and gp91phox caused granulomatous synovitis and increased connective tissue destruction in experimental arthritis models, *Am J Pathol* 163(4):1525, 2003.

AUTHORS: **GLENN G. FORT, M.D., M.P.H.,** and **DENNIS J. MIKOLICH, M.D.**

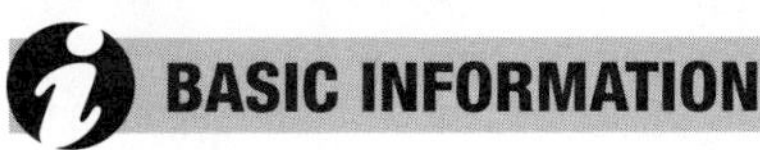

BASIC INFORMATION

DEFINITION

Bacterial arthritis is a highly destructive form of joint disease most often caused by hematogenous spread of organisms from a distant site of infection. Direct penetration of the joint as a result of trauma or surgery and spread from adjacent osteomyelitis may also cause bacterial arthritis. Any joint in the body may be affected.

SYNONYMS

Septic arthritis
Pyogenic arthritis

ICD-9CM CODES

711 Pyogenic arthritis, site unspecified

EPIDEMIOLOGY & DEMOGRAPHICS

INCIDENCE (IN U.S.): Unknown

PEAK INCIDENCE:

- Gonococcal arthritis: young adults
- Other bacterial causes: all ages

PREVALENCE (IN U.S.): Unknown

PREDOMINANT SEX: Gonococcal arthritis in females

PREDOMINANT AGE: Gonococcal arthritis in sexually active adults

PHYSICAL FINDINGS & CLINICAL PRESENTATION

- Hallmark: acute onset of a swollen, painful joint
- Limited range of motion of the joint
- Effusion, with varying degrees of erythema and increased warmth around the joint
- Single joint affected in 80% to 90% of cases of nongonococcal arthritis
- Gonococcal dermatitis-arthritis syndrome
  1. Typical pattern is a migratory polyarthritis or tenosynovitis
  2. Small pustules on the trunk or extremities
- Febrile patient at presentation
- Most commonly affected joints in adult: knee and hip, but any joint may be involved; in children: hip

ETIOLOGY

- Bacteria spread from another locus of infection
  1. Highly vascular synovium is invaded by hematogenously spread bacteria.
  2. WBC enzymes cause necrosis of synovium, cartilage, and bone.
  3. Extensive joint destruction is rapid if infection is not treated with appropriate IV antibiotics and drainage of necrotic material.
- Predisposing factors: rheumatoid arthritis, prosthetic joints, advanced age, immunodeficiency
- The most common nongonococcal organisms are *Staphylococcus aureus,* β-hemolytic streptococci, and gram-negative bacilli
- Staphylococci (*S. aureus* and coagulase-negative staphylococcus species) account for >50% of prosthetic-hip and prosthetic-knee infections. *S. aureus* is very common in patients with rheumatoid arthritis.

Dx DIAGNOSIS

DIFFERENTIAL DIAGNOSIS

- Gout
- Pseudogout
- Trauma
- Hemarthrosis
- Rheumatic fever
- Adult or juvenile rheumatoid arthritis
- Spondyloarthropathies such as reactive arthritis (Reiter's syndrome)
- Osteomyelitis
- Viral arthritides
- Septic bursitis
- Lyme disease

WORKUP

- Joint aspiration, Gram stain, and culture of the synovial fluid
- Immediate arthrocentesis before other studies are undertaken or antibiotics instituted

LABORATORY TESTS

- Joint fluid analysis
  1. Synovial fluid leukocyte count is usually elevated >50,000 cells/mm³ with >80% polymorphonuclear cells.
  2. Counts are highly variable, with similar findings in gout, pseudogout, or rheumatoid arthritis.
  3. The differential diagnosis of synovial fluid abnormalities is described in Section III.
  4. A PCR for Lyme disease on synovial fluid is best test to diagnose Lyme arthritis.
- Blood cultures
- Culture of possible extraarticular sources of infection
- Elevated peripheral WBC count and ESR (nonspecific)

IMAGING STUDIES

- X-ray of the affected joint to rule out osteomyelitis
- CT scan for early diagnosis of infections of the spine, hips, and sternoclavicular and sacroiliac joints
- Technetium and gallium scintigraphic scans (positive, but do not permit differentiation of infection from inflammation)
- Indium-labeled WBC scans (less sensitive, but more specific)

Rx TREATMENT

NONPHARMACOLOGIC THERAPY

- Affected joints aspirated daily to remove necrotic material and to follow serial WBC counts and cultures
- If no resolution with IV antibiotics and closed drainage: open debridement and lavage, particularly in nongonococcal infections
- Prevention of contractures:
  1. After acute stage of inflammation, range-of-motion exercises of the affected joint
  2. Physical therapy helpful

ACUTE GENERAL Rx

- IV antibiotics immediately after joint aspiration and Gram stain of the synovial fluid
- For infections caused by Gram-positive cocci: penicillinase-resistant penicillin, such as nafcillin (2 g IV q4h), unless there is clinical suspicion of methicillin-resistant *Staphylococcus aureus,* in which case vancomycin (1 g IV q12h)
- Infections caused by Gram-negative bacilli: treated with a third-generation cephalosporin or an antipseudomonal penicillin plus an aminoglycoside, pending C&S results
- For suspected gonococcal infection, including young adults when the synovial fluid Gram stain is nondiagnostic: ceftriaxone 1 g IV q24h

CHRONIC Rx

See indications for surgical drainage.

DISPOSITION

- With prompt treatment, complete resolution is expected.
- Delay in treatment may result in permanent destruction of cartilage and loss of function of the affected joint.

REFERRAL

To an orthopedist for open drainage if the infected joint fails to improve on appropriate antibiotics and closed aspiration

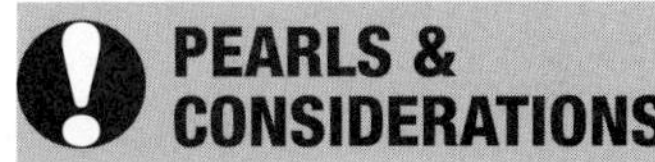

PEARLS & CONSIDERATIONS

COMMENTS

Any patient with acute monoarticular arthritis should undergo an urgent joint aspiration to rule out septic arthritis, even if there is a history of gout.

SUGGESTED READINGS

DelPozo JL, Patel R: Infection associated with prosthetic joints, *N Engl J Med* 361:787-794, 2009.

Margaretten ME: Does this adult patient have septic arthritis? *JAMA* 297:1478-1488, 2007.

Ross JJ: Septic arthritis, *Infect Dis Clin N Am* 19:799-817, 2005.

Yagupsky P: Differentiation between septic arthritis and transient synovitis of the hip in children, *J Bone Joint Surg Am* 87(2):459, 2005.

AUTHORS: **GLENN G. FORT, M.D., M.P.H.,** and **DENNIS J. MIKOLICH, M.D.**

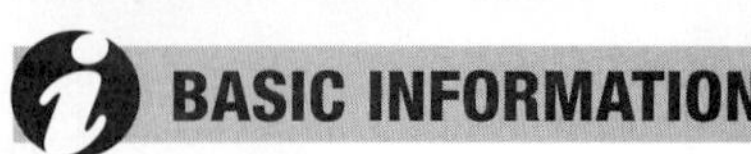

BASIC INFORMATION

DEFINITION

Psoriatic arthritis is an inflammatory spondyloarthritis occurring in patients with psoriasis who are usually seronegative for rheumatoid factor. It is often included in a class of disorders called *rheumatoid variants* or *seronegative spondyloarthropathies.*

ICD-9CM CODES
696.0 Psoriatic arthritis

EPIDEMIOLOGY & DEMOGRAPHICS

PREVALENCE: 5% to 10% of patients with psoriasis (psoriasis affects 1% to 1.5% of general population)
PREDOMINANT SEX: Males and females equally
PREDOMINANT AGE: 30 to 55 yr

PHYSICAL FINDINGS & CLINICAL PRESENTATION

- Usually gradual clinical onset
- Asymmetric involvement of scattered joints
- Selective involvement of the distal interphalangeal (DIP) joints (described in "classic" cases but present in only 5% of patients; Fig. 1-26)
- Symmetric arthritis similar to RA in 15% of patients
- Possible development of predominant sacroiliitis in a small number of cases
- Advanced form of hand involvement (arthritis mutilans) in some patients
- Dystrophic changes in the nails (pitting, ridging) in many patients with DIP involvement
- Fingers often assume a "sausage" appearance (dactylitis)

ETIOLOGY

Unknown. Destructive changes probably caused by release of cytokines and tumor necrosis factor.

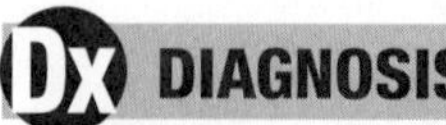

DIAGNOSIS

DIFFERENTIAL DIAGNOSIS

- Rheumatoid arthritis
- Erosive osteoarthritis
- Gouty arthritis
- Ankylosing spondylitis
- The differential diagnosis of spondyloarthropathies is described in Section III

WORKUP

- Early diagnosis may be difficult to establish because the arthritis may develop before skin lesions appear.
- Laboratory studies show no specific abnormalities in most cases.

LABORATORY TESTS

- Slight elevation of erythrocyte sedimentation rate (ESR)
- Possible mild anemia
- Possible HLA-B27 antigen (especially in patients with sacroiliitis)

IMAGING STUDIES

- Peripheral joint findings similar to those in rheumatoid arthritis, but erosive changes in the distal phalangeal tufts characteristic of psoriatic arthritis
- Bony osteolysis; periosteal new bone formation
- Changes in axial skeleton: sacroiliitis, development of vertebral syndesmophytes (osteophytes) that often bridge adjacent vertebral bodies
- Paravertebral ossification
- Spinal changes: do not have same appearance as ankylosing spondylitis; however, spine abnormalities are less common than sacroiliitis

Rx TREATMENT

NONPHARMACOLOGIC THERAPY

- Rest
- Splinting
- Joint protection
- Physical therapy

ACUTE GENERAL Rx

- NSAIDs
- Occasional intraarticular steroid injections
- DMARDs: rarely required

DISPOSITION

- Different from rheumatoid arthritis in both prognosis and response to treatment
- Generally, mild joint symptoms in psoriatic arthritis although some patients develop a more severe form that requires intensive treatment
- Disease-free intervals lasting for several years in many patients

REFERRAL

- Orthopedic surgery consultation for painful joint deformity
- Rheumatology for uncontrolled symptoms

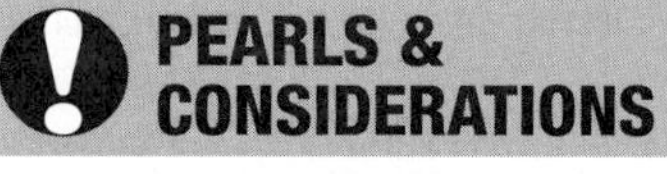

PEARLS & CONSIDERATIONS

- There is often a strong family history of psoriasis in patients with psoriatic arthritis.
- Enthesitis (inflammation of tendon and fascial attachments) is a common feature of the spondyloarthropathies typically involving the plantar fascia and tendo Achilles.

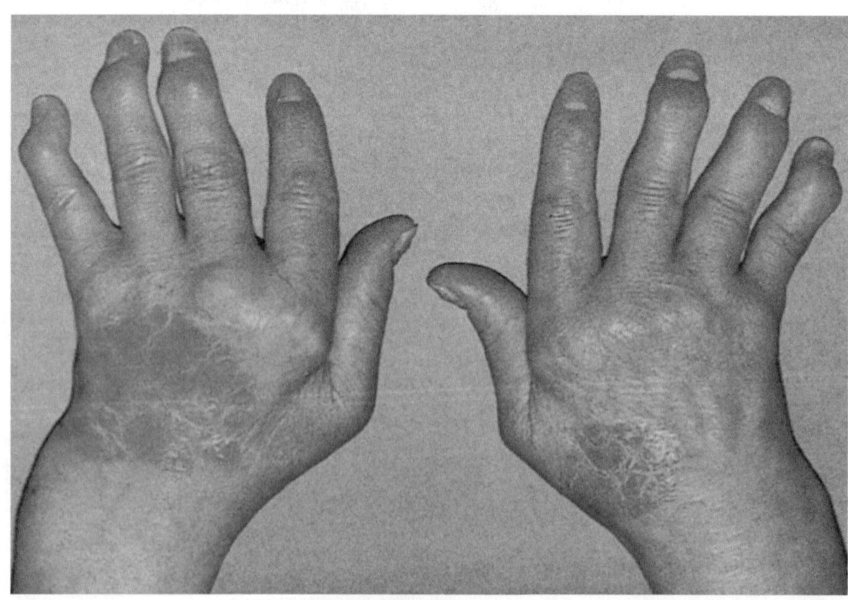

FIGURE 1-26 The hands of a woman with symmetric polyarthritis. Initially, this was indistinguishable from rheumatoid disease, but note the distal interphalangeal joint involvement, which is uncommon in rheumatoid arthritis, as well as the skin psoriasis. (From Klippel J et al [eds]: *Primary care rheumatology,* London, 1999, Mosby.)

SUGGESTED READINGS

Ali Y et al: Improved survival in psoriatic arthritis with calendar time, *Arthritis Rheum* 56(8):2708, 2007.

Gladman DD: Spondyloarthropathies: Targeted therapy for psoriatic arthritis, *Nat Rev Rheumatol* 5:241, 2009.

Griffiths CE, Barker JN: Pathogenesis and clinical features of psoriasis, *Lancet* 370(9583):263, 2007.

Gulliver W: Long-term prognosis in patients with psoriasis, *Br J Dermatol* 159:Suppl 2-9, 2008.

Heiberg MS et al: The comparative one-year performance of anti-tumor necrosis factor alpha drugs in patients with rheumatoid arthritis, psoriatic arthritis, and ankylosing spondylitis: results from a longitudinal, observational, multicenter study, *Arthritis Rheum* 59:234, 2008.

Kataria RK, Brent LH: Spondyloarthropathies, *Am Fam Phys* 69:2853, 2004.

Liu Y et al: Recent advances in the treatment of the spondyloarthropathies, *Curr Opin Rheumatol* 16: 357, 2004.

Scarpa R et al: Early psoriatic arthritis: the clinical spectrum, *J Rheumatol* 57(8):1560, 2007.

Taylor WJ: Assessment of outcome in psoriatic arthritis, *Curr Opin Rheumatol* 16:350, 2004.

AUTHOR: **LONNIE R. MERCIER, M.D.**

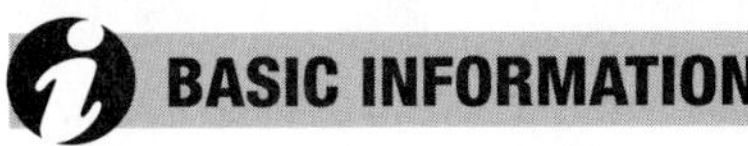

BASIC INFORMATION

DEFINITION

Asbestosis is a slowly progressive diffuse interstitial fibrosis resulting from dose-related inhalation exposure to fibers of asbestos.

ICD-9CM CODES
501 Asbestosis

EPIDEMIOLOGY & DEMOGRAPHICS

- Five to 10 new cases per 100,000 persons per year in U.S.
- Prolonged interval (20 to 30 yr) between exposures to inhaled fibers and clinical manifestations of disease
- Most common in workers involved in the primary extraction of asbestos from rock deposits and in those involved in the fabrication and installation of products containing asbestos (e.g., naval shipyards in World War II; installation of floor tiles, ceiling tiles, acoustic ceiling coverings, wall insulation, and pipe coverings in public buildings)

PHYSICAL FINDINGS & CLINICAL PRESENTATION

- Insidious onset of shortness of breath with exertion is usually the first sign of asbestosis.
- Dyspnea becomes more severe as the disease advances; with time, progressively less exertion is tolerated.
- Cough is frequent and usually paroxysmal, dry, and nonproductive.
- Scant mucoid sputum may accompany the cough in the later stages of the disease.
- Fine end-respiratory crackles (rales, crepitations) are heard more predominantly in the lung bases.
- Digital clubbing, edema, jugular venous distention are present.

ETIOLOGY

Inhalation of asbestos fibers

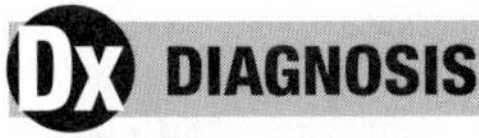

DIAGNOSIS

DIFFERENTIAL DIAGNOSIS

- Silicosis
- Siderosis, other pneumonoconioses
- Lung cancer
- Atelectasis

WORKUP

Documentation of exposure history, diagnostic imaging, pulmonary function testing

LABORATORY TESTS

- Generally not helpful
- Possible mild elevation of erythrocyte sedimentation rate (ESR), positive antinuclear antibody (ANA) and rheumatoid factor (RF) (these tests are nonspecific and do not correlate with disease severity or activity)
- Pulmonary function testing: decreased vital capacity, decreased total lung capacity, decreased carbon monoxide gas transfer
- Arterial blood gases: hypoxemia, hypercarbia in advanced stages

IMAGING STUDIES

Chest radiograph (Fig. 1-27):

- Small, irregular shadows in lower lung zones.
- Thickened pleura, calcified plaques (present under diaphragm and lateral chest wall).
- CT scan of chest confirms diagnosis. Typical findings on high-resolution CT of the chest include increased interstitial markings found mainly at the bases. As the disease progresses, honeycombing is noted.

Rx TREATMENT

NONPHARMACOLOGIC THERAPY

- Smoking cessation, proper nutrition, exercise program to maximize available lung function
- Home oxygen therapy prn
- Removal of patient from further asbestos fiber exposure

GENERAL Rx

- Prompt identification and treatment of respiratory infections
- Supplemental oxygen on a prn basis
- Annual influenza vaccination, pneumococcal vaccination

DISPOSITION

- There is no specific treatment for asbestosis.
- Death is usually from respiratory failure from cor pulmonale.
- Patients with asbestosis have increased risk for mesotheliomas, lung cancer, and tuberculosis. Recent reports indicate that the risk of asbestos-induced lung cancer may be overestimated.
- Survival in patients after development of mesothelioma is 4 to 6 yr.

REFERRAL

To pulmonologist initially

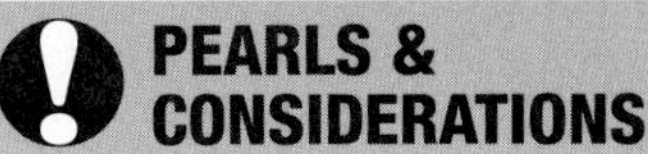

PEARLS & CONSIDERATIONS

COMMENTS

Patient information on asbestosis can be obtained from the American Lung Association, 1740 Broadway, New York, NY 10019.

SUGGESTED READINGS

American Thoracic Society: Diagnosis and initial management of nonmalignant diseases related to asbestos, *Am J Resp Crit Care Med* 170:691, 2004.

O'Reilly K et al: Asbestos-related lung disease, *Am Fam Physician* 75:683, 2007.

AUTHOR: **FRED F. FERRI, M.D.**

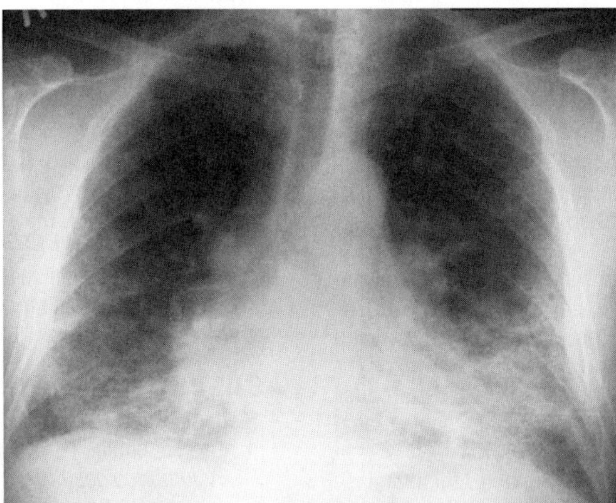

FIGURE 1-27 Asbestosis. Posteroanterior radiograph shows coarse linear opacities at both lung bases obscuring the cardiac borders. (From McLoud TC: *Thoracic radiology: the requisites,* St Louis, 1998, Mosby.)

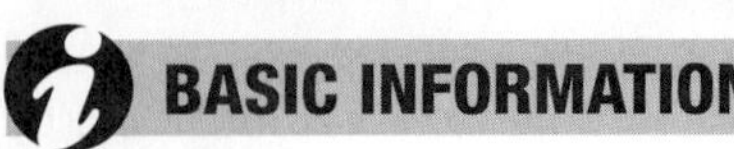

BASIC INFORMATION

DEFINITION

Ascariasis is a parasitic infection caused by the nematode *Ascaris lumbricoides.* The majority of those infected are asymptomatic; however, clinical disease may arise from pulmonary hypersensitivity, intestinal obstruction, and secondary complications.

SYNONYMS

Round worms
Worms

ICD-9CM CODES
127.0 Ascariasis

EPIDEMIOLOGY & DEMOGRAPHICS

INCIDENCE (IN U.S.):
- Unknown
- Three times the infection rates found in blacks as in whites

PEAK INCIDENCE: Unknown
PREVALENCE (IN U.S.): Estimated at 4 million, the majority of which live in the rural southeastern part of the country
PREDOMINANT SEX: Both sexes probably equally affected, with a possible slight female preponderance
PREDOMINANT AGE: Most common in children, with estimated mean age of approximately 5 yr based on surveys in highly endemic areas
NEONATAL INFECTION: Probable transmission, though not specifically studied

PHYSICAL FINDINGS & CLINICAL PRESENTATION

- Occurs approximately 9 to 12 days after ingestion of eggs (corresponding to the larva migration through the lungs)
- Nonproductive cough
- Substernal chest discomfort
- Fever
- In patients with large worm burdens, especially children, intestinal obstruction associated with perforation, volvulus, and intussusception
- Migration of worms into the biliary tree giving clinical appearance of biliary colic and pancreatitis as well as acute appendicitis with movement into that appendage
- Rarely, infection with *A. lumbricoides* producing interstitial nephritis and acute renal failure
- In endemic areas in Asia and Africa, malabsorption of dietary proteins and vitamins as a consequence of chronic worm intestinal carriage

ETIOLOGY

- Transmission is usually hand to mouth, but eggs may be ingested via transported vegetables grown in contaminated soil.
- Eggs are hatched in the small intestine, with larvae penetrating intestinal mucosa and migrating via the circulation to the lungs.
- Larval forms proceed through the alveoli, ascend the bronchial tree, and return to the intestines after swallowing, where they mature into adult worms.
- Estimated time until the female adult worm begins producing eggs is 2 to 3 mo.
- Eggs are passed out of the intestines with feces.
- Within human host, adult worm lifespan is 1 to 2 yr.

Dx DIAGNOSIS

DIFFERENTIAL DIAGNOSIS

Radiologic manifestations and eosinophilia to be distinguished from drug hypersensitivity and Löffler's syndrome

LABORATORY TESTS

- Examination of the stool for *Ascaris* ova
- Expectoration or fecal passage of adult worm
- Eosinophilia: most prominent early in the infection and subsides as the adult worm infestation established in the intestines
- Anti-ascaris IgG4 blood levels by ELISA is a sensitive and specific marker of infection and may be useful in the evaluation of treatment
- Malondialdehyde levels clearly increase in patients infected with *A. lumbricoides*

IMAGING STUDIES

- Chest x-ray examination to reveal bilateral oval or round infiltrates of varying size (Löffler's syndrome); NOTE infiltrates are transient and eventually resolve.
- Plain films of the abdomen and contrast studies to reveal worm masses in loops of bowel.
- Ultrasonography and endoscopic retrograde cholangiopancreatography (ERCP) to identify worms in the pancreaticobiliary tract.

Rx TREATMENT

NONPHARMACOLOGIC THERAPY

Aggressive IV hydration, especially in children with fever, severe vomiting, and resultant dehydration

ACUTE GENERAL Rx

- Mebendazole (Vermox)
  1. Drug of choice for intestinal infection with *A. lumbricoides*
  2. 100 mg PO tid given for 3 days or 500 mg as a single dose
- Albendazole, given as a single 400-mg dose PO
- Both mebendazole and albendazole are contraindicated in pregnancy
- Pyrantel pamoate (Antiminth)
  1. Given at a dose of 11 mg/kg PO (maximum dose of 1 g/day)
  2. Considered safe for use in pregnant women
- Piperazine citrate
  1. Recommended in cases of intestinal or biliary obstruction
  2. Administered as a syrup, given via nasogastric tube, a 150 mg/kg loading dose, followed by six doses of 65 mg/kg q12h
  3. Considered safe in pregnancy, but cannot be given concurrently with chlorpromazine
- Complete obstruction should be managed surgically

DISPOSITION

Overall prognosis is good. Patients should be reevaluated in 2 to 3 months. Reinfection is common.

REFERRAL

- To gastroenterologist in cases of visualized pancreaticobiliary tract or appendiceal obstruction
- To surgeon in cases of complete obstruction or suspected secondary complication (e.g., perforation or volvulus)

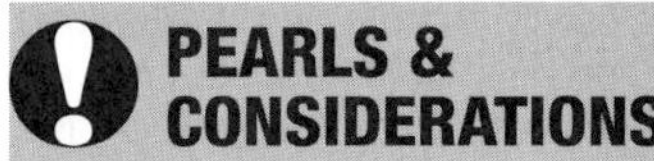

PEARLS & CONSIDERATIONS

COMMENTS

- Hepatic abscess, containing both viable and dead worms, complicating *Ascaris*-induced biliary duct disease has been documented.
- Given the known transmission of the parasite, routine hand washing and proper disposal of human waste would significantly decrease the prevalence of this disease.

SUGGESTED READINGS

Bethony et al: Soil-transmitted helminth infections: Ascariasis, trichriasis, and hookworm, *Lancet* 367(9521):1521-1532, 2006.

Kilic E et al: Serum malondialdehyde level in patients infected with *Ascaris lumbricoides, World J Gastroenterol* 9(10):2332, 2003.

Legesse M et al: Comparative efficacy of albendazole and three brands of mebendazole in the treatment of ascariasis and trichuriasis, *East Afr Med J* 81(3): 134, 2004.

Sangkhathat S et al: Massive gastrointestinal bleeding in infants with ascariasis, *J Pediatr Surg* 38(11): 1696, 2003.

Shah OJ et al: Biliary ascariasis: a review, *World J Surg* 30(8):1500, 2006.

AUTHORS: **GLENN G. FORT, M.D., M.P.H.,** and **DENNIS J. MIKOLICH, M.D.**

BASIC INFORMATION

DEFINITION

Ascites is the accumulation of excess fluid in the peritoneal cavity, most commonly caused by liver cirrhosis.

SYNONYMS

Fluid in peritoneal cavity
Hydroperitoneum
Hydroperitonia
Hydrops abdominis

ICD-9CM CODES
789.5 Ascites

EPIDEMIOLOGY & DEMOGRAPHICS

Ascites is the most common complication of cirrhosis. Ascites occurs in 50% of individuals with cirrhosis within 10 years of diagnosis. Cirrhosis is the cause of 75% of cases of ascites. Other causes include malignancy (10%), cardiac failure (3%), tuberculosis (3%), and pancreatitis (5%).

CLINICAL PRESENTATION

- Important information to elicit within history:
  - Viral hepatitis
  - Alcoholism
  - Increasing abdominal girth
  - Increasing lower extremity edema
  - Intravenous drug use
  - Sexual history (i.e., men who have sex with men)
  - History of transfusions
- Important physical exam findings:
  - Bulging flanks
  - Flank dullness to percussion
  - Fluid wave on abdominal exam
  - Lower extremity edema
  - Shifting dullness on abdominal exam
  - Physical signs associated with liver cirrhosis: spider angiomas, jaundice, loss of body hair, Dupuytren's contracture, muscle wasting, bruising, palmar erythema, gynecomastia, testicular atrophy, hemorrhoids, caput medusae

ETIOLOGY

Pathophysiology of ascites: increased hepatic resistance to portal flow leads to portal hypertension. The splanchnic vessels respond by increased secretion of nitric oxide, causing splanchnic artery vasodilation. Early in the disease increased plasma volume and increased cardiac output compensate for this vasodilation. However, as disease progresses the effective arterial blood volume decreases, causing sodium and fluid retention through activation of the renin-angiotensin system. The change in capillary pressure causes increased permeability and retention of fluid in the abdomen.

Dx DIAGNOSIS

DIFFERENTIAL DIAGNOSIS

- Chronic parenchymal liver disease, leading to portal hypertension
- Peritoneal carcinomatosis
- Congestive heart failure
- Peritoneal tuberculosis
- Nephrotic syndrome
- Pancreatitis

LABORATORY TESTS

- Initial evaluation should always include:
  - Diagnostic paracentesis. Laboratory tests on this fluid should include a CBC with differential, albumin, total protein, culture and Gram stain. Optional tests on paracentesis fluid include amylase, LDH, acid-fast bacilli, and glucose levels.
  - AST, ALT, total and direct bilirubin, albumin, alkaline phosphatase, GGTP
  - CBC, coagulation studies
  - Electrolytes, BUN, creatinine
- A serum to ascites albumin gradient (SAAG) should be calculated in all patients. If the SAAG is greater than 1.1, the cause of ascites can be attributed to portal hypertension. If SAAG is less than 1.1, a non–portal hypertension etiology of ascites must be sought.

IMAGING STUDIES

- Endoscopy of the upper GI tract to evaluate for esophageal varices if ascites is secondary to portal hypertension.
- Abdominal ultrasound is the most sensitive measure for detecting ascitic fluid; a CT scan is a viable alternative.
- Liver biopsy in selected patients (i.e., those with portal hypertension of uncertain etiology).

Rx TREATMENT

NONPHARMACOLOGIC THERAPY

- Sodium-restricted diet (maximum 60 to 90 milliequivalents per day).
- Fluid restriction to 1 liter per day in patients with hyponatremia.

ACUTE GENERAL Rx

- Patients with moderate-volume ascites causing only moderate discomfort may be treated on an outpatient basis with the following diuretic regimen: spironolactone 50 to 200 mg qd or amiloride 5 to 10 mg qd. Add furosemide (Lasix) 20 to 40 mg/day in the first several days of treatment, monitoring renal functions carefully for signs of prerenal azotemia (in patients without edema, goal weight loss is 300 to 500 g/day; in patients with edema it is 800 to 1000 g/day).
- Patients with large-volume ascites causing marked discomfort or decrease in activities of daily living may also be treated as outpatients if there are no complications. There are two options for treatment in these patients: (1) large-volume paracentesis or (2) diuretic therapy until loss of fluid is noted (maximum spironolactone 400 mg qd and furosemide (Lasix) 160 mg qd). No difference in long-term mortality rate was found; however, paracentesis is faster, more effective, and associated with fewer adverse effects.

CHRONIC Rx

5% to 10% of patients with large-volume ascites will be refractory to high-dose diuretic treatment. Treatment strategies include repeated large-volume paracentesis with infusion of albumin every 2 to 4 weeks or placement of a transjugular intrahepatic portosystemic shunt (TIPS).

DISPOSITION

Monitor closely for worsening liver function, development of spontaneous bacterial peritonitis (SBP).

REFERRAL

Referral to gastroenterology for endoscopy in patients with ascites secondary to cirrhosis

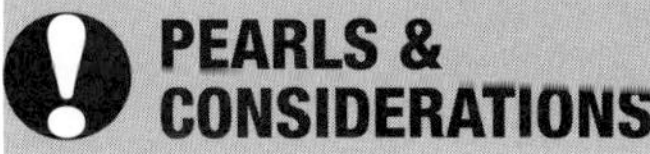

PEARLS & CONSIDERATIONS

COMMENTS

Prevalence of SBP in patients with ascites ranges between 10% and 30%. Presence of at least 250 neutrophils per cubic millimeter of ascitic fluid is diagnostic. Gram negatives such as *E. coli* are the most common isolates. Third-generation cephalosporins are the treatment of choice. By 1 year, 70% of patients have recurrence of SBP and may be prophylaxed with quinolones.

PREVENTION

Prevention of liver cirrhosis through avoidance of long-term use of alcohol, immunization against hepatitis B, and treatment of hepatitis C

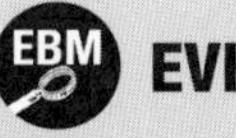

EVIDENCE

Please note: Complete text of EBM for this topic is available online.

SUGGESTED READINGS

Bickley L: *Bates' guide to physical examination and history taking,* Philadelphia, 1999, Lippincott, Williams & Wilkins, pp 53, 374-375.

Gines P et al: Management of cirrhosis and ascites, *N Engl J Med* 350:1646-1654, 2004.

Moore et al: The management of ascites in cirrhosis. Report on the Consensus Conference of the International Ascites Club, *Hepatology* 38:258-266, 2003.

AUTHORS: **JOANNE M. SILVIA, M.D.,** and **PAUL F. GEORGE, M.D.**

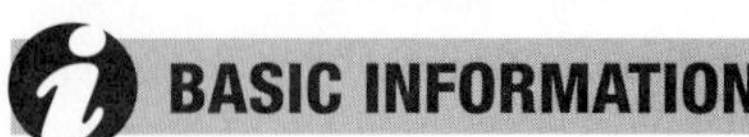

BASIC INFORMATION

DEFINITION

Aseptic necrosis is cell death in components of bone: hematopoietic fat marrow and mineralized tissue. Osteonecrosis is not a specific disease entity but a final common pathway to several disorders that impair blood supply to the femoral head and other locations.

SYNONYMS

Osteonecrosis
Avascular necrosis

ICD-9CM CODES
733.40 Aseptic necrosis
733.43 Aseptic necrosis of femoral condyle
733.42 Aseptic necrosis of femoral head
733.41 Aseptic necrosis of humeral head
733.44 Aseptic necrosis of talus

EPIDEMIOLOGY & DEMOGRAPHICS

- 15,000 new cases per year in the U.S.
- Associated conditions:
  1. Corticosteroid treatment: 35%
  2. Alcohol abuse: 22%
  3. Idiopathic and other: 43%
- Common sites involved
  1. Femoral head
  2. Femoral condyle
  3. Humeral head
  4. Navicular and lunate wrist bones
  5. Talus

PHYSICAL FINDINGS & CLINICAL PRESENTATION

- May be asymptomatic
- Pain in the involved area exacerbated by movement or weight bearing
- Decreased range of motion as the disease progresses
- Functional limitation

ETIOLOGY

Final common pathway of conditions that lead to impairment of the blood supply to the involved bone.

Stages:

- Stage 0
  - Asymptomatic
  - Normal imaging
  - Histologic findings only (i.e., silent osteonecrosis)
- Stage 1
  - Asymptomatic or symptomatic
  - Normal radiographs and CT scan
  - Abnormal bone scan or MRI
- Stage 2
  - Abnormal radiographs or CT scan, including linear sclerosis, focal bead mineralization, cysts; however, the overall architecture of the involved bone is normal
- Stage 3
  - Early evidence of mechanical bone failure (subchondral fracture), but the overall shape of the bone is still intact
- Stage 4
  - Flattening or collapse of the bone
- Stage 5
  - Joint space narrowing
- Stage 6
  - Extensive joint destruction

Dx DIAGNOSIS

DIFFERENTIAL DIAGNOSIS

- None in late stages
- Early: any condition causing focal musculoskeletal pain, including arthritis, bursitis, tendinitis, myopathy, neoplastic bone and joint diseases, traumatic injuries, pathologic fractures

IMAGING STUDIES (Fig. 1-28)

1. Radiography: insensitive early in the course. The earliest changes include diffuse osteopenia, areas of radiolucency with sclerotic border, and linear sclerosis. Later, a subchondral lucency (crescent sign) indicates subchondral fracture. More advanced cases reveal flattening, collapsed bone, and abnormal bone contour. In late disease, osteoarthritic changes are seen.
2. Bone scan:
   - Early: "cold" area.
   - Later: increased radionuclide uptake as a result of remodeling.
   - Sensitivity in early disease is only 70% and specificity is poor.
3. CT scan: may reveal central necrosis and area of collapse before those are visible on radiographs.
4. MRI: the most sensitive technology to diagnose early aseptic necrosis. The first sign is a margin of low signal. An inner border of high signal associated with a low-signal line is specific of aseptic necrosis ("double line sign"). Sensitivity is 75% to 100%.

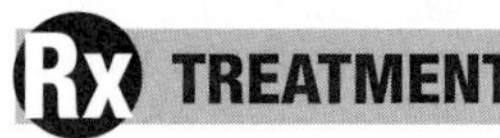

TREATMENT

PREVENTION

- Manage etiologic conditions
- Minimize corticosteroid use

NONPHARMACOLOGIC THERAPY

- Core decompression: effectiveness 35% to 95% in early phases
- Bone grafting
- Osteotomies
- Joint replacement

ACUTE GENERAL Rx

- Decrease weight bearing of affected area.
- Pulsing electromagnetic fields applied externally (still experimental).
- Peripheral vasodilators (e.g., dihydroergotamine) (unproven).

PROGNOSIS

- When diagnosed at an early stage treatment is appropriate in all cases because 85% to 90% can be expected to progress to a more advanced stage.
- Contralateral joint involvement is common (30% to 70%).

SUGGESTED READINGS

Glesby MJ et al: Osteonecrosis in patients infected with HIV, *J Infect Dis* 184:519-523, 2001.
Mont MA et al: Atraumatic osteonecrosis of the knee, *J Bone Joint Surg* 82A:1279-1290, 2000.

AUTHOR: **FRED F. FERRI, M.D.**

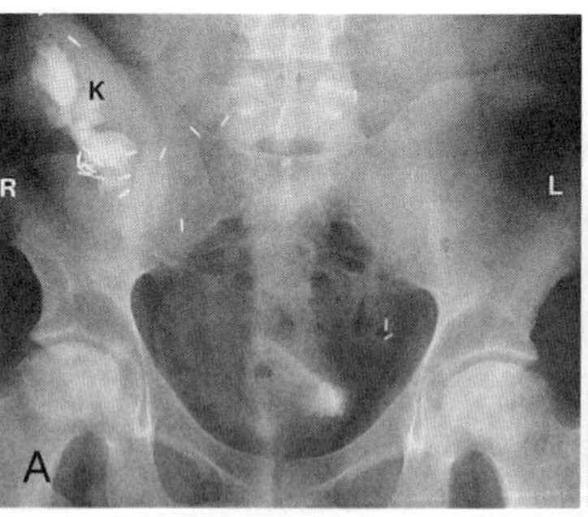

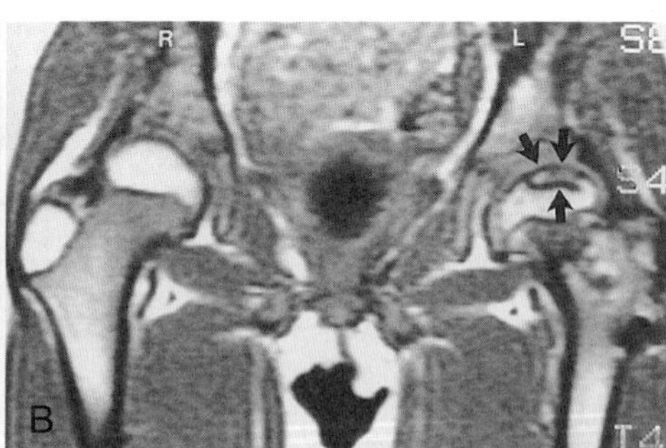

FIGURE 1-28 Aseptic necrosis of the hips. A, Aseptic necrosis can occur from a number of causes, including trauma and steroid use. In this patient, an anteroposterior view of the pelvis shows a transplanted kidney (K) in the right iliac fossa. Use of steroids has caused this patient to have bilateral aseptic necrosis. The femoral heads are somewhat flattened, irregular, and increased in density. **B,** Aseptic necrosis in a different patient is demonstrated on an MRI scan as an area of decreased signal *(arrows)* in the left femoral head. This is the most sensitive method for detection of early aseptic necrosis. (From Mettler FA [ed]: *Primary care radiology,* Philadelphia, 2000, WB Saunders.)

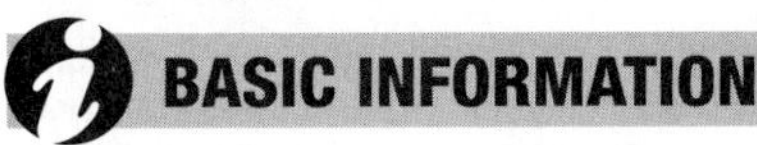

DEFINITION

Aspergillosis refers to several forms of a broad range of illnesses caused by infection with *Aspergillus* species.

ICD-9CM CODES
117.3 Aspergillosis
117.3 Aspergillosis with pneumonia
117.3 *Aspergillus* infection *(A. flavus, fumigatus, terreus)*

EPIDEMIOLOGY & DEMOGRAPHICS

INCIDENCE & PREVALENCE:

- *Aspergillus* species are ubiquitous in the environment internationally and occur as a mold found in soil.
- Cause a variety of illness from hypersensitivity pneumonitis to disseminated overwhelming infection in immunosuppressed patients.
- Frequently cultured from hospital wards from unfiltered outside air circulating through open windows as well as water sources.
- Reach the patient by airborne conidia (spores) that are small enough (2.5 to 3 μm) to reach the alveoli on inhalation.
- Can invade the nose, paranasal sinuses, external ear, or traumatized skin.

RISK FACTORS:

- The clinical syndrome depends on the underlying lung architecture, the host's immune response, and the degree of inoculum.
- Incidence of invasive aspergillosis is increasing with advances in the treatment of life-threatening diseases, such as aggressive chemotherapy or bone marrow and organ transplantation. It also can rarely occur in normal hosts, especially associated with influenza A. Liver and lung transplant recipients are at highest risk for pulmonary disease.
- Patients with AIDS and a CD4 count $<$50 mm^3 have an increased susceptibility to invasive aspergillosis.

ETIOLOGY

- *A. fumigatus* is the usual cause.
- *A. flavus* is the second most important species, particularly in invasive disease of immunosuppressed patients and in lesions beginning in the nose and paranasal sinuses. *A. niger* can also cause invasive human infection.

ALLERGIC ASPERGILLOSIS

- Is a hypersensitivity pneumonitis.
- Presents as cough, dyspnea, fever, chills, and malaise typically 4 to 8 hr after exposure.
- Repeated attacks can lead to granulomatous disease and pulmonary fibrosis.

ALLERGIC BRONCHOPULMONARY ASPERGILLOSIS (ABPA):

- Symptoms occur most commonly in atopic individuals during the third and fourth decades of life.
- Hypersensitivity reaction to *Aspergillus* fungal antigens present in the bronchial tree.
- Results from an initial type I (immediate hypersensitivity) and type III reactions (immune complexes).
- Underdiagnosed pulmonary disorder in patients with asthma and cystic fibrosis.

ASPERGILLOMAS ("FUNGUS BALLS"):

- In the absence of invasion or significant immune response, *Aspergillus* can colonize a preexisting cavity, causing pulmonary aspergilloma.
- Forms masses of tangled hyphal elements, fibrin, and mucus.
- Patients typically have a history of chronic lung disease, tuberculosis, sarcoidosis, or emphysema.
- Manifests commonly as hemoptysis.
- Many are asymptomatic.

INVASIVE ASPERGILLOSIS:

- Patients with prolonged and profound granulocytopenia or impaired phagocytic function are predisposed to rapidly progressive *Aspergillus* pneumonia.
- Typically a necrotizing bronchopneumonia, ranging from small areas of infiltrate to intensive bilateral hemorrhagic infarction.
- Most common presentation: unremitting fever and a new pulmonary infiltrate despite broad-spectrum antibiotic therapy in an immunosuppressed patient.
- Dyspnea and nonproductive cough are common; sudden pleuritic pain and tachycardia, sometimes with a pleural rub, may mimic pulmonary embolism; hemoptysis is uncommon.
- Chest radiograph (CXR) may reveal patchy bronchopneumonic, nodular densities, consolidation, or cavitation.
- Immunocompromised patients: invasive pulmonary *Aspergillus* (IPA) generally is acute and evolves over days to weeks; less commonly, patients with normal or only mild abnormalities of the immune system may develop a more chronic, slowly progressive form of IPA.

EXTRAPULMONARY DISSEMINATION:

- Cerebral infarction from hematogenous dissemination may occur in immunosuppressed individuals.
- Abscess formation from direct extension or invasive disease in the sinuses.
- Esophageal or gastrointestinal ulcerations may occur in the immunosuppressed host.
- Fatal perforation of the viscus or bowel infarction may occur.
- Necrotizing skin ulcers involving the extremities (Fig. 1-29).
- Osteomyelitis.
- Endocarditis in patients who have recently undergone open heart surgery.
- Infection of an implantable cardioverter-defibrillator has been reported.

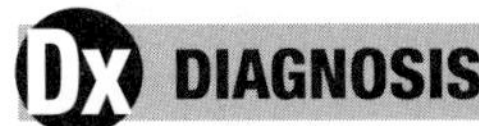

DIFFERENTIAL DIAGNOSIS

- Tuberculosis
- Cystic fibrosis
- Carcinoma of the lung
- Eosinophilic pneumonia
- Bronchiectasis
- Sarcoidosis
- Lung abscess

WORKUP

Physical examination and laboratory data

LABORATORY TESTS

ABPA:

- Peripheral blood eosinophilia and an elevated total serum immunoglobulin E (IgE) level.
- Skin test with *Aspergillus* antigenic extract is usually positive but nonspecific.
- *Aspergillus* serum precipitating antibody is present in 70% to 100% of cases.
- Sputum cultures may be positive for *Aspergillus* spp. but are nonspecific.

ASPERGILLOMAS:

- Sputum culture
- Serum precipitating antibody

Invasive aspergillosis: definitive diagnosis requires the demonstration of tissue invasion (i.e., septate, acute angle branching hyphae) or a positive culture from the tissue obtained by an invasive procedure such as transbronchial biopsy.

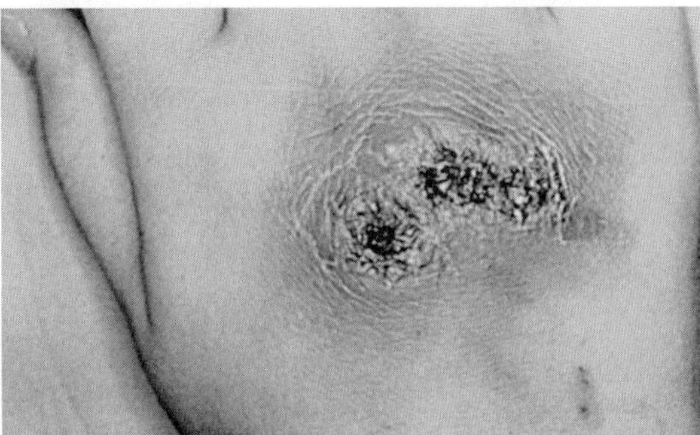

FIGURE 1-29 Cutaneous aspergillosis in a patient with acute leukemia and marked neutropenia. The lesion developed at the site where a steel needle had been left for several days of intravenous infusion. (From Mandell GL [ed]: *Mandell, Douglas, and Bennett's principles and practice of infectious diseases,* ed 6, New York, 2005, Churchill Livingstone.)

 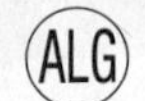

- Sputum and nasal cultures: in high-risk patients a positive culture is strongly suggestive of invasive aspergillosis.
- Serology: the *Platelia Aspergillus* ELISA assay detects a circulating fungal antigen, galactomannan, and is used in some centers in neutropenic patients and for those undergoing stem cell transplantation.
- Blood cultures: usually negative.
- Lung biopsy is necessary for definitive diagnosis.
- Biopsy and culture of extrapulmonary lesions.
- Real-time polymerase chain reaction tests are investigational.

IMAGING STUDIES

ABPA:

- CXRs show a variety of abnormalities, from small, patchy, fleeting infiltrates (commonly in the upper lobes) to lobar consolidation or cavitation.
- A majority of patients eventually develop central bronchiectasis.

ASPERGILLOMAS: CXR or CT scans usually show the characteristic intracavity mass partially surrounded by a crescent of air (Fig. 1-30).

INVASIVE ASPERGILLOSIS: CXR and CT scanning may reveal cavity formation.

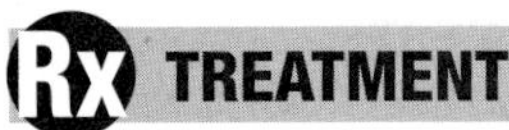

TREATMENT

ACUTE GENERAL Rx

ABPA:

- Prednisone (0.5 to 1 mg/kg PO) until the CXR has cleared, followed by alternate-day therapy at 0.5 mg/kg PO (3 to 6 mo).
- If a patient is corticosteroid dependent, prophylaxis for the prevention of *Pneumocystis jiroveci* infection and maintenance of bone mineralization should be considered.
- Bronchodilators and physiotherapy.
- Serial CXR and serum IgE useful in guiding treatment.
- Itraconazole 200 mg PO bid for 4 to 6 mo, then taper over 4 to 6 mo may be considered as a steroid-sparing agent or if steroids are ineffective.

ASPERGILLOMAS:

- Controversial and problematic; the optimal treatment strategy is unknown.
- Up to 10% of aspergillomas may resolve clinically without overt pharmacologic or surgical intervention.
- Observation for asymptomatic patients.
- Surgical resection/arterial embolization for those patients with severe hemoptysis or life-threatening hemorrhage.
- For those patients at risk for marked hemoptysis with inadequate pulmonary reserve, consider itraconazole 200 to 400 mg/day PO.

INVASIVE ASPERGILLOSIS:

- The guidelines of the Infectious Diseases Society of America recommend the use of voriconazole as the primary therapy for invasive aspergillosis. Voriconazole dose is 6 mg/kg IV bid followed by 4 mg/kg IV q12h or 200 mg PO q12h for body weight >40 kg but 100 mg PO q12h for body weight <40 kg.
- Amphotericin B 0.8 to 1.2 mg/kg IV qd to total dose of 2 to 2.5 g; itraconazole 200 to 400 mg/d PO × 1 yr.
- Amphotericin B lipid complex (ABLC) 5 mg/kg IV qd in those intolerant of or refractory to amphotericin B.
- Amphotericin B colloidal dispersion (ABCD) 3 to 6 mg/kg IV qd; stepwise approach in those who have not responded to amphotericin B.
- Liposomal amphotericin B (L-AMB) 3 to 5 mg/kg IV qd; stepwise approach is indicated as empiric therapy for presumed fungal infection in febrile neutropenic patients who are refractory to or intolerant of amphotericin B.
- Itraconazole 200 mg IV bid × 4 doses followed by 200 mg IV qd or 200 mg tid for 4 days, then 200 mg PO bid—first-line therapy if not taking p450 inducers. Levels may be obtained to ensure compliance and adequate absorption. Approved only for salvage therapy in the United States at this time.
- Posaconazole 200 mg PO tid with food or liquid nutritional supplement to enhance absorption is approved in the European Union, but in the United States is approved only for prophylaxis in leukemic neutropenic patients, those with myelodysplasia, or those who have undergone allogeneic hematopoietic stem cell transplantation; ravuconazole is currently under investigation.
- Caspofungin (Candigas) is the first of a new class of antifungals, the echinocandins, approved for the treatment of invasive aspergillosis in patients who do not respond to or are unable to tolerate other antifungal drugs. Starting dose 70 mg IV over 1 hr on day 1, then 50 mg IV qd thereafter (reduce to 35 mg IV qd in cases with moderate hepatic insufficiency). Can switch to oral voriconazole after 2 to 3 wk if the response is favorable. Micafungin 150 mg IV qd is another alternative.
- Because azoles and echinocandins target different cellular sites, combination therapy may have additive activity against *Aspergillus* species. Although still under investigation, some bone marrow transplant units use caspofungin and voriconazole as the preferred initial treatment, especially in patients receiving high-dose corticosteroids.
- Cytokine therapy may offer future treatment options in conjunction with the currently available antifungals.

REFERRAL

To an infectious diseases specialist

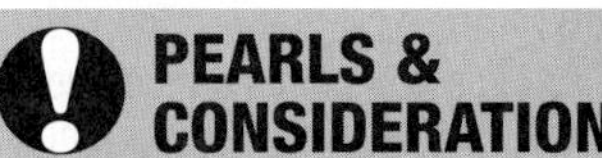

PEARLS & CONSIDERATIONS

- Unlike fluconazole, the potential for drug-drug interactions with voriconazole is high.
- Agitation of hospital buildings by renovations or repairs may increase the incidence of *Aspergillus* infections in immunosuppressed individuals.
- Breakthrough zygomycosis infection may occur with voriconazole treatment.
- *A. terreus* is clinically resistant to amphotericin B.

SUGGESTED READINGS

Cook RJ et al: *Aspergillus* infection of implantable cardioverter defibrillator, *Mayo Clinic Proc* 79(4): 549-552, 2005.

Hasejima N et al: Invasive pulmonary aspergillosis associated with influenza B, *Respirology* 10(1):116-119, 2005.

Marr KA et al: Combination antifungal therapy for invasive aspergillosis, *CID* 39:797, 2004.

Pfaller MA: Anidulafungin: an echinocandin antifungal, *Expert Opin Invest Drugs* 13(9):1183-1197, 2004.

Segal BH: Aspergillosis, *N Engl J Med* 360:1870-1884, 2009.

Steinbach WJ, Stevens DA: Review of newer antifungal and immunomodulatory strategies for invasive aspergillosis, *Clin Infect Dis* 37(suppl 3):S157, 2003.

Walsh JW et al: Treatment of *Aspergillosis:* clinical practice guidelines of the Infectious Diseases Society of America, *Clin Infect Dis* 46:327, 2008.

AUTHOR: **SAJEEV HANDA, M.D.**

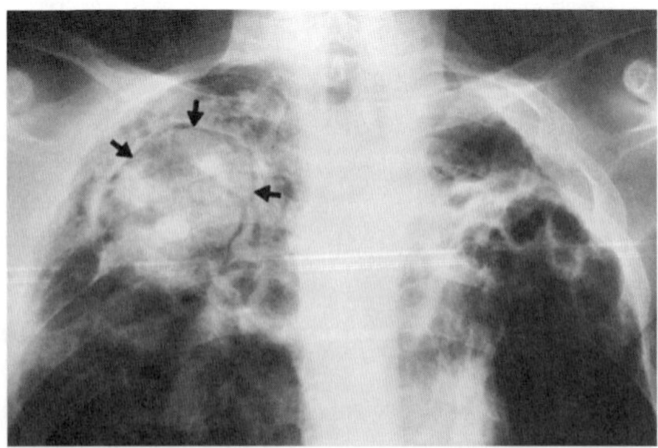

FIGURE 1-30 Fungus ball or mycetoma caused by *Aspergillus.* Coned-down posteroanterior view of the chest of a patient with biapical fibrocavitary tuberculosis accompanied by volume loss. There is a mass in a large right upper-lobe cavity with air dissecting into the cavity producing "air crescents" *(arrows).* (From McLoud TC: *Thoracic radiology: the requisites,* St Louis, 1998, Mosby.)

BASIC INFORMATION

DEFINITION

The National Asthma Education and Prevention Program (NAEPP) guidelines define asthma as "a chronic inflammatory disease of the airways in which many cells and cellular elements play a role: in particular mast cells, neutrophils, eosinophils, T lymphocytes, macrophages, and epithelial cells. In susceptible individuals, this inflammation causes recurrent episodes of coughing (particularly at night or early in the morning), wheezing, breathlessness, and chest tightness. The episodes are usually associated with widespread but variable airflow obstruction that is reversible either spontaneously or as a result of treatment." *Status asthmaticus* can be defined as a severe continuous bronchospasm.

SYNONYMS

Bronchospasm
Reactive airway disease
Bronchial asthma

ICD-9CM CODES
493.9 Asthma, unspecified
493.1 Intrinsic asthma
493.0 Extrinsic asthma

EPIDEMIOLOGY & DEMOGRAPHICS

- Asthma affects 5% to 12% of the population and accounts for more than 450,000 hospitalizations and nearly 2 million emergency department visits yearly in the U.S.
- It is more common in children (10% of children, 5% of adults).
- 50% to 80% of children with asthma develop symptoms before 5 yr of age.
- Overall asthma mortality rate in the U.S. is 20 per 1 million persons.

PHYSICAL FINDINGS & CLINICAL PRESENTATION

Physical examination varies with the stage and severity of asthma and may reveal only increased inspiratory and expiratory phases of respiration. Physical examination during status asthmaticus may reveal:

- Tachycardia and tachypnea
- Use of accessory respiratory muscles
- Pulsus paradoxus (inspiratory decline in systolic blood pressure >10 mm Hg)
- Wheezing: absence of wheezing (silent chest) or decreased wheezing can indicate worsening obstruction
- Mental status changes: generally secondary to hypoxia and hypercapnia and constitute an indication for urgent intubation
- Paradoxic abdominal and diaphragmatic movement on inspiration (detected by palpation over the upper part of the abdomen in a semirecumbent position): important sign of impending respiratory crisis, indicates diaphragmatic fatigue
- The following abnormalities in vital signs are indicative of severe asthma:
    1. Pulsus paradoxus >18 mm Hg
    2. Respiratory rate >30 breaths/min
    3. Tachycardia with heart rate >120 beats/min

ETIOLOGY

- Symptoms are more commonly due to specific (aeroallergens) or nonspecific (dust, cigarette smoke, fumes, cold air, exercise, etc.) exposures.
- Traditionally, intrinsic asthma was described as occurring in patients who have no history of allergies possibly triggered by upper respiratory infections or psychologic stress and extrinsic asthma (allergic asthma) brought on by exposure to allergens (e.g., dust mites, cat allergen, industrial chemicals).
- Exercise-induced asthma: seen most frequently in adolescents; manifests with bronchospasm after beginning exercise and improves with discontinuation of exercise.
- Drug-induced asthma: often associated with use of NSAIDs, β-blockers, sulfites, and certain foods and beverages.
- There is a strong association of the *ADAM 33* gene with asthma and bronchial hyperresponsiveness.

DIAGNOSIS

DIFFERENTIAL DIAGNOSIS

- CHF
- COPD
- Pulmonary embolism (in adult and elderly patients)
- Foreign body aspiration (most frequent in younger patients)
- Pneumonia and other upper respiratory infections
- Rhinitis with postnasal drip
- TB
- Hypersensitivity pneumonitis
- Anxiety disorder
- Wegener's granulomatosis
- Diffuse interstitial lung disease

WORKUP

- The clinician should evaluate for environmental causes (e.g., house dust mites, indoor pets) and exposure to other allergens such as tobacco smoke. For symptomatic adults and children aged >5 yr who can perform spirometry, asthma can be diagnosed after a medical history and physical examination documenting an episodic pattern of respiratory symptoms and from spirometry that indicates partially reversible airflow obstruction (>12% increase and 200 ml in forced expiratory volume in 1 sec [FEV_1] after inhaling a short bronchodilator or receiving a short [2 to 3 wk] course of oral corticosteroids). For children aged <5 yr, spirometry is generally not feasible. Young children with asthma symptoms should be treated as having suspected asthma once alternative diagnoses are ruled out.
- The degree of reversibility measured by spirometry correlates with airway obstruction, and patients with a high degree of reversibility have a greater risk of irreversible airflow obstruction in subsequent years.
- Section III describes an algorithm for diagnosing asthma.
- After diagnosis severity of asthma should be classified during the initial assessment before initiating therapy. The following questions from Asthma Control and endorsed by the American Lung Association are important in assessing patients with asthma:
    1. Has your asthma prevented normal activities at home or work?
    2. Have you had shortness of breath in the past 4 weeks?
    3. Has your asthma kept you awake at night?
    4. How often have you used your asthma inhaler in the last 4 weeks?
    5. Overall, how have kept your asthma in control in the last 4 weeks?
- Once therapy is initiated, the emphasis for clinical management is changed to the assessment of asthma control. The level of asthma control should be used to guide decisions either to maintain or adjust therapy.
- Schedule visits at 2- to 6-wk intervals for patients who are just starting therapy or who require a step up in therapy to achieve or regain asthma control. Schedule visits at 1- to 6-mo intervals, after asthma control is achieved, to monitor whether asthma control is maintained. The interval will depend on factors such as the duration of asthma control or the level of treatment required. Consider scheduling visits at 3-mo intervals if step-down therapy is anticipated.

LABORATORY TESTS

Laboratory tests are usually not necessary and the results can be normal if obtained during a stable period. The following laboratory abnormalities may be present during an acute bronchospasm:

- Arterial blood gases (ABGs) can be used in staging the severity of an asthmatic attack:
    - Mild: decreased Pa_{O_2} and Pa_{CO_2}, increased pH
    - Moderate: decreased Pa_{O_2}, normal Pa_{CO_2}, normal pH
    - Severe: marked decreased Pa_{O_2}, increased Pa_{CO_2}, and decreased pH
- Complete blood count: leukocytosis with left shift may indicate the existence of bacterial infection.
- Spirometry is recommended at the initial assessment and at least every 1 to 2 yr after treatment is initiated and when the symptoms and peak expiratory flow have stabilized. Spirometry as a monitoring measure may be performed more frequently, if indicated, based on severity of symptoms and the disease's lack of response to treatment.
- Pulmonary function studies: during acute severe bronchospasm, FEV_1 is <1 L and peak expiratory flow rate (PEFR) <80 L/min.

IMAGING STUDIES

- Chest radiograph: usually normal, may show evidence of thoracic hyperinflation (e.g., flattening of the diaphragm, increased volume over the retrosternal air space).

- ECG: tachycardia, nonspecific ST-T wave changes are common during an asthma attack; may also show cor pulmonale, right bundle-branch block, right axial deviation, counterclockwise rotation.

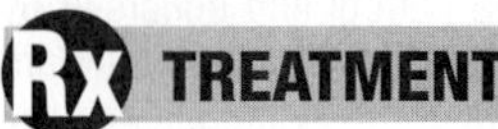

TREATMENT

NONPHARMACOLOGIC THERAPY

- Avoidance of triggering factors (e.g., salicylates, sulfites), environmental or occupational triggers
- Encouragement of regular exercise (e.g., swimming)
- Patient education regarding warning signs of an attack and proper use of medications (e.g., correct use of inhalers)

GENERAL Rx

- The 2007 NAEPP guidelines (see Tables 1-6 to 1-14) broadly classify treatment options by age: 0 to 4 yr, 5 to 11 yr, and >12 yr. When asthma symptoms are mild, short-lived, or infrequent, use of short-acting beta-selective adrenergic agonists (SABA) administered by inhalation is the most effective therapy for quick relief of asthmatic symptoms. They are recommended for use only as needed for relief of symptoms or before anticipated exposure to known triggers such as exercise. When symptoms become more frequent or more severe, step-up treatment includes use of an inhaled steroid or leukotriene receptor antagonist (LTRA). If symptoms persist, recommendations include use of long-acting beta-agonist (LABA) or LTRA plus inhaled steroid. If asthma control remains inadequate, additional treatment consists of inhaled steroid plus LABA plus LTM. The addition of omalizumab, an anti-IgE monoclonal antibody, is indicated for the treatment of moderate and severe persistent asthma refractory to other treatment noted earlier. It is administered subcutaneously every 2 or 4 weeks. This medicine is expensive ($10,000-30,000/yr). Patients should be closely monitored in the first month because omalizumab can result in allergic reactions (anaphylaxis) in 1 to 2 patients/1000.

Treatment of *status asthmaticus* is as follows:

- Oxygen generally started at 2 to 4 L/min by nasal cannula or Venti-Mask at 40% FiO_2; further adjustments are made according to the ABGs.
- Bronchodilators: various agents and modalities are available. Inhaled bronchodilators are preferred when they can be administered quickly. Parenteral administration of sympathomimetics (e.g., SQ epinephrine) when necessary should be accompanied by electrocardiographic monitoring.
- Albuterol: 0.5 to 1 ml (2.5 to 5 mg) in 3 ml of saline solution tid or qid by nebulizer is effective. Other useful medications are levalbuterol nebulizer solution (0.31 mg/3 ml, 0.63 mg/3 ml, 1.25 mg/3 ml), and ipratropium nebulizer solution (0.25/ml [0.025%]).
- Corticosteroids:
  1. Early administration is advised, particularly in patients using steroids at home.
  2. Patients may be started on methylprednisolone 0.5 to 1 mg/kg IV loading dose, then q6h prn; higher doses may be necessary in selected patients (particularly those receiving steroids at home); steroids given by inhalation (e.g., beclomethasone 2 inhalations qid, maximum 20 inhalations/day) are also useful for controlling bronchospasm and tapering oral steroids and should be used in all patients with severe asthma. However, inhaled steroids are less effective than oral steroids in mild to moderate and severe acute asthma.
  3. Rapid but judicious tapering of corticosteroids will eliminate serious steroid toxicity; long-term low-dose methotrexate may be an effective means of reducing the systemic corticosteroid requirement

TABLE 1-6 Classifying Asthma Severity and Initiating Treatment in Youths ≥12 Yr and Adults (Assessing severity and initiating treatment for patients who are not currently taking long-term control medications)

		CLASSIFICATION OF ASTHMA SEVERITY (≥12 yr)			
			PERSISTENT		
Components of Severity		**Intermittent**	**Mild**	**Moderate**	**Severe**
Impairment Normal FEV_1/FVC: 8-19 yr 85% 20-39 yr 80% 40-59 yr 75% 60-80 yr 70%	Symptoms	≤2 days/wk	>2 days/wk but not daily	Daily	Throughout the day
	Nighttime awakenings	≤2×/mo	3-4×/mo	>1×/wk but not nightly	Often 7×/wk
	Short-acting $beta_2$-agonist use for symptom control (not prevention of EIB)	≤2 days/wk	>2 days/wk but not daily, and not more than 1× on any day	Daily	Several times per day
	Interference with normal activity	None	Minor limitation	Some limitation	Extremely limited
	Lung function	Normal FEV_1 between exacerbations			
		FEV_1 >80% predicted	FEV_1 >80% predicted	FEV_1 >60% but <80% predicted	FEV_1 <60% predicted
		FEV_1/FVC normal	FEV_1/FVC normal	FEV_1/FVC reduced 5%	FEV_1/FVC reduced >5%
Risk	Exacerbations requiring oral systemic corticosteroids	0-1 per yr	≥2 per yr →		
		← Consider severity and interval since last exacerbation. Frequency and severity may fluctuate over time for patients in any severity category. →			
		Relative annual risk of exacerbations may be related to FEV_1.			
Recommended Step for Initiating Therapy		Step 1	Step 2	Step 3	Step 4 or 5
				and consider short course of oral systemic corticosteroids	
		In 2-6 wks, evaluate level of asthma control that is achieved and adjust therapy accordingly.			

The stepwise approach is meant to assist, not replace, the clinical decision-making required to meet individual patient needs.

Level of severity is determined by assessment of both impairment and risk. Assess impairment domain by patient's/caregiver's recall of previous 2-4 wks and spirometry. Assign severity to the most severe category in which any feature occurs.

At present, there are inadequate data to correspond frequencies of exacerbations with different levels of asthma severity. In general, more frequent and intense exacerbations (e.g., requiring urgent, unscheduled care, hospitalization, or ICU admission) indicate greater underlying disease severity. For treatment purposes, patients who had ≥2 exacerbations requiring oral systemic corticosteroids in the past year may be considered the same as patients who have persistent asthma, even in the absence of impairment levels consistent with persistent asthma.

To access the complete *Expert Panel Report 3: Guidelines for the Diagnosis and Management of Asthma,* go to www.nhlbi.nih.gov/guidelines/asthma/asthgdln.pdf.

EIB, Exercise-induced bronchospasm; *FEV_1,* forced expiratory volume in 1 second; *FVC,* forced vital capacity; *ICU,* intensive care unit.

From National Asthma Education and Prevention Program: *Expert panel report 3: Guidelines for diagnosis and management of asthma,* National Institutes of Health, National Heart, Lung, and Blood Institute, August 2007, NIH publication 08-4051.

in some patients with severe refractory asthma.

4. The most common errors regarding steroid therapy in acute bronchospasm are the use of "too little, too late" and too-rapid tapering with return of bronchospasm.

- IV hydration: judicious use is necessary to avoid congestive heart failure in elderly patients.
- IV antibiotics are indicated when there is suspicion of bacterial infection (e.g., infiltrate on chest radiograph, fever, or leukocytosis).
- Intubation and mechanical ventilation are indicated when previous measures fail to produce significant improvement.
- General anesthesia: halothane may reverse bronchospasm in a severe asthmatic who cannot be ventilated adequately by mechanical means.
- IV magnesium sulfate supplementation in children with low or borderline-low magnesium levels may improve acute bronchospasm. Several reports in recent literature point to the beneficial effect on bronchospasm with a 20-min infusion of 40 mg/kg, up to a maximum of 2 g of magnesium sulfate in patients with acute asthma attack.

REFERRAL

Box 1-1 describes indications for referral to an asthma specialist.

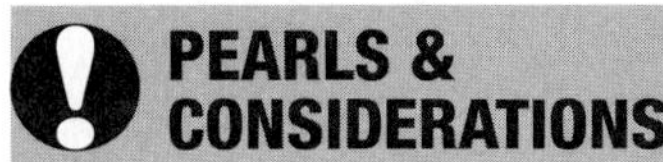

PEARLS & CONSIDERATIONS

COMMENTS

- The differentiation of asthma from COPD can be challenging. A history of atopy and intermittent, reactive symptoms points toward a diagnosis of asthma, whereas smoking and advanced age are more indicative of COPD. Spirometry is useful in distinguishing asthma from COPD.
- In all asthma patients it is important to treat or prevent comorbid conditions (e.g., rhinosinusitis, vocal cord dysfunction, gastroesophageal reflux disease).
- Inhaled low-dose corticosteroids are the single most effective therapy for adult patients with asthma who require more than an occasional use of short-acting beta-2 agonists to control their asthma.
- Leukotriene modifiers/receptor agonists represent a reasonable alternative in adults unable or unwilling to use corticosteroids; however, these agents are less effective than monotherapy with inhaled corticosteroids.
- Patients who remain symptomatic despite inhaled corticosteroids benefit from the addition of long-acting beta-2 agonists.
- In patients with allergies and elevated serum immunoglobulin (Ig) E levels, use of anti-IgE therapy is beneficial.

TABLE 1-7 Assessing Asthma Control and Adjusting Therapy in Youths ≥12 Yr and Adults

Components of Control		CLASSIFICATION OF ASTHMA CONTROL (≥12 yr): Well Controlled	Not Well Controlled	Very Poorly Controlled
Impairment	Symptoms	≤2 days/wk	>2 days/wk	Throughout the day
	Nighttime awakenings	≤2×/mo	1-3×/wk	≥4/wk
	Interference with normal activity	None	Some limitation	Extremely limited
	Short-acting beta$_2$-agonist use for symptom control (not prevention of EIB)	≤2 days/wk	>2 days/wk	Several times per day
	FEV$_1$ or peak flow	>80% predicted/personal best	60%-80% predicted/personal best	<60% predicted/personal best
	Validated questionnaires			
	ATAQ	0	1-2	3-4
	ACQ	≤0.75*	≥1.5	N/A
	ACT™	≥20	16-19	≤15
Risk	Exacerbations requiring oral systemic corticosteroids	0-1 per yr; Consider severity and interval since last exacerbation	≥2 per yr	
	Progressive loss of lung function	Evaluation requires long-term follow-up care		
	Treatment-related adverse effects	Medication side effects can vary in intensity from none to very troublesome and worrisome. The level of intensity does not correlate to specific levels of control but should be considered in the overall assessment of risk.		
Recommended Action for Treatment		Maintain current step. Regular follow-up every 1-6 mos to maintain control. Consider step down if well controlled for at least 3 mos.	Step up 1 step and Reevaluate in 2-6 wks. For side effects, consider alternative treatment options.	Consider short course of oral systemic corticosteroids. Step up 1-2 steps. Reevaluate in 2 wks. For side effects, consider alternative treatment options.

The stepwise approach is meant to assist, not replace, the clinical decision-making required to meet individual patient needs.

The level of control is based on the most severe impairment or risk category. Assess impairment domain by patient's recall of previous 2-4 wks and by spirometry or peak flow measures. Symptom assessment for longer periods should reflect a global assessment, such as inquiring whether the patient's asthma is better or worse since the last visit.

At present, there are inadequate data to correspond frequencies of exacerbations with different levels of asthma control. In general, more frequent and intense exacerbations (e.g., requiring urgent, unscheduled care, hospitalization, or ICU admission) indicate poorer disease control. For treatment purposes, patients who had ≥2 exacerbations requiring oral systemic corticosteroids in the past year may be considered the same as patients who have not-well-controlled asthma, even in the absence of impairment levels consistent with not-well-controlled asthma.

Validated questionnaires for the impairment domain (the questionnaires do not assess lung function or the risk domain)
- ATAQ = Asthma Therapy Assessment Questionnaire
- ACQ = Asthma Control Questionnaire (user package may be obtained at www.qoltech.co.uk or juniper@qoltech.co.uk)
- ACT = Asthma Control Test™
- Minimal Important Difference: 1.0 for the ATAQ; 0.5 for the ACQ; not determined for the ACT

Before step up in therapy:
- Review adherence to medication, inhaler technique, environmental control, and comorbid conditions
- If an alternative treatment option was used in a step, discontinue and use the preferred treatment for that step

*ACQ values of 0.76-1.4 are indeterminate regarding well-controlled asthma.

EIB, Exercise-induced bronchospasm; *FEV$_1$,* forced expiratory volume in 1 second; *ICU,* intensive care unit.

The Asthma Control Test is a trademark of QualityMetric Incorporated.

From National Asthma Education and Prevention Program: *Expert panel report 3: Guidelines for diagnosis and management of asthma,* National Institutes of Health, National Heart, Lung, and Blood Institute, August 2007, NIH publication 08-4051.

TABLE 1-8 Stepwise Approach for Managing Asthma in Youths ≥12 Yr and Adults

Intermittent Asthma	**Persistent Asthma: Daily Medication** Consult with asthma specialist if step 4 care or higher is required. Consider consultation at step 3.					↑
Step 1 *Preferred:* SABA prn	**Step 2** *Preferred:* Low-dose ICS *Alternative:* Cromolyn, LTRA, nedocromil, or theophylline	**Step 3** *Preferred:* Low-dose ICS + LABA OR Medium-dose ICS *Alternative:* Low-dose ICS + either LTRA, theophylline, or zileuton	**Step 4** *Preferred:* Medium-dose ICS + LABA *Alternative:* Medium-dose ICS + either LTRA, theophylline, or zileuton	**Step 5** *Preferred:* High-dose ICS + LABA AND Consider omalizumab for patients who have allergies	**Step 6** *Preferred:* High-dose ICS + LABA + oral corticosteroid AND Consider omalizumab for patients who have allergies	Step up if needed (first, check adherence, environmental control, and comorbid conditions) **Assess control** Step down if possible (and asthma is well controlled at least 3 months)
Each step: Patient education, environmental control, and management of comorbidities Steps 2-4: Consider subcutaneous allergen immunotherapy for patients who have allergic asthma						
Quick-Relief Medication for All Patients • SABA as needed for symptoms. Intensity of treatment depends on severity of symptoms: up to 3 treatments at 20-minute intervals as needed. Short course of oral systemic corticosteroids may be needed. • Use of SABA >2 days a week for symptom relief (not prevention of EIB) generally indicates inadequate control and the need to step up treatment.						↓

The stepwise approach is meant to assist, not replace, the clinical decision-making required to meet individual patient needs.
If alternative treatment is used and response is inadequate, discontinue it and use the preferred treatment before stepping up.
Zileuton is a less desirable alternative due to limited studies as adjunctive therapy and the need to monitor liver function. Theophylline requires monitoring of serum concentration levels.
In step 6, before oral systemic corticosteroids are introduced, a trial of high-dose ICS + LABA + either LTRA, theophylline, or zileuton may be considered, although this approach has not been studied in clinical trials.
Steps 1, 2, and 3 preferred therapies are based on Evidence A; step 3 alternative therapy is based on Evidence A for LTRA, Evidence B for theophylline, and Evidence D for zileuton. Step 5 preferred therapy is based on Evidence B. Step 6 preferred therapy is based on (EPR-2 1997) and Evidence B for omalizumab.
Immunotherapy for steps 2-4 is based on Evidence B for house-dust mites, animal danders, and pollens; evidence is weak or lacking for molds and cockroaches. Evidence is strongest for immunotherapy with single allergens. The role of allergy in asthma is greater in children than in adults.
Clinicians who administer immunotherapy or omalizumab should be prepared and equipped to identify and treat anaphylaxis that may occur.
This information is directly abstracted from the 2007 NAEPP *Expert Panel Report 3: Guidelines for the Diagnosis and Management of Asthma* and is not intended to promote or endorse any of the listed products.
To access the complete *Expert Panel Report 3: Guidelines for the Diagnosis and Management of Asthma,* go to www.nhlbi.nih.gov/guidelines/asthma/asthgdln.pdf.
ICS, Inhaled corticosteroid; *LABA,* inhaled long-acting beta$_2$-agonist; *LTRA,* leukotriene receptor antagonist; *SABA,* inhaled short-acting beta$_2$-agonist.
From National Asthma Education and Prevention Program: *Expert panel report 3: Guidelines for diagnosis and management of asthma*, National Institutes of Health, National Heart, Lung, and Blood Institute, August 2007, NIH publication 08-4051.

BOX 1-1 Possible Indications for Referral to an Asthma Specialist

Severe, acute asthma that has caused loss of consciousness, hypoxia, respiratory failure, convulsions, or near death

Poorly controlled asthma as indicated by admission to a hospital, frequent need for emergency care, need for oral corticosteroids, absence from school or work, disruption of sleep, interference with quality of life

Severe, persistent asthma requiring step 4 care (consider for patients who require step 3 care)

Patient <3 yr who requires step 3 or 4 care (consider for patient <3 yr who requires step 2 care)

Requirement for continuous oral corticosteroids or high-dose inhaled corticosteroids or more than two short courses of oral corticosteroids within 1 yr

Need for additional diagnostic testing such as allergy skin testing, rhinoscopy, provocative challenge, complete pulmonary function testing, bronchoscopy

Consideration for immunotherapy

Need for additional education regarding asthma, complications of asthma and treatment of asthma, problems with adherence to management recommendations, or allergen avoidance

Uncertainty of diagnosis

Complications of asthma, including sinusitis, nasal polyposis, aspergillosis, severe rhinitis, vocal cord dysfunction, gastroesophageal reflux

Modified from National Asthma Education and Prevention Program, National Heart, Lung, and Blood Institute: *Expert Panel Report 2: guidelines for the diagnosis and management of asthma,* Bethesda, MD, 1997, National Institutes of Health, NIH publication No 97-4051.

TABLE 1-9 Classifying Asthma Severity and Initiating Treatment in Children 5-11 Yr (Assessing severity and initiating treatment in children who are not currently taking long-term control medications)

Components of Severity		CLASSIFICATION OF ASTHMA SEVERITY (5-11 yrs of age)			
		Intermittent	PERSISTENT: Mild	PERSISTENT: Moderate	PERSISTENT: Severe
Impairment	Symptoms	≤2 days/wk	>2 days/wk but not daily	Daily	Throughout the day
	Nighttime awakenings	≤2×/mo	3-4×/mo	>1×/wk but not nightly	Often 7×/wk
	Short-acting beta$_2$-agonist use for symptom control (not prevention of EIB)	≤2 days/wk	>2 days/wk but not daily	Daily	Several times per day
	Interference with normal activity	None	Minor limitation	Some limitation	Extremely limited
	Lung function	Normal FEV$_1$ between exacerbations			
		FEV$_1$ >80% predicted	FEV$_1$ = >80% predicted	FEV$_1$ = 60%-80% predicted	FEV$_1$ <60% predicted
		FEV$_1$/FVC >85%	FEV$_1$/FVC >80%	FEV$_1$/FVC = 75%-80%	FEV$_1$/FVC <75%
Risk	Exacerbations requiring oral systemic corticosteroids	0-1 per yr	≥2 per yr ⟶		
		⟵ Consider severity and interval since last exacerbation. Frequency and severity may fluctuate over time for patients in any severity category. ⟶			
		Relative annual risk of exacerbations may be related to FEV$_1$.			
Recommended Step for Initiating Therapy		Step 1	Step 2	Step 3, medium-dose ICS option	Step 3, medium-dose ICS option, or Step 4
				and consider short course of oral systemic corticosteroids	
		In 2-6 wks, evaluate level of asthma control that is achieved and adjust therapy accordingly.			

The stepwise approach is meant to assist, not replace, the clinical decision-making required to meet individual patient needs.

Level of severity is determined by both impairment and risk. Assess impairment domain by patient's/caregiver's recall of previous 2-4 wks and spirometry. Assign severity to the most severe category in which any feature occurs.

At present, there are inadequate data to correspond frequencies of exacerbations with different levels of asthma severity. In general, more frequent and intense exacerbations (e.g., requiring urgent, unscheduled care, hospitalization, or ICU admission) indicate greater underlying disease severity. For treatment purposes, patients who had ≥2 exacerbations requiring oral systemic corticosteroids in the past year may be considered the same as patients who have persistent asthma, even in the absence of impairment levels consistent with persistent asthma.

EIB, Exercise-induced bronchospasm; *FEV$_1$,* forced expiratory volume in 1 second; *FVC,* forced vital capacity; *ICU,* intensive care unit.

From National Asthma Education and Prevention Program: *Expert panel report 3: Guidelines for diagnosis and management of asthma,* National Institutes of Health, National Heart, Lung, and Blood Institute, August 2007, NIH publication 08-4051.

TABLE 1-10 Assessing Asthma Control and Adjusting Therapy in Children 5-11 Yr

Components of Control		CLASSIFICATION OF ASTHMA CONTROL (5-11 yrs of age): Well Controlled	Not Well Controlled	Very Poorly Controlled
Impairment	Symptoms	≤2 days/wk but not more than once on each day	>2 days/wk or multiple times on ≤2 days/wk	Throughout the day
	Nighttime awakenings	≤1×/mo	≥2×/mo	≥2×/wk
	Interference with normal activity	None	Some limitation	Extremely limited
	Short-acting beta$_2$-agonist use for symptom control (not prevention of EIB)	≤2 days/wk	>2 days/wk	Several times per day
	Lung function			
	FEV$_1$ or peak flow	>80% predicted/personal best	60%-80% predicted/personal best	<60% predicted/personal best
	FEV$_1$/FVC	>80% predicted	75%-80%	<75% predicted
Risk	Exacerbations requiring oral systemic corticosteroids	0-1 per yr	≥2 per yr	
		Consider severity and interval since last exacerbation		
	Reduction in lung growth	Evaluation requires long-term follow-up care		
	Treatment-related adverse effects	Medication side effects can vary in intensity from none to very troublesome and worrisome. The level of intensity does not correlate to specific levels of control but should be considered in the overall assessment of risk.		
Recommended Action for Treatment		Maintain current step. Regular follow-up every 1-6 mos. Consider step down if well controlled for at least 3 mos.	Step up 1 step and Reevaluate in 2-6 wks. For side effects, consider alternative treatment options.	Consider short course of oral systemic corticosteroids. Step up 1-2 steps. Reevaluate in 2 wks. For side effects, consider alternative treatment options.

The stepwise approach is meant to assist, not replace, the clinical decision-making required to meet individual patient needs.

The level of control is based on the most severe impairment or risk category. Assess impairment domain by patient's/caregiver's recall of previous 2-4 wks and by spirometry or peak flow measures. Symptom assessment for longer periods should reflect a global assessment such as inquiring whether the patient's asthma is better or worse since the last visit.

At present, there are inadequate data to correspond frequencies of exacerbations with different levels of asthma control. In general, more frequent and intense exacerbations (e.g., requiring urgent, unscheduled care, hospitalization, or ICU admission) indicate poorer disease control. For treatment purposes, patients who had ≥2 exacerbations requiring oral systemic corticosteroids in the past year may be considered the same as patients who have persistent asthma, even in the absence of impairment levels consistent with persistent asthma.

Before step up in therapy:

- Review adherence to medications, inhaler technique, environmental control, and comorbid conditions.
- If an alternative treatment option was used in a step, discontinue it and use preferred treatment for that step.

EIB, Exercise-induced bronchospasm; *FEV$_1$,* forced expiratory volume in 1 second; *ICU,* intensive care unit.

From National Asthma Education and Prevention Program: *Expert panel report 3: Guidelines for diagnosis and management of asthma,* National Institutes of Health, National Heart, Lung, and Blood Institute, August 2007, NIH publication 08-4051.

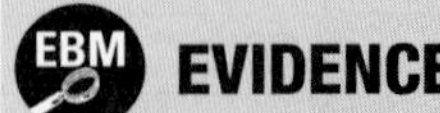

EVIDENCE

Please note: Complete text of evidence-based medicine (EBM) for this topic is available online.

Key trials and commentary:

Attacks of wheezing induced by upper respiratory viral infections are common in preschool children between the ages of 10 months and 6 years. A short course of oral prednisolone is widely used to treat preschool children with wheezing who present to a hospital, but there is conflicting evidence regarding its efficacy in this age group.

One study revealed that in preschool children presenting to a hospital with mild-to-moderate wheezing associated with a viral infection, oral prednisolone was not superior to placebo.

This report and one other that appeared simultaneously in the same issue of the *New England Journal of Medicine* tell us the role of steroids as part of the management for wheezing in preschoolers. Anyone who has been in pediatric practice for more than a few days knows about this problem because about one third of preschool children 4 years of age or younger will have intermittent wheezing, and the most common trigger of this is a respiratory viral infection. Wheezing with viral colds may persist into adult life or may disappear before school age. Some children, particularly those with atopy, have a different clinical phenotype known as "multi-trigger" wheezing. This condition is characterized by wheezing after exposure to multiple triggers, such as exercise and exposure to smoke, allergens, or cold air as well as viral infections.

Although the basis for the treatment of preschool wheezing is pitifully small in terms of evidence in the literature, what studies there are have suggested that the early use of inhaled corticosteroids (either intermittently for viral symptoms or continuously) does not prevent the progression of any type of preschool wheezing to established asthma in childhood. Recognizing this, most believe that treatment should be based solely on relief of symptoms. The current approach to the treatment of acute virus-associated wheezing among preschoolers has been based on the treatment for asthma in school-aged children. Oral corticosteroids are the bedrock of therapy. However, the report of Panickar et al describes an extension of their earlier work on the role of oral corticosteroids in acute virus-induced wheezing. The authors previously reported that in preschool children with an episode of wheezing that was sufficiently severe for admission to a hospital, a parent-initiated course of oral prednisolone made no difference in the outcome. In this report, we see the results of a double-blind, randomized, placebo-controlled trial showing no benefit of

TABLE 1-11 Stepwise Approach for Managing Asthma in Children 5-11 Yr

Intermittent Asthma	**Persistent Asthma: Daily Medication** Consult with asthma specialist if step 4 care or higher is required. Consider consultation at step 3.					↑
Step 1 *Preferred:* SABA prn	**Step 2** *Preferred:* Low-dose ICS *Alternative:* Cromolyn, LTRA, nedocromil, or theophylline	**Step 3** *Preferred:* Low-dose ICS + either LABA, LTRA, or theophylline OR Medium-dose ICS	**Step 4** *Preferred:* Medium-dose ICS + LABA *Alternative:* Medium-dose ICS + either LTRA or theophylline	**Step 5** *Preferred:* High-dose ICS + LABA *Alternative:* High-dose ICS + either LTRA or theophylline	**Step 6** *Preferred:* High-dose ICS + LABA + oral corticosteroid *Alternative:* High-dose ICS + either LTRA or theophylline + oral systemic corticosteroid	Step up if needed (first, check adherence, inhaler technique, environmental control, and comorbid conditions) **Assess control** Step down if possible (and asthma is well controlled at least 3 months)
Each step: Patient education, environmental control, and management of comorbidities Steps 2-4: Consider subcutaneous allergen immunotherapy for patients who have allergic asthma						
Quick-Relief Medication for All Patients • SABA as needed for symptoms. Intensity of treatment depends on severity of symptoms: up to 3 treatments at 20-minute intervals as needed. Short course of oral systemic corticosteroids may be needed. • Caution: Increasing use of SABA or use >2 days a week for symptom relief (not prevention of EIB) generally indicates inadequate control and the need to step up treatment.						↓

The stepwise approach is meant to assist, not replace, the clinical decision-making required to meet individual patient needs.

If alternative treatment is used and response is inadequate, discontinue it and use the preferred treatment before stepping up.

Theophylline is a less desirable alternative due to the need to monitor serum concentration levels.

Step 1 and step 2 medications are based on Evidence A. Step 3 ICS + adjunctive therapy and ICS are based on Evidence B for efficacy of each treatment and extrapolation from comparator trials in older children and adults–comparator trials are not available for this age group; steps 4-6 are based on expert opinion and extrapolation from studies in older children and adults.

Immunotherapy for steps 2-4 is based on Evidence B for house-dust mites, animal danders, and pollens; evidence is weak or lacking for molds and cockroaches. Evidence is strongest for immunotherapy with single allergens. The role of allergy in asthma is greater in children than in adults. Clinicians who administer immunotherapy should be prepared and equipped to identify and treat anaphylaxis that may occur.

This information is directly abstracted from the 2007 NAEPP *Expert Panel Report 3: Guidelines for the Diagnosis and Management of Asthma* and is not intended to promote or endorse any of the listed products.

ICS, Inhaled corticosteroid; *LABA,* inhaled long-acting beta$_2$-agonist; *LTRA,* leukotriene receptor antagonist; *SABA,* inhaled short-acting beta$_2$-agonist.

From National Asthma Education and Prevention Program: *Expert panel report 3: Guidelines for diagnosis and management of asthma,* National Institutes of Health, National Heart, Lung, and Blood Institute, August 2007, NIH publication 08-4051.

TABLE 1-12 Classifying Asthma Severity and Initiating Treatment in Children 0-4 Yr (Assessing severity and initiating treatment in children who are not currently taking long-term control medications)

Components of Severity		CLASSIFICATION OF ASTHMA SEVERITY (0-4 yrs of age)			
			PERSISTENT		
		Intermittent	Mild	Moderate	Severe
Impairment	Symptoms	≤2 days/wk	>2 days/wk but not daily	Daily	Throughout the day
	Nighttime awakenings	0	1-2×/mo	3-4×/mo	>1×/wk
	Short-acting beta$_2$-agonist use for symptom control (not prevention of EIB)	≤2 days/wk	>2 days/wk but not daily	Daily	Several times per day
	Interference with normal activity	None	Minor limitation	Some limitation	Extremely limited
Risk	Exacerbations requiring oral systemic corticosteroids	0-1 per yr	≥2 exacerbations in 6 mos requiring oral systemic corticosteroids, or ≥4 wheezing episodes/1 yr lasting >1 day AND risk factors for persistent asthma.		
		← Consider severity and interval since last exacerbation. → Frequency and severity may fluctuate over time.			
		Exacerbations of any severity may occur in patients in any severity category.			
Recommended Step for Initiating Therapy		Step 1	Step 2	Step 3 and consider short course of oral systemic corticosteroids	
		In 2-6 wks, depending on severity, evaluate level of asthma control that is achieved. If no clear benefit is observed in 4-6 wks, consider adjusting therapy or alternative diagnoses.			

The stepwise approach is meant to assist, not replace, the clinical decision-making required to meet individual patient needs.
Level of severity is determined by assessment of both impairment and risk. Assess impairment domain by patient's/caregiver's recall of previous 2-4 wks. Symptom assessment for longer periods should reflect a global assessment such as inquiring whether the patient's asthma is better or worse since the last visit. Assign severity to the most severe category in which any feature occurs.
At present, there are inadequate data to correspond frequencies of exacerbations with different levels of asthma severity. For treatment purposes, patients who had ≥2 exacerbations requiring oral systemic corticosteroids in the past six months, or ≥4 wheezing episodes in the past year, and who have risk factors for persistent asthma may be considered the same as patients who have persistent asthma, even in the absence of impairment levels consistent with persistent asthma.
To access the complete Expert Panel Report 3: Guidelines for the Diagnosis and Management of Asthma, go to www.nhlbi.nih.gov/guidelines/asthma/asthgdln.pdf.
EIB, Exercise-induced bronchospasm.
From National Asthma Education and Prevention Program: *Expert panel report 3: Guidelines for diagnosis and management of asthma,* National Institutes of Health, National Heart, Lung, and Blood Institute, August 2007, NIH publication 08-4051.

TABLE 1-13 Assessing Asthma Control and Adjusting Therapy in Children 0-4 Yrs of Age

Components of Control		CLASSIFICATION OF ASTHMA CONTROL (0-4 yrs of age)		
		Well Controlled	Not Well Controlled	Very Poorly Controlled
Impairment	Symptoms	≤2 days/wk	>2 days/wk	Throughout the day
	Nighttime awakenings	≤1×/mo	>1×/mo	>1×/wk
	Interference with normal activity	None	Some limitation	Extremely limited
	Short-acting beta$_2$-agonist use for symptom control (not prevention of EIB)	≤2 days/wk	>2 days/wk	Several times per day
Risk	Exacerbations requiring oral systemic corticosteroids	0-1 per yr	2-3 per yr	>3 per yr
	Treatment-related adverse effects	Medication side effects can vary in intensity from none to very troublesome and worrisome. The level of intensity does not correlate to specific levels of control but should be considered in the overall assessment of risk.		
Recommended Action for Treatment		Maintain current step. Regular follow-up every 1-6 mos. Consider step down if well controlled for at least 3 mos.	Step up 1 step. Reevaluate in 2-6 wks. If no clear benefit in 4-6 wks, consider alternative diagnoses or adjusting therapy. For side effects, consider alternative treatment options.	Consider short course of oral systemic corticosteroids. Step up 1-2 steps. Reevaluate in 2 wks. If no clear benefit in 4-6 wks, consider alternative diagnoses or adjusting therapy. For side effects, consider alternative treatment options.

The stepwise approach is meant to assist, not replace, the clinical decision-making required to meet individual patient needs.
The level of control is based on the most severe impairment or risk category. Assess impairment domain by caregiver's recall of previous 2-4 wks. Symptom assessment for longer periods should reflect a global assessment such as inquiring whether the patient's asthma is better or worse since the last visit.
At present, there are inadequate data to correspond frequencies of exacerbations with different levels of asthma control. In general, more frequent and intense exacerbations (e.g., requiring urgent, unscheduled care, hospitalization, or ICU admission) indicate poorer disease control. For treatment purposes, patients who had ≥2 exacerbations requiring oral systemic corticosteroids in the past year may be considered the same as patients who have not-well-controlled asthma, even in the absence of impairment levels consistent with not-well-controlled asthma.
Before step up in therapy:
- Review adherence to medications, inhaler technique, and environmental control.
- If an alternative treatment option was used in a step, discontinue it and use preferred treatment for that step.

EIB, Exercise-induced bronchospasm; *ICU,* intensive care unit.
From National Asthma Education and Prevention Program: *Expert panel report 3: Guidelines for diagnosis and management of asthma,* National Institutes of Health, National Heart, Lung, and Blood Institute, August 2007, NIH publication 08-4051.

oral prednisolone in preschool children hospitalized with acute virus-associated wheezing.

There are a few take-home messages from this report. One is that there can no longer be justification for the administration of prednisolone to preschoolers without atopy who have episodic (viral) wheezing in either a community or hospital setting unless a severe clinical course is anticipated. It is possible that prednisolone might have a role in the treatment of preschool children with atopy who have acute exacerbations, particularly in patients with multitrigger wheezing. The use of steroids in such cases is a study waiting to be done. In a commentary that accompanied this report, it was remarked that it is disturbing to contemplate how many unnecessary courses of prednisolone have been given over the years, in good faith, because we all assume that preschool children are little adults. A wise statement indeed. This same commentary also suggests that on the basis of these new data, we should be rethinking our management of viral-associated wheezing. β2-agonists that are inhaled through an appropriate spacer, with a mask if age appropriate, should be given. Prophylactic or intermittent use of leukotriene receptor antagonists may be beneficial, but comparisons with intermittent inhaled corticosteroids are needed. Prednisolone should be administered to preschoolers only when they are severely ill in the hospital. Intermittent, high-dose inhaled corticosteroids should not be used according to the commentary.

Needless to say, any child enrolled in one of these therapeutic trials should be followed well into adulthood to see if he or she has persistent, atopic, multitrigger wheezing (true asthma). Perhaps, we will learn more about whether those who ultimately develop true asthma fared any better, or worse, with the use of episodic steroids during episodes of viral-associated wheezing early in life.[1] Ⓐ

In another study the open-label phase of the START study was included to determine the effect on lung function and asthma control of adding budesonide to the reference group patients who had not initially received inhaled corticosteroids.

It revealed that in mild persistent asthma early intervention with inhaled budesonide was associated with improved asthma control and less additional asthma medication use.

This report of Inhaled Steroid Treatment as Regular Therapy in Early Asthma (START) study results that includes outcomes from the final 2 years of the study during which all subjects (both the group randomized to 3 years of budesonide [B] and the placebo [P] group), received unblinded inhaled budesonide in addition to usual care for asthma. Interestingly, at 5 years there was no significant difference in pulmonary function (FEV_1). However, there was a statistically significant reduction in time to first serious asthma-related event in the group who had received budesonide during the blinded portion of the study, and a statistically significant reduction in use of additional asthma medications. This suggests that early treatment with inhaled budesonide in new onset, mild asthma has the potential to result in improved early asthma control and a lesser need for additive asthma medications.[2] Ⓐ

A separate trial compared the effect of inhaled budesonide given daily or as-needed on mild persistent childhood asthma. It revealed that regular use of budesonide afforded better asthma control but had a more systemic effect than did use of budesonide as needed. The dose of ICS could be reduced as soon as asthma is controlled. Some children do not seem to need continuous inhaled corticosteroid treatment.

TABLE 1-14 Stepwise Approach for Managing Asthma in Children 0-4 Yr

Intermittent Asthma	**Persistent Asthma: Daily Medication** Consult with asthma specialist if step 3 care or higher is required. Consider consultation at step 2.					↑
Step 1 *Preferred:* SABA prn	**Step 2** *Preferred:* Low-dose ICS *Alternative:* Cromolyn or montelukast	**Step 3** *Preferred:* Medium-dose ICS	**Step 4** *Preferred:* Medium-dose ICS + either LABA or montelukast	**Step 5** *Preferred:* High-dose ICS + either LABA or montelukast	**Step 6** *Preferred:* High-dose ICS + either LABA or montelukast Oral systemic corticosteroid	Step up if needed (first, check adherence, inhaler technique, and environmental control) **Assess control** Step down if possible (and asthma is well controlled at least 3 months)
Patient Education and Environmental Control at Each Step						
Quick-Relief Medication for All Patients • SABA as needed for symptoms. Intensity of treatment depends on severity of symptoms. • With viral respiratory infection: SABA q 4-6 hours up to 24 hours (longer with physician consult). Consider short course of oral systemic corticosteroids if exacerbation is severe or patient has history of previous severe exacerbations. • Caution: Frequent use of SABA may indicate the need to step up treatment. See text for recommendations on initiating daily long-term-control therapy.						↓

The stepwise approach is meant to assist, not replace, the clinical decision-making required to meet individual patient needs.
If alternative treatment is used and response is inadequate, discontinue it and use the preferred treatment before stepping up.
If clear benefit is not observed within 4-6 wk and patient/family medication technique and adherence are satisfactory, consider adjusting therapy or alternative diagnosis.
Studies on children 0-4 yr are limited. Step 2 preferred therapy is based on Evidence A. All other recommendations are based on expert opinion and extrapolation from studies in other children.
This information is directly abstracted from the 2007 NAEPP *Expert Panel Report 3: Guidelines for the Diagnosis and Management of Asthma* and is not intended to promote or endorse any of the listed products.
ICS, Inhaled corticosteroid; *LABA,* inhaled long-acting beta$_2$-agonist; *SABA,* inhaled short-acting beta$_2$-agonist.
From National Asthma Education and Prevention Program: *Expert panel report 3: Guidelines for diagnosis and management of asthma,* National Institutes of Health, National Heart, Lung, and Blood Institute, August 2007, NIH publication 08-4051.

The debate continues. This pediatric asthma study compared outcomes in patients treated with (1) continuous budesonide (BC) (in reducing doses) for 18 months, (2) budesonide continuously for 6 months followed by budesonide (BP) exacerbations through 18 months, and (3) disodium cromoglycate (DSCG) 10 mg three times a day for 18 months with use of budesonide twice a day for 2 weeks for exacerbations. Pulmonary function, growth, and exacerbations were monitored. Following 18 months, pulmonary function did not differ significantly between groups; during months 7 to 18, the group receiving continuous budesonide had significantly fewer exacerbations than the other 2 groups ($P < 0.001$) (Table 3 in the original article). Time to first exacerbation was statistically significantly longer for both the continuous budesonide and the budesonide for 6 months followed by budesonide prn only for exacerbations than for DSCG ($P < 0.001$ for both), and longest for the BC group (Figure 3 in the original article). Growth velocity was similar with BC and BP, but the growth velocity during the P phase of BP was more rapid (Figure 4 in the original article). Bottom line: use of budesonide improved asthma control and reduced exacerbations in the pediatric population studied. Use of budesonide until control is achieved with subsequent conversion to as needed budesonide for exacerbations was well tolerated in some children. The key lies in knowing which children will do well in the budesonide treatment until control is achieved followed by prn budesonide for exacerbations only. For now, the crystal ball is hazy on this question, just as it is in adults.[3] Ⓐ

Long-acting β-agonists (LABAs) and inhaled corticosteroids administered together appear to be complementary in terms of effects on asthma control. The elements of asthma control achieved by LABAs (improved lung function) and leukotriene receptor antagonists (LTRAs; protection against exacerbations) may be complementary as well. This study sought to determine whether the combination of the LTRA montelukast and the LABA salmeterol could provide an effective therapeutic strategy for asthma.

It showed that patients with moderate asthma similar to those we studied should not substitute the combination of an LTRA and an LABA for the combination of inhaled corticosteroid and an LABA.

A study from the American Lung Association's Asthma Clinical Research Center's Network comparing combination therapy with montelukast/salmeterol (M/S) to beclomethasone/salmeterol (B/S) in a 14-week prospective, randomized, placebo-controlled study of moderate asthmatics. The study was stopped early by the data safety monitoring board because of clear inferiority of the M/S treatment arm. By 120 days of study participation, 26% of the M/S group had treatment failure compared with 9% of the B/S group ($P = 0.0008$). Statistically significant improvement in lung function, asthma control scores, and airway markers of inflammation were noted in the B/S group versus the M/S group. The results of this study are consistent with current national/international guidelines that promote combination therapy with inhaled corticosteroids with long-acting β-agonists for moderate asthma.[4] Ⓐ

Evidence-Based References

1. Panickar J et al: Oral prednisolone for preschool children with acute virus-induced wheezing, *N Engl J Med* 360:329-338, 2009. Commentary by J.A. Stockman III, M.D. Ⓐ
2. Busse WW et al: The Inhaled Steroid Treatment As Regular Therapy in Early Asthma (START) study 5-year follow-up: effectiveness of early intervention with budesonide in mild persistent asthma, *J Allergy Clin Immunol* 121:1167-1174, 2008. Commentary by S.K. Willsie, D.O. Ⓐ
3. Turpeinen M et al: Daily versus as-needed inhaled corticosteroid for mild persistent asthma (The Helsinki early intervention childhood asthma study), *Arch Dis Child* 93:654-659, 2008. Commentary by S.K. Willsie, D.O. Ⓐ
4. Deykin A, for the National Heart, Lung, and Blood Institute's Asthma Clinical Research Network: Combination therapy with a long-acting β-agonist and a leukotriene antagonist in moderate asthma, *Am J Respir Crit Care Med* 175:228-234, 2007. Commentary by S.K. Willsie, D.O. Ⓐ

SUGGESTED READINGS

American Lung Association Asthma Clinical Research Centers: Randomized comparison of strategies for reducing treatment in mild persistent asthma, *N Engl J Med* 356:2027, 2007.

Braman SS, Vigg A: The national Asthma Education and Prevention Program (NAEPP) Guidelines: will they improve the quality of care in America? *Medicine Health Rhode Island* 91:166, 2008.

Fanta CH: Asthma, *N Engl J Med* 360:10, 2009.

National Asthma Education and Prevention Program: *Expert panel report 3: guidelines for diagnosis and management of asthma*, Bethesda, MD, 2007, National Institutes of Health, NIH publication 08-4051.

Schatz M, Dombrowski MP: Asthma in pregnancy, *N Engl J Med* 360:1862-1869, 2009.

AUTHOR: **FRED F. FERRI, M.D.**

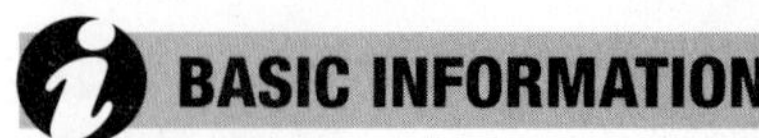

BASIC INFORMATION

DEFINITION

Astrocytoma is a type of neuroepithelial tumor that arises from glial precursor cells (astrocytes, oligodendrocytes, ependymal cells, epithelial cells of the choroids plexus, and others). Astrocytoma arises from astrocytes within the central nervous system (CNS). They are commonly graded by the World Health Organization (WHO) or the Saint Anne–Mayo grading system.

The WHO grades astrocytomas as follows:

- Grade I: pilocytic astrocytoma
- Grade II: low-grade astrocytoma (LGA), fibrillary infiltrating astrocytoma
- Grade III: anaplastic astrocytoma
- Grade IV: glioblastoma multiforme (GBM)
- Grades III and IV are considered high-grade astrocytomas (HGAs) or malignant.

Kernohan system grades astrocytomas based on histologic features: cellularity, mitoses, pleomorphism, vascularity, and necrosis. It has proved to be of prognostic value.

- Grade I: increased cellularity
- Grade II: greater cellularity than grade I plus pleomorphism
- Grade III: greater cellularity and pleomorphism than grade II plus vascular proliferation
- Grade IV: all the above, plus necrosis and pseudopalisading

SYNONYMS

Astroglial neoplasms

ICD-9CM CODES

191.9 Astrocytoma, unspecified site

EPIDEMIOLOGY & DEMOGRAPHICS

- According to SEER registry, the incidence of primary CNS tumor is 2.2 to 8.3/100,000 persons and about 30% of these tumors are astrocytomas.
- Astrocytomas can be found at all ages, with an early peak from birth to 4 yr, followed by a trough between the ages of 15 and 24 yr, and then a steady increase in incidence.
- Male/female ratio is 2:1.
- In adults, glioblastoma is the most common brain tumor.
- In children, astrocytomas are the second most common primary brain tumor and medulloblastoma is the most common.
- LGAs represent approximately 25% of all CNS gliomas in children.
- Peak age of incidence for juvenile pilocytic astrocytomas is 5 to 14 yr.
- Peak age of incidence for glioblastoma is 45 to 70 yr.

GENETICS:

- Alteration of *p53,* a tumor-suppressor gene encoded by the *TP53* gene on chromosome 17, plays a key role in the development of a large number of adult astrocytomas.
- Genetic abnormalities occur in a stepwise manner with accumulation of multiple abnormalities leading to dedifferentiation and transformation into higher grade.
- Abnormalities of the cell cycle regulatory complex that includes p16, cdk6/cyclinD1, cdk4/cyclinD1, and loss of chromosome 9P that targets the CDKN2A locus is thought to play an important role in progression to grade III astrocytoma.
- Transformation to GBM is the result of multiple mitogenic effects, with deregulation of p16-CDK4D1-pRb pathway being an important component. Loss of chromosome 10, which targets the PTEN tumor-suppressor gene, is also a frequent finding.

PHYSICAL FINDINGS & CLINICAL PRESENTATION

The presenting symptoms of astrocytoma depend, in part, on the location of the lesion and its rate of growth. Astrocytomas classically present with any one or more of the following features:

- Headache (less frequent)
- New-onset partial or generalized seizures (>50%)
- Nausea and vomiting
- Focal neurologic deficit (cranial nerve palsy, hemiplegia, ataxia)
- Change in mental status
- Papilledema (rare)

ETIOLOGY

- The specific etiology of astrocytoma is unknown.
- The only proven risk factor for development of astrocytoma has been significant exposure to ionizing radiation.
- Other risk factors, such as increased exposure to certain chemicals (petroleum, solvents, lead, pesticides and herbicides), have been proposed but not proved.

DIAGNOSIS

A provisional diagnosis of astrocytoma is made on clinical grounds and radiographic imaging studies. Tissue pathology is needed to establish the diagnosis and to grade the astrocytoma.

DIFFERENTIAL DIAGNOSIS

The differential diagnosis is vast and includes any cause of headache, seizures, change in mental status, and focal neurologic deficits.

WORKUP

- A CT scan or MRI of the head makes the diagnosis of an intracranial brain tumor. However, tissue is needed to establish a diagnosis of astrocytoma.
- Stereotactic biopsy under CT or MRI guidance has been shown to be a relatively safe and accurate method for diagnosis of LGA.
- In the presence of mass effect, either clinically or radiologically, craniotomy with open biopsy and tumor debulking is more appropriate than stereotactic biopsy to establish a tissue diagnosis.

LABORATORY TESTS

Blood tests are not specific.

IMAGING STUDIES

- MRI is the diagnostic imaging study of choice. MRI with contrast and magnetic resonance angiography are used to locate the margins of the tumor, distinguish vascular masses from tumors, detect LGAs not seen by CT scan, and provide clear views of the posterior fossa.
- Newer imaging modalities like magnetic resonance spectroscopy, dynamic enhance MRI, diffusion perfusion MRI, and functional MRI may lead to improved tumor delineation and functional mapping, and provide information to facilitate resection.

TREATMENT

ACUTE GENERAL Rx

- Once a clinical diagnosis is made on imaging and there is evidence of edema, patients should be started on dexamethasone 10 mg intravenously (IV) followed by 4 mg IV q6h.
- If there is increased intracranial pressure and impending herniation, patient should be started on IV mannitol, and mechanical ventilation with hyperventilation should be considered if there is depressed consciousness.
- Surgery remains the initial treatment of almost all astrocytomas, particularly if the tumor is in an anatomically accessible location. Surgery helps in the following ways:
  1. Establishing a pathologic diagnosis and providing information on grade
  2. Debulking the tumor
  3. Alleviating intracranial pressure
- Grade I astrocytomas are usually circumscribed, and complete resection is possible with a high likelihood of long-term remission.
- In grade II astrocytomas, the extent of surgical resection and amount of postoperative residual disease is an important variable for time to first relapse. Randomized trials have shown that postoperative radiotherapy in grade II astrocytoma increases progression-free survival (PFS), but no increase in median survival occurs.
- In grade III and grade IV astrocytomas, gross total resection is the initial treatment of choice. Patients with no residual enhancing tumor have a longer median survival (17.9 vs 12.9 mo; $P < 0.001$) than patients with residual tumor.
- Use of radiation after surgery in HGAs has shown a clear benefit of survival.
- In a randomized trial of patients with GBM, radiation with concurrent temozolomide followed by six cycles of adjuvant temozolomide increases median and overall survival, and this is considered the standard of care for patients with GBM.

CHRONIC Rx

- Attempt at resection again should be considered in all types of astrocytomas on relapse if possible and in grade I astrocytomas can lead to long-term remissions.

- Radiation therapy can be considered in the relapsed setting in grade II astrocytomas if not given in the adjuvant setting. Chemotherapy has been tried but has no proven role in these tumors.
- Chemotherapy in anaplastic astrocytomas that have relapsed after radiation does have a role, and the active agents are nitrosourea-based regimen and temozolomide. Grade III anaplastic astrocytomas that have 1p and 19q deletions are especially sensitive to chemotherapy.
- Chemotherapy is used in patients with GBM on relapse, but efficacy is limited. Temozolomide is the most commonly used agent, but radiologic response is in the 5% to 10% range. Recently, a number of phase II trials have shown the efficacy of the combination of inrinotecan and avastin with response rates in the 30% range and have provided a new option in the treatment of GBMs.
- Patients presenting with seizures should be treated with anticonvulsants.

DISPOSITION

- Approximately 10% to 35% of astrocytomas (usually grade I pilocytic astrocytomas) are amenable to complete surgical excision and cure. WHO grade I astrocytomas usually do not progress to higher grade tumors.
- Grade II astrocytomas have a median survival of 7.7 yr if they are low risk and 3.2 yr if they are high risk.
- Grade III astrocytomas have a 3-yr survival rate of 55%.
- Median survival for patients with GBM is about 1 yr. Median survival of patients with GBM treated with supportive care is approximately 14 wk. This increases to 20 wk with surgical resection alone, 36 wk with surgery plus x-ray therapy, and 40 to 50 wk with the addition of adjuvant chemotherapy.

REFERRAL

A team of specialty consultations is indicated in patients diagnosed with astrocytoma. A neurosurgeon, radiation oncologist, and neurooncologist are all needed to assist in establishing the diagnosis and to provide immediate and follow-up treatment.

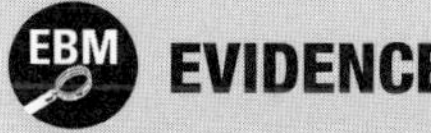

EVIDENCE

Please note: Complete text of EBM for this topic is available online.

Key trials and commentary:

The World Health Organization (WHO) recently updated its classification of central nervous system (CNS) tumors, adding eight entities, as well as defining new variants and morphologic patterns of existing entities. Despite the continued refinement of brain tumor histologic classification and grading, there remain some diagnostic "gray zones" that challenge general surgical pathologists and neuropathologists alike. These include the presence of oligodendroglial features in (mixed) oligoastrocytomas and glioblastomas (GBMs), GBM variants (such as small cell GBM), meningioma classification and grading, medulloblastoma variants, ependymoma grading, the presence of "neuronal features" in otherwise morphologically classic gliomas, and low-grade gliomas with high Ki-67 labeling indices. This current review discusses these issues and offers some practical guidelines for dealing with problematic cases.

The diagnosis and grading of the multiple variations of primary glial, neuronal, and glioneuronal CNS tumors are challenging and require distinction among the various types of tumors. Distinction is critical for both appropriate classification and then treatment of an individual patient's neoplasm and for optimizing the research of CNS tumors.

The WHO-sponsored working group of neurooncology experts apply a uniform, consensus classification and grading system to CNS neoplasms, based on peer-reviewed studies, for use in clinical and research settings throughout the world. The CNS tumor "Blue Book" provides concisely compiled clinicopathologic, histologic, immunohistochemical, and genetic data about CNS neoplasms. Critically, the WHO CNS tumor working group has, over the years, helped to establish criteria for the diagnosis and grading of these tumor entities and their variants and histologic patterns of differentiation. As an example, the provision of specific diagnostic criteria for the grading of meningiomas has immensely facilitated the consistent sign-out of such neoplasms. New in the 2007 edition, identification of "brain invasion" by meningioma on histologic examination is sufficient in and of itself to confer a "WHO grade II" on a tumor, regardless of other features identified in the neoplasm, clearing up an issue that had been contentious for years.

Nevertheless, despite the excellent guidance of the WHO text, multiple "gray zones" exist in the diagnosis and grading of tumors. This article provides an excellent overview and illustration of remaining controversies and offers suggestions about how to approach tumors within this zone. Critical topics include (1) identification of an oligodendroglial component within a glial neoplasm sufficient to make the diagnosis of oligoastrocytoma or glioblastoma with oligodendroglial features; (2) identification of variants of glioblastoma distinction including the small-cell variant and distinction from oligodendroglioma (and small-cell astrocytoma); (3) distinction of variants of medulloblastoma; (4) grading of ependymomas; (5) classification of neuronal features in otherwise classic gliomas; and (6) dealing with high MIB-1/Ki-67 labeling indices in low-grade neoplasms. This article provides a succinct review of these topics and offers practical guidance when they are encountered.

GBM is the most common form of Astrocytoma and is incurable in nature. An attempt at total resection is the initial treatment of choice. There is evidence that insertion of Gliadel wafer[1] in the resection cavity at the time of surgery increases survival. For adjuvant therapy a randomized trial showed that concurrent temozolomide and radiation followed by six cycles of temozolomide is superior to radiation alone.[2] For relapsed GBM a number of recent trials have shown impressive activity with a combination of irinotecan and avastin[3,4] leading to an FDA approval of Avastin for GBM.[5] Ⓐ

Evidence-Based References

1. Westphal M et al: Gliadel wafer in initial surgery for malignant glioma: long-term follow-up of a multicenter controlled trial, *Acta Neurochir (Wien)* 148(3):269-275, 2006.
2. Stupp R et al: Radiotherapy and concomitant and adjuvant temozolomide for glioblastoma, *N Engl J Med* 352(10):987-996, 2005.
3. Vredenburgh JJ et al: Bevacizumab plus irinotecan in recurrent glioblastoma multiforme, *J Clin Oncol* 25:4722-4729, 2007.
4. Vredenburgh JJ et al: Phase II trial of bevacizumab and irinotecan in recurrent malignant glioma, *Clin Cancer Res* 13:1253-1259, 2007.
5. Trembath D et al: Gray zones in brain tumor classification: evolving concepts, *Adv Anat Pathol* 15:287-297, 2008. Commentary by P. Boyer, M.D., Ph.D. Ⓐ

SUGGESTED READINGS

Batchelor T et al: Management of malignant gliomas. Available at http://www.uptodate.com. Accessed Sep 28, 2008.

Grossman SA, Batara JF: Current management of glioblastoma multiforme, *Semin Oncol* 31(5):635, 2004.

Olson JJ et al: Management of newly diagnosed glioblastoma: guidelines development, value and application, *J Neurooncol* 93(1):1-23, 2009.

Reardon DA et al: Recent advances in the treatment of malignant astrocytoma, *J Clin Oncol* 24:8, 2006.

AUTHOR: **BILAL H. NAQVI, M.D.**

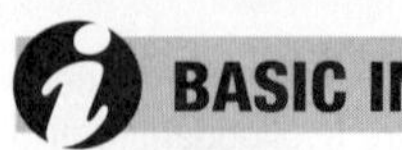

BASIC INFORMATION

DEFINITION

Ataxia telangiectasia (AT) is a rare autosomal recessive disorder of childhood that results from defective DNA damage repair. AT is a multisystemic disease characterized by progressive cerebellar ataxia, choreoathetosis, oculocutaneous telangiectasias (see Fig. 1-31), frequent infections, increased sensitivity to ionizing radiation, and predisposition to malignancies.

ICD-9CM CODES
334.8 Ataxia telangiectasia

EPIDEMIOLOGY & DEMOGRAPHICS

INCIDENCE: 1/40,000 live births; it is estimated that 1.4% to 2% of whites in the United States carry one defective AT gene
PEAK INCIDENCE: Childhood
PREDOMINANT SEX: Sexes are equally affected.
GENETICS: Condition is autosomal recessive, chromosome 11q22.3. Gene product is *ATM,* which is expressed in all tissues and encodes a large protein that is a member of the phosphatidylinositol-3 kinases and another region similar to DNA repair genes.

PHYSICAL FINDINGS & CLINICAL PRESENTATION

- Children show normal early development until they start to walk, when gait and truncal ataxia become apparent. They soon experience development of polyneuropathy, progressive apraxia of eye movements and slurred speech, choreoathetosis, mild diabetes mellitus, delayed physical and sexual development, and signs of premature aging (graying of the hair).
- Children with AT experience deterioration of motor skills; by the second decade of life, most patients rely on wheelchairs for at least part of the day. Progressive oromotor difficulties also develop over time, placing patients at risk for aspiration.
- Telangiectasias, which are characteristic of the disease but not always present, occur in the outer parts of the bulbar conjunctivae, over the surface of the ears and cheeks, on exposed parts of the neck, on the bridge of the nose, and in the flexor creases of the forearms.
- Immunodeficiencies occur in 60% to 80% of individuals with AT. Impaired humoral and cellular immunity lead to recurrent sinopulmonary infections in about 70% of children.
- Beyond 10 yr of age, incidence rate is 1% per yr; overall risk rate is 10% to 20%, of which 85% of cases are leukemia and lymphoma. Predisposition to other cancers (such as breast cancer) may also exist, which is thought to be due to the phosphorylation of the tumor-suppressor/breast cancer susceptibility gene *BRCA1* by *ATM.*
- Typically, individuals with AT have normal intelligence. Deterioration of speech is typically noted after the age of 5 to 8 yr. Slow motor and verbal responses may make traditional timed assessments inaccurate.
- Heterozygotes/carriers of the *ATM* gene are thought to have none of the classic manifestations of AT; however, they may have a greater incidence of malignancy at a younger age.

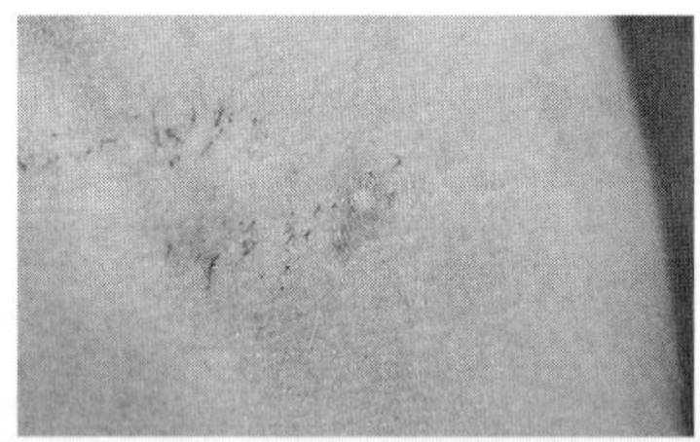

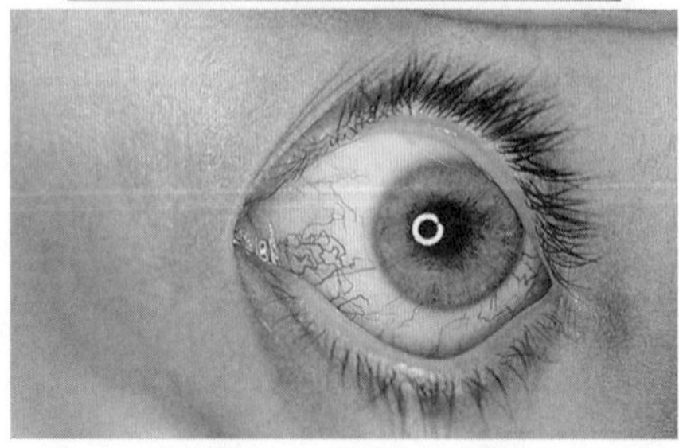

FIGURE 1-31 Ataxia telangiectasia. (From Callen JP [ed]: *Color atlas of dermatology,* ed 2, Philadelphia, 2000, WB Saunders.)

ETIOLOGY

- Cytogenetics show a 7;14 translocation in 5% to 15% of individuals with AT. Cloning and sequencing has identified the *ATM* gene (ataxia telangiectasia, mutated), which is a protein kinase that is missing or defective. This delays accumulation of the tumor-suppressor p53 in response to DNA damage, thereby increasing the risk for cancer. Cells are susceptible to damage by ionizing radiation or chemotherapeutic agents that cause double-stranded DNA breakages.

Dx DIAGNOSIS

DIFFERENTIAL DIAGNOSIS: Early-onset ataxia:
- Friedreich's ataxia
- Abetalipoproteinemia (Bassen-Kornzweig syndrome)
- Acquired vitamin E deficiency
- Early-onset cerebellar ataxia with retained reflexes (EOCA)
- Ataxia-ocular apraxia type 1 (AOA1)
- Ataxia-ocular apraxia type 2

WORKUP

Diagnosis relies on the constellation of clinical findings, including ataxia and speech changes, as well as family history and neuroimaging studies.

LABORATORY TESTS

- Patients should be evaluated for serum immunoglobulin levels (IgA, IgG, IgE, and IgG subclasses) to evaluate for immunoglobulin deficiency, and α-fetoprotein, which is increased in more than 95% of patients.
- Prenatal testing is available. Fibroblasts can be screened for abnormal sensitivity to ionizing radiation.
- Immunoblotting for ATM protein can be done. This determines whether ATM protein is present in cells; approximately 90% of individuals will have no detectable ATM protein.

IMAGING STUDIES

CT or MRI scans will show cerebellar atrophy but may not be obvious in very young children.

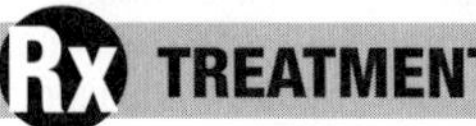

Rx TREATMENT

- There is no proven disease-specific treatment available to delay the progressive ataxia, dysarthria, and oculomotor apraxia. Treatment remains supportive.
- Surveillance for infections and neoplasms is ongoing. Individuals with frequent and severe infections may benefit from intravenous immunoglobulin to supplement immune system.
- The cloning and sequencing of the gene for AT has opened several avenues for intervention, including gene therapy, targeted pharmacologic intervention, and direct protein replacement.

NONPHARMACOLOGIC THERAPY

- Minimize radiation as it may induce further chromosomal damage and lead to neoplasms. Even diagnostic x-rays should be limited because of the theoretical risk that radiation may lead to chromosomal breakages.
- Physical and occupational therapy to maintain flexibility and minimize contractures.

COMPLEMENTARY AND ALTERNATIVE MEDICINE

- Antioxidant treatment with vitamin E is often given empirically, though it has not been formally tested. α-Lipoic acid crosses the blood-brain barrier and may, therefore, have some advantage.

DISPOSITION

- The expected life span has increased considerably; most individuals now live beyond 25 yr of age and some into the fourth and fifth decades of life.

REFERRAL

- Immunology
- Neurology
- Physical and occupational therapy
- Genetic counselor

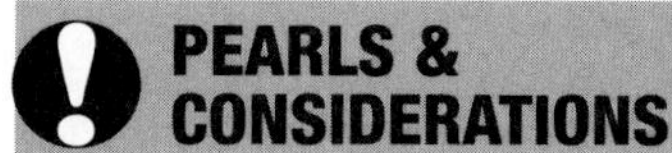

PEARLS & CONSIDERATIONS

COMMENTS

- Most common cause of hereditary ataxia
- Defect in DNA repair
- Predisposition to frequent infections, malignancies, and sensitivity to ionizing radiation

PATIENT/FAMILY EDUCATION

Ataxia Telangiectasia Children's Project: www.atcp.org

National Ataxia Foundation (NAF): www.ataxia.org

SUGGESTED READINGS

Butch AW et al: Immunoassay to measure ataxia-telangiectasia mutated protein in cellular lysates, *Clin Chem* 50:2302-2308, 2004.

Crawford TO et al: Survival probability in ataxia telangiectasia, *Arch Dis Child* 91:610, 2006.

Gatti RA et al: Localization of an ataxia-telangiectasia gene to chromosome 11q22-23, *Nature* 336:577, 1988.

McKinnon PJ: ATM and ataxia telangiectasia, *EMBO Rep* 5(8):772-776, 2004.

Nowak-Wegrzyn A: Immunodeficiency and infections in ataxia-telangiectasia, *J Pediatr* 144:505, 2004.

Renwick A, Thompson D, Seal S et al: ATM mutations that cause ataxia-telangiectasia are breast cancer susceptibility alleles. *Nat Genet* 38:873, 2006.

Sun X et al: Early diagnosis of ataxia-telangiectasia using radiosensitivity testing, *J Pediatr* 140:724-731, 2002.

Taylor AMR, Byrd PJ: Molecular pathology of ataxia telangiectasia, *J Clin Pathol* 58(10):1009-1015, 2005.

AUTHOR: **NICOLE J. ULLRICH, M.D., PH.D.**

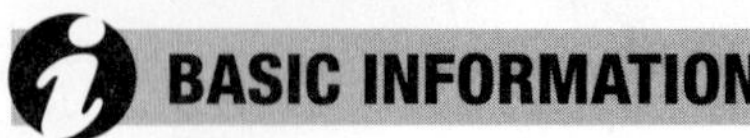

BASIC INFORMATION

DEFINITION

Atelectasis is the collapse of lung volume.

ICD-9CM CODES

518.0 Atelectasis

EPIDEMIOLOGY & DEMOGRAPHICS

- Occurs frequently in patients receiving mechanical ventilation with higher FiO_2
- Dependent regions of the lung are more prone to atelectasis: they are partially compressed, they are not as well ventilated, and there is no spontaneous drainage of secretions with gravity

PHYSICAL FINDINGS & CLINICAL PRESENTATION

- Decreased or absent breath sounds
- Abnormal chest percussion
- Cough, dyspnea, decreased vocal fremitus and vocal resonance
- Diminished chest expansion, tachypnea, tachycardia

ETIOLOGY

- Mechanical ventilation with higher FiO_2
- Chronic bronchitis
- Cystic fibrosis
- Endobronchial neoplasms
- Foreign bodies
- Infections (e.g., TB, histoplasmosis)
- Extrinsic bronchial compression from neoplasms, aneurysms of ascending aorta, enlarged left atrium
- Sarcoidosis
- Silicosis
- Anterior chest wall injury, pneumothorax
- Alveolar injury (e.g., toxic fumes, aspiration of gastric contents)
- Pleural effusion, expanding bullae
- Chest wall deformity (e.g., scoliosis)
- Muscular weaknesses or abnormalities (e.g., neuromuscular disease)
- Mucus plugs from asthma, allergic bronchopulmonary aspergillosis, postoperative state

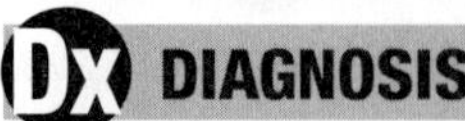

DIAGNOSIS

DIFFERENTIAL DIAGNOSIS

- Neoplasm
- Pneumonia
- Encapsulated pleural effusion
- Abnormalities of brachiocephalic vein and the left pulmonary ligament

WORKUP

- Chest radiograph (Fig. 1-32)
- CT scan and fiberoptic bronchoscopy (selected patients)

IMAGING STUDIES

- Chest radiograph will confirm diagnosis.
- CT scan is useful in patients with suspected endobronchial neoplasm or extrinsic bronchial compression.
- Fiberoptic bronchoscopy (selected patients) is useful for removal of foreign body or evaluation of endobronchial and peribronchial lesions.

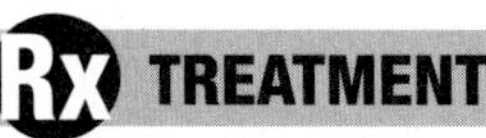

TREATMENT

NONPHARMACOLOGIC THERAPY

- Deep breathing, mobilization of the patient
- Incentive spirometry
- Tracheal suctioning
- Humidification
- Chest physiotherapy with percussion and postural drainage

ACUTE GENERAL Rx

- Positive-pressure breathing (continuous positive airway pressure by face mask, positive end-expiratory pressure for patients on mechanical ventilation)
- Use of mucolytic agents (e.g., acetylcysteine [Mucomyst])
- Recombinant human DNase (dornase alpha) in patients with cystic fibrosis
- Bronchodilator therapy in selected patients

CHRONIC Rx

- Chest physiotherapy
- Humidification of inspired air
- Frequent nasotracheal suctioning

DISPOSITION

Prognosis varies with the underlying etiology

REFERRAL

- Bronchoscopy for removal of foreign body or plugs unresponsive to conservative treatment
- Surgical referral for removal of obstructing neoplasms

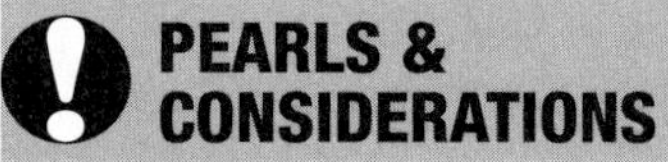

PEARLS & CONSIDERATIONS

COMMENTS

Patients should be educated that frequent changes of position are helpful in clearing secretions. Sitting the patient upright in a chair is recommended to increase both volume and vital capacity relative to the supine position.

AUTHOR: **FRED F. FERRI, M.D.**

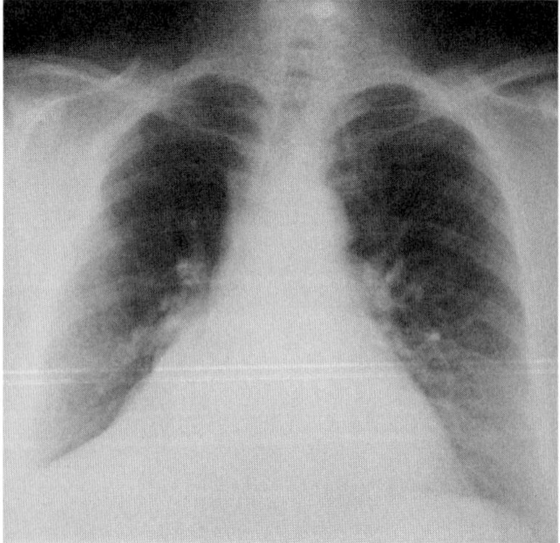

FIGURE 1-32 Right middle and right lower lobe atelectasis that silhouettes the diaphragm and the right heart border. (From Specht N [ed]: *Practical guide to diagnostic imaging,* St Louis, 1998, Mosby.)

BASIC INFORMATION

DEFINITION

Atopic dermatitis is a genetically determined eczematous eruption that is pruritic, symmetric, and associated with personal family history of allergic manifestations (atopy).

SYNONYMS

Eczema
Atopic neurodermatitis
Atopic eczema

ICD-9CM CODES
691.8 Atopic dermatitis

EPIDEMIOLOGY & DEMOGRAPHICS

- Incidence is between 5 and 25 cases/1000 persons.
- Highest incidence is among children (5% to 10%). It accounts for 4% of acute care pediatric visits.
- Onset of disease before age 5 yr in 85% of patients.
- More than 50% of children with generalized atopic dermatitis develop asthma and allergic rhinitis by age 13 yr.
- Concordance in monozygotic twins is 77%.

PHYSICAL FINDINGS & CLINICAL PRESENTATION

- There are no specific cutaneous signs for atopic dermatitis, and there is a wide spectrum of presentations ranging from minimal flexural eczema to erythroderma.
- The primary lesions are a result of itching caused by severe and chronic pruritus. The repeated scratching modifies the skin surface, producing lichenification, dry and scaly skin, and redness.
- The lesions are typically on the neck, face, upper trunk, and bends of elbows and knees (symmetric on flexural surfaces of extremities).
- There is dryness, thickening of the involved areas, discoloration, blistering, and oozing.
- Papular lesions are frequently found in the antecubital and popliteal fossae.
- In children, red scaling plaques are often confined to the cheeks and the perioral and perinasal areas.
- Inflammation in the flexural areas and lichenified skin is a very common presentation in children.
- Constant scratching may result in areas of hypopigmentation or hyperpigmentation (more common in blacks).
- In adults, redness and scaling in the dorsal aspect of the hands or about the fingers are the most common expression of atopic dermatitis; oozing and crusting may be present.
- Secondary skin infections may be present (*Staphylococcus aureus,* dermatophytosis, herpes simplex).

ETIOLOGY

Unknown; elevated T-lymphocyte activation, defective cell immunity, and B cell IgE overproduction may play a significant role.

DIAGNOSIS

DIFFERENTIAL DIAGNOSIS

- Scabies
- Psoriasis
- Dermatitis herpetiform
- Contact dermatitis
- Photosensitivity
- Seborrheic dermatitis
- Candidiasis
- Lichen simplex chronicus
- Other: Wiskott-Aldrich syndrome, PKU, mycosis fungoides, ichthyosis, HIV dermatitis, nonnummular eczema, histiocytosis X

WORKUP

Diagnosis is based on the presence of three of the following major features and three minor features.

MAJOR FEATURES:

- Pruritus
- Personal or family history of atopy: asthma, allergic rhinitis, atopic dermatitis
- Facial and extensor involvement in infants and children
- Flexural lichenification in adults

MINOR FEATURES:

- Elevated IgE
- Eczema-perifollicular accentuation
- Recurrent conjunctivitis
- Ichthyosis
- Nipple dermatitis
- Wool intolerance
- Cutaneous *S. aureus* infections or herpes simplex infections
- Food intolerance
- Hand dermatitis (nonallergic irritant)
- Facial pallor, facial erythema
- Cheilitis
- White dermographism
- Early age of onset (after 2 mo of age)

LABORATORY TESTS

- Lab tests are generally not helpful.
- Elevated IgE levels are found in 80% to 90% of atopic dermatitis.
- Blood eosinophilia correlates with disease severity.

TREATMENT

NONPHARMACOLOGIC THERAPY

- Clip nails to decrease abrasion of skin

Avoidance of triggering factors:

- Sudden temperature changes, sweating, low humidity in the winter
- Contact with irritating substance (e.g., wool, cosmetics, some soaps and detergents, tobacco)
- Foods that provoke exacerbations (e.g., eggs, peanuts, fish, soy, wheat, milk)
- Stressful situations
- Allergens and dust
- Excessive hand washing

GENERAL Rx

- Emollients can be used to prevent dryness. Severely affected skin can be optimally hydrated by occlusion in addition to application of emollients.
- Topical corticosteroids (e.g., 1% to 2.5% hydrocortisone) may be helpful and are generally considered first line therapy. Use intermediate-potency steroids (e.g., triamcinolone, fluocinolone) for more severe cases and limit potent corticosteroids (e.g., betamethasone, desoximetasone, clobetasol) to severe cases.
- The topical immunomodulators pimecrolimus and tacrolimus are especially useful for treatment of the face and intertriginous sites, where steroid-induced atrophy may occur. However, due to concerns about carcinogenic potential, the FDA recommends limiting their use for short periods in patients who are intolerant or unresponsive to other treatments. Pimecrolimus cream (Elidel) 1% is applied bid and has antiinflammatory effects secondary to blockage of activated T-cell cytokine production. Tacrolimus (Protopic) ointment (0.03% or 0.1%) applied bid is a macrolide that suppresses humoral and cell-mediated immune responses.
- Oral antihistamines (e.g., hydroxyzine, diphenhydramine) are effective in controlling pruritus and inducing sedation, restful sleep, and prevention of scratching during sleep. Doxepin and other tricyclic antidepressants also have antihistamine effect, induce sleep, and reduce pruritus.
- Oral prednisone, IM triamcinolone, Goeckerman regimen, PUVA are generally reserved for severe cases.
- Methotrexate, cyclosporine azathioprine, and systemic corticosteroids are sometimes tried for recalcitrant disease in adults.

DISPOSITION

- Resolution occurs in approximately 70% of patients by adulthood.
- Most patients have a course characterized by remissions and intermittent flares.

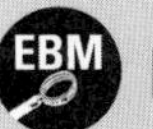

EVIDENCE

Please note: Complete text of EBM for this topic is available online.

SUGGESTED READINGS

Bieber T: Atopic dermatitis, *N Engl J Med* 358:1483-1494, 2008.

Buys LM: Treatment options for atopic dermatitis, *Am Fam Physician* 75:523-528, 2007.

AUTHOR: **FRED F. FERRI, M.D.**

Atrial Fibrillation (PTG) (ALG)

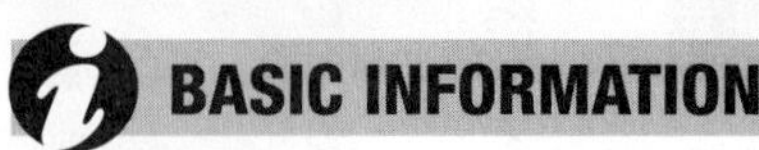

BASIC INFORMATION

DEFINITION

Atrial fibrillation (AF) is chaotic atrial activity caused by simultaneous discharge of multiple atrial foci because of multiple reentrant circuits.

SYNONYMS

AF
A-fib

ICD-9CM CODES
427.31 Atrial fibrillation

EPIDEMIOLOGY & DEMOGRAPHICS

- The prevalence of AF increases with age, from 0.1% in adults <55 yr old to 9% of those ≥80 yr old.
- The prevalence of AF is increasing and is greater in men than in women.
- AF affects 2.3 million people in the U.S. and is a major cause of stroke (fivefold increased risk).
- Chronic AF develops in 25% of patients 5 yr after paroxysmal AF.

PHYSICAL FINDINGS & CLINICAL PRESENTATION

Clinical presentation is variable:

- Palpitations, dizziness, or lightheadedness
- Fatigue, weakness, or impaired exercise tolerance
- Angina
- Dyspnea
- Some patients are asymptomatic
- Cardiac auscultation revealing irregularly irregular rhythm

ETIOLOGY

- Vascular causes: hypertensive heart disease, increased pulse pressure (calculated as the difference between systolic and diastolic pressure), a reflection of aortic stiffness
- Valvular heart disease
- Pulmonary causes: pulmonary embolism, chronic obstructive pulmonary disease, obstructive sleep apnea, carbon monoxide poisoning
- Structural cardiac disease: pericarditis, myocarditis, cardiomyopathy, congestive heart failure, coronary artery disease, myocardial infarction, congenital heart disease (especially those that lead to atrial enlargement such as atrial septal defect), tachycardia-bradycardia syndrome
- Arrhythmias: atrial tachycardia, Wolff-Parkinson-White syndrome
- Endocrine: thyrotoxicosis, hyperthyroidism or subclinical hyperthyroidism, pheochromocytoma
- Surgery: both cardiac and noncardiac
- Electrolytes: hypokalemia, hypomagnesemia
- Systemic stress: fever, anemia, hypoxia, sepsis, infections (e.g., pneumonia)
- Medications/toxins: digitalis, adenosine, theophylline, amphetamines, cocaine, antihistamines, alcohol abuse and/or withdrawal, caffeine

DIAGNOSIS

DIFFERENTIAL DIAGNOSIS

- Multifocal atrial tachycardia
- Atrial flutter
- Frequent atrial premature beats

WORKUP

New-onset AF: ECG, echocardiogram, Holter monitor (selected patients), and laboratory evaluation

LABORATORY TESTS

- Thyroid-stimulating hormone, free T_4
- Serum electrolytes
- Toxicity screen

IMAGING STUDIES

- ECG (see Fig. 1-33 for atrial flutter and fibrillation)
- Absence of P waves
- Fibrillatory or f waves at the isoelectric baseline with varying amplitude, morphology, and intervals
- Irregular ventricular rate
- Echocardiography to rule out structural heart disease (evaluate ventricular size, thickness, and function, atrial size, and valve function)
- Holter monitor: useful only in selected patients to evaluate paroxysmal AF

TREATMENT

NONPHARMACOLOGIC THERAPY

- Avoidance of alcohol in patients with suspected excessive alcohol use
- Avoidance of caffeine and nicotine
- Treatment of underlying source/cause, if any found
- The Maze surgical procedure, with its recent modifications creating electrical barriers to the macroreentrant circuits that are believed to underlie AF, is being performed with good results in several medical centers (preservation of sinus rhythm in >95% of patients without the use of long-term antiarrhythmic medication). Clear indications for its use remain undefined. In general, surgery is reserved for patients with rapid heart rate refractory to pharmacologic therapy or those who cannot tolerate pharmacologic therapy.
- Pulmonary vein ablation for chronic AF: Sinus rhythm can be maintained long term in the majority of patients with chronic AF by circumferential pulmonary vein ablation, independently of the effects of antiarrhythmic drug therapy, cardioversion, or both. The American College of Cardiology/American Heart Association/European Society of Cardiology (ACC/AHA/ESC) guidelines state that catheter ablation is a reasonable alternative to medical therapy to prevent recurrent AF in symptomatic patients in the absence of significant left atrial enlargement (class 2A recommendation).

ACUTE GENERAL Rx

New-onset AF:

- If the patient is hemodynamically unstable (hypotension, congestive heart failure or angina), perform synchronized cardioversion after immediate conscious sedation with a rapid short-acting sedative (e.g., midazolam). The likelihood of cardioversion-related clinical thromboembolism is low in patients with AF lasting <48 hours. Patients with AF lasting >2 days have a 5% to 7% risk for clinical thromboembolism if cardioversion is not preceded by several weeks of warfarin therapy. However, if transesophageal echocardiography reveals no atrial thrombus, cardioversion may be performed safely after anticoagulation has been achieved. Anticoagulant therapy should be continued for at least 1 mo after cardioversion to minimize the incidence of adverse thromboembolic events. It can be stopped as long as AF has not recurred.
- If the patient is hemodynamically stable, a rate-control strategy is typically pursued initially. Treatment options include the following:
    1. Diltiazem 0.25 mg/kg (maximum of 25 mg) given intravenously (IV) over 2 min followed by a second dose of 0.35 mg/kg (maximum of 25 mg) 15 min later if the rate is not slowed to <100 beats/min. May then follow with IV infusion 10 mg/hour (range, 5 to 15 mg/hour) to achieve a resting heart rate of <100 beats/min. Onset of action after IV administration is usually within 3 min, with peak effect most often occurring within 10 min. After the ventricular rate is slowed, the patient can be changed to oral diltiazem 60 to 90 mg q4-6h.
    2. Verapamil 2.5 to 5 mg IV initially, then 5 to 10 mg IV 10 min later if the rate is still not slowed to <100 beats/min. After the ventricular rate is slowed, the patient can be changed to oral verapamil 80 to 120 mg q6-8h. Main concern is hypotension with this medication.
    3. Esmolol, metoprolol, and atenolol are beta-blockers available in IV preparations that can be used in AF.
    4. Digoxin is not a potent atrioventricular nodal blocking agent, has a potential for toxicity and, therefore, cannot be relied on for acute control of the ventricular response, unless the patient is hypotensive or has a low left ventricular systolic function. When used, give 0.5 mg IV loading dose (slow), then 0.25 mg IV 6 hours later. A third dose may be needed after 6 to 8 hours; daily dose varies from 0.125 to 0.25 mg (decrease dosage in patients with renal insufficiency and elderly patients) depending on the heart rate and signs/symptoms of digoxin toxicity.

- All atrioventricular nodal blocking agents should be avoided in patients with Wolff-Parkinson-White syndrome and AF because they may increase the frequency of atrioventricular conduction through the accessory pathway. Procainamide is the preferred pharmacologic agent in these patients.
- In the acute setting, pharmacologic cardioversion is less commonly used than electrical cardioversion.

CHRONIC Rx

- For patients without symptomatic AF, rate-control strategy with calcium channel blockers, beta-blockers, or digoxin is a reasonable option. In patients with symptomatic AF or with difficult to control heart rate, attempt should be made to maintain sinus rhythm with antiarrhythmic agents. Options of antiarrhythmic agents include amiodarone, dofetilide, flecainide, propafenone, procainamide, or sotalol. The decision of which best strategy to follow should be best made in consultation with cardiology.
- The decision whether to pursue long-term anticoagulation with warfarin must be made in light of the patient's risk for a cardioembolic event vs. risk for a bleeding event. The CHADS2 scoring system is a well-validated model that estimates the risk for stroke in patients with AF based on clinical risk factors (congestive heart failure, hypertension (HTN), age ≥75 yr, and diabetes, which are 1 point each, or ischemic stroke and transient ischemic attack [TIA], which are 2 points each if present). Patients with a CHADS2 score of 0 are considered low risk, 1 to 2 are considered moderate risk, and ≥3 are considered high risk. The ACC/AHA recommends long-term anticoagulation with warfarin in all patients with a prior TIA or stroke (unless contraindicated) and in patients with more than one risk factor for thromboembolism that is not TIA/stroke.
- Anticoagulation with warfarin is generally not recommended in patients with CHADS2 score of zero. For patients with CHADS2 score of 1 who do not want to undergo anticoagulation, low-dose aspirin is an appropriate alternative in these patients.
- For patients in whom anticoagulation with warfarin is contraindicated, aspirin plus clopidogrel has been shown to be of similar benefit in reducing thromboembolic events as warfarin (Coumadin) with a similar bleeding risk.

DISPOSITION

Factors associated with maintenance of sinus rhythm after cardioversion include:

- Left atrium diameter <60 mm
- Absence of mitral valve disease
- Short duration of AF

REFERRAL

Refer to a cardiologist those patients in whom antiarrhythmic therapy or catheter-based/surgical intervention is being considered.

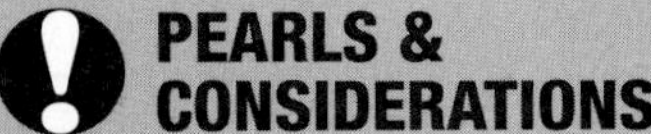

PEARLS & CONSIDERATIONS

COMMENTS

The American Academy of Family Physicians and the American College of Physicians provide the following recommendations for the management of newly detected AF:

- Rate control with chronic anticoagulation is the recommended strategy for the majority of asymptomatic patients with chronic AF. Rhythm control has not been shown to be superior to rate control (with chronic anticoagulation) in reducing morbidity and mortality, and may be inferior in some patient subgroups to rate control. Rhythm control is appropriate when based on other special considerations, such as patient symptoms, exercise tolerance, and patient preference.
- Patients with AF should receive chronic anticoagulation with adjusted-dose warfarin, unless they are at low risk for stroke as stated earlier or have specific contraindications to the use of warfarin (thrombocytopenia, recent trauma or surgery, alcoholism).
- For patients with AF, the following drugs are recommended for their demonstrated efficacy in rate control during exercise and while at rest: atenolol, metoprolol, diltiazem, and verapamil (drugs listed alphabetically by class). Digoxin is effective only for rate control at rest and, therefore, should be used only as a second-line agent for rate control in AF.
- For patients who elect to undergo acute cardioversion to achieve sinus rhythm in AF, both direct-current cardioversion and pharmacologic conversion are appropriate options in an otherwise healthy patient.
- Both transesophageal echocardiography with short-term prior anticoagulation followed by early acute cardioversion (in absence of intracardiac thrombus) with postcardioversion anticoagulation vs. delayed cardioversion with preanticoagulation and postanticoagulation are appropriate management strategies for patients who elect to undergo cardioversion.

EBM EVIDENCE

There is evidence for similar mortality and cardiovascular morbidity in older asymptomatic patients with chronic AF treated with either a rate-controlling therapy or rhythm-controlling therapy.

- Five randomized controlled trials have found similar mortality rates between asymptomatic patients with rate-controlled vs. rhythm control chronic AF.[1]

Warfarin is effective for both the primary and secondary prevention of ischemic stroke and TIA in patients with chronic AF. General recommendations are as follows:

- In people with persistent or intermittent AF with a CHADS2 score of ≥2, anticoagulation with an oral vitamin K antagonist, such as warfarin, is recommended (target international normalized ratio, 2.5; range, 2.0 to 3.0).[2]
- In people with persistent or intermittent AF with a CHADS2 score of 1, anticoagulation with either an oral vitamin K antagonist, such as warfarin, or aspirin therapy is recommended.[2]

Primary prevention of stroke in patients at high risk:

- Adjusted-dose warfarin is significantly more effective than placebo in reducing the risk for stroke in people at high risk for stroke.[3]
- Adjusted-dose warfarin is significantly more effective than aspirin in reducing the risk for ischemic stroke or systemic embolism in patients at high risk for stroke.[3]

Primary prevention of stroke in patients at lower risk:

- Adjusted-dose oral anticoagulation is significantly more effective than placebo in reducing overall stroke, disabling or fatal stroke, and death in patients with nonvalvular AF and no prior history of strokes or TIA. The combined end point of all stroke, myocardial infarction, or vascular death was also reduced. The observed rates of intracranial and extracranial hemorrhage were not significantly increased, but confidence intervals were wide.[4]

Secondary prevention of stroke:

- Anticoagulants are significantly more effective than antiplatelet therapy in reducing all vascular events and also recurrent stroke in patients with nonrheumatic AF and a history of minor ischemic stroke or TIA. The risk for major extracranial bleeds, but not intracranial bleeds, appears to be increased in patients on anticoagulants.[5]
- Dronedarone is a newer, recently approved agent that is pharmacologically similar to amiodarone with less toxicity. A recent multicenter, double blind trial showed that dronedarone was more effective than placebo in maintaining normal sinus rhythm[6] and in reducing cardiovascular events.[7] However, dronedarone is not indicated in patients with severe heart failure and left ventricular systolic dysfunction (ejection fraction <35%), because it was associated with increased early mortality related to the worsening of heart failure.[8]
- In patients with AF and congestive heart failure, a routine strategy of rhythm control does not reduce the rate of death from cardiovascular causes compared with a rate-control strategy.[9]

Evidence-Based References

1. Cadwallader K, Jankowski TA: Other than anticoagulation, what is the best therapy for those with AF? *J Fam Pract* 53:581, 2004.

2. Singer DE et al: Antithrombotic therapy in atrial fibrillation: the seventh ACCP conference on antithrombotic and thrombolytic therapy, *Chest* 126(3 Suppl):429S, 2004.

A

Diseases and Disorders

I

3. Lip GY, Edwards SJ: Stroke prevention with aspirin, warfarin and ximelagatran in patients with non-valvular atrial fibrillation: a systematic review and meta-analysis, *Thromb Res* 118:321, 2006.
4. Aguilar MI, Hart R: Oral anticoagulants for preventing stroke in patients with non-valvular atrial fibrillation and no previous history of stroke or transient ischemic attacks, *Cochrane Database Syst Rev* 3:CD001927, 2005.
5. Saxena R, Koudstaal PJ: Anticoagulants versus antiplatelet therapy for preventing stroke in patients with nonrheumatic atrial fibrillation and a history of stroke or transient ischemic attack, *Cochrane Database Syst Rev* 4:CD000187, 2004.
6. Singh BN et al: Dronedarone for maintenance of sinus rhythm in atrial fibrillation or flutter, *N Engl J Med* 357:987, 2007.
7. Hohnloser SH et al: Effect of dronedarone on cardiovascular events in atrial fibrillation, *N Engl J Med* 360:668, 2009.
8. Kober L et al: Increased mortality after dronedarone therapy for severe heart failure, *N Engl J Med* 358:2678, 2008.
9. Roy D et al: Rhythm control versus rate control for atrial fibrillation and heart failure. *N Engl J Med* 358:2667-2677, 2008.

SUGGESTED READINGS

Calkins H et al: HRS/EHRA/ECAS expert Consensus Statement on catheter and surgical ablation of atrial fibrillation: recommendations for personnel, policy, procedures and follow-up. A report of the Heart Rhythm Society (HRS) Task Force on catheter and surgical ablation of atrial fibrillation, *Heart Rhythm* 4(6):816-861, 2007 Epub 2007. Apr 30.

Hart RG et al: Meta-analysis: antithrombotic therapy to prevent stroke in patients who have non-valvular atrial fibrillation, *Ann Intern Med* 146:857, 2007.

Lip G, Tse H: Management of atrial fibrillation, *Lancet* 370:604, 2007.

Snow V et al: Management of newly detected atrial fibrillation: a clinical practice guideline from the Academy of Family Physicians and the American College of Physicians, *Ann Intern Med* 139:1009, 2003.

AUTHORS: **THOMAS J. EARL, M.D., FRED F. FERRI, M.D.,** and **WEN-CHIH WU, M.D.**

BASIC INFORMATION

DEFINITION

Atrial flutter is characterized by an ectopic atrial focus with rapid, regular atrial depolarizations caused by a macroreentrant circuit (usually in the right atrium), typically at a rate of 250 to 350 beats/min.

ICD-9CM CODES
427.32 Atrial flutter

EPIDEMIOLOGY & DEMOGRAPHICS

- Atrial flutter is the second most common atrial tachyarrhythmia after atrial fibrillation, with an estimated 200,000 new cases annually in the U.S.
- Atrial flutter is common during the first week after open-heart surgery.
- Atrial flutter is more common in men than women.
- Atrial flutter is typically seen in patients with underlying structural heart disease.

PHYSICAL FINDINGS & CLINICAL PRESENTATION

- Palpitations
- Dizziness, lightheadedness, syncope, or near syncope
- Angina
- Congestive heart failure
- Embolic phenomena from intracardiac thrombus

ETIOLOGY

- Rheumatic heart disease
- Congenital heart disease
- Left ventricular dysfunction
- Acute myocardial infarction (rarely)
- Thyrotoxicosis
- Pulmonary embolism
- Mitral valve disease
- Cardiac surgery
- Chronic obstructive pulmonary disease
- Obesity
- Pericarditis
- Atrial flutter can also occur spontaneously or as a result of organization of atrial fibrillation from antiarrhythmic therapy

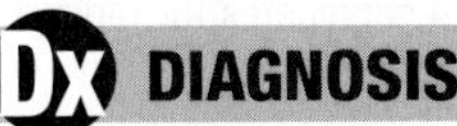

DIAGNOSIS

DIFFERENTIAL DIAGNOSIS

- Atrial fibrillation
- Paroxysmal atrial tachycardia

WORKUP

- ECG
- Laboratory evaluation

LABORATORY TESTS

- Thyroid function studies
- Serum electrolytes

IMAGING STUDIES

ECG (Fig. 1-33)

- Absence of P waves
- Regular, "sawtooth," or "F (flutter)" wave pattern in the isoelectric baseline, best seen in leads II, III, and AVF
- There is rarely 1:1 atrioventricular (AV) conduction in atrial flutter (unless preexcitation is present). Rather, AV conduction is usually in a 2:1, 3:1, or 4:1 fashion, with corresponding usual ventricular rates of 150, 100, or 75 beats/min, respectively (assuming an atrial rate of 300 beats/min)
- Echocardiography to evaluate for structural heart disease (ventricular size, thickness, and function, atrial size, and valve function)

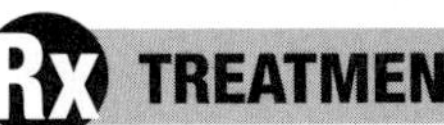

TREATMENT

NONPHARMACOLOGIC THERAPY

- Valsalva maneuver or carotid sinus massage usually slows the ventricular rate (increases grade of AV block) and may make flutter waves more evident. Adenosine may be similarly helpful.
- Direct current cardioversion is the treatment of choice for acute management of atrial flutter associated with hemodynamic instability or debilitating symptoms such as angina or congestive heart failure. Electrical cardioversion is typically successful at low energy levels (20 to 25 J). Sedation of a conscious patient is highly recommended before cardioversion is performed. The use of external defibrillators with biphasic waveforms decreases the amount of energy required for cardioversion and improves cardioversion success rate.
- Overdrive pacing in the atrium may also terminate atrial flutter. This method is especially useful in patients who have recently undergone cardiac surgery and still have temporary atrial pacing wires.
- Radiofrequency ablation to interrupt the atrial flutter is highly effective for patients with chronic or recurring atrial flutter and is generally considered first-line therapy in those with recurrent episodes of atrial flutter.

ACUTE GENERAL Rx

- Treatment choices are based on clinical circumstances. If the patient is unstable, proceed directly to electrical cardioversion.
- In the hemodynamically stable patient, proceed with rate control or rhythm control strategy.
- AV blocking agents such as calcium channel blockers, beta-blockers, or digitalis may all be used for rate control. Atrial flutter may spontaneously convert to normal sinus rhythm with this strategy.
- Ibutilide is the first-line medication for chemical cardioversion of atrial flutter in patients with normal systolic function and QT intervals.

CHRONIC Rx

- Fewer data exist to decide on the choice of rate control vs. rhythm control in patients with atrial flutter. There are several options to help maintain sinus rhythm after cardioversion of atrial flutter, such as dofetilide, amiodarone, flecainide, propafenone, or sotalol. The choice of antiarrhythmic therapy is, in part, dictated by the presence or absence of

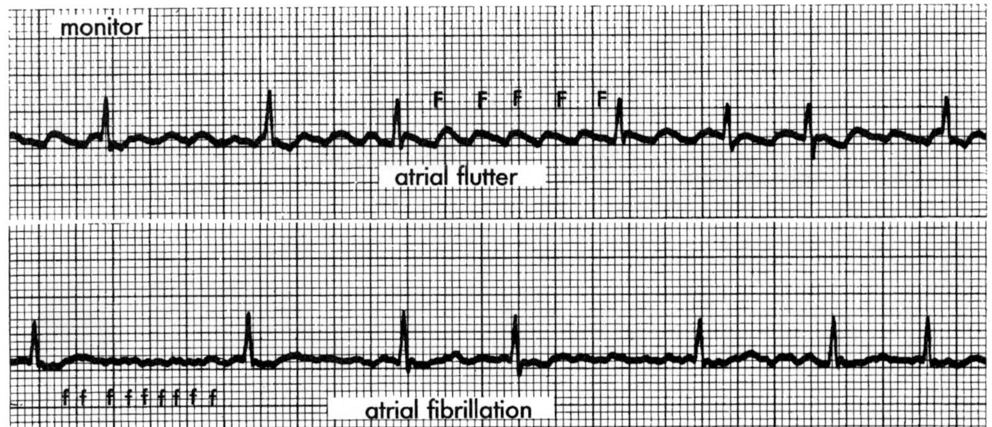

FIGURE 1-33 Atrial flutter and fibrillation. Notice the sawtooth waves with atrial flutter *(F)* and the irregular fibrillatory waves with atrial fibrillation *(f)*. (From Goldberger AL [ed]: *Clinical electrocardiography,* ed 5, St Louis, 1994, Mosby.)

underlying structural heart disease. In patients who have chronic atrial flutter, rate control (to rates as physiologic as possible) can be achieved using AV blocking agents, to prevent occurrence of tachycardia-mediated cardiomyopathy.

- Although data are much less convincing than in atrial fibrillation, current consensus is to treat atrial flutter similar to atrial fibrillation in terms of the risk for thromboembolic events and the need for anticoagulation. In this case, CHADS2 scoring system (see "Atrial Fibrillation") can be used to risk-stratify patients for their need to stay on long-term anticoagulation.

DISPOSITION

More than 85% of patients convert to regular sinus rhythm after cardioversion with as little as 25 to 50 J.

REFERRAL

Refer patients who are considered for rhythm control of atrial flutter to cardiologists, especially patients who are candidates for radiofrequency ablation.

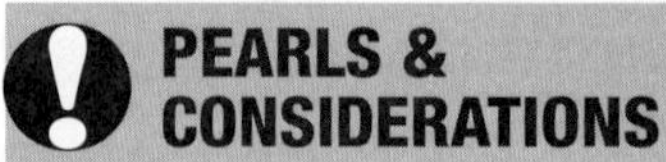

PEARLS & CONSIDERATIONS

COMMENTS

- Atrial flutter has a stroke risk at least as high as atrial fibrillation and carries a greater risk for subsequent development of atrial fibrillation than in the general population.
- Anticoagulation should be considered for all patients whose CHADS2 score is ≥ 2.
- Anticoagulation with warfarin is generally not recommended in patients with CHADS2 score of zero. For patients with CHADS2 score of 1 who do not want to undergo anticoagulation, low-dose aspirin is an appropriate alternative in these patients.

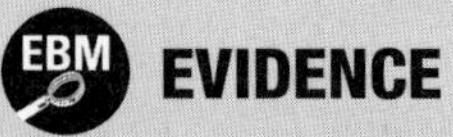

EVIDENCE

Please note: Complete text of EBM for this topic is available online.

SUGGESTED READINGS

Ghali WA et al: Atrial flutter and the risk of thromboembolism: a systematic review and meta-analysis, *Am J Med* 118(2):101-107, 2005.

Natale A et al: Prospective randomized comparison of antiarrhythmic therapy versus first-line radiofrequency ablation in patients with atrial flutter. *J Am Coll Cardiol* 35(7):1898-1904, 2007.

AUTHORS: **THOMAS J. EARL, M.D., FRED F. FERRI, M.D.,** and **WEN-CHIH WU, M.D.**

BASIC INFORMATION

DEFINITION

Atrial myxoma is a benign neoplasm of mesenchymal origin and is the most common primary tumor of the heart.

SYNONYMS

Cardiac myxoma

ICD-9CM CODES

212.7 Benign neoplasm, heart

EPIDEMIOLOGY & DEMOGRAPHICS

- Primary cardiac tumors are extremely rare, with an autopsy frequency of 0.001% to 0.03%. The most frequent cardiac tumors are metastases, occurring 30 times more frequently than primary tumors.
- Benign atrial myxomas account for 70% of all primary tumors of the heart. The remaining 30% are composed of a variety of benign and malignant tumors.
- 65% of sporadic cases occur in females.
- Average age of incidence of sporadic cases is 30 to 50 yr but can occur at any age.
- Average age of incidence of familial cases is 25 yr.

PHYSICAL FINDINGS & CLINICAL PRESENTATION

Patients with atrial myxomas characteristically present in one of three ways:

1. Atrioventricular valve obstruction (e.g., mitral or tricuspid valve): dyspnea, orthopnea, paroxysmal nocturnal dyspnea, edema, dizziness, syncope, elevated jugular venous pressure, widely split loud S2, secondary pulmonary hypertension, murmurs of regurgitation (holosystolic) or stenosis (rumbles), third heart sound "tumor plop," atrial fibrillation, and sudden death (rarely)
2. Systemic embolization: leading to cerebrovascular accidents, pulmonary embolism, paradoxical embolism
3. Constitutional symptoms: fever, weight loss, arthralgias, Raynaud's phenomenon

ETIOLOGY

- Most cases (90%) of atrial myxomas are sporadic with no known cause
- In the remaining 10% of cases, a familial pattern occurs having an autosomal-dominant transmission, known as the Carney complex or syndrome myxoma (cardiac and noncardiac myxomas, pigmented nevi, endocrine tumors, and schwannomas)

DIAGNOSIS

DIFFERENTIAL DIAGNOSIS

- Primary valvular diseases: mitral stenosis, mitral regurgitation, tricuspid stenosis, tricuspid regurgitation
- Pulmonary hypertension
- Endocarditis
- Vasculitis
- Atrial thrombus
- Pulmonary embolism
- Cerebrovascular accidents
- Collagen-vascular disease
- Carcinoid heart disease

WORKUP

A high index of suspicion is needed because the clinical manifestations are nonspecific and similar to many common cardiovascular and pulmonary diseases.

LABORATORY TESTS

Although not very specific, the following laboratory findings may be abnormal in patients with atrial myxomas:

- Complete blood count: anemia, polycythemia, thrombocytopenia may occur
- Erythrocyte sedimentation rate, C-reactive protein, and serum immunoglobulins are commonly elevated
- Electrocardiogram: left or right atrial enlargement, atrial fibrillation, premature ventricular depolarizations, or ventricular tachycardia

IMAGING STUDIES

- Echocardiography: initial test of choice in suspected cases of atrial myxoma
- Chest radiograph: altered cardiac contour and chamber enlargement
- Transesophageal echocardiography: may better define cardiac masses not clearly visualized by transthoracic echocardiography
- CT: often used for diagnosis; defines tumor extension and evaluates adjacent cardiac structures
- MRI: delineates size, shape, and tissue characteristics, helping distinguish thrombus from tumor
- Cardiac catheterization: will show neovascularization in 50% of the cases and may be required to rule out concomitant coronary artery disease in anticipation of surgical excision

TREATMENT

ACUTE GENERAL THERAPY

- Surgical excision is the treatment of choice
- Surgery should be done promptly because systemic embolization and/or sudden death can occur while waiting for the procedure

CHRONIC Rx

Postoperative arrhythmias and conduction abnormalities were present in 26% of patients and can be treated accordingly.

DISPOSITION

- Surgical results have reported a 95% survival rate after a follow-up of 3 yr.
- Careful follow-up is necessary because up to 5% of sporadic cases and 20% of familial cases of atrial myxoma may recur within the first 6 yr after surgery.
- Sudden death in untreated patients may occur in up to 15%, resulting from coronary or systemic embolization or obstruction of the mitral or tricuspid valve.

REFERRAL

- Consultation with a cardiologist is recommended.
- Once the presence of cardiac tumor is confirmed, consultation with a cardiovascular surgeon is needed for prompt surgical excision.

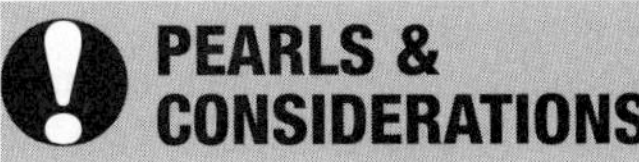

PEARLS & CONSIDERATIONS

- Approximately two thirds of patients present with cardiovascular symptoms, specifically dyspnea, often suggestive of valvular obstruction.
- Nearly one third of patients have evidence of systemic embolization.

COMMENTS

Annual echocardiograms should be performed to monitor for recurrence of atrial myxomas after surgical excision.

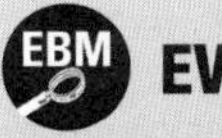

EVIDENCE

Major investigations are lacking given the low incidence of cardiac tumors. Most of the current data have been obtained through clinical series and case reports. 83% of myxomas arise from the left atrium and 13% from the right atrium. Biatrial or ventricular myxomas are rare. Once the diagnosis is made, excision is the treatment of choice, with a surgical mortality rate less than 5%.[1] The recurrence rate can be up to 5%, which merits close follow-up in the future.[2,3]

Evidence-Based References

1. Kuon E et al: The challenge presented by right atrial myxoma, *Herz* 29:702, 2004.
2. Keeling IM et al: Cardiac myxomas: 24 years of experience in 49 patients, *Eur J Cardiothorac Surg* 22:971, 2002.
3. Selkane C et al: Changing management of cardiac myxoma based on a series of 40 cases with long-term follow-up, *Ann Thorac Surg* 76:1935, 2003.

SUGGESTED READINGS

Ipek G et al: Surgical management of cardiac myxoma, *J Card Surg* 20(3):300, 2005.

Swartz MF et al: Atrial myxomas: pathologic types, tumor location, and presenting symptoms, *J Card Surg* 21(4):435, 2006.

Vasquez A, et al: Atrial myxomas in the elderly: a case report and review of the literature, *Am J Geriatr Cardiol* 13(1):39-44, 2004.

AUTHORS: **ROBERTO PACHECO, M.D., FRED F. FERRI, M.D.,** and **WEN-CHIH WU, M.D.**

Atrial Septal Defect (PTG)

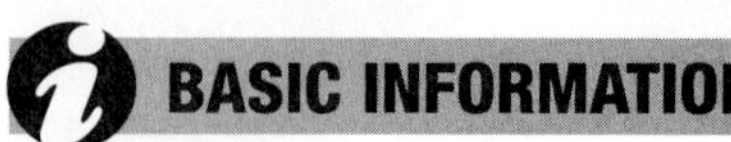

BASIC INFORMATION

DEFINITION

Atrial septal defect (ASD) is an abnormal opening in the atrial septum that allows blood flow between the atria. It should be distinguished from patent foramen ovale, which is a persistent patency of the flaplike communication in which the septum primum covering the fossa ovalis overlaps the superior limbic band of the septum secundum. There are several forms (Fig. 1-34):

- Ostium primum: This type of ASD represents a deficiency of the endocardial cushion contribution to the atrial septum. It usually involves the atrioventricular valves.
- Ostium secundum: This is the most common form; it represents a deficiency of the septum primum or a septum secundum, or both. This defect most often occurs in the region of the fossa ovalis.
- Sinus venosus defect: This defect is located at the junction of the right atrium and superior vena cava, and is not a "true ASD" as it does not involve the true atrial septum. In a sinus venusus defect, the wall separating the pulmonary veins and the right atrium is deficient, causing a left-to-right shunt. Most commonly this defect involves the right upper pulmonary vein, which is still connected to the left atrium, but the drainage is anomalous. Less commonly, the right lower pulmonary vein is involved.
- Coronary sinus septal defect (unroofed coronary sinus): This defect results when the wall separating the coronary sinus from the left atrium is deficient, causing a right-to-left shunt. This is not a "true ASD" because it is not a defect in the atrial septum. This defect is often associated with a persistent left superior vena cava.

SYNONYMS

ASD

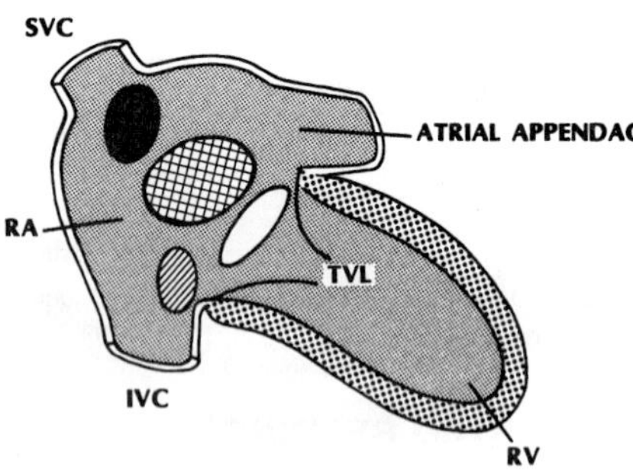

Sinus venosus defect
Secundum defect
Primum defect
Coronary sinus defect

FIGURE 1-34 Location of the four types of atrial septal defect. *IVC,* Inferior vena cava; *RA,* right atrium; *RV,* right ventricle; *SVC,* superior vena cava; *TVL,* tricuspid valve leaflet. (From Noble J [ed]: *Primary care medicine,* ed 2, St Louis, 1996, Mosby.)

ICD-9CM CODES
429.71 Atrial septal defect

EPIDEMIOLOGY & DEMOGRAPHICS

- 80% of cases of ASD involve persistence of ostium secundum
- Incidence is greater in female sex
- Accounts for 8% to 10% of congenital heart abnormalities

PHYSICAL FINDINGS & CLINICAL PRESENTATION

- Pansystolic murmur best heard at apex secondary to mitral regurgitation (ostium primum defect)
- Widely split S_2
- Visible and palpable pulmonary artery pulsations
- Ejection systolic flow murmur (pulmonary valve flow murmur)
- Diastolic rumble (atrioventricular valve flow murmur)
- Prominent right ventricular (RV) impulse
- Increased jugular venous pressure (with RV failure)
- Cyanosis and clubbing (severe cases)
- Exertional dyspnea
- Patients with small defects: generally asymptomatic

ETIOLOGY

Unknown

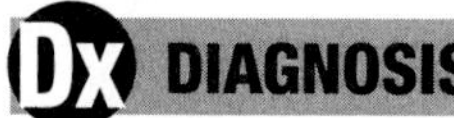

DIAGNOSIS

DIFFERENTIAL DIAGNOSIS

- Primary pulmonary hypertension
- Pulmonary stenosis
- Rheumatic heart disease
- Mitral valve prolapse
- Cor pulmonale

WORKUP

- ECG:
  - Ostium primum defect: left axis deviation, incomplete or total right bundle branch block, prolongation of PR interval
  - Sinus venous defect: left axis deviation, abnormal P axis
  - Ostium secundum defect: right axis deviation, incomplete or total right bundle branch block
- Chest x-ray examination
- Echocardiography
- Cardiac catheterization
- Cardiac magnetic resonance imaging (MRI), CT, or both

IMAGING STUDIES

- Chest x-ray examination: cardiomegaly, enlargement of right atrium and right ventricle, increased pulmonary vascularity, small aortic knob
- Echocardiography with saline bubble contrast and Doppler flow studies: may demonstrate the size of the defect, the direction of shunting, presence of anomalous pulmonary return (in sinus venosus ASD), right heart volume overload, and pulmonary artery pressures; transesophageal echocardiography is much more sensitive than transthoracic echocardiography in identifying sinus venous defects and is preferred by some for the initial diagnostic evaluation
- Cardiac catheterization: not usually a diagnostic necessity; is useful unless the coronaries need to be assessed before surgery
- Cardiac MRI and CT: may be useful if echo is not diagnostic; MRI is gold standard for assessing RV size and function, and it can determine whether the right-sided chambers are, in fact, enlarged; it is also good to assess pulmonary venous return; cardiac CT can offer similar information

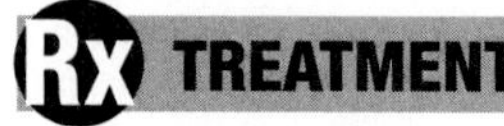

TREATMENT

NONPHARMACOLOGIC THERAPY

- Symptomatic patients should avoid strenuous activity.
- Patients with small shunts (<10 mm) without pulmonary artery hypertension and normal RV size are generally asymptomatic and require no medical therapy. Routine assessment of these patients includes symptoms, arrhythmias, and embolic events. A repeat echocardiogram should be obtained every 2 to 3 years to assess RV size and function, and pulmonary pressure.

GENERAL Rx

- Children and infants: Closure of ASD before age 10 yr is indicated if pulmonary to systemic flow ratio is $>1.5:1$.
- Adults: Closure is indicated in symptomatic patients with shunts $>1.5:1$.
- Closure of an ASD either percutaneously or surgically is indicated with size ≥ 10 mm and signs of RV enlargement with or without symptoms.
- Closure of an ASD, either percutaneously or surgically, is reasonable in the presence of:
  - Paradoxical embolism (class 2a indication)
  - Documented orthodeoxia-platypnea (class 2a indication)
- Percutaneous catheter device closure is advocated in patients with secundum ASDs (with proper size and location), with $\sim 95\%$ success rate. A combination of low-dose aspirin and clopidogrel is usually prescribed for 3 mo after the procedure to prevent thrombus formation.
- Surgical closure is indicated in all patients with ostium primum defect and sinus venosus defects.
- Closure should be avoided in patients with pulmonary hypertension with reversed shunting (Eisenmenger's syndrome) because of increased risk for right-heart failure (the ASD acts as a "pop-off" valve for the right heart) in patients with severe left ventricular dysfunction (the ASD functions as a "pop-off" valve for the systemic ventricle).

DISPOSITION

- Mortality rate is high in patients with significant ostium primum defect if left untreated.
- Patients with small shunts (<10 mm) have a normal life expectancy.
- Surgical mortality rate varies with the age of the patient and the presence of cardiac failure and pulmonary artery hypertension; mortality rate ranges from <1% in young patients (<45 yr) to >10% in elderly patients with presence of heart failure and pulmonary hypertension.
- Preoperative atrial fibrillation is a risk factor for immediate postoperative and long-term atrial fibrillation. Patients with a repaired ASD still have an increased risk for development of atrial fibrillation that directly correlates with the age at which the defect is corrected (later correction = greater risk).
    - After closure, anticipated benefits include improved functional status and exercise capacity, improved survival after closure as a child, improved quality of life, prevention of right-heart failure, and prevention of pulmonary arterial hypertension.
    - Potential mid- to long-term complications after ASD closure in adulthood include tachyarrhythmias (atrial fibrillation or atrial flutter), bradyarrhythmias (sinus node dysfunction or heart block), stroke (greater risk in older patients), residual ASDs (small usually close spontaneously, large may be because of patch dehiscence), right-heart failure or pulmonary artery hypertension (risk is inversely related to age at time of closure), left atrioventricular valve regurgitation or subaortic stenosis (usually in patients with primum ASDs), device migration/erosion, and pulmonary venous congestion (uncommon).
    - Pregnancy is usually well tolerated in women with ASDs. Follow-up is recommended because of small risk for paradoxical embolus, stroke, arrhythmia, and heart failure. If known, ASDs should be closed before pregnancy if indicated. The sole contraindication to pregnancy in women with an ASD is severe pulmonary arterial hypertension.
- In regard to infective endocarditis prophylaxis:
    - Prophylaxis is not indicated for isolated secundum ASDs.
    - Prophylaxis is not indicated for patients ≥6 mo after successful surgical or percutaneous repair of an ASD.
    - Prophylaxis is reasonable for a completely repaired ASD with prosthetic material or device whether placed by surgery or by catheter intervention, during the first 6 mo after the procedure.
    - Prophylaxis is reasonable for repaired ASDs with residual defects at the site or adjacent to the site of a prosthetic patch or prosthetic device (both of which inhibit endothelialization).

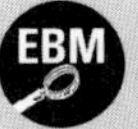

EVIDENCE

One randomized controlled trial of 400 patients >40 yr assessed whether surgical treatment of secundum ASD improves long-term outcome. After a median follow-up of 7.3 years, surgical closure was associated with lower rates of mortality and cardiovascular events.[1]

Evidence-Based Reference

1. Attie F et al: Surgical treatment for secundum atrial septal defects in patients >40 years old. A randomized clinical trial, *J Am Coll Cardiol* 38:2035, 2001.

SUGGESTED READINGS

Krasuski RA: When and how to fix a “hole in the heart”: approach to ASD and PFO, *Cleve Clin J Med* 74:137, 2007.

Warnes CA et al: ACC/AHA 2008. guidelines for the management of adults with congenital heart disease: a report of the American College of Cardiology/American Heart Association Task Force on Practice Guidelines (Writing Committee to Develop Guidelines for the Management of Adults With Congenital Heart Disease), *J Am Coll Cardiol* 52: e143-e263, 2008.

Webb G, Gatzoulis MA: Atrial septal defects in the adult: recent progress and overview, *Circulation* 114:1645-1653, 2006.

AUTHORS: **SCOTT COHEN, M.D., FRED F. FERRI, M.D.,** and **WEN-CHIH WU, M.D.**

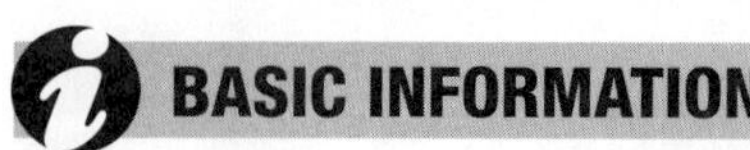

BASIC INFORMATION

DEFINITION

Attention deficit hyperactivity disorder (ADHD) is a chronic disorder of attention/concentration and/or hyperactivity/impulsivity. Symptoms must be present in early childhood, last at least 6 mo, and cause functional impairment in multiple settings.

SYNONYMS

Hyperactivity, attention deficit disorder (ADD)

ICD-9CM CODES
ICD-9: 314.XX
ICD-10: F90.X

EPIDEMIOLOGY & DEMOGRAPHICS

PEAK INCIDENCE: Diagnosis is usually first made in school-aged children (6 to 9 yr).

PREVALENCE: 3% to 9% of school-aged children and 2% to 5% of adults

PREDOMINANT SEX: Among children, male predominance with ratio of 3:1 to 9:1. Among adults, ratio is closer to 1:1 (sex difference may reflect referral bias).

PREDOMINANT AGE: Some symptoms must occur before age 7 yr. Symptoms (especially hyperactivity) tend to diminish with age. More than 70% continue to meet criteria in adolescence, and an estimated 40% to 65% have some symptoms in adulthood.

GENETICS: Strong polygenetic component. First-degree relatives of ADHD patients have 5 times greater risk of ADHD relative to controls. Studies suggest potential involvement of several genes, including those associated with dopamine metabolism and transmission.

RISK FACTORS: Possible environmental and epidemiologic risk factors include in utero tobacco/drug exposure or hypoxia, low birth weight, prematurity, pregnancy complications, lead exposure (though most children with elevated lead levels do not develop ADHD), family dysfunction, low socioeconomic status.

PHYSICAL FINDINGS & CLINICAL PRESENTATION

- Three types:
  1. Predominantly inattentive: difficulty organizing, planning, remembering, concentrating, starting/completing tasks; symptoms may not be present during preferred activities.
  2. Predominantly hyperactive-impulsive: edgy/restless, talkative, disruptive/intrusive, disinhibited, impatient.
  3. Combined.
- Usually diagnosed in elementary school when achievement is compromised and behavioral problems are not tolerated. Children with academic underproductivity, problems with peer and family relations, or discipline issues are often referred for evaluation.
- Adults with substance abuse or other addictions, multiple traffic violations, or frequent life failures should be screened.
- Up to 50% may have associated disorders such as psychiatric diagnoses (oppositional defiant disorder, conduct disorder, depression, anxiety), learning disabilities, substance abuse, and criminal behavior.

ETIOLOGY

Strongest evidence exists for genetic inheritance. Other theories include abnormal metabolism of brain catecholamines, structural brain abnormalities, and environmental factors (see earlier).

Dx DIAGNOSIS

DIFFERENTIAL DIAGNOSIS

- Medical: visual/hearing impairment, seizure disorder, head injury, sleep disorder, medication interactions, mental retardation, developmental delay, thyroid abnormalities, lead toxicity.
- Psychiatric: depression, bipolar disorder, anxiety, obsessive-compulsive disorder, conduct disorder, posttraumatic stress disorder, substance abuse, antisocial personality disorder, Tourette syndrome, tics.
- Psychosocial: mismatch of learning environment with ability, family dysfunction, abuse/neglect.

WORKUP

- Clinical interview should include assessment of symptoms and impact on work/school and relationships; developmental history; personal and family psychiatric history, including substance abuse; social history, including family dysfunction; medical history.
- Physical examination should be performed to investigate medical causes for symptoms, coexisting conditions, and contraindications to treatment.
- Many patients will not display symptoms during an office visit and may underreport or overreport symptoms. Therefore information from collateral sources (parents, partners, teachers) is crucial to diagnosis.
- Self-rating scales and standardized symptom-specific questionnaires from collateral sources can help diagnose and assess response to treatment.
- Laboratory or imaging studies should be undertaken only if indicated by history or physical examination.
- Ancillary testing (e.g., IQ/achievement testing, language evaluation, and mental health assessment) may be indicated based on clinical findings and may require referral.

Rx TREATMENT

NONPHARMACOLOGIC THERAPY

- Data comparing the efficacy of behavioral or educational therapy versus pharmacologic management are limited. Prevailing opinion favors a multimodal approach in which nonpharmacologic therapies can be used to target comorbid conditions or behaviors that have not responded to medication.
- Educational interventions are recommended, particularly in the setting of learning disabilities. Children with AD/HD are entitled to reasonable educational accommodations under a 504 Plan or the Individuals with Disabilities Education Act.
- Behavioral interventions (e.g., goal setting and rewards systems) show short-term efficacy and are endorsed by most national organizations (e.g., American Academy of Pediatrics, American Medical Association). Time management and organizational skills appear useful.
- Psychotherapy (cognitive behavioral, group, social skills, and parent training) may be beneficial, particularly with coexisting psychiatric disease.
- Many support and advocacy groups provide education and other resources (e.g., Children and Adolescents with ADHD, National ADD Association, American Academy of Child and Adolescent Psychiatry).

ACUTE GENERAL Rx

- Most studies on treatment of ADHD are performed in children; limited data available on adults.
- Mainstay of treatment is drug therapy, particularly stimulants. Second-line therapies include antidepressants and alpha-agonists.
- Stimulants:
  1. Release or block uptake of dopamine and norepinephrine.
  2. Include short- and long-acting methylphenidate and dextroamphetamine/amphetamine combinations.
  3. Do not cause euphoria or lead to addiction when taken as directed.
  4. Improve cognition, inattention, impulsiveness/hyperactivity, and driving skills. Limited impact on academic performance, learning, and emotional problems.
  5. Side effects are mild, reversible, and dose dependent, including anorexia, weight loss, sleep disturbances, increased heart rate and blood pressure, nervousness/irritability, headache, onset or worsening of motor tics, reduction of growth velocity (but not adult height). Do not worsen seizures in patients on adequate anticonvulsant therapy. Rebound of symptoms can occur with withdrawal of medication.
  6. All equally effective; however, not all patients improve with stimulants. Patients who do not respond well to one stimulant may respond to another.
- Atomoxetine (Strattera):
  1. Selective norepinephrine reuptake inhibitor.
  2. Efficacy and safety of long-term use has not been studied. Reports of behavioral abnormalities and increased suicidality in children.
  3. Side effects: gastrointestinal upset, sleep disturbance, decreased appetite, dizziness, sexual side effects in men.
  4. Monitor liver function because of reports of severe liver injury in adults and children.

- Antidepressants (bupropion, imipramine, nortriptyline):
    1. May be useful in patients with coexisting psychiatric disorders.
    2. Studies comparing efficacy versus stimulants are inconclusive.
    3. Side effects: arrhythmias, anticholinergic effects, lowering of seizure threshold.
- Use of medications, particularly stimulants (which are monitored under the Controlled Substance Act), requires frequent monitoring.
- Stimulants have been associated with cardiovascular events and death. Patients should be carefully evaluated for cardiovascular disease before beginning therapy and be periodically monitored, including blood pressure checks, while they are treated.

DISPOSITION

- Although symptoms may change over time, for many patients ADHD represents a chronic condition that requires lifelong management.
- Patients are at higher risk for academic underachievement, lower socioeconomic status, work and relationship difficulties, high-risk behavior, and psychiatric comorbidities.

REFERRAL

- Diagnosis complicated by difficult-to-treat comorbid psychiatric conditions, developmental disorders, or mental retardation
- Lack of adequate response to stimulants/atomoxetine

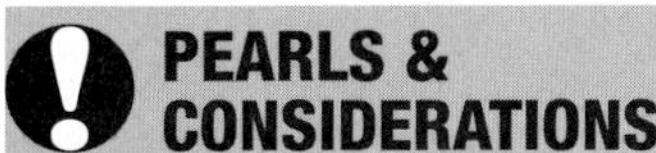

PEARLS & CONSIDERATIONS

The World Health Organization's Adult Self-Report Scale (ASRS) v1.1 has good sensitivity and adaptability to the primary care setting.

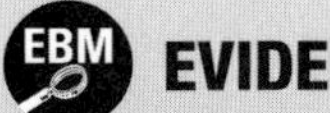

EVIDENCE

Please note: Complete text of EBM for this topic is available online.

Key trials and commentary:

The extant literature does not provide definite answers pertaining to whether stimulant treatment increases, decreases, or does not affect the risk for subsequent substance use disorders in youths with attention deficit hyperactivity disorder (ADHD). This study examined the association between stimulant treatment in childhood and adolescence and subsequent substance use disorders (alcohol, drug, and nicotine) into the young adult years. This study revealed no evidence that stimulant treatment increases or decreases the risk for subsequent substance use disorders in children and adolescents with ADHD when they reach young adulthood.

Despite several previous studies to the contrary, the concern that stimulant use in ADHD promotes risk for substance use disorders is a persistent worry. The basic understanding has been that properly treating ADHD mitigates the risk for substance use that is naturally higher among those with ADHD. This study is further evidence of this tenet. The authors gathered data on a large number of males with ADHD and reviewed previous exposure to stimulants. Figure 1 in the original article includes the Kaplan-Meier curves for substance use as an outcome stratified by previous exposure to stimulant medications, which leads to no significant differences. In general, the risks of abuse do seem to be mitigated by proper ADHD treatment, even if at a young age. The authors had, in past years, promoted that stimulant treatment imparted a reduced risk; there is a need to find further data coordinating these two perspectives.

It should be remembered that this study is focused on males only.[1] Ⓐ

In another study response to atomoxetine, a nonstimulant norepinephrine-specific reuptake inhibitor, was compared with the effect of osmotic-release oral methylphenidate, a long-acting methylphenidate preparation, in patients with ADHD.

This study showed that response was significantly greater with osmotically released methylphenidate than with atomoxetine. One-third of patients who received methylphenidate followed by atomoxetine responded better to one or the other, suggesting that there may be preferential responders.

This report provides data about atomoxetine, a norepinephrine transporter-blocking agent that is indicated and widely used for ADHD. It is a large, randomized placebo-controlled study that compares doses of a form of methylphenidate (MPH, "Concerta") with atomoxetine and with placebo. Furthermore, it uses a crossover assessment for those who responded to MPH. The study demonstrates that MPH has the highest effect on ADHD outcome measures with atomoxetine slightly less efficacious, but greater than placebo. The study also provides data to support the concept that some ADHD patients will respond to specific medications—the idea being that atomoxetine might be the right medication for some patients, or that it, at least, should be considered as a second-line medication in MPH failure. But the clinician should remember that, after MPH, there are several different classes to switch to, including stimulants of different mechanism (e.g., Dexedrine following methylphenidate) or different neurotransmitter systems altogether. In fact, another study, using the same rating scale as outcome measure, found that an extended release formulation of guanfacine (an alpha-2 agonist that is preferential to alpha-2 agonist receptors in the prefrontal cortex) led to significant improvement in ADHD subscales as well. Stimulant medications are the primary mainstay of treatment for ADHD, but there is a growing list of stimulants and other efficacious medications to keep in the armamentarium.[2] Ⓐ

A separate trial sought to investigate the effect of melatonin treatment on sleep, behavior, cognition, and quality of life in children with ADHD and chronic sleep onset insomnia.

It revealed that melatonin advanced circadian rhythms of sleep-wake and endogenous melatonin and enhanced total time asleep in children with ADHD and chronic sleep onset insomnia; however, no effect was found on problem behavior, cognitive performance, or quality of life.

Although not listed as a diagnostic criterion for ADHD, sleep problems are not uncommon in children with ADHD. Parents describe their ADHD child as a restless or fretful sleeper, often having trouble falling asleep and staying asleep. Some clinicians propose that many of the behavior problems associated with ADHD are attributed to sleep problems. Not infrequently, sleep improves with the appropriate dosing of stimulant medication or with the prescription of atomoxetine, and if sleep problems persist, a low dose of an α-adrenergic agent is often added.

This article investigates the use of melatonin in stimulant-free children with diagnosed ADHD and chronic sleep insomnia. The results of this well-controlled, double-blind, placebo study demonstrated that sleep onset was advanced and total sleep time was increased, but there was no change in the behavior problems, cognitive performance, or quality of life of these ADHD children. Thus, the stimulants and the nonstimulants remain the first-line pharmacologic treatment for children with ADHD. If sleep problems persist, melatonin may be added without significant side effects. So, sleep is a problem for many children with ADHD, but it is not *the* problem.[3] Ⓐ

The primary objective of another trial was to determine if the abuse liability of methylphenidate is governed by formulation differences that affect rates of drug delivery.

Although requiring epidemiological confirmation, the results suggest that OROS methylphenidate, with its characteristic slow ascending plasma concentration profile, may have lower abuse potential. This conclusion is reflected by lower subjective responses during early hours as compared with the IR formulation with its rapid drug delivery and accompanying greater subjective effects.

The large numbers of young people placed on stimulants for treatment of ADHD and the potential of these medications being abused underlines the importance of this study. Finding safer ways of formulating medications and finding ADHD medications with less abuse potential would help to reduce the growing controversy about how useful these medications are and whether as reported in the literature they can actually lower substance abuse when used appropriately with patients who are properly diagnosed. The problem of diversion and misuse of these medications initially often for the stated goal of performance enhancement but then leading to recreational use, abuse, and dependence in others is being widely reported and is of great concern, especially among high school and college students. The use of longer-acting preparations of methylphenidate is a promising strategy, and this study found they had lower abuse potential than those that have shorter-acting properties. The need for epidemiological studies in this is very important. The objectivity of some researchers in this area of research, who receive large support from the pharmaceutical industry, has also been called into question and may have the unfortunate consequence of frightening families who follow this data, and who have seen their children benefit from these stimulant medications.[4] Ⓐ

Evidence-Based References

1. Biederman J et al: Stimulant therapy and risk for subsequent substance use disorders in male adults with ADHD: a naturalistic controlled 10-year follow-up study, *Am J Psychiatry* 165:597-603, 2008. Commentary by A. Mack, M.D. Ⓐ
2. Newcorn JH et al: Atomoxetine and osmotically released methylphenidate for the treatment of attention deficit hyperactivity disorder: acute comparison and differential response, *Am J Psychiatry* 165:721-730, 2008. Commentary by A. Mack, M.D. Ⓐ
3. Van der Heijden KB et al: Effect of melatonin on sleep, behavior, and cognition in ADHD and chronic sleep-onset insomnia, *J Am Acad Child Adolesc Psychiatry* 46:233-241, 2007. Commentary by R.M. Sarles, M.D. Ⓐ
4. Parasrampuria DA et al: Do formulation differences alter abuse liability of methylphenidate? A placebo-controlled, randomized, double-blind, crossover study in recreational drug users, *J Clin Psychopharmacol* 27:459-467, 2007. Commentary by R. Frances, M.D. Ⓐ

SUGGESTED READINGS

American Academy of Pediatrics/American Heart Association clarification of statement on cardiovascular evaluation and monitoring of children and adolescents with heart disease receiving medications for ADHD: May 16, 2008. *J Dev Behav Pediatr* 29(4): 335, 2008.

Babcock T, Ornstein CS: Comorbidity and its impact in adult patients with attention-deficit/hyperactivity disorder; a primary care perspective, *Postgrad Med* 121(3):73-82, 2009.

Dopheide JA, Pliszka SR: Attention-deficit/hyperactivity disorder: an update, *Pharmacotherapy* 29(6):656-679, 2009.

Rader R et al: Current strategies in the diagnosis and treatment of childhood attention-deficit/hyperactivity disorder, *Am Fam Physician* 79(8):657-665, 2009.

AUTHOR: **MITCHELL D. FELDMAN, M.D., M.PHIL.**

BASIC INFORMATION

DEFINITION

Autism spectrum disorders encompass a spectrum of developmental disorders characterized by impairment in several behavioral domains. There is usually impairment in the development of language, communication, and reciprocal social interaction, together with a restricted behavioral repertoire. Onset is typically before age 3 yr.

SYNONYMS

Autism
Early infantile autism
Childhood autism
Kanner's autism
Pervasive developmental disorder

ICD-9CM CODES
F84.0 Autistic disorder

DSM-IV-TR CODES
299.00 Autistic disorder
299.80 Asperger's disorder
299.80 Pervasive developmental disorder NOS

EPIDEMIOLOGY & DEMOGRAPHICS

INCIDENCE (IN U.S.): 3 to 6/1000 of autism spectrum disorders (2 to 5/10,000 if restricted to autism alone)
PREVALENCE: 1/166 to 1/250
PREDOMINANT SEX: Male:female ratio of 2.1 to 6.5:1.0
PREDOMINANT AGE: Lifelong
PEAK INCIDENCE: Before age 3 yr
GENETICS:
- Autism is highly heritable.
- Defined and de novo mutations account for 10% to 20% of autism spectrum disorder cases. Active research into common biologic mechanisms underlying autism spectrum disorders (including defective synaptic function) has identified chromosomal abnormalities in multiple genetic loci, including glutamate-related genes.
- 2% to 8% risk rate for sibling of affected individual.
- 60% to 92% concordance for classic autism in monozygotic twins and 0% to 10% for dizygotic pairs.

PHYSICAL FINDINGS & CLINICAL PRESENTATION

- Common triad of impairment in social interactions, impaired and atypical verbal and nonverbal communication, and repetitive and usual behavior or play
- Marked impairment in the understanding and use of both verbal and nonverbal communication (likely underlies the profound impairment in social interaction)
- Stereotypic behavior or language
- Sensory overload and avoidance of novel stimuli

ETIOLOGY

- Majority of cases are not associated with a medical condition
- Significant increase in comorbid seizure disorder (25%) and developmental delay (45% to 60%)
- Autism is sometimes associated with other neurologic conditions (e.g., encephalitis, tuberous sclerosis, phenylketonuria [PKU], fragile X syndrome), suggesting that it may result from nonspecific neuronal injury

Dx DIAGNOSIS

DIFFERENTIAL DIAGNOSIS

- Rett's syndrome: autism spectrum disorder; occurs in females individual; characterized by head growth deceleration, loss of previously acquired motor skills, and incoordination
- Childhood disintegration disorder: normal development until age 2 yr, followed by regression
- Childhood-onset schizophrenia: follows period of normal development
- Asperger's syndrome: lacks the language developmental abnormalities of autism
- Isolated symptoms of autism: when occurring in isolation, defined as disorders (i.e., selective mutism, expressive language disorder, mixed receptive-expressive language disorder, or stereotypic movement disorder)

WORKUP

- Rule out underlying medical condition.
- Administer age-appropriate diagnostic instruments based on questionnaires and observation noting scales. Validated autism spectrum disorder–specific screening tools are available for children age $\geq$18 mo (e.g., Modified Checklist for Autism in Toddlers) and are being developed for younger children. General developmental screening tools are currently used in children $<$18 mo.

LABORATORY TESTS

- PKU screen (usually done at birth in the U.S.)
- Lead exposure screening
- Audiology testing for young children with autism spectrum disorders; school-based hearing screening may be sufficient in older children with autism spectrum disorders and without significant language or learning deficits
- Karyotype and DNA testing for fragile X in both boys and girls (carrier girls may exhibit mild symptoms)

IMAGING STUDIES

- EEG to diagnose coexisting seizure disorder if seizure is suspected or if language regression is present
- Brain MRI if tuberous sclerosis is suspected

Rx TREATMENT

NONPHARMACOLOGIC THERAPY

- A consistent behavioral training program in both the home and school environments
- A number of programs are currently being used; many are based on applied behavioral analysis (ABA)
- An educational program focused on language and social development
- A highly structured environment
- Education for families and teachers; the Autism Speaks™ website may be helpful in this regard: http://www.autismspeaks.org/about_us.php

ACUTE GENERAL Rx

- Obsessive or ritualistic behaviors: selective serotonin reuptake inhibitors (SSRIs), atypical antipsychotics, valproic acid
- Aggression, irritability, self-injury: atypical antipsychotic agents (e.g., risperidone), α-agonists, anticonvulsant mood stabilizers, SSRIs, beta-blockers
- Hyperactivity, impulsivity, inattention: stimulants, α-agonists, atypical antipsychotics
- Anxiety: SSRIs, buspirone, mirtazapine
- Depression: SSRIs, mirtazapine

CHRONIC Rx

- Extended use of medications used for acute management
- Pharmacotherapy is palliative, not curative

DISPOSITION

- Most children will require some degree of assistance as adults.
- Children with Asperger's syndrome may have a very good outcome despite ongoing symptoms.
- Poorer outcomes are associated with a lack of joint attention by 4 yr, a lack of functional speech by 5 yr, mental retardation, seizures, comorbid medical or psychiatric syndromes, and severe autistic symptoms.
- Better outcomes are associated with early identification and treatment, and regular inclusion in settings with typically developing peers.

REFERRAL

Assistance may be needed in diagnosis (geneticist, pediatric neurologist, developmental pediatrician), management (speech language pathologist, occupational therapist), parental teaching (mental health provider), or intervention with the school system.

PEARLS & CONSIDERATIONS

- There appears to be no relation between childhood vaccination and the development of autism.
- University of California Davis M.I.N.D. Institute is devoted to the study of autism (http://www.ucdmc.ucdavis.edu/mindinstitute).

 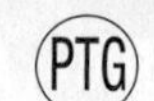

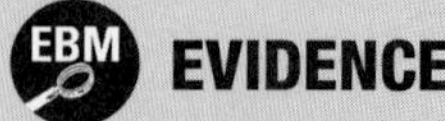

EVIDENCE

Please note: Complete text of EBM for this topic is available online.

Key trials and commentary:

There is increasing evidence that fatty acid deficiencies or imbalances may contribute to childhood neurodevelopmental disorders. The results of this study provide preliminary evidence that omega-3 fatty acids may be an effective treatment for children with autism.

Articles by Amminger et al and Nemets et al both reflect a flurry of activity in the literature regarding various vitamins, minerals, and supplements (notably omega-3 fatty acids) for the treatment of ADHD, depression, dyslexia, and autistic spectrum disorders. Of all of the various supplements, omega-3 fatty acids appear to offer some beneficial results in some studies, although the data are not strong or consistent. Clinicians need to pay attention to this emerging literature, but it would be premature to jump on this bandwagon overenthusiastically at this time.[1] A

Evidence-Based Reference

1. Amminger GP et al: Omega-3 fatty acids supplementation in children with autism: a double-blind randomized, placebo-controlled pilot study, *Biol Psychiatry* 61:551-553, 2007. Commentary by R.M. Sarles, M.D. A

SUGGESTED READINGS

Johnson CP et al, for the Council on Children with Disabilities: Identification and evaluation of children with autism spectrum disorders, *Pediatrics* 120(5):1183-1215, 2007.

Rapin I, Tuchman RF: Autism: definition, neurobiology, screening, diagnosis. *Pediatr Clin North Am* 55(5): 1129-1146, viii, 2008. Review.

Zwaigenbaum L et al: Clinical assessment and management of toddlers with suspected autism spectrum disorder: insights from studies of high-risk infants. *Pediatrics* 123(5):1383-1391, 2009. Review.

AUTHOR: **MITCHELL D. FELDMAN, M.D., M.PHIL.**

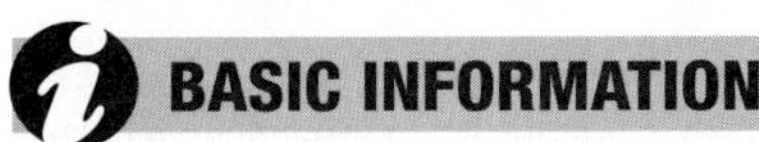

BASIC INFORMATION

DEFINITION

Babesiosis is a tick-transmitted protozoan disease of animals, caused by intraerythrocytic parasites of the genus *Babesia.* Humans are incidentally infected, resulting in a nonspecific febrile illness. The disease can be severe in immunocompromised hosts.

ICD-9CM CODES
088.82 Babesiosis

EPIDEMIOLOGY & DEMOGRAPHICS

INCIDENCE (IN U.S.): Unknown
PREVALENCE (IN U.S.):

- In areas of high endemicity, seropositivity ranging from 9% (Rhode Island) to 21% (Connecticut)
- Highest number of reported cases in New York

PREDOMINANT SEX: Males (most likely through increased exposure to vectors during recreational or occupational activities)
PREDOMINANT AGE: Severity apparently increasing with age >40 yr
PEAK INCIDENCE: Spring and summer months, May through September
GENETICS: None known
CONGENITAL INFECTION: At least one case of probable vertical transmission
NEONATAL INFECTION: At least two cases of perinatal transmission
BLOOD TRANSFUSION: Many instances

PHYSICAL FINDINGS & CLINICAL PRESENTATION

- Incubation period 1 to 4 wk, or 6 to 9 wk in transfusion-associated disease
- Gradual onset of irregular fever, chills, diaphoresis, headache, myalgia, arthralgia, fatigue, and dark urine
- On physical examination: petechiae, frank or mild hepatosplenomegaly, and jaundice
- Infection with *B. divergens* (Europe) producing a more severe illness with a rapid onset of symptoms and increasing parasitemia progressing to massive intravascular hemolysis and renal failure

ETIOLOGY

- Vector: Deer tick, *Ixodes scapularis* (also known as *I. dammini*)
    1. Feeds on rodents during the spring and summer while in its larval and nymphal stages and on deer as an adult
    2. Requires a blood meal to mature to each stage, hence human infection
    3. During the warmer months in endemic areas, humans are readily infected while engaging in outdoor activities
- *B. microti* and *B. divergens* account for most human infections.
- In the U.S., cases caused by *B. microti* are acquired on offshore islands of the northeastern coast, including Nantucket Island, Cape Cod, and Martha's Vineyard in Massachusetts; Block Island in Rhode Island; and Long Island, Fire Island, and Shelter Island in New York; as well as the nearby mainland including Connecticut and New Jersey.
- Sporadic cases reported from California, Georgia, Maryland, Minnesota, Virginia, Wisconsin, and most recently the WA-1 strain from Washington State and the MO-1 strain from Missouri.
- *B. divergens* is implicated in human disease in Europe, where the disease remains rare and predominantly associated with asplenia.
- Majority of cases are asymptomatic.
- May be transmissible by transfusion, through platelets and erythrocytes.
- Mixed infections (*B. microti* and *Borrelia burgdorferi,* the causative agent of Lyme disease) are estimated to occur in 10% (Rhode Island and Connecticut) to 60% (New York) of cases.

Dx DIAGNOSIS

DIFFERENTIAL DIAGNOSIS

- Amebiasis
- Ehrlichiosis
- Hepatic abscess
- Leptospirosis
- Malaria
- Salmonellosis, including typhoid fever
- Acute viral hepatitis
- Hemorrhagic fevers

WORKUP

Should be suspected in any febrile patient living or traveling in an endemic area, irrespective of exposure history to ticks or tick bites, especially if asplenic

LABORATORY TESTS

- CBC to reveal mild to moderate pancytopenia
- Abnormally elevated serum chemistries, including creatinine, liver function profile, lactate dehydrogenase, and indirect and total bilirubin levels; hepatoglobin is low.
- Urinalysis to reveal proteinuria and hemoglobinuria
- Examination of Giemsa- or Wright-stained thin blood films for intraerythrocytic parasites
    1. In its classic, though infrequently seen, form a "tetrad" or "Maltese Cross" composed of four daughter cells attached by cytoplasmic strands is observed (Fig. 1-35).
    2. More commonly, smaller forms composed of a single chromatin dot are eccentrically located within bluish cytoplasm.
    3. Parasitized erythrocytes may be multiply infected but not enlarged.
- Diagnosis achieved serologically by indirect immunofluorescence assay (IFA) is specific for *B. microti.*
    1. Titer of ≥1:64 is indicative of seropositivity, whereas one ≥1:256 is considered diagnostic of acute infection.
    2. Assay is hampered by the inability to distinguish between exposed patients and those who are actively infected.
    3. Immunoglobulin M indirect immunofluorescent-antibody test may be highly sensitive and specific for diagnosis.
    4. Babesial DNA by polymerase chain reaction (PCR) has comparable sensitivity and specificity to microscopic analysis of thin blood smears.

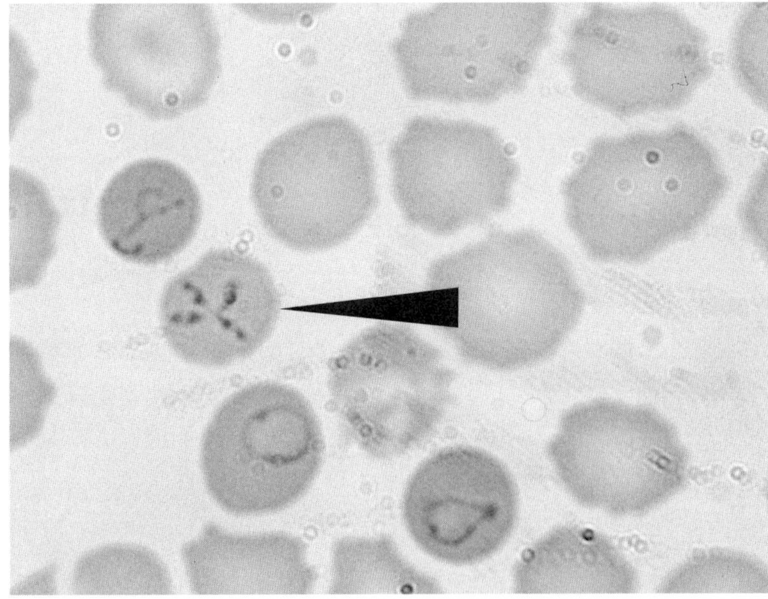

FIGURE 1-35 ***Babesia* spp.** Single and multiple intraerythrocytic parasites can be seen. The *arrow* marks a typical Maltese cross. (From Cohen J, Powderly WG: *Infectious Diseases,* ed 2, St Louis, 2004, Mosby.)

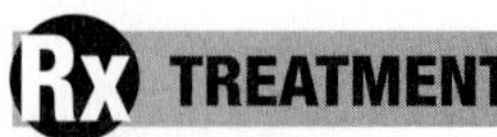

TREATMENT

NONPHARMACOLOGIC THERAPY

Supportive care with adequate hydration

ACUTE GENERAL Rx

- In patients with intact spleens: predominantly asymptomatic or if symptomatic, generally self-limited
- Therapy reserved for the severely ill patient, especially if asplenic, elderly, or immunosuppressed
- Combination of quinine sulfate 650 mg PO tid plus clindamycin 600 mg PO tid (1.2 g parenterally bid) taken for 7 to 10 days: effective but may not eliminate parasites
- Combination of atovaquone 750 mg every 12 hr and azithromycin 500 mg on day 1 and 250 mg per day thereafter for 7 days appears to be as effective as a regimen of clindamycin and quinine with fewer adverse reactions
- Exchange transfusions in addition to antimicrobial therapy: successful treatment for severe infections in asplenic patients associated with high levels of *B. microti* or *B. divergens* parasitemia

DISPOSITION

Prognosis is usually good and fatal outcomes are rare.

REFERRAL

- For prompt consultation with an infectious disease specialist if the diagnosis is acutely suspected, especially in the asplenic, elderly, or immunocompromised patient
- For hospitalization for the severely ill patient who may require exchange transfusions in addition to antibiotic therapy

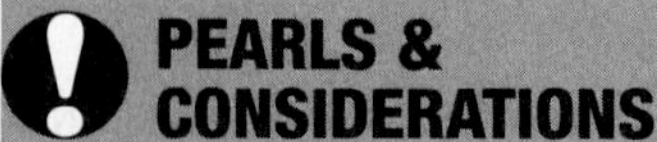

PEARLS & CONSIDERATIONS

COMMENTS

- Prevention of babesiosis in asplenic or immunocompromised hosts is best achieved by avoidance of areas where the vector is endemic, especially during the months of May through September.
- If residence or travel in endemic areas is unavoidable, advise patients to perform daily cutaneous self-examination, wear light-colored clothing (to facilitate removal of ticks), tuck pants into socks, and apply tick repellent (diethyltoluamide and dimethylphthalate) to skin or clothing.
- Advise a daily inspection for ticks in family pets (e.g., cats and dogs).
- Infection with *B. divergens,* especially in the asplenic patient, is often fatal.
- Concurrent babesiosis and Lyme disease has been documented—check for combined infection in severely ill patients.
- Clindamycin and quinine has been successfully used to treat babesiosis during the third trimester of pregnancy without incurring apparent adverse effect on the fetus.

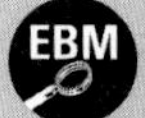

EVIDENCE

Combination therapy with clindamycin and quinine is as effective as the atovaquone and azithromycin combination. Adverse effects from medication may be more common with clindamycin and quinine. Both combinations are effective in eradicating babesiosis parasites at 3 mo after the treatment course.[1] B

Silent infection may persist for months or years when left untreated. Treatment of babesiosis with clindamycin and quinine may reduce the duration of parasitemia.[2] B

Evidence-Based References

1. Krause PJ et al: Atovaquone and azithromycin for the treatment of babesiosis, *N Engl J Med* 343:1454, 2000. B

2. Krause PJ et al: Persistent parasitemia after acute babesiosis, *N Engl J Med* 339:160, 1998. B

SUGGESTED READINGS

Cable RG, Leiby DA: Risk and prevention of transfusion-transmitted babesiosis and other tick-borne diseases, *Curr Opin Hematol* 10(6):405, 2003.

Gelfand JA, Callahan MV: Babesiosis: an update on epidemiology and treatment, *Curr Infect Dis Rep* 5(1):53, 2003.

Gubernot DM et al: Babesia infection through blood transfusions: reports received by the US FDA, 1997-2007, *Clin Infect Dis* 48:25, 2009.

Hunfeld KP et al: Babesiosis: recent insights into an ancient disease, *Int J Parasitol* 38(11):1219-1237, 2008.

Krause PJ: Babesiosis diagnosis and treatment, *Vector Borne Zoonotic Dis* 3(1):45, 2003.

Vannier E et al: Human babesiosis, *Infect Dis Clin North Am* 22:469, 2008.

Wormser GP et al: The clinical assessment, treatment, and prevention of Lyme disease, human granulocytic anaplasmosis, and babesiosis: clinical practice guidelines by the IDSA, *Clin Infect Dis* 43:1089, 2006.

AUTHORS: **PATRICIA CRISTOFARO, M.D., GLENN G. FORT, M.D., M.P.H.,** and **DENNIS J. MIKOLICH, M.D.**

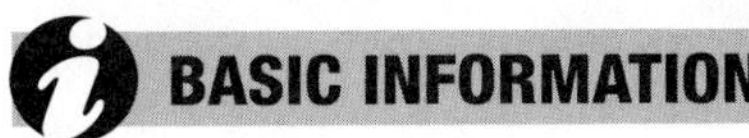

BASIC INFORMATION

DEFINITION

Baker's cyst is a fluid-filled popliteal bursa located along the medial border of the popliteal fossa.

SYNONYMS

Popliteal cyst

ICD-9CM CODES

727.51 Baker's cyst (knee)

EPIDEMIOLOGY & DEMOGRAPHICS

- Occurs at all ages.
- Incidence is unknown.
- Between 2% and 6% of all patients believed to have clinical deep venous thrombosis (DVT) have symptomatic Baker's cysts.
- Approximately 5% of MRIs of the knees reveal popliteal cysts.

PHYSICAL FINDINGS & CLINICAL PRESENTATION

- Pain in the popliteal space
- Knee swelling
- Leg edema
- Prominence of the popliteal fossa
- Decreased range of motion of the knee
- Locking of the knee
- Foucher's sign: The cyst becomes hard with knee extension and soft with knee flexion.
- Neuropathic lancinating pains radiating from the knee down the back of the leg
- Presence of associated DVT

ETIOLOGY

- Believed to represent fluid distention of the bursal sac separating the semimembranous tendon from the medial head of the gastrocnemius.
- May represent a true cyst but more often results from the posterior herniation of a tense knee effusion. Thus a Baker's cyst usually denotes increased intraarticular pressure from underlying joint disease.
- In children, Baker's cysts are believed to result from trauma and irritation of the knee.
- In adults, Baker's cysts are usually associated with pathologic changes of the knee joint, such as the following:
    - Rheumatoid arthritis (RA)
    - Osteoarthritis of the knee
    - Meniscal tears
    - Patellofemoral chondromalacia
    - Fracture
    - Gout
    - Pseudogout
    - Infection (tuberculosis)

Dx DIAGNOSIS

Baker's cyst frequently mimics DVT and is sometimes referred to as *pseudothrombophlebitis syndrome.*

DIFFERENTIAL DIAGNOSIS

- DVT
- Popliteal aneurysm
- Abscess
- Tumor
- Lymphadenopathy
- Varicosity
- Ganglion

WORKUP

Anyone suspected of having a popliteal cyst should undergo imaging studies to exclude other causes.

LABORATORY TESTS

Blood tests are not specific in the diagnosis of Baker's cysts.

IMAGING STUDIES

- Plain radiographs (AP and lateral views) may show calcification in a solid tumor or in the posterior meniscal area.
- Ultrasound is safe, portable, cost effective, and excludes other clinically important causes of popliteal fossa pathology, including DVT.
- MRI of the knee identifies coexisting joint pathology (e.g., osteoarthritis, torn meniscus).

Rx TREATMENT

NONPHARMACOLOGIC THERAPY

- Rest
- Strenuous activity avoidance
- Knee immobilization necessary in some cases

ACUTE GENERAL Rx

- Nonsteroidal antiinflammatory drugs, ibuprofen 400 to 800 mg PO tid or naproxen 250 to 500 mg PO bid, can be used to treat Baker's cyst caused by RA, gout, and pseudogout.
- Intraarticular injection or injection of the cyst with corticosteroids, triamcinolone acetonide 40 mg, is sometimes tried.

CHRONIC Rx

- The majority of Baker's cysts are successfully treated conservatively.
- Surgical procedures addressing the underlying cause include:
    1. Arthroscopic surgery to remove loose cartilaginous fragment
    2. Partial or total meniscectomy
    3. Open excision of the cyst (Fig. 1-36)

DISPOSITION

- Baker's cyst may spontaneously resolve without treatment.
- Complications of Baker's cysts include:
    1. Rupture
    2. DVT
    3. Nerve impingement

REFERRAL

Rheumatology or orthopedics if surgery is contemplated

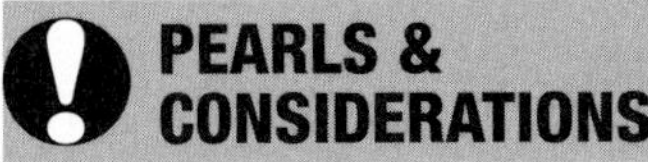

PEARLS & CONSIDERATIONS

- Popliteal cysts were first described in 1840 by Adams, but it is Baker's writing about disease of the knee joint in 1877 that gave rise to the eponym Baker's cyst.
- A Baker's cyst may serve as a protective mechanism for the knee. Intrinsic intraarticular disorders cause joint effusion. The knee effusion is displaced into the Baker's cyst, thus reducing potentially destructive pressure in the joint space.

COMMENTS

Baker's cyst and DVT can coexist. It is imperative to exclude the diagnosis of DVT before discharging the patient.

SUGGESTED READINGS

Handy JR: Popliteal cysts in adults: a review, *Semin Arthritis Rheum* 31(2):108, 2001.

Torreggiani WC et al: The imaging spectrum of Baker's (popliteal) cysts, *Clin Radiol* 57(8):681, 2002.

AUTHORS: **RICHARD REGNANTE, M.D.,** and **IMMAD SADIQ, M.D.**

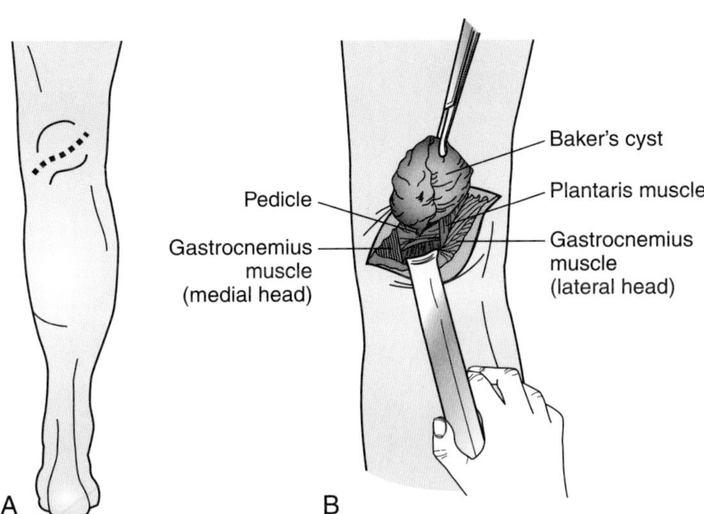

FIGURE 1-36 Removal of midline Baker's cyst. A, Skin incision. **B,** After being exposed, pedicle is clamped, ligated, divided, and inverted. (Redrawn and modified from Meyerding HW, Van Demark GE: Posterior hernia of the knee, *JAMA* 122:858, 1943.)

Balanitis (PTG)

BASIC INFORMATION

DEFINITION

Balanitis is an inflammation of the superficial tissues of the penile head.

ICD-9CM CODES
112.2 Balanitis

EPIDEMIOLOGY & DEMOGRAPHICS

INCIDENCE (IN U.S.): Unknown
PREVALENCE (IN U.S.): Unknown
PREDOMINANT SEX: Exclusive to males
PEAK INCIDENCE: All ages, especially in sexually active men

PHYSICAL FINDINGS & CLINICAL PRESENTATION

- Itching and tenderness
- Pain, dysuria, and local edema
- Rarely, ulceration and lymph node enlargement
- Severe ulcerations leading to superimposed bacterial infections
- Inability to void: unusual, but a more distressing and serious complication

ETIOLOGY

- Poor hygiene, causing erosion of tissue with erythema and promoting growth of *Candida albicans*
- Sexual contact, urinary catheters, and trauma
- Allergic reactions to condoms or medications

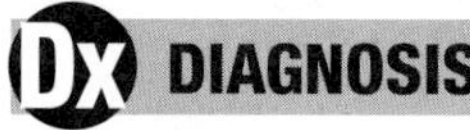

DIAGNOSIS

DIFFERENTIAL DIAGNOSIS

- Leukoplakia
- Reiter's syndrome
- Lichen planus
- Balanitis xerotica obliterans
- Psoriasis
- Carcinoma of the penis
- Erythroplasia of Queyrat
- Nodular scabies

WORKUP

- Sexually active males: assessment for evidence of other sexually transmitted diseases
- Biopsy if lesions do not heal

LABORATORY TESTS

- VDRL
- Serum glucose
- Wet mount
- KOH prep
- Microbial culture

Rx TREATMENT

NONPHARMACOLOGIC THERAPY

- Maintenance of meticulous hygiene
- Retraction and bathing of prepuce several times a day
- Warm sitz baths to ease edema and erythema
- Consideration of circumcision, especially when symptoms are severe or recurrent
- With Foley catheters, strict catheter care strongly advised

ACUTE GENERAL Rx

- Fluconazole 150 mg PO × 1 or itraconazole 200 mg PO bid × 1 day
- Clotrimazole 1% cream applied topically twice daily to affected areas
- Bacitracin or Neosporin ointment applied topically 4 times daily
- With more severe bacterial superinfection: cephalexin 500 mg PO qid
- Topical corticosteroids added 4 times daily if dermatitis severe
- Patients with suspected urinary tract infections: trimethoprim-sulfa DS twice daily or ciprofloxacin 500 mg PO bid after obtaining appropriate cultures

DISPOSITION

Balanitis is often self-limited and usually responds to conservative therapy; if it does not improve, consider circinate balanitis (Reiter's syndrome), nodular scabies, and primary skin lesions including skin carcinoma.

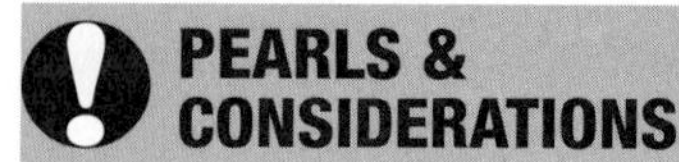

PEARLS & CONSIDERATIONS

Don't forget about nodular scabies involving the prepubic area—examine the region carefully for burrows and tracks of *Sarcoptes scabiei.*

REFERRAL

- For surgical evaluation for circumcision if symptoms are recurrent, especially if phimosis or meatitis occurs (NOTE Severe phimosis with an inability to void may require prompt slit drainage.)
- For biopsy to rule out other diagnosis such as premalignant or malignant lesions if lesions are not healing

SUGGESTED READINGS

Buechner SA: Common skin disorders of the penis, *BJU Int* 90(5):498, 2002.

Bunker CB: Topics in penile dermatology, *Clin Exp Dermatol* 26(6):469, 2001.

Lisboa C et al: Noninfectious balanitis in patients attending a sexually transmitted disease clinic, *Int J Dermato* 48(4):445-446, 2009.

Pandher BS et al: Treatment of balanitis xerotica obliterans with topical tacrolimus, *J Urol* 170(3):923, 2003.

Thiruchelvan M et al: Emergency dorsal slit for balanitis with retention, *J R Soc Med* 97(4):206, 2004.

AUTHORS: **GLENN G. FORT, M.D., M.P.H.,** and **DENNIS J. MIKOLICH, M.D.**

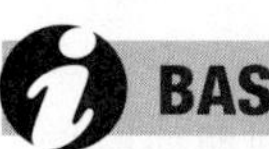

BASIC INFORMATION

DEFINITION

Barrett's esophagus occurs when the squamocolumnar junction is displaced proximal to the gastroesophageal junction, and the squamous lining of the lower esophagus is replaced by metaplastic, intestinalized columnar epithelium. The condition is associated with an increased risk (~0.5%/yr) for development of adenocarcinoma of the esophagus.

SYNONYMS

Intestinal metaplasia of lower esophagus

ICD-9CM CODES
530.85 Barrett's esophagus

EPIDEMIOLOGY & DEMOGRAPHICS

- Male:female ratio of 4:1
- Mean age of onset is 40 yr, with a mean age range of diagnosis of 55 to 60 yr
- Occurs more frequently in white and Hispanic individuals than in African American individuals, with a ratio of 10 to 20:1
- Mean prevalence of 5% to 15% in patients undergoing endoscopy (EGD) for symptoms of gastroesophageal reflux disease (GERD)
- Obesity may be an independent risk factor
- Prevalence rate in asymptomatic cohorts ranges from 5% to 25%

CLINICAL PRESENTATION

SYMPTOMS:

- Chronic heartburn
- Dysphagia with solid food
- May be an incidental finding on EGD in patients without reflux symptoms
- Less frequent: chest pain, hematemesis, melena
- Patients may be asymptomatic

PHYSICAL FINDINGS:

- Nonspecific; can be completely normal
- Epigastric tenderness on palpation

ETIOLOGY

- Metaplasia is thought to result from reepithelialization of esophageal tissue injured as a result of chronic GERD.
- Patients with Barrett's esophagus tend to have more severe esophageal motility disturbances (decreased lower esophageal sphincter pressure, ineffective peristalsis) and greater esophageal acid exposure on 24-hour pH monitoring.
- Intraesophageal bile reflux may also play a role in the pathogenesis.
- Familial clustering of GERD and Barrett's esophagus suggests a genetic predisposition, but no gene has yet been identified.
- Progression from metaplasia to carcinoma is associated with changes in gene structure and expression.

Dx DIAGNOSIS

DIFFERENTIAL DIAGNOSIS

- GERD, uncomplicated
- Erosive esophagitis
- Gastritis
- Peptic ulcer disease
- Angina
- Malignancy
- Stricture or Schatzki's ring

WORKUP

- EGD with biopsy is necessary for diagnosis.
- Wireless esophageal capsule endoscopy may detect Barrett's, but with a lower sensitivity and specificity than EGD.
- Imaging studies are nonspecific and insensitive for the diagnosis.
- Diagnosis requires the presence of intestinal metaplasia in columnar epithelium proximal to the gastroesophageal junction. Longer segment Barrett's esophagus is more readily diagnosed.
- Intestinal metaplasia of the gastric cardia is not Barrett's esophagus and does not have the same risk for malignancy.
- The Practice Parameters Committee of the American College of Gastroenterology (ACG) has suggested that the highest yield for Barrett's esophagus screening is in older (age >50 yr) white men with longstanding heartburn. General population screening is not currently recommended. The benefit of screening in high-risk populations is not established. Although screening has become standard of practice in some communities, the effectiveness of screening using current techniques is controversial because it may not improve mortality rates from adenocarcinoma or be cost-effective.
- Screening for *Helicobacter pylori* infection in patients with GERD and Barrett's esophagus is not recommended.

Rx TREATMENT

Goal is to control GERD symptoms and maintain healed mucosa.

NONPHARMACOLOGIC THERAPY

Lifestyle modifications; elevating head of bed; avoiding chocolate, tobacco, caffeine, mints, and certain drugs (see "Gastroesophageal Reflux Disease")

ACUTE GENERAL Rx

- Proton pump inhibitors are the most effective treatment. Chronic acid suppression is often necessary to control symptoms and promote healing.
- Adequate control of GERD symptoms in patients with Barrett's esophagus may not completely control intraesophageal acid exposure. Some studies suggest that normalization of intraesophageal acid exposure may either lead to regression of Barrett's esophagus or reduce the risk for dysplasia.
- If patient is asymptomatic and incidentally found to have Barrett's esophagus, medication use may be considered.

CHRONIC Rx

- Thermal ablation techniques, photodynamic therapy, and endoscopic mucosal resection are all possible approaches to the treatment of patients with Barrett's esophagus and high-grade dysplasia, either in conjunction with aggressive surveillance or as an alternate to surgery in poor operative candidates. Radiofrequency ablation and cryotherapy are newer techniques currently being evaluated. All these options run the risk for residual intestinal metaplasia or buried glands. Because only a minority of patients with Barrett's esophagus progress to high-grade dysplasia or carcinoma, these techniques cannot be currently recommended in patients with Barrett's esophagus without dysplasia. In recent trials in patients with dysplastic Barrett's esophagus, radiofrequency ablation was associated with high rate of complete eradication of both dysplasia and intestinal metaplasia, and reduced risk for disease progression. Additional studies will need to show that radiofrequency ablation and cryotherapy reduce or eliminate the need for surveillance endoscopy and/or the risk for cancer, and that they are cost-effective in the long term.
- Antireflux surgery may be considered for management of GERD and associated sequelae. Patients should still have endoscopic surveillance of their esophagus. Surgical resection is offered for multifocal high-grade dysplasia or carcinoma.

DISPOSITION

- Overall, increased risk for adenocarcinoma of the esophagus in patients with Barrett's esophagus may be as high as 100 times that of the general population.
- Corresponds to 500 cancers per yr per 100,000 persons with Barrett's esophagus.
- The lifetime cancer risk for patients with nondysplastic Barrett's esophagus is ~5% to 8%.
- Frequency of monitoring is controversial; no studies have proved that surveillance increases life expectancy.
- American College of Gastroenterology recommends that patients with Barrett's esophagus undergo surveillance EGD and systematic four-quadrant biopsy at intervals determined by the presence and grade of dysplasia. All mucosal abnormalities should undergo biopsy. Patients who have had two consecutive EGDs showing no dysplasia should have follow-up every 3 yr. Patients with low-grade dysplasia should have extensive mucosal sampling within 6 mo and follow-up every year. Patients with high-grade dysplasia should have expert confirmation and extensive mucosal sampling. High-grade dysplasia with visible mucosal irregularities should be removed by endoscopic mucosal resection. Consider intensive surveillance every 3 mo for patients with fo-

cal high-grade dysplasia. Patients with multifocal high-grade dysplasia or carcinoma should be considered for resection or ablation if not an operative candidate.
- Patients should be treated aggressively for GERD before surveillance.

REFERRAL

- Consider EGD with biopsy in patients (particularly white men >50 yr old) with chronic GERD who have not had previous EGD.
- Refer for surveillance those with biopsy-proven Barrett's esophagus.
- For those with high-grade dysplasia, refer for intensive surveillance or esophageal resection; ablative therapy may be considered as part of a research protocol or if patient is not an operative candidate.

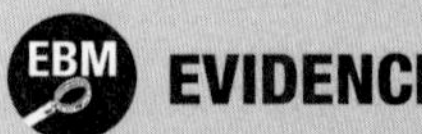

EVIDENCE

Please note: Complete text of EBM for this topic is available online.

Key trials and commentary:

This study sought to determine the efficacy of endoscopic argon plasma coagulation (APC) for ablation of Barrett's esophagus. APC has been used to ablate Barrett's esophagus. However, the long-term outcome of this treatment is unknown. This study reports 5-year results from a randomized trial of APC vs. surveillance for Barrett's esophagus in patients who had undergone a fundoplication for the treatment of gastroesophageal reflux. Regression of Barrett's esophagus after fundoplication is more likely, and greater in extent, in patients who undergo ablation with APC. In most patients treated with APC the neosquamous mucosa remains stable at up to 5-year follow-up. The development of high-grade dysplasia only occurred in patients who were not treated with APC.

The authors present a long-term follow-up of their trial in which they randomize patients who have Barrett's esophagus and fundoplication for continued surveillance vs. APC ablation of the Barrett's esophagus. The median follow-up for this long-term result is 68 months, and 69% of the patients were available at follow-up at this time. The follow-up was equally distributed between the surveillance and APC group. At 5-year follow-up, 70% of the APC patients had continued regression of at least 95% of their metaplastic mucosa compared with only 25% in the surveillance group. Both groups did have shortening in the length of their Barrett's, suggesting that fundoplication without APC ablation is effective in inducing some regression of Barrett's. The additional regression of Barrett's with APC was double the effect, with 40% of patients having completely microscopic progression of Barrett's esophagus compared with only 20% in the surveillance group. Of note, only two patients developed high-grade dysplasia at long-term follow-up, and these are both in the surveillance group. These data provide promising results for the regression of Barrett's esophagus following fundoplication and augmentation of the regression with the addition of APC treatment of the Barrett's mucosa. These results should be corroborated in a larger trial.[1] Ⓐ

Evidence-Based Reference

1. Bright T et al: Randomized trial of argon plasma coagulation versus endoscopic surveillance for Barrett esophagus after antireflux surgery: late results, *Ann Surg* 246:1016-1020, 2007. Commentary by M.T. Hawn, M.D. Ⓐ

SUGGESTED READINGS

Bonino JA, Sharma P: Barrett's esophagus, *Curr Opin Gastroenterol* 22:406, 2006.

Dellon ES, Shaheen NJ: Does screening for Barrett's esophagus and adenocarcinoma of the esophagus prolong survival? *J Clin Oncol* 23:4478, 2005.

Shaheen NJ: Advances in Barrett's esophagus and esophageal adenocarcinoma, *Gastroenterology* 128:1554, 2005.

Shaheen NJ, Richter JE: Barrett's esophagus, *Lancet* 373:850-861, 2009.

Shaheen NJ et al: Radiofrequency ablation in Barrett's esophagus with dysplasia, *N Engl J Med* 360:2277-2288, 2009.

Sharma P: Barrett's esophagus, *N Engl J Med* 361:26, 2009.

Sharma P et al: A critical review of the diagnosis and management of Barrett's esophagus: the AGA Chicago workshop, *Gastroenterology* 127:310, 2004.

Spechler SJ, Barr B: Review article: screening and surveillance of Barrett's esophagus: what is a cost-effective framework? *Aliment Pharmacol Ther* 19(Suppl 1):49, 2004.

Wang KK, Sampliner RE: Updated guidelines 2008. for the diagnosis, surveillance, and therapy of Barrett's esophagus, *Am J Gastroenterol* 103:788, 2008.

AUTHOR: **HARLAN G. RICH, M.D.**

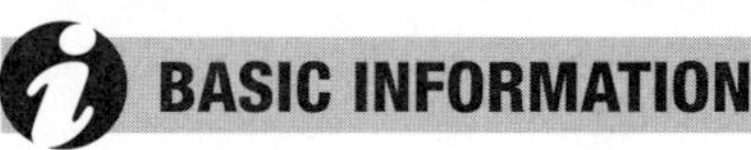

BASIC INFORMATION

DEFINITION

Bartter's syndrome is a group of renal tubular disorders characterized by metabolic alkalosis, hypokalemia, hyperplasia of the juxtaglomerular apparatus, hyperreninemic hyperaldosteronism, and hypercalciuria.

SYNONYMS

Hypokalemic alkalosis with hypercalciuria

ICD-9CM CODES

255.13 Bartter's Syndrome

EPIDEMIOLOGY & DEMOGRAPHICS

- Classic Bartter's syndrome can present with symptoms at 2 years of age or younger.
- Neonatal Bartter's syndrome can be diagnosed at birth.
- The true incidence in the U.S. is not known.
- Incidence is similar in males and in females.

CLINICAL PRESENTATION

- Neonatal Bartter's syndrome involves maternal polyhydramnios, frequent preterm delivery, fotal polyuria, and failure to thrive.
- Classic Bartter's syndrome may include a history of maternal polyhydramnios and premature delivery. The following features are characteristic:
  - Polyuria
  - Polydipsia
  - Hypokalemia
  - Metabolic alkalosis
  - Hypercalciuria
  - Plasma magnesium is normal or mildly reduced
  - Patients are normotensive
  - Patients do not have edema

ETIOLOGY

- Disorder of chloride reabsorption in the thick ascending loop of Henle.
- A couple of defects manifest the same phenotype.
- Tubular pathophysiology is identical to loop diuretic mechanism of action.

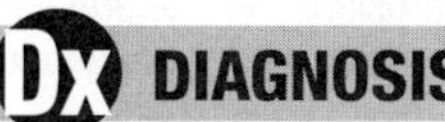

DIAGNOSIS

DIFFERENTIAL DIAGNOSIS

- Diuretic abuse
- Surreptitious vomiting
- Gitelman's syndrome
- Autosomal dominant hypocalcemia
- Hyperprostaglandin E syndrome

WORKUP

- Classic Bartter's syndrome is usually a diagnosis of exclusion.
- Vomiting associated with a low urine chloride and scarring of the dorsum of the hand and dental erosions suggests bulimia nervosa.
- Diuretic abuse can only be excluded by a urinary assay for diuretics.

LABORATORY TESTS

- Serum sodium, potassium, chloride, bicarbonate, calcium, magnesium, phosphorus.
- Urine calcium, chloride, assay for diuretics as above.
- Serum pH can be confirmed by performing ABG.

IMAGING STUDIES

- Renal ultrasonography may show nephrocalcinosis, hydronephrosis, and hydroureter in neonatal Bartter's syndrome.
- Classic signs of hypokalemia may be present on ECG.

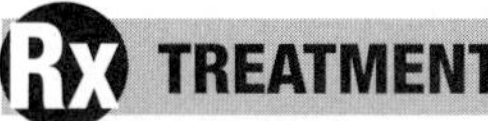

TREATMENT

NONPHARMACOLOGIC THERAPY

None

ACUTE GENERAL Rx

Neonatal Bartter's syndrome requires correction of electrolyte imbalance and volume depletion.

CHRONIC Rx

- Usual treatment includes oral potassium and magnesium supplementation, although achievement of normal serum potassium and magnesium levels is often difficult.
- Potassium-sparing diuretics such as spironolactone/amiloride have also been used effectively in the treatment of Bartter's.

REFERRAL

Consultation with nephrology facilitates diagnosis and management of this condition.

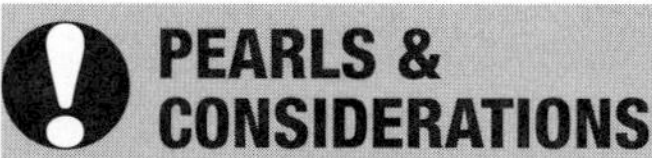

PEARLS & CONSIDERATIONS

COMMENTS

- Just as Bartter's looks like loop diuretic use from the point of view of laboratory testing, Gitelman's syndrome appears identical to thiazide use.
- High urine calcium is the best way to distinguish Bartter's from Gitelman's syndrome.
- Serum magnesium differences have been described but are likely to be low in both syndromes and are probably not useful in distinguishing these syndromes.

PREVENTION

None

PATIENT/FAMILY EDUCATION

- Foods with high potassium content should be emphasized in dietary education.
- Patients with Bartter's syndrome are more vulnerable to volume depletion due to potassium derangement during exercise and exposure.

SUGGESTED READINGS

Hebert SC: Bartter syndrome, *Curr Opin Nephrol Hypertens* 12(5):527, 2003.

Kurtz I: Molecular pathogenesis of Bartter's and Gitelman's syndromes, *Kidney Int* 54:1396, 1998.

AUTHOR: **JONATHAN BURNS, M.A., M.D.**

Basal Cell Carcinoma 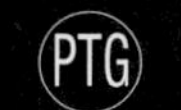

 BASIC INFORMATION

DEFINITION

Basal cell carcinoma (BCC) is a malignant tumor of the skin arising from basal cells of the lower epidermis and adnexal structures. It may be classified as one of six types: nodular, superficial, pigmented, cystic, sclerosing or morpheaform, and nevoid. The most common type is nodular (21%); the least common is morpheaform (1%). A mixed pattern is present in approximately 40% of cases. BCC advances by direct expansion and destroys normal tissue.

SYNONYMS

BCC

ICD-9CM CODES
179.9 Basal cell carcinoma, site unspecified
173.3 Basal cell carcinoma, face
173.4 Basal cell carcinoma, neck, scalp
173.5 Basal cell carcinoma, trunk
173.6 Basal cell carcinoma of the limb
173.7 Basal cell carcinoma, lower limb

EPIDEMIOLOGY & DEMOGRAPHICS

- Most common cutaneous neoplasm
- 85% of cases appear on the head and neck region
- Most common site: nose (30%)
- Increased incidence with age >40 yr
- Increased incidence in men
- Risk factors: fair skin, increased sun exposure, use of tanning salons with ultraviolet A or B radiation, history of irradiation (e.g., Hodgkin's disease), personal or family history of skin cancer, impaired immune system

PHYSICAL FINDINGS & CLINICAL PRESENTATION

Variable with the histologic type:
- Nodular: dome-shaped, painless lesion that may become multilobular and frequently ulcerates (rodent ulcer); prominent telangiectatic vessels are noted on the surface. Border is translucent, elevated, pearly white (Fig. 1-37). Some nodular BCCs may contain pigmentation, giving an appearance similar to a melanoma.
- Superficial: circumscribed, scaling, black appearance with a thin, raised, pearly-white border; a crust and erosions may be present. Occurs most frequently on the trunk and extremities.
- Morpheaform: flat or slightly raised yellowish or white appearance (similar to localized scleroderma); appearance similar to scars; surface has a waxy consistency.

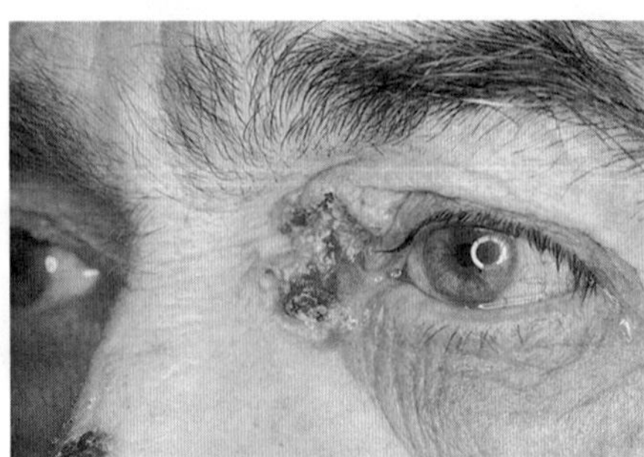

FIGURE 1-37 Basal cell carcinoma. Note rolled translucent border and central ulceration in typical facial location. (From Noble J et al: *Textbook of primary care medicine,* ed 3, St Louis, 2001, Mosby.)

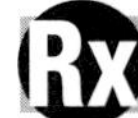 DIAGNOSIS

DIFFERENTIAL DIAGNOSIS

- Keratoacanthoma
- Melanoma (pigmented BCC)
- Xeroderma pigmentosa
- Basal cell nevus syndrome
- Molluscum contagiosum
- Sebaceous hyperplasia
- Psoriasis

WORKUP

Biopsy to confirm diagnosis

Rx TREATMENT

Variable with tumor size, location, and cell type:
- Excision surgery: preferred method for large tumors with well-defined borders on the legs, cheeks, forehead, and trunk.
- Mohs' micrographic surgery: preferred for lesions in high-risk areas (e.g., nose, eyelid), very large primary tumors, recurrent BCCs, and tumors with poorly defined clinical margins.
- Electrodesiccation and curettage: useful for small (<6 mm) nodular BCCs.
- Cryosurgery with liquid nitrogen: useful in BCCs of the superficial and nodular types with clearly definable margins; no clear advantages over the other forms of therapy; generally reserved for uncomplicated tumors.
- Radiation therapy: generally used for BCCs in areas requiring preservation of normal surrounding tissues for cosmetic reasons (e.g., around lips); also useful in patients who cannot tolerate surgical procedures or for large lesions and surgical failures.
- Imiquimod 5% cream can be used for treatment of small, superficial BCCs of the trunk and extremities. Efficacy rate is approximately 80%. Its main advantage is lack of scarring, which must be weighed against higher cure rates with surgical intervention.
- GDC-0449, an orally active small molecule that targets the hedgehog pathway, appears to have antitumor activity in locally advanced or metastatic basal-cell carcinoma.

DISPOSITION

- More than 90% of patients are cured; however, periodic evaluation for at least 5 yr is necessary because of increased risk of recurrence of another BCC (>40% risk within 5 yr of treatment).
- A lesion is considered low risk if it is <1.5 cm in diameter, is nodular or cystic, is not in a difficult-to-treat area (H zone of face), and has not been previously treated.
- Nodular and superficial BCCs are the least aggressive.
- Morpheaform lesions have the highest incidence of positive tumor margins (>30%) and the greatest recurrence rate.

EBM EVIDENCE

Please note: Complete text of EBM for this topic is available online.

Key trials and commentary:

Basal-like breast cancer is associated with high grade, poor prognosis, and younger patient age. Clinically, a triple-negative phenotype definition [estrogen receptor, progesterone receptor, and human epidermal growth factor receptor (HER)-2, all negative] is commonly used to identify such cases. EGFR and cytokeratin 5/6 are readily available positive markers of basal-like breast cancer applicable to standard pathology specimens. This study directly compares the prognostic significance between three- and five-biomarker surrogate panels to define intrinsic breast cancer subtypes, using a large clinically annotated series of breast tumors. It revealed that the expanded surrogate immunopanel of estrogen receptor, progesterone receptor, human HER-2, EGFR, and cytokeratin 5/6 provides a more specific definition of basal-like breast cancer that better predicts breast cancer survival.

The concept of a distinct subtype of breast carcinoma with basal cell-like features first began 20 years ago. From its inception, several features were noted to correlate including characteristic morphologic features, expression of basal-type cytokeratins, and poor prognosis. Additional features include the important observation that these tumors typically do not express estrogen and progesterone receptor or human epidermal growth factor receptor 2 (HER-2/neu), resulting in a so-called triple negative phenotype. Despite 20 years of development of the basal-like carcinoma concept including the advent of gene expression pattern analysis, a widely accepted consensus definition for basal cell carcinoma based on immunohistochemistry still does not exist. Some have proposed that the triple negative phenotype is sufficient to define basal-like carcinoma. The authors of this study make an evidenced argument that using an expanded panel of immunohistochemical markers, a group of tumors can be identified that more closely approximates the basal-like carcinoma entity as defined by gene expression analysis. The practicing pathologist should remain aware of the basal-like carcinoma concept development, as it may ultimately become an important distinction with unique genetic, immunohistochemical, and prognostic implications.[1] Ⓐ

This study sought to compare the efficacy and cosmetic outcome (CO) of photodynamic therapy with topical methyl aminolevulinate (MAL-PDT) with simple excision surgery for sBCC over a 1-year period. It revealed that MAL-PDT offers a similarly high efficacy and a much better CO than simple excision surgery in the treatment of sBCC.

This is an interesting study comparing results of a nonsurgical method of treatment for sBCC, photodynamic therapy with topical methyl aminolevulinate, with standard surgical excision therapy. Although at the end of 12 months the recurrence rate with the photodynamic therapy was 9.3% as compared with no recurrences following surgical excision, the cosmetic results were deemed more favorable, excellent/good, with the photodynamic therapy, compared with 59.8% after surgical excision. Cosmetic results were judged by patients and physicians alike. Although the treatment was randomized, it was clearly not double blinded for either patients or physicians. Photodynamic treatment required at least one cycle of at least two treatments 7 days apart, and, if no response, a second cycle of two treatments 7 days apart. The use of photodynamic therapy should be confined to the treatment of small (8-20 mm) superficial basal cell cancers, and not used for nodular, multifocal, or cicatricial BCC. The major problem with this study is that the follow-up period is far too short, and future studies should be extended out to 36 months to assess the real recurrence rate after photodynamic therapy.[2] Ⓐ

Evidence-Based References

1. Cheang MC et al: Basal-like breast cancer defined by five biomarkers has superior prognostic value than triple-negative phenotype, *Clin Cancer Res* 14:1368-1376, 2008. Commentary by G. Azabdaftari, M.D. Ⓐ

2. Szeimies RM et al: A clinical study comparing methyl aminolevulinate photodynamic therapy and surgery in small superficial basal cell carcinoma (8-20mm), with a 12-month follow-up, *J Eur Acad Dermatol Venereol* 22:1302-1311, 2008. Commentary by S. Miller, M.D. Ⓐ

SUGGESTED READING

Von Hoff DD et al: Inhibition of the hedgehog pathway in advanced basal cell carcinoma, *N Engl J Med* 361:1164-1172, 2009.

AUTHOR: **FRED F. FERRI, M.D.**

Bedbug Bite

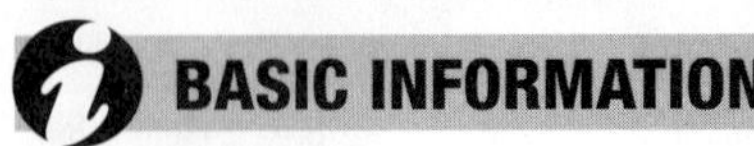

BASIC INFORMATION

DEFINITION

A bedbug's bite is a wound caused by the penetration of the bedbug mouthpiece into the skin as the insect feeds on blood from vessels or extravasated blood from the damaged surrounding tissue. The saliva of the bedbug contains pharmacologically active substances responsible for a spectrum of undesirable skin reactions depending on the individual.

SYNONYMS

Insect bite
Bedbug *Cimex lectularius* bite

ICD-9CM CODES

919.4 Insect bite w/o infection (may also code based on bite location)

EPIDEMIOLOGY & DEMOGRAPHICS

- Traditionally, bedbugs were considered more common in poorer areas, but they are now increasingly found in areas of frequent travel.
- Bedbug infestations may spread among multifamily and institutional facilities with shared walls and are consequently difficult to eradicate.
- Reports of bedbug infestations have increased dramatically in the U.S., as well as worldwide, likely because of the decreased use of pesticides and increased international travel.
- Bedbugs are attracted to carbon dioxide gas and warm bodies.
- Bedbugs do not have a preference for specific age groups, ethnicity, or sex.
- Studies have shown increased sensitivity of cutaneous reaction in previous bite victims.

PHYSICAL FINDINGS AND CLINICAL PRESENTATION

- Firm, purpuric or erythematous macules, urticaria, or bullae may be present. Bites are often inflammatory and pruritic, although bedbug naive individuals may be asymptomatic to their first bites.
- Bite may have a central hemorrhagic punctum.
- Victim may observe a linear series of three bites ("breakfast, lunch, and dinner").
- As bedbug bites usually do not penetrate clothing, bite distribution is generally on areas of exposed skin. Otherwise, there is no preferential distribution.

ETIOLOGY

- The *Cimex lectularius* species, also known as the common bedbug, feeds on mammals and birds. *Cimex hemipterus* is a tropical species that bites mostly humans, and hybrid species of the two insects exist. Both generally feed nocturnally on the blood of sleeping humans. The adult bedbug is wingless and about 5 to 7 mm in length. It has a modified mouthpart for piercing and sucking that usually leaves a bite mark of papular urticarial presentation to exposed areas of skin. Bedbugs have weak appendages for latching on to their hosts and are not usually transported from person to person.
- The saliva of the bedbug contains nitrophorin that enables vasodilation, an anticoagulant that interferes with production of coagulation Factor Xa, a salivary apyrase that inhibits platelet aggregation, and an anesthetic. Consequently, the host often does not feel the bite until the effects have worn off.

Dx DIAGNOSIS

DIFFERENTIAL DIAGNOSIS

Scabies, flea and mite bites, vesicular disorders, delusional parasitosis, dermatitis herpetiformis, pemphigus herpetiformis, ecthyma, drug eruptions

WORKUP

- Workup begins with history and physical for clinical symptoms and environmental findings.
- Victims should carefully scrutinize the bedroom for signs of bedbug infestation. One may encounter fecal smears or flecks of blood on bed linens, inside furniture cracks and crevices, and behind peeling wallpaper. Bedbugs may travel as far as 20 feet for a meal. Densely infested rooms may also have a distinctive, pungent, soda syrup–like odor.

LABORATORY TESTS

- No specific tests recommended except for identification of the insect.
- The histology of bedbug bites is similar to other insect bites. Perivascular infiltrate of lymphocytes, histiocytes, eosinophils, and mast cells are seen within the upper dermis. One may also observe collagen bundles with interstitial eosinophils, dermal edema, and extravasated erythrocytes.

IMAGING STUDIES

None

Rx TREATMENT

- Treatment of bites is often not necessary. Bites may self-resolve within a week for milder cases and a few weeks for more severe cases.
- Topical glucocorticoids or systemic antihistamines are appropriate in patients with severe pruritus from the bedbug bite.
  - triamcinolone cream 0.1%, apply thin film to affected areas bid
  - chlorpheniramine 4 mg PO hs (adults), 2 mg PO hs (children)
- Insecticides may be effective in eradicating the bedbug, but growing resistance has been seen and multi-insecticide therapy is recommended.
  - Use permethrin spray for clothing and bedsheets or bednets
  - Diethyltoluamide (DEET): Be wary of toxic levels in children when used at high concentrations.
  - Deltamethrin and chlorfenapyr are two common insecticides used.
  - Please consult a pest control professional for safe eradication.

NONPHARMACOLOGIC THERAPY

Vacuuming is effective in removing bedbugs but does not remove the eggs. Wash bedsheets and clothing in hot water with detergent with at least 20 minutes in a dryer. Bedbugs have a high thermal death point of 45° C and also may survive at temperatures as low as 7° C. Coating bedposts with antifriction or adhesive substances such as petrolatum or duct tape may hinder bedbugs from gaining access to the bed.

ACUTE GENERAL Rx

Immunologic response is dependent on immunocompetence and individual sensitivity to the salivary components of the bedbug bite. Often, patients with papular urticaria have IgG antibodies to specific bedbug proteins. IgE antibodies may also mediate bullae formation. Anaphylaxis and death from bites is rare but documented in literature.

DISPOSITION

Patient may resume normal activity and lifestyle. Travelers should inspect their clothing and suitcases before returning home.

BEDBUGS AS POTENTIAL VECTORS

The bedbug has been studied extensively as a potential vector for human pathogens such as HIV and viral hepatitis, as well as many other diseases. To date, there is no evidence of transmission from an infected bedbug to a human.

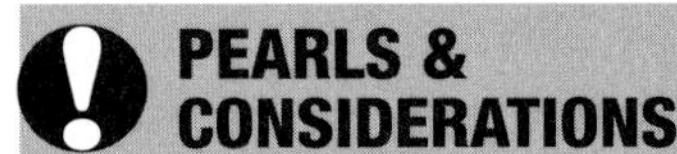

PEARLS & CONSIDERATIONS

COMMENTS

- Bedbugs are an increasing source of anguish and frustration for humans, and clinicians should evaluate for signs of stress and depression.
- A combination of chemical and physical intervention is often necessary for complete eradication. All hiding areas must be carefully inspected and cleaned. Treatment may include pesticides plus laundering, heat, freezing, and vacuuming.

SUGGESTED READINGS

Goddard J, deShazo R: Bedbugs (Cimex lectularius) and clinical consequences of their bites. *JAMA* 301(13):1358-1366, 2009.

Kolb A et al: Bedbugs. *Dermatologic Therapy* 22(4):347-352, 2009.

AUTHOR: **STEPHANIE W. CHOW, M.D.**

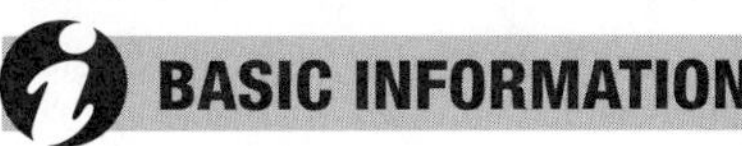

BASIC INFORMATION

DEFINITION

Behçet's disease is a chronic, relapsing, inflammatory disorder characterized by the presence of recurrent oral aphthous ulcers, genital ulcers, uveitis, and skin lesions (Figs. 1-38 and 1-39).

SYNONYMS

Behçet's syndrome

ICD-9CM CODES
136.1 Behçet's syndrome

EPIDEMIOLOGY & DEMOGRAPHICS

PREVALENCE:

- Behçet's disease is observed in two different geographic locations.
  1. One region consists of Eastern Asia, Turkey, and the Mediterranean basin.
     - Prevalence ranges from 13 to 17 cases per 100,000 persons.
     - Turkey has the highest prevalence at up to 300 cases per 100,000 persons.
  2. The second region consists of North America and Northern Europe.
     - Prevalence ranges from 0.5 to 17 cases per 100,000 persons. Germany has the greatest prevalence.
     - Prevalence of Behçet's disease in the U.S. is 6.6 cases per 100,000 persons.
- In these regions, the prevalence of HLA-B51 is greater in patients with Behçet's disease.

PREDOMINANT SEX: Equal sex distribution

GENETICS: No clear pattern of inheritance can be determined. Familial disease was noted in 15% of affected children.

PHYSICAL FINDINGS & CLINICAL PRESENTATION

- Behçet's disease typically affects individuals in the third to fourth decade of life and primarily presents with painful aphthous oral ulcers. The ulcers occur in crops measuring 2 to 12 mm and are found on the mucous membrane of the cheek, gingiva, tongue, pharynx, and soft palate.
- Genital and perianal ulcers are similar to the oral ulcers. They may result in scarring.
- Decreased vision secondary to uveitis, keratitis, and retinal artery occlusion with ischemia may be followed by neovascularization, vitreous hemorrhage and contraction, glaucoma, and retinal detachment. Younger male individuals are at greater risk for ocular involvement.
- Skin findings (41% to 97%) include nodular lesions, which are histologically divided to erythema nodosum-like lesions, pseudofolliculitis, papulopustular lesions, acneform nodules, or pyoderma gangrenosum-like lesions (cutaneous aphthosis).
- Intermittent, symmetric oligoarthritis (40% to 70%) is the most common; ankylosing spondylitis or arthralgias may occur.
- Central nervous system (CNS; 30% in U.S. and 5% in Turkey) meningeal findings including headache, fever, and stiff neck can occur. Cerebellar ataxia, pseudobulbar palsy, and dementia occur with involvement of the brainstem.
- Vascular involvement (25% to 30%), arterial and venous, of all sizes may cause systemic arterial vasculitis (aneurysms and occlusions), pulmonary artery vasculitis, venous occlusions (including superficial, deep, cerebral, portal, and mesenterial veins), pulmonary embolus, right ventricle thrombosis, and Budd-Chiari syndrome.
- GI involvement is more common in Japanese individuals; ulcerative lesions primarily involve distal ileum and cecum, but any region can be affected. GI lesions tend to perforate or bleed and may recur after surgery.

ETIOLOGY

The etiology of Behçet's disease is unknown. An immune-related vasculitis, a perivascular inflammation, or both are thought to lead to many of the manifestations of Behçet's disease. Multiple triggers for this process have been investigated, including herpes simplex virus infection, streptococcal antigen, and others.

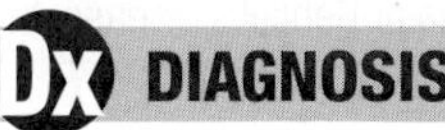

DIAGNOSIS

According to the International Study Group for Behçet's disease, the diagnosis of Behçet's disease is established when oral ulcerations recur at least three times in one 12-mo period plus at least two of the following conditions in the absence of other systemic diseases:

- Recurrent genital ulceration
- Eye lesions
- Skin lesions
- Positive pathergy test (erythematous papules or pustules [>2 mm in diameter] at sterile needle injection sites after 24 to 48 hours)

DIFFERENTIAL DIAGNOSIS

- Inflammatory bowel disease (ulcerative colitis and Crohn's disease)
- Sprue disease
- Herpes simplex infection
- Benign aphthous stomatitis
- Cyclic neutropenia
- Acquired immune deficiency syndrome (AIDS)
- Systemic lupus erythematosus
- Reiter's syndrome
- Ankylosing spondylitis
- Hypereosinophilic syndrome
- Sweet's syndrome
- Lichen planus
- Pemphigoid

WORKUP

The diagnosis of Behçet's disease is a clinical diagnosis. Laboratory tests and x-ray imaging may be helpful in working up the complications of Behçet's disease or excluding other diseases in the differential.

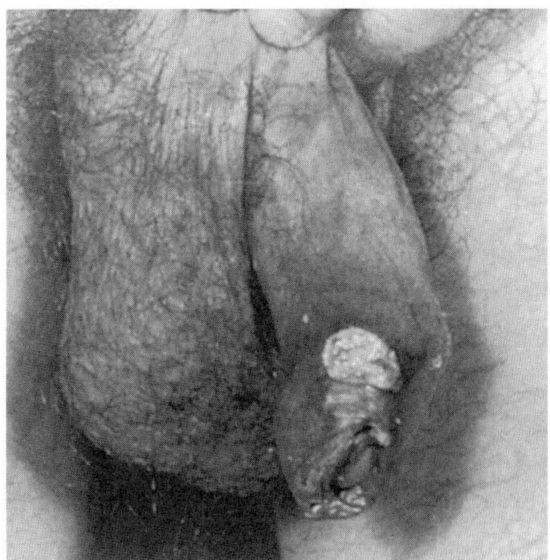

FIGURE 1-38 Behçet's syndrome. Painful preputial ulcer in a male patient with superficial thrombophlebitis, oral ulcers, and bowel vasculitis. (From Canoso J: *Rheumatology in primary care,* Philadelphia, 1997, WB Saunders.)

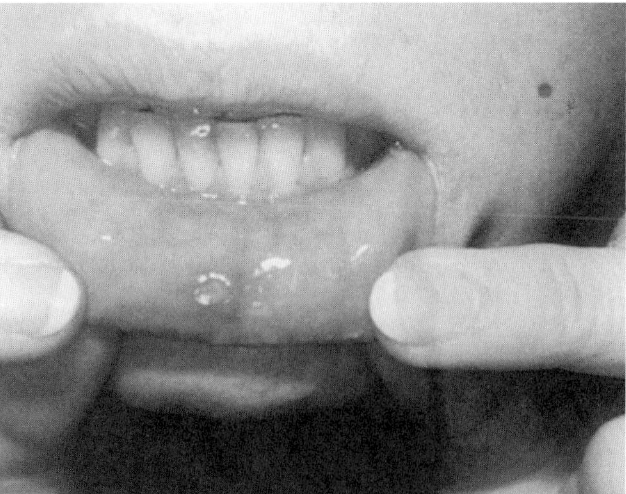

FIGURE 1-39 Behçet's syndrome. Painful aphthous inner lower lip ulcer in a 30-yr-old Chinese woman with relapsing oral and genital ulcers and uveitis. She responded well to low-dose prednisone plus colchicine. (From Canoso J: *Rheumatology in primary care,* Philadelphia, 1997, WB Saunders.)

LABORATORY TESTS

No diagnostic laboratory tests for Behçet's disease exist. The measurements of T cell proliferative response to heat shock protein (HSP) and impaired fibrinolytic activity have been proposed for the diagnosis of Behçet's disease, but the value of testing has not been confirmed.

IMAGING STUDIES

CT scan, MRI, and angiography are useful for detecting CNS and vascular lesions.

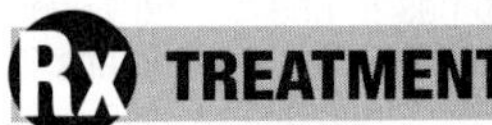

TREATMENT

Treatment is directed at the patient's clinical presentation and complications (e.g., mucocutaneous lesions, ocular lesions, arthritis, GI, CNS, or vascular lesions).

NONPHARMACOLOGIC THERAPY

Supportive care and rest during flares, and moderate exercises such as swimming or walking when symptoms improve or disappear

ACUTE GENERAL Rx

- Oral and genital ulcers:
  1. Topical and intralesional corticosteroids (e.g., triamcinolone acetonide ointment applied tid)
  2. Tetracycline tablets 250 mg dissolved in 5 cc water and applied to the ulcer for 2 to 3 min
  3. Colchicine 0.5 to 1.5 mg/day PO
  4. Thalidomide 100 to 300 mg PO daily
  5. Dapsone 100 mg PO daily
  6. Pentoxifylline 300 mg/day PO
  7. Azathioprine 1 to 2.5 mg/kg/day PO
  8. Methotrexate 7.5 to 25 mg/wk PO or intravenously
  9. Interferon alfa-2a and interferon alfa-2b (generally given 3 to 19 million units three times weekly)
- Ocular lesions:
  1. Anterior uveitis is treated by an ophthalmologist with topical corticosteroids (e.g., betamethasone drops 1 to 2 drops tid); topical injection with dexamethasone 1 to 1.5 mg has also been tried
  2. Infliximab 5 mg/kg single dose
  3. Cyclosporine A (5 mg/kg/day) with or without prednisone or azathioprine 1 to 2.5 mg/kg/day PO
- CNS disease:
  1. Chlorambucil 0.1 mg/kg/day is used in the treatment of posterior uveitis, retinal vasculitis, or CNS disease; patients not responding to chlorambucil can be tried on cyclosporine 5 to 7 mg/kg/day.
  2. In CNS vasculitis, cyclophosphamide 2 to 3 mg/kg/day is used. Prednisone can be used as an alternative.
- Arthritis:
  1. NSAIDs (e.g., ibuprofen 400 to 800 mg tid PO or indomethacin 50 to 75 mg/day PO)
  2. Sulfasalazine 1 to 3 g/day PO is an alternative treatment
- GI lesions:
  1. Sulfasalazine 1 to 3 g/day PO
  2. Prednisone 40 to 60 mg/day PO
- Vascular lesions:
  1. Prednisone 40 to 60 mg/day PO
  2. Cytotoxic agents as mentioned previously
  3. Heparin 5000 to 20,000 U/day followed by oral warfarin

CHRONIC Rx

- Chronic therapy is usually continued for approximately 1 yr after remission.
- Surgery may be indicated in patients with complications of bowel perforation, vascular occlusive disease, and aneurysm formation.

DISPOSITION

- The aphthous oral ulcers last 1 to 2 wk, recurring more frequently than genital ulcers.
- 25% of Japanese patients with ocular lesions become blind.
- The disease course is unpredictable.
- The morbidity of Behçet's disease comes primarily from ocular and cutaneous involvement; however, mortality relates primarily to large-size vessel involvement and CNS diseases.

REFERRAL

If the diagnosis of Behçet's disease is suspected, a referral to dermatology, rheumatology, and ophthalmology is indicated because the disease is so rare.

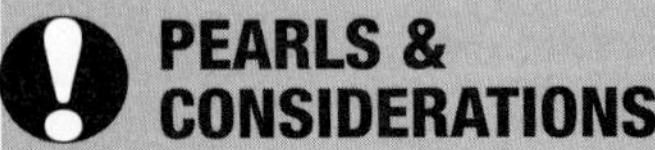

PEARLS & CONSIDERATIONS

COMMENTS

- The pathergy test refers to the formation of an erythematous papule or pustule of ≥2 mm after oblique insertion of a sterile 20- or 25-gauge needle into the skin after 24 to 48 hours.
- Because of the rarity of this disease, data from controlled, prospective, randomized clinical trials are lacking.

SUGGESTED READINGS

Al-Otaibi LM et al: Behcet's disease: a review, *J Dent Res* 84(3):209, 2005.

Bonfioli AA, Orefice F: Behcet's disease, *Semin Ophthalmol* 20(3):199, 2005.

Evereklioglu C: Managing the symptoms of Behcet's disease, *Expert Opin Pharmacother* 5(2):317, 2004.

Kurokawa MS et al: Behcet's disease, *Semin Respir Crit Care Med* 25(5):557, 2004.

Yazici H: Behçet's syndrome: an update, *Curr Rheumatol Rep* (5):195, 2003.

AUTHORS: **MONZR M. AL MALKI, M.D., GLENN G. FORT, M.D., M.P.H.,** and **DENNIS J. MIKOLICH, M.D.**

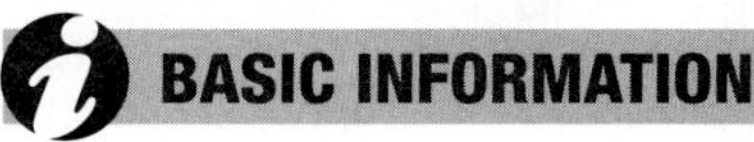

BASIC INFORMATION

DEFINITION

Bell's palsy is an idiopathic, isolated, usually unilateral facial weakness in the distribution of the seventh cranial nerve (<1% are bilateral).

SYNONYMS

Idiopathic facial paralysis

ICD-9CM CODES
351.0 Bell's palsy

EPIDEMIOLOGY & DEMOGRAPHICS

INCIDENCE: 20 to 30 cases/100,000; occurs at any age, median age 45 yr

RISK FACTORS:

- Pregnancy (especially third trimester/first postpartum week)
- Diabetes (5% to 10% of patients)
- Travel to area endemic for Lyme disease

PHYSICAL FINDINGS & CLINICAL PRESENTATION

- Unilateral paralysis of the upper and lower facial muscles (asymmetric eye closure, brow, and smile).
- Ipsilateral loss of taste
- Ipsilateral ear pain, usually 2 to 3 days before presentation
- Increased or decreased unilateral eye tearing
- Hyperacusis
- Subjective ipsilateral facial numbness
- In approximately 8% of cases, other cranial neuropathies may occur

ETIOLOGY

- Most cases are idiopathic, although the cause is often viral (herpes simplex).
- Herpes zoster can cause Bell's palsy in association with herpetic blisters affecting the outer ear canal or the area behind the ear (Ramsay-Hunt syndrome).
- Bell's palsy can also be one of the manifestations of Lyme disease.

Dx DIAGNOSIS

DIFFERENTIAL DIAGNOSIS

- Neoplasms affecting the base of the skull or the parotid gland
- Infectious process (meningitis, syphilis, otitis media, osteomyelitis of the skull base)
- Brain stem stroke
- Multiple sclerosis
- Head trauma/temporal bone fracture
- Other: sarcoidosis, Guillain-Barré syndrome, carcinomatous or leukemic meningitis, leprosy, Melkersson-Rosenthal syndrome

WORKUP

Bell's palsy is a clinical diagnosis. A focused history and neurologic examination confirm the diagnosis.

LABORATORY TESTS

- Consider CBC, fasting glucose, VDRL, ESR, ACE in selected patients.
- Lyme titer in endemic areas.

IMAGING STUDIES

- Contrast-enhanced MRI to exclude neoplasms is indicated only in patients with atypical features or course.
- Chest x-ray may be useful to exclude sarcoidosis or rule out TB in selected patients before treating with steroids.

Rx TREATMENT

NONPHARMACOLOGIC THERAPY

- Reassure patient that the prognosis is usually good and the disease is most likely a result of a virus attacking the nerve, not a stroke.
- Avoid corneal drying by patching the eye. Lacri-Lube ophthalmic ointment at night and artificial tears during the day are also useful to prevent excessive drying.

ACUTE GENERAL Rx

- A short course of oral prednisone is commonly used even though the evidence from randomized, controlled trials demonstrating efficacy is inadequate.
- If used, prednisone therapy should be started within 24 to 48 hr of symptom onset. Optimal steroid dose is unknown.
- Combination therapy with acyclovir and prednisone may be effective in improving clinical recovery, although robust evidence from high-quality randomized controlled trials is lacking.
- Surgical decompression remains controversial, and data from randomized trials are lacking to compare medical and surgical therapy.
- Some data suggest that methylcobalamin (active form of vitamin B_{12}) and hyperbaric oxygen may be of benefit, but these have not yet received widespread acceptance.
- Botulinum toxin may be helpful for treatment of synkinesis and hemifacial spasm, two late sequelae of Bell's palsy.

CHRONIC Rx

Patients should be monitored for evidence of corneal abrasion and ulceration. Physical therapy, including moist heat and massage, may be beneficial.

DISPOSITION

- 71% of patients should recover completely. Prognosis is better for those with less severity of symptoms at onset and clinical improvement within 3 wk.
- Recovery begins within 3 wk in 85% of patients. The remaining patients have some improvement within 3 to 6 mo.
- Recurrence occurs in 5% of cases.

REFERRAL

- Persistent eye irritation or redness requires referral to ophthalmology.
- Neurology referral is recommended if diagnosis is unclear or if clinical course is atypical.
- Consider plastic surgery referral if there is persistent, severe difficulty in closing the eye (6 mo).

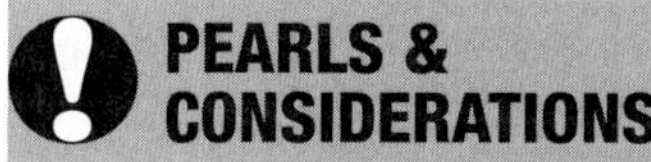

PEARLS & CONSIDERATIONS

Ensure that both upper and lower aspects of the face are involved (as this suggests a peripheral lesion). Lower facial asymmetry alone is more likely central (e.g., stroke) and further workup is necessary.

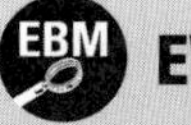

EVIDENCE

Please note: Complete text of EBM for this topic is available online.

SUGGESTED READINGS

de Almeida JR et al: Combined corticosteroid and antiviral treatment for Bell Palsy, *JAMA* 302(9): 985-993, 2009.

Sullivan FM et al: Early treatment with prednisolone or acyclovir in Bell's palsy, *N Engl J Med* 357:1598, 2007.

AUTHOR: **RICHARD S. ISAACSON, M.D.**

 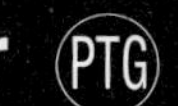

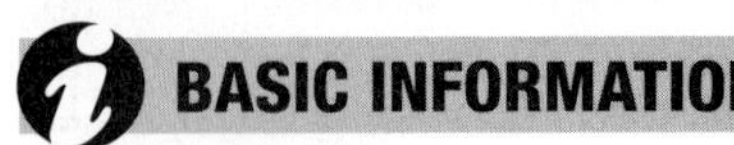

BASIC INFORMATION

DEFINITION

Bipolar disorder is an episodic, recurrent, and frequently progressive condition in which the afflicted individual experiences at least one episode of mania, characterized by at least 1 wk of continuous symptoms of elevated, expansive, or irritable mood, in association with three or four of the following symptoms:

- Decreased need for sleep
- Grandiosity
- Pressured speech
- Subjective or objective flight of ideas
- Distractibility
- Increased level of goal-directed activity
- Problematic behavior

Most individuals with bipolar disorder also experience one or more episodes of major depression over their lifetimes or have symptoms of a depressive episode commingled with those of mania (mixed episode).

SYNONYMS

Manic-depression
Cycloid psychosis

ICD-9CM CODES
296.4-6 Circular manic, circular depressed, circular type mixed

EPIDEMIOLOGY & DEMOGRAPHICS

INCIDENCE: 0.016% to 0.021%

PREVALENCE (IN U.S.): 0.4% to 1.6%; bipolar spectrum disorders: 2.8% to 6.5%

PREDOMINANT SEX: Equal distribution among male and female

PREDOMINANT AGE: Lifelong condition with age of onset 14 to 30 yr

PEAK INCIDENCE: Onset in 20s

GENETICS:

- Concordance rates for monozygotic twins: 0.7 to 0.8; for dizygotic twins: 0.2
- Risk of affective disorder in offspring with one affected parent with bipolar disorder: 27% to 29%; with two affected parents: 50% to 74%
- Heritability estimate of 0.85
- Although no specific causal mutations have been identified, genome-wide association analyses have suggested a role for ANK3 and CACNA1C and implicated ion channelopathies in pathogenesis of bipolar disorder.

PHYSICAL FINDINGS & CLINICAL PRESENTATION

- Mania associated with psychomotor activation that is usually goal directed but not necessarily productive; increase in goal-directed activity and excessive involvement in activities leading to unexpected adverse outcomes
- Elevated, euphoric, and frequently labile mood
- Decreased need for sleep
- Flight of ideas with rapid, loud, pressured speech
- Psychosis may occur, with delusions, hallucinations, and formal thought disorder
- Depressive episodes resembling major depressive disorder (see Depression, Major); however, atypical features (hypersomnia, weight gain) may be present
- Mixed states, characterized by activation, irritability, and dysphoria, also possible

ETIOLOGY

Hypotheses:

1. Abnormalities of receptor and membrane function
2. Alteration of cAMP, MAP kinase, protein kinase C, and glycogen synthase kinase-3 signal transduction pathways
3. Alteration in cell survival pathways

Dx DIAGNOSIS

DIFFERENTIAL DIAGNOSIS

- Secondary manias caused by medical disorders (e.g., hyperthyroidism, AIDS, stroke, Cushing's syndrome) are frequent.
- First onset of mania after age 50 yr is suggestive of secondary mania.
- Less severe, and possibly distinct, conditions of bipolar type II and cyclothymia are possible.
- Comorbidity with substance abuse or dependency may confound diagnostic assessment and treatment.
- Cross-sectional examination of acutely manic patient can be confused with schizophrenia or a paranoid psychosis.

WORKUP

- History
- Physical examination
- Mental status examination
- Mood Disorder Questionnaire (MDQ)

LABORATORY TESTS

Because of high rate of secondary manias, initial evaluation to confirm health of all major organ systems (routine chemistries, complete blood count, urinalysis, sedimentation rate)

IMAGING STUDIES

- Consider brain imaging if late onset or if neurologic examination is abnormal.
- Neuroimaging may show evidence of ventricular enlargement or increased white matter hyperintensities; changes in amygdala, frontal cortex, and striatal volume have also been reported.

Rx TREATMENT

NONPHARMACOLOGIC THERAPY

- Cognitive-behavioral and family-focused psychoeducational psychotherapy to help patients cope with consequences of the disease, improve adherence with medications, and identify possible environmental triggers
- Bright light therapy in the northern latitudes in individuals exhibiting a seasonal pattern of winter depression
- Lifestyle "regularization"

ACUTE GENERAL Rx

- First-line agents for acute mania: lithium 1500-1800 mg/day (0.8-1.2 mEq/L), valproate 1000-1500 mg/day (50-125 ng/ml), carbamazepine 600-800 mg/day (4-12 mcg/ml), oxcarbazepine 900-2400 mg/day, olanzapine 10-20 mg/day, risperidone 2-4 mg/day, quetiapine 350-800 mg/day, ziprasidone 80-120 mg/day, and aripiprazole 10-30 mg/day.
- Useful adjuncts to acute treatment: benzodiazepines: lorazepam 1-2 mg/q4h, clonazepam 1-2 mg/q4h.
- Traditional antidepressants can induce manic episodes and exacerbate mania in mixed episodes.
- Lamotrigine can have acute antidepressant benefit.

CHRONIC Rx

- Goal of long-term treatment: prevention of relapse or episode recurrence
- Best agents for prophylaxis of mania: lithium, valproate, and olanzapine (carbamazepine/oxcarbazepine possibly beneficial)
- Best agents for prophylaxis of depression: lamotrigine and lithium
- Role of atypical antipsychotics in maintenance unclear
- Long-term use of antidepressants: frequently destabilizes patient and leads to more frequent relapses

DISPOSITION

- Course is variable.
- More than 90% of patients having a single manic episode are likely to experience others.
- Uncontrolled manic or depressive episodes can lead to additional episodes ("illness begets illness").
- Lithium treatment shown to specifically decrease suicidal risk.
- Psychosocioeconomic consequences of both mania and depression can be severe and disabling.

REFERRAL

- If use of antidepressant contemplated
- If patient is severely manic, rapid cycling, or suicidal or is in a bipolar, mixed episode

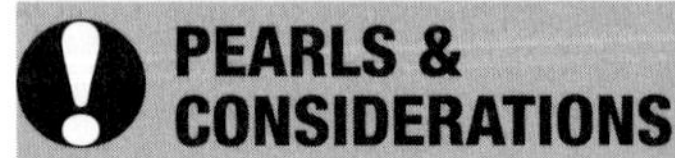

PEARLS & CONSIDERATIONS

COMMENTS

- All patients presenting with depression should be asked about past personal and family history of mania and hypomania; 70% of bipolar patients have previously been misdiagnosed.
- Prompt recognition of the earliest signs of mania in a given individual (e.g., decreased need for sleep, increased rate of speech) al-

lows earlier intervention and a better likelihood of preventing a full episode.

- Bipolar disorder in children frequently manifests as behavioral disinhibition.
- Patients treated with atypical antipsychotic agents should be carefully monitored for development of metabolic syndrome.

PATIENT/FAMILY EDUCATION

Information available at www.NMHA.org/ and www.dbsalliance.org/.

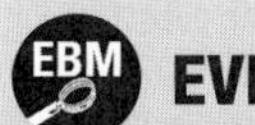

EVIDENCE

Please note: Complete text of EBM for this topic is available online.

Key trials and commentary:

This study sought to determine whether advanced paternal age is associated with an increased risk of BPD in the offspring and to assess if there was any difference in risk when analyzing patients with early-onset BPD separately. It revealed that advanced paternal age is a risk factor for BPD in the offspring. The results are consistent with the hypothesis that advancing paternal age increases the risk for de novo mutations in susceptibility genes for neurodevelopmental disorders.

This is a provocative and interesting study of an area that has been barely examined in bipolar disorder. The relationship between advanced paternal age and risk for the development of schizophrenia has been fairly well established by several studies similar to this study. In one of these, bipolar disorder was buried in the "Other" category, but an effect was still seen for advanced paternal age in that heterogeneous group. Here, this study focuses on bipolar disorder alone and applies a strong methodology with rigorous control for subject variation. The effect (1.37 times above expected) among males is actually similar to that observed in schizophrenia studies. The association appears all the more credible because it was most pronounced for individuals with early-onset bipolar disorder. Thus, this association may be generalized across putative neurodevelopmental disorders because it has now been reported for schizophrenia, bipolar disorder, and autism. This article is a great read about this risk factor, as well as the methodological nuances in this epidemiological research.[3] Ⓐ

Another trial sought to examine the benefits of family-focused treatment for adolescents (FFT-A) and pharmacotherapy in the 2-year course of adolescent bipolar disorder. It revealed that family-focused therapy is effective in combination with pharmacotherapy in stabilizing bipolar depressive symptoms among adolescents. To establish full recovery, FFT-A may need to be supplemented with systematic care interventions effective for mania symptoms.

This study addresses the role of family psychotherapy vs. medication treatment for adolescents with bipolar disorder. The study design is exemplary and the results are important. This study also complements previous, similar research by this team in the long-term care of adults with bipolar disorder. As perhaps might not be anticipated, the family therapy and extended "care" group did not differ much in relapse over the 2-year follow-up. Moreover, family therapy was not effective for patients with persistent manic symptoms. Perhaps, the most sobering aspect of this study is the high relapse rate over 2 years (in excess of 60%) in pediatric bipolar disorder—even when treated with medications. Bipolar disorder with onset in childhood/adolescence is, by very definition, a more severe form of mood disorder than mood problems that emerge later in adulthood. Because of the high toll of personal and familial "damage" caused by relapse in adolescents with bipolar disorder, this study could be viewed as evidence that we must use all the available tools to provide comprehensive care to adolescents who have bipolar disorder.[4] Ⓐ

Psychotherapy has long been recommended as adjunctive to pharmacotherapy for bipolar disorder, but it is unclear which interventions are effective for which patients, over what intervals, and for what domains of outcome. An article on adjunctive psychotherapy reviews randomized trials for bipolar disorder.

This study revealed that adjunctive psychotherapy enhances the symptomatic and functional outcomes of bipolar disorder over 2-year periods. The various modalities differ in content, structure, and associated mediating mechanisms. Treatments that emphasize medication adherence and early recognition of mood symptoms have stronger effects on mania, whereas treatments that emphasize cognitive and interpersonal coping strategies have stronger effects on depression. The placement of psychotherapy within chronic care algorithms and its role as a preventive agent in the early stages of the disorder deserve investigation.

This is an extremely useful review article that explores the impact of 18 trials of various types of psychosocial interventions for the treatment of bipolar disorder. It shows that psychosocial treatments definitely have an important role to play in the treatment of bipolar disorder, a condition that is primarily thought of in terms of pharmacological treatment. It also shows that there is a long way to go in successfully helping people who suffer from this illness.

The article answers an important question about which treatments work most effectively at which stage of the illness. There are clear differences in which treatments are more effective for a manic phase and which work best in a depressive phase of the illness, and this is crucial information for clinicians who work with this population. Table 1 included in the article summarizes the specific groups for which a given intervention is effective and can be used as a quick reference guide.

Even with the progress that has been made in tailoring treatments to this specific disorder, this article makes clear that existing treatment options go only so far. It was alarming to read, "even with optimal psychotherapy and pharmacotherapy, recurrence occurred in 50% to 75% of patients in 1 year." Bipolar disorder remains a considerable challenge to the field. This article goes a long way, however, in advising readers how to be most helpful to their patients from a psychosocial perspective.[5] Ⓐ

Given high rates of suicide and suicide attempts in bipolar disorder and the data suggesting a suicide-protective effect of lithium, a separate study evaluated the impact of pharmacotherapy on prospectively observed suicides and suicide attempts in subjects in the Systematic Treatment Enhancement Program for Bipolar Disorder (STEP-BD).

The data from this study are not consistent with a suicide-protective effect of lithium. The association between suicide events and SSRI prescriptions requires cautious interpretation because of the complex relationships between treatment, severity, and suicidality.

This study provides data from the large STEP-BD trial of 4360 bipolar individuals. The results provide some light but continued confusion of the issues of the relationship between medicines and suicidal ideation and attempts. The authors did not find an antisuicide effect for lithium, valproate, carbamazepine, lamotrigine, and SGA. This is disappointing because other data sets have shown a protective effect for lithium. Even more confusing is that the authors found a positive association between the use of SSRIs and suicide events that was highly statistically significant. They do warn that there needs to be cautious interpretation of that relationship because of the complexity of the issues. One thing that we should remember in evaluating this study is that it was conducted in bipolar patients, not unipolar patients. The issues are complex in unipolar about whether the SSRIs are associated with increased suicidality, whereas the issues are different in bipolar illness. We now know that the SSRIs are not effective antidepressants and that they worsen the course in about a third of bipolar patients. This could be the primary explanation for why this association was observed.[6] Ⓐ

Recent studies demonstrate the poor psychosocial outcomes associated with bipolar disorder. Occupational functioning, a key indicator of psychosocial disability, is often severely affected by the disorder. This study describes the effect of acute treatment with interpersonal and social rhythm therapy on occupational functioning over a period of approximately 2.5 years. In this study, interpersonal and social rhythm therapy, with its emphasis on amelioration of interpersonal and role functioning, improved occupational functioning significantly more rapidly than did a psychoeducational and supportive approach with no such emphasis on functional capacities.

In the past, far too many studies were concerned only with reduction of symptoms in treatment outcome studies. This makes this exploration of the role of interpersonal and social rhythm therapy in improving occupational functioning a welcome addition to the literature on psychotherapy outcome.

The ability to work is one of the most social roles that individuals have, and the role played by psychotherapy in affecting this capacity is of crucial importance to patients, their families, and society.

As the authors point out, bipolar illness is associated with significant problems in the work arena. Thus, a treatment, whether primary or adjunctive, that could help enhance work functioning could make a big difference in the lives of individuals with a potentially seriously disabling condition.

The finding that patients who were randomly assigned to interpersonal and social rhythm therapy showed more rapid improvements in occupational functioning relative to those who were assigned to clinical management during the acute phase suggests that adding this type of intervention to pharmacological treatment during the acute phase offers important benefits. The fact that this type of intervention targets the kinds of behaviors that can lead to difficulty for individuals with bipolar disorder (e.g., addressing potentially disruptive stressful life events and emphasizing the importance of maintaining routines) is the likely source of added benefit. Findings from this study also suggest the importance of the timing of an intervention. In this case, providing this type of treatment was important during the acute phase, in which it had its significant impact.

It is unfortunate that of the 125 participants who entered the maintenance phase of treatment, only 70 participants completed assessments at the end of 2 years. This creates some problems about generalizability regarding the maintenance phase.[7] Ⓐ

Evidence-Based References

1. Gijsman HJ et al: Antidepressants for bipolar depression: a systematic review of randomized controlled trails, *Am J Psychiatry* 161:1537-1547, 2004.
2. Vieta E et al: Effectiveness of aripiprazole v. haloperidol in acute bipolar mania: double-blind, randomized, comparative 12-week trial, *Br J Psychiatry* 187:235-242, 2005.
3. Frans EM et al: Advancing paternal age and bipolar disorder, *Arch Gen Psychiatry* 65:1034-1040, 2008. Commentary by P. Buckley, M.D. Ⓐ
4. Miklowitz DJ et al: Family-focused treatment for adolescents with bipolar disorder: results of a 2-year randomized trial, *Arch Gen Psychiatry* 65:1053-1061, 2008. Commentary by P. Buckley, M.D. Ⓐ
5. Miklowitz DJ: Adjunctive psychotherapy for bipolar disorder: state of the evidence, *Am J Psychiatry* 165:1408-1419, 2008. Commentary by J.L. Krupnick, Ph.D. Ⓐ
6. Marangell LB et al: Case-control analyses of the impact of pharmacotherapy on prospectively observed suicide attempts and completed suicides in bipolar disorder: findings from STEP-BD, *J Clin Psychiatry* 69:916-922, 2008. Commentary by J.C. Ballenger, M.D. Ⓐ
7. Frank E et al: The role of interpersonal and social rhythm therapy in improving occupational functioning in patients with bipolar i disorder, *Am J Psychiatry* 165:1559-1565, 2008. Commentary by J.L. Krupnick, Ph.D. Ⓐ

SUGGESTED READINGS

Fornito A et al: Reconciling neuroimaging and neuropathological findings in schizophrenia and bipolar disorder, *Curr Opin Psychiatry* 22(3):312-319, 2009.

Gershon S et al: Lithium specificity in bipolar illness: a classic agent for the classic disorder, *Bipolar Disord* 11(2):34-44, 2009.

Goodwin FK, Redfield JK: *Manic-depressive illness: bipolar disorders and recurrent depression,* ed 2, New York, 2007, Oxford University Press.

Newberg AR et al: Neurobiology of bipolar disorder, *Expert Rev Neurother* 8(1):93-110, 2008.

Pompili M et al: Assessment and treatment of suicide risk in bipolar disorders, *Expert Rev Neurother* 9(1): 109-136, 2009.

Proudfoot JG et al: What happens after diagnosis? Understanding the experiences of patients of newly-diagnosed bipolar disorder, *Health Expect* 12(2):120-129, 2009.

Sanches M et al: Neurodevelopmental basis of bipolar disorder: a critical appraisal, *Prog Neuropsychopharmacol Biol Psychiatry* 32(7):1617-1627, 2008.

Soreca I et al: The phenomenology of bipolar disorder: what drives the high rate of medical burden and determines long-term prognosis? *Depress Anxiety* 26(1):73-82, 2009.

Wingo AP et al: Neurocognitive impairment in bipolar disorder patients: functional implications, *Bipolar Disord* 11(2):113-125, 2009.

AUTHOR: **VICTOR I. REUS, M.D.**

BASIC INFORMATION

DEFINITION

A bite wound can be animal or human, accidental or intentional.

ICD-9CM CODES

879.8 Bite wound, unspecified site

EPIDEMIOLOGY & DEMOGRAPHICS

- Bite wounds account for 1% of emergency department visits.
- More than 1 million bites occur in human beings annually in the U.S.
- Dog bites account for 85% to 90% of all bites and result in 10 to 20 fatalities yearly in the U.S.; cat bites account for 10% to 20%. The animal typically is owned by the victim.
- Infection rates are highest for cat bites (30% to 50%), followed by human bites (15% to 30%) and dog bites (5%).
- The extremities are involved in 75% of bites.

PHYSICAL FINDINGS & CLINICAL PRESENTATION

- The appearance of the bite wound is variable (e.g., puncture wound, tear, avulsion).
- Cellulitis, lymphangitis, and focal adenopathy may be present in infected bite wounds.
- Patient may have fever and chills.

ETIOLOGY

- Increased risk of infection: human and cat bites, closed-fist injuries, wounds involving joints, puncture wounds, face and lip bites, bites with skull penetration, bites in immunocompromised hosts
- Most frequent infecting organisms:
  1. *Pasteurella* spp.: responsible for majority of infections within 24 hr of dog *(P. canis)* and cat *(P. multocida, P. septica)* bites
  2. *Capnocytophaga canimorsus* (formerly DF-2 bacillus): a gram-negative organism responsible for late infection, usually after dog bites
  3. Gram-negative organisms *(Pseudomonas, Haemophilus)*: often found in human bites
  4. *Streptococcus* spp., *Staphylococcus aureus*
  5. *Eikenella corrodens* in human bites

Dx DIAGNOSIS

DIFFERENTIAL DIAGNOSIS

- Bite from a rabid animal (often the attack is unprovoked)
- Factitious injury

WORKUP

- Determination of the time elapsed since the patient was bitten, status of rabies immunization of the animal, and underlying medical conditions that might predispose the patient to infection (e.g., DM, immunodeficiency)
- Documentation of bite site, notification of appropriate authorities (e.g., police department, animal officer)

LABORATORY TESTS

- Generally not necessary
- Hct if there has been significant blood loss
- Wound cultures (aerobic and anaerobic) if there is evidence of sepsis or victim is immunocompromised; cultures should be obtained before irrigation of the wound but after superficial cleaning

IMAGING STUDIES

Radiographs are indicated when bony penetration is suspected or if there is suspicion of fracture or significant trauma; they are also useful for detecting foreign bodies (when suspected).

Rx TREATMENT

NONPHARMACOLOGIC THERAPY

- Local care with debridement, vigorous cleansing, and saline irrigation of the wound; debridement of devitalized tissue
- High-pressure irrigation to clean bite wound and ensure removal of contaminants (e.g., use saline solution with a 30- to 35-ml syringe equipped with a 20-gauge needle or catheter with tip of syringe placed 2 to 3 cm above the wound)
- Avoid blunt probing of wounds (increased risk of infection)
- If the animal is suspected to be rabid: infiltrate wound edges with 1% procaine hydrochloride, swab wound surface vigorously with cotton swabs and 1% Benz alcuronium solution or other soap, and rinse wound with normal saline

ACUTE GENERAL Rx

- Avoid suturing of hand wounds and any wounds that appear infected
- Puncture wounds should be left open
- Give antirabies therapy and tetanus immune globulin (250 to 500 units IM in limb contralateral to toxoid) and toxoid (adult or child older than 5 yr: 0.5 ml DT given IM, child $<$5 yr 0.5 ml DPT IM) as needed
- Use empiric antibiotic therapy in high-risk wounds (e.g., cat bite, hand bites, face bites, genital area bites, bites with joint or bone penetration, human bites, immunocompromised host): amoxicillin-clavulanate 875 to 1000 mg bid for 7 days or cefuroxime 500 mg bid for 7 days
- In hospitalized patients, IV antibiotics of choice are cefoxitin 1 to 2 g q6h, ampicillin-sulbactam 1.5 to 3 g q6h, ticarcillin-clavulanate 3 g q6h, or ceftriaxone 1 to 2 g q24h
- Penicillin allergy: animal bite (doxycycline or moxifloxacin or trimethoprim/sulfamethoxazole with either clindamycin or metronidazole); human bite (moxifloxacin plus clindamycin trimethoprim/sulfamethoxazole plus metronidazole)
- Prophylactic therapy for persons bitten by others with HIV and hepatitis B (see Section V)

DISPOSITION

- Prognosis is favorable with proper treatment.
- Important prognostic factors are type and depth of wound, which compartments are entered, and pathogenicity of inoculated bacteria.
- Punctures that are difficult to irrigate adequately, carnivore bites over vital structures (arteries, nerves, joints), and tissue crushing that cannot be debrided have a worse prognosis.
- In general, human bites have a higher complication and infection rate than do animal bites.
- Nearly 50% of the anaerobic gram-negative bacilli isolated from human bite wounds may be penicillin resistant and beta-lactamase positive.

REFERRAL

- Hospitalization and IV antibiotic therapy for infected human bites; bites with injury to joints, nerves, or tendons; or any animal bites unresponsive to oral therapy.
- Human bites with tendon involvement should go to operating room for washout.
- In the outpatient setting, bite wounds should be reevaluated within 48 hr to assess for signs of infection.

SUGGESTED READING

Broder J et al: Human bites, *Am J Med* 22:10, 2004.

AUTHOR: **FRED F. FERRI, M.D.**

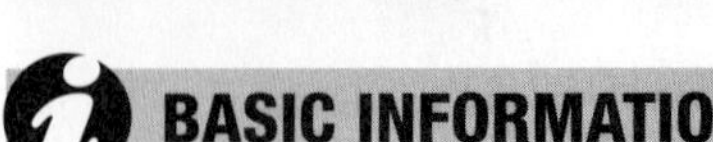

BASIC INFORMATION

DEFINITION

There are two major classes of arthropods: insects and arachnida. This chapter focuses on the class arachnida. Arachnid bites consist of bites caused by:
- Spiders
- Scorpions
- Ticks

ICD-9CM CODES

E905.1 Venomous spiders (black widow spider, brown spider, tarantula)
E905.2 Scorpion
989.5 Bites of venomous snakes, lizards, and spiders; tick paralysis
E906.4 Bite of nonvenomous arthropod; insect bite NOS

EPIDEMIOLOGY & DEMOGRAPHICS

- Spiders—ubiquitous; only three types potentially significantly harmful:
  1. Sydney funnel web spider—Australia
  2. Black widow—worldwide (excluding Alaska)
  3. Brown recluse—most common (South Central U.S.)
- Scorpions—various warm climates: Africa, Central South America, Middle East, India; Texas, New Mexico, California, and Nevada in the U.S.
- Ticks—woodlands

PHYSICAL FINDINGS & CLINICAL PRESENTATION

Spiders:
- Sydney funnel web—natracotoxin toxin
  1. Piloerection, muscle spasms leading to tachycardia, hypertension, increased intracranial pressure, coma
- Black widow—females toxic
  1. Initial reaction: local swelling, redness (two fang marks) leading to local piloerection, edema, urticaria, diaphoresis, lymphangitis
  2. Pain in limb leading to rest of body (chest pain, abdominal pain), compartment syndrome
- Brown recluse
  1. Minor sting or burn.
  2. Wound may become pruritic and red with a blanched center with vesicle. Can necrose, especially in fatty areas. Leaves eschar, which sloughs and leaves ulcer; can take months to heal.
  3. Systemic symptoms: headache, fever, chills, gastrointestinal upset, hemolysis, renal tubular necrosis, disseminated intravascular coagulation possible.

Scorpions:
- Sting leading to sympathetic and parasympathetic stimulation: hypertension, bradycardia, vasoconstriction, pulmonary edema, reduced coronary blood flow, priapism, inhibition of insulin
- Also possible: tachycardia, arrhythmia, vasodilation, bronchial relaxation, excessive salivation, vomiting, sweating, bronchoconstriction, pancreatitis.
- Clinically significant scorpion envenomation by Centruroides sculpturatus produces a severe neuromotor syndrome and respiratory insufficiency that often requires ICU admission.

Ticks: U.S., Europe, Asia
- Very small (<1 mm). Must be attached >36 hr to transmit disease.
- Lyme disease—most common
  1. Early: erythema migrans in 60% to 80% of cases
  2. 7 to 10 days: mild to moderate constitutional symptoms—disseminated—secondary skin lesions, fever, adenopathy, constitutional symptoms, facial palsy, peripheral neuropathy, lymphocytic meningitis, meningoencephalitis, cardiac manifestations (heart block)
  3. Late: chronic arthritis, dermatitis, neuropathy, keratitis

Dx DIAGNOSIS

DIFFERENTIAL DIAGNOSIS

- Cellulitis
- Urticaria

Other tick-borne illnesses:
- Babesiosis
- Tick-borne relapsing fever
- Tularemia
- Rocky Mountain spotted fever
- Ehrlichiosis
- Colorado tick fever
- Tick paralysis
- Community-acquired cutaneous methicillin-resistant *Staphylococcus aureus*

WORKUP

Physical examination: thorough skin examination may reveal fang marks, attached ticks, black eschar.

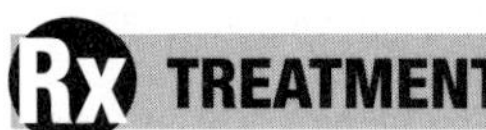

TREATMENT

ACUTE GENERAL Rx

Spiders:
- Sydney funnel web
  1. Pressure, immediate immobilization, supportive care, antivenin
- Black widow
  1. Treatment based on severity of symptoms; bite is rarely fatal.
  2. All should receive oxygen, IV, cardiac monitor, tetanus prophylaxis.
  3. Symptomatic/supportive therapy.
  4. 10% calcium gluconate for muscle cramps (controversial).
  5. Antivenin only for more severe reactions; it carries a risk of anaphylaxis.
     - Dose: one vial in 100 ml 0.9% saline over 20 to 30 min.
     - Skin test before use.
     - Give antihistamines with use.
- Brown recluse
  1. Pain management, tetanus, supportive treatment
  2. No consensus regarding best treatment; some evidence for hyperbaric oxygen

Scorpions:
- Fluids, supportive care, species-specific antivenin (equine based, risk of serum sickness) is controversial.
- IV administration of scorpion-specific F(ab')2 antivenom has been reported effective in resolving the clinical syndrome within 4 hours and reducing the need for concomitant sedation with midazolam and reducing the levels of circulating unbound venom.

Ticks:
- Prophylactic: tick >36 hr: single dose of doxycycline 200 mg
- Early localized disease
  1. Treatment of choice in children: amoxicillin for 14 days.
  2. Doxycycline preferred in patients with possible concurrent ehrlichiosis.
  3. Early disseminated: treatment depends on manifestation.
  4. Late disease: may require longer term or IV therapy; controversial for neurologic disease (see chapter on Lyme disease).

DISPOSITION

- For patients with systemic reactions, send home with emergency epinephrine kit.
- If severe or anaphylactic reaction, admit and observe for 48 hr for cardiac, renal, or neurologic problems.

REFERRAL

For patients with systemic reactions, refer to allergist for immunotherapy; 95% to 98% effective in preventing anaphylaxis.

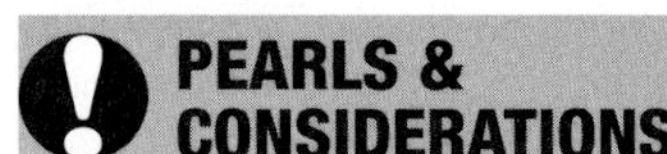

PEARLS & CONSIDERATIONS

Identification of spider should not be based on patient history (many lookalikes); spider should be brought to medical facility to be identified. Bedbugs becoming more prevalent, repeated exposure increases severity of reaction.

SUGGESTED READINGS

Boyer LV et al: Antivenom for critically ill children with neurotoxicity from scorpion stings, *N Engl J Med* 360:2090-2098, 2009.

Diaz JH, LeBlanc KE: Common spider bites, *Am Fam Physician* 75:869-873, 2007.

AUTHOR: **GAIL M. O'BRIEN, M.D.**

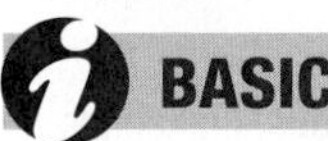

BASIC INFORMATION

DEFINITION

Most stinging insects belong to the Hymenoptera order and include yellow jackets (most common cause of reactions), hornets, bumblebees, sweat bees, wasps, harvester ants, fire ants, and the Africanized honey bee ("killer bee"). Brown recluse spiders, although not insects, are another common cause of bites (see Bites and Stings, Arachnids). The usual effect of a sting is intense local pain, some immediate erythema, and often a small area of edema from the injecting venom. Allergic reactions can be either local or generalized, leading to anaphylactic shock. The majority of reactions occur within the first 6 hr after the sting or bite, but a delayed presentation may occur up to 24 hr.

SYNONYMS Venom allergy

ICD-9CM CODES
989.5 Stings (bees, wasps)
989.5 Bites (fire ant, brown recluse spider)

EPIDEMIOLOGY & DEMOGRAPHICS

PREVALENCE (OF BEE STINGS AND INSECT BITES):

- Unknown.
- From 0.5% to 3.3% of the population is allergic to the venom of one or more stinging insects.
- Most anaphylactic reactions occur during summer months in those most likely to be exposed, including children, males, outdoor workers.
- Approximately half of fatal reactions occur without prior allergic response.
- Bites by fire ants and brown recluse spiders are less likely to cause systemic disease.

INCIDENCE (IN U.S.): Forty to 100 people die each year from insect sting anaphylaxis; anaphylaxis occurs more often within 10 to 30 min of a sting. Delayed reactions are rare, occurring only in <0.3% of stings.

PHYSICAL FINDINGS & CLINICAL PRESENTATION

Stings:

- Cutaneous: the skin is the most common site of an allergic reaction. Manifestations include flushing, urticaria, pruritus, and angioedema.
- Respiratory: hoarseness, difficulty speaking, choking, throat tightness or tingling may progress to stridor, laryngeal edema, laryngospasm, and bronchoconstriction. This is the leading cause of anaphylactic death.
- Cardiovascular: tachycardia, hypotension, and arrhythmia can progress to profound hypovolemic shock. Myocardial infarction is rare. Cardiac manifestations are the second leading cause of death from anaphylaxis.
- Other symptoms: abdominal pain, nausea, vomiting, and diarrhea.

Fire ant bites:

- Initial wheal and flare response.
- Subsequent development of circularly arrayed blisters within 24 hr.
- Blisters may develop appearance of pustules, but they are not infected.

ETIOLOGY

Stings:

- Most systemic reactions to insect stings are classic immunoglobin E (IgE)–mediated reactions.
- Reactions occur in previously sensitized patients who have produced high titers of IgE antibody to insect venom antigens.
- Sensitization to wasp venom requires only a few stings and can occur after a single sting.
- Sensitization to bee venom occurs mainly in people who have been stung frequently by bees.

Bites:

- Fire ant venom contains proteins toxic to the skin.

Dx DIAGNOSIS

DIFFERENTIAL DIAGNOSIS

- Stings: cellulitis, bites
- Bites: stings, cellulitis

WORKUP

History is essential for accurate diagnosis including timing of sting or bite and type of insect (bee, wasp, spider, or ant) if known.

LABORATORY TESTS

- Skin test: either skin prick test or intradermal method with fire ant or hymenoptera venom.
- Venom skin tests and occasionally radioallergosorbent tests (RAST) to provide additional information.

Rx TREATMENT

ACUTE GENERAL Rx

Sting:

- Removal of the stinger most easily performed with a flat tool such as a credit card, followed by cleansing and application of ice.
- Treatment with oral antihistamines and nonsteroidal antiinflammatory medications for limited reactions. Topical corticosteroids may provide some relief of inflammation.
- Patients with previous reactions or multiple stings to the mouth or neck should be evaluated in an emergency department.
- Larger swellings may benefit from oral steroids.
- Generalized reactions should be treated with epinephrine. Antihistamines, oxygen, IV corticosteroids, beta-agonists, pressors, and IV fluids may also be beneficial for anaphylaxis.

Bite:

- Supportive care
- Application of ice
- Surveillance for secondary infection

DISPOSITION

Sting:

- Prognosis for a limited reaction is excellent.
- Subsequent anaphylaxis may occur in 35% to 65% of patients stung again.
- There is no evidence that the next sting will necessarily cause a more severe reaction. The reasons for the variable outcome include patient's age, comorbidities, time elapsed since prior exposure, dose of venom injected, and site of sting.
- Patients with a history of sting allergies should carry syringes preloaded with epinephrine (EpiPen) and oral antihistamines to take if they are stung again.
- Patients should seek additional medical care after using an autoinjector.
- Patients at risk should wear shoes and socks outdoors, remove nests near homes, keep food containers closed, and avoid wearing perfume or flowered print clothing.

Bite:

- Prognosis for fire ant bite is excellent.
- Large lesions from brown recluse spider bites may take months to heal.

REFERRAL

- Consider a referral to an allergist for venom immunotherapy (VIT).
- Risk of subsequent anaphylaxis with immunotherapy falls to <3%.
- VIT for 3 to 5 yr induces long term protection in most patients.

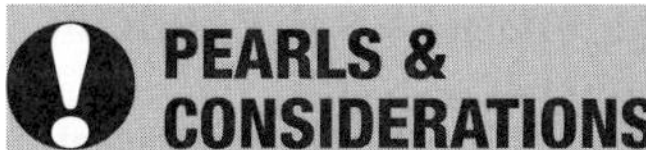

PEARLS & CONSIDERATIONS

Hypersensitivity to stings is common. Reactions range from local nonallergic reaction to venom to life-threatening anaphylaxis. Venom-specific immunotherapy is highly effective in decreasing subsequent reactions.

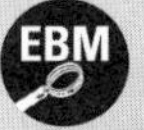

EVIDENCE

VIT can significantly reduce risk of subsequent sting reactions. Patients who would benefit from VIT should undergo immediate hypersensitivity skin tests with stinging insect venoms.

Evidence-Based Reference

Clark S: Multicenter study of emergency department visits for insect sting allergies, *J Allergy Clin Immunol* 116(3):643, 2005.

SUGGESTED READINGS

Annila I: Bee venom allergy, *Clin Exp Allergy* 30(12):1682, 2000.

Bilo B: Epidemiology of insect-venom anaphylaxis, *Curr Opin Allergy Clin Immunol* 8:330-337, 2008.

Freeman TM: Hypersensitivity to hymenoptera stings, *N Engl J Med* 351(19):1978, 2004.

Graft D: Insect sting allergy, *Med Clin North Am* 1(90):211, 2006.

Greco LK: Hymenoptera stings, *Top Emerg Med* 22(2):37, 2000.

Neugut AI et al: Anaphylaxis in the United States: an investigation into its epidemiology, *Arch Intern Med* 161(1):15, 2001.

Weinstein SA et al: Envenomations: an overview of clinical toxinology for the primary care physician, *Am Fam Physician* 80(8):793-802, 2009.

AUTHOR: **JENNIFER JEREMIAH, M.D.**

Bites, Snake (PTG) (ALG)

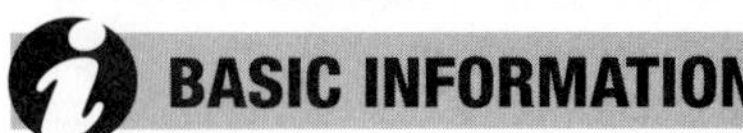

BASIC INFORMATION

DEFINITION

Injury resulting from snake biting a human.

ICD-9CM CODES
989.5 Venomous poisoning

EPIDEMIOLOGY & DEMOGRAPHICS

- 45,000 snakebites occur annually in the U.S. Of the 8000 caused by poisonous snakes, approximately 5 to 12 result in fatality (i.e., $<$ 1% to 2%). Children, the elderly, and those in whom treatment has been delayed are at highest risk.
- In the U.S. at least one species of poisonous snake has been identified in every state except Alaska, Hawaii, and Maine (Fig. 1-40). The majority of venomous snakes are members of the family Crotalidae, which includes rattlesnakes, copperheads, and cottonmouths. The Elapidae family, which includes the coral snake, accounts for the remainder.

PHYSICAL FINDINGS & CLINICAL PRESENTATION

In addition to local tissue injury, envenomation may affect the renal, neurologic, gastrointestinal, vascular, and coagulation systems. Species-specific signs and symptoms include:

CROTALIDAE (PIT VIPERS): Signs and symptoms:

- Fang punctures (see "Diagnosis")
- Pain within 5 min
- Edema within 30 min
- Erythema of site and adjacent tissues/serous or hemorrhagic bullae, ecchymosis and/or lymphangitis over the ensuing hours

If no edema or erythema is manifested within 8 hr after a confirmed Crotalid snakebite, it is safe to assume envenomation did not occur. (Roughly 25% of cases do not involve envenomation.)

Systemic manifestations may include:

- Mild to moderate manifestations: nausea/vomiting, perioral paresthesias, metallic taste, tingling of fingers or toes (especially with rattlesnake bites) and/or fasciculations (local or generalized).
- Severe manifestations: hypotension (due to increased vascular permeability), mental status change, respiratory distress, tachycardia, acute renal failure, rhabdomyolysis, intravascular hemolysis, disseminated intravascular coagulation.

ELAPIDAE (CORAL SNAKES): Signs and symptoms:

- Local symptoms are far less pronounced (little or no pain/swelling immediately after the bite).
- Systemic symptoms predominate, but onset may be delayed for up to 12 hr. Examples include:
    - Cranial nerve palsies featuring ptosis, dysphagia, or dysarthria
    - Tremors
    - Intense salivation
    - Loss of DTRs and respiratory depression (late manifestations)

ETIOLOGY

- The majority of victims are young men who purposefully attempt to handle or harm a snake that formerly had no intention of biting them.
- Victims are frequently intoxicated at the time of the bite.

Dx DIAGNOSIS

DIFFERENTIAL DIAGNOSIS

- Harmless snakebite
- Scorpion bite
- Insect bite
- Cellulitis
- Laceration or puncture wound

NOTE: Harmless snakebites are usually characterized by four rows of small scratches (teeth in upper jaw) separated from two rows of scratches (teeth in lower jaw). This is in distinction to venomous snakebites, which should have puncture wounds produced by the snake's fangs, whether other teeth marks are noted.

FIGURE 1-40 Comparison of pit vipers and nonvenomous snakes. Rattle in **D** (top panel) applies to rattlesnakes only. (**A** to **D**, From Sullivan JB et al: North American venomous reptile bites. In Auerbach PS [ed]: *Wilderness medicine: management of wilderness and environmental emergencies,* ed 3, p. 684, St Louis, 1995, Mosby.)

WORKUP

An estimated 25% of venomous snakebites do not result in envenomation, but observation is critical in all suspected cases:

- Clinical and laboratory evaluation are used to assess the severity of envenomation.
- A nonstandardized classification system for grading envenomations was developed by Russell in 1964:
    - Minimal: confined to the site of the bite, no significant systemic symptoms or signs, no laboratory abnormalities
    - Moderate: manifestations extend beyond the site of the bite, but no life-threatening systemic symptoms
    - Severe: extensive limb involvement, severe systemic symptoms and signs, or significant laboratory abnormalities (including abnormal coagulation studies)

Determination of severity is based on the most severe symptom, sign, or laboratory result. Continual reassessment is indicated throughout the observation period because grading may change.

LABORATORY TESTS

- For all suspected envenomations, obtain CBC (with peripheral smear and platelet count), DIC screen (PT/INR, PTT, fibrinogen, fibrin degradation products, D-dimer), ECG, serum electrolytes, BUN, Cr, and urinalysis.
- For more severe bites, consider LFTs, sedimentation rate, creatine kinase (r/o rhabdomyolysis), ABG, and type and cross-match.
- Other: consider CXR in cases with severe envenomation or in patients $>$40 yr with underlying cardiopulmonary disease; x-ray of bite site for retained fangs (poor sensitivity); head CT if concern is raised for intracranial hemorrhage.

Rx TREATMENT

ACUTE GENERAL Rx

IN THE FIELD: For a suspected snakebite:

- Immobilize affected part below level of the heart.
- Remove any constricting items. Local pressure has been advocated for elapid bites, particularly in Australia, as a means of delaying absorption of neurotoxins. However, crotalid bites are far more common in the U.S., and these frequently have tissue-necrosing venom, which will yield more damage with local pressure. Thus, as with incision and suction techniques, use by those without specialized training in snakebite management is discouraged.
- *Do not* apply ice; keep victim warm.
- Avoid alcohol, stimulants (caffeine), or agents that can suppress mental status.
- Transport immediately to nearest medical facility and contact poison control center.

IN THE HOSPITAL:

- Establish intravenous access.
- Initiate reconstitution of appropriate antivenom. (Antivenoms are typically supplied in

- Indwelling catheters
- Bladder diverticula

Miscellaneous causes:
- Phenacetin abuse
- Cyclophosphamide
- Pelvic irradiation
- Tuberculosis

Adenocarcinomas are associated with:
- Exstrophy
- Endometriosis
- Neurogenic bladder
- Urachal abnormalities
- As a secondary site for distant metastases from other organs (e.g., colon cancer)

Dx DIAGNOSIS

- History and physical examination.
- Urinalysis.
- Cystoscopy with bladder barbotage and biopsy. Fluorescence cystoscopy offers improvement in the detection of flat neoplastic lesions such as carcinoma in situ.
- Transurethral resection of bladder tumor(s).
- There is insufficient evidence to determine whether a decrease in mortality rate from bladder cancer occurs with hematuria testing, urinary cytology, or a variety of other tests on exfoliated urinary cells or other substances.
- In addition to urinary cytology and bladder barbotage, BTA, NMP22, and fibrin degradation products have been approved by the FDA as bladder cancer tumor markers. No marker has general, widespread acceptance because the results are affected by the presence of stents, recent urologic manipulation, stones, infection, bowel interposition, and prostatitis, creating false-positive results.

DIFFERENTIAL DIAGNOSIS

- Urinary tract infection
- Frequency-urgency syndrome
- Interstitial cystitis
- Stone disease
- Endometriosis
- Neurogenic bladder

LABORATORY TESTS

- Urine cytology.
- Urine telomerase: telomerase activity in voided urine or bladder washings determined by the telomeric repeat amplification protocol (TRAP) assay. This test has been reported to accurately detect the presence of bladder tumors in men. It represents a potentially useful noninvasive diagnostic innovation for bladder cancer detection in high-risk groups such as habitual smokers or in symptomatic patients.

RADIOLOGIC TESTS:
- IVP, renal ultrasound, retrograde pyelography, CT scan, and MRI.
- One or a combination of studies can be used. In the absence of skeletal symptoms, bone scan is not recommended.

Rx TREATMENT

NONPHARMACOLOGIC THERAPY

- Initially, transurethral resection of bladder tumor (TURBT)
- Loop biopsy of the prostatic urethra if high-grade TCCa is suspected
- If superficial disease, follow-up protocol with repeat TURBT and/or the use of intravesical agents is recommended
- For advanced bladder cancer, radical cystectomy with urethrectomy (unless orthotopic diversion is planned) and either ileal loop conduit or orthotopic diversion

BLADDER PRESERVATION APPROACHES: After cystectomy for muscle invasive disease, 50% or more of the patients will develop metastases. Most patients develop metastases at distant sites, a third relapse locally. Bladder preservation management is offered in individuals who refuse surgery or who might not be suitable radical cystectomy patients. Bladder-sparing protocols include extensive TURBT or partial cystectomy with external-beam or interstitial radiotherapy and systemic chemotherapy. Radiotherapy as a single treatment modality is not effective. The best predictor of successful bladder preservation is a complete response after the combination of initial TURBT and two cycles of CMV (cisplatin, methotrexate, vinblastine) chemotherapy used with stages T_2 to T_{3a}.

INDICATIONS FOR PARTIAL CYSTECTOMY:
- Tumor within a bladder diverticulum
- Solitary, primary, and muscle-invasive or high-grade lesion of a region of the bladder that allows complete excision with adequate surgical margins
- Inability to adequately resect tumor by TURBT alone because of size or location
- Tumor overlying a ureteral orifice requiring ureteral reimplantation
- Biopsy of a radiation-induced ulceration
- Palliation of severe local symptoms
- Patient refusal of urinary diversion
- Poor-risk patient who is not a diversion candidate

CONTRAINDICATIONS:
- Multiple tumors
- CIS
- Cellular atypia on biopsy
- Prostatic invasion
- Invasion of the trigone
- Inability to achieve adequate surgical margins
- Prior radiotherapy
- Inability to maintain adequate bladder volume after resection
- Evidence of extravesical tumor extension
- Poor surgical risk

ACUTE GENERAL Rx

INDICATIONS FOR INTRAVESICAL CHEMOTHERAPY:
- High-grade tumor
- Tumor size >5 cm
- Tumor multiplicity
- Presence of CIS
- Positive urinary cytologic findings after a resection
- Incomplete tumor resection

Intravesical agents: thiotepa, Adriamycin, mitomycin C, AD-32, BCG, interferon, bropirimine, Epodyl, interleukin-2, and keyhole-limpet hemocyanin. Photodynamic therapy with hematoporphyrin derivatives has also been used.

INDICATIONS FOR CYSTECTOMY:
- Large tumors not amenable to complete TURBT
- High-grade tumor
- Multiple tumors with frequent recurrences
- Diffuse CIS not responsive to intravesical chemotherapy
- Prostatic urethra involvement
- Irritative bladder symptoms with upper tract deterioration
- Muscle-invasive disease
- Disease outside the bladder

SYSTEMIC CHEMOTHERAPY: Used as neoadjuvant and adjuvant therapy for systemic disease. The most effective agents are cisplatin, methotrexate, vinblastine, Adriamycin (MVAC). Other agents include mitoxantrone, vincristine, etoposide (VP16), 5-fluoruracil, ifosfamide, Taxol, gemcitabine, Piritrexim, and gallium nitrate. Chemotherapy in combination can provide palliation and modest survival benefit.

RADIOTHERAPY: Conflicting reports suggest that superficial bladder cancer is more sensitive to radiotherapy. Squamous changes within the tumor and secretion of human chorionic gonadotropin by the lesion are associated with poor response to radiotherapy. Only 20% to 30% of patients with invasive bladder cancer can be cured by external-beam radiation therapy alone. It is used in combination with surgery or with systemic agents to treat bladder cancer primarily in patients who are not surgical candidates or who refuse surgery.

CHRONIC Rx

FOLLOW-UP RECOMMENDATIONS FOR SUPERFICIAL BLADDER CANCER:
- Cystoscopy, bladder barbotage, and bimanual examination every 3 mo for 2 yr, then every 6 mo for 2 yr, and annually thereafter.
- Upper tract studies are based on the risk of upper tract tumor development, generally every 2 to 5 yr.

FOLLOW-UP RECOMMENDATIONS FOR ADVANCED DISEASE: Bladder preservation:
- Cystoscopy, barbotage, bimanual examination, biopsy (when indicated), every 3 mo for 2 yr, then every 6 mo for 2 yr, yearly thereafter
- CT scan of abdomen and pelvis every 6 mo for 2 yr in addition to chest x-ray examination, liver function testing, and serum creatinine

Cystectomy with ileal loop/orthotopic bladde
- Neobladder endoscopy and IVP yearly
- CT scan of abdomen and pelvis every for 2 yr in addition to chest x-ray ex tion, liver function tests, and serum nine
- Loopogram every 6 mo for 2 yr, th ally

powder form and must be reconstituted before administration. The process can take up to 1 hr, so it is recommended that it be initiated as soon as the patient arrives in the ED). While this is being done:
- Obtain time of bite and description of snake if possible.
- Obtain past medical history; ask about allergies to horse serum in those previously treated for snake bite.
- Record vital signs: BP, HR, T, RR.
- Inspect site of bite for fang marks, local symptoms.
- Delineate margins of erythema/edema with a marker.
- Measure circumference of bitten part at two or more proximal sites and compare with unaffected limb; repeat every 15 to 20 min; assess for extension of erythema/edema.
- Neurologic examination.
- Gauge the severity of the bite and decide whether administration of antivenom is necessary.
- For minimal envenomation without progressive manifestations:
  1. Clean and immobilize affected part.
  2. Immunize against tetanus.
  3. Observe patient for at least 8 hr. If, at the end of this interval, local and systemic sequelae are absent and lab values remain normal, the likelihood of significant envenomation is low, and the patient can be discharged from the acute setting.
- Patients who have progressive symptoms (local or systemic) or moderate to severe envenomation should be considered for antivenom. The high incidence of allergic reactions argues against its use in less severe cases.
- Since the introduction of antivenoms in the U.S. in the 1950s, mortality rates from snakebites have dropped from as high as 25% (when no treatment was available) to 0.5% in patients who receive timely administration of antivenom.
- Antivenom is most effective when given within 4 hr of the bite and least effective if delayed beyond 12 hr. Systemic symptoms (coagulopathy, CNS effects, etc.) respond better to treatment than local symptoms (erythema/edema, bullae, etc.).
- It is recommended that patients be monitored in an ICU setting during administration of antivenom.

Once the decision is made to use antivenom:
- Prepare epinephrine 0.5 to 1.0 ml of a 0.1% solution to be administered in case of a hypersensitivity reaction to the antivenom. (Prophylactic antihistamines are not efficacious.)

TREATMENT OF CROTALID (PIT VIPER) BITES WITH SHEEP IMMUNOGLOBULIN–BASED ANTIVENOM:
- Most centers now have sheep immunoglobulin-based antivenom (Crofab) for crotalid bites. (A potent, safe, sheep-based antivenom for elapid bites exists but is not yet approved in the U.S.) Sheep-based antivenoms are very safe, but repeat administration may be necessary owing to a short half-life. An initial IV loading dose of 4 to 6 vials (depending on the size and age of the patient and the severity of the bite) is infused over 60 min. If the patient has not responded after 1 hr, a repeat dose of 4 to 6 vials is indicated.
- Because of the short half-life of sheep-based antivenom, relapse may occur in up to two thirds of patients after an initial response. Consequently, it is recommended that three maintenance doses—each consisting of 2 vials—be given at 6, 12, and 18 hours following the patient's initial response to the loading dose.
- Help in using the antivenom is available 24/7 by calling (877) 377-3784.

TREATMENT OF CROTALID (PIT VIPER) OR ELAPID (CORAL SNAKE) BITES WITH HORSE SERUM–BASED ANTIVENOM:
- Horse serum–based antivenoms were previously available for both crotalid and elapid (coral snake) bites, but are being phased out due to much higher risk of hypersensitivity reactions such as anaphylaxis and serum sickness. (Skin testing is available, but it is not recommended because it is not completely reliable and may delay time to administration beyond the most effective period.) For treatment considerations, see "Complications." Wyeth stopped distributing horse serum–based crotalid antivenom in 2007, but unexpired stock is still available for cases where sheep serum–based antivenom is not available. Guidelines to dosage of horse serum–based antivenom are as follows:
- For pit viper bites
  - Mild 5 vials
  - Moderate 10 vials
  - Severe 15 vials
  - Shock 20 vials
- Production of horse serum–based coral snake antivenom was discontinued in 2006. All stock is expired as of October 31, 2008, except for lot 4030026, which received a one-year extension until October 31, 2009. After that date, one option will be to seek compassionate release of expired stock in conjunction with your local poison control center. Prior experience suggests that translucent samples are more likely to have retained potency than cloudy samples. Another option is to contact a zoo that cares for exotic snakes and obtain Mexican coral snake or Australian Tiger snake antivenom, although efficacy for North American coral snake envenomation is unproven.
- For confirmed coral snake bites, antivenom should be administered immediately if available. If coral snake bite is only suspected, the patient should be monitored for 12 hr for evidence of envenomation, and treated if it occurs.
- If there are no systemic symptoms at the time of administration, start with 3 vials. If symptoms evolve, repeat with 5 vials.
- If systemic symptoms are already present, an initial dose of 6 to 10 vials is recommended.

TREATMENT OF NONNATIVE (EXOTIC) SNAKE BITES:
- For bites by exotic or nonnative snakes, contact a poison control center or your local zoo. (Zoos with exotic snakes are required to maintain a supply of snake-specific antivenom on their premises.)

Other considerations:
- Initial dose of antivenom should be repeated until progression of symptoms has abated, but observation of bitten part should be continued for another 48 hr.
- Dosage of antivenom is based on typical envenomation rather than age or weight, so dose is the same for children and adults.
- Pregnancy is not a contraindication to antivenom.
- Immunize against tetanus if no booster within past 5 yr; if never immunized, give immunoglobulin as well as toxoid.
- Manage pain as needed (acetaminophen, codeine, meperidine).
- Avoid sedation in Mojave rattlesnake, eastern diamondback rattlesnake, and coral snake bites.
- Antibiotics reserved for moderate to severe contamination or definite infection; broad-spectrum coverage to include gram negatives preferred (i.e., amp-sulbactam or quinolone derivatives).

DISPOSITION

Prognosis is good with prompt evaluation and treatment.

REFERRAL

To medical facility with ICU for administration of antivenom

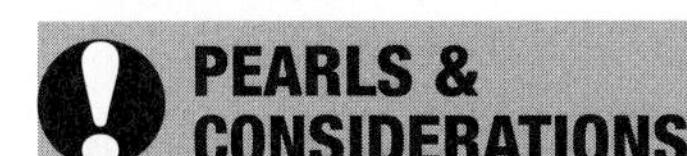

PEARLS & CONSIDERATIONS

COMPLICATIONS

Most frequent complication of treated envenomations is serum sickness; occurs 7 to 14 days after antivenom administration and is characterized by fever, rash, arthralgias, and lymphadenopathy. It can be treated with PO prednisone 60 mg/day, tapered over 7 to 10 days. Acutely, there is the risk of anaphylaxis to antivenom as mentioned previously. This occurs within 30 min and is treated with:
- IV epinephrine
- IV diphenhydramine
- IV hydrocortisone

Injuries also result from:
- Tourniquet placement
- Cryotherapy

National poison control hotline: (800) 222-1222

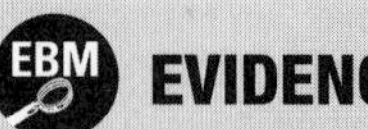

EVIDENCE

There are no controlled trials of postexposure tetanus vaccination versus placebo in circumstances where vaccination is appropriate but a consensus opinion that vaccination should be given. Ⓒ

Evidence-Based Reference

Centers for Disease Control and Prevention. Recommended adult immunization schedule, *MMWR* 55(40):Q1-4, 2006. Ⓒ

SUGGESTED READINGS

Cheng AC: Snake bite management in the United States, *Up To Date Online*, May 2009.

Dart RC: Efficacy, safety and use of snake antivenoms in the United States, *Ann Emerg Med* 37:181-188, 2001.

Gold BS et al: Bites of venomous snakes, *N Engl J Med* 347:347, 2002.

Juckett G, Honcox JG: Venomous snakebites in the United States: management review and update, *Am Fam Physician* 65:1367, 2002.

LoVecchio F et al: Antibiotics after rattlesnake envenomation, *J Emerg Med* 23:327-328, 2002.

The Medical Letter: a new snake antivenom, *Med Lett Drugs Ther* 43:55, 2001.

Offerman SR et al: Crotaline Fab antivenom for the treatment of children with rattlesnake envenomation, *Pediatrics* 110:968-971, 2002.

Ries NL, Dart RC: New developments in antidotes, *Med Clin North Am* 89(6):1379, 2005.

Weinstein SA et al: Envenomations: an overview of clinical toxinology for the primary care physician, *Am Fam Physician* 80(8):793-802, 2009.

AUTHORS: **JACK L. SCHWARTZWALD, M.D.,** and **REBECCA A. GRIFFITH, M.D.**

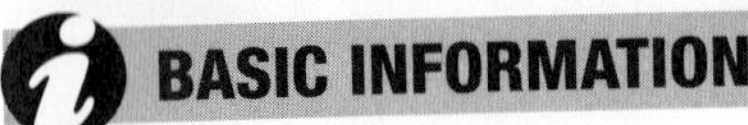

BASIC INFORMATION

DEFINITION

Bladder cancer is a heterogeneous spectrum of neoplasms ranging from non–life-threatening, low-grade, superficial papillary lesions to high-grade invasive tumors, which often have metastasized at the time of presentation. It is a field change disease in which the entire urothelium from the renal pelvis to the urethra may be susceptible to malignant transformation. The three types of bladder cancer are transitional cell carcinoma (TCCa), squamous cell carcinoma, and adenocarcinoma.

ICD-9CM CODES	
Primary:	188.9
Secondary:	198.1
CIS:	233.7
Benign:	223.3
Uncertain behavior:	236.7
Unspecified:	239.4

EPIDEMIOLOGY & DEMOGRAPHICS

Each year approximately 54,000 new cases are diagnosed and more than 12,000 deaths are attributed to bladder cancer. Overall, bladder cancer is the sixth most prevalent malignancy in the U.S.

Until 1990, the incidence of bladder cancer in the U.S. was rising. Since 1990, the incidence of bladder cancer is decreasing at a rate of 0.8% per year (1.2% among men and 0.4% among women).

PREDOMINANT SEX: In males, it is the fourth most common cancer, accounting for 10% of all cancers. In females, it is the eighth most common cancer, accounting for 4% of all cancers.

RISK: The lifetime risk of developing bladder cancer is 2.8% in white males, 0.9% in black males, 1% in white females, and 0.6% in black females.

Smoking:
- Users of "black" tobacco in place of "blond" tobacco have a twofold to threefold increase in developing bladder cancer.
- Smoking risk is based on consumption:
  - A twofold to threefold increase for subjects smoking at least 10 cigarettes per day
  - The risk increases again when the daily consumption rises above 40 to 60 cigarettes per day
- Smokers of low-tar and nicotine cigarettes have a lower risk when compared with higher tar and nicotine cigarettes.
- Those who smoke unfiltered cigarettes have a 50% increased risk of bladder cancer compared with those who smoke filtered cigarettes.
- Pipe smokers have a lower risk of bladder cancer compared with cigarette smokers.
- Cigars, snuff, and chewing tobacco, although implicated in nonurologic cancers, are not believed to influence bladder cancer risk.

Diet:
- Diets rich in beef, pork, and animal fat increase risk of bladder cancer.
- There is no indication that consumption of non-beer alcoholic drinks contributes to bladder cancer development.
- Beer consumption has been linked to bladder cancer development as a result of the presence of nitrosamines in the beer. Nitrosamines have also been implicated in the development of rectal cancer.
- Drinking coffee is not believed to contribute to bladder cancer risk. There is additional evidence that coffee consumption is protective for colorectal cancers, possibly by diminishing fecal transit time.

PEAK INCIDENCE: Incidence increases with age: higher after age 60 yr, uncommon younger than 40 yr.

GENETICS: It is thought to be multifactorial in etiology, involving both genetic and environmental interactions. Overall, approximately 20% to 25% of the male population in the U.S. with bladder cancer is estimated to have the disease as a result of occupational exposure.

DISTRIBUTION: In North America, transitional cell carcinomas comprise 93%, squamous cell carcinomas comprise 6%, and adenocarcinomas account for 1% of bladder cancers.

PATHOGENESIS: Two pathways exist for bladder cancer (TCCa):
1. Papillary superficial disease occasionally leading to invasive cancer (75%)
2. Carcinoma-in-situ (CIS) and solid invasive cancer with high risk of disease progression (25%)

Two distinct forms of "superficial cancer" exist:
1. T_a: Papillary low-grade tumor with a high rate of recurrence; disease progression occurs in 5%.
2. T_1: Higher grade papillary tumor that infiltrates the lamina propria; often associated with flat CIS that may involve the urothelium diffusely. Disease progression occurs in 30% to 50%.

Subdivided into:
- T_{1a}: Penetration of tumor up to the muscularis mucosa; disease progression in 5.3%
- T_{1b}: Penetration of tumor through the muscularis mucosa; disease progression 53%

Flat CIS:
- Entirely different and separate pathway of cancer development whose mechanism is manifested by dysplasia, which leads to the occurrence of poorly differentiated malignant cells that replace or undermine the normal urothelium and extend along the plane of the bladder wall. It penetrates the basement membrane and lamina propria in 20% to 30% of cases and is associated with the development of solid tumor growth. A defect in chromosome 17p53 occurs in 50% of the cases.

At presentation, 72% of cancers are localized to the bladder, 20% of the cancers extend to the regional lymph nodes, and 3% present with distant metastases. Eighty percent of superficial TCCa recur, with up to 30% progressing to a higher stage or grade. Younger patients most commonly develop low-grade papillary noninvasive TCCa and are less likely to have recurrences when compared with older patients with similar lesions. Involvement of the with tumor occurs in 25% to 50% o

STAGING (BASED ON THE TNM SYS

T_0	No tumor in specimen
T_{is}	CIS
T_a	Papillary TCCa noninvasive
T_1	Papillary TCCa into lamina prop
T_2	TCCa invasive of superficial mus
T_{3a}	Invasive of deep muscle
T_{3b}	Invasive of perivesical fat
T_{4a}	Invasive of adjacent pelvic organ
T_{4b}	Invasive of pelvic wall with fixation

Invasive of nodal status:

N_0	No nodal involvement
N_{1-3}	Pelvic nodes
N_4	Nodes above bifurcation
N_x	Unknown

Invasive of metastatic status:

M_0	No distant metastases
M_1	Distant metastases
M_x	Unknown

MOLECULAR EPIDEMIOLOGY: TCCa is usually a field change disease with tumors arising at different times and sites in the urothelium, suggesting a polyclonal etiology of bladder cancer. Bladder cancers have been associated with abnormalities on chromosomes 1, 4, 11, 5, 7, 3, 9, 21, 18, 13, 8; with alterations in suppressor genes *P53*, retinoblastoma gene, and *P16;* and with alterations in oncogenes H-ras and epidermal growth factor receptor.

PHYSICAL FINDINGS & CLINICAL PRESENTATION

- Gross, painless hematuria
- Microhematuria
- Frequency, urgency, occasional dysuria

With locally invasive to distant metastatic disease, the presentation can include:
- Abdominal pain
- Flank pain
- Lymphedema
- Renal failure
- Anorexia
- Bone pain

ETIOLOGY

Bladder cancer is a potentially preventable disease associated with specific etiologic factors:
- Cigarette smoking is associated with 25% to 65% of cases. The risk of developing a TCCa is two to four times higher in smokers than in nonsmokers, and that risk persists for many years, being equal to nonsmokers only after 12 to 15 yr of smoking abstinence. Smoking tobacco is associated with tumors that are characterized by higher histologic grade, increased tumor stage, increase in the numbers of tumor present, and increased tumor size.
- Occupational exposures: dye workers, textile workers, tire and rubber workers, petroleum workers.
- Chemical exposure: O-toluidine, 2-naphthylamine, benzidine, 4-amino-biphenyl, and nitrosamines.
- Exposure to herpes papilloma virus type 16.

Squamous carcinomas are associated with:
- Schistosomiasis
- Urinary calculi

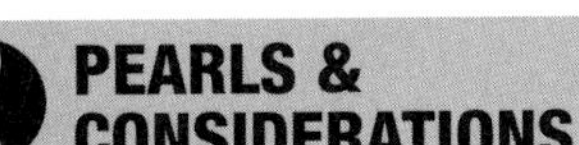

PEARLS & CONSIDERATIONS

COMMENTS

- The most useful prognostic parameters for bladder tumor recurrence and subsequent cancer progression are tumor grade, depth of tumor penetration, multifocal tumors, frequency of recurrence, tumor size, CIS, lymphatic invasion, papillary or solid tumor configuration.
- Box 1-2 describes the American Urological Association Guideline Recommendations for bladder cancer.

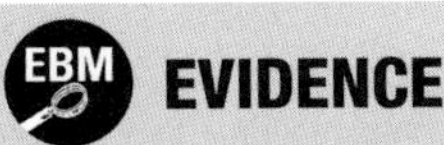

EVIDENCE

Superficial bladder tumors:

Although randomized controlled trials are lacking, the use of TURBT in the treatment of bladder cancer is endorsed by expert opinion.

Guidelines from the National Comprehensive Cancer Network Panel on Bladder Cancer include the following statements regarding TURBT in the treatment of non-muscle-invasive bladder cancer:

- Transurethral resection without intravesical therapy is the standard treatment for Ta, G1 and Ta, G2 tumors.[1] Ⓒ
- Primary Tis is a high-grade lesion that is believed to be a precursor of invasive bladder cancer. Standard therapy for this lesion is a complete endoscopic resection, followed by intravesical therapy with BCG.[1] Ⓒ
- If progression to an invasive lesion is documented at any point during follow-up, a radical cystectomy is recommended.[1] Ⓒ
- T1 lesions, those invading lamina propria, are considered to be potentially dangerous (usually T1, G2 or T1, G3) and have a high risk for recurrence and progression. These tumors may occur as solitary lesions or as multifocal tumors with or without an associated in situ component. These are also treated with a complete endoscopic resection followed by intravesical therapy (this is optional for G1 or G2 lesions).[1] Ⓒ

The use of intravesical therapy following TURBT is effective in reducing recurrence of Ta and T1 bladder cancer. Data suggests that bacillus Camlette-Guérin (BCG) is superior to mitomycin as intravesical therapy

- However, sub-group analyses of systematic reviews have found that BCG is superior to mitomycin as intravesical therapy to reduce tumor recurrence only in those studies where BCG maintenance therapy was used.[2]

Muscle-invasive bladder tumors:

Although randomized controlled trials are lacking, the use of radical cystectomy as the primary treatment for muscle-invasive bladder cancer is endorsed by expert opinion.

Guidelines from the National Comprehensive Cancer Network panel on bladder cancer include the following statements regarding radical cystectomy in the surgical treatment of muscle-invasive disease:

- Surgical treatment with radical cystectomy is still the most effective local therapy in muscle-invasive bladder cancer. The appropriate surgical procedure involves a cystoprostatectomy in men and, in women, a cystectomy and usually a hysterectomy, followed by the formation of a urinary diversion.[1] Ⓒ
- Primary surgical treatment for T2 lesions include radical cystectomy with the consideration of neoadjuvant chemotherapy, and segmental cystectomy only in patients with a single tumor (solitary lesion in a suitable location) and no any presence of CIS, or previous multifocal bladder cancers.[1] Ⓒ
- For non-organ confined disease primary surgical treatment for a tumor that extends beyond the confines of the bladder wall and is still considered resectable, based on the mobility of the bladder, is radical cystectomy with consideration of neoadjuvant chemotherapy.[1] Ⓒ

Data from retrospective studies suggests that overall and recurrence-free survival following radical cystectomy is highly dependant upon pathological stage.

- A recent study collected retrospective and prospective data on 888 consecutive patients with bladder transitional cell carcinoma treated by radical cystectomy and pelvic lymphadenectomy in the U.S. This study reported that, at 5 years, 58% of patients were recurrence-free. Patients with organ-confined disease had a lower risk of for bladder cancer recurrence and death compared with patients with extravesical tumor extension who in turn fared better than patients with loco-regional lymph node metastases.[3] Ⓑ

Data from RCTs and meta-analyses have found that cisplatin-based neoadjuvant chemotherapy improves overall survival in patients with invasive bladder cancer.

- A Cochrane review and related systematic reviews identified 11 RCTs comparing neoadjuvant chemotherapy plus definitive treatment vs definitive treatment alone in-

BOX 1-2 American Urological Association Guideline Recommendations

For all index patients:
- Standard: Physicians should discuss with the patient the treatment options and the benefits and harms, including side effects, of intravesical treatment.

For a patient who presents with an abnormal growth on the urothelium but who has not yet been diagnosed with bladder cancer:
- Standard: If the patient does not have an established histologic diagnosis, a biopsy should be obtained for pathologic analysis.
- Standard: Under most circumstances, complete eradication of all visible tumors should be performed.
- Standard: If bladder cancer is confirmed, periodic surveillance cystoscopy should be performed.
- Option: An initial single dose of intravesical chemotherapy may be administered immediately postoperatively.

For a patient with small volume, low-grade Ta bladder cancer:
- Recommendation: An initial single dose of intravesical chemotherapy may be administered immediately postoperatively.

For a patient with multifocal and/or large volume, histologically confirmed, low-grade Ta or a patient with recurrent low-grade Ta bladder cancer:
- Recommendation: An induction course of intravesical therapy with bacillus Calmette-Guérin or mitomycin C is recommended for the treatment of these patients with the goal of preventing or delaying recurrence.
- Option: Maintenance bacillus Calmette-Guérin or mitomycin C may be considered.

For a patient with initial histologically confirmed high-grade Ta, T1, and/or carcinoma in situ bladder cancer:
- Standard: For patients with lamina propria invasion (T1) but without muscularis propria in the specimen, repeat resection should be performed prior to additional intravesical therapy.
- Recommendation: An induction course of bacillus Calmette-Guérin followed by maintenance therapy is recommended for treatment of these patients.
- Option: Cystectomy should be considered for initial therapy in select patients.

For a patient with high-grade Ta, T1, and/or carcinoma in situ bladder cancer that has recurred after prior intravesical therapy:
- Standard: For patients with lamina propria invasion (T1) but without muscularis propria in the specimen, repeat resection should be performed prior to additional intravesical therapy.
- Recommendation: Cystectomy should be considered as a therapeutic alternative for these patients.
- Option: Further intravesical therapy may be considered for these patients.

From the American Urological Association, Guideline Division, http://www.auanet.org.

volving 3005 patients with invasive (i.e. clinical stage T2-T4a) transitional cell carcinoma of the bladder. This study found that platinum-based combination neoadjuvant chemotherapy significantly improved overall survival, irrespective of local therapy, compared with such therapy alone, with an absolute benefit of 5% improvement in survival and 9% improvement in disease free survival at 5 years.[4,5] Ⓐ

- Another systematic review with meta-analysis of RCTs examined the effect of neoadjuvant chemotherapy on overall survival, and more closely the effect of cisplatin-based combination therapy. This study found that neoadjuvant cisplatin-based chemotherapy resulted in an absolute survival benefit of 6.5% (from 50% to 56.5%).[6] Ⓐ

Data for the use of adjuvant chemotherapy is less robust than that for chemotherapy prior to surgical treatment.

- The role of adjuvant chemotherapy in invasive bladder cancer is unclear because no randomized comparisons of adequate sample size have definitively shown a survival benefit. Limited data suggests that adjuvant chemotherapy can delay recurrences, which may justify the routine administration of chemotherapy in those at a high risk for relapse (nodal involvement, vascular invasion, high grade histology).[1]
- A Cochrane review and related sytematic review analysed individual patient data (491 patients) from six RCTs comparing local treatment plus adjuvant chemotherapy versus the same local treatment alone in the treatment of invasive bladder cancer. Meta-analysis found that the overall hazard ratio for survival was 0.75 suggesing a 25% relative reduction in the risk of death for patients treated with adjuvant chemotherapy. However, the authors commented that at present there is insufficient evidence on which to reliably base treatment decisions regarding the use of adjuvant chemotherapy.[7,8]

Metastatic disease:

For patients with advanced disease the use of chemotherapy improves survival. Historically MVAC has been used, although data suggests that gemcitabine plus cisplatin is equally effective with a better toxicity profile.

- An RCT compared high-dose intensity MVAC with growth factor support vs conventional MVAC in 266 patients with advanced transitional cell cancer. This study found that although median survival was similar between the two regimens, high-dose intensity MVAC was associated with a borderline statistically significant relative reduction in the risk of progression and death compared to conventional M-VAC.[9] Ⓐ
- Follow-up data confirmed that overall and progression-free survival was similar between the two regimens with 5-year overall survival rates of 13% to 15%. The presence of visceral metastases was a significant negative prognostic factor.[10] Ⓐ

Evidence-Based References

1. National Comprehensive Cancer Network: NCCN Clinical Practice Guidelines in Oncology, *Bladder Cancer* 2007. Ⓒ
2. Bohle A, Bock PR: Intravesical bacille Calmette-Guerin versus mitomycin C in superficial bladder cancer: formal meta-analysis of comparative studies on tumor progression, *Urology* 63:682-686, 2004.
3. Shariat SF et al: Outcomes of radical cystectomy for transitional cell carcinoma of the bladder: a contemporary series from the Bladder Cancer Research Consortium, *J Urol* 176(6 Pt 1):2414-2422, 2006. Ⓑ
4. Advanced Bladder Cancer Overview Collaboration: Neoadjuvant chemotherapy for invasive bladder cancer, *Cochrane Rev* (1), 2004. Ⓐ
5. Advanced Bladder Cancer (ABC) Meta-analysis Collaboration: Neoadjuvant chemotherapy in invasive bladder cancer: update of a systematic review and meta-analysis of individual patient data advanced bladder cancer (ABC) meta-analysis collaboration, *Eur Urol* 48:202-205, 2005. Ⓐ
6. Winquist E et al: Genitourinary Cancer Disease Site Group, Cancer Care Ontario Program in Evidence-based Care Practice Guidelines Initiative. Neoadjuvant chemotherapy for transitional cell carcinoma of the bladder: a systematic review and meta-analysis, *J Urol* 171(2 Pt 1):561-569, 2004. Ⓐ
7. Advanced Bladder Cancer (ABC) Meta-analysis Collaboration. Adjuvant chemotherapy for invasive bladder cancer (individual patient data), *Cochrane Rev* (2), 2006.
8. Advanced Bladder Cancer (ABC) Meta-analysis Collaboration. Adjuvant chemotherapy in invasive bladder cancer: a systematic review and meta-analysis of individual patient data Advanced Bladder Cancer (ABC) Meta-analysis Collaboration, *Eur Urol* 48:189-199, 2005.
9. Sternberg CN et al: EORTC Genito-Urinary Cancer Group. Seven year update of an EORTC phase III trial of high-dose intensity M-VAC chemotherapy and G-CSF versus classic M-VAC in advanced urothelial tract tumours, *Eur J Cancer* 42:50-54, 2006. Ⓐ
10. von der Maase H et al: Long-term survival results of a randomized trial comparing gemcitabine plus cisplatin, with methotrexate, vinblastine, doxorubicin, plus cisplatin in patients with bladder cancer, *J Clin Oncol* 23:4602-4608, 2005. Ⓐ

SUGGESTED READINGS

Sanchini MA et al: Relevance of urine telomerase in the diagnosis of bladder cancer, *JAMA* 294:2052, 2005.

Sharma S et al: Diagnosis and treatment of bladder cancer, *Am Fam Physician* 80(7):717-723, 2009.

AUTHORS: **PHILIP J. ALIOTTA, M.D., M.S.H.A.,** and **RUBEN ALVERO, M.D.**

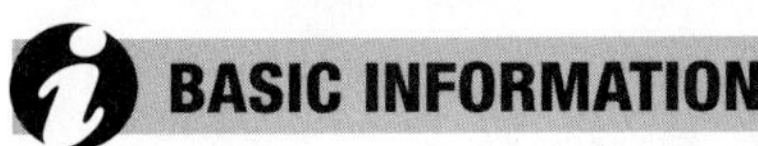

BASIC INFORMATION

DEFINITION

Blastomycosis is a systemic pyogranulomatous disease caused by a dimorphic fungus, *Blastomyces dermatitidis.*

ICD-9CM CODES
116.0 Blastomycosis

EPIDEMIOLOGY & DEMOGRAPHICS

INCIDENCE & PREVALENCE:

- Most patients reside in the southeastern and south central states, especially those bordering the Mississippi and Ohio River valleys, the Midwestern states, and Canadian provinces bordering the Great Lakes.
- Rare cases reported outside the U.S.

RISK FACTORS:

- Widely disseminated disease is most common in immunocompromised hosts, especially those with acquired immunodeficiency syndrome (AIDS).
- Initial infections result from inhalation of conidia into the lungs, although primary cutaneous blastomycosis has been reported after dog bites.

PHYSICAL FINDINGS & CLINICAL PRESENTATION

- Acute infection: <50% symptomatic, median incubation 30 to 45 days. Symptoms are nonspecific: mimic influenza or bacterial infection with abrupt onset of myalgias, arthralgias, chills and fever; transient pleuritic pain, cough that is initially nonproductive. Resolution within 4 wk is usual.
- Chronic or recurrent infection: indolent, progressive; includes pulmonary or extrapulmonary disease.

PULMONARY MANIFESTATIONS: Symptoms and signs of chronic pneumonia: productive cough, hemoptysis, pleuritic chest pain, weight loss, low-grade pyrexia

EXTRAPULMONARY MANIFESTATIONS:

1. Cutaneous: most common; may occur with or without pulmonary disease. Two different lesions:
   - *Verrucous:* beginning as a small papulopustular lesion on exposed body areas that may develop into an eschar with peripheral microabscesses (Fig. 1-41)
   - *Ulcerative:* Subcutaneous nodules (cold abscesses) and rarely cutaneous inoculation blastomycosis may occur
2. Bone and joint: 10% to 50% have osteolytic lesions; affects long bones, vertebrae, and ribs; lesions may present with contiguous soft tissue abscess or draining sinus that spreads to a joint, resulting in pyarthrosis
3. Genitourinary: 10% to 30%; prostatic involvement is most common and may present as obstruction; epididymis and testes may also be affected
4. Central nervous system: 5% normal host; 40% AIDS patients; meningitis and abscess formation

ETIOLOGY

Blastomyces dermatitidis exists in warm, moist soil that is rich in organic material. When these microfoci are disturbed, the aerosolized spores or conidia are inhaled into the lungs. Disease at other sites is a result of dissemination from the initial pulmonary infection; the latter may be acute or chronic.

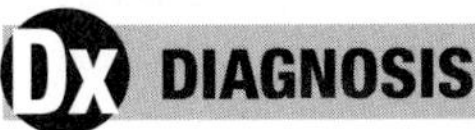

DIAGNOSIS

DIFFERENTIAL DIAGNOSIS

PULMONARY INFECTION:

- Tuberculosis
- Bronchogenic carcinoma
- Histoplasmosis
- Bacterial pneumonia

CUTANEOUS INFECTION:

- Bromoderma
- Pyoderma gangrenosum
- *Mycobacterium marinum* infection
- Squamous cell carcinoma
- Giant keratoacanthoma

WORKUP

- Physical examination and laboratory data
- Definitive diagnosis established by culture

LABORATORY TESTS

- Presumptive diagnosis can be made by visualizing the distinctive yeast forms in clinical specimens
- Culture: on Sabouraud medium or more enriched media
  1. Aspirated material from abscesses
  2. Skin scrapings
  3. Prostatic secretions (urine culture with prostatic massage)
- Direct examination of specimens
  1. Wet preparation with 10% KOH (Fig. 1-42)
  2. Histopathology: typically demonstrates pyogranulomas; yeast identification requires special stains
- A commercial test for *Blastomyces* antigen in specimens of urine, blood, and other fluids is available
- Serologic tests: a negative test cannot exclude blastomycosis, and a positive titer should not be an indication to start treatment

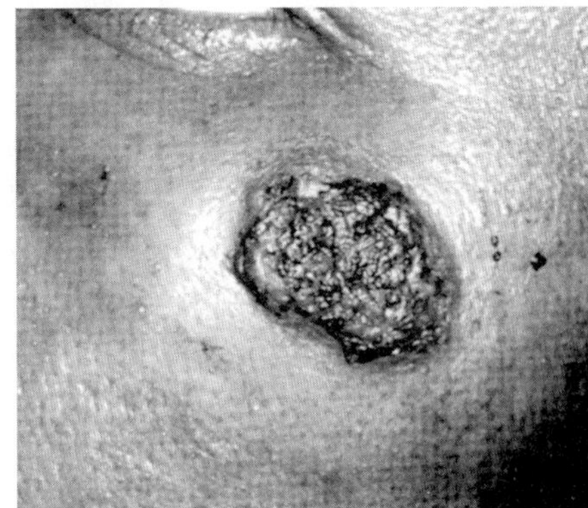

FIGURE 1-41 The typical verrucous skin lesion of blastomycosis on the cheek. Note the circumscribed edges. (From Mandell GL, Bennett JE, Dolin R: *Principles and practice of infectious diseases,* ed 6, Philadelphia, 2005, Elsevier.)

IMAGING STUDIES

In chronic disease, chest radiographic findings are nonspecific, but lobar or segmental alveolar infiltrates, especially of the upper lobes, are most common and may progress to cavitation.

TREATMENT

ACUTE BLASTOMYCOSIS GENERAL Rx

- Treatment remains controversial for acute pulmonary blastomycosis.
- Because the acute form may be benign and self-limited, patients may be closely observed.
- Some patients progress to chronic infection with significant morbidity and therefore may require treatment.
- Patients who are immunocompromised or who have extrapulmonary disease or progressive pulmonary disease should be treated.

PULMONARY BLASTOMYCOSIS

- Amphotericin B (AmB) lipid formulation 3-5 mg/kg/day or AmB deoxycholate at 0.7-1 mg/kg/day for 1-2 wk or until improvement is noted, followed by oral itraconazole 200 mg PO three times a day for 3 days and then 200 mg PO twice a day for a total of 6-12 mo.
- Itraconazole 200 mg PO three times a day for 3 days and then once or twice per day for 6-12 mo for mild to moderate diseases.
- Fluconazole 400-800 mg PO once a day for those intolerant to itraconazole.

DISSEMINATED EXTRAPULMONARY BLASTOMYCOSIS

- Lipid formulation AmB 3-5 mg/kg/day or AmB dexoycholate 0.7-1 mg/kg/day for 1-2 wk or until improvement is noted followed by oral itraconazole 200 mg PO three times a day for 3 days and then 200 mg PO twice a day for a total of at least 12 mo for moderately severe to severe disease

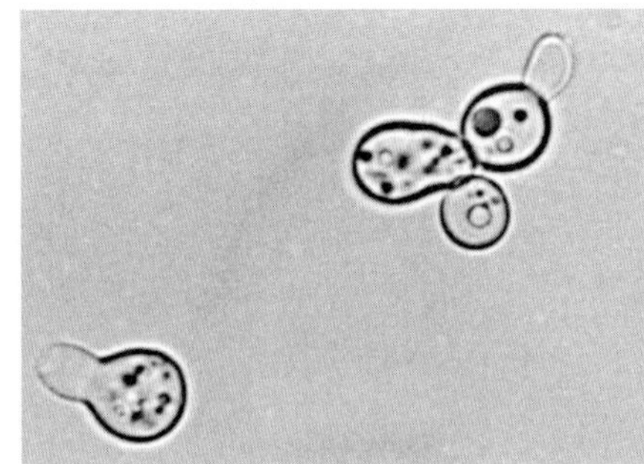

FIGURE 1-42 Yeast cells of *Blastomyces dermatitidis* in wet smear (×1000). (From Mandell GL, Bennett JE, Dolin R: *Principles and practice of infectious diseases,* ed 6, Philadelphia, 2005, Elsevier.)

- Itraconazole 200 mg PO three times a day for 3 days and then once or twice per day for 6-12 mo for mild to moderate diseases

CENTRAL NERVOUS SYSTEM BLASTOMYCOSIS

AmB lipid formulation at a dosage of 5 mg/kg/day over 4-6 wk followed by either fluconazole 800 mg/day or itraconazole 200 mg PO two to three times per day or voriconazole 200-400 mg PO twice a day for at least 12 mo and until resolution of CSF abnormalities.

BLASTOMYCOSIS IN IMMUNOSUPPRESSED INDIVIDUALS

- AmB as a lipid formulation 3-5 mg/kg/day or AmB deoxycholate 0.7-1 mg/kg/day for 1-2 wk or until improvement is noted followed by itraconazole 200 mg PO three times a day for 3 days and then twice per day as step-down therapy for at least 12 mo. Lifelong suppressive therapy with oral itraconazole 200 mg/day may be required.
- Serum itraconazole levels should be determined in all patients after they have received treatment with this agent for 2 wk.
- Surgery may be indicated for drainage of large abscesses.

DISPOSITION

- Before antifungal therapy, the disease had a progressive course with eventual extrapulmonary disease and a mortality rate >60%.
- Relapse rate for patients treated with AmB is 5%; relapse is more common in AIDS patients.

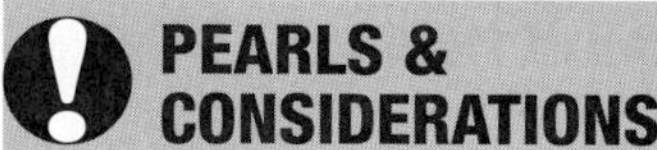

PEARLS & CONSIDERATIONS

- *Blastomyces dermatitidis* may mimic other diseases.
- Colonization does not occur as with *Candida* and *Aspergillus* species.

SUGGESTED READINGS

Bradsher RW et al: Blastomycosis, *Infect Dis Clin N Am* 17:21, 2003.

Martynowicz MA et al: Pulmonary blastomycosis: an appraisal of diagnostic techniques, *Chest* 121(3): 768, 2002.

Stanley WC et al: Clinical practice guidelines for the management of blastomycosis: 2008 update by the Infectious Diseases Society of America, *Clin Infect Dis* 46:1801-1812, 2008.

AUTHOR: **SAJEEV HANDA, M.D.**

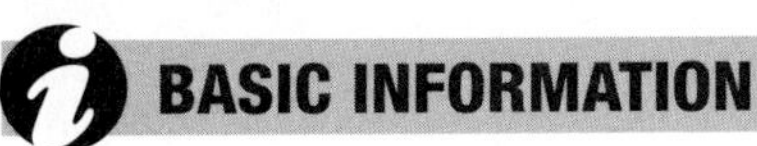

BASIC INFORMATION

DEFINITION

Blepharitis is an acute or, most often, chronic inflammation of the eyelid margins that is often refractory to treatment.

SYNONYMS

Eye lid infection or inflammation
Eczema of the eye lids
Dermatoblepharitis
Angular blepharitis

ICD-9CM CODES
373.0 Blepharitis

EPIDEMIOLOGY & DEMOGRAPHICS

- Common in children, particularly those with atopic dermatitis and eczema
- Adults with seborrhea involving the eyelids

PHYSICAL FINDINGS & CLINICAL PRESENTATION

- Chronically infected lids are usually diffusely erythematous, with collarettes (fibrin exudate) at the base of the lashes (Fig. 1-43).
- Lid margins thicken over time, with associated loss of eyelashes (madarosis), misdirected growth of lashes (trichiasis), and overflow or inspissation of the meibomian glands.
- Associated conjunctivitis with erythema, edema but no discharge.
- Chalazia may develop.
- Superficial punctate erosions of the inferior corneal epithelium are common.
- More severe findings, such as corneal pannus, ulcerative keratitis, or lid ectropion, are less common.

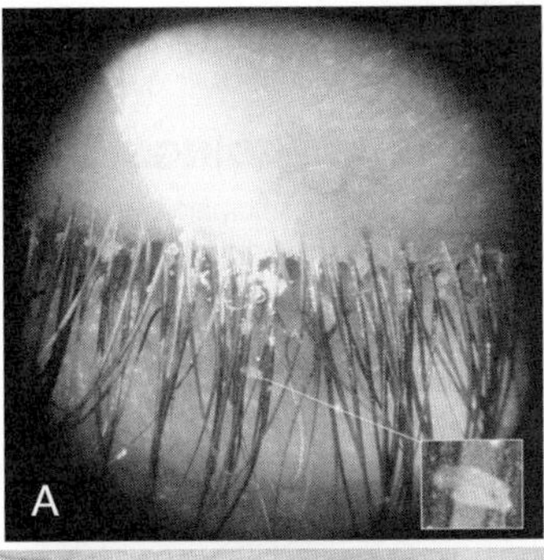

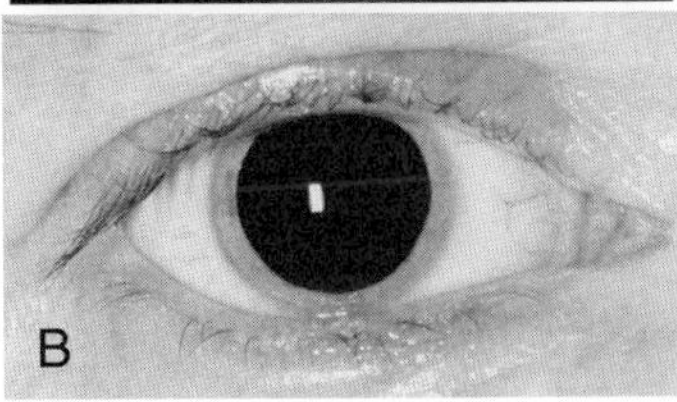

FIGURE 1-43 A, Seborrheic blepharitis. The typical scales (scurf) are translucent and easily removed. **B,** Staphylococcal blepharitis showing the typical lid margin erythema and discharge. (From Palay D [ed]: *Ophthalmology for the primary care physician,* St Louis, 1997, Mosby.)

ETIOLOGY

Multiple: bacterial and nonbacterial causes

- Staphylococcal infection most common but streptococcal, Moraxella, and other bacterial infections; viral infections (e.g., herpes simplex, herpes zoster, *Molluscum contagiosum*); and a number of ecoparasites, including pediculosis, may cause blepharitis
- Seborrheic dermatitis
- Rosacea
- Dry eye (keratoconjunctivitis sicca): decrease in tear volume
- Meibomian gland dysfunction
- Two categories of blepharitis:
  1. Anterior blepharitis, most often associated with staphylococcal infection or seborrheic dermatitis
  2. Posterior blepharitis, associated with meibomian gland dysfunction

NOTE: Blepharitis patients have normal skin microflora in greater amounts (mostly *S. epidermidis* and *P. acnes*). (*S. aureus* and *S. epidermidis* can be cultured in 10% to 35% and 90% to 95% of healthy persons, respectively.)

DIAGNOSIS

DIFFERENTIAL DIAGNOSIS

- Keratoconjunctivitis sicca
- Eyelid malignancies
- Herpes simplex blepharitis
- Molluscum contagiosum
- Phthiriasis palpebrarum
- Phthirus pubis (pubic lice)
- Demodex folliculorum (transparent mites)
- Allergic blepharitis

WORKUP

Scrapings of the eyelids to show polymorphonuclear leukocytes and gram-positive cocci

LABORATORY TESTS

Eyelid cultures and antibiotic sensitivity testing (usually not done unless patient fails to respond to initial treatment regimen)

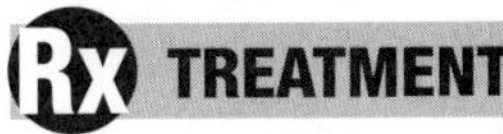

TREATMENT

NONPHARMACOLOGIC THERAPY

- Alkaline soaps may be beneficial; alcohol and some detergents remove surface lipids and microflora.
- Hot compresses applied to closed lids for 5 to 10 min: heat loosens debris from lid margins and increases meibomian gland fluidity.
- Firm massage of the lid margins to enhance the flow of secretions from glands, followed by cleansing of the lids with cotton-tipped applicators dipped in a 50:50 mixture of baby shampoo and water.
- Lashes and lid margins scrubbed vigorously while the eyelids are closed, followed by thorough rinsing.
- Following local massage and cleansing, the mainstay of treatment is application of topical antibiotic ointment to the eyelid margins.
  1. Most effective topical antibiotics include bacitracin, erythromycin, aminoglycoside and fluoroquinolone ophthalmic ointments.
  2. Ointment is applied 1 to 4 times daily, depending on the severity, for 1 to 2 wk, followed by once daily, at bedtime, for another 4 to 8 wk until all signs of inflammation have disappeared.

For patients with rosacea:

1. Tetracycline 250 mg orally 4 times daily or doxycycline 100 mg orally bid along with local treatment for several months

Recalcitrant cases with antibiotic resistance:

1. Vancomycin eye drops 1%
2. Ciprofloxacin or ofloxacin eyedrops

CHRONIC Rx

By definition, this is a chronic condition for which there is frequently no cure.

Some newer agents being evaluated are antioxidant flavonoid-type compounds (resveratrol, silymarin); azelaic acid and glycolic acid (antikeratinizing effects); and adapalene gel (anti-inflammatory properties and an antiproliferative effect on keratinocytes).

DISPOSITION

This condition may be refractory to treatment.

REFERRAL

To an ophthalmologist if patient fails to respond to local therapy.

SUGGESTED READINGS

Mathers WD, Choi D: Cluster analysis of patients with ocular surface disease, blepharitis and dry eye, *Arch Ophthalmol* 122:1700, 2004.

McCann LC et al: Tear and meibomian gland function in blepharitis and normals, *Eye Contact Lens* 35(4):203-208, 2009.

Saccà SC: Prevalence and treatment of *Helicobacter pylori* in patients with blepharitis, *Invest Ophthalmol Vis Sci* 47(2):501, 2006.

AUTHORS: **GLENN G. FORT, M.D., M.P.H.,** and **DENNIS J. MIKOLICH, M.D.**

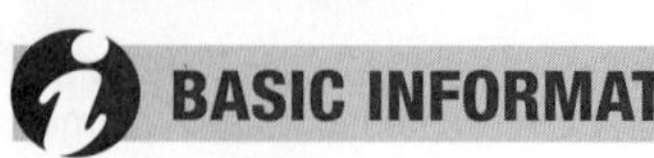

BASIC INFORMATION

DEFINITION

Body dysmorphic disorder (BDD) is a somatoform disorder characterized by preoccupation with a minor or imagined defect in physical appearance that causes significant impairment in social or occupational functioning. Although other psychiatric conditions such as anorexia nervosa or depression may occur with BDD, diagnosis requires a preoccupation not otherwise explained by another mental disorder.

SYNONYMS

Dysmorphophobia
Dysmorphic syndrome
Body dysmorphia

ICD-9CM CODES

306.9 Unspecified psychophysiologic malfunction
DSM-IV: 300.7

EPIDEMIOLOGY & DEMOGRAPHICS

- Affects approximately 1% to 2% of the general population
- Incidence among cosmetic surgery patients is 2% to 15%
- Onset generally in adolescence or young adulthood
- Equal prevalence among males and females
- No known genetic predisposition

PHYSICAL FINDINGS & CLINICAL PRESENTATION

- Patients have an excessive preoccupation (obsession) with a perceived or minor defect in their appearance. Any part of the body may be a focus of concern, although skin, hair, body odor, and nose shape and size are the most common.
- The patient usually appears physically normal; if a defect is present, the patient's reaction to it is disproportionate to its severity.
- Most patients have poor insight or are delusional.
- Many patients engage in compulsive behaviors such as frequent mirror checking, excess grooming, camouflaging, skin picking, and repeatedly measuring or feeling the perceived defect and seek constant reassurance about the perceived defect.
- Most patients experience some impairment in functioning.

ETIOLOGY

Unknown, though comorbid mental disorders associated with BDD include major depression, obsessive-compulsive disorder (OCD), generalized anxiety disorder, agoraphobia, trichotillomania, eating disorders.

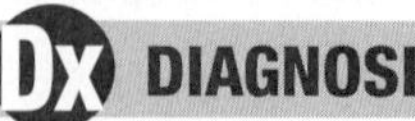

DIAGNOSIS

- Psychiatric interview
- Ask:
  1. Have you ever been worried about your appearance in any way?
  2. Did this concern preoccupy you?
  3. What effect did this have on your life?

DIFFERENTIAL DIAGNOSIS

- Often goes unrecognized and undiagnosed because of patient's reluctance to divulge symptoms.
- BDD has many features in common with OCD.
- Anorexia nervosa.
- Obsessive-compulsive disorder.
- Anxiety disorder.
- Social phobia.
- Hypochondriasis.
- Many patients have comorbid personality disorder.

WORKUP

- Organic etiology should be assessed with Mini-Mental Status Examination.
- Body Dysmorphic Disorder Examination Self-Report used in clinical trials.

TREATMENT

NONPHARMACOLOGIC THERAPY

- Cognitive behavioral therapy (particularly exposure and response prevention).
- Do not try to talk patients out of their concern; it is ineffective.
- Avoid cosmetic procedures.

ACUTE GENERAL Rx

Precautions/hospitalization if actively suicidal

CHRONIC Rx

- High-dose selective serotonin reuptake inhibitors (SSRIs).
- Other agents (neuroleptic, tricyclic antidepressant, anticonvulsants) not as beneficial.
- Cognitive behavioral therapy highly recommended as stand-alone or along with SSRIs.
- Support groups if available.

DISPOSITION

- Untreated BDD tends to be chronic and can lead to social isolation, school dropout, major depression, unnecessary surgery, and even suicide.
- With early diagnosis and treatment patients appear to have a favorable course (though prospective trials not completed).

REFERRAL

Refer for psychiatric evaluation and treatment if diagnosis is suspected.

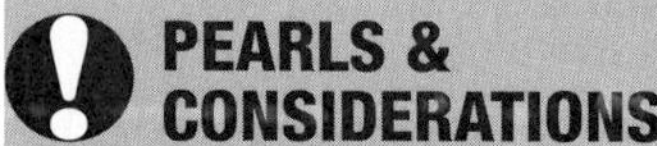

PEARLS & CONSIDERATIONS

- In clinical settings, up to 60% of patients with BDD have major depression.
- Reassurance rarely lessens the patient's fear or dislike of his or her appearance.
- Patients often have an unrealistic expectation of improvement regarding plastic surgery, and surgery itself provides little to no relief.
- All patients should be screened for suicidality.

PATIENT/FAMILY EDUCATION

- Family behavioral treatment can be useful, especially if the affected individual is an adolescent.
- Consider therapy with family members, spouse, significant others.
- Body Dysmorphic Disorder Central: http://www.BDDCentral.com

SUGGESTED READINGS

Cerand CE et al: Body dysmorphic disorder: diagnosis and approach, *Plast Reconstr Surg* 119(6):1924, 2007.

Ipser JC et al: Pharmacotherapy and psychotherapy for body dysmorphic disorder, *Cochrane Database Sys Rev* (1)CD005332, 2009.

Phillips KA: Body dysmorphic disorder: a guide for primary care physicians, *Prim Care* 29(1):99, 2002.

AUTHOR: **MITCHELL D. FELDMAN, M.D., M.PHIL.**

BASIC INFORMATION

DEFINITION

Primary malignant bone tumors are invasive and anaplastic and have the ability to metastasize. Most arise from the marrow (myeloma), but tumors may develop from bone, cartilage, fat, and fibrous tissues. Leukemia and lymphoma are excluded from this discussion.

FIBROSARCOMA AND LIPOSARCOMA: Extremely rare. They are similar to tumors arising in soft tissue.

OSTEOSARCOMA: A rare primary malignant tumor of bone characterized by malignant tumor cells that produce osteoid or bone. Several variants have been described: parosteal sarcoma, periosteal sarcoma, multicentric, and telangiectatic forms.

CHONDROSARCOMA: A malignant cartilage tumor that may develop primarily or secondarily from transformation of a benign osteocartilaginous exostosis or enchondroma.

EWING'S SARCOMA: A malignant tumor of unknown histogenesis.

MULTIPLE MYELOMA: A neoplastic proliferation of plasma cells.

SYNONYMS

Multiple myeloma:
1. Plasma cell myeloma
2. Plasmacytoma

ICD-9CM CODES	
203.0	Multiple myeloma
170.9	Neoplasm, bone (periosteum), primary malignant
M9180/3	Osteosarcoma
N9220/3	Chondrosarcoma
M9260/3	Ewing's sarcoma

EPIDEMIOLOGY & DEMOGRAPHICS

MULTIPLE MYELOMA:
- The most common tumor in bone
- Age at onset: usually >40 yr
- Male/female ratio of 2:1

OSTEOGENIC SARCOMA:
- Average age at onset: 10 to 20 yr
- Males afflicted more often than females
- Parosteal sarcoma in older patients

CHONDROSARCOMA:
- Age at onset: 40 to 60 yr
- Male/female ratio of 2:1

EWING'S SARCOMA: Age at onset: 10 to 15 yr

PHYSICAL FINDINGS & CLINICAL PRESENTATION

MULTIPLE MYELOMA:
- May present as a systemic process or, less commonly, as a "solitary" lesion
- Early manifestations: anorexia, weight loss, and bone pain; majority of cases present initially with back pain that often leads to the detection of a destructive skeletal lesion
- Other organ systems eventually become involved, resulting in more bone pain, anemia, renal insufficiency, and/or bacterial infections, usually as a result of the dysproteinemia typical of this disorder
- Possible secondary amyloidosis, leading to cardiac failure or nephrotic syndrome

OSTEOSARCOMA:
- Most originating in the metaphysis
- 50% to 60% around the knee
- Possible pain and swelling, but otherwise healthy patient
- Osteosarcoma in conjunction with Paget's disease, manifested primarily as a sudden increase in bone pain

CHONDROSARCOMA:
- Tumor most commonly involving the pelvis, upper femur, and shoulder girdle
- Painful swelling

EWING'S SARCOMA:
- Painful soft tissue mass often present
- Possibly increased local heat
- Midshaft of a long bone usually affected (in contrast to other tumors)
- Weight loss, fever, and lethargy

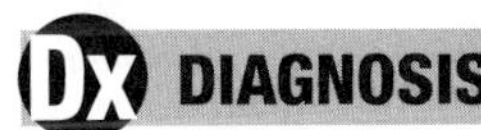

DIAGNOSIS

DIFFERENTIAL DIAGNOSIS

- Osteomyelitis
- Metastatic bone disease

LABORATORY TESTS

- Slightly elevated alkaline phosphatase in osteosarcoma
- In Ewing's sarcoma: reflective of systemic reaction; include anemia, an increase in white blood cell count, and an elevated sedimentation rate
- In multiple myeloma:
  1. Bence Jones protein in the urine
  2. Anemia and elevated sedimentation rate
  3. Characteristic dysproteinemia on serum protein electrophoresis
  4. Diagnostic feature: peak in the electrophoretic pattern suggestive of a monoclonal gammopathy
  5. Rouleaux formation in the peripheral blood smear
  6. Often presence of hypercalcemia, but alkaline phosphatase levels usually normal

IMAGING STUDIES

- Classic osteogenic sarcoma penetrates the cortex early in many cases.
  1. A blastic (dense), lytic (lucent), or mixed response may be seen in the affected bone.
  2. An aggressive perpendicular sunburst pattern may be present as a result of periosteal reaction, and peripheral Codman's triangles are often noted.
  3. Margins of the tumor are poorly defined.
- Speckled calcifications in a destructive radiolucent lesion are usually suggestive of chondrosarcoma.
- Ewing's sarcoma is characterized radiographically by mottled, irregular destructive changes with periosteal new bone formation. The latter may be multilayered, producing the typical "onion skin" appearance.
- Typical roentgenographic finding in multiple myeloma is the "punched out" lesion with sharply demarcated edges.
  1. Multiple lesions are usual.
  2. Diffuse osteoporosis may be the only finding in many cases.
  3. Pathologic fractures are common.

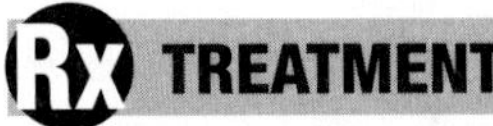

TREATMENT

The evaluation and treatment of malignant bone tumors are complicated. Diagnostic studies and treatment should be supervised by an orthopedic cancer specialist and oncologist.

DISPOSITION

- In the past 20 yr, dramatic improvements have been made in the treatment protocols for osteosarcoma with the use of adjuvant multidrug regimens and limb-sparing surgery.
- Prognosis of multiple myeloma remains poor despite new therapies.
- Prognosis for Ewing's sarcoma has improved with a combination of chemotherapy, local resection, and radiation therapy.
- Chondrosarcomas are not sensitive to chemotherapy or radiation, and prognosis depends on the grade of the tumor and the ability to obtain an adequate resection.

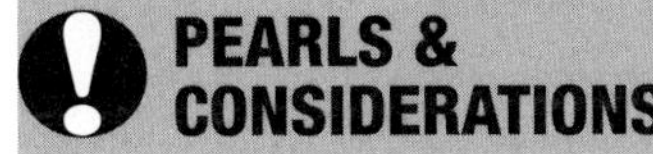

PEARLS & CONSIDERATIONS

Early diagnosis is important because most tumors have not metastasized at the time of initial presentation.

SUGGESTED READINGS

Dormans JP, Moroz L: Infection and tumors of the spine in children, *J Bone Joint Surg* 89A:79, 2007.

Futani H et al: Long-term follow-up after limb salvage in skeletally immature children with a primary malignant tumor of the distal end of the femur, *J Bone Joint Surg* 88A:595, 2006.

Hoffmann C et al: Functional results and quality of life after treatment of pelvic sarcomas involving the acetabulum, *J Bone Joint Surg Am* 88A:575, 2006.

Lewis VO: What's new in musculoskeletal oncology? *J Bone Joint Surg Am* 89:1399, 2007.

Messerschmitt PJ et al: Osteosarcoma, *J Am Acad Orthop Surg* 17:515, 2009.

Plate AM et al: Malignant tumors of the hand and wrist, *J Am Acad Orthop Surg* 14:680, 2006.

Staals EL et al: Dedifferentiated chondrosarcomas arising in preexisting osteochondromas, *J Bone Joint Surg Am* 89A:987, 2007.

van Kampen M et al: Replacement of the hip in children with a tumor in the proximal part of the femur, *J Bone Joint Surg Am* 90:785-795, 2008.

Worch J et al: Ethnic and racial differences in patients with Ewing sarcoma, *Cancer* 116:983, 2010.

AUTHOR: **LONNIE R. MERCIER, M.D.**

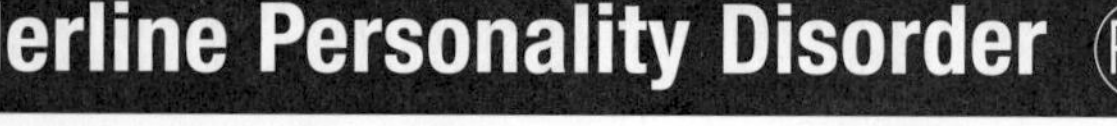

Borderline Personality Disorder (PTG)

BASIC INFORMATION

DEFINITION

Borderline personality disorder (BPD) is characterized by a pervasive pattern of instability in interpersonal relationships, self-image, affect regulation, and impulse control that causes significant subjective distress or impairment of functioning. The individual must meet five or more of the following criteria:

1. Frantic efforts to avoid real or imagined abandonment
2. Unstable and intense personal relationships characterized by alternating between extremes of idealization and devaluation
3. Identity disturbance characterized by an unstable self-image
4. Impulsivity in at least two areas that are potentially self-damaging (e.g., overspending, sex, substance abuse, binge eating, reckless driving)
5. Recurrent suicidal behavior, gestures, threats, or self-mutilating behavior
6. Affective instability due to a marked reactivity of mood
7. Chronic feelings of emptiness
8. Inappropriate, intense anger or difficulty controlling anger
9. Transient, stress-related paranoid ideation or severe dissociative symptoms

ICD-9CM CODES
301.83 Borderline personality

EPIDEMIOLOGY & DEMOGRAPHICS

PREVALENCE: Affects approximately 1% to 2% of the general population and up to 10% of psychiatric outpatients
PREDOMINANT SEX: Female (3:1)
PREDOMINANT AGE: 20s
GENETICS: BPD is five times as likely if disorder is present in a first-degree relative. An increased prevalence of mood disorders and substance abuse disorders is also found in first-degree relatives of persons with BPD.
RISK FACTORS: Association with childhood physical, sexual, or emotional abuse and/or neglect

PHYSICAL FINDINGS & CLINICAL PRESENTATION

- There are no specific physical findings associated with BPD.
- Mental status examination may reveal affective lability.
- Clinical presentation may reveal the following:
  - Patients experience a pervasive sense of loneliness and emptiness. In addition to affective instability, persons with BPD often demonstrate an underlying negative affect with dysphoria.
  - Intense emotions with difficulty returning to emotional baseline.
  - All-or-nothing, either/or cognitive style that is represented by a phenomenon known as "splitting," in which patient sees situations or people as all good or all bad.
  - Difficulty in maintaining commitment to long-term goals; history of numerous stormy relationships and multiple jobs.
  - Reacts with rage, panic, despair to actual or perceived abandonment; may present with suicidality or self-mutilating behavior in response to recent stressor.
  - Attempts to block the experience of pain, which may induce feelings of derealization, depersonalization, changes in consciousness, and/or brief psychotic reactions with delusions and hallucinations.
  - Substance use, gambling, overspending, eating binges, and/or self-mutilation as a way to escape intensely painful affect.
  - Some patients may display psychotic symptoms.

ETIOLOGY

- Interaction of psychosocial adversity plus genetic factors
- Hypotheses:
  1. Genetic: increased risk if first-degree relative with BPD.
  2. Biologic: abnormalities in limbic system and other areas of the brain cause emotional dysregulation. Serotonergic functioning appears to be disturbed.
  3. Environmental: history of childhood abuse or neglect.

Dx DIAGNOSIS

DIFFERENTIAL DIAGNOSIS

- Histrionic and narcissistic personality disorders share some common features.
- Dysthymia and other depressive disorders: requires a stability of affective symptoms not seen in BPD.
- Bipolar disorder: mood changes in BPD are often triggered by stressors and are less sustained than in bipolar disorder.
- Substance abuse or dependence: often induces impulsive, emotionally labile behavior.
- Posttraumatic stress disorder (PTSD): individuals with BPD often have history of trauma but do not avoid the feared stimulus or reexperience the trauma, as do individuals with PTSD.
- Mild cases of schizophrenia may superficially resemble BPD.

WORKUP

- History (often helpful to gather collateral information from family and friends)
- Physical examination
- Mental status examination

LABORATORY TESTS

- Toxicology screen; substance use is common and can mimic features of personality disorders.
- Screen for HIV and other sexually transmitted illnesses. Patients with personality disorders often exhibit poor impulse control.

IMAGING STUDIES

Structural and functional MRI demonstrate abnormalities in the amygdala and hippocampus. PET scans reveal altered metabolism in prefrontal cortex. Imaging is not recommended as part of routine evaluation.

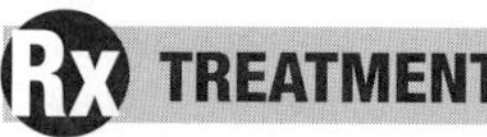

Rx TREATMENT

NONPHARMACOLOGIC THERAPY

- Few randomized trials have assessed psychosocial interventions for BPD.
- Dialectical behavior therapy (DBT), a variation of cognitive behavior therapy (CBT), and transference-focused psychotherapy, a type of psychodynamic therapy, have the most empirical support from randomized trials. The goal of DBT is to help patients control impulses and angry outbursts and to develop social skills. The focus of transference-focused psychotherapy is on examining the affect-laden themes that emerge in the relationship between patient and therapist.

ACUTE GENERAL Rx

Low-dose antipsychotics to control impulsivity, brief psychotic episodes.

CHRONIC Rx

- Medications have low-to-moderate effectiveness and are most effective in improving symptoms of impulsivity, mood instability, and self-destructive behavior. Effectiveness of medications for BPD has only been studied within the first 3 mo of treatment.
- SSRIs if concurrent mood disorder. Higher doses of antidepressants may be required than for patients with major depression alone.
- Low-dose antipsychotics.
- Mood stabilizers (lithium, valproate, carbamazepine, topiramate).
- In preliminary studies, daily omega-3 fatty acids improve symptoms of irritability.

DISPOSITION

- Course is variable. The most unstable period is typically in early adulthood; the majority of patients achieve greater stability in social/occupational functioning later in life but often continue to have difficulty maintaining intimate relationships.
- There is no evidence of progression to schizophrenia, but patients have a high incidence of episodes of major depressive disorder and other Axis I disorders. This highlights the importance of evaluating for Axis I pathology in patients with BPD to identify potentially treatable illness.

REFERRAL

- Referral to mental health specialty care advised to confirm diagnosis and assist in management.
- Referral recommended if:
  - Use of pharmacotherapy contemplated
  - Patient is severely impaired in daily function or suicidal

PEARLS & CONSIDERATIONS

COMMENTS

Guidelines for physician management of patients with BPD:

- Consider frequent, brief, scheduled visits for needy, demanding, or somaticizing patients with BPD.
- Validate the patient's feelings while stating the expectation of behavior control.
- Be matter-of-fact; avoid expressing extreme emotions.
- Be alert to the risk of suicide and assess suicide risk often.
- Convey a demeanor of competence but openly acknowledge minor errors.
- Have a low threshold for seeking psychiatric consultation.

PREVENTION

There are no known ways to prevent BPD and other personality disorders. Attempts may be made to prevent the deleterious consequences of personality disorders:

- Suicidality should be actively and consistently monitored.
- Benzodiazepines, narcotic analgesics, and other drugs with potential for dependency should be used rarely and with great caution. Nearly all personality disorders are marked by impaired impulse control and consequent risk of addictive behavior.
- Patients with personality disorder who have children should be asked frequently and in detail about their parenting practices. Their low frustration tolerance, externalization of blame for psychological distress, and impaired impulse control put the children of these patients at risk for neglect or abuse.

PATIENT & FAMILY EDUCATION

National Alliance for the Mentally Ill (NAMI; http://www.nami.org) provides patient information, online chat groups, and information on support groups throughout the U.S. for people with BPD and their families.

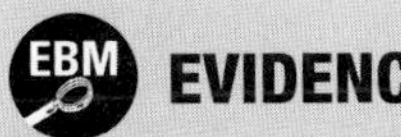

EVIDENCE

Please note: Complete text of EBM for this topic is available online.

Key trials and commentary:

One study examined three year-long outpatient treatments for borderline personality disorder (BPD): dialectical behavior therapy (DBT), transference-focused psychotherapy, and a dynamic supportive treatment. It revealed that patients with BPD respond to structured treatments in an outpatient setting with change in multiple domains of outcome. A structured dynamic treatment, transference-focused psychotherapy was associated with change in multiple constructs across six domains; DBT and supportive treatment were associated with fewer changes. Future research is needed to examine the specific mechanisms of change in these treatments beyond common structures.

BPD remains one of the most difficult conditions for clinicians to treat. These authors did an excellent study comparing the three most frequently applied psychotherapies: DBT, transference-focused psychotherapy, and a dynamic supportive treatment. They randomly assigned 90 patients and rated them blindly at 4-month intervals during a year. Interestingly, all three groups had significant positive changes in global functioning and social adjustment, as well as in depression and anxiety. Transference-focused therapy and DBT were associated with significant decreases in suicidality but only transference-based therapy and supportive therapy with decreases in anger. Transference-based and supportive treatments also had decreases in impulsivity but only transference-based psychotherapy led to decreases in irritability and verbal and direct assaults. Interestingly, this result is what I was taught many years ago and again in recent years, largely by Glen Gabbard and his group. This is one area in which transference-based psychotherapy appears to have an edge and in many ways appears to be the best treatment. It is interesting that DBT was less effective in certain areas than the other two treatments, but it is certainly reassuring that all three were effective.[1] Ⓐ

Another trial investigated the quality and development of the therapeutic alliance as a mediator of change in schema-focused therapy (SFT) and transference-focused psychotherapy (TFP) for BPD. 78 patients were randomly allocated to 3 years of biweekly SFT or TFP. Scores of both therapists and patients for the therapeutic alliance were higher in SFT than in TFP. Negative ratings of therapists and patients at early treatment were predictive of dropout, whereas increasingly positive ratings of patients in the first half of treatment predicted subsequent clinical improvement. Dissimilarity between therapist and patients in pathological personality characteristics had a direct effect on growth of the therapeutic alliance but showed no relationship with clinical improvement. The authors conclude that the therapeutic alliance and specific techniques interact with and influence one another and may serve to facilitate change processes underlying clinical improvement in patients with BPD.

The therapeutic alliance is a perpetual factor in psychotherapy outcome research, the variable most repeatedly shown to correlate with treatment outcome. As the authors of this thoughtful and carefully written report note, however, most research on the therapeutic alliance has come from short-term studies of psychotherapy for Axis I disorders, which generally have shown that a positive early alliance predicts better outcome. Here the authors elaborate on the results of a longer Dutch study of an Axis II diagnosis.

The 3-year randomized controlled trial for BPD showed gains in both treatments, but advantages for cognitively-based SFT over psychodynamic TFP. BPD is a challenging field on which to test the effects of the therapeutic alliance. The two quite different psychotherapeutic approaches were expected to vary in degree of therapist support and expressed warmth. The investigators also explored the congruency and dissimilarity of patient and therapist characterological traits as factors that might contribute to the alliance. Such attributes, particularly those of the therapists, have received little previous research attention.

Data on the alliance were collected at 3 mo, 15 mo, and 33 mo. (More frequent ratings might have been helpful.) Patients, who ranged between the ages of 18 and 60 years and met DSM-IV criteria for BPD, answered personality questionnaires at the start of the study, whereas therapists did so after 3 months of treatment. Therapists remained generally adherent to their approaches over 3 years of twice-weekly individual therapy. Data were analyzed to control for early outcomes that might themselves influence the therapeutic alliance, thereby creating a circular, tautological association.

Poor alliance was associated with dropout, although unfortunately no patient ratings of the alliance were available before the 3-month assessment, by which time eight subjects had already terminated TFP. Patients who remained in the study reported increasing levels of therapeutic alliance over time in both therapies. Patients and therapists in SFT rated their therapeutic alliance consistently higher than did their TFP counterparts. (The authors might have elaborated on what a one-point difference on the Working Alliance Inventory might mean.) TFP therapists reported increasing frustration over time, whereas SFT therapists recorded less. Although therapists' frustration might be presumed to reflect their patients' relative clinical success, the differing associations for the two treatments persisted even after controlling for outcome.

Interestingly, dissimilarity in the maladaptive schemas and personality organizations of therapists and patients was associated with better alliance from the patients', but not the therapists', viewpoint across treatment conditions. On the other hand, these associations did not significantly influence treatment outcome. The authors underscore that the treatment alliance is necessary but not necessarily sufficient for treatment outcome; differences in therapeutic conception and technique may also play a role.

For clinicians, take-home points may include the following:

1. A therapeutic alliance is a sine qua non for treatment: it is crucial to develop an emotional engagement and shared treatment goals with patients.

2. A supportive approach may effect this more easily than a confrontational approach.
3. It may complicate treatment if your own blind spots coincide with those of your patient.[2] Ⓐ

There is conflicting evidence about comorbid personality pathology in depression treatments. A separate trial sought to test the effects of antidepressant drugs and cognitive therapy in people with depression distinguished by the presence or absence of personality disorder. It revealed that comorbid personality disorder was associated with differential initial response rates and sustained response rates for two well-validated treatments for depression.

The question of whether and how personality disorder affects the outcome of major depressive disorder is an important one. As the authors note, it has received inconsistent answers and at times confused interpretation in the past. Researchers conducting a randomized controlled trial of cognitive behavioral therapy (CBT) and paroxetine for patients with moderate to severe major depression analyzed their data to examine this question. Not all personality disorders were involved: antisocial, schizotypal, and borderline personality disorders were study exclusion criteria. Nonetheless, 48% of subjects met criteria for a DSM-IV personality disorder. The presence or absence of personality disorder made a considerable difference in interacting with treatment assignment. A number of the findings reported are surprising and counterintuitive: (1) Patients with comorbid personality disorders had a lower attrition rate than patients without personality disorders in the paroxetine subsample, whereas the reverse was true in CBT. We generally think of psychotherapy as having greater flexibility than medication in addressing personality issues, but this seems not to have been the case here. (2) Similarly, there was a trend for patients with comorbid personality disorder to have a better outcome than noncomorbid patients treated with paroxetine, whereas in CBT patients without Axis II diagnoses fared better than those who had them. Controlling for potential confounding variables did not alter these outcomes. The effect appeared greatest for the "dramatic" cluster B of Axis II. Less surprisingly, medication patients switched to placebo had high relapse rates. These interesting findings should make us rethink our preconceived notions about the medication and psychotherapy for personality disorders. Of course, for many patients with high levels of depressive severity and comorbid personality and other disorders, the combination of medication and an empirically validated psychotherapy might be optimal.[3] Ⓐ

Another study evaluated the effect of mentalization-based treatment by partial hospitalization compared to treatment as usual for BPD 8 years after entry into a randomized, controlled trial and 5 years after all mentalization-based treatment was complete. It revealed that patients with 18 months of mentalization-based treatment by partial hospitalization followed by 18 months of maintenance mentalizing group therapy remain better than those receiving treatment as usual, but their general social function remains impaired.

Clinicians have long considered BPD a frightening diagnosis with a dangerous and violent prognosis. BPD is surely a debilitating and potentially lethal condition, but hopeless it is not. A series of studies have shown that many patients with this diagnosis and with considerable comorbidity improve over time in naturalistic follow-up and in treatment studies. As the authors note, follow-up of patients from treatment studies has been limited. This important article presents long-term, controlled follow-up data on one of the best such studies. Patients in the United Kingdom with BPD were treated either with mentalization therapy in a partial hospitalization program for 18 months, with 18 subsequent months of twice-weekly maintenance outpatient group mentalization therapy; or with treatment as usual (TAU). Mentalization, a treatment based on psychodynamic principles and delivered largely by psychiatric nurses rather than by psychoanalysts, showed impressive benefits both at the end of acute treatment and in previous follow-up reports. For a condition like BPD, follow-up data are crucial. It is not enough to know that patients improve; we need to know whether they stay better. In this landmark report, we learn that they do. The researchers compared patients treated in the mentalization condition ($N = 22$) with those in TAU ($N = 19$) 8 years after they had entered and 5 years after they had completed the active phase of treatment. Raters were blind to treatment condition and used state-of-the-art assessments at 6-month intervals. Suicide attempts, hospitalizations, emergency room visits, employment, Global Assessment of Functioning Scale (GAF) score, interpersonal, and occupational functioning—indeed, all of the outcome measures greatly favored the experimental condition. It also appears that TAU was the more expensive condition, inasmuch as subjects in that group continued to heavily use medication and treatment services in comparison with the mentalization group. At the end of follow-up, only 13% of mentalization but 87% of TAU subjects still met criteria for BPD. Every study has some limitations. (1) Selecting patients who were willing to attend a lengthy partial hospitalization program may have yielded subjects who were atypical of patients with BPD in general. (2) The structure of treatment makes it hard to gauge whether it was mentalization itself or other aspects of the partial hospitalization program that yielded such benefits. (3) "Treatment as usual" is a hard-to-define and highly variable condition. It often means little treatment for some patients, intensive but low-quality treatment for others. Here it included inpatient, partial hospital, and outpatient treatment with medication and supportive treatment, but no focused psychotherapy. Thus, patients in the two groups were not matched for psychotherapy "dosage," and psychotherapy is generally considered central to treatment of BPD. Nonetheless, the sample comprised a severely and chronically ill group of patients, and they both improved dramatically and stayed much better than the control group.[4] Ⓐ

Another study evaluated whether DBT was more efficacious than treatment by nonbehavioral psychotherapy experts in reducing co-occurring Axis I disorders among suicidal individuals with BPD.

This is a nicely conducted study, comparing the efficacy of DBT with treatment by nonbehavioral psychotherapy experts in reducing co-occurring Axis I disorders in patients with BPD. There is a good sample size, and appropriate measures and statistics are used.

However, it would be helpful to know which treatment approaches were used among the community therapists. The author's note that this condition was used to "control for expertise, treatment allegiance, availability of clinical supervision group," etc., but it is not clear what the theoretical orientation of these therapists happened to be. All that the reader learns is that the community therapists were not self-identified as cognitive or behavioral in orientation. In the absence of this information, one may imagine that all or many may have used a psychodynamic or interpersonal approach. If this is the case, the finding that DBT fared much better than expert community therapy with patients who had co-occurring substance use disorders is not surprising. The research literature suggests that cognitive and behavioral treatments are more effective with substance dependence than psychodynamically oriented treatments. Furthermore, as the authors note, DBT has been adapted to treat co-occurring substance use disorders in patients with BPD. It is also likely that therapists who have been trained in DBT would have received more training in working with patients with substance dependency than many other therapists in the community.

What is surprising is that there were no significant differences between DBT and community treatment in the reduction of anxiety disorders, eating disorders, or major depressive disorder. The surprising aspect of this is that it is likely that the DBT therapists who were selected for this study have a great deal of experience in treating patients with BPD, possibly more experience than even the expert therapists in the community. This finding may be due, as the authors suggest, to inadequate power to detect differences because the subgroups of patients with these Axis I disorders were too small. Alternatively, approaches other than cognitive and behavioral therapies are comparable in addressing both BPD and other co-occurring disorders.

Existing literature on treatments for depression, eating disorders, and anxiety disorders does confirm that there are a variety of approaches, including psychodynamic, interpersonal, and humanistic therapies, that might be quite effective in the treatment of these disorders as well as evidence of the efficacy of psychodynamic therapy in addressing borderline and other personality disorders.

This study provides more data to the referring clinician about which treatments have an evidence base for addressing specific disorders. Clearly, if a patient has co-occurring BPD and substance dependence, DBT or possibly other cognitive or behavioral treatments, such as seeking safety, would be appropriate choices. If a patient has BPD and another co-occurring Axis I disorder, such as an anxiety disorder, an eating disorder, or depression, there would be a wider range of approaches that could be considered.[5] Ⓐ

Evidence-Based References

1. Clarkin JF et al: Evaluating three treatments for borderline personality disorder: a multiwave study, *Am J Psychiatry* 164:922-928, 2007. Commentary by J.C. Ballenger, M.D. Ⓐ

2. Spinhoven P et al: The therapeutic alliance in schema-focused therapy and transference-focused psychotherapy for borderline personality disorder, *Consult Clin Psychol* 75:104-115, 2007. Commentary by J.C. Markowitz, M.D. Ⓐ

3. Fournier JC et al: Antidepressant medications v. cognitive therapy in people with depression with or without personality disorder, *Br J Psychiatry* 192: 124-129, 2008. Commentary by J.C. Markowitz, M.D. Ⓐ

4. Bateman A, Fonagy P: 8-year follow-up of patients treated for borderline personality disorder: mentalization-based treatment versus treatment as usual, *Am J Psychiatry* 165:631-638, 2008. Commentary by J.C. Markowitz, M.D. Ⓐ

5. Harned MS et al: Treating co-occurring Axis I disorders in recurrently suicidal women with borderline personality disorder: a 2-year randomized trial of dialectical behavior therapy versus community treatment by experts, *J Consult Clin Psychol* 76:1068-1075, 2008. Commentary by J.L. Krupnick, Ph.D. Ⓐ

SUGGESTED READINGS

American Psychiatric Association: Practice guidelines for the treatment of patients with BPD. Available at http://www.psychiatryonline.com/pracGuide/pracGuideTopic_13.aspx.

Choi-Kain LW, Gunderson JG: Mentalization: ontogeny, assessment, and application in the treatment of borderline personality disorder, *Am J Psychiatry* 165(9):1127-1135, 2008.

Gunderson JG: Borderline personality disorder: ontogeny of a diagnosis, *Am J Psychiatry* 166(5):530-539, 2009.

Kendall T et al: Borderline and antisocial personality disorders: summary of NICE guidance, *BMJ* 338: B93, 2009.

AUTHOR: **MITCHELL D. FELDMAN, M.D., M.PHIL.**

BASIC INFORMATION

DEFINITION

Botulism is an illness caused by a neurotoxin produced by *Clostridium botulinum.* Three types of disease can occur: foodborne botulism, wound botulism, and infant intestinal botulism. Recent concern has increased about a possible fourth type of disease: inhalational botulism, which does not occur naturally, but may occur as a result of bioterrorism.

SYNONYMS

Clostridium botulinum food poisoning
Botulinum toxin food poisoning
Wound botulism
Infantile botulism

ICD-9CM CODES

005.1 Botulism

EPIDEMIOLOGY & DEMOGRAPHICS

INCIDENCE (IN U.S.): Approximately 24 cases/yr of foodborne illness, 3 cases/yr of wound botulism, and 71 cases/yr of infant botulism

PHYSICAL FINDINGS & CLINICAL PRESENTATION

- Symptoms usually begin 12 to 36 hr following ingestion.
- Severity of illness is related to the quantity of toxin ingested.
- Significant findings:
    1. Cranial nerve palsies, with ocular and bulbar manifestations being most frequent (diplopia, ophthalmoplegia, ptosis, dysphagia, dysarthria, fixed and dilated pupils, and dry mouth)
    2. Usually bilateral nerve involvement that may progress to a descending flaccid paralysis
    3. Typically, absence of sensory findings; sensorium intact
    4. GI symptoms (nausea, vomiting, diarrhea, or cramps)
    5. Usually no fever
- Wound botulism
    1. Occurs mostly in injecting drug users (subcutaneous heroin injection—"skin popping") or with traumatic injury.
    2. Presentation is similar to that of foodborne disease, except for a longer incubation period and the absence of GI symptoms.
    3. Wound infection is not always apparent, but injection sites frequently reveal cellulitis, draining pus, or abscess formation.

ETIOLOGY

- Cause is one of several types of neurotoxins (usually A, B, or E) produced by *C. botulinum,* an anaerobic, gram-positive bacillus. Spore production guarantees survival of the organism in extreme conditions. Botulinum toxin is the most powerful neurotoxin known.
- Disease results from absorption of toxin into the circulation from a mucosal surface or wound. Botulinum toxin does not penetrate intact skin.
- In foodborne variety, disease is caused by ingestion of preformed toxin. Although rapidly inactivated by heat, the toxin can survive the proteolytic environment of the stomach.
- In wound botulism, toxin is elaborated by organisms that contaminate a wound. Most cases reported are from California.
- In infant botulism, toxin is produced by organisms in the GI tract.
- Inhalational botulism has been demonstrated experimentally in primates. This manufactured form results from aerosolized toxin and has been attempted by bioterrorists.

Dx DIAGNOSIS

DIFFERENTIAL DIAGNOSIS

- Myasthenia gravis
- Guillain-Barré syndrome
- Tick paralysis
- CVA

WORKUP

- Search made for toxin and the organism (see "Laboratory Tests")
- Electrophysiologic studies (e.g., EMG) may aid in the diagnosis

LABORATORY TESTS

- Samples of food and stool are cultured for the organism.
- Food, serum, and stool are sent for toxin assay.

Rx TREATMENT

NONPHARMACOLOGIC THERAPY

- Supportive care with intubation if respiratory failure occurs
- Debridement of the wound in wound botulism

ACUTE GENERAL Rx

- Give trivalent equine serum botulinum antitoxin as early as possible. Once a clinical diagnosis is made, antitoxin should be administered before laboratory confirmation.
    1. Give one vial by IM injection and one vial IV.
    2. The antitoxin is available from the Centers for Disease Control and Prevention [(404) 639-2206 or (404) 639-2888]; it is derived from horse serum, so there is a significant incidence of serum sickness. A human-derived antitoxin immunoglobin is now available for infants less than 1 yr of age (BIG-IV).
    3. Skin testing (conjunctival instillation and observation for 15 min), and possible desensitization, is recommended before treatment.
- Give wound botulism patients penicillin 2 million U IV q4h.
- Babies with infantile intestinal botulism may benefit from a cathartic to mechanically clear the number of *C. botulinum* vegetative forms and spores residing in the gastrointestinal tract.

CHRONIC Rx

- Supportive
- Rehabilitation/physical therapy

DISPOSITION

- Highest mortality in the first case in an outbreak, with subsequent cases receiving rapid treatment
- Complete recovery for most individuals (this may take several weeks in severely affected individuals)

REFERRAL

Immediate for all cases to an ER and an infectious disease consultant

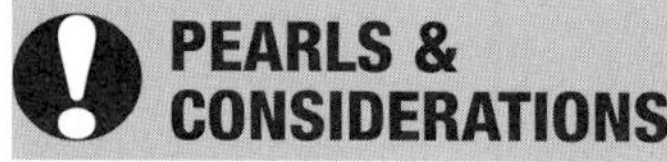

PEARLS & CONSIDERATIONS

COMMENTS

- Routine cooking inactivates the toxin, but spores are resistant to environmental factors. At room temperature, spores can germinate and produce toxin.
- Most outbreaks are associated with home-canned foods, especially vegetables.
- Patients must be closely monitored for progression to respiratory paralysis.
- There is increasing concern over the potential use of botulinum toxin as a biologic weapon, either by the enteric route or by aerosolization.
- Notify public health authorities immediately to alert other health care services of possible additional cases and to initiate investigation into cause and scope of outbreak.
- Recent botulism food recalls have involved canned chili, cut green beans, and olives.

SUGGESTED READINGS

Amon SS et al: Botulinum toxin as a biological weapon, *JAMA* 285(8):1059, 2001.
Arnon SS et al: Human botulism immune globulin for the treatment of infant botulism, *N Engl J Med* 354(5):462, 2006.
Bleck TP: *Clostridium botulinum* (botulism). In Mandell GL, Bennett JE, Dolin R (eds): *Principles and practice of infectious diseases,* ed 6, New York, 2005, Churchill Livingstone.
Cherington M: Botulism: update and review, *Semin Neurol* 24:155, 2004.
Sobel J: Botulism, *Clin Infect Dis* 41(8):1167, 2005.

AUTHORS: **GLENN G. FORT, M.D., M.P.H.,** and **DENNIS J. MIKOLICH, M.D.**

BASIC INFORMATION

DEFINITION

Brain neoplasms are a diverse group of primary (nonmetastatic) tumors arising from one of many different cell types within the central nervous system (CNS). Specific tumors subtypes and prognosis depend on the tumor cell of origin and pattern of growth.

SYNONYMS

Low-grade glioma
Glioneuronal tumor
Meningioma
Primary brain tumor

ICD-9CM CODES
225.0 Brain neoplasm (benign)
239.2 Brain neoplasm (unspecified)

EPIDEMIOLOGY & DEMOGRAPHICS

INCIDENCE: Approximately 18.2 cases/100,000 persons per yr for all primary brain tumors. Incidence of primary nonmalignant tumors ranges from 6.3 to 16.68 cases/100,000 persons per yr from 2004 to 2005. Primary brain neoplasms account for ~2% of all cancers, with a disproportionate share of cancer morbidity and mortality. It is the most common cause of cancer death in children up to 15 yr.

PEAK INCIDENCE: Depends on histology, though highest peak at ~age 50 yr

PREDOMINANT SEX AND AGE: Slight male preponderance (8.0 vs. 5.5/100,000 person/yr)

GENETICS: Most primary CNS neoplasms are sporadic; 5% is associated with hereditary syndromes that predispose to neoplasia. The most common of these include:

- Li-Fraumeni syndrome: *p53* mutation on chromosome 17q13, gliomas
- Von Hippel-Lindau: VHL, chromosome 3p25, hemangioblastoma
- Tuberous sclerosis: TSC1/TSC2 (chromosome 9q34/16p13), subependymal giant cell astrocytoma
- Neurofibromatosis type 1: NF1, chromosome 17q11, neurofibroma, optic nerve glioma, low-grade glioma
- Neurofibromatosis type 2: NF2, chromosome 22q12, schwannoma, meningioma, ependymoma
- Retinoblastoma: pRB, chromosome 13q, retinoblastoma
- Gorlin's syndrome: chromosome 9q31, desmoplastic medulloblastoma

RISK FACTORS: Exposure to ionizing radiation has been implicated in meningiomas, gliomas, and nerve sheath tumors. No convincing evidence has shown a link with trauma, occupation, diet, or electromagnetic fields.

PHYSICAL FINDINGS & CLINICAL PRESENTATION

- In general, the location, size, and rate of growth will determine the symptoms and signs of a brain tumor.
- Headache is common and is the worst symptom in nearly half of all patients. Symptoms of intracranial pressure may also be present, including nausea and vomiting. Headache may be localizing. Papilledema is suggestive of obstructive hydrocephalus.
- Seizures occur in 33% of patients and are among the most common symptoms, particularly with brain metastases and low-grade gliomas. The type of seizure and clinical presentation depends on location. Seizures are more common in low-grade compared with high-grade gliomas. It is thought that patients with seizures typically have smaller tumors at time of diagnosis compared with those with other symptoms, because the onset of seizures prompts an imaging study, leading to an earlier diagnosis.
- Focal neurologic signs and symptoms, including muscle weakness, sensory changes, or visual disturbances are also quite frequent. In addition, cognitive dysfunction, accompanied by changes in memory or personality change, may be recounted, often in retrospect.

ETIOLOGY

Most cases are idiopathic, though specific chromosomal abnormalities have been implicated in some tumor types.

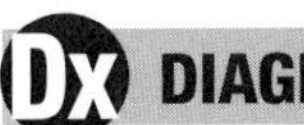

DIAGNOSIS

- Most common tumors in children: low-grade astrocytoma, medulloblastoma, ependymoma
- Most common adult tumors: glioblastoma multiforme, anaplastic astrocytoma, meningioma

LABORATORY

- Ultimately, only histologic examination can provide the exact diagnosis. Information may also be gleaned from additional features such as proliferative index, immunohistochemical stains, and electron microscopy.
- The current classification schema for gliomas is based on pathologic and microscopic criteria.
- Genetic analysis of tumors is rapidly becoming important for genetic classification, stratification of treatments, and predicting outcome. Different subtypes of gliomas have distinct gene-expression profiles, which can be distinguished from one another and from normal tissue; these differences typically involve pathways of cell proliferation, energy metabolism, and signal transduction. In adults, global expression profiling identified differences in 360 genes between low-grade and high-grade tumors.

DIFFERENTIAL DIAGNOSIS

- Stroke/cerebral hemorrhage
- Abscess/parasitic cyst
- Demyelinating disease: multiple sclerosis, postinfectious encephalomyelitis
- Metastatic tumors
- Primary CNS lymphoma

WORKUP

- Neuroimaging studies and pathologic sampling are the most important diagnostic modalities in evaluation of brain tumors and may be critical for preoperative planning.

IMAGING STUDIES

- MRI with gadolinium enhancement is highly sensitive, though CT scanning is useful if calcification or hemorrhage suspected. MRI permits visualization of the tumor, as well as the relation to the surrounding tissue. Enhancing tumor can be distinguished from surrounding edema. Low-grade tumors often present as an infiltrating lesion without mass effect. MRI is superior to CT scanning to evaluate the meninges, subarachnoid space, and posterior fossa, and for defining relation to major intracranial vessels.
- Magnetic resonance spectroscopy is increasingly being used as a diagnostic tool to define metabolic composition of an area of interest and may be useful to contrast areas of tumor progression from radiation necrosis. N-acetylaspartate is often decreased in brain tumors, whereas choline, a component of cell membranes, is increased because of high cellular turnover.
- PET scan is helpful to distinguish neoplastic lesions (with high rate of metabolism) from other lesions such as demyelination or radiation necrosis (with a much lower metabolic rate). Such lesions take up greater amounts of glucose than surrounding tissues or tumors with slower metabolic rates. May be useful to help map functional areas of the brain before surgery or radiation.
- Functional MRI is now used as an adjunct in perioperative planning for patients whose lesion is in vital regions, such as those responsible for speech, language, and motor control.

TREATMENT

NONPHARMACOLOGIC THERAPY

- Maximal surgical removal or debulking is the initial treatment of choice and provides tissue for diagnosis and molecular characterization. Maximal safe resection is often favored with a trend toward improved survival with this approach.
- Biopsy alone is performed if the tumor is located in eloquent regions of brain or is inaccessible; this is essential for histopathologic diagnosis. Biopsy can be performed under CT or MRI guidance using stereotactic localization.
- If the tumor is benign (e.g., meningioma, acoustic neuroma), often no further therapy is required.

ACUTE GENERAL Rx

Antiseizure medications have been used perioperatively and to control seizures resulting from focal lesions. Prophylactic use of anticonvulsants is not typically recommended without clear history of seizures.

CHRONIC Rx

- Chemotherapy (combination or single agent) may be used before, during, or after surgery and radiation therapy. (In children, chemotherapy is often used to delay radiation therapy.) Radiosensitizers may help increase the therapeutic effect of radiation therapy.
- Radiation is useful for certain types of tumors and is often used if there is residual tumor after surgery; conventional radiation uses external beams over a period of weeks, whereas stereotactic radiosurgery delivers a single, high dose of radiation to a well-defined area (usually <1 cm). Long-term effects of radiation therapy include radiation necrosis (particularly of white matter), blood vessel hyalinization, and secondary tumors (usually meningiomas, sarcomas, and malignant astrocytomas).
- Experimental therapies are continually in development and are typically based on molecular characterization of tumors and small molecule blockers of signal transduction cascades. Some of these therapies involve antisense molecules, biologic agents, immunotherapies, or angiogenesis inhibitors. Intratumoral drug infusions and convection-enhanced delivery of novel agents are currently under study.

DISPOSITION

- Tumor histology/histologic diagnosis (World Health Organization [WHO] grading system), including number of mitoses, capillary endothelial proliferation, and necrosis (*Note:* There can be a high degree of morbidity based on tumor location, even with more benign histology.)
- In general, younger age, high performance status, and lower pathologic grade have more favorable prognosis. For all histologic subtypes of brain tumors, pediatric and young adult patients have a better survival rate.

REFERRAL

- All cases warrant evaluation by an oncologist and neurosurgeon.
- Patients should be evaluated for physical and occupational therapy.
- Children should undergo neuropsychologic evaluations and screening for learning disabilities.

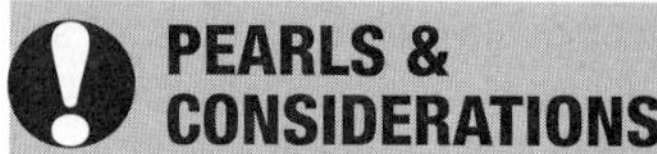

PEARLS & CONSIDERATIONS

COMMENTS

In general, younger age, high performance status, and lower pathologic grade have more favorable prognosis. For all histologic subtypes of brain tumors, pediatric and young adult patients have a better survival.

PATIENT/FAMILY EDUCATION

American Brain Tumor Association

National Brain Tumor Society (http://www.braintumor.org)

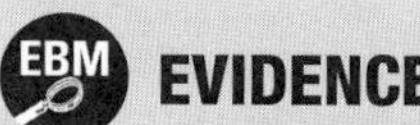

EVIDENCE

Please note: Complete text of EBM for this topic is available online.

SUGGESTED READINGS

Bogomolny DL et al: Functional MRI in the brain tumor patient, *Top Magn Reson Imaging* 15(5):325-335, 2004.

Bradley KA, Mehta MP: Management of brain metastases, *Semin Oncol* 31(5):693-701, 2004.

Glantz MJ et al: Practice parameter: anticonvulsant prophylaxis in patients with newly diagnosed brain tumors. Report of the Quality Standards Subcommittee of the American Academy of Neurology, *Neurology* 54:1886, 2000.

Jemel A et al: Cancer statistics, 2007. *CA Cancer J Clin* 57:43, 2007.

Kleihues P: Pathology and genetics of tumors of the nervous system. In Kleihues P, Cavenee WK (eds): *International agency for research on cancer,* Lyon, 2000, Harcourt, p. 22.

Mischel PS et al: DNA-microarray analysis of brain cancer: molecular classification for therapy, *Nat Rev Neurosci* 5(10):782-792, 2004.

Purow B, Fine HA: Progress report on the potential of angiogenesis inhibitors for neuro-oncology, *Cancer Invest* 22(4):577-587, 2004.

Riva M: Brain tumoral epilepsy: a review, *Neurol Sci* 26(Suppl 1):S40-S42, 2005.

Ullrich NJ, Pomeroy SL: Pediatric brain tumors, *Neurol Clin NA* 21:897-913, 2003.

Wen PY, Marks PW: Medical management of patients with brain tumors, *Curr Opin Oncol* 14:299, 2002.

Wrensch M: Epidemiology of primary brain tumors: current concepts and review of the literature, *Neuro-oncol* 4:278, 2002.

AUTHOR: **NICOLE J. ULLRICH, M.D., PH.D.**

BASIC INFORMATION

DEFINITION

Brain neoplasms are a diverse group of primary (nonmetastatic) tumors arising from one of the many different cell types within the central nervous system. Malignant brain tumors are defined by histopathologic features and a rapidly progressive pattern of growth. Glioblastoma is the most common primary brain tumor in adults, accounting for 50% to 60% of primary brain tumors.

SYNONYMS

Glioblastoma
GBM

ICD-9CM CODES
191.9

EPIDEMIOLOGY & DEMOGRAPHICS

INCIDENCE: Annual incidence rate of glioblastoma is approximately 2 to 3 cases/100,000 persons. High-grade/malignant astrocytomas are slightly more common in whites than in blacks, Latinos, and Asians.
PREDOMINANT SEX AND AGE: Glioblastoma is slightly more common in men than women with a male:female ratio of 3:2. Peak incidence is between 45 and 70 yr. Approximately 10% of glioblastomas occur in children.
PEAK INCIDENCE: High-grade gliomas, such as anaplastic astrocytoma and glioblastoma, tend to originate in the fourth to fifth decade of life and beyond.
RISK FACTORS: Prior radiation may increase risk for primary brain tumor.
GENETICS: Malignant progression is associated with inactivation of *PTEN* tumor-suppressor gene and amplification of epidermal growth factor receptor *(EGFR)* gene.

PHYSICAL FINDINGS & CLINICAL PRESENTATION

- In general, the location, size, and rate of growth will determine the symptoms and signs. Clinical history of patients with glioblastoma is typically brief, <3 mo in the majority of patients with primary glioblastoma.
- Most frequent symptoms include:
  - Headache occurs in the majority of cases. The headache can be localizing or may result from increased intracranial pressure.
  - Seizures occur in 30% to 60% depending on tumor location and grade.
  - Symptoms and signs of hydrocephalus and raised intracranial pressure (headache, vomiting, clouding of consciousness, papilledema).
  - Other symptoms seen in 20% or more of patients include memory loss, focal motor weakness, visual changes, language deficits, and cognitive disturbances or memory changes.

ETIOLOGY

- Glioblastomas are classified as primary or secondary. Primary glioblastoma constitutes the majority of cases (60%) in adults older than 50 yr and are considered de novo tumors. Secondary glioblastoma typically involves malignant progression from a lower grade (grade II or III) glioma. Overexpression of *EGFR* gene occurs in 40% to 50% of primary glioblastoma cases. Loss of heterozygosity on chromosome 10q occurs in 60% to 90% of both primary and secondary glioblastoma cases and is associated with poor prognosis. The pathway involving mutations of the tumor-suppressor gene *p53* is typically associated with secondary glioblastoma. Other genetic mutations have also been recognized as potential contributors in the pathogenesis of glioblastoma, including *PTEN* and *MDM2.*

Dx DIAGNOSIS

DIFFERENTIAL DIAGNOSIS

- Stroke
- Arteriovenous malformations
- Abscess/parasitic cyst (neurocysticercosis)
- Demyelinating disease: multiple sclerosis, postinfectious encephalomyelitis
- Metastatic tumors
- Primary central nervous system lymphoma

LABORATORY TESTS

- Routine laboratory studies are not typically helpful.
- Lumbar puncture is generally contraindicated; cerebrospinal fluid studies do not add much specific additional information for the diagnosis for glioblastoma.
- Ultimately, only a histologic examination can provide the exact diagnosis. Information may also be gleaned from additional features such as proliferative index, immunohistochemical stains, and electron microscopy, as well as molecular markers.

IMAGING STUDIES

- MRI with and without contrast is the imaging study of choice, though CT scanning is useful if calcification or hemorrhage is suspected. MRI permits visualization of the tumor, as well as the relation to the surrounding tissue. Enhancing tumor can be distinguished from surrounding edema. MRI is superior to CT scanning to evaluate the meninges, subarachnoid space, and posterior fossa, and for defining relation to major intracranial vessels.
- Magnetic resonance spectroscopy is increasingly being used as a diagnostic tool to define metabolic composition of an area of interest and may be useful to contrast areas of tumor progression from radiation necrosis. N-acetylaspartate is often decreased in brain tumors, whereas choline, a component of cell membranes, is increased because of high cellular turnover.
- PET scan is helpful to distinguish neoplastic lesions (with high rate of metabolism) from other lesions such as demyelination or radiation necrosis (with a much lower metabolic rate). Such lesions take up greater amounts of glucose than surrounding tissues or tumors with slower metabolic rates. May be useful to help map functional areas of the brain before surgery or radiation.
- Functional MRI is now used as an adjunt to in perioperative planning for patients whose lesion is in vital regions, such as those responsible for speech, language, and motor control.

Rx TREATMENT

- Current standard-of-care therapies include surgery, radiation, and palliative chemotherapy, which have significant adverse effects and limited efficacy. Median time to recurrence after standard therapy is 6.9 mo.

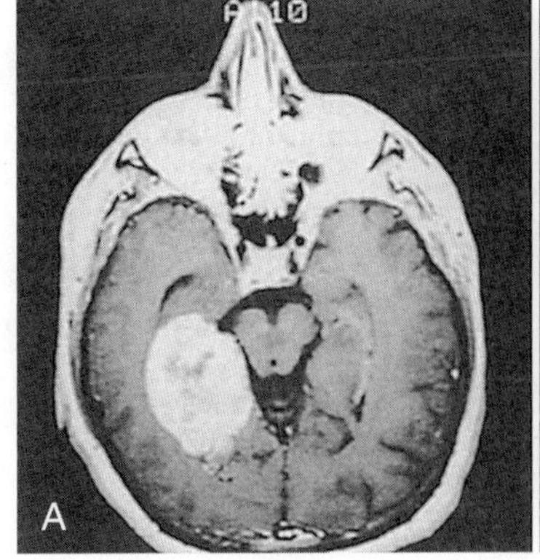

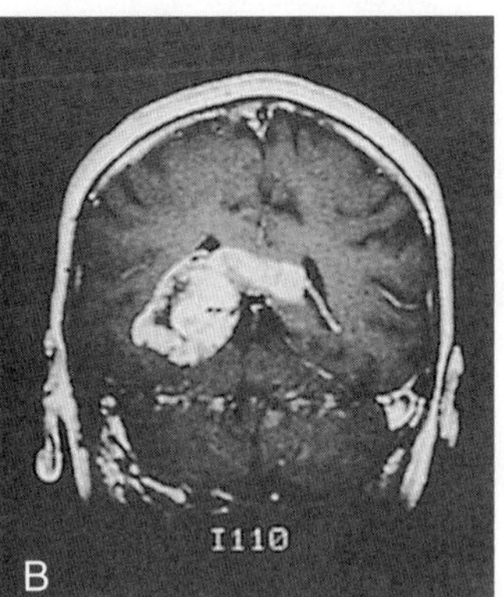

FIGURE 1-44 Glioblastoma multiforme. Axial **(A)** and coronal **(B)** postcontrast enhanced T1-weighted image showing a large homogenously contrast-enhancing mass in the right medial temporal lobe with extension across the midline. (From Specht N [ed]: *Practical guide to diagnostic imaging,* St Louis, 1998, Mosby.)

 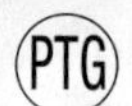

NONPHARMACOLOGIC THERAPY

- Maximal surgical removal or debulking is the initial treatment of choice.
- Biopsy alone is performed if the tumor is located in eloquent regions of brain or is inaccessible; this is essential for histopathologic diagnosis. Biopsy can be performed under CT or MRI guidance using stereotactic localization.

ACUTE GENERAL Rx

- Steroids are used to reduce edema and may also be used perioperatively or during radiation therapy.
- Antiseizure medications have been used perioperatively and to control seizures resulting from focal lesions. Prophylactic use of anticonvulsants is not typically recommended without clear history of seizures.

CHRONIC Rx

- After surgery, radiation therapy remains the most effective adjuvant therapy for patients with glioblastoma.
- Chemotherapy (combination or single agent) may be used before, during, or after surgery and radiation therapy. (In children, chemotherapy is often used to delay radiation therapy.) Radiosensitizers may help increase the therapeutic effect of radiation therapy.
- Experimental therapies are continually in development and are typically based on molecular characterization of tumors and small molecule blockers of signal transduction cascades. Some of these therapies involve antisense molecules, biologic agents, immunotherapies, or angiogenesis inhibitors. Intratumoral drug infusions and convection-enhanced delivery of novel agents are currently under study.

DISPOSITION

- The most important prognostic factors are extent of resection, patient age, tumor grade/histology, and performance status. In general, younger age, high performance status, and lower pathologic grade have more favorable prognosis. For all histologic subtypes of brain tumors, pediatric and young adult patients have a better survival.
- Terminal events typically result from increased intracranial pressure.

REFERRAL

Treatment involves a multispecialty team. Consultations from oncology, neurosurgery, neurology, radiation oncology, psychiatry, and physical therapy are all warranted.

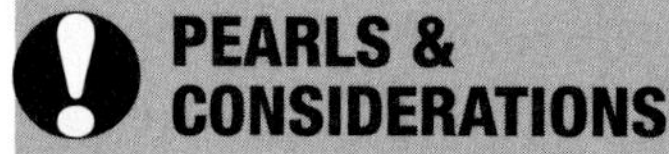

PEARLS & CONSIDERATIONS

COMMENTS

Glioblastoma distinguished pathologically by the presence of vascular proliferation and necrosis. The most important prognostic factors are age, tumor grade, and performance status. The extent of surgical resection also appears to impat prognosis.

PATIENT/FAMILY EDUCATION

American Brain Tumor Association

National Brain Tumor Society (http://www.braintumor.org)

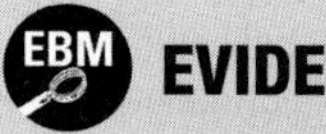

EVIDENCE

Please note: Complete text of EBM for this topic is available online.

SUGGESTED READINGS

Bogomolny DL et al: Functional MRI in the brain tumor patient, *Top Magn Reson Imaging* 15(5):325-335, 2004.

Chao ST: The sensitivity and specificity of FDG PET in distinguishing recurrent brain tumor from radionecrosis in patients treated with stereotactic radiosurgery, *Int J Cancer* 96:191, 2001.

Chang SM et al: Glioma Outcomes Project, *JAMA* 293:557, 2005.

Glantz MJ et al: Practice parameter: anticonvulsant prophylaxis in patients with newly diagnosed brain tumors. Report of the Quality Standards Subcommittee of the American Academy of Neurology, *Neurology* 54:1886, 2000.

Jemel A et al: Cancer statistics, 2007. *CA Cancer J Clin* 57:43, 2007.

Kesari S et al: Targeted molecular therapy of malignant gliomas, *Curr Neurol Neurosci Rep* 5(3):186-197, 2005.

Kleihues P: Pathology and genetics of tumors of the nervous system. In Kleihues P, Cavenee WK (eds): *International agency for research on cancer,* Lyon, 2000, Harcourt, p. 22.

Mischel PS et al: DNA-microarray analysis of brain cancer: molecular classification for therapy, *Nat Rev Neurosci* 5(10):782-792, 2004.

Purow B, Fine HA: Progress report on the potential of angiogenesis inhibitors for neuro-oncology, *Cancer Invest* 22(4):577-587, 2004.

Riva M: Brain tumoral epilepsy: a review, *Neurol Sci* 26(Suppl 1):S40-S42, 2005.

Ullrich NJ, Pomeroy SL: Pediatric brain tumors, *Neurol Clin NA* 21:897-913, 2003.

Wen PY, Marks PW: Medical management of patients with brain tumors, *Curr Opin Oncol* 14:299, 2002.

Wrensch M: Epidemiology of primary brain tumors: current concepts and review of the literature, *Neuro-oncol* 4:278, 2002.

AUTHOR: **NICOLE J. ULLRICH, M.D., PH.D.**

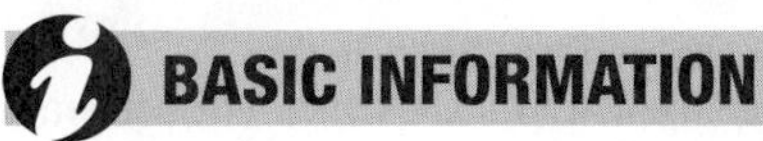

BASIC INFORMATION

DEFINITION

The term *breast cancer* refers to invasive carcinoma of the breast, whether ductal or lobular.

SYNONYMS

Carcinoma of the breast

ICD-9CM CODES
174.9 Malignant neoplasm female breast

EPIDEMIOLOGY & DEMOGRAPHICS

- Nearly exclusively the disease of women, with only 1% of breast cancers in males
- Steady increase in its incidence in the U.S., with 205,000 new patients annually
- Annual mortality of 40,000
- Risk steadily increases with age
- Genetically defined group of women with *BRCA-1* or *BRCA-2* genes identified to carry lifetime risk as high as 85%

PHYSICAL FINDINGS & CLINICAL PRESENTATION

- Increasing number of small breast cancers found by mammograms
- Patients usually completely free of physical findings
- Palpable tumors possibly as small as 1 cm or even smaller
- Size of the mass and its location measured and documented
- Skin and/or nipple retraction and skin edema, erythema, ulcer, satellite nodule
- Nodal enlargement in axilla and supraclavicular areas
- Advanced disease: clinical signs of pleural effusion and/or hepatomegaly
- Rare instances: clear, serous, or bloody discharge only symptom
- Nipple evaluation (see "Paget's Disease of the Breast")

ETIOLOGY

- Precise mechanism of carcinogenesis not understood
- Possibly interaction of ovarian estrogen, nonovarian estrogen, estrogens of exogenous origin with breast tissue of varied carcinogenic susceptibility to develop cancer
- Other known or suspected variables: childbearing, breastfeeding practice, diet, physical activities, body mass, alcohol intake
- Have identified families with known high risk
- Women with *BRCA-1* and *BRCA-2* genes associated with high risk

Dx DIAGNOSIS

DIFFERENTIAL DIAGNOSIS

The following nonmalignant breast lesions can simulate breast cancer on both physical and mammogram examinations:

- Fibrocystic changes
- Fibroadenoma
- Hamartoma

WORKUP

- Physical examination:
  1. Mass detected by patient or medical professional: workup required
  2. Negative mammogram: breast cancer not ruled out
  3. Sonogram: to demonstrate mass to be cyst, usually eliminating need for further workup
  4. Screening with both MRI and mammography might rule out cancerous lesions better than mammography alone in women who are known or likely to have an inherited predisposition to breast cancer
- To establish diagnosis:
  1. Positive aspiration cytology on a clinically and mammographically malignant mass—highly accurate but still requires open biopsy confirmation
  2. Stereotactic core needle biopsy diagnosis: reliable with invasive carcinoma identified, but negative or equivocal results require careful evaluation
  3. Atypical hyperplasia or in situ carcinoma found by core needle biopsy: open surgical biopsy confirmation still required
  4. Excisional or incisional biopsy: establishes diagnosis
- NOTE: Do not rely on negative mammogram or negative aspiration cytology findings to exclude malignancy. Make appropriate referral. Obtain imaging studies such as bone scan, chest x-ray examination, CT scan of abdomen, or CT scan of liver.
- Breast radiologic evaluation and an algorithm for breast cancer screening and evaluation are described in Section III. The differential diagnosis of breast lumps is described in Section II.

IMAGING STUDIES

Mammograms: 30% to 50% of breast cancers detected by screening mammograms only as a spiculated mass, a mass with or without microcalcifications, or a cluster of microcalcifications. MRI is an excellent modality that is particularly useful in patients with breast implants and when there is a strong family history of breast cancer.

Rx TREATMENT

NONPHARMACOLOGIC THERAPY

- Early breast cancer: primarily surgical or surgical and radiotherapeutic
- Choice in 60% to 70% of women between modified mastectomy and breast-conserving treatment, which consists of lumpectomy, axillary staging with sentinel node biopsy or axillary dissection, and breast irradiation

ACUTE GENERAL Rx

- May require adjuvant chemotherapy or endocrine therapy. Standard chemotherapy consists of either cyclophosphamide, methotrexate, and fluorouracil or cyclophosphamide plus doxorubicin. Endocrine therapy is recommended after chemotherapy in patients with hormone-receptor positive tumors.
- Weekly paclitaxel after standard adjuvant chemotherapy with doxorubicin and cyclophosphamide improves disease-free and overall survival in women with breast cancer. However, patients with HER2-negative, estrogen-receptor-positive, node-positive breast cancer may gain little benefit from administration of paclitaxel after adjuvant chemotherapy with doxorubicin plus cyclophosphamide.
- Initial therapy of metastatic breast cancer with paclitaxel plus bevacizumab prolongs progression-free survival, but not overall survival.
- Evaluation and treatment by medical oncologist

CHRONIC Rx

Follow-up required after proper treatment of primary breast cancer includes:

- Periodic clinical evaluations as delineated by medical oncologist or surgeon
- Annual mammograms
- Other tests as indicated
- Patient instruction in monthly breast self-examination technique

DISPOSITION

- Prognosis after curative therapy: depends on size of tumor, extent of nodal metastasis, and pathologic grade of tumor
  1. Patient with 1-cm tumor with no axillary node metastasis: 10-yr disease-free survival rate of 90%
  2. Patient with 3-cm tumor with metastasis in four nodes: 10-yr disease-free survival rate of 15% if no systemic adjuvant therapy given
  3. Outlook for most patients is between these extremes
- Systemic adjuvant therapy: improves prognosis significantly
- Isolated tumor cells or micrometastases in regional lymph nodes is associated with a reduced 5-year rate of disease-free survival among women with favorable early-stage breast cancer who do not receive adjuvant therapy. Survival is improved in patients with isolated tumor cells or micrometastases who received adjuvant therapy.
- The addition of zoledronic acid to adjuvant endocrine therapy improves disease-free survival in premenopausal patients with estrogen-responsive early breast cancer.
- Figure 1-45 illustrates frequency of breast cancer metastases.

REFERRAL

Referral is necessary as soon as breast cancer is even remotely suspected.

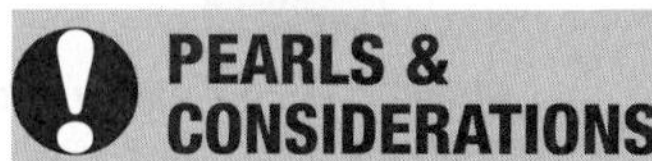

PEARLS & CONSIDERATIONS

Breast cancer in pregnancy and lactation:

1. Frequency in women 40 yr or younger reported to be 15%
2. May carry worse prognosis because disease discovery delayed by engorged and nodular

breast changes and/or because disease progression more rapid in pregnancy
3. Survival rates similar to those for nonpregnant early-stage breast cancer patients in same age group
4. Mass usually found by patient or obstetrician
5. Expedient workup recommended, including mammography and sonography
6. Diagnosis to be made without delay
7. Choice of mastectomy or lumpectomy with axillary dissection for treatment
8. Adjuvant chemotherapy delayed until third trimester or after delivery
9. Irradiation to breast after lumpectomy delayed until after delivery

Ductal carcinoma in situ (DCIS, intraductal carcinoma):

1. "New" disease mostly found by mammogram as cluster of microcalcifications and/or density
2. Presents less often as a palpable mass or nipple discharge
3. Before mammogram screening, DCIS accounted for 1% of all breast cancers
4. Now 15% to 20% or even higher proportion have DCIS
5. Formerly treated with mastectomy, now lumpectomy
6. Cure rates 98% to 99%
7. No axillary dissection required
8. With radiation, breast recurrences reduced
9. Mastectomy possibly required with extensive and/or high-grade DCIS
10. Systemic adjuvant treatment is not indicated

Inflammatory carcinoma:

1. Rare but rapidly progressive and often lethal form of breast cancer
2. Presents as erythematous and edematous breast resembling mastitis
3. Biopsy required, including skin
4. Treatment with combination chemotherapy followed by surgery and radiation therapy
5. Prognosis once dismal, now 5-yr disease-free survival in 50% of patients

COMMENTS

- Patient education material can be obtained from the following:
  1. SHARE: Self-Help for Women with Breast Cancer, 19 W 44th Street, No 415, New York, NY 10036-5902
  2. Y-ME National Organization of Breast Cancer Information and Support, 18220 Harwood Avenue, Homewood, IL 80430
- Breast radiologic evaluation, evaluation of nipple discharge, and evaluation of palpable mass are described in Section III.

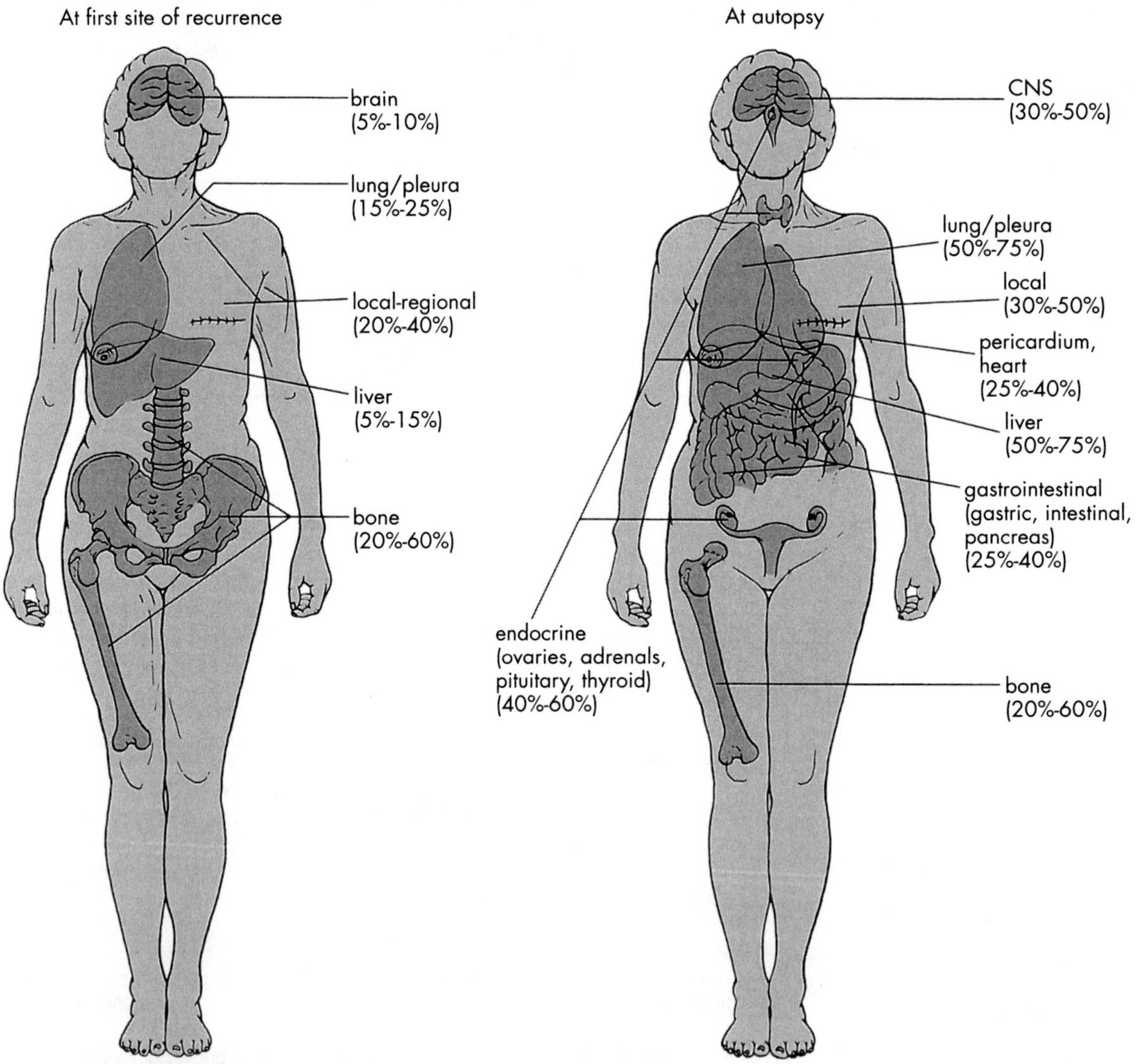

At first site of recurrence

brain (5%-10%)
lung/pleura (15%-25%)
local-regional (20%-40%)
liver (5%-15%)
bone (20%-60%)

At autopsy

CNS (30%-50%)
lung/pleura (50%-75%)
local (30%-50%)
pericardium, heart (25%-40%)
liver (50%-75%)
gastrointestinal (gastric, intestinal, pancreas) (25%-40%)
endocrine (ovaries, adrenals, pituitary, thyroid) (40%-60%)
bone (20%-60%)

FIGURE 1-45 Frequency of breast cancer metastases. The most common first sites of recurrent breast cancer are the chest wall, the regional lymph nodes, and/or bone. Liver, lung, and central nervous system (CNS) are less common sites of recurrence. In patients with well-advanced disease, breast cancer can be found in almost any organ. Autopsy studies show that metastases are most commonly found in the chest wall and in the surrounding lymph nodes, as well as in the bones, liver, lung, pleura, and CNS (brain, spinal cord, meninges). Metastases may also occur in gastrointestinal organs (pancreas, stomach, large and small intestine), endocrine organs (ovaries, adrenals, pituitary, thyroid), and in the cardiovascular system (pericardium, endocardium, myocardium). (From Skarin AT: *Atlas of diagnostic oncology,* ed 3, St. Louis, 2003, Mosby.)

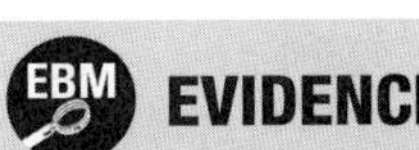

EVIDENCE

Please note: Complete text of EBM for this topic is available online.

Key trials and commentary:

High insulin and insulin-like growth factor-1 (IGF-1) levels may be associated with an increased breast cancer risk and/or death. Given the need to identify modifiable factors that decrease insulin, IGF-1, and breast cancer risk and death, This study investigated the effects of a 6-month randomized controlled aerobic exercise intervention vs. usual care on fasting insulin, IGF-1, and its binding protein (IGFBP-3) in postmenopausal breast cancer survivors. It revealed that moderate-intensity aerobic exercise, such as brisk walking, decreases IGF-1 and IGFBP-3. The exercise-induced decreases in IGF may mediate the observed association between higher levels of physical activity and improved survival in women diagnosed with breast cancer.

The study by Irwin and colleagues investigates circulating insulin and insulin-like growth factors as potential links between physical activity, breast cancer recurrence, and death. In women with breast cancer, moderate-intensity physical activity initiated after diagnosis has been associated with reduced risk of death. In this randomized clinical trial, previously sedentary women with a history of stage 0-IIIA breast cancer engaged in supervised and home-based cardiovascular exercise or usual activities for 6 months. Serum insulin, IGF-1, and IGFBP-3 decreased in the exercise group, whereas they increased in the usual care group. The between-group changes reached statistical significance for IGF-1 and IGFBP-3. An interesting finding was that the effects of exercise on insulin and IGF were modified by age, with a stronger exercise effect in older women. Obesity is another potential moderator of an exercise-insulin interaction in women with breast cancer. Although body mass index was not a significant modifier of the exercise effect in this study, a review of the relevant literature suggests more potent effects of exercise to reduce insulin and IGF-1 in obese as compared with lean women. To the contrary, it remains plausible that favorable changes in circulating growth factors in response to cardiovascular endurance exercise are independent of body composition because muscle contraction alone stimulates several insulin-sparing mechanisms, including postreceptor insulin signaling, increased glucose delivery, and increased clearance of free fatty acids. Large-scale studies will be needed to test the significance of age, adiposity, or other potential moderators of the exercise and growth factor interaction among breast cancer survivors.[1] Ⓐ

Ovarian suppression plus tamoxifen is a standard adjuvant treatment in premenopausal women with endocrine-responsive breast cancer. Aromatase inhibitors are superior to tamoxifen in postmenopausal patients, and preclinical data suggest that zoledronic acid has antitumor properties.

One study revealed that the addition of zoledronic acid to adjuvant endocrine therapy improves disease-free survival in premenopausal patients with estrogen-responsive early breast cancer.

This trial looks at the comparative efficacy of tamoxifen vs. anastrozole and the role of bisphosphonates in premenopausal women on adjuvant endocrine therapy for limited breast cancer. None of the patients had known bone involvement at the time of initiation of therapy on study. A statistically significant 36% reduction in the likelihood of disease progression was observed in the group assigned to receive zoledronic acid 4mg every 6 months (the first 254 patients received 4mg every 4 weeks). There was no observed difference between tamoxifen and anastrozole. No improvement in overall survival was noted, but there were only 42 events for survival at the time of this report. No osteonecrosis was observed on the study. These data show that the observed advantage of aromatase inhibitors over antiestrogens in postmenopausal women could not be confirmed in premenopausal women; hence, the use of tamoxifen in premenopausal remains reasonable first hormonal therapy. The data also suggest that a bisphosphonate should be included in the management of these patients who do not have observable bone involvement.[2] Ⓐ

Quality of life (QL) is an important consideration when comparing adjuvant therapies for early breast cancer, especially if they differ substantially in toxicity. We evaluated QL and Q-TWiST among patients randomized to adjuvant dose-intensive epirubicin and cyclophosphamide administered with filgrastim and progenitor cell support (DI-EC) or standard-dose anthracycline-based chemotherapy (SD-CT). Despite greater initial toxicity, This study showed that quality-adjusted survival was similar or better with dose-intensive treatment as compared to standard treatment. Thus, QL considerations should not be prohibitive if future intensive therapies show superior efficacy.

On the basis of well-designed randomized controlled trials,[1-4] high-dose chemotherapy (HDC) with stem cell support has proven to be more toxic and no more efficacious than standard-dose chemotherapy for cases of both high-risk and metastatic breast cancer. This approach of hitting the most serious cases of breast cancer with the most aggressive or intense form of chemotherapy was initially viewed as promising based on the results of single-arm trials demonstrating results that appeared superior to historical outcomes from standard therapy.[5] Accrual to randomized trials was difficult due to patients' and physicians' preferences, with the majority of patients treated off-protocol or in single-arm studies.

In this context, two recent publications, one by Bernhard and colleagues in the *British Journal of Cancer* and one by Crump and colleagues[1] in the *Journal of Clinical Oncology* present results that are important both for the clinical information they provide and for their fulfillment of the obligation between researcher and trial participants to analyze and publicize trial results, even when the trial is negative.

The article by Crump and colleagues presented the results of a randomized multicenter trial conducted by the National Cancer Institute Clinical Trials Group, in which 386 patients with metastatic breast cancer were treated with induction chemotherapy, and those with a significant response (224) were randomized to HDC versus standard-dose chemotherapy. Although this trial was underpowered and closed early because of poor accrual following negative results from similar randomized trials, it provided further evidence that there was no benefit in terms of survival from HDC and a substantial cost, in this case a 6% increased incidence of 100-day mortality over the more intensive approach. Scant details of the longitudinal quality of life analysis are provided, but it appears that quality of life was substantially worse during chemotherapy although comparable between study arms by 6 mo after treatment.

The message of higher toxicity and worse quality of life during therapy with recovery to baseline or better by several months after treatment is mirrored in the study by Bernhard and colleagues. This publication reported the QL and Q-TWiST analysis for a randomized trial of HDC versus standard-dose adjuvant chemotherapy conducted by the International Breast Cancer Study Group. This trial also failed to show a significant benefit for HDC over standard-dose therapy, but quality of life improved to better than baseline by several months after completion of either therapy.[7]

In general, the principle that "more is better" when it comes to cytotoxic chemotherapy for breast cancer has been discredited; however, given the emerging understanding of the heterogeneity of this disease, it is not impossible that there will be a subset of patients for whom this hypothesis merits further testing in the future among carefully selected patients in a well-designed randomized clinical trial. If so, these trials suggest that quality of life differences should not preclude a more intense, but more effective therapy. Of course, the hope is that we will identify pathways and targeted agents that will allow us to improve outcomes with little additional toxicity, as has been demonstrated for patients with HER2–positive breast cancer in both the metastatic and adjuvant settings. These HDC studies highlight the importance of randomized trials, even when the experimental therapy seems promising and the need for continued efforts to find better strategies to improve outcomes for women with high-risk and metastatic breast cancer.[3] Ⓐ

Worldwide, approximately 750,000 new cases of breast cancer are diagnosed annually in premenopausal women with limited economic resources. Longer-term survival benefits from adjuvant therapies in such women with operable breast cancer are unknown.

Another study showed that in premenopausal women with operable breast cancer not selected for estrogen receptor status or with estrogen receptor–positive tumors, 5- and 10-year DFS and OS rates are significantly improved following adjuvant oophorectomy and tamoxifen.

Love et al made two points in their conclusion. First, they stated that "the survival of adjuvant-treated patients in this trial . . . supports use of [surgical oophorectomy and tamoxifen] in many circumstances." *Probably.* However, whereas ovarian function suppression (OFS) by oophorectomy has clear advantages in a resource-poor population, its exact role in the treatment of hormone receptor-positive breast cancer in premenopausal women remains unclear. Adjuvant tamoxifen is now routinely recommended. The benefit of OFS when added to 5 years of tamoxifen is unproven. Previous trials frequently used 2 years of tamoxifen. The one randomized European Cooperative Oncology Group trial addressing the issue in node-negative breast cancer was underpowered and did not show a significant benefit. Chemotherapy followed by tamoxifen is commonly recommended in high-risk patients, and the advantage of adding OFS to this combination is uncertain. OFS can add significantly to toxicity and should not be added without solid evidence of benefit. The international Suppression of Ovarian Function Trial, which randomly assigns premenopausal women with hormone receptor–positive breast cancer to tamoxifen vs. OFS plus tamoxifen vs. OFS plus an aromatase inhibitor, remains open to accrual and has the potential to answer the question definitively.

The second conclusion Love and colleagues drew was that "the increase in the hazard function for recurrence between years 5 and 10 supports investigation of intervention and treatment strategies directed to this hazard." *Definitely.* The risk of recurrence for women with estrogen receptor–positive breast cancer after 5 years of tamoxifen therapy remains substantial. Few data have specifically addressed the issue in premenopausal women. In the study by Love and colleagues, the hazard for recurrence after year 5 appears to increase for women who were treated (despite permanent ovarian function ablation), whereas women not treated appear to have a continued decline in risk. However, the confidence intervals on these estimates are large. Over time, an increasing proportion of the untreated women would naturally undergo menopause, which may have influenced their risk of late relapse. A recent abstract presenting preliminary results of the Adjuvant Tamoxifen, Longer against Shorter (ATLAS) trial suggested that, contrary to previous publication of smaller trials, the recurrence rate was lower among women allocated to continue tamoxifen. It would be interesting to see an analysis of outcomes in the premenopausal women from the ATLAS trial.[4] Ⓐ

The international standard radiotherapy schedule for early breast cancer delivers 50 Gy in 25 fractions of 2.0 Gy over 5 weeks, but there is a long history of non-standard regimens delivering a lower total dose using fewer, larger fractions (hypofractionation). This study aimed to test the benefits of radiotherapy schedules using fraction sizes >2.0 Gy in terms of local-regional tumor control, normal tissue responses, quality of life, and economic consequences in women prescribed post-operative radiotherapy.

This study revealed that a radiation schedule delivering 40 Gy in 15 fractions seems to offer rates of local-regional tumour relapse and late adverse effects at least as favourable as the standard schedule of 50 Gy in 25 fractions.

The START Trial B is a prospective, randomized clinical trial comparing 50 Gy in 25 fractions of 2.0 Gy over 5 weeks to 40 Gy in 15 fractions of 2.67 Gy over 3 weeks for early-stage breast cancer. Whereas whole-breast fractionation of 1.8-2.0 Gy daily to 46-50 Gy has been the standard in clinical practice in the United States for over 30 years, alternative schedules using hypofractionation, or greater than 2.0 Gy per daily fraction, have been commonly used in the United Kingdom and Canada.

In this study, there was no statistically significant difference in local relapse at 5 years, but there was a trend favoring hypofractionation over conventional fractionation (2.0% vs. 3.3%). The 5-year distant relapse, disease-free survival, and overall survival rates were superior in the hypofractionation arm. Patient self-assessments, including changes in breast or skin appearance, edema, and hardness, were also consistently better with the hypofractionated regimen.

Areas for future research include determining the optimal method of integrating a supplemental tumor bed boost with a hypofractionated radiation schedule and whether results of hypofractionated radiation would have been better with intensity-modulated radiation therapy (IMRT) compared with conventional radiation. Promising results have been demonstrated with new protocols in the United States that combine hypofractionation with IMRT and a concurrent breast boost.

The present study is now one of four prospective randomized trials from Canada and the United Kingdom that have shown hypofractionation schedules to be noninferior in local control and late effects with 5-year and 10-year results. In fact, the number of patients treated in these four trials of hypofractionated radiation (7095 patients) now exceeds the number treated in the six major trials comparing breast-conserving surgery and radiation with mastectomy (approximately 4100 patients). It is time we overcame physician practice inertia and offered these shortened treatment schedules more widely to women in the United States.[5] Ⓐ

Most invasive breast cancers are classified as invasive ductal carcinoma not otherwise specified (IDC NOS), whereas about 25% are defined as histological "special types." These special-type breast cancers are categorized into at least 17 discrete pathological entities; however, whether these also constitute discrete molecular entities remains to be determined. Current therapy decision-making is increasingly governed by the molecular classification of breast cancer (luminal, basal-like, HER2 positive). The molecular classification is derived from mainly IDC NOS and it is unknown whether this classification applies to all histological subtypes. We aimed to refine the breast cancer classification systems by analyzing a series of 11 histological special types (invasive lobular carcinoma [ILC], tubular, mucinous A, mucinous B, neuroendocrine, apocrine, IDC with osteoclastic giant cells, micropapillary, adenoid cystic, metaplastic, and medullary carcinoma) using immunohistochemistry and genome-wide gene expression profiling. Hierarchical clustering analysis confirmed that some histological special types such as micropapillary carcinoma constitute discrete entities but also revealed that others, including tubular and lobular carcinoma, are very similar at the transcriptome level. When classified by expression profiling, IDC NOS and ILC contain all molecular breast cancer types (i.e., luminal, basal-like, HER2+), whereas histological special-type cancers, apart from apocrine carcinoma, are homogeneous and only belong to one molecular subtype. Our analysis also revealed that some special types associated with a good prognosis, such as medullary and adenoid cystic carcinomas, display a poor prognosis basal-like transcriptome, providing strong circumstantial evidence that basal-like cancers constitute a heterogeneous group. Taken together, our results imply that the correct classification of breast cancers of special histological type will allow a more accurate prognostication of breast cancer patients and facilitate the identification of optimal therapeutic strategies.

In 2000, Perou et al published the results of a study subclassifying breast carcinomas based on the expression pattern of 8102 genes. Based on this molecular classification approach, three general categories of breast carcinoma have been proposed, including luminal, basal-like, and HER2 positive. This landmark study was, however, limited predominantly to invasive ductal carcinoma. This study applies the concept of gene expression profile-based taxonomy to include 11 subtypes of breast cancer, which are well known to pathologists, and of these only invasive lobular was included in the original

Perou study. This wide-reaching study suggests an overall classification scheme that could potentially encompass all epithelial breast neoplasms based on gene expression profiles. The practicing pathologist, who has relied on histopathologic and immunohistochemical features for classification, may find it interesting how the gene expression data validate the unique characterization of some subtypes (pleomorphic lobular) and demonstrate relationships between others (adenoid cystic, metaplastic, and basal-like). As acknowledged by the authors, this classification model is far from complete, but this study gives a workable indication of what a future arrangement may look like.[6] Ⓐ

This study reviewed (1) the epidemiological literature on physical activity and the risk of breast cancer, examining the effect of the different parameters of activity and effect modification within different population subgroups; and (2) the biological mechanisms whereby physical activity may influence the risk of breast cancer.

This study showed that the effect of physical activity on the risk of breast cancer is stronger in specific population subgroups and for certain parameters of activity that need to be further explored in future intervention trials.

It has been known for a number of years that, in common with several other forms of carcinoma, the risk of developing a cancer of the breast is substantially lower in physically active individuals. It is theoretically possible that those with a low risk of cancer choose to exercise, but a causal relationship appears more probable. The association seems strongest for those who undertake moderate rather than extreme forms of physical activity. Prolonged but moderate exercise is the most effective way of controlling obesity, and this suggests that one of the mechanisms of benefit may be a limitation of fat accumulation. Certainly, carcinogenic steroids can be synthesized in body fat depots following the menopause. Dr. Friedenreich and her colleagues at the Alberta Cancer Board have been accumulating information on the relationship between breast cancer and physical activity throughout the past decade, and their current review offers a competent meta-analysis of 62 published case-control and cohort trials. An association was found in only about three-quarters of the studies, but many of these showed the previously noted dose/response relationship typical of a causal relationship. Nevertheless, as in earlier analyses of this question, the advantage of vigorous over moderate physical activity (26% vs 22% reduction in risk) was not very impressive. The association of a reduced cancer risk was greater for long-term than for recent physical activity. This probably implies a need to be active throughout much of the life cycle, although it is also conceivable that lifetime habits can be assessed more accurately than the current behavior. Perhaps, the most useful feature of the present review is the accumulation of sufficient data to assess benefit in terms of the individual's body mass index. The risk reduction associated with physical activity showed a clear gradation through lean (0.73) and normal (0.76), to overweight (0.81) and obese (1.04) individuals. This would seem to point to benefit from the estrogen-suppressing effect of a combination of low body fat and physical activity in premenopausal women. There are many other potential mechanisms that merit further exploration, including the reduction of blood glucose levels, and modulation of inflammatory and immune responses associated with regular physical activity. As our knowledge of these other factors grows, one may hope that the beneficial effects of regular physical activity will grow beyond the current 25% reduction in risk.[7] Ⓐ

A separate trial conducted a meta-analysis of randomized trials that evaluated the efficacy of incorporating taxanes into anthracycline-based regimens for early breast cancer (EBC). We aimed to determine whether this approach improves disease-free survival (DFS) and overall survival (OS) and whether benefits are maintained across relevant patient subgroups.

This study revealed that the addition of a taxane to an anthracycline-based regimen improves the DFS and OS of high-risk EBC patients. The DFS benefit was independent of ER expression, degree of nodal involvement, type of taxane, age/menopausal status of patient, and administration schedule.

A large number of clinical trials have been conducted worldwide in the past decade to test the benefit of taxanes combined with traditional adjuvant anthracyclines and non-anthracycline polychemotherapy in patients with EBC.

The debate over the benefit of taxanes in EBC has now been settled with these first-generation taxane trials. We should now focus our attention on the second- and third-generation taxane trials in order to optimally combine taxanes with anthracyclines, including determining the proper sequencing, dose, frequency of administration, and optimal duration of therapy, and to explore measures for decreasing toxicities. Methods to predict response to taxanes and to identify patients who may benefit from anthracyclines, the development of novel taxanes, and the combination of taxanes with biologic agents are urgently needed in order to offer individualized therapy tailored to the biology of each patient with EBC that requires adjuvant chemotherapy.[8] Ⓐ

Another study is a comprehensive comparison of biomarker expression between patients' primary breast carcinoma (PBC) and their metastatic breast carcinomas (MBC).It showed that Therapeutic targets identified in the PBC or even some MBC may not reflect targets present in all metastatic sites.

This study used a rapid autopsy protocol to study the biological changes between primary breast carcinomas and their associated metastatic deposits. With this methodology the investigators were able to construct tissue microarrays for each patient, which were composed of the primary tumor and metastases from different sites. This allowed direct evaluation and comparison of clinically important biomarker expression. Markers that were evaluated include estrogen receptor, progesterone receptor, E-cadherin, cyclooxygenase-2, EGFR, mesothelin, and HER-2/neu. The important finding for the practicing pathologist is that metastatic lesions frequently demonstrate altered biological activity from the primary tumor. Some markers, notably ER and PR were often down-regulated in the metastatic disease, whereas others such as EGFR and MET were often relatively overexpressed in the metastasis. Given the current use of therapeutic modalities targeted to specific proteins, these and similar findings will become important as pathologists evaluate samples from metastatic disease. The article also addresses fundamental issues in the biology of metastatic disease, notably that the promoter methylation profile for selected genes is not altered, thus the authors furthered the concept that "a cancer's genetic makeup and, therefore, its clinical behavior are likely determined at its primary site."[9] Ⓐ

Evidence-Based References

1. Irwin ML et al: Randomized controlled trial of aerobic exercise on insulin and insulin-like growth factors in breast cancer survivors: the Yale Exercise and Survivorship Study, *Cancer Epidemiol Biomarkers Prev* 18:306-313, 2009. Commentary by C.M. Jankowski, Ph.D. Ⓐ
2. Gnant M et al: Endocrine therapy plus zoledronic acid in premenopausal breast cancer, *N Engl J Med* 360:679-691, 2009. Commentary by J.T. Thigpen, M.D. Ⓐ
3. Bernhard J et al: Quality of life and quality-adjusted survival (Q-TWiST) in patients receiving dose-intensive or standard dose chemotherapy for high-risk primary breast cancer, *Br J Cancer* 98: 25-33, 2008. Commentary by J. Peppercorn, M.D., MPH Ⓐ
4. Love RR et al: Survival after adjuvant oophorectomy and tamoxifen in operable breast cancer in premenopausal women, *J Clin Oncol* 26:253-257, 2008. Commentary by G.F. Fleming, M.D., P. Francis, M.D. Ⓐ
5. The START Trialists' Group: The UK Standardisation of Breast Radiotherapy (START) Trial B of radiotherapy hypofractionation for treatment of early breast cancer: a randomised trial, *Lancet* 371:1098-1107, 2008. Commentary by G.M. Freedman, M.D. Ⓐ
6. Weigelt B et al: Refinement of breast cancer classification by molecular characterization of histological special types, *J Pathol* 216:141-150, 2008. Commentary by G. Azabdaftari, M.D. Ⓐ
7. Friedenreich CM, Cust AE: Physical activity and breast cancer risk: impact of timing, type and dose of activity and population subgroup effects, *Br J*

Sports Med 42:636-647, 2008. Commentary by R.J. Shephard, M.D., Ph.D., D.P.E. Ⓐ

8. De Laurentiis M et al: Taxane-based combinations as adjuvant chemotherapy of early breast cancer: a meta-analysis of randomized trials, *J Clin Oncol* 26:44-53, 2008. Commentary by S.-C. Tang, M.D., Ph.D. Ⓐ

9. Wu JM et al: Heterogeneity of breast cancer metastases: comparison of therapeutic target expression and promoter methylation between primary tumors and their multifocal metastases, *Clin Cancer Res* 14:1938-1946, 2008. Commentary by G. Azabdaftari, M.D. Ⓐ

SUGGESTED READINGS

Berry DA et al: Estrogen-receptor status and outcomes of modern chemotherapy for patients with node-positive breast cancer, *JAMA* 295:1658-1667, 2006.

Buchholz T: Radiation therapy for early-stage breast cancer after breast conserving surgery, *N Engl J Med* 360:63-70, 2009.

De Boer M et al: Micrometastases or isolated tumor cells and the outcome of breast cancer, *N Engl J Med* 361:653-663, 2009.

Gnant M et al: Endocrine therapy plus zoledronic acid in premenopausal breast cancer, *N Engl J Med* 360: 679-691, 2009.

Hayes DF et al: HER2 and response to paclitaxel in node-positive breast cancer, *N Engl J Med* 357: 1496-1506, 2007.

Knutson D, Steiner E: Screening for breast cancer: current recommendations and future directions, *Am Fam Physician* 5:1660-1666, 2007.

Marchionni L et al: Systematic review: gene expression profiling assays in early stage breast cancer, *Ann Intern Med* 148:358-368, 2008.

Miller K et al: Paclitaxel plus bevacizumab versus paclitaxel alone for metastatic breast cancer, *N Engl J Med* 357:2666-2676, 2007.

Muss HB et al: Adjuvant chemotherapy in older women with early-stage breast cancer, *N Engl J Med* 360: 2055-2065, 2009.

Punglia RS et al: Local therapy and survival in breast cancer, *N Engl J Med* 356:2399-2405, 2007.

Robson M, Offit K: Management of an inherited predisposition to breast cancer, *N Engl J Med* 357: 154-162, 2007.

Smith RA: The evolving role of MRI in the detection and evaluation of breast cancer, *N Engl J Med* 256: 13, 2007.

Sparano JA et al: Weekly paclitaxel in the adjuvant treatment of breast cancer, *N Engl J Med* 358:1663-1671, 2008.

Warner E et al: Systematic review: using magnetic resonance imaging to screen women at risk for breast cancer, *Ann Intern Med* 148:671-679, 2008.

Whelan TJ et al: Long-term results of hypofractionated radiation therapy for breast cancer, *N Engl J Med* 362:513-520, 2010.

Woolf SH: The 2009 breast cancer screening recommendations of the US Preventive Services Task Force, *JAMA* 303:162, 2010.

AUTHORS: **TAKUMA NEMOTO, M.D.,** and **RUBEN ALVERO, M.D.**

BASIC INFORMATION

DEFINITION

Breech presentation occurs when the fetal longitudinal axis is such that the cephalic pole occupies the uterine fundus. Three types exist, with respective percentages at term: frank (48% to 73%, flexed hips, extended thighs), complete (4.6% to 11.5%, flexed hips and knees), and footling (12% to 38%, hips extended).

ICD-9CM CODES
652.2 Breech presentation without mention of version

EPIDEMIOLOGY & DEMOGRAPHICS

INCIDENCE: Gestational age dependent: 3% to 4% overall, 14% at 29 to 32 wk, 33% at 21 to 24 wk

PERINATAL MORTALITY: 9% to 25%, or three to five times increase over vertex presentation at term. When correcting for the associated increase in congenital anomalies and complications of prematurity, the morbidity and mortality rates approach those of the vertex presentation at term regardless of route of delivery.

PHYSICAL FINDINGS & CLINICAL PRESENTATION

- Lack of presenting part on vaginal examination
- Fetal heart tones heard above the umbilicus
- Leopold maneuvers revealing mobile fetal part in the uterine fundus

ETIOLOGY

- Abnormal placentation (fundal), uterine anomalies (fibroids, septa), pelvic or adnexal masses, alterations in fetal muscular tone, or fetal malformations
- Associated conditions: trisomy 13, 18, 21; Potter syndrome; myotonic dystrophy; prematurity

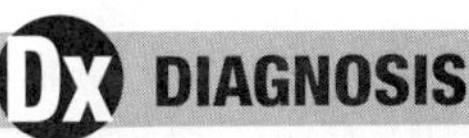

DIAGNOSIS

DIFFERENTIAL DIAGNOSIS

Vertex, oblique, or transverse lie

WORKUP

- Determine reason for breech presentation, history of uterine anomalies, gestational age, or associated fetal congenital anomalies
- Assess fetal status by continuous fetal heart rate monitoring or ultrasound
- Assess pelvis to determine feasibility of vaginal delivery
- Assess risk for safety of vaginal versus abdominal delivery

IMAGING STUDIES

Ultrasound to evaluate for:

- Fetal anomalies, such as hydrocephalus
- Placental location
- Position of fetal head relative to spine (check for hyperextension)
- Estimated fetal weight (2500 to 3800 g)
- Type of breech (frank, complete, footling)

TREATMENT

ACUTE GENERAL Rx

- Vaginal delivery in selected patients (see "Comments" section): allow maternal expulsive forces to deliver fetus until scapula visible (avoiding traction); with flexion and/or Piper forceps, deliver fetal head
- Perform cesarean section (see "Comments")
- External cephalic version: success 60% to 75% after 37 wk, contraindicated with placental abruption, low-lying placenta, maternal hypertension, previous uterine incision, multiple gestation, nonreassuring fetal status
- Adequate pelvic/cervical relaxation essential for vaginal breech (i.e., need anesthesia in-room during birth [delivery] with uterine relaxants on hand [nitroglycerin, terbutaline])

COMPLICATIONS

- Head entrapment: leading cause of death (with the exception of anomalous fetuses), 88 cases per 1000 deliveries; avoid by maintaining flexion of fetal head, use of Piper forceps or Dührssen's incisions. Before 36 wk, HC > AC, thus fetal predisposition. Tentorial tears from hyperextended head. Association with trisomy 21 in 3% to 5% of cases. Avoid hyperextension of head during delivery.
- Cord prolapse: usually occurs late in the course of labor. Incidence depends on type of breech: frank (0.5%), complete (4% to 5%), footling (10%).
- Nuchal arm: arm extended above fetal head, occurs when there is undue traction before delivery of fetal scapulas. Treatment depends on bringing trapped arm across infant's face.

DISPOSITION

If confounding variables are corrected for, such as prematurity and associated congenital anomalies (6.3% of breeches vs. 2.4% in general population), route of delivery plays a less important role in fetal outcome than previously believed.

REFERRAL

An obstetrician trained in delivery of the vaginal breech is a prerequisite for attempting vaginal route, although it must be explained to the patient that with cesarean section certain risks (such as hyperextension of the fetal head with resultant spinal cord injury) may be minimized but not eliminated.

PEARLS & CONSIDERATIONS

COMMENTS

In general, for breech presentation, mortality rate is increased 13-fold and morbidity sevenfold. The main reasons are an increase in congenital anomalies, perinatal hypoxia, birth injury, and prematurity.

There is no contraindication to induction of labor in the breech presentation, and labor is not prohibited in a primigravida.

CRITERIA FOR TRIAL OF LABOR:

- Estimated fetal weight 2000 to 3800 g
- Frank breech
- Adequate pelvis
- Flexed fetal head
- Continuous fetal monitoring
- Normal progress of labor
- Bedside availability of anesthesia and capability for immediate cesarean section
- Informed consent
- Obstetrician trained in vaginal breech delivery

CRITERIA FOR CESAREAN SECTION:

- Estimated fetal weight <1500 g or >4000 g
- Footling presentation (20% risk of cord prolapse, usually late in course of labor)
- Inadequate pelvis
- Hyperextended fetal head (21% risk of spinal cord injury)
- Nonreassuring fetal status
- Abnormal progress of labor
- Lack of trained obstetrician

AUTHORS: **SCOTT J. ZUCCALA, D.O.,** and **RUBEN ALVERO, M.D.**

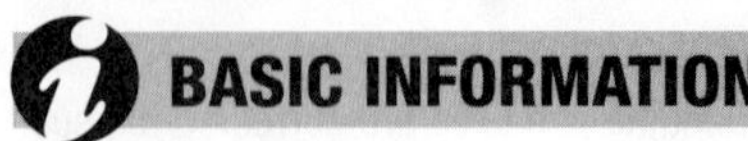

BASIC INFORMATION

DEFINITION

Bronchiectasis is the abnormal dilation and destruction of bronchial walls, which may be congenital or acquired.

ICD-9CM CODES
494.0 Bronchiectasis

EPIDEMIOLOGY & DEMOGRAPHICS

- Cystic fibrosis is responsible for nearly 50% of all cases of bronchiectasis.
- Acquired primary bronchiectasis is uncommon because of rapid diagnosis of pulmonary infections and frequent use of antibiotics.
- Effective childhood immunizations have led to a significant decrease in the incidence of bronchiectasis resulting from pertussis.

PHYSICAL FINDINGS & CLINICAL PRESENTATION

- Moist crackles at lung bases
- Cough with expectoration of large amount of purulent sputum
- Fever, night sweats, generalized malaise, weight loss
- Hemoptysis
- Halitosis, skin pallor
- Clubbing (infrequent)

ETIOLOGY

- Cystic fibrosis
- Lung infections (pneumonia, lung abscess, TB, fungal infections, viral infections)
- Abnormal host defense (panhypogammaglobulinemia, Kartagener's syndrome, AIDS, chemotherapy)
- Localized airway obstruction (congenital structural defects, foreign bodies, neoplasms)
- Inflammation (inflammatory pneumonitis, granulomatous lung disease, allergic aspergillosis)

Dx DIAGNOSIS

DIFFERENTIAL DIAGNOSIS

- TB
- Asthma
- Chronic bronchitis or chronic sinusitis
- Interstitial fibrosis
- Chronic lung abscess
- Foreign body aspiration
- Cystic fibrosis
- Lung carcinoma

LABORATORY TESTS

- Sputum for Gram stain, culture and sensitivity, and acid-fast bacteria
- Complete blood count with differential (leukocytosis with left shift, anemia)
- Serum protein electrophoresis to evaluate for hypogammaglobulinemia
- Antibody test for aspergillosis
- Sweat test in patients with suspected cystic fibrosis

IMAGING STUDIES

- Chest radiograph: hyperinflation, crowded lung markings, small cystic spaces at the base of the lungs.
- High-resolution CT scan of the chest has become the best tool to detect cystic lesions and exclude underlying obstruction from neoplasm. The CT study should be a noncontrast study with the use of 1- to 1.5-mm window every 1 cm with acquisition time of 1 sec. Typical findings on CT include dilation of airway lumen, lack of tapering of an airway toward periphery, ballooned cysts at the end of bronchus, and varicose constrictions along airways.
- Bronchoscopy may be helpful to evaluate hemoptysis, rule out obstructive lesions, and remove mucus plugs.

Rx TREATMENT

NONPHARMACOLOGIC THERAPY

- Postural drainage (reclining prone on a bed with the head down on the side) and chest percussion with use of inflatable vests or mechanical vibrators applied to the chest may enhance removal of respiratory secretions.
- Adequate hydration.
- Supplemental oxygen for hypoxemia.

ACUTE GENERAL Rx

- Antibiotic therapy is based on the results of sputum, Gram stain, and culture and sensitivity; in patients with inadequate or inconclusive results, empiric therapy with amoxicillin/clavulanate 500 mg to 875 mg q12h, TMP-SMX q12h, doxycycline 100 mg bid, or cefuroxime 250 mg bid for 10 to 14 days is recommended.
- Bronchodilators are useful in patients with demonstrable airflow obstruction.

CHRONIC Rx

- Avoidance of tobacco
- Maintenance of proper nutrition and hydration
- Prompt identification and treatment of infections
- Pneumococcal vaccination and annual influenza vaccination

DISPOSITION

Prognosis is variable with severity of the disease and underlying etiology of bronchiectasis.

REFERRAL

Surgical referral for partial lung resection in patients with localized severe disease unresponsive to medical therapy or in patients with massive hemoptysis

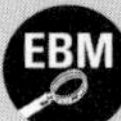

EVIDENCE

There is evidence that inspiratory muscle training compared with placebo improves endurance exercise capacity in patients with bronchiectasis.[1] Ⓐ

A systematic review found a small benefit for the use of prolonged antibiotics (given with prophylactic intent) in the treatment of bronchiectasis compared with placebo. Response rates showed a significant benefit, but exacerbation rates and lung function showed no difference to placebo.[2] Ⓑ

Inhaled tobramycin may result in bacterial eradication and clinical improvement for patients infected with *Pseudomonas aeruginosa.* Further studies are required to evaluate the use of inhaled tobramycin.[3] Ⓑ

Although there is no clear evidence sufficient to guide clinical practice, regular inhaled corticosteroids may improve lung function in patients with bronchiectasis. Further studies are required.[4] Ⓐ

There is not enough evidence to evaluate the routine use of mucolytics for bronchiectasis.[5]

We are unable to cite any evidence that meets our criteria for the effectiveness of long-acting bronchodilator or short-acting bronchodilator therapy in the management of bronchiectasis.

The evidence for bronchopulmonary hygiene physical therapy is insufficient. No effect on pulmonary function was seen in most comparison studies apart from improved sputum clearance.[6] Ⓑ

We were unable to cite any evidence that meets our criteria concerning the efficacy of surgical intervention for bronchiectasis.

Evidence-Based References

1. Bradley J et al: Physical training for bronchiectasis, *Cochrane Rev* 1, 2000. Ⓐ
2. Evans DJ et al: Prolonged antibiotics for purulent bronchiectasis, *Cochrane Rev* 2, 2002. Ⓑ
3. Barker AF et al: Tobramycin solution for inhalation reduces sputum *Pseudomonas aeruginosa* density in bronchiectasis, *Am J Respir Crit Care Med* 162:481, 2000. Ⓑ
4. Ram FSF et al: Inhaled steroids for bronchiectasis, *Cochrane Rev* 2, 2000. Ⓐ
5. Crockett AJ et al: Mucolytics for bronchiectasis, *Cochrane Rev* 1, 2001.
6. Jones AP, Rowe BH: Bronchopulmonary hygiene physical therapy for chronic obstructive pulmonary disease and bronchiectasis, *Cochrane Rev* 4, 1998. Ⓑ

SUGGESTED READING

Barker AF: Bronchiectasis, *N Engl J Med* 346:1383, 2002.

AUTHOR: **FRED F. FERRI, M.D.**

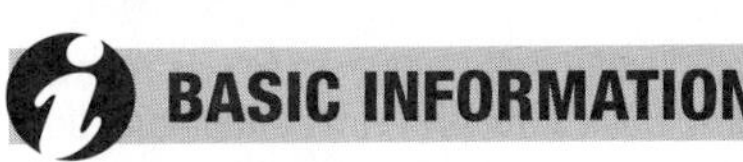

BASIC INFORMATION

DEFINITION

Brucellosis is a zoonotic infection caused by one of four species of *Brucella.* It commonly presents as a nondescript febrile illness.

SYNONYMS

Malta fever, ungulate fever
Bang's disease

ICD-9CM CODES

023.9 Brucellosis

EPIDEMIOLOGY & DEMOGRAPHICS

INCIDENCE (IN U.S.): About 100 cases/yr (may be underreported)
PREDOMINANT SEX: Male
PREDOMINANT AGE: Adult
CONGENITAL INFECTION: Recent evidence suggests a high rate of spontaneous abortions in untreated pregnant women during the first and second trimesters.
NEONATAL INFECTION: Can occur if mother is infected during pregnancy.

PHYSICAL FINDINGS & CLINICAL PRESENTATION

- Incubation period is 1 wk to 3 mo.
- Patients may be asymptomatic or have nonspecific symptoms such as fever, sweats, malaise, weight loss, depression, arthralgia, and arthritis.
- Fever is the most common finding.
- Hepatomegaly, splenomegaly, or lymphadenopathy is possible.
- Localized disease includes endocarditis, meningitis, spondylitis, sacroiliitis, and osteomyelitis (especially vertebral).

Chronic hepatosplenic suppurative brucellosis (CHSB) presents with hepatic or splenic abscesses. This form is thought to be a reactivation and can occur years after the acute infection.

ETIOLOGY

- Caused by infection with *Brucella* species:
  1. Most commonly *B. melitensis,* but also *suis, abortus,* or *canis*
  2. A small, gram-negative coccobacillus
- Acquired through ingestion of organisms (unpasteurized goat or cow's milk), breaks in the skin, or by inhalation.
- Most cases occur after exposure to animals (sheep, goats, swine, cattle, or dogs), or animal products (i.e., milk, hides, tissue).
- Most cases (in U.S.) occur in men with occupational exposure to animals (farmers, ranchers, laboratory workers, veterinarians, abattoir workers).
- Laboratory workers, especially those in microbiology, are also at increased risk. Guidelines for post-exposure prophylaxis are available from *MMWR Surveill Summ* 57:39, 2009.

DIAGNOSIS

DIFFERENTIAL DIAGNOSIS

Many febrile conditions without localizing manifestations (i.e., TB, endocarditis, typhoid fever, malaria, autoimmune diseases)

WORKUP

- Cultures of blood, bone marrow, or other tissue (lymph node, liver) should be sent and held for 4 wk, because *Brucella* spp. grow slowly in vitro.
- Granulomas on biopsy are suggestive of diagnosis.

LABORATORY TESTS

- WBC count: normal or low
- Serology:
  1. Serum agglutination test (SAT) to detect antibodies to *B. abortus, melitensis,* and *suis.*
  2. Specific antibody test to identify antibodies to *B. canis.*
  3. False-negative SAT possibly resulting from a prozone effect.
  4. PCR (polymerase chain reaction) for *Brucella* spp. specific 16S rRNA or DNA sequences are increasingly used for the diagnosis of brucellosis from blood, tissue samples, and bone marrow.

IMAGING STUDIES

- Radiographs to show splenic or hepatic calcifications in chronic disease
- Bone scan, MRI, and radiographs of the spine to suggest osteomyelitis
- Ultrasound or CT scan of the abdomen to show an enlarged liver or spleen
- Echocardiogram to reveal vegetations in endocarditis

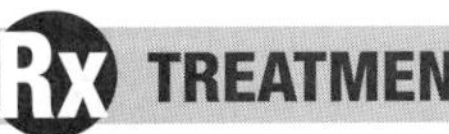

TREATMENT

NONPHARMACOLOGIC THERAPY

- Drainage of abscesses
- Valve replacement for endocarditis

ACUTE GENERAL Rx

Combination antibiotics required:

- Doxycycline 100 mg PO bid plus streptomycin 15 mg/kg IM qd for 6 wk
- Less effective: doxycycline 100 mg PO bid plus rifampin 600 mg PO qd or sulfamethoxazole 800 mg/trimethoprim 160 mg one DS tablet PO qid, ciprofloxacin 500 mg bid for 6 wk along with doxycycline or rifampin as an alternative regimen

Courses <6 wk are associated with higher relapse rates; longer courses are recommended for complicated disease (e.g., osteomyelitis, endocarditis, and neurobrucellosis).

DISPOSITION

- Relapse is possible weeks to months after the completion of therapy.
- Reactivation with CHSB has been reported up to 35 yr after initial illness.

REFERRAL

For all cases to an infectious disease specialist

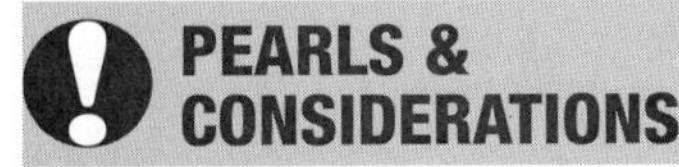

PEARLS & CONSIDERATIONS

COMMENTS

- Alert the microbiology laboratory to the possibility of *Brucella* spp. (prolonged incubation needed and biohazard for laboratory personnel).
- Do not use doxycycline in children or pregnant women.
- Avoid aminoglycosides in pregnant women.
- Fluoroquinolones have good in vitro activity against *Brucella* spp. and are under study as components of complex regimens. Monotherapy is not effective.

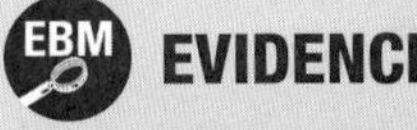

EVIDENCE

A doxycycline-rifampin combination therapy for 45 days is as effective as the classic doxycycline-streptomycin combination in most patients with brucellosis.[1]

Doxycycline-rifampin therapy may be less effective in patients with spondylitis.[1]

Streptomycin plus doxycycline therapy is associated with higher success rates (judged by the frequency of treatment failure and relapse following therapy) than combinations of rifampin and doxycycline.[2]

Oral rifampin plus oral doxycycline for 45 days has a high cure rate, as does oral doxycycline for 45 days plus intramuscular streptomycin for 21 days.[3]

Regimens containing streptomycin yielded favorable results in clinical study.[4]

Rifampin plus trimethoprim-sulfamethoxazole is associated with low relapse rates ranging from 4% to 8% in patients receiving therapy for 3 or 5 wk and no relapses in patients treated for 8 wk.[5]

Evidence-Based References

1. Ariza J et al: Treatment of human brucellosis with doxycycline plus rifampin or doxycycline plus streptomycin, *Ann Intern Med* 117:25-30, 1992.
2. Luzzi GA et al: Brucellosis: imported and laboratory acquired cases, and an overview of treatment trials, *Trans R Soc Trop Med Hyg* 87:138-141, 1993.
3. Acocella G et al: Comparison of three different regimens in the treatment of acute brucellosis: a multinational study, *J Antimicrob Agents Chemother* 23:433-439, 1989.
4. Montejo JM et al: Open, randomized therapeutic trial of six antimicrobial regimens in the treatment of human brucellosis, *Clin Infect Dis* 16:671-676, 1993.
5. Lubani et al: A multicenter therapeutic study of 1100 children with brucellosis, *Ped Infect Dis J* 8:75-78, 1989.
6. Skalsky K et al: Treatment of human brucellosis: systematic review and meta-analysis of randomized controlled trials, *BMJ* 336:701, 2008.

SUGGESTED READINGS

Navarro E et al: Use of real-time quantitative PCR to monitor the evolution of Brucella melitensis DNA load during therapy and post-therapy follow-up in patients with brucellosis, *Clin Infect Dis* 42:1266, 2006.
Pappas G et al: The new global map of human brucellosis, *Lancet* 6:91, 2006.
Pappas et al: Brucellosis, *N Engl J Med* 352:2335, 2005.

AUTHORS: **PATRICIA CRISTOFARO, M.D., GLENN G. FORT, M.D., M.P.H.,** and **DENNIS J. MIKOLICH, M.D.**

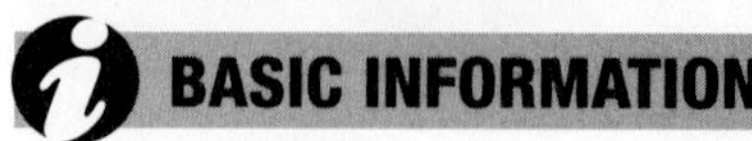

BASIC INFORMATION

DEFINITION

Forcible clenching or grinding of the teeth during sleep or wakefulness, often leading to damage of the teeth.

ICD-9CM CODES

306.8 Bruxism

EPIDEMIOLOGY & DEMOGRAPHICS

- Occurs in 15% of children and 75% of adults
- Familial cases have occasionally been described.
- Bruxism often presents between age 10 and 20 yr but may persist throughout life.
- Nocturnal bruxism is noted most often during stages I and II NREM sleep and REM sleep.

PHYSICAL FINDINGS & CLINICAL PRESENTATION

Complaints of grinding of teeth from a sleep partner or members of the family are common. In many cases the masticatory system will adapt to the phenomenon, but in severe cases nearly every part of the masticatory system may be damaged. Excessive wearing of dentition is the most common physical finding. Tender or hypoatrophied masticatory muscles may also be observed.

ETIOLOGY

- Cause is controversial.
- Possible causes include occlusal discrepancies, anatomy of the bony structures of the orofacial region, part of the sleep arousal response, disturbances of the central dopaminergic system, smoking, alcohol, drugs, stress, and personality.

DIAGNOSIS

DIFFERENTIAL DIAGNOSIS

- Dental compression syndrome
- Temporomandibular joint disorders
- Chronic orofacial pain disorders
- Oral motor disorders
- Malocclusion

WORKUP

- History should have an emphasis on sleep habits, including excessive snoring, pain in the temporal mandibular region, interview with close family members, health habits, personality quirks.
- Physical examination of the teeth and masticatory muscles is mandatory.
- Sleep studies in selected cases may be helpful.

LABORATORY TESTS

None indicated unless a systemic disease is suspected (e.g., infection, autoimmune disorder)

IMAGING STUDIES

X-ray studies of teeth and temporomandibular joints

TREATMENT

NONPHARMACOLOGIC THERAPY

Biofeedback, psychological counseling, and elimination of harmful health habits have been used with limited success.

GENERAL Rx

- Oral splints (Fig. 1-46); nightguard to protect teeth may be useful
- Correction of malocclusion
- Pain management (e.g., gabapentin, ibuprofen)
- Medication to relieve anxiety and improve sleep (e.g., benzodiazepine or trazodone at bedtime)
- Local injections of botulinum toxin into masseter muscles to prevent dental and temporomandibular joint complications

DISPOSITION

Referral to dentist mandatory if damage to teeth evident

PEARLS & CONSIDERATIONS

- Like any poorly understood disease, treatment is often unsatisfactory and subject to quackery.
- Both diurnal and nocturnal bruxism may be associated with various movement and degenerative disorders (e.g., Huntington disease, oromandibular dystonia) and are quite common in children with cerebral palsy and mental retardation.

SUGGESTED READINGS

Attansio R: An overview of bruxism and its management, *Dent Clin North Am* 41(2):229, 1997.

Dae TT, Lavigne EJ: Oral splints: the crutches for temporomandibular disorders and bruxism, *Crit Rev Oral Biol Med* 9(3):345, 1998.

Lopbezoo F, Naeije M: Bruxism is mainly regulated centrally, not peripherally, *J Oral Rehabil* 28(12): 1085, 2001.

Tan EK, Jankovic J: Treating severe bruxism with botulinum toxin, *J Am Dent Assoc* 131:211, 2000.

AUTHOR: **FRED F. FERRI, M.D.**

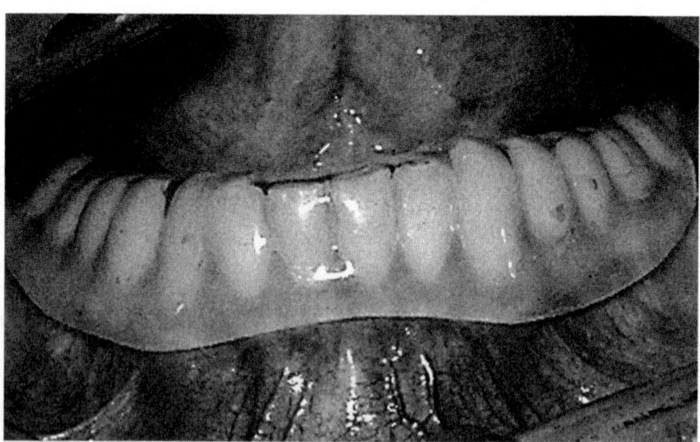

FIGURE 1-46 Occlusal splint. (From Hochberg MC et al [eds]: *Rheumatology,* ed 3, St Louis, 2003, Mosby.)

BASIC INFORMATION

DEFINITION

Budd-Chiari syndrome (BCS) is a rare disease defined by the obstruction of hepatic venous outflow anywhere from the small hepatic veins to the junction of the inferior vena cava (IVC) and the right atrium. Primary BCS is defined by endoluminal obstruction as seen in thromboses or webs. Secondary BCS occurs when the obstruction is caused by compression or invasion by a lesion originating outside the veins (tumor, abscess, cyst, etc.). It can also be a postoperative complication of orthotopic liver transplantation.

SYNONYMS

Hepatic vein thrombosis
Obliterative endophlebitis of the hepatic veins
IVC thrombosis (obliterative hepatocavopathy)

ICD-9CM CODES

453.0 Budd-Chiari syndrome

EPIDEMIOLOGY & DEMOGRAPHICS

INCIDENCE: 1/2.5 million persons per yr
PREDOMINANT SEX: In Western countries, women are more commonly affected
PREDOMINANT AGE: Presentation is usually in the third and fourth decades of life.

PHYSICAL FINDINGS & CLINICAL PRESENTATION

Clinical presentation and characteristics vary with geography. In Africa and South Asia, intravascular webs are more often associated with IVC thrombosis with a stronger association with subsequent hepatocellular carcinoma. In the U.S., BCS is more commonly associated with primary myeloproliferative disorders and underlying hypercoagulable states. Underlying factors that contribute to BCS can be identified in ~85% of cases, and multiple causative factors are identified in 50% of cases.

- Need two of three hepatic veins to be compromised to see clinical manifestations.
- Variable according to the degree, location, acuity of obstruction, and presence of collateral circulation:
  - Fulminant/acute (20%): severe right upper quadrant abdominal pain, fever, nausea, vomiting, jaundice, hepatomegaly, ascites, marked elevation in serum aminotransferases, elevation of alkaline phosphatase to 300 to 400 IU/L, decrease in coagulation factors, and encephalopathy within 8 wk of onset of jaundice; early recognition and treatment are essential for survival
  - Subacute/chronic (60%): vague abdominal discomfort, gradual progression to caudate lobe hypertrophy with atrophy of the rest of the liver, portal hypertension with or without cirrhosis and its sequelae, ascites, lower extremity edema, esophageal varices, splenomegaly, coagulopathy, hepatorenal syndrome in up to half of patients, hepatopulmonary syndrome in up to 28% of patients, and rarely, encephalopathy
  - Asymptomatic (5% to 20%): usually discovered incidentally by abnormal liver function tests

ETIOLOGY

- Primary myeloproliferative diseases: 20% to 53%
  - Polycythemia vera, responsible for 10% to 40% of cases
  - Essential thrombocythemia and idiopathic myelofibrosis are less common causes
  - *JAK2* mutations associated with many myeloproliferative disorders are now being implicated in cases of idiopathic BCS
- Hypercoagulable states: often coexist with other causes, up to 31%
  - Factor V Leiden (25%)
  - Factor II gene mutation (5%)
  - Anticardiolipin antibodies (25%)
- Protein C deficiency, protein S deficiency, and antithrombin III deficiency are difficult to interpret because of acute thrombus and liver disease; need familial studies to prove
- Heterozygosity for G20210A prothrombin gene mutation or methylene-tetrahydrofolate reductase (MTHFR) mutation may be seen in BCS
- Hyperhomocysteinemia
- Pregnancy and oral contraceptive pills
- Rare but reported: sickle cell anemia, infections with liver abscess, hydatid cyst (echinococcosis), schistosomiasis, malignancies, sarcoidosis, Behçet's disease (<5%), paroxysmal nocturnal hemoglobinuria (leading cause of mortality in this condition), IVC membrane/congenital web, abdominal trauma, ulcerative colitis, celiac disease, idiopathic (10% to 20%)

DIAGNOSIS

DIFFERENTIAL DIAGNOSIS

- Hepatitis from ischemia, viral infection, toxin, alcohol
- Cholecystitis
- Hepatic venoocclusive disease (sinusoidal obstruction syndrome)
- Congestive hepatopathy, also known as *cardiac cirrhosis,* from tricuspid regurgitation, right atrial myxoma, constrictive pericarditis
- Cirrhosis from any etiology

LABORATORY TESTS

- Assessment of liver injury and function: serum aminotransferases, alkaline phosphatase, prothrombin time (PT), albumin, bilirubin
- Exclusion of another form of liver disease: viral hepatitis panel, autoantibodies (antinuclear antibody, anti–smooth muscle antibody, anti-mitochondrial antibody), serum iron, transferrin saturation, ferritin, ceruloplasmin, and α-1 antitrypsin
- Ascites protein content >3.0 g/dl and serum ascites albumin gradient $\geq$1.1 g/dl are suggestive of ascites from BCS, cardiac or pericardial disease
- Evaluation for underlying myeloproliferative disorder and hypercoagulable state: CBC, bone marrow biopsy, tests for hypercoagulable states (Factor V Leiden, prothrombin gene G20210A mutation, protein C, protein S, and antithrombin deficiencies, antiphospholipid antibodies, hyperhomocystinemia, paroxysmal nocturnal hemoglobinuria, and MTHFR C677T mutation); protein C, protein S, and antithrombin deficiencies may be difficult to interpret in the setting of liver dysfunction, but levels <20% of normal are suggestive of a true deficiency; thrombophilia screening for the JAK2 V617F mutation may be useful

IMAGING STUDIES

- Diagnosis of BCS is made by radiographic imaging.
- Ultrasound and color and pulsed Doppler are the first-line tests. Diagnostic sensitivity and specificity are 85% to 90%. Findings include large hepatic vein with an absent flow signal, or with reversed or turbulent flow; large intrahepatic collateral vessels; enlarged, stenotic, or tortuous hepatic veins; and caudate lobe hypertrophy.
- MRI with gadolinium contrast—better than contrast-enhanced CT (Fig. 1-47), with a sensitivity and specificity of approximately 90%—is the second-line test. Findings include obstructed hepatic veins or IVC, large, intrahepatic, or subcapsular collaterals, and caudate lobe hypertrophy. Three-dimensional contrast-enhanced magnetic resonance angiography rivals hepatic venography in sensitivity.
- CT image reconstruction of vasculature is becoming available.
- Venography: This is not essential for diagnosis, but when done with measurement of pressure gradients is mainly indicated to predict success of percutaneous or surgical shunt intervention. Confirms the pathognomonic web pattern caused by collateral venous flow.
- Liver biopsy: This is not necessary to diagnose BCS but may be helpful in patients with cirrhosis in whom the diagnosis remains uncertain and critical for differentiating from hepatic venoocclusive disease. Findings in-

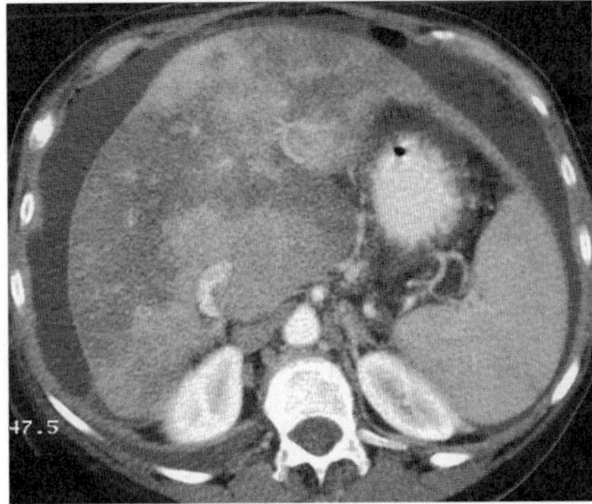

FIGURE 1-47 CT scan of Budd-Chiari syndrome. The appearances are not immediately diagnostic for the nonexpert, and infiltrative disease is sometimes suspected. (From Forbes A et al [eds]: *Atlas of clinical gastroenterology*, ed 3, 2005, Mosby.)

clude hepatic congestion, hepatocyte necrosis and fibrosis in centrilobular areas, and compensatory nodular regenerative hyperplasia with progression to fibrosis and cirrhosis. In advanced BCS, may also see infarction caused by concomitant thrombosis of the intrahepatic, extrahepatic, and portal veins.

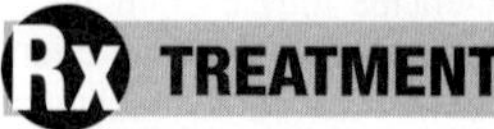

TREATMENT

NONPHARMACOLOGIC THERAPY

- Goal of therapy is decompression of hepatic congestion.
- In general, therapeutic procedures should be introduced by order of increasing invasiveness based on response/failure to therapy rather than disease severity.
- Hypercoagulable states should be investigated in all patients.

ACUTE GENERAL Rx

- Anticoagulation, first with low-molecular-weight heparin (LMWH), followed by warfarin, even in the absence of an underlying hypercoagulable disorder
- In situ thrombolysis: can be successful when performed in recently thrombosed veins, and high blood flow can be restored by angioplasty or stenting
- Balloon angioplasty: complicated by 50% restenosis rate
- Stenting: may improve long-term patency rates to 90%, but if placed above the intrahepatic IVC, may complicate future liver transplantation
- Transjugular intrahepatic portosystemic shunt (TIPS) has been increasingly used in recent years; usually performed in patients with no improvement on anticoagulation therapy; TIPS has replaced surgical shunting as the most common invasive therapeutic procedure
- Surgical portal systemic shunts: feasibility depends on technical factors, as well as on locating a center with well-trained surgeons
- Liver transplant may be indicated in patients with fulminant hepatic failure and in patients who fail to respond to TIPS
- Supportive measures

CHRONIC Rx

- Lifelong anticoagulation: Warfarin therapy with a target international normalized ratio of (INR) 2 to 3 lessens, but does not completely prevent, recurrence.
- In patients with an underlying myeloproliferative disorder, treatment with hydroxyurea and aspirin, or anagrelide, may be given instead of traditional anticoagulation.
- Treat liver dysfunction and complications related to portal hypertension, such as ascites.
- Invasive interventions should be reserved for symptomatic patients who do not improve with medical therapy.
- Manage shunt thrombosis, which is a common complication.
- Liver transplantation is another treatment option.
- Monitor for development of hepatocellular carcinoma and transformation of myeloproliferative disease in patients with longstanding, well-controlled BCS.

DISPOSITION

Prognosis is variable and depends on multiple factors, including time to recognition and treatment, etiology, acuity, the type of intervention, and the condition of the patient at the time of treatment. Overall mortality rates are decreasing with the use of anticoagulation and early diagnosis of asymptomatic cases. Survival rates have been reported as 77%, 65%, and 57% at 1, 5, and 10 yr from diagnosis. A prognostic index called the *Rotterdam BCS Index* has been described: 1.27 × Encephalopathy + 1.04 × Ascites + 0.72 × PT + 0.004 × Bilirubin. Encephalopathy and ascites are scored as 1 for present or 0 as absent, and PT is scored as greater (1) or less than (0) an INR of 2.3. An index of $<$1.1 correlates to low risk (5-yr survival rate, 89%), 1.1 to 1.5 with intermediate risk (5-yr survival rate, 74%), and $>$1.5 with high risk (5-yr survival rate, 42%).

REFERRAL

Fulminant presentations should immediately be referred to a center capable of liver transplantation. All cases benefit from referral to a hepatologist, a hematologist, an interventional radiologist, and a surgeon specializing in hepatobiliary disease.

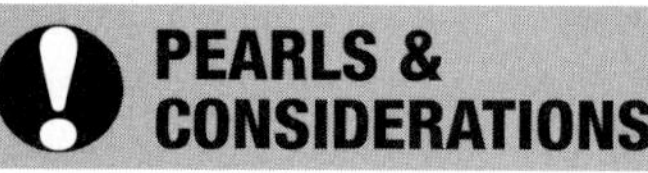

PEARLS & CONSIDERATIONS

COMMENTS

- Look for one or more underlying causes, especially hypercoagulable or hematologic disorders.
- Myeloproliferative disorders are most common.
- Diagnosis relies on imaging, beginning with Doppler ultrasound.
- Treatment with anticoagulation comes first, followed by invasive interventions as needed.
- Referral for liver transplantation may be necessary.
- Prognosis depends on presence of ascites, encephalopathy, PT, and serum bilirubin levels.

PREVENTION

In the setting of known risk factors, such as a hypercoagulable state or myeloproliferative disorder, any additional risks, such as smoking or oral contraceptive therapy, should be avoided.

SUGGESTED READINGS

Darwish Murad S et al; EN-Vie (European Network for Vascular Disorders of the Liver): Etiology, management, and outcome of the Budd-Chiari syndrome, *Ann Intern Med* 151:167-175, 2009.

DeLeve LD et al; American Association for the Study Liver Diseases: Vascular disorders of the liver, *Hepatology* 49(5):1729-1764, 2009.

Garcia-Pagán JC et al; Budd-Chiari Syndrome-Transjugular Intrahepatic Portosystemic Shunt Group: TIPS for Budd-Chiari syndrome: long-term results and prognostics factors in 124 patients, *Gastroenterology* 135(3):808-815, 2008.

Murad SD et al: Etiology, management, and outcome of the Budd-Chiari syndrome, *Ann Intern Med* 151:167-175, 2009.

Plessier A, Valla DC: Budd-Chiari syndrome, *Semin Liver Dis* 28(3):259-269, 2008.

AUTHORS: **KITTICHAI PROMRAT, M.D.,** and **JENNIFER ROH HUR, M.D.**

BASIC INFORMATION

DEFINITION

Bulimia nervosa is a prolonged illness characterized by a specific psychopathology.

ICD-9CM CODES
783.6 Bulimia

EPIDEMIOLOGY & DEMOGRAPHICS

INCIDENCE/PREVALENCE: Affects 1% to 3% of female adolescents and young adults
PREDOMINANT SEX: Female/male ratio of 10:1
PREDOMINANT AGE: Adolescence to young adulthood; mean age of onset: 17 yr

PHYSICAL FINDINGS & CLINICAL PRESENTATION

- Parotid and salivary gland swelling
- Scars on the back of the hand and knuckles (Russell sign) from rubbing against the upper incisors when inducing vomiting
- Eroded enamel, particularly on the lingual surface of the upper teeth; pyorrhea and other gum disorders possible
- Petechial hemorrhages of the cornea, soft palate, or face possibly noted after vomiting
- Loss of gag reflex, well-developed abdominal musculature
- Often no emaciation; normal physical examination possible

ETIOLOGY

- Etiology is unknown but likely multifactorial (sociocultural, psychologic, familial factors).
- Bulimia is much more common in Western societies, where there is a strong cultural pressure to be slender.
- According to the American Psychiatric Association, patients with eating disorders display a broad range of symptoms that occur along a continuum between those of anorexia nervosa and bulimia.

Dx DIAGNOSIS

DIFFERENTIAL DIAGNOSIS

- Schizophrenia
- Gastrointestinal disorders
- Neurologic disorders (seizures, Kleine-Levin syndrome, Klüver-Bucy syndrome)
- Brain neoplasms
- Psychogenic vomiting

WORKUP

- The following questions are useful to screen patients for bulimia:
  1. "Are you satisfied with your eating habits?"
  2. "Do you ever eat in secret?"
- Answering "no" to the first question and/or "yes" to the second question has 100% sensitivity and 90% specificity for bulimia. The SCOFF questionnaire can also be used as a screening tool for eating disorders (see Anorexia Nervosa).
- A diagnosis can be made using the following DSM-IV diagnostic criteria for bulimia nervosa:
  1. Recurrent episodes of binge eating (rapid consumption of a large amount of food in a discrete period)
  2. A feeling of lack of control over eating behavior during the eating binges
  3. Self-induced vomiting, use of laxatives or diuretics, strict dieting or fasting, or rigorous exercise to prevent weight gain
  4. A minimum of two binge-eating episodes a week for at least 3 mo
  5. Persistent overconcern with body shape and weight

LABORATORY TESTS

- Electrolyte abnormalities from vomiting (hypokalemia and metabolic alkalosis) or diarrhea from laxative abuse (hypokalemia and hyperchloremic metabolic acidosis)
- Hyponatremia, hypocalcemia, hypomagnesemia (caused by laxative abuse)
- Elevated cortisol, decreased luteinizing hormone, decreased follicle-stimulating hormone

Rx TREATMENT

NONPHARMACOLOGIC THERAPY

- Cognitive behavioral therapy, particularly interpersonal therapy to control abnormal behaviors
- Use of food diaries, nutritional counseling, and planning meals at least 1 day in advance are useful measures to counter abnormal eating behaviors
- Correction of electrolyte abnormalities

ACUTE GENERAL Rx

- Selective serotonin reuptake inhibitors are generally considered to be the safest medication option in these patients. They are useful in severely depressed patients and in those who do not benefit from cognitive behavioral therapy.
- Prompt recognition and treatment of complications:
  1. Ipecac cardiotoxicity from laxative abuse
  2. Electrolyte abnormalities (see "Laboratory Tests" above)
  3. Esophagitis and Mallory-Weiss tears; esophageal rupture from repeated vomiting
  4. Aspiration pneumonia and pneumomediastinum
  5. Menstrual irregularities (including amenorrhea)
  6. Gastrointestinal abnormalities: acute gastric dilatation, pancreatitis, abdominal pain, constipation

CHRONIC Rx

- Psychotherapy continued for years and focused specifically on self-image and family and peer interactions is an integral part of successful recovery.
- Family therapy is also recommended, especially in younger patients.

DISPOSITION

Course is variable and marked by frequent recurrence of exacerbations.

REFERRAL

- In addition to the primary care physician, the multidisciplinary team should include a dietician, a psychiatrist, and a family therapist.
- Hospitalization should be considered for patients with severe electrolyte abnormalities or those with suicidal thoughts.

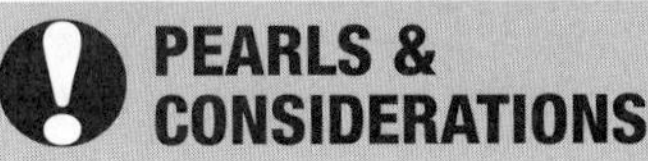

PEARLS & CONSIDERATIONS

COMMENTS

- Bulimia has a close association with depression, bipolar disorder, obsessive-compulsive disorder, alcoholism, and substance abuse.
- Bulimia should be considered in all patients (especially adolescents) with unexplained hypokalemia and metabolic alkalosis.

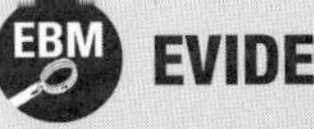

EBM EVIDENCE

Please note: Complete text of EBM for this topic is available online.

Key trials and commentary:

The aim of this study was to compare two cognitive-behavioral treatments for outpatients with eating disorders, one focusing solely on eating disorder features and the other a more complex treatment that also addresses mood intolerance, clinical perfectionism, low self-esteem, or interpersonal difficulties.

This study showed that these two transdiagnostic treatments appear to be suitable for the majority of outpatients with an eating disorder. The simpler treatment may best be viewed as the default version, with the more complex treatment reserved for patients with marked additional psychopathology of the type targeted by the treatment.

This is a nicely conducted study that addresses highly prevalent disorders. What makes it particularly clinically relevant is that it extends the work of Fairburn et al with patients with bulimia nervosa to eating disorders NOS, the big "catch-all" category for the many patients who do not fit criteria for anorexia or bulimia. There is already a good deal of evidence for Fairburn's cognitive-behavioral therapy (CBT) approach for bulimia, so the finding that two variants of this approach also work well for the more expanded group adds to the evidence base.

It was interesting to learn that while the simpler version and the more complex version of the treatment were not significantly different in their outcomes, patients with mood intolerance, clinical perfectionism, low-self-esteem, or interpersonal difficulties did better with the variant that addressed those issues rather than simply focusing on issues specific to eating (e.g., concerns about body shape and weight). It seems likely that the vast majority of patients with eating disorders would suffer from at least one of those non–eating-related issues, however. It would have been helpful to know a bit more about the prevalence of eating disorder patients who do not suffer from comorbid mood disorders or interpersonal problems.

A major concern about this study is that 40% of potentially eligible patients refused to take part, mainly because they would not be available for the 28 weeks required for participation in the study or because they did not wish to participate in research. This is an extremely high number and the authors should have determined if there were significant demographic or other types of relevant differences between the group that agreed to participate and the group that did not. If the nonparticipants had more severe disorders, would their outcomes have been as good?

Overall, the specific adaptations that have been made to make CBT specifically relevant to eating disorders (with the exception of anorexia nervosa, which requires a different type of approach) appear to be quite effective. The follow-up of 60 weeks is also a strength given the high rate of relapse with this type of problem.[1] Ⓐ

Evidence-Based Reference

1. Fairburn CG et al: Transdiagnostic cognitive-behavioral therapy for patients with eating disorders: a two-site trial with 60-week follow-up, *Am J Psychiatry* 166:311-319, 2009. Commentary by J.L. Krupnick, Ph.D. Ⓐ

SUGGESTED READINGS

American Psychiatric Association: Practice guideline for the treatment of patients with eating disorders, *Am J Psychiatry* 157(suppl):4, 2000.

Mehler PS: Bulimia nervosa, *N Engl J Med* 349:875, 2003.

Williams PM et al: Treating eating disorders in primary care, *Am Fam Physician* 77(2):187, 2007.

AUTHOR: **FRED F. FERRI, M.D.**

BASIC INFORMATION

DEFINITION

Bullous pemphigoid is an autoimmune, subepidermal blistering disease commonly seen in the elderly. A related entity is cicatricial pemphigoid, which predominantly affects the mucous membranes.

SYNONYMS

Pemphigoid

ICD-9CM CODES
694.5 Pemphigoid

EPIDEMIOLOGY & DEMOGRAPHICS

- Mostly occurs in people older than 60 yr, with peak incidence in those aged ≥80 yr
- Incidence 10 cases per 1 million persons
- No gender or racial predilection
- Most common of the autoimmune bullous dermatoses

PHYSICAL FINDINGS & CLINICAL PRESENTATION

History:
- Skin lesions typically start as eczematous or urticarial plaques on the extremities with significant associated pruritus
- Taut blisters form between 1 wk and several months

Physical findings:
- Anatomic distribution
  1. Flexor surfaces of the arms and legs, groin, axilla, chest, and abdomen; generally spares the head and neck
  2. Rare involvement of mucous membranes
- Lesion configuration
  1. May be localized to the extremities or generalized
  2. Lesions irregularly grouped but may sometimes be serpiginous (Fig. 1-48)
- Lesion morphology
  1. Taut blisters (bullae) measuring 5 mm to 2 cm in diameter filled with clear or bloody fluid on normal or erythematous skin are characteristic
  2. Heal without scarring but may leave postinflammatory hyperpigmentation

ETIOLOGY

- Autoimmune disease with immunoglobulin (Ig) G and/or C3 complement targeting hemidesmosomal antigens located in the epidermal basement membrane zone
- Drug-induced pemphigoid, although rare, can occur in patients taking penicillamine, furosemide, captopril, penicillin, or sulfasalazine

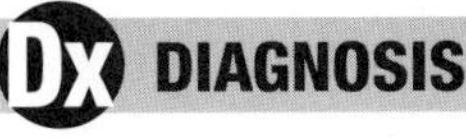

DIAGNOSIS

Skin biopsy aids in the diagnosis, and specimens should be sent for routine histochemical staining and direct immunofluorescence.

DIFFERENTIAL DIAGNOSIS

- Cicatricial pemphigoid
- Epidermolysis bullosa acquisita
- Pemphigus
- Linear IgA disease

LABORATORY TESTS

- Indirect immunofluorescence detects anti–basement membrane antibodies in 70% of patients with bullous pemphigoid.
- Histology of lesional skin shows a subepidermal blister with a superficial inflammatory infiltrate, often with eosinophils.
- Direct immunofluorescence of perilesional skin shows C3 and IgG linearly arranged along the epidermal basement membrane.
- Approximately half of patients will have a peripheral blood eosinophilia.

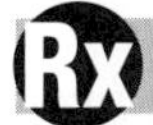

TREATMENT

Bullous pemphigoid may be a self-limited disease, but its course may last from months to years. Treatment is based on the degree of disease involvement and the rate of disease progression.

NONPHARMACOLOGIC THERAPY

- Mild soaps with emollients to wet skin after bathing
- Topical antipruritic creams

ACUTE GENERAL Rx

Localized disease:
- Potent topical steroids (e.g., clobetasol) until blistering ceases with gradual tapering over several weeks
- Oral antihistamines to control pruritus

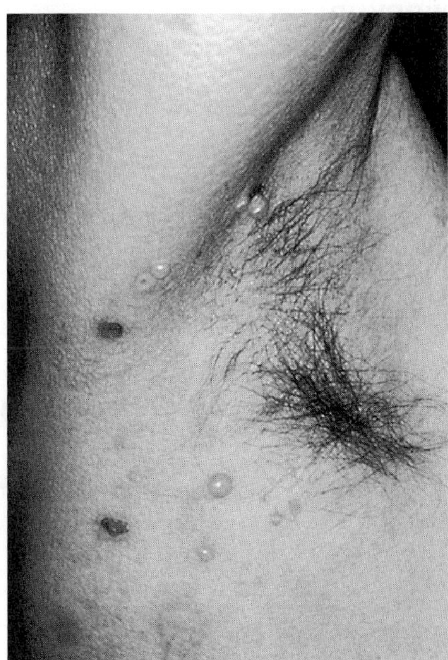

FIGURE 1-48 Bullous pemphigoid. Note intact bullae with erosions in a flexural distribution. (From Goldstein BG, Goldstein AO: *Practical dermatology,* ed 2, St Louis, 1997, Mosby.)

Generalized disease:
- Mainstay of therapy is prednisone, usually beginning with a minimal dose of 1 mg/kg/day
- Steroid-sparing agents, such as azathioprine or mycophenolate mofetil, may be started with prednisone or shortly after prednisone therapy is initiated and may be continued once prednisone is discontinued
- Tetracyclines
- Low-dose methotrexate has recently been suggested to be an optimal therapy in the elderly

CHRONIC Rx

- Prednisone combined with steroid-sparing agents with the goal of limiting oral corticosteroid intake
- Other immunosuppressive agents, such as cyclophosphamide or cyclosporine, are occasionally used

DISPOSITION

Mortality rates are estimated at between 10% and 40% after 1 yr. Approximately 50% of treated patients experience remission within 2 to 6 yr.

REFERRAL

Dermatology

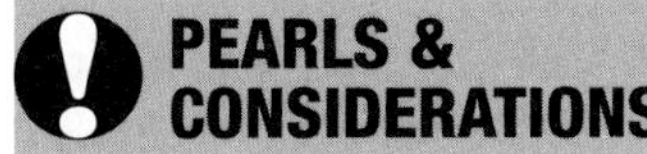

PEARLS & CONSIDERATIONS

COMMENTS

- Bullous pemphigoid has been associated with diabetes, multiple sclerosis, pernicious anemia, rheumatoid arthritis, lichen planus, psoriasis, and vitiligo.
- Not believed to represent a paraneoplastic process.

SUGGESTED READINGS

Bickle KM, Roark TR: Autoimmune bullous dermatoses: a review, *Am Fam Physician* 65:1861-1870, 2002.

Kolanko E et al: Subepidermal blistering disorders: a clinical and histopathologic review, *Semin Cutan Med Surg* 23(1):10-18, 2004.

Stanley JR: Bullous pemphigoid. In Wolff K et al (eds): *Fitzpatrick's dermatology in general medicine,* New York, 2008, McGraw Hill, pp 475-480.

Walsh SR et al: Bullous pemphigoid: from bench to bedside, *Drugs* 65(7):905, 2005.

Wojnarowska F et al: Guidelines for the management of bullous pemphigoid, *Br J Dermatol* 147:214-221, 2002.

AUTHORS: **JESSICA RISSER, M.D., M.P.H.,** and **KACHIU LEE, B.A.**

BASIC INFORMATION

DEFINITION

Burning mouth syndrome (BMS) is characterized by burning pain in the tongue or oral mucous membranes, usually occurring without any identifiable precipitating factor. Patients may also have the sensation of dryness or a bitter or metallic taste in their mouth.

SYNONYMS

Scalded mouth syndrome
Glossodynia
Glossopyrosis

ICD-9CM CODES
529.6 Glossodynia

EPIDEMIOLOGY & DEMOGRAPHICS

- Most prevalent in postmenopausal women; reported in 10% to 40% of women presenting for treatment of menopausal symptoms.
- Epidemiologic studies report 0.7% to 2.6% in the general population of both men and women.
- Typically occurs in middle-aged or older adults.

PHYSICAL FINDINGS & CLINICAL PRESENTATION

- For the majority of patients, the onset of pain is spontaneous without an identifiable precipitating factor.
- One third of patients relate the time of onset to a dental procedure, recent illness, or medication.
- Often persists for many years.
- The burning sensation often occurs in more than one oral site, most frequently in the anterior two thirds of the tongue, the anterior hard palate, and the lower lip mucosa.
- Pain is often absent at night but will increase in severity progressively throughout the day.
- Associated with sleep disturbances as well as difficulty falling asleep.
- Also associated with mood changes such as irritability, anxiety, and depression.
- Up to two thirds of patients report a spontaneous partial recovery within 6 to 7 years from onset with the pain changing from constant to intermittent.

ETIOLOGY

Because of its complex clinical picture, many different hypotheses have been suggested for its etiology. Possible causes include:

- Psychologic dysfunction: many patients concomitantly have personality or mood changes, report more adverse life events, somatization, anxiety, and depression.
- Chronic pain conditions, such as headaches.
- Local irritants such as smoking.
- Dry mouth: however, most salivary flow rate studies in affected patients have not shown a decrease in unstimulated or stimulated salivary flow.
- Oral candidal infections.
- Medications: e.g., angiotensin-converting enzyme (ACE) inhibitors.
- Nerve damage.
- Nutritional deficiencies: iron, zinc, folate, and vitamin B.

There may be an association between supertasters (those with enhanced ability to taste) and those with BMS due to their increased density of taste buds that are surrounded by bundles of trigeminal nerve neurons.

Dx DIAGNOSIS

DIFFERENTIAL DIAGNOSIS

- Mucosal disease such as lichen planus or candidiasis
- Nutritional deficiency in zinc, iron, folate, or vitamins B_1, B_2, B_6, B_9, B_{12}
- Dry mouth from Sjögren's syndrome or after chemo/radiation therapy
- Cranial nerve injury
- Medication effect

WORKUP

- Clinical history is the most important in diagnosing BMS.
- Very important to rule out other pathologic conditions first.

LABORATORY TESTS

There is no test for BMS, but consider testing for vitamin B or zinc deficiency.

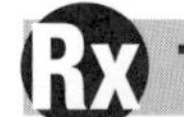

TREATMENT

NONPHARMACOLOGIC THERAPY

Capsaicin (hot pepper powder) can be used as a topical desensitizing agent.

- Rinse mouth with 1 tsp of a 1:2 solution of hot pepper and water; increase strength of capsaicin as tolerated to a maximum 1:1 dilution.

ACUTE GENERAL Rx

Given the chronic nature of BMS, there is a need to identify effective treatments. However, the current evidence does not provide clear guidance.

Possibly effective treatments:

- Low-dose benzodiazepines:
  - Clonazepam (Klonopin) 0.25 to 2 mg/day; start with 0.25 mg qhs and increase dose q 4 to 7 days until oral burning is relieved or side effects
  - Chlordiazepoxide (Librium) 10 to 30 mg/day; start with 5 mg qhs and increase dose q 4 to 7 days until oral burning is relieved or side effects
- Low-dose tricyclic antidepressants:
  - Amitriptyline or nortriptyline 10 to 150 mg/day; start with 10 mg qhs and increase dose by 10 mg q 4 to 7 days.
- Low-dose gabapentin (Neurontin) 300 to 1600 mg/day; start with 100 mg qhs and increase dose by 100 mg q 4 to 7 days (take in divided doses).

REFERRAL

To a subspecialist, such as a dentist or ENT, in this area if initial therapy fails to resolve symptoms.

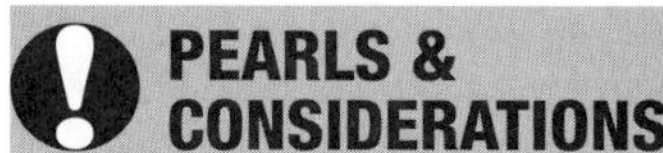

PEARLS & CONSIDERATIONS

COMMENTS

Burning mouth syndrome is a rare but possibly debilitating disease. Other diseases should be ruled out.

SUGGESTED READINGS

Gao J et al: A case-control study on etiological factors involved in patients with burning mouth syndrome, *J Oral Pathol Med* 38(1):24-28, 2009.

Grushka M et al: Burning mouth syndrome, *Am Fam Physician* 65:615, 2002.

Grushka M et al: Burning mouth syndrome: evolving concepts, *Oral Maxillofac Surg Clin North Am* 12:287, 2000.

MayoClinic.com: http://www.mayoclinic.com/invoke.cfm?id=DS00462.

Zakrzewska JM et al: Interventions for the treatment of burning mouth syndrome, *Cochrane Database* (1):CD002779, 2005.

AUTHOR: **MADHAVI SHAH, M.D.**

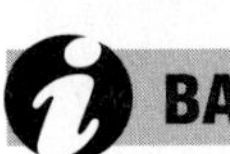

BASIC INFORMATION

DEFINITION

Burn injuries include thermal injuries (flames, scalds, cigarettes), as well as chemical, electrical, and radiation burns.

SYNONYMS Thermal injury

ICD-9CM CODES
942-949 (by region, % burn)

EPIDEMIOLOGY & DEMOGRAPHICS

PREVALENCE (IN U.S.): Burn injuries account for approximately 500,000 emergency department visits, 40,000 hospitalizations, and 4000 deaths annually.

PREDOMINANT SEX: Occur in males more often than females

PHYSICAL FINDINGS & CLINICAL PRESENTATION

- Burns are defined by surface area and depth of skin involved.
- *First-degree burns (superficial)* involve the epidermis only and appear painful and red.
- *Second-degree burns* involve the dermis and appear blistered, moist, and red with two-point discrimination intact *(superficial partial-thickness)* or red and blanched white with only sensation of pressure intact *(deep partial thickness).*
- *Third-degree burns (full-thickness)* extend through the dermis with associated destruction of hair follicles and sweat glands. The skin is charred, pale, *painless,* and leathery. These burns are caused by flames, immersion scalds, and chemical and high-voltage injuries.

DIAGNOSIS

CLASSIFICATION

Burns are classified by extent of the burn or total burn surface area (TBSA). The TBSA is best classified by using age-specific burn charts.

Major burns: Partial-thickness burns ≥25% TBSA (or 20% if younger than 10 yr or older than 50 yr); full-thickness burns ≥10% TBSA; burns crossing major joints or involving the hands, face, feet, or perineum; electrical or chemical burns; those complicated by inhalation injury or involving high-risk patients (extremes of age/comorbid diseases)

Moderate burns: Partial-thickness burns ≥15% to 25% TBSA (or 10% in children and older adults); full-thickness burns ≥2% to 10% TBSA and not involving the specific conditions of major burns

Minor burns: Partial-thickness burns <15% TBSA or full-thickness burns <2% TBSA

LABORATORY STUDIES

- CBC, electrolytes, BUN, creatinine, and glucose
- Serial ABG and carboxyhemoglobin if smoke inhalation suspected
- Urinalysis, urine myoglobin, and CPK levels if concern for rhabdomyolysis

IMAGING STUDIES

Chest radiograph and bronchoscopy if smoke inhalation suspected

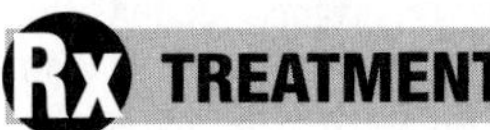

TREATMENT

ACUTE GENERAL Rx

- Establish airway: inspect for inhalation injury and intubate for suspected airway edema (often seen 12 to 24 hr later); supplemental O_2
- Remove jewelry and clothing and place one or two large-bore peripheral IVs (if TBSA >20%)
- Fluid resuscitation with Ringer's lactate at 2 to 4 ml/kg per %TBSA per 24 hr with half the calculated fluid given in the first 8 hr
- Foley catheter and NG tube (20% of patients develop an ileus)
- Tetanus update
- Treat pain and anxiety
- Stress ulcer prophylaxis in high-risk patients
- Address adequate nutritional support
- ECG monitoring for high-voltage burns given increased risk for arrhythmias
- Routine systemic prophylactic antibiotic treatment is not recommended for the prevention of burn wound infections; however, burn victims should be considered immunosuppressed. Of note, early use of topical antibiotics such as silver sulfadiazine has been associated with decreased incidence of burn infections.

BURN WOUND Rx

First-degree burns (e.g., sunburns):

- Can be treated with cool compresses, antihistamines, emollients, and, at times, a rapidly tapering dose of steroids.

Second-degree and third-degree burns:

- Wash burned skin with cool tap water or saline (15° to 25° C; immerse approximately 30 min if able) and cleanse with mild soap. Ice or ice water may increase tissue injury and should not be used.
- Sharp debridement of ruptured blisters (except palms and soles). Leave unruptured blisters intact.
- Several approaches to burn dressings after cleansing and debriding:
  1. Apply thin layer of antibiotic ointment (silver sulfadiazine can be used unless sulfa allergy or facial burn) and cover with a nonadherent dressing (e.g., Telfa or petroleum-soaked gauze) followed by a sterile gauze wrap. Wash wound and change dressing when dressing soaked.
  2. Apply saline-soaked gauze (Xeroform, Owen's), cover with 4 × 4 dressing and a bulky absorbent dressing such as Kerlex. Reevaluate in 5 to 7 days.
  3. Apply occlusive dressing (DuoDerm, Tegasorb), remove in 7 to 10 days.
- Specialized care, such as excision and autografting, is required for some deep second-degree and most third-degree burns.

DISPOSITION

- Respiratory injury, sepsis, and multiorgan failure may complicate severe burns.
- Scarring can be expected in many second-degree and all third-degree burns.

REFERRAL

Major and some moderate burns require referral to specialized burn centers for surgical debridement, grafting evaluation, and rehabilitation.

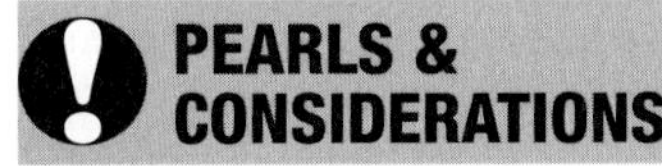

PEARLS & CONSIDERATIONS

COMMENTS

Burn victims must be reassessed frequently because the patient's condition can change significantly in the first 24 to 72 hr.

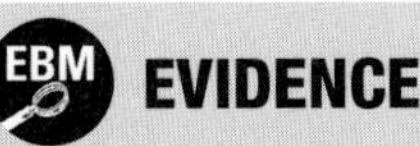

EVIDENCE

Please note: Complete text of EBM for this topic is available online.

Key trials and commentary:

Use of colloids in acute burn resuscitation may reduce fluid requirements, but effect on mortality is unknown. This study hypothesized that patients who received albumin would have similar mortality to patients who did not receive albumin. This study showed that despite more severe systemic dysfunction, burn patients who received albumin did not suffer increased mortality. A novel finding is the decreased likelihood of mortality associated with the administration of albumin during burn resuscitation.

Another study adds to the confusion over the proper composition of fluids to be administered for resuscitation after thermal injury. These authors observed a decreased mortality in patients who were administered albumin. In fairness, however, they make a plea for a multicenter trial to settle the issue of whether colloids should be given as part of a resuscitation regimen. It is extraordinary that, given the advances in burn care, this one issue cannot be resolved. The bibliography is outstanding.[1] Ⓐ

Acute burn wounds often require early excision and adequate coverage to prevent further hypothermia, protein and fluid losses, and the risk of infection. Meshed autologous skin grafts are generally regarded as the standard treatment for extensive full-thickness burns. Graft take and rate of wound healing, however, depend on several endogenous factors. This paper describes a standardized reproducible porcine model of burn and skin grafting that can be used to study the effects of topical treatments on graft take and re-epithelialization.

Procedures provide a protocol for successful porcine burn wound experiments with special focus on preoperative care, anesthesia, burn allocation, excision and grafting, postoperative treatment, dressing application, and specimen collection. Selected outcome measurements include percent area of wound closure by planimetry, wound assessment using a clinical assessment scale, and histological scoring.

The use of this standardized model provides burn researchers with a valuable tool for the comparison of different topical drug treatments and dressing materials in a setting that closely mimics clinical reality.

This article is a multidisciplinary effort from three fine institutions and provides an excellent attempt at a working model to study burn wound healing. Unfortunately, much of the experimental work has been done in animal skin that is nonautologous to the human situation. The pig is an outstanding model but is difficult to work with as noted by the authors. Hopefully, this preliminary study on acute wound healing will be followed by others, but the clear description by the authors of why they chose the pig and how they were able to successfully work with the animal should be instructional for other investigators.[2] Ⓐ

Another trial sought to investigate and evaluate the clinical efficacy and safety of Acticoat with nanocrystalline silver for external use on the management of the residual wounds post-burn.

It revealed that Acticoat with nanocrystalline silver promotes the healing process of residual wounds post-burn effectively. No adverse reaction of Acticoat was found during the study.

This prospective study is nicely organized and deals with the clinical issues of the burn wound in a logical fashion. The points the authors make about Acticoat have been confirmed by others, and it is noteworthy that they are not denigrating the use of silver sulfadiazine. The authors are merely demonstrating that Acticoat is a superior treatment for specific wound types.[3] Ⓐ

For pediatric burn patients with the symptoms of acute stress disorder (ASD), a first-line medication is not widely agreed upon. A prospective, randomized, placebo-controlled, double-blind design was used to test the efficacy of imipramine and fluoxetine.

This separate study showed that within the parameters of this study design and sample, placebo was statistically as effective as either drug in treating symptoms of ASD.

This beautifully designed, prospective, randomized, double-blind study did not show any efficacy of medications over placebo in treating children. Its importance for the surgeon is that there should be a familiarity with the present agents suggested for use in the burn patient for pain, anxiety, loss of sleep, and depression. Patient care should not be left to the rotating resident of the month who may have his or her own limited grasp of a particular "cocktail." The complications and side effects of many of these agents can be significant. Professionals who do not consult regularly in a burn center have a steep learning curve in appreciating that these traumatized children may respond very differently to drugs than children with cancer or other disease processes.[4] Ⓐ

Another trial is one of the largest prospective studies of patients with major burn injuries to use psychometrically sound methods to track and predict posttraumatic stress disorder (PTSD) across 2 years after burn. In conclusion, ASD and PTSD are prevalent following major burn injuries, ASD symptomatology can reliably predict PTSD up to 24 months later, and, once established, PTSD usually persists. Research is needed to determine whether early recognition and treatment of persons with in-hospital ASD can improve long-term outcomes.

Survival following a major burn injury has improved significantly in the last several decades because of advances in surgical management, critical care, nutritional management, and control of infection. This progressive decline in mortality demands that we focus not only on physical recovery as an endpoint, but focus on the psychological health and well-being of these burn survivors. Both ASD and PTSD are common among adults and children surviving burn injuries. This study was chosen because it is comprehensive and has the largest number of cases reported in the literature on this subject. It also represents the first prospective cohort research study to examine the prevalence, and course of these conditions in patients with major burns with follow-up to 24 months after injury. The authors found that both ASD and PTSD were common and that most symptoms are very stable for the first 2 years following a major burn. The present study also shows that in those persons with major burn injuries, a diagnosis of in hospital ASD significantly predicts the development of PTSD up to 12 months after discharge. An important direction for future research is to test the effectiveness of beginning treatment for those patients with high levels of ASD symptoms to prevent subsequent development of PTSD.[5] Ⓐ

Evidence-Based References

1. Cochran A et al: Burn patient characteristics and outcomes following resuscitation with albumin, *Burns* 33:25-30, 2007. Commentary by R.E. Salisbury, M.D. Ⓐ
2. Branski LK et al: A porcine model of full-thickness burn, excision and skin autografting, *Burns* 34:1119-1127, 2008. Commentary by R.E. Salisbury, M.D. Ⓐ
3. Huang Y et al: A randomized comparative trial between Acticoat and SD-Ag in the treatment of residual burn wounds, including safety analysis, *Burns* 33:161-166, 2007. Commentary by R.E. Salisbury, M.D. Ⓐ
4. Robert R et al: Treating thermally injured children suffering symptoms of acute stress with imipramine and fluoxetine: a randomized, double-blind study, *Burns* 34:919-928, 2008. Commentary by R.E. Salisbury, M.D. Ⓐ
5. McKibben JB et al: Acute stress disorder and posttraumatic stress disorder: a prospective study of prevalence, course, and predictors in a sample with major burn injuries, *J Burn Care Res* 29:22-35, 2008. Commentary by D.W. Mozingo, M.D. Ⓐ

SUGGESTED READINGS

Orgill DP: Excision and skin grafting of thermal burns, *N Engl J Med* 360:893-901, 2009.

Sheridan R: Burn care: results of technical and organizational progress, *JAMA* 290(6):719, 2003.

Singer AJ: Management of local burn wounds in the ED, *Am J Emerg Med* 25(6):666, 2007.

AUTHORS: **SRIVIDYA ANANDAN, M.D.,** and **MICHELLE STOZEK ANVAR, M.D.**

BASIC INFORMATION

DEFINITION

Bursitis is an inflammation of a bursa and is usually aseptic. A *bursa* is a closed sac lined with a synovial-like membrane that sometimes contains fluid that is found or that develops in an area subject to pressure or friction.

SYNONYMS

Housemaid's knee (prepatellar bursitis)
Weaver's bottom (ischial gluteal bursitis)
Baker's cyst (gastrocnemius-semimembranosus bursa)

ICD-9CM CODES

726.19	Subacromial bursitis
726.33	Olecranon bursitis
726.5	Ischiogluteal bursitis (hip)
726.5	Iliopsoas bursitis (hip)
726.61	Anserine bursitis
726.5	Trochanteric bursitis
726.65	Prepatellar bursitis
727.51	Baker's cyst
726.79	Retrocalcaneal bursitis

PHYSICAL FINDINGS & CLINICAL PRESENTATION

- Swelling, especially if bursa is superficial (olecranon, prepatellar)
- Local tenderness with pain on pressure against bursa
- Pain with joint movement
- Referred pain
- Palpable occasional fibrocartilaginous bodies (most common in olecranon and prepatellar bursae)

ETIOLOGY

- Acute trauma
- Repetitive trauma
- Sepsis
- Crystalline deposit disease
- Rheumatoid arthritis

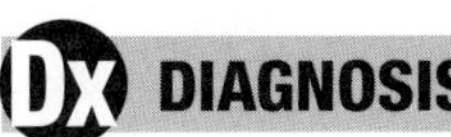

DIAGNOSIS

DIFFERENTIAL DIAGNOSIS

- Degenerative joint disease
- Tendinitis (sometimes occurs in conjunction with bursitis)
- Cellulitis (if bursitis is septic)
- Infectious arthritis

WORKUP

Aspiration with Gram stain and C&S if infection suspected

IMAGING STUDIES

- Plain radiography to rule out other potential or coexisting bone or joint problems (Fig. 1-49)
- MRI

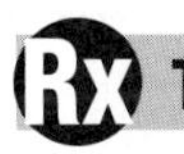

TREATMENT

NONPHARMACOLOGIC THERAPY

- If chronic, elimination of cause of pressure or irritation
- Use of relief pads, avoidance of direct pressure
- Rest
- Elevation
- Ice for acute trauma

ACUTE GENERAL Rx

- Septic:
  1. Appropriate antibiotic coverage and drainage
  2. Aspiration of purulent fluid with a large-bore needle (if there is no rapid clinical response, incision and drainage are indicated)
- Nonseptic:
  1. Aspiration of blood from acute trauma
  2. Application of compression dressing

CHRONIC Rx

- Aspiration if excessive fluid volume present, followed by application of compression dressing to prevent fluid reaccumulation (repeat aspiration may be required)
- Steroid injection into bursa (1 ml of triamcinolone, 40 mg, mixed with 1 to 3 ml of Xylocaine depending on size of bursa)
- NSAIDs

DISPOSITION

- Many bursal sacs "dry up" eventually.
- Nonsurgical treatment is effective in most cases.

REFERRAL

For orthopedic consultation to assist in treatment of sepsis or for excision of chronic enlarged bursa when indicated

PEARLS & CONSIDERATIONS

COMMENTS

- Injection of trochanteric bursa may require spinal needle in a large patient.
- Sterile bursae should not be incised and drained because a chronic draining sinus tract may develop.
- Involvement of the iliopsoas bursa may cause groin pain, although the diagnosis is difficult to make because of the inaccessibility of the area to direct examination. (This also makes steroid injection impossible even if the diagnosis could be established.)

SUGGESTED READINGS

Beaman FD, Peterson JJ: MR imaging of cysts, ganglia and bursae about the knee, *Radiol Clin North Am* 45:969, 2007.

Floemer F et al: MRI characteristics of olecranon bursitis, *Am J Roentgenol* 183:29, 2004.

Metz JP: Helpful tips for performing musculoskeletal injections, *Am Fam Physician* 78:971, 2008.

Pateder DB et al: Masquerade: nonspinal musculoskeletal disorders that mimic spinal conditions, *Cleve Clin J Med* 75:50, 2008.

Sofka CM, Adler RS: Sonography of cubital bursitis, *Am J Roentgenol* 183:51, 2004.

Tortolani PJ et al: Greater trochanteric pain syndrome in patients referred to orthopedic spine specialists, *Spine* 2:251, 2002.

Van Mieghem IM et al: Ischiogluteal bursitis: an uncommon type of bursitis, *Skeletal Radiol* 33:413, 2004.

Webner D, Drezner JA: Lesser trochanteric bursitis: a rare cause of anterior hip pain, *Clin J Sport Med* 14:242, 2004.

Woodley SJ et al: Morphology of the bursae associated with the greater trochanter of the femur, *Am J Bone Joint Surg* 90:284, 2008.

AUTHOR: **LONNIE R. MERCIER, M.D.**

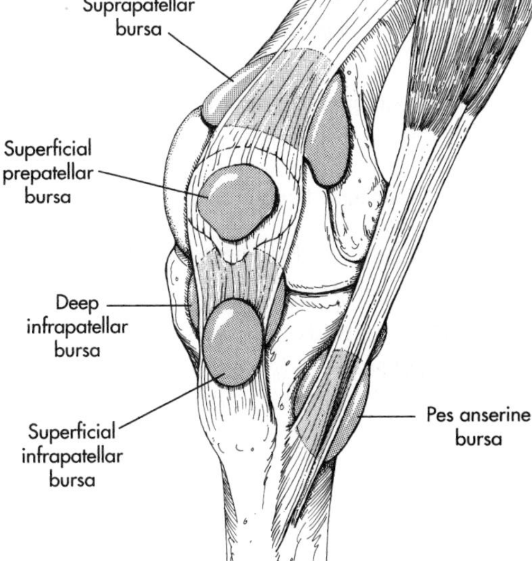

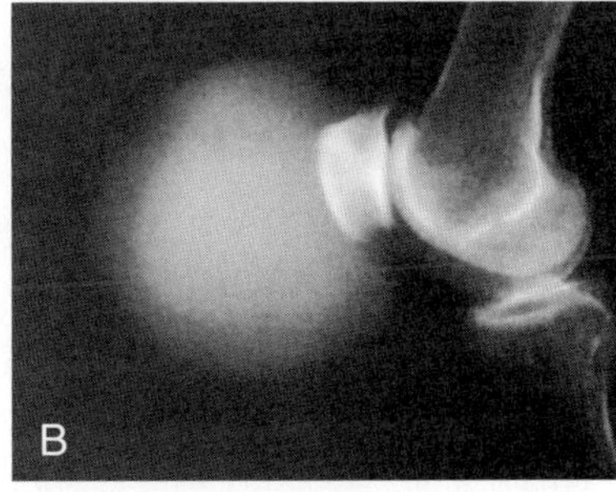

FIGURE 1-49 A, Bursae around the knee. **B,** Markedly swollen prepatellar bursa. (From Scudieri G [ed]: *Sports medicine principles of primary care,* St Louis, 1997, Mosby.)

Candidiasis, Vulvovaginal (PTG) (ALG)

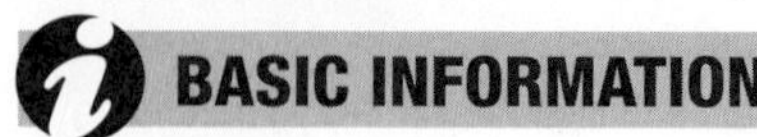

BASIC INFORMATION

DEFINITION

Candidiasis is an inflammatory process involving the vulva or the vagina caused by superficial invasion of epithelial cells by *Candida* species.

SYNONYMS

Moniliasis
Thrush

ICD-9CM CODES
112.1 Moniliasis
112.0 Thrush
112 Candidosis

EPIDEMIOLOGY & DEMOGRAPHICS

- This is the second most common form of vaginitis in the U.S.; 75% of women will have at least one episode of vulvovaginal candidiasis (VVC) during their childbearing years and approximately 45% will have a second attack. A small subpopulation of <5% of adult women has recurrent, often intractable episodes. *Candida* may be isolated in up to 20% of asymptomatic women of childbearing age.
- Factors that predispose to development of symptomatic VVC include pregnancy, antibiotic use, and diabetes. Antibiotic use disturbs normal vaginal flora and allows overgrowth of fungi; pregnancy and diabetes are associated with decrease in cell-mediated immunity.
- Factors associated with increased rates of asymptomatic vaginal colonization: pregnancy, high-estrogen oral contraceptives, uncontrolled diabetes mellitus, treatment at sexually transmitted disease clinics.

UNCOMPLICATED VVC

- Infrequent VVC
- Mild-to-moderate vaginitis and candida
- Likely to be *C. albicans*
- Nonimmunocompromised women

COMPLICATED VVC

- Recurrent VVC
- Severe VVC
- Non-*albicans* candidiasis
- Women with uncontrolled diabetes, immunosuppression, or pregnancy

PHYSICAL FINDINGS & CLINICAL PRESENTATION

Symptoms of VVC consist of:

- Vulvar pruritus with vaginal discharge that typically resembles cottage cheese.
- Erythema and edema of labia and vulvar skin; possible discrete papular peripheral lesions (satellite lesions) (Fig. 1-50).
- Vagina may be erythematous with an adherent, whitish discharge.
- Cervix may appear normal.
- Symptoms characteristically exacerbated in the week preceding menses with some relief after onset of menstrual flow.

ETIOLOGY

- *Candida* are dimorphic fungi (spores and mycelial forms).
- *C. albicans* is responsible for 85% to 90% of vaginal yeast infections.
- *C. glabrata, C. tropicalis* (non-*albicans* species) also cause vaginitis and may be more resistant to conventional therapy.

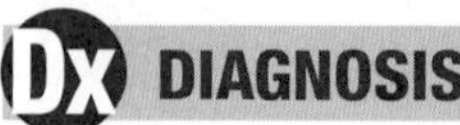

DIAGNOSIS

DIFFERENTIAL DIAGNOSIS

- Bacterial vaginosis
- Trichomoniasis

WORKUP

- Usually normal vaginal pH (<4.5).
- Budding yeast forms or mycelia will appear in as many as 80% of cases. Saline wet prep of vaginal secretions usually is normal; may be increased in inflammatory cells in severe cases.
- Whiff test negative (KOH).
- 10% KCl useful and more sensitive than wet mount for microscopic identification.
- Can make a presumptive diagnosis based on symptomatology in the absence of microscopy-proven fungal elements if the pH and wet prep are normal. Fungal culture is recommended to confirm diagnosis.
- In chronic/recurrent VVC, burning replaces itching as prominent symptom. Confirm diagnosis with direct microscopy and culture. Many may actually have chronic or atrophic dermatitis. Test for HIV.

LABORATORY TESTS

If sending cultures, send on Nickerson's media or semiquantitative Slide-Stix cultures. There is no reliable serologic technique for diagnosis.

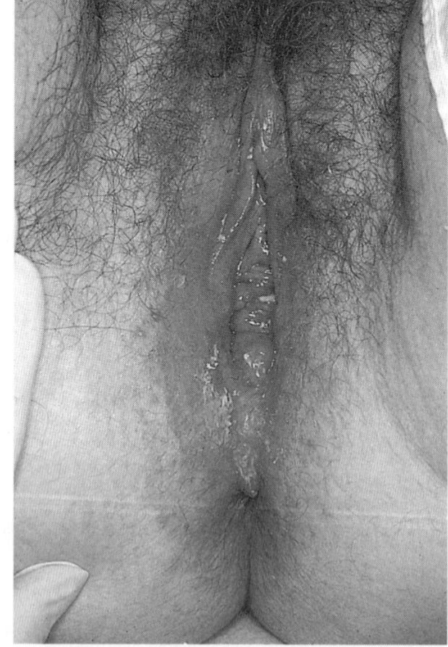

FIGURE 1-50 Candidiasis. Vaginal candidiasis is common, and lesions often spread to the vulva. Peeling and erosions are seen in tertriginous areas, and satellite pustules are scattered at the periphery. In contrast, tinea infections do not have satellite lesions; tiny vesiculopustules occur along the lesional border. (From Black M, McKay M: *Obstetrics and gynecological dermatology,* ed 2, St Louis, 2002, Mosby.)

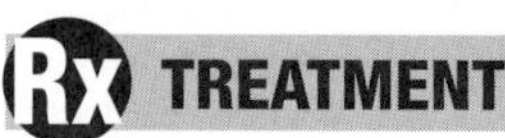

TREATMENT

ACUTE GENERAL Rx (UNCOMPLICATED VVC)

ORAL FLUCONAZOLE:
- 150-mg single PO dose

TOPICAL BUTOCONAZOLE:
- 2% vaginal cream 5 g intravaginally for 3 days
- Butoconazole (sustained release) 5 g intravaginally for 1 dose

TOPICAL CLOTRIMAZOLE
- 1% cream 5 g intravaginally for 7 to 14 days
- 100-mg vaginal tablet for 7 days
- 100-mg vaginal tablets, 2 tablets for 3 days
- 500-mg vaginal tablet, single dose

TOPICAL MICONAZOLE:
- 2% cream 5 g intravaginally for 7 days
- 200-mg vaginal suppository for 3 days
- 100-mg vaginal suppository for 7 days

TOPICAL TIOCONAZOLE:
- 6.5% ointment 5 g intravaginally, single dose

TOPICAL TERCONAZOLE:
- 0.4% cream 5 g intravaginally for 7 days
- 0.8% cream 5 g intravaginally for 3 days
- 80-mg suppository for 3 days

(COMPLICATED VVC)

- 150 mg fluconazole orally, repeat in 3 days
- Recurrent VVC: 7 to 14 days of topical therapy
- Maintenance regimen:
  1. Clotrimazole: 500-mg vaginal suppositories once weekly
  2. Ketoconazole: 100 mg qd
  3. Fluconazole: 100 to 150 mg orally once weekly
  4. Itraconazole 400 mg/mo or 100 mg/day
  5. Continue one of the above regimens for 6 mo

(COMPROMISED HOST)

- Treat with traditional antimycotics for at least 7 to 14 days
- Pregnancy: topical azoles recommended for 7 days
- Women with HIV: fluconazole 200 mg/wk
- Not usually a sexually transmitted disease

CHRONIC Rx

Ketoconazole 400 mg PO qd or fluconazole 200 mg PO qd until symptoms resolve. Then maintenance on prophylactic doses of these agents for 6 mo (ketoconazole 100 mg/day, fluconazole 150 mg/wk).

DISPOSITION

If chronic or recurrent, consider screening for diabetes, HIV, or other immune deficiencies.

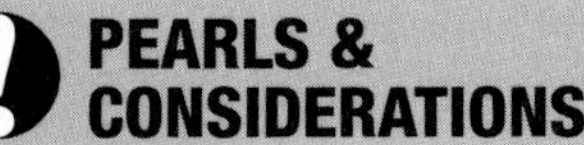

PEARLS & CONSIDERATIONS

COMMENTS

- Azoles are more effective than nystatin. Symptoms usually take 2 to 3 days to resolve. Adjunctive treatment with weak topical steroid such as 1% hydrocortisone cream may help with relief of symptoms.
- Creams and suppositories are oil based and may weaken latex condoms and diaphragms.
- Invasive candidosis is discussed in the EBM section.

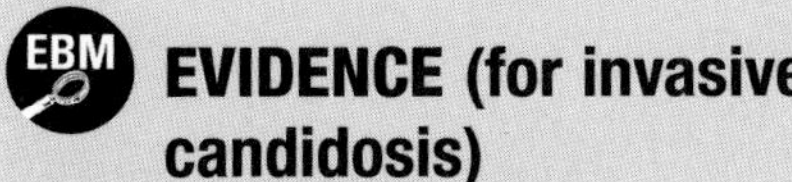

EVIDENCE (for invasive candidosis)

Please note: Complete text of EBM for this topic is available online.

Key trials and commentary:

Anidulafungin, a new echinocandin, has potent activity against *Candida* spp. This study compared anidulafungin with fluconazole in a randomized, double-blind, noninferiority trial of treatment for invasive candidiasis. Anidulafungin was shown to be noninferior to fluconazole in the treatment of invasive candidiasis.

The results of this study by Reboli et al, which compared anidulafungin with fluconazole for the treatment of invasive candidiasis, failed to show a clear winner. Whether echinocandins are superior to azoles for the treatment of invasive *Candida* infections is highly controversial. The new echinocandin antifungal agents provide practitioners with a broader choice for prophylaxis and therapy, but evidence is lacking to prove their superiority to older drugs.[1] Ⓐ

Invasive infection with *Candida* spp. is an important cause of morbidity and mortality in intensive care unit (ICU) patients. Optimal preventive strategies have not been clearly defined.

One study showed that in critically ill adults with risk factors for invasive candidiasis, empirical fluconazole did not clearly improve a composite outcome more than placebo.

ICU presence of invasive *Candida* infection in critically ill ICU patients is associated with a marked increase in morbidity and mortality. Although only 1% to 2% of all ICU patients ever develop invasive candidiasis, *Candida* infections can account for as many as 5% to 10% of all blood isolates or cases of septic shock in the ICU. *Candida* infections may be substantially underdiagnosed given the difficulty in determining the presence of invasive infection with this organism. *Candida* are often thought to be present as colonizers at a variety of sites in critically ill infected patients. However, it is possible that these isolates may represent true but unrecognized invasive infection.

In this randomized study, Schuster et al test the possibility that empirical fluconazole administration in high-risk patients with fever unresponsive to broad-spectrum antibiotics leads to improved fever resolution and decreased subsequent documentation of invasive *Candida*. Unfortunately, the small improvement in fever resolution and decreased occurrence of invasive *Candida* infection failed to even approach statistical significance. However, this question may not be fully resolved. Closer examination of the study suggests an unusually low rate of *Candida* infection in the control group, suggesting that a larger study may have been required to adequately examine this question. For the present, though, there is no documented benefit of empirical antifungal therapy in high-risk antibiotic-treated ICU patients with unresolving fever.[2] Ⓐ

Invasive candidosis is increasingly prevalent in seriously ill patients. The aim of another trial was to compare micafungin with liposomal amphotericin B for the treatment of adult patients with candidemia or invasive candidosis. It revealed that micafungin was as effective as—and caused fewer adverse events than—liposomal amphotericin B as first-line treatment of candidemia and invasive candidosis.

Serious infections caused by *Candida* spp. have in the past been treated with amphotericin B, which is well known for its potential toxicity, and fluconazole, which often has a limited spectrum of activity. Newer generation drugs such as liposomal amphotericin B, voriconazole, and the echinocandins caspofungin and anidulafungin have largely overcome these limitations. Micafungin, another echinocandin, has high success rates against candidemia in open-label studies. Kuse et al compared the efficacy of micafungin with liposomal amphotericin B in the treatment of adult patients with candidemia or invasive candidosis and found the drug to be as effective with fewer adverse events. Because micafungin appears to have broad-spectrum activity against *Aspergillus* spp., future studies should assess its efficacy in the treatment of invasive aspergillosis. The improved safety profile of micafungin likely results from its mechanism of action, which involves rather specific inhibition of fungal cell wall synthesis with little impact on human cells.[3] Ⓐ

Invasive *Candida* infections are a major cause of morbidity and mortality in preterm infants. One study performed a multicenter, randomized, double-blind, placebo-controlled trial of fluconazole for the prevention of fungal colonization and infection in very-low-birth-weight neonates. It revealed that prophylactic fluconazole reduces the incidence of colonization and invasive *Candida* infection in neonates weighing less than 1500 g at birth. The benefit of treating *Candida* colonization is unclear.

Until this report appeared, this editor did not realize how problematic systemic fungal infection had become in the tiny infant nurseries of this country. The significant majority of very-low-birth-weight neonates (less than 1500 g) are colonized with *Candida* spp. About 1 in 5 colonized neonates will develop an invasive fungal infection. Many of these infections are recognized late largely because of the poor sensitivity of the diagnostic tools available to us. The consequence of such an infection is significant in that these infections increase the rate of death from all causes (25% vs. 7% for infants without such infections) and death that is attributable to fungal infection itself (up to 44% of deaths). Even early diagnosis and successful treatment have not been shown to prevent significantly longer stays in the neonatal ICU, remarkably increased cost of care, or neurodevelopmental impairment.

Because treatment after the problem has occurred has an inherently limited success rate, the concept of prophylaxis with antifungal drugs is an attractive consideration in the nursery setting. Such prophylaxis has its roots in the management of adult and pediatric patients with hematologic cancers and immune deficiency syndromes. Very-low-birth-weight neonates, in fact, are at added risk for fungal infection because of their immature immune system. It was on this basis that the Italian Task Force for the Study and Prevention of Neonatal Fungal Infections and the Italian Society of Neonatology decided to undertake a multicenter, prospective, randomized, double-blind, placebo-controlled evaluation of fluconazole prophylaxis in very-low-birth-weight infants in the neonatal intensive care unit. What was found was that fluconazole prophylaxis did reduce fungal colonization and infection in preterm babies. The reduction was quite dramatic. It should be noted that once a baby is colonized, however, fluconazole prophylaxis has no effect on the subsequent development of an invasive fungal infection.

We have come a long way since amphotericin B was the sole drug of choice to manage invasive candidiasis. A new class of agents known as echinocandins has emerged as important agents for the treatment of this infection. The newest echinocandin is anidulafungin, which has shown some effectiveness in the management of this problem.

Evidence-Based References

1. Reboli AC, for the Anidulafungin Study Group: Anidulafungin versus fluconazole for invasive candidiasis, *N Engl J Med* 356:2472-2482, 2007. Commentary by B.H. Thiers, M.D. Ⓐ
2. Schuster MG et al: Empirical fluconazole versus placebo for intensive care unit patients: a randomized trial, *Ann Intern Med* 149:83-90, 2008. Commentary by A. Kumar, M.D. Ⓐ
3. Kuse E-R, for the Micafungin Invasive Candidiasis Working Group: Micafungin versus liposomal amphotericin B for candidaemia and invasive candidosis: a phase III randomised double-blind trial,

 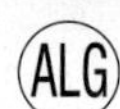

Lancet 369:1519-1527, 2007. Commentary by B.H. Thiers, M.D. Ⓐ

4. Manzoni P: A multicenter, randomized trial of prophylactic fluconazole in preterm neonates, *N Engl J Med* 356:2483-2495, 2007. Commentary by J.A. Stockman III, M.D. Ⓐ

SUGGESTED READINGS

Centers for Disease Control and Prevention: 2006 sexually transmitted diseases treatment guidelines, *MMWR* 55(RR-11), 2006.

Sheary B, Dayan L: Recurrent vulvovaginal candidiasis, *Aust Fam Physician* 34(3):147-150, 2005.

Spence D: Candidiasis (vulvovaginal), *Clin Evid* (12): 2493-2511, 2004.

AUTHORS: **MARIA A. CORIGLIANO, M.D.,** and **RUBEN ALVERO, M.D.**

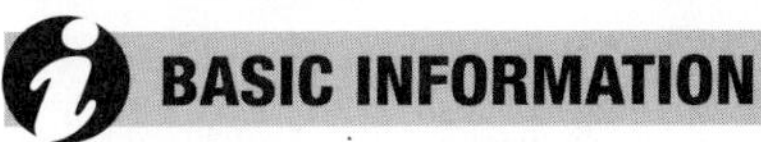

BASIC INFORMATION

DEFINITION

Carbon monoxide (CO) is a colorless, odorless, tasteless, nonirritating gas. When inhaled it produces toxicity by causing cellular hypoxia and damage.

ICD-9CM CODES
986 Carbon monoxide poisoning

EPIDEMIOLOGY & DEMOGRAPHICS

- A leading cause of accidental and intentional poisoning in the United States.
- CO poisoning is seen more frequently during the fall and winter months in cold climates. Frequently seen after storm-related power outages, mostly because of the use of portable gasoline-powered electrical generators.
- In adults, 20% of CO poisonings occur in occupational settings.

PHYSICAL FINDINGS & CLINICAL PRESENTATION

- Depends on the severity and duration of exposure. The brain and heart are most sensitive to CO poisoning.
- Presentation is often nonspecific and may be mistaken for a flulike illness.
- Mild to moderate poisoning may present with headache, malaise, dizziness, nausea, dyspnea, difficulty concentrating, confusion, and blurred vision. Patients may have tachypnea and tachycardia.
- Severe poisoning may present with hypotension, arrhythmias, myocardial ischemia, pulmonary edema, lethargy, ataxia, loss of consciousness, seizure, coma, or rarely, cherry-red skin.
- Severity of poisoning does not correlate with carboxyhemoglobin (COHgb) levels.
- Delayed neurologic sequelae may develop days to weeks after recovery from acute poisoning. Patients may present with neurologic or psychiatric symptoms (cognitive deficits, memory loss, personality changes, movement disorders, Parkinson's, psychosis, neurologic deficits).

ETIOLOGY

- CO results from the incomplete combustion of carbon-containing compounds. CO poisoning occurs from inhaling smoke from fires, motor vehicle exhaust, or the burning of fuel (oil, wood, coal, natural gas) in poorly functioning or improperly ventilated devices (heating systems, stoves/grills, portable generators, etc.). Methylene chloride (paint stripper) fumes are converted to CO by the liver.
- CO toxicity results from tissue hypoxia and direct CO-mediated damage at the cellular level. This may explain why COHgb levels alone are not predictive of clinical toxicity. The mechanisms of CO toxicity are not completely understood.
- CO impairs oxygen delivery. CO binds hemoglobin with an affinity 250 times greater than oxygen, displacing oxygen from hemoglobin and decreasing the oxygen-carrying capacity of blood. By binding to hemoglobin, CO changes the structure of the hemoglobin molecule and decreases oxygen release to tissue.
- CO also interferes with peripheral oxygen utilization. Cellular respiration is depressed by inhibition of the mitochondrial cytochrome oxidase system. By binding to myoglobin, CO decreases its ability to use and store oxygen.
- Neurologic toxicity is not explained by hypoxia alone and is related to the complex intracellular actions of CO. CO precipitates an inflammatory cascade that results in oxidative damage and brain lipid peroxidation.

Dx DIAGNOSIS

DIFFERENTIAL DIAGNOSIS

- Viral syndromes
- Cyanide, hydrogen sulfide
- Methemoglobinemia
- Amphetamines and derivatives
- Cocaine, phencyclidine (PCP)
- Cyclic antidepressants
- Phenothiazines
- Theophylline

WORKUP

History (duration and source of CO exposure, loss of consciousness), physical examination (detailed neurologic examination), laboratory and imaging tests

LABORATORY TESTS

- COHgb level (measured by co-oximetry of blood gas sample): COHgb level >3% in nonsmokers confirms exposure. Heavy smokers may have baseline levels of up to 10%. Levels may be low if the patient has already received supplemental oxygen or if delay occurs between exposure and testing.
- Direct measurement of arterial oxyhemoglobin (by co-oximetry): Pulse oximetry and arterial blood gas (ABG) may be falsely normal because neither measures oxygen saturation of hemoglobin directly. Pulse oximetry is inaccurate because of the similar absorption characteristics of oxyhemoglobin and COHgb. An ABG is inaccurate because it measures oxygen dissolved in plasma (which is not affected by CO) and then calculates oxygen saturation of hemoglobin.
- Electrolytes, glucose, BUN, creatinine, cardiac biomarkers, ABG (lactic acidosis and rhabdomyolysis may develop), CBC (polycythemia from hypoxia in chronic CO poisoning).
- ECG (ischemia, arrhythmia).
- Pregnancy test (fetus at high risk).
- Consider toxicology screen.

IMAGING STUDIES

- Chest radiograph (noncardiogenic edema)
- CT, MRI if neurologic abnormalities are present

Rx TREATMENT

ACUTE GENERAL Rx

- Remove from site of CO exposure.
- Ensure adequate airway.
- Continuous ECG monitor.
- Fetal monitoring if pregnant.
- 100% oxygen by nonrebreather mask or endotracheal tube (decreases half-life of COHgb from 4 to 6 hr to 60 to 90 min) until COHgb level is <10% and patient is asymptomatic.
- Hyperbaric oxygen (2.5 to 3 atm).
  - Decreases half-life of COHgb to 20 to 30 min; increases amount of oxygen dissolved in plasma
  - Questionable beneficial effect over normobaric oxygen
  - May reduce incidence of neurologic sequelae of CO poisoning
  - Consider for individuals with:
    1. Severe intoxication (COHgb >25%, history of loss of consciousness, neurologic symptoms or signs, cardiovascular compromise, severe metabolic acidosis)
    2. Pregnant women with COHgb >20% or signs of fetal distress: CO elimination slower in fetus than mother, fetal Hgb has greater affinity for CO than adult Hgb
  - Should be instituted quickly if deemed necessary
- Consider concomitant poisoning with other toxic/irritant gases that may be present in smoke (e.g., cyanide) or thermal injury to airway. Toxic effects of CO and cyanide are synergistic.
- Identify source of exposure and determine if poisoning was accidental.

DISPOSITION

- Patients with mild accidental poisoning can be treated in an ambulatory setting. Those with moderate/severe poisoning or coexisting illness require hospitalization.
- Survivors of severe poisoning are at 14% to 40% risk for neurologic sequelae.
  - Deficits usually apparent within 3 wk of poisoning but may present months later.
  - Risk of developing sequelae is greater if patient lost consciousness during acute poisoning and with older age.
  - Brain MRI may reveal changes; damage is seen most often in the globus pallidus and deep white matter
  - Recovery may occur over months to years.
- CO-mediated cardiac damage is associated with increased long-term mortality rate.
- High risk of fetal demise.

REFERRAL

- United States Poison Control Network, 1-800-222-1222
- Hyperbaric unit; facilities are listed on the Undersea & Hyperbaric Medical Society website (www.uhms.org)
- Psychiatric evaluation if intentional poisoning

PEARLS & CONSIDERATIONS

- Severity of poisoning and prognosis do not correlate with COHgb levels.
- Neuropsychometric testing is an objective measure of cognitive function but is not universally used.
- Contact local Fire Department to assess environment and identify source of CO.

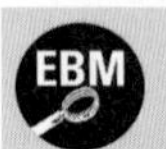

EVIDENCE

Please note: Complete text of EBM for this topic is available online.

Key trials and commentary:

Elevated blood carboxyhemoglobin (COHb) levels are used to confirm a clinical diagnosis of exposure to carbon monoxide (CO) and, in some instances, assess severity of poisoning. However, many hospital laboratories cannot measure COHb because they do not have CO-oximeters. In such instances, blood samples are often sent to outside laboratories or with a transported patient for measurement at the receiving hospital. This study was conducted to assess the stability of COHb in stored and mailed blood samples anticoagulated with heparin. This study showed that carboxyhemoglobin levels in whole blood samples anticoagulated with heparin are stable with or without refrigeration for up to 4 weeks. If COHb measurement capability is not available, such samples may be shipped or transported with patients with confidence that the COHb level will be stable when measured at a later time.

This is a useful bit of information, also valuable in retrospectively establishing the diagnosis of CO poisoning. Stored specimens from admission can be sampled days later if the opportunity to get a COHb level was missed.[1] Ⓐ

Evidence-Based Reference

1. Hampson NB: Stability of carboxyhemoglobin in stored and mailed blood samples, *Am J Emerg Med* 26:191-195, 2008. Commentary by R.J. Hamilton, M.D. Ⓐ

SUGGESTED READINGS

Domachevsky L et al: Hyperbaric oxygen in the treatment of carbon monoxide poisoning, *Clin Toxicol* 43(3):181, 2005.

Graber J et al: Results from a state-based surveillance system for carbon monoxide poisoning, *Public Health Reports* 122(2):145, 2007.

Hampson N: Storm-related carbon monoxide poisoning: lessons learned from recent epidemics, *Undersea Hyperb Med* 33(4):257, 2006.

Henry CR et al: Myocardial injury and long-term mortality following moderate to severe carbon monoxide poisoning, *JAMA* 295(4):398, 2006.

Kao LW et al: Toxicity associated with carbon monoxide, *Clin Lab Med* 26:99, 2006.

Weaver LK: Carbon monoxide poisoning, *N Engl J Med* 360:1217-1225, 2009.

AUTHOR: **SUDEEP KAUR AULAKH, M.D.**

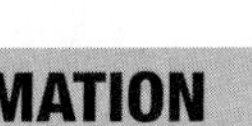

BASIC INFORMATION

DEFINITION

Carcinoid syndrome is a symptom complex characterized by paroxysmal vasomotor disturbances, diarrhea, and bronchospasm. It is caused by the action of amines and peptides (serotonin, bradykinin, histamine) produced by tumors arising from neuroendocrine cells.

SYNONYMS

Flush syndrome
Argentaffinoma syndrome

ICD-9CM CODES
259.2 Carcinoid syndrome

EPIDEMIOLOGY & DEMOGRAPHICS

INCIDENCE:

- Carcinoid tumors are found incidentally in 0.5% to 0.75% of autopsies.
- Carcinoid tumors are principally found in the following organs: appendix (40%); small bowel (20%; 15% in the ileum); rectum (15%); bronchi (12%); esophagus, stomach, and colon (10%); and ovary, biliary tract, and pancreas (3%).
- The incidence of carcinoids is 2.47 to 4.48/100,000, depending on race and sex, and is highest in black men. The overall incidence has increased over the last 30 years due in part to improved diagnostic modalities.

PHYSICAL FINDINGS & CLINICAL PRESENTATION

- Cutaneous flushing (75% to 90%)
  1. The patient usually has red-purple flushes starting in the face, then spreading to the neck and upper trunk.
  2. The flushing episodes last from a few minutes to hours (longer lasting flushes may be associated with bronchial carcinoids).
  3. Flushing may be triggered by emotion, alcohol, or foods or may occur spontaneously.
  4. Dizziness, tachycardia, and hypotension may be associated with the cutaneous flushing.
- Diarrhea (>70%): often associated with abdominal bloating and audible peristaltic rushes
- Intermittent bronchospasm (25%): characterized by severe dyspnea and wheezing
- Facial telangiectasia
- Tricuspid insufficiency, pulmonic stenosis from carcinoid heart lesions

ETIOLOGY

- Carcinoid syndrome is caused by neoplasms originating from neuroendocrine cells.
- Carcinoid tumors do not usually produce the syndrome unless liver metastases are present or the primary tumor does not involve the gastrointestinal tract.

DIAGNOSIS

DIFFERENTIAL DIAGNOSIS

- Flushing: Carcinoid syndrome must be distinguished from idiopathic flushing (IF); patients with IF more often are female, are younger, and have a longer duration of symptoms; palpitations, syncope, and hypotension occur primarily in patients with IF. Additional causes of flushing that need to be ruled out are menopause, medications (niacin, nitrates), alcohol, renal cell carcinoma, medullary cancer of thyroid, VIPoma, mastocytosis, and chronic use of food additives (nitrites, sulfites)
- Diarrhea: IBD, IBS, laxative abuse, infectious colitis
- Bronchospasm: Asthma, foreign body, GERD, lung neoplasm

LABORATORY TESTS

- The biochemical marker for carcinoid syndrome is increased 24-hr urinary 5-hydroxyindoleacetic acid, a metabolite of serotonin (5-hydroxytryptamine).
- False elevations can be seen with ingestion of certain foods (bananas, pineapples, eggplant, avocados, walnuts) and certain medications (acetaminophen, caffeine, guaifenesin, reserpine); therefore patients should be on a restricted diet and avoid these medications when the test is ordered.
- Falsely low results can occur with use of alcohol, aspirin, MAO inhibitors, and St. John's wort.
- Liver function studies are an unreliable indicator of liver involvement.

IMAGING STUDIES

- Chest x-ray is useful to detect bronchial carcinoids.
- CT scan of abdomen or a liver and spleen radionuclide scan is useful to detect liver metastases (palpable in >50% of cases).
- Iodine-123–labeled somatostatin can detect carcinoid endocrine tumors with somatostatin receptors.
- Scanning with radiolabeled octreotide can visualize previously undetected or metastatic lesions.

TREATMENT

NONPHARMACOLOGIC THERAPY

Avoidance of ethanol ingestion (may precipitate flushing)

GENERAL Rx

- Surgical resection of the tumor can be curative if the tumor is localized or palliative and results in prolonged asymptomatic periods if metastases are present. Surgical manipulation of the tumor can, however, cause severe vasomotor abnormalities and bronchospasm (carcinoid crisis).
- Percutaneous embolization and ligation of the hepatic artery can decrease the bulk of the tumor in the liver and provide palliative treatment of tumors with hepatic metastases.
- Cytotoxic chemotherapy: combination chemotherapy with 5-fluorouracil and streptozocin can be used in patients with unresectable or recurrent carcinoid tumors; however, it has only limited success.
- Control of clinical manifestations:
  1. Somatostatin analogues (octreotide and lancreotide) are effective for both flushing and diarrhea in most patients. Interferon alfa may be useful as an additive therapy for persistent symptoms despite use of somatostatin analogues; however, data remains inconclusive.
  2. Flushing may be controlled by the combination of H_1- and H_2-receptor antagonists (e.g., diphenhydramine 25 to 50 mg PO q6h and ranitidine 150 mg bid).
  3. Diarrhea may respond to diphenoxylate with atropine (Lomotil).
  4. Bronchospasm can be treated with aminophylline and/or albuterol.
- Nutritional support: supplemental niacin therapy may be useful to prevent pellagra because the tumor uses dietary tryptophan for serotonin synthesis, resulting in a nutritional deficiency in some patients.
- Interferon alfa may be useful as an additive to control symptoms unresponsive to somatostatin analogues.
- Echocardiography and monitoring for right-sided congestive heart failure are recommended for patients with unresectable disease because endocardial fibrosis, involving predominantly the endocardium, chordae, and valves of the right side of the heart, can occur.

DISPOSITION

Carcinoids of the appendix and rectum have a low malignancy potential and rarely produce the clinical syndrome; metastases are also uncommon if the size of the primary lesion is <2 cm in diameter.

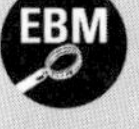

EVIDENCE

A study among patients with endocrine gastroenteropancreatic tumors found no significant difference in progression-free and long-term survival rates between patients treated with octreotide versus octreotide plus interferon-alfa.[1] A

We are unable to cite evidence that meets our criteria for the other therapies for carcinoid syndrome.

Evidence-Based Reference

1. Arnold R et al: Octreotide versus octreotide plus interferon-alpha in endocrine gastroenteropancreatic tumors: a randomized trial, *Clin Gastroenterol Hepatol* 3:761, 2005. A

AUTHOR: **FRED F. FERRI, M.D.**

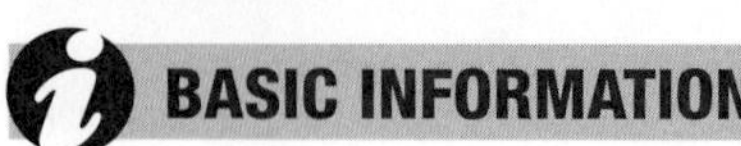

BASIC INFORMATION

DEFINITION

Cardiac tamponade is a life-threatening condition where an accumulation of fluid within the pericardial sac impairs filling of the ventricles during diastole and causes a decline in cardiac output.

SYNONYMS

None

ICD-9CM CODES
423.9 Unspecified diseases of the pericardium

PHYSICAL FINDINGS & CLINICAL PRESENTATION

1. Chest pain
2. Tachypnea/dyspnea
3. Beck's triad
   a. Absolute or relative hypotension
   b. Elevated jugular venous pressure (with prominent *x* descent and blunted *y* descent)
   c. Muffled heart sounds
4. Tachycardia (except in uremia or hypothyroid patients)
5. Pulsus paradoxus (decrease in systolic arterial pressure of 10 mm Hg or more during normal inspiration while in normal sinus rhythm)
6. Pericardial friction rub may be present
7. Reduced or absent apical cardiac impulse

ETIOLOGY

Acute (rapidly accumulating pericardial effusion leading to cardiac tamponade): does not need a large amount of effusion to cause tamponade

1. Penetrating trauma
2. Aortic dissection
3. Following treatment of myocardial infarction with thrombolytics and/or heparin because of myocardial rupture and/or hemorrhagic pericarditis
4. Iatrogenic (central line and pacemaker insertions, post–coronary bypass surgery or post–percutaneous coronary intervention)

Subacute or chronic (effusion is usually large):

1. Malignancy (e.g., lung, breast, lymphoma)
2. Viral pericarditis (e.g., Coxsackie, human immunodeficiency virus)
3. Bacterial, fungal, or tuberculous pericarditis
4. Uremia
5. Myxedema (rare)
6. Collagen vascular disease (e.g., lupus, rheumatoid arthritis, scleroderma)
7. Radiation
8. Idiopathic

Dx DIAGNOSIS

Cardiac tamponade is a clinical diagnosis made at the bedside from history and physical examination. The echocardiogram will help confirm or reject the clinical diagnosis. Tamponade can be confirmed invasively by the measurement of elevated intrapericardial pressures with an intrapericardial catheter and lowering of the intrapericardial pressure in response to pericardial fluid drainage. Thereafter, the underlying etiology must be determined with specific laboratory work (see "Laboratory Tests" below).

DIFFERENTIAL DIAGNOSIS

Other conditions that can also lead to elevated jugular venous pressure, decreased systemic pressure, and pulsus paradoxus include:

- Chronic obstructive pulmonary disease
- Constrictive pericarditis
- Restrictive cardiomyopathy
- Right ventricular infarction
- Pulmonary embolism
- Chronic biventricular heart failure

LABORATORY TESTS

- Electrolytes, blood urea nitrogen, creatinine, erythrocyte sedimentation rate, thyroid function tests, antinuclear antibody, rheumatoid factor, PPD, blood cultures, viral titers, and pericardial fluid analysis and cultures
- Possible 12-lead ECG findings:
  1. Sinus tachycardia
  2. PR depression and/or diffuse ST elevations if acute pericarditis is present
  3. Electrical alternans
  4. Low voltage if massive effusion is present

IMAGING STUDIES

- Chest radiograph (enlarged cardiac silhouette with clear lung fields)
- Echocardiogram (collapse of the right atrium and/or right ventricle during diastole, respiratory variation in transvalvular blood flow)
- Right-sided heart catheterization and intrapericardial pressure measurements confirm the diagnosis
- Typical findings are diastolic equalization of pressures, usually ranging from 15 to 30 mm Hg (diastolic pulmonary artery pressure = right ventricular diastolic pressure = right atrial pressure = intrapericardial pressure)

Rx TREATMENT

NONPHARMACOLOGIC THERAPY

- Cardiac tamponade should be treated emergently.
- Avoid drugs that reduce preload (e.g., nitrates, diuretics).
- Large pericardial effusions without hemodynamic compromise (tamponade) can be managed conservatively with careful monitoring, treatment of the underlying cause, and frequent serial surveillance echocardiography.

ACUTE GENERAL Rx

- Aggressive intravascular volume expansion (saline or blood)
- Emergency pericardial fluid removal by pericardiocentesis or surgical pericardiotomy by way of the subxiphoid pericardial window
- Pericardiocentesis should be performed under fluoroscopic or echocardiographic guidance when available
- Inotropic or vasopressor support if above measures cannot be performed immediately

CHRONIC Rx

- Depends on etiology.
- Pericardiocentesis with draining catheter: the catheter can be left inside the pericardium to allow continued drainage for 24 to 48 hr. If residual fluid still persists with hemodynamic compromise, surgical drainage should be sought. In the absence of hemodynamic compromise or significant residual fluid, discontinuation of the draining catheter can be done with periodic postprocedure echocardiographic monitoring of reaccumulation (e.g., 24 hr, 7 days, 30 days, 3 mo, 6 mo, 12 mo) depending on the etiology and rate of reaccumulation.
- Other surgical drainage procedures include:
  1. Subxiphoid pericardiotomy drainage
  2. Limited pericardiectomy draining the pericardial fluid into the left hemithorax
  3. Complete pericardiectomy, especially in patients with effusive-constrictive pericarditis or bacterial pericarditis (see "Pearls & Considerations" below).

DISPOSITION

The prognosis of cardiac tamponade depends on the underlying cause.

REFERRAL

- Cardiology consultation should be made if cardiac tamponade is suspected.
- Cardiothoracic surgery consultation should also be considered if surgical pericardial drainage is indicated.

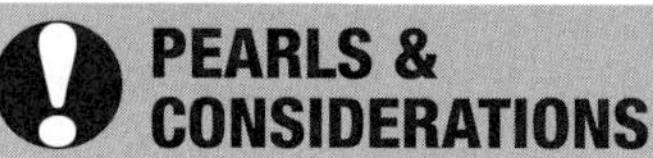

PEARLS & CONSIDERATIONS

- Cardiac tamponade should always be considered during pulseless electrical activity arrest and may require emergent pericardiocentesis.
- Evaluation for pulsus paradoxus should always be performed during normal respiration because deep inspiration may render a false positive finding.
- Strong consideration should be given to performing early pericardiocentesis in patients who have pericardial effusion associated with bacterial pneumonia or empyema because the incidence of bacterial pericarditis is especially high in this clinical situation and the subsequent development of cardiac tamponade and severe chronic constrictive pericarditis occurs frequently.

COMMENTS

As little as 100 ml of fluid can lead to acute cardiac tamponade, whereas with gradual accumulation, the pericardial sac can hold up to 5 L of fluid before tamponade occurs.

EVIDENCE

Please note: Complete text of EBM for this topic is available online.

SUGGESTED READINGS

Holmes DR et al: Iatrogenic pericardial effusion and tamponade in the percutaneous intracardiac intervention era, *J Am Coll Cardiol Intv* 2(8):705, 2009.

Meltser H, Kalaria VG: Cardiac tamponade, *Catheter Cardiovasc Interv* 64(2):245, 2005.

Roy CL et al: Does this patient with pericardial effusion have cardiac tamponade? *JAMA* 297(16):1810, 2007.

Sagristà-Sauleda J et al: Hemodynamic effects of volume expansion in patients with cardiac tamponade, *Circulation* 117(12):1545, 2008.

Spodick DH: Acute cardiac tamponade, *N Engl J Med* 349(7):684, 2003.

AUTHORS: **ROBERTO PACHECO, M.D.,** and **WEN-CHIH WU, M.D.**

Cardiomyopathy, Dilated (PTG) (ALG)

BASIC INFORMATION

DEFINITION

Dilated cardiomyopathy describes a group of diseases involving the myocardium and characterized by myocardial dysfunction that is not primarily the result of hypertension, coronary atherosclerosis, valvular dysfunction, or congenital heart disease. As a result, the heart is enlarged and the ventricles are dilated with impaired systolic function.

SYNONYMS

Congestive cardiomyopathy

ICD-9CM CODES
425.4 Other primary cardiomyopathies

EPIDEMIOLOGY & DEMOGRAPHICS

- The prevalence rate of dilated cardiomyopathy in the general adult population is approximately 1%.
- Incidence increases with age and approaches 10% at age 80 yr.

PHYSICAL FINDINGS & CLINICAL PRESENTATION

- Increased jugular venous pressure
- Narrow pulse pressure
- Pulmonary rales, hepatomegaly, peripheral edema
- S_3, S_4
- Mitral regurgitation, tricuspid regurgitation (less common)

ETIOLOGY

- Idiopathic (most common)
- Alcoholism (15% to 40% of all cases in Western countries)
- Infections (viral [Coxsackie B, adenovirus, parvovirus, HIV], rickettsial, mycobacterial, toxoplasmosis, trichinosis, Chagas' disease)
- Uncontrolled tachyarrhythmia ("tachycardia-mediated")
- Peripartum (greatest risk from last trimester of pregnancy to 6 mo postpartum)
- Toxins (cobalt, lead, phosphorus, carbon monoxide, mercury)
- Nutritional (selenium deficiency, carnitine deficiency, thiamine deficiency)
- Drug induced (antiretrovirals, phenothiazines, cocaine, heroin, organic solvents "glue-sniffer's heart," doxorubicin, daunorubicin)
- Collagen-vascular disease (systemic lupus, rheumatoid arthritis, polyarteritis, dermatomyositis, sarcoidosis)
- Postmyocarditis
- Heredofamilial neuromuscular disease (e.g., muscular dystrophy)
- Excess hormones (acromegaly, osteogenesis imperfecta, myxedema, thyrotoxicosis, diabetes)
- Hematologic (e.g., sickle cell anemia, hemochromatosis)

Dx DIAGNOSIS

Dilated cardiomyopathy is a diagnosis of exclusion, after ruling out other causes of myocardial dysfunction.

DIFFERENTIAL DIAGNOSIS

- Coronary atherosclerosis
- Valvular dysfunction (especially aortic and mitral regurgitation)
- Pulmonary disease
- Pericardial abnormalities
- Anemia
- Hypothyroidism/myxedema

WORKUP

- Chest x-ray examination, ECG, echocardiogram; myocardial biopsy is not routinely recommended, unless acute myocarditis requiring immunosuppressive therapy is considered (e.g., giant cell myocarditis)
- Medical history with emphasis on the following symptoms:
  1. Dyspnea on exertion, orthopnea, paroxysmal nocturnal dyspnea
  2. Palpitations
  3. Systemic and pulmonary embolism
- Persistently increased cardiac troponin T levels are a marker of poor outcome in cardiomyopathy patients

IMAGING STUDIES

Chest x-ray examination:
- Massive cardiac enlargement
- Interstitial pulmonary edema (Kerley B lines), Pleural effusion (more often on right side)

ECG:
- Left ventricular (LV) hypertrophy with ST-T wave changes
- Right or left bundle branch block
- Arrhythmias (atrial fibrillation, premature ventricular or atrial contractions, ventricular tachycardia)

Echocardiogram:
- Low ejection fraction with global hypokinesis
- Four-chamber enlargement
- Regurgitation from atrioventricular valves (from malposition of valves caused by dilation of ventricle)

Rx TREATMENT

NONPHARMACOLOGIC THERAPY

- Treatment of underlying disease (systemic lupus, alcoholism)
- Avoidance of dietary salt
- Exercise training has been shown to be associated with reduced risk for hospitalization and death in patients with history of heart failure in limited trials; enrollment in a formal cardiac rehabilitation program may be beneficial in improving patient's functional status

ACUTE GENERAL Rx

- Diuretics are indicated for all patients with current symptoms or history of heart failure and reduced left ventricular ejection fraction (LVEF) with evidence of volume overload (peripheral edema, orthopnea, paroxysmal nocturnal dyspnea).
- ACE inhibitors (and angiotensin receptor blockers) have been shown to have favorable effects on ventricular remodeling in patients with cardiomyopathy and have shown a demonstrable mortality benefit in these patients, and are therefore recommended in all patients with reduced LV systolic function, unless specific contraindications exist.
- Beta-blockers (in particular, carvedilol, long-acting metoprolol, and bisoprolol) work by inhibiting the adverse effects of the sympathetic nervous system in patients with ventricular systolic dysfunction, and have likewise shown a mortality benefit in patients with LV systolic dysfunction and should be used unless specifically contraindicated.
- Additional medical therapies (aldosterone antagonists, hydralazine/nitrates, digitalis) can be considered in certain patient subpopulations with persistent symptoms on otherwise optimal medical management.
- Patients with associated coronary atherosclerosis (angina, ECG changes, reversible defects on myocardial perfusion imaging) may benefit from percutaneous or surgical revascularization.

DISPOSITION

Annual mortality rate is 20% in patients with moderate heart failure, and it exceeds 50% in patients with severe heart failure.

REFERRAL

- Patients with dilated cardiomyopathy are at increased risk for sudden cardiac death, and implantation of acardiac defibrillator for primary prevention of sudden cardiac death can be considered for patients with heart failure symptoms and LVEF <35% on optimal medical therapy.
- Patients with LVEF <35%, wide QRS duration by ECG (>−0.12 sec), and persistent heart failure symptoms may benefit from cardiac resynchronization therapy via a biventricular pacemaker.
- Consider heart transplantation for young patients (<60 yr) who are no longer responsive to medical therapy. Dilated cardiomyopathy is the reason for 45% of heart transplantations.

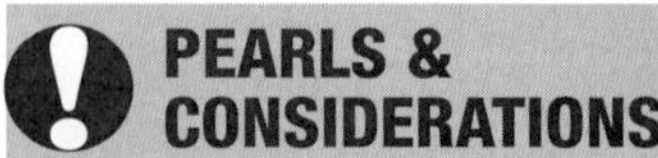

PEARLS & CONSIDERATIONS

COMMENTS

- Patients should be encouraged to restrict or eliminate alcohol and reduce sodium intake (<2 g daily).
- Patients may benefit from daily weight checks as a means of early detection of volume overload and decompensated heart failure.
- Vulnerability to cardiomyopathy among chronic alcohol abusers is partially genetic and related to the presence of the ACE *DD* genotype.

- Idiopathic dilated cardiomyopathy is often familial, and apparently healthy relatives may have latent, early, or undiagnosed disease. Echocardiographic evaluation of family members is recommended.

EVIDENCE

Please note: Complete text of EBM for this topic is available online.

SUGGESTED READINGS

Hunt SA et al: 2009 focused update incorporated into the ACC/AHA 2005. Guidelines for the Diagnosis and Management of Heart Failure in Adults, *Circulation* 119:e391, 2009.

Kadish A et al: Prophylactic defibrillator implantation in patients with non-ischemic dilated cardiomyopathy, *N Engl J Med* 350:2151, 2004.

Mahon NG et al: Echocardiographic evaluation in asymptomatic relatives of patients with dilated cardiomyopathy reveals preclinical disease, *Ann Intern Med* 143:108, 2005.

AUTHORS: **ANTHONY S. GEMIGNANI, M.D., FRED F. FERRI, M.D.,** and **WEN-CHIH WU, M.D., M.P.H.**

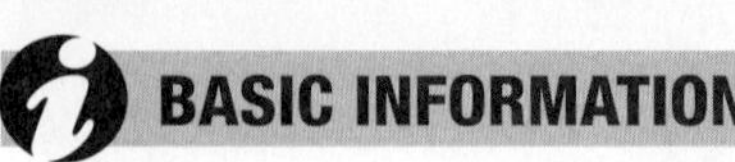

DEFINITION

Cardiomyopathy describes a group of diseases that involve the myocardium and are characterized by myocardial dysfunction that is not primarily the result of hypertension, coronary atherosclerosis, valvular dysfunction, or congenital heart disease. Hypertropic cardiomyopathy (HCM) describes a spectrum of diseases characterized by disorganized myocyte architecture and thickening of the left ventricular wall beyond 15 mm that is out of proportion of the afterload. The interventricular septum is the most common site of enlargement, though hypertrophy may involve other focal regions or may be concentric. HCM may result in hemodynamically significant obstruction within the left ventricular outflow tract and/or impairment in the diastolic function of the ventricle.

SYNONYMS

Hypertrophic cardiomyopathy
Idiopathic hypertrophic subaortic stenosis (IHSS)
Hypertrophic obstructive cardiomyopathy (HOCM)
Asymmetric septal hypertrophy (ASH)

ICD-9CM CODES

425.4	Cardiomyopathy, hypertrophic nonobstructive
425.1	Cardiomyopathy, hypertrophic obstructive
746.84	Cardiomyopathy, hypertrophic congenital

EPIDEMIOLOGY & DEMOGRAPHICS

- The disease occurs in two major forms:
  1. A familial form, usually diagnosed in young patients and gene mapped to chromosome 14q, is caused by a missense mutation in 1 of at least 10 genes that encode the proteins of the cardiac sarcomere (60%-70% of cases of hypertrophic cardiomyopathy are familial)
  2. A sporadic form usually found in elderly patients
- To date, more than 200 different HCM-causing mutations have been reported.
- The prevalence rate of phenotypically expressed HCM in the adult general population is 0.2% (most common genetic cardiovascular disease).
- It is the most common cause of sudden cardiac death in young athletes.

PHYSICAL FINDINGS & CLINICAL PRESENTATION

- HCM may be suspected on the basis of abnormalities found on physical examination. Classic findings include:
  - Harsh, systolic, crescendo-decrescendo murmur at the left sternal border or apex that increases with any maneuver that reduces volume in the left ventricle (e.g., Valsalva)
  - Paradoxic splitting of S_2 (if left ventricular obstruction is present)
  - S_4 may be present
  - Double or triple apical impulse ("Triple ripple": atrial contraction, early rapid ejection, and late slow ejection)
  - Pulsus bisferiens (double pulsation on palpation of the carotid pulse)
- Increased obstruction can occur with:
  - Drugs: digitalis, β-adrenergic stimulators (isoproterenol, dopamine, epinephrine), nitroglycerin, vasodilators, diuretics, alcohol
  - Hypovolemia
  - Tachycardia
  - Valsalva maneuver
  - Standing position
- Decreased obstruction is seen with:
  - Drugs: β-adrenergic blockers, calcium channel blockers, disopyramide, α-adrenergic stimulators
  - Volume expansion
  - Bradycardia
  - Hand grip exercise
  - Squatting position
- Clinical manifestations are as follows:
  - Dyspnea
  - Syncope (usually seen with exercise)
  - Angina (decreased angina in recumbent position)
  - Palpitations

ETIOLOGY

- Autosomal dominant trait with variable penetrance caused by mutations in any of 1 to 10 genes, each encoding proteins of cardiac sarcomere
- Sporadic occurrence

Dx DIAGNOSIS

DIFFERENTIAL DIAGNOSIS

- Hypertensive heart disease
- Valvular disease, especially aortic stenosis
- Cardiac amyloidosis
- Fabry disease
- Athlete's heart

WORKUP

- ECG is abnormal in 75% to 95% of patients: left ventricular hypertrophy, abnormal Q waves in lateral and inferior leads, and taller than normal R waves in the right precordial leads. T wave changes may also be present especially in patients with predominantly apical hypertrophy.
- Echocardiography may be useful as up to 95% of patients will have asymmetric wall thickening, most often within the septum. Up to 30% of patients will manifest systolic anterior motion of the anterior leaflet of the mitral valve, which leads to obstruction.
- 24-hour Holter monitor to screen for potential lethal arrhythmias (principal cause of syncope or sudden death in obstructive cardiomyopathy) should be performed initially and annually.
- Exercise testing is indicated to evaluate for symptoms related to obstruction and can also provide prognostic information.
- Screening for sarcomere protein gene mutations in family members of patients with HCM can identify a broad subgroup of patients with increased propensity toward long-term impairment of left ventricular function and adverse outcome, irrespective of the myofilament (thick, intermediate, or thin) involved.

IMAGING STUDIES

- Chest x-ray examination may be normal or show cardiomegaly.
- Two-dimensional echocardiography is used to establish the diagnosis. Findings include ventricular hypertrophy, which can be symmetric or asymmetric hypertrophy (ratio of septum thickness to left ventricular wall thickness, >1.3:1), presence of a narrow LV outflow tract with a pressure gradient suggestive of obstruction, systolic anterior motion of anterior leaflet, or the chordae of the mitral valve.
- Magnetic resonance imaging (MRI) may be of diagnostic value when echocardiographic studies are technically inadequate. MRI is also useful in identifying unusual segmental hypertrophy undetectable by standard echocardiography.

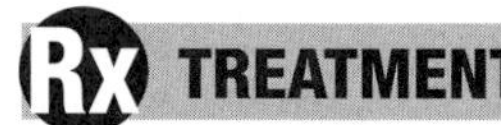

NONPHARMACOLOGIC THERAPY

Advise avoidance of alcohol; alcohol use (even in small amounts) results in increased obstruction of the left ventricular outflow tract. Patients should also be advised to avoid dehydration and strenuous exertion.

GENERAL Rx

- Therapy for HCM is directed at blocking the effect of catecholamines that can exacerbate dynamic left ventricular outflow tract obstruction and avoiding vasodilator or diuretic agents that can worsen the obstruction.
- Beta-blockers: The beneficial effects of beta-blockers on symptoms (principally dyspnea and chest pain) and exercise tolerance appear to be largely a result of a decrease in the heart rate with consequent prolongation of diastole and increased passive ventricular filling. By reducing the inotropic response, beta-blockers may also reduce myocardial oxygen demand and decrease the outflow gradient during exercise, when sympathetic tone is increased.
- Verapamil also decreases left ventricular outflow obstruction by improving filling and probably reducing myocardial oxygen demand. It is used mainly as a second-line agent in patients who cannot tolerate beta-blockers. It should be used with caution in patients with symptomatic obstruction. Administration in the hospital setting is recommended in these patients.
- Disopyramide is an antiarrhythmic that is also a negative inotrope, resulting in further decrease in outflow gradient.
- Prophylactic antibiotics before dental, GI, and genitourinary procedures are no longer rec-

ommended according to the 2007 American Heart Association (AHA) guidelines.

- Avoid use of digitalis, diuretics, nitrates, and vasodilators.
- Dual-chamber pacing has been recommended for hemodynamic and symptomatic benefit in patients with drug-resistant hypertrophic obstructive cardiomyopathy; however, it has not been shown to result in significant improvement in objective measures of exercise capacity.
- Implantable cardiac defibrillators (ICDs) are a safe and effective therapy in HCM patients prone to ventricular arrhythmias. Their use is strongly warranted for patients with prior cardiac arrest or sustained spontaneous ventricular tachycardia. The use of ICDs to prevent sudden death in HCM is a class IIa recommendation according to AHA/American College of Cardiology/Heart Rhythm Society 2008 Guidelines for Device Based Therapy in Cardiac Rhythm Abnormalities for patients with HCM with at least one high-risk feature (see list in "Disposition").

DISPOSITION

HCM is not a static disease. Some adults may experience subtle regression in wall thickness, whereas others (~5% to 10%) paradoxically evolve into an end-stage cardiomyopathy resembling dilated cardiomyopathy, characterized by cavity enlargement, left ventricular wall thinning, and diastolic dysfunction. Patients with HCM are at increased risk for sudden death, especially if onset of symptoms began during childhood. Severe left ventricular outflow obstruction at rest is also a strong, independent predictor of severe symptoms of heart failure and death. Adult patients can be considered low risk if they have no symptoms or mild symptoms and also if they have none of the following:

- A family history of premature death caused by HCM
- Nonsustained ventricular tachycardia during Holter monitoring
- A marked outflow tract gradient (≥50 mm Hg)
- Substantial hypertrophy (>20 mm)
- Marked left atrial enlargement
- Abnormal blood pressure response during exercise

REFERRAL

- Surgical treatment (myotomy-myectomy involving resection of the basal septum) is reserved for patients who have both a large outflow gradient (≥50 mm Hg) and severe symptoms of heart failure unresponsive to medical therapy. The risk for sudden death from arrhythmias is not altered by surgery. When this operation is performed by experienced surgeons in tertiary referral centers, the operative mortality rate is <2%, and many patients are able to achieve near-normal exercise capacity after surgery.
- Nonsurgical reduction of the interventricular septum can be used in patients with HCM refractory to pharmacologic treatment who are at a greater surgical risk (e.g., >40 yr old). This technique involves the injection of ethanol in the septal perforator branch of the left anterior descending coronary artery, producing a controlled myocardial infarction of the interventricular septum, and thereby reducing septal mass and consequently the left ventricular outflow tract gradient. This method may lead to improvement in both subjective and objective measures of exercise capacity, but results are not as effective as surgery and are associated with a high incidence of heart block, requiring permanent pacing in approximately one fourth of patients and/or recurrence of obstruction and symptoms.

PEARLS & CONSIDERATIONS

COMMENTS

- Screening of first-degree relatives with two-dimensional echocardiography and ECG is indicated, particularly if adverse HCM-related events have occurred in the family. Annual screening is recommended for all adolescents from age 12 to 18 yr. Periodic screening of all first-degree adult family members at 5-yr intervals is recommended because hypertrophy may not be detected until the sixth decade of life. It is advisable to have a trained clinical genetic counselor see the patient and obtain consent before genetic testing.
- Future screening techniques may involve identification of mutations in the gene encoding the sarcomeric proteins. The most common sarcomeric subtype is MYBPC3-HCM, affecting one in five patients. Clinical predictors of positive genotype, such as the presence of ventricular arrhythmias, age at diagnosis, degree of left ventricular wall hypertrophy, and family history of HCM, may aid in patient selection for genetic testing and increase the yield of cardiac sarcomere gene screening.
- The mortality rate in HCM is approximately 1% to 2%.
- It is important to remember that HCM is predominantly a nonobstructive disease (75% of patients do not have a sizable resting outflow tract gradient).
- Section III describes an algorithm for the management of symptoms and risks in patients with HCM.

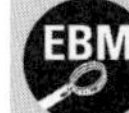

EVIDENCE

Please note: Complete text of EBM for this topic is available online.

Key trials and commentary:

Hypertrophic cardiomyopathy (HCM) is often accompanied by atrial fibrillation (AF) due to diastolic dysfunction, elevated left atrial pressure, and enlargement. Although catheter ablation for drug-refractory AF is an effective treatment, the efficacy in HCM remains to be established.

This study showed that outcomes after AF ablation in patients with HCM are favorable. Diastolic dysfunction, left atrial enlargement, and AF subtype influence outcomes. Future studies of rhythm management approaches in HCM patients are required to clarify the optimal clinical approach.

This patient population has been difficult to manage in general, and particularly difficult to manage in the presence of AF. This study confirms that radiofrequency ablation for symptomatic AF is an effective approach in patients with HCM. These findings are similar to previous studies, which also found that most of these patients respond favorably to a radiofrequency ablation approach to treat atrial fibrillation. In aggregate, the reported success rates have ranged from 70% to 77%. Of note, and pretty much like most other studies, there is a high recurrence rate, 39% in this study. Thus, this approach appears to be reasonable in the treatment of HCM patients with AF.[1] Ⓐ

Evidence-Based Reference

1. Bunch TJ et al: Substrate and procedural predictors of outcomes after catheter ablation for atrial fibrillation in patients with hypertrophic cardiomyopathy, *J Cardiovasc Electrophysiol* 19:1009-1014, 2008. Commentary by A.L. Waldo, M.D. Ⓐ

SUGGESTED READINGS

Fifer MA, Vlahakes GJ: Management of symptoms in hypertrophic cardiomyopathy, *Circulation* 117:429, 2008.

Maron BJ: Hypertrophic cardiomyopathy, a systematic review, *JAMA* 287:1308, 2002.

Maron BJ et al: Implantable cardioverter-defibrillators and prevention of sudden cardiac death in hypertrophic cardiomyopathy, *JAMA* 298(4):405, 2007.

Maron MS et al: Effect of left ventricular outflow tract obstruction on clinical outcome in hypertrophic cardiomyopathy, *N Engl J Med* 348:295, 2003.

Montgomery JV et al: Relation of electrocardiographic pattern to phenotypic expression and clinical outcome in hypertrophic cardiomyopathy, *Am J Cardiology* 96:270, 2005.

Nagueh SF, Mahmarian JJ: Noninvasive cardiac imaging in patients with hypertropic cardiomyopathy, *J Am Coll Cardiol* 48:2410, 2006.

Nishimura RA, Holmes DR: Hypertrophic obstructive cardiomyopathy, *N Engl J Med* 350:1320, 2004.

Olivotto I et al: Myofilament protein gene mutation screening and outcome of patients with hypertrophic cardiomyopathy, *Mayo Clin Proc* 83(60):630-638, 2008.

Wilson W et al: Prevention of infectious endocarditis: guidelines from the American Heart Association, *Circulation* 116:1736, 2007.

AUTHORS: **ANTHONY S. GEMIGNANI, M.D., FRED F. FERRI, M.D.,** and **WEN-CHIH WU, M.D., M.P.H.**

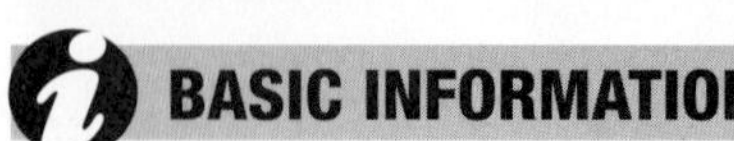

BASIC INFORMATION

DEFINITION

Cardiomyopathy describes a group of diseases involving the myocardium and characterized by myocardial dysfunction that is not primarily the result of hypertension, coronary atherosclerosis, valvular dysfunction, or congenital heart disease. Restrictive cardiomyopathy is characterized by decreased ventricular compliance, with impaired ventricular filling and generally normal systolic function.

ICD-9CM CODES
425.4 Other primary cardiomyopathies

EPIDEMIOLOGY & DEMOGRAPHICS

- Relatively uncommon cardiomyopathy, accounting for 5% of all primary myocardial diseases
- Most frequently caused by amyloidosis (Fig. 1-51), myocardial fibrosis (after open heart surgery), and radiation
- Patients classified as having "idiopathic" restrictive cardiomyopathy may have mutations in the gene for cardiac troponin I, and restrictive cardiomyopathy may represent an overlap with hypertrophic cardiomyopathy in many familial cases.

PHYSICAL FINDINGS & CLINICAL PRESENTATION

Restrictive cardiomyopathy presents with symptoms of progressive left-sided and right-sided heart failure:

- Fatigue, weakness (caused by low output as patients are unable to augment cardiac output by increasing heart rate without compromising ventricular filling)
- Edema, ascites, hepatomegaly, distended neck veins
- Kussmaul's sign may be present
- Regurgitant murmurs
- Apical impulse may be palpable (can help distinguish it from constrictive pericarditis)

ETIOLOGY

Disease may be classified according to pathophysiologic processes:

Infiltrative:
- Amyloidosis
- Sarcoidosis (usually results in a dilated cardiomyopathy with regional wall motion abnormalities)
- Gaucher's disease
- Hurler's disease

Noninfiltrative:
- Idiopathic (familial subtypes may have genetic overlap with hypertrophic cardiomyopathy)
- Scleroderma
- Diabetic cardiomyopathy
- Pseudoxanthoma elasticum

Storage diseases:
- Hemochromatosis (unusual as it is commonly associated with a dilated cardiomyopathy)
- Fabry disease
- Glycogen storage diseases

Endomyocardial:
- Endomyocardial fibrosis
- Hypereosinophilic syndrome (Loeffler's)
- Carcinoid heart disease
- Radiation
- Metastatic cancers
- Drug related (anthracyclines, serotonin, ergotamine, busulfan, methylsergide)

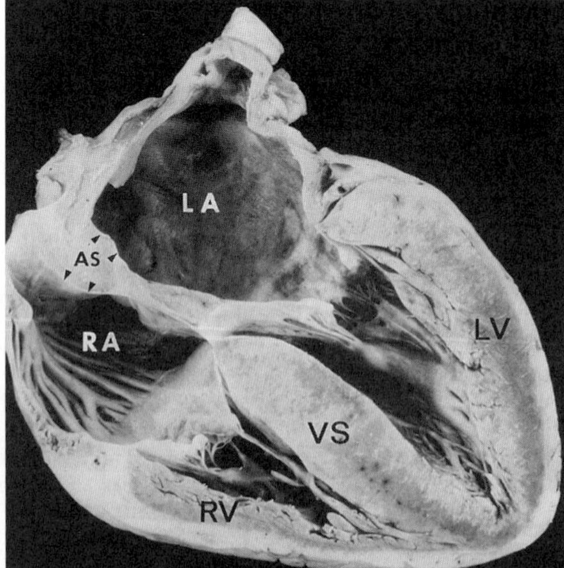

FIGURE 1-51 Necropsy specimen of an amyloid heart demonstrating the thickened ventricular septum *(VS)*, atrial septum *(AS)*, and free wall of the left ventricle *(LV)* and right ventricle *(RV)*, and the dilated left atrium *(LA)*. *RA*, Right atrium. (Courtesy Dr. William Edwards, Mayo Clinic, Rochester, MN. From Goldman L, Ausiello D [eds]: *Cecil textbook of medicine,* ed 22, Philadelphia, 2004, WB Saunders.)

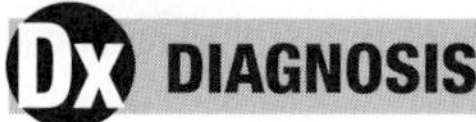

DIAGNOSIS

DIFFERENTIAL DIAGNOSIS

- Constrictive pericarditis
- Valvular dysfunction (especially aortic stenosis)
- Hypertrophic cardiomyopathy
- Hypertension
- Coronary atherosclerosis
- Chronic lung disease

WORKUP

- Blood count (to identify eosinophilia), chest x-ray examination, ECG, echocardiogram
- Cardiac catheterization, magnetic resonance imaging, and computed tomography (selected cases)

IMAGING STUDIES

- Chest x-ray examination:
  1. Ranges from normal cardiomediastinal silhouette to moderate cardiomegaly (primarily because of biatrial enlargement).
  2. Evidence of heart failure may be present.
  3. Presence of pericardial calcification favors alternate diagnosis of constrictive pericarditis.
- ECG:
  1. Nonspecific ST-T wave abnormalities are the most common finding. Voltage may be low in infiltrative etiologies such as amyloidosis.
  2. Frequent atrial and ventricular ectopy are often present. Atrial fibrillation may be present.
  3. High-degree atrioventricular block, intraventricular conduction delay may be seen in advanced cases.
- Echocardiogram:
  1. Biatrial enlargement almost always present.
  2. Wall thickness depends on etiology, often normal but may be thickened in infiltrative disease such as amyloidosis.
  3. Ventricular chamber sizes and systolic function are often normal or reduced.
- Cardiac catheterization:
  - Characteristic hemodynamic finding is a dip and plateau, or square-root sign in the left ventricular tracing, where deep and rapid decline in ventricular pressure at the onset of diastole is immediately followed by rapid rise and plateau in early diastole phase. To distinguish restrictive cardiomyopathy from constrictive pericarditis:
    1. Constrictive pericarditis: Usually involves both ventricles and leads to equalization of diastolic pressures between all four cardiac chambers to within 5 mm Hg.
    2. Restrictive cardiomyopathy: Impairs the left ventricle more than the right, often with left-sided end-diastolic pressures of 5 mm Hg greater than the right. The presence of increased pulmonary arterial systolic pressures is also suggestive of restrictive disease.

- Cardiac computed tomographic scan may be helpful to identify a thickened and calcified pericardium, consistent with constrictive pericarditis.
- Magnetic resonance imaging may also be useful to distinguish restrictive cardiomyopathy from constrictive pericarditis (thickness of the pericardium less than 5 mm in the latter).

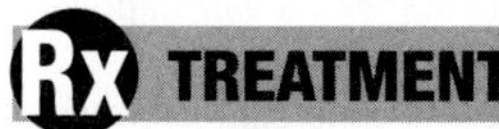

TREATMENT

NONPHARMACOLOGIC THERAPY

Control heart failure by restricting salt.

ACUTE GENERAL Rx

Treatment of volume overload and heart failure symptoms with diuretic therapy.

CHRONIC Rx

Treatment involves management of the underlying disease if it exists (hemochromatosis may respond to repeated phlebotomy to decrease iron deposition in the heart, sarcoidosis may respond to corticosteroid therapy, and eosinophilic cardiomyopathy may respond to corticosteroid and cytotoxic drugs). There is no effective therapy for other causes of restrictive cardiomyopathy.

Death usually results from heart failure or arrhythmias; therefore, therapy should be aimed at controlling symptoms of heart failure by restricting salt, administering diuretics, and treating potentially fatal arrhythmias.

DISPOSITION

Prognosis varies with the etiology of the cardiomyopathy but is poor overall as disease is rarely detected before advanced stages.

REFERRAL

Cardiac transplantation can be considered in patients with refractory symptoms and idiopathic or familial restrictive cardiomyopathies.

SUGGESTED READINGS

Kushwaha SS et al: Restrictive cardiomyopathy, *N Engl J Med* 336:267, 1997.

Maron BJ et al: Contemporary definitions and classification of the cardiomyopathies: an American Heart Association Scientific Statement from the Council on Clinical Cardiology, Heart Failure and Transplantation Committee; Quality of Care and Outcomes Research and Functional Genomics and Translational Biology Interdisciplinary Working Groups; and Council on Epidemiology and Prevention, *Circulation* 113:1807, 2006.

AUTHORS: **ANTHONY S. GEMIGNANI, M.D., FRED F. FERRI, M.D.,** and **WEN-CHIH WU, M.D., M.P.H.**

Carotid Sinus Syndrome (ALG)

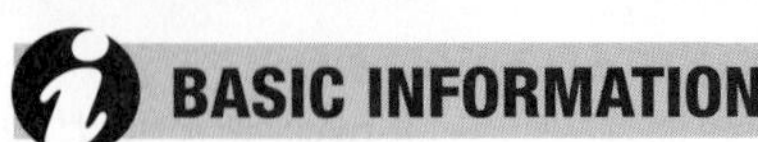

BASIC INFORMATION

DEFINITION

Light-headedness, dizziness, presyncope, or syncope in a patient with carotid sinus hypersensitivity is defined as carotid sinus syndrome (CSS). Carotid sinus hypersensitivity is the exaggerated response to carotid stimulation resulting in bradycardia, hypotension, or both. CSS is often considered a variant of neurocardiogenic syncope.

SYNONYMS

Carotid sinus syncope
CSS
Carotid sinus hypersensitivity

ICD-9CM CODES
337.0 Idiopathic peripheral autonomic neuropathy
780.2 Syncope or collapse

EPIDEMIOLOGY & DEMOGRAPHICS

- Carotid sinus hypersensitivity accounts for 10% to 20% of presyncopal and syncopal episodes.
- Carotid sinus hypersensitivity is frequently associated with atherosclerosis and diabetes mellitus.
- Incidence increases with age, with an average age of onset at 61 to 74 yr.
- Men are affected more often than women (2:1).
- Carotid sinus syndrome is rarely found in patients younger than 50 yr.

PHYSICAL FINDINGS & CLINICAL PRESENTATION

- Usually associated with sudden neck movements or tight-fitting collars
- Usually associated with prodrome of nausea, warmth, pallor, or diaphoresis
- Light-headedness or presyncopal symptoms
- Syncope

Properly performed carotid sinus massage (CSM) at the bedside is diagnostic. This maneuver can elicit three types of responses in patients with carotid sinus hypersensitivity (see "Diagnosis").

1. CSM should be performed with the patient in the supine and upright position while monitoring the patient's blood pressure by cuff and heart rate by ECG.
2. CSM should be performed on only one carotid artery at a time.
3. Vigorous circular pressure is applied over one carotid artery at the level of the cricoid cartilage for approximately 5 to 10 sec and repeated on the opposite side if no effect is produced.
4. Contraindications to CSM include the presence of carotid artery bruits, documented carotid artery stenosis >70%, history of stroke or transient ischemic attack <3 mo, history of myocardial infarction <6 mo, history of serious ventricular arrhythmia, or prior carotid endarterectomy.
5. Complications of transient visual disturbance or transient paresis occur in <1% of patients.

ETIOLOGY

- Idiopathic
- Head and neck tumors (e.g., thyroid)
- Significant lymphadenopathy
- Carotid body tumors
- Prior neck surgery

Dx DIAGNOSIS

- The diagnosis of CSS is made when carotid sinus hypersensitivity is demonstrated by CSM and no other cause of syncope is identified.
- CSM can elicit three types of responses diagnostic of carotid sinus hypersensitivity:
  1. Cardioinhibitory type: CSM producing (1) asystole for at least 3 sec in the absence of symptoms or (2) reproduction of symptoms occurring with a decline in heart rate of 30% to 40% or asystole of up to 2 sec in duration. Symptoms should not recur when CSM is repeated after atropine infusion.
  2. Vasodepressor type: CSM producing (1) a decrease in systolic blood pressure of 50 mm Hg in the absence of symptoms or 30 mm Hg in the presence of neurologic symptoms; (2) no evidence of asystole; or (3) neurologic symptoms that persist after infusion of atropine.
  3. Mixed type: CSM producing both types of responses.

DIFFERENTIAL DIAGNOSIS

All causes of syncope

WORKUP

- CSS is a diagnosis of exclusion.
- Exclude other causes of syncope or presyncope: detailed history, physical examination including orthostatic vital signs, ECG. Other tests should be considered depending on the clinical setting.

Rx TREATMENT

NONPHARMACOLOGIC THERAPY

Avoid applying neck pressure from tight collars, shaving, or rapid head turning.

ACUTE GENERAL Rx

Treatment will vary according to the type of carotid hypersensitivity response and symptoms present (see "Chronic Rx").

CHRONIC Rx

Therapy is divided into three classes: medical, surgical (carotid denervation), and cardiac pacing. Surgical therapy has been largely abandoned except in cases of compressing tumors or masses responsible for CSS.

For infrequent and mildly symptomatic carotid sinus hypersensitivity of either the cardioinhibitory or vasodepressor type, treatment is generally not necessary.

For symptomatic patients with a cardioinhibitory response to CSM:

- A dual-chamber permanent pacemaker is a class I indication.

For symptomatic patients with a vasodepressor response to CSM:

- Sympathomimetics: midorine 2.5 to 10 mg tid
- Serotonin-specific reuptake inhibitors
- Fludrocortisone
- Elastic knee-high or thigh-high stockings
- Carotid sinus denervation

For symptomatic patients with CSS with a mixed response to CSM:

- Combination of dual-chamber permanent pacemaker and agents used to treat vasodepressor response

DISPOSITION

- Up to 50% of the patients have recurrent symptoms.
- No increased mortality rate in patients with idiopathic CSS compared with the general population.

REFERRAL

Cardiology referral is indicated if cardiac testing, such as tilt-table test, or pacemaker placement is being considered.

Neurology referral is indicated if neurologic causes of syncope are suggested by history or physical examination findings.

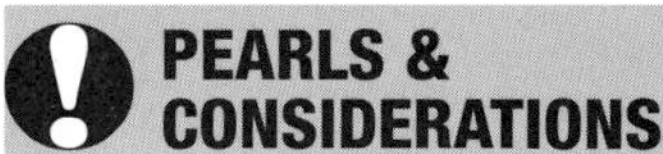

PEARLS & CONSIDERATIONS

CSS accounts for syncope in 6% to 14% of patients.

The most common type of CSS is cardioinhibitory, followed by mixed and vasodepressor responses.

COMMENTS

Prognosis depends on the underlying cause.

SUGGESTED READINGS

AHA/ACCF scientific statement on the evaluation of syncope, *J Am Coll Cardiol* 47(2):473, 2006.

Brignole M et al: Task Force on Syncope, European Society of Cardiology. Guidelines on management (diagnosis and treatment) of syncope—update 2004, *Europace* 6:467, 2004.

Grubb BP: Clinical practice: neurocardiogenic syncope, *N Engl J Med* 352:1004, 2005.

Kerr SR et al: Carotid sinus hypersensitivity in asymptomatic older persons: implications for diagnosis of syncope and falls, *Arch Intern Med* 166(5):515, 2006.

AUTHORS: **SCOTT BRANCATO, M.D.,** and **WEN-CHIH WU, M.D.**

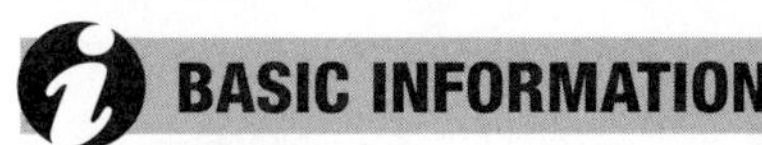

BASIC INFORMATION

DEFINITION

Carotid stenosis is narrowing of the arterial lumen within the carotid artery that is typically a result of atherosclerosis.

SYNONYMS

Atherosclerotic disease of the carotid artery

ICD-9CM CODES
433.1 Carotid stenosis

EPIDEMIOLOGY & DEMOGRAPHICS

INCIDENCE: 2.2 to 8/1000 persons per yr
PREVALENCE: 1.1 to 77/100,000 persons; it is estimated that 5/1000 persons ages 50 to 60 yr and 100/1000 persons >80 yr have carotid stenosis >50%. (*Note:* The incidence of carotid stenosis is unknown as screening is not routine. However, the incidence of transient ischemic attack [TIA], a common presenting symptom of carotid stenosis, is well-known.)
PREDOMINANT SEX AND AGE: Male:female ratio of 2:1; more common in whites than African Americans and Asians
PEAK INCIDENCE: Peak incidence is between 50 and 60 yr of age.
GENETICS: Multifactorial; twin studies (monozygous vs. dizygous) suggest a familial influence
RISK FACTORS: Hypertension, dyslipidemia, diabetes mellitus, and smoking are the four major risk factors.

PHYSICAL FINDINGS & CLINICAL PRESENTATION

Patients with carotid stenosis are often asymptomatic, but many have presence of a carotid bruit or TIA.

- Carotid bruit: In general, the presence of a carotid bruit is a better indicator of generalized atherosclerosis and as such, is a better predictor of ischemic heart disease than future stroke.
- TIA: Carotid stenosis is classically heralded by ipsilateral transient monocular blindness (Amaurosis fugax), contralateral numbness or weakness, contralateral homonymous hemianopsia, aphasia, or *syncope (if bilateral disease is present).*

ETIOLOGY

The primary etiology of carotid stenosis is atherosclerosis. Less common etiologies include aneurysm, arteritis, carotid dissection, fibromuscular dysplasia, postradiation necrosis, and vasospasm.

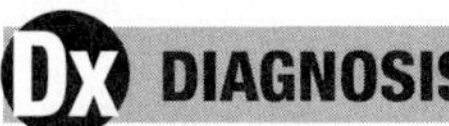

DIAGNOSIS

DIFFERENTIAL DIAGNOSIS

Aneurysm, arteritis, and carotid dissection

WORKUP

Systematic history, examination, and diagnostic studies to assess for carotid stenosis and other risk factors of TIA

LABORATORY TESTS

CBC, basic metabolic panel, fasting lipid profile, prothrombin time/international normalized ratio, activated partial thromboplastin time, C-reactive protein

IMAGING STUDIES

- Four imaging modalities exist for the evaluation of carotid stenosis (see Table 1-14).
- General guidelines state that patients who have neurologic sequelae suggestive of carotid stenosis should be screened via carotid duplex. If carotid stenosis is suspected on carotid duplex, but inconclusive, magnetic resonance angiography, computed tomography angiography, or angiography should be obtained to confirm the degree of stenosis (Fig. 1-52).

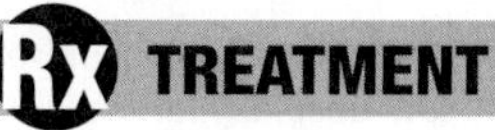

TREATMENT

NONPHARMACOLOGIC THERAPY

Carotid endarterectomy (CEA) and carotid artery stenting (CAS) are available.

CEA is the surgical removal of atherosclerotic plaque from the lining of the carotid artery. Several studies have proved the efficacy of this procedure. The selection of surgical candidates should be guided primarily by the presence or absence of symptoms and the degree of stenosis.

Asymptomatic patients: Four major trials have investigated the benefit of CEA in an asymptomatic patient with carotid stenosis: Carotid Artery Surgery Asymptomatic Narrowing Operation vs Aspirin (CASANOVA), Veterans Affairs Cooperative Study Group, Asymptomatic Carotid Atherosclerosis Study (ACAS), and Asymptomatic Carotid Surgery Trial (ACST). In addition, a meta-analysis was subsequently performed.

Pearls:

Most studies have shown that a benefit from CEA in asymptomatic patients is not seen until 2 yr after surgery.

CEA should be considered in asymptomatic patients only if the perioperative risk for stroke and death at the given surgical institution is less than 3%.

The studies failed to show a benefit in the presence of contralateral carotid occlusion.

Recommendations for asymptomatic patients with carotid stenosis:

CEA should be considered in patients between the ages of 40 and 75 yr

TABLE 1-14 Imaging Modalities for Carotid Stenosis

Imaging Modality	Benefit	Drawback
Cerebral angiography	• Gold standard • Assesses plaque morphology • Assesses presence of collaterals	• Invasive • High cost • 4% incidence rate of complications • 1% incidence rate of serious complications or death
Carotid duplex	• Sensitive in detecting high-grade stenosis (>70%) • Less invasive • Lower cost	• Can be limited by body habitus • Technician dependent • Overestimates degree of stenosis
Magnetic resonance angiography (MRA)	• Sensitive in detecting high-grade stenosis (>70%) • Less operator dependent	• Overestimates degree of stenosis • Cannot be performed in patients who are critically ill, unable to tolerate supine positioning, have pacemaker or other ferromagnetic hardware, or are claustrophobic* • Expensive • Takes much longer to obtain compared with other modalities
Computed tomography angiography (CTA)	• Sensitive for high-grade stenosis	• Contraindicated in patients with serum creatinine concentration >1.5 mg/dl

*One study revealed that ~17% of patients are unable to tolerate MRA secondary to claustrophobia or are unable to lie still for procedure.

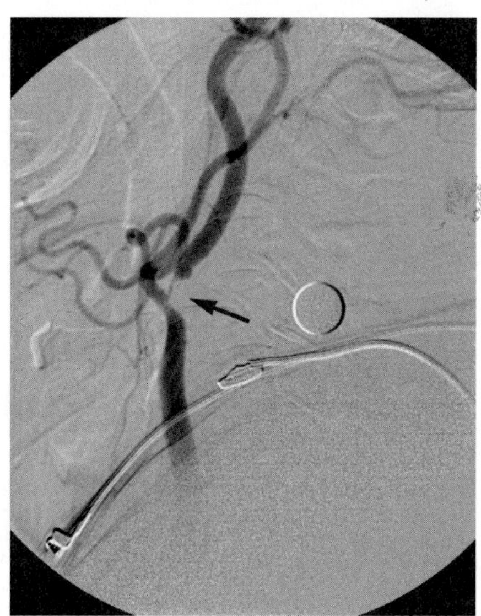

FIGURE 1-52 Conventional angiography demonstrating severe stenosis of the internal carotid artery at the bifurcation.

with asymptomatic 60% to 99% stenosis if their life expectancy is greater than 5 yr and the perioperative stroke and mortality rates are <3%.

All patients undergoing CEA should be started on low-dose aspirin (ASA; 81 or 325 mg daily) before surgery and should be continued indefinitely. Although variations exist among surgeons, aspirin is typically continued during the perioperative period.

Symptomatic patients: Two major trials (North American Symptomatic Carotid Endarterectomy Trial [NASCET] and European Carotid Surgery Trial [ECST]) and subsequent pooled analysis have shown the benefit of CEA in patients with symptomatic carotid stenosis.

Pearls:

There is improved outcome in patients with mild stroke or TIA if surgical treatment is within 2 wk of the symptomatic event.

Men seem to benefit more when compared with women.

CEA does not appear to be beneficial in women with 50% to 69% stenosis.

Despite increased perioperative risk, patients with contralateral carotid occlusion who undergo CEA have benefit in terms of stroke and death rate when compared with patients undergoing medical management alone.

Recommendations:

CEA is recommended for recently symptomatic patients with 70% to 99% stenosis if their life expectancy is >5 yr and perioperative risk for mortality is <6%. Number needed to treat (NNT) at 5 yr = 6.3.

CEA is beneficial for recently symptomatic men with 50% to 69% stenosis if their life expectancy is >5 yr and perioperative risk of mortality is <6%. NNT at 5 yr = 22.

Medical management is recommended for patients with stenosis <50%.

Low-dose ASA (81 or 325 mg daily) should be initiated before CEA and continued after surgery.

CAS:

CAS is recommended only for patients who are "high risk" for CEA. Three major studies have compared stenting and CEA (Stent-Protected Angioplasty vs. Carotid Endarterectomy [SPACE], endarterectomy vs. stenting in patients with symptomatic severe carotid stenosis [EVA-3S], and Stenting and Angioplasty with Protection in Patients at High Risk for Endarterectomy [SAPPHIRE]).

Recommendations:

CAS may be considered for symptomatic patients with >70% carotid stenosis who have either difficult surgical access or medical risk that increases the risk of surgery (those with severe cardiac or pulmonary disease, contralateral carotid occlusion, prior neck surgery, prior neck irradiation, contralateral laryngeal nerve palsy, recurrent stenosis after prior CEA, age >80 yr).

CAS should be considered only if operators have periprocedural morbidity and mortality rates between 4% and 6%.

ASA should be given before procedure and indefinitely after procedure.

Clopidogrel should be given for 6 mo to 2 yr after stent placement.

Risk for CAS:

Minor or major stroke related to hyperperfusion syndrome, periprocedural bradycardia, hypotension, and restenosis.

Hyperperfusion syndrome: 1.1%

Restenosis: 0.5% to 2%

ACUTE GENERAL Rx

General medical therapy should be aimed at risk factor reduction. As stated earlier, the major risk factors for carotid stenosis are hypertension (HTN), diabetes mellitus (DM), dyslipidemia (HL), and smoking.

Antiplatelet therapy:

Three antiplatelet options are available for patients with carotid stenosis: ASA, ASA plus dipyridamole, and clopidogrel.

DISPOSITION

Disposition and prognosis depend on several variables (Table 1-15): the degree of stenosis, the presence of symptoms, medication compliance, and the type of intervention (if any).

REFERRAL

Patients with carotid stenosis should be referred to a neurologist with vascular neurology experience.

TABLE 1-15 Carotid Stenosis Management

Degree of Carotid Stenosis	<50%	50-69%	70-99%
Asymptomatic	• Medical management	• Men: CEA if stenosis >60% and age <75 yr; otherwise, medical management • Women: medical management	• Men <75 yr: CEA • Women: medical management
Symptomatic	• Medical Management	• Men: CEA • Women: medical management	• Men: CEA • Women: CEA

CEA, Carotid endarterectomy.

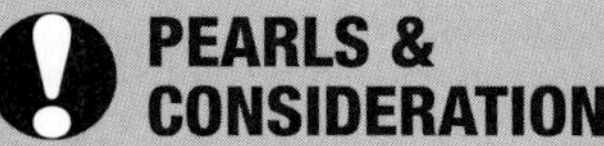

PEARLS & CONSIDERATIONS

Additional stenting trials are under way. Keep abreast of these as treatment recommendations may change suddenly.

SPECIAL CONSIDERATION

Some studies have shown that in patients with bilateral hemodynamically significant stenosis (>70%), reduction of blood pressure resulted in worse outcome in terms of stroke. These patients would likely be candidates for CEA.

Carotid artery occlusion (100% blockage), for which there is no routine treatment, is being reexamined in the national Carotid Occlusion Surgery Study (http://www.cosstrial.org). Consider referring symptomatic carotid occlusion patients for consideration of this study.

PREVENTION

Prevention of carotid stenosis should be guided at pursuing a healthy lifestyle and management of risk factors for development of atherosclerosis.

PATIENT/FAMILY EDUCATION

Patients should be counseled on pursuing a healthy lifestyle to include exercise and smoking cessation. In addition, patients should take an active role in controlling blood pressure and blood glucose. Further educational materials can be found online at: http://www.strokecenter.org/education.

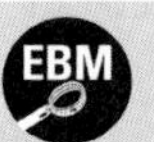

EVIDENCE

- According to the VA Study and ACAS, asymptomatic patients with carotid stenosis undergoing CEA plus medical management have improved outcomes when compared with medical management alone (4.7% vs. 9.4% for VA and 5% vs. 11% for ACAS).
- Patients with symptomatic carotid stenosis who undergo CEA have a smaller risk for stroke when compared with patients with medical management alone (9% vs. 26% for NASCET and 2.8% vs. 16.8% for ECST).[1]
- Patients undergoing CEA and CAS have a risk for reacquiring clinically significant stenosis after the procedure (restenosis). The risk for restenosis varies widely among studies but is generally thought to be between 0.5% and 2%. One study reported the 1-yr risk for restenosis to be 6% for CAS and 5.2% to 11.4% for CEA.[2]

Evidence-Based References

1. Chaturvedi S et al: Carotid endarterectomy—an evidence-based review: report of the Therapeutics and Technology Assessment Subcommittee of the American Academy of Neurology, *Neurology* 65(6), 2005.

2. Roubin GS et al: Carotid stent-supported angioplasty: a neurovascular intervention to prevent stroke, *Am J Cardiol* 78(3A), 1996.

SUGGESTED READINGS

Caplan LR: Large artery occlusive disease of the anterior circulation. In Caplan LR (ed): *Caplan's stroke: a clinical approach,* Philadelphia, 2009, Saunders, pp. 221-257.

Sacco RL et al: Guidelines for prevention of stroke in patients with ischemic stroke or transient ischemic attack: a statement for healthcare professionals from the American Heart Association/American Stroke Association Council on Stroke: co-sponsored by the Council on Cardiovascular Radiology and Intervention: the American Academy of Neurology affirms the value of this guideline, *Stroke* 37(2), 2006.

AUTHOR: **JOSEPH R. OWENS, M.D.**

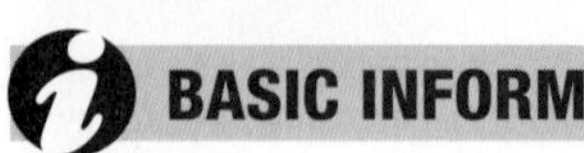

BASIC INFORMATION

DEFINITION

Carpal tunnel syndrome is an entrapment neuropathy involving the median nerve at the wrist (Fig. 1-53). It is the most common entrapment neuropathy in the upper extremity.

ICD-9CM CODES
354.0 Carpal tunnel syndrome

EPIDEMIOLOGY & DEMOGRAPHICS

PREVALENT AGE: 30 to 60 yr (bilateral up to 50%)

PREVALENT SEX: Females are affected two to five times as often as males.

PHYSICAL FINDINGS & CLINICAL PRESENTATION

- Nocturnal pain
- Occasional median nerve sensory impairment (often only index and long fingers)
- Positive Tinel's sign at wrist (tapping over the median nerve on the flexor surface of the wrist produces a tingling sensation radiating from the wrist to the hand)
- Positive Phalen's test (reproduction of symptoms after 1 min of gentle, unforced wrist flexion)
- Carpal compression test: Pressure with the examiner's thumb over the patient's carpal tunnel for 30 sec elicits symptoms
- Thenar atrophy in longstanding cases

ETIOLOGY

- Idiopathic in most cases
- Space-occupying lesions in carpal tunnel (tenosynovitis, ganglia, aberrant muscles)
- Often associated with hypothyroidism, hormonal changes of pregnancy
- Job-related mechanical overuse may be a risk factor
- Traumatic injuries to wrist

DIAGNOSIS

DIFFERENTIAL DIAGNOSIS

- Cervical radiculopathy
- Chronic tendinitis
- Vascular occlusion
- Reflex sympathetic dystrophy
- Osteoarthritis
- Other arthritides
- Other entrapment neuropathies

IMAGING STUDIES

Routine roentgenograms may be helpful in establishing cause or ruling out other conditions.

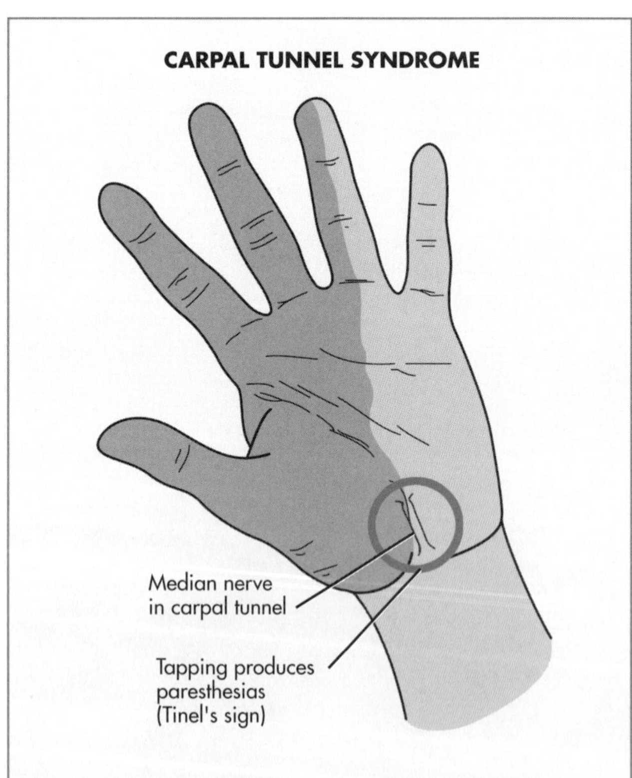

FIGURE 1-53 Distribution of pain and/or paresthesias *(dark-shaded area)* when the median nerve is compressed by swelling in the wrist (carpal tunnel). (From Arnett FC: Rheumatoid arthritis. In Andreoli TE [ed]: *Cecil essentials of medicine,* ed 4, Philadelphia, 1997, WB Saunders.)

ELECTRODIAGNOSTIC STUDIES

Nerve conduction velocity tests and electromyography are useful in establishing the diagnosis and ruling out other syndromes.

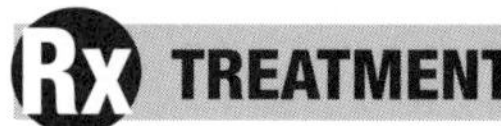

TREATMENT

ACUTE GENERAL Rx

- Elimination of repetitive trauma
- Occupational splints or braces
- NSAIDs
- Injection of carpal canal on ulnar side of palmaris longus tendon at wrist flexor crease (avoiding median nerve) (Fig. 1-54)
- Low-dose oral corticosteroids (e.g., prednisolone 20 mg qd for 2 wk, followed by 10 mg qd for 2 more wk) are also effective for symptom relief in selected patients
- Stretching exercises

DISPOSITION

Prognosis is variable. Some cases resolve spontaneously. Relief from local injection appears transient and symptoms recur in the majority of cases after injection.

Carpal tunnel syndrome is common in the third trimester of pregnancy, but symptoms subside after delivery in most cases, often dramatically. Symptoms may recur with subsequent pregnancies. Surgery is not recommended in pregnant patients because of the likelihood of spontaneous recovery.

REFERRAL

Surgical referral in cases of failed medical management or signs of motor weakness. Results of surgery are usually excellent, with return to full activity in 4 to 6 wk.

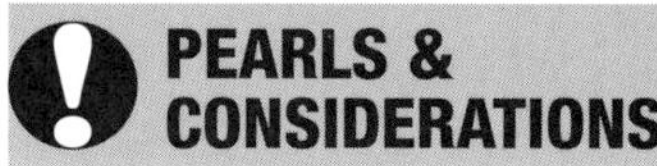

PEARLS & CONSIDERATIONS

- Carpal tunnel syndrome may occur in conjunction with cervical nerve root compression, a situation sometimes termed "double-crush syndrome." Compression at a more proximal level has been suggested to decrease the ability of the nerve to tolerate distal compression.
- Whether computer keyboard use is a risk factor is controversial.

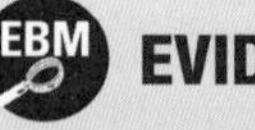

EVIDENCE

Please note: Complete text of EBM for this topic is available online.

Key trials and commentary:

There is no clear-cut consensus on the best diagnostic criteria for carpal tunnel syndrome (CTS). The objective of this study was to compare the probability of CTS being present following electrodiagnostic testing with the probability of it being present after the diagnosis was established on the basis of a clinical evaluation alone.

This study showed that for the majority of patients who are considered to have CTS on the basis of their history and physical examination alone, electrodiagnostic tests do not change the probability of diagnosing this condition to an extent that is clinically relevant.

The authors performed a clinical test using the CTS-6 instrument before an electrodiagnostic test on all patients who had been referred to an electrodiagnostic laboratory in a tertiary care center for the evaluation of any upper extremity peripheral nerve problem. They found that the probability of diagnosing CTS was lowered after the electrophysiological testing for a majority of the patients. This means that the electrophysiological studies are not necessary to make a diagnosis of CTS. This result is also preferable from the economic point of view.

The authors measured the sensory latency of the median nerve in the palm in the electrodiagnostic testing. Hand surgeons who are familiar with electrophysiological studies usually perform the studies on not only the median nerve but also the ulnar nerve. The motor and sensory latencies of the nerves are also measured below and above the wrist joint of bilateral upper extremities. Because the probability for diagnosing CTS with use of the CTS-6 instrument was extremely high, the probability would not change, even if such additional electrophysiological studies were performed. However, the additional studies provide us with some useful information, including unrecognized neuropathies hidden behind CTS such as cervical neuropathy, ulnar nerve neuropathy, and peripheral neuropathies due to metabolic abnormality. Although electrophysiological studies are not likely to add to the diagnosis of CTS, they may be helpful to treat patients with suspicion of CTS where the clinical examination is not entirely clear.[1] Ⓐ

The purpose of a separate investigation was to extend the previously reported short-term randomized trial of open and endoscopic carpal tunnel release in patients with CTS to compare outcomes 5 years after surgery.

This study showed that the improvements in symptoms of CTS and hand-related disability 5 years after open and two-portal endoscopic carpal tunnel release were equivalent.

This comprehensive prospective randomized trial comparing open with two-portal endoscopic carpal tunnel release has the longest term follow-up of any study to date, and expands upon the short-term results previously reported. The study is important, because few prospective long-term studies comparing the two techniques have been reported; hand surgeons are usually firmly entrenched in one camp or the other, seemingly basing their convictions on surgical technique preference and familiarity, and patient perceptions and demands, rather than on hard outcome data. One can glean favorable or unfavorable data from any number of short-term studies that would correctly support one's convictions for either technique. This study shows that over the long term (5 years) the two methods are comparatively similar with respect to reoperation rate, pain, symptom severity score, and functional status.[2] Ⓐ

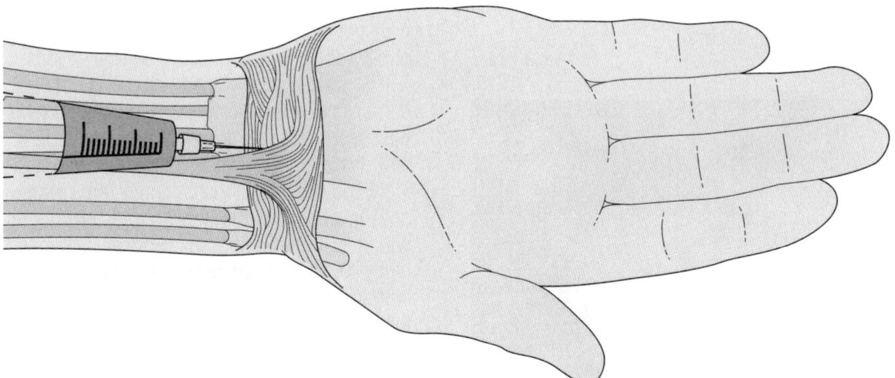

FIGURE 1-54 Injection of the carpal tunnel. (From Hochberg MC et al [eds]: *Rheumatology,* ed 3, St Louis, 2003, Mosby.)

Evidence-Based References

1. Graham B: The value added by electrodiagnostic testing in the diagnosis of carpal tunnel syndrome, *J Bone Joint Surg Am* 90:2587-2593, 2008. Commentary by J. Yao, M.D. Ⓐ
2. Atroshi I et al: Open compared with 2-portal endoscopic carpal tunnel release: a 5-year follow-up of a randomized controlled trial, *J Hand Surg* 34:266-272, 2009. Commentary by S. Trigg, M.D. Ⓐ

SUGGESTED READINGS

Atroshi I et al: Carpal tunnel syndrome and keyboard use at work: a population-based study, *Arthritis Rheum* 56:3620, 2007.

Burke FD et al: Primary care management of patients with carpal tunnel syndrome referred to surgeons: are non-operative interventions effectively utilized? *Postgrad Med J* 83:498, 2007.

Cranford CS et al: Carpal tunnel syndrome, *J Am Acad Orthop Surg* 15:537, 2007.

Dias JJ et al: Carpal tunnel syndrome and work, *J Hand Surg* 29:329, 2004.

Geoghegan JM et al: Risk factors in carpal tunnel syndrome, *J Hand Surg* 29:315, 2004.

Gerritsen AM et al: Splinting vs surgery in the treatment of carpal tunnel syndrome, *JAMA* 288:1245, 2002.

Goodyear-Smith F, Arroll B: What can family physicians offer patients with carpal tunnel syndrome other than surgery? A systematic review of nonsurgical management, *Ann Fam Med* 2:267, 2004.

Graham B: The value added by electrodiagnostic testing in the diagnosis of carpal tunnel syndrome, *J Bone Joint Surg Am* 90:2587, 2008.

Hui AC et al: Long-term outcome of carpal tunnel syndrome after conservative treatment, *Int J Clin Pract* 58:337, 2004.

Katz JN, Simmons BP: Carpal tunnel syndrome, *N Engl J Med* 346:1807, 2002.

Keith MW et al: Diagnosis of carpal tunnel syndrome, *J Am Acad Orthop Surg* 17:389, 2009.

Keith MW et al: Treatment of carpal tunnel syndrome, *J Am Acad Orthop Surg* 17:397, 2009.

Lee DH et al: Clinical nerve conduction and needle electromyography studies, *J Am Acad Orthop Surg* 12:276, 2004.

Piszzini DB et al: A systematic review of conservative treatment of carpal tunnel syndrome, *Clin Rehabil* 21:299, 2007.

Rich JT et al: Carpal tunnel syndrome due to tophaceous gout, *Orthopedics* 27:862, 2004.

Schnetzler KA: Acute carpal tunnel syndrome, *J Am Acad Orthop Surg* 16:276, 2008.

Uchiyama S et al: Current concepts of carpal tunnel syndrome: pathophysiology, treatment and evaluation, *J Orthop Sci* 15:1, 2010.

Vjera AJ: Management of carpal tunnel syndrome, *Am Fam Physician* 68:265, 2003.

AUTHOR: **LONNIE R. MERCIER, M.D.**

BASIC INFORMATION

DEFINITION

Cataracts are the clouding and opacification of the normally clear crystalline lens of the eye. The opacity may occur in the cortex, the nucleus of the lens, or the posterior subcapsular region, but it is usually in a combination of areas.

SYNONYMS

Congenital cataracts (e.g., from rubella)
Metabolic cataracts (e.g., caused by diabetes)
Collagen-vascular disease cataracts (caused by lupus)
Hereditary cataracts
Age-related senile cataracts
Traumatic cataracts
Toxic or drug-induced cataracts (e.g., caused by steroids)
Lenticular opacities

ICD-9CM CODES
366 Cataract

EPIDEMIOLOGY & DEMOGRAPHICS

INCIDENCE (IN U.S.): Most common cause of treatable blindness; cataract removal is the most frequent surgical procedure in patients >65 yr (1.3 million operations per year, with an annual cost of approximately $3 billion). By year 2020 more than 30 million Americans will have cataracts. Of Americans >40 yr, 20.5 million (17.2%) have cataracts. Of these, 5% have had surgery.

PEAK INCIDENCE:
- In early life: congenital and hereditary causes predominant; consider drug related and trauma
- In older age group: senile cataracts (after 40 yr)

PREDOMINANT AGE: Elderly; some stage of cataract development is present in >50% of persons 65 to 74 yr and in 65% of those >75 yr. Lens clouding begins at 39 to 40 yr and then usually progresses either slowly or rapidly depending on individual and health.

GENETICS: Hereditary with syndromes such as galactosemia, homocystinuria, diabetes

PHYSICAL FINDINGS & CLINICAL PRESENTATION

Cloudiness and opacification of the crystalline lens of the eye (Fig. 1-55)

ETIOLOGY

- Heredity
- Trauma
- Toxins
- Age related
- Drug related
- Congenital
- Inflammatory
- Diabetes
- Collagen vascular disease

DIAGNOSIS

DIFFERENTIAL DIAGNOSIS

- Corneal lesions
- Retinal lesions, detached retina, tumors
- Vitreous disease, chronic inflammation

WORKUP

- Complete eye examination, including slit lamp examination, funduscopic examination, and brightness acuity testing
- Complete physical examination for other underlying causes

LABORATORY TESTS

- Rarely, urinary amino acid screening and central nervous system imaging studies with congenital cataracts
- Fasting glucose in young adults with cataracts
- Diabetes, collagen vascular disease, other metabolic diseases in younger patients
- Genetic and hereditary evaluation

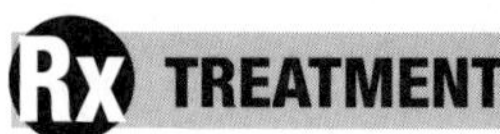

TREATMENT

There is no evidence that antioxidants or drugs will slow or treat cataracts.

NONPHARMACOLOGIC THERAPY

- Wait until vision is compromised before doing surgery.
- Surgery is indicated when corrected visual acuity in the affected eye is >20/30 in the absence of other ocular disease; however, surgery may be justified when visual acuity is better in specific situations (especially disabling glare, monocular diplopia). Surgery indicated when vision in one eye is greatly different from the other and affects the patient's life.

ACUTE GENERAL Rx

None necessary except when acute glaucoma or inflammation occurs

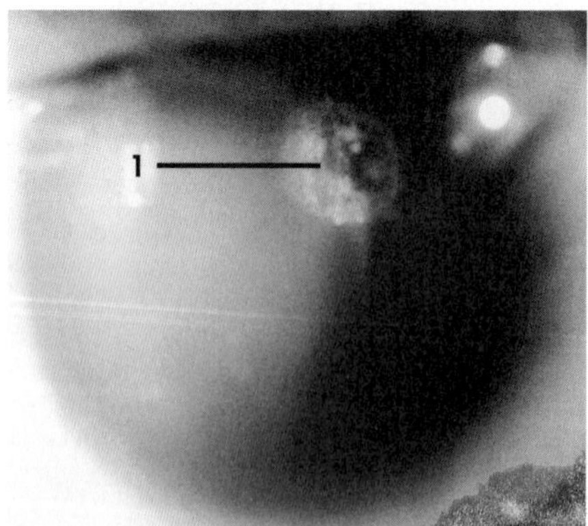

FIGURE 1-55 The central location of a posterior subcapsular cataract *(1)*. (From Palay D [ed]: *Ophthalmology for the primary care physician,* St Louis, 1997, Mosby.)

CHRONIC Rx

- Change glasses as cataracts develop.
- Myopia is common, and glasses can be adjusted until surgery is contemplated.

DISPOSITION

Refer if sight is compromised or the eye is red or inflamed.

REFERRAL

Refer to ophthalmologist for evaluation for extraction when vision is compromised (see "Nonpharmacologic Therapy").

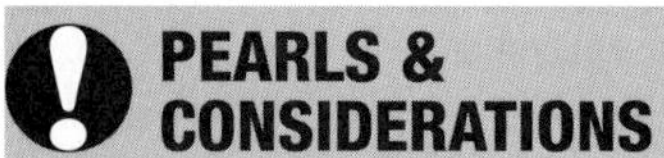

PEARLS & CONSIDERATIONS

Patients want to know five things about cataracts:
1. Chance for vision improvement
2. When vision will improve
3. Risk from surgery
4. Effect of surgery
5. Types of complications

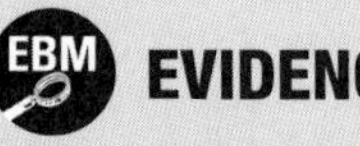

EVIDENCE

Please note: Complete text of EBM for this topic is available online.

Key trials and commentary:

Cataract surgery is the most common operative procedure performed in Canada, and how patients are affected by wait times for this surgery has important clinical, public health, and health policy considerations. This study conducted a systematic review to understand the relation between wait time for cataract surgery and patient outcomes and the variables that modify this relation.

This study showed that patients who wait more than 6 months for cataract surgery may experience negative outcomes during the wait period, including vision loss, a reduced quality of life, and an increased rate of falls.

This study out of Canada stratifies cataract surgery patients into two groups: Those who have a surgery with a wait of 6 weeks or less, and those with a wait of 6 months. Interestingly, the group that waits longer fares worse both in quality of life and number of falls. It would be interesting to perform a similar study looking at patients who defer cataract surgery despite visually significant cataracts. Every clinician encounters patients with bilateral cataracts and combined vision 20/100 or poorer. Typically, in this situation if the patient does not have any visual complaints, conservative management is still recommended. One wonders based on the results of this study if this is always in the patient's best interest.[1] Ⓐ

Another study sought to evaluate the effect of a multivitamin/mineral supplement on development or progression of age-related lens opacities.

This study showed that lens events were less common in participants who took the multivitamin/mineral formulation, but treatment had opposite effects on the development or progression of nuclear and PSC opacities, the two most visually important opacity subtypes.

This article is important because it helps address a question that patients frequently ask: typically a day doesn't go by in the office when I am not queried whether taking vitamins will have any beneficial effect to reduce the chances of developing cataracts. I usually try to tell patients that healthy eating and healthy lifestyle are probably the most important controllable factors in their general health as well as their ocular health.

Some patients are highly motivated to learn more about their general health and nutrition. If patients were extremely motivated to "delve deeper," I would refer them to this article. Otherwise, based on this study I would probably tell patients that there is no statistically significant difference with regard to cataract surgery but that again common sense basics (sunglasses, proper diet, and exercise) were probably even more important than vitamins alone.[2] Ⓐ

Evidence-Based References

1. Hodge W et al: The consequences of waiting for cataract surgery: a systematic review, *CMAJ* 176: 1285-1290, 2007. Commentary by R. Tipperman, M.D. Ⓐ

2. Clinical Trial of Nutritional Supplements and Age-Related Cataract Study Group: A randomized, double-masked, placebo-controlled clinical trial of multivitamin supplementation for age-related lens opacities. Clinical Trial of Nutritional Supplements and Age-Related Cataract Report No. 3, *Ophthalmology* 115:599-607.e1, 2008. Commentary by R. Tipperman, M.D. Ⓐ

SUGGESTED READINGS

Congdon N et al: Prevalence of cataract and pseudophakia/aphakia among adults in the US, *Arch Ophthalmol* 122(4):487, 2004.

Solomon R, Donninfeld ED: Recent advances and future frontiers in treating age-related cataracts, *JAMA* 290:248, 2003.

AUTHOR: **MELVYN KOBY, M.D.**

Cat-Scratch Disease (PTG)

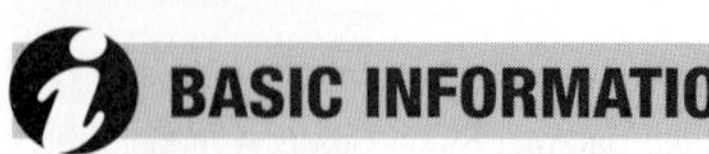

BASIC INFORMATION

DEFINITION

Cat-scratch disease (CSD) is a syndrome consisting of gradually enlarging regional lymphadenopathy occurring after contact with a feline. Atypical presentations are characterized by a variety of neurologic manifestations as well as granulomatous involvement of the eye, liver, spleen, and bone. The disease is usually self-limiting, and recovery is complete; however, patients with atypical presentations, especially if immunocompromised, may suffer significant morbidity and mortality.

SYNONYMS

Cat-scratch fever
Benign inoculation lymphoreticulosis
Nonbacterial regional lymphadenitis

ICD-9CM CODES

078.3 Cat-scratch disease

EPIDEMIOLOGY & DEMOGRAPHICS

PREVALENCE: Unknown
INCIDENCE (IN U.S.):
- Unknown
- Majority of reported cases in children

PEAK INCIDENCE: August through January
GENETICS: Unknown

PHYSICAL FINDINGS & CLINICAL PRESENTATION

- Classic, most common finding: regional lymphadenopathy occurring within 2 wk of a scratch or contact with felines; usually a new kitten in the household
- Tender, swollen lymph nodes most commonly found in the head and neck, followed by the axilla and the epitrochlear, inguinal, and femoral areas
- Erythematous overlying skin, showing signs of suppuration from involved lymph nodes
- On careful examination; evidence of cutaneous inoculation in the form of a nonpruritic, slightly tender pustule or papule (Fig. 1-56)
- Fever in most patients
- Malaise and headache in fewer than a third of patients
- Atypical presentations in fewer than 15% of cases
  1. Usually in association with lymphadenopathy and a low-grade or frank fever (>101° F, >38.3° C)
  2. Include granulomatous involvement of the conjunctiva (Parinaud's oculoglandular syndrome) and focal masses in the liver, spleen, and mesenteric nodes
- CNS involvement: neuroretinitis, encephalopathy, encephalitis, transverse myelitis, seizure activity, and coma
- Osteomyelitis in adults and children

ETIOLOGY

- Major cause: *Bartonella henselae,* possibly *Afipia felis* and *B. clarrigeiae*
- Mode of transmission: predominantly by direct inoculation through the scratch, bite, or lick of a cat, especially a kitten
- Limited evidence in support of an arthropod (flea) as an alternative vector of infection arising from bacteremic felines
- Rarely, associated with dogs, monkeys, and inanimate objects with which a feline has been in recent contact
- Approximately 2 wk after introduction of the bacteria into the host, regional lymphatic tissues displaying granulomatous infiltration associated with gradual hypertrophy
- Possible dissemination to distant sites (e.g., liver, spleen, and bone), usually characterized by focal masses or discrete parenchymal lesions

Dx DIAGNOSIS

DIFFERENTIAL DIAGNOSIS

Granulomas of this syndrome must be differentiated from those associated with:
- Tularemia
- Tuberculosis or other myobacterial infections
- Brucellosis
- Sarcoidosis
- Sporotrichosis or other fungal diseases
- Toxoplasmosis
- Lymphogranuloma venereum
- Benign and malignant tumors such as lymphoma

WORKUP

Diagnosis should be considered in patients who present with a predominant complaint of gradually enlarging regional (focal) lymphadenopathy, often with fever and a recent history of having contact with a cat. A primary ulcer at the site of the cat scratch may or may not be present at the time lymphadenopathy becomes manifest.

LABORATORY TESTS

- CSD skin test is no longer used for clinical purposes.
- Biopsied lymph node histology consistent with CSD.
- Enhanced culture techniques and serologies augment establishment of the diagnosis. An IFA *Bartonella* serology is commercially available. A PCR is used in research settings.
- Histopathologically, Warthin-Starry silver stain has been used to identify the bacillus.
- Routine laboratory findings:
  1. Mild leukocytosis or leukopenia
  2. Infrequent eosinophilia
  3. Elevated ESR or CRP
- Abnormalities of bilirubin excretion and elevated hepatic transaminases are usually secondary to hepatic obstruction by granuloma, mass, or lymph node.
- In patients with neurologic manifestations, lumbar puncture usually reveals normal CSF, although there may be a mild pleocytosis and modest elevation in protein.

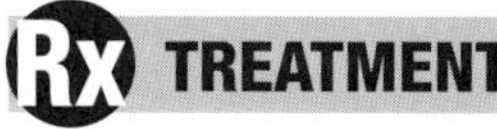

TREATMENT

NONPHARMACOLOGIC THERAPY

- Warm compresses to the affected nodes
- In cases of encephalitis or coma: supportive care

ACUTE GENERAL Rx

- There is no consensus over therapy, especially as the disease is self-limited in a majority of cases.
- It would be prudent to treat severely ill patients, especially if immunocompromised, with antibiotic therapy, because these patients tend to suffer dissemination of infection and increased morbidity.
- *Bartonella* is usually sensitive to a 5-day course of azithromycin, or alternatively aminoglycosides, tetracycline, and the quinolones can be used.
- When the isolate is proven by culture, the patient should receive antibiotic therapy as directed by the obtained susceptibilities.
- Antipyretics and NSAIDs may also be used.

DISPOSITION

Overall prognosis is good.

REFERRAL

- To an appropriate subspecialist to evaluate specific lesions
- For diagnostic aspiration or excision in presence of regional lymphadenopathy, bone lesions, and mesenteric lymph nodes and organs

FIGURE 1-56 Primary lesion of cat-scratch disease is a tender papule occurring 3 to 10 days after a scratch. (From Noble J [ed]: *Primary care medicine,* ed 2, St Louis, 1996, Mosby.)

- To ophthalmologist for ocular granulomas
  1. Usually diagnosed clinically
  2. Rarely require excision

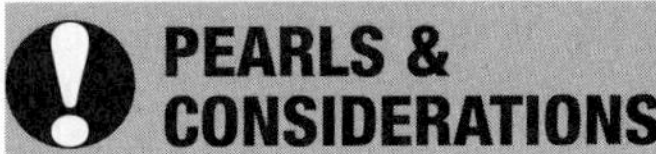

PEARLS & CONSIDERATIONS

COMMENTS

- A presentation of this syndrome, especially in patients with HIV infection or impaired cellular immunity, may be fever of unknown origin.
- Hepatic and splenic granulomas, coronary valve infections may offer few physical clues to diagnosis, emphasizing the need for a complete history.
- CSD should be considered in the differential diagnosis of school-aged children presenting with status epilepticus.
- Chronically immunocompromised patients considering the acquisition of a young feline should be made aware of the possible risk of infection.
- No signs of illness may be apparent in bacteremic kittens.

SUGGESTED READINGS

Arvand M, Schäd SG: Isolation of Bartonella henselae DNA from the peripheral blood of a patient with cat scratch disease up to 4 months after the cat scratch injury, *J Clin Microbiol* 44(6):2288, 2006.

Batts S, Demers DM: Spectrum and treatment of cat-scratch disease, *Pediatr Infect Dis J* 23(12):1161, 2004.

Koehler JE et al: Prevalence of Bartonella infection among human immunodeficiency virus-infected patients with fever, *Clin Infect Dis* 37(4):559, 2003.

Massel F et al: The expanded spectrum of bartonellosis in children, *Infec Dis Clin North Am* 19(3):691-711, 2005.

Tsuneoka H, Isukahara M: Analysis of data in 30 patients with cat scratch disease without lymphadenopathy, *J Infect Chemother* 12(4):224, 2006.

AUTHORS: **GLENN G. FORT, M.D., M.P.H.,** and **DENNIS J. MIKOLICH, M.D.**

 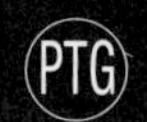

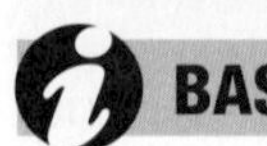 BASIC INFORMATION

DEFINITION

Cavernous sinus thrombosis (CST) is a late complication of facial or paranasal sinus infection, resulting in thrombosis of the cavernous sinus and inflammation of its surrounding anatomic structures, including cranial nerves III, IV, V (ophthalmic and maxillary branch), and VI, and the internal carotid artery.

SYNONYMS

Intracranial venous sinus thrombosis or thrombophlebitis

ICD-9CM CODES
325 Phlebitis and thrombophlebitis of intracranial venous sinuses

EPIDEMIOLOGY & DEMOGRAPHICS

- Cavernous sinus thrombosis is rare in the postantibiotic era.
- Before antibiotics the mortality rate was 80% to 100%.
- With antibiotics and early diagnosis, mortality rates have fallen to ~20%.
- Reported morbidity rates have also declined from between 50% and 70% to only 22% with advances in imaging modalities and aggressive medical care.

PHYSICAL FINDINGS & CLINICAL PRESENTATION

- Can be either an acute and fulminant disease or an indolent and subacute presentation.
- Headache, though not specific, is the most common presenting symptom and may precede fever and periorbital edema by several days. Elderly patients, however, may only demonstrate alteration in mental status without antecedent headache. A classic presentation is abrupt onset of unilateral periorbital edema progressing to bilateral eye involvement, headache, photophobia, and proptosis. These signs and symptoms are related to the anatomic structures affected within the cavernous sinus, notably cranial nerves III to VI, as well as impaired venous drainage from the orbit and the eye.

Other common signs and symptoms include:

- Ptosis
- Chemosis
- Cranial nerve palsies (III, IV, V, VI)
  1. Sixth nerve palsy is the most common (abducens nerve is located medially in the cavernous sinus and is surrounded by blood, making it more susceptible to inflammatory changes).
  2. Hypoesthesia or hyperesthesia of the ophthalmic and maxillary branch of the fifth nerve is common. Periorbital sensory loss and impaired corneal reflex may be noted.
- Papilledema, retinal hemorrhages, and decreased visual acuity to blindness may occur from venous congestion within the retina.
- Pupil may be dilated and sluggishly reactive.
- Fever, tachycardia, and sepsis may be present.
- Headache with nuchal rigidity and changes in mental status may occur.

Infection can spread to the contralateral cavernous sinus through the intercavernous sinuses within 24 to 48 hr of initial presentation.

ETIOLOGY

- CST most commonly results from contiguous spread of an infection from the sinuses (sphenoid, ethmoid, or frontal) or the medial third of the face (areas around the eyes and nose that drain to the ophthalmic vein). Nasal furuncles are the most common facial infection to produce this complication. Less-common primary sites of infection include dental abscess, tonsils, soft palate, middle ear, or orbit (orbital cellulitis).
- CST also can result from hematogenous spread of infection to the cavernous sinus by the superior and inferior ophthalmic veins or through the lateral and sigmoid sinuses. It can spread in a retrograde direction depending on the pressure gradients, because the dural sinuses are valveless.
- *Staphylococcus aureus* is the most common infectious microbe, found in 60% to 70% of the cases.
- *Streptococcus* is the second leading cause.
- Gram-negative rods and anaerobes may also lead to cavernous sinus thrombosis.
- Rarely, *Aspergillus fumigatus* and mucormycosis cause CST.

Dx DIAGNOSIS

- The diagnosis of CST is made by clinical suspicion and confirmed by appropriate imaging studies.
- Proptosis, ptosis, chemosis, and cranial nerve palsy beginning in one eye and progressing to the other eye establish the diagnosis.

DIFFERENTIAL DIAGNOSIS

- Orbital or periorbital cellulitis
- Internal carotid artery aneurysm or fistula
- Cerebrovascular disease
- Migraine headache
- Allergic blepharitis
- Thyroid ophthalmopathy
- Orbital neoplasm
- Meningitis
- Epidural and subdural infections
- Epidural and subdural hematoma
- Subarachnoid hemorrhage
- Acute angle-closure glaucoma
- Trauma

WORKUP

CST is a clinical diagnosis, with laboratory tests and imaging studies confirming the clinical impression.

LABORATORY TESTS

- Complete blood count, erythrocyte sedimentation rate, blood cultures, and sinus cultures help establish and identify an infectious primary source.
- Lumbar puncture (LP) helps to distinguish CST from more localized processes (e.g., sinusitis, orbital cellulites). LP reveals inflammatory cells in 75% of cases. In half of these cases, the cerebrospinal fluid profile is typical for a parameningeal focus (high white blood cells with polymorphonuclear and/or mononuclear cells, normal glucose, normal protein, culture negative), and in one third may be similar to that of a bacterial meningitis.

IMAGING STUDIES

- Contrast-enhanced CT or MRI venography can show evidence of CST.
- Noncontrast CT scan of the head and orbits may demonstrate increased density in the region of the cavernous sinus but has relatively low sensitivity. Contrast-enhanced CT scan may reveal underlying sinusitis, thickening of the superior ophthalmic vein, and irregular filling defects within the cavernous sinus; however, findings may be normal early in the disease course.
- MRI with gadolinium, including magnetic resonance angiography, is more sensitive than CT scan and is the imaging study of choice to diagnose CST. Findings may include deformity of the internal carotid artery within the cavernous sinus and an obvious signal hyperintensity within thrombosed vascular sinuses on all pulse sequences.
- Cerebral angiography can be performed, but it is invasive and not very sensitive.
- Orbital venography is difficult to perform, but it is excellent in diagnosing occlusion of the cavernous sinus.

Rx TREATMENT

NONPHARMACOLOGIC THERAPY

Recognizing the primary source of infection (i.e., facial cellulitis, middle ear, and sinus infections) and treating the primary source expeditiously is the best way to prevent CST.

ACUTE GENERAL Rx

- Appropriate therapy should take into account the primary source of infection as well as possible associated complications such as brain abscess, meningitis, or subdural empyema.
- Broad-spectrum intravenous antibiotics are used as empiric therapy until a definite pathogen is found. Treatment should include a penicillinase-resistant penicillin at maximum dose plus a third- or fourth-generation cephalosporin:
  1. Nafcillin (or oxacillin) 2 g IV q4h plus either ceftriaxone (2 g q12h) or cefepime (2 g q8-12h).
  2. Metronidazole 500 mg IV q6h should be added if anaerobic bacterial infection is suspected (dental or sinus infection).
- Vancomycin (1 g q12h with normal renal function) may be substituted for nafcillin if

significant concern exists regarding infection by methicillin-resistant *Staphylococcus aureus* or resistant *Streptococcus pneumoniae.*

- Anticoagulation with heparin is controversial. Cerebral infarction or intracranial hemorrhage should first be ruled out by noncontrast CT scan before initiating heparin therapy. Early heparinization has been suggested in patients with unilateral cavernous sinus thrombosis to prevent clot propagation. Coumadin therapy should be avoided in the acute phase of the illness but should ultimately be instituted to achieve an INR of 2 to 3 and continued until the infection, symptoms, and signs of CST have resolved or significantly improved. There are no reports of low-molecular-weight heparin being used in this setting.
- Steroid therapy is also controversial but may prove helpful in reducing cranial nerve dysfunction or when progression to pituitary insufficiency occurs. Corticosteroids should only be instituted after appropriate antibiotic coverage. Dexamethasone 10 mg q6h is the treatment of choice.
- Emergent surgical drainage with sphenoidotomy is indicated if the primary site of infection is believed to be the sphenoid sinus.

CHRONIC Rx

- Patients with CST are usually treated with prolonged courses (3 to 4 wk) of IV antibiotics. If there is evidence of complications such as intracranial suppuration, 6 to 8 wk of total therapy may be warranted.
- All patients should be monitored for signs of complicated infection, continued sepsis, or septic emboli while antibiotic therapy is being administered.

DISPOSITION

- CST can be a life-threatening, rapidly progressive infectious disease with high morbidity and mortality rates (30%) despite antibiotic use. Morbidity and mortality rates are increased in cases of sphenoid sinus infection.
- Complications of untreated CST include extension of thrombus to other dural sinuses, carotid thrombosis with concomitant strokes, subdural empyema, brain abscess, or meningitis. Septic embolization may also occur to the lungs, resulting in acute respiratory distress syndrome, pulmonary abscess, empyema, and pneumothorax.
- Thirty percent of treated patients develop long-term sequelae, including cranial nerve palsies, blindness, pituitary insufficiency, and hemiparesis.

REFERRAL

If CST is suspected, it should be considered a medical emergency. Depending on the primary site of infection, appropriate consultation should be made (i.e., ear-nose-throat, ophthalmology, and infectious disease).

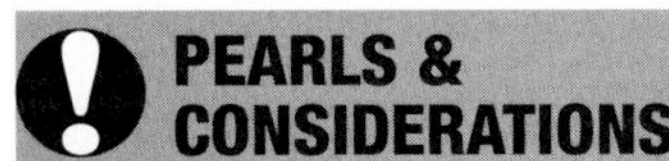

PEARLS & CONSIDERATIONS

COMMENTS

Realizing the cavernous sinus lies just above and lateral to the sphenoid sinus and drains the middle portion of the face by the superior and inferior ophthalmic veins and knowing that cranial nerves III, IV, V, and VI pass alongside or through the cavernous sinus make the clinical findings and diagnosis easier to understand.

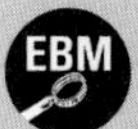

EVIDENCE

We were unable to cite any evidence that meets our criteria regarding the use of antibiotics in CST.

A systematic review concluded that heparin treatment appeared safe and was associated with an important reduction in the risk of death or dependency, which did not reach statistical significance in cases of CST.[1] Ⓐ

Evidence-Based Reference

1. Stam J et al: Anticoagulation for cerebral sinus thrombosis, *Cochrane Rev* 4, CD002005, 2002. Ⓐ

SUGGESTED READINGS

Agayev A, Yilmaz S: Images in clinical medicine. Cavernous sinus thrombosis, *N Engl J Med* 359(21): 2266, 2008.

Ferro JM et al: Cerebral vein and dural sinus thrombosis in elderly patients, *Stroke* 36:1927, 2005.

Hoshino CH et al: Septic cavernous sinus thrombosis complicated by narrowing of the internal carotid artery, subarachnoid abscess and multiple pulmonary septic emboli, *Intern Med* 46:317, 2007.

Leach JL et al: Imaging of cerebral venous thrombosis: current techniques, spectrum of findings, and diagnostic pitfalls, *Radiographics* 26:S19-41, 2006.

Southwick FS: *Septic dural sinus thrombosis.* Available from http://www.uptodate.com. Accessed Aug 30, 2009.

Stam J: Thrombosis of the cerebral veins and sinuses, *N Engl J Med* 352(17):1791-1798, 2005.

AUTHORS: **MARK F. BRADY, M.D., M.P.H.,** and **WEN Y. WU-CHEN, M.D.**

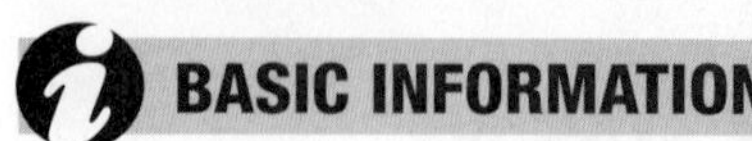

BASIC INFORMATION

DEFINITION

Celiac disease is a chronic disease characterized by malabsorption and diarrhea precipitated by ingestion of food products containing gluten.

SYNONYMS

Gluten-sensitive enteropathy
Celiac sprue
Nontropical sprue

ICD-9CM CODES

579.0 Celiac disease

EPIDEMIOLOGY & DEMOGRAPHICS

- The prevalence of celiac disease is 1% in the general population in North America and Western Europe and 5% in high-risk groups such as first-degree relatives of persons with the disease.
- Incidence is highest during infancy and the first 36 mo of life (after introduction of foods containing gluten), in the third decade (frequently associated with pregnancy and severe anemia during pregnancy), and in the seventh decade.
- There is a slight female predominance.

PHYSICAL FINDINGS & CLINICAL PRESENTATION

- Physical examination may be entirely within normal limits.
- Weight loss, dyspepsia, short stature, and failure to thrive may be noted in children and infants.
- Weight loss, fatigue, and diarrhea are common in adults.
- Abdominal pain, nausea, and vomiting are unusual.
- Pallor as a result of iron-deficiency anemia is common.
- Atypical forms of the disease are being increasingly recognized and include osteoporosis, short stature, anemia, infertility, and neurologic problems. Manifestations of calcium deficiency, such as tetany and seizures, are rare and can be exacerbated by coexistent magnesium deficiency.
- Angular cheilitis, aphthous ulcers, atopic dermatitis, and dermatitis herpetiformis are frequently associated with celiac disease.

ETIOLOGY

- Celiac sprue is considered an autoimmune-type disease, with tissue transglutaminase (tTG) suggested as a major autoantigen. It results from an inappropriate T-cell–mediated immune response against ingested gluten in genetically predisposed individuals who carry either *HLA-DQ2* or *HLA-DQ8* genes. There is sensitivity to gliadin, a protein fraction of gluten found in wheat, rye, and barley. In patients with celiac disease, immune responses to gliadin fractions promote an inflammatory reaction, mainly in the upper small intestine, manifested by infiltration of the lamina propria and the epithelium with chronic inflammatory cells and villous atrophy.
- Timing of introduction of gluten into the infant diet is associated with the appearance of celiac disease in children at risk. Children initially exposed to gluten in the first 3 mo of life have a fivefold increased risk.

Dx DIAGNOSIS

DIFFERENTIAL DIAGNOSIS

- Inflammatory bowel disease
- Laxative abuse
- Intestinal parasitic infestations
- Other: irritable bowel syndrome, tropical sprue, chronic pancreatitis, Zollinger-Ellison syndrome, cystic fibrosis (children), lymphoma, eosinophilic gastroenteritis, short bowel syndrome, Whipple's disease

LABORATORY TESTS

- Iron-deficiency anemia (microcytic anemia, low ferritin level)
- Folic acid deficiency
- Vitamin B_{12} deficiency, hypomagnesemia, hypocalcemia
- IgA tTG antibody by enzyme-linked immunosorbent assay (tissue transglutaminase [tTG] test) is the best screening serologic test for celiac sprue. IgA antiendomysial antibodies (EMA) test is also a good screening test for celiac disease, except in the case of patients with IgA deficiency.
- Biopsy of the small bowel is the standard for diagnosing celiac disease. It is, however, invasive and not always necessary. It may be reasonable in children with significant elevations of tTG levels ($>$100 U) to first try a gluten-free diet and consider biopsy in those who do not improve with diet.
- The *HLA-DQ2* allele is identified in $>$ 90% of patients with celiac disease, and *HLA-DQ8* is identified in most of the remaining patients. These genes occur in only 30% to 40% of the general population. Their greatest diagnostic value is in their negative predictive value, making them useful when negative in ruling out the disease.

IMAGING STUDIES

Capsule endoscopy can be used to evaluate mucosa of the small intestine, especially if future innovations will allow mucosal biopsy.

Rx TREATMENT

NONPHARMACOLOGIC THERAPY

Patients should be instructed on a gluten-free diet (avoidance of wheat, rye, and barley). Safe grains (gluten-free) include rice, corn, oats, buckwheat, millet, amaranth, quinoa, sorghum, and teff (an Ethiopian cereal grain).

GENERAL Rx

- Correct nutritional deficiencies with iron, folic acid, calcium, and vitamin B_{12} as needed.
- Prednisone 20 to 60 mg qd gradually tapered is useful in refractory cases.
- Lifelong gluten-free diet is necessary.

DISPOSITION

- Prognosis is good with adherence to a gluten-free diet. Rapid improvement is usually seen within a few days of treatment.
- Serial antigliadin or antiendomysial antibody tests can be used to monitor the patient's adherence to a gluten-free diet.
- Repeat small-bowel biopsy after treatment generally reveals significant improvement. It is also useful to evaluate for increased risk of small-bowel T-cell lymphoma in these patients, especially untreated patients.

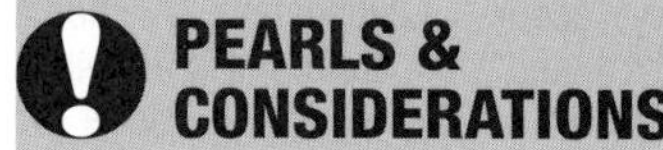

PEARLS & CONSIDERATIONS

COMMENTS

- Some experts recommend a repeat biopsy only in selected patients who have an unsatisfactory response to a strict gluten-free diet.
- Celiac disease should be considered in patients with unexplained metabolic bone disease, osteoporosis, or hypocalcemia, especially because gastrointestinal symptoms may be absent or mild. Clinicians should also consider testing children and young adults for celiac disease if unexplained weight loss, abdominal pain or distention, or chronic diarrhea is present.
- The prevalence of celiac disease in patients with dyspepsia is twice that of the general population. Screening for celiac disease should be considered in all patients with persistent dyspepsia.
- Patients with celiac disease have an overall risk of cancer that is almost twice that of the general population. The risk of adenocarcinoma of the small intestine is increased manifold compared with the risk in the general population. Celiac disease is also associated with an increased risk for non-Hodgkin's lymphoma, especially of T-cell type and primarily localized in the gut. Lymphoma is four to 40 times more common, and death from lymphoma is 11 to 70 times more common in patients with celiac disease.

SUGGESTED READINGS

Green PH, Cellier C: Celiac disease, *N Engl J Med* 357: 1731-1743, 2007.

Ludvigsson JF et al: Small intestinal histopathology and mortality risk in celiac disease, *JAMA* 302(11): 1171-1178, 2009.

AUTHOR: **FRED F. FERRI, M.D.**

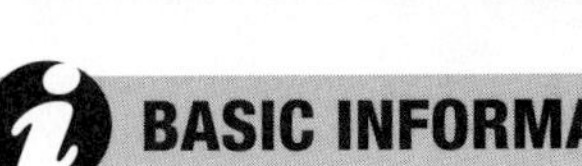

BASIC INFORMATION

DEFINITION

Cellulitis is a superficial inflammatory condition of the skin and underlying tissues characterized by erythema, warmth, and tenderness of the involved area.

SYNONYMS

Erysipelas (cellulitis generally caused by group A β-hemolytic streptococci)

ICD-9CM CODES
682.9 Cellulitis

EPIDEMIOLOGY & DEMOGRAPHICS

- Occurs most frequently in diabetics, immunocompromised hosts, and patients with venous and lymphatic compromise.
- Frequently found near skin breaks (trauma, surgical wounds [surgical site infections develop in 2% to 5% of all surgical procedures], ulcerations, tinea infections). Edema, animal or human bites, subadjacent osteomyelitis, and bacteremia are potential sources of cellulitis.

PHYSICAL FINDINGS & CLINICAL PRESENTATION

Variable with the causative organism:

- Erysipelas: superficial-spreading, warm, erythematous lesion distinguished by its indurated and elevated margin; lymphatic involvement and vesicle formation are common.
- Staphylococcal cellulitis: area involved is erythematous, hot, and swollen; differentiated from erysipelas by nonelevated, poorly demarcated margin; local tenderness and regional adenopathy are common; up to 85% of cases occur on the legs and feet.
- *Haemophilus influenzae* cellulitis: area involved is a blue-red/purple-red color; occurs mainly in children; generally involves the face in children and the neck or upper chest in adults.
- *Vibrio vulnificus:* larger hemorrhagic bullae, cellulitis, lymphadenitis, myositis; often found in critically ill patients in septic shock.

ETIOLOGY

- Group A β-hemolytic streptococci (may follow a streptococcal infection of the upper respiratory tract)
- Staphylococcal cellulitis: Diabetics, athletes, men who have sex with men, people living in public housing, and incarcerated men are at greater risk for methicillin-resistant *S. aureus* (MRSA) infection. A community-acquired MRSA strain, USA 300, is replacing nosocomial strains of MRSA in hospitals.
- IV drug use: MRSA, *P. aeruginosa.*
- *V. vulnificus:* higher incidence in patients with liver disease (75%) and in immunocompromised hosts (corticosteroid use, diabetes mellitus, leukemia, renal failure). *V. vulnificus* infection is the leading cause of death related to seafood consumption in the United States.
- *Erysipelothrix rhusiopathiae:* common in people handling poultry, fish, or meat.
- *Aeromonas hydrophila:* generally occurs in contaminated open wounds in fresh water.
- Fungi *(Cryptococcus neoformans):* may be present in immunocompromised granulopenic patients.
- Gram-negative rods *(Serratia, Enterobacter, Proteus, Pseudomonas):* may be present in immunocompromised or granulopenic patients.
- Hot tub exposure: *P. aeruginosa*; fish tank exposure: *Mycobacterium marinum.*
- Bites: Human *(eikenella corrodens),* dog *(P. multicida, C. canimorsus),* cat *(P. multicida),* rat *(Streptobacillus moniliformis).*

Dx DIAGNOSIS

DIFFERENTIAL DIAGNOSIS

- Necrotizing fasciitis (reddish-purple discoloration of skin, rapid increase in size, woody induration and pale appearance rather then erythema, violaceous bullae, pain out of proportion to appearance, sepsis)
- Deep vein thrombosis
- Peripheral vascular insufficiency
- Paget disease of the breast
- Thrombophlebitis
- Acute gout
- Psoriasis
- Candida intertrigo
- Pseudogout
- Osteomyelitis
- Insect bite
- Fixed drug eruption
- Lymphedema
- Contact dermatitis
- Olecranon bursa infection
- Herpetic whitlow, early herpes zoster (before blisters)
- Erythema migrans (Lyme disease)
- Rare: *Vaccinia* vaccination, Kawasaki disease, pyoderma gangrenosum, Sweet syndrome, carcinoma erysipeloides, anaerobic myonecrosis, erythromelalgia, eosinophilic cellulitis (Well's syndrome), familial Mediterranean fever

LABORATORY TESTS

- Gram stain and culture (aerobic and anaerobic):
  1. Aspirated material from:
     a. Advancing edge of cellulitis
     b. Any vesicles
  2. Swab of any drainage material
  3. Punch biopsy (in selected patients)
- Blood cultures in hospitalized patients, in patients who have cellulitis superimposed on lymphedema, in patients with buccal or periorbital cellulitis, and in patients suspected of having a salt-water or fresh-water source of infection. Bacteremia is uncommon in cellulitis (positive blood cultures in only 4% of patients).
- Anti-streptolysin O (ASLO) titer (in suspected streptococcal disease)

Despite the previous measures, the cause of cellulitis remains unidentified in most patients. Patients with recurrent lower-extremity cellulites should be inspected for tinea pedis. If found it should be treated.

IMAGING STUDIES

CT or MRI in patients with suspected necrotizing fasciitis (deep-seated infection of the subcutaneous tissue that results in the progressive destruction of fascia and fat).

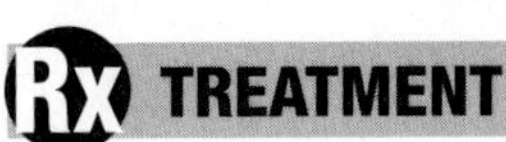

TREATMENT

NONPHARMACOLOGIC THERAPY

Immobilization and elevation of the involved limb. Cool sterile saline dressings to remove purulence from any open lesion. Support stockings in patients with peripheral edema.

ACUTE GENERAL Rx

Erysipelas:

- PO: dicloxacillin 500 mg PO q6h
- IV: cefazolin 1 g q6-8h or nafcillin 1.0 or 1.5 g IV q4-6h

NOTE: Use erythromycin, clindamycin, or vancomycin in patients allergic to penicillin.

Staphylococcal cellulitis:

- PO: dicloxacillin 250 to 500 mg qid
- IV: nafcillin, 1 to 2 g q4-6h
- Cephalosporins (cephalothin, cephalexin, cephradine) also provide adequate antistaphylococcal coverage, except for MRSA.
- Trimethoprim-sulfamethoxazole (Bactrim DS 1 PO bid) may be appropriate in mild MRSA infections. Use vancomycin 1.0 to 2.0 g IV qd or linezolid 0.6 g IV q12h in patients allergic to penicillin or cephalosporins and in patients with moderate/severe MRSA. Daptomycin (Cubicin), a cyclic lipopeptide, can be used as an alternative to vancomycin for complicated skin and skin structure infections. Usual dose is 4 mg/kg IV given over 30 min every 24 hr.

H. influenzae cellulitis:

- PO: cefixime or cefuroxime
- IV: cefuroxime or ceftriaxone

Vibrio vulnificus:

- Doxycycline 100 mg IV bid plus ceftazidime 2 g IV q8h or IV ciprofloxacin 400 mg bid. Mild cases can be treated with oral antibiotics (doxycycline 100 mg bid plus ciprofloxacin 750 mg bid).
- IV support and admission into intensive care unit (mortality rate >50% in septic shock).

E. rhusiopathiae:

- Penicillin

A. hydrophila:

- Aminoglycosides
- Chloramphenicol
- Complicated skin and skin structure infections in hospitalized patients can be treated with daptomycin (Cubicin) 4 mg/kg IV q24h

REFERRAL

For surgical debridement in addition to antibiotics in patients with suspected necrotizing fasciitis

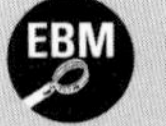

EVIDENCE

Please note: Complete text of EBM for this topic is available online.

SUGGESTED READINGS

Daum RS: Skin and soft-tissue infections caused by methicillin-resistant staphylococcus aureus, *N Engl J Med* 357:380-390, 2007.

Swartz MN: Cellulitis, *N Engl J Med* 350:904, 2004.

AUTHOR: **FRED F. FERRI, M.D.**

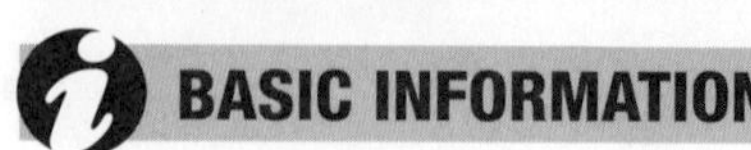

BASIC INFORMATION

DEFINITION

Cerebral palsy (CP) is a group of disorders of the central nervous system characterized by aberrant control of movement or posture, present since early in life and not the result of a progressive or degenerative disease.

SYNONYMS

Little's disease
Congenital static encephalopathy
Congenital spastic paralysis

ICD-9CM CODES
343 Infantile cerebral palsy

EPIDEMIOLOGY & DEMOGRAPHICS

INCIDENCE (IN U.S.): 2 to 2.5 persons per 1000 live births
PREDOMINANT SEX: Males and females affected equally
PREDOMINANT AGE: Diagnosis typically made at 3 to 5 yr

PHYSICAL FINDINGS & CLINICAL PRESENTATION

- Monoplegia, diplegia, quadriplegia, hemiplegia
- Often hypotonic in newborn period, followed by development of hypertonia
- Spasticity
- Athetosis
- Delay in motor milestones
- Hyperreflexia
- Seizures
- Mental retardation

ETIOLOGY

Multifactorial, including low birth weight, congenital malformation, asphyxia, multiple gestation, intrauterine exposure to infection, neonatal stroke, hyperbilirubinemia and maternal thyroid malfunction

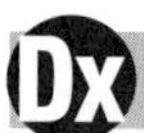

DIAGNOSIS

A motor deficit is always present. The usual presenting complaint is that child is not reaching motor milestones at the appropriate age. Medical history establishes that the child is not losing function. This history, combined with a neurologic examination establishing that motor deficit is due to a cerebral abnormality, establishes the diagnosis of CP. Serial examinations may be necessary if the history is unreliable.

DIFFERENTIAL DIAGNOSIS

Other causes of neonatal hypotonia include muscular dystrophies, spinal muscular atrophy, Down syndrome, and spinal cord injuries.

WORKUP

- Laboratory tests are not necessary to establish the diagnosis.
- Workup is helpful for assessment of recurrence risk, implementation of prevention programs, and medicolegal purposes.

LABORATORY TESTS

- Metabolic and genetic testing should be considered if on follow-up the child has (1) evidence of deterioration or episodes of metabolic decompensation, (2) no etiology determined by neuroimaging, (3) family history of childhood neurologic disorder associated with CP, or (4) developmental malformation on neuroimaging.
- If previous stroke seen on neuroimaging, consider evaluation for coagulopathy.
- An EEG should be obtained when a child with CP has a history suggestive of seizures.
- Children with CP should be screened for ophthalmologic and hearing impairments, as well as speech and language disorders. Nutrition, growth, and swallowing function should be monitored.

IMAGING STUDIES

- Neuroimaging is recommended if the etiology has not been established previously, for example by perinatal imaging.
- MRI, when available, is preferred to CT scanning because of higher yield in suggesting an etiology and timing of the insult leading to CP.

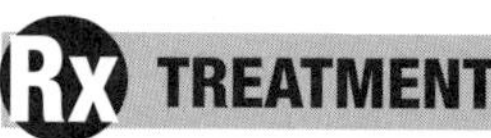

TREATMENT

NONPHARMACOLOGIC THERAPY

- Physical therapy, occupational therapy, and speech therapy.
- Orthotics and casting are used to increase musculotendinous length.

ACUTE GENERAL Rx

If present, treatment of seizures

CHRONIC Rx

- Treatment of seizures, as directed by seizure type.
- Medical treatment of spasticity includes baclofen (oral and intrathecal), as well as botulinum toxin A.
- Surgical treatments of spasticity include dorsal rhizotomy, tendon lengthening, and osteotomy.

DISPOSITION

Most children with cerebral palsy live at home. Those children with severely impaired mobility or other disabilities often live in chronic-care nursing facilities.

REFERRAL

If the child has difficulty with spasticity, physical medicine and rehabilitation referrals are especially helpful.

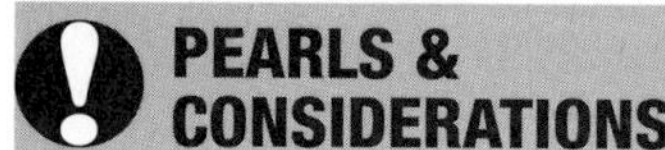

PEARLS & CONSIDERATIONS

In full-term infants, there is usually no history of traumatic delivery.

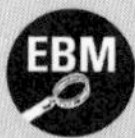

EVIDENCE

Please note: Complete text of EBM for this topic is available online.

Key trials and commentary:

Research suggests that fetal exposure to magnesium sulfate before preterm birth might reduce the risk of cerebral palsy (CP). This study showed that fetal exposure to magnesium sulfate before anticipated early preterm delivery did not reduce the combined risk of moderate or severe CP or death, although the rate of CP was reduced among survivors.

CP remains a considerable dilemma for obstetricians and pediatricians. Although there are well-known etiologies for cerebral palsy that include severe fetal hypoxia and genetic predisposition, the etiology of most cases of CP is not clear. Indeed, this has given rise to the theory that many cases of CP result from intrauterine events that are not associated with conventional signs and symptoms of fetal distress. Accordingly, a lack of a clear etiology makes research into effective preventive measures more challenging. Results from earlier research have suggested that maternal exposure to magnesium sulfate ($MgSO_4$) may reduce the risk for cerebral palsy. To this end, the authors sought to more vigorously test this hypothesis through a randomized controlled trial. Unfortunately, the authors found that the combined rate of moderate or severe CP or death was not reduced among women randomized to the $MgSO_4$ cohort, although the rate of CP was reduced in this cohort among all survivors. Although this is disappointing, it does provide some evidence with which to pursue more research into the etiology, and eventually, into the reduction and prevention of CP.[1] Ⓐ

Randomized trials indicate that mild therapeutic hypothermia reduces the risk of cerebral palsy in term infants.[2] Magnesium sulfate administered to women about to give birth very preterm,[3] or administered soon after birth to term infants with serious neonatal neurological depression[4] have improved neurological outcomes.

Intensive (weekly) neurodevelopmental therapy has been demonstrated to lead to improved motor and functional outcomes after 6 months when compared with monthly therapy in children under age 18 months.[5] Children receiving constraint-induced therapy demonstrated significant gain in use of the more-affected arm when compared to controls.[6] There is not strong or controlled evidence to support or refute the use of botulinum toxin A for the treatment of lower leg spasticity.[7] For upper limb spasticity, however, injections of botulinum toxin A provide a supplementary benefit to upper-limb training approaches (such as occupational and constraint-induced movement therapy).[8,9]

Evidence-Based References

1. Rouse DJ et al: A randomized, controlled trial of magnesium sulfate for the prevention of cerebral palsy, *N Eng J Med* 359:895-905, 2008. Commentary by L.P. Shulman, M.D. Ⓐ

2. Gluckman PD et al: Selective head cooling with mild systemic hypothermia after neonatal encephalopathy: multicentre randomised trial, *Lancet* 365: 663-670, 2005.

3. Rouse DJ: Magnesium sulfate for the prevention of cerebral palsy, *Am J Obstet Gynecol* 200:610-612, 2009.

4. Bhat MA et al: Magnesium sulfate in severe perinatal asphyxia: a randomized, placebo-controlled trial, *Pediatrics* 123:e764-e769, 2009.

5. Mayo NE: The effect of physical therapy for children with motor delay and cerebral palsy. A randomized clinical trial, *Am J Phys Med Rehabil* 70: 258-267, 1991.

6. Taub E et al: Efficacy of constraint-induced movement therapy for children with cerebral palsy with asymmetric motor impairment, *Pediatrics* 113: 305-312, 2004.

7. Ade-Hall RA, Moore AP: Botulinum toxin type A in the treatment of lower limb spasticity in cerebral palsy, *Cochrane Database Syst Rev* CD001408, 2000.

8. Wasiak J et al: Botulinum toxin A as an adjunct to treatment in the management of the upper limb in children with spastic cerebral palsy, *Cochrane Database Syst Rev* CD003469, 2004.

9. Sakzewski L et al: Systematic review and meta-analysis of therapeutic management of upper-limb dysfunction in children with congenital hemiplegia, *Pediatrics* 123:e1111-e1122, 2009.

SUGGESTED READINGS

Ashwal S et al: Practice parameter: diagnostic assessment of the child with cerebral palsy: report of the Quality Standards Subcommittee of the American Academy of Neurology and the Practice Committee of the Child Neurology Society, *Neurology* 62(6):851, 2004.

Nelson KB: The epidemiology of cerebral palsy in term infants, *Ment Retard Dev Disabil Res Rev* 8(3):146, 2002.

AUTHOR: **MAITREYI MAZUMDAR, M.D., M.P.H., M.SC.**

Cerebral Vasculitis

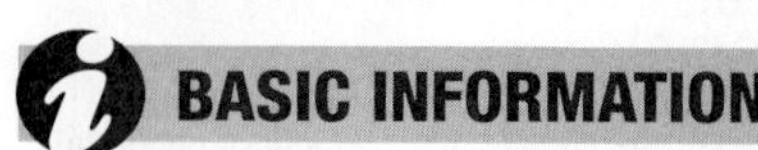

BASIC INFORMATION

DEFINITION

Cerebral vasculitis refers to a group of heterogenous disorders characterized by pathologic inflammation and leukocytoclastic changes in the blood vessel walls.

SYNONYMS

Central nervous system angiitis/cerebral arteritis

ICD-9CM CODES
Diagnosis 437.4 Cerebral arteritis

EPIDEMIOLOGY & DEMOGRAPHICS

INCIDENCE: Average annual incidence rate is 2.4 cases per 1,000,000 person-yr.
PEAK INCIDENCE: Fourth decade of life
PREDOMINANT SEX: Males are affected twice as often as females.
PREDOMINANT AGE: Usual age of presentation is in the third and fourth decades of life, but can present in age ranging from 17 to 70 yr.
GENETICS: Multifactorial
RISK FACTORS: Infections, connective tissue disorders, systemic vasculitis, and substance abuse are the prominent risk factors for secondary cerebral vasculitis.
CLASSIFICATION:

- Primary cerebral vasculitis/primary angiitis of the central nervous system (CNS): Is due to primary involvement of the blood vessels in brain or spinal cord. It does not involve blood vessels or organs beyond the CNS.
- Secondary CNS vasculitis (Table 1-16): Is secondary involvement of the brain or spinal cord blood vessels by a systemic disorder such as systemic vasculitis, connective tissue disorders, infections, malignancy, or substance abuse.

PHYSICAL FINDINGS & CLINICAL PRESENTATION

- The range of manifestations of cerebral vasculitis is diverse. It can present with nonspecific symptoms like weight loss, lethargy, vomiting, headache, and confusion in the early course of the disease. As the disease progresses, multifocal neurologic deficits appear in 80% of the patients.
- Clinical presentations of primary vasculitis can mimic atypical multiple sclerosis, predominantly relapsing and remitting course. Stroke can occur in 40% of the patients; transient ischemic attacks have been reported in 30% to 50% of patients. Aphasia and visual field deficits are commonly seen as well. Seizures have been reported in 25% of the patients. Other common presentations include intracerebral hemorrhage (11%) and intracranial space-occupying lesions (15%).
- Most of the cases of secondary vasculitis present with stroke-like symptoms. Sjögren's syndrome and Behçet's disease can present with variety of symptoms including multiple sclerosis–like presentation, seizures, movement disorders, encephalopathy, dementia, and aseptic meningitis.

ETIOLOGY

The exact etiology of primary cerebral vasculitis is unknown. It has been associated with various infectious agents such as herpes zoster, mycoplasma, HIV, and unknown viruses. Amyloid angiopathy has been described with primary cerebral vasculitis.

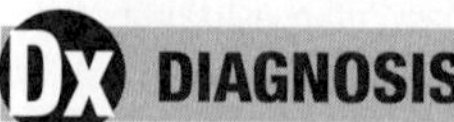

DIAGNOSIS

DIFFERENTIAL DIAGNOSIS

- Reversible cerebral vasoconstriction syndromes
- Intracranial vessels atherosclerosis
- Cerebral emboli
- Intravascular lymphoma
- Sarcoidosis
- Cerebral autosomal dominant arteriopathy with subcortical infarcts and leukoencephalopathy (CADASIL)

WORKUP

Brain biopsy (nondominant temporal lobe tip along with overlying leptomeninges) is the gold standard for the diagnosis of cerebral vasculitis. Cerebral angiography also supports the diagnosis of CNS vasculitis but has low sensitivity and specificity (Fig. 1-57).

LABORATORY TESTS

Cerebrospinal fluid analysis should be part of the workup for diagnosis of cerebral vasculitis (common findings include increased opening pressure, raised proteins, lymphocytic pleocytosis, negative cultures).

TABLE 1-16 Common Causes of Secondary Cerebral Vasculitis and Associated Features

Cause	Features
Giant cell arteritis/Takayasu's arteritis	"Pulseless disease," fever, weight loss, syncope, visual field defects
Polyarteritis nodosa	Fever, weight loss, arthralgia, renal failure, myocardial infarction
Churg-Strauss syndrome	Asthma-like features followed by multiple-organ system involvement including GI, skin, kidneys, CNS, heart
Wegener's granulomatosis	Rhinitis, epistaxis, hemoptysis, hematuria, chronic renal failure
Behçet's disease	Oral ulcers, genital ulcers, skin lesions, uveitis, iritis
Systemic lupus erythematosus	Malar rash, oral ulcers, photosensitivity, arthralgia, renal failure, anemia, ANA positive
Rheumatoid arthritis	Arthritis involving hand joints, radiological evidence of joint erosion, rheumatoid factor positive
Sjögren's syndrome	Dry mouth, dry eyes, involvement of lung, liver, pancreas, joints
Lymphoma	Fever, weight loss, night sweats, lymph node enlargement, hepatosplenomegaly

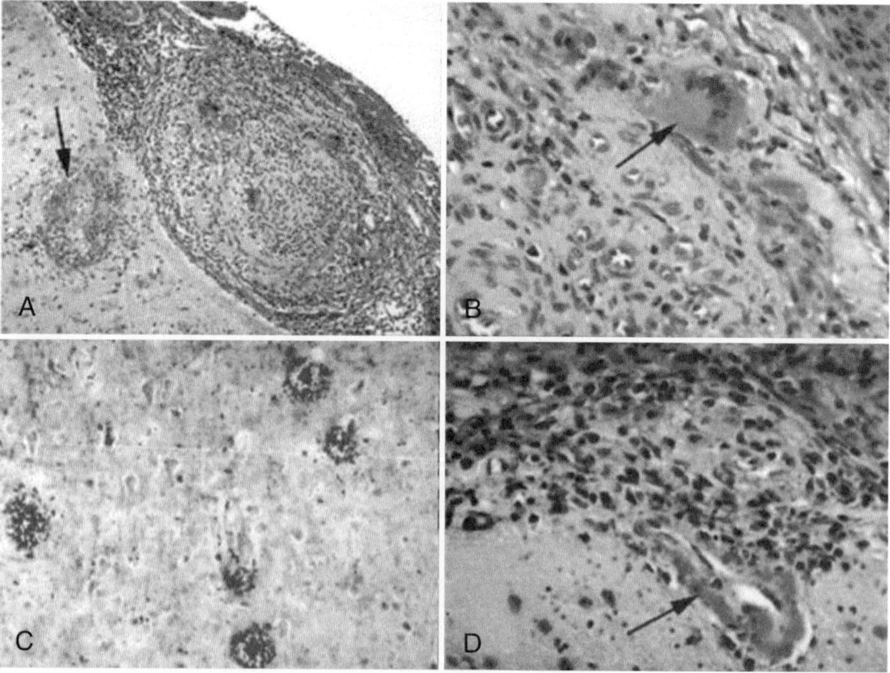

FIGURE 1-57 A, Low-power hematoxylin and eosin stain (10×) demonstrates diffuse inflammation in the leptomeninges with infiltration of lymphocytes, eosinophils, and macrophages with destruction of the vessel wall. **B,** A multinucleated giant cell *(arrow).* **C,** Multiple neuritic plaques are seen on this silver stain. **D,** Congo red stain demonstrating the presence of amyloid within a vessel wall *(arrow).* (From Jacobs DA et al: Primary central nervous system angiitis, amyloid angiopathy and Alzheimer's pathology presenting with Balint's syndrome, *Surv Ophthalmol* 49(4):454-459, 2004, Elsevier Inc.)

Basic laboratory testing should include CBC with differential, blood urea nitrogen and serum creatinine, hepatic functions and enzymes, erythrocyte sedimentation rate, C-reactive protein, and urine analysis.

Specific tests for systemic causes include ANA, rheumatoid factor, anti–double-stranded DNA, anti SS-A, anti SS-B, anti–neutrophil cytoplasmic antibody (ANCA), complement 3 and 4, cryoglobulins, serum immunoglobulins, HIV testing, and blood cultures.

IMAGING STUDIES

Magnetic resonance imaging (MRI) is the neuroimaging of choice. Abnormal findings are seen in 90% to 100% of the patients. Cerebral cortex, deep white and gray matter changes are commonly reported (Fig. 1-58).

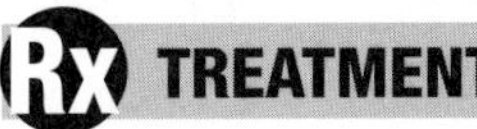

TREATMENT

No prospective studies suggesting specific guidelines for treatment of cerebral vasculitis are available. Most of the treatment is similar to the therapies used for other systemic vasculitis.

NONPHARMACOLOGIC THERAPY

Patients with permanent deficits are provided with physical and occupational therapy.

ACUTE GENERAL Rx

If cerebral vasculitis is suspected, after ruling out infections, empiric therapy with glucocorticoids is started while the workup is completed. Intravenous pulse glucocorticoid, methylprednisolone 1 g daily is given for 3 days, if patient has immediate life-threatening condition; otherwise, oral prednisone is started at 1 mg/kg/day.

CHRONIC Rx

Oral prednisone is continued at high dose (1 mg/kg/day) for 4 to 6 wk and then tapered over 12 mo. As a part of remission induction strategy, cyclophosphamide is given orally daily for 3 to 6 mo, then switched to milder and relatively safer immunosuppressants like azathioprine, methotrexate, or mycophenolate for 2 to 3 yr.

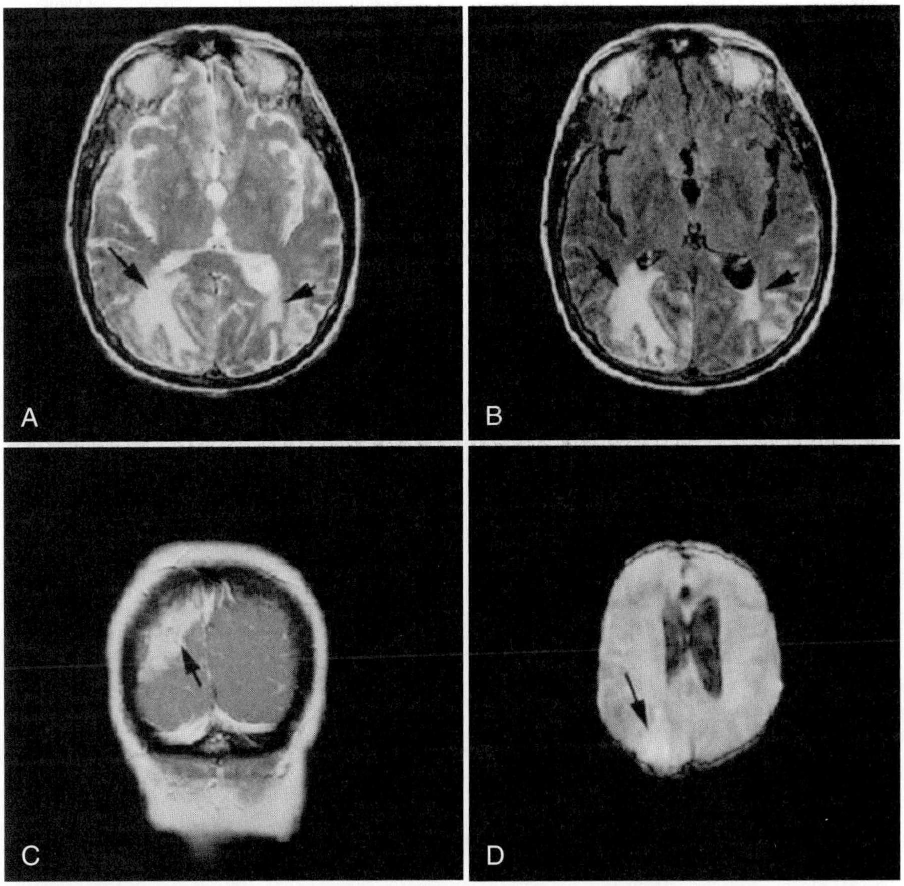

FIGURE 1-58 A, Axial T2-weighted image shows abnormal signal in bilateral parietooccipital lobes, greater on the right than left *(arrows).* **B,** Axial fluid attenuated inversion recovery image further delineating the extent of bilateral parietooccipital lesions *(arrow).* **C,** Coronal T1-gadolinium study demonstrating nodular leptomeningeal enhancement in the lesion *(arrow).* **D,** Diffusion-weighted magnetic resonance imaging shows bright signal in the right parietooccipital region, suggesting ischemic changes *(arrow).* (From Jacobs DA et al: primary central nervous system angiitis, amyloid angiopathy and Alzheimer's pathology presenting with Balint's syndrome, *Surv Ophthalmol* 49(4):454-459, 2004, Elsevier Inc.)

DISPOSITION

Course and prognosis of the disease is variable. It depends on the extent of neurologic involvement, severity of deficits, and response to treatment. Neurologic deficits may resolve acutely, slowly, or not at all. Some patients have symptomatic improvement with resolution of headache or altered mental status. Some have improvement in laboratory values, and others have improved MRI scans.

REFERRAL

Refer to neurology if diagnosis is uncertain or patients have neurologic deficits of uncertain etiology, at younger age, or with headaches not responding to medical therapy.

Refer to neurosurgery for brain biopsy.

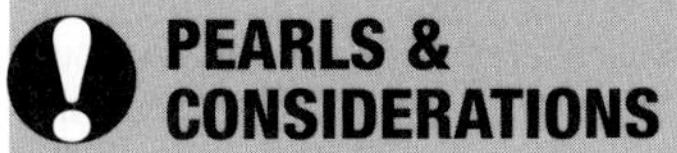

PEARLS & CONSIDERATIONS

COMMENTS

Cerebral vasculitis is a rare disorder that is difficult to identify because of variable presentation. Early recognition of the clinical symptoms and signs is important to prevent long-term morbidity and mortality. Response to the treatment should be assessed periodically by repeated evaluation of the clinical symptoms, examination, and neuroimaging.

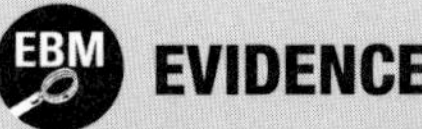

EVIDENCE

Brain biopsy remains the gold standard for establishing the diagnosis.[1]

Most patients show favorable response to prednisone in combination with cyclophosphamide, with an early response rate of 80%.[2,3]

Mycophenolate mofetil in combination with prednisone has been found to be effective in some patients experiencing cytotoxic side effects of cyclophosphamide.[4]

Evidence-Based References

1. Volcy M et al: Primary angiitis of the central nervous system: report of five biopsy-confirmed cases from Colombia, *J Neurol Sci* 227(1):85-89, 2004.
2. Molloy ES, Hajj Ali RA: Primary angiitis of the central nervous system, *Curr Treat Options Neurol* 9(3):169-175, 2007.
3. Hajj Ali RA, Calabrese LH: Central nervous system vasculitis, *Curr Opin Rheumatol* 21:10-18, 2009.
4. Chenevier F et al: Primary angiitis of the central nervous system: response to mycophenolate mofetil, *J Neurol Neurosurg Psychiatry* 80:1159-1161, 2009.

SUGGESTED READINGS

Birnbaum J, Hellmann DB: Primary angiitis of the central nervous system, *Arch Neurol* 66(6):704-709, 2009.

Salvarani C et al: Primary central nervous system vasculitis: analysis of 101 patients, *Ann Neurol* 62(5):442-451, 2007.

AUTHOR: **FARIHA ZAHEER, M.D.**

BASIC INFORMATION

DEFINITION

Cervical cancer is penetration of the basement membrane and infiltration of the stroma of the uterine cervix by malignant cells.

ICD-9CM CODES
180 Malignant neoplasm of cervix uteri

EPIDEMIOLOGY & DEMOGRAPHICS

INCIDENCE: There are approximately 15,000 new cases annually, with 4000 to 5000 associated deaths. The U.S. has an age-adjusted mortality rate of 2.6 per 100,000 persons for cervical cancer.

PREDOMINANCE: Higher incidence rates occur in developing countries. Among the U.S. population, Hispanics have a higher incidence than African Americans, who likewise have a higher incidence than whites.

RISK FACTORS: Smoking, early age at first intercourse, multiple sexual partners, immunocompromised state, nonbarrier methods of birth control, infection with high-risk human papillomavirus (HPV; types 16 and 18), and multiparity.

PHYSICAL FINDINGS & CLINICAL PRESENTATION

- Unusual vaginal bleeding, particularly postcoital
- Vaginal discharge and/or odor
- Advanced cases may present with lower extremity edema or renal failure
- In early stages there may be little or no obvious cervical lesion; more advanced cases may present with large, bulky, friable lesions encompassing the majority of the vagina (Fig. 1-59)

ETIOLOGY

- Dysplastic cells progress to invasive carcinoma.
- Believed to be linked to the presence of HPV 16, 18, 45, and 56 by interaction of E6 oncoprotein on p53 gene product.
- There may be an association with past infection with *Chlamydia trachomatis.*

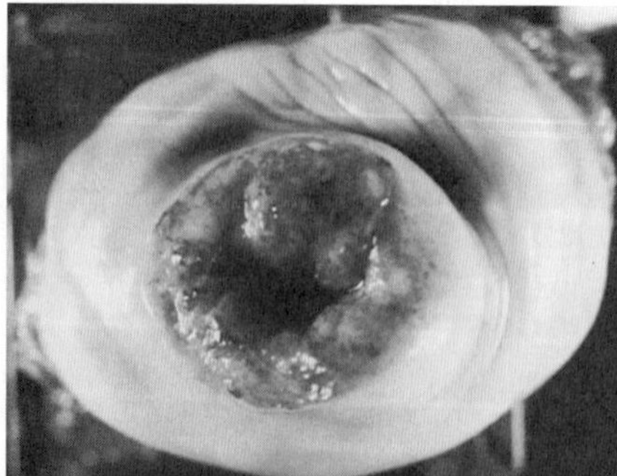

FIGURE 1-59 Carcinoma of cervix (gross specimen). (From Mishell D [ed]: *Comprehensive gynecology,* ed 3, St Louis, 1997, Mosby.)

DIAGNOSIS

DIFFERENTIAL DIAGNOSIS

- Cervical polyp or prolapsed uterine fibroid
- Preinvasive cervical lesions
- Neoplasia metastatic from a separate primary neoplasia

WORKUP

- Thorough history and physical examination.
- Pelvic examination with careful rectovaginal examination.
- Compared with Pap testing, HPV testing has a greater sensitivity for the detection of cervical intraepithelial neoplasia. The addition of an HPV test to the Pap test to screen women in their mid-30s for cervical cancer reduces the incidence of grade 2 or 3 cervical intraepithelial neoplasia or cancer detected by subsequent screening examinations.
- Colposcopy with directed biopsy and endocervical curettage.
- Clinically staged, not surgically staged.

LABORATORY TESTS

- Complete blood count, chemistry profile
- Squamous cell carcinoma antigen in research setting
- Carcinoembryonic antigen

IMAGING STUDIES

- Chest x-ray
- Depending on stage, may need cystoscopy, sigmoidoscopy or barium enema, CT scan or MRI, lymphangiography
- Intravenous pyelogram

TREATMENT

NONPHARMACOLOGIC THERAPY

- FIGO stage IA: cone biopsy or simple hysterectomy
- FIGO stage IB or IIA: type III radical hysterectomy and pelvic lymphadenectomy *or* pelvic radiation therapy
- Advanced or bulky disease: multimodality therapy (radiation, chemotherapy, and/or surgery); platinum use before radiation therapy

ACUTE GENERAL Rx

Cervical cancer may present with massive and acute vaginal bleeding requiring volume and blood replacement, vaginal packing or other hemostatic modalities, and/or high-dose local radiotherapy.

CHRONIC Rx

- Physical examination with Pap smear every 3 mo for 2 yr, every 6 mo during the third to fifth year, and annually thereafter
- Chest x-ray examination annually

DISPOSITION

Five-year survival varies by stage:
- Stage I: 60% to 90%
- Stage II: 40% to 80%
- Stage III: <60%
- Stage IV: <15%

Early detection by Pap smear is imperative to long-term improvements in survival.

REFERRAL

Gynecologic oncologist for all invasive disease

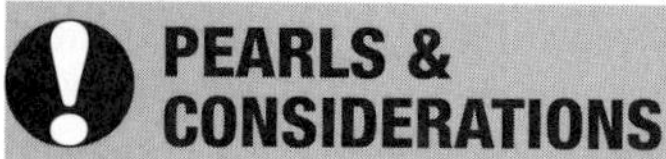

PEARLS & CONSIDERATIONS

Gardasil is a vaccine indicated in girls and women aged 9 to 26 yr for the prevention of cervical cancer caused by HPV types 6, 11, 16, and 18.

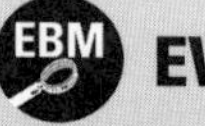

EVIDENCE

Please note: Complete text of EBM for this topic is available online.

Key trials and commentary:

Human papillomavirus types 16 (HPV-16) and 18 (HPV-18) cause approximately 70% of cervical cancers worldwide. A phase 3 trial was conducted to evaluate a quadrivalent vaccine against HPV types 6, 11, 16, and 18 (HPV-6/11/16/18) for the prevention of high-grade cervical lesions associated with HPV-16 and HPV-18.

This study showed that in young women who had not been previously infected with HPV-16 or HPV-18, those in the vaccine group had a significantly lower occurrence of high-grade cervical intraepithelial neoplasia related to HPV-16 or HPV-18 than did those in the placebo group.

This report and one that appeared simultaneously with it in the *New England Journal of Medicine* launched the data demonstrating the value of HPV vaccination while simultaneously creating a firestorm of controversy about whether this vaccine should be mandated in its use. The HPV vaccine is the first vaccine explicitly designed to prevent cancer induced by a virus. The hepatitis B vaccine may also reduce the risk of cancer in the long run, but it was not primarily designed to prevent cancer. The potential ability to reduce the burden of HPV-related disease by vaccination against certain disease-inducing strains of the virus has created a volatile intersection between the community's interest in limiting the transmission of infectious diseases and promoting health on one hand and social mores on the other. The resulting firestorm has created a smoke cloud that has blurred our vision of just how effective this vaccine can be.

HPV is known to be the major cause of cervical cancer. Recognize, however, that not all cervical cancer is caused by HPV-16 or HPV-18. Also, if one is going to prevent the related risk of cervical cancer, the vaccine has to be given before infection occurs. The report of the Future II Study Group clearly tells us that the vaccine will significantly lower the occurrence of high-grade cervical intraepithelial neoplasia related to HPV-16 or HPV-18. Only time will tell whether the prevention of cervical dysplasia aborts the long-term development of cancer, but it should. Please note, however, that cervical dysplasia does not always transition to cancer. In fact, grade 2 cervical intraepithelial neoplasia spontaneously resolves in as many as 40% of cases. Grade 3 cervical intraepithelial dysplasia, on the other hand, has the lowest likelihood of regression and the strongest potential to be invasive. The FDA does consider grade 2 and grade 3 cervical intraepithelial neoplasia and adenocarcinoma in situ to be acceptable surrogate outcomes for cervical cancer in studies of the HPV vaccine.

Please recognize that the HPV vaccine is not the magic bullet for the prevention of cervical cancer. At least 15 oncogenic HPV types have been identified, so targeting only 2 types may not lead to a complete effect on the prevention of cervical cancer. Nonetheless, including types 16 and 18 in the vaccine does produce a sizable decrease in the development of cervical dysplasia. As far as the implications of these reports on screening for cervical cancer, it is clear that screening should continue even in vaccinated women, given the cumulative lifetime risk of exposure to other oncogenic HPV types and the unknown duration of anti-HPV immunity.

For more on the topic of the debate about mandating the HPV vaccine, an analysis of private rights vs. public good, see the superb commentary on this topic by Charo. Unfortunately, experience shows that the alternative to the HPV vaccine ("just say no") has a marginal effect on delaying the age of sexual initiation. Data from the CDC show that with or without sex education, 13% of American girls are sexually experienced by 15 years of age; by 17, the proportion grows to 43%, and by 19 to 70%.[3] Thus, it is important for this vaccine to be given to preteens and to do so without the backlash that the governor of Texas received when he issued an executive order that the HPV vaccine be required.[1] Ⓐ

A separate trial sought to compare the accuracy of conventional cytology with liquid-based cytology for primary screening of cervical cancer.

This study showed that liquid-based cytology showed no statistically significant difference in sensitivity to conventional cytology for detection of cervical intraepithelial neoplasia of grade 2 or more. More positive results were found, however, leading to a lower positive predictive value. A large reduction in unsatisfactory smears was evident.

This large randomized trial from Italy adds to the literature of determining the optimal screening intervention for cervical dysplasia. Specifically, this study compares performance of liquid-based cytology with conventional Pap cytology for detection of cervical lesions. This study is a subset of another larger trial investigating long-term outcomes from a cervical screening program. Key conclusions from this prospective trial are that liquid-based cytology results in fewer uninterpretable smears, thus diminishing recall of patients to repeat the Pap smear for this reason. This reduction was sizable—40% reduction in uninterpretability for any reason, and 80% reduction specifically for obscuring inflammation. Whether this benefit justifies the increased cost of liquid-based cytology awaits additional study. The women undergoing liquid-based cytology were significantly more likely to receive an atypical squamous cells of undetermined significance (ASCUS) or low-grade squamous intraepithelial lesion (LSIL) result, only to have cervical squamous intraepithelial neoplasia 1 (CIN 1) detected at colposcopy, thus lowering the positive predictive values (PPV) of this technology for detecting higher-grade lesions. There was no difference in the ability to detect high-grade lesions. This study would seem to indicate that liquid-based cytology does not achieve a level of specificity that would be desirable by most systems paying for cervical cytology screening. The conclusions from the full trial, examining the long-term impact of liquid-based cytology in this population, may help answer that question.[2] Ⓐ

Cervical cancer and its obligate precursors, cervical intraepithelial neoplasia grades 2 and 3 (CIN2/3), and adenocarcinona in situ (AIS), are caused by oncogenic HPV. In a combined analysis of four clinical trials, we assessed the effect of prophylactic HPV vaccination on these diseases.

This study showed that administration of HPV vaccine to HPV-naive women, and women who are already sexually active, could substantially reduce the incidence of HPV-16/18-related cervical precancers and cervical cancer.

This article by the Future II Study Group presents additional evidence documenting the efficacy of the Merck vaccine in preventing high-grade vulvar and vaginal lesions associated with HPV-16 or HPV-18. The maximum effect is achieved in girls who are vaccinated in early adolescence, and it is anticipated that widespread use of this vaccine will reduce morbidity, mortality, and health care costs associated with cervical cancer. Nevertheless, a number of important questions about the use of these vaccines remain and are discussed explicitly in an accompanying commentary. These include the duration of protection from HPV infection after immunization, the best age at which to vaccinate, the possible benefits of vaccinating boys and young men, the need for protection against infection by other virus types that might lead to cervical neoplasia, and the cost barrier to widespread use of the vaccine, especially, in the developing world. Other important hurdles include the absence of a health-delivery infrastructure in many countries, the political debate surrounding the issue of voluntary vs. mandatory vaccination, the unsubstantiated claims that HPV vaccination will encourage promiscuity, and the belief by some that vaccination may be unnecessary, given the effectiveness of cervical screening strategies.

Evidence-Based References

1. Koutsky LA: Quadrivalent vaccine against human papillomavirus to prevent high-grade cervical lesions, *N Engl J Med* 356:1915-1927, 2007. Commentary by J.A. Stockman III, M.D. Ⓐ
2. Ronco G et al: Accuracy of liquid based versus conventional cytology: overall results of new technologies for cervical cancer screening: randomised controlled trial, *BMJ* 335:28, 2007. Commentary by J.S. Dungan, M.D. Ⓐ
3. The Future II Study Group: Effect of prophylactic human papillomavirus L1 virus-like-particle vaccine on risk of cervical intraepithelial neoplasia grade 2, grade 3, and adenocarcinoma in situ: a combined analysis of four randomised clinical trials, *Lancet* 369:1861-1868, 2007. Commentary by B.H. Thiers, M.D. Ⓐ

SUGGESTED READINGS

Kahn JA: HPV vaccination for the prevention of cervical intraepithelial neoplasia, *N Engl J Med* 361:271-278, 2009.

Long HJ et al: Prevention, diagnosis, and treatment of cervical cancer, *Mayo Clin Proc* 82(12):1566-1574, 2007.

Mayrand MH et al: Human papillomavirus DNA versus Papanicolaou screening tests for cervical cancer, *N Engl J Med* 357:1579-1588, 2007.

McCreath S: Cervical cancer: current management of early/late disease, *Surg Oncol Clin North Am*, 14(2): 249, 2005.

Naucler P et al: Human papillomavirus and Papanicolaou tests to screen for cervical cancer, *N Engl J Med* 357:1589-1597, 2007.

AUTHORS: **GIL M. FARKASH, M.D.,** and **RUBEN ALVERO, M.D.**

Cervical Disk Syndromes 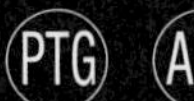 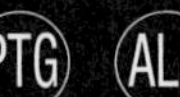

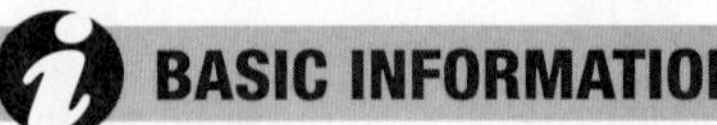

BASIC INFORMATION

DEFINITION

Cervical disk syndromes refer to diseases of the cervical spine resulting from disk disorder, either herniation or degenerative change (spondylosis). When posterior osteophytes compress the anterior spinal cord, lower extremity symptoms may result, a condition called *cervical spondylotic myelopathy.*

ICD-9CM CODES

722.4 Degenerative intervertebral cervical disk

722.71 Degenerative cervical disk with myelopathy

EPIDEMIOLOGY & DEMOGRAPHICS

PREVALENCE: 10% of general adult population (symptoms in 50% of population at some time in their life)

PREDOMINANT SEX: Males and females affected equally

PREDOMINANT AGE: 30 to 60 yr

PHYSICAL FINDINGS & CLINICAL PRESENTATION

- Neck pain, radicular symptoms, or myelopathy, either alone or in combination
- Limited neck movement
- Pain with neck motion, especially extension
- Referred unilateral interscapular pain, resulting in a local trigger point
- Radicular arm pain (usually unilateral), numbness, and tingling possible, most commonly involving the C6 (C5-C6 disk) or C7 (C6-C7 disk) nerve root
- Weakness and reflex changes (C6, biceps; C7, triceps)
- Myelopathy, possibly resulting in gait disturbance, weakness, and even spasticity
- Sensory examination usually not helpful

ETIOLOGY

Unknown

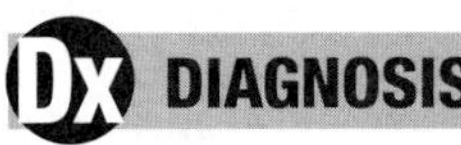

DIAGNOSIS

DIFFERENTIAL DIAGNOSIS

- Rotator cuff tendinitis
- Carpal tunnel syndrome
- Thoracic outlet syndrome
- Brachial neuritis

A differential diagnosis for evaluation of neck pain is described in Section II.

WORKUP

In most cases, the diagnosis can be established on a clinical basis alone.

Cervical Disk Syndrome in Section III describes an algorithm for a workup of suspected cases.

IMAGING STUDIES

- Plain roentgenograms within the first few weeks
  1. Usually normal in soft disk herniation
  2. With chronic degenerative disk disease, usually loss of height of the disk space, anterior and posterior osteophyte formation, and encroachment on the intervertebral foramen by osteophytes
- Myelography, CT scanning, and MRI indicated in patients whose symptoms do not resolve or when other spinal pathology suspected
- Electrodiagnostic studies to confirm the diagnosis or rule out peripheral nerve disorders

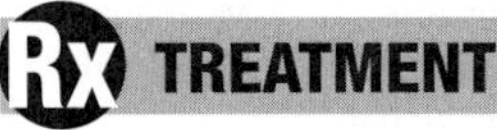

TREATMENT

NONPHARMACOLOGIC THERAPY

- Rest and cervical collar if needed
- Local modalities such as heat
- Physical therapy (Fig. 1-60)
- Avoid extreme range-of-motion exercises in degenerative disk disease

ACUTE GENERAL Rx

- Nonsteroidal anti-inflammatory drugs
- "Muscle relaxants" for their sedative effect
- Analgesics as needed
- Epidural steroid injection for radicular pain

DISPOSITION

- Usually improves with time
- Surgical intervention in <5%

REFERRAL

Orthopedic or neurosurgical consultation for intractable pain or neurologic deficit

PEARLS & CONSIDERATIONS

Myelopathy from cervical spondylosis is the most common cause of acquired spastic paralysis in the adult and is usually progressive. Whether to intervene surgically is a complicated decision in these patients.

COMMENTS

- Pain relief with physical therapy seems anecdotal and short lived; any overall improvement usually parallels what would have probably occurred naturally.
- Sometimes carpal tunnel syndrome and cervical radiculopathy occur together; this is called *double-crush syndrome* and results from nerve compression at two separate levels. Proximal compression may decrease the ability of the nerve to tolerate a second, more distal compression.
- Surgical intervention is indicated primarily for relief of radicular pain caused by nerve root compression or for the treatment of myelopathy; it is generally not helpful when the chief complaint is neck pain alone.
- In many cases of cervical spondylosis with myelopathy, the lower extremity symptoms are much more disabling than the neck symptoms, a situation that can cause some difficulty in determining their etiology.

SUGGESTED READINGS

Gorski JM, Schwartz LH: Shoulder impingement presenting as neck pain, *J Bone Joint Surg Am* 85A: 635, 2003.

King JT et al: Preference-based quality of life measurement in patients with cervical spondylotic myelopathy, *Spine* 29:1271, 2004.

Nasca RJ: Cervical radiculopathy: current diagnostic and treatment options, *J Surg Orthop Adv* 18:13, 2009.

Nowak DD et al: Central cord syndrome, *J Am Acad Orthop Surg* 17:756, 2009.

Rao RD et al: Operative treatment of cervical spondylotic myelopathy, *J Bone Joint Surg Am* 88A:1619, 2006.

Rao RD et al: Degenerative cervical spondylosis: clinical syndromes, pathogenesis, and management, *J Bone Joint Surg Am* 89A:1360, 2007.

Rhee JM et al: Cervical radiculopathy, *J Am Acad Orthop Surg* 15:486, 2007.

Seo M, Choi D: Adjacent segment disease after fusion for cervical spondylosis: myth or reality? *Br J Neurosurg* 22:195, 2008.

AUTHOR: **LONNIE R. MERCIER, M.D.**

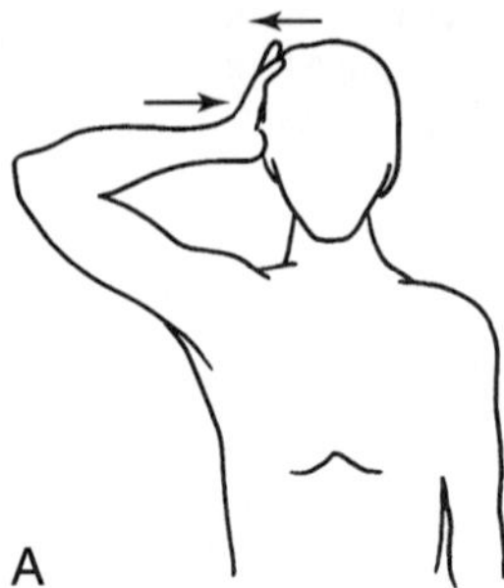

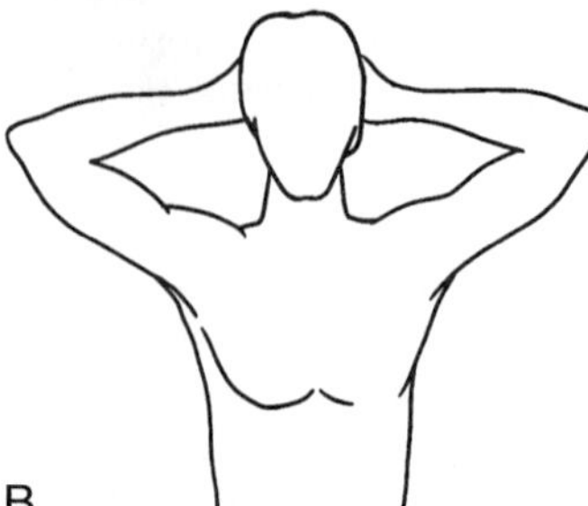

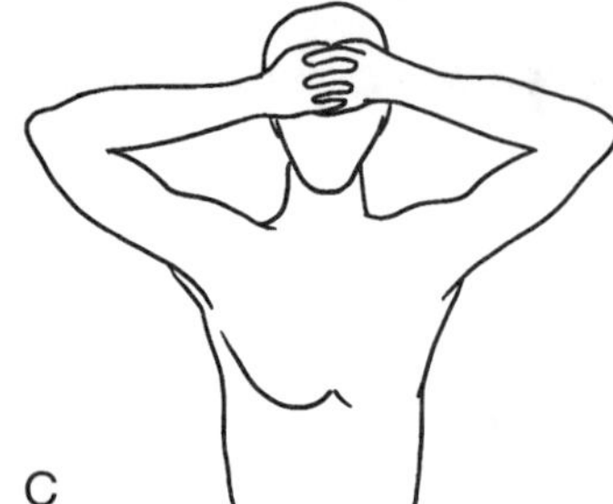

FIGURE 1-60 Isometric neck exercises. A, The hand is placed against the side of the head slightly above the ear, and pressure is gradually increased while resisting with the neck muscles and keeping the head in the same position. The position is held 5 sec, relaxed, and repeated five times. **B,** The exercise is performed on the other side and then from the back and front **(C).** The exercise should be performed three to four times daily. (From Mercier LR [ed]: *Practical orthopedics,* ed 4, St Louis, 1995, Mosby.)

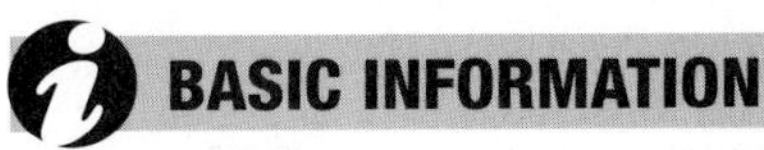

BASIC INFORMATION

DEFINITION

Cervical dysplasia refers to atypical development of immature squamous epithelium that does not penetrate the basement epithelial membrane. Characteristics include increased cellularity, nuclear abnormalities, and increased nuclear:cytoplasm ratio. A progressive polarized loss of squamous differentiation exists beginning adjacent to the basement membrane and progressing to the most advanced stage (severe dysplasia), which encompasses the complete squamous epithelial layer thickness (Fig. 1-61). The revised 2001 Bethesda System terminology was used in a National Institutes of Health consensus conference, sponsored by the American Society for Colposcopy and Cervical Pathology (ASCCP) and its partner professional organizations in 2006. The conference updated therapeutic options for women based on studies such as the **A**SC-US (atypical squamous cells of undetermined significance)/**L**SIL (low-grade squamous intraepithelial lesions) **T**riage **S**tudy (ALTS) that appeared after revision of the Bethesda classification.

BETHESDA 2001 UPDATED CLASSIFICATION: The Bethesda 2001 System was the result of a year-long iterative process held to update the original 1991 system and to broaden participation in the consensus process, clarify reporting of abnormalities and incorporating data that had been collected since the initial system was created.

The reporting system includes the following areas:

Specimen adequacy: The system defines the specimen as either satisfactory for evaluation or unsatisfactory and then specifies the reason for inadequacy if necessary.

General categorization (optional): This serves to triage the specimen into normal finding (negative for intraepithelial lesion or malignancy) or identifies it as an "epithelial abnormality." The descriptions are meant to be mutually exclusive.

Interpretation/result: Makes a distinction between "interpretation" and "diagnosis" of the specimen so that the interpretation may be incorporated into the overall clinical context for the particular patient being evaluated.

Negative for intraepithelial lesion or malignancy: In this screening test, no intraepithelial lesion or malignancy is identified. Non-neoplastic findings such as organisms or reactive cellular findings may be specified but are still considered to be a negative result.

- Epithelial cell abnormalities:
  - Squamous cell:
    - Atypical squamous cell (ASC) of undetermined significance (ASC-US) emphasizing the unusual but still possible association with underlying cervical intraepithelial neoplasia (CIN) II/III and extremely rare possibility of squamous cell carcinoma
    - ASC cannot exclude high-grade squamous intraepithelial lesion (HSIL) (ASC-H), suggesting a risk for CIN II/III that is intermediate between ASC-US and HSIL
    - Low-grade squamous intraepithelial lesion (LSIL) suggests a transient viral infection with a greater likelihood for regression, more likely to encompass human papillomavirus (HPV) infection and CIN I histologically
    - HSIL suggestive of a more persistent viral infection and with a greater risk for progressive disease, more likely to encompass CIN II/III and carcinoma in situ (CIS) histologically
    - Squamous cell carcinoma
  - Glandular cell
    - Atypical glandular cells (should specify endocervical, endometrial, or not otherwise specified)
    - Atypical glandular cell, favor neoplasia (should specify endocervical or not otherwise specified)
    - Endocervical adenocarcinoma in situ (AIS)
    - Adenocarcinoma

Other: Endometrial cells in a woman ≥40 yr of age. Because menopausal status is sometimes uncertain, age was chosen to discriminate women who might, with the findings of endometrial cells on cytology, warrant further evaluation with endometrial sampling

KEY POINTS:

1. The cytologic distinction of low grade (LSIL) and high grade (HSIL) do not necessarily equate to the histologic classifications CIN I and CIN II/III.
2. The 2006 conference notes that one cytologic abnormality can have different histologic risk in different women and highlights "special populations" such as adolescent and young women, and those women who are pregnant. In young women, spontaneous HPV clearance rates are exceptionally high; therefore, it is worthwhile to defer aggressive evaluative and therapeutic steps to assess whether spontaneous remission has taken place. In pregnant women, colposcopy

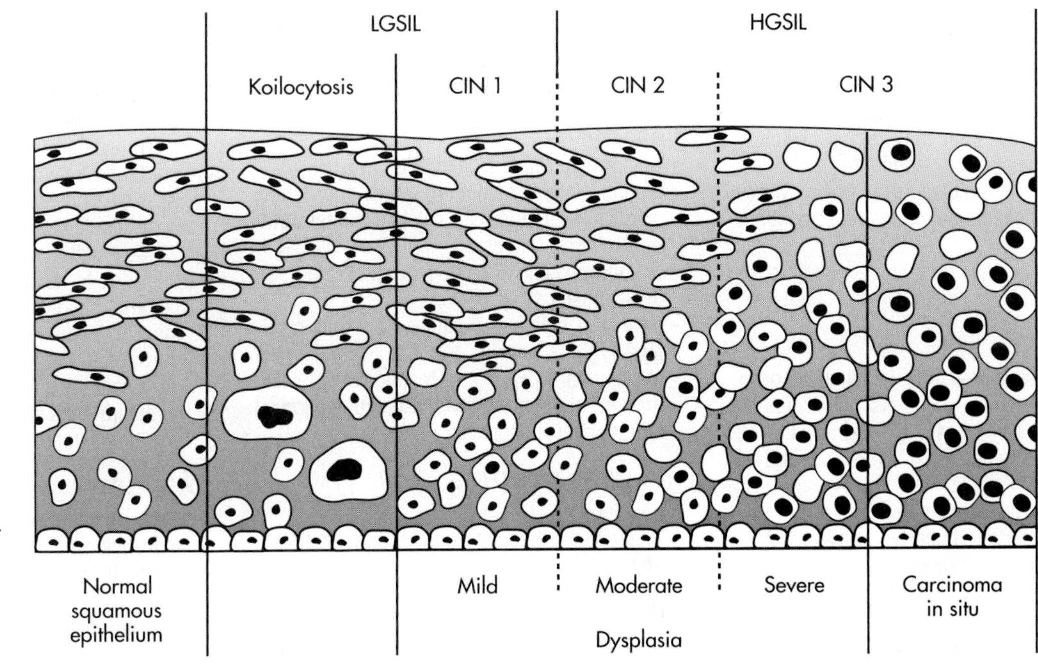

FIGURE 1-61 Diagram of cervical epithelium showing various terminologies used to characterize progressive degrees of cervical epithelium. (From Mishell D [ed]: *Comprehensive gynecology,* ed 3, St Louis, 1997, Mosby.)

may be deferred if the patient is at low risk for invasive cancer, and therapy should take place only if there is a strong suspicion for carcinoma.

3. DNA testing for high-risk HPV types is incorporated into the evaluation and treatment algorithms for women with cytologic cervical abnormalities.

Histologically, a two-tiered system is developed in this guideline that distinguishes between the lower risk CIN I and higher risk CIN II/III diagnoses.

ICD-9CM CODES
622.1 Dysplasia of cervix (uteri)

EPIDEMIOLOGY & DEMOGRAPHICS

PREDOMINANT AGE:
- Dysplasia: peak age, 26 yr (3600 cases/100,000 persons)
- CIS: peak age, 32 yr (1100 cases/100,000 persons)
- Invasive cancer: peak age >60 yr (800 cases/100,000 persons)

PEAK INCIDENCE:
- Age 35 yr
- Abnormal Pap smear rate revealing dysplasia approximates 2% to 5% depending on population risk factors and false-negative rate variance
- False-negative rate approaching 40%
- Average age-adjusted incidence of severe dysplasia is 35 cases/100,000 persons

PHYSICAL FINDINGS & CLINICAL PRESENTATION

- Cervical lesions associated with dysplasia often are not visible to the naked eye; therefore, physical findings are best viewed by colposcopy of a 3% acetic acid–prepared cervix.
- Patients evaluated by colposcopy are identified by abnormal cervical cytology screening from Pap smear screening.
- Colposcopic findings:
  1. Leukoplakia (white lesion seen by the unaided eye that may represent condyloma, dysplasia, or cancer)
  2. Acetowhite epithelium with or without associated punctation, mosaicism, abnormal vessels
  3. Abnormal transformation zone (abnormal iodine uptake, "cuffed" gland openings)

ETIOLOGY

- Strongly associated and initiated by oncogenic HPV infection (high-risk HPV types are 16, 18, 31, 33, 35, 45, 51, 52, 56, and 58; low-risk HPV types are 6, 11, 42, 43, and 44)
- Risk factors:
  - Any heterosexual coitus
  - Coitus during puberty (transformation-zone metaplasia peak)
  - Diethyl stilbestrol exposure
  - Multiple sexual partners
  - Lack of prior Pap smear screening
  - History of STD
  - Other genital tract neoplasia
  - HIV
  - Tuberculosis
  - Substance abuse
  - "High-risk" male partner (HPV)
  - Low socioeconomic status
  - Early first pregnancy
  - Tobacco use
  - HPV

Dx DIAGNOSIS

DIFFERENTIAL DIAGNOSIS

- Metaplasia
- Hyperkeratosis
- Condyloma
- Microinvasive carcinoma
- Glandular epithelial abnormalities
- AIS
- Vulvar intraepithelial neoplasm
- Vaginal intraepithelial neoplasm
- Metastatic tumor involvement of the cervix

WORKUP

- Periodic history and physical examination (including cytologic screening) depending on age, risk factors, and history of preinvasive cervical lesions
- Consider screening for sexually transmitted disease (gonorrhea, chlamydia, herpes, HIV, HPV)
- Abnormal cytology (HSIL/LSIL, initial ASC/ASC-US/ASC-H in high-risk patients, recurrent in low-risk/postmenopausal patients) and grossly evident suspicious lesions; refer for colposcopy and possible directed biopsy/endocervical curettage (ECC) (examination should include cervix, vagina, vulva, and anus)
- For glandular cell abnormalities (AGCs): refer for colposcopy and possible directed biopsy/ECC, and consider endometrial sampling
- In pregnancy: abnormal cytology followed by colposcopy in the first trimester and at 28 to 32 wk; only high-grade lesions suspect for cancer biopsied; ECC contraindicated

LABORATORY TESTS

- Gonorrhea, *Chlamydia* to rule out STD
- Pap cytology screening (requires appropriate sampling, preparation, cytologist interpretation, and reporting)
- Colposcopy and directed biopsy, ECC for indications (see "Workup")
- HPV DNA typing if identified abnormal cytology
- As compared with Pap testing, HPV testing has greater sensitivity for the detection of intraepithelial neoplasia

IMAGING STUDIES

- Cervicography
- Computer-enhanced Pap cytology screening (e.g., PAPNET)

MANAGEMENT

Refer to the literature for a more comprehensive approach. The following treatment paradigms give a general outline for care. Where identified below, HPV status refers to oncogenic types (e.g., 16, 18, 31, 33, 35, 45, 51, 52, 56, 58)

- *ASC-US:* Patients with ASC-US who are HPV negative can repeat cytologic screen in 12 mo. Women who have oncogenic HPV type should have colposcopy performed. Adolescent women should not have HPV testing performed and can be followed with cytologic screen, with colposcopy performed if ASC-US persists after 24 mo or if HSIL is found. Pregnant women can be followed as with nonpregnant women; but if colposcopy is recommended, it can be deferred until at least 6 wk after delivery. Pregnant women should not have endocervical curettage performed.
- *ASC-H:* Patients with ASC-H should have a colposcopic evaluation.
- *LSIL:* Colposcopy with endocervical biopsy is recommended for women with LSIL. Adolescent women with LSIL may be followed with cytology at 12 and 24 mo, and referred for colposcopy if they retain a finding of ASC-US or greater. Postmenopausal women may have DNA testing and be referred for colposcopy if this test is positive for oncogenic HPV type. Pregnant women should have colposcopy, but this procedure may be deferred until the patient is postpartum, particularly if there is no other clinical suspicion for higher grade lesions.
- *HSIL:* Either colposcopy with endocervical curettage or immediate loop electrosurgical excision procedures (LEEPs) are acceptable with HSIL. If CIN II/III is not found by either method, the patient may followed colposcopically or a LEEP performed if only colposcopy was initially used. If CIN II/III is identified by adequate colposcopy, a LEEP or ablation may be performed. Adolescent girls in whom CIN II/III is not identified may be observed by colposcopy and cytology at 6-mo intervals up to 24 mo. If CIN II/III persists for 24 mo, then the adolescent girl may be treated by excisional or ablative therapy. Pregnant women should have colposcopy and biopsies performed where CIN II/III or cancer is suspected. Colposcopy should be performed 6 wk or later after delivery when CIN II/III is not found antepartum.
- *AGC/AIS:* Colposcopy with endocervical biopsy should be performed in these women. In women older than 35 and in women with high risk for endometrial hyperplasia or carcinoma (oligo-ovulation, unscheduled bleeding), an endometrial biopsy should also be performed. Pregnant women should also be colposcoped, but endocervical and endometrial curettings should not be performed during the gestation.

DISPOSITION

- Because of the large number of women in high-risk groups, the prevalence of HPV, and the high false-negative Pap smear rate, routine Pap smear screening should be strongly encouraged for all women, especially those with a history of cervical dysplasia. The addition of an HPV test to the Pap test reduces the

incidence of CIN II or III, or cancer detected by subsequent screening.
- Success rates for treatment approach 80% to 90%.
- Detection of persistence of recurrence requires careful follow-up.
- Cervical treatment possibly results in infertility (cervical stenosis or incompetence), which requires careful consideration and discretion for use of LEEP and cone biopsy.
- Appropriate counseling and informed consent are needed when considering any form of management of cervical dysplasia.

REFERRAL

- Patients with abnormal Pap cytology should not be monitored by repeat Pap smear screening.
- Patients with identified abnormal cytology should be evaluated by a skilled colposcopist (defined as documented didactic and preceptorship training, including 50 cases of identified pathology, ongoing colposcopy activity with a minimum of 2 cases/wk, quality-assurance log, and periodic continuing medical education).
- If treatment is required, patient should be referred to a gynecologist or gynecologic oncologist skilled in the diagnosis and treatment of preinvasive cervical disease.

PEARLS & CONSIDERATIONS

COMMENTS

- Patient education material is available from American College of Obstetricians and Gynecologists.
- Gardasil is a vaccine indicated in girls and women aged 9 to 26 yr for the prevention of CIN caused by HPV types 6, 11, 16, and 18.

EBM EVIDENCE

Please note: Complete text of EBM for this topic is available online.

Ablative therapies include cryotherapy, laser therapy, and other techniques that do not involve the resection and histologic examination of tissues. Excisional methods include LEEPs and cold knife cone procedures. The available evidence suggests that there is no obviously superior surgical technique for the treatment of CIN, but excisional methods allow the additional benefit of histological assessment.[1]

Evidence-Based Reference

1. Martin-Hirsch PL et al: Surgery for cervical intraepithelial neoplasia, *Cochrane Rev* 3, 1999.

SUGGESTED READINGS

Apgar BS et al: Update on ASCCP Consensus Guidelines for abnormal cervical screening tests and cervical histology, *Am Fam Physician* 80(2):147-155, 2009.

Kahn JA: HPV vaccination for the prevention of cervical intraepithelial neoplasia, *N Engl J Med* 361:271-278, 2009.

Mayrand M et al: Human papillomavirus DNA versus Papanicolaou screening tests for cervical cancer, *N Engl J Med* 357:1579, 2007.

Naucler P et al: Human papillomavirus and Papanicolaou tests to screen for cervical cancer, *N Engl J Med* 357:1589-1597, 2007.

Solomon D et al: The 2001. Bethesda system terminology for reporting results of cervical cytology, *JAMA* 287:2114, 2002.

Stoler MH: New Bethesda terminology and evidence-based management guidelines for cervical cytology findings, *JAMA* 287:2140, 2002.

Wright TC et al: 2006 consensus guidelines for the management of women with abnormal cervical cancer screening tests, *Am J Obstet Gynecol* 197:346, 2007.

Wright TC et al: 2006 consensus guidelines for the management of women with cervical intraepithelial neoplasia or adenocarcinoma in situ, *Am J Obstet Gynecol* 197:340, 2007.

AUTHORS: **DENNIS M. WEPPNER, M.D.,** and **RUBEN ALVERO, M.D.**

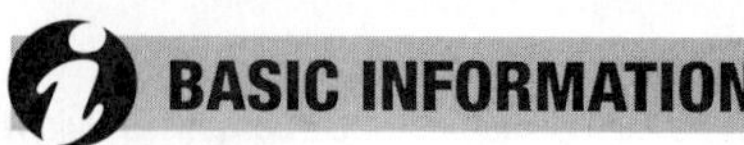

BASIC INFORMATION

DEFINITION

A cervical polyp is a growth protruding from the cervix or endocervical canal. Polyps that arise from the endocervical canal are called *endocervical polyps.* If they arise from the ectocervix, they are called *cervical polyps.*

ICD-9CM CODES
622.7 Mucous polyp of cervix

EPIDEMIOLOGY & DEMOGRAPHICS

Cervical polyps are found in approximately 4% of all gynecologic patients. They most commonly present in perimenopausal and multigravida women between the ages of 30 and 50 yr. Endocervical polyps are more common than cervical polyps and are almost always benign (Fig. 1-62). Malignant degeneration is extremely rare.

PHYSICAL FINDINGS & CLINICAL PRESENTATION

Polyps may be single or multiple and vary in size from being extremely small (a few mm) to large (4 cm). They are soft, smooth, and reddish-purple to cherry-red in color. They bleed easily when touched. Very large polyps can cause some cervical dilation. There may be vaginal discharge associated with cervical polyps if the polyp has become infected.

ETIOLOGY

- Most unknown
- Inflammatory
- Traumatic
- Pregnancy

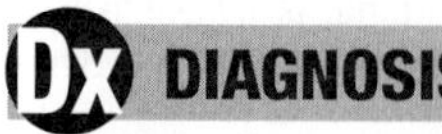

DIAGNOSIS

DIFFERENTIAL DIAGNOSIS

- Endometrial polyp
- Prolapsed myoma
- Retained products of conception
- Squamous papilloma
- Sarcoma
- Cervical malignancy

WORKUP

Polyps are most commonly asymptomatic and are usually found at the time of annual gynecologic pelvic examination. Polyps are also found in women who present for evaluation of intermenstrual or postcoital bleeding and for profuse vaginal discharge. Polyps are painless. Unless a patient has a bleeding abnormality that necessitates evaluation by a physician, polyps would go undiagnosed until the next Pap smear was obtained.

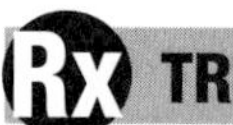

TREATMENT

NONPHARMACOLOGIC THERAPY

Simple surgical excision can be done in the office. The physician should be prepared for bleeding, which can easily be controlled with silver nitrate or Monsel's solution. Most commonly a polyp is excised by grasping it at the stalk and twisting it off. Polyps can also be excised by electrocautery or, in the case of very large polyps, in an outpatient surgical suite. Sexual intercourse and tampon use are to be avoided until the patient's follow-up visit. Douching is not to be performed.

ACUTE GENERAL Rx

Generally no medication is needed.

CHRONIC Rx

Patient is followed up in 2 wk for recheck of the surgical excision site unless there is active bleeding, in which case she would be seen immediately. The cervix should be checked at the patient's routine gynecologic visits.

DISPOSITION

Because these are almost always benign, no further treatment is usually needed. Annual gynecologic examinations should be performed to check for any regrowths.

REFERRAL

To a gynecologist for removal of polyps

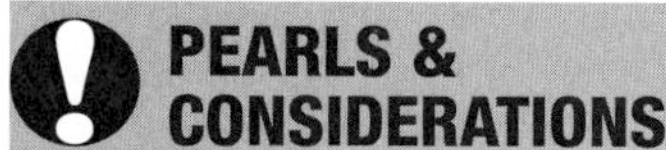

PEARLS & CONSIDERATIONS

COMMENTS

A Pap smear should be obtained before removing the polyp. If an abnormal Pap smear is obtained, it is highly probable that the cause will be the polyp. If a colposcopic evaluation is needed, this should also be performed. During pregnancy the cervix is highly vascularized. If the polyps are stable and benign appearing, they should be observed during the pregnancy and removed only if they cause bleeding.

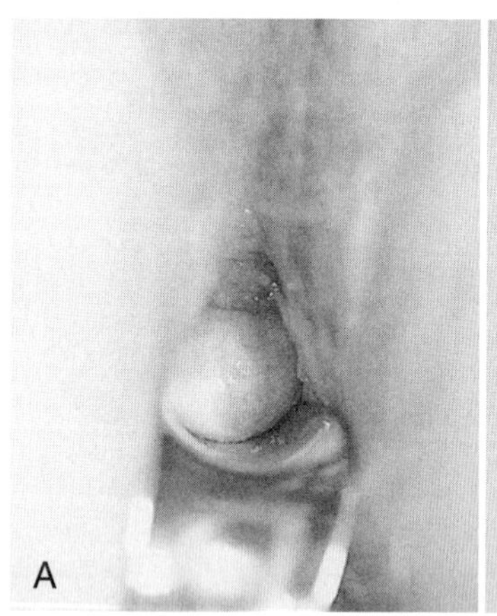

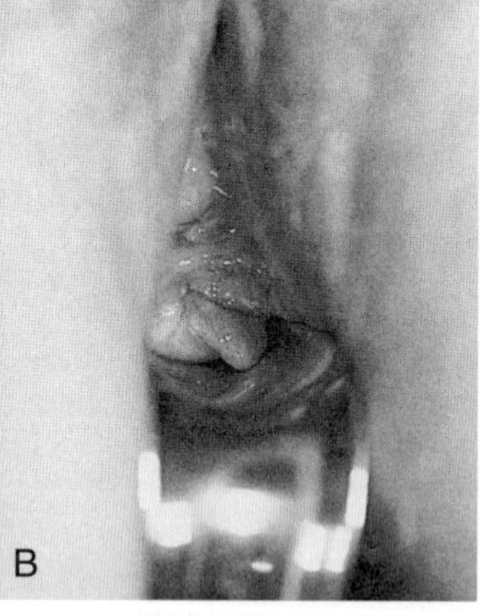

FIGURE 1-62 A, Fibroid polyp protruding through the external cervical os. **B,** Small endocervical polyp. (From Symonds EM, Macpherson MBA: *Color atlas of obstetrics and gynecology,* St Louis, 1994, Mosby.)

SUGGESTED READINGS

Endo H et al: Cervical polyp with eccrine syringofibroadenoma-like features, *Histopathology* 42(3):301, 2003.

Rupke S: Family practice forum: clinical medicine. Evaluation and management of cervical polyps, *Hosp Pract* 33(6):81, 1998.

Scott PM: Procedures in family practice. Performing cervical polypectomy, *JAAPA* 12(6):81, 1999.

Spiewankiewicz B: Hysteroscopy in cases of cervical polyps, *Eur J Gynaecol Oncol* 24(1):67, 2003.

AUTHORS: **GEORGE T. DANAKAS, M.D.,** and **RUBEN ALVERO, M.D.**

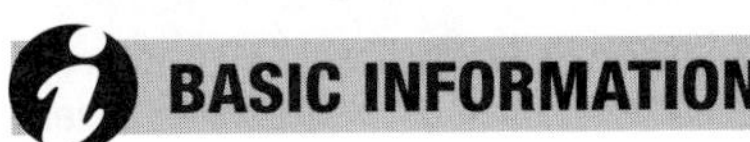

BASIC INFORMATION

DEFINITION

Cervicitis is an infection of the cervix. It may result from direct infection of the cervix, or it may be secondary to uterine or vaginal infection.

SYNONYMS

Endocervicitis
Ectocervicitis
Mucopurulent cervicitis

ICD-9CM CODES
616.0 Cervicitis
098.15 Acute gonococcal cervicitis
079.8 Chlamydia infection

EPIDEMIOLOGY & DEMOGRAPHICS

Cervicitis accounts for 20% to 25% of patients with abnormal vaginal discharge. It is most common in adolescents, but it can be found in any sexually active woman. Practicing unsafe sex with multiple partners increases the risk of developing cervicitis as well as other sexually transmitted diseases.

PHYSICAL FINDINGS & CLINICAL PRESENTATION

Cervicitis is usually asymptomatic or associated with mild symptoms. Copious purulent or mucopurulent vaginal discharge (Fig. 1-63), pelvic pain, and dyspareunia may be present if cervicitis is severe. The cervix can be erythematous and tender on palpation during bimanual examination. The cervix may also bleed easily when obtaining cultures or a Pap smear. Patients may have postcoital bleeding.

ETIOLOGY

- *Chlamydia*
- Trichomonas
- *Neisseria gonorrhoeae*
- Herpes simplex
- *Trichomonas vaginalis*
- Human papillomavirus

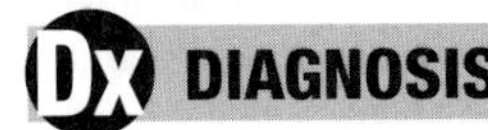

DIAGNOSIS

DIFFERENTIAL DIAGNOSIS

- Carcinoma of the cervix
- Cervical erosion
- Cervical metaplasia

WORKUP

The patient usually presents with a vaginal discharge or history of postcoital bleeding. Otherwise the patient is asymptomatic and diagnosed during routine examination. On examination there is gross visualization of yellow, mucopurulent material on the cotton swab.

LABORATORY TESTS

On a smear there will be 10 or more polymorphonuclear leukocytes per microscopic field. Positive Gram stain is found. Cultures should be obtained for *Chlamydia* and *N. gonorrhoeae.* Use a wet mount to look for trichomonads. Obtain a Pap smear.

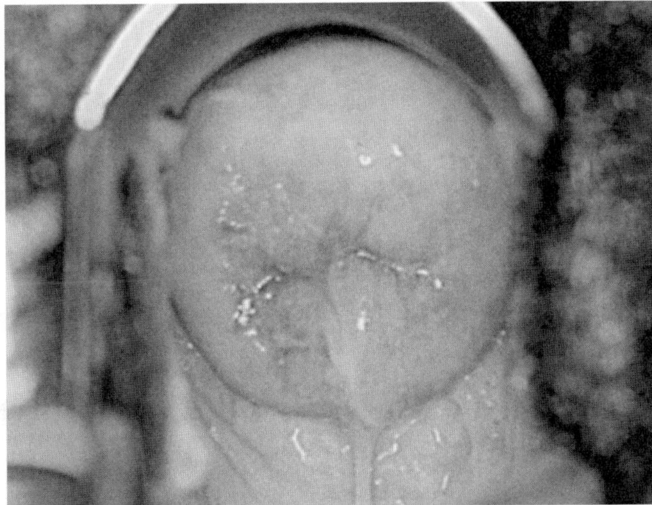

FIGURE 1-63 Colposcopy of a woman with mucopurulent cervicitis and purulent discharge from endocervical os. (Courtesy Dr. David Soper, Richmond, VA. From Mandell GL [ed]: *Mandell, Douglas, and Bennett's principles and practice of infectious diseases,* ed 5, New York, 2000, Churchill Livingstone.)

Rx TREATMENT

NONPHARMACOLOGIC THERAPY

- Cervicitis is treated in an outpatient setting. Cryosurgery is an option for treatment of cervicitis with negative cultures and negative biopsies. Safe sex should be practiced with the use of condoms.
- Partners should be treated in all cases of infection proven by culture.

ACUTE GENERAL Rx

Because *Chlamydia* and *N. gonorrhoeae* cause >50% of cases of infectious cervicitis, if it is suspected treat without waiting for culture results. Administer ceftriaxone 125-mg IM single dose followed by doxycycline 100 mg PO bid for 7 days. If the patient is pregnant, treat with azithromycin (Zithromax) 1-g single dose instead of using doxycycline, which is contraindicated in pregnant or nursing mothers. Alternative treatments include erythromycin base 500 mg PO qid for 7 days, erythromycin ethylsuccinate 800 mg PO qid for 7 days, ofloxacin 300 mg PO bid for 7 days, or levofloxacin 500 mg PO qd for 7 days. If *Trichomonas* is the etiologic agent, treat with metronidazole 2-g single dose. For herpes, treat with acyclovir 200 mg PO five times daily for 7 days.

DISPOSITION

Cervicitis responds well to antibiotics. Possible complications to watch for are a subsequent pelvic inflammatory disease (PID) and infertility (found in 5% to 10% of patients). Repeat cultures should be performed after treatment. Sexual relations can be resumed after negative cultures.

REFERRAL

If subsequent PID develops, consider hospital admission for IV antibiotics.

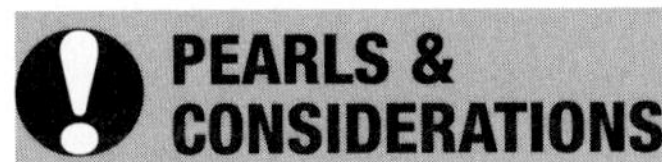

PEARLS & CONSIDERATIONS

COMMENTS

Patient educational material can be obtained from local health clinics and clinics for sexually transmitted diseases.

SUGGESTED READINGS

Centers for Disease Control and Prevention: 2006 sexually transmitted diseases treatment guidelines, *MMWR* 55(RR-11), 2006.

Marrazzo JM: Mucopurulent cervicitis: no longer ignored, but still misunderstood, *Infect Dis Clin North Am* 19(2):333, 2005.

Simpson T: Urethritis and cervicitis in adolescents, *Adolesc Med Clin* 15(2):253, 2004.

AUTHORS: **GEORGE T. DANAKAS, M.D.,** and **RUBEN ALVERO, M.D.**

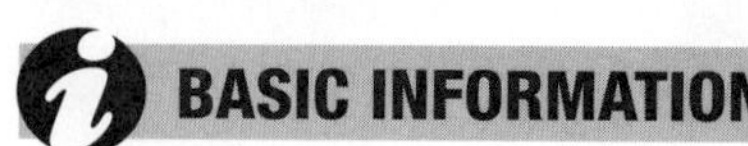

Chagas' Disease (PTG)

BASIC INFORMATION

DEFINITION

Chagas' disease is an infection caused by the protozoan parasite *Trypanosoma cruzi.* This is a vector-borne disease transmitted by reduviid bugs from multiple wild and domesticated animal reservoirs. The disease is characterized by an acute nonspecific febrile illness that may be followed, after a variable latency period, by chronic cardiac, GI, and neurologic sequelae.

SYNONYMS

American trypanosomiasis

ICD-9CM CODES

086.2 Chagas' disease

EPIDEMIOLOGY & DEMOGRAPHICS

INCIDENCE (IN U.S.):

- Five cases of autochthonous transmission in California and Texas
- In the last 2 decades, six cases of laboratory-acquired infection, three cases of transfusion-associated transmission, and nine cases of imported disease reported to the Centers for Disease Control and Prevention (none of the imported cases involving returning tourists)
- Infection has been transmitted by organ transplantation

PREVALENCE (IN U.S.): Based on regional seroprevalence studies in Hispanic blood donors, it is estimated that between 50,000 and 100,000 persons infected with *T. cruzi* are currently residing in the U.S.

PREDOMINANT SEX: Male = female

PREDOMINANT AGE:

- In highly endemic areas, mean age of acute infection: approximately 4 yr
- Variable age distribution for both types of chronic disease, depending on geography
- Mean age of onset: usually between 35 and 45 yr

PEAK INCIDENCE: Unknown

GENETICS:

Congenital infection: Congenital transmission has been documented with attendant high fetal mortality and morbidity in surviving infants.

Neonatal infection: In rural areas, within substandard housing, transmission is likely to occur.

PHYSICAL FINDINGS & CLINICAL PRESENTATION

- Inflammatory lesion that develops about 1 wk after contamination of a break in the skin with infected insect feces (chagoma)
  1. Area of induration and erythema
  2. Usually accompanied by local lymphadenopathy
- Presence of Romaña's sign, which consists of unilateral painless palpebral and periocular edema, when conjunctiva is portal of entry
- Constitutional symptoms of fever, fatigue, and anorexia, along with edema of the face and lower extremities, generalized lymphadenopathy, and mild hepatosplenomegaly after the appearance of local signs of disease
- Myocarditis in a small portion of patients, sometimes with resultant CHF
- Uncommonly, CNS disease, such as meningoencephalitis, which carries a poor prognosis
- Symptoms and signs of disease persisting for weeks to months, followed by spontaneous resolution of the acute illness; patient then in the indeterminate phase of the disease (asymptomatic with attendant subpatent parasitemia and reactive antibodies to *T. cruzi* antigens)
- Chronic disease may become manifest years to decades after the initial infection:
  1. Most common organ involved: heart, followed by GI tract, and to a much lesser extent the CNS
     a. Cardiac involvement takes the form of arrhythmias or cardiomyopathy, but rarely both.
     b. Cardiomyopathy is bilateral but predominantly affects the right ventricle and is often accompanied by apical aneurysms and mural thrombi.
     c. Arrhythmias are a consequence of involvement of the bundle of His and have been implicated as the leading cause of sudden death in adults in highly endemic areas.
     d. Right-sided heart failure, thromboembolization, and rhythm disturbances associated with symptoms of dizziness and syncope are characteristic.
  2. Patients with megaesophagus: dysphasia, odynophagia, chronic cough, and regurgitation, frequently resulting in aspiration pneumonitis
  3. Megacolon: abdominal pain and chronic constipation, which, when severe, may lead to obstruction and perforation
  4. CNS symptoms: most often secondary to embolization from the heart or varying degrees of peripheral neuropathy

ETIOLOGY

- *T. cruzi*
  1. Found only in the Americas, ranging from the southern U.S. to southern Argentina
  2. Transmitted to humans by various species of bloodsucking reduviid ("kissing") insects, primarily those of the genera *Triatoma, Panstrongylus,* and *Rhodnius*
  3. Usually found in burrows and trees where infected insects transmit the parasite to natural reservoirs (e.g., opossums and armadillos)
  4. Intrusion into enzootic areas for farmland, allowing insects to take up residence in rural dwellings, thus including humans and domestic animals in the cycle of transmission
  5. Initial infection of insects by ingesting blood from animals or humans that have circulating flagellated trypanosomes (trypomastigotes)
  6. Multiplication in the insect midgut as epimastigotes, then differentiation into metacyclic trypomastigotes discharged with the feces during subsequent blood meals
  7. Transmission to the second mammalian host through contamination of mucous membranes, conjunctivae, or wounds with insect feces containing infected forms
- In the vertebrate host
  1. Movement of parasites into various cell types, intracellular transformation into amastigotes, and thereafter differentiation into trypomastigotes
  2. Following rupture of the cell membrane, parasitic invasion of local tissues or hematogenous spread to distant sites, maintaining a parasitemia infective for vectors
- In addition to insect vectors, *T. cruzi* is transmitted through blood transfusions, transplacentally, and, occasionally, secondary to laboratory accidents

DIAGNOSIS

DIFFERENTIAL DIAGNOSIS

Acute disease

- Early African trypanosomiasis
- New World cutaneous and mucocutaneous leishmaniasis

Chronic disease

- Idiopathic cardiomyopathy
- Idiopathic achalasia
- Congenital or acquired megacolon

WORKUP

Principal considerations in diagnosis:

- A history of residence where transmission is known to occur
- Recent receipt of a blood product while in an endemic area
- Occupational exposure in a laboratory

LABORATORY TESTS

For acute diagnosis:

- Demonstration of *T. cruzi* in wet preparations of blood (Fig. 1-64), buffy coat, or Giemsa-stained smears

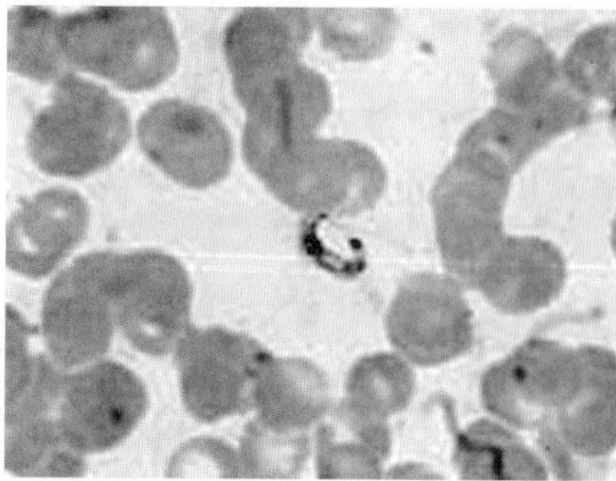

FIGURE 1-64 ***T. cruzi* in human blood film.** The causative agent occurs in blood films characteristically as short C-shaped or S-shaped trypomastigotes with a prominent kinetoplast. It is otherwise monomorphic *(Giemsa × 950).* (From Hoffmann R et al: *Hematology: basic principles and practice,* ed 5, Philadelphia, 2009, Churchill Livingstone.)

- Xenodiagnosis, a technique involving laboratory-reared insect vectors fed on subjects with suspected infection thereafter examined for parasites, and culture of body fluids in liquid media to establish diagnosis
  1. Hampered by the length of time required for completion
  2. Of limited use in clinical decision making with regard to drug therapy
  3. Although xenodiagnosis and broth culture are considered to be more sensitive than microscopic examination of body fluids, sensitivities may not exceed 50%
- Recent advances in serologic testing include immunoblot assay, in situ indirect fluorescent antibody, PCR-based techniques, and an immunochromatographic assay (Chagas Stat Pak)

For chronic *T. cruzi* infection:

- Traditional serologic tests including: complement fixation (CF), indirect immunofluorescence (IIF), indirect hemagglutination, and enzyme-linked immunosorbent assay (ELISA)
- Serologic tests have variable sensitivity and specificity and frequent false-positive results
- Saliva ELISA may be useful as a screening diagnostic test in epidemiologic studies of chronic trypanosomiasis infection in endemic areas

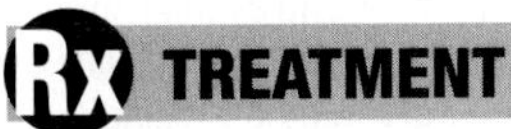

TREATMENT

NONPHARMACOLOGIC THERAPY

- Chronic chagasic heart disease: mainly supportive
- Megaesophagus: symptoms usually amenable to dietary measures or pneumonic dilation of the esophagogastric junction
- Chagasic megacolon: in its early stages responsive to a high-fiber diet, laxatives, and enemas

ACUTE GENERAL Rx

Nifurtimox (Lampit, Bayer 2502):

- Only drug available in the U.S. for the treatment of acute, congenital, or laboratory-acquired infection
- Recommended oral dosage for adults: 8 to 10 mg/kg/day given in 4 divided daily doses and continued for 90 to 120 days
- Parasitologic cure in approximately 50% of those treated; should be begun as early as possible

Benznidazole, a nitroimidazole derivative:

- Has demonstrated similar efficacy as nifurtimox in limited trials
- Recommended oral dosage: 5 mg/kg/day for 60 days

CHRONIC Rx

- In patients with indeterminate phase or chronic disease: Some evidence of benefit in a recent uncontrolled trial with benznidazole in patients with chagasic cardiomyopathy
- In patients exhibiting bradyarrhythmias: pacemakers
- In individuals with congestive heart failure:
  1. Treat with standard modalities for dilated, right-sided, cardiomyopathic disease.
  2. Cardiac transplant is an option for end-stage cardiomyopathy; moreover, reactivation rate found to be low and amenable to therapy without subsequent infection of the allograft.
  3. Myotomy or esophageal resection is reserved for patients with advanced disease.
- In advanced chagasic megacolon associated with chronic fecal impaction, perforation, or, less commonly, volvulus: surgical resection

DISPOSITION

Based on few prospective studies, most patients infected with *T. cruzi* will not develop symptomatic Chagas' disease.

REFERRAL

- For consultation with an infectious disease specialist or communication with the Centers for Disease Control and Prevention when the disease is acutely suspected
- To a cardiologist for pacemaker implantation for patients with bradyarrhythmias
- To a surgeon for symptomatic disease with chagasic megaesophagus or megacolon

PEARLS & CONSIDERATIONS

COMMENTS

- In recipients of solid organ or bone marrow transplants, patients with AIDS, or those receiving chemotherapy, there may be reactivation of indeterminate phase disease.
- Mortality predictors associated with chagasic cardiomyopathy include CHF, QT-interval dispersion, left ventricular (LV) end-systolic dimension, the presence of pathological Q waves, frequent PVCs, and isolated LAFB on ECG.
- Chagasic esophageal disease has an increased incidence of esophageal malignancy.
- The use of pyrethroid-impregnated curtains may represent an option for the reduction or elimination of Chagas' disease transmission in certain endemic areas.

SUGGESTED READINGS

Benchimol Barbosa PR: The oral transmission of Chagas' disease: an acute form of infection responsible for regional outbreaks, *Int J Cardiol* 112(1):132-133, 2006.

Bern C et al: Evaluation and treatment of Chagas disease in the United States, *JAMA* 298:2171-2181, 2007.

Garcia S et al: Treatment with benznidazole during the chronic phase of experimental Chagas' disease decreases cardiac alterations, *Antimicrob Agents Chemother* 49(4):1521, 2005.

Golgher D, Gazzinelli RT: Innate and acquired immunity in the pathogenesis of Chagas disease, *Autoimmunity* 37(5):399, 2004.

Kirchhoff LV et al: Transfusion-associated Chagas disease (American trypanosomiasis) in Mexico: implications for transfusion medicine in the United States, *Transfusion* 46(2):298, 2006.

Leiby DA et al: Trypanosoma cruzi parasitemia in US blood donors with serologic evidence of infection, *J Infect Dis* 198:609, 2008.

Reyes P et al: Trypanocidal drugs for late stage, symptomatic Chagas disease (Trypanosoma cruzi infection), *Cochrane Database Syst Rev* 2005.

Villar R et al: Trypanocidal drugs for chronic asymptomatic Trypanosoma cruzi infection, *Cochrane Database Sys Rev* 2002.

Viotti R et al: Long-term cardiac outcomes of treating chronic Chagas disease with benznidazole versus no treatment: a nonrandomized trial, *Ann Intern Med* 144(10):724, 2006.

AUTHORS: **PATRICIA CRISTOFARO, M.D., GLENN G. FORT, M.D., M.P.H.,** and **DENNIS J. MIKOLICH, M.D.**

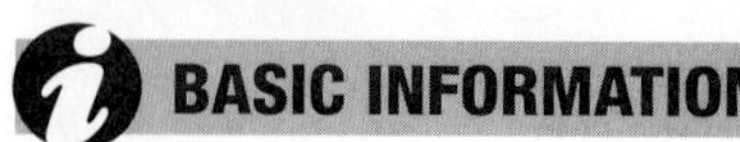

BASIC INFORMATION

DEFINITION

Chancroid is a sexually transmitted disease characterized by painful genital ulceration and inflammatory inguinal adenopathy.

SYNONYMS

Soft chancre
Ulcus molle

ICD-9CM CODES
099.0 Chancroid

EPIDEMIOLOGY & DEMOGRAPHICS

- Exact incidence is unknown.
- Occurs more frequently in men (male/female ratio of 10:1).
- Clinical infection is rare in women.
- There is a higher incidence in uncircumcised men and in tropical and subtropical regions.
- Incubation period is 4 to 7 days but may take up to 3 wk.
- High incidence of HIV infection associated with chancroid.

PHYSICAL FINDINGS & CLINICAL PRESENTATION

- One to three extremely painful ulcers (Fig. 1-65) accompanied by tender inguinal lymphadenopathy (especially if fluctuant)
- May present with inguinal bubo and several ulcers
- In women: initial lesion in the fourchette, labia minora, urethra, cervix, or anus; inflammatory pustule or papule that ruptures, leaving a shallow, nonindurated ulceration, usually 1- to 2-cm diameter with ragged, undermined edges
- Unilateral lymphadenopathy develops 1 wk later in 50% of patients

ETIOLOGY

Haemophilus ducreyi, a bacillus

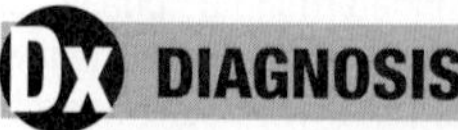

DIAGNOSIS

DIFFERENTIAL DIAGNOSIS

- Other genitoulcerative diseases such as syphilis, herpes, lymphogranuloma venereum (LGV), granuloma inguinale.
- A clinical algorithm for the initial management of genital ulcer disease is described in Section III.

WORKUP

Diagnosis based on history and physical examination is often inadequate. Must rule out syphilis in women because of the consequences of inappropriate therapy in pregnant women. Base initial diagnosis and treatment recommendations on clinical impression of appearance of ulcer and most likely diagnosis for population. Definitive diagnosis is made by isolation of organism from ulcers by culture or Gram stain.

LABORATORY TESTS

Darkfield microscopy, RPR, HSV cultures, *H. ducreyi* culture, HIV testing recommended

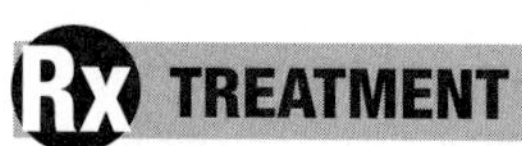

TREATMENT

NONPHARMACOLOGIC THERAPY

Fluctuant nodes should be aspirated through healthy adjacent skin to prevent formation of draining sinus. Incision and drainage not recommended because it delays healing. Use warm compresses to remove necrotic material.

ACUTE GENERAL Rx

- Azithromycin 1 g PO (single dose) *or*
- Ceftriaxone 250 mg IM (single dose) *or*
- Ciprofloxacin 500 mg PO bid for 3 days *or*
- Erythromycin 500 mg PO qid for 7 days

NOTE: Ciprofloxacin is contraindicated in patients who are pregnant, lactating, or <18 yr.

- HIV-infected patients may need more prolonged therapy

DISPOSITION

- All sexual partners should be treated with a 10-day course of one of the regimens (see "Acute General Rx").
- Patients should be reexamined 3 to 7 days after initiation of therapy. Ulcers should improve symptomatically within 3 days and objectively within 7 days after initiation of successful therapy.

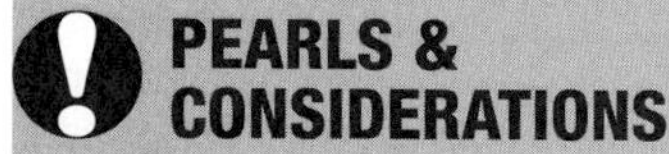

PEARLS & CONSIDERATIONS

COMMENTS

In the U.S. herpes simplex-1 and syphilis are the most common causes of genital ulcers, followed by chancroid, LGV, and granuloma inguinale.

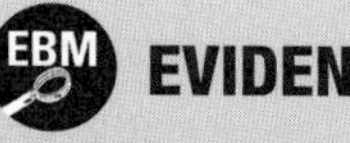

EVIDENCE

Despite the absence of an extensive clinical trial database, these therapies have gained acceptance and are in accordance with Centers for Disease Control and Prevention (CDC) guidelines.[1]

The CDC recommends oral azithromycin, intramuscular ceftriaxone sodium, oral ciprofloxacin, or oral erythromycin as first-line therapies for treatment of chancroid caused by *H. ducreyi.*

All regimens are effective for treating chancroid in patients who are HIV negative or HIV positive.

Azithromycin and ceftriaxone are offered as single-dose therapies.

Evidence-Based Reference

1. Centers for Disease Control and Prevention: Sexually transmitted diseases treatment guidelines, *MMRW* 55(RR-11):1, 2006.

SUGGESTED READINGS

Lewis DA: Chancroid: clinical manifestations, diagnosis and management, *Sex Transm Infect* 79(1):68, 2003.

Sehgal VN, Srivastave G: Chancroid: contemporary appraisal, *Int J Dermatol* 42(3):182, 2003.

AUTHORS: **MARIA A. CORIGLIANO, M.D.,** and **RUBEN ALVERO, M.D.**

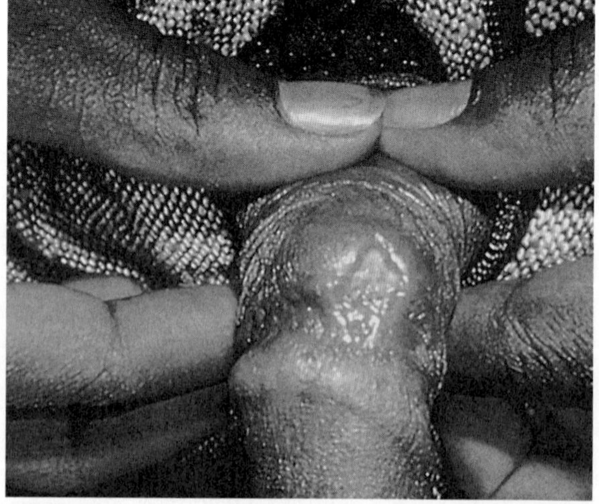

FIGURE 1-65 Chancroid. Note shaggy, ragged-edged ulcer with edema and exudative base. (Courtesy Beverly Sanders. From Goldstein B [ed]: *Practical dermatology,* ed 2, St Louis, 1997, Mosby.)

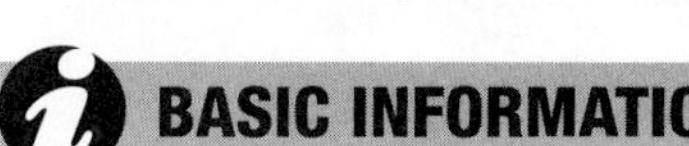

BASIC INFORMATION

DEFINITION

Charcot-Marie-Tooth disease is a heterogeneous group of noninflammatory inherited peripheral neuropathies. It is the most common inherited neuromuscular disorder (See also "Neuropathy, Hereditary.")

SYNONYMS

Peroneal muscular atrophy
Hereditary motor and sensory neuropathy (HMSN)
Idiopathic dominantly inherited hypertrophic polyneuropathy

ICD-9CM CODES
356.1 Charcot-Marie-Tooth disease, paralysis, or syndrome

EPIDEMIOLOGY & DEMOGRAPHICS

PREDOMINANT AGE: Onset usually 10 to 20 yr but can be delayed to 50 to 60 yr
PREDOMINANT SEX: Male/female ratio of 3:1

PHYSICAL FINDINGS & CLINICAL PRESENTATION

- Variable presentation from family to family, but affected individuals in a family tend to have similar symptoms
- Usually gradual onset, with slowly progressive disorder
- Foot deformity producing a high arch (cavus) and hammertoes
- Atrophy of the lower legs producing a stork-like appearance (muscle wasting does not involve the upper legs) (Fig. 1-66)
- Nerve enlargement
- Sensory loss or other neurologic signs, although the sensory involvement is usually mild
- Scoliosis
- Decreased proprioception that often interferes with balance and gait
- Painful paresthesias
- In late cases, possible involvement of hands
- Absence of deep tendon reflexes in many cases
- Poorly healing foot ulcers in some patients

ETIOLOGY

Chronic segmental demyelination of peripheral nerves with hypertrophic changes caused by remyelination

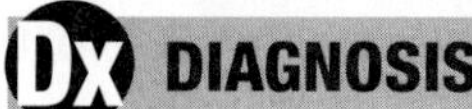

DIAGNOSIS

DIFFERENTIAL DIAGNOSIS

- Other inherited neuropathies
- Toxic, metabolic, and nutritional polyneuropathies

WORKUP

- The early onset, slow progression, and familial nature of the disorder are usually sufficient to establish diagnosis.
- Electrophysiologic studies are often diagnostic and may also be helpful in defining various subtypes of this group of neuropathies.
- Occasionally muscle and nerve (sural) biopsy may be required.

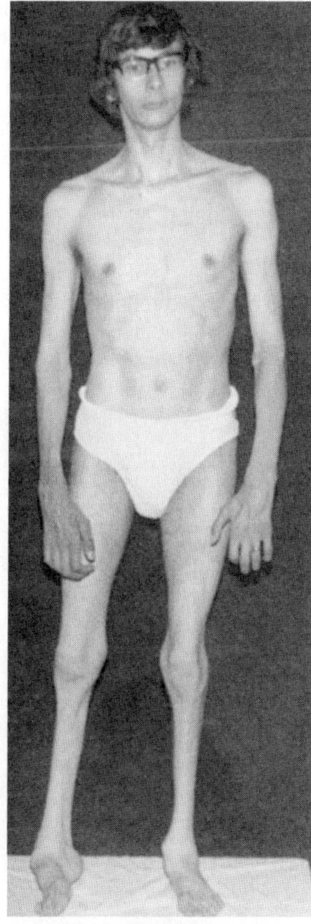

FIGURE 1-66 Patient with Charcot-Marie-Tooth disease showing marked wasting of calf muscles and intrinsic foot muscles. (From Dubowitz V: *Muscle disorders in childhood,* London, 1995, WB Saunders. In Goetz CG: *Textbook of clinical neurology,* Philadelphia, 1999, WB Saunders.)

Rx TREATMENT

ACUTE GENERAL Rx

- Genetic counseling
- Supportive physical therapy and occupational therapy
- Prevention of injury to limbs with diminished sensibility
- Bracing

CHRONIC Rx

Occasionally, surgery to add stability and restore a plantigrade foot

DISPOSITION

- Disability is usually mild and compatible with a long life.
- 10% to 20% of patients are asymptomatic.
- A small number of cases are nonambulators by the sixth or seventh decade.
- The condition is usually not life threatening.

REFERRAL

- For orthopedic consultation for bracing and treatment of deformity
- For genetic counseling

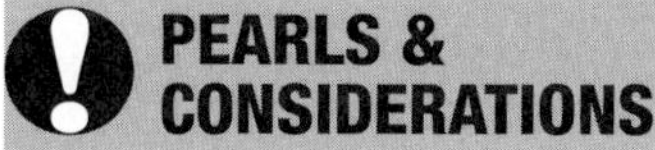

PEARLS & CONSIDERATIONS

COMMENTS

Patient information on Charcot-Marie-Tooth disease is available from the Muscular Dystrophy Association, 3300 East Sunrise Drive, Tucson, AZ 85718; phone: 800-572-1717.

SUGGESTED READINGS

Bennett CL: Late-onset hereditary axonal neuropathies: *Neurology* 71:14, 2008.

Chetlin RD et al: Resistance training exercise and creatine in patients with Charcot-Marie-Tooth disease, *Muscle Nerve* 30:69, 2004.

Gemignani F, Marbini A: Charcot-Marie-Tooth disease (CMT) distinctive phenotypic and genotypic features in CMT type 2, *J Neurol Sci* 184:1, 2001.

Karol LA, Elerson E: Scoliosis in patients with Charcot-Marie-Tooth disease, *J Bone Joint Surg Am* 89A: 1504, 2007.

Nave KA et al: Mechanisms of disease: inherited demyelinating neuropathies—from basic to clinical research, *Nat Clin Pract Neurol* 3:453, 2007.

Pareyson D: Differential diagnosis of Charcot-Marie-Tooth disease and related neuropathies, *Neurol Sci* 25:72, 2004.

Parman Y: Hereditary neuropathies, *Curr Opin Neurol* 20:542, 2007.

Redmond AC et al: Factors that influence health-related quality of life in Australian adults with Charcot-Marie-Tooth disease, *Neuromuscul Disord* 18:619-625, 2008.

AUTHOR: **LONNIE R. MERCIER, M.D.**

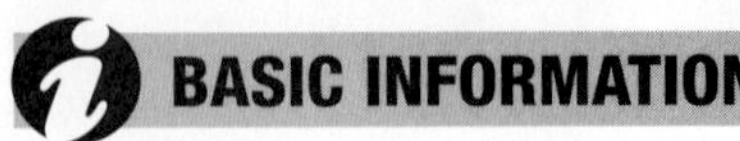

BASIC INFORMATION

DEFINITION

Charcot's joint is a chronic, often devastating, progressive joint degeneration seen most commonly in peripheral weight-bearing joints and vertebrae, which develops as a result of the loss of normal sensory innervation of the joint. It was described by Charcot as a result of tabes dorsalis.

SYNONYMS

Neuropathic arthropathy

ICD-9CM CODES

094.0 Charcot's arthropathy

EPIDEMIOLOGY & DEMOGRAPHICS

PREVALENCE:

- One case per 750 patients with diabetes mellitus; five cases per 100 of those with peripheral neuropathy (foot is most commonly involved)
- 20% to 40% of patients with syringomyelia (shoulder most commonly involved)
- 5% to 10% of patients with tabes dorsalis; usually >60 yr (spine, hip, and knee most commonly involved)

PHYSICAL FINDINGS & CLINICAL PRESENTATION

Neuropathic joint disease is relatively painless, often despite considerable destruction

- Diffusely warm, swollen, and occasionally erythematous involved joint is often found, the latter suggesting sepsis
- Possible progression of joint instability; palpable osseous debris; crepitus common
- Frank dislocation leading to bony deformity often found, especially in more superficial joints

ETIOLOGY

The most widely accepted theory is the "neurotraumatic" theory:

- Impairment and loss of joint sensitivity decrease the protective mechanism around the joint.
- Rapid destruction occurs.
- Chronic inflammation and repetitive effusions develop, eventually contributing to joint instability and incongruity.

DIAGNOSIS

DIFFERENTIAL DIAGNOSIS

- Osteomyelitis, cellulitis, abscess
- Infectious arthritis
- Osteoarthritis
- Rheumatoid and other inflammatory arthritides

WORKUP

- An underlying neurologic disorder must always be present.
- Diabetes mellitus with peripheral neuropathy is the most common cause (Fig. 1-67).
- Syringomyelia, tabes dorsalis, Charcot-Marie-Tooth disease, congenital indifference to pain, alcoholism, and spinal dysraphism can all lead to the disorder.

LABORATORY TESTS

In questionable cases, aspiration, sometimes including biopsy, to rule out sepsis

IMAGING STUDIES

Plain roentgenography:

- Sufficient to establish diagnosis in most cases, especially if etiology is known
- Findings: variable degrees of destruction and dislocation

TREATMENT

ACUTE GENERAL Rx

- Protection of effusions, sprains, and fractures until all hyperemic response has resolved
- Braces, special shoes with molded inserts, and elevation of the extremity
- Patient education with avoidance of weight bearing when lower extremity joints are involved
- Surgery: only limited value

DISPOSITION

Once the full-blown neuropathic joint has developed, treatment is difficult.

SUGGESTED READINGS

Choski P et al: Charcot arthropathy: an often overlooked complication of diabetes mellitus, *Am J Ark Med Soc* 103:229, 2007.

Desouza LJ: Charcot arthropathy and immobilization in a weight-bearing total contact cast, *Am J Bone Joint Surg* 90:754, 2008.

Guyton GP, Saltzman CL: The diabetic foot: basic mechanisms of disease, *Instr Course Lect* 51:169, 2002.

Herbst SA et al: Pattern of diabetic neuropathic arthropathy associated with peripheral bone mineral density, *Br J Bone Joint Surg* 86:378, 2004.

Neves FS et al: Syringomyelia, neuropathic arthropathy and rheumatoid arthritis as diagnostic dilemmas in two different cases: confounding factor and true coexistence, *Clin Rheumatol* 26:98, 2007.

Pakarinen TK et al: Charcot arthropathy of the diabetic foot: current concepts and review of 36 cases, *Scand J Surg* 91:195, 2002.

Pinzur MS: Current concepts review: Charcot arthropathy of the foot and ankle, *Foot Ankle Int* 28:952, 2007.

Slater RA et al: The diabetic Charcot foot, *1st Med Assoc J* 6:280, 2004.

van der Ven A: Charcot neuropathy of the foot and ankle, *J Am Acad Orthop Surg* 17:562, 2009.

AUTHOR: **LONNIE R. MERCIER, M.D.**

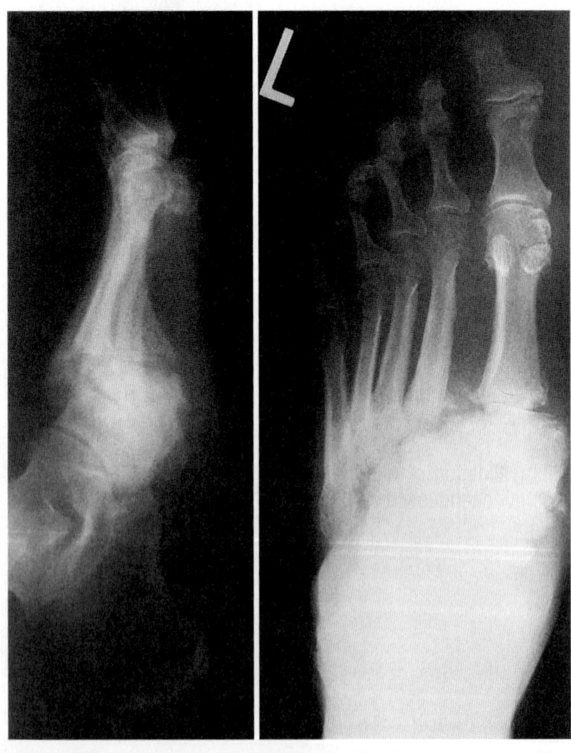

FIGURE 1-67 Diabetes mellitus and neuropathic arthritis. Note lateral displacement of metatarsals *(left)* and fragmentation and osseous debris *(right)*. (From Goldman L, Ausiello D [eds]: *Cecil textbook of medicine,* ed 22, Philadelphia, 2004, WB Saunders.)

BASIC INFORMATION

DEFINITION

Chemotherapy-induced nausea and vomiting (CINV) refers to adverse effects of drugs used to treat cancer. There are three recognized subtypes: acute-phase CINV, where nausea and vomiting begin minutes to hours after administration of the drug(s); delayed-phase CINV, where symptoms can begin or return 24 hours or more after taking the medication(s); and anticipatory CINV, where nausea and vomiting begin before receiving treatment.

SYNONYMS

Drug-induced nausea and vomiting
Chemotherapy-induced emesis

ICD-9CM CODES
787.01 Nausea with vomiting
787.02 Nausea alone
787.03 Vomiting alone
E933.1 Adverse effect of antineoplastic and immunosuppressive drugs
V58.11-V58.12 Encounter for antineoplastic chemotherapy and immunotherapy

EPIDEMIOLOGY & DEMOGRAPHICS

- The patient's risk for development of nausea and vomiting is most strongly dependent on the drugs used.
- With certain medications, nausea and vomiting will occur in almost 100% of patients. With other drugs, the risk for symptoms can be as low as 10%.
- Symptoms may be dose dependent (the higher the dose, the greater the risk for symptoms).
- CINV is more likely to affect female and younger patients.
- Those patients expecting CINV from medications are more likely to have it (anticipatory emesis).
- Those patients with a history of alcohol consumption are at lower risk.
- Patients with a history of motion sickness are at greater risk.

PHYSICAL FINDINGS & CLINICAL PRESENTATION

- For acute-phase CINV, nausea and vomiting start within minutes to hours after receiving chemotherapy.
- For delayed-phase CINV, nausea and vomiting begin or return 24 hours or more after receiving chemotherapy.
- With anticipatory CINV, symptoms begin before receiving the medication.
- Other symptoms may include anxiety and lightheadedness.
- Physical findings are most commonly elevated pulse and abnormal blood pressure (high if the person is highly anxious, low if the patient is getting dehydrated).
- Symptoms such as diarrhea, fever, headache, and abdominal pain may suggest an etiology of symptoms other than chemotherapy; physical examination findings such as increased blood pressure, abdominal tenderness, or focal neurologic deficits may suggest symptoms caused by cancer progression or other acute illness such as infection.

ETIOLOGY

CINV is probably the result of chemotherapy drugs acting in two places: in the gastrointestinal tract directly and in the vomiting center of the brain. In both areas, nausea and vomiting are mediated by the actions of certain neurotransmitters, with serotonin, dopamine, and neurokinin being the most important.

DIAGNOSIS

DIFFERENTIAL DIAGNOSIS

- The two main considerations are progression of cancer and infection
- Intestinal/gastric: obstruction or partial obstruction of the digestive tract from tumor
- Neurologic: metastases to the brain causing vomiting; infiltration of nerves affecting the digestive tract
- Infectious: acute bacterial, viral, or parasitic infectious of the digestive tract causing symptoms (usually diarrhea will be present)
- Renal: dehydration leading to kidney failure, causing a worsening of nausea and vomiting

WORKUP

No workup is indicated if patient's symptoms and timeframe of nausea and vomiting fit the usual presentation for CINV. If other symptoms or unexpected physical examination findings are present, then other causes need to be ruled out. A combination of blood work and imaging may be helpful.

LABORATORY TESTS

- If the onset of symptoms is not typical for CINV, then blood tests such as a CBC, liver tests, and kidney tests may be indicated.
- Stool studies looking for infections from bacteria or parasites may be ordered if diarrhea is also present.

IMAGING STUDIES

- Abdominal radiographs may be ordered to look for obstruction of the digestive tract but will not give any information about tumor progression.
- Abdominal CT scan will give more detailed information about cancer in the proximity of the digestive tract and whether obstruction of the digestive tract is present.
- Brain CT scan or magnetic resonance imaging (MRI) will give information about possible metastases to the brain.

TREATMENT

- Treatment depends on the likelihood of a given drug or drug regimen to cause CINV and is preventative in nature.
- For those medications with a high probability of causing CINV, a combination of antinausea medications has proved to be highly effective.
- Which combination of drugs is used and for how many days is dependent on the chemotherapy regimen used.
- The most common combination includes a serotonin-receptor antagonist (ondansetron, granisetron, dolasetron, tropisetron, or palonosetron), a corticosteroid (methylprednisolone or dexamethason), and a neurokinin-1 receptor antagonist (aprepitant).
- Many other drugs are available, such as prochlorperazine, metochlopramide, haloperidol, and marinol, but most are less effective and have greater potential for adverse effects.
- Benzodiazepines (usually lorazepam) may help in patients with high anxiety levels leading to anticipatory CINV.
- Patients with uncontrolled symptoms may require hospitalization for supportive care including intravenous fluids.

NONPHARMACOLOGIC THERAPY

For those patients with a significant anxiety component to their CINV, behavior therapy may help.

DISPOSITION

Although CINV is one of the most feared complications of cancer therapy, its treatment has been revolutionized in the last 20 years, with most patients achieving adequate symptom control.

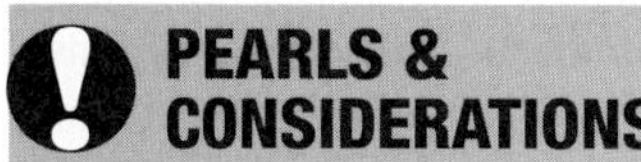

PEARLS & CONSIDERATIONS

COMMENTS

- Aggressive attempts to control the acute phase of CINV are the key to symptom control. Prevention of the acute phase has led to much greater control of the delayed phase, which, in turn, has greatly decreased the incidence of anticipatory CINV.
- Prevention of symptoms is much easier to achieve than controlling/treating symptoms once they have begun.

SUGGESTED READINGS

Hesketh P: Chemotherapy-induced nausea and vomiting, *N Engl J Med* 358:2482-2494, 2008.

Markman M: Progress in preventing chemotherapy-induced nausea and vomiting, *Cleve Clin J Med* 69: 609-617, 2002.

AUTHOR: **CHARLES WOLFF, M.D.**

Chlamydia Genital Infections (PTG)

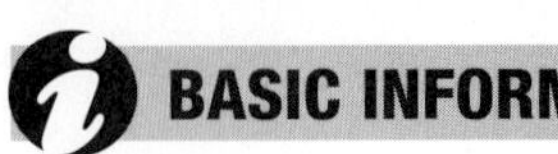

BASIC INFORMATION

DEFINITION

Genital infection with *Chlamydia trachomatis* may result in urethritis, epididymitis, cervicitis, and acute salpingitis, but often it is asymptomatic in women (see "Pelvic Inflammatory Disease"). In men, urethritis, mucopurulent discharge, dysuria, and urethral pruritus are noted.

ICD-9CM CODES
597.80 Urethritis
604.0 Epididymitis
616.0 Cervicitis
381.51 Acute salpingitis

EPIDEMIOLOGY & DEMOGRAPHICS

- *Chlamydia trachomatis* is the most common sexually transmitted disease in the U.S. More than 4 million infections occur annually, although the exact number is unknown because reporting is not required in all states. Occurrence is common worldwide and has been increasing steadily over the last 2 decades in the U.S., Canada, Australia, and Europe.
- Most women with endocervical or urethral infections are asymptomatic.
- Up to 45% of cases of gonococcal infection may have concomitant chlamydial infection.
- Infertility or ectopic pregnancy can result as a complication from symptomatic or asymptomatic chronic infections of the endometrium and fallopian tubes.
- Conjunctival and pneumonic infection of the newborn may result from infection in pregnancy.
- In men 15% to 55% of cases are caused by *C. trachomatis*. Complications of nongonococcal urethritis in men infected with *C. trachomatis* include epididymitis and Reiter's syndrome.

PHYSICAL FINDINGS & CLINICAL PRESENTATION

Clinical manifestations may be similar to those of gonorrhea: mucopurulent endocervical discharge, with edema, erythema, and easily induced endocervical bleeding caused by inflammation of endocervical columnar epithelium. Less-frequent manifestations may include bartholinitis, urethral syndrome with dysuria and pyuria, and perihepatitis (Fitz-Hugh–Curtis syndrome).

ETIOLOGY

- *Chlamydia trachomatis,* serotypes D through K
- Obligate, intracellular bacteria

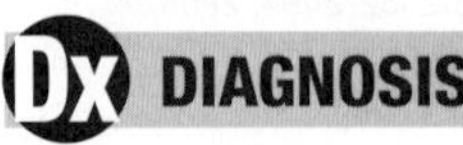

DIAGNOSIS

DIFFERENTIAL DIAGNOSIS

Gonorrhea, nongonococcal urethritis (nonchlamydial etiologies)

WORKUP

Diagnosis based on laboratory demonstration of evidence of infection in intraurethral or endocervical swab by various tests. The intracellular organism is less readily recovered from the discharge.

LABORATORY TESTS

- Cell culture is the reference method for diagnosis (single culture sensitivity 80% to 90%), but it is labor intensive and takes 48 to 96 hr; it is not suited for large screening programs.
- Nonculture methods:
  - Direct fluorescent antibody tests
  - Enzyme immunoassay
  - DNA probes
  - Polymerase chain reaction (PCR)
- With the exception of PCR, the other tests are probably less specific than cell culture and may yield false-positive results.
- Because this is an intracellular organism, purulent discharge is not an appropriate specimen. An adequate sample of infected cells must be obtained.
- Ten white blood cells per high-power field.

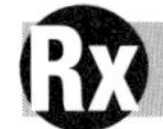

TREATMENT

ACUTE GENERAL Rx

Nongonococcal urethritis, urethritis, cervicitis, conjunctivitis (except for lymphogranuloma venereum):
- Azithromycin 1 g PO × 1 *or*
- Doxycycline 100 mg PO bid for 7 days
- Alternatives
  1. Erythromycin base 500 mg PO qid for 7 days *or*
  2. Erythromycin ethylsuccinate 800 mg PO qid for 7 days *or*
  3. Ofloxacin 300 mg PO bid for 7 days
  4. Levofloxacin 500 mg PO qd for 7 days

Infection in pregnancy:
- Erythromycin base 500 mg PO qid for 7 days *or*
- Amoxicillin 500 mg PO tid for 7 days

Alternatives:
1. Erythromycin base 250 mg PO qid for 7 days *or*
2. Erythromycin ethylsuccinate 800 mg PO qid for 7 days *or*
3. Erythromycin ethylsuccinate 400 mg PO qid for 14 days *or*
4. Azithromycin 1 g PO (single dose)

NOTE: Doxycycline and ofloxacin are contraindicated in pregnancy. Safety and efficacy of azithromycin are not established in pregnancy and lactation, although preliminary data indicate that it may be safe and effective. Erythromycin estolate is contraindicated in pregnancy because of drug-related hepatotoxicity.

FOLLOW-UP: Reculture after therapy completion and refer partners for evaluation and treatment.

RECURRENT AND PERSISTENT URETHRITIS: Retreat noncompliant patients with the above regimens. If patient was initially compliant, recommended regimens: metronidazole 2 g PO in single dose plus erythromycin base 500 mg PO qid for 7 days or erythromycin ethylsuccinate 800 mg PO qid for 7 days.

CLINICAL PEARL

When treating *Chlamydia,* it is best to assume concomitant gonorrhea because co-infection is common. Combination of cetriaxone 125 mg IM single dose plus azithromycin 1 g PO single dose will treat both.

REFFERAL

Refer to infectious disease specialist if persistent infection or gynecologist if salpingitis is suspected.

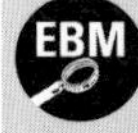

EVIDENCE

Doxycycline is effective in the treatment of genital chlamydial infections in men and nonpregnant women. Small randomized controlled trials (RCTs) with short-term follow-up have found microbiologic cure rates of at least 95%.[1] (A)

Another systematic review found no significant difference between azithromycin and doxycycline in terms of microbiologic cure rates in males and nonpregnant females with genital chlamydial infections.[2] (A)

In small, short-term RCTs including men and nonpregnant women with genital chlamydial infection, cure rates achieved with erythromycin ranged from 77% to 100%.[1] (A)

No significant difference was found in two unblinded RCTs between azithromycin and amoxicillin in terms of microbiologic cure in pregnant women with chlamydial infections.[3] (B)

Evidence-Based References

1. Low N: Chlamydia (uncomplicated, genital), *Clin Evidence* 12:2203, 2004. (A)
2. Lau CY, Qureshi AK: Azithromycin versus doxycycline for genital chlamydial infections: a meta-analysis of randomized clinical trials, *Sex Transm Dis* 29:497, 2002. (A)
3. Jacobson GF: A randomized controlled trial comparing amoxicillin and azithromycin for the treatment of *Chlamydia trachomatis* in pregnancy, *Am J Obstet Gynecol* 184:1352, 2001. (B)

SUGGESTED READINGS

Centers for Disease Control and Prevention: 2006 sexually transmitted diseases treatment guidelines, *MMWR* 55(RR-11), 2006.

Spiliopoulou A et al: Chlamydia trachomatis: time for screening? *Clin Microbiol Infect* 11(9):687, 2005.

AUTHORS: **MARIA A. CORIGLIANO, M.D.,** and **RUBEN ALVERO, M.D.**

BASIC INFORMATION

DEFINITION

Cholangitis refers to an inflammation and/or infection of the hepatic and common bile ducts associated with obstruction of the common bile duct.

SYNONYMS

Biliary sepsis
Ascending cholangitis
Suppurative cholangitis

ICD-9CM CODES
576.1 Cholangitis

EPIDEMIOLOGY & DEMOGRAPHICS

INCIDENCE (IN U.S.): Complicates approximately 1% of cases of cholelithiasis
PEAK INCIDENCE: Seventh decade
PREVALENCE (IN U.S.): 2 cases/1000 hospital admissions
PREDOMINANT SEX:

- Females, for cholangitis secondary to gallstones
- Males, for cholangitis secondary to malignant obstruction and HIV infection

PREDOMINANT AGE: Seventh decade and older; unusual <50 yr of age

PHYSICAL FINDINGS & CLINICAL PRESENTATION

- Usually acute onset of fever, abdominal pain (RUQ), and jaundice (Charcot's triad)
- All signs and symptoms in only 50% to 85% of patients
- Often, dark coloration of the urine resulting from bilirubinuria
- Complications:
  1. Bacteremia (50%) and septic shock
  2. Hepatic abscess and pancreatitis

ETIOLOGY

Obstruction of the common bile duct causing rapid proliferation of bacteria in the biliary tree

- Most common cause of common bile duct obstruction: stones, usually migrated from the gallbladder
- Other causes: prior biliary tract surgery with secondary stenosis, tumor (usually arising from the pancreas or biliary tree), and parasitic infections from *Ascaris lumbricoides* or *Fasciola hepatica*
- Iatrogenic after contamination of an obstructed biliary tree by endoscopic retrograde cholangiopancreatoscopy (ERCP) or percutaneous transhepatic cholangiography (PTC)
- Primary sclerosing cholangitis (PSC)
- HIV-associated sclerosing cholangitis: associated with infection by CMV, *Cryptosporidium,* Microsporidia, and *Mycobacterium avium* complex

DIAGNOSIS

DIFFERENTIAL DIAGNOSIS

- Biliary colic
- Acute cholecystitis
- Liver abscess
- Peptic ulcer disease (PUD)
- Pancreatitis
- Intestinal obstruction
- Right kidney stone
- Hepatitis
- Pyelonephritis

WORKUP

- Blood cultures
- CBC
- Liver function tests

LABORATORY TESTS

- Usually, elevated WBC count with a predominance of polymorphonuclear forms
- Elevated alkaline phosphatase and bilirubin in chronic obstruction
- Elevated transaminases in acute obstruction
- Positive blood cultures in 50% of cases, typically with enteric gram-negative aerobes (e.g., *E. coli, Klebsiella pneumoniae*), enterococci, or anaerobes

IMAGING STUDIES

- Ultrasound:
  1. Allows visualization of the gallbladder and bile ducts to differentiate extrahepatic obstruction from intrahepatic cholestasis
  2. Insensitive but specific for visualization of common duct stones
- CT scan:
  1. Less accurate for gallstones
  2. More sensitive than ultrasound for visualization of the distal part of the common bile duct
  3. Also allows better definition of neoplasm
- ERCP:
  1. Confirms obstruction and its level
  2. Allows collection of specimens for culture and cytology
  3. Indicated for diagnosis if ultrasound and CT scan are inconclusive
  4. May be indicated in therapy (see "Treatment")

TREATMENT

NONPHARMACOLOGIC THERAPY

Biliary decompression

- May be urgent in severely ill patients or those unresponsive to medical therapy within 12 to 24 hr
- May also be performed semielectively in patients who respond
- Options:
  1. ERCP with or without sphincterotomy or placement of a draining stent
  2. Percutaneous transhepatic biliary drainage for the acutely ill patient who is a poor surgical candidate
  3. Surgical exploration of the common bile duct

ACUTE GENERAL Rx

- Nothing by mouth
- Intravenous hydration
- Broad-spectrum antibiotics directed at gram-negative enteric organisms, anaerobes, and enterococcus such as ampicillin/sulbactam or piperacillin/tazobactam; if infection is nosocomial, post-ERCP, or the patient is in shock, broaden antibiotic coverage.

CHRONIC Rx

Repeated decompression may be necessary, particularly when obstruction is related to neoplasm.

DISPOSITION

Excellent prognosis if obstruction is amenable to definitive surgical therapy; otherwise relapses are common.

REFERRAL

- To biliary endoscopist if obstruction is from stones or a stent needs to be placed
- To interventional radiologist if external drainage is necessary
- To a general surgeon in all other cases
- To an infectious disease specialist if blood cultures are positive or the patient is in shock or otherwise severely ill

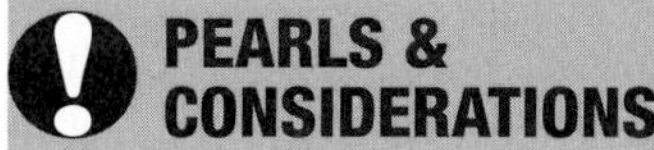

PEARLS & CONSIDERATIONS

- Cholangitis is a life-threatening form of intra-abdominal sepsis, though it may appear to be rather innocuous at its onset.
- Antibiotics alone will not resolve cholangitis in the presence of biliary obstruction because high intrabiliary pressures prevent antibiotic delivery. Decompression and drainage of the biliary tract to alleviate the obstruction with antimicrobial therapy is the therapy of choice.

SUGGESTED READINGS

Kumar R et al: Endoscopic biliary drainage for severe acute cholangitis in biliary obstruction as a result of malignant and benign diseases, *J Gastroenterol Hepatol* 19(9):994, 2004.

Lee JG: Diagnosis and management of acute cholangitis, *Nat Rev Gastroenterol Hepatol* 6(9):553-541, 2009.

Ozden I et al: Endoscopic and radiologic interventions as the leading causes of severe cholangitis in a tertiary referral center, *Am J Surg* 189(6):702, 2005.

AUTHORS: **GLENN G. FORT, M.D., M.P.H.,** and **DENNIS J. MIKOLICH, M.D.**

BASIC INFORMATION

DEFINITION

Cholecystitis is acute or chronic inflammation of the gallbladder generally caused by gallstones (>95% of cases).

SYNONYMS

Gallbladder attack

ICD-9CM CODES
575.0 Acute cholecystitis
574.0 Calculus of the gallbladder with acute cholecystitis
575.1 Cholecystitis without mention of calculus

EPIDEMIOLOGY & DEMOGRAPHICS

- Acute cholecystitis occurs most commonly in women during the fifth and sixth decades. Approximately 120,000 cholecystectomies are performed for acute cholecystitis annually in the U.S.
- The incidence of gallstones is 0.6% in the general population and much higher in certain ethnic groups (>75% of Native Americans by age 60 yr). Most patients with gallstones are asymptomatic. Of such patients, biliary colic develops in 1% to 4% annually.

PHYSICAL FINDINGS & CLINICAL PRESENTATION

- Pain and tenderness in the right hypochondrium or epigastrium; pain possibly radiating to the infrascapular region
- Palpation of the right upper quadrant (RUQ) eliciting marked tenderness and stoppage of inspired breath (Murphy's sign)
- Guarding
- Fever (33%)
- Jaundice (25% to 50% of patients)
- Palpable gallbladder (20% of cases)
- Nausea and vomiting (>70% of patients)
- Fever and chills (>25% of patients)
- Medical history often revealing ingestion of large, fatty meals before onset of pain in the epigastrium and RUQ

ETIOLOGY

- Gallstones (>95% of cases)
- Ischemic damage to the gallbladder, critically ill patient (acalculous cholecystitis)
- Infectious agents, especially in patients with AIDS (cytomegalovirus, *Cryptosporidium*)
- Strictures of the bile duct
- Neoplasms, primary or metastatic

Dx DIAGNOSIS

DIFFERENTIAL DIAGNOSIS

- Hepatic: hepatitis, abscess, hepatic congestion, neoplasm, trauma
- Biliary: neoplasm, stricture
- Gastric: pelvic ulcer disease, neoplasm, alcoholic gastritis, hiatal hernia
- Pancreatic: pancreatitis, neoplasm, stone in the pancreatic duct or ampulla
- Renal: calculi, infection, inflammation, neoplasm, ruptured kidney
- Pulmonary: pneumonia, pulmonary infarction, right-sided pleurisy
- Intestinal: retrocecal appendicitis, intestinal obstruction, high fecal impaction
- Cardiac: myocardial ischemia (particularly involving the inferior wall), pericarditis
- Cutaneous: herpes zoster
- Trauma
- Fitz-Hugh-Curtis syndrome (perihepatitis)
- Subphrenic abscess
- Dissecting aneurysm
- Nerve root irritation caused by osteoarthritis of the spine

WORKUP

Workup consists of detailed history and physical examination coupled with laboratory evaluation and imaging studies. No single clinical finding or laboratory test is sufficient to establish or exclude cholecystitis without further testing.

LABORATORY TESTS

- Leukocytosis (12,000 to 20,000) is present in >70% of patients.
- Elevated alkaline phosphatase, ALT, AST, bilirubin; bilirubin elevation >4 mg/dl is unusual and suggests presence of choledocholithiasis.
- Elevated amylase may be present (consider pancreatitis if serum amylase elevation exceeds 500 U).

IMAGING STUDIES

- Ultrasound of the gallbladder is the preferred initial test; it will demonstrate the presence of stones and also dilated gallbladder with thickened wall and surrounding edema in patients with acute cholecystitis.
- Nuclear imaging (HIDA scan) is useful for diagnosis of cholecystitis when sonogram is inconclusive: sensitivity and specificity exceed 90% for acute cholecystis. This test is only reliable when bilirubin is <5 mg/dl. A positive test result (absence of gallbladder filling within 60 min after the administration of tracer) will demonstrate obstruction of the cystic or common hepatic duct; the test will not demonstrate the presence of stones.
- CT scan of abdomen is useful in cases of suspected abscess, neoplasm, or pancreatitis.
- Plain radiograph of the abdomen generally is not useful because <25% of stones are radiopaque.

Rx TREATMENT

NONPHARMACOLOGIC THERAPY

Provide IV hydration; withhold oral feedings.

ACUTE GENERAL Rx

- Laparoscopic cholecystectomy is considered the treatment of choice for most patients. The rate of conversion to open cholecystectomy is higher when laparoscopic cholecystectomy is performed for acute cholecystitis rather than for uncomplicated cholelithiasis; conservative management with IV fluids and antibiotics (ampicillin-sulbactam [Unasyn] 3 g IV q6h *or* piperacillin-tazobactam [Zosyn] 4.5 g IV q8h) may be justified in some high-risk patients to convert an emergency procedure into an elective one with a lower mortality rate.
- Endoscopic retrograde cholangiopancreatoscopy with sphincterectomy and stone extraction can be performed in conjunction with laparoscopic cholecystectomy for patients with choledochal lithiasis; approximately 7% to 15% of patients with cholelithiasis also have stones in the common bile duct.

DISPOSITION

- Prognosis is good; elective laparoscopic cholecystectomy can be performed as outpatient procedure.
- Hospital stay (when necessary) varies from overnight with laparoscopic cholecystectomy to 4 to 7 days with open cholecystectomy.
- Complication rate is approximately 1% (hemorrhage and bile leak) for laparoscopic cholecystectomy and <0.5% (infection) with open cholecystectomy.

REFERRAL

Surgical referral in all patients with acute cholecystitis

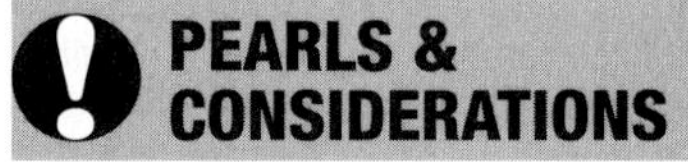

PEARLS & CONSIDERATIONS

COMMENTS

- Patients should be instructed that stones may recur in bile ducts.
- Gallbladder aspiration, in which all fluid visualized by ultrasound is aspirated, represents a nonsurgical treatment when patients who are at high operative risk develop acute cholecystitis. Salvage cholecystectomy is reserved for nonresponders.

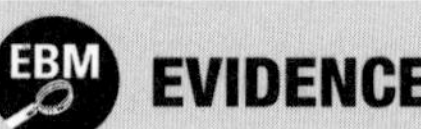

EVIDENCE

Please note: Complete text of EBM for this topic is available online.

SUGGESTED READING

Strasberg SM: Acute calculous cholecystitis, *N Engl J Med* 358:2804, 2008.

AUTHOR: **FRED F. FERRI, M.D.**

BASIC INFORMATION

DEFINITION

Cholelithiasis is the presence of stones in the gallbladder.

SYNONYMS

Gallstones

ICD-9CM CODES

574.2 Calculus of the gallbladder without mention of cholecystitis

574.0 Calculus of the gallbladder with acute cholecystitis

EPIDEMIOLOGY & DEMOGRAPHICS

- Gallstone disease can be found in 12% of the U.S. population. Of these, 2% to 3% (500,000 to 600,000) are treated with cholecystectomies each year.
- Annual medical expenditures for gallbladder surgeries in the U.S. exceed $5 billion.
- Incidence of gallbladder disease increases with age. Highest incidence is in the fifth and sixth decades. Predisposing factors for gallstones are female sex, pregnancy, age >40 yr, family history of gallstones, obesity, ileal disease, oral contraceptives, diabetes mellitus, rapid weight loss, estrogen replacement therapy.
- Patients with gallstones have a 20% chance of developing biliary colic or its complications at the end of a 20-yr period.

PHYSICAL FINDINGS & CLINICAL PRESENTATION

- Physical examination is entirely normal unless patient is having biliary colic; 80% of gallstones are asymptomatic.
- Typical symptoms of obstruction of the cystic duct include intermittent, severe, cramping pain affecting the right upper quadrant.
- Pain occurs mostly at night and may radiate to the back or right shoulder. It can last from a few minutes to several hours.

ETIOLOGY

- 75% of gallstones contain cholesterol and are usually associated with obesity, female sex, and diabetes mellitus; mixed stones are most common (80%); pure cholesterol stones account for only 10% of stones.
- 25% of gallstones are pigment stones (bilirubin, calcium, and variable organic material) associated with hemolysis and cirrhosis. These tend to be black-pigmented stones that are refractory to medical therapy.
- 50% of mixed-type stones are radiopaque.

DIAGNOSIS

DIFFERENTIAL DIAGNOSIS

- Pelvic ulcer disease
- Gastroesophageal reflux disease
- Irritable bowel disease
- Pancreatitis
- Neoplasms
- Nonnuclear dyspepsia
- Inferior wall myocardial infarction
- Hepatic abscess

LABORATORY TESTS

Generally normal unless patient has biliary obstruction (elevated alkaline phosphatase, bilirubin).

IMAGING STUDIES

- Ultrasound of the gallbladder will detect small stones and biliary sludge (sensitivity, 95%; specificity, 90%); the presence of dilated gallbladder with thickened wall is suggestive of acute cholecystitis.
- Nuclear imaging (HIDA scan) can confirm acute cholecystitis (>90% accuracy) if gallbladder does not visualize within 4 hr of injection and the radioisotope is excreted in the common bile duct.
- Common bile duct stones can be detected noninvasively by magnetic resonance cholangiopancreatography or invasively by endoscopic retrograde cholangiopancreatography (ERCP) and intraoperative cholangiography.

TREATMENT

NONPHARMACOLOGIC THERAPY

Lifestyle changes (avoidance of diets high in polyunsaturated fats, weight loss in obese patients; however, avoid rapid weight loss)

ACUTE GENERAL Rx

- The management of gallstones is affected by the clinical presentation.
- Asymptomatic patients do not require therapeutic intervention.
- Surgical intervention is generally the ideal approach for symptomatic patients. Laparoscopic cholecystectomy is generally preferred over open cholecystectomy because of the shorter recovery period and lower mortality rate. Between 5% and 26% of patients undergoing elective laparoscopic cholecystectomy will require conversion to an open procedure. Most common reason is the inability to clearly identify the biliary anatomy.
- Laparoscopic cholecystectomy after endoscopic sphincterectomy is recommended for patients with common bile duct stones and residual gallbladder stones. Where possible, single-stage laparoscopic treatments with removal of duct stones and cholecystectomy during the same procedure are preferable.
- Patients who are not appropriate candidates for surgery because of coexisting illness or patients who refuse surgery can be treated with oral bile salts: ursodiol (Actigall) 8 to 10 mg/kg/day in two to three divided doses for 16 to 20 mo, or chenodiol (Chenix) 250 mg bid initially, increasing gradually to a dose of 60 mg/kg/day. Candidates for oral bile salts are patients with cholesterol stones (radiolucent, noncalcified stones), with a diameter of ≤15 mm and having three or fewer stones. Candidates for medical therapy must have a functioning gallbladder and must have absence of calcifications on CT scans.
- Direct solvent dissolution with methyl *tert*-butyl ether (MTBE) is rarely used. Administration of the solvent is either through percutaneous transhepatic placement of a catheter into the gallbladder or endoscopic retrograde catheter placement with subsequent continuous infusion and aspiration of the solvent either manually or by automatic pump system.
- Extracorporeal shock wave lithotripsy (ESWL) is another form of medical therapy. It can be used in patients with stone diameter of ≤3 cm and having three or fewer stones.

DISPOSITION

- Recurrence rate after bile acid treatment is approximately 50% in 5 yr. Periodic ultrasound is necessary to assess the effectiveness of treatment.
- Gallstones recur after dissolution therapy with MTBE in >40% of patients within 5 yr.
- After ESWL, stones recur in approximately 20% of patients after 4 yr.
- Patients with at least one gallstone <5 mm in diameter have a greater than fourfold increased risk of presenting with acute biliary pancreatitis. A policy of watchful waiting in such cases is generally unwarranted.
- A potential serious complication of gallstones is acute cholangitis. ERCP and endoscopic sphincterectomy followed by interval laparoscopic cholecystectomy are effective in acute cholangitis.

SUGGESTED READINGS

Bellows CF et al: Management of gallstones, *Am Fam Physician* 72:637, 2005.

Moon JH et al: The detection of bile duct stones in suspected biliary pancreatitis: comparison of MRCP, ERCP, and intraductal US, *Am J Gastroenterol* 100: 1051, 2005.

AUTHOR: **FRED F. FERRI, M.D.**

Cholera

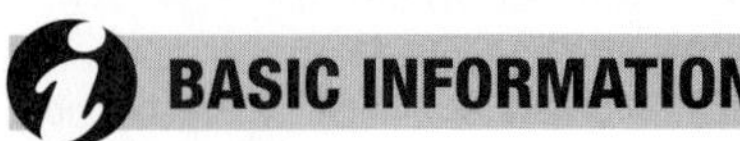

BASIC INFORMATION

DEFINITION

Cholera is an acute diarrheal illness caused by *Vibrio cholerae.*

ICD-9CM CODES
001.0 Cholera

EPIDEMIOLOGY & DEMOGRAPHICS

INCIDENCE (IN U.S.): Previously, approximately 50 cases per yr, mostly in travelers returning from endemic areas. From 1995 to 2000, 61 cases reported, 37 (61%) of which acquired outside the U.S.

PEAK INCIDENCE:
- None in the U.S.
- Summer and fall in endemic areas

PREDOMINANT SEX: None

PREDOMINANT AGE: In nonendemic areas, attack rates are equal in all age groups. In epidemic areas, children over the age of 2 yr are most commonly infected. Neonatal infection: illness is uncommon before the age of 2 yr, likely because of passive immunity.

PHYSICAL FINDINGS & CLINICAL PRESENTATION

Infection may result in asymptomatic illness or a mild diarrhea. The classic illness is described as the abrupt onset of voluminous watery diarrhea, which may lead to severe dehydration, acidosis, shock, and death. Vomiting may occur early in the illness, but fever and abdominal pain are usually absent. The typical "rice water" stools are pale with flecks of mucus and contain no blood. Muscle cramps may be prominent and are the result of loss of fluid and electrolytes. Untreated illness results in hypovolemic shock, and death may occur in hours to days. With adequate fluid and electrolyte repletion, cholera is a self-limited illness that resolves in a few days. The use of antimicrobials can shorten the course of illness.

ETIOLOGY The organism responsible for this illness is one of several strains of *V. cholerae.* Most infections result from the 01 serotype, the El Tor biotype. In the U.S., one outbreak occurred from the ingestion of illegally imported crab, and sporadic infection has been associated with the consumption of contaminated shellfish in Gulf Coast states. Most cases are seen in returning travelers. Transmission during epidemics is the result of the ingestion of contaminated water and, in some instances, contaminated food.

Dx DIAGNOSIS

DIFFERENTIAL DIAGNOSIS

- Mild illness may mimic gastroenteritis resulting from a variety of etiologies.
- Sudden, voluminous diarrhea causing marked dehydration is uncommon in other illnesses.

WORKUP Stool should be sent for culture and microscopy. Treatment should not be delayed while awaiting culture results.

LABORATORY TESTS

- WBC may be elevated, and hemoglobin may be increased as a result of hemoconcentration.
- Elevated BUN and creatinine suggests prerenal azotemia. Hypoglycemia may occur. Stool cultures on appropriate media may grow the organism. Wet mount of stool under dark field or phase contrast microscopy shows organisms with characteristic darting motility.

Rx TREATMENT

NONPHARMACOLOGIC THERAPY

The mainstay of therapy is adequate fluid and electrolyte replacement. This can usually be achieved using oral rehydration solutions containing salts and glucose. Some patients may require intravenous fluid and electrolyte replacement.

ACUTE GENERAL Rx

- Antimicrobial therapy can decrease shedding of fluid and organisms and can shorten the course of illness:
  1. Doxycycline 100 mg PO bid for 5 days *or*
  2. SMX-TMP, one DS tablet PO bid for 5 days *or*
  3. Azithromycin two 500 mg tablets PO as a single dose
- Resistance to SMX-TMP is increasing in travel-associated infections.

CHRONIC Rx It is likely that asymptomatic chronic carriers exist; however, because they are difficult to identify, and their role in transmission of disease appears to be rather limited, there is no recommendation for treatment of these individuals.

DISPOSITION The mortality of adequately hydrated patients is less than 1%.

REFERRAL If more than mild illness occurs

REPORTING In the U.S., all cases of cholera must be reported to the local and state health departments. Bacterial isolates must be sent to the state health department and the CDC.

PEARLS & CONSIDERATIONS

COMMENTS

- There is currently no indication for vaccination of travelers to endemic areas. The risk of infection is small, protection from available vaccines is limited, and side effects are prominent and frequent.
- Doxycycline should not be used to treat children or pregnant women.
- A recent study indicates a single dose treatment strategy with azithromycin is significantly better than ciprofloxacin for the management of cholera.

EBM EVIDENCE

Please note: Complete text of EBM for this topic is available online.

Key trials and commentary:

Infections due to *Vibrio* species cause an estimated 8000 illnesses annually, often through consumption of undercooked seafood. Like foodborne *Vibrio* infections, nonfoodborne *Vibrio* infections (NFVI) also result in serious illness, but awareness of these infections is limited.

This study showed that NFVIs, especially those due to *V. vulnificus*, demonstrate high morbidity and mortality. Persons with liver disease should be advised of the risks associated with seawater exposure if a wound is already present or is likely to occur. Clinicians should consider *Vibrio* species as an etiologic agent in infections occurring in persons with recent seawater exposure, even if the individual was only exposed during recreational marine activities. Immediate antibiotic treatment with aggressive monitoring is advised in suspected cases.

The awareness of serious illness from NFVI is limited. The Gulf Coast Vibrio Surveillance System (1988-1996) reported the largest case series of 189 *V. vulnificus* wound infections. Wound infections from *V. vulnificus* in this series were fatal in 17% of the cases. Subsequent to Hurricane Katrina, 22 cases of *Vibrio* wound infection and 5 deaths were reported. This study analyzed illnesses caused by *Vibrio* species reported to the CDC between 1997 and 2006. A total of 1210 (25%) of the *Vibrios* reported were NFVIs, *V. vulnificus* being the most common. The soft tissue infections, caused by *V. vulnificus,* demonstrated high morbidity and mortality. Risk factors include seawater exposure and liver disease. In patients suspected to have NFVI, immediate and appropriate antibiotic therapy should be instituted in addition to supportive care. Antimicrobial susceptibility of *Vibrio* species differs from that of common pathogens involved in skin and skin structure infections. Tetracycline and gentamicin are most useful.[1] Ⓐ

Evidence-Based Reference

1. Dechet AM et al: Nonfoodborne vibrio infections: an important cause of morbidity and mortality in the United States, 1997-2006, *Clin Infect Dis* 46:970-976, 2008. Commentary by N. Khardori, M.D. Ⓐ

SUGGESTED READINGS

Centers for Disease Control: Two cases of Vibrio cholera 01 infection after Hurricanes Katrina and Rita–Louisiana, October 2005, *MMWR Morb Mortal Wkly Rep* 55(2):31-32, 2006.

Hill DR et al: Oral cholera vaccines: use in clinical practice, *Lancet Infect Dis* 6(6):361, 2006.

Sack PD et al: Cholera, *Lancet* 363:223, 2004.

Saha D et al: Single dose azithromycin for the treatment of cholera in adults, *N Engl J Med* 354(23): 2452, 2006.

Tobin-D'Angelo M et al: Severe diarrhea caused by cholera toxin-producing vibrio cholerae serogroup 075 infections acquaired in the southeastern United States, *Clin Infect Dis* 47(8):1035-1040, 2008.

AUTHORS: **PATRICIA CRISTOFARO, M.D., GLENN G. FORT, M.D., M.P.H.,** and **DENNIS J. MIKOLICH, M.D.**

BASIC INFORMATION

DEFINITION

Chronic fatigue syndrome (CFS) is characterized by four or more of the following symptoms, present concurrently for at least 6 mo:

- Impaired memory or concentration
- Sore throat
- Tender cervical or axillary lymph nodes
- Muscle pain
- Multijoint pain
- New headaches
- Unrefreshing sleep
- Postexertion malaise

SYNONYMS

Yuppie flu
CFS
Chronic Epstein-Barr syndrome

ICD-9CM CODES
780.7 Chronic fatigue syndrome
300.8 Neurasthenia

EPIDEMIOLOGY & DEMOGRAPHICS

PREVALENCE IN U.S.: 10 to 300 cases per 100,000 persons
PREDOMINANT AGE: Young adulthood and middle age
PREDOMINANT SEX: Females affected more often than males

PHYSICAL FINDINGS & CLINICAL PRESENTATION

- There are no physical findings specific for CFS.
- The physical examination may be useful to identify fibromyalgia and other rheumatologic conditions that may coexist with CFS.

ETIOLOGY

- The etiology of CFS is unknown.
- Many experts suspect that a viral illness may trigger certain immune responses that lead to the various symptoms. Most patients often report the onset of their symptoms with a flulike illness.

DIAGNOSIS

DIFFERENTIAL DIAGNOSIS

- Psychosocial depression, dysthymia, anxiety-related disorders, and other psychiatric diseases
- Infectious diseases (subacute bacterial endocarditis, Lyme disease, fungal diseases, mononucleosis, HIV, chronic hepatitis B or C, TB, chronic parasitic infections)
- Autoimmune diseases: SLE, myasthenia gravis, multiple sclerosis, thyroiditis, RA
- Endocrine abnormalities: hypothyroidism, hypopituitarism, adrenal insufficiency, Cushing's syndrome, diabetes mellitus, hyperparathyroidism, pregnancy, reactive hypoglycemia
- Occult malignant disease
- Substance abuse
- Systemic disorders: chronic renal failure, chronic obstructive pulmonary disease, cardiovascular disease, anemia, electrolyte abnormalities, liver disease
- Other: inadequate rest, sleep apnea, narcolepsy, fibromyalgia, sarcoidosis, medications, toxic agent exposure, Wegener's granulomatosis

LABORATORY TESTS

- No specific laboratory tests exist for diagnosing CFS. Initial laboratory tests are useful to exclude other conditions that may mimic or may be associated with CFS.
  1. Screening laboratory tests: CBC, ESR, ALT, total protein, albumin, globulin, alkaline phosphatase, calcium, phosphorus, glucose, BUN, creatinine, electrolytes, TSH, and urinalysis are useful.
  2. Serologic tests for Epstein-Barr virus, *Candida albicans,* human herpesvirus 6, and other studies for immune cellular abnormalities are not useful; these tests are expensive and generally not recommended.
- Other tests may be indicated depending on the history and physical examination (e.g., ANA, RF in patients presenting with joint complaints or abnormalities on physical examination, Lyme titer in areas where Lyme disease is endemic).

IMAGING STUDIES

Generally not recommended unless history and physical examination indicate specific abnormalities (e.g., chest radiography in any patient suspected of TB or sarcoidosis)

TREATMENT

NONPHARMACOLOGIC THERAPY

- Patients should be reassured that the illness is not fatal and that most patients improve over time.
- An initially supervised exercise program to preserve and increase strength is beneficial for most patients and can improve symptoms.

GENERAL Rx

Therapy is generally palliative. The following medications may be helpful; however, evidence is conflicting:

- Antidepressants: The choice of antidepressant varies with the desired side effects. Patients with difficulty sleeping or fibromyalgia-like symptoms may benefit from low-dose tricyclics (doxepin 10 mg hs or amitriptyline 25 mg qhs). When sedation is not desirable, low-dose SSRIs (paroxetine 20 mg qd) often help alleviate fatigue and associated symptoms.
- NSAIDs can be used to relieve muscle and joint pain and headaches.

"Alternative" medications (herbs, multivitamins, nutritional supplements) are very popular with many CFS patients but are generally not very helpful.

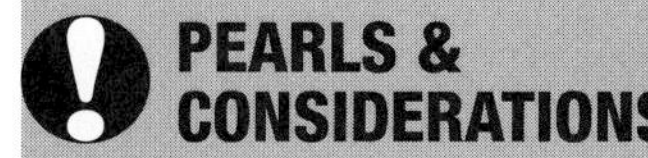

PEARLS & CONSIDERATIONS

COMMENTS

- In CFS the symptoms are serious enough to reduce daily activities by >50% in the absence of any other medically identifiable disorders.
- Moderate to complete recovery at 1 yr occurs in 22% to 60% of patients with CFS.

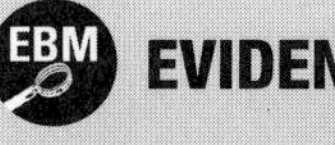

EVIDENCE

Graded aerobic exercise has been shown to result in improvements in fatigue and physical functioning in patients with CFS.[1] Ⓐ

A randomized, controlled trial compared graded exercise plus fluoxetine, graded exercise plus placebo, general advice to exercise plus fluoxetine, and general advice to exercise plus placebo. After 26 wk significantly fewer patients in the active exercise groups experienced fatigue.[2] Ⓐ

Cognitive-behavioral therapy appears to be an effective treatment for adult outpatients with CFS. Physical functioning is significantly improved, and the treatment is highly acceptable to patients.[3] Ⓐ

There is insufficient evidence for the benefit of corticosteroids, nicotinamide adenine dinucleotide, immunoglobulins, prolonged rest, or antidepressants in the treatment of CFS.[4]

Evidence-Based References

1. Edmonds M et al: Exercise therapy for chronic fatigue syndrome, *Cochrane Rev* 3:CD003200, 2004. Ⓐ
2. Wearden AJ et al: Randomised, double-blind, placebo controlled treatment trial of fluoxetine and a graded exercise programme for chronic fatigue syndrome, *Br J Psychiatry* 172:485, 1998. Ⓐ
3. Price JR, Couper J: Cognitive behaviour therapy for chronic fatigue syndrome in adults *Cochrane Rev* 2:CD001027, 2000. Ⓐ
4. Reid S et al: Chronic fatigue syndrome. In: *Clinical evidence*, 12, London, 2003, BMJ Publishing Group.

SUGGESTED READING

Hickie I et al: Post-infective and chronic fatigue syndromes precipitated by viral and non-viral pathogens: prospective cohort study, *BMJ* 333:575, 2006.

AUTHOR: **FRED F. FERRI, M.D.**

BASIC INFORMATION

DEFINITION

A chronic demyelinating disease of the spinal nerve roots and peripheral nerves that is marked by sensory deficits and muscle weakness.

SYNONYMS

CIDP

RELATED DISORDERS

- Multifocal motor neuropathy with conduction block
- Lewis-Sumner syndrome
- Multifocal acquired demyelinating sensory and motor (MADSAM) neuropathy

ICD-9CM CODES
357.8 Inflammatory and toxic neuropathy, other (use for chronic inflammatory demyelinating polyneuropathy)

EPIDEMIOLOGY & DEMOGRAPHICS

PREVALENCE: 1.0 to 1.9 per 100,000
PREDOMINANT SEX: Male predominance
PREDOMINANT AGE: Most common in the fifth to seventh decade, although may also occur in children

PHYSICAL FINDINGS & CLINICAL PRESENTATION

- Onset is over weeks, months, or years.
- Symptoms may be both sensory (paresthesias, neuropathic pain, and numbness of the hands and feet) and motor (weakness).
- Postural instability, gait abnormalities, and proximal muscle weakness may become prominent late in the disease.
- Sensory findings on examination include impaired vibration and joint position sense more commonly than impaired light touch, pinprick, and temperature sensation.
- Muscle weakness is usually distal and symmetric, although may occasionally be asymmetric and more proximal than distal.
- Reflexes are usually reduced or absent.
- Cranial nerve abnormalities as well as bowel and bladder dysfunction are highly unusual.
- Autonomic dysfunction is rare, but may occur.

ETIOLOGY

CIDP occurs as a primary (idiopathic) form and may also occur in association with a number of systemic disorders.

- The idiopathic variety is most common and an autoimmune process is likely.
- The most common systemic disorder associated with CIDP is a monoclonal gammopathy of undetermined significance (MGUS).
- Occasionally an underlying plasma cell dyscrasia such as Waldenstrom's macroglobulinemia, multiple myeloma, or osteosclerotic myeloma may be identified.
- An association with diabetes mellitus has been recognized more recently.
- CIDP may occasionally occur in the context of human immunodeficiency virus (HIV) and hepatitis B or C virus infection.

DIAGNOSIS

DIFFERENTIAL DIAGNOSIS

- Guillain-Barré syndrome (GBS)—the difference being that GBS evolves over a maximum of 4 wk and CIDP usually progresses over at least 8 wk.
- Diabetic neuropathy—the distinction can often be made with electrodiagnostic studies, which typically show axonal physiology in diabetic neuropathy.
- Mononeuritis multiplex.
- Monoclonal gammopathy of undetermined significance, plasma cell dyscrasia, osteosclerotic myeloma, and HIV infection are not so much part of the differential diagnosis, but may coexist and so should always be sought.

WORKUP

Nerve conduction studies and electromyography—these should show evidence of primary demyelination (with or without secondary axonal loss).

LABORATORY TESTS

- Lumbar puncture
  1. Shows increased CSF protein
  2. There is little or no pleocytosis (<10 white cells)
- Serum protein electrophoresis and immunofixation electrophoresis to search for M-protein
- Urine protein electrophoresis
- Hepatitis and HIV serology
- Fasting blood sugar and/or glucose tolerance test
- Bone marrow biopsy if a monoclonal gammopathy is identified to exclude myeloma or other plasma cell dyscrasias

IMAGING STUDIES

Long bone skeletal survey to identify osteosclerotic myeloma

TREATMENT

NONPHARMACOLOGIC THERAPY

- Physical and occupational therapy
- Ankle foot orthoses if there is significant weakness of ankle dorsiflexion

ACUTE GENERAL Rx

- The three primary treatment modalities for CIDP include high-dose oral corticosteroids, intravenous immunoglobulin (IVIg), and plasma exchange (PE).
- The benefit of each of these primary treatment modalities has been proven in randomized controlled trials, but their relative efficacies have not been evaluated.
- These three options for therapy should be discussed with the patient and a decision made to initiate therapy with one modality based on patient preference, tolerability of potential side effects, and cost (IVIg and PE are extremely expensive).
- IVIg is usually administered at a dose of 2 g/kg divided over 3 to 5 days. Initial improvement is observed in two thirds of patients. If there has been incomplete improvement or no major improvement, it is advised to repeat the course of IVIg in 1 to 2 months. If there continues to be further improvement of symptoms after repeated administration of IVIg, monthly infusions may be necessary to maintain a response.
- PE is usually performed every other day for approximately 4 to 6 weeks. Like IVIg, plasma exchanges may be repeated on a regular basis if therapeutic benefit has been established.
- Oral prednisone is usually initiated at a dose of ~1 mg/kg/day. High-dose prednisone dosing should be maintained until a clinical response is achieved, typically within 4 to 8 wk, after which the dose may be slowly tapered. The goal is to maintain a clinical response with the lowest possible dose administered on an alternate-day regimen.

CHRONIC Rx

- IVIg, PE, and/or prednisone are usually required on a chronic basis to maintain a clinical response. The frequency and dosing requirements must be determined on an individual basis.
- Steroid-sparing agents such as azathioprine, mycophenolate mofetil, methotrexate, cyclosporine, or cyclophosphamide may sometimes be necessary to reduce the maintenance dose of steroids or the frequency with which IVIg or PE is administered.

DISPOSITION

- Prognosis for functional recovery is quite variable, although most patients (70% to 80%) will be left with only minor disability (some difficulty with premorbid activities, but functionally independent) if treated aggressively with immunosuppressive therapy.
- Approximately 15% to 30% of patients will be left with moderate disability (i.e., require significant assistance with activities of daily living or with ambulation).
- In terms of the neuropathy, there is no clear evidence that the prognosis differs for patients with idiopathic forms of CIDP compared with those with CIDP associated with monoclonal proteins.
- Overall prognosis (not related to the neuropathy) may be worse in patients with multiple myeloma.
- Younger age, female gender, and the presence of a relapsing-remitting (rather than a monophasic progressive) course may portend a better prognosis.

REFERRAL

- Neurologist
- Physical therapy
- Occupational therapy
- Hematologist for further evaluation and management of associated plasma cell dyscrasia

PEARLS & CONSIDERATIONS

COMMENTS

- Electrophysiology (nerve conduction studies) offer the best combination of sensitivity and specificity for the diagnosis of CIDP.
- Lumbar puncture for CSF analysis is also helpful, especially if a markedly elevated protein without associated pleocytosis is found.

PREVENTION

There is no known preventative therapy.

PATIENT/FAMILY EDUCATION

CIDP is a chronic and often lifelong illness that may be punctuated by long periods of remission and significant improvement. With appropriate therapy, patients often return to previous baseline level of functioning. Relapses, however, do occur. Complications of chronic steroid use are significant causes of morbidity in patients with CIDP.

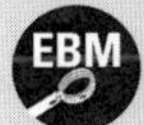

EVIDENCE

There is no evidence that steroid treatment given alone is beneficial in the treatment of GBS, but there is weak evidence that it can be of benefit in the treatment of CIDP.

Expert opinion and systematic reviews of trials comparing the use of steroids vs. placebo provide no evidence that the use of steroids in the treatment of GBS is beneficial.[1] Ⓐ Ⓒ

The authors of a systematic review concluded that the results of a small randomized controlled trial provided weak evidence to support the experience from large nonrandomized studies, which suggests that steroids are beneficial in reducing impairment from CIDP.[2] Ⓐ

The available evidence is inadequate to assess whether azathioprine, interferon beta, or any other immunosuppressive drug or interferon is beneficial for the treatment of CIDP.

A systematic review of cytotoxic drugs and interferons identified only one small, open trial of azathioprine and one small trial of interferon beta for the treatment of CIPD. Neither trial showed any significant beneficial effect on any of the outcomes measured. The authors of the review concluded that the evidence is inadequate to assess whether these or any other immunosuppressive drug or interferon is beneficial for the treatment of CIDP.[3] Ⓐ

Evidence-Based References

1. Hughes RAC et al: Corticosteroids for Guillain-Barré syndrome, *Cochrane Rev,* 2, 2006. Ⓐ Ⓒ
2. Mehndiratta MM et al: Plasma exchange for chronic inflammatory demyelinating polyradiculoneuropathy, *Cochrane Rev,* 3, 2004. Ⓐ
3. Hughes RAC, Swan AV, van Doorn PA: Cytotoxic drugs and interferons for chronic inflammatory demyelinating polyradiculoneuropathy, *Cochrane Rev,* 4, 2004. Ⓐ

SUGGESTED READINGS

Adams R, Victor M: *Principles of neurology,* New York, 1993, McGraw-Hill.

Bouchard C et al: Clinicopathologic findings and prognosis of chronic inflammatory demyelinating polyneuropathy, *Neurology* 52:498, 1999.

Hughes RAC, Swan AV, van Doorn PA: Cytotoxic drugs and interferons for chronic inflammatory demyelinating polyradiculoneuropathy, *Cochrane Database Sys Rev* 3, 2005.

Koller H et al: Chronic inflammatory demyelinating polyneuropathy, *N Engl J Med* 352:1343, 2005.

Mehndriatta M, Hughes R: Corticosteroids for chronic inflammatory demyelinating polyradiculopathy, *Cochrane Database Sys Rev* 2, 2004.

Mehndriatta M, Hughes R, Agarwal P: Plasma exchange for chronic inflammatory demyelinating polyradiculoneuropathy, *Cochrane Database Sys Rev* (3):CD003906, 2004.

Noseworthy J et al: *Neurological therapeutics principles and practice,* London and New York, 2003, Martin Dunitz.

Van Schaik IN et al: Intravenous immunoglobulin for chronic inflammatory demyelinating polyradiculoneuropathy, *Cochrane Database Sys Rev* 3, 2005.

AUTHOR: **GENNA GEKHT, M.D.**

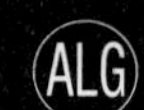

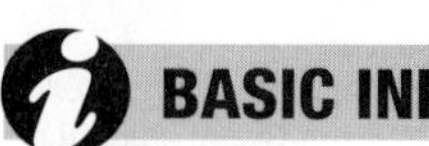

BASIC INFORMATION

DEFINITION

- Chronic obstructive pulmonary disease (COPD) is an inflammatory respiratory disease caused by exposure to tobacco smoke. It is characterized by the presence of airflow limitation that is not fully reversible. The pathophysiology of COPD is related to chronic airway irritation, mucus production, and pulmonary scarring. Traditionally, COPD was described as encompassing *emphysema,* characterized by loss of lung elasticity and destruction of lung parenchyma with enlargement of air spaces, and *chronic bronchitis,* characterized by obstruction of small airways and productive cough >3 mo for more than 2 successive years. These terms are no longer included in the formal definition of COPD, although they are still used clinically.
- Patients with COPD have also been classically subdivided in two major groups based on their appearance:
  1. *Blue bloaters* are patients with chronic bronchitis; the name is derived from the bluish tinge of the skin (as a result of chronic hypoxemia and hypercapnia) and from the frequent presence of peripheral edema (from cor pulmonale); chronic cough with production of large amounts of sputum is characteristic.
  2. *Pink puffers* are patients with emphysema; they have a cachectic appearance but pink skin color (adequate oxygen saturation); shortness of breath is manifested by pursed-lip breathing and use of accessory muscles of respiration.

SYNONYMS

COPD
Emphysema
Chronic bronchitis

ICD-9CM CODES
496 COPD
492.8 Emphysema

EPIDEMIOLOGY & DEMOGRAPHICS

- COPD affects 16 million Americans and is responsible for >80,000 deaths annually.
- COPD is the fourth leading cause of death in the U.S. and is expected to become the third leading cause of death by 2020.
- Highest incidence is in males >40 yr.
- 16 million office visits, 500,000 hospitalizations, 120,000 deaths annually, and >$18 billion in direct health care costs annually can be attributed to COPD.

PHYSICAL FINDINGS & CLINICAL PRESENTATION

- Peripheral cyanosis, productive cough, tachypnea, tachycardia.
- Dyspnea, pursed-lip breathing with use of accessory muscles for respiration, decreased breath sounds, wheezing.
- Acute exacerbation of COPD is mainly a clinical diagnosis and generally manifests with worsening dyspnea, increase in sputum purulence, and increase in sputum volume.

ETIOLOGY

- Tobacco exposure
- Occupational exposure to pulmonary toxins (e.g., dust, noxious gases, vapors, fumes, cadmium, coal, silica). The industries with the highest exposure risk are plastics, leather, rubber, and textiles.
- Atmospheric pollution.
- Alpha-1-antitrypsin deficiency (rare; <1% of COPD patients).

Dx DIAGNOSIS

DIFFERENTIAL DIAGNOSIS

- Congestive heart failure
- Asthma
- Respiratory infections
- Bronchiectasis
- Cystic fibrosis
- Neoplasm
- Pulmonary embolism
- Sleep apnea, obstructive
- Hypothyroidism

WORKUP

Chest radiograph, pulmonary function testing (spirometry), oxygen saturation, blood gases (in selected patients with acute exacerbation)

LABORATORY TESTS

- Complete blood count may reveal leukocytosis with left shift during acute exacerbation.
- Sputum may be purulent with bacterial respiratory tract infections. Sputum staining and cultures are usually reserved for cases refractory to antibiotic therapy.
- Arterial blood gases: normocapnia, mild to moderate hypoxemia may be present.
- Spirometry: pulmonary function testing (PFT) reveals that the primary physiologic abnormality in COPD is an accelerated decline in forced expiratory volume in 1 sec (FEV_1) from the normal rate in adults >30 yr of approximately 30 ml/yr to nearly 60 ml/yr. PFT results in COPD reveal abnormal diffusing capacity, increased total lung capacity and/or residual volume, and fixed reduction in FEV_1 in patients with emphysema; normal diffusing capacity and reduced FEV_1 are found in patients with chronic bronchitis. PFTs can be used to estimate disease severity in COPD as follows (where FEV is forced vital capacity):
  Mild COPD: FEV_1/FVC < 0.70; FEV_1 ≥80% of predicted
  Moderate COPD: FEV_1/FVC < 0.70; FEV_1 50% to 79% of predicted
  Severe COPD: FEV_1/FVC < 0.70; FEV_1 30% to 49% of predicted
  Very severe COPD: FEV_1/FVC < 0.70; FEV_1 <30% of predicted or <50% of predicted with chronic respiratory failure (SaO_2 <88%)
- Patients with COPD can generally be distinguished from asthmatics by their incomplete response to albuterol (change in FEV_1 <200 ml and 12%) and absence of an abnormal bronchoconstrictor response to methacholine or other stimuli. However, nearly 40% of patients with COPD respond to bronchodilators.

IMAGING STUDIES

Chest x-ray:
- Hyperinflation with flattened diaphragm, tenting of the diaphragm at the rib, and increased retrosternal chest space (Fig. 1-68)
- Decreased vascular markings and bullae in patients with emphysema
- Thickened bronchial markings and enlarged right side of the heart in patients with chronic bronchitis

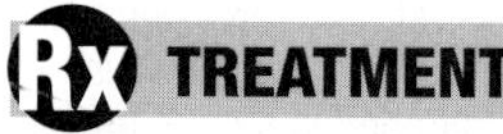

TREATMENT

NONPHARMACOLOGIC THERAPY

- Weight loss in obese patients.
- Avoidance of tobacco and elimination of air pollutants.
- Supplemental oxygen, usually through a face mask, to ensure oxygen saturation >90% as measured by pulse oximetry.
- Pulmonary clearing: careful nasotracheal suction is indicated only in patients with excessive secretions and an inability to expectorate. Mechanical percussion of the chest as applied by a physical or respiratory therapist is ineffective with acute exacerbations of COPD.

GENERAL Rx

- Pharmacologic treatment should be administered in a stepwise approach according to

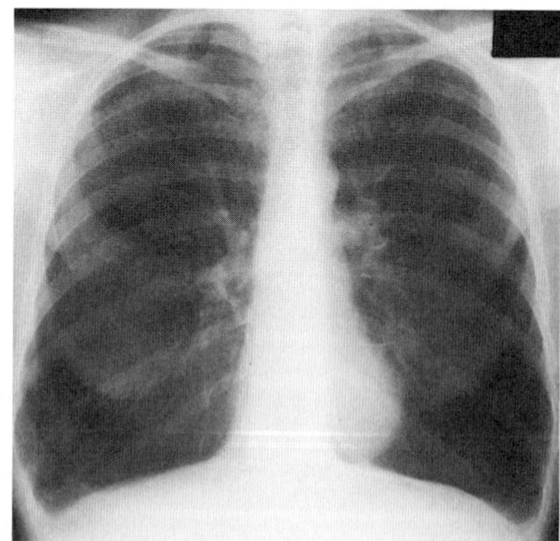

FIGURE 1-68 Severe diffuse emphysema. The posteroanterior chest radiograph shows the right hemidiaphragm to be flattened and located below the anterior aspect of the eighth rib. Left lung parenchyma is seen between the heart and the left hemidiaphragm. Arterial depletion is present in the lung bases. (From Grainger RG et al [eds]: *Grainger & Allison's diagnostic radiology,* ed 4, Philadelphia, 2001, Churchill Livingstone.)

the severity of disease and patient's tolerance for specific drugs.

1. Bronchodilators improve symptoms, quality of life, and exercise tolerance and decrease incidence of exacerbations.
2. Short-acting beta-2 agonists (e.g., albuterol metered-dose inhaler 1 to 2 puffs q4-6h prn) are acceptable in patients with mild, variable symptoms. Long-acting inhaled agents (e.g., salmeterol or formoterol 1 or 2 puffs bid) are preferred in patients with mild to moderate or continuous symptoms.
3. Anticholinergics (e.g., ipratropium inhaler 2 puffs qid) are also effective and are available in combination with albuterol (Combivent). Tiotropium (Spiriva handihaler) is a newer long-acting bronchodilator. It is very effective for the long-term, once-a-day maintenance treatment of bronchospasm.
4. Addition of inhaled steroids (fluticasone, budesonide, triamcinolone) is used to reduce exacerbations in patients with moderate to severe COPD.

- Acute exacerbation of COPD can be treated with:
  1. Aerosolized beta-2 agonists (e.g., metaproterenol nebulizer solution 5% 0.3 ml or albuterol nebulized 5% solution 2.5 to 5 mg).
  2. Anticholinergic agents, which have equivalent efficacy to inhaled beta-adrenergic agonists. Inhalant solution of ipratropium bromide 0.5 mg can be administered every 4 to 8 hr.
  3. Short courses of systemic corticosteroids have been shown to improve spirometric and clinical outcomes. In the hospital setting give IV methylprednisolone 50- to 100-mg bolus, then 40 mg q6-8h; taper as soon as possible. In the outpatient setting, oral prednisone 40 mg/day initially, decreasing the dose by 10 mg every other day is generally effective.
  4. Use of noninvasive positive pressure ventilation (NIPPV) decreases the risk of endotracheal intubation and decreases intensive care unit admission rates. Contraindications to its use are uncooperative patient, decreased level of consciousness, hemodynamic instability, inadequate mask fit, and severe respiratory acidosis. Increased airway pressure can be delivered by using inspiratory positive airway pressure, continuous positive airway pressure, or bilevel positive airway pressure, which combines the other modalities. When using NIPPV, the nasal mask is usually tolerated the best; however, patients must be instructed to keep their mouths closed while breathing with the nasal apparatus. Oxygen can be delivered at 10 to 15 L/min and started in spontaneous ventilation mode with an initial expiratory positive airway pressure setting of 3 to 5 cm H_2O and an inspiratory positive airway pressure setting of 8 to 10 cm H_2O. Adjustments in these settings should be made in 2-cm H_2O increments. It is important to monitor patients with frequent vital signs measurements, arterial blood gases, or pulse oxymetry. Intubation and mechanical ventilation may be necessary if previous measures fail to provide improvement.
  5. The role of inhaled corticosteroids (ICS) in COPD is controversial. Although some trials have demonstrated mild improvement in patients' symptoms and decreased frequency of exacerbations, most pulmonologists believe that these drugs are ineffective in most patients with COPD but should be considered for patients with moderate to severe airflow limitation who have persistent symptoms despite optimal bronchodilator therapy. ICS therapy does not affect 1-year all-cause mortality among patients with COPD and is associated with a higher risk of pneumonia.
  6. IV aminophylline administration is controversial and generally not recommended. When used, serum levels should be closely monitored (keep level 8 to 12 mcg/ml) to minimize risks of tachyarrhythmias.
- Appoximately 50% of COPD exacerbations are caused by bacterial infection. Antibiotics are indicated in suspected respiratory infection (e.g., increased purulence and volume of phlegm).
  1. *Haemophilus influenzae* and *Streptococcus pneumoniae* are frequent causes of acute bronchitis.
  2. Oral antibiotics of choice are azithromycin, levofloxacin, amoxicillin-clavulanate, and cefuroxime.
  3. The use of antibiotics is beneficial in exacerbations of COPD presenting with increased dyspnea and sputum purulence (especially if the patient is febrile).
- Guaifenesin may improve cough symptoms and mucus clearance; however, mucolytic medications are generally ineffective. Their benefits may be greatest in patients with more advanced disease.
- Lung volume reduction surgery has been proposed as a palliative treatment for severe emphysema. Overall it increases the chance of improved exercise capacity but does not confer a survival advantage over medical therapy. It is most beneficial in patients with both predominantly upper-lobe emphysema and low baseline exercise capacity.

In patients with end-stage emphysema who have an FEV_1 <25% of predicted normal value after administration of bronchodilator and additional complications such as severe hypoxemia, hypercapnia and pulmonary hypertension single-lung transplantation should be considered a surgical option.

DISPOSITION

- After the initial episode of respiratory failure, 5-yr survival is approximately 25%.
- Development of cor pulmonale or hypercapnia and persistent tachycardia are poor prognostic indicators.

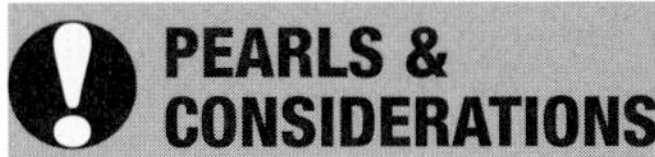

PEARLS & CONSIDERATIONS

COMMENTS

- All patients with COPD should receive pneumococcal vaccine and yearly influenza vaccine.
- In assessing the severity of COPD, the FEV_1 is limited by the fact that it does not take into account the systemic manifestations of COPD. The BODE index (***b***ody mass index, degree of ***o***bstruction, ***d***yspnea, and ***e***xercise capacity) has been proposed as a multidimensional scale to better assess the morbidity and mortality associated with COPD. It is better than the FEV_1 at predicting the risk of death from any cause and from respiratory causes among patients with COPD.

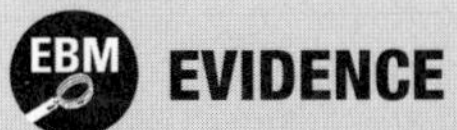

EVIDENCE

Please note: Complete text of evidence-based medicine (EBM) for this topic is available online.

Key trials and commentary:

This study sought to evaluate hospital readmission rates and mortality at 6-month follow-up in selected elderly patients with acute exacerbation of chronic obstructive pulmonary disease (COPD).

This study showed that physician-led substitutive hospital-at-home care as an alternative to inpatient care for elderly patients with acute exacerbations of COPD is associated with a substantial reduction in the risk of hospital readmission at 6 months, lower healthcare costs, and better quality of life.

In this Italian study, patients aged 75 years and older with COPD exacerbations (increased breathlessness, increased sputum production, and increased sputum purulence) were randomized to an organized home hospitalization service or the general medical ward for care. Patients receiving home care had to have good support systems and could not have severe hypoxemia, acidosis or alkalemia, or significant comorbid illness. Outcomes were similar in the two groups. However, the home-managed patients did not have to endure the disorienting experience of hospitalization, exposure to all the hazards older patients face in the hospital, and the cost of care was slightly less. This was reflected in improvements in depression and quality of life in this group compared with the hospitalized group. Unfortunately, home hospital programs are not well developed in the United States, but this study and others suggest that this may well be the best approach to management of many elderly patients who need acute care and have a baseline limited disease burden.[1] Ⓐ

Skeletal muscle strength and bulk are reduced in patients with COPD and influence quality of life, survival, and utilization of health care resources. Exercise training during pulmonary rehabilitation (PR) can reverse some of these effects. In athletes and healthy elderly individuals, dietary creatine supplementation (CrS) has been shown to augment high-intensity exercise training, thereby increasing muscle mass. This adequately powered, randomized, placebo-controlled trial shows that CrS does not augment the substantial training effect of multidisciplinary PR for patients with COPD.

A number of different approaches—hormonal therapy, dietary therapy, and supplements—have been tried as adjunctive treatments to try to improve the physical status and exercise capacity of patients with advanced COPD. Creatine is one supplement that has been shown in healthy subjects to increase muscle mass, enhance high-intensity exercise, and has been proposed as a candidate for doing the same in COPD patients. There is evidence (by muscle biopsy) in COPD patients that phosphocreatine is lower than normal. This group of authors has demonstrated a correlation between phosphocreatine preexercise and the incremental shuttle walking distance. This, along with other data, seems to make a case that creatine supplementation would be useful in patients with advanced COPD. To determine if creatine would impact exercise capacity, the authors performed a double-blind, randomized trial with one group of patients receiving a placebo supplement and the other creatine supplement. They found that both groups improved with endurance and strength training programs, but there was no appreciable difference caused by creatine. This study is a negative study, but it is important because good, adequately powered, double-blind trials are uncommon in evaluating proposed adjunctive treatments for these very ill patients. Physicians often are tempted to try the latest fad treatment to offer something to these desperate patients. Good scientific evaluations can help physicians make the right decisions.[2] Ⓐ

A separate study sought to determine whether combining tiotropium with salmeterol or with fluticasone-salmeterol improves clinical outcomes in adults with moderate to severe COPD compared with tiotropium alone.

This study showed that addition of fluticasone-salmeterol to tiotropium therapy did not statistically influence rates of COPD exacerbation but did improve lung function, quality of life, and hospitalization rates in patients with moderate-to-severe COPD.

This study is included here for several reasons. It is one of the first well-designed studies to directly compare respiratory medications that are commonly used in day-to-day treatment in terms of outcomes. Although some studies have looked at the impact of these drugs or drug combinations individually on outcome parameters, this study compares them to each other in terms of outcomes. Outcomes are measured by proportion of patients with an exacerbation within the year of the study, mean number of COPD exacerbations per patient-year, parameters around health care use, and measures of health-related quality of life. Readers should be aware that during the year of the study a number of patients (between 52% and 74%) in each arm failed to complete the assigned drug treatment. In addition, the period of follow-up was only 1 year, which, although a common follow-up period for COPD drug trials, allows for only limited conclusions. This study should be followed by others with similarly well-designed trials that address the limitations noted here and that will help to ultimately define the roles of the various medications and medication combinations.[3] Ⓐ

Treatment with systemic corticosteroids for exacerbations of COPD results in improvement in clinical outcomes. On hospitalization, corticosteroids are generally administered intravenously (IV). It has not been established whether oral administration is equally effective. de Jong and colleagues conducted a study to demonstrate that therapy with oral prednisolone was not inferior to therapy with IV prednisolone using a double-blind, double-dummy design.

This study showed that therapy with oral prednisolone is not inferior to IV treatment in the first 90 days after starting therapy. We suggest that the oral route is preferable in the treatment of COPD exacerbations.

A number of studies have confirmed the benefit of corticosteroids in acute exacerbations of COPD, but less data are available on whether oral medicines are as effective as IV medicines. In this study from the Netherlands, the authors found no difference in outcomes whether you use oral or IV drugs. For both oral and IV groups, prednisolone 60 mg was administered for 5 days in addition to placebo medication to blind the administration route; after 5 days, all were placed on 30 mg oral prednisolone daily, then tapered by 5 mg each day to 0 mg or their previous stable baseline dose. All also received bronchodilators and antibiotics. It is important to note that the sickest patients (pH <7.26) were excluded from the study. The outcomes were the same for oral and IV groups, although the 90-day failure rate in both groups was quite high. This high failure rate may be related to the definition of failure, which in addition to including the usual death and readmission or readmission to intensive care unit (ICU) parameters also included that the patient's primary care physician had to increase the patient's medication (without admission). This makes the treatment failure rate seem somewhat larger than that of other studies. Overall, this study supports the noninferiority of oral corticosteroids in the managements of most COPD patients with exacerbations. Oral drugs are cheaper, easier to administer, take less nursing care, and allow more patient mobility among other things. Clearly this is the preferable way to go.[4] Ⓐ

Evidence-Based References

1. Aimonino Ricauda N et al: Substitutive "hospital at home" versus inpatient care for elderly patients with exacerbations of chronic obstructive pulmonary disease: a prospective randomized, controlled trial, *J Am Geriatr Soc* 56:493-500, 2008. Commentary by J. Maurer, M.D.

2. Deacon SJ et al: Randomized controlled trial of dietary creatine as an adjunct therapy to physical training in chronic obstructive pulmonary disease, *Am J Respir Crit Care Med* 178:233-239, 2008. Commentary by J. Maurer, M.D. Ⓐ

3. Aaron SD, for the Canadian Thoracic Society/Canadian Respiratory Clinical Research Consortium: Tiotropium in combination with placebo, salmeterol, or fluticasone-salmeterol for treatment of chronic obstructive pulmonary disease: a randomized trial, *Ann Intern Med* 146:545-555, 2007. Commentary by J.R. Maurer, M.D., M.B.A. Ⓐ

4. de Jong YP et al: Oral or IV prednisolone in the treatment of COPD exacerbations: a randomized, controlled, double-blind study, *Chest* 132:1741-1747, 2007. Commentary by J. Maurer, M.D. Ⓐ

SUGGESTED READINGS

Cosio MG et al: Immunologic aspects of chronic obstructive pulmonary disease, *N Engl J Med* 360: 2445-2454, 2009.

Drummond MB et al: Inhaled corticosteroids in patients with stable chronic obstructive pulmonary disease, *JAMA* 300(20): 2407-2416, 2008.

Eisner MD et al: COPD as a systemic disease: impact on physical functional limitations, *Am J Med* 121: 789, 2008.

Gross NJ: Chronic obstructive pulmonary disease: an evidence-based approach to treatment with a focus on anticholinergic bronchodilation, *Mayo Clin Proc* 83(11):1241-1250, 2008.

Rodriguez J et al: The association of pipe and cigar use with cotinine levels, lung function, and airflow obstruction, *Ann Int Med* 152:201-210, 2010.

Sethi S, Murphy TF: Infection in the pathogenesis and course of chronic obstructive pulmonary disease, *N Engl J Med* 359:2355-2365, 2008.

Stephens MB, Yew KS: Diagnosis of chronic obstructive pulmonary disease, *Am Fam Physician* 78(1): 87, 2008.

Tashkin DP et al: Comparing COPD treatment: nebulizer, metered dose inhaler, and concomitant therapy, *Am J Med* 120:435, 2007.

U.S. Preventive Services Task Force: Screening for chronic obstructive pulmonary disease using spirometry: U.S. Preventive Services Task Force recommendation statement, *Ann Intern Med* 148:529, 2008.

Wedzicha J, Seemungal TA: COPD exacerbation: defining their cause and prevention, *Lancet* 370:786, 2007.

AUTHOR: **FRED F. FERRI, M.D.**

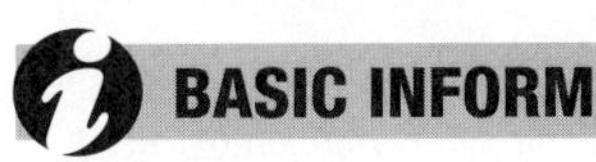

BASIC INFORMATION

DEFINITION

Chronic pain is pain that persists for longer than the expected time frame or that is associated with progressive, nonmalignant disease. Pain is an unpleasant sensory and emotional experience associated with actual or potential tissue damage or described in terms of such damage. The perception of pain is influenced by physiological, psychological, and social factors.

SYNONYMS

Nonmalignant chronic pain

ICD-9CM CODES

v15.89	Chronic pain
304.7x/304.8x	Opioid dependence

EPIDEMIOLOGY & DEMOGRAPHICS

The National Center for Health Statistics estimates that 32.8% of the U.S. population suffers from some form of chronic pain. Chronic pain is the third leading cause of physical impairment in the U.S., and related costs are estimated to be tens of billions annually. Patients with chronic pain may also experience changes in mood, depression, sleep disturbances, and fatigue, and decreased overall physical functioning.

CLINICAL PRESENTATION

- History: Comprehensive patient assessment, including history of present illness (cause of pain, location timing, characteristics, exacerbating/relieving factors, triggers, past therapies (pharmacologic and nonpharmacologic), medical history, family and social history, psychiatric history, substance use history, allergies, and current medications, should be performed on initial evaluation.
- Pain assessment: Performed at each visit; includes pain intensity (1 to 10), response to medication, attributes of pain, and assessment of function (cognitive, emotional, employment, sleep, mobility, and self-care).
- Physical examination: Directed at systems affected by pain and neurologic examination.

ETIOLOGY

Etiologies of chronic pain may include headache, low back pain, previous trauma, arthritis, neurogenic (e.g., trigeminal neuralgia), psychogenic (related to depression or anxiety), fibromyalgia, reflex sympathetic dystrophy, myofascial pain syndrome, phantom limb pain, idiopathic, or unknown.

DIAGNOSIS

DIFFERENTIAL DIAGNOSIS

- Based on proposed etiology
- Depression and anxiety disorders can be both a cause and a result of chronic pain, so temporal association of these disorders is important

WORKUP

- Laboratory testing, imaging studies, and/or electromyographic studies should be used when etiology of chronic pain is unknown or unclear, when comorbidities are suspected, and as the history and physical examination directs.
- Consider use of urine drug screen or other tests to screen for presence of illegal drugs, unreported prescribed medications, or alcohol use.

TREATMENT

- Studies increasingly support the application of a multidisciplinary approach that addresses the multiple facets of pain (e.g., physical, psychologic, social aspects).
- Therapeutic goal is the reduction of pain (elimination of chronic pain is generally unlikely and providers need to discuss these limitations with patients at outset).

NONPHARMACOLOGIC THERAPY

- Exercise
- Modalities: heat therapy, cold therapy, transcutaneous electrical nerve stimulation (TENS) units, cognitive behavioral therapy, psychologic counseling, physical therapy
- Electrostimulation therapy: TENS units
- Behavioral therapies: cognitive behavioral therapy, hypnosis, biofeedback, relaxation therapy
- Music therapy (in conjunction with other types of therapy)
- Surgery

ACUTE GENERAL Rx

- Short-acting anti-inflammatory and analgesic medications (e.g., acetaminophen/NSAIDs/opioids)
- Trigger point or joint injections (immediate anesthetic + long-acting corticosteroids)
- Epidural steroid injections
- Nerve blocks

CHRONIC Rx

- Pain management with long-acting pharmacologic agents is considered a key aspect of therapy but often underused; Figure 1-69 illustrates a strategy for pharmacologic management of pain using the World Health Organization (WHO) analgesic ladder
- Long-acting NSAIDs
- Sustained-release opioids (used for moderate-to-severe pain that has failed other therapeutic interventions): oxycodone, morphine SR, methadone (use with caution), or Duragesic patch; short-acting opioids can be used in conjunction with these agents for management of breakthrough pain; conversion to a long-acting opioid should be based on an equianalgesic conversion (http://www.acpinternist.org/archives/2008/01/extra/pain_charts.pdf)
- Antidepressants (tricyclic and selective serotonin reuptake inhibitor)
- Anticonvulsant medications: particularly helpful for neuropathic conditions
- Implantable methods: epidural and intrathecal drug delivery systems, dorsal column stimulators

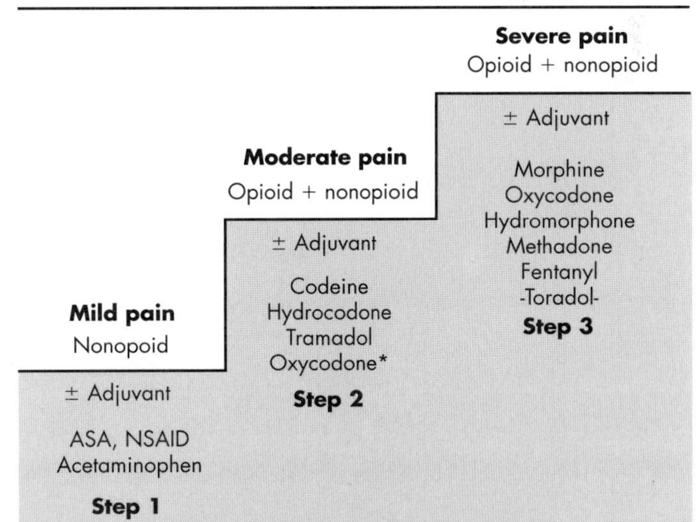

FIGURE 1-69 Strategy for pharmacologic management of pain using the World Health Organization (WHO) analgesic ladder. Multiagent therapy is usually required for optimal pain management. Patients with mild pain should be started on a nonopioid analgesic, and those with moderate pain on a step 2 opioid. Many patients can benefit from the addition of a nonopioid to the opioid (e.g., for bone pain) or an adjuvant agent to the opioid (e.g., for neuropathic pain). If this combination does not produce adequate relief or the patient has severe pain, step 3 opioids should be started initially. Toradol (Ketorolac) is a nonsteroidal anti-inflammatory drug (NSAID) with the pain-relieving potency of a step 3 opioid. Many patients can benefit from the addition of nonopioid analgesics or adjuvants, if indicated. *ASA,* Aspirin. (From Hoffman R et al: *Hematology, basic principles and practice,* ed 5, Philadelphia, 2009, Churchill Livingstone.)

COMPLEMENTARY & ALTERNATIVE MEDICINE

Acupuncture and massage (evidence based for some indications). Acupuncture is most likely to benefit patients with low back pain, neck pain, chronic idiopathic or tension headache, migraine, and knee osteoarthritis.

REFERRAL

- Pain medicine specialist or multidisciplinary pain clinic: useful when primary therapies fail, in patients with complex pain conditions, or for invasive therapies
- Consider referral to an addiction specialist if patient has a history of substance abuse or addiction
- Psychiatry/psychologic services for counseling, if needed

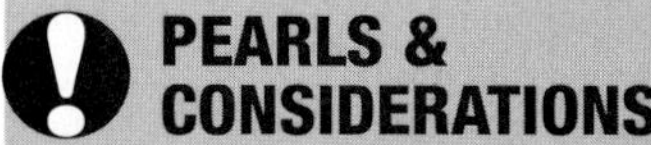

- Patient consent should be obtained in the form of a *written treatment agreement* before initiating treatment. This agreement should outline the goals of therapy, use of a single provider or treatment team, limitations on dose and number of prescribed medications, prohibition on use with alcohol or sedating medications, keeping medication safe and secure, prohibition on selling or sharing medication, limitations on refills, compliance with all components of the treatment plan, the role of drug screening, and consequences of nonadherence.
- Follow-up assessment should occur every 1 to 6 mo and include a complete pain assessment (see earlier), review of the type of long-acting analgesic used and dosage, use of breakthrough analgesics, side effects and their management, use of nonpharmacologic therapies, and adjunct medication use.

COMMENTS

- Medication dependence and addiction should not be confused. Most patients receiving chronic opioid therapy can become dependent on these medications for pain relief but opioid addiction does not occur. Patients exhibiting signs of addiction often will seek escalating doses of medication, request refills of prescriptions earlier than planned, and engage in drug-seeking activities (e.g., emergency department visits between prescriptions, seeking multiple prescriptions).
- Side effects need not preclude use of opioid medications and should be anticipated. Antiemetics can aid in controlling nausea. Constipation can be managed with increased fiber and water in diet, stool softeners, and laxatives.

PATIENT/FAMILY EDUCATION

National Pain Foundation (http://www.painconnection.org)
American Pain Foundation (http://www.painfoundation.org)
National Institutes of Health (http://www.nih.gov)

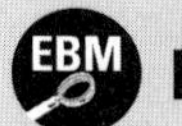

EVIDENCE

Please note: Complete text of EBM for this topic is available online.

Key trials and commentary:

Approximately 30% to 80% of postoperative patients complain about moderate to severe postsurgical pain, indicating that postoperative pain treatment is still a problem.

This study demonstrated that PCEA, IV-PCA, and CPNB are safe and efficient. Although all of these treatment strategies provide effective analgesia, PCEA and CPNB provided superior pain relief compared with IV-PCA. We demonstrated that serious complications of analgesic techniques are rare but possibly disastrous necessitating a close supervision by an acute pain service. This study found a low rate of adverse effects including hypotension and motor impairment and a low incidence of epidural hematoma for thoracic PCEA compared with lumbar PCEA

This study will be helpful for acute pain service personnel when convincing surgeons and patients of the safety and efficacy of continuous regional anesthetic techniques. The most obvious benefit was the reduction in pain with movement. Serious complications were rare, and the morbidity associated with these complications was remarkably low.

There is already substantial data that demonstrate improved functional outcomes, and there is some evidence that regional anesthetic techniques reduce the risk of persistent neuropathic pain after thoracotomy, amputation, and other surgeries that predispose to chronic pain development. However, cost-benefit studies are still needed. It is no longer enough to show improved medical outcomes.[1] Ⓐ

Evidence-Based Reference

1. Pöpping DM et al: Effectiveness and safety of postoperative pain management: a survey of 18 925 consecutive patients between 1998 and 2006 (2nd revision): a database analysis of prospectively raised data, *Br J Anaesth* 101:832-840, 2008. Commentary by S. Abram, M.D. Ⓐ

SUGGESTED READINGS

American Academy of Pain Medicine Web site. Available at www.painmed.org

American College of Physicians: ACP internist supplements, internist extra, chronic pain management: an appropriate use of opioid analgesics, January 2008: http://www.acpinternist.org/supplements. Last accessed March 2010.

Ashburn MA et al: Management of chronic pain, *Lancet* 353:1865-1869, 1999.

Chang G et al: Opioid tolerance and hyperalgesia, *Med Clin North Am* 91(2):199-211, 2007.

Kelly RB: Acupuncture for pain, *Am Fam Physician* 80(5):481-484, 2009.

Marcus D: Treatment of non-malignant chronic pain, *Am Fam Physician* 61:1331-1338, 2000.

AUTHOR: **ANNGENE A. GIUSTOZZI, M.D., M.P.H.**

BASIC INFORMATION

DEFINITION

Churg-Strauss syndrome (CSS) refers to a systemic necrotizing vasculitis accompanied by severe asthma (core clinical feature) and hypereosinophilia (HES).

SYNONYMS

Allergic angiitis
Allergic granulomatosis

ICD-9CM CODES
446.4 Angiitis, allergic granulomatous

EPIDEMIOLOGY & DEMOGRAPHICS

- Overall incidence of 2.4 cases per 1 million persons in the U.S. Among asthma patients, the annual incidence of CSS is estimated to average 34.6 per 1 million patients.
- Usually occurs at a mean age of 50 yr but may present as young as 4 yr or in the elderly
- Slight male/female predominance (1.3:1).
- Before steroid therapy, 50% of untreated patients with CSS died within 3 months of the onset of vasculitis. With treatment, 5-year survival exceeds 90%.

PHYSICAL FINDINGS & CLINICAL PRESENTATION

The clinical picture of CSS typically consists of three partially overlapping phases, which may or may not be sequential:

1. Prodromal phase:
    - Severe adult-onset asthma, with or without allergic rhinitis, sinusitis, headache, cough, and wheezing
    - Precedes development of systemic vasculitis by several years
2. Eosinophilic/tissue infiltration phase:
    - Peripheral eosinophilia and eosinophilic infiltration of the lungs, myocardium, and gastrointestinal (GI) tract, with or without granulomas
    - Signs and symptoms of cough, fever, anorexia, weight loss, sweats, malaise, nausea, vomiting, abdominal pain, and diarrhea
3. Systemic vasculitic phase:
    - Development of necrotizing vasculitis that is clinically apparent primarily in peripheral nerves, skin, and kidneys
    - Any organ can be affected, with skin involvement present in 50% to 67% of patients

Skin involvement is divided into three categories:

1. Erythematous maculopapules (can resemble erythema multiforme)
2. Hemorrhagic lesions (associated with wheals)
3. Cutaneous and subcutaneous nodules

ETIOLOGY

- Etiology unknown, but believed to be an autoimmune-mediated process
- Triggering factors implicated in CSS include inhaled allergens, vaccinations, infections, and drugs such as macrolides (see "Comments").

Dx DIAGNOSIS

- Clinical findings and biopsy showing eosinophilia vasculitis
- The American College of Rheumatology (ACR) has established the criteria for CSS diagnosis in patients without vasculitis:
    - Asthma
    - Eosinophilia >10% on white blood cell count
    - Mononeuropathy or polyneuropathy
    - Migratory pulmonary infiltrates
    - Paranasal sinus abnormalities
    - Extravascular eosinophils on biopsy

The presence of any four or more of the six criteria yields a sensitivity of 85% and a specificity of 99.7%. For patients with vasculitis, the presence of asthma and eosinophilia was 90% sensitive and 99% specific for CSS.

DIFFERENTIAL DIAGNOSIS

- Polyarteritis nodosa (PAN)
- Wegener's granulomatosis (WG)
- Goodpasture syndrome
- Loeffler syndrome
- Hypereosinophilia syndrome
- Rheumatoid arthritis
- Leukocytoclastic vasculitis

Although similar and at times grouped with patients with PAN or WG, CSS differs in that:

- CSS vasculitis involves small-sized arteries, veins, and venules.
- CSS, unlike PAN, predominantly involves the lung. Other organs affected include heart, GI system, central nervous system, kidney, and skin
- Kidney involvement is much less common in CSS than in WG. Pulmonary lesions in WG usually involve the upper respiratory tract rather than the peripheral lung parenchyma in CSS.
- CSS shows necrotizing vasculitis along with eosinophilic granulomas.

LABORATORY TESTS

- Complete blood count with differential: eosinophilia >10% is an American College of Rheumatology (ACR) diagnostic criterion.
- Blood urea nitrogen and creatinine may be mildly elevated, suggesting renal involvement.
- Urinalysis may show mild hematuria and proteinuria.
- 24-hour urine for protein; greater than 1 g/day is a poor prognostic factor.
- Perinuclear antineutrophilic cytoplasmic antibody (ANCA) is found in 13% to 70% of patients. Negative ANCA does not rule out CSS.
- Stools may be positive for occult blood (enteric involvement during eosinophilic phase).
- Elevation of aspartate aminotransferase, alanine aminotransferase, and creatine phosphokinase may indicate liver or muscle (skeletal or cardiac) involvement.
- Rheumatoid factor and antinuclear antibody may be positive. Erythrocyte sedimentation rate is usually elevated.
- Biopsy confirms the diagnosis. Surgical lung biopsy is the gold standard. Transbronchial biopsy is rarely helpful. Necrotizing vasculitis and extravascular necrotizing granulomas, usually with eosinophilic infiltrates, are suggestive of CSS. The presence of eosinophils in extravascular tissues is most specific for CSS.

IMAGING STUDIES

- Chest radiograph is abnormal in eosinophilic and vasculitic phases: asymmetrical bilateral patchy migratory infiltrates, interstitial lung disease, or nodular infiltrates (Fig. 1-70). Small pleural effusions are found in 29% of cases.

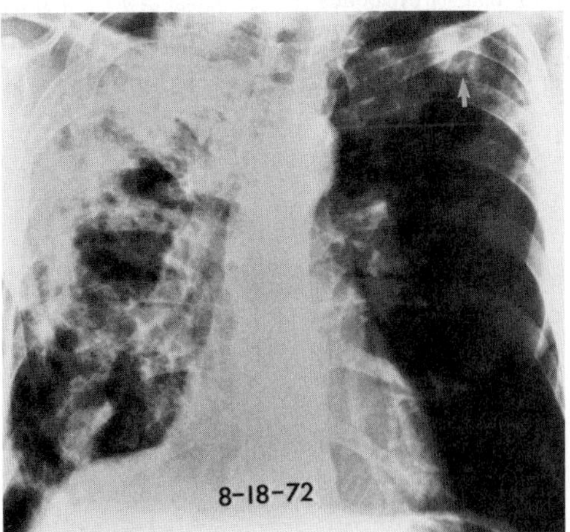

FIGURE 1-70 Allergic angiitis and granulomatosis. Posteroanterior chest radiograph demonstrates peripheral air space consolidation in the right lung and a nodule *(arrow)* in the left upper lobe in this asthmatic patient. (From McLoud TC [ed]: *Thoracic radiology: the requisites,* St Louis, 1998, Mosby.)

- Lung lesions in CSS are noncavitating, as opposed to those in WG.
- Paranasal sinus films may reveal sinus opacification, which is an ACR diagnostic criterion.
- Angiography is sometimes done in patients with mesenteric ischemia or renal involvement.

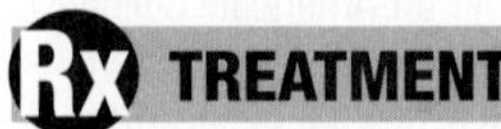

TREATMENT

NONPHARMACOLOGIC THERAPY

Oxygen therapy in severe asthmatic exacerbations

PHARMACOLOGIC THERAPY

The following five factors suggest poor prognosis (five-factor score) and determine the aggressiveness of the immune suppressive therapy:

1. Proteinuria >1 g/day
2. Creatinine >1.58 mg/dl
3. Cardiomyopathy
4. GI tract involvement
5. Central nervous system involvement

ACUTE GENERAL Rx

- Corticosteroids are the treatment of choice if no poor prognostic factors are present. Prednisone 1 mg/kg/day is the starting dose and is continued for 6 to 12 wk and then tapered to 10 mg/day at 1 yr as clinical disease resolves. Response to steroids may be dramatic. Patients with extensive disease may require IV corticosteroids.
- A drop in the patient's eosinophil count and the erythrocyte sedimentation rate indicates a response to treatment. ANCA does not reliably correspond with disease activity.

CHRONIC Rx

- In patients with one or more poor prognostic factors, immunosuppressant agents (cyclophosphamide 1 to 2 mg/kg/day) are used with corticosteroids as first-line therapy. Limit duration of cyclophosphamide to a maximum of 6 mo.
- In patients who do not respond to corticosteroid treatment or in CSS relapse, cyclophosphamide therapy is indicated as a second-line therapy.
- Azathioprine (2 mg/kg/day) or high-dose intravenous immunoglobulin has shown benefit in patients with severe disease and in patients unresponsive to corticosteroids.
- Corticosteroids, in combination with interferon-alpha, have also been used in refractory cases but may be difficult to tolerate.
- Patients with persistent symptoms of asthma will require long-term corticosteroids even if vasculitis is no longer present.
- Maintenance therapy using methotrexate (15 to 25 mg/wk) or azathioprine (2 mg/kg/day) is an alternative to cyclophosphamide.

DISPOSITION

- Clinical remission is obtained in more than 90% of patients after treatment. Relapse is common on cessation of therapy (approximately 26%).
- 5-yr survival rate with treatment is 90% and decreases to 50% at 7 yr. Asthma generally remains persistent, and ischemic damage to peripheral nerves can be permanent.
- The 5-yr survival rate of untreated CSS is 25%.
- Death usually occurs from progressive refractory vasculitis, myocardial involvement (approximately 50% of deaths), or severe GI involvement (mesenteric ischemia, pancreatitis).

REFERRAL

- A pulmonary referral for diagnosis and management is appropriate.
- Patients should be followed up closely by rheumatology. Patients usually need long-term immunosuppressive medications.

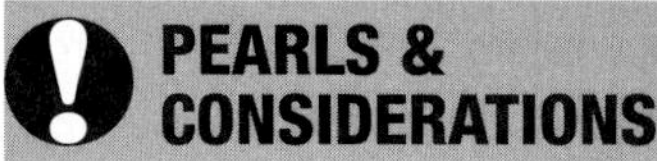

PEARLS & CONSIDERATIONS

COMMENTS

- CSS is a rare disease that is less common than other ANCA-associated vasculitides.
- CSS is distinguished from other vasculitides by the nearly universal presence of adult-onset asthma that typically precedes all other symptoms. Family history is often negative for allergies or asthma.
- Up to 77% of patients in the prodromal phase of CSS require oral steroids for asthma control.
- Patients often have constitutional symptoms of weight loss, fever, and malaise before specific organ involvement is clinically evident.
- Peripheral nerve involvement from vasculitis of the vasa vasorum commonly manifests as mononeuritis multiplex. Patients may present with sudden foot or wrist drop, along with sensory deficits in the distribution of one or more distal nerves.
- Most patients with GI involvement are symptomatic. Gastroenteritis, acute abdomen, cholecystitis, hemorrhage, bowel perforation, and mesenteric ischemia have all been reported in patients with CSS.
- Most patients with CSS respond to corticosteroid treatment and do not require cytotoxic therapy.
- Symptoms of CSS typically appear as oral corticosteroids are being decreased or discontinued for the treatment of asthma and not triggered by leukotriene receptor-1 antagonists, as previously reported.
- Compared to WG, patients more often present with history of atopy, asthma, or allergic rhinitis. When present, eosinophilia in CSS is often >1000 eosinophils/mm^3 compared with WG, where eosinophilia is much milder (<500 eosinophils/mm^3).
- The heart is involved in up to 60% of patients with CSS and represents a major cause of death.

SUGGESTED READINGS

Kallenberg CG: Churg-Strauss syndrome: just one disease entity? *Arthritis Rheum* 52(9):2589-2593, 2005.

Masi A et al: American College of Rheumatology 1990 criteria for the classification of Churg-Strauss syndrome, *Arthritis Rheum* 33:1094, 1990.

Pagnoux C et al: Churg Strauss syndrome, *Curr Opin Rheumatol* 19(1):25-32, 2007.

Seo P et al: Small-vessel and medium-vessel vasculitis, *Arthritis Rheum* 57(8):1552-1559, 2007.

AUTHORS: **KACHIU LEE, B.A.,** and
JESSICA RISSER, M.D., M.P.H.

BASIC INFORMATION

DEFINITION

Cirrhosis is defined histologically as the presence of fibrosis and regenerative nodules in the liver. It can be classified as micronodular, macronodular, or mixed; however, each form may be seen in the same patient at different stages of the disease. Cirrhosis manifests clinically with portal hypertension, hepatic encephalopathy, and variceal bleeding.

ICD-9CM CODES
571.5 Cirrhosis of the liver
571.2 Cirrhosis of the liver secondary to alcohol

EPIDEMIOLOGY & DEMOGRAPHICS

- Cirrhosis is the eleventh leading cause of death in the U.S. (nine per 100,000 persons annually).
- Alcohol abuse and viral hepatitis are the major causes of cirrhosis in the U.S.

PHYSICAL FINDINGS & CLINICAL PRESENTATION

SKIN: Jaundice, palmar erythema (alcohol abuse), spider angiomata, ecchymosis (thrombocytopenia or coagulation factor deficiency), dilated superficial periumbilical vein (caput medusae), increased pigmentation (hemochromatosis), xanthomas (primary biliary cirrhosis), needle tracks (viral hepatitis)
EYES: Kayser-Fleischer rings (corneal copper deposition seen in Wilson's disease; best diagnosed with slit lamp examination), scleral icterus
BREATH: Fetor hepaticus (musty odor of breath and urine found in cirrhosis with hepatic failure)
CHEST: Possible gynecomastia in men
ABDOMEN: Tender hepatomegaly (congestive hepatomegaly), small, nodular liver (cirrhosis), palpable, nontender gallbladder (neoplastic extrahepatic biliary obstruction), palpable spleen (portal hypertension), venous hum auscultated over periumbilical veins (portal hypertension), ascites (portal hypertension, hypoalbuminemia)
RECTAL EXAMINATION: Hemorrhoids (portal hypertension), guaiac-positive stools (alcoholic gastritis, bleeding esophageal varices, peptic ulcer disease, bleeding hemorrhoids)
GENITALIA: Testicular atrophy in males (chronic liver disease, hemochromatosis)
EXTREMITIES: Pedal edema (hypoalbuminemia, failure of right side of the heart), arthropathy (hemochromatosis)
NEUROLOGIC: Flapping tremor, asterixis (hepatic encephalopathy), choreoathetosis, dysarthria (Wilson's disease)

ETIOLOGY

- Alcohol abuse
- Secondary biliary cirrhosis, obstruction of the common bile duct (stone, stricture, pancreatitis, neoplasm, sclerosing cholangitis)
- Drugs (e.g., acetaminophen, isoniazid, methotrexate, methyldopa)
- Hepatic congestion (e.g., CHF, constrictive pericarditis, tricuspid insufficiency, thrombosis of the hepatic vein, obstruction of the vena cava)
- Primary biliary cirrhosis
- Hemochromatosis
- Chronic hepatitis B or C
- Wilson's disease
- Alpha-1-antitrypsin deficiency
- Infiltrative diseases (amyloidosis, glycogen storage diseases, hemochromatosis)
- Nutritional: jejunoileal bypass
- Others: parasitic infections (schistosomiasis), idiopathic portal hypertension, congenital hepatic fibrosis, systemic mastocytosis, autoimmune hepatitis, hepatic steatosis, inflammatory bowel disease (IBD)

Dx DIAGNOSIS

WORKUP

In addition to an assessment of liver function, the evaluation of patients with cirrhosis should also include an assessment of renal and circulatory function. Diagnostic workup is aimed primarily at identifying the most likely cause of cirrhosis. The history is extremely important:

- Alcohol abuse: alcoholic liver disease
- History of hepatitis B (chronic active hepatitis, primary hepatic neoplasm, or hepatitis C)
- History of IBD (primary sclerosing cholangitis)
- History of pruritus, hyperlipoproteinemia, and xanthomas in a middle-aged or elderly woman (primary biliary cirrhosis)
- Impotence, diabetes mellitus, hyperpigmentation, arthritis (hemochromatosis)
- Neurologic disturbances (Wilson's disease, hepatolenticular degeneration)
- Family history of "liver disease" (hemochromatosis [positive family history in 25% of patients], alpha-1-antitrypsin deficiency)
- History of recurrent episodes of right upper quadrant pain (biliary tract disease)
- History of blood transfusions, IV drug abuse (hepatitis C)
- History of hepatotoxic drug exposure
- Coexistence of other diseases with immune or autoimmune features (immune thrombocytopenic purpura, myasthenia gravis, thyroiditis, autoimmune hepatitis)

LABORATORY TESTS

- Decreased hemoglobin and hematocrit, elevated mean corpuscular volume, increased blood urea nitrogen (BUN) and creatinine (the BUN may also be "normal" or low if the patient has severely diminished liver function), decreased sodium (dilutional hyponatremia), and decreased potassium (as a result of secondary aldosteronism or urinary losses). Evaluation of renal function should also include measurement of urinary sodium and urinary protein from a 24-hr urine collection.
- Decreased glucose in a patient with liver disease, indicating severe liver damage.
- Other laboratory abnormalities:
  1. Alcoholic hepatitis and cirrhosis: possible mild elevation of alanine aminotransferase (ALT) and aspartate aminotransferase (AST), usually $<$500 IU; AST $>$ ALT (ratio $>$2:3).
  2. Extrahepatic obstruction: possible moderate elevations of ALT and AST to levels $<$500 IU.
  3. Viral, toxic, or ischemic hepatitis: extreme elevations ($>$500 IU) of ALT and AST.
  4. Transaminases may be normal despite significant liver disease in patients with jejunoileal bypass operations or hemochromatosis or after methotrexate administration.
  5. Alkaline phosphatase elevation can occur with extrahepatic obstruction, primary biliary cirrhosis, and primary sclerosing cholangitis.
  6. Serum lactate dehydrogenase is significantly elevated in metastatic disease of the liver; lesser elevations are seen with hepatitis, cirrhosis, extrahepatic obstruction, and congestive hepatomegaly.
  7. Serum gamma-glutamyl transpeptidase is elevated in alcoholic liver disease and may also be elevated with cholestatic disease (primary biliary cirrhosis, primary sclerosing cholangitis).
  8. Serum bilirubin may be elevated; urinary bilirubin can be present in hepatitis, hepatocellular jaundice, and biliary obstruction.
  9. Serum albumin: significant liver disease results in hypoalbuminemia.
  10. Prothrombin time/INR: elevation in patients with liver disease indicates severe liver damage and poor prognosis.
  11. Presence of hepatitis B surface antigen implies acute or chronic hepatitis B.
  12. Presence of antimitochondrial antibody suggests primary biliary cirrhosis, chronic hepatitis.
  13. Elevated serum copper, decreased serum ceruloplasmin, and elevated 24-hr urine may be diagnostic of Wilson's disease.
  14. Protein immunoelectrophoresis may reveal decreased α-1 globulins (alpha-1-antitrypsin deficiency), increased IgA (alcoholic cirrhosis), increased IgM (primary biliary cirrhosis), increased IgG (chronic hepatitis, cryptogenic cirrhosis).
  15. An elevated serum ferritin and increased transferrin saturation are suggestive of hemochromatosis.
  16. An elevated blood ammonia suggests hepatocellular dysfunction; serial values, however, are generally not useful in monitoring patients with hepatic encephalopathy because there is poor correlation between blood ammonia level and degree of hepatic encephalopathy.
  17. Serum cholesterol is elevated in cholestatic disorders.
  18. Antinuclear antibodies (ANA) may be found in autoimmune hepatitis.

19. Alpha fetoprotein: levels >1000 pg/ml are highly suggestive of primary liver cell carcinoma.
20. Hepatitis C viral testing identifies patients with chronic hepatitis C infection.
21. Elevated level of serum globulin (especially gamma-globulins) and positive ANA test may occur with autoimmune hepatitis.

IMAGING STUDIES

- Ultrasonography is the procedure of choice for detecting gallstones and dilation of common bile ducts.
- CT scan is useful for detecting mass lesions in liver and pancreas, assessing hepatic fat content, identifying idiopathic hemochromatosis, diagnosing Budd-Chiari syndrome early, assessing dilation of intrahepatic bile ducts, and detecting varices and splenomegaly.
- MRI can be used to identify hemangiomas.
- Technetium-99m sulfur colloid scanning is rarely used but can be useful for diagnosing cirrhosis (there is a shift of colloid uptake to the spleen and bone marrow), identifying hepatic adenomas (cold defect is noted), and diagnosing Budd-Chiari syndrome (there is increased uptake by the caudate lobe).
- Endoscopic retrograde cholangiopancreatography can be used for diagnosing periampullary carcinoma and common duct stones; it is also useful in diagnosing primary sclerosing cholangitis.
- Percutaneous transhepatic cholangiography is useful when evaluating patients with cholestatic jaundice and dilated intrahepatic ducts by ultrasonography; presence of intrahepatic strictures and focal dilation is suggestive of primary sclerosing cholangitis.
- Percutaneous liver biopsy is useful in evaluating hepatic filling defects; diagnosing hepatocellular disease or hepatomegaly; evaluating persistently abnormal liver function tests; and diagnosing hemachromatosis, primary biliary cirrhosis, Wilson's disease, glycogen storage diseases, chronic hepatitis, autoimmune hepatitis, infiltrative diseases, alcoholic liver disease, drug-induced liver disease, and primary or secondary carcinoma.

Rx TREATMENT

NONPHARMACOLOGIC THERAPY

Avoid any hepatotoxins (e.g., ethanol, acetaminophen), improve nutritional status

GENERAL Rx

- Remove excess body iron with phlebotomy and deferoxamine in patients with hemochromatosis.
- Remove copper deposits with D-penicillamine in patients with Wilson's disease.
- Long-term ursodiol therapy will slow the progression of primary biliary cirrhosis. It is, however, ineffective in primary sclerosing cholangitis.
- Glucocorticoids (prednisone 20 to 30 mg/day initially or combination therapy or prednisone and azathioprine) is useful in autoimmune hepatitis.
- Liver transplantation may be indicated in otherwise healthy patients (age <65 yr) with sclerosing cholangitis, chronic hepatitis cirrhosis, or primary biliary cirrhosis with prognostic information suggesting <20% chance of survival without transplantation. Contraindications to liver transplantation are AIDS, most metastatic malignancies, active substance abuse, uncontrolled sepsis, and uncontrolled cardiac or pulmonary disease.
- Treatment of complications of portal hypertension (ascites, esophagogastric varices, hepatic encephalopathy, and hepatorenal syndrome).

DISPOSITION

- Prognosis varies with the etiology of the patient's cirrhosis and whether there is ongoing hepatic injury. Regression of cirrhosis has been demonstrated after antiviral therapy in some patients with chronic hepatitis C. Regression is associated with decreased disease-related morbidity and improved survival. Mortality rate exceeds 80% in patients with hepatorenal syndrome.
- If advanced cirrhosis is present and transplantation is not feasible, survival is 1 to 2 yr.

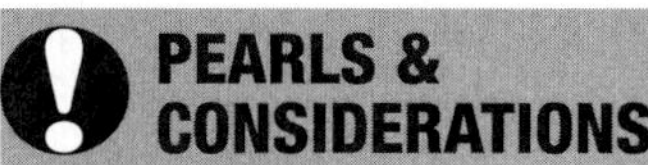

PEARLS & CONSIDERATIONS

COMMENTS

- Thrombocytopenia and advanced Child-Pugh cases are associated with the presence of varices. These factors are useful to identify cirrhotic patients who benefit most from referral for endoscopic screening for varices.
- A combination of endoscopic and drug therapy reduces overall and variceal rebleeding in cirrhosis more than either therapy alone.

EBM EVIDENCE

Please note: Complete text of EBM for this topic is available online.

Key trials and commentary:

Norfloxacin is highly effective in preventing spontaneous bacterial peritonitis (SBP) recurrence in cirrhosis, but its role in the primary prevention of this complication is uncertain.

This study showed that primary prophylaxis with norfloxacin has a great impact in the clinical course of patients with advanced cirrhosis. It reduces the incidence of SBP, delays the development of hepatorenal syndrome (HRS), and improves survival.

The organisms that cause SBP originate in the intestinal lumen, which translocate and cause infection and HRS, leading to mortality. SBP's mortality has decreased, as outlined in the elegant editorial by Runyon. This is likely because of our heightened index of suspicion for SBP and our performance of a diagnostic paracentesis on almost all hospitalized patients who could possibly be manifesting SBP, that is, those with abdominal pain, elevated temperature, altered mental status, or laboratory abnormalities of leukocytosis, acidosis, or azotemia. Early recognition of SBP and use of a cefotoxin regimen has reduced mortality from acute episodes. We use antibiotic prophylaxis in these patients who have had an episode of SBP, so-called secondary prophylaxis, and this has, again, decreased recurrence. However, the role of primary prophylaxis for prevention of SBP and HRS was unclear until the Fernandez et al study. They included a study population that was at high risk for developing SBP and HRS because of their advanced liver failure with serum bilirubin ≥3 mg/dl, and low ascites fluid protein concentration (<1.5 g/dl), impaired renal function with a creatinine ≥1.2 mg/dl or ≤130 mEq/L. These patients were randomly selected to be given norfloxacin or placebo, and survival was the primary end point. If SBP occurred, albumin was effective in preventing development of HRS. They found that administration of norfloxacin resulted in a significant decrease in the 1-year probability of developing SBP and HRS and an increase in survival. The authors postulated that the mechanism of preventing HRS was improvement in systemic hemodynamics by norfloxacin, probably via decreasing endotoxemia. The effect of norfloxacin on HRS development is mostly in the first 3 months.

The take-home message is that we need to use norfloxacin prophylaxis in patients who are at high risk for SBP and HRS, especially for those who are awaiting transplantation.[1] Ⓐ

Evidence-Based Reference

1. Fernández J et al: Primary prophylaxis of spontaneous bacterial peritonitis delays hepatorenal syndrome and improves survival in cirrhosis, *Gastroenterology* 133:818-824, 2007. Commentary by J.S. Barkin, M.D. Ⓐ

SUGGESTED READINGS

Garcia-Tsao G, Bosch J: Management of varices and variceal hemorrhage in cirrhosis, *N Engl J Med* 362:823-832, 2010.

Gines P, Schrier RW: Renal failure in cirrhosis, *N Engl J Med* 361:1279-1290, 2009.

Gonzalez R et al: Meta-analysis: combination endoscopic and drug therapy to prevent variceal rebleeding in cirrhosis, *Ann Intern Med* 149:109, 2008.

Heidelbaugh JJ, Bruderly M: Cirrhosis and chronic liver failure, *Am Fam Physician* 74:756, 2006.

AUTHOR: **FRED F. FERRI, M.D.**

BASIC INFORMATION

DEFINITION

Primary biliary cirrhosis (PBC) is a chronic, variably progressive cholestatic liver disease most often affecting women and characterized by destruction of the small intrahepatic bile ducts leading to portal inflammation, fibrosis, cirrhosis, and ultimately, liver failure.

SYNONYMS

Biliary cirrhosis
Nonsuppurative destructive cholangitis
Autoimmune cholangiopathy

ICD-9CM CODES
571.6 Biliary cirrhosis
698 Pruritus
780.7 Malaise and Fatigue

EPIDEMIOLOGY & DEMOGRAPHICS

INCIDENCE:

- PBC affects all races and accounts for 0.6% to 2% of deaths from cirrhosis worldwide.
- Annual incidence rates range from 0.7 to 49 cases per million.

PREVALENCE: Prevalence is greatest in the U.K., Scandinavia, Canada, and the U.S., and varies tremendously by geographic areas, ranging from 6.7 to 402 cases per million.

PREDOMINANT SEX: Approximately 95% of patients are female.

PREDOMINANT AGE: Onset typically occurs between the ages of 30 and 65 yr, and it is uncommon before age 25 yr.

GENETICS:

- Although there are no clearly identified genetic factors associated with PBC, there is a clear familial occurrence. Prevalence among first-degree relatives is 5% to 6%, and 1% to 6% of all patients have at least one affected family member. The concordance rate among monozygotic twins is 63%.
- Up to 84% of patients with PBC have at least one other autoimmune disorder, such as thyroiditis, Sjögren's syndrome, rheumatoid arthritis, Raynaud's phenomenon, or scleroderma. A variant form of PBC exists as an overlap syndrome with autoimmune hepatitis (AIH).

ETIOLOGY

- Although the cause of PBC remains unknown, it is believed to be attributable to an environmental insult that modifies mitochondrial proteins triggering persistent T lymphocyte–mediated attack on intralobular bile duct epithelial cells in genetically susceptible individuals.
- PBC is associated with the DRB1*08 family of alleles, but there is a great deal of variation among ethnicities.
- Possible environmental triggers include cigarette smoking, urinary tract infections, reproductive hormone replacement, nail polish, and toxic waste sites, as well as xenobiotics in animal models of PBC.
- Recent studies have identified a peptide, an enzyme complex subunit (PDC-E2) in the mitochondrial membrane, as a major autoantigen in the early pathogenesis of PBC. Patients with PBC have a tenfold increased concentration of cytotoxic $CD8^+$ lymphocytes recognizing this peptide in their livers compared with their blood, and anti–mitochondria antibodies (AMA), especially the PDC-E2 subunit, are the serologic hallmark of this disease. In addition, bile duct epithelial cells handle PDC-E2 in a unique way that exposes them to immune-mediated attack by PDC-E2–oriented cytotoxic T cells. Future therapies may be specific immunomodulation directed at these peptides.
- In addition to the T lymphocyte–mediated direct destruction of small bile ducts, secondary damage to hepatocytes results from the accumulation of noxious substances such as bile acids.
- Recent data show a significant association between PBC and common genetic variants at the human leukocyte antigen (HLA) class II, IL12A, and IL12RB2 loci, and suggest that the interleukin-12 immunoregulatory signaling axis is relevant to pathophysiology of PBC.

PHYSICAL FINDINGS & CLINICAL PRESENTATION

Clinical stages:

- Asymptomatic
- Symptomatic
- Cirrhotic
- Hepatic failure

Symptoms:

- 48% to 60% of patients may be asymptomatic; 40% to 100% of these patients will develop symptoms, and nearly 25% of symptomatic patients at diagnosis will progress to liver failure within 10 yr without treatment.
- Fatigue (78% of patients) and pruritus (20% to 70% of patients) are the usual presenting symptoms.
- Pruritus is worse at night, under constricting, coarse garments; in association with dry skin; and in hot, humid weather. The cause is unknown; it is no longer believed to be a result of the retention of bile acids in skin. Pruritus may first occur during pregnancy but is distinguished from pruritus of pregnancy because it persists into the postpartum period and beyond.
- Other common symptoms include hepatomegaly, jaundice, unexplained right upper quadrant pain (10%), splenomegaly, manifestations of portal hypertension, sicca symptoms, and scleroderma-like lesions.
- Musculoskeletal complaints caused by inflammatory arthropathy in 40% to 70% of patients: 5% to 10% experience development of chronic rheumatoid arthritis and 10% experience development of "arthritis of PBC."
- Steatorrhea may be seen in advanced disease.

Physical:

- Variable: Results depend on stage of disease at time of presentation; patients at the early stage may be completely unaffected.
- Excoriations may be present.
- Hepatomegaly (70%) and splenomegaly (initially 35%) may be present in more advanced disease.
- Xanthomas and jaundice appear in advanced disease. Kayser-Fleischer rings are rare and result from copper retention.
- Late physical findings mirror those of cirrhosis: spider nevi, temporal and proximal limb wasting, ascites, and edema.

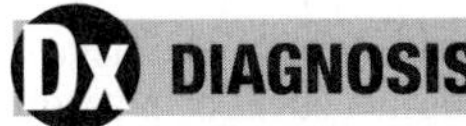

DIAGNOSIS

Based on three criteria:

- Positive serum AMA, titer >1:40
- Biochemical evidence of cholestasis (mainly alkaline phosphatase elevation)
- Characteristic liver histology: nonsuppurative destructive cholangitis and destruction of interlobar bile ducts

Two criteria indicate a probable diagnosis, and all three criteria are required for a definite diagnosis.

DIFFERENTIAL DIAGNOSIS

- Drug-induced cholestasis
- PBC-AIH overlap syndrome: reported in almost 10% of adults with AIH or PBC; transition from stable PBC to AIH and vice versa also seen
- Other etiologies of chronic liver disease and cirrhosis, such as alcoholic cirrhosis, chronic viral hepatitis, primary sclerosing cholangitis, AIH, sarcoidosis, chemical/toxin-induced cirrhosis, other hereditary or familial disorders (e.g., cystic fibrosis, α-1-antitrypsin deficiency)
- Biliary obstruction

WORKUP

History, physical examination, laboratory evaluation, liver biopsy

LABORATORY TESTS

- AMAs found in 95% of patients with PBC and are 98% specific.
- Antinuclear antibodies (ANAs) and anti–smooth muscle antibody (AMA) found in approximately 50% of patients. In approximately 5% of patients, AMAs are absent or present only in low titer (AMA-negative PBC). Nearly all of these patients have ANA or anti–smooth muscle antibodies, or both.
- Cholestatic pattern of liver biochemical markers, that is, markedly increased alkaline phosphatase (of hepatic origin).
- γ-Glutamyl transpeptidase is increased.
- Serum IgM levels are increased (lower in AMA-negative PBC).
- Bilirubin level is normal early; increases with disease progression (direct and indirect) in 60% of patients. Increased serum bilirubin level is a poor prognostic sign.
- Aminotransferase level may be normal and, if increased, is rarely more than five times the upper limit of normal.
- Markedly increased serum lipids in more than 50% of patients. Total cholesterol may

exceed 1000 mg/dl. No increased risk for death from atherosclerosis seen, possibly because of high levels of LP-X, an antiatherogenic low-density lipoprotein particle, very-high-density lipoprotein levels, and low serum levels of lipoprotein(a).
- Percutaneous liver biopsy confirms or rules out the diagnosis, allows staging, but is not essential to initiate medical therapy in patients with typical liver chemistry and positive AMA test.
- Histology is not uniform, so histologic stage is based on the most advanced lesion present.
  - Stage I: Lymphocytic infiltration of the epithelial cells of the small bile ducts with granuloma-like lesions, limited to portal triads
  - Stage II: Extension of inflammatory cells to periportal parenchyma, invasion by foamy macrophages, and development of biliary piecemeal necrosis
  - Stage III: Fibrous septa link portal triads
  - Stage IV: Frank cirrhosis; hyaline deposits and accumulation of stainable copper are also seen

IMAGING STUDIES

If history, physical examination, blood tests, and liver biopsy are all consistent with PBC, neither imaging nor cholangiography is necessary.

PROGNOSIS

- Median survival was 10 yr but may be getting longer with earlier diagnosis and initiation of treatment.
- Mean time of progression from stage I or II disease to cirrhosis with no medical treatment is 4 to 6 yr.
- Neither presence nor titer of antimitochondrial antibodies predicts survival, disease progression, or response to therapy.
- Prognostic laboratory measures: Serum bilirubin is most important.
- Response to ursodiol therapy can be prognostic: Patients with a decrease in alkaline phosphatase level of at least 40% or to the reference range after 1 yr of treatment with ursodeoxycholic acid (UDCA) may have a prognosis similar to an age-matched healthy population. Similarly, the Mayo Risk score, a predictor of short-term survival probability (http://www.mayoclinic.org/gi-rst/mayomodel1.html), can also reliably predict life expectancy when calculated after 6 mo of ursodiol therapy.
- Poorer prognosis exists with jaundice, advanced histologic stage, advanced age, edema, coagulopathy, and ascites.

Rx TREATMENT

- Treatment is according to the clinical stage of the disease.
- Asymptomatic stage: Follow bilirubin every 3 mo. Once liver function test results become abnormal, begin UDCA at 13 to 15 mg/kg/day in a twice-daily divided dose regardless of histologic stage. Side effects may include weight gain of approximately 5 lbs during the first 1 to 2 yr and, less commonly, thinning of hair and loose stools. Watch for interactions with cholestyramine and other bile-acid sequestrants, as well as antacids, which may interfere with UDCA absorption. Efficacy is best if started during stage I or II disease but should be started at any stage of disease. Lifelong therapy is currently recommended, but benefits are still observed if therapy is interrupted and restarted.
- Treatment also includes treatment of associated conditions such as pruritus, osteoporosis, increased low-density lipoprotein level, and any eventual complications of cirrhosis.
- 20% of patients will not respond to medical therapy and will proceed to liver transplantation, which is the only definitive treatment for this disease.

ACUTE GENERAL Rx

- Symptomatic stage: Goals of treatment are resolution of pruritus, decrease of alkaline phosphatase levels, and delay of progression to liver failure.
- Ursodiol can significantly improve bilirubin and alkaline phosphatase levels, prolong survival without liver transplantation, and delay progression of liver fibrosis and development of portal hypertension.
- The addition of colchicine (0.6 mg bid) or methotrexate (15 mg/wk) has not been found to be of benefit in controlled trials.
- Prednisone, azathioprine, penicillamine, and cyclosporine are no longer used because of limited efficacy and significant toxicity.
- For the pruritus of PBC, cholestyramine resin (4 g/dose; maximum, 16 g/day) reduces pruritus in most patients but must be given at least 2 to 4 hr apart from ursodiol to avoid reducing the efficacy of that drug. Antihistamines at bedtime help nighttime symptoms. Rifampin (150 to 300 mg bid) or oral opiate antagonists such as naltrexone (50 mg daily) can be used for pruritus refractory to bile acid sequestrants. Intractable pruritus can be an indication for liver transplantation.

CHRONIC Rx

- Management of Sicca syndrome: Artificial tears can be used initially for dry eyes. Saliva substitutes can be used for xerostomia and dysphagia; pilocarpine or cevimeline for refractory cases. Moisturizers can be given for vaginal dryness.
- Treatment for osteopenia/osteoporosis: Patients with PBC should be provided 1000 to 1500 mg calcium and 1000 IU of vitamin D daily in the diet and as supplements if needed. Alendronate (70 mg weekly) should be considered if patients are osteopenic in the absence of acid reflux or known varices.
- Hyperlipidemia is common in patients with cholestatic liver disease. Statins are safe in patients who may need treatment even if liver chemistry is abnormal.
- Vitamin A, K, and E deficiencies can be clinically important in advanced cases and respond to oral replacement.
- Upper endoscopy to assess for varices should be done every 2 to 3 yr in patients with cirrhosis or Mayo risk score >4.1. Nonselective beta-blockers or endoscopic banding can be considered for prevention of variceal hemorrhage.
- Regular screening for hepatocellular carcinoma with ultrasound and α-fetoprotein every 6 to 12 mo is recommended for patients with cirrhosis.
- Liver transplantation is the only effective treatment for patients with liver failure. Indications for transplantation include hepatic decompensation (ascites, encephalopathy, jaundice), hepatocellular carcinoma fulfilling Milan criteria (see "Hepatocellular Carcinoma"), and intractable pruritus.
- The outcome of liver transplantation for patients with PBC is more favorable than that of nearly all other liver disease categories. The survival rates are 85% to 90% and 80% to 85% at 1 and 5 yr, respectively. Although recurrent disease may develop in 20% to 25% of patients after liver transplantation over 10 yr, patient and graft survival is usually not affected.

DISPOSITION

Definitive treatment requires liver transplantation; survival is 7 to 16 yr depending on symptoms at time of diagnosis.

REFERRAL

Gastroenterology and/or hepatology for treatment, evaluation for liver transplantation, and management of portal hypertension

PEARLS & CONSIDERATIONS

- Anti–mitochondrial antibody (AMA) is the serologic hallmark of PBC.
- The prototypical patient with PBC is a middle-aged, white woman reporting fatigue and pruritus.
- Ursodiol should be started as soon as liver biochemical markers begin to increase and is most effective when started early in the course of the disease.
- Associated illnesses must be detected and treated.
- Liver transplantation is the only effective treatment for PBC with end-stage liver failure.

SUGGESTED READINGS

Hirschfield GM et al: Primary biliary cirrhosis associated with HLA, IL12A, aqnd IL12RB2 variants, *N Engl J Med* 360:2544-2555, 2009

Jones DEJ: Pathogenesis of primary biliary cirrhosis, *Gut* 56:1615-1624, 2007.

Lindor K: Ursodeoxycholic acid for the treatment of primary biliary cirrhosis, *N Engl J Med* 357:1524-1529, 2007.

Lindor KD et al; American Association for Study of Liver Diseases: Primary biliary cirrhosis, *Hepatology* 50(1):291-308, 2009.

AUTHORS: **KITTICHAI PROMRAT, M.D.,** and **JENNIFER ROH HUR, M.D.**

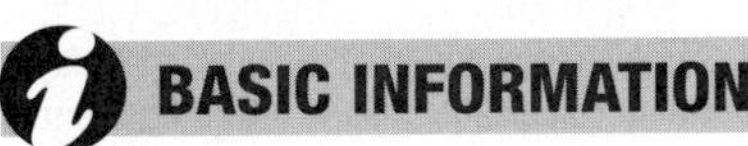

DEFINITION

Claudication refers to reproducible discomfort of limb muscles brought on by exertion and relieved with rest.

SYNONYMS

Intermittent claudication

ICD-9CM CODES
443.9 Peripheral vascular disease, unspecified
440.21 Intermittent claudication due to atherosclerosis

EPIDEMIOLOGY & DEMOGRAPHICS

- The prevalence rate is 2% to 4% in the general population and increasing with age, especially after age 40 yr.
- The risk factors associated with development of intermittent claudication are similar to coronary artery disease. Cigarette smoking and diabetes mellitus are the strongest risk factors, followed by hypertension and dyslipidemia.
- There is an association between peripheral artery disease (PAD) and cardiovascular disease.
- In 2005, the American College of Cardiology/American Heart Association (ACC/AHA) guidelines suggested the following distribution of clinical presentation of PAD in patients >50 yr of age:
  1. asymptomatic: 20%-50%
  2. atypical leg pain: 40%-50%
  3. classic claudication: 10%-35%
  4. critical limb ischemia: 1%-2%

PHYSICAL FINDINGS & CLINICAL PRESENTATION

- The severity of claudication symptoms varies with severity of stenoses, collateral blood supply, and exertional demand.
- Classic symptoms include calf pain brought on by exertion, causing patient to stop exertion and pain resolves within 10 min of rest. Claudication can present in buttock and hip, thigh, calf, or foot, with one or more of the following findings:
  1. Diminished or absent pedal pulses, cool skin temperature
  2. Bruits over the distal aorta, iliac or femoral arteries
  3. Pallor of the distal extremities on elevation
  4. Rubor with prolonged capillary refill on dependency
  5. Trophic changes of hair loss and muscle atrophy
  6. Nonhealing ulcers, necrotic tissue, and gangrene
  7. Weakness, numbness, or heaviness feeling in legs

ETIOLOGY

The primary cause of claudication is peripheral atherosclerosis, resulting in inability to supply blood to meet the metabolic demand of limb muscles.

Dx DIAGNOSIS

DIFFERENTIAL DIAGNOSIS

- Spinal stenosis (neurogenic or pseudoclaudication)
- Musculoskeletal disorders
- Degenerative osteoarthritic joint disease, particularly of the lumbar spine and hips
- Compartment syndrome
- Peripheral neuropathy

WORKUP

History and physical findings suggest the diagnosis of claudication. Noninvasive studies help confirm the diagnosis.

- Measurement of resting ankle–brachial index (ABI): the ratio of highest ankle systolic pressure to brachial pressure
- The severity of PAD is based on the ABI at rest and during treadmill exercise (1 to 2 miles/hour, 5 min, or symptom limited). It is classified as follows:
  - Mild: ABI at rest 0.71 to 0.90 or ABI during exercise 0.50 to 0.90
  - Moderate: ABI at rest 0.41 to 0.70 or ABI during exercise 0.20 to 0.50
  - Severe: ABI at rest <0.40 or ABI during exercise <0.20
- Segmental systolic pressures are measured from thigh, calf, ankle, metatarsal, and toes. Normally, there should not be >20 mm Hg difference in pressures between adjacent segments. If the gradient is >20 mm Hg, significant narrowing is suspected in the intervening segment.
- Both ABI and segmental pressures can be taken before and after exercise for objective characterization of severity of claudication symptoms.
- ABI >1.3 may represent significant PAD. In such cases, measuring a toe–brachial index can increase the sensitivity of testing, as patients with highly calcified arteries may have a normal or increased ABI. A toe–brachial index <0.7 is abnormal.

IMAGING STUDIES

- Duplex ultrasound can be used to assess occlusion location and patency of the distal arterial system or prior vein grafts.
- Magnetic resonance angiography and spiral CT angiography are effective modalities for imaging of the aorta and peripheral lower extremity arteries above the knee.
- Angiography remains the gold standard for diagnosing peripheral arterial occlusion, especially below the knee, and before revascularization.

Rx TREATMENT

NONPHARMACOLOGIC THERAPY

- Smoking cessation is vital.
- Aggressive risk factor modification for hypertension, dyslipidemia and diabetes mellitus, including diet and weight loss counseling.
- Walking 30 to 60 min/day at approximately 2 miles/hour to near-maximal pain for 6 mo is recommended.
- New prospective data point to intermittent pneumatic compression as a promising adjunctive therapy.

ACUTE GENERAL Rx

Revascularization by endovascular or surgical approach is usually reserved for patients with symptoms refractory to medical therapy or impending ischemic limb loss.

CHRONIC Rx

- Aspirin 75 to 325 mg daily; thienopyridines (clopidogrel and ticlodipine) can be considered as alternatives, especially for those intolerant of aspirin.
- Cilostazol 100 mg bid may be used in conjunction with aspirin or clopidogrel. It has been shown to increase walking distance by 50% in symptomatic patients.
- Revascularization is indicated in patients with refractory rest pain or claudication that limits their lifestyle, nonhealing ulcers, or gangrene, and in a select group of patients with functional disability. Common procedures include:
  1. Aortoiliofemoral reconstruction or bypass or infrainguinal bypass (e.g., femoropopliteal, femorotibial)
  2. Angioplasty, often with stenting, is used primarily on short, discrete stenotic lesions in the iliac or femoropopliteal artery

COMPLEMENTARY & ALTERNATIVE MEDICINE

- A meta-analysis found that over 12 to 24 wk, *Ginkgo biloba* increased pain-free walking distance by 34 m compared with placebo, although the benefit is not well established according to ACC/AHA guidelines.
- Estrogen replacement therapy and chelation therapy are ineffective in the treatment of intermittent claudication.

DISPOSITION

- Intermittent claudication progressing to an ischemic leg or limb loss is unusual, especially if maintaining the conservative treatment of exercise and smoking cessation.
- The 5-yr risk for development of ischemic ulceration in patients treated for diabetes and with ABI <0.5 was 30% compared with only 5% in patients with neither characteristic.

REFERRAL

Consultation with physicians specializing in vascular medicine is recommended in the patient with threatened limb loss, rest pain, nonhealing ulcers, functional disability from pain, and gangrene.

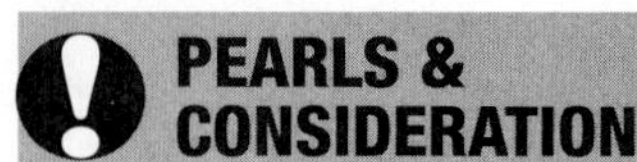

PEARLS & CONSIDERATIONS

- Approximately 70% of patients with peripheral vascular disease will have concomitant coronary artery disease.
- Beta-blockers may worsen claudication symptoms in some patients, although their underuse is associated with excess cardiovascular death.
- Patients with peripheral vascular disease may benefit from secondary cardiovascular prevention with clopidogrel vs. aspirin more than other high-risk patients (CAPRIE trial).

COMMENTS

- Claudication is a marker for generalized atherosclerosis. This group of patients has a greater risk for death from cardiovascular events than from limb loss. Patients with claudication experience diminished overall quality of life similar to patients with coronary or cerebrovascular disease.
- The ABI is more closely associated with leg function in persons with peripheral arterial disease than is intermittent claudication or other leg symptoms.

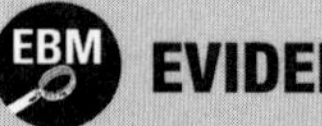

EVIDENCE

Please note: Complete text of EBM for this topic is available online.

SUGGESTED READINGS

Aboyans V et al: Risk factors for progression of peripheral arterial disease in large and small vessels, *Circulation* 113:2623, 2006.

Abramson B et al: Canadian Cardiovascular Society Consensus Conference: peripheral arterial disease—executive summary, *Can J Cardiol* 21(12):997-1006, 2005.

Hirsch AT et al: ACC/AHA Guidelines for the Management of Patients with Peripheral Arterial Disease (Lower Extremity, Renal, Mesenteric, and Abdominal Aortic): a collaborative report from the American Association for Vascular Surgery/Society for Vascular Surgery, Society for Cardiovascular Angiography and Interventions, Society of Interventional Radiology, Society for Vascular Medicine and Biology, and the American College of Cardiology/American Heart Association Task Force on Practice Guidelines (Writing Committee to Develop Guidelines for the Management of Patients with Peripheral Arterial Disease), *J Am Coll Cardiol* 47:1239-1312, 2006.

Kakkos S et al: Improvement of the walking ability in intermittent claudication due to superficial femoral artery occlusion with supervised exercise and pneumatic foot and calf compression: a randomized controlled trial, *Eur J Endovasc Surg* 302(2):164, 2005.

McDermott MM et al: Leg symptoms in peripheral arterial disease: associated clinical characteristics and functional impairment, *JAMA* 286:1599, 2001.

McDermott MM et al: Treadmill exercise and resistance training in patients with peripheral arterial disease with and without intermittent claudication: a randomized controlled trial, *JAMA* 301:165, 2009.

Met R et al: Diagnostic performance of computed tomography angiography in peripheral arterial disease, *JAMA* 301(4):415-424, 2009.

Simon RW et al: Intermittent claudication, *BMJ* 334: 746, 2007.

Sobel M et al: Antithrombotic therapy for peripheral arterial occlusive disease: American College of Chest Physicians Evidence-Based Clinical Practice guidelines (8th Edition), *Chest* 133(Suppl 6):815S-843S, 2008.

White C: Clinical practice: intermittent claudication, *N Engl J Med* 356:1241-1250, 2007.

AUTHORS: **GARY S. MAK, M.D.,** and **PRANAV M. PATEL, M.D.**

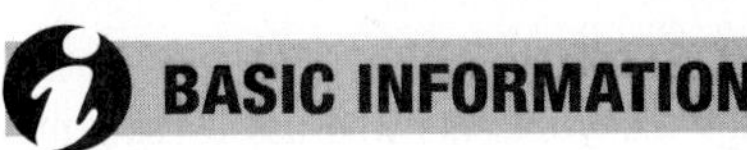

BASIC INFORMATION

DEFINITION

Cocaine is an alkaloid derived from the coca plant *Erythroxylum coca,* native to South America, which contains approximately 0.5% to 1% cocaine. The drug produces physiologic and behavioral effects when administered orally, intranasally, intravenously, or by inhalation after smoking. Cocaine has potent pharmacologic effects on dopamine, norepinephrine, and serotonin neurons in the central nervous system (CNS) involving alteration and blockade of cellular membrane transport and prevention of reuptake. Cocaine's second action involves the blockage of voltage-gated sodium ion membrane channels, which is responsible for its anesthetic effect.

SYNONYMS

Cocaine hydrochloride: topical solution (FDA approved as a topical anesthetic)

Freebase: aqueous solution of cocaine hydrochloride converted to a more volatile base state by the addition of alkali, thereby extracting the cocaine base in a residue or precipitate

Crack: potent, purified smokable form; produces effects similar to those of intravenous administration

Street names include Bernice, Bernies, C, Cadillac or Champagne of drugs, Carrie, Cecil, Charlie, Coke, Dust, Dynamite, Flake, Gin, Girl, Gold dust, Green gold, Jet, Powder, Star dust, Paradise, Pimp's drug, Snowflake, Stardust, White girl

Liquid lady = alcohol + cocaine

Speedball = heroin + cocaine

Street measures: hit (2 to 200 mg), snort, line, dose, spoon (approximately 1 g)

ICD-9CM CODES
304.2 Cocainism

EPIDEMIOLOGY & DEMOGRAPHICS

- The 1993 National Household Survey on Drug Abuse estimated that 4.5 million Americans used cocaine in 1992, with 1.3 million reporting use at least monthly. By 1998 this had not significantly changed.
- Between 1993 and 1994, intravenous cocaine and heroin abusers accounted for a major new group of persons with HIV in several metropolitan areas.
- In 1999 an estimated 25 million Americans admitted that they used cocaine at least once—3.7 million the previous year and 1.5 million currently. It is the most frequent cause of drug-related death reported by medical examiners and is increasing more sharply in women than in men.
- The 2006 National Survey on Drug Use and Health indicates that there were 2.4 million users aged ≥12 yr, which was the same in 2005 but greater than in 2002, when there were an estimated 2 million.

PHYSICAL FINDINGS & CLINICAL PRESENTATION

PHASE I:

- CNS: euphoria, agitation, headache, vertigo, twitching, bruxism, unintentional tremor
- Nausea, vomiting, fever, hypertension, tachycardia

PHASE II:

- CNS: lethargy, hyperreactive deep tendon reflexes, seizures (status epilepticus)
- Sympathetic overdrive: tachycardia, hypertension, hyperthermia
- Incontinence

PHASE III:

- CNS: flaccid paralysis, coma, fixed dilated pupils, loss of reflexes
- Pulmonary edema
- Cardiopulmonary arrest

Psychologic dependence manifests with habituation, paranoia, and hallucinations (cocaine "bugs"):

CNS: Cerebral ischemia and infarction, cerebral arterial spasm, cerebral vasculitis, cerebral vascular thrombosis, subarachnoid hemorrhage, intraparenchymal hemorrhage, seizures, cerebral atrophy, movement disorders

Cardiac: Acute myocardial ischemia and infarction, arrhythmias and sudden death, dilated cardiomyopathy and myocarditis, infective endocarditis, aortic rupture

Pulmonary: Inhalation injuries (secondary to smoking crack cocaine): cartilage and nasal septal perforation, oropharyngeal ulcers; immunologically mediated diseases: hypersensitivity pneumonitis, bronchiolitis obliterans; pulmonary vascular lesions and hemorrhage, pulmonary infarction, pulmonary edema secondary to left ventricular failure, pneumomediastinum, and pneumothorax

Gastrointestinal: Gastroduodenal ulceration and perforation; intestinal infarction or perforation, colitis

Renal: Acute renal failure secondary to rhabdomyolysis and myoglobinuria; renal infarction; focal segmental glomerulosclerosis

Obstetric: Placental abruption, low infant weight, prematurity, microcephaly

Psychiatric: Anxiety, depression, paranoia, delirium, psychosis, suicide

ETIOLOGY

Cocaine may be absorbed through different routes with varying degrees of speed:

- Nasal insufflation/snorting: 2.5 min
- Smoking: <30 sec
- Oral: 2 to 5 min
- Mucosal: <20 min
- Intravenous injection: <30 sec

Dx DIAGNOSIS

DIFFERENTIAL DIAGNOSIS

- Methamphetamine ("speed") abuse
- Methylenedioxyamphetamine ("ecstasy") abuse
- Cathione ("khat") abuse
- Lysergic acid diethylamide (LSD) abuse

WORKUP

Physical examination and laboratory evaluation

LABORATORY TESTS

- Toxicology screen (urine): cocaine is metabolized within 2 hr by the liver to major metabolites, benzoylecgonine and ecgonine methyl ester, which are excreted in the urine. Metabolites can be identified in urine within 5 min of IV use and up to 48 hr after oral ingestion.
- Blood: CBC, electrolytes, glucose, BUN, creatinine, calcium.
- Arterial blood gas analysis.
- ECG.
- Serum creatinine kinase and troponin concentration.

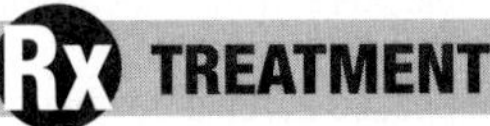

TREATMENT

There is no specific antidote and, at present, no drug therapy is uniquely effective in treating cocaine abuse and dependence. In addition, adulterants, contaminants, and other drugs may be admixed with street cocaine. Amantadine may provide effective treatment for cocaine-dependent patients with severe cocaine withdrawal symptoms, as well as the other dopamine agonist bromocriptine (1.5 mg PO tid), which may alleviate some of the symptoms of craving associated with acute cocaine withdrawal.

ACUTE GENERAL Rx

Acute cocaine toxicity requires following advanced poisoning treatment and life support. A suspected "body packer" should have an abdominal radiograph to detect the continued presence of cocaine-containing condoms in the intestinal tract. If present, gentle catharsis with charcoal and mineral oil should be performed with ICU admission and monitoring.

SPECIFIC TREATMENT

INHALATION: Wash nasal passages

AGITATION:

- Check STAT glucose
- Diazepam 15 to 20 mg PO or 2 to 10 mg IM or IV for severe agitation

HYPERTHERMIA:

- Check rectal temperature, creatine kinase, electrolytes
- Monitor with continuous rectal probe; bring temperature down to 101° F within 30 to 45 min

RHABDOMYOLYSIS:

- Vigorous hydration with urine output at least 2 ml/kg
- Mannitol or bicarbonate for rhabdomyolysis resistant to hydration

SEIZURE MANAGEMENT (STATUS EPILEPTICUS):

- Diazepam 5 to 10 mg IV over 2 to 3 min; may be repeated every 10 to 15 min.
- Lorazepam 2 to 3 mg IV over 2 to 3 min; may be repeated.

- Phenytoin loading dose 15 to 18 mg/kg IV at a rate not to exceed 25 to 50 mg/min under cardiac monitoring.
- Phenobarbital loading dose 10 to 15 mg/kg IV at a rate of 25 mg/min; an additional 5 mg/kg may be given in 30 to 45 min if seizures are not controlled.
- For refractory seizures, consider:
  1. Pancuronium 0.1 mg/kg IV
  2. Halothane general anesthesia
  3. Both require EEG monitoring to determine brain seizure activity.

HYPERTENSION: Cocaine-induced hypertension usually responds to benzodiazepines. If this fails:
- Consider arterial line for continuous blood pressure monitoring
- Avoid the use of calcium channel blockers because they may potentiate the incidence of seizures and death, especially in body packers.
- The use of beta-blockers may exacerbate cocaine-induced vasoconstriction.
- Phentolamine (unopposed adrenergic effects) or nitroglycerin may be required.
- If diastolic pressure >120 mm Hg: hydralazine hydrochloride 25 mg IM or IV; may repeat q1h.
- If hypertension is uncontrolled or hypertensive encephalopathy is present: sodium nitroprusside initially at 0.5 μg/kg/min not to exceed 10 μg/kg/min.

CHEST PAIN:
- Chest radiograph, ECG, cardiac enzymes.
- Benzodiazepines for agitation.
- Acetylsalicylic acid and nitroglycerin for ischemic pain.
- Percutaneous transluminal coronary angioplasty possibly better than thrombolysis for cocaine-associated myocardial infarction.
- The use of beta-adrenergic blockers remains controversial because of the unopposed alpha-adrenergic effects of cocaine.
- The combination of nitroprusside and a beta-adrenergic blocking agent or phentolamine alone or in addition to a beta-adrenergic blocking agent may successfully treat myocardial ischemia and hypertension.

VENTRICULAR ARRHYTHMIAS:
- Antiarrhythmic agents should be used with caution during the early period after cocaine exposure as a result of their proarrhythmic and proconvulsant effects.
- Propranolol 1 mg/min IV for up to 6 mg.
- Lidocaine 1.5 mg/kg IV bolus followed by IV infusion (controversial: may be proarrhythmic and proconvulsant).
- Termination of ventricular arrhythmias may be resistant to lidocaine and even cardioversion.
- $NaHCO_3^-$ is under investigation in cocaine-mediated conduction abnormalities and rhythm disturbances.

DISPOSITION

Although many patients who use cocaine may not require treatment because of the short half-life of the drug, others may require specific treatment for possible cocaine-related complications.

REFERRAL

Consider psychotherapy or behavioral therapy once stable.

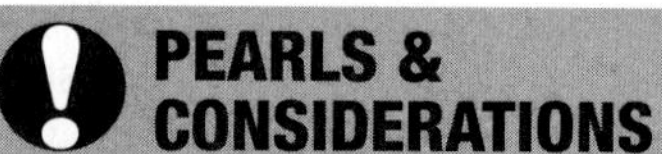

PEARLS & CONSIDERATIONS

- Cocaine-induced vasoconstriction may be exacerbated by the use of selective and nonselective beta-adrenergic blocking agents.
- The use of lidocaine in treating ventricular arrhythmias may precipitate seizures and further arrhythmias.

SUGGESTED READINGS

Jones JH, Wier WB: Cocaine associated chest pain, *Med Clin North Am* 89(6):1323, 2005.

Lange RA, Hillis LD: Cardiovascular complications of cocaine use, *N Engl J Med* 345:351, 2001.

Mokhlesi B, Corbridge T: Adult toxicology in critical care: part II: specific poisonings, *Clin Chest Med* 123(3):897, 2003.

AUTHOR: **SAJEEV HANDA, M.D.**

BASIC INFORMATION

DEFINITION

Coccidioidomycosis is an infectious disease caused by the fungus *Coccidioides immitis.* It is usually asymptomatic and characterized by a primary pulmonary focus with infrequent progression to chronic pulmonary disease and dissemination to other organs.

SYNONYMS

San Joaquin Valley fever

ICD-9CM CODES

114.0 Coccidioides pneumonia
114.1 Cutaneous or extrapulmonary (primary) coccidioidomycosis
114.3 Disseminated or prostate coccidioidomycosis
114.5 Pulmonary coccidioidomycosis
114.2 Coccidioidal meningitis
114.4 Chronic coccidioidomycosis

EPIDEMIOLOGY & DEMOGRAPHICS

INCIDENCE (IN U.S.): Estimated annual infection rate 100,000 persons, predominantly in southwest U.S.
PEAK INCIDENCE: Unknown
PREVALENCE: Unknown
PREDOMINANT SEX: Males, between the ages of 25 and 55 yr
Clinical disease more severe in older children and adults

PHYSICAL FINDINGS & CLINICAL PRESENTATION

- Asymptomatic infections or illness consistent with a nonspecific upper respiratory tract infection in at least 60%.
- Symptoms of primary infection—cough, malaise, fever, chills, night sweats, anorexia, weakness, and arthralgias (desert rheumatism)—in remaining 40% within 3 wk of exposure.
- Erythema nodosum and erythema multiforme more common in women.
- Scattered rales and dullness on percussion.
- Spontaneous improvement within 2 wk of illness, with complete recovery usual.
- Pulmonary nodules and cavities in <10% of those patients with primary infection; half of these patients asymptomatic.
- In a small portion of these patients: a progressive pneumonitis, often with a fatal outcome.
- Immunocompromised or diabetic patients may progress to chronic pulmonary disease.
- Over many years, granulomas rupture, leading to new cavity formation and continued fibrosis, often accompanied by hemoptysis.
- Disseminated or extrapulmonary disease in approximately 0.5% of acutely infected patients.
  1. Early signs of probable dissemination: fever, malaise, hilar adenopathy, and elevated ESR persisting in the setting of primary infection.
  2. Most organs are susceptible to dissemination, with heart and GI tract generally spared.
- Musculoskeletal involvement: bone lesions often unifocal, ribs, long bones, and vertebral lesions are common.
  1. Joint lesions predominantly unifocal, most commonly involving the ankle and knee, and often accompanying adjacent sites of osteomyelitis.
- Meningeal involvement: headache, fever, weakness, confusion, lethargy, cranial nerve defects, seizures; meningeal signs often minimal or absent.
- Cutaneous involvement: variable lesions—pustules, papules, plaques, nodules, ulcers, abscesses, or verrucous proliferative lesions.
  1. Dissemination and fatal outcomes most common in men, pregnant women, neonates, immunocompromised hosts, and individuals of dark-skinned races, especially those of African, Filipino, Mexican, and Native American ancestry.

ETIOLOGY

- *Coccidioides immitis* is endemic to North and South America.
- In the U.S., endemic areas coincide with the Lower Sonoran Life Zone, with semiarid climate, sparse flora, and alkaline soil in Arizona, California, New Mexico, and Texas.
- Fungus exists in the mycelial phase in soil, having barrel-shaped hyphae (arthroconidia). Arthrospores are aerosolized and deposit in the alveoli, then fungus converts to thick-walled spherule.
- Internal spherical spores (endospores) are released through spherule rupture and mature into new spherules (parasitic cycle).
- Fungus incites a granulomatous reaction in host tissue, usually with caseation necrosis.

DIAGNOSIS

DIFFERENTIAL DIAGNOSIS

- Acute pulmonary coccidioidomycoses:
  1. Community-acquired pneumonias caused by *Mycoplasma* and *Chlamydia*
  2. Granulomatous diseases, such as *Mycobacterium tuberculosis* and sarcoidosis
  3. Other fungal diseases, such as *Blastomyces dermatitidis* and *Histoplasma capsulatum*
- Coccidioidomas: true neoplasms

WORKUP

Suspected in patients with a history of residence or travel in an endemic area, especially during periods favorable to spore dispersion (e.g., dust storms and drought followed by heavy rains)

LABORATORY TESTS

- CBC to reveal eosinophilia, especially with erythema nodosum
- Routine chemistries: usually normal but may reveal hyponatremia
- Elevated serum levels of IgE; associated with progressive disease
- CSF cell counts and chemistry: pleocytosis with mononuclear cell predominance associated with hypoglycorrhachia and elevated protein level
- Definitive diagnosis based on demonstration of the organism by culture from body fluids or tissues
  1. Greatest yield with pus, sputum, synovial fluid, and soft tissue aspirations, varying with the degree of dissemination
  2. Possible positive cultures of blood, gastric aspirate, pleural effusion, peritoneal fluid, and CSF, but less frequently obtained
- Serologic evaluations
  1. Latex agglutination and complement fixation
  2. Elevated serum complement-fixing antibody (CFA) titers ≥1:32 strongly correlated with disseminated disease, except with meningitis where lower titers seen
  3. In meningeal disease: CFA detected in CSF except with high serum CFA titers secondary to concurrent extraneural disease
  4. Enzyme-linked immunosorbent assay (ELISA) against a 33-kDa spherule antigen to detect and monitor CNS disease
- Skin test: coccidioidin, the mycelial phase antigen, and spherulin, the parasitic phase antigen
  1. Positive (>5 mm) 1 mo following onset of symptomatic primary infection
  2. Useful in assessing prior infection
  3. Negative skin test with primary infection: latent or future dissemination

IMAGING STUDIES

Chest radiograph examination:

- Reveals unilateral infiltrates, hilar adenopathy, or pleural effusion in primary infection
- Shows areas of fibrosis containing usually solitary, thin-walled cavities that persist as residua of primary infection
- Possible coccidioidoma, a coinlike lesion representing a healed area of previous pneumonitis

TREATMENT

NONPHARMACOLOGIC THERAPY

- Supportive care in mild symptomatic disease
- In patients with extrapulmonary manifestations involving draining skin, joint, and soft tissue infection: local wound care to avoid possible bacterial superinfection

ACUTE GENERAL Rx

- In general, drug therapy is not required for patients with asymptomatic pulmonary disease and most patients with mild symptomatic primary infection.
- Chemotherapy is indicated under the following circumstances:
  1. Severe symptomatic primary infection
  2. High serum CFA titers

3. Persistent symptoms >6 wk
4. Prostration
5. Progressive pulmonary involvement
6. Pregnancy
7. Infancy
8. Debilitation
9. Concurrent illness (e.g., diabetes, asthma, COPD, malignancy)
10. Acquired or induced immunosuppression
11. Racial group with known predisposition for disseminated disease

- Fluconazole
  1. Most commonly, oral therapy with 400 mg/day up to 1.2 g/day appears to be the drug of choice for meningeal and deep-seated mycotic infections.
  2. In patients with AIDS, fluconazole may be considered the drug of choice for initial and maintenance therapy.
  3. All patients with coccidioidal meningitis should continue azole therapy indefinitely.
- Itraconazole
  1. 400 to 600 mg/day achieves 90% response rate in bone, joint, soft tissue, lymphatic, and genitourinary infections.
  2. Itraconazole may be more efficacious than fluconazole in the treatment of skeletal (bone) infections.
- Posaconazole is a new triazole that has recently been approved for use for systemic mycoses such as coccidioidomycosis; its relative efficacy compared to other agents will need additional clinical study.
- For pulmonary infections, treatment with either fluconazole or itraconazole, given for 6 to 12 wk, appears to be equal in efficacy.
- Amphotericin B is the classic therapy for disseminated extraneural disease, dose 0.6 to 1 mg/kg/day, qd for the first week then 0.8 mg/kg every other day, for a total dose of 1 to 2.5 g or until clinical and serologic remission is accomplished.
  1. Local instillation into body cavities such as sinuses, fistulae, and abscesses has been adjunct to therapy.
  2. Liposomal amphotericin B is probably equally effective.
  3. Duration of therapy for extraneural disease is undefined but probably about 1 yr.
- With meningeal disease: fluconazole 400 to 1000 mg PO q24h indefinitely
  1. Intrathecal amphotericin B is the alternate treatment modality, given alone or preceding the use of oral agents.
  2. Begin in doses of 0.01 to 0.025 mg/day, gradually increasing the dose as tolerated, to 0.5 mg/day with the patient in Trendelenburg's position.
  3. If given via Ommaya reservoir, as in ventriculitis, dose may be increased to 1.5 mg/day if tolerated.
  4. Concomitant parenteral therapy with amphotericin B is used for simultaneous extraneural disease as standard doses and with purely meningeal disease in smaller doses, although not strictly indicated.
  5. Intrathecal therapy is usually given three times a week for at least 3 mo, then discontinued or gradually tapered until once every 6 wk through 1 yr of therapy.
  6. Patients need routine monitoring of CSF, CFA, cell count, and chemistries for at least 2 yr following cessation of therapy.
- For osteomyelitis, soft tissue closed-space infections, and pulmonary fibrocavitary disease: surgical debridement, drainage, or resection, respectively, in addition to oral azole therapy or parenteral administration of amphotericin B.

CHRONIC Rx

For chronically immunocompromised patients, lifelong therapy with oral azoles or amphotericin B

DISPOSITION

- Prognosis for primary symptomatic infection is good.
- Immunocompromised patients are most likely to have disseminated disease and higher morbidity and mortality.

REFERRAL

- To surgeon for the evaluation of chronic hemoptysis, enlarging cavitary lesions despite chemotherapy and intrapleural rupture, osteomyelitis, and other synovial or soft tissue closed space infections
- For neurosurgical consultation in patients with meningeal disease to establish the delivery route of intrathecal drug therapy

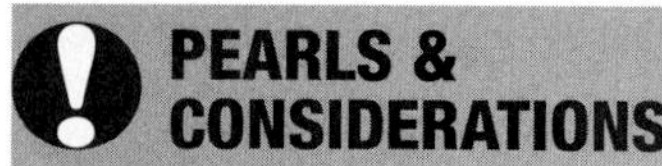

PEARLS & CONSIDERATIONS

COMMENTS

- Infected body fluids contained within a closed moist environment (e.g., sputum in a specimen cup) provide the opportunity for the fungus to revert to its hyphal form whereby spores may be made airborne on opening of the container. This is a biohazard for laboratory personnel. Purulent drainage into a cast, allowing conversion of fungus to the saprophytic phase, has been responsible for acute disease when the cast was opened and the spores were unintentionally made airborne.
- Patients with a remote history of exposure, especially if immunosuppressed by medication or disease, may reactivate primary disease and suffer rapid dissemination.
- Although cardiac disease is rare, constrictive pericarditis in the setting of disseminated coccidioidomycosis has been documented and is potentially fatal.
- Organ transplant recipients may develop disease if the transplant donor has unrecognized active coccidioidomycosis at the time of death.

SUGGESTED READINGS

Adam RD et al: The spectrum and presentation of disseminated coccidioidomycosis, *Am J Med* 122:770-777, 2009.

Ampel NM et al: The mannose receptor mediates the cellular immune response in human coccidioidomycosis, *Infect Immun* 73(4):2554-2555, 2005.

Blair JE, Smilack JD, Caples SM: Coccidioidomycosis in patients with hematologic malignancies, *Arch Intern Med* 165(1):113-117, 2005.

Parish JM, Blair JE: Coccidioidomycosis, *Mayo Clin Proc* 83(3):343-349, 2008.

Wang CY et al: Disseminated coccidioidomycosis, *Emerg Infect Dis* 11(1):177-179, 2005.

AUTHORS: **GLENN G. FORT, M.D., M.P.H.,** and **DENNIS J. MIKOLICH, M.D.**

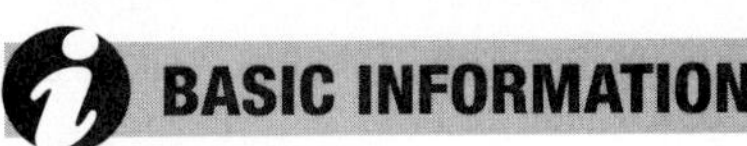

BASIC INFORMATION

DEFINITION

Acute, self-limited febrile illness caused by infection with a Coltivirus.

ICD-9CM CODES
066.1 Colorado tick fever

EPIDEMIOLOGY & DEMOGRAPHICS

- Incidence: approximately 330 cases reported per year in the U.S.
- Demographics: children and adults of both genders.
- Geography: Rocky Mountains at elevations of 4000 to 10,000 feet. Sporadic cases have been reported from areas of California outside the range of *Dermacentor andersoni.*
- Colorado has the highest incidence (Fig. 1-71).

PHYSICAL FINDINGS & CLINICAL PRESENTATION

- Incubation: 3 to 4 days is usual but can be up to 14 days
- First symptoms: fever, chills, severe headache, severe myalgias, and hyperesthetic skin
- Initial signs and symptoms:
  1. Tick bite
  2. Fever and chills
  3. Headache
  4. Myalgias
  5. Weakness
  6. Prostration and indifference
  7. Injected conjunctivae
  8. Erythematous pharyngitis
  9. Lymphadenopathy
  10. Maculopapular or petechial rash

These first symptoms last for 1 wk or less but 50% of patients have a febrile relapse 2 to 3 days after an initial remission. Weakness and fatigue may persist for several months after the acute phase(s). This chronic phase is more likely in older patients.

In children, 5% to 10% of cases are complicated by aseptic meningitis. In adults, rare complications include pneumonia, hepatitis, myocarditis, and epididymo-orchitis. Vertically transmitted fetal infection is possible.

ETIOLOGY

- Infectious agent: Coltiviruses; 7 species, including three in the U.S.
- Vector: wood tick, *D. andersoni.*
- Pathogenesis: human transmission occurs by tick bite. Tick season spans from March to September. The virus infects marrow erythrocytic precursors, explaining the protracted disease course because viremia lasts for the lifespan of the infected red blood cell.

Dx DIAGNOSIS

DIFFERENTIAL DIAGNOSIS

- Rocky Mountain spotted fever
- Influenza
- Leptospirosis
- Infectious mononucleosis
- CMV infection
- Pneumonia
- Hepatitis
- Meningitis
- Endocarditis
- Scarlet fever
- Measles
- Rubella
- Typhus
- Lyme disease
- Immune thrombocytopenic purpura (ITP)
- Thrombotic thrombocytopenic purpura (TTP)
- Kawasaki disease
- Toxic shock syndrome
- Vasculitis

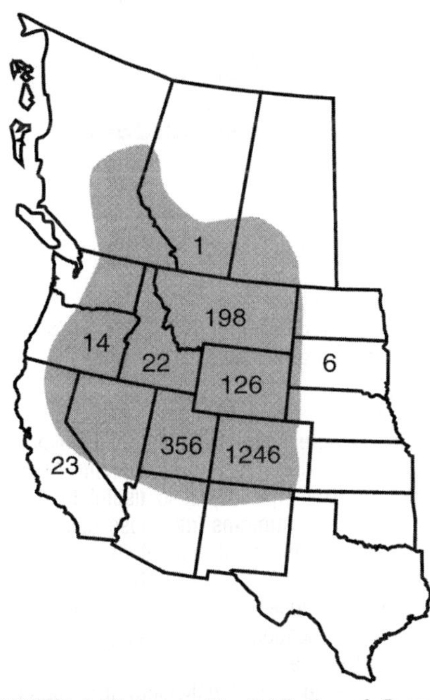

FIGURE 1-71 Geographic distribution of *Dermacentor andersoni* (wood ticks) and reported cases of Colorado tick fever, 1990-1996, United States and Canada. (From Mandell GL: *Mandell, Douglas, and Bennett's principles and practice of infectious diseases,* ed 6, New York, 2005, Churchill Livingstone.)

WORKUP

Consider Colorado tick fever in the presence of the above symptoms associated with travel to an endemic area coupled with a history of tick exposure.

LABORATORY TESTS

- Complete blood count
  1. Leukopenia
  2. Atypical lymphocytes
  3. Moderate thrombocytopenia
- Virus identification in red blood cells by indirect immunofluorescence
- Serology with enzyme-linked immunosorbent assay, neutralization, or complement fixation

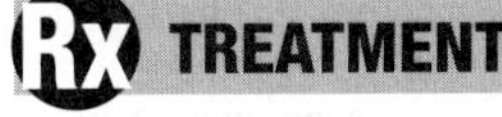

TREATMENT

- No specific therapy, although Coltiviruses are sensitive to ribavirin
- Bedrest, fluids, acetaminophen
- Avoid aspirin because of thrombocytopenia
- Prevention: tick avoidance measures

SUGGESTED READINGS

Jaffar FM et al: Recombinant VP-7-based enzyme-linked immunosorbent assay for detection of immunoglobulin G antibodies to Colorado tick fever virus, *J Clin Microbiol* 41:2102, 2003.

Tsai TF: Coltiviruses (Colorado tick fever). In Mandell GL et al (eds): *Principles and practice of infectious diseases,* ed 6, Philadelphia, 2005, Churchill Livingstone.

AUTHOR: **FRED F. FERRI, M.D.**

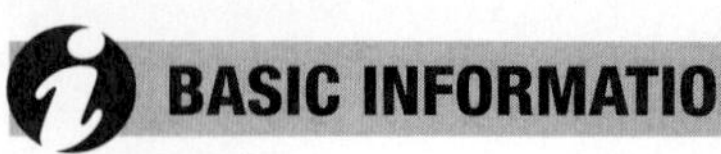

BASIC INFORMATION

DEFINITION

Colorectal cancer (CRC) is a neoplasm arising from the luminal surface of the large bowel; locations include descending colon (40% to 42%), rectosigmoid and rectum (30% to 33%), cecum and ascending colon (25% to 30%), and transverse colon (10% to 13%).

ICD-9CM CODES
154.0 Colorectal cancer

EPIDEMIOLOGY & DEMOGRAPHICS

CRC is the second leading cause of cancer deaths in the U.S. (>135,000 new cases and >50,000 deaths/yr).

Peak incidence is in the seventh decade of life. The lifetime risk for development of CRC is 1 in 17, with 90% of cases occurring after the age of 50 yr.

50% of rectal cancers are within reach of the examiner's finger, and 50% of colon cancers are within reach of the flexible sigmoidoscope.

CRC accounts for 14% of all cases of cancer (excluding skin malignancies) and 14% of all yearly cancer deaths.

Risk factors:

1. Hereditary polyposis syndromes
   a. Familial polyposis (high risk)
   b. Gardner's syndrome (high risk)
   c. Turcot's syndrome (high risk)
   d. Peutz-Jeghers syndrome (low to moderate risk)
2. Inflammatory bowel disease (IBD), both ulcerative colitis and Crohn's disease
3. Family history of "cancer family syndrome"
4. Heredofamilial breast cancer and colon carcinoma
5. History of previous colorectal carcinoma
6. Women undergoing irradiation for gynecologic cancer
7. First-degree relatives with colorectal carcinoma
8. Age >40 yr
9. Possible dietary factors (diet high in fat or meat, beer drinking, reduced vegetable consumption); prolonged high consumption of red and processed meat may increase the risk for cancer of the large intestine
10. Hereditary nonpolyposis colon cancer (HNPCC): autosomal dominant disorder characterized by early age of onset (mean age, 44 yr) and right-sided or proximal colon cancers, synchronous and metachronous colon cancers, mucinous and poorly differentiated colon cancers; accounts for 1% to 5% of all cases of CRC
11. Previous endometrial or ovarian cancer, particularly when diagnosed at an early age

PHYSICAL FINDINGS & CLINICAL PRESENTATION

- Physical examination may be completely unremarkable.
- Digital rectal examination can detect approximately 50% of rectal cancers.
- Palpable abdominal masses may indicate metastasis or complications of colorectal carcinoma (abscess, intussusception, volvulus).
- Abdominal distention and tenderness are suggestive of colonic obstruction.
- Hepatomegaly may be indicative of hepatic metastasis.

ETIOLOGY

CRC can arise through two mutational pathways: microsatellite instability or chromosomal instability. Germline genetic mutations are the basis of inherited colon cancer syndromes; an accumulation of somatic mutations in a cell is the basis of sporadic colon cancer.

Dx DIAGNOSIS

DIFFERENTIAL DIAGNOSIS

- Diverticular disease
- Strictures
- IBD
- Infectious or inflammatory lesions
- Adhesions
- Arteriovenous malformations
- Metastatic carcinoma (prostate, sarcoma)
- Extrinsic masses (cysts, abscesses)

WORKUP

The clinical presentation of colorectal malignancies is initially vague and nonspecific (weight loss, anorexia, malaise). It is useful to divide colon cancer symptoms into those usually associated with the right side of the colon and those commonly associated with the left side of the colon because the clinical presentation varies with the location of the carcinoma.

1. Right side of colon:
   a. Anemia (iron deficiency from chronic blood loss)
   b. Dull, vague, and uncharacteristic abdominal pain may be present, or patient may be completely asymptomatic
   c. Rectal bleeding is often missed because blood is mixed with feces
   d. Obstruction and constipation are unusual because of large lumen and more liquid stools
2. Left side of colon:
   a. Change in bowel habits (constipation, diarrhea, tenesmus, pencil-thin stools)
   b. Rectal bleeding (bright red blood coating the surface of the stool)
   c. Intestinal obstruction is frequent because of small lumen

Early diagnosis of patients with surgically curable disease (Dukes A/B) is necessary because survival time is directly related to the stage of the carcinoma at the time of diagnosis. Appropriate screening recommendations are discussed in Section V.

CLASSIFICATION AND STAGING: Dukes and UICC classification for CRC:

A. Confined to the mucosa-submucosa (stage I)
B. Invasion of muscularis propria (stage II)
C. Local node involvement (stage III)
D. Distant metastasis (stage IV)

TNM Classification:

Stage	TNM classification
I	$T_{1\text{-}2}$, N_0, M_0
IIA	T_3, N_0, M_0
IIB	T_4, N_0, M_0
IIIA	$T_{1\text{-}2}$, N_1, M_0
IIIB	$T_{3\text{-}4}$, N_1, M_0
IIIC	T(any), N_2, M_0
IV	T(any), N(any), M_1

LABORATORY TESTS

- Positive fecal occult blood test (FOBT): Many primary care physicians use single digital FOBT as their primary screening test for CRC. Single FOBT has low specificity for detecting human hemoglobin, is a poor screening method for CRC (sensitivity, 4.9%), and is inappropriate as the only test because negative results do not decrease the odds of advanced neoplasia. The American College of Gastroenterology recommends fecal immunochemical test as a replacement for guaiac-based FOBT for CRC detection. Annual Hemoccult SENSA and fecal DNA testing every 3 yr are alternative cancer detection tests.
- Microcytic anemia on CBC may be indicative of chronic blood loss.
- Increased plasma carcinoembryonic antigen (CEA) level: CEA should not be used as a screening test for CRC because it can be increased in patients with many other conditions (smoking, IBD, alcoholic liver disease). A normal CEA result does not exclude the diagnosis of CRC.
- Liver function tests should be ordered.

IMAGING STUDIES

- Colonoscopy with biopsy (primary assessment tool): The American College of Physicians recommends that patients should be offered a colonoscopy beginning at age 50 yr and repeated every 10 yr in average-risk patients. Screening is recommended in African Americans beginning at 45 yr of age. Persons with only one first-degree relative with CRC or advanced adenomas diagnosed at 60 yr or older may be screened as at average risk. A family history of small tubular adenomas in first-degree relatives is not considered to increase the risk for CRC. The U.S. Preventive Services Task Force guidelines state that screening should not be routinely recommended in persons older than 75 yr, and it should be not recommended at all in persons older than 85 yr. If persons between the ages of 75 and 85 yr have never undergone screening, the decision about screening should be individualized according to health status.
- Computed tomography colonoscopy (CTC) virtual colonoscopy (VC) uses helical (spiral) CT scanning to generate a two- or three-

dimensional virtual colorectal image. CTC does not require sedation; but, like optical colonoscopy, it requires some bowel preparation (either bowel cathartics or ingestion of iodinated contrast medium with meals during the 48 hours before CT) and air insufflation. It also involves substantial exposure to radiation. In addition, patients with lesions detected by VC will require traditional colonoscopy. Compared with colonoscopy, CTC sensitivity for detection of polyps >10 mm ranges from 70% to 96%, and specificity ranges from 72% to 96%. CTC has replaced double-contrast barium enema as the radiographic screening alternative when patients decline colonoscopy.

- Capsule endoscopy allows visualization of the colonic mucosa but is not recommended as a screening procedure because its sensitivity for detecting colonic lesions is low compared with colonoscopy.
- CT scanning of the abdomen, pelvis, and chest assists in preoperative staging.
- PET scanning can display functional information and is accurate in the detection of CRC and its distant metastases. Combined PET/CT scanners are increasingly more available, and are useful to detect and characterize malignant lesions. Colonography composed of a combined modality of PET and CT is a newer diagnostic modality that can provide whole-body tumor staging in a single session.

Rx TREATMENT

GENERAL Rx

- Surgical resection: 70% of CRCs are resectable for cure at presentation; 45% of patients are cured by primary resection.
- The backbone of treatment of CRC is fluorouracil (FU). Leucovorin (folinic acid) enhances the effect of FU and is given concomitantly. Adjuvant chemotherapy with combination of 5-FU and levamisole substantially increases cure rates for patients with stage III colon cancer and should be considered standard treatment for all such patients and selected patients with high-risk stage II colon cancer (adherence of tumor to an adjacent organ, bowel perforation, or obstruction).
- Radiation therapy is a useful adjunct to FU and leucovorin therapy for stage II or III rectal cancers.
- When given as adjuvant therapy after a complete resection in stage III disease, FU increases overall 5-yr survival rate from 51% to 64%. The use of adjuvant FU in stage II disease (no involvement of regional nodes) is controversial because 5-yr overall survival is 80% for treated or untreated patients, and the addition of FU only increases the probability of a 5-yr disease-free interval from 72% to 76%. For patients with standard-risk stage III tumors (e.g., involvement of one to three regional lymph nodes), both FU alone and FU with oxaliplatin (Eloxatin, an inhibitor of DNA synthesis) are reasonable choices. In general, reversible peripheral neuropathy is the main side effect of FU plus oxaliplatin. The oral fluoropyrimidine capecitabine (Xeloda) is a prodrug that undergoes enzymatic conversion to FU. It is an effective alternative to IV FU as adjuvant treatment for stage III colon cancer because it has a lower incidence of mouth sores and bone marrow suppression. It does, however, have an increased incidence of palmar-plantar erythrodysesthesia (hand-foot syndrome).
- Irinotecan (Camptosar), a potent inhibitor of topoisomerase I, a nuclear enzyme involved in the unwinding of DNA during replication, can be used to treat metastatic CRC refractory to other drugs, including 5-FU; it may offer a few months of palliation but is expensive and is associated with significant toxicity.
- Oxaliplatin (Eloxatin), a third-generation platinum derivative, can be used in combination with FU and leucovorin (FL) for patients with metastatic CRC whose disease has recurred or progressed despite treatment with FL plus irinotecan. FL plus oxaliplatin should be considered for high-risk patients with stage III cancers (e.g., more than three involved regional nodes [N_2] or tumor invasion beyond the serosa [T_4 lesion]).
- Laboratory studies have identified molecular sites in tumor tissue that may serve as specific targets for treatment by using epidermal growth factor receptor (EGFR) antagonists and angiogenesis inhibitors. The monoclonal antibodies cetuximab (Erbitux), panitumumab (Vectibix), and bevacizumab (Avastatin) have been approved by the FDA for advanced CRC. Bevacizumab is an angiogenesis inhibitor that binds and inhibits the activity of human vascular endothelial growth factor. Cetuximab and panitumumab are EGFR blockers that inhibit the growth and survival of tumor cells that overexpress EGFR. Cetuximab has synergism with irinotecan, and its addition to irinotecan in patients with advanced disease resistant to irinotecan increases the response rate from 10% when cetuximab is used alone to 22% with combination of cetuximab and irinotecan. The addition of bevacizumab to FL in patients with advanced CRC has been reported to increase the response rate from 17% to 40%. Severe dermatologic toxicity can occur with both cetuximab and panitumumab.
- The liver is generally the initial and most common site of CRC metastases. Resection of metastases limited to the liver is curative in more than 30% of selected patients. In patients who undergo resection of liver metastases, postoperative treatment with a combination of hepatic arterial infusion of floxuridine and IV FU improves the outcome at 2 yr.

CHRONIC Rx

Follow-up is indicated with:

- Physician visits with a focus on the clinical and disease-related history, directed physical examination guided by this history, coordination of follow-up, and counseling every 3 to 6 mo for the first 3 yr, then decreased frequency thereafter for 2 yr
- Colonoscopy yearly for the initial 2 yr, then every 3 yr
- Baseline CEA level should be obtained; if elevated, it can be used after surgery as a measure of completeness of tumor resection or to monitor tumor recurrence. If used to monitor tumor recurrence, CEA should be obtained every 3 to 6 mo for up to 5 yr. The role of CEA for monitoring patients with resected colon cancer has been questioned because of the small number of cures attributed to CEA monitoring despite the substantial cost in dollars and physical and emotional stress associated with monitoring.

DISPOSITION

The 5-yr survival rate varies with the stage of the carcinoma:

- Dukes:
  1. Dukes A 5-yr survival rate: >80%
  2. Dukes B 5-yr survival rate: 60%
  3. Dukes C 5-yr survival rate: 20%
  4. Dukes D 5-yr survival rate: 3%
- TNM classification:

Stage	TNM Classification	5-yr Survival Rate
I	T_{1-2}, N_0, M_0	>90%
IIA	T_3, N_0, M_0	60-85%
IIB	T_4, N_0, M_0	60-85%
IIIA	T_{1-2}, N_1, M_0	25-65%
IIIB	T_{3-4}, N_1, M_0	25-65%
IIIC	T(any), N_2, M_0	25-65%
IV	T(any), N(any), M_1	5-7%

- Overall 5-yr disease-free survival rate has increased from 50% to 63% during the past two decades.
- High-frequency microsatellite instability in CRC is independently predictive of a relatively favorable outcome and reduces the likelihood of metastases.
- In patients with Dukes C (stage III) CRC, there is improved 5-yr survival among women treated with adjuvant chemotherapy (53% with chemotherapy vs. 33% without) and among patients with right-sided tumors treated with adjuvant chemotherapy.
- Retention of 18q alleles in microsatellite-stable cancers and mutation of the gene for the type I receptor for tumor growth factor B1 in cancers with high levels of microsatellite instability point to a favorable outcome after adjuvant chemotherapy with FU-based regimens for stage II colon cancer.
- Expression patterns of microRNA are systemically altered in colon adenocarcinomas. High *miR-21* expression is associated with poor survival and poor therapeutic outcome.
- Guanylyl cyclase 2 C (GUCY2C) has been identified as a marker expressed by colorectal tumors that could reveal occult metastases in lymph nodes. Expression of GUCY2C in histologically negative lymph nodes appears to be independently associated with time to recurrence and disease-free survival in patients with lymph nodes free of tumor cells by histopathology (pNO) in CRC.

 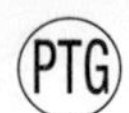

- Regular aspirin use after the diagnosis of CRC has been reported to be associated with lower risk for CRC-specific and overall mortality, especially among individuals with tumors that overexpress cyclooxygenase-2.

REFERRAL

- Surgical referral for resection
- Oncology referral for adjuvant chemotherapy in selected patients
- Radiation oncology referral for patients with stage II or III rectal cancers

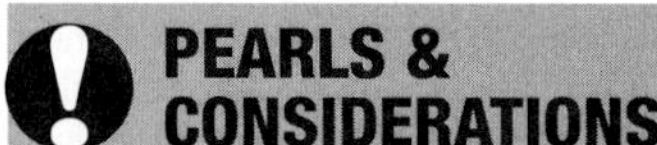

PEARLS & CONSIDERATIONS

COMMENTS

- Metastases of tumor cells to regional lymph nodes is the single most important prognostic factor in patients with colon cancer.
- Decreased fat intake to 30% of total energy intake, increased fiber, and fruit and vegetable consumption may reduce CRC risk. Recent literature reports, however, do not support a protective effect from dietary fiber against CRC in women.
- Chemoprophylaxis with aspirin (81 mg/day) reduces the incidence of colorectal adenomas in persons at risk.
- Statins inhibit the growth of colon cancer lines. Use of statins is associated with a 47% relative reduction in the risk for CRC. Additional trials are necessary to investigate the overall benefits of statins in preventing CRC.
- The National Cancer Institute has published consensus guidelines for universal screening for HNPCC in patients with newly diagnosed CRC. Tumors in mutation carriers of HNPCC typically exhibit microsatellite instability, a characteristic phenotype caused by expansion or contraction of short nucleotide repeat sequences. These guidelines (Bethesda Guidelines) are useful for selective patients for microsatellite instability testing. Screening patients with newly diagnosed CRC for HNPCC is cost effective, especially if the benefits to their immediate relatives are considered.
- Expression of guanylyl cyclase C mRNA in lymph nodes is associated with recurrence of CRC in patients with stage II disease. Analysis of guanylyl cyclase mRNA expression by reverse transcription polymerase chain reaction may be useful for CRC staging.
- The use of either annual or biennial FOBT significantly reduces the incidence of CRC.
- The detection of mutations in the *APC* gene from stool samples is a promising new modality for early detection of colorectal neoplasms.

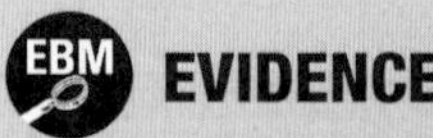

EVIDENCE

The principle that appropriate surgical therapy is the foundation for optimal management of CRC is supported by guidelines from professional bodies.

Surgery is the preferred treatment for CRC. Primary surgical resection is indicated in nearly all patients with newly diagnosed CRC, unless survival is unlikely or life expectancy is very short. If curative surgery is not possible, palliative surgery should be performed to prevent obstruction and further bleeding.[1]

Abdominoperineal resection is generally indicated for tumors of the lower third of the rectum or for higher lesions when tumor characteristics and anatomic factors favor such a resection.[2]

Sphincter-preserving resection is possible for most patients with rectal carcinoma.[3]

Open and laparoscopically assisted colectomy for adenocarcinoma of the colon result in similar rates of recurrence.

In a recent multiinstitutional study, 872 patients with adenocarcinoma of the colon were randomly assigned to 2 groups receiving open or laparoscopically assisted colectomy performed by credentialed surgeons. At 3 yr, the rates of recurrence were similar in the two groups.[3]

A systematic review of randomized trials comparing laparoscopic and conventional resection found that, although methodologic quality of the studies was considered moderate, there was some evidence that laparoscopic surgery may offer some advantages for select patients.[4]

Postoperative adjuvant chemotherapy based on FU and FL offers an overall survival benefit in stage III (Dukes C) colon carcinoma. The survival benefit for stage II (Dukes B) colon carcinoma and for rectal carcinoma has not yet been fully established.

The addition of oxaliplatin to adjuvant FU and FL in patients with stage II and III colon cancer has been shown to improve disease-free survival at 3 yr compared with treatment with FL alone. Patients with stage III disease appear to respond most favorably.[5]

In colon cancer, the use of additional chemotherapy agents alongside FU plus FL (including oxaliplatin or irinotecan) and adjunctive immunotherapy is recommended in certain circumstances.[6]

Although specific regimens continue to evolve, the evidence is that the use of FU-based chemoradiation is superior to radiation therapy alone as an adjunct to surgical resection of rectal carcinoma. The optimal timing for chemoradiation remains uncertain.

A recent randomized controlled trial compared preoperative chemoradiotherapy (FU) with postoperative chemoradiotherapy in 823 patients with clinical stage T_3 or T_4 or node-positive rectal cancer. This study found that, at 5-yr follow-up, preoperative chemoradiotherapy significantly improved local control and was associated with reduced toxicity compared with the postoperative regimen. However, there was no difference in overall survival between the two patient groups.[7]

Monoclonal antibodies can have a useful role in treatment in some circumstances. The FDA recently approved cetuximab (a monoclonal antibody that inhibits the EGFR pathway) for the treatment of advanced CRC. A phase II, open-label clinical trial found that patients who had tumors with EGFR expression and who also demonstrated clinical failure with irinotecan had modest results with a once-weekly cetuximab regimen.[8]

A recent randomized controlled clinical trial compared the addition of the monoclonal antibody against vascular endothelial growth factor bevacizumab with an FU-based combination chemotherapy regimen vs. the addition of placebo to the same regimen in patients with untreated metastatic CRC. It found that the addition of bevacizumab resulted in a statistically significant and clinically meaningful improvement in survival.[9]

Evidence-Based References

1. Otchy D et al; Standards Practice Task Force; American Society of Colon and Rectal Surgeons: Practice parameters for colon cancer, *Dis Colon Rectum* 47:1269-1284, 2004.
2. Tjandra JJ et al; The Standards Practice Task Force; The American Society of Colon and Rectal Surgeons: Practice parameters for the management of rectal cancer (revised), *Dis Colon Rectum* 48:411-423, 2005.
3. Clinical Outcomes of Surgical Therapy Study Group: A comparison of laparoscopically assisted and open colectomy for colon cancer, *N Engl J Med* 350:2050-2059, 2004.
4. Schwenk W et al: Short term benefits for laparoscopic colorectal resection, *Cochrane Rev* 2, 2005.
5. Andre T et al; Multicenter International Study of Oxaliplatin/5-Fluorouracil/Leucovorin in the Adjuvant Treatment of Colon Cancer (MOSAIC) investigators: Oxaliplatin, fluorouracil, and leucovorin as adjuvant treatment for colon cancer, *N Engl J Med* 350:2343, 2004.
6. National Comprehensive Cancer Network: NCCN clinical practice guidelines in oncology, *Colon Cancer* 2006.
7. Sauer R et al; German Rectal Cancer Study Group: Preoperative versus postoperative chemoradiotherapy for rectal cancer, *N Engl J Med* 351:1731, 2004.
8. Saltz LB et al: Phase II trial of cetuximab in patients with refractory colorectal cancer that expresses the epidermal growth factor receptor, *J Clin Oncol* 22:1201-1208, 2004.
9. Hurwitz H et al: Bevacizumab plus irinotecan, fluorouracil, and leucovorin for metastatic colorectal cancer, *N Engl J Med* 350:2335-2342, 2004.

SUGGESTED READINGS

Chan AT et al: Aspirin use and survival after diagnosis of colorectal cancer, *JAMA* 302(6):649-659, 2009.

Gill S et al: Colorectal cancer, *Mayo Clin Proc* 82:114-129, 2007.

Johnson CD et al: Accuracy of CT colonography for detection of large adenomas and cancers, *N Engl J Med* 359:1207-1217, 2008.

Jonker DJ et al: Cetuximab for the treatment of colorectal cancer, *N Engl J Med* 357:2040-2048, 2007.

Levi Z et al: A qualitative immunochemical fecal occult blood test for colorectal neoplasia, *Ann Intern Med* 146:244-255, 2007.

Liebman DA: Screening for colorectal cancer, *N Engl J Med* 361:1179-1187, 2009.

Markowitz SD, Bertagnolli M: Molecular basis of colorectal cancer, *N Engl J Med* 361:2449-2460, 2009.

Rex DK et al; for the American College of Gastroenterology: American College of Gastroenterology guidelines for colorectal cancer screening, *Am J Gastroenterology* 104(3): 740, 2009.

Schetter AJ et al: MicroRNA expression profiles associated with prognosis and therapeutic outcome in colon adenocarcinoma, *JAMA* 299(4):425-436, 2008.

Van Gossum et al: Capsule endoscopy versus colonoscopy for the detection of polyps and cancer, *N Engl J Med* 361:264-270, 2009.

Waldman SA et al: Association of GUCY2C expression in lymph nodes with time to recurrence and disease-free survival in PNO colorectal cancer, *JAMA* 301(7): 745-752, 2009.

AUTHOR: **FRED F. FERRI, M.D.**

BASIC INFORMATION

DEFINITION

Condyloma acuminatum is a sexually transmitted viral disease of the vulva, vagina, and cervix caused by the human papillomavirus (HPV).

SYNONYMS

Genital warts
Venereal warts
Anogenital warts

ICD-9CM CODES
078.11 Condyloma acuminatum

EPIDEMIOLOGY & DEMOGRAPHICS

- Seen mostly in young adults, with a mean age of onset of 16 to 25 yr
- A sexually transmitted disease spread by skin-to-skin contact
- Highly contagious, with 25% to 65% of sexual partners developing it
- Virus shed from both macroscopic and microscopic lesions
- Average incubation time is 2 mo (range, 1 to 8 mo)
- Predisposing conditions: diabetes, pregnancy, local trauma, and immunosuppression (e.g., transplant recipients, those with HIV infection)

PHYSICAL FINDINGS & CLINICAL PRESENTATION

- Usually found in genital area but can be present elsewhere
- Lesions usually in similar positions on both sides of perineum
- Initial lesions pedunculated, soft papules about 2 to 3 mm in diameter, 10 to 20 mm long; may occur as single papule or in clusters
- Size of lesions varies from pinhead to large cauliflower-like masses
- Usually asymptomatic, but if infected can cause pain, odor, or bleeding
- Vulvar condyloma more common than vaginal and cervical
- Four morphologic types: condylomatous, keratotic, papular, and flat warts

ETIOLOGY

- HPV DNA types 6 and 11 usually found in exophytic warts and have no malignant potential
- HPV types 16 and 18 usually found in flat warts and are associated with increased risk of malignancy
- Recurrence associated with persisting viral infection of adjacent normal skin in 25% to 50% of cases

Dx DIAGNOSIS

DIFFERENTIAL DIAGNOSIS

- Abnormal anatomic variants or skin tags around labia minora and introitus
- Dysplastic warts

WORKUP

- Colposcopic examination of lower genital tract from cervix to perianal skin with 3% to 5% acetic acid
- Biopsy of vulvar lesions that lack the classic appearance of warts and that become ulcerated or do not respond to treatment
- Biopsy of flat, white, or ulcerated cervical lesions

LABORATORY TESTS

- Pap smear
- Cervical cultures for *Neisseria gonorrhoeae* and *Chlamydia*
- Serologic test for syphilis
- HIV testing offered
- Wet mount for trichomoniasis, *Candida albicans,* and *Gardnerella vaginalis*
- Testing for diabetes (blood glucose)

Rx TREATMENT

NONPHARMACOLOGIC THERAPY

- Keep genital area dry and clean.
- If present, keep diabetes well controlled.
- Advise use of condoms to prevent spread of infection to sexual partner.

ACUTE GENERAL Rx

Keratolytic agents:

- Podophyllin
  1. Acts by poisoning mitotic spindle and causing intense vasospasm
  2. Applied directly to lesion weekly and washed off in 6 hr
  3. Used in minimal vulvar or anal disease
  4. Applied cautiously to nonkeratinized epithelial surfaces
  5. Contraindicated in pregnancy
  6. Discontinued if lesions do not disappear in 6 wk; switch to other treatment
- Trichloroacetic acid (30% to 80% solution)
  1. Acts by precipitation of surface proteins
  2. Applied twice monthly to lesion
  3. Indicated for vulvar, anal, and vaginal lesions; can be used for cervical lesions
  4. Less painful and irritating to normal tissue than podophyllin
- Fluorouracil
  1. Causes necrosis and sloughing of growing tissue
  2. Can be used intravaginally or for vulvar, anal, or urethral lesions
  3. Better tolerated; 3 g (two thirds of vaginal applicator) applied weekly for 12 wk
  4. Possible vaginal ulceration and erythema
  5. Patient's vagina examined after four to six applications
  6. 80% cure rate

Physical agents:

- Cryotherapy
  1. Can be used weekly for 3 to 6 wk
  2. 62% to 79% success rate
  3. Not suitable for large warts
- Laser therapy
  1. Done by physician with necessary expertise and equipment
  2. Painful; requires anesthesia
- Electrocautery or excision
  1. For recurrent, very large lesions
  2. Local anesthesia needed

Immunotherapy:

- Interferon
  1. Injected intralesionally at a dose of 3 million U/m^2 three times weekly for 8 wk
  2. Side effects: fever, chills, malaise, headache
- Imiquimod 5% cream at hs, 3× wk up to 16 wk increases wart clearance after 3 mo
- Interferon, topical: increases wart clearance at 4 wk

DISPOSITION

Follow-up exam every 6 to 12 mo, as needed.

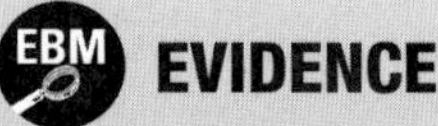

EVIDENCE

Podofilox and imiquimod have been shown to be more effective than placebo.[1,2] A

Trichloroacetic acid and cryotherapy appear to be equally effective at producing clearance of warts.[3,4] A

Evidence-Based References

1. Wiley DJ: Genital warts, *Clin Evid* 8:1620, 2002. A
2. Moore RA et al: Imiquimod for the treatment of genital warts: a quantitative systematic review, *BMC Infect Dis* 1:3, 2001. A
3. Abdullah AN et al: Treatment of external genital warts comparing cryotherapy (liquid nitrogen) and trichloroacetic acid, *Sex Transm Dis* 20:344, 1993. A
4. Godley MJ et al: Cryotherapy compared with trichloroacetic acid in treating genital warts, *Genitourin Med* 63:390, 1987. A

SUGGESTED READING

Centers for Disease Control and Prevention: Sexually transmitted diseases guidelines, 2006, *MMR* 55/RR-11, 2006.

AUTHORS: **GEORGE T. DANAKAS, M.D.,** and **RUBEN ALVERO, M.D.**

BASIC INFORMATION

DEFINITION

Congenital adrenal hyperplasia (CAH) refers to several different genetic mutations in the enzymes responsible for cortisol synthesis, which are each inherited in an autosomal-recessive fashion.

SYNONYMS

21-hydroxylase deficiency (equivalent to CYP21A2 deficiency)
11B-hydroxylase deficiency
3B-hydroxysteroid dehydrogenase deficiency
17-hydroxylase deficiency
Lipoid adrenal hyperplasia
CYP 17 deficiency

ICD-9CM CODES
255.2 Adrenogenital disorders; hyperplasia, congenital adrenal

EPIDEMIOLOGY & DEMOGRAPHICS

- Between 90% and 95% of cases of CAH are caused by "classic" 21-hydroxylase deficiency, of which 75% of cases represent the salt-wasting form.
- Inheritance pattern is autosomal recessive.
- Prevalence of 21-hydroxylase deficiency is one in every 16,000 infants in the U.S. but may be higher among other groups, such as Hispanics and Ashkenazi Jews (1% to 2%).
- The frequency of heterozygous carriers is controversial; estimates range between 1:5 and 1:80 persons.

CLINICAL PRESENTATION

"Classic" salt-wasting form (impaired cortisol and aldosterone synthesis):
- Infants are acutely ill with poor weight gain, hypovolemia, hyponatremia, hyperkalemia, and elevated plasma renin.
- If patients survive infancy, their overall life expectancy is not compromised.
- Females are born with ambiguous genitalia and may have irregular menses and infertility as adults.
- Males may have greater penile size and smaller testes than expected during childhood. Males may also develop adrenal rests, or ectopic islands of adrenal cortical tissue in the testes, in childhood and may experience infertility as adults.
- Both males and females may exhibit rapid growth in childhood (due to early epiphyseal closure, which then results in short stature in adulthood).
- Precocious puberty is common in both males and females.

"Classic" non-salt-wasting or simple virilizing form (impaired cortisol synthesis only):
- Females present with ambiguous genitalia at birth.
- The normal appearance of male genitalia in the simple virilizing form makes this a difficult diagnosis in male infants.
- Characterized by precocious puberty, short stature, and testicular adrenal rests, as in the salt-wasting form.

"Nonclassic" or mild, late-onset form (varying degrees of androgen excess):
- Usually presents in adolescence or adulthood and is not detected on newborn screening.
- Often asymptomatic but can be associated with mild virilization.
- Symptoms similar to polycystic ovarian syndrome occur in women (hirsutism, oligomenorrhea, acne, infertility, insulin resistance, abnormal menses).
- Associated with infertility in males.

ETIOLOGY

In 21-hydroxylase deficiency, the pathways for aldosterone production (from the conversion of progesterone to deoxycorticosterone) and cortisol production (from the conversion of 17-hydroxyprogesterone to 11-deoxycortisol) by the cP450 enzyme 21-hydroxylase are interrupted. The production of adrenocorticotropic hormone is thus stimulated by a negative feedback mechanism, leading to adrenal hyperplasia and mineralocorticoid deficiency as the intermediaries in aldosterone and cortisol synthesis are shunted to the androgen biosynthesis pathway (Fig. 1-72). A recombination event between the active *CYP21A2* gene on chromosome 6p21.3 and the *CYP21A1* pseudogene is thought to create the deficient 21-hydroxylase enzyme.

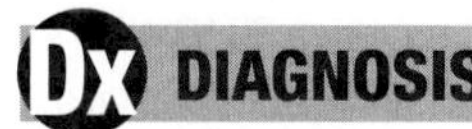

DIAGNOSIS

DIFFERENTIAL DIAGNOSIS

- Precocious puberty
- Polycystic ovarian syndrome
- Androgen resistance syndromes
- Pseudohermaphroditism
- Mixed gonadal dysgenesis
- Testicular carcinoma

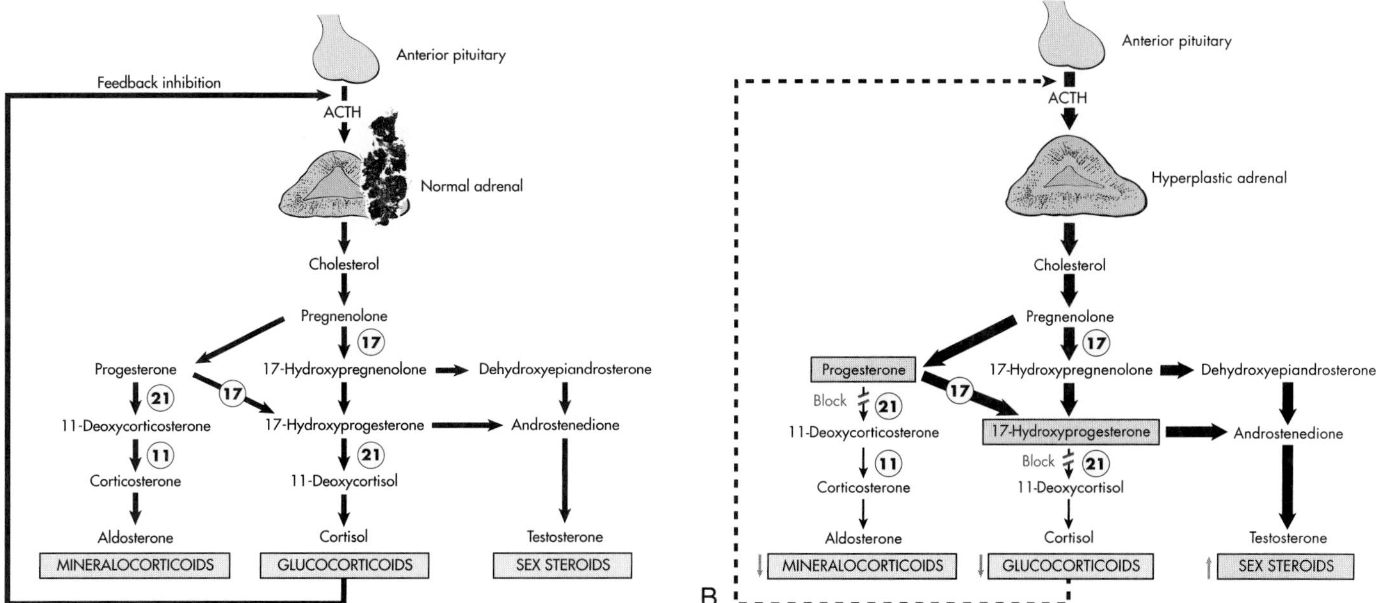

FIGURE 1-72 **A,** Normal adrenal steroidogenesis. **B,** Consequences of C-21 hydroxylase deficiency. (From Cotran R et al [eds]: *Robbins pathologic basis of disease,* ed 6, Philadelphia, 1999, WB Saunders, p 1158.)

- Leydig cell tumors
- Adrenocortical carcinoma
- Addison's disease
- Pituitary adenoma

LABORATORY TESTS

Laboratory tests (for 21-hydroxylase deficiency):

- Prenatal: chorionic villus sampling for genetic testing or measurement of 17-hydroxyprogesterone
- Neonates, children, and adults: screening for elevated 17-hydroxyprogesterone levels (not done by all states), high-dose cosyntropin stimulation test, and genotyping

IMAGING STUDIES

- Ultrasound to identify a uterus in cases of ambiguous genitalia.
- Ultrasound is preferred to rule out testicular adrenal rest tumors (found in classic and nonclassic forms) and should be done beginning in adolescence. MRI and color-flow Doppler may also be used for this purpose.

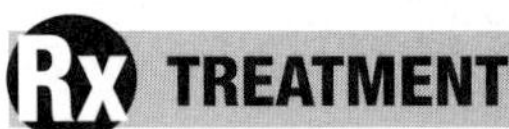

TREATMENT

NONPHARMACOLOGIC THERAPY

- Surgical correction of ambiguous genitalia is recommended by age 6 mo.
- Bilateral laparoscopic adrenalectomy with lifelong glucocorticoid and mineralocorticoid replacement (controversial).
- Gene therapy (hypothetical).

ACUTE GENERAL Rx

Overall goal is suppression of adrenocorticotropic hormone.

- Prenatal: dexamethasone 20 to 25 mcg/kg/day in the first trimester in female fetuses only (controversial because long-term studies are unavailable).
- Infants: fludrocortisone 0.1 to 0.2 mg/day, hydrocortisone 5 to 15 mg/day, NaCl 1 to 2 g/day.
- Stress states (e.g., major illness) require increased glucocorticoid dosing.

CHRONIC Rx

- Long-term treatment:
  - Children: hydrocortisone 10 to 30 mg/day (minimizes the risk of iatrogenic short stature found in other corticosteroids with longer half-lives).
  - Adolescents/adults: dexamethasone 0.25 to 0.75 mg PO qhs (also use to treat adrenal rests) or prednisone 5 to 7.5 mg/day.
  - Fludrocortisone: 0.1 to 0.2 mg/day (may decrease glucocorticoid requirement).
  - Experimental four-drug regimen: flutamide and testolactone in addition to hydrocortisone and fludrocortisone.
  - Psychological counseling.
  - Monitoring: serum 17-hydroxyprogesterone and androstenedione, renin, electrolytes, blood pressure, bone age and density, Tanner staging, growth velocity, weight.
- Treatment of simple virilizing form: similar to salt-wasting form but mineralocorticoid replacement is unnecessary.
- Treatment of nonclassic form:
  - In adolescent and adult women: oral contraceptives, glucocorticoids, and/or antiandrogens.
  - In children and adult males, usually no treatment is necessary.

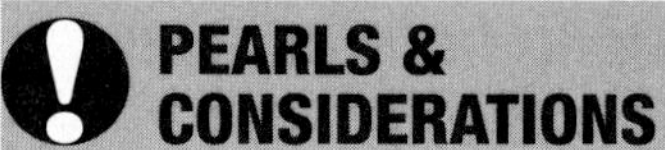

PEARLS & CONSIDERATIONS

COMMENTS

- Consider the diagnosis of classic salt-wasting CAH in infants with failure to thrive.
- There is believed to be an increased prevalence of CAH in patients diagnosed with adrenal "incidentalomas"—adrenal gland lesions detected unexpectedly on imaging, usually by MRI or CT scanning.
- Cushing's syndrome may result from overtreatment of CAH with glucocorticoids.
- Treatment of CAH in pregnancy with dexamethasone will confound newborn screening for 17-hydroxyprogesterone; these infants should be screened 1 to 2 wk postpartum.
- Patients with CAH may have gender identity disorders and sexual dysfunction.

PREVENTION

- Early chorionic villus sampling and maternal glucocorticoid administration (see above)
- Neonatal screening
- Genetic counseling

SUGGESTED READINGS

Levine L, DiGeorge A: Adrenal disorders and genital abnormalities: congenital adrenal hyperplasia. In Behrman R et al (eds): *Nelson's textbook of pediatrics*, Philadelphia, 2000, WB Saunders, pp 1729-1737.

Merke DP et al: NIH conference: future directions in the study and management of congenital adrenal hyperplasia due to 21-hydroxylase deficiency, *Ann Intern Med* 136:320, 2002.

Speiser PW et al: Congenital adrenal hyperplasia, *N Engl J Med* 349:776, 2003.

AUTHOR: **TIMOTHY W. FARRELL, M.D.**

BASIC INFORMATION

DEFINITION

Heart failure (HF) is a clinical syndrome that can result from any structural or functional cardiac disorder that impairs the ability of the ventricle to fill with or eject blood at normal filling pressures. Congestive heart failure (CHF) usually denotes a volume overloaded status as a result of HF. Because not all patients have volume overload at the time of the evaluation, CHF should be distinguished from the broader term *heart failure.*

CLASSIFICATION

The American College of Cardiology and the American Heart Association describe the following four stages of HF:

A. At high risk for HF but without structural heart disease or symptoms of HF (e.g., hypertension)
B. Structural heart disease but without symptoms of HF (e.g., left ventricular [LV] dysfunction)
C. Structural heart disease with prior or current symptoms of HF
D. Refractory HF requiring specialized interventions

The New York Heart Association (NYHA) defines the following functional classes:

I. Asymptomatic
II. Symptomatic with moderate exertion (2 city blocks or 1 flight of stairs in a faster than usual pace)
III. Symptomatic with minimal exertion (<2 city blocks or <1 flight of stairs)
IV. Symptomatic at rest

The ACC/AHA stages of HF are designed to emphasize preventability of symptomatic HF, to recognize the progressive nature of LV dysfunction, and to have direct implications on the therapy of HF. It should be distinguished from NYHA classification, which is dynamic and reversible.

SYNONYMS

Congestive heart failure (CHF)
Cardiac failure
Heart failure

ICD-9CM CODES
428.0 Congestive heart failure

EPIDEMIOLOGY & DEMOGRAPHICS

- CHF is the most common inpatient diagnosis in the U.S. for patients >65 yr of age.
- HF occurs in 4.7 million persons in the U.S. and is the discharge diagnosis in 3.5 million hospitalizations annually.
- There are 100 to 400 new cases of HF per 100,000 of the population per yr, and 1000 or more new cases per 100,000 of the population per yr for people >65 yr of age (20%).
- Occurs in approximately 1000 to 2000 per 100,000 of the population.
- It leads to a total of 12 to 15 million office visits per yr.
- Prevalence is greater in African American than white individuals.
- More common in male than female individuals between 40 and 75 yr of age.
- Both sexes equally affected in age >75 yr.

PHYSICAL FINDINGS & CLINICAL PRESENTATION

The findings on physical examination in patients with CHF vary depending on the severity and whether the failure symptoms are predominantly right or left sided.

- Common clinical manifestations are:
  1. Dyspnea on exertion initially, then with progressively less strenuous activity, and eventually manifesting when patient is at rest; caused by increasing pulmonary congestion
  2. Orthopnea caused by increased venous return in the recumbent position
  3. Wheezing may accompany dyspnea in patients with pulmonary congestion
  4. Paroxysmal nocturnal dyspnea resulting from multiple factors (increased venous return in the recumbent position, decreased Pa_{O_2} during sleep, decreased adrenergic stimulation of myocardial function during sleep)
  5. Nocturnal angina resulting from increased cardiac work (secondary to increased venous return) in patients with concomitant coronary artery disease
  6. Cheyne-Stokes respiration: alternating phases of apnea and hyperventilation caused by prolonged circulation time from lungs to brain
  7. Fatigue, lethargy resulting from low cardiac output
- Physical examination: pulmonary rales, tachypnea, S_3 gallop, paradoxic splitting of S_2, jugular venous distention, peripheral edema (initially feet, ankle in ambulatory, and sacrum in bedridden patients), perioral and peripheral cyanosis in patients with low cardiac output, congestive hepatomegaly (occasionally), ascites (occasionally), and hepatojugular reflux
- In patients with HF, low functional status and LV systolic dysfunction are each independently associated with adverse outcomes
- Acute precipitants of CHF exacerbations are noncompliance with salt restriction, pulmonary infections, arrhythmias, medications (e.g., calcium channel blockers/antiarrhythmic agents), NSAIDs, kidney dysfunction, and inappropriate reductions in CHF therapy

ETIOLOGY

LEFT VENTRICULAR FAILURE:

- Ischemic heart disease (most common cause of HF in the U.S.)
- Systemic hypertension
- Valvular heart disease (aortic stenosis, aortic regurgitation, mitral regurgitation)
- Cardiomyopathy, myocarditis
- Bacterial endocarditis
- Amyloidosis
- Sarcoidosis
- Hemochromatosis
- Obesity
- Diabetes

HF is further differentiated according to LV systolic dysfunction (low ejection fraction [EF]) and preserved systolic function (LVEF ≥50%). It is important to make this distinction because treatment is significantly different (see "Treatment"). Patients with HF and a normal EF may have significant abnormalities in active relaxation and passive stiffness of the LV, renal function, and/or arterial vasoreactivity.

RIGHT VENTRICULAR FAILURE:

- Valvular heart disease (mitral stenosis)
- Primary pulmonary hypertension
- Chronic hypoxemic pulmonary disease
- Severe pulmonary hypertension
- Right-to-left shunts that causes systemic hypoxemia
- Bacterial endocarditis (right sided)
- Right ventricular infarction

BIVENTRICULAR FAILURE:

- LV failure
- Cardiomyopathy
- Myocarditis
- Arrhythmias
- Anemia
- Thyrotoxicosis
- Atrioventricular fistula
- Paget's disease
- Beriberi
- Excessive alcohol consumption

Dx DIAGNOSIS

DIFFERENTIAL DIAGNOSIS

- Cirrhosis
- Nephrotic syndrome
- Venous occlusive disease
- Chronic obstructive pulmonary disease, asthma
- Pulmonary embolism
- Acute respiratory distress syndrome
- Heroin overdose
- Pneumonia

WORKUP

- Echocardiography plays a critical diagnostic role in patients with HF. Doppler echocardiography, which measures the velocity of intracardiac blood flow, is also helpful in the assessment of diastolic function.
- Standard 12-lead ECG is useful to diagnose ischemic heart disease and obtain information about rhythm abnormalities. More than 25% of patients with CHF have some form of intraventricular conduction abnormality that is manifested as an increased QRS duration on ECG. The most common pattern is left bundle branch block.
- Cardiac catheterization provides direct measurement of ventricular diastolic pressure and can demonstrate impaired relaxation and filling; however, it is invasive and indicated only in selected patients.

LABORATORY TESTS

- CBC (to rule out anemia, infections), blood urea nitrogen, creatinine, electrolytes (including calcium and magnesium), liver enzymes

- Thyroid-stimulating hormone (TSH) levels should be measured in every patient older than 65 yr with HF without any clear etiology and patients with atrial fibrillation or other indicators for thyroid disease.
- Beta-type natriuretic peptide (BNP) is a cardiac neurohormone specifically secreted from the ventricles in response to volume expansion and pressure overload. Increased levels are indicative of LV volume overload. Bedside measurement of beta-type natriuretic peptide is useful in establishing or excluding the diagnosis of CHF in patients with acute dyspnea. Increased BNP levels are also strong predictors of survival in patients with HF.
- In patients with acute decompensated HF, a positive cardiac troponin test is associated with higher in-hospital mortality, independently of other predictable variables.

IMAGING STUDIES

- Chest x-ray examination:
  - Pulmonary venous congestion
  - Cardiomegaly with dilation of the involved heart chamber
  - Pleural effusions
- Two-dimensional echocardiography is useful to assess global and regional LV function and estimate EF.
- Exercise stress testing may be useful for evaluating concomitant coronary disease and to assess degree of disability. The decision to perform exercise stress testing should be individualized.
- Cardiac catheterization remains an excellent method to evaluate ventricular diastolic properties, significant coronary artery disease, or valvular heart disease; however, it is invasive. The decision to perform cardiac catheterization should be individualized.

Rx TREATMENT

NONPHARMACOLOGIC THERAPY

- Determine the etiology of HF and treat accordingly.
- Identify and correct precipitating factors (i.e., anemia, thyrotoxicosis, infections, increased sodium load, medical noncompliance).
- Decrease cardiac workload: aggressive reduction of the blood pressure and heart rate, restrict patients' activity only during periods of acute decompensation; the risk for thromboembolism during this period can be minimized by using prophylactic heparin in hospitalized patients. In patients with mild-to-moderate symptoms, aerobic training may improve symptoms and exercise capacity.
- Restrict sodium intake to <2 g/day.
- Restricting fluid intake to 2 L or less may be useful in patients with hyponatremia.
- Caloric supplementation should be provided with patients with advanced HF with weight loss and muscle wasting secondary to cardiac cachexia.
- For patients with concomitant HF with obstructive sleep apnea, continuous positive airway pressure is recommended after polysomnography, which reduces systolic blood pressure and improves LV function.

ACUTE GENERAL Rx

1. Oxygen: given initially for patients in acute decompensation and continued to improve arterial oxygenation
2. Diuretics: indicated in patients with volume overload; the most useful approach to selecting the dose of, and monitoring the response to, diuretic therapy is by measuring body weight, preferably daily
   a. Furosemide: 20 to 80 mg produces prompt venodilation and diuresis. Intravenous (IV) therapy may produce diuresis when oral therapy has failed; when changing from IV to oral furosemide, doubling the dose is usually necessary to achieve an equal effect. Administering smaller doses of short-acting loop diuretics two or three times a day is preferable to a single large dose because it results in greater diuresis and less physiological disruption.
   b. Thiazides are not as powerful as furosemide but are useful in the outpatient management of mild CHF.
   c. The addition of metolazone to furosemide enhances diuresis.
   d. Frequent monitoring of renal function and electrolytes is recommended in all patients receiving diuretics.

TREATMENT OF CONGESTIVE HEART FAILURE SECONDARY TO SYSTOLIC DYSFUNCTION:

1. ACE inhibitors:
   a. They cause dilation of the arteriolar resistance vessels and venous capacity vessels, thereby reducing both preload and afterload.
   b. They are associated with decreased mortality and improved clinical status when used in patients with chronic HF caused by systolic dysfunction.
   c. They can be used as first-line therapy or they can be added to diuretics.
   d. Therapy with ACE inhibitors should be initiated at low dose (e.g., captopril 6.25 mg tid or enalapril 2.5 mg bid) to prevent hypotension and rapidly titrated up to high doses if tolerated.
   e. Contraindications to use of ACE inhibitors are renal insufficiency (creatinine >3.0 or creatinine clearance <30 ml/min), bilateral renal artery stenosis, persistent hyperkalemia, symptomatic hypotension, and history of adverse reactions (e.g., angioedema).
2. Beta-blockers: reduce hospitalizations, sudden death, and overall mortality in CHF. All patients with stable HF caused by LV systolic dysfunction should receive a beta-blocker unless they have a contraindication to its use or are intolerant to it. Carvedilol 3.125 mg bid initially, titrated upward as tolerated, is an effective agent. An effective dose will usually be reached in 8 to 12 wk. Caution is advised in patients with recurrent hypoglycemia, asthma, resting limb ischemic pain, and particularly in patients with symptomatic bradycardia or hypotension <80 mm Hg systolic. Other beta-blockers proved effective in increasing survival for HF patients with LV systolic dysfunction are metoprolol succinate (25 to 200 mg daily) and bisoprolol (2.5 to 10 mg daily).
3. Angiotensin II receptor blockers (ARBs) block the A-II type 1 (AT) receptor, which is responsible for many of the deleterious effects of angiotensin II. These receptors are potent vasoconstrictors that may contribute to the impairment of LV function. ARBs are useful in patients unable to tolerate ACE inhibitors because of angioedema or intractable cough. They can also be used in combination with a beta-blocker.
4. Aldosterone antagonists: Low-dose spironolactone or eplerenone therapy should be considered in patients with NYHA class III or IV who remain symptomatic despite therapy with ACE inhibitors and beta-blockers. Spironolactone (12.5 to 25 mg bid) used in conjunction with ACE inhibitors reduces both mortality and morbidity in patients with severe CHF. Serum electrolytes and renal function should be closely monitored after initiation of therapy and when changing doses. Concomitant therapy with an angiotensin receptor antagonist, ACE inhibitor, and an aldosterone antagonist is not recommended because of risk for hyperkalemia.
5. Direct vasodilating drugs (hydralazine and isosorbide) are useful in the therapy of systolic dysfunction with CHF because they can reduce the systemic vascular resistance and pulmonary venous pressure. Trials in African American patients revealed that the combination of hydralazine and isosorbide is effective in advanced HF when added to ACE inhibitors and beta-blockers. Tolerability is an issue, with more than 20% of patients stopping the medications because of adverse effects. Hydralazine and nitrates are especially useful for patients who are intolerant to both ACE inhibitors and ARBs. They should also be considered in African American patients as an add-on to standard therapy with ACE and ARBs with NYHA grade II, III, or IV HF.
6. Digitalis has been traditionally used because of its positive inotropic and vagotonic effects on patients with CHF secondary to systolic dysfunction. It can alleviate symptoms and decrease hospitalizations. When used, it should be reserved for patients with symptomatic NYHA class II to IV CHF and systolic dysfunction. Digoxin has a narrow therapeutic window. Dose should be based on lean body mass, creatinine clearance, and concomitant medications. Its beneficial effects are found with a low dose that results in a serum concentration of approximately 0.5 to 0.8 ng/ml. Usually, dosage will be 0.125 mg daily in majority of the patients. Higher doses (maintenance dose >0.25 mg daily) could be detrimental.

7. Intracardiac defibrillators (ICDs) monitor heart rate and rhythm and correct arrhythmias. ICDs should be considered in patients with previous myocardial infarction and EF <30%, or in patients with CHF with EF <35% and NYHA class II or III HF. It should be placed in patients whose life expectancy exceeds 1 yr.
8. Placement of a biventricular pacemaker is beneficial in symptomatic patients (NYHA class 3 or 4) with EF <35% and QRS interval >130 ms on ECG despite maximal medical therapy.
9. Other agents: Use of inotropic agents (dobutamine, milrinone) should be reserved for patients with severe HF unresponsive to other therapies noted earlier and used as a palliative therapy for patients with end-stage disease.
10. Anticoagulants and antiplatelet agents:
    a. Anticoagulation is not recommended for patients in sinus rhythm and no prior history of stroke, LV thrombi, or arteriolar emboli.
    b. Anticoagulation therapy is appropriate for patients with HF and atrial fibrillation or a history of embolism.
    c. Antiplatelet agents like aspirin and/or clopidogrel are recommended for patients with coronary artery disease. Low-dose aspirin (75 or 81 mg) is recommended in most patients in which anticoagulation with warfarin is not specifically indicated because some data suggest worsening of HF with higher doses.
11. Surgical revascularization should be considered in patients with both HF and severe limiting angina.

TREATMENT OF CONGESTIVE HEART FAILURE WITH PRESERVED SYSTOLIC FUNCTION: The initial treatment of CHF should be directed at reducing the congestive state with the use of diuretics, being careful to avoid excessive diuresis. Long-term goals are to control hypertension, tachycardia, congestion, and ischemia. Therapeutic options are determined by the cause.

- Control of hypertension, diabetes, or both
- Control of the heart rate in atrial fibrillation
- Treatment of the underlying coronary artery disease or valvular disease if it is severe.

DISPOSITION

- Annual mortality rate ranges from 10% in stable patients with mild symptoms to >50% in symptomatic patients with advanced disease.
- Sudden death secondary to ventricular arrhythmias occurs in >40% of patients with HF.
- Cardiac transplantation has a 5-yr survival rate of >70% in many centers and represents a viable option in selected patients.
- The use of a LV assist device in patients with advanced HF can result in a clinically meaningful survival benefit and improve quality of life. It is an acceptable alternative therapy in selected patients who are not candidates for cardiac transplantation.
- In patients with advanced HF and a prolonged QRS interval, cardiac-resynchronization therapy decreases the combined risk for death from any cause or first hospitalization and, when combined with an implantable defibrillator, significantly reduces mortality.

COMMENTS

- Diabetes and obesity are established risk factors for CHF, and both are associated with insulin resistance. Insulin resistance predicts CHF incidence independently of established risk factors, including diabetes.
- Sudden death from cardiac causes remains a leading cause of death among patients with CHF. In patients with NYHA class II or III CHF and LVEF <35%, amiodarone has no favorable effect on survival, whereas single-lead, shock-only ICD therapy reduces overall mortality by 23%.
- HF therapy guided by N-terminal BNP did not improve overall clinical outcomes or quality of life compared with symptom-guided treatment.
- Always look for underlying causes for HF that could be treatable, like anemia, thyrotoxicosis, valvular disorders, and myocardial ischemia.

EBM EVIDENCE

Please note: Complete text of EBM for this topic is available online.

Key trials and commentary:

A direct comparison of survival benefits between cardiac resynchronization therapy-pacemaker (CRT-P) and defibrillator (CRT-D) was not yet performed, leaving clinicians to question whether CRT-P alone is enough to protect congestive heart failure (CHF) patients from sudden cardiac death and whether CRT-D should be implanted to all CHF patients indicated for biventricular pacing. This study attempts to make this type of comparison in a large CHF population and seeks to identify predictors of death in patients with different comorbidities. Data from this nonrandomized study indicate that CRT-D has additional survival benefits over CRT-P. Given these findings, CRT-D should be recommended to most CHF patients with indications for biventricular pacing. After CRT implant, chronic renal failure, diabetes mellitus, and history of atrial fibrillation are strong independent predictors of death.

This nonrandomized study does clearly show that CRT-D (combined CRT/ICD) therapy has long-term survival superiority over CRT-P (CRT/pacing) therapy in heart failure patients who were considered for biventricular pacing.[1] Ⓐ

Atrial fibrillation (AF) is a common comorbidity in heart failure (HF) patients and is classically associated with acceleration in the rate of HF progression. The precise mechanism for this interaction is unclear, but comprises "bidirectional" aspects in which AF promotes HF and HF also increases the likelihood of AF. A study by Byrne and colleagues analyzed the relationship between AF in an ovine model of pacing-induced congestive HF, in an attempt to identify the mechanisms that underpin the apparent synergistic relationship between AF and HF.

This study showed that AF induction significantly depresses left ventricular function and causes activation of myocardial neurohormones. In conjunction, the presence of functional MR increases susceptibility to AF and this may be attenuated by MR reduction by percutaneous mitral annular reduction.

This study of a sheep model of HF is of interest because of the key role of mitral regurgitation. This also seems to be an important connection between HF and AF in patients as well, and as a clinician, suggests to this editor that careful attention should be paid to repair mitral regurgitation early on as an important part of preventive treatment for AF.[2] Ⓐ

Evidence-Based References

1. Bai R et al: Mortality of heart failure patients after cardiac resynchronization therapy: identification of predictors, *J Cardiovasc Electrophysiol* 19:1259-1265, 2008. Commentary by A.L. Waldo, M.D. Ⓐ
2. Byrne M et al: The synergism between atrial fibrillation and heart failure, *J Card Fail* 14:320-326, 2008. Commentary by A.L. Waldo, M.D. Ⓐ

SUGGESTED READINGS

Dickstein K et al: ESC guidelines for the diagnosis and treatment of acute and chronic heart failure 2008. the Task Force for the Diagnosis and Treatment of Acute and Chronic Heart Failure 2008. of the European Society of Cardiology. Developed in collaboration with the Heart Failure Association of the ESC (HFA) and endorsed by the European Society of Intensive Care Medicine (ESCIM), *Eur Heart J* 29: 2388, 2008.

Hunt SA et al: 2009 focused update incorporated into the ACC/AHA 2005. Guidelines for the Diagnosis and Management of Heart failure in Adults: a report of the American College of Cardiology Foundation/ American Heart Association Task Force on Practice Guidelines: developed in collaboration with the International Society for Heart and Lung Transplantation. *Circulation* 119:e391, 2009.

McMurry J: Systolic heart failure, *N Engl J Med* 362: 228-238, 2010.

AUTHORS: **SYEDA M. SAYEED, M.D., FRED F. FERRI, M.D.,** and **WEN-CHIH WU, M.D.**

Conjunctivitis (PTG)

BASIC INFORMATION

DEFINITION

The term *conjunctivitis* refers to an inflammation of the conjunctiva resulting from a variety of causes, including allergies and bacterial, viral, and chlamydial infections.

SYNONYMS

"Red eye"
Pink eye
Acute conjunctivitis
Subacute conjunctivitis
Chronic conjunctivitis
Purulent conjunctivitis
Pseudomembranous conjunctivitis
Papillary conjunctivitis
Follicular conjunctivitis
Newborn conjunctivitis

ICD-9CM CODES
372.30 Conjunctivitis, unspecified

EPIDEMIOLOGY & DEMOGRAPHICS

INCIDENCE (IN U.S.): 1.6% to 12% in newborns

PREVALENCE (IN U.S.):
- Allergic conjunctivitis, the most common form of ocular allergy, is usually associated with allergic rhinitis and may be seasonal or perennial.
- Bacterial or viral conjunctivitis is often seasonal and can be extremely contagious.

PREDOMINANT AGE: Occurs at any age

PEAK INCIDENCE: More common in the fall, when viral infections and pollens increase

PHYSICAL FINDINGS & CLINICAL PRESENTATION

- Infection and chemosis of conjunctivae with discharge (Fig. 1-73)
- Cornea is clear or can be involved
- Vision is often normal but can be blurred

ETIOLOGY

- Bacterial
- Viral
- Chlamydial
- Allergic
- Traumatic

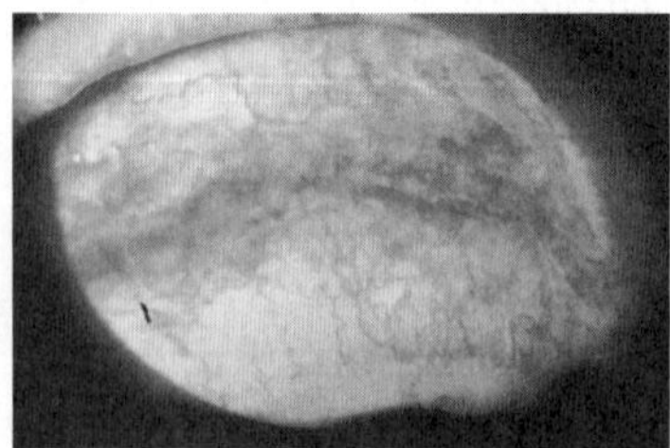

FIGURE 1-73 Conjunctival infection from viral conjunctivitis. (From Marx JA [ed]: *Rosen's emergency medicine,* ed 5, St Louis, 2002, Mosby.)

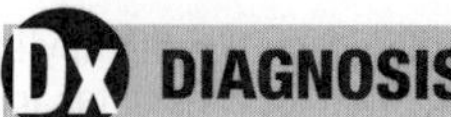

DIAGNOSIS

DIFFERENTIAL DIAGNOSIS

- Acute glaucoma
- Corneal lesions
- Acute iritis
- Episcleritis
- Scleritis
- Uveitis
- Canalicular obstruction

WORKUP

- History and physical examination
- Reports of itching, pain, visual changes

LABORATORY TESTS

Cultures are useful if not successfully treated with antibiotics; initial culture is usually not necessary.

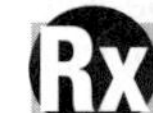

TREATMENT

NONPHARMACOLOGIC THERAPY

- Warm compresses if infective conjunctivitis.
- Cold compresses if irritative or allergic conjunctivitis.
- Contact lenses should be taken out until an infection is completely resolved. Nondisposable lenses should be cleaned thoroughly as recommended by the manufacturer, and a new lens case should be used. Disposable contact lenses should be thrown away.

ACUTE GENERAL Rx

- Antibiotic drops (e.g., levofloxacin, ofloxin, ciprofloxacin, tobramycin, gentamicin ophthalmic solution, 1 or 2 drops q2-4h) are indicated for suspected bacterial conjunctivitis.
- Caution: be careful with ophthalmic corticosteroid treatment and avoid unless sure of diagnosis; corticosteroids can exacerbate infections and have been associated with increased intraocular pressure and cataract formation.
- An oral antihistamine (cetirizine, loratadine, desloratadine, or fexofenadine) is effective in relieving itching.
- Mast cell stabilizers (e.g., cromolyn [4%, 1 to 2 drops q4-6h], lodoxamide [Alomide, 0.1%, 1 to 2 drops qid]) are effective for allergic conjunctivitis. Others include Elestat, Optivar, and Patanol.
- The topical NSAID ketorolac (Voltaren, 0.5%, 1 drop qd) is also useful in allergic conjunctivitis but expensive.
- Antihistamine/decongestant combinations such as pheniramine/naphazoline (Visine A), available over the counter, are more effective than either agent alone but have a short duration and can result in rebound vasodilatation with prolonged use. Others include Naphcon-A, Albacon-A, and Opcon-A.

CHRONIC Rx

- Depends on cause.
- If allergic, nonsteroidals such as Voltaren, Acular, and Xibrom ophthalmic solution; mast cell stabilizers such as Elestat, Alocril, Patanol, Zaditor are useful for improving ocular itching in patients with allergic conjunctivitis.
- If an infection, use antibiotic drops (see "Acute General Rx").
- Dry eyes need artificial tears (Restasis) or lacrimal duct plugs when indicated.

DISPOSITION

Follow carefully for the first 2 wk to ensure secondary complications do not occur.

REFERRAL

To ophthalmologist if symptoms are refractory to initial treatment. Indications for urgent referral are severe eye pain or headache, photophobia, decreased vision, and contact lens use.

PEARLS & CONSIDERATIONS

COMMENTS

- Red eyes are not simply conjunctivitis when the patient has significant pain or loss of sight. However, it is usually safe to treat pain-free eyes and the normal seeing red eye with lid hygiene and topical treatment.
- Use caution with patients wearing soft contact lenses, infants, and the elderly.
- Do not use steroids indiscriminately; use only when the diagnosis is certain.

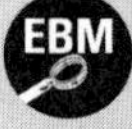

EVIDENCE

Acute bacterial conjunctivitis is often self-limiting, but treatment with topical antibiotics improves the time to clinical recovery and rates of microbiologic remission. The randomized controlled trials included in this systematic review were conducted in specialist centers, so the results may not be generalizable to a primary care population.[1] Ⓐ

One randomized controlled trial found that combination treatment with naphazoline plus pheniramine and pheniramine alone were both effective in relieving symptoms associated with allergic conjunctivitis.[2] Ⓑ

Evidence-Based References

1. Sheikh A et al: Antibiotics versus placebo for acute bacterial conjunctivitis, *Cochrane Rev* 2: CD001211, 2000. Ⓐ

2. Dockhorn RJ, Duckett TG: Comparison of Naphcon-A and its components (naphazoline and pheniramine) in a provocative model of allergic conjunctivitis, *Curr Eye Res* 13:319, 1994. Ⓑ

AUTHOR: **MELVYN KOBY, M.D.**

BASIC INFORMATION

DEFINITION

Contact dermatitis is an acute or chronic skin inflammation, usually eczematous dermatitis resulting from exposure to substances in the environment. It can be subdivided into "irritant" contact dermatitis (nonimmunologic physical and chemical alteration of the epidermis) and "allergic" contact dermatitis (delayed hypersensitivity reaction).

SYNONYMS

Irritant contact dermatitis
Allergic contact dermatitis

ICD-9CM CODES

692 Contact dermatitis and other eczema

EPIDEMIOLOGY & DEMOGRAPHICS

- 20% of all cases of dermatitis in children are caused by allergic contact dermatitis.
- Rhus dermatitis (poison ivy, poison oak, and poison sumac) is responsible for most cases of contact dermatitis.
- Frequent causes of irritant contact dermatitis are soaps, detergents, and organic solvents.

PHYSICAL FINDINGS & CLINICAL PRESENTATION

IRRITANT CONTACT DERMATITIS:

- Mild exposure may result in dryness, erythema, and fissuring of the affected area (e.g., hand involvement in irritant dermatitis caused by exposure to soap, genital area involvement in irritant dermatitis caused by prolonged exposure to wet diapers).
- Eczematous inflammation may result from chronic exposure.

ALLERGIC CONTACT DERMATITIS:

- Poison ivy dermatitis can present with vesicles and blisters; linear lesions (as a result of dragging of the resins over the surface of the skin by scratching) are a classic presentation.
- The pattern of lesions is asymmetric; itching, burning, and stinging may be present.
- The involved areas are erythematous, warm to touch, swollen, and may be confused with cellulitis.

ETIOLOGY

- Irritant contact dermatitis: cement (construction workers), rubber, ragweed, malathion (farmers), orange and lemon peels (chefs, bartenders), hair tints, shampoos (beauticians), rubber gloves (medical, surgical personnel)
- Allergic contact dermatitis: poison ivy, poison oak, poison sumac, rubber (shoe dermatitis), nickel (jewelry), balsam of Peru (hand and face dermatitis), neomycin, formaldehyde (cosmetics)

DIAGNOSIS

DIFFERENTIAL DIAGNOSIS

- Impetigo
- Lichen simplex chronicus
- Atopic dermatitis
- Nummular eczema
- Seborrheic dermatitis
- Psoriasis
- Scabies

WORKUP

- Medical history: gradual onset vs. rapid onset, number of exposures, clinical presentation, occupational history
- Physical examination: contact dermatitis in the neck may be caused by necklaces, perfumes, after-shave lotion; involvement of the axillae is often secondary to deodorants, clothing; face involvement can occur with cosmetics, airborne allergens, aftershave lotion

LABORATORY TESTS

Patch testing is useful to confirm the diagnosis of contact dermatitis; it is indicated particularly when inflammation persists despite appropriate topical therapy and avoidance of suspected causative agent; patch testing should not be used for irritant contact dermatitis because this is a nonimmunologic-mediated inflammatory reaction.

TREATMENT

NONPHARMACOLOGIC THERAPY

Avoidance of suspected allergens

ACUTE GENERAL Rx

- Removal of the irritant substance by washing the skin with plain water or mild soap within 15 min of exposure is helpful in patients with poison ivy, poison oak, or poison sumac dermatitis.
- Cold or cool water compresses for 20 to 30 min five to six times a day for the initial 72 hr are effective during the acute blistering stage.
- Oral corticosteroids (e.g., prednisone 20 mg bid for 6 to 10 days) are generally reserved for severe, widespread dermatitis.
- IM steroids (e.g., Kenalog) are used for severe reactions and in patients requiring oral corticosteroids but unable to tolerate PO.
- Oral antihistamines (e.g., hydroxyzine 25 mg q6h) will control pruritus, especially at night; calamine lotion is also useful for pruritus; however, it can lead to excessive drying.
- Colloidal oatmeal (Aveeno) baths can also provide symptomatic relief.
- Patients with mild to moderate erythema may respond to topical steroid gels or creams.
- Patients with shoe allergy should change their socks at least once a day; use of aluminum chloride hexahydrate in a 20% solution (Drysol) qhs will also help control perspiration.
- Use hypoallergenic surgical gloves in patients with rubber and surgical glove allergy.

DISPOSITION

Allergic contact dermatitis generally resolves within 2 to 4 wk if reexposure to allergen is prevented.

REFERRAL

For patch testing in selected patients (see Laboratory Tests)

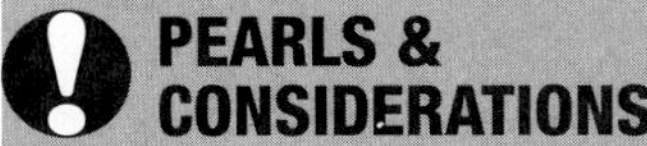

PEARLS & CONSIDERATIONS

COMMENTS

Commercially available corticosteroid dose packs should be avoided, because they generally provide an inadequate amount of medication.

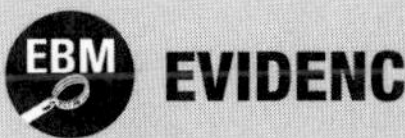

EVIDENCE

A double-blind, intra-individual comparative study with 18 volunteers comparing 0.05% clobetasone butyrate vs its emollient carrier base alone vs 1% hydrocortisone cream vs no treatment in nickel-induced contact dermatitis found that 0.05% clobetasone butyrate had a significantly better response in terms of a physician's global assessment than hydrocortisone 1% cream or no treatment, though it was not significantly better than its emollient base alone.[1] B

There is evidence that tacrolimus 0.1% ointment is significantly better than placebo in the treatment of nickel-induced contact dermatitis.

A double-blind, randomized, controlled, bilateral paired comparison study of topical 0.1% tacrolimus ointment in the treatment of nickel-induced allergic contact dermatitis found evidence that tacrolimus was significantly more effective than placebo in ameliorating the nickel reaction in volunteers and patient groups.[2] B

Evidence-Based References

1. Parneix-Spake A et al: Eumovate (clobetasone butyrate) 0.05% cream with its moisturizing emollient base has better healing properties than hydrocortisone 1% cream: a study in nickel-induced contact dermatitis, *J Dermatol Treat* 12:191, 2001. B
2. Saripalli YV et al: Tacrolimus ointment 0.1% in the treatment of nickel-induced allergic contact dermatitis, *J Am Acad Dermatol* 49:477, 2003. B

AUTHOR: **FRED F. FERRI, M.D.**

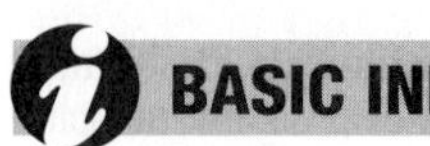

BASIC INFORMATION

DEFINITION

Contraception refers to the various modalities that a sexually active couple use to prevent pregnancy. These options can be either medical or nonmedical and used by men or women or both. The options are as follows:

- No contraception: failure rate 85% both typical use and perfect use
- Abstinence
  1. 12.4% of unmarried men
  2. 13.2% of unmarried women
  3. More frequently practiced before age 17 yr
  4. No intercourse experienced by 13% of women ages 30 to 34 yr
  5. Failure rate 0%
- Withdrawal
  1. Used in only 2% of sexually active women
  2. Failure rate with perfect use, 4%; with typical use, 19%
- Rhythm method (natural family planning)
  1. Failure rate with perfect use, 1% to 9%; with typical use, 20%
  2. Symptothermal type: mucus method and ovulation pain combined with basal body temperature
  3. Ovulation (Billings' method): takes into account mucus quality
  4. Basal body temperature method: uses biphasic temperature chart
  5. Lactation amenorrhea method: effective in fully breastfeeding women, especially 70 to 100 days after delivery; depends on number of feedings per day
- Barriers
  1. Diaphragm and cervical cap: failure rate 5% to 9% in nulliparous women, 20% in multiparous women
  2. Female condom: failure rate with perfect use, 5.1%; with typical use, 12.4%; FDA labeling states 25% failure rate
  3. Male condom: failure rate with perfect use, 3%; with typical use, 12%
  4. Spermicides (aerosols, foam, jellies, creams, tabs): failure rate with perfect use, 3%; with typical use, 21%
- Oral contraceptives
  1. Failure rate with perfect use, <1%; with typical use, 3%
  2. Come in combinations of estrogen/progestin or as progestin only
- Hormonal implants and injectables
  1. Norplant
     a. Most typically used in U.S.
     b. Failure rate in first 5 yr: 1%
     c. Failure rate after 6 yr: 2%
     d. May be extended to 7 yr use
  2. Depo-Provera: failure rate 0.3% in first year of use
  3. Lunelle: failure rate 0.2% in first year
  4. Etonogestrel implant: 2-yr cumulative pregnancy rate 0%
  5. Nestorone-releasing single implant: not yet available
  6. Jadelle implant
- Mini pill (progesterone only pill)
  1. Failure rate with typical use, 1.1% to 13.2%
  2. With perfect use, five pregnancies per 1000 women
- Emergency postcoital contraception
  1. Decreases pregnancy rate by 75% with women treated immediately postcoitally
  2. Involves hormonal use or intrauterine device (IUD) insertion
- IUD (available over the counter in some states)
  1. Progestasert: failure rate with perfect use, 2%; with typical use, 3%
  2. Copper T (380-A): failure rate with perfect use, 0.8%; with typical use, 3%
  3. Levonorgestrel Intrauterine System (Mirena)
     a. 1-yr failure rate, 1%
     b. 5-yr cumulative failure rate, 0.71 per 100 women
- Female sterilization (tubal ligation): failure rate with perfect use, 0.2%; with typical use, 3%
- Male sterilization (vasectomy): failure rate of 0.1% in first year
- Vaginal ring (Nuva ring): failure rate pearl index 0.77
- Contraceptive patch (Ortho Evra): failure rate 0.4% to 0.7%

SYNONYMS

Birth control
Family planning

ICD-9CM CODES
V25.01 Oral contraceptives
V25.02 Other contraceptive measures
V25.09 Family planning
V25.1 IUD
V25.2 Sterilization

EPIDEMIOLOGY & DEMOGRAPHICS

For women at risk for pregnancy, ranges for *use* of most commonly used birth control are age dependent, as follows:

- Oral contraceptives: 3% (40 to 44 yr) to 60% (20 to 24 yr)
- Condoms: 9% (40 to 44 yr) to 26% (15 to 19 yr)
- Diaphragm: 0.8% (15 to 19 yr) to 8% (30 to 34 yr)
- Periodic abstinence: 0.7% (15 to 19 yr) to 3% (35 to 39 yr)
- Withdrawal: 1.1% (40 to 44 yr) to 3% (20 to 30 yr)
- IUD: 0% (15 to 19 yr) to 3% (30 to 34 yr)
- Spermicides: 0.8% (15 to 19 yr) to 2.7% (35 to 39 yr)
- No method: 6.3% (35 to 39 yr) to 19.8% (15 to 19 yr)
- Sterilization:
  - Female: 0.2% (15 to 19 yr) to 47% (40 to 44 yr)
  - Male: 0.2% (15 to 19 yr) to 21% (40 to 44 yr)

Women are more likely to use contraception. The only two male forms available are condoms and vasectomy (sterilization).

DIAGNOSIS

WORKUP

- Thorough medical history
- Thorough surgical history
- Obstetric history (fertility desired?)
- Gynecologic history, including:
  1. History of previous sexually transmitted diseases
  2. Number of partners
  3. Previous difficulties with contraception
  4. Frequency of intercourse
- Family history

LABORATORY TESTS

- Pap smear
- Cultures, aerobic and *Chlamydia*
- Pregnancy test if suspected pregnancy
- Lipid profile if family history of premature vascular event

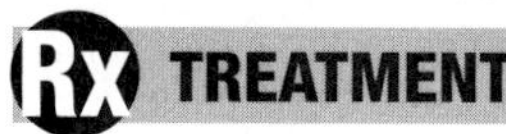

TREATMENT

NONPHARMACOLOGIC THERAPY

- Male condoms
  1. 95% latex (rubber), 5% skin or natural membrane
  2. Proper use: place on an erect penis and leave one-half-inch empty space at the tip of the condom; use with non–oil-based lubricants
  3. Effectiveness increased when used with spermicides
- Female condoms
  1. Composed of polyurethane, with one end open and one end closed
  2. Proper use: place closed end over cervix, open end hanging out of vagina to cover penis and scrotum
  3. Highly effective against HIV
- Spermicides
  1. Types: nonoxynol, octoxynol
  2. Forms: jellies, creams, foams, suppositories, tablets, soluble films
  3. Proper use: put in immediately before intercourse; may be used with other barrier methods
- Diaphragm and cervical cap
  1. Must be fitted by practitioner, used with contraceptive gels, and refitted with weight gain or loss
  2. Diaphragm sizes: 50 to 95 mm; cervical cap sizes: 22, 25, 28, and 31 mm
  3. Proper use of diaphragm: put in immediately before intercourse and keep in for 6 hr after intercourse; must not remain in the vagina for longer than 24 hr
  4. Proper use of cervical cap: fit over the cervix exactly; must not remain in place for longer than 48 hr
- Lactation amenorrhea method
  1. Depends on number of feedings per day; effective as birth control for 6 mo if 15 or more feedings, lasting 10 min each, are accomplished daily
  2. Not a common practice in the U.S.

- Withdrawal
  1. Withdrawal of the penis from the vagina before ejaculation
  2. Depends on self-control
- Rhythm method
  1. Depends on awareness of physiology of male and female reproductive tracts
  2. Sperm viable in vagina for 2 to 7 days
  3. Ovum life span 24 hr
- Sterilization
  1. Male:
     a. Vasectomy to interrupt vas deferens and block passage of sperm to seminal ejaculate
     b. Scalpel and nonscalpel techniques available
     c. More easily performed procedure than female sterilization and does not require general anesthesia
  2. Female:
     a. Leading method of birth control in U.S. in women older than 30 yr
     b. Interrupts fallopian tubes, blocking passage of ovum proximally and sperm distally through tube
     c. Several types; modified Pomeroy done during cesarean section or laparoscopic done in nonpregnant females most common
     d. Essure-tubal occlusion through hysteroscopic placement of micro-inserts into the fallopian tubes.

ACUTE GENERAL Rx

- Combination oral contraceptives
  1. Taken daily for 21 days, pill-free interval of 7 days
  2. Less than 50 mcg ethynyl estradiol in most common combination oral contraceptives; progestins most commonly used in combination pills are norethindrone, levonorgestrel, norgestrel, norethindrone acetate, ethynodiol diacetate, norgestimate, or desogestrel; triphasic combination oral contraceptives (give varying doses of progestin and estrogens throughout cycle); monophasic oral contraceptives: offer same dose of progestin and estrogen throughout cycle, taken daily at same time; estrophasic pill (constant progesterone with variation of estrogen throughout the cycle)
  3. If pill taken with antibiotics, efficacy affected by inadequate gastrointestinal absorption in most cases; only rifampin truly reduces pill's effectiveness
  4. Increased body weight decreases effectiveness
- Mini pill
  1. Progestin only; taken without a break
  2. Causes much irregular bleeding because of the lack of estrogen effect on the lining of the uterus
- Hormonal implants and injectables
  1. Norplant
     a. Progestin only; inserted under the skin
     b. Six levonorgestrel implants placed subcutaneously in upper inner arm effective for 5 yr
  2. Depo-Provera
     a. Medroxyprogesterone acetate given every 3 mo in IM injection form
     b. Major side effect: irregular bleeding
     c. Fertility return possibly delayed up to 18 mo after discontinuation
  3. Lunelle: monthly injectable administered intramuscularly. Contains 0.5 ml aqueous, 5 mg estradiol cypionate and 25 mg medroxyprogesterone acetate
  4. Etonogestrel implant: single-rod release etonogestrel for 3 yr placed subdermally
- Postcoital contraception
  1. Done on emergency basis, usually as a result of noncompliance with birth control or failure of birth control (e.g., condom breakage) at the time of ovulation
  2. Methods:
     a. IUD insertion within 7 days of coitus
     b. Hormonal methods (combination pills and danazol) given within 48 hr of coitus
- IUD
  1. Device inserted into uterus to prevent sperm and ovum from uniting in fallopian tube
  2. Types available in the U.S.:
     a. Progestasert: a T-shaped device that is an ethylene vinyl acetate copolymer T; vertical stem contains 38 mg progesterone and must be changed yearly
     b. ParaGard (Copper T/380-A): a polyethylene T wrapped with a fine copper wire effective for 10 yr
     c. Mirena Levonorgestrel Intrauterine System (LNGIUS): a T-shaped system with a chamber that contains levonorgestrel. Releases 20 mcg/day; is effective for 5 yr
- Vaginal ring (NuvaRing)
  1. Provides daily dose of 120 mcg of etonogestrel and 15 mcg ethinyl estradiol
  2. Stays in vagina 3 wk and is removed the fourth
  3. Increased body weight decreases effectiveness
- Contraceptive patch (Evra)
  1. Provides low daily dose of steroids
  2. Releases a progestin and estrogen (ethinyl estradiol)
  3. Patch size 20 cm^2
  4. Each patch contains 6 mg norelgestromin and delivers an estimated continuous systemic dose of 150 mcg norelgestromin and 20 mcg of ethinyl estradiol; common dose 250 mcg/day progestin and 25 mcg/day estrogen
  5. Worn 3 out of 4 wk
  6. Increased body weight decreases effectiveness

CHRONIC Rx

- With all the previously mentioned types of birth control, patient is followed up at least yearly, or as necessary, if problems arise.
- Full history, physical examination, and Pap smear, including cultures when needed, are performed yearly.
- Patients with medical problems are followed up approximately every 6 mo when taking hormonal therapy.

DISPOSITION

- Follow yearly or more frequently according to patient's side effects.
- Tailor birth control to patient according to different needs or side effects present at different times in life.

REFERRAL

With hormonal contraception, if neurologic or cardiac symptoms arise, stop method immediately, evaluate, and refer to internist when appropriate.

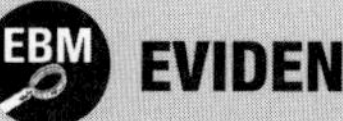

Please note: Complete text of EBM for this topic is available online.

Key trials and commentary:

This study sought to estimate whether young women taking the first pill on the day of prescription had higher continuation rates and lower pregnancy rates than women who waited until menses to start the oral contraceptive pill (OCP).

This study showed that protocols that require a woman to wait until the next menses to start hormonal contraceptives are an obstacle to contraceptive initiation. Directly observed, immediate initiation of the pill improves short-term continuation.

Too often, the practice of medicine involves a continuation of practice based not on evidence but rather on anecdote. For many of us, a stern stare and a "just do it" were the reasons used to teach us clinical care and why we continue these practices today. In this article, Westhoff et al show that protocols in which women wait to initiate contraception until their next menstrual flow are fraught with challenges and present obstacles to contraceptive initiation and success. The "quick start" method has women initiating their pill in the clinician's office and is shown to be associated with a higher short-term continuation rate and a lower overall pregnancy rate compared with a conventional use protocol. We have used the "Sunday start" for decades without the benefit of a study demonstrating its clinical benefit. This study shows that there is a better approach to initiate contraceptive pills and that clinicians need to consider such changes in the face of a continuing high and unacceptable rate of unintended and unplanned pregnancy.[1] Ⓐ

Evidence-Based Reference

1. Westhoff C, for the Quick Start Study Group: Initiation of oral contraceptives using a quick start compared with a conventional start: a randomized controlled trial, *Obstet Gynecol* 109:1270-1276, 2007. Commentary by L.P. Shulman, M.D. Ⓐ

AUTHORS: **MARIA A. CORIGLIANO, M.D.,** and **RUBEN ALVERO, M.D.**

BASIC INFORMATION

DEFINITION

Conversion disorder involves symptoms or deficits affecting voluntary motor or sensory function that cannot be explained by a neurologic or other medical condition. The symptom or deficit is not intentionally produced, distinguishing conversion disorder from factitious disorder or malingering. Conversion disorder is usually characterized by a single symptom that is sporadic, as opposed to somatization or somatoform disorder, and is presumed to be preceded by a psychological conflict or stressor. The conversion symptom functions to express and manage the unconscious psychological conflict. There is no well validated neurobiological model for conversion disorder, but advances in neuroscience and neuroimaging may reveal new etiologies in the future.

SYNONYMS

Dissociative conversion
Hysterical conversion
Hysteria
Medically unexplained symptom
Psychogenic, nonorganic, or functional symptoms

ICD-10
Dissociative (Conversion) Disorders

EPIDEMIOLOGY & DEMOGRAPHICS

- Incidence estimated at 5 to 10/100,000 in general population, 20 to 100/100,000 in hospital inpatients
- All ages, including early childhood
- Affects women more than men (ratios range from 2:1 to 5:1)
- Highest in rural areas, among undereducated, and in lower socioeconomic classes
- Associated with axis I disorders (depression more than anxiety) and axis II disorders (most commonly histrionic, passive dependent, and passive aggressive)

PHYSICAL FINDINGS & CLINICAL PRESENTATION

- Presents with a motor symptom (e.g., paralysis, aphonia, difficulty swallowing), a sensory symptom (loss of sensation, double vision, blindness, deafness), a psychogenic seizure, or "mixed" (symptoms from more than one category).
- Symptoms tend to occur in isolation (compared with multisystem involvement in somatization disorder).
- The symptoms or signs persist whether the patient is observed or unobserved, though are typically worse when the patient is attentive to them.
- May last from hours to years and tends to be sporadic.
- May occur in the context of documented medical illness (e.g., a patient with epileptic seizure may also have psychogenic seizure).
- May have comorbid axis I or axis II disorders, commonly depression, panic attacks, generalized anxiety, and PTSD.

ETIOLOGY

- The concept of the conversion symptom originated in the 1800s when neurologists such as Charcot and Bernheim demonstrated that symptoms such as "glove anesthesia" and "hysterical blindness" could not be explained neurologically and could sometimes be altered by hypnosis.
- Complex interplay of neurologic and psychologic factors.
- Symptom is preceded by psychological conflict or stressor that is completely or partially unconscious.
- Functional brain imaging studies suggest alterations in processing of sensory and motor signals. Hypotheses include an association with right-sided brain lesions and dysfunction in signals between the anterior cingulated and prefrontal cortex.

Dx DIAGNOSIS

DIFFERENTIAL DIAGNOSIS

Broad differential diagnosis depending on presenting signs and symptoms, including multiple sclerosis, CNS neoplasm, myasthenia gravis, Guillain-Barré syndrome, amyotrophic lateral sclerosis, Parkinson's disease, seizure disorder, systemic lupus erythematosus, spinal cord compression, intracerebral infarct, drug-induced dystonia, and HIV.

WORKUP

Thorough history and physical examination, including careful neurologic examination

LABORATORY TESTS

- No gold standard diagnostic tests exist; no single associated finding is pathognomonic.
- Laboratory tests or procedures may be needed to rule out other etiologies (e.g., EEG for seizures, EMG for lower motor neuron paralysis, optokinetic drum test in blindness).

IMAGING STUDIES

As indicated by presenting signs and symptoms

Rx TREATMENT

NONPHARMACOLOGIC THERAPY

- No good evidence exists demonstrating the efficacy of any treatment.
- Cognitive behavioral therapy is often the treatment of choice, although evidence is mixed.
- A long tradition of psychodynamic therapy exists but has not been validated by controlled trials.
- Treatment success has been associated with a caring, long-term relationship between patient and physician and a safe, nonconfrontational approach, with the exception of psychogenic seizure for which empathic confrontation and acceptance of disease is advocated as a foundation of treatment.
- Physical and occupational therapy can help "retrain" the patient in normal behaviors.
- Studies have shown no additional benefit to hypnosis, although case records describe treatment with hypnosis dating back to at least the 1800s, more recently using barbiturate-induced hypnosis as a psychotherapeutic aid.

ACUTE GENERAL Rx

- Antidepressants may be helpful in treating underlying mood or anxiety disorders.
- Patients with longstanding symptoms may require inpatient treatment.

CHRONIC Rx

See "Nonpharmacologic Therapy" and "Acute General Rx."

DISPOSITION

Long-term follow-up is essential to address recurrent conversion symptoms and underlying mood disorders.

REFERRAL

Refer to rule out other psychiatric disorders and for psychotherapy.

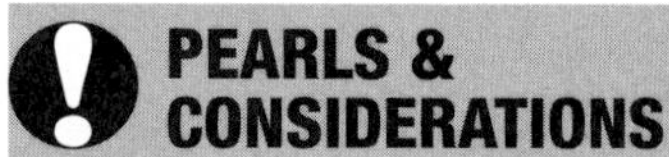

PEARLS & CONSIDERATIONS

COMMENTS

- Good prognostic factors: sudden onset, presence of psychological stressors at onset of symptoms, short duration between diagnosis and treatment, high level of intelligence, absence of other psychiatric or medical disorders, and no ongoing compensation litigation.
- Poor prognostic factors: severe disability, long duration of symptoms, age >40 yr at symptom onset, and convulsions and paralysis as presenting symptoms.
- Differentiation between conversion, somatization, dissociative, factitious, and malingering disorders, as well as organic versus functional etiologies, may be challenging.
- Studies show an association between sexual trauma and conversion symptoms, although evidence does not support causality because of confounding and methodological factors.
- Significant controversy exists regarding the categorization of conversion symptoms as somatoform as opposed to dissociative. Conversion disorder was categorized as somatoform originally in the DSM-III where, by presuming unconscious intent, it became a remnant of psychoanalytic theory otherwise removed from the DSM-III.
- Although not well demonstrated, some argue that conversion and somatized symptoms are more prevalent in cultures without an articulated concept of affective disorder or in which mental illness is highly stigmatized.

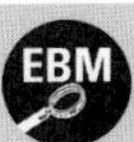

EVIDENCE

Evidence for the treatment of conversion disorder is sparse. Although some randomized controlled trials suggest that cognitive behavioral therapy is effective,[1] a 2007 review of randomized controlled trials for the treatment of somatoform disorders concluded that cognitive-behavioral therapy was the best established treatment for somatoform disorders with the exception of conversion disorder and pain disorder.[2] Regarding psychogenic seizure specifically, a 2007 Cochrane review stated, "There is currently no sound evidence on which to base treatment decisions for people with non-epileptic attacks."[3]

A 2005 meta-analysis of the misdiagnosis of conversion symptoms noted that reported misdiagnoses have declined from approximately 17% in the 1960s to 4% in the 1970s, predating the widespread introduction of computed tomography and likely the result of poor study design and vague definitions. They also noted that the most common misdiagnoses were of gait and movement disorders.[4]

A 2008 review suggests that a history of physical injury may play a previously underappreciated and not well understood role in some cases of conversion disorder.[5]

Evidence-Based References

1. Speckens AEM et al: Cognitive behavioural therapy for medically unexplained physical symptoms: a randomised controlled trial, *BMJ* 311:1328, 1995.
2. Kroenke K: Efficacy of treatment for somatoform disorders: a review of randomized controlled trials, *Psychosomat Med* 69:881, 2007.
3. Baker GA et al: Treatment for non-epileptic attack disorder, *Cochrane Database Review* 1, CD006370, 2007.
4. Stone J et al: Systematic review of misdiagnosis of conversion symptoms and "hysteria," *BMJ* 10: 1136, 2005. Ⓑ
5. Stone J et al: The role of physical injury in motor and sensory conversion symptoms: a systematic and narrative review, *J Psychosom Res* 66(5):383-390, 2008.

SUGGESTED READINGS

Abyek S et al: The neuropsychiatry of conversion disorder, *Curr Opin Psychiatry* 21(3):275-280, 2008.

Ballmeier M et al: Conversion disorder revisited, *Functional Neurology* 20:105, 2005.

Binder M et al: Psychogenic nonepileptic seizures, *Neuropsychol Rev* 17:405, 2007.

Halligan PW et al (eds): *Contemporary approaches to the study of hysteria,* Oxford, 2001, Oxford University Press.

AUTHOR: **KAILA COMPTON, M.D., PH.D.**

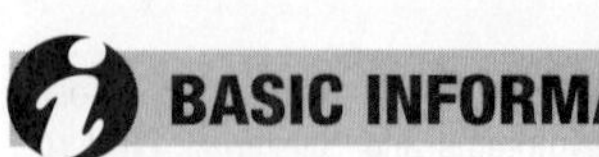

BASIC INFORMATION

DEFINITION

Cor pulmonale is an alteration in the structure and function of the right ventricle from pulmonary hypertension caused by diseases of the lungs or pulmonary vasculature. It is a state of cardiopulmonary dysfunction that may result from multiple etiologies rather than a specific disease state. Right-sided heart failure resulting from primary disease of the left heart and congenital heart disease are not considered in this disorder.

SYNONYMS

Acute cor pulmonale
Chronic cor pulmonale

ICD-9CM CODES
415.0 Cor pulmonale, acute
416.9 Cor pulmonale, chronic

ETIOLOGY

Most conditions that cause cor pulmonale are chronic. Acute cor pulmonale is often life threatening but transient. For example, acute pulmonary embolus may present with acute cor pulmonale, cardiogenic shock, or death, but if the patient survives the initial event, then the right ventricle often recovers and cor pulmonale is no longer existent after several weeks.

Mechanisms leading to pulmonary hypertension and predisposing to the development of cor pulmonale include:

- Pulmonary vasoconstriction resulting from any condition causing alveolar hypoxia and/or acidosis
- Anatomic reduction of the pulmonary vascular bed (e.g., emphysema, interstitial lung disease, pulmonary emboli)
- Increased blood viscosity (e.g., polycythemia vera, Waldenström's macroglobulinemia)

PHYSICAL FINDINGS & CLINICAL PRESENTATION

No symptoms are specific for cor pulmonale. Typically, the symptoms depend on the underlying disease process. The symptoms are most often a result of right ventricular failure:

- Dyspnea, fatigue, chest pain, or syncope with exertion (from pulmonary hypertension)
- Right upper quadrant abdominal pain and anorexia (from passive hepatic congestion)
- Hoarseness (caused by compression of the left recurrent laryngeal nerve by dilation of the main pulmonary artery; known as *Ortner's syndrome*)
- Signs of right ventricular failure: jugular venous distention, peripheral edema, hepatic congestion, ascites, and a right ventricular third heart sound
- Signs of associated tricuspid regurgitation: holosystolic murmur heard best along the left parasternal border (augments during inspiration), prominent V-wave on jugular venous pulse, and pulsatile hepatomegaly (in severe tricuspid regurgitation)
- Pulmonary hypertension will increase the intensity of the pulmonic component of S2, which may be narrowly split
- Rarely, cough and hemoptysis

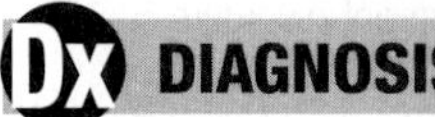

DIAGNOSIS

WORKUP

Search for an underlying pulmonary process resulting in pulmonary hypertension:

- Left ventricular dysfunction should be excluded in initial assessment.
- 80% to 90% of cor pulmonale cases are attributable to chronic obstructive pulmonary disease (COPD).
- Consideration of alveolar hypoventilation, chronic thromboembolic disease, and neuromuscular disease should be given in the absence of parenchymal lung disease.

LABORATORY TESTS

- Complete blood count may show erythrocytosis from chronic hypoxia.
- Arterial blood gas levels confirm hypoxemia and acidosis or hypercapnia.
- Pulmonary function tests.

IMAGING STUDIES

- Chest radiograph may show underlying pulmonary disease and evidence of pulmonary hypertension (e.g., enlargement of the pulmonary arteries or right atrium and right ventricular dilation) (Fig. 1-74).
- ECG may reveal right ventricular hypertrophy, right atrial enlargement (P-pulmonale), right-axis deviation, or incomplete/complete right bundle branch block.
- Echocardiogram to detect right ventricular enlargement and/or hypertrophy and estimate pulmonary artery pressure.
- Radionuclide ventriculography to measure right ventricular ejection fraction, which may be reduced.
- Cardiac MRI can accurately measure right ventricular dimensions and function.
- Right-sided heart catheterization measures pulmonary artery pressures and pulmonary vascular resistance. It can also determine response to oxygen or vasodilators.
- Chest CT can assess for pulmonary parenchymal disease and embolus in the pulmonary vasculature.

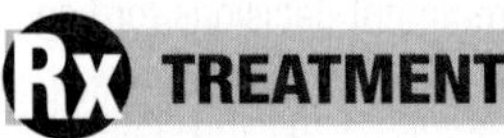

TREATMENT

The treatment of cor pulmonale is directed toward the underlying etiology while also reversing hypoxemia, improving right ventricular contractility, decreasing pulmonary artery vascular resistance, and improving pulmonary hypertension

NONPHARMACOLOGIC THERAPY

- Continuous positive airway pressure is used in patients with obstructive sleep apnea.
- Phlebotomy is reserved as adjunctive therapy in patients with polycythemia (hematocrit >55%) who have acute decompensation of cor pulmonale or remain polycythemic despite long-term oxygen therapy. Phlebotomy has been shown to decrease mean pulmonary artery pressure and pulmonary vascular resistance.

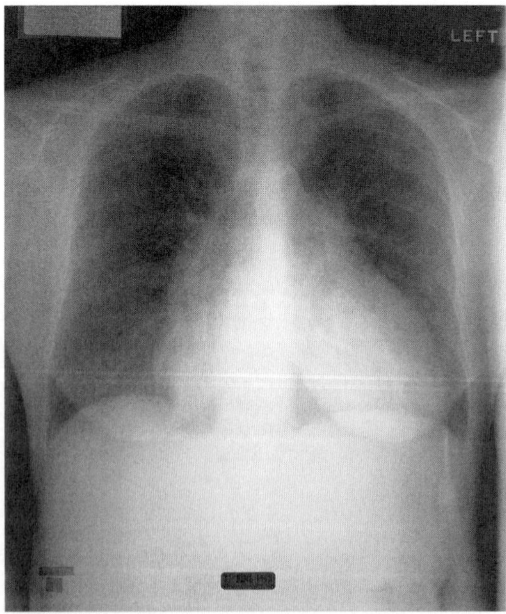

FIGURE 1-74 Chest radiography in a patient with severe intrinsic pulmonary vascular disease demonstrating enlargement of the main pulmonary artery, right ventricle, and right atrium. (From Crawford MH et al [eds]: *Cardiology,* ed 2, St Louis, 2004, Mosby.)

ACUTE GENERAL Rx

- Pulmonary embolism is the most common cause of acute cor pulmonale (see "Pulmonary Embolism"). The treatment is anticoagulation, hemodynamic support, and consideration of thrombolytics.
- In patients with preexisting cor pulmonale, acute pulmonary illnesses or hypoxia can increase pulmonary hypertension and worsen right ventricular function. The underlying exacerbating conditions should be treated.

CHRONIC Rx

- Long-term oxygen supplementation improves survival in hypoxemic patients with COPD.
- Right ventricular volume overload should be treated with diuretics (e.g., furosemide). However, excessive diuresis can reduce right ventricular filling and decrease cardiac output.
- Theophylline and sympathomimetic amines may improve diaphragmatic excursion, myocardial contraction, and pulmonary artery vasodilation.
- The long-term use of nonselective vasodilators including nitrates, calcium channel blockers, and angiotensin-converting enzyme inhibitors has not resulted in significant survival improvement. This is probably because of a lack of vasoreactivity in patients with COPD as well as the risk of worsening of ventilation/perfusion mismatch and systemic vasodilation. Vasodilators to combat pulmonary hypertension should not be administered empirically in the absence of a right-sided heart catheterization.

DISPOSITION

The level of pulmonary artery pressure in COPD patients with cor pulmonale is a good indicator of prognosis. Right ventricular function may provide additional information.

REFERRAL

Patients with pulmonary disease who have progressed to cor pulmonale should be followed up by a pulmonologist.

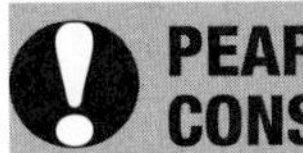

PEARLS & CONSIDERATIONS

- There is no differential diagnosis, but rather an evaluation of the patient to identify the underlying cause.
- Prognosis and treatment are related to the underlying cause, whereas the presence of cor pulmonale is merely a marker of the underlying disease severity.

COMMENTS

There is increasing interest in selective pulmonary vasodilators to improve right ventricular heart function in patients with cor pulmonale.

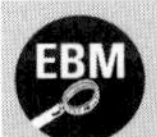

EVIDENCE

A randomized controlled trial (RCT) found that domiciliary oxygen given at a rate of 2 L/min for at least 15 hr/day to patients with COPD who were extremely hypoxic significantly reduced mortality rate compared with no oxygen therapy over 5 yr.[1] A

A systematic review concluded that long-term oxygen therapy improved survival rate in patients with COPD and severe hypoxemia but not in those with moderate hypoxemia or only arterial desaturation at night. Four of five of the RCTs included did not specifically include those diagnosed with cor pulmonale.[2] A

Evidence-Based References

1. Medical Research Council Working Party: Long-term domiciliary oxygen therapy in chronic hypoxic cor pulmonale complicating chronic bronchitis and emphysema, *Lancet* 1:681, 1981. A
2. Cranston JM et al: Domiciliary oxygen for chronic obstructive pulmonary disease, *Cochrane Rev,* Issue 4, Chichester, UK, 2005, John Wiley & Sons, pp 27. A

SUGGESTED READINGS

Lehrman S et al: Primary pulmonary hypertension and cor pulmonale, *Cardiol Rev* 10(5):265-278, 2002.

Weitzenblum E: Chronic cor pulmonale, *Heart* 89(2): 225-230, 2003.

AUTHORS: **DOUGLAS W. MARTIN, M.D.,** and **GAURAV CHOUDHARY, M.D.**

Corneal Abrasion (PTG) (ALG)

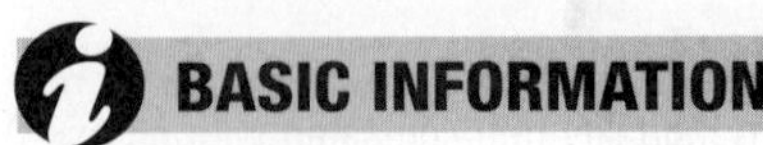

BASIC INFORMATION

DEFINITION

A corneal abrasion is a loss of surface epithelial tissue of the cornea caused by trauma.

SYNONYMS

Corneal erosion
Corneal contusion

ICD-9CM CODES
918.1 Corneal abrasion

EPIDEMIOLOGY & DEMOGRAPHICS

INCIDENCE (IN U.S.): A universal problem
PEAK INCIDENCE: Childhood through active adulthood and older and debilitated patients
PREDOMINANT AGE: Any age

PHYSICAL FINDINGS & CLINICAL PRESENTATION

- Haziness of the cornea
- Disruption of the corneal surface (Fig. 1-75)
- Redness and infection of the conjunctiva
- Pain
- Light sensitivity
- Tearing
- Gritty feeling
- Pain on opening or closing eyes
- Sensation of a foreign body

ETIOLOGY

- Trauma (direct mechanical event)
- Foreign body
- Contact lenses
- Unknown

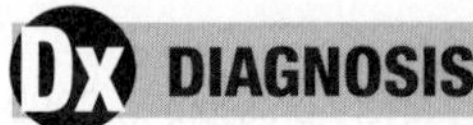

DIAGNOSIS

DIFFERENTIAL DIAGNOSIS

- Acute-angle glaucoma
- Herpes ulcers and other corneal ulcers
- Foreign body in the cornea (be certain it is not a keratitis)

WORKUP

- Fluorescein staining, slit lamp evaluation
- Assessment of visual acuity
- Intraocular pressure
- Rule out corneal laceration
- Rule out other eye pathology

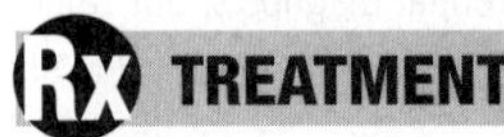

TREATMENT

NONPHARMACOLOGIC THERAPY

- Patching is controversial (see below).
- Bandage.
- Contact lenses.
- Warm compresses.
- Pressure dressing is controversial. Although eye patching traditionally has been recommended in the treatment of corneal abrasions, several studies show that patching does not help and may hinder healing.
- Removal of any foreign particles if present.

ACUTE GENERAL Rx

- Topical antibiotics such as 10% sulfacetamide or ofloxacin 0.3% solution 2 drops qid.
- Pressure patching of eye with eyelid closed is no longer recommended because it can result in decreased oxygen delivery, increased moisture, and a higher chance of infection.
- Cycloplegics such as 5% homatropine are often prescribed to relieve ciliary muscle spasm; however, their benefit has been questioned and they are no longer routinely recommended.
- Topical nonsteroidal antiinflammatory drugs (e.g., diclofenac 0.1% or ketorolac 0.5%) 1 drop qid.
- Topical antibiotics to prevent secondary infection.

DISPOSITION

Follow-up in 24 hr and then every 3 days until abrasion has cleared and vision has returned to normal

REFERRAL

To ophthalmologist if patient has no relief within 24 hr or for patients with deep eye injuries, foreign bodies that cannot be removed, or suspected recurrent corneal erosion.

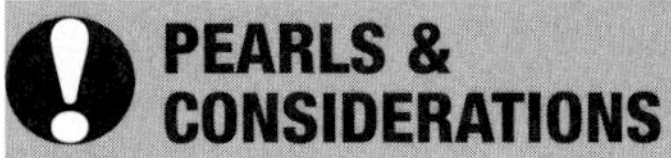

PEARLS & CONSIDERATIONS

COMMENTS

- Never give the patient topical anesthetic to use at home because these can cause decomposition of the cornea and permanent damage.
- Most corneal abrasions heal in 24 to 48 hr and rarely progress to corneal erosion or infection.

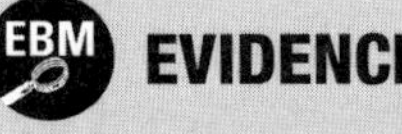

EVIDENCE

In patients with uncomplicated corneal abrasions, the application of an eye patch does not improve the rate of corneal healing, reduce pain, or reduce complications compared with wearing no patch.[1] (B)

Evidence-Based Reference

1. Flynn CA et al: Should we patch corneal abrasions? A meta-analysis, *J Fam Pract* 47:264, 1998. (B)

SUGGESTED READING

Wilson SA, Last A: Management of corneal abrasions, *Am Fam Physician* 70(1):123, 2004.

AUTHOR: **MELVYN KOBY, M.D.**

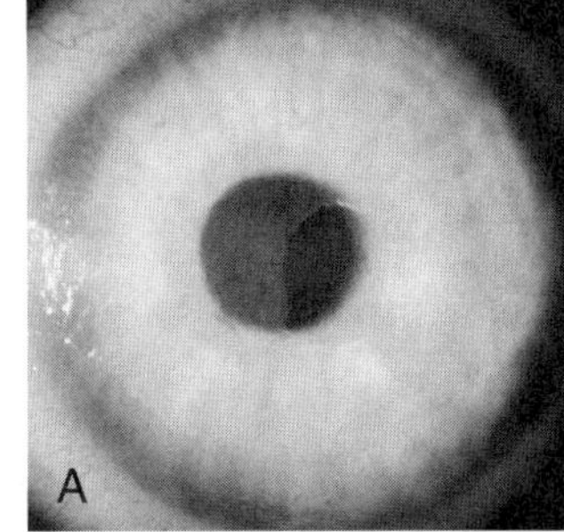

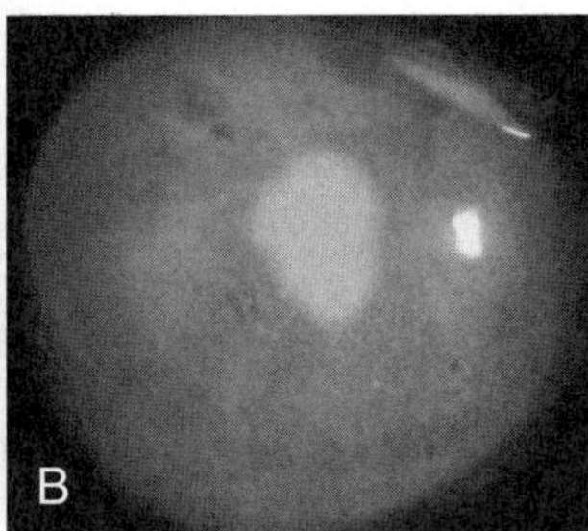

FIGURE 1-75 Corneal epithelial abrasion. A, Epithelial defect without fluorescein highlighting the defect. An irregularity in the otherwise smooth corneal surface is the key to identifying the defect if no fluorescein is available. **B,** Classic fluorescein staining of an epithelial defect. (From Palay D [ed]: *Ophthalmology for the primary care physician,* St Louis, 1997, Mosby.)

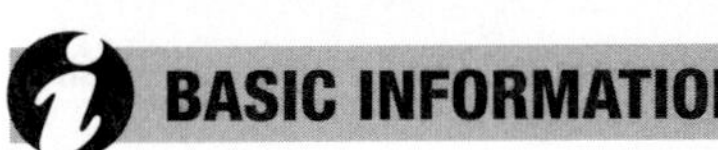

BASIC INFORMATION

DEFINITION

Corneal ulceration refers to the disruption of the corneal surface and/or deeper layers caused by trauma, contact lenses infection, degeneration, or other means.

SYNONYMS

Infectious keratitis with ulceration
Bacterial keratitis with ulceration
Viral keratitis with ulceration
Fungal keratitis with ulceration

ICD-9CM CODES
370.0 Corneal ulcer NOS

EPIDEMIOLOGY & DEMOGRAPHICS

INCIDENCE (IN U.S.): Four to six cases per month seen by an average general ophthalmologist
PREVALENCE (IN U.S.): Common
PREDOMINANT SEX: Either
PREDOMINANT AGE: All ages

PHYSICAL FINDINGS & CLINICAL PRESENTATION

- Localized, well-demarcated, infiltrative lesion with corresponding focal ulcer (Fig. 1-76) or oval, yellow-white stromal suppuration with thick mucopurulent exudate and edema. Usually red, angry-looking eye with infiltration in surrounding area of cornea.
- Eye possibly painful, with conjunctival edema and infection.
- Sterile neurotrophic ulcers with tissue breakdown and no pain.

ETIOLOGY

- Complication of contact lens wear, trauma, or diseases such as herpes simplex keratitis or keratoconjunctivitis sicca. Often associated with collagen vascular disease and severe exophthalmus and thyroid disease.
- Viral causes often contagious.

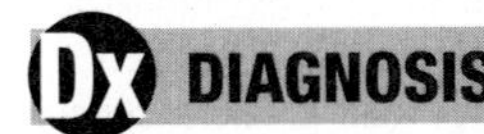

DIAGNOSIS

DIFFERENTIAL DIAGNOSIS

- *Pseudomonas* and pneumococcus and other bacterial infection—virulent
- *Moraxella, Staphylococcus, α-Streptococcus* infection—less virulent
- Herpes simplex infection or disease caused by other viruses
- Contact lens ulcers differ

WORKUP

- Fluorescein staining, slit lamp
- Appearance often typical
- Differentiate carefully with contact lens wearers
- Note previous eye surgery or laser vision correction

LABORATORY TESTS

Microscopic examination and culture of scrapings

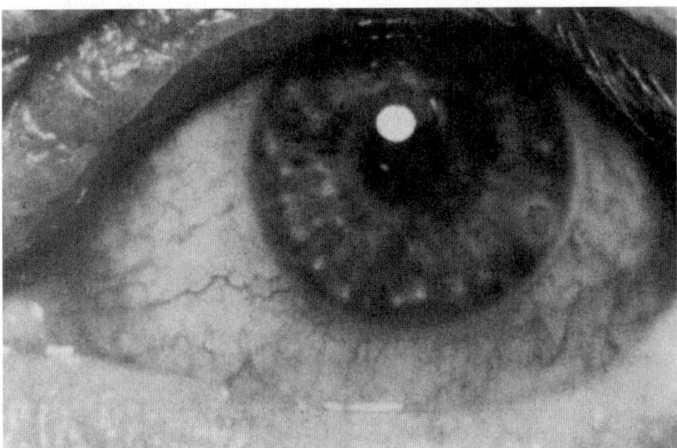

FIGURE 1-76 Peripherally located corneal ulcer. (From Marx JA [ed]: *Rosen's emergency medicine,* ed 5, St Louis, 2002, Mosby.)

Rx TREATMENT

NONPHARMACOLOGIC THERAPY

- Warm compresses
- Bandage contact lenses
- Patching
- Stop contact lens wearing
- Remove eyelid crusting

ACUTE GENERAL Rx

- An ophthalmic emergency
- Intense antibiotic and antiviral therapy
- Nonsteroidal antiinflammatory drugs
- Viroptic/Zymar
- Bacterial infection: subconjunctival cefazolin or gentamicin (topical Zymar, Vigomax, etc.)
- Fungal infection: hospitalization and topical application of antifungal agents
- Herpes: Viroptic and oral therapy

DISPOSITION

Ideally treated by an ophthalmologist if the patient does not rapidly respond to antibiotics (within 24 hr)

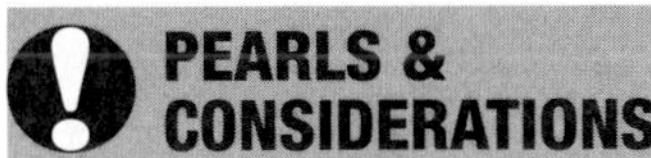

PEARLS & CONSIDERATIONS

- Always stop contact lens wearing.
- Always refer ulcers to ophthalmologist.
- Never treat with topical anesthetics or steroids.

COMMENTS

Do not use topical steroids because herpes, fungal, or other ulcers may be aggravated, leading to perforation of the cornea. Antibiotics may delay response and result in overgrowth of nonbacterial (fungal and amoebic) pathogens.

SUGGESTED READINGS

Price FW: New pieces for the puzzle: nonsteroidal anti-inflammatory drugs and corneal ulcers, *J Cataract Refract Surg* 26(9):1263, 2000.

Schaefer F et al: Bacterial keratitis: a prospective clinical and microbiological study, *Br J Ophthalmol,* 85(7):42, 2001.

Stretton S et al: Corneal ulceration in pediatric patients: a brief overview of progress in topical treatment, *Paediatr Drugs* 4(2):95, 2002.

Varaprasathan G et al: Trends in the etiology of infectious corneal ulcers at the F. I. Proctor Foundation, *Cornea* 23(4):360, 2004.

AUTHOR: **MELVYN KOBY, M.D.**

Costochondritis

BASIC INFORMATION

DEFINITION

Costochondritis is an inflammation of costochondral junctions of ribs or chondroternal joints of the anterior chest wall.

SYNONYMS

Benign chest wall pain syndrome
Costosternal syndrome
Costosternal chondrodynia

ICD-9CM CODES
733.6 Costochondritis

EPIDEMIOLOGY & DEMOGRAPHICS

PREVALENCE: Unknown
PREDOMINANT SEX: Women afflicted more often than men
PREDOMINANT AGE: >40 yr

PHYSICAL FINDINGS & CLINICAL PRESENTATION

- Tenderness of costochondral junctions (second through fifth) and/or sternum
- Pain with coughing and deep breathing
- Both sides of chest equal in frequency of involvement
- Often associated with anxiety, headache, and hyperventilation

ETIOLOGY

- Unknown
- May be a form of regional fibrositis
- May be referred pain from cervical or thoracic spine
- Emotional factors often involved

DIAGNOSIS

DIFFERENTIAL DIAGNOSIS

- Tietze's syndrome
- Cardiovascular disease
- Gastrointestinal disease
- Pulmonary disease
- Osteoarthritis of sternoclavicular, sternomanubrial, or shoulder joints (Table 1-17)
- Cervical disc syndrome
- Fibromyalgia
- Herpes zoster of thorax
- Destruction of costal cartilage by infections or neoplasms
- Slipping rib syndrome
- Tramatic muscle pain and overuse myalgia

WORKUP

- There are no laboratory or radiographic abnormalities.
- Testing to rule out or rule in more serious disorders is performed on a case-by-case basis. Coronary artery disease is present in 3 to 6% of adult patients with chest pain and chest wall tenderness on palpation. Consider ECG and chest x-ray in patients older than 35 years, in those with risk factors of heart disease, and in patients with cardiopulmonary symptoms.

TREATMENT

ACUTE GENERAL Rx

- Explanation, reassurance
- Application of heat with compresses or heating pad is helpful in case of muscle overuse
- Minimize activities that provoke symptoms
- Nonsteroidal antiinflammatory drugs or acetaminophen for analgesia
- Refractory cases can be treated with local injections of combined lidocaine/corticosteroid into costochondral areas

DISPOSITION

- The duration of the disorder is variable.
- Spontaneous remission is the rule.

REFERRAL

- Cardiologist to rule out primary cardiac disease when indicated.
- Gastroenterologist to rule out gastrointestinal disorders when indicated.

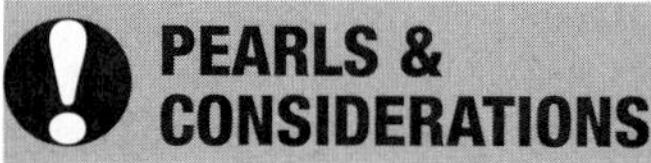

PEARLS & CONSIDERATIONS

One of a large number of nonspecific musculoskeletal diagnoses based strictly on subjective symptoms and lacking any objective abnormalities.

COMMENTS

Despite the name, no inflammation is present. After other, more serious conditions are ruled out, the treatment is strictly symptomatic and supportive.

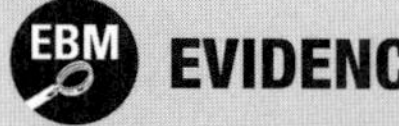

EVIDENCE

Evidence supporting these treatments is lacking. However, clinical experience indicates that one or more of these treatments may be helpful for many patients.

SUGGESTED READINGS

Freeston J et al: Can early diagnosis and management of costochondritis reduce acute chest pain admissions? *J Rheumatol* 31:2269, 2004.

Gregory PL et al: Musculoskeletal problems of the chest wall in athletes, *Sports Med* 32:325, 2002.

Hiramuro-Shoji F et al: Atraumatic conditions of the sternoclavicular joint, *J Shoulder Elbow Surg* 12:79, 2003.

Jenson S: Musculoskeletal causes of chest pain, *Am Fam Physician* 30:834, 2001.

Proulx AM, Zryd T: Costochondritis: diagnosis and treatment, *Am Fam Physician* 80(6):617-620, 2009.

Rumball JS et al: Rowing injuries, *Sports Med* 35:537, 2005.

Sik EC et al: Atypical chest pain in athletes, *Curr Sports Med Rep* 8:52, 2009.

AUTHOR: **LONNIE R. MERCIER, M.D.**

TABLE 1-17 Musculoskeletal Chest Pain

Disorder	Clinical Features	Comments
Tietze's syndrome	Pain and swelling of sternoclavicular joint or second or third costochondral junctions (usually left). Worse with cough and deep breathing. Local tenderness.	Traumatic cause? Rare.
Costochondritis	Pain and tenderness but no swelling. Costochondral junctions of ribs 2 to 5. Increased pain with cough and sneeze.	Sometimes associated with headache and hyperventilation.
Seronegative spondyloarthropathy (ankylosing spondylitis)	Sternoclavicular or manubriosternal joint. Worse in morning. Relieved by activity. May be associated with swelling.	Local chest findings usually associated with other symptoms of ankylosing spondylitis such as sacroiliitis. May need HLA-B27 antigen testing.
Cervical, thoracic disc disease	Referred regional pain from affected area. No local swelling. Often aggravated by spine motion and may be accompanied by radicular pain into arm if cervical or along intercostal nerve if thoracic.	May mimic chest disease if spinal complaints are minimal and referred or radicular symptoms predominate.
Fibromyalgia	Widespread pain with other sites involved. Symptoms often change in location. Local tender points but no swelling or objective findings.	Female/male ratio of 9:1. Prevalent age 30-50 yr.
Osteoarthritis, sternoclavicular or manubriosternal joint	Dull, aching local pain with tenderness. Occasional bony joint enlargement with soft tissue swelling.	Crepitus may rarely be present.

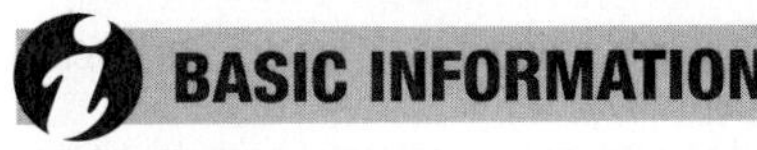

BASIC INFORMATION

DEFINITION

Craniopharyngiomas are tumors arising from squamous cell remnants of Rathke's pouch, located in the infundibulum or upper anterior hypophysis.

SYNONYMS

Subset of nonadenomatous pituitary tumors

ICD-9CM CODES
237.0 Craniopharyngioma

EPIDEMIOLOGY & DEMOGRAPHICS

PEAK INCIDENCE: Occurs at all ages; peak during the first 2 decades of life, with a second small peak occurring in the sixth decade.

PREDOMINANT SEX:
- Both sexes are usually equally affected.
- Craniopharyngiomas are the most common nonglial tumors in children and account for 3% to 5% of all pediatric brain tumors.

PHYSICAL FINDINGS & CLINICAL PRESENTATION

- The typical onset is insidious and a 1- to 2-year history of slowly progressive symptoms is common.
- Presenting symptoms are usually related to the effects of a sella turcica mass. Approximately 75% of patients report headache and have visual disturbances.
- The usual visual defect is bitemporal hemianopsia. Optic nerve involvement with decreased visual acuity and scotomas and homonymous hemianopsia from optic tract involvement may also occur.
- Other symptoms include mental changes, nausea, vomiting, somnolence, or symptoms of pituitary failure. In adults, sexual dysfunction is the most common endocrine complaint, with impotence in men and primary or secondary amenorrhea in women. Diabetes insipidus is found in 25% of cases. In children, craniopharyngiomas may present with dwarfism.
- More than 70% of children at the time of diagnosis present with growth hormone deficiency, obstructive hydrocephalus, short-term memory deficits, and psychomotor slowing.

ETIOLOGY

Craniopharyngiomas are believed to arise from nests of squamous epithelial cells that are commonly found in the suprasellar area surrounding the pars tuberalis of the adult pituitary.

Dx DIAGNOSIS

DIFFERENTIAL DIAGNOSIS

- Pituitary adenoma
- Empty sella syndrome
- Pituitary failure of any cause
- Primary brain tumors (e.g., meningiomas, astrocytomas)
- Metastatic brain tumors
- Other brain tumors
- Cerebral aneurysm

LABORATORY TESTS

- Hypothyroidism (low FT_4, FT_3 with high thyroid-stimulating hormone).
- Hypercortisolism (low cortisol) with low adrenocorticotropic hormone.
- Low sex hormones (testosterone, estriol) with low follicle-stimulating hormone and luteinizing hormone.
- Diabetes insipidus (hypernatremia, low urine osmolarity, high plasma osmolarity).
- Prolactin may be normal or slightly elevated.
- Pituitary stimulation tests may be required in some cases.

IMAGING STUDIES

- Visual field testing for bitemporal hemianopsia.
- Skull film.
  - Enlarged or eroded sella turcica (50%)
  - Suprasellar calcification (50%)
- MRI (Fig. 1-77) or head CT. MRI features include a multicystic and solid enhancing suprasellar mass. Hydrocephalus may also be present if the mass is large. CT usually reveals intratumoral calcifications.

Rx TREATMENT

GENERAL Rx

- Surgical resection (curative or palliative).
  - Transsphenoidal surgery for small intrasellar tumors
  - Subfrontal craniotomy for most patients
- Postoperative radiation.
- Intralesional ^{32}P irradiation or bleomycin for unresectable tumors. Long-term complications of radiation include secondary malignancies, optic neuropathy, and vascular injury.

PROGNOSIS

- Operative mortality rate: 3% to 16% (higher with large tumors).
- Postoperative recurrence rate: 30% of cases after total resection and 57% of cases after subtotal resection.
- 5-yr and 10-yr survival: 88% and 76%, respectively, with surgery and radiation.
- The most important factors that correlate with prognosis are the extent of resection and postoperative radiation.

AUTHORS: **FRED F. FERRI, M.D.,** and **TOM J. WACHTEL, M.D.**

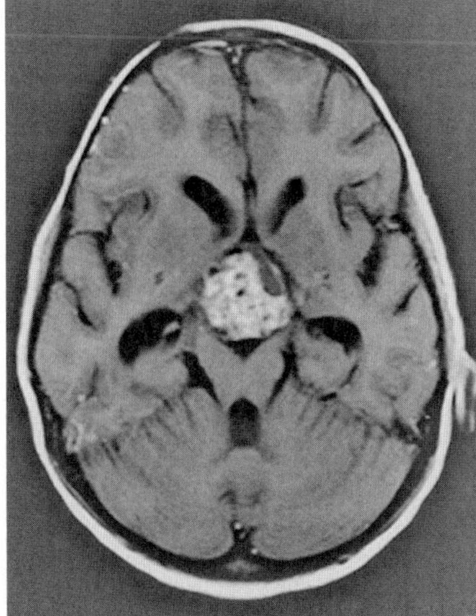

FIGURE 1-77 MRI scan of a craniopharyngioma, demonstrating a cystic contrast-enhancing mass in the suprasellar area extending upward and compressing the hypothalamus. (From Goetz CG: *Textbook of clinical neurology,* Philadelphia, 1999, WB Saunders.)

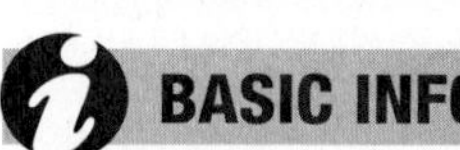

BASIC INFORMATION

DEFINITION

Creutzfeldt-Jakob disease (CJD) is a progressive, fatal, dementing illness caused by an infectious protein agent known as a *prion.*

SYNONYMS

Transmissible spongiform encephalopathy
Mad cow disease
Prion disease

ICD-9CM CODES
046.1 Creutzfeldt-Jakob disease

EPIDEMIOLOGY & DEMOGRAPHICS

- Incidence of one per 1 million population per year
- Peak age 60 yr (range, 16 to 82 yr)
- 5% to 10% familial, remaining cases are sporadic; iatrogenic cases (corneal transplants, dura mater allograft, human pituitary extract) are very rare
- Normal prion protein (PRNP) gene found on human chromosome 20
- Methionine and valine distribution on codon 129 of the PRNP determines the six clinical phenotypes of CJD

PHYSICAL FINDINGS & CLINICAL PRESENTATION

- All patients present with cognitive deficits (dementing illness—memory loss, behavioral abnormalities, higher cortical function impairment).
- More than 80% will have myoclonus.
- Pyramidal tract signs (weakness), cerebellar signs (clumsiness), and extrapyramidal signs (parkinsonian features) are seen in more than 50% of the cases.
- Less common features include cortical visual abnormalities, abnormal eye movements, vestibular dysfunction, sensory disturbances, autonomic dysfunction, lower motor neuron signs, and seizures.

ETIOLOGY

Small proteinaceous infectious particle (prion). Noninfectious prion protein (PrP) is a cellular protein found on the surfaces of neurons. Normal function is not known. Protein is converted to protease-resistant and infectious agent by infectious prion protein.

DIAGNOSIS

- Definite CJD: Neuropathologically confirmed spongiform encephalopathy in a case of progressive dementia.
- Probable CJD: History of rapidly progressive dementia (<2 yr) with typical EEG and with at least two of the following clinical features: myoclonus, visual or cerebellar dysfunction, pyramidal or extrapyramidal features, akinetic mutism.
- Possible CJD: Same as probable CJD without EEG findings.

DIFFERENTIAL DIAGNOSIS

- Other dementias (Alz, FTD, DLBD, vascular)
- Infectious (viral, HIV, fungal, TB)
- Inflammatory/Autoimmune (CNS vasculitis, Hashimoto's encephalopathy)
- Metabolic (vitamin deficiency, endocrine)
- Cancers (CNS lymphoma, gliomatosis cerebri, paraneoplastic)

A clinical algorithm for the evaluation of dementia is described in Section III, "Dementia."

WORKUP

- Evaluate for treatable causes of dementia (see "Alzheimer's Disease").
- Brain biopsy can be diagnostic, but it is usually not performed because there is no treatment or cure.

LABORATORY TESTS

- Presence of periodic sharp wave complexes on EEG in cases of rapidly progressive dementia has a sensitivity of 67% and a specificity of 86%.
- In cases of probable or possible CJD, presence of the 14,3,3 protein in CSF has a 95% positive predictive value with its absence having a 92% negative predictive value.

IMAGING STUDIES

MRI scan can show areas of restricted diffusion in the basal ganglia and cerebral cortex. MRI diffusion-weighted imaging has a sensitivity of 92.3% and a specificity of 93.8% only in cases of rapidly progressive dementia.

TREATMENT

NONPHARMACOLOGIC THERAPY

Full-time caregiver and/or nursing home. Social work can be helpful with end-of-life discussions, family counseling, and optimizing appropriate home services.

ACUTE GENERAL Rx

No known therapy

CHRONIC Rx

No known therapy

DISPOSITION

The disease is fatal. Mean duration of illness is 8 mo (range, 1 to 130 mo). One in 7 survives to 1 yr, and 1 in 30 survives to 2 yr. Better survival found in younger age at onset of disease and female gender.

REFERRAL

- Neurology for evaluation of any rapidly progressive dementia
- Social work

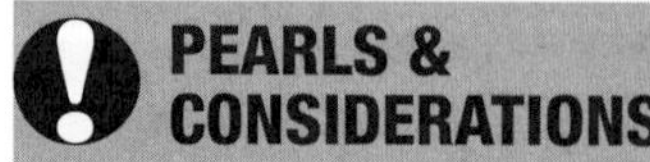

PEARLS & CONSIDERATIONS

COMMENTS

- Related diseases in human beings: kuru, fatal familial insomnia, Gerstmann-Sträussler-Scheinker syndrome, new-variant Creutzfeldt-Jakob disease.
- Related diseases in animals: scrapie, bovine spongiform encephalopathy (mad cow disease).

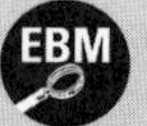

EVIDENCE

Please note: Complete text of EBM for this topic is available online.

Key trials and commentary:

The E200K mutation of the *PRNP* (prion protein) gene is the most common cause of familial Creutzfeldt-Jakob disease (fCJD), which has imaging and clinical features that are similar to the sporadic form. The purpose of this study was to conduct a controlled and blinded evaluation of the sensitivity and specificity of MRI in this unique population.

This study showed that FLAIR and DWI abnormalities in the caudate nucleus and putamen offer the best sensitivity and specificity for diagnosing fCJD. Our findings support recent recommendations that MR imaging should be added to the diagnostic evaluation of CJD.

Familial CJD is one of the rare forms of CJD, being much less common than sCJD, without many larger patients samples to date for the purposes of determining the imaging findings. This study confirms that FLAIR and DWI can be used with a relatively high sensitivity and specificity (around 90%) for detection of involved regions in fCJD, most commonly the caudate and putamen (70%-80%) and less commonly the thalamus and cingulate gyrus (40%) and other cortical areas. These were compared with controls from the same families.

The importance is that similar locations are involved in sCJD but with differing frequencies of regional involvement depending on the subtype. In the most common (MM1 subtype), the near-midline frontal cortical and cingulate gyral and other regions are involved in the majority on FLAIR and DWI, whereas the deep structures, including the basal ganglia and thalami, are less likely to be involved. However, in the MV2 and VV2 subtypes (the second and third most common subtypes of sCJD), the basal ganglia are less likely to be involved. Of note is that in variant CJD (commonly associated with "mad cow disease") the "pulvinar sign" on FLAIR or DWI is considered highly sensitive, but is not unique for it. To elucidate, signal intensity greater in the thalami relative to the caudate/putamen is considered to be suggestive of vCJD, whereas in fCJD and sCJD the thalamus is less likely to be involved and the pulvinar/thalamus has lesser signal intensity than the caudate/putamen.

Hence, because the interpreting neuroradiologist may not know the underlying variant or subtype of CJD at the presenting scan, I would submit that, given the appropriate clinical scenario, the general diagnosis of CJD should be in the differential diagnosis of a patient with an MRI (FLAIR and/or DWI) demonstrating symmetrical abnormalities in the caudate, putamen, thalami/pulvinar, frontal cortical, insular cortical, or cingulate cortical regions.[1] Ⓐ

Evidence-Based Reference

1. Fulbright RK et al: MR Imaging of familial Creutzfeldt-Jakob disease: a blinded and controlled study, *AJNR Am J Neuroradiol* 29:1638-1643, 2008. Commentary by A. McKinney, M.D. Ⓐ

SUGGESTED READINGS

Knight RSG, Will RG: Prion disease, *J Neurol Neurosurg Psychiatry* 75:36, 2004.

Masters CL et al: Creutzfeldt-Jakob disease: patterns of worldwide occurrence and the significance of familial and sporadic clustering, *Ann Neurol* 5:177, 1979.

Shiga Y et al: Diffusion-weighted MRI abnormalities as an early diagnostic marker for Creutzfeldt Jakob disease, *Neurology* 63:443, 2004.

Steinhoff BJ et al: Accuracy and reliability of periodic sharp wave complexes in Creutzfeldt Jakob disease, *Arch Neurol* 53:162, 1996.

AUTHOR: **CHUN LIM, M.D., PH.D.**

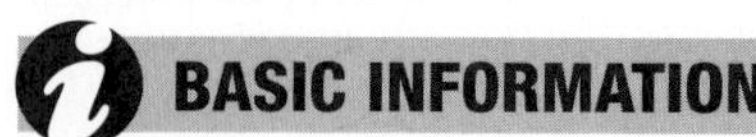

BASIC INFORMATION

DEFINITION

Crohn's disease is an inflammatory disease of the bowel of unknown etiology, most commonly involving the terminal ileum and manifesting primarily with diarrhea, abdominal pain, fatigue, and weight loss.

SYNONYMS

Regional enteritis
Inflammatory bowel disease (IBD)

ICD-9CM CODES
555.9 Crohn's disease, unspecified site
555.0 Crohn's disease, small intestine
555.1 Crohn's disease involving large intestine

EPIDEMIOLOGY & DEMOGRAPHICS

PREVALENCE:
- One case per 1000 persons; most common in whites and Jews
- Crohn's disease affects approximately 380,000 to 480,000 persons in the U.S.
- Incidence: bimodal with a peak in the third decade of life and another in the fifth decade

PHYSICAL FINDINGS & CLINICAL PRESENTATION

- Abdominal tenderness, mass, or distention
- Chronic or nocturnal diarrhea
- Weight loss, fever, night sweats
- Hyperactive bowel sounds in patients with partial obstruction, bloody diarrhea
- Delayed growth and failure of normal development in children
- Perianal and rectal abscesses, mouth ulcers, and atrophic glossitis
- Extraintestinal manifestations: joint swelling and tenderness, hepatosplenomegaly, erythema nodosum, clubbing, tenderness to palpation of the sacroiliac joints
- Symptoms may be intermittent with varying periods of remission

ETIOLOGY

Unknown. Pathophysiologically, Crohn's disease involves an immune system dysfunction.

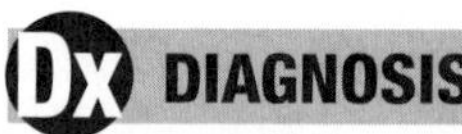

DIAGNOSIS

DIFFERENTIAL DIAGNOSIS

- Ulcerative colitis
- Infectious diseases (tuberculosis, *Yersinia, Salmonella, Shigella, Campylobacter*)
- Parasitic infections (amebic infection)
- Pseudomembranous colitis
- Ischemic colitis in elderly patients
- Lymphoma
- Colon carcinoma
- Diverticulitis
- Radiation enteritis
- Collagenous colitis
- Fungal infections *(Histoplasma, Actinomyces)*
- Gay bowel syndrome (in homosexual patient)
- Carcinoid tumors
- Celiac sprue
- Mesenteric adenitis

LABORATORY TESTS

- Decreased hemoglobin and hematocrit from chronic blood loss, effect of inflammation on bone marrow, and malabsorption of vitamin B_{12}
- Hypokalemia, hypomagnesemia, hypocalcemia, and low albumin in patients with chronic diarrhea
- Vitamin B_{12} and folate deficiency
- Elevated erythrocyte sedimentation rate
- Positive antisaccharomyces cerevisiae antibodies (ASCA)
- Elevated INR (due to vitamin K malabsorption)

ENDOSCOPIC EVALUATION

Endoscopic features of Crohn's disease include asymmetric and discontinued disease, deep longitudinal fissures, cobblestone appearance, and presence of strictures. Crypt distortion and inflammation are also present. Granulomas may be present.

IMAGING STUDIES

- Barium imaging studies are essentially outdated examinations. When performed, they reveal deep ulcerations (often longitudinal and transverse) and segmental lesions (skip lesions, strictures, fistulas, cobblestone appearance of mucosa caused by submucosal inflammation); "thumbprinting" is common, and "string sign" in terminal ileum may be noted. Although the diagnosis may be suggested by radiographic studies, it should be confirmed by endoscopy and biopsy when possible.
- CT of abdomen is helpful in identifying abscesses and other complications.
- Magnetic resonance enterography (MRe) is superior to other imaging modalities in its ability to distinguish active from chronic fibrotic disease. It is, however, more expensive.
- In 5% to 10% of patients with IBD, a clear distinction between ulcerative colitis and Crohn's disease cannot be made. In general, Crohn's disease can be distinguished from ulcerative colitis by the presence of transmural involvement and the frequent presence of noncaseating granulomas and lymphoid aggregates on biopsy.

Rx TREATMENT

The medical management of Crohn's disease is based on disease activity. According to Hanauer and Sanborn, disease activity can be defined as follows:
- Mild to moderate disease: The patient is ambulatory and able to take oral alimentation. There is no dehydration, high fever, abdominal tenderness, painful mass, obstruction, or weight loss of $>10\%$.
- Moderate to severe disease: Either the patient has not responded to treatment for mild to moderate disease *or* has more pronounced symptoms, including fever, significant weight loss, abdominal pain or tenderness, intermittent nausea and vomiting, or significant anemia.
- Severe fulminant disease: Either the patient has persistent symptoms despite outpatient steroid therapy *or* has high fever, persistent vomiting, evidence of intestinal obstruction, rebound tenderness, cachexia, or evidence of an abscess.
- Remission: The patient is asymptomatic *or* without inflammatory sequelae, including patients responding to acute medical intervention.

NONPHARMACOLOGIC THERAPY

- Nutritional supplementation is needed in patients with advanced disease. Total parenteral nutrition may be necessary in selected patients.
- Low-residue diet is necessary when obstructive symptoms are present.
- If diarrhea is prominent, increased dietary fiber and decreased fat in the diet are sometimes helpful.
- Psychotherapy is useful for situational adjustment crises. A trusting and mutually understanding relationship and referral to self-help groups are very important because of the chronicity of the disease and the relatively young age of the patients.
- Avoid oral feedings during acute exacerbation to decrease colonic activity: a low-roughage diet may be helpful in early relapse.

ACUTE GENERAL Rx

- Traditionally, sulfasalazine, 500 mg PO qid initially, increased qd or qod by 1 g until therapeutic dosages of 4 to 6 g/day are achieved, has been used. Individuals with sulfa allergies should avoid sulfasalazine. Folate supplementation is recommended because sulfasalazine inhibits folate absorption. Oral salicylates, such as mesalamine (Asacol, Rowasa), are as effective as sulfasalazine and better tolerated and have become preferred agents despite their higher cost.
- Corticosteroids have been the mainstay for treating moderate to severe active Crohn's disease. Prednisone 40 to 60 mg/day is useful for acute exacerbation. Steroids are usually tapered over approximately 2 to 3 mo. Some patients require a low dose for a prolonged period of maintenance.
- Steroid analogues are locally active corticosteroids that target specific areas of inflammation in the gastrointestinal tract. Budesonide (Entocort EC) is available as a controlled-release formulation and is approved for mild to moderate active Crohn's disease involving the ileum and/or ascending colon. The adult dose is 9 mg qd for a maximum of 8 wk.
- Immunosuppressants such as azathioprine (Imuran) 150 mg/day, methotrexate, or cyclosporine can be used for severe, progressive disease. In patients with Crohn's disease who enter remission after treatment with methotrexate, a low dose of methotrexate maintains remission.

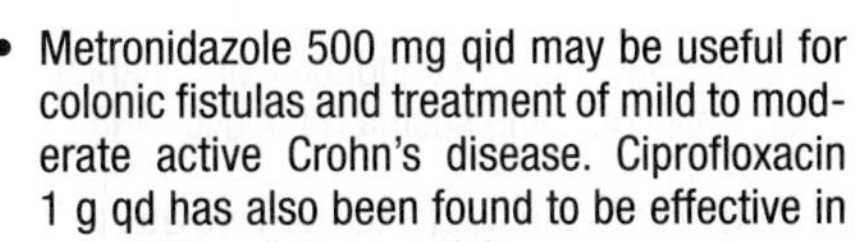

- Metronidazole 500 mg qid may be useful for colonic fistulas and treatment of mild to moderate active Crohn's disease. Ciprofloxacin 1 g qd has also been found to be effective in decreasing disease activity.
- TNF inhibitors: Infliximab, a chimeric monoclonal antibody targeting tumor necrosis factor-α, is effective in the treatment of enterocutaneous fistulas. This medication can induce clinical improvement in 80% of patients with Crohn's disease refractory to other agents. Its mechanism of action is incompletely understood. It is very costly. A PPD test should be done before using this medication. Adalimumab and certolizumab are other TNF inhibitors also effective in inducing remissions and may be useful in adult patients with Crohn's disease who cannot tolerate infliximab or have symptoms despite receiving infliximab therapy.
- Natalizumab, a selective adhesion-molecule inhibitor, has been reported to be effective in increasing the rate of remission and response in patients with active Crohn's disease. Recent trials with pegylated antibody fragments in patients with moderate to severe Crohn's disease involving certolizumab pegol revealed a modest improvement in response rates but no significant improvement in remission rates.
- Hydrocortisone (Cortenema) enema bid or tid is useful for proctitis.
- Most patients who have anemia associated with Crohn's disease respond to iron supplementation. Erythropoietin is useful in patients with anemia refractory to treatment with iron and vitamins.

CHRONIC Rx

- Monitor disease activity with symptom review and laboratory evaluation (complete blood count and sedimentation rate)
- Liver tests and vitamin B_{12} levels monitored on a yearly basis

DISPOSITION

One tenth of patients have prolonged remission, three quarters have a chronic intermittent disease course, and one eighth have an unremitting course.

REFERRAL

- Surgical referral is needed for complications such as abscess formation, obstruction, fistulas, toxic megacolon, refractory disease, or severe hemorrhage. A conservative surgical approach is necessary because surgery is not curative. Multiple surgeries may also result in short bowel syndrome.

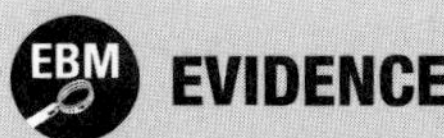

EVIDENCE

Please note: Complete text of EBM for this topic is available online.

Key trials and commentary:

The purpose of this study was to analyze long-term recurrence rates and complications in patients previously enrolled in a prospective randomized trial comparing laparoscopic (LC) and open ileocolectomy (OC) for ileocolic Crohn's disease (CD).

This study showed that long-term data from this prospective randomized trial confirm that LC is at least comparable to OC in the treatment of ileocolic CD.

In an attempt to analyze long-term recurrence rates in complications of a prospectively studied, randomized trial comparing LC vs. OC for ileocolic CD, Stocchi and associates of the Cleveland Clinic and Cornell University continue the follow-up of 56 of 60 patients. The authors validate that the overall recurrence rate was 52% with comparable numbers of these recurrences from both surgical groups experiencing endoscopic, radiologic, or surgical recurrence.

Preoperatively, all anastomotic recurrences had evidence of same radiologically (CT and/or small bowel follow-through) or colonoscopy or both. Of interest, one significant advantage, despite the small total numbers of patients in each cohort, is the fact that OC patients required operation in follow-up of a significantly more frequent rate than did the laparoscopic group ($P = 0.006$). Importantly, the authors have also acknowledged one major flaw of the paper—the lack of evidence to evaluate quality of life (QoL) after either technique. As noted, however, previous evaluations of QoL in prospective, randomized trials that compared the two surgical techniques for colon carcinoma and ileal resection for CD suggest minimal, if any, appreciable advantage and short-term benefits for the laparoscopic approach.[1] Ⓐ

CD commonly recurs after intestinal resection. A separate study evaluated whether the administration of infliximab after resective intestinal surgery for CD reduces postoperative recurrence.

This study showed that administration of infliximab after intestinal resective surgery was effective at preventing endoscopic and histologic recurrence of CD.

Though only a small study, the findings are very important. Recurrence rates among patients with CD who undergo surgery for treatment-refractory disease are significant. One important marker for the likelihood of recurrence is ulceration at the anastomotic site post operatively. Whereas clinical recurrence could not be measured, endoscopic score is an acceptable surrogate of eventual clinical recurrence. In this study nearly all the patients had surgery for penetrating (fistulizing) disease, a group that is difficult to treat and has a high risk of recurrence. Infliximab had a dramatic effect in preventing endoscopic recurrence. Although the findings are provocative, they should not be interpreted as meaning that all patients who have surgery for CD should be given biologic therapy postoperatively to prevent recurrence. The study was small and there were differences in immunomodulator use and smoking between the placebo and infliximab groups. The group selected has a high rate of recurrence and therefore would most likely benefit from this therapy. Many patients had been treated with immunomodulators before surgery suggesting that these patients were a more refractory group. Clearly patient selection is important. Those having nonpenetrating nonstricturing disease may benefit less because many have a more benign course whereas those with fibrostenotic disease would be unlikely to benefit compared with penetrating disease. Unresolved questions remain. Which patients will benefit most from this therapy? When should it be initiated and can it be stopped? These issues are very important because of the significant long-term failure rate of infliximab and other biologic therapies. Are there patient-specific characteristics that can be used to predict who will benefit most to justify the risk of treatment failure?[2] Ⓐ

Recurrence after surgery to treat CD is frequent and unpredictable. The efficacy of postsurgery capsule endoscopy in detecting recurrence in patients with CD is yet to be confirmed. Another study sought to assess the safety, accuracy, and therapeutic impact of capsule endoscopy in these patients.

It showed that capsule endoscopy is more effective in the evaluation of recurrence after surgery for CD and is better tolerated than colonoscopy. This is of significant therapeutic relevance.

Postsurgical recurrence of CD is well characterized and recognized to be frequent and unpredictable. The ability of capsule endoscopy to detect CD recurrence has yet to be determined. The authors thus conducted this study to ascertain the safety, accuracy, and therapeutic impact of capsule endoscopy in these patients. All patients had a patency capsule assessment initially and then underwent evaluation with capsule endoscopy.

All patients had colonoscopy and capsule endoscopy performed. The authors note that all patients preferred capsule endoscopy. Additionally, the authors noted that therapeutic management was modified in 16 patients.

The study, as it was designed, did not answer the question as to whether capsule endoscopy is better than small bowel radiographic imaging. Most individuals who treat patients with inflammatory bowel disease (IBD) prefer to do a small bowel radiographic study—given this can detect the presence of fistulas, whereas capsule endoscopy is unlikely to do so. Additionally, individuals need to do two capsule endoscopy studies now—one via the patency capsule and if this is not suggestive of obstruction, then a second standard capsule study is done. In addition, in capsule endoscopy there is no validated standard that discusses lesion size, number configuration, and other features that identify which of these are confirmed to be caused by CD. This is important because it is well recognized that normal individuals may have mucosal breaks, as well patients with celiac sprue and also individuals who are using nonsteroidal anti-inflammatory drugs.[3] Ⓐ

Endogenous opioids and opioid antagonists have been shown to play a role in healing and repair of tissues. In an open-labeled pilot prospective trial, the safety and efficacy of low-dose naltrexone (LDN), an opioid antagonist, was tested in patients with active CD.

This study showed that LDN therapy appears effective and safe in subjects with active CD. Further studies are needed to explore the use of this compound.

This study was a prospective, randomized, non–placebo-controlled evaluation of patients with active CD using 4.5 mg of naltrexone per day. The individuals were maintained on continued therapy before this study, and the end point evaluated was that of clinical response of which 67% achieved remission. There was no placebo in this particular study. The study suggests that there should be a randomized placebo-controlled phase II study of the low-dose naltrexone compared with placebo. This study presented, herein, that individuals were unchanged and did improve 4 wk after cessation of naltrexone. As it was suggested by the authors, the longer file period should be observed to determine the durability of response. It would also be important to look at the effect of LDN on the enkephalins, both in the serum and even in the mucosa, as an effort to better explain the changes that have occurred. Opioids have been shown to increase release of peritoneal cytokines and naltrexone has been shown to block TNF production in a previous murine model. It is potentially possible that the therapy with low-dose opioid antagonist, that is, naltrexone, may have affected a different endogenous opioid substance such as endorphins. This is certainly an area of interest; however, to date this particular area has not been studied adequately to make firm conclusions to use particular medications in clinical practice.[4] Ⓐ

Inflammatory bowel disease (IBD) has a typical onset during the peak reproductive years. Evidence of the risk of adverse pregnancy outcomes in IBD is important for the management of pregnancy to assist in its management.

A separate trial has shown a higher incidence of adverse pregnancy outcomes in patients with IBD. Further studies are required to clarify which women are at higher risk, because this was not determined in the present study. The results of this study should affect management of patients with IBD during pregnancy, who should be treated as a potentially high-risk group.

There is growing concern about adverse pregnancy outcomes in women who have IBD. It is uncertain which patients are at risk for this outcome. In an effort to better define these risks, the researchers searched the Medline literature. In women with IBD, there was a 1.9-fold increase in prematurity compared with controls, a 2.37-fold risk of congenital abnormalities, a 1.87-fold increase in prematurity, and the incidence of low birth weight was over twice that of normal controls. In this study, women with IBD were more likely to undergo a cesarean section.

The authors of this study are to be congratulated for identifying these problems. It remains undetermined who is likely to develop these problems. This particular study did identify the at-risk population for these problems, but was unable to identify which patients would develop these problems.

It is unlikely that a meta-analysis will help identify these patients. The authors will need patient level data from studies to identify who will develop these problems. Another approach to this problem is to develop a database—the Crohn's and Colitis Foundation of America is currently compiling such a database.[5] Ⓐ

Evidence-Based References

1. Stocchi L et al: Long-term outcomes of laparoscopic versus open ileocolic resection for Crohn's disease: follow-up of a prospective randomized trial, *Surgery* 144:622-628, 2008. Commentary by K.I. Bland, M.D. Ⓐ
2. Regueiro M et al: Infliximab prevents Crohn's disease recurrence after ileal resection, *Gastroenterology* 136:441-450.e1, 2009. Commentary by M.F. Picco, M.D. Ⓐ
3. Beltrán VP et al: Evaluation of postsurgical recurrence in Crohn's disease: a new indication for capsule endoscopy? *Gastrointest Endosc* 66:533-540, 2007. Commentary by G.R. Lichtenstein, M.D. Ⓐ
4. Smith JP et al: Low-dose naltrexone therapy improves active Crohn's disease, *Am J Gastroenterol* 102:820-828, 2007. Commentary by G.R. Lichtenstein, M.D. Ⓐ
5. Cornish J et al: A meta-analysis on the influence of inflammatory bowel disease on pregnancy, *Gut* 56:830-837, 2007. Commentary by G.R. Lichtenstein, M.D. Ⓐ

SUGGESTED READINGS

Abraham C, Cho JH: Inflammatory bowel disease, *N Engl J Med* 361:2066-2078, 2009.

Baumgart DC, Carding SR: Inflammatory bowel disease: cause and immunobiology, *Lancet* 369:1627, 2007.

Baumgart DC, Carding SR: Inflammatory bowel disease: clinical aspects and established and evolving therapies, *Lancet* 369:1641, 2007.

Sandborn WJ et al: Adalimumab induction therapy for Crohn disease previously treated with infliximab, *Ann Intern Med* 146:829, 2007.

Sandborn WJ et al: Certolizumab pegol for the treatment of Crohn's disease, *N Engl J Med* 357:228, 2007.

AUTHOR: **FRED F. FERRI, M.D.**

BASIC INFORMATION

DEFINITION

Cryoglobulins are serum immunoglobulins that precipitate when cooled and redissolve when heated. Cryoglobulinemia is a clinical syndrome that results from systemic inflammation caused by cryoglobulin-containing immune complexes.

SYNONYMS

Cryoglobulinemic vasculitis
Cryoproteinemia
Mixed cryoglobulinemia
Essential cryoglobulinemia

ICD-9CM CODES
273.2 Cryoglobulinemia, cryoglobulinemic vasculitis (CV), mixed cryoglobulinemia (MC)

EPIDEMIOLOGY & DEMOGRAPHICS

INCIDENCE: Unknown
PREVALENCE:
- Prevalence of mixed cryoglobulinemia is approximately 1:100,000
- More than 50% of patients with HCV are found to have mixed cryoglobulinemia
- Three types: types I (monoclonal), II (IgM monoclonal and IgG polyclonal), and III (polyclonal)

PREDOMINANT SEX AND AGE: Femaie:male ratio of 3:1
PREDOMINANT AGE: Mean age reported is 42 to 52 yr
RISK FACTORS: Hepatitis C virus (HCV) infection, connective tissue disorders, lymphoproliferative disorders

PHYSICAL FINDINGS & CLINICAL PRESENTATION

- Meltzer triad of purpura, arthralgias/myalgia, and weakness
- Other symptoms include dyspnea, cough, numbness, abdominal pain, acrocyanosis
- Hypertension, hepatosplenomegaly, Raynaud's phenomenon, and in severe cases, distal necrosis and ulcerations of lower limbs

ETIOLOGY

- Intravascular deposition of cryoglobulins leads to ischemic insults in territory supplied by vasa nervorum
- Necrotizing vasculitis caused by cryoglobulin precipitation
- Infections: HCV, mycosis fungoides, HBV, Epstein-Barr virus, cytomegalovirus, Treponema pallidum, Mycobacterium leprae, and in post-streptococcal glomerulonephritis
- Lymphoproliferative disorders: chronic lymphocytic leukemia, Waldenström's macroglobulinemia, multiple myeloma
- Connective tissue disorders: rheumatoid arthritis, systemic lupus erythematosus (SLE), scleroderma, Sjögren's syndrome, vasculitis
- Renal diseases including proliferative glomerulonephritis

Dx DIAGNOSIS

DIFFERENTIAL DIAGNOSIS

Antiphospholipid syndrome, SLE, lupus, Churg-Strauss syndrome, cirrhosis, glomerulonephritis, Goodpasture syndrome, hemolytic uremic syndrome, hepatitis, lymphoma, sarcoidosis, Waldenström's hypergammaglobulinemia

WORKUP

History and physical examination; laboratory tests; imaging tests depending on patients' presentations

LABORATORY TESTS

- Serum cryoglobulins, rheumatoid factor, serum complement, hepatitis C titers, urinalysis, CBC, chem
- Electromyogram/nerve conduction studies may demonstrate axonal changes and distal muscle denervation
- Sural nerve and skin biopsy

IMAGING STUDIES

Chest x-ray examination for pulmonary involvement, CT to study for malignancy, and angiography for vasculitis

Rx TREATMENT

- Immunosuppressive therapies such as corticosteroids are the mainstay treatment for mixed cryoglobulinemia.
- In patients with HCV, IFN-α can be added.
- Combination of pegylated IFN-α with ribavirin results in 77% remission.
- Variable success rate with plasma exchange, intravenous immunoglobulin, and anti-CD20 (rituximab) treatments

NONPHARMACOLOGIC THERAPY

Avoidance of cold exposure

ACUTE GENERAL Rx

NSAIDS in those with general fatigue and arthralgia; see "Treatment" for further management

DISPOSITION

Overall prognosis is worse with concomitant renal disease. Mean survival rate is ~50% at 10 yr.

REFERRAL

Nephrologist if there is renal involvement, hematologist in those with lymphoproliferative disorders, gastroenterologist/hepatologist in hepatitis, rheumatologist in connective tissue disease cases, and consider clinical immunologist in severe cases.

PEARLS & CONSIDERATIONS

COMMENTS

Always look for underlying causes for cryoglobulinemia.

PREVENTION

Avoidance of cold exposure, avoidance of late complications

PATIENT/FAMILY EDUCATION

Inform patients about early signs/symptoms of cryoglobulinemia so that treatments can be rendered before the development of complications.

SUGGESTED READINGS

Cacoub P et al: Anti-CD 20 monoclonal Ab (Rituximab) for tx for cryoglobulinemic vasculitis: where do we stand? *Ann Rheum Dis* 67(3):283-287, 2008.

Carlson JA et al: Cutaneous vasculitis update: small vessel neutrophilic vasculitis syndromes, *American Journal of Dermatopathology* 28(6):486-506, 2006.

Chacko JM et al: Paraproteinemic neuropathies, *J Clin Neuromuscul Dis* 7(4):185-197, 2006.

Crowson AN et al: Small vessel cutaneous vasculitis, *Pathol Case Rev* 12(5):205-213, 2007.

Edgerton CE et al: Cryoglobulinemia, *eMedicine Journal*, last updated July 4, 2009. Available at www.emedicine.com.

AUTHOR: **QUANG P. LE, M.D., M.P.H.**

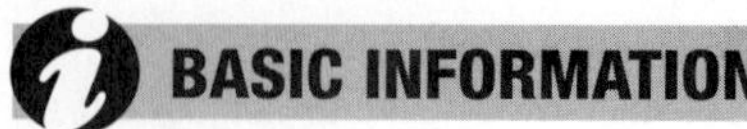

BASIC INFORMATION

DEFINITION

Cryptococcosis is an infection caused by the fungal organism *Cryptococcus neoformans.*

SYNONYMS

C. neoformans var. *neoformans* infection
C. neoformans var. *gatti* infection
C. neoformans var. *grubii* infection

ICD-9CM CODES
117.5 Cryptococcosis

EPIDEMIOLOGY & DEMOGRAPHICS

INCIDENCE (IN U.S.)

- 1 to 2 cases/1 million (non–HIV-infected) persons annually
- 6% to 7% in HIV-infected persons

PEAK INCIDENCE: 20 to 40 yr (parallel to AIDS epidemic)

PREDOMINANT SEX: Equal sex distribution when corrected for HIV status

PREDOMINANT AGE: Less than 2 yr of age; 20 to 40 yr of age

NEONATAL INFECTION: Very uncommon

PHYSICAL FINDINGS & CLINICAL PRESENTATION

- More than 90% present with meningitis; almost all have fever and headache.
- Meningismus, photophobia, mental status changes are seen in approximately 25%.
- Increased intracranial pressure.
- Most common infections outside the CNS:
  1. In the lungs (fever, cough, dyspnea)
  2. In the skin (cellulitis, papular eruption)
  3. In the lymph nodes (lymphadenitis)
  4. Potential involvement of virtually any organ

ETIOLOGY

- Caused by the fungal organism *C. neoformans*

There are 3 varieties of *Cryptococcus spp.* and 4 capsular serotypes: Serotype A is *Cryptococcus neoformans* var. *grubii* and Serotype D is known as *Cryptococcus neoformans* var. *neoformans.* Both cause disease primarily in immunocompromised patients. Serotype B and C are known as *C. neoformans* var. *gatti.* This organism causes disease primarily in normal hosts.

- Infection originates by inhalation into the respiratory tract followed by dissemination to the CNS in most cases, usually without recognizable lung involvement
- Almost always in the setting of AIDS or other disorders of cellular immune function
- Neutropenia alone poses a much lower risk of significant cryptococcal infection

DIAGNOSIS

DIFFERENTIAL DIAGNOSIS

- Subacute meningitis (caused by *Listeria monocytogenes, Mycobacterium tuberculosis, Histoplasma capsulatum,* viruses)
- Intracranial mass lesion (neoplasms, toxoplasmosis, TB)
- Pulmonary involvement confused with *Pneumocystis jiroveci* pneumonia when diffuse or confused with TB or bac-terial pneumonia when focal or involving the pleura
- Skin lesions confused with bacterial cellulitis or molluscum contagiosum

WORKUP

- Lumbar puncture to exclude cryptococcal meningitis.
- CT scan of the head when focal lesion or increased intracranial pressure is suspected.
- Biopsy of enlarged lymph nodes and skin lesions if feasible.

LABORATORY TESTS

- Culture and India ink stain (60% to 80% sensitive in culture-proven cases [Fig. 1-78]) examination of the CSF in all cases when CNS involvement is suspected
- Blood and serum cryptococcal antigen assay (>90% sensitivity and specificity)
- Culture and histologic examination of biopsy material

IMAGING STUDIES

- CT scan or MRI of the head if focal neurologic involvement is suspected
- Chest x-ray examination to exclude pulmonary involvement

TREATMENT

ACUTE GENERAL Rx

- Therapy for CNS disease is initiated with IV Amphotericin B (0.7 to 1 mg/kg/day) with flucytosine, 100 mg/kg/day (assuming normal renal function), for 2 weeks.
- After stabilization, fluconazole (400 to 800 mg qd PO) for a minimum of 10 wk.
- Alternative: IV fluconazole for initial therapy in patients unable to tolerate amphotericin B.
- If symptomatic increased intracranial pressure, consider therapeutic lumbar taps or intraventricular shunt.

CHRONIC Rx

- Fluconazole (200 to 400 mg PO qd) is highly effective in preventing a relapse in HIV-infected patients; development of resistance may occur. Itraconazole is an alternative agent.
- Immune reconstitution syndrome following the institution of HARRT can cause transient worsening of meningitis and necessitate the use of a short course of corticosteroids.

DISPOSITION

Without maintenance therapy, relapse rate is >50% among AIDS patients.

REFERRAL

- For consultation with infectious diseases specialist in all cases
- For neurologic consultation if level of consciousness is depressed or focal lesion is present

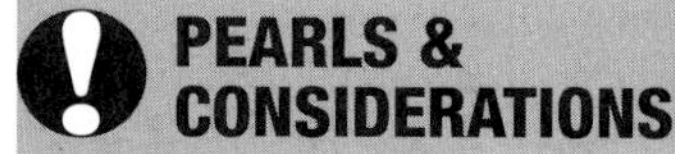

PEARLS & CONSIDERATIONS

Cryptococcal meningitis can be remarkably insidious in nonimmunocompromised patients.

COMMENTS

Cryptococcosis is considered an AIDS-defining infection; thus all patients should be HIV tested.

SUGGESTED READINGS

Chayakulkeeree M, Perfect JR: Cryptococcosis, *Infect Dis Clin N Am* 20:507-544, 2006.

Lui G et al: Cryptococcosis in apparently immunocompetent patients, *QJM* 99(3):143, 2006.

AUTHORS: **GLENN G. FORT, M.D., M.P.H.,** and **DENNIS J. MIKOLICH, M.D.**

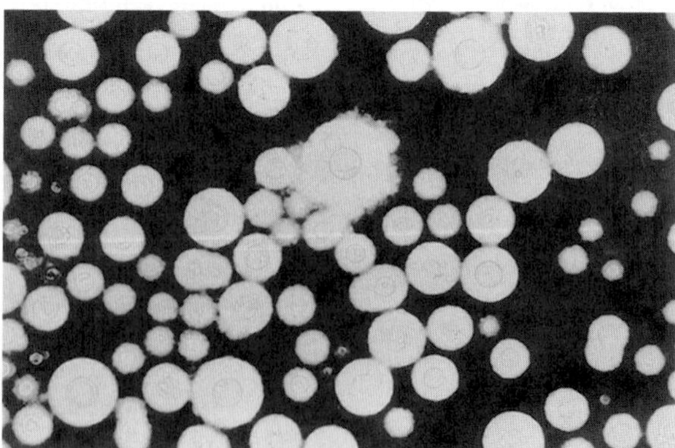

FIGURE 1-78 India ink preparation of cerebrospinal fluid revealing encapsulated cryptococci. Note the large capsules surrounding the smaller organisms. (From Andreoli TE [ed]: *Cecil essentials of medicine,* ed 4, Philadelphia, 1997, WB Saunders.)

BASIC INFORMATION

DEFINITION

Cryptorchidism is the incomplete or improper descent of the testis (testes) into the scrotum during fetal development. Testes that can be manually manipulated into the scrotum and which remain there without traction until cremasteric reflexes are induced are called *retractile.* Testes previously located but no longer palpable in the scrotum are called *ascended testes.*

SYNONYMS Undescended testis

ICD-9CM CODES
752.51 Cryptorchidism

EPIDEMIOLOGY & DEMOGRAPHICS

- Cryptorchidism is the most common genitourinary disorder of male children.
- Occurs in approximately 30% of premature and 5% of term male infants. In 10%, it can be bilateral.
- Within the first year of life, most cryptorchid testes descend into the scrotum so that incidence becomes approximately 1% in boys.
- Increased rates with premature birth, low birth weight, twins, and family history of cryptorchidism.
- Associated with Kallman's and Prader-Willi syndromes, pituitary hypoplasia, testicular feminization, prune belly syndrome, cystic fibrosis, myelomeningocele, and Reifenstein syndrome.
- With retractile testes there is up to a 32% risk of subsequent ascent leading to an undescended testis.

CLINICAL PRESENTATION

- Typically asymptomatic and is noted incidentally on screening examination. Undescended testes are at risk for testicular torsion.
- The testis may be nonpalpable or palpable in a location along the path of normal descent (Fig. 1-79) or less commonly ectopic and located in the perineum, femoral canal, superficial inguinal pouch, suprapubic area, or contralateral hemiscrotum.
- In 80% the undescended testis is palpable in the inguinal canal.
- Associated with infertility and a sevenfold increased risk of testicular cancer. Risk of infertility is the greatest for a child with bilateral intraabdominal testes and longer duration of cryptorchidism.

ETIOLOGY

Normal testicular descent is a complex interplay among mechanical (gubernaculums, vas deferens and testicular vessel length, cremasteric muscles, and abdominal pressure), hormonal (gonadotropin, testosterone, dihydrotestosterone, and mullerian inhibiting substance), and neural (ilioinguinal and genitofemoral nerves) factors.

DIAGNOSIS

DIFFERENTIAL DIAGNOSIS

- Retractile testis
- Ascended testis
- Atrophic testis
- Vanished testis

WORKUP

- Physical examination:
    - When done in a warm room with warm hands, can identify presence, absence, and location of palpable testes.
    - Should be done with the patient in the supine, sitting, and standing positions with adequate cremasteric relaxation to differentiate true cryptorchidism from retractile testes.
    - Often associated with an indirect inguinal hernia as the tunica vaginalis fails to close above the testis.
    - An enlarged contralateral testis in the presence of a nonpalpable undescended testis is suggestive of but not definitive for testicular atrophy/absence.
- Hormonal challenge:
    - Human chorionic gonadotropin (hCG) will confirm the presence of functioning testicular tissue and is useful in the setting of bilateral nonpalpable undescended testes.
    - If the follicular stimulating hormone level is three times normal and there is no increase in testosterone in response to hCG, functional testes are absent.

IMAGING

- Ultrasound: sensitivity of 76%, specificity of 100%, accuracy of 84%.
- MRI: sensitivity of 86% and specificity of 79%. CT results are inconsistent.

TREATMENT

- Repeat examination at 3 mo of age because many testes will descend spontaneously. Spontaneous descent is rare after 3 mo of age.

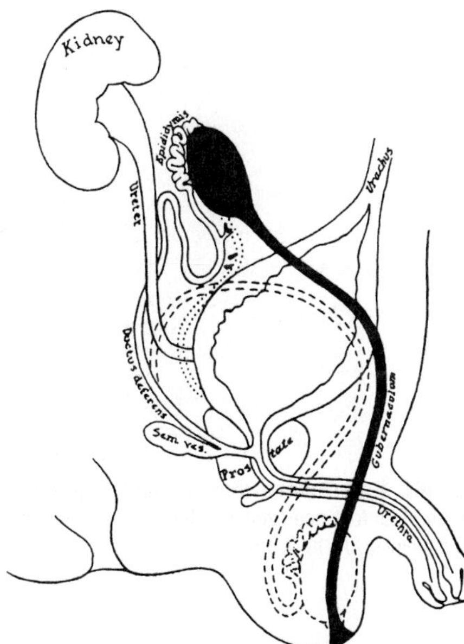

FIGURE 1-79 The path of testicular descent. (Reproduced with permission from Sarnat HB, Sarnat MS: Disorders of muscle in the newborn. In Moss AJ, Stern L [eds]: *Pediatrics update,* ed 4, New York, 1983, Elsevier-North Holland.)

- Treatment can be hormonal, surgical, or both.
- Treatment recommended as early as 6 mo and should be completed before 2 yr because histologic changes have been identified as early as age 1.5 yr.
- Earlier orchidopexy may improve testicular function and decrease the risk of testicular cancer. Orchidopexy allows testicular self-examination and detection of testicular cancer should it occur.

HORMONAL Rx

- Results of hCG are variable for undescended testes but good for retractile testes.
- The International Health Foundation recommends biweekly injections of 250 IU hCG for infants, 500 IU for children up to 6 yr, and 100 IU for children 6 yr and older, for a total of 5 wk. Therapy may induce precocious puberty.
- Administration of gonadotropin-releasing hormone before orchiopexy may improve fertility in adulthood.

SURGICAL Rx

- For the palpable undescended testis, orchiopexy, the surgical placement of an undescended testis into the scrotum, is the standard approach.
- In the setting of a nonpalpable undescended testis, laparoscopy is recommended to identify the presence or absence of a testis and the location of the testis if present and to determine the length of the testicular vessels.
- A two-stage approach is recommended for an intraabdominal testis with short vessels. The testicular vessels are clipped laparoscopically in the first stage, and the testis is brought into the scrotum in the second stage.
- Although the risk of testicular cancer is higher, the removal of all intraabdominal testes is not warranted.

DISPOSITION

- Earlier orchidopexy may decrease the risk of malignancy and infertility.
- Lifelong testicular examinations after puberty.

REFERRAL

Early referral to a pediatric urologist

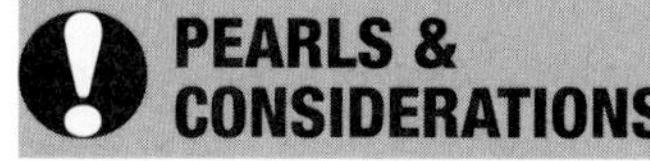

PEARLS & CONSIDERATIONS

Regular testicular examinations should be performed in infants and children, particularly those with retractile testes, because ascent of scrotal testis can occur.

SUGGESTED READINGS

Agarwal P, Diaz M, Elder J: *J Urol* 175(4):1496, 2006.
Cortes D: *Scan J Nephrol* 9:54, 1998.
Dawson C, Whitfield H: *BMJ* 312(7041):1291, 1996.
Docimo S et al: *Am Fam Physician* 62:2037, 2000.
Giannopoulos MD et al: *Horm Res* 55(1):33, 2001.
Lee P: *Urology* 66:427, 2005.
Leissner J et al: *Br J Urol Int* 83(8):885, 1999.
Patik K et al: *BJU* 95:704, 2005.
Schwentner C et al: *J Urol* 173:974, 2005.
Thayyil S et al: *Arch Dis Child* 89:890, 2004.

AUTHORS: **PAMELA ELLSWORTH, M.D.,** and **IRIS TONG, M.D.**

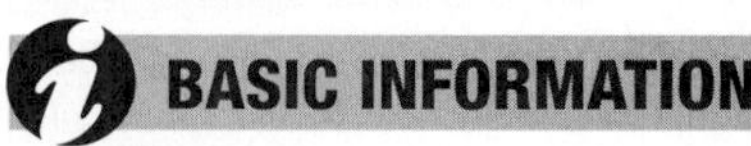

BASIC INFORMATION

DEFINITION

The intracellular protozoan parasite *Cryptosporidium parvum* is associated with gastrointestinal disease and diarrhea, especially in AIDS patients or immunocompromised hosts. It is also associated with sporadic infections and waterborne outbreaks in immunocompetent hosts.

Other species, including *C. hominus, C. felis, C. muris,* and *C. meleagridis,* are now described to be pathogens as well.

SYNONYMS

Cryptosporidiosis

ICD-9CM CODES

007.4 Cryptosporidia infection

EPIDEMIOLOGY & DEMOGRAPHICS

INCIDENCE (IN U.S.):

- Approximately 2% in industrial countries, 5% to 10% in third world countries
- 10% to 20% of HIV patients in U.S. may excrete cyst

PREVALENCE: Worldwide, especially third world countries; associated with poor hygiene as a waterborne pathogen

PREDOMINANT SEX: Male = female

TRANSMISSION:

- Person to person (daycare, family members)
- Animal to person (pets, farm animals)
- Environmental (water-associated outbreaks, including travel associated with swimming in or drinking contaminated water)
- May be significant pathogen causing diarrhea in AIDS

PHYSICAL FINDINGS & CLINICAL PRESENTATION

- Usually limited to gastrointestinal tract
- Diarrhea, severe abdominal pain (2 to 28 days)
- Impaired digestion, dehydration
- Fever, malaise, fatigue, nausea, vomiting
- Pneumonia if aspirated

ETIOLOGY

Cryptosporidium hominis, C. parvum, C. felis, C. muris, C. meleagridis

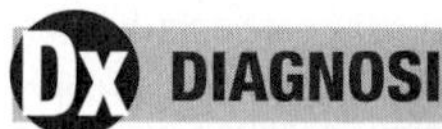

DIAGNOSIS

Clinical presentation of acute gastrointestinal illness, especially associated with HIV or with travel and waterborne outbreaks.

DIFFERENTIAL DIAGNOSIS

- *Campylobacter*
- *Clostridium difficile*
- *Entamoeba histolytica*
- *Giardia lamblia*
- *Salmonella*
- *Shigella*
- Microsporidia
- Cytomegalovirus
- *Mycobacterium avium*

Disease may cause cholecystitis, reactive arthritis, hepatitis, pancreatitis, pneumonia in immunocompromised or HIV-infected patients.

WORKUP

- Stool evaluation looking for characteristic oocyst by modified acid-fast stain (Fig. 1-80).
- Direct immunofluorescence using monoclonal antibodies is the gold standard for stool exams.

Rx TREATMENT

- May be self-limited in normal host—often requiring hydration. Antidiarrhea agents Pepto-Bismol, Kaopectate, or loperamide may give symptomatic relief.
- Pharmacologic treatment with antibiotics has been largely unsatisfactory in AIDS patients. Oocyst excretion reduction has been shown with nitazoxanide 500 mg PO bid for 3 days. If treatment fails, consider a trial of paromomycin, metronidazole, or Bactrim.
- Nitazoxanide elixir has been approved for the treatment of cryptosporidiosis in children ages 1 to 11 yr.
- Biliary cryptosporidiosis can be treated with antiretroviral therapy in the HIV setting.

DISPOSITION

- A self-limited disease in immunocompetent patients with complete recovery over 2 to 3 weeks.
- Chronic arthralgia, headache, malaise, and weakness may persist after cryptosporidial infection even in immunologically normal people.
- If severe and prolonged (>30 days), testing for HIV and other immunocompromised states is appropriate along with a referral to an infectious disease specialist or gastroenterologist.

REFERRAL

- To an infectious disease specialist if symptoms persist and if HIV infection is found
- To a gastroenterologist if chronic malabsorption, or biliary or pancreatic complications occur

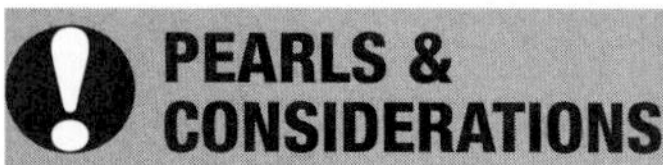

PEARLS & CONSIDERATIONS

- Chronic cryptosporidiosis (>30 days of diarrhea from *Cryptosporidium* spp. infection) in a patient with HIV is an AIDS-qualifying opportunistic infection.
- *Cryptosporidium hominis* has a limited host range (humans), whereas *Cryptosporidium parvum* has a wide host range including humans, horses, cattle, other domesticated animals, and wild animals—both species present a similar illness in humans.

SUGGESTED READINGS

Hunter PR et al: Health sequelae of human cryptosporidiosis in immunocompetent patients, *Clin Infect Dis* 39(4):504-510, 2004.

Smith HV, Corcoran GD: New drugs and treatment for cryptosporidiosis, *Curr Opin Infect Dis* 17(6):557, 2004.

AUTHORS: **GLENN G. FORT, M.D., M.P.H.,** and **DENNIS J. MIKOLICH, M.D.**

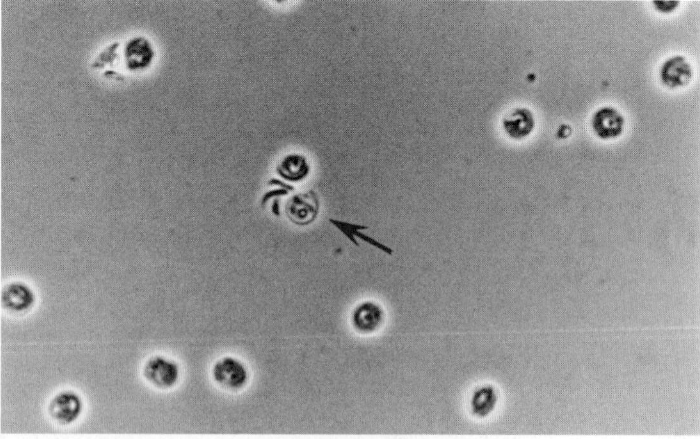

FIGURE 1-80 Human stool-derived *Cryptosporidium* oocysts. Excysting oocyst *(arrow)* is releasing three of its four sporozoites. (Phase-control microscopy ×630.) (From Gorbach SL: *Infectious diseases,* ed 2, Philadelphia, 1998, WB Saunders.)

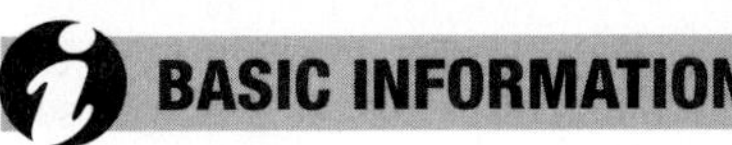

BASIC INFORMATION

DEFINITION

Compression of the ulnar nerve behind the elbow (cubitus)

SYNONYMS

Tardy ulnar palsy

ICD-9CM CODES

354.2 Cubital tunnel syndrome

EPIDEMIOLOGY & DEMOGRAPHICS

Prevalent sex: Males and females affected equally

PHYSICAL FINDINGS & CLINICAL PRESENTATION

- Paresthesias and numbness along distribution of ulnar nerve (ulnar one and one-half fingers)
- Positive Tinel's sign at elbow
- Positive elbow flexion test (flexion of elbow with wrist extended for 30 sec may reproduce symptoms)
- May be diminished sensation to tip of small finger
- Ulnar nerve may be subluxable with elbow motion or by manipulation
- Cubitus valgus may be present if prior bony injury
- Interosseous weakness in longstanding cases with atrophy (Fig. 1-81)

ETIOLOGY

- Direct pressure
- Cubitus valgus deformity
- Subluxation of ulnar nerve
- Repeated stretching during throwing motion
- Elbow synovitis
- Local muscular hypertrophy

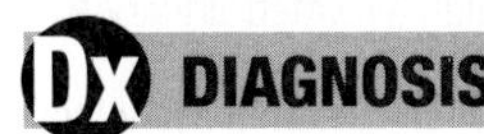

DIAGNOSIS

DIFFERENTIAL DIAGNOSIS

- Medial epicondylitis
- Medial elbow instability
- Carpal tunnel syndrome
- Cervical disc syndrome with radicular arm symptoms
- Ulnar nerve compression at wrist (Guyon's canal)

WORKUP

Diagnosis can usually be established clinically

IMAGING STUDIES

- Routine roentgenograms may be helpful in establishing cause or ruling out other conditions.
- Electrodiagnostic studies: nerve conduction tests and electromyography are useful in establishing diagnosis and ruling out other syndromes.

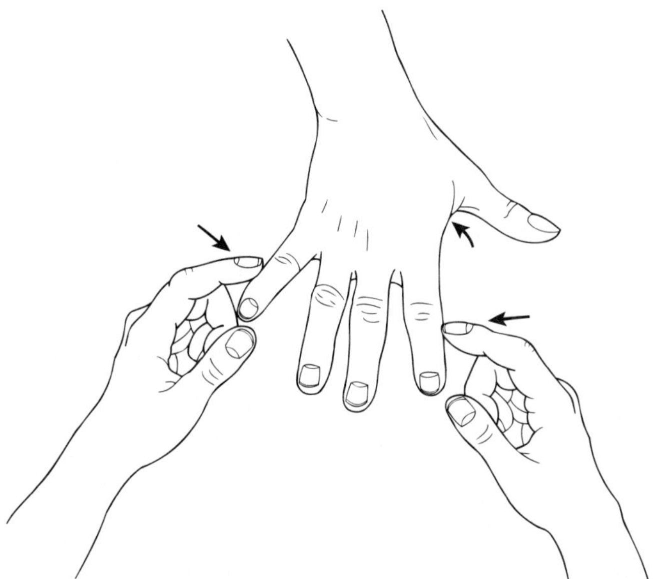

FIGURE 1-81 Testing for intrinsic (ulnar) motor weakness (fanning the fingers against resistance). Always look for atrophy of the first dorsal interosseus *(curved arrow)* when ulnar nerve lesions are suspected. (From Mercier LR: *Practical orthopedics,* ed 5, St Louis, 2000, Mosby.)

Rx TREATMENT

ACUTE GENERAL Rx

- Protect nerve from pressure
- Elbow pads
- Avoid prolonged elbow flexion (talking on phone with elbow bent)

DISPOSITION

- Prognosis is variable.
- Mild to moderate cases recover well if offending activity can be eliminated. If muscle atrophy has developed, recovery of strength may be incomplete despite treatment.
- Medical management may be continued as long as symptoms are controlled and no motor deficit has developed.

REFERRAL

Surgical referral in cases of failed medical management or if signs of motor impairment are present

SUGGESTED READINGS

Creighton RA et al: Evaluation of the medial elbow in the throwing athlete, *Am J Orthop* 35:266, 2006.

Cutts S: Cubital tunnel syndrome, *Postgrad Med J* 83:28, 2007.

Elhassan B, Steinmann SP: Entrapment neuropathy of the ulnar nerve, *J Am Acad Orthop Surg* 15:672, 2007.

Gellman H: Compression of the ulnar nerve at the elbow: cubital tunnel syndrome, *Instr Course Lect* 57:187, 2008.

Kato H et al: Cubital tunnel syndrome associated with medial elbow ganglia and osteoarthritis of the elbow, *J Bone Joint Surg Am* 84(A):1413, 2002.

Lee DH et al: Clinical nerve conduction and needle electromyography studies, *J Am Acad Orthop Surg* 12:276, 2004.

Palmer BA, Hughes TB: Cubital tunnel syndrome, *J Hand Surg Am* 35:153, 2010.

Park GY et al: The ultrasonographic and electro-diagnostic findings of ulnar neuropathy at the elbow, *Arch Phys Med Rehabil* 85:1000, 2004.

Sasaki J et al: Ultrasonographic assessment of ulnar collateral ligament and medial elbow laxity in college baseball players, *J Bone Joint Surg Am* 84(A):525, 2002.

Shin R, Ring D: The ulnar nerve in elbow trauma, *J Bone Joint Surg Am* 89:1108, 2007.

Svernlov B et al: Conservative treatment of the cubital tunnel syndrome, *J Hand Surg Eur* 34:201, 2009.

Szabo RM, Kwak C: Natural history and conservative management of cubital tunnel syndrome, *Hand Clin* 23:311, 2007.

AUTHOR: **LONNIE R. MERCIER, M.D.**

BASIC INFORMATION

DEFINITION

- Cushing's syndrome is the occurrence of clinical abnormalities associated with glucocorticoid excess as a result of exaggerated adrenal cortisol production or long-term glucocorticoid therapy.
- Cushing's disease is Cushing's syndrome caused by pituitary adrenocorticotropic hormone (ACTH) excess.

ICD-9CM CODES
255.0 Cushing's disease or syndrome

PHYSICAL FINDINGS & CLINICAL PRESENTATION

- Hypertension
- Central obesity with rounding of the facies (moon facies); thin extremities
- Hirsutism, menstrual irregularities, hypogonadism
- Skin fragility, ecchymoses, red-purple abdominal striae, acne, poor wound healing, hair loss, facial plethora, hyperpigmentation (with ACTH excess)
- Psychosis, emotional lability, paranoia
- Muscle wasting with proximal myopathy

NOTE: The previous characteristics are not commonly present in Cushing's syndrome caused by ectopic ACTH production. Many of these tumors secrete a biologically inactive ACTH that does not activate adrenal steroid synthesis. These patients may have only weight loss and weakness.

ETIOLOGY

- Iatrogenic from long-term glucocorticoid therapy (common)
- Pituitary ACTH excess (Cushing's disease; 60%)
- Adrenal neoplasms (30%)
- Ectopic ACTH production (neoplasms of lung, pancreas, kidney, thyroid, thymus; 10%)

DIAGNOSIS

DIFFERENTIAL DIAGNOSIS

- Alcoholic pseudo-Cushing's syndrome (endogenous cortisol overproduction)
- Obesity associated with diabetes mellitus
- Adrenogenital syndrome

WORKUP

- In patients with a clinical diagnosis of Cushing's syndrome the initial screening test is the overnight dexamethasone suppression test:
  1. Dexamethasone 1 mg PO given at 11 PM
  2. Plasma cortisol level measured 9 hr later (8 AM)
  3. Plasma cortisol level <5 mcg/100 ml excludes Cushing's syndrome
- Serial measurements (two or three consecutive measurements) of 24-hr urinary free cortisol and creatinine (to ensure adequacy of collection) are undertaken if overnight dexamethasone test is suggestive of Cushing's syndrome. Persistent elevated cortisol excretion (>300 mcg/24 hr) indicates Cushing's syndrome.
- The low-dose (2 mg) dexamethasone suppression test is useful to exclude pseudo-Cushing's syndrome if the previous results are equivocal. Corticotropic-releasing hormone (CRH) stimulation after low-dose dexamethasone administration (dexamethasone-CRH test) is also used to distinguish patients with suspected Cushing's syndrome from those who have mildly elevated urinary free cortisol level and equivocal findings.
- The high-dose (8 mg) dexamethasone test and measurement of ACTH by radioimmunoassay are useful to determine the etiology of Cushing's syndrome.
  1. ACTH undetectable or decreased and lack of suppression indicate adrenal cause of Cushing's syndrome.
  2. ACTH normal or increased and lack of suppression indicate ectopic ACTH production.
  3. ACTH normal or increased and partial suppression suggest pituitary excess (Cushing's disease).
- A single midnight serum cortisol level (normal diurnal variation leads to a nadir around midnight) >7.5 mcg/dl has been reported as 96% sensitive and 100% specific for the diagnosis of Cushing's syndrome.

LABORATORY TESTS

- Hypokalemia, hypochloremia, metabolic alkalosis, hyperglycemia, hypercholesterolemia
- Increased 24-hr urinary free cortisol (>100 mcg/24 hr)

IMAGING STUDIES

- CT scan or MRI of adrenal glands in suspected adrenal Cushing's syndrome
- MRI of pituitary gland with gadolinium in suspected pituitary Cushing's syndrome
- Additional imaging studies to localize neoplasms of the lung, pancreas, kidney, thyroid, or thymus in patients with ectopic ACTH production

TREATMENT

GENERAL Rx

The treatment of Cushing's syndrome varies with its cause:

- Pituitary adenoma: transsphenoidal microadenomectomy is the therapy of choice in adults. Pituitary irradiation is reserved for patients not cured by transsphenoidal surgery. In children, pituitary irradiation may be considered as initial therapy because 85% of children are cured by radiation. Stereotactic radiotherapy (photon knife or gamma knife) is effective and exposes the surrounding neuronal tissues to less irradiation than conventional radiotherapy. Total bilateral adrenalectomy is reserved for patients not cured by transsphenoidal surgery or pituitary irradiation.
- Adrenal neoplasm:
  1. Surgical resection of the affected adrenal
  2. Glucocorticoid replacement for approximately 9 to 12 mo after the surgery to allow time for the contralateral adrenal gland to recover from its prolonged suppression
- Bilateral micronodular or macronodular adrenal hyperplasia: bilateral total adrenalectomy
- Ectopic ACTH:
  1. Surgical resection of the ACTH-secreting neoplasm
  2. Control of cortisol excess with metyrapone, aminoglutethimide, mifepristone, or ketoconazole
  3. Control of the mineralocorticoid effects of cortisol and 11-deoxycorticosteroid with spironolactone
  4. Bilateral adrenalectomy: a rational approach to patients with indolent, unresectable tumors

DISPOSITION

Prognosis is favorable in patients with surgically amenable disease.

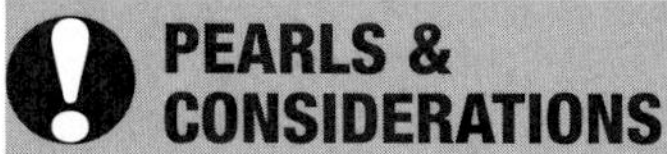

PEARLS & CONSIDERATIONS

COMMENTS

Screening for multiple endocrine neoplasia type I should be considered in patients with Cushing's disease.

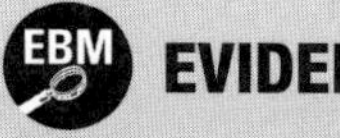

EVIDENCE

Please note: Complete text of EBM for this topic is available online.

Key trials and commentary:

The objective of this study was to evaluate the published literature and reach a consensus on the treatment of patients with ACTH-dependent Cushing's syndrome, because there is no recent consensus on the management of this rare disorder.

This study showed that ACTH-dependent Cushing's syndrome is a heterogeneous disorder requiring a multidisciplinary and individualized approach to patient management. Generally, the treatment of choice for ACTH-dependent Cushing's syndrome is curative surgery with selective pituitary or ectopic corticotroph tumor resection. Second-line treatments include more radical surgery, radiation therapy (for Cushing's disease), medical therapy, and bilateral adrenalectomy. Because of the significant morbidity of Cushing's syndrome, early diagnosis and prompt therapy are warranted.

ACTH-dependent Cushing's syndrome is caused by an ACTH-producing tumor typically located in the pituitary but occasionally located elsewhere in the body (e.g., from a lung carcinoid). The workup and treatment of ACTH-dependent hypercortisolemia can be perplexing at times and there has been an outstanding need for a good consensus statement on the workup and management of this often poorly understood disease. This statement was generated by 32 leading endocrinologists, neurosurgeons, and other experts in the field. These authors outline and analyze the most compelling data defining our understanding of the disease and its management. Areas reviewed include the criteria for cure and remission of Cushing's syndrome, the surgical treatment for Cushing's disease, treatment options when pituitary surgery fails, and management of ectopic tumors, Nelson's syndrome, and other populations. The statement was generated through a systematic process of synthesizing data and expert opinion. The statement is thorough, well written, and rigorously based on the literature.[1] Ⓐ

Chronic exposure to hypercortisolism has significant impact on patients' health and health-related quality of life (HRQoL), as demonstrated with generic questionnaires. A separate study developed a disease-generated questionnaire to evaluate HRQoL in patients with Cushing's syndrome (CS; CushingQoL).

Although there are many treatment modalities to normalize the high cortisol levels seen in Cushing's syndrome, altered physical and psychological parameters are much slower to normalize. Historically, there has been no standardized Cushing's specific quality of life (QoL) assays to help in following the physical and psychosocial parameters of treatment. Although many treatment modalities are known to normalize hypercortisolemia, it is not well established which treatments for Cushing's syndrome are best for restoring QoL. The aim of this observational, international, and cross-sectional study is to validate a Cushing's-specific QoL questionnaire (see Table 2 in the original article). 125 patients recruited by 14 investigators from five countries were evaluated. Clinical and hormonal data, as well as information on a SF-36 questionnaire, a questionnaire on self-perceived health status, and the CushingQoL score questionnaire were collected. There was excellent correlation between the three questionnaires. The CushingQoL questionnaire was validated and was determined to be a useful tool in the assessment of QoL in Cushing's patients. Its score correlated closely with biochemical parameters of the Cushing's patient it was assessing. This tool will be very useful in assessing the impact on QoL of the different options for treating Cushing's syndrome.[2] Ⓐ

Evidence-Based References

1 Biller BMK et al: Treatment of adrenocorticotropin-dependent Cushing's syndrome: a consensus statement, *J Clin Endocrinol Metab* 93:2454-2462, 2008. Commentary by W.H. Ludlam, M.D., Ph.D. Ⓐ

2. Webb SM et al: Evaluation of health-related quality of life in patients with Cushing's syndrome with a new questionnaire, *Eur J Endocrinol* 158:623-630, 2008. Commentary by W.H. Ludlam, M.D., Ph.D. Ⓐ

SUGGESTED READING

Boscaro M et al: The diagnosis of Cushing's syndrome, *Arch Intern Med* 160:3045, 2000.

AUTHOR: **FRED F. FERRI, M.D.**

Cutaneous Larva Migrans

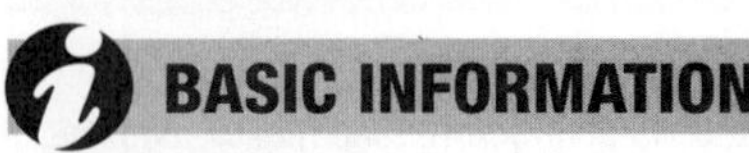

BASIC INFORMATION

DESCRIPTION

Cutaneous larva migrans (CLM) is a syndrome defined clinically and parasitologically by subcutaneous larval migration of nematodes. Creeping eruption is the cardinal manifestation. It includes neither diseases in which creeping eruption is due to non-larval forms of parasites nor diseases without creeping eruptions from subcutaneous migration of larval parasites. As animal hookworms are the most common cause, some people use the term "hookworm-related cutaneous larva migrans" (HrCLM) instead. Table 1-18 describes other clinical syndromes associated with unusual helminth infections in humans.

SYNONYMS

Creeping eruption
Plumber's itch
Creeping verminous dermatitis
Sand worm eruption
Duck hunter's itch

ICD-9CM CODES
126.9

EPIDEMIOLOGY & DEMOGRAPHICS

- Commonly seen in tropical and subtropical countries. In U.S. it is most prevalent in southeastern states. Florida tops among these states.
- More often seen in children than adults.
- Has no racial or sexual predilection.
- Peak incidence is seen during rainy season.
- Second to pinworm among helminth infection in developed countries.
- Most common tropically acquired dermatosis.
- Most common imported ectoparasites in travelers returning to U.S. after holiday.

RISK FACTORS

Hobbies and occupations that involve contact with warm, moist, sandy soil
- Tropical/subtropical climate travels
- Barefoot beach goers/sunbathers
- Children playing in sandboxes
- Carpenter, electrician, plumber, farmer, gardener, pest exterminator

ETIOLOGY

- Animal hookworms
- *Ancylostoma Braziliense* (commonest cause)
- *Ancylostoma caninum*
- *Uncinaria stenocephala*
- *Bunostomum phlebotomum*
- *Pelodera strongyloides*
- *Gnathostoma* species
- *Strongyloides stercoralis*
- *Spirurina* species

PATHOGENESIS

The infection is usually acquired via skin contact with the soil or sand contaminated with feces of infected dogs or cats. The filariform larva is the infective form. It penetrates the skin and migrates within the epidermis by releasing protease and hyaluronidase. The inflammatory reaction along the cutaneous tract of their migration results in creeping eruptions. The larvae are believed to lack the collagenase enzymes required to penetrate the basement membrane to invade the dermis. In contrast to cats or dogs, humans are incidental host. Thus the larvae are unable to complete their natural cycles in humans. The larvae die without treatment and are resorbed within weeks to months of invasion. This explains why CLM is a self-limiting disease and rarely has systemic features.

CLINICAL FEATURES

- Often associated with a history of sunbathing, walking barefoot on a beach, or similar activity in a tropical location.
- Incubation period is around 1 to 6 days.
- Intense pruritus at the site of invasion within hours of invasion.
- Many patients report a stinging sensation, which they may misinterpret as a puncture or insect bite.
- Erythematous papules develop at the larval penetration site. Feet, buttocks, and thighs are most commonly affected anatomical locations.
- The most frequent and cardinal finding of HrCLM is *creeping dermatitis,* which takes few days to develop. It is defined as an erythematous, slightly elevated, linear, or serpiginous track that is 3 mm in width and may be up to 15 to 20 cm in length. The mean number of lesions per person varies from 1 to 3. The creeping track associated with the larva migration may extend a few millimeters to few centimeters daily. These eruptions last 2 to 8 wk without treatment.
- Edema and vesicobullous lesions along the course of the larva.
- Rare presentation is hookworm folliculitis. It is characterized by numerous (20-100) follicular, erythematous, and pruritic papules and pustules, located mainly in the buttocks. Generally numerous short tracks are seen arising from these follicular lesions.
- In case of rare pulmonary involvement, dry cough and wheezing develop a week after the dermal invasion.

TABLE 1-18 Clinical Syndromes Associated with Unusual Helminth Infections in Humans

Clinical Syndrome	Parasite	Usual Host
Visceral larva migrans	Toxocara canis Toxocara cati Baylisascaris procyonis	Canines Felines Raccoons
Eosinophilic gastroenteritis	*Anisakis* spp. *Phocanema* spp. Ancylostoma caninum	Sea mammals Sea mammals Canines
Cutaneous larva migrans	Ancylostoma braziliense Ancylostoma caninum Uncinaria stenocephala	Canines, felines Canines, felines Canines, felines
Eosinophilic meningitis	Angiostrongylus cantonensis Gnathostoma spinigerum	Rats Felines, other mammals
Pulmonary or cutaneous nodules	*Dirofilaria* spp.	Canines, other mammals
Abdominal angiostrongyliasis	Angiostrongylus costaricensis	Cotton rats
Capillariasis	Capillaria philippinensis	Birds
Diarrhea	Nanophyetus salmincola	Mammals, birds
Swimmer's itch	*Trichobilharzia* spp.	Birds

DIAGNOSIS

Diagnosis is made on clinical grounds and history of potential exposure. Clinical characteristics of the creeping trails (length, width, speed of migration, location, duration) help differentiate HrCLM from other causes of creeping dermatitis.

- Blood tests are not necessary for diagnosis. Theoretically, blood test could detect eosinophilia and elevated IgE level.
- Biopsy specimens usually show an eosinophilic inflammatory infiltrate, but not the migratory parasite. For this reason, biopsy is not indicated to establish the diagnosis. Nonetheless, in case of hookworm folliculitis, skin biopsy specimens may reveal nematode larvae in the follicular canal.
- Stool studies and serology are not helpful.
- Radiograph of chest is indicated when migratory pulmonary infiltrates are suspected.
- A new technology, optical coherence tomography, has been found to identify the larva in the epidermis, allowing direct removal.

DIFFERENTIAL DIAGNOSIS

- Superficial thrombophlebitis
- Mondor's disease
- Lichen striatus
- Phytophotodermatitis
- Herpes zoster
- Migratory myiasis
- Scabies
- Loiasis
- Dracunculiasis
- Cercarial dermatitis

- Onchocerciasis
- Dirofilariasis
- Contact dermatitis
- Creeping hair
- Jelly fish stings
- Fascioliasis
- Bacterial folliculitis
- Tenia pedis/corporis
- Impetigo
- Erytherma chronicum migrans of Lyme disease
- Ground itch
- Toxocariasis

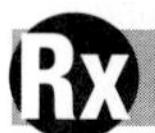

TREATMENT

- Oral Albendazole and Ivermectin are the first line of drugs.
- Oral administration is preferred in presence of extensive lesions or when topical application fails.
- Topical application should cover the tracks and area covering up to 2 cm from the leading edge.
- Albendazole should be given (400 mg orally per day for 3-5 days).
- At times, when oral drugs are contraindicated, topical 10% albendazole creams are applied twice a day for a period of 10 days.
- Ivermectin should be given (200 mcg/kg given as a single dose).
- Thiabendazole should be given (25-50 mg/kg divided into twice-daily doses for 2 days).
- Because of its higher side effect profile when given orally, it is more often applied topically (10-15% cream or aqueous suspension of 500 mg/5 ml) four times a day for 5-10 days.
- Mebendazole should be given (100 mg orally twice for 3 days).
- Cryotherapy with liquid nitrogen is obsolete. It is ineffective as the larva is usually located 1 to 2 cm beyond the visible end of the trail, and the larva is capable of withstanding temperature as low as -21° C for more than 5 minutes. Moreover, this procedure is painful and can lead to chronic ulcerations.
- Specific antihelminthic therapy for pulmonary involvement is generally not required since the illness is usually mild and self-limiting.
- In the case of hookworm folliculitis, treatment is more difficult than traditional form and necessitates repeated courses of oral antihelmintic agents.
- Antihistamines and topical steroids relieve intense pruritus.
- Antibiotics are indicated for bacterial superinfection.
- Generally there should be no attempt to extract the worm.

COMPLICATIONS

- Secondary bacterial infection
- Erythema multiform
- Migratory eosinophilic pneumonitis (Loeffler syndrome)
- Eosinophilic enteritis

PROGNOSIS

Self-limiting benign disease. Even without treatment most cases resolve within 4-8 weeks.

PREVENTION

- Prohibit pets such as dogs and cats walking on the beaches in tropical areas.
- Avoid allowing pets in the sandbox.
- Deworm household pets.
- Clean up pet droppings.
- Protective foot wear while walking on the beach.
- Avoiding tropical beaches frequented by dogs and cats.
- When lying on tropical beaches potentially frequented by dogs and cats, areas of sand washed by the tide are preferable to dry sand, and mattresses are preferable to towels.
- Towels and clothes should not touch the ground when hung up for drying.

SUGGESTED READINGS

Epidemiological and clinical characteristics of hookworm related cutaneous larva migrans, *Lancet Infect Dis* 8:302-309, 2008.

Hookworm-related cutaneous larva migrans, *J Travel Med* 14(5):326-333, 2007.

AUTHOR: **HEMANT K. SATPATHY, M.D.**

Cystic Fibrosis (PTG)

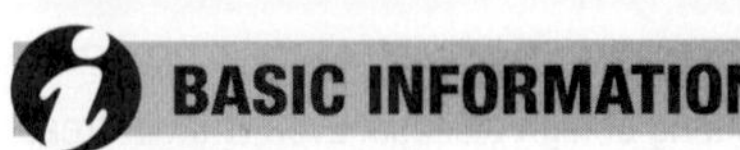

BASIC INFORMATION

DEFINITION

Cystic fibrosis (CF) is an autosomal recessive disorder characterized by dysfunction of exocrine glands.

ICD-9CM CODES
277.0 Cystic fibrosis

EPIDEMIOLOGY & DEMOGRAPHICS

- CF is the most common fatal hereditary disorder of whites in the U.S. (one case per 2500 whites) and second most common life-shortening childhood-onset inherited disorder in the U.S., behind sickle cell disease.
- Median age at diagnosis is 5.3 mo. Median survival is 30 yr.
- Carrier screening is associated with a decrease in incidence of CF.

PHYSICAL FINDINGS & CLINICAL PRESENTATION

- Failure to thrive in children
- Increased anterior/posterior chest diameter
- Basilar crackles and hyperresonance to percussion
- Digital clubbing
- Chronic cough
- Abdominal distention
- Greasy, smelly feces

ETIOLOGY

Chromosome 7 gene mutation (*CFTR* gene) resulting in abnormalities in chloride transport and water flux across the surface of epithelial cells; the abnormal secretions cause obstruction of glands and ducts in various organs and subsequent damage to exocrine tissue (recurrent pneumonia, atelectasis, bronchiectasis, diabetes mellitus, biliary cirrhosis, cholelithiasis, intestinal obstruction, increased risk of gastrointestinal malignancies).

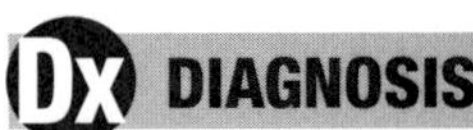

DIAGNOSIS

DIFFERENTIAL DIAGNOSIS

- Immunodeficiency states
- Celiac disease
- Asthma
- Recurrent pneumonia

WORKUP

A diagnosis of CF requires a positive quantitative pilocarpine iontophoresis test with one or more phenotypic features consistent with CF [illegible]g., chronic suppurative obstructive lung dis[illegible], pancreatic insufficiency) or documented [illegible]a sibling or first cousin.

[illegible]ATORY TESTS

- Pi[illegible] iontophoresis (sweat test): diagnostic[illegible] in children if sweat chloride is >60 m[illegible] (>80 mmol/L in adults) on two separate te[illegible] on consecutive days. Repeat testing may b[illegible]necessary because not all infants have sufficient quantities of sweat for reliable testing.
- DNA testing may be useful for confirming the diagnosis and providing genetic information for family members.
- Sputum culture and sensitivity and Gram stain (frequent bacterial infections with *Staphylococcus aureus, Pseudomonas aeruginosa* [most common virulent respiratory pathogen], *Haemophilus influenzae*).
- Low albumin level, increased 72-hr fecal fat excretion.
- Pulse oximetry or arterial blood gases: hypoxemia.
- Pulmonary function studies: decreased total lung capacity, forced vital capacity, pulmonary diffusing capacity.

IMAGING STUDIES

- Chest radiograph: may reveal focal atelectasis, peribronchial cuffing, bronchiectasis, increased interstitial markings, hyperinflation
- High-resolution chest CT scan: bronchial wall thickening, cystic lesions, ring shadows (bronchiectasis)

Rx TREATMENT

NONPHARMACOLOGIC THERAPY

- Postural drainage and chest percussion
- Encouragement of regular exercise and proper nutrition
- Psychosocial evaluation and counseling of patient and family members

ACUTE GENERAL Rx

- Antibiotic therapy based on results of Gram stain and culture and sensitivity of sputum (PO ciprofloxacin or floxacillin for *Pseudomonas,* cephalosporins for *S. aureus,* IV aminoglycosides plus ceftazidime for life-threatening *Pseudomonas* infections). Macrolides are also active against *Pseudomonas aeruginosa.* A recent study using azithromycin maintenance in children with CF for 6 mo found less use of additional antibiotics and improvement in some aspects of pulmonary function. Additional studies may be necessary to determine if azithromycin should be used as a primary therapy or rescue treatment.
- Bronchodilators for patients with airflow obstruction.
- Long-term pancreatic enzyme replacement.
- Alternate-day prednisone (2 mg/kg) possibly beneficial in children with CF (decreased hospitalization rate, improved pulmonary function); routine use of corticosteroids not recommended in adults; among children with CF who have received alternate-day treatment with prednisone, boys, but not girls, have persistent growth impairment after treatment is discontinued.
- Proper nutrition and vitamin supplementation.
- Recombinant human deoxyribonuclease (DNase [Dornase alpha]) 2.5 mg qd or bid given by aerosol for patients with viscid sputum. It is useful to improve mucociliary clearance by liquefying difficult-to-clear pulmonary secretions. It is, however, very expensive (annual cost to the pharmacist is >$10,000); most beneficial in patients with forced vital capacity values >40% of predicted. Its cost can be decreased by using alternate-day rhDNase therapy.
- Intermittent administration of inhaled tobramycin has been reported beneficial in CF.
- Treatment of impaired glucose tolerance and diabetes mellitus.

CHRONIC Rx

Pneumococcal vaccination, yearly influenza vaccination

DISPOSITION

- More than 50% of children with CF live beyond age 20 yr.
- Lung transplantation is the only definitive treatment; 3-yr survival after transplantation exceeds 50%.
- Obstructive azoospermia is present in >98% of postpubertal males.
- The SERPINA Z allele is a risk factor for liver disease in CF. Patients that carry the Z allele are at a greater risk of developing severe liver disease with portal hypertension.

REFERRAL

- To regional ambulatory care CF center.
- For lung transplantation in selected patients. Indications for lung transplantation are FEV_1 <30% of predicted, rapidly progressive respiratory deterioration, increasing number of hospital admissions, massive hemoptysis, recurrent pneumothorax, arterial partial pressure of oxygen <55 mm Hg, arterial partial pressure of carbon dioxide >50 mm Hg, multiresistant organisms, wasting. Young female patients should be referred earlier because of overall poor prognosis.
- For screening of family members with DNA analysis.

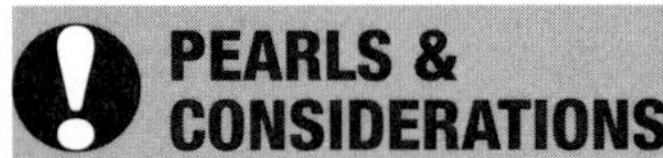

PEARLS & CONSIDERATIONS

COMMENTS

- Clinicians should think of CF in any patient with bronchiectasis plus any of the following: male infertility, recurrent idiopathic pancreatitis, recurrent nasal polyposis.
- Genetic testing for CF should be offered to adults with a positive family history of CF, to couples currently planning a pregnancy, and to couples seeking prenatal care.
- Inhalation of hypertonic saline (5 ml of 7% sodium chloride qid) has been reported to produce a sustained acceleration of mucus clearance and improved lung function.

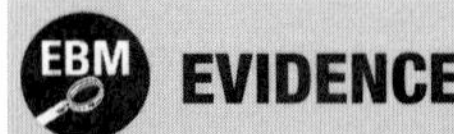

EVIDENCE

Please note: Complete text of EBM for this topic is available online.

Key trials and commentary:
Four randomized, placebo-controlled trials have previously documented the clinical benefits of azithromycin (AZM) in cystic fibrosis (CF) patients. The present study examined whether the beneficial effect of AZM is equivalent when administered daily or weekly.

This is an interesting 6-month, double-blind, placebo-controlled trial of daily (250 mg) vs. weekly (1200 mg) Azithromycin (A) in 208 CF patients, inclusive of 54 children <14 years of age. Not surprisingly, gastrointestinal side effects were the most common adverse event and more common in the group receiving the weekly dose of 1200 mg ($P = 0.02$). The primary endpoint studied (forced expiratory volume in one second [FEV_1] % predicted), was comparable in both groups over the time studied. Children were more likely to have positive changes in height and weight z-scores, but not BMI, over time, when receiving the daily dose of AZM. Over time, mean numbers of hospital admissions and days in the hospital were decreased for both groups (compared to with 6 months pretrial), but only daily therapy was associated with reduced numbers of patients admitted to the hospital. The next step is a long-term study of a 250 mg dose in children (12 months perhaps) to determine whether improved nutritional status as indicated by weight/height is preserved over a longer period of study is needed.[1] Ⓐ

Evidence-Based Reference

1. McCormack J et al: Daily versus weekly azithromycin in cystic fibrosis patients, *Eur Respir J* 30: 487-495, 2007. Commentary by S.K. Willsie, D.O. Ⓐ

SUGGESTED READINGS

Bartlett JR et al: Genetic modifiers of liver disease in cystic fibrosis, *JAMA* 302(10):1076-1083, 2009.

Castellani C et al: Association between carrier screening and incidence of cystic fibrosis, *JAMA* 302(23): 2573-2579, 2009.

AUTHOR: **FRED F. FERRI, M.D.**

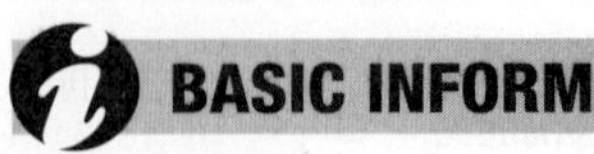

BASIC INFORMATION

DEFINITION

Cysticercosis is an infection caused by the tissue deposition of larval forms of the pork tapeworm *Taenia solium. T. solium* cysts, or cysticerci, which may accumulate in any human tissue, including the eyes, spinal cord, skin, muscle, heart, and brain.

Central nervous system (CNS) involvement is common and is known as neurocysticercosis. Humans acquire cysticercosis by fecal-oral transmission of *T. solium* eggs from human tapeworm carriers, often by ingesting tapeworm eggs or cysts in contaminated food or water. Undercooked pork is the most commonly identified food source. The eggs hatch in the gastrointestinal tract, and larvae migrate hematogenously to tissues where they encyst, forming cysticerci.

SYNONYMS

Cysticerciasis
Taeniasis
Pork tapeworm

ICD-9CM CODES
123.1 Cysticercosis

EPIDEMIOLOGY & DEMOGRAPHICS

- *T. solium* infection is worldwide in distribution. Tapeworm infection and cysticercosis are endemic in rural, developing countries where pigs are raised as a food source.
- Serologic studies from endemic areas of Latin America have demonstrated seroprevalences of 4.9% to 24%.
- Neurocysticercosis is the most common cause of acquired epilepsy worldwide and has become an important parasitic disease in the U.S., especially in states with large immigrant populations from countries where the disease is endemic.

PHYSICAL FINDINGS & CLINICAL PRESENTATION

- After ingestion of *T. solium* eggs or cysts, human beings may remain asymptomatic for years.
- The symptoms vary and depend on the location of cysticerci. Cysticerci in muscles and skin may form "cold" nodules, which are usually asymptomatic but may calcify.
- Neurocysticercosis, or the presence of cysts within the brain parenchyma, is usually asymptomatic. Symptoms stem from inflammation associated with the degeneration of cysts.
- Seizures are the most common manifestation of neurocysticercosis, occurring in 70% to 90% of symptomatic cases. Headache is also common.
- Inflammation around degenerating cysts may result in focal encephalitis, vasculitis, chronic meningitis, and cranial nerve palsies.
- In 10% to 20% of cases of neurocysticercosis, cysts lodge within the ventricular system and result in obstructive hydrocephalus, causing acute intracranial hypertension. This syndrome is related to the location of the parasites in the cerebral ventricles or basal cisterns, blocking the circulation of cerebrospinal fluid, and is caused by the presence of the parasite itself, ependymal inflammation, and/or fibrosis. Death may occur from progressive hydrocephalus, cerebral edema, or intractable seizures.
- Ocular cysticercosis occurs in less than 5% of infections and is generally asymptomatic. Inflammation in response to degenerating cysticerci may result in chorioretinitis, vasculitis, or retinal detachment, threatening vision.

ETIOLOGY

- *T. solium* has a complex two-host life cycle.
- Human beings are the only definitive host and harbor the adult worm in the intestine (taeniasis). However, both human beings and pigs can serve as intermediate hosts and harbor the larvae or cysticerci (Fig. 1-82).

Dx DIAGNOSIS

DIFFERENTIAL DIAGNOSIS

- Idiopathic epilepsy
- Migraine
- CNS vasculitis
- Primary neoplasia of CNS
- Chronic CNS infections, including toxoplasmosis, coccidioidomycosis, tuberculosis, and cryptococcosis
- Brain abscess
- CNS sarcoidosis, Systemic Lupus Erythematosus (SLE)

WORKUP

Comprehensive clinical history: obtain information on area and sanitary conditions of residence, previous travel, and dietary habits, most importantly consumption of undercooked pork.

LABORATORY TESTS

- Definitive diagnosis is based on the histopathologic demonstration of cysticerci in the tissue involved.
- Peripheral eosinophilia is usually absent.
- Stool examination for ova and proglottids of *T. solium* is insensitive and not specific for the diagnosis of cysticercosis.
- Cerebrospinal fluid (CSF) examination may demonstrate pleocytosis, with lymphocytic or eosinophilic predominance, low glucose, and elevated protein with neurocysticercosis. However, CSF is normal in most cases.
- Serologic testing is supportive of a suspected diagnosis of cysticercosis. An enzyme-linked immunoelectrotransfer blot (EITB) assay is the test of choice for detecting anticysticercal antibodies. This assay uses affinity purified glycoprotein antigens and has higher sensitivity (83% to 100%) and specificity (93% to 98%) than other enzyme-linked antibody (e.g., ELISA) tests. However, the diagnostic performance of the EITB can vary in different patient populations depending on the activity of the cysts and number of lesions. Single calcified

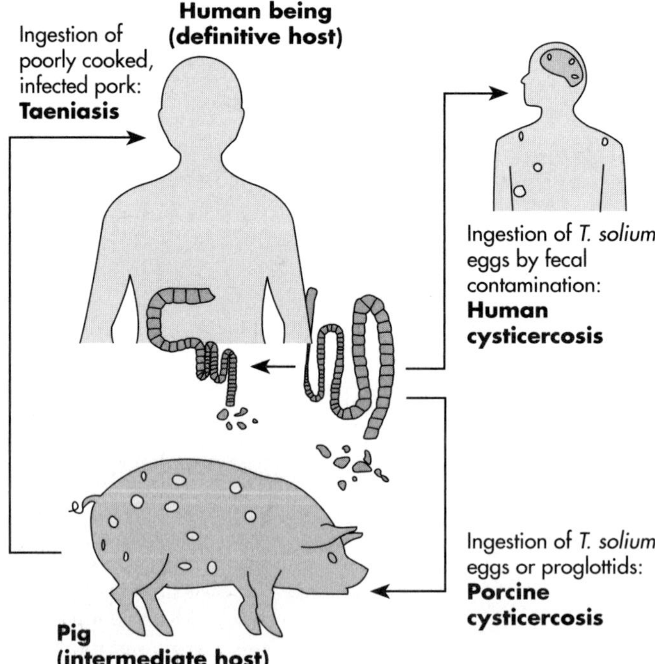

FIGURE 1-82 Cysticercosis is most commonly acquired by ingesting undercooked pork infected with *Taenia solium* cysticerci. Adult worms develop in the small intestine, forming proglottids that produce many fertilized eggs. Eggs and proglottids are intermittently shed in the stools of the persons infected with an adult tapeworm, where they can be ingested by pigs (the intermediate host) or transmitted by fecal-oral contamination to other human beings. In the small intestine of the host, the eggs hatch and release larvae that travel through the bloodstream to various organs, where they develop into fluid-filled cystic larvae within months. Skeletal muscle, subcutaneous tissue, the eyes, and the central nervous system are most commonly invaded.

lesions are more likely to be associated with a false-negative assay result. This test can be run on CSF, although its sensitivity is limited.

- Antigen detection tests are also being developed. Serum and urine, monoclonal antibody based ELISA has been used to detect circulating antigens and was shown to be 85-92% sensitive for viable parasites. Sensitivity, however, decreases in patients with a single cyst. This method may be particularly useful in monitoring patients following therapy. Parasite antigen levels usually fall by three months of treatment.
- More recently, amplification of *Taenia solium* DNA, with the method of polymerase chain reaction, has been achieved (sensitivity 96.7%).

IMAGING STUDIES

- Plain radiographs of the extremities may reveal calcified cysts in patients with soft tissue or muscle involvement.
- For diagnosis of neurocysticercosis, CT and MRI are most commonly used.
- Brain CT has a sensitivity and specificity of 95% and can identify living cysticerci, which appear as hypodense lesions, as well as degenerating cysts, which appear as isodense or hyperdense lesions. It is the best method for detecting calcification associated with prior infection, which suggests inactivity.
- Brain MRI is the most accurate technique to assess the extent of infection, location, and evolutionary stage of the parasites. MRI provides detailed images of living and degenerating cysts, perilesional edema, as well as small cysts or those located in the ventricles, brainstem, and cerebellum.

Rx TREATMENT

ACUTE GENERAL Rx

Asymptomatic cysticercosis:

- There is no evidence that administering antiparasitic therapy is beneficial.

Symptomatic cysticercosis:

- Patients with active lesions, with evidence of surrounding edema and/or inflammation, generally warrant treatment with antiparasitics, corticosteroids, and anticonvulsants.
  1. Anticonvulsant therapy:
     - Patients who have seizures or are considered at risk for recurrent seizures based on imaging should be treated with anticonvulsants.
  2. Antiparasitic therapy:
     - Pharmacologic therapy is indicated in the treatment of symptomatic patients with multiple viable brain parenchymal cysticerci.
     - Calcified cysticerci are inactive and do not warrant antiparasitic treatment.
     - Antiparasitic therapy is often unnecessary in patients with single cysts because treatment does not alter the natural history of single-cyst disease.
  3. Cysticidal therapy:
     - Antiparasitic therapy hastens the disappearance of cysts and should initially be given in conjunction with corticosteroids to control the inflammation associated with dying organisms.
     - Patients with viable parenchymal or subarachnoid cysts should be treated with albendazole 15 mg/kg/day for 8 days or praziquantel 50 mg/kg/day for 15 days. Antiparasitics should be used cautiously in patients with massive cysticercal infection of the brain parenchyma (≥50 cysts) or cysticercal encephalitis. These patients should be managed initially with corticosteroids, and perhaps mannitol, to control intracranial hypertension. Once the inflammation and the edema have resolved by MRI, antiparasitics can be administered.
     - Praziquantel may cause drug interactions with other agents metabolized by the cytochrome p450 systems, including phenytoin and phenobarbital.
     - Albendazole has no significant drug interactions with anticonvulsants.
  4. Surgical therapy:
     - Surgery may be indicated in patients with obstructive hydrocephalus or giant cysts with associated intracranial hypertension.
     - Surgical interventions may include craniotomy, with cyst extraction, stereotactic cyst aspiration, and/or ventriculoperitoneal shunt placement to control hydrocephalus.
     - Extraparenchymal cysticercosis, including ocular, subarachnoid, and intraventricular disease, carries a poor prognosis and requires a more aggressive approach. When feasible, complete surgical excision of lesions remains the definitive therapy.

CHRONIC Rx

- A recently published study suggests that prolonged antiparasitic therapy does not improve outcomes in patients with neurocysticercosis and seizures. Antiparasitic therapy, in fact, delayed calcification of lesions. Antiepileptic medications may need to be continued indefinitely.
- Rare patients with neurocysticercosis develop chronic or recurrent perilesional inflammation, requiring long-term, high-dose steroid therapy. Methotrexate has been reported to be of use as a steroid-sparing agent in this setting.

DISPOSITION

- In seizure-free, stable neurocysticercosis, outpatient management is appropriate.
- Patients with seizures should be restricted from driving.

REFERRAL

- Infectious diseases consultation
- Neurology consultation in patients with seizures
- Neurosurgical consultation if extraparenchymal neurocysticercosis or obstructive hydrocephalus is present

PREVENTION

- Eradication of taeniasis/cysticercosis is possible with implementation of meat inspection, improvement of pig husbandry, and improvement of socioeconomic conditions in endemic areas.
- A porcine vaccine against *T. solium* has been developed and successfully implemented in Peru, Mexico, and Australia.
- There is currently no human vaccine to prevent tapeworm infection or cysticercosis.

PATIENT & FAMILY EDUCATION

- Pork should be inspected for the presence of cysticerci, which are visible in raw meat.
- Pork must be well cooked.
- Proper disposal of human excreta and handwashing are of utmost importance to break the transmission cycle in households.

SUGGESTED READINGS

Almeida CR et al: Taenia solium DNA is present in the cerebrospinal fluid of neurocysticercosis and can be used for diagnosis, *Eur Arch Psyciatry Clin Neurosci* 256(5):307-310, 2006.

Castillo Y et al: Urine antigen detection for the diagnosis of human neurocysticercosis, *Am J Trop Med Hyg Hyg* 80(3):379-383, 2009.

Das K et al: Role of antiparasitic therapy for seizures and resolution of lesions in neurocysticercosis patients: an 8 year randomized study, *J Clin Neurosci* 14:1172-1177, 2007.

Del Brutto OH et al: Meta-analysis: cysticidal drugs for neurocysticercosis: albendazole and praziquantel, *Ann Intern Med* 145:43, 2006.

Garcia HH et al: A trial of antiparasitic treatment to reduce the rate of seizures due to cerebral Cysticercosis, *N Engl J Med* 350:249, 2004.

Garcia HH et al: Strategies for the elimination of taeniasis/cysticercosis, *J Neurological Sci* 262:153-157, 2007.

Garcia HH et al: New concepts in the diagnosis and management of neurocysticercosis *(Taenia solium)*, *Am J Trop Med Hyg* 72:3, 2005.

Garcia HH et al: Taenia solium cysticercosis, *Lancet* 362:547-556, 2003.

Gonzalez AE et al: Short report: vaccination of pigs to control human neurocysticercosis, *Am J Trop Med Hyg* 72:837-839, 2005.

Kraft R: Cysticercosis: An emerging parasitic disease, *Am Fam Physician* 75:91-96, 2007.

Mitre E et al: Methotrexate as a corticosteroid-sparing agent in complicated neurocysticercosis, *Clin Infect Dis* 44:449-553, 2007.

Nash TE et al: Treatment of neurocysticercosis: current status and future research needs, *Neurology* 67: 1120-1127, 2006.

Sorvillo FJ et al: Deaths from cysticercosis, United States, *Emerg Infect Dis* 13(2):230-235, 2007.

Takayanagui OM et al: Clinical aspects of neurocysticercosis, *Parasitol Int* 55:S111-S115, 2006.

White AC: Neurocysticercosis: A major cause of neurological disease worldwide, *Clin Infect Dis* 24:101-115, 1997.

AUTHORS: **ELENI PATROZOU, M.D.,** and **STACI A. FISCHER, M.D.**

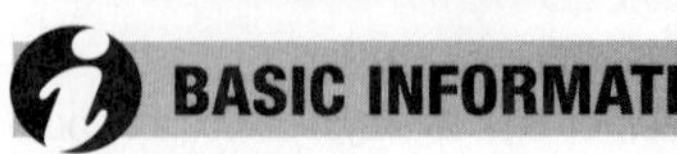

BASIC INFORMATION

DEFINITION

Infection with cytomegalovirus (CMV), a herpes virus, is common in the general population, with multiple mechanisms for transmission, often during childhood and adolescence. CMV is associated with pregnancy and can be a congenital disease. CMV is also associated with immunocompromised states and may be life threatening.

SYNONYMS

CMV
Heterophil-negative mononucleosis
Cytomegalic inclusion disease virus

ICD-9CM CODES
078.5 CMV infection
771.1 Congenital or perinatal CMV infection
V01.7 Exposure to CMV

EPIDEMIOLOGY & DEMOGRAPHICS

- Seroprevalence is widespread: 40% to 100% antibody positivity in adults.
- Increased infection develops perinatally, in day care exposure, and then during reproductive age, related to sexual activity.

ROUTES OF TRANSMISSION

- Blood transfusions
- Sexually (STDs) via uterus, cervix, and semen
- Perinatally via breast milk
- Transplant of organs—bone marrow, kidneys, liver, heart, or lung

PHYSICAL FINDINGS & CLINICAL PRESENTATION

CHILDREN: Congenital—25% of infected children with symptoms if congenital:
- Petechial rash
- Jaundice and/or hepatosplenomegaly
- Lethargy
- Respiratory distress
- CNS involvement, seizures

Postnatal acquisition:
- CMV mononucleosis
- Pharyngitis, croup, bronchitis, pneumonia

HEALTHY ADULTS:
Common
- May be asymptomatic
- CMV mononucleosis similar to EBV mononucleosis
- Fever—lasting 9 to 30 days—mean of 19 days

Less common
- Exudative pharyngitis
- Lymphadenopathy, hepatitis, splenomegaly
- Interstitial pneumonia (rare)
- Nonspecific rash
- Thrombocytopenia/hemolytic anemia

Rare
- Guillain-Barré syndrome
- Meningoencephalitis
- Myocarditis

IMMUNOSUPPRESSED PATIENTS:
- Febrile mononucleosis
- GI ulcerations, hepatitis, pneumonitis, retinitis, encephalopathy, meningoencephalopathy
- HIV associated—dementia, demyelination, retinitis (Fig. 1-83), acalculous cholecystitis, adrenalitis, diarrhea, enterocolitis, esophagitis
- Diabetes associated with pancreatitis
- Adrenalitis associated with HIV

ETIOLOGY

Cytomegalovirus infection can remain latent, reactive with immunosuppression.

DIAGNOSIS

DIFFERENTIAL DIAGNOSIS

Congenital:
- Acute viral, bacterial, parasitic infections including other congenitally transmitted agents (toxoplasmosis, rubella, syphilis, pertussis, croup, bronchitis)

Acquired:
- EBV mononucleosis
- Viral hepatitis—A, B, C
- Cryptosporidiosis
- Toxoplasmosis
- *Mycobacterium avium* infections
- Human herpesvirus 6
- Acute HIV infection

WORKUP

- Laboratory confirmation combined with clinical findings often with leukopenia, thrombocytopenia, lymphocytosis
- Demonstration of virus in tissue or serologic testing including CMV IgM antibodies, rising titers of complement fixation (CF), and indirect fluorescent antibody (IFA) or anticomplement IFA
- Funduscopic—necrotic patches with white granular component of retina
- Cultures—(viral) human fibroblast from urine, cervical swab, tissue buffy coat
- Biopsy—"owl's eye" inclusion bodies on tissue sample

IMAGING STUDIES

- Chest radiograph—if pneumonitis suspected, consider bronchoscopy
- Endoscopy—if GI involvement
- CT scan/MRI—if CNS involvement

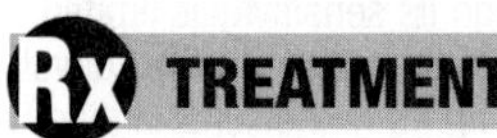

TREATMENT

NONPHARMACOLOGIC THERAPY

- Strict hand washing and standard precautions limit CMV transmission in health care facilities
- Highly active antiretroviral therapy (HAART) in patients with CD4 count $<50/mm^3$ for the goal of CD4 $>100/mm^3$ for a 3- to 6-mo period

ACUTE GENERAL Rx

For compromised hosts with CMV retinitis or pneumonitis:
- Ganciclovir 5 mg/kg bid IV × 21 days, then 5 mg/kg/day IV, or 1 g PO tid or ocular implant
- Foscarnet 60 mg/kg tid × 3 wk, then 90 mg/kg/day
- Cidofovir 5 mg/kg IV, repeat 1 wk later, then q2 wk IV
- Fomivirsen-salvage therapy for CMV retinitis 300 μg injected into vitreous

DISPOSITION

- CMV infection in patients who are immunocompromised (especially those with AIDS, bone marrow and solid organ transplant recipients, and disorders of cell-mediated immune function) will need expert, long-term follow-up by an infectious disease specialist or immunologist familiar with the care of such patients.
- CMV mononucleosis, hepatitis, pharyngitis, etc. in immunologically normal hosts are usually self-limiting infections requiring no special follow-up plans.

REFERRAL

- To an ophthalmologist if CMV retinitis is present
- To an infectious disease specialist or AIDS specialist for patients who are HIV-positive with CMV disease
- To a cellular immunologist or transplant specialist in the case of CMV infection in a transplant recipient

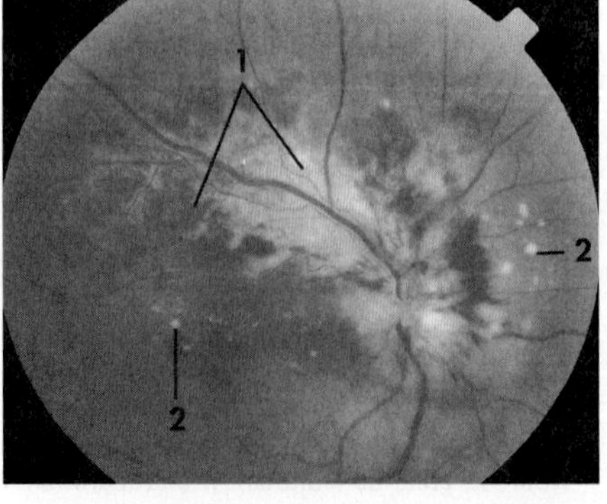

FIGURE 1-83 Sight-threatening CMV retinitis involves the macula and optic nerve of this HIV-positive young man. White, infected retina with intraretinal hemorrhage is present in the arcuate distribution of the nerve fiber layer *(1)*. A small amount of lipid exudation near the fovea and nasal to the optic nerve is also seen *(2)*. (From Palay D [ed]: *Ophthalmology for the primary care physician,* St Louis, 1997, Mosby.)

- To a pediatric infectious disease specialist for congenital CMV infection

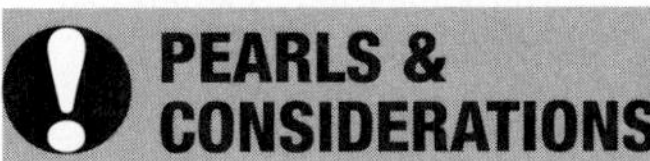

PEARLS & CONSIDERATIONS

CMV is ubiquitous in the environment and is asymptomatically shed by latently infected persons with CMV infection, making it difficult to protect patients who are immunocompromised from acquiring this infection.

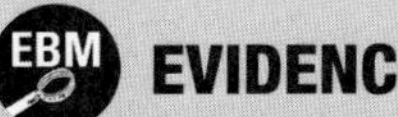

EVIDENCE

Please note: Complete text of EBM for this topic is available online.

SUGGESTED READINGS

Hodson E et al: Antiviral medications to prevent cytomegalovirus disease and early death in recipients of solid-organ transplants: a systematic review of randomised controlled trials. *Lancet* 365: 2105-2115, 2005.

Nichols W et al: Recent advances in the therapy and prevention of CMV infections. *J Clin Virology* 16(1): 25-40, 2000.

Razonable R: Cytomegalovirus infection after liver transplantation: current concepts and challenges, *World J Gastroenterol* 14(31): 4849-4860, 2008.

AUTHORS: **GLENN G. FORT, M.D., M.P.H.,** and **DENNIS J. MIKOLICH, M.D.**

BASIC INFORMATION

DEFINITION

Decubitus ulcers (pressure ulcers) are any damage to the skin and the underlying tissue or both that results from pressure, friction, or shearing forces that usually occur over bony prominences.

SYNONYMS

Pressure ulcers
Pressure sores
Bedsores
Decubiti

ICD-9CM CODES
707.0X Decubitus ulcers (X defines location)
707.2X Stages of decubitus ulcers (X defines specific staging)

EPIDEMIOLOGY & DEMOGRAPHICS

- Present in 5% to 10% of patients in all health care settings: hospitals, nursing homes, and home confined.
- Associated with significant morbidity and mortality. One-year mortality rate approaches 40%.
- Pain occurs in two thirds of patients with stage II or greater pressure ulcers.
- Complicated by cellulitis, osteomyelitis, abscesses, and sepsis.

CLINICAL PRESENTATION

A new pressure ulcer staging system was developed in 2007, adding the last two stages.

Stage I: Nonblanchable erythema of intact skin or boggy, mushy feeling of skin

Stage II: Partial-thickness skin loss involving the epidermis, dermis, or both

Stage III: Full-thickness skin loss involving damage or necrosis of subcutaneous tissue that may extend down to, but not through, underlying fascia or muscle

Stage IV: Full-thickness skin loss with extensive destruction and tissue damage to muscle, bone, or supporting structures (e.g., tendons, joint capsule) (Fig. 1-84)

Deep tissue injury: Purple or maroon skin overlying an area of dead tissue (muscle or fat), which usually develops into a stage III or IV.

Unstageable: Ulcer base is covered by slough and eschar and cannot be staged.

ETIOLOGY

Decubitus ulcers are caused by constant, unrelieved pressure in tissues where circulation is diminished, leading to necrosis of the tissues. Shearing and friction forces can also contribute or cause damage to the tissues, leading to an ulcer. Risk factors include malnutrition, bowel or bladder incontinence, and dry or damaged skin.

DIAGNOSIS

DIFFERENTIAL DIAGNOSIS

- Venous stasis ulcers
- Arterial ulcers
- Diabetic ulcers
- Skin cancer
- Cellulitis
- Kennedy ulcers (rapidly progressing ulcers that occur at the end of life)

WORKUP

Describe ulcer, including the stage, location, and size. For stages III and IV, describe the wound bed (epithelialization, granulation tissue, necrotic tissue, eschar); presence of any exudates, including type and amount; depth and wound edges (undermining, sinus tracts, tunneling, or fistulas); any signs of infection (purulent drainage, odor, surrounding cellulitis); and pain. In addition, pressure ulcer risk factors and causes should be reassessed.

LABORATORY TESTS

- Directed at identifying cause of risk factors or any complications arising from the pressure ulcer (e.g., abscess or osteomyelitis).
- Cultures of wound bed are often not helpful and should not be routinely performed.
- Low prealbumin levels may reveal malnutrition.
- Complete blood count if infection is suspected.

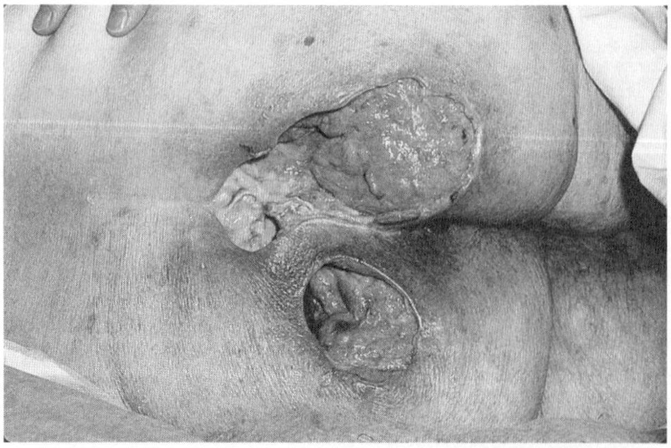

FIGURE 1-84 Natural debridement of pressure injury at 2 weeks. (From Tallis R, Fillit H: *Brockelhurst's textbook of geriatric medicine and gerontology,* ed 6, London, 2003, Churchill Livingstone.)

IMAGING STUDIES

- Ultrasound not proven to be effective.
- MRI or bone scans may help identify osteomyelitis when clinically suspected.

TREATMENT

PREVENTION

- Identify high-risk patients by using standardized risk assessment scales such as the Braden scale.
- Routine skin inspection and good skin care for high-risk patients.
- Minimize prolonged skin exposure to moisture, urine, or stool.
- Treat dry, cracking skin.
- Use repositioning and pressure-reducing devices (e.g., foam mattresses, low–air loss beds, pillows, or foam wedges when in bed or in a chair).
    - Patient repositioning
        1. Although there is clinical consensus that repositioning is critical, three randomized controlled trials (RCTs) found no evidence that regular manual repositioning prevented pressure ulcers.
    - Bed surface
        1. Air-fluidized beds
            a. Two RCTs found that use of air-fluidized beds contributed to the healing of a greater number of ulcers after 15 days compared with standard care.
            b. Systematic review revealed no differences in rate of pressure ulcer healing with use of either alternating-pressure mattresses or low–air loss beds compared with standard care.
        2. Pressure-relieving overlays
            a. One RCT demonstrated that viscoelastic pad on the operating table significantly reduced incidence of postoperative pressure ulcers compared with a standard operating table.
            b. One RCT found that sheepskin overlays plus standard care compared with standard care alone significantly reduced incidence of pressure sores in elderly patients recuperating from hip fracture.
        3. Foam alternatives
            a. Four RCTs revealed that foam alternatives versus standard hospital mattresses reduced the incidence of pressure ulcer development in elderly patients in orthopedic hospital wards.
            b. Forty-one RCTs demonstrated that patients lying on standard hospital mattresses are more likely to develop pressure ulcers than those patients lying on higher specification foam mattresses.
- Use adequate support surfaces while in bed or in a chair to prevent "bottoming out" (defined as less than 1 inch between patient and

support surface; measured by putting hand under support surface and feeling thickness to patient).
- Recent systematic review of pressure ulcer prevention strategies showed poor methodology in most studies. Use of support surfaces, repositioning, optimized nutrition, and sacral skin moisturizing were most appropriate.

NONPHARMACOLOGIC THERAPY

- Should be cleaned at each dressing change; necrotic tissue should be debrided quickly because it delays wound healing (except for heel ulcers).
- Wound irrigation should not exceed 15 psi and is best done with an 18-gauge angiocatheter.
- No single dressing or product is superior; should be used to keep ulcer bed moist and protect it from urine/stool.
- Avoid agents that are cytotoxic to epithelial cells (e.g., iodine, iodophor, sodium hypochlorite, hydrogen peroxide, acetic acid, alcohol).
- Reduce pressure by using foam mattress, dynamic support surface (e.g., low–air loss bed), and frequent repositioning (e.g., q2h).
- Hyperbaric oxygen, ultrasound, ultraviolet, and low-energy radiation either are ineffective or have not been extensively evaluated for efficacy.
- Negative pressure devices (Vac devices) may help in wounds that have significant drainage.
- Correct poor nutrition.
- Minimize urinary and/or fecal incontinence.
- Use a standardized assessment tool (e.g., PUSH tool) to monitor wound healing on weekly basis.
- No RCTs have compared debridement versus no debridement in the treatment of pressure ulcers.
- Thirty-two RCTs have compared different debridement agents, but there is insufficient evidence to promote the use of one particular agent.
- One RCT demonstrated ulcers treated with collagenase healed significantly more quickly than those treated with hydrocolloid.
- A meta-analysis and one RCT found significant benefit in rates of healing with use of hydrocolloid dressings versus traditional saline gauze dressings but not over other forms such as hydrogels, foam dressings, or collogenase.
- No benefit was found with nutritional supplements, artificial nutrition, or ultrasound therapy.

ACUTE GENERAL Rx

- Pain medications may be necessary because 50% of decubitus ulcers are painful.
- Growth factors appear promising but are second-line treatments if traditional approaches are ineffective.

CHRONIC Rx

- Continue vigilance with pressure reduction because decubitus ulcers can recur with minimal trauma.
- Consider evaluation for infected ulcer bed, occult osteomyelitis, or abscess.

COMPLEMENTARY & ALTERNATIVE MEDICINE

Vitamin C, zinc, and multivitamin supplements may be of benefit to optimize nutrition.

DISPOSITION

- When systematic risk assessments are done and preventive measures are followed, most pressure ulcers can be prevented. Most heal when appropriate management strategies are followed.
- Stage IV ulcers in high-risk patients (e.g., paraplegics) can take months or years to heal.

REFERRAL

- Physical and occupational therapists to improve bed and chair mobility.
- Wounds with necrotic tissue need referral to persons trained in sharp debridement.
- To plastic surgeons for operative repair for large stage III or IV ulcers that do not respond to optimal care.
- To a specialty wound center for nonhealing ulcers.

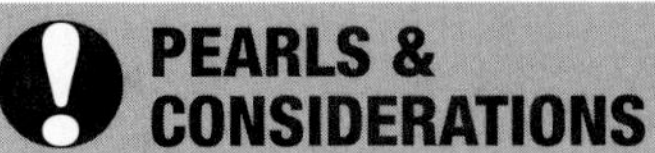

PEARLS & CONSIDERATIONS

COMMENTS

- Up to 10% of older persons will have a pressure ulcer.
- Identify and reduce all risk factors for pressure ulcers.
- Treat the pain associated with pressure ulcers.
- Proper skin care, use of support surfaces, mobilization, and attention to nutrition are key for prevention and treatment.
- Clinical studies have not revealed if any one dressing product is superior.
- Nonhealing ulcers require assessment for debridement, infection, abscess, and/or referral to a wound center.

PATIENT & FAMILY EDUCATION

- Educate patient and family members on the risk factors for pressure ulcers.
- Encourage mobility and adequate nutritional intake and avoid bed rest.

SUGGESTED READINGS

Black J et al: National Pressure Ulcer Advisory Panel's updated pressure ulcer staging system, *Dermatological Nursing* 19(4):343, 2007.

Bluestein D, Javaheri A: Pressure ulcers: prevention, evaluation, and management, *Am Fam Physician* 78(10):1186-1194, 2008.

Heyneman A et al: A systematic review of the use of hydrocolloids in the treatment of pressure ulcers, *J of Clin Nurs* 17(9):1164, 2008.

Lyder C: Pressure ulcer prevention and management, *JAMA* 289(2):223, 2003.

National Pressure Ulcer Advisory Panel 9 (NPUAP): Pressure Ulcer Scale for Healing (PUSH), PUSH tool version 3.0. Available at http://www.npuap.org/PDF/push3.pdf.

Reddy M et al: Preventing pressure ulcers: a systematic review, *JAMA* 296(8):974, 2006.

Reddy M et al: Treatment of pressure ulcers: a systematic review, *JAMA* 300(22):2647-2662, 2008.

AUTHORS: **DAVID R. GIFFORD, M.D., M.P.H.,** and **LYNN MCNICOLL, M.D., F.R.C.P.C.**

Deep Vein Thrombosis 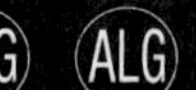

BASIC INFORMATION

DEFINITION

Deep venous thrombosis (DVT) is the development of thrombi in the deep veins of the extremities or pelvis.

SYNONYMS

DVT
Venous thromboembolism (VTE) (VTE includes DVT and pulmonary embolism [PE])
Deep venous thrombosis

ICD-9CM CODES

451.1	Thrombosis of deep vessels of lower extremities
451.83	Thrombosis of deep veins of upper extremities
541.9	Deep vein thrombosis of unspecified site

EPIDEMIOLOGY & DEMOGRAPHICS

- Annual incidence in urban population is 1.6 cases/1000 persons.
- The risk of recurrent thromboembolism is higher among men than women.

PHYSICAL FINDINGS & CLINICAL PRESENTATION

- Pain and swelling of the affected extremity
- In lower extremity DVT: leg pain on dorsiflexion of the foot (Homans' sign)
- Physical examination may be unremarkable in early DVT

ETIOLOGY

The etiology is often multifactorial (prolonged stasis, coagulation abnormalities, vessel wall trauma). The following are risk factors for DVT:

- Prolonged immobilization (≥3 days)
- Postoperative state
- Trauma to pelvis and lower extremities for lower extremity DVT; central line placement for upper extremity DVT
- Birth control pills, high-dose estrogen therapy; conjugated equine estrogen but not esterified estrogen is associated with increased risk of DVT; estrogen plus progestin is associated with doubling the risk of venous thrombosis. The use of bevacizumab is also significantly associated with an increased risk of developing DVT in cancer patients receiving this drug
- Visceral cancer (lung, pancreas, alimentary tract, genitourinary tract)
- Age >60 yr
- History of thromboembolic disease
- Hematologic disorders (e.g., factor V Leiden mutation [FVL], antithrombin III deficiency, protein C deficiency, protein S deficiency, heparin cofactor II deficiency, sticky platelet syndrome, G20210A prothrombin mutation, lupus anticoagulant, dysfibrinogenemias, anticardiolipin antibody, hyperhomocystinemia, concurrent homocystinuria, high levels of factors VIII, XI, and single nucleotide polymorphisms [SNPs] such as CYP4V2)
- Pregnancy and early puerperium
- Obesity (BMI >30)
- Congestive heart failure
- Surgery, fracture, or injury involving lower leg or pelvis
- Surgery requiring >30 min of anesthesia
- Gynecologic surgery (particularly gynecologic cancer surgery)
- Recent travel (within 2 wk, lasting >8 hours)
- Smoking and abdominal obesity
- Central venous catheter or pacemaker insertion
- Superficial vein thrombosis, varicose veins
- Long-term exposure to particulate air pollution is also associated with altered coagulation function and DVT risk

Dx DIAGNOSIS

DIFFERENTIAL DIAGNOSIS

- Postphlebitic syndrome
- Superficial thrombophlebitis
- Ruptured Baker's cyst
- Cellulitis, lymphangitis, Achilles tendinitis
- Hematoma
- Muscle or soft tissue injury, stress fracture
- Varicose veins, lymphedema
- Arterial insufficiency
- Abscess
- Claudication
- Venous stasis

WORKUP

- The clinical diagnosis of DVT is inaccurate. Pain, tenderness, swelling, or color changes are not specific for DVT.
- Clinical prediction rules can be used to establish pretest probability of DVT. The Wells prediction rules for DVT and for pulmonary embolism are described in Box 1-3. These rules perform better in younger patients without a history of DVT and in those without comorbidities. In younger patients without associated comorbidities and a low pretest probability using Wells criteria and a negative high-sensitivity D-dimer test, the diagnosis of DVT can be reasonably excluded.
- Compression ultrasonography is preferred as the initial study to diagnose DVT in patients with intermediate to high pretest probability. An initial negative test should be repeated after 5 days (if the clinical suspicion of DVT persists) to detect propagation of any thrombosis to the proximal veins. Comprehensive ultrasonography is a more extensive test that examines the deep veins from the inguinal ligament to the level of the malleolus. Recent literature reports indicate that it may be safe to withhold anticoagulation after negative results on comprehensive duplex ultrasonography in nonpregnant patients with a suspected first episode of symptomatic DVT of the leg.

LABORATORY TESTS

- Laboratory tests are not specific for DVT. Baseline prothrombin time (INR), partial thromboplastin time, and platelet count should be obtained on all patients before starting anticoagulation.
- Use of D-dimer assay by ELISA may be useful in the management of suspected DVT. The combination of a normal D-dimer study on presentation together with a normal compression venous ultrasound is useful to exclude DVT and generally eliminate the need to do repeat ultrasound at 5 to 7 days. Recent trials indicate that DVT can be ruled out in patients who are clinically unlikely to have DVT and who have a negative D-dimer test. Compressive ultrasonography can be safely omitted in such patients. An algorithm for the diagnosis of deep vein thrombosis is described in Section III.
- Laboratory evaluation of young patients with DVT, patients with recurrent thrombosis without obvious causes, and those with a family history of thrombosis should include protein S, protein C, fibrinogen, antithrombin III level, lupus anticoagulant, anticardiolipin antibodies, factor V Leiden, factor VIII, factor IX, and plasma homocysteine levels.

BOX 1-3 Wells Prediction Rule for Diagnosing Deep Venous Thrombosis: Clinical Evaluation Table for Predicting Pretest Probability of Deep Venous Thrombosis*

Clinical Characteristic	Score
Active cancer (treatment ongoing, within previous 6 mo, or palliative)	1
Paralysis, paresis, or recent plaster immobilization of the lower extremities	1
Recently bedridden >3 days or major surgery within 12 wk requiring general or regional anesthesia	1
Localized tenderness along the distribution of the deep venous system	1
Entire leg swollen	1
Calf swelling 3 cm larger than asymptomatic side (measured 10 cm below tibial tuberosity)	1
Pitting edema confined to the symptomatic leg	1
Collateral superficial veins (nonvaricose)	1
Alternative diagnosis at least as likely as deep venous thrombosis	−2

*Clinical probability: low, ≤0; intermediate, 1-2; high, ≥3. In patients with symptoms in both legs, the more symptomatic leg is used.

Reprinted from Wells PS et al: Value assessment of pretest probability of deep-vein thrombosis in clinical management, *Lancet* 351:1795-1798, 1997. With permission from Elsevier.

D

IMAGING STUDIES

Compression ultrasonography is generally preferred as the initial study because it is noninvasive and can be repeated serially (useful to monitor suspected acute DVT); it offers good sensitivity for detecting proximal vein thrombosis (in the popliteal or femoral vein). Its disadvantages are poor visualization of deep iliac and pelvic veins and poor sensitivity in isolated or nonocclusive calf vein thrombi.

Contrast venography is the gold standard for evaluation of DVT of the lower extremity. It is, however, invasive and painful. Additional disadvantages are the increased risk of phlebitis, new thrombosis, renal failure, and hypersensitivity reaction to contrast media; it also gives poor visualization of the deep femoral vein in the thigh and the internal iliac vein and its tributaries.

Magnetic resonance direct thrombus imaging (MRDTI) is an accurate noninvasive test for diagnosis of DVT. Current limitations are its cost and lack of widespread availability.

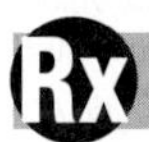 TREATMENT

NONPHARMACOLOGIC THERAPY

- Gradual resumption of normal activity. Immobility promotes stasis and propagation of DVT. Patients should get up and walk as tolerated. The theoretical risk that ambulation may dislodge thrombi in the legs, precipitating PE, is unfounded.
- Patient education on anticoagulant therapy and associated risks.

ACUTE GENERAL Rx

- Low-molecular-weight heparin (LMWH) for 4 to 7 days followed by warfarin therapy. Recommended dose of enoxaparin is 1 mg/kg q12h SC and continued for a minimum of 5 days and until a therapeutic INR (2 to 3) has been achieved with warfarin. Once-daily fondaparinux, a synthetic analog of heparin, is also as effective and safe as twice daily enoxaparin in the initial treatment of patients with symptomatic DVT. Warfarin therapy should be initiated when appropriate (usually within 72 hr of initiation of heparin). A 5-mg loading dose of warfarin is recommended in inpatients because it produces less excess anticoagulation than does a 10-mg dose; the smaller dose also avoids the development of a potential hypercoagulable state caused by precipitous decreases in levels of protein C during the first 36 hr of warfarin therapy. In the outpatient setting, a warfarin nomogram using 10-mg loading doses may be more effective in reaching a therapeutic INR. Long term LMWH may be preferable to warfarin in patients with cancer or those whose INR is difficult to control.
- Outpatient treatment of DVT is appropriate for patients without prior DVT, thrombophilic conditions, or substantial comorbidity, but not for those who are pregnant or likely not to adhere to therapy.
- Exclusions from outpatient treatment of DVT include patients with potential high complication risk (e.g., hemoglobin <7, platelet count <75,000, guaiac-positive stool, recent cerebrovascular accident or noncutaneous surgery, noncompliance).
- Compression stockings are effective in reducing the incidence of postthrombotic syndrome and should be used starting within 1 month of proximal DVT and for at least 1 yr after diagnosis.
- Insertion of an inferior vena cava filter to prevent pulmonary embolism is recommended in patients with contraindications to anticoagulation.
- Thrombolytic therapy (streptokinase) can be used in rare cases (unless contraindicated) in patients with extensive iliofemoral venous thrombosis and a low risk of bleeding.
- Preliminary trials reveal that idraparinux, a long-acting inhibitor of activated factor X given once weekly SC as a fixed dose for 3 or 6 months has efficacy similar to that of heparin plus a vitamin K antagonist in the treatment of DVT and causes less bleeding. However, in patients with PE, idraparinux was less efficacious than standard therapy.

CHRONIC Rx

- Conventional-intensity warfarin therapy is more effective than low-intensity warfarin therapy for the long-term prevention of recurrent DVT. The low-intensity warfarin regimen does not reduce the risk of clinically important bleeding.
- The optimal duration of anticoagulant therapy varies with the cause of DVT and the patient's risk factors:
- Therapy for 3 to 6 months is generally satisfactory in patients with reversible risk factors (low-risk group). A high D-dimer level measured after 3 months of anticoagulation in patients with unprovoked DVT should favor a longer duration of therapy.
- Anticoagulation for at least 6 months is recommended for patients with idiopathic venous thrombosis or medical risk factors for DVT (intermediate-risk group).
- Indefinite anticoagulation is necessary in patients with DVT associated with active cancer; long-term anticoagulation is also indicated in patients with inherited thrombophilia (e.g., deficiency of protein C or S antibody), antiphospholipid antibody, and those with recurrent episodes of idiopathic DVT (high-risk group).
- Measurement of D-dimer after withdrawal of oral anticoagulation may be useful to estimate the risk of recurrence. Patients with a first spontaneous DVT and a D-dimer level <250 mg/ml after withdrawal of oral anticoagulation have a low risk of DVT recurrence. The presence of residual thrombosis on ultrasonography when warfarin therapy is discontinued is also associated with an increased risk for subsequent recurrent DVT; a recent trial showed that tailoring the duration of anticoagulation on the basis of the persistence of residual thrombi on ultrasonography may reduce the rate of recurrent DVT. Additional trials are needed before this approach can be adapted for all patients.
- Recent trials show that in patients who have completed at least 3 months of anticoagulation for a first episode of unprovoked DVT and after approximately 2 yr of follow-up, a negative D-dimer result was associated with a 3.5% annual risk of recurrent disease, whereas a positive D-dimer result was associated with an 8.9% annual risk for recurrence.

PEARLS & CONSIDERATIONS

COMMENTS

- When using heparin, there is a risk of heparin-induced thrombocytopenia (with unfractionated more so than with LMWH). Platelet count should be obtained initially and repeated every 3 days while on heparin.
- Prophylaxis of DVT is recommended in all patients at risk (e.g., low-molecular-weight heparin [enoxaparin 30 mg SC bid] after major trauma, post surgery of hip and knee; enoxaparin 40 mg SC qd post–abdominal surgery in patients with moderate to high DVT risk; gradient elastic stockings alone or in combination with intermittent pneumatic compression [IPC] boots following neurosurgery). Graduated compression stockings are effective for preventing air-travel-related DVT.
- Fondaparinux, a synthetic analog of heparin, can also be used for prevention of DVT after hip fracture surgery, hip replacement, or knee replacement. Initial dose is 2.5 mg SC given 6 to 8 hr postoperatively and continued daily. Its bleeding risk is similar to enoxaparin; however, it is more effective in preventing DVT.
- The risk of recurrent venous thromboembolism in heterozygous carriers of factor V Leiden and a first spontaneous venous thromboembolism is similar to that of noncarriers of factor V Leiden; therefore, heterozygous patients should receive secondary thromboprophylaxis for a similar length of time as patients without factor V Leiden.
- Approximately 20% to 50% of patients with DVT develop *postthrombotic syndrome* characterized by leg edema, pain, venous ectasia, skin induration, and ulceration. Patients with extensive DVT and those with more severe postthrombotic manifestations 1 month after DVT have poorer long-term outcomes.
- Exercise following DVT is reasonable because it improves flexibility of the affected leg and does not increase symptoms in patients with postthrombotic syndrome.
- Previously undiagnosed cancer is frequent in patients with newly diagnosed DVT. A cancer screening strategy should be considered in all patients with unprovoked venous thromboembolism.
- Vitamin K (1 mg PO or 2 mg IV) can be used to reverse elevated INR (3 to 6) when elective or urgent procedures are needed.

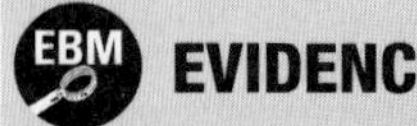

EVIDENCE

Please note: Complete text of EBM for this topic is available online.

Key trials and commentary:

Measures to prevent deep venous thrombosis (DVT), including low-dose subcutaneous heparin, low-molecular-weight heparin, or sequential compression devices, may be considered in high-risk patients, specifically those with a previous history of thromboembolic disease, and in patients with significant burns of the lower extremities. The purpose of this guideline is to review the principles of prophylaxis for DVT in burn patients and to present a reasonable approach for the treatment of patients during burn resuscitation. This guideline is designed to aid those physicians who are responsible for the triage and initial management of burn patients. DVT in the burn patient is a more common event than previously reported, with incidence ranging from 1% to 23% in the few available studies. The suspected risk of bleeding using low-dose heparin has deterred most burn surgeons from using heparin routinely in all burn patients. Much remains unknown, however, regarding the real risks and benefits of this complication and its treatment. A Medline search of all English language citations from 1966 through 2006 was undertaken using the key words "deep vein thrombosis" and "deep venous thrombosis" with "burns." This produced 18 references. The addition of the key words "pulmonary embolism" with "burns" produced a total of 82 references, of which 7 were felt to be relevant to this topic based on evidentiary classification of the data. There are no prospective, randomized, controlled studies evaluating the effectiveness of any prophylactic preventive measures against DVT in burn patients. The apparently low incidence of this condition in burn patients would appear to preclude its evaluation in a single-center study, and no multicenter studies have been conducted.

Faucher and Conlon do a nice job of reviewing the current data regarding thromboembolic prevention in burn patients during the early part of their care. Unfortunately, there are few studies available to guide our interventions, and none of them involve class I data. This article should propel the members of the Multi-institutional Trials Committee of the American Burn Association to encourage a randomized, prospective, double-blind study to obtain class I data for this issue. The numbers necessary to conduct such a study will require coordination among multiple burn centers and a central funding source that is adequate for the task. Such a study could definitively answer the questions of the true incidence of DVT in burn patients, the best diagnostic methods, and the best therapeutic options.[1] Ⓐ

Evidence-Based Reference

1. Faucher LD, Conlon KM: Practice guidelines for deep venous thrombosis prophylaxis in burns, *J Burn Care Res* 28:661-663, 2007. Commentary by B.A. Latenser, M.D. Ⓐ

SUGGESTED READINGS

Baccarelli A et al: Exposure to particulate air pollution and risk of deep vein thrombosis, *Arch Intern Med* 168(9):920, 2008.

Bezemer ID et al: Gene variants associated with deep vein thrombosis, *JAMA* 299:1306, 2008.

Carrier M et al: Systematic review: the Trousseau Syndrome revisited: should we screen extensively for cancer in patients with venous thromboembolism, *Ann Intern Med* 149:323-333, 2008.

Chan WS et al: A red blood cell agglutination D-dimer test to exclude deep venous thrombosis in pregnancy, *Ann Intern Med* 147:165-170, 2007.

Francis CW: Prophylaxis for thromboembolism in hospitalized medical patients, *N Engl J Med* 356:1438-1444, 2007.

Kahn SR et al: Determinants and time course of the postthrombotic syndrome after acute deep venous thrombosis, *Ann Intern Med* 149:698-707, 2008.

Landerfeld CS: Noninvasive diagnosis of deep vein thrombosis, *JAMA* 300:1696, 2008.

Marik PE, Plante LA: Venous thromboembolic disease and pregnancy, *N Engl J Med* 359:2025-2033, 2008.

Nallur SR et al: Risk of venous thromboembolism with the angiogenesis inhibitor bevacizumab in cancer patients, *JAMA* 300(19):2277-2285, 2008.

Piazza G, Goldhaber SZ: Improving clinical effectiveness in thromboprophylaxis for hospitalized medical patients, *Am J Med* 122:230-232, 2009.

Polareti G et al: D-dimer testing to determine the duration of anticoagulation therapy, *N Engl J Med* 355:1780-1789, 2006.

Prandoni P et al: Residual thrombosis on ultrasonography to guide the duration of anticoagulation in patients with deep vein thrombosis, *Ann Intern Med* 150:577-585, 2009.

Qaseem A et al: Current diagnosis of venous thromboembolism in primary care: a clinical practice guideline from the American Academy of Family Physicians and the American College of Physicians, *Ann Intern Med* 146:454-458, 2007.

Segal JB et al: Management of venous thromboembolism: a systematic review for a practice guideline, *Ann Intern Med* 146:211-222, 2007.

Snow V et al: Management of venous thromboembolism: a clinical practice guideline from the American College of Physicians and the American Academy of Family Physicians, *Ann Intern Med* 146:204-210, 2007.

The van Gogh investigators: Idraparinux versus standard therapy for venous thromboembolic disease, *N Engl J Med* 357:1094-1104, 2007.

Verhovsek M et al: Systematic review: D-Dimer to predict recurrent disease after stopping anticoagulant therapy for unprovoked venous thromboembolism, *Ann Intern Med* 149:481-490, 2008.

AUTHOR: **FRED F. FERRI, M.D.**

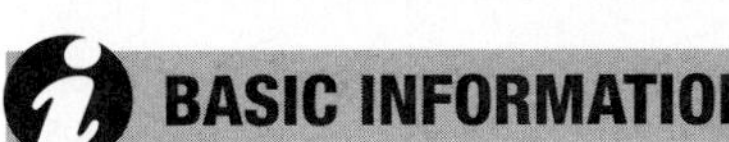

BASIC INFORMATION

DEFINITION

The key to delirium is that it has an acute/subacute onset. The American Psychiatric Association's *Diagnostic and Statistical Manual*, 4th edition (DSM-IV) defines delirium as:

A. Disturbance of consciousness (i.e., reduced clarity of awareness about the environment) with reduced ability to focus, sustain, or shift attention.
B. A change in cognition (e.g., memory deficit, disorientation, language disturbance) or development of a perceptual disturbance that is not better accounted for by a preexisting, established, or evolving dementia.
C. The disturbance develops over a short period of time (usually hours to days) and tends to fluctuate during the course of a day.
D. Evidence from the history, physical examination, or laboratory findings indicates that the disturbance is caused by direct physiologic consequences of a general medical condition.

SYNONYMS

Acute confusional state
Acute brain syndrome
Toxic or metabolic encephalopathy

ICD-9CM CODES
780.09 Delirium

EPIDEMIOLOGY & DEMOGRAPHICS

Approximately 10% to 30% of hospitalized patients experience delirium during the course of their treatment, but the rates can be even higher, especially in intensive care units where it can affect up to 60% to 80%. Risk factors include extremes of age, severe pain, illicit substance use, surgery, dementia, and kidney or liver failure.

PHYSICAL FINDINGS & CLINICAL PRESENTATION

- Pay particular attention to reversible causes for delirium.
- Start with a careful history, especially including the time course of the symptoms. Symptoms may differ both among and within one patient. Thus history from various caregivers may conflict because delirium implies a mental status that is frequently in flux. Symptoms may include poor attention, sleepiness, agitation, or psychosis. Take notice of new medications, recent surgeries or illnesses, and treatments.
- Next perform a physical examination focusing on signs of infection, dehydration, or chronic disease that may be exacerbated. Vital signs are key. Be sure to include the Mini-Mental Status Exam.

ETIOLOGY

Can be multifactorial; often falls into one of the following categories:

- Drugs: psychiatric and neurologic, narcotics, anticholinergics, beta-blockers, steroids, nonsteroidal anti-inflammatory drugs, digoxin, cimetidine
- Infection or inflammation: any, including abdominal processes
- Metabolic: kidney or liver failure, thyroid, adrenal or glucose dysregulation, anemia, vitamin deficiency
- Stress: surgery, sleep problems, pain, fever, hypoxia, anesthesia, environmental changes, fecal or urinary retention
- FEN: dysregulation of calcium, magnesium, potassium, or sodium; dehydration; volume overload; altered pH

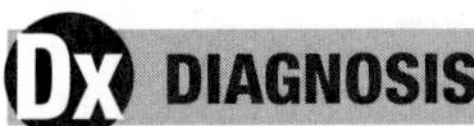

DIAGNOSIS

DIFFERENTIAL DIAGNOSIS

- Psychosis
- Dementia
- Depression or mania

LABORATORY TESTS

- Complete blood count, blood urea nitrogen, creatinine, and electrolytes
- Toxicology screen, liver function tests, ammonia
- Thyroid function tests, vitamin B_{12}, and folate levels
- Rapid plasma reagin for syphilis, blood, urine, and spinal culture
- Arterial blood gas measurement

IMAGING STUDIES

- Consider head CT (to look for bleed, trauma, tumor, atrophy, dementia, stroke)
- Chest radiograph (to look for tumor, infection)

Rx TREATMENT

NONPHARMACOLOGIC THERAPY

- The most important consideration is to keep the patient safe by using a variety of methods, including frequent reorientation.
- A quiet, restful, simplified environment with cues to time and location such as clock or calendar are helpful, as well as consistent staff providing both personal and medical care.
- Physical restraints if necessary to ensure safety.

ACUTE GENERAL Rx

- Reverse any treatable cause.
- Haloperidol can be used to control agitation, with doses ranging from 0.25 to 2 mg IM/IV twice daily, repeating the dose every 20 to 30 min until patient has calmed and using lower doses for the elderly.
- Risperidone 0.5 mg twice daily can also be used with a slow increase to desired dose.

CHRONIC Rx

Delirium is not a chronic condition; if assessing a more long-term mental status change, consider other diagnoses.

DISPOSITION

Requires frequent monitoring, often necessitating hospital level of care to ensure safety and assess etiology.

REFERRAL

Consider neurologic or psychiatric consultation if not improved in several days or in complicated cases.

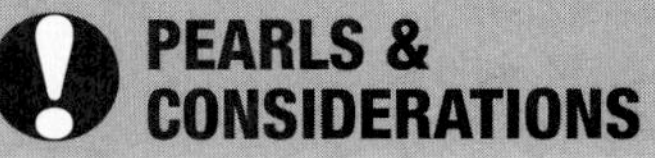

PEARLS & CONSIDERATIONS

COMMENTS

Although benzodiazepines are frequently used in hospitalized patients for sedation and are the mainstay of therapy for alcohol withdrawal, they must be used with caution in the elderly because they can have a paradoxic effect on agitation.

PREVENTION

- Avoid polypharmacy as much as possible.
- Optimize chronic medical conditions.
- Provide frequent reorientation and a soothing environment for high-risk patients (e.g., lights on during the day, off at night; open curtains during the day so patient can see the weather).
- A recent Cochrane review concluded more studies are needed to determine effective ways to prevent delirium.

PATIENT & FAMILY EDUCATION

Inform about the above preventative techniques, especially polypharmacy risks.

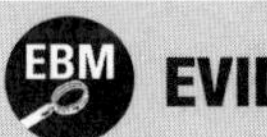

EVIDENCE

Please note: Complete text of EBM for this topic is available online.

SUGGESTED READINGS

American Psychiatric Association: *Diagnostic and statistical manual of mental disorders*, ed 4, Washington DC, 2000, American Psychiatric Association Press.

Gleason O: Delirium, *Am Fam Physician* 67:5, 2003.

Pandharipande P et al: Delirium: acute cognitive dysfunction in the critically ill, *Curr Opin Crit Care* 11, 2005.

Siddiqi N et al: Interventions for preventing delirium in hospitalized patients. *Cochrane Rev* 2, 2007.

AUTHOR: **CRISTINA ANTONIO PACHECO, M.D.**

Delirium Tremens

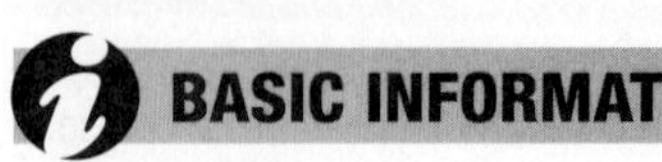

BASIC INFORMATION

DEFINITION

Delirium tremens is overactivity of the central nervous system after cessation of alcohol intake. The time interval is variable; it usually occurs within 1 wk after reduction or cessation of heavy alcohol intake and persists for 1 to 3 days.

SYNONYMS

Alcohol withdrawal syndrome
DTs
Alcoholic delirium

ICD-9CM CODES
291.00 Alcohol withdrawal delirium

EPIDEMIOLOGY & DEMOGRAPHICS

INCIDENCE (IN U.S.): Up to 500,000 cases annually
PEAK INCIDENCE: 30 yr and older
PREDOMINANT SEX: Male
PEAK AGE: Teenage years and older
GENETICS: More common with patients who have relatives who are alcoholics

PHYSICAL FINDINGS & CLINICAL PRESENTATION

- Initially: anxiety, insomnia, tremulousness
- Early: tachycardia, sweating, anorexia, agitation, headache, gastrointestinal distress
- Late: seizures, visual hallucinations, delirium

ETIOLOGY

Alcoholism

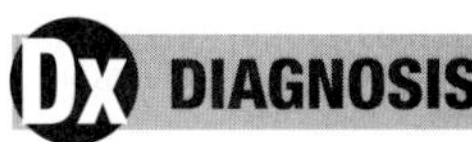

DIAGNOSIS

DIFFERENTIAL DIAGNOSIS

- Coexisting illness
- Trauma
- Drug use

WORKUP

- Frequent rating of symptoms (hallucinations, tremor, sweating, agitation, orientation).
- The Clinical Institute Withdrawal Assessment-Alcohol (CIWA-A) scale can be used to measure the severity of alcohol withdrawal. It consists of the 10 following items:
  1. Nausea
  2. Tremor
  3. Autonomic hyperactivity
  4. Anxiety
  5. Agitation
  6. Tactile disturbances
  7. Visual disturbances
  8. Auditory disturbances
  9. Headache
  10. Disorientation

The maximum score is 67.

LABORATORY TESTS

- Electrolytes (including magnesium, phosphate)
- Close monitoring of glucose levels
- Drug screen (blood and urine)

IMAGING STUDIES

CT scan of head if there is a history of head trauma.

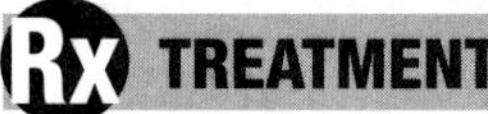

TREATMENT

NONPHARMACOLOGIC THERAPY

Refer to drug rehabilitation program after patient recovers.

ACUTE GENERAL Rx

1. Admission to a detoxification unit where patient can be observed closely.
2. Vital signs q30min initially (neurologic signs, if necessary).
3. Use of lateral decubitus or prone position if restraints are necessary.
4. Nothing by mouth: nasogastric tube for abdominal distention may be necessary but should not be routinely used.
5. Vigorous hydration (4 to 6 L/day): IV with glucose (Na^+, K^+, PO_4^{-3}, and Mg^{2+} replacement). Use with caution in patients with CHF.
6. Vitamins: thiamine 100 mg IV qd. The initial dose of thiamine should precede the administration of IV dextrose; multivitamins (may be added to the hydrating solution).
7. Sedation:
   a. Initially: lorazepam 2 to 5 mg IM/IV repeated prn
   b. Maintenance (individualized dosage): chlordiazepoxide, 50 to 100 mg PO q4-6h, lorazepam 2 mg PO q4h, or diazepam 5 to 10 mg PO tid; withhold doses or decrease subsequent doses if signs of oversedation are apparent.
   c. Midazolam is also effective for managing DTs. Its rapid onset (sedation within 2 to 4 min of IV injection) and short duration of action (approximately 30 min) make it an ideal agent for titration in continuous infusion.
8. Treatment of seizures: diazepam 2.5 mg/min IV until seizure is controlled (check for respiratory depression or hypotension) may be beneficial for prolonged seizure activity; IV lorazepam 1 to 2 mg q2h can be used in place of diazepam. In general, withdrawal seizures are self-limited and treatment is not required; the use of phenytoin or other anticonvulsants for short-term treatment of alcohol withdrawal seizures is not recommended.
9. Diagnosis and treatment of concomitant medical, surgical, or psychiatric conditions.

CHRONIC Rx

Alcoholics Anonymous has the best record in breaking addiction, but the results are still disappointing.

DISPOSITION

Refer to drug rehabilitation program.

REFERRAL

If cardiac arrhythmias are prominent or respiratory distress develops

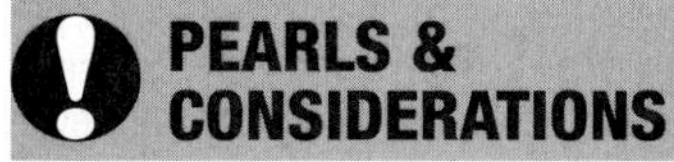

PEARLS & CONSIDERATIONS

COMMENTS

This is a potentially lethal disease if not carefully treated. Mortality rate is 15% in untreated patients.

SUGGESTED READING

Kosten TR, O'Connor PG: Management of drug and alcohol withdrawal, *N Engl J Med* 348:1786, 2003.

AUTHOR: **FRED F. FERRI, M.D.**

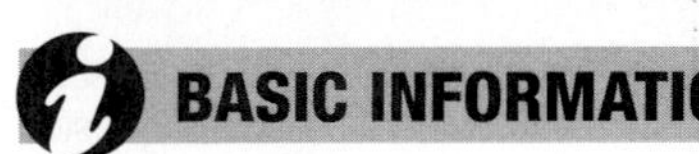

BASIC INFORMATION

DEFINITION

A progressive neurodegenerative disease with core features of dementia accompanied or followed by parkinsonism.

SYNONYMS

Diffuse Lewy body disease, dementia with parkinsonism

ICD-9CM CODES
331.82 Dementia with Lewy bodies (DLB)

EPIDEMIOLOGY & DEMOGRAPHICS

- Now thought to be the second most common primary degenerative dementia, accounting for 10% to 15% of cases at autopsy
- Prevalence at age 65 estimated at 0.7%; at age 85 rises to 5.0%

PHYSICAL FINDINGS & CLINICAL PRESENTATION

- Dementia typically precedes appearance of parkinsonism by months to years. Occasionally parkinsonism precedes dementia; especially in this case there is clinical overlap between DLB and Parkinson's disease with dementia (PDD). There is debate whether DLB and PDD are actually a spectrum of the same disease, as pathologic findings are quite similar.
- Dementia is superficially quite similar to Alzheimer's disease. Early visual hallucinations (outside the setting of dopaminergic therapy) occur in up to 80% and are the major differentiating feature from AD. Typically the hallucinations are well formed and detailed.
- Fluctuations in performance, especially with regards to attention and alertness, are another key feature of the presentation. Can occur acutely, leading to misdiagnosis of vascular dementia presenting with stroke. These fluctuations may last hours or days.
- Parkinsonism is typically symmetrical and axially predominant, with little tremor but prominent gait impairment and postural instability.
- Parkinsonism is not ubiquitous; up to 25% of cases diagnosed by autopsy had mild or no reported parkinsonian features.
- Rapid eye movement (REM) sleep behavior disorder and other related sleep abnormalities are common.

ETIOLOGY

- Uncertain; it is felt that DLB probably results from abnormal alpha-synuclein with resulting aggregation of the protein inside neurons.
- Lewy bodies are eosinophilic intracellular inclusions, which contain alpha-synuclein and ubiquitin; it is not clear whether they are pathogenic.

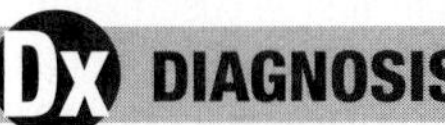

DIAGNOSIS

DIFFERENTIAL DIAGNOSIS

- Parkinson's disease dementia (PDD)—differentiated from DLB in which dementia usually precedes parkinsonism. A somewhat arbitrary "1-year" rule is sometimes used to differentiate DLB from PDD in that if dementia presents within first year after the parkinsonism, DLB can still be diagnosed.
- Alzheimer's disease (AD)—differs from DLB in which visual hallucinations and parkinsonism are prominent.
- Atypical parkinsonian syndromes (multiple systems atrophy, progressive supranuclear palsy, corticobasal degeneration)—these syndromes have other features such as cerebellar degeneration, supranuclear gaze palsy, or asymmetrical limb apraxia that are not seen in DLB.
- Vascular dementia—differs from DLB in that despite the fluctuations in performance seen in DLB, there is no clear history of multiple strokes.
- Frontotemporal dementia (FTD, a.k.a. Pick's disease).
- Creutzfeldt-Jacob disease (CJD)—differs from DLB in that it is usually more rapidly progressive, can have cerebellar signs and symptoms, and often has distinctive EEG abnormalities.
- Toxic/metabolic/pharmacologic-related delirium.

WORKUP

- Diagnosis is largely clinical.
- Although dementia may be clinically similar to AD, detailed neuropsychologic testing can be helpful in bringing out prominent frontosubcortical and visuospatial deficits more typical of DLB.

LABORATORY TESTS

- Routine blood tests are normal but should be done to rule out treatable causes of dementia (e.g., B_{12}, TSH). In the setting of a fluctuation in performance, laboratory studies to rule out metabolic causes of delirium are appropriate.
- Spinal fluid analysis is normal; this may be helpful in more rapidly progressive cases if CJD is suspected.
- EEG may be helpful in the setting of fluctuations in performance to look for subclinical status epilepticus or other evidence of seizures, or if CJD is suspected.

IMAGING STUDIES

- Brain MRI is indicated mostly to look for multiple prior strokes suggestive of vascular dementia. In the setting of a sudden deterioration in performance, MRI with diffusion-weighted imaging may be needed to rule out acute stroke.
- Conventional neuroimaging is not diagnostic of DLB. Functional neuroimaging such as PET and SPECT show promise but are not yet routinely indicated or available.

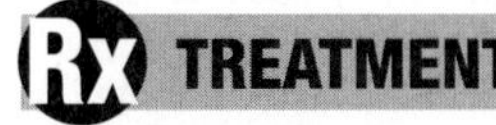

TREATMENT

NONPHARMACOLOGIC THERAPY

Dementia-care education with physical and occupational therapy may be of benefit to both patients and caregivers.

ACUTE GENERAL Rx

None available

CHRONIC Rx

- Treatment of parkinsonism with levodopa can be partially successful, but because of risk of hallucinations the lowest effective dose should be used.
- Cholinesterase inhibitors are modestly effective for treating cognitive impairment (possibly better than in AD), as well as hallucinations, sleep impairments, and anxiety.
- Antipsychotic medications are helpful in treating hallucinations; however, older neuroleptic agents should be avoided in favor of low doses of newer "atypical" antipsychotics.

DISPOSITION

Median survival similar to AD.

REFERRAL

Referral to a general neurologist, dementia specialist, or movement disorders center is appropriate.

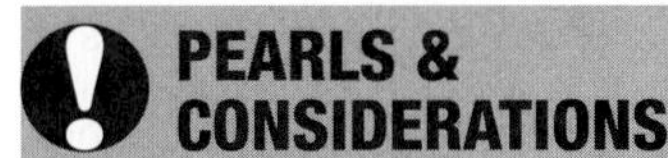

PEARLS & CONSIDERATIONS

COMMENTS

- REM sleep behavior disorder is common in DLB (as it is in PD and multiple systems atrophy) but uncommon in Alzheimer's disease and frontotemporal dementia.
- DLB patients are unusually susceptible to extrapyramidal reactions to traditional neuroleptics, with sensitivity reactions in up to 50% of patients.

PREVENTION

None known

AUTHOR: **DAVID P. WILLIAMS, M.D.**

BASIC INFORMATION

DEFINITION

Dengue fever (DF) is an infectious disease endemic in most tropical and subtropical countries (Fig. 1-85). The causative agent is the dengue virus, a single positive-stranded RNA virus of the Flaviviridae family, which has four distinct but closely related serotypes (DEN-1, DEN-2, DEN-3, DEN-4). Dengue virus is transmitted by the *Aedes* mosquito, principally *Aedes aegypti*.

SYNONYMS

Classic dengue fever
Dengue hemorrhagic fever
Dengue shock syndrome

ICD-9CM CODES
061 Dengue
065.4 Mosquito-borne hemorrhagic fever

EPIDEMIOLOGY & DEMOGRAPHICS

INCIDENCE: Attack rates during epidemics range from 1 to 10/1000.

PEAK INCIDENCE: In hyperendemic countries, rates among children are as high as 22 to 292 per 1000 per yr.

PREVALENCE: Worldwide, more than 50 million cases of dengue infection are diagnosed yearly. DF is confirmed in up to 8% of febrile travelers returning from the tropics.

PREDOMINANT AGE: All ages are susceptible.

RISK FACTORS: Travel to endemic regions. Locally acquired cases have been reported in Mexico, Hawaii, and Texas.

ETIOLOGY

After bite by infected mosquito, the virus replicates in regional lymph nodes, then spreads by blood and the lymphatic system to other tissues. Incubation period is typically 4 to 7 days (range, 3 to 14 days). Most important risk factors for development of severe disease (dengue hemorrhagic fever/dengue shock syndrome [DHF/DSS]) are age, viral genotype, genetic background of the host, and prior infection. Majority of DHF/DSS cases occur during secondary heterologous (different from first exposure) infection, in which T memory cells from the primary infection are preferentially expanded because of a lower threshold of activation compared with naïve T cells of higher affinity to the current serotype. This results in suboptimal clearance of the virus and quicker, more robust cytokine production leading to changes in vascular permeability and plasma leakage. Severe disease during primary infection is most commonly seen in infants in whom DENV-specific antibodies transferred transplacentally from their DENV-immune mothers facilitate viral entry into cells through an antibody-dependent enhancement mechanism, increasing viral load and inducing immune activation.

PHYSICAL FINDINGS & CLINICAL PRESENTATION

Clinical presentation ranges from asymptomatic infection to shock syndrome and vary according to age of patient and previous infection with dengue virus.

Symptomatic DF infection can be classified into three categories:

1. Undifferentiated fever
2. Classic DF: characterized by acute febrile illness accompanied by symptoms such as headache, retroorbital pain, fatigue, mild respiratory and gastrointestinal symptoms, and myalgias/arthralgias ("break bone fever"); DF usually follows an incubation period of 3 to 14 days and fever typically lasts 5 to 7 days; physical findings may include a maculopapular rash, lymphadenopathy, pharyngeal erythema, and injected conjunctivae; some patients may experience development of hemorrhagic manifestations with petechiae, purpura, and rarely, epistaxis, gum bleeding, and gastrointestinal bleeding; during pregnancy, DF has been associated with increased risk for premature labor and birth, uterine hemorrhage, intrautero death, neonatal death, and maternofetal transmission
3. DHF/DSS: occurs in less than 3% of infected individuals; early course is similar to presentation of classic dengue, but 4 to 7 days after onset of illness, plasma leakage with hemorrhagic manifestations develops; plasma leakage may result in hypoproteinemia, peripheral edema, ascites, and pleural and cardiac effusions, and is suggested by a hematocrit increase of 20% during course of illness; thrombocytopenia is also a hallmark, with resultant clinical manifestations such as petechiae, echymosis, mucosal hemorrhage, and GI bleeding; may progress to DSS with circulatory collapse, including rapid/weak pulse, profound hypotension, and pulse pressure of <20 mm Hg; warning signs for DHF/DSS include abdominal pain, persistent vomiting, abrupt defervescence, change in mental status, and respiratory distress

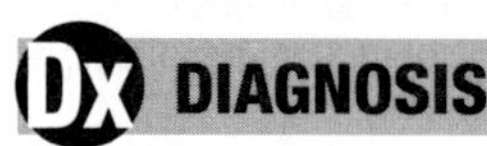

DIAGNOSIS

DIFFERENTIAL DIAGNOSIS

- Influenza
- Measles
- Rubella
- Epstein-Barr virus
- West Nile virus
- HIV conversion
- Malaria
- Typhoid
- Leptospirosis
- Chikungunya
- Rickettsial diseases
- Early severe acute respiratory syndrome
- Other viral hemorrhagic fevers

DHF is defined by the following World Health Organization (WHO) criteria:

1. Fever lasting 2 to 7 days
2. Hemorrhagic tendency (spontaneous bleeding or positive tourniquet test)
3. Thrombocytopenia
4. Evidence of plasma leakage

WORKUP

- Suspicion for DF based on travel, exposure history, and clinical presentation
- Tourniquet test can be performed to look for hemorrhagic manifestations; inflate blood pressure cuff midway between systolic and diastolic blood pressure for 5 min; the test result is positive when more than 20 petechial hemorrhages per square inch are counted on the forearm

LABORATORY TESTS

- CBC, liver function tests, chemistries
- Additional laboratory tests based on differential diagnoses (e.g., malaria smears, monospot/Epstein-Barr virus titers, HIV testing)
- With compatible exposure history and symptom profile, positive anti–dengue IgM suggests recent infection, whereas positive anti–dengue IgG may indicate past infection
- Confirm diagnosis with a fourfold increase of IgG and IgM between acute (<6 days after illness onset) and convalescence titers; IgM capture enzyme-linked immunosorbent as-

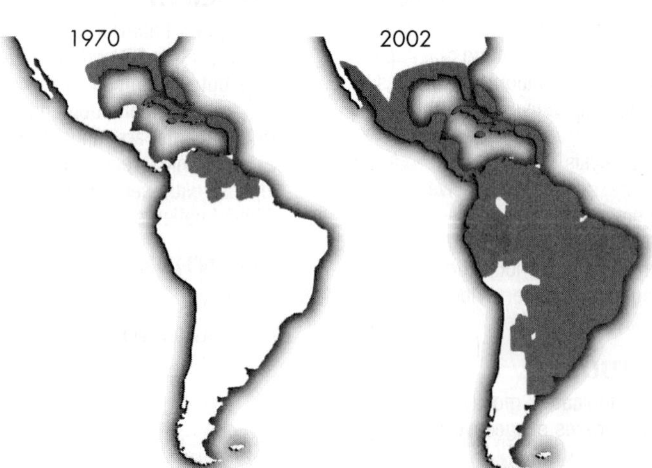

FIGURE 1-85 Distribution of *Aedes aegypti* in the Americas in 1970 (at the end of the mosquito eradication program) and in 2002. (Source: CDC and PAHO; from Mandell GL et al: *Principles and practice of infectious diseases,* ed 6, Philadelphia, 2005, Elsevier.)

say (ELISA) commonly used, but test is negative early in the course of disease
- Identification of DENV from serum by reverse transcriptase polymerase chain reaction

IMAGING STUDIES

As dictated by clinical course

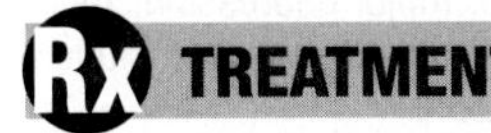

TREATMENT

No specific pharmacologic treatment for dengue.

NONPHARMACOLOGIC THERAPY

- Treatment is based on supportive measures.
- Mortality rate from DHS/DSS is improved by early and correct fluid replacement.

ACUTE GENERAL Rx

- Monitor platelet count and hematocrit at least daily.
- Patients with platelet counts $<$100,000 have increased risk for DHF and should be monitored as inpatients.
- Hematocrit increase of 20% suggests substantial plasma loss for which patients should be admitted for intensive care and intravenous fluid replacement.
- Fever should be managed with acetaminophen; aspirin and NSAIDs should be avoided because of their anticoagulant properties.

DISPOSITION

- Classic dengue is usually self-limiting and rarely fatal.
- Of an estimated 500,000 cases of DHF/DSS admitted early, the mortality rate is approximately 2.5%.
- Mortality rate for DHF/DSS is as high as 20% without proper treatment but decreases to $<$1% with prompt recognition and appropriate treatment.

REFERRAL

- Infectious disease consultation for suspicion of DF
- Referral/transfer to center experienced with DHF/DSS if available

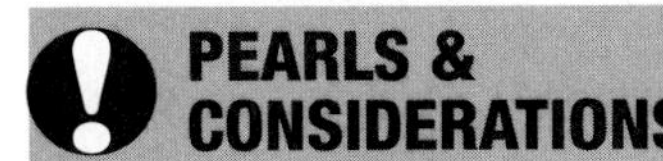

PEARLS & CONSIDERATIONS

COMMENTS

- Health care providers should consider dengue infection in any traveler returning from endemic areas who presents with fever.
- Given the incubation period, dengue infection can be ruled out if onset of symptoms begins 2 wk after individual leaves endemic area.
- Asymptomatic dengue infections are common; however, immunity that results from primary infection increases the risk for DHF/DSS during subsequent infections.
- Serologic testing is complicated by cross-reactions with over flaviviruses (including vaccines for yellow fever and Japanese encephalitis).
- Contact the Dengue Branch at the Centers for Disease Control and Prevention for additional information and testing (http://www.cdc.gov/ncidod/dvbid/misc/db.htm).

PREVENTION

- There is no vaccine for dengue.
- For travelers, the most effective preventive measure is avoidance of mosquito bites by using protective clothing and insect repellents containing DEET.
- *Aedes* mosquitoes primarily bite during the day and typically live indoors.

SUGGESTED READINGS

Basurko C et al: Maternal and fetal consequences of dengue fever during pregnancy, *Eur J Obstet Gynecol Reprod Biol* 147:29-32, 2009.

Freedman DO et al; for the GeoSentinel Surveillance Network: Spectrum of disease and relation to place of exposure among ill returned travelers, *N Eng J Med* 354:119, 2006.

Mathew A, Rothman A: Understanding the contribution of cellular immunity to dengue disease pathogenesis, *Immunological Reviews* 225:300, 2008.

Tomashek K: Dengue fever (DF) and dengue hemorrhagic fever (DHF), CDC traveler's health yellow book. Available at http://wwwn.cdc.gov/travel/yellowbook/2010/chapter-5. Accessed Sept 2009.

Wider-Smith A, Schwartz E: Dengue in travelers, *N Engl J Med* 353:924, 2005.

World Health Organization: Dengue and dengue hemorrhagic fever. Available at http://www.who.int/mediacentre/factsheets/fs117/en. Accessed Sept 2009.

AUTHORS: **VALERIA FABRE, M.D., CLAUDIA RODRIGUEZ CABRERA, M.D.,** and **JOSEPH DIAZ, M.D.**

Dependent Personality Disorder

BASIC INFORMATION

DEFINITION

Dependent personality disorder (DPD) is characterized by a pervasive and excessive need to be taken care of that leads to submissive and clinging behavior and fears of separation. DPD begins by early adulthood and causes significant distress or impairment in multiple domains of functioning. Individuals must meet five or more of the following criteria:

1. Difficulty making routine decisions without an excessive amount of advice and reassurance from others.
2. Need others to assume responsibility for most major areas of their life.
3. Difficulty expressing disagreement with others because of fear of loss of support or approval.
4. Difficulty initiating or completing projects on own because of a lack of self-confidence in abilities rather than lack of motivation or energy.
5. Excessive attempts to obtain nurturance and support from others.
6. Feel uncomfortable or helpless when alone because of exaggerated fears of being unable to care for self.
7. Urgently seek another relationship when a close relationship ends.
8. Unrealistically preoccupied with being left to take care of self.

SYNONYMS

None

ICD-9CM CODES
301.6

EPIDEMIOLOGY & DEMOGRAPHICS

PREVALENCE: 0.5% in general population. Dependent traits, as opposed to the disorder itself, are among the most frequently reported in outpatient mental health clinics.

PREDOMINANT SEX: Female (2:1) in clinical settings.

CLINICAL PRESENTATION

- Early onset and chronic course. Impairment is frequently mild.
- On interview, will defer excessively to partner or parent.
- Indecision in routine decisions.
- Depend on a parent or spouse to decide where they should live, work, and recreate and who they should befriend.
- Need for others to function for them goes beyond age-appropriate and situation-appropriate requests for assistance.
- Will agree with objectionable opinions, submit to unreasonable requests, and not express appropriate anger or disappointment for fear of alienating the person without whom they believe they cannot function.
- Convinced that they are not capable of independent function and present themselves as inept.
- Often do not develop independent living skills, perpetuating their dependency.
- Social relations tend to be limited to those few people on whom the person depends.

ETIOLOGY

Chronic physical illness or separation anxiety disorder may predispose for DPD.

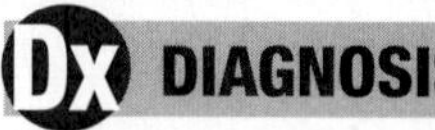

DIAGNOSIS

DIFFERENTIAL DIAGNOSIS

- Dependency and personality changes arising as a consequence of an Axis I disorder.
- Dependency arising as a consequence of a general medical condition.
- Most common comorbid Axis I conditions are major depressive and other mood disorders, anxiety disorders, including social phobia, and adjustment disorder.
- Most common comorbid personality disorders are histrionic, avoidant, and borderline. Each of these disorders is characterized by dependent features. DPD is distinguished by its predominantly submissive, reactive, and clinging behavior.

WORKUP

- History: collateral information is essential to establishing the presence of longstanding interpersonal pattern in multiple domains of the patient's life.
- Physical examination.
- Mental status examination.

LABORATORY TESTS

Tests necessary to rule out medical causes of personality changes

IMAGING STUDIES

Tests necessary to rule out medical causes of personality changes

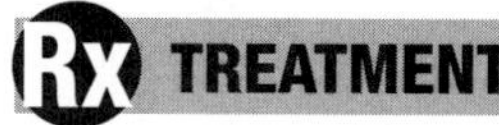

TREATMENT

NONPHARMACOLOGIC THERAPY

- Cognitive-behavioral and psychodynamic psychotherapy to diminish and better contain anxiety and to help patients develop sense of self as competent and requisite assertiveness skills
- Psychodynamic psychotherapy to help develop improved self-concept and interpersonal functioning

ACUTE GENERAL Rx

Benzodiazepines to control highly anxious states

CHRONIC Rx

- Selective serotonin reuptake inhibitors (SSRIs) and selective serotonin-norepinephrine reuptake inhibitors (SNRIs) for anxiety
- SSRIs and SNRIs for comorbid depression, social phobia, other anxiety disorders, and agoraphobia

DISPOSITION

- Chronic course; severity is variable
- Impairments often mild
- At increased risk for major depression, social phobia, and other anxiety disorders, including panic and agoraphobia

REFERRAL

- If pharmacotherapy or psychotherapy is contemplated
- If patient's functioning is impaired

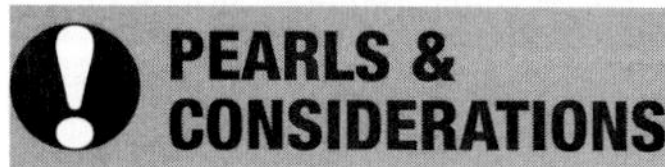

PEARLS & CONSIDERATIONS

COMMENTS

- DPD patients fear illness will lead to abandonment by others.
- This fear of simultaneous helplessness and abandonment intensifies neediness and may lead to dramatic demands for urgent medical attention.
- When physicians do not respond as wanted, angry outbursts may ensue.
- Medical care can also become a means by which dependency needs are met. As a result, some of these patients may unconsciously or consciously prolong their illness for primary gain.
- Physicians often react to the extreme neediness with avoidance or overengagement, leading to burnout.
- Management guidelines:
  1. Overall strategy is to provide reassurance and allay fear of abandonment.
  2. Specific strategies include scheduling frequent visits, noncontingent care (i.e., scheduling visits regardless of whether ill or not).
  3. Establish firm and realistic limits to availability as early as possible in treatment.
  4. Enlist other members of health care team for support.
  5. Encourage patient to develop additional "outside" support systems.

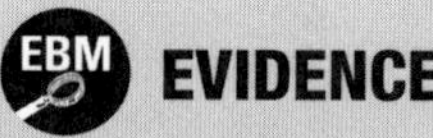

EVIDENCE

Please note: Complete text of EBM for this topic is available online.

SUGGESTED READINGS

Livesley J: Integrated therapy for complex cases of personality disorder, *J Clin Psychol* 64(2):207-221, 2008.

Ward RK: Assessment and management of personality disorders, *Am Fam Physician* 15;70(8):1505-1512, 2004.

AUTHOR: **JOHN Q. YOUNG, M.D., M.P.P.**

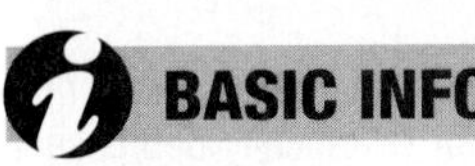

BASIC INFORMATION

DEFINITION

Major depression is an episodic, frequently recurring syndrome. Diagnosis of major depression requires that five of nine symptoms be present daily for 2 wk. One of these nine symptoms must be either a persistent depressed mood and/or pervasive anhedonia (loss of interest or pleasure in living). Other symptoms include sleep disorder (insomnia or hypersomnia), appetite loss/gain or weight loss/gain, fatigue, psychomotor retardation or agitation, difficulty concentrating, feelings of guilt or low self-esteem, and recurrent thoughts of death or suicidal ideation.

SYNONYMS

Unipolar affective disorder
Melancholia
Manic-depressive illness, depressed type
Depressive episode

ICD-9CM CODES
296.2
296.3
311

EPIDEMIOLOGY & DEMOGRAPHICS

LIFETIME RISK (IN U.S.): 10% of men, 20% of women
PREVALENCE (IN U.S.): Point prevalence in a community sample is 3% of men, 4.5% to 9.3% of women, and 1% of children. Prevalence of 20% to 40% in patients with comorbid medical conditions.
PREDOMINANT SEX: Female/male ratio 2:1
PREDOMINANT AGE: 25 to 44 yr; 5% of adolescents
PEAK INCIDENCE: 30 to 40 yr; 13% of postpartum women
GENETICS:
- Clear evidence of familial predominance
- Prevalence is two to three times greater among first-degree relatives of patients with major depression
- Concordance among monozygotic twins approximately 50%
- No established pattern of inheritance

PHYSICAL FINDINGS & CLINICAL PRESENTATION

- Clinical evaluation can be facilitated by organizing the major symptoms into four hallmarks: (1) depressed mood, (2) anhedonia, (3) physical symptoms (sleep disorder, appetite problem, fatigue, psychomotor changes), and (4) psychologic symptoms (difficulty concentrating or indecisiveness, guilt or low self-esteem, and hopelessness).
- A stressful life event, typically a serious loss, may trigger a depressive episode; however, the presence or absence of identifiable precipitants is irrelevant to the diagnosis of major depression.
- Patients often present with somatic complaints such as pain, fatigue, insomnia, dizziness, headache, or gastrointestinal problems.
- May be associated with mood-congruent delusional thinking (paranoid and melancholic themes) in approximately 15% of individuals.
- May be associated with active or passive suicidal ideation.
- Serious misconduct may appear in adolescents.
- Major depression may be misdiagnosed in elderly patients, with signs and symptoms attributed to normal aging.

ETIOLOGY

- Major depression is a heterogeneous group of disorders probably arising from a variety of etiologic determinants.
- Genetic and family experiences both play roles, though neither is a determining factor.
- Significant psychosocial stressors, especially involving loss, often trigger depression.
- Numerous biologic markers have been identified, including endocrine and central nervous system factors, though none is considered causative.

Dx DIAGNOSIS

DIFFERENTIAL DIAGNOSIS

- Other mental disorders such as anxiety disorders, somatoform disorders, obsessive-compulsive disorder, substance abuse, and personality disorders often present with symptoms similar to depression.
- Important to distinguish between a depressive episode occurring as part of a major depression and a depressive episode that is part of bipolar disorder.
- Approximately 10% to 15% of depression is caused by general medical illness. General medical conditions with high prevalence of depression include Alzheimer's disease, Parkinson's disease, stroke, end-stage renal failure, cardiac disease, HIV infection, and cancer.
- Some medical conditions can present as depression, such as hypothyroidism or hyperthyroidism and neurosyphilis.
- Premenstrual dysphoric disorder.
- In elderly patients, depression often coexists with dementia.

WORKUP

- A careful medical history is required
- Physical examination reveals no specific diagnostic signs of depression
- Mental status examination
- The Patient Health Questionnaire (PHQ-9) has documented high sensitivity and specificity for the diagnosis of depression (http://www.depression-primarycare.org)

LABORATORY TESTS

- No laboratory studies can definitively diagnose depression.
- The following can be done to rule out other major organ system disease:
  1. Routine blood chemistry evaluation
  2. CBC with differential
  3. Thyroid function studies
  4. Vitamin B_{12} levels

IMAGING STUDIES

With unusual presentations (e.g., associated with new-onset severe headache, focal neurologic signs, a cognitive or sensory disturbance), the following may be performed:
- EEG (diffuse slowing indicates metabolic encephalopathy)
- Anatomic brain imaging (CT scan or MRI)

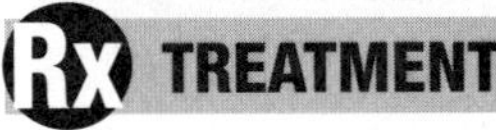

TREATMENT

NONPHARMACOLOGIC THERAPY

- Good evidence that cognitive-behavioral therapy is as effective as antidepressant medication in achieving a significant reduction or remission of depression.
- Problem solving and interpersonal psychotherapies have efficacy rates of 50% to 60%.
- By 12 wk, psychotherapy and medication are equally effective.
- Patients with severe symptoms should generally not be treated exclusively with nonpharmacological therapy.

ACUTE GENERAL Rx

- The patient's concurrent medical or psychiatric illnesses, history of prior response, cost, and side effects should be taken into account when selecting an initial treatment.
- Antidepressants are effective in approximately 60% to 70% of cases.
- Selective serotonin reuptake inhibitors (SSRIs) generally are first-line agents.
- According to the STAR-D trial, approximately one third of patients achieve remission with the first prescribed medication. Treatment-refractory patients should be switched to another SSRI or to another class of medication, offered adjunctive medication such as bupropion, or referred for evidence-based counseling. Approximately 25% more patients will achieve remission with this secondary intervention.
- Therapy should be continued for 4 to 9 mo after the full remission of symptoms.
- Electroconvulsive therapy is the most effective means available for the treatment of severe, refractory depression.

CHRONIC Rx

Long-term treatment, in some cases, lifelong treatment, is recommended for individuals with multiple depressive episodes, a severe episode or significant suicidality, or a strong family history of severe depression or bipolar disorder.

DISPOSITION

- Major depression is a relapsing and remitting illness characterized by recurrent episodes for many patients.
- Physical symptoms predict a favorable response to biologic intervention.
- Additional episodes are experienced by >50% of individuals having one depressive episode.

- Without treatment, episodes last an average of 6 to 12 mo; risk of recurrence is higher without treatment.

REFERRAL

- If treatment refractory
- If patient suicidal or psychotic
- For suspected bipolar depression

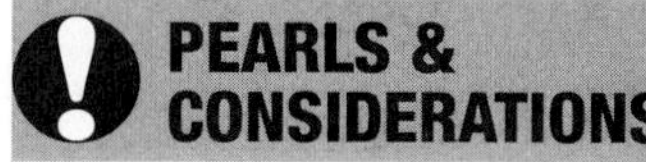

PEARLS & CONSIDERATIONS

COMMENTS

All threats of suicide should be taken very seriously. Clinicians can use the mnemonic SAL: Is the method ***s***pecific? Is it ***a***vailable? Is it ***l***ethal?

- Rule out bipolar affective disorder before initiating treatment with an antidepressant medication.
- Many patients and families are reluctant to accept the diagnosis of depression because of associated stigma.
- A two-question screener is as effective as longer screening instruments. A positive answer to one of the following two questions should lead to a full diagnostic assessment for depression.
    1. Over the past 2 weeks, have you ever felt down, depressed, or hopeless?
    2. Over the past 2 weeks, have you felt little interest or pleasure in doing things?

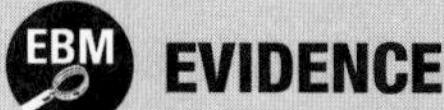

EVIDENCE

Please note: Complete text of EBM for this topic is available online.

Key trials and commentary:

There is a paucity of controlled trials examining the efficacy of brief dynamic psychotherapy (BDT) in the treatment of major depressive disorder, especially in a long-term perspective. The aim of this study was to evaluate recurrence rates in unipolar major depressed patients who are responsive to acute phase combined treatment with BDT plus pharmacotherapy in comparison with patients initially treated with pharmacotherapy alone.

This study showed that the significant lower recurrence rates in a 48-month follow-up in the group of patients treated with the addition of BDT to medication in the acute phase support the view of the advantage in the long-term outcome of adding psychotherapeutic intervention to pharmacotherapy in the acute therapy of unipolar major depression.

What is particularly valuable about this study is that it represents treatment as it is frequently practiced, yet rarely studied. There are far too few studies of psychodynamic psychotherapy, although this is one of the main treatment modalities that are taught, particularly in psychiatry and social work programs. (Cognitive-behavioral therapy tends to be the primary modality taught in many clinical psychology programs.) The other main strength is the assessment of patients over the course of 48 months, a very long-term follow-up compared with most studies.

Although the selection of patients who have had only a unipolar single episode with complete remission to acute treatment is a good selection in terms of the credibility of research findings, it poses a problem of generalizability. Given the recurrent nature of depression, many patients who seek care for depression have a history of previous episodes and many have residual symptoms.

An interesting feature of this study was that the number of sessions, which ranged from 15 to 30, was determined at intake by the therapist on the basis of focus characteristics. It's not clear how the therapist could determine at intake how many sessions a given patient would need because this is typically a conclusion that a therapist would reach after working with a patient for a while. The other usual course of action for a research study would be to predetermine that every research participant receives the same number of sessions. It is also curious that the number of brief dynamic therapy sessions ranged from 15 to 30. Proponents of this type of treatment (e.g., Mann, Horowitz) propose a 12-session model. Theorists such as Habib Davanloo will use as many as 30 sessions, but typically only for patients with entrenched character disorders. It would have been useful to know more about how the researchers determined their length of treatment.

Studies such as this one would be useful for consideration for an update of treatment guidelines for primary care providers. In their guidelines, it is recommended that patients not receive referrals for psychotherapy until 2 antidepressant medications have been tried. Given the long-term advantage of adding dynamic psychotherapy to medication, it would be helpful to make such referrals much sooner.[1] Ⓐ

Clinical guidelines recommend the combination of pharmacotherapy and psychotherapy for the treatment of chronic depression, although there are only a few studies supporting an additive effect of psychotherapy.

This study showed that intensive combined treatment provides superior acute and long-term effects over standard treatment in chronically depressed inpatients.

Although there is ample evidence that IPT is efficacious in the treatment of acute depression, including severe cases (e.g., Elkin et al, 1989), IPT has not been shown to be more effective than medication in studies of patients with chronic depression. In addition, most, if not all, studies of IPT have been conducted in outpatient settings. This study is remarkable in that it shows evidence of significantly greater gains in chronically depressed inpatients who received IPT plus medication than in patients who received CM and medication. In addition, the greater treatment gains were maintained over a 1-year period. This is an impressive showing for the use of adapted IPT for chronically depressed patients in inpatient settings.

The authors raise some interesting points about the different responses of chronically depressed patients in this study vs. earlier studies. They note that most previous trials of psychotherapy for chronic depression included only dysthymic patients, whereas this study included predominantly severely depressed patients. Thus, the patient populations are different. In addition, previous studies used standard IPT, whereas this study adapted the treatment for this population, using a combination of individual and group treatment. Most patients in this study also continued medication and/or psychotherapy after hospital discharge, whereas previous studies used a short-term model of treatment.

As the authors note, one reason for the differential response may be that therapists spent a good deal more time with IPT patients than the patients who received CM. IPT patients received treatment that was the length of a full psychotherapy session, whereas the CM patients saw their therapists for only 15 to 20 minutes. This means that clinical management patients received only one half or one third the amount of time with their clinicians as those being treated with IPT.

Although this study provides useful information, it is doubtful that IPT will be added to many inpatient regimens. An important caveat is that this study was conducted in Germany, a country with a health care system that is quite different from that in the U.S. Given that many inpatients in the U.S. spend only a few days in the hospital, it is unlikely that many units would have the time or the resources to implement a program with as intensive a psychotherapy program as this study recommends.[2] Ⓐ

In the population at large, regular exercise is associated with reduced anxious and depressive symptoms. Results of experimental studies in clinical populations suggest a causal effect of exercise on anxiety and depression, but it is unclear whether such a causal effect also drives the population association. We cannot exclude the major contribution of a third underlying factor influencing exercise behavior and symptoms of anxiety and depression.

This study sought to test causal effects of exercise on anxious and depressive symptoms in a population-based sample.

This study showed that regular exercise is associated with reduced anxious and depressive symptoms in the population at large, but the association is not because of causal effects of exercise.

Ever since the running boom of the 1970s, there has been a belief in the running and psychiatric running communities that exercise can help, indeed perhaps cure depression. Because of this belief, and what I had thought before now were published studies, a well-known New York runner-psychiatrist used to take his depressed patients running in Central Park. So when I read in the *New York Times* that the *Archives of General Psychiatry* had published this study I was dumbstruck. How could so many have gotten it so wrong for all these years? What the authors call "folk wisdom" was more than that; it was a belief system. Now I wonder what it was about running with patients that worked? Was it sunshine, being with one's psychiatrist in an out-of-the-office experience, or just wishful thinking? This raises a question in selecting and rating articles such as these, which may be more suitable to *Runner's World* than the *Archives of General Psychiatry*—just because a finding smashes a widely held belief, is it important?[3] Ⓐ

Evidence-Based References

1. Maina G et al: Brief dynamic therapy combined with pharmacotherapy in the treatment of major depressive disorder: long-term results, *J Affect Disord* 114:200-207, 2009. Commentary by J.L. Krupnick, Ph.D. Ⓐ

2. Schramm E et al: Efficacy of interpersonal psychotherapy plus pharmacotherapy in chronically depressed inpatients, *J Affect Disord* 109:65-73, 2008. Commentary by J.L. Krupnick, Ph.D. Ⓐ

3. De Moor MHM et al: Testing causality in the association between regular exercise and symptoms of anxiety and depression, *Arch Gen Psychiatry* 65:897-905, 2008. Commentary by J.A. Talbott, M.D. Ⓐ

SUGGESTED READINGS

Belmaker RH, Agam G: Major depressive disorder, *N Engl J Med* 358:55-68, 2008.

Feldman MD et al: Let's not talk about it: suicide inquiry in primary care, *Ann Fam Medicine* 5(5):412, 2007.

Mitchell A et al: Clinical diagnosis of depression in primary care: a meta-analysis, *Lancet* 374:609-619, 2009.

Trivedi MD et al: Medication augmentation after the failure of SSRIs for depression, *N Engl J Med* 354: 1243, 2006.

AUTHOR: **MITCHELL D. FELDMAN, M.D., M.PHIL.**

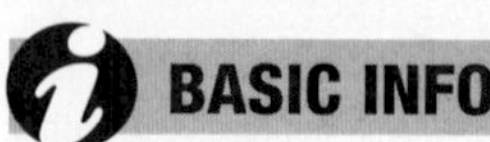

BASIC INFORMATION

DEFINITION

De Quervain's tenosynovitis refers to an inflammatory process of the first dorsal retinacular compartment containing the tendons of the abductor pollicis longus (APL) and extensor pollicis brevis (EPB).

SYNONYMS

Stenosing tenosynovitis of the radial styloid process
Stenosing tenovaginitis of the first dorsal compartment
De Quervain's disease
De Quervain's tendonitis
De Quervain's stenosinig tenosynovitis

ICD-9CM CODES
727.04 Tenosynovitis radial styloid

EPIDEMIOLOGY & DEMOGRAPHICS

- More common in women than in men (10:1)
- Usually occurs between the ages of 30 and 50
- Associated with rheumatoid arthritis
- Seen more frequently in certain occupations involving repetitive wrist motion (e.g., clerical, assembly, and manual labor)

PHYSICAL FINDINGS & CLINICAL PRESENTATION

- Pain over the styloid process of the radius with grasping and isometric thumb abduction
- Swelling compared to the contralateral side
- Tenderness in the anatomic snuffbox
- Positive Finkelstein's test (Fig. 1-86)
- Crepitance

ETIOLOGY

- The cause is usually repetitive use or overuse of the hands (e.g., typing, writing, nailing, new mothers who hold or pick up their babies with poor form, etc.).
- Acute trauma can also cause tenosynovitis of the radial styloid.

DIAGNOSIS

- The diagnosis of de Quervain's tenosynovitis is based on the clinical triad of:
  1. Tenderness over the radial styloid
  2. Swelling over the first dorsal retinacular compartment
  3. Positive Finkelstein's test (see Fig. 1-86)
- Sometimes 1.5 ml of 1% Xylocaine can be injected into the tenosynovial sac, and if all three physical signs resolve, the diagnosis is confirmed, allowing for differentiation from carpometacarpal osteoarthritis.

DIFFERENTIAL DIAGNOSIS

- Carpal tunnel syndrome
- Arthritis (e.g., degenerative osteoarthritis or rheumatoid arthritis)
- Gout
- Infiltrative tenosynovitis
- Radiculopathy
- Compression neuropathy (e.g., superficial branch of the radial nerve "bracelet syndrome")
- Infection (e.g., tuberculosis, bacterial)

LABORATORY TESTS

- Erythrocyte sedimentation rate (ESR) is usually normal in patients with de Quervain's tenosynovitis
- Aspiration to rule out gout
- Gram stain and culture of aspirate

IMAGING STUDIES

- Radiograph studies of the hand if fracture is suspected

TREATMENT

NONPHARMACOLOGIC THERAPY

- Rest
- Splinting (thumb spica)
- Icing
- Physiotherapy

ACUTE GENERAL Rx

- Corticosteroid injection using 20 to 40 mg triamcinolone acetonide and 1% Xylocaine is effective in relieving pain.
- Nonsteroidal anti-inflammatory drugs (NSAIDs) ibuprofen 800 mg tid or naproxen 500 mg bid.

CHRONIC Rx

Surgical release is generally reserved for patients not responding to NSAIDs and corticosteroid injection therapy.

DISPOSITION

- Approximately 90% of patients have relief of symptoms with either single or multiple steroid injections.
- Surgical control of symptoms achieved in 90% of referred cases.
- Complications of surgery include:
  1. Radial nerve damage
  2. Paresthesia (~10%)
  3. Neuroma

REFERRAL

Rheumatologist or orthopedist

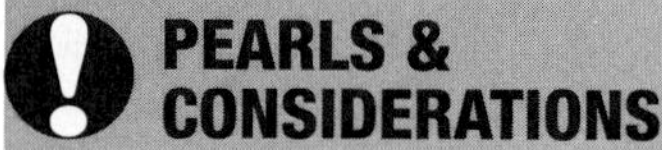

PEARLS & CONSIDERATIONS

- Steroid injection is generally recommended after failure of conservative treatment for 2 to 6 wk.
- Pain relief is usually noted within 48 hr with patient becoming asymptomatic by the first or second week after corticosteroid injection.
- If there is no improvement by 6 wk post second corticosteroid injection, referral to an orthopedic hand surgeon is recommended.
- Avoid repetitive activities.

SUGGESTED READINGS

Chin DH, Jones NF: Repetitive motion hand disorder, *J Calif Dent Assoc* 30(2):149, 2002.
Graham JB, Hulkower SD, Bosworth M: Are steroid injections effective for tenosynovitis of the hand? *J Fam Pract* 56(12):1045-1047, 2007.
Ilyas AM et al: De Quervain tenosynovitis of the wrist, *J Am Acad Orthop Surg* 15(12): 757-764, 2007.
Jirarttanphochai K et al: Treatment of de Quervain disease with triamcinolone injection with or without nimesulide. A randomized, double-blind, placebo-controlled trial, *J Bone Joint Surg Am* 86-A: 2700, 2004.
Richie CA, Briner WW Jr: Corticosteroid injection for treatment of de Quervain's tenosynovitis: a pooled quantitative literature evaluation, *J Am Board Fam Pract* 16:102, 2003.

AUTHOR: **MARK BRADY, M.D., M.P.H., M.M.S.**

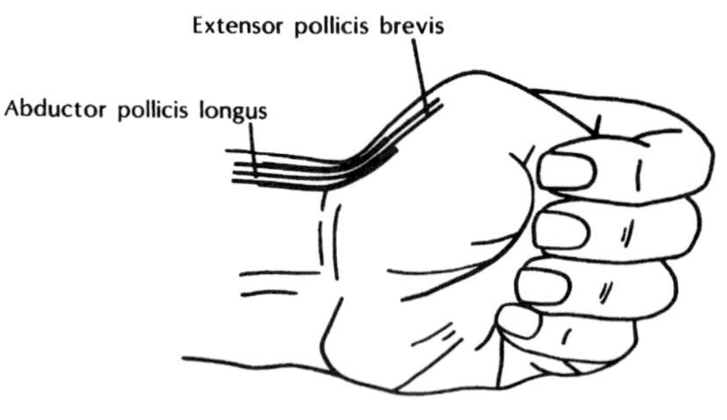

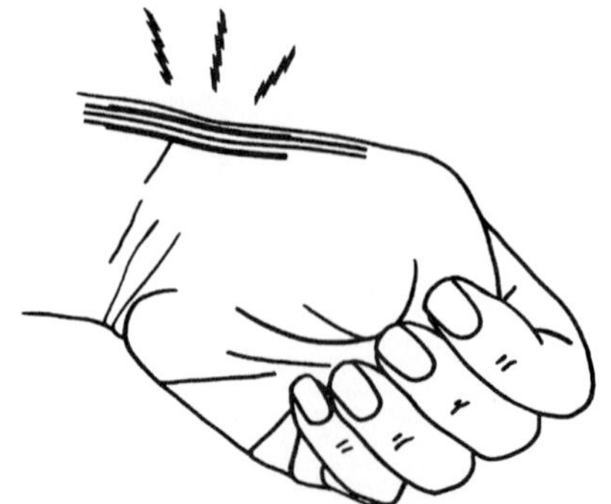

FIGURE 1-86 Finkelstein's test is positive in de Quervain's stenosing synovitis. Ulnar flexion of the wrist produces pain over the dorsal compartment containing the extensor pollicis brevis and abductor pollicis longus. (From Noble J [ed]: *Textbook of primary care medicine,* ed 2, St Louis, 1996, Mosby.)

D

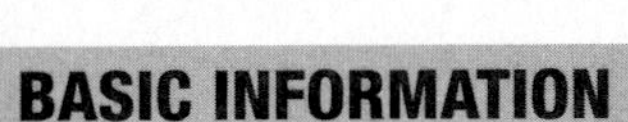

BASIC INFORMATION

DEFINITION

Dermatitis herpetiformis (DH) is a rare, chronic skin disorder characterized by an intensely burning, pruritic, vesicular rash. It is strongly associated with gluten-sensitive enteropathy. Twenty percent to 70% of patients with DH will have gastrointestinal symptoms, whereas approximately 10% of patients with celiac sprue will have DH.

SYNONYMS

None

ICD-9CM CODES
694.0 Dermatitis herpetiformis

EPIDEMIOLOGY & DEMOGRAPHICS

PREVALENCE (IN U.S.): 11.2 cases per 100,000 persons; prevalence for celiac disease is one in 133 adults
PREDOMINANT SEX: Slight male predominance
PREDOMINANT AGE: Third to fifth decades
PREDOMINANT RACE: Rarely seen in blacks/African Americans or Asians
GENETICS: A specific HLA type, DQ2, is present in 90% of patients with celiac disease with or without DH. DQ8 is present in the remaining 10%. DQ2 is present in 16% to 18% of the normal population. Eleven percent of patients with DH have a first-degree relative with either DH or celiac disease.

PHYSICAL FINDINGS & CLINICAL PRESENTATION

- Pruritic, burning vesicles initially, frequently grouped (hence the name "herpetiform") (Fig. 1-87)
- Symmetrically distributed on extensor surfaces: elbows, knees, scalp, nuchal area, shoulder, and buttocks; rarely found in mouth
- May evolve in time to intensely burning urticarial papules, vesicles, and rarely bullae
- Celiac-type enamel defects to permanent teeth found in 53% of patients

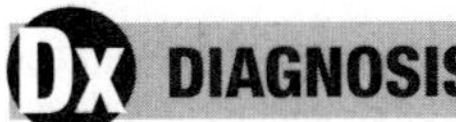

DIAGNOSIS

Diagnosis is confirmed histologically by the demonstration of granular deposition of immunoglobulin (Ig) A at the dermal-epidermal junction, which is specific to the diagnosis of DH.

DIFFERENTIAL DIAGNOSIS

- Linear IgA bullous dermatosis (not associated with gluten-sensitive enteropathy)
- Herpes simplex infection
- Herpes zoster infection
- Bullous erythema multiforme
- Bullous pemphigoid

WORKUP

History of chronic diarrhea and pruritic, vesicular rash highly suggestive of diagnosis

LABORATORY TESTS

- Skin biopsy for immunofluorescence studies. Diagnosis is confirmed by granular IgA deposits at the dermal-epidermal junction. More than 90% will have granular or fibrillar IgA deposits in the dermal papillae. Multiple specimens may be needed to obtain positive findings because of the focal nature of deposits. Biopsies are taken from adjacent normal skin because the diagnostic IgA deposits are usually destroyed by the blistering process.
- Circulating antibody levels
  1. IgA antiendomysial antibody is found:
     a. In 70% of patients with rash and who are not on gluten-free diet and
     b. In 100% of patients with rash and grade 3 to 4 flattening of intestinal mucosa or with untreated celiac disease. Levels decrease to 0% when gluten is avoided for 3 mo.
  2. IgA antigliadin antibodies: found in 66% of patients with DH; also present in patients with pemphigus and pemphigoid
  3. IgA reticulin antibody: found in 36% of patients with DH
  4. IgA antitissue transglutaminase: elevated levels in 75% patients with DH and in 90% to 100% of patients with celiac disease
  5. IgA antiepidermal transglutaminase: elevated in adult patients with DH or celiac disease but may be more specific for DH

Rx TREATMENT

- Spontaneous remission of DH in patients on a normal diet has been described in 10% to 15% of cases.
- Adherence to a gluten-free diet has been associated with sustained remission of DH.
- Patients may be given a trial of pharmacologic therapy if they are extremely uncomfortable. Symptoms are often dramatically relieved within hours or days of initiation of medical therapy.

NONPHARMACOLOGIC THERAPY

- Gluten-free diet: for at least 6 mo, which will allow most patients to begin to decrease or discontinue sulfone therapy (see "Acute General Rx" below). The diet usually needs to be followed for 2 yr before medications can be discontinued. Although intestinal villous architecture improves, symptoms and lesions recur in 1 to 3 wk if a normal diet is resumed. Most patients need to follow the diet indefinitely. Gluten is found in grains, such as wheat, barley, rye, and oats, but not rice or corn.
- A recent small study demonstrated that a gluten-free diet alone was comparable to a gluten-free diet plus dapsone in the treatment of DH.
- Elemental diet: other dietary factors may also be important in DH. Antigens stimulate the production of antibodies, leading to the formation of immune complexes. Most antigens that elicit a humoral immune response are proteins. Thus a diet without full proteins, an elemental diet, is not likely to contain major antigens. A diet of amino acids, fat, and carbohydrates can produce a rapid benefit and allow a decrease in the dosage of dapsone within 2 wk.

ACUTE GENERAL Rx

- Dapsone:
  - Initial dose of 50 mg PO bid. Itching and burning are controlled in 12 to 48 hr and new lesions stop appearing.
  - Adjust dose to the lowest level that provides adequate relief, which can range from 25 to 400 mg/day.
  - Peripheral motor neuropathy, such as paresthesias and weakness of the distal upper

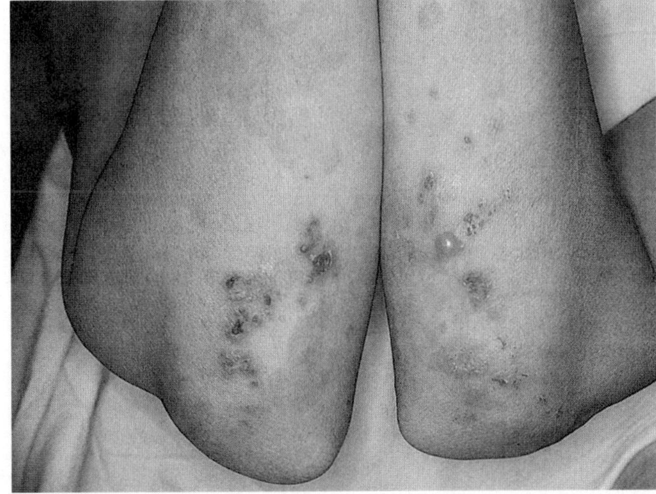

FIGURE 1-87 Dermatitis herpetiformis is an immunologically mediated blistering disease. There is a strong association of dermatitis herpetiformis with HLA-B8, DR3. Gluten-sensitive enteropathy is a common associated finding. The lesions are grouped (herpetiform) and extremely pruritic. (From Callen JP [ed]: *Color atlas of dermatology,* ed 2, Philadelphia, 2000, WB Saunders.)

Diseases and Disorders I

and lower extremities and footdrop, can occur in the first few months of therapy. Symptoms slowly improve over months to years after dapsone is discontinued.
  - Hemolysis, anemia, and methemoglobinemia occur to some degree in all patients receiving dapsone therapy. Vitamin E 800 IU daily may be helpful in preventing methemoglobinemia. Patients at risk for G6PD deficiency should have levels drawn before initiation because dapsone may cause severe hemolytic anemia in these patients.
  - Probenecid blocks the renal excretion of dapsone, and rifampin increases the rate of its clearance.
- Sulfapyridine:
  - Initial dosage 500 to 1500 mg/day.
  - Sulfapyridine is associated with agranulocytosis and aplastic anemia. It also may cause severe hemolysis in patients with G6PD deficiency.
- Sulfasalazine:
  - 500 to 1000 mg bid.
  - Sulfasalazine is metabolized to sulfapyridine and has been demonstrated to be effective in patients who are unable to tolerate dapsone in case reports.
- Tetracycline:
  - Successful treatment has been reported with tetracycline 500 mg PO qd to tid and minocycline 100 mg PO bid. Cessation resulted in a flare of the rash.
- Nicotinamide:
  - Successful treatment has been reported with nicotinamide 500 mg PO bid to tid. Cessation resulted in a flare of the rash.
- Topical steroids: may help but can cause skin irritation and atrophy with prolonged use.
- Nonsteroidal anti-inflammatory drugs and iodide can worsen skin inflammation.

CHRONIC Rx

Gluten-free diet

DISPOSITION

- DH is considered to represent an intolerance to gluten, which requires lifelong avoidance of gluten.
- Some patients may be able to reintroduce gluten into their diet without experiencing a recurrence of DH.
  - A study of 38 patients demonstrated that seven (18%) could resume a normal diet without relapse of cutaneous or gastrointestinal symptoms.
  - Patients who did not relapse after resumption of a normal diet were all diagnosed in childhood, had poor adherence to a gluten-free diet, and were more likely to have been treated with dapsone.
- There is an increased incidence of other autoimmune disorders, including thyroid disease, type 1 diabetes mellitus, systemic lupus erythematosus, vitiligo, and Sjögren's syndrome in patients with DH.
- Small bowel lymphoma and nonintestinal lymphoma have been reported in patients with DH and celiac disease. Patients adhering strictly to a gluten-free diet can reduce their risk of gut-related lymphomas within 5 yr to that of the baseline population.

REFERRAL

To dermatologist for skin biopsy and to nutritionist to educate patients about gluten-free diet

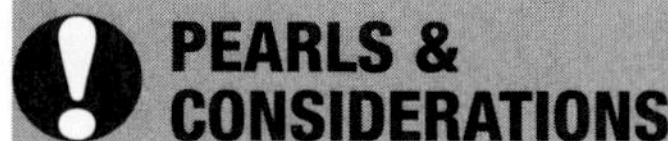

PEARLS & CONSIDERATIONS

- Treatment with a gluten-free diet alone was found comparable to dapsone plus a gluten-free diet in a recent small study.
- Maintaining a gluten-free diet has been demonstrated to have a protective effect against the development of lymphoma in patients with celiac disease.

SUGGESTED READINGS

Bardella MT et al: Long-term remission in patients with dermatitis herpetiformis on a normal diet, *Br J Dermatol* 149:968-971, 2003.

Dieterich W et al: Antibodies to tissue transglutaminase as serologic markers in patients with dermatitis herpetiformis, *J Invest Dermatol* 113(1):133, 1999.

Eedy DJ et al: Updates from the British Association of Dermatologists 84th Annual Meeting, *Br J Dermatol* 152:13-28, 2005.

Hull CM et al: Elevation of IgA antiepidermal transglutaminase antibodies in dermatitis herpetiformis, *Br J Dermatol* 159:120, 2008.

Nino M et al: A long-term gluten-free diet as an alternative treatment in severe forms of dermatitis herpetiformis, *J Dermatol Treat* 13:10-12, 2007.

Turchin I, Barankin B: Dermatitis herpetiformis and gluten-free diet, *Dermotol Online J* 11(1):6, 2005.

Willsteed E et al: Sulfasalazine and dermatitis herpetiformis, *Australas J Dermatol* 26(2):101, 2005.

Zone JJ et al: Warning: bread may be harmful to your health, *J Am Acad Dermatol* 51(suppl 1):S27, 2004.

AUTHOR: **IRIS TONG, M.D.**

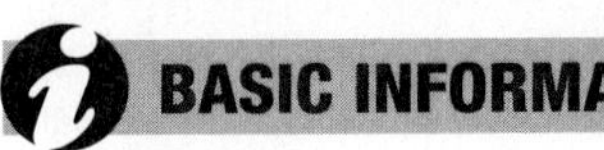

BASIC INFORMATION

DEFINITION

Diabetes insipidus is a polyuric disorder resulting from insufficient production of antidiuretic hormone (ADH) (pituitary [neurogenic] diabetes insipidus) or unresponsiveness of the renal tubules to ADH (nephrogenic diabetes insipidus).

ICD-9CM CODES
253.5 Diabetes insipidus

EPIDEMIOLOGY & DEMOGRAPHICS

GENETICS:

- Nephrogenic diabetes insipidus can be inherited as a sex-linked recessive trait.
- There is also a rare autosomal-dominant form of neurogenic diabetes insipidus.

PHYSICAL FINDINGS & CLINICAL PRESENTATION

- Polyuria: urinary volumes ranging from 2.5 to 6 L/day
- Polydipsia (predilection for cold or iced drinks)
- Neurologic manifestations (seizures, headaches, visual field defects)
- Evidence of volume contractions

NOTE: The physical findings and clinical manifestations are generally not evident until vasopressin secretory capacity is reduced to <20% of normal.

ETIOLOGY

Neurogenic diabetes insipidus:

- Idiopathic
- Neoplasms of brain or pituitary fossa (craniopharyngiomas, metastatic neoplasms from breast or lung)
- Posttherapeutic neurosurgical procedures (e.g., hypophysectomy)
- Head trauma (e.g., basal skull fracture)
- Granulomatous disorders (sarcoidosis or tuberculosis)
- Histiocytosis (Hand-Schüller-Christian disease, eosinophilic granuloma)
- Familial (autosomal dominant)
- Other: interventricular hemorrhage, aneurysms, meningitis, postencephalitis, multiple sclerosis

Nephrogenic diabetes insipidus:

- Drugs: lithium, amphotericin B, demeclocycline, methoxyflurane anesthesia
- Familial: X-linked
- Metabolic: hypercalcemia or hypokalemia
- Other: sarcoidosis, amyloidosis, pyelonephritis, polycystic disease, sickle cell disease, postobstructive, low-protein diets (protein malnourishment)

Dx DIAGNOSIS

DIFFERENTIAL DIAGNOSIS

- Diabetes mellitus, nephropathies
- Primary polydipsia, medications (e.g., chlorpromazine)
- Osmotic diuresis (glucose, mannitol, anticholinergics)
- Psychogenic polydipsia, electrolyte disturbances

WORKUP

- The diagnostic workup is aimed at showing that polyuria is caused by the inability to concentrate urine and determining whether the problem is the result of decreased ADH or insensitivity to ADH. This is done with the water deprivation test:
  1. After baseline measurement of weight, ADH, plasma sodium, and urine and plasma osmolarity, the patient is deprived of fluids under strict medical supervision.
  2. Frequent (q2h) monitoring of plasma and urine osmolarity follows.
  3. The test is generally terminated when plasma osmolarity is >295 mOsm/kg or the patient loses ≥3.5% of initial body weight.
  4. Diabetes insipidus is confirmed if the plasma osmolarity is >295 mOsm/kg and the urine osmolarity is <500 mOsm/kg.
  5. To distinguish nephrogenic from neurogenic diabetes insipidus, the patient is given 5 U of vasopressin (ADH) and the change in urine osmolarity is measured. A significant increase (>50%) in urine osmolarity after administration of ADH is indicative of neurogenic diabetes insipidus.
- A diagnostic algorithm for diabetes insipidus is described in Section III.

LABORATORY TESTS

- Decreased urinary specific gravity (≤1.005)
- Decreased urinary osmolarity (usually <200 mOsm/kg) even in the presence of high serum osmolality
- Hypernatremia, increased plasma osmolarity, hypercalcemia, hypokalemia

IMAGING STUDIES

MRI of the brain if neurogenic diabetes insipidus is confirmed

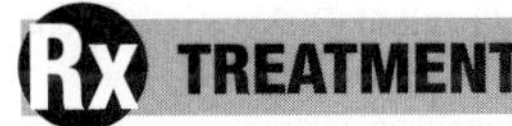

Rx TREATMENT

NONPHARMACOLOGIC THERAPY

- Patient education regarding control of fluid balance and prevention of dehydration with adequate fluid intake
- Daily weight

ACUTE GENERAL Rx

Therapy varies with the degree and type of diabetes insipidus.

- Neurogenic diabetes insipidus:
  1. Desmopressin acetate (DDAVP) 10 to 40 mcg qd intranasally in one to three divided doses or in tablet form 0.1 or 0.2 mg. Usual oral dose is 0.1 to 1.2 mg/day in two to three divided doses. Desmopressin is also available in injectable form given as 2 to 4 mcg/day SC or IV in two divided doses.
  2. Vasopressin tannate in oil: 2.5 to 5 U IM q24-72h; useful for long-term management because of its long half-life.
  3. In mild cases of neurogenic diabetes insipidus, polyuria may be controlled with HCTZ 50 mg qd (decreases urine volume by increasing proximal tubular reabsorption of glomerular infiltrate).
- Nephrogenic diabetes insipidus:
  1. Removal of the underlying cause. However, prolonged lithium therapy can lead to irreversible nephrogenic diabetes insipidus even after lithium therapy is withdrawn.
  2. Adequate hydration.
  3. Low-sodium diet and chlorothiazide to induce mild sodium depletion. Indomethacin may also be useful to reduce urine volume.

CHRONIC Rx

Patients should be aware of the danger of dehydration and the need for liberal water intake.

REFERRAL

Endocrinology consultation for diagnostic testing

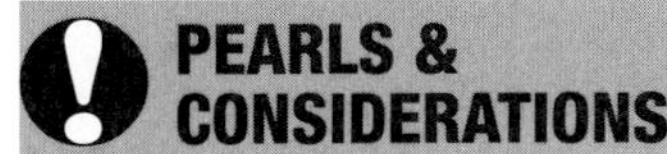

PEARLS & CONSIDERATIONS

COMMENTS

- Patients should be instructed to wear a medical identification tag or bracelet identifying their medical illness.
- In central diabetes insipidus, the use of DDAVP has become the standard of care. Extensive clinical experience has shown it to be both safe and effective in the treatment of this disorder.
- The treatment of nephrogenic diabetes insipidus is more complicated than the central form, and opinion varies among experts in the field. Consultation with a specialist is always recommended in this setting.

SUGGESTED READING

Sands JM, Bichet DG: Nephrogenic diabetes insipidus, *Ann Intern Med* 144:186, 2006.

AUTHOR: **FRED F. FERRI, M.D.**

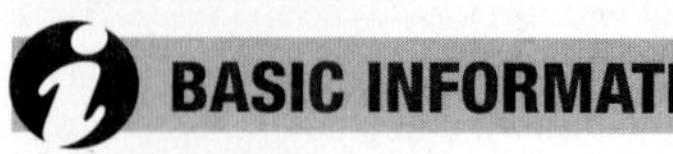

DEFINITION

- Diabetes mellitus (DM) refers to a syndrome of hyperglycemia resulting from many different causes (see "Etiology"). It can be classified into type 1 and type 2 DM. Because "insulin-dependent" and "non–insulin-dependent" refer to stage at diagnosis, when a person with type 2 diabetes needs insulin, he or she remains classified as type 2 and does not revert to type 1. Table 1-19 provides a general comparison of the two types of DM.
- The American Diabetes Association (ADA) defines DM as follows:
  1. A fasting plasma glucose (FPG) ≥126 mg/dl, which should be confirmed with testing on a different day; fasting is defined as no caloric intake for at least 8h
  2. Symptoms of hyperglycemia and a casual (random) plasma glucose ≥200 mg/dl, random plasma glucose is defined as any time of the day without regard to time since last meal; classic symptoms of hyperglycemia include polyuria, polydipsia, and unexplained weight loss
  3. An oral glucose tolerance test (OGTT) ≥200 mg/dl in the 2-hour sample; OGTT using glucose load containing the equivalent of 75 g (100 g for pregnant women) anhydrous glucose dissolved in water; furthermore, the ADA also defines a value <100 mg/dl on fasting blood sugar as the upper limit of normal for glucose; a fasting glucose level between 100 and 126 mg/dl is classified as "impaired fasting glucose" (IFG); when results of the OGTT are between 140 and 199 mg/dl, the patient is classified as "impaired glucose tolerance" (IGT)

SYNONYMS

IDDM (insulin-dependent diabetes mellitus)
NIDDM (non–insulin-dependent diabetes mellitus)
Type 1 diabetes mellitus (insulin-dependent diabetes mellitus)
Type 2 diabetes mellitus (non–insulin-dependent diabetes mellitus)

ICD-9CM CODES
250.0 Diabetes mellitus (NIDDM)
250.1 Insulin-dependent diabetes mellitus without complication (IDDM)

EPIDEMIOLOGY & DEMOGRAPHICS

- DM affects 7% to 9% of the U.S. population. Prevalence rate in Pima Indians is 35%.
- Incidence rate increases with age, with 2% in persons age 20 to 44 yr to 18% in persons 65 to 74 yr. Type 2 DM is often present at least 4 to 7 yr before diagnosis.
- Diabetes accounts for 8% of all legal blindness and is the leading cause of end-stage renal disease (ESRD) in the U.S.
- Patients with diabetes are twice as likely as nondiabetic patients to experience development of cardiovascular disease.

PHYSICAL FINDINGS & CLINICAL PRESENTATION

1. Physical examination varies with the presence of complications and may be normal in early stages
2. Diabetic retinopathy:
   a. Nonproliferative (background diabetic retinopathy):
      (1) Initially: microaneurysms, capillary dilation, waxy or hard exudates, dot and flame hemorrhages, atrioventricular shunts
      (2) Advanced stage: microinfarcts with cotton wool exudates, macular edema
   b. Proliferative retinopathy: characterized by formation of new vessels, vitreal hemorrhages, fibrous scarring, and retinal detachment
3. Cataracts and glaucoma occur with increased frequency in patients with diabetes
4. Peripheral neuropathy: patients often report paresthesias of extremities (feet more than hands); the symptoms are symmetric, bilateral, and associated with intense burning pain (particularly during the night)
   a. Mononeuropathies involving cranial nerves III, IV, and VI, intercostal nerves, and femoral nerves are also common.
   b. Physical examination may reveal:
      (1) Decreased pinprick sensation, sensation to light touch, and pain sensation
      (2) Decreased vibration sense
      (3) Loss of proprioception (leading to ataxia)
      (4) Motor disturbances (decreased deep tendon reflexes [DTRs], weakness and atrophy of interossei muscles); when the hands are affected, the patient has trouble picking up small objects, dressing, and turning pages in a book
      (5) Diplopia, abnormalities of visual fields
5. Autonomic neuropathy:
   a. GI disturbances: esophageal motility abnormalities, gastroparesis, diarrhea (usually nocturnal)
   b. Genitourinary (GU) disturbances: neurogenic bladder (hesitancy, weak stream, and dribbling), impotence
   c. Orthostatic hypotension: postural syncope, dizziness, light-headedness

TABLE 1-19 General Comparison of the Two Most Common Types of Diabetes Mellitus

	Type 1	Type 2
Previous terminology	Insulin-dependent diabetes mellitus (IDDM), type I, juvenile-onset diabetes	Non–insulin-dependent diabetes mellitus, type II, adult-onset diabetes
Age of onset	Usually <30 yr, particularly childhood and adolescence, but any age	Usually >40 yr, but any age
Genetic predisposition	Moderate; environmental factors required for expression; 35%-50% concordance in monozygotic twins; several candidate genes proposed	Strong; 60%-90% concordance in monozygotic twins; many candidate genes proposed; some genes identified in maturity-onset diabetes of the young
Human leukocyte antigen associations	Linkage to DQA and DQB, influenced by DRB (3 and 4) (DR2 protective)	None known
Other associations	Autoimmune; Graves' disease, Hashimoto's thyroiditis, vitiligo, Addison's disease, pernicious anemia	Heterogenous group, ongoing subclassification based on identification of specific pathogenic processes and genetic defects
Precipitating and risk factors	Largely unknown; microbial, chemical, dietary, other	Age, obesity (central), sedentary lifestyle, previous gestational diabetes
Findings at diagnosis	85%-90% of patients have one and usually more autoantibodies to ICA512/IA-2/IA-2β, GAD_{65}, insulin (IAA)	Possibly complications (microvascular and macrovascular) caused by significant preceding asymptomatic period
Endogenous insulin levels	Low or absent	Usually present (relative deficiency), early hyperinsulinemia
Insulin resistance	Only with hyperglycemia	Mostly present
Prolonged fast	Hyperglycemia, ketoacidosis	Euglycemia
Stress, withdrawal of insulin	Ketoacidosis	Nonketotic hyperglycemia, occasionally ketoacidosis

GAD, Glutamic acid decarboxylase; *IA-2/IA-2β,* tyrosine phosphatases; *IAA,* insulin autoantibodies; *ICA,* islet cell antibody; *ICA512,* islet cell autoantigen 512 (fragment of IA-2).
From Andreoli TE (ed): *Cecil essentials of medicine,* ed 6, Philadelphia, 2005, WB Saunders.

6. Nephropathy: pedal edema, pallor, weakness, uremic appearance
7. Foot ulcers: occur in 15% of individuals with diabetes (annual incidence rate, 2%) and are the leading causes of hospitalization; they are usually secondary to peripheral vascular insufficiency, repeated trauma (unrecognized because of sensory loss), and superimposed infections; if a diabetic foot ulcer has been present for weeks and foot pulses are palpable, neuropathy should be considered a major cause; neuropathy can be detected with a simple examination of the lower extremities using a 10-g monofilament to test sensation; prevention of foot ulcers in individual with diabetes includes strict glucose control, patient education, prescription footwear, intensive podiatric care, and evaluation for surgical interventions
8. Neuropathic arthropathy (Charcot's joints): bone or joint deformities from repeated trauma (secondary to peripheral neuropathy; Fig. 1-88)
9. Necrobiosis lipoidica diabeticorum: plaque-like reddened areas with a central area that fades to white-yellow found on the anterior surfaces of the legs (Fig. 1-89); in these areas, the skin becomes very thin and can ulcerate readily

ETIOLOGY

IDIOPATHIC DIABETES: Type 1 DM:

- Hereditary factors:
  1. Islet cell antibodies (found in 90% of patients within the first yr of diagnosis)
  2. Higher incidence of human leukocyte antigen (HLA) types DR3, DR4
  3. 50% concordance rate in identical twins
- Environmental factors: viral infection (possibly Coxsackie virus, mumps virus)

Type 2 DM:

- Hereditary factors: 90% concordance rate in identical twins
- Environmental factor: obesity, sedentary lifestyle, high carbohydrate content in food

DIABETES SECONDARY TO OTHER FACTORS:

- Hormonal excess: Cushing's syndrome, acromegaly, glucagonoma, pheochromocytoma
- Drugs: glucocorticoids, diuretics, oral contraceptives
- Insulin receptor unavailability (with or without circulating antibodies)
- Pancreatic disease: pancreatitis, pancreatectomy, hemochromatosis
- Genetic syndromes: hyperlipidemias, myotonic dystrophy, lipoatrophy
- Gestational diabetes

Dx DIAGNOSIS

DIFFERENTIAL DIAGNOSIS

- Diabetes insipidus
- Stress hyperglycemia
- Diabetes secondary to hormonal excess, drugs, pancreatic disease

LABORATORY TESTS

- Diagnosis is made on the basis of the following tests:
  1. Fasting glucose $\geq$126 mg/dl (ADA criterion), should be confirmed by repeated testing on a different day
  2. Non-FPG $\geq$200 mg/dl and symptoms of DM
  3. OGTT (75-g glucose load for nonpregnant individuals)
  4. Glycosylated hemoglobin (HbA1c) $\geq$6.5% (International Expert Committee [IEC], 2009 recommendation)
  5. Testing for prediabetes and diabetes in asymptomatic patients:
     - Should be considered in adults of any age who are overweight or obese (body mass index [BMI] $>$25 kg/m^2) and who have one or more additional risk factors for diabetes. In those who are without these risk factors, testing should begin at age 45 yr.
     - If normal, repeat testing should be carried out at least at 3-yr intervals.
  6. Detection and diagnosis of gestational diabetes mellitus (GDM)
     - Screen for GDM using risk factor analysis and, if appropriate, use of an OGTT
     - Women with GDM should be screened for diabetes 6 to 12 wk postpartum and should be followed with subsequent screening for the development of diabetes or prediabetes
- Screening for diabetic nephropathy by measuring microalbuminuria is recommended in all patients with diabetes. It can be accomplished by any of the following three methods:
  1. Measurement of the albumin:creatinine ratio in random spot urine collection. This is the easiest method to administer in the office setting because it is an easy assay to perform in most laboratories. To perform this test, the physician simply orders "Urine for microalbumin level."
  2. Measurement of a 24-hour urine collection for albumin, creatinine clearance.
  3. Timed (4 hours or overnight) urine collection.
- The diagnosis of microalbuminuria (30 to 299 mg/24 hours) should be based on 2 to 3 elevated levels within a 3- to 6-mo period because there is a marked variability in day-to-day albumin excretion and possible transient elevations in urine albumin from short-term hyperglycemia, exercise, severe hypertension, and other illnesses such as sepsis and congestive heart failure. Patients with overt nephropathy do not need screening for microalbuminuria because the level of protein in the urine is high enough to be detected on routine urinalysis.
- A fasting serum lipid panel, serum creatinine, and electrolytes should be obtained yearly on all adult patients with diabetes.

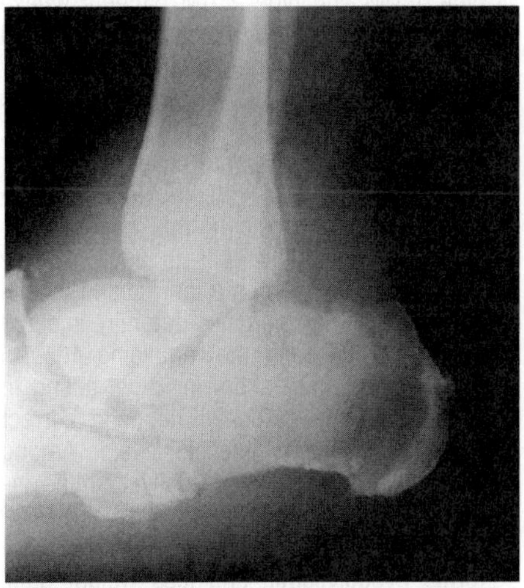

FIGURE 1-88 Diabetic neuropathy of the hindfoot. Destruction of the joint with collapse and fragmentation. (From Hochberg MC et al [eds]: *Rheumatology*, ed 3, St Louis, 2003, Mosby.)

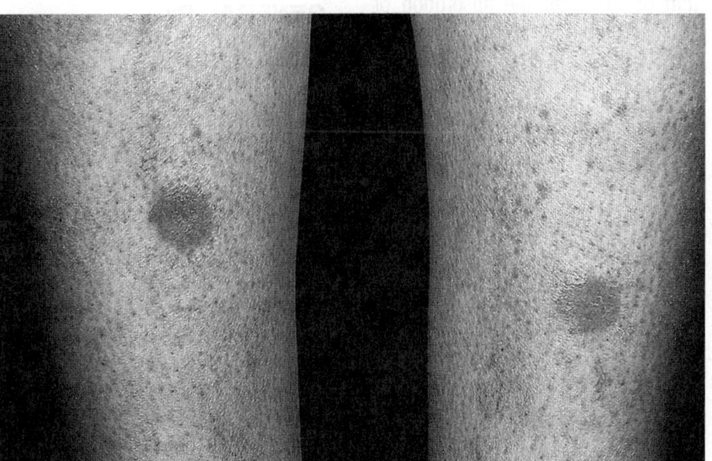

FIGURE 1-89 Necrobiosis lipoidica: symmetrical early lesions with erythema. (Courtesy of the Institute of Dermatology; from McKee PH, Calonje E, Granter SR [eds]: *Pathology of the skin with clinical correlations,* ed 3, St Louis, 2005, Mosby.)

Rx TREATMENT

ADA and European Association for the Study of Diabetes recommends: "Intervention at the time of diagnosis with metformin in combination with life style changes (diet and exercise) and continuing timely augmentation of therapy with additional agents (including early initiation of insulin therapy) as a means of achieving and maintaining recommended levels of glycemic control of A1C <7%."

NONPHARMACOLOGIC THERAPY

1. Diet
   a. Calories
      (1) The patient with diabetes can be started on 15 calories/lb of ideal body weight; this number can be increased to 20 calories/lb for an active person and 25 calories/lb if the patient does heavy physical labor.
      (2) The calories should be distributed as 45% to 65% carbohydrates, <30% fat, with saturated fat limited to <7% of total calories, and 10% to 30% protein. Daily cholesterol intake should not exceed 300 mg.
      (3) The emphasis should be on complex carbohydrates rather than simple and refined starches, and on polyunsaturated instead of saturated fats in a ratio of 2:1.
   b. Seven food groups
      (1) The exchange diet of the ADA includes protein, bread, fruit, milk, and low- and intermediate-carbohydrate vegetables.
      (2) The name of each exchange is meant to be all-inclusive (e.g., cereal, muffins, spaghetti, potatoes, rice are in the bread group; meats, fish, eggs, cheese, peanut butter are in the protein group).
      (3) The *glycemic index* compares the increase in blood sugar after the ingestion of simple sugars and complex carbohydrates with the increase that occurs after the absorption of glucose; equal amounts of starches do not give the same increase in plasma glucose (pasta equal in calories to a baked potato causes less of an increase than the potato); thus, it is helpful to know the glycemic index of a particular food product.
      (4) Fiber: Insoluble fiber (bran, celery) and soluble globular fiber (pectin in fruit) delay glucose absorption and attenuate the postprandial serum glucose peak; they also appear to reduce the increased triglyceride level often present in patients with uncontrolled diabetes. A diet high in fiber should be emphasized (20 to 35 g/day of soluble and insoluble fiber).
   c. Other principles
      (1) Modest sodium restriction to 2400 to 3000 mg/day. If hypertension is present, restrict to <2400 mg/day; if nephropathy and hypertension are present, restrict to <2000 mg/day.
      (2) Moderation of alcohol intake recommended (≤2 drinks/day in men, ≤1 drink/day in women).
      (3) Non-nutritive artificial sweeteners are acceptable in moderate amounts.
2. Exercise: increases the cellular glucose uptake by increasing the number of cell receptors. The following points must be considered:
   a. Exercise program must be individualized and built up slowly. Consider beginning with 15 min of low-impact aerobic exercise 3 times per wk and increasing the frequency and duration to 30 to 45 min of moderate aerobic activity (50% to 70% of maximum age predicted heart rate) to 3 to 5 days/wk
      In the absence of contraindications, resistance training three times per wk should be encouraged.
   b. Insulin is more rapidly absorbed when injected into a limb that is then exercised, and this can result in hypoglycemia.
3. Weight loss: to ideal body weight if the patient is overweight
4. Screening for nephropathy, neuropathy, and retinopathy: annual serum creatinine and urine albumin excretion; initial comprehensive eye examination and at least annually thereafter
5. Diabetes self-management education: could also address psychosocial issues
6. Self-monitoring of blood glucose should occur three to four times per day for patients using multiple insulin injections or on insulin pump therapy
7. Perform A1C at least two times a year in patients who are meeting treatment goals and who have stable glycemic control
   - A1C quarterly in patients whose therapy has changed or who are not meeting glycemic goals
   - The A1c goal for nonpregnant adults in general is <7%

GENERAL Rx

- When the previous measures fail to normalize the serum glucose, oral hypoglycemic agents should be added to the regimen in type 2 DM. Table 1-20 describes commonly used oral hypoglycemic agents.
- The primary mechanism of metformin is to decrease hepatic glucose output. Because metformin does not produce hypoglycemia when used as a monotherapy, it is preferred for most patients. It is contraindicated in patients with severe renal insufficiency with an estimated glomerular filtrate rate <30 ml/min or in patients with significant liver disease.
- Sulfonylureas work best when given before meals because they increase the postprandial output of insulin from the pancreas. All sulfonylureas are contraindicated in patients who are allergic to sulfa.
- Sitagliptin inhibits the enzyme DPP-4, responsible for inactivation and degradation of glucagon-like peptide-1 (GLP-1) and glucose-dependent insulinotropic polypeptide (GIP), which potentiate insulin synthesis, and release and decrease glucagon production.
- Pioglitazone and rosiglitazone increase insulin sensitivity and are useful in addition to other agents in patients with type 2 diabetes, whose hyperglycemia is inadequately controlled. Serum transaminase levels should be obtained before starting therapy and monitored periodically. Glitazones, in general, may increase the risk for heart failure, whereas rosiglitazone may increase the incidence of myocardial infarction.
- Acarbose and miglitol work by competitively inhibiting pancreatic amylase and small intestinal glucosidases, which delay gastrointestinal absorption of carbohydrates, thereby reducing alimentary hyperglycemia. The major side effects are flatulence, diarrhea, and abdominal cramps.
- Exenatide, a synthetic peptide that stimulates release of insulin from pancreatic beta cells, can be used as adjunctive therapy for patients with type 2 DM. It is an incretin mimetic. Incretins are endogenous proteins that modulate the glycemic response. Exenatide is not indicated in type 1 DM and is contraindicated in patients with severe renal impairment. Starting dose is 5 μg subcutaneously (SC) bid before morning and evening meals.
- Pramlintide, a synthetic analog of human amylin (a hormone synthesized by pancreatic beta cells and cosecreted with insulin in response to food intake) can be used as an adjunctive treatment for patients with type 1 or type 2 DM who inject insulin at mealtime. In type 1 DM, initial dose is 15 μg SC before major meals. In type 2 DM, initial dose is 60 μg before major meals. Nausea is its major side effect.
- Combination therapy of various hypoglycemic agents is commonly used when monotherapy results in inadequate glycemic control.
- Insulin is indicated for the treatment of all type 1 DM and type 2 DM patients whose condition cannot be adequately controlled with diet and oral agents. Table 1-21 describes commonly used types of insulin. The risks of insulin therapy include weight gain, hypoglycemia, and in rare cases, allergic or cutaneous reactions. Replacement insulin therapy should mimic normal release patterns. Approximately 50% to 60% of daily insulin can be given as a long-acting insulin (NPH, ultralente, glargine, detemir) injected once or twice daily, the remaining 40% to 50% can be short-acting or rapid-acting to cover mealtime carbohydrates and correct increased current glucose levels. Among long-acting insulins, once-daily bedtime insulin glargine is as effective as once- or twice-daily NPH but has a lower risk for nocturnal hypoglycemia and less weight gain. Insulin detemir is a newer, long-acting insulin analog approved as basal therapy for treatment of DM. It is indicated for use in adults and children in combination with short-acting

TABLE 1-20 Non-Insulin Antidiabetic Agents

	Sulfonylureas	Biguanides	α-Glucosidase Inhibitors	Thiazolidinediones	Meglitinides	Dipeptidyl Peptidase-4 Inhibitors	Incretin Mimetics	Amylin Analogue
Generic name	Glimepiride, glyburide, glipizide,	Metformin	Acarbose, miglitol	Rosiglitazone, pioglitazone	Repaglinide, nateglinide	Sitagliptin, saxagliptin	Exenatide	Pramlintide
Mode of action	↑↑ Pancreatic insulin secretion chronically	↓↓HGP; ↓ peripheral IR; ↓ intestinal glucose absorption	Delays PP digestion of carbohydrates and absorption of glucose	↓↓ Peripheral IR; ↑↑ glucose disposal; ↓ HGP	↑↑ Pancreatic insulin secretion acutely	Potentiate insulin synthesis and release	Mimics incretin action by increasing glucose dependent insulin secretion	Amylinomimetic agent; modulates gastric emptying, prevents postprandial glucagon secretion, and promotes satiety
Preferred patient type	Type 2 DM	Overweight, IR, fasting hyperglycemia, dyslipidemia	PP hyperglycemia	Overweight, IR, dyslipidemia, renal dysfunction	PP hyperglycemia	Type 2 DM	DM type 2 as monotherapy or adjunct, overweight	As an adjunct type 1 and type 2 DM
Therapeutic Effects								
↓ HBA_{1c}* (%) decrease	1-2	1-2	0.5-1	0.8-1	1-2	0.5	24 wks of monotherapy with 5mcg reduces HbA1c by 0.7% and 10mcg reduces by 0.9%	With the start of pramlintide, reduce preprandial, rapid acting or short acting insulin dosages by 50%
↓ FPG* (mg/dl) decrease	50-70	50-80	15-30	25-50	40-80			
↓ PPG* (mg/dl) decrease	~90	80	40-50	—	30			
Insulin levels	↑	—	—	—	↑			
Weight	↑	—/↓	—	—/↑	↑		↓	↓
Lipids	—	↓ LDL ↓↓ TG		↑ Large "fluffy" LDL ↓↓ TG ↑ HDL	—			
Side effects	Hypoglycemia	Diarrhea, lactic acidosis	Abdominal pain, flatulence, diarrhea	Heart failure; edema	Hypoglycemia (low-risk)		Hypoglycemia, nausea, vomiting, diarrhea, headache, pancreatitis	Severe hypoglycemia, abdominal pains, loss of appetite, nausea, vomiting, headache, cough
Dose(s)/day	1-2	1-3	1-3	1-2	+−2		Initial: 5 mcg SUBQ twice a day; maintenance: 10 mcg SUBQ twice a day after one month of start of therapy	Type 1 initial: 15 mcg SUBQ prior to major meals; maintenance: titrate 15-mcg increments to 30-60 mcg; type 2 initial 60 mcg SUBQ immediately prior to major meals; maintenance, 120 mcg SUBQ as tolerated
Maximum daily dose	Glimepiride 8 mg, glyburide 20 mg, glipizide 40 mg	2550 mg	150 mg (<60-kg bw), 300 mg (>60-kg bw or above)	45 mg for pioglitazone, 8 mg for rosiglitazone	16 mg (repaglinide), 360 mg (nateglinide)	Sitagliptin 100 mg; saxagliptin 5 mg	10 mcg SUBQ twice a day	Type 1: 60 mcg as tolerated; type 2: 120 mcg as tolerated
Renal impairment	Glipizide preferred—no adjustment needed	Can be used in creatinine clearance > 30 ml/min	Can be used when serum creatinine < 2 mg/dl	No dose adjustment needed	Repaglinide: CrCl 20-40 ml/min start lower at 0.5 mg, avoid if CrCl < 20 ml/min; Nateglinide: no adjustment needed	50% of the dose when CrCl < 50 ml/min	No dose adjustment needed	No dose adjustment needed when CrCl > 20 ml/min, not studied < 20 ml/min
Optimal administration time	~30 min premeal	After meal	With first bite of meal	With meal (breakfast)	Preferably <15 (0-30 min) premeals (omit if no meal)		Within 30-60 min period before meals twice a day	Immediately prior to major meals
Main site of metabolism/excretion	Hepatic/renal, fecal	Not metabolized/renal	Only 2% absorbed/fecal	Hepatic/fecal	Hepatic/fecal		Renal	Renal

*Values combined from numerous studies; values are also dose dependent.
↑, Increased; ↓, decreased; —, unchanged; *bw,* body weight; *FPG,* fasting plasma glucose; *HDL,* high-density lipoprotein; *HGP,* hepatic glucose production; *IR,* insulin resistance; *LDL,* low-density lipoprotein; *PP,* postprandial; *PPG,* postprandial plasma glucose; *TG,* triglyceride.
Modified from Andreoli TE (ed): *Cecil essentials of medicine,* ed 6, Philadelphia, 2005, WB Saunders.

insulin for type 1 diabetes and oral agents or short-acting insulin for adults with type 2 DM. Unlike NPH insulin, its use has not been associated with weight gain. Short-acting insulins include insulin aspart and insulin lispro, which are more effective in lowering postprandial glucose levels than regular insulin.

- Continuous subcutaneous insulin infusion (CSII, or insulin pump) provides better glycemic control than does conventional therapy and comparable with or slightly better control than multiple daily injections. It should be considered for diabetes presenting in childhood or adolescence and during pregnancy.
- The Diabetes Control and Complications Trial (DCCT) showed that intensive treatment for glucose control decreases the development and progression of complications of type 1 DM. In this trial, the risks for retinopathy, nephropathy, and neuropathy were decreased by 35% to 90%.
- Low-dose aspirin (ASA; 81 mg/day) to decrease the risk for cerebrovascular disease is beneficial for patients with diabetes older than 40 yr with other risk factors (hypertension, dyslipidemia, smoking, obesity).
- Measure fasting lipid profile at least annually in adults with low-risk lipid values (low-density lipoprotein [LDL] cholesterol <100 mg/dl, high-density lipoprotein [HDL] cholesterol >50 mg/dl, and triglycerides <150 mg/dl). All patients with diabetes older than 40 yr with one or more additional risk factors for cardiovascular disease should be on statin therapy together with lifestyle modification regardless of baseline lipid levels. The primary goal is an LDL cholesterol level <100 mg/dl without overt coronary artery disease (CAD), and in patients with overt CAD, a goal of <70 mg/dl is an option. In patients for whom target goals cannot be easily reached on maximal tolerated therapy, an alternative therapeutic goal should be the reduction in LDL of ~30% to 40% from baseline.
- Becaplermin is a recombinant human platelet-derived growth factor useful for diabetic foot ulcers. It is applied as a topical gel to promote wound healing by enhancing the formation of granulation tissue in stage III and IV diabetic peripheral ulcers of the lower extremities.
- Aggressive antihypertensive therapy is recommended to keep systolic blood pressure (BP) <130 and diastolic BP <80 mm Hg. Use of angiotensin-converting enzyme (ACE) inhibitors or angiotensin receptor blockers (ARBs) to decrease albuminuria and for prevention of progression of kidney disease should be considered regardless of BP level; kidney function and serum potassium levels should be closely monitored.
- Bariatric surgery should be considered in adults with BMI >35 kg/m^2 and type 2 diabetes, especially if the diabetes is difficult to control with lifestyle and pharmacologic therapy.
- Treat hypoglycemia in a conscious person with glucose tab or gel 15 to 20 g, and intramuscular injection of glucagon if unconscious. Patient and family members should be instructed on the administration of glucagon for individuals at significant risk for severe hypoglycemia.

TABLE 1-21 Types of Insulin

Preparation	Brand	Onset (hr)*	Peak (hr)	Duration (hr)[†]	Route
Insulin Aspart	NovoLog[‡]	<0.25	1-3	3-5	SC, IV, CSII
Insulin Aspart Protamine/ Insulin Aspart	NovoLog Mix 70/30[‡]	<0.25	1-4	24	SC
Insulin Detemir	Levemir[§]	1	None	24	SC
Insulin Glargine	Lantus[‡]	1.1	None	≥24	SC
Insulin Glulisine	Apidra[‡]	≤0.25	1	2-4	SC, IV
Insulin Lispro	Humalog[‡]	<0.25	1	3.5-4.5	SC
Insulin Lispro Protamine/ Insulin Lispro	Humalog Mix 75/25[‡]	≤0.25	0.5-1.5	24	SC
	Humalog Mix 50/50[‡]	≤0.25	1	16	SC
Insulin Injection Regular (R)	Humulin R[¶]	0.5	2-4	6-8	SC, IM, IV
	Novolin N[§]	0.5	2.5-5	8	SC, IM, IV
Insulin Isophane Suspension (NPH)/Regular Insulin (R)	Humulin 70/30[¶]	0.5	2-12	24	SC
	Humulin 50/50[¶]	0.5	3-5	24	SC
	Novolin 70/30[§]	0.5	2-12	24	SC
Insulin Isophane Suspension (NPH)	Humulin N[¶]	1-2	6-12	18-24	SC
	Novolin N[§]	1.5	4-12	24	SC

*Onset for injectable formulations is always for the subcutaneous (SC) route. All times are approximate.
†Maximum effect occurs between these times; actual effect may last longer.
‡Recombinant human insulin analogue (using *E. coli*).
§Recombinant (using *S. cerevisiae*).
Injectable insulins listed are available in a concentration of 100 U/ml; Humulin R, in a concentration of 500 U/ml for SC injection. SC injection only, is available by prescription from Lilly for insulin-resistant patients who are hospitalized or in need of medical supervision.
¶Recombinant (using *E. coli*).
CSII, Continuous subcutaneous infusion; *IM*, intramuscularly; *IV*, intravenously.

DISPOSITION

- Diabetic retinopathy occurs in ~15% of patients with diabetes after 15 yr of diagnosis and increases 1%/yr after diagnosis. Retinal laser photocoagulation and vitrectomy are effective treatment modalities. Prevention is best accomplished by strict glucose and BP control.
- The frequency of neuropathy in patients with type 2 diabetes approaches 70% to 80%. It can be subdivided in sensorimotor neuropathy (distal symmetric polyneuropathy, focal neuropathy [diabetic mononeuropathy, mononeuropathy multiplex], diabetic amyotrophy) and autonomic neuropathy (vasomotor neuropathy, GI autonomic neuropathy [gastric atony, diabetic diarrhea or constipation, fecal incontinence], genitourinary autonomic neuropathy [bladder dysfunction, sexual dysfunction], hypoglycemic unawareness, sudomotor neuropathy). Duloxetine, a selective serotonin and norepinephrine reuptake inhibitor, is effective and FDA approved for relief of diabetic peripheral neuropathy. Pregabalin and gabapentin (900 to 3600 mg/day) are also effective for the symptomatic treatment of peripheral neuropathic pain. Topical capsaicin, 5% lidocaine transdermal patches, amitriptyline, and carbamazepine are also modestly effective.
- Diabetic gastroparesis is most often seen in patients who have had diabetes for at least 10 yr and typically have retinopathy, neuropathy, and nephropathy. Major manifestations are postprandial fullness, nausea, vomiting, and bloating. Pharmacologic therapy involves prokinetic agents (metoclopramide). Endoscopic injection of botulinum toxin into the pylorus and gastric electrical stimulation (using f electrodes placed laparoscopically in the muscle wall of the stomach antrum and connected to a neurostimulator) represent newer approaches to nonpharmacologic therapy.
- Nephropathy: The first sign of renal involvement in patients with DM is most often microalbuminuria, which is classified as incipient nephropathy. Without specific intervention, 50% of patients with diabetes with type 1 DM with overt diabetic nephropathy (urine protein ≥300 mg/24 hr) progress to ESRD within 10 yr of onset. More than 75% of type 1 DM and 20% of type 2 DM cases progress to ESRD over a 20-yr period.
- Infections are generally more common in patients with diabetes because of multiple factors, such as impaired leukocyte function, decreased tissue perfusion secondary to vascular disease, repeated trauma because of loss of sensation, and urinary retention secondary to neuropathy.
- Diabetic ketoacidosis and hyperosmolar nonketotic state are described in detail in Section I.
- Prevention/delay of type 2 diabetes: Patients with IGT or IFG should achieve weight loss of 5% to 10% of body weight and increase physical activity to at least 150 min/wk of moderate activity such as walking.

REFERRAL

- Patients with diabetes should be advised to have annual ophthalmologic examinations. In type 1 DM, ophthalmologic visits should begin within 3 to 5 yr of diagnosis, whereas type 2 DM patients should be seen from disease onset.
- Podiatric care can significantly reduce the rate of foot infections and amputations in patients with DM. Noninfected neuropathic foot ulcers require debridement and reduction of pressure.
- Nephrology consultation in all cases of proteinuria, hyperkalemia, uncontrolled BP, and when GFR has decreased to <30 ml/min/1.73 m^2.

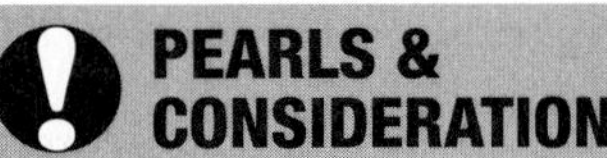

PEARLS & CONSIDERATIONS

COMMENTS

- Because normalization of serum glucose level is the ultimate goal, every patient should measure his or her blood glucose unless contraindicated by senility or blindness.
- For blood glucose monitoring, glucose oxidase strips are used in conjunction with a meter to give a digital reading. The testing can be done once a day, but the time should be varied each day so that over time the serum glucose level before meals and at bedtime can be assessed frequently without pricking the patient's fingers four times daily.
- Underinsured children and those with psychiatric illness are at greater risk for acute complications in type 1 DM and require frequent monitoring and aggressive risk management with diet, exercise, and periodic laboratory evaluation.
- Vascular endothelial growth factor and erythropoietin have been identified as factors involved in angiogenesis in proliferative diabetic retinopathy.
- Significant sustained weight loss using bariatric surgery has been reported as effective in achieving remission of type 2 diabetes in morbidly obese patients.
- Cigarette smoking predicts incident type 2 diabetes. For a smoker at risk for diabetes, smoking cessation should be coupled with strategies for diabetes prevention and early detection.

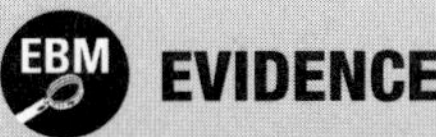

EVIDENCE

Please note: Complete text of EBM for this topic is available online.

Key trials and commentary:

Intensified multifactorial intervention—with tight glucose regulation and the use of renin–angiotensin system blockers, aspirin, and lipid-lowering agents—has been shown to reduce the risk of nonfatal cardiovascular disease among patients with type 2 diabetes mellitus and microalbuminuria. This study evaluated whether this approach would have an effect on the rates of death from any cause and from cardiovascular causes.

This study showed that in at-risk patients with type 2 diabetes, intensive intervention with multiple drug combinations and behavior modification had sustained beneficial effects with respect to vascular complications and on rates of death from any cause and from cardiovascular causes.

This study is an observational follow-up study of the participants of the Steno-2 Study, a randomized, controlled trial.

The Steno-2 Study randomly assigned 160 subjects with type 2 diabetes and microalbuminuria to an intensive therapy or a conventional arm for a total of almost 8 years. In this observational follow-up study, subjects were followed for over 5 years after finishing the active treatment period.

After the end of the active study period, all patients and their primary care physicians were informed of the study finding. Their treatment then became much more similar, and both groups were then managed with the same degree of intensity. Although the groups' glucose, blood pressure, and lipid control were similar during the follow-up period, their cardiovascular outcomes and mortality were very different, almost half in the previously intensively treated group.

These findings are consistent with those of the Diabetes Control and Complications Trial (DCCT), (Epidemiology of Diabetes Interventions and Complications [EDIC]), and UK Prospective Diabetes Study (UKPDS) follow-up studies underscoring the need and significant benefit of early aggressive treatment in diabetes. The reason for the continued and progressively larger difference in cardiovascular and mortality outcomes is not well understood, but has been ascribed to a so-called metabolic memory or legacy effect.[1] Ⓐ

Trials have found no significant clinical differences in efficacy and harmful effects between human and purified animal (mainly porcine) insulin. A systematic review was unable to find any significant difference in metabolic control or hypoglycemic episodes between the various types of insulin, although the authors comment that most studies were of poor methodological quality.[2]

There is limited evidence for the benefit of insulin analogs in patients with type 1 diabetes who are prone to frequent episodes of severe hypoglycemia or nocturnal hypoglycemia. There is evidence that short-acting insulin analogs seem to reduce the incidence of severe hypoglycemia but not the overall likelihood of hypoglycemia.[3]

The longer-acting insulin analogs, insulin detemir and insulin glargine, seem to result in glycemic control that is at least as good as isophane insulin. Both analogs appear to reduce nocturnal hypoglycemia compared with isophane insulin.[3]

Pancreas transplantation

Guidelines based on a technical review, concerning the indications for possible pancreas transplantation in patients with type 1 diabetes, have been produced by the American Diabetes Association.[4]

Medical nutrition therapy

Medical nutrition therapy for people with diabetes should be individualized, with consideration given to the individual's usual food and eating habits, metabolic profile, treatment goals, and desired outcomes.[5]

- Intensive vs. conventional glucose control in critically ill patients showed that intensive glucose control increased mortality : a blood glucose target of 180mg/dl or less resulted in lower mortality than did a target of 81-108 mg/dl. (The NICE-SUGAR study Investigators).[6]

  A Meta-analysis also showed that a tight glycemic control in critically ill patients is not associated with significantly reduced mortality but is associated with an increased risk of hypoglycemia.[7]
- In patients with type 2 DM and stable ischemic heart disease, rates of survival did not differ significantly between the revascularized group and the medical therapy group. (The BARI 2D Study Group)[8]
- Long-term follow-up the Diabetes Control and Complications Trial (DCCT-EDIC) and UK Prospective Diabetes Study (UKPDS) cohorts suggests that treatment to A1C targets below or around 7% in the years soon after the diagnosis of diabetes is associated with long-term reduction in the risk of macrovascular disease (legacy effect).[9,10] Ⓑ
- In a UKPDS follow-up trial, mortality was reduced after metformin therapy among overweight patients.[10]
- Subgroup analysis of clinical trials such as DCCT and UKPDS and the microvascular evidence from the ADVANCE (Action in Diabetes and Vascular Disease: Preterax and Diamicron MR controlled Evaluation) trial suggests a small but incremental benefit in microvascular outcomes with A1C target of <6.5% as opposed to 7.5%. Such patients might include those with short duration of diabetes, long life expectancy, and no significant cardiovascular disease at baseline. Ⓑ
- Conversely, less stringent A1C goals than the general goal of <7% may be appropriate for patients with a history of severe hypoglycemia, limited life expectancy, advanced microvascular or macrovascular complications, and extensive comorbid conditions and those with longstanding diabetes in whom the general goal is difficult to attain despite self-management education, appropriate glucose monitoring, and effective doses of multiple glucose lowering agents including insulin.[11] Ⓒ
- The Action to Control Cardiovascular Risk in Diabetes study (ACCORD) trial: as compared with standard therapy, the use of intensive therapy to achieve A1C levels of 6% or less increased mortality after 3.5 years of follow-up.[12]

- Glucose Control and Vascular complications in Veterans with longstanding type 2 Diabetes (VADT) failed to show that intensive glucose control to median A1C levels of 6.9% translated into significant effect on the rates of major cardiovascular events, death, or microvascular complications vs. a median A1C of 8.4%.[13]

Evidence-Based References

1. Gæde P, Lund-Andersen H, Parving H-H: Effect of a Multifactorial Intervention on Mortality in Type 2 Diabetes, *N Engl J Med* vol. 358, 580-591, 2008. Commentary by F. Ovalle, M.D.

2. Richter B, Neises G: 'Human' insulin versus animal insulin in people with diabetes mellitus. *Cochrane Database Rev* (1), 2005.

3. Update on insulin analogues. In: *Drug and Therapeutics Bulletin* 42:77-80, 2004.

4. American Diabetes Association: Pancreas transplantation in type 1 diabetes, *Diabetes Care* 27: S105, 2004.

5. Franz MJ et al; American Diabetes Association: Nutrition principles and recommendations in diabetes, *Diabetes Care* 27(Suppl 1):S36-46, 2004.

6. NICE-SUGAR Study Investigators et al: Intensive versus conventional glucose control in critically ill patients, *N Engl J Med* 360:1283-1297, 2009.

7. Weiner et al: A Meta-analysis Benefits and Risks of Tight Glucose Control in Critically ill Adults, *JAMA* 300(8):933-944, 2008.

8. The BARI 2D study group. A randomized Trial of Therapies for Type 2 Diabetes and Coronary Artery Disease, *N Engl J Med* 360:2503-15, 2009.

9. Diabetes Control and Complications Trial (DCCT)/Epidemiology of Diabetes Interventions and Complications Research Group: Effect of intensive therapy on the microvascular complications of type 1 diabetes mellitus, *JAMA* 287:2563, 2002.

10. 10-Year Follow-up of Intensive Glucose Control in Type 2 Diabetes, (UKPDS), *N Engl J Med* 359: 1577-89, 2008.

11. Intensive Blood Glucose Control and Vascular Outcomes in Patients with Type 2 Diabetes. The ADVANCE Collaborative Group, *N Engl J Med* 358: 2560-72, 2008.

12. Effects of Intensive Glucose Lowering in Type 2 Diabetes. The action to Control Cardiovascular Risk in Diabetes Study Group (ACCORD) *N Engl J Med* 358:2545-59, 2008.

13. Duckworth W et al: Glucose control and vascular complications in veterans with type 2 diabetes, *N Engl J Med* 360:129-39, 2009.

SUGGESTED READINGS

American Diabetes Association Position Statement: Standards of medical care for patients with diabetes mellitus, *Diabetes Care* 32:S 1, January 2009.

Guidelines on diabetes, pre-diabetes, and cardiovascular disease: executive summary. The Task Force on Diabetes and Cardiovascular Diseases of the European Society of Cardiology (ESC) and of the European Association for the Study of Diabetes (EASD) *European Heart Journal* 28:88-136, 2007.

Inzucchi SE: Management of hyperglycemia in the hospital setting, *N Engl J Med* 355:1903, 2006.

Kelly TN: Systematic review: Glucose control and cardiovascular disease in type 2 diabetes, *Ann Intern Med* 151:394-403, 2009.

Mooradian A et al: Narrative review: a rational approach to starting insulin therapy, *Ann Intern Med* 145:125, 2006.

Ripsin CM et al: Management of blood glucose in type 2 diabetes mellitus, *Am Fam Phys* 79(1):29-36, 2009.

Yeh HC et al: Smoking, smoking cessation, and risk for type 2 diabetes mellitus, *Ann Intern Med* 152:10-17, 2010.

AUTHORS: **SHAHNAZ PUNJANI, M.D., FRED F. FERRI, M.D.,** and **WEN-CHIH WU, M.D.**

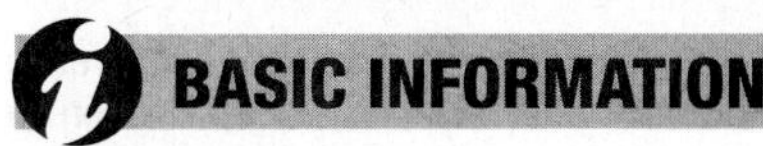

BASIC INFORMATION

DEFINITION

Diabetic ketoacidosis (DKA) is a life-threatening complication of diabetes mellitus resulting from severe insulin deficiency or insulin resistance with relative insulin deficiency and manifested clinically by severe dehydration and alterations in sensorium.

SYNONYMS

DKA

ICD-9CM CODES
250.1 Diabetic ketoacidosis

EPIDEMIOLOGY & DEMOGRAPHICS

INCIDENCE/PREVALENCE: 6 episodes per 10,000 individuals with diabetes; it accounts for 8% to 29% of all hospital admissions of patients with diabetes
PREDOMINANT AGE: 1 to 25 yr

PHYSICAL FINDINGS & CLINICAL PRESENTATION

- Evidence of dehydration (tachycardia, hypotension, dry mucous membranes, sunken eyeballs, poor skin turgor)
- Altered mental status
- Tachypnea with air hunger (Kussmaul's respiration)
- Fruity breath odor (caused by acetone)
- Lipemia retinalis in some patients
- Possible evidence of precipitating factors (infected wound, pneumonia)
- Abdominal tenderness in some patients

ETIOLOGY

- Metabolic decompensation in individuals with diabetes is usually precipitated by an infectious process (up to 40%).
- Poor compliance with insulin therapy and severe medical illness are other common causes.
- Delay in seeking medical attention and protein energy malnutrition may add to the problem in developing countries.
- Cocaine abuse has been reported as a risk factor for DKA in adult and teenage patients, particularly in patients with multiple admissions.
- Lack of education of primary caregiver (mother, sibling), proper monitoring of blood glucose, correct administration of insulin, supervision of insulin pump maintenance, and monitoring of diabetic caloric retraints are causes of recurrences of DKA.

DIAGNOSIS

DIFFERENTIAL DIAGNOSIS

- Hyperosmolar nonketotic state (Table 1-22)
- Alcoholic ketoacidosis
- Uremic acidosis
- Metabolic acidosis caused by methyl alcohol or ethylene glycol
- Salicylate poisoning

WORKUP

- Laboratory evaluation (see "Laboratory Tests") to confirm diagnosis and evaluate precipitating factors
- ECG to evaluate electrolyte abnormalities and rule out myocardial ischemia or infarction as a contributing factor

LABORATORY TESTS

- Glucose level demonstrates severe hyperglycemia (serum glucose generally >250 mg/dl)
- Arterial blood gases demonstrate acidosis: arterial pH usually <7.30 with Pco_2 <40 mm Hg
- Serum ketonemia (β-hydroxybutyrate > 300 μmol/L), ketonuria, and glycosuria
- Serum electrolytes:
    1. Serum bicarbonate is usually <15 mEq/L.
    2. Serum potassium (K^+) may be low, normal, or high. There is always significant total body potassium depletion regardless of the initial potassium level.
    3. Serum sodium is usually decreased as a result of hyperglycemia, dehydration, and lipemia. Assume 1.6-mEq/L decrease in extracellular sodium for each 100-mg/dl increase in glucose concentration. Initially, a modest degree of hypernatremia is advantageous to help prevent the fast fall of effective plasma osmolality when glycemia is under control.
    4. Calculate the anion gap (AG):

    $$AG = Na^+ - (Cl^- + HCO^-{}_3)$$

    In DKA, the anion gap is increased (generally >10) because of high levels of ketones; hyperchloremic metabolic acidosis may be present in unusual circumstances when both the glomerular filtration rate and the plasma volume are well maintained.

    Mixed metabolic disturbances demonstrate an anion gap metabolic acidosis overlapping metabolic alkalosis may be present; this is common in patients with DKA with persistent vomiting.
- CBC with differential, urinalysis, and urine and blood cultures to rule out infectious precipitating factor
- Serum calcium, magnesium, and phosphorus; the plasma phosphate and magnesium levels may be significantly depressed and should be rechecked within 24 hours because they may decrease further with correction of DKA
- Blood urea nitrogen and creatinine generally reveal significant dehydration
- Amylase and liver enzymes should be checked in patients with abdominal pain

IMAGING STUDIES

Chest radiographs are helpful to rule out infectious process. The initial chest film may be negative if the patient has significant dehydration. Repeat chest x-ray after 24 hours if pulmonary infection is strongly suspected.

TABLE 1-22 Comparison of Diabetic Ketoacidosis and Hyperosmolar Nonketotic Syndrome

Feature	DKA	HNKS
Age of patient	Usually <40 yr	Usually >60 yr
Duration of symptoms	Usually <2 days	Usually >5 days
Serum glucose concentration	Usually <800 mg/dl	Usually >800 mg/dl
Serum sodium concentration (Na^+)	More likely to be normal or low	More likely to be normal or high
Serum bicarbonate concentration ($HCO^-{}_3$)	Low	Normal
Ketone bodies	At least 4 + 1:1 dilution	<2 + in 1:1 dilution
pH	Low	Normal
Serum osmolality	Usually <350 mOsm/kg	Usually >350 mOsm/kg
Cerebral edema	Occasionally clinical symptoms	Rarely (never?) clinical
Prognosis	3-10% mortality rate	10-20% mortality rate
Subsequent course	Insulin therapy required in almost all cases	Insulin therapy not required in most cases

DKA, Diabetic ketoacidosis; *HNKS,* hyperosmolar nonketotic syndrome.
From Andreoli TE (ed): *Cecil essentials of medicine,* ed 6, Philadelphia, 2005, WB Saunders.

TREATMENT

NONPHARMACOLOGIC THERAPY

- Monitor mental status, vital signs, and urine output hourly until improved, then monitor q2-4h.
- Monitor electrolytes, renal function, and glucose level (see "Acute General Rx").

ACUTE GENERAL Rx

Fluid replacement (usual deficit is 6 to 8 L):

1. Do not delay fluid replacement until laboratory results have been received. Fluid deficits are typically 100 ml/kg of body weight. The normalization of hypotension is imperative within the initial hour of presentation while avoiding the use of hypotonic fluids. The total fluid administered should not exceed 4 L/m²/24 hours for fear of causing cerebral edema (CE). One rule of thumb is to deliver fluids (deficit and maintenance) over

a period of 48 hours if serum osmolality is >360 mOsm/L.

2. The initial fluid replacement should be with 0.9% normal saline (NS) until blood pressure and organ perfusion are restored. In patients with severe hypernatremia (serum sodium >160 mEq/L), 0.45% saline infusion can be used. Careful monitoring for fluid overload is necessary in elderly patients and those with a history of congestive heart failure.
3. The rate of fluid replacement varies with the age of the patient and the presence of significant cardiac or renal disease.
    - The usual rate of infusion is 500 ml to 1 L over the first hour and 300 to 500 ml/hour for the next 12 hours.
    - Continue the infusion at a rate of 200 to 300 ml/hour, using 0.45% NS until the serum glucose level is <300 mg/dl, then change the hydrating solution to D_5W to prevent hypoglycemia, replenish free water, and introduce additional glucose substrate (necessary to suppress lipolysis and ketogenesis).

Insulin administration:

1. The patient should be given an initial loading IV bolus of 0.15 to 0.2 U/kg regular insulin followed by a constant infusion at a rate of 0.1 U/kg/hour (e.g., 25 U of regular insulin in 250 ml of 0.9% saline solution at 70 ml/hour equals 7 U/hour for a 70-kg patient). Insulin replacement should generally not be started until serum potassium is >3.3 mEq/L to prevent life-threatening hypokalemia.
2. Monitor serum glucose hourly for the first 2 hours, then monitor q2-4h.
3. The goal is to decrease serum glucose level by 80 mg/dl/hour (after an initial decline because of rehydration); if the serum glucose level is not decreasing at the expected rate, double the rate of insulin infusion.
4. When the serum glucose level approaches 250 mg/dl, decrease the rate of insulin infusion to 2 to 3 U/hour and continue this rate until the patient has received adequate fluid replacement, HCO^-_3 is close to normal, and ketones have cleared. After target glucose levels are achieved, it usually takes 5 to 7 hours for ketosis to clear. In young children and adolescents who have high growth rate, they have greater levels of human growth hormones so that there is a prolonged time lag for plasma glucose to reach to above levels. Patients with fever or infections and higher metabolic requirements need 15% to 20% more insulin than the usual starting dose.
5. Approximately 30 to 60 min before stopping the IV insulin infusion, administer an SC dose of regular insulin (dose varies with the patient's demonstrated insulin sensitivity); this SC dose of regular insulin is necessary because of the extremely short life of the insulin in the IV infusion.
6. When the patient is able to eat, long-acting insulin such as NPH insulin is given in the morning and/or at bedtime, and shorter-acting insulin such as aspart insulin is administered before each meal by using a sliding scale. In individuals with newly diagnosed diabetes, the total daily dose to maintain metabolic control ranges from 0.5 to 0.8 U/kg/day.

Electrolyte replacement:

- Potassium replacement: the average total potassium loss in DKA is 300 to 500 mEq.
- K^+ can be supplemented as chloride- and phosphate-containing solutions.
    1. The rate of replacement varies with the patient's serum potassium level, degree of acidosis (decreased pH, increased potassium level), and renal function (potassium replacement should be used with caution in patients with renal failure).
    2. As a rule of thumb, potassium replacement may be started when there is no ECG evidence of hyperkalemia (tall, narrow, or tent-shaped T waves; decreased or absent P waves; short QT intervals; widening of QRS complex).
    3. In patients with normal renal function, potassium replacement can be started by adding 20 to 40 mEq KCl/L of IV hydrating solution if serum potassium is 4 to 5 mEq/L, and more if serum potassium level is lower than 4 mEq/L. In patients with severe hypokalemia (potassium <3.3 mEq/L), give 40 mEq/hour potassium until potassium is >3.3 mEq/L.
    4. Monitor serum potassium level hourly for the first 2 hours, then monitor q2-4h.
- Phosphate replacement: If the serum PO_4 is <1.5 mEq/L, give 2.5 mg/kg IV over 6 hours of elemental phosphate. Routine replacement of phosphate (in the absence of laboratory evidence of significant hypophosphatemia) is not indicated. Rapid IV phosphate administration can cause hypocalcemia.
- Magnesium replacement: Replacement is indicated only in the presence of significant hypomagnesemia or refractory hypokalemia.

Bicarbonate therapy:

- Routine use of bicarbonate in DKA is contraindicated because it can worsen hypokalemia and intracellular acidosis, and cause CE. Bicarbonate therapy should be considered only if the arterial pH is <6.9 and HCO^-_3 is <5.
- In these patients, 44 to 88 mEq sodium bicarbonate can be added to 1 L of 0.45% NS q2-4h until pH increases to >7.
- Use of bicarbonate therapy is particularly dangerous in the pediatric population. Children with DKA who have a low $Paco_2$ and high serum urea nitrogen concentration at presentation and who are treated with bicarbonate are at increased risk for CE. Bicarbonate therapy in children with DKA should be limited to those with severe circulatory failure and a high risk for cardiac decompensation resulting from profound acidosis.

PREVENTION

- Provide information/education for teachers, parents, school staff, and caregivers on how to recognize children with undiagnosed diabetes.
- Review sick day management; increase home blood glucose monitoring, education on how to measure urinary or fingerstick ketones, compliance with insulin; and maintain adequate hydration and nutrition.

DISPOSITION

- Average mortality rate in DKA is 5% to 10%.
- In children <10 yr, DKA causes 70% of diabetes-related deaths.
- CE occurs in 1% of episodes of DKA in children and is associated with a mortality rate of 40% to 90%.

REFERRAL

Patients with DKA should be admitted to the intensive care unit. Alert patients who are able to take fluids orally and have mild DKA occasionally can be treated under observation and sent home. The American Diabetes Association admission guidelines are a plasma glucose level >250 mg/dl, with arterial pH <7.30, a serum bicarbonate level <15 mEq/L, and a moderate or greater level of ketones in the serum or urine.

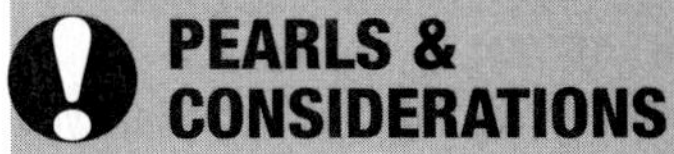

PEARLS & CONSIDERATIONS

COMMENTS

- Although DKA occurs more commonly in type 1 diabetes mellitus, a significant proportion (>20%) occurs in patients with type 2 diabetes.
- 30% to 40% of DKA admissions involve patients with newly diagnosed diabetes.
- Potential complications of DKA therapy include hypoglycemia, CE, cardiac arrhythmias, shock, myocardial infarction, and acute pancreatitis.
- Risk factors for CE include age <5 yr, high initial BUN reflecting severe prolonged state of dehydration, hyperventilation to a $Paco_2$ of <22 mm Hg, and presenting arterial pH of <7.00. It presents 4 to 8 hours after start of rehydration therapy. Presentation may be abrupt with sudden severe headache, vomiting, sudden hypertension, and obtunded sensorium. First management response to CE is to elevate head of the patient to 30-degree angle, followed by IV mannitol and intubation and hyperventilation, finally cutting back of the maintenance fluid to 75% of the amount required.
- Underinsured children and those with psychiatric illness are at greater risk for DKA.
- Subcutaneous administration of rapid-acting insulin analogues may be reasonable alternatives to IV regular insulin infusion for treating uncomplicated DKA.
- DKA can occur with blood glucose <350 mg/dl in the setting of poor oral intake or pregnancy.
- Ketones can be positive in starvation or with heavy alcohol intake; DKA can coexist with other causes of metabolic acidosis such as lactic acidosis.

- Euglycemic DKA is reported to occur in 1% to 17% of cases; normal or minimally elevated blood sugar levels seen in starvation, especially if insulin is continued or in the presence of severe hepatic disease.
- Use of low-level IV unfractionated herapin has been reported as effective in reducing severe elevations of plasma triglicerides in DKA.

SUGGESTED READINGS

Argus MS et al: Continuous non invasive end tidal CO2 monitoring in pediatrics patients with DKA, *Pediatr Diabetes* 7:196, 2006.

Cole RP: Herapin treatment for severe hypertriglyceridemia in diabetic ketoacidosis, *Arch Intern Med* 169(15):1439-1441, 2009.

Halperin M et al: Strategies to diminish the danger of cerebral edema in pediatric diabetes, *Pediatr Diabetes* 7:191, 2006.

Kitabchi AE et al: Hyperglycemic crises in diabetes mellitus: diabetic ketoacidosis and hyperglycemic hyperosmolar state, *Endocrinol Metab Clin North Am* 35:725-751, 2006.

Koul PB: Diabetic ketoacidosis: a current appraisal of pathophysiology and management, *Clin Pediatr (Phila)* 48:135, 2009.

Mazer M et al: Is subcutaneous administration of rapid-acting insulin as effective as intravenous insulin for treating diabetic ketoacidosis? *Ann Emerg Med* 53:259-263, 2009.

Newton CA, Raskin P: Diabetic ketoacidosis in type 1 and type 2 diabetes mellitus, *N Engl J Med* 164:1925, 2004.

AUTHORS: **SHAHNAZ PUNJANI, M.D., FRED F. FERRI, M.D.,** and **WEN-CHIH WU, M.D.**

Diabetic Polyneuropathy (ALG)

BASIC INFORMATION

DEFINITION

Diabetic polyneuropathy (DPN) is an insidious and progressive length-dependent disorder of peripheral nerves (large, small, and autonomic fibers) that is secondary to diabetes and is characterized by distal and symmetric pain, numbness, tingling, or autonomic dysfunction. Other diabetic neuropathies may present with proximal or asymmetric pain and weakness.

SYNONYMS

Chronic distal symmetric polyneuropathy
Diabetic peripheral neuropathy

ICD-9CM CODES

250.6 Diabetic polyneuropathy

EPIDEMIOLOGY & DEMOGRAPHICS

PREVALENCE (IN U.S.): 7.5% of diabetics at initial diagnosis and 40% (type 2 diabetics) after 10 years of diabetes. Overall, 10% to 64% of all diabetics.

PREDOMINANT SEX: Male diabetics have a higher incidence than females.

PREDOMINANT AGE: More common in patients older than 50 years of age.

PHYSICAL FINDINGS & CLINICAL PRESENTATION

- Tingling, buzzing, numbness, tightness, electric shock-like, hot, cold, or burning sensations starting in the feet bilaterally and slowly progressing to involve the hands. The level of impairment in the legs usually reaches above the knees before the hands are affected and in severe cases the sensory disturbances may involve the anterior trunk and the head. Symptoms are typically worse at night.
- Some patients report difficulties in opening jars, turning keys, difficulty with stairs, getting up from a sitting or lying position, raising their arms above the shoulders, and falling.
- Autonomic dysfunction presents as dry skin, lack of or excessive sweating, sensitivity to bright lights, postural light-headedness, fainting, urinary urgency, incontinence, nocturnal diarrhea, constipation, vomiting, erectile and ejaculatory dysfunction in men, and loss of ability to reach sexual climax in women.
- Examination shows decreased pinprick, light touch, temperature, vibration, and proprioceptive sensations in a stocking or glove distribution with absent or reduced ankle reflexes. Gait abnormalities (sensory ataxia), anhidrosis, and poorly reactive pupils can be seen. Muscle weakness (of the distal muscles) may be seen in later stages.

OTHER DIABETIC NEUROPATHIES

Generalized:

- *Hyperglycemic neuropathy:* tingling, pain, or hyperesthesia in the feet of a patient with poor glycemic control that rapidly resolves with improving hyperglycemia.
- *Insulin neuritis:* severe pain (worse at night) that is difficult to control, which is seen in patients who are on insulin.
- *Chronic inflammatory demyelinating polyneuropathy (CIDP):* more common in those with type 1 diabetes. DPN differs from CIDP in that patients with DPN are older, imbalance is more common, duration of symptoms at time of presentation is longer, and there is more prominent secondary axonal loss on nerve conduction studies and less response to therapy.

Focal:

- *Cranial neuropathies:* abrupt painless sixth or third nerve palsy. Third nerve palsy is less common than sixth and half of the patients complain of retroorbital pain and headache. The pupil is also spared due to central rather than peripheral ischemia of the nerve fascicle. Symptoms usually resolve within 6 mo.
- *Somatic mononeuropathies:* focal neuropathies in the extremities caused by entrapment or compression of nerves including the median at the wrist (carpal tunnel syndrome), the ulnar at the elbow, or the common peroneal at the fibular head.
- *Diabetic truncal radiculoneuropathy (thoracoabdominal radiculopathy):* patients present with a unilateral (later becomes bilateral) focal contact hyperesthesia and stabbing, burning, beltlike pain in the same area (worse at night), focal weakness of the anterior abdominal wall muscles, and weight loss. Sensory deficits seen in a dermatomal distribution. Most recover within months.
- *Diabetic lumbosacral radiculoplexus neuropathy (Bruns-Garland syndrome or diabetic amyotrophy):* patients present with an abrupt onset of severe unilateral low back, hip, or anterior thigh pain. Asymmetric proximal weakness and muscle atrophy develop a few days to weeks later (initially unilateral then becomes bilateral) with marked weight loss.

ETIOLOGY

- Not fully understood.
- *The polyol pathway theory:* high blood glucose leads to high nerve glucose, which causes overactivity of the polyol pathway and a disturbance of axoplasmic transport.
- *Microvascular ischemia and hypoxia theory:* hyperglycemia causes endothelial cell hypertrophy of the blood vessel walls and capillary damage, which eventually causes ischemia of the central portion of the nerve fascicle.
- *Nonenzymatic glycosylation theory:* increased low-density lipoproteins (LDL) that promote smooth muscle proliferation and atheroma formation.

Dx DIAGNOSIS

DIFFERENTIAL DIAGNOSIS

Various other causes of neuropathy

WORKUP

- *Nerve conduction studies:* distal symmetric predominantly sensory polyneuropathy with axonal features (reduced response amplitudes)
- *Electromyography:* denervation (positive sharp waves and fibrillations) and reinnervation (high-amplitude, long-duration, and polyphasic motor unit potentials) changes in the distal muscles
- *Other diagnostic testing* (MRI and CT of the spine and or brain) to rule out other diseases as indicated
- *Skin biopsy:* checks intraepidermal nerve fiber density, which measures the sensory and sympathetic innervation to the skin. Used in some university centers and in drug trials to measure regenerative capacity of peripheral nerves (Herrmann et al).

LABORATORY TESTS

- Serum protein electrophoresis, immunofixation electrophoresis
- Screening laboratory tests for other treatable causes of neuropathy
- Fasting blood sugar, hemoglobin A1c, or glucose tolerance test

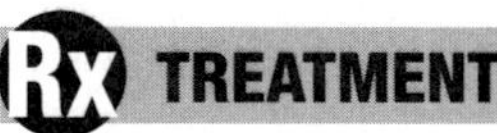

TREATMENT

NONPHARMACOLOGIC THERAPY

- Tight glucose control from the time of diagnosis of diabetes is the most important measure taken (69% reduction in risk of developing neuropathy in type 1 diabetes).
- Frequent follow-up visits, foot inspection for ulcers, and education on foot care.

GENERAL Rx

- Treatment of pain and paresthesias
- Anticonvulsants:
  - Gabapentin (Neurontin): 100-1200 mg tid
  - Pregabalin (Lyrica): 75-300 mg bid
  - Oxcarbazepine (Trileptal): 300-1800 mg bid
  - Carbamazepine (Tegretol): 100-200 mg bid or tid
- Antidepressants:
  - Nortriptyline (Pamelor): 25-150 mg qhs or bid
  - Amitriptyline (Elavil) 25-150 mg qhs or bid
  - Duloxetine (Cymbalta): 30-60 mg qd
- Others:
  - Tramadol (Ultram): 50-400 mg qd-qid (short-term)
  - Lidocaine patch: 5% 1-4 patches 12 hours on 12 hours off
  - Capsaicin extract: 7.5% 3-4 times per day
  - Opiates

DISPOSITION

Diabetes carries significant morbidity and complications. Patients with untreated diabetic peripheral neuropathy have higher morbidity and complication rates than those without neuropathy or those with treated neuropathy.

REFERRAL

- A neurologist or a neuromuscular specialist for neurophysiologic testing and assistance in managing pain and paresthesias

- Podiatrist for yearly foot examination
- Ophthalmologist for yearly eye examination

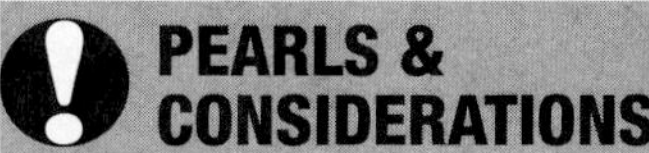

PEARLS & CONSIDERATIONS

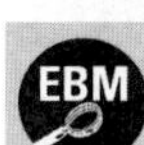

EVIDENCE

There is evidence for a significant improvement in glycemic control and slower development and progression of microvascular diabetic complications with intensive versus conventional insulin regimens in patients with type 1 diabetes at the expense of increased episodes of severe hypoglycemia.

The evidence for a reduction in the development of macrovascular disease or in macrovascular mortality in patients treated with intensive regimes versus conventional regimes is not clear, although a systematic review found intensive insulin regimes were associated with a reduction in macrovascular events vs conventional regimes.[1] Ⓐ

Trials have found no significant clinical differences in efficacy and harmful effects between human and purified animal (mainly porcine) insulin.

A systematic review was unable to find any significant difference in metabolic control or hypoglycemic episodes between the various types of insulin, although the authors comment that most studies were of poor methodological quality.[2] Ⓑ

There is limited evidence for the benefit of insulin analogs in patients with type 1 diabetes who are prone to frequent episodes of severe hypoglycemia or nocturnal hypoglycemia.

There is evidence that short-acting insulin analogs seem to reduce the incidence of severe hypoglycemia but not the overall likelihood of hypoglycemia.[3] Ⓑ

The longer-acting insulin analogs, insulin detemir and insulin glargine, seem to result in glycemic control that is at least as good as isophane insulin. Both analogs appear to reduce nocturnal hypoglycemia compared with isophane insulin.[3] Ⓑ

Pancreas transplantation

Guidelines based on a technical review, concerning the indications for possible pancreas transplantation in patients with type 1 diabetes, have been produced by the American Diabetes Association.[4]

Medical nutrition therapy

Medical nutrition therapy for people with diabetes should be individualized, with consideration given to the individual's usual food and eating habits, metabolic profile, treatment goals, and desired outcomes.[5] Ⓒ

Evidence-Based References

1. Campbell A: Glycaemic control in type 1 diabetes, *Clin Evid* 2007. Ⓐ
2. Richter B, Neises G: "Human" insulin versus animal insulin in people with diabetes mellitus, *Cochrane Database Rev* (1), 2005. Ⓑ
3. Update on insulin analogues, *Drug and Therapeutics Bulletin* 42:77-80, 2004. Ⓑ
4. American Diabetes Association: Pancreas transplantation in type 1 diabetes, *Diabetes Care* 27:S105, 2004.
5. Franz MJ et al: American Diabetes Association. Nutrition principles and recommendations in diabetes, *Diabetes Care* 27(Suppl 1):S36-46, 2004. Ⓒ

SUGGESTED READINGS

DCCT Research Group: The effect of intensive treatment of diabetes on the development and progression of long-term complications in insulin-dependent diabetes mellitus, *N Engl J Med* 329:14: 977-986, 1993.

Herrmann DN et al: Epidermal nerve fiber density and sural nerve morphometry in peripheral neuropathies, *Neurology* 53:1634-1640, 1999.

Katirji B et al: *Neuromuscular disorders in clinical practice,* Boston, 2002, Butterworth-Heinemann, pp. 598-621.

Llewelyn G: The diabetic neuropathies: types, diagnosis and management, *J Neurol Neurosurg Psychiatry* 74:ii15, 2003.

Rosenstock J et al: Pregabalin for the treatment of painful diabetic peripheral neuropathy: a double-blind, placebo-controlled trial, *Pain* 110(3):628-638, 2004.

AUTHOR: **MUSTAFA A. HAMMAD, M.D.**

Digoxin Overdose

BASIC INFORMATION

DEFINITION

Digoxin, a cardiac glycoside, is used for the treatment of symptomatic heart failure and ventricular rate control in atrial fibrillation.

Chronic digoxin therapy or acute overdose can cause toxicity. Toxicity can occur even when serum levels are within the therapeutic range.

SYNONYMS

Digitalis overdose
Cardiac glycoside toxicity

ICD-9CM CODES
972.1 Digitalis overdose

PHARMACOKINETICS

Steady-state levels (not peak levels) correlate with toxicity; digoxin reaches steady state 6 to 8 hr after ingestion.
BIOAVAILABILITY: Approximately 80%
VOLUME OF DISTRIBUTION: 5 to 7 L/kg, highly tissue bound
HALF-LIFE: 36 hr
EXCRETION: Predominantly renal
THERAPEUTIC LEVEL: 0.5 to 2 ng/ml (0.5 to 1.0 ng/ml suggested in heart failure); check level one week after starting therapy or changing dose. Sample should be drawn at least 8 hr after last dose.

EPIDEMIOLOGY & DEMOGRAPHICS

- Digoxin toxicity occurs in up to 5% of individuals on therapy.
- Factors that potentiate toxicity (may increase level or modify cardiac sensitivity): advanced age, female gender, renal insufficiency, cardiac or pulmonary disease, drugs that affect elimination (ACE inhibitors, amiodarone, clarithromycin, cyclosporine, diltiazem, erythromycin, itraconazole, NSAIDs, rifampin, spironolactone, SSRIs, tetracyclines, quinidine, verapamil, and herbal supplements), coingestion of cardiotoxic drugs (beta-blockers, calcium channel blockers, tricyclic antidepressants), hypokalemia, hypomagnesemia, hypercalcemia, acid-base disturbance, hypoxia, hypothyroidism, and volume depletion.

PHYSICAL FINDINGS & CLINICAL PRESENTATION

Cardiac, gastrointestinal, and central nervous systems are affected. Fatigue, malaise, and weakness are common symptoms.
CARDIAC: The most common and often first finding is an increase in premature ventricular complexes. Can present with almost any dysrhythmia or conduction block.
GASTROINTESTINAL: Anorexia, nausea, vomiting, diarrhea, abdominal pain
CENTRAL NERVOUS SYSTEM:
- Headache, dizziness, visual disturbance (flashing lights, halos, blurred vision, change in color perception, decreased visual acuity), confusion, hallucinations, delirium, syncope
- Hyperkalemia often seen in acute poisoning; hypokalemia more common in chronic toxicity

ETIOLOGY

Digoxin reversibly inhibits the function of sodium-potassium adenosine triphosphatase, increasing extracellular K^+ and intracellular Na^+. This reduces the activity of the Na-Ca exchanger, leading to intracellular accumulation of calcium. This results in increased myocardial contractility and cardiac output, the positive inotropic effect associated with digoxin therapy. Cardiac glycosides also decrease the heart rate (effect on SA node) and slow conduction throughout the AV node by increasing parasympathetic tone. Sympathetic activity is decreased at therapeutic levels but increased in toxicity. Enhanced automaticity of cardiac tissue and depressed conduction lead to the extrasystoles and arrhythmias seen in toxicity.

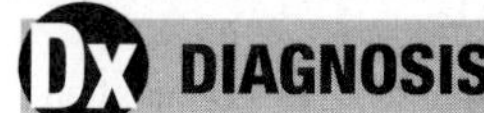

DIAGNOSIS

DIFFERENTIAL DIAGNOSIS

Medications:
- Beta-blockers
- Calcium channel blockers
- Clonidine
- Cyclic antidepressants
- Encainide and flecainide
- Procainamide
- Propoxyphene
- Quinidine

Plants producing digitalis-like glycosides:
- Foxglove
- Oleander
- Lily of the valley

Cardiac conduction abnormalities:
- Sick sinus syndrome
- AV node dysfunction

Electrolyte abnormalities:
- Hyperkalemia

WORKUP

- History: medication changes, herbal supplements, deliberate overdose
- Physical examination

LABORATORY TESTS

- Stat digoxin level (in acute ingestion high levels may not be toxic, as tissue redistribution will occur)
- Electrolytes, BUN, creatinine, magnesium, calcium
- ECG (Figs. 1-90 and 1-91)
- Almost any dysrhythmia can occur, but simultaneous increased automaticity of cardiac tissue and conduction delay in the AV node should raise suspicion. Findings suggestive of toxicity include the following:
  - Frequent premature ventricular complexes (bigeminy)
  - Bradydysrhythmias
  - AV block (Mobitz type 1)

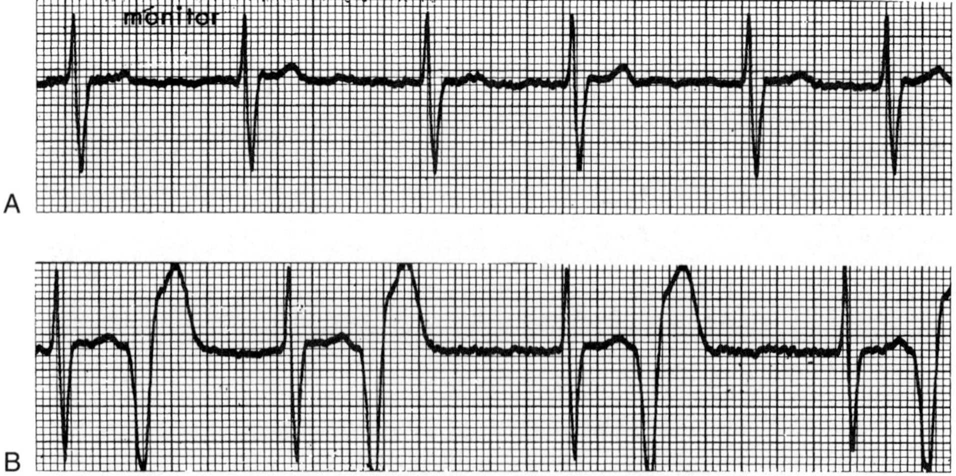

FIGURE 1-90 Ventricular bigeminy caused by digoxin toxicity. Ventricular ectopy is one of the most common signs of digoxin toxicity. The underlying rhythm in **A** is atrial fibrillation. In **B** each normal QRS is followed by a ventricular premature beat. (Reprinted from Goldberger AL [ed]: *Clinical electrocardiography,* ed 5, St Louis, 1994, Mosby.)

- ○ Atrial tachycardia with AV block
- ○ Junctional tachycardia
- ○ Venticular arrhythmias: Bidirectional ventricular tachycardia, ventricular tachycardia, ventricular fibrillation

Rx TREATMENT

NONPHARMACOLOGIC THERAPY

- Ensure adequate airway
- Cardiac monitor

ACUTE GENERAL Rx

DECREASE TOXICITY:

- Acute toxicity: activated charcoal if within 1 hr of ingestion.
- Treat hyperkalemia
- Treat hypokalemia and hypomagnesemia, both potentiate toxicity
- Digoxin-specific Fab fragments (Digibind):
  1. Specific antibodies that bind to digoxin and to a lesser extent other cardiac glycosides
  2. Initial response usually seen in 30 min, and complete reversal usually occurs within 4 hr
  3. Indications: hyperkalemia ($\geq$5 mEq/L), hemodynamic instability, severe arrhythmias, massive overdose (acute ingestion of $\geq$10 mg digoxin or digoxin serum level $\geq$10 ng/ml), coingestion of cardiotoxic drugs or plants containing cardiac glycosides
  4. Dosing: 1 vial (38 mg) of Fab fragments binds 0.5 mg of digoxin
     a. Digoxin
        (i) Acute ingestion: number of vials = (ingested digoxin [mg] $\times$ 0.8)/0.5
        (ii) Chronic ingestion: number of vials = (serum digoxin level [ng/ml] $\times$ weight [kg]/100
     b. If neither the amount ingested nor serum level is known, treat empirically:
        (i) Acute intoxication: 10 vials and repeat if needed
        (ii) Chronic toxicity: 6 vials
        NOTE: Underdosing of Fab fragments may result in rebound toxicity as free digoxin is released from tissue stores.
  5. After use of Fab fragments, the free digoxin level decreases, but the measured digoxin level may increase because most assays measure free and bound digoxin levels. Serum levels are unreliable for days.
  6. Renal elimination: half-life of inactive complex is 15 to 20 hr. In renal failure, consider plasma exchange or plasmapheresis to remove Fab-digoxin complex; theoretically, complexes may dissociate before excretion and toxicity may reoccur.
  7. Class C for pregnancy.
  8. Adverse effects of treatment:
     a. May undo desirable action of digoxin and exacerbate heart failure or increase ventricular response in previously controlled atrial fibrillation.
     b. Hypokalemia: monitor potassium level hourly for several hours. The hyperkalemia seen in toxicity reflects a change in potassium distribution, not an increase in total body stores. As toxicity resolves, the potassium moves back into the cell and hypokalemia can occur.
     c. Allergic reactions (<1%): Skin testing appropriate for high-risk individuals (history of sheep protein allergy or prior use).
- Hemodialysis and hemoperfusion: not useful because of extensive tissue binding and large volume of distribution.

COMPLICATIONS:

Hyperkalemia:

- Sodium bicarbonate
- Glucose and insulin
- Sodium polystyrene sulfonate (Kayexalate)
- Do not use calcium because it may worsen ventricular arrhythmias

Bradycardia and heart block:

- Atropine
- Transcutaneous external cardiac pacemaker

Supraventricular and ventricular tachycardia:

- Lidocaine or phenytoin: decrease ventricular automaticity without slowing AV node conduction
- Avoid quinidine, bretylium, procainamide, and verapamil; may increase ventricular arrhythmias/AV node block
- Elective electrocardioversion is relatively contraindicated because it may precipitate ventricular fibrillation

DISPOSITION

- Good with prompt treatment
- Chronic poisoning is associated with higher mortality rate than acute poisoning

REFERRAL

U.S. Poison Control network: 800-222-1222

PEARLS & CONSIDERATIONS

- High index of suspicion is necessary; the signs and symptoms of toxicity often are similar to those of the underlying disease.
- To minimize toxicity, digoxin levels should be checked if the patient's condition changes (e.g., weight loss, worsening renal function) or an interacting drug is started or stopped.
- Hyperkalemia in acute toxicity is suggestive of significant poisoning (reflects the amount of poisoning of Na^+-K^+ ATPase) and is associated with increased mortality rate.
- Falsely elevated digoxin levels may be seen in pregnant women, renal failure, hepatobiliary disease, and CHF as a result of the presence of an endogenous digoxin-like substance.
- Severe toxicity from ingestion of nondigoxin cardiac glycosides (plants, etc.) may present with low digoxin levels because of low cross-reactivity between these substances and the digoxin assay.

SUGGESTED READINGS

Antman EM et al: Treatment of 150 cases of life-threatening digitalis intoxication with digoxin-specific Fab antibody fragments. Final report of a multicenter study, *Circulation* 81:1744, 1990.

Bauman JL et al: Mechanisms, manifestations, and management of digoxin toxicity in the modern era, *Am J Cardiovasc Drugs* 6(2):77, 2006.

AUTHOR: **SUDEEP KAUR AULAKH, M.D.**

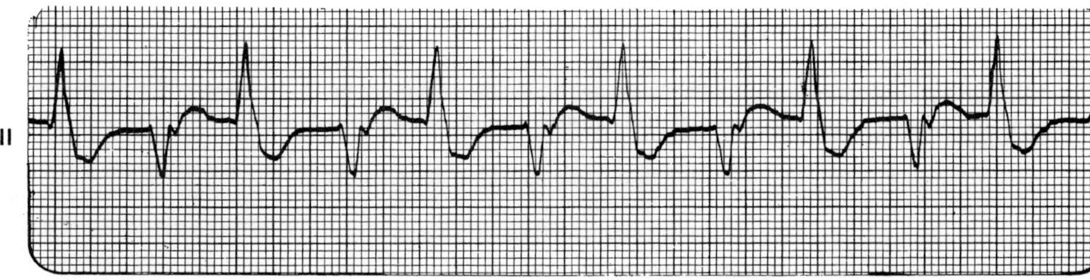

FIGURE 1-91 This digoxin-toxic arrhythmia is a special type of ventricular tachycardia (bidirectional tachycardia) with QRS complexes that alternate in direction from beat to beat. No P waves are present. (Reprinted from Goldberger AL [ed]: *Clinical electrocardiography,* ed 5, St Louis, 1994, Mosby.)

BASIC INFORMATION

DEFINITION

Diphtheria is an infection of the mucous membranes or skin caused by *Corynebacterium diphtheriae.*

SYNONYMS

Pharyngeal diphtheria
Wound diphtheria
Diphtheric cardiomyopathy
Diphtheric polyneuropathy

ICD-9CM CODES
032.9 Diphtheria

EPIDEMIOLOGY & DEMOGRAPHICS

INCIDENCE (IN U.S.): Since 2000 only 5 cases in the U.S. due to widespread vaccination
PREDOMINANT AGE: Adult years

PHYSICAL FINDINGS & CLINICAL PRESENTATION

RESPIRATORY DIPHTHERIA:

- Commonly presenting as pharyngitis, but any part of the respiratory tract may be involved, including the nasopharynx, larynx, trachea, or bronchi
- Areas of gray or white exudate coalescing to form a "pseudomembrane" that bleeds when removed
- Possible fever and dysphagia
- Complications: respiratory tract obstruction and pneumonia
- Systemic effects of the toxin: myocarditis and polyneuritis (frequently involving a bulbar distribution), less often nephritis
- Occurs mostly in nonimmune individuals; usually milder and less likely to be complicated in those adequately immunized

CUTANEOUS DIPHTHERIA:

- Usually complicates existing skin lesion (i.e., impetigo or scabies)
- Resembles the underlying condition or presents as a nonhealing ulcer with a grayish membrane

ETIOLOGY

- Caused by *C. diphtheriae,* an aerobic, gram-positive rod
- Transmitted by close contact through droplets of nasopharyngeal secretions
- Symptomatic disease of the respiratory system caused by toxin-producing strains (tox$^+$)
- Systemic effects of toxin: ranging from nausea and vomiting to polyneuropathy, nephritis, myocarditis, and vascular collapse
- Presence of strains not producing toxin (tox$^+$) in the respiratory tract of asymptomatic carriers and in skin lesions of cutaneous diphtheria

DIAGNOSIS

DIFFERENTIAL DIAGNOSIS

- Streptococcal pharyngitis
- Viral pharyngitis
- Mononucleosis

WORKUP

- Presence of a pseudomembrane in the oropharynx suggestive of diagnosis (not always present)
- Gram stains of secretions to show club-shaped organisms, which appear as "Chinese letters"
- Nasolaryngoscopy to identify lesions in the nares, nasopharynx, larynx, or tracheobronchial tree

LABORATORY TESTS

- Cultures of mucosal lesions or of nasal discharge
  1. Positive culture for *C. diphtheriae* confirms the diagnosis.
  2. Laboratory is notified of the suspected diagnosis so that appropriate culture medium (Tinsdale agar) is used.
- Testing of all isolated organisms for toxin production

IMAGING STUDIES

Chest radiograph examination to rule out pneumonia

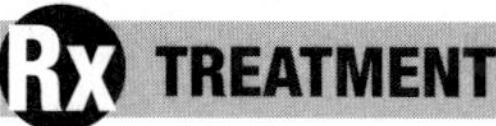

TREATMENT

NONPHARMACOLOGIC THERAPY

- Intubation or tracheostomy if signs of respiratory distress occur
- Nasogastric or parenteral nutrition in those with bulbar signs
- ICU monitoring for patients with signs of systemic toxicity
- Cardiac pacing in patients with heart block
- Respiratory isolation

ACUTE GENERAL Rx

- Administration of diphtheria antitoxin once a clinical diagnosis is made
- If tests for hypersensitivity to horse serum are negative: 20,000 to 40,000 units for pharyngeal/laryngeal disease present less than 48 hr, 40,000 to 60,000 units for nasopharyngeal disease, and 80,000 to 120,000 units for greater than 3 days of illness or diffuse neck swelling ("bull-neck") (available via the CDC)
- IV infusion of antitoxin over 60 min
- Serum sickness in 10% of treated individuals; those with hypersensitivity to horse serum should be desensitized before administration of antitoxin
- Antibiotics to eradicate the organism in carriers or patients
- For respiratory diphtheria:
  1. Erythromycin 500 mg qid PO or IV (clarithromycin and azithromycin are acceptable alternatives) or IM penicillin G 600,000 U bid for 14 days
  2. Carriers or patients with cutaneous disease: erythromycin 500 mg PO qid or rifampin 600 mg PO qd for 7 days

CHRONIC Rx

Antibiotics to limit toxin production and eradicate carrier state, thereby preventing transmission

DISPOSITION

Complete recovery with adequate supportive measures and antitoxin

REFERRAL

- Hospitalization and referral to an infectious disease specialist for all suspected patients
- To an otolaryngologist for evaluation in cases of respiratory diphtheria
- All cases reported to the public health authorities

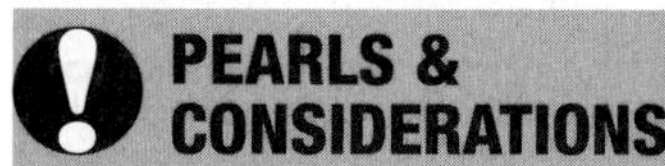

COMMENTS

- Most cases are imported by travelers in epidemic areas, so recent epidemics in Eastern Europe are a cause for concern. A widespread epidemic of diphtheria began in 1990 in the former Soviet Union.
- Vaccination with diphtheria toxoid (attenuated toxin) is safe and effective in the form of DPT or Td; Td boosters should be given to adults every 10 yr. A new formulation of Tdap vaccine with reduced amounts of diphtheria toxoid and acellular pertussis antigens is available; it is well tolerated in clinical trials and provides excellent protection in adolescents and adults.
- According to serologic studies, 20% to 60% of U.S. adults $>$20 yr of age are susceptible to diphtheria.

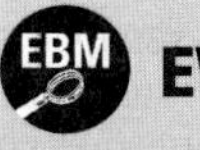

EVIDENCE

Antiserum has been used for the treatment of diphtheria for over 100 years and has stood the test of time as an effective treatment strategy. It was tested in one of the first controlled trials in clinical medicine.[1] Ⓑ

Evidence-Based Reference

1. Fibiger JA: Om Serumbehandling af Difteri, *Hospitalstidende* 6:309, 1898. Reviewed in: The controlled clinical trial turns 100 years: Fibiger's trial of serum treatment of diphtheria, *BMJ* 317:1243, 1998. Ⓑ

SUGGESTED READINGS

Berrington J, Fenton A: Immunization responses in preterm infants who receive postnatal steroid treatment, *Pediatrics* 114(4):1127, 2004.

Broder KR et al: Preventing tetanus, diphtheria, and pertussis among adolescents: use of tetanus toxoid, reduced diphtheria toxoid and acellular pertussis vaccines recommendations of the Advisory Committee on Immunization Practices (ACIP), *MMWR Recomm Rep* 55(RR-3):1, 2006.

Kadirova R et al: Clinical characteristics and management of 676 hospitalized diphtheria cases, Kyrgyz Republic, 1995, *J Infect Dis* 181(1):S110, 2000.

Kneen R et al: Penicillin vs. erythromycin in the treatment of diphtheria, *Clin Infect Dis* 27:845, 1998.

Tiwari TS et al: Investigations of two cases of diphtheria-like illness due to toxigenic Corynebacterium ulcers, *Clin Infect Dis* 46:395, 2008.

AUTHORS: **PATRICIA CRISTOFARO, M.D., GLENN G. FORT, M.D., M.P.H.,** and **DENNIS J. MIKOLICH, M.D.**

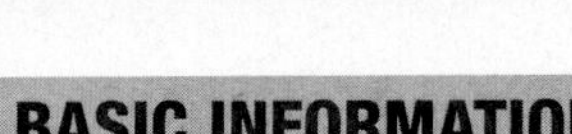

BASIC INFORMATION

DEFINITION

Discoid lupus erythematosus (DLE) refers to a chronic inflammatory autoimmune skin disorder that can lead to significant disfiguration and scarring. It can be associated with systemic lupus erythematosus (SLE).

SYNONYMS

Chronic cutaneous lupus erythematosus (CLE)

ICD-9CM CODES

695.4 Lupus erythematosus erythematodes (discoid) erythematosus (discoid), not disseminated

EPIDEMIOLOGY & DEMOGRAPHICS

- Slightly more common in African Americans than in Asians or whites
- Cutaneous lupus erythematosus is two to three times more likely in women than in men
- Approximately 5% to 10% of patients presenting with DLE will develop SLE; those with widespread, numerous lesions are more likely to progress

PHYSICAL FINDINGS & CLINICAL PRESENTATION

General:

- Early lesions: single or multiple erythematous or violaceous, discrete papules or plaques with scale, often extending into dilated hair follicles (Figs. 1-92 and 1-93)
- Older lesions: peripheral hyperpigmentation with scarring, central depigmentation, and telangiectasia

Anatomic distribution:

- Commonly involves the scalp, face, ears, and extensor surface of the arms
- Mucosal and nail involvement is also possible

Lesion configuration:

- Irregularly grouped, confluent and disfiguring plaques

Lesion morphology:

- Plaque lesions with scale
- Follicular plugging
- Atrophy
- Irreversible, scarring alopecia (34%)
- May be associated with other clinical findings of SLE (e.g., oral ulcers, arthritis, pleuritis, pericarditis)

ETIOLOGY

Unknown, but thought to be an autoimmune-mediated disorder

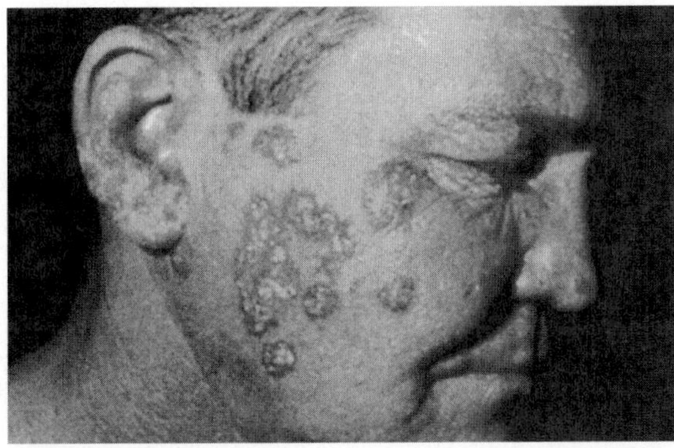

FIGURE 1-92 Scaling plaques with thick scales on the ear and face of a patient with discoid lupus. (Courtesy Department of Dermatology, University of North Carolina at Chapel Hill. From Goldstein BG, Goldstein AO [eds]: *Practical dermatology,* ed 2, St Louis, 1977, Mosby.)

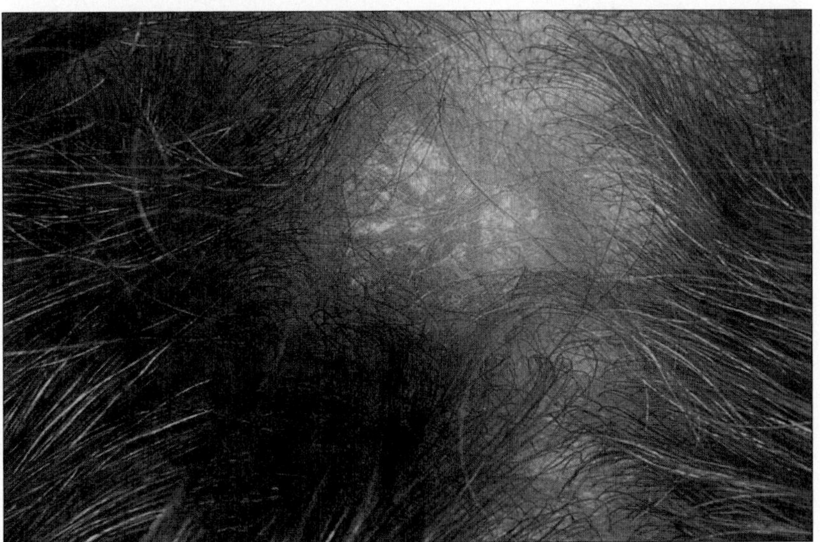

FIGURE 1-93 Discoid lupus erythematosus. There is considerable scaling and conspicuous background erythema. (Courtesy of the Institute of Dermatology, London, UK. From Granter SR [ed]: *Pathology of the skin with clinical correlations,* St Louis, Mosby.)

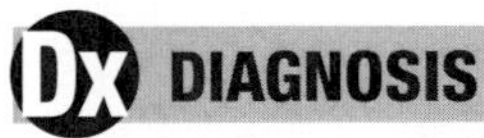

DIAGNOSIS

Clinical findings and skin biopsy are used to establish the diagnosis of DLE

DIFFERENTIAL DIAGNOSIS

Psoriasis, lichen planus or lichen planopilaris, dermatophyte infections, photosensitivity eruption, sarcoidosis, subacute CLE, rosacea, dermatomyositis, subcutaneous lymphoma

LABORATORY TESTS

- Complete blood count is usually normal in isolated DLE, but a small percentage of patients may show low-grade anemia
- Blood urea nitrogen and creatinine are normal in isolated DLE
- Erythrocyte sedimentation rate is elevated in active disease
- Urinalysis may show proteinuria
- Antinuclear antibody positive in 30% to 40% of patients with isolated DLE
- Anti-Ro (SS-A) autoantibodies are present in 1% to 3% of patients
- dsDNA antibodies are uncommon
- Complement levels may be low in rare instances
- Histology of skin reveals hyperkeratosis with follicular plugging, a thickened basement membrane, and a perivascular, interstitial, and appendageal lymphocytic infiltrate

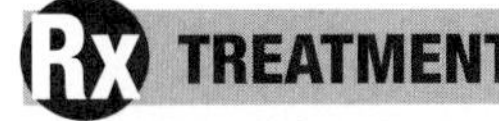

TREATMENT

NONPHARMACOLOGIC THERAPY

Avoid sun exposure by using protective clothing and a broad-spectrum sunscreen of SPF >30

ACUTE GENERAL Rx

1. Topical steroids: intermediate- to high-potency steroids are needed; use caution when applying to the face
2. Intralesional steroids: triamcinolone acetonide 2.5 to 5.0 mg/ml with 1% Xylocaine
3. Topical calcineurin inhibitors: pimecrolimus 1% cream and tacrolimus 0.1% ointment
4. Hydroxychloroquine sulfate 400 mg PO qd
5. Avoid use of systemic glucocorticoids in patients with isolated DLE because of risks of side effects

CHRONIC Rx

1. Chloroquine 250 to 500 mg PO qd
2. Auranofin 6 mg/day PO qd or divided bid; after 3 mo, may increase to 9 mg/day divided tid
3. Thalidomide 100 to 300 mg PO before sleep, with water, and >1 hr after meals for refractory CLE

4. Azathioprine 1 mg/kg/day PO for 6 to 8 wk, increase by 5 mg/kg q4 wk until response is seen or dose reaches 2.5 mg/kg/day
5. Dapsone: 100 mg/day

DISPOSITION

If untreated, DLE can lead to significant and permanent atrophy and scarring of the skin.

REFERRAL

Dermatology, rheumatology

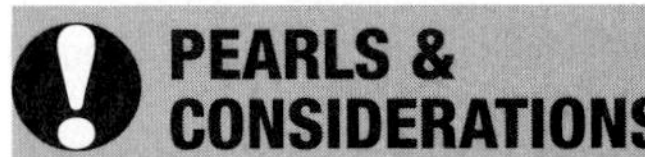

PEARLS & CONSIDERATIONS

- Cutaneous lesions account for four of the 11 criteria in the diagnosis of SLE (e.g., malar rash, discoid rash, photosensitivity, and oral ulcers).
- Rarely, patients with DLE may develop non-melanoma skin cancer in areas of disease.

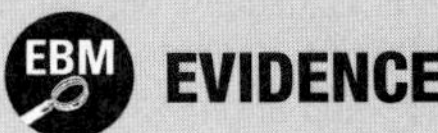

EVIDENCE

A systematic review identified one randomized controlled trial comparing topical fluocinonide vs. hydrocortisone in 78 patients with DLE. Clinical improvement was low for both treatments, although improvement was seen in a greater number of patients treated with fluocinonide.[1] Ⓐ

A systematic review identified one randomized controlled trial that compared hydroxychloroquine vs. acitretin in 58 patients with DLE. Improvement was similar in both treatment groups (hydroxychloroquine 50% vs. 46% with acitretin), but patients treated with hydroxychloroquine had fewer adverse reactions.[1] Ⓐ

A recent study evaluated the efficacy of thalidomide in 48 patients with DLE ($n = 18$), subacute cutaneous lupus ($n = 6$), or systemic lupus erythematosus with skin involvement ($n = 24$) refractory to other therapies. Treatment with thalidomide resulted in complete remission in 60% of patients and partial remission in 21%. However, in patients with a complete/partial response, the relapse rate after stopping thalidomide was 67%.[2] Ⓑ

Evidence-Based References

1. Jessop S et al: Drugs for discoid lupus erythematosus, *Cochrane Database Syst Rev* 2, 2000. Ⓐ

2. Cuadrado MJ et al: Thalidomide for the treatment of resistant cutaneous lupus: efficacy and safety of different therapeutic regimens, *Am J Med* 118:246, 2005. Ⓑ

SUGGESTED READINGS

Callen JP: Lupus erythematosus, discoid, *e-Medicine Journal* June 20, 2007. Available at http://www.emedicine.com.

Fabri P et al: Cutaneous lupus erythematosus: diagnosis and management, *Am J Clin Dermatol* 4(7):449, 2003.

Pramatorov KD: Chronic cutaneous lupus erythematosus—clinical spectrum, *Clin Dermatol* 22(2):113, 2004.

Rothfield NR et al: Lupus erythematosus: systemic and cutaneous manifestations, *Clin Dermatol* 24(5):348, 2006.

Werth V: Clinical manifestations of cutaneous lupus erythematosus, *Autoimmune Rev* 4(5):296, 2005.

AUTHORS: **KACHIU LEE, B.A.,** and **JESSICA RISSER, M.D., M.P.H.**

 BASIC INFORMATION

DEFINITION

Disseminated intravascular coagulation (DIC) is an acquired thromboembolic disorder characterized by generalized activation of the clotting mechanism, which results in the intravascular formation of fibrin and ultimately thrombotic occlusion of small and midsize vessels.

SYNONYMS

Consumptive coagulopathy
DIC
Defibrination syndrome

ICD-9CM CODES
286.6 Disseminated intravascular coagulation

EPIDEMIOLOGY & DEMOGRAPHICS

More than 50% of cases are associated with gram-negative sepsis or other septicemic infections.

PHYSICAL FINDINGS & CLINICAL PRESENTATION

- Wound site bleeding, epistaxis, gingival bleeding, hemorrhagic bullae
- Petechiae, ecchymosis, purpura
- Dyspnea, localized rales, delirium
- Oliguria, anuria, gastrointestinal bleeding, metrorrhagia

ETIOLOGY

- Infections (e.g., gram-negative sepsis, Rocky Mountain spotted fever, malaria, viral or fungal infection)
- Obstetric complications (e.g., dead fetus, amniotic fluid embolism, toxemia, abruptio placentae, septic abortion, eclampsia, placenta previa, uterine atony)
- Tissue trauma (e.g., burns, hypothermia rewarming)
- Neoplasms (e.g., adenocarcinomas [gastrointestinal, prostate, lung, breast], acute promyelocytic leukemia)
- Quinine, cocaine-induced rhabdomyolysis
- Liver failure
- Acute pancreatitis
- Transfusion reactions
- Respiratory distress syndrome
- Toxins (snake bites, amphetamine overdose)
- Other: systemic lupus erythematosus (SLE), vasculitis, aneurysms, polyarteritis, cavernous hemangiomas

Dx DIAGNOSIS

DIFFERENTIAL DIAGNOSIS

- Hepatic necrosis: normal or elevated Factor VIII concentrations
- Vitamin K deficiency: normal platelet count
- Hemolytic uremic syndrome
- Thrombotic thrombocytopenic purpura
- Renal failure, SLE, sickle cell crisis, dysfibrinogenemias
- HELLP syndrome (***h***emolysis, ***e***levated ***l***iver function tests, and ***l***ow ***p***latelets)
- Section III describes an algorithm for the differential diagnosis of deep vein thrombosis

WORKUP

Diagnostic workup includes laboratory screening to confirm the diagnosis and exclude conditions noted in the differential diagnosis. Workup is also aimed at distinguishing DIC progression (acute vs. chronic), chief manifestations (thrombotic or hemorrhagic), and extent (localized or systemic).

LABORATORY TESTS

- Peripheral blood smear generally shows red blood cell fragments (schistocytes) and low platelet count.
- Coagulation factors are consumed at a rate in excess of the capacity of the liver to synthesize them, and platelets are consumed in excess of the capacity of the bone marrow megakaryocytes to release them. Diagnostic characteristics of DIC are decreased fibrinogen level; thrombocytopenia; and increased prothrombin time (PT), partial thromboplastin time (PTT), TT, fibrin split products, and D-dimer.
- Coagulopathy secondary to DIC must be differentiated from that secondary to liver disease or vitamin K deficiency.
  1. Vitamin K deficiency manifests with prolonged PT and normal PTT, TT, platelet, and fibrinogen level; PTT may be elevated in severe cases.
  2. Patients with liver disease have abnormal PT and PTT; TT and fibrinogen are usually normal unless severe disease is present; platelets are usually normal unless splenomegaly is present.
  3. Factors V and VIII are low in DIC, but they are normal in liver disease with coagulopathy.

IMAGING STUDIES

Imaging studies are generally not useful. Chest radiographs may be helpful to exclude infectious processes in patients with pulmonary symptoms such as dyspnea, cough, or hemoptysis.

Rx TREATMENT

NONPHARMACOLOGIC THERAPY

No specific precautions regarding activity level are necessary unless thrombocytopenia is severe.

ACUTE GENERAL Rx

- Correct and eliminate underlying cause (e.g., antimicrobial therapy for infection, removal of necrotic bowel, evacuation of uterus in obstetric emergencies).
- Give replacement therapy with fresh frozen plasma (FFP) and platelets in patients with significant hemorrhage:
  1. FFP 10 to 15 ml/kg can be given with a goal of normalizing International Normalized Ratio.
  2. Platelet transfusions are given when platelet count is $<$10,000 (or higher if major bleeding is present).
  3. Cryoprecipitate 1 U/5 kg is reserved for hypofibrinogen states.
  4. Antithrombin III treatment may be considered as a supportive therapeutic option in patients with severe DIC. Its modest results and substantial cost are limiting factors.
- Heparin therapy at a dose lower than that used in venous thrombosis (300 to 500 U/hr) may be useful in selected cases to increase neutralization of thrombin (e.g., DIC associated with acute promyelocytic leukemia, purpura fulminans, acral ischemia).

CHRONIC Rx

Follow-up management includes coagulation screening to assess factor replacement therapy. Laboratory abnormalities generally correct with treatment of the underlying disorder. Long-term laboratory monitoring is not required.

DISPOSITION

Mortality rate in severe DIC exceeds 75%. Death generally results from progression of the underlying disease and complications such as acute renal failure, intracerebral hematoma, shock, or cardiac tamponade.

REFERRAL

Hematology consultation is recommended in all cases of DIC.

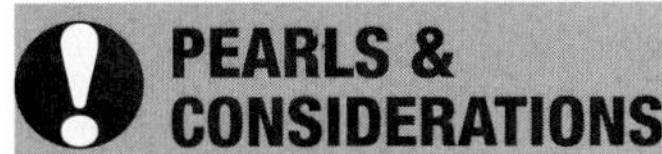

COMMENTS

The treatment of chronic DIC is controversial. Low-dose SC heparin and/or combination antiplatelet agents such as aspirin and dipyridamole may be useful.

AUTHOR: **FRED F. FERRI, M.D.**

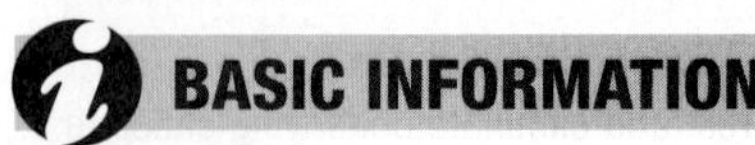

BASIC INFORMATION

DEFINITION

- Colonic diverticula are herniations of mucosa and submucosa through the muscularis. They are generally found along the colon's mesenteric border at the site where the vasa recta penetrates the muscle wall (anatomic weak point).
- *Diverticulosis* is the asymptomatic presence of multiple colonic diverticula.
- *Diverticulitis* is an inflammatory process or localized perforation of diverticulum.

ICD-9CM CODES
562.10 Diverticulosis of colon
562.11 Diverticulitis of colon

EPIDEMIOLOGY & DEMOGRAPHICS

- Incidence of diverticulosis in the general population is 35% to 50%.
- Diverticulosis is more common in Western countries, affecting >30% of people >40 yr and >50% of people >70 yr.

PHYSICAL FINDINGS & CLINICAL PRESENTATION

- Physical examination in patients with diverticulosis is generally normal.
- Painful diverticular disease can present with LLQ pain, often relieved by defecation; location of pain may be anywhere in the lower abdomen because of the redundancy of the sigmoid colon.
- Diverticulitis can cause muscle spasm, guarding, and rebound tenderness predominantly affecting the LLQ.

ETIOLOGY

Diverticular disease is believed to be secondary to low intake of dietary fiber.

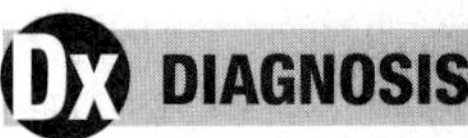

DIAGNOSIS

DIFFERENTIAL DIAGNOSIS

- Irritable bowel syndrome
- IBD
- Carcinoma of colon
- Endometriosis
- Ischemic colitis
- Infections (pseudomembranous colitis, appendicitis, pyelonephritis, PID)
- Lactose intolerance

LABORATORY TESTS

- WBC count in diverticulitis reveals leukocytosis with left shift.
- Microcytic anemia can be present in patients with chronic bleeding from diverticular disease. MCV may be elevated in acute bleeding secondary to reticulocytosis.

PROCEDURES: Colonoscopy should be avoided during acute diverticulitis due to the risk of perforation. It can generally be performed after 6 wk to rule out the presence of cancer and IBD.

IMAGING STUDIES

- A CT scan of the abdomen is recommended as the initial radiologic examination to diagnose acute diverticulitis; It has a sensitivity of 93% to 97% and a specificity approaching 100%. Typical findings are thickening of the bowel wall, fistulas, or abscess formation. CT may also reveal other disease processes (e.g., appendicitis, tubo-ovarian abscess, Crohn's disease) accounting for lower abdominal pain
- Evaluation of suspected diverticular bleeding:
  1. Arteriography if the bleeding is faster than 1 ml/min (advantage: the possible infusion of vasopressin directly into the arteries supplying the bleeding, as well as selective arterial embolization; disadvantages: its cost and invasive nature)
  2. Technetium-99m sulfa colloid
  3. Technetium-99m labeled RBC (can detect bleeding rates as low as 0.12 to 5 ml/min)

Rx TREATMENT

NONPHARMACOLOGIC THERAPY

- Increase in dietary fiber intake and regular exercise to improve bowel function
- NPO and IV hydration in severe diverticulitis; NG suction if ileus or small bowel obstruction is present

ACUTE GENERAL Rx

TREATMENT OF DIVERTICULITIS:

- Mild case: broad-spectrum PO antibiotics (e.g., Ciprofloxacin 500 mg bid to cover aerobic component of colonic flora and metronidazole 500 mg q6h for anaerobes) and liquid diet for 7 to 10 days
- Severe case: NPO and aggressive IV antibiotic therapy
  a. Ampicillin-sulbactam 3 g IV q6h *or*
  b. Piperacillin-tazobactam 4.5 g IV q8h *or*
  c. Ciprofloxacin 400 mg IV q12h plus metronidazole 500 mg IV q6h *or*
  d. Cefoxitin 2 g IV q8h plus metronidazole 500 mg IV q6h
- Life-threatening case: Imipenem 500 mg IV q6h *or* meropenem 1 g IV q8h
- Surgical treatment consisting of resection of involved areas and reanastomosis (if feasible); otherwise a diverting colostomy with reanastomosis performed when infection has been controlled; surgery should be considered in patients with:
  1. Repeated episodes of diverticulitis (two or more)
  2. Poor response to appropriate medical therapy (failure of conservative management)
  3. Abscess or fistula formation
  4. Obstruction
  5. Peritonitis
  6. Immunocompromised patients, first episode in young patient (<40 yr old)
  7. Inability to exclude carcinoma (10% to 20% of patients diagnosed with diverticulosis on clinical grounds are subsequently found to have carcinoma of the colon)

DIVERTICULAR HEMORRHAGE:

1. Bleeding is painless and stops spontaneously in the majority of patients (60%); it is usually caused by erosion of a blood vessel by a fecalith present within the diverticular sac.
2. Medical therapy consists of blood replacement and correction of volume and any clotting abnormalities.
3. Colonoscopic treatment with epinephrine injections, bipolar coagulation, or both may prevent recurrent bleeding and decrease the need for surgery.
4. Surgical resection is necessary if bleeding does not stop spontaneously after administration of 4 to 5 U of PRBCs or recurs with severity within a few days; if attempts at localization are unsuccessful, total abdominal colectomy with ileoproctostomy may be indicated (high incidence of rebleeding if segmental resection is performed without adequate localization).

CHRONIC Rx

Asymptomatic patients with diverticulosis can be treated with a high-fiber diet or fiber supplements.

DISPOSITION

- Most patients with diverticulitis respond well to antibiotic management and bowel rest. Up to 30% of patients with diverticulitis will eventually require surgical management.
- Diverticular bleeding can recur in 15% to 20% of patients within 5 yr.

REFERRAL

GI referral for colonoscopy. Surgical referral when considering resection.

SUGGESTED READING

Jacobs DO: Diverticulitis, *N Engl J Med* 357:2057-2066, 2007.

AUTHOR: **FRED F. FERRI, M.D.**

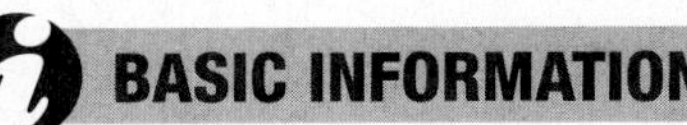

BASIC INFORMATION

DEFINITION

Down syndrome is a disorder characterized by mental retardation and multiple organ defects that is caused by a chromosomal abnormality (trisomy 21).

SYNONYMS

Trisomy 21

ICD-9CM CODES

758.0 Down Syndrome

EPIDEMIOLOGY & DEMOGRAPHICS

INCIDENCE (IN U.S.): 1 in 800 births
PEAK INCIDENCE: Newborn
PREVALENCE (IN U.S.): 300,000 persons
PREDOMINANT SEX: Male:female ratio of 1.3:1.0
PREDOMINANT AGE: Newborn to early adulthood
GENETICS: Nondisjunction causing trisomy 21

PHYSICAL FINDINGS & CLINICAL PRESENTATION

(Fig. 1-94)

- Microcephaly
- Flattening of occiput and face
- Upward slant to eyes with epicanthal folds
- Brushfield spots in iris
- Broad, stocky neck
- Small feet, hands, digits
- Single palmar crease
- Hypotonia
- Short stature
- Associated with congenital heart disease, malformations of the GI tract, cataracts, hypothyroidism, hip dysplasia, obstructive sleep apnea, and myeloproliferative disorders
- About half of children with Down syndrome are born with congenital heart disease, with the most common lesions being atrial septal defect and ventricular septal defect
- Persistent primary congenital hypothyroidism is found in 1 in 141 newborns with Down syndrome, as compared with 1 in 4000 in the general population
- Ophthalmologic disorders increase in frequency with age; >80% of children aged 5 to 12 yr have disorders that need monitoring or intervention, such as refractive errors, strabismus, or cataracts
- Renal and urinary tract abnormalities

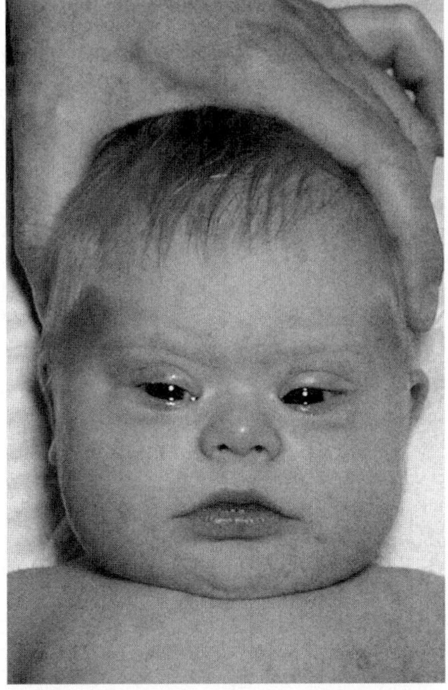

FIGURE 1-94 Down syndrome. Note depressed nasal bridge, epicanthal folds, mongoloid slant of eyes, low-set ears, and large tongue. (From Zitelli BJ, Davis HW: *Atlas of pediatric physical diagnosis,* ed 3, St Louis, 1997, Mosby.)

ETIOLOGY

Nondisjunction of chromosome 21

Dx DIAGNOSIS

- Prenatal cytogenic diagnosis by amniocentesis or chorionic villus sampling
- Combined use of serum screening and fetal ultrasound testing for thickened nuchal fold has 85% detection rate with 5% false-positive results
- Postnatal chromosomal karyotype

DIFFERENTIAL DIAGNOSIS

- Congenital hypothyroidism
- Other chromosomal abnormalities

WORKUP

Postnatal chromosomal karyotype

Rx TREATMENT

- Thyroid screen at birth, at age 6 mo, and yearly thereafter
- Echocardiogram in all newborns and cardiac assessment of adolescents for development of mitral valve prolapse
- Treatment consists of vigilant monitoring for comorbid states, such as obesity, hypothyroidism, leukemia, hearing loss, and valvular heart disease
- Prevention of obesity with low-calorie, high-fiber diet
- Auditory brain stem responses in all newborns and aggressive testing for hearing loss in children with chronic otitis media
- Ophthalmologic assessment by age 6 mo for congenital cataracts and annual examinations for monitoring of refractive errors and strabismus
- Regular dental care
- Pelvic examination of women who are sexually active or who have menstrual problems
- Dermatologic issues such as folliculitis can become problematic in adolescents, and require topical antibiotics and careful attention to hygiene

DISPOSITION

Most children with Down syndrome live at home. As these individuals reach adulthood, those with higher functioning sometimes live in supervised settings away from their families.

REFERRAL

Down syndrome clinics use a preventive checklist to anticipate many clinical challenges.

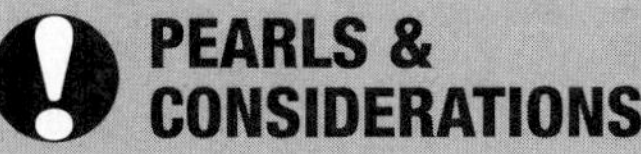

PEARLS & CONSIDERATIONS

COMMENTS

- Screening for atlantoaxial subluxation is controversial.
- Most patients experience neuropathologic changes typical of Alzheimer's disease. Presenting symptoms include seizures, focal neurologic signs, and apathy. If Alzheimer's disease is suspected, screen for treatable diseases such as depression or hypothyroidism.
- This syndrome accounts for approximately one third of moderate-to-severe cases of mental retardation.
- Individuals with Down syndrome have a wide range of function, but all will have decrease in intelligence quotient (IQ) in first decade of life.
- Deficiency of language production relative to other areas of development often causes substantial impairment.
- Individuals with Down syndrome have more behavioral and psychiatric problems than other children, but fewer than other individuals with mental retardation.
- Though increased maternal age is a risk factor, most children with Down syndrome are born to women younger than 35 yr.

SUGGESTED READINGS

Ball RH et al: First- and second-trimester evaluation for Down syndrome, *Obstset Gynecol* 110(1):10-17, 2007.

Lott IT, Head E: Down syndrome and Alzheimer's disease: a link between development and aging, *Ment Retard Dev Disabil Res Rev* 7(3):172, 2001.

Patterson D, Costa AC: Down syndrome and genetics—a case of linked histories, *Nat Rev Genet* 6(2):137, 2005.

Roizen NJ: Medical care and monitoring for the adolescent with Down syndrome, *Adolesc Med* 13(2): 345, 2002.

AUTHOR: **MAITREYI MAZUMDAR, M.D., M.P.H.**

Dumping Syndrome

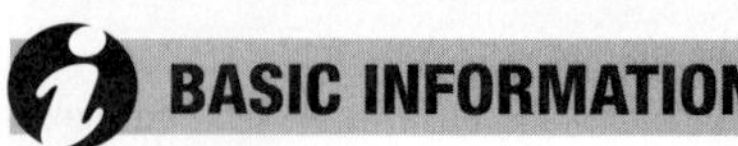

BASIC INFORMATION

DEFINITION

Dumping syndrome refers to a constellation of postprandial symptoms resulting from rapid delivery of hypertonic stomach contents into the small bowel that is most often caused by gastric surgery, such as procedures for peptic ulcer disease and gastric bypass.

SYNONYMS

Postgastrectomy syndrome
Rapid gastric emptying

ICD-9CM CODES

564.2 Postgastric surgery syndromes

EPIDEMIOLOGY & DEMOGRAPHICS

Incidence is 10% of all patients having gastric surgery.

- Vagotomy and pyloroplasty (8.5% to 20%)
- Vagotomy and antrectomy (4% to 27%)
- Subtotal gastrectomy (10% to 40%)
- Parietal cell vagotomy (3% to 5%)
- Gastric bypass surgeries (up to 50%)
- Males and females are affected equally

PHYSICAL FINDINGS & CLINICAL PRESENTATION

1. Early dumping syndrome: symptoms start within 1 hr after eating food:
   - No symptoms in fasting state
   - Nausea, vomiting, and belching
   - Epigastric fullness, cramping, and diarrhea
   - Dizziness, flushing, diaphoresis, and syncope
   - Palpitations and tachycardia
2. Late dumping syndrome: symptoms occurring 1 to 3 hr after eating:
   - Diaphoresis
   - Irritability
   - Difficulty in concentration
   - Tremulousness

ETIOLOGY

Dumping syndrome occurs almost exclusively in patients who have had gastric surgery.

- Systemic symptoms in early dumping syndrome are thought to be partially due to hypovolemia caused by rapid shifts of fluid from the intravascular space into the lumen of the bowel.
- Increase in vasoactive substances related to rapid gastric emptying is thought to play a role in dumping syndrome.
- Late dumping symptoms are thought to be due to reactive hypoglycemia.

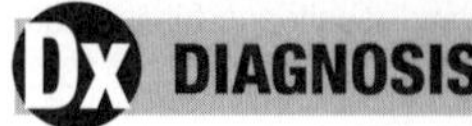

DIAGNOSIS

A detailed clinical history and evidence of prior gastric surgery are necessary for the diagnosis.

DIFFERENTIAL DIAGNOSIS

- Pancreatic insufficiency
- Inflammatory bowel disease
- Afferent loop syndromes
- Bile acid reflux after surgery
- Bowel obstruction
- Gastroenteric fistula

WORKUP

Diagnosis is typically made on clinical grounds. In certain clinical settings, where patients exhibit symptoms with no prior history of gastric surgery, oral glucose challenge and imaging studies may be pursued and aid in establishing the diagnosis.

LABORATORY TESTS

Oral glucose challenge test:

- Oral intake of 50 g of glucose is followed by serial measurements of heart rate, serum glucose, and hydrogen breath test every 15 min for 6 hr.
- An increase in the heart rate >12 beats/min and a rise in hydrogen breath excretion have a sensitivity of 94% and specificity >92%. A nadir blood glucose <3.3 mmol/L (<59 mg/dl) was present in 75% of late dumpers.

IMAGING STUDIES

- Upper GI series properly defines anatomy.
- Scintigraphic imaging documents rapid gastric emptying and may be useful in patients with dumping syndrome and no prior history of gastric surgery.

Rx TREATMENT

NONPHARMACOLOGIC THERAPY

- Diet modification
  1. Divide caloric intake over six small meals
  2. Limit fluid intake with meals (try to avoid fluids 30 min before meals and following meals)
  3. Decrease carbohydrate intake and avoid simple sugars
  4. Increase/supplement dietary fibers
  5. Avoid milk/milk products

ACUTE GENERAL Rx

- Acarbose 50 mg PO daily can be tried if dietary modification does not help.
- Octreotide 25 to 50 μg SC 30 min before meals is effective in relieving symptoms of dumping syndrome.
- Pectin and Guar have been used to increase viscosity of intraluminal contents and relieve symptoms from rapid emptying and absorption.

CHRONIC Rx

- Surgery is considered in patients with severe symptoms refractory to the above mentioned dietary and acute general treatment.
- Surgical procedures include: reconstruction of the pylorus, converting Billroth II to a Billroth I anastomosis, and a Roux-en-Y reconstruction.
- In severe cases, can consider depot long acting release octreotide, given as 10 mg intramuscularly every 4 wk for symptom relief.

DISPOSITION

- Dumping syndrome improves with time. Approximately 1% to 2% of patients will continue to have significant symptoms several months after surgery.
- Dietary modification effectively treats the majority of patients.

REFERRAL

- A gastrointestinal specialist consult is recommended in patients suspected of having dumping syndrome.
- If medical management is unsuccessful, a general surgical consultation is warranted.

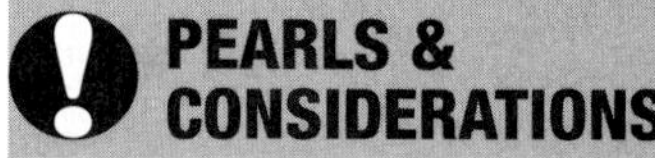

PEARLS & CONSIDERATIONS

COMMENTS

- The majority of patients usually manifest with early dumping symptoms or combination of early and late symptoms. Few have late dumping symptoms alone.
- Octreotide has an inhibitory effect on the release of insulin and other vasoactive substances released by the gut. It also works by decreasing gastric emptying.

SUGGESTED READINGS

Hasler WL: Dumping syndrome, *Current Treat Options Gastroenterol* 5(2):139, 2002.

Li-Ling J, Irving M: Therapeutic value of octreotide for patients with severe dumping syndrome: a review of randomized controlled trials, *Postgrad Med J* 77(909):441, 2001.

Parrish CR, Lin HC, Parkman H: Dietary nutritional recommendations for patients with dumping syndrome (rapid gastric emptying), *Digestive Health Matters* 15(02):15, 2006.

Tack J: Gastric motion disorders, *Best Pract Res Clin Gastroenterol* 21(4):633, 2007.

Ukleja A: Dumping syndrome: pathophysiology and treatment, *Nutr Clin Pract* 20(5):517, 2005.

AUTHOR: **MARK BRADY, M.D., M.P.H., M.M.S.**

BASIC INFORMATION

DEFINITION

Dupuytren's contracture is a disease of the palmar fascia characterized by nodular fibroblastic proliferation that often results in progressive contractures of the fascia and flexion deformity of the fingers.

ICD-9CM CODES
728.6 Dupuytren's contracture

EPIDEMIOLOGY & DEMOGRAPHICS

PREVALENCE: Varies depending on nationality
PREVALENT SEX: Male/female ratio of 10:1
PREVALENT AGE: 40 to 60 yr

PHYSICAL FINDINGS & CLINICAL PRESENTATION

- Usually asymptomatic
- Most common complaints: deformity and interference with the use of the hand by the flexed, contracted fingers (Fig. 1-95)
- Process usually begins on the ulnar side of the hand, often starting at the ring finger
- Isolated, painless nodules that eventually harden and mature into a longitudinal cord that extends into the finger
- Lesion often begins in the distal palmar crease
- Overlying skin adherent to the fascia
- Later stages: fibrous cord begins to contract and pull the finger into flexion
- Possible involvement of other fingers, particularly small finger

ETIOLOGY

Unknown. Pathologically, the contracture consists of proliferating vascular tissue that later develops into mature collagen.

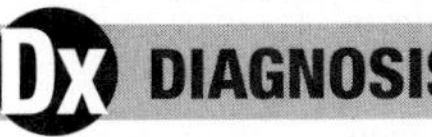

DIAGNOSIS

DIFFERENTIAL DIAGNOSIS

- Soft tissue tumor
- Tendon cyst

WORKUP

The typical case is easily diagnosed clinically. Plain radiographs may be useful to rule out bony abnormalities.

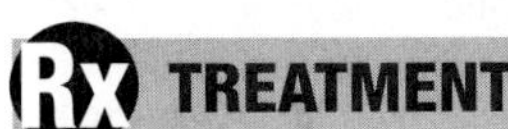

TREATMENT

NONPHARMACOLOGIC THERAPY

- Stretching exercises
- Local heat
- Surgical referral is indicated when metacarpophalangeal joint contracture occurs at any degree.
- Surgery is usually performed when the metacarpophalangeal joint contracture exceeds 40 degrees or when the proximal interphalangeal joint contracture exceeds 20 degrees.
- Percutaneous needle aponeurotomy performed in the office represents an alternative to surgery.

DISPOSITION

Rate of development is variable.

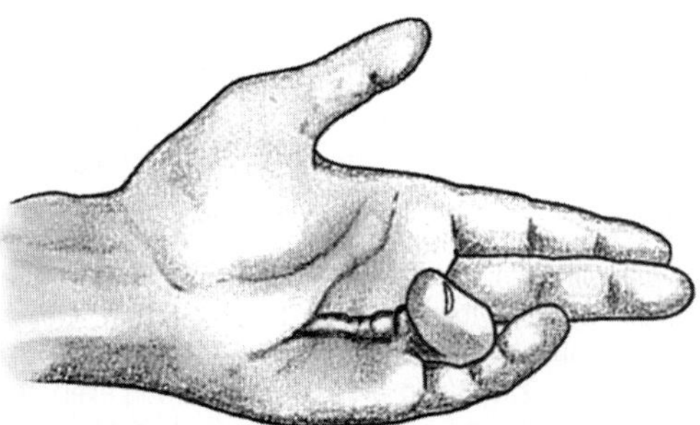

FIGURE 1-95 Dupuytren's contracture. A flexion deformity of the finger is present, with nodular thickening of the fascia to the ring finger.

REFERRAL

- If joint contracture begins to develop
- For excision of rare nodule that is painful (at any stage)

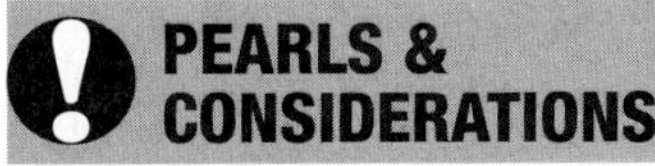

PEARLS & CONSIDERATIONS

COMMENTS

- Dupuytren's contracture develops earlier and more often in certain families.
- The disorder is more common in Scandinavians; some Northern Europeans have a 25% prevalence after age 60 yr.
- Approximately 5% of patients develop a similar condition elsewhere, such as Peyronie's disease or Ledderhose disease (involvement of the plantar fascia).
- Soft tissue "pads" in the knuckles may also be present.
- Individuals with these additional findings are considered to have Dupuytren's diathesis, and their disease is generally more severe and recurrent.

SUGGESTED READINGS

Bayat A: Connective tissue diseases: a nonsurgical therapy for Dupuytren disease, *Nat Rev Rheumatol* 6:7, 2010.

Frank PL: An update on Dupuytren's contracture, *Hosp Med* 62:678, 2001.

Khan AA et al: The role of manual occupation in the aetilogy of Dupuytren's disease in men in England and Wales, *J Hand Surg* 299(1):12, 2004.

Loos B et al: 50 years experience with Dupuytren's contracture in the Erlangen University Hospital—a retrospective analysis of 2919 operated hands from 1956 to 2006, *BMC Musculo Skelet Disord* 8:60, 2007.

McFarlane RM: On the origin and spread of Dupuytren's disease, *J Hand Surg* 27:385, 2002.

Ragsowansi RH, Britto JA: Genetic and epigenetic influence on the pathogenesis of Dupuytren's disease, *J Hand Surg* 26:1157, 2001.

Rayan GM: Dupuytren's disease: anatomy, pathology, presentation, and treatment, *J Bone Joint Surg Am* 89A:189, 2007.

Schechtman AD: Combining triamcinolone and lidocaine for soft tissue injections, *Am Fam Physician* 77:1372, 2008.

Thurston AJ: Dupuytren's disease, *J Bone Joint Surg Br* 85B(4):469, 2003.

Trojian TH, Chu SM: Dupuytren's disease: diagnosis and treatment, *Am Fam Physician* 76:86, 2007.

AUTHOR: **LONNIE R. MERCIER, M.D.**

BASIC INFORMATION

DEFINITION

Dysfunctional uterine bleeding (DUB) describes abnormal uterine bleeding in the absence of disease in the pelvis, pregnancy, or medical illness. Specific types of abnormal bleeding include the following:

- Hypermenorrhea: excessive bleeding amount during normal duration of regular menstrual cycles
- Hypomenorrhea: decreased bleeding amount in regular menstrual cycles
- Menorrhagia: regular normal intervals, excessive flow and duration
- Metrorrhagia: irregular intervals, excessive flow and duration
- Menometrorrhagia: irregular or excessive bleeding during menstruation and between periods
- Oligomenorrhea: intervals >35 days
- Polymenorrhea: intervals <21 days

SYNONYMS

DUB

ICD-9CM CODES

626 Disorders of menstruation and other abnormal bleeding from female genital tract
626.2 Hypermenorrhea
626.1 Hypomenorrhea
626.2 Menorrhagia
626.6 Metrorrhagia
626.2 Menometrorrhagia
626.1 Oligomenorrhea
626.2 Polymenorrhea

EPIDEMIOLOGY & DEMOGRAPHICS

- Most cases of DUB occur in postmenarchal and perimenopausal age groups.
- During reproductive age, <20% of abnormal bleeding results from anovulatory DUB.

PHYSICAL FINDINGS & CLINICAL PRESENTATION

- A clinical diagnosis of exclusion
- Thorough physical and pelvic examination to exclude the other causes of abnormal bleeding
  1. Includes thyroid, breast, liver, presence or absence of ecchymotic lesions
  2. Patient possibly obese and hirsute (polycystic ovarian disease)
  3. No evidence of any vulvar, vaginal, cervical lesions, uterine (fibroid) or ovarian tumor, urethral caruncle, urethral diverticula, hemorrhoids, anal fissure, colorectal lesions
  4. Bimanual pelvic examination: normal-sized or slightly enlarged uterus

ETIOLOGY

- 90% is caused by anovulation.
- 10% is ovulatory in origin; can be caused by dysfunction of corpus luteum or midcycle bleeding.
- Section II describes the various causes of abnormal uterine bleeding.

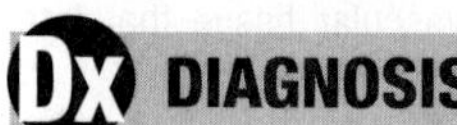

DIAGNOSIS

DIFFERENTIAL DIAGNOSIS

- Pregnancy-related cause
- Anatomic uterine causes:
  1. Leiomyomas
  2. Adenomyosis
  3. Polyps
  4. Endometrial hyperplasia
  5. Cancer
  6. Sexually transmitted diseases
  7. Intrauterine contraceptive devices
- Anatomic nonuterine causes:
  1. Cervical neoplasia, cervicitis
  2. Vaginal neoplasia, adhesions, trauma, foreign body, atrophic vaginitis, infections, condyloma
  3. Vulvar trauma, infections, neoplasia, condyloma, dystrophy, varices
  4. Urinary tract: urethral caruncle, diverticulum, hematuria
  5. Gastrointestinal tract: hemorrhoids, anal fissure, colorectal lesions
- Systemic diseases:
  1. Exogenous hormone intake
  2. Coagulopathies: von Willebrand's disease, thrombocytopenia, hepatic failure
  3. Endocrinopathies: thyroid disorder, hypothyroidism and hyperthyroidism, diabetes mellitus
  4. Renal diseases
- Section II describes a differential diagnosis of vaginal bleeding abnormalities.

WORKUP

- A detailed history and thorough physical examination, including a pelvic examination to exclude causes mentioned above.
- Clinical algorithms for the evaluation of vaginal bleeding are described in Section III, "Bleeding, Vaginal."

LABORATORY TESTS

- Complete blood count with platelets; possible iron-deficiency anemia or thrombocytopenia
- Prothrombin; partial thromboplastin and bleeding time if coagulopathy is suspected
- Serum human chorionic gonadotropin
- Chemistry profile, including liver function tests
- Thyroid profile
- Stool testing for occult blood
- Urinalysis for hematuria
- Pap smear
- Cultures for gonorrhea and *Chlamydia*
- Serum gonadotropins and prolactin
- Serum androgens
- Endometrial biopsy in women >35 yr or earlier if longstanding history of anovulatory bleeding
- Hysterogram and hysteroscopy

IMAGING STUDIES

- Pelvic ultrasound, including measurement of endometrial thickness
- Hydrosonogram (also known as fluid contrast ultrasound, saline sonogram)

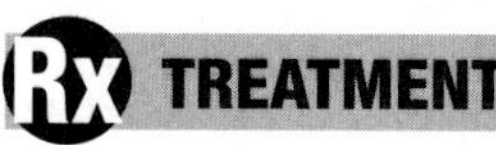

TREATMENT

NONPHARMACOLOGIC THERAPY

Increase iron intake in the form of pills and in a diet rich in iron.

ACUTE GENERAL Rx

- Progestational agents
  1. Progesterone in oil, 100 to 200 mg
  2. Medroxyprogesterone acetate, 20 to 40 mg qd for 15 days
  3. Megestrol acetate, 40 to 120 mg daily in divided doses for 15 days
  4. Oral contraceptives: any oral contraceptive pill, 1 tablet qid for 5 to 7 days, followed by 1 tablet low-dose estrogen qd for 21 days; causes heavy withdrawal bleeding; should then be on cyclical Provera or continue on oral contraceptives
- Estrogens
  1. Conjugated estrogen (Premarin) 25 mg IV q4h until bleeding is under control (in cases of severe or life-threatening bleeding); maximum three doses
  2. For prolonged bleeding that is not life threatening: Premarin 1.25 mg (Estrace 2 mg) q4h for 24 hr, followed by Provera to bring on withdrawal bleeding; then sequential regimen of estrogen and progestin (Premarin 1.25 mg qd for 24 days, Provera 10 mg for last 10 days) or oral contraceptives
- Surgical treatment
  1. Dilation and curettage (D&C) and hysteroscopy
  2. Endometrial ablation
  3. Hysterectomy

CHRONIC Rx

- Progestational agents
  1. Medroxyprogesterone acetate 10 mg qd for 12 days, then cyclically to induce monthly withdrawal bleeding
  2. Norethindrone 2.5 to 10 mg qd for 12 days
  3. Depo-Provera 150 mg IM and then 150 mg every 3 mo
  4. Oral contraceptives, 1 tablet qd
  5. Levonorgestrel-releasing intrauterine device (Mirena)
- Clomiphene citrate: patients with anovulatory bleeding who want to become pregnant
- Others
  1. Antiprostaglandins
  2. Danazol (rarely used due to side-effect profile)
  3. Gonadotropin-releasing hormone analogs (GNRH)
  4. Human menopausal gonadotropin (HMG) (desire pregnancy)
- Surgical treatment
  1. D&C and hysteroscopy
  2. Endometrial ablation
  3. Hysterectomy

D

Diseases and Disorders

DISPOSITION

Cyclical treatment on birth control pills or Provera for several cycles, then discontinue pill and watch patient for onset of regular menses

REFERRAL

To gynecologist in case of failure of treatment

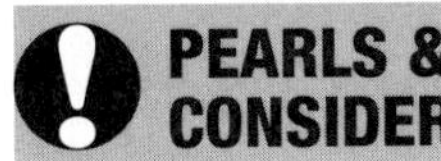

PEARLS & CONSIDERATIONS

COMMENTS

Patient education material may be obtained from the American College of Obstetricians and Gynecologists, 409 12th Street SW, Washington, DC 20024-2188; phone 202-638-5577.

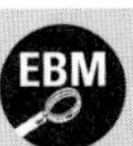

EVIDENCE

Estrogens can be used intravenously for the emergency treatment of acute uterine bleeding; or orally for the management of long-term uterine bleeding, usually in the form of the combined contraceptive pill or alongside cyclical medroxyprogesterone.

Another RCT compared the efficacy of multidose medroxyprogesterone and a multidose monophasic combined oral contraceptive (COC), containing norethindrone and ethinyl estradiol, for hemodynamically stable women with nongestational acute uterine bleeding. Emergency surgical procedures were avoided in 100% of the medroxyprogesterone group, and 95% of the COC group. Cessation of bleeding had occurred in 88% of the COC group, and 76% of the medroxyprogesterone group (median time to bleeding cessation = 3 days for both groups). Although the trial was limited by sample size, it concluded that both regimens may be effective and reasonably well tolerated.[1] B

Progesterones, either alone or in combination with estrogens, can be used for the long-term treatment, coordination, and regulation of dysfunctional uterine bleeding.

A systematic review analyzed the efficacy of progesterone or progestogen-releasing intrauterine devices in achieving a reduction in heavy menstrual bleeding. It found that the levonorgestrel-releasing intrauterine device (LNG IUS) is more effective than cyclical norethisterone (for 21 days).[2]

The same review also compared the LNG IUS to endometrial ablation: either transcervical resection of the endometrium (TCRE) or balloon ablation. It found that the LNG IUS resulted in a smaller mean reduction in menstrual blood loss than endometrial ablation. Women with an LNG IUS, however, experienced more progestogenic side effects compared to women having TCRE for treatment of their heavy menstrual bleeding—but there is no evidence of a difference in their perceived quality of life.[2] A

Another systematic review comparing the efficacy of surgery versus medical therapy for heavy menstrual bleeding found that surgery, especially hysterectomy, reduces menstrual bleeding at one year more than medical treatments. The intrauterine medical device LNG IUS, however, improves quality of life as effectively as surgery. Furthermore, although all treatments have potential side effects, hysterectomy is more likely to cause serious complications. It concluded that oral medication suits a minority of women long term.[3] A

Another systematic review analyzed the efficacy of progestogens, gonadotrophin-releasing hormone (GNRH) analogues, and danazol, when used for endometrial thinning prior to endometrial destruction for menorrhagia, at improving the intrauterine operating environment and treatment outcome after surgery. Three RCTs identified by the review provided insufficient evidence about the effects of oral progestogens compared with placebo, no preoperative treatment, or the other medical treatments.[4] A

A further systematic review found that luteal-phase progesterone (from day 15 or 19, to 26) was less effective in reducing menstrual blood loss than danazol, tranexamic acid, and levonorgestrel intrauterine system. 21-day progesterone, however, resulted in significant blood flow reduction, though women found this treatment less acceptable than the levonorgestrel intrauterine system.[5] A

A small RCT compared the efficacy of multidose medroxyprogesterone and a multidose monophasic COC, containing norethindrone and ethinyl estradiol, for hemodynamically stable women with nongestational acute uterine bleeding. Emergency surgical procedures were avoided in 100% of those taking medroxyprogesterone, and 95% of the COC group. Cessation of bleeding had occurred in 88% of the COC group and 76% of the medroxyprogesterone group (median time to bleeding cessation = 3 days for both groups). Although the trial was limited by sample size, it concluded that both regimens may be effective and reasonably well tolerated.[1] B

Goserelin, given in combination with cyclical hormone replacement therapy, significantly reduces bleeding in women with heavy menstrual loss of no known cause (includes dysfunctional uterine bleeding).

A small RCT compared the efficacy of adding combined estradiol/norethisterone acetate therapy (CENT), vs placebo, to goserelin, for the treatment of dysfunctional uterine bleeding in perimenopausal women. It found that abdominal pain, number of bleeding days and endometrial thickness decreased in both groups, but the between-group difference in decrease was not statistically significant.[6] B

Hysterectomy offers a definitive solution to dysfunctional uterine bleeding. Patients need to be carefully selected, however, as the side effects and potential complications of this surgery may outweigh its benefits.

A systematic review compared the efficacy, safety, and acceptability of surgery versus medical (oral or intrauterine) therapy for heavy menstrual bleeding. It found that surgery, especially hysterectomy, reduces menstrual bleeding at one year more than medical treatments; but the levonorgestrel-releasing intrauterine device appears equally effective in improving quality of life. The evidence for longer-term comparisons is weak and inconsistent. Oral medication suits a minority of women long term.[3] A

An RCT included in the first review compared clinical outcomes after hysterectomy versus medical treatment in patients with chronic abnormal uterine bleeding (which encompasses dysfunctional uterine bleeding) refractory to medroxyprogesterone acetate. It concluded that hysterectomy is superior to expanded efforts with oral medications for alleviating clinical symptoms but may lead to more days of restricted activity.[7] B

A prospective study analyzed the efficacy of a policy of performing a vaginal hysterectomy for as many cases of dysfunctional uterine bleeding, without uterine prolapse, as possible during a seven year period. It concluded that the vaginal approach is possible for an average gynecologist, with no additional complications and an improved recovery rate for patients (compared with abdominal hysterectomy).[8] B

Endometrial ablation is less invasive and simpler than hysterectomy, but does not always offer a long-term solution to women with dysfunctional uterine bleeding.

A systematic review comparing endometrial ablation techniques for the management of heavy menstrual bleeding found newer non-hysteroscopic techniques were less difficult to perform than transcervical resection of the endometrium. Overall, the newer techniques took less time to perform and were more likely to be performed under local anesthesia but had a greater chance of equipment failure.[9] A

A further systematic review comparing the efficacy and acceptability of surgery versus medical therapy for heavy menstrual bleeding found that endometrial resection, compared to oral medication, was significantly more effective in controlling bleeding and significantly less likely to cause side effects.[3] A

Evidence-Based References

1. Munro MG et al: Oral medroxyprogesterone acetate and combination oral contraceptives for acute uterine bleeding: a randomized controlled trial, *Obstet Gynecol* 108:924-929, 2006. B

2. Lethaby AE et al: Progesterone or progestogen-releasing intrauterine systems for heavy menstrual bleeding, *Cochrane Database Rev* (4), 2005. A

3. Marjoribanks J et al: Surgery versus medical therapy for heavy menstrual bleeding, *Cochrane Database Rev* (2), 2006. A

4. Lethaby A et al: Preoperative GnRH analogue therapy before hysterectomy or myomectomy for uterine fibroids, *Cochrane Database Rev* (2), 2001. A

5. Lethaby A et al: Endometrial destruction techniques for heavy menstrual bleeding, *Cochrane Database Rev* 4, 2005. Ⓐ
6. Franke HR et al: Treatment of dysfunctional uterine bleeding in the perimenopause: the effects of adding combined estradiol/norethisterone acetate therapy to goserelin acetate treatment—a randomized, placebo-controlled, double-blind trial, *Gynecol Endocrinol* 22:692-697, 2006. Ⓑ
7. Learman LA et al; Medicine or Surgery Research Group: Hysterectomy versus expanded medical treatment for abnormal uterine bleeding: clinical outcomes in the medicine or surgery trial, *Obstet Gynecol* 103:824-833, 2004. Ⓑ
8. Olah KS, Khalil M: Changing the route of hysterectomy: the results of a policy of attempting the vaginal approach in all cases of dysfunctional uterine bleeding, *Eur J Obstet Gynecol Reprod Biol* 125: 243-247, 2006. Ⓑ
9. Lethaby A et al: Endometrial destruction techniques for heavy menstrual bleeding. *Cochrane Database Rev* (4), 2005. Ⓐ

SUGGESTED READING

Mihm LM et al: The accuracy of endometrial biopsy and saline sonohysterography in the determination of the cause of abnormal uterine bleeding, *Am J Obstet Gynecol* 186:858, 2002.

AUTHORS: **MANDEEP K. BRAR, M.D.,** and **RUBEN ALVERO, M.D.**

BASIC INFORMATION

DEFINITION

Dysmenorrhea is pain with menstruation, usually cramping and usually centered in the lower abdomen. It is defined as *primary dysmenorrhea* when there is no associated organic pathology and *secondary dysmenorrhea* when there is demonstrable organic pathology.

SYNONYMS

Menstrual cramps
Painful periods

ICD-9CM CODES

625.3 Dysmenorrhea

EPIDEMIOLOGY & DEMOGRAPHICS

Approximately 50% of menstruating women are affected by dysmenorrhea, with approximately 10% of them having severe dysmenorrhea with incapacitation for 1 to 3 days/mo. Dysmenorrhea is most common in the age group from 20 to 24 yr, and primary dysmenorrhea usually appears within 6 to 12 mo after menarche.

PHYSICAL FINDINGS & CLINICAL PRESENTATION

- Sharp, crampy, midline, lower abdominal pain without a lower quadrant or adnexal component but possible radiation to the lower back and upper thighs
- Unremarkable pelvic examination in nonmenstruating patient
- Accompanying symptoms: nausea, vomiting, headaches, anxiety, fatigue, diarrhea, fainting, and abdominal bloating
- Cramps usually lasting <24 hr and seldom lasting >2 to 3 days
- Secondary dysmenorrhea: dyspareunia is a common complaint, and bimanual pelvic-abdominal examination may demonstrate uterine or adnexal tenderness, fixed uterine retroflexion, uterosacral nodularity, a pelvic mass, or an enlarged, irregular uterus

ETIOLOGY

Prostaglandin $F_2\alpha$ is the agent responsible for dysmenorrhea. It stimulates uterine contractions and cervical stenosis (narrowing) and increases vasopressin release. Behavior and psychological factors have also been implicated in the etiology of primary dysmenorrhea. Primary dysmenorrhea only occurs in ovulatory cycles. Secondary dysmenorrhea is usually caused by endometriosis, adenomyosis, leiomyomas and, less commonly, chronic salpingitis, intrauterine device (IUD) use, or congenital or acquired outflow tract obstruction, including cervical stenosis.

DIAGNOSIS

DIFFERENTIAL DIAGNOSIS

- Adenomyosis
- Adhesions
- Allen-Masters syndrome
- Cervical structures or stenosis
- Congenital malformation of müllerian system
- Ectopic pregnancy
- Endometriosis, endometritis
- Imperforate hymen
- IUD use
- Leiomyomas
- Ovarian cysts
- Pelvic congestion syndrome, pelvic inflammatory disease
- Polyps
- Transverse vaginal septum

WORKUP

- Primary dysmenorrhea: characteristic history, physical examination normal with the absence of an identifiable cause of pelvic pain
- Secondary dysmenorrhea: history of onset generally >2 yr after menarche; physical examination may reveal uterine irregularity, cul-de-sac tenderness, or nodularity or pelvic masses

LABORATORY TESTS

- No specific tests diagnostic for dysmenorrhea
- Elevated white blood cell count in the presence of infection
- Human chorionic gonadotropin to rule out ectopic pregnancy

IMAGING STUDIES

- Ultrasound scan of the pelvis to evaluate the presence of leiomyomas, ovarian cysts, or ectopic pregnancy
- Hysterosalpingogram or saline ultrasonography to assess the uterine cavity to rule out endometrial polyps or submucosal or intraluminal leiomyomas

TREATMENT

NONPHARMACOLOGIC THERAPY

- Applying heat to the lower abdomen with hot compresses, heating pads, or hot water bottles seems to offer some relief.
- Other reassurance that this is a treatable condition.

ACUTE GENERAL Rx

- Nonsteroidal anti-inflammatory drugs such as ibuprofen 400 to 600 mg q4-6h or naproxen sodium 550 mg q12h, mefenamic acid 500 mg initial dose followed by 250 mg q6h prn, aspirin 650 mg q4-6h, or oral contraceptives
- Nifedipine 30 mg qd in difficult cases of dysmenorrhea
- Magnesium supplements have been found likely to be beneficial
- Thiamine supplements may reduce pain
- Secondary dysmenorrhea: treatment directed to the specific underlying condition; surgery plays a greater role

CHRONIC Rx

Acupuncture and transcutaneous electrical nerve stimulation may be tried. In cases in which medical therapy has not worked, laparoscopy or other surgical treatments should be considered depending on the secondary cause of the dysmenorrhea.

DISPOSITION

The majority of patients are satisfactorily treated with good outcomes. Possible chronic complications with primary dysmenorrhea that has not been adequately treated can lead to anxiety and depression. With certain causes of secondary dysmenorrhea, infertility can become a problem.

REFERRAL

If a secondary cause of dysmenorrhea is revealed, refer to the appropriate specialist for further medical or surgical treatment (e.g., gynecologist, pain management center).

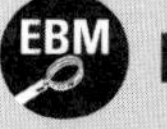

EVIDENCE

Two RCTs have found topical heat treatment to be as effective as either ibuprofen or paracetamol.[1] Ⓐ

A systematic review concluded that overall there is no evidence to suggest that spinal manipulation is effective in the treatment of primary or secondary dysmenorrhea.[2]

A systematic review concluded that there is insufficient evidence to recommend the use of nerve interruption in the management of dysmenorrhea, regardless of the cause.[3]

Evidence-Based References

1. Akin M et al: Continuous, low-level, topical heat wrap therapy as compared to acetaminophen for primary dysmenorrhea, *J Reprod Med* 49:739-745, 2004. Ⓐ
2. Proctor ML et al: Spinal manipulation for primary and secondary dysmenorrhoea, *Cochrane Database Rev* (4), 2006.
3. Proctor ML et al: Surgical interruption of pelvic nerve pathways for primary and secondary dysmenorrhoea, *Cochrane Database Rev* (4), 2005.
4. Bitner M et al: Efficacy and tolerability of lumiracoxib in the treatment of primary dysmenorrhoea, *Int J Clin Pract* 58:340-345, 2004.

AUTHORS: **GEORGE T. DANAKAS, M.D.,** and **RUBEN ALVERO, M.D.**

Dyspareunia

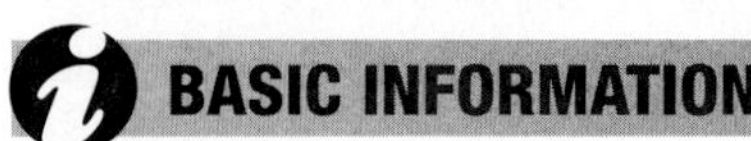

BASIC INFORMATION

DEFINITION

Persistent and/or recurrent pain associated with sexual intercourse

SYNONYMS

Painful intercourse

ICD-9CM CODES
625.0 Pain associated with female genital organs
302.76 Sexual deviations and disorders with functional dyspareunia, psychogenic dyspareunia

EPIDEMIOLOGY & DEMOGRAPHICS

PREVALENCE: 7% to 60% depending on definition
PREDOMINANT SEX: Female
AT-RISK POPULATION: No consistent findings regarding:
- Age
- Parity
- Educational status
- Race
- Income
- Marital status

RISK FACTORS: Lower:
- Frequency of intercourse
- Levels of desire and arousal
- Orgasmic response
- Physical and emotional satisfaction
- General happiness

HISTORICAL FACTORS:
- Pain parameters
  1. Character
  2. Location (Introital, middle, deep)
  3. Onset
  4. Duration
  5. Timing
  6. Chronicity
  7. Cyclicity
  8. Recurrence
- Gynecologic history
  1. History of STD
  2. History of HSV or HPV
  3. Other sexual dysfunctions
  4. Prior abdominal or gynecologic surgery
  5. Prior pelvic or abdominal radiation
  6. History of endometriosis, fibroids
  7. History of genital or uterine prolapse
  8. History of gynecologic infection
  9. History of pelvic pain
  10. History of menopausal symptoms
  11. Sexual misinformation
- OB history
  1. Lacerations
  2. Episiotomy
- General medical causes
  1. History of chronic diseases
  2. GI or GU symptoms
  3. Medications
  4. History of psychological disorders
  5. History of dermatologic condition
  6. Religious beliefs
  7. Generalized anxiety

PHYSICAL FINDINGS & CLINICAL PRESENTATION

- Primary versus secondary dyspareunia
  1. Latter with history of pain-free coitus
- Visual inspection
  1. Discoloration
  2. Ulcerations
  3. Discharge
  4. Prolapse
  5. Dysplastic changes
  6. Infestations
- Physical examination
  1. Sensitivity to light touch
  2. Tenderness to palpation
  3. Genital prolapse
     a. Uterus
     b. Bladder
     c. Cervix
     d. Vagina
     e. Adnexa
     f. Rectum
     g. Bowel
  4. Ridges, septum
  5. Levator muscle tone
  6. Evidence of previous surgery
  7. Vaginal length, depth, caliber constrictions

ETIOLOGY

- Pathology or alteration or reduction of genital-associated tissue
- Psychosocial factors
- Marital or relationship discord
- History of sexual abuse

DIAGNOSIS

DIFFERENTIAL DIAGNOSIS

- Congenital deformities (septa/agenesis)
- Imperforate hymen
- Menopausal changes
- Atrophic tissue
- Impaired lubrication
- Psychogenic
- Vaginismus
- Inadequate foreplay
- Endometriosis
- Levator ani myalgia
- Chronic pelvic pain
- Previous surgery (posterior colporrhaphy, perineorrhaphy)
  1. Alteration in vaginal length, depth, caliber
  2. Adhesions
- Infectious
  1. Human papillomavirus
  2. Herpes simplex virus
  3. Candidiasis
  4. Tinea cruris
  5. Acute or chronic salpingitis or endometritis
- Pelvic carcinoma
- Previous radiation
- Adnexal attachment or tubal prolapse
- Pelvic tumor
- Uterine prolapse, malposition, enlargement, or retroversion
- Genital prolapse
- Cystocele, rectocele, enterocele
- Urethral or bladder pathology
- Pelvic congestion
- Vulvar vestibulitis
- Postcoital cystitis
- Broad ligament pathology
- Neuroma at the site of previous episiotomy
- Previous sexual abuse
- Vulvodynia
- Contact or allergic dermatitis
- Vitamin A, B, or C deficiency
- Equestrian dyspareunia
- Interstitial cystitis
- Pudendal neuralgia
- Myofascial pain syndrome
- Rectal pathology
- Structural abnormalities or alterations
  1. Muscle
  2. Bone
  3. Ligament

WORKUP

- History and physical examination are key
- If needed:
  1. Colposcopy
  2. Cystoscopy
  3. Consider laparoscopy for unexplained deep dyspareunia

LABORATORY TESTS

- Erythrocyte sedimentation rate
- White blood cell count
- Wet mount
- Cultures
  1. Cervical
     a. Gonorrhea
     b. *Chlamydia*
  2. Vaginal
  3. Lesions
  4. Urine
- Vulva, vaginal, or cervical biopsy
- Pap smear
- Herpes simplex virus antibodies
- Gonadotropin levels

IMAGING STUDIES

Pelvic or abdominal ultrasonography

TREATMENT

NONPHARMACOLOGIC THERAPY

- Patient education
- Discontinue exacerbating activity and irritants
- Lubrication with coitus
- Coital position changes: female superior position
- Warm or cool soaks
- Reassurance to patient of nonmalignant condition
- Psychosocial interventions
  1. Systemic desensitization techniques
  2. Behavior modification
- Vaginal dilators
- Vaginal muscle exercises and relaxation techniques
- Excision of pathologic tissue
- Surgical correction of altered, reduced, or deformed tissues

ACUTE GENERAL Rx

- Topical lidocaine
- Corticosteroids
- Antiinfective agents
- Trigger point injections
- Massage
- Acupuncture
- Transcutaneous electrical nerve stimulation
- Stress reduction techniques
- Safe sexual practices
- Hormonal replacement therapy
- Antiviral agents
- Intralesional interferon
- Mild analgesics
- Antidepressants

CHRONIC Rx

All the previous plus:

- Set supportive visits as needed
- Oral contraceptives
- Regular sexual activity
- Balanced diet
- Vitamin supplementation
- Proper hygiene

DISPOSITION

Most patients will have a reduction and/or resolution of their symptoms by using the appropriate therapeutic approaches.

REFERRAL

A multidisciplinary approach using the expertise of psychologists, dermatologists, gynecologic surgeons, infectious disease specialists, or urologists is helpful.

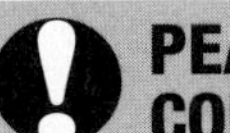

PEARLS & CONSIDERATIONS

- Dyspareunia is a symptom complex resulting from a multitude of etiologies, some of which act simultaneously.
- Uncovering the etiology of dyspareunia is predominantly based on a comprehensive history and physical examination.
- The differential diagnoses can be sorted into superficial, intermediate, and deep dyspareunia categories.
- As with the physical evaluation of any painful condition, attempt—by precise touching (moistened cotton swab), palpation, or applied pressure—to reproduce the patient's chief complaint.
- Performing a one-finger pelvic examination without concurrent abdominal palpation allows a more precise assessment of the source of genital pain.
- Individualize therapy.
- Initiate and maintain an honest diagnosis and compassionate demeanor with the patient and her partner.
- Be open minded, approachable, nonjudgmental, and diligent in your search for a solution to help these often silently suffering patients.

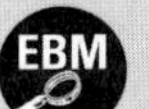

EVIDENCE

We are unable to cite evidence that meets our criteria for most of the recommended therapies.

Although the management recommendations are not evidence-based, they have been found to be successful clinically.

A Cochrane systematic review found that perineal repair with synthetic absorbable suture material vs. catgut following childbirth was associated with less pain in the subsequent 3 days. However, there was no significant difference in long-term rates of dyspareunia experienced.[1] Ⓐ

Another Cochrane systematic review concluded that there is not enough evidence to evaluate the use of ultrasound in treating perineal pain and/or dyspareunia following childbirth.[2] Ⓐ

Evidence-Based References

1. Kettle C, Johanson RB: Absorbable synthetic versus catgut suture material for perineal repair, *Cochrane Database Rev* (3), 1999. Ⓐ

2. Hay-Smith EJC: Therapeutic ultrasound for postpartum perineal pain and dyspareunia, *Cochrane Database Rev* (3), 1998. Ⓐ

SUGGESTED READINGS

Hawton RL: Female dyspareunia, *BMJ* 328(7452):1357, 2004.

Helm LJ: Evaluation and differential diagnosis of dyspareunia, *Am Fam Physician* 63:1535, 2001.

Nichols D: *Reoperative gynecologic and obstetric surgery,* ed 2, St Louis, 1997, Mosby.

AUTHORS: **DAVID I. KURSS, M.D.,** and **RUBEN ALVERO, M.D.**

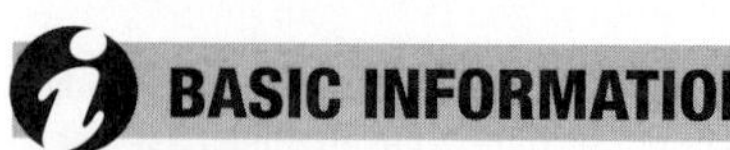

BASIC INFORMATION

DEFINITION

Nonulcerative dyspepsia is persistent or recurrent dyspepsia centered in the upper abdomen without evidence of organic disease.

SYNONYMS

Functional dyspepsia
Idiopathic dyspepsia

ICD-9CM CODES
536.8 Nonulcerative dyspepsia

EPIDEMIOLOGY & DEMOGRAPHICS

- Annual prevalence of dyspepsia approximately 25% of population.
- Dyspepsia, GERD, PUD account for 2% to 5% of all primary care visits.

CLINICAL PRESENTATION

An international committee of clinical investigators developed the Rome II criteria to define nonulcerative dyspepsia for both research purposes and clinical practice:

- Having at least 12 weeks (may be nonconsecutive) within preceding 12 months of:
  1. Persistent or recurrent dyspepsia
  2. No evidence of organic disease that is likely to explain symptoms
  3. No evidence that dyspepsia is exclusively relieved by defecation or associated with the onset of a change in stool frequency or form
- Additional symptoms include:
  - Bloating
  - Early satiety
  - Indigestion
  - Nausea, vomiting
  - Weight loss/anorexia

ETIOLOGY

Pathophysiology is still unclear but research is focused on the following factors:

- Abnormalities of gastric motor function—especially in delayed gastric emptying, antral hypomotility, the relationship between low fasting gastric volumes and faster gastric emptying, and lower gastric compliance
- Visceral hypersensitivity
- *Helicobacter pylori* infection
- Psychosocial factors—associated with anxiety and depression

DIAGNOSIS

DIFFERENTIAL DIAGNOSIS

Made from the exclusion of other causes of dyspepsia

Other possible etiologies for dyspepsia:

- Peptic ulcer disease
- Gastroesophageal reflux
- Gastric/esophageal/all abdominal cancers
- Biliary tract disease
- Gastroparesis
- Pancreatitis
- Medications (i.e., NSAIDs, erythromycin, steroids)
- Infiltrative diseases of the stomach (i.e., Crohn's or sarcoidosis)
- Metabolic disturbances (i.e., hypercalcemia or hyperkalemia)
- Ischemic bowel disease
- System disorders (i.e., diabetes, thyroid disorders, or connective tissue diseases)

LABORATORY TESTS

WORKUP:

- The pattern of symptoms overlap considerably for all types of dyspepsia; therefore, the history should focus on finding specific symptoms that help exclude other causes of dyspepsia.
- However, the specific etiology of dyspepsia often cannot be identified by history and physical exam alone and much controversy surrounds the optimal approach for further testing and treatment.

IMAGING STUDIES

ENDOSCOPY: The American Gastroenterological Association as well as the Maastricht European consensus report both recommend:

- Patients older than age 45 or those with alarming symptoms (weight loss, bleeding, anemia, or dysphagia) should have early upper endoscopy for tissue sampling to evaluate for gastric malignancy, as well as *H. pylori* testing. Patients whose symptoms have failed to respond to empiric therapeutic approaches should also undergo endoscopy.
- AGA also recommends empiric trial of antisecretory therapy or prokinetic agent for 1 mo in patients younger than 45 years without alarming symptoms who are *H. pylori* negative. *H. pylori* testing includes serology, stool antigen, or urea breath test.

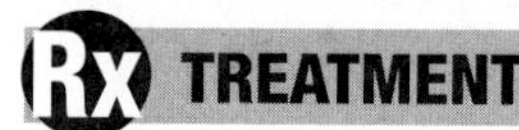

TREATMENT

NONPHARMACOLOGIC THERAPY

Controversial and often disappointing. Goal should be to help patients accept, diminish, and cope with symptoms rather than eliminate them.

ACUTE GENERAL Rx

PHARMACOLOGIC THERAPY: Treatment sometimes depends on the predominant symptoms.

Predominant Symptom	Possible Etiology	Recommended Medication
Nausea	Motility dysfunction	Prokinetic agent
Bloating	Motility dysfunction	Prokinetic agent
Pain	Mucosal disease or *H. pylori* infection	Trial of medications listed below or *H. pylori* regimen
Somatic complaints	Psychosocial	Psychotropic medication

Medication categories

Antacids (i.e., aluminum hydroxide, calcium carbonate)
H2-receptor antagonists (i.e., cimetidine)
Proton pump inhibitors (PPIs) (i.e., omeprazole)
Prokinetic agents (i.e., metoclopramide)
Antidepressants (i.e., selective serotonin receptor inhibitors)
H. pylori therapy/antibiotic therapy (clarithromycin + amoxicillin or metronidazole + PPI)

REFERRAL

- Referral to gastroenterology if patient with alarming symptoms or when endoscopy is indicated
- Alarming symptoms include GI bleeding, dysphagia, odynophagia, unexplained anemia, change in appetite, and weight loss.
- Referral to cardiology if cardiac etiology suspected.

SUGGESTED READINGS

Dickerson LM et al: Evaluation and management of nonulcer dyspepsia, *Am Fam Physician* 70:1, 2004.
Fennerty MB et al: Short- and long-term management of heartburn and other acid-related disorders, *J Fam Prac* 58:S1-S12, 2009.

AUTHOR: **HANNAH VU, D.O.**

BASIC INFORMATION

DEFINITION

The term "dysphagia" is derived from the Greek words dys (with difficulty) and phagia (to eat). It is characterized by abnormal transfer of food from mouth to the stomach, which may involve the oral, pharyngeal, or esophageal stages of swallowing.

ICD-9CM Code
782.2 Dysphagia

EPIDEMIOLOGY & DEMOGRAPHICS

- This is seen in 10% of individuals above the age of 50 yr. Its prevalence increases with advancing age.
- Nearly 12% of hospitalized patients have symptoms of dysphagia.
- Up to 30% to 60% of nursing home patients have some form of dysphagia.
- Special populations, including patients with head injury, stroke, or Parkinson's disease, have 30% to 50% prevalence of oropharyngeal dysphagia.

ETIOLOGY

- Oropharyngeal
  1. Neuromuscular causes
     - Stroke
     - Parkinson's disease
     - Multiple sclerosis
     - Myasthenia gravis
     - Amyotrophic lateral sclerosis
     - CNS tumors
     - Muscular dystrophy
     - Thyroid dysfunction
     - Polymyositis and dermatomyositis
     - Sarcoidosis
     - Cerebral palsy
     - Head trauma
     - Metabolic encephalopathy
     - Dementia
     - Bell's palsy
  2. Structural causes
     - Oropharyngeal tumors
     - Zenker's diverticulum
     - Infection of pharynx or neck (mucositis from candida, herpes, and CMV)
     - Thyromegaly
     - Prior surgery or radiotherapy
     - Osteophytes and other spinal disorders
     - Proximal esophageal webs
     - Congenital anomalies (e.g., cleft palate)
     - Poor dentition
- Esophageal
  1. Neuromuscular disorders
     - Achalasia
     - Diffuse esophageal spasm
     - Nutcracker esophagus
     - Hypertensive lower esophageal sphincter
     - Ineffective esophageal motility
     - Scleroderma
     - Reflex associated dysmotility
  2. Structural disorder
     - Peptic stricture
     - Esophageal rings and webs
     - Diverticuli
     - Carcinoma and benign tumors
     - Foreign bodies
     - Vascular compression
     - Mediastinal masses
     - Spinal osteophytes
     - Mucosal injury (from pills, infection, GERD, etc.)

PATHOGENESIS

The inability to swallow is caused either by a problem in strength or coordination of the muscles required to move material from the mouth to stomach or by a fixed obstruction somewhere between the mouth and the stomach.

CLINICAL FEATURES

Oropharyngeal dysphagia

- Problem arises within 2 seconds of initiating the voluntary phase of swallowing.
- Typical symptoms include drooling, spillage of food, postnasal regurgitation, difficulty in initiation of swallowing, sialorrhea, sensation of food stuck in the neck, coughing or choking during swallowing, the need to swallow repeatedly to clear food or fluid from the pharynx, dysphonia, nasal speech, hoarseness of voice, and dysarthria.
- A thorough physical examination including that of the nervous system, oral cavity, and the head/neck is very important in patients with oropharyngeal dysphagia.

Esophageal dysphagia

- Problem usually arises several seconds after swallowing.
- Patients often complain of food being stuck in lower substernal area.
- Dysphagia to solids suggests mechanical obstruction.
- Neuromuscular causes result in dysphagia to both solids and liquids. Particularly, patients with achalasia tend to drink a lot of fluids while eating or apply maneuvers such as straightening the back, raising their arms over their heads, or standing to increase intraesophageal pressure to facilitate the emptying of food into the stomach.
- Often times, ingestion of very cold or very hot foods precipitate the dysphagia associated with neuromuscular disorder.
- Delayed regurgitation of food, heartburn, and chest pain are usually present.
- Weight loss is usually associated with malignancy or achalasia.
- Symptoms are intermittent in patients with esophageal dysphagia from benign causes of structural obstruction or diffuse esophageal spasm. However, it is progressive in patients with peptic stricture, esophageal carcinoma, scleroderma, and achalasia.
- In patients with structural obstruction, when the luminal diameter is more than 18 to 20 mm, they are rarely symptomatic, whereas those with a diameter of less than 13 mm are nearly always symptomatic.
- These patients with esophageal dysphagia usually do not have any characteristic physical findings.

Dx DIAGNOSIS

Laboratory evaluation

- CBC
- Thyroid studies
- Nutritional assessment by checking serum protein and albumin levels
- Other studies based on specific clinical conditions

Special studies

- Oropharyngeal dysphagia
  1. Videofluoroscopy is the first test often ordered in evaluation of patients with oropharyngeal dysphagia
  2. Double contrast modified barium swallow study
  3. Fiberoptic flexible nasopharyngeal laryngoscopy is mandatory in all cases when a structural lesion, particularly malignancy, is suspected.
  4. Pharyngeal and upper esophageal manometry (Fig. 1-96) are occasionally of value to predict which patients will have a favorable outcome from cricopharyngeal myotomy or dilatation.
  5. Radiography of head and neck when indicated
- Esophageal dysphagia
  1. Barium esophagography should precede upper endoscopies to identify patients at risk from potential perforation with an endoscopy and to help plan fluoroscopically guided dilatation. It is often the first step in evaluating patients with dysphagia, especially if an obstructive lesion is suspected.
  2. EGD
  3. Esophageal manometry is indicated if no abnormality is identified by barium study or EGD.
  4. Esophageal pH monitoring in patients with suspected reflux disease
  5. Endoscopic ultrasonography
  6. Radiograph, CT, and MRI of chest

DIFFERENTIAL DIAGNOSIS

- Globus pharyngeus
- Odynophagia
- Phagophobia
- GERD

Rx TREATMENT

- Treatment should be approached with the help of specialists of multiple disciplines (ENT, head and neck surgeon, radiologist, speech pathologist, physical therapist, dietitian, gastroenterologist, physical medicine and rehabilitation specialist, dentist, neurologist, etc.).
- Goal of therapy is airway protection and maintenance of nutrition.
- Alteration of food consistency, volume, and delivery rate plays a major role.

- The goal of direct therapy is to change swallowing physiology with medical treatment of primary disease, maxillofacial prosthesis, and cricopharyngeal myotomy
- Indirect therapies include exercise programs for tongue coordination and chewing under the guidance of a speech therapist.
- Maintenance of oral feeding often requires compensatory techniques such as chin-tuck position, rotation of head to the affected side, tilting of head to the strong side, and lying on one's back or on one's side during swallowing.
- Some of the voluntary maneuvers applied include supraglottic swallow, effortful swallow, Mendelson maneuver, Shaker exercise, and the Heimlich maneuver.
- Placement of nasogastric tube, jejunostomy tube, or percutaneous endoscopic gastrotomy (PEG) tube is considered for enteral feeding when other measures fail and the patient remains at significant risk for aspiration or nutrition becomes compromised.
- Treatment of associated GERD should not be forgotten.
- Surgery for chronic aspiration may involve tracheostomy, medialization, laryngeal suspension, laryngeal closure, and/or laryngotracheal separation-diversion.
- Other measures include esophageal dilatation, removal of foreign body, esophagel resection, chemotherapy, radiotherapy, endoscopic ablation of tumor, phodynamic therapy, esophageal prosthesis/stents, diverticulectomy, intrasphincteric injection of botulinum toxin, surgical myotomy, and others. Smooth muscle relaxants such as nitrates and calcium channel blockers have been used to effectively treat patients with diffuse esophageal spasm and nutcracker esophagus.
- Several scales have been suggested to determine patients' functional outcome. One of them is the "Swallowing Rating Scale."

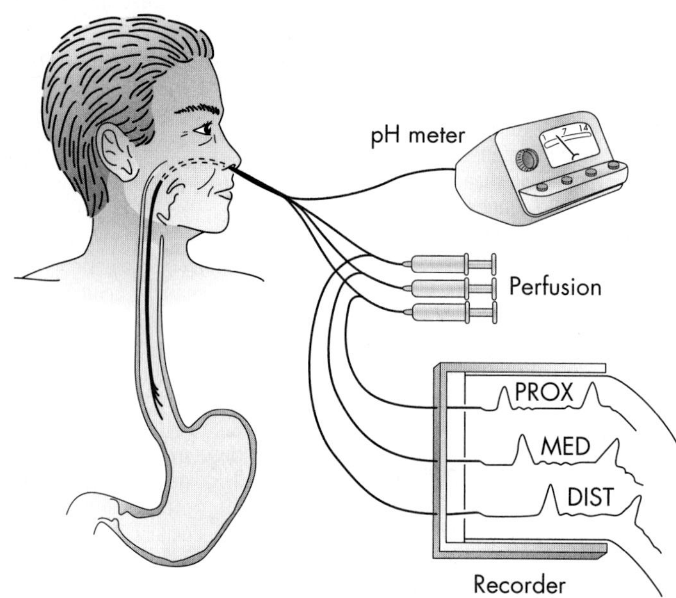

FIGURE 1-96 Combined manometric-pH recording system used in the evaluation of esophageal function. The triple-lumen perfused recording catheter measures intraluminal pressures from three levels in the esophagus. Measurements are made in terms of centimeters from the nostrils to the proximal opening of the recording catheter (PROX). The medial catheter (ED) records pressures 5 cm distal to the proximal opening and the distal catheter (DIST) 5 cm below this. The intraesophageal pH electrode is used to document gastroesophageal reflux. (From Townsend CM et al: *Sabiston textbook of surgery,* ed 17, Philadelphia, 2004, Saunders.).

COMPLICATIONS

- Dehydration
- Malnutrition
- Aspiration pneumonia
- Airway obstruction
- Death resulting from pulmonary complications

PROGNOSIS

- Depends on the etiology.
- Nursing home patients with oropharyngeal dysphagia and a history of aspiration have an approximately 45% mortality rate over one year.
- All patients, especially the elderly, should take their medications with a full glass of water while in upright position well before bedtime.
- Dysphagia should be considered an alarm symptom, indicating the need for immediate evaluation.

PATIENT EDUCATION

Elderly patients with dysphagia should not attribute their symptoms to aging.

SUGGESTED READINGS

Lind C: Dysphagia: evaluation and treatment, *Gastroenterol Clin N Am* 32(2):553-575, 2003.

Logemann J: Oropharyngeal dysphagia and nutritional management, *Curr Opin Clin Nutr Metab Care* 10(5): 611-614, 2007.

Saud BM, Szyjkowski RD: A diagnostic approach to dysphagia, *Clin Fam Prac* 6(3):525-546, 2004.

AUTHOR: **HEMANT K. SATPATHY, M.D.**

BASIC INFORMATION

DEFINITION

Dystonia is characterized by involuntary muscle contractions (sustained or spasmodic) that lead to abnormal body movements or postures. Dystonia can be generalized or focal, of early (<20 yr) or late onset, and primary or secondary.

SYNONYMS

Blepharospasm
Oromandibular (orofacial) dystonia
Spasmodic (limb or axial) dystonia
Torticollis
Writer's cramp

ICD-9CM CODES

333.6	Genetic torsion dystonia
335.7	Acquired torsion dystonia
333.7	Acute dystonia due to drugs
333.85	Subacute dyskenesia due to drugs

EPIDEMIOLOGY & DEMOGRAPHICS

PREVALENCE: Estimated at one in 3000 persons.
PREDOMINANT SEX: Cervical dystonia has a 3:2 female preponderance.
PREDOMINANT AGE:
- Onset of focal cervical dystonia is usually in the fifth decade.
- Hereditary forms may have an onset in childhood or adulthood and tend to be more severe.

GENETICS: Autosomal-dominant, autosomal-recessive, and X-linked forms of dystonia have been identified. Ashkenazi Jews are particularly susceptible to primary early-onset dystonia.

CLINICAL PRESENTATION

Focal dystonias produce abnormal sustained muscle contractions in a single region of the body:
- Neck (torticollis): most commonly affected site with a tendency for the head to turn to one side
- Eyelids (blepharospasm): involuntary closure of the eyelids
- Mouth (oromandibular dystonia): involuntary contraction of muscles of the mouth, tongue, or face
- Hand (writer's cramp) (Fig. 1-97)

Generalized dystonia affects multiple areas of the body and can lead to marked joint deformities.

ETIOLOGY

- Exact pathophysiology of primary dystonia is unknown but believed to involve abnormalities of basal ganglia. Specifically, reduced and abnormal patterns of neuronal activity in the basal ganglia result in disinhibition of the motor thalamus and cortex, leading to abnormal movement.
- Fifteen hereditary forms have been described, including the severe progressive form, dystonia musculorum deformans.
- Secondary dystonia results from central nervous system (CNS) disease of the basal ganglia (stroke, demyelination, hypoxia, trauma), Huntington's disease, Wilson's disease, Parkinson syndromes, and lysosomal storage diseases.
- Acute dystonia can occur with drugs that block dopamine receptors, such as phenothiazines or butyrophenones.
- Tardive dyskinesia can result from long-term treatment with antiemetics (e.g., phenothiazines), antipsychotics (e.g., haloperidol), levodopa, anticonvulsants, or ergots.

DIAGNOSIS

DIFFERENTIAL DIAGNOSIS

- Parkinson's disease
- Progressive supranuclear palsy
- Wilson's disease
- Huntington's disease
- Drug effects

WORKUP

History (family history, birth history, trauma, medication use), physical examination

LABORATORY TESTS

- Usually not helpful for diagnosis
- Serum ceruloplasmin if Wilson's disease is suspected

IMAGING STUDIES

- Primary dystonias are generally not associated with structural CNS abnormalities. CT scan or MRI of brain if a CNS lesion is suspected as a cause of secondary dystonia.
- Electrophysiologic testing can provide diagnostic support for the diagnosis.

TREATMENT

NONPHARMACOLOGIC THERAPY

- Heat, massage, physical therapy to relieve pain
- Splints to prevent contractures

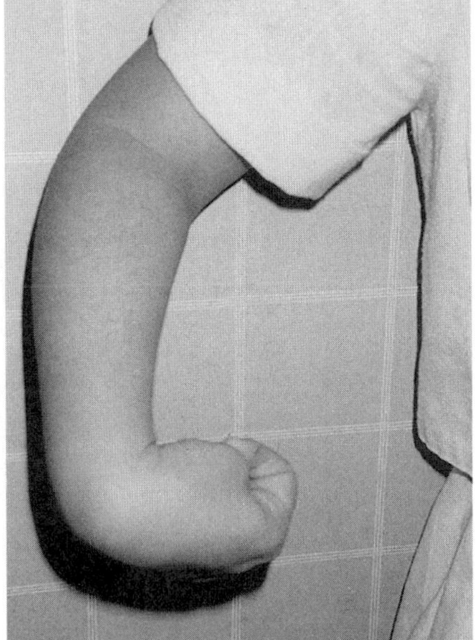

FIGURE 1-97 Focal dystonia of the distal right arm. (From Goldman L, Ausiello D [eds]: *Cecil textbook of medicine,* ed 22, Philadelphia, 2004, WB Saunders.)

ACUTE GENERAL Rx

For acute dystonic reactions to phenothiazines/butyrophenones, use diphenhydramine 50 mg IV or benztropine 2 mg IV.

CHRONIC Rx

- Pharmacologic treatment is often ineffective.
- Slowly withdraw offending agents.
- Diazepam, baclofen, or carbamazepine may be helpful.
- Intrathecal baclofen is most useful for spastic or truncal dystonia.
- Trihexyphenidyl or benztropine may be helpful in up to 50% of tardive dystonias.
- For generalized dystonia, a trial of carbidopa/levodopa may be beneficial.
- Injections of botulinum toxin into the affected muscles is the standard treatment for focal dystonias.
- Surgical procedures, including denervation, myectomy, rhizotomy, thalamotomy (pallidotomy), or functional stereotactic surgery may be helpful for severe, refractory cases.
- Deep brain stimulation is becoming more promising, especially for refractory primary generalized dystonias.

DISPOSITION

Spontaneous remission of focal cervical dystonia can occur, but dystonia is generally progressive and pharmacologic therapy is often ineffective.

REFERRAL

Neurology and/or neurosurgery for severe or refractory cases.
Physical therapy for maintaining flexibility.

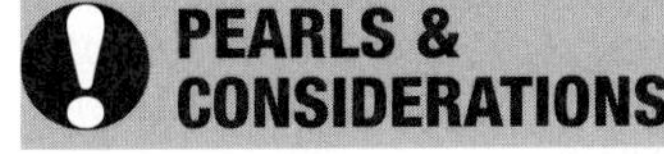

PEARLS & CONSIDERATIONS

COMMENTS

- Avoid triggers/exacerbating factors.
- Early physical therapy and splinting to prevent contractures.
- Consider botulism injections or deep brain stimulation surgery for severe or refractory dystonia.
- Botulism injections remain the treatment of choice for focal dystonias.

SUGGESTED READINGS

Bhidaya Siri R: Dystonia: genetics and treatment update, *Neurologist* 12:74, 2006.

Defazio G et al: Epidemiology of primary dystonia, *Lancet Neurol* 3:673, 2004.

Simpson D et al: Assessment: Botulism neurotoxin for the treatment of movement disorders (an evidence-based review): report of the Therapeutics and Technology Assessment Subcommittee of the American Academy of Neurology, *Neurology* 70:1699, 2009.

Tarsy D, Simon DK: Dystonia, *N Engl J Med* 355:818, 2006.

AUTHORS: **LYNN MCNICOLL, M.D., F.R.C.P.C.,** and **MARK J. FAGAN, M.D.**

Echinococcosis

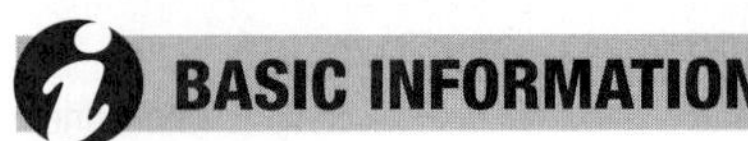

BASIC INFORMATION

DEFINITION

Echinococcosis is a chronic infection caused by the larval stage of several animal cestodes (tapeworms) of the genus *Echinococcus.*

SYNONYMS

Hydatid disease

ICD-9CM CODES
122.9 *Echinococcus* infection

EPIDEMIOLOGY & DEMOGRAPHICS

INCIDENCE (IN U.S.): Seen primarily in immigrants.
PEAK INCIDENCE: Presumed to be acquired in childhood or early adulthood in most cases.
PREVALENCE (IN U.S.): See Incidence
PREDOMINANT SEX: Male = female
PREDOMINANT AGE: 0 to 50 yr of age

PHYSICAL FINDINGS & CLINICAL PRESENTATION

- Signs of an enlarging mass lesion in a visceral site such as the liver, lungs, kidneys, bone, or CNS
- Occasional cyst rupture causing allergic manifestations such as urticaria, angioedema, or anaphylaxis that bring the patient to medical attention
- Incidental discovery of cysts by abdominal or thoracic imaging studies performed for other reasons

ETIOLOGY

- Four species of *Echinococcus: E. granulosus, E. multilocularis, E. oligarthrus,* and *E. vogeli.*
  1. *E. granulosus* is the cause of cystic hydatid disease.
  2. *E. multilocularis* and *E. vogeli* are the causes of alveolar and polycystic disease.
- The disease is transmitted to humans by infected canines (domestic or wild dogs, wolves, foxes) and seen most commonly in livestock-producing areas of the Middle East, Africa, Australia, New Zealand, Europe, and the Americas, including the southwestern U.S.
- Eggs are present in the feces of infected canines; human infection occurs by ingestion of viable eggs in contaminated food.
- It is common in many areas of the world, especially the Middle East.

DIAGNOSIS

DIFFERENTIAL DIAGNOSIS

- Cystic neoplasms
- Abscess (amebic or bacterial)
- Congenital polycystic disease

WORKUP

- Antibody assay
- Imaging study (CT scan, ultrasonography)
- Histologic examination of cyst or contents obtained by aspiration or resection (if possible) to confirm diagnosis

LABORATORY TESTS

Antibody assays (ELISA, Latex agglutination, and Western blot): >90% sensitive and specific for liver cysts, but less accurate for cysts in other sites. A PCR assay is now available for problematic cases.

IMAGING STUDIES

Ultrasonography and/or CT scan:

- Both are extremely sensitive for the detection of cysts, especially in the liver (Fig. 1-98).
- Both lack specificity and are inadequate to establish the diagnosis of echinococcosis with certainty.

TREATMENT

NONPHARMACOLOGIC THERAPY

- Treatment of choice for echinococcal cysts is surgical resection, when feasible.
- If resection is not feasible, perform percutaneous drainage with instillation of 95% ethanol to prevent dissemination of viable larvae.
- Surgical therapy is followed by medical therapy with albendazole (see "Acute General Rx").

ACUTE GENERAL Rx

For echinococcosis confined to the liver:

- Albendazole (400 mg bid for 28 days followed by 14 days of rest for at least three cycles)
- Mebendazole (50 to 70 mg/kg qd) if albendazole not available

CHRONIC Rx

See "Acute General Rx."

DISPOSITION

- Long-term follow-up is necessary following surgical or medical therapy because of the high incidence of late relapse.
- Antibody assays and imaging studies are repeated every 6 to 12 mo for several years following successful surgical or medical therapy.

REFERRAL

All patients for evaluation for possible surgical resection of cysts

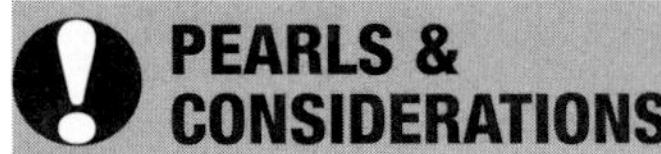

PEARLS & CONSIDERATIONS

COMMENTS

Cyst resection, if indicated, should be performed by surgeons experienced with this procedure.

SUGGESTED READINGS

Eckert J, Deplazes P: Biological, epidemiological, and clinical aspects of echinococcosis, a zoonosis of increasing concern, *Clin Microbiol Rev* 17(1):107, 2004.

Yang YR et al: A hospital-based retrospective survey of human cystic and alveolar echinococcosis in Ningxia Hui Autonomous Region, PR China, *Acta Trop* 97(3):284, 2006.

Zhang W, McManus DP: Recent advances in the immunology and diagnosis of echinococcosis, *FEMS Immunol Med Microbiol* 47(1):24, 2006.

AUTHORS: **GLENN G. FORT, M.D., M.P.H.,** and **DENNIS J. MIKOLICH, M.D.**

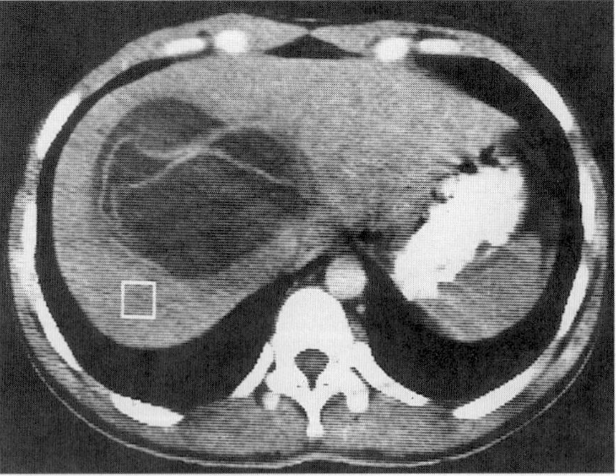

FIGURE 1-98 Computed tomographic scan of an echinococcal cyst in a 25-year-old man, demonstrating the complex structure of the wall and the interior. (From Goldman L, Ausiello D [eds]: *Cecil textbook of medicine,* ed 22, Philadelphia, 2004, WB Saunders.)

BASIC INFORMATION

DEFINITION

Eclampsia is the occurrence of seizures or coma in a woman with preeclampsia, occurring at >20 wk of gestation or <48 hr postpartum. Atypical eclampsia occurs at <20 wk of gestation or as much as 14 days postpartum.

SYNONYMS

Toxemia
Seizures of pregnancy

ICD-9CM CODES
642.6 Eclampsia

EPIDEMIOLOGY & DEMOGRAPHICS

INCIDENCE: One case per 150 to 3000 pregnancies; 2% to 4% of those with preeclampsia
GENETICS: Increased incidence with a first-degree relative (sister or mother) having had eclampsia
RISK FACTORS: Multifetal gestation (3.6% in twin gestation), molar pregnancy, nonimmune hydrops fetalis, uncontrolled hypertension, preexisting hypertension, renal disease

PHYSICAL FINDINGS & CLINICAL PRESENTATION

- Seizure begins as facial twitching, then spreads to generalized clonicotonic state, with cessation of respiration followed by a postictal period of amnesia, agitation, and confusion.
- 40% have severe hypertension, 40% have mild to moderate hypertension, and 20% are normotensive.
- Generalized edema with rapid weight gain (>2 lb/wk) may be one of the earliest signs of eclampsia.
- Persistent occipital headache and hyperreflexia with clonus occur in 80% of patients with eclampsia; epigastric pain occurs in 20% of these patients.

ETIOLOGY

- Exact etiology unknown.
- Common pathway relates to abnormalities in autoregulation of cerebral blood flow. This may involve transient vasospasm, ischemia, cerebral hemorrhage, and edema occurring by a mechanism involving hypertensive encephalopathy, decreased colloid osmotic pressure, and prostaglandin imbalance.

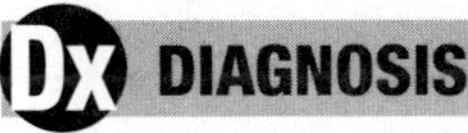

DIAGNOSIS

DIFFERENTIAL DIAGNOSIS

- Preexisting seizure disorder
- Metabolic abnormalities (hypoglycemia, hyponatremia, hypocalcemia)
- Substance abuse
- Head trauma, infection (meningitis, encephalitis)
- Intracerebral bleeding or thrombosis
- Amniotic fluid embolism
- Space-occupying brain lesions or neoplasms
- Pseudoseizure

WORKUP

- Rule out other causes of seizures during pregnancy.
- Atypical presentations such as prolonged postictal state; status epilepticus; gestational age <20 wk or >48 hr postpartum; or signs of meningitis, substance abuse, or severe uncontrolled hypertension should prompt a search for other seizure etiologies.

LABORATORY TESTS

- Proteinuria: severe (49%), mild to moderate (29%), absent (22%)
- HCT: elevated as a result of hemoconcentration
- Platelet count: decreased; LFTs elevated in HELLP syndrome (hemolysis, elevated liver enzymes, and low platelet count)
- BUN and creatinine: elevated with renal involvement
- Serum electrolytes, glucose, calcium, toxicology profile: rule out other causes of seizures
- Hyperuricemia: >6.9 mg/dl found in 70% of eclamptics
- ABG: maternal acidemia and hypoxia

IMAGING STUDIES

- CT scan or MRI indicated in atypical presentation, suspected intracerebral bleeding, or focal neurologic deficit.
- There are abnormal findings, including cerebral edema, hemorrhage, and infarction, in 50% of patients.

TREATMENT

NONPHARMACOLOGIC THERAPY

- Airway protection (risk of aspiration)
- Supportive care during acute event

ACUTE GENERAL Rx

- Maintain airway, adequate oxygenation, and IV access.
- Fetal resuscitation, involving maternal oxygenation, left lateral positioning, and continuous fetal heart rate monitoring, is needed.
- Magnesium sulfate is the drug of choice. Give magnesium sulfate 6 g IV load over 20 min, then 3 g/hr maintenance, for recurrent seizure prophylaxis. If repeated convulsions, may give an additional 2 g IV over 3 to 5 min. Approximately 10% to 15% of patients will have a second seizure after initial loading dose. Check magnesium level 1 hr after loading dose, then q6h (therapeutic range 4 to 6 mg/dl). Antidote for toxicity is calcium gluconate 10 ml of 10% solution. Phenytoin has been used as an alternative in patients in whom magnesium sulfate is contraindicated (renal insufficiency, heart block, myasthenia gravis, hypoparathyroidism).
- Give sodium amobarbital 250 mg IV over 3 min for persistent seizures.
- Treat blood pressure if >160 mm Hg/110 mm Hg with labetalol 20- to 40-mg IV bolus, hydralazine 10 mg IV, or nifedipine 10 to 20 mg sublingual q20min.
- Evaluate patient for delivery.

CHRONIC Rx

- The first priority is stabilization of the mother in terms of adequate oxygenation, hemodynamics, and laboratory abnormalities, such as associated coagulopathies.
- Cervical status and gestational age should be assessed. If unfavorable cervix and <30 wk of gestation, consider C-section; otherwise consider induction.
- Controlled epidural is the anesthesia of choice for labor or C-section.
- Avoid general anesthesia in uncontrolled hypertension to minimize risk of catastrophic cerebral events.

DISPOSITION

The maternal mortality rate for eclampsia averages 5% to 6%. Morbidity rate is 25%, including placental abruption (10%), maternal apnea with fetal asphyxia, aspiration pneumonia, pulmonary edema (4%), renal failure, cardiopulmonary arrest, and coma.

REFERRAL

Because of the potential for serious permanent maternal and fetal sequelae, all cases should be managed by a team approach of obstetrician, neonatologist, and intensivist.

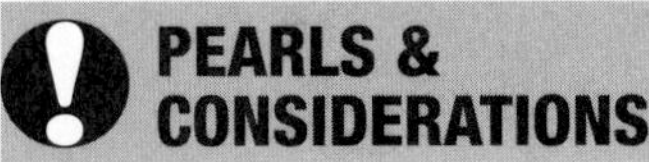

PEARLS & CONSIDERATIONS

COMMENTS

- Eclampsia antepartum, 50%; intrapartum, 20%; and postpartum, 30%.
- Postseizure there is an associated period of fetal bradycardia from 1 to 9 min; if there is evidence of fetal compromise beyond that time, consider alternative etiologies such as placental abruption (23% incidence).

SUGGESTED READINGS

Duley L: Evidence and practice: the magnesium sulphate story, *Best Pract Res Clin Obstet Gynaecol* 19(1):57, 2005.

Schroeder BM: ACOG practice bulletin on diagnosing and managing preeclampsia and eclampsia, *Am Fam Physician* 66:330, 2002.

Sibai BM: Diagnosis, prevention, and management of eclampsia, *Obstet Gynecol* 105(2):402, 2005.

AUTHORS: **SCOTT J. ZUCCALA, D.O.,** and **RUBEN ALVERO, M.D.**

BASIC INFORMATION

DEFINITION

An ectopic pregnancy (EP) occurs when a fertilized ovum implants outside the endometrial lining of the uterus.

SYNONYMS

Abdominal pregnancy (1% to 2%)
Cervical pregnancy (0.5%)
Interstitial pregnancy (2% to 3%)
Ovarian pregnancy (1%)
Tubal pregnancy (97%)

ICD-9CM CODES
633 Ectopic pregnancy

EPIDEMIOLOGY & DEMOGRAPHICS

- 1% to 2% of pregnancies
- 13% of maternal deaths

PREVALENCE (IN U.S.): Increasing number of EPs; 17,800 reported cases in 1970 and 108,000 reported cases in 1992.

RISK FACTORS: Previous salpingitis, previous EP, previous tubal ligation, previous tuboplasty, intrauterine device use, progestin-only pill, assisted reproductive techniques

PHYSICAL FINDINGS & CLINICAL PRESENTATION

- Abdominal tenderness: 95%
- Adnexal tenderness: 87% to 99%
- Peritoneal signs: 71% to 76%
- Adnexal mass: 33% to 53%
- Enlarged uterus: 6% to 30%
- Shock: 2% to 17%
- Amenorrhea or abnormal vaginal bleeding: 75%
- Shoulder pain: 10%
- Tissue passage: 6% to 7%

ETIOLOGY

- Anatomic obstruction to zygote passage
- Abnormalities in tubal motility
- Transperitoneal migration of the zygote

DIAGNOSIS

DIFFERENTIAL DIAGNOSIS

- Corpus luteum cyst
- Rupture or torsion of ovarian cyst
- Threatened or incomplete abortion
- Pelvic inflammatory disease
- Appendicitis
- Gastroenteritis
- Dysfunctional uterine bleeding
- Degenerating uterine fibroids
- Endometriosis

WORKUP

1. The classic presentation of EP includes the triad of abnormal vaginal bleeding, pelvic pain, and an adnexal mass. Consider in all women with abdominopelvic pain and a positive pregnancy test
2. Transvaginal ultrasound
3. Laparoscopy in equivocal situations and possibly for treatment

LABORATORY TESTS

- Quantitative human chorionic gonadotropin (QhCG): if normal intrauterine pregnancy (IUP), 85% have doubling time of 2 days. If abnormal gestation, will show <66% increase of QhCG within 2 days. However, 13% of ectopic pregnancies have a normal doubling time (see Section III, "Ectopic Pregnancy").
- Progesterone: decreased production in EP; <5 ng/ml strongly predictive of abnormal pregnancy. If >25 ng/ml, strongly predictive of normal IUP.
- Dropping hematocrit associated with tubal rupture, resolving ectopic pregnancy, or abnormal intrauterine pregnancy.
- Leukocytosis.

IMAGING STUDIES

- Ultrasound (Fig. 1-99): presence of an IUP makes EP extremely unlikely. A repeat ultrasonographic examination 2 to 7 days after presentation may identify the location of a pregnancy that was not identified on initial ultrasonographic examination.
- If QhCG >6000 mIU/ml, should see IUP on abdominal scan; QhCG >1500 mIU/ml for transvaginal scan.
- Findings on ultrasound in EP include:
  1. Empty uterus
  2. Adnexal mass
  3. Cul-de-sac fluid
  4. Fetal sac in tube
  5. Fetal cardiac activity in adnexa

TREATMENT

NONPHARMACOLOGIC THERAPY

Surgery can be performed by laparoscopy if patient is stable or by laparotomy if patient is unstable. Salpingiosis is the direct injection of chemotherapy into the EP by laparoscopy, transvaginal ultrasound, or hysteroscopy.

- Conservative surgery, salpingostomy or segmental resection, depends on tubal location and size of EP.
- Salpingectomy should be considered in the following circumstances:
  1. Ruptured tube
  2. Future fertility not desired
  3. Recurrent EP in the same tube
  4. Uncontrolled hemorrhage

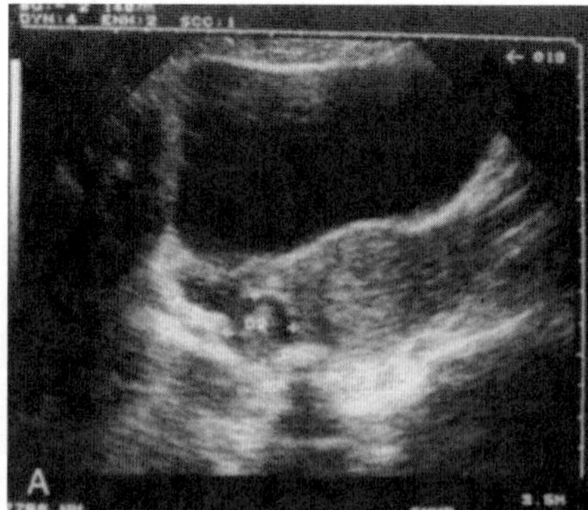

FIGURE 1-99 Ultrasound scan showing ectopic pregnancy. This transabdominal scan shows empty uterus with a complex mass in the right adnexa. The mass measures 21 × 22 mm. (From Greer IA et al: *Mosby's color atlas and test of obstetrics and gynecology,* London, 2001, Harcourt.)

ACUTE GENERAL Rx

- If the patient is stable and compliant, consider medical management with methotrexate. Patient should not have contraindications to methotrexate such as hepatic or renal disease, thrombocytopenia, leukopenia, or significant anemia. There should be no evidence of hemoperitoneum on transvaginal ultrasound. EP should be <4 cm mass with QhCG <30,000 mIU/ml. Presence of cardiac activity in the fetus is a relative contraindication to methotrexate.
- Most common regimen is methotrexate 50 mg/m^2 of body surface area. May require second dose or surgical intervention if QhCG increases or plateaus (<15% drop) when comparing values from the fourth through seventh day after treatment. Absolute contraindications to methotrexate include breast feeding, preexisting blood dyscrasias, known sensitivity to methotrexate, active pulmonary disease, chronic liver disease, alcoholism, laboratory evidence of immunodeficiency, renal disease, and peptic ulcer disease.

CHRONIC Rx

Persistent EP results from residual trophoblastic tissue or secondary implantation after conservative surgery. There is a 5% incidence of persistent EP with conservative treatment.

DISPOSITION

If diagnosed and treated early (before rupture), prognosis is excellent for good recovery. Monitor QhCG weekly until negative. Use reliable contraception until hCG is negative. With subsequent pregnancies, follow QhCG and perform early ultrasound to confirm IUP. There is a 12% recurrence rate for EP.

REFERRAL

Should obtain gynecologic consultation if EP is suspected.

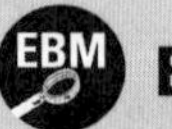

EVIDENCE

Methotrexate is a therapeutic option for women with tubal ectopic pregnancy who have no signs of bleeding, and whose pregnancy hormone blood levels are relatively low.

A systematic review analyzing the efficacy of surgery, medical treatment, and expectant management of tubal ectopic pregnancy found that single dose methotrexate was significantly less effective than salpingotomy (by laparoscopy) in primary treatment success (elimination of tubal pregnancy), but found no significant difference in tubal patency, subsequent intrauterine pregnancy, and repeat ectopic pregnancy rates. It concluded that systemic methotrexate is an option for women with tubal ectopic pregnancy with no signs of bleeding, whose pregnancy hormone blood levels are relatively low.[1] Ⓐ

Besides a high serum human chorionic gonadotropin (hCG) concentration, large tubal size (3.5 cm), and fetal cardiac activity, trials suggest that the presence of a yolk sac is associated with an increased risk of medical treatment failure.[2] Ⓑ

A review analyzing the efficacy of single-dose methotrexate stratified outcomes according to initial hCG concentration. Patients with an initial hCG level of 5000 mIU/ml or more had significantly higher failure rates with medical treatment, compared to those with initial hCG levels of less than 5000 mIU/ml. It concluded that methotrexate should be used with caution in patients with ectopic pregnancy who present with hCG levels above 5000 mIU/ml.[3] Ⓑ

Laparoscopic conservative surgery is superior to laparotomy, even though there is a higher rate of persistent trophoblast associated with it.

A systematic review identified two RCTs that compared laparoscopic vs open (laparotomy approach) salpingostomy. It found that laparoscopy is significantly less successful than open surgery in the elimination of ectopic pregnancy, owing to a higher rate of persistent trophoblast. Both approaches have similar long-term tubal patency rates, and subsequent intrauterine pregnancy rates, but laparoscopy shows a tendency to reduce subsequent ectopic pregnancy rates, although this difference is not significant. Laparoscopy is cheaper, quicker to perform, and involves a shorter hospital stay and shorter convalescence.[1] Ⓐ

The review also found that laparoscopic salpingostomy is significantly more effective than a single local or systemic methotrexate injection at eliminating ectopic pregnancy—but comparable to methotrexate when given as a multiple intramuscular injection regime.[1] Ⓐ

Salpingostomy by laparoscopy results in a higher initial treatment failure than salpingostomy by laparotomy. Subsequent fertility or repeat ectopic pregnancy, however, is no different between the two groups.

A systematic review identified two randomized controlled trials that compared laparoscopic vs open salpingostomy in the treatment of ectopic pregnancy. The review found that open salpingostomy significantly increased rates of elimination of tubal pregnancies, compared with laparoscopic salpingostomy.[1] Ⓐ

This review also found that laparoscopic salpingostomy is significantly more effective than a single local or systemic methotrexate injection at eliminating ectopic pregnancy, but is comparable to methotrexate when given as a multiple intramuscular injection regime. However, methotrexate was associated with a significantly decreased health related quality of life.[1] Ⓐ

Evidence-Based References

1. Hajenius PJ et al: Interventions for tubal ectopic pregnancy, *Cochrane Database Rev* (1), 2007. Ⓐ
2. Bixby S et al: Presence of a yolk sac on transvaginal sonography is the most reliable predictor of single-dose methotrexate treatment failure in ectopic pregnancy, *J Ultrasound Med* 24:591-598, 2005. Ⓑ
3. Menon S et al: Establishing a human chorionic gonadotropin cutoff to guide methotrexate treatment of ectopic pregnancy: a systematic review, *Fertil Steril* 87:481-484, 2007. Ⓑ

SUGGESTED READINGS

Barnhart KH: Ectopic pregnancy, *N Engl J Med* 361: 379-387, 2009.

Della-Giustina D, Denny M: Ectopic pregnancy, *Emerg Med Clin North Am* 21(3):565, 2003.

Gracia CR, Barnhart KT: Diagnosing ectopic pregnancy: decision analysis comparing six strategies, *Obstet Gynecol* 97(3):464, 2001.

AUTHORS: **GEORGE T. DANAKAS, M.D.**, and **RUBEN ALVERO, M.D.**

Ehlers-Danlos Syndrome (PTG)

BASIC INFORMATION

DEFINITION

Ehlers-Danlos syndrome (EDS) refers to a group of inherited, clinically variable, and genetically heterogeneous connective tissue disorders. EDS is characterized by skin hyperextensibility, skin fragility, joint laxity, and joint hyperextensibility.

ICD-9CM CODES
756.83 Ehlers-Danlos syndrome

EPIDEMIOLOGY & DEMOGRAPHICS

- The prevalence of EDS is estimated to be approximately one in 5000 births, although it is somewhat higher in African Americans.
- There are six distinct forms of EDS according to the revised classification system established at the Villefranche Consensus Conference, 1997 (see "Physical Findings & Clinical Presentation").
- Classic and hypermobility EDS are most prevalent. Classic EDS accounts for approximately 80% of reported cases.
- Vascular EDS is the most dangerous because it is associated with spontaneous rupture of medium and large arteries and hollow organs, especially the large intestine and uterus; occurs in 4% of patients with EDS. Vascular events typically occur between the third and fifth decade.
- In most cases, transmission is autosomal dominant except for some unclassified forms of EDS (previously known as type V and type IX, which are x-linked; type X is autosomal recessive).

PHYSICAL FINDINGS & CLINICAL PRESENTATION

- Classic (previously types I and II): patients have moderate-to-severe skin hyperelasticity (easy scarring and bruising ("cigarette-paper scars"); smooth, velvety skin and subcutaneous spheroids (small, firm, cystlike nodules) along shins or forearms, hyperextensibility ("Gorlin's sign": ability to touch tip of tongue to nose), and joint hypermobility and dislocation; patients have complications such as hernias, pelvic organ prolapsed, premature arthritis, and cervical insufficiency
- Hypermobility (type III): most frequent form, causing recurrent joint dislocations, often leaving a patient unable to walk; chronic limb/joint pain is a prominent feature; skin involvement is less prominent
- Vascular (type IV): cardinal features include distinctive facial features (pinched nose, thin lips, tight skins hollow cheeks, lobeless ears), acrogeria, thin, translucent skin, excessive bruising, and most importantly, rupture of vessels and viscera including arterial, intestinal, and uterine walls; spontaneous rupture of organs occurs in the sigmoid colon, spleen, liver, and uterus; facial features are often not prominent in children, and vascular EDS is usually not diagnosed until adulthood
- Kyphoscoliotic (type VI): rare; characterized by marked muscular hypotonia, osteopenia, joint hypermobility, progressive scoliosis, ocular fragility and possible globe rupture, mitral valve prolapse, and aortic dilation
- Arthrochalasia (types VIIA and VIIB): prominent joint hypermobility with subluxations, congenital hip dislocation, skin hyperextensibility, and tissue fragility
- Dermatosparaxis (type VIIC): severe skin fragility with decreased elasticity, bruising, hernias
- Unclassified types: type V—X-linked recessive, similar to classic EDS with skin fragility but less joint hypermobility and bruising; type IX—classic characteristics; type VIII—classic characteristics and severe periodontal disease; type X—mild classic characteristics, mitral valve prolapse; type XI—joint instability

ETIOLOGY

- Defects of collagen in extracellular matrices of multiple tissues (skin, tendons, blood vessels, and viscera) underlie all forms of EDS.
- Classic EDS is associated with defects in type V collagen, corresponding to mutations of *COL5A* genes.
- Vascular EDS involves a deficiency in type III collagen, and several studies suggest that mutations of gene *COL3A1* lead to this deficiency.
- Arthrochalasia EDS results from a defect in type I collagen, caused by mutations in the *COL1A1* and *COL1A2* genes.

Dx DIAGNOSIS

Diagnosis is based solely on clinical criteria. It is important to identify patients with vascular EDS because of the grave consequences of the disease.

- Clinical criteria for vascular EDS: two of four major diagnostic criteria establish the diagnosis; ≥1 minor criterion supports but is not sufficient to establish the diagnosis.
- Major criteria:
  1. Easy bruising
  2. Arterial, intestinal, or uterine fragility
  3. Thin, translucent skin
  4. Characteristic facial features (thin, delicate, and pinched nose, hollow cheeks, prominent staring eyes): occur in <30% of patients with vascular EDS
- Minor criteria:
  - Small joint hypermobility
  - Skin hyperextensibility
  - Spontaneous pneumothorax/hemothorax
  - Tendon or muscle rupture
  - Early-onset varicose veins
  - Carotid-cavernous fistula
  - Talipes equinovarus (clubfoot)

DIFFERENTIAL DIAGNOSIS

- Marfan's syndrome
- Osteogenesis imperfecta
- Autosomal dominant cutis laxa
- Familial joint hypermobility

WORKUP

Diagnosis is based solely on clinical criteria.

LABORATORY TESTS

- Biochemical and gene testing for known molecular defects recommended to confirm the diagnosis in vascular EDS.
- Plain radiographs may reveal calcified nodules along the shin or forearms corresponding to the subcutaneous spheroids.
- Echocardiogram can identify mitral valve prolapse and aortic dilation.

Rx TREATMENT

- All patients should receive genetic counseling about the mode of inheritance of their EDS.
- Management of most skin and joint problems should be conservative and preventive. Joint hypermobility and pain in EDS usually does not require surgical intervention. Physical therapy to strengthen muscles is helpful. Surgical repair and tightening of joint ligaments can be performed, but ligaments frequently will not hold sutures. Surgical intervention should be considered on an individual basis.
- For patients with vascular EDS:
  - Special surgical care is required because of increased tissue friability.
  - Patients should be advised to avoid contact sports.
  - Elevated blood pressure should be aggressively treated with beta-blockers, given the risk of arterial dissection.

DISPOSITION

Prognosis varies according to type of EDS. For vascular EDS:

- 25% will have a complication by age 25 yr; >80% will have a complication by age 40 yr.
- Most vascular complications consist of arterial dissections.
- Vascular events typically occur between the third and fifth decade.
- Median age of survival is 48 years. Most deaths are related to arterial rupture.

REFERRAL

Referral to dermatology for skin biopsy to confirm diagnosis of vascular EDS and to cardiology, orthopedic surgery, general surgery, and physical therapy as needed.

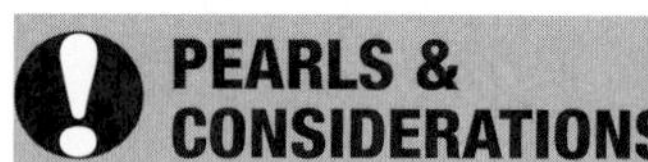

PEARLS & CONSIDERATIONS

- Women with vascular EDS should be counseled about the risk of uterine, intestinal, and arterial rupture.
  - Pregnancy is associated with up to a 25% mortality rate; however, successful childbirth is possible.
  - There is a 50% chance that the child will be affected.
- Family members of patients with EDS should be recommended for evaluation for EDS and genetic testing/counseling.

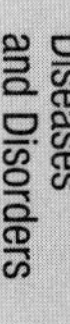

SUGGESTED READINGS

Fernandes NF, Schwartz RA: A "hyperextensive" review of Ehlers-Danlos syndrome, *Pediatric Dermatology* 82:242, 2008.

Gawthrop G et al: Ehlers-Danlos syndrome, *BMJ* 335: 448-50, 2008.

Oderich GS: Current concepts in the diagnosis and management of vascular Ehlers-Danlos syndrome, *Perspect Vasc Surg Endovasc Ther* 18(3):206, 2006.

Pepin M et al: Clinical and genetic features of Ehlers-Danlos syndrome type IV, the vascular type, *N Engl J Med* 342:673, 2000.

Prahlow JA: Death due to Ehlers-Danlos syndrome type IV, *Am J Forensic Med Pathol* 26(1):78, 2005.

Pyeritz R: Ehlers-Danlos syndrome, *N Engl J Med* 342(10):730, 2000.

Pyeritz RE: Ehlers-Danlos syndromes. In Goldman L, Bennett JC (eds): *Cecil textbook of medicine,* ed 21, vol 1, Philadelphia, 2000, WB Saunders.

Shapiro JR: Heritable disorders of structural proteins, *Kelley's textbook of rheumatology,* ed 6, Philadelphia, 2001, WB Saunders.

AUTHOR: **IRIS TONG, M.D.**

BASIC INFORMATION

DEFINITION

The clinically significant disorders of ejaculation are failure of emission, retrograde ejaculation, premature ejaculation, hematospermia, and anorgasmia. Failure of emission occurs when semen is not propulsed into the urethra during orgasm, resulting in a dry ejaculate. Retrograde ejaculation is a backward flow of semen into the bladder. Premature ejaculation exists when there is an inability to delay ejaculation such that ejaculation occurs sooner than desired, either before or shortly after penetration, causing distress to either one or both partners. Hematospermia is the appearance of blood in the ejaculate. Anorgasmia is the inability to achieve orgasm in a timely manner.

SYNONYMS

Ejaculatory dysfunction
Early or rapid ejaculation
Inhibited ejaculation
Retarded ejaculation

ICD-9CM CODES

608.87	Ejaculation, retrograde
608.82	Hematospermia
306.59	Ejaculation, psychogenic
302.75	Ejaculation, premature
302.74	Orgasm inhibited male (psychosexual)

EPIDEMIOLOGY & DEMOGRAPHICS

Premature ejaculation is the most prevalent male sexual complaint, affecting 20% to 30% of men.

CLINICAL PRESENTATION

- Failure of emission: No ejaculate is expelled either antegrade or retrograde during orgasm. Physical findings may be normal or may reveal nervous system dysfunction (e.g., spinal cord injury); may present with infertility.
- Retrograde ejaculation: Little or no ejaculate is expelled at orgasm. Patients may report cloudy postcoital urine. Physical examination is usually normal; may present with infertility.
- Premature ejaculation: Ejaculation occurs sooner than desired, either before or shortly after penetration. Physical examination is normal. Sexual and psychologic history may be revealing. Patients often incorrectly report erectile dysfunction because they lose the erection after orgasm.
- Hematospermia: Bloody ejaculate, may be associated with pain. Physical findings are usually normal; not associated with malignancy.
- Anorgasmia: Patient is not able to achieve orgasm despite appropriate stimulation.

ETIOLOGY

- Retrograde ejaculation may be caused by anatomic abnormalities of the bladder neck or nerve injury affecting the bladder neck sphincter.
- Either retrograde ejaculation or failure of emission may result from functional abnormalities. These include spinal cord injury, diabetes mellitus, retroperitoneal surgery, transurethral prostate surgery, urethral strictures, alpha-blocker therapy, antipsychotics, multiple sclerosis, peripheral neuropathies, or other neurologic abnormalities.
- The exact etiology of premature ejaculation is unknown, but there is evidence for psychological and biologic contributions.
- Hematospermia may be idiopathic or secondary to infection or inflammation of the genitourinary tract.
- Anorgasmia may be caused by medications, particularly serotonin reuptake inhibitors. Patients with spinal cord injuries may be unable to achieve orgasm. Additional causes include psychogenic factors and dysfunctional sexual techniques.

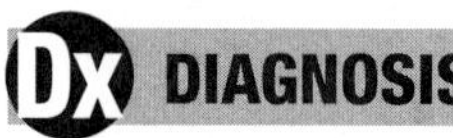

DIAGNOSIS

DIFFERENTIAL DIAGNOSIS

- Erectile dysfunction
- Low seminal fluid volume attributable to hypogonadism or ejaculatory duct obstruction

LABORATORY TESTS

- In the case of a dry or low-volume ejaculate, postejaculate urine should be evaluated for spermatozoa to differentiate failure of emission from retrograde ejaculation.
- A urine analysis in the setting of hematospermia can help rule out hematuria. The presence of hematuria requires a hematuria evaluation.
- A fasting blood glucose test may be considered if diabetes is suspected as a cause of lack of emission or retrograde ejaculation.

IMAGING STUDIES

Transrectal ultrasonography to rule out ejaculatory duct obstruction or absence of the seminal vesicles, if these diagnoses are suspected as a cause of low-volume ejaculate

Rx TREATMENT

NONPHARMACOLOGIC THERAPY

- Retrograde ejaculation and failure of emission do not require treatment unless fertility is desired. Retrograde ejaculation may rarely be converted to antegrade ejaculation if intercourse occurs when the bladder is full. Viable sperm can be recovered from the postejaculate urine and used for intrauterine insemination or in vitro fertilization.
- Premature ejaculation can improve with sex therapy (e.g., "coronal squeeze" or "start-and-stop" technique) and effective partner communication. These approaches may be more effective when combined with pharmacologic therapy.
- Although alarming to the patient, idiopathic hematospermia may be followed expectantly.
- Anorgasmia caused by serotonin reuptake inhibitors usually improves with withdrawal of the medication or change to another medication. Sexual therapy and counseling can improve anorgasmia caused by dysfunctional sexual techniques or psychological issues. Vibratory or electrical stimulation of emission is helpful in selected cases.

ACUTE GENERAL Rx

- Retrograde ejaculation: It is crucial to distinguish between anatomic and functional causes because pharmacologic treatment is likely to be effective only in patients who do not have an anatomic disturbance of the bladder neck. Sympathomimetic medications (phenylpropanolamine, ephedrine, pseudoephedrine) and imipramine may be useful in converting retrograde ejaculation to antegrade ejaculation.
- Failure of emission: May be converted to retrograde ejaculation by oral sympathomimetic therapy.
- Premature ejaculation: Selective serotonin reuptake inhibitors (sertraline, fluoxetine) and clomipramine have shown success in delaying premature ejaculation. Initially, these are taken only on the days of intercourse. If no improvement occurs, they may be taken daily. Topical anesthetics such as lidocaine cream have also been used.

SURGICAL THERAPY

There is currently no role for surgery for ejaculatory disorders.

DISPOSITION

Prognosis varies with etiology. Ejaculatory dysfunction attributable to sexual techniques or psychological issues can improve with therapy and counseling. Pharmacologic treatment may be helpful in certain cases of premature ejaculation.

REFERRAL

All fertility issues and suspected anatomic problems should be referred to a urologist. Professional psychotherapy and sex therapy should be considered for some patients. Endocrine input should be considered for patients with diabetes.

SUGGESTED READINGS

McMahon CG et al: An evidence-based definition of lifelong premature ejaculation: report of the International Society for Sexual Medicine Ad Hoc Committee for the Definition of Premature Ejaculation, *J Sex Med* 5(7):1590-606, 2008.

Ohl DA: Anejaculation and retrograde ejaculation, *Urol Clin North Am* 35(2):211-220, 2008.

Waldinger MD: Premature ejaculation: State of the Art, *Urol Clin N Am* 34:591-599, 2007.

AUTHORS: **AKANKSHA MEHTA, M.D.,** and **MARK SIGMAN, M.D.**

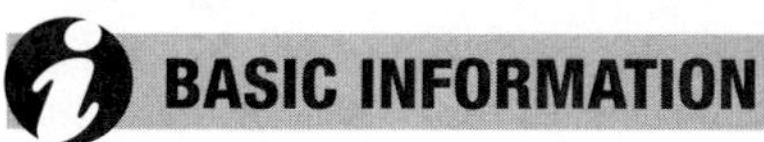

BASIC INFORMATION

DEFINITION

Premature ejaculation is a persistent or recurrent problem in which a male experiences orgasm or ejaculation in the early phases of sexual contact and before he and his partner wish it. Other definitions have emphasized elapsed time after intromission (with durations of 30 sec to several min), number of thrusts, or rate of partner satisfaction. However, no absolute measure is applicable to the diverse numbers of men with this problem.

SYNONYMS

Rapid ejaculation
Early ejaculation
Inadequate ejaculatory control

ICD-9CM CODES
F52.4 Premature ejaculation
(DSM-IV Code 302.75)

EPIDEMIOLOGY & DEMOGRAPHICS

PEAK INCIDENCE: Adolescence and young adulthood

PREVALENCE (IN U.S.):
- 7% to 40% of adult men, most with no underlying physical condition
- Often present more or less since start of sexual life
- Most prevalent sexual disorder in men; more common than low libido and erectile dysfunction

PREDOMINANT AGE: None defined

GENETICS: No identifiable genetic factors

PHYSICAL FINDINGS & CLINICAL PRESENTATION

- Complaint of ejaculation before, upon, or shortly after penetration
- Frequently associated with anxiety related to either sexual activity or more generalized anxiety disorder
- Premature ejaculation caused by a medical condition frequently associated with low desire and/or erectile insufficiency

ETIOLOGY

- Increasingly believed to be a neurobiologic phenomenon particularly related to serotonergic pathway
- Different theoretical frameworks emphasize anxiety related to performance or personal interactions, behavioral concepts of learned expectations related to early experience, or heightened penile sensitivity
- Organic factors are contributory in some individuals (e.g., abdominal or pelvic trauma or surgery, neuropathies, or urologic pathology such as prostatic urethritis)
- Biologic causes include penile hypersensitivity, hyperexcitable ejaculatory reflex, increased sexual arousability, possible endocrinopathy, a genetic predisposition, and central 5-hydroxytryptamine receptor dysfunction

DIAGNOSIS

DIFFERENTIAL DIAGNOSIS

- In as many as 25% of men with complaints of premature ejaculation, partner is anorgasmic
- In young adolescents, premature ejaculation may be normally experienced as a consequence of heightened excitation

WORKUP

- History with a specific emphasis on sexual activities and beliefs
- Factors to be assessed include patient's subjective evaluation, degree of sexual satisfaction, sense of control, and personal or interpersonal distress related to ejaculation
- Collateral information from sexual partner when possible
- Additional history regarding surgery, trauma, and neurologic symptoms
- History of prescribed and recreational drugs (e.g., antidepressants, alcohol, opiates)

LABORATORY TESTS

Urinalysis and urine culture after prostatic massage to rule out prostatic infection

IMAGING STUDIES

None routinely indicated

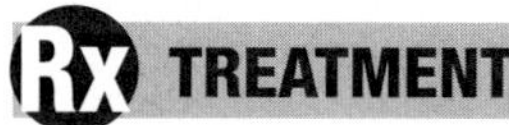

TREATMENT

NONPHARMACOLOGIC THERAPY

- Behavioral and psychotherapeutic interventions: strongly guided by a specific theoretical framework; often inadequate data to suggest the superiority of any particular approach
- Use of condoms may reduce penile sensitivity
- Use of "pause-squeeze" technique (in which 4 sec of moderate pressure is applied to the frenulum to reduce ejaculatory urge) or "stop-start" technique may be helpful for some patients

ACUTE GENERAL Rx

- Topical anesthetic, such as lidocaine-prilocaine cream, increases ejaculatory latency if applied <20 minutes before intercourse.
- Anxiolytics (benzodiazepines) may be useful in individuals with anxiety.
- Daily selective serotonin reuptake inhibitors (SSRIs), such as paroxetine (most potent) or setraline, delay ejaculation. May take several weeks for response to occur. If one SSRI does not work, may try a different SSRI. Clomipramine (tricyclic antidepressant) has also been found to delay orgasm in men. Discontinuation of daily SSRIs often leads to recurrence of premature ejaculation.
- Sildenafil may be superior to antidepressants in delaying ejaculation, especially in premature ejaculation accompanied by erectile dysfunction.

DISPOSITION

There is gradual improvement with age, but it is frequently a chronic, lifelong problem with few spontaneous remissions.

REFERRAL

Behavioral sex therapy or psychotherapy may be helpful; if recurrent prostate infection, referral to urology is indicated.

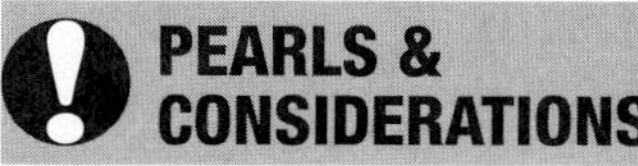

PEARLS & CONSIDERATIONS

Various psychological risk factors are cited for premature ejaculation, including lack of sexual experience, infrequent sexual intercourse, fear, anxiety, social phobia, relationship problems, and a lack of sexual education.

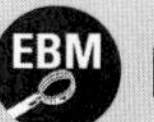

EVIDENCE

Please note: Complete text of EBM for this topic is available online.

Key trials and commentary:
This study sought to evaluate the efficacy and safety of pindolol 7.5 mg/day in delaying of ejaculation in paroxetine-refractory patients. The findings support that a single high dose of pindolol (7.5 mg) is an effective augmentation strategy in paroxetine-refractory patients.

The lack of a widely accepted and approved drug for the management of premature ejaculation (PE) remains a serious deficit in our ability to manage men with this troublesome sexual dysfunction. Selective serotonin reuptake inhibitors (SSRIs) are efficacious but do not work in all cases, and the gains made with their use are often minor. In this study, the 5-hydroxytryptamine $(5\text{-HT})_{1A}$ autoreceptor antagonist pindolol was used to enhance the serotonergic effect of paroxetine. Marked enhancement in intravaginal ejaculatory latency time (IELT) was noted in the pindolol-treated group; this was accompanied by significant increases in sexual satisfaction and intercourse frequency in the pindolol group. Unfortunately, this increase in efficacy came at the cost of significantly higher rates of adverse events, including nausea, headache, dizziness, and mild blood pressure decrease (5 mm Hg). Despite the higher incidence of side effects in the pindolol group, the rate of drug discontinuation was low in both groups. Although the development of a drug specifically designed to treat PE remains a goal, augmentation therapy with a drug such as pindolol may merit further investigation.[1] Ⓐ

Evidence-Based Reference

1. Safarinejad MR: Once-daily high-dose pindolol for paroxetine-refractory premature ejaculation: a double-blind, placebo-controlled and randomized study, *J Clin Psychopharmacol* 28:39-44, 2008. Commentary by A. Shindel, M.D. Ⓐ

SUGGESTED READINGS

Giulano F, Hellstrom WJ: The pharmacological treatment of premature ejaculation, *BJU Int* 102(6):668, 2008.
Patrick DL et al: The Premature Ejaculation Profile: validation of self-reported outcome measures for research and practice, *BJU Int* 103(3):358-364, 2008.

AUTHORS: **CINDY LAI, M.D., NICOLE APPELLE, M.D.,** and **MITCHELL D. FELDMAN, M.D., M.PHIL.**

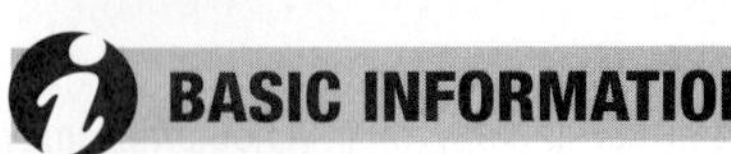

BASIC INFORMATION

DEFINITION

Injuries or wounds that occur as a result of contact with an electrical current.

ICD-9CM CODES
994.8 Electrical shock, nonfatal

EPIDEMIOLOGY & DEMOGRAPHICS

- Causes approximately 1000 deaths annually, with two thirds occurring in persons between ages 15 and 40 yr.
- Most electrical injuries in children occur at home (e.g., oral burns from electrical appliances).
- Most electrical injuries in adults are occupationally related. It ranks fifth as a cause of occupational death.
- Accounts for 4% to 6.5% of all admissions to burn units.
- Lightning strikes kill on average 100 people annually.
    - Eight of every 10 lightning strike victims are male; 75% of lightning deaths in the U.S. occur in the South and Midwest.
    - 25% of lightning deaths are work related.
- Electronic weapons (stun gun and Taser) are capable of causing fatal cardiac arrhythmias.

PHYSICAL FINDINGS & CLINICAL PRESENTATION

- Cognitive changes: depending on the extent of injury, the patient may be unconscious, seizing, or confused and unable to present a history
- Extensive skin burns (>10% of the body surface)
    1. Located over the entry and exit sites (Fig. 1-100)
    2. Most common entry sites are the hands and skull
    3. Most common exit sites are the heels
    4. "Kissing burns" over the flexor creases
    5. Oral burns are common in children; bleeding from the labial artery may present 7 to 10 days after the injury
- Asystole or ventricular fibrillation may be the initial cardiac rhythm
- Bone fractures and periosteal burns
- Compartment syndrome from severe muscle tissue damage
- Headaches, memory disturbances
- Weakness and paresthesias
- Otologic injury, conductive hearing loss from tympanic membrane rupture or ossicular disruption
- Rhabdomyolysis and myoglobin-induced acute tubular necrosis
- Vascular injury from coagulation of small vessels or compartment syndrome

ETIOLOGY

- Electricity causes tissue injury by converting electrical energy into heat or by blunt trauma from being thrown from the electrical source or from continuous muscle contraction (tetany).
- The effects of electricity are determined by seven factors: type of current, amount of current, pathway of current, duration, area of contact, resistance of the body, and voltage.
- Tissue damage is greater with higher voltage and longer duration of contact.
- Direct current (DC) contact causes a single muscle contraction, throwing the patient away from the source. Alternating current (AC) contact precipitates a tetanic contraction, not allowing the patient to withdraw from the source and prolonging the duration of contact. AC contact is more ominous than DC contact.
- Electrical injuries are arbitrarily divided into high-voltage (>1000 volts) and low-voltage (<1000 volts) burns. Low-voltage burns involve almost exclusively either the hands or oral cavity. High-voltage injuries have a wide variety of systemic manifestations.
- The entry and exit path of the electrical current determines which tissues are affected.

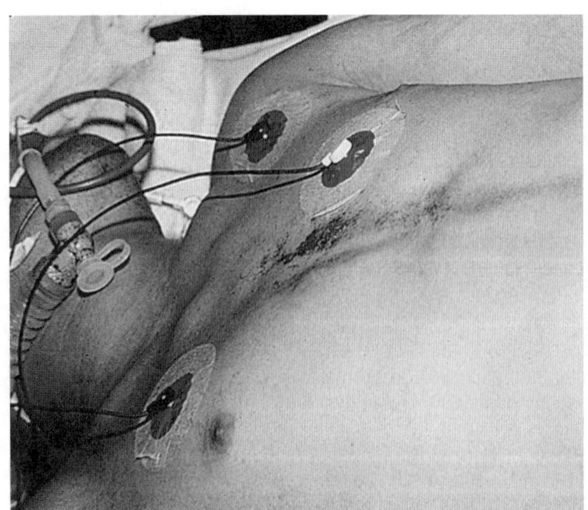

FIGURE 1-100 Linear burns from lightning injury. (From Auerbach P: *Wilderness medicine,* ed 4, St Louis, 2001, Mosby.)

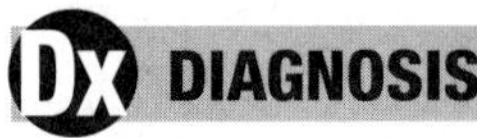

DIAGNOSIS

WORKUP

Physical examination may not reveal the extent of damage that has occurred. Detailed testing to determine the extent of internal organ damage is indicated. In lightning injuries, male victims may have scrotal (on the undersurface of the scrotum) and penile burns, which may often be overlooked. Hemorrhage behind the eardrum with or without perforation is not uncommon. An otoscopic examination is indicated in all lightning strike victims.

LABORATORY TESTS

- Complete blood count
- Blood chemistry profile including electrolytes
- Blood urea nitrogen and creatinine
- Arterial blood gas analysis
- Myoglobin
- Creatinine kinase with isoenzyme fractionation
- Urinalysis, including screening for myoglobinuria
- Liver function tests
- Type and cross-match
- ECG

IMAGING STUDIES

- Radiographs: any suspicious area for bone fractures
- CT scan of the head and cervical spine in patients with suspected head injury, coma, or neurologic deficit

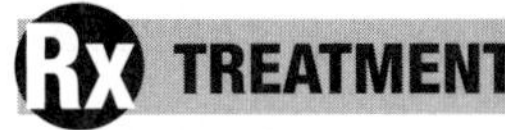

TREATMENT

NONPHARMACOLOGIC THERAPY

- At the scene: ensure the electrical power source of injury is turned off before approaching patients.
- Basic and advanced cardiac life support with cervical spine precautions. Prolonged cardiopulmonary resuscitation should be undertaken regardless of the initial cardiac rhythm.
- Cardiac monitoring.
- Oxygen.
- Tetanus prophylaxis.

ACUTE GENERAL Rx

- IV fluids to maintain urine output of 50 to 100 ml/hr (IV hydration should be reassessed with central nervous system expert in patients at risk of developing cerebral edema).
- Alkalinization of the urine (sodium bicarbonate 50 mEq in 1 L of normal saline) in patients with or at risk of myoglobinuria.
- Furosemide 20 to 40 mg PO or IV and/or mannitol 12.5 g/kg/hr may be used to force diuresis.
- Seizures are treated in the standard fashion.
- Treat burns with sulfadiazine silver dressings.

CHRONIC Rx

- Hospitalization is indicated in patients with high-voltage injuries, extensive burns, central nervous system symptoms, myonecrosis (creatine kinase level more than twice normal, high serum myoglobin levels, or myoglobinuria), new cardiac arrhythmia or ECG changes, or any internal organ damage.
- Ophthalmology consultation at the follow-up to screen for cataract formation (occurs within 1 to 24 mo of a high-voltage electrical injury in 5% to 20% of patients).

DISPOSITION

- Patients with severe burns should be transferred to the regional burn center.
- Complications of electrical injuries include:
  1. Infection
  2. Renal failure from rhabdomyolysis
  3. Seizure disorder
  4. Fasciotomies
  5. Amputation
- Delayed neurologic damage may present as ascending paralysis, amyotrophic lateral sclerosis, or transverse myelitis weeks to years after the injury.
- Vascular damage may also present in a delayed fashion.

REFERRAL

- Referrals to general surgery, burn surgery, trauma surgery, orthopedic surgery, and/or critical care specialists as appropriate in any patient that meets hospitalization criteria. Ophthalmology and ear-nose-throat specialist referral may be indicated.
- Plastic surgery is recommended in children with oral burns.

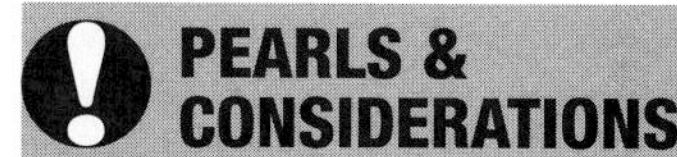

PEARLS & CONSIDERATIONS

COMMENTS

- The size of external skin burns can often underestimate the degree of internal injury.
- Lightning Strike and Electric Shock Survivors International is a support group that serves people from around the world who have sustained an electric injury (http://www.lightning-strike.org).
- Home safety education provided one to one in a clinical setting or at home, especially with the provision of safety equipment, is effective in increasing the range of safety practices.

SUGGESTED READINGS

Bailey B et al: Cardiac monitoring of high-risk patients after an electrical injury: a prospective multicentre study, *Emerg Med J* 24(5):348-352, 2007.

Edlich RF et al: Modern concepts of treatment and prevention of electrical burns, *J Long Term Eff Med Implants* 15(5):511-532, 2005.

Kendrick D et al: Home safety education and provision of safety equipment for injury prevention, *Cochrane Rev* 1:CD005014, 2007.

Spies C, Trohman RG: Narrative review: electrocution and life-threatening electrical injuries, *Ann Intern Med* 145(7):531, 2006.

Zafren K et al: Lightning injuries: prevention and on-site treatment in mountains and remote areas. Official guidelines of the International Commission for Mountain Emergency Medicine and the Medical Commission of the International Mountaineering and Climbing Federation (ICAR and UIAA MEDCOM), *Resuscitation* 65(3):369-372, 2005.

AUTHORS: **ROBERT M. KIRCHNER, M.D.,** and **PAUL GORDON, M.D.**

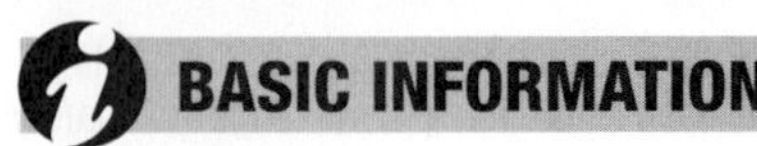

BASIC INFORMATION

DEFINITION

Emergency contraception (EC) can prevent pregnancy soon after unprotected intercourse, sexual assault, or failure or improper use of a birth control method. EC reduces the risk of pregnancy when used up to 120 hr (5 days) after unprotected sex but is more effective if used earlier.

Emergency contraceptive pills (Table 1-23):

- Levonorgestrel EC products:
  - 3 dedicated emergency contraceptive products available in U.S.
  - Women and men age $\geq$17 can purchase EC without a prescription.
  - Women $<$17 require a prescription.
- Combined oral contraceptives:
  - Higher doses of available oral contraceptive pills containing ethinyl estradiol plus levonorgestrel or norgestrel can be used for EC.
- Copper-bearing intrauterine device (IUD):
  - Emergency insertion of the copper-bearing IUD (Paraguard) can be used for EC.

MECHANISM: Current evidence indicates that the primary mechanism of levonorgestrel EC is inhibition or delay of ovulation. Emergency insertion of the copper IUD may prevent fertilization or implantation.

EFFECTIVENESS: Levonorgestrel prevents an estimated 89% of unexpected pregnancies after unprotected intercourse, combined hormonal EC prevents 75%, and the copper IUD prevents 99%.

SYNONYMS

Morning-after pill, postcoital contraception

ICD-9CM CODES

V25.03 Emergency contraceptive counseling and treatment
V25.09 Family planning

EPIDEMIOLOGY & DEMOGRAPHICS

Approximately 49% of all pregnancies and more than 82% of teen pregnancies in the U.S. are unintended. An estimated 1.7 million unintended pregnancies could be prevented annually if emergency contraception use were widespread.

LABORATORY TESTS

- If there is doubt about whether a patient is already pregnant from intercourse that occurred more than 1 wk previously, a pregnancy test may be helpful. However, there is no need for a pregnancy test before administering EC pills. Delays in administration of the medication will reduce its efficacy. The medications in EC pills will not harm an established pregnancy.
- A pregnancy test should be done before insertion of a copper IUD.

TABLE 1-23 Emergency Contraceptive Pills Available in the United States

Emergency Contraception Pills (Levonorgestrel Only)[1]

Brand	Dose	Levonorgestrel per Dose (mg)
Next Choice	2 peach pills	1.5
Plan B	2 white pills	1.5
Plan B One-Step	1 white pill	1.5

Combined Oral Contraceptive Pills for Emergency Contraception[2]

Brand	First Dose	Second Dose (12 hours later)	Ethinyl Estradiol per Dose (mcg)	Levonorgestrel per Dose (mg)
Aviane	5 orange pills	5 orange pills	100	0.50
Cryselle	4 white pills	4 white pills	120	0.60
Enpresse	4 orange pills	4 orange pills	120	0.50
Jolessa	4 pink pills	4 pink pills	120	0.60
Lessina	5 pink pills	5 pink pills	100	0.50
Levora	4 white pills	4 white pills	120	0.60
Lo/Ovral	4 white pills	4 white pills	120	0.60
LoSeasonique	5 orange pills	5 orange pills	100	0.50
Low-Ogestrel	4 white pills	4 white pills	120	0.60
Lutera	5 white pills	5 white pills	100	0.50
Lybrel	6 yellow pills	6 yellow pills	120	0.54
Nordette	4 light-orange pills	4 light-orange pills	120	0.60
Ogestrel	2 white pills	2 white pills	100	0.50
Portia	4 pink pills	4 pink pills	120	0.60
Quasense	4 white pills	4 white pills	120	0.60
Seasonale	4 pink pills	4 pink pills	120	0.60
Seasonique	4 light-blue-green pills	4 light-blue-green pills	120	0.60
Sronyx	5 white pills	5 white pills	100	0.50
Trivora	4 pink pills	4 pink pills	120	0.50

[1]Package instructions for Plan B and Next Choice recommend 1 pill per dose, 12 hours apart, but research shows similar efficacy and side effects with taking both pills at the same time.

[2]For combined oral contraceptive pills as EC, take two doses, 12 hours apart. The FDA has declared these products safe for use as EC.

TREATMENT

ACUTE GENERAL Rx

- Administer EC as soon as possible after unprotected intercourse. EC reduces the risk of pregnancy when used up to 120 hr (5 days) after unprotected intercourse but is more effective if used earlier. NOTE: *Package inserts recommend EC use within 72 hours, but research supports some efficacy up to 120 hours.*
- Use of EC
  1. Levonorgestrel (Plan B, Next Choice, Plan B One-Step)
     - Total dose 1.5 mg levonorgestrel (see Table 1-23)
     - A single dose is equally effective and causes no more side effects than two divided doses.
     - Levonorgestrel EC is preferable to combined estrogen-progestin EC because of greater efficacy and lower incidence of nausea and vomiting.

     NOTE: *For women $<$17 yr, a doctor's prescription is necessary to obtain EC pills.*
  2. Combined oral contraceptive pills:
     - Two doses, 12 hours apart, of 100 to 120 mcg ethinyl estradiol and 0.5 to 0.6 mg levonorgestrel (or 1.0 to 1.2 mg norgestrel) per dose.
     - See Table 1-23 for dosing.
- Side effects:
  - Nausea occurs in 50% of women taking combined estrogen-progestin EC pills, vomiting in 20%. Levonorgestrel EC is associated with approximately half the incidence of nausea and vomiting. Side effects resolve within 1 to 2 days. Antinausea medication such as meclizine 25 mg orally is recommended 1 hr before taking combined EC pills.
- Contraindications:
  - Few contraindications to EC exist other than hypersensitivity to the product. EC pills will not affect an established pregnancy.
  - There are no other evidence-based medical contraindications to the use of EC pills. The benefits of EC in preventing pregnancy generally outweigh the theoretical risks for women with contraindications to long-term use of combined hormonal contraception, such as thromboembolic disease, smoking after age 35, heart disease, or liver disease. Use of progestin-only EC may be preferable to use of combined estrogen-progestin EC for women with any of these conditions or who are breastfeeding. EC is not indicated for breastfeeding

women <6 weeks postpartum as ovulation is extremely unlikely.

- Alternative EC option: copper IUD.
  - Emergency insertion of the copper IUD is highly effective for EC up to 5 days after unprotected intercourse. This option may be preferable for women who desire effective long-term contraception and have no contraindications to IUD insertion. A pregnancy test should be done before IUD insertion.

CHRONIC Rx

Because EC pills are less effective than other forms of contraception, they are not recommended as an ongoing method of contraception. The copper IUD is highly effective for emergency contraception and can be kept in place to prevent pregnancy for 10 years.

DISPOSITION

After using EC, for most women menses will occur within 3 days of the expected onset date. If a woman's next expected menses are delayed by more than 1 wk, a pregnancy test should be done.

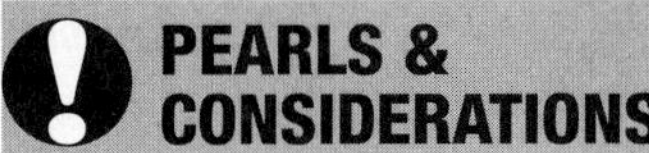

PEARLS & CONSIDERATIONS

COMMENTS

- EC is effective in preventing pregnancy up to 120 hr (5 days) after unprotected intercourse.
- A pregnancy test is not necessary before administering EC pills because the medicines in EC will not harm an existing pregnancy.
- Advanced prescription of EC pills at routine visits may increase timely use of EC and does not decrease the use of more reliable means of contraception.
- Men and women ≥17 can purchase EC pills without a prescription.

PREVENTION

- Patients should begin an effective method of birth control immediately after using EC. Hormonal contraceptives can be started the day after EC is administered. A backup method should be used for 7 days.
- Emergency contraception should be offered to all women after sexual assault.

PATIENT & FAMILY EDUCATION

- Emergency contraception website: http://ec.princeton.edu

SUGGESTED READINGS

Cheng L et al: Interventions for emergency contraception, *Cochrane Database Syst Rev*, 2008.

Stewart F et al: Emergency contraception. In Hatcher R et al (eds): *Contraceptive technology*, New York, 2004, Ardent Media, Inc., pp 279-298.

AUTHORS: **MELISSA NOTHNAGLE, M.D., M.SC.,** and **JENNIFER BUCKLEY, M.D.**

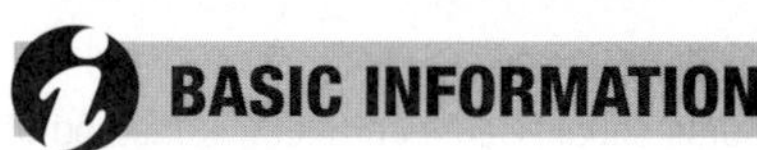

BASIC INFORMATION

DEFINITION

An accumulation of pus in the pleural space, most often caused by bacterial infection.

SYNONYMS

Infected pleuritis
Infected pleural effusion
Purulent pleural effusion

ICD-9CM CODES
510.9 Empyema Lung

EPIDEMIOLOGY & DEMOGRAPHICS

- Empyema most commonly a complication of bacterial pneumonia, especially in association with pneumococcal or anaerobic infection
- Occur as a complication of thoracic surgery
- Penetrating chest trauma
- Bronchopleural fistulae resulting from malignancy or lung biopsy

PHYSICAL FINDINGS & CLINICAL PRESENTATION

- May be abrupt or chronic and insidious depending on the etiologic agent and host factors.
- Typically presents as progressive pleuritic chest pain, persistent fever, and other sustained signs and symptoms of infection.
- In anaerobic empyema, particularly that caused by the actinomycetes, the clinical picture is dominated by systemic symptoms and signs: weight loss, malaise, and low grade fever.
- A slowly enlarging chest wall mass.
- As a complication of thoracic trauma or surgery, empyema typically results from contamination of blood within the pleural space several days following the event.
- The physical findings of empyema are those of pleural effusion. Decreased breath sounds and dullness to percussion over the involved part of the thorax is typical. Systemic signs include fever, tachycardia, leukocytosis, and warmth and erythema over the involved area.

ETIOLOGY

Infection of the lung parenchyma spreading to pleural space caused by

- *Streptococcus pneumoniae*
- *Haemophilus influenzae*
- *Staphylococcus aureus*
- *Legionella species*
- *Mycobacterium tuberculosis*
- *Actinomyces* spp.
- A variety of oral anaerobic bacteria have been cultured in 36% to 37% of empyemas

Dx DIAGNOSIS

DIFFERENTIAL DIAGNOSIS

- Uninfected parapneumonic effusion
- Congestive heart failure
- Malignancy involving the pleura
- Tuberculous pleurisy
- Collagen vascular disease (particularly rheumatoid lung and systemic lupus erythematosus)

LABORATORY TESTS

- Complete blood count; arterial blood gas.
- Blood cultures.
- Pleural fluid analysis in empyema has the characteristics of an exudate with a ratio of pleural fluid to serum protein >0.5 or pleural fluid to serum LDH >0.6. Characteristically, empyema fluid is grossly purulent with visible organisms on Gram stain with glucose <50 mg/dl and pH <7. These findings justify immediate drainage by chest tube or surgery because of the high risk of loculation and progressive systemic infection.

IMAGING STUDIES

- Chest roentgenogram
- Lateral decubitus view to establish the presence of free fluid in the pleural space
- Computed tomography to establish the presence of fluid loculation, underlying mass lesions, and other intrathoracic pathology

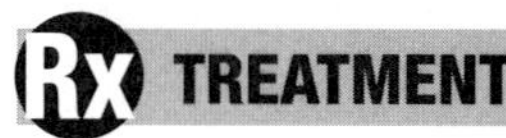

TREATMENT

NONPHARMACOLOGIC THERAPY

Prompt drainage by thoracostomy (chest tube) or open thoracotomy

ACUTE GENERAL Rx

- Maintenance of drainage until infection controlled.
- Antibiotics directed at suspected or proven bacterial or fungal pathogens.
- Thoracoscopy or instillation of thrombolytic agents (streptokinase or urokinase) may be considered in refractory, loculated empyema.

CHRONIC Rx

- If thorough drainage cannot be accomplished, open thoracotomy with pleural decortication may be required.
- Lung function should be monitored following completion of therapy.

DISPOSITION

Hospitalization with supplemental oxygen with ventilatory support if necessary

REFERRAL

Consultation by infectious diseases, pulmonary, or thoracic surgery specialists as needed.

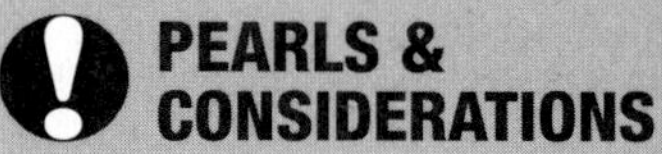

PEARLS & CONSIDERATIONS

COMMENTS

- Empyema caused by actinomycetes may present with erosion through the chest wall and formation of a fistulous tract.
- Nosocomial infection caused by relatively resistant bacterial or fungal pathogens may result in empyema in patients with indwelling thoracostomy tubes.

SUGGESTED READINGS

Jaffe A, Cohen G: Thoracic empyema, *Arch Dis Child* 88(10):839, 2003.

Lardinois D et al: Delayed referral and gram-negative organisms increase the conversion thoracotomy rate in patients undergoing video-assisted thoracoscopic surgery for empyema, *Ann Thorac Surg* 79(6):1851, 2005.

Melloni G et al: Decortication for chronic parapneumonic empyema: results of a prospective study, *World J Surg* 28(5):488, 2004.

Schiza S, Siafakas NM: Clinical presentation and management of empyema, lung abscess and pleural effusion, *Curr Opin Pulm Med* 12(3):205, 2006.

AUTHORS: **GLENN G. FORT, M.D., M.P.H.,** and **DENNIS J. MIKOLICH, M.D.**

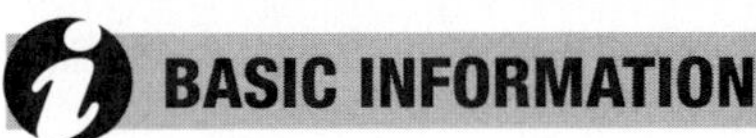

BASIC INFORMATION

DEFINITION

Acute viral encephalitis is an acute febrile syndrome with evidence of meningeal involvement and of derangement of the function of the cerebrum, cerebellum, or brain stem.

SYNONYMS

Arboviral encephalitis
Brain stem encephalitis
Acute necrotizing encephalitis
Rasmussen encephalitis
Encephalitis lethargica

ICD-9CM CODES
049.9 Viral encephalitis, NOS

EPIDEMIOLOGY & DEMOGRAPHICS

INCIDENCE (IN U.S.): About 20,000 cases/yr are reported to the CDC.
PEAK INCIDENCE: Any age
PREVALENCE (IN U.S.): Unknown
PREDOMINANT SEX: Male = female
PREDOMINANT AGE: Any age
GENETICS: No specific genetic or congenital predisposition

ETIOLOGY

- Can be caused by a host of viruses, with herpes simplex the most common virus identified.
- Arboviruses transmitted by mosquitoes include Eastern equine encephalitis, Western equine encephalitis, St. Louis encephalitis, Venezuelan equine encephalitis, California virus encephalitis, Japanese B encephalitis, Murray Valley and West Nile encephalitis. Tick-borne diseases include Russian spring-summer encephalitis, Powassan encephalitis, and other lesser known agents.
- Also implicated: rabies-causing agents, CMV, Epstein-Barr, varicella-zoster, echo virus, mumps, adenovirus, coxsackie, rubeola, and herpes viruses.
- Meningoencephalitis: acute retroviral infection
- In the U.S., the most commonly identified etiologies are herpes simplex virus, West Nile virus, and the enteroviruses.

PHYSICAL FINDINGS & CLINICAL PRESENTATION

- Initially, fever and evidence of meningeal irritation
- Headache and stiff neck
- Later, development of signs of cortical dysfunction: lethargy, coma, stupor, weakness, seizures, facial weakness, as well as brainstem findings
- Cerebellar findings: ataxia, nystagmus, hypotonia, myoclonus, cranial nerve palsies, and abnormal tendon reflexes
- Patients with rabies: hydrophobia, anxiety, facial numbness, psychosis, coma, or dysarthria
- Rarely, movement disorders, such as chorea, hemiballismus, or dystonia
- Recall of a prodromal viral-like illness (this finding is not at all uniform)

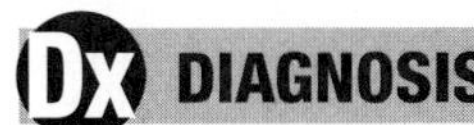

DIAGNOSIS

DIFFERENTIAL DIAGNOSIS

- Bacterial infections: brain abscess, toxic encephalopathies, TB
- Protozoal infections
- Behçet's disease
- Lupus encephalitis
- Sjögren's syndrome
- Multiple sclerosis
- Syphilis
- Cryptococcus
- Toxoplasmosis
- Brucellosis
- Leukemic or lymphomatous meningitis
- Other metastatic tumors
- Lyme disease
- Cat-scratch disease
- Vogt-Koyanagi-Harada syndrome
- Mollaret's meningitis

WORKUP

- Lumbar puncture to reveal pleocytosis, usually lymphocytic, although neutrophils may be seen early on
- Usually, elevated CSF protein
- Normal or low CSF glucose
- In herpes simplex encephalitis: RBCs and xanthochromia
- EEG changes showing periodic high-voltage sharp waves in the temporal regions and slow wave complexes suggestive of herpes encephalitis (Fig. 1-101)
- CT scan and MRI to reveal edema and hemorrhage in the frontal and temporal lobes
- Temporal lobe involvement suggests herpes simplex encephalitis
- Basal ganglia and thalami are areas involved as generally seen in Eastern equine encephalitis
- With West Nile infection, MRI changes have shown changes in basal ganglia, thalami, mesial temporal structures, brainstem, and cerebellum
- Arboviral infections suspected during outbreaks in specific areas
- Rising titers of neutralizing antibodies from the acute to the convalescent stage demonstrated but often not helpful in the acutely ill patient
- Polymerase chain reaction that amplifies DNA from the CSF for herpes simplex encephalitis
- Rarely, brain biopsy to assist in the diagnosis; viral culture of cerebral tissue obtained if biopsy done
- Classic herpetic skin lesions suggestive of herpes encephalitis
- In diagnosing arboviral encephalitis:
  1. Presence of antiviral IgM within the first few days of symptomatic disease; detected and quantified by ELISA
  2. Unusual to recover an arbovirus from the blood or CSF

LABORATORY TESTS

- Aside from the lumbar puncture, most other laboratory studies are nonspecific.
- Skin lesions and urine may be cultured for herpes simplex and CMV.

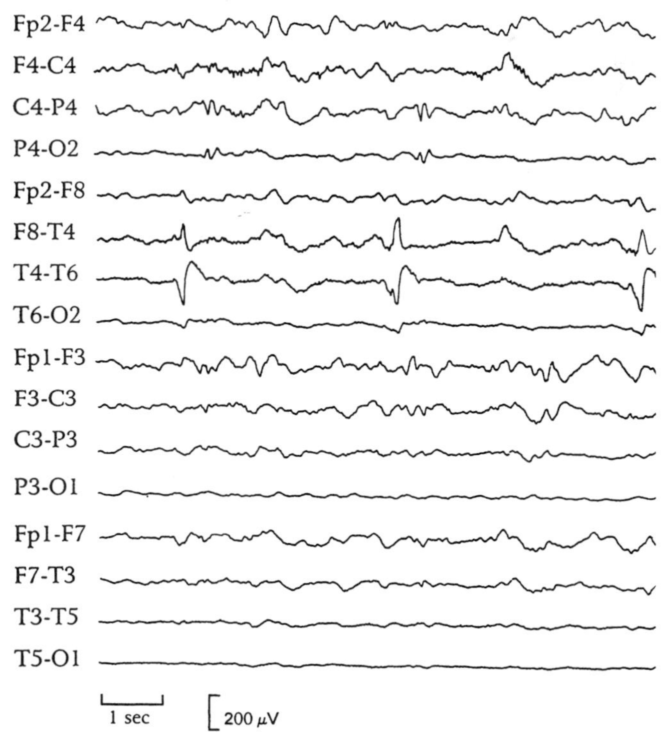

FIGURE 1-101 Repetitive complexes occurring in the right temporal region of a child with herpes simplex encephalitis. (From Goetz CG, Pappert EJ: *Textbook of clinical neurology,* Philadelphia, 1999, Saunders.)

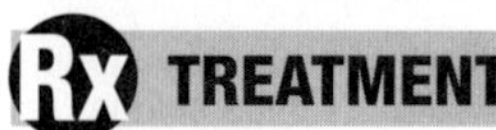

TREATMENT

ACUTE GENERAL Rx

- Supportive care, frequent evaluation, and neurologic examination
- Ventilatory assistance for patients who are moribund or at risk for aspiration
- Avoidance of infusion of hypotonic fluids to minimize the risk of hyponatremia
- For patients who develop seizures: anticonvulsant therapy and follow-up in a critical care setting
- For comatose patients:
  1. Aggressive care to avoid decubitus ulcers, contractures, and DVT
  2. Close attention to weights, input/output, and serum electrolytes
- Acyclovir 30 mg/kg/day IV total dose divided in q8 hour intervals for 14 days for herpes simplex encephalitis
- Short courses of corticosteroids to control brain edema and prevent herniation
- In patients with suspected rabies:
  1. Human rabies immune globulin (HRIG) should be given at a dose of 20 U/kg.
  2. Active immunization may be stimulated by recently developed rabies vaccine, which is grown on a human diploid cell line (HDCV) and has reduced the number of doses needed to five.
  3. If suspect animal is a dog or cat and can be found, observe closely for 10 days to detect rabid behavior; any significant illness in the animal should promptly initiate humane sacrifice of the animal with the brain submitted to local or state health departments for pathology and immunologic testing for rabies. Any wild animal suspected of rabies should be humanely sacrificed, if possible, and submitted for rabies testing immediately.
  4. If signs are seen, animal should be euthanized and its brain examined for signs of rabies.
- No specific pharmacologic therapy for most other viral pathogens

CHRONIC Rx

Some patients may develop permanent neurologic sequelae; these patients will benefit from intensive rehabilitation programs, including physical, occupational, and speech therapy.

DISPOSITION

- Patients with suspected encephalitis of any cause should generally be admitted for initial diagnostic workup and specific treatment (if available).
- Long-term management of patients with significant neurologic sequelae from encephalitis (e.g., memory defects, depression, difficulty with organization of thoughts, movement disorders) may benefit from rehabilitation services, home care, or nursing home placement.

REFERRAL

- To a neurologist for initial workup and management
- To an infectious disease specialist for diagnostic and therapeutic plan
- To a rehabilitation service for long-term evaluation and convalescent services

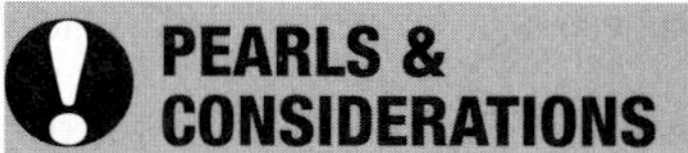

PEARLS & CONSIDERATIONS

- West Nile virus encephalitis occurs primarily in elderly patients >65 years of age.
- Rabies may occur months after contact with the rabid animal, and the exposure (especially bat rabies) may have been seemingly insignificant and even inapparent.
- Experimental therapies are worthy of consideration for some forms of viral encephalitis (e.g., immune plasma, ribavirin, interferons), and expert consultation should be obtained early on for possible treatment interventions with promising experimental therapies.

SUGGESTED READINGS

Beckwith WH et al: Isolation of eastern equine encephalitis virus and West Nile virus from crows during increased arbovirus surveillance in Connecticut, 2000, *Am J Trop Med Hyg* 66(4):422, 2002.

De Tiege X et al: Postinfectious immune-mediated encephalitis after pediatric herpes simplex encephalitis, *Brain Dev* 27(4):304-307, 2005.

Frenkel LM: Challenges in the diagnosis and management of neonatal herpes simplex virus encephalitis, *Pediatrics* 115(3):795-797, 2005.

Kennedy PG: Viral encephalitis, *J Neurol* 252(3):268, 2005.

Roos KL: Fatal encephalitis due to rabies virus transmitted by organ transplantation, *Arch Neurol* 62(6): 855-856, 2005.

Sellal F, Stoll-Keller F: Rabies: ancient yet contemporary cause of encephalitis, *Lancet* 365(9463):921-923, 2005.

Steiner I et al: Viral encephalitis: a review of diagnostic methods and guidelines for management, *Eur J Neurol* 12(5):331-343, 2005.

Tunkel AR et al: The management of encephalitis: Clinical Practice Guidelines by the Infectious Diseases Society of America, *CID* 47, 2008.

AUTHORS: **GLENN G. FORT, M.D., M.P.H.,** and **DENNIS J. MIKOLICH, M.D.**

BASIC INFORMATION

DEFINITION

Encephalopathy is a clinical syndrome of global cognitive impairment characterized by impaired arousal, inattention, and disorientation.

SYNONYMS

Delirium, acute confusional state

ICD-9CM CODES

348.3 Encephalopathy, NOS
348.30 Encephalopathy, unspecified
348.31 Encephalopathy, metabolic
348.39 Encephalopathy, other
349.82 Encephalopathy, toxic

EPIDEMIOLOGY & DEMOGRAPHICS

POINT PREVALENCE: 1.1% of adults in the general population >55 yr, 10% to 40% of hospitalized elderly, and 60% of nursing home patients >75 yr; 100,000 to 200,000 cases annually with anoxic encephalopathy

RISK FACTORS: Age, cancer, AIDS, terminal illness, bone marrow transplant, surgery

PHYSICAL FINDINGS & CLINICAL PRESENTATION

- The essential feature of encephalopathy is the patient's inability to maintain a coherent stream of thought or action.
- The history may often suggest a waxing and waning of the level of arousal and general cognitive ability.
- Because toxins and metabolic disturbances are common causes of encephalopathy, the history should focus on exposure to toxins (especially medications) and symptoms suggesting a concurrent illness such as a urinary tract infection or pneumonia.
- Common to all encephalopathies is a fluctuating level of arousal, poor attention, and disorientation.
- Some patients may appear agitated and others lethargic.
- Delusions (fixed false beliefs) and hallucinations are common.
- Asterixis (negative myoclonus) is extremely common.
- Other physical findings may vary depending on the underlying cause of encephalopathy, such as fever, ascites, jaundice, or tachycardia.

ETIOLOGY

- The final common pathway of all causes of encephalopathy is widespread cortical and subcortical neuronal dysfunction. The causes may be structural or functional.
- Many conditions are reversible and carry a good prognosis if treated in a timely manner.
- Organ failure (e.g., hepatic encephalopathy, hypoxia, hypercapnia, uremia).
- Infection: systemic (e.g., urinary tract, pneumonia) or involving the central nervous system (e.g., meningitis, encephalitis).
- Toxin ingestion or withdrawal (e.g., alcohol, medications, recreational drugs).
- Metabolic disturbances: hyperosmolar states, hypernatremia, hyponatremia, hyperglycemia, hypoglycemia, hypercalcemia, hypophosphatemia, acidosis, alkalosis, inborn errors of metabolism.
- Endocrinopathy: hyperthyroidism, hypothyroidism, Cushing's syndrome, adrenal insufficiency, pituitary failure.
- Neoplasm: tumors of the central nervous system, primary or metastatic. Also effect of distant tumors (e.g., paraneoplastic limbic encephalitis).
- Nutritional deficiency, mostly in alcoholics and chronically ill patients, such as vitamin B_1 deficiency (Wernicke's encephalopathy).
- Seizures: postictal state, nonconvulsive status epilepticus, complex partial seizures, absence seizures.
- Trauma: concussion, contusion, subdural hematoma, epidural hematoma, diffuse axonal injury.
- Vascular: both ischemic and hemorrhagic strokes, vasculitis, venous thrombosis.
- Postanoxic encephalopathy.
- Other: hypertensive encephalopathy, postoperative status, sleep deprivation.

Dx DIAGNOSIS

DIFFERENTIAL DIAGNOSIS

- Dementia: distinguished from encephalopathy by a history of slowly progressive cognitive decline over time (fluctuating cognitive function is rare except in diffuse Lewy body disease).
- Hypersomnia.
- Aphasia: distinguished from encephalopathy by virtue of it representing a specific disorder of language rather than a global disturbance of cognitive function.
- Depression.
- Psychosis: some overlap with encephalopathy because delusions and hallucinations may be common to both.
- Mania.
- Vegetative state from cerebral injury; these patients appear awake (eyes are open) but there is no content to their consciousness.
- Akinetic mutism: these patients do not talk and do not move; there is little fluctuation in their state and there is no asterixis.
- Locked-in syndrome: may be distinguished from encephalopathy by the presence of fixed neurologic deficits (e.g., paralysis of all four limbs).

WORKUP

- Electroencephalography is helpful to confirm the presence of encephalopathy (diffuse slowing) and also to exclude nonconvulsive seizures.
- Chest radiograph to rule out pneumonia.

LABORATORY TESTS

- General chemistry: electrolytes, glucose, creatinine, ammonia, blood urea nitrogen, transaminases, amylase, lipase
- Arterial blood gases
- Complete blood count
- Drug screen and alcohol level (must order ethylene glycol separately if suspected)
- Lumbar puncture if meningitis, encephalitis, or subarachnoid hemorrhage with negative imaging is suspected
- HIV testing
- Endocrine testing: cortisol level, thyroid function test
- Urinalysis and microscopy

IMAGING STUDIES

- CT to rule out bleeding, hydrocephalus, tumors
- MRI with diffusion-weighted images for suspected encephalitis, tumors, and acute strokes
- Magnetic resonance angiography/venography for strokes, arterial dissection, venous thrombosis
- Conventional angiography for central nervous system (CNS) vasculitis and aneurysms

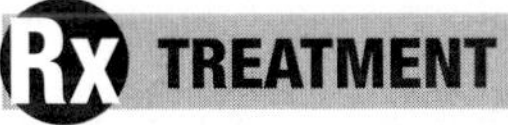

NONPHARMACOLOGIC THERAPY

The best approach is to treat the underlying toxic or metabolic disturbance. The encephalopathy itself is a symptom of these underlying problems. In general, it is best to avoid treating the symptom of encephalopathy with antipsychotics or sedatives.

GENERAL Rx

- Glucose if hypoglycemia
- Antibiotics in cases of infections (choice of an agent with good CNS penetration in cases of primary CNS infections)
- Insulin in hyperglycemic conditions (e.g., diabetic ketoacidosis, hyperosmolar nonketosis, and sepsis)
- Lactulose in hepatic encephalopathy
- Thiamine (vitamin B_1) and folate replacement when deficiency is suspected
- Anticonvulsants if seizures likely
- Librium or diazepam for delirium tremens (alcohol withdrawal)
- Ensure hemodynamic stability (blood pressure and heart rate)

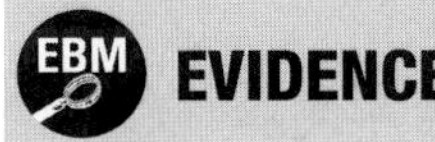

Please note: Complete text of EBM for this topic is available online.

AUTHOR: **ACHRAF A. MAKKI, M.D., M.SC.**

Encopresis (PTG)

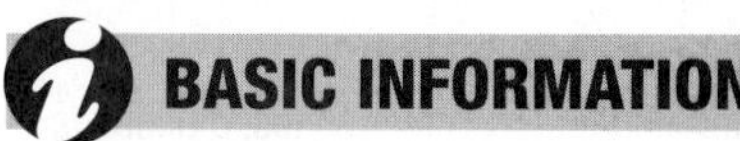

BASIC INFORMATION

DEFINITION

Encopresis is the voluntary or involuntary passage of stool in inappropriate places, in children over the developmental age of 4 yr, with the absence of direct physiologic causes. Occurs at least once per month for at least 3 months.

SYNONYMS

Functional incontinence of stool

ICD-9CM CODES
787.6 Incontinence of feces
307.7 Encopresis

EPIDEMIOLOGY & DEMOGRAPHICS

PEAK INCIDENCE: 4 to 5 yr of age
PREVALANCE (IN U.S.): 1% to 1.5% of children ages 5 to 8 yr
PREDOMINANT SEX: Occurs in males more often than females (4:1)
PREDOMINANT AGE: 4 to 9 yr
GENETICS: Factors that contribute to slow gut motility may predispose to encopresis.

PHYSICAL FINDINGS & CLINICAL PRESENTATION

- Most children attain fecal continence by the age of 4 yr. In primary encopresis continence is never fully established, whereas in secondary encopresis incontinence is preceded by a year or more of continence.
- In secondary encopresis, constipation is generally severe, causing an overflow incontinence in which soft or liquid stool flows around the retained feces, often several times per day.
- When constipation and overflow incontinence are causative, defecation is usually uncomfortable or painful, so patient avoids defecation with consequent stool retention.
- Stool is usually poorly formed and leakage is continuous (occurring during sleep and wakefulness).
- Encopresis resolves when the constipation is resolved.
- In primary encopresis, stool is more likely to be normal in character.
- Soiling is intermittent and usually in a prominent location.
- Coexisting oppositional-defiant or conduct disorders are frequent.

ETIOLOGY

- Children with encopresis exhibit abnormal anorectal dynamics.
- Primary encopresis may be related to developmental delay of sphincter control, whereas secondary encopresis develops in the setting of constipation.
- Approximately 96% of children will have bowel movements between three times daily to once every other day. When bowel movements are less frequent, stool becomes drier and harder and much more uncomfortable to pass. Children may avoid the discomfort by avoiding elimination, but this only results in worsening constipation. Soiling results from more liquid stool that leaks around the main stool mass.
- Constipation may begin gradually as a result of a slow decrease in elimination frequency or more acutely after an illness, dehydration, or prolonged bed rest.
- In encopresis without constipation and overflow incontinence, soiling is often intentional. This may occur in the setting of oppositional-defiant disorder or conduct disorder.
- Harsh or inconsistent toilet training and resultant anxiety may lead to retention of stool, constipation, and eventually encopresis.

Dx DIAGNOSIS

DIFFERENTIAL DIAGNOSIS

- Hirschsprung's disease
- Endocrine disease (hypothyroidism)
- Cerebral palsy
- Myelomeningocele
- Pseudoobstruction
- Anorectal lesions (rectal stenosis)
- Malformations
- Trauma
- Rectal prolapse
- Hypothyroidism
- Medications

WORKUP

- History: pay particular attention to frequency of elimination, character of the stool, associated pain, and presence of enuresis (with which it is frequently associated).
- Evaluate child for other developmental or psychiatric problems.
- Physical examination: pay particular attention to the abdomen, anus, rectum, and saddle sensation.

LABORATORY TESTS

Consider thyroid function tests, electrolytes, calcium, urinalysis, and culture.

IMAGING STUDIES

- Abdominal imaging to determine extent of obstruction or megacolon
- Anorectal manometric studies to determine sphincter function if Hirschsprung's disease is suspected

Rx TREATMENT

NONPHARMACOLOGIC THERAPY

- Behavioral and/or individual psychotherapy and family therapy
- Biofeedback advocated by some to improve sphincter function

ACUTE GENERAL Rx

- In secondary encopresis, disimpaction with hypertonic phosphate (30 ml/5 kg body weight) or isotonic saline enemas
- Resistant cases: repeated instillation of 200 to 600 ml of milk of magnesia enemas
- If child does not permit enemas: oral disimpaction with large doses of mineral oil or lactulose until stool mass is cleared (NOTE: this is frequently more painful and more uncomfortable than an enema)

CHRONIC Rx

- Prevent recurrence of constipation by increased dietary fiber and bulk agents and the use of laxatives (Senokot) and stool softeners (Colace).
- In immediate postdisimpaction period (3 mo after acute treatment) laxatives are needed because bowel tone remains low.
- In primary encopresis, continue with nonpunitive toilet training and encourage regular toilet times (the latter is also helpful in secondary encopresis).

DISPOSITION

In most cases encopresis is self-limited and of relatively brief duration.

REFERRAL

If patient is resistant to treatment, complicated family factors are involved, or encopresis is purposeful.

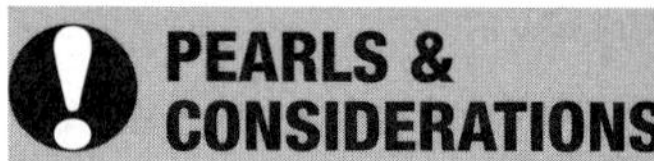

PEARLS & CONSIDERATIONS

It is important to educate parents and children regarding the nature of the problem and to defuse hostile or negative interactions between them.

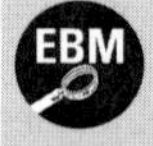

EVIDENCE

A systematic review of the use and efficacy of stimulant laxatives for constipation and soiling in children found insufficient evidence that met the selection criteria.[1] Ⓐ

A systematic review found some evidence that behavioral intervention plus laxative therapy, rather than behavioral therapy or laxative therapy alone, improves continence in children with primary and secondary encopresis. There was no evidence that biofeedback adds any benefit to conventional management of encopresis and constipation in children.[1] Ⓐ

Evidence-Based References

1. Price KJ, Elliott TM: Stimulant laxatives for constipation and soiling in children, *Cochrane Database Rev* (3), 2001. Ⓐ

2. Brazelli M, Griffiths P: Behavioural and cognitive interventions with or without other treatments for defaecation disorders in children, *Cochrane Database Rev* (4), 2001. Ⓐ

SUGGESTED READINGS

Culbert TP, Banez GA: Integrative approaches to childhood constipation and encopresis, *Pediatr Clin North Am* 54(6):927,2007.

Levitt M, Peña A: Update on pediatric faecal incontinence, *Eur J Pediatr Surg* 19(1):1-9, 2009.

AUTHOR: **MITCHELL D. FELDMAN, M.D., M.PHIL.**

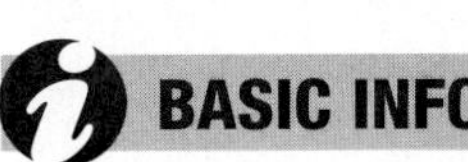

BASIC INFORMATION

DEFINITION

Infective endocarditis is an infection of the endocardial surface of the heart or mural endocardium.

ACUTE ENDOCARDITIS: Usually caused by *Staphylococcus aureus, Streptococcus pyogenes, Streptococcus pneumoniae,* and *Neisseria* organisms; classic clinical presentation of high fever, positive blood cultures, vascular and immunologic phenomenon

SUBACUTE ENDOCARDITIS: Usually caused by viridans streptococci in the presence of valvular pathology; less toxic, often indolent presentation with lower fevers, night sweats, fatigue

ENDOCARDITIS IN INJECTION DRUG USERS: Often involving *S. aureus* or *Pseudomonas aeruginosa* with variation that may be geographically influenced; tricuspid (Fig. 1-102) or multiple valvular involvement; high mortality rate of 50% to 60%

PROSTHETIC VALVE ENDOCARDITIS (EARLY): Usually caused by *S. aureus* (leading cause of PVE) within 2 mo of valve replacement; other organisms include *S. epidermis,* gram-negative bacilli, diphtheroids, *Candida* organisms

PROSTHETIC VALVE ENDOCARDITIS (LATE): Typically develops >60 days after valvular replacement; involved organisms similar to early prosthetic valve endocarditis, including viridans streptococci, enterococci, and group D streptococci

NOSOCOMIAL ENDOCARDITIS: Secondary to intravenous catheters, TPN lines, pacemakers; coagulase-negative staphylococci, *S. aureus,* and streptococci most common

Non-HACEK gram-negative bacillus endocarditis is not primarily a disease of injection drug users. More than half of all cases are associated with health care contact

SYNONYMS

Bacterial endocarditis
Subacute bacterial endocarditis (SBE)
Endocarditis

ICD-9CM CODES

421.0 Infective endocarditis
996.61 Prosthetic valve endocarditis

EPIDEMIOLOGY & DEMOGRAPHICS

INCIDENCE (IN U.S.): 1.7 to 3.8 cases/100,000 persons/yr
PEAK INCIDENCE: Females: often <35 yr old; males: 45 to 65 yr old
NOSOCOMIAL ENDOCARDITIS: 14% to 28% of cases
PREVALENCE (IN U.S.): 0.3 to 3 cases/1000 hospital admissions
PREDOMINANT SEX: Male > female
PREDOMINANT AGE: 45 to 65 yr

PHYSICAL FINDINGS & CLINICAL PRESENTATION

- Fever may be variable in presentation; may be high, hectic, or absent.
- Fever, chills, fatigue, and rigors occur in 25% to 80% of patients.
- Heart murmur may be absent in right-sided endocarditis.
- Embolic phenomenon with peripheral manifestations is found in 50% of patients.
- Skin manifestations include petechiae, Osler nodes, splinter hemorrhages, Janeway lesions.
- Splenomegaly is more common with subacute course.

ETIOLOGY

Streptococcal and staphylococcal infections are the most common causes of infective endocarditis. Variation in incidence may occur that is influenced by the patient's risk for developing infection.

ACUTE ENDOCARDITIS:
- *S. aureus*
- *Streptococcus pneumoniae*
- Streptococcal species and groups A through G
- *Haemophilus influenzae*

SUBACUTE ENDOCARDITIS:
- Viridans streptococci (alpha-hemolytic)
- *S. bovis*
- Enterococci
- *S. aureus*

ENDOCARDITIS IN INJECTION DRUG USERS:
- *S. aureus*
- *P. aeruginosa*
- *Candida* species
- Enterococci

PROSTHETIC VALVE ENDOCARDITIS (EARLY):
- *S. epidermidis*
- *S. aureus*
- Gram-negative bacilli
- Group D streptococci

PROSTHETIC VALVE ENDOCARDITIS (LATE):
- *S. epidermidis*
- Viridans streptococci
- *S. aureus*
- Enterococci and group D streptococci

NOSOCOMIAL ENDOCARDITIS:
- Coagulase-negative staphylococci
- *S. aureus*
- Streptococci: viridans, group B, enterococcus

HACEK ORGANISMS:
- Fastidious gram-negative bacilli
- *Haemophilus parainfluenzae*
- *Haemophilus aphrophilus*
- *Actinobacillus actinomycetemcomitans*
- *Cardiobacterium hominis*
- *Eikenella corrodens*
- *Kingella kingae*

RISK FACTORS

- Poor dental hygiene
- Long-term hemodialysis
- Diabetes mellitus
- HIV infection
- Mitral valve prolapse

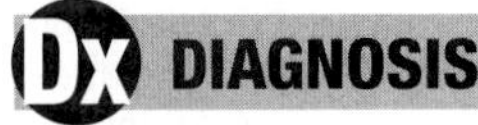

DIAGNOSIS

DIFFERENTIAL DIAGNOSIS

- Brain abscess
- FUO
- Pericarditis
- Meningitis
- Rheumatic fever
- Osteomyelitis
- Salmonella
- TB
- Bacteremia
- Pericarditis
- Glomerulonephritis

WORKUP

Physical examination to evaluate for the previous physical findings followed by laboratory testing (see "Laboratory Tests")

LABORATORY TESTS

- Blood cultures: three sets in first 24 hr
- More culturing if patient has received prior antibiotic
- CBC (anemia possibly present, subacute)
- WBC (leukocytosis is higher in acute endocarditis)
- ESR and C-reactive protein (elevated)
- Positive rheumatoid factor (subacute endocarditis)
- False-positive VDRL
- Proteinuria, hematuria, RBC casts
- Electrocardiogram: look for cardiac conduction abnormalities, injury pattern, or evidence of pericarditis—any such new findings are suggestive of myocardial abscess.

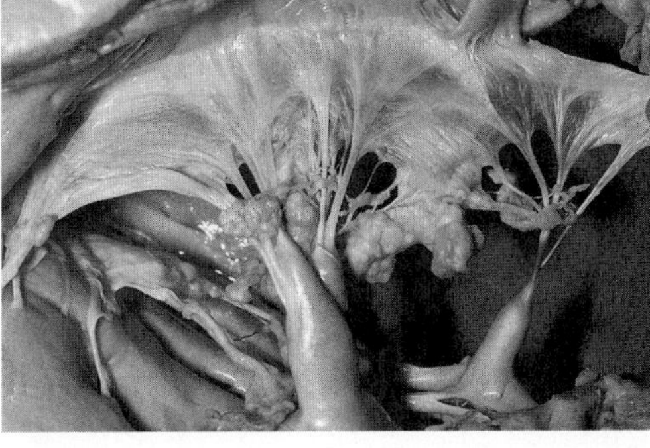

FIGURE 1-102 Tricuspid valve endocarditis. There are large vegetations on the leaflets and the chordae tendineae. (From Crawford MH et al (eds): *Cardiology,* ed 2, St Louis, 2004, Mosby.)

IMAGING STUDIES

- Echocardiogram: two-dimensional
- Transesophageal echocardiography (TEE): more sensitive in detecting vegetations if two dimensional is negative, especially helpful with prosthetic valves or in detecting perivalvular disease

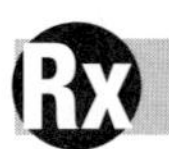

TREATMENT

Initial IV antibiotic therapy (before culture results) is aimed at the most likely organism:

- In patients with prosthetic valves or patients with native valves who are allergic to penicillin: vancomycin (1 g IV every 12 hr for 4 wk) plus rifampin 600 mg PO daily and gentamicin (1mg/kg IV every 8 hr for 2 wk)—assuming normal renal function in adult patients.
- In IV drug users: nafcillin or oxacillin (2 g IV every 4 hr) plus gentamicin (1 mg/kg every 8 hr for 3 to 5 days until blood cultures are negative); if MRSA, vancomycin (1 g IV every 12 hr for 4 wk) plus gentamicin (1 mg/kg every 8 hr for 3 to 5 days until blood cultures are negative).
- In native valve endocarditis with a penicillin-susceptible streptococcal isolate: combination of penicillin (18 to 24 million units/day IV for 4 wk) and gentamicin (1 mg/kg every 8 hr for 2 wk) assuming normal renal function. Extend the gentamicin therapy for 4 wk if a relatively penicillin-resistant strain of streptococcus is isolated (penicillin MIC $>$0.5 microgram/ml); a penicillinase-resistant penicillin (oxacillin or nafcillin—2 g IV every 4 hr for 4 to 6 wk plus gentamicin 1mg/kg IV every 8 hr for 3 to 5 days) can be used if acute bacterial endocarditis is present or if *S. aureus* is suspected as one of the possible causative organisms; for HACEK organisms, treat with third-generation cephalosporin (ceftriaxone—2 g IV every 24 hr for 4 to 6 wk).
- Ceftriaxone: 2 g IV every 24 hr and an aminoglycoside (e.g., gentamicin 1 mg/kg IV every 8 hr for 2 wk) effective for *Streptococcus viridans* endocarditis.
- Daptomycin (6 mg/kg/day for 4 to 6 wk) has recently been approved for use in *S. aureus* bacteremia and right-sided endocarditis; may prove useful in MRSA infections.

Antibiotic therapy after identification of the organism should be guided by susceptibility testing—preferably by formal testing by MIC (minimum inhibitory testing).

DISPOSITION

- The patient may need outpatient IV antibiotic therapy, and arrangements need to be made to ensure safe vascular access and continuity of care with outpatient IV therapy team.
- Long-term follow-up is essential after therapy has ended; relapse of endocarditis may occur.
- Prophylaxis with antibiotics will be needed before dental procedures as a previous episode of endocarditis increases the risk of recurrent endocarditis associated with transient bacteremia from dental procedures.

REFERRAL

- To an infectious disease specialist for an optimal antibiotic regimen
- To a cardiologist or a cardiac surgeon if evidence of heart failure, refractory infection, myocardial abscess, valve disruption, or major embolic events occur
- To a dentist or oral surgeon if dental work needs to be conducted with appropriate use of prophylactic antibiotics to prevent recurrent endocarditis

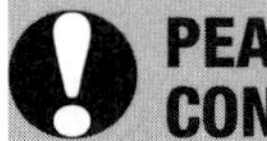

PEARLS & CONSIDERATIONS

COMMENTS

For endocarditis prophylaxis refer to Section V.

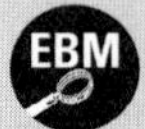

EVIDENCE

There is a lack of randomized trials that have evaluated the use of specific agents in the treatment of infective endocarditis. The rationale for their use in specific situations, as described in the sections above, is based upon clinical consensus and expert recommendations.[1,2] Ⓒ

Evidence-Based References

1. Baddour LM et al; Committee on Rheumatic Fever, Endocarditis, and Kawasaki Disease; Council on Cardiovascular Disease in the Young; Councils on Clinical Cardiology, Stroke, and Cardiovascular Surgery and Anesthesia; American Heart Association; Infectious Diseases Society of America: Infective endocarditis: diagnosis, antimicrobial therapy, and management of complications: a statement for healthcare professionals from the Committee on Rheumatic Fever, Endocarditis, and Kawasaki Disease, Council on Cardiovascular Disease in the Young, and the Councils on Clinical Cardiology, Stroke, and Cardiovascular Surgery and Anesthesia, American Heart Association: endorsed by the Infectious Diseases Society of America, *Circulation* 11(23):e394-434, 2005.
2. Wilson W et al: Prevention of Infective Endocarditis. Guidelines from the American Heart Association. A guideline from the American Heart Association Rheumatic Fever, Endocarditis, and Kawasaki Disease Committee, Council on Cardiovascular Disease in the Young, and the Council on Clinical Cardiology, Council on Cardiovascular Surgery and Anesthesia, and the Quality of Care and Outcomes Research Interdisciplinary Working Group, *Circulation* 116(5): 1736-1754, 2007.

SUGGESTED READINGS

Cecchi E et al: Are the Duke criteria really useful for the early bedside diagnosis of infective endocarditis? Results of a prospective multicenter trial, *Ital Heart J* 6(1):41-48, 2005.

Cha R, Brown WJ, Rybak MJ: Bactericidal activities of daptomycin, quinupristin-dalfopristin, and linezolid against vancomycin-resistant *Staphylococcus aureus* in an in vitro pharmacodynamic model with simulated endocardial vegetations, *Antimicrob Agents Chemother* 47(12):3960-3963, 2003.

Fowler VG et al: Daptomycin versus standard therapy for bacteremia and endocarditis caused by *Staphylococcus aureus*, *N Engl J Med* 355(7):653, 2006.

McDonald JR et al: Enterococcal endocarditis: 107 cases from the international collaboration on endocarditis merged database, *Am J Med* 118(7):759, 2005.

Morpeth S et al: Non-HACEK gram-negative bacillus endocarditis, *Ann Intern Med* 147:829-835, 2007.

Morris AJ et al: Gram stain, culture, and histopathological examination findings for heart valves removed because of infective endocarditis, *Clin Infect Dis* 36(6):697-704, 2003.

Patrick T et al: Complexity and subtlety of infective endocarditis, *Mayo Clin Pro* 82(5):615-621, 2007.

Wang A et al: Contemporary clinical profile and outcome of prosthetic valve endocarditis, *JAMA* 297:1354-1361, 2007.

AUTHORS: **GLENN G. FORT, M.D., M.P.H.,** and **DENNIS J. MIKOLICH, M.D.**

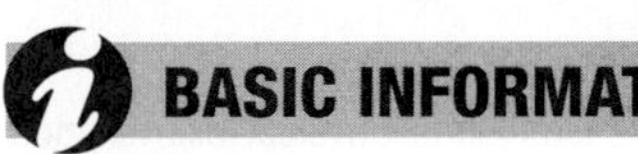

BASIC INFORMATION

DEFINITION

Endometrial cancer (EC) is a malignant transformation of endometrial stroma and/or glands typified by irregular nuclear membranes, nuclear atypia, mitotic activity, loss of glandular pattern, and irregular cell size (Fig. 1-103). The two main histologic subcategories of EC, endometrioid and nonendometrioid EC, show unique molecular aberrations and differing clinical behaviors.

SYNONYMS

Uterine cancer (some forms)
EC

ICD-9CM CODES
182 Malignant neoplasm of body of uterus

EPIDEMIOLOGY & DEMOGRAPHICS

INCIDENCE: 21.2 cases per 100,000 persons; approximately 30,000 new cases annually. It is the most common gynecologic malignancy in the U.S.

PREDOMINANCE: Median age at onset: 60 yr; only 5% occur in women <40 yr

RISK FACTORS: Obesity, diabetes, nulliparity, early menarche and late menopause, unopposed estrogen therapy, tamoxifen use, endometrial atypical hyperplasia

PHYSICAL FINDINGS & CLINICAL PRESENTATION

- Abnormal uterine bleeding or postmenopausal bleeding in 90%
- Pyometra or hematometra
- Abnormal Pap smear

ETIOLOGY

Endogenous or exogenous chronic unopposed estrogen stimulation of the endometrium

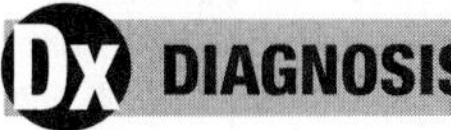

DIAGNOSIS

DIFFERENTIAL DIAGNOSIS

- Atypical hyperplasia
- Other genital tract malignancy
- Polyps
- Atrophic vaginitis
- Granuloma cell tumor
- Fibroid uterus

WORKUP

- Complete history and physical examination
- Endometrial biopsy or dilation and curettage
- Assessment of operative risk

LABORATORY TESTS

- Complete blood count
- Chemistry profile including liver function tests
- Consider CA-125 level

IMAGING STUDIES

- Chest x-ray examination
- CT scan, and/or pelvic ultrasound
- Endovaginal ultrasound in postmenopausal women with vaginal bleeding

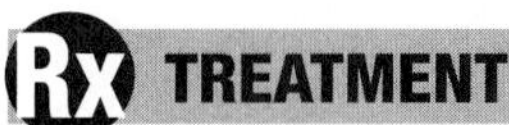

TREATMENT

NONPHARMACOLOGIC THERAPY

- Surgery is the mainstay of treatment, with or without radiation, depending on tumor stage and grade.
- Surgery consists of pelvic washings, total abdominal hysterectomy and bilateral salpingo-oophorectomy, omental biopsy, and selective pelvic and periaortic lymphadenectomy, depending on stage and grade.
- Brachytherapy and/or teletherapy are added in an advanced stage.
- Chemotherapy (cisplatin, Adriamycin) or tamoxifen may also be used.
- Hormonal therapy is an option for some young women with EC who wish to preserve fertility.

ACUTE GENERAL Rx

- A thorough workup should be completed before any therapy for endometrial cancer.
- Surgery is the treatment of choice.

CHRONIC Rx

- Physical and pelvic examination every 3 mo for 2 yr, then every 6 mo for 2 yr, annually thereafter
- Yearly Pap smear
- Hormone replacement (combination) a consideration in low-risk patients (stage I or early stage II)

DISPOSITION

The majority of cases present early, and the 5-yr survival is generally good:

Stage I	75% to 100%
Stage II	60%
Stage III	50%
Stage IV	20%

Some histologic types (clear cell, serous papillary) have worse survival rates.

REFERRAL

Refer to a gynecologic oncologist.

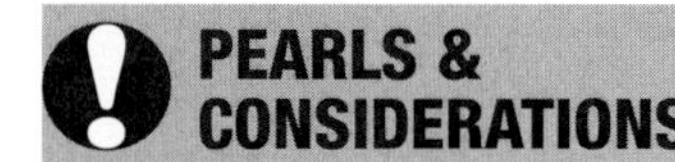

PEARLS & CONSIDERATIONS

COMMENTS

Estrogen replacement therapy after surgery for endometrial cancer remains controversial. Recent data suggest that it does not increase endometrial cancer recurrence rates.

SUGGESTED READINGS

Amant et al: Endometrial cancer, *Lancet* 366 (9484): 491, 2005.

Bakkum-gamez JN et al: Current issues in the management of endometrial cancer, *Mayo Clin Proc* 83(1):97-112, 2008.

Tabor A et al: Endometrial thickness as a test for endometrial cancer in women with postmenopausal vaginal bleeding, *Obstet Gynecol* 99:529, 2002.

AUTHORS: **GIL M. FARKASH, M.D.,** and **RUBEN ALVERO, M.D.**

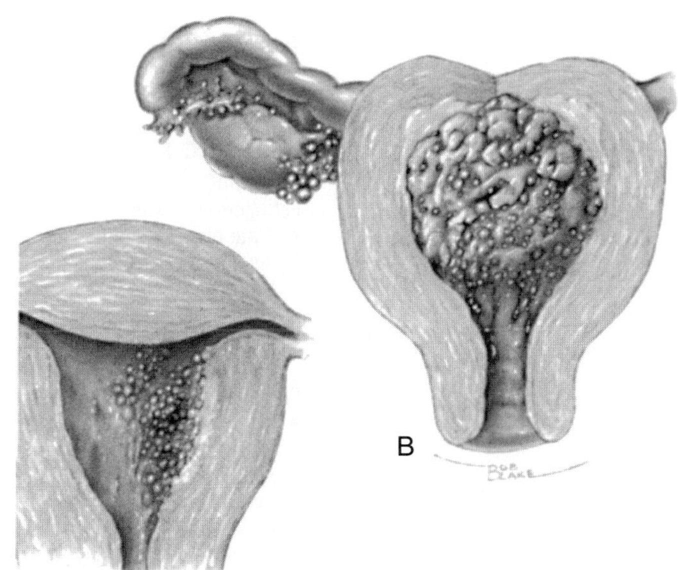

FIGURE 1-103 Carcinoma of the endometrium. A, Stage I. **B,** Stage III, myometrial invasion. (From Sabiston D: *Textbook of surgery,* ed 17, Philadelphia, 2006, WB Saunders.)

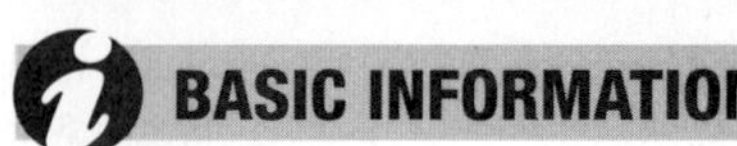

BASIC INFORMATION

DEFINITION

Endometriosis is defined as the presence of functioning endometrial glands and stroma outside the uterine cavity (Fig. 1-104).

ICD-9CM CODES
617.9 Endometriosis

EPIDEMIOLOGY & DEMOGRAPHICS

PREVALENCE:

- In asymptomatic women: 2% to 22%
- Women with dysmenorrhea: 40% to 60%
- Subfertile women: 20% to 30%
- Incidence peaks at approximately 40 yr

MOST COMMON AGE AT DIAGNOSIS: 25 to 29 yr

GENETICS:

- Multifactorial inheritance pattern
- 6.9% occurrence rate in first-degree female relatives

PHYSICAL FINDINGS & CLINICAL PRESENTATION

- Classic triad is dysmenorrhea, dyspareunia, and infertility.
- Presence of pelvic pain *not correlated* with the total area of endometriosis, type of lesion, or volume of disease, but *is correlated* with the depth of infiltration.
- Other symptoms include abnormal bleeding (premenstrual spotting, menorrhagia), cyclic abdominal pain, intermittent constipation/diarrhea, dyschezia, dysuria, hematuria, and urinary frequency.
- Rare manifestations: catamenial hemothorax, bloody pleural effusion, massive ascites occurring during menses.
- Most severe discomfort is associated with lesions >1 cm in depth.
- Bimanual examination may reveal tender uterosacral ligaments, cul-de-sac nodularity, induration of the rectovaginal septum, fixed retroversion of the uterus, adnexal mass, and generalized or localized tenderness.

ETIOLOGY

- Reflux and direct implantation theory: retrograde menstruation with implantation of viable endometrial cells to surrounding pelvic structures
- Coelomic metaplasia theory: transformation of multipotential cells of the coelomic epithelium into endometrium-like cells
- Vascular dissemination theory: transport of endometrial cells to distant sites by the uterine vascular and lymphatic systems
- Autoimmune disease theory: disorder of immune surveillance allows growth of endometrial implants

Dx DIAGNOSIS

DIFFERENTIAL DIAGNOSIS

- Ectopic pregnancy
- Acute appendicitis
- Chronic appendicitis
- Pelvic inflammatory disease (PID)
- Pelvic adhesions
- Hemorrhagic cyst
- Hernia
- Psychologic disorder
- Irritable bowel syndrome
- Uterine leiomyomata
- Adenomyosis
- Nerve entrapment syndrome
- Scoliosis
- Muscular/skeletal strain
- Interstitial cystitis

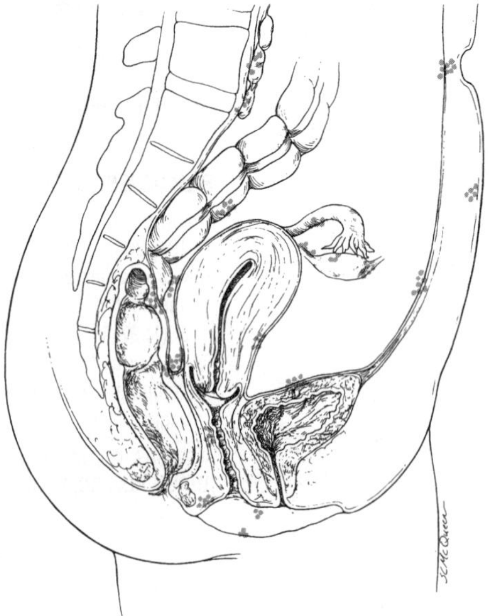

FIGURE 1-104 Common pelvic sites of endometriosis. (From Mishell D [ed]: *Comprehensive gynecology,* ed 3, St Louis, 1997, Mosby.)

WORKUP

- Thorough history and physical examination, including inquiry about physical and emotional abuse
- Colonoscopy if rectal bleeding present
- Laparoscopy for definitive diagnosis
- Revised American Fertility Society scale to classify endometriosis (since 1985):

Stage I	Minimal
Stage II	Mild
Stage III	Moderate
Stage IV	Severe

LABORATORY TESTS

Cancer antigen 125 (CA125):

- Also elevated in ovarian epithelial neoplasm, myomas, adenomyosis, acute PID, ovarian cysts, pancreatitis, chronic liver disease, menstruation, and pregnancy
- CA125 value >35 U/ml: positive predictive value of 0.58 and a negative predictive value of 0.96 for the presence of endometriosis

IMAGING STUDIES

- Ultrasound: for evaluating adnexal mass; cannot reliably distinguish endometriomas from other benign or malignant ovarian conditions
- MRI:
  1. Highly accurate in detecting endometriomas
  2. Limited sensitivity in detecting diffuse pelvic endometriosis

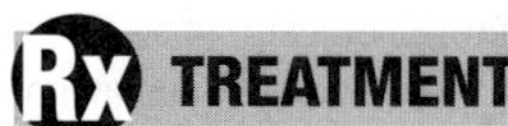

TREATMENT

NONPHARMACOLOGIC THERAPY

Expectant management (observation for 5 to 12 mo) for stage I or stage II endometriosis-associated infertility

ACUTE GENERAL Rx

Nonsteroidal anti-inflammatory drugs for symptomatic relief of dysmenorrhea

CHRONIC Rx

PHARMACOLOGIC MANAGEMENT:

Estrogen-progesterone:

- State of "pseudopregnancy" created by continuous use of combination oral contraceptives for 6 to 12 mo
- Breakthrough bleeding treated by administering conjugated estrogens 1.25 mg/day for 2 wk

Progestins:

- Medroxyprogesterone acetate 10 to 30 mg PO qd and occasionally up to 100 mg PO qd
- Alternatively, 100 mg IM q2wk for four doses, followed by 200 mg IM monthly for 4 mo
- Breakthrough bleeding treated with ethinyl estradiol (20 mcg/day) or conjugated estrogens (1.25 mg/day) for 1 to 2 wk
- Comparison with danazol: progestins cost less, have a more tolerable side-effect profile, and have comparable efficacy with regard to pain relief and so are often the first-line drug

Gonadotropin-releasing hormone (GnRH) agonists:
- Use usually limited to 6 mo
- Leuprolide acetate depot 3.75 mg IM monthly *or* 11.25 mg IM q3mo *or* nafarelin 200 mcg nasal puffs bid *or* goserelin 3.6 mg SC monthly
- As effective as danazol for relief of pelvic pain
- Add-back therapy for protection against vasomotor symptoms and bone loss: norethindrone acetate 5 mg PO qd alone *or* in combination with conjugated estrogen 0.625 mg PO qd
- Add-back therapy allows gonadotropin-releasing hormone (GnRH) agonist use to be extended to 1 yr

Alternative therapies for inhibition of estrogen action currently under investigation are:
- Aromatase inhibitors: anastrozole, letrozole
- SERM: raloxifene
- Agents enhancing cell-mediated immunity are cytokines (interleukin-12 and interferon-α-2b)
- Immunomodulators (loxoribine, levamisole)
- Antiinflammatory: pentoxifylline

SURGICAL MANAGEMENT:

Conservative:
- Directed at enhancing fertility or treating pain unresponsive to first-line medical treatment
- Usually accomplished through laparoscopy
- Removal or destruction of endometriotic implants by excision, electrocautery, or laser
- Cystectomy for endometrioma
- Laparoscopic uterosacral nerve ablation for midline pain such as dysmenorrhea or dyspareunia (evidence does not support its use)
- Unless pregnancy is desired, patient is usually started on GnRH agonist therapy immediately after surgery
- For those desiring pregnancy, surgery alone results in significant increase in fertility

Definitive:
- Directed at relieving endometriosis-associated pain
- Total abdominal hysterectomy with bilateral salpingo-oophorectomy and complete excision or ablation of endometriosis
- Thorough abdominal exploration to ensure removal of all disease
- Must be prepared to manage possible gastrointestinal and urinary tract endometriosis
- 90% effective in pain relief; patient must be counseled that pain relief is not guaranteed
- Estrogen replacement therapy (ERT) to be considered in all women undergoing definitive surgical management; after ERT, recurrence rate is 0% to 5% in women with endometriosis confined to the pelvis but 18% in women with bowel involvement

MANAGEMENT OF ENDOMETRIOSIS-ASSOCIATED INFERTILITY:

Conservative surgery:
- Yields significantly increased pregnancy rate than does expectant management, in part because of correction of mechanical factors such as adhesions

Assisted reproductive technologies:
- Can be used to circumvent unknown mechanism of endometriosis-associated infertility
- Superovulation with clomiphene citrate or human menopausal gonadotropins; clomiphene citrate results in threefold pregnancy rate over either danazol or expectant management
- Further improvement with intrauterine insemination combined with superovulation
- In vitro fertilization if above procedures are unsuccessful

DISPOSITION

Tends to recur unless definitive surgery is performed and should be considered a chronic condition

REFERRAL

To a reproductive endocrinologist for advanced surgical management or infertility management

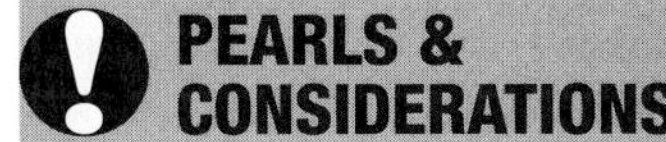

PEARLS & CONSIDERATIONS

COMMENTS

Patient information can be obtained through the following organizations: Endometriosis Association, 8585 North 76th Place, Milwaukee, WI 53223, 414-355-2200 or 800-992-ENDO; Women's Reproductive Health Network, P.O. Box 30167, Portland, OR 97230-9067 or 503-667-7757.

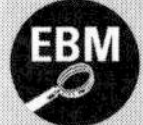

EVIDENCE

Progestogens effectively reduce endometriosis-associated pain but with less impact on bone mineral density than gonadorelin analogs.

Another systematic review analyzed the efficacy of postoperative use of a levonorgestrel-releasing intrauterine system (LNG-IUS) in women with endometriosis to see if it improves pain symptoms associated with menstruation. It also analyzed whether it reduces recurrence, compared to treatment with surgery only, placebo, or systemic hormones. It found only one small study, which showed that postoperative use reduces the recurrence of painful periods in women who have had surgery for endometriosis.[1] Ⓑ

A randomized controlled trial (RCT) compared the efficacy of subcutaneous depot medroxyprogesterone acetate and leuprolide acetate in treatment of patients with endometriosis. It concluded that the efficacy of the depot therapy was equivalent to that of leuprolide for reducing endometriosis-associated pain. Furthermore, it had less impact on bone mineral density (BMD) and fewer hypoestrogenic side effects but more bleeding.[2] Ⓑ

Another RCT compared the efficacy of depot medroxyprogesterone acetate and leuprolide for endometriosis-associated pain. It also concluded that medroxyprogesterone reduces endometriosis-associated pain as effectively as leuprolide and improves productivity with significantly less BMD decline.[3] Ⓑ

An RCT excluded from the second review compared the efficacy of a levonorgestrel-releasing intrauterine system (LNG-IUS) and a depot-GnRH-analogue in the control of endometriosis-related pain over a period of six months. It concluded that both the LNG-IUS and the GnRH-analogue were effective in the treatment of chronic pelvic pain-associated endometriosis, although no differences were observed between the two treatments. Among the additional advantages of the LNG-IUS is the fact that it does not provoke hypoestrogenism and that it requires only one medical intervention for its introduction every 5 yr. This device could therefore become the treatment of choice in women who do not wish to conceive.[4] Ⓐ

A further RCT analyzed the efficacy of an estrogen-progestogen combination versus low-dose norethindrone acetate in the treatment of persistent pain after surgery for symptomatic rectovaginal endometriosis. It concluded that low-dose norethindrone acetate could be considered an effective, tolerable, and inexpensive first-choice medical alternative to repeat surgery for treating symptomatic rectovaginal endometriotic lesions in patients who do not seek conception.[5] Ⓐ

GnRH analogs are effective in reducing endometriosis-associated pain, but any benefit needs to be balanced against their potentially significant side effects.

GnRH analogs versus combined oral contraceptives:

A subsequent RCT found that gonadorelin analogues (with and without add-back estrogen/progestogen) for 12 mo significantly reduced dysmenorrhea, pelvic pain, and dyspareunia compared with combined oral contraceptive for 12 mo.[6] Ⓐ

GnRH analogs versus danazol:

An RCT found no significant difference in the improvement of total symptom severity score, which included pelvic pain, dysmenorrhea, and dyspareunia, after 180 days of treatment for the gonadorelin analogue nafarelin, compared with danazol.[7] Ⓐ

GnRH analogs versus medroxyprogesterone:

An RCT comparing medroxyprogesterone versus gonadorelin analogues found that both treatments significantly improved symptoms attributable to endometriosis, sleep disturbances, and anxiety-depression scores, from baseline measurements. And there was no significant difference between the two.[2] Ⓐ

GnRH analogs versus levonorgestrel-releasing intrauterine system:

An RCT found no significant difference between levonorgestrel-releasing intrauterine system and a depot gonadorelin analogue, leuprorelin, in reduction of a visual analogue scale for chronic pelvic pain throughout the 6-mo treatment.[4] Ⓐ

GnRH analogs preoperatively and postoperatively:

A systematic review analyzed the efficacy of systemic medical therapies used for hormonal suppression before or after surgery for endometriosis, or before and after surgery for endometriosis in the eradication of endometriosis, improvement of symptoms, pregnancy rates, and overall tolerability by comparing them with no treatment or placebo. It found insufficient evidence from the studies identified to conclude that hormonal suppression, in association with surgery for endometriosis, is associated with a significant benefit with regard to any of the outcomes identified.[9] Ⓐ

Danazol is effective in reducing endometriosis-associated pain, but any benefit needs to be balanced against its potential side effects.

An additional RCT found no significant difference in the improvement of total symptom severity score, which included pelvic pain, dysmenorrhea, and dyspareunia after 180 days of treatment for the gonadorelin analogue nafarelin compared with danazol.[7] Ⓐ

A third systematic review analyzed the efficacy of systemic medical therapies used for hormonal suppression before or after surgery for endometriosis or before and after surgery for endometriosis in the eradication of endometriosis, improvement of symptoms, pregnancy rates, and overall tolerability by comparing them with no treatment or placebo. It found insufficient evidence from the studies identified to conclude that hormonal suppression, in association with surgery for endometriosis, is associated with a significant benefit with regard to any of the outcomes identified.[9] Ⓐ

An additional RCT found no significant difference in pain control and American Fertility Society score between triptorelin and danazol.[10] Ⓐ

Conservative surgical management seems to be effective in the treatment of women with endometriosis-associated pain, but perceived benefit(s) may be due to a "placebo" effect.

Another systematic review identified four RCTs comparing laparoscopic ablation plus LUNA versus laparoscopic removal alone. It found no significant difference in dysmenorrhea pain relief at up to 6, 12, or 36 mo between the two procedures.[13] Ⓐ

The same systematic review identified three RCTs comparing laparoscopic ablation plus presacral neurectomy (PSN) versus laparoscopic removal alone. It found limited evidence of improvement in midline dysmenorrhea pain relief at both 6 and 12 mo after laparoscopic removal plus PSN compared with laparoscopic removal alone.[11] Ⓐ

An additional RCT compared laparoscopic removal of endometriotic deposits alone (by excisional surgery) versus diagnostic laparoscopy in women with pain attributed to endometriosis. It found that laparoscopic excision significantly improved pain symptoms, compared with diagnostic laparoscopy, at 6 mo.[12] Ⓐ

Another small RCT compared laparoscopic excision versus laparoscopic ablation of endometriotic lesions. It found no differences between the two groups, with 67% of women in both treatment groups reporting good symptomatic relief.[13] Ⓐ

A further RCT compared laparoscopic ablation or excision with helium thermal coagulator, versus 6 mo of treatment with the gonadorelin analogue Zoladex. At 12 mo follow-up, more women treated surgically than treated medically were symptom free.[8] Ⓐ

Assisted reproductive technologies are sometimes necessary for women with endometriosis who are trying to become pregnant.

A systematic review analyzing the efficacy of administering GnRH agonists for 3 to 6 mo prior to IVF or ICSI in women with endometriosis found that it increases the odds of clinical pregnancy by fourfold.[14] Ⓐ

Expectant management may have a role in the ongoing care of women post-surgery; but evidence is lacking for its role as a primary management strategy.

A systematic review identified an RCT of women with mild to moderate symptomatic endometriosis who had had laparoscopic conservative surgery. It compared 6 mo of open label allocation of subcutaneous goserelin versus expectant management with 2 yr of follow-up. It found that goserelin reduced recurrence of pain over 2 yr, but the difference was not significant.[9] Ⓐ

Evidence-Based References

1. Abou-Setta AM et al: Levonorgestrel-releasing intrauterine device (LNG-IUD) for symptomatic endometriosis following surgery, *Cochrane Database Rev* (4), 2006. Ⓑ
2. Schlaff WD et al: Subcutaneous injection of depot medroxyprogesterone acetate compared with leuprolide acetate in the treatment of endometriosis-associated pain. *Fertil Steril* 85:314-325, 2006. Ⓑ
3. Crosignani PG et al: Subcutaneous depot medroxyprogesterone acetate versus leuprolide acetate in the treatment of endometriosis-associated pain, *Hum Reprod* 21:248-256, 2006. Ⓑ
4. Petta CA et al: Randomized clinical trial of a levonorgestrel-releasing intrauterine system and a depot GnRH analogue for the treatment of chronic pelvic pain in women with endometriosis, *Hum Reprod* 20:1993-1998, 2005. Ⓐ
5. Vercellini P et al: Treatment of symptomatic rectovaginal endometriosis with an estrogen-progestogen combination versus low-dose norethindrone acetate, *Fertil Steril* 84:1375-1387, 2005. Ⓐ
6. Zupi E et al: Add-back therapy in the treatment of endometriosis-associated pain, *Fertil Steril* 82: 1303-1308, 2004. Ⓐ
7. Cheng MH et al: A randomized, parallel, comparative study of the efficacy and safety of nafarelin versus danazol in the treatment of endometriosis in Taiwan, *J Chin Med Assoc* 68:307-314, 2005. Ⓐ
8. Lalchandani S: Is helium thermal coagulator therapy for the treatment of women with minimal to moderate endometriosis cost-effective? A prospective randomised controlled trial, *Gynecol Surg* 2: 255-258, 2005. Ⓐ
9. Yap C et al: Pre and post operative medical therapy for endometriosis surgery, *Cochrane Database Rev* (3), 2004. Ⓐ
10. Wong AYK, Tang L: An open and randomized study comparing the efficacy of standard danazol and modified triptorelin regimens for postoperative disease management of moderate to severe endometriosis, *Fertil Steril* 81:1522-1527, 2004. Ⓐ
11. Proctor ML et al: Surgical interruption of pelvic nerve pathways for primary and secondary dysmenorrhoea, *Cochrane Database Rev* (4), 2005. Ⓐ
12. Abbott J et al: Laparoscopic excision of endometriosis: a randomized, placebo-controlled trial, *Fertil Steril* 82:878-884, 2004. Ⓐ
13. Wright J et al: A randomized trial of excision versus ablation for mild endometriosis, *Fertil Steril* 83:1830-1836, 2005. Ⓐ
14. Sallam HN et al: Long-term pituitary down-regulation before in vitro fertilization (IVF) for women with endometriosis, *Cochrane Database Rev* (1), 2006. Ⓐ

SUGGESTED READINGS

Bulun SE: Endometriosis, *N Engl J Med* 360:268-279, 2009.

Olive DL: Gonadotropin-releasing hormone agonists for endometriosis, *N Engl J Med* 359:1136, 2008.

Winkel CA: Evaluation and management of women with endometriosis, *Obstet Gynecol* 102(2):397, 2003.

AUTHORS: **WAN J. KIM, M.D.,** and **RUBEN ALVERO, M.D.**

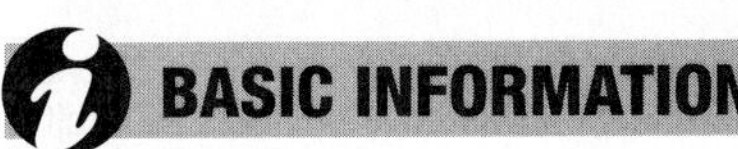

BASIC INFORMATION

DEFINITION

Endometritis is defined as a uterine infection after delivery or abortion.

SYNONYMS

Endomyometritis
Metritis

ICD-9CM CODES

615.9 Endometritis

EPIDEMIOLOGY & DEMOGRAPHICS

- Overall rate of postpartum infection: estimated between 1% and 8%
- Most common genital tract infection after delivery
- Usually presents early in postpartum period; more commonly seen after cesarean section than vaginal delivery; also seen with an incomplete abortion (spontaneous abortion, legal abortion, or illegal abortion)
- More common in preterm deliveries
- Possible after any uterine manipulation in the presence of undiagnosed cervicitis or vaginitis

PHYSICAL FINDINGS & CLINICAL PRESENTATION

- Postpartum oral temperature >37.8° C
- Localized uterine tenderness, purulent or foul lochia; physical examination revealing uterine or parametrial tenderness
- Nonspecific signs and symptoms such as malaise, abdominal pain, chills, and tachycardia

ETIOLOGY

Endometritis is usually associated with multiple organisms: group A or B streptococci, *Staphylococcus aureus* and *Bacteroides* species, *Neisseria gonorrhoeae, Chlamydia trachomatis,* enterococci, *Gardnerella vaginalis, E. coli,* and *Mycoplasma.*

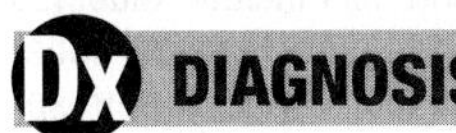

DIAGNOSIS

DIFFERENTIAL DIAGNOSIS

Causes of postoperative or postprocedural infections

WORKUP

Diagnosis based on symptoms of fever, malaise, abdominal pain, uterine tenderness, and purulent, foul vaginal discharge

LABORATORY TESTS

Complete blood count, blood cultures, and uterine culture

IMAGING STUDIES

Ultrasound may be useful if retained products are considered a possible source of infection.

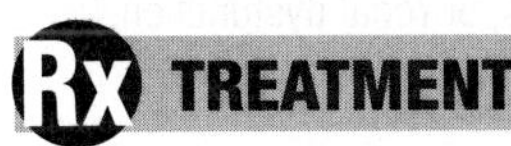

TREATMENT

ACUTE GENERAL Rx

- In treating endometritis after a vaginal delivery, ampicillin 2 g IV q6h plus gentamicin loading dose IV or IM (2 mg/kg of body weight) followed by a maintenance dose (1.5 mg/kg of body weight) q8h are used.
- Regimen should be continued for at least 48 hr after substantial clinical improvement. If response is not adequate, check cultures and treat with appropriate antibiotics (Table 1-24).
- Endometritis after cesarean section should be treated with ampicillin 2 g IV q6h plus gentamicin loading dose IV or IM (2 mg/kg of body weight) followed by a maintenance dose (1.5 mg/kg of body weight) q8h and clindamycin 900 mg IV q8h. If *Chlamydia* is one of the etiologic agents, add doxycycline 100 mg PO bid for completion of a 14-day course of therapy (if breastfeeding, use erythromycin).

CHRONIC Rx

Watch for recurrent infection.

DISPOSITION

With appropriate antibiotic therapy, 95% to 98% cure rate

REFERRAL

For patients who do not respond within 48 to 72 hr of appropriate antibiotic therapy, obtain an infectious disease consult or gynecologic consultation.

TABLE 1-24 Identified Causes of Poor Response to Antibiotic Therapy in Patients with Endometritis

Cause	Approximate Prevalence (%)
Infected mass, including abscess, hematoma, septic pelvic thrombophlebitis, pelvic cellulitis, retained placenta	40-50
Resistant organisms, commonly enterococci, in a patient receiving clindamycin-aminoglycoside or a cephalosporin	20
Additional cause, including catheter phlebitis, inadequate dose of antibiotics	10
No cause evident but response to empirical change in antibiotic therapy	20-30

From Gorbach SL: *Infectious diseases,* ed 2, Philadelphia, 1998, WB Saunders.

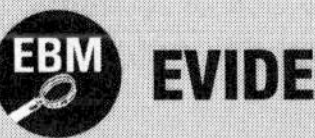

EVIDENCE

There is good evidence that antibiotics are effective in the treatment of postpartum endometritis.

A systematic review of randomized controlled trials found that treatment with clindamycin and an aminoglycoside was associated with fewer treatment failures than alternative regimens in the treatment of postpartum endometritis following cesarean or vaginal delivery. The review found that combined gentamicin and clindamycin is an appropriate treatment, and regimens with activity against penicillin-resistant anaerobic bacteria are better than those without such activity. After clinical improvement of uncomplicated endometritis with intravenous therapy, oral therapy is unnecessary.[1] Ⓐ

Evidence-Based Reference

1. French LM, Smaill FM: Antibiotic regimens for endometritis after delivery, *Cochrane Database Rev* (4), 2004.

AUTHORS: **GEORGE T. DANAKAS, M.D.,** and **RUBEN ALVERO, M.D.**

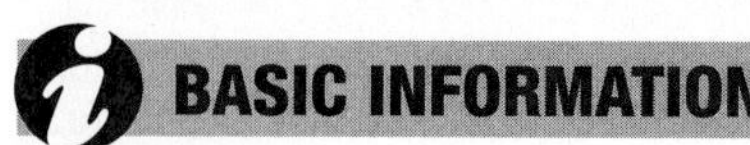

BASIC INFORMATION

DEFINITION

Enuresis refers to the voiding of urine into clothes or in bed that is usually involuntary in individuals who are expected to be continent (>5 yr of age). The diagnosis is made if voiding occurs at least twice a week for 3 mo. Primary enuresis refers to enuresis without a period of continence, whereas secondary enuresis occurs after a period of normal bladder control.

SYNONYMS

Urinary incontinence
Bed-wetting

ICD-9CM CODES
788.36 Nocturnal Enuresis
DMS-IV Code 307.6 Enuresis Primary/Secondary of Nonorganic Origin

EPIDEMIOLOGY & DEMOGRAPHICS

PEAK INCIDENCE: Ages 5 to 10 yr
PREVALENCE (IN U.S.):
- Age 5 yr: 7% of males and 3% of females
- Age 10 yr: 3% of males and 2% of females
- Age 18 yr: 1% of males

PREDOMINANT SEX: Twice as many males as females at all ages
PREDOMINANT AGE: By definition, enuresis does not begin before age 5 yr, at which time the prevalence is highest, and decreases steadily thereafter at a rate of approximately 15% per year.
GENETICS:
- Approximately 75% of children with enuresis have a first-degree relative with enuresis.
- Almost twice as common in monozygotic than dizygotic twins.

PHYSICAL FINDINGS & CLINICAL PRESENTATION

Three enuresis subtypes are defined:
- Nocturnal only: usually occurs in first third of sleep, frequently during REM sleep; child may recall a dream with voiding
- Diurnal only: more frequent in girls and rarely after age 9 yr; voiding occurs in early afternoon on school days
- Combined nocturnal and diurnal enuresis; often called complex or complicated enuresis

ETIOLOGY

- Enuresis correlates with other maturational delays, particularly language, motor skills, and social development
- May be related to lax toilet training, stress, inability to concentrate urine, and altered smooth muscle physiology
- Diurnal enuresis associated with a higher rate of urinary tract infections

Dx DIAGNOSIS

DIFFERENTIAL DIAGNOSIS

- May be associated with encopresis and sleep disorders such as sleep terrors; much less likely to be a primary psychological disorder.
- Organic causes of enuresis include diabetes mellitus, diabetes insipidus, bladder outlet obstruction, small bladder capacity, detrusor instability, urethral valves, meatal stenosis, cerebral palsy, spina bifida, pelvic mass, impacted stool, sedating medications, nocturnal seizures.

WORKUP

- History and physical examination to rule out anatomic abnormalities. Fluid intake and voiding diaries may be useful.
- Children frequently experience shame, so gentleness and care must be exercised when questioning or examining the child.

LABORATORY TESTS

- Urinalysis with specific gravity and urine culture if white cells or nitrites on analysis.
- Serum studies to rule out diabetes, electrolyte abnormalities, or renal dysfunction.

IMAGING STUDIES

- In complicated cases, sleep studies may be useful.
- If an anatomic abnormality suspected, renal ultrasound or intravenous pyelogram is possibly indicated; MRI of the spine if evidence of abnormalities of lower spine or perineum is found on examination.

Rx TREATMENT

NONPHARMACOLOGIC THERAPY

Behavioral treatment:
- Alarm and pad technique: up to 80% cure rate, although 30% relapse
- Scheduled voiding to reduce the frequency of enuretic episodes
- Star charts to reward child for dry nights
- Punishment for enuresis is not effective

ACUTE GENERAL Rx

- Desmopressin (DDAVP) administered intranasally at bedtime significantly reduces the incidence of bedwetting.
- Tricyclic antidepressants (imipramine): efficacy supported by randomized control trials. Use with care in children.
- Serotonin reuptake inhibitors: lack of adequate trials is notable.
- Indomethacin suppositories may reduce normal prostaglandin inhibitory effects on antidiuretic hormone.

DISPOSITION

- After age 5 yr, the rate of spontaneous remissions is approximately 15% per year.
- The disorder usually resolves by adolescence.
- Fewer than 1% will have enuresis as adults.

REFERRAL

If coexisting, a psychiatric condition complicates the course of treatment.

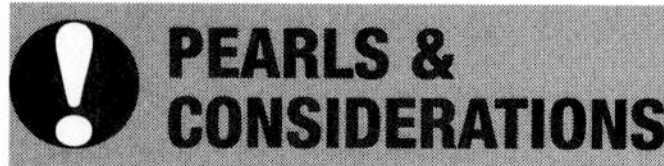

PEARLS & CONSIDERATIONS

Illness, hospitalization, and family stressors may precipitate recurrent enuresis after a period of dryness.

PATIENT & FAMILY EDUCATION

Bedwetting: Jasper to the Rescue! video available from Disney Educational Productions (http://dep.disney.go.com/educational/index)

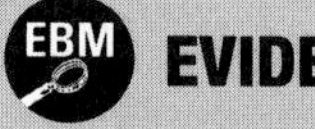

EVIDENCE

An enuresis alarm is an effective intervention for nocturnal enuresis in children.[1] Ⓐ

An alarm may be less effective initially than desmopressin, but an alarm appears to be more effective by the end of a treatment course and possibly in the long term. It appears to be more effective than tricyclic drugs both during treatment and afterward.[1] Ⓑ

Relapse rates are reduced when overlearning (giving the child extra fluids at bedtime after he or she has become dry using the alarm) is added to the use of an alarm.[1] Ⓐ

Complex lifestyle interventions such as dry bed training including an alarm are more effective than no-treatment control groups, but there is insufficient evidence on the effect of lifestyle intervention alone.[2] Ⓐ

A complex lifestyle intervention coupled with an alarm might reduce relapse rate compared with the alarm alone.[2] Ⓑ

Penalties for bedwetting appear to be counterproductive.[1] Ⓐ

Evidence-Based References

1. Glazener CMA et al: Alarm interventions for nocturnal enuresis in children, *Cochrane Database Rev* (2), 2005. Ⓐ Ⓑ
2. Glazener CMA et al: Complex behavioural and educational interventions for nocturnal enuresis, *Cochrane Database Rev* (1), 2004. Ⓐ Ⓑ

SUGGESTED READINGS

Makari J, Ruston HG: Nocturnal enuresis, *Am Fam Physician* 73(9):1611, 2006.

Ramakrishnan K: Evaluation and treatment of enuresis, *Am Fam Physician* 78(4):489-496, 2008.

Robson WL: Clinical practice. Evaluation and management of enuresis, *N Engl J Med* 360(14):1429-1436, 2009.

Van Dommelen P et al: The short- and long-term effects of simple behavioral interventions for nocturnal enuresis in young children: a randomized controlled trial, *J Pediatr* 154(5):662-666, 2009.

AUTHOR: **MITCHELL D. FELDMAN, M.D., M.PHIL.**

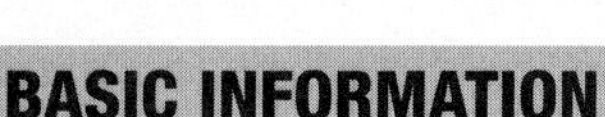

BASIC INFORMATION

DEFINITION

Eosinophilic fasciitis (EF) is a rare inflammatory disease of the skin and subcutaneous tissue that is initially characterized by pain, edema, and eosinophilia in peripheral blood. This condition starts with symmetrical erythema, edema, and induration of an extremity or trunk and later may progress to sclerosis of the dermis and subcutaneous fascia leading to contractures.

SYNONYMS

Shulman's syndrome
Diffuse fasciitis with eosinophilia

ICD-9CM CODES
728.89 Eosinophilic fasciitis

EPIDEMIOLOGY & DEMOGRAPHICS

- Males and females are affected equally.
- Most common in the fourth and fifth decades.

CLINICAL PRESENTATION

- Initial presentation consists of acute erythema, swelling, and induration of the skin that is accompanied by eosinophilia.
  - Extremities usually symmetrically involved.
  - Upper more commonly affected than lower extremities.
  - Face, fingers, and toes are spared.
  - Sunken veins may be seen when the extremity is elevated (Fig. 1-105). The groove sign marks the borders of different muscle groups.
  - Skin may appear deeply rippled (peau d'orange).
- Arthritis was found in 40% of cases in one series.
- Cranial and peripheral neuropathy (mononeuritis multiplex) may occur.
- Myalgia and weakness are common.
- Hematologic abnormalities are present in 10% of cases, including aplastic anemia, amegakaryocytic thrombocytopenia, myeloproliferative disorders, and hematologic malignancies.
- The presence of Raynaud's phenomenon and visceral involvement is more suggestive of systemic sclerosis or other scleroderma-like disorders than EF.
- Spontaneous resolution or improvement has been reported after 2 to 5 yr.

ETIOLOGY

The etiology is unknown. Most cases are considered idiopathic. Vigorous exercise, initiation of hemodialysis, and infection with *Borrelia burgdorferi* have been suggested as possible causes of EF.

DIAGNOSIS

DIFFERENTIAL DIAGNOSIS

- Systemic or localized sclerosis
- Systemic or localized scleroderma
- Scleroderma-like disorders
- Chemical-induced sclerosis
- Generalized lichen sclerosus et atrophicus
- Eosinophilia-myalgia syndrome
- Porphyria cutanea tarda
- Chronic Lyme borreliosis

WORKUP

- Physical examination to confirm characteristic distribution.
- Skin biopsy that penetrates to muscle is optimal for diagnosis:
  - Epidermis is usually normal.
  - Dermis may demonstrate mild inflammation with lymphocytes, histiocytes, plasma cells, and eosinophils with some fibrosis.
  - Moderate inflammation of subcutaneous tissue and sclerosis of fat septa.
  - Muscle demonstrates perivascular mixed inflammatory cell infiltrate.

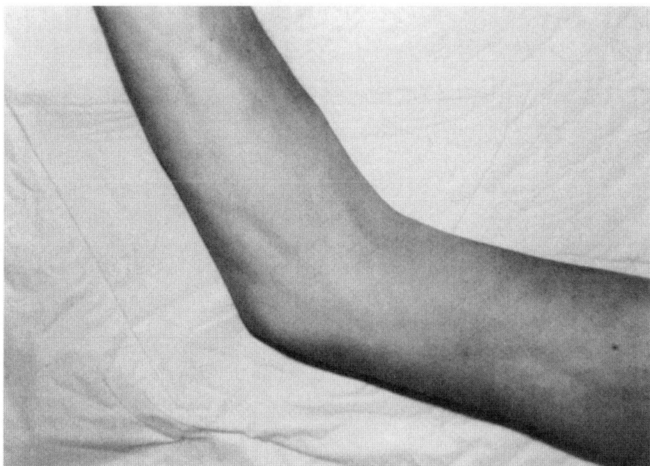

FIGURE 1-105 Eosinophilic fasciitis. This 29-year-old butcher had to stop working because of a generalized painful induration of his skin. Fingers were spared. As he raised his forearms, the collapsed veins appeared as grooves (the "groove sign"), which is pathognomonic of eosinophilic fasciitis. His condition subsided 4 years later, leaving joint contractures. (Reprinted from Canoso J: *Rheumatology in primary care,* Philadelphia, 1997, WB Saunders.)

LABORATORY TESTS

- Peripheral eosinophilia in up to 70% during the acute phase of the disease
- Elevated erythrocyte sedimentation rate (29%)
- Hypergammaglobulinemia (35%)
- Creatine kinase is usually normal even in patients with myalgia
- Occasional thrombocytopenia, anemia
- Serum antinuclear antibodies are negative

IMAGING STUDIES

- MRI may be useful in assessing patients with suspected EF
- Increased T2 signal in the subcutaneous and deep fascia with enhancement of these structures on T1 images after gadolinium administration

TREATMENT

ACUTE GENERAL Rx

- Although no controlled trials exist, corticosteroids (prednisone 1 mg/kg/day) are effective in most patients, but the duration and extent of symptom reduction are variable.
- Hydroxychloroquine is an alternative that may be as effective as steroids.
- In resistant cases, ultraviolet A photochemotherapy, cyclosporine, antithymocyte globulin, methotrexate, D-penicillamine, and sulfasalazine have been successfully used.

CHRONIC Rx

Surgery is sometimes required to reduce contractures and maintain function.

DISPOSITION

- Prognosis is generally good with frequent spontaneous regression and response to steroids.
- Contractures are common.
- 10% may develop blood dyscrasias.

REFERRAL

To dermatology for biopsy to make definitive diagnosis. Functional impairment requires surgical evaluation.

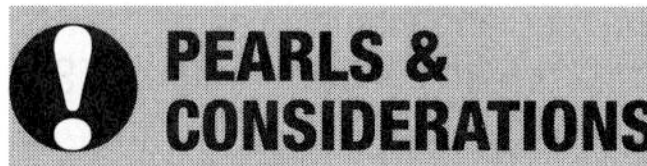

PEARLS & CONSIDERATIONS

COMMENTS

- EF is a rare inflammatory disorder of unknown etiology with symmetric painful edema and induration of the arms and legs with peripheral eosinophilia.
- Rapid onset, progression, and good response to systemic corticosteroids are characteristic of the disease.
- Prognosis is usually good.

SUGGESTED READINGS

Mosconi S et al: Eosinophilic fasciitis (Shulman syndrome), *Dermatology* 205(2):204, 2002.

Moulton SJ et al: Eosinophilic fasciitis: spectrum of MRI findings, *AJR Am J Roentgenol* 184(3):975, 2005.

AUTHOR: **ETSUKO AOKI, M.D., PH.D.**

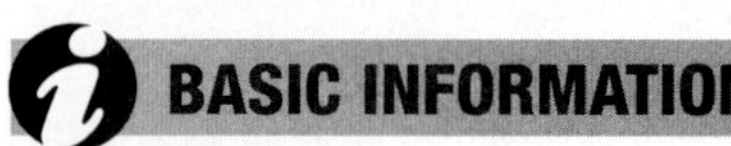

BASIC INFORMATION

DEFINITION

Eosinophilic pneumonias (EPs) are a group of disorders characterized by pulmonary infiltrates, pulmonary parenchymal eosinophilia, and possibly peripheral blood eosinophilia. They manifest by different radiologic and clinical syndromes.

SYNONYMS

Simple pulmonary eosinophilia
Chronic eosinophilic pneumonia
Acute eosinophilic pneumonia
Churg-Strauss syndrome
Idiopathic hypereosinophilic syndrome
Allergic bronchopulmonary aspergillosis
Parasite-induced, fungal-induced, and drug-induced pulmonary eosinophilia

ICD-9CM CODES

518.3 Eosinophilic pneumonia

EPIDEMIOLOGY & DEMOGRAPHICS

Vary depending on the specific cause

PHYSICAL FINDINGS & CLINICAL PRESENTATION

- Fever, cough, and shortness of breath
- Vary depending on the specific cause

ETIOLOGY

SIMPLE PULMONARY EOSINOPHILIA (LÖFFLER'S SYNDROME):

- Transient pulmonary infiltrates
- Symptoms range from asymptomatic to dyspnea and dry cough
- Usually idiopathic
- May be secondary to parasitic infection or drugs (nitrofurantoin, penicillin)
- Remove the offending agent
- If idiopathic and severe symptoms, then give glucocorticoid therapy

IDIOPATHIC ACUTE EP:

- Absence of infection or other cause
- Acute onset of fever, cough, dyspnea (<1 mo); often presents with acute respiratory failure, requiring intensive care
- Erythrocyte sedimentation rate (ESR), C-reactive protein (CRP), and IgE may be elevated but nonspecific
- Bilateral diffuse infiltrates on chest radiograph
- High-resolution CT scan of the chest may demonstrate patchy ground glass with reticular infiltrates; small pleural effusions present in two thirds of cases
- Pleural fluid analysis reveals elevated pH and high eosinophil count
- Hypoxemia (PaO_2 <60)
- Lung eosinophilia >25% on bronchoalveolar lavage (BAL)
- Pulmonary function test can demonstrate restrictive dysfunction with reduction in diffusion capacity
- Associations: recent onset of tobacco smoking, World Trade Center dust, Scotchguard inhalation, tear gas, gasoline, indoor renovation work, multiple medications, firework smoke, cocaine
- Steroids lead to rapid improvement, though there is no consensus about ideal dosing strategy

IDIOPATHIC CHRONIC EP:

- Absence of infection or other cause
- Presentation over weeks to months
- Productive cough, dyspnea, malaise, weight loss, night sweats, and fever (with or without hemoptysis/chest pain)
- Progressive pulmonary infiltrates
- "Photographic negative" pulmonary edema (peripheral alveolar infiltrates) is pathognomonic but only present in 25% of cases; high-resolution CT of the chest may reveal atelectasis, pleural effusions, lymphadenopathy, and septal line thickening
- Blood eosinophilia not always present
- ESR, CRP, platelets, and IgE may be elevated but are nonspecific
- Diagnose by BAL (up to 90% of cases will have 60% eosinophils) or lung biopsy
- Spontaneous remission in 10% of cases
- Treatment with glucocorticoids is rapidly effective
- Relapses are common when glucocorticoids tapered
- Prevalence of patients with asthma

ALLERGIC BRONCHOPULMONARY ASPERGILLOSIS (ABPA):

- Hypersensitivity reaction to *Aspergillus fumigatus*
- Occurs most often in patients with asthma and atopy (up to 13% of the asthma population)
- Fever, flulike symptoms, myalgias, lassitude, persistent cough and wheezing, hemoptysis, and/or expectoration of brown-black mucous plugs
- A patient with chronic asthma with a component of bronchiectasis and pulmonary infiltrates should be evaluated carefully for ABPA
- Chest radiograph: infiltrates (sometimes migratory) and atelectasis, reflecting endobronchial mucous inspissation ("finger in glove")
- Blood and sputum eosinophilia
- Diagnosis by
  1. *Aspergillus* isolation from multiple sputum samples
  2. Positive skin test to *Aspergillus* (Fig. 1-106)
  3. Elevated serum IgE
  4. *Aspergillus*-specific IgE and IgG
  5. Serum eosinophilia >1000 cells/μl

The disease has been characterized by a staging system:

Patients do not necessarily proceed from one stage to another.

Stage I	Acute phase
Stage II	Remission
Stage III	Exacerbation
Stage IV	Glucocorticoid-dependent ABPA
Stage V	End-stage (fibrotic) ABPA

- Treatment: systemic corticosteroids are the mainstay of treatment. Antifungals may provide additional benefit in modulating airway fungal burden and are recommended for use in patients with relapse or glucocorticoid-dependent disease
- Development of bronchiectasis portends a worse prognosis
- Response to therapy and activity of disease may be monitored by measuring IgE levels,

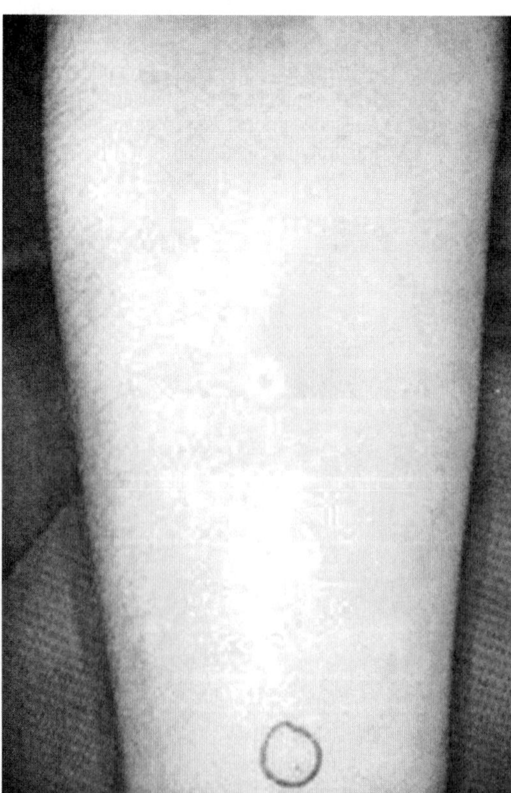

FIGURE 1-106 A positive prick test with *Aspergillus fumigatus* in a patient with allergic bronchopulmonary aspergillosis. The wheal and erythema reaction at 15 min after performing the skin test. (From Fireman P: *Atlas of allergies and immunology,* ed 3, St Louis, 2006, Mosby.

which will decrease by 35% to 50% when a patient is in remission

TROPICAL PULMONARY EOSINOPHILIA:
- Onset of asthma, fever, paroxysmal cough and bronchospasm, marked blood eosinophilia
- Basilar reticulonodular and alveolar infiltrates
- High serum IgE levels
- Presumed etiology: filariasis

PULMONARY VASCULITIS (ALLERGIC GRANULOMATOSIS AND ANGIITIS OR CHURG-STRAUSS SYNDROME):
- Vasculitis and necrotizing granulomatous inflammation that involves many organ systems in the setting of asthma
- Blood eosinophilia and elevated IgE
- Antineutrophilic cytoplasmic antibody may be positive in up to two thirds of patients; antinuclear antibody, rheumatoid factor, and ESR also may be elevated
- Common symptoms include cough, dyspnea, sinusitis, allergic rhinitis; other symptoms depend on other organs involved
- Pulmonary function test may reveal obstructive dysfunction
- Organ and systems involved include lungs, heart, skin, gastrointestinal, renal, neurologic

HYPEREOSINOPHILIC SYNDROME:
- A disease of persistently elevated eosinophils (>6 mo) with no known cause
- Cardiac problems are the prominent clinical feature with mural thrombi and endocardial/myocardial fibrosis
- Hepatosplenomegaly is common
- Fever, cough, weight loss, wheezing
- Diagnosis of exclusion
- Check echocardiogram
- Treat with steroids if symptoms or cardiac abnormalities

DRUG- OR TOXIN-INDUCED EP:
- Can have several different clinical presentations, including simple pulmonary eosinophilia, chronic, or acute
- Symptoms resolve when offending drug is removed
- Common drug/toxin causes: antibiotics, NSAIDs, amiodarone, bleomycin, captopril, gold salts, iodine, methotrexate, smoke, illicit drugs, radiation exposure
- BAL to exclude infection or other lung disease
- Laboratory evaluation rarely diagnostic

Dx DIAGNOSIS

- Diagnosis varies depending on specific cause of pneumonia
- Usually involves chest radiograph, CT, peripheral eosinophil count, BAL, and possibly lung biopsy

DIFFERENTIAL DIAGNOSIS

- Tuberculosis
- Brucellosis
- Fungal diseases
- Parasitic infection (ascaris, strongyloides)
- Idiopathic pulmonary fibrosis
- Bronchiolitis obliterans and organizing pneumonia
- Radiation pneumonitis
- Bronchogenic carcinoma
- Hodgkin's disease
- Immunoblastic lymphadenopathy
- Rheumatoid lung disease
- Sarcoidosis

WORKUP

Physical examination, laboratory tests, imaging, bronchoscopy

LABORATORY TESTS

- WBC counts are often normal
- Often blood eosinophilia
- Elevated eosinophil count on BAL

IMAGING STUDIES

Chest radiograph may show a variety of infiltrates depending on the cause of EP. CT demonstrates a more characteristic pattern and distribution of parenchymal opacities than chest radiograph.

Rx TREATMENT

- Varies depending on the cause.
- Remove offending agent or treat with appropriate antibiotic.
- Steroids may be helpful in many cases; doses and length of treatment depend on etiology of symptoms and response to treatment.
- Supportive respiratory care.

DISPOSITION

Prognosis is good if offending agent can be removed or an infectious etiology treated. Glucocorticoids have a good effect, but relapse often recurs with tapering in chronic idiopathic cases.

REFERRAL

To pulmonologist if a BAL is needed to establish the diagnosis

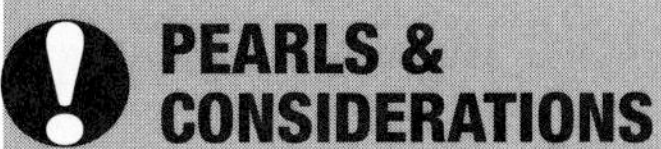

PEARLS & CONSIDERATIONS

- History (including travel) and physical examination are most important. Temporal association of eosinophilia and pulmonary abnormalities is an important diagnostic clue.
- Coccidioidomycosis and *Aspergillus* can present as eosinophilic lung disease and are important to recognize because steroid therapy can produce progressive infection.
- *Aspergillus* from respiratory specimens does not always indicate true infection and may be colonization.
- Blood eosinophilia $>1 \times 10^9$ eosinophils/L or BAL >25% is helpful in narrowing diagnosis.
- Integrating the clinical, radiologic, and pathologic findings facilitates the initial and differential diagnoses of various eosinophilic lung diseases.

SUGGESTED READINGS

Agarwal R: Allergic bronchopulmonary aspergillosis, *Chest* 135:805, 2009.

Alam M: Chronic eosinophilic pneumonia: a review, *South Med J* 100(1):49, 2007.

Allen J: Acute eosinophilic pneumonia, *Semin Resp Crit Care Med* 27(2):142, 2006.

Allen JN et al: The eosinophilic pneumonias, *Semin Resp Crit Care Med* 23(2):127, 2002.

Janz DR et al: Acute eosinophilic pneumonia: a case report and review of the literature, *Crit Care Med* 37:1470, 2009.

Jeong YJ: Eosinophilic lung diseases: a clinical, radiologic and pathologic overview, *Radiographics* 27: 617, 2007.

Leslie KO: Transbronchial biopsy interpretation in a patient with diffuse parenchymal lung disease, *Arch Pathol Lab Med* 131:407, 2007.

Marchand E: Idiopathic chronic eosinophilic pneumonia, *Semin Resp Crit Care Med* 27(2):134, 2006.

Mochimaru H et al: Clinicopathological differences between acute and chronic eosinophilic pneumonia, *Respirology* (10)1:76-85, 2005.

Solomon J: Drug, toxin, and radiation therapy-induced eosinophilic pneumonia, *Semin Resp Crit Care Med* 27(2):192, 2006.

Uchiyama H et al: Alterations in smoking habits are associated with acute eosinophilic pneumonia, *Chest* 133:1174, 2008.

Wechsler ME: Pulmonary eosinophilic syndromes, *Immunol Allergy Clin North Am* 27:477-492, 2007.

AUTHORS: **CAROLYN J. O'CONNOR, M.D.,** and **KRISTINA KRAMER, M.D.**

BASIC INFORMATION

DEFINITION

Epicondylitis is inflammation (tendinosis) of the musculotendinous origin of the common extensors at the lateral elbow or the flexor pronator group at the medial elbow.

SYNONYMS

Tennis elbow (lateral epicondylitis)
Golfer's elbow (medial epicondylitis)

ICD-9CM CODES	
726.31	Medial epicondylitis
726.32	Lateral epicondylitis
723.4	Radial nerve neuralgia

EPIDEMIOLOGY & DEMOGRAPHICS

PREVALENCE:

- 10% to 15% of regular (2 hr/wk) tennis players
- Lateral side is involved five times more often than the medial

PREVALENT AGE AND SEX: Affects men and women equally and is more common in persons 40 yr and older

PHYSICAL FINDINGS & CLINICAL PRESENTATION

- Local tenderness over affected epicondyle
- Reproduction of pain by resistance against wrist extension (lateral) (Fig. 1-107) or flexion (medial)

ETIOLOGY

- Unknown
- Overuse probably causing minor tendinous tears, resulting in inflammation
- Posterior interosseous nerve syndrome: compression of this nerve has occasionally been cited as a possible etiology, especially in cases that have not responded to traditional medical and surgical treatment. In this disorder the site of tenderness is 2 to 3 cm distal to the epicondyle.

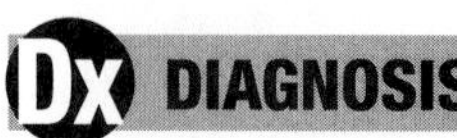

DIAGNOSIS

DIFFERENTIAL DIAGNOSIS

- Cervical radiculopathy
- Intraarticular elbow pathology (osteoarthritis, osteochondritis dissecans, loose body)
- Radial nerve compression
- Ulnar neuropathy
- Medial collateral ligament instability

IMAGING STUDIES

Traction spur or minor soft tissue calcification may be present on plain radiography. Other studies are not usually needed.

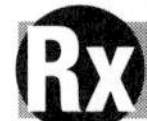

TREATMENT

- Rest, restricted activities
- Ice after exercise
- Stretching exercise program
- Nonsteroidal anti-inflammatory drugs (NSAIDs)
- Local steroid/lidocaine injection (Table 1-25; Fig. 1-108)
- Counterforce brace
- Proper technique in sports activities
- Intermittent immobilization
- Patients with refractory symptoms may benefit from surgical intervention

DISPOSITION

Disorder is self-limited in most cases. Resolution of symptoms may take months to years.

REFERRAL

- If symptoms do not respond to medical management
- For surgical consideration

PEARLS & CONSIDERATIONS

Concepts are changing regarding the underlying pathology of epicondylitis and similar musculoskeletal conditions, which were always thought to be inflammatory in nature. Many are now considered more degenerative, as evidenced by tissue specimens that lack the cellular changes expected with inflammation.

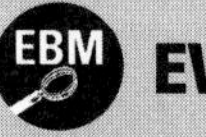

EVIDENCE

Please note: Complete text of EBM for this topic is available online.

Key trials and commentary:

The aims of this double-blind, randomized, placebo-controlled trial were to determine whether ultrasound-guided extracorporeal shock wave therapy (ESWT) reduced pain and improved function in patients with lateral epicondylitis (tennis elbow) in the short term and intermediate term. This study found little evidence to support the use of ESWT for the treatment of lateral epicondylitis and is in keeping with recent systematic reviews of ESWT for lateral epicondylitis that have drawn similar conclusions.

This is a well-designed, randomized controlled trial looking at one treatment modality for lateral elbow pain, that is, lateral epicondylitis. The fact that this article shows no effect on the outcome between the two groups is important. This is important information for the clinician treating this particular entity, which is a hard population of patients to treat. We need to know what works, and what does not work. The power analysis is very important; it substantiates the "no effect" results. The addition of a third group would have been helpful: one that received no treatment (vs. a subtherapeutic-dose treatment). Because there was no effect at 3 or 6 months, most likely we can assume that there would also be no effect at 1 year. Therefore, I commend the authors on not following these patients out to 1 year.[1] Ⓐ

Radial epicondylitis (tennis elbow) is the most frequent type of myotendinosis. Patients can experience substantial loss of function, especially when this condition becomes chronic. A successful therapy has not yet been established. A preliminary study of injections of botulinum toxin A in patients with chronic epicondylitis has shown promising results. This study concluded that local injection of botulinum toxin A is a beneficial treatment for radial epicondylitis (tennis elbow). The treatment can be performed in an outpatient setting and does not impair the patient's ability to work.

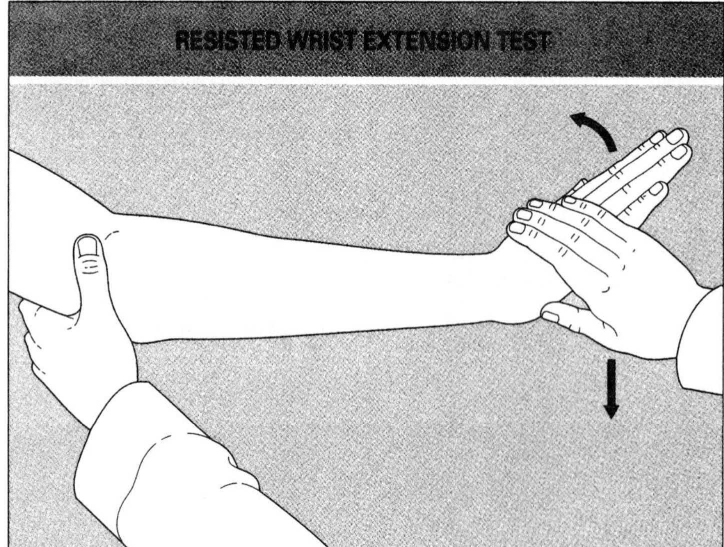

FIGURE 1-107 Resisted wrist extension to test for lateral epicondylitis. The examiner asks the patient to try to extend the wrist but prevents movement by fixing the wrist; this puts tension on the lateral epicondyle without moving the elbow and reproduces the pain of lateral epicondylitis. (From Klippel J et al [eds]: *Primary care rheumatology,* London, 1999, Mosby.)

The most common clinical condition of the elbow continues to be that of tennis elbow and is the most commonly addressed issue in the orthopedic literature referable to this joint. This article is included simply to apprise the reader of the ongoing efforts to manage this ubiquitous condition. Botulinum toxin A is being used in numerous clinical settings. In the elbow, I have used this as an adjunct for the management of chronic refractory elbow stiffness. I think it is of interest to see the application to the patient with tennis elbow. It is of particular interest to note that there was a significant improvement of the patients with botulinum toxin A compared with the placebo. The conclusion that it is a beneficial treatment in this prospective, randomized study is based on this group of patients followed for a relatively short period of time (18 wk). Yet, statistically significant improvement in virtually every category of assessment was realized in this short period. Other modalities have also shown short-term benefit but little value compared with placebo in the long term. Additional studies are indicated to determine whether this treatment modality does, in fact, provide long-term relief or even a cure of this condition.[2] Ⓐ

TABLE 1-25 Guidelines for Common Steroid Injections

Site	Diagnosis	Needle Size (Gauge, Inches)	Anesthetic Volume (ml)
Subacromial bursa	Rotator cuff tendinitis	22, 1½	4-5
Bicipital groove	Biceps tendinitis	22, 1½	2-3
A-C joint	Arthritis	25, 1½	1-2
Lateral medial epicondyle	Epicondylitis	25, ⅝	1.5
First extensor sheath	De Quervain's disease	25, ⅝	1.5
Trochanteric bursa	Tendinitis	22, spinal	4-5
Knee joint	Arthritis	22, 1½	5-10
Knee, soft tissue	Tendinitis	25, 1½	3-4
Plantar fascia	Fasciitis	25, 1½	1.0
Toe metatarsophalangeal	Arthritis	25, ⅝	1.5

From Mercier LR: *Practical orthopedics*, ed 5, St Louis, 2000, Mosby.

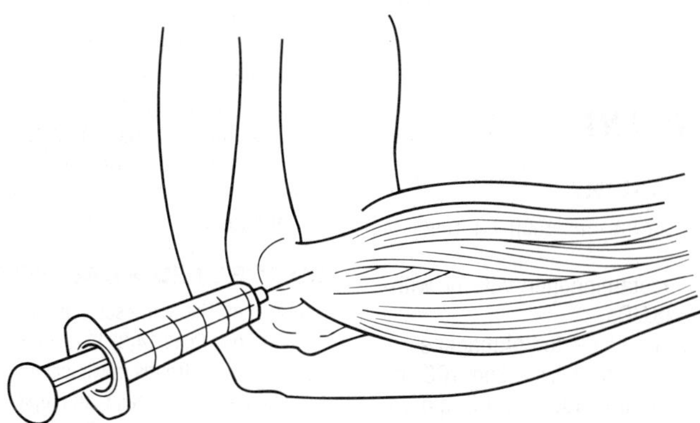

FIGURE 1-108 Soft-tissue injection for lateral epicondylitis. The patient is supine and the elbow is flexed 90 degrees. A 25-gauge needle is used to inject the tender spot, which is usually approximately 1 cm distal to the bony epicondyle. (From Mercier L: *Practical orthopedics*, ed 6, St Louis, 2005, Mosby.)

Evidence-Based References

1. Staples MP et al: A randomized controlled trial of extracorporeal shock wave therapy for lateral epicondylitis (tennis elbow), *J Rheumatol* 35:2038-2046, 2008. Commentary by S.P. Steinman, M.D. Ⓐ
2. Placzek R et al: Treatment of chronic radial epicondylitis with botulinum toxin A: a double-blind, placebo-controlled, randomized multicenter study, *J Bone Joint Surg Am* 89:255-260, 2007. Commentary by B.F. Morrey, M.D. Ⓐ

SUGGESTED READINGS

Ashe MC et al: Tendinopathies in the upper extremity: a paradigm shift, *J Hand Ther* 17(8):329, 2004.

Bunata RE et al: Anatomic factors related to the cause of tennis elbow, *J Bone Joint Surg* 89:1955, 2007.

Calfee RP et al: Management of lateral epicondylitis: current concepts, *J Am Acad Orthop Surg* 16:19, 2008.

Cole BJ, Schumacher HR: Injectable corticosteroids in modern practice, *J Am Acad Orthop Surg* 13:37, 2005.

David TS: Medial elbow pain in the throwing athlete, *Orthopedics* 26:94, 2003.

Haake M et al: Extracorporeal shock wave therapy in the treatment of lateral epicondylitis, *J Bone Joint Surg Am* 84(A):1982, 2002.

Johnson GW et al: Treatment of lateral epicondylitis, *Am Fam Physician* 76:843-48, 2007.

Kohia M et al: Effectiveness of physical therapy treatments of lateral epicondylitis, *J Sports Rehabil* 17:119, 2008.

Nirschl RP, Ashman ES: Tennis elbow tendinosis (epicondylitis), *Instr Course Lect* 53:587, 2004.

Placzek R et al: Treatment of chronic radial epicondylitis with botulinum toxin A: a double-blind, placebo-controlled randomized multicenter study, *J Bone Joint Surg Am* 89A:255, 2007.

Rineer CA, Ruch DS: Elbow tendinopathy and tendon ruptures: epicondylitis, biceps and triceps ruptures, *J Hand Surg Am* 34:566, 2009.

Rompe JD et al: Repetitive low-energy shock wave treatment for chronic lateral epicondylitis in tennis players, *Am J Sports Med* 32:734, 2004.

Sems A et al: Extracorporeal shock wave therapy in the treatment of chronic tendinopathies, *J Am Acad Orthop Surg* 14:195, 2006.

Smidt N et al: Corticosteroid injections, physiotherapy, or wait-and-see policy for lateral epicondylitis: a randomized controlled trial, *Lancet* 359:657, 2002.

Tsai P, Steinberg DR: Median and radial nerve compression about the elbow, *Instr Course Lect* 57:177-185, 2008.

Walz DM et al: Epicondylitis: pathogenesis, imaging, and treatment, *Radiographics* 30:167, 2010.

AUTHOR: **LONNIE R. MERCIER, M.D.**

Epididymitis (PTG)

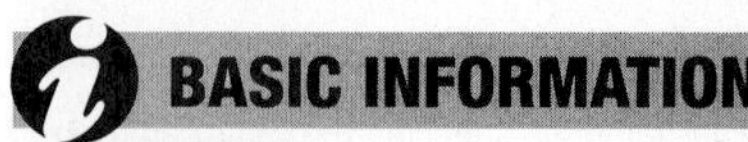

BASIC INFORMATION

DEFINITION

Epididymitis is an inflammatory reaction of the epididymis caused by either an infectious agent or local trauma.

SYNONYMS

Nonspecific bacterial epididymitis
Sexually transmitted epididymitis

ICD-9CM CODES
604.90 Nonvenereal epididymitis
098.0 Gonococcal epididymitis

EPIDEMIOLOGY & DEMOGRAPHICS

INCIDENCE (IN U.S.): Cause of >600,000 visits to physicians per year
PEAK INCIDENCE: Sexually active years
PREDOMINANT SEX: Exclusive to males
PREDOMINANT AGE: All ages affected but usually in sexually active men or older males
CONGENITAL: Congenital urologic structural disorders possibly predisposing to infections

PHYSICAL FINDINGS & CLINICAL PRESENTATION

- Tender swelling of the scrotum with erythema, usually unilateral testicular pain and tenderness
- Dysuria and/or urethral discharge
- Fever and signs of systemic illness (less common)
- Pain and redness on scrotal examination
- Hydrocele or even epididymoorchitis, especially late
- Chronic draining scrotal sinuses with a "beadlike" enlargement of the vas deferens in tuberculous disease

ETIOLOGY

- In young, sexually active men, the most common infectious agents isolated are *N. gonorrhoeae* and *Chlamydia trachomatis.*
- In men >35 yr or with underlying urologic disease:
  1. Gram-negative aerobic rods are predominant.
  2. Similar organisms are found in men following invasive urologic procedures.
  3. Gram-positive cocci are rarely seen in these groups.
  4. Mycobacteria are also a cause of epididymitis.
- Young, prepubertal boys may present with epididymitis caused by coliform bacteria; almost always a complication of underlying urologic disease such as reflux.
- Recently, in AIDS patients, CMV and *Salmonella* epididymitis have been described. CMV may have a negative urine culture. Toxoplasmosis should also be considered as a cause of epididymitis in AIDS patients.

Dx DIAGNOSIS

DIFFERENTIAL DIAGNOSIS

- Orchitis
- Testicular torsion, trauma, or tumor
- Epididymal cyst
- Hydrocele
- Varicocele
- Spermatocele
- Testicular torsion should be considered in all cases.

WORKUP

- Consideration of a full assessment of the urologic tract in patients with bacterial infection, especially if recurrent
- Imaging with sonogram or IVP (possibly procedures of choice)
- If discharge is present: cultures and Gram stain smear of urethral exudate
- In sexually active men: gonococcal cultures of the throat and rectum possibly of value
- If testicular torsion a consideration: radionuclear imaging
- Examination of first void uncentrifuged urine for leukocytes if the urethral Gram stain is negative. A culture and Gram-stained smear of this urine specimen should be obtained along with nucleic acid amplifications studies (ligase chain reaction [LCR]) from urine samples for gonorrhea and *Chlamydia spp.*

LABORATORY TESTS

- Urinalysis and urine culture if dysuria is present or if urinary tract infection is suspected
- VDRL in sexually active men
- PPD placed and chest x-ray viewed if TB suspected
- Rarely, biopsy to assure the diagnosis of tuberculous epididymitis
- HIV testing and counseling

Rx TREATMENT

ACUTE GENERAL Rx

- Ice packs and scrotal elevation for relief of pain
- Analgesia with acetaminophen with or without codeine or NSAIDs
- Antibiotics to cover suspected pathogens
- In sexually active men, doxycycline 100 mg PO bid or tetracycline 500 mg PO qid for 10 days to cover both gonococci and chlamydia; ceftriaxone 250 mg IM as a single dose may be adequate for gonococci alone
- Best treatment for older men with gram-negative bacteriuria: ofloxacin 300 mg PO bid for 10 days or levofloxacin 500 mg PO qd for 10 days
- *Pseudomonas* covered by ciprofloxacin or cefepime (2 g IV q12h)
- Gentamicin in toxic-appearing patients (1 mg/kg IV q8h following a loading dose of 2 mg/kg): doses must be adjusted for renal function and these agents may be more toxic
- Vancomycin (1 g IV q12h) to cover suspected gram-positive infections
- Surgical aspiration of local abscesses or even open surgical drainage
- Diabetics: especially prone to develop more extensive scrotal infections, including Fournier's gangrene
- Reinforcement of compliance with antibiotics to avoid partial treatment

CHRONIC Rx

- Repair of underlying structural defects is considered especially if infections are severe or recur.
- Surgical repair of reflux in young boys should be undertaken promptly and at a young age when possible.
- Sex partners of patient should be referred for evaluation and treatment.

DISPOSITION

Usually self-limited

REFERRAL

- If abscess or chronic structural problems suspected
- If other diagnosis, such as testicular torsion, strongly considered

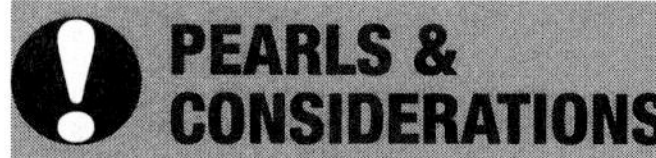

PEARLS & CONSIDERATIONS

- Recurrent epididymitis in sexually active men is usually related to failure to simultaneously treat sexual partners for STDs.
- Recurrent epididymitis in non-sexually active men is generally related to structural-anatomic defects in the genitourinary system or relapsing disease from inadequate initial treatment or antimicrobial resistance.
- Tuberculous epididymitis fails to respond to seemingly adequate antimicrobial therapy even without characteristic radiographic changes on chest films.

SUGGESTED READINGS

Abul F et al: The acute scrotum: a review of 40 cases, *Med Princ Pract* 14(3):177, 2005.

Chen MY et al: Trends in clinical encounters for pelvic inflammatory disease and epididymitis in a national sample of Australian general practices, *Int J STD AIDS* 17(6):384, 2006.

Drury NE et al: Management of acute epididymitis: are European guidelines being followed? *Eur Urol* 46(4): 522, 2004.

Nickel JC et al: Prevalence, diagnosis, characterization, and treatment of prostatitis, interstitial cystitis, and epididymitis in outpatient urological practice: the Canadian PIE Study, *Urology* 66(5):935, 2005.

AUTHORS: **GLENN G. FORT, M.D., M.P.H.,** and **DENNIS J. MIKOLICH, M.D.**

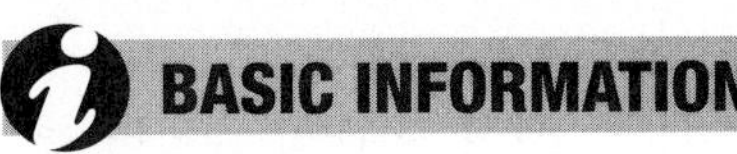

BASIC INFORMATION

DEFINITION

Bleeding in the potential space surrounding the brain, between the dura mater and the inner surface of the skull

SYNONYMS

Extradural hematoma/hemorrhage

ICD-9CM CODES
432.0 Nontraumatic extradural hemorrhage
852.5 Extradural hemorrhage following injury without intracranial wound
852.5 Extradural hemorrhage following injury with open intracranial wound

EPIDEMIOLOGY & DEMOGRAPHICS

INCIDENCE: Exact incidence is unknown, however, it is found in 1% to 4% of traumatic head injury cases and 5% to 15% of autopsy series
PREDOMINANT SEX AND AGE: Male > female
PEAK INCIDENCE: Peak incidence among adolescents and young adults
GENETICS: There is a role for genetics in spontaneous (nontraumatic) epidural hematoma caused by coagulopathies and vascular malformations.
RISK FACTORS: Head trauma associated with skull fracture

PHYSICAL FINDINGS & CLINICAL PRESENTATION

- History of head trauma is present.
- Transient loss of consciousness, followed by a "lucid interval" in 47% of cases, where the patient is free of any neurologic signs or symptoms. This is followed by clinical deterioration.
- Signs and symptoms vary depending on severity.
- Symptoms: headache, vomiting, drowsiness, confusion, aphasia, seizures, paralysis, and even coma are found.
- Signs: external signs of skull fracture—lacerations, ecchymoses, cerebrospinal fluid (CSF) rhinorrhea or otorrhea are observed.
- Altered mental status, nuchal rigidity, photophobia, focal neurologic deficit—paralysis of one limb, unequal pupils, decerebrate posture, coma—are seen.

ETIOLOGY

- Traumatic: commonly caused by arterial injury (the middle meningeal artery) but may also be injury of the anterior meningeal artery, a dural arteriovenous (AV) fistula at the vertex, or from venous bleeding
- Nontraumatic: caused by an infection/eroding abscess, coagulopathy, hemorrhagic tumors, vascular malformations, postsurgical procedures, and in special populations (e.g., pregnant women, patients receiving hemodialysis)

Dx DIAGNOSIS

DIFFERENTIAL DIAGNOSIS

In the setting of head trauma: subdural hematoma, subarachnoid hemorrhage, cerebral contusion, brain laceration, diffuse brain swelling

WORKUP

- Imaging is the mainstay of diagnosis.
- Head CT is the test most commonly used due to its simplicity, widespread use and availability. Typical appearance is a "lens shaped," or "lentiform" hyperdensity (Fig. 1-109).
- Note: Head CT is not conclusive in 8% of cases due to severe anemia, early scanning, and severe hypotension.
- Brain MRI: more sensitive. Indicated in situations in which there is a strong clinical suspicion but no evidence of epidural hematoma on head CT (Fig. 1-110). Preferred in spinal as opposed to intracranial pathology due to higher resolution.
- Angiography: rarely necessary but may be used to evaluate an underlying vascular lesion.
- Note: lumber puncture (LP) is contraindicated in epidural hematoma due to risk of brain stem herniation.

LABORATORY TESTS

- Laboratory tests are helpful as adjunct to diagnosis but are not the mainstay of diagnosis or treatment.
- CBC may be helpful to evaluate for anemia.
- Other tests: renal functions, electrolytes, liver functions may be helpful depending on the case scenario.

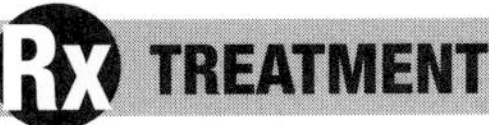

Rx TREATMENT

Acute symptomatic epidural hematoma is a neurologic emergency that requires surgical treatment to prevent permanent brain injury.

NONPHARMACOLOGIC THERAPY

- Burr hole evacuation: this involves drilling a hole in the skull to evacuate the hematoma. It is a lifesaving procedure that is indicated if surgical expertise is limited.
- Craniotomy and hematoma evacuation is the mainstay of treatment. When indicated, identification and ligation of the bleeding vessel.

ACUTE GENERAL Rx

- ABCD: Airway, breathing (may need intubation), circulation, and assess for disability.
- Medical resuscitation maneuvers: head elevation, hyperventilation, monitoring of vital signs and avoidance of hypotension and hyperthermia, sedation if necessary.
- Medications: osmotic diuresis with IV mannitol, antiepileptics may be used to treat or, in some situations, prevent seizures.
- Note: glucocorticoid therapy is *not* indicated following head injury and may be related to increased mortality.
- Evaluation for surgery: nonoperative treatment is only indicated if the patient has no symptoms, no focal neurologic deficit, no coma (Glasgow coma score >8), and epidural hematoma volume is less than 30 ml by CT scan, with clot thickness <15 mm and midline shift of less than 5 mm.
- Nonoperative treatment involves close monitoring, hourly neurologic checks, and serial head CT scans.

CHRONIC Rx

- There is a risk of permanent brain damage whether the disorder is treated or not. Most recovery occurs in the first 6 months with some improvement over 2 years.
- Children recover more quickly.
- Patients should be educated on rehabilitative exercises and to alert medical professionals in the event of new neurologic symptoms.

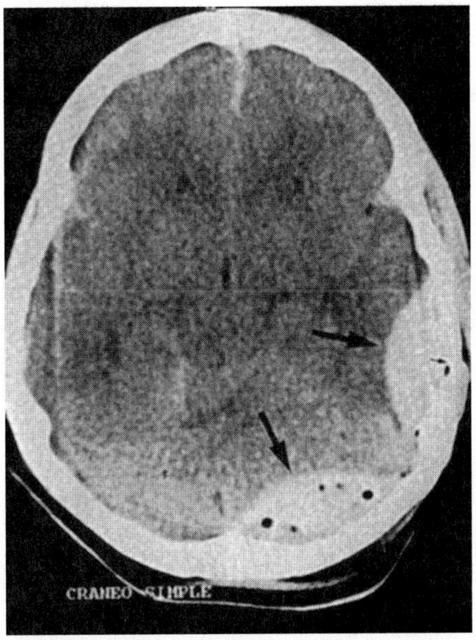

FIGURE 1-109 Head CT showing two epidural hematomas in 23-year-old involved in a motor vehicle accident. Note air bubbles that are a result of linear fracture in the left temporal bone (short arrow).

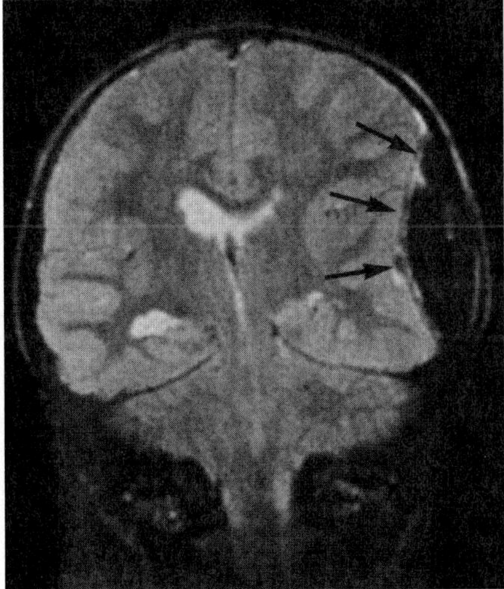

FIGURE 1-110 Epidural hematoma on MRI. Coronal T2-weighted images show hypointense biconvex extraaxial collection in the left temporal region.

- Support and encouragement to patient and family should always be provided.

REFERRAL

Clinical nurse practitioners, pastoral care staff, and social workers to help patients and families are also appropriate.

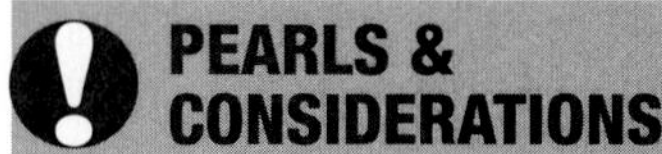

PEARLS & CONSIDERATIONS

- Acute symptomatic epidural hematoma is a neurologic emergency.
- Epidural hematoma should be suspected in any patient with a history of blow to the head leading to a period of loss of consciousness.
- Initial resuscitation is extremely important, but surgery is the mainstay of treatment for acute symptomatic epidural hematoma.

PREVENTION

Should be directed toward preventing head trauma: use of appropriate safety equipment (e.g., helmets, hard hats, safe driving, avoiding to dive into unknown depths)

PATIENT/FAMILY EDUCATION

Online head injury support groups are helpful: www.headinjury.com/linktbisup.htm, www.headinjury.com/, www.dailystrength.org/c/Brain-Injury/support-group.

SUGGESTED READINGS

Bullock MR et al: Surgical management of acute epidural hematomas, *Neurosurgery* 58:S7, 2006.

Kucharczyk J, Moseley E: Imaging of head trauma. In *Imaging of the nervous system diagnostic and therapeutic applications,* vol II, Philadelphia, 2005, Elsevier Mosby.

AUTHOR: **HODA ELTOMI, M.D.**

BASIC INFORMATION

DEFINITION

Epiglottitis is a rapidly progressive cellulitis of the epiglottis and adjacent soft tissue structures with the potential to cause abrupt airway obstruction.

SYNONYMS

Supraglottitis
Cherry-red epiglottitis

ICD-9CM CODES
464.30 Epiglottitis

EPIDEMIOLOGY

INCIDENCE (IN U.S.): Highest in young children, 2 to 4 yr
INCIDENCE (IN U.S.): Unknown
PEAK INCIDENCE: Peaks in young boys ages 2 to 4 yr, but it is reported in adults as well
PREDOMINANT SEX: Males

PHYSICAL FINDINGS & CLINICAL PRESENTATION

- Irritability, fever, dysphonia, and dysphagia
- Respiratory distress, with child tending to lean up and forward
- Often, drooling or oral secretions
- Often, presence of tachycardia and tachypnea
- On visualization, edematous and cherry-red epiglottis
- Often, no classic barking cough as seen in croup
- Possibly fulminant course (especially in children), leading to complete airway obstruction

ETIOLOGY

- In children, *Haemophilus influenzae* type b is usual.
- In adults, *H. influenzae* can be isolated from blood and/or epiglottis (about 26% of cases).
- Pneumococci, streptococci, and staphylococci are also implicated.
- Role of viruses in epiglottitis unclear.

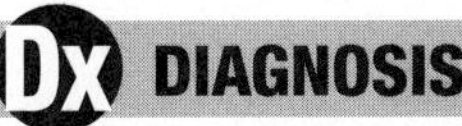

DIAGNOSIS

DIFFERENTIAL DIAGNOSIS

- Croup
- Angioedema
- Retropharyngeal or peritonsillar abscess
- Diphtheria
- Foreign body aspiration
- Lingual tonsillitis

WORKUP

- Cultures of blood and urine
- Lateral neck radiograph to show an enlarged epiglottis, ballooning of the hypopharynx, and normal subglottic structures (Fig. 1-111)
  1. Radiographs are of only moderate sensitivity and specificity and take time to perform.
  2. Visualization of the epiglottitis may be safer in adults than in children.
- Cultures of the epiglottitis

LABORATORY TESTS

- CBC: may reveal a leukocytosis with a shift to the left
- Chest radiograph examination: may reveal evidence of pneumonia in close to 25% of cases
- Cultures of blood, urine, and the epiglottis, as noted previously

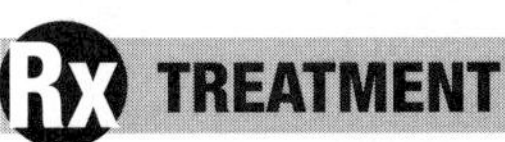

TREATMENT

ACUTE GENERAL Rx

- Maintenance of adequate airway is critical.
- Early placement of an endotracheal or nasotracheal tube in a child is advised.
- Closely follow the adult patient, if no signs of airway obstruction, and defer intubation.
- In children, visualization and intubation are best done in the most controlled environment.
- *H. influenzae* in children is less common thanks to the HIB vaccine.
- Use antibiotics such as ceftriaxone (80 to 100 mg/kg/day in two divided doses), cefotaxime (50 to 180 mg/kg/day in four divided doses), or ampicillin (200 mg/kg/day in four divided doses) with chloramphenicol (75 to 100 mg/kg/day in four divided doses).
- If possible, obtain cultures before initiating antibiotics.
- Treat adult patients with similar antibiotic regimens.
- If there is an unvaccinated child at home (or in a day care center) who is >4 yr and living with an index case, give close family contacts of the patient (including adults) rifampin 20 mg/kg/day for 4 days (up to 600 mg/day) for prophylaxis.
- Role of epinephrine or corticosteroids in the management of epiglottitis is not firmly established.

DISPOSITION

Invasive *Haemophilus influenzae* infections and epiglottitis are reportable illnesses; this may be particularly important in recognizing an outbreak in a day care center with unvaccinated children.

REFERRAL

- Close cooperation between the pediatrician or internist, anesthesiologist, and otorhinolaryngologist, especially when epiglottis is visualized and when the patient requires endotracheal intubation
- Best managed in a critical care setting or ICU

PEARLS & CONSIDERATIONS

The incidence of epiglottitis has diminished markedly since the introduction of the conjugate vaccine against *H. influenzae* serotype B into routine childhood immunization.

SUGGESTED READINGS

Hafidh MA et al: Acute epiglottitis in adults: a recent experience with 10 cases, *J Laryngol Otol* 120(4): 310, 2006.

Wood N et al: Epiglottitis in Sydney before and after the introduction of vaccination against Haemophilus influenzae type b disease, *Intern Med J,* 35(9): 530, 2005.

AUTHORS: **GLENN G. FORT, M.D., M.P.H.,** and **DENNIS J. MIKOLICH, M.D.**

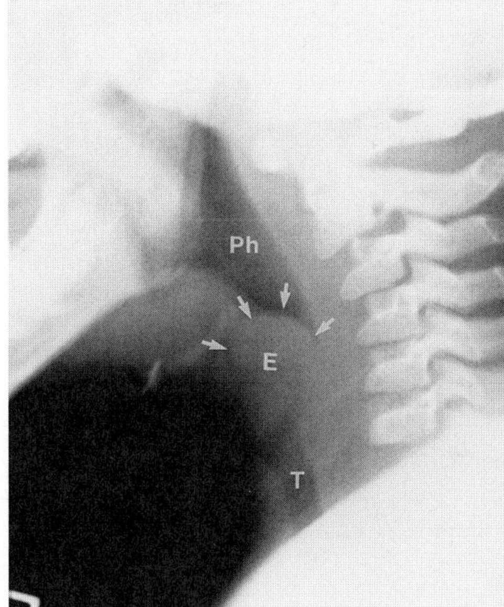

FIGURE 1-111 Epiglottitis. A lateral soft tissue view of the neck shows a ballooned pharynx *(Ph)* with swollen epiglottis *(E)* in the shape of a large thumbprint *(arrows). T,* Trachea. (From Mettler FA [ed]: *Primary care radiology,* Philadelphia, 2000, WB Saunders.)

E
Diseases and Disorders I

Episcleritis

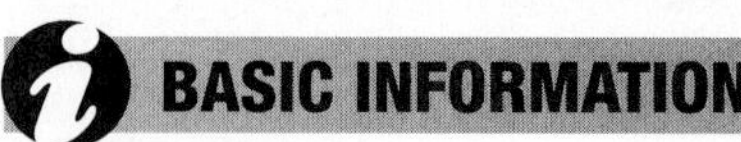

BASIC INFORMATION

DEFINITION

Episcleritis is an inflammation of the episclera, the thin layer of vascular elastic tissue between the sclera and conjunctiva.

ICD-9CM CODES
379.0 Scleritis and episcleritis

EPIDEMIOLOGY & DEMOGRAPHICS

INCIDENCE (IN U.S.): Relatively rare in an ophthalmologic practice
PEAK INCIDENCE: Most common in middle and old age
PREDOMINANT SEX: None
PREDOMINANT AGE: 43 yr

PHYSICAL FINDINGS & CLINIAL PRESENTATION

- Red, vascular injection of conjunctiva with engorged and enlarged blood vessels beneath the conjunctions (Fig. 1-112)
- Pain in area of inflammation that is usually localized

ETIOLOGY

Associated with collagen-vascular diseases, vasculitis, trauma; often nonspecific

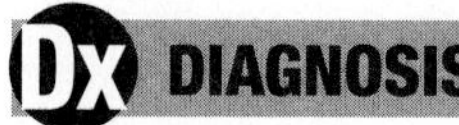

DIAGNOSIS

DIFFERENTIAL DIAGNOSIS

- Acute glaucoma
- Conjunctivitis
- Scleritis
- Subconjunctival hemorrhage
- Congenital or lymphoid masses
- The differential diagnosis of "red eye" is described in Section II

WORKUP

Eye examination, general check-up for collagen-vascular disease or other autoimmune diseases

LABORATORY TESTS

Studies for collagen-vascular disease (e.g., ANA, ESR, RF)

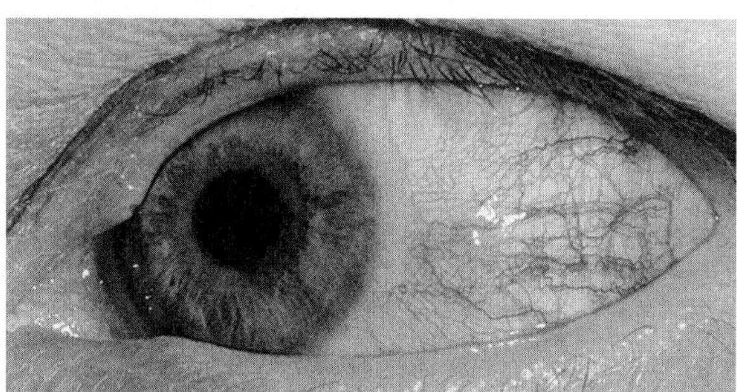

FIGURE 1-112 Nodular episcleritis in a patient with gout. (From Palay D [ed]: *Ophthalmology for the primary care physician,* St Louis, 1997, Mosby.)

Rx TREATMENT

NONPHARMACOLOGIC THERAPY

Warm compresses

ACUTE GENERAL Rx

- Topical steroids, 1% prednisolone if no glaucoma; nonsteroidals if there is a tendency for glaucoma
- Nonsteroidal anti-inflammatory drugs (NSAIDs): treat underlying systemic disease

CHRONIC Rx

NSAIDs such as Voltaren or Acular qd

DISPOSITION

Close follow-up needed

REFERRAL

To ophthalmologist if patient unresponsive to treatment after a few days

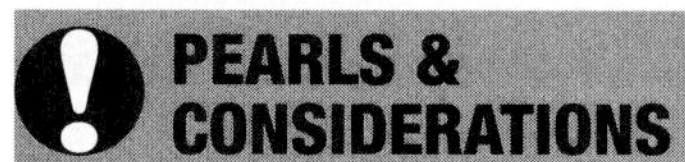

PEARLS & CONSIDERATIONS

COMMENTS

- Often associated with collagen-vascular disease
- Usually related to systemic disease

SUGGESTED READINGS

Jabs DA et al: Episcleritis and scleritis: clinical features and treatment results, *Am J Ophthalmol* 130(4):469, 2000.

Paresio CE, Meier FM: Systemic disorders associated with episcleritis and scleritis, *Curr Opin Ophthalmol* 12(6):471, 2002.

Shaw C et al: Rheumatoid arthritis and ocular involvement, *J Indian Med Assoc* 101(9)537, 2003.

AUTHOR: **MELVYN KOBY, M.D.**

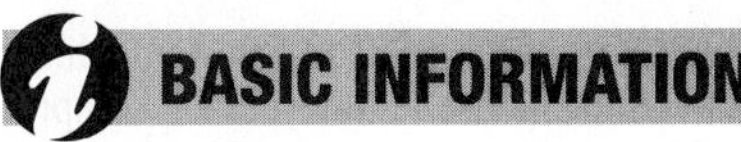

BASIC INFORMATION

DEFINITION

Epistaxis is defined as bleeding from the nose or nasal hemorrhage and is classified as either anterior or posterior.

SYNONYMS

Nosebleed

ICD-9CM CODES
784.7 Epistaxis

EPIDEMIOLOGY & DEMOGRAPHICS

- Epistaxis accounts for one of every 200 emergency department visits in the U.S. annually.
- It increases in frequency after age 20 yr and reaches the highest levels among the elderly population.
- More than 80% of cases of epistaxis are anterior in origin (Little's area) and occur from Kiesselbach's plexus (Fig. 1-113).
- Only 5% of patients with epistaxis have posterior bleeds.

PHYSICAL FINDINGS & CLINICAL PRESENTATION

- Nosebleed
- Hypotension and hemodynamic instability with acute, severe epistaxis

ETIOLOGY

- Approximately 90% of epistaxis events are idiopathic.
- Common identifiable causes are:
  1. Cold, dry environment
  2. Trauma (nose picking, accidents, and physical altercations)
  3. Structural deformities (septal deviations or spurs, chronic perforations)
  4. Inflammatory (rhinosinusitis, nasal polyposis)
  5. Allergies
  6. Foreign bodies in the nasal cavity
  7. Tumors (juvenile angiofibroma)
  8. Irritants
  9. Hypertension
  10. Coagulopathy (hemophilia, von Willebrand's disease, thrombocytopenia)
  11. Osler-Weber-Rendu disease
  12. Renal failure
  13. Drugs: aspirin, nonsteroidal antiinflammatory drugs, warfarin, alcohol, sildenafil, and tadalafil
  14. Blood vessel disorders (connective tissue disease, hereditary hemorrhagic telangiectasia)
  15. Pseudoaneurysm and aneurysm of the internal carotid artery might present as epistaxis

DIAGNOSIS

A good attempt should be made to directly visualize the source of bleeding to confirm the diagnosis and determine the best treatment.

DIFFERENTIAL DIAGNOSIS

Pseudoepistaxis must be ruled out. Common extranasal sites of bleeding that can simulate epistaxis include:

1. Pulmonary hemoptysis
2. Bleeding esophageal varices
3. Tumor bleeding from the pharynx, larynx, or trachea

WORKUP

The workup should include laboratory blood testing to exclude obvious causes. Type and cross in anticipation of transfusion if the bleeding is severe.

LABORATORY TESTS

- Hemoglobin and hematocrit
- Platelet count
- Blood urea nitrogen and creatinine
- Coagulation studies (prothrombin time and partial thromboplastin time)
- Type and crossmatching of blood products

IMAGING STUDIES

Radiographic studies are usually not helpful.

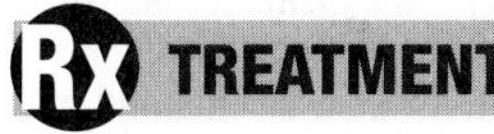

TREATMENT

NONPHARMACOLOGIC THERAPY

- Digital compression or pinching of the lower soft cartilaginous part of the nose for 10 min is the method of choice.
- Use cotton or tissue plug.
- The patient should be sitting and leaning forward, breathing through the mouth, allowing blood to flow out of the nostrils as opposed to bending backward, which would allow the blood to flow down the throat.
- Application of cold compresses to the bridge of the nose to cause a vasoconstrictive effect; the patient may also suck on ice to achieve this effect.

ACUTE GENERAL Rx

Anterior epistaxis:

- Local vasoconstriction is performed by moistening a cotton pledget with either:
  1. 4% lidocaine with 1:1000 epinephrine
  2. 4% lidocaine with 1% phenylephrine (Neo-Synephrine)
  3. 4% lidocaine with 0.05% oxymetazoline (Afrin)
  4. 4% cocaine or cocaine 25% in paraffin base ointment and inserting the pledget into the nasal cavity with bayonet forceps.
- Cauterization with silver nitrate or trichloroacetic acid is performed once hemostasis is achieved.
- Anterior nasal packing is needed when local measures are unsuccessful. Nasal packing is performed under local anesthesia and is done by inserting Vaseline gauze strips in layers from the floor of the nasal cavity to the front entrance of the nasal orifice. Enough pressure is placed to tamponade the epistaxis (Fig. 1-114).
- Other commercially available nasal packing uses sponge packs that expand when exposed to blood or moisture and can be used for anterior epistaxis.

Posterior epistaxis:

- Posterior nasal packing
  1. Commercially available nasal sponge packing can be applied
  2. Rolled gauze technique (see Dai, Jurges, 2005)
- Foley catheter balloon insertion into the nasopharynx can be tried in patients with posterior epistaxis (for the proper technique, see reference)

CHRONIC Rx

- If acute treatment fails to stop the bleeding or the site of bleeding cannot be located, electrocautery or endoscopic cauterization can be used.

FIGURE 1-113 Kiesselbach's plexus on the anterior septum derives blood supply from the superior labial, descending palatine, and sphenopalatine arteries. (From Noble J: *Primary care medicine,* ed 3, St Louis, 2001, Mosby.)

- Electrocautery is performed after suitable anesthesia, such as application of a topical anesthetic followed by local anesthetic injection. Only one side of the nasal septum should be cauterized at a time because perforation can result from bilateral cauterization.
- Arterial ligation or embolization has been used in refractory posterior epistaxis.
- For cases involving irritated or inflamed mucosa, a conservative regimen of triamcinolone 0.025%, Nemdyn, Nasalate, or equivalent cream should be applied once a week, combined with nightly application of a small quantity of petroleum jelly to the septum before bedtime.

DISPOSITION

- Most cases of anterior epistaxis from Kiesselbach's plexus can be stopped by nasal compression and local vasoconstriction or cauterization.
- Nasal packing with gauze or sponge can control 90% of anterior epistaxis.
- Anterior and posterior packs are removed in 2 to 3 days. Hospital admission should be considered in patients who cannot be expected to return for prompt follow-up because prolonged packing increases the risk of pressure necrosis, toxic shock syndrome, sinus infections, and other complications.

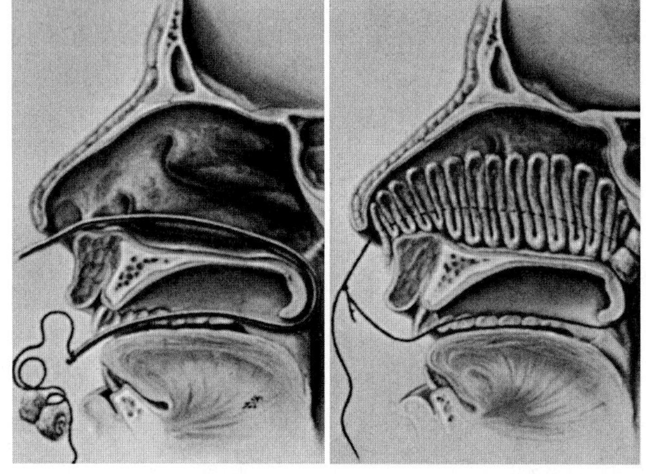

FIGURE 1-114 Packing of the nose for epistaxis with a postnasal pack and an anterior nose pack. (From Boies LR et al: *Fundamentals of otolaryngology: a textbook of ear, nose, and throat diseases,* ed 4, Philadelphia, 1964, WB Saunders.)

- Although rare, epistaxis can lead to death by aspiration of blood, hemodynamic compromise from rapid excessive blood loss, or toxic shock syndrome.

REFERRAL

- If epistaxis cannot be controlled, an ear-nose-throat (ENT) specialist should be called for assistance.
- ENT specialist should be consulted in any patient with posterior epistaxis requiring posterior packing.

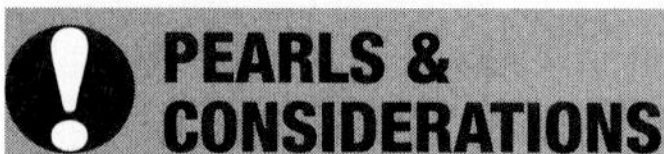

PEARLS & CONSIDERATIONS

COMMENTS

- Silver nitrate cauterization, if done on both sides of the nasal septum, can lead to septal perforation and should be discouraged.
- If anterior nasal packing is done, broad-spectrum antibiotics (e.g., amoxicillin-clavulanate 250 mg PO tid or trimethoprim-sulfamethoxazole 1 tablet PO bid) are used until the anterior packs are removed.
- Complications of nasal packing include:
  1. Aspiration
  2. Dislodged packing
  3. Infection
  4. Nasal trauma

SUGGESTED READINGS

Dai A, Jurges E: The problem with nose bleeds, *Emerg Med J* 22(8):596, 2005.

Leong SC et al: No frills management of epistaxis, *Emerg Med J* 22(7):470, 2005.

Pallin DJ et al: Epidemiology of epistaxis in U.S. emergency departments, 1992 to 2001, *Ann Emerg Med* 46(1):77, 2005.

Pope LE, Hobbs CG: Epistaxis: an update on current management, *Postgrad Med J* 81(955):309, 2005.

AUTHOR: **TANYA ALI, M.D.**

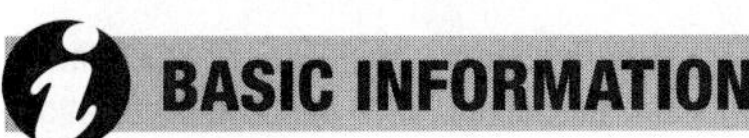

DEFINITION

Epstein-Barr virus infection refers to a disease caused by Epstein-Barr virus (EBV), a human herpesvirus.

SYNONYMS

Infectious mononucleosis (IM)
Kissing disease

ICD-9CM CODES
075 Mononucleosis

EPIDEMIOLOGY & DEMOGRAPHICS

INCIDENCE (IN U.S.): 5 cases/100,000 persons per yr of IM

PREDOMINANT SEX: Neither, although peak incidence occurs about 2 yr earlier in women

PREDOMINANT AGE:
- Clinical evidence of IM: occurs most commonly at ages 15 to 24 yr
- EBV infection: occurs earlier in life in lower socioeconomic groups

PHYSICAL FINDINGS & CLINICAL PRESENTATION

- Most EBV infections either are asymptomatic or cause a nonspecific viral illness.
- Incubation period is 1 to 2 mo, possibly followed by a prodrome of anorexia, low-grade fever, malaise, headache, and chills; after several days, clinical triad of pharyngitis, moderate to high fever, and adenopathy may appear, accompanied by fatigue and malaise.
- Pharyngitis is usually the most severe symptom; white or necrotic appearance exudates are common.
- Symmetrical lymphadenopathy is most prominent in the posterior more than anterior cervical region but may be diffuse.
- Splenomegaly (50% of cases) is possible, most commonly during the second week of illness.
- Maculopapular or morbilliform rash is uncommon but will occur in patients who receive ampicillin. Patients may have palatal petechiae, periorbital, or palpebral edema. Mucocutaneous oral hairy leukoplakia (OHL), which is associated with intense EBV replication and the action of EBV-encoded proteins such as latent membrane protein-1, may occur.
- Possible IM presentation: fever and adenopathy without pharyngitis.
- Nausea, vomiting, and anorexia are frequent in patients with IM, probably reflecting mild hepatitis encountered in 90% of infected individuals.
- Although complications such as spleen rupture, airway obstruction, and malignancy may be severe and fatal, they are uncommon and tend to resolve completely.
- Hematologic involvement includes hemolytic or aplastic anemia, thrombocytopenia, thrombotic thrombocytopenic purpura/hemolytic-uremic syndrome, and disseminated intravascular coagulation (DIC). Pneumonia, myocarditis, pancreatitis, mesenteric adenitis, myositis, and glomerulonephritis may occur as well. Nervous system involvement includes Guillain-Barré syndrome, facial nerve palsy, meningoencephalitis, aseptic meningitis, transfer myelitis, peripheral neuritis and optic neuritis.
- IM is usually a self-limited illness. Acute symptoms resolve in 1 to 2 wk, but symptoms of malaise and fatigue often persist for months.
- EBV is related to lymphoproliferative syndromes in transplant recipients and in AIDS patients.
- Increasing evidence showing an association between EBV infection and African Burkitt's, B-cell, T-cell lymphoma, and nasopharyngeal carcinoma.

ETIOLOGY

- EBV is a ubiquitous virus.
- Infection during childhood is much less likely to cause significant illness.
- Frequency of IM in late adolescence is attributed to the onset of social contact between the sexes.
- Close personal contact is usually necessary for transmission, although EBV is occasionally transmitted by blood transfusion; transfer via saliva while kissing may be responsible for many cases.

Dx DIAGNOSIS

DIFFERENTIAL DIAGNOSIS

- Heterophile-negative IM caused by cytomegalovirus (CMV)
- Although clinical presentation similar, CMV more frequently follows transfusion
- Bacterial and viral causes of pharyngitis
- Toxoplasmosis
- Acute retroviral syndrome of HIV
- Lymphoma
- Lyme disease

WORKUP

Heterophile antibody and CBC with blood smear

LABORATORY TESTS

- Increased WBC common, with a relative lymphocytosis of more than 50% and neutropenia are identified.
- Hallmark of IM: atypical lymphocytes of more than 10% (not pathognomonic) are found.
- Mild thrombocytopenia is present.
- Falling hematocrit signals the possibility of splenic rupture or immune hemolytic anemia.
- Elevated hepatocellular enzymes and cryoglobulins are found in most cases.
- Heterophile antibody:
  - As measured by the monospot test, may be positive at presentation or may appear later in the course of illness.
  - Negative test is repeated in 1 wk if clinical suspicion is high.
  - A positive test has been reported with primary HIV infection.
- Viral capsid antigen (VCA) IgG and IgM are rarely used for diagnosis, but better value in children because heterophile antibody is negative in most of children younger than 8 years.
- PCR DNA for CMV is the test of choice in transplant recipients who develop lymphoproliferative syndromes.

IMAGING STUDIES

Chest radiograph examination:
- May rarely show infiltrates
- Possible elevated left hemidiaphragm with splenic rupture

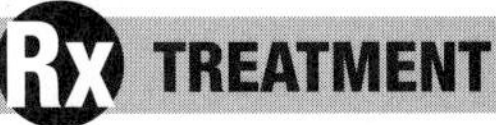

NONPHARMACOLOGIC THERAPY

- Supportive including rest
- Splenectomy if rupture occurs
- Transfusions for severe anemia or thrombocytopenia

ACUTE GENERAL Rx

- Pharmacologic therapy is not indicated in uncomplicated illness.
- Avoid aspirin due to the risk of Reye's syndrome.
- Avoid ampicillin and amoxicillin as their use can frequently precipitate a nonallergic rash.
- Use of steroids is suggested in patients who have severe thrombocytopenia, hemolytic anemia, impending airway obstruction resulting from enlarged tonsils, or fulminant liver failure. Prednisone 60 to 80 mg PO qd for 3 days, then tapered over 1 to 2 wk.
- Although it may reduce initial viral shedding, there is little evidence to support the use of antiviral agents such as acyclovir in the management of IM.

CHRONIC Rx

An extremely rare, chronic form of IM with persistent fevers and fatigue has been described and should be differentiated from chronic fatigue syndrome, which is not related to EBV.

DISPOSITION

Eventual resolution of all symptoms

REFERRAL

If more than mild illness

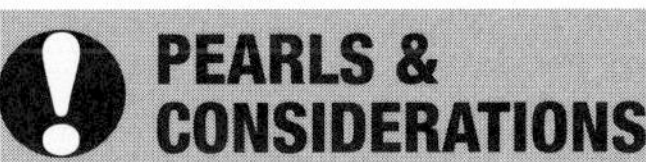

COMMENTS

Avoidance of contact sports during the first month of illness because splenic rupture can occur even in the absence of clinically detectable splenomegaly.

SUGGESTED READINGS

Bauer CC et al: Serum Epstein-Barr virus DNA load in primary Epstein-Barr virus infection, *J Med Virol* 75(1):54, 2005.

Crum NF: Epstein Barr virus hepatitis: case series and review, *South Med J* 99(5):544, 2006.
Ebell MH: Epstein-Barr virus: infectious mononucleosis, *Am Family Physician* 70:1279, 2004.
Kaygusuz I et al: The role of viruses in idiopathic peripheral facial palsy and cellular immune response, *Am J Otolaryngol* 25(6):401, 2004.
Ozyar E et al: Prognostic role of Ebstein-Barr virus latent membrane protein-1 and interleukin-10 expression in patients with nasopharyngeal carcinoma, *Cancer Invest* 22(4):483, 2004.
Thorley-Lawson DA, Gross A: Persistence of the Epstein-Barr virus and the origins of associated lymphomas, *N Engl J Med* 350:1328, 2004.
Vernon SD et al: Preliminary evidence of mitochondrial dysfunction associated with post-infective fatigue after acute infection with Epstein Barr virus, *BMC Infect Dis* 6:15, 2006.

AUTHORS: **MONZR M. AL MALKI, M.D., DENNIS J. MIKOLICH, M.D.,** and **GLENN G. FORT, M.D., M.P.H.**

BASIC INFORMATION

DEFINITION

Erectile dysfunction (ED) is the persistent inability to achieve or sustain a penile erection of adequate rigidity to make intercourse possible or satisfactory.

SYNONYMS

Impotence
Male erectile disorder
Sexual dysfunction (a nonspecific term)

ICD-9CM CODES

F52.2 Male erectile disorder (DSM-IV Code: 302.72 Male erectile disorder)

EPIDEMIOLOGY & DEMOGRAPHICS

PREVALENCE (IN U.S.):

- Increases with age and presence of vascular comorbidities.
- Approximately 7% for men in their 20s, 18% for men in their 50s, 25% for men in their 60s, 80% for men in their 80s.

PREDOMINANT SEX: By definition, only in males

PREDOMINANT AGE: Increases with age

RISK FACTORS: Coronary artery disease, peripheral vascular disease, hypertension, diabetes mellitus, hypercholesterolemia, numerous medications, alcohol, smoking or drug abuse

PHYSICAL FINDINGS & CLINICAL PRESENTATION

- Psychogenic impotence: inability to obtain erection, inability to obtain or maintain an adequate erection, or the loss of erection before completion of sexual intercourse; nocturnal penile tumescence usually normal
- Organic impotence: inability to obtain an erection or inability to obtain an adequate erection; nocturnal penile tumescence usually abnormal

ETIOLOGY

- Most cases are caused by organic problems related to neurologic, hormonal, or vascular abnormalities or prescription or recreational drugs.
- Psychogenic erectile dysfunction results from mental stress, depression, widower syndrome, and performance anxiety. Characterized objectively by nocturnal and morning erections and otherwise negative test results.
- Vascular disease: History of hypertension (HTN), peripheral vascular disease, ischemic heart disease, diabetes, smoking. In approximately 40% of men >50 yr, the primary cause of ED is related to atherosclerotic disease, diabetes mellitus (DM), neuropathy, or vascular disease.
- Medication side effects: Antihypertensives such as thiazides and clonidine (consider change to ACE inhibitors and calcium channel blockers with lower reported incidence of ED); antiandrogens such as spironolactone, finasteride, ketoconazole; cimetidine; antidepressants such as selective serotonin reuptake inhibitors [SSRIs]; and antipsychotics.
- Alcohol and nicotine use.
- Recreational drugs, including cocaine, heroin, amphetamines, and marijuana. These may increase libido but impair performance.
- Hormonal dysfunction such as testosterone deficiency (decreases libido and erection), hypothyroidism or hyperthyroidism, hyperprolactinemia, and adrenal insufficiency.
- Neurogenic causes including spinal cord lesions, cortical lesions, and peripheral neuropathies.
- Pelvic surgeries such as radical prostatectomy or cystectomy.

Dx DIAGNOSIS

DIFFERENTIAL DIAGNOSIS

- A useful tool to diagnose and evaluate ED severity is the Sexual Health Inventory for Men.
- Psychogenic dysfunction distinguished from organic.
- Determine etiology of organic dysfunction.
- ED possible in the setting of another psychiatric condition (e.g., depression or obsessive-compulsive disorder).

WORKUP

- Clinical history should include time course (abrupt onset may correlate with reversible cause such as medication, psychosocial stress, psychiatric complaint), cause (psychogenic vs. organic), and change in libido.
- Report of spontaneous nocturnal or morning erections indicate intact neurologic reflexes and penile blood flow.
- Decreased libido may indicate endocrinologic or psychogenic cause.
- Medical and social history (including partner report) should address cardiac disease symptoms and risk factors (HTN, DM, hyperlipidemia, smoking, and substance abuse), pelvic surgery, medications, and mental health.
- Physical examination to check blood pressure, femoral and peripheral pulses, femoral bruits; gynecomastia; neuronal damage (genital sensation, cremasteric reflex); direct penile damage (e.g., plaque formation such as Peyronie's disease); prostate examination; or testicular atrophy and other secondary sexual characteristics.

LABORATORY TESTS

- Only pursue serologic evaluation if suspect organic cause.
- Screen with fasting glucose in all men. Consider lipid panel, thyroid-stimulating hormone, morning serum testosterone. If decreased testosterone, check prolactin, follicle-stimulating hormone, and luteinizing hormone.
- If normal libido and examination results, unlikely to be testosterone deficiency, so no need to check serum testosterone.

IMAGING STUDIES

Imaging studies are rarely performed except in situations of pelvic trauma or surgery.

OTHER STUDIES

- Nocturnal penile tumescence testing very specific for distinguishing psychogenic versus organic causes.
- Neurogenic etiologies examined by the cremasteric reflex (inner-thigh touch elicits scrotal contraction), the bulbocavernosus reflex, or the pudendal-evoked response.
- Intracorporeal injection of prostaglandin E_1 to distinguish vascular and nonvascular etiologies (erection is achieved in patients with normal vascular systems). If no erection with direct injection of vasoactive substance, consider duplex ultrasound of penile vasculature.

Rx TREATMENT

NONPHARMACOLOGIC THERAPY

- Various psychotherapeutic approaches: cognitive-behavioral therapy preferred because it is the most focused; success rates decrease with advancing age and duration of symptoms.
- Psychosexual therapy (sex therapy and couples therapy) is first line for psychogenic ED and for adjunctive therapy in ED from any cause. Therapy is used to address social issues that contribute to impotence.
- Mechanical vacuum devices (function by drawing blood into corpus cavernosum) are 70% to 90% effective, but they are difficult to use and cumbersome.
- Incorporate vascular risk factor reduction including counsel on diet, exercise, smoking cessation, ETOH intake and screening/treatment for HTN, insulin resistance, and hypercholesterolemia as appropriate.

ACUTE GENERAL Rx

- First-line treatment: In setting of sexual stimulation, three selective phosphodiesterase type 5 (PDE5) inhibitors prolong nitric oxide–induced vasodilation by increase of intracavernosal cyclic guanosine monophosphate levels. All three PDE5 inhibitors have similar efficacy and tolerability. Sildenafil (Viagra) 30 to 60 min before sexual activity is the most common first-line therapy and lasts 4 hr. Vardenafil (Levitra) is taken 30 to 60 min before sexual activity and lasts 4 hr. Patient must avoid food and excessive amounts of alcohol with sildenafil and vardenafil. Tadalafil (Cialis), with longer period of responsiveness (to 36 hr), gives enhanced patient convenience. Patients can take tadalafil several hours before sexual activity, although about half of men respond by 30 min.
- With PDE5 inhibitors, avoid concomitant use of nitrates (absolute contraindication), alpha-adrenergic blockers, drugs that inhibit or induce cytochrome P450 CYP3A4, and drugs that prolong the QT interval. Caution in men who have had myocardial infarction in the past

6 mo, resting hypotension or uncontrolled hypertension, unstable angina, positive exercise stress test or poor exercise tolerance. Counsel on side effects of headache, flushing, dyspepsia, nasal congestion, changes in color perception, and priapism (rare).
- Second-line treatment if PDE5 inhibitors fail: intraurethral alprostadil (prostaglandin E_1 [medicated urethral suppository]) applied into meatus of penis before intercourse; other more invasive intracavernosal injections of vasodilators (e.g., papaverine or prostaglandin E_1 pellet). Consider combining intraurethral alprostadil with sildenafil.
- Second-line treatment alternative: vacuum constriction pump; has variable satisfaction rate.

CHRONIC Rx

- Psychosexual therapy is helpful as an adjunctive treatment in all cases. Sexual therapists can also re-motivate patients in whom PDE5 inhibitors initially failed.
- Psychogenic impotence: PDE5 inhibitors are effective in patients with depression because tissues, nerves, hormones, and vasculature are normal. Full psychologic evaluation is recommended before starting treatment so underlying problem is addressed.
- For men not responding to other approaches: penile prosthesis.
- Testosterone therapy in elderly hypogonadal men; must rule out prostate cancer before use.

DISPOSITION

- When ED has an organic cause it does not remit unless the cause is corrected; therefore it is usually a chronic condition.
- Psychogenic-acquired ED will remit spontaneously in 15% to 30% of cases.
- Lifelong ED is usually a chronic and unremitting condition.
- Situational ED may remit with changes in social environment but usually recurs.

REFERRAL

- If psychotherapy, sex therapy, or invasive organic treatment required
- To urology if PDE5 inhibitors fail

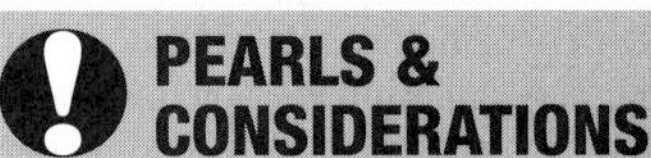

PEARLS & CONSIDERATIONS

- Commonly evaluated and treated by primary care physician; refer to urologist if oral therapy fails or surgery is required.
- PDE5 inhibitors are treatment of choice for most causes of ED. Main contraindications include HTN, nitrate use, decompensated cardiac disease, and alpha-adrenergic blockers.
- For optimal response, patients should be appropriately informed of proper use, precautions, and adverse effects of PDE5 inhibitors. Try six to eight times at optimal doses before declaring PDE5 inhibitors a failure. Consider switching among the three PDE5 inhibitors if one fails.

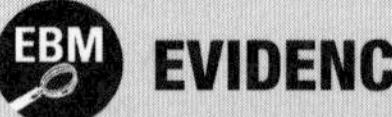

EVIDENCE

Please note: Complete text of EBM for this topic is available online.

Key trials and commentary:

With once-daily administration of tadalafil, dosing and sexual activity would no longer need to be temporally linked for patients with erectile dysfunction (ED).This study sought to evaluate long-term safety and efficacy of tadalafil 5 mg dosed once daily for the treatment of ED. This study showed that in these long-term, open-label, once-daily dosing studies, tadalafil 5 mg was well tolerated and effective, making it a viable alternative to the current on-demand dosing of tadalafil for men with ED.

Daily dose tadalafil appears to be safe and efficacious in the management of ED. This new regimen for use of tadalafil represents the first time that a pharmacological treatment for ED has been recommended as a daily supplement. Although somewhat similar to the concept of penile rehabilitation after radical pelvic surgery, the principle of this treatment is restoration of sexual function rather than prevention of end organ damage.

This new approach suggests a paradigm shift in our pharmacological management of ED. Previous pharmacological treatments have used a reactive, on-demand management scheme. Daily dosing makes ED a chronic disease to be managed with a chronic, steady-state dosing of medication. The long half-life of tadalafil makes attainment of baseline steady-state concentrations of the drug feasible. The significance of this change in concept is not immediately clear but may signify a change in how ED is perceived both by patients and providers.

Daily dosing is most likely to benefit men for whom sexual activity is frequent and unpredictable. Men who engage in intercourse less frequently than twice a week may minimize their exposure to the drug by using on-demand therapy. Interestingly, total drug dosing may be lower with a 5 mg daily dose than it would be with a higher on-demand dose in men who engage in intercourse more than twice a week.[1] Ⓐ

Cynics may argue that this new dosing regimen is a ploy by which to sell more drugs. Certainly, there may be some truth to that assertion, but that does not eliminate the possibility that daily dosing may be preferable for some men with ED.[1] Ⓐ

A separate study compared the efficacy of testosterone gel (T-gel) vs. placebo as adjunctive therapy to sildenafil in hypogonadal men with ED who do not respond to sildenafil alone. This study showed that T-gel taken with sildenafil may be beneficial in improving erectile function in hypogonadal men with erectile dysfunction who are unresponsive to sildenafil alone.

In this randomized and blinded study of hypogonadal men with ED refractory to phosphodiesterase type 5 (PDE5) inhibitor monotherapy, a significant improvement in International Index of Erectile Function (IIEF) was noted in the group treated with a daily topical testosterone preparation (5 g) as an adjunct therapy to PDE5 inhibitor. Significant improvements were also noted in orgasmic function and overall sexual satisfaction in the testosterone-treated group. Interestingly, there was no correlation between serum testosterone at study end point and improvement in IIEF scores. Although a definitive conclusion on what this means cannot be gleaned from these data, it may be hypothesized that there is a minimum level of serum testosterone, which is necessary for normal erectile function. This value is likely to vary between individuals.

This study speaks for the importance of assessing for hypogonadism in the ED population, particularly in cases of PDE5 inhibitor failure. Supplementation of testosterone may obviate the need for progression to more invasive erectogenic therapies in some select men with ED. Controversy still exists, however.[2] Ⓐ

Another trial showed that in men with mild to moderate ED, responsiveness to sildenafil may persist much longer than 4 hours.

PDE5 inhibitors with a long half-life offer the theoretical advantage of increased flexibility with respect to interval between when the drug is taken and when intercourse is attempted. This advantage may be useful for couples who wish to have intercourse more than once in a prolonged interval of time, couples who may be interrupted at the time intercourse is planned, and those who wish to dissociate medication use from sexual expression.

This interesting article suggests that even PDE5 inhibitors with short half-life may exert a prolonged positive effect on erections. In this double-blind study, roughly 75% of men with mild-to-moderate ED given sildenafil at a dosage of 100 mg were able to have intercourse at 8 and 12 hours postdose, compared with a successful intercourse rate of roughly 50% in similar men treated with placebo.

Maximal efficacy is still likely to occur when intercourse is attempted early after medication ingestion. Nevertheless, research such as this suggests that the therapeutic window for PDE5 inhibitor may be much longer than elimination half-lives suggest.[3] Ⓐ

A separate study sought to investigate the effect of early postoperative dosing with vardenafil, administered either nightly or on demand, compared with placebo on recovery of erectile function in men with ED following bilateral nerve-sparing radical prostatectomy (NSRP) surgery.

In this study of men with ED following bilateral NSRP, vardenafil was efficacious when used on demand, supporting a paradigm shift towards on-demand dosing with PDE5 inhibitors in this patient group.

The debate on clinical efficacy of PDE5 inhibitors as penile rehabilitation after surgical prostatectomy continues. Many animal studies and small studies enlisting humans have supported the role of various erectogenic therapies in prompting restoration of normal erectile function after prostatectomy. The general theory is that corporal oxygenation, prompted by venous engorgement brought on by the various therapies, will maintain corporal tissue integrity.

Unfortunately, this large, multicenter, randomized, real-world study of a PDE5 inhibitor for the treatment of postprostatectomy ED did not show any discernible benefit with respect to preservation of unmedicated penile erections after 9 months of treatment. These conclusions are important because this multicenter study is perhaps more indicative of results that can be expected from practitioners outside of the "centers of excellence" that have provided much of the previous data on PDE5 inhibitor as rehabilitation.

Fortunately, this study did indicate that PDE5 inhibitors are an effective on-demand therapy for postprostatectomy ED, so the condition remains a manageable one in most cases. Further research and studies are required to better our understanding of means by which to preserve erectile function after cavernous nerve injury.[4] Ⓐ

Evidence-Based References

1. Porst H et al: Long-term safety and efficacy of tadalafil 5mg dosed once daily in men with erectile dysfunction, *J Sex Med* 5:2160-2169, 2008. Commentary by A. Shindel, M.D. Ⓐ

2. Shabsigh R et al: Randomized study of testosterone gel as adjunctive therapy to sildenafil in hypogonadal men with erectile dysfunction who do not respond to sildenafil alone, *J Urol* 179:97-102, 2008. Commentary by A. Shindel, M.D. Ⓐ

3. McCullough AR et al: Randomized, double-blind, crossover trial of sildenafil in men with mild to moderate erectile dysfunction: efficacy at 8 and 12 hours postdose. *Urology* 71:686-692, 2008. Commentary by A. Shindel, M.D. Ⓐ

4. Montorsi F et al: Effect of nightly versus on-demand vardenafil on recovery of erectile function in men following bilateral nerve-sparing radical prostatectomy, *Eur Urol* 54:924-931, 2008. Commentary by A. Shindel, M.D. Ⓐ

SUGGESTED READINGS

Beckman T et al: Evaluation and medical management of erectile dysfunction, *Mayo Clin Proc* 81(3):385-390, 2006.

McVary KT: Erectile dysfunction, *N Engl J. Med* 357: 2472-2481, 2007.

McVary KT: Clinical practice. Erectile dysfunction, *N Engl J Med* 357(24):2472-2481, 2007.

Melnik T et al: Psychosocial interventions for erectile dysfunction, *Cochrane Database Syst Rev* 3: CD004825, 2007.

Rosenberg MT: Diagnosis and management of erectile dysfunction in the primary care setting, *Int J Clin Pract* 61:1198, 2007.

AUTHORS: **CINDY LAI, M.D.,** and
NICOLE APPELLE, M.D.

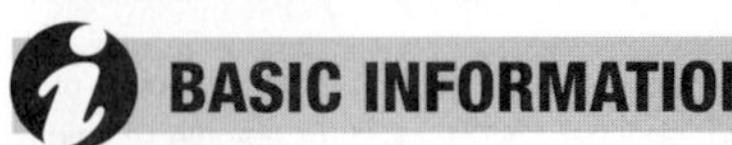

BASIC INFORMATION

DEFINITION

Erysipelas is a type of cellulitis caused by infection of the superficial layers of the skin and cutaneous lymphatics. Erysipelas is characterized by redness, induration, and a sharply demarcated, raised border.

SYNONYMS

St. Anthony's fire

ICD-9CM CODES
035 Erysipelas

EPIDEMIOLOGY & DEMOGRAPHICS

PREDOMINANT AGE: Occurs most often in the young or old
RISK FACTORS: Patients with impaired lymphatic or venous drainage (mastectomy, saphenous vein harvesting) and immunocompromised patients. Athlete's foot is a common portal of entry.
RECURRENCE RATE: Relatively common

PHYSICAL FINDINGS & CLINICAL PRESENTATION

- Distinctive red, warm, tender skin lesion with induration and a sharply defined, advancing, raised border (Fig. 1-115).
- Most common sites are lower extremities and face.
- Systemic signs of infection (fever) are often present.
- Vesicles or bullae may develop.
- After several days lesions may appear ecchymotic.
- After 7 to 10 days desquamation of affected area may occur.

ETIOLOGY

- Usually group A β-hemolytic streptococci
- Less often group B, C, or G streptococci
- Rarely *Staphylococcus aureus*

COMPLICATIONS

- Abscess
- Necrotizing fasciitis
- Thrombophlebitis
- Gangrene
- Metastatic infection

Dx DIAGNOSIS

DIFFERENTIAL DIAGNOSIS

- Other types of cellulitis
- Necrotizing fasciitis
- Deep vein thrombosis
- Contact dermatitis
- Erythema migrans (Lyme's disease)
- Insect bite
- Herpes zoster
- Erysipeloid
- Acute gout
- Pseudogout

WORKUP

History, physical examination, and laboratory evaluation

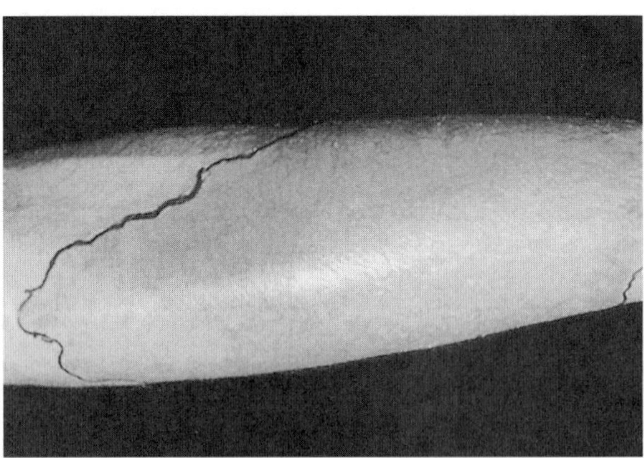

FIGURE 1-115 Erysipelas. Note well-demarcated erythematous plaque on arm. (From Goldstein B [ed]: *Practical dermatology,* ed 2, St Louis, 1997, Mosby. Courtesy Department of Dermatology, University of North Carolina at Chapel Hill.)

LABORATORY TESTS

Diagnosis is usually made by characteristic clinical setting and appearance.
- Complete blood count and white blood cell count often elevated
- Blood cultures positive in 5% of patients
- Gram stain and culture of any drainage from skin lesions
- Culture of aspirated fluid from leading edge of skin lesion has low yield

IMAGING STUDIES

- Duplex ultrasound for patients suspected of having deep vein thrombosis
- CT scan or MRI for patients with suspected necrotizing fasciitis

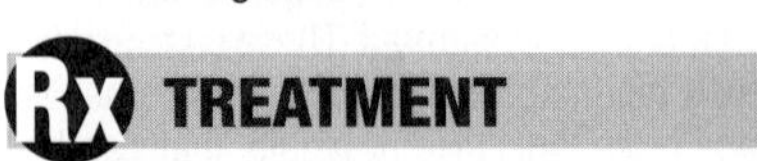

TREATMENT

NONPHARMACOLOGIC THERAPY

- Elevation of the affected limb
- Warm compresses

ACUTE GENERAL Rx

Typical erysipelas of extremity in nondiabetic patient:
- PO: penicillin V 250 mg to 500 mg qid
- IV: penicillin G (aqueous) 1 to 2 million units q6h

NOTE: Use erythromycin or cephalosporin in patients allergic to penicillin.
Facial erysipelas (include coverage for *Staphylococcus aureus*):
- PO dicloxacillin 500 mg q6h
- IV nafcillin or oxacillin 2 g q4h

DISPOSITION

Prognosis is good with antibiotic treatment but recurrence is common.

REFERRAL

For surgical debridement for patients with necrotizing fasciitis or for drainage of abscess

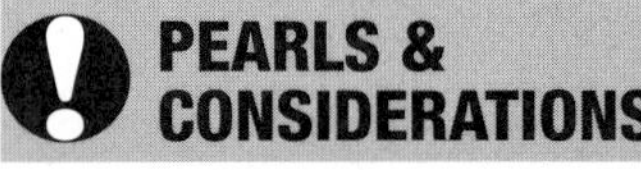

PEARLS & CONSIDERATIONS

Consider early surgical referral when necrotizing fasciitis suspected. Consider skin biopsy when not responding to appropriate antibiotics.

SUGGESTED READINGS

Falagas M et al: Narrative review: diseases that masquerade as infectious cellulites, *Ann Intern Med* 142(1):47, 2005.
Guisto J, Meislin H: Soft tissue infections. In *Rosen's emergency medicine,* ed 6, Philadelphia, 2006, Mosby.

AUTHORS: **GAIL M. O'BRIEN, M.D.,** and **MARK J. FAGAN, M.D.**

BASIC INFORMATION

DEFINITION

Erythema multiforme is an inflammatory disease believed to be caused by immune complex formation and subsequent deposition in the skin and mucous membranes. It is considered a hypersensitivity reaction to infection or drugs.

SYNONYMS

EM

ICD-9CM CODES
695.1 Erythema multiforme

EPIDEMIOLOGY & DEMOGRAPHICS

PREDOMINANT AGE: 20 to 40 yr
RISK FACTORS: Often associated with herpes simplex and other infectious agents, drugs, or connective tissue diseases.

PHYSICAL FINDINGS & CLINICAL PRESENTATION

- Prodromal symptoms are mild or absent. Itching or burning at the site of eruption may occur.
- Symmetric skin lesions with a classic "target" appearance (caused by the centrifugal spread of red maculopapules to circumference of 1 to 3 cm with a purpuric, cyanotic, or vesicular center) are present (Fig. 1-116). The papules may enlarge into plaques measuring a few centimeters in diameter with a dark or red central portion. Target lesions may not be apparent for several days.
- Lesions are most common in the back of the hands and feet and extensor aspect of the forearms and legs. Trunk involvement can occur in severe cases.
- Urticarial papules, vesicles, and bullae may also be present and generally indicate a more severe form of the disease.
- Individual lesions heal in 1 to 2 wk without scarring.
- Bullae and erosions may also be present in the oral cavity.

ETIOLOGY

- Immune complex formation and subsequent deposition in the cutaneous microvasculature may play a role in the pathogenesis of erythema multiforme.
- The majority of cases follow outbreaks of herpes simplex virus 1 and 2.
- Mycoplasma pneumoniae, fungal infections, medications (bupropion, sulfonamides, penicillins, nonsteroidal anti-inflammatory drugs, barbiturates, phenothiazines, hydantoins).
- In >50% of patients no specific cause is identified.

DIAGNOSIS

DIFFERENTIAL DIAGNOSIS

- Chronic urticaria
- Secondary syphilis
- Pityriasis rosea
- Contact dermatitis
- Pemphigus vulgaris
- Lichen planus
- Serum sickness
- Drug eruption
- Granuloma annulare
- Polymorphic light eruption
- Viral exanthem

WORKUP

- Medical history with emphasis on drug ingestion
- Laboratory evaluation in patients with suspected collagen-vascular diseases
- Skin biopsy when diagnosis is unclear

LABORATORY TESTS

- Complete blood count with differential
- Antinuclear antibody
- Serology for *Mycoplasma pneumoniae,* HSV-1, HSV-2
- Urinalysis

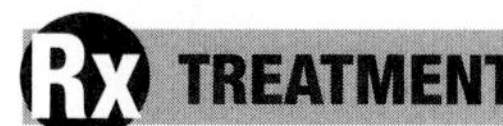

TREATMENT

NONPHARMACOLOGIC THERAPY

- Mild cases generally do not require treatment; lesions resolve spontaneously within 1 mo.
- Potential drug precipitants should be removed.

ACUTE GENERAL Rx

- Treatment of associated diseases (e.g., acyclovir for herpes simplex, erythromycin for *Mycoplasma* infection).
- Prednisone 40 to 80 mg/day for 1 to 3 wk may be tried in patients with many target lesions; however, the role of systemic steroids remains controversial.
- Levamisole, an immunomodulator, may be effective in the treatment of patients with chronic or recurrent oral lesions (dose is 150 mg/day for 3 consecutive days used alone or in combination with prednisone).

DISPOSITION

The rash generally evolves over a 2-wk period and resolves within 3 to 4 wk without scarring. A severe bullous form can occur (see entry for Stevens-Johnson Syndrome).

REFERRAL

Hospital admission in patients with suspected Stevens-Johnson syndrome

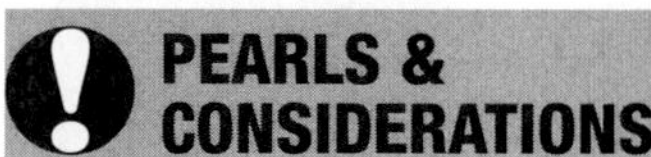

PEARLS & CONSIDERATIONS

COMMENTS

The risk of recurrence of erythema multiforme exceeds 30%. Recurrence may be treated with valacyclovir 500 to 1000 mg/day, famciclovir 125 to 250 mg/day, or acyclovir 400 mg bid. Dapsone, antimalarials, azathioprine, or cyclosporine use is reserved for cases resistant to antivirals.

SUGGESTED READING

Lamoreux M et al: Erythema multiforme, *Am Fam Phys* 74:1883, 2006.

AUTHOR: **FRED F. FERRI, M.D.**

FIGURE 1-116 Iris and arcuate lesions of erythema multiforme. Note erythematous lesions with multiform configurations: target, arcuate, and vesicles. (From Noble J et al: *Textbook of primary care medicine,* ed 2, St Louis, 1995, Mosby.)

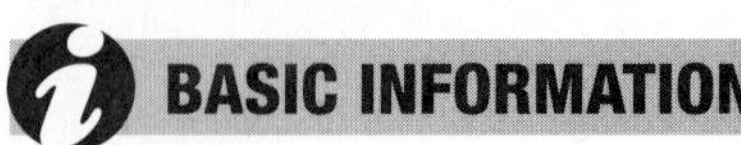

BASIC INFORMATION

DEFINITION

Erythema nodosum is an acute, tender, erythematous, nodular skin eruption resulting from inflammation of subcutaneous fat, often associated with bruising. It is the most common form of panniculitis.

ICD-9CM CODES
695.2 Erythema nodosum
017.10 Erythema nodosum, tuberculous, NOS

EPIDEMIOLOGY & DEMOGRAPHICS

INCIDENCE: Two to three cases/100,000 persons per yr

PREDOMINANT SEX: Female/male ratio of 3 to 4:1

PREDOMINANT AGE: 25 to 40 yr

PHYSICAL FINDINGS & CLINICAL PRESENTATION

- Acute onset of tender nodules typically located on the shins (Fig. 1-117) and occasionally seen on the thighs and forearms.
- The nodules are usually ⅛ to 1 inch in diameter but can be as large as 4 inches; they begin as light red lesions, then become darker and often ecchymotic. The nodules heal within 8 wk without ulceration.

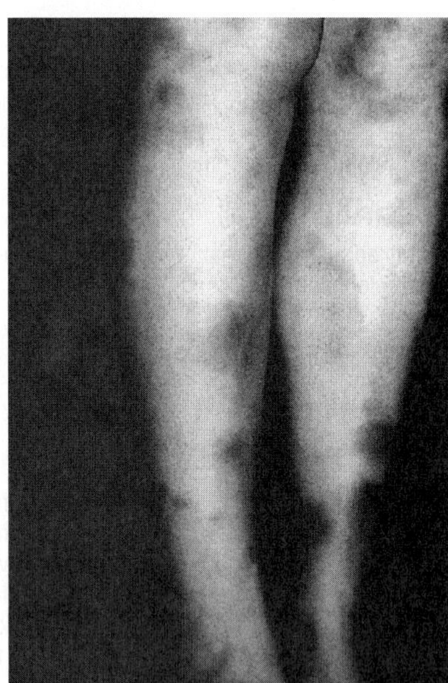

FIGURE 1-117 Erythema nodosum. (From Arndt KA et al: *Cutaneous medicine and surgery, vol 1,* Philadelphia, 1997, WB Saunders.)

- Associated findings:
  1. Fever
  2. Lymphadenopathy
  3. Arthralgia
  4. Signs of the underlying illness

ETIOLOGY

Cell-mediated hypersensitivity reaction is seen more frequently in persons with human leukocyte antigen (HLA) B8. The lesion results from an exaggerated interaction between an antigen and cell-mediated immune mechanisms leading to granuloma formation. Up to 55% of cases of erythema nodosum are idiopathic.

Infections:

- Bacteria
  - Streptococcal pharyngitis (28% to 48%)
  - *Salmonella* enteritis
  - *Yersinia* enteritis
  - Psittacosis
  - *Chlamydia pneumoniae* infection
  - *Mycoplasma* pneumonia
  - Meningococcal infection
  - Gonorrhea
  - Syphilis
  - Lymphogranuloma venereum
  - Tularemia
  - Cat-scratch disease
  - Leprosy
  - Tuberculosis
- Fungi
  - Histoplasmosis
  - Coccidioidomycosis
  - Blastomycosis
  - *Trichophyton verrucosum*
- Viruses
  - Cytomegalovirus
  - Hepatitis B
  - Epstein-Barr virus
- Drugs (3% to 10%)
  - Sulfonamides
  - Penicillins
  - Oral contraceptives
  - Gold salts
  - Prazosin
  - Aspirin
  - Bromides
- Sarcoidosis (11% to 25%)
- Cancer, usually lymphoma
- Ankylosing spondylosis and reactive arthropathies (e.g., associated with inflammatory bowel disease)

Dx DIAGNOSIS

DIFFERENTIAL DIAGNOSIS

- Insect bites
- Posttraumatic ecchymoses
- Vasculitis
- Weber-Christian disease
- Fat necrosis associated with pancreatitis
- Necrobiosis lipoidica
- Scleroderma
- Lupus panniculitis
- Subcutaneous granuloma
- Alpha-1 antitrypsin deficiency

WORKUP

- Physical examination
- Diagnosis of underlying illness by history, physical examination, and laboratory tests as indicated

LABORATORY TESTS

- Erythrocyte sedimentation rate
- Throat culture and antistreptolysin O titer
- PPD
- Others depending on index of suspicion (e.g., stool culture and evaluation for ova and parasites in patients with diarrhea and gastrointestinal symptoms)
- Skin biopsy in doubtful cases:
  1. Early lesion: inflammation and hemorrhage in subcutaneous tissue
  2. Late lesion: giant cells and granulomata

IMAGING STUDIES

Chest radiograph to rule out sarcoidosis and tuberculosis

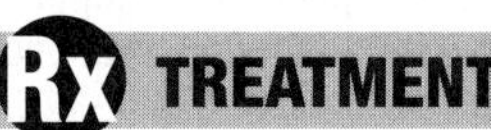

Rx TREATMENT

- The disease is self-limited and treatment is symptomatic. Erythema nodosum nodules develop in pretibial locations and resolve spontaneously over several weeks without scarring or ulceration.
- Treatment of underlying disorders.
- Avoidance of contact irritation of affected areas.
- Nonsteroidal anti-inflammatory drugs for pain.
- Systemic steroids (prednisone 1 mg/kg of body weight/day, tapered over several days) may be useful in severe cases if underlying risk of sepsis and malignancy have been excluded.

PROGNOSIS

Typical case:

- Pain for 2 wk
- Resolution within 8 wk

SUGGESTED READING

Schwartz RA, Nervi S: Erythema nodosum: a sign of systemic disease, *Am Fam Physician* 75: 695-700, 2007.

AUTHOR: **FRED F. FERRI, M.D.**

BASIC INFORMATION

DEFINITION

Approximately 15% of esophageal tumors arise in the proximal esophagus, 50% in the middle third of the esophagus, and 35% in the lower third. Eighty-five percent of esophageal tumors are squamous cell carcinoma mostly in the proximal and mid-esophagus. Adenocarcinomas arise from dysplastic columnar epithelium in the distal esophagus; Barrett's metaplasia from chronic gastric reflux.

SYNONYMS

Neoplasm of the esophagus
Malignancy of the esophagus

ICD-9CM CODES
150.8 Esophageal cancer, NEC
150.9 Esophageal cancer, NOS
230.1 Carcinoma of esophagus, in situ

EPIDEMIOLOGY & DEMOGRAPHICS

Carcinomas of the esophageal epithelium, both squamous cell and adenocarcinoma, are by far the most common tumors of the esophagus. Benign neoplasms are much less common (leiomyoma, papilloma, and fibrovascular polyps).

PREVALENCE: Varies widely worldwide. It is the sixth leading cause of cancer death. Rates are highest in the Asian esophageal cancer belt, extending from the Caspian Sea to northern China, with certain high-incidence pockets in Finland, Ireland, southeast Africa, and northwest France. In the U.S., 16,500 new cases and 14,300 deaths are expected in 2008, making it the seventh leading cause of death by cancer among men. Incidence has increased sixfold since 1975.

AGE & SEX PREDOMINANCE: Esophageal cancer is more common among blacks than whites and has a high male/female ratio of 3:1. It usually develops in the seventh and eighth decades and is associated with lower socioeconomic status. The majority are diagnosed at an advanced stage (unresectable or metastatic disease).

GENETICS: Increasing evidence shows that genetics may play a role by increasing susceptibility to esophageal cancer.

CLINICAL PRESENTATION

Symptoms and signs:

- Dysphagia (74%): initially occurs with solid foods and gradually progresses to include semisolids and liquids; latter signs usually indicate incurable disease with tumor involving more than 60% of the esophageal circumference.
- Weight loss: usually of short duration. Losing >10% of body mass predicts poor outcome.
- Hoarseness: suggests recurrent laryngeal nerve involvement.
- Odynophagia: an unusual symptom.
- Cervical adenopathy: usually involving supraclavicular lymph nodes.
- Dry cough: suggests tracheal involvement.
- Aspiration pneumonia: caused by development of a fistula between the esophagus and trachea.
- Massive hemoptysis or hematemesis: results from the invasion of vascular structures.
- Advanced disease spreads to lymph nodes, liver, lungs, peritoneum, and pleura.
- Hypercalcemia: associated with squamous cell carcinoma from secretion of a parathyroid-like tumor peptide.

ETIOLOGY

Pathogenesis of esophageal cancers is attributable to chronic recurrent oxidative damage from any of the following etiologic agents, which cause inflammation, and esophagitis, increased cell turnover, and, ultimately, initiation of the carcinogenic process.

ETIOLOGIC AGENTS:

- Excess alcohol consumption accounts for 80% to 90% of esophageal cancer in the U.S.; whiskey is associated with a higher incidence than wine or beer.
- Tobacco and alcohol use combined increases risk substantially for squamous cell cancer.
- Obesity.
- Other ingested carcinogens:
  - Nitrates (converted to nitrites): South Asia, China
  - Smoked opiates: Northern Iran
  - Fungal toxins in pickled vegetables
- Mucosal damage:
  - Long-term exposure to extremely hot tea
  - Lye ingestion
- Radiation-induced strictures
- Chronic achalasia: incidence of esophageal cancer is seven times greater in this population
- Host susceptibility as a result of precancerous lesions:
  - Plummer-Vinson syndrome (Paterson-Kelly): glossitis with iron deficiency
  - Congenital hyperkeratosis and pitting of palms and soles
- Chronic GERD leading to Barrett's esophagus and adenocarcinoma (whites are affected more than blacks).
- Possible association with celiac sprue or dietary deficiencies of molybdenum, zinc, vitamin A.

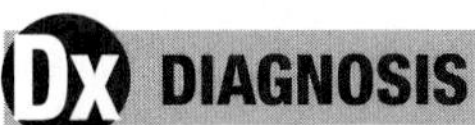

DIAGNOSIS

DIFFERENTIAL DIAGNOSIS

- Achalasia
- Scleroderma of the esophagus
- Diffuse esophageal spasm
- Esophageal rings and webs

LABORATORY TESTS

Complete blood cell count, blood chemistry, liver enzymes. No biomarkers are available currently to diagnose, monitor, or predict outcomes.

IMAGING STUDIES

- Double-contrast esophagogram effectively identifies large esophageal lesions (Fig. 1-118).
  - In contrast to benign esophageal leiomyomata, which cause narrowing with preservation of normal mucosal pattern, esophageal carcinomas cause ragged ulcerating mucosal changes in association with deeper infiltration.

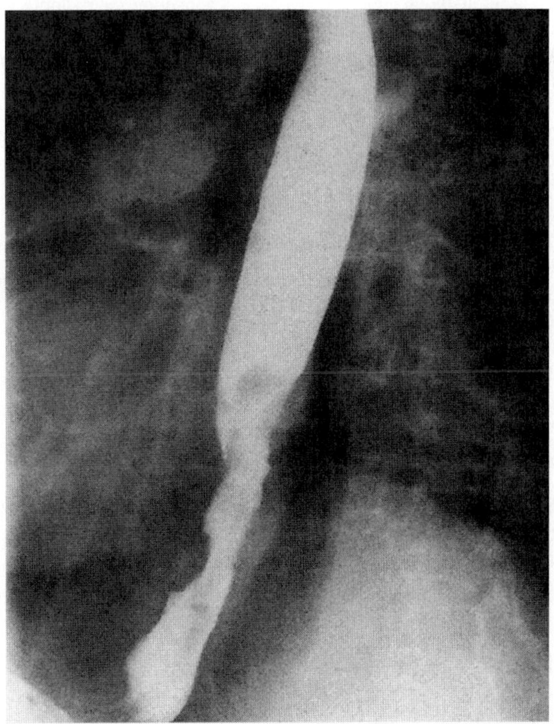

FIGURE 1-118 Barium swallow demonstrating the classic findings in cancer of the distal third of the esophagus. (Reprinted from Noble J [ed]: *Primary care medicine,* ed 2, St Louis, 1996, Mosby.)

 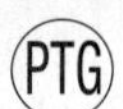

- Esophagoscopy may be performed initially if suspicion is high and to visualize smaller tumors missed by esophagogram and allow histopathologic confirmation. In conjunction, an endoscopic sonogram is often performed to determine the depth of tumor invasion.
  - Endoscopic inspection of the larynx, trachea, and bronchi may identify concomitant cancers of head, neck, and lung.
  - Endoscopic biopsies fail to recover malignant tissue one third of the time; thus cytologic examination of tumor brushings should be routinely performed.
  - Examination of the fundus of the stomach by retroflexion of the endoscope is imperative.
- Chest and abdominal CT or integrated CT-PET scan can determine tumor spread.

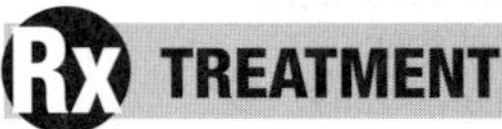

TREATMENT

ACUTE GENERAL Rx

SURGICAL RESECTION:

- Surgical resection of squamous cell carcinoma and adenocarcinoma of the lower third of the esophagus is indicated if no widespread metastasis is detected by CT-PET. Stomach or colon typically is used for esophageal replacement.
- Endoscopic resection may replace radical surgical resection in early tumors with no lymph node involvement, but a recent Cochrane review found no studies comparing endoscopic treatment vs. surgery.
- Complications of surgery:
  - Anatomic fistula (usually with colon interposition, subphrenic abscesses)
  - Respiratory complications
  - Cardiovascular complications are most common, including MI, CVA, and PE

RADIATION THERAPY:

- Squamous cell carcinomas are more radiosensitive than adenocarcinoma. Radiation achieves good local control and is an excellent palliative modality for obstructive symptoms but is rarely curative. It is best used for upper esophageal tumors.
- Approximately 40% of tumors cannot be destroyed even after 6000 rads.
- Palliative radiation therapy for bone metastasis is also effective.
- Complications of radiation therapy:
  - Esophageal stricture, radiation-induced pulmonary fibrosis, and transverse myelitis are the most feared.
  - Radiation-induced cardiomyopathy and skin changes are rare.

COMBINATION CHEMOTHERAPY, RADIATION Rx, & SURGICAL Rx:

- Single-agent chemotherapy resulted in significant tumor regression in 15%-25% of patients.
- Most beneficial chemotherapy appeared to be a cisplatin/5-fluorouracil–based combination.
- Combination chemotherapy including cisplatin achieved significant tumor reduction in 30% to 60% of patients.
- Capecitabine and oxaliplatin are as effective as fluorouracil and cisplatin, respectively, in patients with previously untreated esophagogastric cancer
- Complications of chemotherapy include mucositis, GI toxicity, myelosuppression, nephrotoxicity; ototoxicity and neurotoxicity occur with cisplatin.
- 2-year survival is improved with chemoradiotherapy (30%) versus radiotherapy alone (10%).
- Preoperative chemoradiotherapy plus surgery significantly reduced the 3-year mortality rate compared with surgery alone in patients with resectable esophageal cancer. Trimodal therapy is the standard of care for most esophageal cancers.

CHRONIC Rx

Palliative procedures such as repeated endoscopic dilation, surgical placement of feeding tube, or polyvinyl prosthesis to bypass tumors have been used for unresectable patients.

DISPOSITION

- Overall 5-yr survival is 13%
- Surgery: 5-yr survival rate is 48% in stages I and II, 20% in advanced stages
- Radiation therapy: 5-yr survival rate of 6%-20%
- Chemotherapy: Single-agent response rate of 15% to 38%; combination response rate 80%
- Combined modality: 18% response rate
- Patients with stage IV disease receive palliative chemotherapy with a median survival of less than 1 year

REFERRAL

- To gastroenterologist or general surgeon for endoscopy for patients with chronic dysphagia, odynophagia, or unexplained weight loss
- To medical oncologist for evaluation of preoperative chemotherapy
- To radiation oncologist for palliative therapy if tumor is unresectable or obstruction is present
- To hospice if appropriate

PEARLS & CONSIDERATIONS

COMMENTS

More than 50% of patients with esophageal cancer are diagnosed when the disease is metastatic or unresectable.

PREVENTION

- A diet high in fruits and vegetables is associated with lower risk of esophageal cancer.
- Avoid tobacco and excessive alcohol use.
- Avoid ingested toxins known to cause esophageal cancers.
- Endoscopic evaluation of persons with chronic dysphagia or GERD symptoms with regularly scheduled surveillance endoscopies if Barrett's esophagus is detected.

PATIENT/FAMILY EDUCATION

Provide education and support about the likely prognosis because most esophageal cancers are diagnosed at an advanced stage.

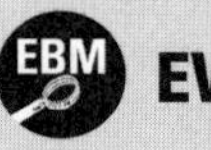

EVIDENCE

Please note: Complete text of EBM for this topic is available online.

Key trials and commentary:

This article updates Radiation Therapy Oncology Group trial 8911 (USA Intergroup 113), a comparison of chemotherapy plus surgery vs. surgery alone for patients with localized esophageal cancer. The relationship between resection type and between tumor response and outcome was also analyzed.

This study showed that for patients with localized esophageal cancer, whether or not preoperative chemotherapy is administered, only an R0 resection results in substantial long-term survival. Even microscopically positive margins are an ominous prognostic factor. After an R1 resection, postoperative chemoradiotherapy therapy offers the possibility of long-term disease-free survival to a small percentage of patients.

This is a long-term follow-up of a randomized control trial comparing neoadjuvant chemotherapy with cisplatin and 5-fluorouracil vs. no neoadjuvant chemotherapy for patients with localized esophageal cancer. The main end point was survival. Preoperative chemotherapy did not increase the likelihood of having an R0 resection. Patients with an R0 resection had significantly greater survival than those without R0 resection, which mitigated any long-term survival benefit of preoperative chemotherapy. Patients who did have a clinical response to preoperative neoadjuvant chemotherapy had a slight improvement in postoperative survival compared with those without chemotherapy. There was also a slight benefit to those with R1 resections who received postoperative chemotherapy and radiation. Overall, 5-year survival for esophageal cancer remains grim, especially in the absence of a complete resection. The role of neoadjuvant chemotherapy remains unclear based on the data.[1] Ⓐ

The primary treatment modality for patients with carcinoma of the esophagus or gastroesophageal junction has been surgery, although primary radiation therapy with concurrent chemotherapy produces similar results. As both have curative potential, there has been great interest in the use of trimodality therapy. To this end, one study compared survival, response, and patterns of failure of trimodality therapy to esophagectomy alone in patients with nonmetastatic esophageal cancer.

The results from this trial reflect a long-term survival advantage with the use of chemoradiotherapy followed by surgery in the treatment of esophageal cancer, and support trimodality therapy as a standard of care for patients with this disease.

Induction chemoradiation followed by surgery has been advocated as a viable treatment option for patients with locoregional advanced esophageal cancer. Although a number of single-institution trials examining this trimodality approach have been performed, no randomized phase III trial has been reported until this study from the Cancer and Leukemia Group B (CALGB). Briefly, patients were randomly assigned to either esophagectomy with nodal dissection alone or combined cisplatin and 5-fluorouracil (FU) with concurrent radiation therapy (50.4 Gy) followed by esophagectomy with node dissection. 56 patients were enrolled in this study between 1997 and 2000, after which time the trial was closed secondary to poor accrual. Mean follow-up was 6 years. Using an intent-to-treat analysis, the median survival of trimodality therapy was 4.5 years compared with 1.8 years for patients who underwent an isolated esophagectomy. This translated into a 5-year survival of 39% for trimodality patients vs. 16% for primary esophagectomy therapy. 10 patients had a complete pathologic response, with 3 of the 6 patients with known N1 disease being downstaged to N0 with preoperative therapy. Distant recurrence was the most common initial site of recurrence in both arms of the study.

The results of this study indicated benefit in overall and progression-free survival. Importantly, there is no suggestion that operative mortality was increased by the use of trimodality therapy. Certainly, a major limitation of this study is the small sample size. Strength of the study was the very long follow-up period and low lost to follow-up rate (5%). In summary, I believe this is the best available data we have to suggest that in appropriate selected patients trimodality therapy is superior to esophagectomy alone. Taken together with all other single-institution trials, I think the overwhelming evidence supports the use of this multimodality approach for patients with more advanced-stage esophageal cancer.[2] Ⓐ

Evidence-Based References

1. Kelsen DP et al: Long-term results of RTOG trial 8911 (USA intergroup 113): a random assignment trial comparison of chemotherapy followed by surgery compared with surgery alone for esophageal cancer, *J Clin Oncol* 25:3719-3725, 2007. Commentary by M.T. Hawn, M.D. Ⓐ

2. Tepper J et al: Phase III trial of trimodality therapy with cisplatin, fluorouracil, radiotherapy, and surgery compared with surgery alone for esophageal cancer: CALGB 9781, *J Clin Oncol* 26:1086-1092, 2008. Commentary by D.R. Jones, M.D. Ⓐ

SUGGESTED READINGS

Arnott SJ et al: Preoperative radiotherapy for esophageal carcinoma, *Cochrane Database Syst Rev* 4: CD001799, 2005.

Cunningham D et al: Capecitabine and oxaliplatin for advanced esophagogastric cancer, *N Engl J Med* 358:36-46, 2008

Green S et al: Surgery versus radical endotherapies for early cancer and high grade dysplasia in Barrett's oesophagus, *Cochrane Database Syst Rev* 2: CD007334, 2009.

Layke JC, Lopez PP: Esophageal cancer: A review and update, *Am Fam Physician* 73:2187-92, 2006

Wong R, Malthaner R: Combined chemotherapy and radiotherapy (without surgery) compared with radiotherapy alone in localized carcinoma of the esophagus, *Cochrane Database Syst Rev* 1:CD002092, 2006.

AUTHOR: **LYNN MCNICOLL, M.D., F.R.C.P.C.**

BASIC INFORMATION

DEFINITION

A predominantly postural and action tremor that is bilateral and tends to progress slowly over the years in the absence of other neurological abnormalities.

SYNONYMS

Benign essential tremor
Familial tremor

ICD-9CM CODES
333.1 Essential tremor

EPIDEMIOLOGY & DEMOGRAPHICS

PREDOMINANT AGE: Can begin at any age, but incidence increases over the age of 40 yr. Prevalence is 6% to 9% for those >60 yr.
GENETICS: No gender or racial predominance.

PHYSICAL FINDINGS & CLINICAL PRESENTATION

- Patients complain of tremor that is most bothersome when writing or holding something such as a newspaper or trying to drink from a cup. Worsens under emotional distress.
- Tremor, 4 to 12 Hz, bilateral postural and action tremor of the upper extremities. May also affect the head, voice, trunk, and legs. Typically it is the same amplitude throughout the action, such as bringing a cup to the mouth. No other neurologic abnormalities on examination except difficulty with tandem gait. Patients often note improvement with intake of small amounts of alcohol.

ETIOLOGY

Often an inherited disease, autosomal dominant; sporadic cases without a family history are frequently encountered

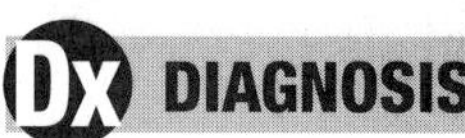

DIAGNOSIS

DIFFERENTIAL DIAGNOSIS

- Parkinson's disease—tremor is usually asymmetric, especially early on in the disease, and is predominantly a resting tremor. Patients with Parkinson's disease will often also have increased tone, decreased facial expression, slowness of movement, and shuffling gait.
- Cerebellar tremor—an intention tremor that increases at the end of a goal-directed movement (such as finger to nose testing). Other associated neurologic abnormalities include ataxia, dysarthria, and difficulty with tandem gait.
- Drug-induced—there are many drugs that enhance normal, physiologic tremor. These include caffeine, nicotine, lithium, levothyroxine, β-adrenergic bronchodilators, amiodarone, valproate, and SSRIs.
- Wilson's disease—wing-beating tremor that is most pronounced with shoulders abducted, elbows flexed, and fingers pointing towards each other. Usually there are other neurologic abnormalities including dysarthria, dystonia, and Keyser Fleischer rings on ophthalmologic examination.
- Physiologic tremor.

WORKUP

- All imaging studies normal (MRI, CT) and are usually unnecessary unless there are other associated neurologic abnormalities
- Check TSH
- In patients younger than 40 yrs with other neurologic abnormalities, send ceruloplasmin, serum Cu, 24-hr urine Cu to rule out Wilson's disease

Rx TREATMENT

Treat essential tremor when it is functionally impairing. Treatments are up to 75% effective.

NONPHARMACOLOGIC THERAPY

Reduction of stress. Minimize use of caffeine. Small quantities of alcohol at social functions may be beneficial.

ACUTE GENERAL Rx

Can take a dose of propranolol (20-40 mg) in preparation for specific event.

CHRONIC Rx

First-line agents:
- Propranolol/Propranolol LA: Usual starting dose is 30 mg. The usual therapeutic dose is 160-320 mg. Although not contraindicated, they must be used with caution in those with asthma, depression, cardiac disease, and diabetes.
- Primidone: Usual starting dose is 12.5 to 25 mg qhs. Usual therapeutic dose is between 62.5 and 750 mg daily (assuming side effects are tolerated). Sedation and nausea when first begin medication are biggest side effects.
- Topiramate: 25 mg qhs, may titrate up to about 400 mg

Other agents:
- Gabapentin: 400 mg qhs, usual therapeutic dose is 1200-3600 mg
- Alprazolam: 0.75-2.75 mg
- Botulinum toxin injected focally may decrease tremor

SURGICAL Rx

Thalamic deep brain stimulation (or possibly thalamotomy) contralateral to side of tremor

DISPOSITION

Patients should be reassured that the condition is not associated with other neurologic disabilities; however, it can become quite functionally disabling over time.

REFERRAL

This is a condition that usually can be treated by the primary care physician; however, if patient fails first-line therapies then patient should be referred to specialists for other drug trials and other possible surgical options.

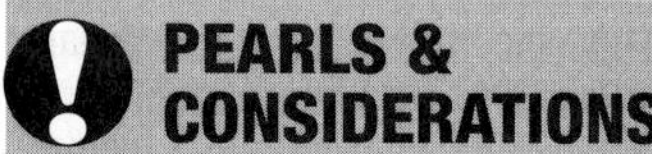

PEARLS & CONSIDERATIONS

Essential tremor is the most common of all movement disorders.

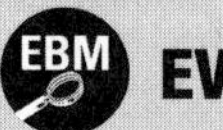

EVIDENCE

A recent American Academy of Neurology Practice Parameter was released in June 2005.[1] They found that propranolol, propranolol LA, and primidone are effective in reducing limb tremor in ET. There is high-quality evidence to recommend the use of these agents. The magnitude of effect of propranolol and primidone is roughly equivalent, and either can be tried as initial therapy. There is only fair evidence for the other drugs listed. Based on available studies, these agents are either "probably" or "possibly" effective in the treatment of limb tremor in ET.

Evidence-Based Reference

1. Zesiewicz TA et al: Practice parameter: therapies for essential tremor. Report of the Quality Standards Subcommittee of the American Academy of Neurology, *Neurology* 64:2008, 2005.

SUGGESTED READINGS

Deuschel G, Volkmann J: Tremors: Differential diagnosis, pathophysiology, and therapy. In Jankovic J, Tolosa E (eds): *Parkinson's disease and movement disorders,* ed 4, 2002, pp. 270-291.

Louis ED: Essential tremor, *N Engl J Med* 345(12):887, 2001.

Zesiewicz TA et al: Phenomenology and treatment of tremor disorders. In Hurtig H, Stern M (eds): *Neurologic clinics: Movement disorders* 19:3, 2001, pp. 651-680.

AUTHOR: **CINDY ZADIKOFF, M.D.**

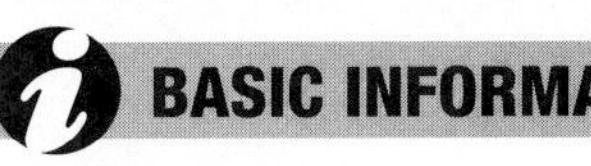

BASIC INFORMATION

DEFINITION

Factitious physical disorder is when an individual intentionally strives to create signs or symptoms of disease. The individual may create signs or symptoms by (1) lying, (2) simulating (e.g., putting drops of blood into a urine sample), or (3) actually creating disease (e.g., injecting bacteria or medications). The primary aim is to achieve the patient role, and the individual may seek invasive diagnostic testing, surgery, and treatment. Munchausen's syndrome is the most severe variant of factitious physical disorder and is characterized by exaggerated lying (pseudologia fantastica), sociopathy, geographic wandering from hospital to hospital, and a continuous life of patienthood.

SYNONYMS

Factitious disorder
Munchausen's syndrome (the most severe variant of factitious disorder)
Munchausen by proxy (factitious disorder created in another person, usually a child)
Deliberate disability
Hospital addiction syndrome
Artifactual illness
Peregrinating problem patients
Dermatitis artefacta
Surreptitious illness

ICD-9CM CODES
300.19 Factitious disorder

EPIDEMIOLOGY & DEMOGRAPHICS

INCIDENCE (IN U.S.): Unknown
PEAK INCIDENCE: 30 to 40 yr
PREVALENCE (IN U.S.): Unknown but considerable in specific illnesses. For example, 3.3% of patients with fever of unknown origin have a factitious disorder.
PREDOMINANT SEX: Male/female ratio of 2:1 for Munchausen's syndrome but 1:2 for individuals with non-Munchausen type of factitious physical disorder.
PREDOMINANT AGE: 30 to 40 yr
GENETICS: No genetic predisposition known

PHYSICAL FINDINGS & CLINICAL PRESENTATION

- False complaints or self-inflicted injury or symptoms without clear secondary gain. The intentional aspect of the disorder is often evident, such as injecting bacteria to produce infection or taking medication to produce an abnormality.
- Presentation may be acute and dramatic, but the condition can be a chronic, recurring problem.
- Workup is usually negative for naturally occurring organic etiology.
- Clinical picture is atypical for the natural history of disease (e.g., an infection that does not respond to multiple courses of appropriate antibiotics).

ETIOLOGY

- A history of significant childhood illness; physical or sexual abuse are thought to predispose.
- Personality disorders and psychodynamic factors often play a significant role.

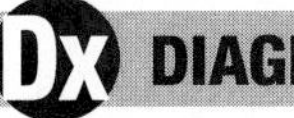

DIAGNOSIS

The diagnosis can be made by (1) direct observation of fabrication, (2) the presence of signs or symptoms that contradict laboratory testing, (3) nonphysiologic response to treatment, (4) the presence of physical evidence of fabrication (e.g., syringes), and (5) recurrent patterns of illness exacerbation (e.g., just before discharge) or failure to follow the natural history of disease (e.g., a wound that does not heal for no apparent reason).

DIFFERENTIAL DIAGNOSIS

- Malingering: falsifying an illness for a clear secondary gain (e.g., financial gain or avoidance of unwanted duties).
- Somatoform disorders or hypochondriasis: these disorders are produced unconsciously and are not intentionally produced.
- Self-injurious behavior is common in many other psychiatric conditions; in those conditions the patients confess the intentional self-harm and describe motivating factors. The main intent is the self-harm and not to attain the patient role, as occurs in factitious disorder.
- May also present as Munchausen by proxy, in which a mother (86% of time) or other caregiver induces illness in a child (52% between ages of 3 and 13 yr) for the purpose of obtaining medical attention or some other psychological need. Mothers often have a history of somatoform, factitious, or personality disorder themselves.

WORKUP

- Dictated by the presenting complaints.
- No specific tests for Munchausen's syndrome.
- Diagnosis may be made when the patient is caught in the act of lying or inducing an injury. The diagnosis often rests on organic workup failing to reveal a plausible natural organic disease. The failure of usual, or even extensive, treatment to ameliorate a condition is an important clue.

LABORATORY TESTS

- Laboratory testing often reveals inconsistencies.
- Other laboratory abnormalities may reflect the underlying factitious behavior (e.g., hypokalemia in an individual surreptitiously taking furosemide).

Rx TREATMENT

NONPHARMACOLOGIC THERAPY

Two major approaches:

- Nonpunitive confrontation. Primary physician and psychiatrist conjointly meet with patient and say, "You must be in a lot of distress to be harming yourself as we believe you have been. We would like to help you deal with your distress more adaptively and get you into psychiatric treatment."
- Avoid overt confrontation with patient but provide him or her with a face-saving way to recover. For example, a therapeutic double bind would involve saying, "There are two possibilities here, one is that you have a medical problem that should respond to the next intervention we do, or two, you have a factitious disorder. The outcome will give us the answer."
- Munchausen's syndrome is the most severe variant and may be virtually impossible to treat except to avoid further invasive and iatrogenic disease.

ACUTE GENERAL Rx

Treatment of comorbid psychiatric disorders may be helpful. Treatment with antidepressants or psychotherapy may ameliorate the factitious behavior. Multidisciplinary staff meetings are useful to ventilate feelings and develop cohesive treatment plans.

DISPOSITION

- After being confronted with their behavior, patients may cease factitious behavior, but they more commonly seek other physicians or hospitals, as in the Munchausen variant. Other factitious disorder patients may enter psychotherapy, particularly when they have been given a face-saving approach with an avoidance of a humiliating confrontation.
- Extensive medical workups and exploratory surgery are frequent.

REFERRAL

Always obtain psychiatric referral. Risk management attorneys and hospital ethicists may contribute to challenging decision making in these patients.

PEARLS & CONSIDERATIONS

Think of factitious disorders whenever there is an unexplained medical course that continues to repeat despite appropriate treatment, particularly in patients associated with the health care field. There is current consideration of whether factitious disorders should be classified in the upcoming DSM-V as a subset of somatoform disorders. This possibility is related to the challenge of discriminating whether an illness state is being consciously (factitious) or unconsciously (somatoform) produced. Future research will investigate the utility of this possible change in classification.

SUGGESTED READINGS

Eisendrath SJ, Telischak KS: Factitious disorders: potential litigation risks for plastic surgeons, *Ann Plast Surg* 60(1):64-69, 2008.

Eisendrath SJ, Young J: Factitious physical disorders. In Maj M et al (eds): *Somatoform disorders,* West Sussex, UK, 2005, John Wiley and Sons, pp 325-338.

Krahn LE et al: Looking toward DSM-V: should factitious disorder become a subtype of somatoform disorder? *Psychosomatics* 49(4):277-282, 2008.

AUTHOR: **STUART J. EISENDRATH, M.D.**

Falls in the Elderly

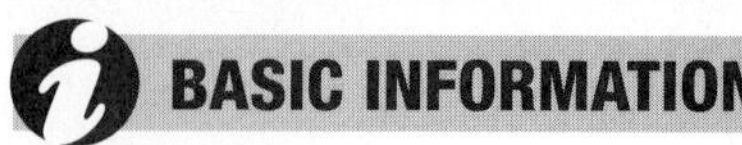

BASIC INFORMATION

DEFINITION

A fall is an "event which results in a person coming to rest inadvertently on the ground and other than a consequence of the following: loss of consciousness, sudden onset of paralysis, or epileptic seizure" (Kellogg International Work Group, *Danish Medical Bulletin,* 34, 1-24).

SYNONYMS

Syncope
Collapse

ICD-9CM CODES
Accidental fall (E880-E888.9)

EPIDEMIOLOGY & DEMOGRAPHICS

INCIDENCE:
- Falls are the leading cause of accidental death among older adults.
- The incidence of falls among community-dwelling older adults is 35% to 40%.
- The incidence of falls for nursing home and hospitalized older adults is three times the rate of community-dwelling older adults.
- Twenty to thirty percent of older adults who fall suffer significant injury leading to immobility and dependence.

PREDOMINANT SEX & AGE:
- Fall-related mortality is highest among older white men followed by white women, black men, and black women.
- The incidence rates of falls increase with advancing age.
- Older adults aged 85 years and over are 10 to 15 times more likely to have a fracture compared with those aged 60 to 65 years.

RISK FACTORS: Three groups of risk factors for falls have been identified (Table 1-26):
1. Intrinsic factors inherent in the older adult who falls
2. Extrinsic factors circumstantial to the older adult who falls
3. Situational or the activity in which the older adult is engaged in when a fall occurs

CLINICAL PRESENTATION

- Older adults who fall may present with minor soft tissue injuries, such as lacerations or bruising, hip fracture or head trauma; however, most falls are not reported unless an injury has occurred.
- A detailed history of events and circumstances surrounding fall, risk factors, medications, chronic illnesses, and a review of systems for acute medical illnesses, cognitive status, and functional status should be obtained.
- Physical examination should focus on the identified risk factors and include:
  - Cardiovascular examination: heart rate and rhythm, orthostatics, carotid pulses
  - Neurologic examination: mental status, visual screen, lower extremity assessment of strength, tone, proprioception, sensation, reflexes and testing of cortical and cerebellar function
  - Gait and balance assessment: "Get up and go test"

ETIOLOGY

- Falls are a multifactorial syndrome resulting from the cumulative effects of impaired gait and balance, aging, polypharmacy, depression, cognitive impairment, acute medical illness, or environmental factors (Fig. 1-119).
- Most falls among community-dwelling older adults are due to environmental factors, whereas falls among nursing home residents are a result of confusion, gait impairment, or postural hypotension.

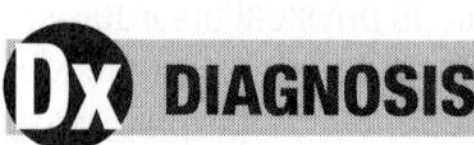

DIAGNOSIS

DIFFERENTIAL DIAGNOSIS

Falls are often a nonspecific symptom of an acute illness (such as a UTI, acute anemia, or pneumonia) or an exacerbation of a chronic disease (CHF or COPD).

WORKUP

- Older adults presenting with a noninjurious fall need a detailed history and physical exam to identify acute medical illnesses and potential modifiable risk factors. Laboratory and neuroimaging studies may be necessary if the history and physical exam indicate a specific problem. ECG and Holter monitoring may be considered if cardiac arrhythmia is suspected.
- See Fig. 1-119

LABORATORY TESTS

CBC, chemistries, thyroid function, drug levels, and urinalysis depending on physical/historical findings

IMAGING STUDIES

- CT or MRI of the brain or cervical spine films in the presence of neurologic or gait impairment.
- Consider ECG, echocardiography, or Holter monitor if suspicious for structural cardiac abnormality or syncope.

TREATMENT

NONPHARMACOLOGIC THERAPY

- Assisted devices such as a cane, walker to improve mobility
- Fall prevention equipment including bed alarms, low beds, and hip protectors
- Physical therapy evaluation for gait and balance training and home safety assessment
- Discontinuation of certain medications associated with falls
- Exercise program to improve strength and balance
- Evaluation of proper footwear, hard sole, and low heel height

ACUTE GENERAL Rx

Hospitalization may be necessary for treatment of hip fracture, subdural hematoma, lacerations,

TABLE 1-26 Risk Factors for Falls in the Elderly

Intrinsic
Aging Age-related decline in vestibular function might lead to increased sway, dizziness, and falls. Aging of the vision system may result in decreased visual acuity, inability to discriminate dark/light, and decreased spatial perception.
Cardiac Cardiac arrhythmias, carotid sinus hypersensitivity
Neurologic Parkinson's disease, normal pressure hydrocephalus (NPH), sensory neuropathy, dementia/impaired cognition, cervical myelopathy, senile gait disorder, prior stroke
Musculoskeletal Lower extremity weakness, deconditioning, arthritis, foot abnormalities (such as bunions, calluses, or nail abnormalities)
Vascular Vertebrobasilar insufficiency, postural hypotension, postprandial hypotension
Metabolic Hypoglycemia, hypothyroidism, hyponatremia
Psychiatric Depression
Extrinsic
Medications Use of more than four medications may be associated with an increased risk of falls. Medications that may increase fall risk include benzodiazepines, sleeping medications, neuroleptics, antidepressants, anticonvulsants, class I antiarrhythmics, and antihypertensives (Rao, 2005).
Environmental Inadequate lighting, ill-fitting shoes, slippery floor surfaces, loose rugs, uneven steps
Situational
Tripping over obstacles, carrying heavy items, descending/ascending stairs, rapid turning, reaching overhead, climbing ladders

or trauma as well as the treatment of underlying cause of the fall such as infection, metabolic disturbances, cardiovascular or neurologic abnormality.

CHRONIC Rx

- Screen and treat for osteoporosis as low bone density increases the risk of hip or other fractures.
- Optimize treatment of chronic illnesses such as CHF, COPD, OA, Parkinson's disease, dementia, and visual problems.

COMPLEMENTARY & ALTERNATIVE MEDICINE

T'ai chi has been shown to reduce the risk of falls in community-dwelling study participants.

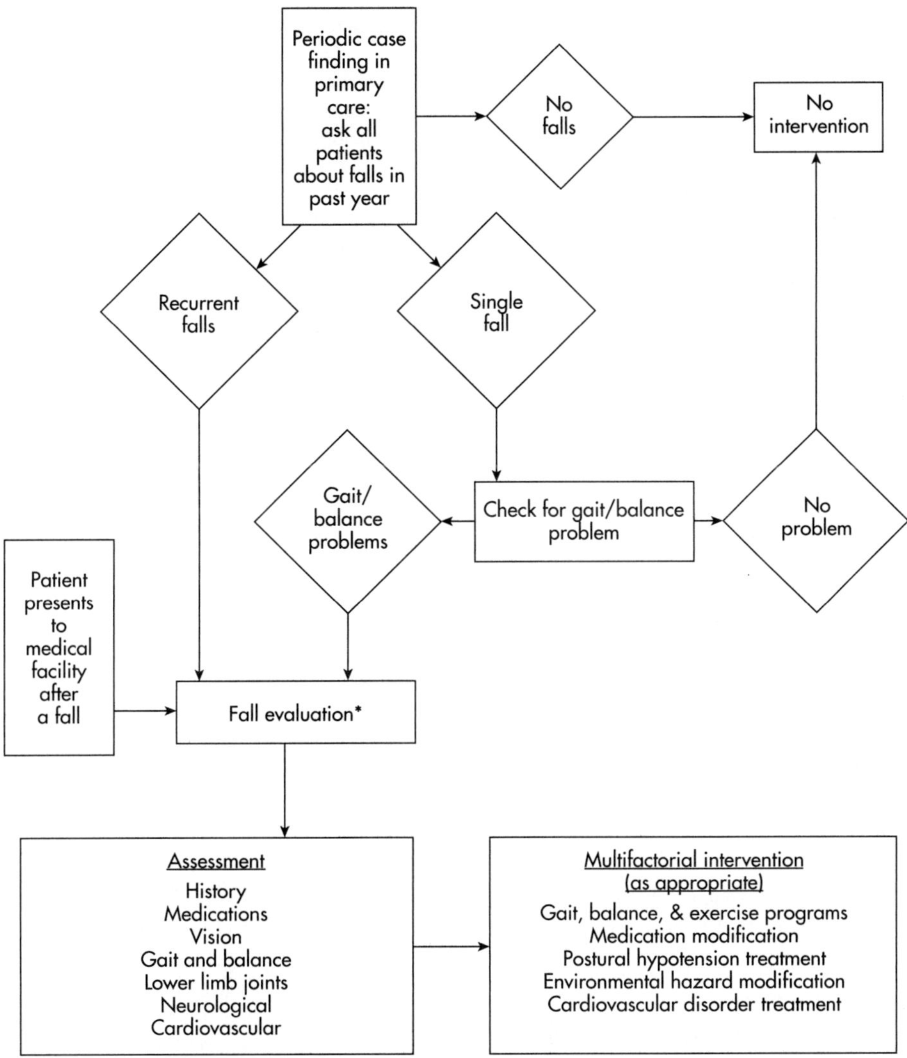

FIGURE 1-119 Guideline for the prevention of falls in older persons. Algorithm summarizing the assessment and management of falls. (From American Geriatrics Society, British Society, and American Academy of Orthopaedic Surgeons Panel on Falls Prevention.)

DISPOSITION

Falls increase the older adult's risk of hospitalization, institutionalization, and mortality.

REFERRAL

- Referral may be appropriate to cardiologist, ophthalmologist, neurologist, or podiatrist depending on the presence of a specific condition.
- Consider referral to physical therapist for gait and balance training, evaluation for assisted device, or strengthening program.

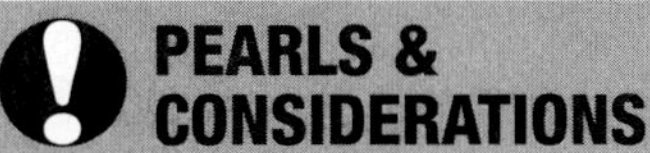

PEARLS & CONSIDERATIONS

COMMENTS

- Fear of falling may lead to restriction of activities, social isolation, and dependence.
- Older adults with four or more risk factors have a 78% chance of falling.

PREVENTION

The USPSTF does recommend counseling elderly patients about fall prevention during routine visits as well as arranging individualized multifactorial home interventions for high-risk elders (USPSTF Guidelines, 1996).

PATIENT/FAMILY EDUCATION

Counseling patient and family about reducing the risks of falling

SUGGESTED READINGS

American Geriatrics Society, British Geriatrics Society, and American Academy of Orthopedic Surgeons Panel on Falls Prevention: Guideline for the prevention of falls, *J Am Geriatr Soc* 49:664-672, 2001.

Centers for Disease Control and Prevention: http://www.cdc.gov/ncipc/factsheets/falls.htm

Rao S: Prevention of falls in older patients, *Am Fam Physician* 72:81-88, 2005.

Sherrington C et al: Effective exercise for the prevention of falls: a systematic review and meta-analysis, *J Am Geriatr Soc* 56(12):2234-2243, 2008.

Tinetti ME: Preventing falls in the elderly, *N Engl J Med* 348:42-49, 2003.

Wolf SL et al: Intense tai chi exercise training and fall occurrences in older, transitionally frail adults: a randomized, controlled trial, *J Am Geriatr Soc* 51: 1693-1697, 2003.

AUTHORS: **SEAN H. UITERWYK, M.D.,** and **ALICIA J. CURTIN, PH.D., G.N.P.**

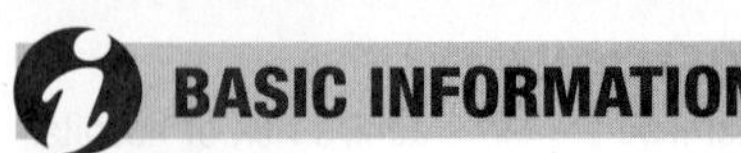

BASIC INFORMATION

DEFINITION

Acute fatty liver of pregnancy (AFLP) is characterized histologically by microvesicular fatty cytoplasmic infiltration of hepatocytes with minimal hepatocellular necrosis.

SYNONYMS

Acute fatty metamorphosis
Acute yellow atrophy

ICD-9CM CODES
646.7 Liver disorders in pregnancy

EPIDEMIOLOGY & DEMOGRAPHICS

INCIDENCE:
- Approximately one in 10,000 pregnancies
- Equal frequencies in all races and at all maternal ages

AVERAGE GESTATIONAL AGE: 37 wk (range 28 to 42 wk)

RISK FACTORS:
- Primiparity
- Multiple gestation
- Male fetus

GENETICS: Some with a familial deficiency of long-chain 3-hydroxyacyl-coenzyme A dehydrogenase (LCHAD)

PHYSICAL FINDINGS & CLINICAL PRESENTATION

- Initial manifestations:
    1. Nausea and vomiting (70%)
    2. Pain in right upper quadrant or epigastrium (50% to 80%)
    3. Malaise and anorexia
- Jaundice often in 1 to 2 wk
- Late manifestations:
    1. Fulminant hepatic failure
    2. Encephalopathy
    3. Renal failure
    4. Pancreatitis
    5. Gastrointestinal and uterine bleeding
    6. Disseminated intravascular coagulation
    7. Seizures
    8. Coma
- Liver:
    1. Usually small
    2. Normal or enlarged in preeclampsia, eclampsia, HELLP syndrome (hemolysis, elevated liver enzymes, and low platelets), and acute hepatitis
    3. Coexistent preeclampsia in up to 46% of patients

ETIOLOGY

- Postulated that inhibition of mitochondrial oxidation of fatty acids may lead to microvesicular fatty infiltration of liver
- Fatty metamorphosis of preeclamptic liver disease believed to be of different etiology

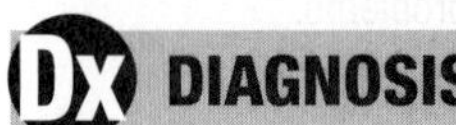

DIAGNOSIS

DIFFERENTIAL DIAGNOSIS

- Acute gastroenteritis
- Preeclampsia or eclampsia with liver involvement
- HELLP syndrome
- Acute viral hepatitis
- Fulminant hepatitis
- Drug-induced hepatitis caused by halothane, phenytoin, methyldopa, isoniazid, hydrochlorothiazide, or tetracycline
- Intrahepatic cholestasis of pregnancy
- Gallbladder disease
- Reye's syndrome
- Hemolytic-uremic syndrome
- Budd-Chiari syndrome
- Systemic lupus erythematosus

WORKUP

- A clinical diagnosis is based predominantly on physical and laboratory findings.
- Most definitive diagnosis is through liver biopsy with oil red O staining and electron microscopy.
- Liver biopsy is reserved for atypical cases only and only after any existing coagulopathy corrected with fresh frozen plasma.

LABORATORY TESTS

Tests to determine the following:
- Hypoglycemia (often profound <60 mg/dl)
- Hyperammonemia
- Elevated aminotransferases (usually <500 U/ml)
- Thrombocytopenia
- Leucocytosis (white blood cell count >15,000)
- Hyperbilirubinemia (usually <10 mg/dl)
- Low albumin
- Hypofibrinogenemia (<300 mg/dl)
- Disseminated intravascular coagulation (DIC) (in 75%)

IMAGING STUDIES

- Ultrasound: best used to rule out other diseases in the differential diagnosis such as gallbladder disease
- CT scan: plays minimal role because of a high false-negative rate

Rx TREATMENT

NONPHARMACOLOGIC THERAPY

- Patient is admitted to intensive care unit for stabilization.
- Fetus is delivered; spontaneous resolution usually follows delivery.
- Mode of delivery is based on obstetric indications and clinical assessment of disease severity.

ACUTE GENERAL Rx

- Decrease in endogenous ammonia through dietary protein restriction; neomycin 6 to 12 g/day PO to decrease presence of ammonia-producing bacteria; magnesium citrate 30 to 50 ml PO or enema to evacuate nitrogenous wastes from colon
- Administration of IV fluids with glucose to keep glucose levels >60 mg/dl
- Coagulopathy corrected with fresh frozen plasma
- Avoidance of drugs metabolized by liver
- Aggressive avoidance and treatment for nosocomial infections; consideration of prophylactic antibiotics
- Monitor closely for development of complications such as hepatic encephalopathy, pulmonary edema, DIC, and respiratory arrest

CHRONIC Rx

Orthotopic liver transplantation is the only treatment for irreversible liver failure.

DISPOSITION

- Before 1980, both maternal and fetal mortality rates were approximately 85%
- Since 1980, both maternal and fetal mortality rates are less than 20%
- Usually rapid return of liver function to normal after delivery
- Minimal risk of recurrence with future pregnancies

REFERRAL

- To tertiary health care facility as soon as diagnosis is suspected.
- Infants of mothers with AFLP should be evaluated for LCHAD deficiency.

SUGGESTED READINGS

Cunningham FG et al: Gastrointestinal disorders. In Cunningham FG et al (eds): *Williams' obstetrics,* ed 20, Stamford, CT, 1997, Appleton & Lange.

Davidson KM: Acute fatty liver of pregnancy, *Postgrad Obstet Gynecol* 15:1, 1995.

Steingrub JS: Pregnancy-associated severe liver dysfunction, *Crit Care Clin* 20(4):763, 2004.

Toro Ortiz JC et al: Acute fatty liver of pregnancy, *J Matern Fetal Neonatl Med* 12(4):277, 2003.

AUTHORS: **ARUNDATHI G. PRASAD, M.D.,** and **RUBEN ALVERO, M.D.**

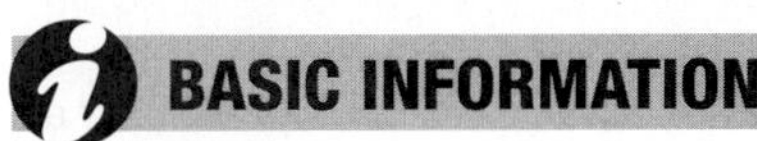

BASIC INFORMATION

DEFINITION

Felty's syndrome (FS) is defined as the triad of rheumatoid arthritis (RA), splenomegaly, and neutropenia. The hallmark of FS is a persistent, idiopathic neutropenia, which is defined as a neutrophil count $<2000/mm^3$. Splenomegaly is extremely variable in its extent and no longer required as an absolute diagnostic requirement. It is an extraarticular manifestation of seropositive RA in which recurrent local and systemic infections are the major source of morbidity and mortality.

ICD-9CM CODES
714.1 Felty's syndrome

EPIDEMIOLOGY & DEMOGRAPHICS

- The lifetime risk of FS for a patient initially diagnosed with RA is estimated to be 1% to 3%.
- 60% to 80% are women.
- Recognized in patients in their late 40s or early 50s who have had RA for 10 yr or more.
- Patients with FS are more likely to have a family history of RA and HLA-DRB1*0401.
- Rare in African Americans (low frequency of HLA-DRB1*0401).

CLINICAL PRESENTATION

- Rarely, splenomegaly and neutropenia are present before the arthritis.
- Articular involvement is usually more severe in patients with FS compared with other patients with RA; however, one third may have relatively inactive synovitis with elevated erythrocyte sedimentation rate (ESR).
- Degree of splenomegaly varies and may be detectable only by imaging studies; degree of splenomegaly has no correlation with the degree of neutropenia.
- Patients with FS have a greater frequency of extraarticular manifestations (rheumatoid nodules, vasculitis, skin lesions, pleuropericarditis, etc.) than other patients with RA.
- Mild hepatomegaly is common (up to 68%).
- Patients with FS have a twentyfold increased frequency of bacterial infections compared with other RA patients.

ETIOLOGY

The pathogenesis of FS is probably multifactorial, and no clear explanation has been elucidated.

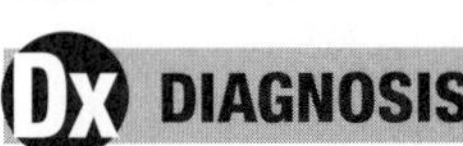

DIAGNOSIS

DIFFERENTIAL DIAGNOSIS

- Systemic lupus erythematosus
- Large granular lymphocytic (LGL) leukemia
- Drug reaction
- Myeloproliferative disorders
- Lymphoma/reticuloendothelial malignancies
- Cirrhosis with portal hypertension
- Sarcoidosis
- Tuberculosis
- Amyloidosis
- HIV infection

LABORATORY TESTS

- There is no diagnostic test for FS.
- Complete blood count with differential to detect neutropenia, mild to moderate anemia, and mild to moderate thrombocytopenia.
- High ESR, C-reactive protein (CRP).
- Rheumatoid factor: positive in 98%, usually high titer.
- Antinuclear antibody (ANA): positive in 67%.
- Antihistone antibody: positive in 83%.
- Antineutrophil cytoplasmic antibodies (ANCA): positive in 77%.
- HLA-DRB1*0401: positive in 98%.
- Immunoglobulins: level may be higher than in RA patients.
- Complement level may be lower than in RA patients.
- Bone marrow examination is often necessary to exclude other cause of neutropenia.
- Clonal cytogenetic abnormalities or clonal *TCR* gene recombination in patients with characteristic lymphocyte phenotypes suggests LGL leukemia.

IMAGING STUDIES

Ultrasonography or CT scan may be useful in diagnosing splenomegaly.

Rx TREATMENT

ACUTE GENERAL Rx

- Splenectomy
  - It was the principal treatment therapy for FS but has now been replaced by drug therapy.
  - Usually reserved for patients with profound neutropenia ($<1000/mm^3$) and severe recurrent infections.
  - Acutely reverses hematologic abnormalities.
  - 25% to 30% will have recurrent neutropenia, but the granulocyte count usually remains above the presplenectomy level.
  - Improvement in frequency of recurrent infection is variable and not correlated with degree of hematologic improvement.
- Antirheumatic drugs: second-line drugs for RA may improve the neutropenia in FS.
  - Gold salt injections: good hematologic response in 60%, partial response in 20%. The recovery of neutrophil count is usually slow.
  - Methotrexate: series of studies with small numbers of patients suggest the efficacy in FS. Follow-up durations are still short. Granulocyte count may begin to rise within several weeks in responders.
  - Penicillamine, sulfasalazine: limited experience; not first choice for FS.
- Corticosteroids
  - Overwhelming infection is the main barrier to the use of corticosteroids.
  - Prednisone 30 mg/day or more can elevate the neutrophil count, but this effect is often not sustained when the dose is reduced.
  - Pulse dosing is a potential alternative for short-term elevation of neutrophils.
- Others
  - Limited experience with cyclophosphamide, cyclosporine, azathioprine, leflunomide, anti–tumor necrosis factor-alpha antibody, rituximab, lithium, and testosterone.
- Recombinant granulocyte colony-stimulating factor/granulocyte-macrophage colony-stimulating factor
  - Improves neutrophil count but not arthritis and anemia of FS.
  - May be useful as adjunctive therapy during serious infection or in preparation for surgery.

DISPOSITION

- Poor prognosis with recurrent infections because of neutropenia.
- Articular involvement can be severe in FS.

REFERRAL

- To hematologist for treatment of neutropenia
- To rheumatologist for treatment of RA

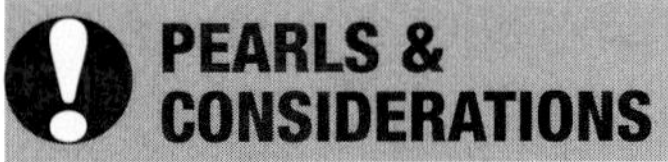

PEARLS & CONSIDERATIONS

COMMENTS

- Recurrent infections are the major cause of death.
- Neutropenia of FS can be effectively treated with disease-modifying antirheumatic drugs, the widest experience being with methotrexate.

SUGGESTED READINGS

Balint GP et al: Felty's syndrome, *Best Pract Res Clin Rheumatol* 18:631, 2004.

Bowman SJ: Hematological manifestations of rheumatoid arthritis, *Scand J Rheumatol* 31:251, 2002.

Burks EJ et al: Pathogenesis of neutropenia in large granular lymphocyte leukemia and Felty's syndrome, *Blood Rev* 20:245, 2006.

Capsoni F et al: Primary and secondary autoimmune neutropenia, *Arthritis Res Ther* 7:208, 2005.

Starkebaum G et al: Chronic neutropenia associated with autoimmune disease, *Semin Hematol* 39:121, 2002.

AUTHOR: **ETSUKO AOKI, M.D., PH.D.**

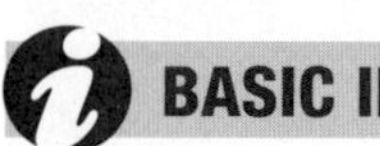

BASIC INFORMATION

DEFINITION

A femoral neck fracture occurs within the capsule of the hip joint between the base of the head and the intertrochanteric line.

SYNONYMS

Intracapsular fracture
Subcapital fracture

ICD-9CM CODES
820.8 Femoral neck fracture

EPIDEMIOLOGY & DEMOGRAPHICS

PREVALENCE: Lifetime risk in women approximately 16%
PREDOMINANT SEX: Female/male ratio of 3:1
PREDOMINANT AGE: 90% >60 yr

PHYSICAL FINDINGS & CLINICAL PRESENTATION

- Hip or groin pain
- Affected limb usually shortened and externally rotated in displaced fractures
- Impacted fractures: possibly no deformity and only mild pain with hip motion
- Mild external bruising

ETIOLOGY

- Trauma
- Age-related bone weakness, usually caused by osteoporosis
- Increased risk of fractures in elderly (decline in muscle function, use of psychotropic medication, etc.)

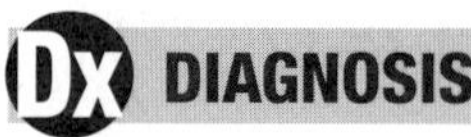

DIAGNOSIS

DIFFERENTIAL DIAGNOSIS

- Osteoarthritis of hip
- Pathologic fracture
- Lumbar disc syndrome with radicular pain
- Insufficiency fracture of pelvis

WORKUP

Diagnosis is usually obvious based on clinical and radiographic findings.

IMAGING STUDIES

- Standard roentgenograms consisting of an anteroposterior view of the pelvis and a cross-table lateral view of the hip to confirm the diagnosis (Fig. 1-120).
- If initial roentgenograms are negative and diagnosis of an occult femoral neck fracture is suspected, hospital admission and further radiographic assessment with either bone scanning or MRI are recommended.
- Bone scanning is sensitive after 48 to 72 hr.

Rx TREATMENT

- Orthopedic consultation
- Surgery indicated in most cases, usually within 24 hr
- Deep vein thrombosis prophylaxis

DISPOSITION

- Mortality rate within 1 yr in elderly patients is 25% to 30%.
- Dementia is a particularly poor prognostic sign.

REFERRAL

For surgical consideration when the diagnosis is made

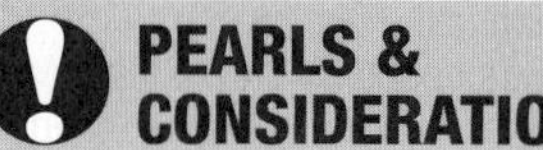

PEARLS & CONSIDERATIONS

COMMENTS

- Complications: nonunion and avascular necrosis
- Intracapsular fractures: occasionally occur in nonambulatory patients
  1. Usually treated nonsurgically, especially in the patient with dementia and limited pain perception
  2. Early bed-to-chair mobilization and vigilant nursing care to avoid skin breakdown
  3. Fracture usually pain free in a short time even if solid bony healing does not occur
- As a result of the increasing life span of the female population, femoral neck fractures are becoming more common. The initial physical examination and roentgenographic studies may be completely negative. Groin pain, sometimes quite severe, may be the only early clue to the diagnosis.
- The rate of hip fracture could be reduced by:
  1. Elimination of environmental hazards (poor lighting, loose rugs)
  2. Regular exercise for balance and strength
  3. Patient education about fall prevention
  4. Medication review to minimize side effects
  5. Prevention and treatment of osteoporosis
- In the U.S., hip fracture rates and subsequent mortality among persons 65 yr and older are declining, and comorbidities among patients with hip fractures have increased. Hip fractures are also very expensive ($40,000 in the first year following hip fracture for direct medical costs and $5,000 in subsequent years).

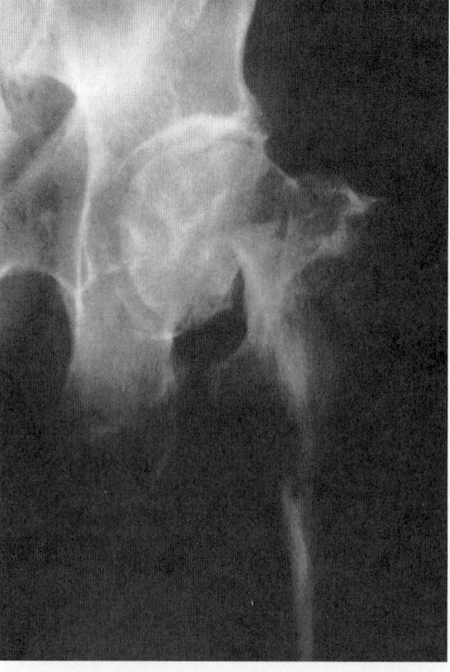

FIGURE 1-120 Femoral neck fracture. (From Scudieri G [ed]: *Sports medicine: principles of primary care,* St Louis, 1997, Mosby.)

SUGGESTED READINGS

Amer NA et al: Early operation on patients with a hip fracture improved the ability to return to independent living, *J Bone Joint Surg Am* 90A:1436, 2008.

Bettelli G et al: Relationship between mortality and proximal femur fractures in the elderly, *Orthopedics* 26:1045, 2003.

Bogoch ER et al: Effective initiation of osteoporosis diagnosis and treatment for patients with a fragility fracture in an orthopedic environment, *J Bone Joint Surg Am* 88A:25, 2006.

Brauer CA et al: Incidence and mortality of hip fractures in the United States, *JAMA* 302(14):1573-1579, 2009.

Clinton J et al: Proximal humeral fracture as a risk factor for subsequent hip fractures, *J Bone Joint Surg Am* 91:503, 2009.

Feldstein AC et al: Older women with fractures: patients falling through the cracks of guideline recommended osteoporosis screening and treatment, *J Bone Joint Surg Am* 85A:2294, 2003.

Gardner MJ et al: Interventions to improve osteoporosis treatment following hip fracture, *J Bone Joint Surg Am* 87A:3, 2005.

Kaufman JD et al: Barriers and solutions to osteoporosis care in patients with a hip fracture, *J Bone Joint Surg Am* 85A:1837, 2003.

Lawrence VA et al: Medical complications and outcomes after hip fracture repair, *Ann Intern Med* 162:2053, 2003.

Logan K: Stress fractures in the adolescent athlete, *Pediatr Ann* 36:738, 2007.

Mirchandani S et al: The effects of weather and seasonality on hip fracture incidence in older adults, *Orthopedics* 28:149, 2005.

Parker MJ et al: Effectiveness of hip protectors for preventing hip fractures in elderly people, *BMJ* 332:571, 2006.

Radcliff TA et al: Patient risk factors, operative care, and outcomes among older community-dwelling male veterans with hip fracture, *J Bone Joint Surg* 90:34, 2008.

Schoofs MW et al: Thiazide diuretics and the risk for hip fractures, *Ann Intern Med* 139:476, 2003.

Tosi LL, Kyle RF: Fragility fractures: the fall and decline of bone health, *J Bone Joint Surg Am* 87A:1, 2005.

Van Helden S et al: Bone and fall-related fracture risks in women and men with a recent clinical fracture, *J Bone Joint Surg* 90:241, 2008.

AUTHOR: **LONNIE R. MERCIER, M.D.**

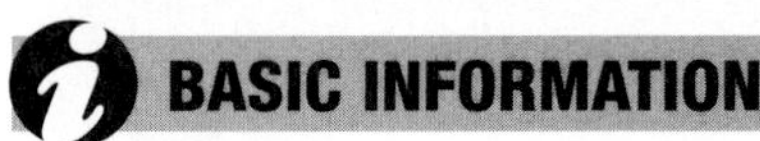

BASIC INFORMATION

DEFINITION

- The adverse effects of alcohol on the developing human represent a spectrum of structural anomalies and behavioral and neurocognitive disabilities, most accurately termed fetal alcohol spectrum disorder (FASD) (Table 1-27).
- Children at the severe end of the spectrum have been defined as having the fetal alcohol syndrome (FAS).

ICD-9CM CODES
760.71 Fetal alcohol syndrome

EPIDEMIOLOGY & DEMOGRAPHICS

- Alcohol is considered to be the most common major teratogen to which the fetus is liable to be exposed.
- 10% report drinking alcohol during pregnancy and 2% to 4% admit to binge drinking.
- FAS represent the most common form of mental retardation in U.S.
- Its prevalence is 1 to 2 per 1000 live births across United States.
- Each year 40,000 babies are born with fetal alcohol spectrum disorder.

RISK FACTORS

- Advance maternal age (>30 yr)
- High parity
- African-American, Alaskan Natives, and Native Indian race
- Binge drinking (more than four drinks per occasion)
- History of prior affected child
- Genetic susceptibility
- Undernutrition
- Low socioeconomic group

PHYSICAL FINDINGS & CLINICAL PRESENTATION

Typical features:

- Growth retardation
  - Prenatal or postnatal
  - Height and/or weight <10%
- Facial dysmorphia
  - Smooth philtrum
  - Thin vermilion border
  - Small palpebral fissure (<10%)
  - Others: epicanthic folds, ptosis of eyelids, flat nasal bridge and midface, upturned nose, railroad track ears, and so forth
- CNS abnormalities
  - Structural
    - Head circumference ,10%
    - Clinically significant brain abnormalities observable through imaging
  - Neurologic
    - Neurologic problems not due to a postnatal insult or fever
  - Functional
    - Intellectual deficit
    - Cognitive or developmental deficits
    - Executive function deficits
    - Motor function delays
    - Problem with attention and hyperactivity
    - Social skills
    - Other problems such as sensory, pragmatic language, and memory

Rare birth defects:

- Cardiac
  - Ventricular septal defect (VSD)
  - Atrial septal defect (ASD)
  - Tetralogy of Fallot
  - Aberrant great vessels
- Skeletal
  - Radioulnar synostosis
  - Hypoplastic nails
  - Clinodactyly
  - Shortened fifth digit
  - Pectus excavatum and carinatum
  - Klippel-Feil syndrome
  - Hemivertebrae
  - Camptodactyly
  - Scoliosis
- Renal
  - Aplastic kidneys
  - Dysplastic kidneys
  - Ureteral duplication
  - Hypoplastic kidneys
  - Hydronephrosis
  - Horseshoe kidneys
- Ocular
  - Strabismus
  - Refractive problems
  - Retinal vascular abnormalities
- Auditory
  - Conductive hearing loss
  - Neurosensory hearing loss
- Others
  - Hockey stick–like palmar crease

TABLE 1-27 The Institute of Medicine's Diagnostic Criteria for Fetal Alcohol Related Abnormalities

Category	Criteria
Category 1 FAS with confirmed maternal alcohol exposure	Presence of classic triad of growth retardation, characteristic facial dysmorphology and neurodevelopmental abnormalities. This is often defined as full-blown FAS
Category 2 FAS without confirmed maternal alcohol exposure	Triad in category 1 is present without confirmed maternal drinking
Category 3 Partial FAS with confirmed maternal alcohol exposure	Presence of some of the characteristic facial anomalies plus growth retardation or central nervous system neurodevelopmental abnormalities or behavioral/cognitive abnormalities
Category 4 FAS with confirmed maternal alcohol exposure and alcohol-related birth defects	These patients will have some congenital anomalies as a result of alcohol toxicity
Category 5 FAS with confirmed maternal alcohol exposure and alcohol-related neurodevelopmental disorder	There is evidence of CNS neurodevelopmental abnormalities or a complex patter of behavioral/cognitive abnormalities or both, but not necessarily any obvious physical changes

ETIOLOGY

- Prenatal damage as a result of chronic alcoholism comes about primarily because of direct action of ethanol or its metabolites (e.g., acetaldehyde) on the fetus.
- The exact damaging mechanism is not clear.
- Although the damaging effect of alcohol is different in the various phases of pregnancy, it is by no means limited to first trimester.
- There is no exact dose-response relationship between the amount of alcohol consumed during the prenatal period and the extent of damage inflicted on the infant.
- An occasional drink during pregnancy carries no risk to the fetus, but no level of drinking is known to be safe during pregnancy.
- The least significant effect recognized at two drinks per day has been slightly smaller birth weight (160 g smaller than average).
- It is not until four to six drinks per day are consumed that additional subtle clinical features are evident.
- Most of the children believed to have FAS have been born to frankly alcoholic mothers whose intake is eight to ten drinks or more per day, and those who engage in binge drinking.
- The risk of serious problem in the offspring of a chronically alcoholic woman has been estimated to be 30% to 50%, the greatest risk being varying degree of mental retardation.

SECONDARY DISABILITIES

- Mental health problems
- Dependent living
- Employment problems
- Disruptive school problems
- Trouble with law
- Confinement
- Inappropriate sexual behavior
- Alcohol or drug problems

Dx DIAGNOSIS

- It is a diagnosis of exclusion.
- Diagnosis is difficult both prenatally and at birth. Unfortunately, most cases are not diagnosed until school age.
- As the characteristic facial features tend to become decreasingly recognizable as the child reaches adolescence, the diagnosis becomes increasingly difficult with advancing age.
- Prenatal exposure to alcohol is not sufficient to warrant a diagnosis. According to the Centers for Disease Control and Prevention the diagnosis of FAS requires three specific findings along with the history of prenatal alcohol exposure:
  - Growth restriction (intrauterine or postnatal)
  - Central nervous system involvement

- Documentation of all three facial abnormalities (smooth philtrum, thin vermilion border, and short palpebral fissure)
- Imaging recommendation during pregnancy with alcohol exposure:
  - High-risk anatomy scan
  - Serial growth scan
  - Fetal echocardiogram at 22 to 24 weeks' intrauterine pregnancy
- Measurement of the ethyl esters of fatty acids in the meconium and hair of the newborn can substantiate maternal alcohol exposure.
- In school-aged children, the diagnostic process should include a through psychologic evaluation that assesses multiple domains. Also, supplement the observation by obtaining standardized testing through early intervention programs, public schools, and psychologists in private practice.

DIFFERENTIAL DIAGNOSIS

- Other causes of symmetrical growth retardation including intrauterine infection and aneuploidy
- Aneuploidy (T21, T18, T13)
- Syndromes with overlapping features of FAS:
  - Fetal anticonvulsant syndrome
  - Maternal phenylketonuria
  - Toluene embryopathy
  - Velocardiofacial syndrome (deletion 22q11)
  - William syndrome
  - Dubowitz syndrome
  - Cornelia de Lange syndrome

Rx TREATMENT

- As there is no cure for FAS, we need to emphasize prevention.
- For those women who are planning pregnancy or who have the potential to become pregnant, the U.S. Surgeon General has recommended that the safest course is to avoid alcohol entirely during pregnancy.
- Women of childbearing age who are not pregnant should drink no more than seven alcoholic drinks per week and no more than three drinks on any one occasion.
- Preconception counseling should be offered to women of childbearing age who are at risk for an alcohol-exposed pregnancy.
- Screen all pregnant women for alcohol use.
- The National Institute on Alcohol Abuse and Alcoholism recommend that any woman who reports drinking more than seven drinks per week or more than three drinks on any given day be further assessed for alcohol-related problems.
- The following two questionnaires are used to identify women drinking sufficiently to potentially damage the fetus. The CAGE questionnaire is less sensitive for screening pregnant women:
  - T-ACE (Table 1-28)
  - TWEAK (Table 1-29)
- Effective treatment alternatives for women who screen positive for hazardous alcohol use include brief interventions to promote reductions in alcohol use and that facilitate referral to specialized treatment programs.
- Discontinuation or reduction of alcohol consumption at any point in pregnancy may be beneficial.
- The use of alcohol-containing tonics and medications with an alcohol base should be avoided. This applies to medications with an alcohol base, at least when the concentration exceeds 10%.
- Alcoholism is one of the few situations in which pregnancy interruption may be discussed with the patient as it may result in FAS.
- Early diagnosis and appropriate treatment may decrease secondary disabilities and recurrence in future pregnancies.
- A child should be referred for full FAS evaluation when substantial prenatal alcohol use by the mother has been confirmed (more than seven drinks per week, or more than three drinks on multiple occasions, or both).
- If substantial prenatal exposure is known, in the absence of any other positive criteria, the physician should document this exposure and closely monitor the child's ongoing growth and development.
- When information about prenatal exposure is unknown, a child should be referred for full FAS if any of the following conditions are present: (1) all three dysmorphic facial features (smooth philtrum, thin vermilion border, and small palpebral fissure), (2) one or more of these facial features with growth deficit, (3) one or more facial features with one or more CNS abnormalities, (4) one or more dysmorphic facial features with growth deficit and one or more CNS abnormalities, or (5) any report of concern by a caregiver or parent that a child has or may have FAS.
- Infants and children who are diagnosed with FAS should be evaluated by a physician who is knowledgeable and competent in the evaluation of neurodevelopment and psychosocial problems associated with the diagnosis.
- A multidisciplinary team including a clinical geneticist, developmental pediatrician, mental health professional, social worker, and education specialist is often necessary for management.
- Treatment options include:
  - Medications to help with symptoms
  - Behavior and education therapy
    Friendship training
    Specialized math training
    Executive function training
    Parent-child interaction training
    Parenting and behavior management training
- Parenting training
  Concentrate on child's strengths and talents
  Accept child's limitations
  Be consistent with everything
  Use concrete language and examples
  Use stable routine that does not change daily
  Keep everything simple
  Be specific (i.e., say exactly what you mean)
  Structure your child's world to provide a foundation for daily living
  Use visualized aids, music, and hands-on activities to help your child learn
  Use positive reinforcement often
  Supervise
  Repeat, repeat, and repeat
- Emphasis on the following protective factors helps reduce the effects and also assists people with this condition to reach their full potential:
  Diagnosing before 6 yr
  Living in stable nurturing home environment in school years
  Absence of violence
  Involvement in special education and social services
- Alternative approaches such as biofeedback, auditory training, relaxation therapy, visual imagery, yoga/exercise, acupuncture/acupressure, massage, Reiki, energy healing, animal-assisted therapy, and so forth may play a role.

TABLE 1-28 T-ACE Questions*

T (tolerance)	How many drinks does it take to make you feel high? (3 or more drinks = 2 points)
A (annoyed)	Have people annoyed you by criticizing your drinking? (Yes = 1 point)
C (cut down)	Have you felt you ought to cut down on your drinking? (Yes = 1 point)
E (eye opener)	Have you ever had to drink first thing in the morning to steady your nerves or to get rid of a hangover? (Yes = 1 point)

* A score of 2 or more indicates heavy or problem drinker. Its sensitivity is 70% and specificity is 85%.

SUGGESTED READINGS

Koren G et al: Fetal alcohol spectrum disorder, *CMAJ* 169:1181-1185, 2003.

Online resources: http://fascenter.samhsa.gov, http://www.cdc.gov/ncbddd/fas, http://depts.washington.edu/fasdpn, http://www.nofas.org

AUTHOR: **HEMANT SATPATHY, M.D.**

TABLE 1-29 TWEAK*

T (tolerance)	How many drinks does it take before you begin to feel the first effects of alcohol? (3 or more drinks = 2 points)
W (worried)	Have close friends or relatives worried about your drinking in the past year? (Yes = 2 point)
E (eye opener)	Do you sometimes take a drink in the morning when you first get up? (Yes = 1 point)
A (amnesia)	Has a friend or family member ever told you about things you said or did while you were drinking that you could not remember? (Yes = 1 point)
K (kut down)	Do you sometimes feel the need to cut down on your drinking? (Yes = 1 point)

*A total of 3 or more points indicate the woman is likely to be a heavy or problem drinker. Its sensitivity is 79% and specificity is 83%.

BASIC INFORMATION

DEFINITION

Fever of undetermined origin (FUO) was defined by Petersdorf and Beeson in 1961 as an illness characterized by temperatures >101° F on several occasions for >3 wk with no known cause despite extensive workup.

- Persistence for >2 wk separates an FUO from an insignificant viral illness.
- Traditionally, diagnosis was made only after a 1-wk inpatient workup. In contemporary practice, much of the workup is performed as an outpatient.

SYNONYMS

Fever of unknown origin

ICD-9CM CODES
780.6 Pyrexia of undetermined origin

EPIDEMIOLOGY & DEMOGRAPHICS

- The incidence of undiagnosed FUO dropped to <10% in the 1950s but increased to approximately 30% in the 1990s.
- True FUOs are uncommon.

CLINICAL PRESENTATION

Fever (101° F or more) >3 wk.

ETIOLOGY

(Most common etiologies italicized)

- Infection (16%)
  - *Abscess: abdominal, pelvic*
  - *Tuberculosis*
  - HIV infection
  - Nosocomial (febrile for 3 days in hospital): urinary tract infection, pneumonia, line-related bacteremia, *Clostridium difficile* diarrhea, sinusitis
  - Bacterial endocarditis (especially caused by difficult-to-isolate organisms)
  - Biliary tract infection
  - Osteomyelitis, vertebral and mandibular
  - Less common infections: Q fever, leptospirosis, psittacosis, tularemia, secondary syphilis, gonococcemia, chronic meningococcemia, Whipple's disease, yersiniosis, fungal infections
- Malignancy (7%): *lymphoma* and *leukemia,* renal cell carcinoma, hepatocellular carcinomas, other tumors metastatic to liver
- Noninfectious inflammatory disease (22%)
  - Juvenile rheumatoid arthritis (younger patients)
  - Temporal arteritis (elderly patients)
  - Other vasculitis: polyarteritis nodosa, Takayasu's arteritis, Wegener's granulomatosis, mixed cryoglobulinemia, adult Still's disease
- Other (4%)
  - Drug-induced fever
  - Inflammatory bowel disease
  - Sarcoidosis
  - Granulomatous hepatitis
  - Deep venous thrombosis
  - Alcoholic hepatitis
- No diagnosis (51%)

Dx DIAGNOSIS

DIFFERENTIAL DIAGNOSIS

Factitious fever

WORKUP

- Accurate history and careful physical examination are essential.
- Laboratory tests and imaging dependent on medical history clues and physical findings.
- When in doubt, perform another complete history and physical examination.

MEDICAL HISTORY CLUES

- Fever duration, tempo; inciting factors
- Rash, myalgia, weight loss, pain
- Sick contacts
- Past medical history: tuberculosis, HIV, malignancies, surgeries
- Medications
- Family history: tuberculosis, malignancies, familial Mediterranean fever
- Social history: daily routine, rural versus urban, pets and animal contacts, arthropod bites, recent and remote travel, socioeconomic status, occupation, military service, sexual history

PHYSICAL FINDINGS

- HEENT (head, ears, eyes, nose, throat): sinus tenderness, dental abscesses, funduscopic lesions
- Neck: adenopathy, palpable thyroid
- Lungs: auscultate for rales
- Heart: murmur
- Abdomen: organomegaly
- Rectal: prostate tenderness
- Pelvic: cervical motion tenderness, fundal or adnexal masses or pain; inguinal adenopathy
- Extremities: clubbing, splinter hemorrhages; tenderness or fluctuance at IV access site
- Musculoskeletal: joint effusions
- Skin: rashes, wounds

LABORATORY TESTS

- Most FUO workups include:
  - Blood cultures
  - Complete blood count with differential
  - Erythrocyte sedimentation rate or C-reactive protein
  - Urinalysis
  - Transaminases
  - Serum lactate dehydrogenase
  - PPD testing
- Consider
  - HIV antibody testing
  - Creatinine phosphokinase
  - Rheumatoid factor
  - Serum protein electrophoresis
  - Lumbar puncture
  - Thyroid function testing
  - Stool culture and *C. difficile* assay
  - Bone marrow biopsy
  - Skin biopsy
  - Antinuclear antibody testing

May need to repeat tests at regular intervals until diagnosis is established.

IMAGING STUDIES

- Most workups eventually include chest radiograph and abdominal CT scan.
- Further imaging is based on medical history clues and physical findings.

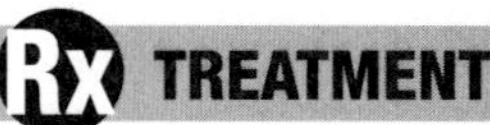

TREATMENT

ACUTE GENERAL Rx

Antibiotics and other treatment indicated only after definitive or highly probable diagnosis is established unless patient is severely ill or septic.

DISPOSITION

Diagnoses are found in majority of cases of FUO. In some cases a diagnosis is not made for years. At 5-yr follow-up, mortality rate among patients with undiagnosed FUO was only 3.2% in one study.

REFERRAL

To an infectious disease specialist, hematologist, or rheumatologist if no diagnosis after thoughtful workup

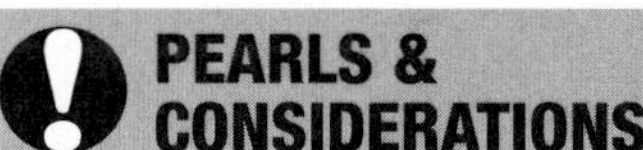

PEARLS & CONSIDERATIONS

COMMENTS

Because of improvements in imaging and laboratory tests, fewer cases of FUO are attributed to infectious causes and more are diagnosed as attributable to tumors and collagen-vascular diseases.

SUGGESTED READINGS

Bleeker-Rovers CP et al: A prospective multicenter study on fever of unknown origin: the yield of a structured diagnostic approach, *Medicine (Baltimore)* 86:26, 2007.

Knockaert DC et al: Long-term follow-up of patients with undiagnosed fever of unknown origin, *Arch Intern Med* 156:6, 1996.

Mourad O et al: A comprehensive evidence-based approach to fever of unknown origin, *Arch Intern Med* 163:5, 2003.

Vanderschueren S et al: From prolonged febrile illness to fever of unknown origin: the challenge continues, *Arch Intern Med* 163, 2003.

AUTHOR: **ETSUKO AOKI, M.D., PH.D.**

Fibrocystic Breast Disease 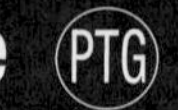

BASIC INFORMATION

DEFINITION

Fibrocystic breast disease (FCD) is a "nondisease" that includes nonmalignant breast lesions such as microcystic and macrocystic changes, fibrosis, ductal or lobular hyperplasia, adenosis, apocrine metaplasia, fibroadenoma, papilloma, papillomatosis, and other changes. Atypical ductal or lobular hyperplasia is associated with a moderate increase in breast cancer risk.

SYNONYMS

Cystic changes
Chronic cystic mastitis
Mammary dysplasia

ICD-9CM CODES
610.0 Solitary cyst of the breast
610.1 Fibrocystic disease of the breast

EPIDEMIOLOGY & DEMOGRAPHICS

- Ubiquitous in premenopausal women after 20 yr of age
- Palpable nodular changes in the breast termed FCD clinically; such changes observable in more than half of adult women 20 to 50 yr of age

PHYSICAL FINDINGS & CLINICAL PRESENTATION

- Tender breasts
- Nodular areas
- Dominant mass
- Thickening
- Nipple discharge
- Can vary with menstrual cycle

ETIOLOGY

- Although it is frequently seen and diagnosed, mechanism of development is not understood.
- Because it is found in the majority of healthy breasts, it is regarded as a nonpathologic process.
- With hormone replacement therapy, the condition may be carried into menopause.

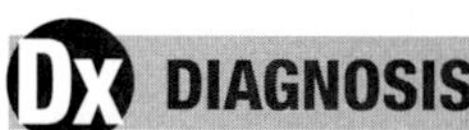

DIAGNOSIS

DIFFERENTIAL DIAGNOSIS

- If presenting as dominant mass or masses, exclude possible carcinoma.
- Carcinoma: detection is difficult with FCD, particularly among premenopausal women.
- If presenting with nipple discharge, differentiate from discharge of possible malignant origin.

WORKUP

- Exclude breast carcinoma if breast mass, thickening, discharge, and/or pain are present.
- Perform biopsy of suspected area for histologic confirmation.

IMAGING STUDIES

Mammography and ultrasound studies required:
- For mammographic changes (suspicious densities, microcalcifications, architectural distortion): careful evaluation, including possibly biopsy to exclude breast cancer
- Ultrasound study: to establish cystic nature of clinical or mammographic mass lesion

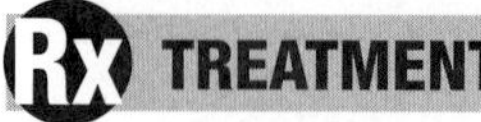

TREATMENT

NONPHARMACOLOGIC THERAPY

- Not considered a "disease" and does not require treatment
- Surgical intervention diagnostic to eliminate possibility of breast cancer
- Periodic physician examination to monitor patients with FCD who have pronounced nodular features
- Aspiration for palpable cysts (NOTE: Cysts often recur; repeat aspiration is not always required unless pain is a problem.)

ACUTE GENERAL Rx

The majority of women require no treatment.

CHRONIC Rx

For breast pain:
- Danocrine (Danazol): limited success reported
- Bromocriptine or tamoxifen: used less frequently
- Limited caffeine intake: not as successful in controlling pain or nodularity as originally suggested

DISPOSITION

- Careful evaluation to exclude suspicious changes for breast cancer, then reassurance and periodic reevaluation as required
- Regular self-examination, annual physician examination, and annual mammograms for women with atypical ductal or lobular hyperplasia

REFERRAL

- For further evaluation and/or biopsy if there are suspicious changes that may be associated with FCD (including changing of dominant mass or thickening, persistent or spontaneous discharge, suspicious mammographic changes or lesions)
- To alleviate anxiety associated with breast symptoms or changes

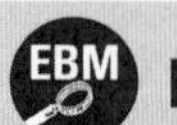

EVIDENCE

There is evidence that both danazol and tamoxifen are effective at relieving breast pain in benign breast conditions, but their benefit needs to be balanced with their side effects.

A randomized controlled trial (RCT) found that danazol and tamoxifen were both significantly more effective than placebo in relieving pain in women with severe cyclical mastalgia. There was no significant difference in pain relief between the two active treatments.[1,2] Ⓐ

A small RCT compared tamoxifen versus placebo in premenopausal women with cyclical breast pain. Significantly more women in the tamoxifen group reported pain relief.[3] Ⓐ

Another RCT compared tamoxifen versus placebo for the treatment of mastalgia and found that the number of women who achieved complete recovery was increased in the tamoxifen group (90% with tamoxifen versus 0% with placebo).[4] Ⓐ

There is limited evidence that bromocriptine is effective in relieving breast pain. However, a high incidence of intolerable side effects is reported, which may outweigh any benefit.

One RCT found that bromocriptine significantly improved breast pain, tenderness, and heaviness compared with placebo in premenopausal women with diffuse fibrocystic breast changes. However, bromocriptine was associated with a significantly higher incidence of adverse effects. The high rate of withdrawal from this study means that the results should be interpreted with caution.[5] Ⓑ

There is evidence that advice to eat a low-fat, high-carbohydrate diet leads to decreased self-reported breast tenderness.

A small RCT compared advice to follow a low-fat, high-carbohydrate diet versus general dietary advice in women with severe cyclical mastalgia. There was a significant reduction in the severity of self-reported breast swelling and tenderness in patients in the low-fat, high-carbohydrate diet group after 6 mo. However, there was no significant reduction in breast swelling, tenderness, or nodularity at physical examination.[6] Ⓑ

Evidence-Based References

1. Kontostolis E et al: Comparison of tamoxifen with danazol for treatment of cyclical mastalgia, *Gynecol Endocrinol* 11:393-397, 1997. Ⓐ

2. Mansel RE et al: Controlled trial of the antigonadotropin danazol in painful nodular benign breast disease, *Lancet* 1:928-930, 1982.

3. Fentiman IS et al: Double-blind controlled trial of tamoxifen therapy for mastalgia, *Lancet* 1:287-288, 1986. Ⓐ

4. Grio R et al: Clinical efficacy of tamoxifen in the treatment of premenstrual mastodynia, *Minerva Ginecol* 50:101-103, 1998. Ⓐ

5. Mansel RE, Dogliotti L: European multicentre trial of bromocriptine in cyclical mastalgia, *Lancet* 335:190-193, 1990. Ⓑ

6. Boyd NF et al: Effect of a low-fat high-carbohydrate diet on symptoms of cyclical mastopathy, *Lancet* 2:128-132, 1988. Ⓑ

AUTHORS: **TAKUMA NEMOTO, M.D.,** and **RUBEN ALVERO, M.D.**

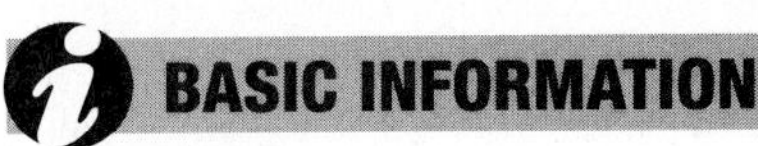

BASIC INFORMATION

DEFINITION

Fibromyalgia is a poorly defined disorder characterized by multiple trigger points and referred pain.

SYNONYMS

Myofascial pain syndrome
Fibrositis
Psychogenic rheumatism
Nonarticular rheumatism
Fibromyalgia syndrome (FS)

ICD-9CM CODES
729.0 Rheumatism, unspecified and fibrositis
729.1 Myalgia and myositis, unspecified

EPIDEMIOLOGY & DEMOGRAPHICS

PREVALENCE: 1% to 2% of the general population
PREDOMINANT SEX: Female/male ratio of 9:1
PREDOMINANT AGE: 30 to 50 yr

PHYSICAL FINDINGS

Tender "nodules" and tender points (Fig. 1-121)

ETIOLOGY

- Unknown. Genetic, environmental, and psychosocial factors appear to influence its expression.
- Pain magnification may play a role

Dx DIAGNOSIS

DIFFERENTIAL DIAGNOSIS

- Polymyalgia rheumatica
- Referred discogenic spine pain
- Rheumatoid arthritis
- Localized tendinitis
- Connective tissue disease
- Osteoarthritis
- Thyroid disease
- Spondyloarthropathies

WORKUP

- Subsets of this disorder are often described:
  1. If symptoms develop in conjunction with other conditions (rheumatoid disease or acute stress)
  2. If findings are more regionally distributed, such as those in the neck after motor vehicle accidents
- The primary condition is often suggested by the following criteria from the American College of Rheumatology:
  1. History of widespread pain
  2. Pain in 11 of 18 selected tender spots on digital palpation (mainly in the spine, elbows, and knees)

LABORATORY TESTS

There are no abnormalities in fibromyalgia, but laboratory assessment may be required to rule out other conditions and may include:

- Complete blood count, erythrocyte sedimentation rate, rheumatoid factor, antinuclear antibody
- Creatine phosphokinase, T_4

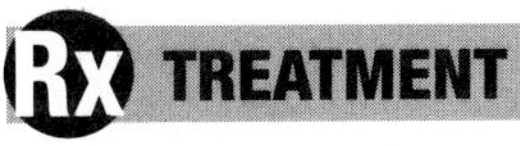

Rx TREATMENT

ACUTE GENERAL Rx

- Self-management
- Explanation, reassurance
- Aerobic and stretching exercise, particularly swimming
- Mild analgesics; avoidance of chronic narcotic use
- Pregabalin 120 mg/day may be effective in symptom control (Lyrica), a GABA analog (75 mg bid), duloxetine (Cymbalta), an SNRI (60-120 mg/day), and milnacipam (Savella), an SNRI (50 mg bid), may be effective in symptom control
- Low-dose tricyclic antidepressants for sleep disturbance (amitriptyline 10 to 25 mg)
- Tricyclic antidepressants for sleep disturbance (amitriptyline 10 to 25 mg)
- Trigger point injections
- Physical therapy

DISPOSITION

- Prognosis is uncertain.
- Symptoms come and go for years despite an aggressive, multifaceted approach to treatment.

REFERRAL

Consultation with rheumatology, psychiatry, and physical medicine may all be helpful.

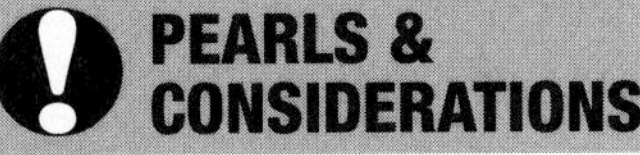

PEARLS & CONSIDERATIONS

Some investigators consider myofascial pain syndrome to be a separate condition, perhaps with a better prognosis.

COMMENTS

- Before making this diagnosis, all other more likely disorders should be ruled out.
- The term "fibrositis" is often used, but no inflammation has ever been found.
- The number of trigger points needed to establish the diagnosis is debated.

SUGGESTED READINGS

Abeles M et al: Update on fibromyalgia therapy, *Am J Med* 121:555-561, 2008.

Bieber C et al: A shared decision-making communication training program for physicians treating fibromyalgia patients: effects of a randomized controlled trial, *J Psychom Res* 64:13, 2008.

Chakrabarty S, Zoorob R: Fibromyalgia, *Am Fam Physician* 76:247-254, 2007.

Freidberg F et al: Publication trends in chronic fatigue syndrome: comparisons with fibromyalgia and fatigue, *J Psychom Res* 63:143, 2007.

Hauser W et al: Treatment of fibromyalgia syndrome with antidepressants, *JAMA* 301(2):198-209, 2009.

Jones KD, Liptan GL: Exercise interventions in fibromyalgia: clinical applications from the evidence, *Rheum Dis Clin North Am* 35(2):373-391, 2009.

Lavergne MR et al: Functional impairment in chronic fatigue syndrome, fibromyalgia, and multiple chemical sensitivity, *Can Fam Physician* 56:57, 2010.

Valkeinen H et al: Acute heavy-resistance exercise-induced pain and neuromuscular fatigue in elderly women with fibromyalgia and in healthy controls: effects of strength training, *Arthritis Rheum* 54:1334, 2006.

Van Middendorp H et al: Emotions and emotional approach and avoidance strategies in fibromyalgia, *J Psychom Res* 64:159, 2008.

Van Wilgen et al: Characteristics and healthcare costs of patients with fibromyalgia implemented in the primary care, *Disabil Rehabil* 29:1207, 2007.

AUTHOR: **LONNIE R. MERCIER, M.D.**

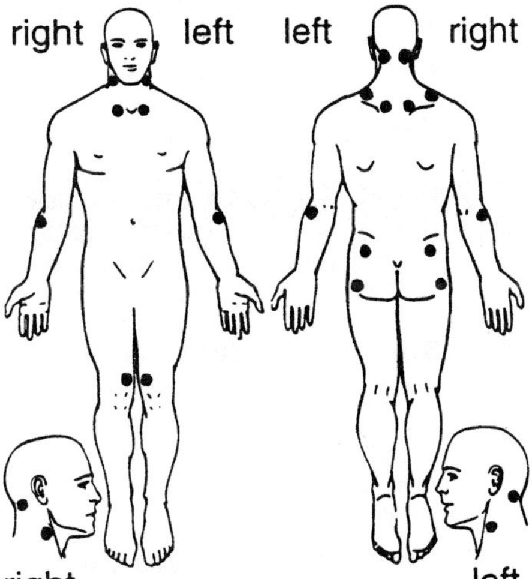

FIGURE 1-121 The sites of the 18 tender points of the 1990 American College of Rheumatology criteria for the classification of fibromyalgia. (From Conn R: *Current diagnosis,* ed 9, Philadelphia, 1997, WB Saunders.)

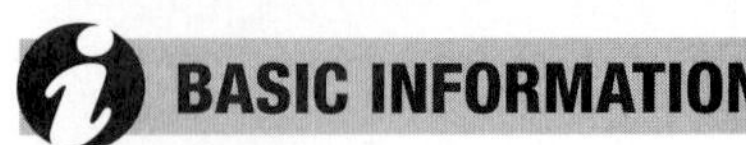

Fifth Disease (PTG)

BASIC INFORMATION

DEFINITION

Fifth disease is a viral exanthem of childhood primarily affecting school-age children that is caused by parvovirus B-19. Historically, erythema infectiosum was the "fifth" in a series of described viral exanthems of childhood and is the most common clinical syndrome associated with parvovirus B-19.

SYNONYMS

Erythema infectiosum

ICD-9CM CODES
057.0 Fifth disease (eruptive)

EPIDEMIOLOGY & DEMOGRAPHICS

PEAK INCIDENCE: Late winter and spring, especially April and May

PREDOMINANT AGE: 5 to 18 yr

GENETICS: Fifty percent to 60% of adults have demonstrated protective antibodies to parvovirus B-19.

PHYSICAL FINDINGS & CLINICAL PRESENTATION

- Typical bright red, nontender maxillary rash with circumoral pallor over cheeks, producing the classic "slapped cheek" appearance (Fig. 1-122)

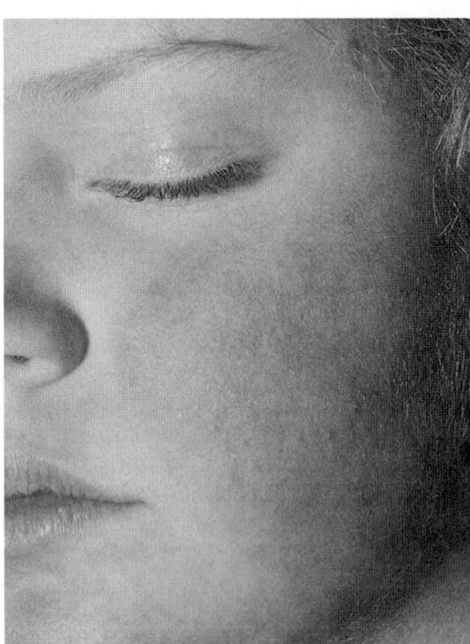

FIGURE 1-122 Fifth disease (erythema infectiosum). Facial erythema "slapped cheek." The red plaque covers the cheek and spares the nasolabial and the circumoral region. (From Habif TP: *Clinical dermatology: a color guide to diagnosis and therapy,* ed 3, St Louis, 1996, Mosby.)

- Reticular, nonpruritic, lacy, erythematous, maculopapular rash over trunk and extremities lasting for up to several weeks after the acute episode. May be worsened by heat or sunlight.
- Polyarthritis and arthralgias are commonly seen in older patients and less commonly in children. Arthritis involves small joints of the extremities in symmetric fashion.
- Mild fever is seen in up to one third of patients.

ETIOLOGY

Syndrome caused by parvovirus B-19, a single-stranded DNA virus, which has been reclassified in the new genus Erythrovirus.

- It remains the only accepted member of this genus, although new variants have recently been described.
- Designation as "parvovirus" is still common in recent literature.

DIAGNOSIS

DIFFERENTIAL DIAGNOSIS

- Juvenile rheumatoid arthritis (Still's disease)
- Rubella, measles (rubeola), and other childhood viral exanthems
- Mononucleosis
- Lyme disease
- Acute HIV infection
- Drug eruption

WORKUP

- Diagnosis made by typical clinical picture
- Parvovirus B-19 immunoglobulin (Ig) M antibody seen in 90% of patients with acute illness

LABORATORY TESTS

- Complete blood count
  1. Transient aplastic crisis is a syndrome distinct from fifth disease, which may be seen in patients with chronic hematologic illness (described with sickle cell disease, spherocytosis, and other hemolytic processes) or AIDS, who are infected with parvovirus B-19.
     a. Usually self-limited and associated with prodrome of fever and malaise. Lasts for 1 to 2 wk followed by marrow recovery.
     b. Rash is usually absent.
     c. These patients are highly infective.
- Human chorionic gonadotropin in women of childbearing age
  - Infection during early pregnancy may result in fetal death (10%) or severe anemia but is usually asymptomatic and not associated with congenital malformations.
- Antibody testing is usually not necessary. IgM levels may be elevated early in the course of the illness.
- Lyme titers, monospot Ab.
- Testing for other viral diseases as indicated by clinical picture.
- Polymerase chain reaction has been used for early, rapid diagnosis in immunocompromised patients.

TREATMENT

ACUTE GENERAL Rx

- Treatment is supportive only
- Nonsteroidal anti-inflammatory drugs for arthralgias and arthritis
- IV immunoglobulin and transfusion support may be used in patients with immunocompromised state with red cell aplasia
- Consider immunoglobulin treatment or prophylaxis in pregnancy

DISPOSITION & PROGNOSIS

- Self-limited illness lasting 1 to 2 wk.
- Arthritis lasts for weeks. In some patients it may be chronic and develop into rheumatoid arthritis as adults.
- Pregnant women should avoid contact with patients who have marrow suppression. Maternal parvovirus infection in pregnancy may have a wide range of fetal effects, including hydrops fetalis, and warrants close monitoring of fetal development and health.
- Patients with transient aplastic crisis or chronic parvovirus B-19 infection pose a risk for nosocomial spread and, when hospitalized, should be isolated with contact and respiratory precautions.
- Children with fifth disease are not contagious and may attend school and day care.
- A vaccine is under development.

REFERRAL

- To hematologist for signs of marrow suppression
- To rheumatologist for signs of severe or erosive arthritis

PEARLS & CONSIDERATIONS

- Self-limited disease lasting 1-2 wk
- Symmetric arthritis involving small joints is common in adults, whereas facial rash is common in children
- Can cause aplastic anemia in patients with an underlying hematologic disorder such as sickle cell disease, in an immunocompromised state, and after transplantation.

SUGGESTED READINGS

Servey JT et al: Clinical presentations of parvovirus B19 infections, *Am Fam Physician* 75(3):373-276, 2007.

Young NS: Parvovirus B19, *New Engl J Med* 350(6): 586, 2004.

AUTHOR: **DOMINICK TAMMARO, M.D.**

BASIC INFORMATION

DEFINITION

Filariasis is a general term for an infection caused by subcutaneous nematodes (roundworms) of the genera *Wuchereria* and *Brugia,* found in the tropical and subtropical regions of the world. The disease is variably characterized by acute lymphatic inflammation or chronic lymphatic obstruction associated with intermittent fevers or recurrent episodes of dyspnea and bronchospasm.

SYNONYMS

Lymphatic filariasis
Elephantiasis

ICD-9CM CODES
125.0 Bancroftian
125.1 Brugian
125.9 Filariasis

EPIDEMIOLOGY & DEMOGRAPHICS

INCIDENCE (IN U.S.): Unknown
PEAK INCIDENCE: Unknown
PREDOMINANT SEX: Male
PREDOMINANT AGE: For both males and females, risk is greatest between the ages of 15 and 35 yr.

PHYSICAL FINDINGS & CLINICAL PRESENTATION

- Clinical manifestations result from acute lymphatic inflammation or chronic lymphatic obstruction.
- Many patients are asymptomatic despite the presence of microfilaremia.
- Episodes of lymphangitis and lymphadenitis are associated with fever, headache, and back pain.
- Acute funiculitis and epididymitis or orchitis may also be present; all usually resolve within days to weeks but tend to recur.
- Chronic infections may be associated with lymphedema, most commonly manifested by hydrocele.
- It is a progressive disease, leading to nonpitting edema and brawny changes that may involve a whole limb (Fig. 1-123).
- Elephantiasis occurs in about 10% of patients, with skin of the scrotum or leg becoming thickened and fissured; patient is thereafter plagued by recurrent ulceration and infection.
- Chyluria, a condition that develops when lymphatic vessels rupture into the urinary tract, may occur.

ETIOLOGY

Caused by one of three types of nematode parasite, all of which are transmitted to humans by *Culex* spp. mosquitoes.
- *W. bancrofti:* distributed in Africa, areas of Central and South America, the Pacific Islands, and the Caribbean Basin
- *B. malayi:* restricted to Southeast Asia
- *B. timori:* confined to the Indonesian archipelago

After bite of an infected mosquito:
- Filarial larvae move into lymphatic vessels and nodes, settling and maturing over 3 to 15 mo into adult male and female worms.
- After fertilization, the female nematode produces large numbers of larvae or microfilariae that enter into the bloodstream via the lymphatics.
- Nocturnal periodicity, characteristic of *B. malayi,* is an increased presence of microfilariae in the circulation during the night.
- Microfilariae of *W. bancrofti* are maximal during late afternoon.
- Most microfilariae remain in the body as immature forms for 6 mo to 2 yr.
- Infected larvae are ingested by mosquitoes, then transmitted to humans, where the microfilariae mature into new adult worms.

Acute and chronic inflammatory and granulomatous changes in the lymphatic channels:
- Result from complex interaction of adult worms and host's immune systems
- Eventually lead to fibrosis and obstruction
- Most likely to develop into obstructive lymphatic disease with recurrent exposure over many years

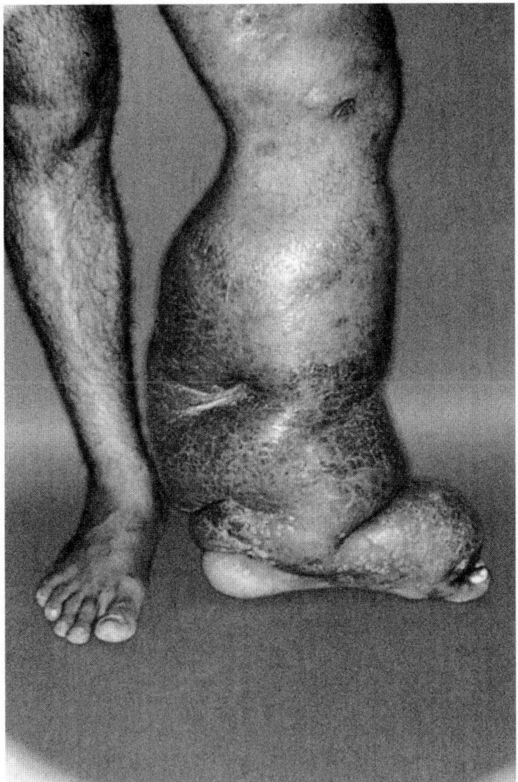

FIGURE 1-123 Filariasis that eventually leads to elephantiasis. Note massive swelling of the extremity. (From Goldstein B [ed]: *Practical dermatology,* ed 2, St Louis, 1997, Mosby.)

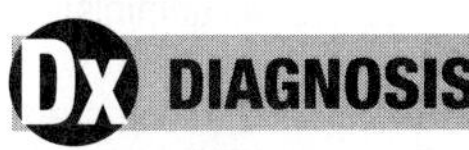

DIAGNOSIS

DIFFERENTIAL DIAGNOSIS

Elephantiasis is distinguished from other causes of chronic lymphedema, including Milroy's disease, postoperative scarring, and lymphedema of malignancy.

WORKUP

Diagnosis is suspected in individuals who have resided in endemic areas for at least 3 to 6 mo or more and complain of recurrent episodes of lymphangitis, lymphadenitis, scrotal edema, or thrombophlebitis, with or without fever.

LABORATORY TESTS

- Demonstration of microfilariae on a blood smear for definitive diagnosis
- For patients from southeastern Asia: blood sample drawn at night, especially between midnight and 2 A.M.
- Occasionally, microfilaremia in chylous urine or hydrocele fluid
- Prominent eosinophilia only during periods of acute lymphangitis or lymphadenitis
- Serologic tests for antibody, including enzyme-linked immunosorbent assay and indirect fluorescent antibody (often unable to distinguish among the various forms of filariasis or between acute and remote infection)
- Immunoassays (such as circulating filaria antigen [CFA]): more successful in antigen detection in patients who are microfilaremic than in those who are amicrofilaremic

IMAGING STUDIES

- Chest radiograph: reticular nodular infiltrates (tropical pulmonary eosinophilia syndrome)
- In men proven to be microfilaremic, scrotal ultrasonography to aid in the detection of adult worms
- Compared with adults, children with FS have more sleep disturbances, fewer tender points, and a better prognosis

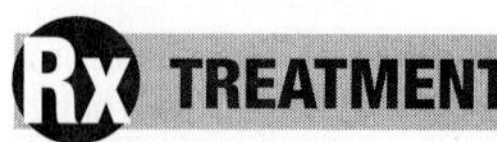

TREATMENT

NONPHARMACOLOGIC THERAPY

- Standard of care for elephantiasis:
  1. Elevation of the affected limb
  2. Use of elastic stockings
  3. Local foot care
- General wound care for chronic ulcers and prevention of secondary infection

ACUTE GENERAL Rx

- Diethylcarbamazine citrate (DEC) to reduce microfilaremia by 90%
  1. Effect on adult worms, especially those of the *Wuchereria* species, less certain
  2. Given in an oral dose of 6 mg/kg qd for 12 to 14 days
- Ivermectin alone or in combination with diethylcarbamazine citrate to decrease microfilaremia
- Both drugs are similar in efficacy and tolerability; advantage of ivermectin: administration in a single oral dose of 200 μg/kg
- World Health Organization (WHO) recommendation: DEC given as a single dose, alone or (preferably) in combination with ivermectin as treatment in endemic areas
- Antibacterial agents (a penicillin or cephalosporin) may be indicated to treat co-existing bacterial soft tissue infection (cellulitis or lymphangiitis), which frequently complicates filariasis of the lower extremities.

CHRONIC Rx

- Surgical drainage of hydroceles
- No satisfactory therapy for those patients with chyluria

DISPOSITION

Rarely fatal, but the psychologic impact of limb and scrotal deformities associated with elephantiasis is substantial.

REFERRAL

To a surgeon for management of hydrocele

PEARLS & CONSIDERATIONS

- Studies in endemic areas suggest that filarial-specific IgG1 is associated with amicrofilaremic states highest in children, regardless of sex.
- Levels of IgE and IgG4 increase with age and are associated with increased levels of microfilaremia.

COMMENTS

Individuals who intend to travel or reside in endemic areas should be advised to institute preventive measures such as the use of netting and insect repellents, especially at night.

SUGGESTED READINGS

Kerketta AS et al: A randomized clinical trial to compare the efficacy of three treatment regimens along with footcare in the morbidity management of filarial lymphoedema, *Trop Med Int Health* 10(7): 698, 2005.

Malhotra I et al: Influence of maternal filariasis on childhood infection and immunity to Wuchereria bancrofti in Kenya, *Infect Immun* 71(9):5231, 2003.

Pal BK et al: Lymphatic filariasis: possible pathophysiological nexus with oxidative stress, *Trans R Soc Trop Med Hyg* 100(7):650, 2006.

Ramaiah KD et al: The prevalences of Wuchereria bancrofti antigenemia in communities given six rounds of treatment with diethylcarbamazine, ivermectin or placebo tablets, *Ann Trop Med Parasitol* 97(7):737, 2003.

Walther M, Muller R: Diagnosis of human filariases (except onchocerciasis), *Adv Parasitol* 53:149, 2003.

Watanabe K et al: Bancroftian filariasis in Nepal: a survey for circulating antigenemia of Wuchereria bancrofti and urinary IgG4 antibody in two rural areas of Nepal, *Acta Trop* 88(1):11, 2003.

AUTHORS: **GLENN G. FORT, M.D., M.P.H.,** and **DENNIS J. MIKOLICH, M.D.**

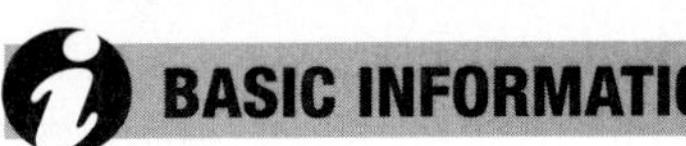

BASIC INFORMATION

DEFINITION

Exaggerated tone, which displays a velocity-dependent increase in resistance of muscles to a passive stretch stimulus

SYNONYMS

Hypertonicity

ICD-9CM CODES

782.85 Spasm of muscle
342.1, 343.0-344.9 Spastic paralysis
781.0 Abnormal involuntary movements/ Spasms NOS
781.2 Abnormality of gait/spastic
342.1 Spastic hemiplegia
344.0-344.9 Spastic paralysis specified as noncongenital or noninfantile
343 Infantile cerebral palsy/spastic infantile paralysis

EPIDEMIOLOGY & DEMOGRAPHICS

INCIDENCE: Spasticity affects between 47% and 70% of people with multiple sclerosis, 32% to 36% of those with spinal cord injury, approximately 20% of those with stroke, more than 90% with cerebral palsy, and approximately 50% of patients with traumatic brain injury.

PREDOMINANT SEX AND AGE: Spasticity is not affected by sex, race, or age group, nor is it more prevalent in any of those groups.

RISK FACTORS: Multiple sclerosis, stroke, spinal cord injury, cerebral palsy, traumatic brain injury

PHYSICAL FINDINGS & CLINICAL PRESENTATION

- Patient may present with impaired gait, impaired limb function, decreased mobility, or discomfort due to increased muscle tone.
- Examine active and passive motion, reflexes, and function:
  - Strength may be normal to decreased. Isometric strength is typically greater than concentric strength.
  - Tone may be slightly to severely (modified Ashworth scale see Table 1-30) increased to passive range of motion.
  - Reflexes are typically brisk.
  - Patient may have accompanied extensor plantar signs, clonus, or spontaneous flexor spasms.
  - Function may be impaired or enhanced due to increased tone.

ETIOLOGY

Upper motor neuron injury, most commonly due to multiple sclerosis, stroke, spinal cord injury, cerebral palsy, traumatic brain injury

TABLE 1-30 Modified Ashworth Scale

0	No increase in muscle tone
1	Slight increase in muscle tone, manifested by a catch and release or by minimal resistance at the end range of motion when the part is moved in flexion or extension/abduction or adduction
1+	Slight increase in muscle tone, manifested by a catch, followed by minimal resistance throughout the remainder (less than half) of the range of motion
2	More marked increase in muscle tone through most of the range of motion, but the affected part is easily moved
3	Considerable increase in muscle tone, passive movement is difficult
4	Affected part is rigid in flexion or extension (abduction or adduction)

From Stein J: Spasticity. In Frontera (ed): *Essentials of physical medicine and rehabilitation,* ed 2, Philadelphia, 2008, Saunders.

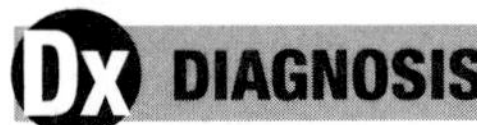

DIAGNOSIS

DIFFERENTIAL DIAGNOSIS

Rigidity, clonus, dystonia, dyskinesia, myotonia, tetanus, muscle contracture, cramps

WORKUP

- The diagnosis of spasticity can be established on a clinical basis alone.
- Investigate for reversible exacerbating causes of spasticity: underlying infection, bladder distention, bowel impaction, fracture, pain.

LABORATORY TESTS

Urinalysis, complete blood count, metabolic panel

IMAGING STUDIES

Chest x-ray, abdominal x-ray series, bladder ultrasound

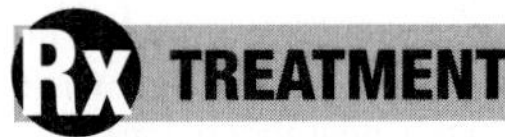

TREATMENT

First treat reversible causes of worsened spasticity (see "Workup"), then proceed to physical and pharmacologic therapeutics. Lastly, consider surgical intervention in severe, refractory cases.

NONPHARMACOLOGIC THERAPY

- Physical therapeutics include range of motion and muscle stretching, serial casting or orthotics, muscle cooling, electrical stimulation.
- Surgical procedures include tenotomy, tendon lengthening, and tendon transfers. More invasive surgical interventions include peripheral neurectomy, myelotomy, and rhizotomy.

ACUTE GENERAL Rx

- Oral medications: baclofen, tizanidine, diazepam, dantrolene (see Table 1-31)
- Other interventions: intrathecal baclofen, botulism toxin intramuscular injections, chemical nerve blocks (with bupivacaine, phenol, or ethyl alcohol)

COMPLEMENTARY & ALTERNATIVE MEDICINE

EMG biofeedback

DISPOSITION

Typically nonprogressive, but medications may lose efficacy after long duration of use. Drug holidays (with use of alternate spasmolytic) may be beneficial.

REFERRAL

- Physicians: neurologist or physiatrist with expertise in botulism toxin injection and/or intrathecal spasmolytic therapy is recommended in cases where oral medication is ineffective or not tolerated.
- Therapists: physical or occupational are recommended.

TABLE 1-31 Commonly Used Oral Spasmolytic Medications

Medication	Mechanism of Action	Starting Dose	Maximum Dose	Common Side Effects	Considerations†
Baclofen	GABA-B agonist	5 mg tid	20 mg qid*	Sedation, rare hepatotoxicity	Cognitive impairment
Diazepam	GABA-A agonist	2 mg bid	10 mg qid	Sedation, dependence or tolerance	History of substance abuse, cognitive impairment
Tizanidine	α-2 agonist	2 mg tid	12 mg tid	Sedation, hypotension, hepatotoxicity	Cognitive impairment
Dantrolene	Blocks Ca^{2+} release from sarcoplasmic reticulum	25 mg daily	100 mg qid	Weakness, hepatotoxicity	Liver disease

*Approved by the U.S. Food and Drug Administration only up to 80 mg/day, but many clinicians exceed this in patients who tolerate this medication well but do not respond to smaller doses.
†Baclofen, diazepam, and tizanidine are centrally acting and may exacerbate cognitive impairment. Dantrolene acts peripherally; however, it has the rare but fatal side effect of hepatotoxicity.
Modified from Stein J: Spasticity. In Frontera (ed): *Essentials of physical medicine and rehabilitation,* ed 2, Philadelphia, 2008, Saunders.

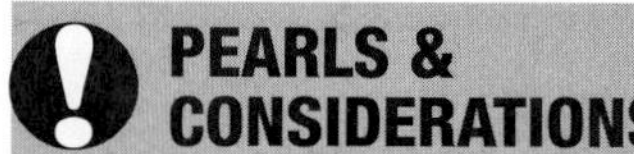

- Assess whether the spasms recently increased in severity or intensity (as would occur with reversible exacerbating causes).
- Consider whether patient's tone is beneficial or detrimental to patient's functionality or overall health status.
- Spasticity may contribute to posture and mobility, as well as maintain muscle mass and bone mineralization, reduce dependent edema, and prevent deep venous thromboses.
- Spasticity may impair patient's functionality, interfere with activities of daily living, interfere with sleep, and cause discomfort.
- Monitor liver function with dantrolene and tizanidine, as these drugs may cause hepatotoxicity.

SUGGESTED READINGS

Bovend'Eerdt T et al: The effects of stretching in spasticity: a systematic review, *Arch Phys Med Rehabil* 89(7):1395-1406, 2008.

Gupta A et al: Non-traumatic spinal cord lesions: epidemiology, complications, neurological and functional outcome of rehabilitation, *Spinal Cord* 47:307-311, 2009.

Little J, Massagli T: Spasticity and associated abnormalities of muscle tone. In Delisa J, Gans B (eds): *Rehabilitation medicine: principles and practice,* ed 3, Philadelphia, 1998, Lippincott-Raven.

New P et al: Nontraumatic spinal cord injury: demographic characteristics and complications, *Arch Phys Med Rehabil* 83(7):996-1001, 2002.

Stein, J: Spasticity. In Frontera (ed): *Essentials of physical medicine and rehabilitation,* ed 2, Philadelphia, 2008, Saunders.

Wedekind C, Lippert-Gruner M: Long-term outcome in severe traumatic brain injury is significantly influenced by brainstem involvement, *Brain Inj* 19:681-684, 2005.

Wichers MJ et al: Clinical presentation, associated disorders and aetiological moments in cerebral palsy: a Dutch population-based study, *Disabil Rehabil* 27:583-589, 2005.

AUTHOR: **KARA A. KENNEDY, D.O.**

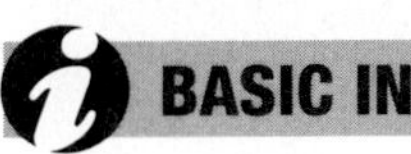

BASIC INFORMATION

DEFINITION

Folliculitis is inflammation of the hair follicle as a result of infection, physical injury, or chemical irritation.

SYNONYMS

Sycosis barbae

ICD-9CM CODES

704.8 Other specified diseases of hair and hair follicles

EPIDEMIOLOGY & DEMOGRAPHICS

PREVALENCE: Staphylococcal folliculitis is the most common form of infectious folliculitis; it occurs most commonly in persons with diabetes.

PREDOMINANT SEX: Sycosis barbae occurs most frequently in men who have commenced shaving.

PHYSICAL FINDINGS & CLINICAL PRESENTATION

- The lesions generally consist of painful yellow pustules surrounded by erythema; a central hair is present in the pustules.
- Patients with sycosis barbae may initially present with small follicular papules or pustules that increase in size with continued shaving; deep follicular pustules may occur surrounded by erythema and swelling; the upper lip is frequently involved (Fig. 1-124).
- "Hot tub" folliculitis occurs within 1 to 4 days after the use of a hot tub with poor chlorination. It is characterized by pustules with surrounding erythema generally affecting the torso, buttocks, and limbs.

ETIOLOGY

- *Staphylococcus* infection (e.g., sycosis barbae), *Pseudomonas aeruginosa* ("hot tub" folliculitis)
- Gram-negative folliculitis *(Klebsiella, Enterobacter, Proteus)* associated with antibiotic treatment of acne
- Chronic irritation of the hair follicle (use of cocoa butter or coconut oil, chronic irritation from workplace)
- Initial use of systemic corticosteroid therapy (steroid acne), eosinophilic folliculitis (AIDS patients), *Candida albicans* (immunocompromised patients)
- *Pityrosporum orbiculare*

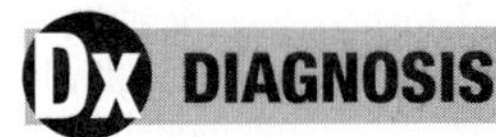

DIAGNOSIS

DIFFERENTIAL DIAGNOSIS

- Pseudofolliculitis barbae (ingrown hairs)
- Acne vulgaris
- Dermatophyte fungal infections
- Keratosis biliaris
- Cutaneous candidiasis
- Superficial fungal infections
- Miliaris

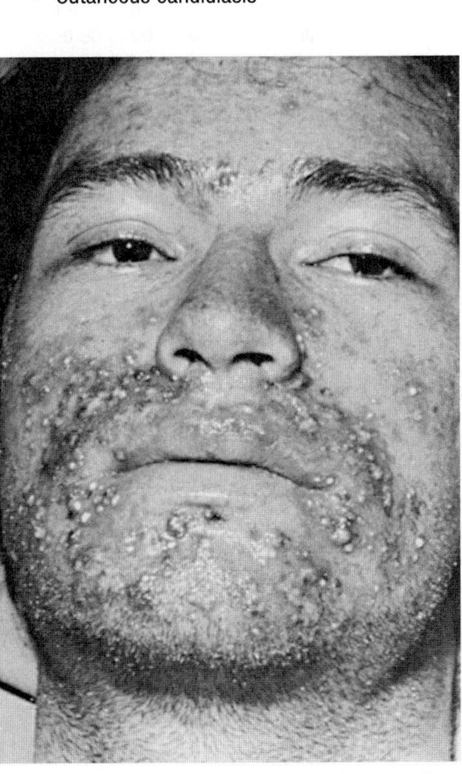

FIGURE 1-124 Folliculitis. Note the pustular eruption with small abscess formation in the hair-bearing areas of the face. General symptoms are usually absent. (From Mandell GL: *Mandell, Douglas, and Bennett's principles and practice of infectious diseases,* ed 6, New York, 2004, Churchill Livingstone.)

WORKUP

Physical examination and medical history (e.g., use of hot tub: "hot tub" folliculitis; adolescent patients who have started shaving: sycosis barbae; use of occlusive topical steroid therapy: *Staphylococcus* folliculitis).

LABORATORY TESTS

- Generally not necessary.
- Gram stain is useful to identify the infective organisms in infectious folliculitis and to differentiate infectious folliculitis from noninfectious.

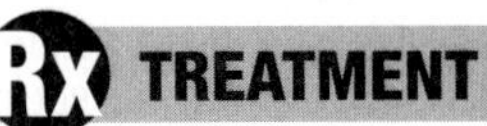

TREATMENT

NONPHARMACOLOGIC THERAPY

- Prevention of chemical or mechanical skin irritation
- Glycemic control in diabetics
- Proper chlorination of hot tubs and spas
- Shaving with a clean razor

ACUTE GENERAL Rx

- Cleansing of the area with chlorhexidine and application of saline compresses to involved area
- Application of 2% mupirocin ointment or 1% Retapamulin ointment for bacterial folliculitis affecting a limited area (e.g., sycosis barbae)
- Treatment of severe cases of *Pseudomonas* folliculitis with ciprofloxacin
- Treatment of *S. aureus* folliculitis with dicloxacillin 250 mg qd for 10 days

CHRONIC Rx

- Chronic nasal or perineal *S. aureus* carriers with frequent folliculitis can be treated with rifampin 300 mg bid for 5 days.
- Mupirocin or Retapamulin ointment applied to nares bid is also effective for nasal carriers.

DISPOSITION

- Most cases of bacterial folliculitis resolve completely with proper treatment.
- Steroid folliculitis responds to discontinuation of steroids.

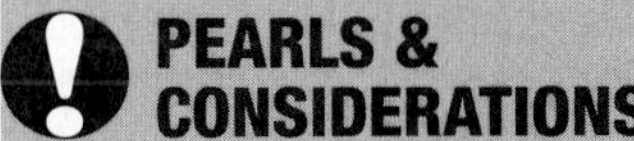

PEARLS & CONSIDERATIONS

COMMENTS

Patients should be instructed in good personal hygiene and avoidance of sharing razors, towels, and washcloths.

AUTHOR: **FRED F. FERRI, M.D.**

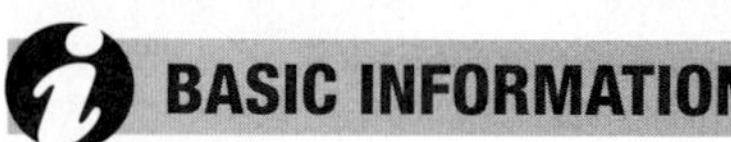

BASIC INFORMATION

DEFINITION

Food allergy is an adverse immune response to food proteins. Food allergies are categorized into IgE-mediated or non–IgE-mediated processes.

ICD-9CM CODES
693.1 Food allergy-ICD

EPIDEMIOLOGY & DEMOGRAPHICS

INCIDENCE: Food allergies have a cumulative incidence of 6% to 8% for the first 3 yr of life.

PREVALENCE:
- Food allergies affect 5% to 7% of children and 1% to 2% of adults. Thirty percent of food allergies are self-reported.
- Cow's milk allergy is found in 2.5% infants. IgE-mediated allergy occurs in 1% of children and non–IgE-mediated allergy occurs in 1.5 % of children.
- Egg allergy occurs in 1.5% to 3.2% children and 1% to 6% of infants have soy allergy.
- There is no predilection for race.

PREDOMINANT SEX: Males are more affected than females among children and among adults females are more frequently affected.

GENETICS: Children with parents or close relatives with allergies may have a tendency to become allergic to foods.

PHYSICAL FINDINGS & CLINICAL PRESENTATION

- IgE-mediated reactions: (immediate) pruritus, urticaria or angioedema, atopic dermatitis, GI symptoms, conjunctival injection, sneezing, nasal congestion, rhinorrhea, bronchospasm, and anaphylaxis
- Non–IgE-mediated reactions: food-induced enterocolitis, celiac disease, Crohn's disease, dermatitis herpetiformis, and pulmonary reactions such as Heiner syndrome
- Assess overall nutritional status, growth parameters, and signs of other allergic diseases such as atopic dermatitis, allergic rhinitis, or asthma
- Skin: eczema (dermatitis), angioedema, urticaria
- HEENT: nasal congestion, boggy mucous membranes, lymphoid tissue hypertrophy, postnasal mucous discharge, conjunctival injection
- Oropharyngeal: cobblestoning
- Lungs: stridor or wheezing.
- Tachycardia or hypotension may indicate anaphylactic shock

ETIOLOGY

There is insufficient evidence to support the hypothesis that early exposure to food allergens may cause an immature immune system to produce IgE. Eight common foods have been found to be responsible for >90% of food allergies. Foods allergies with the greatest likelihood of spontaneous resolution are those involving milk, soy, egg, and wheat. Allergies least likely to resolve spontaneously are peanut, tree nuts, fish, and shellfish.

DIAGNOSIS

- Thorough history and physical exam should be performed.
- Differential diagnosis should include toxic reactions (food poisoning), psychologic reactions (strongly held beliefs), and carbohydrate malabsorption.
- Skin testing: simple, inexpensive, with excellent sensitivity and negative predictive value. A wheal of 3 mm or greater is considered a positive test. Skin testing if negative can reliably exclude food allergies, but as it has variable specificity and positive predictive value, it does not confirm food allergies when the test is positive. In such cases a food challenge is often necessary.
- In vitro testing: RAST testing: Historically it is less sensitive than skin testing, but sensitivity has improved with cut off points indicating a positive predictive value of 95% for allergies to eggs, milk, peanuts, wheat, and fish.
- Atopy patch test: used in conjunction with RAST and skin testing in multiallergic children to plan widen the elimination diet.
- Double-blind, placebo-controlled food challenges are the gold standard test for determining food allergies. These need to be done in a supervised and controlled setting.
- In summary, if the history and lab tests are suggestive of specific food allergy, that food should be eliminated from the diet. If reaction involves various food allergens then positive skin tests or specific IgE measurements should be confirmed by double-blind, placebo-controlled food challenge.

DIFFERENTIAL DIAGNOSIS

- Gastrointestinal disorders
- Irritable bowel syndrome
- Carcinoid syndrome
- Giardiasis
- Structural abnormalities like hiatal hernia, pyloric stenosis, Hirschsprung's disease, tracheoesophageal fistula
- Disaccharidase deficiencies: lactase, sucrase-isomaltase complex, glucose-galactose complex
- Pancreatic insufficiency: cystic fibrosis
- Gallbladder disease
- Peptic ulcer disease
- Malignancy
- Metabolic disorders
- Galactosemia
- Phenylketonuria
- Pharmacologic-related conditions
- Gustatory rhinitis
- Auriculotemporal syndrome (facial flush from tart food)

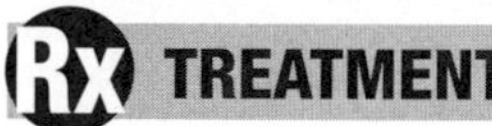

TREATMENT

NONPHARMACOLOGICAL THERAPY

- Elimination diet should be used.
- Formula-fed infants: brief trial of hydrolyzed milk formula as most children with milk allergy induced skin symptoms will respond to the change of formula. Nonresponders may require amino acid–based formula.
- In older children: elimination of one to two suspected foods are appropriate for 2 wk or longer and then reintroducing the foods to determine if symptoms recur.
- Epinephrine and antihistamines should be readily available during food challenges should anaphylactic reactions occur.

ACUTE GENERAL Rx

Antihistamines (both H_1 and H_2 antihistamines), albuterol if wheezing, epinephrine and glucocorticoids in patients with anaphylaxis.

NEW TREATMENTS FOR FOOD ALLERGIES

- Oral and sublingual immunotherapy may play a role in management of food allergies, but this is currently under investigation.
- Recombinant vaccines and other immunomodulatory strategies are under development, although monoclonal anti-IgE antibody has shown benefit in adults with peanut allergy.

PEARLS & CONSIDERATIONS

- Eczema that develops in first 6 to 12 mo of life is usually the first manifestation of atopy.
- Egg allergy or sensitization is the strongest recognized predictor of respiratory allergies in children and asthma in adults.
- Consultation with trained dietitian is critical to avoid potentially adverse nutritional consequences in children with multiple food allergies.
- Skin testing is the preferred method for identifying food-specific IgE. RAST is useful if there is chance of severe food reaction causing risk to the patient.
- American Academy of Pediatrics recommends avoiding influenza vaccine in patients with severe systemic allergic reactions to egg. Skin prick testing using influenza vaccine containing egg is recommended before vaccination in children with egg allergy and asthma. Skin prick testing not required before MMR vaccine in children with egg allergy.

COMMENTS

- Milk allergy usually resolves by age 5. Risk factors for persistence are early cutaneous manifestations following milk ingestion, development of other atopic conditions, and persistence of milk-specific high IgE titers. Soy milk is recommended for these children, keeping in mind that about 15% risk of these children can develop soy allergy.
- Egg allergy has been thought to resolve in 66% of children by 5 yr of age and in 75% of children by 7 yr of age.
- Wheat allergy found to resolve by 5 yr of age and soybean allergy by 2 yr of age.

PREVENTION

- There is conflicting evidence regarding the protective effect of breastfeeding on food allergies.
- There is no evidence to suggest that exclusive breastfeeding for 6 mo or more is superior to exclusive breastfeeding for 4 to 6 mo in terms of developing food allergies.
- In high-risk infants that are not exclusively breast fed, there is limited evidence to suggest that feeding with hydrolyzed formula compared to cow's milk formula reduces allergies.
- Currently there is no evidence to support the use of prebiotics, probiotics, or synbiotics for the prevention of allergic diseases.
- No current evidence exists to support delaying the introduction of solid foods beyond 4 to 6 mo.

PATIENT/FAMILY EDUCATION

Information can be found on American Academy of Allergy Asthma and Immunology (www.aaaai.org), the Food Allergy and Anaphylaxis Network (www.foodallergy.org), and the Anaphylaxis Campaign (www.anaphylaxis.org.uk).

SUGGESTED READINGS

Bock SA: Diagnostic evaluation, *Pediatrics* 111(6 pt. 3):1638-1644, 2003.

Bock SA, Sampson HA: Double blind placebo controlled food challenge as an office procedure: a manual, *J Allergy Clin Immunol* 82(6):986-997, 1988.

Grimshaw KE et al: Infant feeding and allergy prevention: a review of current knowledge and recommendations. A EuroPrevall state of the art paper, *Allergy* 64(10):1407-1416, 2009.

Kagan RS: Food allergy: an overview, *Environ Health Perspect* 111(2):223-225, 2003.

Lack G: Clinical practice: food allergy, *N Engl J Med* 359(12):1252-1260, 2008.

Muraro A et al: The management of anaphylaxis in childhood: position paper of the European Academy of Allergology and Clinical Immunology, *Allergy* 62(8):857-871, 2007.

Sampson HA: Atopic dermatitis, *Ann Allergy* 69:469-479, 1992.

AUTHOR: **DIVJOT SOOCH, M.D.**

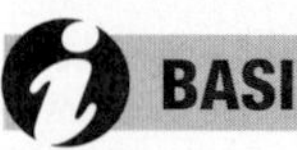

BASIC INFORMATION

DEFINITION

Food poisoning is an illness caused by ingestion of food contaminated by bacteria and/or bacterial toxins.

SYNONYMS

Enterotoxin-poisoning
Epidemic vomiting disease

ICD-9CM CODES

See specific illness.

EPIDEMIOLOGY & DEMOGRAPHICS

INCIDENCE (IN U.S.):
- Estimated range of 6 to 8 million cases/yr
- Majority of identifiable causes are bacterial, although more than 250 known diseases can be transmitted through food

PEAK INCIDENCE: Varies with specific organism
- Summer: *Staphylococcus aureus, Salmonella, Shigella* spp.
- Summer and fall: *Clostridium botulinum, Vibrio parahaemolyticus*
- Spring and fall: *Campylobacter jejuni*
- Winter: *Clostridium perfringens, Yersinia enterocolitica*

PREDOMINANT AGE: Varies with specific agent
NEONATAL INFECTION: Rare but severe with *Shigella* and *Salmonella* spp.

PHYSICAL FINDINGS & CLINICAL PRESENTATION

- Any combination of GI symptoms and fever
- Specific organisms suspected on the basis of the incubation period and predominant symptoms, although a great deal of overlap exists
  1. Short incubation period (1 to 6 hr): involve the ingestion of preformed toxin; noninvasive
     a. *S. aureus:* nausea, profuse vomiting, and abdominal cramps common; diarrhea possible, but fever uncommon; usually resolves within 24 hr; foods implicated in outbreaks include meats, mayonnaise, and cream pastries
     b. *B. cereus:* two forms, a short incubation (emetic) form (characterized by vomiting and abdominal cramps in virtually all patients, diarrhea in one third of patients, fever uncommon) and a long incubation (diarrheal) form; illness usually mild, resolves within 12 hr; unrefrigerated rice most often implicated as vehicle
  2. Moderate incubation period (8 to 16 hr): involves the in vivo production of toxin; noninvasive
     a. *C. perfringens:* severe crampy abdominal pain and watery diarrhea common; fever and vomiting unlikely; symptoms usually resolving within 24 hr; outbreaks invariably related to cooked meat or poultry that is allowed to cool without refrigeration; most cases in the fall and winter months
     b. *B. cereus:* diarrheal (or long incubation) form most commonly beginning with diarrhea, abdominal cramps, and occasionally vomiting; fever uncommon; usually resolves within 24 hr; the responsible food is usually fried rice
  3. Long incubation period (>16 hr): some toxin-mediated, some invasive
     a. Toxin-producing organisms include:
        (1) *C. botulinum:* should be considered when a diarrheal illness coincides with or precedes paralysis; severity of illness related to the quantity of toxin ingested; characteristic cranial nerve palsies progressing to a descending paralysis; fever usually absent; usually associated with home-canned foods
        (2) Enterotoxigenic *E. coli* (ETEC): most common cause of travelers' diarrhea; after 1- to 2-day incubation period, abdominal cramps and copious diarrhea occur; vomiting and fever uncommon; usually resolves after 3 to 4 days; vehicle usually unbottled water or contaminated salad or ice
        (3) Enterohemorrhagic *E. coli* (EHEC): can cause severe abdominal cramps and watery diarrhea, which may eventually become bloody; bacteria (strain 0157:H7) are noninvasive; no fever; illness may be complicated by hemolytic-uremic syndrome; associated with contaminated beef
        (4) *V. cholerae:* varies from a mild, self-limited illness to life-threatening cholera; diarrhea, nausea and vomiting, abdominal cramps, and muscle cramps; no fever; severe cases may progress to shock and death within hours of onset; survivors usually have resolution of symptoms in 1 wk; U.S. cases are either imported or result from ingestion of imported food
     b. Invasive organisms include:
        (1) *Salmonella:* associated most often with nontyphoidal strains; incubation period generally 12 to 48 hr; nausea, vomiting, diarrhea, and abdominal cramps typical; fever possible; outbreaks of gastroenteritis related to contaminated poultry, meat, and dairy products
        (2) *Shigella:* asymptomatic infection possible, but some with fever and watery diarrhea that may progress to bloody diarrhea and dysentery; with mild illness, usually self-limited, resolves in a few days; with severe illness, may develop complications; transmission usually from person to person but can occur via contaminated food or water
        (3) *C. jejuni:* the most common food-borne bacterial pathogen; incubation period is about 1 day, then a prodrome of fever, headache, and myalgias; intestinal phase marked by diarrhea associated with fever, malaise, and abdominal pain; diarrhea mild to profuse and bloody; usually resolves in about 7 days, but relapse is possible; associated with undercooked meats and poultry, unpasteurized dairy products, and drinking from freshwater streams
        (4) *Y. enterocolitica* and *Y. pseudotuberculosis:* infrequent causes of enteritis in U.S.; children affected more often than adults; fever, diarrhea, and abdominal pain lasting 1 to 3 wk; some with mesenteric adenitis that mimics acute appendicitis; contaminated food or water is usually responsible
        (5) *V. parahaemolyticus:* In U.S., most outbreaks in coastal states or on cruise ships during the summer months; incubation period usually <1 day, followed by explosive watery diarrhea in the majority of cases; nausea, vomiting, abdominal cramps, and headache also common; fever less common; usually resolves by 1 wk; related to ingestion of seafood
        (6) Enteroinvasive *E. coli* (EIEC): a rare cause of disease in the U.S.; high incidence of fever and bloody diarrhea; may resemble bacillary dysentery
        (7) *V. vulnificus:* may cause serious, often fatal illness in persons with chronic liver disease; GI symptoms usually absent, but fever, chills, hypotension, and hemorrhagic skin lesions possible; patients with liver disease or at increased risk of developing liver disease should avoid eating raw oysters

ETIOLOGY

Classically categorized as either inflammatory (invasive) or noninflammatory:
- Noninflammatory: *B. cereus, S. aureus, C. botulinum, C. perfringens, V. cholerae,* enterotoxigenic *E. coli* (ETEC), and enterohemorrhagic *E. coli* (EHEC); toxin-producing organisms that are noninvasive; fecal leukocytes are not seen.
- Inflammatory: *Campylobacter,* enteroinvasive *E. coli* (EIEC), *Salmonella, Shigella, V. parahaemolyticus,* and *Yersinia;* cause disease by invasion of intestinal tissue; fecal leukocytes are seen.

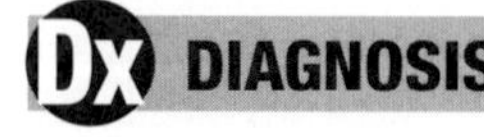

DIAGNOSIS

DIFFERENTIAL DIAGNOSIS

Gastroenteritis caused by viruses (Norwalk, Noro, or rotavirus), parasites *(Amoeba histolyt-*

ica, Giardia lamblia),* or toxins (ciguatoxins, mushrooms, heavy metals)

LABORATORY TESTS

- Test stool for fecal leukocytes to help narrow the differential diagnosis:
  1. Send stool for culture and for ova and parasites.
  2. Send stool for *C. difficile* toxin in patients with current or recent antibiotic use.
  3. NOTE: Some pathogens are not identified on routine stool culture; laboratory should be advised if *Yersinia, C. botulinum, Vibrio,* or enterohemorrhagic *E. coli* (O157:H7) are suspected.
  4. Finding *B. cereus, C. perfringens,* or *E. coli* in stool is of little value, because these may be part of the normal bowel flora.
- If botulism suspected, send food, serum, and stool for toxin assay.
- Blood cultures are needed for all febrile patients.

Rx TREATMENT

NONPHARMACOLOGIC THERAPY

Adequate rehydration is the mainstay of therapy.

ACUTE GENERAL Rx

- Gastroenteritis caused by the following organisms requires no antimicrobial treatment: *B. cereus, S. aureus, C. perfringens, V. parahaemolyticus, Yersinia,* and enterohemorrhagic and enteroinvasive *E. coli.*
- The usual cause of traveler's diarrhea is enterotoxigenic *E. coli.* Although usually a self-limited illness, antibiotics can shorten the course.
  1. SMX/TMP one DS tab bid for 3 days
  2. Ciprofloxacin 500 mg PO bid for 3 days
- The mainstay of therapy for cholera is fluid replacement. Antibiotics should be given to decrease shedding and duration of illness.
  1. Doxycycline 100 mg PO bid for 3 days
  2. SMX/TMP one DS tab bid for 3 days
- Treatment is not indicated for *Salmonella* gastroenteritis. Patients who are at high risk of developing bacteremia may be treated for 48 to 72 hr (see "Salmonellosis").
- Although shigellosis tends to be a self-limited illness, antibiotics shorten the course of illness and may limit transmission of the illness (see "Shigellosis").
- Those with moderate or severe *Campylobacter* diarrhea may benefit from treatment.
  1. Erythromycin 500 mg PO qid for 5 days
  2. Ciprofloxacin 500 mg PO bid for 5 days
- *V. vulnificus* sepsis should be treated with:
  1. Doxycycline 100 mg IV bid for 2 wk
  2. Ceftazidime 2 g IV q8h for 2 wk
- For suspected botulism, antitoxin should be administered early (see "Botulism").

CHRONIC Rx

Patients with *Salmonella* infections may become carriers and may require treatment (see "Salmonellosis").

DISPOSITION

- Most infections are self-limited and do not require therapy.
- In immunocompromised host or patient with underlying disease, serious complications are possible.
- Postinfectious syndromes are important with some infections:
  1. Reiter's syndrome: *Salmonella, Shigella, Campylobacter, Yersinia* spp.; more common in genetically susceptible host (HLA-B27+)
  2. Guillain-Barré syndrome: *Campylobacter spp.*

REFERRAL

If more than a mild illness

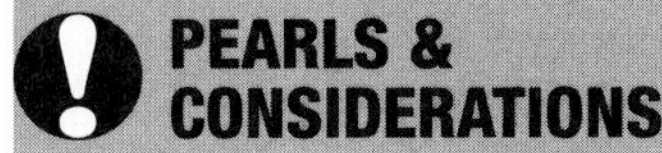

PEARLS & CONSIDERATIONS

COMMENTS

- Grossly underreported and undiagnosed
- All cases to be reported to the local health department

SUGGESTED READINGS

Allos BM et al: Surveillance for sporadic foodborne disease in the 21st century: the FoodNet perspective, *Clin Infect Dis* 38 (suppl 3)pS115, 2004.

Chiang YC et al: PCR primers for the detection of staphylococcal enterotoxins K, L, and M and survey of staphylococcal enterotoxin types in *Staphylococcus aureus* isolates from food poisoning cases in Taiwan, *J Food Prot* 69(5):1072, 2006.

Ikeda T et al: Mass outbreak of food poisoning disease caused by small amounts of staphylococcal enterotoxins A and H, *Appl Environ Microbiol* 71(5): 2793, 2005.

Saito N et al: An outbreak of food poisoning caused by an enteropathogenic Escherichia coli O115:H19 in Miyagi Prefecture, *Jpn J Infect Dis* 58(3):189, 2005.

AUTHORS: **DENNIS J. MIKOLICH, M.D.,** and **GLENN G. FORT, M.D., M.P.H.**

 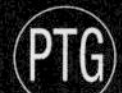

BASIC INFORMATION

DEFINITION

Friedreich's ataxia is the most common neurodegenerative hereditary ataxic disorder, caused by degeneration of dorsal root ganglions, posterior columns, spinocerebellar and corticospinal tracts, and large sensory peripheral neurons.

ICD-9CM CODES
334.0 Friedreich's ataxia

EPIDEMIOLOGY & DEMOGRAPHICS

INCIDENCE (IN U.S.): Estimated at one in 30,000 whites

PEAK INCIDENCE: 8 to 15 yr

PREVALENCE (IN U.S.): Two to four per 100,000. Carrier rate 1:120 to 1:160. Lower prevalence in Asians and people of African descent.

PREDOMINANT SEX: Males and females affected equally

GENETICS: Autosomal recessive; 96% of affected patients are homozygous and 4% are compound heterozygous (two different mutations). Trinucleotide repeat expansion accounts for 94% to 98% of cases, whereas point mutations account for 2% to 6% of cases.

PHYSICAL FINDINGS & CLINICAL PRESENTATION

- Onset of progressive appendicular and gait ataxia, with absent muscle stretch reflexes in the lower extremities.
- With disease progression (within 5 yr): dysarthria, distal loss of position and vibration sense, pyramidal leg weakness, areflexia in all four limbs, and extensor plantar responses.
- Common findings: progressive scoliosis, distal atrophy, pes cavus, and cardiomyopathy (symmetric concentric hypertrophic form in most cases).
- Insulin-requiring diabetes mellitus may occur in 10% of patients, with glucose intolerance occurring in an additional 10% to 20%.

ETIOLOGY

- Genetic: frataxin gene is localized to the centromeric region of chromosome 9q13.
- Normal sequence has six to 27 repeats; abnormal sequence has 120 to 1700 GAA repeats.
- Frataxin deficiency leads to impaired mitochondrial iron homeostasis.

DIAGNOSIS

DIFFERENTIAL DIAGNOSIS

- Charcot-Marie-Tooth disease type
- Abetalipoproteinemia
- Severe vitamin E deficiency with malabsorption
- Early-onset cerebellar ataxia with retained reflexes
- Autosomal-dominant cerebellar ataxia (spinocerebellar ataxia)

WORKUP

- Diagnostic criteria include electrophysiologic evidence for a generalized axonal sensory neuropathy.
- ECG may show widespread T-wave inversion and evidence of left ventricular hypertrophy. ECG abnormalities are present in 65% of patients.
- Sural nerve biopsy shows loss of large myelinated fibers.
- Specific gene testing for the expanded GAA trinucleotide repeat.

LABORATORY TESTS

- Electromyography or nerve conduction study
- ECG and echocardiogram
- Peripheral blood smear for acanthocytes
- Lipid profile
- Two-hour glucose tolerance test
- Vitamin E levels (if necessary)

IMAGING STUDIES

MRI of the spinal cord may demonstrate spinal cord atrophy with essentially normal cerebrum, brainstem, and cerebellum (Fig. 1-125).

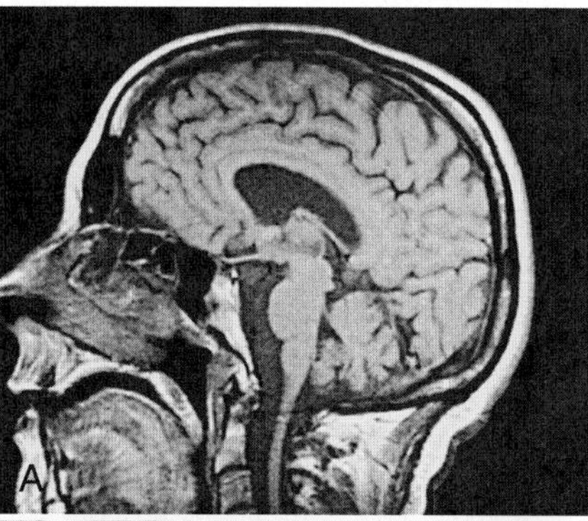

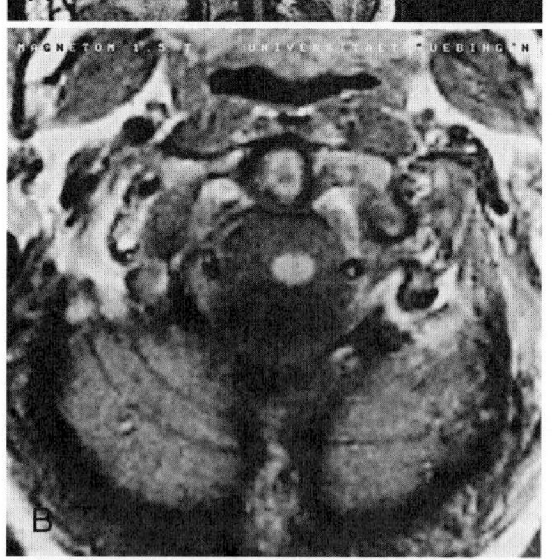

FIGURE 1-125 T1 MRI of the brain (midsagittal section) and spinal cord (axial slice at level of the dens) showing severe shrinkage of the cervical cord, but the cerebellum and brain stem are of normal size. (From Goetz CG: *Textbook of clinical neurology,* Philadelphia, 1999, WB Saunders.)

TREATMENT

NONPHARMACOLOGIC THERAPY

- Surgical correction of scoliosis and foot deformities in selected patients
- Prosthetic devices as required (e.g., ankle-foot orthosis for foot drop)
- Physical therapy
- Communication devices for patients with severe dysarthria

ACUTE GENERAL Rx

None established.

- An antioxidant, idebenone (short-chain analogue of coenzyme Q10), administered orally at 5 to 10 mg/kg/day with or without vitamin E may improve outcomes in patients with cardiomyopathy without clinical deterioration. This treatment is experimental, and research may be reviewed at http://www.idebenone.org.
- Further research with various antioxidants and iron chelators is ongoing. An open-label pilot study of antioxidants (coenzyme Q10, 400 mg/day, and vitamin E, 2100 U/day) suggested slowing in progression in generalized ataxia and kinetic function and significant improvement in cardiac function with unaltered deterioration in posture, gait, and hand dexterity.

CHRONIC Rx

Chronic management of congestive heart failure is required. Cardiac arrhythmias will warrant pacemaker implantation.

DISPOSITION

- Loss of ambulation typically occurs within 15 yr of symptom onset, and 95% are wheelchair bound by age 45 yr.
- Life expectancy is reduced, particularly if heart disease with or without diabetes mellitus is present.

REFERRAL

- If uncertain about diagnosis
- For genetic counseling (recommended if available)

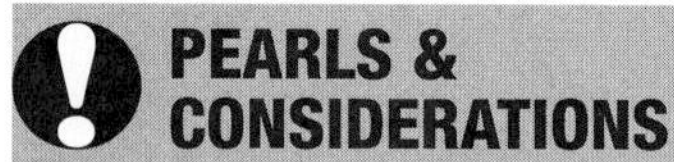

PEARLS & CONSIDERATIONS

Friedreich's ataxia should be considered in all preadolescent and adolescent children presenting with progressive ataxia. Early recognition of cardiac failure and arrhythmias and institution of appropriate therapy helps prolong survival.

SUGGESTED READING

Hart PE et al: Antioxidant treatment of patients with Friedreich ataxia: four-year follow-up, *Arch Neurol* 62:621, 2005.

AUTHOR: **EROBOGHENE E. UBOGU, M.B.B.S. (HONS.)**

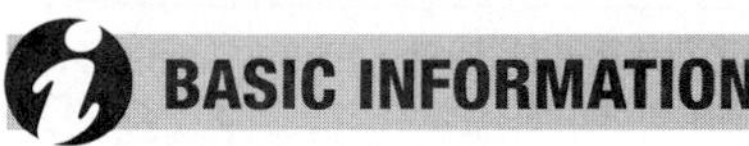

BASIC INFORMATION

DEFINITION

Frostbite represents tissue injury (or death) from freezing and vasoconstriction induced by severe environmental cold exposure.

SYNONYMS

Cold-induced tissue injury

ICD-9CM CODES

991.3 Frostbite

EPIDEMIOLOGY & DEMOGRAPHICS

- Environmental factors include wind chill factor, temperature, duration of exposure, altitude, and degree of wetness. Hands and feet account for 90% of injuries; earlobes, nose, and male genitalia are also more susceptible.
- Host factors include older age, psychiatric illness, neuroleptic and sedative drugs (especially alcohol), immobility, previous frostbite, skin damage, malnutrition, tobacco use, peripheral neuropathy, peripheral vascular disease, hypothyroidism, fatigue, and constricting clothing and footwear.

PHYSICAL FINDINGS & CLINICAL PRESENTATION

- Frostbite may be classified into grades I to IV of injury severity or, more practically, into *superficial* and *deep* groups.
- *Superficial* frostbite involves the skin and subcutaneous tissue. The frozen part is waxy, white (or mottled), and firm but soft and resilient below the surface when gently depressed. After rewarming, there is an initial hyperemia that may be followed by swelling and formation of superficial blisters with clear or milky fluid within 6 to 24 hr (Fig. 1-126). There is no ultimate tissue loss.
- *Deep* frostbite also involves muscles, nerves, tendons, or bones. The skin may be hard or wooden, without tissue resilience. Nonblanching cyanosis, hemorrhagic blisters (after 3 to 7 days), tissue necrosis, and gangrene may develop. Affected tissue has a poor prognosis and debridement or amputation is generally required.

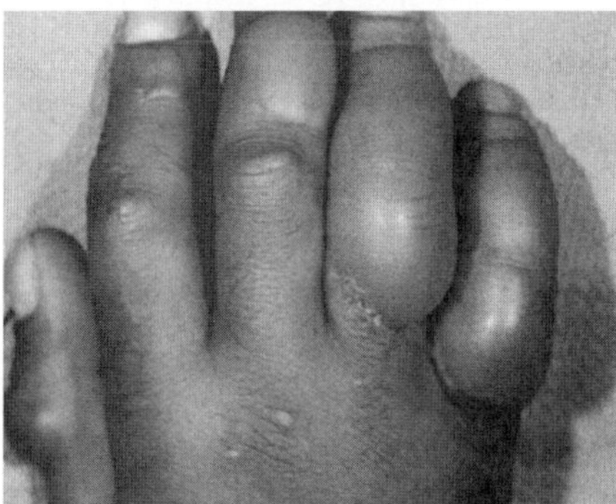

FIGURE 1-126 Large, clear frostbite blisters on the right hand. (From Rosen P [ed]: *Emergency medicine,* ed 4, St Louis, 1998, Mosby.)

- Patients initially feel numbness, prickling, and itching. More severe injury can produce paresthesias and stiffness, with burning or throbbing pain on thawing.

ETIOLOGY

Two mechanisms of tissue injury:

1. Cellular death occurring at time of exposure from intracellular water crystallization and temperature-induced protein changes.
2. Vascular impairment from vasoconstriction and endothelial injury result from tissue thawing and associated edema. On a cellular level, Prostaglandin F and Thromboxane AZ are involved in platelet aggregation and thrombosis leading to ischemia. Most frostbite injury occurs in this phase. Hemorrhage, necrosis, and gangrene may develop.

DIAGNOSIS

DIFFERENTIAL DIAGNOSIS

- Frostnip: transient tingling and numbness without associated permanent tissue damage
- Pernio (chilblains): self-limited, cold-induced vasculitis associated with purple plaques or nodules, often affecting dorsum of hands and feet; seen with prolonged cold exposure to above-freezing temperatures
- Cold immersion (trench foot): caused by ischemic injury resulting from sustained, severe vasoconstriction in appendages exposed to wet cold at temperatures above freezing

WORKUP

- Laboratory work is not indicated unless the patient has systemic hypothermia.
- No reliable predictors of tissue viability. MRI/MRA and triple-phase bone scanning (with technetium) are the most promising modalities. (Some centers have reduced amputation rates by imaging within 24 hr of injury and giving thrombolytics to those with impaired blood flow.)

TREATMENT

FIELD MANAGEMENT

- Remove constricting or wet clothing. Gently insulate, splint, and elevate affected area.
- Avoid thawing if there is any risk of refreezing.
- Never rub or massage the affected area. Avoid dry heat (e.g., fires and heaters) and exercising the affected area.
- If hypothermic (core body temperature <32° C), initiate active core rewarming (e.g., pleural and peritoneal irrigation, hemodialysis or cardiopulmonary bypass) and adjunctive treatment with warmed, humidified oxygen, heated IV saline (45° C), and warming blankets before thawing frostbitten extremities.

ACUTE GENERAL Rx

- Rapid rewarming is the main objective.
- Immerse affected area in circulating warm water bath with a mild antibacterial agent (e.g., chlorhexidene or povidone-iodine) maintained at 40 to 42° C for 15 to 30 min. Repeat until capillary refill returns and tissue is supple and flushed. Active motion during rewarming is advisable; massage is not.
- IV narcotics for pain during thawing.
- Tetanus prophylaxis and topical antibiotics if potentially contaminated skin wound.
- Streptococcal prophylaxis for 48 to 72 hr with IV penicillin for severe cases.
- Thrombolytic therapy followed by short-term anticoagulation appears to considerably improve reperfusion and reduce subsequent digit amputations.
- Dextran, heparin, vasodilators, hyperbaric oxygen, reserpine, and sympathectomy are of unproven benefit.

POST-THAW Rx

- Daily dressing changes with dry, sterile, noncompressive, and nonadherent dressings. Splint and elevate hands and feet to reduce edema and separate digits with cotton gauze. Avoid even slightest abrasion to limit risk of infection.
- Whirlpool hydrotherapy with warm water (38° C) and an antiseptic for 20 to 30 min bid to tid for several weeks.
- Debride broken clear vesicles and avoid disrupting intact blisters (especially hemorrhagic ones) unless they interfere with mobility.
- Topical aloe vera q6h and ibuprofen 400 to 600 mg tid for 1 wk may be beneficial as thromboxane inhibitors.
- Gentle, progressive physical therapy after edema resolves.
- Avoid all vasoconstrictors, including nicotine.

DISPOSITION

A majority of patients have long-term residual symptoms, including neuropathic pain, sensory deficits, hyperhidrosis, secondary Raynaud's disease, edema, hair or nail deformities, and (rarely) arthritis. Treatment with antiadrenergics or calcium channel blockers and careful protection from further cold exposure are often helpful.

REFERRAL

- Hospitalize for hypothermia or deep frostbite; a burn unit is best.
- Surgical decisions regarding amputation should be deferred until demarcation of viable tissue is clear (1 to 3 mo) unless refractory pain, sepsis, or gangrene occurs.

SUGGESTED READINGS

Bruen KJ et al: Reduction of the incidence of amputation in frostbite injury with thrombolytic therapy, *Arch Surg* 142(6):546, 2007.

Imray C et al: Cold damage to the extremities: frostbite and non-freezing cold injuries, *Postgrad Med J* 85:481, 2009.

Jurkovich GJ: Environmental cold-induced injury, *Surg Clin North Am* 87(1):247, 2007.

Patel NN, Patel DN: Frostbite, *Am J Med* 121(9):765, 2008.

AUTHOR: **MICHAEL P. JOHNSON, M.D.**

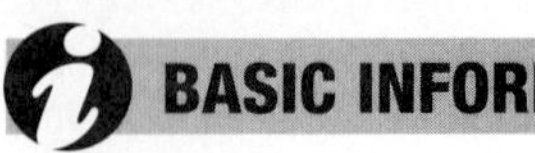

BASIC INFORMATION

DEFINITION

Frozen shoulder is a condition unique to the shoulder and characterized by pain and restricted passive and active range of motion (Fig. 1-127).

SYNONYMS

Adhesive capsulitis
Periarthritis
Pericapsulitis
Check-rein shoulder

ICD-9CM CODES
726.0 Adhesive shoulder capsulitis

EPIDEMIOLOGY & DEMOGRAPHICS

PREDOMINANT SEX: Females affected more often than males
PREDOMINANT AGE: >40 yr

PHYSICAL FINDINGS & CLINICAL PRESENTATION

- Arm held protectively at the side with apprehension caused by pain
- Varying degrees of deltoid and spinatus atrophy
- Generalized shoulder tenderness
- Restricted active and passive shoulder motion of varying degrees

ETIOLOGY

- Unknown
- Fig. 1-127 illustrates the sequence of events terminating in frozen shoulder.

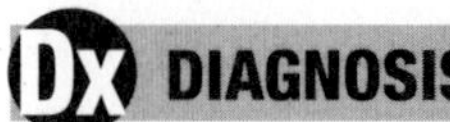

DIAGNOSIS

DIFFERENTIAL DIAGNOSIS

- Secondary causes of shoulder stiffness (prolonged immobilization after trauma or surgery)
- Posterior shoulder dislocation
- Ruptured rotator cuff
- Glenohumeral osteoarthritis
- Rotator cuff inflammation
- Superior sulcus tumor
- Cervical disk disease
- Brachial neuritis

WORKUP

Laboratory and radiographic studies are generally normal.

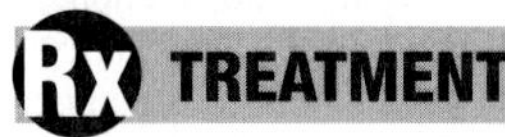

TREATMENT

NONPHARMACOLOGIC THERAPY

Prevention is important. Shoulder motion should be maintained when the patient may be inactive as a result of illness or injury.

ACUTE GENERAL Rx

- Moist heat, sedation, and analgesics as needed.
- A local steroid/lidocaine mixture injected into the subacromial space and joint (see "Epicondylitis" entry for guidelines to common steroid injections).
- Home exercise program. Should be performed on an hourly basis, if possible, at least in the early stages of treatment. Physical therapy may be needed.
- Manipulation of shoulder under anesthesia (rarely needed).

DISPOSITION

- The initial stage of pain followed by stiffness may last several months; recovery phase may also last several months; complete recovery is typical.
- Recurrence in the same shoulder is rare, although the opposite limb may develop the same symptoms.
- Some patients have mild residual loss of movement but without any significant functional impairment.

REFERRAL

Orthopedic consultation in patients with resistant disease

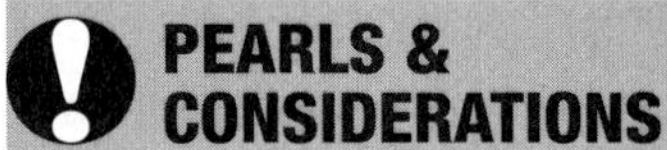

PEARLS & CONSIDERATIONS

COMMENTS

- "Capsulitis" with an inflammatory infiltrate is not consistently found pathologically.
- Frozen shoulder is more common in patients with diabetes, thyroid disease, and recent cardiopulmonary conditions.
- Some cases have findings of reflex sympathetic dystrophy.

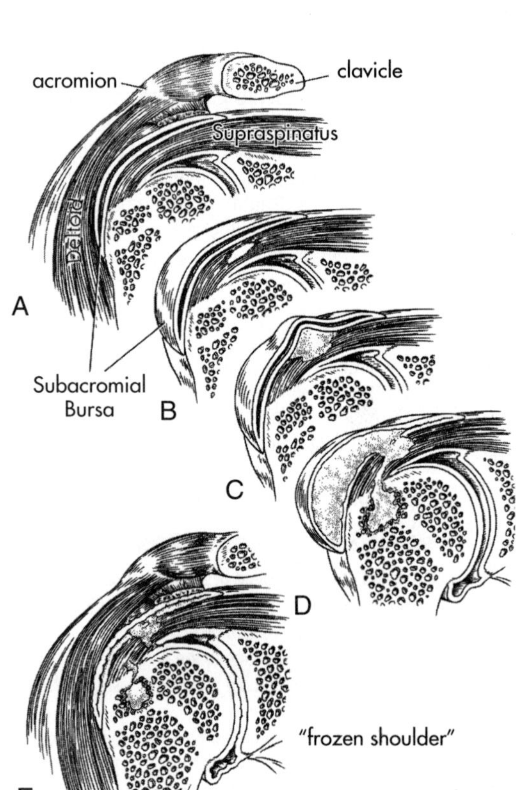

FIGURE 1-127 Sequence of events terminating in frozen shoulder. A, Normal structures of the shoulder. **B,** Supraspinatus tendonitis, sometimes calcific, in the "critical zone." **C,** Spread of inflammation to the tendon sheath and a bulge into the floor of the subacromial bursa. **D,** Rupture into the subacromial bursa and extension of the inflammatory process as an osteitis into the humeral head and greater tuberosity. **E,** Frozen shoulder with involvement of tendons, bursa, capsule, synovium, and muscle with fibrous contracture and markedly diminished volume of the shoulder joint space. (From Noble J [ed]: *Primary care medicine,* ed 2, St Louis, 1996, Mosby.)

SUGGESTED READINGS

Cheville AL, Tchou J: Barriers to rehabilitation following surgery for primary breast cancer, *J Surg Oncol* 95(5):409, 2007.
Cohen BL: Treatment of shoulder complaints, *Lancet* 363:492, 2004.
Hand GC et al: The pathology of frozen shoulder, *J Bone Joint Surg Br* 89(B):928, 2007.
Harrast MA, Rao AG: The stiff shoulder, *Phys Med Rehabil Clin North Am* 15(3):557, 2004.
Klauser A, Frauscher F: Treatment of shoulder complaints, *Lancet* 363:491, 2004.
Milgrom C et al: Risk factors for idiopathic frozen shoulder, *Isr Med Assoc J* 10:361, 2008.
Placzek JD et al: Theory and technique of translational manipulation for adhesive capsulitis, *Am J Orthop* 33:173, 2004.
Tasto JP, Elias DW: Adhesive capsulitis, *Sports Med Arthrosc* 15:216, 2007.
Thomas SJ et al: Prevalence of symptoms and signs of shoulder problems in people with diabetes mellitus, *J Shoulder Elbow Surg* 16:748, 2007.
Tonino PM et al: Complex shoulder disorders: evaluation and treatment, *J Am Acad Orthop Surg* 17(3): 125-136, 2009.

AUTHOR: **LONNIE R. MERCIER, M.D.**

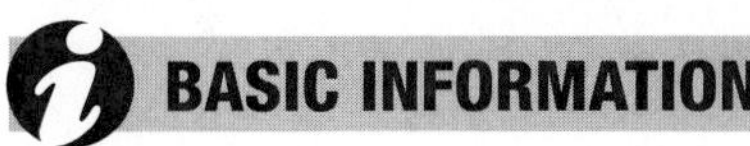

BASIC INFORMATION

DEFINITION

Galactorrhea can be defined as inappropriate lactation (in the absence of pregnancy or postpartum state) as a result of nonphysiologic augmentation of prolactin release.

ICD-9CM CODES
611.6 Galactorrhea

PHYSICAL FINDINGS & CLINICAL PRESENTATION

- Milky discharge from nipples usually occurring bilaterally
- Evidence of chest wall irritation from ill-fitting clothing, herpes zoster, or atopic dermatitis may be present
- Visual field defects may be present with prolactinomas
- Evidence of acromegaly, Cushing's disease, or hypothyroidism when galactorrhea is caused by these disorders

ETIOLOGY

- Medications (phenothiazines, metoclopramide, selective serotonin reuptake inhibitors, anxiolytics, buspirone, atenolol, valproic acid, conjugated estrogen and medroxyprogesterone, methyldopa, verapamil, H_2 receptor blockers, octreotide, danazol, tricyclic antidepressants, isoniazid, amphetamine, reserpine, opiates, sumatriptan, rimantadine, oral contraceptive formulations); after infancy, galactorrhea is usually medication induced
- Breast stimulation (prolonged suckling), sexual intercourse
- Pituitary tumors (prolactinomas, craniopharyngiomas)
- Chest wall irritation from ill-fitting clothing, herpes zoster, atopic dermatitis, burns
- Hypothyroidism (elevated thyroid-stimulating hormone [TSH] increases thyroid-releasing hormone [TRH], which increases prolactin)
- Increased stress, major trauma
- Chronic renal failure (decreased prolactin clearance)
- Cushing's disease
- Herbs (e.g., fennel, red clover, anise, red raspberry, marshmallow)
- Cannabis
- Spinal cord surgery or injury, or tumors
- Severe gastroesophageal reflux disease, esophagitis (stimulation of thoracic nerves by the cervical and thoracic ganglia)
- Breast surgery
- Idiopathic
- Neonatal ("witch's milk" produced by 2% to 5% of neonates because of precipitous drop in maternal estrogen and progesterone post-delivery)
- Lymphomas, Hodgkin's disease, bronchogenic carcinoma, renal adenocarcinomas
- Sarcoidosis and other infiltrative disorders
- Tuberculosis affecting pituitary gland
- Pituitary stalk resection
- Multiple sclerosis
- Empty sella syndrome
- Acromegaly

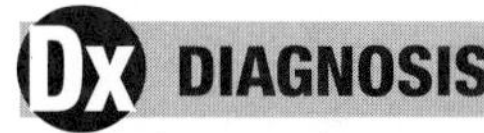

DIAGNOSIS

DIFFERENTIAL DIAGNOSIS

- Intraductal papilloma
- Breast cancer
- Paget's disease of breast
- Breast abscess

WORKUP

- Complete history focusing on menstrual irregularity, infertility, previous pregnancies, duration of galactorrhea, medications, visual complaints, fatigue. Age of onset is also significant (e.g., prolactinoma most common between ages 20 and 35 yr; neonatal galactorrhea is usually secondary to transplacental transfer of maternal estrogen)
- Physical examination: hirsutism, acne, obesity, visual field defects, goiter
- Breast examination for presence of nodules, evaluation of discharge (milky versus serosanguineous versus purulent)
- Laboratory testing and imaging studies (see "Laboratory Tests")

LABORATORY TESTS

- Prolactin level (elevated, usually $>$200 ng/ml in prolactinoma)
- Human chorionic gonadotropin level (positive in pregnancy)
- TSH, TRH (both elevated in hypothyroidism)
- Blood urea nitrogen, creatinine (elevated in renal failure), glucose (elevated in Cushing's syndrome)
- Urinalysis (hematuria in renal cell carcinoma)
- Microscopic examination of nipple discharge (scant cellular material, numerous fat globules)

IMAGING STUDIES

- MRI of brain if prolactin level is elevated, amenorrhea is present, or visual field defects are detected on physical examination.
- High-resolution CT of brain with special coronal cuts through the pituitary region may be helpful in patients with contraindications to MRI; however, it may miss small lesions.

TREATMENT

- Discontinuation of potential offending agents.
- Avoidance of excessive breast stimulation.
- Galactorrhea resulting from prolactinoma can be managed medically, surgically, or with careful surveillance depending on size and growth of tumor, associated symptoms, and prolactin level. Please refer to "Prolactinoma" in Section I for additional information.

REFERRAL

Endocrine and surgical consultation if prolactinoma is detected

SUGGESTED READINGS

Leung A, Pacaud D: Diagnosis and management of galactorrhea, *Am Fam Physician* 70:543, 2004.

Pena KS, Rosenfeld JA: Evaluation and treatment of galactorrhea, *Am Fam Physician* 63:1763, 2001.

AUTHOR: **FRED F. FERRI, M.D.**

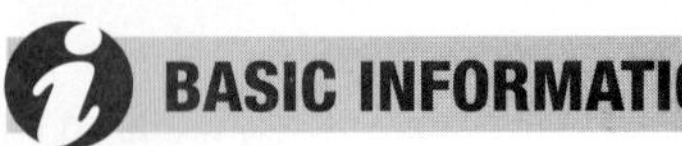

BASIC INFORMATION

DEFINITION

A fluid filled sac (cyst) overlying a tendon sheath or joint

SYNONYMS

Ganglion

ICD-9CM CODES

727.43 Ganglion

EPIDEMIOLOGY & DEMOGRAPHICS

- Ganglia are more common in women than men (3:1)
- Can occur at any age, but usually between second and fourth decades of life
- Most common soft tissue tumor of the hand and wrist

PHYSICAL FINDINGS & CLINICAL PRESENTATION

- Most ganglia occur on the dorsum of the wrist (50% to 70%) (Fig. 1-128).
- The volar wrist (18% to 20%) is the next most common site.
- Can also involve the proximal digital flexor tendons and the distal interphalangeal joints.
- Left and right hands are equally affected.
- Ganglia are usually solitary, firm, smooth, round, and fluctuant.
- Pain from mass effect or compression against nearby structure may be present (e.g., median nerve and radial nerve).
- Hand numbness may be present.
- Patient may have hand muscle weakness.
- Ganglia usually develop over a period of months but may arise suddenly.

ETIOLOGY

Ganglia are believed to derive from synovial herniation or expansion from the joint capsule or tendon sheath. Repetitive movement as an etiology is uncertain, although it may cause enlargement of the lesion or worsen symptoms.

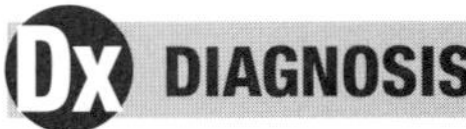

DIAGNOSIS

Direct inspection and localization of the cyst often is enough to make the diagnosis of ganglia. Transillumination is an easy method of differentiating ganglia from solid tumors; ganglia transilluminate while solid tumors do not.

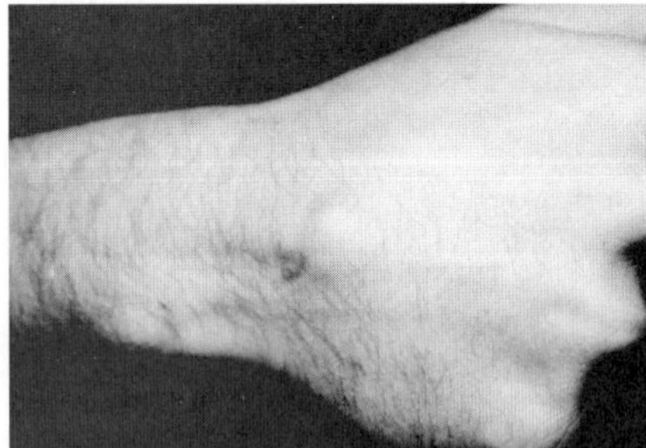

FIGURE 1-128 Round and firm ganglion cyst bulging from the dorsal aspect of the hand. (From Kelly WN: *Textbook of rheumatology,* ed 5, Philadelphia, 1997, WB Saunders.)

DIFFERENTIAL DIAGNOSIS

- Lipoma
- Fibroma
- Epidermoid inclusion cyst
- Osteochondroma
- Hemangioma
- Infection (tuberculosis, fungi, and secondary syphilis)
- Gout
- Rheumatoid nodule
- Radial artery aneurysm

WORKUP

The workup of ganglia usually consists of history, physical examination, and x-ray imaging.

LABORATORY TESTS

Blood tests are not specific in the diagnosis of ganglia.

IMAGING STUDIES

- Radiographs of the hand and wrist are taken to rule out other bone or joint abnormalities.
- Ultrasound studies are helpful in the diagnosis of ganglia by demonstrating smooth cystic walls that may be septated.
- CT scan can be done if the ultrasound is equivocal.
- MRI helps differentiate malignant bone lesions from cystic structures.
- Arthrography may demonstrate a communication between the joint and ganglia (not commonly done).

Rx TREATMENT

Expectant treatment is appropriate if the mass is not painful or interfering with motor function.

NONPHARMACOLOGIC THERAPY

- Attempts to rupture the cyst by sharp blows with a book or with finger compression are not recommended.
- Aspiration, heat, and sclerotherapy have been tried but have met with high recurrence rates (60%).

ACUTE GENERAL Rx

- Aspiration at the base with a large-bore needle (18-gauge) followed by injection of 20 to 40 mg of triamcinolone acetonide can be tried.
- This may be repeated if the ganglia recurs (35% to 40%).

CHRONIC Rx

Total ganglionectomy and repair of the defect after tracing its connection to the tendon sheath is effective and the surgical procedure of choice.

DISPOSITION

- Ganglia spontaneously resolve in approximately 40% to 50% of cases.
- Aspiration with steroid injection is successful in approximately 65% of cases.
- Surgery provides cure in 85% to 95% of the cases.
- Complications of ganglia include:
  1. Carpal tunnel syndrome with pain and muscle atrophy
  2. Radial nerve impingement
  3. Radial artery compression
- Complications of ganglion surgery include:
  1. Infection
  2. Recurrence (5% to 15%), usually from inadequate excision
  3. Reflex sympathetic dystrophy
  4. Scar formation

REFERRAL

It is best to refer patients with symptomatic ganglia to a hand surgeon.

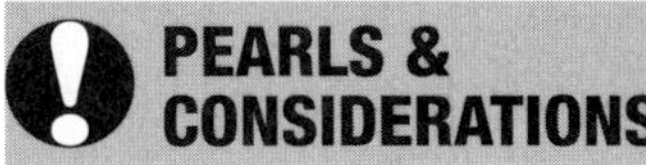

PEARLS & CONSIDERATIONS

- Dorsal ganglia usually originate from the scapholunate ligament.
- Volar ganglia typically originate between the tendons of the flexor carpi radialis and brachioradialis.

COMMENTS

A ganglion's synovial membrane maintains its secretory function. Aspiration of ganglia often demonstrates a viscous, mucinous, clear fluid containing albumin, globulin, and hyaluronic acid.

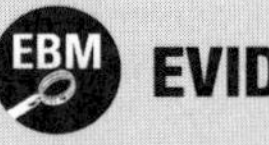

EVIDENCE

Single versus multiple needle punctures were compared in one study, which showed similar efficacy for symptom relief.[1] Intralesional hyaluronidase injection resulted in a 95% cure rate at 6 mo in hand and wrist ganglia.[2]

Evidence-Based References

1. Stephen AB et al: A prospective study of two conservative treatments for ganglia of the wrist. *J Hand Surg [Br]* 24:104, 1999.

2. Otu AA: Wrist and hand ganglion treatment with hyaluronidase injection and fine needle aspiration: a tropical African perspective, *J R Coll Gen Pract* 37:405, 1992.

SUGGESTED READINGS

Ho PC et al: Current treatment of ganglion of the wrist, *Hand Surg* 6(1):49, 2001.

Nahra ME, Bucchieri JS: Ganglion cysts and other tumor related cysts of the hand and wrist, *Hand Clin* 20(3):249, 2004.

Wang AA, Hutchinson DT: Longitudinal observation of pediatric hand and wrist ganglia, *J Hand Surg* 26(4):599, 2001.

AUTHORS: **RYAN W. ZUZEK, M.D.,** and **IMMAD SADIQ, M.D.**

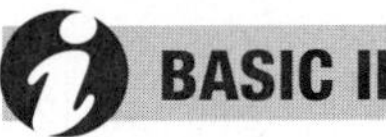

BASIC INFORMATION

DEFINITION

Gardner's syndrome is a variant of familial adenomatous polyposis (FAP), with prominent extraintestinal manifestations. It is a highly penetrant autosomal-dominant condition characterized by the following:

- Adenomatous intestinal polyps
- Soft tissue tumors
- Osteomas

SYNONYMS

Familial adenomatous polyposis

ICD-9CM CODES
211.3 Familial adenomatous polyposis

EPIDEMIOLOGY & DEMOGRAPHICS

- FAP occurs in approximately 1 in 10,000 births.
- FAP accounts for about 1% of all colorectal cancers.
- Individuals develop hundreds to thousands of adenomatous colorectal polyps.
- Polyps usually present in adolescence.
- 100% lifetime risk for colorectal cancer; most diagnosed by 40 yr of age.
- Gastric, duodenal, and small bowel polyps occur but have lower malignant potential.
- Increased risk for other tumors: desmoid (15%), duodenal-ampullary (7%), thyroid (2%), brain (1%), childhood hepatoblastoma (1%), nasopharyngeal angiofibroma, pancreatic, adrenal, and gastric.

PHYSICAL FINDINGS & CLINICAL PRESENTATION

Phenotypic variability is seen in individuals and families with the same mutation. Soft tissue and bone abnormalities may precede intestinal disease.

- Congenital hypertrophy of the retinal pigment epithelium (CHRPE): benign fundus lesions, usually present at birth
- Dental abnormalities: supernumerary or unerupted teeth
- Soft tissue lesions: epidermal or sebaceous cysts, fibromas, lipomas, desmoid tumors (benign, locally invasive, connective tissue tumors)
- Skull, mandible, long bone osteomas (benign bony growths)
- Anemia, occult blood in stool, bowel obstruction, weight loss

ETIOLOGY

- Caused by mutations of the tumor suppressor gene adenomatous polyposis coli *(APC)* on chromosome 5q21-q22; more than 700 diseases causing mutations identified. The site of the mutation may explain the prominent extraintestinal lesions found in Gardner's syndrome.
- De novo mutations are responsible for approximately 20% of FAP cases.

Dx DIAGNOSIS

In individuals with a family history, more than 100 adenomatous colorectal polyps, CHRPE lesions, or genetic testing confirms diagnosis. In those without a family history, more than 100 adenomatous colorectal polyps suggest the diagnosis and genetic testing confirms it.

DIFFERENTIAL DIAGNOSIS

- Turcot's syndrome
- Attenuated familial adenomatous polyposis
- MYH-associated polyposis
- Peutz-Jeghers syndrome
- Juvenile polyposis syndrome
- Hereditary mixed polyposis syndrome
- Hyperplastic polyposis

WORKUP

History, physical examination, laboratory tests, imaging studies

DIAGNOSTIC SCREENING OPTIONS

GENETIC TESTING

- Should be offered to first-degree relatives of affected individuals (with an identified mutation) at age 10 to 12 yr and clinically suspected individuals.
- Able to identify a mutation in approximately 80% of families. To ensure that the family has a detectable mutation, test an affected family member first.
- If positive in the affected individual, the test can differentiate with 100% accuracy affected and unaffected family members. If negative in the affected individual, screening family members will not be useful in determining disease status.
- If no known family history exists, screening the clinically suspected individual is reasonable. A positive test rules in FAP but a negative test does not rule it out.
- May require multiple tests to identify the mutation.

NOTE: Genetic counseling should be performed and written informed consent obtained before testing.

SIGMOIDOSCOPY

- Individuals with a positive genetic test: annual flexible sigmoidoscopy beginning at 10 to 12 yr of age.
- Untested at-risk family members or patients from families with an unidentified *APC* mutation: annual flexible sigmoidoscopy beginning at 10 to 12 yr until 25 yr of age, then decreasing frequency until age 50 yr, when age-appropriate guidelines may be followed.
- Once adenomatous polyps are detected, patients should undergo colonoscopy and evaluation for colectomy.
- Negative genetic test in patients from families with an identified mutation: average risk screening.

CHRPE: Lesions occur in approximately 80% of families and are a reliable indicator of affected status in these families.

Rx TREATMENT

- Prophylactic colectomy or proctocolectomy: timing determined by polyp number, size, and degree of dysplasia.
- Consider celecoxib therapy to reduce polyposis.
- Screening of remaining GI tract and screening for extraintestinal manifestations must continue after colectomy.
  - Annual physical examination: history, examination (including thyroid), and blood tests
  - Upper endoscopy to screen for duodenal polyps: baseline at age 20 yr and repeated every 1 to 5 yr based on findings
  - Some recommend annual thyroid ultrasound
  - Other possible cancer sites imaged if symptoms occur or if these cancers have occurred in relatives
- Treat soft tissue lesions and osteomas for symptoms or cosmetic concerns. Treat desmoid tumors if they pose a risk to adjacent structures.

DISPOSITION

- 100% chance of colorectal cancer in untreated individuals. Many other neoplasms occur at higher rates.
- Metastatic colorectal cancer is the leading cause of death (58%), followed by desmoid tumors (11%) and duodenal-ampullary adenocarcinoma (8%).

REFERRAL

- Patients should be managed at centers with expertise in FAP, including a gastroenterologist, medical geneticist, and surgeon.
- Genetic counseling and testing sites can be found at GeneTests (www.ncbi.nlm.nih.gov/sites/GeneTests).

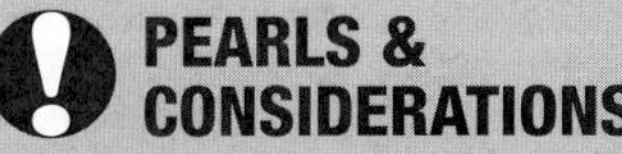

PEARLS & CONSIDERATIONS

- Management should be individualized based on genotype, phenotype, and individual preferences.
- Sulindac (nonselective NSAID) and celecoxib (cyclooxygenase-2 inhibitor) cause polyp regression in individuals with FAP. Celecoxib is FDA approved for this indication. Cancer risk remains; neither replaces colon resection for cancer prevention.
- Desmoid tumors frequently occur in the abdomen and are difficult to treat with high rates of recurrence. Growth is stimulated by surgery and estrogen.
- Screen children of affected parents yearly (from infancy to age 7 yr) with alpha-fetoprotein level and liver ultrasound to rule out hepatoblastoma.

SUGGESTED READINGS

Cunningham D et al: Perioperative chemotherapy versus surgery alone for respectable gastroesophageal cancer, *N Engl J Med* 355(1):11, 2006.

Galiatsatos P et al: Familial adenomatous polyposis, *Am J Gastroenterol* 101:385, 2006.

Macrae F et al: Familial adenomatous polyposis, *Best Pract Res Clin Gastroenterol* 23:197, 2009.

Vasen HF et al: Guidelines for the clinical management of familial adenomatous polyposis (FAP), *Gut* 57: 704, 2008.

Winawer S et al: Colorectal cancer screening and surveillance: clinical guidelines and rationale–update based on new evidence, *Gastroenterology* 124:544, 2003.

AUTHOR: **SUDEEP KAUR AULAKH, M.D.**

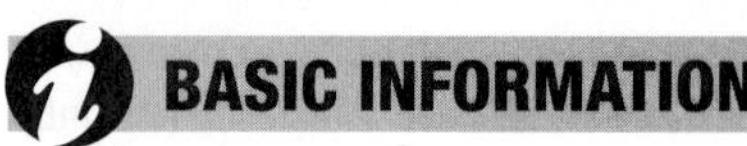

DEFINITION

Gastric cancer is an adenocarcinoma arising from the stomach.

SYNONYMS

Stomach cancer
Linitis plastica

ICD-9CM CODES
451 Malignant neoplasm of stomach

EPIDEMIOLOGY & DEMOGRAPHICS

- Annual incidence of gastric cancer in the U.S. is seven cases per 100,000 persons. The incidence is much higher in Japan, with rates as high as 80 cases per 100,000 persons.
- Most gastric cancers arise in the antrum (35%).
- The incidence of distal stomach tumors has greatly declined, whereas that of proximal tumors of the cardia and fundus is on the rise.
- Gastric cancer occurs most commonly in male patients >65 yr (70% of patients are >50 yr).
- Incidence of gastric cancer has been declining over the past 30 yr.
- Male/female ratio is 3:2.
- Familiar diffuse gastric cancer is a disease with autosomal-dominant inheritance in which gastric cancer develops at a young age. Germ-line truncating mutations in the E-cadherin gene *(CDH1)* are found in these families.

PHYSICAL FINDINGS & CLINICAL PRESENTATION

- Medical history may reveal complaints of postprandial fullness with significant weight loss (70% to 80%), nausea/emesis (20% to 40%), dysphagia (20%), and dyspepsia, usually unrelieved by antacids; epigastric discomfort, usually lessened by fasting and exacerbated by food intake, is also common.
- Epigastric or abdominal mass (30% to 50%), epigastric pain.
- Skin pallor from anemia.
- Hard, nodular liver: generally indicates metastatic disease to the liver.
- Hemoccult-positive stools.
- Ascites, lymphadenopathy, or pleural effusions: may indicate metastasis.

ETIOLOGY

Risk factors:

- Chronic *Helicobacter pylori* gastritis. Gastric cancer develops in persons infected with *H. pylori* but not in uninfected persons. Those with histologic findings of severe gastric atrophy, corpus-predominant gastritis, or intestinal metaplasia are at increased risk. Persons with *H. pylori* infection and duodenal ulcer are not at risk, whereas those with gastric ulcers, nonulcer dyspepsia, and gastric hyperplastic polyps are. Eradication of *H. pylori* reduces gastric cancer risk.
- Tobacco abuse, alcohol consumption.
- Food additives (nitrosamines), smoked foods, occupational exposure to heavy metals, rubber, asbestos.
- Chronic atrophic gastritis with intestinal metaplasia, hypertrophic gastritis, and pernicious anemia.

Dx DIAGNOSIS

DIFFERENTIAL DIAGNOSIS

- Gastric lymphoma (5% of gastric malignancies)
- Hypertrophic gastritis
- Peptic ulcer
- Reflux esophagitis

WORKUP

Upper endoscopy with biopsy will confirm diagnosis. Endoscopic ultrasonography in combination with CT scanning and operative lymph node dissection can be used in staging of the tumor.

LABORATORY TESTS

- Microcytic anemia
- Hemoccult-positive stools
- Hypoalbuminemia
- Abnormal liver enzymes in patients with metastasis to the liver
- Mutation-specific predictive genetic testing by polymerase chain reaction amplification followed by restriction: enzyme digestion and DNA sequencing for truncating mutations in *CDH1* is recommended in families of patients with familiar diffuse cancer because gastric cancer develops in three of every four carriers of a mutant *CDH1* gene.

IMAGING STUDIES

Abdominal CT scan to evaluate for metastasis (70% accurate for regional node metastases)

Rx TREATMENT

ACUTE GENERAL Rx

- Gastrectomy with regional lymphadenectomy is performed in patients with curative potential (<30% of patients at time of diagnosis). In patients with operable gastric cancer, a perioperative regimen of epirubicin, cisplatin, and infused fluorouracil (ECF) decreases tumor size and stage and significantly improves progression-free and overall survival. Postoperative adjuvant chemoradiation therapy using 5-fluorouracil and leucovorin is now the standard of care for resected patients able to tolerate such treatment. Postoperative chemotherapy and radiotherapy, compared with surgical resection alone, can extend the survival rate of patients with gastric cancer in those who are able to complete adjuvant therapy.
- When surgical cure is not possible, palliative resection may prolong duration and quality of life.
- Chemotherapy (FAM: 5-***f***luorouracil, ***A***driamycin, and ***m***itomycin C) may provide some palliation; however, it generally does not prolong survival. Chemotherapy with docetaxel, cisplatin, and 5-fluorouracil can be used for chemotherapy-naive patients with metastatic or locally recurrent gastric cancer.

DISPOSITION

- 5-yr survival rate of gastric carcinoma is 12% overall.
- 5-yr survival for early gastric cancers (usually detected incidentally with endoscopy in populations where screening is recommended) is >35%.

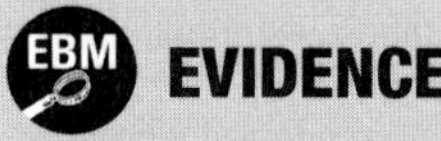

PEARLS & CONSIDERATIONS

COMMENTS

- Gastrectomy patients will need vitamin B_{12} replacement. They are also at risk for dumping syndrome and should be advised to ingest frequent, small meals.
- Prophylactic gastrectomy should be considered in young, asymptomatic carriers of germ-line truncating *CDH1* mutations who belong to families with highly penetrant heredity diffuse gastric cancer.

EBM EVIDENCE

Please note: Complete text of EBM for this topic is available online.

Key trials and commentary:

Gastrectomy with D2 lymphadenectomy is the standard treatment for curable gastric cancer in eastern Asia. Whether the addition of para-aortic nodal dissection (PAND) to D2 lymphadenectomy for stage T2, T3, or T4 tumors improves survival is controversial. This study conducted a randomized controlled trial at 24 hospitals in Japan to compare D2 lymphadenectomy alone with D2 lymphadenectomy plus PAND in patients undergoing gastrectomy for curable gastric cancer.

This study showed that as compared with D2 lymphadenectomy alone, treatment with D2 lymphadenectomy plus PAND does not improve the survival rate in curable gastric cancer.[1] Ⓐ

One of the major issues with gastric cancer is the extent of dissection of lymph nodes. This is a randomized prospective trial that is multi-institutional and compares a large number of patients. There is no difference between a D2 lymphadenectomy and the addition of peri-aortic nodal dissection. In addition, there is no apparent difference in the site of first tumor recurrence. As in previous published studies, pathologic stage and pathologic nodal status seem most predictive of outcome in these patients.

Evidence-Based Reference

1. Sasako M et al: D2 lymphadenectomy alone or with para-aortic nodal dissection for gastric cancer, *N Engl J Med* 359:453-462, 2008. Commentary by T.J. Eberlein, M.D. Ⓐ

SUGGESTED READING

Fuccio L et al: Meta-analysis: Can *Helicobactor pylori* eradication treatment reduce the risk for gastric cancer? *Ann Intern Med* 151:121-128, 2009.

AUTHOR: **FRED F. FERRI, M.D.**

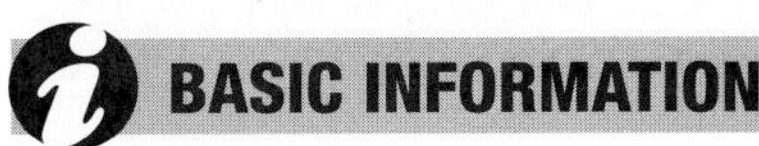

BASIC INFORMATION

DEFINITION

Histologically, gastritis refers to inflammation in the stomach. Endoscopically, gastritis refers to a number of abnormal features such as erythema, erosions, and subepithelial hemorrhages. Gastritis can also be subdivided into erosive, nonerosive, and specific types of gastritis with distinctive features both endoscopically and histologically.

SYNONYMS

Erosive gastritis
Hemorrhagic gastritis
Helicobacter pylori gastritis

ICD-9CM CODES
535.5 Gastritis (unless otherwise specified)
535.0 Gastritis, acute
535.3 Alcoholic gastritis
535.1 Atrophic (chronic) gastritis
535.4 Erosive gastritis
535.2 Hypertrophic gastritis

EPIDEMIOLOGY & DEMOGRAPHICS

- Erosive and hemorrhagic gastritis is most commonly seen in patients taking nonsteroidal anti-inflammatory drugs (NSAIDs), alcoholics, and critically ill patients (usually on ventilator support).
- *H. pylori* infection with gastritis is believed to be present in 30% to 50% of the population; however, the majority are asymptomatic.
- The prevalence of *H. pylori* infection increases with age from <10% in whites <40 yr to >50% in patients >50 yr.

PHYSICAL FINDINGS & CLINICAL PRESENTATION

- Patients with gastritis generally present with nonspecific clinical signs and symptoms (e.g., epigastric pain, abdominal tenderness, bloating, anorexia, nausea [with or without vomiting]). Symptoms may be aggravated by eating.
- Epigastric tenderness in acute alcoholic gastritis (may be absent in chronic gastritis).
- Foul-smelling breath.
- Hematemesis ("coffee grounds" emesis).

ETIOLOGY

- Alcohol, NSAIDs, stress (critically ill patients usually on mechanical respiration), hepatic or renal failure, multiorgan failure
- Infection (bacterial, viral)
- Bile reflux, pancreatic enzyme reflux
- Gastric mucosal atrophy, portal hypertension gastropathy
- Irradiation

Dx DIAGNOSIS

DIFFERENTIAL DIAGNOSIS

- Peptic ulcer disease
- Gastroesophageal reflux disease
- Nonulcer dyspepsia
- Gastric lymphoma or carcinoma
- Pancreatitis
- Gastroparesis

WORKUP

Diagnostic workup includes a comprehensive history and endoscopy with biopsy.

LABORATORY TESTS

- *H. pylori* testing by urea breath test, stool antigen test (*H. pylori* stool antigen), endoscopic biopsy, or specific antibody test is recommended.
  1. The urea breath test documents active infection (sensitivity and specificity >90%). A new card test for ^{14}C urea has recently been developed, providing a testing option in primary care settings. It uses a flat breath card read by a small analyzer.
  2. The stool antigen test is an enzymatic immunoassay (ELISA) that identifies *H. pylori* antigen in a stool specimen with a polyclonal anti–*H. pylori* antibody. It is as accurate as the urea breath test for diagnosis of active infection and follow-up evaluation of patients treated for *H. pylori.* A negative result on the stool antigen test 8 wk after completion of therapy identifies patients in whom eradication of *H. pylori* was unsuccessful.
  3. Histologic evaluation of endoscopic biopsy samples is considered by many the gold standard for accurate diagnosis of *H. pylori* infection. However, detection of *H. pylori* depends on the site and number of biopsy samples, the method of staining, and experience of the pathologist.
  4. Serologic testing for antibodies to *H. pylori* is easy and inexpensive; however, the presence of antibodies demonstrates previous but not necessarily current infection. Antibodies to *H. pylori* can remain elevated for months to years after infection has cleared; therefore antibody levels must be interpreted in light of patient's symptoms and other test results (e.g., peptic ulcer disease (PUD) seen on upper gastrointestinal series).
- Vitamin B_{12} level in patients with atrophic gastritis.
- Hematocrit (low if significant bleeding has occurred).

Rx TREATMENT

NONPHARMACOLOGIC THERAPY

- Avoidance of mucosal irritants such as alcohol and NSAIDs
- Lifestyle modifications with avoidance of tobacco and foods that trigger symptoms

ACUTE GENERAL Rx

Eradication of *H. pylori,* when present, can be accomplished with various regimens:

1. Proton pump inhibitor (PPI) bid *plus* amoxicillin 500 mg bid *plus* metronidazole 500 mg for 10 days.
2. PPI bid *plus* clarithromycin 500 mg bid *and* metronidazole 500 mg bid for 10 days. This regimen is useful in those with penicillin allergy.
3. A 1-day quadruple-therapy regimen may be as effective as a 7-day triple-therapy regimen. The 1-day quadruple-therapy regimen consists of two tablets of 262 mg bismuth subsalicylate qd, one 500-mg metronidazole tablet qd, 2 g of amoxicillin suspension qd, and two capsules of 30 mg of lansoprazole.
4. A 5-day treatment with three antibiotics (amoxicillin 1 g bid, clarithromycin 250 mg bid, and metronidazole 400 mg bid) plus either lansoprazole 30 mg bid or ranitidine 300 mg bid is an efficacious, cost-saving option for patients >55 yr with no history of PUD.
5. A combination of levofloxacin 250 mg bid, amoxicillin 1000 mg bid, and a PPI bid for 10 to 14 days can be used as salvage therapy after unsuccessful attempts to eradicate *H. pylori* using other regimens.
   - A 10-day sequential therapy has been reported to be superior to standard triple therapy for eradication of *H. pylori.* It consists of 5 days of treatment with a PPI and one antibiotic (usually amoxicillin) followed by 5-day treatment with the PPI and two other antibiotics (usually clarithromycin and metronidazole).
6. Prophylaxis and treatment of stress gastritis with sucralfate suspension 1 g orally q4-6h, H_2-receptor antagonists, or PPIs in patients on ventilator support.

CHRONIC Rx

- Omeprazole 20 mg/qd in patients receiving long-term NSAIDs
- Avoidance of alcohol, tobacco, and prolonged NSAID or corticosteroid use

DISPOSITION

- Undetectable stool antigen 4 wk after therapy accurately confirms cure of *H. pylori* infection in initially seropositive healthy subjects with reasonable sensitivity.
- Surveillance gastroscopy in patients with atrophic gastritis (increased risk of gastric cancer).

AUTHOR: **FRED F. FERRI, M.D.**

Gastroesophageal Reflux Disease

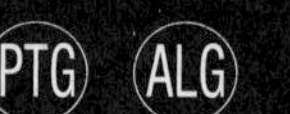

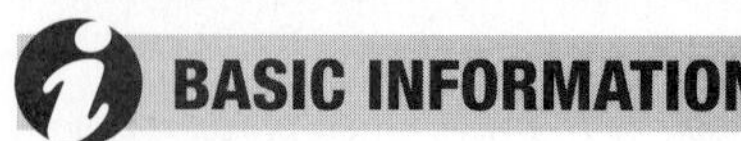

BASIC INFORMATION

DEFINITION

Gastroesophageal reflux disease (GERD) is a motility disorder characterized primarily by heartburn and caused by the reflux of gastric contents into the esophagus. A current definition is a condition that develops when the reflux of stomach contents causes at least two heartburn episodes per week and/or complications.

SYNONYMS

Peptic esophagitis
Reflux esophagitis
GERD

ICD-9CM CODES

530.81 Gastroesophageal reflux disease
530.1 Esophagitis
787.1 Heartburn

EPIDEMIOLOGY & DEMOGRAPHICS

- GERD is one of the most prevalent gastrointestinal disorders. It is the most common GI diagnosis recorded during visits to outpatient clinics. From 14% to 20% of adults are affected.
- Nearly 7% of persons in the U.S. have heartburn daily, 20% have it monthly, and 60% have it intermittently. Incidence in pregnant women exceeds 80%.
- Nearly 20% of adults use antacids or over-the-counter H_2 blockers at least once a week for relief of heartburn.

PHYSICAL FINDINGS & CLINICAL PRESENTATION

- Physical examination: generally unremarkable
- Clinical signs and symptoms: heartburn, dysphagia, sour taste, regurgitation of gastric contents into the mouth
- Chronic cough and bronchospasm
- Chest pain, laryngitis, early satiety, abdominal fullness, and bloating with belching
- Dental erosions in children

ETIOLOGY

- Incompetent lower esophageal sphincter (LES)
- Medications that lower LES pressure (calcium channel blockers, alpha-adrenergic antagonists, nitrates, theophylline, anticholinergics, sedatives, prostaglandins)
- Foods that lower LES pressure (chocolate, yellow onions, peppermint)
- Tobacco abuse, alcohol, coffee
- Pregnancy
- Gastric acid hypersecretion
- Hiatal hernia (controversial) present in >70% of patients with GERD; however, most patients with hiatal hernia are asymptomatic
- Obesity is associated with a statistically significant increase in the risk for GERD symptoms, erosive esophagitis, and esophageal carcinoma

DIAGNOSIS

DIFFERENTIAL DIAGNOSIS

- Peptic ulcer disease
- Unstable angina
- Esophagitis (from infections such as herpes, *Candida*), medication induced (doxycycline, potassium chloride)
- Esophageal spasm (nutcracker esophagus)
- Cancer of esophagus

WORKUP

- Aimed at eliminating the conditions noted in the differential diagnosis and documenting the type and extent of tissue damage. Generally, when symptoms of GERD are typical and the patient responds to therapy, there is no need for further diagnostic tests to verify the diagnosis.
- Upper GI endoscopy is useful to document the type and extent of tissue damage in persistent GERD and to exclude potentially malignant conditions such as Barrett's esophagus. The American College of Gastroenterology recommends endoscopy to screen for Barrett's esophagus in patients who have chronic GERD symptoms. The data demonstrating the cost-effectiveness of endoscopic screening remain controversial. Also, there is imperfect correspondence between symptoms attributed to the condition and endoscopic features of the disease.

LABORATORY TESTS

- 24-hr esophageal pH monitoring and Bernstein test are sensitive diagnostic tests; however, they are not practical and generally not done. They are useful in patients with atypical manifestations of GERD, such as chest pain or chronic cough.
- Esophageal manometry is indicated in patients with refractory reflux in whom surgical therapy is planned.

IMAGING STUDIES

An upper GI series is useful in patients unwilling to have endoscopy or with medical contraindications to the procedure. It can identify ulcerations and strictures; however, it may miss mucosal abnormalities. Only one third of patients with GERD have radiographic signs of esophagitis on an upper GI series.

TREATMENT

NONPHARMACOLOGIC THERAPY

- Lifestyle modifications with avoidance of foods (e.g., citrus- and tomato-based products, onions, spicy foods, carbonated beverages, mint, chocolate, fried foods) and drugs that exacerbate reflux (e.g., caffeine, β-blockers, calcium channel blockers, α-adrenergic agonists, theophylline)
- Avoidance of tobacco and alcohol use
- Elevation of head of bed (4 to 8 in) with blocks
- Avoidance of lying down directly after late or large evening meals, consumption of smaller and more frequent meals
- Weight reduction to BMI <25, decreased fat intake
- Avoidance of clothing that is tight around the waist

GENERAL Rx

- Proton pump inhibitors (PPIs) (esomeprazole 40 mg qd, omeprazole 20 mg qd, lansoprazole 30 mg qd, rabeprazole 20 mg qd, or pantoprazole 40 mg qd, or dexlansoprazole 30 mg) are safe, tolerated, and highly effective in most patients.
- H_2 blockers (nizatidine 300 mg qhs, famotidine 40 mg qhs, ranitidine 300 mg qhs, or cimetidine 800 mg qhs) can be used but are generally much less effective than PPIs.
- Antacids (may be useful for relief of mild symptoms; however, they are generally ineffective in severe cases of reflux).
- Prokinetic agents (metoclopramide) are indicated only when PPIs are not fully effective. They can be used in combination therapy; however, side effects limit their use.
- For refractory cases: surgery with Nissen fundoplication. Potential surgical candidates should have reflux esophagitis documented by esophagogastroduodenoscopy and normal esophageal motility as evaluated by manometry. Surgery generally consists of reduction of hiatal hernia when present and placement of a gastric wrap around the gastroesophageal (GE) junction (fundoplication). Although laparoscopic fundoplication is now widely used, surgery should not be advised with the expectation that patients with GERD will no longer need to take antisecretory medications or that the procedure will prevent esophageal cancer among those with GERD and Barrett's esophagus.
- Endoscopic radiofrequency heating of the GE junction (Stretta procedure) is a newer treatment modality for GERD patients unresponsive to traditional therapy. Its mechanism of action remains unclear. Endoscopy gastroplasty (EndoCinch procedure) is also aimed at treating GERD. Initial results appear encouraging; however, long-term studies are needed before recommending these procedures.
- Lifestyle modification must be followed for life because this is generally an irreversible condition.

DISPOSITION

- The majority of patients respond well to therapy.
- Recurrence of reflux is common if treatment is discontinued.
- Postsurgical complications occur in nearly 20% of patients (dysphagia, gas, bloating, diarrhea, nausea). Long-term follow-up studies also reveal that within 3 to 5 yr, 52% of patients who had undergone antireflux surgery are taking antireflux medications again.

REFERRAL

- There is a strong and probably causal relation between symptomatic prolonged and untreated GERD, Barrett's esophagus, and esophageal adenocarcinoma. GI referral for upper endoscopy is needed when there are concerns about associated peptic ulcer disease, Barrett's esophagus, or esophageal cancer.
- Patients with Barrett's esophagus should undergo surveillance endoscopy with mucosal biopsy every 2 yr or less because the risk of developing adenocarcinoma of esophagus is at least 30 times greater than that of the general population.
- Testing and treating for *Helicobacter pylori* in patients with GERD has not been shown to improve symptoms.
- All children with dental erosions should be evaluated for GERD.

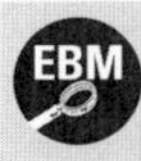

EVIDENCE

Adults

H_2 receptor antagonists are more effective than placebo but less effective than PPIs. Antagonists, compared with placebo, are more likely to relieve heartburn in patients with endoscopy-negative reflux disease.[1] Ⓐ

Antagonists are less effective than PPIs in the empirical treatment of typical GERD symptoms, although the difference is not significant for heartburn remission.[1] Ⓐ

Antagonists are more effective than placebo but less effective than PPIs at reducing the risk of persistent esophagitis.[2] Ⓐ

Ranitidine is less effective at 6 mo than are PPIs at reducing relapse rate in people with healed esophagitis.[3] Ⓐ

Ranitidine is less effective than omeprazole at maintaining remission at 12 mo in patients with healed esophagitis and no reflux symptoms.[4] Ⓐ

There is some evidence that esomeprazole may be more effective than other PPIs at promoting healing from esophagitis at 4 wk. Otherwise, there is little or no evidence to suggest that some PPIs are more effective than others.

A systematic review that compared various PPIs in people with reflux esophagitis found that esomeprazole was more effective than omeprazole at promoting healing at 4 wk. There were no significant differences between lansoprazole and omeprazole, pantoprazole and omeprazole, or rabeprazole and omeprazole.[5] Ⓐ

Another systematic review and three randomized controlled trials (RCTs) also compared various PPIs in people with reflux esophagitis. There were no significant differences in clinical benefit between other PPIs.[6] Ⓐ

Open surgery appears to be more effective than medical therapy in severe or complicated GERD in the short term; there may be no difference in the long term. No evidence suggests a difference between open and laparoscopic fundoplication.

A systematic review of RCTs showed that open surgery, compared with medical therapy, in patients with severe or complicated GERD significantly reduced symptoms and produced endoscopic improvements in esophagitis.[7] Ⓐ

However, a 10-year follow-up of one of the RCTs in this review found no significant difference in endoscopic appearance between those who had been treated with open surgery and those who had received medical therapy.[8] Ⓐ

There appears to be no clear difference in efficacy between open and laparoscopic fundoplication.[9,10] Ⓐ

Children

Cimetidine has been found to be more effective than placebo for the treatment of children with GERD and esophagitis in a small RCT.[11] Ⓐ

Another small RCT found that significantly more children achieved healing of esophagitis and symptomatic improvement when treated with nizatidine compared with placebo.[12] Ⓐ

There is insufficient evidence for the use of metoclopramide in the treatment of GERD in children.[13] Ⓐ

A systematic review found that adults and children with asthma and GERD did not achieve an overall improvement in asthma after antireflux treatment. The patients were not specifically recruited on the basis of reflux-associated respiratory symptoms. Subgroups of patients may benefit, but it appears difficult to predict responders.[14] Ⓐ

Evidence-Based References

1. van Pinxteren B et al: Short-term treatment with proton pump inhibitors, H_2-receptor antagonists and prokinetics for gastro-oesophageal reflux disease-like symptoms and endoscopy negative reflux disease, *Cochrane Rev* 3, 2004. Ⓐ
2. Delaney B, Moayyedi P: Dyspepsia. In Stevens A, Raftery J (eds): *Health care needs assessment,* ed 4, 2002, NHS Executive. Ⓐ
3. Caro JJ et al: Healing and relapse rates in gastro-oesophageal reflux disease treated with the newer proton-pump inhibitors lansoprazole, rabeprazole and pantoprazole compared with omeprazole, ranitidine and placebo: evidence from randomized controlled trials, *Clin Ther* 23:998, 2001. Ⓐ
4. Festen HPM et al: Omeprazole versus high-dose ranitidine in mild gastro-oesophageal reflux disease: short- and long-term treatment, *Am J Gastroenterol* 94:931, 1999. Ⓐ
5. Edwards SJ et al: Systematic review of proton pump inhibitors for the acute treatment of reflux oesophagitis, *Aliment Pharmacol Ther* 15:1729, 2001. Ⓐ
6. Moayyedi P et al: Gastro-oesophageal reflux disease, *Clin Evid* 10:518, 2003. Ⓐ
7. Allgood PC, Bachmann M: Medical or surgical treatment for chronic gastro-oesophageal reflux? A systematic review of published evidence of effectiveness, *Eur J Surg* 166:713, 2000. Ⓐ
8. Spechler SJ et al: Long-term outcome of medical and surgical therapies for gastroesophageal reflux disease, *JAMA* 285:2331, 2001. Ⓐ
9. Bias JE et al: Laparoscopic or conventional Nissen fundoplication for gastro-oeosophageal reflux disease: randomized clinical trial, *Lancet* 355:170, 2000. Ⓐ
10. Heikkinen T-J et al: Comparison of laparoscopic and open Nissen fundoplication 2 years after operation, *Surg Endosc* 14:1019, 2000. Ⓐ
11. Cucchiara S et al: Cimetidine treatment of reflux esophagitis in children: an Italian multicenter study, *J Pediatr Gastroenterol Nutr* 8:150, 1989. Ⓐ
12. Simeone D et al: Treatment of childhood peptic esophagitis: a double-blind placebo-controlled trial of nizatidine, *J Pediatr Gastroenterol Nutr* 25:51, 1997. Ⓐ
13. Kumar Y, Sarvananthan R: Gastro-oesophageal reflux in children, *Clin Evid* 11:414, 2004. Ⓐ
14. Gibson PG et al: Gastro-oesophageal reflux treatment for asthma in adults and children, *Cochrane Rev* 1, 2003. Ⓐ

SUGGESTED READINGS

Hampel H et al: Meta-analysis: obesity and the risk for gastroesophageal reflux disease and its complications, *Ann Intern Med* 143(3):199, 2005.

Heidelbaugh JL et al: Management of gastroesophageal reflux disease, *Am Fam Physician* 68:1311, 2003.

Kahrilas PJ: Gastroesophageal reflux disease, *N Engl J Med* 359:1700-7, 2008.

AUTHOR: **FRED F. FERRI, M.D.**

Gestational Diabetes Mellitus (GDM) (PTG)

BASIC INFORMATION

DEFINITION

Glucose intolerance that begins, or is first recognized, during pregnancy. Women are first screened with a 1-hr, nonfasting glucose tolerance test. If the result is >130 mg/dl, a 3-hr glucose tolerance test is ordered. The diagnosis is made if two or more of the glucose values are met or exceeded:

Fasting: 95 mg/dl
1-hr: 180 mg/dl
2-hr: 155 mg/dl
3-hr: 140 mg/dl

Pregnant women with diabetes mellitus (DM) (gestational or preexisting) are classified according to White's classification (Table 1-32).

SYNONYMS

Gestational diabetes
Sugar of pregnancy
Diet-controlled gestational diabetes (A1)
Insulin-treated gestational diabetes (A2)

ICD-9CM CODES

648.8; if using insulin to treat, add V58.67

EPIDEMIOLOGY & DEMOGRAPHICS

INCIDENCE: Approximately 7% of all pregnancies (may range from 1% to 14% in the U.S. depending on the population studied and the diagnostic tests used)

PREDOMINANT SEX AND AGE: Women of childbearing age

GENETICS: Higher rate in women with family history of gestational DM (GDM) or type 2 diabetes; specific HLA alleles (DR3 or DR4) predispose to the development of DM type 1 after delivery

RISK FACTORS

- Obesity
- Family history of GDM or type 2 diabetes
- Glycosuria at first prenatal visit
- Polycystic ovarian syndrome
- Twin gestation
- Hypertension
- Chronic systemic steroid use
- Maternal birth weight >9 lb or <6 lb
- Age >25 y
- Previous infant weighing >9 lb or with shoulder dystocia
- Unexplained perinatal loss or malformation
- Personal history of abnormal glucose tolerance or GDM
- Latin American, Native American, African American, or Asian ethnicity

POTENTIAL RISK FACTORS

- Mixing or applying agricultural pesticides in the first trimester
- Limited physical activity the year before pregnancy
- Prepregnancy diet low in fiber and high in glycemic load

PHYSICAL FINDINGS & CLINICAL PRESENTATION

Suspect GDM if:

- Fetal size greater than dates
- Macrosomia on ultrasound
- Marked maternal obesity or weight gain

ETIOLOGY

- During normal pregnancy there is increased insulin resistance because of placental secretion of diabetogenic hormones in the late second and third trimesters. Pancreatic beta-cell secretion increases to compensate for the increased insulin resistance. GDM occurs when this need cannot be met.
- Insulin resistance is also exacerbated by an increase in maternal adipose deposition, decreased exercise, and increased caloric intake.

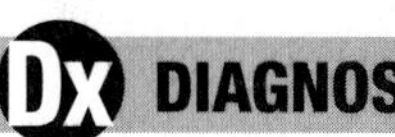

DIAGNOSIS

DIFFERENTIAL DIAGNOSIS

Preexisting type 1 or 2 DM not previously diagnosed

WORKUP

- History with focus on personal medical history, prior pregnancy history, and family history
- Routine prenatal examination
- Laboratory evaluation

LABORATORY TESTS

- Screening with 1-hr glucose tolerance test (Nonfasting; 50-g oral glucose load)
  - For screening without risk factors, order at 24 to 28 wk
  - For screening with risk factors, order at first prenatal visit, then repeat at 24 to 28 wk if initial screen was normal. If abnormal at intake, consider possibility of undiagnosed preexisting DM and check hemoglobin A1c.
- If 1-hr test result is abnormal (>130 mg/dl), order 3-hr glucose tolerance test
  - Performed after 3 days of unrestricted diet (carbohydrate load is probably not necessary)
  - Fasting
  - 100-g oral glucose load
- If one fourth of values on 3-hr glucose tolerance test is abnormal, repeat in 1 month and consider beginning a diabetic diet
- The U.S. Preventive Services Task Force (USPSTF) concludes that the evidence is insufficient to recommend for or against routine screening for gestational diabetes. The current evidence is insufficient to assess the balance between the benefits and harms of screening women for GDM either before or after 24 weeks gestation. Harms of screening include short-term anxiety in some women with positive screening results and inconvenience to many women and medical practices because most positive screening tests are likely false-positives. Until there is better evidence, clinicians should discuss screening for GDM with their patients and make case-by-case decisions. The discussion should include information about the uncertain benefits and harms as well as the frequency and uncertain meaning of a positive screening test result.

IMAGING STUDIES

Ultrasound for fetal size at least once at 36 to 37 wk; more frequently if macrosomia suspected

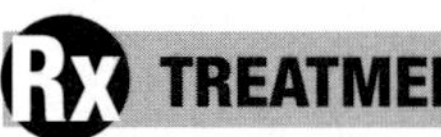

TREATMENT

NONPHARMACOLOGIC THERAPY

- Glucose monitoring:
  - Four times daily: fasting and 2-hr postprandial
  - Goals: fasting <95 to 105 mg/dl; 2-hr postprandial <110 to 120 mg/dl
  - Can also use 1-hr postprandial goal of <130 to 140 mg/dl
- Dietary modifications aimed at glycemic control:
  - Follow a low-fat, high-fiber diet; avoid sugar and concentrated sweets; and eat small, frequent meals.
  - Nutrition counseling for diet that adequately meets the needs of pregnancy but restricts carbohydrates to 35% to 40% of daily calories.

TABLE 1-32 White's Classification for Pregnant Women with Diabetes (Gestational or Preexisting)

Class	Description
A1	DM diagnosed during pregnancy and controlled by diet
A2	DM diagnosed during pregnancy and requiring medication
B	Insulin-requiring DM diagnosed before pregnancy, age >20 yr, lasting <10 yr
C	Insulin-requiring DM, onset at age 10 to 19 yr, with a duration 10 to 19 yr
D	Onset >10 yr or duration >20 yr, or associated with hypertension or background retinopathy
F	DM with renal disease
H	DM with coronary artery disease
R	DM with proliferative retinopathy
T	DM with renal transplant

- For women with a body mass index >30, restrict calories to 25 kcal/kg actual weight per day.
- Regular moderate exercise

PHARMACOLOGIC Rx

Begin if >20% of glucose values are elevated after trial of diet control:

- Oral hypoglycemics:
  - Glyburide: begin at 2.5 mg qd and titrate up to a maximum of 20 mg qd (10 mg bid). Increase dose as needed by 2.5 to 5 mg/wk.
  - Metformin use in pregnancy remains controversial because it crosses the placenta.
- Insulin:
  1. One commonly used regimen:
     - Insulin 0.7 U/kg/day SQ, with two thirds of the total daily dose given in the morning and one third of the total daily dose given in the evening
     - One third of each dose is given as short-acting insulin and the remaining two thirds as NPH insulin
  2. Another option:
     - If fasting values are elevated, use NPH at bedtime with initial dose of 0.2 U/kg
     - If postprandial values are elevated, use rapid-acting insulin before meals with initial dose 1.5 U/10 g carbohydrate at breakfast and 1 U/10 g carbohydrate at lunch and dinner
  3. Long-acting insulin such as Lantus does not have sufficient data to determine whether it crosses the placenta; it may be continued in persons with preexisting diabetes who are well controlled but is not recommended in patients with newly diagnosed GDM
  4. Glyburide and insulin have overall similar rates of clinical effectiveness and fetal safety

ANTENATAL TESTING

Routine blood pressure and urine protein monitoring:

- Class A1: NST/AFI at 40 wk
- Class A2: weekly NST/AFI beginning at 32 wk or when insulin is started
- Poorly controlled diabetes, vascular complications, or hypertension: biweekly NST/AFI beginning at 28 wk and consider admission for initial glycemic control

TIMING AND ROUTE OF DELIVERY

- Class A1 (well controlled): deliver by 41 wk
- Class A2: deliver by 40 wk
- Offer elective cesarean section at 38 wk if estimated fetal weight >4500 g
- Consider delivery by 37 wk if poor control or intrauterine growth retardation after confirmed fetal lung maturity by amniocentesis

INTRAPARTUM MANAGEMENT

- Goal is normoglycemia (80 to 110 mg/dl) using insulin and D5 lactated Ringer's IV fluid
- Monitor glucose hourly
- Preparation for shoulder dystocia
- If on glyburide, discontinue in labor or 12 hr before a scheduled induction

NEONATAL MANAGEMENT

- Check 30- and 60-min glucose
- Watch for signs of hypoglycemia, hypocalcemia, hyperbilirubinemia, and polycythemia

POSTPARTUM MANAGEMENT

- Class A2: check fasting level before discharge; if abnormal, continue checking at home and early follow up with primary care physician to confirm diagnosis of DM
- 6-wk postpartum visit: screen for diabetes with 2-hr glucose tolerance test or two fasting values
- If no evidence of DM, screen annually for DM and counsel on risk factor modification

REFERRAL

- Nutritionist
- High-risk obstetrician
- Maternal-fetal medicine
- Diabetes educator

COMPLICATIONS

- Maternal: preeclampsia, future type 2 DM or GDM, operative delivery
- Fetal: polyhydramnios, macrosomia, shoulder dystocia, birth trauma, congenital malformations
- Neonatal: hypoglycemia, hypocalcemia, hyperbilirubinemia, polycythemia, perinatal death, future obesity and DM, impaired fine and gross motor functions; increased rates of inattention and hyperactivity

PEARLS & CONSIDERATIONS

PREVENTION

Regular exercise, maintenance of ideal body weight, and high-fiber low-glycemic diet

PATIENT & FAMILY EDUCATION

Gestational Diabetes Patient Information
American Academy of Family Physicians
http://www.aafp.org/afp/20031101/1775ph.html

American Dietetic Association
Consumer Nutrition Information and Referrals
http://www.eatright.org
Telephone: 800-366-1655

American Diabetes Association: Gestational Diabetes
http://www.diabetes.org
800-DIABETES (800-342-2383)

NOAH: New York Online Access to Health
http://www.noah-health.org

National Institute of Child Health and Human Development
Managing Gestational Diabetes: A Patient's Guide to a Healthy Pregnancy
http://www.nichd.nih.gov/publications/pubs/gest_diabetes/
800-370-2943

Food and Nutrition Information Center
Food Guide Pyramid
http://www.nal.usda.gov.

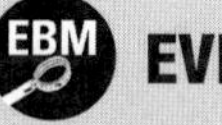

EVIDENCE

ACOG Practice Bulletin: *Clinical management guidelines for obstetrician-gynecologists,* Number 30, 2001, ACOG.

American Diabetes Association: Gestational diabetes position statement, *Diabetes Care* 27(suppl 1): S88, 2004.

Crowther CA et al: Effect of treatment of gestational diabetes mellitus on pregnancy outcomes, *N Engl J Med* 24:2477, 2005.

Lo JC et al: Increased prevalence of gestational diabetes mellitus among women with diagnosed polycystic ovary syndrome, *Diabetes Care* 29(8): 1915, 2006.

Rochon M et al: Glyburide for the management of gestational diabetes: risk factors predictive of failure and associated pregnancy outcomes, *Am J Obstet Gynecol* 195:1090, 2006.

Saldana TM et al: Pesticide exposure and self-reported gestational diabetes mellitus in the agricultural health study, *Diabetes Care* 30(3):529, 2007.

SUGGESTED READINGS

AACE Diabetes Mellitus Clinical Practice Guidelines Task Force: AACE diabetes mellitus guidelines. Diabetes and pregnancy, *Endocrinol Pract* 13(suppl 1):55, 2007.

Meneghini L, McDonough B: at www.clinicalmedicinetoday.com

Turok et al: Management of gestational diabetes mellitus, *Am Fam Physician* 68:1767, 2003.

AUTHORS: **JORDAN WHITE, M.D., NIRALI BORA, M.D., HEIDI H. PETERSON, M.D.,** and **SUSANNA R. MAGEE, M.D., M.P.H.**

Giant Cell Arteritis

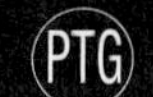

BASIC INFORMATION

DEFINITION

Giant cell arteritis (GCA) is a segmental systemic granulomatous arteritis affecting medium and large arteries in individuals >50 yr. Peak incidence is in patients aged 60 to 80 yr. Inflammation primarily targets extracranial blood vessels, and although the carotid system is usually affected, pathology in the posterior cerebral artery has been reported.

SYNONYMS

Temporal arteritis
Cranial arteritis

ICD-9CM CODES

446.5 Temporal arteritis

EPIDEMIOLOGY & DEMOGRAPHICS

INCIDENCE: 17 to 23.3 new cases per 100,000 persons >50 yr

PREVALENCE: 200 cases per 100,000 persons; female/male predominance of twofold to fourfold

PHYSICAL FINDINGS & CLINICAL PRESENTATION

GCA can present with the following clinical manifestations:

- Headache, often associated with marked scalp tenderness
- Constitutional symptoms (fever, weight loss, anorexia, fatigue)
- Polymyalgia syndrome (aching and stiffness of the trunk and proximal muscle groups)
- Visual disturbances (transient or permanent monocular visual loss)
- Intermittent claudication of jaw and tongue on mastication

Important physical findings in GCA:

- Vascular examination: tenderness, decreased pulsation, and nodulation of temporal arteries; diminished or absent pulses in upper extremities

ETIOLOGY

Vasculitis of unknown etiology

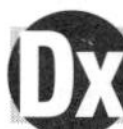

DIAGNOSIS

Clinical history and vascular examination are cornerstones of diagnosis.

- Age of onset >50 yr
- New-onset or new type of headache
- Temporal artery tenderness or decreased pulsation
- Westergren erythrocyte sedimentation rate (ESR) elevated (typically >50 mm/hr)
- Jaw claudication
- Temporal artery biopsy with vasculitis and mononuclear cell infiltrate or granulomatous changes

DIFFERENTIAL DIAGNOSIS

- Other vasculitic syndromes
- Nonarteritic anterior ischemic optic neuropathy (AION)
- Primary amyloidosis
- Transient ischemic attack, stroke
- Infections
- Occult neoplasm, multiple myeloma

LABORATORY TESTS

- ESR elevated; up to 22.5% patients with GCA have normal ESR before treatment.
- C-reactive protein is typically included in laboratory investigation; it may have greater sensitivity than ESR.
- Mild to moderate normochromic normocytic anemia, elevated platelet count.

IMAGING STUDIES

- Reliability of color duplex ultrasonography of temporal artery is controversial because it is believed to not improve diagnostic accuracy over careful physical examination.
- Fluorescein angiogram of ophthalmic vessels may be warranted to differentiate between arteritic AION (i.e., GCA) and nonarteritic AION.

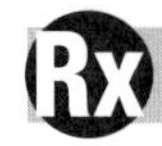

TREATMENT

ACUTE GENERAL Rx

- IV methylprednisolone (250 to 1000 mg qd for 3 to 5 days) is indicated in those with significant clinical manifestations (e.g., visual loss).
- Oral prednisone (1 mg/kg/day). High-dose oral regimen should be continued at least until symptoms resolve and ESR returns to normal. Prednisone treatment may last up to 2 yr and is tapered over several weeks to months.
- Other immunosuppressive agents may be used when steroids are contraindicated.

DISPOSITION

If steroid therapy is initiated early, GCA has excellent prognosis; however, once there is visual loss, improvement is dismal. In one study only 4% of eyes improved in both visual acuity and central visual field.

REFERRAL

- Surgical referral for biopsy of temporal artery
- Ophthalmology referral in patients with visual disturbances and after initiation of corticosteroid therapy
- Rheumatology referral for patients in whom steroids are contraindicated

PEARLS & CONSIDERATIONS

The diagnostic utility of temporal artery biopsy is not compromised if performed within days of starting steroid therapy.

COMMENTS

- The relation between polymyalgia rheumatica and GCA is unclear, but the two frequently coexist.
- Clinical picture rather than ESR should be the prime yardstick for continuing prednisone therapy. A rising ESR in a clinically asymptomatic patient with normal hematocrit should raise suspicion for alternate explanations (e.g., infections, neoplasms).
- GCA is associated with a markedly increased risk for the development of aortic aneurysm, which is often a late complication and may cause death. Annual chest radiograph in chronic CGA patients has been suggested, as well as emergent chest CT or MRI for clinical suspicion.

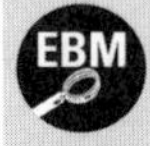

EVIDENCE

The recommendation to perform temporal artery biopsy before beginning long-term corticosteroid therapy is based on consensus rather than evidence.

The recommendation that daily high-dose corticosteroid therapy should not be delayed pending confirmation of the diagnosis from temporal artery biopsy is similarly based on consensus rather than evidence.

The efficacy of adding methotrexate or azathioprine to the steroid regimen for their steroid-sparing effect is unproven.

SUGGESTED READINGS

Gold R et al: Therapy of neurological disorders in systemic vasculitis, *Semin Neurol* 23(2):207, 2003.

Gonzalez-Gay MA: The diagnosis and management of patients with giant cell arteritis, *J Rheumatol* 32: 1186, 2005.

Hayreh SR et al: Visual improvement with corticosteroid therapy in giant cell arteritis. Report of large study and review of the literature, *Acta Opththalmol Scand* 80:355, 2002.

Hoffman GS et al: A multicenter, randomized, double-blind, placebo-controlled trial of adjuvant methotrexate for giant-cell arteritis, *Arthritis Rheum* 46(5): 1309, 2002.

Karassa FB et al: Meta-analysis: test performance of ultrasonography for giant cell arteritis, *Ann Intern Med* 142:359-369, 2005.

Norborg E, Norborg C: Giant cell arteritis: epidemiological clues to its pathogenesis and an update on its treatment, *Rheumatology* 42:413, 2003.

Salvarani C et al: Polymyalgia rheumatica and giant-cell arteritis, *N Engl J Med* 347(4):261, 2002.

Smetana GW, Shmerling RH: Does this patient have temporal arteritis? *JAMA* 287:92, 2002.

AUTHOR: **U. SHIVRAJ SOHUR, M.D., PH.D.**

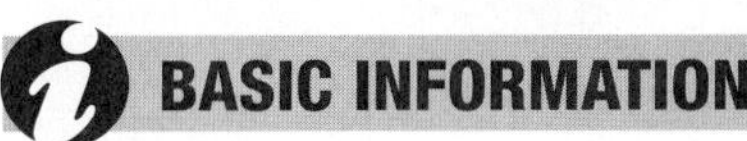

BASIC INFORMATION

DEFINITION

Giardiasis is an intestinal and/or biliary tract infection caused by the protozoal parasite *Giardia lamblia.* The organism is a widespread zoonotic parasite and frequently contaminates fresh water sources worldwide.

SYNONYMS

Giardiasis
Giardia duodenalis
Giardia intestinalis

ICD-9CM CODES

007.1 Giardiasis

EPIDEMIOLOGY & DEMOGRAPHICS

INCIDENCE (IN U.S.):

- Exact incidence unknown
- Frequently occurs in outbreaks

PREVALENCE (IN U.S.): 4%

PREDOMINANT SEX: Male = female

PREDOMINANT AGE:

- Preschool children, especially if in day care
- 20 to 40 yr of age, especially among sexually active homosexual men

PEAK INCIDENCE:

- Varies with risk factors, outbreaks
- All age groups affected

GENETICS: Familial disposition: Patients with common variable immunodeficiency or X-linked agammaglobulinemia are at increased risk of infection.

PHYSICAL FINDINGS & CLINICAL PRESENTATION

- More than 70% with one or more intestinal symptoms (diarrhea, flatulence, cramps, bloating, nausea)
- Fever in <20%
- Chronic diarrhea, malabsorption, and weight loss
- GI bleeding is unusual
- Continuous or intermittent symptoms, lasting for weeks
- Of infected patients, 20% to 25% are asymptomatic

ETIOLOGY

Infection is acquired by ingestion of viable cysts of the organism, typically in contaminated water or by fecal-oral contact.

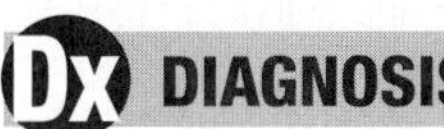

DIAGNOSIS

DIFFERENTIAL DIAGNOSIS

- Other agents of infective diarrhea (amebae, *Salmonella* sp., *Shigella* sp., *Staphylococcus aureus, Cryptosporidium,* etc.)
- Noninfectious causes of malabsorption

WORKUP

- Stool specimen (three specimens yield 90% sensitivity) or duodenal aspirate for microscopic examination to establish diagnosis and exclude other pathogens (Fig. 1-129)
- Immunoassays for *Giardia* sp. Antigens in stool samples are now routinely used in most clinical laboratories

LABORATORY TESTS

Serum albumin, vitamin B12 levels, and stool fat test to exclude malabsorption

IMAGING STUDIES

- Not necessary unless biliary obstruction is suspected
- In detection of organism, possible interference by barium in stool from radiographic studies

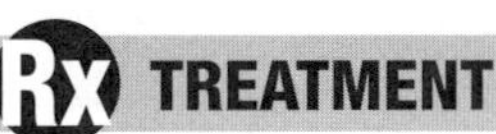

TREATMENT

NONPHARMACOLOGIC THERAPY

Avoidance of milk products to reduce symptoms of transient lactase deficiency that occur in many patients

ACUTE GENERAL Rx

Adults:

- Nitazoxanide 500 mg PO twice daily for 3 days
- Metronidazole 250 mg PO three times daily for 7 days (metronidazole avoided in pregnancy) or Tinidazole 2 mg PO once
- Paromomycin 25 to 30 mg/kg/day in three doses for 5 to 10 days

CHRONIC Rx

May require retreatment.

DISPOSITION

Reinfection is possible.

REFERRAL

For evaluation by gastroenterologist if malabsorption and persistent weight loss

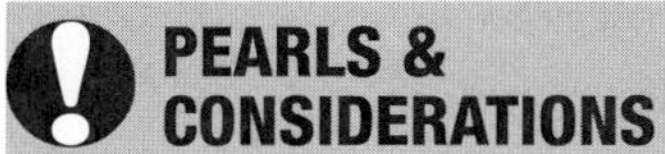

PEARLS & CONSIDERATIONS

COMMENTS

Travelers to endemic areas (developing world, wilderness areas) should be cautioned to boil drinking water or use water purification tablets.

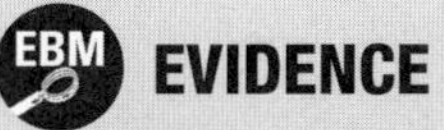

EVIDENCE

Randomized controlled trials (RCTs) have shown cure rates of 80% to 90% at 7 to 14 days follow-up, after 5 to 7 days' treatment with metronidazole, in children with giardiasis.[1] B

An RCT comparing the efficacy and safety of furazolidone and metronidazole in liquid suspension found no significant differences between the treatments in children with giardiasis.[2] B

An RCT comparing the efficacy and safety of albendazole and metronidazole in suspension found no significant differences between the treatments in children with giardiasis.[3] B

Evidence-Based References

1. Ortiz JJ et al: Randomized clinical study of nitazoxanide compared to metronidazole in the treatment of symptomatic giardiasis in children from Northern Peru, *Aliment Pharmacol Ther* 15:1409, 2001. B
2. Quiros-Buelna E: Furazolidone and metronidazole for treatment of giardiasis in children, *Scand J Gastroenterol Suppl* 169:65, 1989. B
3. Misra PK et al: A comparative clinical trial of albendazole versus metronidazole in children with giardiasis, *Indian Pediatr* 32:779, 1995. B

SUGGESTED READINGS

Hlavsa MC et al: Giardiasis surveillance—United States, 1998. 2002, *MMWR Surveill Summ* 54(1):9, 2005.

Lalle M et al: Genotyping of Giardia duodenalis from humans and dogs from Mexico using a beta-giardin nested polymerase chain reaction assay, *J Parasitol* 91(1):203, 2005.

Yakoob J et al: Giardiasis in patients with dyspeptic symptoms, *World J Gastroenterol* 11(42):6667, 2005.

AUTHORS: **GLENN G. FORT, M.D., M.P.H.,** and **DENNIS J. MIKOLICH, M.D.**

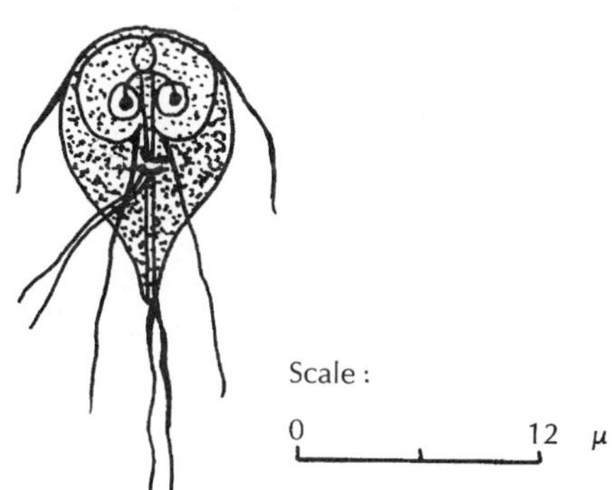

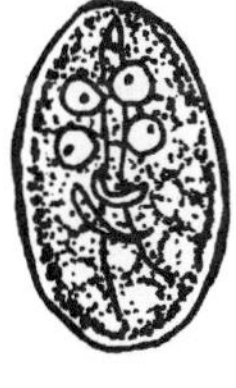

FIGURE 1-129 ***Giardia*** **organisms.** The trophozoite *(left)* is 12 to 15 μm long and has four pairs of flagella. This form is not commonly seen in stools. Cysts *(right)* are 9 to 19 μm long and may have two to four nuclei. (From Hoekelman R [ed]: *Primary pediatric care,* ed 3, St Louis, 1997, Mosby.)

Gilbert's Disease

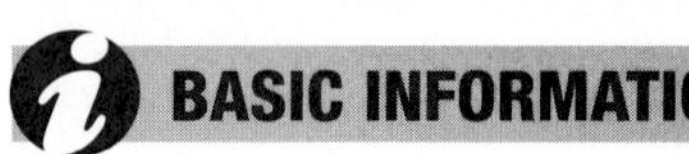

BASIC INFORMATION

DEFINITION

Gilbert's disease is an autosomal-dominant disease characterized by indirect hyperbilirubinemia caused by impaired glucuronyl transferase activity.

SYNONYMS

Gilbert's syndrome

ICD-9CM CODES
277.4 Gilbert's syndrome

EPIDEMIOLOGY & DEMOGRAPHICS

INCIDENCE (IN U.S.): Probable autosomal-dominant disease affecting >5% of the U.S. population
PREDOMINANT SEX: Male/female ratio of 3:1
GENETICS: Most common hereditary hyperbilirubinemia (genotypic prevalence 12%)

PHYSICAL FINDINGS & CLINICAL PRESENTATION

- No abnormalities on physical examination other than mild jaundice when bilirubin exceeds 3 mg/dl.
- A family history of unconjugated hyperbilirubinemia may be present.

ETIOLOGY

- Decreased elimination of bilirubin in bile is caused by inadequate conjugation of bilirubin.
- Alcohol consumption and starvation diet can increase bilirubin level.
- The pathogenesis of Gilbert's syndrome has been linked to a reduction in the bilirubin UGT-1 gene *(HUG-Brl)* transcription, resulting from a mutation in the promoter region.

Dx DIAGNOSIS

DIFFERENTIAL DIAGNOSIS

- Hemolytic anemia
- Liver disease (chronic hepatitis, cirrhosis)
- Crigler-Najjar syndrome

WORKUP

- Most patients are diagnosed during or after adolescence, when isolated hyperbilirubinemia is detected as an incidental finding on routine biochemical testing.
- Laboratory evaluation to exclude hemolysis and liver diseases as a cause of the elevated bilirubin level (Table 1-33).

LABORATORY TESTS

Elevated indirect (unconjugated) bilirubin (rarely exceeds 5 mg/dl)

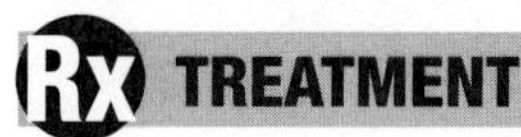

TREATMENT

ACUTE GENERAL Rx

Treatment is generally unnecessary. Phenobarbital (if clinical jaundice is present) can rapidly decrease serum indirect bilirubin level.

DISPOSITION

Prognosis is excellent. Treatment is generally unnecessary.

REFERRAL

Referral is generally not necessary.

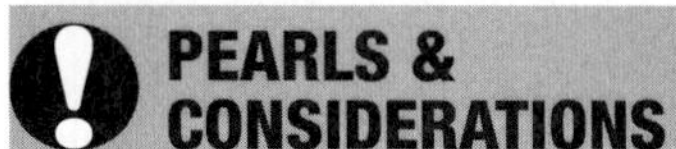

PEARLS & CONSIDERATIONS

COMMENTS

- Patients should be reassured about the benign nature of their condition.
- Fasting for 2 days or significant dehydration may raise the bilirubin level and result in the clinical recognition of jaundice.

AUTHOR: **FRED F. FERRI, M.D.**

TABLE 1-33 Characteristic Patterns of Liver Function Tests

Disorder	Bilirubin	Alkaline Phosphatase	AST	ALT	Prothrombin Time	Albumin
Gilbert's syndrome (abnormal bilirubin metabolism)	↑	NL	NL	NL	NL	NL
Bile duct obstruction (pancreatic cancer)	↑↑↑	↑↑↑	↑	↑	↑-↑↑	NL
Acute hepatocellular damage (toxic, viral hepatitis)	↑-↑↑↑	↑-↑↑	↑↑↑	↑↑↑	NL-↑↑↑	NL-↓↓
Cirrhosis	NL-↑	NL-↑	NL-↑	NL-↑	NL-↑↑	NL-↓↓

From Andreoli TE (ed): *Cecil essentials of medicine,* ed 6, Philadelphia, 2005, WB Saunders.
ALT, Alanine aminotransferase; *AST,* aspartate aminotransferase; *NL,* normal; ↑, increase; ↓, decrease (arrows indicate extent of change: ↑-↑↑↑, slight to large).

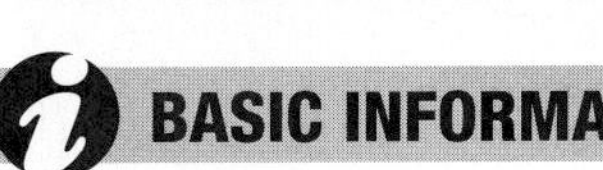

BASIC INFORMATION

DEFINITION

Inflammation of the gums covering the maxilla and mandible

SYNONYMS

None

ICD-9CM CODES
523.1 Chronic gingivitis
523.01 Acute gingivitis

EPIDEMIOLOGY & DEMOGRAPHICS

Gingivitis generally occurs in adults.

PHYSICAL FINDINGS & CLINICAL PRESENTATION

- Inflammation is usually painless.
- Bleeding may occur with minor trauma such as brushing teeth.
- A bluish discoloration of the gums and halitosis are sometimes present.
- Subgingival plaque may be seen on close examination, and in time, there is detachment of soft tissue from the tooth surface.
- Longstanding infection may lead to destructive periodontal disease, which may involve teeth and bones.
- A dramatic form of gingivitis called acute ulcerative necrotizing gingivitis (ANUG or "trench mouth") can occur. This is manifested by acute, painful inflammation of the gingivae, with bleeding, ulceration, and halitosis. At times this is accompanied by fever and lymphadenopathy.
- Linear gingival erythema ("HIV Gingivitis") presents as a brightly inflamed band of marginal gingiva. It may be painful, with easy bleeding and rapid destruction.
- Severe periodontitis can occur in patients with diabetes mellitus or HIV infection and in primary HIV infection (acute retroviral syndrome).
- Pregnancy may be associated with an acute form of gingivitis. Gingivae become inflamed and hypertrophic; this is likely the result of hormonal shifts.

ETIOLOGY

- A variety of organisms may be found in the environment of plaque. Anaerobes play a predominant role in periodontal disease.
- Improper hygiene and poorly fitting dentures may contribute to the development of gingivitis.
- Excessive use of tobacco and alcohol may predispose individuals to gingival disease.
- In patients with HIV infection, gram-negative anaerobes, enteric organisms, and yeast predominate.
- Appropriate oral hygiene, such as flossing and tooth brushing, can prevent the accumulation of bacterial plaque; once dense plaque is present, adequate hygiene becomes more difficult.

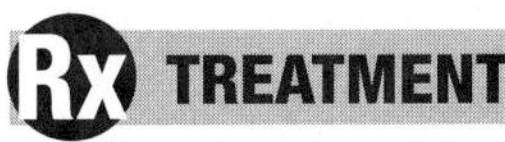

DIAGNOSIS

DIFFERENTIAL DIAGNOSIS

Gingival hyperplasia, which may be caused by long-term use of phenytoin or nifedipine

WORKUP

Oral examination

LABORATORY TESTS

Elevated serum glucose in diabetics

IMAGING STUDIES

Radiographs of the teeth and facial bones may reveal extension of infection to these structures.

Rx TREATMENT

NONPHARMACOLOGIC THERAPY

Removal of plaque, and at times, debridement of soft tissue

ACUTE GENERAL Rx

- Penicillin VK, 500 mg PO qid for 1 to 2 wk or
- Clindamycin, 300 mg PO qid for 1 to 2 wk
- For linear gingival erythema, chlorhexidine gluconate rinses and nystatin rinses or troches may be used

CHRONIC Rx

Extensive or recurrent infection may require periodic evaluation and debridement.

DISPOSITION

Continued inflammation can eventually lead to destruction of teeth and bone.

REFERRAL

Patients should be referred to a dentist or periodontist.

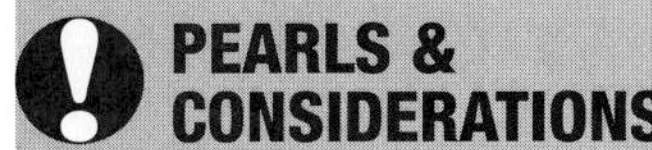

PEARLS & CONSIDERATIONS

COMMENTS

- Presence of periodontal disease is associated with an increased incidence of anaerobic pleuropulmonary infections.
- Existing data support the recommendation to change a toothbrush every 3 mo. Worn brushes seem to be less effective in plaque reduction.

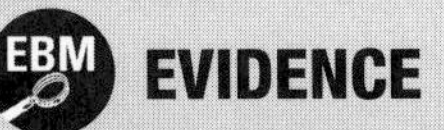

EVIDENCE

Professional cleaning and scaling reaches subgingival areas not usually accessible to the patient through toothbrushing and flossing.[1]

Failure by the patient to remove plaque deposits regularly between visits will result in extension of plaque to subgingival crevices and accumulation of calculus.

Parameter on plaque-associated gingivitis. Chicago: American Academy of Periodontology, National Guideline Clearinghouse recommends patient education, including oral hygiene instruction; debridement of tooth surfaces to remove plaque and calculus; correction of restorations hindering oral hygiene; surgical correction of the gums where indicated; and outcomes assessment.[2]

Evidence-Based References

1. Axelsson P, Lindhe J: Effect of controlled oral hygiene procedures on caries and periodontal disease in adults: results after 6 years, *J Clin Periodontol* 8:239, 1981.

2. American Academy of Periodontology: Guidelines for periodontal therapy, *J Periodontol* 69:405, 1998.

SUGGESTED READINGS

Rudiger SG et al: Dental biofilms at healthy and inflamed gingival margins, *J Clin Periodontol* 29(6): 524, 2002.

Sharma NC et al: Antiplaque and antigingivitis effectiveness of a hexetidine mouthwash, *J Clin Periodontol* 30(7):590, 2003.

AUTHORS: **GLENN G. FORT, M.D., M.P.H.,** and **DENNIS J. MIKOLICH, M.D.**

Gingivitis, Necrotizing Ulcerative (NUG)

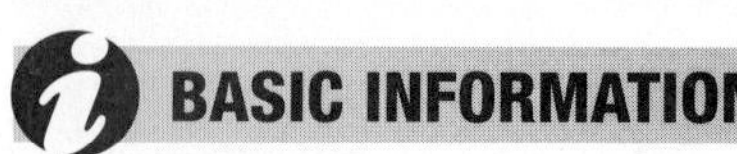

BASIC INFORMATION

DESCRIPTION

Necrotizing ulcerative gingivitis (NUG) is a distinct painful infectious disease primarily of the interdental and marginal gingiva. It is characterized by a symptom triad that includes gingival pain, ulcer, and bleeding.

SYNONYMS

Trench mouth
Acute necrotizing ulcerative gingivitis (ANUG)
Vincent's stomatitis
Fusospirochetal gingivitis
Acute ulcerative gingivitis

ICD-9CM CODES

101 Acute necrotizing ulcerative gingivitis

EPIDEMIOLOGY

- Unlike in the developing world, NUG is seen rarely in developed countries.
- Occurs in the 2nd and 3rd decade of life in the developed world.
- In contrast, it affects young children more often in developing countries.
- Slightly more prevalent in males than in females because the latter group tend to have a better oral hygiene.

RISK FACTORS

- Poor oral hygiene
- Smoking/chewing tobacco
- Alcohol use
- Drug addiction
- Poor socioeconomic status
- Psychological stress
- Preexisting gingivitis
- Lack of sleep
- Malnutrition
- Overcrowding
- Living near livestock
- History of prior NUG
- Recent illness
- Underlying systemic diseases
- Acatalasia
- Various infections such as measles, malaria, and infestation with intestinal parasites
- Trauma
- Immunosuppression
  - Dermatomyositis (DM)
  - Steroid use
  - HIV/AIDS
  - Use of chemotherapeutic drugs
  - Leukemia and other malignancies

ETIOLOGY

- Polymicrobial
- Often caused by both Fusobacterium and spirochetes

PATHOGENESIS

- Unknown
- For the most part it appears to result from an opportunistic infection in a host with lowered resistance.

CLINICAL FEATURES

- Onset of the disease is usually sudden
- Severe gingival pain
- Gingival tissue is inflamed, edematous, friable, and necrotic; the normal pointed interdental papillae are blunted, but there is no loss of attachment
- Gingival bleeding with little or no provocation
- Punched out ulcerations are seen along the interdental papillae around the anterior incisors and posterior molars. A grayish-white pseudomembrane often covers these ulcers. These punched out ulcers along the pseudomembrane are pathognomonic of NUG.
- Other features include
  - Halitosis
  - Alteration in taste, such as a metallic flavor
  - Wooden teeth feeling
  - Odynophagia
  - Fever and fatigue
  - Cervical lymphadenopathy

Dx DIAGNOSIS

- Based on the clinical features
- WBC may be elevated
- Gram stain and aerobic/anaerobic culture
- Dental x-ray or x-ray of face to check on the extent of the disease
- HIV testing is recommended for patients refractory to antibiotic therapy

DIFFERENTIAL DIAGNOSIS

- Gingivitis
- Acute herpetic gingivostomatitis
- Aphthous stomatitis
- Chronic periodontal disease
- Desquamative gingivitis
- Gonococcal and streptococcal gingivostomatitis
- Oral candidiasis
- Ludwig's angina
- HIV-associated idiopathic ulcerations

Rx TREATMENT

- Improve oral hygiene by flushing and brushing at least twice a day.
- Improve nutrition and hydrations.
- Eliminate contributing factors such as smoking, alcohol, carbonated beverages, spicy/hot foods, poor nutrition, stress, and so on.
- Antibiotics coverage for 5 to 10 days. Most recommend oral penicillin V 250 to 500 mg orally every 6 to 8 hr and metronidazole 250 to 500 mg orally every 8 hr. Tetracycline is given instead of penicillin in patients allergic to the latter. As an alternative one could give only clindamycin instead of the drug combination of penicillin and metronidazole.
- Rinsing the mouth at least twice a day with warm saline (1/2 teaspoon of salt in 1 cup of water), 0.12% chlorhexidine, or dilute 3% hydrogen peroxide (mixed half and half with water).
- Pain is controlled with oral pain medications and topical application of 2% viscous lidocaine (15 ml oral rinse every 6 to 8 hr as needed) to the inflamed gum.
- Surgical debridement is needed in severe cases.
- Scaling and root planning following the resolution of infection and the acute inflammation.
- At times reconstructive surgery may be needed.

COMPLICATIONS

- Cancrum oris (noma) results when NUG involves the deeper tissue
- Vincent's angina from the involvement of tonsils and pharynx
- Necrotizing ulcerative periodontitis
- Loss of teeth
- Periodontal abscess
- Alveolar bone destruction
- Disfigurement
- Cellulitis
- Dehydration/malnutrition

PROGNOSIS

- Dramatic relief of symptoms within 24 hr of initiating antibiotics and supportive treatment is characteristic.
- Risk of recurrence is high.

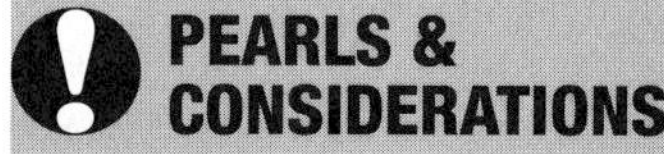

PEARLS & CONSIDERATIONS

PREVENTION

- Good oral hygiene
- Use of power toothbrush is better than a manual brush
- Good general health including proper nutrition, sleep, and exercise
- Routine dental checks
- Avoidance of smoking and alcohol
- Stress management

PATIENT EDUCATION

Not a communicable disease

SUGGESTED READING

Necrotizing ulcerative gingivitis. *Ann Periodontol* 4:65-73, 1999

AUTHOR: **HEMANT K. SATPATHY, M.D.**

BASIC INFORMATION

DEFINITION

Primary angle-closure glaucoma (PACG) occurs when elevated intraocular pressure is associated with closure of the filtration angle or obstruction in the circulating pathway of the aqueous humor.

SYNONYMS

Acute glaucoma, angle-closure
Pupillary block glaucoma
Narrow-angle glaucoma

ICD-9CM CODES
365.2 Primary angle-closure glaucoma (PACG)

EPIDEMIOLOGY & DEMOGRAPHICS

INCIDENCE (IN U.S.):
- 2% to 8% of all patients with glaucoma
- Higher incidence among those with hyperopia, small eyes, dense cataracts, shallow anterior chambers

PEAK INCIDENCE: Greater >50 yr; high association with hypopia, cataracts, and eye trauma
PREDOMINANT SEX: Females are affected more often than males
PREDOMINANT AGE: 50 to 60 yr
GENETICS: High family history

PHYSICAL FINDINGS & CLINICAL PRESENTATION

- Hazy cornea (Fig. 1-130)
- Narrow angle
- Red eyes
- Pain
- Injection of conjunctiva
- Shallow anterior chamber
- Thick cataract
- Old trauma
- Chronic eye infections

ETIOLOGY

- Narrow angles with acute closure: blockage of circulatory path of the aqueous humor causing increase in interior ocular pressure
- Secondary angle-closure glaucoma (SACG) resulting from neovascularization of iris, iris tumors, pharmacology, lens induced, iris scarring, trauma, chronic inflammation with scarring, malignant glaucoma with aqueous misdirection

DIAGNOSIS

DIFFERENTIAL DIAGNOSIS

- High pressure
- Optic nerve cupping
- Field loss
- Shallow chamber
- Open-angle glaucoma
- Conjunctivitis
- Corneal disease, keratitis
- Uveitis
- Scleritis
- Allergies
- Contact lens wearing with irritation

WORKUP

- Intraocular pressure
- Gonioscopy
- Slit lamp examination
- Visual field examination
- GDx examination (laser scan of nerve fiber layer), OCT
- Optic nerve evaluation
- Anterior chamber depth
- Cataract evaluation
- High hyperopia
- Dilantin provocative testing

LABORATORY TESTS

- Blood sugar and complete blood count (if diabetes or inflammatory disease is suspected)
- Visual field
- GDx nerve fiber analysis, OCT, Heidelberg retinal tomography

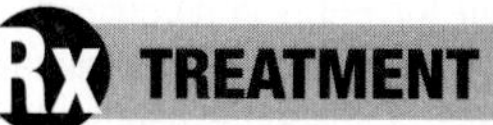

IMAGING STUDIES

- Fundus photography
- Fluorescein angiography for neurovascular disease

TREATMENT

The goal of treatment is to acutely lower pressure on the eye and keep it down.

NONPHARMACOLOGIC THERAPY

Laser iridotomy early in disease process

ACUTE GENERAL Rx

- IV mannitol
- Pilocarpine
- β-blockers
- Diamox
- Laser iridotomy
- Anterior chamber paracentesis (as emergency treatment)

CHRONIC Rx

- Iridotomy
- Trabeculectomy
- Filter valves
- Other laser procedures

DISPOSITION

Refer to ophthalmologist immediately.

REFERRAL

This is an emergency; refer immediately to an ophthalmologist.

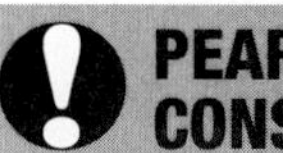

PEARLS & CONSIDERATIONS

COMMENTS

- Do not use antihistamines or vasodilators with narrow-angle glaucoma.
- After iridotomy, the majority of patients will be totally cured and will need no further medication and have no visual loss.
- Lower socioeconomic status and higher levels of social deprivation are risk factors for delayed detection and probable worse outcomes in glaucoma.

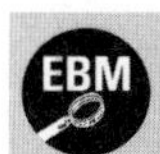

EVIDENCE

Medical Therapies

There is consensus that medical treatment with pressure-lowering drugs (especially those that can be given parenterally, such as IV acetazolamide) are effective in PACG.[1]

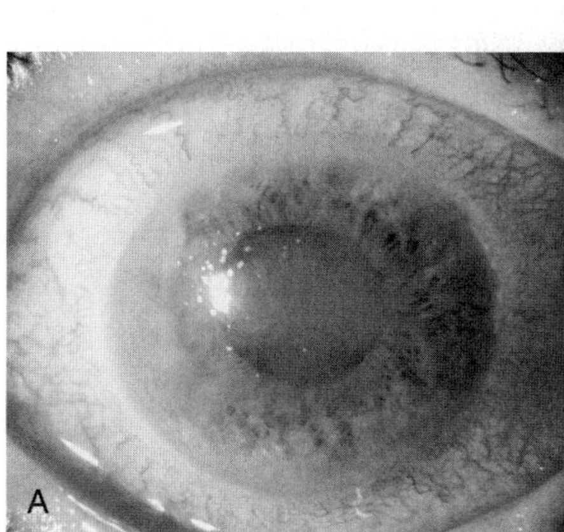

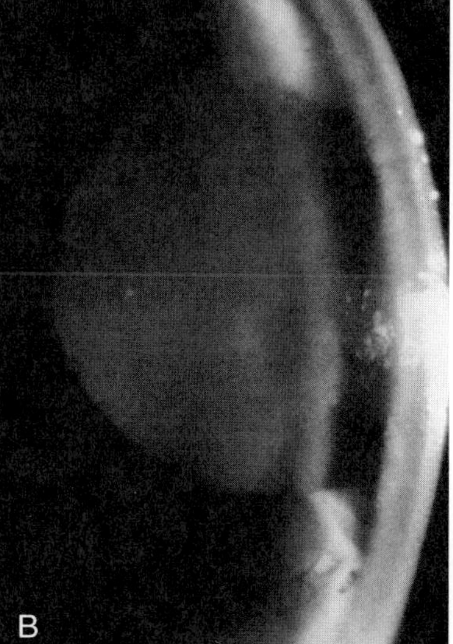

FIGURE 1-130 Acute angle-closure glaucoma. A, Acutely elevated pressure produces an inflamed eye with corneal edema (note fragmented light reflex) and a mid-dilated pupil. **B,** Slit lamp examination shows a very shallow central anterior chamber (space between cornea and iris) and no peripheral chamber. (From Palay D [ed]: *Ophthalmology for the primary care physician,* St Louis, 1997, Mosby.)

Recommendations from the American Academy of Ophthalmology state that in PACG attacks, medical therapy is usually initiated first to lower the intraocular pressure to reduce pain and clear corneal edema in preparation for iridectomy.[2] **C**

Surgical Therapies

There is a lack of randomized studies that evaluate the efficacy of surgical therapies for PACG. Consensus suggests that surgical treatments are effective for PACG.[1]

Recommendations from the American Academy of Ophthalmology state that the definitive treatment for PACG is surgical, either by means of laser iridectomy or incisional iridectomy if a laser iridectomy cannot be successfully performed.[2] **C**

Systematic reviews have found that the use of intraoperative mitomycin C and postoperative 5-fluorouracil reduces the risk of surgical failure in eyes that have undergone no previous surgery and in eyes at high risk of failure.[3] **A**

Further recommendations from the American Academy of Ophthalmology include:

- Laser iridectomy is the preferred surgical treatment because it has a favorable risk/benefit ratio.[2] **C**
- When laser iridectomy is not possible or if the acute angle-closure attack cannot be medically broken, incisional iridectomy remains an effective alternative.[2] **C**
- Patients who require bilateral incisional iridectomy should have surgery on one eye at a time (several days apart) whenever feasible to avoid simultaneous bilateral complications.[2] **C**
- The fellow eye should receive a prophylactic iridectomy if the chamber angle is anatomically narrow because approximately half of fellow eyes of PACG patients will have acute attacks within 5 yr.[2] **C**

Evidence-Based References

1. Shah R, Wormald R: Glaucoma, *Clin Evid* 14:776, 2005.

2. American Academy of Ophthalmology: *Primary angle closure, preferred practice pattern,* San Francisco, 2005, American Academy of Ophthalmology. **C**

3. Wilkins M et al: Intra-operative mitomycin C for glaucoma surgery, *Cochrane Rev* 4, 2005. **A**

SUGGESTED READINGS

Foster PJ et al: Defining "occludable" angles in population surveys: drainage angle width, peripheral anterior synechiae, and glaucomatous optic neuropathy in East Asian people, *Br J Opthalmol* 88(4): 486, 2004.

Fraser S et al: Deprivation and late presentation of glaucoma: case control study, *BMJ* 322:638, 2001.

Gazzard G et al: Intraocular pressure and visual field loss in primary angle closure and primary open angle glaucomas, *Br J Ophthalmol* 87(6):720, 2003.

Kapur SB: The lens and angle-closure glaucoma, *J Cataract Refract Surg* 27(2):176, 2001.

Lam DS et al: Angle-closure glaucoma, *Opthalmology* 109:1, 2002.

AUTHOR: **MELVYN KOBY, M.D.**

BASIC INFORMATION

DEFINITION

Glenohumeral dislocation is complete separation or displacement of the humeral head from the glenoid surface (partial separation is termed *subluxation*). Most often the cause is traumatic, and the humeral head dislocates anteriorly and inferiorly. This may cause a tear of the glenoid labrum (the Bankart lesion). Less commonly the head dislocates posteriorly.

Rarely, multidirectional instability may be present in which dislocation or subluxation, often bilateral, may occur in multiple directions, usually the result of excessive joint laxity and generally without trauma.

ICD-9CM CODES
831.01 Anterior
831.02 Posterior
831.03 Inferior
718.31 Recurrent
718.81 Instability

PHYSICAL FINDINGS & CLINICAL PRESENTATION

Traumatic:

- The arm is held in external rotation with anterior dislocation and internal rotation with posterior dislocation.
- Little movement is possible without pain.
- The acromion may appear more prominent, and there is absence of the normal "fullness" beneath the acromion.
- The status of the axillary nerve must always be checked (sensation to the mid-deltoid should be assessed).
- The apprehension test may become positive if anterior instability persists (pain and apprehension that the shoulder will dislocate when the relaxed arm is manually placed in the "throwing position" of external rotation and abduction).
- Recurrent episodes of anterior dislocation may occur with minor movement, such as putting on a coat or turning off a light.

Multidirectional:

- Often difficult to diagnose, especially if only subluxation occurs.
- Recurrent episodes of giving out and weakness, often bilateral and without trauma.
- Sulcus sign is often positive (the arms are pulled downward with the patient standing; a sulcus [indentation] will form between the acromion and humeral head, indicating excessive inferior movement of the head).
- Other signs of generalized joint laxity may be present, such as joint hyperextensibility and the ability of the patient to touch the thumb against the flexor aspect of the forearm.

ETIOLOGY

- Trauma
- Generalized joint laxity (multidirectional)
- Seizures (posterior dislocations)

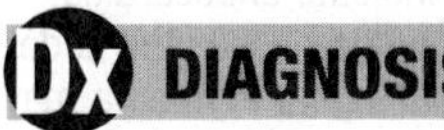

DIAGNOSIS

DIFFERENTIAL DIAGNOSIS

- Rotator cuff rupture
- Frozen shoulder (posterior dislocation)
- Suprascapular nerve paralysis
- Anterior instability

IMAGING STUDIES

- Acute shoulder injury: true anteroposterior roentgenogram plus lateral view of the glenohumeral joint, either transaxillary or transcapular
- MRI: to determine soft tissue status, especially the presence of Bankart lesion or rotator cuff tear; may be indicated after a second episode of dislocation

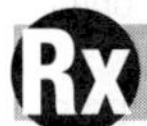

TREATMENT

- Reduction of the acute dislocation by gentle straight traction in the relaxed patient followed by light immobilization
- Gentle limited range-of-motion exercises as pain subsides followed by strengthening exercises at 2 wk

DISPOSITION

- Recurrence of anterior dislocation is common in the young; these patients may have to avoid the arm position associated with dislocation (external rotation with abduction).
- Primary dislocations in patients >40 yr are not generally complicated by recurrence but may result in shoulder stiffness and associated rotator cuff injuries.
- There is an almost 100% recurrence after the third dislocation.

REFERRAL

Surgical reconstruction may be required in the recurrent dislocator.

PEARLS & CONSIDERATIONS

COMMENTS

- It is important to know if there was an injury involved in the first episode and if a radiograph was taken to determine direction of the dislocation.
- Up to 50% of posterior dislocations are missed by the first examiner, usually the result of an inadequate lateral radiograph of the glenohumeral joint.
- "Voluntary" posterior dislocators should always be treated nonsurgically.
- Sports activities may be resumed when there is pain-free full flexibility and normal strength.
- Multidirectional instabilities are usually treated nonsurgically with strengthening exercises.
- Dislocations in either direction are occasionally overlooked. If the injury is over 2 to 4 weeks old, enough tissue healing will have occurred to make closed reduction fail. Open reduction or arthroplasty will then be needed in the young. Older patients may improve with therapeutic exercises, and the resultant disability is often acceptable.

SUGGESTED READINGS

Caplan J et al: Multidirectional instability of the shoulder in elite female gymnasts, *Am J Orthop* 36:660, 2007.

Cicak N: Posterior dislocation of the shoulder, *J Bone Joint Surg Br* 86B(3):324, 2004.

Hovelius L et al: Nonoperative treatment of primary anterior shoulder dislocation in patients forty years of age and younger, *J Bone Joint Surg Am* 90(A):945, 2008.

Matsen III FA et al: Principles for the evaluation and management of shoulder instability, *J Bone Joint Surg Am* 88A:648, 2006.

McFarland EG et al: The effect of variation in definition on the diagnosis of multidirectional instability of the shoulder, *J Bone Joint Surg Am* 85A:2138, 2003.

O'Connor DR et al: Painless reduction of acute anterior shoulder dislocations without anesthesia, *Orthopedics* 29:528, 2006.

Owens BD et al: Incidence of shoulder dislocation in the United States Military: demographic consideration from a high-risk population, *J Bone Joint Surg Am* 91:791, 2009.

Robinson CM, Dobson RJ: Anterior instability of the shoulder after trauma, *J Bone Joint Surg Br* 86B(4): 469, 2004.

Robinson CN et al: Redislocation of the shoulder during the first 6 weeks after a primary anterior dislocation: risk factor and results of treatment, *J Bone Joint Surg* 84:1552, 2002.

Sachs RA et al: Can the need for future surgery for acute traumatic anterior dislocation be predicted? *J Bone Joint Surg Am* 89A:1665, 2007.

Sahajpal DT, Zuckerman JD: Chronic glenohumeral dislocation, *J Am Acad Orthop Surg* 16:385, 2008.

Sayegh FE et al: Reduction of acute anterior dislocations: a prospective randomized study comparing a new technique with the Hippocratic and Kocher methods, *J Bone Joint Surg Am* 91:2775, 2009.

Sileo MJ et al: Management of acute glenohumeral dislocations, *Am J Orthop* 38(6):282-290, 2009.

te Slaa RL et al: The prognosis following acute primary glenohumeral dislocation, *J Bone Joint Surg Br* 1B(86):58, 2004.

AUTHOR: **LONNIE R. MERCIER, M.D.**

Glomerulonephritis, Acute (PTG)

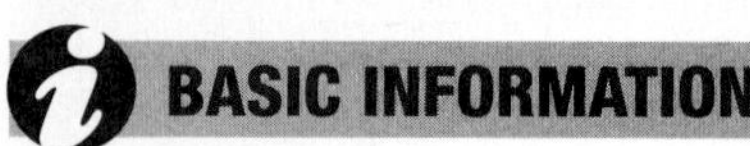

BASIC INFORMATION

DEFINITION

Acute glomerulonephritis is an immunologically mediated inflammation primarily involving the glomerulus that can result in damage to the basement membrane, mesangium, or capillary endothelium. Table 1-34 summarizes primary renal diseases that present as acute glomerulonephritis.

SYNONYMS

Postinfectious glomerulonephritis
Acute nephritic syndrome

ICD-9CM CODES

583.9 Glomerulonephritis, acute

EPIDEMIOLOGY & DEMOGRAPHICS

- More than 50% of cases involve children <13 yr.
- Glomerulonephritis is the most common cause of chronic renal failure (25%).
- Immunoglobulin A (IgA) nephropathy glomerulonephritis (Berger's disease) is the most common glomerulonephritis worldwide.

PHYSICAL FINDINGS & CLINICAL PRESENTATION

- Edema (peripheral, periorbital, or pulmonary)
- Joint pains, oral ulcers, malar rash (frequently seen with lupus nephritis)
- Dark urine
- Hypertension
- Findings of palpable purpura in patients with Henoch-Schönlein purpura
- Heart murmurs may indicate endocarditis
- Impetigo, skin pallor, tenderness in the abdomen and/or back, pharyngeal erythema may be present

ETIOLOGY

Acute glomerulonephritis may be caused by primary renal disease or a systemic disease. A number of pathogenic processes (e.g., antibody deposition, cell-mediated immune mechanisms, complement activation, hemodynamic alterations) have been implicated in the pathogenesis of glomerular inflammation. Medical disorders generally associated with glomerulonephritis are:

- Group A beta-hemolytic *Streptococcus* infection (other infectious etiologies including endocarditis and visceral abscess)
- Collagen-vascular diseases (systemic lupus erythematosus [SLE])
- Vasculitis (Wegener's granulomatosis, polyarteritis nodosa)
- Idiopathic glomerulonephritis (membranoproliferative, idiopathic, crescentic, IgA nephropathy)
- Goodpasture's syndrome
- Other cryoglobulinemia (Henoch-Schönlein purpura)
- Drug-induced (gold, penicillamine)

Table 1-34 summarizes primary renal diseases that present as acute glomerulonephritis.

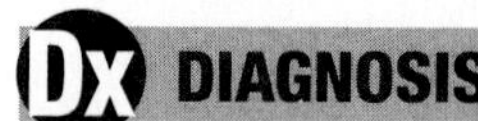

DIAGNOSIS

DIFFERENTIAL DIAGNOSIS

- Cirrhosis with edema and ascites
- Congestive heart failure
- Acute interstitial nephritis
- Severe hypertension
- Hemolytic-uremic syndrome
- SLE, diabetes mellitus, amyloidosis, preeclampsia, sclerodermal renal crisis

WORKUP

Initial evaluation of suspected glomerulonephritis consists of laboratory testing.

LABORATORY TESTS

- Urinalysis (hematuria [dysmorphic erythrocytes and red cell casts], proteinuria)
- Serum creatinine (to estimate glomerular filtration rate [GFR]), blood urea nitrogen
- 24-hr urine for protein excretion and creatinine clearance (to document degree of renal dysfunction and amount of proteinuria). Proteinuria in acute glomerulonephritis typically ranges from 500 mg/day to 3 g/day, but nephrotic-range proteinuria (>3.5 g/day) may be present.
- Streptococcal tests (Streptozyme), antistreptolysin O (ASO) quantitative titer (highest in 3 to 5 wk); ASO titer, however, is not related to severity of renal disease, duration, or prognosis.

TABLE 1-34 Summary of Primary Renal Diseases that Present as Acute Glomerulonephritis

Diseases	PSGN	IgA Nephropathy	Membranoproliferative Glomerulonephritis	Idiopathic RPGN
Clinical manifestations	All ages; mean, 7 yr, 2:1 male	15-35 yr; 2:1 male	15-30 yr; 6:1 male	Mean, 58 yr; 2:1 male
Age and sex	90%	50%	90%	90%
Acute nephritic syndrome	Occasionally	50%	Rare	Rare
Asymptomatic hematuria	10%-20%	Rare	Rare	10%-20%
Nephrotic syndrome	70%	30%-50%	Rare	25%
Hypertension	50% (transient)	Very rare	50%	60%
Acute renal failure	Latent period of 1-3 wk	Follows viral syndromes	Pulmonary hemorrhage; iron-deficiency anemia	None
Other				
Laboratory findings	↑ ASO titers (70%) Positive streptozyme (95%) ↓ C3-C9; Normal C1, C4	↑ Serum IgA (50%) IgA in dermal capillaries	Positive anti-GBM antibody	Positive ANCA
Immunogenetics	HLA-B12, D "EN" (9)*	HLA-Bw 35, DR4 (4)*	HLA-DR2 (16)*	None established
Renal Pathology				
Light microscopy	Diffuse proliferation	Focal proliferation	Focal → diffuse proliferation with crescents	Crescentic GN
Immunofluorescence	Granular IgG, C3	Diffuse mesangial IgA	Linear IgG, C3	No immune deposits
Electron microscopy	Subepithelial humps	Mesangial deposits	No deposits	No deposits
Prognosis	95% resolve spontaneously 5% RPGN or slowly progressive	Slow progression in 25%-50%	75% stabilize or improve if treated early	75% stabilize or improve if treated early
Treatment	Supportive	None established	Plasma exchange, steroids, cyclophosphamide	Steroid pulse therapy

Modified from Goldman L, Ausiello D (eds): *Cecil textbook of medicine,* ed 22, Philadelphia, 2004, WB Saunders.
ANCA, Antineutrophil cytoplasm antibody; *ASO,* antistreptolysin O; *GBM,* glomerular basement membrane; *GN,* glomerulonephritis; HLA, human leukocyte antigen; *Ig,* immunoglobulin; *PSGN,* poststreptococcal glomerulonephritis; *RPGN,* rapidly progressive glomerulonephritis.
*Relative risk.

- Additional useful tests depending on the history: anti-DNA antibodies (rule out SLE), CH_{50} level (if elevated, obtain C_3, C_4 levels), triglycerides, cryoglobulins, hepatitis B and C serologies, antineutrophil cytoplasmic antibody (ANCA), c-ANCA (in suspected cases of Wegener's granulomatosis), p-ANCA found in pauciimmune (lack of immune deposits) idiopathic rapidly progressive glomerulonephritis with or without systemic vasculitis, and antiglomerular basement membrane (type alpha[3] IV collagen) antibodies.
- Hematocrit (decrease in glomerulonephritis) and platelet count (thrombocytopenia in cases of lupus nephritis).
- Anti–glomerular basement membrane antibody (in Goodpasture's syndrome).
- Blood cultures are indicated in all febrile patients.

IMAGING STUDIES

- Chest x-ray: pulmonary congestion, Wegener's granulomatosis, and Goodpasture's syndrome.
- Renal ultrasound if GFR is depressed to evaluate renal size and determine extent of fibrosis. A kidney size of <9 cm is suggestive of extensive scarring and low likelihood of reversibility.
- Echocardiogram in patients with new cardiac murmurs or positive blood cultures to rule out endocarditis and pericardial effusion.
- Renal biopsy and light (Fig. 1-131), electron, and immunofluorescent microscopy to confirm diagnosis.
- Kidney biopsy: generally reveals a granular pattern in poststreptococcal glomerulonephritis and a linear pattern in Goodpasture's syndrome; absence of immune deposits suggests vasculitis. Renal biopsy, although helpful to define the etiology of glomerulonephritis, is not usually essential. It is useful to determine the degree of inflammation and fibrosis. It is also especially important for patients with rapidly progressive glomerulonephritis, in whom prompt diagnosis and treatment are essential.
- Immunofluorescence: generally reveals C_3. Negative immunofluorescence suggests Wegener's granulomatosis, idiopathic crescentic glomerulonephritis, or polyarteritis nodosa.
- Angiography or biopsy of other affected organs if systemic vasculitis is suspected.

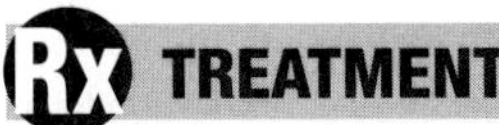

TREATMENT

NONPHARMACOLOGIC THERAPY

- Avoidance of salt if edema or hypertension is present
- Low-protein intake (approximately 0.5 g/kg/day) in patients with renal failure
- Fluid restriction in patients with significant edema
- Avoidance of high-potassium foods

ACUTE GENERAL Rx

- Correction of electrolyte abnormalities (hypocalcemia, hyperkalemia) and acidosis (if present)
- Treatment of streptococcal infection with penicillin (or erythromycin in penicillin-allergic patients)
- Furosemide in patients with significant hypertension and/or edema; hydralazine or nifedipine in patients with hypertension
- Immunosuppressive treatment in patients with heavy proteinuria or rapidly decreasing GFR (high-dose steroids, cyclosporin A, cyclophosphamide); corticosteroids generally not useful in poststreptococcal glomerulonephritis
- Fish oil (n-3 fatty acids) 12 g/day; may prevent or slow loss of renal function in patients with IgA nephropathy
- Plasma exchange therapy and immunosuppressive drugs (prednisone and cyclophosphamide); effective in Goodpasture's syndrome
- Short-term therapy with IV cyclophosphamide followed by maintenance therapy with mycophenolate mofetil or azathioprine is more efficacious and safer than long-term therapy with IV cyclophosphamide in patients with proliferative lupus nephritis

CHRONIC Rx

- Frequent monitoring of urinalysis, serum creatinine, and blood pressure in the initial 12 mo
- Monitoring for onset of hypertensive retinopathy, encephalopathy
- Aggressive treatment of infections, particularly streptococcal infections
- Dosage adjustment of all renally excreted medications

DISPOSITION

- Prognosis is generally related to histology, with excellent prognosis in patients with minimal change in glomerulonephritis and focal segmental proliferative glomerulonephritis. Between 25% and 30% of patients with mesangial IgA disease and membranous glomerulonephritis generally progress to chronic renal failure; >70% of patients with mesangial capillary glomerulonephritis will develop chronic renal failure.
- In general, prognosis is worse in patients with heavy proteinuria, severe hypertension, and significant elevations of creatinine.
- Recovery of renal function occurs within 8 to 12 wk in 95% of patients with poststreptococcal glomerulonephritis.

REFERRAL

- Nephrology consultation. The urgency for referral depends on the GFR. Urgent consultation is recommended if GFR is significantly abnormal or rapidly deteriorating or if the patient has systemic symptoms.
- Surgical referral for biopsy in selected cases.

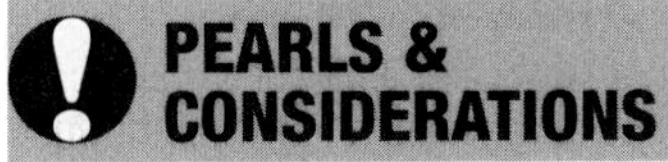

PEARLS & CONSIDERATIONS

COMMENTS

- Anticoagulation to prevent deep vein thrombosis should be considered in patients with a low level of physical activity.
- Monitoring of lipids and aggressive treatment of hyperlipidemias are recommended.
- Close monitoring of side effects of immunosuppressive drugs and complications of corticosteroids is necessary.

SUGGESTED READINGS

Contreras G et al: Sequential therapies for proliferative lupus nephritis, *N Engl J Med* 350:971, 2004.

Hricik D et al: Glomerulonephritis, *N Engl J Med* 339:888, 1998.

Madaio MP, Harrington JT: The diagnosis of glomerular diseases, *Arch Intern Med* 161:25, 2001.

AUTHOR: **FRED F. FERRI, M.D.**

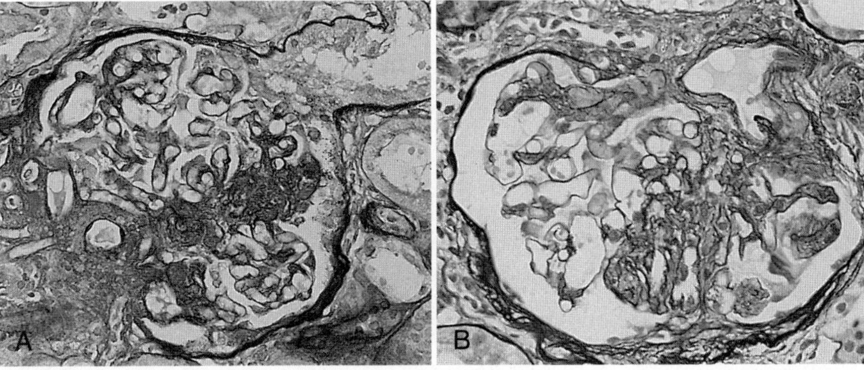

FIGURE 1-131 Light microscopic appearances in focal segmental glomerulosclerosis. Segmental scars with capsular adhesions in otherwise normal glomeruli. A, Periodic acid-Schiff, ×300. **B,** Methenamine silver stain, ×300. (Courtesy Dr. D. Davies. From Johnson RJ, Feehally J: *Comprehensive clinical nephrology,* ed 2, St Louis, 2000, Mosby.)

Glossitis (PTG)

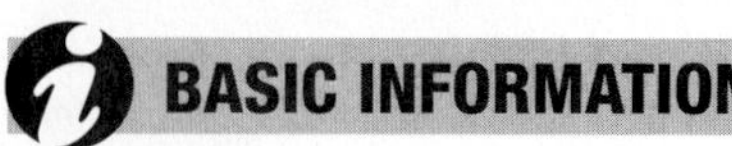

BASIC INFORMATION

DEFINITION

Glossitis is an inflammation of the tongue that can lead to loss of filiform papillae.

ICD-9CM CODES
529.0 Glossitis

EPIDEMIOLOGY & DEMOGRAPHICS

Glossitis is seen more frequently in patients of lower socioeconomic status, malnourished patients, alcoholics, smokers, elderly patients, immunocompromised patients, and patients with dentures.

PHYSICAL FINDINGS & CLINICAL PRESENTATION

- The appearance of the tongue varies depending on the etiology of the glossitis. Loss of filiform papillae results in a red, smooth-surfaced tongue (Fig. 1-132).
- The tongue may appear pale in patients with significant anemia.
- Pain and swelling of the tongue may be present when glossitis is associated with infections, trauma, or lichen planus.
- Ulcerations may be present in patients with herpetic glossitis, pemphigus, or streptococcal infection.
- Excessive use of mouthwash may result in a "hairy" appearance of the tongue.

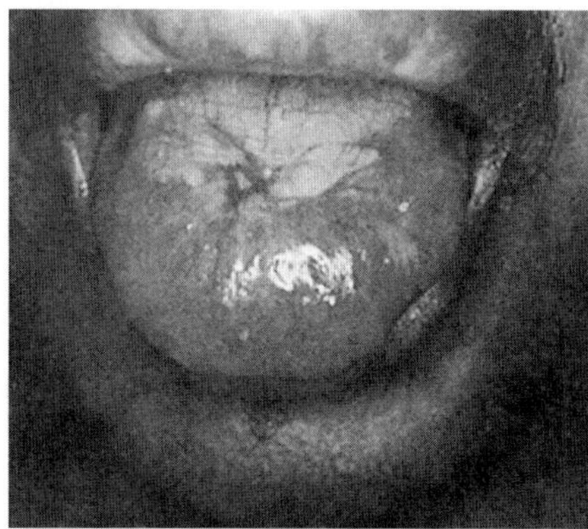

FIGURE 1-132 Glossitis. (From Seidel HM [ed]: *Mosby's guide to physical examination,* ed 4, St Louis, 1999, Mosby.)

ETIOLOGY

- Nutritional deficiencies (vitamin E, riboflavin, niacin, vitamin B_{12}, iron)
- Infections (viral, candidiasis, tuberculosis, syphilis)
- Trauma (generally caused by poorly fitting dentures)
- Irritation of the tongue from toothpaste, medications, alcohol, tobacco, citrus
- Lichen planus, pemphigus vulgaris, erythema multiforme
- Neoplasms

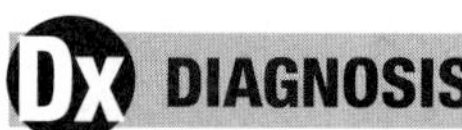

DIAGNOSIS

DIFFERENTIAL DIAGNOSIS

- Infections
- Use of chemical irritants
- Neoplasms
- Skin disorders (e.g., Behçet's syndrome, erythema multiforme)

WORKUP

- Laboratory evaluation to exclude infectious processes, vitamin deficiencies, and systemic disorders
- Biopsy of lesion only when there is no response to treatment

LABORATORY TESTS

- Complete blood count: decreased hemoglobin and hematocrit, low mean corpuscular volume (MCV) (iron-deficiency anemia), elevated MCV (vitamin B_{12} deficiency)
- Vitamin B_{12} level
- 10% KOH scrapings in patients with white patches suspect for candidiasis

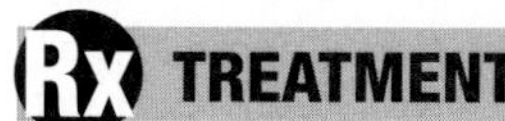

TREATMENT

NONPHARMACOLOGIC THERAPY

Avoidance of primary irritants such as hot foods, spices, tobacco, and alcohol

ACUTE GENERAL Rx

Treatment varies with the etiology of the glossitis.

- Malnutrition with avitaminosis: multivitamins
- Candidiasis: fluconazole 200 mg on day 1, then 100 mg/day for at least 2 wk or nystatin 400,000 U suspension qid for 10 days or 200,000 pastilles dissolved slowly in the mouth four to five times qd for 10 to 14 days
- Painful oral lesions: rinsing of the mouth with 2% lidocaine viscous, 1 to 2 tablespoons q4h prn; triamcinolone 0.1% applied to painful ulcers prn for symptomatic relief

CHRONIC Rx

- Lifestyle changes with elimination of tobacco, alcohol, and other primary irritants
- Dental evaluation for correction of ill-fitting dentures
- Correction of associated metabolic abnormalities such as hyperglycemia from diabetes mellitus

DISPOSITION

Most patients experience prompt improvement with identification and treatment of the cause of the glossitis.

REFERRAL

Surgical referral for biopsy of solitary lesions unresponsive to treatment to rule out neoplasm

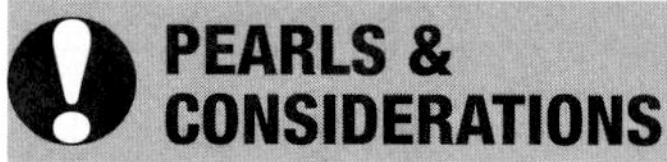

PEARLS & CONSIDERATIONS

COMMENTS

If the primary cause of glossitis is not identified or cannot be corrected, enteric nutritional replacement therapy should be considered in malnourished patients.

AUTHOR: **FRED F. FERRI, M.D.**

BASIC INFORMATION

DEFINITION

Gonorrhea is a sexually transmitted bacterial infection with a predilection for columnar and transitional epithelial cells. It commonly manifests as urethritis, cervicitis, or salpingitis. Infection may be asymptomatic. It differs in males and females in course, severity, and ease of recognition.

SYNONYMS

Gonococcal urethritis
Gonococcal vulvovaginitis
Gonococcal cervicitis
Gonococcal bartholinitis
Clap; GC

ICD-9CM CODES

098 Gonococcal infections

EPIDEMIOLOGY & DEMOGRAPHICS

- The disease is common worldwide, affects both sexes and all ages, especially younger adults; highest incidence is in inner-city areas, with an estimated 3 million new cases annually.
- Asymptomatic anterior urethral carriage may occur in 12% to 50% of cases in men.
- Asymptomatic in 50% to 80% of cases in women. Most common dissemination by mucosal passage to fallopian tubes, resulting in pelvic inflammatory disease (PID) in 10% to 15% of infected women. Hematogenous spread may result in septic arthritis and skin lesions. Conjunctivitis rarely occurs but may result in blindness if not rapidly treated. Infection can occur in both men and women in oropharynx and anorectally.
- 600,000 new infections per year.

PHYSICAL FINDINGS & CLINICAL PRESENTATION

- Males: purulent discharge from anterior urethra with dysuria appearing 2 to 7 days after infecting exposure. May have rectal infection causing pruritus, tenesmus, and discharge or may be asymptomatic.
- Females: initial urethritis or cervicitis may occur a few days after exposure, frequently mild. In approximately 20% of cases uterine invasion occurs after menstrual period with signs and symptoms of endometritis, salpingitis, or pelvic peritonitis. The patient may have purulent discharge or inflamed Skene's or Bartholin's glands.
- Classic presentation of acute gonococcal PID is fever, abdominal and adnexal tenderness, and often absence of purulent discharge. Physical examination may be normal if asymptomatic.

ETIOLOGY

Neisseria gonorrhoeae is the gonococcus. Plasmids coding for β-lactamase render some strains resistant to penicillin or tetracycline. There is an increasing frequency of chromosomally mediated resistance to penicillin, tetracycline, and cefoxitin. In the Far East, high-level resistance to spectinomycin is endemic.

There are a rising number of cases of quinolone-resistant *N. gonorrhoeae* worldwide, with the expected number to rise in the U.S. from importation.

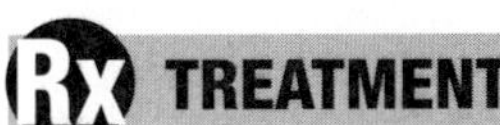

DIAGNOSIS

DIFFERENTIAL DIAGNOSIS

- Nongonococcal urethritis (NGU)
- Nongonococcal mucopurulent cervicitis
- *Chlamydia trachomatis*

WORKUP

- Diagnosis depends on bacteriologic investigation.
- Gram-negative intracellular diplococci are diagnostic in male urethral smears. There is a false-negative rate of 60% to 70% in female cervical or urethral smears. Culture is essential in women.

LABORATORY TESTS

- Gonorrhea culture on Thayer-Martin medium (organism is fastidious; requires aerobic conditions with increased carbon dioxide atmosphere; incubate ASAP)
- Serologic testing for syphilis on all patients
- *Chlamydia* testing on all patients
- Offer of HIV counseling and testing

Rx TREATMENT

ACUTE GENERAL Rx

Uncomplicated infections of the cervix, urethra, and rectum:

- Cefixime 400 mg PO × 1 dose *or*
- Ceftriaxone 125 mg IM × 1 dose *or*
- Doxycycline 100 mg PO bid × 7 days
- Dual treatment with azithromycin and doxycycline may prevent the development of antimicrobial resistant *N. gonorrhoeae.*

Alternatives:

- Cefpodoxime 400 mg single dose or
- Cefuroxime 1 gm PO single dose

Uncomplicated pharyngeal infection:

- Ceftriaxone 125 mg IM × 1 dose

DISPOSITION

- Pregnant patients require test of cure (as do those treated with regimens other than ceftriaxone/doxycycline); reculture 4 to 7 days after treatment.
- Treatment failure in nonpregnant patients is rare, and test of cure is not required. Rescreening in 1 to 2 mo detects treatment failures and reinfections.
- All sexual partners should be identified, examined, cultured, and receive presumptive treatment.

REFERRAL

PID requiring hospitalization, disseminated gonococcal infection

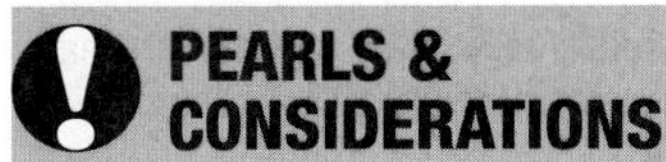

PEARLS & CONSIDERATIONS

COMMENTS

This is a reportable disease.

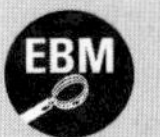

EVIDENCE

Treatment of uncomplicated gonococcal infections of the cervix, urethra, and rectum in men and nonpregnant women.

The CDC currently includes ceftriaxone 125 mg intramuscularly in a single dose or cefixime 400 mg orally in a single dose as recommended treatment options for uncomplicated gonococcal infections of the cervix, urethra, and rectum, plus treatment for *Chlamydia* if chlamydial infection is not ruled out.[1] Ⓒ

The CDC has published an update to the 2006 guidelines on Sexually Transmitted Diseases Treatment. They no longer recommend the use of fluoroquinolones for the treatment of gonococcal infections and associated conditions such as pelvic inflammatory disease. This is based on evidence for the increasing prevalence of fluoroquinolone resistance in *Neisseria gonorrhoeae* in the U.S.[2] Ⓒ

Spectinomycin is useful for the treatment of people with uncomplicated gonococcal infections of the cervix, urethra, and rectum who cannot tolerate cephalosporins or quinolones.[1] Ⓒ

Spectinomycin is currently unavailable in the U.S. Check the Centers for Disease Control and Prevention website for updates on availability.

Resistance to penicillins, tetracyclines, and sulfonamides is now widespread, and resistance to fluoroquinolones has become common in some geographic areas.[3]

Dual treatment with an antimicrobial effective against gonorrhea and *Chlamydia* infections is based on theory and expert opinion rather than on evidence from randomized controlled trials (RCTs).[3]

Treatment of gonorrhea in pregnancy.

Pregnant women should not be treated with quinolones or tetracyclines. Those infected with *Neisseria gonorrhoeae* should be treated with a recommended or alternate cephalosporin.[1] Ⓒ

Effective strategies for increasing treatment rates of patients' sexual partners are crucial in reducing the rates of persistent or recurrent gonorrhea.

An RCT analyzed the efficacy of "expedited treatment" versus "standard referral" of the sexual partners of 1860 patients with gonorrhea or chlamydial infection. Patients in the expedited-treatment group were offered medication to give to their sex partners, or if they preferred, study staff members contacted partners and provided them with medication without a clinical examination. Patients assigned to standard partner referral were advised to refer their partners for treatment and were offered assistance in notifying partners.[4]

Persistent or recurrent gonorrhea or chlamydial infection occurred in 13% assigned to standard partner referral and in 10% assigned to expedited treatment of sexual partners. It concluded that expedited treatment of sex partners reduces the rates of persistent or recurrent gonorrhea or chlamydial infection.[4] Ⓐ

Evidence-Based References

1. Centers for Disease Control and Prevention; Workowski KA, Berman SM: Sexually transmitted diseases treatment guidelines, *MMWR Recomm Rep* 55(RR-11):1-94, 2006.

2. Centers for Disease Control and Prevention (CDC): Update to CDC's sexually transmitted diseases treatment guidelines, 2006: fluoroquinolones no longer recommended for treatment of gonococcal infections, *MMWR Morb Mortal Wkly Rep* 56(14): 332-336, 2007.

3. Moran J: Gonorrhoea, *Clin Evid,* 2007.

4. Golden MR et al: Effect of expedited treatment of sex partners on recurrent or persistent gonorrhea or chlamydial infection, *N Engl J Med* 352:676-685, 2005.

AUTHORS: **MARIA A. CORIGLIANO, M.D.,** and **RUBEN ALVERO, M.D.**

BASIC INFORMATION

DEFINITION

Goodpasture's syndrome is characterized by idiopathic recurrence of alveolar hemorrhage and rapidly progressive glomerulonephritis. It can also be defined by the triad of glomerulonephritis, pulmonary hemorrhage, and antibody to basement membrane antigens.

ICD-9CM CODES
446.2 Goodpasture's syndrome

EPIDEMIOLOGY & DEMOGRAPHICS

- Goodpasture's syndrome affects predominantly young, white, male smokers.
- Male/female ratio is 6:1.
- Goodpasture's syndrome accounts for 5% of all cases of rapidly progressive glomerulonephritis.
- 80% of patients are HLA-BR2 positive.

PHYSICAL FINDINGS & CLINICAL PRESENTATION

- Dyspnea, cough, hemoptysis
- Skin pallor, fever, arthralgias (may be mild or absent at the time of initial presentation)

ETIOLOGY

Presence of glomerular basement membranes (GBM) antibody deposition in kidneys and lungs with subsequent pulmonary hemorrhage and glomerulonephritis

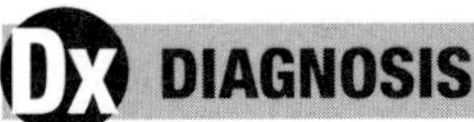

DIAGNOSIS

DIFFERENTIAL DIAGNOSIS

- Wegener's granulomatosis
- Systemic lupus erythematosus
- Systemic necrotizing vasculitis
- Idiopathic rapidly progressive glomerulonephritis
- Drug-induced renal pulmonary disease (e.g., penicillamine)

WORKUP

Laboratory evaluation, diagnostic imaging, immunofluorescence studies of renal biopsy

LABORATORY TESTS

- Presence of circulating serum anti-GBM antibodies
- Absence of circulating immunocomplexes, antineutrophils, cytoplasmic antibodies, and cryoglobulins
- Urinalysis revealing microscopic hematuria and proteinuria
- Elevated blood urea nitrogen and creatinine from rapidly progressive glomerulonephritis
- Immunofluorescence studies of renal biopsy material: linear deposits of anti-GBM antibody, often accompanied by C3 deposition
- Anemia from iron deficiency (from blood loss and iron sequestration in the lungs)

IMAGING STUDIES

Chest radiograph: fluffy alveolar infiltrates, evidence of pulmonary hemorrhage (Fig. 1-133)

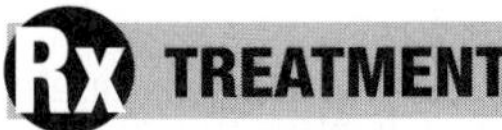

TREATMENT

ACUTE GENERAL Rx

- Plasma exchange therapy
- Immunosuppressive therapy with prednisone (1 mg/kg/day) and cyclophosphamide (2 mg/kg/day)
- Dialysis support in patients with renal failure

DISPOSITION

Life-threatening pulmonary hemorrhage and irreversible glomerular damage are the major causes of death.

REFERRAL

- Referral for renal biopsy to guide the management
- Referral of patients with renal failure to dialysis center
- Consideration for renal transplantation in patients with end-stage renal failure

SUGGESTED READINGS

Levy JB et al: Long-term outcome of anti-glomerular basement membrane antibody disease treated with plasma exchange and immunosuppression, *Ann Intern Med* 134:1033, 2001.

Turner AN: Goodpasture's disease, *Nephrol Dial Transplant* 16:52, 2001.

AUTHOR: **FRED F. FERRI, M.D.**

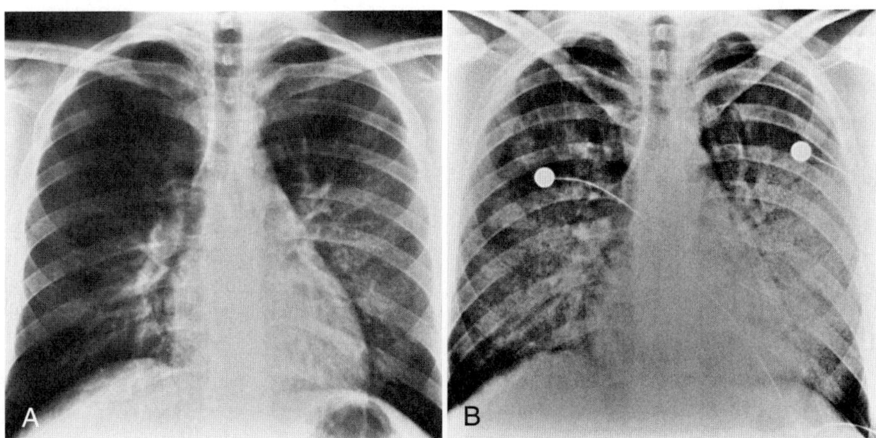

FIGURE 1-133 Goodpasture's syndrome. Posteroanterior chest radiographs several days apart demonstrate consolidation in the left lung **(A),** which progressed to diffuse alveolar disease (consolidation) **(B).** (From McLoud TC [ed]: *Thoracic radiology: the requisites,* St Louis, 1998, Mosby.)

Gout

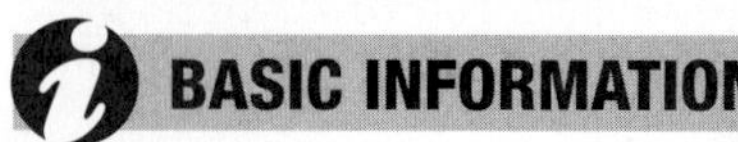

BASIC INFORMATION

DEFINITION

Gout is a clinical disorder in which crystals of monosodium urate are deposited in tissue as a result of hyperuricemia. Gout and hyperuricemia can be classified as either primary or secondary if resulting from another disorder.

ICD-9CM CODES
274.9 Gout

EPIDEMIOLOGY & DEMOGRAPHICS

PREVALENCE: Three cases per 1000 persons
PREDOMINANT SEX: 95% males, rare in females before menopause
PREDOMINANT AGE: 30 to 50 yr

PHYSICAL FINDINGS & CLINICAL PRESENTATION

- Usually, initial attack in a single joint or an area of tenosynovium
- Mainly a disease of the lower extremities
- First site of involvement: classically, metatarsophalangeal joint of the great toe
- Another common site of acute attack: extensor tenosynovium on the dorsum of the midfoot
- Severe pain and inflammation, which may be precipitated by exercise, dietary indiscretions, and physical or emotional stress
- Attacks after illness or surgery
- Presence of swelling, heat, redness, and other signs of inflammation (physical findings simulating cellulitis)
- Exquisite soft tissue tenderness
- Fever, tachycardia, and other constitutional symptoms
- Eventually, deposits of urate crystals (tophi) in the subcutaneous tissue (Fig. 1-134)

ETIOLOGY

- Hyperuricemia and gout develop from excessive uric acid production, a decrease in the renal excretion of uric acid, or both.

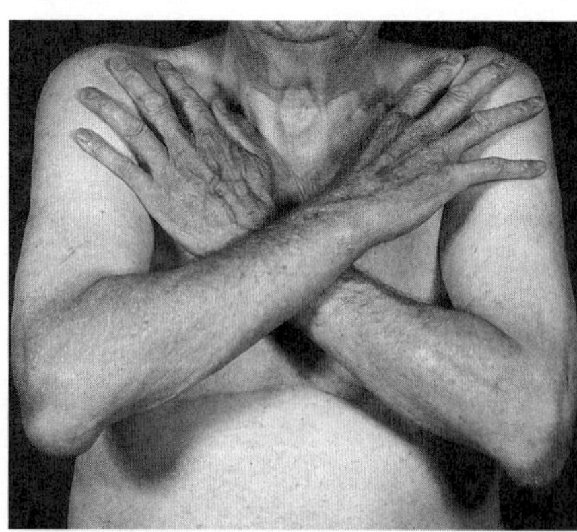

FIGURE 1-134 Tophi on the elbows in a patient with chronic polyarthritis affecting the fingers. He was thought to have nodular rheumatoid arthritis and was treated with sodium aurothiomalate injections despite a negative test for rheumatoid factor. (From Hochberg MC et al [eds]: *Rheumatology,* ed 3, St Louis, 2003, Mosby.)

- Primary gout results from an inborn error of metabolism and may be attributed to several biochemical defects.
- Secondary hyperuricemia may develop as a complication of acquired disorders (e.g., leukemia) or as a result of the use of certain drugs (e.g., diuretics).

DIAGNOSIS

DIFFERENTIAL DIAGNOSIS

- Pseudogout
- Rheumatoid arthritis
- Osteoarthritis
- Cellulitis
- Infectious arthritis

Section II describes the differential diagnosis of acute monoarticular and oligoarticular arthritis.

WORKUP

Hyperuricemia accompanying a typical history of monoarticular acute arthritis is usually sufficient to establish the diagnosis.

LABORATORY TESTS

- Mild leukocytosis
- Elevated erythrocyte sedimentation rate
- Hyperuricemia. A normal serum uric acid does not exclude gout as the cause of an acutely inflamed joint since about 1/3 of patients with acute gouty arthritis have serum uric acid levels <8 mg/dl
- Synovial aspirate: usually cloudy and markedly inflammatory in nature; urate crystals in fluid: needle-shaped and birefringent under polarized light

IMAGING STUDIES

- Plain radiography to rule out other disorders
- No typical findings in early gouty arthritis but late disease possibly associated with characteristic punched-out lesions and joint destruction

TREATMENT

NONPHARMACOLOGIC THERAPY

- Modification of diet (avoidance of foods high in purines [e.g., anchovies, organ meat, liver, spinach, mushrooms, asparagus, oatmeal, cocoa, sweetbreads]) and lifestyle
- Treatment for obesity
- Moderation in alcohol intake, no more than two drinks per day
- Hypertension and its management requiring careful assessment and possibly nondiuretic drugs

ACUTE GENERAL Rx

- Quick-acting nonsteroidal anti-inflammatory drugs (NSAIDs) such as ibuprofen.
- Colchicine (given PO or IV). One oral dose of 1.2 mg followed by a second dose of 0.6 mg one hour later is as effective and less toxic than older regimens.
- Corticosteroids or adrenocorticotropic hormone for those who are intolerant of NSAIDs or colchicine.
- Intraarticular cortisone when oral medication cannot be given.
- General measures such as rest, elevation, and analgesics as needed until acute pain subsides.
- Table 1-35 describes treatment options for gout.

CHRONIC Rx

- Prevention is achieved through normalization of serum urate concentration.
- Uricosuric agents (e.g., probenecid) or xanthine oxidase inhibitors (allopurinol or febuxostat) are used in patients with recurrent attacks despite adequate dietary restrictions.
- A 24-hr urine collection is useful in deciding which antihyperuricemic agent is indicated. Allopurinol is generally used if the uric acid output is >900 mg/day on a regular diet. However, hyperuricemic therapy should not be started for at least 2 wk after the acute attack has resolved because it may prolong the acute attack and also precipitate new attacks by rapidly lowering the serum uric acid level.
- Urinary uric acid hypoexcretors (<700 mg/day) can be given, such as probenecid (250 mg bid for 1 wk, then increased to 500 mg bid), to block absorption of uric acid. Probenecid should be started only after the acute attack of gout has completely subsided.
- Colchicine 0.6 mg bid is indicated for acute gout prophylaxis before starting hyperuricemic therapy. It is generally discontinued 10 to 12 wk after normalization of serum urate levels. Long-term colchicine therapy (0.6 mg qd or bid) may be necessary in patients with frequent gout attacks despite the use of uricosuric agents.
- Surgery usually limited to excision of large tophi and, occasionally, arthroplasty.

DISPOSITION

- Musculoskeletal complications are usually limited to joint disease.
- Surgical intervention may occasionally be indicated.
- Renal disease is the most frequent complication of gout after arthritis; most gouty patients develop renal disease as a result of parenchymal urate deposition but the involvement is only slowly progressive and often has no effect on life expectancy.
- Incidence of urolithiasis is increased, with 80% of calculi being uric acid stones.

REFERRAL

For orthopedic consultation when joint destruction has occurred

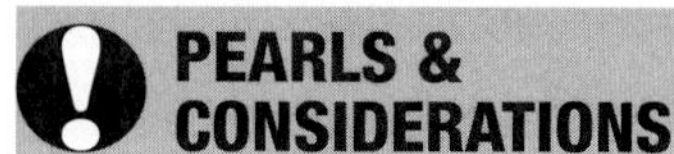

PEARLS & CONSIDERATIONS

COMMENTS

- No significant correlation between coronary artery disease and gout

- No indication to treat asymptomatic hyperuricemia
- Acute attacks of gout occasionally associated with normal levels of uric acid
- The main indication for prophylaxis is recurrent attacks of gouty joint inflammation (three or more per year)

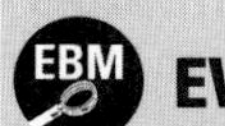

EVIDENCE

Limited evidence suggests nonsteroidal anti-inflammatory drugs may be effective in relieving pain in acute gout, but no one drug can be recommended over another. Systematic reviews and randomized controlled trials relating to the prevention of the recurrence of gout are lacking.

No systematic review has compared nonsteroidal anti-inflammatory drugs versus placebo, or versus each other, in the management of acute gout.[1]

We are unable to cite evidence that meets our criteria for any other treatment, or lifestyle intervention, used in the management or prevention of acute gout.

Evidence-Based Reference

1. Underwood M: Gout. *Clin Evid,* 2007.

SUGGESTED READINGS

Eggbeen AT: Gout: an update, *Am Fam Physician* 76: 801, 2007.

Fitzgerald BT et al: Gout affecting the hand and wrist, *J Am Acad Orthop Surg* 15:625, 2007.

Fox R: Management of recurrent gout, *BMJ* 336:329, 2008.

Liote F, Ea HK: Recent developments in crystal-induced inflammation: pathogenesis and management, *Curr Rheumatol Rep* 9(3):243, 2007.

Rosenthal AK: Crystal arthropathies and other unpopular rheumatic diseases, *Curr Opin Rheumatol* 16: 262, 2004.

Schlesinger N et al: Serum urate during acute gout, *J Rheumatol* 36:(6)1287-1289, 2009.

Schumacher HR et al: Outcome evaluations in gout, *J Rheumatol* 34(6):1381, 2007.

Turkeltaub R: Update on gout: new therapeutic strategies and options, *Nat Rev Rheumatol* 6:30, 2010.

Wizenberg T, Buchbinder R: Cochrane Musculoskeletal Group review: acute gout. Steroids or NSAIDs? *J Fam Pract* 58(7):E1, 2009.

AUTHOR: **LONNIE R. MERCIER, M.D.**

TABLE 1-35 Treatment of Gout

Acute Gout	Interval Gout	Long-Term Treatment
NSAIDs (preferred): Indomethacin, 50 mg qid, or ibuprofen, 800 mg tid (or other NSAID in full doses); lower dose in renal insufficiency; contraindicated with peptic ulcer disease. ***or***	**Colchicine, oral:** 0.6-1.2 mg/day as prophylaxis against recurrent attacks.	**Colchicine, oral:** 0.6-1.2 mg/day for 1-2 wk before initiating hypouricemic therapy and for several months afterward to prevent recurrent attacks during initial period of hypouricemic therapy.
Colchicine, oral: 1.2 mg followed by a second dose of 0.6 mg 1 hr later.	**Hypouricemic agent:** Start only if indicated by frequent attacks, severe hyperuricemia, presence of tophi, urolithiasis, or urate overexcretion.	**Allopurinol:** Dose variable; usually 300 mg qd, but up to 900 mg may be needed in occasional patient; dose should be reduced to 100 mg/day or every other day in patients with renal insufficiency. ***or***
Colchicine, IV (only if oral medication is precluded): 1-2 mg in 20 ml 0.9% saline infused slowly (extravasation causes tissue necrosis); dose may be repeated q6h. Few GI symptoms with IV use. Maximum total dose, 4 mg per attack. Monitor blood counts.	**Other:** Diet—moderate protein, low fat; avoid excessive alcohol. Treat hypertension if present. High fluid intake to promote uric acid excretion in a dilute urine (for uric acid overexcretors).	**Uricosuric agent** (reduced efficacy if creatinine clearance $<$80 ml; ineffective if $<$30 ml): probenecid, 0.5-1 g bid, or sulfinpyrazone, 100 mg tid or qid; usually well tolerated but may cause headache, GI upset, rash.
Steroids (if NSAIDs or colchicines are contraindicated or if oral medication is precluded, e.g., postoperatively): Triamcinolone acetonide, 60 mg IM, or ACTH, 40 U IM or 25 U by slow IV infusion, or prednisone, 20-40 mg daily. Intraarticular steroids may be used to treat a single inflamed joint: triamcinolone hexacetonide, 5-20 mg, or dexamethasone phosphate, 1-6 mg.		**Other:** Diet—moderate protein, low fat; avoid excessive alcohol. Treat hypertension if present. For uric acid overexcretors or when initiating uricosuric agent: high fluid intake, particularly at night, to promote uric acid excretion in a dilute urine. Acetazolamide, 250 mg at bedtime, may be used to keep urine pH $>$6.
Hypouricemic agents: Of no benefit for inflammatory attack and may initiate recurrent attack. Should not be started until attack has resolved, but ongoing use should not be interrupted during an attack.		

From Goldman L, Ausiello D (eds): *Cecil textbook of medicine,* ed 22, Philadelphia, 2004, WB Saunders.
ACTH, Adrenocorticotropic hormone; *GI,* gastrointestinal; *IM,* intramuscularly; *IV,* intravenously; *NSAIDs,* nonsteroidal anti-inflammatory drugs.

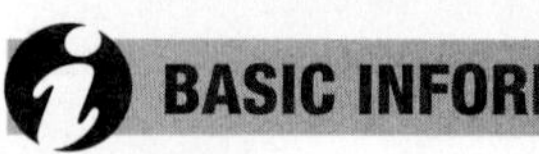

BASIC INFORMATION

DEFINITION

Granuloma annulare (GA) is a chronic, usually self-limited, inflammatory disorder of the dermis that classically presents as arciform to annular plaques located on the extremities.

SYNONYMS

Pseudorheumatoid nodule—subcutaneous granuloma annulare
GA

ICD-9CM CODES
695.89 Granuloma annulare

EPIDEMIOLOGY & DEMOGRAPHICS

- Most common in children and young adults; most cases of localized granuloma annulare are diagnosed in patients <30 yr
- Female predominance (2:1)
- Disseminated form associated with diabetes mellitus
- Recurrent in 40% of affected individuals
- A generalized form of GA can occur in up to 15% of patients

PHYSICAL FINDINGS & CLINICAL PRESENTATION

- The four main clinical variants of granuloma annulare are localized (75%), disseminated (>10 lesions), subcutaneous (occurring primarily in children aged 2 to 5 yr), and perforating (rare form manifesting with 1- to 4-mm papules with a central crust).
- Localized granuloma annulare starts as a small ring of colored skin or pale erythematous papules.
- Lesions coalesce and evolve into annular plaques over several weeks.
- Plaques undergo central involution and increase in diameter over several months (0.5 to 5 cm) (Fig. 1-135).
- Most frequently found on the lateral and dorsal surfaces of the hands and feet.
- Most lesions resolve spontaneously after several months.
- The generalized form of GA is characterized by hundreds to thousands of small, flesh-colored papules in a symmetric distribution on the trunk and extremities.
- Deep dermal (subcutaneous GA) presents as large, painless, skin-colored nodules that are frequently mistaken for rheumatoid nodules.

ETIOLOGY

Unknown, but may be related to vasculitis, trauma, monocyte activation, or delayed hypersensitivity.

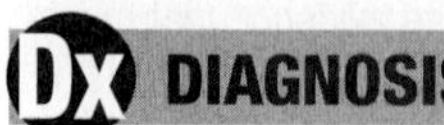

DIAGNOSIS

DIFFERENTIAL DIAGNOSIS

- Tinea corporis
- Lichen planus
- Necrobiosis lipoidica diabeticorum
- Sarcoidosis
- Rheumatoid nodules
- Late secondary or tertiary syphilis
- Arcuate and annular plaques of mycosis fungoides
- Papular GA can simulate insect bites, secondary syphilis, xanthoma
- Annular elastolytic giant cell granuloma

WORKUP

- Diagnosis based on clinical appearance and presentation
- Biopsy when diagnosis is unclear

LABORATORY TESTS

- No laboratory tests will help confirm the diagnosis.

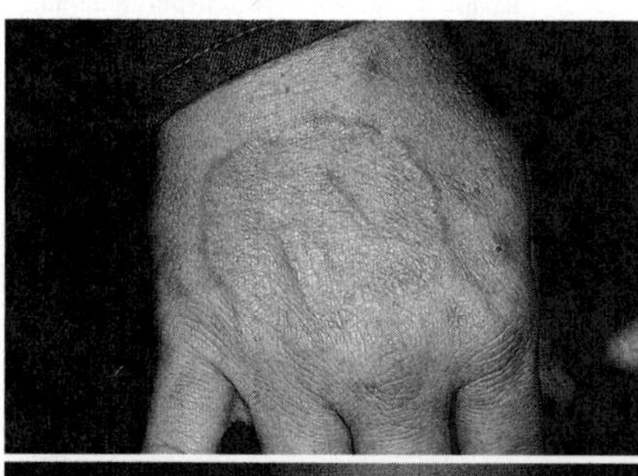

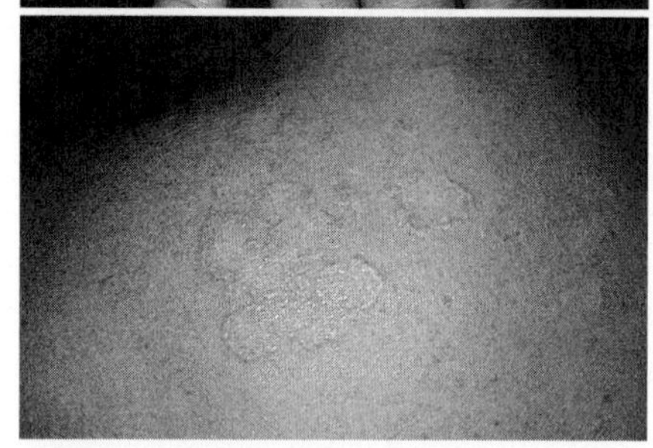

FIGURE 1-135 Granuloma annulare. (From Callen JP [ed]: *Color atlas of dermatology,* ed 2, Philadelphia, 2000, WB Saunders.)

- Biopsy shows focal degeneration of collagen and elastic fibers, mucin deposition, and perivascular and interstitial lymphohistiocytic infiltrate in the upper and middle dermis.

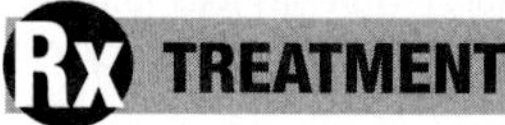

TREATMENT

NONPHARMACOLOGIC THERAPY

Reassurance, given the self-limited and benign nature of GA

CHRONIC Rx

High-potency topical corticosteroids with or without occlusion and intralesional steroid injection into elevated border with triamcinolone 2.5 to 10 mg/ml are useful first-line local therapies.

- Cryosurgery, psoralen ultraviolet-A (UVA) range or UVA-1 therapy, and carbon dioxide laser treatment can also be used.
- Systemic agents (e.g., niacinamide, hydroxychloroquine, chloroquine, cyclosporine, dapsone) are generally reserved for severe cases. Recent case reports indicate positive outcomes with tacrolimus and pimecrolimus and the tumor necrosis factor infliximab.

DISPOSITION

Most lesions resolve spontaneously within 2 yr.

REFERRAL

Dermatology referral recommended for symptomatic, disseminated disease

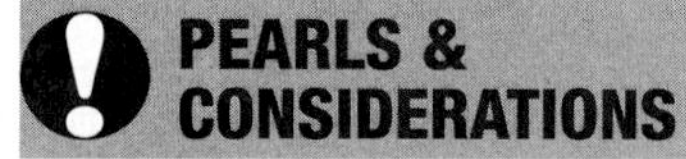

PEARLS & CONSIDERATIONS

COMMENTS

GA has been described as a paraneoplastic granulomatous reaction to Hodgkin's disease, non-Hodgkin's lymphoma, solid organ tumors, and mycosis fungoides.

SUGGESTED READING

Cyr PR: Diagnosis and management of granuloma annulare, *Am Fam Physician* 74:1729-1734, 2006.

AUTHOR: **JENNIFER R. SOUTHER, M.D.**

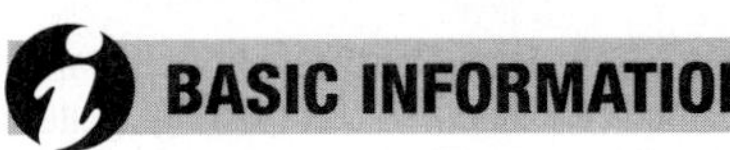

BASIC INFORMATION

DEFINITION

Granuloma inguinale is caused by a gram-negative bacterium, *Calymmatobacterium granulomatis,* which may be sexually transmitted, possibly by anal intercourse. It can also be spread through close, long-term, nonsexual contact.

SYNONYMS

Donovanosis

ICD-9CM CODES
099.2 Granuloma inguinale

EPIDEMIOLOGY & DEMOGRAPHICS

INCIDENCE: Rare in the U.S. ($<$100 cases reported annually) and other developed countries
PREVALENCE: Endemic in Australia, India, Caribbean, and Africa; incubation period is variable (1 to 2 wk)
PREDOMINANT SEX: Can affect both males and females

PHYSICAL FINDINGS & CLINICAL PRESENTATION

- Indurated nodule is the primary lesion and is usually painless.
- Lesion erodes to granulomatous-heaped ulcer (Fig. 1-136); progresses slowly.
- Pathogenic features:
  1. Large, infected mononuclear cell containing many Donovan bodies
  2. Intracytoplasmic location

ETIOLOGY

C. granulomatis is a gram-negative bacillus that reproduces within polymorphonuclear cells, plasma cells, and histiocytes, causing the infected cells to rupture 20 to 30 organisms.

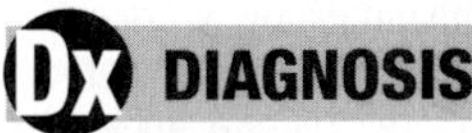

DIAGNOSIS

DIFFERENTIAL DIAGNOSIS

- Carcinoma
- Secondary syphilis: condylomata lata
- Amebiasis: necrotic ulceration
- Concurrent infections
- Lymphogranuloma venereum
- Chancroid
- Genital herpes

WORKUP

- Check for clinical manifestations.
  1. Lesions bleed easily.
  2. Lesions sharply defined and painless.
  3. Secondary infection may ensue.
  4. Inguinal involvement may cause pseudobuboes.
  5. Elephantiasis can result from obstruction of lymphatics.
  6. Suppuration and sinus formation are rare in female patients.
- Screen for other sexually transmitted diseases.
- Exclude other causes of lesions.
- Obtain stained, crushed prep from lesion.

A clinical algorithm for evaluation of genital ulcer disease is described in Section III.

Section II describes the differential diagnosis of genital sores.

LABORATORY TESTS

Wright stain: observation of Donovan bodies (intracellular bacteria); organisms in vacuoles within macrophages

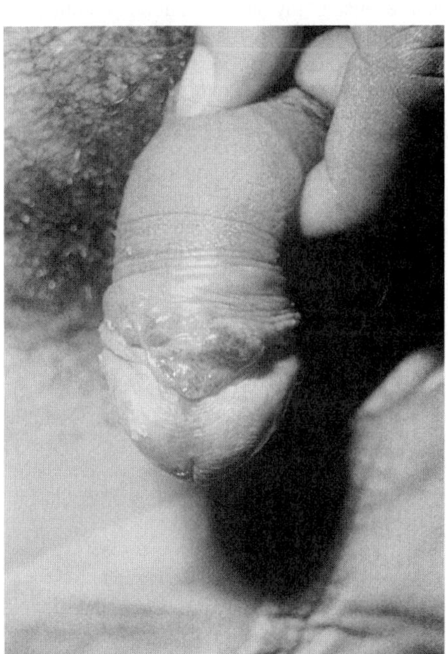

FIGURE 1-136 Involvement of the penis, with a beefy red, granulomatous ulceration in a patient with granuloma inguinale. (From Goldstein B [ed]: *Practical dermatology,* ed 2, St Louis, 1997, Mosby.)

Rx TREATMENT

ACUTE GENERAL Rx

Recommended regimen:
- Doxycycline 100 mg orally bid × 3 wk minimum

Alternative regimens:
- Ciprofloxacin 750 mg PO bid × 3 wk
- Erythromycin base 500 mg PO daily × 3 wk
- Trimethoprim/sulfamethoxazole, one double-strength tablet PO bid × 3 wk minimum
- Azithromycin 1 g PO/wk × 3 wk
- All gentamicin 1 mg/kg IV q8h if no improvement within the first few days of therapy

CHRONIC Rx

If there is a poor initial response, extend treatment. Treatment of relapses is often necessary. Patients should be counseled to avoid risky sex practices and not resume having sex until infection is cleared.

DISPOSITION

Follow up clinically until signs and symptoms have resolved, then routine annual or semiannual visits

REFERRAL

If response is poor, consider referral to infectious disease specialist.

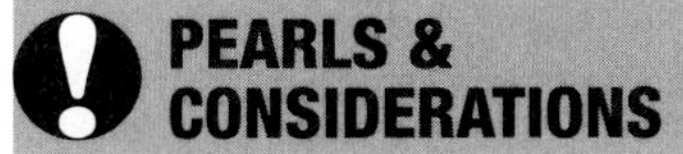

PEARLS & CONSIDERATIONS

COMMENTS

- Sexual partners should be examined and offered therapy.
- Pregnant women should be treated with erythromycin regimen.
- Patient education material can be obtained from local and state health clinics and also from American College of Obstetricians and Gynecologists.

SUGGESTED READING

Centers for Disease Control and Prevention: 2006. sexually transmitted diseases treatment guidelines, *MMWR* 55(RR-11), 2006.

AUTHORS: **GEORGE T. DANAKAS, M.D.,** and **RUBEN ALVERO, M.D.**

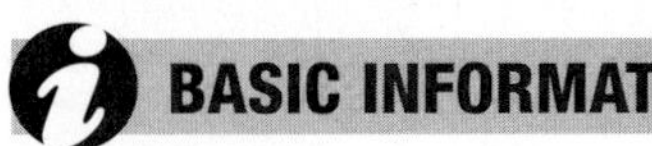

BASIC INFORMATION

DEFINITION

Graves' disease is a hypermetabolic state caused by circulating immunoglobulin (Ig) G antibodies that bind to and activate the G-protein–coupled thyrotropin receptor. This activation stimulates follicular hypertrophy and hyperplasia, causing thyroid enlargement as well as increases in thyroid hormone production. It is characterized by thyrotoxicosis, diffuse goiter, and infiltrative ophthalmopathy (edema and inflammation of the extraocular muscles and an increase in orbital connective tissue and fat); infiltrative dermopathy characterized by lymphocytic infiltration of the dermis; accumulation of glycosaminoglycans; and occasionally edema.

SYNONYMS

Thyrotoxicosis

ICD-9CM CODES
242.0 Toxic diffuse goiter

EPIDEMIOLOGY & DEMOGRAPHICS

INCIDENCE/PREVALENCE: Hyperthyroidism affects 2% of women and 0.2% of men in their lifetimes. More than 80% of these cases are caused by Graves' disease.

PREDOMINANT AGE: Peak incidence is between 40 and 60 yr.

GENETICS: Increased prevalence of HLA-B8 and HLA-DR3 in whites with Graves' disease. Concordance rate is 20% among monozygotic twins.

PHYSICAL FINDINGS & CLINICAL PRESENTATION

- Tachycardia, palpitations, tremor, hyperreflexia
- Goiter, exophthalmos (50% of patients), lid retraction, lid lag
- Nervousness, weight loss, heat intolerance, atrial fibrillation
- Increased sweating, brittle nails, clubbing of fingers
- Localized dermopathy (1% to 2% of patients) is most frequent over the anterolateral aspects of the skin but can be found at other sites (especially after trauma)
- Men may have gynecomastia, reduced libido, and erectile dysfunction. Women often have irregular menses

ETIOLOGY

Autoimmune etiology: the activity of the thyroid gland is stimulated by the action of T cells, which induce specific B cells to synthesize antibodies against thyroid-stimulating hormone (TSH) receptors in the follicular cell membrane.

DIAGNOSIS

DIFFERENTIAL DIAGNOSIS

- Anxiety disorder
- Premenopausal state
- Thyroiditis
- Other causes of hyperthyroidism (e.g., toxic multinodular goiter, toxic adenoma)
- Other: metastatic neoplasm, diabetes mellitus, pheochromocytoma

WORKUP

The diagnostic workup includes a detailed medical history followed by laboratory and imaging studies and ECG. Patients often present with anxiety, heat intolerance, menstrual dysfunction, increased appetite, and weight loss. Elderly patients can have an atypical presentation (apathetic hyperparathyroidism). For additional information, refer to the topic "Hyperthyroidism."

LABORATORY TESTS

- Increased free thyroxine (T_4) and free triiodothyronine (T_3)
- Decreased TSH
- Presence of thyroid-stimulating immunoglobulin or thyrotropin-receptor antibodies (useful in selected patients to differentiate Graves' disease from toxic nodular goiter)

IMAGING STUDIES

- 24-hr radioactive iodine uptake (RAIU): increased homogeneous uptake
- CT or MRI of the orbits is useful if there is uncertainty about the cause of ophthalmopathy

TREATMENT

NONPHARMACOLOGIC THERAPY

- Patient education and discussion of therapeutic options
- Smoking cessation: smoking is associated with an increased risk of progression of Graves' ophthalmopathy.

ACUTE GENERAL Rx

- Antithyroid drugs (ATDs) to inhibit thyroid hormone synthesis or peripheral conversion of T_4 to T_3:
  1. Methimazole or propylthiouracil (PTU) are available. Methimazole is generally preferred because it has a longer half-life, allowing for once-daily dosing. PTU is preferred during pregnancy.
  2. Side effects: skin rash (3% to 5%), arthralgias, myalgias, granulocytopenia (0.5%); rare side effects: aplastic anemia, hepatic necrosis (PTU), cholestatic jaundice.
- Radioactive iodine (RAI):
  1. Treatment of choice for patients >21 yr and younger patients who have not achieved remission after 1 yr of ATD therapy
  2. Contraindicated during pregnancy and lactation
- Surgery: near-total thyroidectomy is rarely performed. Indications: obstructing goiters despite RAI and ATD therapy, patients who refuse RAI and cannot be adequately managed with ATDs, and pregnant women inadequately managed with ATDs.
- Adjunctive therapy: Beta-adrenergic receptor blockers (e.g. atenolol 25 to 100 mg/day) to alleviate the β-adrenergic symptoms of hyperthyroidism (tachycardia, tremor); contraindicated in patients with bronchospasm.
- Graves' ophthalmopathy: methylcellulose eye drops to protect against excessive dryness, sunglasses to decrease photophobia, intraocular and systemic high-dose corticosteroids for severe exophthalmos. Worsening of ophthalmopathy after RAI therapy is often transient and can be prevented by the administration of prednisone. Other treatment options include antiinflammatory and immunosuppressive agents, radiation, and corrective surgical procedures.

CHRONIC Rx

Patients undergoing treatment with ATDs should be seen every 1 to 3 mo until euthyroidism is achieved and every 3 to 4 mo while they are receiving ATDs.

DISPOSITION

- ATDs induce sustained remission in <60% of cases.
- The incidence of hypothyroidism after RAI is >50% within the first year and 2% per year thereafter.
- Complications of surgery include hypothyroidism (28% to 43% after 10 yr), hypoparathyroidism, and vocal cord paralysis (1%).
- Successful treatment of hyperthyroidism requires lifelong monitoring for the onset of hypothyroidism or the recurrence of thyrotoxicosis.
- RAI therapy is followed by the appearance or worsening of ophthalmopathy more often than is therapy with methimazole, particularly in patients who are cigarette smokers. It can be prevented with the administration of prednisone 0.5 mg/kg body weight per day starting 2 to 3 days after RAI, continued for 1 mo, then tapered off over 2 mo.
- Mild to moderate ophthalmopathy often improves spontaneously. Severe cases can be treated with high-dose glucocorticoids, orbital irradiation, or both. Orbital decompression may be used in patients with optic neuropathy and exophthalmos (see "Hyperthyroidism").

SUGGESTED READINGS

Bartalena L, Tanda ML: Graves' ophthalmopathy, *N Engl J Med* 360:994-1001, 2009.

Brent GA: Graves' disease, *N Engl J Med* 358:2594, 2008.

AUTHOR: **FRED F. FERRI, M.D.**

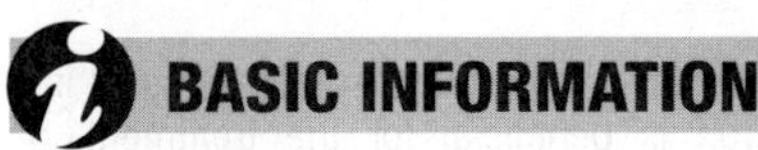

BASIC INFORMATION

DEFINITION

Guillain-Barré syndrome (GBS) is an acute immune-mediated polyradiculoneuropathy (affects nerve roots and peripheral nerves), with predominant motor involvement. It is the most common cause of acute flaccid paralysis in the Western hemisphere and probably worldwide. By definition, maximal clinical weakness occurs within 4 wk of disease onset.

SYNONYMS

AIDP (acute inflammatory demyelinating polyradiculoneuropathy)
Acute polyneuropathy
Ascending paralysis
Postinfectious polyneuritis

ICD-9CM CODES
357.0 Guillain-Barré

EPIDEMIOLOGY & DEMOGRAPHICS

INCIDENCE:

- 0.6 to 1.9 cases/100,000 persons annually without geographic variation. Incidence increases with age. A slight peak in incidence occurs between late adolescence and early adulthood. A slight male preponderance (1.25:1) also exists.
- GBS consists of several clinical variants based on the pattern of clinical involvement and electrophysiologic findings. These include:
  - AIDP (most common form in Europe and North America)
  - Acute motor axonal neuropathy (AMAN; most prevalent form in China and Japan)
  - Acute motor and sensory axonal neuropathy (AMSAN; has more severe sensory involvement and is associated with more severe clinical course and poorer prognosis)
  - Miller Fisher syndrome (MFS; triad of ophthalmoplegia, ataxia, and areflexia)
  - Acute pandysautonomia (rapid onset of parasympathetic and sympathetic failure without motor or sensory involvement)
  - Regional variants (e.g., pharyngeal-cervical-brachial GBS, pure ataxic GBS)

PREDISPOSING FACTORS: Viral (HIV, CMV, EBV, influenza) and bacterial *(Campylobacter jejuni, Mycoplasma pneumonia)* infections; systemic illness (Hodgkin's lymphoma, immunizations)

PHYSICAL FINDINGS & CLINICAL PRESENTATION

- Symmetric weakness, most commonly involving proximal muscles initially, subsequently involving both proximal and distal muscles; difficulty in ambulating, getting up from a chair, or climbing stairs.
- Depressed or absent reflexes bilaterally.
- Minimal to moderate glove and stocking paresthesias/dysesthesia/anesthesia or back pain.
- Pain (caused by involvement of posterior nerve roots) may be prominent.
- Autonomic abnormalities (brady- or tachyarrhythmias, hypo- or hypertension).
- Respiratory insufficiency (caused by weakness of bulbar/intercostal muscles).
- Facial paresis, ophthalmoparesis, dysphagia (secondary to cranial nerve involvement).

ETIOLOGY

- Unknown
- Preceding infectious illness 1 to 4 wk before disease onset in 66% of patients
- Humoral and cell-mediated immune attack of peripheral nerve myelin, Schwann cells; sometimes with axonal involvement

Dx DIAGNOSIS

DIFFERENTIAL DIAGNOSIS

- Toxic peripheral neuropathies: heavy metal poisoning (lead, thallium, arsenic), medications (vincristine, disulfiram), organophosphate poisoning, hexacarbon (glue sniffer's neuropathy)
- Nontoxic peripheral neuropathies: acute intermittent porphyria, vasculitic polyneuropathy, infectious (poliomyelitis, diphtheria, Lyme disease, West Nile virus); tick paralysis
- Neuromuscular junction disorders: myasthenia gravis, botulism, snake envenomations
- Myopathies such as polymyositis, acute necrotizing myopathies caused by drugs
- Metabolic derangements such as hypermagnesemia, hypokalemia, hypophosphatemia
- Acute CNS disorders such as basilar artery thrombosis with brain stem infarction, brain stem encephalomyelitis, transverse myelitis, or spinal cord compression
- Hysterical paralysis or malingering

WORKUP

1. Exclude other causes based on clinical history, examination, and laboratory tests.
2. Lumbar puncture (may be normal in the first 1 to 2 wk of the illness).
   Typical findings include elevated CSF protein with few mononuclear leukocytes (albuminocytologic dissociation) in 80% to 90% of patients. Elevated CSF cell counts is an expected feature in cases associated with HIV seroconversion.
3. EMG/NCS: may be normal in the first 10 to 14 days of the disease. The earliest electrodiagnostic abnormality is prolongation or absence of H-reflexes. EMG/NCS evidence of demyelination (prolonged distal latency, conduction velocity slowing, conduction block, temporal dispersion, and prolonged F-waves) in two or more motor nerves confirms diagnosis of AIDP in the appropriate clinical context.

LABORATORY TESTS

- CBC may reveal early leukocytosis with left shift. Electrolytes are tested to exclude metabolic causes.
- Heavy metal testing, urine porphyria screen, creatine kinase, HIV titers, neuroimaging of the brain and spinal cord if diagnosis uncertain. Nerve root enhancement may be seen on MRI of the lumbosacral spine.
- Antibodies against ganglioside GQ1b may be present in up to 90% of patients with MFS. IgG antibodies against ganglioside GM1 may be associated with AMAN. There are no antiganglioside antibodies commonly associated with AIDP.
- In equivocal cases (especially if peripheral nerve vasculitis is a concern), nerve biopsy may aid in confirming a diagnosis of GBS. Sensory nerve biopsy demonstrates segmental demyelination with infiltration of monocytes and T cells into the endoneurium. Axonal loss is commonly seen in sensory nerve biopsy specimens in GBS.

Rx TREATMENT

NONPHARMACOLOGIC THERAPY

- Close monitoring of respiratory function (frequent measurements of vital capacity, negative inspiratory force, and pulmonary toilet), because respiratory failure is the major complication in GBS
- Frequent repositioning of patient to minimize formation of pressure sores
- Prevention of thromboembolism with antithrombotic stockings and SC heparin (5000 U q12h) in nonambulatory patients
- Emotional support and social counseling

ACUTE GENERAL Rx

- Infusion of IV immunoglobulins (IVIG; 0.4 g/kg/day for 5 days). Always check serum IgA levels before infusion to prevent anaphylaxis in deficient patients.
- Early therapeutic plasma exchange (TPE or plasmapheresis: 200 to 250 ml/kg over five sessions every other day), started within 7 days of onset of symptoms, is beneficial in reducing the need for mechanical ventilation in patients with rapidly progressive disease and results in improved rate of recovery. It is contraindicated in patients with cardiovascular disease (recent MI, unstable angina), active sepsis, and autonomic dysfunction.
- There is no proven benefit from combining IVIG and plasma exchange.
- Mechanical ventilation may be needed if FVC is $<$12 to 15 ml/kg, vital capacity is rapidly decreasing or is $<$1000 ml, negative inspiratory force <-20 cm H_2O, PaO_2 is $<$70, the patient is having significant difficulty clearing secretions or is aspirating.

CHRONIC Rx

- Ventilatory support: may be necessary in 10% to 20% of patients. Adequate fluid/electrolyte support and nutrition are necessary, especially in patients with dysautonomia or bulbar dysfunction.
- Aggressive nursing care to prevent decubitus, infections, fecal impactions, and pressure nerve palsies.
- Monitoring and treatment of autonomic dysfunction (bradyarrhythmias or tachyarrhyth-

 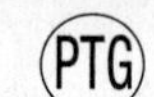

mias, orthostatic hypotension, systemic hypertension, altered sweating).

- Treatment of back pain and dysesthesia with low-dose tricyclics, gabapentin, and so on. Opiate narcotics can be used cautiously in the short term but may compound dysautonomia.
- Stress ulcer prevention in patients receiving ventilator support.
- Physical and occupational therapy rehabilitation, including supportive devices.

DISPOSITION

- Mortality is approximately 5% to 10%. Causes of death include cardiac arrest, pulmonary embolism, and fulminant infections. A recent study showed 62% complete motor recovery, 14% mild weakness, 9% moderate weakness, 4% bed-bound or ventilated, and 8% dead at 1 yr. Another study suggested that about 33% of patients were free from sensory symptoms at 1 yr, with residual sensory loss present in the lower extremities in 67% and 36% in the upper extremities. About 32% had to change their work, 30% were unable to function at home as well as they could before the disease, and 52% had to alter their leisure activities 1 yr after GBS onset. Excessive fatigue is a common complaint in patients during the recovery phase of GBS. This may be treated with exercise therapy (e.g., bicycle exercise training).
- Predictors for poor recovery (inability to walk independently at 1 yr): age >60 yr, preceding diarrheal illness, recent CMV infection, fulminant or rapidly progressing course, ventilatory dependence, reduced motor amplitudes (<20% normal), or inexcitable nerves on NCS. Outcomes may also be influenced by complications of medical therapy.
- GBS is typically a monophasic illness. Recurrence may occur in <5% of patients following full recovery.

REFERRAL

Tracheostomy may be necessary in patients with prolonged ventilatory support. Percutaneous endoscopic gastrostomy may be temporarily required.

PEARLS & CONSIDERATIONS

- GBS is the most common cause of acute flaccid paralysis.
- Close monitoring of ventilatory function with respiratory mechanics (FVC and NIF) is of paramount importance in all patients with suspected GBS.

COMMENTS

Patient education information may be obtained from the Guillain-Barré Foundation International, Box 262, Wynnewood, PA 19096; phone: (610) 667-0131.

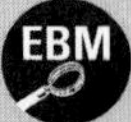

EVIDENCE

Expert opinion and evidence from randomized controlled trials (RCTs) suggests plasmapheresis and IVIG therapy are equivalently effective in the treatment of GBS and significantly hasten recovery. Combining the two treatments is not beneficial.

Six RCTs comparing IVIG with plasmapheresis in the management of GBS have shown that IVIG is equally effective in hastening patient recovery as plasmapheresis. No additional benefit from the use of IVIG following plasmapheresis has been found.[1] Ⓐ

There is no evidence that steroid treatment given alone is beneficial in the treatment of GBS, but there is weak evidence that it can be of benefit in the treatment of CIDP.

Expert opinion and systematic reviews of trials comparing the use of steroids to placebo provide no evidence that the use of steroids in the treatment of GBS is beneficial.[2] Ⓐ Ⓒ

The authors of a systematic review concluded that the results of a small RCT provided weak evidence to support the experience from large nonrandomized studies, which suggests that steroids are beneficial in reducing impairment from CIDP.[3] Ⓐ

The available evidence is inadequate to assess whether azathioprine, interferon beta, or any other immunosuppressive drug or interferon is beneficial for the treatment of CIDP.

A systematic review of cytotoxic drugs and interferons identified only one small, open trial of azathioprine and one, small trial of interferon beta for the treatment of CIPD. Neither trial showed any significant beneficial effect on any of the outcomes measured. The authors of the review concluded that the evidence is inadequate to assess whether these or any other immunosuppressive drug or interferon is beneficial for the treatment of CIDP.[4] Ⓐ

Evidence-Based References

1. Hughes RAC et al: Intravenous immunoglobulin for Guillain-Barré syndrome *Cochrane Database Syst Rev* 1, 2006. Ⓐ
2. Hughes RAC et al: Corticosteroids for Guillain-Barré syndrome. *Cochrane Database Syst Rev* 2: 2006. Ⓐ Ⓒ
3. Mehndiratta MM et al: Plasma exchange for chronic inflammatory demyelinating polyradiculoneuropathy, *Cochrane Database Syst Rev* 3, 2004. Ⓐ
4. Hughes RAC et al: Cytotoxic drugs and interferons for chronic inflammatory demyelinating polyradiculoneuropathy. *Cochrane Database Syst Rev* 4: 2004. Ⓐ

SUGGESTED READINGS

Bernsen RA et al: How Guillain-Barré patients experience their functioning after 1 year, *Acta Neurol Scand* 112:51-56, 2005.

Garssen MP et al: Physical training and fatigue, fitness, and quality of life in Guillain-Barré syndrome and CIDP, *Neurology* 63:2393-2395, 2004.

Hughes RA et al: Multidisciplinary Consensus Group: supportive care for patients with Guillain-Barré syndrome, *Arch Neurol* 62:1194-1198, 2005.

Kieseier BC et al: Advances in understanding and treatment of immune-mediated disorders of the peripheral nervous system, *Muscle Nerve* 30: 131-156, 2004.

Kuwabara S: Guillain-Barré syndrome: epidemiology, pathophysiology and management, *Drugs* 64:597, 2004.

AUTHOR: **EROBOGHENE E. UBOGU, M.B.B.S. (HONS.)**

BASIC INFORMATION

DEFINITION

Hand-foot-mouth (HFM) disease is a viral illness characterized by superficial lesions of the oral mucosa and skin of the extremities. HFM is transmitted primarily by the fecal-oral route and is highly contagious. Although children are predominantly affected, adults are also at risk. This disease is usually self-limited and benign.

SYNONYMS

Vesicular stomatitis with exanthem
Coxsackievirus infection

ICD-9CM CODES
074.0 Hand-foot-mouth disease

EPIDEMIOLOGY & DEMOGRAPHICS

- Children <5 yr are at the highest risk and have the most severe cases.
- HFM is usually found in children <10 yr.
- HFM is contagious. Close contacts of affected children, including family members and health care workers, are the most commonly affected adults.
- Infection is spread from person to person by direct contact with nasal discharge or stool.
- A person is most contagious during the first week of illness.
- Outbreaks tend to occur during the summer.
- Infection leads to immunity, but a second episode may occur after infection with a different agent.

PHYSICAL FINDINGS & CLINICAL PRESENTATION

Symptoms:
- After a 4- to 6-day incubation period, patients may report odynophagia, sore throat, malaise, and fever (38.3° to 40° C).
- One to 2 days later the characteristic oral lesions appear.
- In 75% of cases skin lesions on the extremities accompany these oral manifestations.
- 11% of adults have cutaneous findings.
- Lesions appear over the course of 1 or 2 days.

Physical findings:
- Oral lesions, usually between five and ten, are commonly found on the tongue, buccal mucosa, gingivae, and hard palate.
- Oral lesions initially start as 1- to 3-mm erythematous macules and evolve into gray vesicles on an erythematous base.
- Vesicles are frequently broken by the time of presentation and appear as superficial gray ulcers with surrounding erythema.
- Skin lesions of the hands and feet start as linear erythematous papules (3 to 10 mm in diameter) that evolve into gray vesicles that may be mildly painful (Fig. 1-137). These vesicles are usually intact at presentation and remain so until they desquamate within 2 wk.
- Involvement of the buttocks and perineum is present in 31% of cases.
- In rare cases, encephalitis, meningitis, myocarditis, poliomyelitis-like paralysis, and pulmonary edema may develop. Sporadic acute paralysis and long term neurologic sequelae have been reported with Enterovirus 71.
- Although information is limited, there is no clear evidence that pregnancy outcomes are affected.

ETIOLOGY

- Coxsackievirus group A, type 16, was the first and is the most common viral agent isolated.
- Coxsackie viruses A5, A7, A9, A10, B1, B2, B3, B5, and Enterovirus 71 have also been implicated.
- Enterovirus 71 infection rates have been rising in the Asian Pacific region. This virus may lead to more severe cases of the disease including CNS involvement.

DIAGNOSIS

DIFFERENTIAL DIAGNOSIS

- Aphthous stomatitis
- Herpes simplex infection
- Herpangina
- Behçet's disease
- Erythema multiforme
- Pemphigus
- Gonorrhea
- Acute leukemia
- Lymphoma
- Allergic contact dermatitis

WORKUP

The diagnosis is usually made on the basis of history and characteristic physical examination.

LABORATORY TESTS

- Not indicated unless the diagnosis is in doubt.
- Throat culture or stool specimen may be obtained for viral testing but may take from 2 to 4 wk for results.

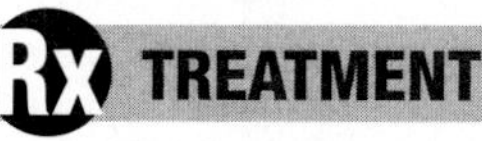

TREATMENT

ACUTE GENERAL Rx

- Palliative therapy is given for this usually self-limited disease.
- Limited data suggest acyclovir may have a role in treatment of certain cases.

DISPOSITION

Prognosis is excellent except in rare cases of central nervous system or cardiac involvement. Most are managed as outpatients.

REFERRAL

Not usually needed

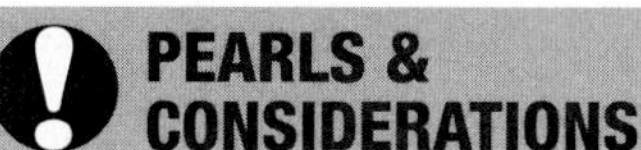

PEARLS & CONSIDERATIONS

- Frequent handwashing, disinfection of contaminated surfaces, and washing of soiled articles of clothing can help reduce transmission.
- HFM has no relation to hoof and mouth disease in cattle.

SUGGESTED READINGS

Chang LY et al: Clinical features and risk of pulmonary edema after enterovirus-related hand, foot, and mouth disease, *Lancet* 354(9191):1682, 1999.

Chang LY et al: Neurodevelopment and cognition in children after enterovirus 71 infection, *N Engl J Med* 356:1226-1234, 2007.

Chang LY et al: Transmission and clinical features of Enterovirus 71 infections in household contacts in Taiwan, *JAMA* 291(2):222, 2004.

Weir E: Foot-and-mouth disease in animals and humans, *Can Med Assoc J* 164(9):1338, 2001.

AUTHORS: **JAMES J. NG, M.D.**, and **JENNIFER JEREMIAH, M.D.**

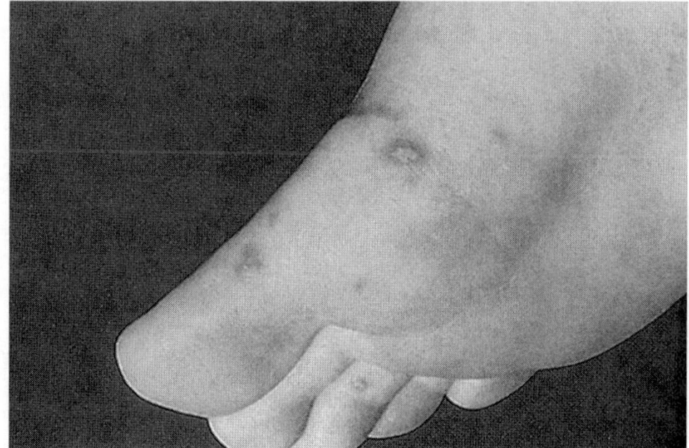

FIGURE 1-137 Hand-foot-mouth disease. Note oval lesions on an erythematous base. (From Goldstein B [ed]: *Practical dermatology,* ed 2, St Louis, 1997, Mosby.)

Hantavirus Pulmonary Syndrome

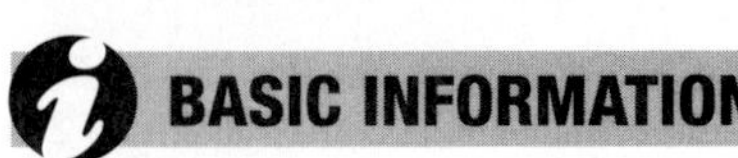

DEFINITION

Hantavirus pulmonary syndrome (HPS) is a severe infectious cardiopulmonary illness usually caused by the Sin Nombre virus (SNV), whose main vector is the deer mouse.

SYNONYMS

Four Corners disease
Hantavirus cardiopulmonary syndrome

ICD-9CM CODES
079.81

EPIDEMIOLOGY & DEMOGRAPHICS

- First identified in the U.S. in 1993, Hantavirus has been found throughout the Continental U.S. and the Americas.
- As of 2005, 396 cases have been identified in 31 states with a mortality rate of 37%.
- The peak incidence to date was in June and July 1993 in the Four Corners region of the U.S.
- HPS is more common in the spring and summer.
- HPS is more prevalent among males, most likely because of increased environmental exposure.
- Mean age is 38 yr.
- HPS has not been found at the extremes of age.
- Risk factors include exposure to rodent populations, rural locales, occupations with increased exposure to rodents, and entering infrequently opened structures.

CLINICAL PRESENTATION

- The most common symptoms are fever, headache, nausea, vomiting, cough, shortness of breath, and myalgia. It is not associated with rhinorrhea or nasal congestion.
- The most common signs on physical examination include fever, hypoxemia, and tachypnea. Rash, mucosal bleeding, or peripheral edema is not found with HPS.
- There are two phases of HPS, the prodromal phase and the cardiopulmonary phase. The prodromal phase is characterized by:
  - Fever, chills, headache, and myalgias, especially in the legs and back
  - Cough, nausea, vomiting, and general malaise
  - Tachypnea, tachycardia, hypoxemia
- The cardiopulmonary phase has the following characteristics:
  - Cough and dyspnea
  - Acute pulmonary edema
  - Hypotension
  - Decreased cardiac output

ETIOLOGY

- HPS is most often caused by the Sin Nombre virus.
- The main vector is the deer mouse.
- It is transmitted by inhalation of aerosolized feces, urine, or saliva from infected rodents.
- No cases of person-to-person transmission have been reported.

Dx DIAGNOSIS

DIFFERENTIAL DIAGNOSIS

- Acute respiratory distress syndrome
- Pneumonia
- Congestive heart failure
- Pulmonary edema
- Acute bacterial endocarditis
- Gastroenteritis
- Plague
- Tularemia ("rabbit fever")
- Histoplasmosis
- Coccidioidomycosis
- Cardiogenic shock
- HIV/AIDS
- Myocardial infarction
- Goodpasture's syndrome—an autoimmune pulmonary disease

WORKUP

- Complete blood count q8h.
  1. All patients manifest thrombocytopenia, and its progression is the most consistent indicator heralding the cardiopulmonary phase of HPS.
  2. Differential usually reveals a left shift. White blood cell counts are an unreliable indicator of severity of infection.
- Lactate level >4 mg/dl is associated with a high mortality rate.
- Rapid immunoblot strip assay for SNV antibodies.
- Diagnosis is confirmed by identification of immunoglobulin M and G antibodies to SNV.

IMAGING STUDIES

Chest radiograph: pulmonary edema

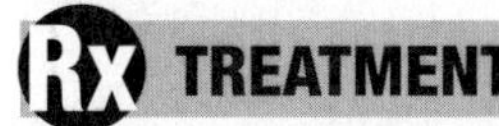

NONPHARMACOLOGIC THERAPY

- Intensive care unit admission in tertiary care center
- Mechanical ventilation with high pulmonary end-expiratory pressure and high Fio_2
- Pulmonary artery catheterization
- Extracorporeal membrane oxygenation (ECMO)

ACUTE GENERAL Rx

- Supportive measures
- Supplemental oxygen
- Intubation when indicated
- Fluid resuscitation
- Hemodynamic monitoring
- Initial broad-spectrum antibiotics
- Pressors
- No medication is effective against SNV

DISPOSITION

- Patients who survive cardiopulmonary phase of HPS have rapid clinical improvement.
- There are no serious sequelae.

REFERRAL

University of New Mexico Hospital is the only facility with experience in ECMO for treatment of HPS. This modality is only for hemodynamically unstable, critically ill patients who do not respond to conventional therapies.

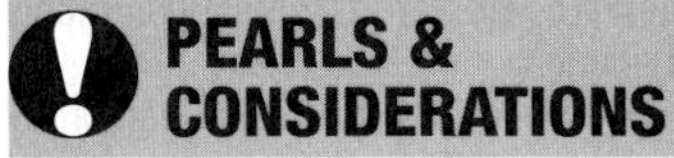

COMMENTS

Although rare, HPS should be a consideration in those with acute respiratory illness and a history suggestive of HPS exposure. The combination of thrombocytopenia, left shift, circulating immunoblasts, and hemoconcentration is rare in other viral illnesses.

PREVENTION

Rodent control is the primary way to prevent Hantavirus infection.

SUGGESTED READINGS

Graziano KL et al: Hantavirus pulmonary syndrome: a zebra worth knowing, *Am Fam Physician* 66(6): 1015-1020, 2002.

Mertz GJ et al: Diagnosis and treatment of new world Hantavirus infections, *Curr Opin Infect Dis* 19(5):437, 2006.

Mills JN et al: Hantavirus pulmonary syndrome—United States: updated recommendations for risk reduction, *MMWR* 51(RR09):1-12, 2002.

National Center for Infectious Diseases, Special Pathogens Branch: All about Hantaviruses. Available at http://www.cdc.gov/ncidod/diseases/hanta/hps/index.htm. Accessed Nov. 2009.

AUTHOR: **CATHERINE SHAFTS, D.O.**

BASIC INFORMATION

DEFINITION

The term *cluster headache* refers to attacks of severe, unilateral pain that is orbital, supraorbital, temporal, or any combination of these sites, lasting 15 to 180 minutes, and occurring from once every other day to eight times a day. The attacks are associated with one or more of the following, all of which are ipsilateral: conjunctival injection, lacrimation, nasal congestion, rhinorrhea, forehead and facial sweating, miosis, ptosis, and eyelid edema. Most patients are restless or agitated during an attack.

SYNONYMS

Ciliary neuralgia
Erythromelalgia of the head
Erythroprosopalgia of Bing
Horton's headache

ICD-9CM CODES
346.2 Variants of migraine

EPIDEMIOLOGY & DEMOGRAPHICS

INCIDENCE: Estimated to occur in 0.05% to 1% of the population
PREDOMINANT SEX: Occurs in males at least five times more commonly than in females
PREDOMINANT AGE: Peak age of onset between 20 and 40 yr
GENETICS: May be inherited (autosomal dominant) in approximately 5% of cases

PHYSICAL FINDINGS & CLINICAL PRESENTATION

- During attack: ipsilateral conjunctival injection, lacrimation, nasal congestion, rhinorrhea, facial sweating, Horner's syndrome.
- In contrast to migraine sufferers, patients are agitated and active during an attack.
- Permanent partial Horner's syndrome in 5% of patients; otherwise examination is normal.

ETIOLOGY

Activation of the posterior hypothalamic grey matter resulting in trigeminal activation coupled with parasympathetic activation. The pathophysiology remains controversial.

DIAGNOSIS

- Severe or very severe unilateral orbital, supraorbital, and/or temporal pain lasting 15 to 180 minutes.
- Frequency of every other day to eight per day; they may cluster seasonally or at a certain time in a patient's life.
- Headache is accompanied by at least one of the following (ipsilateral):
  1. Conjunctival injection and/or lacrimation
  2. Nasal congestion and/or rhinorrhea
  3. Eyelid edema
  4. Forehead and facial sweating
  5. Miosis and/or ptosis
  6. Restlessness or agitation

DIFFERENTIAL DIAGNOSIS

- Migraine
- Trigeminal neuralgia
- Temporal arteritis
- Postherpetic neuralgia
- Venous sinus thrombosis
- Carotid-cavernous fistula or other cavernous sinus lesions
- Other trigeminal autonomic cephalalgias
- Section II describes the differential diagnosis of headaches

WORKUP

Diagnosis is usually established by characteristic history.

IMAGING STUDIES

None, unless history or examination suggests focal neurologic deficit or headaches change in character or are of new onset.

TREATMENT

NONPHARMACOLOGIC THERAPY

Avoidance of alcohol, histamine, nitroglycerine, and tobacco during clusters

ABORTIVE Rx

- Inhalation of 100% oxygen by face mask for 15 min often aborts an attack.
- About 75% of users of triptans (sumatriptan, zolmatriptan) will be pain free within 20 minutes.
- Cafergot, octreotide, intranasal lidocaine, or dihydroergotamine may abort an attack or prevent one if given just before a predictable episode. Acute episode is typically resolved before oral analgesics become effective, although indomethacin and other NSAIDs may also be effective in prolonged attacks.
- Acute episode is typically resolved before oral analgesics become effective, although indomethacin and other NSAIDs may also be effective in prolonged attacks.

PROPHYLAXIS Rx

Various medications have been tried without great success, although good responses may be obtained in up to 50% of cases. Examples include:

- Valproic acid: start at 500 mg/day
- Topiramate: up to 50 mg bid
- Verapamil: up to 480 mg/day as tolerated
- Lithium: 200 mg tid with frequent monitoring and adjustment to maintain therapeutic serum level of 0.4 to 1 mEq/L. Equally effective as verapamil, but more side effects
- Methysergide: 1 to 2 mg tid; requires familiarity with the potential adverse effects and use of "drug holidays" to decrease risk of fibrosis
- Ergotamine tartrate: 3 to 4 mg/day during clusters
- Prednisone: 60 mg PO qd for 1 wk followed by taper; headaches can return during taper

DISPOSITION

Headache-free periods tend to increase with increasing age.

REFERRAL

Refractory cluster headaches may require referral to a headache specialist.

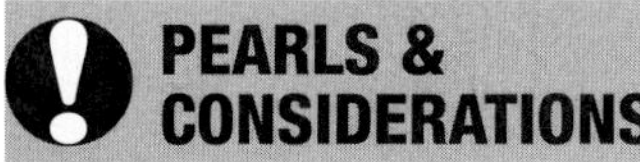

PEARLS & CONSIDERATIONS

COMMENTS

- Cluster headaches are divided into episodic (attacks lasting up to 1 yr with more than 1 mo pain-free periods) and chronic (>1 yr without remission).
- Home oxygen therapy is reasonable for cluster headache sufferers.

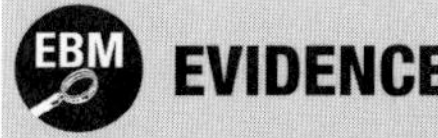

EVIDENCE

Treatments for cluster headache can be considered in terms of acute or abortive treatments and prophylactic treatments.

Abortive treatments should be started as soon as possible.

A randomized, double-blind, placebo-controlled crossover trial of subcutaneous sumatriptan found a significant increase in pain-free rates 10 to 15 minutes after administration of sumatriptan compared with placebo.[1] B

A double-blind, placebo-controlled, randomized trial of intranasal sumatriptan found a significant benefit in favor of sumatriptan over placebo in response rates and pain-free rates at 30 minutes, with benefits also seen in initial response, meaningful relief, and relief of associated symptoms.[2] B

A small, double-blind, placebo-controlled trial showed a significant effect on the intensity of single pain attacks with dihydroergotamine nasal spray.[3] B

Nitroglycerin-induced pain in cluster headache showed a prompt response with cessation of pain after local application of cocaine hydrochloride or lidocaine in the area corresponding to the sphenopalatine fossa under anterior rhinoscopy.[4] B

A double-blind crossover study compared oxygen versus air inhalation at 6 L/min via nonrebreathing face masks for 15 minutes or less for up to 6 headaches. Oxygen-treated patients showed a significantly higher pain-relief score.[5] B

Prophylactic therapy should also be started as soon as possible after the start of a cluster episode. Chronic cluster headache may require longer-term therapy.

A randomized controlled trial assessing the efficacy and safety of gabapentin versus placebo in people with chronic daily headache found gabapentin to produce a small but significant increase in the number of headache-free days and a reduction of indicators such as severity, nausea, and photophobia.[6] Ⓑ

In a study of 19 patients with cluster headaches whose pain was not mitigated by standard treatment, a double-blind control study with single crossover showed sustained improvement on oral prednisone compared with placebo in 17 cases.[7] Ⓑ

A small, randomized, controlled trial compared the efficacy of verapamil versus placebo in the prophylaxis of episodic cluster headache. There was a significant reduction in the frequency of attacks and in the consumption of abortive agents in the verapamil-treated group, suggesting that verapamil is effective in episodic cluster headache prophylaxis.[8] Ⓑ

In a double-dummy, double-blind, crossover comparison of verapamil with lithium carbonate in preventing chronic cluster headache (CCH) attacks, both agents were found to be effective in preventing CCH attacks, but verapamil caused fewer side effects and had a shorter latency period.[9] Ⓑ

In a double-blind, placebo-controlled pilot study, oral melatonin significantly reduced headache frequency compared with placebo.[10] Ⓑ

A systematic review of acupuncture for idiopathic headache included 26 trials and a total of 1151 patients. Sixteen trials were conducted with patients with migraine, 6 among patients with tension headache and 4 among patients with various types of headache. The reviewers' conclusion was that overall the existing evidence supports the value of acupuncture for the treatment of idiopathic headaches; however, they noted that quality and amount of evidence are not fully convincing.[11] Ⓑ

In a randomized, controlled trial, 401 patients with chronic headache were randomized to receive up to 12 acupuncture treatments over 3 mo or a usual care control intervention. Headache scores, SF-36 health status, and use of medication were assessed at baseline, 3, and 12 mo. A 34% reduction in headache scores were seen in the acupuncture group at 12 mo compared to a 16% reduction in the control group, and patients in the acupuncture group required 15% less medication than the control group.[12] Ⓑ

A Cochrane review of 18 studies including 808 patients reviewed studies of psychological treatments, especially relaxation and cognitive behavioral therapy, in children and adolescents with various types of pain, including headache. The conclusion was that these therapies were effective in reducing pain severity and frequency in chronic headaches.[13] Ⓐ

Evidence-Based References

1. Sumatriptan Cluster Headache Study Group: Treatment of acute cluster headache with sumatriptan, *N Engl J Med* 325:322-326, 1991. Ⓑ
2. van Vliet JA et al: Intranasal sumatriptan in cluster headache: randomized placebo-controlled double-blind study, *Neurology* 60:630-633, 2003. Ⓑ
3. Andersson PG, Jespersen LT: Dihydroergotamine nasal spray in the treatment of attacks of cluster headache. A double-blind trial versus placebo, *Cephalalgia* 6:51-54, 1986. Ⓑ
4. Costa A et al: The effect of intranasal cocaine and lidocaine on nitroglycerin-induced attacks in cluster headache. *Cephalalgia* 20:85-91, 2000. Ⓑ
5. Fogan L: Treatment of cluster headache. A double-blind comparison of oxygen v air inhalation, *Arch Neurol* 42:362-363, 1985. Ⓑ
6. Spira PJ, Beran RG; Australian Gabapentin Chronic Daily Headache Group: Gabapentin in the prophylaxis of chronic daily headache: a randomized, placebo-controlled study, *Neurology* 61:1753-1759, 2003. Ⓑ
7. Jammes JL: The treatment of cluster headaches with prednisone, *Dis Nerv Syst* 36:375-376, 1975. Ⓑ
8. Leone M et al: Verapamil in the prophylaxis of episodic cluster headache: a double-blind study versus placebo, *Neurology* 54:1382-1385, 2000. Ⓑ
9. Bussone G et al: Double blind comparison of lithium and verapamil in cluster headache prophylaxis, *Headache* 30:411-417, 1990. Ⓑ
10. Leone M et al: Melatonin versus placebo in the prophylaxis of cluster headache: a double-blind pilot study with parallel groups, *Cephalalgia* 16:494-496, 1996. Ⓑ
11. Melchart D et al: Acupuncture for idiopathic headache, *Cochrane Database Rev* (1), 2001. Ⓑ
12. Vickers AJ et al: Acupuncture for chronic headache in primary care: large, pragmatic, randomised trial, *BMJ* 328:744, 2004. Ⓑ
13. Eccleston C et al: Psychological therapies for the management of chronic and recurrent pain in children and adolescents, *Cochrane Database Rev* (1), 2003. Ⓐ

SUGGESTED READINGS

Ekbom K, Hardebo JE: Cluster headache: aetiology, diagnosis and management, *Drugs* 62(1):61, 2002.

Goadsby PJ: Trigeminal autonomic cephalalgias. Pathophysiology and classification, *Rev Neurol* (Paris) 161: 692, 2005.

Headache Classification Committee of the International Headache Society: The international classification of headache disorders, *Cephalgia* 24:s1, 2004.

May A: Cluster headache: pathogenesis, diagnosis, and management, *Lancet* 366:843, 2005.

AUTHOR: **CHUN LIM, M.D., PH.D.**

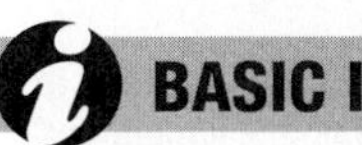

BASIC INFORMATION

DEFINITION

Migraine headaches are recurrent headaches preceded by a focal neurologic symptom (migraine with aura), occur independently (migraine without aura), or have atypical presentations (migraine variants). The migraine aura typically is characterized by visual or sensory symptoms that develop over a period of 5 to 20 min. In both migraine with and without aura the headache is typically unilateral, pulsatile, and associated with nausea and vomiting, photophobia, and phonophobia.

ICD-9CM CODES
346 Migraine

EPIDEMIOLOGY & DEMOGRAPHICS

INCIDENCE: Increases from infancy, peaks during the third decade of life, then decreases
PREVALENCE (IN U.S.): Females: 18%; males: 6%
PREDOMINANT SEX: Female/male ratio of 3:1
GENETICS:
- Familial predisposition, with more than 50% of migraine sufferers having an affected family member
- Autosomal-dominant transmission for some rare migraine variants (familial hemiplegic migraine; cerebral autosomal-dominant arteriopathy with subcortical infarcts and leukoencephalopathy [CADASIL])

PHYSICAL FINDINGS & CLINICAL PRESENTATION

- Normal between episodes.
- Normal for migraine without aura. Focal motor or sensory abnormalities possible with migraine with aura or migraine variants.
- Common aura types include scintillating scotomata, bright zigzags, homonymous visual disturbance such as paresthesias, speech disturbances, or hemiparesis (familial or sporadic hemiplegic migraine).

ETIOLOGY

The pathophysiology of migraines is not clearly understood. It is believed that a primary neuronal event results in a trigeminovascular reflex causing neurogenic inflammation. Serotonin, substance P, nitric oxide, and calcitonin-gene-related peptide also play a role, but the exact mechanism is unknown. Cortical spreading depression is probably responsible for the aura.

Dx DIAGNOSIS

Migraine without aura:
- Five attacks fulfilling criteria
- Headache attacks lasting 4 to 72 hours
- Headache has at least two of the following characteristics:
  1. Unilateral location
  2. Pulsating quality
  3. Moderate or severe pain intensity
  4. Aggravation or causing avoidance of routine physical activity
- During headache at least one of the following:
  1. Nausea and/or vomiting
  2. Photophobia and phonophobia

Migraine with aura:
- At least two attacks
- Aura consisting of at least one of the following, but no motor weakness:
  1. Fully reversible visual symptoms, including positive features and/or negative features
  2. Fully reversible sensory symptoms, including positive and/or negative features
- At least two of the following:
  1. Homonymous visual symptoms and/or unilateral sensory symptoms
  2. At least one aura symptom develops gradually over >5 min and/or different aura symptoms occur in succession over >5 min
- A migraine occurring during or within 60 min of the aura

DIFFERENTIAL DIAGNOSIS

- Subarachnoid hemorrhage
- Cluster headache
- Chronic daily headaches
- Arteriovenous malformation
- Vasculitis
- Intracranial mass lesion
- Section II describes the differential diagnosis of headaches

WORKUP

- In general, no additional investigation is needed with recurrent, typical attacks with usual age of onset, family history, and a normal physical examination.
- If there is an unusual presentation and/or unexpected findings on examination, investigation for other causes is required.

LABORATORY TESTS

Lumbar puncture for history of abrupt-onset headaches and uncertain diagnosis of migraine

IMAGING STUDIES

- Imaging should be done in patients with headaches and an unexplained abnormal finding on the neurologic examination.
- Imaging should be considered in patients with rapidly increasing headache frequency, history of dizziness or incoordination, headache causing wakening from sleep, or headaches worsening with Valsalva maneuver.

Rx TREATMENT

Consider the use of a headache log/diary to identify triggers of headaches, record efficacy of treatments, and track history of the headaches.

NONPHARMACOLOGIC THERAPY

- Avoid any identifiable provoking factors: caffeine, tobacco, and alcohol may trigger attacks, as may dietary or other environmental precipitants (less common)
- Avoid stressors in life and minimize variations in daily routine with regular sleep, meals, and exercise
- Relaxation training, behavioral therapy, and biofeedback

ACUTE ANALGESIC Rx

- Many oral agents are ineffective because of poor absorption from migraine-induced gastric stasis. Non-oral route of administration should be selected in patients with severe nausea or vomiting.
- Acetaminophen, NSAIDS, combination analgesics, benzodiazepines, opioids, barbiturates.

ACUTE ABORTIVE Rx

- IV antiemetics (prochlorperazine, metoclopramide, domperidone). Acute dystonic reactions and akathisia are rare side effects. These are generally not used as monotherapy.
- Ergotamine and ergotamine combinations (PO/PR) and dihydroergotamine (DHE 45) (SC, IV, IM, intranasal) have well-documented efficacy against migraines. DHE is usually administered in combination with an antiemetic drug (Table 1-36).
- Triptans (SC, PO, and intranasal) are now considered the drug class of choice for abortive therapy. Meta-analysis suggests that 10 mg rizatriptan, 80 mg eletriptan, and 12.5 mg almotriptan are most effective.
- Early administration improves effectiveness.

PROPHYLAXIS Rx

- Prophylactic treatment is generally indicated when headaches occur more than once a week or when symptomatic treatments are contraindicated or not effective. They are most effective when initiated during a headache-free period. All prophylaxis should be maintained for at least 3 mo before deeming the medication a failure.
- Well-established options for prophylactic treatment include β-blockers (propranolol, timolol, atenolol, metoprolol), tricyclic antidepressants (amitriptyline), and the antiepileptic drug valproic acid.
- Less-established options include calcium channel blockers, selective serotonin reuptake inhibitors, and the antiepileptic drugs gabapentin and topiramate.

DISPOSITION

After age 30 yr, 40% of patients are migraine free.

REFERRAL

If uncertain about diagnosis or treatment not effective

 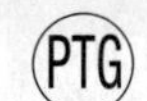

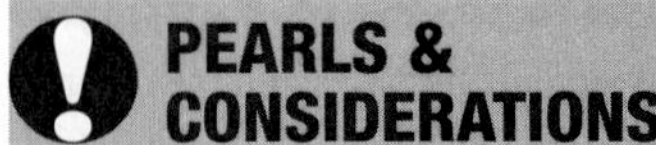

PEARLS & CONSIDERATIONS

- Avoid overuse of narcotics, barbiturates, caffeine, and benzodiazepines because they are habit-forming.
- Long-term use of analgesic medications can result in drug-induced or rebound headaches.

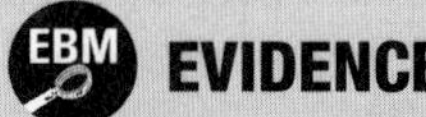

EVIDENCE

Evidence for therapies used to treat acute attacks:

The combination of acetaminophen, aspirin, and caffeine has been shown to be more effective than placebo for the treatment of acute, nondisabling migraine.[1] A

Evidence for acetaminophen alone in the management of acute migraine is limited.[2] B

There is some evidence that improved headache relief may be achieved with ibuprofen.[3-5] A

Multiple RCTs have shown the efficacy of triptans in relieving migraine headache.[6-10] A

There is some evidence that oral ergotamine is more effective than placebo for the acute treatment of migraine headache—three of seven trials in a systematic review reported efficacy.[11] A

Ergotamine is less effective than triptans in the acute treatment of migraine.[6,12-14]

In general, acupuncture for the management of idiopathic headaches is supported by the existing evidence, but the overall amount and quality of evidence are not fully convincing.[15] A

Evidence for therapies used to prevent attacks:

Propranolol as a prophylactic treatment for migraine confers a short-term benefit compared with placebo. There is, as yet, a lack of evidence for its benefit in the long-term.[16] A

Anticonvulsants appear to be effective in reducing migraine frequency and are reasonably well tolerated. However, there are wide variations among individual agents.[17] A

Feverfew appears to confer no clear benefit compared with placebo for the prevention of migraine.[18] A

Selective serotonin reuptake inhibitors have not been shown to be more effective than placebo in preventing migraine, although results are based on short-term trials.[19] A

TABLE 1-36 Abortive and Analgesic Therapy for Migraine*

Drug	Route	Dose
Triptans (Serotonin Agonists)		
Sumatriptan	Subcutaneous	6 mg, repeat in 2 hr (max 2 doses/day)
Sumatriptan	Oral	25 mg, 50 mg, repeat in 2 hr (max 200 mg/day)
Sumatriptan	Nasal spray	5 mg and 20 mg, repeat in 2 hr (max 40 mg/day)
Zolmitriptan	Oral	1.25, 2.5 mg, 5 mg, repeat in 2 hr (max 10 mg/day)
Zolmitriptan	Nasal spray	5 mg, repeat in 2 hr (max 10 mg/day)
Zolmitriptan	Orally disintegrating tab	2.5, 5 mg, repeat in 2 hr (max 10 mg/day)
Naratriptan	Oral	1 mg, 2.5 mg, repeat in 4 hr (max 5 mg/day)
Rizatriptan	Oral	5 mg, 10 mg, repeat in 2 hr (max 30 mg/day)
Almotriptan	Oral	6.25 mg, 12.5 mg, may repeat in 2 hr (max 25 mg/day)
Eletriptan	Oral	20 mg, 40 mg, may repeat in 2 hr (max 80 mg/day)
Frovatriptan	Oral	2.5 mg, may repeat in 2 hr (max 7.5 mg/day)
Ergotamine Preparations		
Ergotamine and caffeine	Oral	2 tablets, may repeat 1 tab q30 min; max 6/day
Ergotamine and caffeine	Rectal	1 suppository, repeat in 1 hr; max 2/day
Ergotamine	Sublingual	1 tablet, repeat in 1 hr; max 2/day
Dihydroergotamine	Intramuscular Subcutaneous Intravenous Nasal spray	0.5-1.0 mg, repeat twice at 1-hr intervals (max 3 mg/attack)
Sympathomimetics (with or without Barbiturates or Codeine)		
Isometheptene+dichloralphenazone+acetaminophen	Oral	1 to 2 capsules, repeat in 4 hr, max 8/day
Nonsteroidal Antiinflammatory Drugs		
Acetaminophen+	Oral	2 tablets, repeat in 6 hr, max 8/day aspirin+caffeine
Naproxen	Oral	550-750 mg, repeat in 1 hr; max 3 times/wk
Meclofenamate	Oral	100-200 mg, repeat in 1 hr; max 3 times/wk
Flurbiprofen	Oral	50-100 mg, repeat in 1 hr; max 3 times/wk
Ibuprofen	Oral	200-300 mg, repeat in 1 hr; max 3 times/wk
Antiemetics		
Promethazine	Oral Intramuscular	50-125 mg
Prochlorperazine	Oral Rectal Intramuscular	1-25 mg 2.5-25 mg (suppository) 5-10 mg
Chlorpromazine	Oral Rectal Intravenous	10-25 mg 50-100 mg (suppository) Up to 35 mg
Trimethobenzamide	Oral Rectal	250 mg 200 mg
Metoclopramide	Oral Intramuscular Intravenous	5-10 mg 10 mg 5-10 mg
Dimenhydrinate	Oral	50 mg

Modified from Wiederholt WC: *Neurology for non-neurologists,* ed 4, Philadelphia, 2000, WB Saunders.
*For side effects and contraindications consult the manufacturer's drug insert before prescribing any of these drugs.

Evidence-Based References

1. Lipton RB et al: Efficacy and safety of acetaminophen, aspirin, and caffeine in alleviating headache pain: three double-blind, randomized, placebo controlled trials, *Arch Neurol* 55:210-217, 1998. A
2. Paracetamol for acute migraine. In: Migraine and Headache, *Bandolier.* www.medicine.ox.ac.uk/bandolier/booth/Migraine/Paracute.html. Accessed May 2007. B
3. Kellstein D et al: Evaluation of a novel solubilized formulation of ibuprofen in the treatment of migraine headache: a randomized, double-blind, placebo-controlled, dose-ranging study, *Cephalalgia* 20:233-243, 2000. A
4. Havanka-Kanniainen H: Treatment of acute migraine attack: ibuprofen and placebo compared, *Headache* 29:507-509, 1989. A
5. Kloster R et al: A double-blind study of ibuprofen versus placebo in the treatment of acute migraine attacks, *Cephalalgia* 12:169-171, 1992. A
6. Tfelt-Hansen P: Efficacy and harms of subcutaneous, oral, and intranasal sumatriptan used for migraine treatment: a systematic review based on number need to treat, *Cephalalgia* 18:532-538, 1998. A
7. McCrory DC, Gray RN: Oral sumatriptan for acute migraine, *Cochrane Database Rev* (3), 2003. A
8. Ferrari MD et al: Triptans (serotonin, 5-HT1B/1D agonists) in migraine: detailed results and methods of a meta-analysis of 53 trials, *Cephalalgia* 22:633-658, 2002. A

9. Mathew NT et al: AEGIS Investigator Study Group. Early intervention with almotriptan: results of the AEGIS trial (AXERT Early Migraine Intervention Study), *Headache* 47:189-198, 2007. Ⓐ

10. Morillo LE: Migraine headache, *Clin Evid* 12: 1817-1840, 2004. Ⓐ

11. Dahlof C: Placebo-controlled clinical trials with ergotamine in the acute treatment of migraine, *Cephalalgia* 13:166-171, 1993. Ⓐ

12. Christie S et al: Crossover comparison of efficacy and preference for rizatriptan 10mg versus ergotamine/caffeine in migraine, *Eur Neurol* 49:20-29, 2003.

13. Multinational Oral Sumatriptan Cafergot Comparative Study Group: A randomized, double-blind comparison of sumatriptan and Cafergot in the acute treatment of migraine, *Eur Neurol* 31:314-322, 1991.

14. Boureau F et al: A clinical comparison of sumatriptan nasal spray and dihydroergotamine nasal spray in the acute treatment of migraine, *Int J Clin Pract* 54:281-286, 2000.

15. Melchart D et al: Acupuncture for idiopathic headache, *Cochrane Database Rev* (1), 2001. Ⓐ

16. Linde K, Rossnagel K: Propranolol for migraine prophylaxis, *Cochrane Database Rev* (2), 2004. Ⓐ

17. Chronicle E, Mulleners W: Anticonvulsant drugs for migraine prophylaxis, *Cochrane Database Rev* (3), 2004. Ⓐ

18. Freitag FG et al: A randomized trial of divalproex sodium extended-release tablets in migraine prophylaxis, *Neurology* 58:1652-1659, 2002. Ⓐ

19. Moja PL et al: Selective serotonin re-uptake inhibitors (SSRIs) for preventing migraine and tension-type headaches, *Cochrane Database Rev* (3), 2005. Ⓐ

SUGGESTED READINGS

Buse DC et al: Assessing and managing all aspects of migraine: migraine attacks, migraine-related functional impairment, common comorbidities, and quality of life, *Mayo Clin Proc* 84(5):422-435, 2009.

Ferrari MD et al: Oral triptans (serotonin 5-HT1B/1D agonist) in acute migraine treatment: a meta-analysis of 53 trials, *Lancet* 358:1668, 2001.

Ferrari MD et al: Migraine—current understanding and treatment, *N Engl J Med* 346:257, 2002.

Headache Classification Committee of the International Headache Society: The international classification of headache disorders, *Cephalgia* 24:s1, 2004.

Laine CL et al: In the clinic: migraine, *Ann Intern Med* ITC11, 2007.

Matchar DB et al: Evidence-based guidelines for migraine headache in the primary care setting: pharmacological management of acute attacks. American Academy of Neurology Practice Guideline, available at http://www.aan.com/professionals/practice/pdfs/gl0087.pdf.

AUTHOR: **CHUN LIM, M.D., PH.D.**

BASIC INFORMATION

DEFINITION

Tension-type headaches (TTH) are recurrent headaches lasting 30 min to 7 days without nausea or vomiting and with at least two of the following characteristics: pressing or tightening quality (nonthrobbing), mild or moderate intensity, bilateral, and not aggravated by routine physical activity.

SYNONYMS

Muscle contraction headache
Tension headache
Stress headache
Essential headache

ICD-9CM CODES
307.81 Tension headache

EPIDEMIOLOGY & DEMOGRAPHICS

INCIDENCE (IN U.S.): Most common type of headache; as high as 70% of all headaches presenting to primary care physician
PEAK INCIDENCE: Occurs at all ages
PREVALENCE (IN U.S.): Males: 63%/yr; females: 86%/yr
PREDOMINANT SEX: Females are affected more often than males

PHYSICAL FINDINGS & CLINICAL PRESENTATION

Pressure or "bandlike" tightness all around the head; may be worse at the vertex. Cervical, paracervical, and trapezius muscle spasm and/or tenderness on palpation may be present. Scalp tenderness or hypersensitivity to pain also occurs. Symptoms suggestive of migraine are usually not present (e.g., throbbing pain, nausea/vomiting, visual complaints, aura). Either one symptom of photo or phonophobia does not exclude the diagnosis of TTH.

ETIOLOGY

- Unclear; little data to support postulated muscle contraction component. More recently has been thought of as a multifactorial disorder with several possible concurrent pathophysiologic mechanisms.
- No recent data to support the longstanding belief that these headaches arise from stress or other psychological factors. However, components of stress, sleep deprivation, hunger, and eyestrain may exacerbate symptoms.

DIAGNOSIS

DIFFERENTIAL DIAGNOSIS

- Migraine (would expect associated symptoms; see entry "Headache, Migraine")
- Cervical spine disease
- Intracranial mass (may present with focal neurologic signs, seizures, or headache awakening patient from sleep)
- Idiopathic intracranial hypertension (found more often in obese women of child-bearing age, may have papilledema, visual loss, or diplopia)
- Rebound headache from overuse of analgesics
- Secondary headache (e.g., temporomandibular joint syndrome, thyrotoxicosis, polycythemia, drug side effects)
- Migraine and TTH may often coexist and may be difficult to differentiate (suggest headache calendar)
- Section II describes the differential diagnosis of headaches

WORKUP

- Thorough history and physical examination for any new-onset headache.
- Neuroimaging should be performed when unexplained neurologic findings are present on examination or in cases of atypical new-onset sudden and severe headaches.

LABORATORY TESTS

- No routine tests
- Erythrocyte sedimentation rate in elderly patients suspected of having cranial arteritis

IMAGING STUDIES

CT scan and/or MRI may be used to exclude intracranial pathology. MRI is better for imaging the posterior fossa. Contrast should be used if mass lesion is suspected.

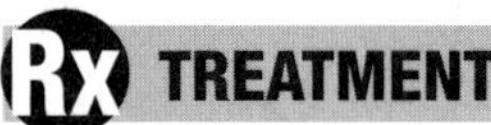

TREATMENT

NONPHARMACOLOGIC THERAPY

- Relaxation and cognitive behavioral therapy (especially in adolescents and children), Schultz-type autogenic training (relaxation technique based on passive concentration and body awareness of specific sensations), transcutaneous electrical nerve stimulation, heat
- Physical therapy, including stretching exercises, massage, and ultrasound

ACUTE GENERAL Rx

Nonnarcotic analgesics with limited frequency to prevent drug-induced and/or rebound headache

CHRONIC Rx

- Tricyclic antidepressants (e.g., amitriptyline 10 to 150 mg hs) and SSRIs
- Avoid narcotics, limit NSAIDs, consider indomethacin; if related to cervical muscle spasm, may consider trial of muscle relaxants (e.g., Skelaxin 400 to 800 mg tid)

DISPOSITION

May not respond fully to treatment

REFERRAL

If uncertain about diagnosis or unexplained focal neurologic findings on examination

PEARLS & CONSIDERATIONS

It is imperative to avoid overuse of caffeine- and barbiturate-containing medications because of the risk of rebound headaches.

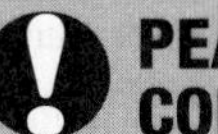

EVIDENCE

There is a lack of quality clinical trials for many of the treatments for tension-type headache. Most studies involve small patient numbers and are heterogeneous regarding the nature of the headache and other clinical parameters. In addition, many of the standard medications commonly used, including simple analgesics, have not been subjected to randomized controlled trials, and their use is governed by clinical experience. As such, the evidence for many of the therapies is limited.

There is some evidence that amitriptyline is beneficial in the management of tension-type headache.

A systematic review and randomized controlled trials (RCTs) have found that, in patients with moderate to severe tension-type headache, amitriptyline significantly reduces the duration and frequency of symptoms compared with placebo.[1-4] Ⓐ

Another systematic review found that tricyclic antidepressants (including amitriptyline) were more effective than SSRIs in the prevention of tension-type headache.[5] Ⓐ

There is some evidence for noninvasive physical treatments for tension-type headache.

A systematic review compared the short-term and long-term effects of noninvasive physical treatments for chronic and recurrent headaches. It failed to find any high-quality evidence of therapeutic effect but concluded that weak evidence supported a number of therapies, which appeared to have little risk of adverse effect.[6] Ⓑ

Systematic reviews have found that acupuncture is probably effective in the treatment of idiopathic headaches. The overall quality and amount of evidence assessed was said by the reviewers not to be fully convincing.[7,8] Ⓑ

Evidence-Based References

1. Bendtsen L et al: A non-selective (amitriptyline), but not a selective (citalopram), serotonin reuptake inhibitor is effective in the prophylactic treatment of chronic tension-type headache, *J Neurol Neurosurg Psychiatry* 61:285-1290, 1996. Ⓐ
2. Bogaards MC et al: Treatment of recurrent tension-type headache: a meta-analytic review, *Clin J Pain* 10:174-190, 1994. Ⓐ
3. Gobel H et al: Chronic tension-type headache: amitriptyline reduces clinical headache-duration and experimental pain sensitivity but does not alter pericranial muscle activity readings, *Pain* 59:241-249, 1994. Ⓐ

4. Holroyd KA et al: Management of chronic tension-type headache with tricyclic antidepressant medication, stress management therapy, and their combination: a randomized controlled trial, *JAMA* 285:2208-2215, 2001. Ⓐ
5. Moja PL et al: Selective serotonin re-uptake inhibitors (SSRIs) for preventing migraine and tension-type headaches, *Cochrane Database Rev* (3), 2005. Ⓐ
6. Bronfort G et al: Non-invasive physical treatments for chronic/recurrent headache, *Cochrane Database Rev* (3), 2004. Ⓑ
7. Melchart D et al: Acupuncture for idiopathic headache, *Cochrane Database Rev* (1), 2001. Ⓑ
8. Vernon H et al: Systematic review of randomised clinical trials of complementary/alternative therapies in the treatment of tension-type and cervicogenic headache, *Complement Ther Med* 7:142-155, 1999. Ⓑ

SUGGESTED READINGS

Bendtsen L, Jensen R: Mirtazapine is effective in the prophylactic treatment of chronic tension-type headache, *Neurology* 62:1706, 2004.

Bronfort G et al: Non-invasive physical treatments for chronic/recurrent headache, *Cochrane Database Rev* 3, 2004.

Goadsby P: Headache (chronic tension-type), *BMJ* 12: 1808, 2004.

Headache Classification Committee of the International Headache Society: The international classification of headache disorders, *Cephalalgia* 24:1, 2004.

Holroyd KA et al: Management of chronic tension-type headache with tricyclic anti-depressant medication, stress management therapy, and their combination: a randomized controlled trial, *JAMA* 285(17):2208, 2001.

Jensen R: Pathophysiological mechanisms of tension-type headache: a review of epidemiological and experimental studies, *Cephalalgia* 19(6):602, 1999.

Lipton RB et al: Classification of primary headaches, *Neurology* 63:427, 2004.

Millea P, Brodie J: Tension-type headache, *Am Fam Physician* 66:797, 2002.

Silberstein, SD, Rosenberg, J: Multispecialty consensus on diagnosis and treatment of headache, *Neurology* 54:1553, 2000.

Zsombok T et al: Effect of autogenic training on drug consumption in patients with primary headache: an 8-month follow-up study, *Headache* 43:251, 2003.

AUTHOR: **RICHARD S. ISAACSON, M.D.**

Heart Block, Complete

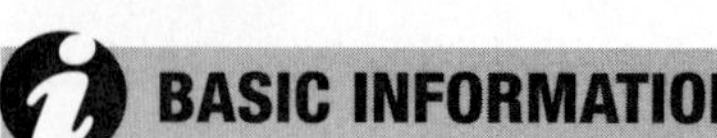

BASIC INFORMATION

DEFINITION

Complete heart block (CHB) is the absence of electrical impulse transmission from the atria to the ventricles.

SYNONYMS

Third-degree AV block

ICD-9CM CODES
426.0 Complete heart block

EPIDEMIOLOGY & DEMOGRAPHICS

- The prevalence of CHB is 0.04%.
- The prevalence of CHB increases with age.

PHYSICAL FINDINGS & CLINICAL PRESENTATION

Physical examination may be normal. Patients may present with the following clinical manifestations:

- Dizziness, palpitations
- Syncope or presyncope
- Fatigue, impaired exercise tolerance
- Mental status changes
- Congestive heart failure
- Angina pectoris
- Some patients may be asymptomatic (e.g., congenital CHB)

ETIOLOGY

- Fibrosis or sclerosis of the conduction system
- Acute myocardial infarction (may be seen in inferior or anterior wall MI)
- Drug effect (digitalis, calcium channel blockers, beta-blockers, amiodarone)
- Cardiomyopathy and myocarditis
- Infiltrative processes of the myocardium (amyloidosis, sarcoidosis, tumor)
- Metabolic abnormalities (hyperkalemia, hypoxia, hypothyroidism)
- Lyme carditis
- Neuromuscular disorders (Becker muscular dystrophy, myotonic muscular dystrophy)
- Congenital (birth from mothers with systemic lupus)
- Iatrogenic (cardiac surgery, catheter ablation of arrhythmias, percutaneous coronary intervention)

DIAGNOSIS

DIFFERENTIAL DIAGNOSIS

The differential diagnosis includes lesser degree of atrioventricular (AV) block, junctional rhythms, and nonconducted premature atrial contractions.

WORKUP

- Workup such as routine labs, cardiac biomarkers, and cardiac imaging should be dictated by the clinical circumstances.
- ECG: diagnostic of the disease (Fig. 1-138):
  - P waves are present with a regular atrial rate that is faster than the ventricular rate.
  - P waves are not related to the QRS complexes. The PR intervals are variable.
  - RR intervals are regular.
  - QRS complexes may be of normal width or abnormally wide, depending on the location of the block in the conduction system.

TREATMENT

ACUTE GENERAL Rx

- Initial treatment should focus on the hemodynamic stability and symptoms of the patient.
- Consider temporary pacemaker insertion if ventricular escape rate is slow (<40 beats per minute [bpm]) and associated with symptoms or hemodynamic compromise.
- Withdraw AV-nodal blocking agents if any.
- Atropine may be used to increase the rate of the escape rhythm.
- Isoproterenol may be used as a bridge to pacer insertion.
- Symptomatic CHB in the absence of a condition that is likely to resolve is an ACC/AHA/HRS Class I indication for permanent pacemaker placement.
- Class 1 indications for permanent pacing in asymptomatic patients according to the ACC/AHA guidelines include:
  - Patients in sinus rhythm, with documented asystolic pauses greater than or equal to 3.0 seconds or an escape rate less than 40 bpm, or with an escape rhythm that is below the AV node
  - Patients with atrial fibrillation and bradycardia with one or more pauses of at least 5 seconds or longer
  - After catheter ablation of the AV junction
  - If cardiomegaly or LV dysfunction is present or if the site of CHB is below the AV node
  - CHB after cardiac surgery block that is not expected to resolve
  - When it is associated with neuromuscular diseases, such as: Erb dystrophy (limb-girdle muscular dystrophy), Kearns-Sayre syndrome, myotonic muscular dystrophy, and peroneal muscular atrophy
  - CHB present during exercise in the absence of myocardial ischemia
- Therapy is directed toward the underlying etiology if there is a reversible source.

CHRONIC Rx

Patients with permanent pacemakers need regular follow-up and pacemaker monitoring to ensure proper device functioning.

DISPOSITION

- Prognosis is favorable after insertion of pacemaker and related to the underlying etiology of complete AV block (e.g., myocardial infarction, cardiomyopathy).
- Nonrandomized studies have shown that permanent pacemaker insertion improves survival in patients with CHB.

REFERRAL

All patients with CHB should be referred to a cardiologist for consideration of temporary and/or permanent pacemaker implantation.

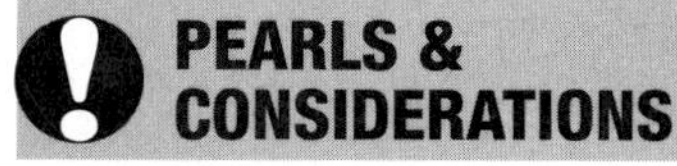

PEARLS & CONSIDERATIONS

COMMENTS

- Patients should be instructed to avoid activities that may damage the pacemaker (e.g., contact sports).
- Pacemaker manufacturers do not recommend any special restrictions regarding proximity to typical household items.
- The presence of a permanent pacemaker is a strong relative contraindication to MRI.

THIRD-DEGREE (COMPLETE) AV BLOCK

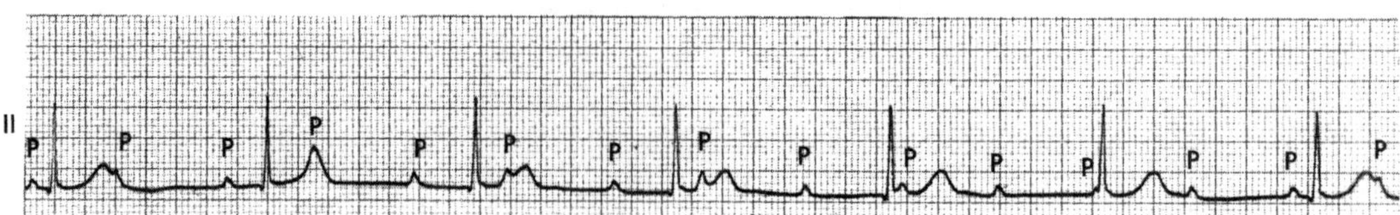

FIGURE 1-138 Third-degree complete atrioventricular heart block is characterized by independent atrial *(P)* and ventricular (QRS) activity. The atrial rate is always faster than the ventricular rate. The PR intervals are completely variable. Some P waves fall on the T wave, distorting its shape. Others may fall in the QRS complex and be "lost." Notice that the QRS complexes are of normal width, indicating that the ventricles are being paced from the atrioventricular junction. (From Goldberger AL [ed]: *Clinical electrocardiography,* ed 5, St Louis, 1994, Mosby.)

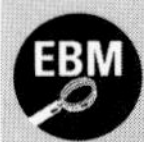

EVIDENCE

A systematic review comparing dual-chamber pacing and single-chamber ventricular pacing for adult patients with AV block, sick sinus syndrome, or both found a trend toward greater effectiveness with dual-chamber pacing compared with single-chamber ventricular pacing.[1]

However, a subsequent large, randomized, controlled trial that compared single-chamber and dual-chamber pacemaker implantation in elderly patients (>70 yr) with high-grade AV block found that the mode of pacing did not influence the all-cause mortality rate during the first 3 yr after implantation.[2]

Evidence-Based References

1. Dretzke J et al: Dual chamber versus single chamber ventricular pacemakers for sick sinus syndrome and atrioventricular block, *Cochrane Database Rev* 2, 2004.

2. Toff WD et al: Single-chamber versus dual-chamber pacing for high-grade atrioventricular block, *N Engl J Med* 353:145, 2005.

SUGGESTED READINGS

Epstein AE et al: ACC/AHA/HRS 2008. Guidelines for device-based therapy of cardiac rhythm abnormalities: a report of the American College of Cardiology/American Heart Association Task Force on Practice Guidelines (Writing Committee to Revise the ACC/AHA/NASPE 2002. Guideline Update for Implantation of Cardiac Pacemakers and Antiarrhythmia Devices): developed in collaboration with the American Association for Thoracic Surgery and Society of Thoracic Surgeons, *Circulation* 117:e350, 2008.

Kojic EM et al: The prevalence and prognosis of third-degree atrioventricular conduction block: the Reykjavik study, *J Intern Med* 246(1):81-86, 1999.

AUTHORS: **THOMAS J. EARL, M.D., FRED F. FERRI, M.D.,** and **WEN-CHIH WU, M.D.**

BASIC INFORMATION

DEFINITION

Second-degree heart block is the blockage of some (but not all) impulses from the atria to the ventricles. There are three types of second-degree atrioventricular (AV) block:

- Mobitz type I (Wenckebach):
  - There is a progressive prolongation of the PR interval before an impulse is completely blocked; the cycle repeats periodically.
  - Site of block is usually AV node (proximal to the bundle of His).
- Mobitz type II:
  - There is a sudden interruption of AV conduction without prior prolongation of the PR interval.
  - Site of block is usually infranodal.
- Advanced or high-degree second-degree block is the term used to describe the block of two or more consecutive P waves with some beats conducted (in contrast to third degree or complete heart block), indicating some preservation of AV conduction.
- 2:1 AV block:
  - Every other P wave is conducted in an alternate fashion.
  - It may become either a Mobitz I or II at faster atrial rates.

SYNONYMS

Wenckebach block (Mobitz type I block)
Mobitz type II block

ICD-9CM CODES
426.13 Mobitz type I
426.12 Mobitz type II

EPIDEMIOLOGY & DEMOGRAPHICS

Mobitz type I block is more common and may occur in individuals with heightened vagal tone or as a side effect of some medications, such as β-blockers or calcium channel blockers.

PHYSICAL FINDINGS & CLINICAL PRESENTATION

- Patients with Mobitz type I are usually asymptomatic.
- Sudden loss of consciousness without warning (Adams-Stokes attack) can occur in patients with Mobitz type II; however, it is much more common in patients with complete heart block.
- Irregular pulse with dropped beats is present (Mobitz type I).
- Irregular pulse with occasional dropped beats is present (Mobitz type II).

ETIOLOGY

- High vagal tone (young patients, athletes at rest)
- Degenerative changes in the AV conduction system
- Ischemia at the AV nodes (particularly in inferior wall myocardial infarction [MI])
- Drugs (digitalis, quinidine, procainamide, adenosine, calcium channel blockers, β-blockers)
- Cardiomyopathies
- Myocarditis (infectious, e.g., Lyme disease, and noninfectious, e.g., systemic lupus erythematosus)
- Hyperkalemia
- Hypothyroidism
- Cardiac valve surgery
- Catheter ablation for arrhythmias

Dx DIAGNOSIS

DIFFERENTIAL DIAGNOSIS

The ECG will distinguish between Mobitz type I and Mobitz type II block and other conduction abnormalities.

WORKUP

ECG, 24-hr Holter monitor (selected patients)

- Mobitz type I (Fig. 1-139) ECG shows:
  1. Gradual prolongation of PR interval leading to a blocked beat
  2. Shortened PR interval after dropped beat
  3. The cycle length with the dropped beat is less than the previous two cycle lengths.
  4. Usually see "grouped beating" pattern.
- Mobitz type II ECG shows:
  1. Fixed duration of PR interval
  2. Sudden appearance of blocked beats
- In 2:1 AV block, it cannot be determined based on the 12-lead EKG whether there is Mobitz type I or type II AV block, although a wide QRS complex is suggestive of Mobitz type II.

Rx TREATMENT

NONPHARMACOLOGIC THERAPY

Elimination of drugs that may induce AV block

ACUTE GENERAL Rx

Mobitz type I:

- Treatment is usually not necessary unless the resting heart rate is less than 40 beats per min while awake.
- If symptomatic (e.g., dizziness), atropine 1 mg (may repeat once after 5 min) may be tried to increase AV conduction; if no response, trial of dobutamine or isoproterenol may be helpful prior to insertion of temporary pacemaker.
- If block is the result of drugs (e.g., digitalis), discontinue the drug.
- If associated with anterior wall MI and wide QRS escape rhythm, consider insertion of a temporary pacemaker.
- Permanent pacemaker implantation is indicated for second-degree AV block with symptomatic bradycardia regardless of the site of the block.

Mobitz type II:

- Pacemaker insertion is usually needed if the patient is symptomatic or if the resting heart rate is less than 40 beats per min while awake because this type of block is usually permanent and often progresses to complete AV block.

DISPOSITION

Prognosis is good with insertion of a pacemaker.

REFERRAL

Referral for pacemaker insertion (see "Acute General Rx")

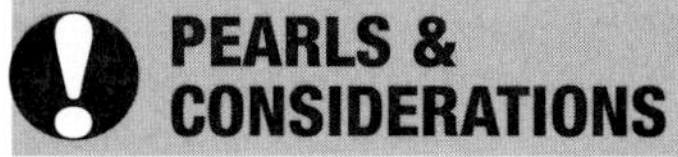

PEARLS & CONSIDERATIONS

COMMENTS

Patients with Mobitz type I should be followed up routinely for potential development of high-grade AV block.

SUGGESTED READINGS

Barold S, Hayes D: Second-degree atrioventricular block: a reappraisal, *Mayo Clin Proc* 76:44, 2001.

Epstein et al: ACC/AHA/HRS 2008. guidelines for device-based therapy of cardiac rhythm abnormalities, *J Am Coll Cardiol* 51:1-62, 2008.

AUTHORS: **SCOTT BRANCATO, M.D., FRED F. FERRI, M.D.,** and **WEN-CHIH WU, M.D.**

WENCKEBACH (MOBITZ TYPE I) SECOND-DEGREE AV BLOCK

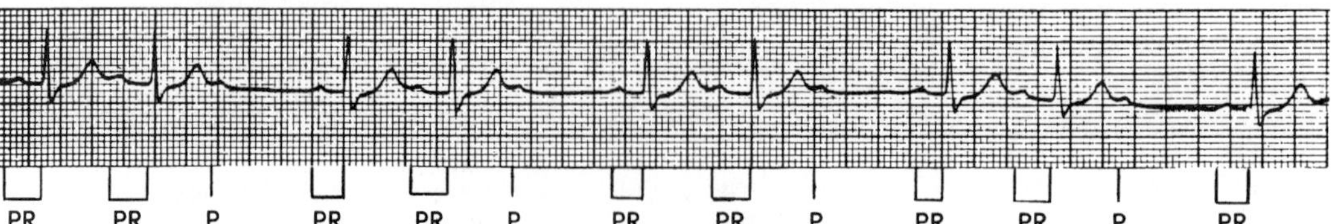

FIGURE 1-139 Wenckebach (Mobitz type I) second-degree atrioventricular block. Notice the progressive increase in PR intervals, with the third P wave in each sequence not followed by a QRS. Wenckebach block produces a characteristically syncopated rhythm with grouping of the QRS complexes (group beating). (From Goldberger AL [ed]: *Clinical electrocardiography,* ed 5, St Louis, 1994, Mosby.)

BASIC INFORMATION

DEFINITION

Heat exhaustion and heat stroke are part of a continuum of heat-related illness, and unless factors leading to heat exhaustion are corrected swiftly, affected patients can progress to heat stroke.

- Heat exhaustion: an illness resulting from prolonged, heavy activity in a hot environment with subsequent dehydration, electrolyte depletion, and rectal temperature >37.8° C but ≤40° C.
- Heat stroke: a life-threatening heat illness characterized by extreme hyperthermia, dehydration, and neurologic manifestations (core temperature >40° C).

SYNONYMS

Heat illness
Hyperthermia

ICD-9CM CODES
992.0 Heat stroke
992.5 Heat exhaustion

EPIDEMIOLOGY & DEMOGRAPHICS

INCIDENCE (IN U.S.): Incidence of heat stroke is approximately 20 cases/100,000 population.

PREDOMINANT AGE: Heat exhaustion and stroke occur more frequently in elderly patients, especially those taking diuretics or medications that impair heat dissipation (e.g., phenothiazines, anticholinergics, antihistamines, β-blockers).

PHYSICAL FINDINGS & CLINICAL PRESENTATION

Heat exhaustion:

- Generalized malaise, weakness, headache, muscle and abdominal cramps, nausea, vomiting, hypotension, tachycardia
- Rectal temperature is usually normal
- Sweating is usually present

Heat stroke:

- Neurologic manifestations (seizures, tremor, hemiplegia, coma, psychosis, other bizarre behavior)
- Evidence of dehydration (poor skin turgor, sunken eyeballs)
- Tachycardia, hyperventilation
- Skin is hot, red, and flushed
- Sweating is often (not always) absent, particularly in elderly patients

ETIOLOGY

- Exogenous heat gain (increased ambient temperature)
- Increased heat production (exercise, infection, hyperthyroidism, drugs)
- Impaired heat dissipation (high humidity, heavy clothing, neonatal or elderly patients, drugs [phenothiazines, anticholinergics, antihistamines, butyrophenones, amphetamines, cocaine, alcohol, β-blockers])
- Diuretics, laxatives

DIAGNOSIS

DIFFERENTIAL DIAGNOSIS

- Infections (meningitis, encephalitis, sepsis)
- Head trauma
- Epilepsy
- Thyroid storm
- Acute cocaine intoxication
- Malignant hyperthermia
- Heat exhaustion can be differentiated from heat stroke by the following:
    1. Essentially intact mental function and lack of significant fever in heat exhaustion
    2. Mild or absent increases in creatine phosphokinase (CPK), aspartate aminotransferase (AST), lactate dehydrogenase (LDH), and alanine aminotransferase (ALT) in heat exhaustion

WORKUP

- Heat stroke: comprehensive history, physical examination, and laboratory evaluation
- Heat exhaustion: in most cases, laboratory tests are not necessary for diagnosis

LABORATORY TESTS

Laboratory abnormalities may include the following:

- Elevated blood urea nitrogen, creatinine, hematocrit
- Hyponatremia or hypernatremia, hyperkalemia or hypokalemia
- Elevated LDH, AST, ALT, CPK, bilirubin
- Lactic acidosis, respiratory alkalosis (from hyperventilation)
- Myoglobinuria, hypofibrinogenemia, fibrinolysis, hypocalcemia

TREATMENT

- Treatment of heat exhaustion consists primarily of placing the patient in a cool, shaded area and providing rapid hydration and salt replacement.
    1. Fluid intake should be at least 2 L q4h in patients without history of CHF.
    2. Salt replacement can be accomplished by using one-quarter teaspoon of salt or two 10-grain salt tablets dissolved in 1 L of water.
    3. If IV fluid replacement is necessary, young athletes can be given normal saline IV (3 to 4 L over 6 to 8 hr); in elderly patients, consider using D5½NS IV with the rate titrated to cardiovascular status.
- Patients with heat stroke should undergo rapid cooling.
    1. Remove the patient's clothes and place the patient in a cool and well-ventilated room.
    2. If patient is unconscious, position on his or her side and clear the airway. Protect airway and augment oxygenation (e.g., nasal O_2 at 4 L/min to keep oxygen saturation >90%).
    3. Monitor body temperature every 5 min. Measurement of the patient's core temperature with a rectal probe is recommended. The goal is to reduce the body temperature to 39° C (102.2° F) in 30 to 60 min.
    4. Spray the patient with a cool mist and use fans to enhance airflow over the body (rapid evaporation method).
    5. Immersion of the patient in ice water, stomach lavage with iced saline solution, intravenous administration of cooled fluids, and inhalation of cold air are advisable only when the means for rapid evaporation are not available. Immersion in tepid water (15° C, 59° F) is preferred over ice water immersion to minimize risk of shivering.
    6. Use of ice packs on axillae, neck, and groin is controversial because they increase peripheral vasoconstriction and may induce shivering.
    7. Antipyretics are ineffective because the hypothalamic set point during heat stroke is normal despite the increased body temperature.
    8. Intubate a comatose patient, insert a Foley catheter, and start nasal O_2. Continuous ECG monitoring is recommended.
    9. Insert at least two large-bore IV lines and begin IV hydration with NS or Ringer's lactate.
    10. Draw initial laboratory studies: electrolytes, complete blood count, blood urea nitrogen, creatinine, AST, ALT, CPK, LDH, glucose, PT (INR), PTT, platelet count, Ca^{2+}, lactic acid, and arterial blood gases.
    11. Treat complications as follows:
        a. Hypotension: vigorous hydration with normal saline or Ringer's lactate.
        b. Convulsions: diazepam 5 to 10 mg IV (slowly).
        c. Shivering: chlorpromazine 10 to 50 mg IV.
        d. Acidosis: use bicarbonate judiciously (only in severe acidosis).
    12. Observe for evidence of rhabdomyolysis and hepatic, renal, or cardiac failure and treat accordingly.

DISPOSITION

Most patients recover completely within 48 hr. Central nervous system injury is permanent in 20% of cases. Mortality rate can exceed 30% in patients with prolonged and severe hyperthermia.

SUGGESTED READING

Glazer JL: Management of heat stroke and exhaustion, *Am Fam Physician* 71:2133, 2005.

AUTHOR: **FRED F. FERRI, M.D.**

Helicobacter Pylori Infection 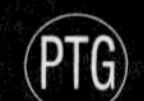

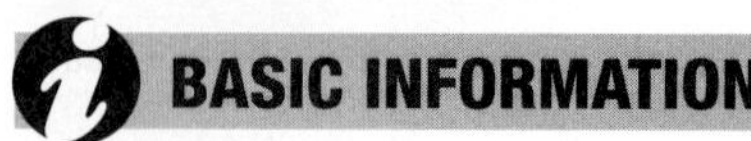

BASIC INFORMATION

DEFINITION

Infection of the human gastric mucosa with the organism *Helicobacter pylori,* a spiral-shaped gram-negative organism with unique features that allow it to survive in the hostile gastric environment.

SYNONYMS

Previously known as *Campylobacter pylori*

ICD-9CM CODES

041.86 *Helicobacter pylori (H. pylori)*

EPIDEMIOLOGY & DEMOGRAPHICS

H. pylori is the most common chronic bacterial infection in human beings, probably affecting 50% of the earth's population in all age groups and probably 30% to 40% of the U.S. population. Infection is acquired at an earlier age and occurs more frequently in developing nations.

CLINICAL PRESENTATION

- *H. pylori* causes histologic gastritis in all affected individuals. The majority of cases are asymptomatic and unlikely to proceed to serious consequences.
- *H. pylori* is a causative agent in peptic ulcer disease (PUD), gastric adenocarcinoma, and gastric mucosa-associated lymphoid tissue lymphoma, and may be a risk factor for iron-deficiency anemia and chronic idiopathic thrombocytopenic purpura. It may present with the signs and symptoms of these disorders, including abdominal pain, bloating, anorexia, and early satiety. Figure 1-140 describes association of *H. pylori* infection and disease states.
- Weight loss, dysphagia, protracted nausea or vomiting, anemia, melena, and palpable abdominal mass are "alarm symptoms" and should prompt more immediate and aggressive workup.

ETIOLOGY

- Route of acquisition is unknown but is presumed to be person to person by oral-oral or fecal-oral exposure.
- The majority of cases are acquired in childhood. Socioeconomic status and living conditions in childhood affect risk of acquisition of infection. These factors include housing density, number of siblings, overcrowding, sharing a bed, and lack of running water.
- *H. pylori* does not invade gastroduodenal tissue, but disrupts the mucous layer, causing the underlying mucosa to be more vulnerable to acid peptic damage.
- What differentiates the subset of patients with *H. pylori* who go on to develop ulcers or cancer remains unclear.

Dx DIAGNOSIS

DIFFERENTIAL DIAGNOSIS

- Infection with *H. pylori* should be considered in the face of PUD, gastric cancer, gastritis, and gastric MALT lymphoma.
- Upper gastrointestinal (GI) tract disease, including nonulcer dyspepsia, reflux esophagitis, biliary tract disease, gastroparesis, pancreatitis, and ischemic bowel, may be considered in the differential diagnosis of *H. pylori.*

WORKUP

- Workup is indicated in patients with active PUD, a past history of documented peptic ulcer, or gastric MALT lymphoma. A test-and-treat strategy may be used in patients <55 yr who have no alarm symptoms.
- The role of routine screening in high-risk population is not clear. However, numerous studies suggest that *H. pylori* eradication is protective against progression of premalignant lesions. Consider a test-and-treat approach in asymptomatic first-degree relatives of gastric cancer patients.
- Routine identification and treatment of *H. pylori* in cases of nonulcer dyspepsia, gastroesophageal reflux disease (GERD), nonsteroidal anti-inflammatory drug (NSAID) use, and in asymptomatic individuals in populations at high risk for gastric cancer is considered controversial, although it may be indicated in specific cases.
- Efficacy of testing is related to the individual patient's likelihood of *H. pylori* infection based on demographic risk factors. In the U.S. population increased probability of infection exists in African Americans, Hispanics/Latinos, immigrants from developing nations, patients with poor socioeconomic status, Native Americans from Alaska, and persons >50 yr.
- Routine screening for *H. pylori* is not indicated in asymptomatic patients who are at low risk of infection.
- There is no evidence that *H. pylori* causes symptoms of nonulcer dyspepsia.

LABORATORY TESTS

- Testing may be invasive or noninvasive depending on the need for endoscopy. There is no indication for endoscopy solely to diagnose *H. pylori.*
- Tests for *H. pylori* may be differentiated as active or passive. Active tests provide direct evidence that *H. pylori* infection is currently present and include urea breath testing and stool antigen testing. Passive testing, which includes all serologic testing for *H. pylori,* gives indirect evidence of its presence by detecting the presence of antibodies to the organism. Serologic testing is limited by its inability to distinguish between current, active infection and prior infection that has resolved.
- Tests that use urease as a marker (urea breath and stool antigen tests and biopsy for urease activity) may result in false-negative results in patients taking antibiotics, bismuth, or antisecretory therapy as well as those with active ulcer bleeding. Patients should be off

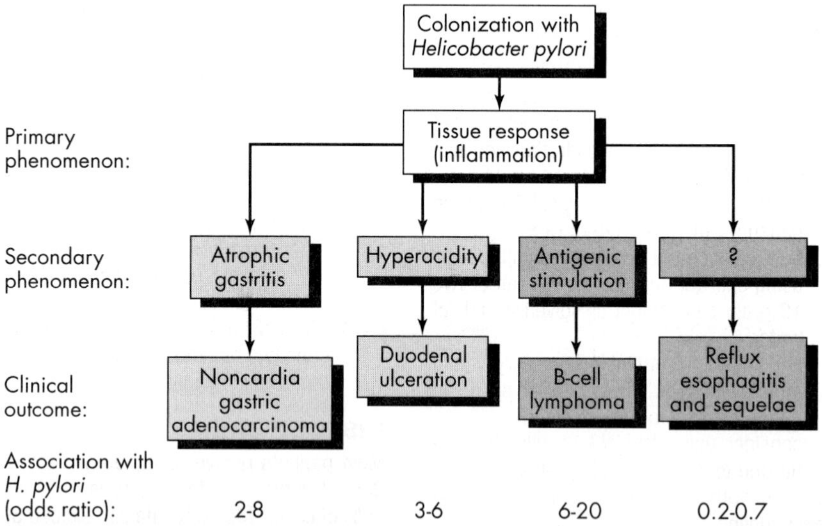

Colonization with *Helicobacter pylori*

Primary phenomenon: Tissue response (inflammation)

Secondary phenomenon: Atrophic gastritis | Hyperacidity | Antigenic stimulation | ?

Clinical outcome: Noncardia gastric adenocarcinoma | Duodenal ulceration | B-cell lymphoma | Reflux esophagitis and sequelae

Association with *H. pylori* (odds ratio): 2-8 | 3-6 | 6-20 | 0.2-0.7

FIGURE 1-140 Association of *Helicobacter pylori* colonization and disease states. After *H. pylori* acquisition, virtually all persons develop persistent colonization that lasts for life. Colonization induces tissue responses termed *chronic gastritis.* This process affects gastric physiology, including glandular structure, acid secretion, and antigen processing, which in turn affect disease risk. Colonization with *H. pylori* increases the risk for certain diseases (duodenal ulcer, gastric ulcer, noncardia gastric adenocarcinoma, and B-cell lymphomas) but appears to decrease the risk for gastroesophageal reflux disease and its complications, including Barrett's esophagus, and adenocarcinoma of the esophagus or gastric cardia. (Mandell GL et al: *Principles and practice of infectious diseases,* ed 7, Philadelphia, 2010, Elsevier.)

antibiotics for 4 wk and off protein pump inhibitors for 2 wk before urea breath or stool antigen testing.

- When diagnostic endoscopy is indicated (for suspicion or follow-up of PUD or gastric MALT), antral biopsy should be tested for urease activity. If urease testing is likely to show a false-negative result because of recent proton pump inhibitor (PPI), bismuth, or antibiotic use or active ulcer bleeding, the sample should undergo histologic examination.
- In cases in which biopsy is not indicated, urea breath testing or stool antigen testing are indicated to evaluate for active infection. The sensitivities and specificities of these two tests are similar (>90%). Urea breath testing is slightly more expensive than stool antigen testing, but both costs are in the modest range. Choice can be made based on patient preference and availability.
- Serologic testing may be useful in cases in whom the pretest probability of infection is high or when it is impractical or contraindicated to stop antisecretory therapy for the required duration. It cannot be used to document eradication of infection.

Rx TREATMENT

ACUTE GENERAL Rx

- Test only patients whom you intend to treat if positive (see "Workup" above). At this time, the value of eradicating *H. pylori* infection is proven in patients with PUD or gastric MALT lymphoma.
- The optimal antibiotic regimen has not been defined. In addition to efficacy, side effects, cost, and ease of administration must be considered.
- The following regimens are effective in 85% of patients (see Chey and Wong under "Suggested Reading" below for specific dosages):
  - PPI twice daily, with twice-daily clarithromycin and amoxicillin.
  - In cases of penicillin allergy, metronidazole may be substituted for amoxicillin. This may reduce effectiveness of treatment because metronidazole resistance has increased.
  - PPI twice daily, combined with bismuth four times daily, as well as tetracycline and metronidazole four times daily.
- Available data suggest that extending triple therapy beyond 7 days is unlikely to be a clinically useful strategy.
- Prior exposure to a macrolide or metronidazole, for any reason, is associated with increased resistance. A preferable regimen would include medications to which the patient has not been previously exposed.
- Diarrhea and abdominal cramping are commonly observed with many of the regimens. Other side effects may include a metallic taste with metronidazole or clarithromycin, neuropathy, seizures, and disulfiram-like reaction with metronidazole, diarrhea with amoxicillin, photosensitivity with tetracycline, and *Clostridium difficile* infection with any antibiotic exposure. Bismuth may cause black stool and constipation. Tetracycline is contraindicated in pregnant patients.
- 20% of patients may not respond to initial therapy. Optimal retreatment regimens are under investigation. Use either an alternative regimen with a different combination of medications or quadruple therapy consisting of twice-daily PPI and bismuth-based triple therapy. Levofloxacin-based triple therapy for persistent infections appears effective in international studies but has not been evaluated in U.S. studies. It is important to reinforce compliance.
- A 10-day sequential therapy has been reported to be superior to standard triple therapy for eradication of *H. pylori.* It consists of 5 days of treatment with a PPI and one antibiotic (usually amoxicillin) followed by 5-day treatment with the PPI and two other antibiotics (usually clarithromycin and metronidazole).

CHRONIC Rx

- Data do not support routine testing for cure. Accepted indications for testing to prove eradication include *H. pylori*–associated ulcers, MALT lymphoma, and early gastric cancer as well as those with persistent dyspepsia despite a test-and-treat management strategy.
- Serology does not reliably revert to undetectable levels after treatment and should not be used to determine eradication.
- Active tests (urea breath test and stool antigen testing) are preferable. They are equally accurate in confirming eradication, and either may be used depending on availability and patient preference. To reduce the likelihood of false-negative results, testing should be performed 4 wk after eradication therapy with PPI and antibiotics or 2 wk after the cessation of PPI therapy.

DISPOSITION

Consider further evaluation in patients with recurrent symptoms after appropriate treatment.

REFERRAL

- Patients with gastric MALT lymphoma should be followed by a gastroenterologist and oncologist with expertise in the care of lymphoid neoplasms.
- Patients with dyspepsia who have tested positive for *H. pylori* and been treated without resolution should be referred for endoscopy.
- Consider referral for biopsy for culture and sensitivity in patients who have not responded to two attempts at treatment.

PEARLS & CONSIDERATIONS

- Whether *H. pylori* eradication reduces the risk of gastric cancer is unclear.
- Outcomes in PUD and gastric MALT lymphoma are improved with treatment of associated *H. pylori* infection.
- Tests that provide direct evidence of active *H. pylori* infection (urea breath and stool antigen testing) are preferred but may result in false-negative results in patients taking antibiotics, bismuth, or antisecretory agents.
- Serologic testing does not differentiate active from prior infection. It may be useful when active tests are not indicated, particularly in high-risk patients.
- Be aware of high-risk populations in low-prevalence settings, including immigrants from Mexico, South America, Southeast Asia, and Eastern Europe.

EBM EVIDENCE

Please note: Complete text of EBM for this topic is available online.

Key trials and commentary:

This study sought to determine the cost effectiveness of *Helicobacter pylori* "test and treat" compared with empirical acid suppression in the initial management of patients with dyspepsia in primary care.

This study showed that test and treat and acid suppression are equally cost effective in the initial management of dyspepsia. Empirical acid suppression is an appropriate initial strategy. As costs are similar overall, general practitioners should discuss with patients at which point to consider *H. pylori* testing.[1] Ⓐ

U.S. guidelines currently recommend either empiric proton pump inhibitor [PPI] therapy or *H. pylori* testing and treatment as the initial management of dyspepsia when there are no alarm features. Canadian data have suggested that *H. pylori* test and treatment may be cost saving. This pragmatic, multicenter, primary care–based, randomized controlled trial assessed the cost-effectiveness of *H. pylori* test and treatment vs. empiric acid suppression. The study was of particularly high quality, and showed that testing and treating *H. pylori* at the initial consultation provided similar outcomes to acid-suppression therapy alone. Indeed, the costs were similar at 1 year for both strategies. Notably, those who were randomized to the *H. pylori* test and treatment arm but were *H. pylori* negative received the same treatment as those randomized to the empiric acid-suppression treatment arm (omeprazole 20 mg once daily for 1 month). Because only 29% of patients randomized to the test and treat arm were infected with *H. pylori*, the results of this trial may not apply to regions where the prevalence of *H. pylori* is higher. However, in relatively low *H. pylori* prevalence regions, either strategy provides similar outcomes, and the choice depends on the clinician's judgment. This reviewer believes that *H. pylori* test and treat makes the most sense, because those in the *H. pylori*–positive arm who have successful eradication will also have the additional benefit of unrecognized peptic ulcer disease being eliminated.

Evidence-Based Reference

1. Delaney BC et al: Helicobacter pylori test and treat versus proton pump inhibitor in initial management of dyspepsia in primary care: multicentre randomised controlled trial (MRC-CUBE trial), *BMJ* 336:651-654, 2008. Commentary by N. Talley, M.D. Ⓐ

SUGGESTED READINGS

Chey W, Wong B: American College of Gastroenterology guideline on the management of *Helicobacter pylori* infection, *Am J Gastroenterol* 102:1808, 2007.

Fuccio L et al: Meta-analysis: duration of first-line proton pump inhibitor-based triple therapy for helicobacter pylori eradication, *Ann Intern Med* 147: 553-562, 2008.

Jafri N et al: Meta-analysis: Sequential therapy appears superior to standard therapy for helicobacter pylori infection in patients naïve to treatment, *Ann Intern Med* 148:923-931, 2008.

Malfertheiner P et al: Current concepts in the management of *Helicobacter pylori* infection : the Maastricht III Consensus Report, *Gut* 56:772, 2007.

AUTHOR: **MARGARET TRYFOROS, M.D.**

BASIC INFORMATION

DEFINITION

The HELLP syndrome is a serious variant of preeclampsia. HELLP is an acronym for ***h***emolysis, ***e***levated ***l***iver function, and ***l***ow ***p***latelet count. It is the most frequently encountered microangiopathy of pregnancy. There are three classes of the syndrome based on the degree of maternal thrombocytopenia as a primary indicator of disease severity:

Class 1: Platelets 50,000/mm^3
Class 2: Platelets >50,000/mm^3 to 100,000/mm^3
Class 3: Platelets >100,000/mm^3

ICD-9CM CODES
642.50 HELLP, episode of care
642.51 HELLP, delivered
642.52 HELLP, delivered with postpartum complications
642.53 HELLP, antepartum complications
642.54 HELLP, postpartum complications

EPIDEMIOLOGY & DEMOGRAPHICS

- Among women with severe preeclampsia, 6% will manifest with one abnormality suggestive of HELLP syndrome, 12% will develop two abnormalities, and approximately 10% will develop all three.
- The HELLP syndrome, like preeclampsia, is rare before 20 wk of gestation.
- One third of all cases occur postpartum; of these, only 80% are typically diagnosed with preeclampsia before delivery.

RISK FACTORS: Women >35 yr, white, multiparity

RECURRENCE RATE: 3% to 25%

PHYSICAL FINDINGS & CLINICAL PRESENTATION

- Definitive laboratory criteria remain to be validated prospectively.
- Most commonly used criteria include hemolysis defined by the presence of an abnormal peripheral smear with schistocytes, lactate dehydrogenase (LDH) >600 U/L, and total bilirubin >1.2 mg/dl; elevated liver enzymes as serum aspartate aminotransferase (AST) >70 U/L and LDH >600 U/L; low platelet count as less than 100,000/mm^3.
- Although many women with HELLP syndrome are asymptomatic, 80% report right upper quadrant pain and 50% to 60% present with excessive weight gain and worsening edema.

ETIOLOGY

As with other microangiopathies, endothelial dysfunction, with resultant activation of the intravascular coagulation cascade, has been proposed as the central pathogenesis of HELLP syndrome.

Dx DIAGNOSIS

DIFFERENTIAL DIAGNOSIS

- Appendicitis
- Gallbladder disease
- Peptic ulcer disease
- Enteritis
- Hepatitis
- Pyelonephritis
- Systemic lupus erythematosus
- Thrombotic thrombocytopenic purpura/hemolytic-uremic syndrome
- Acute fatty liver of pregnancy

WORKUP

Because HELLP syndrome is a disease entity based on laboratory values, initial assessment is detailed below.

LABORATORY TESTS

- Initial assessment of suspected HELLP syndrome should include a complete blood count to evaluate platelets, urinalysis, serum creatinine, LDH, uric acid, indirect and total bilirubin levels, and AST/alanine aminotransferase (ALT).
- Tests of prothrombin time, partial thromboplastin time, fibrinogen, and fibrin split products are reserved for women with a platelet count well below 100,000/mm^3.

IMAGING STUDIES

No imaging modalities aid in diagnosis.

Rx TREATMENT

Treatment depends on gestational age of the fetus, severity of condition, and maternal status. Stabilization of the mother is the first priority.

ACUTE GENERAL Rx

- Assess gestational age thoroughly. Fetal status should be monitored with nonstress tests, contraction stress tests, and/or biophysical profile
- Maternal status should be evaluated by history, physical examination, and laboratory testing
- Magnesium sulfate is administered for seizure prophylaxis regardless of blood pressure
- Blood pressure control is achieved with agents such as hydralazine or labetalol
- Indwelling Foley catheter to monitor maternal volume status and urine output

CHRONIC Rx

- In pregnancies of 34 wk or with class 1 HELLP syndrome, delivery, either vaginal or abdominal, within 24 hr is the goal.
- In the preterm fetus corticosteroid therapy to enhance fetal lung maturation is indicated.
- Some reports have shown temporary amelioration of HELLP severity with the administration of high-dose steroids measured by increased urine output, improvement in platelet count, and liver function test.
- Judicious use of blood products, especially in those requiring surgery.
- The patient requires intensive observation for 48 hr postpartum; laboratory levels should begin to improve during this time.

DISPOSITION

The natural history of this disorder is a rapidly deteriorating condition requiring close monitoring of maternal and fetal well-being.

REFERRAL

Preterm patients with HELLP syndrome should be stabilized hemodynamically and transferred to a tertiary care center. Term patients can be treated at a local hospital depending on the availability of obstetric, neonatal, and blood banking services.

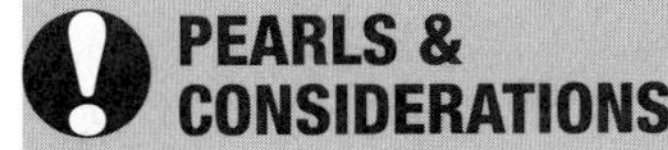

PEARLS & CONSIDERATIONS

Not all women with HELLP have hypertension or proteinuria.

SUGGESTED READINGS

Magann EF, Martin JN: Twelve steps to optimal management of HELLP syndrome, *Clin Obstet Gynecol* 42(3):532, 1999.

Norwitz ER et al: Acute complications of preeclampsia, *Clin Obstet Gynecol* 45(2):308, 2002.

AUTHORS: **SONYA S. ABDEL-RAZEQ, M.D.,** and **RUBEN ALVERO, M.D.**

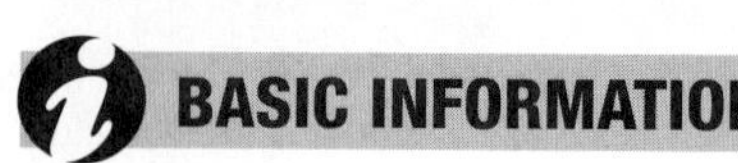

BASIC INFORMATION

DEFINITION

Hemochromatosis is an autosomal-recessive disorder characterized by increased accumulation of iron in various organs (adrenals, liver, pancreas, heart, testes, kidneys, pituitary) and eventual dysfunction of these organs if not treated appropriately.

SYNONYMS

Bronze diabetes

ICD-9CM CODES
275.0 Hemochromatosis

EPIDEMIOLOGY & DEMOGRAPHICS

INCIDENCE: In whites, approximately 1 in 385 persons.

PREDOMINANT SEX AND AGE:

Generally diagnosed in males in their fifth decade. Diagnosis in females is generally not made until 10 to 20 yr after menopause.

GENETICS:

Most common genetic disorder in North European ancestry. Homozygosity for the *C282Y* mutation is now found in approximately 5 of every 1000 persons of European descent.

PHYSICAL FINDINGS & CLINICAL PRESENTATION

- In earlier stages patients completely asymptomatic and diagnosed due to abnormal laboratory tests
- Hepatic dysfunction leading to hepatomegaly, fibrosis, and eventually cirrhosis
- Arthritis
- Gonadal insufficiency leading to loss of libido and testicular atrophy
- Diabetes mellitus: risk greater in patients with family history
- Iron-induced cardiac disease resulting in cardiomyopathy, heart failure, and arrhythmias
- Skin pigmentation

ETIOLOGY

- The majority of the patients diagnosed with hemochromatosis have mutation in the *HFE* gene and are either homozygous for the *C282Y* mutation *(C282Y/C282Y)* or compound heterozygote for the *C282Y* mutation and either the mutation *H63D (C282Y/H63D)* or less commonly the *S65C (C282Y/S65C)*.
- The remainder of the patients are classified as non–*HFE*-associated hemochromatosis.

Dx DIAGNOSIS

DIFFERENTIAL DIAGNOSIS

- Hereditary anemias with defect of erythropoiesis
- Cirrhosis
- Repeated blood transfusions
- The various causes of iron overload are described in Section II

WORKUP

Medical history, physical examination, and laboratory evaluation should be focused on affected organ systems (see "Physical Findings & Clinical Presentation"). Liver biopsy is the gold standard for diagnosis; it reveals iron deposition in hepatocytes, bile ducts, and supporting tissues.

LABORATORY TESTS

- Transferrin saturation is the best screening test. Values >45% are an indication for further testing.
- Elevated serum ferritin is good evidence of iron overload, but other causes like chronic inflammatory conditions, malignancy, and so forth needs to be ruled out as ferritin is also an acute phase reactant.
- Genotypical screening for *C282Y* and *H63D* mutation in *HFE* gene should be done in patients with high transferring saturation, elevated ferritin, or both.
- Liver biopsy is the gold standard but is not needed in somebody who has a persistently elevated transferring saturation, elevated ferritin, or both.
- Hepatic iron index can help differentiate between various causes of iron overload.
- Elevated aspartate aminotransferase, alanine aminotransferase, and alkaline phosphatase are seen.
- Hyperglycemia is found.
- Endocrine abnormalities (decreased testosterone, luteinizing hormone, follicle-stimulating hormone) are noted.

IMAGING STUDIES

Routine radiologic imaging is not needed.

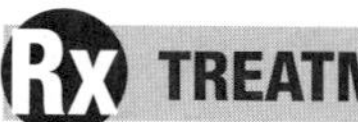

TREATMENT

The goal of therapy is the removal of excess iron and maintaining it at a normal or near normal level.

NONPHARMACOLOGIC THERAPY

Phlebotomy is the treatment of choice.

ACUTE GENERAL Rx

- The timing and frequency of phlebotomy needs to be individualized for each patient.
- For patients with heavy iron overload twice weekly phlebotomies should be started.
- The effectiveness of treatment is monitored by periodic ferritin measurement. The goal is to bring ferritin level below 50 μg.
- Patients with iron overload due to transfusion dependent anemias may not tolerate phlebotomy. For these patients iron chelation may be needed.
- The chelating agent deferoxamine has to be given daily as a 9 to 12 hr IV or SC infusion and compliance is difficult.
- An oral chelating agent deferasirox (Exjade) was approved by the FDA in 2005.

CHRONIC Rx

After the ferritin has been brought to less than 50 μg, phlebotomy is needed on a prn basis to keep the ferritin at that level.

DISPOSITION

Prognosis is good if phlebotomy is started early (before onset of cirrhosis or diabetes mellitus); women can have the full phenotypic expression of the disease, including cirrhosis, and should also be aggressively treated.

REFERRAL

For liver biopsy if diagnosis is uncertain

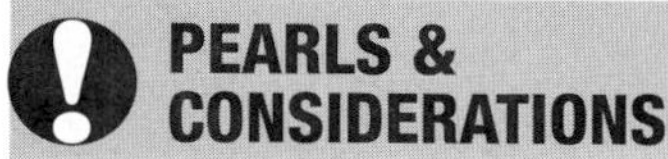

PEARLS & CONSIDERATIONS

COMMENTS

- Patients with hemochromatosis and serum ferritin levels <1000 μg/L are unlikely to have cirrhosis. Liver biopsy to screen for cirrhosis may be unnecessary in such patients.
- Cirrhotic patients must be periodically monitored (ultrasound or CT scan) because of their increased risk of hepatocellular carcinoma.
- *HFE* gene testing for *C282Y* mutation is a cost-effective method of screening relatives of patients with hereditary hemochromatosis. The American College of Gastroenterology recommends genotyping persons who have abnormal iron screening tests and first-degree relatives of those identified with *C282Y* homozygosity.
- Established cirrhosis, hypogonadism, destructive arthritis, and insulin-dependent diabetes mellitus secondary to hemochromatosis cannot be reversed with repeated phlebotomy, but their progress can be slowed.
- In patients who are heterozygotes for *C282Y* or *H63D* mutation, clinically meaningful iron overload does not develop.

SUGGESTED READINGS

Allen KJ et al: Iron-overload related disease in HFE hereditary hemochromatosis, *N Engl J Med* 358:221-230, 2008.

Phatak P et al: Hereditary hemochromatosis: time for targeted screening, *Ann Intern Med* 149:270, 2008.

Whitlock EP et al: Screening for hereditary hemochromatosis: a systematic review for the US Preventive Services task force, *Ann Intern Med* 145:209, 2006.

AUTHORS: **BILAL H. NAQVI M.D.,** and **FRED F. FERRI, M.D.**

BASIC INFORMATION

DEFINITION

Hemolytic-uremic syndrome (HUS) refers to an acute syndrome characterized by microangiopathic hemolytic anemia, thrombocytopenia, and severe renal failure.

SYNONYMS

HUS

ICD-9CM CODES

283.11 Hemolytic-uremic syndrome

EPIDEMIOLOGY & DEMOGRAPHICS

- HUS affects mainly children younger than 5 yr with incidence rate of 6.1 cases/100,000.
- Overall incidence is 1 to 2 cases/100,000.
- May be epidemic, most commonly occurring during the summer months in rural populations.
- Most common cause of acute renal failure in children.
- In the U.S., 300 to 700 new cases occur each year.

PHYSICAL FINDINGS & CLINICAL PRESENTATION

- HUS usually preceded by diarrhea in 90% of cases, bloody in 75%
- Abdominal pain, vomiting, and fever
- Neurologic symptoms principally seizure and somnolence were observed in 20% to 25% of cases. Stroke or coma: may occur and associated with significant mortality
- Hypertension
- Hepatomegaly and abnormality in liver function tests
- Anuria or oliguria
- Glucose intolerance and transient diabetes (10%)

ETIOLOGY

Pathologically, it is thought that thrombin generation (probably the result of accelerated thrombogenesis) and inhibition of fibrinolysis leads to renal arteriolar and capillary microthrombi preceding renal injury.

In children:

- *Escherichia coli* serotype 0157:H7 is the leading cause of HUS.
- The infection is acquired by eating undercooked red meat, nonpasteurized milk or milk products, water, fruits, or vegetables.
- Other causes of HUS in children and adults are:
  - Drugs (cyclosporine, mitomycin, tacrolimus, ticlopidine, clopidogrel, cisplatin, quinine, penicillin, penicillamine, oral contraceptives, and quinine used to treat muscle cramps) and toxins
  - Infection (*Salmonella, Shigella, Yersinia,* Group A streptococci, *Clostridium difficile, Campylobacter,* coxsackievirus, rubella, influenza virus, Epstein-Barr virus)
  - HIV-associated thrombotic microangiopathy
  - Pneumococcal infection
- Complement disorders involving factors H, I, and membrane cofactors protein have been associated with cases of nondiarrhea-associated HUS (atypical HUS).
- Mutations that impair the function of thrombomodulin occur in about 5% of patients with atypical HUS.

DIAGNOSIS

The triad of thrombocytopenia, acute renal failure, and microangiopathic hemolytic anemia establishes the diagnosis of HUS.

DIFFERENTIAL DIAGNOSIS

The differential is vast, including all causes of bloody and nonbloody diarrhea because the GI symptoms usually precede the triad of HUS:

- Thrombotic thrombocytopenic purpura
- Disseminated intravascular coagulation
- Prosthetic valve hemolysis
- Malignant hypertension
- Vasculitis
- Catastrophic antiphospholipid syndrome.
- Postpartum acute renal failure.
- Scleroderma renal crisis

WORKUP

The workup for suspected HUS patients includes blood tests and stool cultures.

LABORATORY TESTS

- Anemia (hemoglobin $<$8 g/dl) with peripheral smear shows the hallmark microangiopathic hemolytic anemia with schistocytes, burr cells, and helmet cells
- Thrombocytopenia (platelet counts usually $<$60,000/mm^3)
- Reticulocyte count high
- LDH level elevated
- Haptoglobin low
- Indirect bilirubin elevated
- Negative Coombs test
- BUN and creatinine elevated
- Urinalysis: proteinuria, microscopic hematuria, and pyuria
- Stool cultures for *E. coli* 0157:H7 are positive in more than 90% of cases if obtained during the first week of illness. After the first week only one third positive

IMAGING STUDIES

Imaging studies are not very helpful in the diagnosis of HUS.

TREATMENT

The treatment of HUS is primarily supportive.

NONPHARMACOLOGIC THERAPY

- Blood transfusions are used for severe anemia.
- Antibiotics and antimotility should be avoided and are not indicated for the treatment of *E. coli* 0157:H7.
- Correction of electrolyte abnormalities and fluid management should be performed.
- Platelet transfusion is preserved only for patients with HUS who have significant bleed or invasive procedure is required.
- Although unproven in patients with HUS, plasma exchange has been used in patients with severe CNS involvement.
- Tissue-type plasminogen activator (PAI-1) may have a role in improving renal function in recent studies.

ACUTE GENERAL Rx

Hypertension and seizure control

CHRONIC Rx

For anuric or oliguric renal failure, dialysis may be required.

DISPOSITION

- Adults presenting with HUS have a worse prognosis than do children with HUS.
- Mortality rate is less than 5%.
- Morbidity includes:
  - Proteinuria (31%)
  - Renal insufficiency (31%)
  - Hypertension (6%)

REFERRAL

- The local health department should be notified if the bacteria *E. coli* 0157:H7 has been isolated; large food-borne outbreaks have occurred with commercial beef products and asparagus.
- Consultation with hematology and nephrology specialist is recommended in patients with HUS.

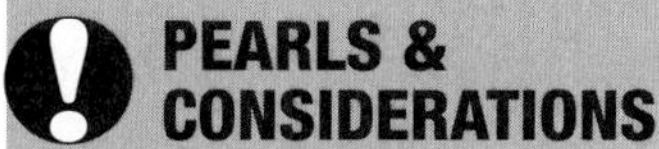

PEARLS & CONSIDERATIONS

COMMENTS

- Children testing positive for the *E. coli* 0157:H7 serotype should not return to school or day care facilities until two consecutive stools test negative for the microorganism.
- *E. coli* 0157:H7 can be transmitted from person to person; therefore universal precautions and hand washing are recommended in preventing the spread of the infection.

SUGGESTED READINGS

Delvaeye M et al: Thrombomodulin mutations in atypical hemolytic-uremic syndrome, *N Engl J Med* 361: 345-357, 2009.

Noris M, Remuzzi G: Atypical hemolytic-uremic syndrome, *N Engl J Med* 361:1676-1678, 2009.

Razzaq S: Hemolytic uremic syndrome: an emerging health risk, *Am Fam Physician* 74:991, 2006.

Zipfel PF, Skerka C: Complement dysfunction in hemolytic uremic syndrome, *Curr Opin Rheumatol* 18(5): 548, 2006.

AUTHORS: **MONZR M. AL MALKI, M.D., GLENN G. FORT, M.D., M.P.H.,** and **DENNIS J. MIKOLICH, M.D.**

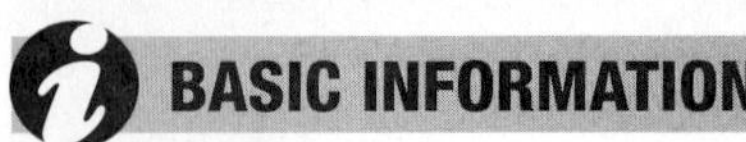

BASIC INFORMATION

DEFINITION

Hemophilia is a hereditary bleeding disorder caused by low factor VIII coagulant activity (hemophilia A) or low levels of factor IX coagulant activity (hemophilia B).

SYNONYMS

Hemophilia A: Classic hemophilia, factor VIII deficiency hemophilia

Hemophilia B: Christmas disease, factor IX hemophilia

ICD-9CM CODES
286.0 Hemophilia A
286.1 Hemophilia B

EPIDEMIOLOGY & DEMOGRAPHICS

INCIDENCE/PREVALENCE (IN U.S.): Hemophilia A: 100 cases per 1 million males; hemophilia B: 20 cases per 1 million males. Approximately 400,000 patients have severe hemophilia worldwide.

GENETIC: Both hemophilias have an X-linked recessive pattern of inheritance with only males affected.

PHYSICAL FINDINGS & CLINICAL PRESENTATION

- The clinical features of hemophilia A and B are generally indistinguishable from each other.
- Bleeding is most commonly seen in joints (knees, ankles, elbows), resulting in hot, swollen, painful joints and subsequent crippling joint deformity.
- Bleeding can also occur into the muscles and the gastrointestinal tract.
- Compartment syndrome can occur from large hematomas.
- Hematuria may be present.

ETIOLOGY

- Hemophilia A: low factor VIII coagulant (VIII:C) activity; can be classified as mild if factor VIII:C levels are >5%, moderate if levels are 1% to 5%, and severe if levels are <1%.
- Hemophilia B: low levels of factor IX coagulant activity.
- Both disorders are congenital.
- Spontaneous acquisition of factor VIII inhibitors (acquired hemophilia) is rare.

Dx DIAGNOSIS

DIFFERENTIAL DIAGNOSIS

- Other clotting factor deficiencies
- Platelet function disorders
- Vitamin K deficiency

WORKUP

Patients with mild hemophilia bleed only in response to major trauma or surgery and may not be diagnosed until young adulthood. Diagnostic workup includes laboratory evaluation (see "Laboratory Tests").

LABORATORY TESTS

- Partial thromboplastin time (PTT) is prolonged.
- Reduced factor VIII:C level distinguishes hemophilia A from other causes of prolonged PTT.
- Factor VIII antigen, prothrombin time, fibrinogen level, and bleeding time are normal.
- Factor IX coagulant activity levels are reduced in patients with hemophilia B.
- Coagulation factor activity measurement is useful to correlate with disease severity. Normal range is 50 to 150 U/dl; 5 to 20 U/dl indicates mild disease, 2 to 5 U/dl indicates moderate disease, and <2 U/dl indicates severe disease with spontaneous bleeding episodes.

Rx TREATMENT

NONPHARMACOLOGIC THERAPY

- Avoidance of contact sports
- Patient education regarding the disease; promotion of exercises such as swimming
- Avoidance of aspirin or other NSAIDs
- Orthopedic evaluation and physical therapy evaluation in patients with joint involvement
- Hepatitis vaccination

ACUTE GENERAL Rx

Hemophilia A:

- Reversal and prevention of acute bleeding in hemophilia A and B are based on adequate replacement of deficient or missing factor protein.
- The choice of the product for replacement therapy is guided by availability, capacity, concerns, and cost. Recombinant factors cost two to three times as much as plasma-derived factors, and the limited capacity to produce recombinant factors often results in periods of shortage. In the U.S., 60% of patients with severe hemophilia use recombinant products.
- Factor VIII concentrates are effective in controlling spontaneous and traumatic hemorrhage in severe hemophilia. The new recombinant factor VIII is stable without added human serum albumin (decreased risk of transmission of infectious agents).
- Recombinant activated factor VII is useful to stop spontaneous hemorrhages and prevent excessive bleeding during surgery in 75% of patients with inhibitors. Recommended dose is 90 μg/mg of body weight every 2 to 3 hr for treatment of life-threatening hemorrhage. It is, however, very expensive ($1 per μg).
- Desmopressin acetate 0.3 μg/kg q24h (causes release of factor VIII:C) may be used in preparation for minor surgical procedures in mild hemophiliacs.
- Aminocaproic acid (EACA, Amicar) 4 g PO q4h can be given for persistent bleeding that is unresponsive to factor VIII concentrate or desmopressin.

Hemophilia B:

- Infuse factor IX concentrates. It is important to remember that factor IX concentrates contain other proteins that may increase the risk of thrombosis with recurrent use. Therefore factor IX concentrates must be used only when clearly indicated.
- Daily administration of oral cyclophosphamide and prednisone without empirical factor VIII therapy is an effective and well-tolerated treatment for acquired hemophilia.

CHRONIC Rx

- The aim of chronic treatment is to prevent spontaneous bleeding and excessive bleeding during any surgical intervention.
- Prophylaxis with recombinant factor VIII can prevent joint damage and decrease the frequency of joint and other hemorrhages in young boys with severe hemophilia A. The estimated annual cost for treatment of one patient with recombinant factor VIII is $300,000.
- Implantation of genetically altered fibroblasts that produce factor VIII is safe and well tolerated. This form is feasible in patients with severe hemophilia. Hemophilia will likely be the first common, severe genetic disease to be cured by gene therapy.

DISPOSITION

- Despite the advent of virally safe blood products and blood treatment programs, nearly 70% of hemophiliacs are HIV seropositive. Survival is of normal expectancy in HIV-negative patients with mild disease.
- Intracranial bleeds are the second most common cause of death in hemophiliacs after AIDS. They are fatal in 30% of patients, occur in 10% of patients, and are generally the result of trauma.

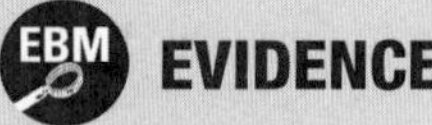

EVIDENCE

Please note: Complete text of EBM for this topic is available online.

SUGGESTED READING

Manco-Johnson MJ et al: Prophylaxis versus episodic treatment to prevent joint disease in boys with severe hemophilia, *N Engl J Med* 357:535, 2007.

AUTHOR: **FRED F. FERRI, M.D.**

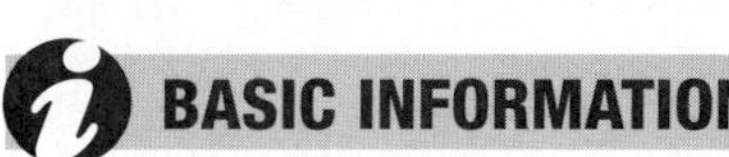

BASIC INFORMATION

DEFINITION

Coughing up of blood originating from the lower respiratory tract, ranging from blood-streaked sputum to gross blood. If greater than 100 to 600 ml in 24 hours, considered massive hemoptysis

ICD-9CM CODES
786.3 Hemoptysis

EPIDEMIOLOGY & DEMOGRAPHICS

INCIDENCE: Unknown, varies based on underlying pathology

RISK FACTORS: Tobacco smoking predisposes to lung cancer, a common cause of hemoptysis. Free-base ("crack") cocaine has been associated with diffuse alveolar hemorrhage. Anticoagulation can worsen bleeding.

PHYSICAL FINDINGS & CLINICAL PRESENTATION

- Presentation of hemoptysis is variable and can range from minimal blood-tinged sputum to more than 500 ml of gross blood in 24 hr. Other symptoms depend on the underlying etiology and can include cough, sputum production, fever, shortness of breath, weight loss, night sweats, wheezing, and chest pain.
- There are no specific exam findings, but clues to the etiology may be present, for example, focal wheezing, rhonchi or rales on pulmonary exam, murmur of mitral stenosis on cardiac exam.

ETIOLOGY

- There are many potential causes of hemoptysis including airway disease (bronchitis, bronchiectasis, lung neoplasm), infection (necrotizing pneumonia, lung abscess, tuberculosis, fungal infection), inflammatory diseases (Wegener's granulomatosis, Goodpasture's syndrome, lupus), cardiac disease (mitral stenosis after rheumatic heart disease, congenital heart diseases), and others (pulmonary embolism, cocaine use, foreign body, airway trauma, iatrogenic and cryptogenic).
- In one study of 208 patients, the most common causes of hemoptysis were bronchiectasis, lung cancer, bronchitis, and pneumonia, respectively.

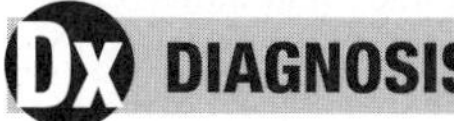

DIAGNOSIS

DIFFERENTIAL DIAGNOSIS

- Various potential causes of lower respiratory tract bleeding
  - Airway disease (bronchitis, bronchiectasis, lung neoplasm)
  - Infection (necrotizing pneumonia, lung abscess, tuberculosis, fungal infection)
  - Inflammatory diseases (Wegener's granulomatosis, Goodpasture's syndrome, lupus)
  - Cardiac disease (mitral stenosis after rheumatic heart disease, congenital heart diseases)
  - Pulmonary embolism
  - Cocaine use
  - Foreign body
  - Airway trauma
- Bleeding from upper respiratory tract
- Hematemesis
- Coagulopathy

WORKUP

Complete history and physical exam may suggest a particular etiology, important to ask about duration and quantity of hemoptysis and smoking history.

LABORATORY TESTS

- Complete blood count
- Coagulation profile
- Serum chemistries including creatinine, urinalysis (these latter studies if pulmonary-renal syndromes are in the differential)
- Arterial blood gas to assess oxygenation
- Sputum for cultures and cytologic studies

IMAGING STUDIES

- Chest x-ray: all patients with hemoptysis should have a chest x-ray but will likely need additional studies to localize site of bleeding.
- Chest CT: chest CT scan combined with flexible bronchoscopy has the highest yield for localizing the site of bleeding.

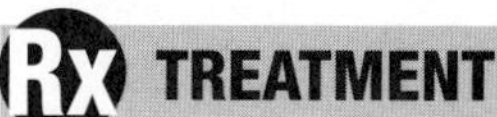

TREATMENT

Varies based on underlying etiology and nonmassive versus massive hemoptysis

NONPHARMACOLOGIC THERAPY

Massive hemoptysis:

- Arteriographic embolization of bronchial arteries and/or collateral systemic vessels
- Surgical resection of affected lung

ACUTE GENERAL Rx

Massive hemoptysis:

- Stabilize hemodynamic status and oxygenation.
- Reverse any coagulopathy.
- If site of bleeding is known, place patient with bleeding lung in dependent position to prevent blood from spilling into nonaffected lung.
- Bronchoscopic lavage with iced saline or topical application of epinephrine can be tried as a temporizing measure.
- Bronchoscopic balloon tamponade of bleeding site can be used as temporizing measure.
- Early consultation with interventional radiology and thoracic surgery for definitive intervention is recommended.

Nonmassive hemoptysis:

For nonmassive hemoptysis, identify and treat underlying condition. Referral to pulmonologist or hematologist if indicated.

CHRONIC Rx

For patients requiring anticoagulation or antiplatelet therapy for another disorder, consider risks/benefits of continued anticoagulation or antiplatelet therapy.

DISPOSITION

Generally, patients have a good prognosis after an episode of hemoptysis, but those with massive bleeding and/or malignancy tend to have a poorer prognosis.

SUGGESTED READINGS

Hirshberg B et al: Hemoptysis: etiology, evaluation and outcome in a tertiary referral hospital, *Chest* 112;440-444, 1997.

Khalil A et al: Severe hemoptysis of pulmonary arterial origin, *Chest* 133;212-219, 2008.

AUTHOR: **SARAH TAPYRIK, M.D.**

BASIC INFORMATION

DEFINITION

A hemorrhoid is a varicose dilation of a vein of the superior or inferior hemorrhoidal plexus, resulting from a persistent increase in venous pressure. External hemorrhoids are below the pectinate line (inferior plexus). Internal hemorrhoids are above the pectinate line (superior plexus) (Fig. 1-141).

SYNONYMS

Piles

ICD-9CM CODES

455.6 Hemorrhoids

EPIDEMIOLOGY & DEMOGRAPHICS

Potential for development of symptomatic hemorrhoids in all adults

PREVALENCE: Estimated 50% of the adult population in the U.S.

PREDOMINANT SEX: Males and females affected equally

PHYSICAL FINDINGS & CLINICAL PRESENTATION

- Painless bleeding with defecation; bleeding is bright red and staining on toilet paper
- Perianal irritation
- Mucofecal staining of underclothes
- Acute external hemorrhoids: painful, swollen, and often thrombosed
- Pain on sitting, standing, or defecating (thrombosed hemorrhoid)
- Prolapse
- Constipation

ETIOLOGY

- Low-fiber, high-fat diet
- Chronic constipation and straining with defecation
- High resting anal sphincter pressures
- Pregnancy
- Obesity
- Rectal surgery (i.e., episiotomy)
- Prolonged sitting
- Anal intercourse

DIAGNOSIS

DIFFERENTIAL DIAGNOSIS

- Fissure
- Abscess
- Anal fistula
- Condylomata acuminata
- Hypertrophied anal papillae
- Rectal prolapse
- Rectal polyp
- Neoplasm

WORKUP

- Inspection
- Digital rectal examination
- Anoscopy
- Sigmoidoscopy

TREATMENT

NONPHARMACOLOGIC THERAPY

- Avoidance of constipation and straining with defecation
- Avoidance of prolonged sitting on toilet
- High-fiber diet (20 to 30 g/day)
- Increased fluid intake (6 to 8 glasses of water per day)
- Cleaning with mild soap and water after defecation
- Warm soaks or ice to soothe
- Sitz baths

ACUTE GENERAL Rx

- Fiber supplements to provide bulk (psyllium extracts or mucilloids)
- Medicated compresses with witch hazel
- Topical hydrocortisone (1%-3% cream or ointment)
- Topical anesthetic spray
- Glycerin suppositories
- Stool softeners
- Surgically remove during first 72 hr after onset

CHRONIC Rx

- Rubber-band ligation
- Injection sclerotherapy
- Photocoagulation
- Cryodestruction
- Hemorrhoidectomy
- Anal dilation
- Laser or cautery hemorrhoidectomy
- Observance for complications: thrombosis, bleeding, infection, anal stenosis or weakness

DISPOSITION

Should resolve, but there is a high rate of recurrence

REFERRAL

To colorectal or general surgeon for any hemorrhoid that does not respond to conservative therapy

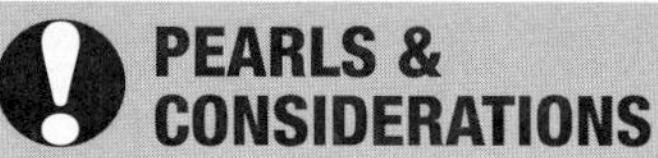

PEARLS & CONSIDERATIONS

COMMENTS

- Patients need to understand the importance of a healthy diet, regular exercise, and rectal hygiene.
- Stress the importance of avoiding prolonged sitting and straining on the toilet.
- Stress the need not to defer the urge to defecate.

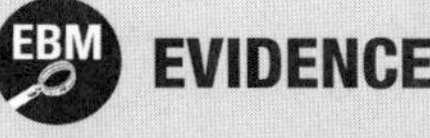

EVIDENCE

Please note: Complete text of EBM for this topic is available online.

Key trials and commentary:

Thrombosed external hemorrhoids are one of the most frequent anorectal emergencies. They are associated with swelling and intense pain. Internal sphincter hypertonicity plays a role in the etiology of the pain. This study evaluated the efficacy and safety of an intrasphincteric injection of botulinum toxin for pain relief in patients with thrombosed external hemorrhoids.

This study showed that a single injection of botulinum toxin into the anal sphincter seems to be effective in rapidly controlling the pain associated with thrombosed external haemorrhoids, and could represent an effective conservative treatment for this condition.

Thrombosed external hemorrhoids are a common cause of severe perianal pain. The intensity of the pain is often determined by the size and extent of the thrombosis and the time from the inciting event. A constant finding is the marked severity of pain at the outset. Treatment for the condition varies from ice packs to emergent excision in either an emergency department or an operating room.

Patti and colleagues from the University of Palermo performed a randomized trial to examine the effect of intrasphincteric botulinum toxin injection in patients with thrombosed

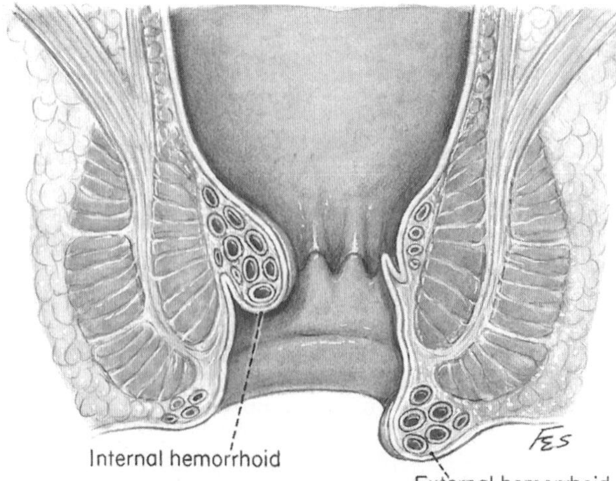

FIGURE 1-141 Anatomy of internal and external hemorrhoids. (From Noble J [ed]: *Textbook of primary care medicine,* ed 2, St Louis, 1996, Mosby.)

external hemorrhoids. They noted rapid control of pain when the toxin was injected when compared with saline controls.

Strengths of this study include its prospective design and inclusion of appropriate controls (saline injected). Additionally, pain control was carefully monitored. An important finding was a significant reduction in the time to return to work in the botulinum toxin group. Surprisingly, anal manometry was tolerated before treatment. In my experience, many of these patients would refuse this evaluation because of the severity of pain.

Study weaknesses include the lack of information concerning the time from onset of symptoms until injection treatment. Additionally, direct injection into the internal sphincter can be somewhat challenging in the office, and it is occasionally difficult to be certain if the toxin is inserted directly into the sphincter rather than extrasphincteric tissue. Finally, there was no significant difference in clot resorption between the two groups.

In summary, the injection of botulinum toxin appears to be effective in reducing pain in patients with thrombosed external hemorrhoids. Other institutions are encouraged to perform similar trials in larger numbers of patients with the hope of replicating these excellent results.[1] Ⓐ

A separate study sought to evaluate the short-term outcomes of hemorrhoidectomy performed using the LigaSure vessel-sealing device (Valleylab, Boulder, Colo.) or the conventional approach.

This study showed that LigaSure hemorrhoidectomy results in a significant reduction in operative time and blood loss, but it may not confer any advantage over the conventional operation in terms of postoperative pain, length of hospital stay, or time taken to return to work or normal activity. The expediency of the device must be weighed against its additional cost. Long-term evaluations of outcomes and morbidity are still needed.

In this analysis, LigaSure was used and provided a superior alternative to conventional diathermy in the therapy of hemorrhoids by reducing the operative operating room time, postoperative pain, and parenteral anesthetic requirements. These superior outcomes were evident in the first 24 hours postoperatively and in the time of complete healing of wounds. When the two techniques were compared, there was no statistical difference in the incidence of postoperative complications between LigaSure and conventional diathermy. In addition, time to return to work and normal activity was significantly superior in the LigaSure group.

In the meta-analysis by Tan et al of short-term outcomes of a randomized controlled trial of LigaSure vs. conventional hemorrhoidal resection approaches, meta-analysis suggests that LigaSure hemorrhoidectomy resulted in a significant reduction in operating room time and blood loss. However, it was unclear of any advantage over conventional operation for postoperative pain, length of hospital stay, or time needed to return to work or normal lifestyle activity. This analysis suggests that although there is expediency with the use of the device intraoperatively, this advantage must be weighed against additional costs. Clearly, long-term evaluations of outcomes and equivalent morbidities will still need to be examined.[2] Ⓐ

Another trial sought to assess the efficacy of internal sphincterotomy compared with application of topical 2% diltiazem ointment after hemorrhoidectomy for pain relief.

This study showed that in patients undergoing hemorrhoidectomy, addition of surgical internal sphincterotomy results in lesser pain in the postoperative period as compared to those receiving topical application of diltiazem.

Excisional hemorrhoidectomy is a painful operation. The rich sensory enervation of the anoderm, increased discomfort associated with pressure from sitting, and perineal friction with walking, all potentiate postoperative pain. Regrettably, there is no panacea for this problem.

Chauhan and colleagues conducted a prospective randomized study in 108 subjects undergoing excisional hemorrhoidectomy over 18 months. Patients received either topical diltiazem ointment or partial, internal anal sphincterectomy at the time of the excisional hemorrhoidectomy. It was concluded that when compared with diltiazem, concomitant internal anal sphincterectomy provided significantly greater relief of postoperative pain.

Several findings in this study merit discussion. The prospective randomized design, the large number of subjects, and the objective measure of pain are all meritorious. Despite these benefits, the study contains several findings that support a more cautious approach to this problem. The significant differences in pain control between treatment groups were not present until the fourth postoperative day. Surgeons performing this operation and patients undergoing surgery frequently acknowledge that the most severe pain occurs during the immediate postoperative period. Additionally, the risk of complications was greater (11.5% vs. 3%) in the internal sphincterectomy group. Finally, cutting even a short segment of the internal sphincter is not without adverse sequelae such as perianal discharge and some minor degrees of incontinence.[3] Ⓐ

More compelling data are needed to justify the addition of internal anal sphincterectomy to patients undergoing excisional hemorrhoidectomy. Until such data are reported, the use of topical and oral postoperative analgesics is justified in these uncomfortable patients.

Evidence-Based References

1. Patti R et al: Randomized clinical trial of botulinum toxin injection for pain relief in patients with thrombosed external haemorrhoids, *Br J Surg* 95: 1339-1343, 2008. Commentary by J. Rombeau, M.D. Ⓐ

2. Tan EK et al: Meta-analysis of short-term outcomes of randomized controlled trials of LigaSure vs. conventional hemorrhoidectomy, *Arch Surg* 142:1209-1218, 2007. Commentary by K.I. Bland, M.D. Ⓐ

3. Chauhan A et al: Comparison of internal sphincterotomy with topical diltiazem for post-hemorrhoidectomy pain relief: a prospective randomized trial, *J Postgrad Med* 55:22-26, 2009. Commentary by J.L. Rombeau, M.D. Ⓐ

SUGGESTED READING

Zuber TJ: Hemorrhoidectomy for thrombosed external hemorrhoids, *Am Fam Physician* 65:1629, 2002.

AUTHORS: **MARIA A. CORIGLIANO, M.D.,** and **RUBEN ALVERO, M.D.**

 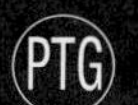

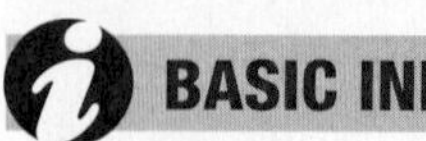

BASIC INFORMATION

DEFINITION

Henoch-Schönlein purpura (HSP) is a systemic, small-vessel, immune complex–mediated leukocytoclastic vasculitis characterized by a triad of palpable purpura, abdominal pain, and arthritis. It may also present with gastrointestinal (GI) bleeding, arthralgias, and renal involvement.

SYNONYMS

Anaphylactoid purpura
Allergic purpura

ICD-9CM CODES

287.0 Henoch-Schönlein purpura

EPIDEMIOLOGY & DEMOGRAPHICS

INCIDENCE: Annual incidence of 14 cases/100,000 population
PEAK INCIDENCE: Spring, although cases are seen throughout the year
PREVALENCE: Most common vasculitis seen in children and younger age groups
PREDOMINANT SEX: 2:1 male/female ratio
PREDOMINANT AGE: Seen mostly from ages 4 to 15 yr, although can be seen in older adolescents and young adults

PHYSICAL FINDINGS & CLINICAL PRESENTATION

- Palpable purpura of dependent areas, especially lower extremities (Fig. 1-142) and areas subjected to pressure, such as the beltline.
- Subcutaneous edema.
- Arthralgias and arthritis in 80%.
- GI symptoms are seen in approximately one third of patients. Common findings are nausea, vomiting, diarrhea, cramping, abdominal pain, hematochezia, and melena.
- Anecdotally may follow upper respiratory infection.
- Renal involvement is seen in up to 80% of older children, usually within the first month of illness. Fewer than 5% progress to end-stage renal failure, a major cause of morbidity.

ETIOLOGY

- Presumptive etiology is exposure to a trigger antigen that causes antibody formation.
- Antigen-antibody (immune) complex deposition then occurs in arteriole and capillary walls of skin, renal mesangium, and GI tract. Immunoglobulin (Ig) A deposition is most common.
- Antigen triggers postulated include drugs, foods, immunization, and upper respiratory and other viral illnesses. Group A streptococcal infection is the most common precipitant in children, seen in up to one third of cases. A recent adult case triggered by pantoprazole has also been reported.
- Serologic and pathologic evidence suggests an association between Parvovirus B19 and HSP, which may explain observed cases of HSP that do not respond to corticosteroids or other immunosuppressive therapy.
- Case reports describing development of HSP after treatment with immunosuppressive agents (e.g., etanercept) have been published.

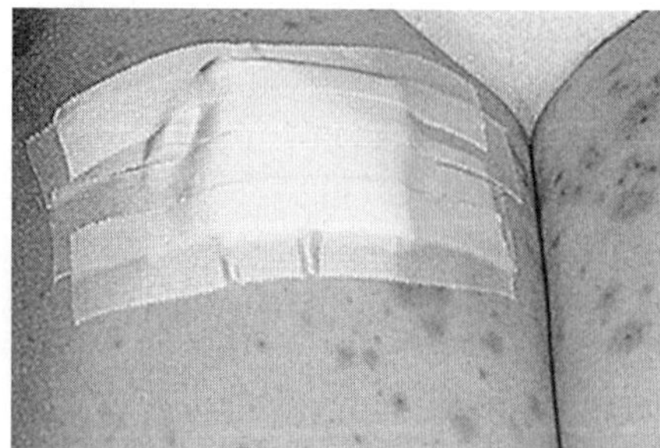

FIGURE 1-142 Henoch-Schönlein purpura on the lower extremities of a child. (Courtesy Medical College of Georgia, Division of Dermatology. From Goldstein B [ed]: *Practical dermatology,* ed 2, St Louis, 1997, Mosby.)

Dx DIAGNOSIS

- Diagnosis is clinical.
- Skin manifestations are most common.
- Palpable purpura is seen in 70% of adult patients, whereas GI symptoms are more common in children.
- Skin biopsy shows leukocytoclastic vasculitis.
- The presence of two of the following four American College of Rheumatology criteria yields a diagnostic sensitivity of 87.1% and specificity of 87.7%:
  - Palpable purpura unrelated to thrombocytopenia
  - Age $<$20 yr at onset of first symptoms
  - Bowel angina or ischemia
  - Granulocytic infiltration of arteriole or venule walls on biopsy

DIFFERENTIAL DIAGNOSIS

- Polyarteritis nodosa
- Meningococcemia
- Thrombocytopenic purpura
- Hypersensitivity vasculitis
- Microscopic polyangitis

WORKUP

History, physical examination, laboratory testing, skin biopsy

LABORATORY TESTS

- Electrolytes, blood urea nitrogen, and creatinine
- Urinalysis
- Complete blood count
- Prothrombin time, fibrinogen, and fibrin degradation products
- Blood cultures

Laboratory abnormalities are not specific for HSP. Leukocytosis and eosinophilia may be seen. IgA levels are elevated in approximately 50% of patients. Glomerulonephritis may be present (microscopic hematuria, proteinuria, and red blood cell casts).

IMAGING STUDIES

Imaging studies are not useful in the diagnosis of HSP. Arteriography or magnetic resonance angiography may be helpful in distinguishing from polyarteritis nodosa.

Rx TREATMENT

- Prednisone 1 mg/kg PO is given if renal or severe GI disease, although clear benefits in renal disease have not been demonstrated according to a recent Cochrane Systematic review.
- A recent double-blind, randomized, controlled trial found that early treatment with prednisone reduced abdominal pain and joint symptoms but did not prevent development of renal disease. It was effective in the treatment of renal disease once it was established.
- Corticosteroids and azathioprine may be beneficial if rapidly progressive glomerulonephritis is present. Pulse methylprednisolone therapy has also been proposed in patients with glomerulonephritis, mesenteric vasculitis, or pulmonary involvement. A recent report described improvement in rapidly progressive glomerulonephritis after treatment with mycophenolate mofetil.
- Nonsteroidal anti-inflammatory drugs for arthritis and arthralgias.

NONPHARMACOLOGIC THERAPY

Supportive care with pain management, adequate hydration, and nutrition

DISPOSITION & PROGNOSIS

- Prognosis excellent, with spontaneous recovery of most patients within 4 wk.
- End-stage renal disease occurs in 1%-5% of patients. Chronic renal insufficiency is the most common long-term morbidity.
- GI complications (mesenteric infarction, perforation, and intussusception).
- Recurrences in up to one third of patients, especially within first 4 to 6 mo after initial episode and most commonly in patients with renal involvement.

REFERRAL

Nephrologist or gastroenterologist

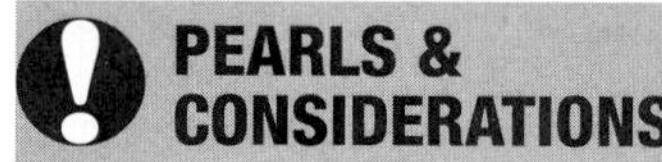

PEARLS & CONSIDERATIONS

- Most with spontaneous recovery within 4 wk of onset of symptoms.
- Organ systems involved are skin, joints, GI tract, and kidneys.
- Palpable purpura more common in adults; GI symptoms more common in children.
- End-stage renal disease occurs in only 5% of patients.
- Steroids and immunosuppressive agents may offer some benefit.

SUGGESTED READINGS

Chartapisak W et al: Prevention and treatment of renal disease in Henoch-Schönlein purpura: a systematic review, *Arch Dis Child* 94:132-137, 2009.

Reamy BV et al: Henoch-Schönlein purpura, *Am Fam Physician* 80(7):697-704, 2009.

Saulsbury FT: Clinical update: v, *Lancet* 369:976, 2007.

AUTHOR: **DOMINICK TAMMARO, M.D.**

BASIC INFORMATION

DEFINITION

Hepatic encephalopathy (HE) is a neuropsychiatric syndrome occurring in patients with severe impairment of liver function and consequent accumulation of toxic products not metabolized by the liver.

SYNONYMS

Hepatic coma

ICD-9CM CODES

572.2 Hepatic encephalopathy

EPIDEMIOLOGY & DEMOGRAPHICS

INCIDENCE/PREVALENCE: Hepatic encephalopathy occurs in >50% of all cases of cirrhosis.

PHYSICAL FINDINGS & CLINICAL PRESENTATION

Hepatic encephalopathy can be classified in stages or grades 1 to 4:

- Grades 1 and 2: mild obtundation
- Grades 3 and 4: stupor to deep coma, with or without decerebrate posturing

The physical examination in hepatic encephalopathy varies with the stage and may reveal the following abnormalities:

- Skin: jaundice, palmar erythema, spider angiomata, ecchymosis, dilated superficial periumbilical veins (caput medusae) in patients with cirrhosis
- Eyes: scleral icterus, Kayser-Fleischer rings (Wilson's disease)
- Breath: fetor hepaticus
- Chest: gynecomastia in men with chronic liver disease
- Abdomen: ascites, small nodular liver (cirrhosis), tender hepatomegaly (congestive hepatomegaly)
- Rectal examination: hemorrhoids (portal hypertension), guaiac-positive stool (alcoholic gastritis, bleeding esophageal varices, peptic ulcer disease, bleeding hemorrhoids)
- Genitalia: testicular atrophy in males with chronic liver disease
- Extremities: pedal edema from hypoalbuminemia
- Neurologic: flapping tremor (asterixis), obtundation, coma with or without decerebrate posturing

ETIOLOGY

- Precipitating factors in patients with underlying cirrhosis (upper gastrointestinal bleeding, hypokalemia, hypomagnesemia, analgesic and sedative drugs, sepsis, alkalosis, increased dietary protein)
- Acute fulminant viral hepatitis
- Drugs and toxins (e.g., isoniazid, acetaminophen, diclofenac and other NSAIDs, statins, methyldopa, loratadine, propylthiouracil, lisinopril, labetalol, halothane, carbon tetrachloride, erythromycin, nitrofurantoin, troglitazone)
- Reye's syndrome
- Shock and/or sepsis
- Fatty liver of pregnancy
- Metastatic carcinoma, hepatocellular carcinoma
- Other: autoimmune hepatitis, ischemic venoocclusive disease, sclerosing cholangitis, heat stroke, amebic abscesses

DIAGNOSIS

DIFFERENTIAL DIAGNOSIS

- Delirium caused by medications or illicit drugs
- Cerebrovascular accident, subdural hematoma
- Meningitis, encephalitis
- Hypoglycemia
- Uremia
- Cerebral anoxia
- Hypercalcemia
- Metastatic neoplasm to brain
- Alcohol withdrawal syndrome

WORKUP

Exclude other etiologies with comprehensive history (obtained from patient, relatives, and others), physical examination, and laboratory and imaging studies. A pertinent history should include exposure to hepatitis, ethanol intake, drug history, exposure to toxins, IV drug abuse, measles or influenza with aspirin use (Reye's syndrome), and history of carcinoma (primary or metastatic).

LABORATORY TESTS

- Alanine aminotransferase, aspartate aminotransferase, bilirubin, alkaline phosphatase glucose, calcium, electrolytes, blood urea nitrogen, creatinine, albumin
- Complete blood count, platelet count, prothrombin time, partial thromboplastin time
- Serum and urine toxicology screen in suspected medication or illegal drug use
- Blood and urine cultures, urinalysis
- Venous ammonia level
- Arterial blood gases

IMAGING STUDIES

CT scan of the head may be useful in selected patients to exclude other etiologies.

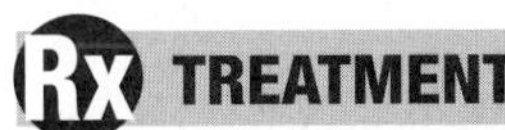

TREATMENT

NONPHARMACOLOGIC THERAPY

- Identification and treatment of precipitating factors
- Restriction of protein intake (30 to 40 g/day) to reduce toxic protein metabolites

ACUTE GENERAL Rx

Reduction of colonic ammonia production:

- Lactulose 30 ml of 50% solution qid initially; dose is subsequently adjusted depending on clinical response. Ornithine aspartate 9 g tid is also effective. Lactulose may improve hepatic encephalopathy but may be less effective than antibiotics.
- Neomycin 1 g PO q4-6h or given as a 1% retention enema solution (1 g in 100 ml of isotonic saline solution); neomycin should be used with caution in patients with renal insufficiency. Metronidazole 250 mg qid may be as effective as neomycin and is not nephrotoxic; however, long-term use can be associated with neurotoxicity. Rifaximin 1200 mg/day is a viable alternative to metronidazole.
- A combination of lactulose and neomycin can be used when either agent is ineffective alone.

Treatment of cerebral edema:

- Cerebral edema is often present in patients with acute liver failure, and it accounts for nearly 50% of deaths. Monitoring intracranial pressure by epidural, intraparenchymal, or subdural transducers and treatment of cerebral edema with mannitol (100 to 200 ml of 20% solution [0.3 to 0.4 g/kg of body weight]) given by rapid IV infusion are helpful in selected patients (e.g., potential transplantation patients).
- Dexamethasone and hyperventilation (useful in head injury) are of little value in treating cerebral edema from liver failure.

CHRONIC Rx

- Avoidance of any precipitating factors (e.g., high-protein diet, medications)
- Consideration of liver transplantation in selected patients with progressive or recurrent encephalopathy

DISPOSITION

Prognosis varies with the underlying etiology of the liver failure and the grade of encephalopathy (generally good for grades 1 or 2; poor for grades 3 or 4).

REFERRAL

The early stages of hepatic encephalopathy can be managed in the outpatient setting, whereas stages 3 or 4 require hospital admission.

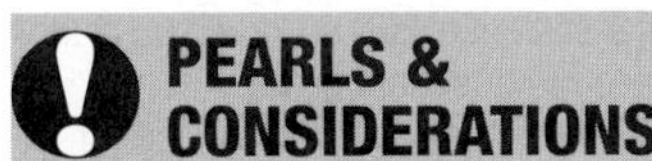

PEARLS & CONSIDERATIONS

COMMENTS

Patients not responding to supportive therapy should be evaluated for liver transplantation.

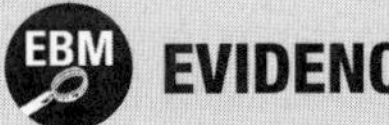

EVIDENCE

Please note: Complete text of EBM for this topic is available online.

AUTHOR: **FRED F. FERRI, M.D.**

Hepatitis A (PTG) (ALG)

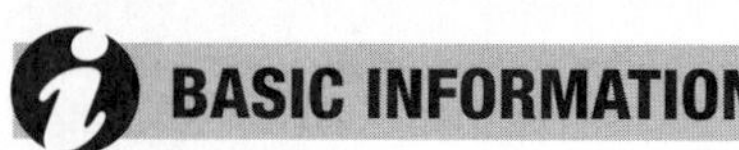

BASIC INFORMATION

DEFINITION

Hepatitis A is generally an acute self-limiting infection of the liver by an enterically transmitted picornavirus, hepatitis A virus (HAV). Infection may range from asymptomatic to fulminant hepatitis.

SYNONYMS

Infectious hepatitis
Short incubation hepatitis
Type A hepatitis
HAV (hepatitis A virus)

ICD-9CM CODES
070.1 Hepatitis A

EPIDIMIOLOGY & DEMOGRAPHICS

INCIDENCE:

- Hepatitis A occurs worldwide, affecting 1.4 million people annually and accounting for 20% to 40% of cases of viral hepatitis in the U.S.
- The seroprevalence increases with age, ranging from 10% in individuals <5 yr to 74% in those >50 yr.
- In the U.S. average disease rate is approximately 15 cases/100,000 persons/yr.
- The incidence is relatively higher in some regions in the U.S., including Arizona, Alaska, California, Idaho, Nevada, New Mexico, Oklahoma, Oregon, South Dakota, and Washington.
- At-risk groups include:
  1. Residents and staff of group homes
  2. Children, employees of day care centers
  3. People who engage in oral-anal contact, regardless of sexual orientation
  4. IV drug abusers
  5. Travel to endemic areas
  6. Areas of overcrowding, poor sanitation, inadequate sewage treatment

PREVALENCE:

- Approximately three fourths of the U.S. population has serologic evidence of prior infection.
- Anti-HAV prevalence has an inverse relation to income and household size.

PREDOMINANT SEX: None, except higher infection rates seen in homosexual males who engage in oral-anal contact.

PREDOMINANT AGE/PEAK INCIDENCE:

- In areas of high rates of hepatitis A, virtually all children are infected while younger than 10 yr, but disease is rare.
- In areas of moderate rates of hepatitis A, disease occurs in late childhood and young adults.
- In areas of low rates of hepatitis A, most cases occur in young adults.

INCUBATION PERIOD: Averages 30 days (15 to 50)

PHYSICAL FINDINGS & CLINICAL PRESENTATION

- Infection with HAV may have acute or subacute presentation, icteric or anicteric. Severity of illness seems to increase with age (90% of infection in children <5 yr may be subclinical).
- A preicteric, prodromal phase of approximately 1 to 14 days. 15% no apparent prodrome. Symptoms are usually abrupt in onset and may include anorexia, malaise, nausea, vomiting, fever, headache, and abdominal pain.
- Less common symptoms are chills, myalgias, arthralgias, upper respiratory symptoms, constipation, diarrhea, pruritus, urticaria.
- Jaundice occurs in >70% of patients.
- The icteric phase is preceded by dark urine.
- Bilirubinuria is typically followed a few days later by clay-colored stools and icterus.

PHYSICAL EXAMINATION

- Jaundice
- Hepatomegaly
- Splenomegaly
- Cervical lymphadenopathy
- Evanescent rash
- Petechiae
- Cardiac arrhythmias

COMPLICATIONS

- Cholestasis
- Fulminant hepatitis
- Arthritis
- Myocarditis
- Optic neuritis
- Transverse myelitis
- Thrombocytopenic purpura
- Aplastic anemia
- Red cell aplasia
- Henoch-Schönlein purpura
- IgA dominant glomerulonephritis

ETIOLOGY

- Caused by HAV, a 27 nm, nonenveloped, icosahedral, positive-stranded RNA virus.
- Transmission is fecal-oral route, from person to person. Transmission occurs with close contact or with food- or water-borne outbreaks with inadequately purified water or cooked foods. Recent outbreaks have involved green onions and tomatoes.
- Parenteral transmission is considered rare.
- Vertical transmission has also been reported.

Dx DIAGNOSIS

DIFFERENTIAL DIAGNOSIS

- Other hepatitis virus (B, C, D, E)
- Infectious mononucleosis
- Cytomegalovirus infection
- Herpes simplex virus infection
- Leptospirosis
- Brucellosis
- Drug-induced liver disease
- Ischemic hepatitis
- Autoimmune hepatitis

WORKUP

- IgM antibody specific for HAV
- Liver function tests; ALT and AST elevations are sensitive for liver damage but not specific for HAV
- Elevated ESR
- CBC; may find mild lymphocytosis

LABORATORY TESTS

- Diagnosis confirmed by IgM anti HAV; it is detectable in almost all infected patients at presentation and remains positive for 3 to 6 mo.
- A fourfold rise in titer of total antibody (IgM and IgG) to HAV confirms acute infection.
- HAV detection in stool and body fluids by electron microscopy.
- HAV RNA detection in stool, body fluids, serum, and liver tissue.
- ALT and AST usually more than 8 times normal in acute infection.
- Bilirubin usually 5 to 15 times normal.
- Alkaline phosphatase minimally elevated but higher level in cholestasis.
- Albumin and prothrombin time are generally normal; if elevated, they may herald hepatic necrosis.
- Fig. 1-143 Illustrates the typical course of hepatis A.

IMAGING STUDIES

- Rarely useful
- Sonogram (fulminant hepatitis)

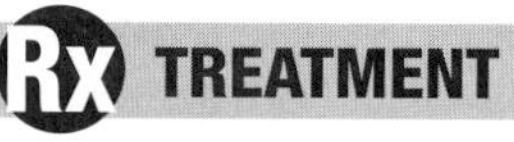

TREATMENT

- Usually self-limited
- Supportive care
- Those with fulminant hepatitis may require hospitalization and treatment of associated complications
- Activity as tolerated
- Advise to avoid alcohol and hepatotoxic drugs
- Patients with fulminant hepatitis should be assessed for liver transplantation

CHRONIC Rx

No chronic HAV and no chronic carrier state

DISPOSITION

Follow-up as outpatient

REFERRAL

- To a hepatologist if severe, fulminant hepatitis develops
- To a transplant surgeon if liver transplant becomes a consideration for fulminant hepatitis and liver failure

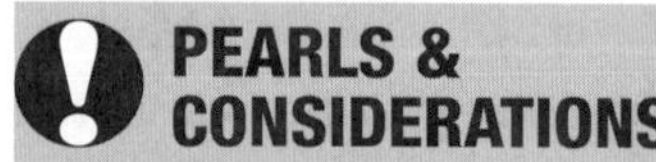

PEARLS & CONSIDERATIONS

- All cases of hepatitis A should be reported to the public heath authorities because food-borne or water-borne outbreaks may occur, and public health efforts (mass vaccination or immunoglobulin therapy) may avert secondary cases.
- Hepatitis A is a common illness in internationally traveled and developing countries. Pretravel vaccination is strongly recommended for travelers who are HAV susceptible.

PREVENTION

- Improvement in hygiene and sanitation
- Heating food
- Avoidance of water and foods from endemic area

PASSIVE IMMUNIZATION

- Immunoglobulin provides protection against HAV through passive transfer of antibody.
- Preexposure prophylaxis indicated for people traveling to endemic areas (Ig 0.02 or 0.06 ml/kg given IM). The lower dose is effective for up to 3 mo, and the higher dose is effective for up to 5 mo.
- Postexposure prophylaxis (Ig 0.02 ml/kg given IM) is indicated for people with recent exposure (within 2 wk) to HAV and who have not been previously vaccinated. In high-risk patients, vaccine may be administered with immunoglobulin.

ACTIVE IMMUNIZATION

- There are several inactivated and attenuated hepatitis vaccines; only the inactivated vaccines are currently available for use and they have been found to be safe and highly immunogenic: HAVRIX or VAQTA. These can be used in adults and children older than 12 mo. A combined hepatitis A and hepatitis B vaccine called TWINRX is also available.
- Protective antibody levels were reached in 94% to 100% of adults 1 mo after the first dose, similar results have been found for children and adolescents.
- Theoretic analyses of antibody levels estimate duration of immunity to be 10 to 20 yr.
- Vaccine should be considered for persons who are at risk: those traveling to or working in endemic areas, homosexual men, illegal drug users, persons with chronic liver disease, children in areas with high rates of hepatitis A infection.

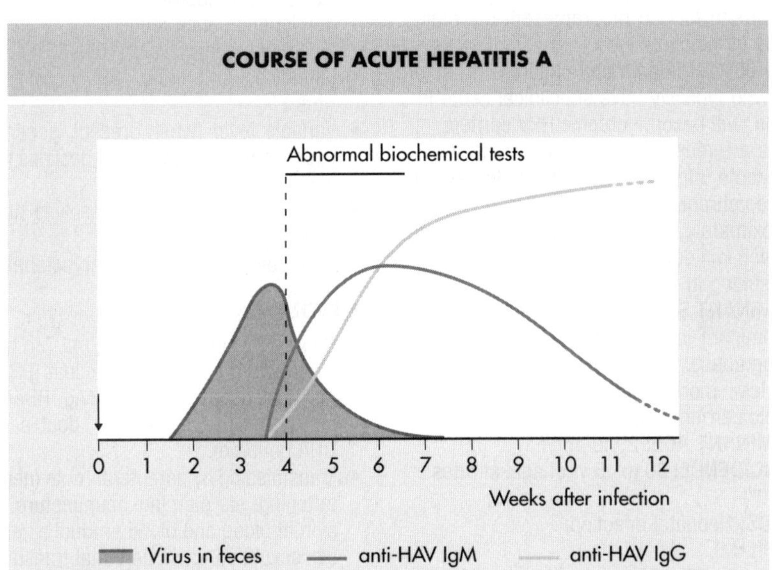

FIGURE 1-143 Course of acute hepatitis A. (From Cohen J, Powderly WG: *Infectious diseases,* ed 2, St Louis, 2004, Mosby.)

SUGGESTED READINGS

Fiore AE et al: Prevention of hepatitis A through active or passive immunization: recommendations of the Advisory Committee on Immunization Practices (ACIP), *MMWR Recomm Rep* 55(RR-7):1, 2006.

Jenson HB: The changing picture of hepatitis A in the United States, *Curr Opin Pediatr* 16(1):89, 2004.

Leach CT: Hepatitis A in the United States, *Pediatr Infect Dis J* 23(6):551, 2004.

Rezende G et al: Viral and clinical factors associated with the fulminant course of hepatitis A infection, *Hepatology* 38:613, 2003.

Victor JC et al: Hepatitis A vaccine versus immune-globulin for postexposure prophylaxis, *N Engl J Med* 357:1685-1694, 2007.

AUTHORS: **GLENN G. FORT, M.D., M.P.H.,** and **DENNIS J. MIKOLICH, M.D.**

H

Diseases and Disorders

I

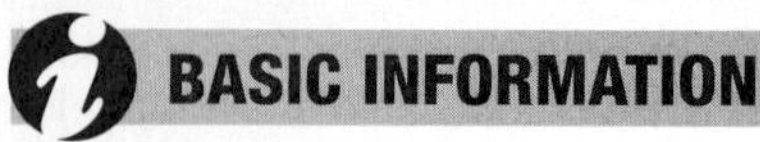

BASIC INFORMATION

DEFINITION

Hepatitis B is an acute infection of the liver parenchymal cells caused by the hepatitis B virus (HBV).

SYNONYMS

Serum hepatitis
Long incubation (30-180 days) hepatitis

ICD-9CM CODES
070.3 Hepatitis B

EPIDEMIOLOGY & DEMOGRAPHICS

INCIDENCE (IN U.S.):

- Approximately 200,000 to 300,000 infections annually in U.S.
- Much higher incidence in Europe (approximately 1 million new cases annually) and in areas of high endemicity.
- In U.S., transmission is mainly horizontal (percutaneous and mucous membrane exposure to infectious blood and other body fluids [e.g., sexual transmission, either homosexual or heterosexual]); also from needle sharing among drug abusers; occupational exposure to contaminated blood and blood products; persons receiving transfusions of blood and blood products; and hemodialysis patients.

NOTE: Improved screening of blood and blood products has greatly reduced, although not eliminated, the risk of posttransfusion HBV infection.

- In areas of high endemicity, transmission is largely vertical (perinatal): HBV exists in the blood and body fluids. Perinatal transmission from HBsAg-positive mothers is as high as 90% unless immunoprophylaxis is given.

PREVALENCE (IN U.S.):

- North America, Western Europe, and Australia are areas of low prevalence, <2%.
- Africa, Asia, and the Western Pacific region are areas of high prevalence, ≥8%.
- Southern and Eastern Europe have intermediate rates, 2% to 7%.
- Chronically infected persons, those with positive HBsAg for >6 mo, represent the major source of infection.
- Up to 95% of infants and children <5 yr of age, who typically have subclinical acute infection, will become chronic HBV carriers.
- Adults are more likely to have clinically evident acute infection, but only 1% to 5% will develop chronic infection.
- Approximately 0.1% of patients with acute infection will develop fulminant acute hepatitis resulting in death.

PREDOMINANT SEX:

- Predominant in males because of increased IV drug abuse, homosexuality
- Females more commonly terminate in chronic carrier state

PREDOMINANT AGE: 20 to 45 yr

PEAK INCIDENCE: 30 to 45 yr of age, at rates of 5% to 20%

GENETICS: Neonatal infection:

- Rare in U.S.
- High (up to 90%) in areas of high endemicity (only 5%-10% of perinatal infections occur in utero)

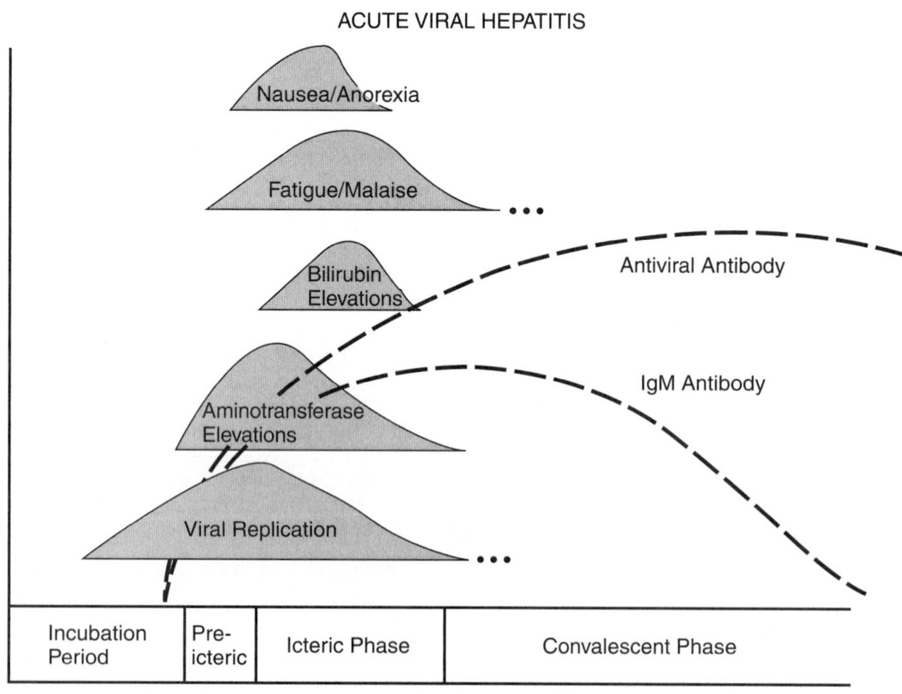

FIGURE 1-144 The typical course of acute viral hepatitis. (From Goldman L, Ausiello D [eds]: *Cecil textbook of medicine,* ed 22, Philadelphia, 2004, WB Saunders.)

PHYSICAL FINDINGS & CLINICAL PRESENTATION (Fig. 1-144)

- Often nonspecific symptoms
- Profound malaise
- Many asymptomatic cases
- Prodrome:
  1. 15% to 20% serum sickness (urticaria, rash, arthralgia) during early HBsAg
  2. HBsAg-Ab complex disease (polyarteritis nodosa–arthritis, arteritis, glomerulonephritis)
- Hepatomegaly (87%) with right upper quadrant (RUQ) tenderness
  1. Hepatic punch tenderness
  2. Splenomegaly: rare (10%-15%)
- Jaundice, dark urine, with occasional pruritus
- Variable fever (when present, generally precedes jaundice and rapidly declines following onset of icteric phase)
- Spider angiomata: rare; resolves during recovery
- Rare polyarteritis nodosa, cryoglobulinemia

ETIOLOGY

- Caused by hepatitis B virus (42-nm hepadnavirus with an outer surface coat [HBsAg], inner nucleocapsid core [HBcAg; HBeAg]; DNA polymerase; and partially double-stranded DNA genome).
- Transmission by parenteral route (needle use, tattooing, ear piercing, acupuncture, transfusion of blood and blood products, hemodialysis, sexual contact), perinatal transmission.
- Infection may result from contact of infectious material with mucous membranes and open skin breaks (e.g., HBV is stable and can be transmitted from toothbrushes, utensils, razors, baby toys, various medical equipment [respirators, endoscopes]).
- Oral intake of infectious material may result in infection through breaks in the oral mucosa.
- Food or water are virtually never found to be sources of HBV infection.
- Infection occurs primarily in liver, where necrosis probably results from cytotoxic T-cell response, direct cytopathic effect of HBcAg (core antigen), high-level HBsAg (surface antigen) expression, or coinfection with delta (D) hepatitis virus (RNA delta core within HBsAg envelope).
- Recovery (>90%):
  1. Fulminant hepatitis occurring in <1% (especially if coinfected with hepatitis D); 80% fatal
  2. Unusual (5%) prolonged acute disease for 4 to 12 mo, with recovery
  3. Overall fatality increases with age and viral inoculation (e.g., transfusions)
- Chronic infection (1%-2%):
  1. Persistent carrier state without hepatitis (HBsAg positive)
  2. Chronic persistent hepatitis (CPH) (clinically well), or chronic active hepatitis (CAH) (HBsAg positive and HBeAg positive)
  3. Cirrhosis
  4. Hepatocellular carcinoma (especially after neonatal infection)

5. Chronic infection: more common following low-dose exposure and mild acute hepatitis, with earlier age of infection, in males, and in immunosuppressed patients
6. One third to one quarter of chronically infected will develop progressive liver disease (cirrhosis, hepatocellular carcinoma)

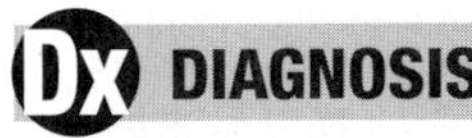

DIAGNOSIS

DIFFERENTIAL DIAGNOSIS

- Acute disease confused with other viral hepatitis infections (A, C, D, E)
- Any viral illness producing systemic disease and hepatitis (e.g., yellow fever, EBV, CMV, HIV, rubella, rubeola, coxsackie B, adenovirus, herpes simplex or zoster)
- Nonviral causes of hepatitis (e.g., leptospirosis, toxoplasmosis, alcoholic hepatitis, drug-induced [e.g., acetaminophen, INH], toxic hepatitis [carbon tetrachloride, benzene])

WORKUP

- Acute serum specimen for hepatitis B serology (HBsAg, HBsAb, HBcAb, HBeAg, HBeAb), HBDNA
- LFTs
- CBC
- Liver biopsy: rarely indicated for diagnosis of fulminant viral hepatitis, chronic hepatitis, cirrhosis, carcinoma

LABORATORY TESTS

- Diagnosis of acute HBV infection is best confirmed by IgM HBcAb in acute or early convalescent serum or by HBDNA.
  1. Generally, IgM present during onset of jaundice
  2. Coexisting HBsAg
- HBsAg and IgG-HBcAb during acute jaundice are strongly suggestive of remote HBV infection and another cause for current illness (Fig. 1-145).
- HBsAb alone is suggestive of immunization response.
- With recovery, HBeAg is rapidly replaced by HBeAb in 2 to 3 mo, and HBsAg is replaced by HBsAb in 5 to 6 mo.
- In chronic HBV hepatitis, HBsAg and HBeAg are persistent without corresponding Ab.
- In chronic carrier state, HBsAg is persistent, but HBeAg is replaced by HBeAb.
- HBcAb develops in all outcomes.
- HBeAg correlation with highest infectivity; appearance of HBeAb heralds recovery.
- LFTs:
  1. ALT and AST: usually more than eight times normal (often 1000 U/L) at onset of jaundice (minimal acute ALT/AST rises often followed by chronic hepatitis or hepatocellular carcinoma)
  2. Bilirubin: variably elevated in icteric viral hepatitis
  3. Alkaline phosphatase: minimally elevated (one to three times normal) acutely
- Albumin and prothrombin time:
  1. Generally normal
  2. If abnormal, possible harbinger of impending hepatic necrosis (fulminant hepatitis)
- WBC and ESR: generally normal

IMAGING STUDIES

- Rarely useful
- Sonogram to document rapid reduction in liver size during fulminant hepatitis or mass in hepatocellular carcinoma

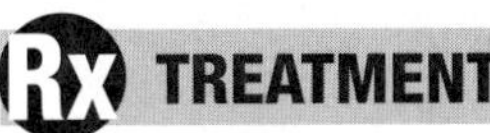

TREATMENT

NONPHARMACOLOGIC THERAPY

- Symptomatic treatment as necessary
- Activity as tolerated
- High-calorie diet preferred; often best tolerated in morning

ACUTE GENERAL Rx

- In most cases of acute HBV infection no treatment necessary; >90% of adults will spontaneously clear infection
- Hospitalization advisable for any patient in danger from dehydration caused by poor oral intake, whose PT is prolonged, who has rising bilirubin level >15 to 20 μg/dl, or who has any clinical evidence of hepatic failure
- IV therapy needed (rarely) for hydration during severe vomiting
- Avoid hepatically metabolized drugs
- No therapeutic measures are beneficial
- Steroids not shown helpful

CHRONIC Rx

- The aim of therapy in chronic HBV infection is to eradicate the virus.
- The two modalities of therapy available to achieve this goal have been immune modulators (interferon alfa) and antiviral agents in the form of nucleoside analogues (e.g., lamivudine).
- Until recently, IFN-α given SQ either daily or thrice weekly for 16 to 24 wk had been the mainstay of therapy. Its mechanism of action is to stimulate the immune system to attack HBV-infected hepatocytes, thus inhibiting viral protein synthesis. Currently, use of pegylated IFN-α offers more convenient administration and more sustained viral suppression as a once-a-wk SQ injection.
- A 4-mo course of treatment results in a 30% to 40% response with significant reduction of serum HBV DNA, normalization of ALT, and loss of HBeAg. Seroconversion from HBeAg to HBeAb occurs in 15% to 20%.
- Factors that increase the likelihood of response to IFN-α therapy include:
  1. Adult onset of infection
  2. High baseline ALT
  3. Low baseline HBV DNA
  4. Absence of cirrhosis
  5. Female
  6. HBeAg positive

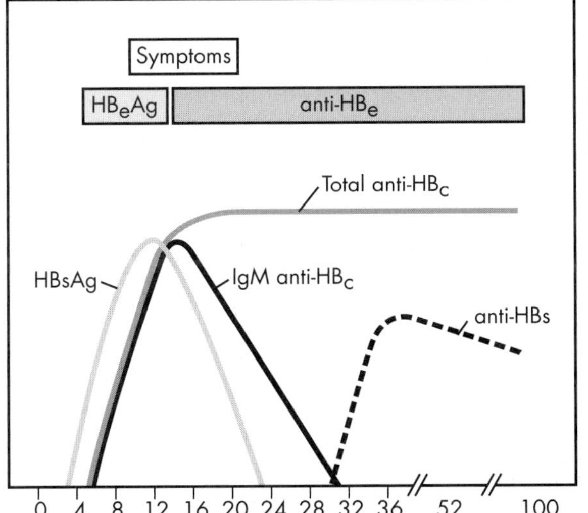

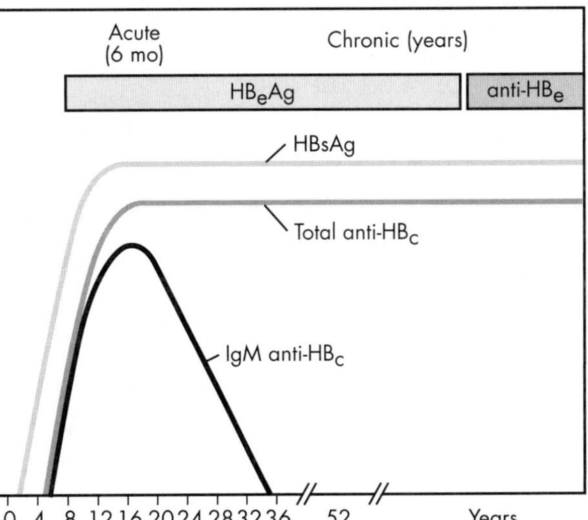

FIGURE 1-145 Typical course of hepatitis B. Left, Typical course of acute hepatitis B. **Right,** Chronic hepatitis B. *HB,* Hepatitis B core; *Hb,* hepatitis B early; *HBsAg,* hepatitis B surface antigen; *IgM,* immunoglobulin M. (From Mandell GL et al: *Principles and practice of infectious diseases,* ed 7, Philadelphia, 2010, Elsevier.)

- Infrequent relapse after successful completion of therapy.
- 80% of patients who lose HBeAg during therapy lose HBsAg in the decade after therapy.
- >50% of patients who do not seroconvert after initial therapy develop a delayed HBeAg seroconversion months to years after therapy.
- Overall incidence of cirrhosis and hepatocellular carcinoma is decreased in those treated with IFN-α.
- IFN-α is successful only in patients with an active immune response; therefore it is not effective in patients with HIV infection and organ transplant patients.
- Asians respond poorly to IFN-α.
- Treatment with IFN-α in general is also poorly tolerated: side effects include flulike symptoms, injection-site reactions, rash, weight loss, anxiety, depression, alopecia, thrombocytopenia, granulocytopenia, and thyroid dysfunction.
- Nucleoside analogues block viral replication by inhibiting HBV polymerase.
- Lamivudine was the first nucleoside analogue approved for treatment of chronic HBV infection; it has been shown to rapidly reduce HBV replication and suppress HBV DNA to undetectable levels after a few wk of treatment, and treatment for 1 yr is as effective as IFN-α with respect to loss of HBeAg seroconversion to HBeAb and loss of HBV DNA. Emergence of resistant HBV strains while on therapy has limited the use of lamivudine (YMDD variants [tyrosine-methionine-aspartate-aspartate]).
- Adefovir dipivoxil is a nucleotide reverse transcriptase inhibitor that also has antiviral activity against HBV. It is a prodrug that is converted to the active drug adefovir. It is highly active against HBV and may be useful as a first-line agent or as salvage therapy for patients who are refractory or intolerant to lamivudine. (Nephrotoxicity is a potential side effect, but emergence of resistant strains is less than with lamivudine.)
- Entecavir is a nucleoside agent approved for the treatment of hepatitis B, and it appears to be more effective and to present fewer concerns than lamivudine or adefovir regarding the emergence of resistant strains.
- Telbivudine, a thymidine nucleosidase analogue, has demonstrated greater and more consistent HBV DNA suppression than adefovir after 24 wk of treatment.
- Combination therapy with two or three nucleoside analogues or combination therapy with IFN-α are currently under investigation.
- Liver transplantation (should be considered for fulminant hepatitis).

DISPOSITION

- Follow-up as outpatient
- Acute disease: usually <6 wk
- Rare fatalities (fulminant hepatitis)
- Possible chronic carrier state, cirrhosis, hepatocellular carcinoma

REFERRAL

To infectious disease specialist and gastroenterologist for consultation regarding fulminant hepatitis or prolonged cholestasis, for cases of uncertain etiology, or for treatment of CAH

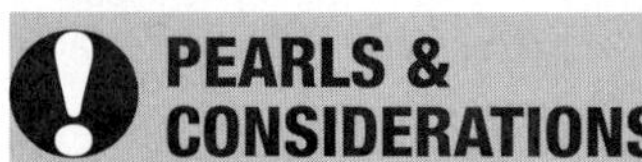

PEARLS & CONSIDERATIONS

COMMENTS

- Virus and HBsAg in high titers in blood for 1 to 7 wk before jaundice and for a variable time thereafter.
- Transmission is possible during entire period of HBsAg (and especially during HBeAg) in serum.
- Universal precautions should be followed for all contacts with blood or secretions/excretions contaminated with blood.
- Preventing before exposure:
  1. Lifestyle changes
  2. Meticulous testing of blood supply (although some chronically infected, infectious donors are HBsAg negative)
  3. Sterilization via steam or hypochlorite
  4. Hepatitis B vaccine for high-risk groups given IM in deltoid to induce HBsAb (response should be confirmed) is protective (>90% effective)
  5. Recommendation for universal childhood immunization with doses at birth, 1 mo, and 6 mo
- Prevention after exposure:
  1. HBV hyperimmune globulin (HBIG) given immediately after needlestick, within 14 days of sexual exposure, or at birth, followed by HBV vaccination
  2. Standard immune globulin: nearly as effective as HBIG
- Preventive therapy with lamivudine for patients who test positive for HBsAg and are undergoing chemotherapy may reduce the risk for HBV reactivation and HBV-associated morbidity and mortality,
- Hepatitis B prophylaxis is described in Section V

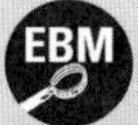

EVIDENCE

Please note: Complete text of EBM for this topic is available online.

Key trials and commentary:

The GLOBE trial compared the efficacy and safety of telbivudine vs. lamivudine treatment over 2 years in patients with chronic hepatitis B.

This study showed that telbivudine is superior to lamivudine in treating patients with chronic hepatitis B over a 2-year period.[1] Ⓐ

The incidence of acute hepatitis B (HBV) in the U.S. is declining according to most recent statistics from the Centers for Disease Control noting an 80% decline from 1987 to 2004. This is largely related to the program of vaccination for HBV. Yet, estimates are that between 1.1 and 2.0 million individuals are chronically infected with HBV in the U.S.

There are now seven drugs available to treat HBV infection. This study together with other studies demonstrates that antiviral agents can reduce the morbidity and improve clinical outcomes in selected individuals with HBV infection as summarized at the recent National Institutes of Health (NIH) consensus conference on HBV.

This study reports the results of the 2-year GLOBE trial demonstrating a significantly better response of telbivudine compared with lamivudine in 921 HBeAg-positive (63% vs. 48%; $P < 0.001$) and 446 HBeAg-negative patients (78% vs. 66%; $P = 0.007$). However, the frequency of telbivudine resistance in HBeAg-positive patients also increased from 5% at 1 year to 25.1% at 2 years. There was also an associated increase in lamivudine resistance of 11% at 1 year and 39.5% at 2 years.

The GLOBE trial demonstrates the importance of ongoing measurement of HBV DNA to ensure drug resistance has not occurred. The trial clearly demonstrated the superiority of telbivudine over lamivudine in treating patients with HBV infection; however, the high resistance rate will likely limit its utility in the management of chronic HBV infection as other agents have been shown to have equal efficacy and less development of resistance.

Evidence-Based Reference

1. 2-Year GLOBE Trial Results: Telbivudine is superior to lamivudine in patients with chronic hepatitis B, *Gastroenterology* 136:486-495, 2009. Commentary by D. Harnois, D.O. Ⓐ

SUGGESTED READINGS

Chan HL et al: Treatment of hepatitis B e antigen-positive chronic hepatitis B with telbivudine or adefovir, *Ann Intern Med* 147:745, 2007.

Chang TT et al: A comparison of entecavir and lamivudine for HbeAg-positive chronic hepatitis B, *N Engl J Med* 354(10):1001, 2006.

Dienstag JL: Hepatitis B virus infection, *N Engl J Med* 359:1486-1500, 2008.

Elgouhari HM et al: Hepatitis B virus infection: understanding its epidemiology, course, and diagnosis, *Cleve Clin J Med* 75:881-889, 2008.

Lai CL et al: Telbivudine versus lamivudine in patients with chronic hepatitis B, *N Engl J Med* 357:2576-2588, 2007.

Lai CL, Yuen MF: Chronic hepatitis B—new goals, new treatment, *N Engl J Med* 359:23, 2008.

Lok AS, McMahon BJ: Chronic hepatitis B (AASLD practice guidelines), *Hepatology* 45:507, 2007.

Loomba R et al: Systematic review: the effect of preventive lamivudine on hepatitis B reactivation during chemotherapy, *Ann Intern Med* 148:519-528, 2008

Pungpapong S et al: Natural history of hepatitis B virus infection: an update for clinicians, *Mayo Clin Proc* 82(8): 967-975, 2007.

Sorrell M et al: National Institutes of Health Consensus Development Conference Statement: management of hepatitis B, *Ann Intern Med* 150:104-110, 2009.

Van der Wielen M et al: Hepatitis A/B vaccination of adults over 40 years old: comparison of three vaccine regimens and effect of influencing factors, *Vaccine* 24(26):5509, 2006.

AUTHORS: **GLENN G. FORT, M.D., M.P.H.,** and **DENNIS J. MIKOLICH, M.D.**

BASIC INFORMATION

DEFINITION

Hepatitis C is an acute liver parenchymal infection caused by hepatitis C virus (HCV).

SYNONYMS

Transfusion-related non-A, non-B hepatitis (incubation period averages 6 wk, intermediate between hepatitis A and B)

ICD-9CM CODES
070.51 Other viral hepatitis

EPIDEMIOLOGY & DEMOGRAPHICS

Hepatitis C infection is the most common chronic blood-borne infection in the U.S.

INCIDENCE (IN U.S.):
- 150,000 new cases/yr (37,500, symptomatic; 93,000, later chronic liver disease; 30,700, cirrhosis)
- Approximately 9000 of these ultimately die of HCV infection; most common (40%) cause of nonalcoholic liver disease in U.S.

PREVALENCE (IN U.S.):
- Overall prevalence of anti-HCV antibody is 1.8% (an estimated 3.9 million persons nationwide)
- Highest prevalence in hemophiliacs transfused before 1987 and users of injection drugs, 72% to 90%
- Among low-risk groups, prevalence 0.6%

PREDOMINANT SEX: Slight male predominance
PREDOMINANT AGE: Highest prevalence in 30- to 49-yr age group (65%)
PEAK INCIDENCE:
- 20 to 39 yr of age
- African Americans and whites have similar incidence of acute disease; Hispanics have higher rates.
- Prevalence is substantially higher among non-Hispanic blacks than among non-Hispanic whites

GENETICS: Neonatal infection is rare; increased risk with maternal HIV-1 coinfection

PHYSICAL FINDINGS & CLINICAL PRESENTATION

- Symptoms usually develop 7 to 8 wk after infection (range of 2 to 26 wk), but 70% to 80% of cases are subclinical.
- 10% to 20% report acute illness with jaundice and nonspecific symptoms (abdominal pain, anorexia, malaise).
- Fulminant hepatitis may rarely occur during this period.
- After acute infection, 15% to 25% have complete resolution (absence of HCV RNA in serum, normal ALT).
- Progression to chronic infection is common, 50% to 84%. 74% to 86% have persistent viremia; spontaneous clearance of viremia in chronic infection is rare. 60% to 70% of patients will have persistent or fluctuating ALT levels; 30% to 40% with chronic infection have normal ALT levels.
- 15% to 20% of those with chronic HCV will develop cirrhosis over a period of 20 to 30 yr; in most others, chronic infection leads to hepatitis and varying degrees of fibrosis.
- 0.4% to 2.5% of patients with chronic infection develop hepatocellular carcinoma.
- 25% of patients with chronic infection continue to have an asymptomatic course with normal LFTs and benign histology.
- In chronic HCV infection, extrahepatic sequelae include a variety of immunologic and lymphoproliferative disorders (e.g., cryoglobulinemia, membranoproliferative glomerulonephritis, and possibly Sjögren's syndrome, autoimmune thyroiditis, polyarteritis nodosa, aplastic anemia, lichen planus, porphyria cutanea tarda, B-cell lymphoma, others).

ETIOLOGY

- Caused by HCV (single-stranded RNA flavivirus).
- Most HCV transmission is parenteral.
- In the U.S., advances in screening of blood and blood products in 1990 and 1992 have made transfusion-related HCV infection rare (the risk is estimated to be 0.001% per unit transfused).
- Injecting-drug use accounts for most HCV transmission in the U.S. (60% of newly acquired cases, 20% to 50% of chronically infected persons).
- Occupational needlestick exposure from an HCV-positive source has a seroconversion rate of 1.8% (range 0% to 7%).
- Nosocomial transmission rates (from surgery and procedures such as colonoscopy and hemodialysis) are extremely low.
- Sexual transmission and maternal-fetal transmission are infrequent (estimated at 5%).
- No identifiable risk in 40% to 50% of community-acquired hepatitis C, but snorting of cocaine by shared use of straw or rolled-up paper has been identified as a risk factor because it causes microscopic bleeding of nasal mucosa.
- HCV infection may stimulate production of cytotoxic T lymphocytes and cytokines (INF-γ), which probably mediate hepatic necrosis.

Dx DIAGNOSIS

DIFFERENTIAL DIAGNOSIS

- Other hepatitis viruses (A, B, D, E)
- Other viral illnesses producing systemic disease (e.g., yellow fever, EBV, CMV, HIV, rubella, rubeola, coxsackie B, adenovirus, HSV, HZV)
- Nonviral hepatitis (e.g., leptospirosis, toxoplasmosis, alcoholic hepatitis, drug-induced hepatitis [acetaminophen, INH], toxic hepatitis)

WORKUP

- Acute hepatitis C antibody (Table 1-37)
- LFTs; CBC

NOTE: ALT is an easy and inexpensive test to monitor infection and efficacy of therapy. However, ALT levels may fluctuate or even be normal in active or chronic infection and even with cirrhosis, and ALT may remain elevated even after clearance of viremia.

- Liver biopsy with histologic staging is the gold standard for assessing the degree of disease activity and the likelihood of disease progression, and also to help rule out other causes of liver disease

LABORATORY TESTS

- Diagnosis is often by exclusion, because it takes 6 wk to 12 mo to develop anti-HCV antibody (70% positive by 6 wk, 90% positive by 6 mo).
- Diagnostic tests include serologic assays for antibodies and molecular tests for viral particles.
  1. Enzyme immunoassay is the test for anti-HCV antibody:
     - The current version can detect antibody within 4 to 10 wk after infection.
     - False-negative rate in low-risk populations is 0.5% to 1%.
     - False-negatives also occur in immune-compromised persons, HIV-1, renal failure, HCV-associated essential mixed cryoglobulinemia.
     - False positives in autoimmune hepatitis, paraproteinemia, and persons with no risk factors
  2. Recombinant immunoblot is used to confirm positive enzyme immunoassays:
     - Recommended only in low-risk settings
  3. Qualitative and quantitative HCV RNA tests using PCR:
     - Lower limit of detection is <100 copies HCV RNA/ml
     - Used to confirm viremia and to assess response to treatment
     - Qualitative polymerase chain reaction (PCR) useful in patients with negative enzyme immunoassay in whom infection is suspected
     - Quantitative tests use either branched-chain DNA or reverse transcription PCR; the latter is more sensitive
  4. Viral genotyping can distinguish among genotypes 1, 2, 3, and 4, which is helpful in choosing therapy; most of these tests use PCR (Note: genotypes 1, 2, 3, and 4 predominate in the U.S. and Europe [1 is especially common in North America])
  5. LFTs:
     - ALT and AST may be elevated to more than eight times normal in acute infection; in chronic infection ALT may be normal or fluctuate
     - Bilirubin may be 5 to 10 times normal
     - Albumin and prothrombin time generally normal; if abnormal, may be harbinger of impending hepatic necrosis
  6. WBC and erythrocyte sedimentation rate (ESR) are generally normal

IMAGING STUDIES

Sonogram: rapid liver size reduction during fulminant hepatitis or mass in hepatocellular carcinoma

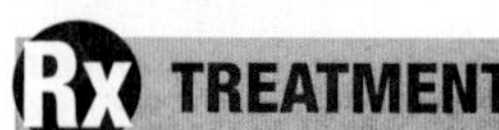

TREATMENT

NONPHARMACOLOGIC THERAPY

Activity and diet as tolerated

ACUTE GENERAL Rx

- Supportive care.
- Avoid hepatically metabolized drugs.
- Specific Rx for acute HCV infection.
- Recent studies demonstrate that early treatment with interferon-alpha-2b during acute HCV infection prevents chronic infection. The aim is to decrease viral load early in infection and allow the patient's immune system to control viral replication, thus preventing progression to chronic infection. The primary end point was sustained virologic response, with absence of HCV RNA in serum 24 wk after completion of therapy.
- Further investigations are in progress.

CHRONIC Rx

- Response to therapy is influenced by HCV genotype. Patients with genotype 1 and genotype 4 have sustained virologic response and cure rates much lower than patients with genotypes 2 and 3. Cure rates for genotypes 1 and 4 are about 45% to 50%, whereas cure rates for genotypes 2 and 3 are as high as 75% to 80%.
- Mainstay of therapy currently is with a pegylated interferon-alpha as a weekly SC injection and oral weight-based ribavirin. For genotypes 1 and 4, the therapy is for 48 wk. For genotypes 2 or 3, the length of therapy is 24 wk.
- Pegylated interferons are interferon-alpha with an attached polyethylene glycol (PEG) molecule. The PEG molecule confers a longer half-life and extended therapeutic activity compared with interferon-alpha and reduced dosing once a wk. A third type of interferon, known as consensus interferon, is also available for treatment of hepatitis C, but it is not a long-acting form like the pegylated interferons.
- Two formulations of PEG interferon are available. Peginterferon alpha-2b (PEG INTRON) uses a weight-based dosage in a once-a-wk SC Redipen injection. Peginterferon alpha-2a (Pegasys) uses a fixed dosage in a once-a-wk premixed syringe, also SC.
- Both PEG interferon-alpha and ribavirin have numerous contraindications (absolute and relative) to use and may cause a variety of side effects. Interferon-alpha can cause flu-like symptoms, thrombocytopenia, granulocytopenia, rash, alopecia, anorexia, psychiatric disturbances, and other side effects. Ribavirin can cause hemolysis, nausea, anemia, nasal congestion, and pruritus. Ribavirin is contraindicated in pregnancy and patients should not get pregnant while on therapy and for 6 mo after therapy.
- In patients who fail to respond to interferon-alpha and ribavirin, <10% will respond to retreatment.
- Treatment trials have shown that pegylated interferon alone achieves higher hepatitis C–specific T-helper-1 response and clinical response rates than does interferon-alpha alone in patients with chronic hepatitis C without cirrhosis, and in patients with chronic hepatitis C with cirrhosis or bridging fibrosis.
- Liver transplantation:
  - Hepatitis C is the main indication for liver transplantation in the U.S.
  - It is the only option for patients with deteriorating HCV-related cirrhosis and for some patients with hepatocellular carcinoma.
  - Recurrent infection occurs in almost all patients with progressive fibrosis and cirrhosis; up to 20% progress to cirrhosis within 5 yr posttransplant.
- Coinfection with HIV:
  - These patients have a poor response to pegylated interferon-alpha and ribavirin if the immune system is depleted, with a low CD4 count as seen in the AIDS category. It is, however, important to treat patients co-infected with HIV and hepatitis C with HAART (highly active antiretroviral therapy). Many co-infected patients are stable from

TABLE 1-37 Tests for Hepatitis C Virus Infection

Test/Type	Application	Comments
Hepatitis C Virus Antibody (anti-HCV)		
EIA	Indicates past or present infection but does not differentiate among acute, chronic, or resolved infection	Sensitivity ≥97%
Supplemental assay (i.e., RIBA)	All positive EIA results should be verified with a supplemental assay	EIA alone has low-positive predictive value in low-prevalence populations
HCV RNA		
Qualitative Tests†*		
RT-PCR amplification of HCV RNA by in-house or commercial assays (e.g., Amplicor HCV)	Detect presence of circulating HCV RNA Monitor patients on antiviral therapy	Detects virus as early as 1-2 wk after exposure Detection of HCV RNA during course of infection might be intermittent; a single negative RT-PCR is not conclusive False-positive and false-negative results might occur
Quantitative Tests†*		
RT-PCR amplification of HCV RNA by in-house or commercial assays (e.g., Amplicor HCV monitor)	Determine concentration of HCV RNA	Less sensitive than qualitative RT-PCR
bDNA assays (e.g., Quantiplex HCV RNA assay)	Might be useful for assessing the likelihood of response to antiviral therapy	Should not be used to exclude the diagnosis of HCV infection or to determine treatment end point
Genotype†*		
Several methodologies available (e.g., hybridization, sequencing)	Group isolates of HCV based on genetic differences, into 6 genotypes and >90 subtypes With new therapies, length of treatment might vary based on genotype	Genotype 1 (subtypes 1a and 1b) most common in U.S. and associated with lower response to antiviral therapy
Serotype*		
EIA based on immunoreactivity to synthetic peptides (e.g., Murex HCV Serotyping 1-6 assay)	No clinical utility	Cannot distinguish among subtypes Dual infections often observed

From *MMWR Morb Mortal Wkly Rep* 47(RR-19), 1998.
*Currently not U.S. Food and Drug Administration approved; lack standardization.
†Samples require special handling (e.g., serum must be separated within 2-4 hours of collection and stored frozen [−20° C or −70° C]; frozen samples should be shipped on dry ice).
bDNA, Branched-chain deoxyribonucleic acid; *EIA,* enzyme immunoassay; *HCV,* hepatitis C virus; *HCV RNA,* hepatitis C virus ribonucleic acid; *RIBA,* recombinant immunoblot assay; *RT-PCR,* reverse transcriptase polymerase chain reaction.

their HIV disease, but have significant morbidity and mortality from their hepatitis C.

DISPOSITION

- Follow-up as outpatient
- Monitor ALT levels as a clue for chronic disease
- Chronic carrier state, cirrhosis, hepatic carcinoma more common than with hepatitis A and B

REFERRAL

- To a hepatologist or infectious disease specialist for treatment for hepatitis C
- To an oncologist if hepatocellular carcinoma develops
- To a transplant surgeon for consideration of liver transplant if indicated

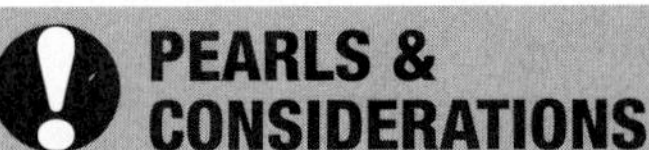

PEARLS & CONSIDERATIONS

- More rapid progression of disease in persons who drink alcohol regularly, persons of advanced age at time of infection, and those co-infected with other viruses (HIV, hepatitis B).
- No preventive vaccine available; postexposure Ig provides minimal protection.
- Preventive measures include use of universal precautions, careful screening of blood and blood products, lifestyle changes.
- Eltrombopag is an orally active thrombopoietin-receptor agonist that stimulates thrombopoiesis. It has been reported effective in increasing platelet counts in patients with thrombocytopenia caused by HCV-related cirrhosis.
- Regression of cirrhosis has been demonstrated after antiviral therapy in some patients with chronic hepatitis C. Regression is associated with decreased disease-related morbidity and improved survival.

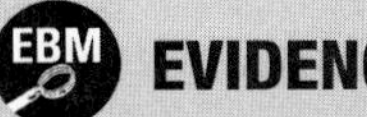

EVIDENCE

Please note: Complete text of EBM for this topic is available online.

Key trials and commentary:

In patients with chronic hepatitis C (HCV) who do not respond to antiviral treatment, the disease may progress to cirrhosis, liver failure, hepatocellular carcinoma, and death. Whether long-term antiviral therapy can prevent progressive liver disease in such patients remains uncertain.

This study showed that long-term therapy with peginterferon did not reduce the rate of disease progression in patients with HCV and advanced fibrosis, with or without cirrhosis, who had not had a response to initial treatment with peginterferon and ribavirin.[1] Ⓐ

The Hepatitis C Antiviral Long-Term Treatment against Cirrhosis (HALT-C) study is a prospective, randomized study to determine whether maintenance therapy with low-dose pegylated interferon alpha in patients with HCV who had failed to clear virus following a standard course of treatment would slow progression of disease. The primary end point of the study was progression of disease as determined by the development of complications of end-stage liver disease including hepatocellular cancer, liver failure, and the need for liver transplant or an increase in fibrosis score (Ishak fibrosis score increase of 2 or more points).

Patients were randomly selected to receive therapy with peginterferon alfa-2a for 3.5 years vs. no treatment. The treatment group had improvement in serum aminotransferases, level of serum HCV RNA, and histology. However, there was no statistical difference in primary end points in the treated and untreated groups. And so the conclusions of the trial are that long-term therapy with peginterferon did not reduce the rate of disease progression in patients with chronic HCV and advanced fibrosis in individuals who had not had an initial response to treatment with peginterferon and ribavirin.

The publication of the results of the HALT-C trial is the final chapter in the use of maintenance therapy as an effective approach in nonresponders with chronic HCV infection. The trial has left us a great deal of knowledge on HCV-related liver disease as yet to be fully understood and has led to the publication of a large number of articles in top-ranking medical journals.

Evidence-Based Reference

1. Di Bisceglie AM, HALT-C Trial Investigators: Prolonged therapy of advanced chronic hepatitis C with low-dose peginterferon, *N Engl J Med* 359: 2429-2441, 2008. Commentary by D. Harnois, D.O.

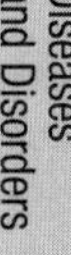

SUGGESTED READINGS

Carrat F et al: Pegylated interferon alfa-2b vs standard interferon alfa-2b, plus ribavirin for chronic hepatitis C in HIV-infected patients: a randomized controlled trial, *JAMA* 292:2839, 2004.

Di Bisceglie AM et al: Prolonged therapy of advanced chronic hepatitis C with low-dose peginterferon, *N Engl J Med* 359:2429-2441, 2008.

Hadziyannis JJ et al: Peginterferon alpha-2a and ribavirin combination therapy in chronic hepatitis C, *Ann Intern Med* 140:346, 2004.

Hezode C et al: Telaprevir and Peginterferon with or without Ribavirin for chronic HCV infection, *N Engl J Med* 360:1839-1850, 2009.

Jensen DM et al: Re-treatment of patients with chronic hepatitis C who do not respond to peginterferon-alpha-2b, *Ann Intern Med* 150:528-540, 2009.

Mallet V et al: Brief communication: the relationship of regression of cirrhosis to outcome in chronic hepatitis C, *Ann Intern Med* 149:399-403, 2008.

McHutchinson JG et al: Eltrombopag for thrombocytopenia in patients with cirrhosis associated with hepatitis C, *N Engl J Med* 357:2227, 2007.

Pardo M et al: Effect of anti-viral therapy for occult hepatitis C virus infection, *Aliment Pharmacol Ther* 23(8):1153, 2006.

Scott JD, Gretch DR: Molecular diagnostics of hepatitis C virus infection, *JAMA* 297:724, 2007.

Torriani FJ et al: Peginterferon alfa-2a plus ribavirin for chronic hepatitis C virus infection in HIV-infected patients, *N Engl J Med* 351:438, 2004.

AUTHORS: **GLENN G. FORT, M.D., M.P.H.,** and **DENNIS J. MIKOLICH, M.D.**

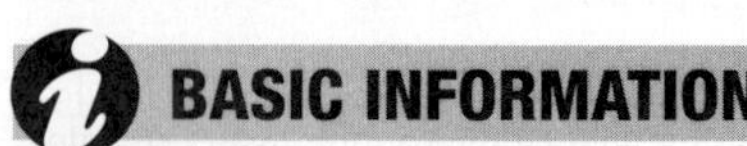

BASIC INFORMATION

DEFINITION

Autoimmune hepatitis is a chronic inflammatory condition of the liver characterized by elevated serum globulin levels and the presence of circulating autoantibodies. Two types have been described:

- Type 1, or "classic," autoimmune hepatitis is the most predominant form in the U.S. and worldwide (80%); patients are positive for antinuclear antibodies (ANA) and/or anti-smooth muscle antibodies (ASMA). Occurs across all age ranges and may be underdiagnosed in the elderly.
- Type 2 is rare in the U.S. and primarily affects young children. Type 2 is characterized by the presence of antibodies to liver/kidney microsomes (anti-LKM-1) or liver cytosol 1.

SYNONYMS

Autoimmune chronic active hepatitis
Chronic active hepatitis
Lupoid hepatitis

ICD-9CM CODES
571.49 Chronic hepatitis

EPIDEMIOLOGY & DEMOGRAPHICS

- Annual incidence (estimated): 1.9 cases per 100,000
- Point prevalence (estimated): 16.9 per 100,000
- Type 1: all age groups; type 2: more common in teenagers and young adults
- Female/male ratio is 3.6:1
- Approximately 100,000 to 200,000 persons affected in the U.S.
- Accounts for 5.9% of liver transplants in U.S.
- Associated with HLA DR3 and HLA DR4

CLINICAL PRESENTATION

- Varies from asymptomatic elevations of liver enzymes to fulminant hepatitis to advanced cirrhosis.
- Symptoms may include fatigue, anorexia, nausea, abdominal pain, pruritus, and arthralgia.
- Jaundice.
- Hepatomegaly/splenomegaly.
- Autoimmune findings may include arthritis, xerostomia, keratoconjunctivitis, cutaneous vasculitis, and erythema nodosum.
- Patients with advanced disease show ascites, edema, abnormal bleeding, and jaundice.

ETIOLOGY

- Exact etiology is unknown; liver histology demonstrates cell-mediated immune attack against hepatocytes.
- Presence of a variety of autoantibodies suggests an autoimmune mechanism.
- Strong genetic predisposition.
- Potential triggering agents such as virus (hepatitis A) or drugs (minocycline, atorvastatin).

Dx DIAGNOSIS

A simplified diagnostic criteria for routine clinical practice has been developed by the International Autoimmune Hepatitis Group (see Table 1-38).

DIFFERENTIAL DIAGNOSIS

- Acute viral hepatitis (A, B, C, D, E, cytomegalovirus, Epstein-Barr, herpes)
- Chronic viral hepatitis (B, C)
- Toxic hepatitis (alcohol, drugs)
- Primary biliary cirrhosis
- Primary sclerosing cholangitis
- Hemochromatosis
- Nonalcoholic steatohepatitis
- SLE
- Wilson's disease
- Alpha-1 antitrypsin deficiency

WORKUP

- History and physical examination with attention to the presence of autoimmune abnormalities such as thyroiditis, Graves' disease, ulcerative colitis, and rheumatoid arthritis
- Liver function tests and serum gamma-globulins
- Tests for autoantibodies
- Liver biopsy for establishing diagnosis and disease severity

LABORATORY TESTS

- Aminotransferases generally elevated, may fluctuate
- Bilirubin and alkaline phosphatase moderately elevated or normal
- Elevation of gamma globulin and immunoglobulin G
- Circulating autoantibodies often present:
  1. Rheumatoid factor
  2. ANAs
     a. Present in two thirds of patients
     b. Typical pattern is homogeneous or speckled
     c. Titer does not correlate with the stage, activity, or prognosis
  3. ASMAs
     a. Present in 87% of patients
     b. Titer does not correlate with course or prognosis
  4. Anti-LKM antibodies
     a. Typically found in patients who are ANA negative and ASMA negative
     b. Found in $<1/25$ of patients in U.S.
     c. Present in pediatric population and up to 20% of adults in Europe; also present in patients with drug-induced hepatitis
  5. Autoantibodies against soluble liver antigen and liver-pancreas antigen (anti-SLA/LP)
     a. Present in 10% to 30% of patients
     b. Associated with higher rate of relapse after corticosteroid therapy
     c. Several studies suggest that patients with anti-SLA/LP have a more severe course
- Hypoalbuminemia and prolonged prothrombin time with advanced disease
- There is a well-described overlap syndrome with primary biliary cirrhosis (7%), primary sclerosing cholangitis (6%), and autoimmune cholangitis (11%)

IMAGING STUDIES

Ultrasound of liver and biliary tree to rule out obstruction or hepatic mass

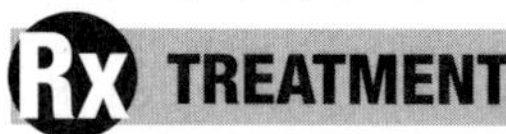

TREATMENT

NONPHARMACOLOGIC THERAPY

- Avoid alcohol and hepatotoxic medications.
- Liver transplantation is an option for end-stage disease or fulminant hepatic failure.

PHARMACOLOGIC THERAPY

- Initial treatment:
  1. Prednisone 60 mg/day PO or combination treatment with prednisone 30 mg/day PO plus azathioprine 50 mg/day PO.
  2. Combination therapy allows lower prednisone doses and fewer steroid side effects.
  3. Goal of therapy is remission (normalization of gamma-globulin and bilirubin, reduction of aminotransferases to less than twice the upper limit of normal).
- Indications for treatment:
  1. Serum aminotransferase >10 times the upper limit of normal
  2. Serum aminotransferase more than five times the upper limit of normal, with serum gamma-globulin level twice the upper limit of normal
  3. Young age

TABLE 1-38 Diagnostic Criteria for Autoimmune Hepatitis

Variable	Cutoff	Points	Cutoff	Points
ANA or SMA	≥1:40	1	≥1:80	2
LKM			≥1:40	2
SLA			Positive	2
IgG	≥ULN	1	≥1.1 × ULN	2
Histology	Compatible with AIH	1	Typical of AIH	2
Absence of viral hepatitis			Yes	2

Maximum number of points for all antibodies = 2, total = 8.
Probable AIH ≥6 points, definite AIH ≥7 points.
AIH, Autoimmune hepatitis; *ANA,* antinuclear antibody; *IgG,* immunoglobulin G; *LKM,* liver/kidney microsomes; *SLA,* soluble liver antigen; *SMA,* smooth muscle antibody; *ULN,* upper limit of normal.

4. Histologic features of bridging necrosis or multiacinar necrosis
5. Compensated cirrhosis:
   a. 3- to 6-mo treatment trial may be beneficial in patients with inflammation on liver biopsy.
   b. Fibrosis may improve during corticosteroid therapy, and treatment may delay or obviate liver transplantation.

- Evaluation of treatment response:
  1. Goal is the absence of symptoms, resolution of liver function test abnormalities, and histologic improvement.
  2. Patients whose transaminase levels normalize may continue to have ongoing active hepatitis involving inflammation and fibrosis. Five percent to 10% of patients with normal transaminase levels progress to cirrhosis.
  3. Histologic improvement may lag behind clinical and laboratory improvement by as much as 6 mo.
  4. Repeat liver biopsy should be considered after normalization of transaminase levels.
  5. Complete normalization on biopsy is associated with a 15% to 20% risk of relapse.
  6. Persistent interface hepatitis is associated with a 90% risk of relapse.

DISPOSITION

- Follow up as outpatient.
- Long-term treatment may be necessary for sustained remission.
- Sixty-five percent of patients achieve remission by 18 mo; 80% achieve remission by 3 yr.
- Approximately 10% of patients do not improve with therapy.
- Patients in whom end-stage liver develops are candidates for liver transplantation. Recurrent disease may occur after liver transplantation.

REFERRAL

Patients with advanced cirrhosis or who progress to end-stage liver disease are candidates for liver transplantation and should be referred to appropriate medical centers that provide liver transplantation services.

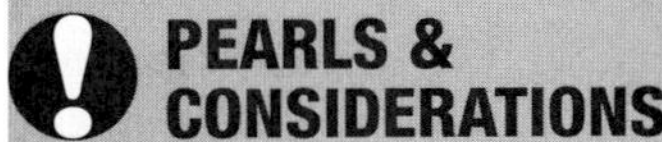

COMMENTS

- A variety of autoimmune conditions can be seen in association with autoimmune hepatitis, including thyroiditis, Graves' disease, ulcerative colitis, rheumatoid arthritis, uveitis, pernicious anemia, Sjögren's syndrome, mixed connective tissue disease, CREST syndrome, and vitiligo.
- Variant forms of autoimmune hepatitis (overlap syndrome) have clinical and serologic findings of autoimmune hepatitis plus features of other forms of chronic liver disease such as primary biliary cirrhosis (PBC) or primary sclerosing cholangitis (PSC).

PREVENTION

None

PATIENT & FAMILY EDUCATION

- American Liver Foundation (ALF) Phone: 800-GO-LIVER (465-4837) E-mail: Internet: www.liverfoundation.org
- National Digestive Diseases Information clearinghouse: http://digestive.niddk.nih.gov/ddiseases/pubs/autoimmunehep

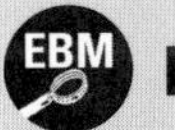

EVIDENCE

The use of prednisone in the treatment of autoimmune hepatitis is based on data from early interventional studies in the 1970s and current expert opinion.

In an early placebo-controlled trial of prednisolone treatment of active chronic hepatitis the 2-yr survival was 86% for the prednisolone group and 66% for placebo.[1] Ⓑ

Prednisone in combination with azathioprine or a higher dose of prednisone alone is considered to be the appropriate treatment for severe autoimmune hepatitis in adults.[2] Ⓒ

The use of azathioprine in the treatment of autoimmune hepatitis is based on current expert opinion and evidence of its use as a steroid-sparing agent and as an aid to long-term maintenance.

Prednisone in combination with azathioprine or a higher dose of prednisone alone is considered to be the appropriate treatment for severe autoimmune hepatitis in adults. Prednisone in combination with azathioprine is the preferred initial treatment because of its lower frequency of side effects.[2] Ⓒ

In a prolonged study many patients with autoimmune hepatitis who had been in complete remission for at least one year with prednisolone and azathioprine were able to remain in remission with a higher dose of azathioprine alone.[3] Ⓑ

The use of liver transplantation in the treatment of patients with autoimmune hepatitis who continue to deteriorate despite conventional corticosteroid treatment, patients who are refractory or intolerant to immunosuppressive therapy, or who have decompensated liver disease is supported by expert opinion.

Evidence-based professional guidelines from the American Association for the Study of Liver Diseases recommend that patients with autoimmune hepatitis who continue to deteriorate despite conventional corticosteroid treatment, patients who are refractory or intolerant to immunosuppressive therapy, or who have decompensated liver disease should be referred for consideration of liver transplantation.[2,4] Ⓒ

Evidence-Based References

1. Cook GC et al: Controlled prospective trial of corticosteroid therapy in active chronic hepatitis, *Q J Med* 40:159-185, 1971. Ⓑ
2. Czaja AJ, Freese DK: Diagnosis and treatment of autoimmune hepatitis, *Hepatology* 36:479-497, 2002. Ⓒ
3. Johnson PJ et al: Azathioprine for long-term maintenance of remission in autoimmune hepatitis, *N Engl J Med* 333:958-963, 1995. Ⓑ
4. Murray KF, Carithers RL Jr; AASLD practice guidelines: evaluation of the patient for liver transplantation, *Hepatology* 41:1407-1432, 2005. Ⓒ

SUGGESTED READINGS

Al-Khalidi JA, Czaja AJ: Current concepts in the diagnosis, pathogenesis, and treatment of autoimmune hepatitis, *Mayo Clin Proc* 76:1237, 2001.

Czaja AJ, Freese AD: American Association for the Study of Liver Diseases guideline: diagnosis and treatment of autoimmune hepatitis, *Hepatology* 36: 479, 2002.

Hennes EM et al: Simplified criteria for the diagnosis of autoimmune hepatitis, *Hepatology* 48:169, 2008.

Krawitt EL: Autoimmune hepatitis, *N Engl J Med* 354: 54, 2006.

AUTHORS: **KITTICHAI PROMRAT, M.D.,** and **CHRISTINE M. DUFFY, M.D., M.P.H.**

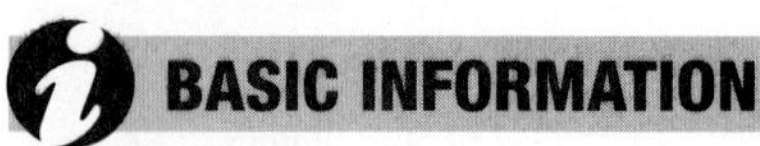

BASIC INFORMATION

DEFINITION

Hepatocellular carcinoma (HCC) is a malignant tumor of the hepatocytes.

SYNONYMS

Hepatoma

ICD-9CM CODES

155.0 Hepatocellular carcinoma

EPIDEMIOLOGY & DEMOGRAPHICS

Fifth most common cancer worldwide and third most common cause of cancer deaths. Incidence varies worldwide:

- Areas with high rates of hepatitis B and C (Asia, sub-Saharan Africa) have high rates of HCC.
- Males more affected than females, with ratios between 2:1 and 4:1.
- Peak incidence: fifth and sixth decades in Western countries, earlier in areas with perinatal transmission of hepatitis B.
- Incidence rapidly growing in U.S. secondary to hepatitis C infection.
  - Incidence: increased more than twofold in the past 20 years; 3.3/100,000 per year between 1999 and 2001
  - Mean age of diagnosis approximately 65 yr
- Risk factors:
  - Hepatitis B infection
  - Chronic hepatitis C infection
  - Cirrhosis from causes other than viral hepatitis: alcoholic liver disease, nonalcoholic steatohepatitis, primary biliary cirrhosis, hemochromatosis, alpha-1-antitrypsin deficiency, and autoimmune hepatitis
  - Hepatotoxins: alcohol and aflatoxin B_1
  - Systemic diseases affecting the liver such as tyrosinemia
  - Obesity and diabetes mellitus

PHYSICAL FINDINGS & CLINICAL PRESENTATION

- One third of patients are asymptomatic. Abdominal pain may be the initial presentation.
- Signs of underlying cirrhosis and portal hypertension are often present.
- Previously compensated cirrhosis with new ascites, encephalopathy, jaundice, or bleeding.
- Paraneoplastic syndromes (hypoglycemia, erythrocytosis, hypercalcemia, severe diarrhea) may be present.

DIAGNOSIS

DIFFERENTIAL DIAGNOSIS

- Metastatic tumor to liver
- Benign liver tumors such as adenomas, focal nodular hyperplasia, and hemangiomas
- Focal fatty infiltration

WORKUP

- History regarding risk factors
- Physical examination with attention to signs of chronic liver disease
- Laboratory evaluation and imaging studies

LABORATORY TESTS

- Liver function tests
- Elevated α-fetoprotein in 70% of patients (sensitivity, 40%-65%; specificity, 80%-94%).
- Paraneoplastic syndromes associated with HCC may cause hypercalcemia, hypoglycemia, and polycythemia
- Elevated serum HBV DNA level ($\geq$10,000 copies/ml) is a strong risk predictor of HCC independent of HBeAg, serum aminotransferase level, and liver cirrhosis

IMAGING STUDIES

Ultrasound (US), CT scan (Fig. 1-146), or MRI. Ultrasound is most commonly used as a screening test for HCC in high-risk patients. Multiphasic CT and MR scans are usually performed when a focal lesion is present on US or strong clinical suspicion of HCC.

BIOPSY

Percutaneous biopsy under ultrasound or CT scan usually is diagnostic. Tissue diagnosis is the gold standard. However, HCC can be reliably diagnosed when:

- Mass >2 cm that shows characteristic arterial vascularization seen on two imaging modalities, or
- Single positive imaging method with AFP >200 μg/ml

SCREENING

Screening high-risk patients with US and AFP every 6 mo may identify HCC at an early stage. The use of AFP alone should be discouraged due to limited sensitivity and specificity. Newer tumor markers (lectin-bound AFP [AFP-L3%] and Des-gamma carboxy-prothrombin [DCP]) have not been shown to be more sensitive than AFP, thus they have very limited clinical utility. Patients on transplant waiting lists should be regularly screened for HCC because in the U.S. the development of HCC gives increased priority for liver transplantation. Screening for HCC is recommended in the following groups:

- Hepatitis B carriers (HBsAg positive): Asian males >40 yr, Asian females >50 yr, all cirrhotic hepatitis B carriers, family history of HCC and Africans over age 20 yr
- Cirrhosis (non-hepatitis B): hepatitis C, alcoholic cirrhosis, hemochromatosis, primary biliary cirrhosis, and possibly α_1-antitrypsin deficiency, autoimmune hepatitis, and nonalcoholic steatohepatitis

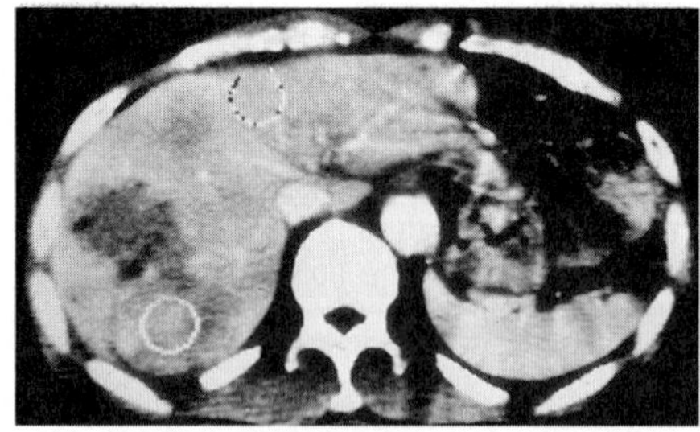

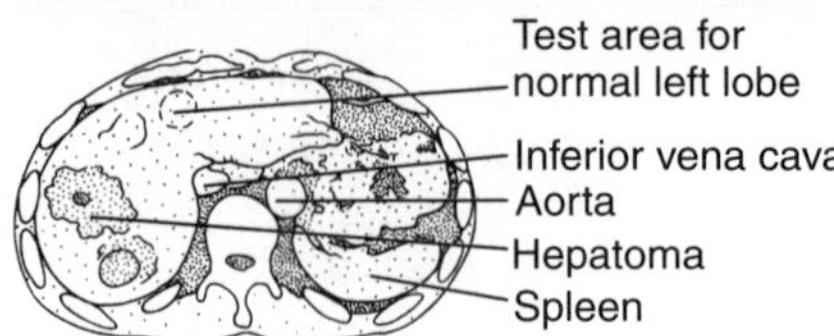

FIGURE 1-146 Hepatoma. CT scan shows a diffuse lesion in the right lobe of an otherwise normal liver. (From Skarin AT: *Atlas of diagnostic oncology,* ed 3, St. Louis, 2003, Mosby.)

STAGING

According to the Barcelona Clinic Liver Cancer (BCLC) staging classification, treatment is determined according to stage:

- Early stage (A): asymptomatic single tumor 5 cm or 3 nodules, each 3 cm (known as Milan criteria)
- Intermediate stage (B): patients with tumors that exceed early criteria but do not yet show cancer-related symptoms, vascular invasion, or metastases
- Advanced stage (C): patients with mild cancer-related symptoms and/or vascular invasion or extrahepatic spread
- End-stage (D): patients with advanced, symptomatic disease

TREATMENT

- Early stage: curative treatment (surgical resection or liver transplantation). Patients who have a single lesion can be offered surgical resection if they are noncirrhotic or have cirrhosis but still have well preserved liver function. Liver transplantation is an effective option for patients with HCC corresponding to the Milan criteria. Local ablation is safe and effective therapy for patients who cannot undergo resection or as a bridge to transplantation. With these options, survival at 5 yr ranges from 50% to 70%.
- Intermediate stage: optimal therapeutic approach is controversial. Outcome may be improved with chemoembolization. Median survival with this option exceeds 2 yr.
- Advanced stage: sorafenib, an oral multikinase inhibitor of the vascular endothelial growth factor receptor (VEGF), the platelet-derived growth factor receptor (PDGF), and Raf, a serine-threonine kinase, has been shown to improve survival and delay disease progression. The SHARP trial included patients with advanced HCC in Child-Pugh A cirrhosis and showed increased median survival from 7.9 to 10.7 mo.
- End stage: palliative care.

DISPOSITION

For unresectable tumors, prognosis is poor; 5-yr survival after surgical resection ranges from 30% to 50%.

REFERRAL

To gastroenterologist for treatment planning

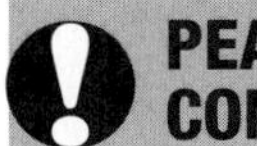

PEARLS & CONSIDERATIONS

Prevention:

- Universal hepatitis B vaccination in children in endemic areas has been shown to decrease the incidence of HCC.
- Treatment of patients with chronic hepatitis B–associated cirrhosis with lamivudine reduces the incidence of HCC.
- For hepatitis C virus–associated HCC, postoperative treatment with interferon-α may decrease the rate of tumor recurrence.
- Eliminate aflatoxin from food.
- HCC screening is recommended in high-risk patients because curative therapies are available for small and early HCC.
- The expression patterns of microRNAs in liver tissue in patients with HCC differ between men and women. The miR-26 expression status of such patients is associated with survival and response to adjuvant therapy with interferon alfa.

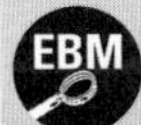

EVIDENCE

Please note: Complete text of EBM for this topic is available online.

Key trials and commentary:

Although the incidence of hepatocellular carcinoma (HCC) is increasing in the U.S., data from large prospective studies are limited. We evaluated the Hepatitis C Antiviral Long-Term Treatment against Cirrhosis (HALT-C) cohort for the incidence of HCC and associated risk factors.

This study showed that maintenance peginterferon did not reduce the incidence of HCC in the HALT-C cohort. Baseline clinical and laboratory features predicted risk for HCC. Additional studies are required to confirm our finding of HCC in patients with chronic hepatitis C (HCV) and bridging fibrosis.[1] Ⓐ

The Hepatitis C Antiviral Long-Term Treatment against Cirrhosis (HALT-C) study is a prospective, randomized study to determine whether maintenance therapy with low-dose pegylated interferon alpha in patients with HCV who had failed to clear virus following a standard course of treatment would slow progression of disease. Progression of disease was determined on biopsy and by the development of complications of end-stage liver disease including HCC, liver failure, and the need for liver transplant.

In this report by Lok et al, the effect of maintenance therapy for HCV was assessed for its impact on the development of HCC. There were a total of 1005 patients studied. Patients received either maintenance peginterferon or placebo for 3.5 years. During the median follow-up of 4.6 years, the cumulative risk for HCC was higher for those patients with cirrhosis (7%) than those with bridging fibrosis (4.1%). The risk of developing HCC was not statistically different for those patients receiving maintenance therapy than for those on placebo.

The results of this study are in direct contrast to previously published reports showing that antiviral therapy did reduce the incidence of HCC in HCV patients. These differences can likely be explained by the fact that the trial reported here involved a large cohort and was a prospective and randomized study.

This study also provided information on the annual incidence of HCC in patients with HCV-related advanced liver disease. The 3-year incidence in the population studied was 1.9% increasing to 5.9% at 5 years, yielding an annual incidence of 1.1%.

A second important outcome of this trial was the development of a predictive model for HCC. A regression formula is reported in this article, stratifying patients into low-, intermediate-, and high-risk groups. The ability for this model to predict the development of HCC in a prospective analysis or to help define screening strategies for HCV patients in the future will require further study.

Evidence-Based Reference

1. Lok AS, The HALT-C Trial Group: Incidence of hepatocellular carcinoma and associated risk factors in hepatitis C-related advanced liver disease, *Gastroenterology* 136:138-148, 2009. Commentary by: D. Harnois, D.O. Ⓐ

SUGGESTED READINGS

Cheng BQ et al: Chemoembolization combined with radio frequency ablation for patients with hepatocellular carcinoma larger than 3 cm: a randomized controlled trial, *JAMA* 299(14):1669-1677, 2008.

Chien-Jen C et al: Risk of hepatocellular carcinoma across a biological gradient of serum hepatitis B virus DNA level, *JAMA* 295:65-73, 2006.

El-Serag H, Rudolph K: Hepatocellular carcinoma: epidemiology and molecular carcinogenesis, *Gastroenterology* 132(7):2557, 2007.

El-Serag H et al: Diagnosis and treatment of hepatocellular carcinoma, *Gastroenterology* 134(6):1752-1763, 2008.

Ji J et al: MicroRNA expression, survival, and response to interferon in liver cancer, *N Engl J Med* 361:1437-47, 2009.

Llovet JM et al: Sorefenib in advanced hepatocellular carcinoma, *N Engl J Med* 359:378-390, 2008.

Parikh S, Hyman D: Hepatocellular cancer: a guide for the internist, *Am J Med* 120:194, 2007.

Perilongo G et al: Cisplatin versus Cisplatin plus Doxorubicin for standard-risk hepatoblastoma, *N Engl J Med* 361:1662-1670, 2009.

Sherman M: Recurrence of hepatocellular carcinoma, *N Engl J Med* 359:19, 2008.

Stravitz RT et al: Surveillance for hepatocellular carcinoma in patients with cirrhosis improves outcome, *Am J Med* 121:119, 2008.

Zhu AX, Ghassan KA: Expanding the treatment options for hepatocellular carcinoma, *JAMA* 299:1716, 2008.

AUTHOR: **KITTICHAI PROMRAT, M.D.**

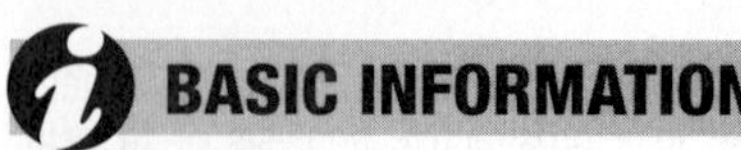

BASIC INFORMATION

DEFINITION

Hepatopulmonary syndrome is characterized by intrapulmonary vascular dilatation in the setting of liver disease causing an increased alveolar-arterial gradient.

SYNONYMS

None

ICD-9CM CODES

417.9 Unspecified disease of pulmonary circulation

EPIDEMIOLOGY & DEMOGRAPHICS

PREVALENCE: Between 4% to 47% of patients with liver disease; wide range due to lack of diagnostic criteria

PREDOMINANT SEX AND AGE: There are no data on gender or age prevalence.

RISK FACTORS: Can occur with any degree or etiology of liver disease but is more common in patients with established cirrhosis and portal hypertension. There is not a clear relationship between severity of hepatic dysfunction and level of hypoxemia.

GENETICS: There are no data on genetic factors in hepatopulmonary syndrome.

PHYSICAL FINDINGS & CLINICAL PRESENTATION

- Dyspnea
- Platypnea: worsened dyspnea when sitting upright compared to supine position due to further ventilation-perfusion mismatch
- Orthodeoxia: decreased PaO_2 when the patient is sitting upright compared to supine position due to ventilation-perfusion mismatch
- Spider angiomata seen in high number
- Signs of severe hypoxemia (e.g., cyanosis and clubbing of the digits)

ETIOLOGY

Dilation of intrapulmonary arterioles and dilated vascular channels between pulmonary arteries and veins leading to a ventilation-perfusion match and right-to-left shunting (Fig. 1-147). Research shows that nitric oxide plays a role in vasodilation. The relationship of vasodilation to liver disease is unclear.

DIAGNOSIS

DIFFERENTIAL DIAGNOSIS

- Portopulmonary hypertension
- Cavo-pulmonary anastomosis
- Hereditary hemorrhagic telangiectasia (Rendu-Osler-Weber syndrome)
- Chronic lung disease (i.e., COPD or pulmonary fibrosis) with coexisting liver disease

WORKUP

Workup includes lab testing and imaging studies (see following), but diagnosis is based on clinical findings.

LABORATORY TESTS

- Arterial blood gas at rest, both supine and erect; $PaO_2 < 80$ mm Hg
- Pulmonary function tests will show nonspecific reduction in DLCO

IMAGING STUDIES

- Chest x-ray may show nonspecific bibasilar interstitial pattern.
- Transthoracic echocardiogram with bubble study to rule out right-to-left cardiac shunt; microbubble opacification in left atrium shows vasodilation of pulmonary vascular bed.
- Scintigraphic perfusion scanning: technetium-99m-labeled albumin found in brain or spleen indicates dilated pulmonary vasculature or cardiac right-to-left shunt.
- Pulmonary angiography rarely used unless there is potential to embolize arteriovenous malformation.

TREATMENT

Ideal treatment would be targeted against pulmonary vasodilation but no effective medications yet exist. Liver transplantation is the only successful treatment, however severe hypoxemia with $PaO_2 < 50$ has been associated with a high posttransplant mortality. Some studies have shown benefit of transjugular portosystemic shunting though it is not currently established treatment. Coil embolization in the setting of pulmonary arteriovenous malformations (AVMs) is another possible area of treatment.

NONPHARMACOLOGIC THERAPY

Oxygen to correct hypoxemia; PaO_2 will partially correct with administration of supplemental O_2.

ACUTE GENERAL Rx

Correct hypoxemia with supplemental O_2.

CHRONIC Rx

Liver transplantation is only successful treatment.

COMPLEMENTARY and ALTERNATIVE MEDICINE

Studies of diets containing low amount of L-arginine have not shown benefit.

DISPOSITION

The diagnosis of hepatopulmonary syndrome confers a poor prognosis. Patients with hepatopulmonary syndrome have high mortality and shorter median survival than other patients with liver disease, even after adjusting for severity of liver disease. According to one natural history study, compared with patients with similar severity of liver disease and comorbidities whose 5-yr survival was estimated at 63%, those patients with the diagnosis of hepatopulmonary syndrome had a 5-yr survival rate of 23%.

REFERRAL

- Referral to pulmonologist to help in establishing diagnosis.
- Referral to a liver transplant center should be considered for patients who would be eligible.

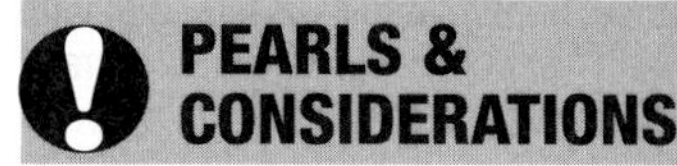

PEARLS & CONSIDERATIONS

COMMENTS

Consider the diagnosis of hepatopulmonary syndrome in patients with cirrhosis who present with dyspnea without signs of pulmonary edema from fluid overload.

SUGGESTED READINGS

Hoeper MM et al: Portopulmonary hypertension and hepatopulmonary syndrome, *Lancet* 363:1461, 2004.

Rodriguez-Roisin R, Krowka MJ: Hepatopulmonary syndrome—a liver-induced lung vascular disorder, *N Engl J Med* 358:2378, 2008.

Swanson KL et al: Natural history of hepatopulmonary syndrome: impact of liver transplantation, *Hepatology* 41:1122, 2005.

AUTHOR: **BEVIN KENNEY, M.D.**

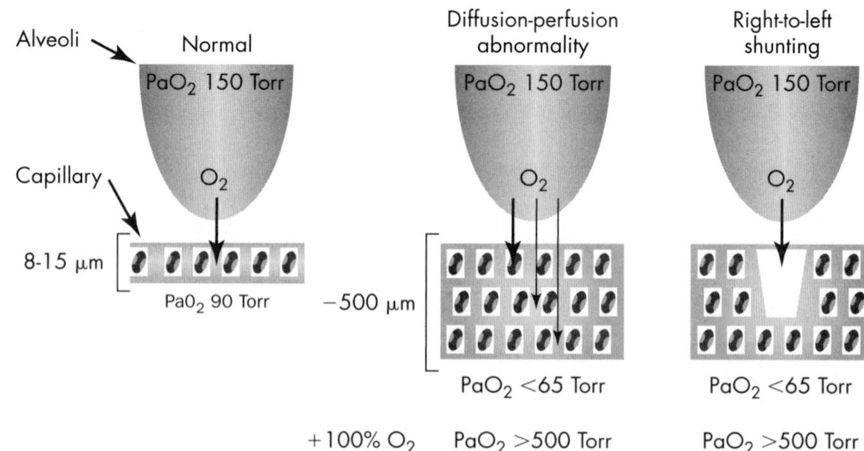

FIGURE 1-147 Pathophysiology of hypoxemia in hepatopulmonary syndrome. Abnormal intrapulmonary vascular dilatation in combination with increased pulmonary blood flow leads to diffusion-perfusion disturbance and arterial hypoxemia, correctable by oxygen supplementation. Most severe intrapulmonary vascular dilatation or formation of arteriovenous malformations causes right-to-left shunting only partially correctable by oxygen administration. (From Hoeper MM et al: Portopulmonary hypertension and hepatopulmonary syndrome, *Lancet* 363:1461, 2004.)

BASIC INFORMATION

DEFINITION

Hepatorenal syndrome (HRS) is a condition of intense renal vasoconstriction resulting from loss of renal autoregulation occurring as a complication of severe liver disease. Criteria for hepatorenal syndrome are:

1. Serum creatinine concentration >1.5 mg/dl or 24-hr creatinine clearance <40 ml/min
2. Absence of shock, ongoing infection, and fluid loss and no current treatment with nephrotoxic drugs
3. Absence of sustained improvement in renal function (decrease in serum creatinine to <1.5 mg/dl after discontinuation of diuretics and a trial of plasma expansion)
4. Absence of proteinuria (<500 mg/day) or hematuria (<50 red blood cells/high power field)
5. Absence of ultrasonographic evidence of obstructive uropathy or parenchymal renal disease
6. Urinary sodium concentration <10 mmol/L

There are two types of hepatorenal syndrome:

1. Type 1: progressive impairment in renal function as defined by a doubling of initial serum creatinine >2.5 mg/dl in <2 wk
2. Type 2: stable or slowly progressive impairment of renal function not meeting the above criteria

SYNONYMS

Hepatic nephropathy
Oliguric renal failure of cirrhosis
HRS

ICD-9CM CODES
572.4 Hepatorenal syndrome

EPIDEMIOLOGY & DEMOGRAPHICS

The probability of HRS in patients with cirrhosis is 18% at 1 yr and 39% at 5 yr.

PHYSICAL FINDINGS & CLINICAL PRESENTATION

- Evidence of cirrhosis is usually present: jaundice, spider angiomas, splenomegaly, ascites, fetor hepaticus, pedal edema
- Hepatic encephalopathy: flapping tremor (asterixis), coma
- Tachycardia and bounding pulse
- Oliguria

ETIOLOGY

An exacerbation of end-stage liver disease, HRS may occur after significant reduction of effective blood volume (e.g., paracentesis, GI bleeding, diuretics) or in the absence of any precipitating factors.

Dx DIAGNOSIS

DIFFERENTIAL DIAGNOSIS

- Prerenal azotemia: response to sustained plasma expansion is good (prompt diuresis with volume expansion). Volume challenge (to increase mean arterial pressure) followed by large-volume paracentesis (to increase cardiac output and decrease renal venous pressure) may be useful to distinguish HRS from prerenal azotemia in patients with FENa <1%. In patients with prerenal azotemia, the increase in renal perfusion pressure and renal blood flow will result in prompt diuresis; the volume challenge can be accomplished by giving a solution of 100 g of albumin in 500 ml of isotonic saline.
- Acute tubular necrosis: urinary sodium >30 mEq/L, fractional excretion of sodium (FENa) >1.5%, urinary/plasma creatinine ratio <30, urine/plasma osmolality ratio = 1, urine sediment reveals casts and cellular debris, no significant response to sustained plasma expansion.

WORKUP

Patients with acute azotemia and oliguria in the setting of liver disease should undergo laboratory evaluation to differentiate HRS from acute tubular necrosis and volume challenge to differentiate HRS from prerenal azotemia if FENa <1%.

LABORATORY TESTS

- Obtain serum electrolytes, blood urea nitrogen, creatinine, osmolality, urinalysis, urinary sodium, urinary creatinine, urine osmolality
- Calculate FENa
- In HRS: urinary sodium <10 mEq/L, FENa <1%, urinary plasma creatinine ratio >30, urinary plasma osmolality ratio >1.5, urine sediment unremarkable

IMAGING STUDIES

Renal ultrasound may be indicated if renal obstruction is suspected.

Rx TREATMENT

NONPHARMACOLOGIC THERAPY

- Avoidance of precipitating factors.
- Transjugular intrahepatic portosystemic shunts may be effective in selected patients, but data are limited.
- Dialysis with molecular adsorbent recirculating systems remains investigational until more data are available.

ACUTE GENERAL Rx

- The only effective treatment of HRS is liver transplantation; ornipressin is used in some liver units to avoid further deterioration of renal function in patients awaiting liver transplantation. In general, dopamine and prostaglandins are ineffective in treating patients with hepatorenal syndrome.
- The best approach to the management of HRS based on its pathogenesis is the administration of vasoconstrictor drugs (terlipressin, norepinephrine, midodrine). Terlipressin may improve renal perfusion by reversing splanchnic vasodilation, which is the hallmark of HRS. Encouraging results were found in a recent study using continuous IV noradrenalin in combination with albumin and furosemide. In this study, reversal of HRS was achieved in 10 of 12 patients.
- Treatment of hepatorenal syndrome with vasoconstrictors for 5 to 15 days in attempt to reduce serum creatinine to <1.5 mg/dl is as follows:
  1. Administration of one of the following drugs or drug combinations:
     a. Norepinephrine (0.5 to 3.0 mg/hr IV)
     b. Midodrine (7.5 mg PO tid, increased to 12.5 mg tid if needed) in combination with octreotide (100 micrograms SC tid, increased to tid prn)
     c. Terlipressin (0.2 to 2.0 mg IV q4-12h)
  2. Concomitant administration of albumin (1 g/kg IV on day 1, followed by 20 to 40 g daily)

DISPOSITION

Mortality rate exceeds 80%; liver transplantation is the only curative treatment.

REFERRAL

Referral for liver transplantation when indicated (see "Comments")

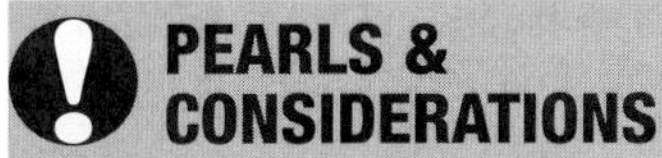

PEARLS & CONSIDERATIONS

COMMENTS

Liver transplantation may be indicated in otherwise healthy patients (age preferably <65 yr) with sclerosing cholangitis, chronic hepatitis with cirrhosis, or primary biliary cirrhosis. Contraindications to liver transplantation are AIDS, most metastatic malignancies, active substance abuse, uncontrolled sepsis, and uncontrolled cardiac or pulmonary disease.

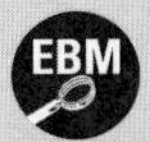

EVIDENCE

Please note: Complete text of EBM for this topic is available online.

SUGGESTED READINGS

Duvoux C et al: Effects of noradrenalin and albumin in patients with type 1 hepatorenal syndrome: a pilot study, *Hepatology* 36:374, 2002.

Gines P et al: Management of cirrhosis and ascites, *N Engl J Med* 350:1646, 2004.

Gines P, Schrier RW: Renal failure in cirrhosis, *N Engl J Med* 361:1279-1290, 2009.

AUTHOR: **FRED F. FERRI, M.D.**

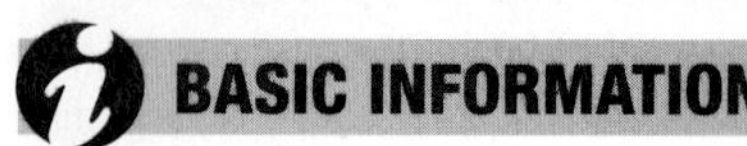

BASIC INFORMATION

DEFINITION

Herpangina is a self-limited upper respiratory tract infection associated with a characteristic vesicular rash on the soft palate.

SYNONYMS

Vesicular stomatitis
Acute lymphonodular pharyngitis

ICD-9CM CODES
074.0 Herpangina

EPIDEMIOLOGY & DEMOGRAPHICS

INCIDENCE (IN U.S.): Unknown
PEAK INCIDENCE: Summer outbreaks common
PREVALENCE (IN U.S.): Unknown
PREDOMINANT SEX: Male = female
PREDOMINANT AGE: 3 to 10 yr

PHYSICAL FINDINGS & CLINICAL PRESENTATION

- Characterized by ulcerating lesions typically located on the soft palate (Fig. 1-148)
- Usually fewer than six lesions that evolve rapidly from a diffuse pharyngitis to erythematous macules and subsequently to vesicles that are moderately painful
- Fever, vomiting, and headache in the first few days of illness but subsiding spontaneously
- Pharyngeal lesions typical for several more days

ETIOLOGY

- Most cases caused by coxsackie A viruses (A2, A4, A5, A6, A10)
- Occasional cases caused by other enteroviruses (Echovirus and Enterovirus 71)

Dx DIAGNOSIS

DIFFERENTIAL DIAGNOSIS

- Herpes simplex
- Bacterial pharyngitis
- Tonsillitis
- Aphthous stomatitis
- Hand-foot-mouth disease

WORKUP

Diagnosis is typically based on characteristic lesions on the soft palate.

LABORATORY TESTS

Viral and bacterial cultures of the pharynx to exclude herpes simplex infection and streptococcal pharyngitis if the diagnosis is in doubt

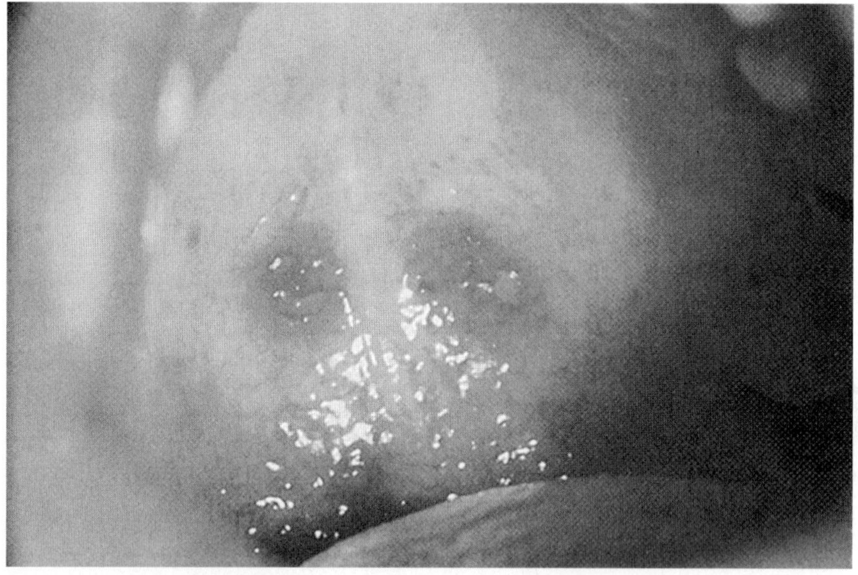

FIGURE 1-148 Herpangina with shallow ulcers in the roof of the mouth. (Courtesy Marshall Guill, M.D. From Goldstein B [ed]: *Practical dermatology,* ed 2, St Louis, 1997, Mosby.)

Rx TREATMENT

- Give symptomatic treatment for sore throat: saline gargles and analgesics, and encourage oral fluids.
- No antiviral therapy indicated; avoid antibacterial agents because they are ineffective, increase cost, might result in side effects, and promote antibiotic resistance.

NONPHARMACOLOGIC THERAPY

Analgesic throat lozenges are helpful in some cases.

ACUTE GENERAL Rx

Antipyretics when indicated

CHRONIC Rx

Self-limited infection

DISPOSITION

- Generally, resolution of symptoms within 1 wk
- Persistence of fever or mouth lesions beyond 1 wk suggestive of an alternative diagnosis (see "Differential Diagnosis")

REFERRAL

For consultation with otolaryngologist or infectious disease specialist if the diagnosis is in doubt

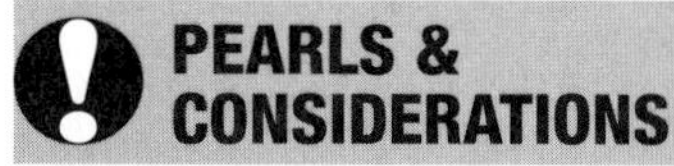

PEARLS & CONSIDERATIONS

COMMENTS

Household outbreaks may occur, especially during the summer months.

SUGGESTED READINGS

Chang LY et al: Outcome of enterovirus 71 infections with or without stage-based management: 1998. to 2002, *Pediatr Infect Dis J* 23(4):327, 2004.

Chang LY et al: Transmission and clinical features of enterovirus 71 infections in household contacts in Taiwan, *JAMA* 291(2):222, 2004.

Stone MS: Viral exanthems, *Dermatol Online J* 9(3):4, 2003.

Urashima M et al: Seasonal models of herpangina and hand-foot-mouth disease to simulate annual fluctuations in urban warming in Tokyo, *Jpn J Infect Dis* 56(2):48, 2003.

AUTHORS: **GLENN G. FORT, M.D., M.P.H.,** and **DENNIS J. MIKOLICH, M.D.**

BASIC INFORMATION

DEFINITION

Herpes simplex is a viral infection caused by the herpes simplex virus (HSV). HSV-1 is associated primarily with oral infections, and HSV-2 causes mainly genital infections. However, either type can infect any site. After the primary infection, the virus enters the nerve endings in the skin directly below the lesions and ascends to the dorsal root ganglia, where it remains in a latent stage until it is reactivated.

SYNONYMS

Genital herpes
Herpes labialis
Herpes gladiatorum
Herpes digitalis

ICD-9CM CODES
054.10 Genital herpes
054.9 Herpes labialis

EPIDEMIOLOGY & DEMOGRAPHICS

- More than 85% of adults have serologic evidence of HSV-1 infection. The seroprevalence of adults with HSV-2 in the U.S. is 25%; however, only approximately 20% of these persons recall having symptoms of HSV infection.
- Most cases of eye or digital herpetic infections are caused by HSV-1.
- Frequency of recurrence of HSV-2 genital herpes is higher than HSV-1 oral labial infection.
- The frequency of recurrence is lowest for oral labial HSV-2 infections.
- The incidence of complications from herpes simplex (e.g., herpes encephalitis) is highest in immunocompromised hosts.
- Male circumcision significantly reduces the incidence of HSV-2.

PHYSICAL FINDINGS & CLINICAL PRESENTATION

Primary infection:

- Symptoms occur from 3 to 7 days after contact (respiratory droplets, direct contact).
- Constitutional symptoms include low-grade fever, headache and myalgias, regional lymphadenopathy, and localized pain.
- Pain, burning, itching, and tingling last several hours.
- Grouped vesicles (Fig. 1-149), usually with surrounding erythema, appear and generally ulcerate or crust within 48 hr.
- The vesicles are uniform in size (differentiating it from herpes zoster vesicles, which vary in size).
- During the acute eruption the patient is uncomfortable; involvement of lips and inside of mouth may make it unpleasant for the patient to eat; urinary retention may complicate involvement of the genital area.
- Lesions generally last from 2 to 6 wk and heal without scarring.

Recurrent infection:

- Generally caused by alteration in the immune system; fatigue, stress, menses, local skin trauma, and exposure to sunlight are contributing factors.
- The prodromal symptoms (fatigue, burning and tingling of the affected area) last 12 to 24 hr.
- A cluster of lesions generally evolves within 24 hr from a macule to a papule and then vesicles surrounded by erythema; the vesicles coalesce and subsequently rupture within 4 days, revealing erosions covered by crusts.
- The crusts are generally shed within 7 to 10 days, revealing a pink surface.
- The most frequent location of the lesions is on the vermilion border of the lips (HSV-1), the penile shaft or glans penis and the labia (HSV-2), buttocks (seen more frequently in women), fingertips (herpetic whitlow), and trunk (may be confused with herpes zoster).
- Rapid onset of diffuse cutaneous herpes simplex (eczema herpeticum) may occur in certain atopic infants and adults. It is a medical emergency, especially in young infants, and should be promptly treated with acyclovir.
- Herpes encephalitis, meningitis, and ocular herpes can occur in patients with immunocompromised status and occasionally in normal hosts.

ETIOLOGY

HSV-1 and HSV-2 are both DNA viruses.

Dx DIAGNOSIS

DIFFERENTIAL DIAGNOSIS

- Impetigo
- Behçet's syndrome
- Coxsackie virus infection
- Syphilis
- Stevens-Johnson syndrome
- Herpangina
- Aphthous stomatitis
- Varicella
- Herpes zoster

WORKUP

Diagnosis is based on clinical presentation. Laboratory evaluation confirms diagnosis.

LABORATORY TESTS

- Direct immunofluorescent antibody slide tests provide a rapid diagnosis.
- Viral culture is the most definitive method for diagnosis; results are generally available in 1 or 2 days. The lesions should be sampled during the vesicular or early ulcerative stage; cervical samples should be taken from the endocervix with a swab.
- Tzanck smear is a readily available test that will demonstrate multinucleated giant cells. However, it is not a highly sensitive test.
- Pap smear will detect HSV-infected cells in cervical tissue from women without symptoms.
- Serologic tests for HSV: immunoglobulin (Ig) G and IgM serum antibodies. Antibodies to HSV occur in 50% to 90% of adults. Routine tests do not discriminate between antibodies that are HSV-1 and HSV-2; the presence of IgM or a fourfold or greater rise in IgG titers indicates a recent infection (convalescent sample should be drawn 2 to 3 wk after the acute specimen is drawn).

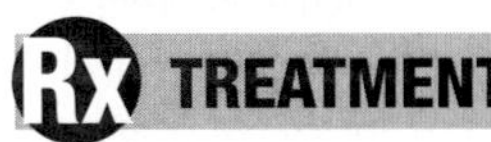

Rx TREATMENT

NONPHARMACOLOGIC THERAPY

Application of topical cool compresses with Burow's solution for 15 min four to six times daily may be soothing in patients with extensive erosions on the vulva and penis (decrease edema and inflammation, debridement of crusts and purulent material).

ACUTE GENERAL Rx

- Acyclovir ointment or cream applied using finger-cot or rubber glove q3-6h (six times daily) for 7 days may be useful for the first

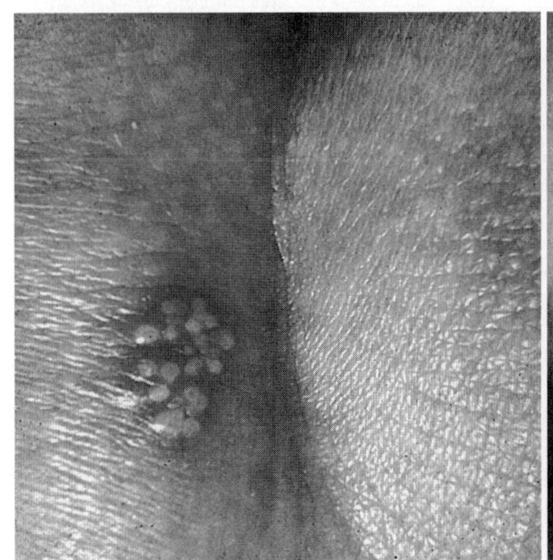

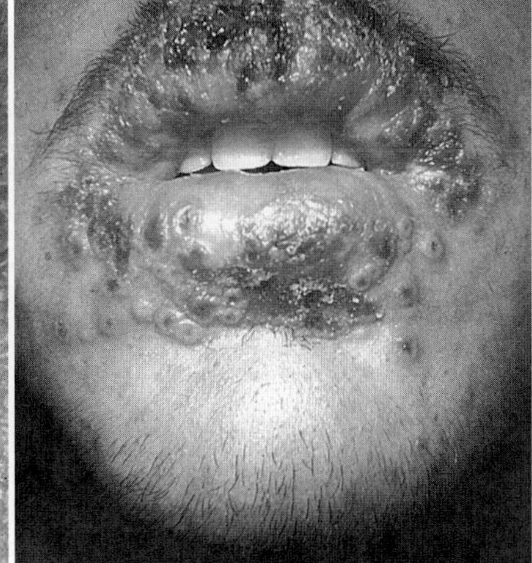

FIGURE 1-149 Herpes simplex. (From Scuderi G [ed]: *Sports medicine: principles of primary care,* St Louis, 1997, Mosby.)

clinical episode of genital herpes. Severe primary genital infections may be treated with IV acyclovir (5 mg/kg infused at a constant rate over 1 hr q8h for 7 days in patients with normal renal function) or oral acyclovir 200 mg five times daily for 10 days. Topical acyclovir 5% cream can also be used for herpes labialis; when started at the prodrome or papule stage, it decreases the duration of an episode by approximately one-half day.
- Valacyclovir caplets can also be used for the initial episode of genital herpes (1 g bid for 10 days).
- Valacyclovir 2 g PO q12h for 1 day begun within the first symptoms of herpes labialis can modestly shorten its duration.
- Penciclovir 1% cream can be used for recurrent herpes labialis on the lips and face. It should be applied q2h while awake for 4 days. Treatment should be started at the earliest sign or symptom. Its use decreases healing time of orolabial herpes by approximately 1 day.
- Docosanol 10% cream, a long-chain saturated alcohol, inhibits fusion between the plasma membrane and the viral envelope, blocking viral entry and subsequent replication. It is available over the counter and, when applied at the first sign of recurrence of herpes labialis, may shorten the duration of the episode by approximately 12 hr.

CHRONIC Rx

- Recurrent episodes of genital herpes can be treated with acyclovir. A short course (800 mg tid for 2 days) is effective. Other treatment options include 800 mg PO bid for 3 to 5 days, generally started during the prodrome or within 2 days of onset of lesions; famciclovir is also useful for treatment of recurrent genital herpes (dose is 125 mg q12h for 5 days in patients with normal renal function) started at the first sign of symptoms, or valacyclovir (dose is 500 mg q12h for 3 days in patients with normal renal function).
- Acyclovir-resistant mucocutaneous lesions in patients with HIV can be treated with foscarnet (40 to 60 mg/kg IV q8h in patients with normal renal function); hydroxypropyl methylcellulose has also been reported to be effective in HSV infections resistant to acyclovir or foscarnet.
- Patients with six recurrences of genital herpes per year can be treated with valacyclovir 1 g qd, acyclovir 400 mg bid, or famciclovir 250 mg bid.

DISPOSITION

Most patients recover from the initial episode or recurrences without complications; immunocompromised hosts are at risk for complications (e.g., disseminated herpes simplex infection, herpes encephalitis).

REFERRAL

- Hospital admission in patients with herpes encephalitis or herpes meningitis and in immunocompromised hosts with diffuse herpes simplex infection
- Ophthalmology referral in patients with suspected ocular herpes

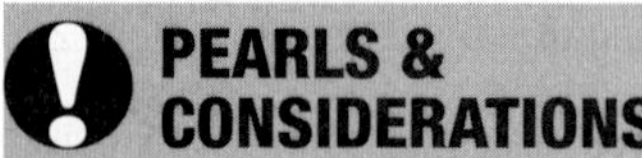

PEARLS & CONSIDERATIONS

COMMENTS

- Provide patient education regarding transmission of HSV.
- Condom use offers significant protection against HSV-1 infection in susceptive women.
- Patients should be instructed on the use of condoms for sexual intercourse and on avoiding kissing or sexual intercourse until lesions are crusted.
- Patients should also avoid contact with immunocompromised hosts or neonates while lesions are present.
- Proper handwashing techniques should be explained.
- Patients with herpes gladiatorum (cutaneous herpes in athletes involved in contact sports) should be excluded from participation in active sports until lesions have resolved.
- Many new HSV-2 infections are asymptomatic, but new symptoms may result from old infections.

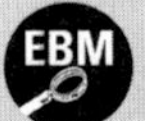

EVIDENCE

Please note: Complete text of EBM for this topic is available online.

Key trials and commentary:

Epidemiologic data suggest that infection with herpes simplex virus type 2 (HSV-2) is associated with increased genital shedding of human immunodeficiency virus type 1 (HIV-1) RNA and HIV-1 transmissibility.

This study showed that HSV suppressive therapy significantly reduces genital and plasma HIV-1 RNA levels in dually infected women. This finding may have important implications for HIV control.

This article shows that HSV-2 prophylactic treatment with Valtrex 500 mg bid is associated with reduced HIV-1 levels, which in turn will delay the development of AIDS and may reduce transmission of HIV. This effect on HIV levels occurs even though Valtrex is not effective against the HIV virus. Advances in the treatment of ocular HSV-1 through the use of prophylactic antiviral treatment were derived from the experience with antivirals in genital HSV-2. An additional, somewhat unexpected, benefit of antiviral prophylaxis of HSV is the effect on HIV in coinfected patients. Antiviral treatment for HSV is much less expensive than drug treatment for HIV/AIDS. This added benefit certainly enhances the cost effectiveness of HSV oral antiviral prophylaxis. When deciding whether to recommend long-term antiviral prophylaxis against ocular and/or facial herpes, one should perhaps ask whether the patient is HIV positive in view of the results of this article.[1] Ⓐ

Across many observational studies, HSV-2 infection is associated with twofold to threefold increased risk for HIV-1 infection. Celum and colleagues investigated whether HSV-2 suppression with aciclovir would reduce the risk of HIV-1 acquisition.

This study showed that that suppressive therapy with standard doses of aciclovir is not effective in reduction of HIV-1 acquisition in HSV-2 seropositive women and MSM. Novel strategies are needed to interrupt interactions between HSV-2 and HIV-1.

Previous studies have suggested an increased risk of HIV-1 acquisition in patients with recently acquired HSV-2 infection. The presumed mechanism for increased HIV-1 susceptibility is thought to involve disruption of the genital epithelium during HSV-2 reactivation. Celum et al hypothesized that a standard suppressive dose of acyclovir might reduce HIV-1 acquisition in high-risk men and women. They performed a randomized, double-blind, placebo-controlled trial of acyclovir 400 mg twice daily in HIV-1–negative, HSV seropositive women to assess whether suppression of genital herpes could reduce the risk of acquisition of HIV-1. Unfortunately, this was not the case, as no reduction in HIV-1 incidence was observed. Even more discouraging was that in addition to acyclovir, study participants received the best available services, including risk-reduction counseling, voluntary counseling, and testing for the prevention, diagnosis, and treatment of sexually transmitted diseases, including HIV. Adherence to the study drug, measured primarily by pill count, was high, and there was no increased rate of serious adverse events. A previously reported trial yielded similar results.[2] Ⓐ

Evidence-Based References

1. Nagot N, for the ANRS 1285 Study Group: Reduction of HIV-1 RNA levels with therapy to suppress herpes simplex virus, *N Engl J Med* 356:790-799, 2007. Commentary by E.J. Cohen, M.D. Ⓐ
2. Celum C et al: Effect of aciclovir on HIV-1 acquisition in herpes simplex virus 2 seropositive women and men who have sex with men: a randomised, double-blind, placebo-controlled trial, *Lancet* 371: 2109-2119, 2008. Commentary by B.H. Thiers, M.D. Ⓐ

SUGGESTED READINGS

Corey L, Wald A: Maternal and neonatal herpes simplex virus infections, *N Engl J Med* 361:1376-1385, 2009.

Tobian AR et al: Male circumcision for the prevention of HSV-2 and HPV infections and syphilis, *N Engl J Med* 360:1298-1309, 2009.

AUTHOR: **FRED F. FERRI, M.D.**

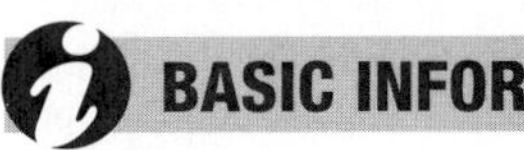

BASIC INFORMATION

DEFINITION

Herpes zoster is a disease caused by reactivation of the varicella-zoster virus (VZV). After the primary infection (chickenpox), the virus becomes latent in the dorsal root ganglia and reemerges when there is a weakening of the immune system (as a result of disease or advanced age).

SYNONYMS

Shingles

ICD-9CM CODES

053.9 Herpes zoster

EPIDEMIOLOGY & DEMOGRAPHICS

- Herpes zoster occurs during the lifetime of 10% to 20% of the population.
- There is an increased incidence in immunocompromised patients (AIDS, malignancy), the elderly, and children who acquired chickenpox when younger than 2 mo.

PHYSICAL FINDINGS & CLINICAL PRESENTATION

- Pain generally precedes skin manifestation by 3 to 5 days and is generally localized to the dermatome that will be affected by the skin lesions.
- Constitutional symptoms are often present (malaise, fever, headache).
- The initial rash consists of erythematous maculopapules generally affecting one dermatome (thoracic region in majority of cases). Typically the rash does not cross the midline. Some patients (<30%) may have scattered vesicles outside the affected dermatome.
- The initial maculopapules evolve into vesicles and pustules by the third or the fourth day.
- The vesicles have an erythematous base, are cloudy, and have various sizes (a distinguishing characteristic from herpes simplex, in which the vesicles are of uniform size).
- The vesicles subsequently become umbilicated and then form crusts that generally fall off within 3 wk; scarring may occur.
- Pain during and after the rash is generally significant.
- Secondary bacterial infection with *Staphylococcus aureus* or *Streptococcus pyogenes* may occur.
- Regional lymphadenopathy may occur.
- Herpes zoster may involve the trigeminal nerve (most frequent cranial nerve involved); involvement of the geniculate ganglion can cause facial palsy and a painful ear, with the presence of vesicles on the pinna and external auditory canal (Ramsay Hunt syndrome).

ETIOLOGY

Reactivation of varicella virus (human herpes virus III)

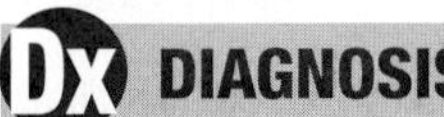

DIAGNOSIS

DIFFERENTIAL DIAGNOSIS

- Rash: herpes simplex and other viral infections
- Pain from herpes zoster: may be confused with acute myocardial infarction, pulmonary embolism, pleuritis, pericarditis, renal colic

LABORATORY TESTS

Laboratory tests are generally not necessary (viral cultures and Tzanck smear will confirm diagnosis in patients with atypical presentation).

Rx TREATMENT

NONPHARMACOLOGIC THERAPY

- Wet compresses (using Burow's solution or cool tap water) applied for 15 to 30 min five to 10 times a day are useful to break vesicles and remove serum and crust.
- Care must be taken to prevent any secondary bacterial infection.

ACUTE GENERAL Rx

- Gabapentin 100 to 600 mg tid is effective in the treatment of pain and sleep interference associated with postherpetic neuralgia. Other effective agents are pregabalin, duloxetine, and tricyclic antidepressants.
- Lidocaine patch 5% (Lidoderm) is also effective in relieving postherpetic neuralgia. Patches are applied to intact skin after resolution of blisters and crusts to cover the most painful area for up to 12 hr within a 24-hr period.
- Oral antiviral agents can decrease acute pain, inflammation, and vesicle formation when treatment is begun within 48 hr of onset of rash. Treatment options are:
  1. Acyclovir (Zovirax) 800 mg five times daily for 7 to 10 days
  2. Valacyclovir (Valtrex) 1000 mg tid for 7 days
  3. Famciclovir (Famvir) 500 mg tid for 7 days
- Immunocompromised patients should be treated with IV acyclovir 500 mg/m^2 or 10 mg/kg q8h in 1-hr infusions for 7 days, with close monitoring of renal function and adequate hydration; vidarabine (continuous 12-hr infusion of 10 mg/kg/day for 7 days) is also effective for treatment of disseminated herpes zoster in immunocompromised hosts.
- Patients with AIDS and transplant recipients may develop acyclovir-resistant varicella-zoster; these patients can be treated with foscarnet (40 mg/kg IV q8h) continued for at least 10 days or until lesions are completely healed.
- Capsaicin cream (Zostrix) can be useful for treatment of postherpetic neuralgia. It is generally applied three to five times daily for several weeks after the crusts have fallen off.
- Sympathetic blocks (stellate ganglion or epidural) with 0.25% bupivacaine and rhizotomy are reserved for severe cases unresponsive to conservative treatment.
- Corticosteroids should be considered in older patients within 72 hr of clinical presentation or if new lesions are still appearing if there are no contraindications. Initial dose is prednisone 40 mg/day decreased by 5 mg/day until finished. When used there is a decrease in the use of analgesics and time to resumption of usual activities, but there is no effect on the incidence and duration of postherpetic neuralgia.

DISPOSITION

- The incidence of postherpetic neuralgia (defined as pain that persists more than 30 days after onset of rash) increases with age (30% by age 40 yr, >70% by age 70 yr); antivirals reduce the risk of postherpetic neuralgia.
- Incidence of disseminated herpes zoster is increased in immunocompromised hosts (e.g., 15% to 50% of patients with active Hodgkin's disease).
- Immunocompromised hosts are also more prone to neurologic complications (encephalitis, myelitis, cranial and peripheral nerve palsies, acute retinal necrosis). The mortality rate is 10% to 20% in immunocompromised hosts with disseminated zoster.
- Motor neuropathies occur in 5% of all cases of zoster; complete recovery occurs in >70% of patients.

REFERRAL

- Hospitalization for IV acyclovir in patients with disseminated herpes zoster.
- Patients with herpes zoster ophthalmicus should be referred to an ophthalmologist.
- Vaccination: immunocompetent adults ≥60 yr are appropriate candidates for a single dose of varicella-zoster vaccine (VZV) whether or not they have had a previous episode of herpes zoster. Immunization with VZV (Zostavax) boosts waning immunity in older adults and reduces the severity and duration of pain caused by herpes zoster by 61%. Adults who are VZV seronegative (never had varicella) should be immunized against varicella with two doses of varicella vaccine (Varivax).

SUGGESTED READING

Kimberlin DW, Whitley RJ: Varicella-zoster vaccine for the prevention of herpes zoster, *N Engl J Med* 356: 1338, 2007.

AUTHOR: **FRED F. FERRI, M.D.**

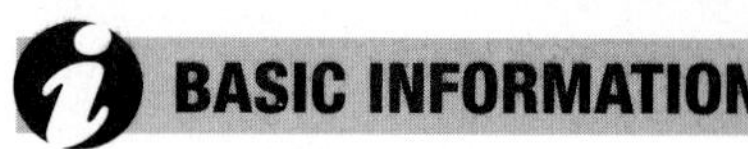

BASIC INFORMATION

DEFINITION

A hiatal hernia is the herniation of a portion of the stomach into the thoracic cavity through the diaphragmatic esophageal hiatus.

SYNONYMS

Hiatus hernia
Diaphragmatic hernia

ICD-9CM CODES
553.3 Diaphragmatic hernia without obstruction or gangrene
750.6 Congenital hiatal hernia
756.6 Congenital diaphragmatic hernia

EPIDEMIOLOGY & DEMOGRAPHICS

- Found in 50% of patients older than 50.
- Prevalence increases with age.
- More prevalent in Western countries than in Africa and Asia.
- Paraesophageal hiatal hernias are more common in women than in men (4:1).
- Associated with diverticulosis (25%), esophagitis (25%), duodenal ulcers (20%), and gallstones (18%).
- More than 90% of patients with endoscopic documentation of esophagitis have hiatal hernias.

PHYSICAL FINDINGS & CLINICAL PRESENTATION

Most patients are asymptomatic. If symptoms are present, they resemble those of gastroesophageal reflux disease (GERD).

- Heartburn
- Dysphagia
- Regurgitation of gastric contents
- Chest pain
- Postprandial fullness
- GI bleed
- Dyspnea
- Hoarseness
- Wheezing with bowel sounds heard over the left lung base

ETIOLOGY

- The repetitive stretching of the gastroesophageal (GE) junction with swallowing and actions (e.g., vomiting) or states (e.g., obesity, pregnancy) that increase intraabdominal pressure may cause widening of the hiatus, rupture of the phrenoesophageal ligament, and onset of the hernia.
- Hiatal hernias are classified as:
  1. Type I: Sliding (Fig. 1-150, A), axial, or concentric hiatal hernia (most common type, 99%). Only the GE junction protrudes into the thoracic cavity and the phrenoesophageal ligament remains intact.
  2. Type II: Paraesophageal or rolling hernia (Fig. 1-150, B) (1%). The GE junction stays at the level of the diaphragm, but part of the stomach bulges into the thoracic cavity through a defect in the phrenoesophageal ligament.
  3. Type III: Mixed (rare), a combination of type I and type II.
  4. Type IV: Large defect in hiatus that allows other intraabdominal organs to enter the hernia sac.

DIAGNOSIS

DIFFERENTIAL DIAGNOSIS

- Peptic ulcer disease
- Unstable angina
- Esophagitis (caused by *Candida,* herpes, NSAIDs, etc.)
- Esophageal spasm
- Barrett's esophagus
- Schatzki's ring
- Achalasia
- Zenker's diverticulum
- Esophageal cancer

WORKUP

- Exclude conditions noted in the differential diagnosis and document the presence of a hiatal hernia. Upper endoscopy may also be needed to exclude abnormal metaplasia, dysplasia, or neoplasia.
- A clinical algorithm for evaluation of heartburn is described in Section III.

LABORATORY TESTS

- Blood tests are not specific.
- Esophageal manometry, although not commonly done, can be used in establishing a diagnosis (low sensitivity, but high specificity when compared with endoscopy).

IMAGING STUDIES

- Barium contrast upper gastrointestinal (UGI) series best defines the anatomic abnormality: Demonstration that the gastric cardia is herniated 2 cm above the hiatus is diagnostic. UGI may also reveal a tortuous esophagus (Fig. 1-151). If endoscopy is performed preoperatively, a barium swallow is generally not necessary.
- UGI endoscopy: documents the presence of a hiatal hernia and also excludes common associated findings of esophagitis and Barrett's esophagus (recommended at least once during the workup). Greater than 2 cm of gastric rugal fold seen above the margins of the diaphragmatic crura is diagnostic.
- Abdominal ultrasonography: simple, well tolerated; a transdiaphragmatic esophageal diameter of more than or equal to 18 mm is highly suggestive of the presence of a sliding hiatal hernia.

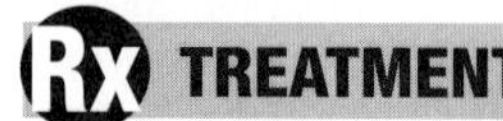

TREATMENT

NONPHARMACOLOGIC THERAPY

- Lifestyle modifications: avoidance of foods and drugs that decrease lower-esophageal pressure (e.g., caffeine, chocolate, mint, calcium channel blockers, and anticholinergics)
- Weight loss
- Avoid large quantities of food with meals
- Sleep with the head of the bed elevated 6 inches

ACUTE GENERAL Rx

- Antacids may be useful to relieve mild symptoms.
- H_2 antagonists (e.g., cimetidine 400 mg bid, ranitidine 150 mg bid, or famotidine 20 mg bid).
- If significant GERD is present with documented esophagitis, proton pump inhibitors (e.g., omeprazole 20 mg qd or lansoprazole 30 mg qd) are used. Refractory symptoms may require higher doses (e.g., bid dosing).
- Prokinetic agents (e.g., metoclopramide 10 mg taken 30 min before each meal) can be added to an H_2 antagonist or proton pump inhibitor.

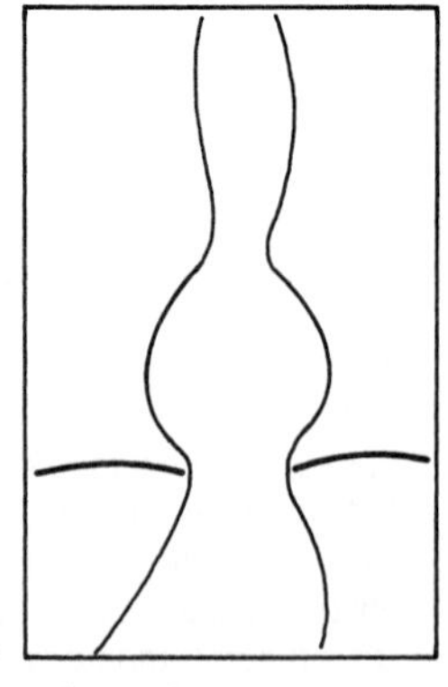

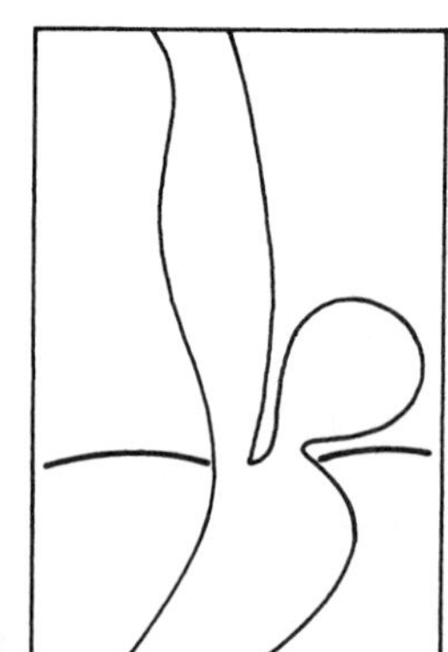

FIGURE 1-150 Types of esophageal hiatal hernia. A, Sliding hiatal hernia, the most common type. **B,** Paraesophageal hiatal hernia. (From Behrman RE: *Nelson textbook of pediatrics,* ed 17, Philadelphia, 2004, WB Saunders.)

CHRONIC Rx

- When indicated, surgery (laparoscopic or open) can be done in patients with refractory symptoms impairing quality of life, or causing intestinal (e.g., recurrent GI bleeds) or extraintestinal complications (e.g., aspiration pneumonia, asthma, or ear-nose-throat complications).
- Prophylactic surgery is a consideration in all paraesophageal hernias because they have a higher incidence of strangulation.

DISPOSITION

- More than 90% of patients having GERD symptoms respond well to medical therapy.
- Complications of hiatal hernias are similar to complications occurring in patients with GERD:
  1. Erosive esophagitis
  2. Ulcerative esophagitis
  3. Barrett's esophagus
  4. Peptic stricture
  5. GI hemorrhage
  6. Extraintestinal complications
  7. Lung collapse or heart failure (severe cases)

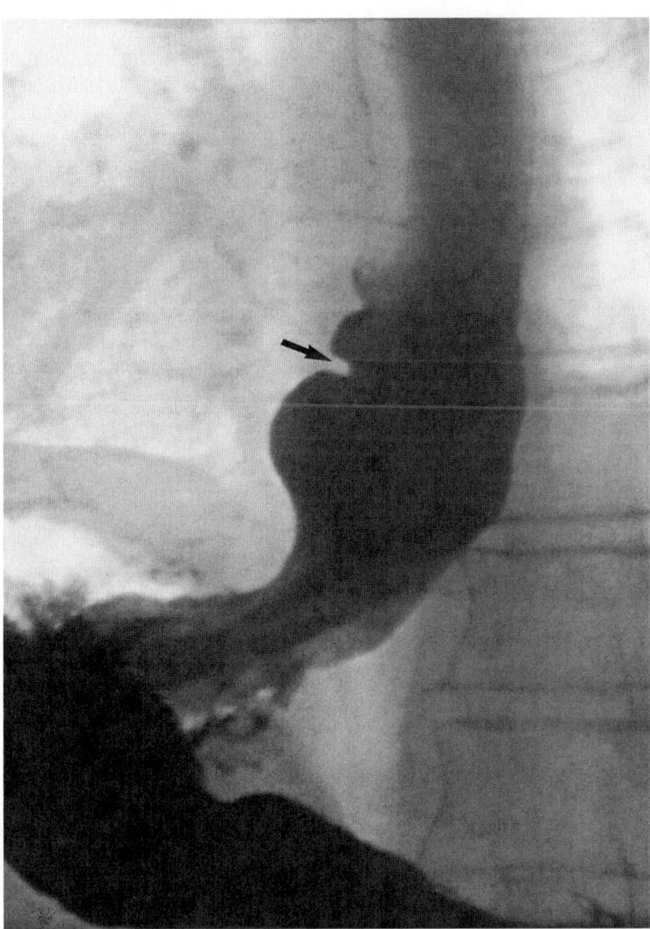

FIGURE 1-151 A sliding hiatal hernia confirmed by the presence of an incisural notch *(arrow)* on the greater curve aspect. (From Grainger RG et al [eds]: *Grainger & Allison's diagnostic radiology,* ed 4, Philadelphia, 2001, Churchill Livingstone.)

REFERRAL

Gastroenterologist: for symptoms refractory to conventional therapy (H_2 antagonists, antacids, and proton pump inhibitors) or having complications previously mentioned.

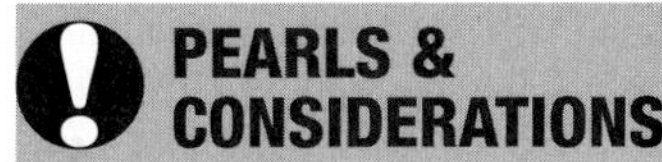

PEARLS & CONSIDERATIONS

COMMENTS

- Gastric ulceration and erosions (Cameron's lesion) can occur in the paraesophageal hernia pouch and are an uncommon cause of UGI bleeding.
- May cause iron deficiency anemia.
- Gastric volvulus or torsion can also occur and presents as dysphagia and postcibal pain.
- High incidence of esophagitis even after the eradication of *Helicobacter pylori.*
- The appearance of hiatal hernia may resemble a left atrial mass by echocardiography.

SUGGESTED READINGS

Andujan JJ et al: Laparoscopic repair of large paraesophageal hernia is associated with low incidence of recurrence and reoperations, *Surg Endosc* 18(3): 444, 2004.

Bawahab M et al: Management of acute paraesophageal hernia, *Surg Endosc Epub* 2008.

Kahrilas PJ et al: Approaches to the diagnosis and grading of hiatal hernia, *Best Pract Res Clin Gastroenterol* 22(4):601, 2008.

Linke GR et al: Is a barium swallow complementary to endoscopy essential in the preoperative assessment of laparoscopic antireflux and hiatal hernia surgery? *Surg Endosc* 22(1):96, 2008.

AUTHOR: **MARK BRADY, M.D., M.P.H., M.M.S.**

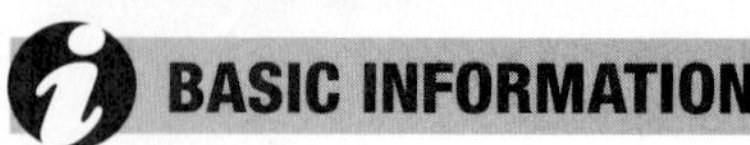

BASIC INFORMATION

DEFINITION

Hidradenitis suppurativa (HS) is a chronic, relapsing condition that occurs within the terminal follicular epithelium of the apocrine glands. Keratinous materials occlude the follicles, causing secondary inflammation of the apocrine glands and resulting in chronic infection and draining abscesses that lead to scarring.

SYNONYMS

Suppurative hidradenitis
Acne inversa
Verneuil's disease
Apocrinitis
Hidradenitis axillaris

ICD-9CM CODES

705.83

EPIDEMIOLOGY & DEMOGRAPHICS

- HS occurs more commonly in women in the U.S.
- It usually begins in the postpubertal age group, with an average age of onset of 23 yr.
- Its overall prevalence in the U.S. is approximately 1% to 2%.
- An increased frequency of this disease is seen in people of African-American descent, though this has not been fully studied. The suspicion is that it is attributable to a greater density of apocrine glands.
- Predisposing factors believed to be involved include hyperandrogenism, obesity, and familial predilection.
- HS has been associated with other endocrine disorders such as diabetes, Cushing's disease, and acromegaly.

PHYSICAL FINDINGS & CLINICAL PRESENTATION

The diagnosis is primarily clinical based on the development of typical lesions. There are three key elements to the diagnosis: typical lesions, characteristic distribution, and relapsing nature.

- Typical lesions:
  - Painful and/or tender erythematous papules and nodules
  - Painful or tender abscesses and inflamed, discharging papules or nodules
  - Dermal contractures and ropelike elevation of the skin
  - Comedones in the apocrine, gland-bearing skin
- Characteristic sites:
  - Axilla (Fig. 1-152)
  - Inguinal perineal region
  - Areola of the breast
  - Submammary folds
- Strong tendency toward relapse and recurrence

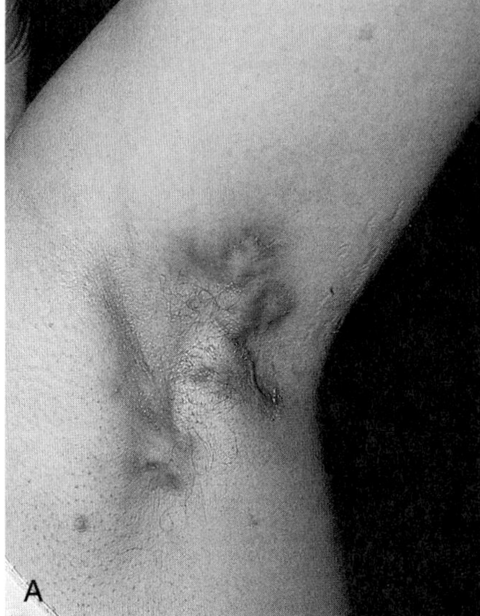

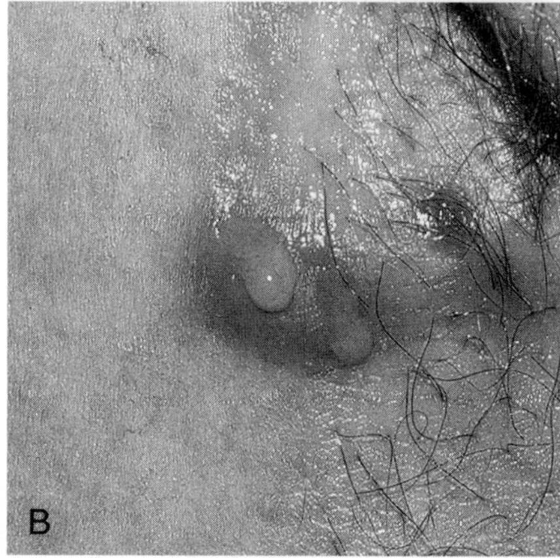

FIGURE 1-152 Hidradenitis suppurativa (HS). A, HS of the axilla. This is the classic appearance with inflammatory nodules and scarred areas. This condition is commonly misdiagnosed as a bacterial infection. **B,** HS of the axilla; a close-up view of the draining pus. When intact, the lesions represent sterile abscesses. Once open, they may become secondarily infected. (From White GM, Cox NH [eds]: *Diseases of the skin: a color atlas and text,* ed 2, St Louis, 2006, Mosby.)

- Other characteristics:
  - Poor response to conventional antibiotics
  - Often no pathogens from routine cultures of pus from boils
  - Personal or family history of acne or pilonidal cysts

ETIOLOGY

The exact cause of HS has not been determined, though a number of theories have been proposed:

1. Folliculitis is observed in almost all patients with HS, though whether this is causative has not been determined.
2. Local friction trauma could be a cause.
3. Infectious agents such as *Streptococcus, Staphylococcus,* and *E. coli* have been identified in cultures, but it is uncertain whether these are a cause or a result.
4. Low levels of estrogen are implicated, as are high levels of androgen.

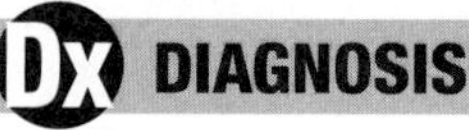

DIAGNOSIS

DIFFERENTIAL DIAGNOSIS

- Follicular pyodermas such as folliculitis, furuncles, carbuncles, and pilonidal cysts
- Granuloma inguinale
- Perianal and vulvar manifestations of Crohn's disease
- Abscess
- Infection of a Bartholin's cyst
- Actinomycosis
- Lymphogranuloma venereum
- Infection of an epidermoid cyst
- Lymphadenitis
- Cat scratch disease
- Tularemia
- Erysipelas
- Ulcerative colitis

WORKUP

This is primarily a clinical diagnosis based on typical lesion (see "Physical Findings & Clinical Presentation").

LABORATORY TESTS

- Patients with acute lesions may have an elevated erythrocyte sedimentation rate or white blood cell count. They also may have serum protein abnormalities on electrophoresis.
- Any pus should be sampled for bacterial culture and sensitivity.

AUTHOR: **CHRISTINE HARTLEY, M.D.**

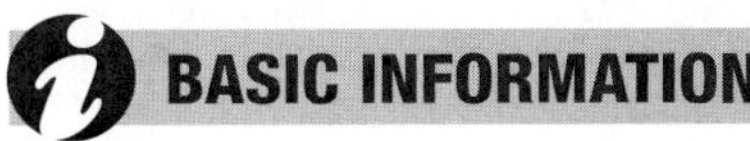

BASIC INFORMATION

DEFINITION

The development of stiff pigmented (terminal) facial and body hair (male distribution) in women as a result of excess androgen production.

SYNONYMS

Excessive hair growth

ICD-9CM CODES
704.1 Hirsutism

EPIDEMIOLOGY & DEMOGRAPHICS

- Overall prevalence unknown, estimated 5% to 10% in reproductive age women.
- Race and genetics should be considered. Some distinct ethnic populations have minimal body hair and others (Mediterranean, Middle Eastern, South Asian) have moderate to large amounts of body hair while serum androgen levels are similar.
- Social norms and culture also determine how much body hair is cosmetically acceptable.
- Half of all cases of mild hirsutism do not have hyperandrogenemia.
- Incidence and presentation of hirsutism is dependent on underlying cause of androgen excess (see "Differential Diagnosis").

PHYSICAL FINDINGS & CLINICAL PRESENTATION

- Timing of symptoms: abrupt onset, short duration, rapid progression, progressive worsening, more severe signs of virilization, or later age of onset suggest androgen-producing tumor, late-onset congenital adrenal hyperplasia, or Cushing's syndrome. Weight increases may produce increased androgen production.
- Menstrual history: menarche, cycle regularity and symptoms of ovulation, fertility, and contraception use. Anovulatory cycles are the most common underlying cause of androgen excess.
- Medication use history: some drugs cause hirsutism or produce androgenic effects (danazol, phenytoin, valproic acid, androgenic progestins (e.g., norgestrel), cyclosporin, minoxidil, metoclopramide, phenothiazines, methyldopa, diazoxide, penicillamine).
- Family history: known or suspected family history of hirsutism, congenital adrenal hyperplasia, insulin resistance, polycystic ovary syndrome (PCOS), infertility, obesity, menstrual irregularity may be found.
- Physical exam reveals deepening voice, body habitus, increased muscle mass, galactorrhea, abdominal and pelvic exam.
- Associated cutaneous manifestations (Fig. 1-153) are acne, acanthosis nigricans, striae, hair distribution, location and quantity, frontotemporal balding, muscle mass, clitoromegaly.

ETIOLOGY

- Presence of hirsutism indicates androgen excess. Total testosterone may be normal, but free testosterone is elevated.
- Androgens induce vellus hair follicles in sex-specific areas to develop into thicker, more heavily pigmented terminal hairs.
- Anovulatory ovaries are usual source of excess androgens through thecal cell steroidogenesis and conversion of androstenedione to testosterone.
- Conditions that decrease hepatic production of sex hormone binding globulin (SHBG) decrease protein-bound testosterone and increase free testosterone fraction (e.g., low estrogen, high androgen, and hyperinsulinemic states).
- Late-onset, congenital adrenal hyperplasia enzyme deficiency (most commonly 21-hydroxylase deficiency) produces excess 17 hydroxy-progesterone (17-OHP) and overproduction of androstenedione.
- Rare ovarian tumors primarily derived from Sertoli-Leydig cells, granulosa theca cells, or hilus cells produce excess androgens.
- Rare adrenal tumors produce excess androgens.
- Rare pituitary or hypothalamic tumors produce excess prolactin and can lead to anovulation.

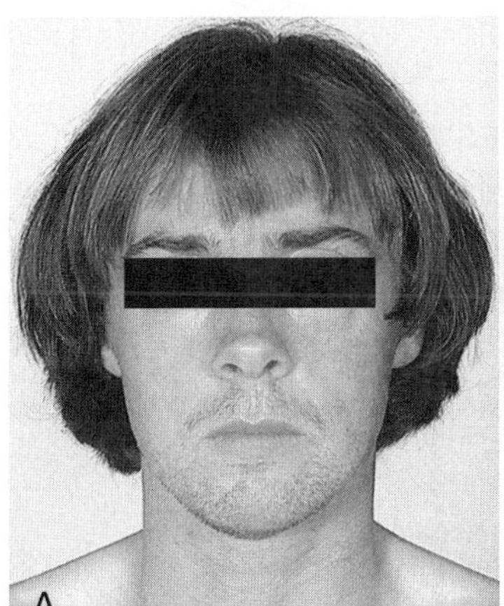

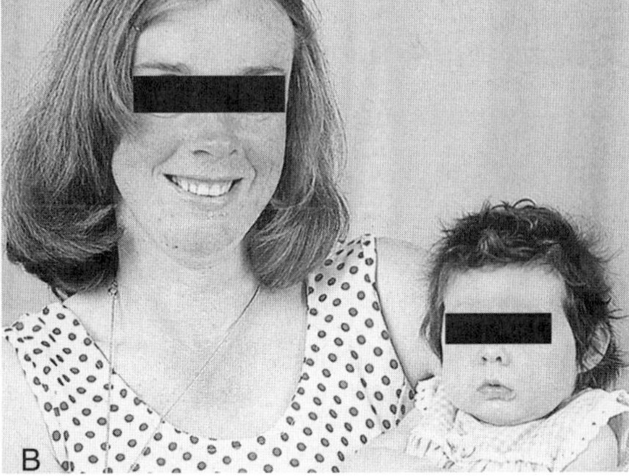

FIGURE 1-153 A patient with an arrhenoblastoma with associated polycystic ovaries before and after treatment. **A,** Before treatment, the patient had marked facial hirsutism. **B,** The patient is shown successfully treated. The tumor was resected and ovulation ensued with clomiphene and human chorionic gonadotropin therapy. (From Besser CM, Thorner MO: *Comprehensive clinical endocrinology,* ed 3, St Louis, 2002, Mosby.)

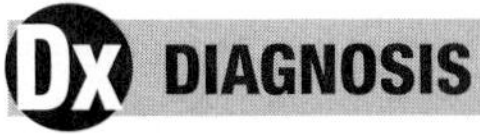

DIAGNOSIS

DIFFERENTIAL DIAGNOSIS

- Androgen-independent vellus hair: soft, unpigmented hair that covers entire body
- Hypertrichosis: diffusely increased total body hair (vellus or lanugo-type) not restricted to androgen-dependent areas often an adverse response to a medication or systemic illness
- PCOS 75%
- Idiopathic 5% to 15%
- Congenital adrenal hyperplasia 1% to 8%
- Insulin resistance syndrome 3% to 4%
- Cushing's syndrome $<1\%$
- Drug induced $<1\%$
- Ovarian tumor $<1\%$
- Adrenal tumor $<1\%$
- Hyperthecosis $<1\%$
- Hyperprolactinemia $<1\%$

WORKUP

- Hirsutism is a clinical diagnosis.
- Management of hirsutism is largely independent of the etiology.
- Workup in selected hirsute women is directed to determine underlying cause of androgen excess.
- Check androgen levels in women with moderate or severe hirsutism, sudden onset, rapid progression, or associated menstrual dysfunction, central obesity, clitoromegaly, or acanthosis nigricans.
- See specific conditions for more detailed workup of individual diagnoses.

LABORATORY TESTS

Total plasma testosterone or free testosterone: early morning on day 4 to 10 of menstrual cycle to screen for testosterone secreting tumors. If markedly elevated may image adrenals and ovaries.

Other laboratory test considerations if appropriate:

- Dehydroepiandrosterone sulfate (DHEA-S): screen for adrenal androgen production as almost entirely produced by adrenals
- Prolactin: moderately elevated values should prompt imaging of pituitary-hypothalamic region
- 17-OHP (17 α-hydroxyprogesterone): screen for adrenal enzyme deficiencies

Other laboratory test considerations if appropriate:
- Follicle-stimulating hormone: (FSH): rule out hypoestrogen state (perimenopausal)
- Luteinizing hormone: (LH): typically elevated in PCOS with low or normal FSH
- Thyroid-stimulating hormone (TSH): rule out hypothyroidism
- 24-hour urinary free cortisol: rule out Cushing's syndrome and overproduction of cortisol
- Overnight single-dose dexamethasone suppression test: rule out Cushing's syndrome and adrenal hyperfunction
- Fasting blood sugar (FBS), 2-hr 75-g oral glucose tolerance test, fasting insulin levels: rule out insulin resistance syndrome

IMAGING STUDIES

Imaging study considerations if appropriate:
- Pelvic ultrasound (high resolution, transvaginal): rule out ovarian tumor
- Abdominal CT/MRI: rule out adrenal tumor
- Pituitary-hypothalamic region CT/MRI: rule out pituitary tumor
- Laparoscopy/laparotomy: rule out small ovarian tumor in cases of elevated testosterone levels without radiologic evidence of adrenal or ovarian pathology

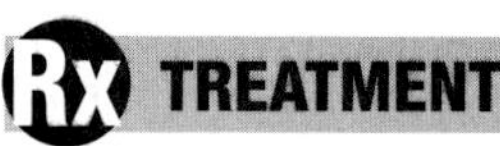

TREATMENT

NONPHARMACOLOGIC THERAPY

- Weight reduction: can reduce androgen production indirectly by reducing insulin-stimulated theca cell androgen production and improve menstrual function, and slow hair growth in obese women.
- Cosmetic: temporary.
  - Shaving: does not stimulate hair growth; lasts days, leaves stubble.
  - Epilation: electronic plucking.
  - Bleaching: removes hair pigment. May cause skin irritation.
  - Mechanical waxing/plucking.
  - Depilatories: gels, lotions, or creams that chemically disrupt sulfide bonds of hair causing dissolution of hair shaft. No stubble.
  - Photoepilation (laser and intense pulsed light [IPL]): hair follicles destroyed by wavelengths of light absorbed by melanin. Good for pigmented hair; lasts 3 to 6 mo as vellus follicles remain and can be converted to terminal pigmented hair under excess androgens.
- Cosmetic: permanent. Electrolysis: destroys individual hair follicles. May be expensive and time consuming.

ACUTE GENERAL Rx

See "Pharmacologic Therapy."

CHRONIC Rx

See "Pharmacologic Therapy."

PHARMACOLOGIC THERAPY

- Usually second-line treatment following nonpharmacologic, physical methods of hair control, and in consideration of patient's comorbidities and risk factors, patient preferences, area of excess hair amenable to treatment, and access and affordability of treatments.
- Pharmacologic treatments categorized as topical, oral contraceptive pills (OCPs), antiandrogens, other treatments directed at underlying etiology.
- Topical: Eflornithine topical cream 13.9%: temporary cosmetic treatment for facial hair. Applied directly to unwanted facial hair bid with at least 8 hr spaced applications. Does not remove hair, rather slows growth. Slow response over 4 to 8 wk. Hair growth returns upon discontinuation of treatment.
- OCPs: Suppress ovarian steroidogenesis and LH through low-dose estrogen and low androgenic progestational agents. Slow response to treatment. Suppresses new hair growth. Established hair unaffected. Low-dose OCPs with low androgenic progestational agents, for example, norethindrone, desogestrel, norgestimate, drospirenone, cyproterone acetate (not available in U.S.). Avoid norgestrel and levonorgestrel (higher androgenic progestational agents).
- Antiandrogens: Spironolactone: when OCPs unacceptable or may be added for disappointing results after 6 mo of OCP treatment.
  - Aldosterone-antagonist diuretic inhibits adrenal and ovarian biosynthesis of androgens. May get ovulation.
  - Slow response usually 6 mo or more.
  - 200 mg PO qd, then decrease to 25 to 50 mg qd maintenance.
  - May cause hyperkalemia.
  - Anovulatory, unopposed estrogen states require progestin management.

REFERRAL

- To endocrinologist if difficulty in determining diagnosis, achieving therapeutic goals, or resistant to first-line therapies
- Consider referral or consultation for following therapies:
  1. Finasteride: antiandrogen, in hair follicle blocks 5 α–reductase conversion of testosterone to intranuclearly active 5 α–dihydrotestosterone (DHT)
     - Use only with reliable contraception because DHT necessary for normal male fetus urogenital development
     - Not FDA approved for treatment of hirsutism
     - 1 to 5 mg PO qd
  2. Flutamide: inhibits androgen uptake and receptor binding
     - Not recommended by Endocrine Society Clinical Practice Guidelines and not FDA approved for treatment of hirsutism, but used by some European endocrinologists
     - Use only with reliable contraception
     - Reserved for women with severe, resistant hirsutism because of risk of hepatic dysfunction
     - 250 mg PO bid
- Other treatments directed at underlying etiology:
  - Metformin/thiazolidinediones: therapy reserved for documented insulin resistant states.
  - GnRH agonists: recommended only in women with severe hyperandrogenemia (e.g., ovarian hyperthecosis) with suboptimal response to combination low-dose estrogen/progestin pills and antiandrogen treatment. Inhibits gonadotropin and consequently ovarian androgen and estrogen secretion.
  - Dexamethasone: adrenal glucocorticoid suppression is reserved for diagnosis of adrenal enzyme deficiency.
  - Total abdominal hysterectomy/bilateral salpingo-oopherectomy reserved for recalcitrant hirsutism in older female with hyperthecosis and undesired fertility.

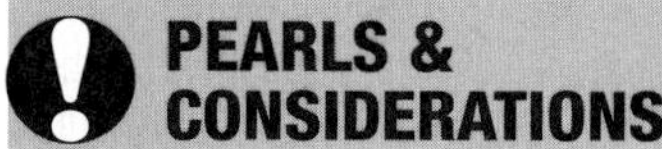

PEARLS & CONSIDERATIONS

COMMENTS

- Hirsutism is both an endocrine and cosmetic problem for patients.
- Ovulation induction therapy is indicated in women desiring pregnancy.
- Evaluation of incidental adrenal mass is warranted.

SUGGESTED READINGS

Koulouri O, Conway G: A systematic review of commonly used medical treatments for hirsutism in women, *Clin Endocrinol* 68(5):800-805, 2008.

Martin KA et al: Evaluation and treatment of hirsutism in premenopausal women: an Endocrine Society Clinical Practice Guideline, *J Clin Endocrinol Metab* 93(4):1105-1120, 2008.

Rosenfield RL: Hirsutism, *N Engl J Med* 353(24):2578-2588, 2005.

AUTHOR: **RICHARD LONG, M.D.**

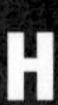

BASIC INFORMATION

DEFINITION

Histiocytosis X, now known as Langerhans cell histiocytosis (LCH), is a rare disorder characterized by the abnormal proliferation of pathologic Langerhans cells. These dendritic cells form characteristic infiltrates with eosinophils, lymphocytes, and other histiocytes found in various organs.

SYNONYMS

Eosinophilic granuloma
Hand-Schüller-Christian disease
Letterer-Siwe disease
Langerhans cell histiocytosis
Langerhans cell granulomatosis
Diffuse reticuloendotheliosis

ICD-9CM CODES
202.5 Acute Histiocytosis X
277.89 Chronic Histiocytosis X

EPIDEMIOLOGY & DEMOGRAPHICS

- LCH is mainly a childhood disorder with a peak incidence from age 1 to 4 yr.
- The annual incidence in the pediatric population is 2 to 5 per million.
- LCH affects males more often than females, 2:1.
- Pulmonary LCH (a localized form more commonly found in adults) has an equal male: female incidence, if not female predominance, probably because of increased prevalence of smoking in women.
- Usually more common in Caucasians.
- Disseminated LCH usually occurs before 2 yr of age.

PHYSICAL FINDINGS & CLINICAL PRESENTATION

- Clinical presentation is variable, and ranges from:
  - A benign isolated bony lesion (eosinophilic granuloma), most often found in children younger than 15 yr of age.
  - Multiple bone lesions with soft tissue gingival and oral mucosal involvement (Hand-Schüller-Christian disease); generally occurs in children younger than 10 yr of age.
  - An aggressive disseminated disease infiltrating organs and causing organ dysfunction (Letterer-Siwe disease). It is the rarest form of LCH, affecting mostly children younger than 2 yr.
- Bone lesions (80% to 100%).
  - May be isolated or multiple
  - Painful, often worse at night
  - Skull most often involved, followed by long bones; lesions rarely seen in small bones of hands and feet
  - Proptosis
  - Mastoiditis
  - Loose teeth
  - Gingival hypertrophy
- Skin is involved in >80% of patients with disseminated disease and in 30% of patients with less extensive disease.
  - Seborrhea-like scaling of scalp, petechial and purpuric lesions, ulcers, and bronzing of the skin may occur.
  - Common sites: scalp, neck, trunk, groin, and extremities.
- Lymphadenopathy (10%): cervical and inguinal.
- Pulmonary disease is very frequent in adults (usually as isolated disease), but can be seen in 23% to 50% of children as well. Lung involvement always occurs as part of the disseminated disease in children.
- Pulmonary involvement may manifest with cough, tachypnea, cyanosis, inspiratory crackles, pleural effusions, or pneumothorax. Diffuse emphysema associated with pulmonary fibrosis is the end stage of a mixed restrictive and obstructive pattern of disease.
- Liver involvement manifesting as hepatomegaly with or without jaundice (50% to 60%).
- Involvement of the biliary tree may be seen as biliary fibrosis or sclerosing cholangitis.
- Splenomegaly (5%).
- CNS involvement occurs in 25% to 35% of patients, most often in those with disseminated disease. The most common cerebral site affected is the hypothalamic-neurohypophyseal region, where infiltration and destruction usually result in diabetes insipidus with insatiable thirst and urination. The second most common site of involvement is the cerebellum.
- Involvement of the thymus, parotid glands, and GI tract has been reported in rare cases.

ETIOLOGY

- The etiology of LCH is unknown, though multiple theories have been proposed.
- Some degree of genetic predisposition has been proposed and recent evidence suggests LCH as a monoclonal proliferative neoplastic disorder in children.
- In adults, pulmonary LCH appears to be primarily an immune-mediated reactive process and has been linked to cigarette smoking. Cigarette smoke had not been observed as a causative factor in other forms of LCH.

DIAGNOSIS

Tissue biopsy of organ lesions reveals pathological Langerhans cells characterized by the presence of multiple surface nucleoproteins including CD1a, the presence of which establishes definitively histological diagnosis of LCH. The infiltration by eosinophils forming pseudoabscesses is characteristic.

DIFFERENTIAL DIAGNOSIS

The differential diagnosis is extensive, including all causes of diabetes insipidus, lytic bone lesions, dermatitis, hepatomegaly, and lymphadenopathy.

WORKUP

Baseline evaluation should include bone scan, chest x-ray, skeletal x-ray, abdominal ultrasound, and routine laboratory to assess the extent of disease involvement.

LABORATORY TESTS

- CBC is not specific but may reveal cytopenias in patients with bone marrow involvement.
- Electrolytes, BUN, creatinine, urinalysis, and urine and serum osmolality are helpful in the diagnosis of diabetes insipidus during fluid deprivation testing.
- Liver function tests (LFTs) may be elevated in patients with liver involvement.
- Bronchoalveolar lavage may show increased numbers of CD1a-positive histiocytes or Langerhans cells in patients with pulmonary LCH.

IMAGING STUDIES

- Radiograph studies of affected areas show lytic lesions with or without sclerotic margins.
- Radiograph bone survey is done searching for other lesions.
- Bone scan complements the bone survey studies.
- Panoramic dental view of the mandible and maxilla for children with oral involvement.
- Chest radiograph can show interstitial reticulonodular infiltrates. This pattern typically progresses toward frank honeycombing fibrosis later in the course of the disease (Fig. 1-154).

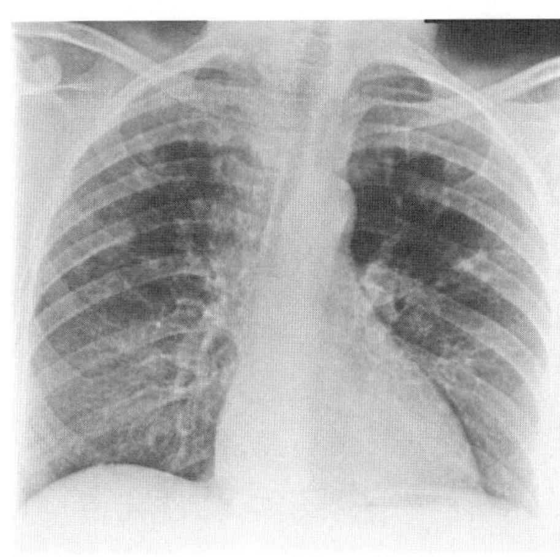

FIGURE 1-154 Langerhans cell histiocytosis (LCH; histiocytosis X). There is a reticular nodular pattern in the upper lobes. The lung volumes are preserved. (From McLoud TC [ed]: *Thoracic radiology, the requisites,* St Louis, 1998, Mosby.)

- High-resolution CT scan of the chest confirms interstitial lung scarring, nodules, and cysts, and represents an excellent noninvasive means for diagnosis and follow-up of pulmonary LCH. Pulmonary cysts are bilateral and symmetric, showing slight upper-lobe predominance with relative sparing of the costophrenic angles.
- CT scans of the temporal bone searching for mastoid, and inner and middle ear involvement.
- Ultrasound of the abdomen may show hepatosplenomegaly.
- Conventional cholangiography or MRI cholangiopancreatography can confirm the presence of disease in patients suspected to have biliary involvement.
- MRI of the brain to visualize the hypothalamic-hypophyseal region in patients suspected of having diabetes insipidus.

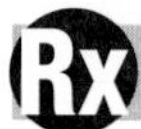

TREATMENT

Treatment is still evolving and is based on organ involvement and the extent of disease.

ACUTE GENERAL Rx

Isolated bone lesions can be treated by:

- Curettage of affected site and implantation of allograft bone chips or polymethylmethacrylate
- Intralesional prednisone or prednisone and vinblastine
- Bisphosphonates
- NSAIDs
- Radiation therapy is useful only for bone lesions of the vertebrae or femoral neck at risk of collapse

Single skin lesions are treated with:

- Topical steroid (e.g., triamcinolone acetonide) applied bid
- Nitrogen mustard in 20% solution
- Surgery
- Intralesional interferon
- Isotretinoin

Treatment of solitary lymph node involvement:

- Excision at the time of diagnosis
- Systemic oral prednisone

Treatment for multiple bone lesions, skull base lesions, or multisystem disease includes:

- Vinblastine 6 mg/m^2 IV bolus every wk for 6 mo or etoposide 150 mg/m^2 IV for 3 days every 3 wk for 6 mo and oral prednisone for 6 mo

CHRONIC Rx

- For severe, high-risk, disseminated patients not responding within 6 wk of initial treatment, salvage therapy, including high dose of the purine analog cladribine along with high-dose cytosine arabinoside followed by allogeneic blood stem cell transplantation, should be considered. Additionally, liver or lung transplantation might be the treatment of choice for terminal liver and lung failure patients.
- Diabetes insipidus is treated with DDAVP 0.1 to 0.8 mg PO or 1 spray bid to tid.
- Adults with isolated pulmonary LCH do not require aggressive treatment, and will benefit from smoking cessation.
- Empirical use of steroids, in either short pulses or longer exposures, has also been implicated in the treatment of pulmonary disease; however, data regarding effectiveness are still limited.
- Lung transplantation has been tried in both children and adults with advanced pulmonary disease and limited lung function, but failure rates are high because of local recurrence after transplantation.

DISPOSITION

- Patients with disease localized to only one organ system have a good prognosis and appear to need minimal, if any, treatment. For patients with isolated pulmonary LCH, the 5-yr survival rate is around 80%.
- Patients with disseminated disease have an increased risk for poor outcome, with a reported mortality rate of 10% to 20%, and 50% risk of life-impairing morbidity. A poor prognostic feature is the failure to respond to therapy in the first 6 wk.
- In patients with disseminated LCH and <2 yr of age, the mortality rate is 30%.

REFERRAL

Multidisciplinary approach: pediatric oncologist, radiation oncologists, oral maxillary surgeons, ear-nose-throat specialists, audiology, dermatology, endocrinology, and family counseling

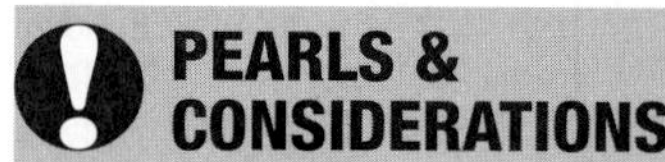

PEARLS & CONSIDERATIONS

COMMENTS

- The course of LCH is often unpredictable and varies from spontaneous resolution to rapid progression and death, or multiple recurrences and regressions with risk for permanent sequelae.
- The association of LCH with other malignancies (e.g., acute lymphocytic leukemia, acute nonlymphoblastic leukemia, and solid tumors) has been cited.

PREVENTION

Effective antismoking measures can prevent pulmonary LCH.

PATIENT/FAMILY EDUCATION

- Instruct patients to promptly report the development of hemoptysis. This symptom may indicate malignancy or superimposed bacterial/fungal infection, such as *Aspergillus* species infection.
- Educate about the likely etiologic role of cigarette smoking.

SUGGESTED READINGS

Dauriat G et al: Lung transplantation for pulmonary Langerhans' cell histiocytosis: a multicenter analysis, *Transplantation* 81:746, 2006.

Gadner H et al: Improved outcome in multisystem Langerhans cell histiocytosis is associated with therapy intensification, *Blood* 111:2556, 2008.

Histiocytosis Association of America: www.histio.org

Hoover KB et al: Langerhans cell histiocytosis, *Skeletal Radiol* 36(2):95-104, 2007.

Stockschlaeder M, Sucker C: Adult Langerhans cell histiocytosis, *Eur J Haematol* 76(5):363-368, 2006.

Weitzman S, Egeler RM: Langerhans cell histiocytosis: update for the pediatrician, *Curr Opin Pediatr* 20:23, 2008.

AUTHOR: **MARK BRADY, M.D., M.P.H., M.M.S.**

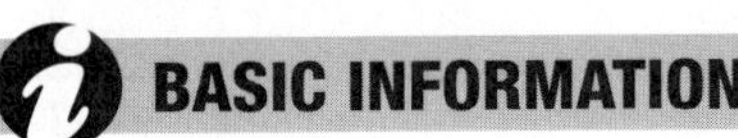

DEFINITION

Histoplasmosis is caused by the fungus *Histoplasma capsulatum* and characterized by a primary pulmonary focus with occasional progression to chronic pulmonary histoplasmosis (CPH) or various forms of dissemination. Progressive disseminated histoplasmosis (PDH) may present with a diverse clinical spectrum, including adrenal necrosis, pulmonary and mediastinal fibrosis, and ulcerations of the oropharynx and GI tract. In those patients coinfected with HIV, it is a defining disease for AIDS.

SYNONYMS

North American histoplasmosis
Ohio Valley fever
Vanderbilt disease

ICD-9CM CODES
115.90 Histoplasmosis
115.94 Histoplasmosis with endocarditis
115.91 Histoplasmosis with meningitis
115.93 Histoplasmosis with pericarditis
115.95 Histoplasmosis with pneumonia
115.92 Histoplasmosis with retinitis

EPIDEMIOLOGY & DEMOGRAPHICS

INCIDENCE (IN U.S.):
- Unknown for acute pulmonary disease
- For CPH, estimated at 1/100,000 cases in endemic areas
- For PDH in immunocompetent adults, estimated at 1/2000 cases of histoplasmosis

PREVALENCE: Unknown

PREDOMINANT SEX: Clinically evident disease is most common in males; male:female ratio of 4:1

PREDOMINANT AGE:
- CPH is most often seen in males >50 yr old with an associated history of COPD.
- Presumed ocular histoplasmosis syndrome (POHS) is seen between ages of 20 and 40 yr.

PEAK INCIDENCE: Unknown

PHYSICAL FINDINGS & CLINICAL PRESENTATION

- Conidia are deposited in alveoli then converted to yeast forms where they spread to regional lymph nodes and other organs, especially liver and spleen.
- 1 to 2 wk later, a granulomatous inflammatory response begins to contain the yeast in the form of discrete granulomas.
- Delayed-type hypersensitivity to *Histoplasma* antigens occurs 3 to 6 wk after exposure.
- Clinical disease manifests in various forms, depending on host cellular immunity and inoculum size:
  1. Acute primary pulmonary histoplasmosis
     a. An overwhelming number of patients are asymptomatic.
     b. Most clinically apparent infections manifest by complaints of fever, headache, malaise, pleuritic chest pain, nonproductive cough, and weight loss.
     c. Less than 10%, mainly women, complain of arthralgias, myalgias, and skin manifestations such as erythema multiforme or erythema nodosum.
     d. Acute pericarditis presents in a smaller percentage of patients.
     e. Hepatosplenomegaly is most commonly observed in children.
     f. With particularly heavy exposure, there is severe dyspnea, marked hypoxemia, impending respiratory failure.
     g. Most patients are asymptomatic within 6 wk.
  2. CPH
     a. Presents insidiously with low-grade fever, malaise, weight loss, cough, sometimes with blood-streaked sputum or frank hemoptysis.
     b. Most patients with cavitary lesions present with associated COPD or chronic bronchitis, masking underlying fungal disease.
     c. Tends to worsen preexisting pulmonary disease and further contribute to eventual respiratory insufficiency.
  3. PDH
     a. In both acute and subacute forms, constitutional symptoms of fever, fatigue, malaise, and weight loss are common.
     b. Acute form (seen in infants and children) presents with respiratory symptoms, fever ≥101° F (38.3° C), generalized lymphadenopathy, marked hepatosplenomegaly, and fulminant course resembling septic shock associated with a high fatality rate.
     c. Subacute form is more common in adults and associated with lower temperatures, hepatosplenomegaly, oropharyngeal ulceration, focal organ involvement (including adrenal destruction, endocarditis, chronic meningitis, and intracerebral mass lesions).
     d. Course of subacute form is relentless, with untreated patients dying within 2 yr.
     e. Chronic PDH is found in adults and marked by gradual symptoms of weight loss, weakness, easy fatigability; low-grade fever when present; oropharyngeal ulcerations and hepatomegaly and/or splenomegaly in one third of patients.
     f. Less clinical evidence of focal organ involvement in chronic form than in subacute form.
     g. Natural history of chronic form is protracted and intermittent, spanning months to years.
- Histoplasmoma
  1. A healed area of caseation necrosis surrounded by a fibrous capsule
  2. Usually asymptomatic
- Mediastinal fibrosis
  1. A rare consequence of a fibroblastic process that encases caseating mediastinal lymph nodes producing severe retraction, compression, and distortion of mediastinal structures
  2. Constriction of the bronchi resulting in bronchiectasis, also esophageal stenosis associated with dysphagia, and superior vena cava syndrome
- POHS
  1. Diagnosis characterized by distinct clinical features, including atrophic choroidal scars and maculopathy in patients with histories suggestive of exposure to the fungus (e.g., residence in an endemic area)
  2. Patient complains of distortion or loss of central vision without pain, redness, or photophobia
  3. Usually no evidence of infection except for a positive skin reaction to histoplasmin
- In patients with AIDS
  1. Possible presentation as overwhelming infection similar to acute PDH seen in children
  2. Constitutional symptoms: fever, weight loss, malaise, cough, dyspnea
  3. About 10% with cutaneous maculopapular, erythematous eruptions or purpuric lesions on face, trunk, and extremities
  4. Up to 20% with CNS involvement, manifesting as intracerebral mass lesions, chronic meningitis, or encephalopathy

ETIOLOGY

- *H. capsulatum* is a dimorphic fungus present in temperate zones and river valleys worldwide.
- In the U.S., it is highly endemic in southeastern, mid-Atlantic, and central states.
- Exists as mold at ambient temperature and favors soils enriched with bird or bat droppings.

Dx DIAGNOSIS

DIFFERENTIAL DIAGNOSIS

- Acute pulmonary histoplasmosis
  1. *Mycobacterium tuberculosis*
  2. Community-acquired pneumonias caused by *Mycoplasma* and *Chlamydia*
  3. Other fungal diseases, such as *Blastomyces dermatitidis* and *Coccidioides immitis*
- Chronic cavitary pulmonary histoplasmosis: *M. tuberculosis*
- Histoplasmomas: true neoplasms

WORKUP

- Suspect diagnosis in patients who present with a history of residence or travel in an endemic area, especially if engaged in occupations (e.g., outside construction or street cleaning) or hobbies (e.g., cave exploring) that increase the likelihood of exposure to fungal spores.
- Suspect diagnosis in immunosuppressed patients with remote history of exposure, especially if associated with characteristic calcifications on chest x-ray examination.

LABORATORY TESTS

- Demonstration of organism on culture from body fluid or tissues to make definitive diagnosis
  1. Especially high yield in patients with AIDS
  2. Characteristic oval yeast cells in neutrophils with Giemsa stain from peripheral smear
  3. Preparations of infected tissue with Gomori's silver methenamine for revealing yeast forms, especially in areas of caseation necrosis
- Serologic tests, including complement-fixing (CF) antibodies and immunodiffusion assays
- Detection of *Histoplasma* antigen in urine: may be influenced by infections with *Blastomyces* and *Coccidioides*
- In PDH
  1. Pancytopenia
  2. Marked elevations in alkaline phosphatase and alanine aminotransferase (ALT) common
- In chronic meningitis (majority of cases)
  1. CSF pleocytosis with either lymphocytes or neutrophils predominating
  2. Elevated CSF protein levels
  3. Hypoglycorrhachia

IMAGING STUDIES

- Chest radiograph examination in acute pulmonary histoplasmosis
  1. Singular or multiple patchy infiltrates, especially in the lower lung fields
  2. Hilar or mediastinal lymphadenopathy with or without pneumonitis
  3. Diffuse nodular or confluent bilateral miliary infiltrates characteristic of heavier exposure
  4. Infrequent pleural effusions, except when associated with pericarditis
- Chest radiograph examination in histoplasmoma: coin lesion displaying central calcification, ranging from 1 to 4 cm in diameter, predominantly located in the subpleural regions
- Chest radiograph examination in CPH:
  1. Upper lobe disease frequently associated with cavities
  2. Preexisting calcifications in the hilum associated with peribronchial streaking extending to the parenchyma
- Chest radiograph examination in acute PDH: hilar adenopathy and/or diffuse nodular infiltrates
- CT scan of adrenals to reveal bilateral enlargement and low-attenuation centers

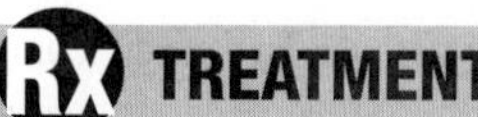

TREATMENT

NONPHARMACOLOGIC THERAPY

For life-threatening disease seen in acute disseminated disease or infection in patients with AIDS: supportive therapy with IV fluids

ACUTE GENERAL Rx

- No drug therapy is required for asymptomatic pulmonary disease.
- A course of therapy with ketoconazole 400 mg/day or itraconazole 200 mg/day PO for 3 to 6 wk may be beneficial in some patients with acute pulmonary distress. Avoid fluconazole because it is not as active.
- Same therapy appropriate for immunocompetent, mild to moderately symptomatic patients with CPH and subacute and chronic forms of PDH, but duration for 6 to 12 mo.
- Use amphotericin B 0.7 to 1 mg/kg IV for 6 to 12 mo in patients hypersensitive to or intolerant of azole therapy.
- Give amphotericin B for life-threatening disease or continued illness as a result of primary failure or relapse of adequate azole therapy. A lipid formulation of amphotericin B can be used to avoid nephrotoxicity.
  1. For acute pulmonary histoplasmosis associated with acute respiratory distress syndrome (ARDS), acute PDH, and histoplasma meningitis: dose of 0.7 to 1 mg/kg IV q24h
  2. End point of therapy for patient with complicated acute pulmonary disease: total dose of 500 mg
  3. End point for patient with acute PDH: total dose 35 mg/kg or 2.5 g total
  4. Prednisone 60 to 80 mg/day beneficial for severe fungal hypersensitivity complicating acute pulmonary disease
- Endocarditis: surgical treatment with excision of infected valve or graft combined with amphotericin for a total dose of 35 mg/kg or 2.5 g.
- For pericardial disease:
  1. Antifungal therapy: no apparent benefit
  2. Best managed with NSAIDs
- For POHS:
  1. Antifungal therapy: no apparent benefit
  2. May respond to laser therapy

CHRONIC Rx

In patients with AIDS: lifelong suppressive therapy with either itraconazole, given 200 mg PO qid, or IV amphotericin B at a dose of 50 mg once weekly; a triazole compound posaconazole (400 mg PO bid) may be useful in refractory cases, but clinical experience is limited at this point.

DISPOSITION

For those with chronic or progressive disease, especially if immunocompromised, prognosis is dependent on prompt recognition and timely administration of appropriate antifungal drugs.

REFERRAL

- To an infectious disease specialist in suspected cases of disseminated disease, especially if immunocompromised
- To a pulmonologist for patients with CPH form because of progressive respiratory compromise
- To a thoracic surgeon for decompression procedures for progressive mediastinal fibrosis

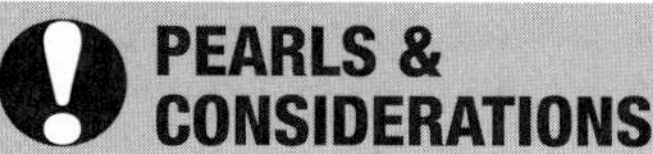

PEARLS & CONSIDERATIONS

- *H. capsulatum,* variety *duboisii,* also known as African histoplasmosis, is restricted to Senegal, Nigeria, Zaire, and Uganda.
- Unlike *H. capsulatum,* pulmonary forms of *duboisii* are not seen, and the disease is limited to the skin, soft tissues, and bone.

COMMENTS

- Patients living in endemic areas, especially if immunocompromised, should take appropriate respiratory precautions when disposing of bird waste from rooftop or home aviaries.
- Appropriate respiratory precautions should also be taken when leisure traveling to areas that act as a natural haven for the fungus, such as bat caves.

SUGGESTED READINGS

Schestatsky P et al: Isolated central nervous system histoplasmosis in immunocompetent hosts: a series of 11 cases, *Scand J Infect Dis* 38(1):43, 2006.

Weinberg M et al: Severe histoplasmosis in travelers to Nicaragua, *Emerg Infect Dis* 9(10):1322, 2003.

Wheat LJ, Kauffman CA: Histoplasmosis, *Infect Dis Clin North Am* 17(1):1, 2003.

AUTHORS: **GLENN G. FORT, M.D., M.P.H.,** and **DENNIS J. MIKOLICH, M.D.**

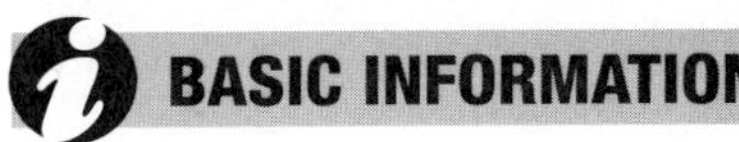

BASIC INFORMATION

DEFINITION

Patients with histrionic personality disorder present with a pervasive pattern of excessive emotionality and attention-seeking behavior that generally begins in early adulthood.

SYNONYMS

Hysterical personality disorder
Psycho-infantile personality disorder
Personality disorder (nonspecific)

ICD-9CM CODES
301.5 Histrionic personality disorder (ICD-9 and DSM IV code)

EPIDEMIOLOGY & DEMOGRAPHICS

PREVALENCE (IN U.S.):

- Diagnosed more often in women; rarely found in men
- Prevalence: 2% to 3% for histrionic personality disorder, 10% to 13% for personality disorders (unspecified)

PREDOMINANT SEX: Predominant in women. Cultural factors (e.g., attention-seeking behavior not as acceptable in men) may lead to more common diagnosis in women.

PREDOMINANT AGE: Generally begins in early childhood

PHYSICAL FINDINGS & CLINICAL PRESENTATION

Features include five or more of the following:

1. Is uncomfortable in situations where he or she is not the center of attention.
2. Interaction with others is often characterized by inappropriate sexually seductive or provocative behavior.
3. Displays rapidly shifting and shallow expression of emotions.
4. Consistently uses physical appearance to draw attention to self.
5. Has a style of speech that is excessively impressionistic and lacking in detail.
6. Shows self-dramatization, theatricality, and exaggerated expression of emotion.
7. Is suggestible (i.e., easily influenced by others or circumstances).
8. Considers relationships to be more intimate than they actually are.

ETIOLOGY

- Unknown
- Hypothesized that childhood events, psychosocial adversity, and genetics are contributory

Dx DIAGNOSIS

DIFFERENTIAL DIAGNOSIS

- Other personality disorders (e.g., borderline personality disorder, antisocial personality disorder, narcissistic personality disorder)
- Personality change attributable to general medical condition
- Symptoms in association with chronic substance abuse

WORKUP

There is no formal test to establish diagnosis.

Rx TREATMENT

NONPHARMACOLOGIC THERAPY

- Long-term individual psychotherapy is treatment of choice.
- Unlike other people who have personality disorders, these individuals often seek treatment and exaggerate their symptoms and difficulties in functioning.
- Patients tend to be more emotionally needy and are often reluctant to terminate therapy.

ACUTE GENERAL Rx

- Four double-blind, placebo-controlled trials suggest that patients with serious personality disorders (especially borderline personality disorder) respond to optimal doses of selective serotonin reuptake inhibitors, with improvements in anger, impulsiveness, aggressive behavior, affective lability, and facilitation of psychotherapy.
- Care should be given when prescribing medications to patients with histrionic personality disorder because of the potential for using the medication to contribute to self-destructive or otherwise harmful behaviors.

DISPOSITION

Therapeutic approaches should not focus on the long-term personality change of the individual, but rather short-term alleviation of difficulties within the person's life.

REFERRAL

Primarily treated by mental health professionals

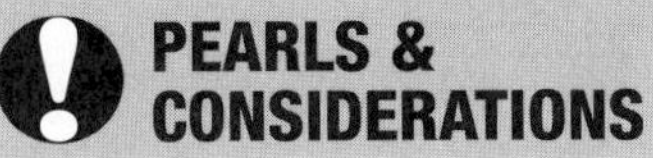

PEARLS & CONSIDERATIONS

- Individuals with this disorder are usually difficult to treat.
- Like most personality disorders, patients present for treatment only when stress or other situational factor within their lives has made their ability to function and cope effectively impossible.
- Suicidality should be assessed on a regular basis, and suicidal threats and self-mutilation should not be ignored or dismissed.

PATIENT & FAMILY EDUCATION

Group and family therapy approaches are generally not recommended because individuals with this disorder often try to draw attention to themselves and exaggerate every action and reaction.

SUGGESTED READINGS

Gabbard GO: Mind, brain and personality disorders, *Am J Psychiatry* 162:4,2005.

Verheul R, Herbrink M: The efficacy of various modalities of psychotherapy for personality disorders: a systematic review of the evidence and clinical recommendations, *Int Rev Psychiatry* 19(1):25, 2007.

AUTHOR: **MITCHELL D. FELDMAN, M.D., M.PHIL.**

BASIC INFORMATION

DEFINITION

Hodgkin's disease is a malignant disorder of lymphoreticular origin, characterized histologically by the presence of multinucleated giant cells (Reed-Sternberg cells) usually originating from B lymphocytes in germinal centers of lymphoid tissue.

ICD-9CM CODES
201.9 Hodgkin's disease, unspecified
201.4 Hodgkin's disease, lymphocyte predominance
201.5 Hodgkin's disease, nodular sclerosis
201.6 Hodgkin's disease, mixed cellularity
201.7 Hodgkin's disease, lymphocyte depletion

EPIDEMIOLOGY & DEMOGRAPHICS

- There is a bimodal age distribution (15 to 34 yr and >50 yr).
- Concordance for Hodgkin's disease in identical twins suggests that a genetic susceptibility underlies Hodgkin's disease in young adulthood.
- The disease is more common in males (in childhood Hodgkin's disease, >80% occur in males), whites, and higher socioeconomic groups.
- Overall incidence of Hodgkin's disease in the U.S. is approximately four per 100,000. There are >8000 new cases of Hodgkin's lymphoma diagnosed annually in the U.S.

PHYSICAL FINDINGS & CLINICAL PRESENTATION

- Palpable lymphadenopathy that is generally painless is the most common presenting symptom
- Most common site of involvement: neck region
- Fever and night sweats: fever in a cyclical pattern (days or weeks of fever alternating with afebrile periods) is known as *Pel-Epstein fever*
- Weight loss, generalized malaise
- Persistent, nonproductive cough
- Pain associated with alcohol ingestion often because of heavy eosinophil infiltration of the tumor sites is relatively uncommon
- Pruritus
- Other: superior vena cava syndrome, spinal cord compression (rare), erythema nodosum, ichthyosis

ETIOLOGY

Unknown; evidence implicating Epstein-Barr virus remains controversial.

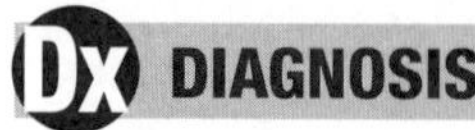

DIAGNOSIS

DIFFERENTIAL DIAGNOSIS

- Non-Hodgkin's lymphoma
- Sarcoidosis
- Infections (e.g., cytomegalovirus, Epstein-Barr virus, toxoplasmosis, HIV)
- Drug reaction

WORKUP

Diagnosis is confirmed by lymph node biopsy. The World Health Organization classifies Hodgkin's lymphoma into two groups: classical Hodgkin's lymphoma (92% to 97%) and nodular lymphocyte-predominant Hodgkin's lymphoma (3% to 8%). Classic Hodgkin's lymphoma has four main histologic subtypes based on the number of lymphocytes, Reed-Sternberg cells (Fig. 1-155), and the presence of fibrous tissue:
1. Nodular sclerosis (60% to 80%)
2. Mixed cellularity (15% to 30%)
3. Lymphocyte predominance (2% to 7%)
4. Lymphocyte depletion (1% to 6%)

Nodular sclerosis occurs mainly in young adulthood, whereas the mixed cellularity type is more prevalent after age 50 yr.

Staging for Hodgkin's disease follows the Ann Arbor staging classification:
- Stage I: Involvement of a single lymph node region
- Stage II: Two or more lymph node regions on the same side of the diaphragm
- Stage III: Lymph node involvement on both sides of diaphragm, including spleen
- Stage IV: Diffuse involvement of external sites
- Suffix A: No systemic symptoms
- Suffix B: Presence of fever, night sweats, or unexplained weight loss of ≥10% body weight over 6 mo
- Suffix X: Indicates bulky disease more than one third of the widening of the mediastinum or >10 cm maximum dimension of nodal mass on a chest film

Proper staging requires the following:
- Detailed history (with documentation of "B symptoms" and physical examination)
- Surgical biopsy
- Laboratory evaluation (complete blood count, erythrocyte sedimentation rate, blood urea nitrogen, creatinine, alkaline phosphatase, liver function tests, albumin, lactate dehydrogenase, uric acid)
- Chest radiograph (posteroanterior and lateral)
- CT scan of chest, abdomen, pelvis, neck
- Positron emission tomography scan
- Bilateral bone marrow biopsy (selected patients)
- Exploratory laparotomy and splenectomy (now rarely performed):
  1. Decision to perform staging laparotomy depends on the therapeutic plan; it is generally not indicated in patients who have a large mediastinal mass (these patients will generally be treated with combined chemotherapy and radiation). Staging laparotomy may also not be required in patients with clinical stage I disease or those who are unlikely to have abdominal disease (e.g., females with supradiaphragmatic disease).
  2. Exploratory laparotomy and splenectomy may be used for selected patients with clinical stage I to IIA or IIB.
  3. It is useful in identifying patients who can be treated with irradiation alone with curative intent.
  4. Polyvalent pneumococcal vaccine should be given prophylactically to all patients before splenectomy (increased risk of sepsis from encapsulated organisms in splenectomized patients).

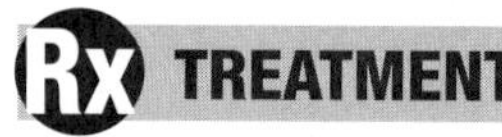

TREATMENT

ACUTE GENERAL Rx

The main therapeutic modalities are radiotherapy and chemotherapy; the indication for which one varies with pathologic stage and other factors. In general, chemotherapy plus involved-field radiotherapy can be used as standard treatment for Hodgkin's disease in early stages with favorable prognostic features. In patients with unfavorable features, four courses of chemotherapy plus involved-field radiotherapy should be the standard treatment. Commonly used therapeutic modalities are:
- Stage I and II: radiation therapy alone (involved-field radiotherapy [35 Gy]) unless a large mediastinal mass is present (mediastinal to thoracic ratio ≥1.3); in the latter case, a combination of chemotherapy and radiation therapy is indicated.

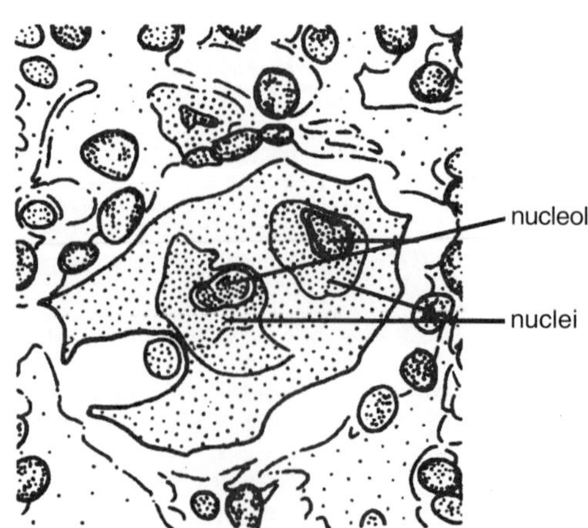

FIGURE 1-155 Hodgkin's disease. High-power photomicrograph demonstrates a binucleate Reed-Sternberg cell exhibiting prominent inclusion-like eosinophilic nucleoli, giving it an "owl's eye" appearance. (From Skarin AT: *Atlas of diagnostic oncology,* ed 3, St Louis, 2003, Mosby.)

- Stage IB or IIB: total nodal irradiation is often used, although chemotherapy is performed in many centers.
- Stage IIIA: treatment is controversial. It varies with the anatomic substage after splenectomy.
  1. III_1A and minimum splenic involvement: radiation therapy alone may be adequate.
  2. III_2 or III_1A with extensive splenic involvement: there is disagreement whether chemotherapy alone or a combination of chemotherapy and radiation therapy is the preferred treatment modality.
  3. IIIB and IVB: the treatment of choice is chemotherapy with or without adjuvant radiotherapy.

Various regimens can be used for combination of chemotherapy. Most oncologists prefer the combination of doxorubicin plus bleomycin plus vincristine plus dacarbazine (ABVD).

- In patients with advanced Hodgkin's disease, increased-dose bleomycin, etoposide, doxorubicin, cyclophosphamide, vincristine, procarbazine, and prednisone (BEACOPP) offers better tumor control and overall survival than COPP-ABVD.
- Monoclonal antibody therapy: SGN-30 and MDX-060 and the anti-CD20 antibody rituximab have shown promising results.

DISPOSITION

- The overall survival at 10 yr is approximately 60%.
- Cure rates as high as 75% to 80% are now possible with appropriate initial therapy.
- Poor prognostic features include presence of B symptoms, advanced age, advanced stage at initial presentation, mixed cellularity, and lymphocyte depletion histology.
- Chemotherapy significantly increases the risk of leukemia.
- The peak in risk of leukemia is seen approximately 5 yr after the initiation of chemotherapy.
- The risk of leukemia is greater for those who undergo splenectomy and patients with advanced stages of Hodgkin's disease; the risk is unaffected by concomitant radiotherapy.
- Involved-field radiotherapy does not improve the outcome in patients with advanced-stage Hodgkin's lymphoma who have a complete remission after MOPP (mechlorethamine, vincristine, procarbazine, and prednisone)-ABV chemotherapy. Radiotherapy may benefit patients with a partial response after chemotherapy.
- Mediastinal irradiation increases the risk of subsequent death from heart disease caused by sclerosis of the coronary artery from irradiation. Risk increases with high mediastinal doses, minimal protective cardiac blocking, young age at irradiation, and increased duration of follow-up.
- Both chemotherapy and radiation therapy increase the risk of developing secondary solid tumors (e.g., carcinoma of the lung, breast, and stomach).

REFERRAL

- To surgery for lymph node biopsy
- Hematology/oncology

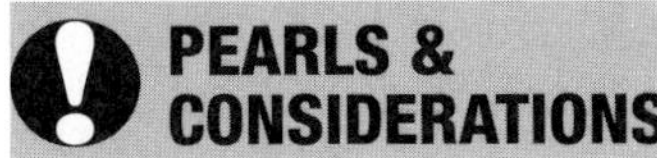

PEARLS & CONSIDERATIONS

COMMENTS

- Young male patients should consider sperm banking before the initiation of therapy.
- Chemotherapy plus involved-field radiotherapy should be the standard treatment for Hodgkin's disease with favorable prognostic features. In patients with unfavorable features, four courses of chemotherapy plus involved-field radiotherapy should be the standard of treatment.

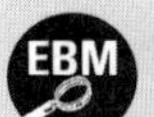

EVIDENCE

Much of the evidence for the benefit of chemotherapy and radiotherapy in the treatment of Hodgkin's disease does not meet our criteria for citation.

The ABVD regimen is superior to the MOPP regimen in the treatment of advanced Hodgkin's disease and is less myelotoxic. ABVD for 6 to 8 mo was as effective as 12 mo of MOPP alternating with ABVD, and both were superior to MOPP alone.[1] B

A systematic review of interventions for early-stage Hodgkin's disease in children found little evidence from randomized, controlled trials (RCTs) to evaluate the consensus approach of short-course chemotherapy and local radiotherapy, although no discernible difference in survival rate was detected between involved-field and extended-field radiotherapy in one RCT.[2] A

A systematic review of radiation therapy trials in Hodgkin's lymphoma showed that in early stages of disease extended-field irradiation is now replaced by short periods of chemotherapy followed by limited radiotherapy. In intermediate stages, two recently reported RCTs indicated that combined-modality treatment is preferable and involved-field could replace extended-field irradiation.[3] A

One RCT found better tumor control and overall survival rate with increased-dose BEACOPP compared with COPP-ABVD followed by local radiotherapy when indicated.[4] A

A systematic review of 12 RCTs comparing prophylaxis with granulocyte colony-stimulating factor (G-CSF) or granulocyte-macrophage CSF (GM-CSF) versus placebo/no prophylaxis in adult patients with malignant lymphoma undergoing chemotherapy found both G-CSF and GM-CSF significantly reduced the relative risk for severe neutropenia, febrile neutropenia, and infection. There was no evidence that either G-CSF or GM-CSF reduced the number of patients requiring IV antibiotics, lowered infection-related mortality rate, or improved complete tumor response.[5] A

Evidence-Based References

1. Cannellos GP et al: Chemotherapy of advanced Hodgkin's disease with MOPP, ABVD, or MOPP alternating with ABVD, *N Engl J Med* 327:1478, 1992.
2. Louw G, Pinkerton CR: Interventions for early stage Hodgkin's disease in children, *Cochrane Rev* 2, 2002.
3. Gustavsson A et al: A systematic overview of radiation therapy effects in Hodgkin's lymphoma, *Acta Oncol* 42:589, 2003.
4. Diehl V et al: Standard and increased-dose BEACOPP chemotherapy compared with COPP-ABVD for advanced Hodgkin's disease, *N Engl J Med* 348: 2386, 2003.
5. Bohlius J et al: Granulopoiesis-stimulating factors to prevent adverse effects in the treatment of malignant lymphoma, *Cochrane Rev* 3, 2004.

SUGGESTED READINGS

Ansell S, Armitage JO: Management of Hodgkin lymphoma, *Mayo Clin Proc* 81(3):419, 2006.

Ferme C et al: Chemotherapy plus involved-field radiation in early-stage Hodgkin's disease, *N Engl J Med* 357:1916, 2007.

Glass C: Role of the primary care physician in Hodgkin lymphoma, *Am Fam Physician* 78(5):615, 2008.

AUTHOR: **FRED F. FERRI, M.D.**

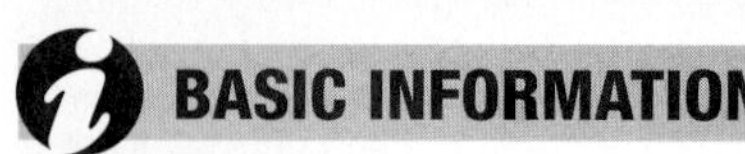

BASIC INFORMATION

DEFINITION

Hookworm is a parasitic infection of the intestine caused by helminths.

SYNONYMS

Ground itch
Ancylostoma duodenale infection
Necator americanus infection

ICD-9CM CODES
126.35 Hookworm

EPIDEMIOLOGY & DEMOGRAPHICS

INCIDENCE (IN U.S.):

- Varies greatly in different areas of the U.S.
- Most common in rural areas of southeastern U.S.
- Poor sanitation and increased rainfall increase incidence

PREVALENCE (IN U.S.): Varies from 10% to 90% in regions where it is found

PREDOMINANT AGE: Schoolchildren

PHYSICAL FINDINGS & CLINICAL PRESENTATION

- Nonspecific abdominal complaints
- Because these organisms consume host RBCs, symptoms related to iron-deficiency anemia, depending on the amount of iron in the diet and the worm burden
- Fatigue, tachycardia, dyspnea, and high-output failure
- Hypoproteinemia and edema from loss of proteins into the intestinal tract
- Unusual for pulmonary manifestations to occur when the larvae migrate through the lungs
- Skin rash at sites of larval penetration in some individuals without prior exposure

ETIOLOGY

Two species can cause this disease: *N. americanus* and *A. duodenale. N. americanus* is the predominant cause of hookworm in the U.S. They are soil nematodes (Geohelminthic infections) that are acquired by skin contact (i.e., bare feet) with contaminated soils in moist, warm climate.

- Infection occurs via penetration of the skin by the larval form, with subsequent migration via the bloodstream to the alveoli, up the respiratory tract, then into the GI tract (Fig. 1-156)
- *Ancylostoma* spp. infection can also occur via the oral route through ingestion of contaminated water supplies
- Sharp mouth parts allow for attachment to intestinal mucosa
- *Ancylostoma* spp. are more likely to cause iron deficiency anemia because they are larger and remove more blood daily from the bowel wall than the other hookworm species, *N. americanus*

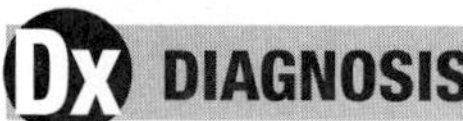

DIAGNOSIS

DIFFERENTIAL DIAGNOSIS

- Strongyloidiasis
- Ascariasis
- Other causes of iron deficiency anemia and malabsorption

WORKUP

Examine stool for hookworm eggs.

LABORATORY TESTS

CBC to show hypochromic, microcytic anemia; possible mild eosinophilia and hypoalbuminemia

IMAGING STUDIES

Chest x-ray examination: occasionally shows opacities

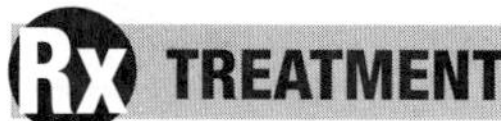

TREATMENT

NONPHARMACOLOGIC THERAPY

Prevention of disease by not walking barefoot and by improving sanitary conditions

ACUTE GENERAL Rx

- Albendazole 400 mg once PO has become preferred treatment.
- Mebendazole 100 mg PO bid for 3 days is also effective.
- Iron supplementation may be helpful in patients with iron deficiency.

DISPOSITION

Easily treated

REFERRAL

If diagnosis uncertain

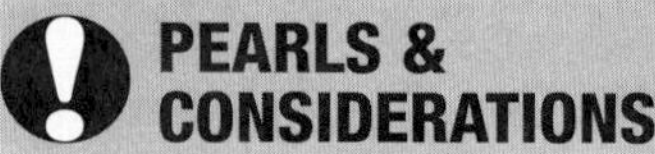

PEARLS & CONSIDERATIONS

COMMENTS

- Appropriate disposal of human wastes is important in controlling the disease in areas with a high prevalence of hookworm infestation.
- Wearing shoes will avoid contact with contaminated soils, and the provision of safe water and sanitation for disposing human excreta is important in control of hookworm.

SUGGESTED READINGS

Brooker S et al: Human hookworm infection in the 21st century, *Adv Parasitol* 58:197, 2004.

Brooker S et al: Epidemiologic, immunologic and practical considerations in developing and evaluating a human hookworm vaccine, *Expert Rev Vaccines* 4(1):35, 2005.

Hotez PJ et al: Hookworm infection, *N Engl J Med* 351(8):799, 2004.

Quinnell RJ et al: The immunoepidemiology of human hookworm infection, *Parasite Immunol* 26(11-12): 443, 2004.

AUTHORS: **STEVEN M. OPAL, M.D.,** and **GLENN G. FORT, M.D., M.P.H.**

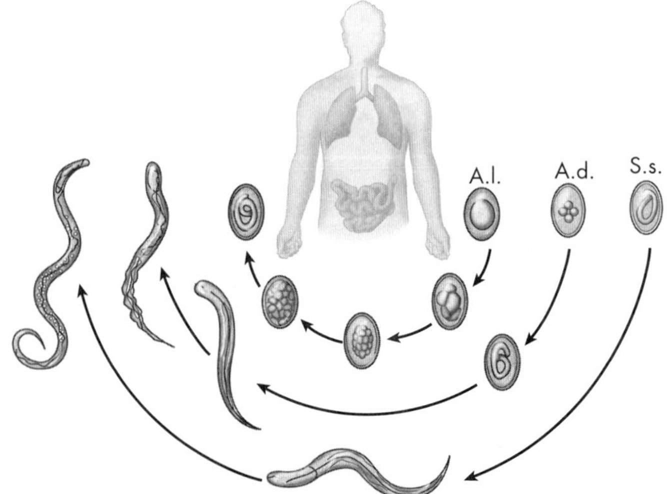

FIGURE 1-156 Life cycle of intestinal nematodes with a migratory phase through the lungs. Eggs are passed with stools in *Ascaris lumbricoides* (A.l.), *Necator americanus,* or *Ancylostoma duodenale* (A.d.), or they hatch on their way out in *Strongyloides stercoralis* (S.s.). Ascaris eggs mature in soil, and humans are infected upon ingestion of these eggs. With hookworm and strongyloidiasis, humans are infected via skin penetration by filariform larvae. In all three infections, larvae pass through a migratory phase via the lungs before reaching maturity at their final habitat in the small intestine. (Mandell GL et al: *Principles and practice of infectious diseases,* ed 7, Philadelphia, 2010, Elsevier.)

BASIC INFORMATION

DEFINITION

A hordeolum is an acute inflammatory process affecting the eyelid and arising from the meibomian (posterior) or Zeis (anterior) glands. It is most often infectious and usually caused by *Staphylococcus aureus.*

SYNONYMS

Stye

ICD-9CM CODES
373.11 External hordeolum
373.12 Internal hordeolum

EPIDEMIOLOGY & DEMOGRAPHICS

INCIDENCE (IN U.S.): Unknown
PREVALENCE (IN U.S.): Unknown
PREDOMINANT SEX: No gender predilection
PREDOMINANT AGE: May occur at any age
NEONATAL INFECTION: Rare in the neonatal period
PEAK INCIDENCE: May occur at any age

PHYSICAL FINDINGS & CLINICAL PRESENTATION

- Abrupt onset with pain and erythema of the eyelid
- Localized, tender mass in the eyelid (Fig. 1-157)
- May be associated with blepharitis
- External hordeolum: points toward the skin surface of the lid and may spontaneously drain
- Internal hordeolum: can point toward the conjunctival side of the lid and may cause conjunctival inflammation

ETIOLOGY

- 75% to 95% of cases are caused by *S. aureus.*
- Occasional cases are caused by *Streptococcus pneumoniae,* other streptococci, gram-negative enteric organisms, or mixed bacterial flora.

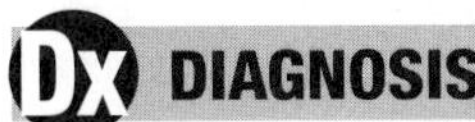

DIAGNOSIS

DIFFERENTIAL DIAGNOSIS

- Eyelid abscess
- Chalazion
- Allergy or contact dermatitis with conjunctival edema
- Acute dacryocystitis
- Herpes simplex infection
- Cellulitis of the eyelid

LABORATORY TESTS

- Generally, none are necessary.
- If incision and drainage are performed, specimens should be sent for bacterial culture.

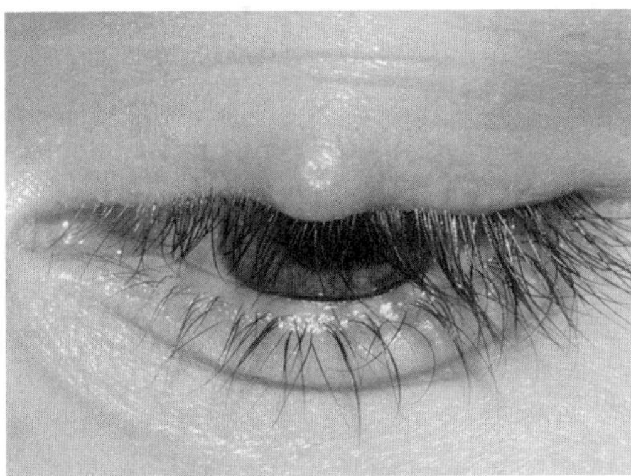

FIGURE 1-157 External stye. (From Palay D [ed]: *Ophthalmology for the primary care physician,* St Louis, 1997, Mosby.)

Rx TREATMENT

NONPHARMACOLOGIC THERAPY

Usually responds to warm compresses

ACUTE GENERAL Rx

- Systemic antibiotics generally not necessary
- In refractory cases, an oral antistaphylococcal agent (e.g., dicloxacillin 500 mg PO qid) possibly helpful
- Topical erythromycin ophthalmic ointment applied to the lid margins two to four times daily until resolution
- Incision and drainage: rarely needed but should be considered for progressive infections

DISPOSITION

- Usually sporadic occurrence
- Possible relapse if resolution is not complete

REFERRAL

- For evaluation by an ophthalmologist if visual acuity or ocular movement is affected or if the diagnosis is in doubt
- For surgical drainage if necessary

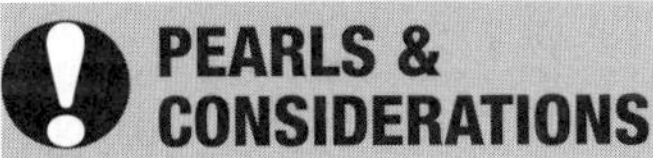

PEARLS & CONSIDERATIONS

COMMENTS

Seborrheic dermatitis may coexist with hordeolum.

SUGGESTED READINGS

Hirunwiwatkul P, Wachirasereechai K: Effectiveness of combined antibiotic ophthalmic solution in the treatment of hordeolum after incision and curettage: a randomized, placebo-controlled trial: a pilot study, *J Med Assoc Thai* 88(5):647, 2005.

Kiratli HK, Akar Y: Multiple recurrent hordeola associated with selective IgM deficiency, *J AAPOS* 5(1):60, 2001.

Miller J: Acinetobacter as a causative agent in preseptal cellulitis, *Optometry* 76(3):176, 2005.

AUTHORS: **GLENN G. FORT, M.D., M.P.H.,** and **DENNIS J. MIKOLICH, M.D.**

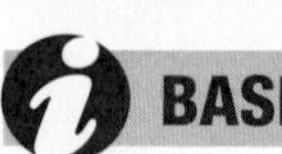

BASIC INFORMATION

DEFINITION

Horner's syndrome is the clinical triad of ipsilateral ptosis, miosis, and sometimes facial anhidrosis. Disruption of any of the three neurons in the oculosympathetic pathway (central, preganglionic, or postganglionic) can cause Horner's syndrome.

SYNONYMS

Oculosympathetic paresis

Raeder's paratrigeminal syndrome: Horner's syndrome of the postganglionic neuron associated with pain in the trigeminal nerve distribution

ICD-9CM CODES

337.9 Horner's syndrome

EPIDEMIOLOGY & DEMOGRAPHICS

Congenital or acquired

PHYSICAL FINDINGS & CLINICAL PRESENTATION

- Ptosis is usually mild. It results from loss of sympathetic tone to Müller's muscle, which contributes approximately 2 mm of upper eyelid elevation. Weakness of the corresponding muscle in the lower eyelid causes it to elevate slightly. This combination causes narrowing of the palpebral fissure. Levator function of the eyelid is preserved.
- Miosis results from loss of sympathetic innervation to the iris dilator muscle (Fig. 1-158). The affected pupil reacts normally to bright light and accommodation. Anisocoria is greater in dim light.
  - Dilation lag: Horner's pupil dilates more slowly than the normal pupil when lights are dimmed (20 versus 5 sec) because it dilates passively as a result of relaxation of the iris sphincter.
- Presence of facial anhidrosis is variable and depends on the site of injury. It occurs with lesions affecting central or preganglionic neurons.
- Congenital Horner's syndrome may result in heterochromia. The affected eye has a lighter colored iris.
- Acute cases may also present with conjunctival injection from the loss of sympathetic vasoconstriction.

ETIOLOGY

Lesions affecting any neuron in the oculosympathetic pathway. Central lesions are least common but are usually caused by pathology in the hypothalamus, brain stem, or cervical spinal cord. Preganglionic lesions are often caused by disease involving the cervicothoracic spinal cord, lung apex, or anterior neck. Postganglionic lesions are usually seen with disease in the internal carotid artery, skull base, cavernous sinus, or orbital apex. Location is often suggested by the presence of associated findings. Vascular disease and neoplasms must be considered.

Mechanical:
- Syringomyelia
- Trauma
- Tumors: benign, malignant (thyroid, Pancoast, mediastinal, metastatic)
- Lymphadenopathy
- Neurofibromatosis
- Cervical rib
- Cervical spondylosis

Vascular (ischemia, hemorrhage or arteriovenous malformation):
- Brain stem lesion: commonly occlusion of the posterior inferior cerebellar artery but other arteries may be responsible (vertebral; superior, middle or inferior lateral medullary arteries; superior or anterior inferior cerebellar arteries)
- Carotid artery aneurysm or dissection. Can also be from injury to other major vessels (internal carotid artery, subclavian artery, ascending aorta)
- Cavernous sinus thrombosis
- Cluster headache, migraine

Miscellaneous:
- Idiopathic
- Congenital
- Demyelination (multiple sclerosis)
- Infection (apical tuberculosis, herpes zoster, Lyme's disease)
- Pneumothorax
- Iatrogenic (angiography, internal jugular/subclavian catheter, chest tube, surgery, epidural spinal anesthesia)
- Radiation

DIAGNOSIS

DIFFERENTIAL DIAGNOSIS

Causes of anisocoria (unequal pupils):
- Normal variant
- Mydriatic use
- Prosthetic eye
- Prior eye surgery
- Unilateral cataract
- Iritis

Causes of ptosis are described in Section II.

WORKUP

History, physical examination, imaging

IMAGING STUDIES

Accompanying signs and symptoms may guide imaging:
- MRI head and neck: evaluate the central and cervical sympathetic pathway
- MR angiography (or ultrasound, CT angiography): assess the vessels in the head and neck
- CT chest and neck: evaluate lung apex, perivertebral areas, mediastinum

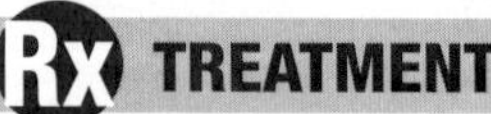

TREATMENT

- Treatment depends on underlying cause.
- Ptosis can be surgically corrected or treated with medication (phenylephrine drops)

DISPOSITION

- Prognosis depends on underlying cause.
- Horner's syndrome is an uncommon presentation for malignancy.
- In one study, 40% of cases were idiopathic.

REFERRAL

- Ophthalmologist to confirm diagnosis and localize lesion.
- Topical cocaine test: confirms sympathetic denervation (drops dilate normal pupil but not Horner's pupil).
- Topical apraclonidine test: confirms diagnosis (drops reverse aniscoria by causing dilatation of Horner's pupil and constriction of normal pupil).
- Topical hydroxyamphetamine test: distinguishes central and preganglionic from postganglionic sympathetic lesions (drops dilate normal pupil and central or preganglionic Horner's pupil, but not postganglionic Horner's pupil).

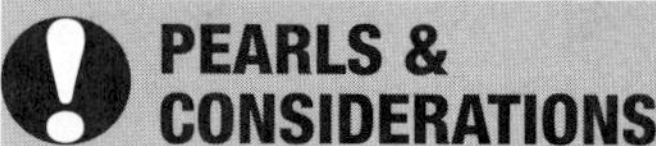

PEARLS & CONSIDERATIONS

- May be the presentation of a life-threatening condition.
- Anisocoria greater in bright light is likely caused by a defect in parasympathetic innervation, and anisocoria greater in dim light is likely caused by a sympathetic defect.
- Normal variant anisocoria:
  - Occurs in 20% of people
  - Usually <1 mm difference between pupils; more apparent in darkness
  - Pupils are round and display a normal, brisk constriction and dilation response to light

SUGGESTED READINGS

Murphy MA et al: Lyme disease associated with postganglionic Horner syndrome and Raeder paratrigeminal neuralgia, *J Neuro-ophthalmol* 27(2):123, 2007.

Walton KA, Buono LM: Horner syndrome, *Curr Opin Ophthalmol* 14(6):357, 2003.

AUTHOR: **SUDEEP KAUR AULAKH, M.D.**

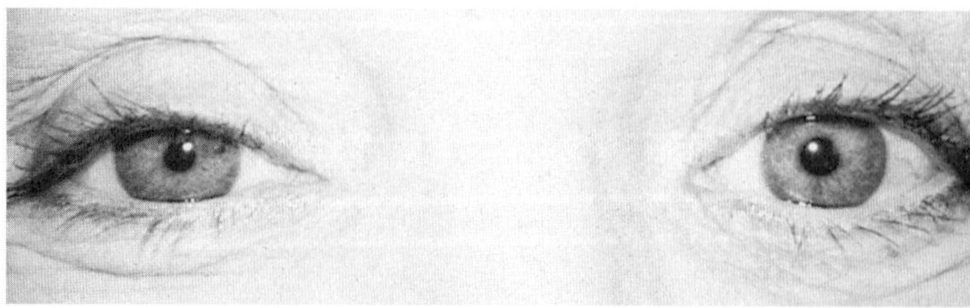

FIGURE 1-158 Horner's syndrome. The mild ptosis (1 to 2 mm) and the smaller pupil (in room light) can be seen on the affected right side. (From Palay D [ed]: *Ophthalmology for the primary care physician,* St Louis, 1997, Mosby.)

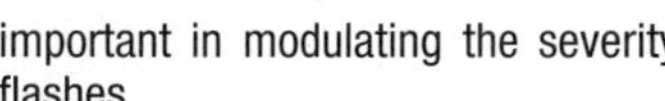

BASIC INFORMATION

DEFINITION

Sudden onset of intense warmth that begins in the neck or face, or in the chest and progresses to the neck and face; often associated with profuse sweating, anxiety, and palpitations.

ICD-9CM CODES
627.2 Hot flashes

EPIDEMIOLOGY & DEMOGRAPHICS

- Hot flashes affect 75% of postmenopausal women.
- Most hot flashes begin 1 to 2 yr before menopause and resolve after 2 yr.
- 15% of women report duration of hot flashes >15 yr.

PHYSICAL FINDINGS & CLINICAL PRESENTATION

- Profuse sweating and red blotching of skin may be noted during the vasomotor event.
- Palpitations and hyperreflexia may be present during the hot flash.
- Hot flashes typically last 1 to 5 min.
- Each hot flash is associated with increase in temperature, increased pulse rate, and increased blood flow into the hands and face.
- Hot flashes during sleep are common and are referred to as *night sweats.*
- There is considerable variation in the frequency of hot flashes. One third of women report more than 10 flashes per day.

ETIOLOGY

- Dysfunction of central thermoregulatory centers caused by changes in estrogen level at the time of menopause
- Tamoxifen use
- Chemotherapy-induced ovarian failure
- Androgen ablation therapy for prostate carcinoma

DIAGNOSIS

DIFFERENTIAL DIAGNOSIS

- Carcinoid syndrome
- Anxiety disorder
- Idiopathic flushing
- Lymphoma (night sweats)
- Hyperthyroidism
- Hyperhidrosis

WORKUP

Evaluation of hot flashes is aimed at excluding the conditions listed in the differential diagnosis.

LABORATORY TESTS

- Follicle-stimulating hormone (FSH), luteinizing hormone, estradiol level. The serum FSH levels rather than estradiol levels are associated with greater severity of hot flashes in older postmenopausal women, suggesting that nonestrogen feedback systems may be important in modulating the severity of hot flashes.
- Thyroid-stimulating hormone.

TREATMENT

NONPHARMACOLOGIC THERAPY

- Behavioral interventions such as relaxation training and paced respiration have been reported effective in reducing symptoms in some women.
- Avoidance of caffeine, alcohol, tobacco, and spicy foods may be beneficial.

GENERAL Rx

- Estrogen replacement therapy reduces hot flashes by 80% to 90%. Estrogen therapy, however, is contraindicated in many women, and others are fearful of its use. Potential risks and side effects should be considered before using estrogen in any patient. When using estrogen, it is best to use low-dose (e.g., Prempro [conjugated equine estrogen 0.45 mg or 0.3 mg plus medroxyprogesterone 1.5 mg]). Femring is an intravaginal ring that is changed every 3 mo and approved to treat vasomotor symptoms in women who have had a hysterectomy. It provides both local and systemic estrogen.
- Megestrol acetate, a progestational agent, is a safer alternative to estrogen in women with a history of breast or uterine cancer and in men receiving androgen ablation therapy for prostate cancer. Usual dose is 20 mg bid.
- The antidepressant venlafaxine has been reported to be 60% effective in reducing hot flashes and represents an alternative treatment modality in women unable or unwilling to use estrogens. Starting dose is 37.5 mg qd, increased as tolerated up to a maximum of 300 mg/day. Other antidepressants such as the selective serotonin reuptake inhibitors fluoxetine and paroxetine are also used by clinicians for hot flashes. However, they appear to be less effective than venlafaxine. A recent trial showed that paroxetine is an effective agent for diminishing hot flashes in men receiving androgen ablation therapy.
- The anticonvulsant gabapentin (300 to 1200 mg/day) represents another nonhormonal alternative in the treatment of hot flashes and can be used alone or in combination with venlafaxine.
- The antihypertensive clonidine is also effective in reducing the frequency of hot flashes. Adverse effects include dry mouth, sedation, and dizziness.
- Vitamin E (800 IU/day) may be effective in patients with mild symptoms that do not interfere with sleep or daily function.
- Soy protein (use of soy extracts that contain plant-derived estrogens [phytoestrogens]) is often used; however, clinical trials have not shown clear efficacy.
- Several classes of herbal remedies are available to patients and are commonly used, generally without significant benefit. Frequently used agents are *Cimicifuga racemosa* (black cohosh, snakeroot, bugbane), *Angelica sinensis,* and evening primrose (evening star). Recent trials using the isopropanolic extract of black cohosh rootstock (Remefemin) did show some improvement in controlling menopausal symptoms.

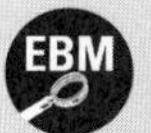

EVIDENCE

Please note: Complete text of EBM for this topic is available online.

Key trials and commentary:

This study sought to determine the immediate and long-term effects of true acupuncture vs. sham acupuncture on hot flash frequency in women with breast cancer.

This study showed that hot flash frequency in breast cancer patients was reduced following acupuncture. However, when compared with sham acupuncture, the reduction by the acupuncture regimen as provided in the current study did not reach statistical significance. We cannot exclude the possibility that a longer and more intense acupuncture intervention could produce a larger reduction of these symptoms.

Hot flashes are common among women receiving treatment for breast cancer. For some patients, symptoms significantly interfere with quality of life and may even be more frequent and severe than those experienced by women during menopause. Because current treatment options for hot flashes in patients with breast cancer are limited, evaluation of complementary therapies, such as acupuncture, is extremely important. To date, few controlled studies have investigated the use of acupuncture to treat hot flashes in patients with breast cancer, and studies in other populations have shown mixed results.[1] Ⓐ

In this randomized, blinded trial, the mean number of hot flashes per day was reduced from 8.7 (SD 3.9) to 6.2 (SD 4.2) in the true acupuncture treatment group and from 10.0 (SD 6.1) to 7.6 (SD 5.7) in the sham group. The differences were not significant (P = 0.3); however, when the sham group was crossed over to true acupuncture at week 7, an additional 20% reduction in the frequency of hot flashes was seen by week 12, and treatment improvements were maintained for up to 6 months after treatment was discontinued. Hot flash frequency was reduced by about 20% in the two groups during the first 2 weeks of treatment. After that, the reduction in frequency in the sham group remained the same, whereas in the true acupuncture treatment group, the frequency decreased by another 10%.

The authors' conclusion that a longer and more intense acupuncture intervention might be necessary to treat hot flashes in this population is consistent with the slow and gentle nature of traditional Chinese medicine. Practitioners of traditional Chinese medicine often recommend multiple courses (1 course equals 8-10 treatments) of acupuncture to effectively treat long-term conditions. The authors also discussed the inherent difficulties in designing an inactive sham treatment in acupuncture trials and the fact that these difficulties could partially explain their findings.

This study by Deng and colleagues is an important step toward evaluating the use of acupuncture to treat hot flashes in patients with breast cancer and substantiates the need for further research.

Hot flashes are a significant problem in women going through the menopausal transition that can substantially affect quality of life. The world of estrogen therapy has been thrown into turmoil with the recent results of the Women's Health Initiative trial report. Pursuant to a growing interest in the use of alternative therapies to alleviate menopausal symptoms and a few pilot trials that suggested that acupuncture could modestly alleviate hot flashes, a prospective, randomized, single-blind, sham-controlled clinical trial was conducted in women experiencing hot flashes.

The results of this study suggest that the used medical acupuncture was not any more effective for reducing hot flashes than was the chosen sham acupuncture.[2] Ⓐ

All that most of us ask is that nonconventional medical approaches undergo the same rigorous clinical assessment as conventional pharmaceuticals, surgical procedures, and devices. It's easy to be a public figure, receive enormous amounts of money from unregulated businesses, expound on the benefits of a particular "natural" or "Eastern medicine" drug or process while chatting with two or three people that have had incredible improvement of their problems. However, this is *not* a clinical trial, or anything that approaches one! In this article by Vincent and colleagues, a rigorous randomized trial comparing acupuncture with a sham trial was undertaken and found no difference in hot flash activities between the two cohorts. I do not revel in such findings—I do believe that medical advances can and should be found outside of conventional research sources. Moreover, when they are being considered for marketing, I want them to undergo the same testing that all of our drugs and devices must undergo before approval. In this way, our patients will be the beneficiaries of a development and scientific process that brings the best products to market and leads to optimal outcomes.

Prior progestin studies treating hot flashes in women have been short duration and single dose. This study tests the progestin megesterol acetate (MA) at two doses vs. placebo over 6 months.

This study showed that MA significantly reduced vasomotor symptoms with durable benefit over 6 months. MA 20 mg/day is the preferred dose. There was no significant impact on other menopausal symptoms.[3] Ⓐ

The vasomotor symptoms of estrogen withdrawal constitute a significant problem for women with previous breast cancers. Previous data from a phase III placebo-controlled trial have shown that venlafaxine can be useful in the prevention of these manifestations. The Southwest Oncology Group trial looks at another commonly used approach to the problem of hot flashes, the use of MA. Progestins were able to significantly reduce the incidence of hot flashes, and the higher dose of 20 mg/day appeared to have an advantage. For women with a substantial problem with hot flashes, the use of MA is a reasonable option.

Hot flashes are experienced by about 52% of perimenopausal women. After breast cancer, this may increase to 70%. The use of hormone replacement therapy is not recommended in women who have had breast cancer; therefore, alternatives are required to help relieve hot flashes. This study was conducted to assess the efficacy of relaxation training in reducing the incidence of hot flashes in women with primary breast cancer. This was a randomized controlled trial of 150 women with primary breast cancer who experienced hot flashes. The intervention group received a single relaxation training session and was instructed to use practice tapes on a daily basis at home for 1 month; the control group received no intervention. Outcomes were incidence and severity of flashes using a diary and validated measures of anxiety and quality of life. The incidence and severity of hot flashes, as recorded by diaries, each significantly declined over 1 month ($P < 0.001$ and $P = 0.01$, respectively), compared with the control group. Distress caused by flashes also significantly declined in the treatment group over 1 month ($P = 0.01$), compared with the control group. There were no significant differences between the treatment group and the control group at 3 months and no changes in anxiety or quality-of-life measures. Relaxation may be a useful component of a program of measures to relieve hot flashes in women with primary breast cancer.

This small but well-designed trial examines the usefulness of programmed relaxation in relieving hot flushes in perimenopausal and fully menopausal women. Previous small trials have shown some efficacy with this type of intervention. These investigators demonstrated a modest reduction in frequency and intensity of hot flush after 1 month, but it was not sustained. Study subjects did not have a statistically significant decrease in hot flushes at the 3-month interval. Reasons for such a minimal response may have to do with the brevity of the relaxation techniques. The 20-minute relaxation session was self-performed by the study patients only once per day. Perhaps more frequent interventions would have had a different outcome. Additionally, this group of women may not be representative of others that could potentially have a different response. All participants had a history of breast cancer, and over half were on tamoxifen. The researchers should be congratulated for focusing on this notoriously challenging problem in this subset of female patients. A motivated woman may want to attempt this kind of intervention for temporary relief, but should do so only with realistic expectations.[4] Ⓐ

Evidence-Based References

1. Deng G et al: Randomized, controlled trial of acupuncture for the treatment of hot flashes in breast cancer patients, *J Clin Oncol* 25:5584-5590, 2007. Commentary by M.K. Garcia, R.N., L.A.c, M.S.N., Ph.D. Ⓐ
2. Vincent A et al: Acupuncture for hot flashes: a randomized, sham-controlled clinical study, *Menopause* 14:45-52, 2007. Commentary by L.P. Shulman, M.D. Ⓐ
3. Goodwin JW et al: Phase III randomized placebo-controlled trial of two doses of megestrol acetate as treatment for menopausal symptoms in women with breast cancer: Southwest Oncology Group Study 9626, *J Clin Oncol* 26:1650-1656, 2008. Commentary by J.T. Thigpen, M.D. Ⓐ
4. Fenlon DR et al: A randomized controlled trial of relaxation training to reduce hot flashes in women with primary breast cancer, *J Clin Oncol* 35:397-405, 2008. Commentary by J.S. Dungan, M.D. Ⓐ

SUGGESTED READINGS

Huang AJ et al: Persistent hot flushes in older postmenopausal women, *Arch Intern Med* 168(8):840-846, 2008.

Loprinzi CL et al: Pilot evaluation of gabapentin for treating hot flashes, *Mayo Clin Proc* 77:1159, 2002.

Loprinzi Cl et al: Pilot evaluation of paroxetine for treating hot flashes in men, *Mayo Clin Proc* 79(10): 1247, 2004.

Nelson HD et al: Nonhormonal therapies for menopausal hot flashes, *JAMA* 295:2057, 2006.

Osmers R et al: Efficacy and safety of isopropanolic black cohosh extract for climacteric symptoms, *Obstet Gynecol* 105:1074, 2005.

Shanafelt TD et al: Pathophysiology and treatment of hot flashes, *Mayo Clin Proc* 77:1207, 2002.

Sikon A, Thacker HL: Treatment options for menopausal hot flashes, *Cleveland Clinic J Med* 71:578, 2004.

Women's Health Initiative Investigators: Risks and benefits of estrogen plus progestin in healthy postmenopausal women: principal results from the Women's Health initiative randomized controlled trial, *JAMA* 288:321, 2002.

AUTHOR: **FRED F. FERRI, M.D.**

BASIC INFORMATION

DEFINITION

Human granulocytic ehrlichiosis (HGE) is a zoonotic infection of granulocytes, caused by *Anaplasma phagocytophilum,* an *Ehrlichia* species closely related to *Ehrlichia chaffeensis* and *E. ewingii,* with multisystem manifestations.

SYNONYMS

Ehrlichiosis
Ehrlichia phagocytophila
Anaplasma phagocytophilum

ICD-9CM CODES

082-8 Other tick-borne rickettsiosis

EPIDEMIOLOGY & DEMOGRAPHICS

INCIDENCE (IN U.S.): Highest overall incidence in Rhode Island, New York, New Jersey, Connecticut, Wisconsin, Minnesota, and northern California; >3000 cases identified in the U.S. since 2006.

PREDOMINANT SEX: Males outnumber females by 2 to 1.

PREDOMINANT AGE: Most severe disease 50 to 70 yr

PEAK INCIDENCE: Occurs throughout the year, with peak incidence between May and July and again in November.

PHYSICAL FINDINGS & CLINICAL PRESENTATION

- Most common initial symptoms
    1. Fever
    2. Chills, rigor
    3. Headache
    4. Myalgia
- Subsequent symptoms
    1. Anorexia, nausea
    2. Arthralgia
    3. Cough
    4. Confusion
    5. Abdominal pain
    6. Rash (erythematous to pustular) rare (<11%)
- Complications
    1. Hepatitis
    2. Interstitial pneumonitis; acute respiratory distress syndrome
    3. Renal and respiratory failure
    4. Demyelinating polyneuropathy
    5. Toxic shock–like syndrome
    6. Life-threatening opportunistic infections

ETIOLOGY

- Obligate intracellular gram-negative bacterium (family Rickettsiaceae, genus *Ehrlichia*), now renamed *Anaplasma phagocytophilum*
- Vector
    1. Almost certainly tick-borne, recently confirmed to be rarely transmitted by infected blood (including nosocomial infection).
    2. Transmitted by *Ixodes scapularis* in the northeastern and upper midwestern states and *Ixodes pacificus* in the Pacific western states.
    3. Tick exposure reported in >90% of patients, with approximately 60% reporting tick bite.
- Mammalian host: deer, horses, dogs, white-footed mice, cattle, sheep, goats, bison
- Host inflammatory and immune responses define final spectrum of disease beyond granulocytes, including hepatitis, interstitial pneumonitis, and nephritis with mild azotemia
- Between 6% and 21% of patients with HGE also have serologic evidence of other *Ixodes* spp. tick-borne diseases: Lyme disease or babesiosis
- Recovery is usual outcome; fatality rate of HGE is <1%
- ICU care required: 7%

DIAGNOSIS

DIFFERENTIAL DIAGNOSIS

- Human monocytic ehrlichiosis (HME)
    1. Caused by *E. chaffeensis* (vector: tick *Amblyomma americanum*)
    2. Rash more common, sometimes petechial
    3. Morulae in monocytes
- Rocky Mountain spotted fever, Colorado tick fever, Q fever, relapsing fever
- Babesiosis
- Leptospirosis
- Lyme disease
- Tularemia
- Typhoid fever, paratyphoid fever
- Brucellosis
- Viral hepatitis
- Meningococcemia
- Infectious mononucleosis
- Hematologic malignancy

WORKUP

- Acute blood samples for Giemsa-stained smears
- CBC, liver function, BUN/Cr
- Acute serum samples for serology
- Chest radiograph examination
- Bone marrow rarely needed

LABORATORY TESTS

- Giemsa-stained smear demonstrating morulae of the organism within granulocytes (sensitivity 20%-75%)
- CBC progressive leukopenia and thrombocytopenia with nadir near day 7
- C reactive protein concentration is generally elevated
- Liver function tests (LFTs): increase in hepatic transaminases, lactate dehydrogenase, and alkaline phosphatase
- Elevated plasma creatinine concentration may be seen
- Serologic titer (IFA) >80 or fourfold increase in titer to *E. equi* antigen
- Polymerase chain reaction (PCR) to facilitate early diagnosis
- Culture on the first 7 days of illness; not readily available in most clinical laboratories

IMAGING STUDIES

- Chest radiograph examination to show interstitial pneumonitis (unusual)
- MRI of the brain

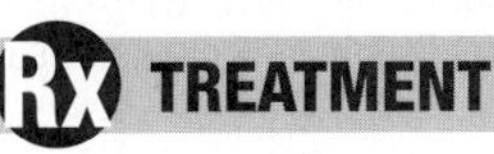

TREATMENT

ACUTE GENERAL Rx

- Immediate therapy to limit extent of acute illness and complication
- Doxycycline: 100 mg twice a day for 10 days is therapy of choice for adults and children >8 years (4 mg/kg/day in 2 divided doses)
- Rifampin: 300 mg twice a day for 7 to 10 days can be used in pregnancy and for children <8 years at 10 mg/kg twice per day
- Most patients defervesce within 24 to 48 hr given appropriate treatment

PROGNOSIS

Poor prognostic indicators include:

- Advanced age
- Concomitant chronic illness (such as diabetes mellitus, collagen-vascular disease)
- Lack of diagnosis recognition
- Delayed onset of specific antibiotic therapy

DISPOSITION

Repeat CBC every 2 to 4 wk until normal

REFERRAL

For consultation with infectious diseases specialist and hematologist in suspected cases

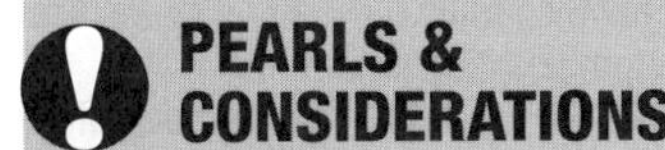

PEARLS & CONSIDERATIONS

COMMENTS

Duration of time tick must be attached to produce illness as few as 4 hr.

SUGGESTED READINGS

Dumier JS et al: Ehrlichioses in humans: epidemiology, clinical presentation, diagnosis, and treatment, *Clin Infect Dis* 45(Suppl 1):S45, 2007.

Moss WJ, Dumler JS: Simultaneous infection with Borrelia burgdorferi and human granulocytic ehrlichiosis, *Pediatr Infect Dis J* 22(1):91, 2003.

Singh-Behl D et al: Tick-borne infections, *Dermatol Clin* 21(2):237, 2003.

Walls JJ et al: Improved sensitivity of PCR for diagnosis of human granulocytic ehrlichiosis using epank1 genes of Ehrlichia phagocytophilia-group ehrlichiae, *J Clin Microbiol* 38:354, 2000.

Wormser GP et al: The clinical assessment, treatment, and prevention of Lyme disease, human granulocytic anaplasmosis, and babesiosis: clinical practice guidelines by the Infectious Diseases Society of America, *Clin Infect Dis* 43:1089, 2006.

AUTHORS: **PATRICIA CRISTOFARO, M.D., GLENN G. FORT, M.D., M.P.H.,** and **DENNIS J. MIKOLICH, M.D.**

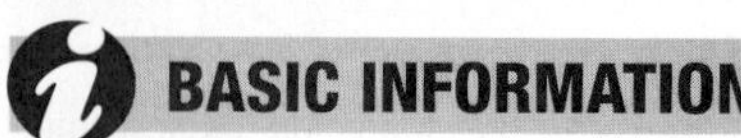

BASIC INFORMATION

DEFINITION

The human immunodeficiency virus, type 1 (HIV) causes a chronic infection that culminates, usually after 5-10 years, in AIDS.

SYNONYMS

AIDS: when a patient with HIV infection meets specific diagnostic criteria (See "Acquired Immunodeficiency Syndrome" in Section I.)

ICD-9CM CODES

044.9 HIV, unspecified

EPIDEMIOLOGY & DEMOGRAPHICS

INCIDENCE (IN U.S.):

- In 2006, there were an estimated 56,300 new HIV infections
- Greatest incidence is in metropolitan areas with population >500,000.

PREVALENCE (IN U.S.): Estimated at 1 to 2 million cases at the end of 2003.

PREDOMINANT SEX:

- Adults: Males accounted for 73% of new infections in 2006.
- Children: male = female

RACIAL DATA:

- In 2006, the rate of HIV diagnosis for black males was 8 times the rate for whites.
- Black females are disproportionately affected by HIV: the rate of HIV diagnosis for black females is 19 times the rate for white females
- The rate for Hispanic women is 5 times that for white females

PEAK INCIDENCE: More than half of new infections in 2006 were in patients ages 25 to 44.

GENETICS:

Familial Disposition:

Although there is no proven genetic predisposition, individuals with deletions in the CCR5 gene are immune from infection with macrophage tropic virus (the predominant virus in sexual transmission).

Congenital Infection:

- 80% of childhood cases are caused by peripartum infection, which may occur in utero, during delivery, or after delivery via breast-feeding.
- No specific congenital abnormalities are associated with HIV infection, although risk of spontaneous abortion and low birth weight is greater.

Neonatal Infection:

- May occur during delivery or via breast-feeding
- Typically asymptomatic

PHYSICAL FINDINGS & CLINICAL PRESENTATION

- Signs and symptoms are variable with stage of disease.
- In acute infection:
  1. May cause a self-limited mononucleosis-like illness characterized by fever, sore throat, lymphadenopathy, headache, and a rash resembling roseola
  2. In a minority of acute cases: frank aseptic meningitis, Bell's palsy, or peripheral neuropathy
  3. Rarely, opportunistic infections such as thrush or *Pneumocystis jiroveci* pneumonia (PJP) may occur.
- Later in the course of infection, after a prolonged asymptomatic phase: nonspecific symptoms of lymphadenopathy, weight loss, diarrhea, and skin changes including seborrheic dermatitis, localized herpes zoster, or fungal infection.
- Advanced disease: characterized by the infections and malignancies associated with AIDS (see specific disorders).
- Some studies suggest that HIV infection in women is associated with lower levels of viral load at comparable degrees of immunosuppression when compared with men. Furthermore, women may, on average, have higher CD4 lymphocyte counts at the time of AIDS diagnosis.
- Another special consideration in women infected with HIV is the high incidence of human papillomavirus (HPV) coinfection and the risk for cervical neoplasm that this presents. Even women with normal Pap smears should have this test repeated after 6 mo and annually thereafter.
- Coinfection with HIV and hepatitis C is common because of common transmission risk. Patients with HIV and hepatitis C progress faster to cirrhosis. Patients may already have signs of advanced liver disease at the time of diagnosis.

ETIOLOGY

- RNA retrovirus (Fig. 1-159) HIV-1 was probably derived from transmission of a simian immunodeficiency virus (SIV) from chimpanzees in Central Africa; a related virus HIV-2 was derived from an SIV found in sooty mangabey monkeys from West Africa.
- HIV-1 is the predominant pathogenic retrovirus in human populations; HIV-2 has limited distribution (primarily in West Africa) and tends to be less rapidly immunosuppressive than HIV-1.
- Transmitted by sexual contact, shared needles, blood transfusion, or from mother to child during pregnancy, delivery, or breast-feeding.
- Primary target of infection: CD4 lymphocyte.
- Direct CNS involvement: manifested as encephalopathy, myelopathy, or neuropathy in advanced cases.
- Renal failure, rheumatologic disorders, thrombocytopenia, or cardiac abnormalities may be seen in association with HIV.

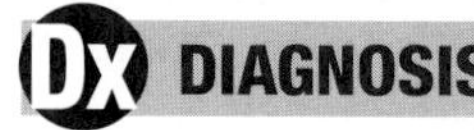

DIAGNOSIS

DIFFERENTIAL DIAGNOSIS

- Acute infection: mononucleosis or other respiratory viral infections
- Late symptoms: similar to those produced by other wasting illnesses such as neoplasms, TB, disseminated fungal infection, malabsorption, or depression
- HIV-related encephalopathy: confused with Alzheimer's disease or other causes of chronic dementia (cognitive impairment in HIV infection is described in Section II); myelopathy and neuropathy possibly resembling other demyelinating diseases such as multiple sclerosis

WORKUP

Since the debut of HIV/AIDS in the 1980s, diagnosis has been established by voluntary testing for antibody to the virus. The CDC is now recommending routine testing for patients in all health care settings unless the patient declines (opt-out screening). This includes routine testing of pregnant women. It is also recommended that separate written consent should no longer be

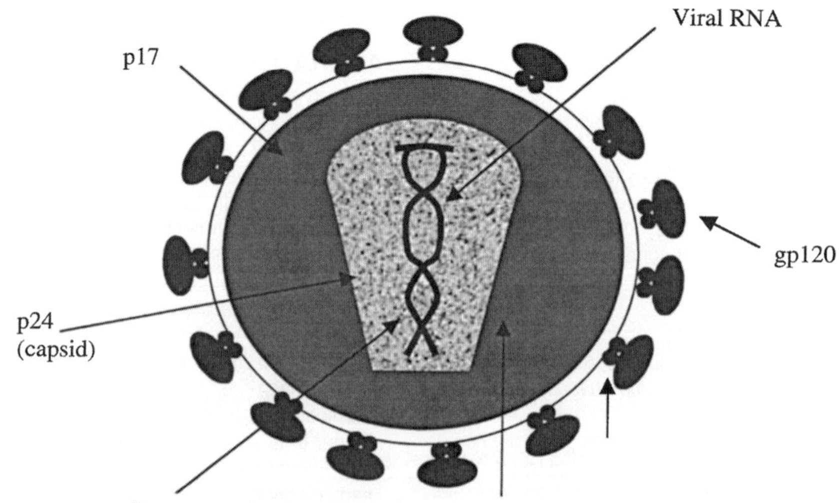

FIGURE 1-159 Locations of viral proteins and nucleic acids in the HIV-1 virion. (From Mandell GL [ed]: *Mandell, Douglas, and Bennett's principles and practice of infectious diseases,* ed 6, New York, 2005, Churchill Livingstone.)

required, although by law this is being addressed on a state-by-state basis.

LABORATORY TESTS

HIV antibody detected by a two-step technique:

- ELISA as a sensitive screening test.
- Confirmation of positive ELISA tests with the more specific Western blot technique.
- The CD4 count and HIV RNA polymerase chain reaction (PCR) should be measured in all patients.
- The CD4 count is a marker of current immune status.

The HIV RNA PCR (viral load) is predictive of disease progression.

- Rapid serologic tests have been increasingly used and are useful in specific settings: occupational exposures, pregnant women in labor without previous testing, and patients in high seroprevalence areas (for immediate results). Specimens are either blood or saliva and results are given within 20 min. Although sensitivity is high (99.1% to 99.7%), false-positive tests are more common in low seroprevalence populations. Thus, all positive results must be confirmed with standard serology, including western blot.

Fig. 1-160 describes the immunologic response to HIV infection.

Rx TREATMENT

NONPHARMACOLOGIC THERAPY

Maintenance of adequate nutrition

ACUTE GENERAL Rx

- Acute management of opportunistic infections and malignancies (see AIDS-associated disorders, "*Pneumocystis carinii* (now *P. jirovecii*) Pneumonia," "Cryptococcosis," "Tuberculosis," "Toxoplasmosis" elsewhere in this text.)

Acute HIV syndrome:

- No definitive evidence supports routine initiation of antiretroviral therapy in primary HIV infection.

CHRONIC Rx

Naïve, chronically infected patients should be considered for therapy based on their current CD4 counts, likelihood for disease progression (viral loads), and ability to remain adherent with combination antiretroviral therapy. Please see current HIV treatment guidelines of the Department of Health and Human Services (www.aidsinfo.nih.gov/guidelines).

1. Therapy is recommended for all patients with symptomatic established HIV disease. Symptomatic HIV disease is defined as the presence of any of the following: thrush, vaginal candidiasis, herpes zoster, peripheral neuropathy, bacillary angiomatosis, cervical dysplasia in situ, constitutional symptoms such as fever or diarrhea for more than 1 mo, ITP, PID, or listeriosis.
2. In asymptomatic individuals, therapy should be initiated before the CD4 count declines below 350 cells/mm^3.
3. For all patients with CD4 count >350, there is insufficient evidence showing clear benefit. Decisions to start treatment above this threshold should be based on several factors: presence of comorbidities or risk factors for cardiovascular and other non-AIDS diseases that favor earlier therapy, rapid decline in CD4 count (>100/yr), or HIV-1 RNA level of >100,000.
4. Antiretroviral therapy using combinations of nucleoside/nucleotide reverse transcriptase inhibitor (NRTI) agents: zidovudine (AZT), lamivudine (3TC), emtricitabine (FTC), tenofovir, abacavir, stavudine (D4T), or didanosine (DDI); in addition to boosted (with ritonavir) protease inhibitors (PI) such as lopinavir/ritonavir, atazanavir, fosamprenavir, darunavir, saquinavir, indinavir, or nonnucleoside reverse transcriptase inhibitors (NNRTI), such as nevirapine or efavirenz. The PI ritonavir is often used, in low dose, in combination with other PIs to obtain more sustained drug levels. Adding a fourth drug to the three-drug regimen does not improve viral suppression or outcome and is not recommended. Treatment interruptions based upon CD4 responses appear harmful in recent comparative studies versus standard continuous treatment protocols and should be avoided.
5. Usual initial dosing regimen consists of two nucleoside/nucleotide reverse transcriptase inhibitors (nRTIs) and a nonnucleoside reverse transcriptase inhibitor (NNRTI) or a PI. Data support inclusion of lamivudine or emtricitabine as 1 of the 2 nRTIs.

Standard nRTIs include:

- Truvada (tenofovir/emtricitabine) 1 tablet once daily.
    - Tenofovir: individuals with underlying renal dysfunction or requiring other nephrotoxic agents may be at increased risk of renal toxicity.
    - Epzicom (abacavir/lamivudine) 1 tablet once daily
- Abacavir: association with increased risk of myocardial infarction. Use with caution in patients with cardiovascular risk.
    - Combivir (Zidovudine/lamivudine) 1 tablet twice daily
    - Zidovudine: associated with lipoatrophy and anemia. GI and CNS side effects.

Standard Backbone Regimens include:

- NNRTI
    - Efavirenz 600mg daily: not recommended for women in the first trimester or those who are contemplating pregnancy
    - Nevirapine 200 mg two times a day: avoid with CD4 count >250 in men and >350 in women because of the risk of hepatitis
- PIs (ritonavir boosted)
    - Lopinavir/ritonavir (200 mg/50 mg) 2 tablets twice a day (or 4 tablets once a day): most likely to cause diarrhea and has the greatest negative effect on triglyceride levels.
    - Atazanavir and ritonavir (300 mg and 100 mg) 2 tablets a day: lower pill burden, but use with caution with acid reducing agents—can alter absorption.
    - Fosamprenavir and ritonavir (700 mg and 100 mg) 2 tablets twice a day (or 4 tablets once a day): cannot take fosamprenavir with sulfa allergy
    - Saquinavir and ritonavir
    - Darunavir and ritonavir: Used more in treatment of experienced patients with multidrug-resistant virus
- All these drugs have their own unique, as well as class-specific, side effects and require careful follow-up to achieve optimal antiviral effects. Compliance with the drug regimen and tolerance of common side effects are critically important to maintain drug efficacy. Antiviral response should be monitored by baseline HIV viral load and CD4 count and repeat measurement at 2 and 4 wk into treatment and then periodically (every 3 mo) to ensure viral suppression.
- All patients should have genotypic resistance testing on entry into medical care.
- Later, an antiretroviral regimen should be constructed based on past antiretroviral experience and the results of genotypic or phenotypic testing.
- Patients with CD4 lymphocyte count <200/mm^3 should be given preventive ther-

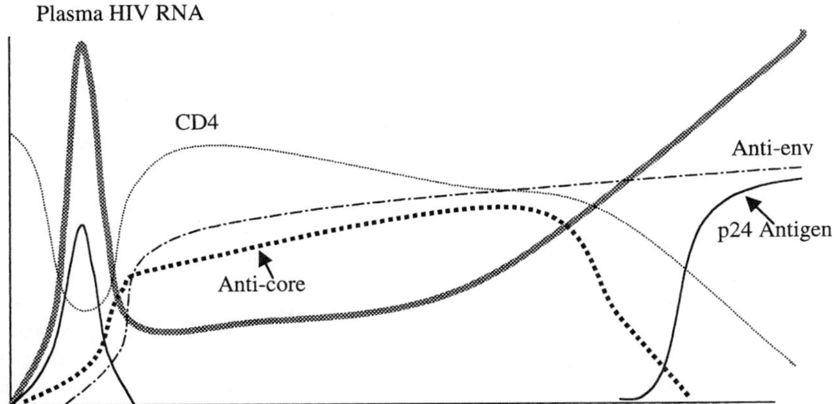

FIGURE 1-160 Course of human immunodeficiency virus infection. (From Mandell GL [ed]: *Mandell, Douglas, and Bennett's principles and practice of infectious diseases*, ed 6, New York, 2005, Churchill Livingstone.)

apy for *Pneumocystis jirovecii* pneumonia (PJP) (see "*Pneumocystis jirovecii [P. carinii]* Pneumonia").

- Evaluation of chronic diarrhea in patients with HIV is described in Section III, "HIV-Infected Patient, Acutely Ill."
- Criteria for discontinuing and restarting opportunistic prophylaxis for adults with HIV infection is described in Section I, "Acquired Immunodeficiency Syndrome."
- HIV infection in a pregnant woman poses special challenges and considerations. Appropriate and timely antiretroviral therapy given to mother and newborn has been shown to dramatically reduce the risk of perinatal transmission of HIV. The goal of therapy is to achieve an undetectable viral load. For HIV-infected pregnant women who are already receiving ART: (1) Continue therapy if suppressing viral replication, but avoid use of efavirenz in the first trimester (substitution is recommended in the first trimester); (2) If viremia on therapy, genotypic testing is recommended; (3) Nevirapine should be continued, regardless of CD4 count, if there is viral suppression. For HIV-infected pregnant women who have never received ART: (1) Women who require ART for their own health should start on ART in the first trimester. Most antiretrovirals are safe in pregnancy, however, Sustiva should be avoided because of tetrogenicity (Class D), DDI and D4T should be avoided (potential of lactic acidosis), and some protease inhibitors may be dose-altered in pregnancy. Nevirapine should not be initiated in an antiretroviral naive pregnant patient with CD4 counts $>$250 because of the risk of hepatotoxicity. (2) Women who do not need ART for their own health should also initiate three-drug therapy, but may do so at the end of the first trimester. (3) Zidovudine (AZT) is recommended as a component of antiretroviral therapy.
- Therapy should continue through the baby's birth. Zidovudine is given intravenously at the time of labor, regardless of whether it is an existing component of her three-drug regimen. In women with viral loads persistently $>$1000 copies/ml despite appropriate ARV, cesarean section may further lower risk of transmission. Zidovudine (AZT) should also be given to the newborn for the first 6 wk of life, and mothers should completely avoid nursing.

DISPOSITION

- Ongoing care consisting of frequent medical evaluations and T-lymphocyte subset analysis along with the plasma HIV load
- Long-term care focused on providing up-to-date antiretroviral therapy and prophylaxis of PJP and other opportunistic infections, as well as early detection of complications (see Section III.)
- Ongoing assessment for cardiovascular risk
- Screening and treatment for Hepatitis B and C
- Yearly screening for STIs (*Chlamydia,* gonorrhea, syphilis)
- Consideration of AIDS (lymphomas, HPV) and non-AIDS related (screening for general population, age specific cancers)

REFERRAL

To a physician knowledgeable and experienced in the management of HIV infection and its complications

PEARLS & CONSIDERATIONS

COMMENTS

- HIV chemoprophylaxis after occupational exposure is described in Section V.
- A recent analysis of the impact of the highly active anti-retroviral therapy (HAART) era indicates that antiretroviral therapy has saved at least 3 million years of life since the introduction of HAART into medicine more than 10 yr ago.
- In persons with HIV infection, screening for TB needs to include questions about combination of symptoms rather than only inquiring about chronic cough.

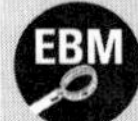

EVIDENCE

Please note: Complete text of EBM for this topic is available online.

Key trials and commentary:

The benefits of continuing antiretroviral therapy are questionable in human immunodeficiency virus (HIV) type 1–infected patients with profound immunodeficiency and multiple treatment failure due to viral resistance.

This study showed that even when effective virological control is no longer achievable, cART still reduces the risk of ADEs in profoundly immunodeficient HIV-infected patients.

The goal of combination antiretroviral therapy (cART) in HIV disease is to improve immune status by suppressing viral replication. Incomplete virologic response is associated with antiretroviral-resistant mutations. Regimens containing five or six drugs or "gigatherapy" are recommended for patients with multiple treatment failures and a highly resistant HIV quasi-species. Gigatherapy has been partially effective. The intervention of treatment interruption to allow wild-type (susceptible to ART) virus to become predominant has not been found to be beneficial in most studies. Immunological, rather than virological factors, may determine progression, particularly in patients with very advanced HIV disease. This study has evaluated the option of continued ART in the most immunosuppressed patients with HIV disease. Compared with patients with virological failure who interrupted cART at least once, profoundly immunodeficient HIV-infected patients, who continued cART, experienced reduced risk of acquired immuno-deficiency syndrome-defining events (ADEs). Continued treatment with cART, even with effective virological control, is no longer achievable; however, it may still be beneficial, unless the drug-related adverse events become unmanageable.[1] Ⓐ

Two recent analyses found that exposure to protease inhibitors (PIs) in the context of antiretroviral (ARV) therapy increased the risk for distal sensory polyneuropathy (DSPN) in subjects with HIV infection. These findings were supported by an in vitro model in which PI exposure produced neurite retraction and process loss in dorsal root ganglion sensory neurons. Confirmation of peripheral nerve toxicity with PIs could substantially limit their long-term use in highly active ARV therapy.

This study showed that evaluation of concomitant risks for HIV DSPN suggests that the independent risk attributable to PIs, if any, is small. This risk must be weighed against the important role of PIs in modern ARV therapy regimens.

HIV disease is currently not curable but it has become manageable with effective ARV therapy. As more people with HIV infection live longer, certain HIV- and ARV-therapy–associated complications have shown a cumulative increase in prevalence in recent years. DSPN tops the list among such neurological complications. DSPN can occur from HIV infection per se or from ARV therapy, mostly from d-drugs. Earlier in vitro studies also indicated peripheral nerve damage from PIs. Our experience in large neuro-HIV clinics does not suggest PIs as a significant cause of DSPN. The findings of this large study involving over 1000 PI-experienced HIV-seropositive patients are reassuring. In univariant and multivariant analyses, the authors document that HIV-seropositive patients with DSPN generally have etiologies other than exposure to PIs to explain the cause of neuropathy. The findings, however, do not obviate the urgent need of effective therapy for HIV- and ARV-therapy–associated common and often disabling neuropathies.[2] Ⓐ

The standard therapy for HIV-associated cryptococcal meningitis of amphotericin B (AmB; 0.7 mg/kg per day) plus flucytosine frequently takes $>$2 weeks to sterilize the cerebral spinal fluid, and acute mortality remains high. A dosage range for AmB of 0.7 to 1 mg/kg per day is noted in current guidelines, but there are no data comparing 0.7 mg/kg per day with 1 mg/kg per day.

AmB, 1 mg/kg per day, plus flucytosine is more rapidly fungicidal than is standard-dose AmB plus flucytosine. Because of its size, this study provides limited data on any difference in toxicity between the regimens, but toxicities were manageable and reversible.

AmB has remained the cornerstone of antifungal therapy for cryptococcal meningitis (CM). AmB is known to have concentration-dependent fungicidal activity.[1] However, the potential of nephrotoxicity and other adverse events led to the use of lower doses of AmB (0.3-0.4 mg/kg/day) in combination with flucytosine in CM. Clinical trials involving cryptococcus in HIV-infected patients have used progressively increasing doses of AmB since the 1980s. Recent trials using 0.7 mg/kg per day of AmB yielded better results than the previously used lower dosages.[2] The current study demonstrated that AmB 1 mg/kg per day plus flucytosine is more rapidly fungicidal than the current standard dose of 0.7 mg/kg per day. This more rapid clearance of infection may reduce the proportion of patients with CM who die before 10 weeks. This incidence of renal toxicity did not differ between the two groups, and the toxicity was manageable in both groups. The data favored the use of AmB at a dosage of 1 mg/kg per day plus flucytosine 25 mg/kg 4 times per day for 2 weeks, followed by oral fluconazole.[3] Ⓐ

Evidence-Based References

1. Kousignian I et al: Maintaining antiretroviral therapy reduces the risk of AIDS-defining events in patients with uncontrolled viral replication and profound immunodeficiency, *Clin Infect Dis* 46:296-304, 2008. Commentary by N. Khardori, M.D. Ⓐ

2. Verma A: Human immunodeficiency virus protease inhibitors and risk for peripheral neuropathy, *Ann Neurol* 64:566-572, 2008. Commentary by A. Verma, M.D. Ⓐ

3. Bicanic T et al: High-dose amphotericin B with flucytosine for the treatment of cryptococcal meningitis in HIV-infected patients: a randomized trial, *Clin Infect Dis* 47:123-130, 2008. Commentary by N. Khardori, M.D. Ⓐ

SUGGESTED READINGS

Bozzette SA: Routine screening for HIV infection—timely and cost-effective, *N Engl J Med* 352:620-621, 2005.

Cain KP et al: An algorithm for tuberculosis screening and diagnosis in people with HIV, *N Engl J Med* 362:707-716, 2010.

Danel C et al: CD4-guided antiretroviral treatment interruption strategy in HIV-infected adults in West Africa (Trivacan ANRS 1269 trial): a randomized trial, *Lancet* 367(9527):1981, 2006.

French N et al: A trial of a 7-valent pneumococcal conjugate vaccine in HIV-infected adults, *N Engl J Med* 362:812-822, 2010.

Gallant JE et al: Tenofir DF, emtricitabine, and efavirenz vs. zidovidine, lamivudine, and efaverenz for HIV, *N Engl J Med* 354(3):251, 2006.

Gulick RM et al: Three- vs four-drug antiretroviral regimens for the initial treatment of HIV-1 infection: a randomized controlled trial, *JAMA* 296(7):769, 2006.

Hammer SM et al: Antiretroviral treatment of adult HIV infection, 2008 recommendations of the international AIDS society-USA panel, *JAMA* 300(5):555, 2008.

Masur H, Kaplan JE: New guidelines for the management of HIV-related opportunistic infections, *JAMA* 301:2378-2382, 2009.

Riddler SA et al: Class-sparing regimens for initial treatment of HIV-1 infection, *N Engl J Med* 358: 2095, 2008

Walensky RP et al: The survival benefits of AIDS treatment in the United States, *J Infect Dis* 194(1):11, 2006. Online at: www.cdc.gov/hiv/topics/surveillance/united_states.html.

Walensky RP et al: Revising expectations from rapid HIV tests in the emergency department, *Ann Intern Med* 149:153, 2008

AUTHORS: **MELISSA GAITANIS, M.D.,** and **DENNIS J. MIKOLICH, M.D.**

Huntington's Disease

BASIC INFORMATION

DEFINITION

Huntington's disease is an inherited neurodegenerative disorder characterized by involuntary movements, psychiatric disturbance, and cognitive decline.

SYNONYMS

Huntington's chorea

ICD-9CM CODES
333.4 Huntington's chorea

EPIDEMIOLOGY & DEMOGRAPHICS

PEAK INCIDENCE: Late 30s and 40s, with onsets from age 2 to 70 yrs of age
PREVALENCE (IN U.S.): 4.1 to 8.4 cases/100,000 persons
PREDOMINANT SEX: Female = male
PREDOMINANT AGE: Adulthood
GENETICS: Autosomal dominant

PHYSICAL FINDINGS & CLINICAL PRESENTATION

- Chorea (irregular, rapid, flowing, nonstereotyped involuntary movements). When there is a writhing quality, it is referred to as *choreoathetosis.* Chorea is present early on and tends to decrease in end stages of disease.
- Dancelike, lurching gait, often caused by chorea.
- Westphal variant: cognitive dysfunction, bradykinesia, and rigidity. This variant is more commonly seen in juvenile-onset Huntington's.
- Oculomotor abnormalities are common early on and include increased latency of response and insuppressible eye blinking.
- Psychiatric disorders (can be present early on): depression is commonly seen as well as obsessive-compulsive behaviors and aggression associated with impaired impulse control.

ETIOLOGY

- Trinucleotide repeat disorder.
- The responsible gene is the Huntington gene located on chromosome 4. Its function is not known.

DIAGNOSIS

DIFFERENTIAL DIAGNOSIS

- Drug-induced chorea: dopamine, stimulants, anticonvulsants, antidepressants, and oral contraceptives have all been known to cause chorea.
- Sydenham's chorea: decreased incidence with decline of rheumatic fever.
- Benign hereditary chorea: autosomal dominant with onset in childhood. There is no progression of symptoms and no associated dementia or behavioral problems.
- Senile chorea: possibly vascular in origin.
- Wilson's disease: autosomal recessive; tremor, dysarthria, and dystonia are more common presentations than chorea. A total of 95% of patients with neurologic manifestations will have Keyser-Fleischer rings.
- Postinfectious.
- Systemic lupus erythematosus: can be the presenting feature of lupus (rare).
- Chorea gravidarum: presents during first 4 to 5 mo of pregnancy and resolves after delivery.
- Paraneoplastic: seen most commonly in small-cell lung cancer and lymphoma.

WORKUP

Onset of symptoms in an individual with an established family history requires no additional investigation.

LABORATORY TESTS

- Genetic testing.
- If normal, obtain complete blood count with smear, erythrocyte sedimentation rate, electrolytes, serum ceruloplasmin, 24-hr urinary copper excretion, TFTs, antinuclear antibody, liver function tests, HIV, and ASO titer. Consider paraneoplastic markers.

IMAGING STUDIES

CT scan or MRI scan will show atrophy, most notably in the caudate and putamen. The cortex is involved to a lesser extent. A normal scan does not exclude the diagnosis.

TREATMENT

NONPHARMACOLOGIC THERAPY

- Supportive counseling
- Physical and occupational therapy
- Home health care
- Genetic counseling

CHRONIC Rx

- Chorea does not need to be treated unless it is disabling.
- Tetrabenazine (TBZ), now available in the U.S., was recently approved by the FDA for the treatment of chorea associated with Huntington's disease. It is a reversible inhibitor of the vesicle monoamine transporter type 2 (VMAT-2). It inhibits primarily dopamine and to a lesser degree serotonin and norepinephrine. Side effects include parkinsonism and depression.
- Neuroleptics at low doses (e.g., haloperidol 1 to 10 mg/day).
- Amantadine (up to 300 to 400 mg divided tid).
- Depression with suicidal ideation is common; may improve with tricyclic antidepressants or SSRI

DISPOSITION

Relentless course of variable duration leading to progressive disability and death

REFERRAL

- Should refer to psychiatry and neurology for treatment of mood disorders and movement disorders
- Genetic counseling

PEARLS & CONSIDERATIONS

- Suicide rate is fivefold that of the general population.
- The number of repeats does correlate with age of onset but does not clearly correlate with disease severity. Interpretation of number of repeats is still difficult at this time; therefore it is debatable whether to disclose this information to patients.

EVIDENCE

Large placebo-controlled studies showing improved outcomes in patients with Huntington's disease are not available. Many drug trials have been undertaken but suffer either from small sample sizes, lack of blinding and placebo control, or negative results. However, amantadine,[1,2] tetrabenazine,[3,4] and fluphenazine[5] have fair (mediocre quality) evidence for symptomatic treatment of chorea when needed. Selective serotonin reuptake inhibitors are used most commonly for depression, although there are small case reports and open-label studies suggesting the use of risperidone and olanzapine,[6] especially if there is aggression or anxiety.

Evidence-Based References

1. Verhagen Metman L et al: Huntington's disease: a randomized, controlled trial using NMDA-antagonist amantadine, *Neurology* 59(5):694, 2002.
2. Heckmann JM et al: IV amantadine improves chorea in Huntington's disease: an acute randomized, controlled study, *Neurology* 10;63(3):597, 2004.
3. Swash M et al: Treatment of involuntary movement disorders with tetrabenazine, *J Neurol Neurosurg Psychiatry* 35:186, 1972.
4. Asher SW, Aminoff MJ: Tetrabenazine and movement disorders, *Neurology* 31:1051, 1981.
5. Terrence CF: Fluphenazine decanoate in the treatment of chorea: a double-blind study, *Curr Ther Res Clin Exp* 20:177, 1976.
6. Bonelli RM et al: Olanzapine for Huntington's disease: an open label study, *Clin Neuropharmacol* 25:263, 2002.

SUGGESTED READINGS

Bonelli RM et al: Huntington's disease: present treatments and future therapeutic modalities, *Intl Clin Psychopharm* 19:51, 2004.
Greenamyre JT: Huntington's disease, making connections, *N Engl J Med* 356:5, 2007.
Higgins D: Chorea and its disorders, *Neuro Clin* 19(3):707, 2001.
Walker FO: Huntington's disease, *Lancet* 369:218-228, 2007.

AUTHOR: **CINDY ZADIKOFF, M.D.**

BASIC INFORMATION

DEFINITION

A hydrocele is a fluid collection in a serous scrotal space, usually between the layers of the tunica vaginalis (Figs. 1-161 and 1-162). A hydrocele that fills with fluid from the peritoneum is termed *communicating.* This is distinguished from a *noncommunicating* hydrocele by history of variation in size throughout the day and palpation of a thickened cord above the testicle on the affected side. A communicating hydrocele is a small inguinal hernia in which fluid, but not peritoneal structures, traverses the processus vaginalis.

ICD-9CM CODES
603.9 Hydrocele

PHYSICAL FINDINGS & CLINICAL PRESENTATION

Symptoms:
- Scrotal enlargement
- Scrotal heaviness or discomfort radiating to the inguinal area
- Back pain

Physical findings:
- Scrotal distention (testicle may be impossible to palpate)
- Transillumination

ETIOLOGY

Hydroceles may occur as a congenital abnormality in which the processus vaginalis fails to close. In this case an inguinal hernia is virtually always associated with the malformation. Congenital hydroceles are most common in infants and children. In adults, hydroceles are more frequently caused by infection, tumor, or trauma. Infection of the epididymis often results in the development of a secondary hydrocele. Tropical infections such as filariasis may produce hydroceles.

DIAGNOSIS

DIFFERENTIAL DIAGNOSIS

- Spermatocele
- Inguinoscrotal hernia
- Testicular tumor
- Varicocele
- Epididymitis

IMAGING STUDIES

Scrotal ultrasound (useful to rule out a testicular tumor as the cause of the hydrocele). The acute development of a hydrocele might be associated with the onset of epididymitis, testicular tumor, trauma, and torsion of a testicular appendage. An ultrasound of the scrotum may provide important diagnostic information.

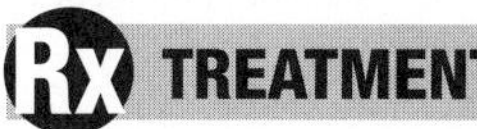

TREATMENT

- No treatment if asymptomatic and testicle is believed to be normal.
- Surgical repair. Communicating hydroceles should be repaired in the same manner as an indirect hernia. The indications for repair of a noncommunicating hydrocele include failure to resolve and increase in size to one that is large and tense.

AUTHOR: **FRED F. FERRI, M.D.**

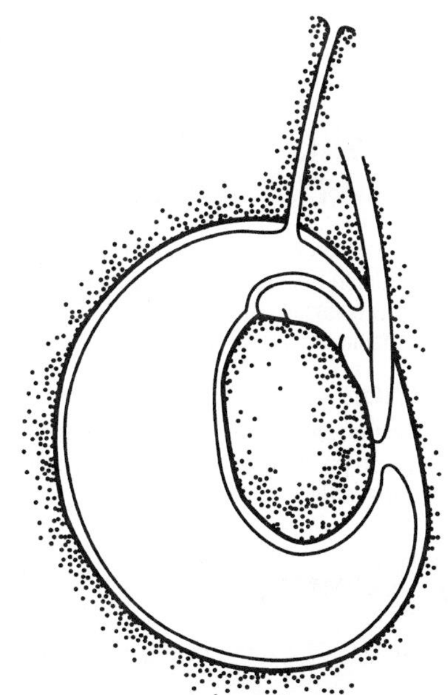

FIGURE 1-161 A hydrocele is a fluid collection in the serous space between the layers of the tunica vaginalis. The tunica vaginalis may or may not remain patent, allowing the hydrocele to communicate with the peritoneum.

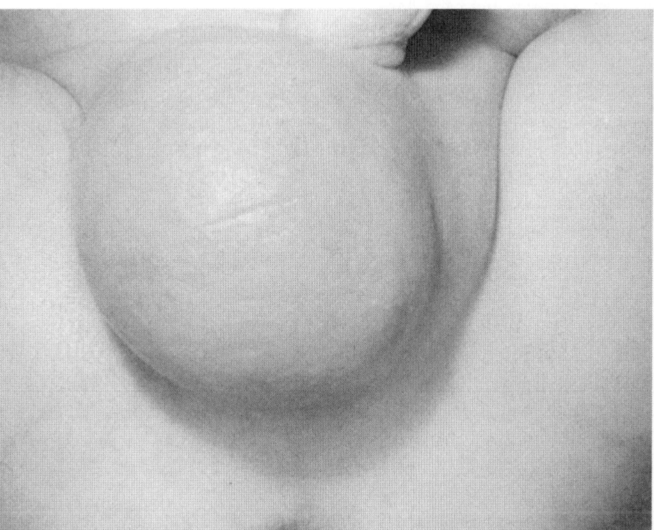

FIGURE 1-162 Newborn with large right hydrocele. (From Behrman RE: *Nelson textbook of pediatrics,* ed 16, Philadelphia, 2000, WB Saunders.)

Hydrocephalus, Normal Pressure (PTG)

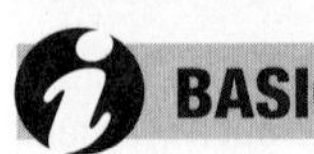

BASIC INFORMATION

DEFINITION

Normal pressure hydrocephalus (NPH) is a syndrome of symptomatic hydrocephalus in the setting of normal cerebrospinal fluid (CSF) pressure. The classic clinical triad of NPH includes gait disturbance, cognitive decline, and incontinence.

SYNONYMS

Occult hydrocephalus
Extraventricular obstructive hydrocephalus
Chronic hydrocephalus

ICD-9CM CODES
331.3 Communicating hydrocephalus

EPIDEMIOLOGY & DEMOGRAPHICS

INCIDENCE: The exact incidence is not known. It may account for up to 5% of dementia in the U.S. Hospital discharge data suggest approximately 11,500 new cases diagnosed annually (may be overestimated).
PREDOMINANT SEX: Males = females
PREDOMINANT AGE: NPH is more common with increasing age.

PHYSICAL FINDINGS & CLINICAL PRESENTATION

- Gait difficulty: patients often have difficulty initiating ambulation, and the gait may be broad based and shuffling, with the appearance that the feet are stuck to the floor ("magnetic gait" or "frontal gait disorder").
- Cognitive decline: mental slowing, forgetfulness and inattention typically without agnosia, aphasia, or other cortical disturbances.
- Incontinence: initially may have urinary urgency; incontinence later develops. Fecal incontinence also occasionally occurs.
- Gegenhalten (paratonia) or other frontal lobe signs may be seen.

ETIOLOGY

- Approximately 50% of cases are idiopathic; the remaining cases have a variety of causes, including prior subarachnoid hemorrhage, meningitis, trauma, or intracranial surgery.
- Symptoms are presumed to result from stretching of sacral motor and limbic fibers that lie near the ventricles as dilation occurs.

Dx DIAGNOSIS

DIFFERENTIAL DIAGNOSIS

- Alzheimer's disease with extrapyramidal features
- Cognitive impairment in the setting of Parkinson's disease or parkinsonism-plus syndromes
- Diffuse Lewy body disease
- Frontotemporal dementia
- Cervical spondylosis with cord compromise in the setting of degenerative dementia
- Multiinfarct dementia
- HIV dementia

WORKUP

- Large-volume lumbar puncture:
  1. Mental status testing and time to walk a prespecified distance (usually 25 feet) are measured, followed by removal of 40 to 50 ml of CSF.
  2. Retest of mental status and timed walking are done later (sometimes at 1 and 4 hr). Patients who have significant improvement in gait or mental status may have a better surgical outcome; those with mild or negative response can have variable outcomes.
  3. Opening and closing pressure are measured; if pressure is elevated, alternative causes must be considered. Higher *normal* pressure may predict a good outcome from CSF shunting.
- Measurement of CSF outflow resistance by an infusion test, CSF pressure monitoring, and prolonged external lumbar drainage are sometimes used to help predict surgical outcome.

LABORATORY TESTS

CSF should be sent for routine fluid analysis to exclude other pathologies.

IMAGING STUDIES

- CT scan or MRI can be used to document ventriculomegaly. The distinguishing feature of NPH is ventricular enlargement out of proportion to sulcal atrophy.
- MRI has advantages over CT, including better ability to visualize structures in the posterior fossa, visualize transependymal CSF flow, and document extent of white matter lesions. On MRI a flow void in the aqueduct and third ventricle ("jet sign") may be seen.
- Isotope cisternography and dynamic MRI studies have not been shown to be superior in predicting shunt outcome.

Rx TREATMENT

There is no evidence that NPH can be effectively treated with medications.

NONPHARMACOLOGIC THERAPY

Response to ventriculoperitoneal shunting is variable. Some patients (variable depending on series reported) show significant improvement from shunting.

Factors that may predict positive outcome with surgery:

- NPH caused by prior trauma, subarachnoid hemorrhage, or meningitis
- History of mild impairment in cognition <2 yr duration
- Onset of gait abnormality before cognitive decline
- Imaging demonstrates hydrocephalus without sulcal enlargement
- Transependymal CSF flow visualized on MRI
- Large-volume tap produces dramatic but temporary relief of symptoms
- High *normal* opening pressure

Factors that may predict negative outcome with surgery:

- Extensive white matter lesions or diffuse cerebral atrophy on MRI
- Moderate to severe cognitive impairment
- Onset of cognitive impairment before gait disorder
- History of alcohol abuse

ACUTE GENERAL Rx

Shunting in selected patients

DISPOSITION

Symptoms of NPH may progress over time. Prompt diagnosis may improve chances for treatment success.

REFERRAL

To neurologist for initial evaluation, including lumbar puncture, followed by neurosurgeon for shunting in appropriate patients

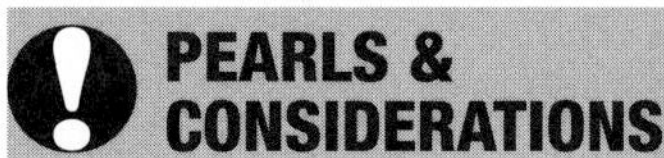

PEARLS & CONSIDERATIONS

Each of the cardinal symptoms of NPH is commonly seen in the elderly and occurs in multiple disease processes; therefore differential diagnoses should always be considered carefully.

CAUTION

Shunt complications, including subdural or intracerebral hematoma, may occur in 30% to 40% of patients.

EBM EVIDENCE

Please note: Complete text of EBM for this topic is available online.

SUGGESTED READINGS

Marmarou A et al: The value of supplemental prognostic tests for the preoperative assessment of idiopathic normal-pressure hydrocephalus, *Neurosurgery* 57(suppl 3):17-28, 2005.

Vanneste JA: Diagnosis and management of normal-pressure hydrocephalus, *J Neurol* 247(1):5, 2000.

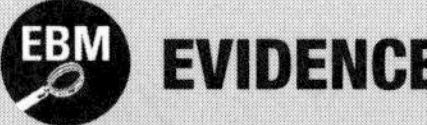

AUTHOR: **TAMARA G. FONG, M.D., Ph.D.**

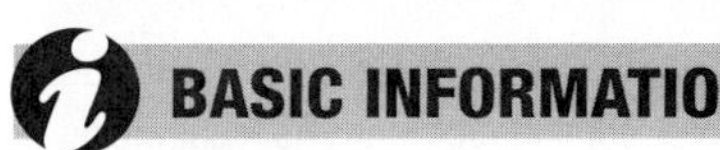

BASIC INFORMATION

DEFINITION

Hydronephrosis is dilation of the renal pyelocalyceal system, most often as a result of impairment of urinary flow.

SYNONYMS

Hydroureter (dilation of ureter, often seen with hydronephrosis when obstruction is in lower urinary tract)
Urinary tract obstruction

ICD-9CM CODES
591 Acquired hydronephrosis
753.2 Congenital hydronephrosis

EPIDEMIOLOGY & DEMOGRAPHICS

Children usually have congenital malformations, whereas adults tend to have acquired defects as etiologies.

CLINICAL PRESENTATION

HISTORY:

- Pain is caused by distention of collecting system or renal capsule and is more related to the rate of onset than the degree of obstruction. It can vary in location from flank to the lower abdomen to the testes/labia. Pain in the flank occurring only on micturition is highly suggestive of vesicoureteral reflux.
- Anuria can occur with total obstruction of urinary flow (bilateral hydronephrosis, or unilateral if only one kidney is present).
- Polyuria or nocturia can occur with chronic (incomplete) obstruction because of deleterious effects on renal concentrating ability (nephrogenic diabetes insipidus).
- Urinary frequency, hesitancy, poor stream, and postvoid dribbling are all symptoms that can occur with obstruction at or below the bladder (e.g., prostatic hyperplasia).
- Chronic urinary infections can either result from chronic urinary obstruction (organisms favoring growth with stasis of urine) or lead to conditions (e.g., urine pH changes) that favor stone formation and subsequent obstruction.

PHYSICAL EXAMINATION:

- Hypertension can be caused by increased renin release in acute or subacute obstruction.
- Fever or costovertebral angle (CVA) tenderness can suggest urinary tract infection.
- Palpate bladder to detect if distention is present.
- Rectal examination to evaluate prostate for size and nodularity and also to check rectal sphincter tone.
- Pelvic examination to assess for vaginal anatomy, pelvic mass, or pelvic inflammatory disease.
- Penile examination to rule out meatal stenosis or phimosis.
- Bladder catheterization to assess postvoid residual volume if urinary tract obstruction is considered. Should rule out postrenal obstruction in unexplained acute renal failure.

ETIOLOGY

MECHANICAL IMPAIRMENTS:

Congenital:

- Ureteropelvic junction narrowing
- Ureterovesical junction narrowing
- Ureterocele
- Retrocaval ureter
- Bladder neck obstruction
- Urethral valve
- Urethral stricture
- Meatal stenosis

Acquired:

- Intrinsic to urinary tract:
  - Calculi
  - Inflammation
  - Trauma
  - Sloughed papillae
  - Ureteral tumor
  - Blood clots
  - Prostatic hypertrophy or cancer
  - Bladder cancer
  - Urethral stricture
  - Phimosis
- Extrinsic to urinary tract:
  - Gravid uterus
  - Retroperitoneal fibrosis or tumor (e.g., lymphoma)
  - Aortic aneurysm
  - Uterine fibroids
  - Trauma (surgical or nonsurgical)
  - Pelvic inflammatory disease
  - Pelvic malignancies (e.g., prostate, colorectal, cervical, uterine, bladder)

FUNCTIONAL IMPAIRMENTS:

- Neurogenic bladder (often with adynamic ureter) can occur with spinal cord disease or diabetic neuropathy.
- Pharmacologic agents such as alpha-adrenergic antagonists and anticholinergic drugs can inhibit bladder emptying.
- Vesicoureteral reflux may occur.
- Pregnancy can cause hydroureter and hydronephrosis (on the right more often than left) as early as the second month. Hormonal effects on ureteral tone combine with mechanical factors.

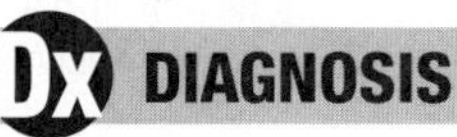

DIAGNOSIS

DIFFERENTIAL DIAGNOSIS

- Urinary stones
- Neoplastic disease
- Prostatic hypertrophy
- Neurologic disease
- Urinary reflux
- Urinary tract infection
- Medication effects
- Trauma
- Congenital abnormality of urinary tract

LABORATORY TESTS

- Serum blood urea nitrogen and creatinine to assess for renal insufficiency (usually implies bilateral obstruction or unilateral obstruction of a solitary kidney).
- Electrolytes may reveal hypernatremia (if nephrogenic diabetes insipidus), hyperkalemia (from renal failure and effects on tubular function), or distal renal tubular acidosis.
- Urinalysis and examination of sediment may reveal white blood cells, red blood cells, or bacteria in the appropriate setting (e.g., infection, stones), but often the sediment is normal in obstructive renal disease.

IMAGING STUDIES

- Assess kidney and bladder size with ultrasound as well as contour of collecting system and ureters. Ultrasound is >90% sensitive and specific for hydronephrosis and is noninvasive; therefore it will not worsen preexisting renal insufficiency.
- Abdominal CT scan without IV contrast provides excellent localization of the site of obstruction (Fig. 1-163).

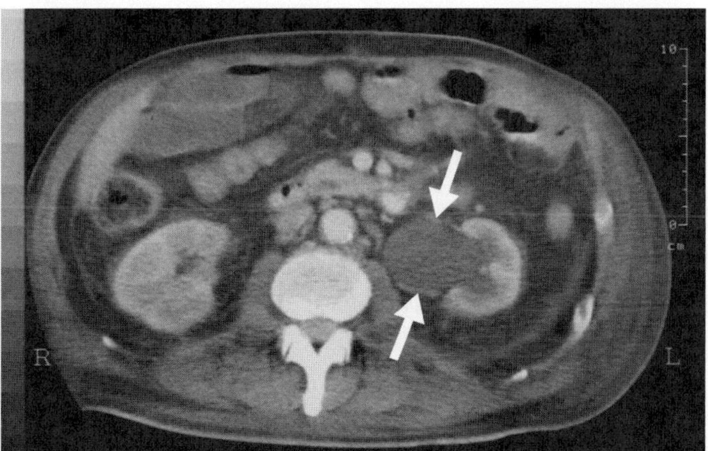

FIGURE 1-163 CT scan of the abdomen showing a grossly hydronephrotic kidney on the left. *Arrows* mark dilated renal pelvis. Dilated loops of small bowel are seen in the right hypochondrium. Sequential sections demonstrated that the ureter was dilated along its length and that there was a pelvic mass, which was responsible for both bowel and left ureteric obstruction. The mass was subsequently shown to be arising from a carcinoma of the colon. (From Johnson RJ, Feehally J: *Comprehensive clinical nephrology,* ed 2, St Louis, 2000, Mosby.)

 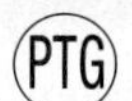

- Once diagnosed, antegrade or retrograde ureterograms can further delineate the point of obstruction.
- Voiding cystourethrogram is helpful in diagnosing vesicoureteral reflux and obstructions of the bladder neck or urethra.

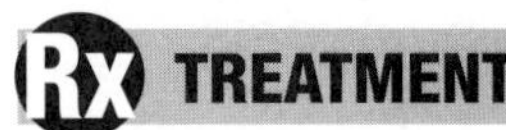

TREATMENT

NONPHARMACOLOGIC THERAPY

- Urgent treatment is required if urinary tract obstruction is associated with urinary tract infection, acute renal failure, or uncontrollable pain.
- Conservative management of calculi with IV fluids, IV antibiotics (if evidence of infection), and aggressive analgesia may be enough to treat acute unilateral urinary tract obstruction depending on the size (90% of stones <5 mm will pass spontaneously).
- Urethral catheter is adequate to relieve most obstructions at or distal to the bladder, but occasionally a suprapubic catheter will be required (e.g., impassable urethral stricture or urethral injury). Neurogenic bladder may require intermittent clean catheterization if frequent voiding and pharmacologic treatments are ineffective.
- Nephrostomy tube can be placed percutaneously to facilitate urinary drainage.
- Extracorporeal shock wave lithotripsy (ESWL) is used to fragment large stones to facilitate spontaneous passage or subsequent extraction. (Note: ESWL is contraindicated in pregnancy.)
- Nephroscopy is performed for extraction of proximal stones under direct visualization.
- Cystoscopy with ureteroscopy is used to remove distal ureteral stones with a loop or basket with or without fragmentation by ultrasonic or laser lithotripsy.
- Ureteral stents can be used for extrinsic and some intrinsic ureteral obstructions.
- Urethral dilation or internal urethrotomy can be used for urethral strictures.
- Nephrectomy or ureteral diversion may be required in severe cases (e.g., malignancy).
- Ureterovesical reimplantation can be used for reflux disease.
- Transurethral retrograde prostatectomy is used for severe obstruction from benign prostatic hypertrophy.
- IV fluid and electrolyte replacement are needed; the patient must be monitored closely during the postobstructive diuresis (usually lasting several days to a week).

ACUTE GENERAL Rx

Antibiotics if indicated

DISPOSITION

Aggressive treatment of infections and early relief of obstruction can usually prevent progressive loss of renal function; however, chronic bilateral obstruction (often from benign prostatic hypertrophy) can lead to chronic renal failure.

REFERRAL

- Urologist consultation early for diagnostic or therapeutic procedures
- Oncologist if a neoplasm is diagnosed
- Gynecologist if pregnancy or female pelvic anatomy is involved

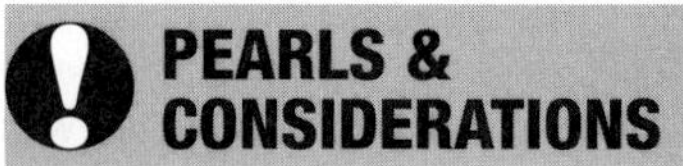

PEARLS & CONSIDERATIONS

COMMENTS

- Not a primary disorder: an underlying etiology should be sought.

PREVENTION

May be achieved through prevention of an underlying potential etiology (e.g., medical or surgical management of benign prostatic hypertrophy before obstruction occurring or medical treatment to avoid formation of renal stones).

SUGGESTED READINGS

Lameire N et al: Acute renal failure, *Lancet* 365:417-430, 2005.

Mostbeck GH et al: Ultrasound of the kidney: obstruction and medical diseases, *Eur Radiol* 11(10):1878-1889, 2001.

AUTHORS: **SHEENAGH M. BODKIN, M.D.,** and **PAUL A. PIRRAGLIA, M.D., M.P.H.**

BASIC INFORMATION

DEFINITION

Primary hyperaldosteronism is a clinical syndrome characterized by hypokalemia, hypertension, low plasma renin activity (PRA), and excessive aldosterone secretion.

SYNONYMS

Hyperaldosteronism
Aldosteronism
Primary aldosteronism
Conn's syndrome

ICD-9CM CODES
255.1 Primary aldosteronism

EPIDEMIOLOGY & DEMOGRAPHICS

INCIDENCE: 1% to 2% of patients with hypertension
PREVALENCE: More common in females

PHYSICAL FINDINGS & CLINICAL PRESENTATION

- Generally asymptomatic
- If significant hypokalemia is present, possible muscle cramping, weakness, paresthesias
- Hypertension
- Polyuria, polydipsia

ETIOLOGY

- Aldosterone-producing adenoma (>60%)
- Idiopathic hyperaldosteronism (>30%)
- Glucocorticoid-suppressible hyperaldosteronism (<1%)
- Aldosterone-producing carcinoma (<1%)

DIAGNOSIS

DIFFERENTIAL DIAGNOSIS

- Diuretic use
- Hypokalemia from vomiting, diarrhea
- Renovascular hypertension
- Other endocrine neoplasm (pheochromocytoma, deoxycorticosterone-producing tumor, renin-secreting tumor)

WORKUP

CT, MRI, and adrenal vein sampling (AVS) are used to distinguish unilateral from bilateral increased aldosterone secretion. This distinction will dictate treatment options since unilateral primary aldosteronism is treated surgically rather than medically. In patients with hypokalemia and a low PRA, confirming tests for primary hyperaldosteronism include the following:

- 24-hr urine test for aldosterone and potassium levels (potassium >40 mEq and aldosterone >15 mcg).
- Captopril test: administer 25 to 50 mg of captopril (an angiotensin-converting enzyme [ACE] inhibitor) and measure plasma renin and aldosterone levels 1 to 2 hr later. A plasma aldosterone level >15 ng/dl confirms the diagnosis of primary aldosteronism. This test is more expensive and is best reserved for situations in which the 24-hr urine test for aldosterone is ambiguous.
- 24-hr urinary tetrahydroaldosterone (<65 mcg/24 hr) and saline infusion test (plasma aldosterone >10 ng/dl) can also be used in ambiguous cases.
- The renin-aldosterone stimulation test (posture test) is helpful in differentiating idiopathic hyperaldosteronism (IHA) from aldosterone-producing adenoma (APA). Patients with APA have a decrease in aldosterone levels at 4 hr, whereas patients with IHA have an increase in aldosterone levels.
- As a screening test for primary aldosteronism, an elevated plasma aldosterone-renin ratio (ARR), drawn randomly from patients taking hypertensive drugs, is predictive of primary aldosteronism (positive predictive value 100% in a recent study). ARR is calculated by dividing plasma aldosterone (mg/dl) by PRA (mg/ml/hr). ARR >100 is considered elevated.
- Bilateral AVS may be done to localize APA when adrenal CT scan is equivocal. In APA, ipsilateral/contralateral aldosterone level is >10:1, and ipsilateral venous aldosterone concentration is very high (>1000 ng/dl).
- A diagnostic evaluation of hypertensive patients with suspected aldosteronism is described in the online version of Section III.

LABORATORY TESTS

Routine laboratory tests can be suggestive but are not diagnostic of primary aldosteronism. Common abnormalities are:

- Spontaneous hypokalemia or moderately severe hypokalemia while receiving conventional doses of diuretics
- Possible alkalosis and hypernatremia

IMAGING STUDIES

- Adrenal CT scans (with 3-mm cuts) or MRI may be used to localize neoplasm.
- Adrenal scanning with iodocholesterol (NP-59) or 6-beta-iodomethyl-19-norcholesterol after dexamethasone suppression. The uptake of tracer is increased in those with aldosteronoma and absent in those with IHA and adrenal carcinoma.

TREATMENT

NONPHARMACOLOGIC THERAPY

- Regular monitoring and control of blood pressure
- Low-sodium diet, tobacco avoidance, maintenance of ideal body weight, and regular exercise

ACUTE GENERAL Rx

- Control of blood pressure and hypokalemia with spironolactone, amiloride, or ACE inhibitors
- Surgery (unilateral adrenalectomy) for APA

CHRONIC Rx

Chronic medical therapy with spironolactone, amiloride, or ACE inhibitors to control blood pressure and hypokalemia is necessary in all patients with bilateral IHA.

DISPOSITION

- Unilateral adrenalectomy normalizes hypertension and hypokalemia in 70% of patients with APA after 1 yr. After 5 yr, 50% of patients remain normotensive.
- Experimental animal studies have suggested that long-term exposure to increased aldosterone levels in untreated aldosteronism may result in renal structural damage. However, clinical trials have shown that primary aldosteronism is characterized by partially reversible renal dysfunction in which elevated albuminuria is a marker of a dynamic rather than structural renal defect.

REFERRAL

Surgical referral for unilateral adrenalectomy after confirmation of unilateral APA or carcinoma

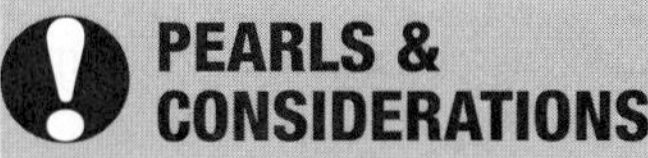

PEARLS & CONSIDERATIONS

- Frequent monitoring of blood pressure and electrolytes postoperatively is necessary because normotension after unilateral adrenalectomy may take up to 4 mo.
- Recent investigations regarding serum aldosterone and the incidence of hypertension in nonhypertensive persons indicate that increased aldosterone levels within the physiologic range predispose to the development of hypertension.

SUGGESTED READINGS

Douma S et al: Prevalence of primary hyperaldosteronism in resistant hypertension: a retrospective observational study, *Lancet* 371:1921, 2008.

Kempers MJ et al: Systematic review: diagnostic procedures to differentiate unilateral from bilateral adrenal abnormality in primary aldosteronism, *Ann Intern Med* 151:329-337, 2009.

Sechi L et al: Long-term renal outcomes in patients with primary aldosteronism, *JAMA* 295:2638, 2006.

AUTHOR: **FRED F. FERRI, M.D.**

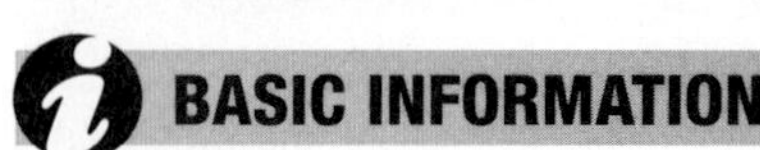

BASIC INFORMATION

DEFINITION

Hypercholesterolemia refers to a blood cholesterol measurement >200 mg/dl. A cholesterol level of 200 to 239 mg/dl is considered borderline high, and a level of >240 mg/dl is considered high.

SYNONYMS

Hypercholesteremia
Hypercholesterinemia
Type II familial hyperlipoproteinemia

ICD-9CM CODES
272.0 Hypercholesterolemia

EPIDEMIOLOGY & DEMOGRAPHICS

- More than half of all U.S. adults have dyslipidemia: 50.4% of men and 50.9% of women.
- Only approximately 12% of people with high cholesterol are being treated.
- Elevated cholesterol requires drug therapy in approximately 60 million Americans.
- Incidence of heterozygous familial hypercholesterolemia: approximately 1:500.
- Incidence of homozygous familial hypercholesterolemia: approximately 1:1 million.
- Prevalence of hypercholesterolemia increases with increasing age.
- Familial hypercholesterolemia: autosomal-dominant disorder.
- Familial combined hyperlipidemia: possibly an autosomal-dominant disorder.
- Multifactorial predilection: apparent in majority of affected individuals.

PHYSICAL FINDINGS & CLINICAL PRESENTATION

- Most patients: no physical findings
- Possible findings, particularly in the familial forms:
  1. Tendon xanthomas
  2. Xanthelasma
  3. Arcus corneae
  4. Arterial bruits (young adulthood)

ETIOLOGY

Primary:
- Genetics
- Obesity
- Dietary intake

Secondary:
- Diabetes mellitus
- Alcohol
- Oral contraceptives
- Hypothyroidism
- Glucocorticoid use
- Most diuretics
- Nephrotic syndrome
- Hepatoma
- Extrahepatic biliary obstruction
- Primary biliary cirrhosis

DIAGNOSIS

DIFFERENTIAL DIAGNOSIS

No real differential diagnosis; however, consider underlying secondary causes for the elevated cholesterol.

LABORATORY TESTS

- Primary prevention without atherosclerosis or diabetes mellitus:
  1. Recommended to get a complete lipoprotein profile (total cholesterol, high-density lipoprotein [HDL], low-density lipoprotein [LDL], and triglycerides) on all adults at 20 yr.
  2. Risk assessment to modify LDL goals: cigarette smoking, hypertension (blood pressure [BP] >140/90 mm Hg on medication), family history of premature congestive heart disease (CHD) (first-degree relative with CHD in male <55 yr or female <65 yr), and age (male at 45 yr, female at 55 yr).
  3. Evaluate for CHD equivalents, including atherosclerosis (peripheral arterial disease, aortic aneurism), diabetes, symptomatic carotid disease, or 10-year rise in CHD >20%.
  4. LDL goal based on modifications:
     - 0 to 1 risk factors, LDL <160 mg/dl
     - Multiple risk factors, LDL <130 mg/dl
     - CHD or equivalents, LDL <100 mg/dl
  5. Fasting lipid profile with LDL <130 mg/dl and no or one risk factor: dietary guidance and repeat every 1 to 5 yrs.
  6. Fasting lipid profile with LDL 130 to 159 mg/dl and less than two risk factors for coronary artery disease (CAD): diet and exercise modification with repeat profile in 12 wk.
  7. Fasting lipid profile with LDL >130 mg/dl and two or more risk factors for CAD: diet and drug therapy.
- Secondary prevention with atherosclerosis or diabetes mellitus:
  1. All patients: fasting lipid profile
  2. If LDL <100 mg/dl: instruction on diet and exercise, repeat annually
  3. If LDL >100 mg/dl: drug therapy required
- Secondary prevention with atherosclerosis and diabetes mellitus:
  1. Now classified as very high risk
  2. Fasting lipid profile for all patients
  3. If LDL >70 mg/dl, drug therapy required
- Metabolic syndrome:
  1. A constellation of lipid and nonlipid risk factors of a metabolic origin
  2. Diagnosed when three or more of the following are present: abdominal obesity; triglycerides >150 mg/dl; HDL <40 mg/dl in males, <50 mg/dl in females; systolic BP >130 mm hg; diastolic BP >85 mm Hg; fasting glucose >110 mg/dl
  3. Needs aggressive treatment with weight loss, increased physical activity, and pharmacologic therapy

TREATMENT

NONPHARMACOLOGIC THERAPY

- First line of treatment: dietary therapy (see "Hyperlipoproteinemia")
- Dietary modifications:
  1. Low-cholesterol, low-fat diet (fat intake to 30% or less of the total caloric intake)
  2. Polyunsaturated fat up to 10% of total calories
  3. Monounsaturated fat up to 20% of total calories
  4. Saturated fats <7% of total calories
  5. No more than 200 mg/day of cholesterol
  6. Fiber 20 to 30 g/day
- Increased activity with aerobic exercise: encourage 20 to 30 min of aerobic exercise three to four times a week
- Smoking cessation encouraged
- Counseling on CAD risk factors

ACUTE GENERAL Rx

No acute treatment needed

CHRONIC Rx

- In primary prevention: needed for patients with LDL >130 mg/dl with two or more risk factors for CAD
- In secondary prevention: needed for patients with known CAD, vascular disease or diabetes mellitus, and LDL >70 mg/dl
- In primary prevention: considered in patients on dietary therapy with LDL >190 mg/dl with no risk factors, LDL >130 mg/dl with two or more risk factors, or HDL <30 mg/dl
- Medications that can be used (Table 1-39):
  1. Bile acid sequestrants (poorly tolerated)
  2. Niacin (poorly tolerated)
  3. HMG-CoA reductase inhibitors ("statins")
  4. Fibric acids
  5. Medication tailored to the patient's lipid profile, lifestyle, and the medication's side-effect profile
- Cholesterol absorption inhibitors (ezetimibe)
- Bile acid sequestrants to lower LDL
- Niacin to lower LDL and triglycerides and raise HDL
- HMG-CoA reductase inhibitors to lower LDL
- Fibric acids work to lower triglycerides more than LDL

DISPOSITION

- After initiation of therapy, repeat laboratory tests in 4 to 6 wk, with modifications as necessary.
- Once goal is achieved, lifelong medication and monitoring are needed at least three to four times a year.
- Dietary modification is needed to continue with drug therapy.
- Repeat review for additional CAD risk factors.

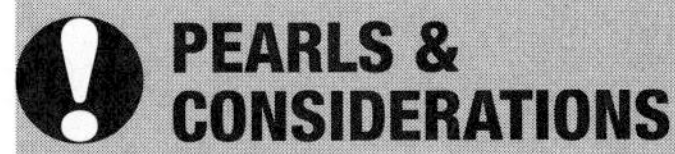

PEARLS & CONSIDERATIONS

COMMENTS

See "Hyperlipoproteinemia."

SUGGESTED READINGS

Barber P et al: HDL cholesterol, very low levels of LDL cholesterol, and cardiovascular events, *N Engl J Med* 357:1301, 2007.

de Lemos JA et al: Early intensive vs a delayed conservative simvastatin strategy in patients with acute coronary syndromes: phase Z of the A to Z trial, *JAMA* 292:1307, 2004.

La Rosa JC et al: Intensive lipid lowering with atorvastatin in patients with stable coronary disease, *N Engl J Med* 352:1425, 2005.

Mosca L et al: National study of physician awareness and adherence to cardiovascular disease prevention guidelines, *Circulation* 111:499, 2005.

National Cholesterol Education Program: Second report on the Expert Panel on Detection, Evaluation, and Treatment of High Cholesterol in Adults (adult treatment panel IV), *JAMA* 285:2486, 2001.

AUTHORS: **BETH J. WUTZ, M.D.**, and **RUBEN ALVERO, M.D.**

TABLE 1-39 Drugs Affecting Lipoprotein Metabolism

Drug Class	Agents and Daily Doses	Lipid/Lipoprotein Effects	Side Effects	Contraindications
HMG-CoA reductase inhibitors (statins)	Lovastatin (20-80 mg) Pravastatin (20-80 mg) Simvastatin (20-80 mg) Fluvastatin (20-80 mg) Atorvastatin (10-80 mg) Rosuvastatin (5-40 mg)	LDL ↓18%-55% HDL ↑5%-15% TG ↓7%-30%	Myopathy; increased liver enzymes	Absolute: • Active or chronic liver disease Relative: • Concomitant use of certain drugs*
Bile acid sequestrants	Cholestyramine (4-16 g) Colestipol (5-20 g) Colesevelam (2.6-3.8 g)	LDL ↓1.5%-30% HDL ↑3%-5% TG No change or increase	Gastrointestinal distress; constipation; decreased absorption of other drugs	Absolute: • Dysbetalipoproteinemia • TG >400 mg/dl Relative: • TG >200 mg/dl
Nicotinic acid	Immediate release (crystalline) nicotinic acid (1.5-3 g), extended-release nicotinic acid (Niaspan) (1-2 g), sustained-release nicotinic acid (1-2 g)	LDL ↓5%-25% HDL ↑15%-35% TG ↓20%-50%	Flushing; hyperglycemia; hyperuricemia (or gout); upper GI distress; hepatotoxicity	Absolute: • Chronic liver disease • Severe gout Relative: • Diabetes • Hyperuricemia • Peptic ulcer disease
Fibric acids	Gemfibrozil (600 mg bid) Fenofibrate (160 mg qd) Clofibrate (1000 mg bid)	LDL ↓5%-20% *(may be increased in patients with high TG)* HDL ↑10%-20% TG ↓20%-50%	Dyspepsia; gallstones; myopathy	Absolute: • Severe renal disease • Severe hepatic disease
Cholesterol absorption inhibitors	Ezetimibe (10 mg qd)	LDL ↓18% HDL ↑1% TG ↓7%-8%	Abdominal pain; myalgias	• Severe renal disease • Severe hepatic disease

Modified from The National Cholesterol Education Program, *JAMA* 285:2486, 2001.
GI, Gastrointestinal; *HDL,* high-density lipoprotein; *HMG-CoA,* 3-hydroxy-3 methylglutaryl coenzyme A; *LDL,* low-density lipoprotein; *TG,* triglyceride.
*Cyclosporine, macrolide antibiotics, various antifungal agents, and cytochrome P-450 inhibitors (fibrates and niacin should be used with appropriate caution).

Hypercoagulable State (PTG)

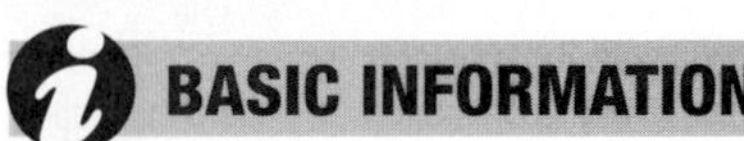

DEFINITION

An inherited or acquired condition associated with an increased risk of thrombosis

SYNONYMS

Thrombophilia

ICD-9CM CODES
289.8 Hypercoagulable state

EPIDEMIOLOGY & DEMOGRAPHICS

See Table 1-40.

- Risk of thrombosis increases with age and with multiple risk factors.
- Most people with a genetic defect will not have thrombotic disease. When thrombosis occurs, it is often associated with an acquired risk factor (e.g., surgery, pregnancy, oral contraceptive [OC] use). Annual risk of thrombosis is <1%.
- Low risk of recurrent thrombosis in patients with a single genetic defect.
- Multiple genetic defects are not uncommon (1%-2% prevalence in patients with idiopathic venous thromboembolism [VTE]); strong synergistic effect when multiple defects are present.
- Approximately half of patients with unprovoked thrombosis have an identifiable inherited thrombophilia.
- Significant variations in the prevalence rates and thrombotic risks for thrombophilia are reported. This may reflect geographic variation in the prevalence of genetic defects, different populations, or the presence of other unidentified thrombophilic risk factors.

HISTORY

A hypercoagulable state is strongly suggested by the following:

- Age <50 yr at first episode of unprovoked thrombosis
- Family history: first-degree relative with thrombosis at age <50 yr
- Recurrent thrombotic events
- Thrombosis in unusual anatomic location (i.e., portal, hepatic, mesenteric, or cerebral vein)
- Thrombosis associated with pregnancy or OC use
- Warfarin-induced skin necrosis
- Adverse pregnancy outcomes may be associated with thrombophilia: recurrent pregnancy loss, preeclampsia, placental abruption, intrauterine growth restriction. Association weak for inherited thrombophilias but strong for antiphospholipid antibodies

PHYSICAL FINDINGS & CLINICAL PRESENTATION

- Inherited thrombophilia is usually associated with VTE, most commonly deep vein thrombosis (DVT)
- Some acquired thrombophilias are associated with arterial thrombosis
- Pregnancy complications
- Medical conditions associated with increased risk of thrombosis

ETIOLOGY

See Table 1-40. The differential diagnosis of the patient presenting with thrombosis or thrombotic diathesis is described in Section II.

- Often it is a multifactorial process with genetic, environmental, and acquired factors.
- Thrombotic risk increases with use of OCs or hormone replacement therapy (HRT) and during the pregnancy/postpartum period.
- Adverse pregnancy outcomes may be caused by thrombosis of the uteroplacental circulation.

INHERITED: Factor V Leiden (FVL) mutation:

- Autosomal-dominant mutation with low penetrance.
- Causes activated protein C resistance (APCR); 90% of APCR is caused by FVL mutation.
- Most common inherited thrombophilia; accounts for 40% to 50% of cases.
- OC use in heterozygous carriers is associated with an eightfold increased risk of VTE compared with noncarriers and a thirty-fivefold increased risk of VTE compared with noncarriers not using OCs.
- May be associated with cardiovascular disease in select high-risk subgroups.

Prothrombin G20210A mutation:

- Autosomal-dominant mutation with low penetrance.
- OC use in heterozygous carriers is associated with a sixteenfold increased risk of VTE compared with noncarriers not using OCs.
- May be associated with cardiovascular disease in select high-risk subgroups and young patients with ischemic stroke.

Protein C, protein S, antithrombin (AT) deficiency:

- Autosomal-dominant inheritance; many mutations identified for each of these conditions.
- Decreased level or abnormal function.
- First episode of thrombosis is usually in young adults.

Protein C and Protein S:

- Homozygous condition is very rare; usually associated with lethal thrombosis in infancy.
- Associated with warfarin-induced skin necrosis, which occurs secondary to depletion of vitamin K–dependent anticoagulant factors sooner than procoagulant factors in the first few days of therapy.

AT deficiency:

- Most thrombogenic of the inherited thrombophilias; 50% lifetime risk of thrombosis.
- Homozygous condition is very rare, probably not compatible with normal fetal development.
- Arterial thrombosis can occur rarely.
- Can cause heparin resistance.

Elevated factor VIII level:

- May be an important risk factor for thrombosis in African-American population.
- Increased risk of recurrent thrombosis.
- Genetic etiology is suspected but not yet identified.

Other possible causes: dysfibrinogenemia, elevated thrombin-activatable fibrinolysis inhibitor, plasminogen deficiency, elevated factor IX and factor XI levels

ACQUIRED: Antiphospholipid antibody syndrome (APS):

- Most common cause of acquired thrombophilia.
- Can present as arterial or venous thrombosis, recurrent pregnancy loss, and adverse pregnancy outcomes.
- Thromboembolic events occur in up to 30% of population; high risk of recurrent thrombosis (up to 70% reported).
- See "Antiphospholipid Antibody Syndrome" for more information.

Hyperhomocysteinemia:

- Can be inherited (most commonly an autosomal recessive mutation in methylene tetrahydrofolate reductase gene) but more fre-

TABLE 1-40 Hypercoagulable Conditions

	Prevalence in General Population (%)	Prevalence in Population with Thrombosis (%)	A/V Events	Relative Risk of Thrombosis
FVL mutation	5% of whites; rare in nonwhites	12%-40%	V	Heterozygous: 3-7; homozygous: 80
Prothrombin G20210A mutation	3% of whites; rare in nonwhites	6%-18%	V	3
AT deficiency	0.02%	1%-3%	V	20-50
PC deficiency	0.2%-0.4%	3%-5%	V	7-15
PS deficiency	0.03%-0.1%	1%-5%	V	5-11
Antiphospholipid antibody syndrome	1%-2%	5%-21%	V + A	2-11
Hyperhomocysteinemia	5%-7%	10%	V + A	3
Elevated factor VIII level	11%	25%		5

A, Arterial; *AT*, antithrombin; *FVL*, factor V Leiden; *PC*, protein C; *PS*, protein S; *V*, venous.

quently acquired; folate, vitamin B_6, or vitamin B_{12} deficiency account for two thirds of cases. Other acquired causes include renal disease, hypothyroidism, malignancy, smoking, and certain medications.
- May be associated with VTE, atherosclerotic disease (cardiovascular, cerebrovascular, and peripheral vascular), and possibly adverse pregnancy outcomes.

Conditions associated with increased risk of thrombosis:
- Prior thrombosis
- Trauma
- Medical illness: heart failure, respiratory failure, infection, diabetes mellitus, obesity, nephrotic syndrome, inflammatory bowel disease, paroxysmal nocturnal hemoglobinuria, sickle cell anemia
- Pregnancy (sixfold increased risk of VTE), postpartum, OC use (fourfold increased risk, higher risk with third-generation OCs), transdermal contraceptive patch, HRT (twofold increased risk), tamoxifen, raloxifene
- Immobilization, travel
- Surgery (especially orthopedic), central venous catheters
- Hyperviscosity syndromes
- Myeloproliferative disorders
- Malignancy: disease or treatment related
- Heparin-induced thrombocytopenia and thrombosis
- Smoking

Dx DIAGNOSIS

WORKUP
- History (presence of conditions or use of medications predisposing to thrombosis, family history of thrombosis), physical examination, laboratory tests, imaging studies.
- Age-appropriate cancer screening.
- No consensus exists regarding screening for thrombophilia; little cost-effectiveness or outcomes data are available. Thrombophilia screening is probably overused, as results usually don't change management.
- Thrombophilia screening is not recommended for primary prevention of VTE, though some advocate testing prior to OC use or pregnancy in women with a strong family history of thrombosis or thrombophilia.
- Screening not recommended if VTE was associated with an identified risk factor. A possible exception is thrombosis associated with pregnancy, the postpartum period or with OC use.
- Unprovoked VTE:
  - Screen individuals for APCR, prothrombin G20210A mutation, protein C, protein S, AT deficiency, and APS if any of the following are present: <50 yr of age at first episode of thrombosis, family history of thrombosis, recurrent thrombosis, thrombosis in unusual anatomic location, life-threatening thrombotic event, warfarin-induced skin necrosis, thrombosis in pregnancy/postpartum period/with OC use, or characteristic pregnancy complications.
  - Screen all Caucasians and all women on HRT for APCR, prothrombin G20210A mutation, and APS.
  - Screen all others for APS.
- Arterial thrombosis: Screen for APS.
- Note: Routine screening for factor VIII level or hyperhomocysteinemia is not recommended.

TIMING OF WORKUP:
- Ideally >2 wk after discontinuation of anticoagulation (except for APS, which requires prolonged anticoagulation).
- Note: Acute thrombosis, anticoagulation, pregnancy, and many medical conditions can affect the results and must be considered in the timing and interpretation of the workup.

LABORATORY TESTS
- CBC with peripheral smear, electrolytes, calcium, renal and liver function tests, prothrombin time/partial thromboplastin time, prostate-specific antigen (in men >50 yr), urinalysis
- Note: Genetic counseling and written informed consent should be obtained before genetic testing. Abnormal nongenetic tests should be repeated after 6 wk to decrease false-positive results.
- APCR: APC-resistance assay (using factor V–deficient plasma) and if positive confirm with genetic test for FVL mutation; use genetic test in pregnancy and if lupus anticoagulant present.
- Prothrombin G20210A mutation test.
- AT deficiency: functional assay (AT-heparin cofactor assay).
- Protein C deficiency: functional assay (activity); may be falsely low in the presence of APCR, elevated factor VIII level, or lupus anticoagulant.
- Protein S deficiency: functional assay (activity) and immunologic assay (free and total level). Functional assay may be falsely low in the presence of APCR, elevated factor VIII level, or lupus anticoagulant.
- APS: any of the following found on two occasions at least 12 wk apart: lupus anticoagulant test or anticardiolipin antibody (IgG and IgM) or anti-B2-glycoprotein-I (IgG and IgM).
- Hyperhomocysteinemia: fasting plasma homocysteine level (if normal but suspicion is high, can proceed with methionine loading test and genotyping for methylene tetrahydrofolate reductase).
- Factor VIII level functional assay.

IMAGING STUDIES
Chest radiograph and other tests as appropriate to diagnose thrombosis and rule out associated conditions

Rx TREATMENT

NONPHARMACOLOGIC THERAPY
OC/HRT use and smoking should be avoided.

PROPHYLAXIS
- Prophylactic anticoagulation in high-risk situations.
- Patients with AT deficiency may benefit from antithrombin concentrates in high-risk situations.
- Although homocysteine levels can be lowered with folic acid, vitamin B_6, and vitamin B_{12} supplements, correcting hyperhomocysteinemia does not decrease risk of thrombosis and routine supplementation is not indicated.
- Vitamin E supplements may decrease risk of VTE in women.
- Pregnancy prophylaxis: timing and intensity of therapy is based on the patient's risk (genetic or acquired defect and clinical history). Women with thrombophilia and recurrent adverse pregnancy outcomes may benefit from prophylaxis with heparin and low-dose aspirin.

ACUTE GENERAL Rx
Initial therapy is the same as for individuals without thrombophilia (exceptions for protein C and AT deficiency).

Venous thrombosis:
- Low-molecular-weight heparin (LMWH) followed by warfarin. Continue heparin for at least 5 days and until international normalized ratio (INR) is therapeutic for 2 consecutive days; continue warfarin for at least 6 to 12 mo. Aim for INR of 2 to 3. Thrombophilia is not associated with a higher risk of recurrent VTE during warfarin therapy. Unfractionated heparin (UH) or Fondaparinux (Factor Xa inhibitor) may be used as alternatives to LMWH. LMWH is preferred over UH (except in patients with massive pulmonary embolism or renal failure) because of equivalent or superior effectiveness and a better safety profile. In cancer patients LMWH for 3 to 6 mo is associated with lower rates of recurrent VTE than warfarin therapy.
- In pregnancy, anticoagulation with heparin throughout pregnancy and for at least 6 wk postpartum. Minimum duration of anticoagulation should be 6 months. LMWH is preferred over UH. Warfarin may be used postpartum.
- Consider thrombolysis or thrombectomy in patients with massive pulmonary embolism or large proximal lower extremity DVT.

Protein C deficiency:
- Warfarin-induced skin necrosis: FFP or protein C concentrates until full anticoagulation with warfarin is achieved.
- After full heparin anticoagulation, begin gradual warfarin loading (2 mg qd for 3 days and increase by 2 to 3 mg qd until target INR is reached). Continue heparin for 5 to 7 days until warfarin-induced anticoagulation is achieved.

AT deficiency:
- AT concentrates may be used if difficulty achieving anticoagulation (heparin resistance), severe thrombosis, or recurrent thrombosis despite adequate anticoagulation.

Arterial thrombosis:

- Anticoagulation and evaluation for thrombolysis or surgery.

Duration of therapy:

- Optimal duration of anticoagulation remains unknown. Length of therapy may be individualized by assessing the risk of recurrence with ultrasonography (looking for residual thrombosis) or D-dimer levels after completion of anticoagulation.
- Must consider risk and benefit; risk of major bleeding 2% to 3% annually in general population on anticoagulation but higher in the elderly (7%-9% per year). Long-term anticoagulation is usually not indicated given the low risk of recurrent thrombosis for most conditions and the bleeding risk associated with anticoagulation.
- Indefinite anticoagulation considered if ≥2 spontaneous thromboses or spontaneous thrombosis associated with any of the following:
  1. Life-threatening thrombosis or thrombosis at an unusual site
  2. More than a single genetic defect
  3. Presence of AT deficiency or APS

DISPOSITION

Depends on underlying condition

REFERRAL

Hematology, maternal-fetal medicine, obstetric medicine

PEARLS & CONSIDERATIONS

- Warfarin therapy effectively reduces the risk of recurrent VTE; when therapy is discontinued VTE risk increases.
- Previous episode of VTE is a major risk factor for recurrence regardless of the presence of thrombophilia. Risk is greatest in the first 2 yr after thrombosis. Approximately 20% of all patients with unprovoked VTE have recurrence within 5 yr.
- Risk of post thrombotic syndrome decreases if compression stockings are worn for at least 1 year, starting in the first month after the DVT.
- Genetic risk factors for thrombosis in non-Caucasians remain largely unknown.
- Interpreting workup: many medical conditions cause acquired abnormalities.
  - Acute thrombosis may be associated with lupus anticoagulant, increased anticardiolipin antibodies, and elevated factor VIII levels
  - Heparin therapy: antithrombin levels decrease by up to 30%; can affect lupus anticoagulant testing
  - Warfarin therapy: cannot measure protein C and protein S (levels and function decrease); antithrombin levels may increase; can affect lupus anticoagulant testing
  - Antithrombin decreases with acute thrombosis (<10 days), surgery, liver disease, disseminated intravascular coagulation (DIC), nephrotic syndrome, chemotherapy, pregnancy, estrogen therapy (HRT, OCs)
  - Protein S levels decrease with acute thrombosis (<10 days), surgery, liver disease, DIC, nephrotic syndrome, HIV infection, chemotherapy, pregnancy (free and total levels may decrease by 60%), estrogen therapy (HRT, OCs)
  - Protein C decreases with acute thrombosis (<10 days), surgery, liver disease, chemotherapy, severe infection, and DIC; levels increase with age and hyperlipidemia
  - APCR is increased with pregnancy, estrogen therapy (HRT, OCs), and certain cancers; elevated factor VIII level and antiphospholipid antibodies can cause APCR

SUGGESTED READINGS

Bates SM et al: Venous thromboembolism, thrombophilia, antithrombotic therapy, and pregnancy: American College of Chest Physicians evidence-based clinical practice guidelines, *Chest* 133(6 Suppl):844S, 2008.

Bauer KA: The thrombophilias: well-defined risk factors with uncertain therapeutic implications, *Ann Intern Med* 135:367, 2001.

Glynn RJ et al: Effects of random allocation to vitamin E supplementation on the occurrence of venous thromboembolism, *Circulation* 116:1497, 2007.

Marques MB, Triplett DA: When to suspect hypercoagulability and how to investigate it, *Ann Diagn Pathol* 5(3):177, 2001.

Minichiello T et al: Diagnosis and management of venous thromboembolism, *Med Clin North Am* 92(2):443, 2008.

Simioni P et al: Inherited thrombophilia and venous thromboembolism, *Semin Thromb Hemost* 32:700, 2006.

AUTHOR: **SUDEEP KAUR AULAKH, M.D.**

BASIC INFORMATION

DEFINITION

Hyperemesis gravidarum is persistent nausea and vomiting with onset in the first trimester of pregnancy, resulting in weight loss and fluid and electrolyte and acid–base imbalances.

ICD-9CM CODES
643.1 Hyperemesis gravidarum

EPIDEMIOLOGY & DEMOGRAPHICS

INCIDENCE: 0.5 to 10 cases per 1000 pregnancies
GENETICS: No genetic disposition

RISK FACTORS:

- Multiple pregnancy
- Molar pregnancy
- Previous history of unsuccessful pregnancy
- Nulliparity
- Hyperemesis gravidarum in a prior pregnancy
- No correlation with race, socioeconomic status, or marital status

PEAK ONSET: 8 to 12 wk of gestation

PHYSICAL FINDINGS & CLINICAL PRESENTATION

- Weight loss
- Rapid heart rate
- Fall in blood pressure
- Dry mucous membranes
- Loss of skin elasticity
- Ketotic odor
- In severe cases, Wernicke's encephalopathy as a result of thiamine deficiency

ETIOLOGY

Specific etiology is unknown.

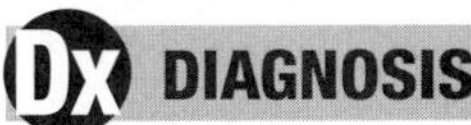

DIAGNOSIS

DIFFERENTIAL DIAGNOSIS

- Pancreatitis
- Cholecystitis
- Hepatitis
- Pyelonephritis

WORKUP

Hyperemesis gravidarum is a diagnosis of exclusion. A detailed history and physical examination along with laboratory tests to rule out other causes of vomiting in early pregnancy are indicated.

LABORATORY TESTS

- Urinalysis to document ketonuria and proteinuria
- Urine culture and sensitivity to rule out pyelonephritis
- Serum electrolytes to rule out electrolyte and acid–base imbalance
- Serum concentration of aminotransferases and bilirubin to rule out hepatitis
- Serum amylase to rule out pancreatitis
- Free T_4 and thyroid-stimulating hormone (TSH). (Elevated T_4 with suppressed TSH levels present in up to 60% of patients with hyperemesis gravidarum. This biochemical hyperthyroidism usually spontaneously resolves after 18 wk.)

IMAGING STUDIES

- Pelvic ultrasound examination to rule out multiple gestation and molar pregnancy
- Ultrasound of the gallbladder to rule out cholecystitis

Rx TREATMENT

NONPHARMACOLOGIC THERAPY

- Reassurance
- Psychologic support
- Avoidance of foods that trigger nausea
- Frequent small meals once oral intake has resumed
- Acupressure with the use of a wrist band
- Ginger has been studied as a promising herbal remedy, but data are relatively sparse

ACUTE GENERAL Rx

- Nothing by mouth order.
- Fluid and electrolyte replacement.
- Parenteral vitamin supplementation.
- Daily supplementation of thiamine 100 mg IM or IV to prevent Wernicke's encephalopathy.
- Pyridoxine (vitamin B_6) 30 mg daily may reduce nausea.
- Antiemetics, such as promethazine (Phenergan) or droperidol (Inapsine), have not been found to be associated with fetal malformations when given in early pregnancy. Promethazine given as a low-dose continuous infusion of 25 mg in each liter of IV fluid has been shown to be effective in controlling nausea and vomiting.
- Restart oral intake gradually no less than 48 hr after vomiting has ceased.

CHRONIC Rx

If the previous acute therapy does not resolve vomiting and oral intake is not feasible, parenteral hyperalimentation may be necessary.

DISPOSITION

- Untreated hyperemesis gravidarum can result in maternal renal and hepatic damage or death from fluid and electrolyte imbalance.
- Hyperemesis gravidarum with severe weight loss has been associated with lower average birth weight and central nervous system malformations in neonates.

REFERRAL

For parenteral hyperalimentation if required

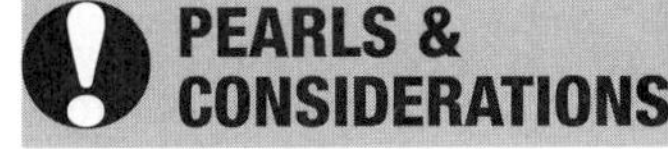

PEARLS & CONSIDERATIONS

COMMENTS

Although the specific etiology of hyperemesis gravidarum is not known, psychogenic causes proposed in older literature have been largely discredited. "Behavioral therapies" for hyperemesis gravidarum are inappropriate.

SUGGESTED READING

Strong T: Alternative therapies of morning sickness, *Clin Obstet Gynecol* 44:653, 2001.

AUTHORS: **LAUREL M. WHITE, M.D.,** and **RUBEN ALVERO, M.D.**

Hypereosinophilic Syndrome

BASIC INFORMATION

DEFINITION

Hypereosinophilic syndrome (HES) refers to a group of disorders of unknown cause characterized by sustained overproduction of eosinophils, in which eosinophilic infiltration and mediators release cause organ dysfunction.

SYNONYMS

Idiopathic hypereosinophilic syndrome (IHES)

ICD-9CM CODES

288.3 Hypereosinophilic syndrome

EPIDEMIOLOGY & DEMOGRAPHICS

PREDOMINANT SEX: Occurs in men more often than women (9:1)

PREDOMINANT AGE: Usually occurs between the ages of 20 and 50 yr

PHYSICAL FINDINGS & CLINICAL PRESENTATION

- Clinical presentation of HES may vary from an incidental finding of eosinophilia to sudden onset of cardiac or neurologic symptoms.
- Early presentation includes fatigue, cough, breathlessness, muscle pain, angioedema, rash, and fever.
- Cardiac manifestations (58%) include dyspnea, orthopnea, and signs and symptoms of congestive heart failure. Including three stages: Acute necrotic stage secondary to endocardial infiltration of eosinophils, Thrombus formation and fibrotic stage. This may result in a restrictive or dilated cardiomyopathy and/or valvular heart disease.
- Neurologic manifestations (54%) may be of three types:
  1. Thromboembolic (e.g., cardiac emboli or local vascular thrombosis)
  2. CNS dysfunction: confusion, loss of memory, ataxia, upper motor neuron signs, seizures, and behavior changes
  3. Peripheral neuropathy (most common) may be symmetric or asymmetric, sensory or mixed sensory and motor deficits
- Pulmonary manifestations (40%) include a chronic persistent nonproductive cough, shortness of breath, and dyspnea on exertion. Diffuse or focal infiltrate may present in 20% of cases. Complications may include pulmonary fibrosis, congestive heart failure (CHF), or pulmonary embolus (PE).
- Cutaneous manifestations (56%) usually include eczema, lichenifications, urticaria, angioedema, or erythematous pruritic papules and nodules.
- GI manifestations (23%) include diarrhea, but findings of gastritis, colitis, pancreatitis, cholangitis, and hepatitis can occur.
- Ocular manifestations (23%) are thought to be the result of retinal microemboli.
- Vascular manifestations include venous or arterial thrombosis of unknown mechanism such as femoral artery occlusion, intracranial sinus thrombosis, and digital gangrene.

ETIOLOGY

- The etiology of HES is unknown and is thought of as a composite of many diseases.
- In some cases, a fusion event generating an abnormal and oncogenic tyrosine kinase (FIP1L1-PDGFRA) appears to be causative especially in males.

Dx DIAGNOSIS

Criteria for the diagnosis of idiopathic HES include:

- Persistent eosinophilia of $>$1500 eosinophils/mm^3 for more than 6 mo
- Exclusion of other conditions causing eosinophilia (e.g., parasites, allergies)
- Signs and symptoms of organ system dysfunction (e.g., heart, liver, lung)

DIFFERENTIAL DIAGNOSIS

The differential includes all causes of peripheral blood eosinophilia. Parasitic infections, coccidioidomycosis, cat-scratch disease, asthma, Churg-Strauss syndrome, allergic rhinitis, atopic dermatitis, drugs-induced eosinophilia, aspergillosis, eosinophilic pneumonia, hypersensitivity pneumonitis, HIV, eosinophilic gastroenteritis, inflammatory bowel disease, leukemias (CML and CMML), systemic mastocytosis with eosinophilia.

WORKUP

The workup of a patient who is suspected of having HES should exclude other causes mentioned in the "Differential Diagnosis" section leading to peripheral eosinophilia.

LABORATORY TESTS

- CBC with differential; often the total WBC ranges from 10,000 to 30,000/mm^3 with eosinophilia of 30% to 70%, anemia is present in 50% of the cases, and either thrombocytopenia or thrombocytosis may be noted
- Erythrocyte sedimentation rate (ESR) and rheumatoid factor
- Liver function tests (LFTs), electrolytes, urinalysis, BUN, and creatinine
- HIV assay
- Stools for ova and parasites $\times$3
- Serologic blood tests for parasitic infections (e.g., Strongyloides)
- Total IgE level
- Bone marrow aspirate and biopsy
- Duodenal aspirate
- ECG
- Tissue biopsies as indicated
- Serum levels of vitamin B_{12}
- Serum levels of tryptase

IMAGING STUDIES

- Chest radiograph may be clear or show infiltrates, effusions, or fibrotic scarring
- CT scan of chest, abdomen, and pelvis
- Echocardiogram (or cardiac MRI for early cardiac involvement) can assess for ventricular function and valvular pathology including regurgitation and thrombi formation

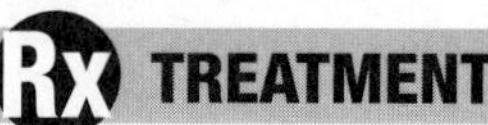

TREATMENT

Treatment is initiated only if there is evidence of organ involvement.

NONPHARMACOLOGIC THERAPY

In patients with hypereosinophilia without organ involvement, serial echocardiograms, blood chemistries, and pulmonary function tests are recommended at 6-mo intervals.

ACUTE GENERAL Rx

- In patients with organ involvement without FIP1L1-PDGFRA fusion, initial therapy is with prednisone 1 mg/kg/day or 60 mg/day in adults.
- Patient's symptoms and peripheral eosinophil counts are monitored.
- Doses may be tapered to alternate-day prednisone use in patients whose eosinophil counts have been suppressed.

CHRONIC Rx

- Patients not responding to corticosteroids, hydroxyurea 1 to 2 g/day may be tried.
- Patient with FIP1L1-PDGFRA fusion with or without organ involvement should be started on tyrosine kinase imatinib or dasatinib for resistant cases.
- If the disease continues to progress, vincristine, etoposide, interferon-α, cyclosporine, and leukapheresis are alternative choices.
- Anticoagulation and/or antiplatelet agents are often used in patients with HES.
- If all else fails, bone marrow transplantation may be considered.

DISPOSITION

- Before the use of cardiac imaging (echo) and cardiac surgeries (valve replacement), patients with HES had a poor prognosis with a mean survival of 9 mo and a 3-yr survival of 12%.
- Deaths usually result from congestive heart failure, endocarditis, and systemic emboli.
- 5-yr and 15-yr survival rates are 80% and 42%, respectively.

REFERRAL

HES is a rare and complicated disorder requiring a multidisciplinary approach.

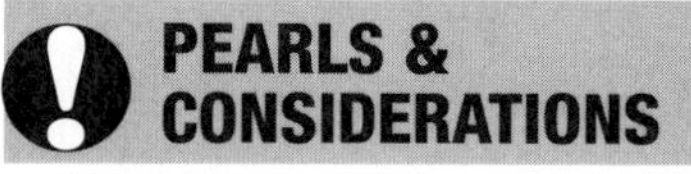

PEARLS & CONSIDERATIONS

COMMENTS

There is still much to be learned about HES. The etiology and exact mechanism of organ damage caused by eosinophils remains unknown.

SUGGESTED READINGS

Katz HT et al: Pediatric hypereosinophilic syndrome (HES) differs from adult HES, *J Pediatr* 146(1):134, 2005.

Tefferi A et al: Hypereosinophilic syndrome and clonal eosinophilia: point-of-care diagnostic algorithm and treatment update, *Mayo Clin Proc* 85(2):158-164, 2004.

AUTHORS: **MONZR M. AL MALKI, M.D., DENNIS J. MIKOLICH, M.D.,** and **GLENN G. FORT, M.D., M.P.H.**

BASIC INFORMATION

DEFINITION

Primary hyperlipoproteinemia is a group of genetic disorders of the lipid transport proteins in the blood that manifests as abnormally elevated levels of cholesterol, triglycerides, or both in the serum of affected patients (Table 1-41).

SYNONYMS

Hyperlipidemia

ICD-9CM CODES
272.4 Hyperlipoproteinemia
272.3 Fredrickson type I
272.0 Fredrickson type IIa
272.2 Fredrickson type IIb, III
272.1 Fredrickson type IV
272.3 Fredrickson type V

EPIDEMIOLOGY & DEMOGRAPHICS

INCIDENCE:
- Variable depending on the genetic defect
- Spectrum spans the common familial hypercholesterolemia, with an incidence of 1:500, to the rare familial lipoprotein lipase deficiency

PREDOMINANT SEX: None

GENETICS:
- Familial lipoprotein lipase deficiency: autosomal recessive, resulting in an elevation in the plasma chylomicrons and triglycerides
- Familial apoprotein CII deficiency: autosomal recessive, resulting in increased serum chylomicrons, very-low-density lipoprotein (VLDL), and hypertriglyceridemia
- Familial type 3 hyperlipoproteinemia: single-gene defect requiring contributory factors to manifest
- Familial hypercholesterolemia: autosomal-dominant defect of the LDL receptor, resulting in an elevated serum cholesterol level and normal triglycerides
- Familial hypertriglyceridemia: common, autosomal-dominant defect resulting in elevated VLDL and triglycerides
- Multiple lipoprotein–type hyperlipidemia: autosomal dominant, manifesting as isolated hypercholesterolemia, isolated hypertriglyceridemia, or hyperlipidemia
- Polygenic hypercholesterolemia: multifactorial
- Polygenic hyperalphalipoproteinemia: autosomal dominant or polygenic, causing an elevated high-density lipoprotein

PHYSICAL FINDINGS & CLINICAL PRESENTATION

- Familial lipoprotein lipase deficiency: recurrent bouts of abdominal pain in infancy, eruptive xanthomas, hepatomegaly, splenomegaly, lipemia retinalis
- Familial apoprotein CII deficiency: occasional eruptive xanthomas
- Familial type 3 hyperlipoproteinemia: after age 20 yr see xanthoma striata palmaris or tuberoeruptive xanthomas, xanthelasmas, arterial bruits at a young age, gangrene of the lower extremities at a young age
- Familial hypercholesterolemia: tendon xanthomas, arcus corneae, xanthelasma
- Familial hypertriglyceridemia: associated obesity; eruptive xanthomas can develop with exacerbations
- Multiple lipoprotein type hyperlipidemia: no discerning physical findings
- Polygenic hypercholesterolemia: no discerning physical findings
- Polygenic hyperalphalipoproteinemia: no discerning physical findings

ETIOLOGY

Genetic defects causing lipid abnormalities

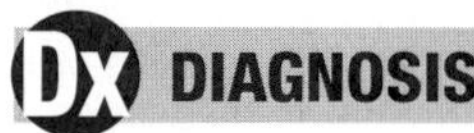

DIAGNOSIS

DIFFERENTIAL DIAGNOSIS

Secondary causes of hyperlipoproteinemias:
- Diabetes mellitus
- Glycogen storage diseases
- Lipodystrophies
- Glucocorticoid use/excess
- Alcohol
- Oral contraceptives
- Renal disease
- Hepatic dysfunction

WORKUP

- Detailed family history for premature cardiac disease
- Recurrent pancreatitis
- Thorough physical examination

LABORATORY TESTS

- Lipoprotein analysis
- Lipoprotein electrophoresis
- Risk factor stratification for medications; see "Hypercholesterolemia"

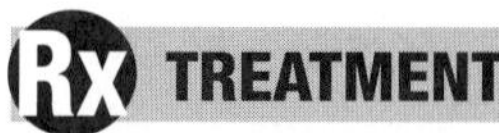

TREATMENT

NONPHARMACOLOGIC THERAPY

- Cornerstone of treatment: dietary therapy
  - TLC diet (*t*herapeutic *l*ifestyle *c*hanges): 7% total calories from saturated fat, ≤10%

TABLE 1-41 Classification of Lipoprotein Disorders by Phenotypes, Genotypes, and Corresponding Clinical Manifestations

	PLASMA LIPID LEVELS				
Phenotype	**Cholesterol**	**Triglyceride**	**Genotype**	**Xanthomas**	**Other Clinical Manifestations**
I	Normal or elevated	Elevated lipemia	Familial lipoprotein lipase deficiency, Apo C-II deficiency	Eruptive, tuberoeruptive	Recurrent abdominal pain, other gastrointestinal symptoms, hepatosplenomegaly
IIA	Normal aortic stenosis (homozygous FHC)	Elevated	FHC, familial combined hyperlipidemia—polygenic and sporadic hypercholesterolemia	Tendinous, xanthelasma, tuberous; planar (homozygous)	Premature CAD, arcus corneae, arthritic symptoms
IIB	Elevated	Elevated	Familial combined hyperlipidemia, FHC		
III	Elevated	Elevated	Familial dysbetalipoproteinemia	Planar (especially palmar), tuberous	Premature CAD and peripheral vascular disease, male > female, obesity, abnormal glucose tolerance, hyperuricemia, aggravated by hypothyroiditis, good response to therapy
IV	Normal or elevated	Elevated symptoms, gallbladder disease	Familial hypertriglyceridemia, familial combined hyperlipidemia, sporadic hypertriglyceridemia	Usually none; rarely eruptive or tuberoeruptive	CAD and peripheral vascular disease, obesity, abnormal glucose tolerance, hyperuricemia, arthritic
V	Normal or elevated	Elevated	Homozygous FHC	Eruptive, tuberoeruptive	Recurrent abdominal pain, other gastrointestinal symptoms, hepatosplenomegaly, peripheral paresthesia

From Graber MA: *The family practice handbook,* ed 4, St Louis, 2001, Mosby.
Apo, Apolipoprotein; *CAD,* coronary artery disease; *FHC,* familial hypercholesterolemia.

total calories from polyunsaturated fat, ≤20% total calories from monounsaturated fat
  - Fat 25% to 30% of total calories
  - Fiber 20 to 30 g/day
  - Cholesterol <200 mg/day
- Risk factor reduction includes smoking cessation, treatment of hypertension, exercise
- Familial lipoprotein lipase deficiency and familial apoprotein CII deficiency: fat-free diet
- Remainder of cases, except those with polygenic hyperalphalipoproteinemia: fat- and cholesterol-restricted diets

ACUTE GENERAL Rx

No acute treatment needed

CHRONIC Rx

- Familial lipoprotein lipase deficiency, polygenic hyperalphalipoproteinemia, or familial apoprotein CII deficiency: no chronic drug therapy
- Familial type 3 hyperlipoproteinemia: usually responds well to secondary causes being treated and diet therapy; if not, fibric acids may be tried
- Familial hypercholesterolemia: bile acid sequestrants, HMG-CoA reductase inhibitors, or niacin
- Familial hypertriglyceridemia: fibric acids
- Multiple lipoprotein–type hyperlipidemia: drug therapy aimed at the predominant lipid abnormality noted
- Recent data suggest in patients with lipoprotein abnormalities that treatment goals should be based on non-HDL cholesterol rather than LDL cholesterol

DISPOSITION

- Those with polygenic hyperalphalipoproteinemia: excellent prognosis for longevity
- Those with familial hypercholesterolemia, familial type 3 hypercholesterolemia, or multiple lipoprotein type hyperlipidemia: even with aggressive treatment, at high risk for accelerated atherosclerosis and coronary artery disease

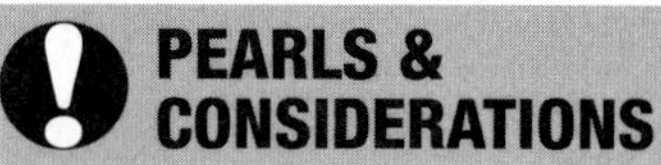

PEARLS & CONSIDERATIONS

COMMENTS

- Patient information is available through the American Heart Association.
- See Tables 1-42 and 1-43 and Boxes 1-4 through 1-8.
- Lipid-lowering drug therapy is recommended for children 10 years and older whose LDL-C levels remain extremely elevated after 6 months to one year of dietary modification.

TABLE 1-42 LDL Cholesterol Goals and Cutpoints for Therapeutic Lifestyle Changes and Drug Therapy in Different Risk Categories

Risk Category	LDL Goal (mg/dl)	LDL Level at Which to Initiate Therapeutic Lifestyle Changes (mg/dl)	LDL Level at Which to Consider Drug Therapy (mg/dl)
CHD or CHD risk equivalents (10-yr risk >20%)	<100	≥100	≥130 (100-129: drug optional)*
2+ risk factors (10-yr risk ≤20%)	<130	≥130	10-yr risk 10%-20%: ≥130 10-yr risk <10%: ≥1600
0-1 risk factor†	<160	≥160	≥190 (160-189: LDL-lowering drug optional)

From National Cholesterol Education Program: Expert Panel on Detection, Evaluation, and Treatment of High Blood Cholesterol in Adults (Adult Treatment Panel III), *JAMA* 285:2486, 2001.
CHD, Coronary heart disease; *LDL,* low-density lipoprotein.
*Some authorities recommend use of LDL-lowering drugs in this category if an LDL cholesterol level of <100 mg/dl cannot be achieved by therapeutic lifestyle changes. Others prefer use of drugs that primarily modify triglycerides and HDL (e.g., nicotinic acid or fibrate). Clinical judgment also may call for deferring drug therapy in this subcategory.
†Almost all people with 0-1 risk factor have a 10-year risk <10%; thus 10-year risk assessment in people with 0-1 risk factor is not necessary.

TABLE 1-43 Comparison of LDL Cholesterol and Non–HDL Cholesterol Goals for Three Risk Categories

Risk Category	LDL Goal (mg/dl)	Non-HDL Goal (mg/dl)
CHD and CHD risk equivalent (10-yr risk for CHD >20%)	<70	<130
Multiple (2+) risk factors and 10-yr risk ≤20%	<130	<160
0-1 risk factor	<160	<190

From National Cholesterol Education Program: Expert Panel on Detection, Evaluation, and Treatment of High Blood Cholesterol in Adults (Adult Treatment Panel III), *JAMA* 285:2486, 2001.
CHD, Coronary heart disease; *HDL,* high-density lipoprotein; *LDL,* low-density lipoprotein.

BOX 1-4 Nutrient Composition of the Therapeutic Lifestyle Changes (TLC) Diet

Nutrient	Recommended Intake
Saturated fat*	<7% of total calories
Polyunsaturated fat	Up to 10% of total calories
Monounsaturated fat	Up to 20% of total calories
Total fat	25%-35% of total calories
Carbohydrate†	50%-60% of total calories
Fiber	20-30 g/day
Protein	Approximately 15% of total calories
Cholesterol	<200 mg/day
Total calories‡	Balance energy intake and expenditure to maintain desirable body weight/prevent weight gain

From National Cholesterol Education Program Expert Panel on Detection, Evaluation, and Treatment of High Blood Cholesterol in Adults (Adult Treatment Panel III), National Institutes of Health, *JAMA* 285:2486, 2001.
*Trans fatty acids are another LDL-raising fat that should be kept at a low intake.
†Carbohydrates should be derived predominantly from foods rich in complex carbohydrates, including grains, especially whole grains, fruits, and vegetables.
‡Daily energy expenditure should include at least moderate physical activity (contributing approximately 200 kcal/day).

Drug therapy also can be considered for children with LDL-C levels of 190 mg/dl or greater. Children who may also require treatment are those whose levels are > 160 mg/dl and who have two or more risk factors for CVD or a family history of premature CVD.

SUGGESTED READINGS

Alawadhi M et al: Genetic lipoprotein disorders and coronary atherosclerosis, *Curr Atheroscler Rep* 7(3): 196, 2005.

American Heart Association: Drug therapy for lipid abnormalities in children and adolescents, *Circulation,* April 10, 2007

Brunzell JD: Hypertriglyceridemia, *N Engl J Med* 357: 1009-17, 2007

National Cholesterol Education Program: Second report on the Expert Panel on Detection, Evaluation and Treatment Of High Cholesterol in Adults (Adult Treatment Panel III), *JAMA* 285:2486, 2001.

Sharma M et al: Systematic review: comparative effectiveness and harms of combination therapy and monotherapy for dysplidemia, *Ann Int Med* 151: 622-630, 2009.

Sveger T, Nordborg K: Apolipoprotein B as a marker of familial hyperlipoproteinemia, *J Atheroscler Thromb* 11(5):286, 2004.

AUTHORS: **BETH J. WUTZ, M.D.,** and **RUBEN ALVERO, M.D.**

BOX 1-5 ATP III Classification of LDL, Total, and HDL Cholesterol (mg/dl)

LDL cholesterol	
<100	Optimal
100-129	Near or above optimal
130-159	Borderline high
160-189	High
≥190	Very high
Total cholesterol	
<200	Desirable
200-239	Borderline high
>240	High
HDL cholesterol	
<40	Low
>60	High

From National Cholesterol Education Program Expert Panel on Detection, Evaluation, and Treatment of High Blood Cholesterol in Adults (Adult Treatment Panel III), National Institutes of Health, *JAMA* 285:2486, 2001.

ATP, Adult treatment panel; *HDL,* high-density lipoprotein, *LDL,* low-density lipoprotein.

BOX 1-6 Major Risk Factors (Exclusive of LDL Cholesterol) That Modify LDL Goals*

Cigarette smoking

Hypertension (blood pressure ≥140/90 mm Hg or on antihypertensive medication)

Low HDL cholesterol (<40 mg/dl)†

Family history of premature CHD (CHD in male first-degree relative) (<55 yr; CHD in female first-degree relative <65 yr)

Age (men ≥45 yr; women ≥55 yr)

From National Cholesterol Education Program Expert Panel on Detection, Evaluation, and Treatment of High Blood Cholesterol in Adults (Adult Treatment Panel III), National Institutes of Health, *JAMA* 285:2486, 2001.

HDL, High-density lipoprotein; *LDL,* low-density lipoprotein.

*Diabetes is regarded as a coronary heart disease (CHD) risk equivalent.

†HDL cholesterol >60 mg/dl counts as a "negative" risk factor; its presence removes 1 risk factor from the total count.

BOX 1-7 Interventions to Improve Adherence

Focus on the Patient

Simplify medication regimens

Provide explicit patient instruction and use good counseling techniques to teach the patient how to follow the prescribed treatment

Encourage the use of prompts to help patients remember treatment regimens

Use systems to reinforce adherence and maintain contact with the patient

Encourage the support of family and friends

Reinforce and reward adherence

Increase visits for patients unable to achieve treatment goal

Increase the convenience and access to care

Involve patients in their care through self-monitoring

Focus on the Physician and Medical Office

Teach physicians to implement lipid treatment guidelines

Use reminders to prompt physicians to attend to lipid management

Identify a patient advocate in the office to help deliver or prompt care

Use patients to prompt preventive care

Develop a standardized treatment plan to structure care

Use feedback from past performance to foster change in future care

Remind patients of appointments and follow up missed appointments

Focus on the Health Delivery System

Provide lipid management through a lipid clinic

Utilize case management by nurses

Deploy telemedicine

Utilize the collaborative care of pharmacists

Execute critical care pathways in hospitals

From National Cholesterol Education Program Expert Panel on Detection, Evaluation, and Treatment of High Blood Cholesterol in Adults (Adult Treatment Panel III), National Institutes of Health, *JAMA* 285:2486, 2001.

BOX 1-8 Clinical Identification of the Metabolic Syndrome

Risk factor	Defining level
Abdominal obesity* (waist circumference)†	
Men	>102 cm (>40 in)
Women	>88 cm (>35 in)
Triglycerides	>150 mg/dl
High-density lipoprotein cholesterol	
Men	<40 mg/dl
Women	<50 mg/dl
Blood pressure	>130/>85 mm Hg
Fasting glucose	>110 mg/dl

From National Cholesterol Education Program Expert Panel on Detection, Evaluation, and Treatment of High Blood Cholesterol in Adults (Adult Treatment Panel III), National Institutes of Health, *JAMA* 285:2486, 2001.

*Overweight and obesity are associated with insulin resistance and the metabolic syndrome. However, the presence of abdominal obesity is more highly correlated with the metabolic risk factors than is an elevated body mass index (BMI). Therefore, the simple measure of waist circumference is recommended to identify the body weight component of the metabolic syndrome.

†Some male patients can develop multiple metabolic risk factors when the waist circumference is only marginally increased, for example, 94-102 cm (37-40 in). Such patients may have strong genetic contribution to insulin resistance, and they should benefit from changes in life habits, similarly to men with categorical increases in waist circumference.

Hyperosmolar Hyperglycemic Syndrome

BASIC INFORMATION

DEFINITION

Hyperosmolar hyperglycemic syndrome (HHS) is a state of extreme hyperglycemia, marked dehydration, serum hyperosmolarity, altered mental status, and absence of ketoacidosis.

SYNONYMS

HHS
Hyperosmolar coma
Nonketotic hyperosmolar syndrome
Hyperosmolar nonketotic state

ICD-9CM CODES
250.2 Hyperosmolar coma

PHYSICAL FINDINGS & CLINICAL PRESENTATION

- Evidence of extreme dehydration (poor skin turgor, sunken eyeballs, dry mucous membranes)
- Neurologic defects (reversible hemiplegia, focal seizures)
- Orthostatic hypotension, tachycardia
- Evidence of precipitating factors (pneumonia, infected skin ulcer)
- Coma (25% of patients), delirium

ETIOLOGY

- Infections, 20% to 25% (e.g., pneumonia, urinary tract infection, sepsis)
- New or previously unrecognized diabetes (30% to 50%)
- Reduction or omission of diabetic medication
- Stress (myocardial infarction, cerebrovascular accident)
- Drugs: diuretics (dehydration), phenytoin, diazoxide (impaired insulin secretion), glucocorticoids, chemotherapeutic agents, calcium channel blockers, total parenteral nutrition, substance abuse (alcohol, cocaine)

Dx DIAGNOSIS

DIFFERENTIAL DIAGNOSIS

- Diabetic ketoacidosis
- The differential diagnosis of coma is described in Section II

LABORATORY TESTS

- Hyperglycemia: serum glucose usually >600 mg/dl, serum/urine ketones absent or "small."
- Hyperosmolarity: serum osmolarity usually >320 mOsm/L.
- Serum sodium: may be low, normal, or high; if normal or high, the patient is severely dehydrated because an elevated glucose draws fluid from intracellular space, decreasing the serum sodium. The corrected sodium can be obtained by increasing the serum sodium concentration by 1.6 mEq/dl for every 100 mg/dl increase in the serum glucose level over normal.
- Serum potassium: may be low, normal, or high; regardless of the initial serum level, the total body deficit is approximately 5 to 15 mEq/kg.
- Serum bicarbonate: usually >15 mEq/L (average 17 mEq/L).
- Arterial pH: usually >7.3; both serum bicarbonate and arterial pH may be lower if lactic acidosis is present.
- Blood urea nitrogen: azotemia (prerenal) is usually present (generally ranges from 60 to 90 mg/dl).
- Phosphorus: hypophosphatemia (average deficit is 70 to 140 mm).
- Calcium: hypocalcemia (average deficit is 50 to 100 mEq).
- Magnesium: hypomagnesemia (average deficit is 50 to 100 mEq).
- Complete blood count with differential, urinalysis, and blood and urine cultures should be performed to rule out infectious etiology.
- ECG to rule out a concomitant myocardial infarction.

IMAGING STUDIES

Chest radiograph is useful to rule out infectious process. The initial radiograph may be negative if the patient has significant dehydration. Repeat chest x-ray after 24 hr of hydration if pulmonary infection is suspected.

Rx TREATMENT

NONPHARMACOLOGIC THERAPY

- Monitor mental status, vital signs, urine output hourly until improved, then monitor q2-4h.
- Monitor electrolytes, renal function, and glucose level (see "Acute General Rx").

ACUTE GENERAL Rx

- Vigorous fluid replacement: the volume and rate of fluid replacement are determined by renal and cardiac function. Typically, infuse 1000 to 1500 ml/hr for the initial 1 to 2 L; then decrease the rate of infusion to 500 ml/hr and monitor urinary output, blood chemistries, and blood pressure. Use 0.9% NS (isotonic solution) if the patient is hypotensive or serum osmolarity is <320 mOsm/L; otherwise use 0.45% NS solution. Slower infusion rate may be used initially in patients with compromised cardiovascular or renal status. When serum glucose reaches 300 mg/dl, change to 5% dextrose with 0.45% NS.
- Replace electrolytes and monitor serum levels frequently (e.g., serum sodium and potassium q2h for the first 12 hr). KCl replacement in patients with normal renal function and adequate urinary output when the serum potassium level is <5.2 mEq/L (e.g., 10 mEq KCl/hr if potassium level is 4 to 5.2 mEq/L). Continuous telemetry monitoring and hourly measurement of urinary output are recommended. In patients with severe hypokalemia (potassium <3.3 mEq/L), give 40 mEq of potassium/hr until potassium is >3.3 mEq/L.
- Correct hyperglycemia. The goal is for plasma glucose to decline by at least 50 to 100 mg/dl/hr.
    1. Vigorous IV hydration will decrease the serum glucose level in most patients by 80 mg/dl/hr; a regular insulin IV bolus (0.15 U/kg of body weight) is often not necessary. Insulin should not be administered until serum potassium is >3.3 mEq/L to prevent life-threatening hypokalemia.
    2. Low-dose insulin infusion at 0.1 U/kg/hr (e.g., 25 U of regular insulin in 250 ml of 0.9% saline solution at 20 ml/hr) until the serum glucose level approaches 300 mg/dl; then the patient is started on regular SC insulin with sliding scale coverage. If the plasma glucose level does not decrease over 2 to 4 hr despite adequate fluid administration and urine output, consider doubling the hourly insulin dose.
    3. Glucose should be monitored q1-2h in the initial 12 hr.
- In the absence of renal failure, phosphate can be administered at a rate of 0.1 mmol/kg/hr (5 to 10 mmol/hr) to a maximum of 80 to 120 mmol in 24 hr. Magnesium replacement, in the absence of renal failure, can be administered IM (0.05 to 0.10 ml/kg of 20% magnesium sulfate) or as IV infusion (4 to 8 ml of 20% magnesium sulfate [0.08 to 0.16 mEq/kg]). Repeat magnesium, phosphate, and calcium levels should be obtained after 12 to 24 hr.
- On day 2 begin or resume feeding if patient is able and glucose is under control (<200 mg/dl). Begin or resume SC insulin. For patients with type 2 diabetes, a mixture of N+R insulin is preferred, timing the injection with a planned meal. Total daily dose (TDD) can be 0.5 U/kg. Insulin proportions are typically 60% in the AM and 40% in the PM.
- AM dose: TDD × 0.4 = AM, NPH insulin
- TDD × 0.2 = AM, regular insulin
- PM dose: TDD × 0.2 = PM, NPH insulin
- TDD × 0.2 = PM, regular insulin
- Individual patients may be appropriate for a trial of oral agents.

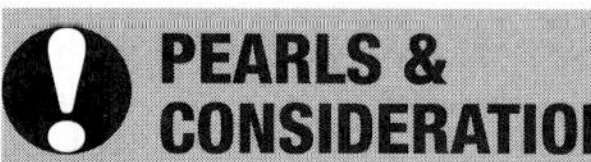

PEARLS & CONSIDERATIONS

COMMENTS

The typical patient is an elderly or bed-confined diabetic with impaired ability to communicate thirst who is evaluated after an interval of 1 to 2 wk of prolonged osmotic diuresis.

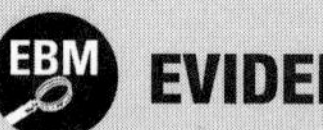

EVIDENCE

Please note: Complete text of EBM for this topic is available online.

SUGGESTED READINGS

Delaney MF et al: Diabetic ketoacidosis and hyperglycemic hyperosmolar nonketotic syndrome, *Endocrinol Metab Clin North Am* 29:683-705, 2000.

Kitabchi AE et al: Hyperglycemic crises in adult patients with diabetes: a consensus statement from the American Diabetes Association, *Diabetes Care* 29:2739-2748, 2006.

Stoner GD: Hyperosmolar hyperglycemic state, *Am Fam Physician* 71:1723, 2005.

AUTHORS: **FRED F. FERRI, M.D.**, **SHAHNAZ PUNJANI, M.D.**, and **WEN-CHIH WU, M.D.**

BASIC INFORMATION

DEFINITION

Hyperparathyroidism is an endocrine disorder caused by excessive secretion of parathyroid hormone (PTH) from the parathyroid glands. Autonomous production of PTH resulting in hypercalcemia defines primary hyperparathyroidism. Secondary hyperparathyroidism occurs when the parathyroid glands appropriately increase PTH production in response to low calcium states. Primary hyperparathyroidism is the focus of this section.

ICD-9CM CODES

252.00	Hyperparathyroidism, unspecified
252.01	Hyperparathyroidism, primary
252.02	Hyperparathyroidism, secondary (non-renal)
588.81	Hyperparathyroidism, secondary (renal)

EPIDEMIOLOGY & DEMOGRAPHICS

INCIDENCE: 2 cases /100,000 person-years
PREVALENCE: 1 case/1000 persons
PREDOMINANT SEX AND AGE: Women:men 2:1, peaks 50 to 60 yr

PHYSICAL FINDINGS & CLINICAL PRESENTATION

The majority of patients with primary hyperparathyroidism are asymptomatic. The development of symptoms varies with severity and rapidity of disease progression and reflects both the hypercalcemic and hyperparathyroid components of the disease process.

- Cardiovascular: hypertension, shortened QT interval, arrhythmia, valvular calcification
- GI: anorexia, nausea, vomiting, constipation, abdominal pain, peptic ulcer disease, pancreatitis
- GU: nephrolithiasis, nephrocalcinosis, renal insufficiency, polyuria, nocturia, nephrogenic diabetes insipidus, renal tubular acidosis
- Musculoskeletal: weakness, myopathy, bone pain, osteoporosis, gout, pseudogout, chondrocalcinosis, osteitis fibrosa cystica
- CNS: confusion, anxiety, fatigue, obtundation, depression, coma
- Other: hypomagnesemia, hypophosphatemia, pruritus, metastatic calcifications, band keratopathy

ETIOLOGY

Most cases of primary hyperparathyroidism are sporadic but it can be associated with rare genetic conditions such as multiple endocrine neoplasia (MEN)-1 and MEN-2. Pathologic characteristics include adenoma (89%), hyperplasia (10%), or carcinomas (<1%).

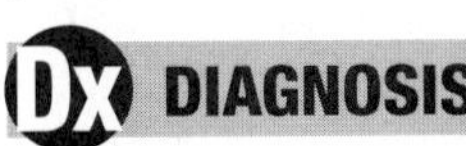

DIAGNOSIS

DIFFERENTIAL DIAGNOSIS

- Other causes of hyperparathyroidism (i.e., secondary hyperparathyroidism) include:
  - Medication: loop diuretics
  - Calcium or vitamin D deficiency
  - Chronic kidney disease
  - Pseudohypoparathyroidism (PTH resistance)
- Other causes of hypercalcemia include:
  - Medications: thiazide diuretics, lithium therapy
  - Vitamin D intoxication, milk-alkali syndrome
  - Familial hypocalciuric hypercalcemia (FHH)
  - Renal failure (tertiary hyperparathyroidism)
  - Granulomatous disorders (e.g., sarcoidosis)
  - Malignancy (e.g., lung cancer, lymphoma, myeloma, bone metastasis)
  - Prolonged immobilization

WORKUP

- Primary hyperparathyroidism is confirmed with an elevated serum calcium and PTH level.
  - Two measurements of serum calcium are required for the confirmation of hypercalcemia. Total calcium should be corrected for low albumin utilizing the formula: Corrected Calcium = (0.8 × [4 – serum albumin]) + serum calcium). If a reliable laboratory is available, an ionized calcium should be considered especially in condition associated with acid-base disturbances or low albumin states.
  - The serum intact PTH (iPTH) level is the single best test to evaluate the etiology of hypercalcemia. PTH is elevated in hyperparathyroidism and decreased in most other conditions associated with elevated calcium.
- Rule out other causes of hypercalcemia. These are typically associated with low PTH levels. Exceptions include lithium use and FHH.
  - Review medication history to determine lithium, thiazide, vitamin D or calcium intake
  - Check 24-hr urine calcium:creatinine to rule out FHH. Urine calcium is usually low in FHH and high in hyperparathyroidism. PTH can be low, normal, or high in FHH.
  - Consider parathyroid hormone–related peptide (PTHrP) to evaluate hypercalcemia related to malignancies and vitamin D1,25 to assess hypercalcemia secondary to glaucomatous diseases or lymphomas. Multiple myeloma and bone metastasis can also result in a high calcium state and therefore must be appropriately evaluated.
- Rule out other causes of elevated PTH (i.e., secondary hyperparathyroidism). Serum calcium is typically low or low-normal in secondary hyperparathyroidism.
  - Check calcium and 25 OH-vitamin D to rule out deficiency states.
  - Assess renal function to evaluate for chronic renal failures.

LABORATORY TESTS

- Elevated serum calcium (ionized or corrected calcium)
- Low or low-normal serum phosphorus
- Elevated PTH
- 24-hr urine calcium to evaluate risk for renal stones and to rule out FHH
- Rule out other etiologies for hypercalcemia by checking PTHrp and 1,25 OH-vitamin D levels.
- Evaluation of 25 OH-vitamin D is recommended in all patients with hyperparathyroidism. Vitamin D deficiency can decrease calcium and increase PTH levels. Due to the clinical impact of vitamin D deficiency, normalization is required prior to making any diagnostic and therapeutic decisions.
- ECG may reveal shortening of the QT interval secondary to severe hypercalcemia (>12 mg/dl)

IMAGING STUDIES

- Parathyroid localization with technetium-99m sestamibi can identify potential adenomas.
- Bone mineral density of the spine, hip, and forearm is recommended for all patients with hyperparathyroidism in order to assess the risk for osteoporosis and fragility fractures. Cortical bone loss (i.e., forearm or hip) is greater in hyperparathyroidism.
- Renal ultrasound can be considered to assess asymptomatic renal stones.
- Plain x-rays may reveal high bone turnover (Fig. 1-164).

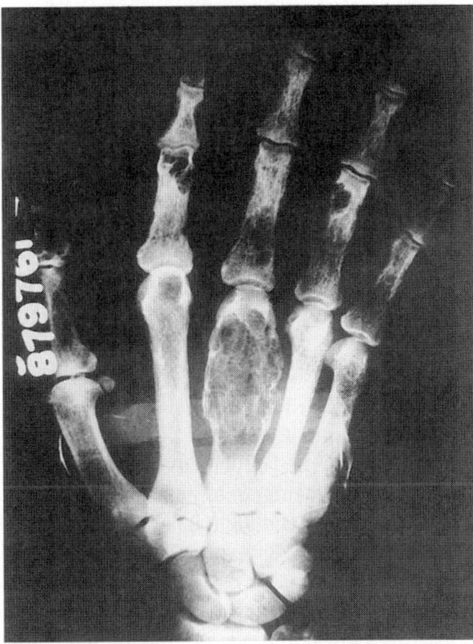

FIGURE 1-164 Radiograph of hand from a patient with severe primary hyperparathyroidism. Note the dramatic remodeling associated with the intense region of high bone turnover in the third metacarpal in addition to widespread evidence of subperiosteal and trabecular resorption. (Courtesy Fuller Albright Collection, Massachusetts General Hospital. From Larsen PR et al [eds]: *Williams textbook of endocrinology,* ed 10, Philadelphia, 2003, WB Saunders.)

Rx TREATMENT

NONPHARMACOLOGIC THERAPY

- Surgery is the only definitive treatment for symptomatic primary hyperparathyroidism. Surgery can normalize calcium levels, decrease the risk for kidney stones, increase bone mineral density, and improve quality of life measures.
  - Indications for parathyroidectomy
    1. All patients younger than 50 yr
    2. Hypercalcemia (Ca > 1 mg/dl above upper limit normal)
    3. Creatinine clearance < 60 ml/min
    4. Osteoporosis (T-score < −2.5 or fragility fracture)
    5. Symptomatic hyperparathyroidism such as nephrolithiasis
  - Surgical approaches include:
    1. The conventional surgical approach is bilateral neck exploration under general anesthesia. An experienced endocrine surgeon cures >95% of patients undergoing bilateral neck exploration and incurs <1% perioperative mortality.
    2. Minimally invasive parathyroidectomy under local anesthesia with intraoperative monitoring of PTH before and after removal is becoming more popular.
- Medical monitoring is recommended for asymptomatic primary hyperparathyroidism. Majority of patients do not manifest disease progression during observation.
  - Indications for medical monitoring
    1. Clinically asymptomatic
    2. Serum calcium level only mildly elevated (<1 mg/dl above upper limit normal)
    3. GFR > 60 ml/min and no nephrolithiasis or nephrocalcinosis
    4. No evidence of osteoporosis
  - Approximately 25% of asymptomatic patients will require surgery over a 10-yr follow-up period. Therefore patients will require regular monitoring of symptoms and assessment of serum calcium and creatinine levels yearly. Bone mineral density can be monitored every 2 yr.
  - Medical management
    1. Avoid medications that precipitate hypercalcemia (e.g., thiazide or lithium)
    2. Since inadequate calcium and vitamin D status stimulates PTH, calcium and vitamin D intake should be the same as for patients without hyperparathyroidism (i.e., 1000 mg of elemental calcium and 600-800 IU of vitamin D daily).
    3. Encourage physical activity since immobilization increases bone resorption.
    4. Recommend adequate hydration (at least 2 L) to minimize the risk of nephrolithiasis.

PHARMACOLOGIC THERAPY

For patients who are not surgical candidates, pharmacologic options are available. Indications include symptomatic hyperparathyroidism or osteopenia associated with an increased fracture risk.

- Agents that inhibit bone resorption such as bisphosphonates (e.g., alendronate, pamidronate, zoledronate), estrogens, and selective estrogen receptor modulators (e.g., Raloxifene) have been shown to improve bone mineral density and decrease calcium levels in patients with hyperparathyroidism.
- Cinacalcet (Sensipar) is an oral calcimimetic agent that activates the calcium sensing receptor in the parathyroid gland. It decreases PTH production and subsequently serum calcium levels. Its role in the management of primary hyperparathyroidism is under evaluation. However, it is indicated for the treatment of secondary hyperparathyroidism associated with chronic kidney disease and hypercalcemia associated with parathyroid carcinoma.

ACUTE GENERAL Rx

Severe and/or symptomatic hypercalcemia may require hospitalization especially if serum calcium >12 mg/dl. Acute management of hypercalcemia includes:

- Vigorous hydration with IV normal saline (2-4 L/day). Fluid status must be monitored in patients with cardiac or renal insufficiency in order to avoid fluid overload.
- Bisphosphonates can effectively decrease calcium levels. Zoledronate (4 mg IV over 15 min) or pamidronate (60-90 mg IV over 4 hr) are both effective. Onset of action after 24 to 48 hr.
- Calcitonin (4 units/kg IM/SC every 12 hr) may be used with bisphosphonates to achieve a more rapid reduction of calcium levels. Onset of action is within hours.

PEARLS & CONSIDERATIONS

COMMENTS

- Parathyroidectomy should be considered for all patients with symptomatic hyperparathyroidism.
- Asymptomatic patients can be monitored with serial creatinine, calcium and bone mineral density measurements. Disease progression may result in surgery. Most patients can be managed medically by limiting factors that result in hypercalcemia (i.e., dehydration, immobilization, thiazide diuretics etc.) and maintaining normal calcium and vitamin D intake. Patients with osteopenia and high fracture risk may require antiresorptive therapy such as bisphosphonates.

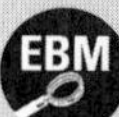

EVIDENCE

A 10-yr prospective study of patients with primary hyperparathyroidism found disease progression in only 25% of individuals with asymptomatic hyperparathyroidism who did not undergo surgery. Disease progression was defined as development of one or more new indications for parathyroidectomy.[1]

A longitudinal study of 71 patients with primary hyperparathyroidism reported that there was no significant effect of dietary calcium (>800 mg/day, mean = 1023 mg/day) on serum PTH levels, calcium, phosphorus, 25-hydroxyvitamin D, 1,25-dihydroxyvitamin D, urinary calcium excretion, or bone mineral density of L-spine, femoral neck, or distal one-third radius.[2]

A prospective study of the effect of vitamin D replacement in 56 patients with primary hyperparathyroidism failed to demonstrate any adverse effects. There was a significant increase in 25-hydroxyvitamin D levels with treatment and no significant changes in serum calcium, PTH levels, or urine Ca:Cr ratios. None of the patients developed any calcium-related adverse effects.[3]

Evidence-Based References

1. Silverberg S et al: A 10-year prospective study of primary hyperparathyroidism with or without parathyroid surgery, *N Engl J Med* 341:1249-1255, 1999.
2. Locker F et al: Optimal dietary calcium intake in primary hyperparathyroidism, *Am J Med* 102:543-550, 1997.
3. Tucci J: Vitamin D therapy in patients with primary hyperparathyroidism and hypovitaminosis D, *Eur J Endocrinol* 161:189-193, 2000.

SUGGESTED READINGS

Bilezikian JP et al: Guidelines for the management of asymptomatic primary hyperparathyroidism: Summary statement from the third international workshop, *J Clin Endocrinol Metab* 94(2):335, 2009.

Farford B et al: Nonsurgical management of primary hyperparathyroidism, *Mayo Clin Proc* 82(3):351, 2007.

Monchik JM et al: Minimally invasive parathyroid surgery in 103 patients with local/regional anesthesia, without exclusion criteria, *Surgery* 131:502, 2002.

Taniegra ED: Hyperparathyroidism, *Am Fam Physician* 69:333, 2004.

Udelsman R: Six hundred fifty-six consecutive explorations for primary hyperparathyroidism, *Ann Surg* 235:665, 2002.

AUTHORS: **ALLISON D. GRAZIADEI, M.D.,** and **GEETHA GOPALAKRISHNAN, M.D.**

BASIC INFORMATION

DEFINITION

Hypersensitivity pneumonitis (HP) is a group of immunologically mediated pulmonary diseases provoked by recurrent exposure to various environmental agents.

SYNONYMS

Extrinsic allergic alveolitis (EAA)
Some specific examples:
- Bird fancier's lung
- Farmer's lung
- Chemical worker's lung
- Humidifier lung
- Hot tub lung
- Sauna taker's lung

ICD-9CM CODES
495.9 Pneumonitis, hypersensitivity

EPIDEMIOLOGY & DEMOGRAPHICS

- Prevalence and incidence of HP vary considerably.
- Depend on definition and methods to establish diagnosis, intensity of exposure, environmental conditions, and genetic risk factors that remain poorly understood.
- More than 300 causative agents have been identified, and the number continues to grow.
- Causative agents in residential and occupational exposures include birds, mold, humidifiers, and organic and inorganic chemicals.
- Likely several genes are involved that cause an exaggerated lung response to an offending agent. The major histocompatibility complex is the most studied thus far.
- A viral connection has been implicated that may enhance clinical exposure to an offending agent.

PHYSICAL FINDINGS & CLINICAL PRESENTATION

Vary depending on frequency and intensity of antigen exposure.
- Acute: fever, cough, malaise, and dyspnea 4 to 6 hr after an intense exposure, lasting 18 to 24 hr
- Subacute: insidious onset of productive cough, dyspnea on exertion, anorexia, and weight loss, usually from a heavy, sustained exposure
- Chronic: gradually progressive cough, dyspnea, malaise, and weight loss, usually from low-grade or recurrent exposure
- Physical examination: cyanosis and crepitant rales, possible fever

ETIOLOGY

- Numerous environmental agents, often encountered in occupational settings
- Common sources of antigens: "moldy" hay, silage, grain, or vegetables; bird droppings or feathers; low-molecular-weight chemicals (e.g., isocyanates); pharmaceutical products

DIAGNOSIS

- Accurate diagnosis is important for differentiating HP from other interstitial disorders because the prognosis and treatment may differ.
- There is no gold standard for diagnosis.
- The clinical syndrome is indistinguishable from an acute respiratory infection without a history of illness occurring within hours of exposure to an antigen.
- Need high index of suspicion.
- Detailed occupational and home exposure history is required.
- Lung biopsy is often necessary for diagnosis.

DIFFERENTIAL DIAGNOSIS

Acute Stages	*Chronic Stages*
Acute bronchopulmonary aspergillosis	Idiopathic pulmonary fibrosis (IPF)
Pulmonary embolism	Bronchiectasis
Asthma	Chronic bronchitis
Aspiration pneumonia	Nonspecific interstitial pneumonia (NSIP)
Recurrent pneumonia	Connective tissue–related lung disease
Bronchiolitis obliterans–organizing pneumonia	
Sarcoidosis	
Churg-Strauss syndrome	
Wegener's granulomatosis	

WORKUP

No single radiologic, physiologic, or immunologic test is specific for the diagnosis of HP. HP must be suspected in any patient presenting with cough, dyspnea, fever, and malaise. A thorough history focusing on potential exposures is essential.

Environmental and occupational history questions should ask about grain dusts; animal handling; food processing; cooling towers; fountains; metalworking fluids; symptom improvement away from exposure; pets (particularly birds); hobbies involving chemicals, feathers, or fur; organic dusts; presence of humidifiers, dehumidifiers, or hot tubs/saunas; leaking or flooding indoors; visible fungal growth in living or working environment; feather pillows or bedding.

Major criteria:
- History of symptoms compatible with HP that appear to worsen within hours after antigen exposure
- Confirmation of exposure to the offending agent by history, investigation of the environment, serum precipitin test, or bronchoalveolar lavage (BAL) antibody
- Compatible changes on chest radiograph or high-resolution CT (HRCT) of the chest
- BAL fluid lymphocytosis (if performed)
- Compatible histologic changes by lung biopsy (if performed)
- Positive natural challenge (reproduction of symptoms and laboratory abnormalities after exposure to the suspected environment) or controlled inhalation challenge

Minor criteria:
- Basilar crackles
- Decreased diffusion capacity
- Arterial hypoxemia (either at rest or with exercise)

LABORATORY TESTS

- Routine laboratory tests do not make the diagnosis, but typically the erythrocyte sedimentation rate, C-reactive protein, lactate dehydrogenase, and leukocyte count are increased; elevated immunoglobulins IgG and IgM are nonspecific; rheumatoid factor (RF) and immune complexes are often positive; peripheral eosinophil count and serum IgE are generally normal.
- Lactate dehydrogenase is increased and tends to decrease with improvement.
- Pulmonary function tests: restrictive ventilatory patterns are typically seen. Decreased FEV_1, decreased forced vital capacity, decreased total lung capacity, decreased diffusing capacity, and decreased static compliance.
- Arterial blood gases show mild hypoxemia (worsens with exercise).
- A-a gradient shows slight increase.
- Serum precipitin test IgG antibody against offending antigen detected in serum. It is sensitive but not specific for HP (asymptomatic patients may have IgG antibodies in serum).
- Skin testing: unclear if helpful. However, some believe it to be a safe, effective, and rapid procedure in the diagnosis and follow-up of patients with HP. Sensitivity is similar to that of the precipitin test but the specificity is higher.

IMAGING STUDIES

Chest radiograph: nonspecific; may be normal in early stage.
- Acute/subacute: bilateral interstitial and alveolar nodular infiltrates (Fig. 1-165) in a patchy or homogeneous distribution. Apices are often spared.
- Chronic: diffuse reticulonodular infiltrates and fibrosis.

High-resolution chest CT scan: no pathognomonic features but demonstrates airspace and interstitial patterns in the acute and subacute stage. The chronic stage reveals honeycombing and bronchiectasis.

 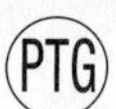

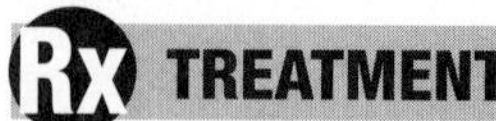

TREATMENT

NONPHARMACOLOGIC THERAPY

Early recognition and avoidance of the causative antigen

ACUTE GENERAL Rx

- Glucocorticoids accelerate initial lung recovery but may have no effect long term (from a controlled study in farmer's lung). No prospective, randomized, placebo-controlled trials for other types of HP or subacute and chronic stages.
- Prednisone 0.5 to 1 mg/kg usually over 1 to 2 wk then tapered over 4 wk. Some patients, particularly those with subacute or chronic presentation, may require a longer course of therapy.

DISPOSITION/PROGNOSIS

Acute: 4 to 48 hr
- Clinical: fever, chills, cough, hypoxia, malaise
- HRCT: ground-glass infiltrates
- Immunopathology: poorly formed, noncaseating granulomas or mononuclear cell infiltration in a peribronchial distribution, frequently with giant cells
- Prognosis: good

Subacute: weeks to 4 mo
- Clinical: dyspnea, cough, episodic flares
- HRCT: micronodules, air trapping
- Immunopathology: more well-formed noncaseating granulomas, bronchiolitis, organizing pneumonia and interstitial fibrosis
- Prognosis: good

Chronic: 4 mo to years
- Clinical: dyspnea, cough, fatigue, weight loss
- HRCT: fibrosis (possible), honeycombing, emphysema
- Immunopathology: granulomatous pneumonitides may be seen in addition to bronchiolitis obliterans (with or without organizing pneumonia) and honeycombing and fibrosis, lymphocytic infiltration, centrilobular and bridging fibrosis, neutrophil-mediated air space destruction, giant cells

REFERRAL

- Bronchoscopy: BAL provides useful supportive data in the diagnosis of HP. Usually reveals intense lymphocytosis (typically T cells >50%) of predominantly CD8+ suppressor cells. In the acute stage neutrophils predominate, but as the disease progresses to chronic form the ratio of CD4+ to CD8+ cells increase. When fibrosis is present the number of neutrophils increases.
- Lung biopsy: the histopathologic features of HP are distinctive but not pathognomonic. Bronchiolitis and interstitial pneumonitis with granuloma formation typically is seen. Variable degrees of interstitial fibrosis are seen in the chronic form. Chronic hypersensitivity pneumonitis may be difficult to distinguish from IPF or NSIP pathologically.
- Laboratory inhalation challenge: testing to prove a direct relation between a suspected antigen and disease; extract of antigen is inhaled by nebulizer.

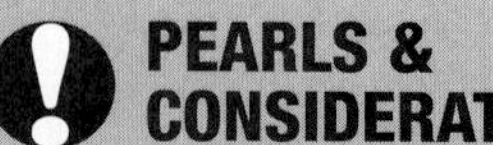

PEARLS & CONSIDERATIONS

A clinical prediction rule using six features has high specificity and sensitivity for the diagnosis of acute and subacute HP:
- Exposure to a known offending agent
- Positive specific precipitating antibody
- Recurrent episodes of symptoms
- Inspiratory crackles
- Symptoms occurring 4 to 8 hr after exposure
- Weight loss

No diagnostic gold standards; requires combination of clinical, environmental, radiologic, physiologic, and pathologic findings that represent a diagnostic challenge.

HP occurs more frequently in smokers than nonsmokers (likely from an immunosuppressive effect).

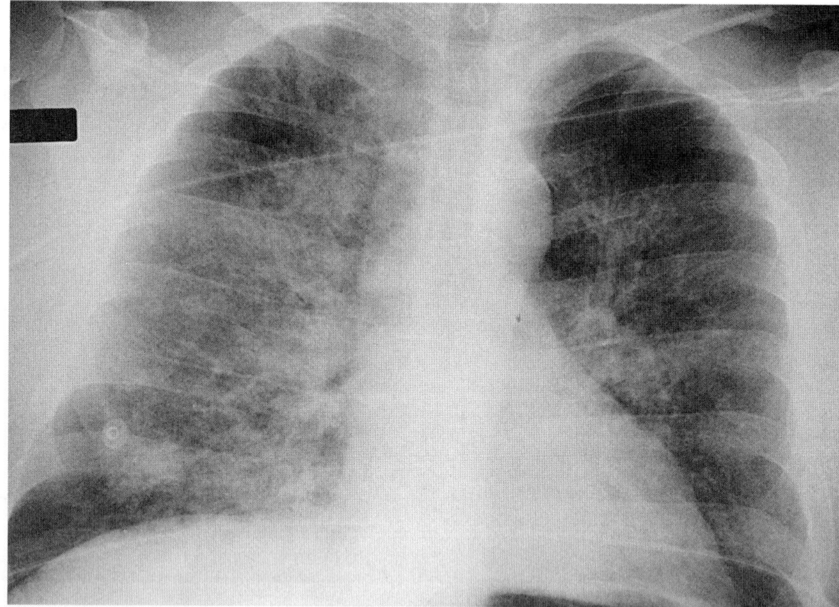

FIGURE 1-165 Chest radiograph of a patient with acute hypersensitivity pneumonitis. Bilateral interstitial infiltrates are evident, more on the right side than the left. Note the absence of pleural effusion, hilar adenopathy, and hyperinflation. (From Altman LV [ed]: *Allergy in primary care,* Philadelphia, 2000, WB Saunders.)

SUGGESTED READINGS

Churg A: Chronic hypersensitivity pneumonitis, *Am J Surg Pathol* 30(2):201, 2006.

Fink JN et al: Needs and opportunities for research in hypersensitivity pneumonitis, *Am J Respir Crit Care Med* 171:792-798, 2005.

Hanak V et al: High resolution CT findings of parenchymal fibrosis correlate with prognosis in hypersensitivity pneumonitis, *Chest* 134(1):133-138, 2008.

Lacasse Y et al: Clinical diagnosis of active hypersensitivity pneumonitis, *Am J Respir Crit Care Med* 168:952-958, 2003.

Morrell F et al: Usefulness of specific skin tests in the diagnosis of hypersensitivity pneumonitis, *J Allergy Clin Immunol* 110(6):939, 2002.

Patel AM et al: Hypersensitivity pneumonitis: current concepts and further questions, *J Allergy Clin Immunol* 108:661, 2001.

Schuyler M, Cormier Y: The diagnosis of hypersensitivity pneumonitis, *Chest* 111:534, 1997.

Selman M: Hypersensitivity pneumonitis: a multifaceted deceiving disorder, *Clin Chest Med* 25:3, 2004.

AUTHORS: **CAROLYN J. O'CONNOR, M.D.,** and **KRISTINA KRAMER, M.D.**

BASIC INFORMATION

DEFINITION

Hypersplenism is a syndrome characterized by splenomegaly, cytopenia (decrease of one or more peripheral cell lines), and compensatory hyperplastic bone marrow. The cytopenias are correctable with splenectomy.

ICD-9CM CODES
289.4 Hypersplenism

EPIDEMIOLOGY & DEMOGRAPHICS

Most often seen in patients with liver disease, hematologic malignancy, and infection

PHYSICAL FINDINGS & CLINICAL PRESENTATION

- Symptoms depend on the size of the spleen, rate of growth, and underlying disease.
- History: early satiety, abdominal discomfort or fullness, left upper quadrant pleuritic pain (abscess, infarction), episodes of acute left upper quadrant pain (sequestration crisis), referred pain to left shoulder
- Physical examination: splenomegaly (normal spleen not palpable), presence of a rub in left upper quadrant (suggestive of a splenic infarct), stigmata of cytopenias

ETIOLOGY

The spleen is an important component of cellular and humoral immunity: antigen recognition, antibody production, and clearance of antibody-coated particles and microorganisms from circulation. It is also responsible for the modification (removal of particles and parasites) and clearance of damaged or old red blood cells (RBCs) from the circulation. The spleen is a platelet reservoir, storing 30% of platelet mass. It can become the site of hematopoiesis in certain disease states. The spleen's normal activities are augmented when enlarged.

- Splenomegaly increases the proportion of blood channeled through the red pulp, causing inappropriate splenic pooling of both normal and abnormal blood cells. The size of the spleen determines the amount of cell sequestration. Up to 90% of platelets may be pooled in an enlarged spleen.
- Splenomegaly leads to increased destruction of RBCs. Platelets and white blood cells (WBCs) have about normal survival time even when sequestered and may be available if needed.
- Splenomegaly causes plasma volume expansion, exacerbating cytopenias by dilution.

Dx DIAGNOSIS

DIFFERENTIAL DIAGNOSIS

Hypersplenism can be caused by splenomegaly of almost any cause.

- Splenic congestion: cirrhosis (portal hypertension); congestive heart failure; portal, splenic, or hepatic vein thrombosis
- Hematologic causes: hemolytic anemia, sickle cell anemia, thalassemia, spherocytosis, elliptocytosis, extramedullary hematopoiesis, following use of granulocyte colony-stimulating factor
- Infections: viral (hepatitis, infectious mononucleosis, cytomegalovirus, HIV), bacterial (abscess, endocarditis, tuberculosis, salmonella, brucella, Lyme's disease), parasitic (babesiosis, malaria, leishmaniasis, schistosomiasis, toxoplasmosis), fungal
- Malignancy: acute or chronic leukemia, lymphoma, myeloproliferative diseases (polycythemia vera, essential thrombocytosis, myelofibrosis), metastatic tumors
- Inflammatory diseases: rheumatic fever, rheumatoid arthritis (Felty's syndrome), systemic lupus erythematosus, sarcoid, serum sickness
- Infiltrative diseases: amyloidosis, Gaucher's disease, Niemann-Pick disease, glycogen storage disease
- Anatomic abnormalities: cyst, pseudocyst, hemangioma, hamartoma

WORKUP

History (including travel), physical examination, laboratory tests, imaging studies

LABORATORY TESTS

- CBC with differential: cytopenia, neutrophilia (infection)
- Peripheral smear: RBC and WBC morphology (abnormal cells may suggest infection, malignancy, bone marrow disease, rheumatologic disease), organisms (bacteria, malaria, babesiosis)
- Bone marrow biopsy: hyperplasia of cytopenic cell lines; hematologic, infiltrative, or infectious disorders
- Tests to diagnose suspected cause of splenomegaly: liver function, hepatitis serology, HIV, rheumatoid factor, antinuclear antibody, tissue biopsy
- Note: red cell mass (^{51}Cr assay) may be used to assess severity of anemia. RBC mass measurement will differentiate true anemia (decrease in RBCs) from dilutional anemia (plasma volume expansion).

IMAGING STUDIES

- Ultrasound: splenic size, presence of cyst or abscess
- CT: estimate volume, obtain structural information: cyst, abscess, tumor, infarct
- MRI: most useful for assessing vascular lesions and infections
- Liver-spleen scan: assess anatomy and function; may suggest presence of portal hypertension
- Consider other studies as suggested by history and examination: chest radiograph, echocardiogram

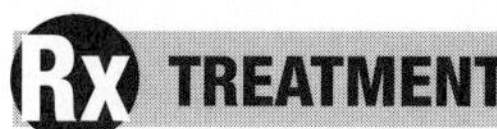

TREATMENT

ACUTE GENERAL Rx

- Treat underlying disease
- Splenectomy is considered if:
  1. Indicated for the management of the underlying cause
  2. Persistent symptomatic disease (severe cytopenia) not responding to therapy
  3. Necessary for diagnosis

Risks:

- Infections (especially encapsulated organisms): risk greatest in the first 2 yr after splenectomy. Mortality rate from sepsis is fiftyfold greater in asplenic patients. Attempts to decrease risk include:
  - Immunization with pneumococcal, meningococcal, and haemophilus influenzae vaccines 3 wk before splenectomy. Revaccination for pneumococcal in 5 yr. Annual influenza vaccination.
  - Prophylactic antibiotics after splenectomy in highest risk patients.
  - Patient education regarding the importance of rapid initiation of antibiotics at the first sign of infection.
- Rapid increase in platelet count may cause thromboembolic complications.
- Possible increased risk of atherosclerotic heart disease.
- Splenectomy should not be performed if the spleen is the main site of hematopoiesis as a result of bone marrow failure (e.g., myelofibrosis).
- Other options include partial splenectomy, partial splenic embolization, portosystemic shunting (for congestive splenomegaly).

DISPOSITION

- Cytopenias are usually correctable with splenectomy; cell counts return to normal within a few weeks.
- Splenectomy may alleviate portal hypertension.
- Prognosis depends on the underlying disease.

REFERRAL

Hematology

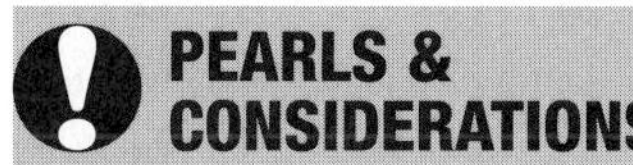

PEARLS & CONSIDERATIONS

- Thrombocytopenia in hypersplenism is usually moderately severe ($>50 \times 10^9$ /L) and asymptomatic; severe thrombocytopenia ($<20 \times 10^9$/L) suggests another diagnosis.
- Neutropenia of hypersplenism is rarely symptomatic.

SUGGESTED READING

Hoffman R et al: *Hematology: basic principles and practice,* ed 5, Philadelphia, Churchill Livingstone Elsevier, 2008.

AUTHOR: **SUDEEP KAUR AULAKH, M.D.**

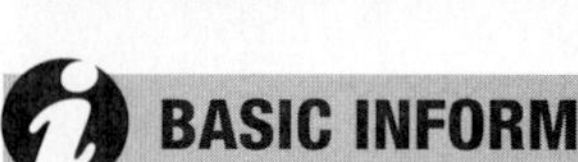

BASIC INFORMATION

DEFINITION

The Joint National Committee on Prevention, Detection, Evaluation, and Treatment of High Blood Pressure (JNC 7) classifies normal blood pressure (BP) in adults as <120 mm Hg systolic and <80 mm Hg diastolic. *Prehypertension* is defined as systolic BP from 120 to 139 mm Hg or diastolic BP from 80 to 89 mm Hg. *Stage 1 hypertension* (HTN) is systolic BP from 140 to 159 mm Hg or diastolic BP from 90 to 99 mm Hg. *Stage 2 hypertension* is systolic BP ≥160 mm Hg or diastolic BP ≥100 mm Hg.

SYNONYMS

Essential hypertension
Idiopathic hypertension
High BP

ICD-9CM CODES

401.1 Essential hypertension (HTN)
401.0-9 with 5th digit 1 Renovascular hypertension
642 Hypertension complicating pregnancy
437.2 Hypertensive encephalopathy

EPIDEMIOLOGY & DEMOGRAPHICS

INCIDENCE: 0% to 15% of adult population
PREVALENCE: 0 million individuals in the U.S. and approximately 1 billion individuals worldwide meet the criteria for diagnosis of HTN.
PEAK INCIDENCE: Males and the elderly

PHYSICAL FINDINGS & CLINICAL PRESENTATION

Physical examination may be entirely within normal limits except for the presence of HTN. A proper initial physical examination on a hypertensive patient should include the following:

- The BP should be measured with an appropriately sized cuff and in both arms (the higher of the readings being used).
- Postural BP change is best assessed by going from the lying to the standing position and should include notation of the changed in heart rate with position change.
- A diagnosis of HTN can be immediately established if the BP is extremely elevated (>180/110 mm Hg).
- Otherwise such a diagnosis should wait until BP is found elevated on at least two occasions where white coat HTN is highly unlikely.
- Measure heart rate, height and weight, body mass index, and waist circumference.
- Evaluate skin for the presence of café-au-lait spots (neurofibromatosis), uremic appearance (congestive renal failure), striae (Cushing's syndrome).
- Perform careful funduscopic examination; check for papilledema, retinal exudates, hemorrhages, arterial narrowing, arteriovenous compression.
- Examine the neck for carotid bruits, distended neck veins, or enlarged thyroid gland.
- Perform extensive cardiopulmonary examination: check for loud aortic component of S_2, S_4, ventricular lift, murmurs, and arrhythmias.
- Check abdomen for masses (pheochromocytoma, polycystic kidneys), periumblical and frank bruit (renal artery stenosis), dilation of the aorta.
- Obtain two or more BP measurements separated by 2 min with the patient either supine or seated and after standing for at least 2 min. Measure BP in both upper extremities (if values differ, use the higher value).
- Examine arterial pulses (dilated or absent femoral pulses and BP greater in upper extremities than lower extremities suggest aortic coarctation).
- Note the presence of truncal obesity (Cushing's syndrome) and pedal edema (congestive heart failure [CHF], nephrosis).
- The clinical evaluation should help determine if the patient has primary or secondary (possibly reversible) HTN, if there is target organ disease present, and if there are cardiovascular risk factors in addition to HTN.

ETIOLOGY

- Essential (primary) HTN (85%)
- Drug induced or drug related (5%)
- Renal HTN (5%)
  1. Renal parenchymal disease (3%)
  2. Renovascular hypertension (RVH) (<2%)
- Endocrine (4%-5%)
  1. Oral contraceptives (4%)
  2. Primary aldosteronism (0.5%)
  3. Pheochromocytoma (0.2%)
  4. Cushing's syndrome and long-term steroid therapy (0.2%)
  5. Hyperparathyroidism or thyroid disease (0.2%)
- Coarctation of the aorta (0.2%)

DIAGNOSIS

WORKUP

- The objective for the initial evaluation of HTN is to establish the diagnosis and stage of HTN.
- By gathering office and nonoffice BP readings, assessing presence of target organ damage (TOD), assessing the level of global cardiovascular disease risk and to produce a plan for individualized monitoring and therapy.
- ECG, CXR, renal imaging, and tests for plasma aldosterone/plasma rennin activity are not routinely recommended at the initial evaluation stage of the patient with newly diagnosed HTN.
- Patient counseling and education should be prominent features of the initial evaluation.

Pertinent history:

- Age of onset of HTN, previous antihypertensive therapy
- Family history of HTN, stroke, cardiovascular disease
- Diet, salt intake, alcohol, drugs (e.g., oral contraceptives, NSAIDs, decongestants, steroids)
- Occupation, lifestyle, socioeconomic status, psychologic factors
- Other cardiovascular risk factors: hyperlipidemia, obesity, diabetes mellitus, carbohydrate intolerance
- Symptoms of secondary HTN:
  1. Headache, palpitations, excessive perspiration (possible pheochromocytoma)
  2. Weakness, polyuria (consider hyperaldosteronism)
  3. Claudication of lower extremities (seen with coarctation of aorta)

An algorithm for investigation of suspected endocrine HTN is described in Section III.

LABORATORY TESTS

- Urinalysis with microscopic evaluation, blood urea nitrogen and creatinine, and an albumin/creatinine ratio; for evidence of renal disease. High-serum creatinine is a predictor of cardiovascular risk in essential HTN.
- Nonoffice (home, workplace, 24-hour ambulatory BP determination to establish the pattern of HTN (sustained, "white coat," or "masked" HTN).
- Serum electrolyte levels: low potassium is suggestive of primary aldosteronism or diuretic use.
- Screening for coexisting diseases that may adversely affect prognosis:
  1. Fasting serum glucose
  2. Serum lipid panel, uric acid, calcium
  3. If pheochromocytoma is suspected: 24-hr urine for VMA and metanephrines

IMAGING STUDIES

- ECG: check for presence of left ventricular hypertrophy (LVH) with strain pattern.
- Magnetic resonance angiography of the renal arteries in suspected RVH (renal artery stenosis).

TREATMENT

NONPHARMACOLOGIC THERAPY

Lifestyle modifications:

- Lose weight if overweight.
- Limit alcohol intake to 1 oz of ethanol per day (<2 drinks/day) in men or 0.5 oz (<1 drink/day) in women.
- Exercise (aerobic) regularly (at least 30 min/day on most days).
- Reduce sodium intake to <100 mmol/day (<2.3 g of sodium/day).
- Maintain adequate dietary potassium (>3500 mg/day) intake in patients with normal kidney function.
- Stop smoking.
- The BP reduction seen ranges from 2 to 20 mm Hg, most significant with substantial weight loss and the implementation of so-called Dietary Approaches to Stop Hypertension (DASH) eating plan, which relies on a diet high in fruits and vegetables, moderate in low-fat dairy products, and low in animal protein, but with substantial amount of plant protein from legumes and nuts.

ACUTE GENERAL Rx

According to the JNC 7:

- For patients with prehypertension and no other complications, recommend lifestyle modifications to prevent progression to sustained HTN.
- For patients with prehypertension and diabetes or chronic kidney disease, aggressive pharmacologic treatment should be undertaken to reduce BP to <130/80 mm Hg.
- Antihypertensive drug therapy should be initiated in patients with stage 1 HTN. Thiazide diuretics are preferred for initial therapy unless there are compelling indications to use other agents for initial therapy.
- Compelling indications for individual drug classes:
    - Congestive heart failure (CHF) due to systolic dysfunction: ACE inhibitors, angiotensin-receptor blockers (ARBs), beta-blockers, diuretics, aldosterone antagonists
    - Post-MI: beta-blockers, ACE inhibitors, aldosterone antagonists
    - High cardiovascular risk: beta-blockers, ACE inhibitors, calcium channel blockers (CCBs), diuretics
    - Diabetes: ACE inhibitors, ARBs, CCBs, beta-blockers, diuretics
    - Chronic kidney disease: ACE inhibitors, ARBs
    - Recurrent stroke prevention: ACE inhibitors, diuretics
- A two-drug combination is necessary for most patients with stage 2 HTN. The combination of a diuretic with another agent is preferred unless there is a compelling indication to use other agents.
- When selecting drugs, also consider the cost of the medication, metabolic and subjective side effects, and drug-drug interactions.
- The major advantages and limitations of each class of drugs are described as follows:
    1. Diuretics:
        a. Advantages: inexpensive, once-daily dosing. Useful in edematous states, CHF, chronic renal disease, elderly patients (decreased incidence of hip fractures in elderly patients)
        b. Disadvantages: significant adverse metabolic effects, increased risk of cardiac arrhythmias, sexual dysfunction, possible adverse effects on lipids and glucose levels
    2. Beta-blockers:
        a. Advantages: ideal in hypertensive patients with ischemic heart disease or status post MI. Favored in hyperkinetic, young patients (resting tachycardia, wide pulse pressure, hyperdynamic heart) and stable CHF patients
        b. Disadvantages: adverse effect on quality of life (increased incidence of fatigue, depression, impotence, bronchospasm, hypoglycemia, peripheral vascular disease, adverse effects on lipids, masking of signs and symptoms of hypoglycemia in diabetics)
    3. Calcium antagonists:
        a. Advantages: helpful in hypertensive patients with ischemic heart disease. Generally favorable effect on quality of life; can be used in patients with bronchospastic disorders, renal disease, peripheral vascular disease, metabolic disorders, and salt sensitivity. CCBs BP-lowering effect is independent of Na+ intake.
        b. Disadvantages: diltiazem and verapamil should be avoided in patients with CHF due to systolic dysfunction because of their negative inotropic effects; pedal edema may occur with nifedipine and amlodipine; constipation can be severe in elderly patients receiving verapamil. CCB-related edema is positional in nature, it improves with lying position, additional strategies include; switching CCB classes; reducing dosage; giving the medication later in the day; and adding a venodilator (nitrates, an ACE, or an ARB); diuretics may improve edema, but at the expense of a reduction in plasma volume.
    4. ACE inhibitors:
        a. Advantages: well tolerated, favorable impact on quality of life; useful in HTN complicated by CHF; helpful in prevention of diabetic renal disease; effective in decreasing left ventricular hypertrophy (LVH).
        b. Disadvantages: cough is a frequent side effect (5%-20% of patients); hyperkalemia may occur in patients with diabetes or severe renal insufficiency; hypotension may occur in volume-depleted patients.
    5. ARBs:
        a. Advantages: well tolerated, favorable impact on quality of life; useful in patients unable to tolerate ACE inhibitors because of persistent cough and in CHF and diabetic patients; single daily dose. An episode of renal insufficiency with ACE inhibitors does not rule out future therapy with an ARB unless high-grade bilateral renal artery stenosis exists.
        b. Disadvantages: excessive cost; hypotension may occur in volume-depleted patients; contraindicated in pregnancy.
    6. Renin inhibitors: newest class of antihypertensives (Aliskiren, Tekturna):
        a. Advantages: generally well tolerated; once-daily dosing; can be used alone or in combination with other antihypertensive agents.
        b. Disadvantages: contraindicated in pregnancy; should not be used in patients with impaired renal function; excessive cost.
    7. α-adrenergic blockers:
        a. Advantages: no adverse effect on blood lipids or insulin sensitivity; helpful in benign prostatic hypertrophy.
        b. Disadvantages: postural hypotension, sedation; syncope can be avoided by giving an initial low dose at bedtime.
    8. Central α-antagonists:
        a. Oral clonidine mainstay of therapy for hypertensive urgencies because of the ease of administration and relative safety.
        b. Transdermal clonidine; useful in management of labile HTN, the hospitalized patient who cannot take medications by mouth, and patients subject to early morning BP surges. At equivalent doses, transdermal clonidine is more apt to precipitate salt and water retention than is the case with oral clonidine.
        c. Dose beyond 0.4 mg causes fatigue, sedation and dry mouth, salt and water retention, and rebound HTN upon abrupt termination of the medication.
    9. Combined α- and β-adrenergic receptor blockers;
       Labetalol and carvedilol: Use is reserved to treat complicated hypertensive patient when an antihypertensive effect beyond β-blockade is sought. IV labetalol is used for hypertensive emergencies. Carvedilol is shown to have less adverse effect on glycemic control than metoprolol and to reduce urinary protein excretion in hypertensive diabetic patients.

TREATMENT OF RVH: The therapeutic approach varies with the cause of the RVH (refer to "Renal Artery Stenosis" for additional information).

1. Young patients with fibromuscular dysplasia can be treated with percutaneous transluminal renal angioplasty (PTRA).
2. Medical therapy is advisable in elderly patients with atheromatous RVH; useful agents are:
    a. Beta-blockers: highly effective in patients with elevated plasma renin
    b. ACE inhibitors: highly effective; however, should be avoided in patients with bilateral renal artery stenosis or with a solitary kidney and renal stenosis
    c. Diuretics: often used in combination with ACE inhibitors
3. Surgical revascularization is generally reserved for atheromatous RVH in patients responding poorly to medical therapy (uncontrolled HTN, deteriorating renal function).

HTN DURING PREGNANCY:

1. HTN complicates 5% to 12% of all pregnancies.
2. The American Obstetrical Committee defines BP of 130/80 mm Hg as the upper limit of normal at any time during pregnancy.
3. A rise of 30 mm Hg systolic or 15 mm Hg diastolic is also considered abnormal regardless of the absolute values obtained.
4. Chronic HTN (occurring before pregnancy) must be distinguished from preeclampsia because the risk to mother and fetus is much greater in the latter.

5. Treatment of chronic HTN during pregnancy is as follows:
   a. Initial treatment with conservative measures (proper nutrition, limited physical activity).
   b. When drug therapy is necessary, initiation of methyldopa, hydralazine, labetalol, or atenolol is preferred.
   c. ACE inhibitors can cause fetal and neonatal complications; their use should be avoided in pregnancy.
   d. The safety of CCBs remains unclear.
   e. Diuretics should be used only if there is a specific reason for initiating and maintaining their use (e.g., HTN associated with severe fluid overload or left ventricular dysfunction).

MALIGNANT HTN, HYPERTENSIVE EMERGENCIES, AND HYPERTENSIVE URGENCIES: Definitions:

1. Malignant HTN is a potentially life-threatening situation caused by elevated BP.
   a. The rate of BP rise is a critical factor.
   b. The clinical manifestations are grade IV hypertensive retinopathy (exudates, hemorrhages, and papilledema), cardiovascular or renal compromise, and encephalopathy.
   c. Requires immediate BP reduction (not necessarily into normal ranges) to prevent or limit target organ disease.
2. Hypertensive emergencies require rapid (within 1 hr) lowering of BP to prevent end-organ damage.
3. Hypertensive urgencies are significant BP elevations that should be corrected within 24 hr of presentation.

Therapy: The choice of therapeutic agents in malignant HTN varies with the cause.

1. Nitroprusside is the drug of choice in hypertensive encephalopathy, HTN and intracranial bleeding, malignant HTN, HTN and heart failure, dissecting aortic aneurysm (used in combination with propranolol); its onset of action is immediate.
2. Fenoldopam is a vasodilator agent useful for the short-term (up to 48 hr) management of severe HTN when rapid but quickly reversible reduction of BP is required.
3. Other commonly used agents are the IV CCBs nicardipine and clevidipine (useful for urgent treatment of HTN in the intensive care unit or operating room), the beta-blocker esmolol (useful in aortic dissection or postoperative HTN), labetalol (combined β-adrenergic and α-blocker useful in patients with coronary disease), phentolamine (useful for catecholamine-related emergencies), IV nitroglycerin (used in patients with cardiac ischemia and hypertensive crisis), and hydralazine (used for hypertensive emergencies in pregnancy).
4. The following are important points to remember when treating hypertensive emergencies:
   a. Introduce a plan for long-term therapy at the time of the initial emergency treatment.
   b. Agents that reduce arterial pressure can cause the kidney to retain sodium and water; therefore the judicious administration of diuretics should accompany their use.
   c. The initial goal of antihypertensive therapy is not to achieve a normal BP, but rather to gradually reduce the BP; cerebral hypoperfusion may occur if the mean BP is lowered $>$40% in the initial 24 hr.

PEARLS & CONSIDERATIONS

COMMENTS

- For patients with prehypertension, every 20/10 mm Hg increase in BP doubles the risk of cardiovascular events.
- Most patients will require at least two medications for BP control.
- Guidelines now suggest that, if BP is greater than 20/10 mm Hg above goal, therapy should be initiated with two drugs.
- A practical approach to multidrug therapy is use of fixed-dose antihypertensive combinations as an alternative to the sequenced addition of two or three drugs.
- Resistant HTN: HTN is considered resistant if the BP cannot be reduced below target levels in patients who are compliant with an optimal triple-drug regimen that includes a diuretic. Terms *refractory* and *resistant* are used interchangeably. Causes include white coat HTN, pseudohypertension, measurement artifact, medication nonadherence, volume overload, and secondary HTN.
  - White coat HTN (clinic BP higher than the levels obtained outside the office setting)
  - Pseudohypertension in elderly: hardened and sclerotic artery is not compressible hence falsely elevates BP measurement artifact
  - Measurement artifact: BP taken with a small cuff in people with large arm diameter. BP should be taken with the patient in the seated position and the arm supported at heart level, the bladder within the cuff should encircle at least 80% of the arm diameter.
- Section III describes an algorithm for patients with resistant HTN.
- Barriers to BP control: system issues, provider issues; patients issues and behavior issues. The rate at which physicians adopt recommended changes based on evidence based findings can be quite slow and has been properly described as "clinical inertia."

EVIDENCE

Please note: Complete text of EBM for this topic is available online.

Key trials and commentary:

Treating hypertension decreases mortality and disability from cardiovascular disease, but most hypertension remains inadequately controlled. This study showed that pharmacist care management delivered through secure patient Web communications improved BP control in patients with hypertension.

Because control of BP is most commonly achieved with antihypertensive drug therapy, pharmacists have had an abiding interest in the process. Meta-analyses of many previous studies have shown an improvement in BP control rates when a pharmacist is added to the health care team, presumably because the pharmacist's background and training in explaining the importance of the medication, assessing and improving adherence, and overcoming barriers to medication taking are typically more extensive than those of other members of the health care team. In the Chronic Care Model, self-management is one of the six domains that are associated with improvements in health. In hypertension, home BP monitoring is the simplest and most direct of the self-management strategies that have been shown to improve BP control. These authors, therefore, combined previous strategies of home BP monitoring, pharmacist input, and secure web-based advice and support in their most intensively supported group, and compared its efficacy with two "control" groups—traditional medical care ("usual care") or web-based training and home BP monitoring (without the pharmacists' advice and assistance).[1] Ⓐ

The fact that those who received pharmacists' assistance, in addition to the web-based training and advice and home BP measurement, had improved BP control is not very surprising, but it does point to the fact that BP control benefits from a multi-faceted intervention. The unanswered question is how well this program can be implemented in the general U.S. population. One inclusion criterion for this study was the availability of Internet and e-mail access, which presumably wasn't a major problem for the health maintenance organization most closely associated geographically with Puget Sound, Microsoft Inc., and the Pacific Northwest technology corridor. The prevalence of BP control at baseline in their cohort was nearly 61%, compared with that of only 44% across the U.S. (in the National Health and Nutritional Examination Survey, 2005-2006[7]). The investigators excluded hypertensives with diabetes, chronic kidney disease, or heart disease from participation, to keep the program "simple," but these individuals have not only a lower BP target, but also a larger pill burden to take on a daily basis, suggesting that these results are a "best-case scenario."[1] Ⓐ

It will be interesting to see if large quality improvement programs are launched by the larger health maintenance organizations, based on these data. As with all things, implementation will likely be thwarted by cost considerations, particularly the effort and expense necessary to keep pharmacists involved in ongoing care of their customers with very frequent monitoring and feedback.

Whether the treatment of patients with hypertension who are 80 years of age or older is beneficial is unclear. It has been suggested that antihypertensive therapy may reduce the risk of stroke, despite possibly increasing the risk of death. The results provide evidence that antihypertensive treatment with indapamide (sustained release), with or without perindopril, in persons 80 years of age or older is beneficial.[2] Ⓐ

This may well be the last ethically defensible, randomized, clinical trial in hypertension to give only placebo to some of its subjects and then to observe them for cardiovascular morbidity/mortality. Therapeutic equipoise for this study was originally provided by a 1999 meta-analysis of 1670 participants over 80 years of age in placebo-controlled clinical trials of various antihypertensive drugs, which showed significant 30% reductions in stroke and heart failure, but these benefits were accompanied by a nonsignificant 14% increase in all-cause mortality. This caused concern among many older people, and authors of guidelines, because recommending antihypertensive drug therapy, thus, could lead to increased mortality. The Hypertension in the Very Elderly Trial (HYVET)-Pilot study randomized 1283 octogenarians to placebo, indapamide, or perindopril, but few cardiovascular events were reported, and the lowest number of deaths was again seen in those given placebo (22 vs. 27 with the ACE-inhibitor vs. 30 with the diuretic). The main HYVET was begun in 2001 in Bulgaria, Poland, Romania, and Russia (55.8% of the 3845 enrolled subjects), China (39.7%), Tunisia (1.8%), Belgium, Finland, France, Ireland, and the United Kingdom (2.2%), and Australia and New Zealand (0.5%). Four clinical centers were closed in the first year because of concerns about data collection. At the second review by the Data Safety and Monitoring Board (after the first 140 strokes were reported by investigators), a significant difference between randomized groups was seen for both the primary end point of stroke and for all-cause mortality. This led to an early termination of the study; close-out visits were quickly arranged and completed within 6 months. During follow-up, BP was reduced more in the actively treated group. Two years after randomization, 48% of the actively treated group and 20% of the placebo-treated group had seated BP <150/90 mm Hg (the predefined target BP). It is likely that these differences would be even greater if BPs were measured standing. About a quarter of the actively treated group needed only sustained-release indapamide at 1.5 mg/day, another quarter needed perindopril 2 mg/day, and nearly half required perindopril at 4 mg/day. At the conclusion of follow-up (median: 1.8 years), the difference in fatal stroke was significant, but the difference between the groups in the incidence of any stroke (the primary end point) just barely missed statistical significance (51 vs. 69, relative risk reduction: 30%, 95% confidence interval: −1%-51%, $P = 0.06$). The difference between this final result and the data evaluated by the Data Safety and Monitoring Board (who saw a 51% relative risk reduction, $P = 0.0007$, based on 140 reported strokes) must be due to reported strokes that were not confirmed at adjudication and reminds us of the hazards of making hasty recommendations to terminate trials based on imperfect information. Nonetheless, the significant difference in all-cause mortality held up (presumably because agreement about death by adjudicators is simpler and easier than agreement about stroke), and the decision to terminate the trial early for safety reasons can be easily justified. The authors are appropriately conservative in their recommendations of how their data should be used in the care of octogenarians. Their subjects were generally healthier than older people in the general population, and extrapolation of their results to more frail elderly is premature. They point out, however, that the survival curves begin to separate after about a year of follow-up, and the absolute benefits of treatment were impressive: one stroke, death, or heart failure episode is prevented if 93, 42, or 49 people are treated for 2 years, respectively. Individuals given active treatment had a significant reduction in serious adverse events, and no significant differences at 2 years with respect to serum potassium, urate, glucose, or creatinine levels, compared with those given placebo. It is likely that the Individual Data Analysis of Antihypertensive Drug Intervention Trials (INDANA) Group will have to redo their meta-analyses, and incorporate the data from both HYVET-Pilot and HYVET (along with the 38 other clinical trials in hypertension completed since 1999), to see if the reported excess risk of death with active antihypertensive drug therapy still holds in octogenarians. Until they do, we should be relatively well-assured that the observational data suggesting harm associated with lowered BP in individuals over age 80 can be refuted by clinical trial evidence, specifically gathered in this population in HYVET, which shows overwhelming benefit of treatment on stroke, cardiovascular events, heart failure, and death.[2] Ⓐ

The number of clinic visits may be reduced with home BP monitoring, making it a potentially cost-effective means for the management of hypertensive patients; Studies have shown that adjustment of antihypertensive treatment based on home BP measurements instead of office BP readings leads to less-intensive drug treatment.[3]

A prudent approach is warranted in patients with concomitant CAD disease, in whom diastolic BP should probably not be brought to < 70 mm Hg.[4]

DASH diet substantially reduces both systolic and diastolic BP among hypertensive and normotensive individuals and adherence to the DASH-style diet lowers risk of coronary heart disease and stoke among middle-aged women during 2 decades of follow-up.[5]

First-line drugs for hypertension—The Cochrane Collaboration review—most of the evidence demonstrated that first-line low-dose thiazide reduce mortality and morbidity (stroke, heart attack, and heart failure).[6]

Evidence-Based References

1. Green BB et al: Effectiveness of home blood pressure monitoring, web communication, and pharmacist care on hypertension control: a randomized controlled trial, *JAMA* 299:2857-2867, 2008. Commentary by W.J. Elliott, M.D., Ph.D. Ⓐ
2. Beckett NS et al: Treatment of hypertension in patients 80 years of age or older. *N Engl J Med* 358:1887-1898, 2008. Commentary by W.J. Elliott, M.D., Ph.D. Ⓐ
3. Verberk et al: Home versus office measurement, reduction of unnecessary treatment study investigators. Self measurement of BP at home reduces the need for antihypertensive drugs; a randomized, controlled trial, *Hypertension* 50:1019-1025, 2007.
4. Figard RH et al: On- treatment diastolic BP and prognosis in systolic hypertension, *Arch Intern Med* 167:1884-1891, 2007.
5. Sacks et al: DASH-sodium Collaborative Research Group. Effects on BP of reduced dietary sodium and the dietary approaches to stop hypertension(DASH) diet, *N Engl J Med* 344:3-10, 2001.
6. Wright Km, Musini VM: First line drugs for hypertension (review), *The Cochrane Collaboration* Issue 3, 2009.

SUGGESTED READINGS

Arguedes JA et al: Treatment blood pressure targets for hypertension (review), *The Cochrane Collaboration*, Issue 3, 2009.

Beckett NS et al: Treatment of hypertension in patients 80 years of age or older. *N Engl J Med* 358:1887-1898, 2008.

Blood Pressure Lowering Treatment Trialist' Collaboration: Effects of different regimens to lower blood pressure on major cardiovascular events in older and younger adults. Meta-analysis of randomized trial. *BMJ* doi:10.1136, 2008.

Moser M, Setaro JF: Resistant or difficult to control hypertension, *N Engl J Med* 355:385, 2006.

Schaer B et al: Risk for incident atrial fibrillation in patients who receive antihypertensive drugs, *Ann Intern Med* 152(2):78-84, 2010.

Seventh Report of the Joint National Committee on Prevention, Detection, Evaluation, and Treatment of High BPBP, *JAMA* 289:2560, 2003.

Sica DA: Management of hypertension in the outpatient setting, *Primary Care Clin Office Pract* 5:451-473, 2008.

Silverstein RL et al: Resistant hypertension, *Primary Care Clin Office Pract* 35:501-513, 2008.

AUTHORS: **SHAHNAZ PUNJANI, M.D., FRED F. FERRI, M.D.,** and **WEN-CHIH WU, M.D.**

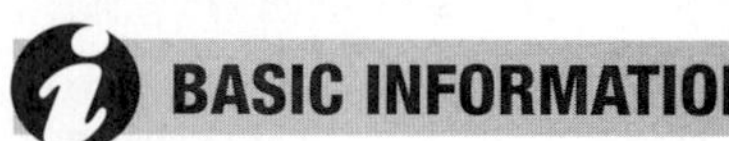

BASIC INFORMATION

DEFINITION

Hyperthyroidism is a hypermetabolic state resulting from excess thyroid hormone.

SYNONYMS

Thyrotoxicosis

ICD-9CM CODES
242.9 Hyperthyroidism
242.0 Hyperthyroidism with goiter
242.2 Hyperthyroidism, multinodular
242.3 Hyperthyroidism, uninodular

EPIDEMIOLOGY & DEMOGRAPHICS

INCIDENCE/PREVALENCE:

- Hyperthyroidism affects 2% of women and 0.2% of men in their lifetimes.
- Toxic multinodular goiter usually occurs in women >55 yr and is more common than Graves' disease in the elderly.

PHYSICAL FINDINGS & CLINICAL PRESENTATION

- Patients with hyperthyroidism generally present with tachycardia, tremor, hyperreflexia, anxiety, irritability, emotional lability, panic attacks, heat intolerance, sweating, increased appetite, diarrhea, weight loss, menstrual dysfunction (oligomenorrhea, amenorrhea). Presentation may be different in elderly patients (see below).
- Patients with Graves' disease may present with exophthalmos, lid retraction (Fig. 1-166, *A*), and lid lag (Graves' ophthalmopathy). The following signs and symptoms of ophthalmopathy may be present: blurring of vision, photophobia, increased lacrimation, double vision, and deep orbital pressure. Clubbing of fingers associated with periosteal new bone formation in other skeletal areas (Graves' acropachy) and pretibial myxedema (Fig. 1-166, *B*) may also be noted.
- Clinical signs of hyperthyroidism in the elderly may be masked by manifestations of coexisting disease (e.g., new-onset atrial fibrillation, exacerbation of congestive heart failure).

ETIOLOGY

- Graves' disease (diffuse toxic goiter): 80% to 90% of all cases of hyperthyroidism
- Toxic multinodular goiter (Plummer's disease)
- Toxic adenoma
- Iatrogenic and factitious
- Transient hyperthyroidism (subacute thyroiditis, Hashimoto's thyroiditis)
- Rare causes: hypersecretion of thyroid-stimulating hormone (TSH) (e.g., pituitary neoplasms), struma ovarii, ingestion of large amount of iodine in a patient with preexisting thyroid hyperplasia or adenoma (Jod-Basedow phenomenon), hydatidiform mole, carcinoma of thyroid, amiodarone therapy

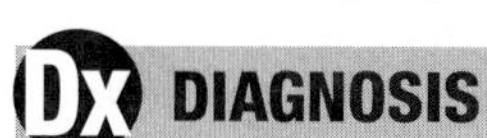

DIAGNOSIS

DIFFERENTIAL DIAGNOSIS

- Anxiety disorder
- Pheochromocytoma
- Metastatic neoplasm
- Diabetes mellitus
- Premenopausal state

WORKUP

Suspected hyperthyroidism requires laboratory confirmation and identification of its etiology because treatment varies with cause. A detailed medical history will often provide clues to the diagnosis and etiology of the hyperthyroidism.

LABORATORY TESTS

- Elevated free thyroxine (T_4)
- Elevated free triiodothyronine (T_3): generally not necessary for diagnosis
- Low TSH (unless hyperthyroidism is a result of the rare hypersecretion of TSH from a pituitary adenoma)
- Thyroid autoantibodies useful in selected cases to differentiate Graves' disease from toxic multinodular goiter (absent thyroid antibodies)

IMAGING STUDIES

- 24-hr radioactive iodine uptake (RAIU) is useful to distinguish hyperthyroidism from iatrogenic thyroid hormone synthesis (thyrotoxicosis factitia) and from thyroiditis.
- An overactive thyroid shows increased uptake, whereas a normal underactive thyroid (iatrogenic thyroid ingestion, painless or subacute thyroiditis) shows normal or decreased uptake.
- The RAIU results also vary with the etiology of the hyperthyroidism:
  - Graves' disease: increased homogeneous uptake
  - Multinodular goiter: increased heterogeneous uptake

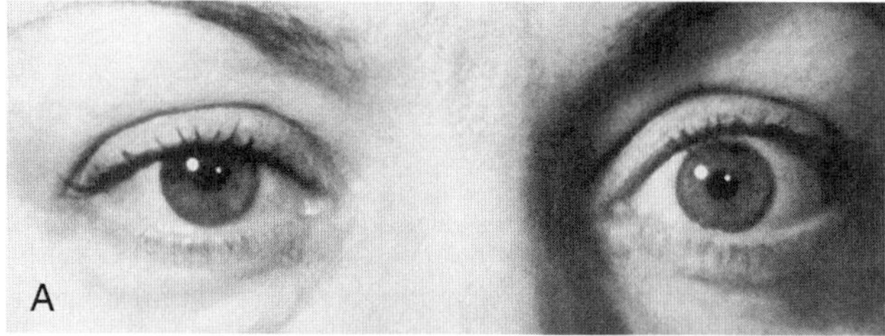

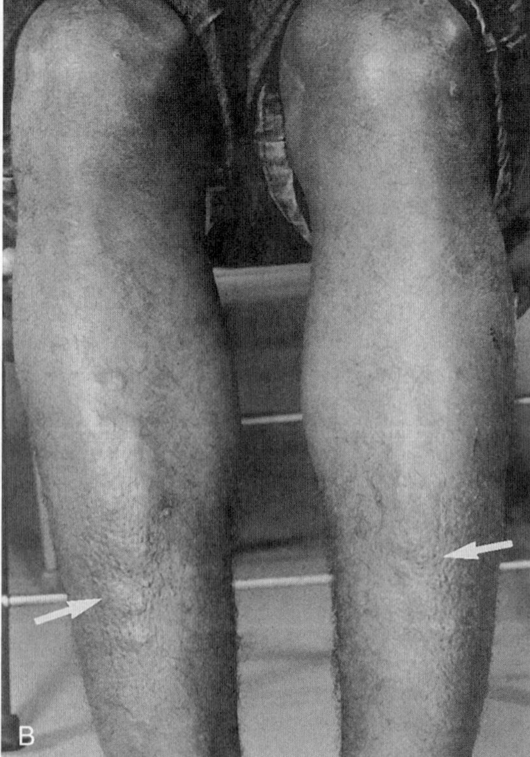

FIGURE 1-166 A, Unilateral *(left)* lid retraction in a patient with hyperthyroidism. **B,** Pretibial myxedema *(arrows)* in a patient with Graves' disease. (From Noble J [ed]: *Textbook of primary care medicine,* ed 2, St Louis, 1996, Mosby.)

- ○ Hot nodule: single focus of increased uptake
- RAIU is also generally performed before the therapeutic administration of radioactive iodine to determine the appropriate dose.

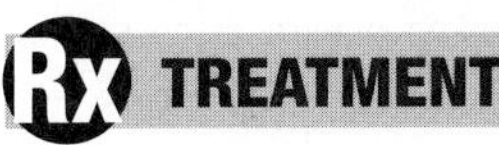

TREATMENT

NONPHARMACOLOGIC THERAPY

Patient education regarding thyroid disease and discussion of the therapeutic options (medications, radioactive iodine, and thyroid surgery)

ACUTE GENERAL Rx

ANTITHYROID DRUGS (THIONAMIDES): Propylthiouracil (PTU) and methimazole (Tapazole) inhibit thyroid hormone synthesis by blocking production of thyroid peroxidase (PTU and methimazole) or inhibit peripheral conversion of T_4 to T_3 (PTU). Methimazole is favored by most endocrinologists. PTU is preferred in pregnant women. Complete blood count and differential should be obtained before their use.

1. Dosage: methimazole 15 to 30 mg/day given as a single dose; PTU 50 to 100 mg PO q8h.
2. Antithyroid drugs can be used as the primary form of treatment or as adjunctive therapy before radioactive therapy or surgery or afterward if the hyperthyroidism recurs.
3. Side effects: skin rash (3% to 5% of patients), arthralgias, myalgias, granulocytopenia (0.5%). Rare side effects are aplastic anemia, hepatic necrosis from PTU, cholestatic jaundice from methimazole.
4. When antithyroid drugs are used as primary therapy, they are usually given for 6 to 18 mo; prolonged therapy may cause hypothyroidism. Monitor thyroid function every 2 mo for 6 mo, then less frequently.
5. The use of antithyroid drugs before radioactive iodine therapy is best reserved for patients in whom exacerbation of hyperthyroidism after radioactive iodine therapy is hazardous (e.g., elderly patients with coronary artery disease or significant coexisting morbidity). In these patients the antithyroid drug can be stopped 2 days before radioactive iodine therapy, resumed 2 days later, and continued for 4 to 6 wk.

RADIOACTIVE IODINE (RAI; ^{131}I):

1. RAI is the treatment of choice for patients >21 yr and younger patients who have not achieved remission after 1 yr of antithyroid drug therapy. RAI is also used in hyperthyroidism caused by toxic adenoma or toxic multinodular goiter.
2. Contraindicated during pregnancy (can cause fetal hypothyroidism) and lactation. Pregnancy should be excluded in women of childbearing age before RAI is administered.
3. A single dose of RAI is effective in inducing a euthyroid state in nearly 80% of patients.
4. There is a high incidence of post-RAI hypothyroidism (>50% within first year and 2%/yr thereafter); these patients should be frequently evaluated for the onset of hypothyroidism (see "Chronic Rx").

SURGICAL THERAPY (SUBTOTAL THYROIDECTOMY):

1. Indicated in obstructing goiters, in any patient who refuses RAI and cannot be adequately managed with antithyroid medications (e.g., patients with toxic adenoma or toxic multinodular goiter), and in pregnant patients who cannot be adequately managed with antithyroid medication or develop side effects to them.
2. Patients should be rendered euthyroid with antithyroid drugs before surgery.
3. Complications of surgery include hypothyroidism (28% to 43% after 10 yr), hypoparathyroidism, and vocal cord paralysis (1%).
4. Hyperthyroidism recurs after surgery in 10% to 15% of patients.

ADJUNCTIVE THERAPY: Propranolol alleviates the β-adrenergic symptoms of hyperthyroidism; initial dose is 20 to 40 mg PO q6h; dosage is gradually increased until symptoms are controlled. Major contraindications to propranolol are congestive heart failure and bronchospasm. Diagnosis and treatment of thyrotoxic storm is also discussed in Section I.

CHRONIC Rx

- Patients undergoing treatment with antithyroid drugs should be seen every 1 to 3 mo until euthyroidism is achieved and every 3 to 4 mo while they remain on antithyroid therapy. After treatment is stopped, periodic monitoring of thyroid function tests with TSH is recommended every 3 mo for 1 yr, then every 6 mo for 1 yr, then annually.
- Orbital decompression surgery can be used to correct Graves' orbitopathy (Fig. 1-167).

DISPOSITION

Successful treatment of hyperthyroidism requires lifelong monitoring for the onset of hypothyroidism or the recurrence of thyrotoxicosis.

REFERRAL

- Endocrinology referral is recommended at the time of initial diagnosis and during treatment.
- Surgical referral in selected patients (see "Surgical Therapy").
- Hospitalization of all patients with thyroid storm.

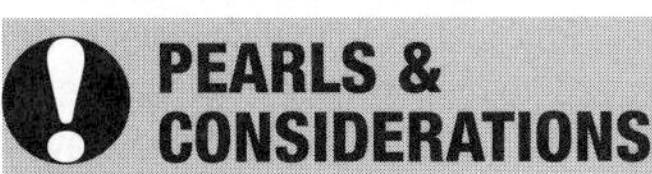

PEARLS & CONSIDERATIONS

COMMENTS

- Elderly hyperthyroid patients may have only subtle signs (weight loss, tachycardia, fine skin, brittle nails). This form is known as ***apathetic hyperthyroidism*** and manifests with lethargy rather than hyperkinetic activity. An enlarged thyroid gland may be absent. Coexisting medical disorders (most commonly cardiac disease) may also mask the symptoms. These patients often have unexplained congestive heart failure, worsening of angina, or new-onset atrial fibrillation resistant to treatment. See the entry on Graves' disease for additional information on diagnosis and treatment.
- Subclinical hyperthyroidism is defined as a normal serum-free thyroxine and free triiodothyronine levels with a TSH level suppressed below the normal range and usually unde-

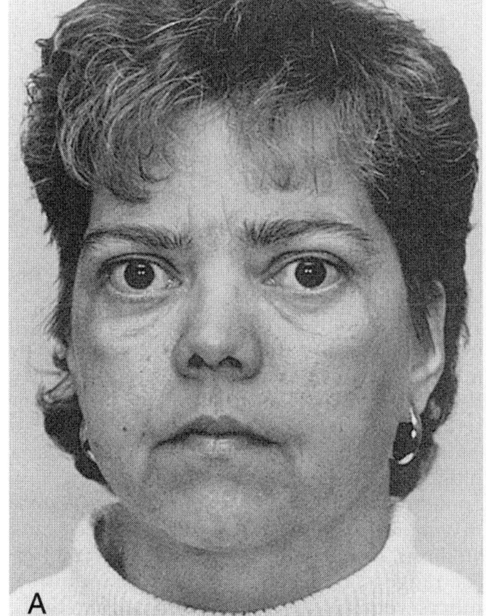

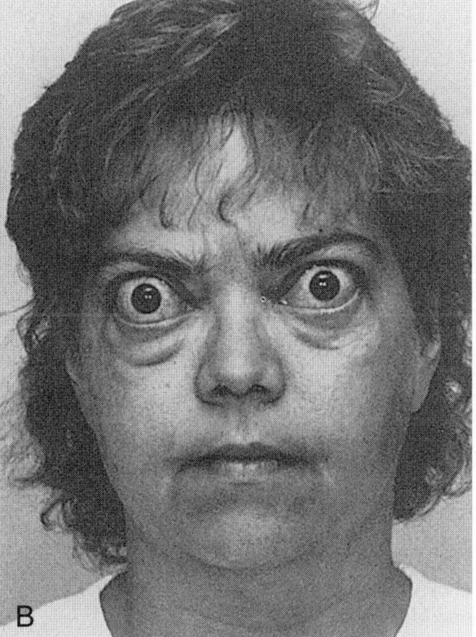

FIGURE 1-167 Characteristic signs of Graves' orbitopathy. A, Subsequently corrected by orbital decompression surgery. **B,** Note the thyroid stare, asymmetry, proptosis, and periorbital edema before correction. (Courtesy Dr. Jack Rootman, University of British Columbia, Vancouver, Canada. From Larsen PR et al [eds]: *Williams textbook of endocrinology,* ed 10, Philadelphia, 2003, Saunders.)

H

Diseases and Disorders I

tectable. These patients usually do not present with signs or symptoms of overt hyperthyroidism. Treatment options include observation or a therapeutic trial of low-dose antithyroid agents for 6 mo to attempt to induce remission.

- ***Thyrotoxic periodic paralysis (TPP)*** is a hyperthyroidism-related hypokalemia and muscle-weakening condition resulting from a sudden shift of potassium into cells. Many patients do not have other symptoms of hyperthyroidism. Typical presentation involves an Asian adult male with acute fatigue and muscle weakness initially presenting in the lower extremities. Physical examination reveals decreased deep tendon reflexes, hypertension, and tachycardia. ECG often reveals U waves, high QRS voltage, and first-degree atrioventricular block. Additional laboratory testing reveals normal acid-base state, hypokalemia with low urinary potassium excretion (spot urinary potassium concentration <20 mEq/L from potassium shift into cells), hypophosphatemia, hypophostaturia, and hypercalciuria. Electromyography during attacks shows low-amplitude compound muscle action potential of the tested muscle. Therapy consists of cautious potassium supplementation (increased risk of rebound hyperkalemia). Use of nonselective beta-blockers (e.g., propranolol) to counteract hyperadrenergic activity, which may be causing TPP, may also be useful.

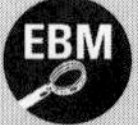

EVIDENCE

PTU and methimazole are both effective at inducing euthyroidism in Graves' disease, although single daily dose methimazole appears to be more effective than single daily dose PTU.[1] **B**

Small trials have found that propranolol and diltiazem effectively lessen the adrenergic symptoms caused by hyperthyroidism.[2,3] **B**

Thyroidectomy (either partial or total) is a successful treatment for hyperthyroidism.[4] **B**

A systematic review of various regimens for medical treatment of Graves' hyperthyroidism found that a titration regimen was as effective as a block-replace regimen and appeared to have fewer side effects. The evidence supported a 12- to 18-mo duration for titration therapy. One trial found that a 6-mo block-replacement regimen was as effective as a 12-mo treatment. In general, there was a high level of loss to follow-up in the trials reviewed.[5] **B**

Evidence-Based References

1. Homsanit M et al: Efficacy of single daily dosage of methimazole vs. propylthiouracil in the induction of euthyroidism, *Clin Endocrinol (Oxf)* 54:385, 2001. **B**
2. Henderson JM et al: Propranolol as an adjunct therapy for hyperthyroid tremor, *Eur Neurol* 37:182, 1997. **B**
3. Kelestimur F, Aksu A: The effect of diltiazem on the manifestations of hyperthyroidism and thyroid function tests, *Exp Clin Endocrinol Diabetes* 104:38, 1996. **B**
4. Palit TK et al: The efficacy of thyroidectomy for Graves' disease: a meta-analysis, *J Surg Res* 90:161, 2000. **B**
5. Abraham P et al: Antithyroid drug regimen for treating Graves' hyperthyroidism, *Cochrane Rev* 2, 2005. **B**

SUGGESTED READINGS

Cooper DS: Antithyroid drugs, *N Engl J Med* 352:905, 2005.

Reid JR, Wheeler SF: Hyperthyroidism, *Am Fam Physician* 72:623, 2005.

Shih HL: Thyrotoxic periodic paralysis, *Mayo Clin Proc* 80(10):99, 2005.

AUTHOR: **FRED F. FERRI, M.D.**

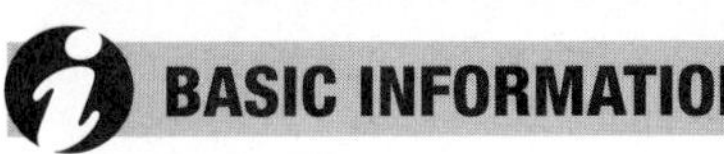

BASIC INFORMATION

DEFINITION

Hypertrophic osteoarthropathy (HOA) is a syndrome of clubbing of the digits, periostitis of long bones, skin changes, and arthritis. HOA may be primary or secondary to other underlying disease processes.

SYNONYMS

- Primary hypertrophic osteoarthropathy:
  1. Pachydermoperiostosis
  2. Idiopathic clubbing
  3. Touraine-Solente-Golé syndrome
- Secondary hypertrophic osteoarthropathy

ICD-9CM CODES
731.2 Hypertrophic osteoarthropathy

EPIDEMIOLOGY & DEMOGRAPHICS

- Primary HOA is a familial autosomal-dominant disease affecting the age group between 1 and 20 yr and is rare.
- Secondary HOA is more common, typically occurs in adults, and is associated with other illnesses, including:
  1. Pulmonary: bronchogenic carcinoma, lung abscesses, bronchiectasis, cystic fibrosis, pulmonary fibrosis, mesothelioma, sarcoidosis
  2. Gastrointestinal: esophageal carcinoma, colon cancer, inflammatory bowel disease (Crohn's disease, ulcerative colitis), hepatocellular carcinoma, liver cirrhosis, amebiasis
  3. Cardiac: infective endocarditis, right-to-left cardiac shunts, aortic aneurysms
  4. Thymoma
  5. Lymphoma
  6. Connective tissue diseases
  7. Thyroid acropachy

PHYSICAL FINDINGS & CLINICAL PRESENTATION

- Primary HOA typically presents with the insidious onset of clubbing of the hands and feet, described as "spadelike." Other signs and symptoms include:
  1. Joint pain and swelling
  2. Decreased use of the fingers and hands
  3. Facial changes, coarse facial skin grooves
  4. Thickening of the arms and legs
  5. Oily skin, diaphoresis, gynecomastia, and acne
- Secondary HOA patients may present with clinical symptoms before the underlying disorder can be detected. Signs and symptoms are similar to the above in addition to findings related to the underlying disease (e.g., bronchogenic carcinoma, infective endocarditis).

ETIOLOGY

The pathogenesis of HOA is not fully understood; current knowledge suggests that HOA results from the activation of one or more growth factors, such as vascular endothelial growth factor (VEGF) and platelet-derived growth factor, that are normally inactivated in the lungs and systemic circulation.

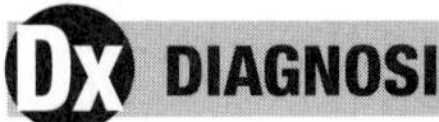

DIAGNOSIS

Diagnosis is primarily clinical; radiographs and bone scans can help confirm the diagnosis.

DIFFERENTIAL DIAGNOSIS

Other causes of HOA include Paget's disease, Reiter's syndrome, psoriasis, syphilis, osteoarthritis, rheumatoid arthritis, and osteomyelitis.

WORKUP

HOA warrants an investigation into any associated illnesses.

LABORATORY TESTS

- Routine laboratory studies such as blood count, electrolytes, and urine studies are typically normal in primary and secondary HOA.
- Erythrocyte sedimentation rate is elevated in secondary HOA.
- Liver function tests may be abnormal in patients with secondary HOA from gastrointestinal pathology.
- Alkaline phosphatase may be elevated as a result of periostitis of long bones.
- Analysis of the synovial fluid from joint effusions reveals a low white blood cell count with normal viscosity, color, and complement levels.

IMAGING STUDIES

- Radiographs of the long bones show periosteal new bone formation.
- A chest radiograph should be obtained to rule out underlying lung cancer.
- Bone scan with technetium-99m reveals uptake along the long bones, phalanges, and periarticular joint spaces.

Rx TREATMENT

ACUTE GENERAL Rx

- Treatment of primary HOA is symptomatic. Nonsteroidal antiinflammatory medications such as aspirin, salicylate, ibuprofen, naproxen, or indomethacin can be used.
- Treatment of secondary HOA is to eradicate the underlying disease (e.g., antibiotics for infective endocarditis, surgery for bronchogenic carcinoma). Correction of heart malformation or removal of an underlying tumor is rapidly followed by regression of HOA.

CHRONIC Rx

In patients with secondary HOA refractory to NSAIDs and aspirin, vagotomy has been tried with some success. However, the definitive treatment is to treat the underlying disease.

DISPOSITION

- Patients with primary HOA typically have symptoms of joint pain and swelling for the early part of their life. However, the disease becomes quiescent thereafter.
- Prognosis and disease course in patients with secondary HOA will depend on the underlying cause. The insidious development of clubbing suggests an infectious process, whereas the rapid progression of clubbing may suggest underlying malignancy.

REFERRAL

Referral should be made to rheumatology when the diagnosis of HOA is suspected and the cause remains unclear.

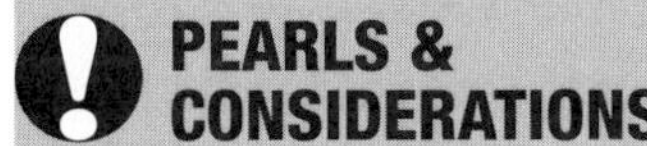

PEARLS & CONSIDERATIONS

Promidronate is a promising agent to relieve intractable pains associated with periosteal proliferation. Some bisphosphonates, including pamidronate, inhibit VEGF expression.

COMMENTS

- Infections and intrathoracic malignancies are the most common causes of secondary HOA.
- Some cases of primary HOA may later be found to be associated with a underlying disease such as patent ductus arteriosus, Crohn's disease, or myelofibrosis, in which case they become secondary.
- The periostosis and the extent of involvement do not depend on the form of the disease (primary or secondary), but rather on its duration.
- HOA secondary to infection of an arterial graft has been reported.
- Primary HOA and polyneuropathy, organomegaly, endocrinopathy, M-protein, and skin changes (POEMS) syndrome share important clinical features.

SUGGESTED READINGS

Amital H et al: Hypertrophic pulmonary osteoarthropathy: control of pain and symptoms with pamidronate, *Clin Rheumatol* 23(4):330, 2004.

Martinez-Lavin M et al: Hypertrophic osteoarthropathy: a palindrome with a pathogenic connotation, *Curr Opin Rheumatol* 20(1):88-91, 2008.

AUTHOR: **SHAHNAZ PUNJANI, M.D.**

Hypoaldosteronism

BASIC INFORMATION

DEFINITION

Hypoaldosteronism is defined as an aldosterone deficiency or impaired aldosterone function.

ICD-9CM CODES
255.4 Hypoadrenalism

EPIDEMIOLOGY & DEMOGRAPHICS

Selective hypoaldosteronism accounts for as many as 10% of cases of unexplained hyperkalemia.

PHYSICAL FINDINGS & CLINICAL PRESENTATION

- Physical examination may be entirely within normal limits.
- Hypertension may be present in some patients.
- Profound muscle weakness and cardiac arrhythmias may be present.

ETIOLOGY

- Hyporeninemic hypoaldosteronism (renin-angiotensin dependent): decreased aldosterone production as a result of decreased renin production; the typical patient has renal disease attributable to various factors (e.g., diabetes mellitus, interstitial nephritis, multiple myeloma).
- Hyperreninemic hypoaldosteronism (renin-angiotensin independent): renin production by the kidneys is intact; the defect is in aldosterone biosynthesis or in the action of angiotensin II. Common causes of this form of hypoaldosteronism are medications (ACE inhibitors, heparin), lead poisoning, aldosterone enzyme defects, and severe illness.

DIAGNOSIS

DIFFERENTIAL DIAGNOSIS

Pseudohypoaldosteronism: renal unresponsiveness to aldosterone. In this condition both renin and aldosterone levels are elevated. Pseudohypoaldosteronism can be caused by medications (spironolactone), chronic interstitial nephritis, systemic disorders (systemic lupus erythematosus, amyloidosis), or primary mineralocorticoid resistance.

WORKUP

Measurement of plasma renin activity after 4 hr of upright posture can differentiate hyporeninemic from hyperreninemic causes. Renin levels in the normal or low range identify cases that are renin-angiotensin dependent, whereas high renin levels identify cases that are renin-angiotensin independent. The diagnosis and etiology of hypoaldosteronism can be confirmed with the renin-aldosterone stimulation test:

- Hyporeninemic hypoaldosteronism: low stimulated renin and aldosterone levels
- End-organ refractoriness to aldosterone action: high stimulated renin and aldosterone levels
- Adrenal gland abnormality: high stimulated renin and low aldosterone levels

LABORATORY TESTS

- Increased potassium, normal or decreased sodium
- Hyperchloremic metabolic acidosis (caused by the absence of hydrogen-secreting action of aldosterone)
- Increased BUN and creatinine (secondary to renal disease)
- Hyperglycemia (diabetes mellitus is common in these patients)

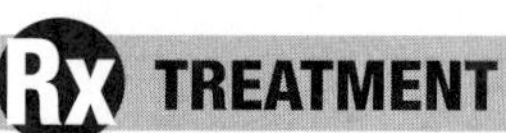

TREATMENT

NONPHARMACOLOGIC THERAPY

- Low-potassium diet with liberal sodium intake (at least 4 g of sodium chloride per day)
- Avoidance of ACE inhibitors and potassium-sparing diuretics

ACUTE GENERAL Rx

- Judicious use of fludrocortisone (0.05 to 0.1 mg PO every morning) in patients with aldosterone deficiency associated with deficiency of adrenal glucocorticoid hormones
- Furosemide 20 to 40 mg qd to correct hyperkalemia of hyporeninemic hypoaldosteronism

DISPOSITION

Prognosis varies with the etiology of hypoaldosteronism and presence of associated disorders.

REFERRAL

Endocrinology referral for renin-aldosterone stimulation test

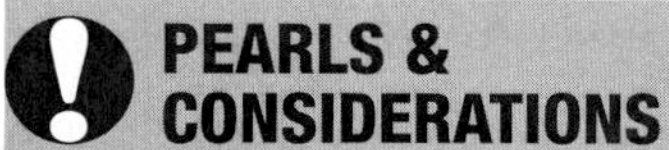

PEARLS & CONSIDERATIONS

COMMENTS

Treatment of pseudohypoaldosteronism is the same as for hypoaldosteronism; however, effect is limited because of impaired renal sensitivity.

AUTHOR: **FRED F. FERRI, M.D.**

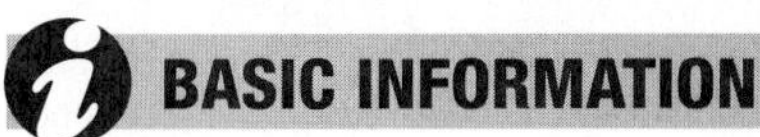

BASIC INFORMATION

DEFINITION

Hypochondriasis is the preoccupation with the fear of having, or the idea that one has, a serious disease. The fear is usually based on a misinterpretation of bodily signs or symptoms and persists despite medical reassurance, although the belief does not have the intensity of a delusion. The preoccupation causes clinically significant distress or impairment in social, occupational, or other important areas of functioning and lasts for at least 6 mo.

SYNONYMS

None

ICD-9CM CODES
300.7 Hypochondriasis

EPIDEMIOLOGY & DEMOGRAPHICS

PREVALENCE: 1% to 5%, but it is thought to be higher in primary care outpatient settings, where estimates range from 3% to 10%.

PREDOMINANT SEX: Occurs with equal frequency in men and women.

PREDOMINANT AGE: Onset can occur at any age, but incidence is most common between 20 and 30 yr of age.

GENETICS/RISK: No genetic component has been identified, and neither socioeconomic nor educational factors appear to predispose people to this disorder. Patients with hypochondriasis are more likely than the general population to have Axis I disorders, such as generalized anxiety, obsessive-compulsive disorder, and depression, as well as Axis II personality disorders.

PHYSICAL FINDINGS & CLINICAL PRESENTATION

- Patient presents with a complaint of a physical symptom or sign (e.g., dizziness, pain) and remains preoccupied with the concern, despite evidence to the contrary, that it represents a serious disease.
- Serious childhood illnesses are common in past medical history.
- There are no specific physical examination findings.
- Degree of insight varies (i.e., recognition that the concern about serious illness is excessive or unreasonable).

ETIOLOGY

Unknown etiology, but psychologic theories include disturbance of perception (amplification of normal somatic sensations), cognition (tendency to attribute sensations to a pathologic process), or interpersonal relationships (learning and then reinforcement of the sick role); or variant of another psychiatric condition such as depression.

Dx DIAGNOSIS

DIFFERENTIAL DIAGNOSIS

- Underlying medical condition, such as multiple sclerosis, hypothyroidism, or systemic lupus erythematosus
- Somatization disorder
- Body dysmorphic disorder (restricted to a circumscribed concern about appearance)
- Factitious disorder or malingering
- Generalized anxiety disorder with health concerns as one worry among many others
- Major depressive disorder with health concerns occurring only during depressive episodes
- Psychosis, as may occur with depression and schizophrenia

WORKUP

- History and physical examination, laboratory and imaging tests as directed by history, as appropriate, to exclude underlying medical condition.
- Symptom measures (e.g., Health Anxiety Inventory, Whiteley Index of Hypochondriasis) may be used for detection and monitoring of severity over time.
- Evaluation for other psychiatric disorders associated with hypochondriasis such as depression and anxiety.

Rx TREATMENT

NONPHARMACOLOGIC THERAPY

- Reassurance and education, including linking the diagnosis to psychologic stressors
- Brief and regularly scheduled appointments with the primary care physician
- Avoidance of laboratory tests, imaging studies, and diagnostic and surgical procedures unless clearly indicated
- Elimination of sources of secondary gain
- Limit on reading medical texts or websites
- Individual or group therapy, including problem-solving (focusing on understanding and coping with the disorder) or cognitive-behavioral (with techniques to alter or restructure hypochondriacal thinking)
- Benign interventions (e.g., exercise, massage, vitamins)

CHRONIC Rx

- Pharmacologic treatment of comorbid psychiatric conditions, if present.
- Antidepressants may be helpful even in patients without features of depression: placebo-controlled trials of fluoxetine and paroxetine suggest benefit; imipramine, fluvoxamine has been studied in small, open-label trials.

DISPOSITION

Waxing and waning course over decades, with relapses often triggered by psychosocial stressors. Recovery rates between 30% and 50%. Good prognostic features include acute onset, absence of secondary gain, lack of comorbid psychiatric disorder, and high socioeconomic status.

REFERRAL

Referral to a therapist and/or psychiatrist may be helpful; however, patients may resist referral given the belief that symptoms are due to an undiagnosed medical illness.

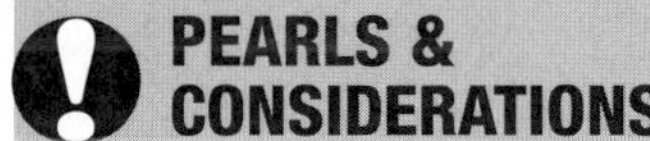

PEARLS & CONSIDERATIONS

- The onset of physical symptoms late in life is almost always the result of a medical disorder.
- Antidepressants and psychoeducational therapy may be helpful treatment modalities, although patients may be resistant to therapy not directed at the perceived illness.

SUGGESTED READINGS

Creed F, Barsky A: A systematic review of the epidemiology of somatisation disorder and hypochondriasis, *J Psychosom Res* 56(4):391, 2004.

Fallon BA et al: A double-masked, placebo-controlled study of fluoxetine for hypochondriasis, *J Clin Psychopharmacol* 28(6):638, 2008.

Fink P et al: A new empirically established hypochondriasis diagnosis, *Am J Psychiatry* 161(9):1680, 2004.

Greeven A et al: Cognitive behavior therapy and paroxetine in the treatment of hypochondriasis: a randomized controlled trial, *Am J Psychiatry* 164(1): 91, 2007.

olde Hartman T et al: Medically unexplained symptoms, somatisation disorder and hypochondriasis: course and prognosis, *J Psychosom Res* 66(5):363, 2009.

AUTHOR: **LUCY KALANITHI, M.D.**

Hypoparathyroidism

BASIC INFORMATION

DEFINITION

A decrease parathyroid hormone (PTH) secretion or function results in hypoparathyroidism. In primary hypoparathyroidism, absence or dysfunction of the parathyroid gland results in under secretion of PTH and subsequent hypocalcemia and hyperphosphatemia. Impaired functions of PTH (i.e., PTH resistance or pseudohypoparathyroidism) can also cause hypocalcemia and hyperphosphatemia but the measured PTH level is elevated in this circumstance. Secondary hypoparathyroidism, a condition in which PTH levels are low in response to hypercalcemic states, is discussed in "Hypocalcemia." The focus of this section is primary hypoparathyroidism.

ICD-9CM CODES
252.1 Hypoparathyroidism

EPIDEMIOLOGY & DEMOGRAPHICS

The incidence and prevalence of primary hypoparathyroidism varies with the etiology of the condition. Postoperative hypoparathyroidism is the most common etiology and has an incidence as high as 3.8% in patients undergoing total or near-total thyroidectomy. Autoimmune polyglandular syndrome type I is reported to have an incidence of 1:100,000 and prevalence 1:25,000. Autoimmune disorders are more common in women (female:male ratio of 1.4:1) and type I syndrome presents in childhood. Other etiologies of primary hypoparathyroidism are very rare.

PHYSICAL FINDINGS & CLINICAL PRESENTATION

The symptoms of primary hypoparathyroidism are related to hypocalcemia (primarily) and the hypoparathyroid state. The presentation of symptoms varies with the severity and duration of illness.

- Cardiovascular: prolonged QT intervals and marked QRS and ST segment changes, ventricular arrhythmias
- Musculoskeletal: muscle cramps, laryngospasm, osteomalacia (adults), rickets (children), weakened tooth enamel, osteosclerosis
- CNS: tetany (Chvostek's sign and Trousseau's sign), seizures, paresthesias, visual impairment from cataract formation, altered mental status, papilledema, and basal ganglia calcifications with longstanding disease
- GI: abdominal pain
- Renal: hypercalciuria and nephrolithiasis
- Other: dry scaly skin, brittle nails, dry hair

ETIOLOGY

There are several etiologies of primary hypoparathyroidism.

- Genetic disorders
  - Branchial dysembryogenesis (DiGeorge's syndrome)
  - Congenital absence of parathyroids
  - Activating mutation of the calcium sensing receptor alters the set point of the receptor and decreases PTH secretion
- Autoimmune
  - Autoimmune polyglandular syndrome type 1 presents in early childhood and is defined by a classic triad of mucocutaneous candidiasis, autoimmune hypoparathyroidism, and Addison's disease.
  - Activating antibodies to calcium sensing receptor alters the set point of the receptor and decreases PTH secretion.
- Postsurgical (most common etiology): can be transient or permanent
  - Parathyroidectomy
  - Complication of neck surgery such as thyroidectomy
- Radiation to the neck
- Infiltration
  - Metastatic carcinoma
  - Wilson's disease
  - Hemochromatosis
  - Granulomas
- Other
  - Hypermagnesemia and hypomagnesemia
  - Severe burns and sepsis

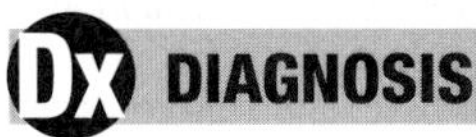

DIAGNOSIS

DIFFERENTIAL DIAGNOSIS

- Other causes of hypoparathyroidism (i.e., secondary hypoparathyroidism) include:
  - Medications: thiazide diuretics
  - Vitamin D intoxication, milk-alkali syndrome
  - Granulomatous disorders (e.g., sarcoidosis)
  - Malignancy (e.g., lung cancer, lymphoma, myeloma, bone metastasis)
  - Prolonged immobilization
- Other causes of hypocalcemia (i.e., secondary hyperparathyroidism) include:
  - PTH resistance (i.e., target organs unresponsive to PTH action)
    1. Pseudohypoparathyroidism: heterogeneous disorder presenting in childhood characterized by hypocalcemia, hyperphosphatemia and elevated PTH levels
    2. Hypomagnesemia
  - Vitamin D deficiency or resistance
  - Hyperphosphatemia (i.e., renal failure, rhabdomyolysis, tumor lysis)
  - Osteoblastic metastasis
  - Acute pancreatitis
  - Drugs: calcium chelators, bisphosphonates, foscarnet, cisplatin

WORKUP

- Primary hypoparathyroidism: serum calcium is usually low and phosphorus is elevated in primary hypoparathyroidism.
  - Two measurements of serum calcium are required for the confirmation of hypocalcemia. Total calcium should be corrected for low albumin utilizing the formula: Corrected Calcium = (0.8 * [4 – serum albumin] + serum calcium). If a reliable laboratory is available, an ionized calcium should be considered especially in conditions associated with acid-base disturbances or low albumin states.
  - The serum intact PTH (iPTH) level is the single best test to evaluate the etiology of hypocalcemia. PTH is decreased in hypoparathyroidism and elevated in most other conditions associated with low calcium levels.
  - Serum phosphorus is usually high normal or elevated in primary hypoparathyroidism.
- Rule out other causes of hypoparathyroidism (i.e., secondary hypoparathyroidism). These conditions are associated with hypercalcemia and subsequent PTH suppression.
- Rule out other causes of hypocalcemia. These conditions are typically associated with elevated PTH levels.

LABORATORY TESTS

- Total and ionized calcium: low in primary hypoparathyroidism and high in secondary hypoparathyroidism
- PTH: low in primary and secondary hypoparathyroidism and high in PTH resistance states like pseudohypoparathyroidism
- Phosphorus: high-normal or high in primary hypoparathyroidism
- Magnesium: both hypomagnesemia and hypermagnesemia can cause hypoparathyroidism
- ECG should be considered in both hypercalcemic and hypocalcemic states. Hypocalcemia associated with prolonged QT interval, rarely ST-segment elevations
- 24-hr urine for calcium to evaluate the risk for renal stones
- Other tests to consider to evaluated conditions discussed in the differential diagnosis includes vitamin D 25, vitamin D 1,25, creatinine, PTHrp, SPEP/UPEP, and amylase

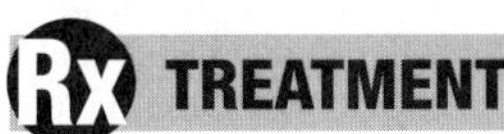

TREATMENT

NONPHARMACOLOGIC THERAPY

Parathyroid autotransplantation:
Hypoparathyroidism and hypocalcemia are common problems after neck exploration for total or near-total thyroidectomy or parathyroidectomy. In cases where there is concern for postoperative hypoparathyroidism, parathyroid autotransplantation of one or two parathyroid glands into the forearm or sternocleidomastoid muscle should be performed to prevent postoperative hypoparathyroidism.

PHARMACOLOGIC THERAPY

The mainstay of treatment for primary hypoparathyroidism is through pharmacologic therapy with calcium and vitamin D supplementation. The goals of therapy are to control symptoms and minimize complications of therapy. The aim should be to obtain low-normal serum calcium, 24-hr urinary calcium <300 mg/day, and a calcium-phosphorus product <55.

- Vitamin D:
  - There are several vitamin D preparations available on the market but the treatment of choice for patients with primary hypoparathyroidism is calcitriol. It is an active metabolite that does not require hydroxylation in the liver or kidney and therefore bypasses the 1-α hydroxylation defect that occurs with hypoparathyroidism.
  - Dose of 0.25 to 1 μg once or twice daily is usually required to correct hypocalcemia and improves symptoms. Its maximal effect is seen after 10 hr and it lasts for 2 to 3 days.
- Calcium:
  - Calcium carbonate or calcium citrates are common oral agents used to treatment hypocalcemia associated with hypoparathyroidism. Calcium carbonate requires an acidic environment for effective absorption, and as a result, it must be taken with food. Its effectiveness is decreased with concomitant use of H_2 blockers or proton pump inhibitors. However, calcium carbonate is cheaper in cost than other calcium supplements and therefore it is first line in the management of hypocalcemia for some patients. The advantage of calcium citrate is that it does not require an acidic environment for effective absorption.
  - Start with a dose of 500 to 1000 mg of elemental calcium TID and adjust the dose for a desired calcium in the low-normal range.
- Magnesium: hypocalcemia is difficult to correct without normalizing magnesium levels. IV magnesium sulfate 2 g over 20 min followed by 1 g/hr infusion can be considered in severe deficiency states. Milder deficiencies can be managed with oral magnesium 100 mg tid.
- Thiazide diuretics: thiazides diuretics decrease urine calcium excretion and decrease kidney stones. They should be considered in individuals with urine calcium $>$250 mg/day.
- PTH replacement:
  - Preliminary studies involving injectable synthetic human PTH (1-34) have been performed with results showing a decrease in urinary calcium excretion and maintenance of serum calcium in the normal range.
  - It is not FDA approved for use in hypoparathyroidism.

ACUTE GENERAL RX

Severe and/or symptomatic hypocalcemia requires hospitalization. Acute management of hypocalcemia includes:

- Telemetry monitoring for arrhythmias associated with severe hypocalcemia
- IV infusion of calcium gluconate 10 ml of 10% solution to receive a bolus of 90 mg of elemental calcium followed by an infusion of 0.5 to 2 mg/kg/hr until ionized calcium levels are equal to or greater than 4 mg/dl.

PEARLS & CONSIDERATIONS

COMMENTS

- The mainstay of treatment for primary hypoparathyroidism is calcitriol and calcium supplementation to maintain a goal serum calcium level in the low-normal range. IV calcium should be considered if calcium $<$7.0 mg/dl. Magnesium levels should be assessed and appropriately replaced in all patients with hypocalcemia. Clinical trials are under way to evaluate the role of recombinant PTH for the treatment of primary hypoparathyroidism.
- In patients undergoing neck exploration, consideration should be given to the parathyroids and autotransplantation of one or more parathyroid glands should be considered when appropriate to prevent postoperative hypoparathyroidism.

EBM EVIDENCE

Key Trials and Commentary:

A long-term follow-up study of patients after total thyroidectomy with parathyroid autotransplantation showed a 1% incidence of hypoparathyroidism. This preventative measure markedly reduced the incidence of hypoparathyroidism.[1]

A randomized, parallel group, open-label trial of patients with hypoparathyroidism studied the effects of twice daily subcutaneous PTH versus conventional therapy with oral calcitriol and calcium supplementation. Serum calcium levels, bone mineral content, and bone mineral density were similar between the two groups. There was a significant difference in urinary calcium excretion, however, with the PTH group showing a normal urinary calcium excretion during the 3-yr study period. In the conventional therapy group, the urinary calcium excretion remained above normal. PTH was found to maintain normal serum calcium levels without hypercalciuria for the 3-yr period.[2]

Evidence-Based References

1. Olson JA et al: Parathyroid autotransplantation during thyroidectomy, *Ann Surg* 223(5):472-480, 1996.
2. Winer KK et al: Long-term treatment of hypoparathyroidism: a randomized controlled study comparing parathyroid hormone (1-34) versus calcitriol and calcium, *J Clin Endocrinol Metab* 88(9):4214-4220, 2003.

SUGGESTED READINGS

Erbil Y et al: The impact of age, vitamin D3 level, and incidental parathyroidectomy on postoperative hypocalcemia after total or near total thyroidectomy, *Am J Surg* 197:439-446, 2009.

Guise TA et al: Clinical review 69: evaluation of hypocalcemia in children and adults, *J Clin Endocrinol Metab* 80(5):1473-1478, 1995.

Husebye ES et al: Clinical manifestations and management of patients with autoimmune polyendocrine syndrome type I. *J Intern Med* 265:514-529, 2009.

Walker Harris V et al: Postoperative hypoparathyroidism: medical and surgical therapeutic options, *Thyroid* 19(9):967-973, 2008.

AUTHORS: **JENNIFER MIRANDA, M.D.,** and **GEETHA GOPALAKRISHNAN, M.D.**

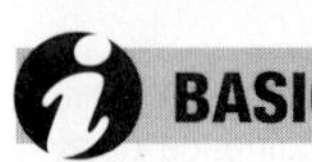

BASIC INFORMATION

DEFINITION

Hypopituitarism (from the Latin *pituita,* meaning phlegm) is the deficiency of one or more of the hormones of the anterior or posterior pituitary gland resulting from diseases of the hypothalamus or pituitary gland. Panhypopituitarism indicates the loss of all the pituitary hormones but is often used in clinical practice to describe patients deficient in growth hormone (GH), gonadotropins, corticotrophin, or thyrotropin in whom posterior pituitary function remains intact.

SYNONYMS

Panhypopituitarism
Pituitary insufficiency

ICD-9CM CODES
253.2 Panhypopituitarism

EPIDEMIOLOGY & DEMOGRAPHICS

Incidence of 4.2 cases per 100,000 persons

PHYSICAL FINDINGS & CLINICAL PRESENTATION

Symptoms depend on type of onset, number and severity of hormone deficiencies, their target organs, and age of onset.

- Mass effect of a pituitary tumor can cause headaches and visual disturbances (typically as bitemporal hemianopsia).
- Rhinorrhea.
- Corticotropin deficiency:
  - Fatigue and weakness, no appetite, abdominal pain, nausea, vomiting, failure to thrive in children, and hyponatremia. If the onset is abrupt, hypotension and shock
- Thyrotropin deficiency:
  - Fatigue and weakness, weight gain, cold intolerance, anemia, constipation
  - Bradycardia, hung-up reflexes, pretibial edema, change in voice, and hair loss
- Gonadotropin deficiency:
  - Loss of libido, erectile dysfunction, amenorrhea, hot flashes, dyspareunia, infertility, gynecomastia, decreased muscle mass, and anemia
- GH deficiency:
  - Growth retardation in children
  - Easy fatigue, hypoglycemia
  - Lean mass is reduced and fat mass is increased, leading to obesity
  - Decreased bone mineral density, increased low density lipoprotein cholesterol, obesity, increased inflammatory cardiovascular markers (interleukin-6 and C-reactive protein)
- Hyperprolactinemia:
  - Galactorrhea, hypogonadism, inability to lactate after delivery
  - Posterior pituitary (vasopressin; antidiuretic hormone [ADH] deficiency): diabetes insipidus with polyuria, polydipsia, nocturia, hypotension, and dehydration

ETIOLOGY

It can be congenital or acquired:

- Congenital: mutations in transcription factors produce multiple hormonal deficiencies. Mutations in genes produce single hormonal deficiency.
- Acquired: the result of destruction of pituitary cells caused by:
  1. Pituitary apoplexy: hemorrhage or infarction of the pituitary gland. Predisposing factors include diabetes mellitus, anticoagulation therapy, head trauma, and radiation therapy. Sheehan's syndrome: postpartum necrosis, a rare complication after pregnancy.
  2. Infiltrative disease, including sarcoidosis, hemachromatosis, histiocytosis X, Wegener's granulomatosis, lymphocytic hypophysitis, and infection of the pituitary (tuberculosis, mycosis, syphilis).
  3. Primary empty sella syndrome: flattening of the pituitary gland caused by extension of the subarachnoid space and filling of cerebrospinal fluid into the sella turcica.
  4. Pituitary tumors: classified by size (microadenomas, $<$10 mm; macroadenomas, $>$10 mm) and function. Prolactin-secreting tumors and nonfunctioning tumors account for the majority of pituitary adenomas.
  5. Suprasellar tumors: craniopharyngiomas are the most common.

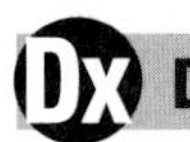

DIAGNOSIS

The diagnosis of hypopituitarism is suspected by clinical history and physical findings and is established by blood tests to confirm the presence of hormone deficiency.

DIFFERENTIAL DIAGNOSIS

The differential diagnosis is as outlined under "Etiology."

WORKUP

Includes baseline determination of each anterior pituitary hormone followed by dynamic provocative stimulation tests, radiograph imaging, and formal visual field testing.

LABORATORY TESTS

- Corticotropin deficiency:
  1. The presence of a 9:00 AM cortisol level $>$20 mcg/dl or $<$4 mcg/dl usually confirms sufficiency or deficiency, respectively.
  2. Corticotropin stimulation test using 250 mcg of corticotropin given IV and measuring serum cortisol before and 30 and 60 min after administration. A normal response is an increase in serum cortisol level $>$20 mcg/dl.
  3. With pituitary disease these test results may be indeterminate, and more dynamic testing such as an insulin-tolerance or metyrapone test may be necessary.
- Thyrotropin deficiency:
  1. Thyroid-stimulating hormone (TSH) and free T_4 measurements
  2. Primary hypothyroidism shows elevated TSH with low free T_4. Secondary hypothyroidism shows normal or low TSH with low free T_4 and low T_3 resin uptake.
- Gonadotropin deficiency:
  1. Follicle-stimulating hormone (FSH), luteinizing hormone (LH), estrogen, and testosterone measurements.
  2. In men, hypogonadotropic hypogonadism is seen with low testosterone levels and normal or low FSH and LH levels (ideally measured at 9:00 AM because of diurnal rhythm). Check free testosterone if patient is obese.
  3. In premenopausal women with amenorrhea, low estrogen with normal or low FSH and LH levels is typically seen.
- GH deficiency:
  1. Insulin-induced hypoglycemia stimulation test using 0.1 to 0.15 unit/kg regular insulin given IV and measuring growth hormone 30, 60, and 120 min after administration. A normal response is a growth hormone level $>$3 mcg/dl. This test is contraindicated in seizure disorder or ischemic heart disease.
  2. Combination of GH-releasing hormone plus arginine is an alternative test, with a diagnostic threshold of 9 mcg/L.
  3. Because the relation between serum insulinlike growth factor (IGF)-1 and GH levels blurs with age, a normal serum IGF-1 does not exclude the diagnosis in older adults.
- Hyperprolactinemia: prolactin levels may be elevated in prolactin-secreting pituitary adenomas.
- Vasopressin deficiency:
  1. Urinalysis shows low specific gravity.
  2. Urine osmolality is low.
  3. Serum osmolality is high.
  4. Fluid deprivation test over 18 hr with inability to concentrate the urine.
  5. Serum vasopressin level is low.
  6. Electrolytes may show hyponatremia and exclude hyperglycemia.

IMAGING STUDIES

- Imaging is the first step in identifying an underlying cause.
- MRI is more sensitive than CT in visualizing the pituitary fossa, sella turcica, optic chiasm, pituitary stalk, and cavernous sinuses. It is also more sensitive in detecting pituitary microadenomas. CT with contrast can be used if MRI is not available.
- Surveillance scan at baseline and 12 mo thereafter depending on protocol and clinical symptoms.

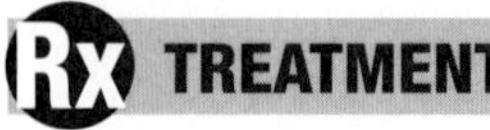

TREATMENT

Threefold: removing underlying cause (surgery or radiation), treating hormonal deficiencies, and addressing any other repercussions from deficiency.

NONPHARMACOLOGIC THERAPY

- IV fluid resuscitation, correction of electrolyte and metabolic abnormalities with potassium bicarbonate, and oxygen therapy.
- Transsphenoidal surgery for tumors causing specific symptoms.
- Radiation or stereotactic radiosurgery ("gamma knife") for medically unresponsive, surgically unresectable tumors and tumors for which other modalities are contraindicated. It is both safe and effective for recurrent or residual pituitary adenomas.

ACUTE GENERAL Rx

Acute situations such as adrenal crisis or myxedema coma can occur in untreated hypopituitarism and should be treated accordingly with IV corticosteroids (e.g., hydrocortisone 100 to 250 mg bolus followed by hydrocortisone 100 mg IV q6h for 24 hr) and levothyroxine (e.g., 5 to 8 mcg/kg IV over 15 min, then 100 mcg IV q24h).

CHRONIC Rx

Treatment is lifelong:

- Adrenocorticotropic hormone (ACTH) deficiency: hydrocortisone 10 mg PO every morning and 5 mg PO every evening or prednisone 5 mg PO every morning and 2.5 mg PO every evening. Dexamethasone or prednisone is often preferred because of longer duration of action.
- LH and FSH deficiency:
  - In men, testosterone enanthate or propionate 200 to 300 mg IM every 2 to 3 wk, or transdermal testosterone scrotal patches can be tried.
  - In women who are not interested in fertility, conjugated estrogen 0.3 to 1.25 mg/day and held the last 5 to 7 days of each month with the addition of medroxyprogesterone 10 mg/day given during days 15 to 25 of the normal menstrual cycle. In those who have secondary hypogonadism and wish to become pregnant, pulsatile gonadotropic-releasing hormone may be of benefit.
- TSH deficiency: levothyroxine 0.05 to 0.15 mg/day.
- GH deficiency:
  - GH replacement in children is universally accepted.
  - GH replacement in adults is not generally recommended and requires careful consideration of each individual case. It may have effects on quality of life, body composition, bone density, and cardiovascular risk factors.
  - Side effects of replacement includes peripheral edema, arthralgia, and headaches.
  - Usual GH dose is between 0.2 and 0.4 mg, determined by the age and gender of a patient and increments of 0.1 mg every 2 to 4 wk until serum IGF-1 is in the upper part of the normal range. Young adults and women taking estrogen require a higher dose.
- ADH deficiency:
  - Desmopressin (DDAVP) 10 to 20 mcg by intranasal spray or 0.05 to 0.1 mg PO bid is used in patients with diabetes insipidus.
  - Vasopressin: 5-10 U given IM or SC q6h.

DISPOSITION

- Hormone replacement therapy is adjusted according to serum hormone monitoring.
- If untreated can lead to adrenal crisis, severe hyponatremia and hypothyroidism, metabolic abnormalities, and death.
- Complications: visual deficit, adrenal crisis, susceptibility to infection and other stressors.
- Prognosis: stable patients have a favorable prognosis with replacement hormone therapy. Patients with acute decompensation are in critical condition with a high mortality rate.

REFERRAL

Consultation with an endocrinologist and neurosurgeon for surgical treatment

PEARLS & CONSIDERATIONS

- All patients sustaining moderate to severe head injury should undergo assessment of anterior pituitary function during the acute phase and at 6 mo.
- IGF-1 can be used as a marker of GH deficiency.
- All tests of GH secretion are more likely to give false-positive results in obese patients.
- The GH axis is the most vulnerable to the effects of radiotherapy; doses as low as 18 Gy in children have caused GH deficiency.
- Sequence of hormonal disruption: GH secretion then gonadotropin secretion. TSH and adrenocorticotropic hormone secretion are somewhat resistant.
- Thyroxine supplementation increases the rate of cortisol metabolism and can lead to adrenal crisis, so corticosteroids should be replaced first.
- All patients receiving glucocorticoid replacement therapy should wear proper identification stating the need for this therapy.
- Stress doses of corticosteroids are indicated before surgery or for any medical emergency (e.g., sepsis, acute myocardial infarction).
- Antidiuretic hormone deficiency may be masked if there is ACTH deficiency with symptoms only appearing when cortisol has been replaced.

COMMENTS

- Mineralocorticoid replacement is not necessary in secondary adrenal insufficiency because the renin-angiotensin-aldosterone system is unaffected by pituitary failure.
- Patients with adult-acquired GH deficiency must meet at least two criteria before replacement therapy: a poor GH response to at least two standard stimuli and hypopituitarism from pituitary or hypothalamic damage. The criteria are different in children in whom GH is required for normal growth.
- Prevention of acute decompensation can be accomplished by reminding patients to increase the dose of hydrocortisone in response to stress.
- Medical therapy should precede surgical therapy.

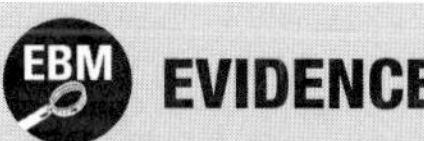

EVIDENCE

Please note: Complete text of EBM for this topic is available online.

SUGGESTED READINGS

American Association of Clinical Endocrinologists: Medical guidelines for clinical practice for growth hormone use in adults and children—2003 update, *Endocr Pract* 9:64, 2003.

Hanberg A: Common disorders of the pituitary gland: hyposecretion versus hypersecretion, *J Infus Nurs* 28(1):36, 2005.

Schneider HJ et al: Hypopituitarism, *Lancet* 369:1461, 2007.

Sheehan JP et al: Stereotactic radiosurgery for pituitary adenomas: an intermediate review of its safety, efficacy, and role in the neurosurgical treatment armamentarium, *J Neurosurg* 102(4):678, 2005.

Tagwood A: Hypopituitarism: clinical features, diagnosis, and management, *Endocrinol Metab Clin North Am* 37:235, 2008.

AUTHOR: **SHAHNAZ PUNJANI, M.D.**

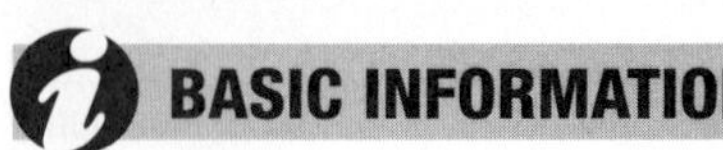

BASIC INFORMATION

DEFINITION

Hypospadias is a developmental abnormality of the penis characterized by:

- Abnormal ventral opening of the urethral meatus anywhere from the ventral aspect of the glans penis to the perineum
- Ventral curvature of the penis (chordee)
- Dorsal foreskin hood

ICD-9CM CODES
752.61
Congenital chordee: 752.63

EPIDEMIOLOGY & DEMOGRAPHICS

PREVALENCE: One male in 250

GENETICS:

- Pertinent familial aspects of hypospadias include the finding of hypospadias in 6.8% of fathers of affected boys and in 14% of male siblings.
- An 8.5-fold higher rate of hypospadias is reported in monozygotic twins, suggesting insufficient production of human chorionic gonadotropin (hCG) by the single placenta.

PHYSICAL FINDINGS & CLINICAL PRESENTATION

- Genetics: normal karyotypes are seen with glandular hypospadias; abnormal karyotypes are noted in more severe forms of hypospadias
- Cryptorchidism: 8% to 9% occurrence
- Inguinal hernia: 9% to 10% occurrence
- Hydrocele: 9% to 16% occurrence

PENILE CURVATURE (CHORDEE): Three theories:

1. Abnormal development of the urethral plate
2. Abnormal fibrotic mesenchymal tissue at the urethral meatus
3. Corporal disproportion

ETIOLOGY

Multifactorial:

- Endocrine factors:
    1. Abnormal androgen production
    2. Limited androgen sensitivity in the target tissues
    3. Premature cessation of androgenic stimulation as a result of Leydig cell dysfunction
    4. Insufficient testosterone-dihydrotestosterone synthesis as a result of deficient 5-alpha reductase enzyme activity
- Arrested development

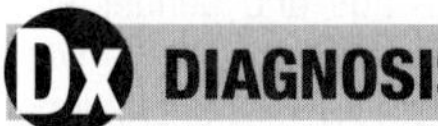

Dx DIAGNOSIS

WORKUP

Made by observation and examination

LABORATORY TESTS

Intersex evaluation should be undertaken if there is associated cryptorchidism. The evaluation should include ultrasound; genitographic studies; and chromosomal, gonadal, biochemical, and molecular studies.

Rx TREATMENT

ACUTE GENERAL Rx

DESIGNATION/CLASSIFICATION:

- Anterior: 33%
- Middle: 25%
- Posterior: 41%

SPECIAL CONSIDERATIONS:

- The only reason for operating on any patient with hypospadias is to correct deformities that interfere with the function of urination and procreation.
- Another reason for intervention is cosmetic concern.
- The American Academy of Pediatrics recommends the best time for surgical intervention to be 6 to 12 mo.

HORMONAL MANIPULATION:

- Controversial.
- hCG administration is given before repair of proximal hypospadias.
- The effect of hCG administration is decreased hypospadias and chordee severity in all patients, increased vascularity and thickness of the proximal corpus spongiosum.
- Application of topical testosterone increases mean penile circumference and length without any lasting side effects.
- Prepubertal exogenous testosterone does not adversely effect ultimate penile growth.

CHRONIC Rx

SURGICAL PROCEDURES:

- Orthoplasty (correcting penile curvature)
- Urethroplasty
- Meatoplasty
- Glanuloplasty
- Skin coverage

There is no single universally acceptable applicable technique for hypospadias repair.

TYPES OF REPAIR:

- Anterior hypospadias: MAGPI, Thiersch-Duplay urethroplasty, glans approximation procedure, tubularized incised plate (TIP) urethroplasty, Mathieu perimeatal flap, Mustarde technique, megameatus intact prepuce, pyramid procedure
- Midlevel hypospadias: TIP, Mathieu flap, onlay island flap (OIF), King procedure
- Posterior hypospadias:
    1. One-stage repair: OIF, double-onlay preputial flap, pedicled preputial flap, transverse preputial island flap
    2. Two-stage repair: orthoplasty to correct chordee followed 6 mo later or longer by Thiersch-Duplay, bladder and/or buccal mucosal hypospadias repair

COMPLICATIONS OF REPAIR: Hematoma, meatal stenosis, fistula, urethral stricture, urethral diverticulum, wound infection, impaired healing, balanitis xerotica obliterans, penile curvature

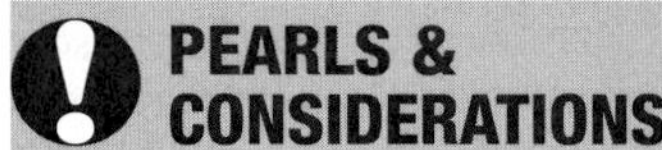

PEARLS & CONSIDERATIONS

- Apparent simple isolated hypospadias may be the only visible indication of an underlying abnormality.
- The dorsal hood of redundant foreskin is used in the repair of hypospadias, so the patient with hypospadias and a dorsal hood should not be circumcised.

SUGGESTED READINGS

American Academy of Pediatrics: Timing of elective surgery on the genitalia of male children with particular reference to the risks, benefits, and psychological effects of surgery and anesthesia, *Pediatrics* 97:590, 1996.

Belman AB: Hypospadias update, *Urology* 49:166, 1997.

Borer JG, Retik AB: Current trends in hypospadias repair, *Urol Clin North Am* 26:1:15, 1999.

Retik AB, Borer JG. In Walsh PC et al (eds): *Campbell's urology,* ed 8, Philadelphia, 2002, WB Saunders.

Zaontz MR, Packer MG: Abnormalities of the external genitalia, *Pediatr Clin North Am* 44:1267, 1997.

AUTHORS: **PHILIP J. ALIOTTA, M.D., M.S.H.A.,** and **RUBEN ALVERO, M.D.**

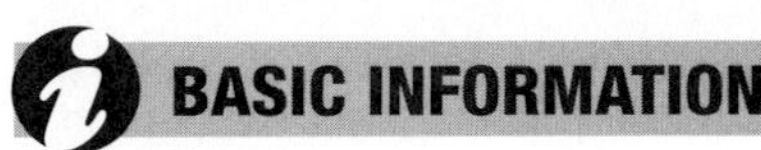

BASIC INFORMATION

DEFINITION

Hypothermia is a rectal temperature <35° C (95.8° F). Accidental hypothermia is an unintentionally induced decrease in core temperature in the absence of preoptic anterior hypothalamic conditions.

ICD-9CM CODES

991.6 Accidental hypothermia
780.9 Hypothermia not associated with low environmental temperature

EPIDEMIOLOGY & DEMOGRAPHICS

- Hypothermia occurs most frequently in the following groups: alcoholics; learning-impaired; patients with cardiovascular, cerebrovascular, or pituitary disorders; those using sedatives or tranquilizers; and elderly patients.
- Approximately 700 persons in the U.S. die from hypothermia annually.

PHYSICAL FINDINGS & CLINICAL PRESENTATION

- The clinical presentation varies with the severity of hypothermia. Shivering may be absent if body temperature is <33.3° C (92° F) or in patients taking phenothiazines.
- Hypothermia may masquerade as cerebrovascular accident, ataxia, or slurred speech, or the patient may appear comatose or clinically dead.
- Physiologic stages of hypothermia:
  1. Mild hypothermia (32.2° to 35° C [90° to 95° F]): arrhythmias, ataxia
  2. Moderate hypothermia (28° to 32.2° C [82.4° to 90° F]):
     a. Progressive decrease of level of consciousness, pulse, cardiac output, and respiration
     b. Fibrillation, dysrhythmias (increased susceptibility to ventricular tachycardia)
     c. Elimination of shivering mechanism for thermogenesis
  3. Severe hypothermia (≤28° C [82.4° F]):
     a. Absence of reflexes or response to pain
     b. Decreased cerebral blood flow, decreased CO_2
     c. Increased risk of ventricular fibrillation or asystole

ETIOLOGY

Exposure to cold temperatures for a prolonged period. Contributing factors include:

1. Drugs: ethanol, phenothiazines, sedative-hypnotics
2. Skin disorders: extensive burns, severe psoriasis, exfoliative dermatitis
3. Metabolic disorders: hypopituitarism, hypothyroidism, hypoadrenalism
4. Neurologic abnormalities: stroke, head trauma, acute spinal cord transaction, impaired shivering
5. Other: lack of acclimatization, aggressive fluid resuscitation, sepsis, heat stroke treatment

DIAGNOSIS

DIFFERENTIAL DIAGNOSIS

- Cerebrovascular accident
- Myxedema coma
- Drug intoxication
- Hypoglycemia

LABORATORY TESTS

1. Metabolic and respiratory acidosis are usually present.
   a. When blood cools, the arterial pH increases, oxygen tension (Po_2) increases, and the Pco_2 falls:
      (1) pH increases 0.008 U/°F (or 0.015 U/°C), causing a decrease in temperature.
      (2) Pao_2 increases 3.3%/°F, causing a decrease in temperature.
      (3) $Paco_2$ decreases 2.4%/°F, causing a decrease in temperature.
   b. Blood gas analyzers warm the blood to 37° C, increasing the partial pressure of dissolved gases, resulting in higher oxygen and carbon dioxide levels and a lower pH than the patient's actual values. Correction of arterial blood gases for temperature is unnecessary as a guide to therapy. The use of uncorrected values also permits reference to the standard acid–base nomograms.
2. A decrease in K^+ initially, then an increase K^+ with increasing hypothermia; extreme hyperkalemia indicates a poor prognosis.
3. Hematocrit increases (caused by hemoconcentration), decreasing leukocytes and platelets (caused by splenic sequestration).
4. Blood viscosity, increased clotting time

IMAGING STUDIES

- Chest radiograph: generally not helpful; may reveal evidence of aspiration (e.g., intoxicated patient with aspiration pneumonia).
- ECG: prolonged PR, QT, and QRS segments, depressed ST segments, inverted T waves, atrioventricular block, and hypothermic J waves (Osborne waves) may appear at 25° to 30° C; characterized by notching of the junction of the QRS complex and ST segments (Fig. 1-168).

TREATMENT

NONPHARMACOLOGIC THERAPY

- Treatment of hypothermia varies with the following:
  1. Degree of hypothermia
  2. Existence of concomitant diseases (e.g., cardiovascular insufficiency)
  3. Patient's age and medical condition (e.g., elderly, debilitated patients vs. young, healthy patients)
- General measures:
  1. Secure an airway before warming all unconscious patients; precede endotracheal intubation with oxygenation (if possible) to minimize the risk of arrhythmias during the procedure.
  2. Peripheral vasoconstriction may impede placement of a peripheral intravenous catheter; consider femoral venous access as an alternative to the jugular or subclavian sites to avoid ventricular stimulation.
  3. A Foley catheter should be inserted, and urinary output should be monitored and maintained >0.5 to 1 ml/kg/hr with intravascular volume replacement.

ACUTE GENERAL Rx

- Continuous ECG monitoring of patients is recommended. Ventricular arrhythmias can be treated with bretylium; lidocaine is generally ineffective, and procainamide is associated with an increased incidence of ventricular fibrillation in hypothermic patients.

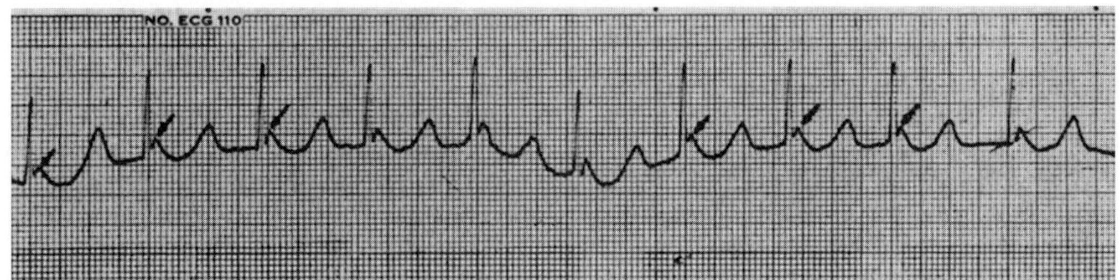

FIGURE 1-168 Hypothermic J waves (Osborne waves) *(arrows)* in an 80-year-old man with core temperature of 86° F (30° C). These waves disappeared with rewarming. (From Morse CD, Rial WY: Emergency medicine. In Rakel RE [ed]: *Textbook of family practice,* ed 4, Philadelphia, 1990, WB Saunders.)

- Correct severe acidosis and electrolyte abnormalities.
- Hypothyroidism, if present, should be promptly treated (see "Myxedema Coma").
- If clinical evidence suggests adrenal insufficiency, administer IV methylprednisolone.
- In patients unresponsive to verbal or noxious stimuli or with altered mental status, 100 mg of thiamine, 0.4 mg of naloxone, and 1 ampule of 50% dextrose may be given.
- Warm (104° to 113° F [40° to 45° C]), humidified oxygen should also be given if available.
- Specific treatment:
  1. Mild hypothermia (rectal temperature $<32.3°$ C [90° F]): passive external rewarming is indicated. Place the patient in a warm room (temperature $>21°$ C [69.8° F]), and cover with insulating material after gently removing wet clothing; recommended rewarming rates vary between 0.5° and 20° C/hr but should not exceed 0.55° C/hr in elderly persons.
  2. Moderate to severe hypothermia:
     a. Active core rewarming
        (1) Delivery of heat by way of fluids: warm gastrointestinal irrigation (with saline enemas and by nasogastric tube); IV fluids (usually D_5NS without potassium) warmed to 104° to 107.6° F (40° to 42° C), peritoneal dialysis with dialysate heated to 40.5° to 42.5° C.
        (2) Inhalation of heated, humidified oxygen (warmed to 40° C [104° F]) increases core temperature by 1° C (1.8° F) per hr and decreases evaporative heat loss from respiration.
     b. Active external rewarming: immersion in a bath of warm water (40° to 41° C); active external rewarming may produce shock because of excessive peripheral vasodilation. Ideal candidates are previously healthy, young patients with acute immersion hypothermia.
     c. Extracorporeal blood warming with cardiopulmonary bypass appears to be an efficacious rewarming technique in young, otherwise healthy persons.

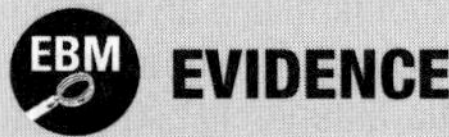

EVIDENCE

Rewarming rates are controversial. Evidence suggests aggressive rewarming is required to gain the best prognosis.[1]

Evidence-Based Reference

1. Walpoth BH et al: Outcome of survivors of accidental deep hypothermia and circulatory arrest treated with extracorporal blood warming, *N Engl J Med* 337:1500, 1997.

SUGGESTED READING

Mccullough L, Arora S: Diagnosis and treatment of hypothermia, *Am Fam Physician* 70:2325, 2004.

AUTHOR: **FRED F. FERRI, M.D.**

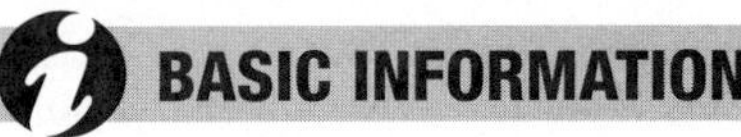

BASIC INFORMATION

DEFINITION

Hypothyroidism is a disorder caused by the inadequate secretion of thyroid hormone.

SYNONYMS

Myxedema

ICD-9CM CODES

244 Acquired hypothyroidism
243 Congenital hypothyroidism
244.1 Surgical hypothyroidism
244.3 Iatrogenic hypothyroidism
244.8 Pituitary hypothyroidism
246.1 Sporadic goitrous hypothyroidism

EPIDEMIOLOGY & DEMOGRAPHICS

INCIDENCE/PREVALENCE: 1.5% to 2% of women and 0.2% of men

PREDOMINANT AGE: Incidence of hypothyroidism increases with age; among persons older than 60 yr, 6% of women and 2.5% of men have laboratory evidence of hypothyroidism (thyroid-stimulating hormone [TSH] more than twice normal level).

PHYSICAL FINDINGS & CLINICAL PRESENTATION

- Hypothyroid patients generally present with the following signs and symptoms: fatigue, lethargy, weakness, constipation, weight gain, cold intolerance, muscle weakness, slow speech, slow cerebration with poor memory.
- Skin: dry, coarse, thick, cool, sallow (yellow color caused by carotenemia); nonpitting edema in skin of eyelids and hands (myxedema) secondary to infiltration of subcutaneous tissues by a hydrophilic mucopolysaccharide substance.
- Hair: brittle and coarse; loss of outer third of eyebrows.
- Facies: dulled expression, thickened tongue, thick and slow-moving lips.
- Thyroid gland: may or may not be palpable (depending on the cause of the hypothyroidism).
- Heart sounds: distant, possible pericardial effusion.
- Pulse: bradycardia.
- Neurologic: delayed relaxation phase of the deep tendon reflexes, cerebellar ataxia, hearing impairment, poor memory, peripheral neuropathies with paresthesia.
- Musculoskeletal: carpal tunnel syndrome, muscular stiffness, weakness.

ETIOLOGY

1. Primary hypothyroidism (thyroid gland dysfunction): the cause of >90% of the cases of hypothyroidism
   - Hashimoto's thyroiditis is the most common cause of hypothyroidism after age 8 yr
   - Idiopathic myxedema (nongoitrous form of Hashimoto's thyroiditis)
   - Previous treatment of hyperthyroidism (radioiodine therapy, subtotal thyroidectomy)
   - Subacute thyroiditis
   - Radiation therapy to the neck (usually for malignant disease)
   - Iodine deficiency or excess
   - Drugs (lithium, para-aminosalicylate, sulfonamides, phenylbutazone, amiodarone, thiourea)
   - Congenital (approximately one case per 4000 live births)
   - Prolonged treatment with iodides
2. Secondary hypothyroidism: pituitary dysfunction, postpartum necrosis, neoplasm, infiltrative disease causing deficiency of TSH
3. Tertiary hypothyroidism: hypothalamic disease (granuloma, neoplasm, or irradiation causing deficiency of TRH)
4. Tissue resistance to thyroid hormone: rare

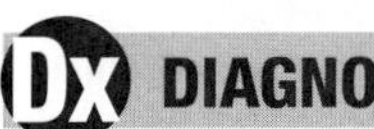

DIAGNOSIS

DIFFERENTIAL DIAGNOSIS

- Depression
- Dementia from other causes
- Systemic disorders (e.g., nephrotic syndrome, congestive heart failure, amyloidosis)

LABORATORY TESTS

- Increased TSH: TSH may be normal if patient has secondary or tertiary hypothyroidism, is receiving dopamine or corticosteroids, or the level is obtained after severe illness
- Decreased free T_4
- Other common laboratory abnormalities: hyperlipidemia, hyponatremia, and anemia
- Increased antimicrosomal and antithyroglobulin antibody titers: useful when autoimmune thyroiditis is suspected as the cause of the hypothyroidism

TREATMENT

NONPHARMACOLOGIC THERAPY

Patients should be educated regarding hypothyroidism and its possible complications. Patients should also be instructed about the need for lifelong treatment and monitoring of their thyroid abnormality.

ACUTE GENERAL Rx

Start replacement therapy with levothyroxine (L-thyroxine) 25 to 100 μg/day, depending on the patient's age and the severity of the disease. Physiologic combinations of L-thyroxine plus liothyronine do not offer any objective advantage over L-thyroxine alone. The levothyroxine dose may be increased every 6 to 8 wk, depending on the clinical response and serum TSH level. Elderly patients and patients with coronary artery disease should be started with 12.5 to 25 μg/day (higher doses may precipitate angina). The average maintenance dose of levothyroxine is 1.7 μg/kg/day (100 to 150 μg/day in adults). The elderly may require <1 μg/kg/day, whereas children generally require higher doses (up to 3 to 4 μg/kg/day). Pregnant patients also have increased requirements. Estrogen therapy may also increase the need for thyroxine. Women with hypothyroidism should increase their levothyroxine dose by approximately 30% as soon as pregnancy is confirmed. Close monitoring of serum thyrotropin levels and adjustment of levothyroxine dose is recommended throughout pregnancy.

CHRONIC Rx

- Periodic monitoring of TSH level is an essential part of treatment. Patients should be evaluated initially with office visit and TSH levels every 6 to 8 wk until the patient is clinically euthyroid and the TSH level is normalized. The frequency of subsequent visits and TSH measurement can then be decreased to every 6 to 12 mo. Pregnant patients should be checked every trimester.
- For monitoring therapy in patients with central hypothyroidism, measurement of serum free thyroxine (free T_4 level) is appropriate and should be maintained in the upper half of the normal range.

REFERRAL

Admission to the hospital intensive care unit is recommended in all patients with myxedema coma. Additional information on the diagnosis and treatment of this life-threatening complication of hypothyroidism is available under "Myxedema Coma" in Section I.

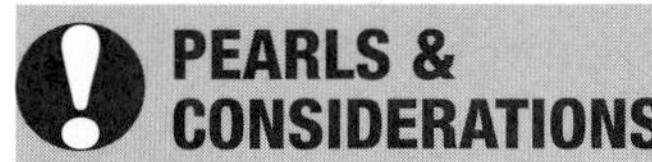

PEARLS & CONSIDERATIONS

COMMENTS

Subclinical hypothyroidism occurs in as many as 15% of elderly patients and is characterized by an elevated serum TSH and a normal free T_4 level. Treatment is individualized. In general, replacement therapy is recommended for all patients with serum TSH >10 mU/L and with presence of goiter or thyroid autoantibodies.

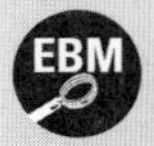

EVIDENCE

There are no randomized, controlled trials comparing levothyroxine with placebo in clinical hypothyroidism for ethical reasons, although there is consensus that this treatment is beneficial.[1]

Evidence-Based Reference

1. Nygaard B: Primary hypothyroidism, *Clinical evidence,* London, 2007, BMJ Publishing Group.

SUGGESTED READING

Escobar-Morreale HF et al: Thyroid hormone replacement therapy in primary hypothyroidism: a randomized trial comparing L-thyroxine plus liothyronine with L-thyronine alone, *Ann Intern Med* 142: 412, 2005.

AUTHOR: **FRED F. FERRI, M.D.**

ID Reaction

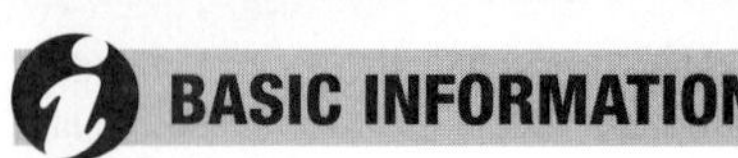

BASIC INFORMATION

DESCRIPTION

The term refers to an acute dermatitis developing at cutaneous sites distant from a primary inflammatory focus and is not explained by the inciting primary inflammation.

SYNONYMS

Autoeczematization

ICD-9CM CODES
692.89 Contact dermatitis and other eczema

EPIDEMIOLOGY

- Exact prevalence in U.S. is unknown.
- Seen in all ages
- Males and females are equally affected
- No particular race or ethnicity is more vulnerable

ETIOLOGY

- Infection with dermatophytes, mycobacterium, histoplasma, viruses, bacteria, or parasites (e.g., lice)
- Dermatitis such as contact, stasis, or eczematous
- Other causes include retained sutures, ionizing radiation, blunt trauma

PATHOGENESIS

- Unknown, but possible explanations include:
  1. Abnormal immune recognition of autologous skin antigens
  2. Stimulation of normal T cells by altered skin constituents
  3. Lowering of the threshold for skin irritation
  4. Dissemination of infectious antigen resulting in a secondary response
  5. Hematogenous dissemination of cytokines from the primary site of inflammation

CLINICAL FEATURES

- Usually associated with exacerbation of primary dermatitis
- Characteristics of the rash in ID reaction include:
  - Sudden onset of rash appearing within a week or two of primary inflammation
  - The rash could not be identified as a common dermatosis
  - Lesions are most commonly seen in the side of the fingers. But, it could be generalized. Particularly in patients with stasis dermatitis, it appears in forearms, thighs, legs, trunk, face, hands, neck, and feet in descending order of frequency.
  - Extremely pruritic
  - Often symmetrical in distribution
  - Most of the time it is vesicular.
- It resolves upon treatment of primary inflammation

Dx DIAGNOSIS

- It is a clinical diagnosis
- Fungus when suspected could be isolated only from the primary site by using potassium hydroxide or by using fungal culture
- At times skin biopsy is done. The biopsy findings are not pathognomonic for ID reaction. These include spongiotic epidermal vesicles associated with superficial perivascular lymphocytic infiltration of dermis, which may also contain scattered eosinophils. Most of the lymphocytes in the epidermis are CD3 and CD8 T cells, whereas those in the dermis are primarily CD4 cells.
- Patch testing may be considered to exclude primary or secondary allergic contact dermatitis.

DIFFERENTIAL DIAGNOSIS

- Atopic dermatitis
- Contact dermatitis
- Drug eruptions
- Dyshidrotic eczema
- Folliculitis
- Scabies
- Dermatophytic infection
- Viral exanthema

Rx TREATMENT

- The treatment is best directed toward the inciting cause.
- Medications used for symptomatic treatment of ID reaction include:
  1. Local or systemic steroids
  2. Local or systemic antihistamines
  3. Topical or systemic antibiotics for secondary bacterial infection
  4. Aluminum sulfate or calcium acetate for weeping skin lesions
  5. Rarely, local or systemic macrolactams (e.g. cyclosporine)

COMPLICATIONS

- Secondary bacterial infection

PROGNOSIS

- It almost always resolves within days when the primary dermatitis is adequately treated.

PATIENT EDUCATION

Treat primary dermatitis promptly.

AUTHOR: **HEMANT K. SATPATHY, M.D.**

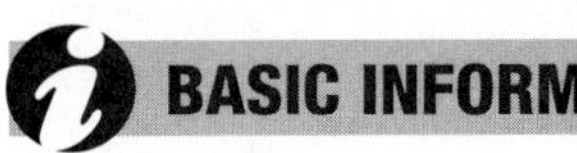

BASIC INFORMATION

DEFINITION

Idiopathic intracranial hypertension (IIH) (pseudotumor cerebri) is a syndrome of increased intracranial pressure without underlying hydrocephalus or mass lesion and with normal cerebrospinal fluid analysis.

SYNONYMS

Pseudotumor cerebri
IIH
Benign intracranial hypertension

ICD-9CM CODES

348.2 Pseudotumor cerebri

EPIDEMIOLOGY & DEMOGRAPHICS

- One case per 100,000 women
- 19 cases per 100,000 women ages 20 to 44 yr and >20% of ideal body weight
- 0.3 to 1.5 cases per 100,000 men
- Female/male ratio from 4.3:1 to 8:1
- More than 90% of IIH patients are obese
- Mean age at diagnosis is 30 yr

PHYSICAL FINDINGS & CLINICAL PRESENTATION

Symptoms:

- Headaches: generalized, throbbing, slowly progressive, worse with straining maneuvers, worse in the morning.
- Transient visual obscurations as a brief blurring of vision or scotomata lasting <30 sec. Occur frequently with Valsalva maneuver and may be monocular.
- Double vision: most often in the horizontal plane (because of pseudo–sixth nerve palsy).
- Pulsatile tinnitus: may be initial symptom.
- Photopsia: lights, sparkles in the eyes.
- Pain: mainly retro-orbital. Pain may also be located in the shoulders or neck. Could be present without a headache. May be associated with Lhermitte's sign.

Signs:

- Papilledema: in virtually all cases; bilateral but may be asymmetric
- Sixth nerve palsy: in approximately 10% to 20% of patients
- Visual field defects: enlarged physiologic blind spot, constricted visual fields
- Loss of vision: end result of longstanding and untreated IIH

ETIOLOGY

IIH may be explained on the basis of decreased cerebrospinal fluid (CSF) absorption and increased intracerebral blood volume.

- Decreased CSF absorption from increased venous sinus pressure: this hypothesis is supported by direct retrograde venography studies and would explain higher incidence of IIH in patients with CHF, hypertension, and obesity.
- Increase in cerebral blood volume: supported by MRI and positron emission tomography, as well as the presence of edema on microscopic evaluation.

Dx DIAGNOSIS

DIFFERENTIAL DIAGNOSIS

- The symptoms and signs of IIH are essentially those of raised intracranial pressure (ICP), and the differential diagnosis includes any condition that may be associated with raised ICP. Here we consider only those disease processes in which elevated ICP occurs in the context of normal CSF analysis and normal MRI. (Of note, venous sinus thrombosis [VST] is on this list despite associated MRI findings. VST should be excluded in all individuals with suspected IIH.)
- Medications: vitamin A and retinoids, steroids (both use and withdrawal), oral contraceptives
- Autoimmune disorders: systemic lupus erythematosus, Behçet's disease
- Vascular disease: venous sinus thrombosis
- Other conditions: hypertension, CHF, pregnancy, obesity, uremia, obstructive sleep apnea

LABORATORY TESTS

- CSF analysis
  1. Shows elevated opening pressure
  2. Shows normal protein, glucose, and cell count
- Hypercoagulability workup if suspicion for VST

IMAGING STUDIES

- MRI of the brain to rule out underlying structural lesions
  1. Empty sella sign often associated with IIH but is not pathognomonic
- Cerebral venography to evaluate venous flow
  1. Magnetic venography
  2. CT venography
  3. Conventional contrast venography
- CT
  1. Slitlike ventricles

Rx TREATMENT

NONPHARMACOLOGIC THERAPY

- Weight loss in obese patients
- Continuous positive airway pressure if obstructive sleep apnea is suspected

ACUTE GENERAL Rx

- Acetazolamide 250 mg to 4 g per day: reduces CSF production by inhibition of carbonic anhydrase, occasionally causing anorexia and resultant weight loss.
- Furosemide 40 to 120 mg/day in divided doses: apparent mechanism of action is by reduced sodium transport, leading to decreased total CSF volume.
- Topiramate 100 to 400 mg/day: antiepileptic medication, recently reported to be effective in treatment of IIH. Weak carbonic anhydrase inhibitor with weight loss as one of its primary side effects.
- Serial lumbar punctures: attempted in patients with severe headaches resistant to medical therapy. Goal is to reduce spinal fluid pressure, allowing immediate reduction in headache severity. This treatment should be reserved only for the most resistant cases and should be used as a conduit to future surgical intervention.

CHRONIC Rx

Surgical intervention is indicated in cases of treatment failure and progressive visual loss.

- Optic nerve fenestration: preferred for patients with visual loss and easily controlled headaches. Proposed mechanism is decompression of the optic nerve. Highly effective; however, has been associated with significant number of failure rates.
- CSF shunting: neurosurgical procedure. Performed in patients with significant visual deterioration and difficult-to-control headaches. Provides rapid improvement in symptoms; however, reported to have significant rates of shunt revisions because of shunt malfunction.

DISPOSITION

- IIH is a self-limiting disease with occasional periods of relapses. Each episode may last from 1 to several years.
- All patients with IIH should undergo MR or CT venography to rule out the possibility of VST.
- The major complication of IIH is visual loss, and treatment should be directed toward reducing ICP to prevent visual loss.

REFERRAL

- Neuro-ophthalmologist for serial evaluation of visual fields and fundus photographs
- Nutritionist for weight loss
- General neurologist for the initial workup and eventual treatment of raised ICP

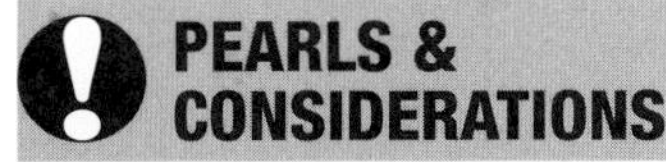

PEARLS & CONSIDERATIONS

COMMENTS

- IIH is a diagnosis of exclusion.
- IIH is a disease of young obese women.
- Ongoing treatment is essential to avoid progressive visual loss, which is the most significant complication of this disorder.

PREVENTION

Maintenance of ideal body weight is one of the best preventative mechanisms for avoidance of IIH. However, it does occur in patients with normal body weight. In these cases there are no known preventable risk factors.

PATIENT & FAMILY EDUCATION

The combination of weight loss and medical therapy is highly effective in treatment of IIH. Given that most patients with IIH are young and otherwise healthy, high success rates can be accomplished. Because IIH is a self-limiting condition, patients with IIH may expect to become both symptom and medication free after intracranial hypertension resolves.

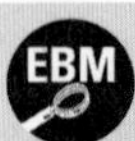

EVIDENCE

Treatment of IIH includes a multitude of approaches, both acute and chronic in nature. Although there have been studies looking specifically at the use of weight loss—acetazolamide therapy, optic nerve sheath fenestration, and ventriculoperitoneal shunting—currently there are no randomized trials to show clear benefits of one treatment over another. Most of the studies are observational and have no well-defined control group. The most comprehensive of studies contained 32 patients, and it was a retrospective case series of patients who underwent bariatric surgery. More research is needed to produce a definitive, evidence-based approach to the treatment of IIH.

SUGGESTED READINGS

Binder D et al: Idiopathic intracranial hypertension, *Neurosurgery* 54:538, 2004.

Friedman D: Pseudotumor cerebri, *Neurol Clin* 22:99, 2004.

Friedman D, Jacobson D: Diagnostic criteria for idiopathic intracranial hypertension, *Neurology* 59: 1492, 2002.

Friedman D, Jacobson D: Idiopathic intracranial hypertension, *J Neuro-opthalmol* 24(2):138, 2004.

Goodwin J: Recent developments in idiopathic intracranial hypertension, *Semin Opthalmol* 18(4):181, 2003.

Lueck C, McIlwaine G: Interventions for idiopathic intracranial hypertension, *Cochrane Rev* 3, 2005.

Mathews M et al: Pseudotumor cerebri, *Curr Opin Ophthalmol* 14:364, 2003.

Miller N: Papilledema. In Miller N, Newman N (eds): *Clinical neuro-ophthalmology,* ed 5, Baltimore, 1998, Williams & Wilkins.

Salman MS et al: Idiopathic "benign" intracranial hypertension: case series and review, *J Child Neurol* 16(7):465, 2001.

Wall M: Papilledema and idiopathic intracranial hypertension (pseudotumor cerebri). In Noseworthy J (ed): *Neurological therapeutics principles and practice,* London, 2003, Martin Dunitz.

AUTHOR: **GENNA GEKHT, M.D.**

BASIC INFORMATION

DEFINITION

Idiopathic pulmonary fibrosis (IPF) is a specific form of chronic fibrosing interstitial pneumonia with histopathologic characteristics of usual interstitial pneumonia (UIP). Disease characterized by progressive parenchymal scarring and loss of pulmonary function.

SYNONYMS

Cryptogenic fibrosing alveolitis
Usual interstitial pneumonia

ICD-9CM CODES
516.3 Idiopathic pulmonary fibrosis

EPIDEMIOLOGY & DEMOGRAPHICS

- Incidence: 7 to 16 cases/100,000 persons worldwide
- Most commonly presents in fifth and sixth decades
- More common in men than women
- Familial forms account for 3% to 25% of cases. Genetic variants: include mutations in surfactant protein C and abnormal telomere shortening
- No distinct geographic distribution; no clear racial predilection

PHYSICAL FINDINGS & CLINICAL PRESENTATION

- Most present with gradual onset (>6 mo) of exertional dyspnea and nonproductive cough. Progressive dyspnea is usually the most prominent symptom.
- Fine bibasilar inspiratory crackles in >80% of patients, with progression upward as the disease advances.
- Clubbing is found in 25% to 50% of patients.
- Cyanosis and right heart failure (cor pulmonale) may occur late in the disease course.
- Extrapulmonary involvement rarely occurs. Fever and wheezing are rare and suggest alternative diagnosis.

ETIOLOGY

- Unknown.
- There are numerous hypotheses, including environmental insults such as metal and wood dust, infectious causes, chronic aspiration, or exposure to certain drugs (antidepressants).
- New research suggests important role of aberrant tissue repair and fibrosis and downplays the importance of generalized inflammation.

Dx DIAGNOSIS

DIFFERENTIAL DIAGNOSIS

- Sarcoidosis
- Drug-induced interstitial lung disease
- Pulmonary manifestations of collagen vascular diseases (e.g., rheumatoid arthritis [RA], systemic sclerosis)
- Bronchoalveolar carcinoma
- Hypersensitivity pneumonitis
- Occupational exposures (e.g., asbestos, silica) may cause pneumoconiosis that mimics IPF
- Other idiopathic interstitial pneumonias:
  - Desquamative interstitial pneumonia
  - Respiratory bronchitis interstitial lung disease
  - Acute interstitial pneumonia
  - Nonspecific interstitial pneumonia
  - Cryptogenic organizing pneumonia

WORKUP

- Almost all patients have abnormal chest radiograph at presentation, with bilateral reticular opacities most prominent in the periphery and lower lobes. Peripheral honeycombing may be seen.
- High-resolution CT scan shows patchy peripheral reticular abnormalities with intralobular linear opacities, irregular septal thickening, subpleural honeycombing, and ground-glass appearance.
- Pulmonary function tests show restrictive pattern and reduced carbon monoxide diffusion into the lung.
- Six-min walk test may show reduced exercise tolerance and/or exertional hypoxia.
- Laboratory abnormalities (nondiagnostic): mild anemia; increases in erythrocyte sedimentation rate, lactate dehydrogenase, C-reactive protein; low titer antinuclear antibody seen in up to 30% of patients.
- There is a limited role for bronchioalveolar lavage either in diagnosis or monitoring IPF.
- Gold standard for diagnosis is lung biopsy (open thoracotomy or video-assisted thoracoscopy). Hallmark features: heterogeneous distribution of parenchymal fibrosis against background of mild inflammation (UIP).
- Lung biopsy is critical to distinguish IPF from diseases with better prognosis and treatment options, especially in patients with any atypical features.
- In absence of or contraindication to lung biopsy, the combination of clinical and radiographic features is often enough to establish the diagnosis.

Rx TREATMENT

- No proven treatment for IPF and little evidence to support the routine use of any specific therapy.
- In patients with mild-moderate disease who desire treatment, conventional treatment includes a trial of corticosteroids combined with azathioprine for 3 to 6 mo; 10% to 30% of patients may respond. The addition of N-acetylcysteine may help to slow the deterioration of lung function, but has not been shown to impact survival.
- Treatment is continued for up to 24 mo if the patient improves or is stable. Long-term treatment only with objective evidence of continued improvement or stabilization.
- In patients with severe disease, treatment options include supportive care (pulmonary rehabilitation, supplemental oxygen) and potential lung transplantation.
- Lung transplantation is the only therapy shown to prolong survival in IPF. Posttransplant 5-yr survival for IPF patients is approximately 40%. Median survival time is longer after bilateral lung transplantation than single lung transplantation but is associated with more complications during the first year.
- Treatment agents designed to target the fibrotic process include pirfenidone, bosentan, Coumadin, and etanercept. These are under investigation and show some initial promise.
- Influenza and pneumonia vaccines should be offered.
- Acute exacerbation of IPF, defined as worsening dyspnea (<1 mo), the presence of new opacities on radiograph, and the lack of evidence of infection, has an incidence of 10% to 57%. Progressive respiratory failure may require mechanical ventilation. Treatment often includes high dose corticosteroids and broad-spectrum antibiotics.

DISPOSITION

- Spontaneous remissions do not occur.
- Natural history includes progressive loss of pulmonary function.
- There is an 8 to 14× increased risk of lung cancer.
- Mean survival after the diagnosis of biopsy-confirmed IPF is 3 to 5 yr.
- Respiratory failure is the most common cause of death.

REFERRAL

To pulmonologist for review of abnormal chest imaging and establishing diagnosis

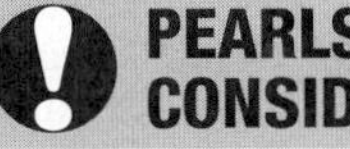

PEARLS & CONSIDERATIONS

- The course is progressive, with a high mortality rate.
- Critical to differentiate IPF from other interstitial lung diseases because prognosis and response to treatment differ.
- There is no proven treatment for IPF. Novel therapeutic agents targeting aberrant epithelial cell activation and repair may prove beneficial.
- Consider early referral for lung transplant.

SUGGESTED READINGS

Armanios MY et al: Telomerase mutations in families with idiopathic pulmonary fibrosis, *N Engl J Med* 356:1317, 2007

Demedts M et al: High-dose acetylcysteine in idiopathic pulmonary fibrosis, *N Engl J Med* 353:2229, 2005.

Thabut G et al: Survival after bilateral versus single-lung transplantation for idiopathic pulmonary fibrosis, *Ann Intern Med* 151:767-774, 2009.

Walter N et al: Current perspectives on the treatment of idiopathic pulmonary fibrosis, *Proc Am Thorac Soc* 3:3308, 2006.

AUTHOR: **MICHAEL BLUNDIN, M.D.**

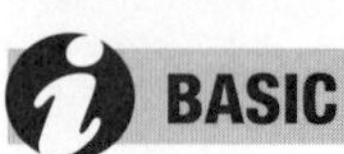

BASIC INFORMATION

DEFINITION

Immunoglobulin A (IgA) nephropathy is a proliferative glomerulonephritis associated with predominant deposition of IgA in the mesangium.

SYNONYMS

Berger's disease

ICD-9CM CODES
583.81 IgA Nephropathy

EPIDEMIOLOGY & DEMOGRAPHICS

INCIDENCE: It is the most common type of glomerulonephropathy worldwide.
PREVALENCE: Prevalence rate is lower in the U.S. (10% to 15%) compared with Asian countries. Lower rates could be explained by a conservative approach by nephrologists in the U.S., who are reluctant to do renal biopsy in asymptomatic patients with minimal renal abnormalities. In most reports prevalence rates are expressed as a percentage of cases of primary glomerulonephritis or as a percentage of total series of renal biopsies.
PREDOMINANT SEX AND AGE: It is most prevalent in the second and third decades of life with a male/female ratio of 6:1 in the U.S.
GENETICS: Although it is considered a sporadic disease, genetic linkage to locus called *IgAN1* on 6q22 and 6q23 has been shown.
RISK FACTORS: It has a higher association with Asians, whites, and Native Americans and is rarely seen in African Americans.

PHYSICAL FINDINGS & CLINICAL PRESENTATION

- Two common presentations include (1) recurrent macroscopic hematuria often associated with upper respiratory infection and (2) persistent microscopic hematuria.
- Loin pain may be associated with macroscopic hematuria.
- Physical findings are usually unremarkable, except hypertension seen in 20% to 30% of patients with chronic disease and edema in 5% of patients with nephrotic range proteinuria.
- Mild proteinuria is common.
- Rarely, IgA nephropathy presents as acute renal failure in 5% of patients and chronic renal failure in 10% to 20% of patients.

ETIOLOGY

- Most cases are idiopathic/primary.
- Secondary causes of IgA nephropathy include Henoch-Schönlein purpura; hepatitis B; alcoholic cirrhosis; celiac disease; inflammatory bowel disease; psoriasis; sarcoidosis; cystic fibrosis; cancer of the lungs, larynx, or pancreas; HIV infection; systemic lupus erythematosus; rheumatoid arthritis; diabetic nephropathy; Sjögren's syndrome; and Reiter's syndrome.

Dx DIAGNOSIS

DIFFERENTIAL DIAGNOSIS

- Henoch-Schönlein purpura
- Hereditary nephritis
- Thin glomerular basement membrane disease
- Lupus nephritis
- Poststreptococcal nephritis
- Secondary causes associated with IgA nephropathy mentioned above

WORKUP

- The diagnosis is suspected on the basis of clinical history and laboratory data but is confirmed by renal biopsy showing IgA deposits in the mesangium.
- Renal biopsy is restricted to patients with sustained proteinuria >1 g/day or worsening renal function.

LABORATORY TESTS

- Urine analysis showing protein, red blood cells and casts, and white blood cells.
- Serum creatinine may be elevated.
- 24-hour urine assay for quantifying proteinuria and to check creatinine clearance.
- Serum IgA is elevated in only 50% of patients and has no clinical utility.

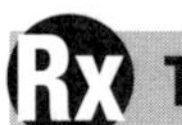

TREATMENT

Although initially considered a benign disease, IgA nephropathy is now recognized as a common cause of renal failure. Currently there is no cure.

NONPHARMACOLOGIC THERAPY

- Moderate dietary protein restriction
- Discourage smoking

ACUTE AND CHRONIC GENERAL Rx

- Aggressive therapy for hypertension, preferably with angiotensin-converting enzyme (ACE) inhibitors. Goal blood pressure is <125/75 mm Hg in the presence of proteinuria >1 g/day.
- Patients with recurrent gross hematuria or isolated microscopic hematuria, no or minimal proteinuria (<1 g/day), normal blood pressure, and normal kidney function should only be monitored every 6 to 12 mo to assess disease progression.
- If bouts of recurrent macroscopic hematuria are associated with tonsillitis, tonsillectomy may benefit these patients.
- Patients with persistent proteinuria >1 g/day with or without hypertension are treated with ACE inhibitors and/or angiotensin receptor blockers (ARBs). Steroids are reserved for patients with persistent proteinuria >1 g/day despite ACE and/or ARB administration.
- Patients with nephrotic syndrome, preserved kidney function, and minimal change in disease are treated with steroids for 6 mo.
- Patients with severe renal disease or crescentic, rapidly progressive glomerulonephritis in the absence of changes of chronic kidney disease in biopsy are treated with steroid and cyclophosphamide combination for the first 2 mo, followed by steroids and azathioprine for 2 yr for maintenance treatment.
- Patients with acute renal failure need renal biopsy to rule out acute tubular necrosis, which needs only supportive therapy, from crescentic IgA nephropathy, which needs aggressive medical management.
- Kidney transplantation is the treatment of choice for end-stage kidney disease. There is no difference in survival in living versus cadaver donors. At present, kidneys with IgA deposits are not used for transplantation.
- Statins are indicated for all IgA nephropathy patients with dyslipidemia, hypertension, and other cardiovascular risks.
- Role of mycophenolate and plasmapheresis is controversial.

COMPLEMENTARY & ALTERNATIVE MEDICINE

Role of fish oil is controversial

DISPOSITION

- Complete remission occurs in <10% of patients.
- End-stage renal failure develops in 15% to 20% of patients within 10 yr of onset and in 30% to 35% of patients within 20 yr. Prognostic markers at presentation in IgA nephropathy are described in Box 1-9.

BOX 1-9 Prognostic Markers at Presentation in IgA Nephropathy

Clinical	Histopathologic
Poor prognosis	Poor prognosis
Increasing age	Glomerular sclerosis
Duration of preceding symptoms	Tubular atrophy
Severity of proteinuria	Interstitial fibrosis
Hyperuricemia	Vascular wall thickening
Hypertension	Capillary-loop IgA deposits
Renal impairment	
Good prognosis	
Recurrent macroscopic hematuria	
No impact on prognosis	No impact on prognosis
Gender	Intensity of IgA deposits
Serum IgA level	

None of the clinical or histopathologic adverse features, except capillary-loop IgA deposits, are specific to IgAN.
From Johnson RJ, Feehaly J: *Comprehensive clinical nephrology,* ed 2, St Louis, 2000, Mosby.

- Poor prognostic indicators include (1) male gender, (2) older age, (3) young age at the onset of the disease, (4) absence of episodes of recurrent macroscopic hematuria, (5) hypertension, (6) extent of renal insufficiency, (7) extent of proteinuria, (8) elevated serum uric acid, and (9) certain histologic changes seen in renal biopsy, such as crescents, glomerulosclerosis, and tubulointerstitial fibrosis or atrophy.

REFERRAL

Patients with IgA nephropathy are commonly referred to nephrologists.

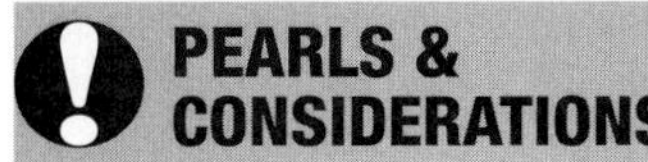

PEARLS & CONSIDERATIONS

COMMENTS

- IgA nephropathy seems to be a kidney-restricted form of Henoch-Schönlein purpura.
- IgA nephropathy is not an entirely benign condition, even when microhematuria is the only clinical presentation.

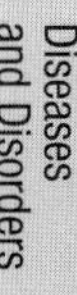

SUGGESTED READINGS

Appel et al: The IgA nephropathy treatment dilemma, *Kidney Int* 69:1939, 2006.

Barrett et al: Treatment of IgA nephropathy, *Kidney Int* 69:1934-1938, 2006.

AUTHOR: **HEMANT K. SATPATHY, M.D.**

Immune Thrombocytopenic Purpura (ALG)

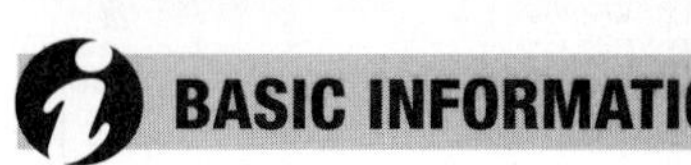

BASIC INFORMATION

DEFINITION

Immune thrombocytopenic purpura (ITP) is an autoimmune disorder in which antibody-coated or immune complex–coated platelets are destroyed prematurely by the reticuloendothelial system, resulting in peripheral thrombocytopenia.

ICD-9CM CODES
287.3 Idiopathic thrombocytopenic purpura (ITP)

EPIDEMIOLOGY & DEMOGRAPHICS

INCIDENCE: 100 cases per 1 million persons annually

PREVALENCE: Five to 10 cases per 100,000 persons

PREDOMINANT SEX: 72% of patients >10 yr are female; in children, males and females are affected equally

PREDOMINANT AGE: Children ages 2 to 4 yr and young women (70% are <40 yr)

PHYSICAL FINDINGS & CLINICAL PRESENTATION

The presentation of ITP is different in children and adults:

- Children generally present with sudden onset of bruising and petechiae from severe thrombocytopenia.
- In adults the presentation is insidious; a history of prolonged purpura may be present; many patients are diagnosed incidentally on the basis of automated laboratory tests that now routinely include platelet counts.
- The physical examination may be entirely normal.
- Patients with severe thrombocytopenia may have petechiae, purpura, epistaxis, or hemepositive stool from gastrointestinal bleeding.
- Splenomegaly is unusual; its presence should alert to the possibility of other etiologies of thrombocytopenia.
- The presence of dysmorphic features (skeletal anomalies, auditory abnormalities) may indicate a congenital disorder as the cause of the thrombocytopenia.

ETIOLOGY

Increased platelet destruction caused by autoantibodies to platelet-membrane antigens. Hundreds of medications can cause thrombocytopenia. Drugs commonly implicated are quinidine, heparin, antibiotics (linezolid, vancomycin, sulfonamides, rifampin), platelet inhibitors (tirofiban, abciximab, eptifibatide), cimetidine, NSAIDs, thiazide diuretics, antirheumatic agents (gold salts, penicillamine), acetaminophen, and chemotherapeutic agents (cyclosporine, fludarabine, oxaliplatin).

Dx DIAGNOSIS

DIFFERENTIAL DIAGNOSIS

- Falsely low platelet count (resulting from EDTA-dependent or cold-dependent agglutinins)
- Viral infections (e.g., HIV, mononucleosis, rubella)
- Drug-induced (e.g., heparin, quinidine, sulfonamides)
- Hypersplenism resulting from liver disease
- Myelodysplastic and lymphoproliferative disorders
- Pregnancy, hypothyroidism
- SLE, TTP, hemolytic-uremic syndrome
- Congenital thrombocytopenia (e.g., Fanconi's syndrome, May-Hegglin anomaly, Bernard-Soulier syndrome)

LABORATORY TESTS

- Complete blood count, platelet count, and peripheral smear: platelets are decreased but are normal in size or may appear larger than normal. Red blood cells and white blood cells have a normal morphology.
- Additional tests may be ordered to exclude other causes of the thrombocytopenia when clinically indicated (e.g., HIV, ANA, TSH, liver enzymes, bone marrow examination).
- The direct assay for the measurement of platelet-bound antibodies has an estimated positive predictive value of 80% to 83%. A negative test cannot be used to rule out the diagnosis.

IMAGING STUDIES

CT scan of abdomen/pelvis in patients with splenomegaly to exclude other disorders causing thrombocytopenia

Rx TREATMENT

NONPHARMACOLOGIC THERAPY

- Minimize activity to prevent injury or bruising (e.g., contact sports should be avoided).
- Stop any potentially offending drugs (see "Etiology"). Avoid medications that increase the risk of bleeding (e.g., aspirin and other NSAIDs).

ACUTE GENERAL Rx

- Treatment varies with the platelet count, patient's age, and bleeding status.
- Observation and frequent monitoring of platelet count are needed in asymptomatic patients with platelet counts >30,000/mm^3.
- Methylprednisolone 30 mg/kg/day IV infused over a period of 20 to 30 min (maximum dose of 1 g/day for 2 or 3 days) plus IV immunoglobulin (1 g/kg/day for 2 or 3 days) and infusion of platelets should be given to patients with neurologic symptoms, internal bleeding, or those undergoing emergency surgery.
- Prednisone 1 to 2 mg/kg qd, continued until the platelet count is normalized then slowly tapered off, is indicated in adults with platelet counts <20,000/mm^3 and those who have counts <50,000/mm^3 and significant mucous membrane bleeding. Response rates range from 50% to 75%, and most responses occur within the first 3 wk. Oral dexamethasone at a dosage of 40 mg/day for 4 consecutive days has also been reported to induce a high response rate (85%).
- High-dose immunoglobulins (IgG 0.4 g/kg/day IV, infused on 3 to 5 consecutive days) or high-dose parenteral glucocorticoids (methylprednisolone 30 mg/kg/day) can be used in children with a platelet count <20,000/mm^3 and significant bleeding or adults with severe thrombocytopenia or bleeding. However, responses are generally transient, lasting no longer than 4 wk.
- Splenectomy should be considered in adults with platelet count <30,000/mm^3 after 6 wk of medical treatment or after 6 mo if more than 10 to 20 mg of prednisone per day is required to maintain a platelet count >30,000/mm^3. In children, splenectomy is generally reserved for persistent thrombocytopenia (>1 yr) and clinically significant bleeding. Appropriate immunizations (pneumococcal vaccine in adults and children, *Haemophilus influenzae* vaccine, meningococcal vaccine in children) should be administered before splenectomy.
- Platelet transfusion is needed only in case of life-threatening hemorrhage.
- Use of danazol, an attenuated androgen, and chemotherapy with cyclophosphamide, vincristine, and prednisone (CVP) has been partially effective in chronic ITP.
- Rituximab, a monoclonal antibody directed against the CD_{20} antigen, has been reported useful for patients with ITP who are resistant to conventional treatment; it may help prevent serious or fatal bleeding. Encouraging results have also been shown in trials involving AMG 531, a thrombopoiesis-stimulating protein in patients with chronic ITP.
- Romiplostim, a recombinant fusion protein, and the oral thrombopoietin-receptor agonist eltrombopag are effective in increasing platelet count in patients with chronic ITP refractory to corticosteroids, immunoglobulins, and/or splenectomy.
- An algorithm for the management of ITP is described in the online version of Section III.

DISPOSITION

- More than 80% of children have a complete remission within 8 wk.
- In adults, the course of the disease is chronic; only 5% of adults have spontaneous remission.
- The principal cause of death from ITP is intracranial hemorrhage (1% of children, 5% of adults).

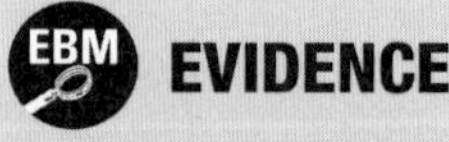

EVIDENCE

Treatment in adults.

The use of high-dose oral dexamethasone has been reported favorably in a small clinical trial of adults with ITP, but randomized controlled trials are lacking.[1] B

Evidence-Based Reference

1. Borst F et al: High-dose dexamethasone as a first- and second-line treatment of idiopathic thrombocytopenic purpura in adults, *Ann Hematol* 83:764-768, 2004. B

AUTHOR: **FRED F. FERRI, M.D.**

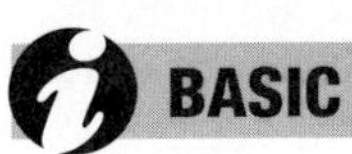

BASIC INFORMATION

DEFINITION

Impetigo is a superficial skin infection generally caused by *Staphylococcus aureus* and/or *Streptococcus* spp.

Common presentations are bullous impetigo (generally caused by staphylococcal disease) and nonbullous impetigo (from streptococcal infection and possible staphylococcal infection); the bullous form is caused by an epidermolytic toxin produced at the site of infection.

SYNONYMS

Impetigo vulgaris
Pyoderma

ICD-9CM CODES

684 Impetigo

EPIDEMIOLOGY & DEMOGRAPHICS

- Bullous impetigo is most common in infants and children. The nonbullous form is most common in children ages 2 to 5 yr with poor hygiene in warm climates.
- The overall incidence of acute nephritis with impetigo varies between 2% and 5%.

PHYSICAL FINDINGS & CLINICAL PRESENTATION

- Nonbullous impetigo begins as a single red macule or papule that quickly becomes a vesicle. Rupture of the vesicle produces an erosion of which the contents dry to form honey-colored crusts. Multiple lesions with golden yellow crusts and weeping areas are often found on the skin around the nose, mouth, and limbs (Fig. 1-169).
- Bullous impetigo is manifested by the presence of vesicles that enlarge rapidly to form bullae with contents that vary from clear to cloudy. There is subsequent collapse of the center of the bullae; the peripheral areas may retain fluid, and a honey-colored crust may appear in the center. As the lesions enlarge and become contiguous with the others, a scaling border replaces the fluid-filled rim; there is minimal erythema surrounding the lesions.
- Regional lymphadenopathy is most common with nonbullous impetigo.
- Constitutional symptoms are generally absent.

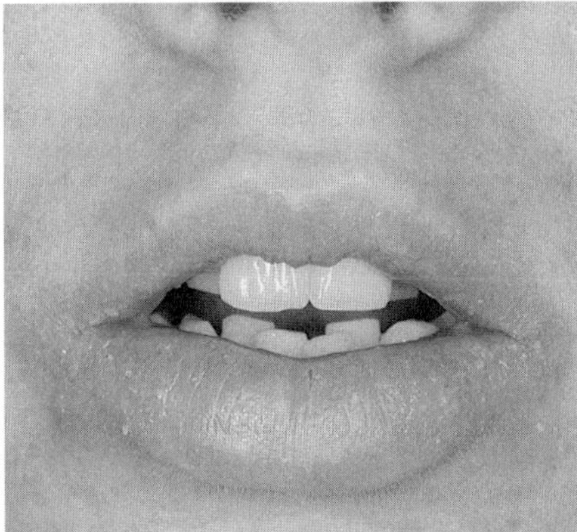

FIGURE 1-169 Impetigo. Serum and crust at the angle of the mouth is a common presentation for impetigo. (From Habif TB: *Clinical dermatology: a color guide to diagnosis and therapy,* ed 4, St Louis, 2000, Mosby.)

ETIOLOGY

- *S. aureus* coagulase positive is the dominant microorganism.
- *S. pyogenes* (group A β-hemolytic streptococci): M-T serotypes of this organism associated with acute nephritis are 2, 49, 55, 57, and 60.

Dx DIAGNOSIS

DIFFERENTIAL DIAGNOSIS

- Atopic dermatitis
- Herpes simplex infection
- Ecthyma
- Folliculitis
- Eczema
- Insect bites
- Scabies
- Tinea corporis
- Pemphigus vulgaris and bullous pemphigoid
- Chickenpox

WORKUP

Diagnosis is clinical.

LABORATORY TESTS

- Generally not necessary
- Gram stain and culture and sensitivity to confirm the diagnosis when the clinical presentation is unclear
- Sedimentation rate parallel to activity of the disease
- Increased anti-DNAse B and antihyaluronidase
- Urinalysis revealing hematuria with erythrocyte casts and proteinuria in patients with acute nephritis (most frequently occurring in children between ages 2 and 4 yr in the southern part of the U.S.)

Rx TREATMENT

NONPHARMACOLOGIC THERAPY

Remove crusts by soaking with wet cloth compresses (crusts block the penetration of antibacterial creams).

GENERAL Rx

- Application of 2% mupirocin ointment tid for 10 days or retapamulin 1% applied bid for 5 days to the affected area or until all lesions have cleared.
- Oral antibiotics are used in severe cases: commonly used agents are dicloxacillin 250 mg qid for 7 to 10 days, cephalexin 250 mg qid for 7 to 10 days, azithromycin 500 mg on day 1, 250 mg on days 2 through 5, amoxicillin/clavulanate 500 mg q8h.
- Impetigo can be prevented by prompt application of mupirocin or triple-antibiotic ointment (bacitracin, Polysporin, and neomycin) to sites of skin trauma.
- Patients who are carriers of *S. aureus* in their nares should be treated with mupirocin ointment applied to their nares bid for 5 days.
- Fingernails should be kept short, and patients should be advised not to scratch any lesions to avoid spread of infection.

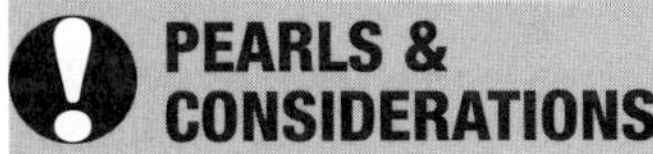

DISPOSITION

Most cases of impetigo resolve promptly with appropriate treatment. Both bullous and nonbullous forms of impetigo heal without scarring.

REFERRAL

Nephrology referral in patients with acute nephritis

PEARLS & CONSIDERATIONS

COMMENTS

- Patients should be instructed on use of antibacterial soaps and avoidance of sharing of towels and washcloths because impetigo is extremely contagious.
- Children attending day care should be removed until 48 to 72 hr after initiation of antibiotic treatment.

EBM EVIDENCE

A systematic review of interventions for impetigo found that topical antibiotics showed better cure rates than placebo, and topical mupirocin was superior to oral erythromycin. Topical and oral antibiotics did not show significantly different cure rates in general, nor did most oral antibiotics. Penicillin was inferior to erythromycin and cloxacillin, and there is little evidence that using disinfectant solutions improved impetigo. Erythromycin is the drug of choice in areas of low resistance because of high efficacy and relatively low cost.[1] A

The same systematic review found oral antibiotic treatment caused more side effects than topical treatment.[1] A

Evidence-Based Reference

1. Koning S et al: Interventions for impetigo, *Cochrane Rev* 3, 2004. A

AUTHOR: **FRED F. FERRI, M.D.**

Inclusion Body Myositis

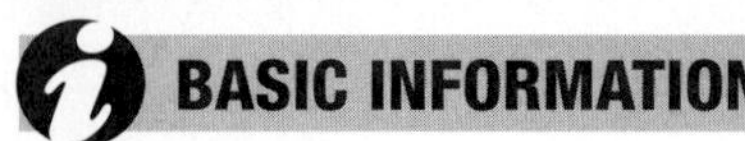

BASIC INFORMATION

DEFINITION

Inclusion body myositis (IBM) is the most common myopathy with onset after the age of 50 yr. Although classified among the inflammatory myopathies, its underlying pathophysiology has not yet been delineated.

SYNONYMS

None

ICD-9CM CODES
728.89 Other disorders of muscle, ligament and fascia

EPIDEMIOLOGY & DEMOGRAPHICS

INCIDENCE: 0.22-0.79 cases/100,000 persons
PREVALENCE: 0.5-7.1 cases/100,000 persons
PREDOMINANT SEX: Male:female ratio 1.2-3:1
PREDOMINANT AGE: 87% older than 50 yr
PEAK INCIDENCE: Seventh decade
RISK FACTORS: None known
GENETICS: Less than 10% of cases familial

PHYSICAL FINDINGS & CLINICAL PRESENTATION

- Insidious onset of slowly progressive proximal and distal weakness.
- Time to diagnosis from symptom onset often lags by years to a decade.
- Functional loss of strength in the legs most often precedes the arms.
- The cardinal clinical features include early weakness and atrophy of quadriceps muscles (difficulty climbing stairs, arising from chairs, and getting out of cars) along with wrist and finger flexor muscles (difficulty grasping, opening jars and turning doorknobs). Ankle dorsiflexion weakness may also be prominent leading to foot drop and tripping.
- When examining strength, side to side asymmetries are seen in one or more muscle groups in the majority of patients. This stands in contrast to the symmetrical, proximal involvement seen in polymyositis and most muscular dystrophies.
- Dysphagia and/or mild facial weakness are present in over half of cases.
- Although sensory symptoms are usually lacking, one third will have evidence for sensory loss in their distal legs on physical examination and electrodiagnostic testing.
- 10% to 15% of patients have concomitant autoimmune disorders such as systemic lupus erythematosus, Sjögren's syndrome, scleroderma, sarcoidosis, or thrombocytopenia. However, different from polymyositis and dermatomyositis, IBM does not portend an increased risk of heart or lung disease nor cancer.

ETIOLOGY

The pathogenesis of IBM is not known. Inflammatory, degenerative, viral and prion etiologies have been postulated, but none substantiated.

Dx DIAGNOSIS

DIFFERENTIAL DIAGNOSIS

- Polymyositis
- Amyotrophic lateral sclerosis
- Late-onset muscular dystrophies
- Acid maltase deficiency

WORKUP

- Thorough neurologic examination with emphasis on the motor exam is important.
- Nerve conduction studies should be performed to exclude other causes and EMG to document a myopathy.
- Muscle biopsy: a diagnosis of definite IBM requires the following features on muscle biopsy: (1) inflammation, (2) inflammatory cells invading healthy muscle fibers, (3) vacuoles, and (4) either amyloid deposits by Congo red staining or tubulofilaments on electron microscopy.

LABORATORY TESTS

Creatine kinase level (labs for collagen vascular diseases may be obtained after the diagnosis). A complete blood count and coagulation studies should be drawn in anticipation of the muscle biopsy.

IMAGING STUDIES

MRI of the forearms to document atrophy and signal abnormalities in volar forearm muscle groups may be performed to increase clinical certainty.

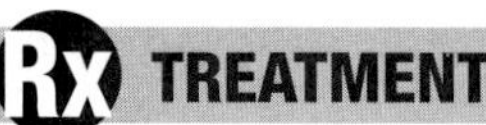

TREATMENT

NONPHARMACOLOGIC THERAPY

- Assistive devices for mobility such as canes, walkers, and wheelchairs are the mainstay of therapy.
- Occasionally knee orthoses or ankle-foot orthoses may improve and prolong ambulation.

ACUTE GENERAL Rx

None

CHRONIC Rx

- Experts have not found clinically significant improvement in functional strength with any pharmacologic therapy. Clinical trials of corticosteroids, methotrexate, intravenous immunoglobulin, anti-T lymphocyte globulin, etanercept, interferon β-1a, and oxandrolone have all failed to demonstrate functional improvements in limb strength.
- A short, small trial of a home exercise program demonstrated mild improvements in strength.
- IBM is generally refractory to therapy.

COMPLEMENTARY & ALTERNATIVE MEDICINE

Some patients choose to self-treat with creatine supplementation, coenzyme Q10, or lithium. There is no evidence supporting these treatments.

REFERRAL

- Patients with suspected IBM should be referred to a neurologist with subspecialty expertise in neuromuscular medicine.
- Physical therapy and occupational therapy consultations help the patient optimize ambulation and fine motor tasks, respectively.
- Speech therapy consultations can assist with symptomatic dysphagia.

PROGNOSIS

Life expectancy is not significantly altered in this late-onset, slowly progressive disorder. Some patients require wheelchair use 10 to 20 yr after disease onset.

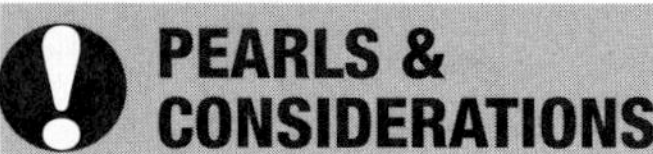

PEARLS & CONSIDERATIONS

COMMENTS

The key to diagnosis rests in finding weakness of finger or wrist flexors on examination (evident in over 95% of patients at initial presentation).

PREVENTION

None known

PATIENT/FAMILY EDUCATION

Patient information and support groups can be found at: www.ninds.nih.gov/disorders/inclusion_body_myositis and http://www.myositis.org.

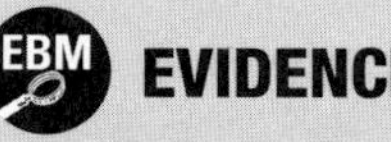

EVIDENCE

There are no Cochrane database reviews related to IBM.

All randomized, placebo-controlled, double-blind studies have failed to demonstrate functional benefit from any pharmacologic agent. Thus unless the patient has a concomitant autoimmune disorder or an overlap syndrome with either dermatomyositis or polymyositis, treatment with immunosuppressive agents, with their deleterious side effects, should be avoided.

SUGGESTED READINGS

Amato AA, Barohn RJ: Inclusion body myositis: old and new concepts, *J Neurol Neurosurg Psychiatry* 80: 1186, 2009.

Amato AA, et al: Inclusion body myositis: clinical and pathological boundaries, *Ann Neurol* 40:581 1996.

Chahin N, Engel AG: Correlation of muscle biopsy, clinical course, and outcome in PM and sporadic IBM, *Neurology* 70:418 2006.

Griggs RC et al: Inclusion body myositis and myopathies, *Ann Neurol* 38:705 1995.

Neuromuscular Home Page: http://neuromuscular.wustl.edu.

AUTHOR: **MATTHEW P. WICKLUND, M.D.**

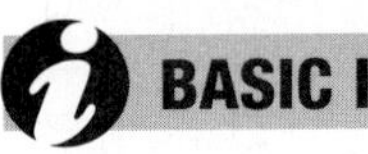

BASIC INFORMATION

DEFINITION

Fecal incontinence is defined as the loss of voluntary bowel control, leading to the inability to hold gas or feces in the rectum.

SYNONYMS

Fecal Incontinence
Anal Incontinence

ICD-9CM CODES
787.6 Incontinence of feces
307.7 Encopresis of non-organic origin

EPIDEMIOLOGY & DEMOGRAPHICS

INCIDENCE: It affects 0.5% to 1.5% of the population younger than age 65 yr but >10% older than age 65. Also more common in institutionalized patients.

PREVALENCE: 2.2% in general population and 21% in older adults. Prevalence increases with age and body mass index (BMI) in women.

PREDOMINANT SEX AND AGE: More common in females as compared to males

RISK FACTORS:

- History of urinary incontinence (present in 50% of the cases)
- Demented or cognitively impaired individuals
- Age >70 yr
- Presence of neurologic or psychiatric disease
- Poor mobility
- Fecal impaction from chronic constipation

PHYSICAL FINDINGS & CLINICAL PRESENTATION

- On inspection and by performing a digital rectal exam to ascertain the presence of fecal material, prolapsed hemorrhoid, dermatitis, scars, absence of perianal creases, or a gaping anus.
- Also assess for anocutaneous reflex. This can be done by stroking skin in each perianal quadrant (normal response is brisk anal wink).
- Assess the length of the anal sphincter.
- Assess resting and squeezing anal tone.
- Assess for rectal prolapsed or excessive perianal descent when patient strains.

ETIOLOGY

- Often multifactorial
- Radiation-induced inflammation and fibrosis
- Rectal inflammation secondary to ulcerative colitis or Crohn's disease
- Neurological disorders:
  - Status post stroke
  - Dementia
  - Multiple sclerosis
  - Dorsal and spinal cord lesions
- Surgery
  - Anorectal surgery for hemorrhoids, fistula, and fissures
- Medicines
  - Narcotics
  - Antidepressants
  - Antipsychotics
  - Calcium channel blockers
- Number of births and episiotomies in females
- Childhood abuse and adult sexual abuse

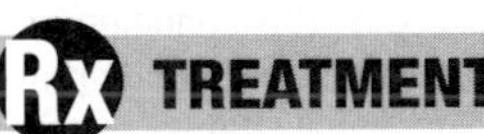

DIAGNOSIS

DIFFERENTIAL DIAGNOSIS

- Fecal encopresis

WORK-UP

- Detailed history taking that includes the onset and precipitating events, duration and severity, stool consistency and urgency, and the presence of coexisting problems including urinary incontinence, surgery, or back injury is important.
- Diagnostic workup includes anal manometry, anorectal ultrasound, proctosigmoidoscopy, and anal electromyography (EMG)

IMAGING STUDIES

- Anal endosonography (most widely used and least expensive)
- MRI

Rx TREATMENT

Loperamide hydrochloride, diphenoxylate/atropine sulphate (mainstay of treatment), estrogen replacement therapy in postmenopausal women (uncontrolled trials)

NONPHARMACOLOGIC THERAPY

- Supportive therapy
  - Education/counseling/habit training
  - Diet (increase fiber, lactulose, and fructose)
- Biofeedback therapy:
  - Anal sphincter muscle strengthening
  - Rectal sensory conditioning
  - Rectoanal coordination training
- Modified Kegel exercises
- Surgery:
  - Sphincteroplasty
  - Anterior repair
  - Artificial bowel sphincter
  - Sacral nerve stimulation
  - Colostomy

REFERRAL

Refer to colorectal surgeon

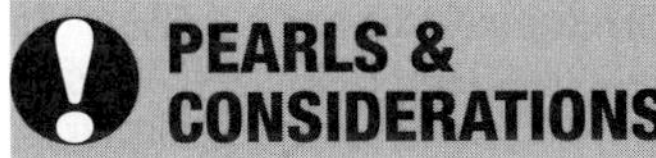

PEARLS & CONSIDERATIONS

COMMENTS

- The shame, embarrassment, and stigma associated with fecal and urinary incontinence pose significant barriers to seeking professional treatment, resulting in many people who suffer from these conditions without help.

PREVENTION

- Endoanal ultrasound to detect and repair anal sphincter tears in women with second-degree perineal tears may reduce severe fecal incontinence (mid-level evidence).
- Routine episiotomy is the most easily preventable risk factor for fecal incontinence in females.

PATIENT/FAMILY EDUCATION

Website: www.familydoctor.org/online/famdocen/home/seniors/common-older/067.html
digestive.niddk.nih.gov/ddiseases/pubs/fecalincontinence

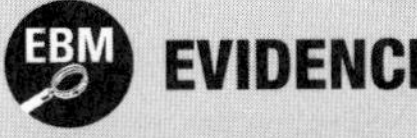

EVIDENCE

There is limited evidence that antidiarrheal drugs and drugs that enhance anal sphincter tone may reduce fecal incontinence in patients with liquid stools.[1] Laxative use in geriatric patients may reduce fecal soiling and the need for help from nurses. However, the trials were small and of short duration.

Anal sphincter injury from childbirth is associated with anal incontinence in women of childbearing ages, most of whom do not seek medical attention secondary to embarrassment.[2] Three A-quality trials including 279 women compared two recognized methods for the anal sphincter repair; the end-to-end repair and the overlap repair. Meta-analysis showed no statistically significant difference in perineal pain, dyspareunia, and flatus incontinence and fecal incontinence between the two repair techniques but showed a statistically significantly lower incidence in fecal urgency and lower anal incontinence score in the overlap group.

Sacral nerve stimulation has been shown to be effective in complete resolution of fecal incontinence in 40% to 75% of patients and improvement of episodes in 75% to 100% of patients with a <10% incidence of adverse events.[3] This was shown in a recent systematic review of the published outcomes of trials investigating sacral nerve stimulation. Ⓐ

Evidence-Based References

1. Cheetham MJ et al: Drug treatment for faecal incontinence in adults, *Cochrane Database Syst Rev* 3, 2002.
2. Fernando R et al: Methods of repair for obstetric anal sphincter injury, *Cochrane Database Syst Rev* 3, 2006.
3. Gladman MA: Surgical treatment of patients with constipation and fecal incontinence, *Gastroenterol Clin North Am* 37(3):605-625, 2008. Ⓐ

SUGGESTED READINGS

Landefeld CS et al: National Institutes of Health State-of-the-Science conference statement: prevention of fecal and urinary incontinence in adults, *Ann Intern Med* 48:449-58, 2008.

Tariq SH: Fecal incontinence in older adults, *Clin Geriatr Med* 23(4), 2007.

AUTHOR: **NADIA MUJAHID, M.D.**

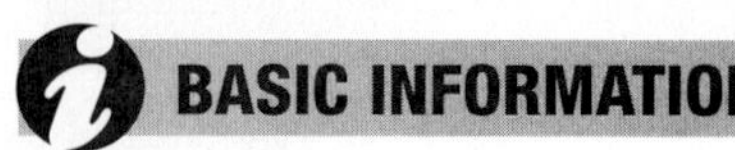

BASIC INFORMATION

DEFINITION

Incontinence is the involuntary loss of urine.

ICD-9CM CODES
788.3 Incontinence
625.6 Stress incontinence
788.33 Mixed stress and urge incontinence
788.32 Male incontinence
788.39 Neurogenic incontinence
307.6 Nonorganic origin

EPIDEMIOLOGY & DEMOGRAPHICS

INCIDENCE/PREVALENCE: In the general population between the ages of 15 and 64 yr, 1.5% to 5% of men and 10% to 25% of women have incontinence. In the nursing home population, 50% of the population has some degree of incontinence. Nearly 20% of children through the mid-teenage years have episodes of urinary incontinence.

CLINICAL, PSYCHOLOGIC, & SOCIAL IMPACT

Fewer than 50% of the individuals with incontinence living in the community consult health care providers, preferring to "suffer silently," turning to home remedies, commercially available absorbent materials, and supportive aids. As their condition worsens, they become depressed, sacrifice their independence, suffer from recurrent urinary tract infection and its sequelae, limit social interaction, refrain from sexual intimacy, and become homebound. In terms of costs, for all ages living in the community, it is estimated that $7 billion is spent for incontinence annually.

MAJOR TYPES OF INCONTINENCE

- **Transient incontinence:** Incontinence occurring as a result or reaction to an acute medical problem affecting the lower urinary tract. Many of these problems can be reversed with treatment of the underlying problem.
- **Urge incontinence:** Involuntary loss of urine associated with an abrupt and strong desire to void. It is usually associated with involuntary detrusor contractions on urodynamic investigation. In neurologically impaired patients, the involuntary detrusor contraction is referred to as *detrusor hyperreflexia*. In neurologically normal patients the involuntary contraction is called *detrusor instability.*
- **Stress incontinence:** The involuntary loss of urine with physical activities that increase abdominal pressure in the absence of a detrusor contraction or an overdistended bladder. Classification of stress incontinence:
  1. Type 0: Report of incontinence without demonstration of leakage.
  2. Type I: Incontinence in response to stress but with little descent of the bladder neck and urethra.
  3. Type II: Incontinence in response to stress with >2 cm descent of the bladder neck and urethra.
  4. Type III: Bladder neck and urethra wide open without bladder contraction; intrinsic sphincter deficiency; denervation of the urethra. The most common causes include urethral hypermobility and displacement of the bladder neck with exertion, intrinsic sphincter deficiency from failed antiincontinence surgery, prostatectomy, radiation, cord lesions, epispadias, and myelomeningocele.
- **Overflow incontinence:** Loss of urine resulting from overdistention of the bladder with resultant overflow or spilling of the urine. Causes include hypotonic-to-atonic bladder resulting from drug effect, fecal impaction, or neurologic conditions such as diabetes, spinal cord injury, surgery, or vitamin B_{12} deficiency. It is also caused by obstruction at the bladder neck and urethra. In this situation prostatism, prostatic cancer, urethral stenosis, antiincontinence surgery, pelvic prolapse, and detrusor-sphincter dyssynergia cause the incontinence.
- **Functional incontinence:** Involuntary loss of urine resulting from chronic impairments of physical and/or cognitive functioning. This is a diagnosis of exclusion. The condition can sometimes be improved or cured by improving the patient's functional status, treating comorbidities, changing medications, and reducing environmental barriers.
- **Mixed stress and urge incontinence.**
- **Sensory urgency incontinence:** Involuntary loss of urine as a result of decreased bladder compliance and increased intravesical pressures accompanied by severe urgency and bladder hypersensitivity without detrusor overactivity. This is seen with radiation cystitis, interstitial cystitis, eosinophilic cystitis, myelomeningocele, and radical pelvic surgery. Nephropathy can occur as a complication of this vesicoureteral reflux.
- **Sphincteric incontinence:**
  1. Urethral hypermobility: The basic abnormality is a weakness of pelvic floor support. Because of this weakness, during increases in abdominal pressure there is rotational descent of the vesical neck and proximal urethra. If the urethra opens concomitantly, stress urinary incontinence ensues. Urethral hypermobility is often present in women who are not incontinent. Its mere presence is not sufficient evidence to make the diagnosis of sphincteric abnormality unless incontinence is shown.
  2. Intrinsic sphincter deficiency: There is an intrinsic malfunction of the sphincter itself. It is characterized by an open vesical neck at rest and a low leak point pressure (<65 cm water). Urethral hypermobility and intrinsic sphincter deficiency may coexist in the same patient. Causes of intrinsic sphincter deficiency are previous pelvic surgery, antiincontinence surgery, urethral diverticulectomy, radical hysterectomy, abdominoperineal resection of the rectum, urethrotomy, Y-V plasty of the vesical neck, myelodysplasia, anterior spinal artery syndrome, lumbosacral disease, aging, and hyperestrogenism.

DIAGNOSIS

HISTORY

- History of present illness, psychosocial factors, congenital disorders, access issues for the physically challenged, neurologic disorders, and disorders pertinent to the urologic tract
- Review of prescription and nonprescription medications
- Voiding diary to assess total voided volume, frequency of micturition, mean volume voided, largest single volume, diurnal distribution, nature and severity of incontinence

WORKUP

- Physical examination including general examination, gait of the patient (neuromuscular deficits), estrogen status, vaginal examination to include the periurethral region, evaluation for cystocele, rectocele, and enterocele
- Pelvic floor strength assessment
- Rectal examination to assess sphincter tone and bulbocavernosus reflex
- Neurologic examination
- Postvoid residual check with bladder scan or catheter

LABORATORY TESTS

Urinalysis, urine culture, urine cytology, blood urea nitrogen, creatinine

IMAGING STUDIES

- Radiographs of the kidney, ureter, and bladder to assess bony skeleton
- Intravenous pyelography to rule out upper tract abnormalities, developmental anomalies, bladder configuration, and fistula
- Renal ultrasound if dye study is contraindicated

SPECIALIZED STUDIES

Simple cystometrogram, complex urodynamics for leak point pressures and uroflowmetry, endoscopic evaluation, cystogram

TREATMENT

- Transient incontinence: Treatment of underlying medical conditions and behavioral therapy to include habit training and timed voiding
- Urge incontinence: Bladder relaxants (tolterodine [Detrol], oxybutynin [Ditropan], imipramine), trospium chloride, estrogen, biofeedback, Kegel exercises, and surgical removal of obstructing or other pathologic lesions. Recent trials reveal promising results with direct intravesical instillation of a botulinum type A toxin/dimethyl sulfoxide (DMSO) solution for the treatment of idiopathic detrusor overactivity in women.
- Stress incontinence: Pelvic floor exercises, Kegel exercises, alpha-adrenergic agonists (e.g., ephedrine), estrogen, biofeedback
  - Cystourethropexy: Marshall-Marchetti-Krantz procedure, Burch procedure, Raz procedure, Stamey-Raz procedure, Gittes

procedure, in situ transvaginal sling, pubovaginal sling with autologous or cadaver graft, laparoscopic Burch procedure, laparoscopic sling, tension-free vaginal tape
    - For intrinsic sphincter deficiency: bulking agents (e.g., collagen), sling, and artificial sphincter
- Overflow incontinence: surgical removal of any obstructing lesions, clean intermittent catheterization, indwelling catheter
- Functional incontinence: behavioral training to include habit training and timed voiding, incontinence undergarments and pads, external collecting devices, environmental manipulation
- Mixed urgency and stress incontinence: use of measures recommended in the management of stress and urge incontinence
- Sensory urgency: bladder relaxants (e.g., anticholinergics, muscle relaxants, and tricyclic antidepressants), behavior therapy to include habit training and timed voiding, cystoscopy and hydrodilation
- Sphincteric deficiency: urethral bulking agents, sling procedure, artificial sphincter, mechanical clamp, external collection devices

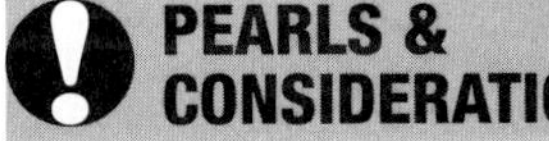

PEARLS & CONSIDERATIONS

COMMENTS

Other forms of incontinence:

- Nocturnal enuresis: (ICD-9CM Code: 788.3) Can be caused by sphincter abnormalities and detrusor overactivity; can occur as idiopathic, neurogenic, and with outlet obstruction
- Postvoid dribble: (ICD-9CM Code: 599.2) A postsphincteric collection of urine seen with urethral diverticulum; can be idiopathic
- Extraurethral incontinence: Enterovesical (ICD-9CM Codes: 596.1 and 596.2), urethral (ICD-9CM Code: 599.1); also known as *fistula*

Conditions that predispose to surgical failure: Advanced age, postmenopausal state, hysterectomy, prior failed incontinence surgery, concurrent detrusor instability, abnormal perineal electromyography, pelvic radiation

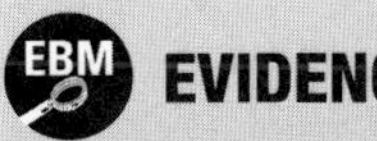

EVIDENCE

Please note: Complete text of EBM for this topic is available online.

Key trials and commentary:

The purpose of this study was to assess patient expectations of surgical outcome after preoperative counseling of surgical procedures in a randomized trial of 655 women in a comparison of the rectus fascial sling and Burch colposuspension.

This study showed that patients who undergo stress incontinence surgery have high expectations regarding the outcome of incontinence surgery, which include the resolution of urgency and frequency.

This is another important article from the NIH/NIDDK sponsored Urinary Incontinence Treatment Network. This is a piece of the rich data collection obtained from the Burch vs. TVT trial, completed and reported on previously. The take-home point from this article is that we are not nearly as good as our patients think we are! Patient expectations are extraordinarily high; however, even the best results published in the literature for any anti-incontinence procedure do not approach the expectations of our patients. It is clear that we either need to improve our surgical outcomes or decrease our patients' expectations into a more realistic range.[1] Ⓐ

Obesity is an established and modifiable risk factor for urinary incontinence, but conclusive evidence for a beneficial effect of weight loss on urinary incontinence is lacking.

This study showed that a 6-month behavioral intervention targeting weight loss reduced the frequency of self-reported urinary-incontinence episodes among overweight and obese women as compared with a control group. A decrease in urinary incontinence may be another benefit among the extensive health improvements associated with moderate weight reduction.

This trial was part of the Program to Reduce Incontinence by Diet and Exercise (PRIDE) study, sponsored by the NIDDK and NIH. A mean weight loss of only 8% resulted in a substantial improvement in urinary incontinence symptoms. It is both surprising and refreshing that such a small degree of weight loss may result in substantial improvements in urinary symptoms. It can be speculated that further weight loss may improve urinary symptoms even more favorably. Although the control group had a substantial reduction in incontinence episodes of almost 28%, this is not necessarily a placebo effect. This is easily explained by the study protocol in which all patients (both controls and subjects) received a self-help behavioral treatment booklet with instructions for improving bladder control. This could be considered a substantial and clinically significant intervention in and of itself in this highly motivated group of patients who entered a study voluntarily with the expectation of weight loss and incontinence improvement. It is also notable that the control group had follow-up sessions monthly for 4 months, which included a 1-hour group session, in which certain behavioral parameters were reinforced, again with potentially significant ramifications with respect to "a placebo response." It is notable in this study that although there was no significant difference in pad-weight testing between the groups, the patient-reported outcomes including satisfaction with and perception of treatment were both significantly greater in the subjects than the controls.[2] Ⓐ

The aim of one study was to determine whether combining antimuscarinic drug therapy with supervised behavioral training, compared with drug therapy alone, improves the ability of women with urge incontinence to achieve clinically important reductions in incontinence episodes and to sustain these improvements after discontinuing drug therapy.

This study showed that the addition of behavioral training to drug therapy may reduce incontinence frequency during active treatment but does not improve the ability to discontinue drug therapy and maintain improvement in urinary incontinence. Combination therapy has a beneficial effect on patient satisfaction, perceived improvement, and reduction of other bladder symptoms.

This is an important study sponsored by the NIDDK at the NIH. This is one of the studies performed as part of the Urinary Incontinence Treatment Network, with this particular study having the acronym BE-DRI (Behavior Enhances Drug Reduction of Incontinence). The results of this trial are no doubt disappointing in that discontinuation of drug therapy and behavioral therapy does not lead to long-term differences in overall outcome. It was hypothesized that the behavioral therapy, which included pelvic floor exercises, fluid management, and other behavioral strategies to diminish urgency, and prevent both stress and urge incontinence, would have a long-term beneficial effect once the drug therapy was discontinued. This unfortunately was not the case, or at least there was no difference between the two groups at the last follow-up. There could be many explanations for this, not the least of which is that the group that was not given reinforced behavioral therapy was nonetheless given a set of written instructions for behavioral therapy. Therefore, it is possible that these individuals were actually doing behavioral therapy and not acting as a "pure" control group. Such an effect could narrow the clinical difference between the two groups. In addition, it is not known whether, and to what extent, each group was compliant with behavioral therapy following the discontinuation of the 10-week active intervention arm.[3] Ⓐ

Do the results of this study mean that there is no benefit to behavioral therapy in addition to drug therapy? The answer is likely no. During active treatment the patients on combined behavioral therapy and drug therapy had greater reduction in incontinence frequency as compared with the group on single therapy. Combination therapy also had a favorable effect on patients' satisfaction and perception of improvement, which after all is what we aim to improve in the field of voiding dysfunction.

Another trial identified baseline demographic and clinical factors associated with treatment failure after surgical treatment of stress urinary incontinence.

This study showed that two years after surgery, risk factors for stress failure are similar after Burch and sling procedures and include greater baseline urge incontinence symptoms, more advanced prolapse, and being menopausal and not on hormone replacement therapy. Higher urge scores predicted failure by nonstress specific outcomes.

The Stress Incontinence Surgical Treatment Efficacy Trial (SISTEr trial) is a multicenter, randomized trial under the auspices of the Urinary Incontinence Treatment Network funded by the NIDDK of the NIH. These 24-month outcome data suggest that many of the variables that were previously felt to correlate with failure of stress urinary incontinence surgery are not significant. Such risk factors as age, body mass index, prior urinary incontinence surgery, previous hysterectomy, and the presence of diabetes mellitus did not affect continence outcomes in this trial. Urodynamic parameters were not reported on in this particular study but had been reported on previously in an article by Nager et al. In this previously reported data, the presence of detrusor overactivity and Valsalva leak point pressure did not statistically correlate with surgical success for the treatments of stress urinary incontinence; however, certain limitations do exist with respect to the data analysis in that particular study. It is interesting and important to note that the three factors in this study that predicted surgical failure (severity of urge incontinence symptoms, prolapse stage, and postmenopausal status without being on hormonal replacement therapy) are essentially modifiable risk factors preoperatively and/or intraoperatively. This suggests that aggressive treatment of vaginal prolapse, replacement with appropriate hormonal therapy, and preoperative treatment of urge incontinence may favorably affect surgical outcomes for stress urinary incontinence surgery. Ideally, this hypothesis would need to be tested in a prospective fashion.[4] Ⓐ

A separate study compared 200 IU intradetrusor botulinum toxin A vs. placebo in women with refractory idiopathic urge incontinence.

Botulinum toxin A continues to be investigated for the treatment of both neurogenic and idiopathic detrusor overactivity, as well as symptomatic urge incontinence. This was a multicenter trial sponsored by the National Institute of Child Health and Human Development as part of the Pelvic Floor Disorders Network research collaboration. It is notable that the study was terminated prematurely because of an interim data analysis that found a much higher than expected incidence of increased post void residual urine requiring intermittent urethral catheterization. The parameters for discontinuation of the study were set by the protocol before the initiation of the study and because the threshold for intermittent urethral catheterization was reached, the study was terminated. It is noteworthy that the vast majority of the patients who were placed on intermittent catheterization were asymptomatic, with only 14% of the patients placed on intermittent catheterization actually having symptoms. The rest of these individuals were placed on intermittent catheterization because of a predetermined limit of a post void residual greater than 200 ml. Nevertheless, despite the premature termination of the study, impressive reductions in urge incontinence were noted as well as improvements in patient satisfaction, which were durable for approximately 1 year. Notably, there was also a significant separation from placebo in this study. It is unclear where this study leaves us with respect to botulinum toxin A as a therapeutic intervention for lower urinary tract dysfunction. The dosage used in the study is somewhat larger than that used in many other studies. Consistent with much of the work that has been done on botulinum toxin A clinically, there appears to be a dose-response relationship with respect to the incidence of urinary retention and voiding dysfunction. The optimal dose of botulinum toxin A, delivery mechanism, dilution, and interval for reinjection remains unclear.[5] Ⓐ

Evidence-Based References

1. Mallett VT et al: The expectations of patients who undergo surgery for stress incontinence, *Am J Obstet Gynecol* 198:308, 2008. Commentary by E.S. Rovner, M.D. Ⓐ

2. Subak LL, for the PRIDE Investigators: Weight loss to treat urinary incontinence in overweight and obese women, *N Engl J Med* 360:481-490, 2009. Commentary by E.S. Rovner, M.D. Ⓐ

3. Burgio KL, for the Urinary Incontinence Treatment Network: Behavioral therapy to enable women with urge incontinence to discontinue drug treatment: a randomized trial, *Ann Intern Med* 149:161-169, 2008. Commentary by E.S. Rovner, M.D. Ⓐ

4. Richter HE et al: Predictors of treatment failure 24 months after surgery for stress urinary incontinence, *J Urol* 179:1024-1030, 2008. Commentary by E.S. Rovner, M.D. Ⓐ

5. Brubaker L, for the Pelvic Floor Disorders Network: Refractory idiopathic urge urinary incontinence and botulinum A injection, *J Urol* 180:217-222, 2008. Commentary by E.S. Rovner, M.D. Ⓐ

SUGGESTED READINGS

Holdroyd-Leduc JM et al: What type of urinary incontinence does this woman have? *JAMA* 299(12): 1446-1456, 2008.

Petrou SP et al: Botulinum A toxin/dimethyl sulfoxide bladder installation for women with refractory idiopathic detrusor overactivity: a phase study, *Mayo Clin Proc* 84(8):702-706, 2009.

Rogers RG: Urinary stress incontinence in women, *N Engl J Med* 358:1029-1036, 2008.

Shamliyan TA et al: Systematic review: randomized controlled trials of nonsurgical treatment for urinary incontinence in women, *Ann Intern Med* 148: 459-473, 2008.

AUTHORS: **PHILIP J. ALIOTTA, M.D., M.S.H.A.,** and **RUBEN ALVERO, M.D.**

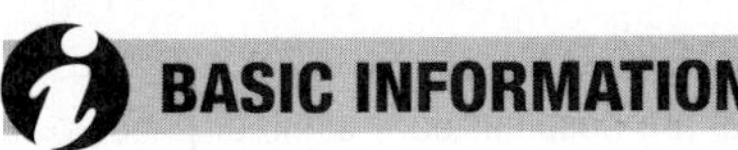

BASIC INFORMATION

DEFINITION

Hypotonia typically describes the inability to move or maintain posture against forces that stretch the body, mainly gravity. The cause can be at any level in the neuroaxis, so the differential is extensive. A detailed history and physical exam are the key tools to localizing the lesion.

SYNONYMS Floppy infant

ICD-9CM CODES
343.8 Infantile cerebral palsy

EPIDEMIOLOGY & DEMOGRAPHICS

Central causes for hypotonia outweigh peripheral causes 3:1

PHYSICAL FINDINGS & CLINICAL PRESENTATION

To assess tone, first observe the fully awake child looking for movement, position, and signs of decreased fetal movement (hip dislocation, arthrogryposis, plagiocephaly, pectus excavatum). When supine, infants with low tone will lay with their extremities extended and abducted, termed the *frog-leg position.* The head needs to be straight to avoid inducing the tonic neck reflex, which can make tone falsely appear to be asymmetric. When pulled gently by the hands toward the sitting position, normal infants will have a *traction response* that involves flexion at the hips, knees, and ankles with the head rising off the bed. Infants with hypotonia will have significant head lag and very little resistance to the examiner. Keep in mind, however, that this response is not present until after 33 wk gestational age. When held under the arms by the axilla in *vertical suspension,* hypotonic infants will start to slip through the examiner's hands, while infants with normal tone will have the same flexion reflex as with the traction response. If held prone with support under the torso in *horizontal suspension,* normal infants will keep their back straight, have flexion at the hips, knees, and ankles, and keep their head up. They will also make efforts to maintain this position, whereas a hypotonic infant will fall limply into an "inverted U" position.

Look for other signs that the hypotonia may have central origin (Table 1-44), for example abnormal head shape or size, decreased level of consciousness, dysmorphic features, other organs with malformations, seizures, apnea, or abnormal sleep-wake cycles. Reflexes should be brisk, but may be decreased acutely after an injury. Infants with peripheral hypotonia (i.e., a lesion in the motor unit) are typically alert and profoundly weak. Reflexes are reduced or absent and muscles may be atrophic. With anterior horn cell disease, the tongue may have fasciculations and the child may have an intention tremor, as well. The rest of the neurologic and general exams can provide pertinent clues to specific diagnoses. Cardiac murmurs, skin lesions, hepatosplenomegaly, and so forth help narrow down the differential.

TABLE 1-44 Localizing Exam Findings

Site of Lesion	Strength	Reflexes	Muscle Mass	Fasciculations
Brain	Normal or slightly impaired	Brisk (low after acute injury)	Normal	None
Anterior horn cell	Weak	Decreased	Significant atrophy	Prominent
Peripheral nerve	Weak	Decreased	Atrophy	None
Neuromuscular junction	Weak	Normal	Normal	None
Muscle	Weak	Decreased or absent	Atrophy or pseudo-hypertrophy	None

DIAGNOSIS

DIFFERENTIAL DIAGNOSIS

Common central causes
- Acquired brain insult
  - Infection
  - Hypoxic encephalopathy
  - Intracranial hemorrhage
- Brain anomalies: neuromigrational disorders
- Genetic disorders
  - Kabuki syndrome
  - Williams syndrome
  - MECP2 duplication syndrome
  - Down syndrome
  - Fragile X syndrome
  - Prader-Willi syndrome
- Congenital syndromes: benign congenital hypotonia

Peripheral causes of hypotonia in infants
- Anterior horn cell disease
  - Spinal muscular atrophy
  - Hypoxic injury
  - Neurogenic arthrogryposis
- Polyneuropathies (motor or sensory)
  - Hereditary motor-sensory neuropathy
  - Charcot-Marie-Tooth disease
  - Guillain-Barré syndrome
  - Congenital hypomyelinating disorder
- Neuromuscular junction disorders
  - Infantile botulism
  - Congenital myasthenia gravis
  - Transient neonatal myasthenia
- Congenital myopathies
  - Central core disease
  - Nemaline rod myopathy
  - Fiber-type disproportion myopathy
  - Multi-Minicore disease
  - Myotubular myopathy
- Muscular dystrophies
  - Congenital dystrophinopathy
  - Congenital muscular dystrophy
  - Congenital myotonic dystrophy
- Metabolic disorders
  - Acid maltase deficiency (Pompe's disease)
  - Cerebrohepatorenal syndrome (Zellweger)
  - Cytochrome-c oxidase deficiency
  - Mitochondrial myopathies
  - Neonatal adrenoleukodystrophy

LABORATORY TESTS

- Evaluate neonate for sepsis
- Electrolytes including glucose, creatinine, calcium
- Liver function tests
- Ammonia level
- Creatinine kinase level
- Lactate
- Consider TORCH titers
- Karyotype or specific genetic testing
- Serum amino acids
- Urine organic acids
- Acylcarnitine/carnitine panel
- Very long chain fatty acids
- EMG/nerve conduction velocity (NCV)
- Muscle biopsy

IMAGING STUDIES

MRI with spectroscopy

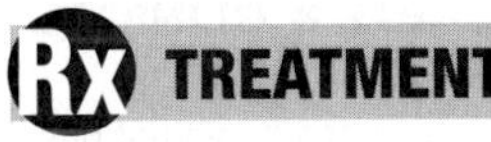

TREATMENT

Most of these disorders have no specific treatment.

CHRONIC Rx

- Physical therapy, occupational therapy, and other therapies tailored to the patient's specific needs can provide significant improvement in quality of life and ability to function.
- Respiratory illnesses are common in these children, so vaccinations should be kept up to date

DISPOSITION

- Long-term outcome varies greatly among different diseases.
- As a general rule, a hypotonic infant that requires mechanical ventilation cannot survive extubation (unless the cause is neonatal myasthenia).

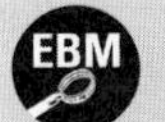

EVIDENCE

Moderate hypothermia for 72 hr after birth has been shown to reduce the risk of cerebral palsy and improve developmental outcomes in neonates with asphyxial encephalopathy.[1]

Evidence-Based Reference

1. Azzopardi DV et al: Moderate hypothermia to treat perinatal asphyxial encephalopathy, *N Engl J Med* 361(14):1349-1358, 2009.

SUGGESTED READINGS

Fenichel GM: *Clinical pediatric neurology: a signs and symptoms approach,* ed 6, Philadelphia, 2009, Saunders Elsevier.

Peredo DE, Hannibal MC: The floppy infant: evaluation of hypotonia, *Pediatr Rev* 30e66-e67, 2009.

AUTHOR: **KIMBERLY JONES, M.D.**

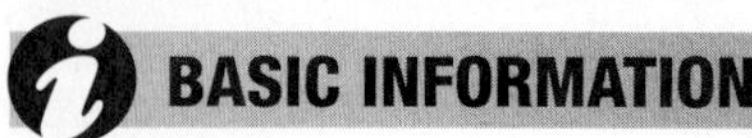

BASIC INFORMATION

DEFINITION

Influenza is an acute febrile illness caused by infection with influenza type A or B virus.

SYNONYMS

Flu

ICD-9CM CODES

487.1 Influenza

EPIDEMIOLOGY & DEMOGRAPHICS

INCIDENCE (IN U.S.): Annual incidence of influenza-related deaths is approximately 20,000 deaths/yr

PEAK INCIDENCE: Winter outbreaks lasting 5 to 6 wk

PREDOMINANT SEX: Male = female

PREDOMINANT AGE: Attack rates are higher among children than adults, although children are less prone to develop pulmonary complications.

PHYSICAL FINDINGS & CLINICAL PRESENTATION

- "Classic flu" is characterized by abrupt onset of fever, headache, myalgias, anorexia, and malaise after a 1- to 2-day incubation period.
- Clinical syndromes are similar to those produced by other respiratory viruses, including pharyngitis, common colds, tracheobronchitis, bronchiolitis, and croup.
- Respiratory symptoms such as cough, sore throat, and nasal discharge are usually present at the onset of illness, but systemic symptoms predominate.
- Elderly patients may experience fever, weakness, and confusion without any respiratory complaints.
- Acute deterioration to status asthmaticus may occur in patients with asthma.
- Influenza pneumonia: rapidly progressive cough, dyspnea, and cyanosis may occur after typical flu onset. This may be caused by primary influenza pneumonia or secondary bacterial pneumonia (often pneumococcal or staphylococcal infection).

ETIOLOGY

- Variation in the surface antigens of the influenza virus, hemagglutinin (HA) and neuraminidase (NA), leading to infection with variants to which resistance is inadequate in the population at risk
- Transmitted by small-particle aerosols and deposited on the respiratory tract epithelium

Dx DIAGNOSIS

DIFFERENTIAL DIAGNOSIS

- Respiratory syncytial virus, adenovirus, parainfluenza virus infection
- Secondary bacterial pneumonia or mixed bacterial-viral pneumonia

WORKUP

- Virus isolation from nasal or throat swab or sputum specimens is the most rapid diagnostic method in the setting of acute illness.
- Specimens are placed into virus transport medium and processed by a reference laboratory.
- For serologic diagnosis:
  1. Paired serum specimens, acute and convalescent, the latter obtained 10 to 20 days later
  2. Fourfold rises or falls in the titer of antibodies (various techniques) considered diagnostic of recent infection

LABORATORY TESTS

Septic syndrome presentation: CBC, ABG analysis, blood cultures

IMAGING STUDIES

- Chest x-ray examination to demonstrate findings of viral pneumonia: peribronchial and patchy interstitial infiltrates in multiple lobes with atelectasis
- Possible progression to diffuse interstitial pneumonitis

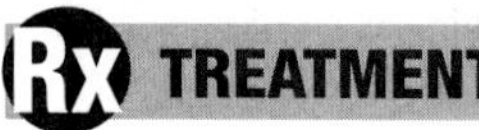

TREATMENT

NONPHARMACOLOGIC THERAPY

- Bed rest
- Hydration

ACUTE GENERAL Rx

- Supportive care: antipyretics; avoid use of aspirin in children because of the association with Reye's syndrome
- Antibiotics if bacterial pneumonia is proven or suspected
- Amantadine (100 mg PO bid for children >10 yr and adults <65 yr; once daily in patients >65 yr) and rimantadine (same dose schedule as amantadine)
  1. Further dose adjustments needed with renal insufficiency
  2. Fewer CNS side effects with rimantadine
- Neuraminidase inhibitors block release of virions from infected cells, resulting in shortened duration of symptoms and decrease in complications; effective against both influenza A and B
  1. Zanamivir, administered via inhaler, 10 mg bid
  2. Oseltamivir, administered orally, 75 mg PO bid for 5 days
- Placebo-controlled studies have suggested that antiviral therapy with any of the previously mentioned agents must be initiated within 1 to 2 days of the onset of symptoms and reduces the duration of illness by approximately 1 day.
- Oseltamivir resistance has developed on therapy in individuals with avian flu (H5, N1) in Asia, and this is associated with poor outcome.

DISPOSITION

Patients are hospitalized if signs of pneumonia are present.

REFERRAL

Infectious disease and/or pulmonary consultation when influenza pneumonia is suspected

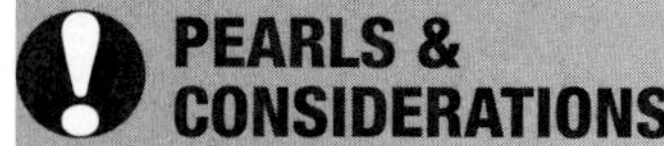

PEARLS & CONSIDERATIONS

COMMENTS

- Prevention of influenza in patients at high risk is an important goal of primary care.
- Vaccines reduce the risk of infection and the severity of illness.
  1. Antigenic composition of the vaccine is updated annually.
  2. Vaccination should be given at the start of the flu season (October) for the following groups:
     a. Adults 50 yr and older
     b. Adults and children with chronic cardiac or pulmonary disease, including asthma
     c. Adults and children with illness requiring frequent follow-up (e.g., hemoglobinopathies, diabetes mellitus)
     d. Children ages 6 to 59 mo and all those receiving long-term aspirin therapy
     e. Immunocompromised patients (including HIV-infected persons)
     f. Household contacts and caregivers of persons in the previous groups
     g. Health care workers, pregnant women
  3. The only contraindication to vaccination is hypersensitivity to hen's eggs.
  4. Special efforts should be made to vaccinate high-risk patients <65 yr, only 10% to 15% of whom are vaccinated each year.
- Chemoprophylaxis:
  1. Table 1-45 describes antiviral agents for influenza. Amantadine and rimantadine approved for prophylaxis against influenza A; they are ineffective against influenza B (NOTE: The avian flu strains [H5N1] are all intrinsically resistant to amantidine and rimantadine)
  2. Consider (after the current circulating strain of influenza has been shown to be sensitive):
     a. For high-risk patients in whom vaccination is contraindicated
     b. When the available vaccine is known not to include the circulating strain
     c. To provide added protection to immunosuppressed patients likely to have a diminished response to vaccination
     d. In the setting of an outbreak, when immediate protection of unvaccinated or recently vaccinated patients is desired
  3. Give for 2 wk in the case of late vaccination and for the duration of the flu season in all other patients

EVIDENCE

Please note: Complete text of EBM for this topic is available online.

Key trials and commentary:

Young infants and pregnant women are at increased risk for serious consequences of influenza infection. Inactivated influenza vaccine is recommended for pregnant women but is not licensed for infants younger than 6 months of age. This study assessed the clinical effectiveness of inactivated influenza vaccine administered during pregnancy in Bangladesh.

This study showed that inactivated influenza vaccine reduced proven influenza illness by 63% in infants up to 6 months of age and averted approximately a third of all febrile respiratory illnesses in mothers and young infants. Maternal influenza immunization is a strategy with substantial benefits for both mothers and infants.[1] Ⓐ

For many women's health care providers, vaccination has been, until recently, a dim and infrequently accessed aspect of our practice of medicine. Aside from the occasional international traveler and the patient who requires a specific vaccine, vaccination is best remembered from our pediatric rotations in medical school. However, with the success of the quadrivalent HPV vaccine (Gardasil), vaccination has become an increasingly important part of the health care of the young girl and woman in reducing the risk of cervical dysplasia, neoplasia, and genital warts. Indeed, vaccination is likely to play a bigger role in the health care of women in years ahead, with the development of new preventive and therapeutic vaccines. One of the occasions on which we are commonly faced with vaccination questions concerns the "flu vaccine." In this study, the authors found that vaccination of pregnant women reduced proven influenza illness in infants by 63% and averted a third of all respiratory illnesses in mothers and infants. We can no longer hide behind a veil of ignorance when it comes to vaccination. The ready availability of thimerosal-free flu vaccines should assuage concerns about short- and long-term safety. Although there are still economic barriers in incorporating these vaccines into our practices, primarily arising from insurance companies unwilling to reimburse us for these vaccinations, our successful incorporation of the HPV vaccine and the results from this well-done study lay a strong foundation for the eventual routine vaccination of pregnant women against current influenza strains. We owe no less to our patients and their newborns.

Evidence-Based Reference

1. Zaman K et al: Effectiveness of maternal influenza immunization in mothers and infants, *N Engl J Med* 359:1555-1564, 2008. Commentary by L.P. Shulman, M.D. Ⓐ

SUGGESTED READINGS

Centers for Disease Control: Prevention and control of influenza, *MMWR* 55(RR-10):1, 2006.

De Jong M et al: Fatal outcome of human influenza A (H5N1) is associated with high viral load and hypercytokinemia, *Nature Med* 10:1038, 2006.

De Jong MD et al: Oseltamivir resistance during treatment of influenza A (H5N1) infection, *N Engl J Med* 353(25):2667, 2006.

WHO Global Influenza Program Surveillance Network: Evolution of H5N1 avian influenza viruses in Asia, *Emerg Infect Dis* 11:1515, 2005.

AUTHORS: **GLENN G. FORT, M.D., M.P.H.,** and **DENNIS J. MIKOLICH, M.D.**

TABLE 1-45 Antiviral Agents for Influenza

	Amantadine	Rimantadine	Zanamivir	Oseltamivir
Protein target	M2	M2	Neuraminidase	Neuraminidase
Activity	A only	A only	A and B	A and B
Side effects	CNS (13%) GI (3%)	GI (6%) GI (3%)	?Bronchospasm	GI (9%)
Metabolism	None	Multiple (hepatic)	None	Hepatic
Excretion	Renal	Renal + others	Renal	Renal (tubular secretion)
Drug interactions	Antihistamines, anticholinergics	None	None	Probenecid (increased levels of oseltamivir)
Dose adjustments needed	≥65 years old CrCl <50 ml/min	≥65 years old CrCl <10 ml/min	None	CrCl <30 ml/min Severe liver dysfunction
Contraindications	Acute-angle glaucoma	Severe liver dysfunction	Underlying airway disease	
FDA-Approved Indications				
Therapy	Adults and children ≥1 yr of age	Adults only	Adults and children ≥7 yr of age	Adults and children ≥1 yr of age*
Prophylaxis	Yes	Yes	No	Adults and children ≥13 yr of age†

CrCl, Creatinine clearance; *FDA,* U.S. Food and Drug Administration; *GI,* gastrointestinal.
*FDA has authorized treatment of S-OIV with oseltamivir in children ≥3 mo of age.
†FDA has authorized prophylaxis for S-OIV with oseltamivir in children ≥1 yr of age.
(From Mandell GL et al: *Principles and practice of infectious diseases,* ed 7, Philadelphia, 2010, Elsevier.)

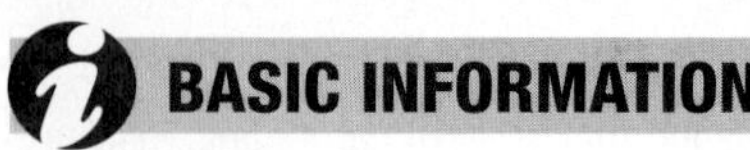

BASIC INFORMATION

DEFINITION

Avian influenza is a virus originating in birds that has the capacity to infect humans. The prior influenza pandemics of the twentieth century (from the devastating 1918 pandemic, in which 40-100 million people died, to the lesser pandemics of 1957 and 1968, of 1-6 million deaths) were caused by highly virulent, efficiently transmitted influenzas that evolved from avian strains. The highly pathogenic avian influenza A (H5N1), which is capable of only incidentally infecting humans but with a near 60% mortality rate, threatens to bring the next pandemic flu. It emerged in 1997 in Hong Kong, and by September 2009 had infected 442 humans as it spread via migrating waterfowl from Asia to Europe and Africa.

SYNONYMS

Bird flu
Pandemic flu

ICD-9CM CODES
488 Avian influenza

EPIDEMIOLOGY & DEMOGRAPHICS

Avian influenza A H5N1 is an influenza virus related to those that bring our yearly flu, against which populations are routinely vaccinated. Influenza viruses are enveloped RNA viruses with segmented genomes and great antigenic diversity. They are categorized by their core proteins (A, B, C), species of origin (avian, swine), geographic site of isolation, serial number, and influenza subtypes based on the major antigenic surface glycoproteins, hemagglutinin (HA) and neuraminidase (NA).

Often human and avian viruses meet and resort in a pig respiratory system. Southeast Asia is often the birthplace of new flu strains because birds, pigs, and people live in close proximity. It is where avian influenza A H5N1 emerged, first infecting domestic poultry, then wild birds that migrated across Eurasia. It is transmitted directly from birds to their keepers. Antigenic drift or shift may allow avian influenza A H5N1 to gain the ability to be easily transmissible from human to human, transforming it from a highly virulent influenza strain to a pandemic flu.

PREDOMINANT SEX AND AGE: Children and young adults

RISK FACTORS: Poultry work, possibly swine work (in case of reassortment), travel to affected areas

PHYSICAL FINDINGS & CLINICAL PRESENTATION

- Presenting features include fever of at least 100.4° F (38° C) with leukopenia or lymphopenia nearly always followed by viral pneumonia with escalating respiratory distress.
- Ventilatory support is often required within 48 hr of hospitalization for acute respiratory distress syndrome (ARDS).
- Symptom onset is 2 to 5 days after exposure, longer than with human influenza.
- Respiratory symptoms may also be accompanied by watery diarrhea and, rarely, encephalopathy.
- Complications include respiratory failure, renal dysfunction, cardiac compromise, pulmonary hemorrhage, pneumothorax, and multiorgan failure. A common cause of death is superinfection with bacterial pneumonias.

ETIOLOGY

H5N1 resists host antiviral cytokines, inducing excessive host pro-inflammatory responses. It may cause death by "cytokine storm" rather than by inherent pathogenicity. It attaches to sialic acid molecules via an α2-3 galactose receptor (common in birds) also found in human alveoli, leading to heavy damage to lower lungs. It causes severe pulmonary injury with diffuse alveolar damage. In the bone marrow, there is a reactive histiocytosis with hemophagocytosis that may lead to pancytopenia.

Dx DIAGNOSIS

DIFFERENTIAL DIAGNOSIS

Atypical pneumonia, typical respiratory virus infections (e.g., influenza, respiratory syncytial virus), severe acute respiratory syndrome, upper respiratory infection with conjunctivitis (e.g., adenovirus). Clinical symptoms indistinguishable from other illnesses

WORKUP

Comprehensive travel, occupational and epidemiologic history

LABORATORY TESTS

- Aspartate aminotransferase, alanine aminotransferase, blood urea nitrogen, creatinine, complete blood count should be performed.
- Throat swab within 3 days of onset of symptoms to be sent for viral culture and polymerase chain reaction assay for avian influenza A (H5N1) RNA with appropriate biosafety precautions. The throat swab is more effective than nasal swabs since avian flu preferentially infects the throat and lower respiratory tract. In the U.S. the FDA has approved the release of influenza H/A5 (Asian lineage) Virus Real-Time Reverse Transcription-PCR Primer and Probe Set for more than 140 labs in 50 states, which will return preliminary results in 4 hr.
- High-risk patients who must be tested include those with history of travel within 10 days of symptom onset to a country with documented H5N1 avian flu as well as patients with radiographically confirmed pneumonia, ARDS, or severe respiratory illness without alternate etiology.
- Low-risk patients are those who have contact with domestic poultry, or contact with people who have traveled to a country with documented H5N1 avian flu, who have fever $>$38° C and cough, sore throat, shortness of breath.

IMAGING STUDIES

- Chest x-rays detect infiltrates a median of 7 days after onset of fever. They may be diffuse, multifocal/patchy infiltrates, or interstitial infiltrates, or segmental/lobular consolidation. Progression to respiratory failure is indicated by diffuse bilateral ground-glass infiltrates.
- See ARDS imaging studies.

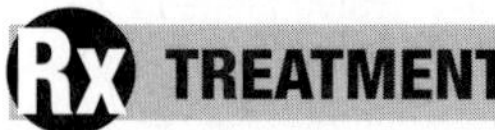

TREATMENT

Vaccines and antivirals are the usual means for preventing and treating flu, but there are limited supplies worldwide. The traditional means of vaccine production using embryonated hens' eggs has been limited because the bird flu kills the eggs. Promising new vaccine production methods are advancing through the experimental stages, but they still fall short of meeting worldwide needs.

NONPHARMACOLOGIC THERAPY

- N95 particulate masks should help prevent person-to-person transmission of H5N1. Surgical masks prevent only large-droplet transmission.
- In preparation for pandemic flu: increase worldwide surveillance and disease reporting, kill infected birds, increase the numbers of available intensive care unit beds with mechanical ventilators and increase emergency capacity, educate medical personnel and the public, produce vaccines.
- In response, use influenza surveillance, social distancing (school closures), travel restrictions, quarantine, respirator masks, communications networking, and international teamwork to cordon off affected areas.

ACUTE GENERAL Rx

- The neuraminidase inhibitor oseltamivir can reduce the severity and duration of symptoms if treatment is initiated in the first 48 hr after symptom onset.
  - Treatment: adults 75 mg PO twice daily for 5 days
  - Postexposure prophylaxis: 75 mg PO daily for 7 to 10 days
- H5N1 demonstrates amantadine and rimantadine resistance.

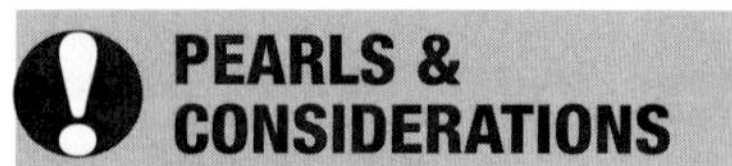

PEARLS & CONSIDERATIONS

The threat of pandemic remains a public health crisis according to the World Health Organization. Health care workers should stay abreast of developments in terms of the epidemiology, preventive measures, and treatments.

PREVENTION

See nonpharmacologic treatment

PATIENT & FAMILY EDUCATION

The American Council on Science and Health: Avian influenza: what you need to know. Available at http://acsh.org/publications/pubid.1294/pub_detail.asp

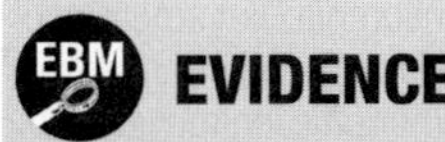

EVIDENCE

Avian H7 influenza viruses, from both the Eurasian and North American lineage, have caused outbreaks in poultry since 2002, with confirmed human infection occurring during outbreaks in the Netherlands, British Columbia, and the United Kingdom. The majority of H7 infections have resulted in self-limiting conjunctivitis, whereas probable human-to-human transmission has been rare. Here, we used glycan microarray technology to determine the receptor-binding preference of Eurasian and North American lineage H7 influenza viruses and their transmissibility in the ferret model. We found that highly pathogenic H7N7 viruses from the Netherlands in 2003 maintained the classic avian-binding preference for α2–3-linked sialic acids (SA) and are not readily transmissible in ferrets, as observed previously for highly pathogenic H5N1 viruses. However, H7N3 viruses isolated from Canada in 2004 and H7N2 viruses from the northeastern United States, isolated in 2002 to 2003, possessed a hemagglutinin (HA) with increased affinity toward α2–6-linked SA, the linkage type found prominently on human tracheal epithelial cells. We identified a low pathogenic H7N2 virus isolated from a man in New York in 2003, A/NY/107/03, which replicated efficiently in the upper respiratory tract of ferrets and was capable of transmission in this species by direct contact. These results indicate that H7 influenza viruses from the North American lineage have acquired sialic acid-binding properties that more closely resemble those of human influenza viruses and have the potential to spread to naïve animals.[1] Ⓐ

Avian influenza viruses of H5 and H7 subtype have caused recent outbreaks of disease in poultry and a limited number of human infections. Unlike most subtypes of influenza, H7 influenza virus frequently causes conjunctivitis in humans but not respiratory disease.[1] Influenza viruses attach through binding of the viral HA to SA glycans present on the host cell surface. Avian influenza viruses bind to α2–3-linked SA, and human influenza viruses bind to α2–6-linked SA, respectively. The pandemic strains of 1918 (H1N1), 1957 (H2N2), and 1968 (H3N2) all possessed HA, with preference for binding to α2–6-linked SA. However, they are all thought to have originated from avian viruses with α2–3-linked SA binding preference, suggesting the evolution of avian viruses with enhanced capability to attach to human cells. So far, avian H5N1 influenza viruses isolated from human cases have retained the classic avian virus binding α2–3-linked SA with few exceptions. The investigators in this study used glycan microassay technology to determine the receptor-binding preference of Eurasian and North American lineage H7 influenza viruses and their transmissibility in the ferret model. The results show that H7N3 viruses, isolated from Canada in 2004, and H7N2 viruses from the northeastern U.S., isolated in 2002-2003, possess an HA with increased affinity to match α2–6-linked SA, the type found predominantly on human tracheal epithelial cells. This finding underscores the pandemic potential of the North American H7 viruses.[1] Ⓐ

Evidence-Based Reference

1. Belser JA et al: Contemporary North American influenza H7 viruses possess human receptor specificity: Implications for virus transmissibility, *Proc Natl Acad Sci USA* 105:7558-7563, 2008. Commentary by N. Khardori, M.D. Ⓐ

SUGGESTED READINGS

Arabi Y et al: The critically ill avian influenza A (H5N1) patient, *Crit Care Med* 35(5):1397-1403, 2007.

Brundage JF: Interactions between influenza and bacterial respiratory pathogens: implications for pandemic preparedness, *Lancet Infect Dis* 6(303):303-312, 2006.

Gambotto A et al: Human infection with highly pathogenic H5N1 influenza virus, *Lancet* 371:1464, 2008.

Juckett G: Avian influenza: preparing for a pandemic, *Am Fam Physician* 74:783, 2006.

Pandey A et al: Egg-independent vaccine strategies for highly pathogenic H5N1 influenza viruses, *Human Vaccin* 6(2), 2010 (epub ahead of print).

Websites: U.S. CDC: avian influenza, http://www.cdc.gov/flu/avian; U.S. government avian and pandemic flu information, http://www.pandemicflue.gov; WHO confirmed cases, http://www.who.int/csr/disease/avian_influenza/country/en/.

AUTHOR: **KOHAR JONES, M.D.**

Insomnia (PTG) (ALG)

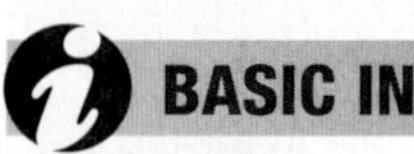

BASIC INFORMATION

DEFINITION

Insomnia is a disturbance of initiating or maintaining sleep. Restless, nonrestorative sleep may also be described as insomnia. The disturbance may be purely subjective without daytime impairment or may be objectively measurable with daytime consequences of sleepiness and functional impairment.

SYNONYMS

Sleeplessness

Sleep disorder, sleep disturbance, dyssomnia (NOTE: The terms *sleep disorder, sleep disturbance,* and *dyssomnia* are generic and can refer to disorders of wakefulness [hypersomnia] or sleep-related behavior disorders [parasomnias]).

ICD-9CM CODES

780.52 Insomnia
780.51 Insomnia with sleep apnea
307.41 Insomnia, nonorganic origin
307.42 Insomnia, persistent (primary)
307.41 Insomnia, transient
307.49 Subjective complaint

DSM IV-TR CODES

307.42 Primary insomnia
307.45 Circadian rhythm disorders
780.52 Insomnia due to a general medical condition
291.89, 292.89 Substance-induced insomnia

EPIDEMIOLOGY & DEMOGRAPHICS

INCIDENCE (IN U.S.): 30% to 45% of adults experience insomnia per year.

PREVALENCE (IN U.S.): 1% to 15% of all adults and 25% of older adults develop persistent insomnia.

PREDOMINANT SEX: More common in women.

PREDOMINANT AGE: Transient insomnia can occur at any age; persistent insomnia is more common after age 60 yr.

GENETICS: Insomnia can run in families and may be genetically influenced. Sleep characteristics in monozygous twins are more similar than in dizygote twins. Some sleep disorders, such as circadian rhythm disorders and narcolepsy, have been traced to specific genes.

PHYSICAL FINDINGS & CLINICAL PRESENTATION

- Difficulty falling asleep, difficulty staying asleep, early morning awakening, restless or nonrestorative sleep, or difficulty sleeping at desired times.
- May have daytime sleepiness or fatigue.
- Symptoms may be acute and self-limited, chronic but intermittent, or chronic and frequent.

ETIOLOGY

- Transient insomnia:
  1. Stress
  2. Illness
  3. Travel (across time zones)
  4. Environmental disruptions (noise, heat, cold, poor bedding, unfamiliar surroundings, etc.)
- Persistent insomnia:
  1. Mood and anxiety disorders (depression, hypomania/mania, PTSD)
  2. Primary or psychophysiologic insomnia (with or without poor sleep hygiene)
  3. Sleep-related breathing disorders (e.g., obstructive apnea and hypopnea, increased upper airway resistance)
  4. Chronobiologic (also known as *circadian rhythm*) disorder (delayed sleep phase, advanced sleep phase, shift work, free-running rhythm secondary to blindness)
  5. Drug and alcohol abuse
  6. Restless legs syndrome and periodic leg movements
  7. Neurodegenerative (Alzheimer's disease, Parkinson's disease, etc.)
  8. Medical (pain, GERD, nocturia, orthopnea, medications, etc.)

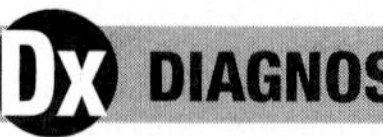

DIAGNOSIS

DIFFERENTIAL DIAGNOSIS

Primary or psychophysiologic insomnia is diagnosed when other etiologies (see "Etiology") are ruled out. Primary insomnia may be related to counterproductive sleep hygiene, hyperarousal, or insufficient sleep drive.

WORKUP

- History (with bed partner interview, if possible)
- Sleep diary for 2 wk to document nightly sleep quality and daytime sleepiness or fatigue (sample sleep diary available at http://www.sleepfoundation.org)
- Validated sleep-quality rating scale (optional)
  1. Pittsburgh Sleep Quality Index or Insomnia Severity Index
  2. Epworth Sleepiness Scale (see Daytime Sleepiness Test at http://www.sleepfoundation.org)

LABORATORY TESTS

- Evaluate for anemia, uremia (for restless legs), thyroid function (if other signs present).
- Polysomnography (in home or in sleep laboratory) for symptoms suggesting something other than primary insomnia: daytime sleepiness (obstructive sleep apnea, narcolepsy), nonrestorative sleep (periodic leg movements), or sleep behavior suggesting parasomnia (somnambulism, REM sleep behavior).

IMAGING STUDIES

- Not generally helpful for insomnia
- Brain CT or MRI for severe daytime sleepiness or acute onset

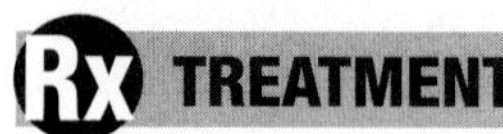

TREATMENT

NONPHARMACOLOGIC THERAPY

- Sleep hygiene measures (Box 1-10)
- Cognitive-behavioral therapy (CBT) can address anxiety and insomnia-perpetuating behaviors. CBT has been shown to reduce time to fall asleep and time awake during the night in placebo-controlled trials and can reduce reliance on sleep medications.
- The cognitive component of CBT involves education about sleep and insomnia to address concerns that might increase anxiety around sleeplessness. The behavioral component attempts to change habits that may perpetuate insomnia. The four components are *relaxation techniques; stimulus control* to address the conditioned cues that create arousal when attempting to sleep; *bed restriction* to sleep and sex and not tossing and turning, watching TV, reading, etc.; and improved *sleep hygiene* practices such as increasing daytime exercise, avoiding heavy meals at night, and reducing or eliminating caffeine, nicotine, and alcohol intake.
- Increased daytime activity improves sleep, especially in people (of any age) who were previously sedentary. Improvements are seen in total sleep duration, sleep-onset latency, and scores on a scale of global sleep quality.
- Insomnia attributable to circadian rhythm disturbances, such as in shift workers, many blind individuals (lack of light–dark cycle to synchronize body clock), adolescents and young adults with delayed sleep phase syndrome, and jet lag can be treated with chronobiologic therapies such as bright light exposure, melatonin, or melatonin agonists. These therapies must be given at specific times of the day or night, and referral to a sleep specialist may be necessary.

BOX 1-10 Sleep Habits (Sleep Hygiene Measures) That May Improve Sleep

1. Reduce caffeine, alcohol, or tobacco late in the day or evening.
2. Avoid heavy meals at night.
3. Increase daytime activity.
4. Increase daytime exposure to natural light.
5. Take warm bath as part of bedtime ritual.
6. Restrict bed to sleep and sex.
7. Get out of bed if not asleep after 30 minutes and return when drowsy.
8. Repeat above if awakened during the night.
9. Maintain regular sleep and wake times.
10. Go to bed with calm mind; resolve arguments or deal with problems earlier in day.

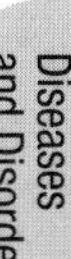

ACUTE GENERAL Rx

- Benzodiazepine sedative-hypnotics (e.g., temazepam 7.5-30 mg, triazolam 0.125-0.25 mg).
- In critical care: lorazepam 0.25-0.5 mg PO, SL, or IV as needed for sleep. In patients with acute delirium, haloperidol 0.25-0.5 mg IV as needed up to 2 mg/day may be less likely to worsen confusion.
- Benzodiazepine receptor agonists zolpidem 5-10 mg and zaleplon 5-10 mg for sleep-onset insomnia, and zolpidem continuous-release formulation 6.25-12.5 mg and eszopiclone 1-3 mg for maintenance insomnia.
- Melatonin agonist ramelteon 8 mg for sleep-onset insomnia when a mild agent without benzodiazepine side effects is desired.
- Avoid antihistamines except for occasional use.
- Optimize treatment of medical symptoms, especially pain.

CHRONIC Rx

- Controlled trials suggest that CBT is superior to medication for chronic insomnia. Long-term management of insomnia needs ongoing attention to sleep hygiene and other cognitive behavioral approaches for best results.
- Three sedative-hypnotics—zolpidem continuous release, eszopiclone, and ramelteon—have been studied in 6-mo controlled trials and are FDA approved for long-term use.
- Some evidence shows that benzodiazepines and benzodiazepine receptor agonists can be used for chronic insomnia on either intermittent or nightly use with moderate risk of tolerance and dependence but low risk of addiction.
- Sedating antidepressants (e.g., trazodone 25-150 mg, mirtazapine 7.5-30 mg, amitriptyline 25-50 mg) are in widespread use, but limited data are available on safety and efficacy for insomnia. Amitriptyline should be avoided if possible in older adults.
- Sedating antipsychotics (e.g., quetiapine 25-200 mg, olanzapine 2.5-10 mg at night) for severe mood or psychotic disorders associated with insomnia.

COMPLEMENTARY & ALTERNATIVE MEDICINE

Melatonin is the only substance that has been studied in larger controlled trials. It may shorten sleep-onset latency in some individuals but not most. Valerian has been studied in small trials but, like melatonin, appears to be of minimal benefit for insomnia in most people.

DISPOSITION

- Transient insomnia: usually self-limited but may require follow-up if stress-related or illness-related because of risk of depression or persistent insomnia.
- Persistent insomnia: patients have a chronic and recurrent disorder and need periodic follow-up to reinforce good sleep hygiene measures and reassess need for pharmacologic therapies. Evidence is growing that insomnia is associated with significant negative health effects over time.

REFERRAL

- Excessive daytime sleepiness not obviously caused by insomnia (e.g., narcolepsy, sleep-related breathing disorder)
- Nighttime behavior suggestive of a parasomnia (e.g., somnambulism, REM behavior disorder)
- Severe insomnia not responsive to basic interventions

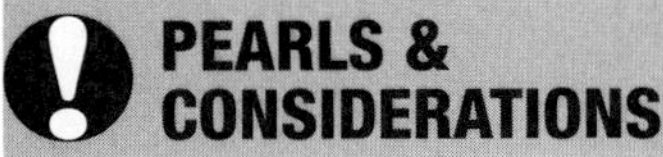

PEARLS & CONSIDERATIONS

COMMENTS

Treatment of insomnia should focus on reducing daytime sleepiness and improving daytime function rather than trying to achieve the elusive goal of uninterrupted nighttime sleep.

PREVENTION

Not much is known about prevention of insomnia. Effective treatment of transient insomnia may reduce the risk of developing persistent insomnia.

PATIENT/FAMILY EDUCATION

The National Sleep Foundation (http://www.sleepfoundation.org) is a comprehensive resource for health care providers and patients.

EBM EVIDENCE

Please note: Complete text of EBM for this topic is available online.

Key trials and commentary:

This study sought to investigate the effect of melatonin treatment on sleep, behavior, cognition, and quality of life in children with attention deficit hyperactivity disorder (ADHD) and chronic sleep onset insomnia.

This study showed that melatonin advanced circadian rhythms of sleep-wake and endogenous melatonin and enhanced total time asleep in children with ADHD and chronic sleep onset insomnia; however, no effect was found on problem behavior, cognitive performance, or quality of life.

Although not listed as a diagnostic criterion for ADHD, sleep problems are not uncommon in children with ADHD. Parents describe their ADHD child as a restless or fretful sleeper, often having trouble falling asleep and staying asleep. Some clinicians propose that many of the behavior problems associated with ADHD are attributed to sleep problems. Not infrequently, sleep improves with the appropriate dosing of stimulant medication or with the prescription of atomoxetine, and if sleep problems persist, a low dose of an α-adrenergic agent is often added.

This article investigates the use of melatonin in stimulant-free children with diagnosed ADHD and chronic sleep insomnia. The results of this well-controlled, double-blind, placebo study demonstrated that sleep onset was advanced and total sleep time was increased, but there was no change in the behavior problems, cognitive performance, or quality of life of these ADHD children. Thus, the stimulants and the nonstimulants remain the first-line pharmacologic treatment for children with ADHD. If sleep problems persist, melatonin may be added without significant side effects. So, sleep is a problem for many children with ADHD, but it is not *the* problem.[1] Ⓐ

The effects of CBT on reduced time to fall asleep are comparable to sleep medication, although they may take several weeks to develop. CBT may be superior to pharmacotherapy for chronic insomnia.[2,3]

Regular, moderate-intensity exercise improves sleep in adults age 60 yr or older with primary insomnia. Improvements are seen in total sleep duration, sleep-onset latency, and scores on a scale of global sleep quality.[4]

Clinical practice guidelines support the use of integrated cognitive-behavioral and medical approaches to chronic insomnia.[5]

Insomnia may be associated with impaired driving, especially at night, in older adults.[6]

Evidence-Based References

1. Van der Heijden KB et al: Effect of melatonin on sleep, behavior, and cognition in ADHD and chronic sleep-onset insomnia, *J Am Acad Child Adolesc Psychiatry* 46:233-241, 2007. Commentary by R.M. Sarles, M.D. Ⓐ
2. Jacobs GD et al: Cognitive behavior therapy and pharmacotherapy for insomnia: a randomized controlled trial and direct comparison, *Arch Intern Med* 164(17):1888, 2004.
3. Silber MH: Chronic insomnia, *N Engl J Med* 353: 803, 2005.
4. Montgomery P, Dennis J: Physical exercise for sleep problems in adults aged 60+, *Cochrane Database Syst Rev* 4, 2002.
5. Schutte-Rodin S et al: Clinical guideline for the evaluation and management of chronic insomnia in adults, *J Sleep Res* 17:3:335-343, 2008.
6. Vaz Fragosos C et al: Prevalence of sleep disturbances in a cohort of older drivers, *J Gerontol Med Sci* 63A:715-723, 2008.

SUGGESTED READINGS

Morin CM et al: Cognitive behavioral therapy, singly and combined with medication, for persistent insomnia: a randomized controlled trial, *JAMA* 20; 301(19):2005-2015, 2009.

Panossian LA, Avidan AY: Review of sleep disorders, *Med Clin North Am* 93(2):407-425, 2009.

Parish JM: Sleep-related problems in common medical conditions, *Chest* 135(2):563-572, 2009.

AUTHORS: **MITCHELL D. FELDMAN, M.D., M.PHIL.**

Diseases and Disorders I

Insulinoma

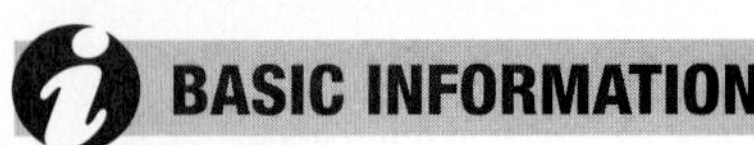

BASIC INFORMATION

DEFINITION

Insulinoma is a pancreatic insulin-secreting tumor that causes symptoms associated with hypoglycemia.

ICD-9CM CODES
M8151/0 Insulinoma

EPIDEMIOLOGY & DEMOGRAPHICS

INCIDENCE: One case per 250,000 persons annually. Ninety percent of insulinomas are benign.

PREDOMINANT SEX AND AGE: Insulinomas occur in both sexes (approximately 60% in women) and at all ages. In a Mayo Clinic series, the median age at diagnosis was 50 yr in sporadic cases but 23 yr in patients with multiple endocrine neoplasia, type 1 (MEN-1).

PHYSICAL FINDINGS & CLINICAL PRESENTATION

Symptoms typically occur in the morning before breakfast (i.e., fasting hypoglycemia as opposed to reactive hypoglycemia, which is not commonly associated with insulinoma)

Neuroglycopenic Symptoms	*%*
Various combinations of diplopia, blurred vision, sweating, palpitations, or weakness	85
Confusion or abnormal behavior	80
Unconsciousness or amnesia	53
Grand mal seizures	12
Adrenergic Symptoms	*%*
Sweating	43
Tremulousness	23
Hunger, nausea	12
Palpitations	10

ETIOLOGY, PATHOLOGY, PATHOPHYSIOLOGY

- Insulinomas are almost always solitary. Malignant insulinomas account for 5% of the total; they tend to be larger (6 cm). Metastases are usually to the liver (47%), regional lymph nodes (30%), or both.
- Insulinomas are evenly distributed in the head, body, and tail of the pancreas; ectopic insulinomas are rare (1% to 3%). Tumor size: 5% are ≤0.5 cm, 34% are 0.5 to 1 cm, 53% are 1 to 5 cm, and 8% are >5 cm.
- Histologic classification includes insulinoma in 86% of patients, adenomatosis in 5% to 15%, nesidioblastosis in 4%, and hyperplasia in 1%. Adenomatosis consists of multiple macroadenomas or microadenomas and occurs especially in patients with MEN-1. Nesidioblastosis is also a diffuse lesion in which islet cells form as buds on ductular structures.

DIAGNOSIS

DIFFERENTIAL DIAGNOSIS (OF FASTING HYPOGLYCEMIA)

Hyperinsulinism:
- Insulinoma
- Nonpancreatic tumors
- Severe congestive heart failure
- Severe renal insufficiency in non-insulin-dependent diabetes

Hepatic enzyme deficiencies or decreased hepatic glucose output (primarily in infants and children):
- Glycogen storage diseases
- Endocrine hypofunction
- Hypopituitarism
- Addison's disease
- Liver failure
- Alcohol abuse
- Malnutrition

Exogenous agents:
- Sulfonylureas, biguanides
- Insulin
- Other drugs (aspirin, pentamidine)

Functional fasting hypoglycemia:
- Autoantibodies to insulin receptor or insulin

LABORATORY TESTS

- An overnight fasting blood sugar level combined with a simultaneous plasma insulin, proinsulin, and/or C peptide level will establish the existence of fasting organic hypoglycemia in 60% of patients.
- If single overnight fasting glucose and insulin levels are nondiagnostic, a 72-hr fast is usually done with blood glucose and insulin levels determined at 2- to 4-hr intervals. A total of 75% of patients with insulinoma develop symptoms and a blood sugar level of <40 mg/dl by 24 hr, 92% to 98% develop these by 48 hr, and virtually all patients develop them by 72 hr. The test is considered positive for insulinoma if the plasma insulin/glucose ratio is more than 0.3. If at any point the patient becomes symptomatic, plasma insulin and glucose values should be obtained and IV glucose should be administered.
- Plasma proinsulin, C-peptide, antibodies to insulin, and plasma sulfonylurea levels may be used to rule out factitious use of insulin or hypoglycemic agents or autoantibodies against the insulin receptor or insulin.
- See Section III, "Hypoglycemia," for a description of the diagnostic approach to patients with documented hypoglycemia and elevated insulin.

IMAGING STUDIES

- Abdominal CT scan or MRI detects half to two thirds of insulinomas (abdominal ultrasound is not effective); should be done only after laboratory tests for insulinoma have confirmed the diagnosis
- Intraoperative ultrasound
- Arteriography
- Octreotide scan

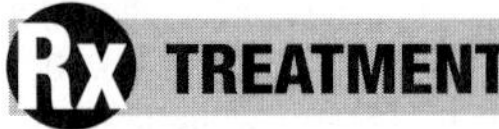

TREATMENT

NONPHARMACOLOGIC THERAPY

- Enucleation of single insulinoma
- Partial pancreatectomy for multiple adenomas

ACUTE GENERAL Rx

- Carbohydrate administration
- Diazoxide directly inhibits insulin release and has an extrapancreatic, hyperglycemic effect that enhances glycogenolysis
- Lanreotide and octreotide (somatostatin analogs)
- Streptozotocin

REFERRAL

At some point in the workup the patient will probably be referred to an endocrinologist and then a surgeon. A combination of fasting hypoglycemia and elevated insulin level is probably a good point at which to refer.

SUGGESTED READING

Axelrod L: Insulinoma: cost-effective care in patients with rare disease, *Ann Intern Med* 123:311, 1995.

AUTHOR: **FRED F. FERRI, M.D.**

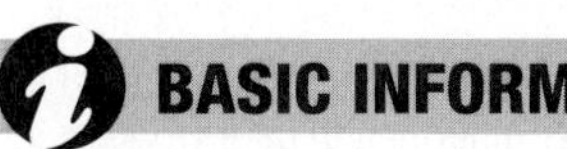

BASIC INFORMATION

DEFINITION

The International Continence Society defines interstitial cystitis (IC), otherwise known as painful bladder syndrome, as a clinical syndrome consisting of suprapubic pain related to bladder filling and accompanied by other symptoms such as increased daytime and nighttime frequency in the absence of proven infection or other obvious pathology.

SYNONYMS

Painful bladder syndrome
Tic douloureux of bladder

ICD-9CM CODES
595.1

EPIDEMIOLOGY & DEMOGRAPHICS

INCIDENCE: 21 cases per 100,000 women and four cases per 100,000 men annually

PREVALENCE:

- 197 per 100,000 women and 41 per 100,000 men in the U.S.
- Because the disease is substantially underdiagnosed, it may actually affect one in five women and one in 20 men.
- More than 81% of women diagnosed with chronic pelvic pain and up to 84% of men initially diagnosed with chronic prostatitis actually have IC.
- More than 90% of patients diagnosed with overactive bladder who do not respond to anticholinergics are subsequently diagnosed with IC.

PREDOMINANT SEX AND AGE:

- White women constitute 95% of patients with IC.
- Female/male ratio of 5 to 10:1.
- Most prevalent in fourth and fifth decades of life.

PHYSICAL FINDINGS & CLINICAL PRESENTATION

- Urinary urgency, frequency (>8 in daytime), nocturia (>2 at night), and suprapubic pain are the most common symptoms.
- Suprapubic pain is worse with bladder filling or urinating and relieved after emptying.
- Dyspareunia.
- Symptoms lasting longer than 6 mo.
- Intensity of symptoms waxes and wanes.
- Insidious onset and worsens to the final stage within 5 to 15 yr.
- Exercise, stress, sexual activity, ejaculation, certain foods with high potassium and acids (beer, spices, bananas, tomatoes, chocolate, strawberries, artificial sweeteners, oranges, cranberries, caffeine), menstruation, prolonged sitting, and activation of allergies exacerbate the symptoms.
- Often associated with irritable bowel syndrome, migraine, endometriosis, skin sensitivities, multiple drug allergies, other allergies, vulvodynia, fibromyalgia, chronic fatigue syndrome, systemic lupus erythematosus, and mood disorders.
- Dysphoric mood.
- Lower abdominal tenderness.
- Tender prostate in digital rectal examination.
- Levator ani tenderness in female.
- Tenderness of anterior vaginal wall/bladder neck in female.

ETIOLOGY

Unknown

DIAGNOSIS

DIFFERENTIAL DIAGNOSIS

- Chronic pelvic pain
- Overactive bladder
- Recurrent urinary tract infection
- Endometriosis
- Pelvic adhesions
- Vulvar vestibulitis
- Vulvodynia
- Urethral pain syndrome
- Chronic nonbacterial prostatitis
- Frequent vaginitis
- Benign prostatic hyperplasia

WORKUP

- Interstitial cystitis can be considered a diagnosis of exclusion when no known cause of painful bladder can be identified.
- There is no definite diagnostic test.
- Validated questionnaires such as Pelvic Pain and Urgency/Frequency scale (PUF), O'Leary-Sant symptoms and problem index, and Wisconsin IC scale. PUF is the most commonly used.
- Voiding diary shows low volume (<100 ml) and high-frequency voiding pattern.
- National Institute of Diabetes and Diseases of the Kidney diagnostic criteria misses 60% of IC patients and is not clinically used any more.
- Anesthetic bladder challenge: with this test the symptoms dissipate on instillation of an anesthetic cocktail into the bladder.
- Cystoscopy and hydrodistension under general anesthesia may show terminal hematuria, glomerulation, Hunner's ulcers, and small bladder capacity of less than 350 ml.
- Bladder biopsy is not essential for diagnosis of IC.
- Parson's potassium sensitivity test (PST).
- Urodynamics are unnecessary in diagnosis of IC.

LABORATORY TESTS

- Urine analysis and culture.
- Urine cytology should be performed if microscopic or gross hematuria is present, or with other risk factors such as smoking, age >40 yr, and other bladder cancer risk factors.
- Culture of sexually transmitted diseases if clinically indicated. Nonbacteriuric patients with pyuria should be screened for *Chlamydia.*
- Urine biomarkers (e.g., antiproliferative factor) are promising but not ready for clinical use.

IMAGING STUDIES

CT or ultrasound of abdomen and pelvis may be considered to rule out other pathology.

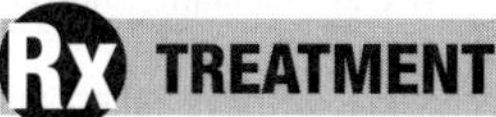

TREATMENT

- There is no consensus for optimal management.
- There is no cure for this disease.

NONPHARMACOLOGIC THERAPY

- Avoidance of activities associated with flare-ups
- Avoidance of smoking
- Dietary restriction
- Physical therapy
- Exercise
- Behavioral therapy
- Bladder retraining
- Biofeedback
- Warm sitz bath, ice, heating pad
- Thiele massage (transrectal and transvaginal manual therapy of pelvic floor muscle) in presence of pelvic floor muscle tenderness and spasm
- Hydrodistension only gives temporary relief, so it is not commonly used anymore

ACUTE AND CHRONIC Rx

- A course of empiric antibiotics if not tried yet.
- Oral therapy is tried first.
- Pentosan polysulfate sodium (Elmiron) is the only FDA approved and most effective oral therapy.
- Most treatment takes 3 to 6 mo before maximum benefit is seen.
- Adjunct oral therapy includes tricyclic antidepressants (amitriptyline), antihistaminics (hydroxyzine, montelukast), neuroleptics (gabapentin, topiramate), analgesics (NSAIDS, opioid analgesics), and occasionally antimuscarinics.
- Oral therapies can be used in combination.
- Antihistaminics are preferred for patients with an allergy history or those who show mast cells in bladder biopsy.
- Oral prednisone is used in presence of Hunner's ulcers.
- Other drugs rarely used for IC are cyclosporin A, interleukin-10, imatinib, methotrexate, suplatast, misoprostol, and quercetin.
- Growth factor inhibitors, gene therapy, RDP 58, and vitamin B_3 analogue (BXL 628) may represent future therapies.
- Intravesical treatment is used when oral medications fail, for acute flare-ups, or before the oral medications take full effect.
- Dimethyl sulfoxide (DMSO), heparin, lidocaine, hyaluronic acid, bacille Calmette-Guérin, capsaicin, resiniferatoxin, botulinum toxin A, chondroitin sulfate, steroids, and Elmiron are drugs used for intravesical treatment.

- DMSO is the only FDA-approved intravesical treatment.
- DMSO is used less often now because of its side effects, specifically a garlic-like odor or taste on breath or skin that lasts 72 hr after treatment.
- Intravesical therapy typically involves mixture of heparin or Elmiron with lidocaine and sodium bicarbonate.
- Silver nitrate and Clorpactin have fallen out of favor.

SURGERY

- Major surgical intervention is not the mainstay of treatment.
- Patients whose condition is extreme and who are miserable may consider surgery if medications fail.
- Sacral neuromodulation (InterStim) is the current preferred surgical intervention.
- Laser ablation, fulguration, or resection is offered when Hunner's ulcers are seen in cystoscopy.
- Augmentation cystoplasty is not recommended.
- Cystourethrectomy with urinary diversion is rarely done.

COMPLEMENTARY & ALTERNATIVE MEDICINE

- Transcutaneous electric nerve stimulation
- Intravaginal electric nerve stimulation
- Acupuncture
- Urinary chelating agents such as Polycitra-K crystals, Urocit-K
- Prelief, an over-the-counter food additive
- Herbal remedies such as Algnot Plus, Cysto-Protek, Cysta-Q, aloe vera

DISPOSITION

- Close follow-up every month for 3 mo and every 3 mo thereafter.
- Voiding diary and symptom questionnaire are helpful to monitor response to treatment.

REFERRAL

- Urologist
- Pain specialist
- Physical therapist

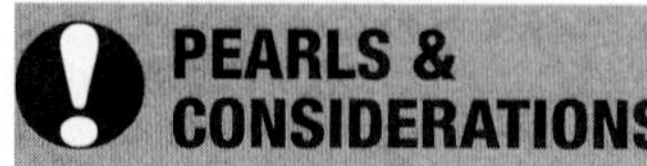

PEARLS & CONSIDERATIONS

COMMENTS

- On average these patients see five physicians and endure irritating voiding symptoms for 5 yr before the disease is identified.
- Besides symptom questionnaire and urine analysis, all other diagnostic tests are optional.
- PST is well tolerated.
- Negative cystoscopy does not rule out IC.

PREVENTION

Early identification and timely intervention improve patient outcome.

PATIENT & FAMILY EDUCATION

- IC support groups
- Interstitial Cystitis Association
- Interstitial Cystitis Network

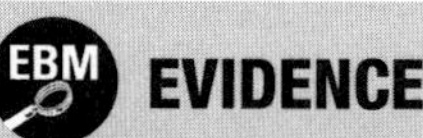

EVIDENCE

Please note: Complete text of EBM for this topic is available online.

Key trials and commentary:

This study sought to determine whether abuse is associated with interstitial cystitis by surveying patients with interstitial cystitis and controls. It corroborated this association in a clinic population.

This study demonstrates an association between interstitial cystitis and abuse. Thus, it is important for clinicians to assess for abuse in women with interstitial cystitis or pelvic pain and provide appropriate referral to psychologists or other health care workers to provide comprehensive care for managing their symptoms. Further research is needed to evaluate the role of biopsychosocial therapies, in addition to traditional interstitial cystitis medical therapies for women with a history of abuse and interstitial cystitis.[1] Ⓐ

There are many proposed etiologies for interstitial cystitis including inflammatory, neurogenic, epithelial, and infectious. These authors present a strong argument for an association of previous emotional, physical, or sexual abuse and a diagnosis of interstitial cystitis. Is this a cause-and-effect relationship? Regardless, it seems incumbent on the practitioner, who is aware of these data, to at least make queries among their patients with interstitial cystitis regarding a previous history of abuse, and, if reported, make the appropriate social, psychological, and medical referrals.

Evidence-Based Reference

1. Peters KM et al: Fact or fiction—is abuse prevalent in patients with interstitial cystitis? Results from a community survey and clinic population, *J Urol* 178:891-895, 2008. Commentary by E.S. Rovner, M.D. Ⓐ

SUGGESTED READINGS

Chronic pelvic pain in women, *J Reprod Med* 51(3), 2006.

Dimitrakon J et al: Pharmacologic management of painful bladder syndrome/interstitial cystitis, *Arch Intern Med* 167(18):1922-1929, 2007.

Interstitial cystitis as a disease: a new paradigm emerges, *J Reprod Med* 69(4):S1, 2007.

Myers DL: Interstitial cystitis, *Med Health R I* 92:22-26, 2009.

AUTHOR: **HEMANT K. SATPATHY, M.D.**

BASIC INFORMATION

DEFINITION

Diffuse interstitial lung disease (ILD) includes a large group of nonmalignant disorders, which are characterized by diffuse damage to the lung parenchyma via inflammation and fibrosis, and/or granulomatous reaction in interstitial or vascular areas.

SYNONYMS

Interstitial lung disease
ILD

ICD-9CM CODES

136.3 Acute interstitial lung disease
515 Chronic interstitial lung disease

EPIDEMIOLOGY & DEMOGRAPHICS

PREVALENCE: Varies with type of ILD. The most common type of ILD is idiopathic interstitial fibrosis, with a prevalence of 20 cases/100,000 people in the general population, increasing with age to 175 cases/100,000 people aged 75 yr or older.

PREDOMINANT SEX & AGE: Some ILDs are more common in women, such as those resulting from connective tissue disorders. One exception is rheumatoid arthritis, which is more common in men. Lymphangiomyomatosis occurs exclusively in postmenopausal women. ILD caused by occupational exposures are more common in men. Generally, ILD occurs in people >50 yr.

RISK FACTORS: History of tobacco abuse; environmental exposures such as to silicone, asbestos, or beryllium; reactions to drugs such as amiodarone, methotrexate, or bleomycin; history of connective tissue disease such as rheumatoid arthritis or systemic lupus erythematosus.

PHYSICAL FINDINGS & CLINICAL PRESENTATION

- Dyspnea
- Tachypnea
- Bibasilar end inspiratory dry crackles
- Pulmonary hypertension
- Cyanosis, clubbing

ETIOLOGY

- The hallmark of ILD is restriction caused by decreased lung compliance. The decreased compliance can be the result of a number of factors depending on the type of ILD. Different types of ILD are characterized by three distinct patterns in the alveolar walls:
  1. Inflammatory changes, which are early and potentially reversible
  2. Fibrotic changes
  3. Lung destruction
- Specific changes may be seen:
  - Granulomatous: accumulation of T lymphocytes, macrophages, and epithelioid cells into granulomas in lung parenchyma
  - Inflammation and fibrosis: injury to epithelium causes inflammation; if chronic, inflammation spreads to interstitium and vascular areas
  - Occupational exposure: pneumoconiosis, asbestosis, silicosis, organic dust
  - Drug induced
  - Connective tissue disorder: systemic lupus erythematosus, rheumatoid arthritis, dermatomyositis, interstitial pneumonitis

DIAGNOSIS

DIFFERENTIAL DIAGNOSIS

- Congestive heart failure
- Chronic renal failure

WORKUP

- Well-defined patterns in pulmonary function tests are usually consistent with restrictive defect (decreased FRC, RV, and TLC) owing to decreased lung compliance caused by alveolar wall thickening as a result of inflammation and fibrosis. Diffusing capacity is usually reduced also because of inflammation and thickening of alveolar walls, though nonspecific. FEV1/FVC is usually normal or increased because lung stiffness keeps small airways open, although some conditions (e.g., sarcoidosis) may reduce air flow.
- Bronchoscopy and BAL may help identify type of ILD. However, their role in defining stage of disease and response to therapy is controversial.
- Biopsy is the most effective method for confirming diagnosis and assessing disease activity.

LABORATORY TESTS

- ABGs may be normal or show respiratory alkalosis.
- Antinuclear antibodies, anti-immunoglobulin antibodies (rheumatoid factors), LDH.
- Serum precipitins confirm exposure if hypersensitivity pneumonitis is suspected.
- Antineutrophil cytoplasmic antibodies or anti-basement membrane antibodies if vasculitis is suspected.
- Elevation in angiotensin-converting enzyme level in sarcoidosis.
- ECG and echocardiogram will check for evidence of pulmonary hypertension.

IMAGING STUDIES

- A chest x-ray may be normal but commonly shows a bibasilar reticular pattern.
- A high-resolution CT is superior to chest x-ray; it is also useful for determining potential biopsy sights.

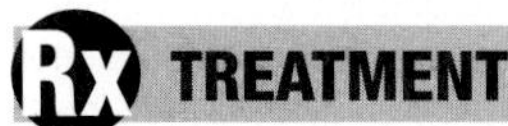

TREATMENT

NONPHARMACOLOGIC THERAPY

Avoidance of tobacco and occupational exposures

ACUTE GENERAL Rx

- Supplemental oxygen in patients with hypoxemia.
- Glucocorticoids are the mainstay of therapy, but success rate is low. Common starting dose is prednisone 0.5 to 1 mg/kg once daily for 4 to 12 wk. Patients should be reevaluated after this initial course of treatment. If they are stable, steroids may be tapered. If not, the same course may be maintained for another 4 to 12 wk. If patient's condition continues to decline, may consider adding second agent (cyclophosphamide, azathioprine).

REFERRAL

- Surgical referral for biopsy
- Pulmonary referral for bronchoscopy or BAL

SUGGESTED READINGS

Grippi MA: *Pulmonary science and medicine,* Philadelphia, 2001, J.B. Lippincott.

Kasper D A et al (eds): *Harrison's principles of internal medicine,* ed 16, 2005, McGraw-Hill Company.

Shah NR et al: A critical assessment of treatment options for idiopathic pulmonary fibrosis, *Sarcoidosis Vasc Diffuse Lung Dis* 22(3):167, 2005.

Swigris JJ et al: Health-related quality of life in patients with idiopathic pulmonary fibrosis: a systematic review, *Thorax* 60:588, 2005.

AUTHORS: **GRACE SHIH, M.D.,** and **CINDY GLEIT, M.D.**

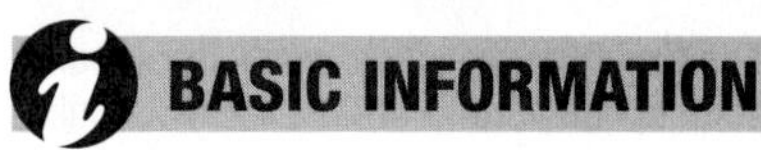

BASIC INFORMATION

DEFINITION

Interstitial nephritis falls into two broad categories: acute and chronic.

- Acute: defined as a decrease in renal function resulting from injury characterized histopathologically with edema and inflammation of the renal interstitium classically sparing the glomeruli and blood vessels. Most often induced by drugs.
- Chronic: represents a large and diverse group of disorders characterized by interstitial fibrosis with mononuclear leukocyte infiltration and tubular atrophy. It is a final common pathway of many chronic kidney diseases including chronic bacterial infections, obstruction, and high-grade vesicoureteral reflux. Histopathologically seen as atrophy and fibrosis of the renal interstitium.

SYNONYMS

Contracted kidney
Cirrhosis of the kidney
Granular kidney
Gouty kidney
Renal sclerosis
Chronic productive nephritis without exudation

ICD-9CM CODES

583 Nephritis and nephropathy not specified as acute or chronic
583.0 With proliferative glomerular nephritis
583.1 With membranous glomerular nephritis
583.2 With membranoproliferative glomerular nephritis
583.4 With rapidly progressive glomerular nephritis
583.9 With unspecified pathological lesions in the kidney

EPIDEMIOLOGY & DEMOGRAPHICS

PEAK INCIDENCE: Median age at presentation is 65 yr.
PREVALENCE: 2% to 3% of all renal biopsies; in cases of acute renal failure, the incidence of acute interstitial nephritis is 7% to 15%.
PREDOMINANT SEX AND AGE: Older patients generally at higher risk given reduced glomerular filtration rates.
RISK FACTORS: Use of drugs known to cause acute interstitial nephritis, increases with age and decreasing glomerular filtration rate, some autoimmune disorders are also risk factors

PHYSICAL FINDINGS & CLINICAL PRESENTATION

Nonspecific, but acutely can present with renal failure, oliguria, hematuria, malaise, mental status changes, rash, nausea, and vomiting. Chronically can be asymptomatic with elevations in BUN or creatinine or the appearance of abnormal urinary sediment.

ETIOLOGY

- Drug induced (71%): antibiotics (penicillins, cephalosporins sulfonamides), nonsteroidal anti-inflammatory drugs, diuretics, proton pump inhibitors, anticonvulsants
- Infection associated (15%):
  - Bacterial: *Corynebacterium diphtheriae,* legionella, staphylococci, streptococci, yersinia
  - Viral: cytomegalovirus, Epstein-Barr virus, hanta viruses, hepatitis C, herpes simplex virus, HIV, mumps, polyoma virus
  - Other: mycobacterium, mycoplasma, rickettsia, syphilis, toxoplasmosis
- Cases associated with immune (systemic lupus erythematosus, Sjögren's, and Wegener's) or neoplastic disorders (5%)

Dx DIAGNOSIS

DIFFERENTIAL DIAGNOSIS

Any other causes of acute renal failure including hypertensive nephrosclerosis, prerenal azotemia, obstructive nephropathy, interstitial nephritis, renal vascular disease, and various electrolyte abnormalities

WORKUP

Medical history with focus on recent infection illness or new medication in the presence of acute to chronic onset of kidney failure; evaluation for underlying infection or insult

LABORATORY TESTS

- Urinalysis, especially eosinophiluria, serum chemistry profile, CBC, liver function tests, 24-hour urine specimen collection, consider serum IgE levels.
- Renal biopsy indicated when diagnosis is unclear, removal of offending agent does not result in improvement, and there are no contraindications to the procedure.

IMAGING STUDIES

Ultrasound; consider Gallium 67 scanning to discriminate acute tubular necrosis (ATN) from acute interstitial nephritis (AIN)

Rx TREATMENT

NONPHARMACOLOGIC THERAPY

Largely supportive, removal of offending agent will resolve 60% of all cases.

ACUTE GENERAL Rx

- Correct fluid and electrolyte imbalances, maintain adequate hydration and urine output but avoid volume overload.
- Identify and treat infection as indicated.
- Remove offending drug, substitute as appropriate.
- Avoid medications that impair renal blood flow.
- If steroids are initiated, a reasonable choice is prednisone 1mg/kg/day for 2 to 3 wk. When using steroids for drug-induced acute interstitial nephrosis, it is best to start them immediately after the diagnosis is made.
- Consider treatment with cyclophosphamide (Cytoxan) if patients fail to respond to corticosteroids.

CHRONIC Rx

- Limit exposure to known nephrotoxic agents.
- Renally adjust medications as indicated by glomerular filtration rate.
- Tight control of blood pressure, diabetes, and cholesterol to preserve kidney function as needed.

DISPOSITION

With acute interstitial nephritis 40% of patients will improve in time.

REFERRAL

Refer to nephrology with question in diagnosis, multiple comorbidities, with failure to respond to supportive care or initial therapies, or with decision to evaluate for biopsy.

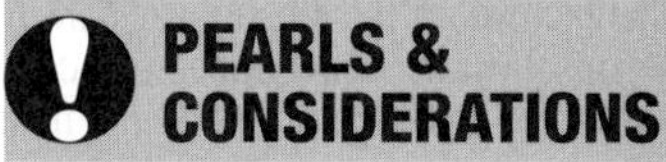

PEARLS & CONSIDERATIONS

COMMENTS

Once known mainly as a complication of streptococcal infection, today acute interstitial nephritis is most often caused by drugs; 88% of the time that drug has been started in the last 30 days. Significant fibrosis of the tubules seen in biopsy is the best predictor of transition to chronic interstitial nephritis. Corticosteroids cannot be recommended as empiric therapy because their efficacy has not been established but may be indicated in specific cases.

PREVENTION

Use known offending agents with care, especially in the elderly and those with known underlying kidney disease.

SUGGESTED READINGS

Clarkston MR et al: Acute interstitial nephritis: clinical features and response to cortical steroid therapy, *Nephol Dial Transplant* 19:2778-2283, 2004.

Gonzalez E et al: Early steroid treatment improves the recovery of renal function in patients with drug-induced acute interstitial nephritis, *Kidney Int* 73: 940, 2008.

Kodner K: Diagnosis and management of acute interstitial nephritis, *AAFP* 12:2527-2534, 2003.

Michael R et al: Acute interstitial nephritis: clinical features response to cortical steroid therapy, *Nephrol Dial Transplant* 19:2778-2783, 2004.

AUTHOR: **JOHN RAGSDALE, M.D.**

BASIC INFORMATION

DEFINITION

Irritable bowel syndrome (IBS) is a chronic functional disorder manifested by alteration in bowel habits and recurrent abdominal pain and bloating. IBS is a symptom complex influenced by a variety of physiologic determinants from gut to brain and back. The ROME III criteria for diagnosis of IBS are:

- Recurrent abdominal pain or discomfort at least 3 days per month in the past 3 mo associated with two or more of the following:
  - Pain is relieved or improved with defecation.
  - Its onset is associated with a change in the frequency of bowel movement.
  - Its onset is associated with a change in the form or appearance of the stool.
- The criteria must be fulfilled for at least the past 3 mo with symptom onset at least 6 mo before the diagnosis.

SYNONYMS

Irritable colon
Spastic colon
IBS

ICD-9CM CODES
564.1 Irritable bowel syndrome

EPIDEMIOLOGY & DEMOGRAPHICS

- IBS is the most common functional bowel disorder. An estimated 15 million people in the U.S. have IBS.
- IBS occurs in 20% of the population of industrialized countries and is responsible for >50% of gastrointestinal (GI) referrals. Worldwide adult prevalence is 12%. Incidence increases during adolescence and peaks in third and fourth decades of life.
- Female:male ratio is 2:1.
- Nearly 50% of patients have psychiatric abnormalities, with anxiety disorders being most common.

PHYSICAL FINDINGS & CLINICAL PRESENTATION

- The clinical presentation of IBS consists of abdominal pain and abnormalities of defecation, which may include loose stools, usually after meals and in the morning, alternating with episodes of constipation.
- Physical examination is generally normal.
- Nonspecific abdominal tenderness and distention may be present.

ETIOLOGY

- Unknown
- Associated pathophysiology includes altered GI motility, alteration in gut flora, and increased gut sensitivity
- Risk factors: anxiety, depression, personality disorders, history of childhood sexual abuse, and domestic abuse in women

DIAGNOSIS

DIFFERENTIAL DIAGNOSIS

- Inflammatory bowel disease (IBD)
- Diverticulitis
- Colon malignancy
- Endometriosis
- Peptic ulcer disease
- Biliary liver disease
- Chronic pancreatitis
- Constipation caused by medications (opiates, calcium channel blockers, anticholinergics)
- Diarrhea caused by medications (metformin, colchicine, proton pump inhibitors, antacids, antibiotics)
- Small-bowel overgrowth
- Celiac disease
- Parasites
- Lymphoma of GI tract

WORKUP

Diagnostic workup is aimed primarily at excluding the conditions listed in the differential diagnoses. It is important to identify red flags of other diseases, such as weight loss, rectal bleeding, onset in patients >50 yr, fever, nocturnal pain, and family history of malignancy or IBD. Additional red flags include abnormal examination (e.g., mass, enlarged lymph nodes, stool positive for occult blood, muscle wasting) and abnormal laboratory values (anemia, leukocytosis, abnormal chemistry).

Common clinical criteria for diagnosis of IBS are >3 mo of symptoms, including abdominal pain that is relieved by a bowel movement, or pain accompanied by a change in bowel pattern, and abnormality in bowel movement 25% of the time, characterized by two of the following features:

- Abdominal distention
- Abnormal consistency
- Abnormal defecation (e.g., straining, sense of incomplete evacuation)
- Abnormal frequency
- Mucus with bowel movement

LABORATORY TESTS

- Blood work is generally normal. CBC is reasonable to evaluate for anemia. The presence of anemia should alert to the possibility of a colonic malignancy or IBD.
- Testing of stool for ova and parasites should be considered only in patients with chronic diarrhea. Evaluation of stool for *Clostridium difficile* may be helpful in patients with predominant diarrhea symptoms who have recently taken antibiotics.

IMAGING STUDIES

Imaging studies (e.g., flat and upright abdominal radiograph, small-bowel series, sonogram or CT of abdomen and pelvis) are normal and not necessary for diagnosis.

Lower endoscopy is generally normal except for the presence of some spasms. Colonoscopic imaging should be performed only in persons who have alarm features to rule out organic disease and in persons older than 50 yr to screen for colorectal cancer.

TREATMENT

NONPHARMACOLOGIC THERAPY

- The patient should be encouraged to maintain an adequate fiber intake and to eliminate foods that aggravate symptoms. Avoidance of caffeine, dairy products, fatty foods, and dietary excesses is also helpful.
- Cognitive-behavioral therapy is also recommended, particularly in younger patients because psychosocial stressors are important triggers of IBS. Reassurance and education about trigger avoidance and stress management are important.
- Importance of regular exercise and adequate fluid intake should be stressed.

GENERAL Rx

- The mainstay of treatment of IBS is a high-fiber diet. Fiber is helpful for relief of constipation but not for relief of pain. Because symptoms are chronic, the use of laxatives should generally be avoided.
- Fiber supplementation with psyllium 1 tbsp bid or calcium polycarbophil (FiberCon) 2 tablets one to four times daily followed by 8 oz of water may be necessary in some patients.
- Patients should be instructed that there might be some increased bloating on initiation of fiber supplementation, which should resolve within 2 to 3 wk. It is important that patients take these fiber products on a regular basis and not only as needed. Fiber is not effective in patients with diarrhea-predominant IBS and may worsen symptoms in these patients.
- Patients who appear anxious can benefit from use of sedatives or selective serotonin reuptake inhibitors (SSRIs). Tricyclic antidepressants in low doses are also effective in some patients with IBS.
- Loperamide is effective for diarrhea. Alosetron, a serotonin type-3 receptor antagonist previously withdrawn because of severe constipation and ischemic colitis, has been reintroduced with limited availability. It is indicated only for women with severe chronic diarrhea-predominant IBS unresponsive to conventional therapy and not caused by anatomic or metabolic abnormality. Starting dose is 1 mg qd.
- C-2 chloride channel activators: Lubiprostone (Amitiza) is a chloride channel activator that stimulates chloride-rich intestinal fluid secretion and accelerates small intestine and colonic transmit time. It may be effective in chronic constipation-predominant IBS unresponsive to conventional treatment. Usual dose is 24 μg qd to bid with food. Side effects include headache and nausea.
- Alterations in gut flora have been identified as potentially contributing to IBS (84% of IBS patients have an abnormal lactulose breath test, suggesting small-intestinal bacterial overgrowth). Rifaximin, a gut-selective antibiotic, has been used in recent trials to eradicate bacterial overgrowth (70% eradication rate). A dose of 400 mg tid for 10 days was reported effective in improving IBS symptoms up to 10 wk after discontinuation of therapy.

Until additional evidence is available, use of rifaximin or other antibiotics in IBS should be reserved for patients with proven bacterial overgrowth.

- Antispasmodics-anticholinergics (e.g., dicyclomine, hyoscyamine) are often used, but efficacy data from clinical trials are inconclusive.
- Probiotics: *Lactobacilli* do not appear to be effective for the treatment of IBS. *Bifidobacteria* and some combinations of probiotics have shown some limited efficacy.
- Antidepressants: SSRIs are more effective than placebo for relief of global IBS symptoms.

DISPOSITION

More than 60% of patients respond successfully to treatment over the initial 12 mo; however, IBS is a chronic, relapsing condition and requires prolonged therapy.

REFERRAL

GI referral is recommended in patients with rectal bleeding, fever, nocturnal diarrhea, anemia, weight loss, or onset of symptoms >40 yr. Consultation is also necessary if specialized diagnostic procedures such as endoscopy are necessary.

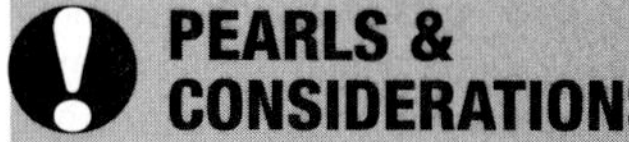

PEARLS & CONSIDERATIONS

COMMENTS

- Patients should be educated regarding maintenance of a high-fiber diet and elimination of stressors, which can precipitate attacks of IBS. They should be reassured that their condition does not lead to cancer.
- Recent drug efforts (alosetron, tegaserod) are aimed at serotonergic receptors in the gut because most of the serotonin in the body is found in the GI tract and is believed to be involved in the mediation of visceral sensation and motility.
- Cognitive-behavioral therapy is effective in the treatment of patients with IBS and should be considered as part of the armamentarium against this disorder.

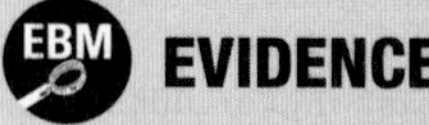

EVIDENCE

Please note: Complete text of EBM for this topic is available online.

Key trials and commentary:

Although multiple clinical trials support the efficacy of psychological treatments for reducing irritable bowel syndrome (IBS) symptoms, the mechanisms responsible for symptomatic improvement are unknown. One hypothesis is that psychological treatments work by alleviating comorbid psychological distress implicated in the worsening of bowel symptoms and quality of life. An alternative hypothesis assumes that changes in distress are not strictly a cause but a consequence of IBS that will decrease with symptomatic improvement.

This study showed that CBT has a direct effect on global IBS symptom improvement independent of its effects on distress. Improvement in IBS symptoms is associated with improvements in the QOL, which may lower distress. Symptom improvements are not moderated by variables reflecting the mental well-being of IBS patients.

This study addresses the role of cognitive dysfunction in the generation of symptoms in IBS. Lackner et al ask the interesting question if the psychological factors that might identify patients who sustain a proven infection with *Campylobacter* are more likely to have prolonged (>6 months) symptoms characteristic of, what we now term, a postinfectious IBS? Their study shows that those who have prolonged symptoms are more likely to be women and have several abnormal psychological variables, including higher levels of stress, anxiety, somatization, perceived stress, and negative illness beliefs. It thus suggests that cognitive-behavioral therapy may be of value in these patients, which has previously been shown to be effective. However, Spence et al give somewhat confusing results. Although we tend to assume that this type of therapy works through identified psychological mechanisms, this study suggests that symptom improvement occurs independent of distress factors and perhaps works through better patient management of GI-specific symptoms. This needs to be sorted out a bit better, but at least these two studies lend further support to psychological cofactors in the occurrence of postinfectious IBS and that cognitive therapy given to these patients might be helpful.[1] Ⓐ

The aim of another study was to determine whether lower visceral pain thresholds in IBS primarily reflect physiological or psychological factors.

This study showed that increased colonic sensitivity in IBS is strongly influenced by a psychological tendency to report pain and urge rather than increased neurosensory sensitivity.

As complicated as the pathophysiology of IBS becomes, one still cannot ignore the psychological factors. This is an excellent study and one worth reading for several reasons. First, it elegantly outlines the "science" of how altered sensory input is differentiated from psychologic alteration of pain perception and reporting through simple physiologic testing and questionnaires. Second, through these methods it nicely demonstrates that those patients who, in general, are more likely to report pain from other forms of stimulation are more likely to report visceral pain from gut stimulation. Third, it reinforces the fact that there are multiple etiologies of pain generation in IBS, all of which are valid but none of which will exclusively explain symptoms in all patients.[2] Ⓐ

One study sought to investigate whether placebo effects can experimentally be separated into the response to three components—assessment and observation, a therapeutic ritual (placebo treatment), and a supportive patient-practitioner relationship—and then progressively combined to produce incremental clinical improvement in patients with IBS. To assess the relative magnitude of these components.

This study showed that factors contributing to the placebo effect can be progressively combined in a manner resembling a graded dose escalation of component parts. Nonspecific effects can produce statistically and clinically significant outcomes and the patient-practitioner relationship is the most robust component.

Maximizing the therapeutic encounter in patients with IBS and other chronic GI is relevant for the clinical practitioner, because this may help to obtain the best outcomes. The data from this novel, randomized controlled trial suggest that the placebo response can be augmented by very simple office techniques. The augmented interaction that was tested comprised asking questions about symptom relationships and lifestyle, assessing nongastrointestinal complaints, probing how the patient understood the causes and meaning of his or her condition, being warm and friendly in manner, listening actively, being empathetic, and communicating a positive expectation and confidence in the outcome. Exactly which of these components has the most effect remains unclear, but presumably a combination of them is required to obtain the best outcome. The patient-physician relationship has been known for a long time to be the centerpiece of the clinical encounter. This randomized trial confirms this belief in a scientific and robust fashion.[3] Ⓐ

Evidence-Based References

1. Lackner JM et al: How does cognitive behavior therapy for irritable bowel syndrome work? A mediational analysis of a randomized clinical trial, *Gastroenterology* 133:433-444, 2007. Commentary by D.A. Katzka, M.D. Ⓐ

2. Dorn SD et al: Increased colonic pain sensitivity in irritable bowel syndrome is the result of an increased tendency to report pain rather than increased neurosensory sensitivity, *Gut* 56:1202-1209, 2007. Commentary by D.A. Katzka, M.D. Ⓐ

3. Kaptchuk TJ et al: Components of placebo effect: randomised controlled trial in patients with irritable bowel syndrome, *BMJ* 336:999-1003, 2008. Commentary by N. Talley, M.D. Ⓐ

SUGGESTED READINGS

Drossman DA: The functional gastrointestinal disorders and the Rome III process, *Gastroenterology* 130:1377-1390, 2006.

Ford AC et al: Will the history and physical examination help establish that irritable bowel syndrome is causing this patient's lower gastrointestinal tract symptoms? *JAMA* 300:1793-1805, 2008.

Mayer EA: Irritable bowel syndrome, *N Engl J Med* 358:1692-1699, 2008.

Mertz HR: Irritable bowel syndrome, *N Engl J Med* 349: 22, 2003.

Pimentel M et al: The effect of a nonabsorbed oral antibiotic (Rifaximin) on the symptoms of the irritable bowel syndrome, *Ann Intern Med* 145:557-563, 2006.

AUTHOR: **FRED F. FERRI, M.D.**

BASIC INFORMATION

DEFINITION

Jaundice is a yellowish discoloration of the sclera, skin, and mucous membranes caused by an excessive amount of bilirubin in the bloodstream. Clinically detectable jaundice in adults is a serum bilirubin of 2.5 to 3 mg/dl.

SYNONYMS

Icterus

ICD-9CM CODES
782.4 Jaundice
283.9 Hemolytic jaundice
576.8 Obstructive jaundice

EPIDEMIOLOGY & DEMOGRAPHICS

The major causes of jaundice by age and sex:
- Young adults: viral hepatitis
- Women over 30: choledocholithiasis
- Middle adulthood (both sexes): drug induced and cirrhosis
- Middle-aged and older men: alcoholic liver disease, pancreatic cancer, hepatoma, primary hemochromatosis
- Women: primary biliary cirrhosis, chronic active hepatitis, choledocholithiasis, carcinoma of the gallbladder

CLINICAL PRESENTATION

Presentation can vary from asymptomatic to acute and life threatening. History and physical examination give important clues to the underlying condition.
Key history:
- Duration of jaundice
- Previous episodes
- Pain
- Color of urine and stool
- Systemic symptoms (fever, chills)
- Alcohol use
- Medications, herbal products
- Injection of illicit drugs
- Blood transfusions
- Hepatitis exposure (e.g., other jaundiced people)
- Shellfish ingestion
- Travel
- Occupation/Exposure to toxins
- Anorexia/weight loss
- Prior abdominal/biliary surgery

Key physical: vital signs
- Fever, signs of chronic liver disease (palmar erythema, spider angiomas, bruising, gynecomastia, testicular atrophy), size of liver, abdominal tenderness (and location), abdominal mass, splenomegaly, ascites, edema, weight loss, Kayser-Fleischer rings (Wilson's disease)

ETIOLOGY

Disruption in any of the three phases of bilirubin metabolism can lead to jaundice:
- Prehepatic phase: bilirubin is produced from the metabolism of heme—80% from red blood cell catabolism, 20% from ineffective erythropoiesis and breakdown of muscle myoglobin and cytochromes—and transported to the liver for conjugation and excretion.
- Intrahepatic phase: unconjugated (indirect) bilirubin, which is fat soluble but water insoluble, is conjugated within the hepatocyte to the water-soluble, conjugated (direct) bilirubin.
- Posthepatic phase: conjugated bilirubin dissolves in the bile and travels through the biliary system to the gallbladder, where it is stored, or passes into the duodenum through the ampulla of Vater. Some bilirubin is excreted in the stool and the rest is converted to urobilinogens by the gut flora and reabsorbed. Most of the urobilinogen is excreted by the kidney. A small amount is reabsorbed by the gut and re-excreted into the bile.

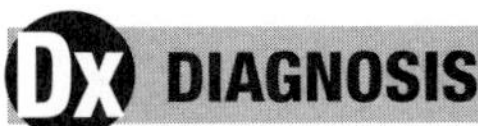

DIAGNOSIS

DIFFERENTIAL DIAGNOSIS

Prehepatic causes:
- Unconjugated hyperbilirubinemia: excessive heme metabolism from hemolysis (e.g., sickle cell disease, spherocytosis, G6PD, immune hemolysis), ineffective erythropoiesis (e.g., thalassemia, folate, severe iron deficiency), or large hematoma reabsorption.

Intrahepatic causes:
- Unconjugated hyperbilirubinemia: disorders of enzyme metabolism such as Gilbert's disease (common, benign), Crigler-Najjar syndrome (rare, severe), or drugs such as rifampin and probenecid
- Conjugated hyperbilirubinemia: intrahepatic cholestasis
  1. Viruses: hepatitis A, B, and C; Epstein-Barr
  2. Alcohol: alcoholic hepatitis, alcoholic cirrhosis
  3. Autoimmune: primary biliary cirrhosis, primary sclerosing cholangitis
  4. Drug induced: acetaminophen, penicillins, oral contraceptives, chlorpromazine (Thorazine), steroids (estrogenic or anabolic), some herbals
  5. Hereditary metabolic: hemochromatosis, Wilson's disease, Dubin-Johnson and Rotor's syndromes, alpha-antitrypsin deficiency
  6. Systemic disease: sarcoidosis, amyloidosis, glycogen storage diseases, celiac disease, tuberculosis, *Mycobacterium avium intracellulare*
  7. Other: sepsis, total parenteral nutrition, pregnancy, graft-versus-host disease, environmental toxins

Posthepatic causes:
- Conjugated hyperbilirubinemia: intrinsic or extrinsic obstruction of the biliary system
  1. Intrinsic blockage: gallstones, cholangitis, strictures, infection (e.g., cytomegalovirus, cryptosporidium in AIDS patients, parasites, cholangiocarcinoma, gallbladder cancer)
  2. Extrinsic blockage: pancreatitis, pancreatic carcinoma, pancreatic pseudocyst
- Pseudojaundice: caused by an excessive ingestion of foods containing beta-carotene (carrots, melons, squash); does *not* result in hyperbilirubinemia or scleral icterus

WORKUP

History and physical examination as above are key to diagnosis.

LABORATORY TESTS

First-line tests:
- Serum total and direct bilirubin
- Urinalysis
- If first-line tests are normal, consider pseudojaundice

If urine is positive for bilirubin and serum has elevated total and direct bilirubin (conjugated hyperbilirubinemia):
- Initial evaluation: liver function tests (AST, ALT, GGTP, alk phos), CBC, liver synthetic function (albumin, PT, PTT), pancreatic function (amylase, lipase).
- Additional tests if diagnosis unclear:
  1. Screen for hepatitis A, B, and C; if still unclear then consider options 2 to 6 below
  2. Other viruses (Epstein-Barr virus, cytomegalovirus)
  3. Autoimmune disorders: antimitochondrial antibody, immunoglobulin (Ig) M (elevated in primary biliary cirrhosis); smooth muscle antibody, antinuclear antibody, IgG (autoimmune chronic active hepatitis); antinuclear cytoplasmic antibody (primary sclerosing cholangitis)
  4. Ceruloplasmin (Wilson's disease)
  5. Alpha-1 antitrypsin deficiency (cirrhosis and emphysema)
  6. Ferritin, Fe saturation (elevated in hemochromatosis)

If urine is negative for bilirubin, increased t. bili and normal d. bili (unconjugated hyperbilirubinemia):
- Hemolysis? (complete blood count, smear for abnormal red blood cell types)
- Genetic syndrome? (e.g., Gilbert's)
- Hematoma?

Liver biopsy: essential in diagnosis of chronic hepatitis. Can be used for diagnosis of liver masses but carries a substantial risk.

IMAGING STUDIES

- Abdominal ultrasound: first-line study. Most sensitive for biliary tract stones and extrahepatic biliary obstruction.
- Abdominal CT: more information on liver, pancreas, and biliary system.
- Endoscopic retrograde cholangiopancreatography: best for lower duct obstruction.
- Percutaneous transhepatic cholangiography: best for hilar obstructions.
- Magnetic resonance cholangiopancreatography: noninvasive visualization of bile and pancreatic ducts; becoming more available.

 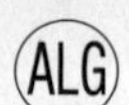

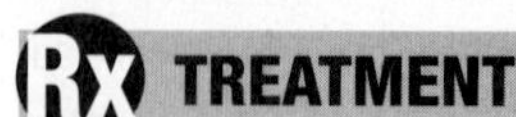

TREATMENT

NONPHARMACOLOGIC THERAPY

Depends on underlying cause of the jaundice, rapidity of onset, and clinical stability of the patient. Generally, obstructive causes require surgical treatment and nonobstructive causes require medical treatment.

ACUTE GENERAL Rx

Acute, life-threatening illness such as acute cholecystitis or ascending cholangitis requires prompt diagnosis and emergent surgical or endoscopic intervention in conjunction with medical management.

CHRONIC Rx

Chronic causes may require such treatment as stopping certain medications; stopping alcohol; antihistamines for pruritus; cholestyramine to bind bilirubin and decrease pruritus; interferon for hepatitis B or C; penicillamine for Wilson's disease; phlebotomy for hemochromatosis; surgical resection for liver for pancreatic cancer; liver transplant for eligible patients with end-stage cirrhosis; and N-acetylcysteine for acetaminophen overdose.

PEARLS & CONSIDERATIONS

COMMENTS

- The key to the management of the jaundiced adult is accurate diagnosis of the underlying cause.
- Prompt diagnosis and treatment of life-threatening illness is essential.
- Careful history and physical examination followed by selective laboratory and imaging studies will lead to accurate diagnosis.
- Collaboration with surgical and gastroenterology colleagues is helpful in complex patient care scenarios.

SUGGESTED READINGS

Beckingham IJ, Ryder SD: ABC of diseases of the liver, pancreas and biliary system: investigation of liver and biliary disease, *BMJ* 322:33-36, 2001.

Braunwald et al (eds): *Harrison's principles of internal medicine,* ed 15, New York, 2001, McGraw-Hill.

Roche SP, Kobos R: Jaundice in the adult patient, *Am Fam Physician* 69:299-304, 2004.

Ryder SD, Beckingham IJ: ABC of diseases of the liver, pancreas and biliary system: other causes of parenchymal liver disease, *BMJ* 322:290-292, 2001.

AUTHOR: **GOWRI ANANDARAJAH, M.D.**

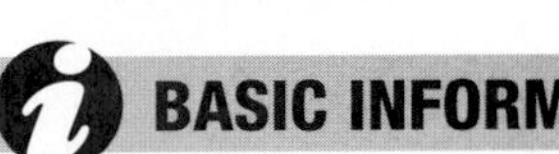

BASIC INFORMATION

DEFINITION

Juvenile rheumatoid (idiopathic) arthritis is arthritis beginning before the age of 16 yr.

SYNONYMS

Still's disease
Juvenile chronic arthritis
Juvenile polyarthritis

ICD-9CM CODES

714.3 Juvenile chronic polyarthritis

EPIDEMIOLOGY & DEMOGRAPHICS

PREVALENCE (IN U.S.): 250,000 to 300,000 cases
PREDOMINANT SEX: Female/male ratio of 2:1
PREDOMINANT AGE: Two peak incidences: between ages of 1 and 3 yr and ages 8 and 12 yr.

PHYSICAL FINDINGS & CLINICAL PRESENTATION

Usually one of three types:

1. Systemic or acute febrile juvenile rheumatoid arthritis (20% of cases):
   - Characterized by extraarticular manifestations, especially spiking fevers and a typical rash that frequently appears in the evening and may be elicited by gently scratching the skin in susceptible areas (Koebner's phenomenon)
   - Possible splenomegaly, generalized lymphadenopathy, pericarditis, and myocarditis
   - Minimal articular findings often overshadowed by systemic symptoms
2. Pauciarticular or oligoarticular form (50% of cases):
   - Involves fewer than five joints
   - Usually involves the larger joints, such as the knees, elbows, and ankles
   - Systemic features often minimal, and only one to three joints usually involved
   - Rarely causes impairment but chronic iridocyclitis develops in approximately 30% of cases with this form, and permanent loss of vision will develop in a high percentage of these patients (Fig. 1-170)
   - Accelerated growth of the affected limb from chronic hyperemia, possibly resulting in a temporary leg-length discrepancy that is eventually equalized in most cases on control of the inflammation
3. Polyarticular juvenile rheumatoid arthritis (30% of cases):
   - Involves five or more joints
   - Resembles adult disease in its symmetric involvement of the small joints of the hands and feet (Fig. 1-171)
   - Cervical spine involvement common and may produce marked loss of motion
   - Early closure of the ossification centers of the mandible, often producing a markedly receding chin, a characteristic of this form
   - Systemic manifestations similar to the febrile variety but not as dramatic

ETIOLOGY

Unknown. There is increasing evidence that the inflammation and destruction of bone and cartilage that occur in many rheumatic diseases are the result of the activation, by some unknown mechanism, of proinflammatory cells that infiltrate the synovium. These cells, in turn, release various substances, such as cytokines and tumor necrosis factor-α, which subsequently cause the pathologic changes typical of this group of diseases. Many of the newer therapeutic agents are directed at the suppression of these final mediators of inflammation.

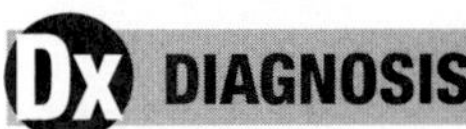

DIAGNOSIS

DIFFERENTIAL DIAGNOSIS

- Infectious causes of fever
- Systemic lupus erythematosus
- Rheumatic fever
- Drug reaction
- Serum sickness
- "Viral arthritis"
- Lyme arthritis

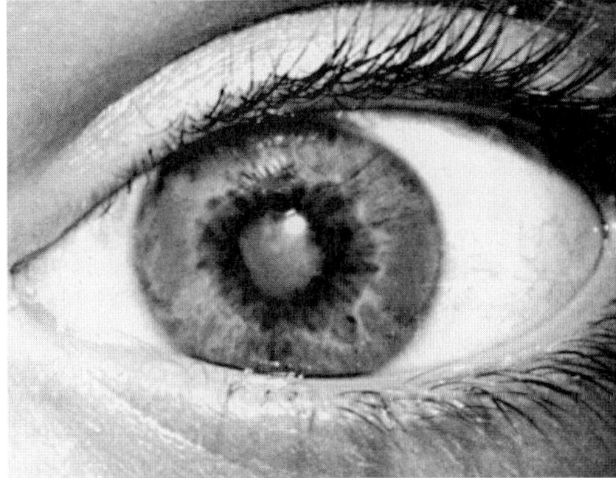

FIGURE 1-170 Chronic iridocyclitis of juvenile rheumatoid arthritis. Extensive posterior synechiae have resulted in a small, irregular pupil. There is a well-developed cataract and early band keratopathy at the medial and lateral margins of the cornea. (From Behrman RE [ed]: *Nelson textbook of pediatrics,* ed 17, Philadelphia, 2004, WB Saunders.)

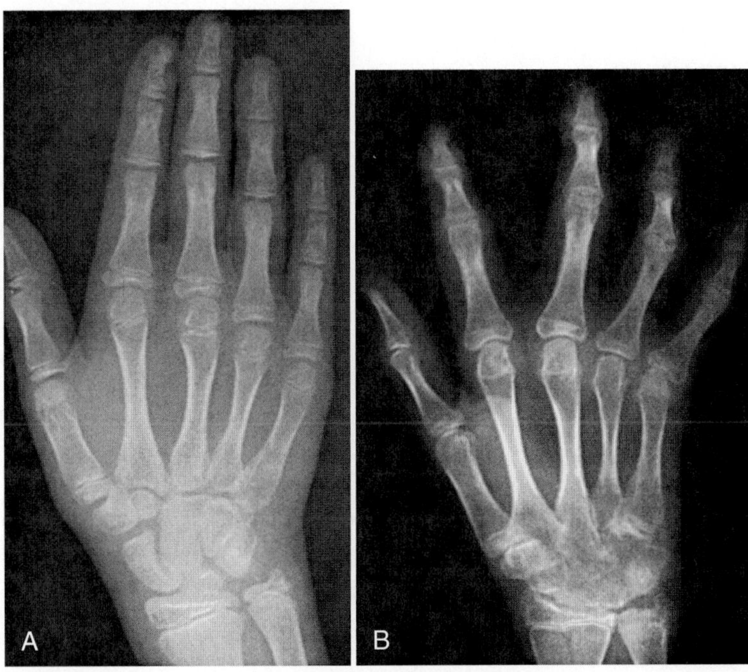

FIGURE 1-171 Progression of joint destruction in a girl with rheumatoid factor–positive juvenile rheumatoid arthritis despite doses of corticosteroids sufficient to suppress symptoms in the interval between **A** and **B.** **A,** Roentgenogram of the hand at onset. **B,** Roentgenogram 4 years later, showing a loss of articular cartilage and destruction changes in the distal and proximal interphalangeal and metacarpophalangeal joints and destruction and fusion of wrist bones. (From Behrman RE [ed]: *Nelson textbook of pediatrics,* ed 17, Philadelphia, 2004, WB Saunders.)

WORKUP

Initial laboratory and imaging studies are often nonspecific in children with rheumatoid arthritis.

LABORATORY TESTS

- Increased erythrocyte sedimentation rate
- Low-grade anemia
- Very high peripheral white blood cell count
- Rheumatoid factor: rarely demonstrable in the serum of children
- Antinuclear antibodies: often found in children with ocular complications

IMAGING STUDIES

- Roentgenographic findings are similar to those in adult, with soft tissue swelling and osteoporosis early in the disease.
- Joint destruction is less frequent.
- Bony erosion and cyst formation may be present as a result of synovial hypertrophy.

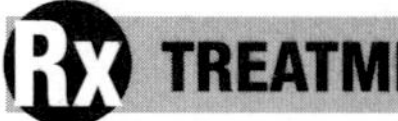

TREATMENT

NONPHARMACOLOGIC THERAPY

Proper management requires close cooperation among primary physician, therapist, rheumatologist, and orthopedist.

- Rest
- Physical and occupational therapy
- Patient and family education
- Proper diet and weight maintenance

ACUTE GENERAL Rx

- NSAIDs
- DMARDs and biologic response modifiers (BMRs)
- Intraarticular steroids
- Systemic corticosteroids

DISPOSITION

- Complete remission occurs in the majority of patients and may occur at any age.
- 70% to 85% of children regain normal function.
- Mortality rate is 2%.
- Children with a protracted systemic phase of the disease are most at risk for developing serious intercurrent infection and potentially fatal amyloidosis.
- Myocarditis may develop in the systemic form.
- Blindness is the most serious complication of the pauciarticular form; joint deformity is the most serious problem of polyarticular disease.

REFERRAL

- Early rheumatology consultation
- Ophthalmology consultation when ocular involvement is suspected (frequent eye examinations, especially in oligoarticular form)
- Orthopedic consultation for corrective surgery

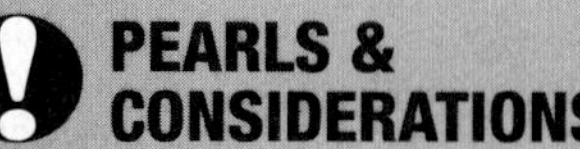

PEARLS & CONSIDERATIONS

COMMENTS

Patient information on juvenile idiopathic arthritis can be obtained from the National Arthritis Foundation, 1330 West Peachtree Street, Atlanta, GA 30309; 800-283-7800.

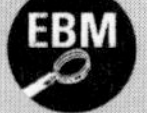

EVIDENCE

Please note: Complete text of EBM for this topic is available online.

Key trials and commentary:

Systemic-onset juvenile idiopathic arthritis (SOJIA) does not always respond to available treatments, including antitumor necrosis factor agents. This study investigated the efficacy and safety of tocilizumab, an anti-interleukin-6-receptor monoclonal antibody, in children with this disorder.[1] Ⓐ

This study showed that trocilizumab is effective in children with SOJIA. It might therefore be a suitable treatment in the control of this disorder, which has so far been difficult to manage.

SOJIA (very similar to adult-onset Still's disease) causes functional disability and growth abnormalities in up to 50% of the affected children. Furthermore, despite significant improvement with TNF inhibition, patients still have had disease progression and develop the potentially fatal macrophage activation syndrome. As a result, the authors performed a multicenter three-phase, randomized, placebo controlled, double-blind trial to evaluate the efficacy and safety of the anti–interleukin-6 (IL-6) antibody tocilizumab.

Evidence-Based Reference

1. Yokota S et al: Efficacy and safety of tocilizumab in patients with systemic-onset juvenile idiopathic arthritis: a randomised, double-blind, placebo-controlled, withdrawal phase III trial, *Lancet* 371:998-1006, 2008. Commentary by S.M. Berney, M.D. Ⓐ

SUGGESTED READINGS

Dhillon S et al: Etanercept: a review of its use in the management of rheumatoid arthritis, *Drugs* 67(8): 1211, 2007.

Edwards JC et al: Efficacy of β-cell-targeted therapy with rituximab in patients with rheumatoid arthritis, *N Engl J Med* 350:2572, 2004.

Feldman DE et al: Effects of adherence to treatment on short-term outcomes in children with juvenile idiopathic arthritis, *Arthritis Rheum* 57(6):905, 2007.

Glueck D, Gellman H: Management of the upper extremity in juvenile rheumatoid arthritis, *J Am Acad Orthop Surg* 13:254, 2005.

Hampton T: Trials reveal promising options for treating juvenile rheumatoid arthritis, *JAMA* 299:27, 2008.

Hashkes PJ et al: Mortality outcomes in pediatric rheumatology in the U.S., *Arthritis Rheum* 62:599, 2010.

Iesaka K et al: Orthopedic surgical management of hip and knee involvement in patients with juvenile rheumatoid arthritis, *Am J Orthop* 35:67, 2006.

Ilowite NT: Update on biologics in juvenile idiopathic arthritis, *Curr Opin Rheumatol* 20:613, 2008.

Long AR, Rouster-Stevens KA: The role of exercise therapy in the management of juvenile idiopathic arthritis, *Curr Opin Rheumatol* 22:213, 2010.

Lovell DJ et al: Adalimumab with or without methotrexate in juvenile rheumatoid arthritis, *N Engl J Med* 359:810-820, 2008.

Olsen NJ, Stein CM: New drugs for rheumatoid arthritis, *N Engl J Med* 350:2167, 2004.

Passo MH, Taylor J: Quality improvement in pediatric rheumatology: what do we need to do? *Curr Opin Rheumatol* 20:625, 2008.

Ravelli A, Martini A: Juvenile idiopathic arthritis, *Lancet* 369:767, 2007.

Reiff AO: Developments in the treatment of juvenile arthritis, *Expert Opin Pharmacother* 5:1485, 2004.

Silverman E et al: Leflunomide of methotrexate for juvenile rheumatoid arthritis, *N Engl J Med* 352: 1655, 2005.

Stinson JN et al: Asking the experts: exploring the self-management needs of adolescents with arthritis, *Arthritis Rheum* 59:65, 2008.

Thomas SL et al: How accurate are diagnoses for rheumatoid arthritis and juvenile idiopathic arthritis in the general practice research database? *Arthritis Rheum* 59:1314, 2008.

AUTHOR: **LONNIE R. MERCIER, M.D.**

BASIC INFORMATION

DEFINITION

Kaposi's sarcoma (KS) is a vascular neoplasm most frequently occurring in AIDS patients. It can be divided into the following four subsets:

1. Classic Kaposi's sarcoma: most frequently found in elderly Eastern European and Mediterranean males. It consists initially of violaceous macules and papules with subsequent development of plaques and red-purple nodules. Growth is slow, and most of the patients die of unrelated causes.
2. Epidemic or AIDS-related Kaposi's sarcoma: most frequently occurs in homosexual men. Lesions are generally multifocal and widespread. Lymphadenopathy may be associated.
3. Endemic Kaposi's sarcoma: usually affects African children and adults. An aggressive lymphadenopathic form affects African children in particular.
4. Immunosuppression-associated, or transplantation-associated, Kaposi's sarcoma: usually associated with chemotherapy.

SYNONYMS

KS

ICD-9CM CODES
173.9 Malignant neoplasm of the skin

EPIDEMIOLOGY & DEMOGRAPHICS

- AIDS-related KS affects >35% of AIDS cases.
- Highest incidence is in homosexual men.

PHYSICAL FINDINGS & CLINICAL PRESENTATION

- AIDS-related KS: multifocal and widespread red-purple or dark plaques and/or nodules on cutaneous or mucosal surfaces (Fig. 1-172).
- Generalized lymphadenopathy at the time of diagnosis is present in >50% of patients with AIDS-related KS; the initial lesions have a rust-colored appearance; subsequent progression to red or purple nodules or plaques occurs.
- Most frequently affected areas are the face, trunk, oral cavity, and upper and lower extremities.

ETIOLOGY

A herpesvirus (HHV-8, Kaposi's sarcoma–associated herpesvirus KSHV) has been isolated from patients with most forms of KS and is believed to be the causative agent. It can be transmitted sexually (homosexual or heterosexual activities) and by other forms of nonsexual contact such as maternal-infant transmission (common in African countries).

Dx DIAGNOSIS

DIFFERENTIAL DIAGNOSIS

- Stasis dermatitis
- Pyogenic granuloma
- Capillary hemangiomas
- Granulation tissue
- Postinflammatory hyperpigmentation
- Cutaneous lymphoma
- Melanoma
- Dermatofibroma
- Hematoma
- Prurigo nodularis

The differential diagnosis of cutaneous lesions in patients with HIV infection is described in Section III.

WORKUP

Diagnosis can generally be made on clinical appearance; tissue biopsy will confirm diagnosis.

LABORATORY TESTS

HIV in patients suspected of AIDS

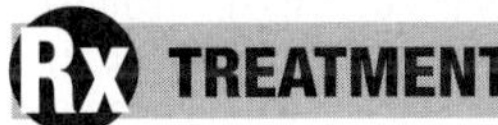

Rx TREATMENT

NONPHARMACOLOGIC THERAPY

Observation is a reasonable option in patients with slowly progressive disease.

GENERAL Rx

- Excisional biopsy often provides adequate treatment for single lesions and resected recurrences in classic Kaposi's sarcoma.
- Liquid nitrogen cryotherapy can result in complete response in 80% of lesions.
- Interlesional chemotherapy with vinblastine is useful for nodular lesions >1 cm in diameter. Intralesional injection of interferon alfa-2b has also been reported as effective and well tolerated.
- Radiation therapy is effective in non-AIDS KS and for large tumor masses that interfere with normal function.
- Systemic therapy with interferon is also effective in AIDS-related KS and is often used in combination with zidovudine.
- Systemic chemotherapy (vinblastine, bleomycin, doxorubicin, and dacarbazine) can be used for rapidly progressive disease and for classic and African endemic KS.
- Sirolimus (rapamycin), an immunosuppressive drug, is effective in inhibiting the progression of dermal Kaposi's sarcoma in kidney transplant recipients.
- Oral etoposide is also effective and has less myelosuppression than vinblastine.
- Paclitaxel is also effective in patients with advanced KS and represents an excellent second-line therapy.
- Thalidomide, retinoids

DISPOSITION

- Prognosis is poor in AIDS-related KS. Death is often a result of other AIDS-defining illnesses.
- Prognosis is better in African cutaneous KS and classic sarcoma (patients usually die of unrelated causes).

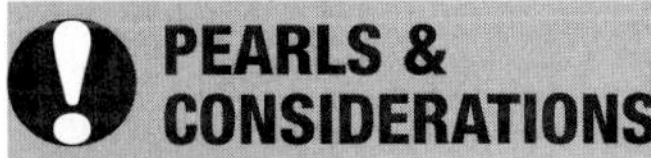

PEARLS & CONSIDERATIONS

COMMENTS

Immunosuppression-associated KS usually regresses with the cessation, reduction, or modification of immunosuppression therapy in most patients. Similarly, in HIV patients KS responds concurrently with the decrease in serum HIV RNA and increase in the CD4 count.

SUGGESTED READING

Stallone et al: Sirolimus for Kaposi's sarcoma in renal-transplant recipients, *N Engl J Med* 352:1317, 2005.

AUTHOR: **FRED F. FERRI, M.D.**

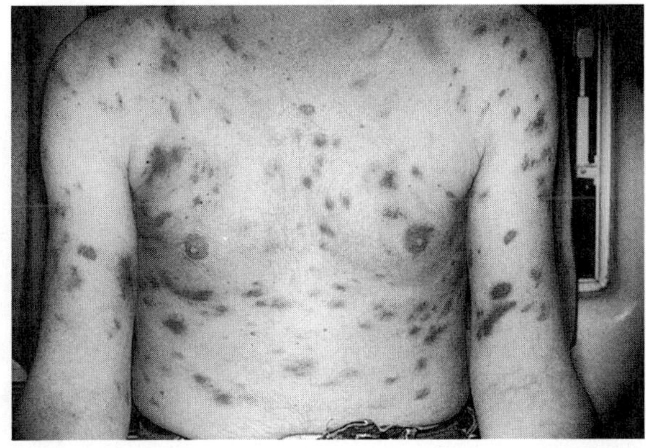

FIGURE 1-172 Kaposi's sarcoma. More advanced lesions. Note widespread hemorrhagic plaques and nodules. (From Noble J [ed]: *Textbook of primary care medicine,* ed 2, St Louis, 1995, Mosby.)

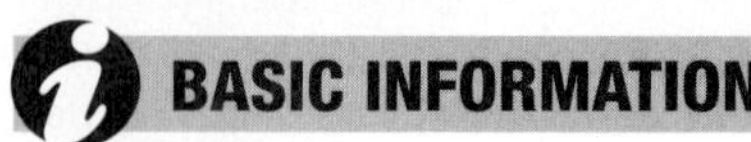

BASIC INFORMATION

DEFINITION

Kawasaki disease (KD) is an acute, febrile, multisystem disease predominantly affecting children that is usually manifested by a self-limited generalized vasculitis of unknown etiology.

SYNONYMS

Kawasaki syndrome
Mucocutaneous lymph node syndrome
Infantile polyarteritis

ICD-9CM CODES
446.1 Kawasaki disease

EPIDEMIOLOGY & DEMOGRAPHICS

- KD is the leading cause of acquired heart disease in children.
- Commonly occurs in children <5 yr (80%); peak age is 18 to 24 mo.
- More prevalent in boys than girls (1.5:1).
- The highest incidence is found in Japan (approximately 174 cases/100,000 children).
- Temporal clustering and seasonality have been observed in KD cases in Japan, supporting an environmental or infectious etiology.
- Incidence of KD in the U.S. is 17 to 18 cases/100,000 children <5 yr.
- Children of Asian descent have the highest incidence of KD compared with those of European or African descent.
- Approximately 4200 new cases are diagnosed each year in the U.S.
- In the U.S., KD has now surpassed acute rheumatic fever as the leading cause of acquired heart disease in children.

PHYSICAL FINDINGS & CLINICAL PRESENTATION

- Diagnosis of KD is based on characteristic clinical signs and symptoms and includes fever persisting for >5 days and the presence of at least four of the following five principal features:
  1. Bilateral, painless bulbar conjunctival injection without exudate
  2. Oral mucosal changes: erythema and fissured lips, strawberry tongue (Fig. 1-173, *B*), diffuse injection of the oropharyngeal mucosae
  3. Polymorphous exanthema (usually in truncal region) (Fig. 1-174, *A* and *B*)
  4. Extremity changes: (a) acute: erythema and edema of hands and feet (Fig. 1-153, *A*); (b) convalescent: membranous desquamation of fingertips
  5. Cervical lymphadenopathy (<1.5 cm in diameter, predominantly unilateral and anterior)
- The fever of KD is usually higher than 102.2° F (39° C) and often >104.0° F (40° C); if untreated, it lasts for an average of 12 days.
- Coronary artery aneurysms can develop in as many as 25% of untreated children and can lead, over time, to ischemic heart disease, myocardial infarction, congestive heart failure, and, occasionally, death. Morbidity and mortality rates are highest if aneurysm diameter is >8 mm.
- Children with KD who are <1 yr or >6 yr are more likely to develop the cardiac sequelae and are most likely to not respond treatment.
- Patients with fever and fewer than four principal symptoms but evidence of coronary artery disease are diagnosed as having atypical KD (10%).
- Cervical lymphadenopathy is the most common physical manifestation absent in atypical KD, followed by exanthema and then extremity changes.
- Oral mucosal changes are the most common manifestations of KD (either typical or atypical).
- On rare occasions aneurysms of peripheral arteries (e.g., axillary) may be seen.
- Beau's lines (transverse grooves of the nails), diarrhea, dyspnea, arthralgia, and myalgia may also been seen.

ETIOLOGY

The cause of KD is not known, although evidence substantiates an environmental or infectious etiology precipitating an immune-mediated reaction in genetically susceptible individuals.

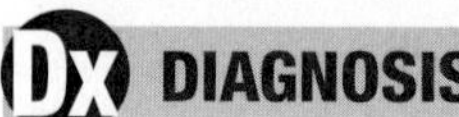

DIAGNOSIS

Diagnosis of KD is made on the basis of clinical features (see "Physical Findings & Clinical Presentation"). The illness begins with the abrupt onset of fever. Typically, the clinical signs appear over the course of several days. Laboratory evaluation may be helpful in making the diagnosis in atypical KD.

DIFFERENTIAL DIAGNOSIS

- Scarlet fever
- Stevens-Johnson syndrome
- Drug eruption
- Henoch-Schönlein purpura
- Toxic shock syndrome
- Measles
- Rocky Mountain spotted fever
- Infectious mononucleosis
- Juvenile rheumatoid arthritis
- Mercury hypersensitivity

WORKUP

Clinical findings in addition to laboratory and imaging studies are useful in searching for multiorgan system involvement and complications (e.g., cardiac, lung, liver).

LABORATORY TESTS

Clinical and laboratory findings observed in patients with this disease are frequently helpful in diagnosis:

- Complete blood count commonly shows a normochromic normocytic anemia, elevated platelet count, and elevated white blood cell count with neutrophil predominance.
- Abnormal liver function tests are found: elevated transaminases (hepatic congestion), elevated bilirubin (gallbladder hydrops), low albumin.
- Elevated erythrocyte sedimentation rate is found (often >40 mm/hr and not uncommonly elevated to levels of >100 mm/hr).
- Elevated C-reactive protein (levels of >3 mg/dl) is identified.
- Urinalysis may show sterile pyuria.

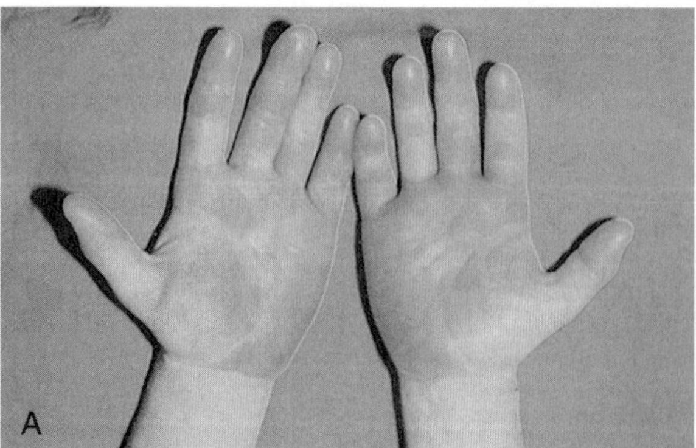

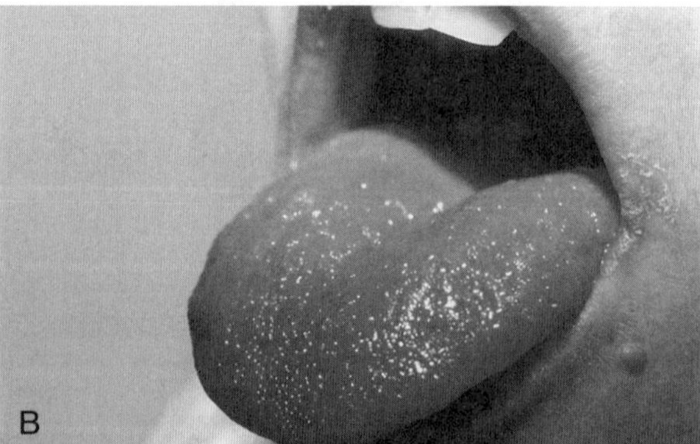

FIGURE 1-173 A, Erythema of the hands, to be followed by desquamation. **B,** Strawberry tongue in a patient with Kawasaki syndrome. (**A** Courtesy Department of Dermatology, University of North Carolina at Chapel Hill. In Goldstein B [ed]: *Practical dermatology,* ed 2, St Louis, 1997, Mosby. **B** Courtesy Marshall Guill, M.D. In Goldstein B [ed]: *Practical dermatology,* ed 2, St Louis, 1997, Mosby.)

IMAGING STUDIES

- Chest radiograph may reveal pulmonary infiltrates; cardiomegaly may also be present.
- Echocardiogram is helpful and may show depressed left ventricular function with regional wall motion abnormalities, pericardial effusion (30%), and mitral valve regurgitation. The echocardiogram is also useful in the long-term follow-up of patients with KD.
- Coronary angiogram, computed tomography angiography, and magnetic resonance angiography can be used to visualize the arterial system and the presence of coronary artery aneurysms. Echocardiography may be able to visualize these aneurysms in infants.
- Intravascular ultrasound can assess for luminal irregularities of the coronary arteries.
- Exercise testing with myocardial perfusion studies can be done to assess for coronary blood flow and the presence of myocardial ischemia.
- ECG changes (arrhythmias, abnormal Q waves, prolonged PR and/or QT intervals, occasionally low voltage, or ST-T wave changes) can be seen.

Rx TREATMENT

Treatment of KD in the acute phase is directed at reducing inflammation in the systemic and coronary arteries and preventing arterial thrombosis. Long-term therapy in individuals who develop coronary aneurysms is aimed at preventing myocardial ischemia or infarction.

NONPHARMACOLOGIC THERAPY

- Oxygen in selected patients
- Salt restriction in patients with congestive heart failure
- Emollient creams for peeling skin and balms for fissured lips

ACUTE GENERAL Rx

- IV immunoglobulin (IVIG) 2 g/kg over 8 to 12 hr is the treatment of choice in children diagnosed with KD and ideally should be given within the first 10 days of the illness.
- Aspirin 80 to 100 mg/kg/day (anti-inflammatory dosing) given in four divided doses until the patient is no longer febrile for 48 hr. Thereafter, aspirin 3 to 5 mg/kg/day (antiplatelet dosing) is continued until laboratory studies (e.g., platelet count, sedimentation rate) return to normal, generally within 6 to 8 wk.
- In patients who do not defervesce within 48 hr or have recrudescent fever after initial IVIG treatment, a second dose of IVIG 2 g/kg IV over 8 to 12 hr should be considered.
- Nonsteroidal anti-inflammatory drugs are not effective in the treatment of KD.
- The effect of corticosteroids on coronary artery aneurysms is unclear. Therefore most experts recommend withholding steroids unless fever persists after at least two courses of IVIG.
- Other therapies, including pentoxifylline, infliximab (monoclonal antibody against tumor necrosis factor-α), plasma exchange, abciximab (platelet glycoprotein IIb/IIIa receptor inhibitor), and immunosuppressive agents (methotrexate, cyclosporine, tacrolimus, antithymocyte globulin, cyclophosphamide) have been used, but data are limited on their success.
- Acute management of patients with coronary artery abnormalities depends on the severity of the lesion.
- Most patients with large or giant coronary artery aneurysms (diameter >8 mm) are maintained on aspirin (or clopidogrel) and warfarin to prevent thrombosis within the aneurysm and myocardial infarction.

CHRONIC Rx

Interventional and surgical procedures can be tried in children who have developed cardiac complications of KD:

- Percutaneous transluminal coronary angioplasty with or without stenting may be performed.
- Coronary bypass graft surgery using the internal mammary artery or the gastroepiploic artery has met with greater patency success than saphenous vein grafts. Patency rates for internal thoracic artery grafts have been shown to be 87% at 20 yr, and patency rates for vein grafts at 1, 10, and 25 yr after surgery have been shown to be 84%, 57%, and 51%, respectively.
- Cardiac transplantation is an option and is indicated in patients with:
  - Severe left ventricular failure
  - Malignant arrhythmias
  - Multivessel coronary artery disease

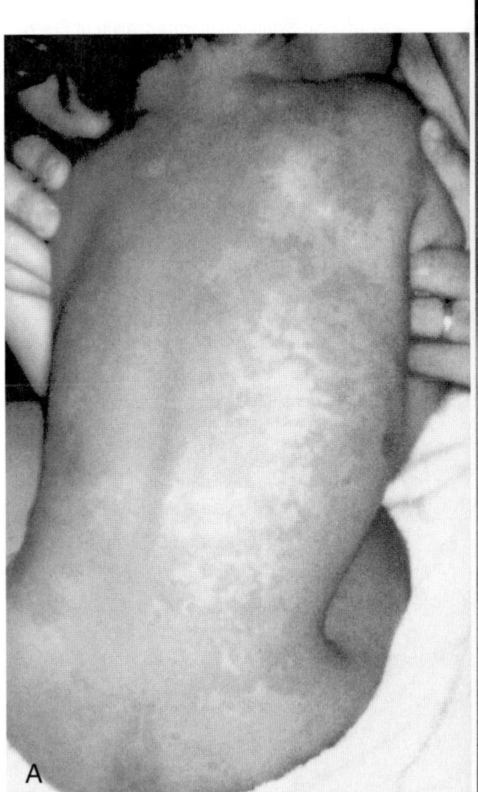

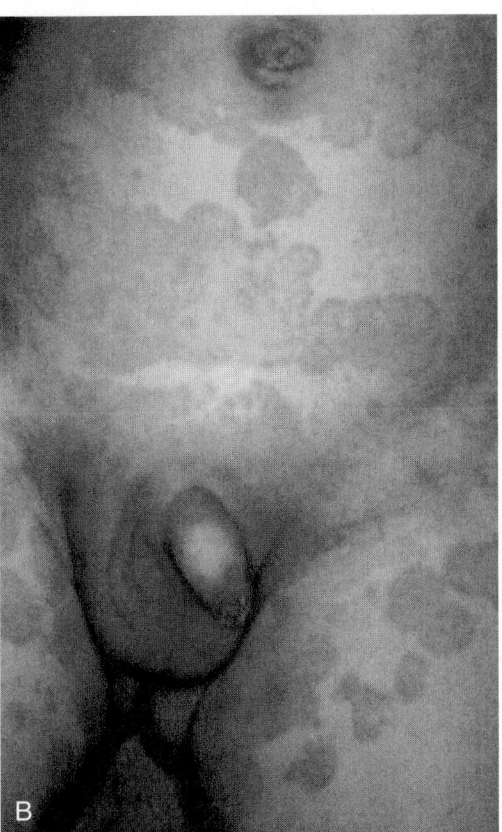

FIGURE 1-174 Clinical manifestations of Kawasaki disease. Polymorphous exanthema **(A, B)**.

DISPOSITION

- Mortality rate of children with KD is 0.5% to 2.8%, usually from coronary aneurysm thrombosis and myocardial infarction.
- Death usually occurs in the third to fourth week of the illness.
- Before the use of IVIG, approximately 20% of all patients with KD developed coronary artery aneurysms.
- Treatment with IVIG has reduced the incidence of coronary aneurysms by 80%.
- IVIG has also been shown to improve left ventricular function during the acute stages of the disease.
- Risk factors for the development of coronary aneurysms or giant coronary aneurysms 8 mm or greater are:
  - Fever lasting >10 days
  - Age <1 yr or >6 yr
  - Male
  - Recurrence of fever
- 1% to 2% of patients have recurrences of KD.

REFERRAL

Multiple specialists may be consulted to assist in the diagnosis of KD, including dermatology, rheumatology, and infectious disease. Cardiology consultation is recommended in any patient with cardiac involvement and in the long-term follow-up of patients with KD.

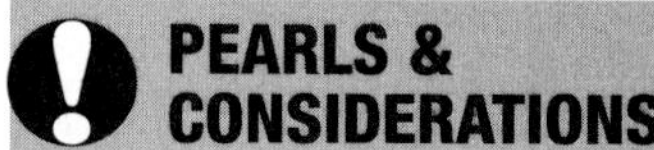

PEARLS & CONSIDERATIONS

COMMENTS

- KD was first described by Dr. Tomisaku Kawasaki in 1967 and published in the *Journal of Allergology.*
- KD is not transmitted from person to person.
- Atypical or incomplete KD can be detected using clinical plus laboratory criteria along with typical findings on echocardiography.
- The mechanism of action of IVIG therapy for KD remains unknown.
- Failure of corticosteroids suggests that the inflammatory response is different compared with other vasculitic conditions.

PREVENTION

- Without a known etiologic agent for KD, primary prevention is not possible.
- Low-dose aspirin (3 to 5 mg/kg/day, given as a single dose) should be continued until 6 to 8 wk after disease onset if there are no coronary artery abnormalities or indefinitely if abnormalities are present.
- Thrombosis leading to myocardial infarction in a stenotic or aneurysmal coronary artery is the leading cause of death in these children and occurs most often in the first year after illness onset. Therefore serial imaging and stress tests are necessary in patients with significant coronary artery abnormalities (by coronary angiography).

PATIENT & FAMILY EDUCATION

- The Kawasaki Disease Foundation, a nonprofit organization dedicated to KD issues (http://www.kdfoundation.org).
- The American Heart Association has developed guidelines for the diagnosis of KD (http://www.americanheart.org).

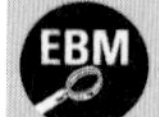

EVIDENCE

Please note: Complete text of EBM for this topic is available online.

Key trials and commentary:

Treatment of acute Kawasaki disease with intravenous (IV) immune globulin and aspirin reduces the risk of coronary-artery abnormalities and systemic inflammation, but despite intravenous immune globulin therapy, coronary-artery abnormalities develop in some children. Studies have suggested that primary corticosteroid therapy might be beneficial and that adverse events are infrequent with short-term use.

This data does not provide support for the addition of a single pulsed dose of IV methylprednisolone to conventional IV immune globulin therapy for the routine primary treatment of children with Kawasaki disease.[1] Ⓐ

You would think by now that we would have figured out the very best way to manage children with Kawasaki disease. At least two generations of us have tackled this problem. As pointed out in a commentary by Burns, "How can an illness look like an infectious disease but not have a recoverable agent, look like an immune-mediated vasculitis but not be easily treated with corticosteroids, and look like a benign, self-limited illness but be the leading cause of acquired heart disease in children?"

With respect to the initial management of Kawasaki disease, our Japanese colleagues have suggested that high doses of intravenously administered immune globulin are most effective in relieving patients of symptoms and reducing the risk of coronary artery disease. From these early Japanese experiences with immune globulin, randomized prospective clinical trials here in the U.S. that took place a quarter of a century ago established that IV immune globulin is, indeed, effective and safe therapy for reducing the rate of coronary artery aneurysms. The mechanism of action of this form of therapy has never been clearly understood, although many theories abound. Aspirin is also administered, usually in high dosages, for its anti-inflammatory effects, and good data exist to support its use as well.

IV immune globulin is not effective in every patient with Kawasaki disease. Failure rates as high as 20% have been described. The findings of Newburger et al suggest that adding corticosteroid therapy to IV immune globulin does not improve the outcome in such children. Why steroids do not work in this form of vasculitis but are the mainstay of therapy for most other vasculitides remains an enigma. Perhaps only when we find out the true etiology of Kawasaki disease will we have a definitive therapy for it. The 4-decade long search for a causative agent has yielded only a long list of ruled-out pathogens. The findings of studies implicating a superantigen in the upregulation of the immune response have not been confirmed. Current evidence suggests the involvement of an oligoclonal antibody response to a conventional antigen.

It is now more than 40 years since the original description of the clinical signs of this illness by the Japanese pediatrician Tomisaku Kawasaki. Hopefully, it will not take another 40 years before we pin down the etiologic agent, if one exists, or understand everything there is to be understood about the pathophysiology of this curious entity.

Evidence-Based Reference

1. Newburger JW, for the Pediatric Heart Network Investigators: Randomized trial of pulsed corticosteroid therapy for primary treatment of Kawasaki disease, *N Engl J Med* 356:663-675, 2007. Commentary by J.A. Stockman III, M.D. Ⓐ

SUGGESTED READINGS

Burns JC et al: Summary of the 8th International Kawasaki Disease Symposium: Presentation of Selected Abstracts. Available at http://americanheart.org/downloadable/heart/11623189833988th%20IKDS%20summary%20revision.pdf. Accessed September 28, 2009.

Freeman A, Shulman S: Kawasaki disease: summary of the American Heart Association guidelines, *Am Fam Physician* 74:1141, 2006.

Newburger JW, Fulton DR: Kawasaki disease, *Curr Opin Pediatr* 16(5):508, 2004.

Newburger JW et al: Diagnosis, treatment, and long-term management of Kawasaki disease: a statement for health professionals from the Committee on Rheumatic Fever, Endocarditis and Kawasaki Disease, Council on Cardiovascular Disease in the Young, American Heart Association, *Circulation* 110:2747-2771, 2004.

Royle J et al: The diagnosis and management of Kawasaki disease, *J Pediatr Child Health* 41(3):87, 2005.

AUTHORS: **SCOTT COHEN, M.D.,** and **WEN-CHIH WU, M.D.**

BASIC INFORMATION

DESCRIPTION

Keloid may be defined as a benign growth of dense fibrous tissue developing from an abnormal healing response to cutaneous injury, extending beyond the original borders of the wound or inflammatory response (Fig. 1-175).

In 1806 Alibert used the term *cheloide,* derived from the Greek *chele,* or crab's claw, to describe lateral growth of tissue into unaffected skin.

ICD-9CM CODES
701.4 Keloid scar

EPIDEMIOLOGY

- Keloid is seen 5 to 15 times more often in pigmented ethnic groups than in whites.
- Its prevalence is 16% in blacks and Hispanics.
- The highest incidence is seen in the second decade.
- It affects both sexes equally.
- Combined incidence of keloid and hypertrophic scar ranges from 40% to 70% following surgery to up to 91% following burns.

ETIOLOGY

- Wounds from trauma, surgery, or body piercing
- Burn
- Other injuries such as insect bites, vaccination, folliculitis, acne, and so on
- Rarely can be spontaneous without obvious injury
- Familial predisposition seen in some patients

RISK FACTORS

- Family history of keloids
- Personal history of keloids
- Blacks, Hispanics, and Asians
- Pregnancy
- Puberty
- Patients with blood group A
- Injury over bones

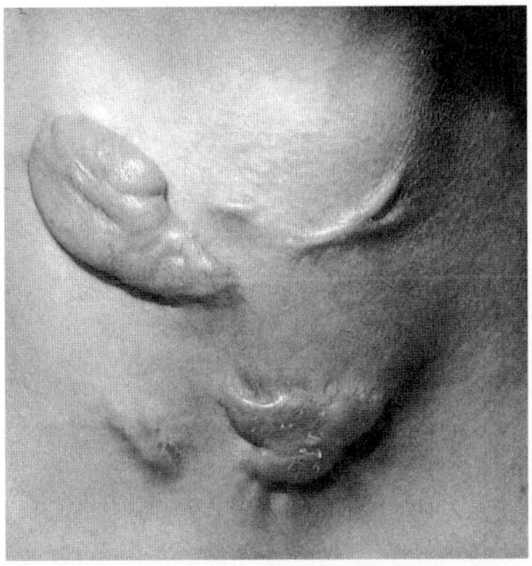

FIGURE 1-175 Keloids. An abnormal reparative reaction to skin injury, keloids are characterized by proliferation of fibroblasts and collagen that extends beyond the margins of the original wound. (From Zitelli BJ, Davis HW: *Atlas of pediatric physical diagnosis,* ed 5, Philadelphia, 2007, Mosby.)

PATHOGENESIS

- Pathophysiology of keloid is not completely understood
- Caused by benign dermal fibroproliferation because of disorder in the regulation of cellularity during the wound healing process

CLINICAL FEATURES

- Keloids usually appear within a few months of the injury, in contrast to the hypertrophic scars, which develop within a few weeks. At times it could take up to a year to appear because the growth is slow.
- Keloids are often symptomatic in the early stages. Common complaints are pruritus, burning, pain, and tenderness.
- Keloids are commonly seen on the shoulders, sternum, upper back, nape of neck, ear lobes, mandibular border, and cheek. Hands and feet are often spared.
- Skin lesions vary from papules to nodules to large tuberous lesions. They have the normal skin color most of the time with well-defined borders. Early on they can appear erythematous, whereas older lesions may be hypo- or hyperpigmented. They can be firm to hard in consistency with smooth surface and are tender to touch. Hair follicles are absent in these keloids.
- Unlike with hypertrophic scar, in keloids the scar extends beyond the margin of the initial wound.

DIAGNOSIS

- Workup is usually not necessary because it is a clinical diagnosis.
- Biopsy is usually avoided because it may increase the keloid size. When biopsy is done, the histology shows randomly organized large collagen fibers in a dense connective tissue matrix. In fact, both major components of extracellular matrix, collagen and glycosaminoglycans, are increased.

DIFFERENTIAL DIAGNOSIS

- Hypertrophic scar
- Dermatofibroma
- Dermatofibrosarcoma protuberance
- Desmoid tumor
- Foreign body granuloma
- Scar with sarcoidosis
- Lobomycosis

TREATMENT

- There is no universally accepted treatment protocol. Prevention is the best strategy.
- Combination treatment is most effective.
- Surgical excision using cold knife followed by intralesional steroids is the preferred method.
- Treatment outcome is the best when it is initiated shortly after the keloid formation.
- Different treatment options include:
  1. Unlike with hypertrophic scars, **surgery** alone is associated with a 55% to 100% recurrence rate in patients with keloids. Results are significantly better when it is followed by intralesional steroids, radiotherapy, pressure therapy, or silicon application. Both complete and near total excision has been advocated. Few recommend core extirpation. Use of Z-plasties or any wound lengthening techniques is strongly discouraged.
  2. **Intralesional steroid** every 2 to 4 wk is administered either alone or following surgery. Duration of treatment depends on the treatment response. Triamcinolone is the most studied steroid and is used at a concentration of 10 to 40 mg/ml. Higher concentration is used for denser, more calcitrant lesions, and those located in trunks or extremities. It could be used in combination with lidocaine to reduce the discomfort. A 27- to 30-gauge needle is used for its administration. To distribute the suspension evenly, it should be injected while continuously advancing the needle. No more than 20 to 30 mg of the drug is used during each treatment. Liquid nitrogen is applied to the injection briefly for 2 to 4 seconds about 10 to 15 min prior to steroid injection for better dispersal of the steroid and to minimize deposition into surrounding normal tissue. Hypopigmentation, skin atrophy, ulceration, and telangiectasia are the side effects associated with this treatment.
  3. **Cryotherapy** has been used for smaller lesions. When this treatment is chosen, the entire lesion is treated with 2 to 3 freeze-thaw cycles of 30 seconds' duration each. Most lesions need 2 to 10 treatment sessions at 4-wk intervals. Pain and hypopigmentation are the main adverse events.
  4. **Silicone gel sheeting or cushioning** can prevent keloids from recurring after surgery. These are applied as soon as re-epithelialization is achieved and are worn for at least 12 hr/day for 2 to 4 mo.
  5. **Application of pressure** by compression devices has been advocated in the treatment of keloids. These compression treatments include button compression, pressure ear rings, pressure gradient garments, ACE bandages, elastic adhesive bandages, compression wraps, Spandex or Elastane bandages, and support bandages. About 24 to 40 mm Hg pressure must be maintained. It must be instituted for long periods (>23 hr/day for 6 to 12 mo) before significant effect can be achieved. Unfortunately many parts of the body are not amenable to this pressure. Patient discomfort frequently reduces compliance.

6. **Radiation** following surgery can also reduce the recurrence rate. X-rays of 700 to 1500 cGy in fractions over 5 to 6 treatments is the most frequently used treatment. It is usually initiated within 10 days, preferably within 24 hr of surgery. It is avoided in pediatric and pregnant patients. At times brachytherapy is used using interstitial iridium 192. Most physicians use radiation only for keloids over the extremities. The reported risk of radiation-induced malignancy is theoretical.
7. **5-Fluorouracil** can be used as an individual agent, following surgery, or in combination with intralesional steroids. Weekly injection of 0.5 to 2 ml at a 50 mg/ml concentration of 5-fluorouracil for 12 wk is the recommended dose.
8. Superiority of **laser** use to simple excision currently has not been demonstrated.
9. Topical 5% **imiquimod** cream has some role when used following surgery locally every night for a minimum of 2 mo.
10. Other treatments include Cordran tape, bleomycin, interferon, vitamin A, nitrogen mustard, antihistamines, zinc, tacrolimus, sirolimus, allantoin, botulinum toxin, colchicine, salicylic acid, calcipotriol, NSAIDs, d-penicillamine, relaxin, quercetin, dinoprostone, doxorubicin, ACE inhibitors, hyaluronidase, pentoxifylline, tranilast, mitomycin-C, tamoxifen, silver sulfadiazine, onion extract, vitamin E, intralesional verapamil.

FOLLOW-UP

Because of the high risk of recurrence, a follow-up of at least 12 mo is necessary to fully evaluate the effectiveness of therapy.

PREVENTION

- Avoid nonessential surgery such as body piercing, which carry a high risk for keloid formation.
- LASIK eye surgery and CO_2 laser resurfacing should be avoided in patients with a tendency for keloids.
- Use a laparoscopic approach when surgery is needed.
- Avoid making incisions over joint spaces or over midchest, and ensure that they follow skin creases.
- Handle tissue gently during surgery.
- Ensure good hemostasis intraoperatively.
- Use tension-free primary wound closure.
- Use monofilament, synthetic permanent sutures.
- Use adhesives instead of sutures when possible for closure of wounds.
- Compressive pressure dressing is preferred in high risk patients following surgery.
- Avoid of wound infection.
- Avoid tattoos.
- Aggressively treat inflammatory acnes.

COMPLICATIONS

- Psychological effects secondary to disfigurement.
- Contracture from keloids may result in loss of function if overlying a joint.

PROGNOSIS

- Unlike with hypertrophic scars, keloids do not regress with time. However, they may continue to expand in size for decades.
- Regardless of the type of treatment there is a high recurrence rate.
- Keloids never become malignant.

SUGGESTED READINGS

Keloids: pathophysiology and management, *Dermatol Online J* 13(3):9, 2007.

Keloid pathogenesis and treatment, *Plast Reconstr Surg* 117(1):286-300, 2006.

Treatment of keloids and hypertrophic scars: a meta-analysis and review of literature, *Arch Facial Plast* 8(6):362-368, 2006.

Keloids and scars: a review of keloids and scars, their pathogenesis, risk factors, and management, *Curr Opin Pediatr* 18(4):396-402, 2006.

Keloids or hypertrophic scar: the controversy: review of the literature, *Ann Plast Surg* 54(6):676-680, 2005.

AUTHOR: **HEMANT K. SAPATHY, M.D.**

BASIC INFORMATION

DEFINITION

Klinefelter's syndrome is a congenital disorder in which a 47,XXY chromosome complement is associated with hypogonadism and infertility.

SYNONYMS

47,XXY Hypogonadism

ICD-9CM CODES
758.7 Klinefelter's syndrome

EPIDEMIOLOGY & DEMOGRAPHICS

INCIDENCE: One in 500 men (most common sex chromosome disorder)

GENETICS: The most common mosaic complement is 46,XY/47,XXY. 47,XXY karyotype 48,XXYY, 48,XXXY, or 49,XXXXY have been reported. The manifestations vary in severity by patient. This sex chromosome mosaicism is believed to account for the variable presentation. Fertility, although very rare, has been reported in men with Klinefelter's syndrome.

PHYSICAL FINDINGS & CLINICAL PRESENTATION

- Classic triad: Small firm testes, azoospermia, and gynecomastia.
- Prepubertal: Small testes; gonadal volume $<$1.5 ml is a result of loss of germ cells before puberty.
- Postpubertal: Gynecomastia (periductal fat growth) with small, firm testes. Exaggerated growth of the lower extremities results in a decreased crown-to-pubis/pubis-to-floor ratio (Fig. 1-176). There is diminished strength, diminished ability to grow a full beard or mustache, and infertility. Decreased intellectual development and antisocial behavior are believed to occur with high frequency.

ETIOLOGY

- Several postulated mechanisms: nondisjunction during meiosis and mitosis and anaphase lag during mitosis or meiosis
- Reason: maternal age
  1. The incidence of Klinefelter's syndrome rises from 0.6% when the maternal age is $\leq$35 yr to 5.4% when the maternal age is $>$45 yr.
  2. Of note, the extra X chromosome has a paternal origin as often as a maternal origin.

Dx DIAGNOSIS

- Markedly elevated follicle-stimulating hormone levels.
- Total plasma testosterone levels are decreased in 50% to 60% of patients.
- Free testosterone levels are decreased.
- Plasma estradiol is increased, stimulating the increase in levels of testosterone-binding globulin with resultant decrease in the testosterone/estradiol ratio, which is believed to be the cause of gynecomastia.

LABORATORY TESTS

- Normal to low serum testosterone.
- Increased sex hormone–binding globulin (acts to further suppress any available free testosterone).
- Normal to increased estradiol (a result of augmented peripheral conversion of testosterone to estradiol).
- Testis biopsy shows azoospermia, Leydig cell hyperplasia, hyalinization, and fibrosis of the seminiferous tubules. Mosaics may have focal areas of spermatogenesis and, on rare occasions, a sperm may appear in the ejaculate. The extra X chromosome is the pivotal factor controlling spermatogenesis and also affects neuronal function directly, leading to the behavioral abnormalities related to decreased IQ.
- Buccal smear: one sex chromatin body.
- Prepubertal male: gonadotropin levels are normal.
- Postpubertal male: Gonadotropin levels are elevated even when the testosterone level is normal.
- Disease associations:
  - Malignancies: breast cancer (20 times greater than XY men and 20% the rate of occurrence in women), nonlymphocytic leukemia, lymphomas, marrow dysplastic syndromes, extragonadal germ cell neoplasms
  - Autoimmune disorders: chronic lymphocytic thyroiditis, Takayasu arteritis, taurodontism (enlarged molar teeth), mitral valve prolapse, varicose veins, asthma, bronchitis, osteoporosis, abnormal glucose tolerance testing, diabetes, varicose veins

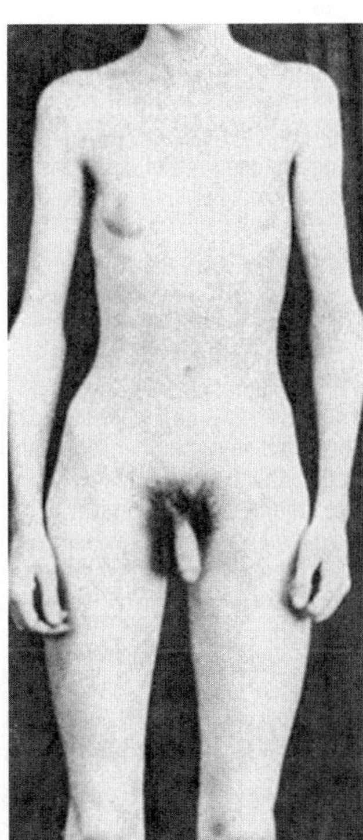

FIGURE 1-176 Klinefelter's syndrome. (From Harrison JH et al: *Campbell's urology,* ed 4, Philadelphia, 1979, WB Saunders.)

Rx TREATMENT

- Revolves around three facets of Klinefelter's syndrome:
  1. Hypogonadism: androgen replacement in the form of testosterone
  2. Gynecomastia: cosmetic surgery
  3. Psychosocial problems: androgen therapy and educational support
- After extensive genetic counseling, intracytoplasmic sperm insertion has been used to treat infertility with limited success in mosaic men

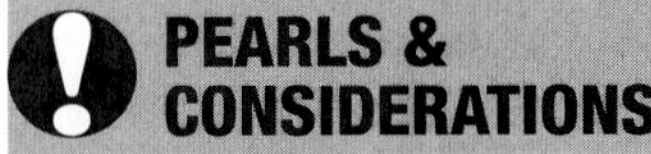

PEARLS & CONSIDERATIONS

COMMENTS

- Androgen therapy should not be used in the case of severe mental retardation.
- Rule out breast and prostate cancer before initiating or continuing androgen therapy.
- Androgen therapy will not improve fertility; it may suppress any spermatogenesis that is taking place within the testes.
- Other causes of primary hypogonadism:
  1. Myotonic muscular dystrophy
  2. Sertoli cell–only syndrome
  3. Kartagener's syndrome
  4. Anorchia
  5. Acquired hypogonadism

SUGGESTED READINGS

Manning MA, Hoyme HE: Diagnosis and management of the adolescent boy with Klinefelter syndrome, *Adolesc Med State Art Rev* 13(2):367, 2002.

Wattendorg D, Muenke M: Klinefelter syndrome, *Am Fam Physician* 72:2259, 2005.

AUTHORS: **PHILIP J. ALIOTTA, M.D., M.S.H.A.,** and **RUBEN ALVERO, M.D.**

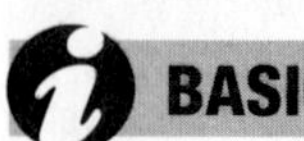

BASIC INFORMATION

DEFINITION

Korsakoff's psychosis is a disorder of learning and memory, out of proportion to other cognitive functions, associated with thiamine deficiency. It is classically seen with chronic alcohol abuse and may follow the presentation of Wernicke's encephalopathy (see relevant entry).

SYNONYMS

Korsakoff's syndrome
Wernicke-Korsakoff syndrome
Alcoholic polyneuritic psychosis

ICD-9CM CODES
291.1 Alcohol amnestic syndrome

EPIDEMIOLOGY & DEMOGRAPHICS

- Formerly seen commonly in chronic alcohol users, but declining in recent years as a result of better nutrition and awareness by health professionals.
- Slightly more common in males.
- Age of onset evenly distributed between ages 30 and 70.

PHYSICAL FINDINGS & CLINICAL PRESENTATION

- Impairment of ability to remember new material.
- Remote memory is relatively better preserved but is commonly impaired on neuropsychologic testing.
- Confabulation (the fabrication of false memories to fill memory gaps) is common.

ETIOLOGY

Thiamine deficiency is the underlying cause. This is most commonly seen in alcoholics and other malnourished populations, although it may be iatrogenic from prolonged infusion of dextrose-containing fluids without thiamine repletion.

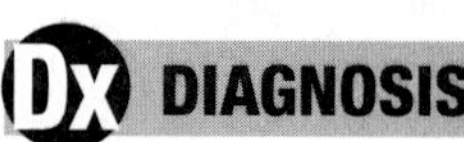

DIAGNOSIS

DIFFERENTIAL DIAGNOSIS

- Stroke, trauma, or tumor affecting the temporal lobes or hippocampus
- Cerebral anoxia
- Transient global amnesia
- Dementia of multiple causes

WORKUP

A high index of suspicion should be maintained in all alcoholics and others in malnourished states.

LABORATORY TESTS

- CBC
- Serum chemistries
- Serum pyruvate is elevated
- Whole-blood or erythrocyte transketolase are decreased; rapid resolution to normal in 24 hr with thiamine repletion

IMAGING STUDIES

MRI may show T_2 hyperintense diencephalic and mesencephalic lesions acutely, but there is no definitive radiologic study for diagnosis.

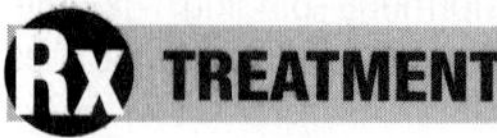

TREATMENT

NONPHARMACOLOGIC THERAPY

A supervised environment may be required.

ACUTE GENERAL Rx

- Thiamine 100 mg IV or IM should be given immediately.
- Thiamine given acutely during Wernicke's phase (disorders of extraocular movements, confusion, and ataxia) may prevent the development of Korsakoff's psychosis.

CHRONIC Rx

- It is impossible to predict acutely the degree of recovery of an individual patient, although the vast majority will have lasting deficits. Decisions regarding long-term institutionalization should therefore be made cautiously.
- Chronic treatment with thiamine.

DISPOSITION

Patient often must live in a protected environment for the rest of his or her life.

REFERRAL

- Neurology to confirm the diagnosis.
- Neuropsychologic testing may be helpful.

PEARLS & CONSIDERATIONS

COMMENTS

- This disease may be underdiagnosed, and memory problems may persist, even in "recovered" patients.
- Replace thiamine in patients at risk, even if clinical symptoms are not evident.
- A preventable cause is prolonged use of dextrose-containing IV fluids without supplemental thiamine.

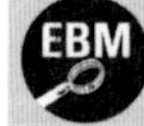

EVIDENCE

The use of thiamine in the management of Korsakoff's psychosis is supported by limited data from randomized studies and endorsed by expert opinion.

A recent Cochrane review identified two RCTs evaluating the use of thiamine in people at risk of Korsakoff's secondary to alcohol excess, of which only one contained sufficient data for quantitative analysis. This review found that although thiamine administration is strongly recommended for alcohol-abusing patients, there is insufficient evidence to make specific recommendations of the dose, frequency, route, or duration of thiamine administration either in the prophylaxis or treatment of Wernicke-Korsakoff syndrome.[1] Ⓐ

The RCT analysis, involving 107 patients detoxifying from alcohol, evaluated the effects of 5 different doses of intramuscular thiamine (ranging from 5 mg daily to 200 mg) over 2 days. This study found that posttreatment performance (the delayed alternation task) was superior in those patients receiving the highest dose compared with all other doses, suggesting a therapeutic relationship between dose and working memory performance.[2] Ⓑ

Recommendations from the American Society of Addiction Medicine are that parenteral administration of thiamine (100 mg daily for at least 3 days, IV or IM) is recommended to prevent or treat Wernicke-Korsakoff syndrome.[3] Ⓒ

Evidence-Based References

1. Day E et al: Thiamine for Wernicke-Korsakoff Syndrome in people at risk from alcohol abuse, *Cochrane Database Rev* 1, 2004. Ⓐ
2. Ambrose ML et al: Thiamin treatment and working memory function of alcohol-dependent people: preliminary findings. *Alcohol Clin Exp Res* 25:112-116, 2001. Ⓑ
3. Mayo-Smith MF et al: Working Group on the Management of Alcohol Withdrawal Delirium, Practice Guidelines Committee, American Society of Addiction Medicine. Management of alcohol withdrawal delirium: an evidence-based practice guideline. *Arch Intern Med* 164:1405-1412, 2004. Ⓒ

SUGGESTED READINGS

Cook CC: Prevention and treatment of Wernicke-Korsakoff syndrome, *Alcohol Suppl* 35(suppl):19, 2000.

Martin PR et al: The role of thiamine deficiency in alcoholic brain disease, *Alcohol Res Health* 27(2):134-142, 2003.

Zubaran C et al: Wernicke-Korsakoff syndrome, *Postgrad Med J* 78(855):27, 1997.

AUTHOR: **DANIEL T. MATTSON, M.S., M.SC. (MED.)**

BASIC INFORMATION

DEFINITION

Labyrinthitis is a peripheral vestibulopathy characterized by acute onset of vertigo usually associated with nausea and vomiting. It may be associated with hearing loss. It may be either serous or purulent.

SYNONYMS

Acute labyrinthitis
Acute vestibular neuronopathy
Vestibular neuronitis
Viral neurolabyrinthitis

ICD-9CM CODES
386.12 Vestibular neuronitis (active and recurrent)
386.3 Labyrinthitis

EPIDEMIOLOGY & DEMOGRAPHICS

INCIDENCE (IN U.S.): Most common cause of prolonged spontaneous vertigo associated with nausea at any age
PREDOMINANT AGE: Any

CLINICAL PRESENTATION

- Vertigo, nausea, and vomiting with onset over several hr.
- Symptoms usually peak within 24 hr, then resolve gradually over several wk.
- During the first day, the patient usually has difficulty focusing the eyes because of spontaneous nystagmus.
- Usually has benign course, with complete recovery within 1 to 3 mo, although older patients may have intractable dizziness that persists for many mo.

PHYSICAL FINDINGS

- Nystagmus
- Nausea
- Vomiting
- Vertigo worsening with head movement
- Abnormal caloric ENG tests
- Possible hearing loss in the affected ear
- Normal otoscopic exam typically
- Otherwise normal neurologic exam, except may possibly have signs of vestibular loss, such as a positive head thrust test

ETIOLOGY

Often preceded for 1 to 2 wk by a viral-like illness. It may be either bacterial or viral, and be either tympanogenic (i.e., resulting from spread of infection into the inner ear from the middle ear, antrum, or petrous apex), meningogenic, or hematogenic from encephalitis or brain abscess. The round window membrane is considered the most likely pathway of inflammatory mediators from the middle to the inner ear that subsequently give rise to labyrinthitis.

Dx DIAGNOSIS

DIFFERENTIAL DIAGNOSIS

- Acute labyrinthine ischemia (vascular insufficiency)
- Other forms of labyrinthitis (bacterial and syphilitic)
- Labyrinthine fistula
- Benign positional vertigo
- Meniere's syndrome
- Cholesteatoma
- Drug induced
- Eighth nerve tumor
- Head trauma
- Vertebrobasilar stroke

WORKUP

- Otoscopic examination
- Neurologic examination, with close attention to cranial nerves
- Bedside test of vestibular function, that is, head thrust or head heave test
- Audiogram if symptoms accompanied by hearing loss
- Caloric test if presentation is atypical

LABORATORY TESTS

- Routine laboratory tests are generally not helpful.
- If there is a history of significant emesis, check electrolytes, BUN, and creatinine.

IMAGING STUDIES

Usually not necessary, but enhancement of bony labyrinth may be seen by MRI after injection of contrast material. Do a head CT with fine cuts through temporal bones if there is a history of trauma or suspicion of cholesteatoma. Use an MRI of the brain with and without contrast with fine cuts through the internal auditory canal if there is an abnormal cranial nerve exam or suspicion of eighth nerve tumor.

Rx TREATMENT

NONPHARMACOLOGIC THERAPY

- Reassurance.
- Initial bed rest, then encourage increase in activity as tolerated.

ACUTE GENERAL Rx

- Phenergan or other antiemetics are typically effective.
- Vestibular suppressant: meclizine 12.5 to 25 mg qid is often used. Scopolamine patch is also effective.
- Methylprednisolone 100 mg per day for 3 days, with slow taper over 3 wk.
- Valacyclovir has not been shown to be helpful.

CHRONIC Rx

No specific chronic therapy

DISPOSITION

Usually does not require hospital admission unless the patient is unable to tolerate oral intake of liquids.

REFERRAL

- Refer if symptoms persist or neurologic abnormalities are present.
- Consider vestibular rehabilitation, particularly in the elderly.

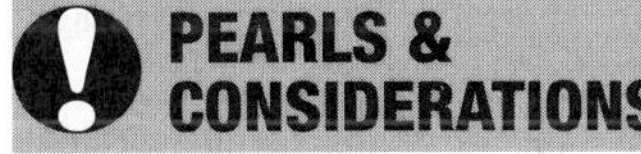

PEARLS & CONSIDERATIONS

COMMENTS

Labyrinthitis is a term that usually implies peripheral vestibulopathy associated with hearing loss. The term vestibular neuronitis is typically used when hearing is not affected. Despite this technical distinction, many physicians use these terms interchangeably.

SUGGESTED READINGS

Baloh RW et al: Neurotology, *Continuum, Lifelong Learning in Neurology* 2(2):37-53, 1996.

Cureoglu S et al: Round window membrane and labyrinthine pathological changes: an overview, *Acta Otolaryngol* 125(1):9-15, 2005.

Nuti D et al: Acute vestibular neuritis: prognosis based upon bedside clinical tests (thrusts and heaves), *Ann N Y Acad Sci* 1039:359-367, 2005.

Strupp M et al: Methylprednisolone, valacyclovir, or the combination for vestibular neuritis, *N Engl J Med* 351(4):322-323, 2004.

AUTHOR: **SHARON S. HARTMAN POLENSEK, M.D., PH.D.**

Lactose Intolerance (PTG)

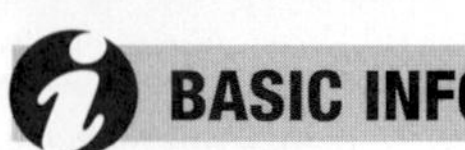

BASIC INFORMATION

DEFINITION

Lactose intolerance is the insufficient concentration of lactase enzyme, leading to fermentation of malabsorbed lactose by intestinal bacteria with subsequent production of intestinal gas and various organic acids.

SYNONYMS

Lactase deficiency
Milk intolerance

ICD-9CM CODES
271.3 Lactose intolerance

EPIDEMIOLOGY & DEMOGRAPHICS

Nearly 50 million people in the U.S. have partial or complete lactose intolerance. There are racial differences, with <25% of white adults being lactose intolerant but >85% of Asian Americans and >60% of African Americans having some form of lactose intolerance.

PHYSICAL FINDINGS & CLINICAL PRESENTATION

- Abdominal tenderness and cramping, bloating, flatulence
- Diarrhea
- Symptoms are directly related to the osmotic pressure of substrate in the colon and occur approximately 2 hr after ingestion of lactose
- Physical examination: may be entirely within normal limits

ETIOLOGY

- Congenital lactase deficiency: common in premature infants; rare in term infants and generally inherited as a chromosomal recessive trait
- Secondary lactose intolerance: usually a result of injury of the intestinal mucosa (Crohn's disease, viral gastroenteritis, AIDS enteropathy, cryptosporidiosis, Whipple's disease, sprue)

Dx DIAGNOSIS

DIFFERENTIAL DIAGNOSIS

- IBD
- IBS
- Pancreatic insufficiency
- Nontropical and tropical sprue
- Cystic fibrosis
- Diverticular disease
- Bowel neoplasm
- Laxative abuse
- Celiac disease
- Parasitic disease (e.g., giardiasis)
- Viral or bacterial infections

WORKUP

- The diagnosis can usually be made on the basis of the history and improvement with dietary manipulation.
- Diagnostic workup may include confirming the diagnosis with hydrogen breath test and excluding other conditions listed in the differential diagnosis that may also coexist with lactase deficiency.

LABORATORY TESTS

- Lactose breath hydrogen test: a rise in breath hydrogen >20 ppm within 90 min of ingestion of 50 g of lactose is positive for lactase deficiency. This test is positive in 90% of patients with lactose malabsorption. Common causes of false-negative results are recent use of oral antibiotics or recent high colonic enema.
- The lactose tolerance test is an older and less accurate testing modality (20% rate of false-positive and false-negative results). The patient is administered an oral dose of 1 to 1.5 g of lactose/kg body weight. Serial measurement of blood glucose level on an hourly basis for 3 hr is then performed. The test is considered positive if the patient develops intestinal symptoms and the blood glucose level rises <20 mg/dl above the fasting baseline level.
- Diarrhea associated with lactase deficiency is osmotic in nature with an osmotic gap and a pH <6.5.

IMAGING STUDIES

Imaging studies are generally not indicated. A small bowel series may be useful in patients with significant malabsorption.

Rx TREATMENT

NONPHARMACOLOGIC THERAPY

A lactose-free diet generally results in prompt resolution of symptoms. Lactose is primarily found in dairy products but may be present as an ingredient or component of common foods and beverages. Possible sources of lactose include breads, candies, cold cuts, dessert mixes, cream soups, bologna, commercial sauces and gravies, chocolate, drink mixes, salad dressings, and medications. Labels should be read carefully to identify sources of lactose.

ACUTE GENERAL Rx

- Addition of lactase enzyme supplement (Lactaid tablets, Dairy Ease) before the ingestion of milk products may prevent symptoms in some patients. However, it is not effective for all lactose-intolerant patients.
- Lactose-intolerant patients must ensure adequate calcium intake. Calcium supplementation is recommended to prevent osteoporosis.

CHRONIC Rx

Patient education regarding foods high in lactose, such as milk, cottage cheese, or ice cream, is recommended.

DISPOSITION

Clinical improvement with restriction or elimination of milk products

REFERRAL

GI referral for endoscopic procedures if concomitant GI disorders are suspected

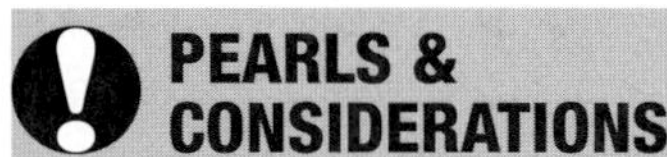

PEARLS & CONSIDERATIONS

COMMENTS

- There is great variability in signs and symptoms in patients with lactose intolerance depending on the degree of lactase deficiency.
- Most patients with lactose intolerance can ingest up to 12 oz of milk daily without symptoms.
- Nondairy synthetic drinks (e.g., Coffee-Mate) and use of rice milk are well tolerated.

SUGGESTED READING

Swagerty DL et al: Lactose intolerance, *Am Fam Physician* 65:1845, 2002.

AUTHOR: **FRED F. FERRI, M.D.**

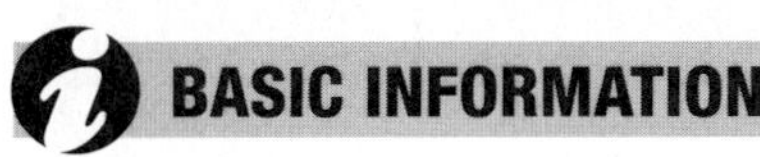

BASIC INFORMATION

DEFINITION

Lambert-Eaton myasthenic syndrome (LEMS) is a disorder of neuromuscular transmission caused by antibodies directed against presynaptic voltage-gated P/Q calcium channels on motor and autonomic nerve terminals. There are two forms: paraneoplastic (most common) and nonparaneoplastic (autoimmune).

SYNONYMS

Eaton-Lambert syndrome

ICD-9CM CODES

199.1 Malignant neoplasm without specification of site, other

EPIDEMIOLOGY & DEMOGRAPHICS

INCIDENCE (IN U.S.): Uncertain; estimated at five cases per 1 million persons annually

PEAK INCIDENCE: Sixth decade

PREVALENCE (IN U.S.): Uncertain; estimated at one per 100,000. Up to 3% of small-cell lung cancer (SCLC) patients are estimated to develop LEMS.

PREDOMINANT SEX: Male/female ratio is 2:1.

PHYSICAL FINDINGS & CLINICAL PRESENTATION

- Weakness with diminished or absent muscle stretch reflexes
- Proximal lower extremity muscles affected most
- Ocular and bulbar muscles less commonly affected
- Transient strength improvement with brief exercise
- Reflexes may be facilitated by repeatedly tapping the tendon
- Autonomic dysfunction common (dry mouth in 75%, sexual dysfunction, blurred vision, constipation, orthostasis, etc.)

ETIOLOGY

- Antibodies directed against presynaptic voltage-gated P/Q calcium channels are present in most patients. The reduction in calcium influx causes a reduction in acetylcholine release at motor and autonomic nerve terminals.
- Paraneoplastic forms, usually associated with SCLC, are present in 50% to 70% of patients.
- Autoimmune forms, usually in patients with other autoimmune diseases, occur in 10% to 30%.

DIAGNOSIS

DIFFERENTIAL DIAGNOSIS

- Myasthenia gravis
- Polymyositis
- Primary myopathies
- Carcinomatous myopathies
- Polymyalgia rheumatica
- Botulism
- Guillain-Barré syndrome

Section II describes the differential diagnosis of muscle weakness.

WORKUP

Confirm diagnosis by characteristic electrodiagnostic (EMG/NCS) findings: reduced motor amplitudes with normal sensory studies; >10% decrement in motor amplitudes on slow repetitive nerve stimulation (RNS) at 2 to 3 Hz, with >100% increment on fast RNS (20 to 30 Hz) or immediately after 10 sec of maximum exercise (postexercise facilitation).

LABORATORY TESTS

Check P/Q calcium channel antibody titers (commercially available).

IMAGING STUDIES

Screen for an underlying malignancy. Presentation with LEMS may precede diagnosis of SCLC by up to 5 yr. Chest radiograph or CT of the chest may be required every 6 to 12 mo for SCLC.

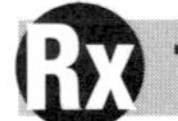

TREATMENT

NONPHARMACOLOGIC THERAPY

Symptomatic treatment for autonomic dysfunction.

ACUTE GENERAL Rx

- Anticholinesterase agents (pyridostigmine 30 to 60 mg q4-6h) may yield some improvement.
- Guanidine hydrochloride: start 5 to 10 mg/kg/day up to 30 mg/kg/day in 3-day intervals.
- Plasma exchange (200 to 250 ml/kg over 10 to 14 days) or IV immunoglobulins (2 g/kg over 2 to 5 days) often produce significant, temporary improvement.
- Prednisone 1.0 to 1.5 mg/kg/day can be gradually tapered over months to minimal effective dose.
- Azathioprine can be given alone or in combination with prednisone. Give up to 2.5 mg/kg/day. If patient is intolerant, can administer cyclosporine up to 3 mg/kg/day instead.
- 3,4-diaminopyridine (3,4-DAP) 10 to 20 mg PO qid (maximum of 100 mg/day) may improve muscle strength and reduce autonomic symptoms in up to 85% of patients in uncontrolled series. It is available in Europe and may be available in the U.S. on a compassionate use basis.

CHRONIC Rx

Treat underlying malignancy if present.

DISPOSITION

- Gradually progressive weakness leading to impaired mobility if untreated
- Clinical remission may occur with chronic immunosuppressive therapy in 43% of cases
- Possible substantial improvement with successful treatment of underlying malignancy

REFERRAL

To a neurologist (recommended) because of infrequency of this disease and risks associated with some treatments. Referral to specialist centers for 3,4-DAP therapy may be warranted in the U.S. Surgical referral for tumor debulking in paraneoplastic forms.

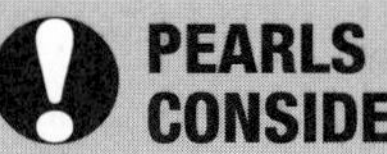

PEARLS & CONSIDERATIONS

COMMENTS

- Prominent autonomic symptoms (dry eyes, dry mouth, impotence, orthostasis) are often the clue to the diagnosis in the appropriate clinical context.
- Many drugs may worsen weakness and should be used only if absolutely necessary. Included are succinylcholine, d tubocurarine, quinine, quinidine, procainamide, aminoglycoside antibiotics, β-blockers, and calcium channel blockers.

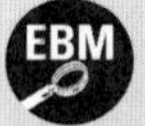

EVIDENCE

Limited evidence from randomized, controlled trials has shown that either 3,4-diaminopyridine or IV immunoglobulin improved muscle strength scores and compound muscle action potential amplitudes in patients with LEMS.[1] However, current data are insufficient to quantify this treatment effect.

Other treatment modalities have not been tested clinically in randomized, controlled trials.

Evidence-Based Reference

1. Maddison P, Newsom-Davis J: Treatment for Lambert-Eaton myasthenic syndrome, *Cochrane Rev* 18:CD003279, 2005.

SUGGESTED READINGS

Dropcho EJ: Remote neurologic manifestations of cancer, *Neurol Clin* 20:85, 2002.

Mareska M, Gutmann L: Lambert-Eaton myasthenic syndrome, *Semin Neurol* 24:149, 2004.

Sanders DB: The Lambert-Eaton myasthenic syndrome diagnosis and treatment, *Ann NY Acad Sci* 998:500, 2003.

AUTHOR: **EROBOGHENE E. UBOGU, M.B.B.S. (HONS.)**

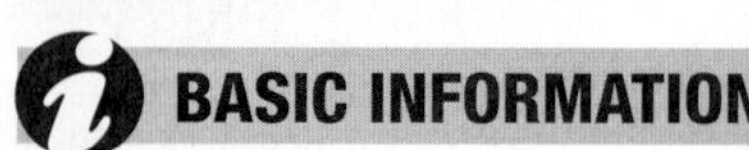

BASIC INFORMATION

DEFINITION

Cancer of the larynx, including the vocal cords (glottis), supraglottis, and subglottis.

SYNONYMS

Laryngeal cancer
Head and neck cancer (subsite); other sites include oral cavity, pharynx, paranasal sinus, and salivary glands

ICD-9CM CODES
231.0 Carcinoma of larynx

EPIDEMIOLOGY & DEMOGRAPHICS

INCIDENCE: 12,000 new cases per year in the U.S.
PEAK INCIDENCE: Sixth decade
PREDOMINANT SEX: 80% male predominance (current, with past and projected increase in female rates as a result of changing smoking habits)

PHYSICAL FINDINGS & CLINICAL PRESENTATION

Glottis:
- Early diagnosis possible because of voice change (hoarseness). Any voice change of more than 2-wk duration should prompt a laryngeal examination.
- Supraglottis:
  1. No early symptom
  2. Cervical lymphadenopathy
  3. Neck pain or ear pain
  4. Discomfort during swallowing
  5. Odynophagia
  6. Later: hoarseness, dysphagia, airway obstruction
- Subglottis: Even more subtle than supraglottic lesion; the same signs occur, only later in the course.

ETIOLOGY

- Smoking (cigarette, cigar, or pipe)
- Alcohol intake/abuse
- Diet and nutritional deficiencies
- Gastroesophageal reflux
- Voice abuse
- Chronic laryngitis
- Exposure to wood dust
- Asbestosis
- Exposure to radiation
- Possible role of human papilloma virus

DIAGNOSIS

DIFFERENTIAL DIAGNOSIS

- Laryngitis
- Allergic and nonallergic rhinosinusitis
- Gastroesophageal reflux
- Voice abuse leading to hoarseness
- Laryngeal papilloma
- Vocal cord paralysis attributable to a neurologic condition or entrapment of the recurrent laryngeal nerve caused by mediastinal compression
- Tracheomalacia

STAGING:
Supraglottic:
- T1: Tumor limited to one subsite with normal cord mobility
- T2: Tumor invades mucosa of more than one subsite (e.g., base of tongue, vallecula, pyriform sinus) without fixation of larynx
- T3: Tumor limited to larynx with vocal cord fixation or invasion of postcricoid area or preepiglottis
- T4: Tumor invades thyroid cartilage or extends into soft tissue of the neck, thyroid, or esophagus

Glottic:
- T1: Tumor limited to vocal cord with normal mobility
- T1a: Tumor limited to one vocal cord
- T1b: Tumor involves both vocal cords
- T2: Tumor extends to supra or subglottis or impairs cord mobility
- T3: Tumor limited to larynx with cord fixation
- T4: Tumor invades through cartilage or other tissues beyond larynx

Stage grouping:
- Stage I: T1, N0, M0
- Stage II: T2, N0, M0
- Stage III: T3, N0, M0
- T1, T2, T3, N1, M0
- Stage IV: T4, N0, N1, M0
- Any T, N2, N3, M0
- Any T, any N or M >0

WORKUP

- Laboratory: none
- Endoscopic laryngeal inspection
- After (and only after) diagnosis of the malignancy, imaging with CT or MRI should be undertaken to stage the disease

HISTOLOGIC CLASSIFICATION

Epithelial cancers:
- Squamous cell carcinoma in situ
- Superficially invasive cancer
- Verrucous carcinoma
- Pseudosarcoma
- Anaplastic cancer
- Transitional cell carcinoma
- Lymphoepithelial cancer
- Adenocarcinoma
- Neuroendocrine tumors, including small cell and carcinoid

Sarcomas:
- Metastatic malignancies

TREATMENT

ACUTE GENERAL Rx

- Early stage (T or T_2) has two options:
  1. Conservative surgery (partial laryngectomy) with neck dissection
  2. Primary radiation
- Intermediate stage has four options:
  1. Primary radiation alone
  2. Supraglottic laryngectomy with neck dissection
  3. Supraglottic laryngectomy with postoperative radiation
  4. Chemotherapy with radiation
- Advanced stage:
  1. Chemotherapy and radiation with total laryngectomy reserved for treatment failure

Glottis:
- Carcinoma in situ
  1. Microexcision
  2. Laser vaporization
  3. Radiation
- Early stage (T or T_2) has two options:
  1. Voice conservation surgery
  2. Radiation
- Intermediate stage (T_3)
  1. Combined radiation and chemotherapy (cisplatin and 5-fluoruracil)
  2. Total laryngectomy for treatment failure
- Advanced stage (T_4)
  1. Combined radiation and chemotherapy
  2. Total laryngectomy and neck dissection followed by postoperative radiation in unfavorable lesion or treatment failure

Subglottis:
- Total laryngectomy and approximate neck surgery to excise the tumor, followed by radiation

Unresected cancers:
- Induction chemotherapy and radiation followed by neck dissection in chemosensitive tumors, or by laryngectomy and neck dissection in chemoresistant tumors
- If hypopharyngeal involvement exists: laryngopharyngectomy, neck dissection, and postoperative radiation

DISPOSITION

Supraglottis 5-yr control:
- T_1 95% to 100%
- T_2 80% to 90%
- T_3 65% to 85%
- T_4 40% to 55%

Glottis 5-yr control:
- T_1 95% to 100%
- T_2 50% to 85%
- T_3 35% to 85%
- T_4 20% to 65%

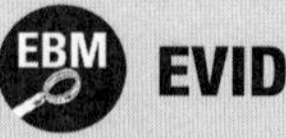

EVIDENCE

Expert opinion supports the use of surgery in the management of laryngeal cancer. Although there have been no definitive studies that compare the primary treatment options for laryngeal cancer, there is a consensus that surgery is effective as a primary treatment.[1] Ⓒ

Expert opinion supports the use of radiation therapy in the treatment of cancer of the head and neck, including laryngeal cancer. Few definitive studies have compared the primary treatment options for laryngeal cancer, but there is a consensus that radiation therapy is effective as a primary treatment of cancer of the larynx. It is also effective as an adjunctive treatment when surgical resection has been carried out as the primary treatment.[1] C

There is good evidence that accelerated/hyperfractionated radiation therapy (RT) regimens are superior to conventional RT in producing locoregional disease control. However, the overall survival benefits are unclear. Randomized, controlled trials (RCTs) have shown that accelerated/hyperfractionated RT regimens significantly increase locoregional disease control compared with conventional RT. However, disease-free survival and overall survival were not significantly different between the two RT regimens.[2] A

A recent analysis within a larger meta-analysis of RCTs in patients with locally advanced squamous cell carcinoma of the head and neck found that, for patients treated with RT as a sole therapy, hyperfractionated RT was superior to other RT protocols.[3] A

Concomitant use of chemotherapy with surgery and radiation therapy is of benefit in the treatment of head and neck cancer. Data suggest that concurrent chemoradiation is superior to alternative schedules. Two RCTs each compared the use of concomitant cisplatin with postoperative radiotherapy versus radiotherapy alone after surgical resection of mucosal squamous cell cancer of the head and neck. Both studies found that the use of cisplatin concurrent to postoperative radiotherapy significantly reduced the incidence of locoregional failure. Both RCTs, however, reported that the use of cisplatin was associated with a greater incidence of adverse effects.[4,5] A

One RCT also demonstrated that the concomitant use of cisplatin significantly improved 5-yr survival rates compared with radiotherapy alone.[4] A

There is some evidence that the addition of cetuximab to treatment regimens is effective in the treatment of head and neck cancer. An RCT compared cetuximab plus high-dose RT with RT alone in 424 patients with locally advanced head and neck cancer (oropharynx, hypopharynx, and larynx). No patients had had previous surgery. This study found that treatment with cetuximab plus RT resulted in significantly increased rates of locoregional control, disease-free survival, and overall survival (median, 49 mo vs. 29 mo; 3-yr survival, 55% vs. 45%) compared with RT alone.[6] A

There is limited evidence that the use of retinoic acid is effective in preventing the development of a new second primary tumor of the aerodigestive tract. Another recent RCT involving 151 patients with primary head and neck cancer compared isotretinoin (at high or moderate doses) with placebo over a 3-yr period. The study found that there were no significant differences in the incidence of new second primary carcinomas between the treatment groups.[7] B

Evidence-Based References

1. National Comprehensive Cancer Network: NCCN Clinical Practice Guidelines in Oncology, *Head Neck Cancer* 2007. C

2. Bourhis J et al: Phase III randomized trial of very accelerated radiation therapy compared with conventional radiation therapy in squamous cell head and neck cancer: a GORTEC trial, *J Clin Oncol* 24: 2873-2878, 2006. A

3. Budach W et al: A meta-analysis of hyperfractionated and accelerated radiotherapy and combined chemotherapy and radiotherapy regimens in unresected locally advanced squamous cell carcinoma of the head and neck, *BMC Cancer* 6:28, 2006. A

4. Bernier J et al: Postoperative irradiation with or without concomitant chemotherapy for locally advanced head and neck cancer, *N Engl J Med* 350: 1945-1952, 2004. A

5. Cooper JS et al: Postoperative concurrent radiotherapy and chemotherapy in high-risk squamous-cell carcinoma of the head and neck, *N Engl J Med* 350:1937-1944, 2004.

6. Bonner JA et al: Radiotherapy plus cetuximab for squamous-cell carcinoma of the head and neck, *N Engl J Med* 354:567-578, 2006.

7. Perry CF et al: Chemoprevention of head and neck cancer with retinoids: a negative result. *Arch Otolaryngol Head Neck Surg* 131:198-203, 2005.

AUTHOR: **FRED F. FERRI, M.D.**

Laryngitis

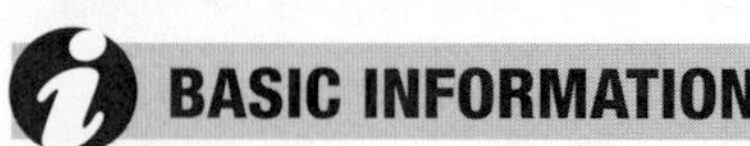

BASIC INFORMATION

DEFINITION

Laryngitis is an acute or chronic inflammation of the laryngeal mucous membranes.

SYNONYMS

Lower respiratory tract infection

ICD-9CM CODES
464.0 Acute laryngitis
476.0 Chronic laryngitis

EPIDEMIOLOGY & DEMOGRAPHICS

It is a common illness in both genders and all age groups, but the diagnosis is imprecise and, therefore, statistics are not readily available with respect to incidence and prevalence.

PHYSICAL FINDINGS & CLINICAL PRESENTATION

ACUTE LARYNGITIS:

- Clinical syndrome characterized by the onset of hoarseness, voice breaks, or episodes of aphonia; may also have accompanying sore throat, cough, nasal congestion, and rhinorrhea
- Usually associated with viral upper respiratory infection
- Larynx with diffuse erythema, edema, and vascular engorgement of the vocal folds, and occasionally mucosal ulceration
- In young children subglottis is often affected, resulting in airway narrowing with marked hoarseness, inspiratory stridor, dyspnea, and restlessness
- Respiratory compromise rare in adults

CHRONIC LARYNGITIS: Characterized by hoarseness or dysphonia persisting for longer than 2 wk

ETIOLOGY

ACUTE LARYNGITIS:

- Most often caused by viruses so treatment consists of supportive measures as outlined in "Nonpharmacologic Therapy" section.
- Studies evaluating the use of antibiotics (erythromycin, penicillin) in acute laryngitis failed to show objective clinical benefit over placebo so they are not routinely recommended. Antibiotics and other antimicrobials may be indicated in cases in which specific treatable pathogens are identified.
- Avoid decongestants because of their drying effect.
- Guaifenesin may be a useful adjunct as a mucolytic agent.
- In GERD-associated laryngitis use acid-suppressive therapy (H_2 blockers, proton pump inhibitors) and nocturnal antireflux precautions.

CHRONIC LARYNGITIS:

- Results from any of the following: tuberculosis, usually through bronchogenic spread; leprosy, from nasopharyngeal or oropharyngeal spread; syphilis, in secondary and tertiary stages; rhinoscleroma, extending from the nose and nasopharynx; actinomycosis; histoplasmosis; blastomycosis; paracoccidiomycosis; coccidiosis; candidiasis; aspergillosis; sporotrichosis; rhinosporidiosis; parasitic infections including leishmaniasis and Clinostomum infection following raw fresh-water fish ingestion.
- Noninfectious causes of both acute and chronic laryngitis include malignancy, voice abuse (singers), GERD, and chemical or environmental irritants such as cigarettes and allergens. Other causes of inflammatory or granulomatous lesions of the larynx include relapsing polychondritis, Wegener's granulomatosis, and sarcoidosis.

Dx DIAGNOSIS

DIFFERENTIAL DIAGNOSIS

- Young children with signs of airway obstruction:
  - Supraglottitis (epiglottitis)
  - Laryngotracheobronchitis
  - Tracheitis
  - Foreign body aspiration
- Adults with persistent hoarseness, consider noninfectious causes of laryngitis as listed previously

WORKUP

- History and physical examination: diagnosis is usually apparent.
- Laryngoscopy for severe or persistent cases.
- Laryngeal cultures should be performed if a cause other than acute viral infection is suspected.
- Imaging not indicated unless there is evidence of airway compromise. Obtain plain radiographs of neck, anteroposterior and lateral views, to differentiate laryngitis from acute laryngotracheobronchitis or supraglottitis.

Rx TREATMENT

NONPHARMACOLOGIC THERAPY

- Rest the voice.
- Use an air humidifier.
- Ensure adequate hydration. Avoid alcohol and caffeine because of diuretic effect.

ACUTE GENERAL Rx

- Antibiotics and other antimicrobials: indicated only when a specific pathogen is isolated; commonly employed antibacterial agents are macrolides (clarithromycin 500 mg by mouth bid for 5 to 7 days or azithromycin 500 mg followed by 250 mg once daily for 4 to 5 days if the cause of laryngitis is found to be *Mycoplasma pneumoniae* or *Chlamydiophila pneumoniae* (the new name for what was formerly known as *Chlamydia pneumoniae*)
- Avoid decongestants because of their drying effect.
- Guaifenesin may be a useful adjunct as a mucolytic agent.
- In GERD-associated laryngitis use acid-suppressive therapy (H_2 blockers, proton pump inhibitors) and nocturnal antireflux precautions.

DISPOSITION

Uncomplicated laryngitis is usually benign, with gradual resolution of symptoms.

REFERRAL

- If symptoms persist for >2 wk, refer to otolaryngologist for laryngoscopy.
- Consider referral to gastroenterologist if GERD is suspected.

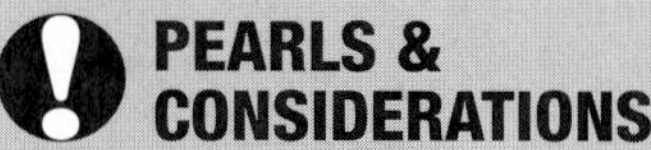

PEARLS & CONSIDERATIONS

- Most cases of uncomplicated acute laryngitis are viral in origin, and bacterial agents should not be routinely administered.
- A recent Cochrane analysis found no evidence for the use of empiric antibiotics in adults with laryngitis.
- The most difficult clinical challenge is often convincing patients with acute laryngitis that they do not need and will not benefit from antibacterial agents.

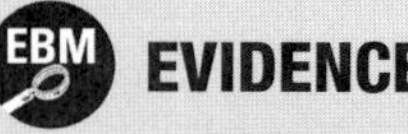

EVIDENCE

Available data in a Cochrane Review indicate that antibiotics are of limited use for most patients with laryngitis.[1] Ⓐ

Evidence-Based Reference

1. Reveiz L et al: Antibiotics for acute laryngitis in adults. *Cochrane Database Syst Rev* 2:CD004783, 2007. Ⓐ

SUGGESTED READINGS

Ebell MH: Antibiotics for acute laryngitis in adults, *Am Fam Physician* 72:76, 2005.

Mehanna HM et al: Fungal laryngitis in immunocompetent patients, *J Laryngol Otol* 118(5):379, 2004.

Reveiz L et al: Antibiotics for acute laryngitis in adults, *Cochrane Database Syst Rev* CD004783, 2005.

AUTHORS: **GLENN G. FORT, M.D., M.P.H.,** and **DENNIS J. MIKOLICH, M.D.**

BASIC INFORMATION

DEFINITION

Acute laryngotracheobronchitis is a viral infection of the upper and lower respiratory tract leading to erythema and edema of the tracheal walls and narrowing of the subglottic region.

SYNONYMS

Croup

ICD-9CM CODES
464.4 Croup

EPIDEMIOLOGY & DEMOGRAPHICS

- Croup is primarily a disease of children occurring between the ages of 1 and 6 yr.
- The peak incidence of croup is the second yr of life (50 cases/1000 children).
- Most cases occur in the fall and represent parainfluenza type 1 viral infection.
- Winter outbreaks usually represent infection by influenza A and B viruses.
- Croup accounts for 10% to 15% of lower respiratory tract infections in young children.
- Boys are affected more often than girls.

PHYSICAL FINDINGS & CLINICAL PRESENTATION

Most children with croup present with symptoms of an upper respiratory infection for several days.

- Rhinorrhea
- Cough
- Low-grade fever
- Barking cough that usually occurs at night and awakes the child
- Sore throat
- Stridor
- Apprehension
- Use of accessory muscles of respiration
- Tachypnea
- Tachycardia
- Wheezing

ETIOLOGY

- Parainfluenza viruses (types 1, 2, and 3) are the most common causes of croup in the U.S.
- Influenza A and B, although not common causes of croup, do lead to more severe cases of the disease.
- Adenovirus.
- Respiratory syncytial virus.
- *Mycoplasma pneumoniae* (rare).

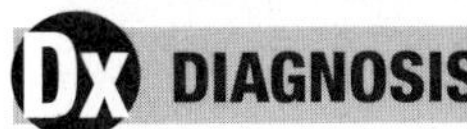

DIAGNOSIS

The diagnosis of croup is usually based on the characteristic clinical presentation of a young child between the ages of 1 and 6 yr waking up with a barking cough ("seal's bark") and stridor.

DIFFERENTIAL DIAGNOSIS

- Spasmodic croup
- Epiglottitis
- Bacterial tracheitis
- Angioneurotic edema
- Diphtheria
- Peritonsillar abscess
- Retropharyngeal abscess
- Smoke inhalation
- Foreign body

WORKUP

- The workup of a child with croup is to differentiate viral laryngotracheobronchitis from noninfectious causes of stridor and epiglottitis caused by *H. influenzae.*
- The clinical presentation and plain films of the soft tissues of the neck assist in differentiating viral from nonviral and noninfectious causes.

LABORATORY TESTS

- Laboratory tests are not often used to make the diagnosis of viral tracheobronchitis.
- CBC, viral serology, and tissue cultures can be ordered and may detect the infecting agent in up to 65% of cases.
- Pulse oximetry and ABG determination for patients with tachypnea and respiratory distress.

IMAGING STUDIES

- Plain (AP and lateral) films of the soft tissues of the neck may show the classic radiographic finding of subglottic stenosis or "steeple" sign.
- CT scan of the soft tissues of the neck may be performed in cases in which the differentiation between croup, epiglottitis, and noninfectious is more difficult.
- Direct visualization via laryngoscopy may be useful in some situations under a controlled setting.

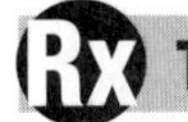

TREATMENT

Treatment of croup focuses on airway management.

NONPHARMACOLOGIC THERAPY

- Oxygen
- Cool mist
- Hot steam

ACUTE GENERAL Rx

- 0.25 to 0.75 ml of 2.25% racemic epinephrine every 20 min is used in children with severe respiratory symptoms, rest stridor, and impending intubation.
- Corticosteroids (e.g., dexamethasone 0.6 mg/kg IV or PO, prednisone 2 mg/kg/day) have been shown to be effective.
- Budesonide, a nebulized corticosteroid given at 4 mg, has been shown to improve symptoms in patients with moderate to severe croup.

DISPOSITION

- Croup is usually benign and self-limited, resolving within 3 to 4 days.
- Complications include:
  1. Airway obstruction
  2. Otitis media
  3. Pneumonia
  4. Dehydration

REFERRAL

If intubation is needed (rarely), an emergency consultation with ENT and/or anesthesiology is recommended.

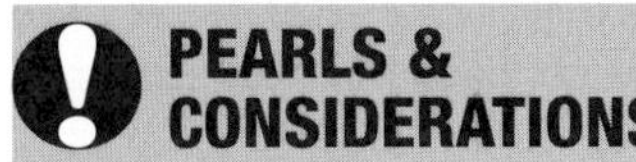

PEARLS & CONSIDERATIONS

COMMENTS

- Most patients with croup can be managed at home (e.g., patients without stridor and in no respiratory distress).
- Hospitalization and observation is required for children with moderate to severe croup (e.g., rest stridor, respiratory distress refractory to the previously mentioned acute treatments).

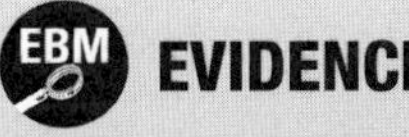

EVIDENCE

There is evidence that corticosteroids are effective in the management of croup.

A systematic review of children with croup treated in pediatric assessment units and hospitals found that corticosteroid treatment is effective in relieving symptoms at 6 hr and 12 hr after administration. Treatment reduced the duration of hospital stay and was associated with fewer return visits and/or readmissions, as well as with reduced use of epinephrine.[1] Ⓐ

Evidence-Based Reference

1. Russell K et al: Glucocorticoids for croup. *Cochrane Database Syst Rev* 1:CD001955, 2004. Ⓐ

SUGGESTED READING

Cherry JD: Croup, *N Engl J Med* 358:384, 2008.

AUTHORS: **GLENN G. FORT, M.D., M.P.H.,** and **DENNIS J. MIKOLICH, M.D.**

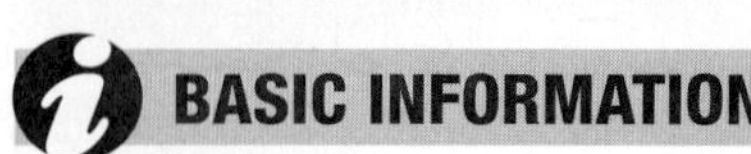

BASIC INFORMATION

DEFINITION

Lead is a potent, pervasive neurotoxicant. Lead poisoning refers to multisystem abnormalities resulting from excessive lead exposure.

SYNONYMS

Plumbism

ICD-9CM CODES
984.0 Lead poisoning

EPIDEMIOLOGY & DEMOGRAPHICS

- Lead poisoning is most common in children ages 1 to 5 yr (17,000 cases/100,000 persons). The highest rates are among blacks, those with low income, and urban children.
- In 1991 the Centers for Disease Control and Prevention (CDC) lowered the definition of a safe blood lead level to <10 μg/dl of whole blood (a blood lead level of 25 μg/dl was considered acceptable before 1991).
- It is estimated that >15% of preschoolers in the U.S. have a blood lead level >15 μg/dl.

PHYSICAL FINDINGS & CLINICAL PRESENTATION

- Findings vary with the degree of toxicity. Examination may be normal in patients with mild toxicity.
- Myalgias, irritability, headache, and general fatigue may be present initially.
- Abdominal cramping, constipation, weight loss, tremor, paresthesias and peripheral neuritis, seizures, and coma may occur with severe toxicity.
- Motor neuropathy is common in children with lead poisoning; learning disorders are also frequent.

ETIOLOGY

Chronic, repeated exposure to paint containing lead, plumbing, storage of batteries, pottery, or lead soldering. Concentration of lead is generally highest in lead-based paint on exterior surfaces. Among interior surfaces, windows are most likely to have the highest lead content.

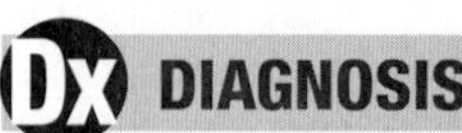

DIAGNOSIS

DIFFERENTIAL DIAGNOSIS

- Polyneuropathies from other sources
- Anxiety disorder, attention deficit disorder
- Malabsorption, acute abdomen
- Iron-deficiency anemia

WORKUP

Laboratory screening: all U.S. children should be considered to be at risk for lead poisoning and should be screened routinely starting at age 1 yr for low-risk children and age 6 mo for high-risk children.

LABORATORY TESTS

- Venous blood lead level: normal level, <10 μg/dl; levels of 50 to 70 μg/dl, indicative of moderate toxicity; levels >70 μg/dl, associated with severe poisoning
- Mild anemia with basophilic stippling on peripheral smear
- Elevated zinc protoporphyrin levels or free erythrocyte protoporphyrin level
- An increased body burden of lead with previous high-level exposure in patients with occupational lead poisoning can be demonstrated by measuring the excretion of lead in urine after premedication with calcium ethylenediamine tetraacetic acid (EDTA) or another chelating agent

IMAGING STUDIES

- Imaging studies are generally not necessary.
- A plain abdominal film can visualize lead particles in the gut.
- "Lead lines" may be noted on x-ray films of long bones.

Rx TREATMENT

NONPHARMACOLOGIC THERAPY

- Provide adequate amounts of calcium, iron, zinc, and protein in patient's diet
- Family education on sources of lead exposure and potential adverse health effects

ACUTE GENERAL Rx

- For children with blood levels of 10 to 19 mcg/dl, the CDC recommends nonpharmacologic interventions (see "Nonpharmacologic Therapy").
- For children with blood levels between 20 and 44 μg/dl, the CDC recommendations include case management by a qualified social worker, clinical management, environmental assessment, and lead hazard control. Chelation therapy should be considered in children with refractory blood lead levels.

Chelation therapy is indicated in children with blood lead levels >45 μg/dl:

- Succimer (DMSA) 10 mg/kg PO q8h for 5 days then q12h for 2 wk can be used in patients with levels between 45 and 70 μg/dl.
- Edetate calcium disodium (EDTA) and dimercaprol (BAL) are effective in patients with severe toxicity.
- Use of both EDTA and DMSA is indicated in children with blood levels >70 μg/dl.
- d-Penicillamine (Cuprimine) can also be used for lead poisoning, but it is not FDA approved for this condition.

CHRONIC Rx

- Reduce exposure, remove any potential lead sources.
- Correct iron deficiency and any other nutritional deficiencies.
- Recheck blood lead level 7 to 21 days after chelation therapy.

DISPOSITION

Patients with mild to moderate toxicity generally improve without any residual deficits. The presence of encephalopathy at diagnosis is a poor prognostic sign. Residual neurologic deficits may persist in these patients. Chelation therapy seems to slow the progression of renal insufficiency in patients with mildly elevated body lead burden.

REFERRAL

If exposure to lead is work related, it should be reported to the Office of the United States Occupational Safety and Health Administration (OSHA). Follow-up testing is mandatory in all patients after an abnormal screening blood lead level.

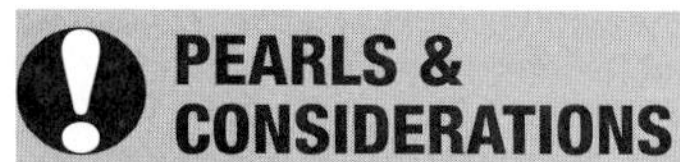

PEARLS & CONSIDERATIONS

COMMENTS

- Even blood lead concentrations <10 mcg/dl are inversely associated with children's IQ scores at age 3 and 5 yr.
- Screening of household members of affected individuals is recommended.
- In children with blood lead levels of >45 mg/dl, treatment with succimer does not improve scores on tests of cognition, behavior, or neuropsychological function.
- Lead toxicity may delay growth and pubertal development in girls.
- Low-level environmental lead exposure may accelerate progressive renal insufficiency in patients without diabetes who have chronic renal disease. Repeated chelation therapy may improve renal function and slow the progression of renal failure.

SUGGESTED READINGS

Canfield RL et al: Intellectual impairment in children with blood lead concentrations below 10 mcg/deciliter, *N Engl J Med* 348:1517, 2003.

Kemper AR et al: Follow-up testing among children with elevated screening blood lead levels, *JAMA* 293:2232, 2005.

Lin JL et al: Environmental lead exposure and progression of chronic renal diseases in patients without diabetes, *N Engl J Med* 348:277, 2003.

Selevan SG et al: Blood lead concentration and delayed puberty in girls, *N Engl J Med* 348:1527, 2003.

AUTHOR: **FRED F. FERRI, M.D.**

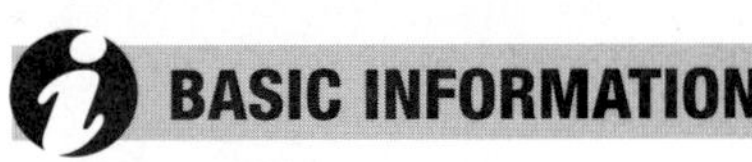

BASIC INFORMATION

DEFINITION

Legg-Calvé-Perthes disease is a self-limited disorder of unknown etiology caused by ischemia of the immature femoral head that leads to bone necrosis and variable amounts of collapse during the reparative process.

SYNONYMS

Coxa plana
Capital femoral osteochondrosis

ICD-9CM CODES
732.1 Perthes' disease

EPIDEMIOLOGY & DEMOGRAPHICS

PREVALENCE: One case in 1300 children
PREDOMINANT SEX: Male/female ratio of 4:1
PREDOMINANT AGE: 3 to 10 yr

PHYSICAL FINDINGS & CLINICAL PRESENTATION

- Initial symptom: usually a mildly painful limp
- Pain referred down the inner aspect of the thigh to the knee
- Moderate restriction of motion resulting from hip synovitis (abduction and internal rotation are especially limited)
- Pain at the extremes of movement and tenderness over anterior hip joint

ETIOLOGY

Unknown

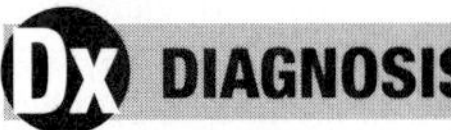

DIAGNOSIS

DIFFERENTIAL DIAGNOSIS

- Transient synovitis
- Low-grade septic arthritis
- Juvenile rheumatoid arthritis

WORKUP

Diagnosis is usually based on the physical findings and eventual radiographic findings.

IMAGING STUDIES

- Plain roentgenography to establish the diagnosis (Fig. 1-177)
- AP and frog-leg lateral radiographs
- Technetlum bone scanning to help confirm the diagnosis in early cases

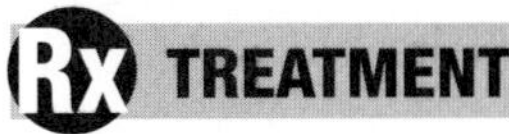

TREATMENT

ACUTE GENERAL Rx

- A brief period of bed rest (1 to 3 days) followed by bracing (except in mild cases)
- Bracing possibly required for 2 to 3 yr in small percent of patients

DISPOSITION

- Prognosis depends on age of patient and degree of involvement of the femoral head at onset.
- Young patients (<6 yr) with minimal involvement do well.
- Older patients (>8 yr) often do poorly.
- A few patients eventually develop degenerative arthritis.

REFERRAL

For orthopedic consultation when diagnosis is suspected

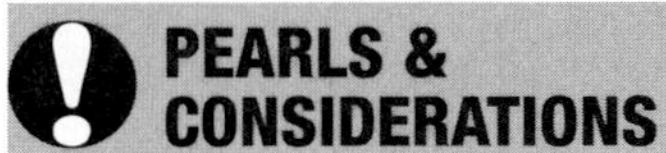

PEARLS & CONSIDERATIONS

Both the etiology and treatment of Legg-Calvé-Perthes disease remain controversial. Treatment recommendations vary widely and continue to evolve.

COMMENTS

There is great uncertainty regarding treatment and its effect on outcome. Bracing may have no effect whatsoever on the end result.

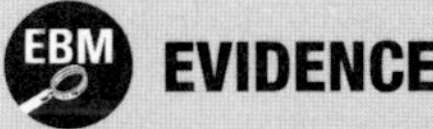

EVIDENCE

A prospective study found no difference in outcome among hips with no treatment, those treated with bracing, and those treated with range-of-motion therapy in children who had a chronological age of 8 years or less or a skeletal age of 6 years or less.[1] B

Evidence-Based Reference

1. Herring JA et al: Legg-Calve-Perthes disease. Part II: Prospective multicenter study of the effect of treatment on outcome, *J Bone Joint Surg Am* 86-A: 2121-2134, 2004. B

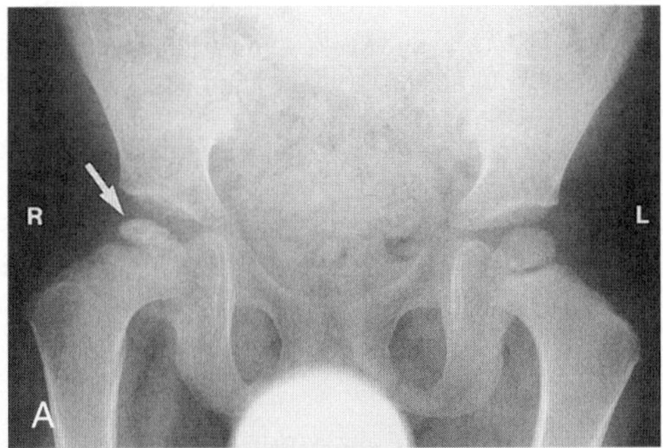

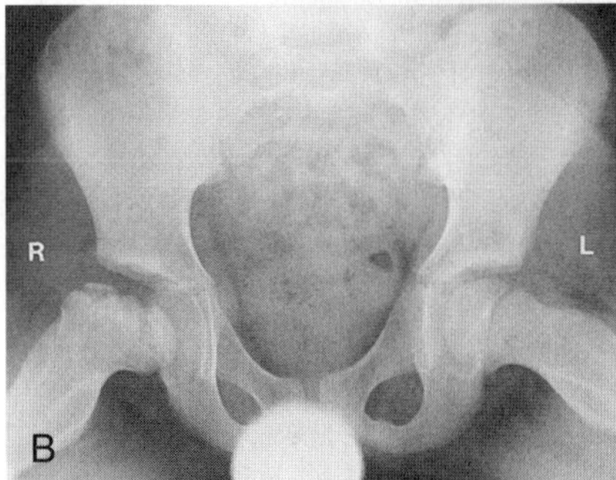

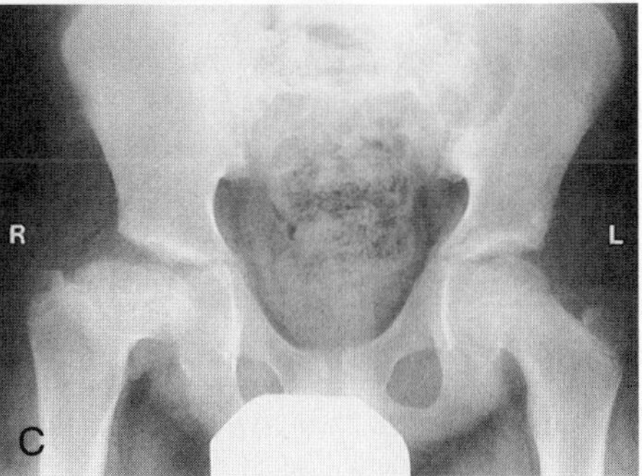

FIGURE 1-177 Legg-Calvé-Perthes disease. A, An anteroposterior view of the pelvis demonstrates fragmentation and sclerosis of the right femoral epiphysis *(arrow)* in this 6-year-old boy. **B,** A follow-up film obtained 8 years later shows continuing deformity resulting from the osteonecrosis. The patient developed significant degenerative arthritis **(C)** by the age of 12 years. (From Mettler FA [ed]: *Primary care radiology,* Philadelphia, 2000, WB Saunders.)

SUGGESTED READINGS

Dillman JR, Hernandez RJ: MRI of Legg-Calvé Perthes disease, *Am J Roentgenol* 193:1394, 2009.
Domzalski ME et al: The proximal femoral growth plate in Perthes disease, *Clin Orthop Relat Res* 458: 150, 2007.
Frick SL: Evaluation of the child who has hip pain, *Orthop Clin North Am* 37:133, 2006.
Gough-Palmer A, McHugh K: Investigating hip pain in a well child, *BMJ* 334:1216, 2007.
Herring JA et al: Legg-Calvé-Perthes disease: part I: classification of radiographs with use of the modified lateral pillar and Stulberg classifications, *J Bone Joint Surg Am* 86A:2103, 2004.
Herring J et al: Legg-Calvé-Perthes disease: part II: prospective multicenter study of the effect of treatment on outcome, *J Bone Joint Surg Am* 86A:2121, 2004.
Rosenfeld SB et al: Legg-Calvé-Perthes disease: a review of cases with onset before six years of age, *J Bone Joint Surg* 89:2712, 2007.
Vosmaer A et al: Coagulation abnormalities in Legg-Calvé-Perthes disease, *J Bone Joint Surg Am* 92: 121, 2010.

AUTHOR: **LONNIE R. MERCIER, M.D.**

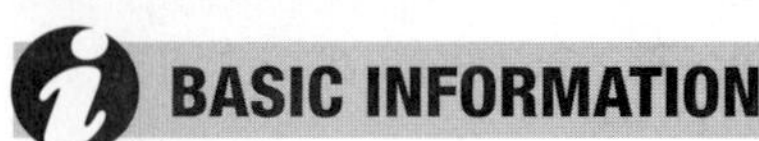

BASIC INFORMATION

DEFINITION

Leishmaniasis is an infectious disease caused by a heterogeneous group of protozoan parasites belonging to the genus *Leishmania* and resulting in a variety of different clinical syndromes.

SYNONYMS

Kala azar
Old world leishmaniasis
New world leishmaniasis

ICD-9CM CODES
085.9 Leishmaniasis

EPIDEMIOLOGY & DEMOGRAPHICS

INCIDENCE: Approximately 2 million total new cases and 500,000 visceral cases occur each yr with almost 400 million people at risk for the disease.

- Can be classified geographically into new world versus old world disease.
- Infection can be divided into cutaneous, mucocutaneous, visceral disease.
- Incubation period: from 1 wk to many mo for cutaneous and mucosal leishmaniasis; 2 to 6 mo (range is 10 days to years) for visceral leishmaniasis.
- Mode of transmission: by the female sandfly vector; can also be spread via shared needles, blood transfusions, vertically from the mother to fetus, or sexually.
- Cutaneous leishmaniasis has been reported in U.S. military personnel in Iraq (more than 500 cases from 2002 to 2004).
- Travelers to endemic areas have become infected after <1 week exposure.

PHYSICAL FINDINGS & CLINICAL PRESENTATION

Cutaneous syndrome

- Localized cutaneous leishmaniasis
- Mucosal leishmaniasis
- Leishmania recidivans
- Diffuse cutaneous leishmaniasis

Visceral syndrome

- Viscerotrophic leishmaniasis: fever, chronic fatigue, malaise, cough, intermittent diarrhea, and abdominal pain. Signs include adenopathy, hepatosplenomegaly, hyperpigmentation of skin, petechiae, jaundice, edema, and ascites
- Post–kala-azar dermal leishmaniasis: generalized cutaneous rash that is often papular or nodular; severe forms with desquamation of skin and mucosa

ETIOLOGY

- Old-world parasite: *Leishmania tropica, L. major, L. aethiopica, L. donovani, L. infantum*
- New-world parasite: *L. braziliensis and L. mexicana complex, L. chagasi, L.b. guyanensis, L.b. panamensis*

Dx DIAGNOSIS

DIFFERENTIAL DIAGNOSIS

- Malaria
- African trypanosomiasis
- Brucellosis
- Enteric fever
- Bacterial endocarditis
- Generalized histoplasmosis
- Chronic myelocytic leukemia
- Hodgkin's disease and other lymphomas
- Sarcoidosis
- Hepatic cirrhosis
- Tuberculosis

WORKUP

- CBC
- LFTs
- Renal panel
- Serology
- Biopsy for histology and culture
- PCR
- Bone marrow bx for visceral disease

LABORATORY TESTS

- CBC: anemia, neutropenia, thrombocytopenia, and eosinopenia
- LFTs: hypergammaglobulinemia, hypoalbuminemia, and hyperbilirubinemia
- Elevated BUN and creatinine
- Specific diagnosis confirmed by intracellular amastigote in Giemsa-stained impression smears or sectioned tissue or culture performed in NMN (Novy, MacNeal, Nicolle) or Schneider's medium
- Serologic diagnosis: ELISA, direct agglutination tests, K39 ELISA, PCR, and monoclonal antibody staining of tissue smears; ELISA and DAT on urine specimens
- Montenegro skin test

Rx TREATMENT

Nonspecific or supportive care

1. Nutritional diet
2. Antimicrobial agents for concurrent infections
3. Blood transfusions
4. Iron and vitamins

Specific antileishmanial therapy

1. Miltefosine (2.5 mg/kg/day orally in two divided doses for 28 days) now the treatment of choice for visceral disease
2. Pentavalent antimonials: sodium stibogluconate and sodium antimony gluconate
3. Lipid formations of Amphotericin B. A single dose of liposomal amphotericin B is as effective as and less expensive than conventional therapy with amphotericin B deoxycholate
4. Fluconazole 200 mg PO daily for 6 wk effective for cutaneous disease
5. Pentamidine 2 to 4 mg/kg/day for 15 doses IV
6. Other agents: allopurinol, ketoconazole, paromomycin (combined with other regimens)
7. Immunotherapy: IFN-γ
8. Local or tropical treatments and physical therapy, including thermal treatments
9. Plastic surgery

DISPOSITION

Follow-up examination is important for the early detection and treatment relapse.

REFERRAL

To infectious disease experts for accurate diagnosis and management

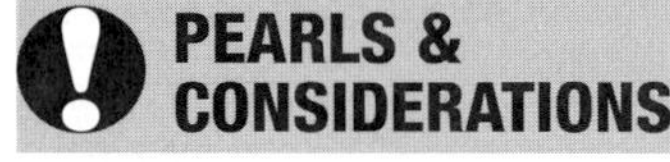

PEARLS & CONSIDERATIONS

COMMENTS

- Prevention by reservoir control-destruction of animal reservoir hosts, mass treatment of human in kala-azar–prevalent areas.
- Prevention by vector control: insecticide spraying in domestic and peridomestic areas.
- Vaccines are in various stages of development and clinical trials. None are licensed or commercially available at this time.

SUGGESTED READINGS

Drugs for parasitic infections, *Med Lett Drugs Ther* August 2004.

Jones J et al: Old world cutaneous leishmaniasis infection in children: a case series, *Arch Dis Child* 90(5):530, 2005.

Murray HW et al: Advances in leishmaniasis, *Lancet* 366:1561, 2005.

Reithinger R et al: Social impact of leishmaniasis, Afghanistan, *Emerg Infect Dis* 11(4):634, 2005.

Reithinger R, Dujardin JC: Molecular diagnosis of leishmaniasis: current status and future applications, *J Clin Microbiol* 45:21, 2007.

Schwartz E et al: New world cutaneous leishmaniasis in travellers, *Lancet Infect Dis* 63:342, 2006.

Sundar S et al: Single-dose liposomal amphotericin B for visceral leishmaniasis in India, *N Engl J Med* 362:504-512, 2010.

AUTHORS: **PATRICIA CRISTOFARO, M.D., GLENN G. FORT, M.D., M.P.H.,** and **DENNIS J. MIKOLICH, M.D.**

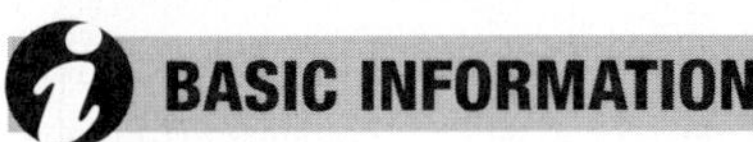

BASIC INFORMATION

DEFINITION

Leprosy is a chronic granulomatous infection of humans that primarily affects the skin and peripheral nerves.

SYNONYMS

Hansen's disease

ICD-9CM CODES

030.9 Leprosy

EPIDEMIOLOGY & DEMOGRAPHICS

- The number of cases worldwide has fallen from more than 5 million cases in 1985 to less than 1 million cases in 1998.
- Nearly 75% of the cases of leprosy are found in India, Brazil, Bangladesh, Indonesia, and Myanmar.
- More than 85% of the cases diagnosed in the U.S. are found among immigrants.
- Worldwide incidence is 650,000 new cases per year.
- Annual incidence in the U.S. is 150 new cases per year.
- Leprosy is more common in men than women (2:1).
- Leprosy can occur at any age but usually is found in young children.

PHYSICAL FINDINGS & CLINICAL PRESENTATION

- A skin lesion: most common initial presentation
- Sensory loss
- Anhidrosis
- Neuritic pain
- Palpable peripheral nerves
- Nerve damage (most commonly affected nerves are ulnar, median, common peroneal, posterior tibial, radial cutaneous nerve of the wrist, facial, and posterior auricular)
- Muscle atrophy and weakness
- Foot drop
- Claw hand and claw toes
- Lagophthalmos, nasal septal perforation, collapse of bridge of nose (Fig. 1-178, *A*), loss of eyebrows resulting in "leonine" facies
- Leprosy can present along a spectrum from simple cutaneous skin lesions with minimal sensory loss (Fig. 1-178, *B*) to severe extensive skin involvement, painful neuritis, muscle wasting and contractures, and multiple peripheral nerve damage.

ETIOLOGY

- Leprosy is caused by *Mycobacterium leprae,* an obligate intracellular acid-fast rod.
- The mode of transmission remains elusive. Spread in humans is thought to occur via the respiratory route or entry through broken skin in patients with multibacillary disease or extensive paucibacillary disease.
- Zoonotic transmission from armadillos has not been proven.
- The majority of people exposed to patients with leprosy do not develop the disease because of their natural immunity. Variants of genes in the NOD2-mediated signaling pathway (which regulates the innate immune response) are associated with susceptibility to infection with *M. leprae.*
- Incubation period is 3 to 5 yr.

Dx DIAGNOSIS

- The diagnosis of leprosy relies on a detailed history and physical examination and is established by the demonstration of acid-fast bacilli in skin smears or skin biopsies of the affected sites.
- Leprosy has been classified according to the WHO system into:
  1. Paucibacillary leprosy is defined as <5 skin lesions with no bacilli on skin smear.
  2. Multibacillary leprosy is defined as >5 skin lesions and may be skin-smear positive.
- Leprosy has also been classified more specifically according to the type of skin lesions, sensory and motor deficits, and biopsy into:
  1. Indeterminate leprosy
  2. Tuberculoid leprosy (paucibacillary [few organisms], intense inflammatory reaction; few, well-demarcated skin lesions)
  3. Borderline tuberculoid leprosy
  4. Borderline lepromatous leprosy
  5. Lepromatous leprosy (multibacillary [numerous organisms], inadequate host response; diffuse, poorly organized skin lesions)

DIFFERENTIAL DIAGNOSIS

The differential diagnosis of leprosy includes: sarcoidosis, rheumatoid arthritis, systemic lupus erythematosus, lymphomatoid granulomatosis, carpal tunnel syndrome, cutaneous leishmaniasis, fungal infections and other causes of hypopigmented, hyperpigmented, and erythematous skin lesions.

WORKUP

Any patient who presents with skin lesions and a sensory or muscle deficit should have a workup for leprosy.

LABORATORY TESTS

- *Mycobacterium leprae* cannot be cultured on artificial media. The bacteria proliferate when

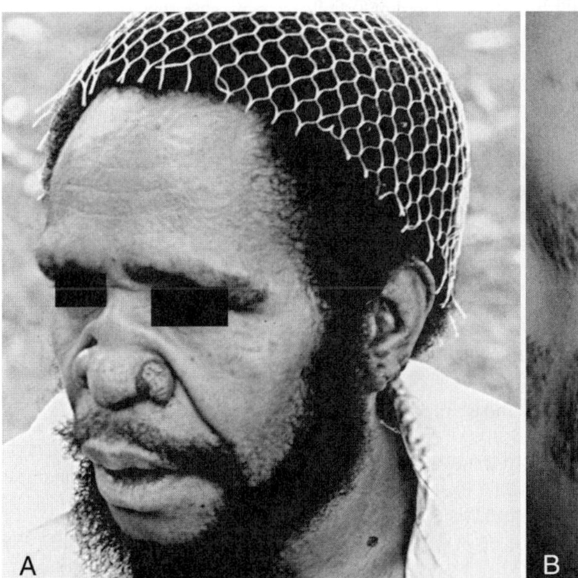

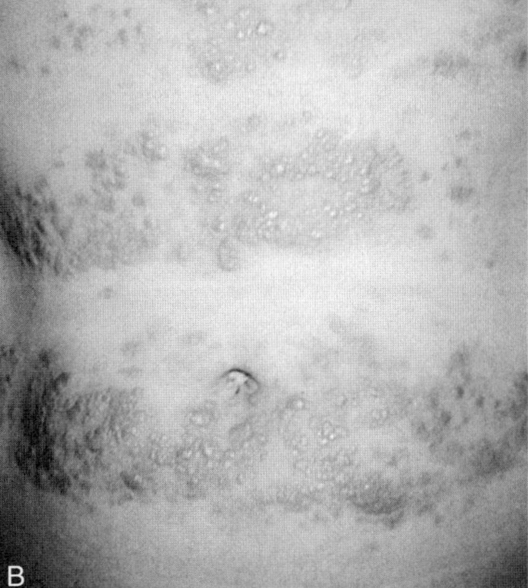

FIGURE 1-178 **A,** Advanced lepromatous leprosy with collapse of the nasal septum. **B,** Lepromatous leprosy characterized by extensive papule formation over abdomen. Minimal or no sensory loss is present in the affected areas. (**A,** From Gorbach SL: *Infectious diseases,* ed 2. Philadelphia, 1998, WB Saunders; **B,** From Mandell GL: *Mandell, Douglas, and Bennett's principles and practice of infectious diseases,* ed 5, New York, 2000, Churchill Livingstone.)

injected into the footpads of mice or armadillos and can be used for drug-sensitivity testing.

- Serologic tests, including the antibody to phenolic glycolipid 1 (PGL-1), are available and used for diagnostic confirmation and research epidemiologic studies.
- Lepromin intradermal skin test is not diagnostic and not for commercial use.
- Skin smears are taken from active sites or most commonly from the earlobe, elbows, or knees and are stained for acid-fast bacilli.
- Skin biopsies of active sites are stained for acid-fast bacilli.
- Peripheral nerve biopsy can be done in patients with sensory loss and no skin lesions. Common nerves biopsied are the radial cutaneous nerve of the wrist and the sural nerve of the ankle.

IMAGING STUDIES

Radiograph studies are usually of no benefit in the diagnosis or treatment of leprosy.

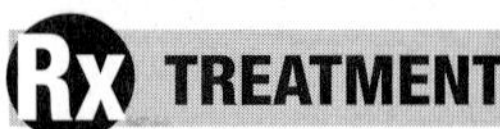

TREATMENT

NONPHARMACOLOGIC THERAPY

- Physical therapy for patients with upper and lower extremity deformities
- Proper foot care and footwear to prevent ulcer formation

ACUTE GENERAL Rx

For paucibacillary leprosy:

- Dapsone 100 mg PO qid for 6 mo in an unsupervised setting is the treatment of choice.
- Rifampin 600 mg PO qid for 6 mo in a supervised setting is the recommendation by WHO.
- Ofloxacin 400 mg qid or minocycline 100 mg qid are other alternatives.

For multibacillary leprosy:

- Rifampin 600 mg PO qid and clofazimine 300 mg PO qid for 24 mo in a supervised setting. Rifampin can be given once monthly without loss of efficacy and at less cost.
- Rifampin 100 mg PO qid and clofazimine 50 mg PO qid for 24 mo in an unsupervised setting.
- Dapsone 100 mg PO qid is sometimes added as triple therapy in this group of patients.
- Clofazimine 50 mg daily is used with dapsone for better bacteriocidal effect.

CHRONIC Rx

- If relapse occurs, the patient is treated with the same medical regimen; drug resistance is low.
- If relapse is from paucibacillary to multibacillary, the medical regimen for multibacillary should be used for therapy.

DISPOSITION

- Relapse is <1% for multibacillary and just over 1% in paucibacillary cases.
- Patients are initially followed up monthly and, when treatment is completed, every 3 to 6 mo for the next 5 to 10 yr.
- Some patients develop reactions known as erythema nodosum leprosum and reversal reaction, usually during treatment.
  1. Erythema nodosum leprosum results in tender nodules and is treated with either prednisolone 40 to 60 mg qid until the reaction is controlled and tapered or thalidomide 300 to 400 mg qid and tapered to 100 mg qid with monthly attempts to wean down further.
  2. Reactive reaction results in the development of new skin lesions with swelling and erythema of existing lesions. Treatment is with either NSAIDs or prednisolone.

REFERRAL

- National Hansen's Disease Programs (NHDP) Center in Baton Rouge, Louisiana, and 15 outpatient clinics in the U.S. offer consultations and treatment. Telephone: 1-800-642-2477.
- Directly observed therapy (DOT), much like DOT for tuberculosis, is highly desirable and should be used if feasible, at least in the first 6 to 12 mo of therapy.
- Any suspected case of leprosy merits an infectious disease consultation. Consultation with orthopedic, podiatry, ophthalmology, physical therapy, plastic surgery, and psychology are all in order for any of the potential sequelae of the disease.

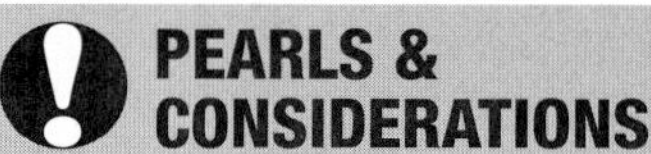

PEARLS & CONSIDERATIONS

COMMENTS

- The risk of transmission is low in patients with leprosy, and therefore no infection control precautions of hospitalized patients is needed.
- Family members and close contacts need to be examined frequently for the development of lesions.
- Dapsone or rifampin prophylaxis is not recommended in the prevention of leprosy.
- BCG vaccination has a 50% efficacy in the prevention of leprosy and may be considered.

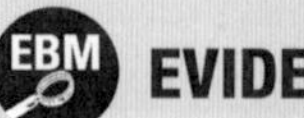

EVIDENCE

There is a relative paucity of randomized controlled trials in antileprosy treatments. The current WHO multidrug regimens have proved so successful that it would likely be deemed unethical to test alternatives, especially in light of the known increase in dapsone resistance.

Multidrug therapy (MDT) regimens, with some regional variations, continue to form the cornerstone of leprosy treatment today.

Observational studies have shown that the WHO MDT regimen, which continues to include dapsone and rifampin (and clofazimine in the case of multibacillary leprosy), improves skin lesions and is associated with low relapse rates.[1] Ⓐ

WHO recommends corticosteroids, with or without clofazimine, for treatment of severe erythema nodosum leprosum (ENL) reactions.

A randomized controlled trial of 636 newly diagnosed multibacillary (MB) leprosy patients examined whether the addition of low-dose prednisolone to MDT prevented reaction and nerve function impairment. It found that low-dose prophylactic prednisolone during the first 4 mo of MDT reduced the incidence of new reactions and nerve function impairment in the short term. The effect, however, was not sustained at 1 yr. It suggested that the presence of nerve function impairment at diagnosis may influence the response to low dose prednisolone.[2] Ⓐ

Thioamides, such as ethionamide, have not been endorsed by WHO for routine use in antileprosy treatments.

Fifty patients with lepromatous leprosy were randomly assigned to directly observed monotherapy with either ethionamide or prothionamide. Clinical improvement was noted in 74% of the patients treated with ethionamide, and in 83% of those treated with prothionamide. Because of the small number of patients included in this study, however, the results must be interpreted with caution. WHO has not endorsed the routine use of thioamides in antileprosy treatment.[3] Ⓑ

Evidence-Based References

1. Lockwood D: Leprosy, *Clin Evid*, 2007. Ⓐ

2. Smith WC et al: Steroid prophylaxis for prevention of nerve function impairment in leprosy: randomised placebo controlled trial (TRIPOD 1), *BMJ* 328:1459-1463, 2004. Ⓐ

3. Fajardo TT et al: A clinical trial of ethionamide and prothionamide for treatment of lepromatous leprosy, *Am J Trop Med Hyg* 74:457-461, 2006. Ⓑ

SUGGESTED READINGS

El-Darouti MA: Histopathological study of apparently normal skin of patients with leprosy, *Int J Dermatol* 45(3):292, 2006.

Moet FJ et al: Physical distance, genetic relationship, age, and leprosy classification are independent risk factors for leprosy in contacts of patients with leprosy, *J Infect Dis* 193(3):346, 2006.

Zhang FR et al: Genomewide association study of leprosy, *N Engl J Med* 361:2609-2618, 2009.

AUTHORS: **GLENN G. FORT, M.D., M.P.H.,** and **DENNIS J. MIKOLICH, M.D.**

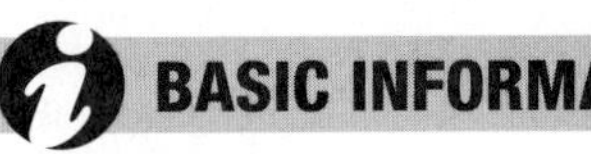

BASIC INFORMATION

DEFINITION

Leptospirosis is a zoonosis caused by the spirochete *Leptospira interrogans.*

SYNONYMS

Weil's disease

ICD-9CM CODES
100.9 Leptospirosis

EPIDEMIOLOGY & DEMOGRAPHICS

INCIDENCE (IN U.S.):

- 0.05 cases/100,000 persons
- Significant underestimation because of underreporting
- Hawaii consistently has the highest reported annual incidence rate in U.S.

PEAK INCIDENCE: Summer months, into the fall
PREDOMINANT SEX: Male (4:1)
PREDOMINANT AGE: Teenagers and young adults
GENETICS: Neonatal infection can occur.

PHYSICAL FINDINGS & CLINICAL PRESENTATION

ANICTERIC FORM:

- Milder and more common presentation of disease
- A self-limited systemic illness with two stages:
    1. Septicemic stage: presents abruptly with fevers, headache, severe myalgias, rigors, prostration, and sometimes circulatory collapse; conjunctival suffusion is common; skin rash, pharyngitis, lymphadenopathy, hepatomegaly, splenomegaly.
    2. Immune stage: occurs a few days after first stage with similar symptoms; hallmark is aseptic meningitis.

ICTERIC LEPTOSPIROSIS (WEIL'S SYNDROME):

1. Denotes severe cases, with symptoms of hepatic, renal, and vascular dysfunction
2. Biphasic course: persistence of fever, jaundice, and azotemia
3. Complications: oliguria or anuria, hemorrhage, hypotension, vascular collapse

ETIOLOGY

Caused by a spirochete, *L. interrogans*

- Infects a variety of animals, including most mammals
- Specific serotypes associated with different hosts—*pomona* in livestock, *canicola* in dogs (Fig. 1-179), and *icterohaemorrhagiae* in rodents
- Organism penetrates skin or mucous membranes through exposure to animal urine or infected water

DIAGNOSIS

DIFFERENTIAL DIAGNOSIS

- Bacterial meningitis
- Viral hepatitis
- Influenza
- Legionnaire's disease

WORKUP

Culture of blood, CSF, and urine:

- Organism can be isolated from blood or CSF during first 10 days of illness.
- Urine should be cultured after first wk and for up to 30 days after onset of illness.

LABORATORY TESTS

- Normal or elevated WBCs, at times with leukemoid reactions up to 70,000/mm^3
- Elevated transaminases or bilirubin
- Anemia, azotemia, hypoprothrombinemia in those with icteric illness
- Elevated CK in first phase
- Meningitis in both phases, but aseptic in second phase

IMAGING STUDIES

Chest radiographs to show interstitial nonlobar infiltrates

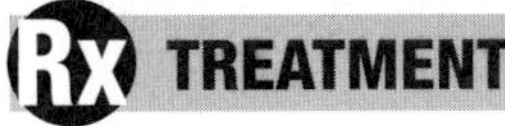

TREATMENT

NONPHARMACOLOGIC THERAPY

- Supportive
- Observation for dehydration, hypotension, renal failure, hemorrhage

ACUTE GENERAL Rx

- IV penicillin G 1 million U q4h
- Doxycycline 100 mg PO bid for 7 days
- Vitamin K administration if hypoprothrombinemia present
- Possible Jarisch-Herxheimer reaction when treated with penicillin

DISPOSITION

- In anicteric leptospirosis, antibiotics can decrease severity and duration of symptoms.
- Icteric leptospirosis, even with supportive therapy, may have a mortality as high as 10%.

REFERRAL

- If more than mild disease
- If no response to treatment

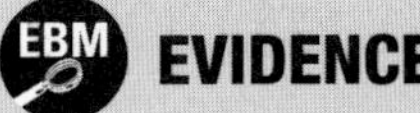

EVIDENCE

Penicillin and doxycycline may be effective in treating leptospirosis but evidence is insufficient to provide clear guidelines for practice.[1] Ⓐ

A randomized controlled trial (RCT) found that prophylactic doxycycline is no better than placebo in reducing infection rate but reduced the rate of clinical illness in those who become infected.[2] Ⓑ

An RCT found that ceftriaxone and penicillin G were equally effective for the treatment of severe leptospirosis.[3] Ⓑ

Evidence-Based References

1. Guidugli F et al: Antibiotics for leptospirosis, *Cochrane Database Rev* CD001306(2), 2000. Ⓐ

2. Sehgal SC et al: Randomized controlled trial of doxycycline prophylaxis against leptospirosis in an endemic area, *Int J Antimicrob Agents* 13:249, 2000. Ⓑ

3. Panaphut T et al: Ceftriaxone compared with sodium penicillin G for treatment of severe leptospirosis, *Clin Infect Dis* 36:1507, 2003. Ⓑ

SUGGESTED READINGS

Karande S et al: Acute aseptic meningitis as the only presenting feature of leptospirosis, *Pediatr Infect Dis J* 24(4):390, 2005.

Segura ER et al: Clinical spectrum of pulmonary involvement in leptospirosis in a region of endemicity, with quantification of leptospiral burden, *Clin Infect Dis* 40(3):343, 2005.

Suputtamongkol Y et al: An open, randomized, controlled trial of penicillin, doxycycline, and cefotaxime for patients with severe leptospirosis, *Clin Infect Dis* 39(10):1417, 2004.

Surveill Simm et al: Surveillance for waterborne diseases and outbreaks associated with recreational water use and other aquatic facility-associated health events. *MMWR Surveil Summ* 57(9):1-29, 2008.

AUTHORS: **DENNIS J. MIKOLICH, M.D.,** and **GLENN G. FORT, M.D.**

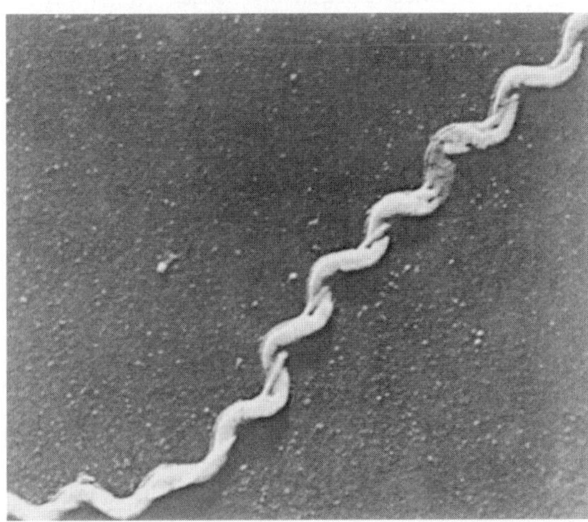

FIGURE 1-179 Electron micrograph of *Leptospira interrogans* (serovar canicola) showing the tightly coiled helicoids rod with the periplasmic axial filament. (Courtesy Armed Forces Institute of Pathology: AFIP No. 60-10941. In Gorbach SL: *Infectious diseases,* ed 2, Philadelphia, 1998, WB Saunders.)

Leukemia, Acute Lymphoblastic (PTG)

BASIC INFORMATION

DEFINITION

Acute lymphoblastic leukemia (ALL) is characterized by uncontrolled proliferation of abnormal, immature lymphocytes and their progenitors, ultimately replacing normal bone marrow elements.

SYNONYMS

Lymphoid leukemia
ALL

ICD-9CM CODES
204.0 Acute lymphoblastic leukemia

EPIDEMIOLOGY & DEMOGRAPHICS

- ALL is primarily a disease of children (peak incidence from ages 2 to 10 yr).
- It is diagnosed in 3000 to 4000 persons in the U.S. each year; two thirds are children.

PHYSICAL FINDINGS & CLINICAL PRESENTATION

- Skin pallor, purpura, or easy bruising
- Lymphadenopathy or hepatosplenomegaly
- Fever, bone pain, oliguria, weakness, weight loss, mental status changes

ETIOLOGY

- Unknown; increased risk in patients with a previous use of antineoplastic agents (e.g., chemotherapy of non-Hodgkin's lymphoma, Hodgkin's disease, ovarian cancer, myeloma)
- Environmental factors (e.g., ionizing radiation), toxins (e.g., benzene)

Dx DIAGNOSIS

DIFFERENTIAL DIAGNOSIS

- Acute myeloid leukemia (AML): the distinction between ALL and AML and the classification of the various subtypes are based on the following factors:
  1. Cell morphology
     - Lymphoblasts: a high nucleus/cytoplasmic ratio; cytoplasmic granules are usually not present.
     - Myeloblasts: abundant cytoplasm; cytoplasmic granules (Auer rods) are often present.
  2. Histochemical stains
     - Peroxidase and Sudan black stains: negative in ALL; useful to distinguish nonlymphoid from lymphoid cells.
     - Chloracetate esterase: a pink cytoplasmic reaction identifies granulocytes; useful to distinguish granulocytes from monocytes in patients with AML.
- Lymphoblastic lymphoma
- Aplastic anemia
- Infectious mononucleosis
- Leukemoid reaction to infection
- Multiple myeloma

WORKUP

- Laboratory evaluation
- Bone marrow examination (with biopsy, cytochemistry, immunophenotyping, and cytogenetics)
- Lumbar puncture and imaging studies

LABORATORY TESTS

- Complete blood count reveals normochromic, normocytic anemia, thrombocytopenia.
- Peripheral smear will reveal lymphoblasts.
- Initial blood work should also include blood urea nitrogen, creatinine, serum electrolytes, uric acid, and lactate dehydrogenase.
- Special diagnostic tests include immunophenotyping, cytogenetics, and cytochemistry.
- The French, American, British (FAB) Cooperative Study Group has classified ALL into three groups (L1 to L3) on the basis of cell size, cytoplasmic appearance, nucleus shape, and chromatin pattern. The most common form is the L2 type.
- Immunologic classification is made on the basis of expression of surface antigens by blast cells: T lineage and B lineage.

IMAGING STUDIES

- Chest x-ray to evaluate for the presence of mediastinal mass
- CT scan or ultrasound of abdomen/pelvis to assess splenomegaly or leukemic infiltration of abdominal organs

Rx TREATMENT

ACUTE GENERAL Rx

- Emergency treatment consisting of one or more of the following is indicated in patients with intracerebral leukostasis:
  1. Cranial irradiation of the whole brain in one- or two-dose fractions
  2. Leukapheresis
  3. Oral hydroxyurea (requires 48 to 72 hr to significantly lower the circulating blast count)
- Urate nephropathy can be prevented by vigorous hydration and lowering uric acid level with allopurinol and urine alkalization with acetazolamide.
- Infections must be aggressively treated with broad-spectrum antibiotics.
  1. Any febrile or neutropenic patients must have cultures taken and be properly treated with IV antibiotics.
  2. If evidence of infection persists despite adequate treatment with antibiotics, amphotericin B may be added to provide coverage against fungal infections *(Candida, Aspergillus).*
- Correct significant thrombocytopenia (platelet counts $<$20,000/mm^3) with platelet transfusion.
- Bleeding secondary to disseminated intravascular coagulation is treated with heparin and replacement of clotting factors.
- Induction therapy is intensive chemotherapy to destroy a significant number of leukemic cells and achieve remission; it usually consists of a combination of vincristine (Oncovin), prednisone, and l-asparaginase (ELSPAR) in children or an anthracene in adults.
- Consolidation therapy consists of an aggressive course of chemotherapy with or without radiotherapy shortly after complete remission has been obtained. Its purpose is to prolong the remission period or cure. Commonly used agents are VM-26, VP-16, HiDAC.
- Dasatinib is a tyrosine kinase inhibitor that can be used as a second line in Philadelphia chromosome–positive ALL.
- Meningeal prophylactic therapy with intrathecal methotrexate with or without cranial irradiation is indicated to prevent meningeal sequestration of leukemic cells. With effective risk-adjusted chemotherapy, prophylactic cranial irridation can in some cases be safely omitted from the treatment of childhood ALL.
- The goal of maintenance therapy is to maintain a state of remission. In patients with ALL, intermittent therapy is continued for at least 3 yr with a combination of methotrexate and 6-mercaptopurine (Purinethol).
- Bone marrow transplantation: patients should receive allograft in the first complete remission if they are between ages 20 and 50 yr and have matched a sibling donor.

DISPOSITION

- Prognosis is generally poorer in adult disease compared with childhood disease (40% adult cure rate versus 80% cure rate in children).
- Five-year leukemia-free survival is $<$40%.
- The different clinical outcomes associated with the various subtypes of ALL can be attributed primarily to drug sensitivity or resistance of leukemic blasts harboring specific genetic abnormalities. For example, cases of ALL expressing the TEL-AML1 fusion protein are very responsive to intensive chemotherapy with asparaginase, whereas the presence of Philadelphia chromosome (Ph{ΣΥ}+{/ΣΥ}), monosomy 5 and 7, and abnormalities of 11q23 are bad prognostic signs in ALL.
- Genetic alteration (deletion) of IKZF1 is associated with a very poor outcome in B-cell-progenitor ALL.

REFERRAL

Referral to a hematologist is indicated in all cases of ALL.

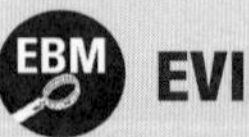

EVIDENCE

Please note: Complete text of EBM for this topic is available online.

SUGGESTED READINGS

Mullighan CG et al: Deletion of IKZF1 and prognosis in acute lymphoblastic leukemia, *N Engl J Med* 360: 470-480, 2009.

Pui CH et al: Treating childhood acute lymphoblastic leukemia without cranial irradiation, *N Engl J Med* 360:2730-2741, 2009.

AUTHOR: **FRED F. FERRI, M.D.**

BASIC INFORMATION

DEFINITION

Acute myelogenous leukemia (AML) is a disorder characterized by uncontrolled proliferation of primitive myeloid cells (blasts), ultimately replacing normal bone marrow elements and frequently resulting in hematopoietic insufficiency (granulocytopenia, thrombocytopenia, or anemia) with or without leukocytosis.

SYNONYMS

Acute nonlymphoblastic leukemia (ANLL)
Acute nonlymphocytic leukemia
Acute myeloid leukemia (AML)

ICD-9CM CODES

205.0 Acute myelogenous leukemia

EPIDEMIOLOGY & DEMOGRAPHICS

- AML usually affects adults (most patients are 30 to 60 yr; median age at presentation is 50 yr).
- Annual incidence is 2 to 4 cases/100,000 persons.

PHYSICAL FINDINGS & CLINICAL PRESENTATION

Patients generally come to medical attention because of the effects of the cytopenias:

- Anemia manifests with weakness or fatigue.
- Thrombocytopenia can manifest with bleeding, petechiae, and ecchymosis.
- Neutropenia can result in infections and fever.
- Physical examination may reveal skin pallor, bruises, petechiae; abdominal examination may reveal hepatosplenomegaly; peripheral lymphadenopathy may also be present.
- Hyperleukocytosis can lead to symptoms of leukostasis, such as ocular and cerebrovascular dysfunction or bleeding.

ETIOLOGY

Risk factors are previous use of antineoplastic agents, chromosomal abnormalities, ionizing radiation, toxins, immunodeficiency states, and chronic myeloproliferative disorders.

DIAGNOSIS

DIFFERENTIAL DIAGNOSIS

- Acute lymphocytic leukemia
- Leukemoid reaction
- Myelodysplastic syndrome
- Infiltrative diseases of the bone marrow
- Epstein-Barr virus, other viral infection

LABORATORY TESTS

- Complete blood count reveals anemia and thrombocytopenia. Peripheral white blood cell count varies from $<5000/mm^3$ to $>100,000/mm^3$.
- Additional laboratory findings may include elevated lactate dehydrogenase and uric acid levels, decreased fibrinogen, and increased fibrin degradation product as a result of disseminated intravascular coagulation (DIC).
- Cytogenetic abnormalities are common (chromosome 8 is most frequently involved in AML).
- The distinction between acute lymphoblastic leukemia (ALL) and AML and the classification of the various subtypes are based on the following factors:
  1. Cell morphology: myeloblasts reveal abundant cytoplasm; cytoplasmic granules are often present (Auer rods).
  2. Histochemical stains:
     - Peroxidase and Sudan black stains are negative in ALL.
     - Chloracetate esterase: a pink cytoplasmic reaction identifies granulocytes; useful to distinguish granulocytes from monocytes in patients with AML.
- AML is diagnosed by the presence of at least 30% blast cells and positive peroxidase or Sudan black histochemical stain in the bone marrow aspirate.
- The French, American, British (FAB) Cooperative Study Group has classified AML into seven categories (M1 to M7) based on the type and percentage of immature cells.
- A stepwise algorithm for diagnosis and classification of AML using cytomorphology, cytochemistry, immunophenotyping, cytogenetics, and molecular genetics is described in Box 1-11 and in the online version of Section III.

BOX 1-11 Stepwise Algorithm for Diagnosis and Classification of Acute Myelogenous Leukemia Using Cytomorphology, Cytochemistry, Immunophenotyping, Cytogenetics, and Molecular Cytogenetics

The criteria are based on Wright-Giemsa–stained blood and marrow smears and biopsy. The percentage of blast cells separates acute myeloid leukemia (AML) from myelodysplastic syndrome (MDS). The World Health Organization (WHO) classification defines AML as greater than 20% blasts in the marrow or blood. The next step is to define the blast population by immunophenotyping and/or immunohistochemistry. The initial evaluation separates AML from ALL. A history of exposure to prior cytoxic chemotherapy or agents associated with AML defines the leukemia as *therapy-related acute myeloid leukemia* (t-AML). The WHO recognizes the unique clinical and biologic features of the therapy-related leukemias (t-AML). This subtype results from prior exposure to cytotoxic chemotherapy and/or radiation therapy. A majority of patients will have clonal cytogenetic abnormalities and now account for more than 40% of all patients with AML. The WHO recognizes two types of t-AML based on the type of prior exposure or treatment: alkylating agent–related AML and topoisomerase II inhibitor–related AML. The WHO classification defines major subgroups of AML that manifest recurring cytogenetic abnormalities. As a group, these AMLs have chromosomal translocations that result in the production of chimeric proteins, which are pivotal in the leukemogenic process. The genetic abnormalities define a specific biology, clinical course, and prognosis and therefore are important to classify them separately. In this group of patients, the diagnosis is defined by the cytogenetic abnormality independent of the percentage of blasts. There are four recurrent translocations in this group. The diagnosis is defined by the cytogenetic abnormalities and is not dependent on the number of blasts: (a) AML with t(8;21)(q22;q22), (AML1/ETO) (RUNX/CBFA2T1); (b) AML with abnormal bone marrow eosinophils and inv[16](p13;q22) or t(16;16)(p13;q22), (CBFB/MYH11); (c) acute promyelocytic leukemia: AML with t(15;17)(q22;q21) (PML/RARA) or t(11;17)(q23;q12) (PLZF/RARA) or t(5;17)(q23;q12)(NPM/RARA), or t(11;17)(q13;q12) (NuMA/RARA); and (d) AML with 11q23 (MLL) abnormalities. If multilineage dysplasia is present, then the leukemia is classified as *acute leukemia with multilineage dysplasia*.

AML with multilineage dysplasia is characterized by the presence of 20% or more blasts in the marrow and dysplasia in at least 50% of the cells of at least two of the three main hemopoietic lines. The leukemia may occur de novo or after a preceding myelodysplastic, myeloproliferative, or overlap myelodysplastic/myeloproliferative syndrome unrelated to prior exposure to chemotherapy. If such a syndrome preceded the development of acute leukemia, the AML is best designated as AML "evolving from a myelodysplastic syndrome." When a leukemia fails to satisfy the cytogenetic, morphologic, or clinical criteria for the newly defined subgroups, it is classified as AML not otherwise categorized. The *not otherwise categorized* designation essentially applies the original FAB classification with some modifications, namely, acute promyelocytic leukemia (M3) is no longer included; a pure erythroleukemia has been distinguished from erythroleukemia, acute erythroid/myeloid type; and acute basophilic leukemia (very rare) has been added, as is a rare entity termed acute panmyelosis with myelofibrosis and the solid tumor myeloid sarcoma.

(From Hoffmann R et al: *Hematology, basic principles and practice*, ed 5, Philadelphia, 2009, Churchill Livingstone.)

CD, Cluster designation; *MPO,* myeloperoxidase; *NEC,* nonerythroid cells; *NSE,* nonspecific esterase; *PAS,* periodic acid–Schiff; *SBB,* Sudan black B; *TdT,* terminal deoxynucleotidyl transferase; *TNC,* total nucleated cells.

IMAGING STUDIES

- Chest x-ray is useful to evaluate for the presence of mediastinal masses.
- CT scan of the abdomen may reveal hepatosplenomegaly or leukemic involvement of other organs.

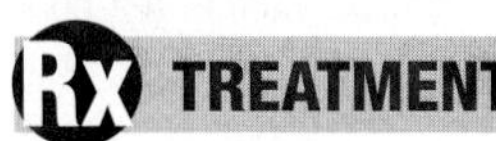

TREATMENT

ACUTE GENERAL Rx

- Emergency treatment consisting of one or more of the following is indicated in patients with intracerebral leukostasis:
  1. Cranial irradiation
  2. Leukapheresis
  3. Oral hydroxyurea
- Urate nephropathy can be prevented by vigorous hydration and lowering uric acid level with allopurinol and urine alkalinization with acetazolamide.
- Infections must be aggressively treated with broad-spectrum antibiotics.
- Correct significant thrombocytopenia with platelet transfusions.
- Bleeding from DIC is treated with heparin and replacement of clotting factors.
- Intensive induction chemotherapy to destroy a significant number of leukemic cells and achieve remission usually consists of cytarabine (Cytosar) and daunorubicin. All-trans retinoic acid is effective for the induction of remission of AML M3 subtype (acute promyelocytic leukemia).
- High-dose cytarabine (ARA-C) (HiDAC) can be used in patients with refractory or relapsed AML. It usually takes 28 to 32 days from the start of therapy to achieve remission. The duration of remission is variable; the median duration of remission in an adult with AML is 1 yr.
- Consolidation therapy consists of an aggressive course of chemotherapy with or without radiation shortly after complete remission has been obtained; its purpose is to prolong the remission period or cure. Complications of consolidation therapy are usually attributable to severe bone marrow suppression (anemia, thrombocytopenia, granulocytopenia).
- Goal of therapy is to maintain a state of remission. A postinduction course of high-dose cytarabine can provide equivalent disease-free survival and somewhat better overall survival than autologous marrow transplantation in adults.
- Autologous bone marrow transplantation is indicated in patients <55 yr without a sibling donor. Allogeneic bone marrow transplantation is generally available to <20% of patients; it is usually performed only in patients <40 yr because of higher incidence of graft-versus-host disease with advancing age.

DISPOSITION

- Remission can be achieved in nearly 80% of patients <55 yr. Remission rates are highest in children.
- Allogeneic stem cell transplantation (SCT) after myoablative conditioning is a curative option in younger patients with AML in first complete remission (CR1). However, concerns related to toxicity limit its use. Cure for allogeneic bone marrow transplantation approaches 60%; cure rates with autologous transplantation are lower. Compared with nonallogeneic SCT therapies, allogeneic SCT has significant relapse-free survival (RFS) and overall survival benefit for intermediate- and poor-risk AML but not for good-risk AML in first complete remission.
- Favorable cytogenics are inv (16) (p13;q22) and t(8;21), t(15;17).

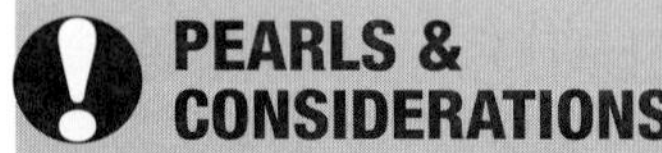

PEARLS & CONSIDERATIONS

- The major complication of chemotherapy is profound marrow depression with pancytopenia lasting 3 to 4 wk. Treatment is aimed at red blood cell and platelet replacement and aggressive monitoring and treatment of suspected infections.
- Low doses of arsenic trioxide can induce complete remission in patients with acute promyelocytic leukemia.

SUGGESTED READING

Koreth J et al: Allogeneic stem cell transplantation for acute myeloid leukemia in first complete remission, *JAMA* 301(22):2349-2361, 2009.

AUTHOR: **FRED F. FERRI, M.D.**

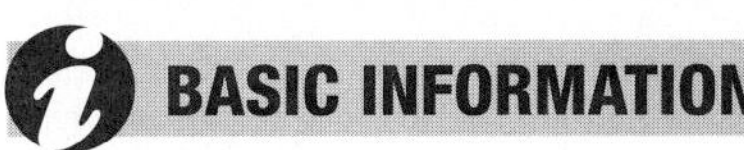

BASIC INFORMATION

DEFINITION

Chronic lymphocytic leukemia (CLL) is a lymphoproliferative disorder characterized by proliferation and accumulation of mature-appearing neoplastic lymphocytes.

SYNONYMS

CLL

ICD-9CM CODES
204.1 Leukemia, chronic lymphocytic

EPIDEMIOLOGY & DEMOGRAPHICS

- Most frequent form of leukemia in Western countries (10,000 new cases annually in the U.S.)
- Generally occurs in middle-aged and elderly patients (median age 65 yr)
- Male/female ratio of 2:1

PHYSICAL FINDINGS & CLINICAL PRESENTATION

- Lymphadenopathy, splenomegaly, and hepatomegaly in the majority of patients
- Variable clinical presentation according to stage of the disease
- Abnormal complete blood count: many cases are diagnosed on the basis of laboratory results obtained after routine physical examination
- Some patients come to medical attention because of weakness and fatigue (as a result of anemia) or lymphadenopathy

ETIOLOGY

CLL is a disease derived from antigen-experienced B lymphocytes that differ in the level of immunoglobulin V-gene mutations.

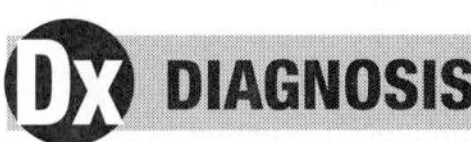

DIAGNOSIS

DIFFERENTIAL DIAGNOSIS

- Hairy cell leukemia
- Adult T-cell lymphoma
- Prolymphocytic leukemia
- Viral infections
- Waldenström's macroglobulinemia

LABORATORY TESTS

- Proliferative lymphocytosis (≥15,000/dl) of well-differentiated lymphocytes is the hallmark of CLL. B-cell clones are early markers for CLL and can be detected in peripheral blood >6 years before a CLL diagnosis.
- There is monotonous replacement of the bone marrow by small lymphocytes (marrow contains ≥30% of well-differentiated lymphocytes).
- Hypogammaglobulinemia and elevated lactate dehydrogenase may be present at the time of diagnosis.
- Anemia or thrombocytopenia, if present, indicates poor prognosis.
- Trisomy-12 is the most common chromosomal abnormality, followed by 14 q+, 13 q, and 11 q; these all indicate a poor prognosis.
- New laboratory techniques (CD 38, fluorescence in situ hybridization) can identify patients with early-stage CLL at higher risk of rapid disease progression. Staining of mononuclear cells by a two-color (fluorescein isothiocyanate/phycoerythrin) flow cytometric assay using antibodies to the chemokine receptors (CXCR1, CXCR2, etc.) can help in the staging and prognosis of patients. Increase in expression of chemokine receptors CXCR4 and CCR7 correlates with advanced Rai stage (stage IV). The presence of V-gene mutations, CD38+, or ZAP-70+ cells also has prognostic relevance. Patients with clones having few or no V-gene mutations or many CD38+ or ZAP-70+ B cells are associated with an aggressive, usually fatal course.
- The percentage of smudge cells (CLL cells ruptured during smear preparation) is associated with mutated IgVH gene status, a favorable prognostic factor. A high percentage of smudge cells on peripheral smear indicates a longer time to treatment from initial diagnosis and better overall survival in patients with early stage CLL.

STAGING:

Rai et al divided CLL into five clinical stages:

- Stage 0: Characterized by lymphocytosis only (>15,000/mm^3 on peripheral smear, bone marrow aspirate ≥40% lymphocytes). The coexistence of lymphocytosis and other factors increases the clinical stage.
- Stage 1: Lymphadenopathy
- Stage 2: Lymphadenopathy/hepatomegaly
- Stage 3: Anemia (hemoglobin [Hgb] <11 g/mm^3)
- Stage 4: Thrombocytopenia (platelets <100,000/mm^3)

Another well-known staging system developed by Binet divides CLL into three stages:

- Stage A: Hgb >10 g/dl, platelets >100,000/mm^3, and fewer than three areas involved (the cervical, axillary, and inguinal lymph nodes [whether unilaterally or bilaterally]; the spleen; and the liver)
- Stage B: Hgb >10 g/dl, platelets >100,000/mm^3, and three or more areas involved
- Stage C: Hgb <10 g/dl, low platelets (<100,000/mm^3), or both (independent of the areas involved)

IMAGING STUDIES

CT scan of abdomen to evaluate for hepatomegaly and splenomegaly

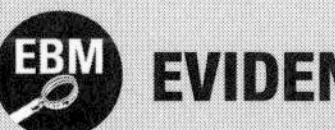

TREATMENT

NONPHARMACOLOGIC THERAPY

- Treatment goals are relief of symptoms and prolongation of life.
- Observation is appropriate for patients in Rai stage 0 or Binet stage A.

ACUTE GENERAL Rx

- Symptomatic patients in Rai stage I or II or Binet stage B: chlorambucil; local irradiation for isolated symptomatic lymphadenopathy and lymph nodes that interfere with vital organs
- Fludarabine is an effective treatment for CLL that does not respond to initial treatment with chlorambucil. Recent reports indicate that when used as the initial treatment for CLL, fludarabine yields higher response rates and a longer duration of remission and progression-free survival than chlorambucil; overall survival, however, is not enhanced.
- Rai stages III or IV, Binet stage C: chlorambucil chemotherapy with or without prednisone:
  1. Fludarabine, CAP (***c***yclophosphamide, ***A***driamycin, ***p***rednisone), or cyclophosphamide, doxorubicin, vincristine, and prednisone (mini-CHOP) can be used in patients who respond poorly to chlorambucil.
  2. Splenic irradiation can be used in selected patients with advanced disease.

CHRONIC Rx

Treatment of systemic complications:

- Hypogammaglobulinemia is frequent in CLL and is the chief cause of infections. Immune globulin (250 mg/kg IV every 4 wk) may prevent infections but has no effect on survival rate. Infections should be treated with broad-spectrum antibiotics. Patients should be monitored for opportunistic infections.
- Recombinant hematopoietic cofactors (e.g., granulocyte-macrophage colony stimulating factor and granulocyte colony stimulating factor) may be useful to overcome neutropenia related to treatment.
- Erythropoietin may be useful to treat anemia that is unresponsive to other measures.

DISPOSITION

The patient's prognosis is generally directly related to the clinical stage (e.g., the average survival in patients in Rai stage 0 or Binet stage A is >120 mo, whereas for RAI stage 4 or Binet stage C it is approximately 30 mo). Overall 5-yr survival is 60%. Measurement of ZAP-70 intracellular protein (where available) is also a useful indicator of prognosis.

EBM EVIDENCE

Please note: Complete text of EBM for this topic is available online.

SUGGESTED READING

Landgren O et al: B-cell clones as early markers for chronic lymphocytic leukemia, *N Engl J Med* 360:659-667, 2009.

AUTHOR: **FRED F. FERRI, M.D.**

Leukemia, Chronic Myelogenous (PTG)

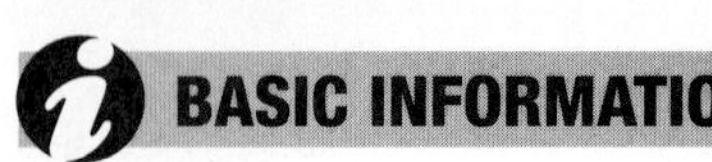

BASIC INFORMATION

DEFINITION

Chronic myelogenous leukemia (CML) is a malignant clonal stem disease caused by an acquired somatic mutation that fuses, through chromosomal translocation, the *ABL* and *BCR* genes on chromosomes 9 and 22 and is characterized by abnormal proliferation and accumulation of immature granulocytes. CML manifests with a chronic phase (CP-CML) lasting months to years, followed by an advanced phase (AP-CML) characterized by poor response to therapy, worsening anemia, or decreased platelet count; the second phase then evolves into a terminal phase (acute transformation) that degenerates into acute leukemia (mostly myeloid and approximately 20% lymphoid subtype), characterized by elevated number of blast cells and numerous complications (e.g., sepsis, bleeding).

SYNONYMS

CML
Chronic granulocytic leukemia
Chronic myeloid leukemia

ICD-9CM CODES
201.1 Chronic myelogenous leukemia

EPIDEMIOLOGY & DEMOGRAPHICS

- CML usually affects elderly patients (median age at presentation is 65 yr) and accounts for 15% of adult cases of leukemia
- Incidence is one to two cases per 100,000 people annually

PHYSICAL FINDINGS & CLINICAL PRESENTATION

- The chronic phase usually reveals splenomegaly; hepatomegaly is not infrequent, but lymphadenopathy is highly unusual and generally indicates the accelerated proliferative phase of the disease.
- Common symptoms at the time of diagnosis are weakness or discomfort from an enlarged spleen (abdominal discomfort or pain). Splenomegaly is present in up to 40% of patients at time of diagnosis.
- 40% of patients are asymptomatic, and diagnosis is based solely on an abnormal blood count.

ETIOLOGY

Current evidence strongly implicates the chromosome translocation t (9;22) (q34;q11.2) as the cause of chronic granulocytic leukemia. This translocation is present in $>95\%$ of patients. The remaining patients have a complex or variant translocation involving additional chromosomes that have the same end result (fusion of the *BCR* [break point cluster region] gene on chromosome 22 to *ABL* [Ableson leukemia virus] gene on chromosome 9).

DIAGNOSIS

DIFFERENTIAL DIAGNOSIS

- Splenic lymphoma
- Chronic lymphocytic leukemia
- Myelodysplastic syndrome

LABORATORY TESTS

- Elevated white blood cell count (generally $>100{,}000/mm^3$) with broad spectrum of granulocytic forms.
- Bone marrow demonstrates hypercellularity with granulocytic hyperplasia, increased ratio of myeloid cells to erythroid cells, and increased number of megakaryocytes. Blasts and promyelocytes constitute $<10\%$ of all cells.
- Philadelphia chromosome (which results from the reciprocal translocation between the long arms of chromosomes 9 and 22) is present in $>95\%$ of patients with CML; its presence (Ph^1) is a major prognostic factor because survival rate of patients with Philadelphia chromosome is approximately eight times better than that of those without it. Some believe that $Ph^1(+)$ defines CML and that those who are $Ph^1(-)$ have another disease.
- Leukocyte alkaline phosphatase is markedly decreased (used to distinguish CML from other myeloproliferative disorders).
- Anemia and thrombocytosis are often present.
- Additional laboratory results are elevated vitamin B_{12} levels (caused by increased transcobalamin 1 from granulocytes) and elevated blood histamine levels (because of increased basophils).

IMAGING STUDIES

Chest radiograph and CT scan of abdomen/pelvis

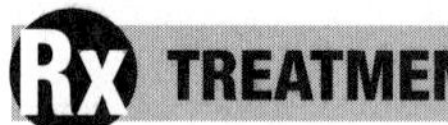

TREATMENT

ACUTE GENERAL Rx

Treatment with a potential to either cure CML or prolong survival should be used during the chronic phase of the disease because it is often futile when administered during the advanced phase. Imatinib mesylate (Gleevec), an oral tyrosine kinase inhibitor, is effective and indicated as first-line treatment for CML myeloid blast crisis, accelerated phase, or CML in its chronic phase. More than 75% of patients have major cytogenetic response ($<35\%$ Philadelphia chromosome-positive cells in the marrow), and more than 80% have progression-free survival after 24 mo. Complete hematologic response usually occurs in <1 mo.

- Symptomatic hyperleukocytosis (e.g., central nervous system symptoms) can be treated with leukapheresis and hydroxyurea; allopurinol should be started to prevent urate nephropathy after the rapid lysis of the leukemia cells.
- Allogeneic stem-cell transplantation (SCT) is the only curative treatment for CML in the chronic phase unresponsive to imatinib. In general only 20% of patients are candidates for SCT given the limitations of age or lack of HLA-matched related donors.
  1. It should be considered in "young" patients (increased survival in patients <55 yr) with compatible siblings.
  2. Early transplantation is also important for patient's survival.
- Nilotinib and dasatinib (Sprycel) are BCR-ABL tyrosine kinase inhibitors active in imatinib-resistant CML.
- Interferon-alfa is an acceptable alternative in the early chronic phase for patients who do not tolerate tyrosine kinase inhibitors.
- Transplantation of marrow from an HLA-matched, unrelated donor is also now recognized as safe and effective therapy for selected patients with chronic myelogenous leukemia.

SUGGESTED READINGS

Hehlmann R et al: Chronic myeloid leukemia, *Lancet* 370:342, 2007.

Kantarjian H et al: Nilotinib in imatinib-resistant CML and Philadelphia chromosome-positive ALL, *N Engl J Med* 354:2542, 2006.

Quintas-Cardam A, Cortes J: Chronic myeloid leukemia: diagnosis and treatment, *Mayo Clin Proc* 81(7): 973, 2006.

Schiffer CA: BCR-ABL tyrosine kinase inhibitors for chronic myelogenous leukemia, *N Engl J Med* 357: 258, 2007.

Talpaz M et al: Dasatinib in imatinib-resistant Philadelphia chromosome-positive leukemias, *N Engl J Med* 354:2531, 2006.

AUTHOR: **FRED F. FERRI, M.D.**

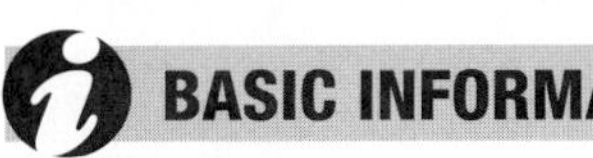

BASIC INFORMATION

DEFINITION

Hairy cell leukemia is a lymphoid neoplasm characterized by the proliferation of mature B cells with prominent cytoplasmic projections (hairs).

SYNONYMS

Leukemic reticuloendotheliosis

ICD-9CM CODES
202.4 Hairy cell leukemia

EPIDEMIOLOGY & DEMOGRAPHICS

PREVALENCE: Occurs predominantly in men between ages 40 and 60 yr. Approximately 2% of leukemia cases are of the hairy cell type.
PREDOMINANT SEX: Male/female ratio of 4:1

PHYSICAL FINDINGS & CLINICAL PRESENTATION

- Usually, splenomegaly (present in >90% of cases) caused by tumor cell infiltration
- Pallor, ecchymosis, and evidence of infection if the pancytopenia is severe
- Weakness, lethargy, and fatigue
- Infections (resulting from impaired resistance caused by neutropenia) and easy bruising (caused by thrombocytopenia) also common

ETIOLOGY

Neoplastic disease of the lymphoreticular system of unknown etiology

Dx DIAGNOSIS

DIFFERENTIAL DIAGNOSIS

- Other forms of leukemia
- Lymphoma
- Viral syndrome

WORKUP

Comprehensive history, physical examination, and laboratory evaluation to confirm the diagnosis

LABORATORY TESTS

- Pancytopenia involving erythrocytes, neutrophils, and platelets is common; anemia is usually present and varies from minimal to severe.
- Hairy cells (Fig. 1-180) can account for 5% to 80% of cells in the peripheral blood. The cytoplasmic projections on the cells are redundant plasma membranes.
- Leukemic cells stain positively for tartrate-resistant acid phosphatase stain.
- Bone marrow may result in a "dry tap" (because of increased marrow reticulin).

Rx TREATMENT

NONPHARMACOLOGIC THERAPY

Approximately 8% to 10% of patients are asymptomatic and have minimal splenomegaly and minor cytopenia. They are usually detected on routine laboratory evaluation and do not require initial therapy. They should, however, be frequently monitored for progression of disease.

ACUTE GENERAL Rx

- Drugs of choice are the purine analogues 2-chloro-2 deoxyadenosine (Cladribine) or 2-deoxycoformycin (DCF, Pentostatin). They induce complete remissions in up to 85% of patients and partial responses in 5% to 25%.
- 2-Chloro-2 deoxyadenosine (CdA) 0.14 mg/kg qd for 7 days has minimal toxicity and is able to induce complete durable responses with a single course of therapy.
- Interferon-α produces a partial remission in 30% to 70% of patients and complete remission, often of short duration, in 5% to 10% of patients.
- The anti-CD 22 recombinant immunotoxin BL 22 can induce complete remission in patients with hairy cell leukemia resistant to treatment with purine analogues.

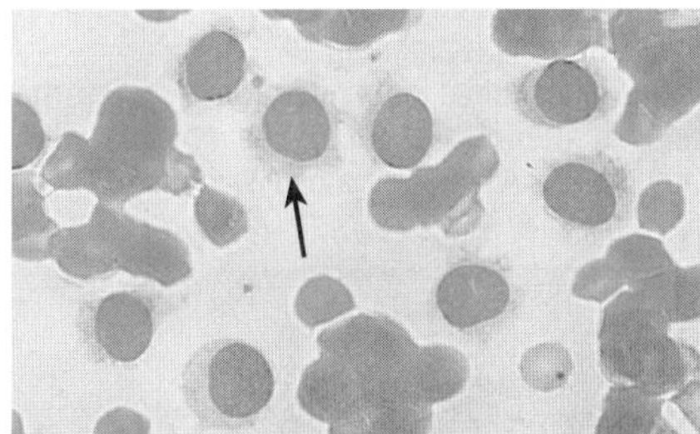

FIGURE 1-180 Hairy cell leukemia. Note the lymphocytes with hairlike cytoplasmic projections surrounding the nucleus. (From Rodak BF: *Diagnostic hematology,* Philadelphia, 1995, WB Saunders.)

CHRONIC Rx

Patients should be monitored with periodic examination and laboratory tests for progression of disease.

DISPOSITION

Prognosis has become increasingly favorable with the newer agents. Approximately 90% of patients who are treated have a complete or partial response.

REFERRAL

Hematology consultation is recommended in all patients.

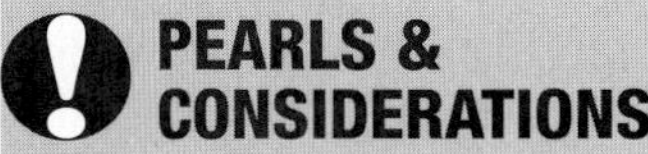

PEARLS & CONSIDERATIONS

COMMENTS

The diagnosis of hairy cell leukemia is occasionally missed and subsequently made by the histopathologist after removal of the spleen for diagnostic purposes.

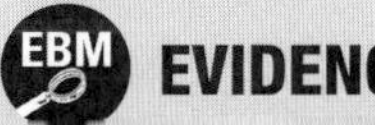

EBM EVIDENCE

We are unable to cite evidence that meets our criteria for some therapies, and there is only limited evidence for other therapies. Initial therapies of choice are cladribine or pentostatin.

In a randomized, controlled trial to compare pentostatin and interferon alpha-2a in previously untreated patients with hairy cell leukemia, 121 of 154 patients treated with pentostatin achieved confirmed complete or partial remission compared with 60 of 159 who received interferon alpha-2a. Response rates were significantly higher and relapse-free survival was significantly longer with pentostatin than interferon.[1] Ⓑ

Evidence-Based Reference

1. Grever M et al: Randomized comparison of pentostatin versus interferon alpha in previously untreated patients with hairy cell leukemia: an intergroup study, *J Clin Oncol* 13:974, 1995. Ⓑ

SUGGESTED READING

Kreitman RJ et al: Efficacy of the anti-CD 22 recombinant immunotoxin BL 22 in chemotherapy resistant hairy-cell leukemia, *N Engl J Med* 345:241, 2001.

AUTHOR: **FRED F. FERRI, M.D.**

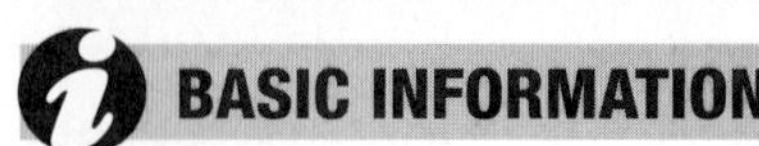

BASIC INFORMATION

DEFINITION

Oral hairy leukoplakia (OHL) is a painless, white, nonremovable, plaquelike lesion typically located on the lateral aspect of the tongue.

ICD-9CM CODES
528.6 Oral hairy leukoplakia

EPIDEMIOLOGY & DEMOGRAPHICS

INCIDENCE AND PREVALENCE: Epstein-Barr virus (EBV) seroprevalence occurs in high incidence in individuals who are HIV seropositive. However, OHL occurs in only 25% of these cases.

RISK FACTORS: OHL is usually found in HIV-seropositive individuals (median CD4 count is 468/μl) but may also be identified in other immunocompromised patients such as transplant recipients (particularly renal) and patients taking steroids. Diagnosing OHL is an indication to institute a workup to evaluate and manage HIV disease.

PHYSICAL FINDINGS & CLINICAL PRESENTATION

- Varying morphology and appearance.
- May be unilateral or bilateral.
- White and can be small with fine, vertical corrugations on the lateral margin of the tongue (Fig. 1-181).
- Irregular surface; may have prominent folds or projection, occasionally markedly resembling hairs.
- May spread to cover the entire dorsal surface or spread onto the ventral surface of the tongue where the lesions usually appear flat.
- Rarely, lesions can manifest on the soft palate, buccal mucosa, or posterior oropharynx.
- Usually asymptomatic, but some patients have mouth pain, soreness, or a burning sensation; impaired taste; or difficulty eating; others complain of its unsightly appearance.
- OHL may progress to oral squamous cell carcinoma, which has a poor prognosis.

ETIOLOGY

EBV is implicated in its etiology, and OHL is a result of replication EBV in the epithelium of keratinized cells. OHL differs from most EBV-related diseases in that infection is predominantly lytic rather than latent.

DIAGNOSIS

DIFFERENTIAL DIAGNOSIS

- *Candida albicans*
- Lichen planus
- Idiopathic leukoplakia
- White sponge nevus
- Dysplasia
- Squamous cell carcinoma

WORKUP

Requires physical examination and evaluation of HIV disease

LABORATORY TESTS

The *provisional* diagnosis is clinical and based on:

- Visual inspection
- Inability to scrape the lesion off the tongue with a blade
- Failure to respond to antifungal therapy

The *presumptive* diagnosis requires biopsy and histologic demonstration of:

- Epithelial hyperplasia with hairs
- Absence of inflammatory cell infiltrate

The *definitive* diagnosis requires:

- In situ hybridization of histologic or cytologic specimens revealing EBV DNA *or*
- Electron microscopy of specimens revealing herpes-like particles
- Measurement of the DNA content in cells of oral leukoplakia may be used to predict the risk of oral carcinoma

NOTE: Specimens obtained from lesions may demonstrate hyphae of *Candida albicans,* which may coexist and potentiate EBV-induced OHL.

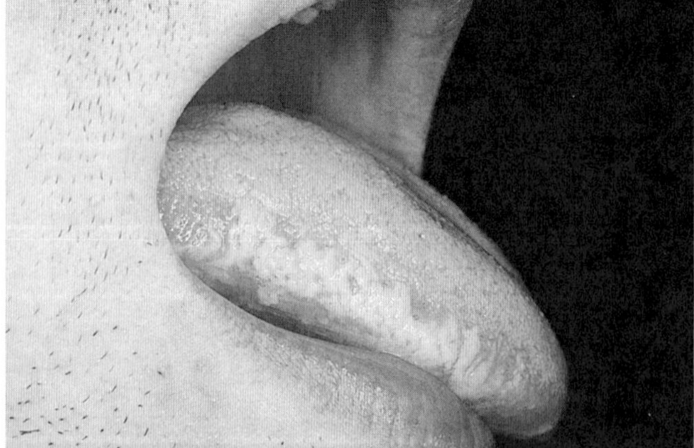

FIGURE 1-181 Oral hairy leukoplakia. Note white verrucoid plaques on the lateral border of the tongue. (From Noble J: *Primary care medicine,* ed 3, St Louis, 2001, Mosby.)

TREATMENT

NONPHARMACOLOGIC THERAPY

OHL is usually asymptomatic and requires no specific therapy. It may resolve spontaneously and has no known premalignant potential.

ACUTE GENERAL Rx

- Highly active antiretroviral therapy (HAART) has considerably changed the frequency of oral lesions caused by opportunistic infections in HIV-seropositive individuals.
- Topical retinoids (0.1% vitamin A) may improve the appearance of OHL-affected oral surfaces through their dekeratinizing and immunomodulation effects; however, they are expensive and prolonged use may result in a burning sensation over the treated area.
- Topical podophyllin resin 25% solution has been reported to induce resolution.
- Surgical excision and cryotherapy may help, but the lesions may recur.
- High-dose acyclovir 800 mg five times per day, valacyclovir 1000 mg tid, famciclovir 500 mg tid, ganciclovir 1000 mg tid, or foscarnet 40 mg/kg IV tid will cause lesions to resolve but only temporarily.

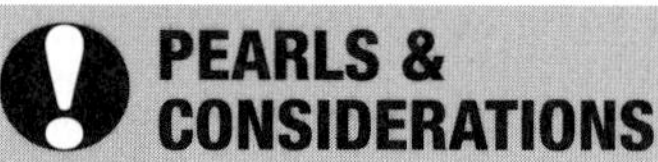

PEARLS & CONSIDERATIONS

- OHL is a nonmalignant lesion seen in patients with AIDS.
- The incidence has decreased significantly in the era of HAART.

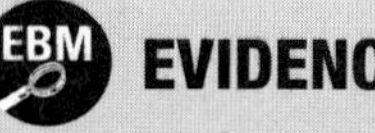

EVIDENCE

A 2006 Cochrane Review found no evidence of effective medical treatment in preventing malignant transformation of leukoplakia.[1] Ⓐ

Surgery is the mainstay of active treatment for leukoplakia, but the possible effectiveness of surgical interventions has never been studied by means of a randomized controlled trial.[1]

Removal of causative lifestyle factors is considered vital in the prevention of progression to oral cancer.[2] Ⓒ

Evidence-Based References

1. Lodi G et al: Interventions for treating oral leukoplakia, *Cochrane Database Rev* (4), 2006. Ⓐ
2. National Cancer Institute (NCI): *Oral cancer: prevention,* Bethesda, 2007, NCI. Ⓒ

SUGGESTED READING

Sudbo J et al: DNA content as a prognostic marker in patients with oral leukoplakia, *N Engl J Med* 344: 1270, 2001.

AUTHOR: **SAJEEV HANDA, M.D.**

BASIC INFORMATION

DEFINITION

Lichen planus refers to a papular skin eruption characteristically found over the flexor surfaces of the extremities, genitalia, and mucous membranes.

SYNONYMS

Lichen
Lichen planus et atrophicus

ICD-9CM CODES

697.0 Lichen planus

EPIDEMIOLOGY & DEMOGRAPHICS

INCIDENCE: One in every 100 new patients seen in dermatology clinics in the U.S. is diagnosed with lichen planus.
PREVALENCE: 440/100,000
PREDOMINANT SEX: Found equally between males and females (1:1)
PREDOMINANT AGE: Usually found in people between the ages of 30 and 60 yr
PREDISPOSING FACTORS:

1. Associated with other autoimmune disorders (e.g., primary biliary cirrhosis, myasthenia gravis, ulcerative colitis, diabetes)
2. Associated with hepatitis C infection
3. Drug-induced form affects any area of the body surface (e.g., beta-blocker, methyldopa, penicillamine, quinidine, nonsteroidal anti-inflammatory drugs, angiotensin-converting enzyme inhibitors, sulfonylurea agents)

PHYSICAL FINDINGS & CLINICAL PRESENTATION

History:

- Usually starts on an extremity and may remain localized or spread to involve other areas over a 1- to 4-mo period
- Pruritic

Physical findings:

- Anatomic distribution:
    1. Flexor surface of wrists, forearms, shins, and upper thighs
    2. Neck and back area
    3. Nails
    4. Scalp (lichen planopilaris)
    5. Oral mucosa, buccal mucosa, tongue, gingiva, and lips
    6. Vulva, penis

Genital mucosa:

- Lesion configuration:
    1. Linear
    2. Annular (more common)
    3. Reticular pattern noted on oral mucosa and genital area
- Lesion morphology:
    1. Papules most common presentation (flat, smooth, shiny)
    2. Hypertrophic
    3. Follicular
    4. Vesicular
- Color:
    1. Dark red, bluish red, purplish-violaceous color is noted in cutaneous lichen planus.
    2. Individual lesions characteristically have white lines visible (Wickham's striae).
    3. Oral and genital lichen planus has a reticular network of white lines that may be raised or annular in appearance.
- Scalp lesions may result in alopecia.

ETIOLOGY

The cause of lichen planus is unknown.

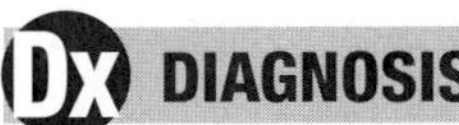

DIAGNOSIS

- Clinical history and physical findings usually establish the diagnosis of lichen planus.
- Skin biopsy (deep shave or punch biopsy of the most developed lesion) can be performed to confirm the diagnosis.

DIFFERENTIAL DIAGNOSIS

Drug eruption, psoriasis, Bowen's disease, leukoplakia, candidiasis, lupus rash, secondary syphilis, seborrheic dermatitis, chronic graft vs. host disease

WORKUP

If the diagnosis is questionable, a skin biopsy is performed.

LABORATORY TESTS

Laboratory tests are not specific for the diagnosis of lichen planus.

IMAGING STUDIES

Imaging studies are not helpful in diagnosing lichen planus.

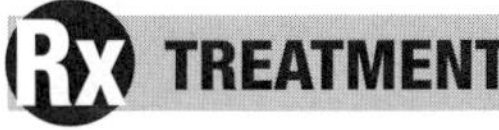

TREATMENT

NONPHARMACOLOGIC THERAPY

- Avoid scratching.
- Use mild soaps and emollients after bathing to prevent dryness.

ACUTE GENERAL Rx

For cutaneous lichen planus:

- Topical steroids (e.g., triamcinolone acetonide 0.1%, fluocinonide 0.05%, clobetasol propionate 0.05% cream or ointment) with occlusion used twice daily.
- Acitretin 30 mg/day PO for 8 wk.
- Systemic prednisone 30 to 60 mg/day as a starting dose and tapered to 15 to 20 mg/day maintenance for 6 wk.
- Intradermal steroid triamcinolone acetonide 5 mg/ml can be tried for thick hyperkeratotic lesions.
- Hydroxyzine 25 mg PO q6h can be used for pruritus.

For oral lichen planus:

- Topical steroid fluocinonide in an adhesive base used six times/day for 9 wk.
- Topical calcineurin in steroid unresponsive cases.
- Topical or systemic retinoids 0.1% retinoic acid in an adhesive base or gel.
- Etretinate 75 mg/day for 2 mo.

CHRONIC Rx

Refer to acute general treatment

DISPOSITION

- Spontaneous remissions of cutaneous lichen planus occur in more than 65% of cases within the first year.
- Spontaneous remission of oral lichen planus usually occurs by 5 yr.
- Approximately 10% to 20% of patients will have recurrence.

REFERRAL

Dermatology

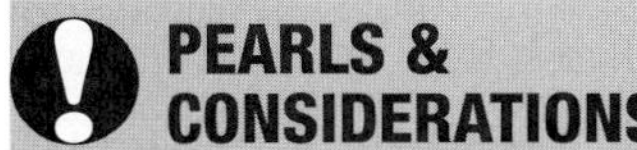

PEARLS & CONSIDERATIONS

COMMENTS

- Lichen planus can be remembered as purple, planar, pruritic, polygonal, papules, and plaques (six P's).
- Lesions can develop at the site of prior skin injury (Koebner's phenomenon).
- Although transformation to skin cancer has been seen in patients with lichen planus, it remains unclear if there is a true correlation.

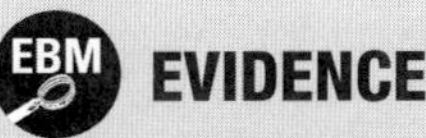

EVIDENCE

There is a lack of quality randomized trials that evaluate the efficacy of the therapies for lichen planus. The rationale for the use of therapies is based upon clinical experience and consensus opinion. However, some brief discussion may be made for the treatment of oral lichen planus:

A meta-analysis of 14 cohort and 5 case-controlled trials evaluated the replacement of dental amalgam restorations in 636 patients with oral lichenoid lesions where amalgam restorations were considered a likely etiological factor and where there was a positive patch test result for at least one mercury compound. This review found that replacement of the amalgam restoration with an alternative restoration resulted in complete healing ranging from 37.5% to 100%. The greatest improvements were seen in those lesions in close contact with amalgam.[1] B

Evidence-Based Reference

1. Issa Y et al: Healing of oral lichenoid lesions after replacing amalgam restorations: a systematic review, *Oral Surg Oral Med Oral Pathol Oral Radi* 98:553-565, 2004. B

SUGGESTED READINGS

Chan ES et al: Interventions for treating oral lichen planus, *Cochrane Rev* 2:CD001168, 2000.
Katta R: Lichen planus, *Am Fam Physician* 61(11):3319, 2000.

AUTHOR: **TANYA ALI, M.D.**

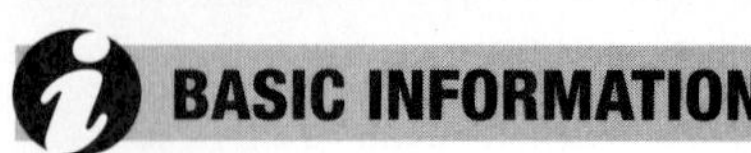

BASIC INFORMATION

DEFINITION

Chronic inflammatory condition of the skin usually affecting the vulva, perianal area, and groin

ICD-9CM CODES
701.0 Lichen sclerosus

EPIDEMIOLOGY & DEMOGRAPHICS

- Most common in postmenopausal women and men between ages 40 and 60 yr
- More common in females
- Can occur in children (usually prepubertal girls with involvement of the vulva and perineum)

PHYSICAL FINDINGS & CLINICAL PRESENTATION

- Erythema may be the only initial sign. A characteristic finding is the presence of ivory-white atrophic lesions on the involved area.
- Close inspection of the affected area will reveal the presence of white-to-brown follicular plugs on the surface (dells).
- When the genitals are involved, the white, parchment-like skin assumes an hourglass configuration around the introital and perianal area ("keyhole" distribution; Fig. 1-182). Inflammation, subepithelial hemorrhages, and chronic ulceration may develop.
- Dyspareunia, genital bleeding, and anal bleeding are common.

ETIOLOGY

Unknown. There may be an autoimmune association and a genetic familial component.

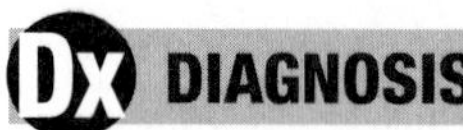

DIAGNOSIS

DIFFERENTIAL DIAGNOSIS

- Localized scleroderma (morphea)
- Cutaneous discoid lupus erythematosus
- Atrophic lichen planus
- Psoriasis

WORKUP

Diagnosis is based on close examination of the lesions for the presence of ivory-white atrophic lesions and typical location.

LABORATORY TESTS

Punch or deep shave biopsy can be used to confirm the diagnosis.

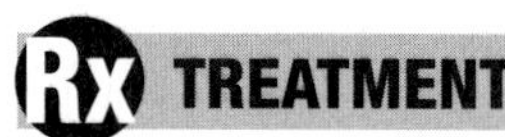

TREATMENT

NONPHARMACOLOGIC THERAPY

Attention to hygiene and elimination of irritants or excessive bathing with harsh soaps

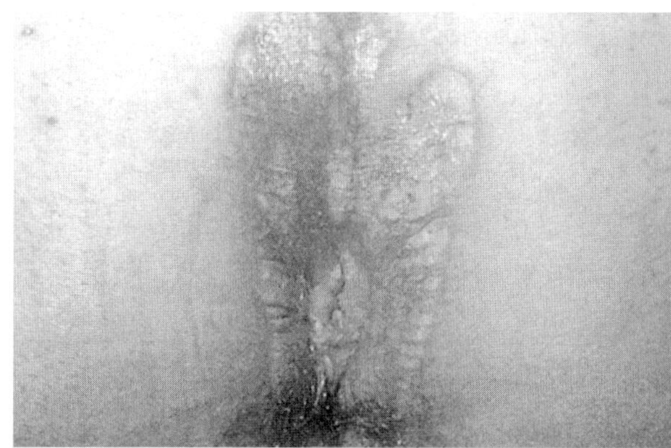

FIGURE 1-182 Lichen sclerosus. Perianal area is thinned and chalk white (keyhole distribution). (Courtesy Department of Dermatology, University of North Carolina at Chapel Hill. From Goldstein BG, Goldstein AO: *Practical dermatology,* ed 2, St Louis, 1997, Mosby.)

GENERAL Rx

- Application of clobetasol propionate 0.05% topically bid for up to 4 wk is usually effective. Repeat courses of corticosteroids may be necessary because of the chronic nature of this disorder. Continual application of topical steroids may lead to atrophy of the vulva.
- Use of topical testosterone (2%) has been found to be less effective than topical corticosteroids.
- Lubricants (e.g., Nutraplus cream) are useful to soothe dry tissues.
- Hydroxyzine 25 mg at bedtime is effective in decreasing nocturnal itching.
- Use of intralesional steroids, etretinate, and surgical management are usually reserved for refractory cases.

DISPOSITION

- The disease persists in approximately one third of patients.
- Most prepubertal girls improve spontaneously at menarche.
- Squamous cell carcinoma can develop within the lesions in 3% to 10% of older patients; therefore periodic examination and biopsy of suspicious areas are indicated.

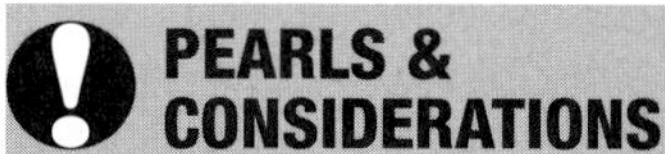

PEARLS & CONSIDERATIONS

COMMENTS

- Prepubertal lichen sclerosus may be confused with sexual abuse in prepubertal girls and may lead to false accusations and investigations.
- Lichen sclerosus of the vulva (kraurosis vulvae) usually occurs after menopause and is generally chronic. It can be painful and interfere with sexual activity.
- Lichen sclerosus of the penis (balanitis xerotica obliterans) is seen more commonly in uncircumcised males. It affects the glans and prepuce and may lead to stricture if it encroaches into the urinary meatus.

AUTHOR: **FRED F. FERRI, M.D.**

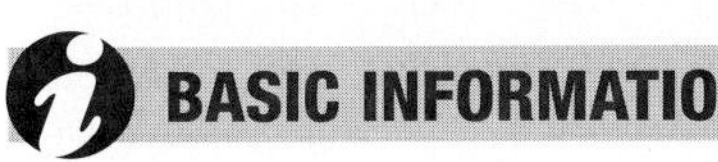

BASIC INFORMATION

DEFINITION

Listeriosis is a systemic infection caused by the gram-positive aerobic bacterium *Listeria monocytogenes.*

SYNONYMS

Listerial infection
Granulomatosis infantisepticum

ICD-9CM CODES
027.0 Listeriosis
771.2 Congenital listeriosis
771.2 Fetal listeriosis
665.4 Suspected fetal damage affecting management of pregnancy

EPIDEMIOLOGY & DEMOGRAPHICS

INCIDENCE (IN U.S.):
- Listeria meningitis: about 0.7 cases/100,000 persons (fourth most common cause of community-acquired bacterial meningitis in adults)
- Perinatal listeriosis: 8.6 cases/100,000 persons
- Nonperinatal listeriosis: 3 cases/1 million persons

PREDOMINANT SEX: Pregnant women are more susceptible to listeria bacteremia, accounting for up to one third of reported cases.

PREDOMINANT AGE:
- Pregnant women
- Immunocompromised patients of any age
- Elderly patients are susceptible even in the absence of recognized immunocompromised states

GENETICS:

Congenital infection:
- With transplacental transmission, syndrome termed *granulomatosis infantisepticum* in neonate
- Characterized by disseminated abscesses in multiple organs, skin lesions, and conjunctivitis
- Mortality: 33% to 100%

Neonatal infection:
- Infant becoming ill after 3 days of age; mother invariably asymptomatic
- Clinical picture of sepsis of unknown origin

PHYSICAL FINDINGS & CLINICAL PRESENTATION

Infections in pregnancy
1. More common in third trimester
2. Usually present with fever and chills without localizing symptoms or signs of infection

Meningoencephalitis
1. More common in neonates and immunocompromised patients, but up to 30% of adults have no underlying condition
2. In neonates: poor appetite with or without fever possibly the only presenting signs
3. In adults: presentation often subacute, with low-grade fever and personality change as only signs
4. Focal neurologic signs seen without demonstrable brain abscess on CT scan

Cerebritis/rhombencephalitis:
1. Headache and fever may be only presenting complaints
2. Progressive cranial nerve palsies, hemiparesis, seizures, depressed level of consciousness, cerebellar signs, respiratory insufficiency may also be seen

Focal infections
1. Ocular infections (purulent conjunctivitis) and skin lesions (granulomatosis infantisepticum) as a result of inadvertent inoculation by laboratory and veterinary personnel
2. Others: arthritis, prosthetic joint infections, peritonitis, osteomyelitis, organ abscesses, cholecystitis

ETIOLOGY

- Direct invasion of skin and eye has been documented, but mechanism of GI entry is unclear.
- Organism's intracellular life cycle explanatory of:
  1. Importance of cell-mediated immunity in host defense
  2. Increased infection in neonates, pregnant women, and immunocompromised hosts

DIAGNOSIS

DIFFERENTIAL DIAGNOSIS

- Meningitis caused by other bacteria, mycobacteria, or fungi
- CNS sarcoidosis
- Brain neoplasm or abscess
- Tuberculous and fungal (especially cryptococcal) meningitis
- Cerebral toxoplasmosis
- Lyme disease
- Sarcoidosis

WORKUP

Dictated by age, end-organ involvement, and immune status

LABORATORY TESTS

- Cultures of blood and other appropriate body fluids
- Variable CSF findings, but neutrophils usually predominate
- Organisms uncommonly seen on Gram stain and may be difficult to identify morphologically
- Monoclonal antibodies, polymerase chain reaction, and DNA probe techniques to detect *Listeria* in foods

IMAGING STUDIES

- If focal cerebral involvement suspected: CT scan or MRI
- MRI most sensitive for evaluation of brainstem and cerebellum

TREATMENT

Empiric therapy should be administered when diagnosis is suspected because overall mortality is 23%.

ACUTE GENERAL Rx

- Drugs of choice:
  1. IV ampicillin 8 to 12 g/day in divided doses
  2. IV penicillin 12 to 24 million U/day in divided doses
- Continuation of therapy for 2 wk
- Alternative (if penicillin allergic): trimethoprim/sulfamethoxazole or vancomycin
- Gentamicin added to provide synergy in meningitis or endocarditis

CHRONIC Rx

Relapses reported, especially in immunocompromised hosts, after 2 wk of therapy.

DISPOSITION

Long-term follow-up of immunodeficiency state

REFERRAL

Infectious disease consultation for all patients

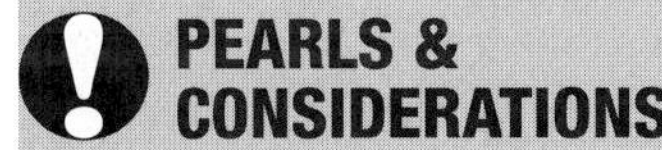

PEARLS & CONSIDERATIONS

COMMENTS

- Foodborne cases have been linked to various products: coleslaw, soft cheeses, unpasteurized milk and milk products, vegetables, undercooked chicken, hot dogs, luncheon meats, refrigerated smoked seafood, and so on.
- Complete decontamination of food products is difficult because *Listeria* is resistant to pasteurization and refrigeration.

SUGGESTED READINGS

Gottlieb SL et al: Multistate outbreak of Listeriosis linked to turkey deli meat and subsequent changes in US regulatory policy, *Clin Infect Dis* 42(1):29, 2006.

Mylonakis E et al: Listeriosis during pregnancy: a case series and review of 222 cases, *Medicine* 81:260, 2002.

Pasche B et al: Sex-dependent susceptibility to *Listeria monocytogenes* infection is mediated by differential interleukin-10 production, *Infect Immun* 73(9):5952, 2005.

Saunders BD et al: Molecular epidemiology and cluster analysis of human Listeriosis cases in three U.S. states, *J Food Prot* 69(7):1680, 2006.

Schlech WF et al: Does sporadic listeria gastroenteritis exist? A 2-year population-based survey in Nova Scotia, Canada, *Clin Infect Dis* 41(6):778, 2005.

AUTHORS: **GLENN G. FORT, M.D., M.P.H.,** and **DENNIS J. MIKOLICH, M.D.**

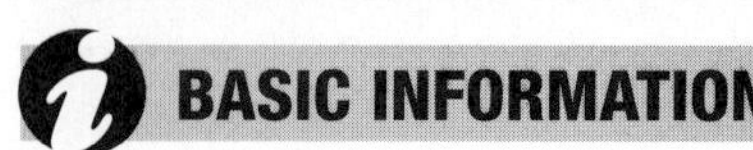

BASIC INFORMATION

DEFINITION

Long QT syndrome is a disorder of myocardial repolarization characterized by a prolonged QT interval on the ECG associated with an increased risk of developing life-threatening ventricular arrhythmias, most commonly torsades de pointes.

SYNONYMS

QT interval prolongation
Congenital forms:
- Jervell and Lange-Nielsen syndrome (associated with deafness)
- Romano-Ward syndrome (associated with normal hearing)

Sporadic forms of long QT syndrome (nonfamilial)

ICD-9CM CODES

427.9 Unspecified cardiac dysrhythmia

EPIDEMIOLOGY & DEMOGRAPHICS

- Congenital long QT syndrome is thought to account for more than 3000 deaths per year in the United States.
- Familial associated with deafness is autosomal recessive.
- Familial associated with normal hearing: autosomal dominant (the incidence is unknown). Although inheritance of long QT syndrome is autosomal dominant, female predominance has often been observed and has been attributed to an increased susceptibility to cardiac arrhythmias in women.
- Long QT syndrome is more common in women than in men.

PHYSICAL FINDINGS & CLINICAL PRESENTATION

- Palpitations, presyncope
- Syncope caused by ventricular tachycardia
- Sudden cardiac death (SCD)
- Seizure
- Family history of long QT syndrome, but a family history of SCD has not been proven to be a risk factor for SCD in patients with long QT syndrome
- Abnormal ECG (prolonged QT) in asymptomatic relatives of known case. Since QT interval shortens with increasing heart rate, the Bazett formula corrects the QT interval by heart rate:
  - QTcorrected (QTc) = QTmeasured divided by the square root of the R-R interval. Calculated QTc should generally be <440 ms in women and <420 ms in men. If the patient has atrial fibrillation, it is reasonable to take the average QTc of the longest and shortest R-R intervals.
- Routine (baseline) ECG finding

ETIOLOGY

- Cardiac repolarization abnormality
- Congenital cause (chromosome 3 or 7 abnormality)
- Acquired causes:
  - Drugs: dofetilide, ibutilide, bepridil, quinidine, procainamide, sotalol, amiodarone, ranolazine, disopyramide, phenothiazines and antiemetic agents (droperidol, domperidone), tricyclic antidepressants, quinolones, astemizole or cisapride given with ketoconazole or erythromycin, clarithromycin, and antimalarials, particularly among patients with asthma or those using potassium-lowering medications; also common in patients receiving methadone
  - Hypokalemia, hypomagnesemia, hypocalcemia (especially in patients with malabsorption syndrome)
  - Liquid protein diet
  - Central nervous system lesions
  - Mitral valve prolapse
  - Hypothyroidism

DIAGNOSIS

DIFFERENTIAL DIAGNOSIS

See "Syncope."

Diagnostic criteria for the congenital long QT syndrome:

ECG Criteria	
Corrected QT >480 ms	3 points
Corrected QT 460 to 480 ms	2 points
Corrected QT 450 to 460 ms (males)	1 point
Torsades de pointes	2 points
T-wave alternans	1 point
Notched T wave in 3 leads	1 point
Bradycardia	0.5 points
History	
Syncope with stress	2 points
Syncope without stress	1 point
Congenital deafness	0.5 points
Definite family history of long QT	1 point
Unexplained cardiac death in first-degree relative <30 yr	0.5 points

Total score = 4: definite long QT syndrome; total score = 2 to 3: intermediate probability; total score = 1: low probability.

WORKUP

Cardiology referral is recommended for all cases.

Genetic analysis is useful for risk stratification of patients with congenital prolonged QT and is important for identification of potential mutation carriers within the proband family.

In relatives of known patients with long QT syndrome or in young patients with syncope:
- Stress test may prolong the QT interval or cause T-wave alternans
- Valsalva maneuver: may prolong the QT interval or cause T-wave alternans
- Prolonged ECG monitoring with various stimulations aimed at increasing catecholamines and assess for QT prolongation (perform in a setting that can provide resuscitation)
- Epinephrine-induced prolongation of the QT interval (epinephrine infusion QT stress test)
- Genetic analysis
  - LQT1 locus of *KCNQ1* potassium channel gene
  - LQT2 locus of *KCNH2* potassium channel gene
  - LQT33 locus of *SCN5A* sodium channel gene
- Risk stratification: QT interval duration was the strongest predictor of risk for cardiac events (syncope, SCD); a QTc exceeding 500 ms identifies patients with the highest risk of becoming symptomatic by age 40; patients with the Jervell Lange-Nielsen and other homozygous syndromes and patients with long QT associated with syndactyly at higher risk
  - High risk (>50% of cardiac event): QTc >500 ms and LQT1 and LQT2 or male with LQT3
  - Moderate risk (30% to 50%): QTc <500 ms in male with LQT3 or in female with LQT2, and female with LQT3
  - Low risk (<30%): QTc <500 ms and LQT1 or male LQT2

TREATMENT

NONPHARMACOLOGIC

- Swimming should be avoided or performed under supervision in patients with LQT1.
- Patients with LQT2 patients should avoid sudden or excessive acoustic stimuli, especially during sleep (e.g., avoid telephone and/or alarm clock in the proximity).
- Avoid competitive sports.
- Implantable defibrillator is recommended according to the ACC/AHA guidelines for patients with a good functional status for more than 1 yr and the following conditions:
  - Survivors of cardiac arrest (class 1)
  - Patients with syncope or ventricular tachycardia while receiving β-blockers (class 2a)
  - Primary prevention in patients with characteristics that suggest high risk, such as LQT2 and LQT3 (class 2b)

PHARMACOLOGIC

- β-blocker at maximum tolerated dose
- Avoidance of medications that may further prolong the QT interval or deplete magnesium or potassium

PROGNOSIS

The timing and frequency of syncope, QTc prolongation, and gender are predictive of risk for aborted cardiac arrest and sudden cardiac death during adolescence. Higher risk is present in those with one or two or more episodes of syncope in the last 10 yr compared with those with no syncopal episodes, those with QTc >530 ms, and males between ages of 10 and 12 yr.

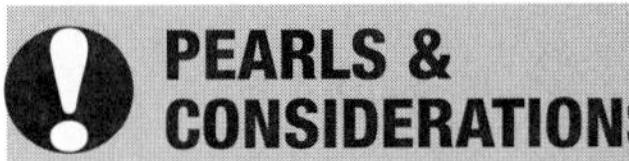

COMMENTS

Family history should be assessed for a history of sudden death and other deaths that may have occurred as manifestations of long QT syndrome (e.g., sudden infant death, drowning, loss of consciousness while driving).

SUGGESTED READINGS

Hobbs et al: Risk of aborted cardiac arrest or sudden cardiac death during adolescence in the long QT syndrome, *JAMA* 296:1249, 2006.

Napolitano C et al: Genetic testing in the long QT syndrome, *JAMA* 294:2975, 2005.

Priori SG et al: Risk stratification in the long-QT syndrome, *N Engl J Med* 348:1866, 2003.

Roden DM: Drug-induced prolongation of the QT interval, *N Engl J Med* 350:1013, 2004.

Roden DM: Long QT syndrome, *N Engl J Med* 358:169-176, 2008.

Zipes DP et al: ACC/AHA/ESC 2006. Guidelines for management of patients with ventricular arrhythmias and the prevention of sudden cardiac death: a report of the American College of Cardiology, American Heart Association Task Force and the European Society of Cardiology Committee for Practice Guidelines (Writing Committee to Develop Guidelines for Management of Patients With Ventricular Arrhythmias and the Prevention of Sudden Cardiac Death), *J Am Coll Cardiol* 48:e247–e346, 2006.

AUTHORS: **THOMAS J. EARL, M.D., FRED F. FERRI, M.D.,** and **WEN-CHIH WU, M.D.**

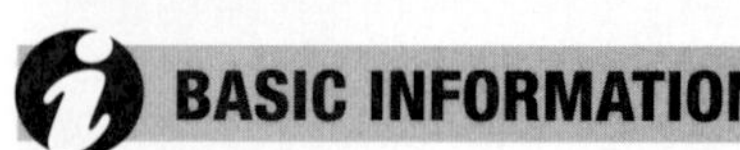

BASIC INFORMATION

DEFINITION

Lumbar disk syndrome includes diseases resulting from disk disorder, either herniation or degenerative change (spondylosis). Massive disk protrusion may rarely lead to paralysis in the lower extremity, a condition termed *cauda equina syndrome.* Gradual narrowing of the spinal canal (lumbar stenosis), usually from spondylosis, may also cause lower extremity symptoms.

SYNONYMS

Lumbago
Sciatica

ICD-9CM CODES
722.10 Lumbar disk displacement
724.02 Lumbar stenosis
344.60 Cauda equina syndrome
721.3 Lumbar spondylosis

EPIDEMIOLOGY & DEMOGRAPHICS

PREVALENCE:
- Variable
- At least one episode in 80% of adults

PREDOMINANT SEX: Approximately equal
PREDOMINANT AGE:
- Herniation: 20 to 40 yr
- Stenosis: >40 to 50 yr
- Disk symptoms: rare <20 yr

PHYSICAL FINDINGS & CLINICAL PRESENTATION

- Overlapping clinical syndromes that may result:
  1. Mild herniation without nerve root compression
  2. Herniation with nerve root compression
  3. Cauda equina syndrome
  4. Chronic degenerative disease with or without leg symptoms
  5. Spinal stenosis
- Low back pain, often worsened by activity or coughing and sneezing
- Local lumbar or lumbosacral tenderness
- Paresthesias, usually unilateral
- Restricted low back motion
- Increased pain on bending toward affected side
- Weakness and reflex changes (L4—knee jerk and quadriceps, L5—extensor hallucis longus, S1—ankle jerk and toe walking)
- Sensory examination usually not helpful
- Lumbar stenosis that possibly produces symptoms (pseudoclaudication), which are often misinterpreted as being vascular (Pseudoclaudication usually recovers quickly with sitting or spine flexion. Vascular disease is unaffected by spine position and is typically associated with atrophic skin changes and diminished pulses.)
- Positive straight leg raising test if nerve root compression is present

ETIOLOGY

Unknown

DIAGNOSIS

DIFFERENTIAL DIAGNOSIS

- Soft tissue strain or sprain
- Tumor
- Degenerative arthritis of hip
- Insufficiency fracture of hip or pelvis

Section II describes the differential diagnosis of common low back pain syndromes.

WORKUP

In most cases the diagnosis can be established on a clinical basis alone.

IMAGING STUDIES

- Plain roentgenograms may be indicated within the first few weeks; they are usually normal in soft disk herniation, but with chronic degenerative disk disease loss of height of the disk space and osteophyte formation can occur.
- Myelography, CT scanning, and MRI (Fig. 1-183) may be indicated in patients whose symptoms do not resolve or when other spinal pathology may be suspected.
- Electrodiagnostic studies may confirm the diagnosis or rule out peripheral nerve disorders.

TREATMENT

NONPHARMACOLOGIC THERAPY

- Short course (3 to 5 days) of bed rest for acute disk herniation with leg pain
- Physical therapy for modalities plus a careful gradual exercise program
- Lumbosacral corset brace during rehabilitation process in conjunction with exercise program
- Percutaneous electrical nerve stimulation may be beneficial in selected patients with chronic back pain

FIGURE 1-183 MRI showing a prolapsed L5/S1 disc. (From Carr A, Hamilton W: *Orthopedics in primary care,* ed 2, Philadelphia, 2005, Elsevier.)

ACUTE GENERAL Rx

- NSAIDs
- Muscle relaxants for sedative effect
- Analgesics
- Epidural steroid injection for leg symptoms in selected patients

DISPOSITION

- Almost all lumbar disk syndromes improve with time.
- Recurrent episodes usually respond to medical management.
- Recovery from the rare paralytic event is often incomplete.

REFERRAL

- For orthopedic or neurosurgical consultation for intractable pain or significant neurologic deficit
- Emergency referral for cauda equina syndrome

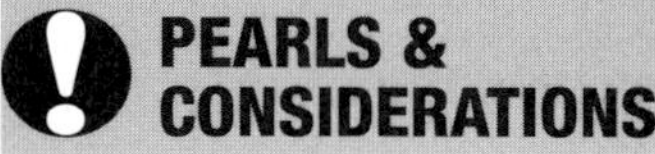

PEARLS & CONSIDERATIONS

Red flags suggesting a more serious condition as a cause of the back pain include:
1. Fever
2. History of malignancy
3. Pain at rest
4. Incontinence
5. Sudden worsening in level of pain
6. Weight loss
7. Significant motor loss, especially if associated with saddle anesthesia

COMMENTS

- Surgery is most consistently helpful when leg pain (not back pain) predominates.
- A clinical algorithm for evaluation of back pain is described in Section III.

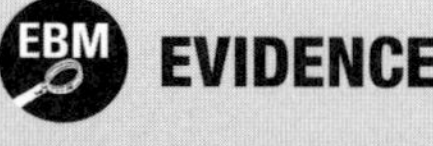

EVIDENCE

Medications for back pain
Two randomized controlled trials (RCTs) have found significant improvements in pain scores and function when etoricoxib 60 mg and 90 mg was compared with placebo for people with chronic back pain.[1] Ⓐ
Other therapies for back pain
A systematic review and additional RCTs have found that advice to stay active (with or without other treatments) is more effective than bed rest (with or without other treatments) in the management of acute low back pain. Patients who remained active had reduced pain, disability, and time away from work.[2] Ⓐ

Evidence from systematic reviews and RCTs suggests that back exercises are either no more effective than conservative or inactive treatments in improving pain and disability associated with acute back pain, or that exercise actually increases pain and disability in people with acute back pain.[2] Ⓐ

A systematic review found that a graded-activity exercise program in people with subacute low back pain in occupational settings had some benefit. Exercise therapy may improve return to normal daily activities and work in patients with chronic low back pain.[3] Ⓐ

A systematic review for chronic low back pain found acupuncture to be more effective than no treatment or sham treatment immediately after treatment and in the short term only but no more effective than other treatments.[4] Ⓐ

There is conflicting evidence about the efficacy of prolotherapy injections in the management of chronic low back pain.[5] Ⓐ

Evidence-Based References

1. Pallay RM et al: Etoricoxib reduced pain and disability and improved quality of life in patients with chronic low back pain: a 3 month, randomized, controlled trial, *Scand J Rheumatol* 33:257-256, 2004. Ⓐ
2. Koes B, van Tulder M: Low back pain (acute), *Clin Evid*, 2007. Ⓐ
3. Hayden JA et al: Exercise therapy for treatment of non-specific low back pain, *Cochrane Database Rev* (3). Ⓐ
4. Furlan AD et al: Acupuncture and dry needling for low back pain, *Cochrane Database Rev* (1), 2005. Ⓐ
5. Dagenais S et al: Prolotherapy injections for chronic low-back pain, *Cochrane Database Rev* (2), 2007. Ⓐ

SUGGESTED READINGS

Anderson PA et al: Randomized controlled trials of the treatment of lumbar-disk herniation: 1983-2007, *J Acad Orthop Surg* 16:566, 2008.

Chou R et al: Diagnosis and treatment of low back pain: a joint clinical practice guideline from the American College of Physicians and the American Pain Society, *Ann Intern Med* 147:478, 2007.

Cole BJ, Schumacher HR: Injectable corticosteroids in modern practice, *J Am Acad Orthop Surg* 13:37, 2005.

Dreyfuss P et al: Sacroiliac joint pain, *J Am Acad Orthop Surg* 12:255, 2004.

Gregory DS et al: Acute lumbar disc pain: navigating evaluation and treatment choices, *Am Fam Physician* 78(7):835-842, 2008.

Haig AJ et al: Electromyographic and magnetic resonance imaging to predict lumbar stenosis, low back pain, and no back symptoms, *J Bone Joint Surg Am* 89A:358, 2007.

Johansson AC et al: A prospective study of cognitive behavioral factors as predictors of pain, disability, and quality of life one year after lumbar disc surgery, *Disabil Rehabil* 32:521, 2010.

Katz JN: Lumbar disc disorders and low-back pain: socioeconomic factors and consequences, *J Bone Joint Surg Am* 88A(suppl 2):21, 2006.

Lee DH et al: Clinical nerve conduction and needle electromyography studies, *J Am Acad Orthop Surg* 12:276, 2004.

Madigan L et al: Management of symptomatic lumbar degenerative disc disease, *J Am Acad Orthop Surg* 17:102, 2009.

Shen FH et al: Nonsurgical management of acute and chronic low back pain, *J Am Acad Orthop Surg* 14: 477, 2006.

Spector LR et al: Cauda equina syndrome, *J Am Acad Orthop Surg* 16:471, 2008.

Thomas KC et al: Outcome evaluation of surgical and non surgical management of lumbar disc protrusion causing radiculopathy, *Spine* 32:1414, 2007.

Tribus CB: Degenerative lumbar scoliosis: evaluation and management, *J Am Acad Orthop Surg* 11:174, 2003.

Young IA et al: The use of lumbar epidural/transforaminal steroids for managing spinal disease, *J Am Acad Orthop Surg* 15:228, 2007.

AUTHOR: **LONNIE R. MERCIER, M.D.**

BASIC INFORMATION

DEFINITION

A primary lung neoplasm is a malignancy arising from lung tissue. The World Health Organization distinguishes 12 types of pulmonary neoplasms. The major types are squamous cell carcinoma, adenocarcinoma, small cell carcinoma, and large cell carcinoma. However, the crucial difference in the diagnosis of lung cancer is between small cell and non–small cell types because the prognosis and therapeutic approach are different.

ADENOCARCINOMA: Represents 35% to 40% of lung carcinomas; frequently located in midlung and periphery; initial metastases are to lymphatics; frequently associated with peripheral scars

SQUAMOUS CELL (EPIDERMOID): 20% to 30% of lung cancers; central location; metastasis by local invasion; frequent cavitation and obstructive phenomena

SMALL CELL (OAT CELL): 20% of lung carcinomas; central location; metastasis through lymphatics; associated with lesion of the short arm of chromosome 3; high cavitation rate

LARGE CELL: 10% to 15% of lung carcinomas; frequently located in the periphery; metastasis to central nervous system and mediastinum; rapid growth rate with early metastasis

BRONCHOALVEOLAR: 5% of lung carcinomas; frequently located in the periphery; may be bilateral; initial metastasis through lymphatic, hematogenous, and local invasion; no correlation with cigarette smoking; cavitation rare

SYNONYMS

Lung cancer

ICD-9CM CODES
162.9 Malignant neoplasm of bronchus and lung, unspecified

EPIDEMIOLOGY & DEMOGRAPHICS

- Lung cancer is responsible for >30% of cancer deaths in males and >25% of cancer deaths in females. It has been the most common cancer in the world since 1985 and is the leading cause of cancer-related death.
- Tobacco smoking is implicated in 85% of cases; second-hand smoke is responsible for approximately 20% of cases.
- There are >200,000 new cases of lung cancer yearly in the U.S., most occurring at age >50 yr (<4% in patients <40 yr).
- Among women there has been a 600% increase in incidence of lung cancer during the past 80 years. The rates of death among women with lung cancer in the U.S. are the highest in the world.

PHYSICAL FINDINGS & CLINICAL PRESENTATION

- Weight loss, fatigue, fever, anorexia, dysphagia
- Cough, hemoptysis, dyspnea, wheezing
- Chest, shoulder, and bone pain
- Paraneoplastic syndromes:
  - Lambert-Eaton syndrome: myopathy involving proximal muscle groups
  - Endocrine manifestations: hypercalcemia, ectopic adrenocorticotropic hormone, syndrome of inappropriate excretion of adrenocorticotropic hormone
  - Neurologic: subacute cerebellar degeneration, peripheral neuropathy, cortical degeneration
  - Musculoskeletal: polymyositis, clubbing, hypertrophic pulmonary osteoarthropathy
  - Hematologic or vascular: migratory thrombophlebitis, marantic thrombosis, anemia, thrombocytosis, or thrombocytopenia
  - Cutaneous: acanthosis nigricans, dermatomyositis
- Pleural effusion (10% of patients), recurrent pneumonias (from obstruction), localized wheezing
- Superior vena cava syndrome:
  - Obstruction of venous return of the superior vena cava is most commonly caused by bronchogenic carcinoma or metastasis to paratracheal nodes.
  - The patient usually reports headache, nausea, dizziness, visual changes, syncope, and respiratory distress.
  - Physical examination reveals distention of thoracic and neck veins, edema of face and upper extremities, facial plethora, and cyanosis.
- Horner's syndrome: constricted pupil, ptosis, facial anhidrosis caused by spinal cord damage between C8 and T1 as a result of a superior sulcus tumor (bronchogenic carcinoma of the extreme lung apex); Pancoast tumor: a superior sulcus tumor associated with ipsilateral Horner's syndrome and shoulder pain

ETIOLOGY

- Tobacco abuse
- Environmental agents (e.g., radon) and industrial agents (e.g., ionizing radiation, asbestos, nickel, uranium, vinyl chloride, chromium, arsenic, coal dust)
- Lung cancer susceptibility and risk increased in inherited cancer syndromes caused by germ-line mutations in p53, retinoblastoma, and germ-line mutation in the epidermal growth factor receptor (EGFR) gene; also an association between single-nucleotide polymorphism variation at 15q24-15q25.1 and susceptibility to lung cancer

Dx DIAGNOSIS

DIFFERENTIAL DIAGNOSIS

- Pneumonia
- Tuberculosis (TB)
- Metastatic carcinoma to the lung
- Lung abscess
- Granulomatous disease
- Carcinoid tumor
- Mycobacterial and fungal diseases
- Sarcoidosis
- Viral pneumonitis
- Benign lesions that simulate thoracic malignancy:
  - Lobar atelectasis: pneumonia, TB, chronic inflammatory disease, allergic bronchopulmonary aspergillosis
  - Multiple pulmonary nodules: septic emboli, Wegener's granulomatosis, sarcoidosis, rheumatoid nodules, fungal disease, multiple pulmonary atrioventricular fistulas
  - Mediastinal adenopathy: sarcoidosis, lymphoma, primary TB, fungal disease, silicosis, pneumoconiosis, drug-induced (e.g., phenytoin, trimethadione)
  - Pleural effusion: congestive heart failure, pneumonia with parapneumonic effusion, TB, viral pneumonitis, ascites, pancreatitis, collagen-vascular disease

WORKUP

Workup generally includes chest radiograph, CT scan of chest, positron-emission tomographic (PET) scan, and tissue biopsy.

LABORATORY TESTS

Obtain tissue diagnosis. Various modalities are available:

- Biopsy of any suspicious lymph nodes (e.g., supraclavicular node)
- Flexible fiberoptic bronchoscopy: brush and biopsy specimens are obtained from any visualized endobronchial lesions
- Transbronchial needle aspiration: done with a special needle passed through the bronchoscope; this technique is useful to sample mediastinal masses or paratracheal lymph nodes
- Transthoracic fine-needle aspiration biopsy with fluoroscopic or CT scan guidance to evaluate peripheral pulmonary nodules
- Mediastinoscopy and anteromedial sternotomy in suspected tumor involvement of the mediastinum
- Pleural biopsy in patients with pleural effusion
- Thoracentesis of pleural effusion and cytologic evaluation of the obtained fluid: may confirm diagnosis

IMAGING STUDIES

- Chest radiograph (Fig. 1-184): The radiographic presentation often varies with the cell type. Pleural effusion, lobar atelectasis, and mediastinal adenopathy can accompany any cell types.
- CT scan of chest is performed to evaluate mediastinal and pleural extension of suspected lung neoplasms.
- PET with 18F-fluorodeoxyglucose (18 FDG-PET), a metabolic marker of malignant tissue, is superior to CT scan in detecting mediastinal and distant metastases in non–small cell lung cancer (NSLC). It is useful for preoperative staging of NSLC.
- The use of PET-CT for preoperative staging of NSLC reduces both the total number of thoracotomies and the number of futile thoracotomies but does not affect overall mortality.

STAGING

After confirmation of diagnosis, patients should undergo staging:

1. The international staging system is the most widely accepted staging system for NSLC. In this system, stage I (N0 [no lymph node involvement]) and stage II (N1 [spread to ipsilateral bronchopulmonary or hilar lymph nodes]) include localized tumors for which surgical resection is the preferred treatment. Stage III is subdivided into IIIA (potentially resectable) and IIIB. The surgical management of stage IIIA disease (N2 [involvement of ipsilateral mediastinal nodes]) is controversial. Only 20% of N2 disease is considered minimal disease (involvement of only one node) and technically resectable. Stage IV indicates metastatic disease. The pathologic staging system uses a tumor/nodal involvement/metastasis system.
2. In patients with small cell lung cancer, a more practical accepted staging system is the one developed by the Veterans Administration Lung Cancer Study Group. This system contains two stages:
   a. Limited-stage disease: confined to the regional lymph nodes and to one hemithorax (excluding pleural surfaces)
   b. Extensive-stage disease: spread beyond the confines of limited-stage disease
3. Pretreatment staging procedures for lung cancer patients, in addition to complete history and physical examination, generally include the following tests:
   a. Chest radiograph (posteroanterior and lateral), ECG
   b. Laboratory evaluation: complete blood count, complete metabolic panel, arterial blood gases, pulse oximetry. The identification of molecular signatures of lung cancer to predict prognosis with data from microarray and/or reverse-transcription polymerase chain reaction analysis has been validated in recent trials. A five-gene signature (*DUSP6, MMD, STAT1, ERBB3,* and *LCK*) is closely associated with relapse-free and overall survival among patients with NSLC. Detection of mutations in epidermal growth factor receptor (EGFR) in circulating tumor cells from the blood of patients with lung cancer offers the possibility of monitoring changes in epithelial tumor genotypes during the course of treatment
   c. Pulmonary function studies
   d. CT scan of chest and PET scan: a recent Dutch trial revealed a 51% relative reduction in futile thoracotomies for patients with suspected NSLC who underwent preoperative assessment with PET with the tracer 18FDG-PET in addition to conventional workup
   e. Mediastinoscopy or anterior mediastinotomy in patients being considered for possible curative lung resection
   f. Biopsy of any accessible suspect lesions
   g. CT scan of liver and brain; radionuclide scans of bone in all patients with small cell carcinoma of the lung and patients with NSLC neoplasms suspected of involving these organs
   h. Bone marrow aspiration and biopsy only in selected patients with small cell carcinoma of the lung. In the absence of an increased lactate dehydrogenase or cytopenia, routine bone marrow examination not recommended
   i. Newer technologies in preoperative staging include endoscopic bronchial ultrasonography and esophageal ultrasonography to guide biopsies; however, cervical mediastinoscopy is criterion standard in preoperative nodal staging (sensitivity $>$ 93%, specificity $>$ 95%)

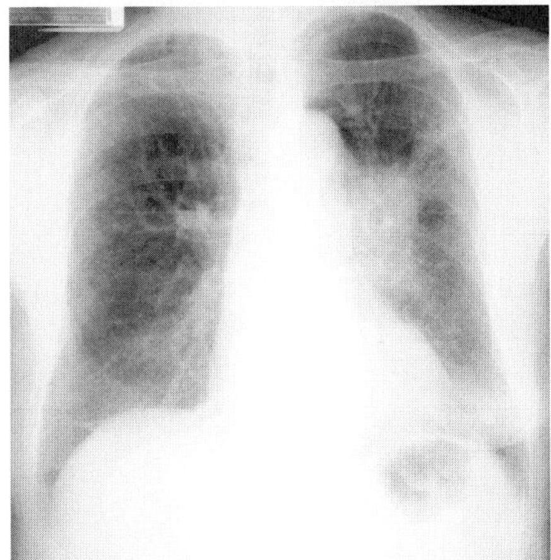

FIGURE 1-184 Chest radiograph shows small cell carcinoma of lung manifesting as left hilar mass. (From Weinberg SE, Cockrill BA, Mandel J: *Principles of pulmonary medicine,* ed 5, Philadelphia, 2008, Saunders.)

Rx TREATMENT

NONPHARMACOLOGIC THERAPY

- Nutritional support
- Avoidance of tobacco and other substances toxic to the lungs
- Supplemental O_2 prn

ACUTE GENERAL Rx

NON–SMALL CELL CARCINOMA:

- Surgical resection is the best hope for cure in patients with operable NSLC.
  1. Surgical resection is indicated in patients with limited disease (not involving mediastinal nodes, ribs, pleura, or distant sites). This represents approximately 15% to 30% of diagnosed cases.
  2. Preoperative evaluation includes review of cardiac status (e.g., recent myocardial infarction, major arrhythmias) and evaluation of pulmonary function (to determine if the patient can tolerate any loss of lung tissue). Pneumonectomy is possible if the patient has a preoperative $FEV_1 = 2$ L or if the maximal voluntary ventilation is $>$50% of predicted capacity. Individuals with $FEV_1 >1.5$ L are suitable for lobectomy without further evaluation unless there is evidence of interstitial lung disease or undue dyspnea on exertion. In that case, carbon dioxide diffusion in the lung (DL_{CO}) should be measured. If the DL_{CO} is $<$80% predicted normal, the individual is not clearly operable.
  3. Preoperative chemotherapy should be considered in patients with more advanced disease (stage IIIA) who are being considered for surgery because it increases the median survival time in patients with NSLC compared with the use of surgery alone. Gene expression profiles that predict the risk of recurrence in patients with early stage (IA) NSLC have been identified. These patients are at high risk of recurrence and may also benefit from adjuvant chemotherapy.
  4. Postoperative adjuvant chemotherapy (chemotherapy given after surgical resection of an apparently localized tumor to eradicate occult metastases) with vinorelbine plus cisplatin significantly increases 5-yr survival (69% vs. 54%) in patients with completely resected stage IB or stage II NSLC and good performance status. Adjuvant chemotherapy is generally indicated for patients with resected stages IIA through IIIA.
- Treatment of unresectable NSLC:
  1. Radiotherapy can be used alone or in combination with chemotherapy; it is used primarily for treatment of central nervous system and skeletal metastases, superior vena cava syndrome, and obstructive atelectasis. Although thoracic radiotherapy is generally considered standard therapy for stage 3 disease, it has limited effect on survival. Palliative radiotherapy should be delayed until symptoms occur because immediate therapy offers no advantage over delayed therapy and results in more adverse events from the radiotherapy.
  2. Chemotherapy: various combination regimens are available. Current drugs of choice are paclitaxel plus either carboplatin or cisplatin, cisplatin plus vinorelbine, gemcitabine plus cisplatin, and carboplatin or cisplatin plus docetaxel. The overall results are disappointing, and none of the standard regimens for NSLC is clearly superior to the others. The addition of bevacizumab to paclitaxel plus carboplatin results in significant survival benefit but carries an increased risk of treatment-related death. Gefitinib and erlotinib are oral inhibitors of EGFR tyrosine kinase. Activating mutations in the *EGFR* gene confer hypersensitivity to these medications. Both agents are currently approved only for patients who have not responded to at least one prior chemotherapy regimen. Sensitivity of lung neoplasms to these agents is seen primarily in tumors with somatic mutations in the tyrosine kinase domain (more common in adenocarcinomas found in patients who never smoked and in Asian patients). Recent

trials revealed that gefitinib is superior to carboplatin-paclitaxel as an initial treatment for pulmonary adenocarcinoma among nonsmokers or former smokers in East Asia. In these patients the presence in the tumor of a mutation of the *EGFR* gene was a strong predictor of a better outcome with gefitinib.

3. The addition of chemotherapy to radiotherapy improves survival in patients with locally advanced, unresectable NSLC. The absolute benefit is relatively small, however, and should be balanced against the increased toxicity associated with the addition of chemotherapy.

SMALL CELL LUNG CANCER:

- Limited-stage disease: standard treatments include thoracic radiotherapy and chemotherapy (cisplatin and etoposide)
- Extensive-stage disease: standard treatments include combination chemotherapy (cisplatin or carboplatin plus etoposide or combination of irinotecan and cisplatin)
- Prophylactic cranial irradiation for patients in complete remission to decrease the risk of central nervous system metastasis

DISPOSITION

- The 5-yr survival of patients with NSLC when the disease is resectable is approximately 30%.
- Median survival time in patients with limited-stage disease and small cell lung cancer is 15 mo; in patients with extensive stage disease, it is 9 mo.
- Methylation of the promoter region of certain genes (*P16, CDH13, APC,* and *RASSF1A*) in a resected NSLC specimen is associated with recurrence of the tumor.

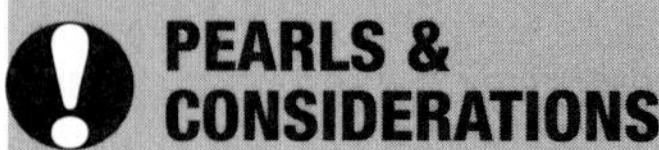

PEARLS & CONSIDERATIONS

COMMENTS

CT screening for detection of lung cancer among persons with a heavy history of smoking increases the percentage of lung cancer cases that are diagnosed in stage 1. However, randomized trials to assess whether such screening reduces mortality rates have not shown a significant benefit for CT screening. Current data do not support screening for lung cancer with any method.

EBM EVIDENCE

Non–Small Cell Lung Cancer (NSLC) Resectable Disease (Stage I-IIIA)

There is evidence that surgical resection is effective in the treatment of NSLC.

A systematic review found that lobectomy with complete resection of the mediastinal lymph nodes was superior (in terms of local recurrence and survival) compared with more limited surgery in the treatment of stage I to IIIA resectable NSLC.[1]

There is evidence for the use of adjuvant chemotherapy in the management of resectable (stage I-IIIA) NSLC. Systematic reviews and meta-analyses of randomized, controlled trials (RCTs) in patients with resectable NSLC have found that the use of postoperative cisplatin-based chemotherapy confers small but significant survival and disease-free survival benefits compared with surgery alone.[2]

Subsequent RCTs have found that the use of postoperative cisplatin-based chemotherapy improves overall and disease-free survival in patients with completely resected stage IB/II NSLC.[3,4]

NSLC: Nonresectable/Advanced Disease (Stage IIIB/IV)

There is evidence that combined chemotherapy plus radiotherapy is of benefit in the treatment of advanced NSLC.

Systematic reviews have found that the use of palliative radiotherapy is superior to supportive care (in terms of increased survival data) in patients with advanced NSLC.[5]

Small Cell Lung Cancer (SCLC)
Treatment for Limited Stage SCLC:

There is good evidence that, for patients undergoing chemotherapy, adjunctive chest irradiation is effective in the treatment of limited stage SCLC.

Systematic reviews have found that the use of concurrent radiation therapy is associated with small but improved survival time compared with later administration.[6,7]

Evidence-Based References

1. Manser R et al: Surgery for early stage non-small cell lung cancer, *Cochrane Rev* 1, 2005.
2. Sedrakyan A et al: Postoperative chemotherapy for non-small cell lung cancer: a systematic review and meta-analysis, *J Thorac Cardiovasc Surg* 128: 414-419, 2004.
3. Arriagada R et al: Cisplatin-based adjuvant chemotherapy in patients with completely resected non-small-cell lung cancer, *N Engl J Med* 350:351-360, 2004.
4. Winton T et al: National Cancer Institute of Canada Clinical Trials Group; National Cancer Institute of the United States Intergroup JBR.10 Trial Investigators. Vinorelbine plus cisplatin vs. observation in resected non-small-cell lung cancer, *N Engl J Med* 352:2589-2597, 2005.
5. Lester JF et al: Palliative radiotherapy regimens for non-small cell lung cancer, *Cochrane Rev* 4, 2006.
6. Pijls-Johannesma MCG et al: Early versus late chest radiotherapy for limited stage small cell lung cancer, *Cochrane Rev* 4, 2004.
7. Fried DB et al: Systematic review evaluating the timing of thoracic radiation therapy in combined modality therapy for limited-stage small-cell lung cancer, *J Clin Oncol* 22:4837-4845, 2004.

SUGGESTED READINGS

Brock MV et al: DNA methylation markers and early recurrence in stage I lung cancer, *N Engl J Med* 358:1118-1128, 2008.

Fisher B et al: Preoperative staging of lung cancer with combined PET-CT, *N Engl J Med* 361:32-9, 2009.

Herbst RS et al: Lung cancer, *N Engl J Med* 359:1367-1380, 2008.

Maheswaran S et al: Detection of mutations in EGFR in circulating lung cancer cells, *N Engl J Med* 359:366, 2008.

Mok TS et al: Gefitinib or carboplatin-paclitaxel in pulmonary adenocarcinoma, *N Engl J Med* 361: 947-57, 2009.

Molina JR et al: Non-small cell lung cancer: epidemiology, risk factors, treatment, and survivorship, *Mayo Clin Proc* 83(5):584-594, 2008.

Mostertz W et al: Age- and sex-specific genomic profiles in non-small cell lung cancer, *JAMA* 303(6): 535-543, 2010.

Shert DY et al: Small cell lung cancer, *Mayo Clin Proc* 83(3):355-367, 2008.

AUTHOR: **FRED F. FERRI, M.D.**

BASIC INFORMATION

DEFINITION

Lyme disease is a multisystem inflammatory disorder caused by the transmission of a spirochete, *Borrelia burgdorferi.* Lyme disease is spread by the bite of infected *Ixodes* ticks, taking 36 to 48 hr for a tick to feed and transmit the infecting organism *B. burgdorferi* to the host.

SYNONYMS

Bannworth's syndrome (Europe)
Acrodermatitis chronica atrophicans

ICD-9CM CODES
088.8 Lyme disease

EPIDEMIOLOGY & DEMOGRAPHICS

INCIDENCE (IN U.S.): 4.4 cases/100,000 persons; 90% of cases in the U.S. are found in: Massachusetts, Connecticut, Rhode Island, New York, New Jersey, Pennsylvania, Minnesota, Wisconsin, and California.
PEAK INCIDENCE: May to November
PREDOMINANT SEX: Male = female
PREDOMINANT AGE: Median age of 28 yr

PHYSICAL FINDINGS & CLINICAL PRESENTATION

Lyme disease may present in the following stages:

- *Early localized:* early Lyme disease, erythema migrans (EM); skin rash, often at site of tick bite; possible fever, myalgias 3 to 32 days after tick bite
- *Early disseminated:* days to weeks later; multiorgan system involvement, including CNS, joints, cardiac; related to dissemination of spirochete
- *Late persistent:* mo to yr after tick exposure; affects central and peripheral nervous system, cardiac, joints

Common presenting signs and symptoms include:

- EM (Fig. 1-185).
- Lymphadenopathy, neck pains, pharyngeal erythema, myalgias, hepatosplenomegaly.
- Patients will complain of malaise, fatigue, lethargy, headache, fever/chills, neck pain, myalgias, back pain.

ETIOLOGY

B. burgdorferi transmitted from bite of an *Ixodes* tick

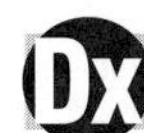

DIAGNOSIS

Clinical presentation, exposure to ticks in endemic area, and diagnostic testing for antibody response to *B. burgdorferi*

DIFFERENTIAL DIAGNOSIS

- Chronic fatigue/fibromyalgia
- Acute viral illnesses
- Babesiosis
- Ehrlichiosis

WORKUP

- ELISA testing-Western blot IgM and IgG
- Immunofluorescent assay
- Early disease often difficult to diagnose serologically secondary to slow immune response
- Culturing of skin lesions (EM) and polymerase chain reaction (PCR) of skin biopsy and blood to give definitive diagnosis (available only in reference laboratories)

IMAGING STUDIES

- Echocardiogram if conduction abnormalities are present with cardiac involvement
- CT scan, MRI of head for CNS involvement

Rx TREATMENT

- Early Lyme disease.
- Doxycycline 100 mg bid or amoxicillin 500 mg tid for 14 days (doxycycline should be avoided in children and pregnant females).
- Alternative treatments: cefuroxime axetil 500 mg bid for 14 to 21 days, azithromycin 500 mg PO for 7 to 10 days but should not be used as a first-line agent.
- Early disseminated and late persistent infection: 30 days of treatment necessary; doxycycline and ceftriaxone appear equally effective for acute disseminated Lyme disease.
- Arthritis: 30 days of doxycycline or amoxicillin plus probenecid.
- Neurologic involvement requires parenteral antibiotics.
- Ceftriaxone 2 g/day for 21 to 28 days; alternative: cefotaxime 2 g q8h; alternative: penicillin G 5 million U qid.
- Cardiac involvement: IV ceftriaxone or penicillin plus cardiac monitoring.
- Prolonged treatment with IV or PO antibiotic therapy for up to 90 days did not improve symptoms more than placebo.

DISPOSITION

The patient often needs careful follow-up and supportive care for the arthralgia-neuritis symptoms.

REFERRAL

- To a neurologist if significant neurologic complications (meningitis, myelitis, ophthalmoplegia, Bell's palsy)
- To a cardiologist if the patient develops evidence of cardiac conduction disturbances or pericarditis

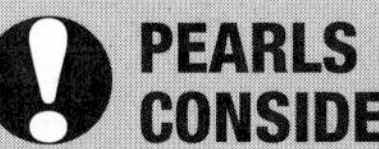

PEARLS & CONSIDERATIONS

- The Lyme disease vaccine was taken off the U.S. market in 2002 because of concerns about possible side effects (arthralgia, arthritis) and its infrequent use.
- A physician diagnosis of classic erythema migrans in an endemic region of Lyme disease is sufficient to make a definitive diagnosis.
- In some patients with Lyme disease, nonspecific complaints such as headache, fatigue, and arthralgia may persist for months after appropriate (and ultimately successful) antibiotic treatment.
- A single dose of 200 mg doxycycline given within 72 hr of *Ixodes* tick bite can prevent development of Lyme disease.

SUGGESTED READINGS

Bratton RL et al: Diagnosis and treatment of Lyme disease, *Mayo Clin Proc* 83(50):566-571, 2008.

Feder HM et al: A critical appraisal of "Chronic Lyme Disease," *N Engl J Med* 357:1422-1430, 2007.

Wormser GP et al: The clinical assessment, treatment, and prevention of Lyme disease, human granulocytic anaplasmosis, and babesiosis: clinical practice guidelines by the Infectious Diseases Society of America, *CID* 43:1089, 2006.

AUTHORS: **GLENN G. FORT, M.D., M.P.H.,** and **DENNIS J. MIKOLICH, M.D.**

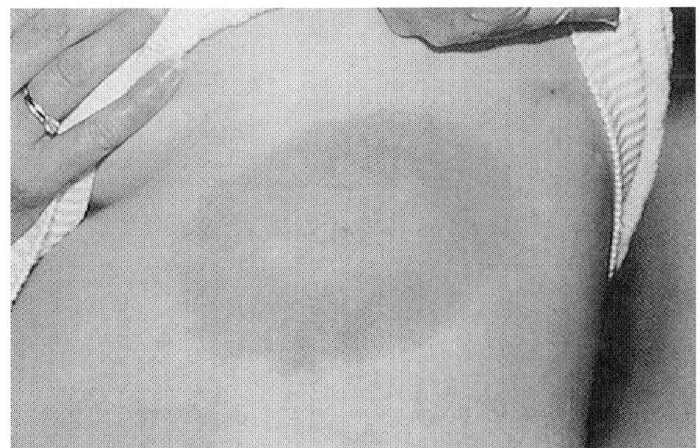

FIGURE 1-185 Erythema migrans. Note expanding erythematous lesion with central clearing on trunk. (Courtesy John Cook, M.D. From Goldstein B [ed]: *Practical dermatology,* ed 2, St Louis, 1997, Mosby.)

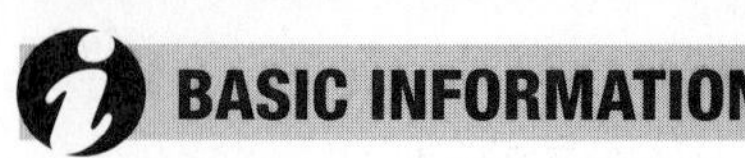

BASIC INFORMATION

DEFINITION

Lymphangitis refers to the inflammation of lymphatic vessels.

SYNONYMS

Nodular lymphangitis
Sporotrichoid lymphangitis

ICD-9CM CODES
457.2 Lymphangitis

EPIDEMIOLOGY & DEMOGRAPHICS

INCIDENCE (IN U.S.): Several hundred cases/yr of sporotrichoid lymphangitis

PHYSICAL FINDINGS & CLINICAL PRESENTATION

ACUTE LYMPHANGITIS:

- Commonly associated with a bacterial cellulitis
- May or may not recognize site of skin trauma (i.e., laceration, puncture, ulcer)
- In hours to days, distal appearance of erythema, edema, and tenderness, with linear erythematous streaks extending proximally to regional lymph nodes
- Possible lymphadenitis and fever
- Predisposition to group A streptococcal infection of the skin in those with chronic lymphedema and superficial fungal infections (e.g., tinea pedis)

SPOROTRICHOID OR NODULAR LYMPHANGITIS:

- Includes subcutaneous nodules that develop along the path of involved lymphatics
- Most commonly results from inoculation of the skin of the hand
- Usually preceded by well-defined episode of cutaneous inoculation or trauma
- Lesions apparent from one to several wk after inoculation
- Initially, nodular or papular lesion; may ulcerate
- May have frank pus or a serosanguineous discharge
- Systemic complaints uncommon, but infection with certain microorganisms associated with fever, chills, myalgias, and headache

ETIOLOGY

- Acute lymphangitis: usually associated with *Streptococcus pyogenes* (group A streptococcus), but staphylococcal organisms are increasingly recognized as a cause of severe soft tissue infections such as lymphangitis, including community-acquired methicillin-resistant *S. aureus* (CA-MRSA)
- Nodular lymphangitis caused by one of several organisms
  1. *Sporothrix schenckii*
     a. Most common recognized cause in the U.S., usually in the Midwest
     b. Found in soil and plant debris
  2. *Nocardia brasiliensis:* found in soil
  3. *Mycobacterium marinum:* associated with trauma related to water (e.g., aquariums, swimming pools, fish)
  4. *Leishmania brasiliensis*
     a. Protozoal parasite transmitted to humans by sandflies, mostly to travelers in endemic areas
     b. Small endemic focus in Texas
  5. *Francisella tularensis*
     a. Most often in Midwestern states
     b. Associated with contact with infected mammals (e.g., rabbits) or tick bites

Dx DIAGNOSIS

DIFFERENTIAL DIAGNOSIS

- Nodular lymphangitis
- Insect or snake bites
- Filariasis

WORKUP

- Acute lymphangitis: blood cultures
- Nodular lymphangitis: various stains and cultures of drainage or biopsy specimens of inoculation sites to make definitive diagnosis

LABORATORY TESTS

- WBCs possibly elevated with cellulitis
- Eosinophilia common with helminthic infections

Rx TREATMENT

NONPHARMACOLOGIC THERAPY

Limb elevation

ACUTE GENERAL Rx

- Penicillin possibly sufficient, but 1 wk of dicloxacillin or cephalexin 500 mg PO qid commonly used to ensure antistaphylococcal coverage; if CA-MRSA suspected, then use oral Bactrim DS: one PO bid is the best oral agent and with vancomycin 1 g IV every 12 hr being reserved for patients requiring IV therapy.
- If allergic to penicillin:
  1. Clindamycin 300 mg PO qid for 7 days *or*
  2. Erythromycin 500 mg PO qid for 7 days
- Nodular lymphangitis: specific therapy directed at etiologic agent.
- For superficial fungal infections: treatment may prevent recurrence of acute lymphangitis.

DISPOSITION

- Acute lymphangitis: usually resolves with therapy
- Recurrent attacks: may lead to chronic lymphedema of limb, rarely resulting in elephantiasis nostras (nonfilarial elephantiasis)
- Nodular lymphangitis: usually responds to appropriate therapy

REFERRAL

- If acute lymphangitis is more than a mild disease or involves the face
- If nodular lymphangitis or filariasis is suspected

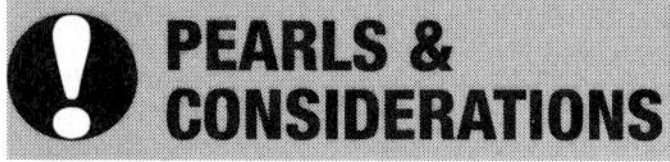

PEARLS & CONSIDERATIONS

COMMENTS

- Outside of the U.S., initial episodes of filariasis caused by *Brugia malayi* resemble acute lymphangitis.
- Chronic lymphedema or elephantiasis results from recurrent episodes.

SUGGESTED READINGS

Eijnden SV et al: Gloves and socks lymphangitis associated with acute parvovirus B19 infection, *Pediatr Dermatol* 20(2):184, 2003.

Kano Y, Inaoka M, Shiohara T: Superficial lymphangitis with interface dermatitis occurring shortly after a minor injury: possible involvement of a bacterial infection and contact allergens, *Dermatology* 203(3):217, 2001.

King MD et al: Emergence of community-acquired methicillin-resistant *Staphylococcus aureus* USA 300 clone as the predominant cause of skin and soft-tissue infections, *Ann Intern Med* 144(5):309, 2006.

Koehler JE, Duncan LM: A 56-year-old man with fever and axillary lymphadenopathy, *N Engl J Med* 355: 1387, 2005.

AUTHORS: **GLENN G. FORT, M.D., M.P.H.,** and **DENNIS J. MIKOLICH, M.D.**

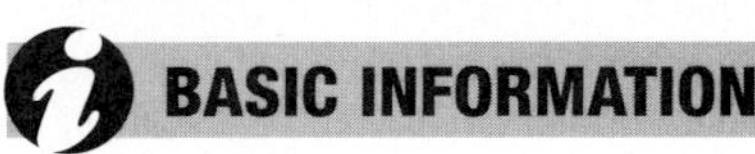

BASIC INFORMATION

DEFINITION

Lymphedema refers to excessive accumulation of interstitial protein-rich fluid typically resulting from impaired regional lymphatic drainage.

SYNONYMS

Elephantiasis

ICD-9CM CODES
457.1 Lymphedema: acquired (chronic), praecox, secondary
457.1 Elephantiasis (nonfilarial)

EPIDEMIOLOGY & DEMOGRAPHICS

PRIMARY LYMPHEDEMA:
- Found in 1.1/100,000 people <20 yr.
- Females outnumber males 3.5:1.
- Incidence peaks between ages 12 and 16 yr.

SECONDARY LYMPHEDEMA: See specific etiology (e.g., filariasis, breast cancer, prostate cancer)

PHYSICAL FINDINGS & CLINICAL PRESENTATION

Edema:
- Painless and progressive
  1. Initially the edema is pitting and smooth (Fig. 1-186); however, with advanced cases, the edema becomes nonpitting (this depends on the extent of fibrosis that has occurred).
  2. Elevation of the leg resolves the swelling in the early stages but not in the advanced stages.
- More often unilateral, but can be bilateral depending on the etiology
- Not always restricted to the lower extremities; may involve the genitals, face, or upper extremities (e.g., arm swelling after mastectomy)
- Stemmer's sign (squaring of the toes caused by edema in the digits)
- "Buffalo hump" appearance of the dorsum of the foot
- Loss of the ankle contour, giving a "tree trunk" appearance of the leg

Skin:
- Hard, thick, leathery skin caused by fibrosis induced by chronic stasis
- Occasional drainage of lymph
- Infections (cellulitis, lymphangitis, onychomycosis)

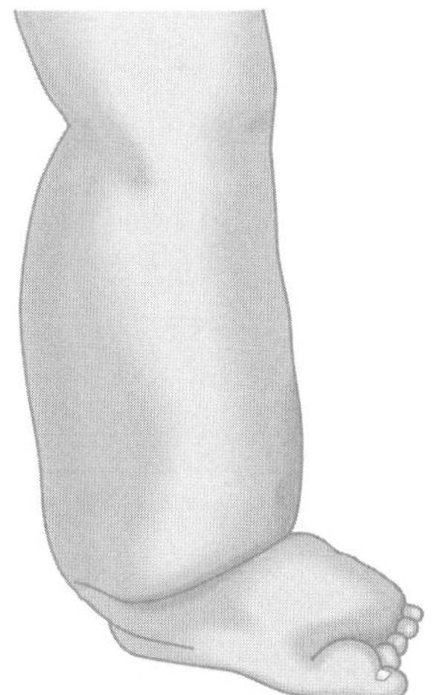

FIGURE 1-186 Lymphedema with characteristic loss of the normal perimalleolar shape resulting in a "tree trunk" pattern. Dorsum of the foot is characteristically swollen, resulting in the appearance of the "buffalo hump." (From Townsend CM, Beauchamp RD, Evers BM, Mattox KL [eds]: *Sabiston textbook of surgery,* ed 17, Philadelphia, 2004, Saunders.)

ETIOLOGY

Lymphedema is caused by a reduction in lymphatic transport and is classified into primary and secondary forms.

Primary idiopathic lymphedema is believed to result from developmental abnormalities such as lymphatic hypoplasia and functional insufficiency or absence of lymphatic valves. Subclasses of this type of lymphedema include:
- Congenital lymphedema:
  1. Detected at birth or recognized within first 2 yr of life
  2. Involves one or both extremities, usually the entire leg
  3. May be familial (Milroy's disease)
- Lymphedema praecox:
  1. Onset in teenage years
  2. Usually unilateral
  3. Most common form of primary lymphedema (up to 94% of cases)
  4. More common in females (10:1), suggesting estrogen has a role in pathogenesis
  5. May be familial (Meige's disease)
- Lymphedema tarda:
  1. Usually occurs after age 30 yr
  2. Uncommon, accounting for <10% of cases of primary lymphedema

Secondary lymphedema develops after disruption or obstruction of the lymphatic system as a consequence of:
- Surgery for malignant tumors (e.g., breast, prostate, lymphoma)
- Edema of the arm after axillary lymph node dissection is the most common cause of lymphedema in the U.S.
- Incidence of lymphedema is approximately 14% in patients after mastectomy with adjuvant radiation treatment
- Inflammation (streptococci, filariasis)
- Filariasis is the most common cause of lymphedema in the world
- Trauma
- Radiation with lymph node removal

Dx DIAGNOSIS

- Lymphedema is primarily a clinical diagnosis made on the basis of physical features that distinguish it from other causes of chronic edema of the extremities, such as the presence of cutaneous and subcutaneous fibrosis (peau d'orange) and the Stemmer sign.
- When physical examination is inconclusive, other available imaging tests can help make the diagnosis: isotopic lymphoscintigraphy, indirect and direct lymphography, lymphatic capillaroscopy, MRI, CT, or ultrasound.

DIFFERENTIAL DIAGNOSIS

Exclude other causes of edema (e.g., cirrhosis, nephrosis, congestive heart failure, myxedema, hypoalbuminemia, chronic venous stasis, reflex sympathetic dystrophy, obstruction from abdominal or pelvic malignancy).

WORKUP

A detailed history and physical examination should help exclude most of the differential diagnoses.

LABORATORY TESTS

- Blood urea nitrogen, creatinine, liver function tests, albumin, urine analysis, and thyroid function tests are obtained to exclude possible systemic causes of edema.
- Noninvasive venous studies help exclude venous insufficiency.
- Genetic testing may be practical in defining a specific hereditary syndrome with a discrete gene mutation such as lymphedema-distichiasis *(FOXC2)* and some forms of Milroy disease *(VEGFR-3).*

IMAGING STUDIES

- Lymphoscintigraphy:
  1. Diagnostic image of choice
  2. Sensitivity and specificity of 100% in diagnosing lymphedema
  3. Currently considered the gold standard for diagnosis of lymphedema
- CT scan: to exclude malignancy leading to obstruction.
- Duplex ultrasound to rule out venous obstruction as a cause for edema.
- Lymphangiography: lymphoscintigraphy is preferred over lymphangiography. Lymphangiography is contraindicated in malignancy.

Rx TREATMENT

NONPHARMACOLOGIC THERAPY

Complex decongestive therapy (CDT) is backed by longstanding experience as the primary treatment of choice for lymphedema in both children and adults. It involves a two-stage treatment program:
1. Reduce leg swelling and size:
   - Leg elevation
   - Limb massage
   - Pneumatic leg compression
2. Maintain edema-free state:
   - Elastic support stockings that are properly fitted according to compression pressure and length are essential to prevent edema from returning.
   - Compression pressures are graduated; most of the pressure is distal with decreasing pressure from the stockings moving proximally.

- Compression pressures range from 20 to 30 mm Hg, 30 to 40 mm Hg, 40 to 50 mm Hg, and 50 to 60 mm Hg. Most prefer 40 to 50 mm Hg for lymphedema.
- The length should cover the edematous site. Choices include below the knee, thigh-high, and pantyhose lengths.

ACUTE GENERAL Rx

- No drugs have been shown to be beneficial. Diuretics, in particular, should not be used because they may promote the development of volume depletion.
- Treat infections, such as lymphangitis (usually caused by group A streptococcus), with penicillin VK 250 mg qd for 10 days or erythromycin 250 mg qd in penicillin-allergic patients. If recurrent episodes of infection occur, consider prophylaxis with penicillin VK 250 mg qd for 10 days at the beginning of each month. Clotrimazole 1% cream should be applied qd to dried, fissured areas in between toes to prevent fungal infections.
- In secondary lymphedema, treating the underlying cause is indicated (e.g., prostate cancer, breast cancer). If the etiology is filariasis caused by the parasites *Wuchereria bancrofti* or *Brugia malayi,* treatment is diethylcarbamazine citrate 5 mg/kg in divided doses for 3 wk.
- Mesotherapy (hyaluronidase), immunological therapy (autologous lymphocyte injection), and fluid restriction all have uncertain benefit in the treatment of lymphedema.
- In children with chylous reflux syndromes, a diet low in long-chain triglycerides and high in short- and medium-chain triglycerides has been shown to be of benefit in treatment.

CHRONIC Rx

Surgery for chronic lymphedema should act as an adjunct to CDT or as an alternative if CDT has proven unsuccessful. Operative treatment is considered with:

- Continued increase in leg size despite medical treatment
- Impaired leg function
- Recurrent infections
- Emotional lability as a result of the cosmetic appearance

Surgical procedures are divided into two types:

- Those performed to improve lymph node drainage (e.g., anastomoses of the lymph system with the venous system)
- Those performed to excise the subcutaneous tissue (e.g., Charles' procedure, Thompson's procedure, and the modified Homans' procedure)
- Liposuction in combination with long-term CDT has been shown to be more effective in reducing edema than long-term CDT alone.

DISPOSITION

- Lymphedema is a slowly progressive disorder that can lead to significant disfigurement of the extremities or other body parts.
- The extent of fibrotic change to the skin of the affected limb increases with the chronicity of lymphatic stasis.
- In many patients the maximum girth of the affected limb is reached within the first year after onset, unless complications such as recurrent cellulitis supervene.
- Patients with lymphedema commonly manifest psychiatric comorbidities as a result of their disease, such as anxiety, depression, adjustment problems, and difficulty in vocational, domestic, or social domains.
- Chronic lymphedema can be complicated by cellulitis or, in rare cases, development of lymphangiosarcomata or other cutaneous malignancies.

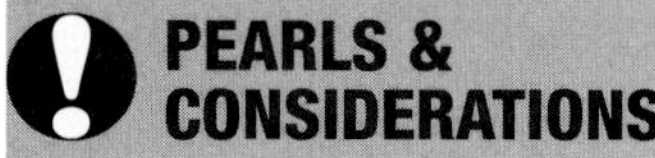

PEARLS & CONSIDERATIONS

- Lymphedema is a chronic, generally incurable ailment that requires lifelong care and attention along with psychosocial support.
- It is important to remember that surgery is not a cure.
- Children and adolescents (along with parents and adults) should be encouraged to pursue a normal life, participating in school activities and sports (preferably noncontact, such as swimming).
- It should also be remembered that cases of lymphangiosarcomas have been associated, although rarely, with postmastectomy lymphedema.
- Gene therapy to develop new lymphangioles in the affected limbs is a potential clinical remedy in the future.

SUGGESTED READINGS

International Society of Lymphology: The diagnosis and treatment of peripheral lymphedema: consensus document of the International Society of Lymphology, *Lymphology* 36(2):84, 2003.

Karkkainen MJ et al: A model for gene therapy of human hereditary lymphedema, *Proc Natl Acad Sci U S A* 98(22):12677, 2001.

O'Brien JG et al: Treatment of edema, *Am Fam Physician* 71(11):2111, 2005.

Rockson SG: Lymphedema, *Am J Med* 110:288, 2001.

AUTHOR: **TANYA ALI, M.D.**

BASIC INFORMATION

DEFINITION

Lymphogranuloma venereum (LGV) is a sexually transmitted, systemic disease caused by *Chlamydia trachomatis.*

SYNONYMS

Tropical bubo
Poradenitis inguinalis
LGV

ICD-9CM CODES

099.1 Lymphogranuloma venereum

EPIDEMIOLOGY & DEMOGRAPHICS

INCIDENCE (IN U.S.): Rare; 285 cases reported in 1993

PREVALENCE: Endemic in Africa, India, parts of Southeast Asia, South America, and the Caribbean

PREDOMINANT SEX: Male/female ratio is 5:1

PHYSICAL FINDINGS & CLINICAL PRESENTATION

Primary stage:

- Primary lesion caused by multiplication of organism at site of infection
- Papule, shallow ulcer
- Herpetiform lesion at site of inoculation (most common)
- Incubation period of 3 to 21 days
- Most common site of lesion in women: posterior wall, fourchette, or vulva
- Spontaneous healing without scarring

Second stage:

- Inguinal syndrome: characteristic inguinal adenopathy
- Begins 1 to 4 wk after primary lesion
- Syndrome is the most frequent clinical sign of the disease
- Unilateral inguinal adenopathy in 70% of cases
- Symptoms: painful, extensive adenitis (bubo) and suppuration may occur with numerous sinus tracts
- "Groove sign" signaling femoral and inguinal node involvement (20%); most often seen in men
- Involvement of deep iliac and retroperitoneal lymph nodes in women may present as a pelvic mass

Third stage (anogenital syndrome):

- Subacute: proctocolitis
- Late: tissue destruction or scarring, sinuses, abscesses, fistulas, strictures of perineum, elephantiasis

ETIOLOGY

Chlamydia trachomatis is the causative agent. There are three serotypes: L1, L2, and L3.

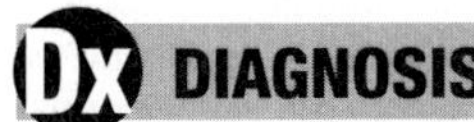

DIAGNOSIS

DIFFERENTIAL DIAGNOSIS

- Inguinal adenitis, suppurative adenitis, retroperitoneal adenitis, proctitis, schistosomiasis.
- Section II describes the differential diagnosis of genital sores.

WORKUP

- Clinical manifestation
- Screening for other STDs
- A clinical algorithm for evaluation of genital ulcer disease is described in Section III, "Genital Lesions."

LABORATORY TESTS

- Positive Frei test:
  1. Intradermal chlamydial antigen
  2. Nonspecific for all *Chlamydia*
  3. No longer available (historical significance only)
- Complement fixation test:
  1. Titer >1:64 in active infection
  2. Convalescent titers no difference
- Cell culture of *Chlamydia* aspiration of fluctuant node yields highest rates of recovery
- Complete blood count: mild leukocytosis with lymphocytosis or monocytosis
- Elevated sedimentation rate
- VDRL and HIV screening to rule out other sexually transmitted diseases

IMAGING STUDIES

- Barium enema: may reveal elongated structure of LGV
- CT scan for retroperitoneal adenitis

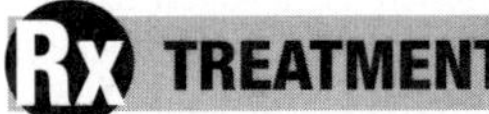

TREATMENT

NONPHARMACOLOGIC THERAPY

- Avoid milk and milk products while taking medication.
- Practice sexual abstinence.
- Treat sexual partners.

ACUTE GENERAL Rx

- Doxycycline 100 mg PO bid × 21 days
- Erythromycin base 500 mg PO qid × 21 days
- Sulfisoxazole 500 mg PO qid × 21 days
- Surgical:
  1. Aspirate fluctuant nodes
  2. Incise and drain abscesses

CHRONIC Rx

- Longer course of therapy will be needed for chronic or relapsing cases, which may be caused by reinfection and/or inadequate treatment.
- A rectal stricture requires a colostomy.
- Surgery should be considered only after antibiotic treatment.

DISPOSITION

Good prognosis with early treatment, usually resulting in complete resolution of symptoms.

REFERRAL

Surgical consultation if patient develops obstruction, fistula, or rectal stricture. May need referral to plastic surgeon if patient has lymphatic obstruction.

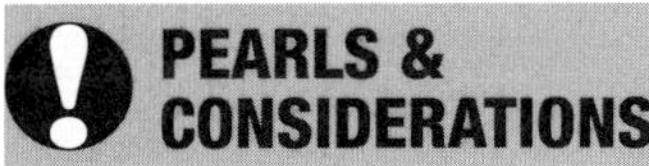

PEARLS & CONSIDERATIONS

COMMENTS

- Pregnant and lactating women should be treated with erythromycin regimen.
- Congenital transmission does not occur, but infection may be acquired through an infected birth canal.
- Patient education materials may be obtained through local and state health clinics.

SUGGESTED READING

Centers for Disease Control and Prevention: 2006 sexually transmitted diseases treatment guidelines, *MMWR* 55(RR-11), 2006.

AUTHORS: **GEORGE T. DANAKAS, M.D.,** and **RUBEN ALVERO, M.D.**

 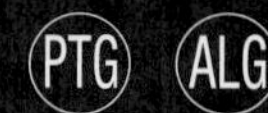

BASIC INFORMATION

DEFINITION

Non-Hodgkin lymphoma (NHL) is a heterogeneous group of malignancies of the lymphoreticular system.

SYNONYMS

NHL

ICD-9CM CODES
201.9 Lymphoma, non-Hodgkin

EPIDEMIOLOGY & DEMOGRAPHICS

INCIDENCE (IN U.S.): Sixth most common neoplasm (56,000 new cases annually). Incidence increases with age. In patients with HIV, NHL is the second most common tumor (after Kaposi's sarcoma).

PREDOMINANT AGE: Median age at time of diagnosis is 50 yr.

PHYSICAL FINDINGS & CLINICAL PRESENTATION

- Patients often present with asymptomatic lymphadenopathy.
- Approximately one third of NHLs originate extranodally. Involvement of extranodal sites can result in unusual presentations (e.g., gastrointestinal tract involvement can simulate peptic ulcer disease).
- NHL cases associated with HIV occur predominantly in the brain.
- Pruritus, fever, night sweats, and weight loss are less common than in Hodgkin's disease.
- Hepatomegaly and splenomegaly may be present.

Dx DIAGNOSIS

DIFFERENTIAL DIAGNOSIS

- Hodgkin's disease
- Viral infections
- Metastatic carcinoma

A clinical algorithm for evaluation of lymphadenopathy is described in Section III. The differential diagnosis of lymphadenopathy is described in Section II.

WORKUP

Initial laboratory evaluation may reveal only mild anemia and elevated lactate dehydrogenase (LDH) and erythrocyte sedimentation rate (ESR). Proper staging of NHL requires the following:

- A thorough history, physical examination, and adequate biopsy. Laparoscopic lymph node biopsy can be used on an outpatient basis for most patients with intraabdominal lymphoma.
- Routine laboratory evaluation (complete blood count, ESR, urinalysis, LDH, blood urea nitrogen, creatinine, serum calcium, uric acid, liver function tests, serum protein electrophoresis).
- Chest x-ray examination (posteroanterior and lateral).
- Bone marrow evaluation (aspirate and full bone core biopsy).
- CT scan of abdomen and pelvis; CT scan of chest if chest x-ray films abnormal.
- Bone scan (particularly in patients with histiocytic lymphoma).
- Depending on the histopathology, the results of the above studies and the planned therapy, some other tests may be performed (e.g., positron-emission tomographic scan).
- β-2 microglobulin levels should be obtained initially (prognostic value) and serially in patients with low-grade lymphomas (useful to monitor therapeutic response of the tumor).
- Serum interleukin levels have prognostic value in diffuse large cell lymphoma.

CLASSIFICATION: The working formulation of NHL for clinical use subdivides lymphomas into low grade, intermediate grade, high grade, and miscellaneous (Table 1-46).

STAGING: The Ann Arbor classification is used to stage NHLs (see "Hodgkin's Disease" in Section I). Histopathology has greater therapeutic implications in NHL than in Hodgkin's disease.

Rx TREATMENT

ACUTE GENERAL Rx

The therapeutic regimen varies with the histologic type and pathologic stage. Following are the commonly used therapeutic modalities:

LOW-GRADE NHL (e.g., NODULAR, POORLY DIFFERENTIATED):

1. Local radiotherapy for symptomatic obstructive adenopathy.
2. Deferment of therapy and careful observation in asymptomatic patients.
3. Single-agent chemotherapy with cyclophosphamide or chlorambucil and glucocorticoids
4. Combination chemotherapy alone or with radiotherapy: generally indicated only when the lymphoma becomes more invasive, with poor response to less aggressive treatment.
5. Monoclonal antibodies directed against B-cell surface antigens can also be used to treat follicular lymphomas resistant to conventional therapy. The anti-CD20 monoclonal antibody rituximab is effective against low-grade NHL in patients who have not received previous treatment.
6. The addition of rituximab to CHOP is generally well tolerated; however, additional studies may be necessary to clarify the role of CHOP plus rituximab in patients with indolent NHL.
7. Ibritumomab tiuxetan (Zevalin), an immunoconjugate that combines the linker-chelator tiuxetan with the monoclonal antibody ibritumomab, can be used as part of a two-step regimen for treatment of patients with relapsed or refractory low-grade, follicular, or transformed B-cell NHL refractory to rituximab.
8. New purine analogs (FLAMP, 2CDA) can be used in salvage treatment of refractory lymphomas. They all have activity in follicular lymphomas.

INTERMEDIATE- AND HIGH-GRADE LYMPHOMAS (e.g., DIFFUSE HISTIOCYTIC LYMPHOMA): Combination chemotherapy regimens (e.g., CHOP, PRO-MACE-CYTABOM, MACOP-B, M-BACOD). An anthracycline-containing regimen (such as CHOP) given in standard doses and schedule is generally best for treatment of older patients with advanced stage, aggressive-histology lymphoma who do not have significant comorbid illness.

1. High-dose sequential therapy is superior to standard-dose MACOP-B for patients with diffuse large-cell lymphoma of the B-cell type.
2. Dose-modified chemotherapy should be considered for most HIV-infected patients with lymphoma.
   - Three cycles of CHOP followed by involved-field radiotherapy may be superior to eight cycles of CHOP alone in patients with localized intermediate- and high-grade NHL.
   - High-dose chemotherapy with autologous stem-cell support has been reported to be superior to CHOP in adults with disseminated aggressive lymphoma.
   - The addition of rituximab against CD20 B-cell lymphoma to the CHOP regimen increases the complete response rate and prolongs event-free and overall survival in elderly patients with diffuse large B-cell lymphoma without a clinically significant increase in toxicity. Bexxar, a combination of the mononuclear antibody tositumomab and radiolabeled iodine-131, can be used for a single treatment of relapsed follicular NHL in patients who are refractory to rituximab.
   - In patients <61 yr, chemotherapy with three cycles of ACVBP (doxorubicin, cyclophosphamide, vindesine, bleomycin, and prednisone) followed by sequential consolidation has been reported to be superior to three cycles of CHOP plus radiotherapy for treatment of newly diagnosed aggressive lymphoma (diffuse mixed, diffuse large cell, or immunoblastic according to the working formulation).
   - Granulocyte-colony stimulating factor: may be effective in reducing the risk of infection in patients with aggressive lymphoma undergoing chemotherapy.
   - Radioimmunotherapy with (^{131}I) anti-B1 antibody therapy for NHL either by itself or in combination with other treatments represents a new modality in the armamentarium against lymphomas.
   - Treatment with high-dose chemotherapy and autologous bone marrow transplant: compared with conventional chemotherapy, increases event-free and overall survival in patients with chemotherapy-sensitive NHL in relapse.
- An algorithm for the management of non-Hodgkin lymphoma in pediatric patients is described in the online version of Section III.

DISPOSITION

- Patients with low-grade lymphoma, despite their long-term survival (6 to 10 yr average), are rarely cured, and the great majority (if not all) eventually die of the lymphoma, whereas patients with a high-grade lymphoma may achieve a cure with aggressive chemotherapy.
- Complete remission occurs in 35% to 50% of patients with intermediate- and high-grade lymphoma. Prognostic factors include the histiologic subtype, age of patient, and bulk of disease.
- Patients who present with AIDS-related NHL and a low CD4 cell count have a poor prognosis (median duration of survival is 15 to 34 mo).

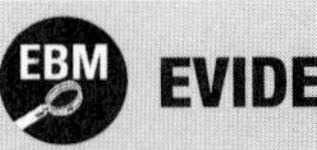

EVIDENCE

A large number of clinical trials have evaluated the efficacy of various therapies used in the management of NHL. Some of these are long-term in nature and others are more recent, evaluating emerging therapies. Many of these trials are heterogeneous in nature (involving different patient age groups, different histological tumor types, and different stages of disease progression) and direct comparisons may not be made. Some trials are in patients undergoing primary treatment and others involve patients with refractory/relapsed disease. As a result, much of the evidence derived from such studies, at present, does not meet our criteria for inclusion. However, some statements may be made:

There is evidence that granulopoiesis-stimulating factors are beneficial in the management of patients with lymphoma undergoing chemotherapy.

A systematic review found that in patients undergoing chemotherapy for aggressive NHL, the use of hematopoietic colony stimulating factors (CSFs) significantly reduced the incidence of both severe and febrile neutropenia and infection. However, there was no evidence that the use of CSFs had any effect on tumor response.[1] Ⓐ

Evidence-Based Reference

1. Bohlius J et al: Granulopoiesis-stimulating factors to prevent adverse effects in the treatment of malignant lymphoma, *Cochrane Rev* 3, 2004. Ⓐ

SUGGESTED READINGS

Kaminski MS et al: ^{131}I-tositumomab therapy as initial treatment for follicular lymphoma, *N Engl J Med* 352:441, 2005.

Milpied N et al: Initial treatment of aggressive lymphoma with high-dose chemotherapy and autologous stem cell support, *N Engl J Med* 350:1287, 2004.

Reyes F et al: ACVBP versus CHOP plus radiotherapy for localized aggressive lymphoma, *N Engl J Med* 352:1197, 2005.

AUTHOR: **FRED F. FERRI, M.D.**

TABLE 1-46 Classification Systems for Grading Lymphomas

Kiel Classification	Working Formulation	Revised European-American Classification
Low-grade malignancy	Low grade	B-cell lymphomas
Lymphocytic, CLL	A. Malignant lymphoma, small lymphocytic	
Lymphocytic, other	Consistent with CLL	B-CLL/SLL
Lymphoplasmacytoid		Lymphoplasmacytoid lymphoma
Centrocytic	B. Malignant lymphoma, follicular, predominantly small cleaved cell	Follicle center lymphomas
Centroblastic/centrocytic		Marginal zone lymphomas (MALT)
Follicular without sclerosis	Diffuse areas	Mantle cell lymphoma
Follicular with sclerosis	Sclerosis	
Follicular and diffuse, without sclerosis	C. Malignant lymphoma, follicular mixed, small cleaved and large cell	
Follicular and diffuse, with sclerosis	Diffuse areas	Diffuse large B-cell lymphoma
Diffuse	Sclerosis	Primary mediastinal large B-cell lymphoma
Low-grade malignant lymphoma, unclassified	Intermediate grade	Burkitt's lymphoma
High-grade malignancy	D. Malignant lymphoma, follicular	T-cell lymphomas
Centroblastic	Diffuse areas	
Lymphoblastic, Burkitt's type	E. Malignant lymphoma, diffuse small cleaved cell	
Lymphoblastic, convoluted cell type		T-CLL
Lymphoblastic, other (unclassified) immunoblastic		Mycosis fungoides/Sézary syndrome
High-grade malignant lymphoma, unclassified	F. Malignant lymphoma, diffuse mixed, small and large cell sclerosis	
Malignant lymphoma unclassified (unable to specify high grade or low grade)	G. Malignant lymphoma diffuse	Peripheral T-cell lymphoma, unspecified
Composite lymphoma	Large cell	Angioimmunoblastic T-cell lymphoma
	Cleaved cell	Angiocentric lymphoma
	Noncleaved cell	Intestinal T-cell lymphoma
	Sclerosis	Adult T-cell lymphoma/leukemia
	High grade	Anaplastic large cell lymphoma
	H. Malignant lymphoma large cell, immunoblastic	Precursor T-lymphoid lymphoma/leukemia
	Plasmacytoid	
	Clear cell	
	Polymorphous	
	Epithelioid cell component	
	I. Malignant lymphoma lymphoblastic	
	Convoluted cell	
	Nonconvoluted cell	
	J. Malignant lymphoma small noncleaved cell	
	Burkitt's	
	Follicular areas	

From Abeloff MD: *Clinical oncology,* ed 3, New York, 2004, Churchill Livingstone.
B-CLL, B-cell chronic lymphoid leukemia; *CLL,* chronic lymphocytic leukemia; *MALT,* mucosa-associated lymphoid tumor; *SLL,* lymphoid leukemia; *T-CLL,* T-cell CLL.

Lynch Syndrome

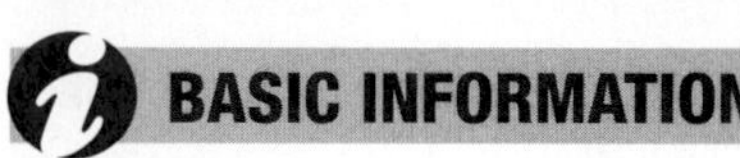

BASIC INFORMATION

DEFINITION

Lynch syndrome is a hereditary predisposition to malignancy of the colon that is explained by a germline mutation in a DNA mismatch repair gene.

SYNONYMS

Hereditary nonpolyposis colorectal cancer
Hereditary site-specific colon cancer

ICD-9CM CODES
1539 Lynch syndrome

EPIDEMIOLOGY & DEMOGRAPHICS

The lifetime risk for developing colon cancer in the U.S. is approximately 6%. Of these cases, 2% to 3% may be attributable to Lynch syndrome. The incidence of Lynch syndrome is estimated to be between 1:660 and 1:2000. The average age of diagnosis for Lynch syndrome is 48 yr, although diagnosis can occur as early as the 20s or as late as the 70s.

RISK FACTORS: Family history of colon cancer or other hereditary nonpolyposis colorectal cancer (HNPCC)-related cancers such as endometrial (up to 43% of women with Lynch syndrome may develop endometrial cancer), biliary tract, ovarian, stomach, or pancreas.

GENETICS: Autosomal-dominant inheritance pattern

ETIOLOGY

Lynch syndrome is thought to be secondary to germline mutations in DNA mismatch repair genes. The predominant genes involved are *MSH2* and *MLH1,* which are tumor suppressor genes, although other genes have documented involvement *(PMS1, PMS2, MSH6, MLH3).* Mutations in these genes prevent repair of DNA mismatches during DNA replication. This is most prevalent in regions of DNA called microsatellites causing DNA microsatellite instability and leading to an increased risk for malignancy, especially colon cancer.

PHYSICAL FINDINGS & CLINICAL PRESENTATION

- Changes in bowel habits (prolonged constipation)
- Melena
- Hematochezia
- Abdominal pain
- Unexplained weight loss
- Decreased appetite

Dx DIAGNOSIS

DIFFERENTIAL DIAGNOSIS

- Familial adenomatosis polyposis
- Peutz-Jeghers syndrome
- Juvenile polyposis
- Nonhereditary colorectal cancer
- Gardner syndrome

WORKUP

If an individual presents with numerous adenomatous polyps or has multiple relatives with cancer at a young age, a family history complete with pedigree must be obtained. Clinical diagnosis of the Lynch syndrome can be made with the Amsterdam criteria or, if these are not met, the Bethesda criteria, which are more sensitive (see following list).

- Amsterdam criteria (must meet all criteria):
  1. Colorectal carcinoma and/or endometrial carcinoma or transitional cell carcinoma of the ureter or carcinoma of the small bowel in at least three individuals in the family
  2. One of the patients is a first-degree family member of two other patients
  3. Involved patients occur in at least two successive generations
  4. At least one of the diagnoses was made before age 50
  5. The diagnoses are histologically confirmed
  6. Familial adenomatous polyposis is excluded
- Bethesda criteria (must meet all criteria):
  1. Colorectal cancer before age 50
  2. Multiple colorectal cancers or other HNPCC-related cancers such as biliary tract, endometrial, stomach, or ovary
  3. Colorectal cancer with microsatellite instability histology <60 years of age
  4. Colorectal cancer or HNPCC-related cancer in first-degree relative <50 years of age
  5. Colorectal cancer or HNPCC-related cancer in at least two first- or second-degree relatives, any age
- If criteria for the Lynch syndrome are not met, no further analysis is necessary (although a genetic syndrome cannot be definitively excluded and genetic referral may be warranted).

LABORATORY TESTS

- If a patient meets criteria for Lynch syndrome, immunohistochemistry can be performed for the presence or absence of mismatch repair genes *MLH1, MSH2, MSH6,* and *PMS2.*
- Microsatellite instability analysis should also be performed if criteria for Lynch syndrome are met.

Rx TREATMENT

- If the mutation has been identified in a family member, screening for this mutation can be performed via genetic testing. Informed consent must be obtained after a thorough explanation has been provided to each individual.
- Surveillance using colonoscopy can be performed in individuals who screen positive, while those who screen negative can be discharged. The mismatch repair gene that is mutated guides screening.
- According to the Netherlands Surveillance Protocol, for example, individuals with mutations in *MLH1, MSH2,* or *MSH6* should have colonoscopies every 1 to 2 yr starting at age 20 to 25 yr; urine cytology every 1 to 2 yr starting at age 30 to 35 yr; gastroscopy every 1 to 2 yr starting at age 30 to 35 yr; and, in females, ultrasound of endometrium and CA-125 every 1 to 2 yr starting at age 30 to 35 yr.

REFERRALS

- To gastroenterology for surveillance colonoscopies
- To genetic counselor if patient satisfies Bethesda criteria
- To psychologist as necessary for psychologic support

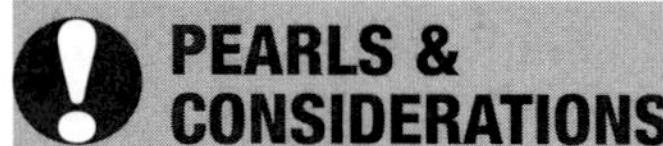

PEARLS & CONSIDERATIONS

- Prior to genetic testing being instituted, informed consent must be obtained because consequences of this testing include the necessity of lifelong screenings such as colonoscopies.
- The risk of pancreatic cancer is increased in families with Lynch syndrome compared with the U.S. population.

PATIENT & FAMILY EDUCATION

- For information on local genetic counselors, visit the National Society of Genetic Counselors Web site at www.nsgc.org.
- For information on Lynch syndrome, visit www.mayoclinic.com/health/lynch-syndrome/DS00669.

SUGGESTED READINGS

Hampel H et al: Screening for the Lynch syndrome (hereditary non-polyposis colorectal cancer), *New Engl J Med* 352:1851, 2005.

Hendriks YM et al: Management of Lynch syndrome (hereditary nonpolyposis colorectal carcinoma): guide for clinicians, *CA Cancer J Clin* 56:213, 2006.

Jass JR: Hereditary non-polyposis colorectal cancer: the rise and fall of a confusing term, *World J Gastroenterol* 12(31):4943, 2006.

Kastrinos F et al: Risk of pancreatic cancer in families with Lynch syndrome, *JAMA* 302(16):1790-1795, 2009.

AUTHORS: **PAUL F. GEORGE, M.D.,** and **JOANNE M. SILVIA, M.D.**

BASIC INFORMATION

DEFINITION

Macular degeneration refers to a group of diseases associated with loss of central vision and damage to the macula. Degenerative changes occur in the pigment, neural, and vascular layers of the macula. Dry macular degeneration is usually ischemic in etiology, and wet macular degeneration is associated with leakage of fluid from blood vessels, usually referred to as *age-related macular degeneration* (ARMD).

ICD-9CM CODES
362.5 Degeneration of macula and posterior pole

EPIDEMIOLOGY & DEMOGRAPHICS

INCIDENCE (IN U.S.):
- Leading cause of irreversible blindness in people ≥50 yr in the developed world.
- Increases with age.
- More than 8 million Americans have age-related macular degeneration. The overall prevalence is projected to increase by >50% by the year 2020.

PEAK INCIDENCE:
- Ages 75 to 80 yr
- Dramatically increases in incidence and prevalence with age until approximately 80% of people ≥75 yr have senile macular degeneration

PREVALENCE (IN U.S.): Varies, but approximately 5% of people >50 yr have some signs of macular degeneration.

PREDOMINANT SEX: Males and females are affected equally (15% of white women >80 yr have severe ARMD).

PREDOMINANT AGE: >50 yr

RISK FACTORS:
- Advancing age
- Genetic factors
- Complement factor H, Tyr402His variant
- LOC387715/ARMS2, Ala69Ser variant
- History of smoking within past 20 yr
- Dietary factors (low intake of antioxidants and zinc, high fat intake)
- Obesity
- White race

PHYSICAL FINDINGS & CLINICAL PRESENTATION

- Decreased central vision
- Macular hemorrhage, pigmentation, edema, atrophy
- The most common abnormality seen in ARMD is the presence of drusen, or yellowish deposits deep to the retina; this may be early in the course of disease
- Choroidal neovascular membrane (CNVM) develops with rapid change in vision

ETIOLOGY

- Subretinal neovascular membrane early
- Pigmentary and vascular changes with exudate, edema, and scar tissue development
- Dry type atrophy of macular pigment epithelium

Dx DIAGNOSIS

DIFFERENTIAL DIAGNOSIS

- Diabetic retinopathy (with neovascularization, can mimic CNVM)
- Hypertension
- Histoplasmosis (less common cause of CNVM)
- Trauma with scar

WORKUP

- Complete eye examination, including visual field and fluorescein angiography
- Optical coherence tomography (OCT)

LABORATORY TESTS

Evaluate for diabetes and other metabolic problems as well as vascular diseases

IMAGING STUDIES

- OCT
- Fluorescein angiography

Rx TREATMENT

NONPHARMACOLOGIC THERAPY

- Laser treatment to stop progression of disease; photodynamic treatment with verteporfin IV
- Laser (Argon) for certain classic membranes (CNVM)
- A high dietary intake of antioxidants, vitamins C and E, and zinc has been reported to substantially reduce the risk of ARMD in elderly persons

ACUTE GENERAL Rx

- Intravitreal steroids; photodynamic treatment with laser.
- Intravitreal administration of ranibizumab, a monoclonal antibody Fab that neutralizes all active forms of vascular endothelial growth factor A, is effective in preventing vision loss and improving mean visual acuity in patients with ARMD. It has also been reported to be superior to photodynamic therapy with verteporfin in the treatment of predominantly classic neovascular age-related macular degeneration. Bevacizumab, a monoclonal antibody to vascular endothelial growth factor, is also often used off-label as intravitreal therapy. Its cost per intravitreal dose is significantly lower than that of ranibizumab.
- Intravitreous injections of pegaptanib (Macugen), an anti–vascular endothelial growth factor, have been reported as effective therapy in slowing vision loss in neovascular ARMD. Pegaptanib is administered once every 6 wk by intravitreous injection into one eye.

CHRONIC Rx

- Repeated laser treatments
- Antioxidants and zinc may slow progression of ARMD

DISPOSITION

- Follow closely by ophthalmologist, retinal specialist
- If vision deteriorates, refer urgently to an ophthalmologist
- Avastin similar to ranibizumab but not yet FDA approved for vitreal injection

REFERRAL

- To ophthalmologist early in the course of the disease if vision is to be saved
- Immediate referral if any change in vision

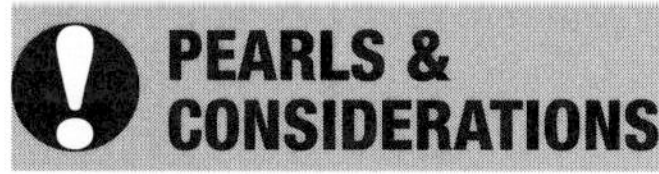

PEARLS & CONSIDERATIONS

COMMENTS

- Sildenafil has no significant effect on macular degeneration.
- Statistically, the vision of only one out of 10 affected persons can be saved, but the disease is so devastating that vigorous therapy should be considered in all patients.
- Statins plus aspirin may slow progression.
- Vitamins with zinc and antioxidants may slow progression of ARMD.

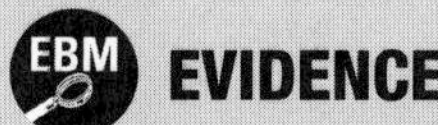

EVIDENCE

Please note: Complete text of EBM for this topic is available online.

SUGGESTED READINGS

Brown DM et al: Ranibizumab versus verteporfin for neovascular age-related macular degeneration, *N Engl J Med* 355:1432, 2006.

Jager RD et al: Age-related macular degeneration, *N Engl J Med* 358:2606-2617, 2008.

Rosenfeld P et al: Ranibizumab for neovascular age-related macular degeneration, *N Engl J Med* 355: 1419, 2006.

AUTHOR: **MELVYN KOBY, M.D.**

BASIC INFORMATION

DEFINITION

Malaria is a protozoan disease caused by the genus *Plasmodium* and transmitted by female *Anopheles* spp. mosquitoes. It is characterized by hectic fever and often presents with classic malarial paroxysm. Four species of genus plasmodium usually infect humans:

- *P. falciparum*
- *P. vivax*
- *P. malariae*
- *P. ovale*

SYNONYMS

Periodic fever
Tertian malaria
Quartan malaria
Tropical splenomegaly

ICD-9CM CODES

084.6 Malaria

EPIDEMIOLOGY & DEMOGRAPHICS

Global:

- 300 to 500 million cases/yr
- 1 to 3 million deaths/yr
- 41% of the world's population lives in endemic area

U.S.:

- Between 1500 and 1800 cases reported by CDC in the last 5 yr.
- 567 cases diagnosed as *P. falciparum.*
- Most infections limited to:
  1. Immigrant population
  2. Returned travelers or troops from endemic area
- Occasionally, transmission through exposure to infected blood product or shared intravenous needles by users of injection drugs.
- Congenital transmission is possible.
- Local mosquito-borne transmission has been reported.
- Competent mosquito vectors are present.
  1. *A. albimanus* in eastern U.S.
  2. *A. freeborni* in western U.S.

Geographic distribution:

- *P. falciparum:* Sub-Saharan Africa, Papua New Guinea, Solomon Islands, Haiti, Indian subcontinent
- *P. vivax:* Central America, South America, North Africa, Middle East, Indian subcontinent
- *P. ovale:* West Africa
- *P. malariae:* worldwide

Parasite life cycle (Fig. 1-187):

- Human infection begins when a female anopheline mosquito bites (only female anopheline mosquito takes blood meal) and inoculates plasmodial sporozoites into bloodstream.
- The sporozoites then travel to liver and invade to hepatocytes.
- In the hepatocytes, the sporozoites mature to tissue schizont or become dormant hypnozoites.
- The tissue schizonts amplify the infection by producing large number of merozoites (10,000 to 30,000).
- Each merozoite is capable of invading an RBC and can establish the asexual cycle of replication in RBCs.
- Asexual cycles produce and release 24 to 32 merozoites at the end of 48- or 72-hr *(P. malariae)* cycles.
- The hypnozoites are only found in relapsing malaria *P. vivax* or *P. ovale* and may remain dormant for up to 5 yr.
- Eventually some intraerythrocytic parasites develop into gametocytes. Male and female gametocytes are taken up by a female anopheline mosquito with a blood meal where they fertilize in the mosquito gut to produce a diploid zygote that matures to an ookinete; haploid sporozoites are generated that migrate to the salivary gland of the mosquito to infect another human.

PHYSICAL FINDINGS & CLINICAL PRESENTATION

- Fever is the hallmark of malaria, known as malarial paroxysm, initially daily until synchronization of infection after several wk, when fever may occur every other day (tertian) in *P. vivax, P. ovale,* or *P. falciparum* malaria or every third day (quartan) in *P. malariae* malaria.
- Classic malarial paroxysm characterized by
  1. Cold stage: abrupt onset of cold feeling associated with rigors, shakes
  2. Hot stage: high fever (~40° C) associated with restlessness
  3. Sweating stage: patient defervesces
- Nonspecific symptoms are
  1. Headache
  2. Cough
  3. Myalgia
  4. Vomiting
  5. Diarrhea
  6. Jaundice
- *P. falciparum*:
  - Most pathogenic of the four species.
  - Rapidly progresses to high-level parasitemia.
  - Important cause of the fatal malaria.
  - Classic malarial paroxysm is usually absent.
  - Incubation period after exposure is 12 days (range: 9 to 60 days).
  - Cytoadherence and resetting of RBCs play central role in pathogenesis.
  - The sequestration of RBCs in vital organs leads to fatal complications.
  - Cerebral malaria is a feared complication.
  - Invades erythrocytes of all ages.
  - Lacks hypnozoites (intrahepatic stage), does not relapse.
  - Blood smear usually shows ring form only.
  - Pigment color is black.

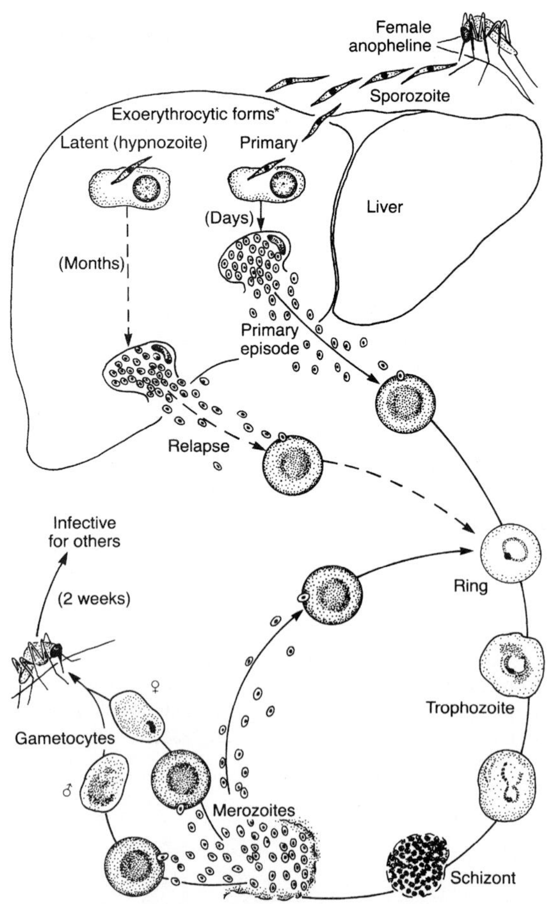

FIGURE 1-187 Life cycle of plasmodia in humans. *Exoerythrocytic forms are also called schizonts. (From Gorbach SL: *Infectious diseases,* ed 2, Philadelphia, 1998, WB Saunders.)

- Banana-shaped gametocytes; if seen in blood, smear is diagnostic.
- Chloroquine resistance is widely present.
- *P. vivax:*
  - Known as tertian malaria: fever occurs every other day.
  - Duffy blood-group antigen FYA- or FYB-related receptor is needed for attachment to RBC.
  - FyFy phenotype (most West African) individuals are resistant to *P. vivax* malaria.
  - Incubation period after exposure is 14 days (range: 8 to 27 days).
  - Hypnozoites may cause relapse of infection after years.
  - Infects mainly reticulocytes.
  - Irregularly shaped large rings and trophozoites, enlarged RBCs, and Schüffner's dot are seen in peripheral blood smear (Fig. 1-188).
  - Pigment color is yellow-brown.
  - *P. vivax* from Papua New Guinea have reduced sensitivity to chloroquine.
  - Primaquine is needed to eradicate the hypnozoites.
- *P. ovale:*
  - Also known as tertian malaria; fever occurs every other day.
  - Occurs mainly in tropical Africa.
  - Incubation period after exposure is 14 days (range: 8 to 27 days).
  - Hypnozoites may cause relapse of infection.
  - Infects mainly reticulocytes.
  - Infected RBC are seen as enlarged, oval shape containing large ring or trophozoites with Schüffner's dot.
  - Pigment color is dark brown.
  - Primaquine needed to eradicate the hypnozoites.
  - No chloroquine resistance has been encountered.
- *P. malariae:*
  - Known as quartan malaria; fever occurs every third day.
  - Common cause of chronic malarial infection.
  - May persist for 20 to 30 yr after leaving the endemic area.
  - Worldwide distribution.
  - Incubation period after exposure is 30 days (range: 16 to 60 days).
  - Lacks hypnozoites (intrahepatic stage).
  - May persist in blood for many years if treated inadequately.
  - Chronic infection may cause soluble immune-complex, resulting in nephritic syndrome.
  - Infects mainly mature RBCs.
  - Band or rectangular forms of trophozoites are commonly seen in peripheral blood smear.
  - Pigment color is brown-black.
- Cerebral malaria:
  - Feared complication of *P. falciparum* infection.
  - Mortality is ~20%.
  - Pathogenesis is poorly understood.
  - Ischemia as a result of sequestration of parasites or cytokines induced by parasite toxin(s) is the key debate.
  - Seizure and altered mental status leading to coma are cardinal manifestation.
  - Hypoglycemia, lactic acidosis, and elevated circulating TNF-α may be present.
  - CSF studies: no increase of WBC count or protein, raised lactate concentrate, and increased opening pressure, especially in children, may be present.

Dx DIAGNOSIS

DIFFERENTIAL DIAGNOSIS

- Typhoid fever
- Dengue fever
- Yellow fever
- Viral hepatitis
- Influenza
- Brucellosis
- UTI
- Leishmaniasis
- Trypanosomiasis
- Rickettsial diseases
- Leptospirosis

WORKUP

- Clinical diagnosis is notoriously inaccurate.
- Demonstration of malarial parasites in blood smear is essential.
- Newer molecular diagnostic techniques are promising.

LABORATORY TESTS

- The thick and thin blood film is required to identify malarial parasites.
- The thick smears are more sensitive and primarily used to detect the presence of parasites.
- The thin smears are used for species differentiation and parasite density estimation.
- A patient who is suspected of having malaria but who has no parasite seen in blood smears should have blood smears repeated every 12 to 24 hr for 3 consecutive days.

PREPARATION OF BLOOD SMEAR:

- Must be prepared from fresh blood obtained by pricking the fingers.
- The thin smear is fixed in methanol before staining.
- The thick smear is stained unfixed.
- The smear should be stained with a 3% Giemsa solution (pH of 7.2) for 30 to 45 min.
- The parasite density should be estimated by counting the percentage of RBCs infected, not the number of parasites, under an oil immersion lens on thin film.

COMMON ERRORS IN READING MALARIAL SMEARS:

- Platelets overlying an RBC
- Misreading artifacts as parasites
- Concern about missing a positive slide

MOLECULAR DIAGNOSIS OF MALARIA:

- Polymerase chain reaction (PCR)
  1. It is useful in accurate species diagnosis.
  2. It can detect the low-level parasitemias.
  3. It is expensive and time consuming.
  4. It needs technical expertise.
- Quantitative buffy coat (QBC)
  1. This test detects nuclear material of parasites using acridine orange stain.
  2. It is unable to speciate the parasites accurately.
  3. It cannot quantitate parasitemias.
- Para Sight F and Malaria PF Test
  1. This test uses a monoclonal antibody to detect *P. falciparum*-specific, histidine-rich protein (HRP)-2.
  2. It can detect *P. falciparum* only.
  3. Past infection may confuse diagnosis.
- OptiMal test
  1. This test detects lactate dehydrogenase (LDH) of parasites.
  2. It can differentiate *falciparum* from non-*falciparum* malaria.

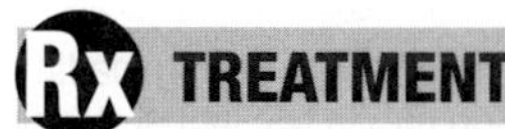

TREATMENT

NONPHARMACOLOGIC THERAPY

ANTIMOSQUITO MEASURES:

1. Eradication of mosquito breeding places by chemical spray
2. Use of mosquito nets properly in the endemic areas
3. Use of protective clothing
4. Use of insect spray (permethrin), mosquito coils, or repellents (diethyltoluamide)

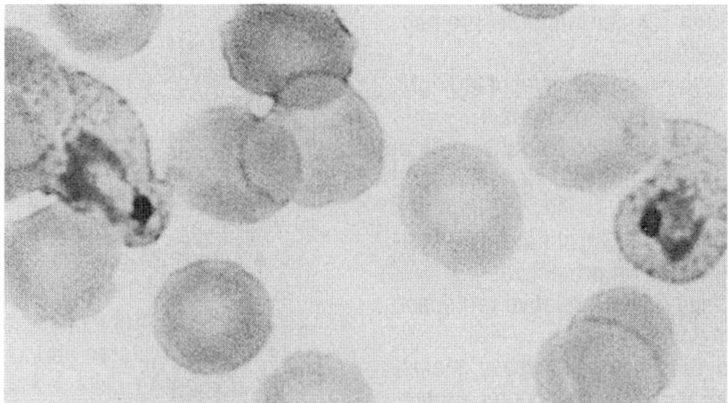

FIGURE 1-188 Giemsa-stained blood smear in *Plasmodium vivax* malaria. Asexual parasites. Note that the parasites are large and ameboid; the infected erythrocytes are the largest cells in the field (because they are reticulocytes), and the erythrocytes contain numerous pink dots (Schüffner's dots) (×2000). (From Klippel JH et al (eds): *Internal medicine,* ed 5, St Louis, 1998, Mosby.)

ACUTE GENERAL Rx

A definitive diagnosis of malaria is essential for specific antimalarial chemotherapy.

NON-*FALCIPARUM* MALARIA:

- Chloroquine 600 mg base (1000 mg chloroquine phosphate) PO loading dose, 6 hr later 300 mg base (500 mg salt), then 300 mg base (500 mg salt) daily for 2 days.
- In the case of *P. vivax* and *P. ovale,* treatment with primaquine 15 mg daily for 14 days is needed to eradicate the exoerythrocytic forms, especially the hypnozoites responsible for relapses.
- G6PD should be measured before primaquine is given.
- Chloroquine-resistant *P. vivax* has been documented; in that case, quinine is given.

FALCIPARUM MALARIA:

- Chloroquine can be used cautiously for *falciparum* malaria acquired in chloroquine-sensitive areas (chloroquine is more rapidly effective than quinine)
- Mainstay of treatment is oral quinine sulfate 10 mg (salt)/kg (usually 650 mg) q8h for 3 to 7 days, followed by pyrimethamine with sulfadoxine (Fansider) 3 tablets (each tablets contains 500 mg sulfadoxine and 25 mg pyrimethamine) or doxycycline 200 mg loading dose, then 100 mg bid for 7 days to eradicate asexual forms of the parasite
- Artemether-Lumefantrine (Coartem), an artemisinin-based drug was recently approved in the U.S. for oral treatment of uncomplicated *Plasmodium falciparum* malaria. It is not approved for prophylaxis. The IV formulation of artesunate, another artemisinin, is available through the CDC.

ALTERNATIVES:

- Quinine followed by clindamycin 900 mg tid for 5 days, or
- Mefloquine 1250 mg as a single dose, or
- Halofantrine 500 mg q6h for 3 doses, repeat 1 wk later, or
- Atovaquone 1000 mg daily for 3 days plus proguanil 400 mg daily for 3 days, or
- Atovaquone 1000 mg daily for 3 days plus doxycycline 100 mg bid for 3 days, or
- Artesunate 4 mg/kg daily for 3 days plus mefloquine 1250 mg single dose

NOTE: Parasitemia may paradoxically rise in the first 24 to 36 hr and is not an indication of treatment failure.

SEVERE *FALCIPARUM* MALARIA: It is a medical emergency; intensive care is preferred.

- Measurement of blood glucose, lactate, ABG is important.
- IV quinidine gluconate 10 mg salt/kg loading dose (maximum 600 mg) in NS; infuse slowly over 1 to 2 hr, followed by continuous infusion of 0.02 mg/kg/min until patient can swallow.
- A cardiac monitor is needed for observation of QT interval.
- Alternatively, artemether 3.2 mg/kg IM then 1.6 mg/kg daily for 3 days can be used.
- Plasmapheresis is an option for parasitemia >30% or in pregnant woman and in elderly with severe malaria.

NOTE: WHO recommends IV artesunate as the treatment of choice for severe malaria in adults and children in area of low transmission. Data on children in high-transmission regions are limited, and WHO recommends treatment with artesunate, artemether, or quinine.

MULTIDRUG-RESISTANT MALARIA:

- Mefloquine 1250 mg as a single dose, or
- Halofantrine 500 mg every 6 hr for 3 doses, repeat same course after 1 wk
- Combination therapy usually preferred

DISPOSITION

RISK FACTORS FOR FATAL MALARIA:

- Failure to take chemoprophylaxis
- Delay in seeking medical care
- Misdiagnosis

COMPLICATIONS OF MALARIA:

- Anemia
- Acidosis
- Hypoglycemia
- Respiratory distress
- DIC
- Blackwater fever
- Renal failure
- Shock

REFERRAL

- To an infectious disease specialist or travel medicine expert for severe malaria complications
- To an intensive care specialist if severe cerebral malaria or other major organ failure develops

PEARLS & CONSIDERATIONS

HOST RESPONSE:

- The specific immune response to malaria confers protection from high-level parasitemia and disease, but not from infection.
- Asymptomatic parasitemia without illness (premunition) is common among adults in endemic areas.
- Immunity is specific for both the species and the strain of infecting malarial parasites.
- Immunity to all strains is never achieved.
- Normal spleen function is an important host factor because of immunologic as well as filtering functions of the spleen.
- Both humoral and cellular immunity are necessary for protection.
- Polyclonal increase in serum level of IgG, IgM, and IgA occur in immune individuals.
- Antibody to antigenically variant protein PfEMP1 is important for protection in case of *P. falciparum* malaria.
- Passively transferred IgG from immune individuals has been shown protective.
- Maternal antibody confers relative protection of infants from severe disease.
- Genetic disorders (sickle cell disease, thalassemia, and G6PD deficiency) confer protection from death because parasites are unable to grow efficiently in low-oxygen tensions, thus preventing high-level parasitemias.
- Individuals deficient of Duffy factor in RBCs are resistant to infection by *P. vivax.*
- Nonspecific defense mechanisms, such as cytokines (TNF-α, IL-1, 6, 8), also play an important role in protection, causing fever (temperatures of 40° C damage mature parasites) and other pathologic effects.

PREVENTION OF MALARIA: Prophylaxis should be taken 1 wk before travel; continue weekly for the duration of stay and for 4 wk after leaving endemic area.

NON-*FALCIPARUM* MALARIA: Chloroquine 300 mg base (500 mg chloroquine phosphate) PO/wk

FALCIPARUM MALARIA:

- Mefloquine 250 mg (228 mg base) PO/wk, or
- Doxycycline 100 mg PO/day, or
- Primaquine 0.5 mg base/kg/day, or
- Chloroquine (300 mg base) plus proguanil (200 mg) PO/day

SPECIAL CONSIDERATIONS:

- Long-term visitors or travelers
- Children <12 yr
- Immunocompromised host
- Pregnant women

VACCINATION:

- No effective and safe vaccine available yet
- A live, attenuated, whole sporozoite vaccine shown to work
- A synthetic peptide (SPf66) vaccine proved ineffective
- New DNA-based vaccines are in development

MALARIA INFORMATION:

- CDC Travelers' Health Hotline (877) 394-8747; CDC Travelers' Health Fax (888) 232–3299
- CDC Malaria Epidemiology (770) 488–7788; internet: www.cdc.gov

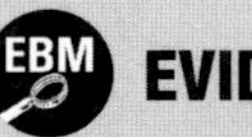

EVIDENCE

Please note: Complete text of EBM for this topic is available online.

Key trials and commentary:

Malaria remains a leading global health problem that requires the improved use of existing interventions and the accelerated development of new control methods. This study aimed to assess the safety, immunogenicity, and initial efficacy of the malaria vaccine RTS,S/AS02D in infants in Africa.

This study showed that the RTS,S/AS02D malaria vaccine was safe, well tolerated, and immunogenic in young infants. These findings set the stage for expanded phase III efficacy studies to confirm vaccine efficacy against clinical malaria disease.[1] Ⓐ

The control of malaria remains a leading global health priority. The endemic countries of sub-Saharan Africa often have weak health systems, and children younger than 2 years have a large and disproportionate incidence of severe disease and death. Aponte et al conducted a randomized trial to test the safety, immunogenicity, and efficacy of a new malaria vaccine in some 200 infants in Mozambique. The children were assigned to receive three doses of either the malaria vaccine or the control hepatitis B vaccine at 10, 14, and 18 weeks of age as well as routine immunization vaccines given at 8, 12, and 16 weeks of age. The investigators reported that the malaria vaccine was safe and conclude that a phase III study is now needed to confirm the impression that the vaccine is effective against the development of clinical malaria.

Previous trials with the RTS,S/AS02D vaccine in humans also showed safety and at least some protective efficacy. In Gambian adults, vaccine efficacy was 71% in the 9 weeks after the last vaccination, but provided little efficacy thereafter. In a cohort of children ages 1 to 4 years in Mozambique, efficacy for delay of first infection in a 6-month follow-up was 45%; however, nearly all had at least one infection, but the rate of acquisition of the first clinical episode was on average 35% lower in infants immunized vs. those in a control group. For severe malaria, the rate of acquisition of the disease was almost 50% less in those who received the vaccine. In this report, efficacy in delaying the time to first infection was 66% when the vaccine was administered to infants.

Thus far, malaria vaccines by definition are known as "partially protective" vaccines. What might be the benefits to a population as a whole of delaying infection and disease? Some experts have predicted that the effect of the introduction of a partly protective vaccine will be reduction in morbidity and mortality at least in the first years of life, but with negligible effect on transmission. Future phase III trials will be critical for determination of the public-health usefulness of the currently available vaccine. Pending licensure, decisions will need to be made about whether or not this vaccine should be widely used and, if so, how best to incorporate it with existing control measures, such as insecticide-treated bed nets and early diagnosis and treatment of malaria.

It seems that we are now closer to having a vaccine for malaria than ever before, at least one that might reduce morbidity and mortality. An ideal vaccine, however, is not at hand that would prevent every child from ever having or dying from this disease. A new vaccine is expected soon. This is a radiation-attenuated sporozoite vaccine that was expected to undergo initial testing in humans very soon. The next 5 to 10 years will probably be the most exciting in the long journey to bring malaria vaccine to the developing world.

Evidence-Based Reference

1. Aponte JJ et al: Safety of the RTS,S/AS02D candidate malaria vaccine in infants living in a highly endemic area of Mozambique: a double blind randomised controlled phase I/IIb trial, *Lancet* 370: 1534-1551, 2007. Commentary by J.A. Stockman III, M.D. A

SUGGESTED READINGS

Baird JK: Effectiveness of antimalarial drugs, *N Engl J Med* 352:1565, 2005.

Griffith KS et al: Treatment of malaria in the United States, a systematic review, *JAMA* 297:2264-2277, 2007.

Marx A et al: Meta-analysis: accuracy of rapid tests for malaria in travelers returning from endemic areas, *Ann Intern Med* 142:836, 2005.

Rosenthal PJ: Artesunate for the treatment of severe falciparum malaria, *N Engl J Med* 358:1829-1836, 2008.

Skarbinski J et al: Malaria surveillance—United States, 2004, *MMWR Surveill Summ* 55(4):23, 2006.

South East Asian Quinine Artesunate Malaria Trial (SEAQUAMAT) group: Artesunate versus quinine for treatment of severe falciparum malaria: a randomized trial, *Lancet* 366:717-725, 2005.

AUTHORS: **GLENN G. FORT, M.D., M.P.H.,** and **DENNIS J. MIKOLICH, M.D.**

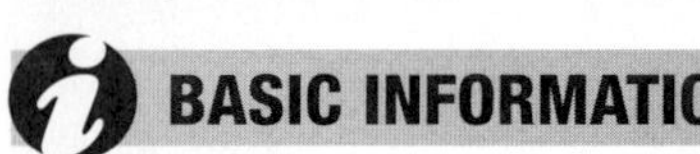

BASIC INFORMATION

DEFINITION

In the setting of recently administered anesthetic agents, most commonly halogenated inhalation agents (halothane) or depolarizing muscle relaxants (succinylcholine), patients with malignant hyperthermia (MH) quickly develop muscle rigidity and elevated temperature.

SYNONYMS

Malignant hyperthermia of anesthesia

ICD-9CM CODES

995.86 Malignant hypothermia of anesthesia

EPIDEMIOLOGY & DEMOGRAPHICS

INCIDENCE: Between 1/200 and 1/250,000. A study by Larach et al demonstrates a mortality rate of 1.4%.

PEAK INCIDENCE: Any age may be affected

PREVALENCE: Difficult to determine because of great variations in both penetrance of gene and severity of illness

PREDOMINANT SEX AND AGE: Any age and either sex may be affected

GENETICS: MH may be considered a pharmacogenetic disorder that is triggered by exposure to anesthetics or depolarizing muscle relaxants in predisposed individuals. Half of cases are autosomal dominant, mostly involving a mutation of the rynodine receptor. Others unknown.

RISK FACTORS: Known family history of malignant hyperthermia or significant problems with general anesthesia. Muscular build increases risk of dying fourteenfold and the risk of cardiac arrest ninteenfold.

PHYSICAL FINDINGS & CLINICAL PRESENTATION

- Within minutes to hours after anesthetic is given, patient develops muscle rigidity (especially masseter spasm), hyperthermia (up to 45° C), tachycardia that may progress to other dysrhythmias, and hypotension. Skin initially reddens but then becomes cyanotic and mottled. There is also increased carbon dioxide production.
- Rhabdomyolysis, acute renal failure, and disseminated intravascular coagulation may soon follow.

ETIOLOGY

- In contrast to fever, in which elevated core temperature is related to hypothalamus set point adjustment by cytokines, malignant hyperthermia results from overproduction of heat via skeletal muscle metabolism in the context of a normal hypothalamic set point.
- In genetically susceptible individuals, administration of anesthetic agents results in release of calcium from the sarcoplasmic reticulum of skeletal muscles, causing muscle rigidity and hypermetabolism. This results in significant heat production that overwhelms the body's normal ability to dissipate heat.

Dx DIAGNOSIS

DIFFERENTIAL DIAGNOSIS

- Neuroleptic malignant syndrome
- Fever
- Heat stroke
- Thyrotoxicosis
- Pheochromocytoma
- Central nervous system infection or space-occupying lesion
- MDMA (Ecstasy), cocaine, alcohol withdrawal, or amphetamine use
- Serotonin syndrome
- Adverse reaction to monoamine oxidase inhibitor or anticholinergic drug
- Strychnine poisoning

WORKUP

Based on history, it is usually easy to distinguish malignant hyperthermia from other causes of hyperthermia. A thorough history, especially including medications and any illicit substances, is important. Consider lumbar puncture to rule out infection.

LABORATORY TESTS

- If the cause of hyperthermia is uncertain, a complete blood count, thyroid function studies, toxicology screen, and urine vanillymandelic acid (VMA) may be useful.
- Once diagnosis is established, it is important to follow electrolytes (especially potassium, calcium, and phosphorus), creatinine, blood urea nitrogen, liver transaminases, and creatinine kinase.
- Prothrombin time and partial thromboplastin time should be followed to evaluate for disseminated intravascular coagulation.

IMAGING STUDIES

CT scan to assess for space-occupying lesion if diagnosis is uncertain

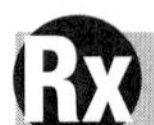

TREATMENT

The most important measures for treatment include stopping the anesthetic agents, starting dantrolene, physical cooling, and preventing sequelae. Antipyretics are not useful because the hypothalamic set point is not altered by cytokines.

NONPHARMACOLOGIC THERAPY

- Cooling by ice bath, ice packs in the groin and axillae, cool spray with fans, or cooling blankets. In severe instances extracorporeal partial bypass or iced peritoneal lavage may be used. Stop cooling when core temperature reaches 38° C to prevent overcooling.
- Careful monitoring of cardiovascular and respiratory status with constant core temperature measurements.

ACUTE GENERAL Rx

- Dantrolene is the mainstay of treatment, starting with a bolus of 5 mg/kg IV, which should be repeated every 5 min until symptoms abate or a maximum of 10 to 20 mg/kg is reached. Then 24 hr of 10 mg/kg/day IV should be given.
- Beta-blockers or lidocaine may be useful for dysrhythmias, but verapamil should be avoided as its use with dantrolene has been shown to depress cardiac function.
- Sodium bicarbonate may be necessary to reverse acidosis.
- Aggressive hydration with forced diuresis and urine alkalinization should be instituted as treatment for rhabdomyolysis.

CHRONIC Rx

This is an acute illness.

COMPLEMENTARY & ALTERNATIVE MEDICINE

None

DISPOSITION

Patient will likely need intensive monitoring, necessitating an intensive care unit bed.

REFERRAL

Anesthesia consultants will likely already be involved. Consider cardiac, renal, or hematologic consult if sequelae are significant.

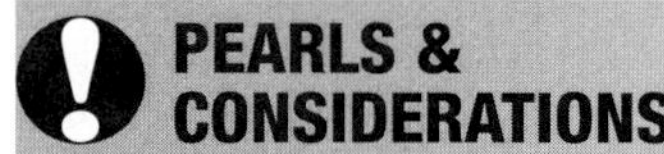

PEARLS & CONSIDERATIONS

COMMENTS

Malignant hyperthermia is a life-threatening condition that requires prompt recognition of the signs and symptoms to minimize illness and end-organ damage.

PREVENTION

- Careful family and personal history of significant adverse effects with general anesthesia are important tip-offs.
- Prophylactic dantrolene therapy is no longer recommended in susceptible individuals.

PATIENT & FAMILY EDUCATION

Because family history is so important in this illness, it is important for patients and families to be aware of a history of problems with general anesthesia.

SUGGESTED READINGS

Hadad E: Drug-induced hyperthermia and muscle rigidity: a practical approach, *Eur J Emerg Med* 10:2, 2003.

Krause T: Dantrolene—a review of its pharmacology, therapeutic use and new developments, *Anaesthesia* 59(4):364-373, 2004.

Larach M et al: Cardiac arrests and deaths associated with malignant hyperthermia in North America from 1987 to 2006, *Anesthesiology* 108:603-611, 2008.

Litman R: Malignant hyperthermia, *JAMA* 293:23, 2005.

Simon H: Hyperthermia, *N Engl J Med* 329:7, 1993.

Stowell KM: Malignant hyperthermia: a pharmacogenetic disorder, *Pharmacogenomics* 9:1657-1672, 2008.

AUTHOR: **CRISTINA ANTONIO PACHECO, M.D.**

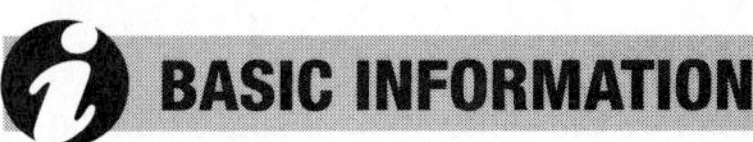

BASIC INFORMATION

DEFINITION

A Mallory-Weiss tear (MWT) is a longitudinal mucosal laceration in the region of the gastroesophageal junction.

SYNONYMS

Mallory-Weiss syndrome

ICD-9CM CODES

530.7 Gastroesophageal laceration-hemorrhage syndrome
530.82 Esophageal hemorrhage

EPIDEMIOLOGY & DEMOGRAPHICS

- Accounts for 5% to 15% of cases of upper gastrointestinal (GI) bleeding
- Reported from early childhood to old age; the majority of patients are age 40 yr to 60 yr
- More common in males
- Alcohol use is present in 30% to 60%

PHYSICAL FINDINGS & CLINICAL PRESENTATION

- Vomiting, retching, or vigorous coughing will often, but not always, precede hematemesis.
- Patients may be clinically stable or present with tachycardia, hypotension, melena, or hematochezia.
- Bleeding may be self-limited or severe.
- Tears may be seen in association with other upper GI tract lesions, including hiatus hernia (present in as many as 90% of patients), ulcers, and esophageal varices, particularly in alcoholics.

ETIOLOGY

- An acute increase in intraabdominal pressure is transmitted to the esophagus, resulting in mucosal laceration.
- Vomiting may be associated with alcohol use, ketoacidosis, ulcer disease, uremia, pancreatitis, cholecystitis, pregnancy (in particular associated with hyperemesis gravidarum), myocardial infarction, or the postoperative period.
- Tears may be iatrogenic, related to endoscopy (especially in struggling or retching patients), esophageal dilation, lower esophageal pneumatic disruption therapy for achalasia, transesophageal echocardiography, or in association with polyethylene glycol electrolyte colonic lavage preparation.

Dx DIAGNOSIS

DIFFERENTIAL DIAGNOSIS

- Esophageal or gastric varices
- Esophagitis or esophageal ulcers (peptic or pill-induced)
- Gastric erosions
- Gastric or duodenal ulcer
- Dieulafoy lesion
- Arteriovenous malformations
- Neoplasms (usually gastric)
- Boerhaave's syndrome

WORKUP

Endoscopy is the diagnostic method of choice.

LABORATORY TESTS

- Complete blood count, prothrombin time, partial thromboplastin time
- Electrolytes, blood urea nitrogen, creatinine, liver function tests, pregnancy test, tests to evaluate for predisposing conditions

IMAGING STUDIES

Upper GI series is usually not sensitive. Patients with concurrent chest pain, dyspnea, shock, or physical examination findings of crepitus or pleural effusion should have a chest radiograph or CT to exclude Boerhaave's syndrome.

Rx TREATMENT

NONPHARMACOLOGIC THERAPY

- Supportive care
- Avoidance of aspirin, nonsteroidal antiinflammatory drugs, and anticoagulants

ACUTE GENERAL Rx

- Patients with active bleeding or hemodynamic instability require large-bore IVs, fluid resuscitation, and transfusion of blood products (red blood cells, fresh frozen plasma, and platelets) as appropriate.
- Nasogastric decompression and antiemetics may be considered.
- Endoscopic therapy for patients with active or ongoing hemorrhage. Therapeutic modalities include electrocoagulation, injection (e.g., 1:10,000 epinephrine, polidocanol), sclerotherapy (for bleeding associated with esophageal varices), band ligation, or endoscopic hemoclips (therapies may be used alone or in combination).
- Arterial embolization in patients with active bleeding who are poor surgical candidates.
- Laparotomy, with gastrotomy and oversewing of the tear, is required in a small percentage of patients with uncontrolled bleeding.

CHRONIC Rx

- Healing will usually occur without specific therapy.
- H_2 blockers or proton pump inhibitors may be given to help facilitate healing but should not be used long term unless appropriate indications are present.

DISPOSITION

- Prognosis is good, with spontaneous cessation of bleeding in upwards of 90% of patients. Endoscopic features can guide treatment.
- Delayed rebleeding is described in patients with high-risk stigmata (shock at initial presentation, spurting or oozing at initial endoscopy).
- Death has been reported in 3% to 12%, often with severe bleeding and underlying comorbid conditions such as coagulopathy, thrombocytopenia, alcohol use, and multisystem organ failure.

REFERRAL

- Gastrointestinal referral for endoscopy
- Surgical referral for bleeding unresponsive to endoscopic treatment or in the setting of coexistent perforation

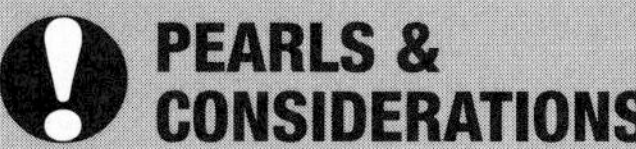

PEARLS & CONSIDERATIONS

Conditions predisposing to retching or vomiting should be identified and treated at presentation.

EBM EVIDENCE

Endoscopic epinephrine treatment

Endoscopic injection of epinephrine and polidocanol versus placebo

- Randomized controlled trial of 32 patients with MWT; hemostasis obtained in all 32 patients.
- Two (6.2%) of 32 patients had minor recurrent bleeding compared with eight (25.8%) of 31 in the control group.
- No major episodes of rebleeding.

Endoscopic hemoclips versus endoscopic injection of epinephrine

- Prospective trial of 35 patients with MWT with spurting vessels or oozing
- Randomized to either treatment
- Primary hemostasis was achieved in 100% of patients in both groups
- Each group had one patient with rebleeding who was successfully re-treated with the same modality; no second episodes of recurrent bleeding
- No procedure-related complications

Endoscopic band ligation versus endoscopic injections of epinephrine

- Prospective trial of 34 patients with actively bleeding MWT
- Randomized to either treatment
- Primary hemostasis achieved in all 17 (100%) patients in band ligation group and 16 (94.1%) of 17 patients in epinephrine injection group
- No major complications or episodes of rebleeding in either group

SUGGESTED READINGS

Huang SP et al: Endoscopic hemoclip placement and epinephrine injection for Mallory-Weiss syndrome with active bleeding, *Gastrointest Endosc* 55:842, 2002.

Kortas DY et al: Mallory-Weiss tear: predisposing factors and predictors of a complicated course, *Am J Gastroenterol* 96:2863, 2001.

Llach J et al: Endoscopic injection therapy in bleeding Mallory-Weiss syndrome: a randomized controlled trial, *Gastrointest Endosc* 54:679, 2001.

Park CH et al: A prospective, randomized trial of endoscopic band ligation vs. epinephrine injection for actively bleeding Mallory-Weiss syndrome, *Gastrointest Endosc* 60:22, 2004.

AUTHOR: **HARLAN G. RICH, M.D.**

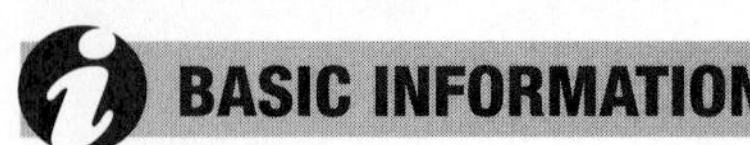

BASIC INFORMATION

DEFINITION

Marfan's syndrome is an inherited disorder of connective tissue involving the skeleton, cardiovascular system, eyes, lungs, and central nervous system.

ICD-9CM CODES
759.82 Marfan's syndrome

EPIDEMIOLOGY & DEMOGRAPHICS

PREVALENCE:
- One case per 10,000 persons.
- Both sexes are affected equally by this autosomal-dominant syndrome.
- Approximately 30% of cases are a new mutation.

PHYSICAL FINDINGS & CLINICAL PRESENTATION

Diagnostic criteria for Marfan's syndrome (Fig. 1-189):
- Skeleton: joint hypermobility, tall stature, pectus excavatum, reduced thoracic kyphosis, scoliosis, arachnodactyly, dolichostenomelia, pectus carinatum, and erosion of the lumbosacral vertebrae from dural ectasia*
- Eye: myopia, retinal detachment, elongated globe, ectopia lentis*
- Cardiovascular: mitral valve prolapse, endocarditis, arrhythmia, dilated mitral annulus, mitral regurgitation, tricuspid valve prolapse, aortic regurgitation, aortic dissection,* dilation of the aortic root*
- Pulmonary: apical blebs, spontaneous pneumothorax
- Skin and integument: inguinal hernias, incisional hernias, striae atrophicae
- Central nervous system: attention deficit disorder, hyperactivity, verbal-performance discrepancy, dural ectasia, anterior pelvic meningocele*

If the family history is positive for a close relative clearly affected by Marfan's syndrome, manifestations should be present in the skeleton and one of the other organ systems and the diagnosis confirmed by linkage analysis or mutation detection.

If the family history is negative or unknown, the patient should have manifestations in the skeleton, the cardiovascular system, and one other system and at least one of the manifestations indicated by an asterisk in the above lists.

Manifestations are listed within each organ system in increasing specificity for Marfan's syndrome; although none is completely specific, those indicated by an asterisk are the most specific.

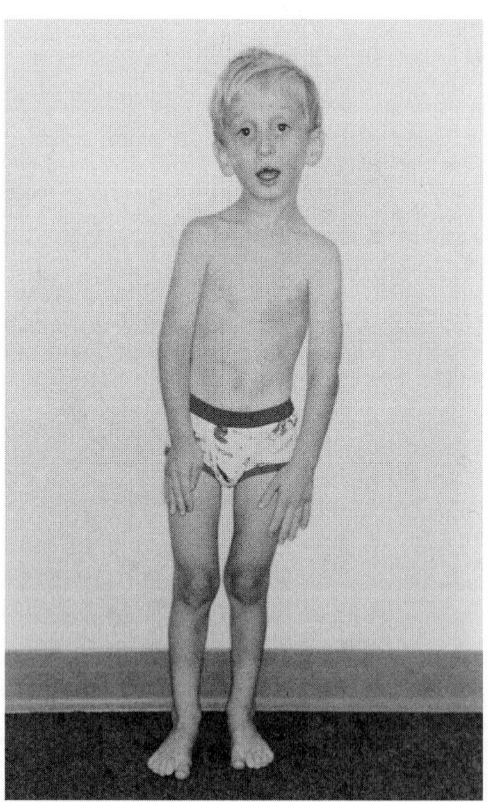

FIGURE 1-189 Marfan's syndrome. Note the elongated facies, droopy lids, apparent dolichostenomelia, and mild scoliosis. (From Behrman RE: *Nelson's textbook of pediatrics,* Philadelphia, 2004, WB Saunders.)

ETIOLOGY

Mutations in the gene that encodes fibrillin-1, the major constituent of microfibrils, which form the frame for elastic fibers. All the manifestations of Marfan's syndrome can be explained by the defective microfibrils.

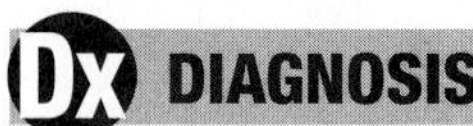

DIAGNOSIS

DIFFERENTIAL DIAGNOSIS

Each of the clinical manifestations of the syndrome may have other causes; however, if the diagnostic criteria are met, the diagnosis is made.

WORKUP

- Echocardiography to establish:
  1. Mitral valve prolapse
  2. Mitral regurgitation
  3. Tricuspid valve prolapse
  4. Aortic regurgitation
  5. Dilation of the aortic root
- Chest radiograph
- Transesophageal echocardiography, chest CT scan, chest MRI, or aortography for suspected aortic dissection
- Chest radiograph for pulmonary apical bullae
- Ophthalmologic examination by ophthalmologist

Rx TREATMENT

- Regular cardiac and aorta monitoring by physical examination and echocardiography.
- Endocarditis prophylaxis.
- Restriction of contact sports, weight lifting, and overexertion.
- Beta-blockers are commonly prescribed to slow the rate of aortic root dilation in children; recent trials, however, have shown that this approach is not effective. Recent reports indicate that use of angiotensin receptor blockers significantly slowed the rate of progressive aortic root dilation.
- Early use of angiotensin-converting enzyme inhibitors in young patients with Marfan's syndrome and valvular regurgitation may lessen the need for mitral valve surgery.
- Genetic counseling.
- Monitor aorta during pregnancy because of the increased risk of dissection.

SUGGESTED READINGS

Brooke BS et al: Angiotensin II blockade and aortic root dilation in Marfan's syndrome, *N Engl J Med* 358:26, 2008.

Selamet Tierney ES et al: Beta-blocker therapy does not alter the rate of aortic root dilation in pediatric patients with Marfan syndrome, *J Pediatr* 150:77, 2007.

AUTHOR: **FRED F. FERRI, M.D.**

BASIC INFORMATION

DEFINITION

Mastitis is the inflammation of breast tissue either from irritation or infection, resulting in subcutaneous cellulitis.

ICD-9CM CODES
611.0 Acute (infective, puerperal, nonpuerperal, diffuse, interstitial)
610.1 Chronic (cystic, fibrocystic)
610.4 Periductal/plasma cell
675.1 Postpartum/puerperal (purulent)
675.2 Postpartum/puerperal (nonpurulent)

EPIDEMIOLOGY & DEMOGRAPHICS

- When present in lactating mothers, mastitis typically occurs in the first 3 mo postpartum (74% to 95% cases). When severe, mastitis can lead to a breast abscess (5% to 11%) or septicemia. Mastitis is a risk factor for vertical transmission of infections as a result of changes in the composition of milk and local immune response.
- In nonlactating women of childbearing age it often presents as granulomatous mastitis (GM).
- In older nonlactating women it is called periductal mastitis (PM) and is caused by inflamed milk ducts near the nipple.
- Mastitis can also occur in early infancy, when breast hypertrophy from maternal hormonal stimulation can lead to infection.
- Recurrent mastitis is typically the result of incomplete or inappropriate antibiotic treatment.

PREVALENCE: 1% to 3% of women to as high as one in three lactating mothers; recurrence 4%

PREDOMINANT SEX: Females

RISK FACTORS:

- Mastitis in the past
- Cracked, fissured, or sore nipples
- Primiparity and improper nursing such that the breast does not empty completely
- Cleft lip or palate or short frenulum in infant
- Milk stasis, engorgement, missed feedings
- Using antifungal nipple cream (presumably for nipple thrush) in the same week
- Plastic-backed breast pads
- Employment outside home
- Tight clothing or bras
- Use of manual breast pump
- Stress or fatigue
- Diabetes
- Use of steroids
- Lumpectomy with radiation
- Breast implants

PHYSICAL FINDINGS & CLINICAL PRESENTATION

- Malaise and myalgia
- Chills and fever >38.3° C
- Warmth, redness, tenderness in breast
- Pain with nursing
- Decreased milk output
- Area of breast is hard, wedge shaped, and swollen
- Breast mass near nipple with retraction or discharge in PM
- Enlarged axillary lymph nodes or sinus tract formation in GM

ETIOLOGY

- Irritation.
- Blocked lactiferous duct and stasis of the duct, leading to engorgement.
- Local adverse immune response to milk proteins.
- Infectious: *Staphylococcus aureus*, coagulase-negative staphylococci, group A- and B-hemolytic streptococci, *Escherichia coli* and *Bacteroides* species, and increasing incidence of methicillin-resistant *S. aureus* (MRSA) mastitis; rare instances with *Salmonella* species, mycobacteria, candida, and Cryptococcus.
  - GM from inflammation with epithelioid histiocytes and multinucleated giant cells can be caused by tuberculosis, sarcoidosis, foreign body reaction, or parasitic and mycotic infections or be idiopathic.
  - Mastitis in neonates is caused by infections with *S. aureus* or gram-negative enteric bacteria.

DIAGNOSIS

DIFFERENTIAL DIAGNOSIS

- Plugged lactiferous ducts.
- Breast abscess.
- Inflammatory breast cancer.
- Mastitis as a symptom of hyperprolactinemia or galactorrhea.
- Other cancers; 3% of women diagnosed with breast cancer are lactating.
- GM can be a manifestation of systemic disease, including sarcoidosis, Wegener's granulomatosis, giant cell arteritis, polyarteritis nodosa, tuberculosis, or syphilis.

WORKUP

- History of signs and symptoms and clinical examination, including thorough breast examination with assessment for axillary nodes and nipple discharge, are sufficient to make the diagnosis.
- Recurrent mastitis should include workup for underlying breast disease.

LABORATORY TESTS

- Simple mastitis requires no milk culture or laboratory studies.
- Obtain midstream sample of milk for culture for antibiotic sensitivities in refractory mastitis or in suspected MRSA.
- Complete blood count and blood cultures in toxic-appearing patients.
- Breast milk analysis reveals raised milk cell counts, increased sodium and protein levels, activation of milk leukocytes, and increased factors such as tumor necrosis factor-alpha and interferon-gamma.
- Gram stain and culture indicated in early childhood mastitis.

IMAGING STUDIES

- Not necessary unless refractory.
- Consider ultrasound to evaluate for abscess or mammogram because carcinoma cannot be excluded.
- In GM, use of mammogram and ultrasound-guided fine-needle aspiration are standard studies.

TREATMENT

NONPHARMACOLOGIC THERAPY

- Warm compresses.
- Continue frequent nursing; change feeding positions to completely empty breasts.
- Increase fluid intake and bed rest.
- Therapeutic ultrasound has been suggested for breast engorgement.
- In abscess formation, drainage is necessary, followed by parenteral antibiotics.
- Surgery in severe periductal mastitis.

ACUTE GENERAL Rx

- Pain medications, including nonsteroidal antiinflammatories and analgesics (e.g., acetaminophen, ibuprofen).
- Antimicrobials:
  - Dicloxacillin or cloxacillin 500 mg PO four times a day for 10 to 14 days.
  - If no response, use cephalexin 500 mg PO four times a day or Augmentin 875 mg PO two times a day.
  - Penicillin-allergic women can use clindamycin 300 mg PO four times per day.
  - Ciprofloxacin 500 mg PO bid.
  - Trimethoprim/sulfamethoxazole 160 mg/800 mg PO two times a day, but sulfa drugs should be avoided in mothers breastfeeding infants <2 mo or compromised infants.
  - In MRSA mastitis, use antimicrobials based on the sensitivity profile.
- Oxytocin nasal spray if letdown reflex os disturbed.
- Mastitis in early infancy should be treated with parenteral antibiotics based on results of Gram stain.

CHRONIC Rx

- Experimental vaccines (especially human staphylococcal vaccine) have shown protection against recurrent mastitis.
- Systemic corticosteroids or wide surgical resection in GM.
- New studies show immunosuppressive therapy (methotrexate, azathioprine) as steroid-sparing agents in GM therapy.

COMPLEMENTARY & ALTERNATIVE MEDICINE

- Belladonna, phytolacca, chamomilla, sulphur, bellis perenis
- Complementary therapies have not been assessed in prospective studies

REFERRAL

Referral to a surgeon for severe periductal mastitis

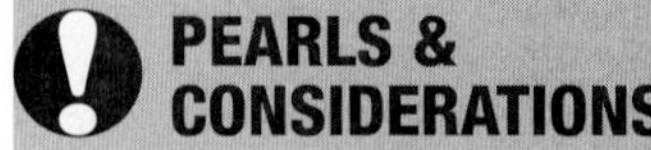

COMMENTS

- Antimicrobials are often not necessary for noninfective mastitis, but 86% of women receive antibiotic treatment.
- Incidence of MRSA mastitis is increasing.
- In reassessing refractory mastitis, the most important consideration is the possibility of cancer.
- Mastitis can be a manifestation of systemic disease.
- Delay in recognition and treatment may result in abscess formation or recurrent mastitis.
- Mastitis is a risk factor for vertical transmission of infections, including increased transmission of retroviruses (especially HIV-1), cytomegalovirus, measles, and hepatitis B and C.
- Mastitis is the major cause of reduction in milk production.
- One quarter of breastfeeding mothers with one episode of mastitis will stop breastfeeding.
- GM mimics breast cancer both clinically and radiologically (>50% of reported cases are initially mistaken for carcinoma). This includes fine-needle aspiration, which is sometimes interpreted as malignant.
- All infants with diagnosis of mastitis should receive parenteral antibiotics.

PATIENT & FAMILY EDUCATION

La Leche League International (http://www.llli.org), International Lactation Consultant Association (http://www.ilca.org)

SUGGESTED READINGS

Academy of Breastfeeding Medicine Protocol Committee: ABM clinical protocol #4: mastitis. Revision, May 2008, *Breastfeed Med* 3(3):177-180, 2008.

Asoglu O et al: Feasibility of surgical management in patients with granulomatous mastitis, *Breast J* 11: 108-114, 2005.

Barbosa-Cesnik C et al: Lactation mastitis, *JAMA* 289: 1609-1612, 2003.

Foxman B et al: Lactation mastitis: occurrence and medical management among 946 breastfeeding women in the United States, *Am J Epidemiol* 55:103, 2002.

Mass S: Breast pain: engorgement, nipple pain and mastitis, *Clin Obstet Gynecol* 47(3):676-682, 2004.

Michie C et al: The challenge of mastitis, *Arch Dis Child* 88:818-821, 2003.

Pouchot J et al: Granulomatous mastitis: an uncommon cause of breast abscess, *Arch Intern Med* 161: 611-612, 2000.

Spencer J et al: Management of mastitis in breastfeeding women, *Am Fam Physician* 78(6):727-731, 2008.

Stricker T et al: Mastitis in early infancy, *Acta Paediatrica* 94:166-169, 2005.

AUTHORS: **AGNIESZKA K. BIALIKIEWICZ, M.D.,** and **JEFFREY BORKAN, M.D.**

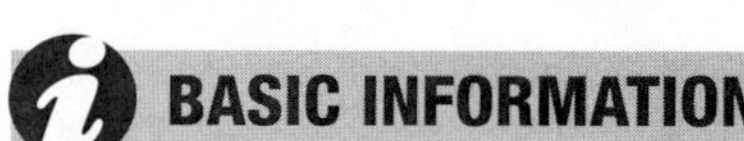

DEFINITION

- Pain in the breast
- Usually cyclical condition but may be noncyclic or extramammary

SYNONYMS

Mastalgia

ICD-9CM CODES
611.71 Mastodynia

EPIDEMIOLOGY & DEMOGRAPHICS

- Mastodynia affects up to 70% of women at some time in their reproductive lives.
- Severe cyclical mastodynia lasting more than 5 days/mo and of sufficient intensity to interfere with sexual, physical, social, and work-related activities is reported among 30% of premenopausal women.
- Underlying fear of breast cancer is the reason most of these women seek medical consultation.
- One tenth of women with mastodynia require pain-relieving therapy.

PHYSICAL FINDINGS & CLINICAL PRESENTATION

- Usually the breasts are normal bilaterally
- Full, tender breasts
- Generalized breast nodularity without discrete lumps
- Chest wall tenderness: extramammary breast pain
- Distinguishing mammary from extramammary pain can be difficult
- With the patient lying on her side so that the breast tissue falls away from the chest wall, tenderness can then be reproduced by direct pressure over the offending site
- Cyclical mastodynia presents in the luteal phase of the menstrual cycle
- Women with cyclical mastodynia tend to have abdominal bloating, leg swelling, and other symptoms of premenstrual syndrome
- Noncyclic mastodynia, on the other hand, is unrelated to the menstrual cycle
- Extramammary breast pain simulates noncyclic mastodynia

ETIOLOGY

- Hormonal imbalance
- Abnormal lipid metabolism
- Premenstrual syndrome (20%)
- Fibrocystic breast disease
- Emotional abuse and anxiety
- Excessive caffeine intake
- Breast cancer (10%)
- Tietze syndrome (idiopathic costochondritis)

Dx DIAGNOSIS

DIFFERENTIAL DIAGNOSIS

- See "Etiology."
- The majority of women with mastodynia have no underlying abnormality.
- Breast fullness and tenderness associated with hormonal changes fluctuate with the menstrual cycle.
- Similarly, breast nodularity, which may or may not be the result of fibrocystic breast disease, also fluctuates with the menstrual cycle.
- Discrete breast lumps need full evaluation to rule out malignancy.
- Tietze syndrome is usually unilateral and may be associated with chest wall swelling.

WORKUP

- Complete history and thorough clinical examination.
- Pain analogue cards may be helpful in establishing the pattern of symptomatology. In patients >35 yr, mammography should be performed as part of the baseline investigation.
- Most women presenting with severe mastodynia are <35 yr. This group has a lower risk of subclinical breast cancer, and their breasts have increased density. In this younger group, radiologic investigations are of limited value unless a discrete breast lump is palpated.

LABORATORY TESTS

Although hormonal imbalance and abnormal lipid metabolism have been implicated in the etiopathogenesis of mastodynia, there is no good evidence to support any consistent pattern of serum hormonal or lipid profile in women with mastodynia. These tests are therefore not recommended.

IMAGING STUDIES

- Mammography should be part of the baseline investigation if the woman is >35 yr.
- Ultrasound can be performed as needed; it is particularly helpful in the assessment of cystic breast lesions.
- In women <35 yr, imaging investigations are not helpful unless a lump has been palpated clinically.
- There are no radiologic features associated with mastodynia: rather, radiologic investigations are performed to exclude the rare presence of a subclinical carcinoma.

Rx TREATMENT

NONPHARMACOLOGIC THERAPY

- 85% of the women with mastodynia can be reassured after full clinical evaluation.
- The remaining 15% require some form of therapy in addition to reassurance.
- A firm, supportive brassiere designed for postpartum use is particularly helpful if mastodynia is associated with breast swelling.
- Follow a low-fat, high-carbohydrate diet.
- Reduce caffeine intake.

ACUTE GENERAL Rx

- Evening primrose oil, which contains gamma-linolenic acid, has been shown to have some effectiveness and is an acceptable treatment for mastodynia.
- Topical NSAID preparations may confer some benefit and can be prescribed for these women.
- Hormonal therapy is the mainstay of treatment.
- Danazol is the only drug approved by the FDA for the treatment of mastodynia. Danazol is an antigonadotropin with some androgenic and peripheral antiestrogenic effects. Its efficacy is well established, with significant relief of mastodynia in 70% to 93% of cases.
- Widespread use of danazol is limited because of its adverse side effects. These include menstrual irregularities, depression, acne, hirsutism and, in severe cases, voice deepening. Women taking danazol should be advised to use effective nonhormonal contraception because of the drug's potential adverse effects on the fetus.
- The side effects of danazol can be significantly reduced by using a low dose (100 mg daily) and confining treatment to 2 wk preceding menstruation.
- Tamoxifen, a synthetic antiestrogen, has also been shown to be effective in the treatment of mastodynia. Although effective in relieving symptoms, its use is extremely limited because of side effects. When used, it should be at a low dosage of 10 mg/day and duration should be limited to 6 mo at a time. In the U.S. this agent is not approved for use in women with mastodynia.
- Bromocriptine is a dopamine-receptor agonist whose primary action is inhibition of prolactin release. It has been used extensively in the treatment of severe cyclical mastodynia and is effective. Again, side effects such as headache and dizziness have limited its use.
- Lisuride maleate was recently found to be effective by one study.
- Other hormonal agents that have been reported to be effective in small studies cannot be recommended. They either have unacceptable side effect profiles or their efficacy is not established. These agents include gestrinone, gonadotropin-releasing hormone analogues, progesterone, and hormone replacement therapy.

CHRONIC Rx

- Longstanding cases of mastodynia can be managed with intermittent low-dose danazol therapy to limit side effects. In between these courses of hormone, nonpharmacologic and nonhormonal therapy can be used.
- Severe, unremitting mastodynia that does not respond to medical treatment may require mastectomy; this is rare.

DISPOSITION

- Cyclical mastodynia resolves spontaneously in 20% to 30% of women.
- Up to 60% of women may develop recurrent symptoms 2 yr after treatment.
- Noncyclic mastodynia responds poorly to treatment but may resolve spontaneously in up to 50% of women.

REFERRAL

- Detection of a breast lump or any other findings suggestive of neoplasm should be fully investigated with an immediate referral.
- Women with chronic, unremitting mastodynia that does not respond to pharmacologic therapy should be referred for possible mastectomy; this is rare.

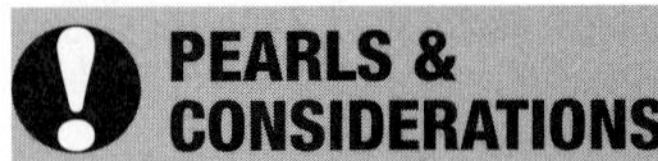

COMMENTS

- There is no good evidence to support the use of vitamin B_6, diuretics, and vitamin E. Mastodynia may represent a presenting symptom of another, more generalized disorder (e.g., premenstrual syndrome, psychologic disturbance).
- In these cases treating mastodynia in isolation will not work; the underlying conditions must be appropriately addressed.

SUGGESTED READINGS

Colgrave S et al: Psychological characteristics of women presenting with breast pain, *J Psychosom Res* 50:303, 2001.

Fentiman IS, Hamed H: Assessment of breast problems, *Int J Clin Pract* 55:458, 2001.

Kaleli S et al: Symptomatic treatment of premenstrual mastalgia in premenopausal women with lisuride maleate: a double-blind placebo-controlled randomized study, *Fertil Steril* 75:718, 2001.

Marchant DJ: Benign breast disease, *Obstet Gynecol Clin North Am* 29:1–20, 2002.

Norlock FE: Benign breast pain in women: a practical approach to evaluation and treatment, *J Am Med Womens Assoc* 57:85, 2002.

AUTHORS: **ALEXANDER B. OLAWAIYE, M.D.,** and **RUBEN ALVERO, M.D.**

BASIC INFORMATION

DEFINITION

Mastoiditis is inflammation of the mastoid process and air cells, a complication of otitis media.

SYNONYMS

Mastoid abscess

ICD-9CM CODES

383.00 Mastoiditis, acute or subacute
383.1 Mastoiditis, chronic

EPIDEMIOLOGY & DEMOGRAPHICS

INCIDENCE (IN U.S.): Widespread use of broad-spectrum antibiotics has led to a marked decline in the incidence of acute mastoiditis.
PREDOMINANT SEX: More common in males
PREDOMINANT AGE: 2 mo to 18 yr
PEAK INCIDENCE: Early childhood

PHYSICAL FINDINGS & CLINICAL PRESENTATION

- Acute mastoiditis is usually a complication of acute otitis media.
- Most common presenting symptom is pain and tenderness in the postauricular region.
- Other signs or symptoms include:
  1. Fever
  2. Postauricular erythema and edema
  3. Protrusion of the pinna inferiorly and anteriorly
  4. Tympanic membrane usually intact with signs of acute otitis media
- Complications of acute mastoiditis include:
  1. Subperiosteal abscess (most common complication)
  2. Hearing loss
  3. Facial nerve palsy
  4. Labyrinthitis
  5. Intracranial complications such as hydrocephalus, meningitis, encephalitis, intracranial abscess, and lateral sinus thrombosis
- Chronic mastoiditis is characterized by chronic otorrhea and chronic tympanic membrane perforation.

ETIOLOGY

- Continuity exists between the middle air space and the mastoid cavity.
- Initial hyperemia and edema of the mucosal lining of the air cells results in accumulation of purulent exudate.
- Dissolution of calcium from bony septae and osteoclastic activity in the inflamed periosteum lead to bone necrosis and coalescence of air cells.
- Most common bacterial isolates are:
  1. *Streptococcus pneumoniae*
  2. *Streptococcus pyogenes*
  3. *Haemophilus influenzae*
  4. *Moraxella catarrhalis*
  5. *Staphylococcus aureus*
- Often, there are multiple organisms in chronic mastoiditis, with predominance of anaerobes and gram-negative bacteria.
- *Mycobacterium tuberculosis,* nontuberculous mycobacteria, *Aspergillus* and *Rhodococcus equi* have been reported in cases of mastoiditis in severely immunocompromised individuals.

DIAGNOSIS

DIFFERENTIAL DIAGNOSIS

- Children
  1. Rhabdomyosarcoma
  2. Histiocytosis X
  3. Leukemia
  4. Kawasaki syndrome
- Adults
  1. Fulminant otitis externa
  2. Histiocytosis X
  3. Metastatic disease

WORKUP

A thorough history and physical examination are important in establishing diagnosis.

LABORATORY TESTS

- Fluid for Gram stain and culture may be obtained by myringotomy.
- If there is a perforation in the tympanic membrane with drainage, cultures of this may be taken after carefully cleaning the external canal.

IMAGING STUDIES

- Plain x-rays of the mastoid region may demonstrate clouding or opacification in areas of pneumatization.
- CT scan can demonstrate early involvement of bone (mastoiditis with bone destruction).
- MRI is more sensitive than CT scan in evaluating soft-tissue involvement and is useful in conjunction with CT scan to investigate other complications of mastoiditis.

TREATMENT

NONPHARMACOLOGIC THERAPY

Myringotomy, if the ear is not already draining

ACUTE GENERAL Rx

- Initiated with IV antibiotics directed against the common organisms *S. pneumoniae* and *H. influenzae.* If the disease in the mastoid has had a prolonged course, coverage for *Staphylococcus aureus* with gram-negative enteric bacilli may be considered for initial therapy until results of cultures become available.
- Continued until all signs of mastoiditis have resolved
- Directed against enteric gram-negative organisms and anaerobes in chronic mastoiditis
- Indications for mastoidectomy:
  1. Failure to improve after 72 hr of therapy
  2. Persistent fever
  3. Imminent or overt signs of intracranial complications
  4. Evidence of a subperiosteal abscess in the mastoid bone

DISPOSITION

Proceed with mastoidectomy when medical therapy fails.

REFERRAL

- To otorhinolaryngologist:
  1. If diagnosis is in doubt
  2. If aural complications present
  3. To evaluate for surgical intervention
- To neurosurgeon if intratemporal or intracranial extension of infection suspected
  1. Aural complications: bone destruction, subperiosteal abscess, petrositis, facial paralysis, labyrinthitis
  2. Intracranial complications: extradural abscess, lateral sinus thrombophlebitis or thrombosis, subdural abscess, meningitis, brain abscess, otitic hydrocephalus

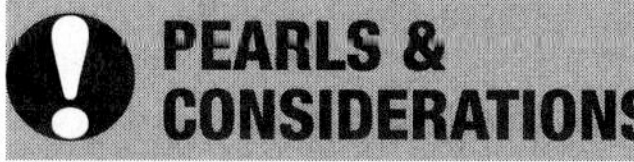

PEARLS & CONSIDERATIONS

Mastoiditis is particularly difficult to eradicate because the mastoid air cells are poorly vascularized and difficult to drain.

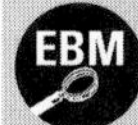

EVIDENCE

According to a retrospective case review of 13 patients with acute mastoiditis, eradication of microorganisms requires appropriate antibiotics based on the infecting microorganism's susceptibility. If there is no improvement despite the use of antibiotics, myringotomy or mastoidectomy may be necessary.[1]

Evidence-Based Reference

1. Lee E-S et al: Clinical experiences with acute mastoiditis—1988 through 1998, *Ear Nose Throat J* 79:884, 2000.

SUGGESTED READINGS

Migirov L et al: Intracranial complications following mastoidectomy, *Pediatr Neurosurg* 40(5):226, 2004.

Oestreicher-Kedem Y et al: Complications of mastoiditis in children at the onset of a new millenium, *Ann Otol Rhinol Laryngol* 114(2):147, 2005.

Taylor MF, Berkowitz RG: Indications for mastoidectomy in acute mastoiditis in children, *Ann Otol Rhinol Laryngol* 113(1):69, 2004.

AUTHORS: **GLENN G. FORT, M.D., M.P.H.,** and **DENNIS J. MIKOLICH, M.D.**

Measles (Rubeola) 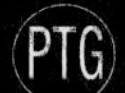

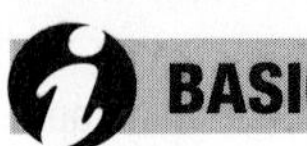

BASIC INFORMATION

DEFINITION

Measles is a childhood exanthem caused by an RNA virus called *Morbillivirus,* belonging to the family *Paramyxoviridae.*

SYNONYMS

Rubeola

ICD-9CM CODES
055.9 Measles
055.0 Encephalitis
055.1 Pneumonia
V04.2 Vaccination

EPIDEMIOLOGY & DEMOGRAPHICS

- Before the introduction of an effective vaccine in 1963, measles was one of the most common childhood illnesses. In developing countries, where it mostly strikes children <5 yr, it remains a leading cause of childhood death.
- 30 million cases occur worldwide each year.
- In developed countries, measles outbreaks occasionally occur in adolescents and young adults who have not been immunized (incidence up to 10 per 100,000 person-years).

PHYSICAL FINDINGS & CLINICAL PRESENTATION

- Incubation: 10 to 14 days (up to 3 wk in adults)
- Prodrome: 2 to 4 days; malaise, fever, rhinorrhea, conjunctivitis, cough
- Exanthem phase: 7 to 10 days
- The fever increases and peaks at 104° to 105° F together with the rash; it persists for 5 or 6 days. The patient's fever decreases over 24 hr.
- Rash: erythematous maculopapular eruption begins behind the ears, progresses to the forehead and neck (Fig. 1-190), then spreads to face, trunk, upper extremities, buttocks, and lower extremities, in that order. After 3 days the rash fades in the same sequence by becoming copper brown and then desquamating.
- Enanthem: *Koplik spots* are white papules 1 to 2 mm in diameter on an erythematous base. They first appear on the buccal mucosa opposite the lower molar 2 days before the rash and spread over 24 hr to involve most of the buccal and lower labial mucosa. They fade after 3 days.
- Other symptoms and signs: malaise, anorexia, vomiting, diarrhea, abdominal pain, pharyngitis, lymphadenopathy, and occasional splenomegaly.

FIGURE 1-190 Rubeola. (From Zitelli BJ, Davis HW: *Atlas of pediatric physical diagnosis,* ed 5, St Louis, 2005, Mosby.)

Atypical measles (in vaccinated persons):
- Incubation: 10 to 14 days
- Prodrome: 1 to 3 days; high fever and headache
- Rash: maculopapular, urticarial, or petechial rash that begins peripherally and progresses centrally
- Modified measles applies to patients who have received immune serum globulin and develop a milder illness
- Complications (30% of all cases):
    - Otitis media
    - Laryngitis, tracheitis
    - Pneumonia (accounts for 90% of measles deaths)
    - Encephalitis with lethargy, irritability, and seizures; 60% recover completely, 25% have neurologic sequelae (mental retardation, hemiplegia, paraplegia, epilepsy, deafness), and 15% die
    - Myocarditis, pericarditis, hepatitis
    - Complications more common in immunocompromised hosts and persons with AIDS

ETIOLOGY & PATHOGENESIS

- The measles virus is transmitted through the respiratory tract by airborne droplets.
- It initially infects the respiratory epithelium; the patient becomes viremic during the prodromal phase and the virus is disseminated to the skin, respiratory tract, and other organs.
- Viral clearance is achieved by cellular immunity.

DIAGNOSIS

DIFFERENTIAL DIAGNOSIS

- Other viral infections by enteroviruses, adenoviruses, human parvovirus B-19, rubella
- Scarlet fever
- Allergic reaction
- Kawasaki disease

WORKUP

Knowledge of outbreak, history and physical findings (Koplik spots are diagnostic), laboratory tests

LABORATORY TESTS

- Complete blood count: leukopenia
- Enzyme-linked immunosorbent assay for measles antibodies, which appear shortly after the onset of the rash and peak 3 to 4 wk later
- Cerebrospinal fluid analysis in encephalitis may reveal pleocytosis (lymphocytes) and an elevated protein

IMAGING STUDIES

Chest radiograph if pneumonia is suspected

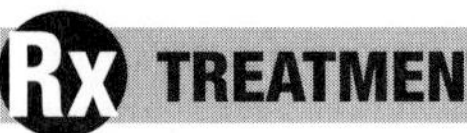

TREATMENT

- Supportive
- Vitamin A
- Ribavirin for severe measles pneumonitis

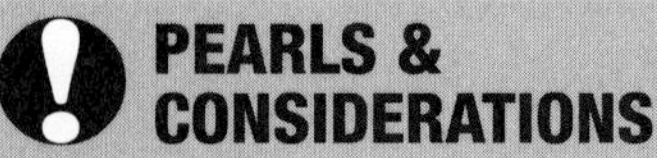

PEARLS & CONSIDERATIONS

PREVENTION

- Passive immunization: human immunoglobulin 0.25 ml/kg IM within 6 days of exposure. Double the dose for immunocompromised persons.
- Active immunization (see Section V).

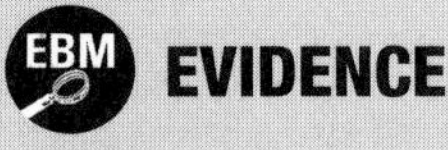

EVIDENCE

Vaccination

Monovalent measles and combined measles, mumps, rubella (MMR) vaccines are highly effective in preventing measles, with both vaccines having similar seroconversion rates at 6 wk.[1] Ⓐ Ⓑ

Existing evidence has failed to show an association between MMR vaccines and any autistic disorder, ulcerative colitis, Crohn's disease, or inflammatory bowel disease.[2] Ⓐ

The MMR vaccine is associated with a number of potential side effects, but recent evidence suggests that the risk of these effects is not significantly greater than when given placebo.[3] Ⓐ

Vitamin A treatment

A single dose of 200,000 international units of vitamin A given to children with measles does not reduce mortality rate, but there is evidence that the same dose given for 2 days is associated with a reduced risk of overall mortality and pneumonia-specific mortality (level of evidence: A).[4]

Evidence-Based References

1. Booy R et al: Measles, mumps and rubella: prevention, *Clin Evid,* 2007. Ⓐ Ⓑ
2. Smeeth L et al: MMR vaccination and pervasive developmental disorders: a case-control study, *Lancet* 364:963, 2004. Ⓐ
3. Demicheli V et al: Vaccines for measles, mumps and rubella in children, *Cochrane Rev* 4, 2005. Ⓐ
4. Huiming Y et al: Vitamin A for treating measles in children, *Cochrane Rev* 4, 2005. Ⓐ

SUGGESTED READING

Mulholland EK: Measles in the United States, *N Engl J Med* 355:5, 2006.

AUTHOR: **FRED F. FERRI, M.D.**

BASIC INFORMATION

DEFINITION

Meckel diverticulum is an ileal diverticulum located 100 cm proximal to the cecum. It results from failure of the omphalomesenteric duct to obliterate completely (as it should by the eighth week of gestation).

SYNONYMS

MD

ICD-9CM CODES
751.0 Meckel diverticulum

EPIDEMIOLOGY & DEMOGRAPHICS

- Meckel diverticulum, based on autopsy studies and intraoperative evidence, occurs in 0.3% to 4% of the population and is the most prevalent congenital anomaly of the gastrointestinal (GI) tract. Complications occur more frequently in males.
- Most patients who develop symptoms are <10 yr.
- The lifetime risk of complications developing in a case of Meckel diverticulum is 4%.
- In adults, complications (small bowel obstruction [25% to 40%], diverticulitis [20%]) are usually attributable to factors other than heterotopic mucosa.
- Tumors have rarely been reported in symptomatic Meckel diverticulum, with carcinoid being the most common type.

PHYSICAL FINDINGS & CLINICAL PRESENTATION

- Painless lower GI bleeding (4%)
- Intestinal obstruction caused by intussusception, volvulus, herniation, or entrapment of a loop of bowel through a defect in the diverticular mesentery (6%)
- Meckel's diverticulitis mimics acute appendicitis (5%)
- Rare primary tumor arising from diverticulum (carcinoid, sarcoma, leiomyoma, adenocarcinoma)
- Asymptomatic (80% to 95%)

ETIOLOGY & PATHOGENESIS

- As a remnant of the omphalomesenteric duct, Meckel diverticulum contains all layers of the intestinal wall and has its own mesentery and blood supply (branch of the superior mesenteric artery).
- The majority of complicated cases of Meckel diverticulum contain ectopic mucosa (75% gastric, 15% pancreatic). It causes ulceration and bleeding of ileal mucosa adjacent to the acidic ectopic gastric secretions. Alkaline secretions of ectopic pancreatic tissue can also cause ulcerations.

Dx DIAGNOSIS

DIFFERENTIAL DIAGNOSIS

- Appendicitis
- Crohn's disease
- All causes of lower GI bleeding (polyp, colon cancer, arteriovenous malformation, diverticulosis, hemorrhoids)

WORKUP

- Diagnosis is often made intraoperatively when the preoperative diagnosis is appendicitis.
- Preoperative detection of symptomatic Meckel diverticulum requires a high index of suspicion.
- In the case of GI bleeding of unknown source, a technetium scan will identify Meckel diverticulum (sensitivity: 85% in children, 62% in adults; specificity: 95% in children, 9% in adults) (Fig. 1-191).
- In patients with suspected small-bowel obstruction, intussusception, or diverticulitis, a CT scan of the abdomen and pelvis is helpful.

Rx TREATMENT

- Surgical resection in symptomatic patients.
- There is controversy regarding the need to remove an incidentally found diverticulum, with most surgeons arguing in favor of resection.

SUGGESTED READINGS

Feller A et al: Meckel diverticulum, *Arch Intern Med* 163:2093, 2003.

Martin JP et al: Meckel's diverticulum, *Am Fam Physician* 61:1037, 2000.

AUTHOR: **FRED F. FERRI, M.D.**

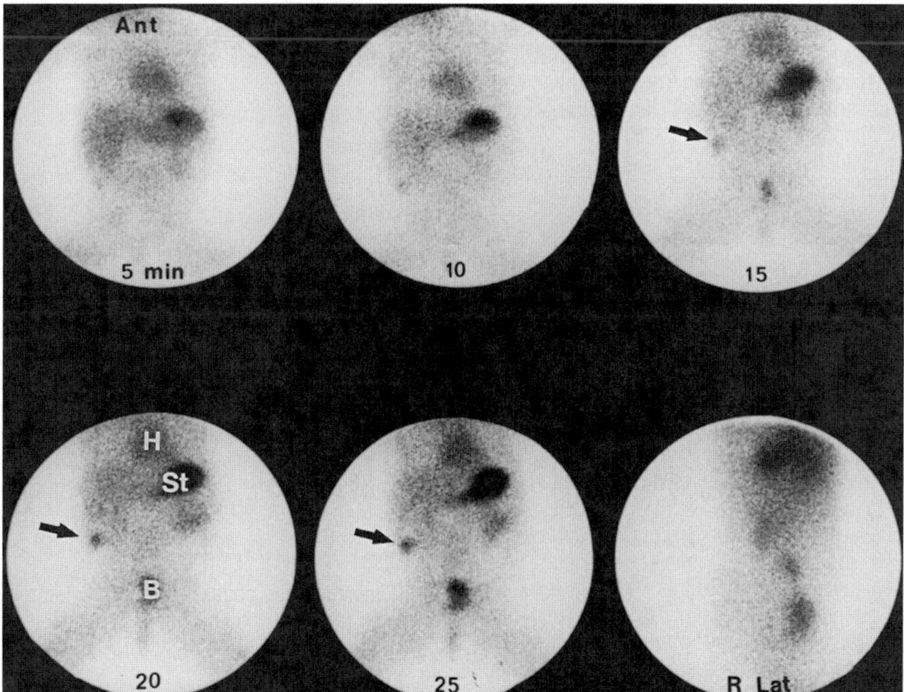

FIGURE 1-191 Meckel diverticulum. In this 2-year-old child who had unexplained rectal bleeding, a nuclear medicine study was performed with radioactive material that concentrates in gastric mucosa (technetium-99m pertechnetate). Sequential 5-min images of the abdomen are obtained. On the 20-min image, the heart *(H),* stomach *(St),* and bladder *(B)* are clearly seen in addition to an ectopic focus of activity *(arrow)* representing a Meckel diverticulum. (From Mettler FA [ed]: *Primary care radiology,* Philadelphia, 2000, WB Saunders.)

Meigs' Syndrome

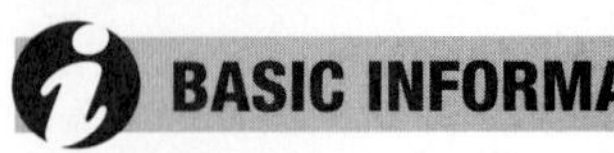

BASIC INFORMATION

DEFINITION

Meigs' syndrome is characterized by the presence of a benign solid ovarian tumor associated with ascites and right hydrothorax that disappear after tumor removal.

ICD-9CM CODES
620.2 Ovarian mass (unspecified)
220.0 Benign ovarian lesion
789.5 Ascites
511.9 Pleural effusion

EPIDEMIOLOGY & DEMOGRAPHICS

- Occurs in <1% of ovarian fibromas (associated with approximately 0.004% of ovarian tumors)
- Most frequently encountered during middle age (average age, approximately 48 yr)

PHYSICAL FINDINGS & CLINICAL PRESENTATION

- Asymptomatic pelvic mass on bimanual examination
- Intermittent pelvic pain (intermittent torsion)
- Acute pelvic tenderness
- Acute abdominal tenderness
- Abdominal pelvic mass
- Abdominal bloating
- Fluid wave
- Shifting dullness
- "Puddle sign"
- Hyperresonance or flatness to chest percussion, absence of tactile and vocal fremitus
- Absent or loud bronchial breath sounds, rales, mediastinal displacement, tracheal shift
- Weight loss and emaciation

ETIOLOGY

- Not specifically known
- Usually associated with "edematous" fibromas (or other benign ovarian solid tumor) in excess of 10 cm
- Plausible that large fibroma with narrow stalk has inadequate lymphatic drainage; when coupled with intermittent torsion, results in backflow transudation into the peritoneal cavity; accumulated peritoneal ascites then pass to the right pleural cavity by the lymphatics (overloaded thoracic duct) or abdominal pleural commutation (i.e., foramen of Bochdalek)

DIAGNOSIS

DIFFERENTIAL DIAGNOSIS

- Abdominal ovarian malignancy
- Various gynecologic disorders:
  1. Uterus; endometrial tumor, sarcoma, leiomyoma ("pseudo-Meigs' syndrome")
  2. Fallopian tube: hydrosalpinx, granulomatous salpingitis, fallopian tube malignancy
  3. Ovary: benign, serous, mucinous, endometrioid, clear cell, Brenner tumor, granulosa, stromal, dysgerminoma, fibroma, metastatic tumor
- Nongynecologic (gastrointestinal tract or genitourinary tract tumor or pathology) causes of pelvic mass
  1. Ascites
  2. Portal vein obstruction
  3. Inferior vena cava obstruction
  4. Hypoproteinemia
  5. Thoracic duct obstruction
  6. Tuberculosis
  7. Amyloidosis
  8. Pancreatitis
  9. Neoplasm
  10. Ovarian hyperstimulation
  11. Pleural effusion
  12. Congestive heart failure
  13. Malignancy
  14. Collagen-vascular disease
  15. Pancreatitis
  16. Cirrhosis

WORKUP

- Clinical condition characterized by ovarian mass, ascites, and right-sided pleural effusion
- Ovarian malignancy and the other causes (see "Differential Diagnosis") of pelvic mass, ascites, and pleural effusion to be considered
- History of early satiety, weight loss with increased abdominal girth, bloating, intermittent abdominal pain, dyspnea, nonproductive cough

LABORATORY TESTS

- Complete blood count to rule out inflammatory process
- Tumor markers (CA-125, hCG, AFP, CEA) to evaluate malignancy
- Chemical and liver function testing profile to evaluate metabolic or hepatic involvement

IMAGING STUDIES

- Pelvic sonography (color-flow Doppler evaluation of adnexal mass) to evaluate pelvic pathology (CT scan or MRI if etiology indeterminate)
- Chest x-ray examination
- Arterial blood gases if respiratory compromise

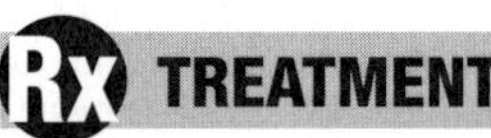

TREATMENT

NONPHARMACOLOGIC THERAPY

- Informed consent and proper preparation of patient for possible staging laparotomy (total abdominal hysterectomy and bilateral salpingo-oophorectomy, omentectomy, possible bowel resection, pelvic/periaortic lymphadenectomy)
- Bowel prep if considering pelvic malignancy

ACUTE GENERAL Rx

Depending on clinical presentation, size of pelvic mass, amount of ascites, and pleural effusion:

- If pelvic mass <10 cm with minimal ascites/pleural effusion: consider diagnostic open laparoscopy (possible exploratory laparotomy) and salpingo-oophorectomy with removal of ovarian fibroma (tumor).
- If pelvic mass >10 cm with moderate/large amount ascites/pleural effusion: consider pleurocentesis if respiratory compromise (cytology: AFB) and exploratory laparotomy with salpingo-oophorectomy and removal of ovarian fibroma (tumor).
- Treat pelvic malignancy, gastrointestinal or genitourinary tumor as indicated.

CHRONIC Rx

- Resolution of ascites and right-sided pleural effusion after removal of ovarian fibroma
- No long-term follow-up for benign ovarian fibroma

DISPOSITION

Excellent progress and complete survival are expected.

REFERRAL

To gynecologist or gynecologic oncologist for evaluation and treatment, especially if malignancy considered or encountered

SUGGESTED READINGS

Abramov Y et al: The role of inflammatory cytokines in Meigs' syndrome, *Obstet Gynecol* 99(5 pt 2):917, 2002.

Buttin BM et al: Meigs' syndrome with an elevated CA 125 from benign Brenner tumors, *Obstet Gynecol* 98(5 pt 2):980, 2001.

Meigs JV, Cass JW: Fibroma of the ovary with ascites and hydrothorax: with a report of seven cases, *Am J Obstet Gynecol* 33:249, 1937.

AUTHORS: **DENNIS M. WEPPNER, M.D.,** and **RUBEN ALVERO, M.D.**

BASIC INFORMATION

DEFINITION

Melanoma is a skin neoplasm arising from the malignant degeneration of melanocytes. It is classically subdivided in four types:

1. Superficial spreading melanoma (70%) (Fig. 1-192, *A*)
2. Nodular melanoma (15% to 20%) (Fig. 1-192, *B*)
3. Lentigo maligna melanoma (5% to 10%)
4. Acral lentiginous melanoma (7% to 10%)

SYNONYMS

Malignant melanoma

ICD-9CM CODES
172.9 Melanoma of the skin, site unspecified

EPIDEMIOLOGY & DEMOGRAPHICS

- Annual incidence of melanoma is 13 cases per 100,000 persons.
- Melanoma has doubled to tripled in incidence over the past 25 yr.
- Melanoma is the most common cancer among women ages 20 to 29 yr.
- Melanoma is much more common in whites (17.2/100,000 white men) than in blacks (one in 100,000 black men).
- Lifetime risk of cutaneous melanoma for white Americans is one in 90.
- Melanoma is the leading cause of death from skin disease.
- Median age at diagnosis is 53 yr.
- Superficial spreading melanoma occurs most often in young adults on sun-exposed areas.
- Acral lentiginous melanoma is most often found in Asian Americans and African Americans and is not related to sun exposure.
- Death rate for white men with melanoma is three per 100,000.
- 8% to 10% of melanomas arise in people with a family history of the disease.

PHYSICAL FINDINGS & CLINICAL PRESENTATION

Variable depending on the subtype of melanoma:

- *Superficial spreading melanoma* is most often found on the lower legs, arms, and upper back. It may have a combination of many colors or may be uniformly brown or black.
- *Nodular melanoma* can be found anywhere on the body, but it most frequently occurs on the trunk on sun-exposed areas. It has a dark-brown or red-brown appearance and can be dome shaped or pedunculated. Lesions are frequently misdiagnosed because they may resemble a blood blister or hemangioma and may also be amelanotic.
- *Lentigo maligna melanoma* is generally found in older adults in areas continually exposed to the sun and frequently arising from lentigo maligna (Hutchinson's freckle) or melanoma in situ. It might have a complex pattern and variable shape; color is more uniform than in superficial spreading melanoma.
- *Acral lentiginous melanoma* frequently occurs on soles, subungual mucous membranes, and palms (sole of the foot is the most prevalent site). Unlike other types of melanoma, it has a similar incidence in all ethnic groups.
- The warning signs that the lesion may be a melanoma can be summarized with the ABCD mnemonic:
  A: Asymmetry (e.g., lesion is bisected and halves are not identical)
  B: Border irregularity (uneven, ragged border)
  C: Color variegation (presence of various shades of pigmentation)
  D: Diameter enlargement (>6 mm)

Recent data regarding small-diameter melanoma suggest that the ABCD criteria for gross inspection of pigmented skin lesions and early diagnosis of cutaneous melanoma should be expanded to ABCDE to include ***e***volving (i.e., lesions that have changed over time).

ETIOLOGY

- Ultraviolet light is the most important cause of malignant melanoma.
- There is a modest increase in melanoma risk in patients with small nondysplastic nevi and a much greater risk in those with dysplastic lesions.
- The *CDKN2A* gene, residing at the 9p21 locus, is often deleted in people with familial melanoma.

DIAGNOSIS

DIFFERENTIAL DIAGNOSIS

- Dysplastic nevi
- Solar lentigo
- Vascular lesions
- Blue nevus
- Basal cell carcinoma
- Seborrheic keratosis

WORKUP

- Perform excisional biopsy with elliptical excision that includes 1 to 2 mm of normal skin surrounding the lesion and extends to the subcutaneous tissue; incisional punch biopsy is sometimes necessary in surgically sensitive areas (e.g., digits, nose).
- Sentinel lymph node dissection should be considered in patients with intermediate (1 to 4 mm) melanomas or high-risk skin tumors to obtain information regarding a patient's subclinical lymph node status with minimal morbidity. It involves the use of radiologic lymphoscintigraphy to map lymphatic drainage from the site of the primary melanoma to the first sentinel lymph node in the region. When properly performed, if the sentinel node is negative the remaining lymph nodes in the region will not have metastases in more than 98% of cases. The staging of intermediate thickness (1.2 to 3.5 mm) primary melanomas, according to the results of sentinel node biopsy, provides important prognostic information and identifies patients with nodal metastases whose survival can be prolonged by immediate lymphadenectomy.
- The staging system for melanoma adapted by the American Joint Committee on Cancer (AJCC) is as follows:

T*	Thickness of primary tumor
Tis	In situ
T1	≤1.0 mm
T2	1.01-2.0 mm
T3	2.01-4.0 mm
T4	>4.0 mm
N†	Number of positive lymph nodes
N0	0
N1	1
N2	2 or 3

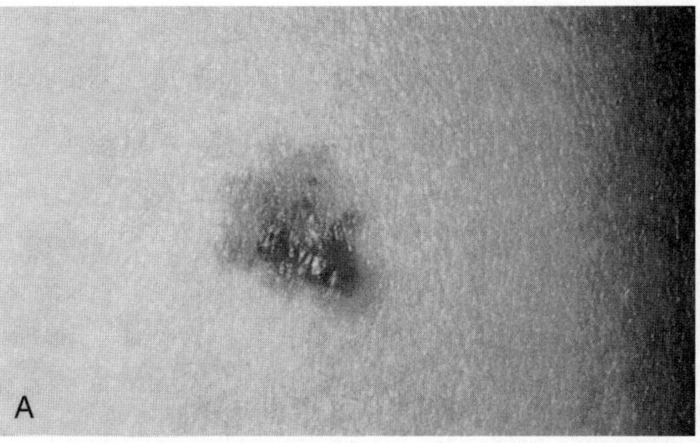

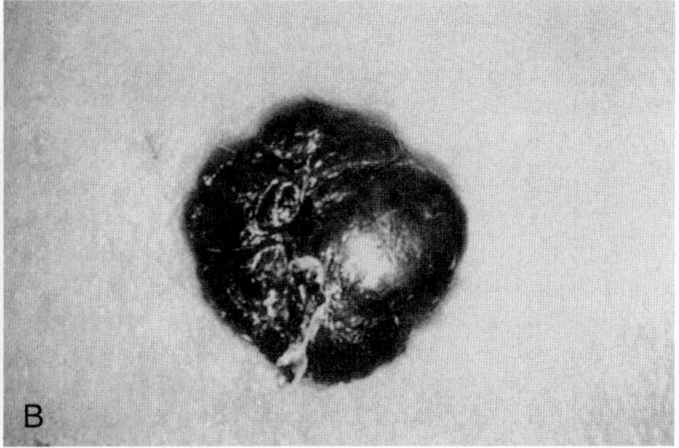

FIGURE 1-192 A, Superficial spreading melanoma. **B,** Nodular melanoma. (From Abeloff MD [ed]: *Clinical oncology,* ed 3, New York, 2004, Churchill Livingstone.)

N3	≥4 (or combination of in-transit metastases, satellite lesions, or an ulcerated primary lesion with any number of nodes)
M	Metastases
M0	0
M1	Distant subcutaneous or lymph node metastases
M2	Lung metastases
M3	All other visceral or any distant metastases or an elevated lactate dehydrogenase level not attributable to another cause
Clinical Stage	
0	(T0N0M0)
IA	(T1aN0M0)
IB	(T1bN0M0) (T2aN0M0)
IIA	(T2bN0M0) (T3aN0M0)
IIB	(T3bN0M0) (T4aN0M0)
IIC	(T4bN0M0)
IIIA	(T1-T4aN1bM0)
IIIB	(T1-T4aN2bM0)
IIIC	(AnyT,N2c,M0) (Any T, N3, M0)
IV	(Any T, Any N, >M1)

*a, Without ulceration; b, with ulceration.
†a, Micrometastasis; b, macrometastases; c, in-transit metastases with metastatic lymph nodes.

LABORATORY TESTS

The pathology report should indicate the following:

- Tumor thickness (Breslow microstage).
- Tumor depth (Clark level): the depth of invasion is the most important histologic prognostic parameter in evaluating the primary tumor.
- Mitotic rate: tabulated as mitoses per square millimeter in the dermal part of the tumor in which most mitoses are identified.
- Radial growth rates versus vertical growth rate: radial growth phase describes the growth of melanoma within the epidermis and along the dermal-epidermal junction.
- Tumor infiltrating lymphocytes have a strong predictive value in vertical growth phase melanomas and are defined as brisk, nonbrisk, or absent.
- Histologic regression: characterized by the absence of melanoma in the epidermis and dermis flanked on one or both sides by melanoma.
- Reverse-transcription polymerase chain reaction assay for tyrosine messenger RNA is a useful marker for the presence of melanoma cells. It is performed on sentinel lymph node biopsy and is useful for detection of submicroscopic metastases.

Rx TREATMENT

- Initial excision of the melanoma
- Reexcision of the involved area after histologic diagnosis:
  1. The margins of reexcision depend on the thickness of the tumor.
  2. Low-risk or intermediate-risk tumors require excision of 1 to 3 cm.
  3. Melanomas of moderate thickness (0.9 to 2.0 mm) can be excised safely with 2-cm margins.
  4. A 1-cm margin of excision for melanoma with a poor prognosis (as defined by a tumor thickness ≥2 mm) is associated with a significantly greater risk of regional recurrence than is a 3-cm margin, but with a similar overall survival rate.
- Lymph node dissection: recommended in all patients with enlarged lymph nodes. Lymph node evaluation is important in patients with melanoma 1 mm in depth because it determines the overall prognosis and need for therapeutic lymph node dissection or adjuvant treatment.
  1. Elective lymph node dissection remains controversial.
  2. It is indicated with positive sentinel node. It may be considered in those with a primary melanoma between 1 and 4 mm thick (especially in patients <60 yr).
- Adjuvant therapy with interferon alfa-2b (intron A) in patients with metastatic melanoma is approved by the FDA for AJCC stages IIb and III melanoma; however, its statistical benefit remains unclear.
- Dacarbazine and interleukin-2 can be used in metastatic melanoma. Results are generally poor, with median survival time in patients with distant metastatic melanoma approximately 6 mo.
- Recent attention has focused on combinations of dacarbazine and cisplatin with interleukin-2 and interferon-alfa (biochemotherapy).
- Novel therapeutics involve cancer vaccines and use of granulocyte-macrophage colony-stimulating factor and angiogenesis inhibitors.
- Patients with a history of melanoma should be followed up with skin examinations every 6 mo or sooner if patient detects any new lesions; the assessments usually consist of medical history, physical examination, laboratory values, and chest radiograph.

DISPOSITION

- Prognosis varies with the stage of the melanoma. The 5-yr survival related to thickness is as follows: <0.76 mm, 99% survival; 0.6 to 1.49 mm, 85%; 1.5 to 2.49 mm, 84%; 2.5 to 3.9 mm, 70%; >4 mm, 44%.
- The 5-yr survival in patients with distant metastasis is <10%.
- Treatment of advanced disease consists (in addition to surgical excision and lymph node dissection) of chemotherapy, immunotherapy, and radiation therapy.

EBM EVIDENCE

Please note: Complete text of EBM for this topic is available online.

Key trials and commentary:

Although attempts to develop any viable chemotherapeutic approaches to combat metastatic cancers have largely failed, potential genetic targets to halt metastatic progression continue to be identified. As drugs are developed to address these targets, there is a need for high-throughput systems that accurately reproduce in vivo microenvironments to gauge their efficacy. Accordingly, there has been developed a three-dimensional in vitro culture system representative of the environment present upon secondary metastasis to quantitatively measure tumor cell invasion in this setting three-dimensionally. Culturing melanomas of different metastatic capacities within the system showed that each cell type invades the matrix in a manner commensurate to its known metastatic potential in vivo. Moreover, the developed quantitative schemes were put to use to characterize the effect of microenvironmental influences (i.e., matrix components, interstitial cell presence) on planar and vertical melanoma invasion. This novel, quantitative system is a useful tool to assess the effects of pharmacologic and/or microenvironmental influences on tumor cell invasion at a metastatic site.[1] Ⓐ

The authors have recognized two crucial problems with developing therapies for melanoma:

1. The most important thing is to stop metastasis; the novel drugs to be developed will be developed with this particular target in mind.

2. Current models that predict metastasis (animal models) are too cumbersome, and it takes too long to evaluate everything that needs to be evaluated.

For us in the trenches, this is of further importance as, down the line, we have to understand what research will be important in the future—research trying to accomplish marriage between cell lines and pathology.

Currently, it is recommended that a sentinel lymph node biopsy (SLNB) be performed only for melanomas >1 mm thick, since the incidence of positivity is otherwise low, unless the lesion is ulcerated or a Clark level IV lesion. In this study, the incidence of positive SLNBs in patients with nonulcerated lesions 0.76 mm to 1 mm thick was 12%, which seems quite high. Unfortunately, we do not have other critical information about the lesions, such as the presence of regression, mitotic rate, and Clark level. However, it was stated that none of these variables predicted SLNB positivity. Moreover, many of the lesions were 0.90 mm to 1 mm thick. When compared to patients with similar lesions who underwent a delayed therapeutic node dissection, patients with a positive SLNB had a better disease-free and disease-specific survival. Interestingly, only 4 of the 10 patients with a positive SLNB underwent a complete node dissection, suggesting that involvement of nonsentinel lymph nodes is uncommon in this subgroup of patients and that, for them, SLNB was "curative." In this reviewer's opinion, additional studies need to be performed before one can recommend routine SLNB for patients with nonulcerated melanomas 0.76 mm to 1.0 mm thick.[2] Ⓐ

Dermoscopy is a noninvasive technique that enables the clinician to perform direct microscopic examination of diagnostic features, not seen by the naked eye, in pigmented skin lesions. Diagnostic accuracy of dermoscopy has previously been assessed in meta-analyses including studies performed in experimental and clinical settings.

One study sought to assess the diagnostic accuracy of dermoscopy for the diagnosis of melanoma compared with naked eye examination by performing a meta-analysis exclusively on studies performed in a clinical setting.

Previous studies have concluded that in the hands of the experienced users, dermoscopy is more effective than naked eye examination at discriminating between melanoma and nonmelanoma These were meta-analyses that included studies performed in an experimental setting and those performed in a clinical setting. Here, Vestergaard et al performed a meta-analysis on prospective studies of a consecutive patient cohort to evaluate the evidence for increased diagnostic accuracy when using dermoscopy in addition to naked eye examination for the diagnosis of melanoma. Patients were examined in a clinical setting. The data provided evidence that clinical examination with the added use of dermoscopy is more accurate than naked eye examination alone. Clearly, the benefits of dermoscopy as a diagnostic adjunct are more pronounced when the technique is used by physicians with training in the technique. Without any formal training, evidence has been presented that dermoscopy may even decrease diagnostic performance when used on pigmented lesions.[3] Ⓐ

Any benefit of adjuvant interferon-alfa-2b for melanoma could depend on dose and duration of treatment. The aim of another study was to determine whether pegylated interferon-alfa-2b can facilitate prolonged exposure while maintaining tolerability.

This study showed that adjuvant pegylated interferon alfa-2b for stage III melanoma has a significant, sustained effect on recurrence-free survival.

The use of interferon alpha in the adjuvant care of patients with melanoma has been confirmed in several randomized controlled trials. The toxicity of the therapy is significant, and as a result many patients will defer the potential benefits in lieu of going on expectant observation. Pegylated interferon-alpha is a modified form of interferon-alpha-2b and exerts similar immunologic effects with less frequent dosing and less subjective toxicity. In this trial, a regimen of weekly pegylated interferon was compared with expectant observation in patients with an indication for adjuvant interferon therapy. The control arm being observation raises the concern that any modest benefit seen may be inferior to that seen with the standard IV followed by thrice weekly subcutaneous (SC) interferon regimen. In this trial, which included patients with microscopically positive solitary nodes, no difference in overall survival was seen, though an improvement in relapse-free survival was identified. The failure to see an overall survival advantage may be related to similar factors that plagued the most recent interferon-based observational studies. In this regard, inclusion of patients with solitary microscopically positive nodes, who may have a better predicted outcome compared with those patients with macroscopic disease, can preclude the identification of an overall survival advantage. In addition, the availability of standard interferon for those patients who may relapse with local/regional disease may improve their secondary outcome. Toxicity of the pegylated interferon was similar to that of the standard interferon dosing regimen, and similar numbers of patients ultimately discontinued therapy. Comparison of this new regimen with the older IV/SC regimen would be required to determine the relative value of one vs. the other.[4] Ⓐ

A separate trial sought to determine the effectiveness of wide vs. narrow excision margins in the treatment of primary cutaneous melanoma.

Although this meta-analysis did not show any statistically significant difference between patients treated with wide or narrow excision margins, insofar as overall mortality and locoregional and local recurrences, current evidence is insufficient to address the optimal excision margins for all types of melanomas. Further research is required to establish the appropriate local treatment for different types of primary melanoma and subgroups of patients.

Fortunately, the surgical management of melanoma has become much more conservative. Gone are the days of elective node dissections and radical excisions. However, it remains unclear as to what margin(s) of excision one should employ when removing a melanoma. As this meta-analysis confirms, for lesions <2 mm thick, 1-cm margins appear to be adequate and are not associated with an increased incidence of local recurrence or mortality. However, for lesions >2 mm thick, the data are conflicting and inconclusive. Moreover, there is still a lack of a consensus definition of true local recurrence. Thus, many studies on margin control include, in their analysis, patients with satellite lesions, which do not reflect inadequate excision and would be associated with an increased mortality. For years, the idea behind wide margins for melanoma has been to encompass satellite lesions. By now, it should be recognized that this is futile and that satellite lesions represent metastatic disease, and thus, even if one was fortunate enough to encompass these, it would be unlikely that the patient would be cured because he or she is likely to already have systemic disease. Nevertheless, the commentaries on this article suggest that wider margins should be employed when dealing with thicker tumors in an attempt to remove all satellite lesions. It is important for physicians who care for melanoma patients to have a clear understanding of the biology of melanoma, and for studies that address excision margins to be uniform in their selection and categorization of patients.[5] Ⓐ

Evidence-Based References

1. Ghajar CM et al: A novel three-dimensional model to quantify metastatic melanoma invasion, *Mol Cancer Ther* 6:552-561, 2007. Commentary by D. Jukic, M.D. Ⓐ
2. Starz H, Balda B-R: Benefit of sentinel lymphadenectomy for patients with nonulcerated cutaneous melanomas in the Breslow range between 0.76 and 1mm: a follow-up study of 148 patients, *Int J Cancer* 121:689-693, 2007. Commentary by B.H. Thiers, M.D. Ⓐ
3. Vestergaard ME et al: Dermoscopy compared with naked eye examination for the diagnosis of primary melanoma: a meta-analysis of studies performed in a clinical setting, *Br J Dermatol* 159:669-676, 2008. Commentary by B.H. Thiers, M.D. Ⓐ
4. Eggermont AMM, for the EORTC Melanoma Group: Adjuvant therapy with pegylated interferon alfa-2b versus observation alone in resected stage III melanoma: final results of EORTC 18991, a randomised phase III trial, *Lancet* 372:117-126, 2008. Commentary by M.S. Gordon, M.D. Ⓐ
5. Lens MB et al: Excision margins for primary cutaneous melanoma: updated pooled analysis of randomized controlled trials, *Arch Surg* 142:885-891, 2007. Commentary by P.G. Lang, Jr., M.D. Ⓐ

SUGGESTED READINGS

Markovic S et al: Malignant melanoma in the 21st century, *Mayo Clin Proc* 82(3):364; 82(4):490, 2007.

Miller AJ, Mihm MC: Melanoma, *N Engl J Med* 355:51, 2006.

AUTHOR: **FRED F. FERRI, M.D.**

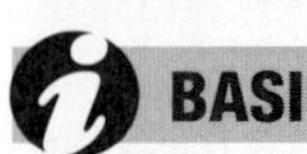

BASIC INFORMATION

DEFINITION

Meniere's disease is a syndrome characterized by recurrent vertigo with fluctuating hearing loss, tinnitus, and fullness in the ear.

SYNONYMS

Endolymphatic hydrops
Lermoyez's syndrome

ICD-9CM CODES
386.01 Meniere's disease, cochleovestibular (active)

EPIDEMIOLOGY & DEMOGRAPHICS

INCIDENCE (IN U.S.): 100 cases/100,000 persons
PREVALENCE (IN U.S.): 15 cases/100,000 persons
PREDOMINANT SEX: Male = female
PEAK INCIDENCE: 20 to 50 yr

PHYSICAL FINDINGS & CLINICAL PRESENTATION

- Hearing may be unilaterally decreased.
- Pallor, sweating, and nausea may occur during a severe attack.
- Usually the patient develops a sensation of fullness and pressure along with decreased hearing and tinnitus in a single ear.
- The patient typically experiences severe vertigo, which peaks within min, then slowly subsides over hr.
- May see spontaneous nystagmus on examination.
- Persistent sense of disequilibrium for days is typical after an acute episode
- May have vestibulopathy demonstrable with a positive head thrust test.

ETIOLOGY

- Unknown; viral and autoimmune causes have been suggested.
- Associated with endolymphatic hydrops.

Dx DIAGNOSIS

Proposed criteria by the American Academy of Otolaryngology-Head and Neck Surgery (AAO-HNS) for diagnosis of Meniere's disease include the following four features, of which (1) and at least one of (2), (3), or (4) must be present:

1. Two spontaneous episodes of vertigo lasting 20 min or longer without loss of consciousness
2. Hearing loss that is usually, but not always, fluctuating
3. Tinnitus in the ear, which may fluctuate
4. Aural fullness in the ear, which may fluctuate

DIFFERENTIAL DIAGNOSIS

- Acoustic neuroma
- Migrainous vertigo
- Multiple sclerosis
- Autoimmune inner ear syndrome
- Otitis media
- Vertebrobasilar disease
- Labyrinthitis

WORKUP

- Electronystagmography may show peripheral vestibular deficit.
- Electrocochleography and glycerol test used by some otoneurologists and ENT specialists.

LABORATORY TESTS

Audiogram may show sensorineural hearing loss, with lower frequencies primarily affected.

IMAGING STUDIES

MRI to rule out acoustic neuroma, especially if cerebellar or CNS dysfunction is present

Rx TREATMENT

NONPHARMACOLOGIC THERAPY

Limit activity during attacks

ACUTE GENERAL Rx

- Prochlorperazine 5 to 10 mg PO q6h or 25 mg PO bid
- Promethazine 12.5 to 25 mg PO q4-6h
- Diazepam 5 to 10 mg IV/PO for acute attack
- Meclizine 25 mg q6h
- Scopolamine patch

CHRONIC Rx

- Diuretics such as hydrochlorothiazide or acetazolamide, salt restriction, and avoidance of caffeine are traditional.
- For refractory cases, surgical interventions.

DISPOSITION

- Patients are usually followed by an otoneurologist or ENT specialist.
- Usual course of disease consists of alternating attacks and remissions.
- Majority of patients can be managed medically. Of patients, 10% to 30% will undergo surgical intervention for persistent incapacitating vertigo.

REFERRAL

To an otolaryngologist for surgical intervention if attacks persist despite medical therapy

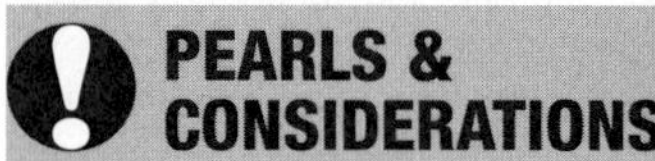

PEARLS & CONSIDERATIONS

COMMENTS

- There are many variations of the classical clinical picture. The essential features for diagnosis are episodic vertigo and sensorineural hearing loss audiometrically documented on at least one occasion.
- In one third of patients, both ears are eventually involved.
- There is some evidence that Meniere's disease and migraines may be pathophysiologically linked.

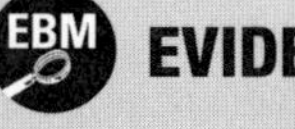

EVIDENCE

There are a variety of medical treatments available for acute attacks and for prophylaxis in the control of symptoms in Menière's disease.

There are no randomized controlled trials on the effects of anticholinergics, benzodiazepines, or betahistine in the treatment of acute attacks in Menière's disease.[1]

Evidence is lacking for other lifestyle measures as a treatment modality.

There is no good quality evidence concerning the effect of dietary modification or psychosocial therapies in the treatment of Menière's disease.[1]

Evidence-Based Reference

1. James A, Thorp M: Menière's disease, *Clin Evid,* 2007.

SUGGESTED READINGS

Committee on Hearing and Equilibrium of the AAO-HNS: Revised guidelines for the diagnosis and evaluation of therapy in Meniere's disease, *Otolaryngol Head Neck Surg* 113:181-185, 1995.

Radtke A et al: Migraine and Meniere's disease: is there a link? *Neurology* 59(11):1700-1704, 2002.

Thai-Von H, Bounaix MJ, Fraysse B: Meniere's disease: pathophysiology and treatment, *Drugs* 61(8): 1089, 2001.

Weber PC, Adkins WY Jr: The differential diagnosis of Meniere's disease, *Otolaryngol Clin North Am* 30(6): 977, 1997.

AUTHOR: **SHARON S. HARTMAN POLENSEK, M.D., PH.D.**

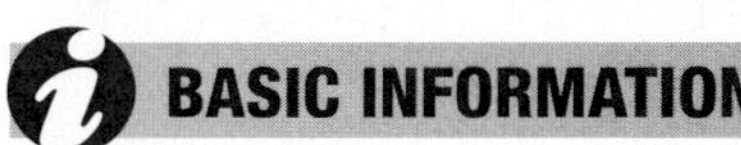

BASIC INFORMATION

DEFINITION

Meningiomas are generally slow-growing tumors arising from arachnoid cells of the arachnoid villi; 90% are benign.

ICD-9CM CODES
225.2 Cerebral meninges

EPIDEMIOLOGY & DEMOGRAPHICS

INCIDENCE: 6/100,000 persons/yr; accounts for 13% to 27% of primary intracranial tumors and are the second most common brain tumor in adults; often underreported

PREDOMINANT SEX AND AGE: Female:male ratio of almost 3:1 in the brain and up to 6:1 in the spinal cord; male > female in childhood and male = female among African Americans

PEAK INCIDENCE: Males: sixth decade, females: seventh decade; rare in childhood

RISK FACTORS: Higher doses of ionizing radiation result in increased incidence and a shorter latency period

GENETICS: Approximately half of meningiomas have allelic losses involving of the *NF2* and *DAL-1* genes. Allelic losses of chromosomes 1p, 2p, 6q, 9q, 10q, 14q, 17p and 18q may be associated with histologic progression.

PHYSICAL FINDINGS & CLINICAL PRESENTATION

- Neurologic symptoms vary with location and size; meningiomas can arise from the dura at any site, although most commonly occur over the cerebral convexities, often associated with the falx. Other common locations include the sphenoid wing, olfactory groove and optic nerve sheath.
- Most common presentation is with a focal or generalized seizure or gradually worsening neurologic deficit. Seizures are present preoperatively in 30% to 40%.
- May be asymptomatic and present incidentally on a neuroimaging study or at autopsy.

ETIOLOGY

- Mutations of the *NF2* gene on chromosome 22 are found in >50% of meningiomas. This gene is thought to act as a tumor suppressor gene; the protein product, merlin, is also involved in cytoskeletal organization.
- Mutations of the *DAL-1* gene, thought to be a meningioma susceptibility gene which is located on chromosome 18p, have been identified in a subset of the approximately 40% of sporadic meningiomas that have neither the *NF2* gene mutations nor allelic loss of chromosome 22q.
- Cranial radiation may be responsible for some cases following an appropriate latency period from 10 to 20 yr. Meningiomas that result from radiation are generally more aggressive.
- The link with steroid hormones and their receptors is suggested by the increase in growth rate and/or development of meningiomas during pregnancy and increased incidence in women who use postmenopausal hormones or in association with breast carcinomas.

Dx DIAGNOSIS

DIFFERENTIAL DIAGNOSIS

Other well-circumscribed intracranial tumors that involve the dura or subdural space.

- Acoustic schwannoma (typically at the pontocerebellar junction)
- Ependymoma, lipoma, and metastases within the spinal cord
- Metastatic disease from lymphoma/adenocarcinoma, inflammatory disease, or infections such as tuberculosis

WORKUP

Imaging studies with CT or MRI, followed by surgical removal with histologic confirmation

LABORATORY TESTS

According to the World Health Organization (WHO) classification, there are nine benign histologic variants and four variants associated with increased recurrence and rates of metastasis. Ninety percent of meningiomas are classified as benign meningiomas or WHO grade I.

IMAGING STUDIES

- Cranial CT scanning or MRI can detect and determine the extent of meningiomas (Fig. 1-193). CT can show hyperostosis and/or intratumoral calcifications. MRI is preferable to show the dural origin of the tumor in most cases, with the characteristic "tail" sign.
- On nonenhanced scans, meningiomas typically are isodense to slightly hyperdense to brain and are homogeneous in appearance. Meningiomas show homogeneous enhancement; gadolinium can facilitate imaging of smaller additional lesions that are missed on unenhanced images.

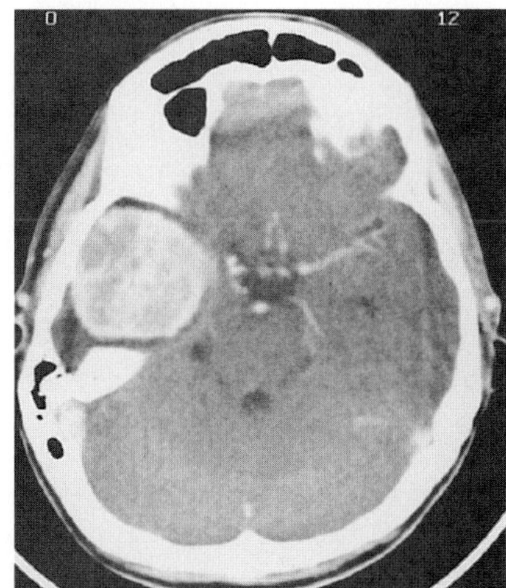

FIGURE 1-193 Contrast-enhanced CT scan demonstrates a large contrast-enhancing right sphenoid wing meningioma. (From Specht N [ed]: *Practical guide to diagnostic imaging,* St Louis, 1998, Mosby.)

- Indistinct margins, marked edema, mushroomlike projections from tumor, brain parenchymal infiltration and heterogeneous enhancement are suggestive of more aggressive behavior.
- PET scan may help in predicting the aggressiveness of the tumor and the potential for recurrence.

Rx TREATMENT

Primary management depends on signs or symptoms, age of patient, and location and size of tumor. Observation may be appropriate if tumors are discovered incidentally and/or if growth is indolent and unlikely to cause symptoms.

NONPHARMACOLOGIC THERAPY

- The mainstay of treatment for meningiomas remains surgical removal. After total excision, recurrence rates of 0 to 20% have been observed, while 20% to 50% of patients recur within 5 yr of a subtotal resection.
- Radiation therapy is the only validated form of adjuvant therapy and may be beneficial in patients with incomplete resections or inoperable tumors. Stereotactic radiosurgery can provide local control with more limited toxicity.

ACUTE GENERAL Rx

- For lesions that cause significant mass effect, steroids are sometimes used to decrease brain edema.
- Anticonvulsants to control seizures. The use of prophylactic anticonvulsants is controversial without a clear history of seizures.

CHRONIC Rx

- Prophylactic use of anticonvulsants is not recommended in patients without a history of seizures.
- There is limited data on the efficacy of traditional chemotherapy and the evidence is largely anecdotal. The most extensively evaluated agents are hydroxyurea, mifepristone (RU486), and interferon alfa-2b.

DISPOSITION

- Estimated surgical mortality is 7%. Significant morbidity and mortality can be observed in meningiomas with otherwise favorable pathology secondary to unfavorable location (e.g., skull base).
- Long-term outcome varies, based on pathology, tumor grade, location, and completeness of resection.
- Most incidentally discovered meningiomas remain asymptomatic and experience a slow rate of growth. Calcified tumors may be less likely to progress than noncalcified ones.
- Meningiomas may recur after surgical resection. In addition, some tumors show histologic progression to a higher grade. Features suggesting increased rate of recurrence include multiple allelic chromosomal losses, local brain invasion, high rate of mitosis and highly anaplastic features.

 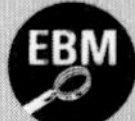

REFERRAL

- Neurosurgical consultation for all cases
- Neurology, radiation oncology, and oncology depending on presence of other sequelae and in setting of recurrence

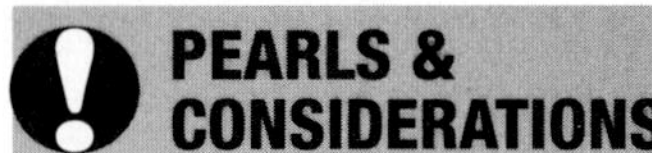

PEARLS & CONSIDERATIONS

COMMENTS

- Many meningiomas are discovered incidentally; most are benign and remain asymptomatic.
- "Dural tail" is classic finding on neuroimaging studies.
- Individuals with neurofibromatosis type 2 are at high risk to develop meningiomas.

PATIENT/FAMILY EDUCATION

Meningioma mommas: www.meninigomamommas.org

Meningioma Support and Patient Information Group:

Meningioma Online Support Group: http://www.brainstrust.org/meningioma.htm

EVIDENCE

Postoperative radiotherapy greatly reduces the risk of recurrence and extends survival in patients with meningiomas who have undergone subtotal tumor resection.[1] B

The use of prophylactic anticonvulsants in patients with newly diagnosed brain tumors remains controversial; because of the lack of defined efficacy and potential for serious side effects, anticonvulsants are not recommended prophylactically in this population.[2] C

Evidence-Based References

1. Blomgren H: Brain tumors, *Acta Oncol* (Suppl 7):16-21, 1996. Reviewed in: DARE Document 978123. York, UK: Centre for Reviews and Dissemination. B
2. Glantz MJ et al: Practice parameter: anticonvulsant prophylaxis in patients with newly diagnosed brain tumors. Report of the Quality Standards Subcommittee of the American Academy of Neurology, *Neurology* 54:1886, 2000. C

SUGGESTED READINGS

Drummond KJ et al: Meningiomas: updating basic science, management, and outcome, *Neurologist* 10(3):113-130, 2004.

Glantz MJ et al: Practice parameter: anticonvulsant prophylaxis in patients with newly diagnosed brain tumors. Report of the Quality Standards Subcommittee of the American Academy of Neurology, *Neurology* 54:1886, 2000.

Perry A et al: Meningiomas. In Louise DN et al (eds): *WHO classification of tumors of the nervous system,* Lyon, France, 2007, IARC Press, p. 164.

Mason WP: Stabilization of disease progression by hydroxyurea in patients with recurrent or unresectable meningioma, *J Neurosurg* 97:341, 2002.

McMullen KP, Stieber VW: Meningioma: current treatment options and future directions, *Curr Treat Options Oncol* 5(6):499-509, 2004.

Perry A et al: Molecular pathogenesis of meningiomas, *J Neurooncol* 70(2):183-202, 2004.

Seizinger JP: Deletion mapping of a locus on human chromosome 22 involved in the oncogenesis of meningioma, *Proc Natl Acad Sci U S A* 84:5419, 1987.

AUTHOR: **NICOLE J. ULLRICH, M.D., PH.D.**

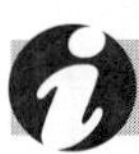

BASIC INFORMATION

DEFINITION

Bacterial meningitis is an inflammation of meninges with increased intracranial pressure, and pleocytosis or increased WBCs in CSF secondary to bacteria in the pia-subarachnoid space and ventricles, leading to neurologic sequelae and abnormalities.

SYNONYMS

Spinal meningitis

ICD-9CM CODES
320 Bacterial meningitis

EPIDEMIOLOGY & DEMOGRAPHICS

INCIDENCE (IN U.S.): 3 cases/100,000 persons
PREDOMINANT SEX: Male = female
PREDOMINANT AGE: All ages, neonate to geriatric

PHYSICAL FINDINGS & CLINICAL PRESENTATION

- Fever
- Headache
- Neck stiffness, nuchal rigidity, meningismus
- Altered mental state, lethargy
- Vomiting, nausea
- Photophobia
- Seizures
- Coma; lethargy, stupor
- Rash: petechial associated with meningococcal infection (Fig. 1-194)
- Myalgia
- Cranial nerve abnormality (unilateral)
- Papilledema
- Dilated, nonreactive pupil(s)
- Posturing: decorticate/decerebrate
- Physical examination findings of Kernig's sign and Brudzinski's sign in adults with meningitis are often not helpful in determining meningeal inflammation

ETIOLOGY

Neisseria meningitidis is now more common than *Haemophilus influenzae* as a cause of bacterial meningitis in children as well as adults. *H. influenzae* is the cause of >30% of cases of meningitis (usually in infants and children <6 yr of age). It is associated with sinusitis, otitis media.

- Neonates: group B streptococci, *Escherichia coli, Klebsiella* sp., *Listeria monocytogenes*
- Infants through adolescence:
  1. *N. meningitidis*
  2. *H. influenzae*
  3. *Streptococcus pneumoniae*
- Adults
  1. *N. meningitidis*
  2. *S. pneumoniae*
- Elderly
  1. *S. pneumoniae*
  2. *N. meningitidis*
  3. *L. monocytogenes*
  4. Gram-negative bacilli

Dx DIAGNOSIS

Diagnostic approach is based on patient presentation and physical examination. Key elements to diagnosis are CSF evaluation and CT scan or MRI if the patient is in a coma or has focal neurologic deficits, pupillary abnormalities, or papilledema.

DIFFERENTIAL DIAGNOSIS

- Endocarditis, bacteremia
- Intracranial tumor
- Lyme disease
- Brain abscess
- Partially treated bacterial meningitis
- Medications
- SLE
- Seizures
- Acute mononucleosis
- Other infectious meningitides
- Neuroleptic malignant syndrome
- Subdural empyema
- Rocky Mountain spotted fever

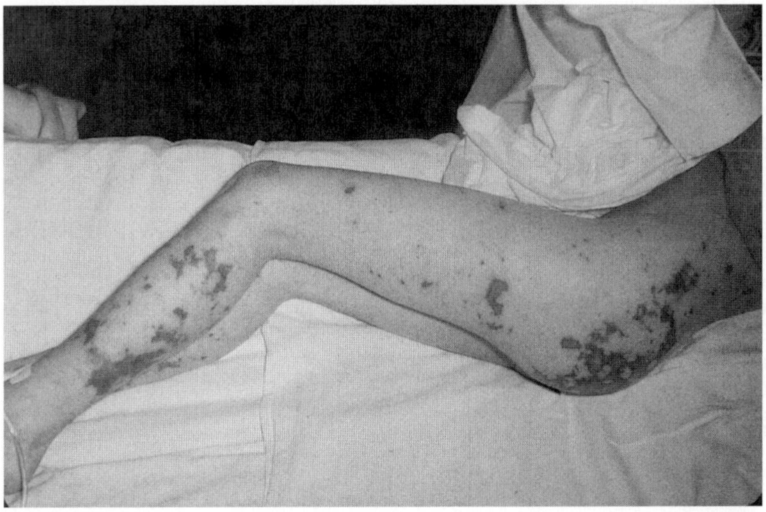

FIGURE 1-194 Fully developed, almost pathognomonic hemorrhagic rash of meningococcal sepsis. (From Cohen J, Powderly WG: *Infectious diseases,* ed 2, St Louis, 2004, Mosby.)

WORKUP

CSF examination:

- Opening pressure >100 to 200 mm Hg
- WBC <5 to >100 mm^3
- Neutrophilic predominance: >80%
- Gram stain of CSF: positive in 60% to 90% of patients
- CSF protein: >50 mg/dl
- CSF glucose: <40 mg/dl
- Culture: positive in 65% to 90% of cases
- CSF bacterial antigen: 50% to 100% sensitivity
- E-test for susceptibility of pneumococcal isolates

LABORATORY TESTS

Blood culturing, WBC with differential, and CSF examination (see "Workup")

IMAGING STUDIES

- CT scan or MRI of head: necessary with increased intracranial pressure, coma, neurologic deficits
- Sinus CT: if sinusitis suspected

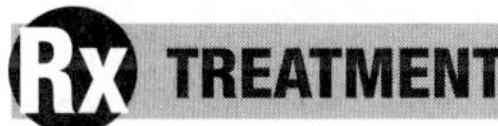

TREATMENT

Empiric therapy is necessary with IV antibiotic treatment if patient has purulent CSF fluid at time of lumbar puncture, is asplenic, or has signs of DIC/sepsis pending Gram stain and culture results. Therapy after Gram stain pending cultures is recommended for the following:

1. Neonates: ampicillin plus cefotaxime
2. Infants/children: ampicillin or third-generation cephalosporin (plus chloramphenicol if purulent or patient compromised)
3. Adults (18 to 50 yr): third-generation cephalosporin
4. Older adults (>50 yr): ampicillin plus third-generation cephalosporin

- Penicillin-resistant pneumococcus: because of an increasing incidence of this organism, empiric treatment with ceftriaxone or cefotaxime plus vancomycin (25 to 50 mg/kg/day) has been recommended.
- Table 1-47 describes common pathogens of bacterial meningitis and their empiric treatment based on age.
- Table 1-48 describes specific antibiotic treatments for known pathogens.
- Steroids: dexamethasone 0.15 mg/kg q6h for first 4 days of therapy should be used in adults with bacterial meningitis and mental status changes or acute neurologic phenomenon. Decreased mortality and neurologic sequelae are seen with adjunct therapy.
- Dexamethasone also benefits children with Hib or pneumococcal meningitis and should be given within the first 2 days of illness.

DISPOSITION

Bacterial meningitis is a reportable disease that needs to be reported to local health authorities.

REFERRAL

- To a neurologist if persistent neurologic sequelae develop after bacterial meningitis

- To an infectious disease consultant if a patient has recurrent bacterial meningitis; such patients deserve a workup for an anatomic (CSF dural leak) or immunologic defect (complement defect, hyposplenism, immunoglobulin deficiency)

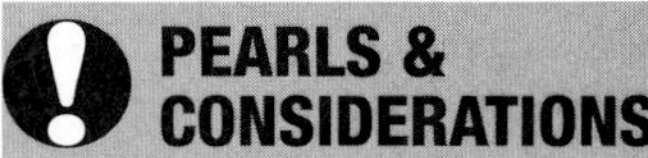

PEARLS & CONSIDERATIONS

COMMENTS

- Nosocomial bacterial meningitis may result from invasive procedures (e.g., placement of ventricular catheters, lumbar puncture, craniotomy, spinal anesthesia). Treatment of this different spectrum of microorganisms requires empirical antimicrobial therapy with vancomycin plus cefepime, ceftazidime, or meropenem. In cases of basilar skull fracture, effective empirical antimicrobial therapy consists of vancomycin plus a third-generation cephalosporin.
- Prevention of meningitis can be achieved through chemoprophylaxis of close contacts (household members and anyone exposed to oral secretions).
- Effective medications are rifampin 10 mg/kg PO bid for 2 days or ceftriaxone 250 mg IM single dose in patients older than age 12; 125 mg IM if age 12 or younger.
- Ciprofloxacin 500 mg for prevention of *Neisseria* meningitis can be given to patients older than 18 yr who cannot tolerate rifampin to eradicate pharyngeal colonization.
- Vaccines against serogroup A, C, Y, W-135 capsular polysaccharides are available for adults and children older than 2 yr; a protein-conjugate vaccine is now available.

TABLE 1-47 Common Pathogens of Bacterial Meningitis and Their Empiric Treatment Based on Age

Age	Common Pathogens	Treatment*	Duration (days)
0-1 mo	Group B streptococcus *Listeria monocytogenes* *Escherichia coli*	Ampicillin and third-generation cephalosporin† or ampicillin and aminoglycoside	14-21 14-21 21
1-3 mo	*Streptococcus pneumoniae* Group B streptococcus, *E. coli, L. monocytogenes* *S. pneumoniae* *Neisseria meningitidis, Haemophilus influenzae*	Ampicillin and third-generation cephalosporin†	10-14 14-21 14-21 10-14 7-10
3 mo-18 yr	*H. influenzae, H. meningitidis, S. pneumoniae*	Third-generation cephalosporin† or meropenem or chloramphenicol	7-10 (*N. influenzae* and *N. meningitidis*) 10-14 *(S. pneumoniae)*
18-50 yr	*H. influenzae, N. meningitidis, S. pneumoniae*	Third-generation cephalosporin† or meropenem or ampicillin and chloramphenicol	Same as above
>50 yr	*S. pneumoniae, L. monocytogenes,* gram-negative bacilli	Ampicillin and third-generation cephalosporin† or ampicillin and fluoroquinolone‡ or meropenem	10-14 *(S. pneumoniae)* 14-21 *(L. monocytogenes)* 21 Gram-negative bacilli other than *H. influenzae*

From Rakel RE (ed): *Principles of family practice,* ed 6, Philadelphia, 2002, WB Saunders.
*Add vancomycin in areas where there is greater than 2% incidence of highly drug-resistant *S. pneumoniae.*
†Ceftriaxone or cefotaxime.
‡Ciprofloxacin or levofloxacin.

TABLE 1-48 Specific Antibiotic Treatments for Known Pathogens

Pathogen	Primary Therapy	Alternative*
Group B streptococcus	Penicillin G or ampicillin	Vancomycin or third-generation cephalosporin†
Streptococcus pneumoniae (MIC < 0.1)	Third-generation cephalosporin†	Meropenem, penicillin
S. pneumoniae (MIC > 0.1)	Vancomycin and third-generation cephalosporin*	Substitute rifampin for vancomycin; or meropenem; or vancomycin as monotherapy if highly allergic to other alternatives
Haemophilus influenzae (β-lactamase-negative)	Ampicillin	Third-generation cephalosporin† or chloramphenicol or aztreonam
H. influenzae (β-lactamase-positive)	Third-generation cephalosporin†	Chloramphenicol or aztreonam or fluoroquinolones‡
Listeria monocytogenes	Ampicillin and gentamicin	Trimethoprim-sulfamethoxazole
Neisseria meningitidis	Penicillin G or ampicillin	Third-generation cephalosporin†
Enterobacteriaceae	Third-generation cephalosporin† and aminoglycoside	Trimethoprim-sulfamethoxazole or aztreonam or fluoroquinolones or antipseudomonal penicillin (or ampicillin) and aminoglycoside
Pseudomonas aeruginosa	Ceftazidime and aminoglycoside	Aminoglycoside and aztreonam or aminoglycoside and antipseudomonal penicillin§
Staphylococcus aureus (methicillin-sensitive)	Antistaphylococcal penicillin¶ and rifampin	Vancomycin and rifampin or trimethoprim-sulfamethoxazole and rifampin
S. aureus (methicillin-resistant)	Vancomycin and rifampin	
Staphylococcus epidermidis	Vancomycin and rifampin	

From Rakel RE (ed): *Principles of family practice,* ed 6, Philadelphia, 2002, WB Saunders.
MIC, Minimum inhibitory concentration.
*If patient is highly allergic or intolerant of primary therapy.
†Ceftriaxone or cefotaxime.
‡Ciprofloxacin or levofloxacin.
§Piperacillin, mezlocillin, or ticarcillin.
¶Nafcillin, oxacillin, or methicillin.

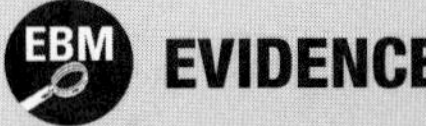

EVIDENCE

Please note: Complete text of EBM for this topic is available online.

Key trials and commentary:

It is uncertain whether all adults with bacterial meningitis benefit from treatment with adjunctive dexamethasone.

This study showed that dexamethasone does not improve the outcome in all adolescents and adults with suspected bacterial meningitis; a beneficial effect appears to be confined to patients with microbiologically proven disease, including those who have received prior treatment with antibiotics.

Animal models of bacterial meningitis suggest that inflammatory response in the subarachnoid space associated with infection contributes to morbidity and mortality; corticosteroids may have a beneficial effect, especially if given early and before antibiotics. A meta-analysis of controlled trials between 1966 and 2001 concluded that corticosteroids reduced mortality as well as hearing loss and neurologic sequelae in children. However, the data were too few to confirm an effect on bacterial meningitis in adults. A study published in 2002 showed an improvement in morbidity and mortality in adult patients with bacterial meningitis treated with adjunct corticosteroid therapy.[1] The current controlled trial of dexamethasone in patients over the age of 14 years with suspected bacterial meningitis looked at reduced risk of death at 1 month and risk of death or disability at 6 months. Bacterial meningitis was confirmed in 69% of the patients. Dexamethasone therapy did not have a beneficial effect on the overall outcome. In patients with confirmed bacterial meningitis, there was a significant reduction in both morbidity and mortality. This beneficial effect included patients who had received treatment with antibiotics. The multivariate analysis of the entire patient group showed that dexamethasone treatment was associated with significant increase in risk of death at 1 month, possibly explained by subsequent diagnosis of tuberculosis meningitis. These data warrant caution in the use of dexamethasone in bacterial meningitis, except in microbiologically proven cases including those who have received antibacterials. The dexamethasone regimen in this study was 0.4 mg per kg every 12 hours for 4 days.[1] Ⓐ

Evidence-Based Reference

1. Mai NTH et al: Dexamethasone in Vietnamese adolescents and adults with bacterial meningitis, *N Engl J Med* 357:2431-2440, 2007. Commentary by: N. Khardori, M.D. Ⓐ

SUGGESTED READINGS

Greenwood BM: Corticosteroids for acute bacterial meningitis, *N Engl J Med* 357:2507, 2007.

Heyderman RS: Early management of suspected bacterial meningitis and meningococcal septicaemia in immunocompetent adults-second edition, *J Infect* 50(5):373, 2005.

Kutz JW et al: Clinical predictors for hearing loss in children with bacterial meningitis, *Arch Otolaryngol Head Neck Surg* 132(9):941, 2006.

Mongelluzzo J et al: Corticosteroids and mortality in children with bacterial meningitis, *JAMA* 299:2048, 2008.

Sinner SW, Tunkel AR: Antimicrobial agents in the treatment of bacterial meningitis. *Infect Dis Clin North Am* 18(3):581, 2004.

Stephens DS et al: Epidemic meningitis, meningococcemia, and neisseria meningitides, *Lancet* 369: 2196, 2007.

van de Beek D et al: Clinical features and prognostic factors in adults with bacterial meningitis, *N Engl J Med* 351:1849, 2004.

van de Beek D et al: Nosocomial bacterial meningitis, *N Engl J Med* 362:146-154, 2010.

Weisfelt M et al: Pneumococcal meningitis in adults: new approaches to management and prevention, *Lancet Neurol* 5(4):332, 2006.

AUTHORS: **GLENN G. FORT, M.D., M.P.H.,** and **DENNIS J. MIKOLICH, M.D.**

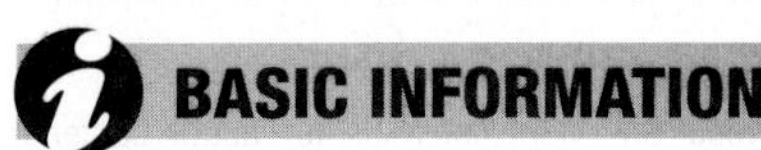

BASIC INFORMATION

DEFINITION

Viral meningitis is an acute aseptic meningitis, usually with lymphocytic pleocytosis and negative CSF stains and cultures.

SYNONYMS

Aseptic meningitis

ICD-9CM CODES
047.8 Meningitis, aseptic

EPIDEMIOLOGY & DEMOGRAPHICS (Table 1-49)

INCIDENCE (IN U.S.): 11 cases/100,000 persons
PREDOMINANT SEX: Male = female
GENETICS: Those with abnormal humoral immunity and agammaglobulinemia have associated difficulty with viral clearance.

PHYSICAL FINDINGS & CLINICAL PRESENTATION

- Fever
- Headache
- Nuchal rigidity
- Photophobia
- Myalgias
- Vomiting
- Rash

ETIOLOGY

- Enterovirus
- Mumps virus
- Measles
- Arboviruses
- Herpes (simplex and zoster)
- HIV
- Lymphocytic choriomeningitis virus
- Adenovirus
- CMV
- Arthropod-borne viruses
- West Nile virus

DIAGNOSIS

The diagnostic approach is similar to that for bacterial meningitis (see "Meningitis, Bacterial"); the foremost need is to rule out bacterial meningitis with CSF evaluation. Presentation may be similar to that of meningitis with bacterial involvement.

DIFFERENTIAL DIAGNOSIS

- Bacterial meningitis
- Meningitis secondary to Lyme disease, TB, syphilis, amebiasis, leptospirosis
- Rickettsial illnesses: Rocky Mountain spotted fever
- Migraine headache
- Medications
- SLE
- Acute mononucleosis/Epstein-Barr virus
- Seizures
- Carcinomatous meningitis

WORKUP

CSF examination:
- Usually shows pleocytosis
- Lymphocytic predominance (neutrophils in early stages)
- Opening pressure: 200 to 250 mm Hg
- WBC: 100 to 1000 mm^3
- Increased CSF protein
- Decreased or normal CSF glucose
- Negative Gram stain, cultures, CIE, latex agglutination
- Viral cultures or serologic testing may be diagnostic
- Polymerase chain reaction for HSV, West Nile, or enterovirus (which could shorten duration of antibiotic treatment and hospitalization if bacterial meningitis was suspected)

LABORATORY TESTS

CBC with differential, blood culturing, and CSF examination (see "Workup")

IMAGING STUDIES

CT scan or MRI: if cerebral edema, focal neurologic findings develop

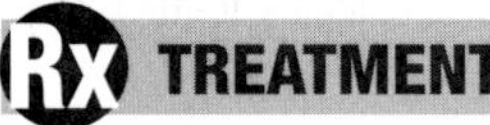

TREATMENT

No specific antiviral therapy for most viruses. Treatment is supportive unless HSV is detected, which would be treated with IV acyclovir.

DISPOSITION

Viral meningitis is almost always an uncomplicated illness that will resolve; however, relapsing headache, myalgia, and weakness may occur for 2 to 3 wk after onset of symptoms.

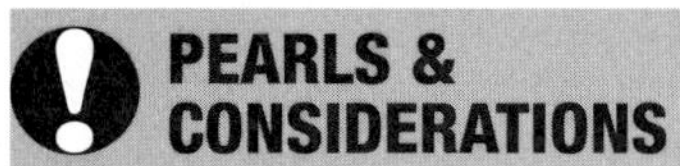

PEARLS & CONSIDERATIONS

Enteroviruses are the most common cause of viral meningitis and are transmitted by fecal-oral and less commonly by the respiratory route.

SUGGESTED READINGS

Ellerin TB et al: Recurrent meningitis of unknown etiology, *Lancet* 363(9423):1772, 2004.
Shah SS et al: Early differentiation of Lyme from enteroviral meningitis, *Pediatr Infect Dis* 24(6):542, 2005.

AUTHORS: **GLENN G. FORT, M.D., M.P.H.,** and **DENNIS J. MIKOLICH, M.D.**

TABLE 1-49 Epidemiology of Acute Viral Meningitis

EPIDEMIOLOGIC FACTORS*

Season	Patient's Age (yr)	Patient's Sex	Risk Factor	Suggested Viral Agent
Summer-fall	Infant	—	Infected mother	Coxsackievirus B
	1-15	—	Swimming pools, closed communities	Enteroviruses
			Geographic area: California, southeastern United States	California serogroup virus
Winter	1-15	—	School exposure	Varicella virus, measles virus
		Male/female 3:1		Mumps virus
	16-21	—	College exposure	Measles virus
		Male/female 3:1		Mumps virus
		—		Epstein-Barr virus (mononucleosis)
	Any	—	Mice, rats, hamsters	Lymphocytic choriomeningitis virus
	Adults	—	Varicella-zoster	Varicella-zoster virus
Any	Any	—	Immunocompromise	Adenovirus
		—	Acquired immunodeficiency syndrome	Human immunodeficiency virus

From Gorbach SI: *Infectious diseases,* ed 2, Philadelphia, 1998, WB Saunders.
*Epidemiologic factors are suggestive but should not be used to exclude diagnoses in individual cases.

BASIC INFORMATION

DEFINITION

Meningomyelocele is the most common type of spina bifida and is characterized by herniation of the spinal cord, nerves, or both through a bony defect of the spine.

SYNONYMS

Myelomeningocele
Spina bifida cystica

ICD-9CM CODES
741.9 Spina bifida without mention of hydrocephalus
741.9 Meningomyelocele

EPIDEMIOLOGY & DEMOGRAPHICS

INCIDENCE (IN U.S.): 4.6/10,000 births
PREDOMINANT SEX: Male = female
PEAK INCIDENCE: Newborn
GENETICS: Environmental and genetic factors have a joint role.

PHYSICAL FINDINGS & CLINICAL PRESENTATION

- Evident at birth—a sac protruding in the lumbar region (Fig. 1-195)
- Severity of neurologic deficits depends on the location of the lesion along the neuroaxis
- Motor dysfunction in the legs
- Lack of bladder or bowel control
- Often associated with Chiari II malformation and resulting obstructive hydrocephalus

ETIOLOGY

- Failure of neural tube to close completely at about 4 wk gestation
- Associated with maternal valproate use
- A small proportion of cases are associated with chromosomal or single-gene disorders

DIAGNOSIS

- Prenatal diagnosis through ultrasound and MRI is being made more frequently
- Coexisting hydrocephalus detected by measurement of head size, ultrasonography, CT, or MRI

DIFFERENTIAL DIAGNOSIS

- Teratoma
- Meningocele

WORKUP

- Evaluate for hydrocephalus
- Evaluate for other congenital abnormalities, such as congenital heart disease, hydronephrosis, intestinal malformation, club foot, and skeletal deformities

LABORATORY TESTS

Prenatal testing often reveals elevated alphafetoprotein in amniotic fluid or maternal serum.

IMAGING STUDIES

- MRI of spine
- X-ray studies of skull exhibit craniolacuna, a honeycombed pattern associated with hydrocephalus
- CT or MRI of head: may reveal hydrocephalus

TREATMENT

- Surgical closure of myelomeningocele is performed soon after birth
- Control of hydrocephalus (shunt)
- Management of urinary incontinence (bladder catheterization)

ACUTE GENERAL Rx

- Immediate goal after delivery is to close defect and prevent infection; surgery usually performed within 24 hr of birth
- Shunt placement for obstructive hydrocephalus
- Treatment of seizures, if present

CHRONIC Rx

- Follow closely for development of hydrocephalus
- Bladder catheterization
- Avoid use of latex-containing products to prevent development of latex allergy

DISPOSITION

Followed by a team of specialists including neurosurgeons, urologists, orthopedists, and myelodysplasia nurses

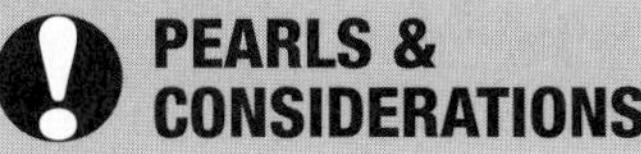

PEARLS & CONSIDERATIONS

All mothers of children with neural tube defects should be instructed on nutritional supplementation with folate for future pregnancies.

COMMENTS

- Intrauterine repair of meningomyelocele decreases the incidence of hindbrain herniation and shunt-dependent hydrocephalus in infants, but increases the incidence of premature delivery.
- U.S. Public Health Service recommends 400 μg of folate intake per day for all women capable of becoming pregnant for primary prevention of neural tube defects.

SUGGESTED READINGS

Adzick NS, Walsh DS: Myelomeningocele: prenatal diagnosis, pathophysiology and management, *Semin Pediatr Surg* 12(3):168, 2003.

Mitchell LE: Epidemiology of neural tube defects, *Am J Med Genet C Semin Med Genet* 135(1):88, 2005.

Spina bifida and anencephaly before and after folic acid mandate—United States, 1995. 1996 and 1999. 2000, *MMWR Morb Mortal Wkly Rep* 53(17):362, 2004.

AUTHOR: **MAITREYI MAZUMDAR, M.D., M.P.H.**

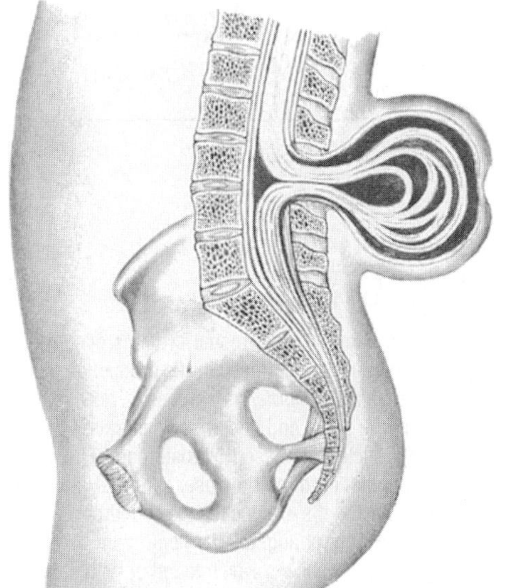

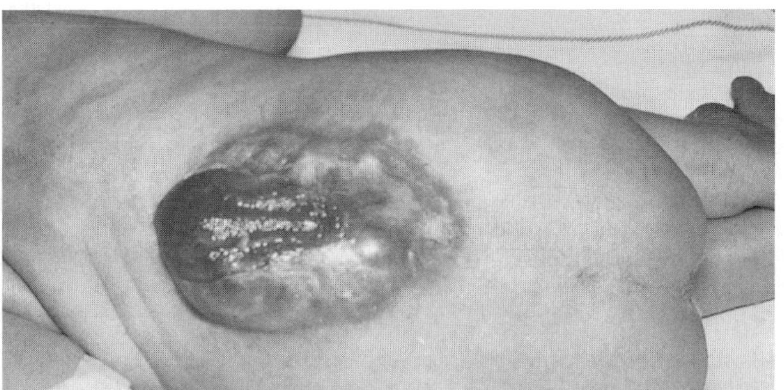

FIGURE 1-195 Meningomyelocele. (From Wong DL: *Whaley's and Wong's nursing care of infants and children,* ed 5, St Louis, 1995, Mosby.)

BASIC INFORMATION

DEFINITION

Menopause is the occurrence of no menstrual periods for 1 yr after age 40 yr or permanent cessation of ovulation after lost ovarian activity. It is a climacteric reproductive stage of life marked by waxing and waning estrogen levels followed by decreasing ovarian function. Premature ovarian failure and no menstrual periods may also occur because of depletion of ovarian follicles before the age of 40 yr.

SYNONYMS

Change of life
Climacteric ovarian failure

ICD-9CM CODES

627 Premenopausal menorrhagia
627.2 Menopausal or female climacteric states
627.4 States associated with artificial menopause
716.3 Climacteric arthritis

EPIDEMIOLOGY & DEMOGRAPHICS

- Average age of menopause in the U.S. is 51 yr.
- Age at which menopause occurs is genetically determined.
- Smokers experience menopause an average of 1.5 yr earlier than nonsmokers.
- More than one third of a woman's life will be spent after menopause.
- Onset of perimenopause is usually in a woman's mid- to late-40s.
- Approximately 4000 women each day begin menopause.

PHYSICAL FINDINGS & CLINICAL PRESENTATION

- Atrophic vaginitis, which can cause burning, itching, bleeding, dyspareunia
- Either complete cessation of menses or a period of irregular cycles and diminished or heavier bleeding
- Osteoporosis
- Psychologic dysfunction:
  1. Anxiety
  2. Depression
  3. Insomnia
  4. Nervousness
  5. Irritability
  6. Inability to concentrate
- Sexual changes, decreased libido, dyspareunia
- Urinary incontinence
- Vasomotor symptoms (hot flashes, flushes), night sweats, cardiovascular disease, coronary artery disease, atherosclerosis, headaches, tiredness, and lethargy

ETIOLOGY

- The most common etiology: physiologic, caused by depleted granulosa and theca cells that fail to react to endogenous gonadotropins, producing less estrogen; decreased negative feedback in the hypothalamic pituitary access, increased follicle-stimulating hormone (FSH), and increased luteinizing hormone (LH), which leads to stromal cells that continue to produce androgens as a result of the LH stimulation (Fig. 1-196)
- Surgical castration
- Family history of early menopause, cigarette smoking, blindness, abnormal chromosomal karyotype (Turner's syndrome, gonadal dysgenesis), precocious puberty, and left-handedness

DIAGNOSIS

DIFFERENTIAL DIAGNOSIS

- Asherman's syndrome
- Hypothalamic dysfunction
- Hypothyroidism
- Pituitary tumors
- Adrenal abnormalities
- Ovarian abnormalities
- Polycystic ovarian syndrome
- Pregnancy

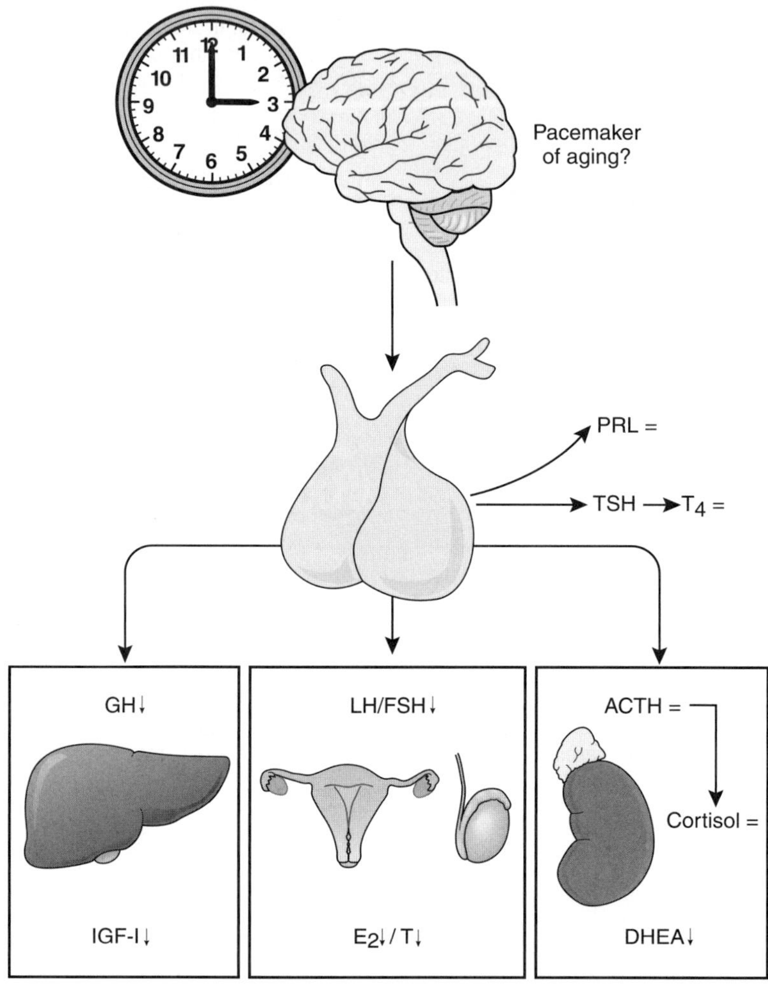

FIGURE 1-196 During aging, declines in the activities of a number of hormonal systems occur. *Left,* A decrease in growth hormone *(GH)* release by the pituitary gland causes a decrease in the production of insulinlike growth factor I *(IGF-I)* by the liver and other organs (somatopause). *Middle,* A decrease in release of gonadotropin luteinizing hormone *(LH)* and follicle-stimulating hormone *(FSH)* and decreased secretion at the gonadal level (from the ovaries, decreased estradiol *[E_2]* from the testicle, decreased testosterone *[T]*) cause menopause and andropause, respectively. (Immediately after the initiation of menopause, serum LH and FSH levels increase sharply.) *Right,* The adrenocortical cells responsible for the production of dehydroepiandrosterone (DHEA) decrease in activity (adrenopause) without clinically evident changes in corticotrophin. A central pacemaker in the hypothalamus or higher brain areas (or both) is hypothesized, which together with changes in the peripheral organs (the ovaries, testicles, and adrenal cortex) regulates the aging process of these endocrine axes. *PRL,* Prolactin; *T4,* thyroxine; *TSH,* thyrotropin. (From Larsen PR et al [eds]: *Williams textbook of endocrinology,* ed 10, Philadelphia, 2003, Saunders.)

- Ovarian neoplasm
- Tuberculosis of the endometrium

WORKUP

- If the clinical picture is highly suggestive of menopause, estrogen can be prescribed. If all symptoms resolve, then diagnosis has essentially been made. Before estrogen is prescribed, a complete history and physical examination are needed. If a patient has estrogen-dependent malignancy, unexplained abnormal uterine bleeding, history of thrombophlebitis, or acute liver disease, estrogen therapy is contraindicated.
- Progesterone challenge test: medroxyprogesterone 10 to 20 mg PO or progesterone 100 mg IM to induce withdrawal bleeding. If no withdrawal bleeding is obtained, a hypoestrogenic state is assumed to be present.
- Physical examination, height, weight, blood pressure, breast examination, and pelvic examination are needed.
- Assess risk for coronary artery disease, osteoporosis, cigarette smoking, personal history, history of breast cancer, liver disease, active coagulation disorder, or any unexplained vaginal bleeding.

LABORATORY TESTS

- FSH, LH, and estrogen levels: markedly elevated FSH and markedly depressed estrogen level constitute laboratory diagnosis of ovarian failure; LH only if polycystic ovarian disease is to be ruled out in a younger patient
- TSH to rule out thyroid dysfunction and prolactin level if patient has symptoms of galactorrhea and if suspicion of pituitary adenoma exists
- A general chemistry profile to check for any systemic diseases
- Pap smear, endometrial biopsy, or dilation and curettage in patients who have had irregular periods or intermenstrual or postmenopausal bleeding
- Mammogram

IMAGING STUDIES

- CT scan or MRI of sella if pituitary tumor is suspected
- Bone density studies if high-risk condition for osteoporosis exists
- Pelvic ultrasound to check endometrial stripe

Rx TREATMENT

NONPHARMACOLOGIC THERAPY

- A balanced diet: low in fat, with total fat intake being <30% of calories; total calories sufficient to maintain body weight or produce weight loss if that is needed
- Avoidance of smoking and excessive alcohol or caffeine intake
- Exercise: weight-bearing exercise for osteoporosis prevention
- Kegel exercises for strengthening the pelvic floor
- Adequate calcium intake: 1500 mg qd is necessary to maintain zero calcium balance in postmenopausal women
- Change in the ambient temperature (may ameliorate hot flashes and reduce night sweats)
- Vitamin E
- Avoidance of caffeine, alcohol, and spicy foods if they trigger hot flashes
- Vaginal lubricants to help with the dyspareunia attributable to vaginal dryness (e.g., Replens, K-Y Jelly, or Gyne-Moistrin cream)

ACUTE GENERAL Rx

Estrogen replacement in symptomatic patients can be done in a variety of forms, including oral estrogen and transdermal estrogen patch. The lowest effective dose should be prescribed.

- Examples of oral estrogen include:
  1. Conjugated estrogens: start with 0.3 mg qd and increase to 1.25 mg qd depending on symptoms.
  2. Estradiol: start with 0.5 mg qd and increase to 2 mg qd.
  3. Esterified estrogens: start with 0.3 to 1.25 mg qd.
  4. Estropipate: start with 0.625 to 2.5 mg qd.
  5. Esterified estrogen/testosterone combination: give 1.25 mg and methyltestosterone 2.5 mg (Estratest) and esterified estrogen 0.625 mg and methyltestosterone 1.25 mg (Estratest HS). May improve sexual enjoyment and libido.
- If the patient has had a hysterectomy for benign disease, estrogen alone is sufficient. However, if she still has her uterus, progestin should be added for its protective effect against endometrial cancer. Progestins can be prescribed as continual daily dose or cyclic fashion. Most commonly prescribed progestins include medroxyprogesterone acetate 2.5 mg, 5 mg, and 10 mg; Prometrium 100 mg, 200 mg, and 400 mg; and Aygestin 5 mg. Continuous hormone replacement therapy is preferred because after time the patient should be amenorrheic. Patients should be counseled that they may experience some irregular spotting for the first 6 to 9 mo after starting the hormone replacement therapy. Cyclic therapy will cause withdrawal bleeding.
- Combination oral preparations Femhrt, Prefest, Prempro, Activella, Premphase.
- Transdermal patches can be either estradiol (Estraderm, Vivelle, FemPatch) 0.025 to 0.1 mg applied twice weekly or Climara 0.025 to 0.1 mg used once a week. With these preparations, progesterone should be used in a similar fashion. Apply CombiPatch twice weekly (combination estrogen and progesterone) or Climara Pro once per week (one patch).
- Vaginal creams can be used; these should be reserved for local therapy of atrophic vaginitis. Systemic absorption does occur; however, blood levels are unpredictable. Usual dose 0.5 to 2 g intravaginally daily, cyclically 3 wk on 1 wk off. When symptoms improve, once to twice weekly is adequate maintenance.
- Vagifem estradiol vaginal tablets. Initial dosage: one Vagifem tablet, inserted vaginally, qd for 2 wk. Maintenance dose: one Vagifem tablet, inserted vaginally, twice weekly.
- Femring vaginal ring delivering the equivalent of 0.5 mg/day inserted every 3 mo or Estring 0.0075 mg/day.
- EstroGel 0.06% (estradiol gel) One Pump (1.25 g/day) applied to one arm from wrist to shoulder.
- For women in whom estrogen is contraindicated or for those who do not wish to take estrogen, the following regimens can be used:
  1. Serotonin reuptake inhibitors
  2. Depo-Provera 150 mg IM every month (may be helpful in alleviating hot flashes)
  3. Clonidine 0.05 to 0.15 mg qd (questionable efficacy)
  4. Bellergal-S (questionable efficacy)
- Tibolone significantly improves vasomotor symptoms, libido, and vaginal lubrication.

CHRONIC Rx

Hormone replacement therapy should be used only for the short term unless benefits outweigh the risks of long-term use.

DISPOSITION

If treated, the patient should have resolution of her symptoms and reduced incidence of osteoporosis. Lifelong medical supervision is necessary to monitor adequacy of treatment and prevention of complications. This should include annual Pap smears, pelvic examinations, breast examinations, mammography, and endometrial sampling of any type of abnormal bleeding. If untreated, the vasomotor symptoms will eventually disappear; however, this may take several years in a small percentage of women. Some women who are in their 80s have experienced hot flashes. Urogenital atrophy will continue to worsen. Osteoporosis and coronary artery disease risks will increase with every passing year. Women using estrogen replacement therapy for >10 yr may have increased risk of developing ovarian cancer.

REFERRAL

Most menopausal women are managed by their gynecologists. However, this condition can be managed adequately by the patient's primary care physician who has an interest in treating menopausal women.

PEARLS & CONSIDERATIONS

COMMENTS

- Short-term risks of hormone replacement therapy (HRT) include an 18-fold increased rise for cholecystitis, 3.5-fold risk of a thrombocardiac event in the first year, and probably increased risk of stroke and myocardial infarction.
- Results of the WHI study found that for every 10,000 women taking HRT for 1 yr (10,000

person-yr), seven more would have coronary events, eight would have more strokes, eight would have more pulmonary emboli, and eight would have earlier breast cancer than would 10,000 women taking placebo. Benefits of HRT were six fewer cases of colorectal cancer and five fewer hip fractures per 10,000 women.

- HRT should not be initiated or continued for the primary or secondary prevention of coronary heart disease.
- Estrogen-replacement therapy or HRT should only be prescribed for patients with sufficient menopausal symptoms that impact the patient's quality of life.

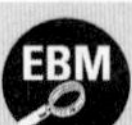

EVIDENCE

Please note: Complete text of EBM for this topic is available online.

Key trials and commentary:

In the Women's Health Initiative Randomized Controlled Trial (WHI RCT), estrogen-only treatment compared with combined estrogen–progestin treatment resulted in less coronary artery disease, no increase in breast cancer and no reduction in colorectal cancer.

This study confirms that postmenopausal women in the overall population respond differently to estrogen-only treatment compared with estrogen–progestin treatment, because of different hormone regimens and/or increased cardiovascular disease in hysterectomized women.[1] Ⓐ

The WHI RCT created controversy over the effects of hormone replacement therapy (HRT) in postmenopausal women on coronary artery disease (CAD). Observational studies had suggested that HRT benefited CAD, whereas the WHI suggested an increased risk for CAD and breast cancer. The controversy has focused on estrogen compared with estrogen plus progestin. In the UK General Practice Research Database (GPRD), estrogen-only adjusted for hazard ratios were lower for CAD and slightly higher for breast cancer and colorectal cancer. When estrogen-only was compared with estrogen plus progestin, the estrogen-alone group had significantly lower myocardial infarctions and breast cancer but higher colorectal cancer. This study confirms the difference in outcome for estrogen alone and estrogen plus progestin. It also suggests that estrogen alone may be safer for HRT than for combination therapy. There are many unanswered questions concerning HRT, which include age, years after menopause, and potential known risk factors for the woman to be treated. We will continue to use HRT cautiously until further clarification is made about the unresolved issues.

Evidence-Based Reference

1. Tannen RL et al: Estrogen affects postmenopausal women differently than estrogen plus progestin replacement therapy, *Hum Reprod* 22:1769-1777, 2007. Commentary by A.W. Meikle, M.D. Ⓐ

SUGGESTED READINGS

Col NF et al: Menopause. In the clinic, *Ann Intern Med* 150(7):ITC4-1-15, April 7, 2009.

Gambrell RD: The Women's Health Initiative Reports: critical review of the findings, the female patient, *Menopause* 29(11):23, 2004.

Lacey JV et al: Menopausal hormone replacement therapy and risk of ovarian cancer, *JAMA* 288:334, 2002.

NIH State of Sciences Panel: NIH State of Sciences Conference Statement: management of menopause related symptoms, *Ann Intern Med* 142:1003, 2005.

Speroff L: Efficacy and tolerability of a novel estradiol vaginal ring for relief of menopausal symptoms, *Obstet Gynecol* 102(4):823, 2003.

Writing Group for the Women's Health Initiative Investigators: Risks and benefits of estrogen plus progestin in healthy postmenopausal women, *JAMA* 288:321, 2002.

AUTHORS: **GEORGE T. DANAKAS, M.D.,** and **RUBEN ALVERO, M.D.**

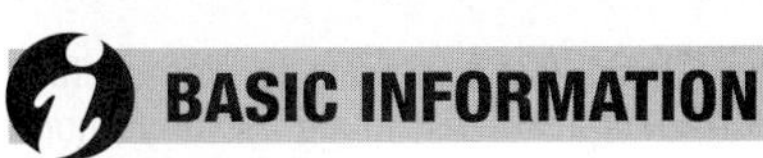

BASIC INFORMATION

DEFINITION

Acute mesenteric lymphadenitis is a syndrome of acute right lower quadrant abdominal pain associated with mesenteric lymph node enlargement and a normal appendix.

ICD-9CM CODES
289.2 Mesenteric adenitis

EPIDEMIOLOGY & DEMOGRAPHICS

- Incidence unknown
- Affects mostly children (<18 yr) with no sex preference
- When *Yersinia* enterocolitis is the cause, boys are more frequently involved

PHYSICAL FINDINGS & CLINICAL PRESENTATION

- Abdominal pain of variable severity (mild ache to severe colic) beginning in upper abdomen or right lower quadrant; eventually localizes in the right side but not in a precise location (unlike appendicitis)
- In *Yersinia* infection outbreaks, symptoms include abdominal pain (84%), diarrhea (78%), fever (43%), anorexia (22%), nausea (13%), and vomiting (8%)
- Physical findings:
  - Other lymphadenopathy (20% of cases)
  - Right lower quadrant tenderness (site of maximal tenderness may vary from one examination to the next)
  - Guarding (rare)
  - Mild fever

ETIOLOGY & PATHOGENESIS

- Reactive hyperplasia of lymph nodes that drain the ileocecal region, similar to that seen in inflammatory or allergic conditions. One study reported that approximately two thirds of cases are secondary (reactive) and one third are primary (no demonstrable associated inflammatory process).
- *Yersinia enterocolitica, Y. pseudotuberculosis, Salmonella* species, *Escherichia coli,* and streptococci have been implicated in mesenteric adenitis.

Dx DIAGNOSIS

In general, the diagnosis is made on exploration of the abdomen of a patient suspected of having acute appendicitis. On examination the appendix appears normal, and enlarged mesenteric lymph nodes are noted (Fig. 1-197). Excision of an enlarged lymph node with culture and nodal histology may provide information regarding the etiology but is not routinely used.

DIFFERENTIAL DIAGNOSIS

- Acute appendicitis (5% to 10% of patients admitted to hospitals with a diagnosis of appendicitis are discharged with a diagnosis of mesenteric adenitis)
- Crohn's disease

Section II describes the differential diagnosis of right lower quadrant abdominal pain.

LABORATORY TESTS

- Complete blood count may show leukocytosis
- Abdominal sonography and helical appendiceal CT scan may be useful
- Laparotomy if appendicitis is suspected

PROGNOSIS

Recurrent bouts are common; therefore if laparotomy is performed and a normal appendix is found, it should be removed.

SUGGESTED READING

Macari M et al: Mesenteric adenitis: CT diagnosis of primary versus secondary causes, incidence, and clinical significance on pediatric and adult patients, *Am J Roentgenol* 178:853, 2002.

AUTHOR: **FRED F. FERRI, M.D.**

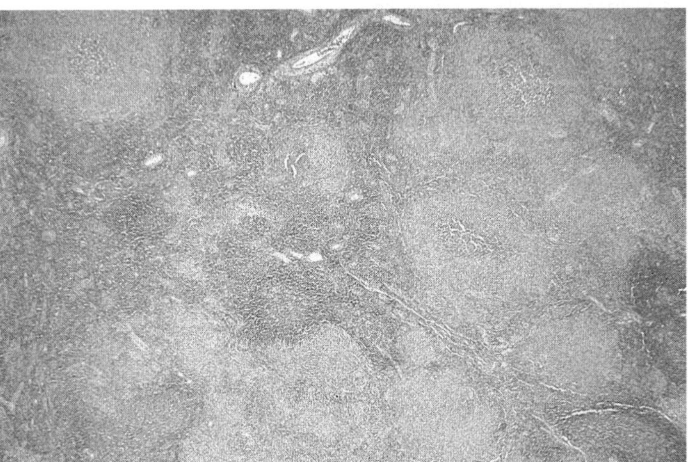

FIGURE 1-197 ***Yersinia* mesenteric lymphadenitis.** Multiple stellate granulomas with central necrosis replace a mesenteric lymph node. The inflammation extends into the surrounding perinodal fat. The preoperative diagnosis was acute suppurativa appendicitis, but the appendix was macroscopically and microscopically normal (hematoxylin and eosin, ×5; *Yersinia pseudotuberloculosis* isolated from cultures). (From Silverberg SG et al [eds]: *Silverberg's principles and practice of surgical pathology and cytopathology,* ed 4, Philadelphia, 2006, Churchill Livingstone.)

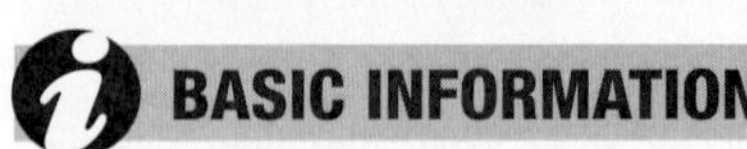

BASIC INFORMATION

DEFINITION

Acute mesenteric ischemia (AMI) is the sudden onset of intestinal hypoperfusion caused by emboli, arterial or venous thrombosis, or vasoconstriction from low-flow states.

ICD-9CM CODES
ICD-557.1 Mesenteric vascular insufficiency

EPIDEMIOLOGY & DEMOGRAPHICS

INCIDENCE:
- AMI accounts for 0.1% of hospital admissions.
- The incidence appears to be increasing, likely due to increased awareness among clinicians and aging of the population.
- Increased use of intensive care units, and longer survival of sicker patients, has allowed mesenteric ischemia to occur more frequently as a complication of their initial illnesses.

PREDOMINANT SEX AND AGE:
- AMI caused by arterial embolism or thrombosis occurs more frequently in the elderly.
- AMI from mesenteric venous thrombosis often presents in younger age groups.

GENETICS: No specific genetic predisposition but may be related to underlying factors such as cardiac disease, atherosclerosis, and hypercoagulable states.

RISK FACTORS:
- Advanced age, atherosclerosis, low cardiac output (especially atrial fibrillation), severe cardiac valvular disease, intraabdominal malignancy.
- In the subgroup of cases caused by venous thrombosis, risk factors include hypercoagulable states, portal hypertension, abdominal infection, blunt trauma, pancreatitis, and portal malignancy.
- Additional risk factors for AMI caused by nonocclusive mesenteric ischemia include recent cardiac surgery, dialysis, and cocaine use.
- AMI may occur rarely in patients with no identifiable risk factors.

PHYSICAL FINDINGS & CLINICAL PRESENTATION

- The classic presentation is rapid onset of severe periumbilical pain out of proportion to physical examination findings.
- Nausea and vomiting are commonly associated.
- Initial abdominal examination may be normal, with no rebound or guarding, or may include minimal distension or stool positive for occult blood.
- Later in the course the patient may present with gross distension, absence of bowel sounds, and peritoneal signs. In the elderly, mental status changes may occur.

ETIOLOGY

The pathophysiologic mechanisms that cause AMI include:
- Mesenteric arterial embolism: typically from the left atrium, left ventricle, or cardiac valves. The superior mesenteric artery is most commonly affected.
- Mesenteric arterial thrombosis: often in patients with prior progressive atherosclerotic stenoses, with superimposed abdominal trauma or infection.
- Mesenteric venous thrombosis may occur in the setting of hypercoagulable states (acquired or inherited), blunt trauma, abdominal infection, portal hypertension, pancreatitis, and portal malignancy.
- Nonocclusive mesenteric ischemia is caused by reduced intestinal perfusion, such as may be seen in a patient with an acute cardiovascular disease process being treated with drugs that reduce intestinal perfusion.

Dx DIAGNOSIS

DIFFERENTIAL DIAGNOSIS

Initially include other causes of abdominal pain of acute onset, including perforated peptic ulcer and early appendicitis. Ultimately, the varied causes of peritonitis.

WORKUP

- Early diagnosis is key. Treatment success is related to the duration of symptoms before diagnosis.
- Consider early laparotomy for diagnosis in cases with a high index of suspicion when angiography is not available.

LABORATORY TESTS

- Laboratory test results are nonspecific, especially early in the course. Later they can include leukocytosis, acidosis, and elevated hematocrit from hemoconcentration. Most abnormalities occur after progression to bowel necrosis.
- When a hypercoagulable state is suspected, workup may include proteins C and S, antithrombin III, and factor V Leiden. This will likely not affect the diagnosis of AMI but may help guide long-term therapy.

IMAGING STUDIES

- The gold standard is mesenteric angiography.
- With strong clinical suspicion, workup should proceed directly to angiography without delay for CT scan or other testing.
- Plain films are normal 25% of the time in the early stages. Suggestive findings may include ileus, bowel wall thickening, or intramural gas. Intraluminal barium should not be used as it is rarely helpful in making a positive diagnosis and will interfere with angiographic studies.
- Doppler ultrasound evaluation of intestinal blood flow is often limited by the presence of air-filled loops of bowel.
- CT findings also are commonly nonspecific and more often found late in the course. Portal venous gas or intramural gas may be seen after the development of gangrene; in many cases, even at that advanced stage CT findings remain nonspecific.
- CT scanning has been found to be more useful in cases of mesenteric vein thrombosis causing AMI, with sensitivity approaching 90%. It has also been found useful in monitoring the progress of patients with superior mesenteric venous thrombosis who are treated nonsurgically.
- Recent studies suggest that multidetector CT angiography may be a useful diagnostic modality.

Rx TREATMENT

- The goal of treatment is to restore blood flow as rapidly as possible to ischemic bowel before the occurrence of infarction.
- Treatment varies depending on etiology.

ACUTE GENERAL Rx

- Initial management should include hemodynamic monitoring and support, correction of acidosis, administration of broad-spectrum antibiotics, and gastric decompression by nasogastric tube.
- Vasoconstricting agents should be avoided.
- Systemic anticoagulation may be started. Optimal timing of initiation is unclear.

NONPHARMACOLOGIC THERAPY

- Signs of peritonitis mandate early laparotomy and resection of infarcted bowel.
- When workup is positive for major superior mesenteric artery (SMA) embolus, embolectomy is considered standard treatment in the absence of peritoneal signs. Depending on the location and degree of occlusion of the embolus, surgical revascularization, intraarterial infusion of thrombolytics or vasodilators, or systemic anticoagulation may be considered.
- In cases of SMA thrombosis, emergency surgical revascularization is the treatment of choice; stent placement may be a viable alternative.
- Angiography is needed to diagnose nonocclusive mesenteric ischemia before infarct and should be followed up by intraarterial vasodilator infusion. This approach has been shown to significantly reduce mortality rate in this situation.
- In patients with mesenteric vein thrombosis, treatment depends on the presence or absence of peritoneal signs. Laparotomy and resection of infarcted bowel is indicated in more advanced cases. If there are no peritoneal signs, immediate anticoagulant therapy with heparin, and ultimately warfarin, may be adequate treatment.

CHRONIC Rx

In the subgroup of patients with mesenteric venous thrombosis, prevention of further thrombosis is indicated. The optimal duration of anticoagulation is unclear.

DISPOSITION

- Prognosis is best in AMI due to mesenteric venous thrombosis and after surgical treatment for acute arterial embolism. It remains poor in cases of arterial thrombosis and nonocclusive ischemia.

- With delayed diagnosis, intestinal infarction—resulting in perforation or gangrenous bowel, sepsis, shock, and death—is typical.

REFERRAL

- Early surgical consultation should be considered. There should be no delay with peritoneal signs.
- If diagnostic angiography is unavailable, surgery may be warranted for diagnostic purposes.

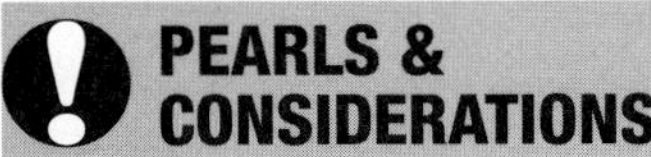

PEARLS & CONSIDERATIONS

COMMENTS

- The diagnosis of AMI should be considered in any patient with acute onset of abdominal pain out of proportion to physical findings, particularly in at-risk patients.
- Early diagnosis, before intestinal infarction occurs, is critical and correlates with improved survival rates.

PREVENTION

Prevention of the underlying factors, most notably atherosclerotic disease

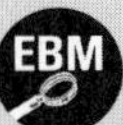

EVIDENCE

Guidelines from the American Heart Association/American College of Cardiology make the following general recommendations:

Surgical treatment of acute obstructive intestinal ischemia includes revascularization, resection of necrotic bowel, and, when appropriate, a "second-look" procedure 24 to 48 hr after the revascularization.[1] Ⓒ

Percutaneous interventions, including transcatheter lytic therapy, balloon angioplasty, and stenting, are appropriate in selected patients with acute intestinal ischemia caused by arterial obstructions. Patients so treated may still require laparotomy.[1] Ⓒ

Treatment of the underlying shock state is the most important initial step in treatment of nonocclusive intestinal ischemia.[1] Ⓒ

Laparotomy and resection of nonviable bowel is indicated in patients with nonocclusive intestinal ischemia who have persistent symptoms despite treatment.[1] Ⓒ

Transcatheter administration of vasodilator medications into the area of vasospasm is indicated in patients with nonocclusive intestinal ischemia who do not respond to systemic supportive treatment and in patients with intestinal ischemia due to cocaine or ergot poisoning.[1] Ⓒ

Evidence-Based Reference

1. Hirsch AT et al: ACC/AHA 2005 guidelines for the management of patients with peripheral arterial disease (lower extremity, renal, mesenteric, and abdominal aortic): A report of the American College of Cardiology/American Heart Association Task Force on Practice Guidelines, *J Am Coll Cardiol* 47: 1239-1312, 2006. Ⓒ

SUGGESTED READINGS

Berland T, Oldenberg WA: Acute mesenteric ischemia, *Curr Gastroenterol Rep* 10(3):341-346, 2008.

Offer A et al: Multidetector CT angiography in the evaluation of acute mesenteric ischemia, *Eur Radiol* 19(1):24-30, 2009.

Schoots IG et al: Systematic review of survival after acute mesenteric ischaemia according to disease aetiology, *Br J Surg* 91(1):17-27, 2004.

AUTHOR: **MARGARET TRYFOROS, M.D.**

Mesenteric Venous Thrombosis

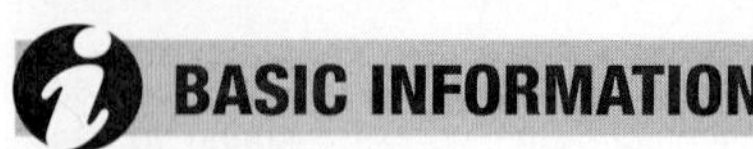

BASIC INFORMATION

DEFINITION

Mesenteric venous thrombosis (MVT) is a thrombotic occlusion of the mesenteric venous system involving major trunks or smaller branches and leading to intestinal infarction in its acute form.

ICD-9CM CODES
557.0 Mesenteric venous thrombosis

EPIDEMIOLOGY & DEMOGRAPHICS

Between 5% and 15% of patients with acute mesenteric infarction have MVT. MVT is slightly more common in men than women. The typical age of occurrence is 50 to 60 yr.

PHYSICAL FINDINGS & CLINICAL PRESENTATION

Acute MVT:
- Symptoms: abdominal pain in 90% of patients, typically out of proportion to the physical findings. Nausea and vomiting occur in 50% and gastrointestinal (GI) bleeding occurs in 50% (occult) and 15% (gross).
- Physical findings:
  - Early: abdominal tenderness, decreased bowel sounds, abdominal distention
  - Later: guarding and rebound tenderness, fever, septic shock

Subacute MVT:
- Symptoms: nonspecific abdominal pain for weeks or months
- Physical findings: none

Chronic MVT:
- Symptoms: upper GI hemorrhage from bleeding varices
- Physical findings: none other than signs of blood loss if significant

ETIOLOGY & PATHOGENESIS

Hypercoagulable states:
- Peripheral deep venous thrombosis
- Neoplasms
- Antithrombin III, protein C, protein S deficiencies
- Lupus anticoagulant (antiphospholipid antibody)
- Oral contraceptive use, pregnancy
- Polycythemia vera
- Thrombocytosis
- Paroxysmal nocturnal hemoglobinuria

Portal hypertension:
- Cirrhosis

Inflammation:
- Pancreatitis
- Peritonitis (e.g., appendicitis, diverticulitis, perforated viscus)
- Inflammatory bowel disease
- Pelvic or intraabdominal abscess
- Intraabdominal cancer

Postoperative state or trauma:
- Blunt abdominal trauma
- Postoperative states (abdominal surgery)

Thrombosis may begin in small mesenteric branches (e.g., in hypercoagulable states) and propagate to the major venous mesenteric trunks or begin in large veins (e.g., in cirrhosis, intraabdominal cancer, surgery) and extend distally. If collateral drainage is inadequate the intestine becomes congested, edematous, cyanotic, and hemorrhagic and eventually may infarct.

Dx DIAGNOSIS

DIFFERENTIAL DIAGNOSIS

All other causes of abdominal pain (e.g., peritonitis, intestinal obstruction, pancreatitis, peptic ulcer disease, gastritis, inflammatory bowel disease, perforated viscus). Also to be considered in the differential diagnosis of GI hemorrhage.

WORKUP

Laboratory tests and imaging studies

LABORATORY TESTS

- Complete blood count: leukocytosis
- Electrolytes: metabolic acidosis (lactic) indicates bowel infarction
- Elevated amylase
- Tests for hypercoagulable status

IMAGING STUDIES

- Abdominal plain radiograph: ileus, ascites, bowel dilation, bowel wall thickening, loop separation, thumbprinting
- Abdominal CT scan (diagnostic in 90%): bowel wall thickening, venous dilation, venous thrombus
- Arteriography if CT scan is not diagnostic
- Diagnosis occasionally made by laparotomy

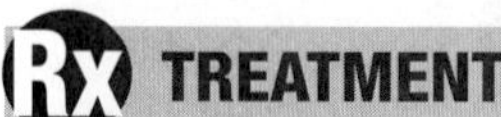

Rx TREATMENT

- Anticoagulation or thrombolytic therapy
- Laparotomy if intestinal infarction is suspected
- Short ischemic segment: resection
- Long ischemic segment:
  1. Nonviable: resection or close
  2. Viable: intraarterial papaverine and/or thrombectomy followed by "second look" intervention
- Treatment of chronic MVT is the same as for portal hypertension

PROGNOSIS

- Mortality rate of acute mesenteric venous thrombosis: 20% to 50%
- Recurrence rate: 15% to 25%

SUGGESTED READINGS

Brandt LJ, Smithline AE: Ischemic lesions of the bowel. In Feldman M et al (eds): *Gastrointestinal and liver disease,* ed 6, Philadelphia, 1998, WB Saunders.

Kumar S et al: Mesenteric venous thrombosis, *N Engl J Med* 345:1683, 2002.

AUTHOR: **FRED F. FERRI, M.D.**

Mesothelioma, Malignant

BASIC INFORMATION

DEFINITION

Malignant mesothelioma is a rare neoplastic lesion associated with asbestos exposure. There are three major histologic subtypes: epithelial (most common), sarcomatous, and mixed (epithelial/sarcomatous).

ICD-9CM CODES
199.1 Malignant mesothelioma, site NOS

EPIDEMIOLOGY & DEMOGRAPHICS

- Associated with asbestos exposure (all fiber types)
- More than 3000 new cases diagnosed in U.S. annually
- More common in men as a result of asbestos exposure in the workplace
- Right-sided involvement is more common
- Incidence of mesothelioma increases with age; median age at presentation is >60 yr
- More than 8 million persons in the U.S. are currently at risk for mesothelioma because of prior asbestos exposure

PHYSICAL FINDINGS & CLINICAL PRESENTATION

- Dyspnea
- Nonpleuritic chest pain
- Fever, weight loss, sweats, fatigue, loss of appetite
- Dysphagia, superior vena cava syndrome, Horner's syndrome in advanced stages
- Auscultation may reveal unilateral loss of breath sounds
- Dullness on percussion may be present

ETIOLOGY

- Asbestos exposure
- Other reported potentially causal factors include prior radiation therapy and extravasated Thorotrast, zeolite, and erionite fibers

DIAGNOSIS

DIFFERENTIAL DIAGNOSIS

Metastatic adenocarcinomas (from lung, breast, ovary, kidney, stomach, prostate)

WORKUP

- Staging evaluation includes complete history (including occupational history), physical examination, and testing to determine potential operability (CT, bone scan, pulmonary function tests [PFTs])
- Thoracoscopy, pleuroscopy, and open-lung biopsy are useful in obtaining adequate tissue samples for diagnosis
- Pulmonary function tests
- Staging: the International Union Against Cancer (UICC) staging uses the TNM categories to organize mesothelioma in stages I to IV in a manner similar to that used for non–small cell lung cancer

LABORATORY TESTS

- Diagnostic thoracentesis is generally insufficient for diagnosis because pleural effusions may only reveal atypical mesothelial cells.
- Immunohistochemistry is useful to distinguish adenocarcinoma from epithelial malignant mesothelioma (mesotheliomas are generally carcinoembryonic antigen negative and cytokeratin positive).
- Thrombocytosis and anemia may be found on initial laboratory evaluation.
- Serum osteopontin levels (when available) can be used to distinguish persons with exposure to asbestos who do not have cancer from those with exposure to asbestos who have pleural mesothelioma.

IMAGING STUDIES

- Chest radiographs may reveal pleural plaques (Fig. 1-198) or calcifications in the diaphragm.
- CT scans of the chest and abdomen and bone scan are used to assess the extent of disease.

TREATMENT

GENERAL Rx

- Operable patient (epithelial type, no positive nodes, confined to pleura, adequate PFTs): the two surgical techniques for therapeutic intervention are decortication (pleurectomy) and extrapleural pneumonectomy. Postoperative chemotherapy with cisplatin, doxorubicin, and cyclophosphamide and subsequent external-beam radiation are used in some centers with limited success.
- Inoperable patient (disease too extensive, sarcomatous or mixed histology type, poor PFTs): supportive care with or without radiation therapy for symptoms or supportive care plus chemotherapy. Combined modality therapies (surgery, radiation therapy, chemotherapy, and biologics) have also been used to reduce both local and distant recurrences. The combination of pemetrexed (an antimetabolite that inhibits enzymes involved in folate metabolism) and cisplatin is used for chemotherapy of unresectable malignant pleural mesothelioma.
- Intrapleural instillation of cisplatin or biologics (e.g., interferons, interleukin-2) is generally limited to very early disease because it can only penetrate a very limited depth of the tumor and there is a propensity of the pleural space to become progressively obliterated with advancing disease.
- The role of radiation therapy in the treatment of mesotheliomas remains uncertain. It is often used for palliation of local pain despite lack of trials to prove its utility.
- Obliteration of the pleural space (pleurodesis) with instillation of tetracycline, bleomycin, or biologic substances such as *Cryptosporidium parvum* into the pleural cavity is often attempted in the treatment of recurrent symptomatic pleural effusions.

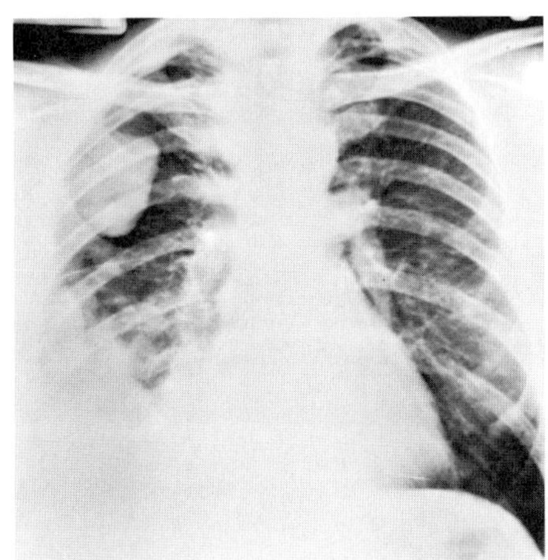

FIGURE 1-198 Chest radiograph of patient with mesothelioma. Note several lobulated, pleural-based masses in right hemithorax accompanied by right pleural effusion. (From Weinberg SE, Cockrill BA, Mandel J: *Principles of pulmonary medicine,* ed 5, Philadelphia, 2008, Saunders.)

DISPOSITION

Median survival is from 6.7 to 21 mo for patients undergoing pleurectomy ranges and from 4 to 21 mo for extrapleural pneumonectomy. Survival is better for patients with the epithelial form.

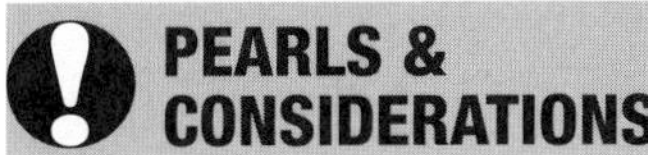

PEARLS & CONSIDERATIONS

COMMENTS

- Patients with early disease should be referred to treatment centers specializing in mesothelioma treatment before attempts are made to obliterate the pleural space with pleurodesis.
- An approach to the evaluation and treatment of mesothelioma is described in Section III, online version.

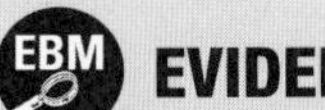

EVIDENCE

Pleurodesis is effective in the management of malignant pleural effusions. Data suggest that talc pleurodesis is more effective than other agents.

A systematic review of pleurodesis for malignant effusion found that talc had a nonsignificant tendency toward fewer recurrences compared with bleomycin and tetracycline. Tetracycline (or doxycycline) was not superior to bleomycin. The authors concluded that talc appears to be effective and should be the agent of choice for pleurodesis. Where thoracoscopic talc insufflation was unavailable, they commented that bedside talc pleurodesis has a high success rate and is the next best option.[1] Ⓐ

A systematic review of pleurodesis for malignant pleural effusions aimed at ascertaining the optimal technique found that sclerosants (mitoxantrone, talc, and tetracycline combined) were associated with a significantly increased efficacy of pleurodesis compared with controls (instillation of isotonic saline or equivalent pH isotonic saline or tube drainage alone). Use of sclerosants significantly reduced the risk of effusion recurrence. Talc was the most efficacious agent, with significant benefit over bleomycin, tetracycline, mustine, and tube drainage alone in terms of risk of recurrence. Pleurodesis achieved by thoracoscopic instillation of sclerosants also significantly reduced risk of recurrence compared with bedside instillation of sclerosants by chest tube. The authors concluded the available evidence supports the need for chemical sclerosants for successful pleurodesis, the use of talc as the sclerosant of choice, and thoracoscopic pleurodesis as the preferred technique.[2] Ⓐ

The role of surgical pneumonectomy procedures in the management of pleural mesothelioma continues to evolve. Its use as part of an integrated approach with adjuvant chemotherapy and radiation therapy (as multimodality treatment) is endorsed by expert opinion.

Recommendations from the European Society of Medical Oncology state that extrapleural pneumonectomy with resection of the hemidiaphragm and the pericardium en bloc has the potential for a radical treatment. This approach is generally combined with chemotherapy and/or adjuvant radiotherapy. Surgery, the appropriateness of which is still under consideration, should only be carried out on selected patients by experienced thoracic surgeons in the context of a multidisciplinary team.[3] Ⓒ

Data from randomized trials have established chemotherapy with cisplatin plus pemetrexed as an effective treatment for pleural mesothelioma. The use of vitamin supplements and agents to reduce treatment toxicity also has a role in such therapy. Studies on the use of alternative chemotherapy combinations are ongoing.

A recent randomized, controlled trial compared cisplatin plus raltitrexed (an antifolate thymidine synthase inhibitor) with cisplatin alone in 250 patients with malignant pleural mesothelioma. This study found that the addition of raltitrexed significantly improved overall survival compared with cisplatin alone.[4] Ⓐ

A recent phase II study evaluated the use of a pemetrexed plus carboplatin combination in 102 patients with malignant pleural mesothelioma. All patients received folic acid and vitamin B_{12} supplementation. This study reported that disease control rate, time to disease progression, and overall survival were similar to results previously reported with the standard regimen of pemetrexed and cisplatin.[5] Ⓑ

Evidence-Based References

1. Tan C et al: The evidence on the effectiveness of management for malignant pleural effusion: a systematic review, *Eur J Cardiothorac Surg* 29:829, 2006. Ⓐ

2. Shaw P, Agarwal R: Pleurodesis for malignant pleural effusions, *Cochrane Rev* 1, 2004. Ⓐ

3. Malignant pleural mesothelioma: ESMO Clinical Recommendations for diagnosis, treatment and follow-up, *Ann Oncol* 18(suppl 2):ii-34, 2007. Ⓒ

4. van Meerbeeck JP et al: European Organisation for Research and Treatment of Cancer Lung Cancer Group; National Cancer Institute of Canada: Randomized phase III study of cisplatin with or without raltitrexed in patients with malignant pleural mesothelioma: an intergroup study of the European Organisation for Research and Treatment of Cancer Lung Cancer Group and the National Cancer Institute of Canada, *J Clin Oncol* 23:6881, 2005. Ⓐ

5. Ceresoli GL et al: Phase II study of pemetrexed plus carboplatin in malignant pleural mesothelioma, *J Clin Oncol* 24:1443, 2006. Ⓑ

SUGGESTED READINGS

Pass H et al: Asbestos exposure, pleural mesothelioma, and serum osteopontin levels, *N Engl J Med* 353:1564, 2005.

Robinson B, Lake R: Advances in malignant mesothelioma, *N Engl J Med* 353:1591, 2005.

AUTHOR: **FRED F. FERRI, M.D.**

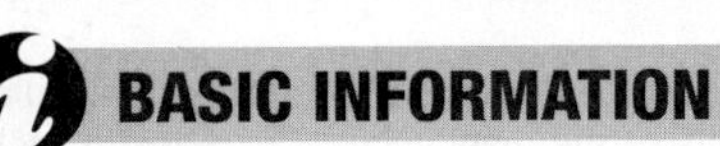

BASIC INFORMATION

DEFINITION

Hyperglycemia, dyslipidemia, abdominal obesity, and hypertension are critical components of most guidelines that define metabolic syndrome. The National Cholesterol Education Program focused its definition on the risk of cardiovascular disease and defined the metabolic syndrome as the presence of any three of the following:

- Abdominal waist circumference >102 cm (40 in) in men and >88 cm (35 in) in women
- Serum hypertriglyceridemia ≥150 mg/dl (1.7 mmol/L) or drug treatment for elevated triglycerides
- Serum high-density lipoprotein (HDL) cholesterol <40 mg/dl (1 mmol/L) in men and <50 mg/dl (1.3 mmol/L) in women or drug treatment for low HDL-C.
- Blood pressure ≥130/85 mm Hg or drug treatment for elevated blood pressure
- Fasting glucose ≥100 mg/dl (5.6 mmol/L) or drug treatment for elevated blood glucose

SYNONYMS

Syndrome X
Insulin resistance syndrome
Obesity dyslipidemia syndrome

ICD-9CM CODES
277.7 Metabolic syndrome

EPIDEMIOLOGY & DEMOGRAPHICS

- Affects 22% of U.S. adults.
- Prevalence increases with age, affecting more than 40% of individuals >60 yr.
- Increasing prevalence among women esp. in the African American and Mexican American populations.
- Weight or body mass index is a major risk factor; 5% of normal weight, 22% of overweight, and 60% of obese individuals have the metabolic syndrome.
- Genetic factors account for up to 50% of the variation noted in the development of metabolic syndrome. Other risk factors include low socioeconomic status, lack of physical activity, high carbohydrate diet, no alcohol intake, smoking, and postmenopausal status.

CLINICAL PRESENTATION

- Obesity, hypertension, dyslipidemia, and hyperglycemia as defined.
  - Blood pressure: ≥130/85 mm Hg
  - Waist circumference: >102 cm (40 in) in men and >88 cm (35 in) in women
  - Triglycerides: ≥150 mg/dl (1.7 mmol/L)
  - HDL: <40 mg/dl (1 mmol/L) in men and <50 mg/dl (1.3 mmol/L) in women
  - High fasting glucose: ≥100 mg/dl (5.6 mmol/L)
- Patients with the metabolic syndrome are at increased risk for diabetes and coronary artery disease. Other complications include cognitive decline, fatty liver disease, polycystic ovary syndrome, obstructive sleep apnea, and chronic kidney disease.
- Focus history on symptoms of diabetes and its complications, obesity and its complications, coronary artery disease (angina), and polycystic ovary syndrome.
- Complete physical examination, including height, weight, waist circumference, and blood pressure.

ETIOLOGY

- Genetic predisposition and environmental factors associated with obesity lead to development of the metabolic syndrome.
- Abdominal obesity is associated with insulin resistance and hyperinsulinemia.
- Elevations in inflammatory markers and cytokines (i.e., plasminogen activator inhibitor [PAI]-1, interleukin-6, and C-reactive protein) have been associated with insulin resistance.
- Insulin resistance results in ineffective glucose and fatty acid utilization leading to type 2 diabetes mellitus. Hyperinsulinemia and cytokines play an important role in development of abnormal lipid profile, hypertension, and vascular endothelial dysfunction, which can lead to the development of atherosclerotic cardiovascular disease.
- Accumulating evidence suggests that the cardiovascular and renal abnormalities associated with insulin resistance are mediated in part by aldosterone acting on the mineralocorticoid receptor

Dx DIAGNOSIS

DIFFERENTIAL DIAGNOSIS

- Other causes of weight gain or obesity (Cushing's syndrome, hypothyroidism)
- Other causes of hyperlipidemia (familial hyperlipidemia, hypothyroidism)
- Other causes of hypertension (Cushing's syndrome, hyperaldosteronism)
- Other forms of diabetes (type 1)

LABORATORY TESTS

- Fasting lipid profile (total cholesterol, low-density lipoprotein [LDL] cholesterol, HDL cholesterol, and triglyceride)
- Fasting glucose

Rx TREATMENT

NONPHARMACOLOGIC THERAPY

- Lifestyle modification:
  - Dietary modifications aimed at weight loss
  - Physical activity of moderate intensity (i.e., brisk walking): 30 min daily
  - Smoking cessation
- Consider bariatric surgery in the management of obesity:
  - Body mass index (BMI) ≥40 kg/m^2 in patients who have not responded to diet and exercise (with or without drug therapy).
  - Individuals with BMI >35 kg/m^2 and comorbidities (hypertension, impaired glucose tolerance, diabetes mellitus, dyslipidemia, sleep apnea) are also potential surgical candidates.

ACUTE GENERAL Rx

- Treat obesity (see "Obesity"): Pharmacologic treatment: consider sibutramine, orlistat, phentermine, diethylpropion, fluoxetine, and bupropion in individuals who have not responded to diet and exercise if BMI >30 kg/m^2 or a BMI of 27 to 30 kg/m^2 with comorbid conditions.
- Treat hypertension (see "Hypertension"): Systolic blood pressures >130/80 mm Hg: consider angiotensin-converting enzyme inhibitors or angiotensin II receptor blocker as first-line therapy.
- Treat hyperlipidemia:
  - Serum LDL cholesterol of <100 mg/dl (2.6 mmol/L) is recommended for secondary prevention (i.e., coronary artery disease [CAD] or CAD equivalent such as diabetes); however, recent studies suggest greater benefit with a more aggressive goal of <80 mg/dl (2.1 mmol/L). For primary prevention, an LDL goal <130 mg/dl (3.4 mmol/L) is recommended for individuals with more than two coronary heart disease risk factors. HMG-CoA reductase inhibitors (statins) are commonly used as first-line agents.
  - Patients with high triglycerides (>200 mg/dl) may benefit from fibric acid derivatives to achieve secondary non-HDL cholesterol target (LDL goal + 30).
- Treat diabetes:
  - Goal fasting blood glucose <100 mg/dl
  - Metformin as first-line therapy to improve insulin sensitivity
- Treat cardiovascular risk factors:
  - Consider aspirin.
  - Risk can be lowered with weight loss, exercise, smoking cessation, blood pressure control, diabetes management, and treatment of hyperlipidemia.

CHRONIC Rx

- Encourage lifestyle modification as above.
- Pharmacologic and surgical management to maintain therapeutic goals described above.

DISPOSITION

Weight loss can prevent disease progression. Appropriate treatment of obesity, hypertension, hyperlipidemia, and diabetes can improve morbidity and mortality rates.

REFERRAL

- To nutritionist for diet counseling
- To weight loss and exercise programs
- To endocrinologist if difficulty reaching therapeutic goals
- To bariatric surgeon if meets surgical criteria (as noted previously)

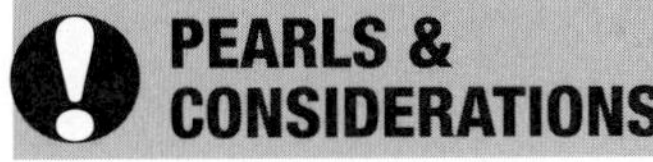

PEARLS & CONSIDERATIONS

PREVENTION

- Weight loss is essential to the prevention and treatment of metabolic syndrome.

- Recommend dietary modifications and moderate physical activity.
- Consider pharmacologic and surgical options in select individuals (as above).

PATIENT & FAMILY EDUCATION

- Weight reduction programs, including Weight Watchers, Curves, etc.
- American Diabetes Association: http://www.diabetes.org
- Polycystic Ovarian Syndrome Association: http://www.pcosupport.org
- The Hormone Foundation: http://www.hormone.org

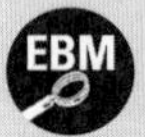

EVIDENCE

Please note: Complete text of EBM for this topic is available online.

Key trials and commentary:

The objective of this study was to compare the effects of two diets on cardiovascular disease risk factors in obese patients with the metabolic syndrome.

This study showed that tailoring diet interventions to the specific presentation of the metabolic syndrome may be the best way of reducing the risk factors for cardiovascular disease.[1] Ⓐ

Calorie-restricted diets are standard treatment for overweight and obese people. Weight loss is frequently associated with metabolic improvement and amelioration of the components of the metabolic syndrome. However, not all diets may have the same effect on the risk factors associated with the metabolic syndrome. This is shown in this article. In a single center trial, 100 obese people with the metabolic syndrome were randomly assigned to a diet with 65% of calories as carbohydrate or a diet with 48% carbohydrate. Both diets had a 500 kcal deficit. Both groups participated in aerobic activities. The study was completed in 5 months. At the end of the study, both groups showed improvement in all the components of the metabolic syndrome, but those on the lower carbohydrate intake had greater decrease in the prevalence of hypertension and hypertriglyceridemia.[1] Ⓐ

The study concluded that tailoring the composition of the diet to the specific presentation of the metabolic syndrome may be the best way of reducing the risk factors for cardiovascular disease. A more sophisticated approach in the future will be to define the metabolic profile of each individual and construct a diet that specifically focuses on each individual's needs.[1] Ⓐ

Clinical use of criteria for metabolic syndrome to simultaneously predict risk of cardiovascular disease and diabetes remains uncertain. One study investigated to what extent metabolic syndrome and its individual components were related to risk for these two diseases in elderly populations.

Metabolic syndrome and its components are associated with type 2 diabetes but have weak or no association with vascular risk in elderly populations, suggesting that attempts to define criteria that simultaneously predict risk for both cardiovascular disease and diabetes are unhelpful. Clinical focus should remain on establishing optimum risk algorithms for each disease.

The concept of the "metabolic syndrome" (i.e., the cluster of xxx) has received substantial attention over the past decades. In particular, this concept has improved our understanding of the interplay of obesity and insulin resistance with comorbidities like diabetes mellitus, arterial hypertension, and dyslipidemia. However, it is not clear whether the definition of the metabolic syndrome allows a prediction of clinical outcome parameters like cardiovascular disease or the manifestation of diabetes mellitus.

In the present report by Sattar et al, approximately 7500 patients were included consisting of two separate prospective studies (PROSPER and BRHS). Notably, the mean age of the patients at entry in the study was 75 years and 68 years, respectively. The patients were screened for components of the metabolic syndrome at the beginning of the study. The diagnosis of diabetes mellitus at the beginning of the study was an exclusion criterion. After follow-up of 3.2 years the authors found a strong correlation of the metabolic syndrome and its individual components (BMI, waist circumference, triglyceride levels, fasting glucose) with the onset of diabetes mellitus. However, the association with cardiovascular disease was only weak. The metabolic syndrome was not a better predictor of cardiovascular disease than the individual components, but predicted future diabetes better than the single components (except for the fasting blood glucose level) in elderly people. Similarly, previous studies showed inferiority of the metabolic to conventional risk scores like the Framingham risk score in predicting cardiovascular disease in middle-aged men. This might be explained by the inclusion of smoking as a major risk factor in conventional cardiovascular risk scores, but not in the metabolic syndrome.[2] Ⓐ

Therefore, the sum of the components defining the metabolic syndrome appears not to be a stronger predictor of cardiovascular events or the manifestation of diabetes mellitus than the individual components.

However, the major limitation of the study is the relatively short follow-up (3.2 years). Other studies with vascular end points pointed out that cardiovascular benefits might take time to develop (see UKPDS 10-year follow-up)

Evidence-Based References

1. Muzio F et al: Effects of moderate variations in the macronutrient content of the diet on cardiovascular disease risk factors in obese patients with the metabolic syndrome, *Am J Clin Nutr* 86:946-951, 2007. Commentary by D.E. Schteingart, M.D. Ⓐ

2. Sattar N et al: Can metabolic syndrome usefully predict cardiovascular disease and diabetes? Outcome data from two prospective studies, *Lancet* 371:1927-1935, 2008. Commentary by S. Schinner, M.D. Ⓐ

SUGGESTED READINGS

Garber A et al: American College of Endocrinology Consensus Statement on the Diagnosis and Management of Pre-Diabetes in the Continuum of Hyperglycemia—when do the risks of diabetes begin? ACE Task Force on the Prevention of Diabetes, *Endocr Pract* 14(7):933-946, 2008.

Genuth S et al: Follow-up report on the diagnosis of diabetes mellitus, *Diabetes Care* 26:3160, 2003.

Grundy SM et al: Definition of metabolic syndrome: report of the National Heart, Lung, and Blood Institute/American Heart Association conference on scientific issues related to definition, *Circulation* 109:433, 2004.

Grundy SM et al: Diagnosis and management of the metabolic syndrome: an American Heart Association/National Heart, Lung, and Blood Institute Scientific Statement, *Circulation* 112:2735, 2005.

Mozaffarian D et al: Metabolic syndrome and mortality in older adults, *Arch Intern Med* 168(9):969-978, 2008.

Park YW et al: The metabolic syndrome: prevalence and associated risk factor findings in the US population from the Third National Health and Nutrition Examination Survey, 1988. 1994, *Arch Intern Med* 163:427, 2003.

Pearson TA et al: AHA guidelines for primary prevention of cardiovascular disease and stroke 2002. Update: consensus panel guide to comprehensive risk reduction for adult patients without coronary or other atherosclerotic vascular diseases. American Heart Association Science Advisory and Coordinating Committee, *Circulation* 106:388, 2002.

Sowers JR et al: Narrative review: the emerging clinical implications of the role of aldosterone in the metabolic syndrome and resistant hypertension, *Ann Intern Med* 150:776-783, 2009

AUTHORS: **GEETHA GOPALAKRISHNAN, M.D.,** and **MICHAEL SCHAEFER, M.D.**

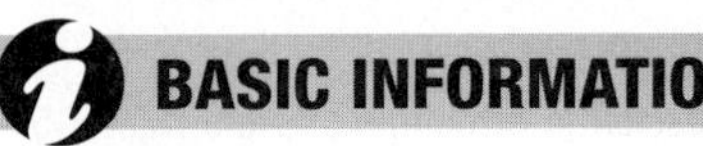

BASIC INFORMATION

DEFINITION

Metatarsalgia refers to pain of the metatarsus, especially of the metatarsophalangeal (MTP) articulation (Fig. 1-199). This is a nonspecific symptom usually involving the lesser toes.

ICD-9CM CODES
726.7 Metatarsalgia

PHYSICAL FINDINGS & CLINICAL PRESENTATION

- Pain beneath the metatarsal heads with ambulation
- Plantar callus formation beneath the metatarsal heads, usually involving one of the middle three toes
- Local tenderness
- Deformity
- Joint stiffness

ETIOLOGY

- Splayfoot
- Osteoarthritis, rheumatoid arthritis
- Freiberg's disease (avascular necrosis of second metatarsal head)
- Cavus foot (high arch)
- Bunion deformity
- Hallux rigidus
- MTP synovitis
- Morton's neuroma
- Often no obvious cause

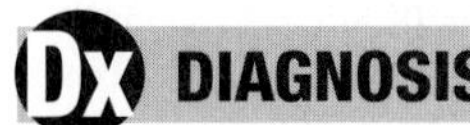

DIAGNOSIS

DIFFERENTIAL DIAGNOSIS

See "Etiology."

WORKUP

Underlying cause should always be sought.

LABORATORY TESTS

Rheumatoid factor may be required to rule out rheumatoid synovitis.

IMAGING STUDIES

- Plain radiography to determine presence or absence of joint disease or deformity
- MRI may be able to detect neuroma

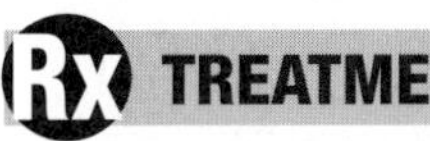

TREATMENT

NONPHARMACOLOGIC THERAPY

- Metatarsal bar or pad proximal to heads to redistribute weight
- Extra-depth shoe for contracture or deformity, if present
- Soft orthotic or well-padded liner to diffuse pressure around metatarsal heads
- Relief pads for plantar keratoses
- Soaks and pumice stone abrasion to decrease callus volume
- Rocker bottom shoe for resistant cases

CHRONIC Rx

- Nonsteroidal antiinflammatory drugs
- Intraarticular injection in selected cases with joint involvement

DISPOSITION

Prognosis is variable depending on etiology.

REFERRAL

Failure to respond to medical management

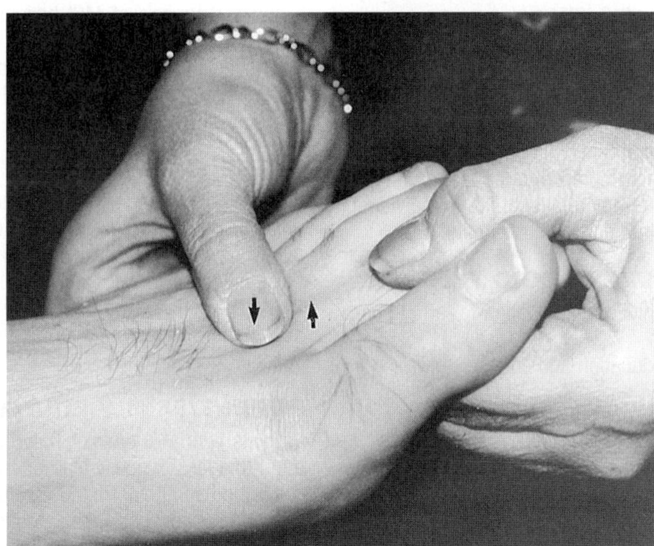

FIGURE 1-199 Vertical stress test for metatarsophalangeal stability. One of the examiner's hands stabilizes the metatarsal head while the other grasps the proximal phalanx. Examiner attempts to displace the proximal phalanx dorsally. A positive test result is the ability to displace dorsally while reproducing symptoms. (From Scuderi G [ed]: *Sports medicine: principles of primary care,* St Louis, 1997, Mosby.)

SUGGESTED READINGS

Espinosa N et al: Current concept review: metatarsalgia, *Foot Ankle Int* 29:871, 2008.

Fuhrmann RA et al: Metatarsalgia: differential diagnosis and therapeutic algorithm, *Orthoade* 34(8):767, 2005.

Gorter K et al: Variation in diagnosis and management of common foot problems by GPs, *Fam Pract* 18(6): 569, 2001.

Hassouna H, Singh D: Morton's metatarsalgia: pathogenesis, aetology and current management, *Acta Orthop Belg* 71(6):43, 2005.

Janisse DJ, Janisse E: Shoe modification and the use of orthotics in the treatment of foot and ankle pathology, *J Am Acad Orthop Surg* 16:152, 2008.

Jarboe NE, Quesada PM: The effects of cycling shoe stiffness on forefoot pressure, *Foot Ankle Int* 24: 784, 2003.

Ko PH et al: Relationship between plantar pressure and soft tissue strain under metatarsal heads with different heel heights, *Foot Ankle Int* 30:1111, 2009.

Latinovic R et al: Incidence of common compression neuropathies in primary care, *J Neurol Neurosurg Psychiatry* 77(2):263, 2006.

Morscher E et al: Morton's intermetatarsal neuroma: morphology and histological substrate, *Foot Ankle Int* 21(7):558, 2000.

Sherry DD, Sapp LR: Enthesalgia in childhood, *J Rheumatol* 30:1335, 2003.

Smith BW, Coughlin MJ: Disorders of the lesser toes, *Sports Med Arthrosc* 17:167, 2009.

Waldecker U: Metatarsalgia in hallux valgus deformity: a pedographic analysis, *J Foot Ankle Surg* 41(5): 300, 2002.

Yu JS, Tanner JR: Considerations in metatarsalgia and midfoot pain: an MR imaging perspective, *Semin Musculoskelet Radiol* 6(2):91, 2002.

AUTHOR: **LONNIE R. MERCIER, M.D.**

Mild Cognitive Impairment

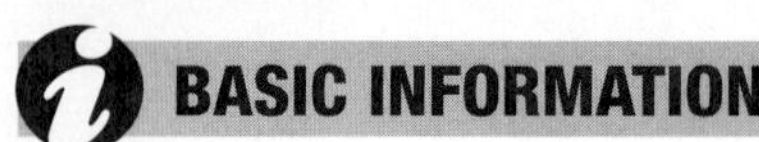

BASIC INFORMATION

DEFINITION

Significant cognitive impairment in the absence of dementia with preserved activities of daily living

SYNONYMS

Minimal dementia
Isolated memory impairment
Cognitive impairment not dementia (CIND)
Predementia

ICD-9CM CODES
331.83 Mild cognitive impairment, so stated

EPIDEMIOLOGY & DEMOGRAPHICS

INCIDENCE:
- 12 to 15/1000 person-year age ≥65
- 54/1000 person-years age ≥75

PREVALENCE: 5% to 25% among community dwelling
PREDOMINANT SEX AND AGE: male, age ≥75
PEAK INCIDENCE: in the elderly
RISK FACTORS: male sex, age, lower socioeconomic status, lower educational level
GENETICS: APOE4 genotype: Various pathways result in amyloid accumulation and deposition.

PHYSICAL FINDINGS & CLINICAL PRESENTATION

- Subjective memory problems, preferably corroborated by another person
- Preserved functional status (ADLs)
- Normal general thinking and reasoning skills
- Subtypes of mild cognitive impairment (MCI): include amnestic versus nonamnestic with involvement of single domain versus multiple domains
- Domains affected in MCI include: memory, visuospatial skills, language, attention, and executive function

ETIOLOGY

Neurodegenerative, vascular, traumatic, depression, or due to underlying medical condition

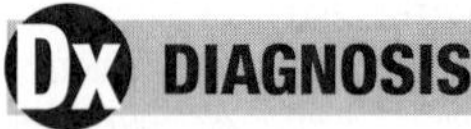

DIAGNOSIS

DIFFERENTIAL DIAGNOSIS

- Delirium
- Dementia
- Depression
- "Reversible" cognitive impairment:
  - Medication related (anticholinergics)
  - Hypothyroidism
  - Vitamin B_{12} deficiency
- Reversible CNS conditions
  - Subdural hematoma
  - Normal pressure hydrocephalus
  - Metastatic disease

WORKUP

History
- Focus on cognitive deficits and impairment
- Review all medications that may impact cognition (i.e. anticholinergics)
- Rule out depression
- Perform functional assessment

Physical exam
- Check blood pressure
- Neurologic exam to rule out reversible CNS causes of cognitive impairment

Cognitive function testing: brief mental status testing using mini-cog, MMSE (Mini-Mental Status Exam), or MOCA (Montreal Cognitive Assessment) for office screening followed by neuropsychological testing if appropriate for specific deficits in cognitive domains

LABORATORY TESTS

- Complete blood count
- Comprehensive metabolic profile
- Thyroid-stimulating hormone (TSH)
- Vitamin B_{12}
- Lipids

IMAGING STUDIES

- CT imaging can detect most reversible CNS conditions leading to cognitive impairment.
- MRI further evaluates vascular, infectious, neoplastic, and inflammatory conditions.

Rx TREATMENT

- There is insufficient evidence to recommend use of cholinesterase inhibitors (Table 1-50) for MCI.
- Consider treatment with these medications only if memory complaints appear to be affecting day-to-day quality of life in individual patients or in amnestic subtypes of MCI.

NONPHARMACOLOGIC THERAPY

- Role of cognitive rehabilitation to target specific deficits
- Caregiver education and counseling

COMPLEMENTARY & ALTERNATIVE MEDICINE

No clear indications for antioxidants, and studies in humans are inconclusive.

DISPOSITION

- Progression to Alzheimer's at the rate of 5% to 15% per year: risk factors for progression to dementia include presence of vascular risk factors, significant cognitive impairment, depression, and presence of extrapyramidal signs.
- Mortality of those with MCI is twice that of those without.
- Twofold to threefold increase in risk of nursing home placement in those with MCI.

REFERRAL

Consider referral to a memory specialist if more than just memory is involved or for further evaluation of specific deficits.

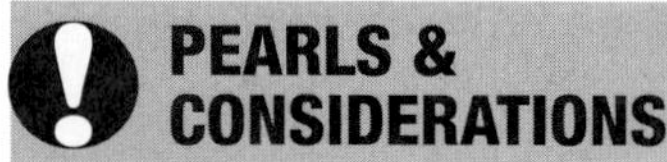

PEARLS & CONSIDERATIONS

COMMENTS

- Patients with MCI usually report short-term memory concerns such as misplacing things, not remembering names of people, or not being able to follow a conversation.
- MCI becomes clinically relevant when quality of life is affected such as problems making financial decisions and problems with personal day-to-day interactions.
- Depression should be ruled out prior to making a diagnosis of MCI because it is highly prevalent in the elderly.
- Anticholinergic medication use should be evaluated carefully prior to making a diagnosis of MCI.

PREVENTION

Patients with MCI should be counseled on strategies to prevent progression to dementia. They should remain physically and mentally active, have a well-balanced diet, continue activities that are socially engaging, reduce stress in their lives, and aggressively pursue treatment of vascular risk factors.

PATIENT/FAMILY EDUCATION

Patients with MCI typically have poor retention and rapid loss of newly learned information.

For additional information for patients, families, and clinicians: Alzheimer's Association (www.alzheimers.org)

TABLE 1-50 Characteristics and Properties of Cholinesterase Inhibitors

Drug Name	Starting Dose	Maintenance Dose	Serum Half-life	Taken With Food?	Elimination
Donepezil	5 mg	10 mg	70 hr	+/−	Hepatic
Rivastigmine pill	1.5 mg bid	6 mg bid	2-8 hr	+	Hepatic
Rivastigmine patch	4.6 mg/24 hr	9.5 mg/24 hr	n/a	n/a	Hepatic
Galantamine	4 mg bid or 8 mg SA daily	12 mg bid or 24 mg SA daily	6-8 hr	+	Hepatic and renal

Adapted from *Physicians' desk reference*, ed 62, Montvale, New Jersey, 2008, Thomson PDR.

EBM EVIDENCE

There is insufficient evidence to recommend cholinesterase inhibitors in all cases of mild cognitive impairment.[1]

Consider use of cholinesterase inhibitors if memory complaints or multiple domains affect day-to-day functioning.[2]

Evidence-Based References

1. Birks J et al: Donepezil for mild cognitive impairment, *Cochrane Database Syst Rev* 3:CD006104, 2006.

2. Petersen RC et al: Vitamin E and donepezil for the treatment of mild cognitive impairment, *N Engl J Med* 352:2379-2388, 2005.

SUGGESTED READINGS

Joshi S, Morley JE: Cognitive impairment, *Med Clin North Am* 90:769-787, 2006.

Kelley BJ, Petersen RC: Alzheimer's disease and mild cognitive impairment, *Neurol Clin* 25:577-609, 2007.

Kelley RE, Minagar A: Memory complaints and dementia, *Med Clin North Am* 93:389-406, 2009.

AUTHORS: **BIRJU B. PATEL, M.D., F.A.C.P.,** and **N. WILSON HOLLAND, M.D., F.A.C.P.**

Milk-Alkali Syndrome

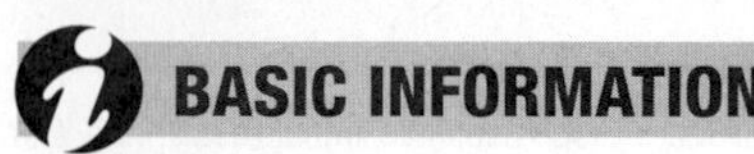

BASIC INFORMATION

DEFINITION

Milk-alkali syndrome is the consumption of large amounts of calcium and alkali, resulting in the triad of hypercalcemia, metabolic alkalosis, and renal insufficiency.

SYNONYMS

Burnett's syndrome (acute form)
Cope's syndrome (subacute form)

ICD-9CM CODES
275.42 Milk-alkali syndrome

EPIDEMIOLOGY & DEMOGRAPHICS

In the early 20th century the milk-alkali syndrome was associated with an antacid regimen created by F.W. Sippy that included large amounts of calcium and bicarbonate. With the development of more effective and less toxic treatments, the syndrome virtually disappeared. Since the 1980s, however, there has been a small resurgence associated with use of calcium-containing products for the prevention of osteoporosis and the use of calcium bicarbonate rather than aluminum bicarbonate in patients with chronic renal failure. More recently, the milk-alkali syndrome was found to be the third leading cause of hypercalcemia (12%) in a review of hypercalcemia in hospitalized patients from 1990 to 1993.

PHYSICAL FINDINGS & CLINICAL PRESENTATION

- Asymptomatic hypercalcemia:
  - Less than half of cases are detected by an incidental finding of hypercalcemia and occasionally renal failure.
- Symptomatic hypercalcemia:
  - Symptoms: nausea, vomiting, anorexia, fatigue, vague abdominal pain, nephrolithiasis- and pancreatitis-related pain, constipation, myalgia, confusion, and psychosis. In more chronic cases polyuria and polydipsia may be reported.
  - Physical examination and further testing: mental status changes such as anxiety, depression, and cognitive dysfunction; shortened QT interval.

ETIOLOGY

Overconsumption of supplemental calcium bicarbonate with reported ranges of 2.5 to 20 g/day, particularly when associated with volume depletion, renal insufficiency, or use of hydrochlorothiazide or calcium-containing substances.

Betel nut chewing, a practice in Asia and the South Pacific, has been associated with a milk-alkali syndrome. Betel nuts are prepared with a compound that can be converted to calcium carbonate.

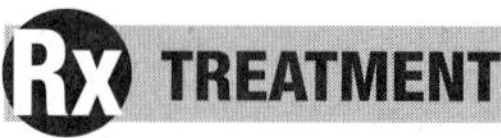

DIAGNOSIS

DIFFERENTIAL DIAGNOSIS

Hypercalcemia secondary to hyperparathyroidism or malignancy

LABORATORY TESTS

- Elevated plasma calcium (wide variation reported).
- Renal insufficiency.
- Elevated plasma bicarbonate and arterial pH, metabolic alkalosis.
- Parathyroid hormone, which is usually suppressed with milk-alkali syndrome, may be elevated, particularly if checked after treatment has begun.
- Phosphate level is variable.

Rx TREATMENT

NONPHARMACOLOGIC THERAPY

Hemodialysis has been indicated for some patients with significant renal failure.

ACUTE GENERAL Rx

- Discontinuation of calcium bicarbonate supplements.
- Aggressive hydration and furosemide if symptomatic hypercalcemia.
- Monitor for rebound hypocalcemia as a result of elevation of parathyroid hormone with treatment.
- Patient education regarding appropriate calcium supplementation. Standard over-the-counter calcium supplements and some antacids contain calcium carbonate.

PROGNOSIS

Hypercalcemia and symptoms resolve with withdrawal of excess calcium supplementation and treatment of hypercalcemia. Acute cases typically resolve in 1 to 2 days while chronic cases will take longer. Patients initially presenting with renal failure may have residual renal insufficiency.

DISPOSITION

Treatment is determined by degree of hypercalcemia and symptoms. Hospital admission is required for patients who require IV hydration and other intensive treatments for hypercalcemia.

REFERRAL

Differentiation from hyperparathyroidism can be difficult and may require the assistance of an endocrinologist. Referral to a nutritionist is generally not required because the excess calcium is from nutritional supplements rather than dietary factors.

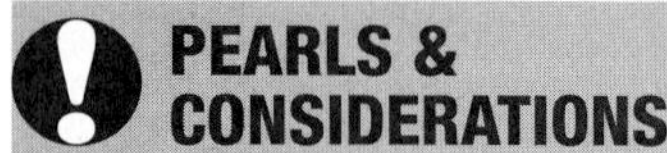

PEARLS & CONSIDERATIONS

COMMENTS

Detailed history of dietary supplements and over-the-counter medications can provide the most important clues. Many patients do not list dietary supplements as a medication.

SUGGESTED READINGS

Abreo K et al: The milk-alkali syndrome: a reversible form of acute renal failure, *Arch Intern Med* 153:1005, 1993.

Beall DP et al: Milk-alkali syndrome: a historical review and description of the modern version of the syndrome, *Am J Med Sci* 331(5):233, 2006.

Medarov B: Milk-alkali syndrome, *Mayo Clin Proc* 84(3):261-267, 2009.

Picolos MK et al: Milk-alkali syndrome is a major cause of hypercalcaemia among non-end-stage renal disease (non-ESRD) inpatients, *Clin Endocrinol* 63(5):566, 2005.

Sippy BW: Gastric and duodenal ulcer: medical cure by an efficient removal of gastric juice corrosion, *JAMA* 64:1625, 1915.

AUTHOR: **MICHELLE STOZEK ANVAR, M.D.**

BASIC INFORMATION

DEFINITION

Mitral regurgitation (MR) is retrograde blood flow into the left atrium resulting from an incompetent mitral valve. This condition can lead to left ventricular (LV) failure as well as increased left atrial and pulmonary pressures, with consequent right heart failure.

SYNONYMS

Mitral insufficiency
MR

ICD-9CM CODES

424.0 Mitral regurgitation

EPIDEMIOLOGY & DEMOGRAPHICS

The incidence of MR has increased over the past 30 yr; however, this may be due to increasing availability of echocardiography and MR diagnosis rather than any real increases in this condition.

PHYSICAL FINDINGS & CLINICAL PRESENTATION

- Many patients with mild to moderate MR will remain asymptomatic and without evidence of hemodynamic compromise for years.
- Symptomatic patients with MR generally present with the following:
  - Symptoms suggestive of heart failure (fatigue, dyspnea, orthopnea, paroxysmal nocturnal dyspnea, edema)
  - Hemoptysis (caused by pulmonary hypertension)
  - Atrial fibrillation
- Hyperdynamic apex, sometimes with palpable LV lift and apical thrill.
- Holosystolic, high-pitched, "blowing" murmur at apex with radiation to base, left axilla, or back; there is a poor correlation between the intensity of the systolic murmur and the degree of regurgitation.
- Apical early diastolic to mid-diastolic rumble suggest severe MR.

ETIOLOGY

- Idiopathic myxomatous degeneration of the mitral valve
- Papillary muscle dysfunction or rupture (as a result of ischemic heart disease)
- Ruptured chordae tendineae
- Infective endocarditis
- Calcified mitral valve annulus
- LV dilation (e.g., secondary to dilated cardiomyopathy)
- Rheumatic valvulitis
- Primary or secondary mitral valve prolapse
- Hypertrophic cardiomyopathy
- Systemic lupus erythematosus (Libman-Sacks endocarditis)
- Fenfluramine, dexfenfluramine, pergolide, cabergoline

DIAGNOSIS

DIFFERENTIAL DIAGNOSIS

- Hypertrophic cardiomyopathy
- Tricuspid regurgitation
- Aortic stenosis
- Aortic sclerosis
- Ventricular septal defect
- Atrial septal defect

WORKUP

Diagnostic workup consists of echocardiography, ECG, and chest radiograph; cardiac catheterization sometimes needed to confirm severity of the disease.

IMAGING STUDIES

- Echocardiography: dilated left atrium, hyperdynamic left ventricle (erratic motion of the leaflet is seen in patients with ruptured chordae tendineae); color flow Doppler will show evidence of MR. The most important aspect of the echocardiographic examination is the quantification of the severity of MR, LV systolic performance, and estimated right ventricular (RV) systolic pressure.
- Chest x-ray:
  - Left atrial enlargement (usually more pronounced in mitral stenosis)
  - LV enlargement
  - Possible pulmonary congestion, though most often normal.
- ECG:
  - Left atrial enlargement
  - LV hypertrophy
  - Atrial fibrillation
- Cardiac catheterization: to confirm severity of MR, or to rule out presence of coronary artery disease in patients being evaluated for surgical replacement

TREATMENT

NONPHARMACOLOGIC THERAPY

Salt restriction

ACUTE GENERAL Rx

- Medical: medical therapy is primarily directed toward treatment of the source or its complications (e.g., atrial fibrillation, ischemic heart disease, infective endocarditis and heart failure).
  - The utility of afterload reduction (to decrease the regurgitant fraction and to increase cardiac output) depends upon the etiology of MR and the administration of afterload reducers. In the acute setting, intravenous nitroprusside has shown some utility. Long term use of oral afterload reducers (such as ACE inhibitors or angiotensin receptor blockers [ARBs]) has shown mixed results in small studies but may be given if another indication for their use exists (hypertension, LV dysfunction, diabetes).
  - Control ventricular response only if atrial fibrillation with rapid ventricular response is present.
  - Anticoagulants if atrial fibrillation occurs.
- Surgery: surgery is the only definitive treatment for MR. Transesophageal echocardiography allows accurate assessment of the feasibility of valve repair and is indicated before surgical intervention. The timing of surgical repair is controversial; surgery should generally be considered early in symptomatic patients despite optimal medical therapy and in patients with moderate to severe MR and minimal symptoms if there is echocardiographic evidence of rapidly progressive increase in LV end-diastolic or end-systolic dimension (end-systolic dimension $\geq$40 mm, end-diastolic dimension $\geq$50 mm or LV ejection fraction $<$0.6). Surgery is also indicated in asymptomatic patients with preserved ventricular function if there is a high likelihood of valve repair or if there is evidence of pulmonary hypertension ($\geq$50 mm Hg at rest or $\geq$60 mm Hg during exercise) or recent atrial fibrillation. Quantitative grading of MR is a powerful predictor of the clinical outcome of asymptomatic mitral regurgitation. In general, patients with regurgitant orifice areas of $>$40 mm^2 should be considered for prompt surgery, whereas those with orifices between 20 and 39 mm^2 can be followed closely.

DISPOSITION

Prognosis is generally good unless there is significant impairment of left ventricle or significantly elevated pulmonary artery pressures. Most patients remain asymptomatic for many years (average interval from diagnosis to onset of symptoms is 16 yr).

REFERRAL

Surgical referral in selected patients (see "Acute General Rx"); emergency surgery may be necessary in patients with MR caused by ruptured chordae tendineae after myocardial infarction.

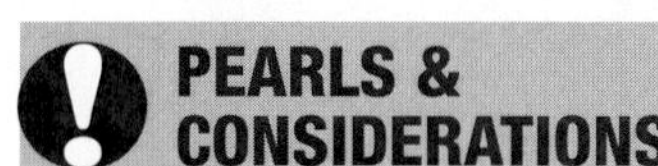

PEARLS & CONSIDERATIONS

COMMENTS

Patients should be counseled regarding weight reduction (if obese), avoidance of tobacco, and maintenance of normal (nonstrenuous) activities.

In 2007, the AHA guidelines for prevention of infectious endocarditis were revised and routine antibiotic prophylaxis to undergo dental or other invasive procedures is no longer recommended, unless the patient has prior endocarditis.

Evidence-Based References

1. Bonow RO et al: 2008 Focused update incorporated into the ACC/AHA guidelines for the management of patients with valvular heart disease, *J Am Coll Cardiol* 52:e1, 2008. Ⓐ

2. Wilson W et al: Prevention of infective endocarditis: a guideline from the American Heart Association, *Circulation* 116:1736, 2007. Ⓐ

3. Salem DN et al: Antithrombotic therapy in valvular heart disease—native and prosthetic: the Seventh ACCP Conference on Antithrombotic and Thrombolytic Therapy, *Chest* 126(3 Suppl):457S, 2004. Ⓐ

SUGGESTED READINGS

Enriquez-Sarano M et al: Quantitative determinants of the outcome of asymptomatic mitral regurgitation, *N Engl J Med* 352:875, 2005.

Otto CM, Salerno CT: Timing of surgery in asymptomatic mitral regurgitation, *N Engl J Med* 352:928, 2005.

AUTHORS: **ANTHONY S. GEMIGNANI, M.D., FRED F. FERRI, M.D.,** and **WEN-CHIH WU M.D., M.P.H.**

BASIC INFORMATION

DEFINITION

Mitral stenosis is a narrowing of the mitral valve orifice. The cross-section of a normal orifice measures 4 to 6 cm^2. A murmur becomes audible when the valve orifice becomes <2 cm^2. When the orifice approaches 1 cm^2, the condition becomes critical and symptoms become more evident.

SYNONYMS

MS

ICD-9CM CODES

394.0 Mitral stenosis

EPIDEMIOLOGY & DEMOGRAPHICS

- The occurrence of mitral valve stenosis has decreased worldwide over the past 30 yr (particularly in developed countries) as a result of declining incidence of rheumatic fever.
- The incidence of MS is higher in women.

PHYSICAL FINDINGS & CLINICAL PRESENTATION

- Dyspnea is the most common symptom along with fatigue and decreased exercise capacity. These occur secondary to an inability to increase cardiac output and elevated pulmonary capillary pressures.
- Paroxysmal nocturnal dyspnea (PND) and orthopnea secondary to elevated left atrial pressure may occur.
- Acute pulmonary edema may occur after an increase in flow across the mitral valve secondary to an increase in cardiac output or heart rate (exertion, tachyarrhythmias, fever).
- Pulmonary hypertension can lead to right ventricular (RV) dysfunction and signs and symptoms of right heart failure (hepatomegaly, pulsatile liver, peripheral edema, ascites).
- Hemoptysis can be present secondary to pulmonary capillary vessel rupture or pulmonary vascular congestion.
- Systemic embolic events are caused by left atrial thrombi. These are associated with atrial fibrillation 80% of the time.
- Chest pain can be caused by RV pressure overload and/or concomitant coronary artery disease in up to 15% of patients.
- Irregularly irregular pulse caused by atrial fibrillation.
- Signs of left and subsequently right heart failure.
- Loud first heart sound (S_1) caused by delayed valve closure and rapid rising left ventricular (LV) pressure.
- A low pitched, rumbling diastolic murmur heard best at the apex. The intensity of the murmur is not related to the severity of the stenosis, but the duration is holodiastolic in severe MS.
- An opening snap (OS) caused by tensing of the valve leaflets after the cusps have opened completely. The OS follows S_2 by 0.03 to 0.14 seconds and the shorter the S_2-OS interval, the more severe the MS, due to higher left atrial pressures.
- Prominent A wave on the venous pulse of patients in normal sinus rhythm.
- A diastolic thrill may be palpable at the apex, especially with the patient in the left lateral recumbent position.
- An RV lift may be palpable at the left sternal border secondary RV hypertrophy and pulmonary hypertension.
- An accentuated P_2 and/or a soft, early diastolic decrescendo murmur (Graham Steell murmur) caused by pulmonary regurgitation may be present in patients with pulmonary hypertension.

ETIOLOGY

- Rheumatic fever (RF) is the predominant cause of MS. Besides the mitral valve, it can affect the aortic, tricuspid, and pulmonary valves in descending order of frequency. RF causes thickening of the leaflet edges, commissure fusion, and chordal shortening and fusion.
- Congenital defect (parachute valve) has the usual two mitral leaflets, but the chordae, instead of diverging to insert into two papillary muscles, converge into one major papillary muscle, which allows little mobility of the leaflets.
- Rare causes are endomyocardial fibroelastosis, malignant carcinoid syndrome, systemic lupus erythematosus, Whipple disease and Fabry disease.

DIAGNOSIS

DIFFERENTIAL DIAGNOSIS

- Left atrial myxoma
- Other valvular abnormalities (e.g., tricuspid stenosis, mitral regurgitation)
- Atrial septal defect

WORKUP

Physical examination and echocardiography

IMAGING STUDIES

- Echocardiography:
  - The characteristic finding on echocardiogram is a markedly diminished E to F slope of the anterior mitral valve leaflet during diastole; there is also fusion of the commissures, resulting in "doming" of the leaflets during diastole.
  - Two-dimensional echocardiogram can measure valve area by direct planimetry or calculate it by Doppler pressure half-time method. The transmitral gradient can also be calculated.
  - Grading of leaflet thickness, mobility, calcification and chordal involvement with a score of 0 to 4 for each characteristic can predict hemodynamic results and outcome of balloon mitral valvuloplasty (a low score of less than 8 is favorable for angioplasty and a high score is unfavorable).
- Chest radiograph:
  - Straightening of the left cardiac border caused by dilated left atrium
  - Left atrial enlargement on lateral chest radiograph
  - Prominence of pulmonary arteries
  - Possible pulmonary congestion and edema (Kerley B lines)
- ECG:
  - RV hypertrophy; right axis deviation caused by pulmonary hypertension
  - Left atrial enlargement (broad, notched P waves)
  - Atrial fibrillation
- Cardiac catheterization:
  - Allows the measurement of transmitral pressure gradient.
  - Allows the measurement of transmitral flow and calculation of the valve area.
  - Is not routinely recommended for the evaluation of MS but is useful when the echocardiographic findings are nondiagnostic or discrepant with the clinical scenario.

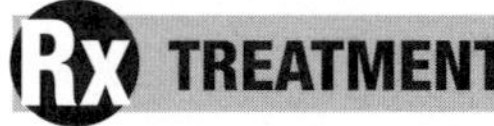

TREATMENT

NONPHARMACOLOGIC THERAPY

Decrease level of activity in symptomatic patients

ACUTE GENERAL Rx

- Medical:
  - Antibiotic prophylaxis to prevent recurrent rheumatic fever is usually not indicated unless presence of high-risk features such as prior endocarditis, prosthetic heart valves, valvulopathy of the transplanted heart, and certain cases of cyanotic congenital heart disease.
  - Anticoagulation for the prevention of systemic embolic events in patients with MS and:
    1. Atrial fibrillation
    2. Prior embolic event
    3. Documented left atrial thrombus
    4. Severe left atrial enlargement and spontaneous echo contrast indicating stagnant blood flow (class 2b indication).
  - Ventricular rate control with beta blockers, calcium channel blockers or digitalis and aggressive treatment of tachyarrhythmias.
  - Treat congestive heart failure with diuretics and sodium restriction.
- Percutaneous balloon mitral valvotomy (BMV) is the therapy of choice for symptomatic patients with moderate to severe MS (valve area <1.5 cm^2) with a favorable valve score, minimal or no mitral regurgitation and no left atrial thrombus. Balloon valvotomy is also indicated in asymptomatic patients with moderate to severe MS that has resulted in pulmonary artery pressures of 50 mm Hg at rest or 60 mm Hg with exercise. In addition, it is a reasonable option for patients who are at high risk for surgery even when their valve morphology is not ideal (class 2a indication).

 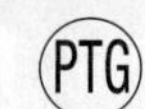

- Surgical intervention is indicated for patients with moderate to severe symptomatic MS when BMV is not available, contraindicated or the valve is calcified and the surgical risk is acceptable. The surgical approaches include closed mitral valvotomy, open valvotomy and repair (preferred) and mitral valve replacement.

DISPOSITION

- Prognosis is generally good except in patients with chronic pulmonary hypertension.
- Operative mortality rates for mitral valve replacement are 1% to 5% at most institutions.

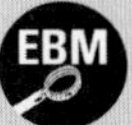

EVIDENCE

Overall, 80% to 95% of patients with MS may have a successful procedure with balloon valvotomy, and overall event-free survival is 90% over 5 to 7 yr. Event-free survival is 80% to 90% for patients with favorable valve morphology.[1,2]

Evidence-Based References

1. Bonow RO et al: Focused update incorporated into the ACC/AHA guidelines for the management of patients with valvular heart disease: a report of the American College of Cardiology/American Heart Association Task Force on Practice Guidelines, *J Am Coll Cardiol* 52:e1-142, 2008.

2. Masakiyo N et al: Percutaneous balloon mitral valvuloplasty: a review, *Circulation* 119:e211-219, 2008.

AUTHORS: **ROBERTO PACHECO, M.D., FRED F. FERRI, M.D.** and **WEN-CHIH WU, M.D.**

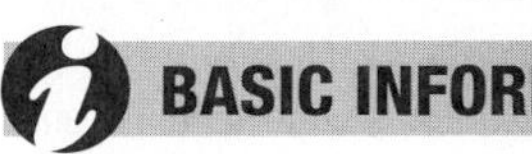

BASIC INFORMATION

DEFINITION

Mitral valve prolapse (MVP) is the bulging of one or both of the mitral valve leaflets into the left atrium during systole. MVP syndrome refers to a constellation of MVP and associated symptoms (e.g., autonomic dysfunction, palpitations) or other physical abnormalities (e.g., pectus excavatum).

SYNONYMS

MVP
Mitral click murmur syndrome

ICD-9CM CODES
424.0 Mitral valve disorders
394.9 Other and unspecified mitral valve diseases

EPIDEMIOLOGY & DEMOGRAPHICS

- MVP can be found by two-dimensional echocardiogram in 1% to 4% of the general population (females more often than males).
- Increased incidence is seen with autoimmune thyroid disorders, Ehlers-Danlos syndrome, Marfan's syndrome, pseudoxanthoma elasticum, pectus excavatum, anorexia nervosa, and bulimia.
- Compared to men, women with MVP have less posterior prolapse (22% vs. 31%), less flail (2% vs. 8%), more leaflet thickening (32% vs. 28%), and less frequent severe regurgitation (10% vs. 23%).
- Although MVP is more common in women than men, men more often develop severe regurgitation requiring surgical intervention.

PHYSICAL FINDINGS & CLINICAL PRESENTATION

- Usually, young female patient with narrow anteroposterior chest diameter, low body weight, low blood pressure
- Mid to late systolic click, heard best at the apex
- Crescendo mid to late systolic murmur, may have a "honking" quality
- Timing of click within the cardiac cycle varies with loading conditions within the left ventricle (i.e., may occur earlier with standing or Valsalva and later with squatting or expiration)
- Most patients with MVP are asymptomatic; symptoms (if present) consist primarily of chest pain and palpitations
- Neurologic abnormalities (e.g., transient ischemic attack [TIA] or stroke) rare
- Patients may also complain of anxiety, fatigue, and dyspnea

ETIOLOGY

- Myxomatous degeneration of connective tissue within mitral valve
- Congenital deformity of mitral valve and supportive structures
- Secondary to other disorders of connective tissue such as Ehlers-Danlos, Marfan, or pseudoxanthoma elasticum; association with other connective tissue disorders suggests MVP result of defective embryogenesis in cells of mesenchymal origin

Dx DIAGNOSIS

DIFFERENTIAL DIAGNOSIS

- Other valvular abnormalities (especially mitral regurgitation [MR])
- Anxiety/panic disorders
- Pulmonary embolism
- Atypical chest pain

WORKUP

- Medical history and physical examination, with increased suspicion in patients with other findings of connective tissue disorder.
- Workup consists primarily of echocardiography in patients with a systolic click or murmur on careful auscultation.
- ECG is most often normal but may show nonspecific ST-T wave changes, prolonged QT interval or prominent Q waves.

IMAGING STUDIES

Echocardiography shows one or more leaflet prolapsing at least 2 mm into the left atrium during systole. Mitral leaflets may be thickened (>5 mm). MR may or may not be present, and sometimes it is only present during exertion. If moderate or severe MR is present, findings of dilated left atrium, LV dilation and/or dysfunction, and elevated estimated RV systolic pressures may also be present. There is an increased incidence of secundum-type atrial septal defects (ASDs) in patients with MVP, which may also be identified with echocardiography.

Rx TREATMENT

NONPHARMACOLOGIC THERAPY

Avoidance of stimulants (e.g., caffeine, nicotine) in patients with palpitations

ACUTE GENERAL Rx

β-blockers may be tried in symptomatic patients (e.g., palpitations, chest pain); they decrease the heart rate and contractility, thus potentially decreasing the stretch on the prolapsing valve leaflets.

CHRONIC Rx

Monitoring for complications:

- Bacterial endocarditis (risk is three to eight times that of the general population)
- TIA or stroke caused by embolic phenomena (from fibrin and platelet thrombi) in patients with thickened leaflets; risk in young patients is <0.05% per year, if present aspirin (75-325 mg) is indicated for secondary prevention
- Cardiac arrhythmias (the vast majority are supraventricular and benign)
- Sudden death (rare occurrence, most often caused by ventricular arrhythmias associated with other structural heart disease)
- MR (most common complication of MVP, on rare occasion may occur acutely due to rupture of chordae tendineae)

DISPOSITION

The incidence of complications of MVP is very low (<1% per year) and generally associated with an increase in mitral leaflet thickness to >5 mm; young patients (age <45 yr) with absence of mitral systolic murmur or MR on Doppler echocardiography are at low risk for any complications.

REFERRAL

Surgical referral may be necessary in patients who develop progressive MR with surgical indications as per guidelines for valvular heart disease (see chapter on MR).

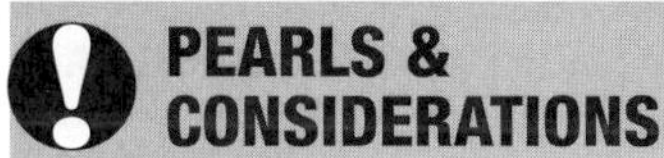

PEARLS & CONSIDERATIONS

COMMENTS

- Recent studies suggest that the prevalence of MVP and its propensity to cause symptoms and serious complications have been overestimated in the past.
- Asymptomatic patients with MVP and mild or no MR can be evaluated clinically every 3 to 5 yr. High-risk patients (those with symptoms, arrhythmias, or significant regurgitation) should undergo a follow-up examination once a year.
- Among patients with severe regurgitation, women have higher mortality and lower surgery rates than men.
- In 2007, the AHA guidelines for prevention of infectious endocarditis were revised and prophylactic antibiotics are no longer recommended for patients with MVP without previous endocarditis.

SUGGESTED READINGS

Avierinos JF et al: Sex differences in morphology and outcomes of mitral valve prolapse, *Ann Intern Med* 149:787-795, 2008.

Bonow RO et al: 2008 focused update incorporated into the ACC/AHA guidelines for the management of patients with valvular heart disease, *J Am Coll Cardiol* 52:e1, 2008.

Verma S, Mesana TG: Mitral-valve repair for mitral valve prolapse, *N Engl J Med* 361:2261-2269, 2009.

Wilson W et al: Prevention of infective endocarditis: a guideline from the American Heart Association, *Circulation* 116:1736, 2007.

AUTHORS: **ANTHONY S. GEMIGNANI, M.D., FRED F. FERRI, M.D.,** and **WEN-CHIH WU, M.D., M.P.H.**

Mixed Connective Tissue Disease

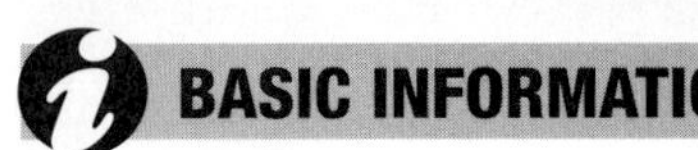

BASIC INFORMATION

DEFINITION

The term *mixed connective tissue disease* (MCTD) describes a set of connective tissue symptoms that sometimes overlap with other known connective tissue diseases (systemic lupus erythematosus [SLE], progressive systemic sclerosis, polymyositis) but whose exact significance remains under debate. The disorder is sometimes referred to as an "overlap syndrome," but many prefer the term *undifferentiated connective tissue disease.*

ICD-9CM CODES
710.9 Diffuse connective tissue disease

EPIDEMIOLOGY & DEMOGRAPHICS

PREVALENCE: Approximately 10 to 15 cases per 100,000 persons
PREDOMINANT SEX: Female/male ratio of 8:1
PREDOMINANT AGE: 4 to 80 yr

PHYSICAL FINDINGS & CLINICAL PRESENTATION

- Polyarthritis, polyarthralgia
- Raynaud's phenomenon, hand swelling, or sclerodactyly
- Esophageal hypomotility, myalgia, and muscle weakness
- Other: pericarditis, facial erythema, psychosis

ETIOLOGY

Autoimmune disorder

DIAGNOSIS

DIFFERENTIAL DIAGNOSIS

Other connective tissue disorders (SLE, progressive systemic sclerosis, polymyositis)

WORKUP

- Diagnosis is not well defined.
- Commonly used diagnostic tests are described in Laboratory Tests.

LABORATORY TESTS (Box 1-12)

- Rheumatoid factor is often present in low titers.
- If myositis is present, muscle enzyme (creatine phosphokinase) levels increase.
- Positive antinuclear antibody is often present with a speckled pattern.
- Erythrocyte sedimentation rate is elevated.
- Anti-ribonucleoprotein antibodies may be present.

TREATMENT

- Except for pulmonary and scleroderma-like symptoms, response to corticosteroids is excellent in most cases.
- Rheumatoid symptoms may respond to nonsteroidal antiiflammatory drugs, but other cases may not even respond to gold or penicillamine.
- Immunosuppressive agents are used on occasion, but the best therapeutic options remain uncertain.

DISPOSITION

- Initially this disorder was believed to be a mild variant of SLE, sometimes called "benign lupus," with an excellent prognosis.
- Further studies suggested, however, that this was not always the case and serious renal, vascular, and neurologic complications were noted.
- Pulmonary involvement is a common clinical manifestation that may even lead to pulmonary hypertension and sometimes death.
- Whether MCTD is a separate entity continues to be debated as concepts about the disorder evolve.
- Long-term outcomes remain uncertain.

REFERRAL

Rheumatology consultation for clarification and assistance in treatment

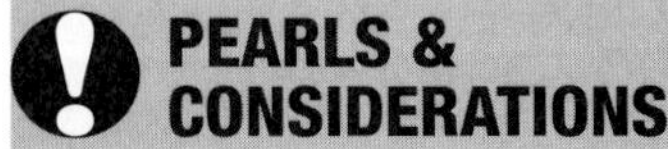

PEARLS & CONSIDERATIONS

COMMENTS

A clinical algorithm for evaluation of a positive ANA titer is described in Section III, "Antinuclear Antibody Testing."

SUGGESTED READINGS

Aringer M, Smolen JS: Mixed connective tissue disease: what is behind the curtain? *Best Pract Res Clin Rheumatol* 21:1037, 2007.

Bodolay E et al: Osteoporosis in mixed connective disease, *Clin Rheumatol* 22:213, 2003.

Chan AT et al: Overlap connective tissue disease, pulmonary fibrosis, and extensive soft tissue calcification, *Ann Rheum Dis* 62:690, 2003.

Hoffman RW, Maldonaldo ME: Immune pathogenesis of mixed connective disease: a short analytical review, *Clin Immunol* 128:8, 2008.

Keith MP et al: Anti-RNP immunity: implications for tissue injury and the pathogenesis of connective tissue disease, *Autoimmun Rev* 6(4):232, 2007.

Ling TC, Johnson BT: Esophageal investigations in connective tissue disease: which tests are most appropriate? *J Clin Gastroenterol* 32:33, 2001.

Lopez-Longo FJ et al: Does mixed connective tissue disease have a less favorable prognosis than systemic lupus erythematosus? *Arthritis Rheum* 44(suppl):119, 2001.

Lowe D et al: Thalidomide: an effective and safe agent for the treatment of pediatric mixed connective tissue disease, *Arthritis Rheum* 43(suppl):117, 2000.

Mosca M et al: A case of undifferentiated connective tissue disease: is it a distinct clinical entity? *Nat Clin Pract Rheumatol* 328, 2008.

Sharp G: The origin of mixed connective disease: a stimulus for autoimmune disease research, *Lupus* 18:1031, 2009.

Tiddens HA et al: Juvenile-onset mixed connective tissue disease: longitudinal follow-up, *J Pediatr* 122(2):191, 2006.

Tsai YY et al: Fifteen-year experience of pediatric-onset mixed connective tissue disease, *Clin Rheumatol* 29:53, 2010.

AUTHOR: **LONNIE R. MERCIER, M.D.**

BOX 1-12 Guidelines for Diagnosing MCTD

General
Clinical features of a diffuse connective tissue disorder

Serologic
1. Positive ANA, speckled pattern, titer >1:1000
2. Antibodies to U1 RNP
3. Absence of antibodies to dsDNA, histones, Sm, Scl-70, and other specificities
4. Commonly: hypergammaglobulinemia and positive rheumatoid factor

Clinical
1. Sequential evolution of overlap features over course of several years, including Raynaud's phenomenon, serositis, gastrointestinal dysmotility, myositis, arthritis, sclerodactyly, skin rashes, and an abnormal DLco on pulmonary function tests
2. Absence of truncal scleroderma, severe renal disease, and severe central nervous system involvement
3. A nail fold capillary pattern identical to that seen in systemic sclerosis (dropout and dilated vessels)

From Bennett RM: Mixed connective tissue disease and other overlap syndromes. In Kelley WN et al (eds): *Textbook of rheumatology,* ed 6, Philadelphia, 2005, WB Saunders.
ANA, Antinuclear antibodies; *dsDNA,* double-stranded DNA; *MCTD,* mixed connective tissue disease; *RNP,* ribonucleoprotein.

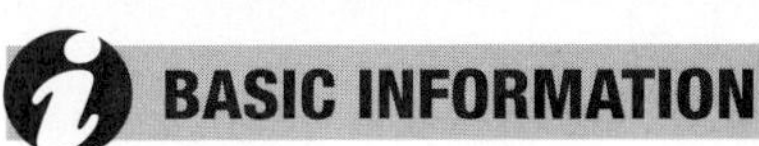

BASIC INFORMATION

DEFINITION

Viral infection characterized by discrete skin lesions with central umbilication (Fig. 1-200).

ICD-9CM CODES
078.0 Molluscum contagiosum

EPIDEMIOLOGY & DEMOGRAPHICS

- Molluscum contagiosum spreads by autoinoculation, scratching, or touching a lesion.
- It usually occurs in young children. It is also common in sexually active adults and patients with HIV infection.
- Incubation period varies between 4 and 8 wk.
- Spontaneous resolution in immunocompetent patients can occur after several months.

PHYSICAL FINDINGS & CLINICAL PRESENTATION

- The individual lesion appears initially as a flesh-colored, firm, smooth-surfaced papule with subsequent central umbilication. Lesions are frequently grouped. The size of each lesion generally varies from 2 to 6 mm in diameter.
- Typical distribution in children involves the face, extremities, and trunk. Mucous membranes are spared.
- Distribution in adults generally involves pubic and genital areas.
- Erythema and scaling at the periphery of the lesions may be present as a result of scratching or hypersensitivity reaction.
- Lesions are not present on the palms and soles.

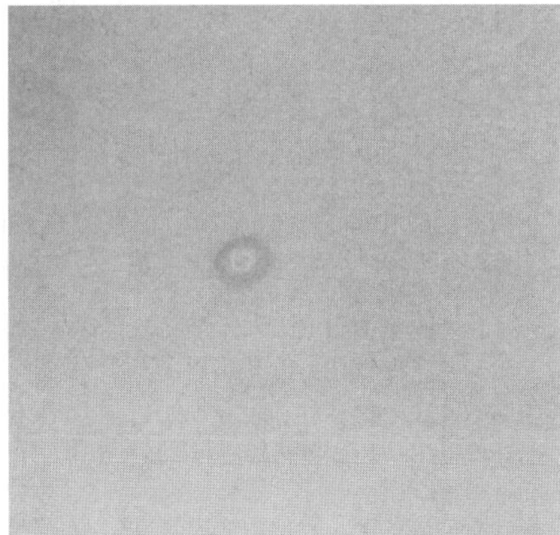

FIGURE 1-200 Molluscum contagiosum. (From Rakel RE: *Textbook of family practice,* ed 6, Philadelphia, 2002, WB Saunders.)

ETIOLOGY

Viral infection of epithelial cells caused by a pox virus

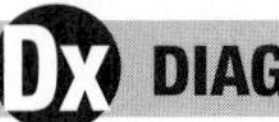

DIAGNOSIS

Diagnosis is usually established by the clinical appearance of the lesions (distribution and central umbilication). A magnifying lens can be used to observe the central umbilication. If necessary, the diagnosis can be confirmed by removing a typical lesion with a curette and examining the content on a slide after adding potassium hydroxide and gentle heating. Staining with toluidine blue will identify viral inclusions.

DIFFERENTIAL DIAGNOSIS

- Verruca plana (flat warts): no central umbilication, not dome shaped, irregular surface, can involve palms and soles
- Herpes simplex: lesions become rapidly umbilicated
- Varicella: blisters and vesicles are present
- Folliculitis: no central umbilication, presence of hair piercing the pustule or papule
- Cutaneous cryptococcosis in AIDS patients: budding yeasts will be present on cytologic examination of the lesions
- Basal cell carcinoma: multiple lesions are absent

WORKUP

Careful examination of the papules

LABORATORY TESTS

Generally not indicated in children. Screening for other sexually transmitted diseases is recommended in all cases of genital molluscum contagiosum.

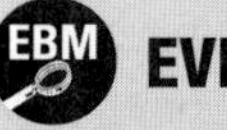

TREATMENT

GENERAL THERAPY

- Therapy is individualized depending on number of lesions, immune status, and patient's age and preference.
- Observation for spontaneous resolution is reasonable in patients with few, small, nonirritated, and nonspreading lesions. Genital lesions should be treated in all sexually active patients.
- Liquid nitrogen cryotherapy.
- Carbon dioxide laser.
- Curettage after pretreatment of the area with combination prilocaine 2.5% with lidocaine 2.5% cream (EMLA) for anesthesia is useful for treatment of a few lesions. Curettage should be avoided in cosmetically sensitive areas because scarring may develop.
- Treatments with liquid nitrogen therapy in combination with curettage are effective in older patients who do not object to some discomfort.
- Application of cantharidin 0.7% to individual lesions covered with clear tape will result in blistering over 24 hr and possible clearing without scarring. This medication should be avoided on facial lesions.
- Other treatment measures include use of imiquimod cream or tretinoin 0.025% gel or 0.1% cream at bedtime, daily use of salicylic acid (Occlusal) at bedtime, and use of laser therapy.
- Trichloroacetic acid peel generally repeated every 2 wk for several weeks is useful in immunocompromised patients with extensive lesions.

DISPOSITION

Most patients respond well to the therapeutic modalities listed previously. Spontaneous resolution can occur after 6 to 9 mo in some immunocompetent patients.

REFERRAL

To dermatology when diagnosis is in doubt or in patients with extensive lesions

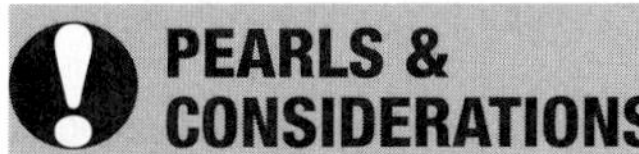

PEARLS & CONSIDERATIONS

COMMENTS

Genital molluscum contagiosum in children may be indicative of sexual abuse.

EBM EVIDENCE

A prospective clinical trial has evaluated the effectiveness of the 585-nm collagen remodeling pulsed-dye laser in the treatment of cutaneous molluscum contagiosum and has found that 96.3% of the lesions healed after the first treatment and the remaining 3.7% healed after the second treatment (2 wk later).[1] B

Evidence-Based Reference

1. Michel JL: Treatment of molluscum contagiosum with 585nm collagen remodeling pulsed dye laser, *Eur J Dermatol* 14:103, 2004. B

AUTHOR: **FRED F. FERRI, M.D.**

Mononucleosis (PTG)

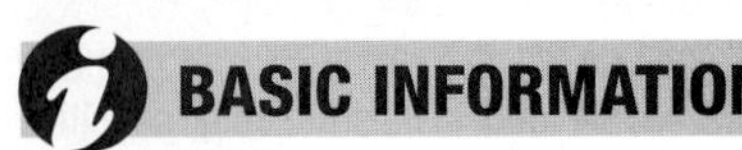

BASIC INFORMATION

DEFINITION

Mononucleosis is a symptomatic infection caused by Epstein-Barr virus (EBV).

SYNONYMS

Infectious mononucleosis (IM)

ICD-9CM CODES
075 Infectious mononucleosis

EPIDEMIOLOGY & DEMOGRAPHICS

INCIDENCE (IN U.S.): 45 cases/100,000 persons/yr
PREDOMINANT SEX: Incidence is the same, but occurs earlier in females.
PREDOMINANT AGE: Most common between the ages of 15 and 24 yr.

PHYSICAL FINDINGS & CLINICAL PRESENTATION

- Following an incubation period of 1 to 2 mo, a prodrome may occur, with fever, chills, malaise, and anorexia for several days. This is followed by the classic triad, which includes pharyngitis, fever, and adenopathy. Although fatigue and malaise may be prominent, pharyngitis is usually the most severe symptom. Exudates are common.
- Lymphadenopathy is most prominent in the cervical region but may be diffuse.
- Splenomegaly may occur, most commonly during the second wk of illness.
- Rash is uncommon but will occur in nearly all patients who receive ampicillin.
- At times, IM can present as fever and adenopathy without pharyngitis. Although complications may be severe, they are uncommon and tend to resolve completely. Involvement of the hematologic, pulmonary, cardiac, or nervous system may occur; splenic rupture is rare. IM is usually a self-limited illness, but symptoms of malaise and fatigue may last months before resolving.

ETIOLOGY

The cause of IM is primary infection with EBV. Primary infection during childhood causes few or no symptoms. Infection during childhood is more common in lower socioeconomic groups. The frequency of IM in late adolescence is attributed to the onset of social contact between the sexes. Close personal contact is usually necessary for transmission, although EBV has occasionally been transmitted by blood transfusion. Transfer via saliva while kissing may be responsible for many cases.

DIAGNOSIS

DIFFERENTIAL DIAGNOSIS

- Heterophile-negative infectious mononucleosis caused by cytomegalovirus (CMV); although clinical presentation may be similar, CMV more frequently follows transfusion
- Bacterial and viral causes of pharyngitis
- Toxoplasmosis
- Acute retroviral syndrome of HIV, lymphoma

WORKUP

Heterophile antibody (monospot) and CBC should be sent.

LABORATORY TESTS

- Increased WBC is common, with a relative lymphocytosis and neutropenia. Atypical lymphocytes are the hallmark of IM, but are not pathognomonic. Mild thrombocytopenia is common. A falling hematocrit may signal splenic rupture or severe immune-mediated hemolytic anemia. Elevated hepatocellular enzymes and cryoglobulins occur in most cases. Heterophile antibody, as measured by the Monospot test, may be positive at presentation, or may appear later in the course of illness. A negative test should be repeated if clinical suspicion is high. If this test remains negative for 8 wk, other causes of IM are likely. The monospot usually remains positive for 3 to 6 mo, but can last for 1 yr.
- A positive test has been reported with primary HIV infection.
- In addition to the heterophile antibody, virus-specific antibodies may result in response to IM. Determination of these EBV-specific antibodies is rarely necessary to diagnose IM, although early diagnosis in monospot negative cases may be made by isolating IgM to the viral capsid antigen (VCA), which is usually positive during the acute illness.

IMAGING STUDIES

Chest radiograph may rarely show infiltrates. An elevated left hemidiaphragm may occur in cases of splenic rupture.

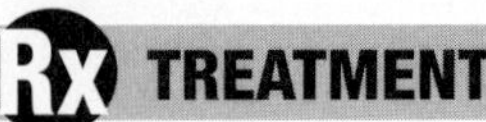

TREATMENT

NONPHARMACOLOGIC THERAPY

- Supportive rest is advocated by some, but effect on outcome is not clear
- Splenectomy if rupture occurs; transfusions for severe anemia or thrombocytopenia

ACUTE GENERAL Rx

- Pharmacologic therapy is not indicated in uncomplicated illness.
- The use of steroids is suggested in patients who have severe thrombocytopenia or hemolytic anemia, or impending airway obstruction as a result of enlarged tonsils. Prednisone, 60 to 80 mg PO qid for 3 days, then tapered over 1 to 2 wk. There is no role for antiviral agents such as acyclovir in the management of IM.

CHRONIC Rx

A rare, chronic form of IM with persistent organ infection and inflammation has been described. This should not be confused with chronic fatigue syndrome, which is unrelated to EBV.

DISPOSITION

Eventual resolution of all symptoms is the rule.

REFERRAL

More than mild illness

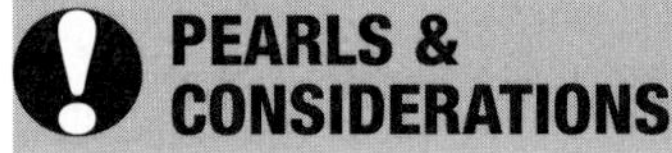

PEARLS & CONSIDERATIONS

COMMENTS

Contact sports should be avoided during the first mo of illness, because splenic rupture can occur, even in the absence of clinically detectable splenomegaly.

SUGGESTED READINGS

Auwaerter PG: Infectious mononucleosis: return to play, *Clin Sports Med* 23:485, 2004.

Bauer CC et al: Serum Epstein-Barr virus DNA load in primary Epstein-Barr virus infection, *J Med Virol* 75(1):54, 2005.

Ebell MH: Epstein-Barr virus: infectious mononucleosis, *Am Family Physician* 70:1279, 2004.

AUTHORS: **GLENN G. FORT, M.D., M.P.H.,** and **DENNIS J. MIKOLICH, M.D.**

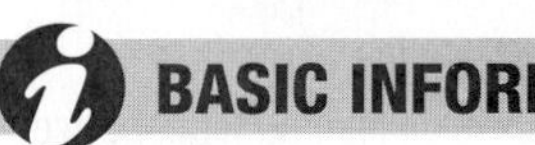

BASIC INFORMATION

DEFINITION

Morton's neuroma refers to an inflammatory fibrosing process of the plantar digital nerve characterized by pain in the sole of the foot. Morton's neuroma is also described as an interdigital plantar neuropathy with or without plantar neuroma.

SYNONYMS

Morton metatarsalgia
Morton toe
Interdigital neuroma

ICD-9CM CODES
355.6 Morton's neuroma

EPIDEMIOLOGY & DEMOGRAPHICS

- Morton's neuroma most commonly involves the plantar digital nerve between the heads of the third and fourth metatarsals.
- May also involve the second and third metatarsal and can involve both simultaneously.
- Commonly occurs in people wearing tight-fitting shoes in toe region and high heels.
- Morton's neuroma is usually unilateral.
- Morton's neuroma is found more often in women than in men.
- Morton's neuroma can occur in both young and old.

PHYSICAL FINDINGS & CLINICAL PRESENTATION

- Pain is usually located in a specific region, usually in the sole of the foot between the third and fourth metatarsal area, and is unilateral in the majority of cases.
- Numbness may occur.
- Pain is exacerbated with exercise and relieved with rest and may radiate to the toes and to the ankle.
- Point tenderness is noted on examination, and palpation reveals fullness at the site of discomfort.
- An audible, painful click called *Murder's click* is noted in patients with Morton's neuroma after compressing and releasing the forefoot.
- Patients may have neuroma but silent lesions without symptoms.

ETIOLOGY

- Morton's neuroma is thought to be caused by nerve thickening from repeated injury.
- The typical finding is swelling of the plantar digital nerve that pathologically resembles other nerve entrapment syndromes (e.g., median nerve compression in carpal tunnel syndrome).

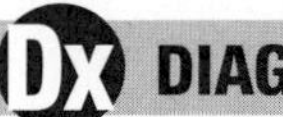

DIAGNOSIS

The diagnosis of Morton's neuroma is strictly made on clinical grounds alone because there are no laboratory tests or x-ray imaging studies that are specific for this disorder.

DIFFERENTIAL DIAGNOSIS

- Diabetic neuropathy
- Alcoholic neuropathy
- Nutritional neuropathy
- Toxic neuropathy
- Osteoarthritis
- Trauma (e.g., fracture)
- Gouty arthritis
- Rheumatoid arthritis

WORKUP

Exclude other causes as mentioned in the "Differential Diagnosis" section.

LABORATORY TESTS

- Laboratory studies are not specific for the diagnosis of Morton's neuroma.
- CBC and ESR are usually normal.
- Blood glucose.
- B_{12} and folic acid level.

IMAGING STUDIES

- X-ray imaging is primarily done to exclude other causes of foot pain (e.g., fractures, osteoarthritis, or gouty arthritis).
- MRI can detect and localize a neuroma but is rarely needed to make the diagnosis. An MRI can also be performed in patients with recurrent pain after surgical excision of a Morton's neuroma.
- Ultrasound imaging is also being used to locate Morton's neuroma but is rarely needed to make the diagnosis.

Rx TREATMENT

NONPHARMACOLOGIC THERAPY

- Changing the type of footwear is the first line of treatment.
- Use open footwear and custom shoe inserts and avoid weight-bearing activities.
- A metatarsal pad with arch support is helpful.
- Participate in ultrasound therapy.

ACUTE GENERAL Rx

- If conservative measures are unsuccessful, injection of the intermetatarsal bursa with hydrocortisone may help. Ultrasound–guided injections of ethyl alcohol plus bupivaine have also been reported effective for Morton's neuroma
- Nonsteroidal anti-inflammatory agents (e.g., ibuprofen 400 to 800 mg PO tid or naproxen 250 to 500 mg bid)

CHRONIC Rx

- If nonpharmacologic and acute treatments do not give sufficient relief, surgical excision of the nerve has been successful in 95% of the cases.
- Surgery can be performed in the physician's office using local anesthesia.
- Numbness in the area where the nerve was excised is a common postoperative finding.

DISPOSITION

- Postoperative patients return to their normal activities in 3 to 6 wk.
- In cases in which pain persists after surgery a "stump neuroma" may be present.
- Approximately 80% of patients who fail to have relief with the initial surgery do find relief with a second procedure.

REFERRAL

If surgery is being considered, a consultation with either a podiatrist or an orthopedic surgeon is indicated.

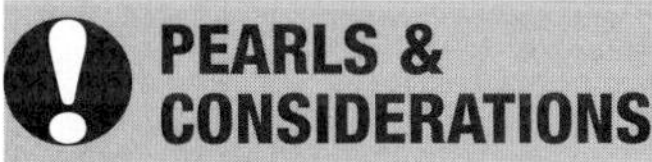

PEARLS & CONSIDERATIONS

COMMENTS

- Dr. Thomas G. Morton is given credit for describing this disorder in 1876.
- Morton's neuroma occurs just before the nerve bifurcates at the metatarsal area to innervate sides of two adjacent toes.
- A recent Cochrane analysis of treatment options for Morton's neuroma found insufficient evidence to support any treatment other than surgical excision for refractory cases.

SUGGESTED READINGS

Hughes RJ et al: Treatment of Morton neuroma with alcohol injection under sonographic guidance: follow-up of 101 cases, *AJR Am J Roentgenol* 188: 1535-1539, 2007.

Kay D, Bennett GL: Morton's neuroma, *Foot Ankle Clin* 8(1):49, 2003.

Sharp RJ et al: The role of MRI and ultrasound imaging in Morton's neuroma and the effect of size of lesion on symptoms, *J Bone Joint Surg Br* 85(7):999, 2003.

Thomson CE, Gibson JN, Martin D: Interventions for the treatment of Morton's neuroma, *Cochrane Database Syst Rev* 3:CD003118, 2004.

Weishaupt D et al: Morton neuroma: MR imaging in prone, supine, and upright weight-bearing body positions, *Radiology* 226(3):849, 2003.

AUTHORS: **GLENN G. FORT, M.D., M.P.H.,** and **DENNIS J. MIKOLICH, M.D.**

Motion Sickness (PTG)

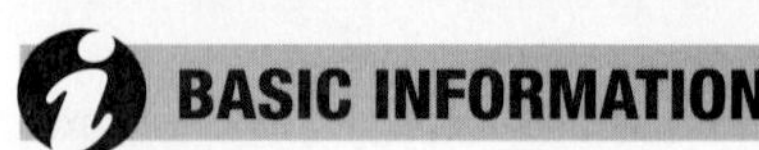

BASIC INFORMATION

DEFINITION
Clinical syndrome associated with motion or perception of motion. Patients with motion sickness suffer perspiration, nausea, vomiting, increased salivation, and generalized malaise in response to movement.

SYNONYMS
Physiologic vertigo

ICD-9CM CODES
994.6 Motion sickness

EPIDEMIOLOGY & DEMOGRAPHICS
INCIDENCE (IN U.S.): Common
PEAK INCIDENCE: Any age
PREVALENCE (IN U.S.): Common
PREDOMINANT SEX: Male = female
PREDOMINANT AGE: Any age
GENETICS: Not known to be genetic

PHYSICAL FINDINGS & CLINICAL PRESENTATION
- Vomiting
- Sweating
- Pallor

ETIOLOGY
- Motion (e.g., amusement rides, rides in automobiles or planes)
- Exacerbated by anxiety, fumes (e.g., industrial pollutants), visual stimuli

DIAGNOSIS

DIFFERENTIAL DIAGNOSIS
- Acute labyrinthitis
- Gastroenteritis
- Metabolic disorders
- Viral syndrome

WORKUP
None necessary in routine case

TREATMENT

NONPHARMACOLOGIC THERAPY
- Fixate on far object
- Cease motion
- Avoid reading
- Avoid alcohol

ACUTE GENERAL Rx
- Scopolamine patch (Transderm Scop) is most effective. It should be applied to a hairless area behind the ear every 3 days prn. It should be applied >4 hr before antiemetic effect is required.
- Over-the-counter oral preparations (e.g., Dramamine) are less effective.
- Meclizine (Antivert) 12.5 to 25 mg q6h may be effective.

CHRONIC Rx
- Rarely chronic
- Symptoms generally resolve completely with cessation of motion exposure

DISPOSITION
Follow-up is not needed.

REFERRAL
If another diagnosis is suspected (e.g., purulent ear, fever, cranial nerve abnormalities)

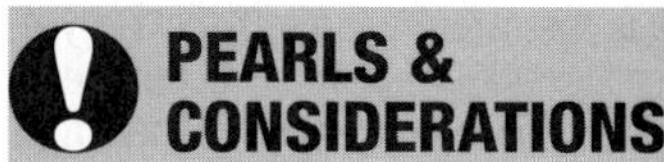

PEARLS & CONSIDERATIONS

COMMENTS
- Many patients with migraine report having severe motion sickness as a child.
- Improved ventilation, avoidance of large meals before travel, semirecumbent sitting, and avoidance of reading while in motion will minimize the risk of motion sickness.

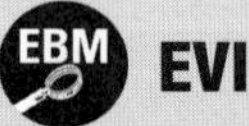

EVIDENCE

A systematic review concluded that scopolamine was more effective than placebo in the prevention of motion sickness, but no conclusions could be drawn from the comparative studies with other agents such as antihistamines and calcium channel antagonists.[1] Ⓐ

Evidence-Based Reference
1. Spinks AB et al: Scopolamine for preventing and treating motion sickness, *Cochrane Rev* 3, 2004. Ⓐ

SUGGESTED READINGS
Koch KL: Illusory self-motion and motion sickness: a model for brain-gut interacting and nausea, *Dig Dis Sci* 48(8 suppl):53S, 1999.

Yates BJ et al: Physiological basis and pharmacology of motion sickness: an update, *Brain Res Bull* 45(5): 395, 1998.

AUTHOR: **FRED F. FERRI, M.D.**

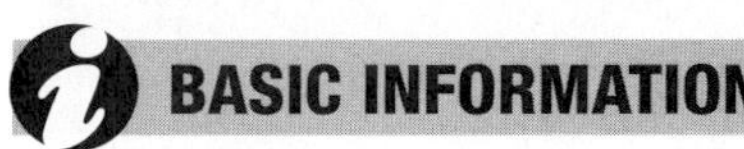

BASIC INFORMATION

DEFINITION

Mucormycosis is a fungal infection by *Zygomycetes fungi,* and includes species in the order Mucorales (*Mucor, Rhizopus, Absidia, Cunninghamella, Mortierella, Saksenaea, Syncephalastrum, Apophysomyces,* and *Thamnidium*) and in the order Entomophthorales (*Conidiobolus* and *Basidiobolus*).

ICD-9CM CODES
117.7 Mucormycosis

EPIDEMIOLOGY & DEMOGRAPHICS

- Infection by these ubiquitous organisms occurs in association with underlying conditions, including diabetes mellitus, lymphoma, severe burns or trauma, prolonged postoperative course, multiple myeloma, hepatitis, cirrhosis, renal failure, steroid treatment, immunodeficiency states (e.g., AIDS), and use of contaminated Elastoplast bandages. Immunocompetent hosts may become infected in tropical climates.
- The fungus gains entry to the body most commonly through the respiratory tract. The spores are deposited in the nasal turbinates and may be inhaled into the pulmonary alveoli. In cases of cutaneous mucormycosis, the spores are introduced directly into the skin lesion.

PHYSICAL FINDINGS & CLINICAL PRESENTATION

- Rhinocerebral-rhinoorbital-paranasal syndrome may present with fever, facial and orbital pain, headache, diplopia, loss of vision, facial or orbital cellulitis, facial anesthesia, cranial nerve dysfunction, black nasal discharge, epistaxis, and seizure. Physical findings in this situation include proptosis; chemosis; nasal, palatal, or pharyngeal necrotic ulcerations; and retinal infarction. Thrombosis of the cavernous sinus or internal carotid artery may occur. This form of mucormycosis is found most commonly in diabetics, primarily in the presence of acidosis, and in patients with leukemia and neutropenia.
- Pulmonary mucormycosis can present with pneumonia, lung abscess, pulmonary infarction, pleurisy, pleural effusion, hemoptysis, chills, and fever. This form of mucormycosis is found most commonly in immunocompromised neutropenic hosts after chemotherapy for hematologic malignancies.
- Gastrointestinal zygomycosis presents with abdominal pain, diarrhea, gastrointestinal hemorrhage, ulcers, peritonitis, and bowel infarction. This form of mucormycosis is found most commonly in patients with extreme malnutrition and is believed to arise from ingestion of the fungi.
- Cutaneous zygomycosis presents as nodular lesions (hematogenous seeding) or a wound infection. It primarily involves the epidermis and dermis after use of occlusive dressings that have not been properly sterilized.
- Cardiac mucormycosis is a form of endocarditis.
- Septic arthritis and osteomyelitis.
- Brain abscess occurs most often from extension of the fungus from the nose or paranasal sinuses through adjacent bones in severely debilitated patients.
- Disseminated zygomycosis (rare but uniformly fatal).
- Physical findings depend on the location of the infection.

ETIOLOGY & PATHOGENESIS

The cause of mucormycosis is infection by a fungus of the *Zygomycetes* class (see "Definition"). Normal host defenses include leukocytes and pulmonary macrophages. Quantitative (e.g., neutropenia) or qualitative (e.g., diabetes mellitus or steroid treatment) disruption in the host defenses predisposes the patient to infection.

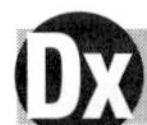

DIAGNOSIS

The hallmark of mucormycosis is vascular invasion and tissue necrosis. Black eschars and discharges should be closely evaluated. Diagnosis depends on the demonstration of the organism in the tissue of a biopsy specimen.

DIFFERENTIAL DIAGNOSIS

- Infection of the sites described previously by other organisms (bacterial [including tuberculosis and leprosy], viral, fungal, or protozoan)
- Noninfectious tissue necrosis (e.g., neoplasia, vasculitis, degenerative) of the sites described previously

WORKUP

- Biopsy of infected tissue with direct-light microscopy examination establishes the diagnosis within minutes of the biopsy in the case of nasopharyngeal infection. Typically the fungi appear as broad (10 to 20 micrometers in diameter) nonseptate hyphae with branches occurring at right angles.
- Bronchoalveolar lavage or bronchoscopy with biopsy for smear, culture, and histologic examination.
- Radiographs and other imaging studies of symptomatic sites may be required before infection is suspected and tissue specimens are obtained.

Rx TREATMENT

Aggressive correction of underlying disease (e.g., hyperglycemia, high steroid doses, use of immunosuppressive drugs) should be undertaken.

Standard therapy for invasive mucormycosis is treatment with amphotericin B given IV at a daily dose of 1.0 to 1.5 mg/kg infused over 2 to 4 hr for a total of 1 to 4 g. Adverse reactions may be managed as follows:

- Fever, chills, headache, myalgias, nausea, and vomiting: premedicate with aspirin (650 mg PO), acetaminophen (650 mg PO), diphenhydramine (25 to 50 mg IV), hydrocortisone (25 to 100 mg IV), or meperidine (25 to 50 mg IV).
- Hypokalemia and hypomagnesemia are treated with potassium and magnesium replacement.
- Nephrotoxicity and renal tubular acidosis can be mitigated to some extent with 500 ml of NS infusion 30 min before and after each dose of amphotericin. Amphotericin dose reduction may also be necessary.
- Renal function and electrolytes should be monitored twice a week during the entire course of amphotericin.
- Lipid preparations of amphotericin B may be less toxic (e.g., amphotericin B lipid complex, amphotericin B colloidal dispersion, and liposomal amphotericin B).
- The role of flucytosine, rifampin, and tetracycline is controversial.
- Surgical debridement or radical resection.
- The role of colony-stimulating factors remains unclear, beyond that of increasing the neutrophil count in patients with neutropenia.

PROGNOSIS

- Sinus infection with no underlying disease: 75% survival.
- Sinus infection with diabetes: 60% survival.
- Sinus infection with renal disease: 25% survival.
- Surgery may increase survival by 5% to 20%.
- Early diagnosis improves survival as well as control of the underlying condition.

SUGGESTED READINGS

Larsen K et al: Unexpected expansive paranasal sinus mucormycosis, *J Otorhinolaryngol Relat Spec* 65:57-60, 2003.

Paydas S et al: Mucormycosis of the tongue in a patient with acute lymphoblastic leukemia: a possible relation with use of tongue depressor, *Am J Med* 114:618-620, 2003.

AUTHOR: **FRED F. FERRI, M.D.**

Multifocal Atrial Tachycardia

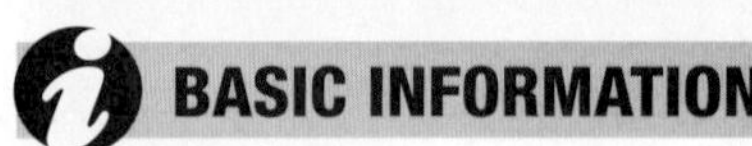

BASIC INFORMATION

DEFINITION

Multifocal atrial tachycardia (MAT) is a supraventricular, moderately rapid arrhythmia (rate 100 to 140 beats/min) with P waves having at least three or more different morphologies and irregular P-P intervals. An isoelectric baseline further differentiates MAT from atrial fibrillation or atrial flutter.

SYNONYMS

Chaotic atrial rhythm

The term *wandering pacemaker* is used for a similar arrhythmia associated with a normal or slow heart rate

ICD-9CM CODES

427.89 Multifocal atrial tachycardia

EPIDEMIOLOGY & DEMOGRAPHICS

Estimated prevalence in hospitalized patients of 0.05% to 0.32%. Average age is 70s. Usually associated with underlying pulmonary disease. COPD is present in approximately 55% of patients with MAT.

PHYSICAL FINDINGS & CLINICAL PRESENTATION

Symptoms:

- Palpitation
- Lightheadedness
- Syncope
- Symptoms of the underlying pulmonary disease
- Physical findings associated with the underlying pulmonary disease

ETIOLOGY

- Exact mechanism unknown
- Associated abnormalities include pulmonary disease, cardiac disease, hypoxia, hypercarbia, acidosis, electrolyte disturbances, digitalis toxicity

Dx DIAGNOSIS

DIFFERENTIAL DIAGNOSIS

- Atrial fibrillation
- Atrial flutter
- Sinus tachycardia
- Paroxysmal atrial tachycardia
- Extrasystole

WORKUP

- ECG (Fig. 1-201)
- Chest x-ray
- Pulmonary function tests
- Electrolytes
- Arterial blood gases
- Digoxin level (if patient on digoxin)

Rx TREATMENT

- Improve the pulmonary or metabolic dysfunction if possible
- Electrolyte repletion, especially magnesium and potassium
- Calcium channel blockers
- β-blockers if not contraindicated by obstructive lung disease or acute heart failure
- If the arrhythmia is asymptomatic, it can be left untreated
- Direct current cardioversion is ineffective

SUGGESTED READING

McCord J, Borzak S: Multifocal atrial tachycardia, *Chest* 113:203-209, 1998.

AUTHORS: **SCOTT BRANCATO, M.D., FRED F. FERRI, M.D.,** and **WEN-CHIH WU, M.D.**

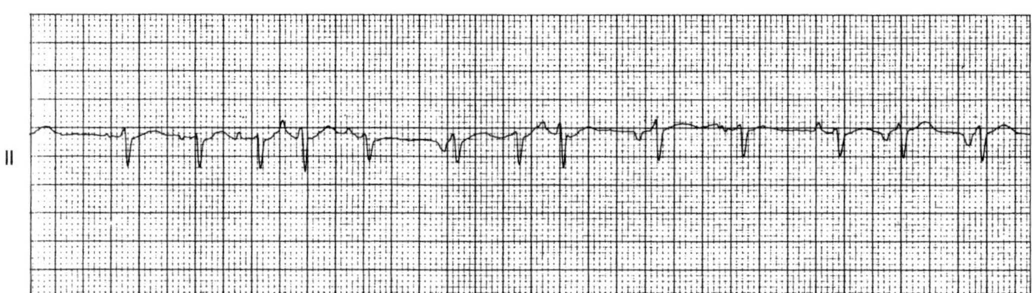

FIGURE 1-201 The P waves show variable shapes, variable PR intervals, or both. (From Goldberger AL: *Clinical electrocardiography,* ed 5, St Louis, 1994, Mosby.)

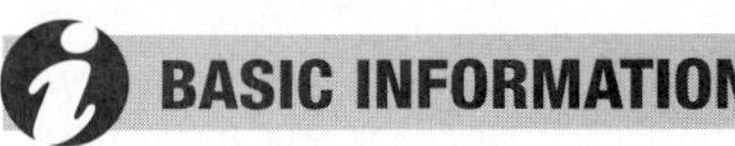

BASIC INFORMATION

DEFINITION

Multiple myeloma is a malignancy of plasma cells characterized by overproduction of intact monoclonal immunoglobulin or free monoclonal kappa or lambda chains. Diagnostic criteria require the following:

1. Presence of ≥10% plasma cells on examination of the bone marrow (or biopsy of a tissue with monoclonal plasma cells).
2. Monoclonal protein in the serum or urine. Occasional patients without detectable monoclonal protein are considered to have nonsecretory myeloma.
3. Evidence of end-organ damage (***c***alcium elevation, ***r***enal insufficiency, ***a***nemia, or ***b***one lesions [CRAB]).

ICD-9CM CODES
203.0 Multiple myeloma

EPIDEMIOLOGY & DEMOGRAPHICS

ANNUAL INCIDENCE: Five cases per 100,000 persons (blacks affected twice as frequently as whites, males more than females); multiple myeloma accounts for 10% of all hematologic cancers. It is the most common primary bone malignancy. There are 16,000 new case diagnosed annually in the U.S.

PREDOMINANT AGE: Peak incidence is in the seventh decade at a median age of 69 yr.

PHYSICAL FINDINGS & CLINICAL PRESENTATION

The patient usually comes to medical attention because of one or more of the following:

- Bone pain (58%) (back, thorax) or pathologic fractures (30%) caused by osteolytic lesions
- Fatigue (32%) or weakness because of anemia from bone marrow infiltration with plasma cells
- Recurrent infections as a result of impaired neutrophil function and deficiency of normal immunoglobulins
- Nausea and vomiting caused by constipation and uremia
- Delirium resulting from hypercalcemia
- Neurologic complications, such as spinal cord or nerve root compression, blurred vision from hyperviscosity
- Pallor and generalized weakness from anemia
- Purpura, epistaxis from thrombocytopenia
- Evidence of infections from impaired immune system
- Paresthesias (5%), weight loss (24%)
- Swelling on ribs, vertebrae, and other bones

Dx DIAGNOSIS

DIFFERENTIAL DIAGNOSIS

- Metastatic carcinoma
- Lymphoma (B-cell NHL)
- Bone neoplasms (e.g., sarcoma)
- Monoclonal gammopathy of undetermined significance
- Primary amyloidosis
- Chronic lymphocytic leukemia
- Waldenström's macroglobulinemia

LABORATORY TESTS

- Normochromic, normocytic anemia; rouleaux formation on peripheral smear.
- Hypercalcemia is present in 15% of patients at diagnosis.
- Elevated blood urea nitrogen, creatinine, uric acid, and total protein.
- Proteinuria from overproduction and secretion of free monoclonal kappa or lambda chains (Bence Jones protein).
- Tall homogeneous monoclonal spike (M spike) on protein immunoelectrophoresis in approximately 75% of patients (Fig. 1-202); decreased levels of normal immunoglobulins (Ig).
  1. The increased immunoglobulins are generally IgG (75%) and IgA (15%).
  2. Approximately 17% of patients have a flat level of immunoglobulins but increased light chains in the urine by electrophoresis.
  3. A small percentage (<2%) of patients have nonsecreting myeloma (no increase in immunoglobulins and no light chains in the urine) but have other evidence of the disease (e.g., positive bone marrow examination).
- Reduced ion gap from the positive charge of the M proteins and the frequent presence of hyponatremia in myeloma patients.
- Hyponatremia, serum hyperviscosity (more common with production of IgA).
- Bone marrow examination: usually demonstrates nests or sheets of plasma cells, which comprise >30% of the bone marrow; ≥10% are immature.
- Serum beta-2 microglobulin has little diagnostic value; it is useful for prognosis because levels >8 mg/L indicate high tumor mass and aggressive disease.
- Elevated serum levels of lactate dehydrogenase at the time of diagnosis define a subgroup of myeloma patients with very poor prognosis.
- Increased interleukin-6 in serum during active stage of myeloma.
- The production of DKK1, an inhibitor of osteoblast differentiation, by myeloma cells is associated with the presence of lytic bone lesions in patients with multiple myeloma.
- Nearly all patients with myeloma present with abnormal chromosomes identified by fluorescence in situ hybridization (FISH). The Mayo Clinic Stratification of Myeloma, for purposes of therapy, identifies high-risk patients (<25% of patients at diagnosis) as those who have any of the following: FISH deletion 17p, FISH translocation 4;14, FISH translocation 14;16, cytogenetic deletion 13q, cytogenetic hypodiploidy, or plasma cell labeling index ≥3%.

IMAGING STUDIES

Radiograph films of painful areas may demonstrate punched-out lytic lesions or osteoporosis (Fig. 1-202). MRI is the preferred technique for suspected spinal compression or soft tissue plasmacytomas. Bone scans are not useful because lesions are not blastic. PET and CT scans are emerging as useful tools.

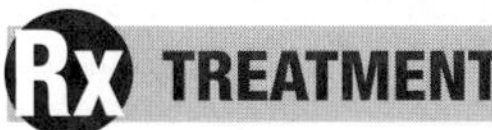

TREATMENT

NONPHARMACOLOGIC THERAPY

Prevention of renal failure with adequate hydration and avoidance of nephrotoxic agents and dye contrast studies

ACUTE GENERAL Rx

- Newly diagnosed patients with good performance status are best treated with autologous stem cell transplantation.
  1. Autologous transplantation is recommended for patients with stage II or III myeloma and good performance status.

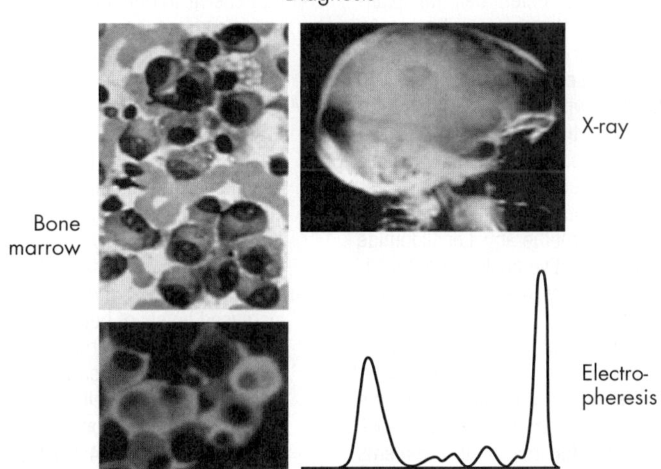

FIGURE 1-202 Common diagnostic features in multiple myeloma. Light chain-restricted plasma cells in a bone marrow aspirate; multiple lytic lesions in a skull radiograph; large monoclonal spike in the γ-globulin area in serum electrophoresis. (From Hoffmann R et al: *Hematology, basic principles and practice,* ed 5, Philadelphia, 2009, Churchill Livingstone.)

2. Induction therapy before stem cell harvest is administered in four cycles. It includes dexamethasone alone or thalidomide-dexamethasone (Thal-Dex).
3. High-dose chemotherapy (HDCT) with vincristine, melphalan, cyclophosphamide, and prednisone (VMCP) alternating with vincristine, carmustine, doxorubicin, and prednisone (BVAP) combined with bone marrow transplantation improves the response rate, event-free survival, and overall survival in patients with myeloma. Current HDCT regimen with autologous stem cell support achieves complete response in approximately 20% to 30% of patients, with the best results seen in good-risk patients, defined as young patients (<50 yr) with good performance status and a low tumor burden (beta-2 microglobulin ≤2.5 mg/L).

- Induction therapy in patients ineligible for transplantation (old age, coexisting conditions, poor physical conditions) includes the following chemotherapeutic agents:
  1. Thalidomide in combination with melphalan and prednisone.
  2. Melphalan and prednisone: the rates of response to this treatment range from 40% to 60%. Adding continuous low-dose interferon to standard melphalan-prednisone therapy does not improve response rate or survival; however, response duration and plateau phase duration are prolonged by maintenance therapy with interferon.
  3. Vincristine, doxorubicin, and dexamethasone (VAD) can be used in patients not responding or relapsing after treatment with melphalan and prednisone; methylprednisolone is substituted for dexamethasone (VAMP) in some centers.
- Therapy for relapsed and refractory myeloma:
  1. If the relapse occurs more than 6 mo after conventional therapy is stopped, the initial chemotherapy regimen can be reinstituted.
  2. Consider autologous stem cell transplantation as salvage therapy in patients who had stem cells cryopreserved early in the course of the disease.
  3. Chemotherapy with vincristine, doxorubicin, and dexamethasone.
  4. Thalidomide, an agent with antiangiogenic properties, is also useful to induce responses in patients with multiple myeloma refractory to chemotherapy. Lenalidomide (CC-5013) is an active analogue of thalidomide developed to overcome the toxic effects of thalidomide.
  5. Bortezomib is a protease inhibitor that is cytotoxic for multiple myeloma. It is indicated for treatment of refractory multiple myeloma. It is superior to high-dose dexamethasone for treatment of patients who have had relapse. Bortezomib plus melphalan-prednisone has also been reported to be superior to melphalan plus prednisone alone as initial therapy for patients with myeloma who are not candidates for hematopoietic stem cell transplantation.
- Approximately 15% of patients with newly diagnosed multiple myeloma are recognized incidentally and present without significant symptoms (smoldering myeloma). The rate of progression of smoldering myeloma to symptomatic disease is 10% per year for the initial 5 yr, decreasing to 5% for the next 5 yr, and decreasing further to 1.5% per year thereafter. Observation alone is reasonable in these patients because no survival advantage has been demonstrated by treating them.

CHRONIC Rx

- Promptly diagnose and treat infections. Common bacterial agents are *Streptococcus pneumoniae* and *Haemophilus influenzae.* Prophylactic therapy against *Pneumocystis jirovecii* with trimethoprim sulfamethoxazole must be considered in patients receiving chemotherapy and high-dose corticosteroid regimens. Vaccinate against *S. pneumoniae,* influenza, and *H. influenzae.*
- Control hypercalcemia with IV fluids and corticosteroids. Monthly infusions of the bisphosphonate pamidronate provide significant protection against skeletal complications and improve the quality of life of patients with advanced multiple myeloma. Zoledronic acid (Zometa) at doses of 2 mg and 4 mg in patients with osteolytic lesions has been shown to be as effective as pamidronate in terms of reducing the need for radiation to bone, increasing bone mineral density, and decreasing bone resorption. It can be infused over 15 min for treatment of hypercalcemia of malignancy. Bisphosphonates (pamidronate, zoledronate, and ibandronate) also appear to have an antitumor effect.
- Control pain with analgesics; radiation therapy to treat painful bone lesions or cord compression. Surgical stabilization of pathologic fractures. Consider vertebroplasty or kyphoplasty for selected vertebral lesions.
- Treat anemia with erythropoietin.
- Aggressive treatment of reversible causes of renal failure such as dehydration, hypercalcemia, and hyperuricemia.

DISPOSITION

- The median length of survival after diagnosis is 3 yr. Prognosis is better in asymptomatic patients with indolent or smoldering myeloma. Median survival time is approximately 10 yr in persons with no lytic bone lesions and a serum myeloma protein concentration <3 g/dl. Adverse outcome is associated with increased levels of beta-2 microglobulin, low levels of serum albumin, circulating plasma cells, plasmablastic features in bone marrow, increased plasma cell labeling index, complete deletion of chromosome 13 or its long arm, t (4;14) or t (14;16) translocation, and increased density of bone marrow microvessels.
- Compared with a single autologous stem cell transplantation, double transplantation (two successive autologous stem cell transplantations) improves survival among patients with myeloma, especially those who do not have a very good partial response after undergoing one transplantation.
- Recent trials reveal that among patients with newly diagnosed myeloma, survival in recipients of a hematopoietic stem cell autograft followed by a stem cell allograft from an HLA-identical sibling is superior to that in recipients of tandem stem cell autografts.

EBM EVIDENCE

Please note: Complete text of EBM for this topic is available online.

Key trials and commentary:

New imaging techniques have been introduced to assess the extent and severity of disease in multiple myeloma (MM) patients. The aim of this study was to compare newer imaging modalities—such as ^{18}F-FDG PET/CT, ^{99m}Tc-methoxyisobutylisonitrile (^{99m}Tc-MIBI) scintigraphy, and MRI—to assess their relative contribution in the evaluation of MM patients at diagnosis.

MM has long been staged using the Durie and Salmon system, which depends on radiographic survey. However, radiographs have long been known to underestimate myelomatous tumor burden. Even worse, radiographic surveys are frequently negative even in the face of diffusely infiltrative disease, giving only the appearance of osteopenia. This article is a well-done study evaluating ^{18}F-fluorodeoxyglucose positron emission tomography and computed tomography (^{18}F-FDG PET/CT), ^{99m}Tc-methoxyisobutylisonitrile (^{99m}Tc-MIBI), and MRI in detection of lesions in patients with multiple myeloma. It shows favorable data regarding the performance of both FDG PET/CT and MRI. This article should be considered an initial foray into this complex topic. Although it validates these imaging methodologies for initial evaluation of disease presence and tumor burden, in this author's opinion it underestimates the use of MRI. Magnetic resonance surveys (evaluating more of the skeleton than demonstrated in this study) for myeloma have been developed and are in use at several institutions, and have proven complementary to FDG PET/CT. More data from large studies are being accumulated which should clarify whether both are needed for initial workup. Even more interesting is the evaluation of these modalities' accuracy in follow-up of treated patients. This is an evolving field that will require sophisticated study of large patient groups. However, it is probably safe to say that the era of radiographic survey for myeloma is over.[1] Ⓐ

A phase III international study compared the efficacy and safety of a combination of pegylated liposomal doxorubicin (PLD) plus bortezomib with bortezomib monotherapy in patients with relapsed or refractory MM.

This study showed that PLD with bortezomib is superior to bortezomib monotherapy for the treatment of patients with relapsed or refractory MM. The combination therapy is associated with a higher incidence of grade 3/4 myelosuppression, constitutional symptoms, and GI and dermatologic toxicities.

Patients with relapsed or refractory MM have numerous options that can include thalidomide, thalidomide successor molecules such as lenalidomide, or bortezomib the proteasome inhibitor. All three of these mentioned drugs are approved for this indication and have varying degrees of benefit. In this study, the investigators assessed patients who had progressed while undergoing prior standard treatments and randomly assigned them to receive either bortezomib monotherapy in the standard twice-weekly IV regimen or bortezomib in combination with PLD. Patients may have previously received anthracycline-based chemotherapy (such as VAD [vincristine, doxorubicin, and dexamethasone] chemotherapy) but may not have progressed actively while being treated. Overall, the regimen of PLD plus bortezomib demonstrated superior activity. Response rates were similar, ranging from 41% for bortezomib monotherapy to 44% for the PLD+bortezomib combination, but the duration of response was significantly longer in the combination arm, ranging from 7.0 to 10.2 months. The 15-month survival for the combination was 76% compared with 65% for bortezomib monotherapy. This again was statistically significant with a *P* value of 0.03. What was not designed into this trial was a crossover in which patients receiving bortezomib monotherapy could be crossed over to PLD; hence, it is unclear whether the survival advantage would have been maintained had all patients by protocol description crossed over. It is well known in many diseases such as breast cancer that sequential single-agent therapies can produce survival rates similar to combination therapies; hence, in this setting, this would have been an important question to have answered, particularly because the combination group had a higher rate of grade 3/4 toxic effects, including neutropenia, thrombocytopenia, and hand-foot syndrome. The combination of PLD and bortezomib does suggest better efficacy, but single-agent bortezomib could still be considered to be reasonable therapy for relapses and refractory disease, particularly in those patients who may not tolerate toxicity well.[2] Ⓐ

The standard treatment for patients with MM who are not candidates for high-dose therapy is melphalan and prednisone. This phase III study compared the use of melphalan and prednisone with or without bortezomib in previously untreated patients with multiple myeloma who were ineligible for high-dose therapy.

This study showed that Bortezomib plus melphalan–prednisone was superior to melphalan–prednisone alone in patients with newly diagnosed myeloma who were ineligible for high-dose therapy. (ClinicalTrials.gov number, NCT00111319).

The treatment of MM has undergone significant evolution with the use of proteasome inhibitors such as bortezomib and imides such as lenalidomide. Newer agents have been approved and are vying for use in earlier stage patients though for most patients the use of high-dose chemotherapy (HDC) with stem cell support has become standard. Despite the fact that the age limit for such treatment options has increased, there are still patients who, because of age or comorbid illnesses, are not candidates for HDC. In this trial, the age-old standard for myeloma, melphalan–prednisone, was tested against this two-drug regimen in combination with bortezomib. Over 600 patients who were not eligible for HDC underwent randomization on the trial and the arm including bortezomib demonstrated statistically significantly greater response rates, duration of response, and most importantly overall survival. Toxicities were those typically associated with bortezomib and were generally manageable. Although similar studies have been carried out with other agents, particularly oral agents such as lenalidomide, this trial impressively demonstrates the ability of a proteasome inhibitor to enhance older standards of care and improve the outcome of patients with myeloma with acceptable safety. Among the newer regimens, melphalan–prednisone, and bortezomib should be considered as a standard for patients who otherwise cannot undergo HDC.[3] Ⓐ

Evidence-Based References

1. Fonti R et al: 18F-FDG PET/CT, 99mTc-MIBI, and MRI in evaluation of patients with multiple myeloma, *J Nucl Med* 49:195-200, 2008. Commentary by: B. J. Manaster, M.D., Ph.D. Ⓐ
2. Orlowski RZ et al: Randomized phase III study of pegylated liposomal doxorubicin plus bortezomib compared with bortezomib alone in relapsed or refractory multiple myeloma: combination therapy improves time to progression, *J Clin Oncol* 25:3892-3901, 2007. Commentary by M.S. Gordon, M.D. Ⓐ
3. San Miguel JF et al: Bortezomib plus melphalan and prednisone for initial treatment of multiple myeloma, *N Engl J Med* 359:906-917, 2008. Commentary by M.S. Gordon, M.D. Ⓐ

SUGGESTED READINGS

Bruno B et al: A comparison of allografting with autografting for newly diagnosed myeloma, *N Engl J Med* 356:1110, 2007.

Dispenzieri A et al: Treatment of newly diagnosed multiple myeloma based on Mayo stratification of myeloma and risk-adapted therapy (mSMART): consensus statement, *Mayo Clin Proc* 82(3):323, 2007.

Facon T et al: Melphalan and prednisone plus thalidomide versus melphalan and prednisone alone or reduced-intensity autologous stem cell transplantation in elderly patients with multiple myeloma (IFM 99-06): a randomized trial, *Lancet* 370:1209-1218, 2007.

Harousseau JL, Moreau P: Autologous hematopoietic stem cell transplantation from multiple myeloma, *N Engl J Med* 360:2645-2654, 2009.

Imrie K et al: The role of high dose chemotherapy and stem-cell transplantation in patients with multiple myeloma: a practice guideline of the Cancer Care Ontario Practice Guidelines Initiative, *Ann Intern Med* 136:619, 2002.

International Myeloma Working Group: Criteria for the classification of monoclonal gammopathies, multiple myeloma, and related disorders: a report of the international Myeloma Working Group, *Br J Haematol* 121:749-757, 2003.

Kyle RA et al: Clinical course and prognosis of smoldering (asymptomatic) multiple myeloma, *N Engl J Med* 356:2582, 2007.

Kyle RA, Rajkumar SV: Multiple myeloma, *N Engl J Med* 351:1860-1873, 2004.

Nau KC, Lewis WD: Multiple myeloma: diagnosis and treatment, *Am Fam Physician* 78(7): 853-859, 2008.

Richardson PG et al: Bortezomib or high dose dexamethasone for relapsed multiple myeloma, *N Engl J Med* 352:2487-2498, 2005.

San Miguel JF et al: Bortezomib plus melphalan and prednisone for initial treatment of multiple myeloma, *N Engl J Med* 359:906-917, 2008.

AUTHOR: **FRED F. FERRI, M.D.**

 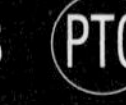

BASIC INFORMATION

DEFINITION

Multiple sclerosis is a chronic autoimmune demyelinating disease of the central nervous system (CNS) characterized by clinical attacks correlated with lesions separated in time and space. A clinical attack or relapse is the subacute onset of neurologic dysfunction that lasts for at least 24 hr. Subtypes include relapsing-remitting MS (RRMS) (relapses followed by complete or near-complete recovery), which often transitions later to secondary progressive MS (SPMS) (progression of disability with few or no relapses), and primary progressive MS (PPMS), which shows progression from the start. Rare MS variants include Balo's concentric sclerosis (neuroimaging and pathology show alternating rings of myelination and demyelination), Marburg's disease (neuroimaging shows a tumorlike lesion with significant edema, and pathology shows severe inflammation with necrosis), and Schilder's diffuse sclerosis (childhood onset with one to two large symmetric lesions). Neuromyelitis optica (NMO; Devic's disease) has recurrent relapses involving only the optic nerves and spinal cord.

SYNONYMS

MS
Disseminated sclerosis

ICD-9CM CODES
340 Multiple sclerosis

EPIDEMIOLOGY & DEMOGRAPHICS

PREVALENCE: Higher in northern latitudes and rare geographic clustering. Prevalence per 10^5 varies from 30 to 70 in parts of Italy and Spain to 100 to 200 in Scandinavia; 100 in the U.S.; 16 to 30 in Middle Eastern Arabs and 30 to 38 in Israeli Jews; and less than five to 10 in Asia, Central America, and most of Africa.

PREDOMINANT SEX & AGE: Female/male ratio is 1.5:1. MS is most commonly a disease of young adults. Mean ages of onset: overall, 30 yr; RRMS, 28 yr; SPMS, 40 yr; and PPMS, 37 yr.

SUBTYPES: 8% RRMS (70% convert to SPMS after 25 yr), 27% SPMS, and 15% PPMS

GENETICS: Frequency of MS in dizygotic twins and siblings is 3% to 5% and 20% to 40% in monozygotic twins. Most common associations include human leukocyte antigen classes I and II (DRB1*1501, DQA1*0102, DQB1*0602), T-cell receptor-beta, CTLA4, ICAM1, and SH2D2A.

PHYSICAL FINDINGS & CLINICAL PRESENTATION

- Common: fatigue, blurred vision, diplopia, vertigo, hemiparesis, paraparesis, monoparesis, numbness, paresthesias, ataxia, cognitive and urinary dysfunction
- Visual abnormalities: nystagmus, visual field defects, Marcus Gunn pupil (see topic "Optic Neuritis" and internuclear ophthalmoplegia)—paresis of the adducting eye on conjugate lateral gaze with horizontal nystagmus of the abducting eye
- Upper motor neuron (UMN) signs: spasticity, increased deep tendon reflexes, extensor plantar responses, clonus and UMN pattern of weakness (shoulder abduction, elbow, hand and finger extension, hip and knee flexion, foot dorsiflexion)
- Sensory loss: dermatomal loss of pain and temperature, loss of vibration and position sense, and a thoracic band of sensory loss
- Ataxia: intention tremor, heel-to-shin ataxia, inability to tandem
- Bladder dysfunction: detrusor hyperreflexia (urge incontinence), flaccidity (neurogenic bladder), and dyssynergia (bladder contracts against a closed sphincter)
- Lhermitte's sign: flexion of the neck elicits an electrical sensation extending down the spine and occasionally into the extremities

ETIOLOGY

The exact etiology of MS is unknown. It is believed to be caused by an interaction between multiple genes influencing the immune system and environmental factors, possibly involving certain viruses, vitamin D, and sun exposure.

DIAGNOSIS

- MS: primarily a clinical diagnosis based on a consistent clinical presentation with evidence of CNS demyelinating lesions disseminated in time and space not better explained by another disease.
- RRMS: a history of two relapses and confirmation on neurologic examination may be sufficient if *both* support the presence of at least two demyelinating lesions separated in time and space. If there is evidence of only one lesion on examination or clinical history of one relapse, MRI and other paraclinical testing may be used to make the diagnosis (Table 1-51).
- PPMS: insidious progression of disability with a positive CSF and both:
  1. Dissemination in space = MRI (nine T2 lesions in brain or two lesions in the spinal cord or four to eight brain lesions plus one spinal cord lesion) *or* visual evoked potential (VEP) (delayed) with four to eight brain lesions or four brain lesions plus one spinal cord lesion.
  2. MRI dissemination in time (as above) *or* continued progression for 1 yr.

DIFFERENTIAL DIAGNOSIS

- Autoimmune: acute disseminated encephalomyelitis (ADEM), postvaccination encephalomyelitis
- Degenerative: subacute combined degeneration of the cord (B_{12} deficiency), inherited spastic paraparesis
- Infections: progressive multifocal leukoencephalopathy, Lyme's disease, syphilis, HIV, human T-lymphotrophic virus 1, Whipple's disease, expanded differential in immunocompromised patients
- Inflammatory: systemic lupus erythematosus, Sjögren's disease, Behçet's disease, vasculitis, sarcoidosis, celiac disease
- Inherited metabolic disorders: leukodystrophies
- Mitochondrial: Leber's hereditary optic neuropathy, mitochondrial encephalopathy lactic acidosis and strokelike episodes
- Neoplasms: metastases, CNS lymphoma
- Vascular: subcortical infarcts, Binswanger's disease

WORKUP

- Lumbar puncture for all first-time relapses and all cases in which the diagnosis of MS is not definite. Possible CSF abnormalities include increased protein and mononuclear white blood cells (both usually only mildly elevated). An elevated CSF immunoglobulin (Ig) G index and positive oligoclonal bands (OCBs; send both with paired serum samples) are present in 70% and 90%, respectively, of clinically definite MS. False-positive results occur with IgG index often in CNS infections and inflammation and rarely with positive OCBs (at least two CSF OCBs with polyclonal or negative serum). Myelin basic protein will typically be elevated in the CSF after an acute exacerbation.
- Serum: recommend complete blood count (CBC), erythrocyte sedimentation rate, CHEM 7, liver function tests (LFTs), antinuclear antibody, vitamin B_{12}. Consider Lyme titer, angiotensin-converting enzyme, other infectious and collagen vascular serologies, thyroid function test, very-long-chain fatty acids, and arylsulfatase A.

TABLE 1-51 Summary of McDonald's Criteria for Diagnosis of MS

Clinical Attacks	Clinical Lesions	Paraclinical Testing Needed
2	2	None
2	1	MRI dissemination in space *or* two lesions on MRI consistent with MS plus positive CSF
1	2	MRI dissemination in time
1	1	MRI dissemination in space *or* two MRI lesions consistent with MS and positive CSF, *and* MRI dissemination in time

Evidence of clinical lesions by physical examination or evoked potentials.
CSF, Cerebrospinal fluid; *MRI,* magnetic resonance imaging; *MRI dissemination in space,* at least three of the following: (1) one enhancing lesion or nine T2 hyperintense lesions, (2) one infratentorial lesion, (3) one juxtacortical lesion, and (4) three periventricular lesions. Note: One spinal cord lesion may be substituted for one brain lesion; *MRI dissemination in time,* a new enhancing at least 3 mo or a new nonenhancing lesion at least 6 mo after the initial attack; *MS,* multiple sclerosis; *positive CSF,* positive oligoclonal bands or elevated immunoglobulin G index.

- Consider evoked potentials (visual, somatosensory, brain stem auditory evoked response). Demyelination will slow conduction velocities.

IMAGING STUDIES

Head imaging (CT or MRI) is strongly recommended. MRI of the head with gadolinium is the most sensitive (Fig. 1-203). MRI of the cervical spine can be helpful. MRI can assess disease load, acute lesions, and atrophy. A normal MRI of the brain does not conclusively exclude MS.

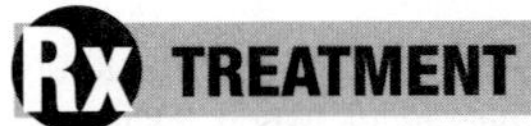

TREATMENT

NONPHARMACOLOGIC THERAPY

Patient education regarding the disease, treatment options, and prognosis

ACUTE GENERAL Rx

Relapses: high-dose IV methylprednisolone (3 to 5 days of 1 g/day; alternative dose is 15 mg/kg/day), often followed by a 7- to 10-day prednisone taper

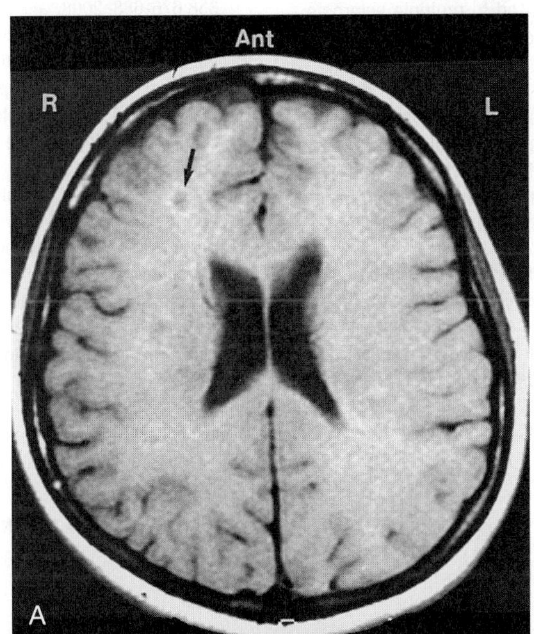

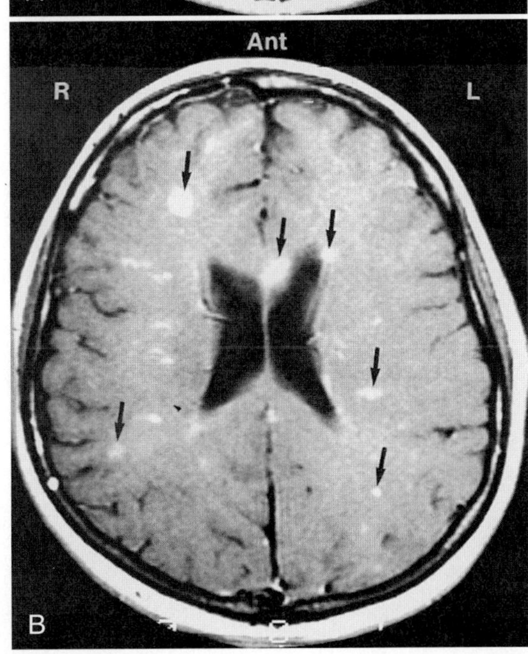

FIGURE 1-203 Multiple sclerosis. The noncontrasted T1-weighted magnetic resonance scan **(A)** shows one hypodensity *(black hole)* in the right frontal lobe *(arrow).* A gadolinium-enhanced scan **(B)** shows many enhancing lesions, only some of which are indicated *(arrows).* (From Mettler FA [ed]: *Primary care radiology,* Philadelphia, 2000, WB Saunders.)

CHRONIC Rx

- Disease-modifying therapy: includes interferon beta-1a (IM Avonex, SC Rebif), interferon beta-1b (SC Betaseron), or glatiramer acetate (SC Copaxone). Interferons need routine CBC and LFT checks (month 1 followed by trimonthly), occasionally thyroid-stimulating hormone. None needed with glatiramer acetate.
- Cytotoxic: methotrexate or azathioprine is occasionally used in RRMS or PPMS. Consider cyclophosphamide or mitoxantrone for frequent relapses with significant disability progression and early secondary progressive MS.
- Monoclonal antibodies: natalizumab (Tysabri) is approved for treatment of relapsing forms of MS by monthly infusion. It has been associated with an increased risk of developing progressive multifocal leukoencephalopathy—a rare but deadly brain infection. Patients taking natalizumab must enter into a registry for monitoring.
- Spasticity: baclofen, tizanidine, diazepam, lorazepam, or intrathecal baclofen.
- Pain: carbamazepine, gabapentin, or amitriptyline.
- Spastic bladder: oxybutynin, tolterodine, or propantheline. Prazosin for spastic sphincter.
- Fatigue: consider amantadine 100 mg bid, modafinil (most effective for somnolence), or fluoxetine.
- Tremor: clonazepam, carbamazepine, or propranolol.

DISPOSITION

Most patients have complete or near-complete recovery weeks to months after a relapse. The rate of disease progression is highly variable.

REFERRAL

- Initial neurology referral is recommended.
- Consider referrals for physical therapy, occupational therapy, social work, and urology.
- Referral to MS specialist if poor response to therapy, for consideration of cytotoxic treatment, or if the diagnosis is in doubt.

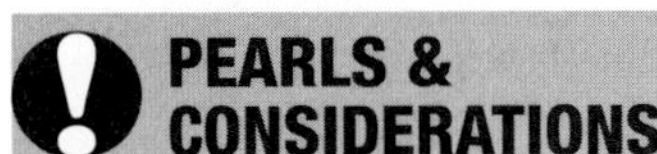

PEARLS & CONSIDERATIONS

- Pseudorelapses may occur with heat, fever, or infections (the Uhtoff phenomenon). Treatment with antipyretic medication or cooling devices may sometimes be appropriate.
- Preliminary trials have shown that cladribine (a drug that provides immunomodulation through selective targeting of lymphocyte subtypes) and fingolimod (a sphingosine-1-phosphate-receptor modulator) significantly reduce relapse rates, the risk of disability progression, and MRI measures of disease activity at 96 weeks.

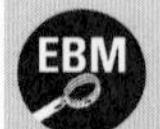

EVIDENCE

Please note: Complete text of EBM for this topic is available online.

Key trials and commentary:

Several controlled studies provide evidence that treatment with interferon-beta in patients with a first event suggestive of multiple sclerosis (MS) delays conversion to clinically definite MS (CDMS). The aim of this study was to determine whether early initiation of treatment with interferon-beta prevents development of confirmed disability in MS.

The data suggest that early initiation of treatment with interferon-beta-1b prevents the development of confirmed disability, supporting its use after the first manifestation of relapsing-remitting MS.

Kappos et al report results of a 3-year follow-up of a clinical trial examining the role of interferon-beta-1b as part of the very initial management of MS in young adults. Although there were no adolescents included in this series, the youngest adult in this series had just passed the adolescent period and therefore one might infer that the important data from this study may very well apply to children. The conclusion of the study was that early initiation of treatment with interferon-beta-1b prevents the development of confirmed disability and alternatively suggests that delaying treatment puts the patient at greater risk for the development of significant disability.[1] Ⓐ

One of the most difficult things an adult or child neurologist has to do when seeing a patient with symptoms suggestive of MS is to decide what to do in terms of therapy. The question is whether watchful waiting in someone with minimal symptoms is reasonable or whether such a delayed approach will compromise long-term outcome. Interferon therapy is expensive and has its side effects. At first look, one might think that the study of Kappos et al at least would solve the dilemma for adult patients, including young adult patients. As noted, however, in an editorial that accompanied this report, caution is warranted about the general applicability of the findings of this report to patients with clinically isolated symptoms related to multiple sclerosis. The concern has to do with the benefit vs. the risk given the fact that the difference between immediate treatment and delayed treatment in terms of long-term disability progression is somewhat small. Nonetheless, it is fair to say that the report of Kappos et al sets a new standard against which future clinical trials will be compared.

Evidence-Based Reference

1. Kappos L, for the BENEFIT Study Group: Effect of early versus delayed interferon beta-1b treatment on disability after a first clinical event suggestive of multiple sclerosis: a 3-year follow-up analysis of the BENEFIT study, *Lancet* 370:389-397, 2007. Commentary by J.A. Stockman III, M.D. Ⓐ

SUGGESTED READINGS

CAMMS 223 Trial Investigators: Alemtuzumab vs. interferon beta-1a in early multiple sclerosis, *N Engl J Med* 359:1786-1801, 2008.

CHAMPS Study Group: MRI predictors of early conversion to clinically definite MS in the CHAMPS placebo group, *Neurology* 59:998, 2002.

Dyment DA et al: Genetics of multiple sclerosis, *Lancet* 3:104, 2004.

Giovannoni G et al: A placebo-controlled trial of oral cladribine for relapsing multiple sclerosis, *N Engl J Med* 362:416-426, 2010.

Goodin DS et al: Disease-modifying therapies in multiple sclerosis, *Neurology* 58:169, 2002.

Hauser SL et al: B-cell depletion with rituximab in relapsing-remitting multiple sclerosis, *N Engl J Med* 358:676-688, 2008.

Jacobs LD et al: Intramuscular interferon beta-1a therapy, initiated during a first demyelinating event in multiple sclerosis, *N Engl J Med* 343:898, 2000.

Kappos L et al: A placebo-controlled trial of oral fingolimod in relapsing multiple sclerosis, *N Engl J Med* 362:387-401, 2010.

Kurtzke JF: Geography in multiple sclerosis, *J Neurol* 215:1, 1977.

McDonald WI et al: Recommended diagnostic criteria for multiple sclerosis, *Ann Neurol* 50:121, 2001.

Ransohoff RM: Natalizumab for multiple sclerosis, *N Engl J Med* 356:2622-2629, 2007.

Renoux C et al: Natural history of multiple sclerosis with childhood onset, *N Engl J Med* 356:2603-2613, 2007.

Weinshenker BG et al: The natural history of multiple sclerosis: a geographically based study, *Brain* 112:1419, 1989.

AUTHOR: **ALEXANDRA DEGENHARDT, M.D.**

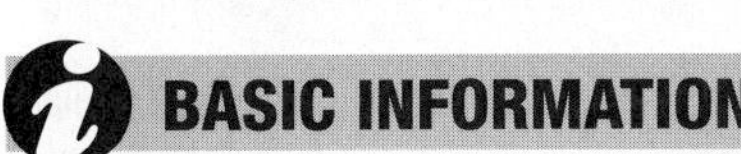

BASIC INFORMATION

DEFINITION

Mumps is an acute generalized viral infection that is usually characterized by nonsuppurative swelling and tenderness of one or both parotid glands. It is caused by mumps virus, a paramyxovirus and member of the paramyxoviridae family.

SYNONYMS

Viral parotitis
Parotitis

ICD-9CM CODES
072.9 Mumps

EPIDEMIOLOGY & DEMOGRAPHICS

INCIDENCE (IN U.S.):
- About 1600 infections/yr
- More than 150,000 cases/yr before licensure of mumps vaccine in 1967

PREDOMINANT SEX: Males = females
PREDOMINANT AGE: 75% of disease in teenage yr
PEAK INCIDENCE: Late winter and early spring months
GENETICS:
Congenital infection:
- First-trimester infection is associated with excessive fetal deaths.
- Second- and third-trimester infection is not associated with increased fetal mortality.

Neonatal infection:
- Uncommon
- Uncommon in infants <1 yr because of passive immunity conferred by placental transfer of maternal antibody

PHYSICAL FINDINGS & CLINICAL PRESENTATION

- Prodromal period:
  1. Low-grade fever
  2. Malaise
  3. Anorexia
  4. Headache
- Parotid swelling and tenderness are often the first signs of infection.
  1. Progresses over 2 to 3 days, then opposite side may become involved
  2. Unilateral parotitis in 25% of cases
  3. Considerable pain with parotid swelling, causing trismus and difficulty with mastication and pronunciation
  4. Pain exacerbated by eating or drinking citrus and other acidic foods
  5. Possible fever with parotid swelling, ranging up to 40° C
  6. Parotid swelling, usually resolving within 1 wk
- CNS involvement:
  1. May occur from 1 wk before to 2 wk after the onset of parotitis or even in its absence
  2. Meningitis:
     a. Occurs in 1% to 10% of patients with mumps parotitis
     b. Occurs 3 times more often in males than females
     c. Symptoms: headache, fever, nuchal rigidity, and vomiting
     d. Full recovery with no sequelae
  3. Encephalitis:
     a. May develop early, as a result of direct viral invasion of neurons, or late, around the second wk after onset of parotitis, and is a postinfectious demyelinating process.
     b. Mumps accounted for only 0.5% of viral meningitis.
     c. Symptoms: fever, alterations in the level of consciousness, possible seizures, paresis or paralysis, and aphasia. Fever can be quite high (40° to 41° C).
     d. Cerebellitis and hydrocephalus are serious complications of mumps encephalitis.
     e. May result in permanent sequelae or death.
  4. Other rare neurologic complications:
     a. Cerebellar ataxia
     b. Transverse myelitis
     c. Gullain-Barré syndrome
     d. Facial palsy
- Epididymoorchitis:
  1. Most common extra salivary gland complication of mumps in adult men
  2. Occurs in 38% of postpubertal males who have mumps
  3. Most often unilateral but is bilateral in 30% of males who develop this complication
  4. May precede development of parotitis
  5. May be only manifestation of mumps
  6. Two thirds of cases develop during first wk of parotitis
  7. One quarter of cases develop in second wk
  8. Symptoms
     a. Severe pain, swelling, and tenderness of the testes and scrotal erythema
     b. Fever and chills
  9. Some degree of testicular atrophy in 50% of cases, mo to yr later
  10. Sterility from bilateral orchitis is rare
- Involvement of pancreas and ovaries:
  1. Abdominal pain
  2. Fever
  3. Vomiting
  4. Oophoritis
     a. Occurs in 5% of postpubertal women with mumps
     b. Symptoms include fever, nausea, vomiting, and lower abdominal pain
     c. May rarely result in decreased fertility and premature menopause
- Transient renal impairment:
  1. Common
  2. Manifested by hematuria and polyuria
- Joint involvement:
  1. Migratory polyarthritis is most frequent
  2. Infrequently affects adults with mumps
  3. Occurs rarely in children
  4. Self-limited, with complete resolution
- Pancreatitis
  1. Uncommon as a severe illness
  2. Milder degree of upper abdominal discomfort
- Deafness:
  1. Most often unilateral, involving high frequencies; may rarely cause bilateral involvement
  2. Most patients recover
  3. Permanent unilateral deafness reported in 1 in 20,000 cases
  4. Labyrinthitis and end lymphatic hydrops also reported
- Myocardial involvement:
  1. Uncommon
  2. Rarely causes progressive and culminant fatal myocarditis with dilated cardiomyopathy
  3. Refractory arrhythmia and congestive heart failure
  4. Coronary artery involvement
- Eye involvement:
  1. Corneal endothelitis following mumps parotitis

ETIOLOGY

- Virus is spread via direct contact, droplet nuclei, fomites, or oral or nasal secretions.
- Patients are contagious from 48 hr before to 9 days after parotid swelling.

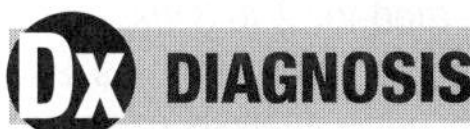

DIAGNOSIS

DIFFERENTIAL DIAGNOSIS

- Other viruses that may cause acute parotitis:
  1. Parainfluenza types 1 and 3
  2. Coxsackie viruses
  3. Influenza A
  4. Cytomegalovirus
- Suppurative parotitis:
  1. Most often caused by *Staphylococcus aureus*
  2. May be differentiated from mumps
     a. Extreme indurations, tenderness and erythema overlying the gland
     b. Ability to express pus from Stensen's duct or massage of parotid
- Other conditions that may occur with parotid enlargement or swelling:
  1. Sjögren's syndrome
  2. Leukemia
  3. Diabetes mellitus
  4. Uremia
  5. Malnutrition
  6. Cirrhosis
- Drugs that cause parotid swelling:
  1. Phenothiazines
  2. Phenylbutazone
  3. Thiouracil
  4. Iodides
- Conditions that cause unilateral swelling:
  1. Tumors
  2. Cysts
  3. Stones causing obstruction
  4. Strictures causing obstruction

WORKUP

- Diagnosis based on history of exposure and physical finding of parotid tenderness with mild to moderate constitutional symptoms.
- Diagnosis is confirmed by a variety of serologic tests or isolation of the virus.

LABORATORY TESTS

- Diagnosis is confirmed by fourfold rise between acute and convalescent sera by CF, ELISA, or neutralization tests.
- Virus can be isolated from the saliva, usually from 2 to 3 days before to 4 to 5 days after the onset of parotitis.
- Virus can be isolated from CSF in patients with meningitis during the first 3 days of meningeal findings. More rapid confirmation of mumps in the CSF is IgM antibody capture immunoassay and nested polymerase chain reaction (PCR) assay.
- Virus can be detected in urine during the first 2 wk of infection.
- WBC:
  1. May be normal or possible mild leucopenia with a relative lymphocytosis
  2. Leucocytosis with left shift with extra salivary gland involvement, such as meningitis, orchitis, or pancreatitis
- Serum amylase:
  1. Elevated in the presence of parotitis
  2. May remain elevated for 2 to 3 wk
  3. May be differentiated from mumps and parotids by isoenzyme analysis or serum pancreatic lipase
- Mumps meningitis:
  1. CSF WBCs from 10 to 2000 WBC/mm^3 with a predominance of lymphocytes
  2. In 20% to 25% of patients, predominance of polymorphonuclear cells
  3. CSF protein normal or mildly elevated
  4. CSF glucose low, <40 mg/dl, in 6% to 30% of patients

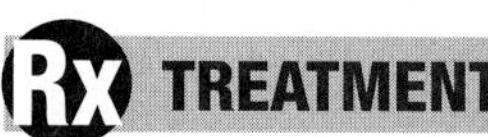

TREATMENT

NONPHARMACOLOGIC THERAPY

- Supportive treatment
- Adequate hydration and nutrition

ACUTE GENERAL Rx

- Analgesics and antipyretics to relieve pain and fever
- Narcotic analgesics, along with bed rest, ice packs, and a testicular bridge, to relieve pain associated with mumps orchitis
- IV fluids for patients with frequent vomiting associated with mumps pancreatitis or meningitis

DISPOSITION

Most patients recover without incident.

REFERRAL

- To a neurologist if significant neurologic complications develop during or following mumps (myelitis, encephalitis, cranial nerve involvement, cerebellar ataxia, etc.)
- To a cardiologist if viral perimyocarditis develops
- To a urologist if orchitis develops

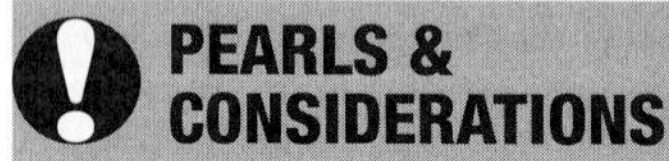

PEARLS & CONSIDERATIONS

COMMENTS

Prevention:

- Attenuated live mumps virus vaccine has been available since 1967.
  1. Usually given in combination with measles and rubella vaccines
  2. Should be given at 15 mo of age, and again at 5 to 12 yr
  3. Seroconversion in about 100% of infants given the vaccine
  4. Contraindicated in pregnant women and immunocompromised patients
  5. Patients with asymptomatic HIV infection and patients with symptomatic HIV infection, in the absence of severe immunosuppression, can safely receive mumps, measles, and rubella (MMR) vaccine
  6. Adverse events of vaccination include: local pain; indurations; thrombocytopenic purpura; Guillain-Barré syndrome; cerebellar ataxia
- Infected patients should be isolated until parotid swelling resolves.
- Because virus may be shed before the onset of parotid swelling, isolation possibly not of great value in limiting spread of infection.

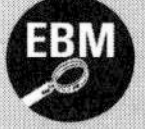

EVIDENCE

Randomized controlled trials and observational studies have shown that mumps vaccination is highly effective, but subsequent outbreak studies have suggested a lower efficacy for the vaccine.

There are no randomized controlled trials comparing the clinical effects of combined MMR vaccine versus no vaccine or placebo.[1]

Randomized controlled trials and observational studies have shown that mumps vaccination is highly effective, with an efficacy rate around 95%.[1] Ⓐ

Outbreak studies have suggested a lower efficacy for the vaccine, and it is unclear whether this reflects true vaccine failure, or is the result of higher transmission rates during outbreaks.[2] Ⓐ

The evidence so far has failed to support the much-publicized hypothesis concerning the link between the MMR vaccine and the development of autistic spectrum disorders or inflammatory bowel disease.

A large proportion of the literature on adverse events after immunization is based on passive reporting, which has major limitations, for example, underreporting events or reporting events that are unassociated with the intervention.[1]

Existing evidence has failed to confirm an association between MMR vaccines and any autistic disorder, ulcerative colitis, Crohn's disease, or inflammatory bowel disease.[3] Ⓐ

A systematic review has found that exposure to the MMR vaccine is likely to be associated with aseptic meningitis if a vaccine containing the Urabe strain of mumps was used, but unlikely to be associated with aseptic meningitis if a vaccine containing the Jeryl-Lynn strain of mumps was used. These findings did not reach statistical significance.[3] Ⓐ

Evidence-Based References

1. Booy R et al: Measles, mumps and rubella: prevention, *Clin Evid* 15:448-468, 2006.
2. Harling R et al: The effectiveness of the mumps component of the MMR vaccine; a case control study, *Vaccine* 23:4070-4074, 2005. Ⓐ
3. Demicheli V et al: Vaccines for measles, mumps and rubella in children, *Cochrane Database Rev* 4, 2005. Ⓐ

SUGGESTED READINGS

Centers for Disease Control and Prevention: Updated recommendations of the Advisory Committee on Immunization Practices (ACIP) for the control and elimination of mumps, *MMWR Morb Mortal Wkly Rep* 55(22):629, 2006.

Dayan GH et al: Recent resurgence of mumps in the United States, *N Engl J Med* 358:1580, 2008.

AUTHORS: **GLENN G. FORT, M.D., M.P.H.,** and **DENNIS J. MIKOLICH, M.D.**

BASIC INFORMATION

DEFINITION

Muscular dystrophy (MD) refers to a heterogeneous group of inherited disorders resulting in characteristic patterns of muscle weakness, some with cardiac involvement. Only disorders with childhood or adult onset are considered here (i.e., excluding congenital myopathies).

ICD-9CM CODES
359 Muscular dystrophies and other myopathies
359.1 Hereditary progressive muscular dystrophy

EPIDEMIOLOGY & DEMOGRAPHICS

INCIDENCE:

- Most common childhood MD is Duchenne's muscular dystrophy (DMD) with an incidence of 1/3500 male births
- Most common adult MD is myotonic dystrophy with an incidence as high as 1/8000

GENETICS:

- **Dystrophinopathies:** X-linked recessive defect in dystrophin gene resulting in either absence (DMD) or reduced/defective (Becker's MD [BMD]) dystrophin.
- **Myotonic Dystrophy:** Autosomal dominant (AD) CTG trinucleotide repeat.
- **Limb-Girdle Muscular Dystrophy:** Autosomal recessive, also autosomal dominant forms with deficiency identified in multiple proteins (sarcoglycan, calpain, dysferlin, telethonin, lamin A/C, myotilin, and caveolin-3).
- **Emery-Dreifuss Muscular Dystrophy:** X-linked recessive defect in nuclear protein emerin or AR defect in inner nuclear lamina proteins lamin A/C.
- **Facioscapulohumeral Muscular Dystrophy:** AD; genetic mutation causes deletion of 3.3 kb repeat.
- **Oculopharyngeal Muscular Dystrophy:** AD GCG trinucleotide repeat resulting in deficient mRNA transfer from nucleus.

PHYSICAL FINDINGS & CLINICAL PRESENTATION

- **Dystrophinopathies:** Proximal arm and leg weakness with hypertrophic calf muscles, delayed motor milestones, cognitive impairment, cardiac involvement, progressive course resulting in respiratory complications and respiratory failure
    - DMD onset at 2 to 3 yr old, typically wheelchair-bound by 12 yr
    - BMD onset at 5 to 15 yr old, ambulatory beyond age 15
- **Myotonic Dystrophy:** Variable age of onset and severity manifesting as predominately distal weakness with long face, percussion and grip myotonia, temporalis and masseter wasting, ptosis, hypersomnolence, cognitive impairment, and cardiac conduction defects. May be associated with frontal balding, cataracts, impaired glucose tolerance, and male infertility.
- **Limb-Girdle MD:** Phenotypically and genetically heterogenous characterized by proximal hip and shoulder girdle weakness, some genotypes featuring cardiac involvement.
- **Emery-Dreifuss MD:** Early adulthood onset with predominately humeroperoneal weakness, early contractures, and cardiac dysfunction.
- **Facioscapulohumeral MD:** Onset typically in late childhood or adolescence with weakness mostly in face and shoulder girdle musculature and possible later, mild involvement of lower extremities.
- **Oculopharyngeal MD:** Symptom onset typically in mid-adult life with ptosis, dysphagia, dysarthria, and proximal muscle weakness.

DIAGNOSIS

DIFFERENTIAL DIAGNOSIS

Myasthenia gravis, inflammatory myopathy, metabolic myopathy, endocrine myopathy, toxic myopathy, mitochondrial myopathy

WORKUP

- CK
- ECG, Holter monitor, echocardiography
- EMG
- Muscle biopsy with immunohistochemistry useful for diagnosis of dystrophinopathies and limb-girdle MD
- DNA analysis helpful if clinical suspicion is for myotonic, Emery-Drefuss, facioscapulohumeral, and oculopharyngeal MDs
- Assessment of respiratory parameters, including forced vital capacity (FVC)

TREATMENT

NONPHARMACOLOGIC THERAPY

- Genetic counseling
- Physical, occupational, respiratory, speech therapy as symptoms dictate
- Screening for sleep-disordered breathing with overnight polysomnogram (PSG) if clinically indicated
- Pacemaker placement may be necessary if cardiac conduction defect present

ACUTE GENERAL Rx

- Prednisone may modestly prolong ambulation in DMD.

CHRONIC Rx

- Vigilance to avoid cardiac and respiratory complications, joint contractures

DISPOSITION

Variable course, because severity of phenotype is contingent upon both diagnosis and genotype

REFERRAL

- Surgical referral for correction of scoliosis or contractures may be necessary.
- Assessment and follow-up in a muscular dystrophy specialty clinic.

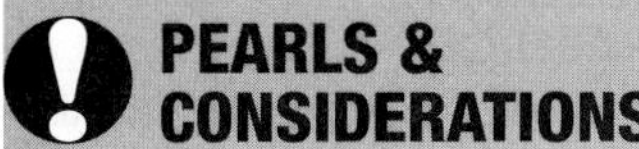

PEARLS & CONSIDERATIONS

Formal evaluation by anesthetist recommended before any operation with general anesthesia in patients with dystrophinopathy

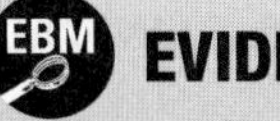

EVIDENCE

There is evidence that corticosteroids are of benefit in the treatment of DMD.

Prednisone has been demonstrated to have a beneficial effect on muscle strength and function in boys with DMD and should be offered (at a dose of 0.75 mg/kg/day) as treatment. Benefits and side effects of corticosteroid therapy need to be monitored.[1] C

A systematic review found that corticosteroid therapy in DMD improves muscle strength and function in the short-term (6 mo to 2 yr). The long-term benefits remain unclear and the review cautioned that any such benefits must be weighed against the long-term side effects of long-term steroid use.[2] A

Evidence-Based References

1. Moxley RT 3rd et al: Practice parameter: corticosteroid treatment of Duchenne dystrophy: report of the Quality Standards Subcommittee of the American Academy of Neurology and the Practice Committee of the Child Neurology Society, *Neurology* 64: 13-20, 2005. C
2. Manzur AY et al: Glucocorticoid corticosteroids for Duchenne muscular dystrophy, *Cochrane Database Syst Rev* 2: 2004. A

SUGGESTED READINGS

Blau HM: Cell therapies for muscular dystrophy, *N Engl J Med* 359:1403-1405, 2008.

Emery AE: Muscular dystrophy into the new millennium, *Neuromuscul Disord* 12(4):843, 2002.

Emery AE: The muscular dystrophies, *Lancet* 359(9307): 687, 2002.

Saperstein DS et al: Clinical and genetic aspects of distal myopathies, *Muscle Nerve* 24(11):1440, 2001.

AUTHOR: **TAYLOR HARRISON, M.D.**

Mushroom Poisoning (PTG)

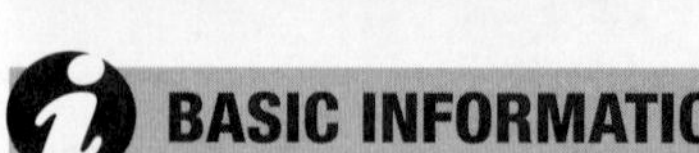

BASIC INFORMATION

DEFINITION

Mushroom poisoning is intoxication resulting from ingestion of poisonous mushrooms.

ICD-9CM CODES
988.1 Mushroom poisoning

EPIDEMIOLOGY & DEMOGRAPHICS

- 5% of all mushrooms are poisonous. Distinction between poisonous and edible mushrooms may be difficult even by experienced persons.
- Common poisonous species include *Amanita, Russula, Gyromitra,* and *Omphalotus.*

PHYSICAL FINDINGS & CLINICAL PRESENTATION (Table 1-52)

- *Russula* causes confusion, delirium, visual disturbance, tachycardia, and diarrhea within a few hours of ingestion. Prognosis: spontaneous recovery (mortality rate <1%).
- *Amanita* and *Gyromitra* intoxication begins with symptoms of gastroenteritis (nausea, vomiting, diarrhea, abdominal cramps) approximately 10 hr after ingestion. *Amanita* then causes cardiomyopathy and hepatic and renal failure. *Gyromitra* produces jaundice and seizures. Both mushrooms are associated with a 50% mortality rate.
- *Omphalotus* causes symptoms of gastroenteritis that subside spontaneously within 24 hr.

ETIOLOGY

- *Amanita* contains cytotoxic substances and isoxazoles that are gamma-aminobutyric acid neurotransmitter analogs.
- *Gyromitra* contains a pyridoxine antagonist that disrupts the gastrointestinal mucosa and causes hemolysis.
- *Russula* contains a cholinergic substance.

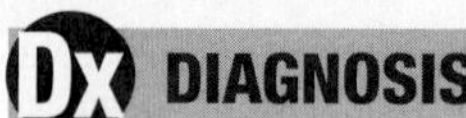

DIAGNOSIS

DIFFERENTIAL DIAGNOSIS

- Food poisoning
- Overdose of prescription or illegal drug
- Other intoxications
- See topic on specific organ failure (e.g., renal or hepatic failure) for differential diagnosis of those conditions

WORKUP

- History
- Inspection and identification of suspected mushrooms
- Mushroom or gastric content analysis (by thin-layer chromatography or radioimmunoassay)

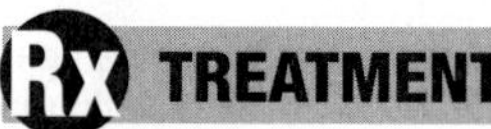

TREATMENT

- Gastric lavage
- Repeated administration of activated charcoal
- Supportive care as needed (may require respiratory assistance, hemodialysis, or emergency liver transplantation)

AUTHOR: **FRED F. FERRI, M.D.**

TABLE 1-52 Mushroom Poisoning Syndromes

Syndrome	Incubation Period (hr)	Species	Toxin
Confusion, restlessness, visual disturbances, lethargy	2	*Amanita muscaria* *Amanita pantherina*	Ibotenic acid, muscimol
Parasympathetic activity	2	*Inocybe* spp. *Clitocybe* spp.	Muscarine
Hallucinations	2	*Psilocybe* spp. *Panacolus* spp.	Psilocybin Psilocin
Disulfiram	2	*Coprinus atramentarius*	Disulfiram-like substances
Gastroenteritis	2	Many	Unknown
Hepatorenal failure	6-24	*Amanita phalloides* *Amanita virosa* *Amanita verna* *Galerina autumnalis* *Galerina marginata* *Galerina venenata*	Amatoxins Phallotoxins
Hepatic failure	6-24	*Gyromitra* spp.	Gyromitrin

From Gorbach SL: *Infectious diseases,* ed 2, Philadelphia, 1998, WB Saunders.

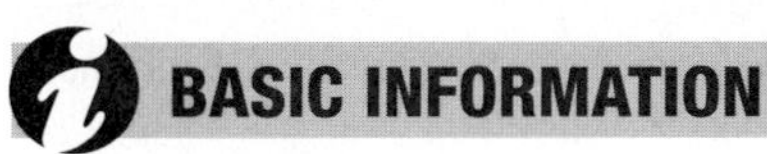

BASIC INFORMATION

DEFINITION

Myasthenia gravis (MG) is an autoimmune disorder of postsynaptic neuromuscular transmission classically directed against the nicotinic acetylcholine receptor (AChR) of the neuromuscular junction, resulting in a decrease in functional postsynaptic ACh receptors and consequent weakness.

ICD-9CM CODES

358.0 Myasthenia gravis

EPIDEMIOLOGY & DEMOGRAPHICS

INCIDENCE (IN U.S.): Two to five cases annually per 1 million persons

PEAK INCIDENCE: Female, second to third decades; male, sixth to seventh decades

PREVALENCE (IN U.S.): One per 20,000 persons

PREDOMINANT SEX: Females are affected more often than males (3:2) in adults; they are equally affected in the elderly

GENETICS: Increased frequency of HLA-B8, DR3

PHYSICAL FINDINGS & CLINICAL PRESENTATION

- The hallmark of MG is fluctuating weakness worsened with exercise and improved with rest.
- Generalized weakness involving proximal muscles, diaphragm, and neck extensors is common.
- Weakness is confined to eyelids and extraocular muscles in approximately 15% of patients.
- Bulbar symptoms of ptosis, diplopia, dysarthria, and dysphagia are common.
- Reflexes, sensation, and coordination are normal.

ETIOLOGY

Antibody-mediated decrease in nicotinic AChR in the postsynaptic neuromuscular junction resulting in defective neuromuscular transmission and subsequent muscle weakness and fatigue

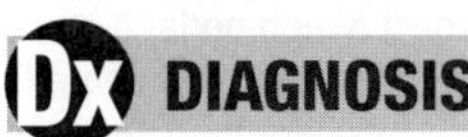

DIAGNOSIS

DIFFERENTIAL DIAGNOSIS

Lambert-Eaton myasthenic syndrome, botulism, medication-induced myasthenia, chronic progressive external ophthalmoplegia, congenital myasthenic syndromes, thyroid disease, basilar meningitis, intracranial mass lesion with cranial neuropathy, Miller-Fisher variant of Guillain-Barré syndrome

WORKUP

- Tensilon test: useful in MG patients with ocular symptoms. Cardiac monitoring and atropine ready at the bedside are essential.
- Repetitive nerve stimulation: successive stimulation shows decrement of muscle action potential in clinically weak muscle; may be negative in up to 50%.
- Single-fiber electromyography: highly sensitive; abnormal in up to 95% of patients.
- Serum AChR antibodies found in up to 80% of patients.
- A subset of patients with seronegative MG may have muscle-specific tyrosine kinase (MUSK) antibodies.

ADDITIONAL TESTS

- Spirometry to document pulmonary function
- CT scan of anterior chest to look for thymoma or residual thymic tissue
- Thyroid-stimulating hormone, free T_4 to rule out thyroid disease

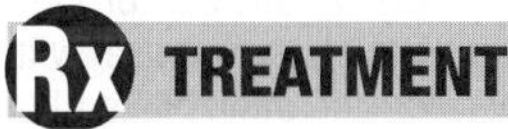

TREATMENT

NONPHARMACOLOGIC THERAPY

- Patient education to facilitate recognition of worsening symptoms and impress need for medical evaluation at onset of clinical deterioration
- Avoidance of selected drugs known to provoke exacerbations of MG (beta-blockers, aminoglycoside and quinolone antibiotics, class I antiarrhythmics)
- Prompt treatment of infections, diet modification, and speech evaluation with dysphagia

ACUTE GENERAL Rx

- Symptomatic treatment with acetylcholinesterase inhibitors:
  1. Pyridostigmine 30 to 60 mg PO q4-6h initially; onset of effects is 30 min, duration 4 hr
- Immunosuppressive treatment with corticosteroids, azathioprine, cyclosporine for long-term disease-modifying therapy
  1. Prednisone initiated at 15 to 20 mg qd titrate by 5-mg increments to effect or dose of 1 mg/kg/day with improvement in 2 to 4 wk and maximal response by 3 to 6 mo
  2. Azathioprine initiated at 50 mg qd titrated to 2 to 3 mg/kg/day with clinical effect in 6 to 12 mo
  3. Cyclosporine initiated at 5 mg/kg/day with clinical effect within 1 to 2 mo
- Plasmapheresis and IV immunoglobulin are short-term options for immunotherapy, including during an exacerbation.
- Mechanical ventilation is lifesaving in setting of a myasthenic crisis. Consider elective intubation if forced vital capacity <15 ml/kg, maximal expiratory pressure <40 cm H_2O, or negative inspiratory pressure <25 cm H_2O.

SURGICAL Rx

- In thymomatous MG, thymectomy is indicated in all patients.
- For nonthymomatous autoimmune MG, thymectomy is an option in select patients, typically <40 yr.

DISPOSITION

Course of disease is highly variable.

REFERRAL

Surgical referral for thymectomy in selected cases (see "Surgical Rx")

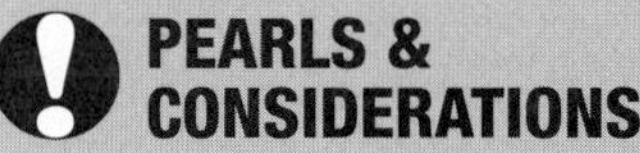

PEARLS & CONSIDERATIONS

- Sustained upward or lateral gaze and arm abduction for 120 sec may be necessary to elicit subtle signs on examination.
- Myasthenic patients can worsen rapidly and warrant close, careful observation during an exacerbation.

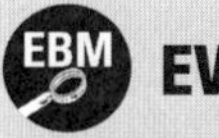

EVIDENCE

A systematic review concluded that limited evidence from randomized controlled trials (RCTs) suggests that corticosteroid treatment offers significant short-term benefit in myasthenia gravis compared with placebo. Limited evidence from RCTs does not show any difference in efficacy between corticosteroids and either azathioprine or intravenous immunoglobulin.[1] Ⓐ

Evidence-Based Reference

1. Schneider-Gold C et al: Corticosteroids for myasthenia gravis, *Cochrane Database Rev* 2, 2005. Ⓐ

SUGGESTED READINGS

Hampton T: Trials assess myasthenia gravis therapies, *JAMA* 298:29-30, 2007.

Keesey JC: Clinical evaluation and management of myasthenia gravis, *Muscle Nerve* 29(4):484, 2004.

AUTHOR: **TAYLOR HARRISON, M.D.**

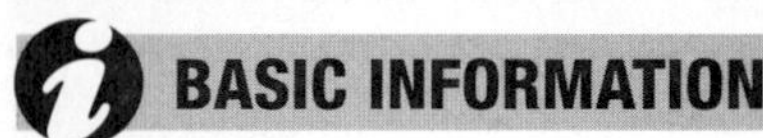

BASIC INFORMATION

DEFINITION

Mycosis fungoides refers to a T-cell lymphoproliferative disorder with characteristic cutaneous skin lesions and the potential to disseminate into lymph nodes and viscera.

SYNONYMS

Cutaneous T-cell lymphoma

ICD-9CM CODES
202.1 Mycosis fungoides

EPIDEMIOLOGY & DEMOGRAPHICS

- Incidence of mycosis fungoides is four cases per 1 million persons.
- Approximately 1000 new cases are diagnosed annually in the U.S.
- More commonly affects males than females (2:1).
- Affects blacks more often than whites (2:1).
- Usually found in males ages 40 to 60 yr.

PHYSICAL FINDINGS & CLINICAL PRESENTATION

Mycosis fungoides characteristically progresses through three phases:

- A *premycotic phase* featuring scaly, erythematous patches that can last from months to years. During this stage the diagnosis can only be suspected because the histopathologic features are not definitive for mycosis fungoides. Lesions are pruritic and can appear anywhere but are usually found in sun-shielded areas. Parapsoriasis in plaques, poikilodermatous parapsoriasis, parapsoriasis lichenoides, and variegata are skin lesions suspicious of representing premycotic cutaneous T-cell lymphoma.
- The *infiltrative plaque phase* features raised, indurated erythematous palpable plaques that are pruritic and may be associated with alopecia.
    - Stage IA disease is defined as a patch or plaque skin disease involving <10% of the skin surface area and with absence of blood involvement or with low blood tumor burden (<5% of atypical T cells [Sézary cells] in the peripheral blood).
    - Stage IB disease (Fig. 1-204) is defined as a patch or plaque skin disease involving ≥10% of the skin surface area with absence of blood involvement or low blood tumor burden (<5% Sézary cells)
- The *tumor phase* is characterized by large, lumpy nodules arising from a premycotic patch, plaque, or unaffected skin and represents systemic infiltration and spreading. The tumors can be pruritic and large (>10 cm) and ulceration can occur.
    - Stage IIA and stage IIB diseases are defined by the presence of tumors with or without clinically abnormal peripheral lymph nodes with absence of blood involvement or low blood tumor burden. In approximately 5% of cases of mycosis fungoides, the presentation may be a diffuse, painful, pruritive erythroderma with Sézary cells in the peripheral blood (known as Sézary syndrome).
    - Stage III disease is defined by the presence of generalized erythroderma from the spread of cancer cells through the skin but not yet to the lymph nodes.
- Lymphadenopathy can occur during the plaque or tumor stages and may be regional or diffuse.
    - Stage IVA disease is defined by a lymph node biopsy showing large clusters of atypical cells, more than six cells, or total effacement by atypical cells.
- Infiltration of the liver, spleen, lungs, bone marrow, kidney, stomach, and brain can occur.
    - Stage IVB disease is defined by the presence of visceral involvement.

ETIOLOGY

The specific cause of mycosis fungoides is not known. Infection with the retrovirus HTLV-1 has been suspected, given the association of individuals infected with HTLV-1 and those with T-cell leukemia. Other considerations listed but unsubstantiated include environmental toxins (e.g., tobacco, pesticides, herbicides, and solvents) and genetic predisposition.

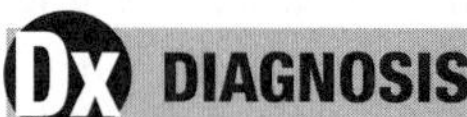

DIAGNOSIS

The diagnosis of mycosis fungoides is established by skin biopsy. This may be difficult to differentiate from other skin lesions in the early phases of the disease (e.g., premycotic patch or early plaque lesions); therefore the diagnosis can only be suspected.

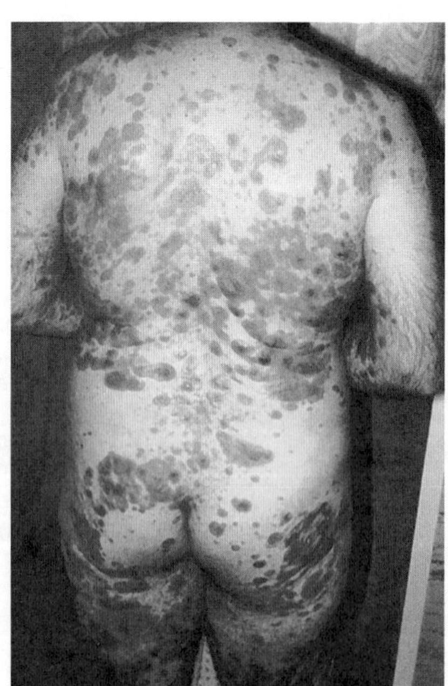

FIGURE 1-204 Cutaneous T-cell lymphoma (mycosis fungoides). Note patch, plaque, and tumor stages. (From Noble J [ed]: *Textbook of primary care medicine,* ed 2, St Louis, 1996, Mosby.)

DIFFERENTIAL DIAGNOSIS

- Contact dermatitis
- Atopic dermatitis
- Nummular dermatitis
- Parapsoriases
- Superficial fungal infections
- Drug eruptions
- Psoriasis
- Photodermatitis
- Alopecia mucinosa
- Lymphomatoid papulosis

WORKUP

Any patient who is suspected of having mycosis fungoides should have a staging workup. Prognosis in patients with mycosis fungoides depends on the type of skin lesions and the extent of disease. The workup should focus on:

1. Complete physical examination:
    - The type of skin lesion and the extent of skin involvement of the body (e.g., skin involvement is >10% or <10% of the skin surface)
    - Identification of palpable lymph node (especially those >1.5 cm in largest diameter)
    - Identification of organomegaly (e.g., lungs, liver)
2. Skin biopsy:
    - Biopsy of the most indurated area
    - Immunophenotyping
    - Evaluation for clonality
3. Blood test:
    - Complete blood count with differential, liver function tests, lactate dehydrogenase, chemistry
    - T-cell receptor gene rearrangement
    - Determination of Sézary cell count and/or flow cytometry
4. Radiologic tests
    - Depending on the stage of the disease, chest radiograph; ultrasound; and CT scan of the chest, abdomen, and pelvis alone, with or without fluorodeoxyglucose positron emission tomography scan
5. Lymph node biopsy
    - Excisional biopsy
    - Biopsy of the largest lymph node
    - If multiple nodes enlarged, order of preference is cervical, axillary, and inguinal areas
    - Histopathology, flow cytometry, T-cell receptor gene rearrangement

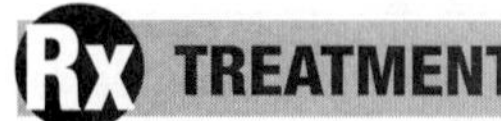

TREATMENT

Treatment is guided according to the stage of disease. A treatment algorithm is described in the online version of Section III.

NONPHARMACOLOGIC THERAPY

- For dry, cracking skin, emollients (e.g., lanolin and petrolatum) are applied bid.
- Moisturizing lotion (e.g., ammonium lactate) applied bid.

- Topical antibiotics (e.g., bacitracin) are used on ulcerative tumors.

ACUTE GENERAL Rx

- Treatment of patients with stage IA limited patch or plaque phase include:
  - Topical nitrogen mustard 10 to 20 mg per 100 ml in water or ointment base applied to affected areas daily until cleared (usually 1 to 2 mo).
  - Psoralen ultraviolet A (PUVA) light therapy where 0.6 mg/kg of 8-methoxypsoralen is ingested 1 to 2 hr before exposure of the skin to UVA light (320 to 400 nm). This is done three times per wk and tapered to twice per wk until all the lesions have cleared. This is typically continued for 6 mo with a 90% complete remission rate.
- Treatment of patients with stage IB and IIA disease is similar to stage IA, with topical nitrogen mustard or PUVA.
  - Total skin electron beam therapy is considered in patients with thick plaques.
  - Interferon-alpha 5 million units SQ three times weekly can be considered in patients with stage IB or IIA disease.
  - Retinoids in combination with PUVA are used in refractory cases. Isotretinoin 1 mg/kg per day or acitretin 25 to 50 mg per day is the standard dosing.
- Treatment of patients with stage IIB disease with generalized tumor and plaque disease includes:
  - Total skin electron beam therapy in doses of 3000 to 3600 cGy given over 8 to 10 wk followed by adjuvant therapy with topical mustard can be used.

CHRONIC Rx

- In patients developing diffuse erythroderma, stage III disease (e.g., Sézary syndrome, extracorporeal photophoresis), 8-methoxypsoralen is ingested and peripheral blood is exposed to UVA through a membrane filter.
- In stage IV disease, interferon and other systemic chemotherapeutic agents (e.g., methotrexate, cyclophosphamide, doxorubicin, vincristine, prednisone) are considered.

DISPOSITION

- The median survival in patients with early patch or plaque phase disease and no extradermal involvement is 12 yr.
- The median survival of patients with skin involvement and lymph node involvement, but no visceral involvement, is approximately 5 yr.
- The median survival in patients with visceral involvement is 2.5 yr.

REFERRAL

Any patient with suspected mycosis fungoides should be referred to a dermatologist for definitive diagnosis and initial therapy. Oncology consultation is also indicated in patients with more advanced disease.

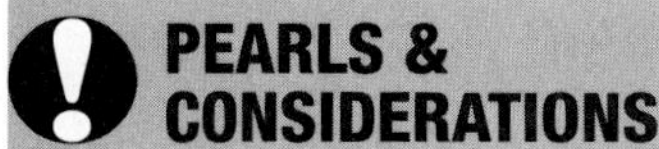

PEARLS & CONSIDERATIONS

A TNM staging classification of mycosis fungoides has been in use for guiding therapy since 1979. The International Society for Cutaneous Lymphomas (ISCL) and the Cutaneous Lymphoma Task Force of the European Organization of Research and Treatment of Cancer (EORTC) recommended revisions to the TNM classification and staging system of cutaneous T-cell lymphoma in 2007.

COMMENTS

Mycosis fungoides is thought to represent one class of the spectrum of cutaneous T-cell lymphomas.

SUGGESTED READINGS

Foss F: Mycosis fungoides and the Sézary syndrome, *Curr Opin Oncol* 16(5):421, 2004.

Girardi M et al: The pathogenesis of mycosis fungoides, *N Engl J Med* 350(19):1978, 2004.

Lundin J, Osterborg A: Therapy for mycosis fungoides, *Curr Treat Options Oncol* 5(3):203, 2004.

Olsen E: Revisions to the staging and classification of mycosis fungoides and Sézary syndrome: a proposal of the International Society for Cutaneous Lymphomas (ISCL) and the Cutaneous Lymphoma Task Force of the European Organization of Research and Treatment of Cancer (EORTC), *Blood* 110(6):1713, 2007.

AUTHOR: **TANYA ALI, M.D.**

Myelodysplastic Syndrome (ALG)

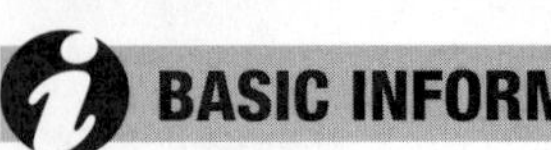

BASIC INFORMATION

DEFINITION

Myelodysplastic syndrome (MDS) is a group of acquired clonal disorders affecting the hemopoietic stem cells and characterized by cytopenias with hypercellular bone marrow and various morphologic abnormalities in the hemopoietic cell lines. MDS shows abnormal (dysplastic) hemopoietic maturation. Marrow cellularity is increased, reflecting an effective hematopoiesis, but inadequate maturation results in peripheral cytopenias.

CLASSIFICATION

- Myelodysplasia encompasses several heterogenous syndromes. The French-American-British (FAB) classification of MDSs is based on the proportion of immature blast cells in the blood and marrow and on the presence or absence of ringed sideroblasts or peripheral monocytosis (Table 1-53). It includes refractory anemia, refractory anemia with ringed sideroblasts, refractory anemia with excess blasts, chronic myelomonocytic leukemia, and refractory anemia with excess blasts in transformation.
- In 1999 the World Health Organization modified the FAB by incorporating newer morphologic insights and cytogenetic findings. It includes the disease subtypes refractory anemia, refractory anemia with ringed sideroblasts, refractory cytopenia with multilineage dysplasia, refractory cytopenia with multilineage dysplasia and ringed sideroblasts, refractory anemia with excessive blasts (1, 2), unclassified MDS, and MDS associated with isolated del(5q).

SYNONYMS

MDS
Preleukemia
Dysmyelopoietic syndrome

ICD-9CM CODES
238.7 Myelodysplastic syndrome

EPIDEMIOLOGY & DEMOGRAPHICS

INCIDENCE (IN U.S.): Approximately 82 cases/100,000 persons per yr. An estimated 7000 to 12,000 new cases are diagnosed annually in the U.S.

PREDOMINANT AGE: More common in elderly patients; median age, >65 yr

PHYSICAL FINDINGS & CLINICAL PRESENTATION

- Splenomegaly, skin pallor, mucosal bleeding, and ecchymosis may be present.
- Patients often present with fatigue.
- Fever, infection, and dyspnea are common.

ETIOLOGY

Unknown. However, exposure to radiation, chemotherapeutic agents, benzene, or other organic compounds is associated with myelodysplasia.

Dx DIAGNOSIS

DIFFERENTIAL DIAGNOSIS

- Hereditary dysplasias (e.g., Fanconi's anemia, Diamond-Blackfan syndrome)
- Vitamin B_{12}/folate deficiency
- Exposure to toxins (drugs, alcohol, chemotherapy)
- Renal failure
- Irradiation
- Autoimmune disease
- Infections (tuberculosis, viral infections)
- Paroxysmal nocturnal hemoglobinuria

WORKUP

Diagnostic workup includes laboratory evaluation and bone marrow examination. Cytogenetic analysis by conventional metaphase karyotyping should be performed in patients with MDS.

Rx TREATMENT

NONPHARMACOLOGIC THERAPY

Red blood cell transfusions in patients with severe symptomatic anemia

ACUTE GENERAL Rx

- Erythropoietin (10,000 to 40,000 U/week) in patient with symptomatic anemia
- DNA methyltransferase inhibitors: Azacitidine (Vidaza), a pyrimidine nucleoside analog of cytidine, has been shown to improve the quality of life for patients with MDS and probably prolong survival. Decitabine (Dacogen), another nucleoside analog, has also been FDA approved for patients with MDS. These agents may also be useful in preventing the transition of MDS to AML.
- Immunomodulators: Lenalidomide (Revlimid), a novel analogue of thalidomide, has demonstrated hematologic activity in patients with low-rise MDS who have no response to erythropoietin or who are unlikely to benefit from conventional therapy. Lenalidomide can also reduce transfusion requirements and reverse cytologic and cytogenetic abnormalities in patients who have MDS with the 5q31 deletion.
- Allogeneic stem cell transplantation should be considered in patients ≤60 yr because this is the established procedure with cure potential.
- Results of chemotherapy are generally disappointing. Combination chemotherapy regimens (e.g., cytarabine plus doxorubicin) generally induce a complete response in only a minority of patients, and the average duration of response is <1 yr.
- The role of myeloid growth factors (granulocyte colony-stimulating factor (G-CSF), granulocyte-macrophage CSF) and immunotherapy is undefined. In a recent trial, 34% of patients treated with antithymocyte globulin (40 mg/kg for 4 days) became transfusion independent. Response was also associated with a statistically significantly longer survival.

CHRONIC Rx

Monitor for infections, bleeding, and complications of anemia. Supportive measures include blood transfusions and erythropoietin for anemia and antibiotics to treat opportunistic infections. Iron overload from frequent transfusions may require iron chelation therapy.

DISPOSITION

- Cure rates in young patients with allogeneic bone marrow transplantation approach 30% to 50%.
- The risk of transformation to acute myelogenous leukemia varies with the percentage of blasts in the bone marrow.
- Advanced age, male sex, and deletion of chromosomes 5 and 7 are associated with a poor prognosis.
- The 1997 International Prognostic Scoring System uses the following three elements for staging: (1) the proportion of myeloblasts in the patient's marrow, (2) the number of blood cell lineage deficits, and (3) the type of chromosomal abnormality present (e.g., poor risk includes abnormalities of chromosome 7; good risk includes clonal loss of the Y chromosome). According to the International Myelodysplastic Syndrome Risk Analysis Workshop, the most important variables in disease outcome are the specific cytogenetic abnormalities, the percentage of blasts in the bone marrow, and the number of hematopoietic lineages involved in the cytopenias.

TABLE 1-53 French-American-British Classification Criteria

Subtype	Abbreviation	Peripheral Blood	Bone Marrow
Refractory anemia	RA	Blasts <1%	Blasts <5%
Refractory anemia with ringed sideroblasts	RARS	Blasts <1%	Blasts <5%, and >15% ringed sideroblasts
Refractory anemia with excess blasts	RAEB	Blasts <5%	Blasts 5%-20%
Refractory anemia with excess blasts in transformation	RAEB-T	Blasts >5%	Blasts 20%-30% or Auer rods
Chronic myelomonocytic leukemia	CMML	Monocytes $>1 \times 10^9$/L	Any of the above
Acute myelogenous leukemia	AML	Blasts >30%	

From Hoffmann R et al: *Hematology, basic principles and practice*, ed 5, Philadelphia, 2009, Churchill Livingstone.

REFERRAL

Hematology referral in all patients with MDS

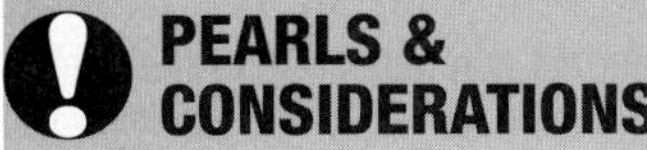

PEARLS & CONSIDERATIONS

COMMENTS

- Patients with cytogenetic abnormalities associated with poor prognosis should be considered for aggressive treatment with high-dose chemotherapy and stem cell transplantation.
- Nearly 50% of the deaths that result from MDS are the result of cytopenia associated with bone marrow failure.

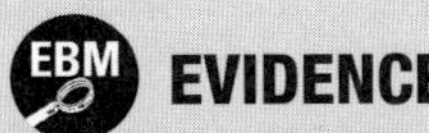

EVIDENCE

Please note: Complete text of EBM for this topic is available online.

Key trials and commentary:

Patients with neutropenia resulting from chemotherapy for acute myelogenous leukemia or the myelodysplastic syndrome are at high risk for difficult-to-treat and often fatal invasive fungal infections.

This study showed that in patients undergoing chemotherapy for acute myelogenous leukemia or the myelodysplastic syndrome, posaconazole prevented invasive fungal infections more effectively than did either fluconazole or itraconazole and improved overall survival. There were more serious adverse events possibly or probably related to treatment in the posaconazole group.[1] Ⓐ

Cornely et al, in a prospective, randomized trial, compared the efficacy of posaconazole with either fluconazole or itraconazole for the prevention of invasive fungal disease in patients who were undergoing chemotherapy for acute leukemia or myelodysplastic syndromes. They found the incidence of proven and probable invasive fungal diseases to be significantly lower in the posaconazole group than in the fluconazole or itraconazole groups. Fewer cases of invasive aspergillosis occurred after posaconazole prophylaxis than after fluconazole or itraconazole prophylaxis. On the basis of currently available data, it now seems that posaconazole is the drug of choice for prophylaxis of invasive aspergillosis, whereas voriconazole remains the preferred treatment for proven or probable aspergillosis. Caspofungin and liposomal amphotericin B remain as options for empirical therapy.

Evidence-Based Reference

1. Cornely OA et al: Posaconazole vs. fluconazole or itraconazole prophylaxis in patients with neutropenia, *N Engl J Med* 356:348-359, 2007. Commentary by B.H. Thiers, M.D. Ⓐ

SUGGESTED READINGS

Griffiths EA, Gore SD: DNA methyltransferase and histone deacetylase inhibitors in the treatment of myelodysplastic syndromes, *Semin Hematol* 45:23-30, 2008.

Haase D: Cytogenetic features in myelodysplastic syndrome, *Ann Hematol* 87:515-26, 2008.

Tefferi A, Vardiman JW: Myelodysplastic syndromes, *N Engl J Med* 361:1872-1885, 2009.

AUTHOR: **FRED F. FERRI, M.D.**

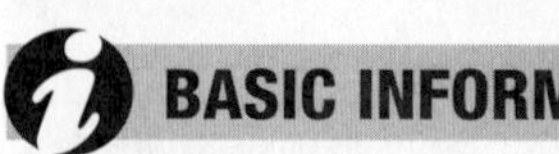

BASIC INFORMATION

DEFINITION

- Acute coronary syndromes are manifestations of ischemic heart disease and represent a broad clinical spectrum that includes non–ST segment elevation acute coronary syndrome (NSTEACS) (collectively unstable angina [UA]/non–ST elevation myocardial infarction [NSTEMI]) and ST-elevation MI (STEMI).
  1. MI is characterized by necrosis resulting from an insufficient supply of oxygenated blood to an area of the heart. According to the joint European Society of Cardiology/American College of Cardiology, either one of the following criteria for acute evolving or recent MI satisfies the diagnosis:
     a. Typical rise and gradual fall (troponin) or more rapid rise and fall (creatine kinase MB fraction [CK-MB]) of biochemical markers of myocardial necrosis with at least one of the following:
        i. Ischemic symptoms
        ii. Development of pathologic Q waves on ECG
        iii. ECG changes indicative of ischemia (ST-segment elevation or depression)
        iv. Coronary artery intervention (e.g., coronary angioplasty)
     b. Pathologic findings of acute MI
  2. STEMI: area of ischemic necrosis that penetrates the entire thickness of the ventricular wall and results in ST-segment elevation.
  3. Unstable angina: coronary arterial plaque rupture with fragmentation and distal arterial embolization resulting in myocardial necrosis. Usually occurs without ST elevation and is thus termed non–ST elevation MI.
- The *European Heart Journal* and the *Journal of the American College of Cardiology* have recently published a new definition of acute MI (see below) to account for advances in diagnosis and management. It includes subtypes of acute MI, imaging tests supporting the diagnosis, and biomarker thresholds after PCI or bypass grafting.
  - Type 1: Spontaneous MI related to ischemia due to a primary coronary event such as plaque erosion and/or rupture, fissuring, or dissection
  - Type 2: MI secondary to ischemia due to either increased oxygen demand or decreased supply (e.g., coronary artery spasm, coronary embolism, anemia, arrhythmias, hypertension, or hypotension)
  - Type 3: Sudden unexpected cardiac death, including cardiac arrest, often with symptoms suggestive of myocardial ischemia, accompanied by presumably new ST elevation, new left bundle branch block, or evidence of fresh thrombus in a coronary artery by angiography and/or at autopsy, but death occurring before blood samples could be obtained or at a time before the appearance of cardiac biomarkers in the blood
  - Type 4a: MI associated with percutaneous coronary intervention
  - Type 4b: MI associated with stent thrombosis as documented by angiography or at autopsy
  - Type 5: MI associated with coronary artery bypass grafting

SYNONYMS

MI
Myocardial infarction
Non–ST elevation MI
ST-elevation MI
Heart attack
Coronary thrombosis
Coronary occlusion

ICD-9CM CODES
410.9 Acute myocardial infarction, unspecified site

EPIDEMIOLOGY & DEMOGRAPHICS

INCIDENCE/PREVALENCE (IN U.S.):

- >500 cases/100,000 persons.
- >500,000 MIs in the U.S. annually.
- More prominent in males between the ages of 40 and 65 yr; no predominant sex after age 65 yr.
- Women experience more lethal and severe first acute MIs than men regardless of comorbidity, previous angina, or age.
- At least one fourth of all myocardial infarctions are clinically unrecognized.

PHYSICAL FINDINGS & CLINICAL PRESENTATION

Clinical presentation:

- Crushing substernal chest pain usually lasts longer than 30 min.
- Pain is unrelieved by rest or sublingual nitroglycerin or is rapidly recurring.
- Pain radiates to the left or right arm, neck, jaw, back, shoulders, or abdomen and is not pleuritic in character.
- Pain may be associated with dyspnea, diaphoresis, nausea, or vomiting.
- There is no pain in approximately 20% of infarctions (usually in diabetic or elderly patients).

Physical findings:

- Skin may be diaphoretic, with pallor (because of decreased oxygen).
- Rales may be present at the bases of lungs (indicative of congestive heart failure [CHF]).
- Cardiac auscultation may reveal an apical systolic murmur caused by mitral regurgitation from papillary muscle dysfunction; S_3 or S_4 may also be present.
- Physical examination may be completely normal.

ETIOLOGY

- Coronary atherosclerosis.
- Coronary artery spasm.
- Coronary embolism (caused by infective endocarditis, rheumatic heart disease, intracavitary thrombus).
- Periarteritis and other coronary artery inflammatory diseases.
- Dissection into coronary arteries (aneurysmal or iatrogenic).
- Congenital abnormalities of coronary circulation.
- MI with normal coronaries: more frequent in younger patients and cocaine addicts. The risk of acute MI is increased by a factor of 24 during the 60 min after the use of cocaine in persons who are otherwise at relatively low risk. Most patients with cocaine-related MI are young, nonwhite, male cigarette smokers without other risk factors for arteriosclerotic heart disease who have a history of repeated cocaine use. Blood and urine toxicology screen for cocaine is recommended in all young patients who present with acute MI.
- Hypercoagulable states, increased blood viscosity (polycythemia vera).

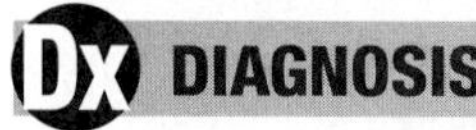

DIAGNOSIS

DIFFERENTIAL DIAGNOSIS

The various causes of myocardial ischemia are described in Section II along with the differential diagnosis of chest pain.

LABORATORY TESTS

- Cardiac troponin levels: cardiac-specific troponin T (cTnT) and cardiac-specific troponin I (cTnI) are generally indicative of myocardial injury. Increases in serum levels of cTnT and cTnI may occur relatively early after muscle damage (3 to 12 hr), peak within 24 hr, and may be present for several days after MI (up to 7 days for cTnI and up to 10 to 14 days for cTnT). cTnT tests can be falsely positive in patients with renal failure. The threshold level of cTnT considered positive for MI is 0.1 ng/ml in patients with normal renal function or 0.5 ng/ml in patients with renal impairment. Although troponin is a sensitive biomarker to rule out NSTMI, it is less useful to "rule in" this event because many other diseases such as sepsis, hypovolemia, atrial fibrillation, CHF, pulmonary embolism, myocarditis, myocardial contusion, and renal failure can be associated with an increase in troponin level.
- CK-MB isoenzyme is a useful marker for MI. It is released in the circulation in amounts that correlate with the size of the infarct.
- Neither CK-MB nor troponin consistently appear in the blood within 6 hr after an ischemic event; therefore serial testing (e.g., on presentation and after 8 hr) is necessary to definitely rule out MI.
- ECG:
  1. In STEMI, there is development of:
     a. Inverted T waves, indicating an area of ischemia.
     b. Elevated ST segment, indicating an area of injury. Significant ST-segment elevation of $\geq$0.10 mV measured 0.02 sec after the J point is evident in two contiguous leads. The presence of this finding in leads V1 to V6 indicates anterior or anterolateral MI, a lateral MI in leads I and aVL, and inferior wall MI in leads II, III, or aVF.

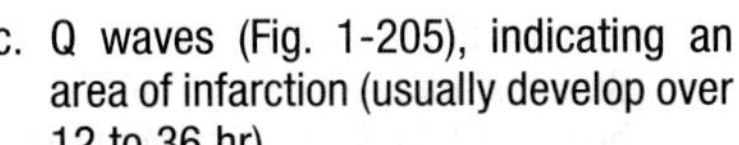

c. Q waves (Fig. 1-205), indicating an area of infarction (usually develop over 12 to 36 hr).

2. In NSTEMI:
   a. History and myocardial enzyme elevations are compatible with MI.
   b. ECG shows no ST-segment elevation and sometimes shows a small depression of the ST segment.

IMAGING STUDIES

- Chest radiograph is useful to evaluate for pulmonary congestion and exclude other causes of chest pain.
- Echocardiography can evaluate wall motion abnormalities and identify mural thrombus or mitral regurgitation, which can occur acutely after MI.

RISK ASSESSMENT

Several risk assessment models are available. The Thrombolysis in Myocardial Infarction risk score uses the seven following variables: age ≥65 yr, at least three conventional risk factors for coronary artery disease, prior coronary stenosis ≥50%, ST-segment deviation on ECG at presentation, two or more anginal events in the preceding 24 hr, use of aspirin in the prior 7 days, and elevated serum cardiac markers.

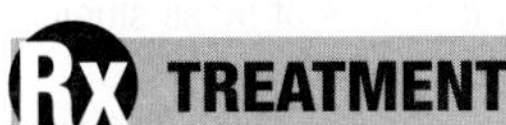

TREATMENT

NONPHARMACOLOGIC THERAPY

- Limit patient's activity: bed rest for the initial 12 to 24 hr; if the patient remains stable, gradually increase activity.
- Diet: nothing by mouth until stable, then no added salt and a low-cholesterol diet.
- Patient education to decrease the risk of subsequent cardiac events (proper diet, cessation of smoking, regular exercise) should be initiated when the patient is medically stable.

ACUTE GENERAL Rx

- Any patient with suspected acute MI should immediately receive the following:
  - Antiplatelet therapy: aspirin, 160 to 325 mg PO unless true aspirin allergy is suspected. If the first dose is chewed, a blood level is achieved more rapidly than if it is swallowed. Clopidogrel 75 mg qd may be substituted if true allergy is present or given in addition to aspirin.
  - Nitrates: increase the supply of oxygen by reducing coronary vasospasm and decreasing consumption of oxygen by reducing ventricular preload. Sublingual nitroglycerin (0.4 mg) can be administered immediately on suspicion of MI (unless systolic blood pressure is <90 mm Hg or ≤30 mm Hg below baseline or heart rate is <50 beats/min or >100 beats/min); IV nitroglycerin can be subsequently used. Nitroglycerin should be used with great caution in patients with inferior wall MI; nitrate use can result in hypotension because these patients are sensitive to change in preload. It should also be avoided in patients suspected of having right ventricular infarction (increased risk of preload reduction) and if a patient has used sildenafil or vardenafil within the previous 24 hr or tadalafil in the previous 48 hr.
  - Adequate analgesia: morphine sulfate 2 to 4 mg IV initially with increments of 2 to 8 mg IV at 5 to 15 min intervals can be given for severe pain unrelieved by nitroglycerin. Hypotension from morphine can be treated with careful IV hydration with saline solution. If sinus bradycardia accompanies hypotension, use atropine (0.5 to 1.0 mg IV every 5 min prn to a total dose of 2.5 mg). Respiratory depression caused by morphine can be reversed with naloxone 0.8 mg.
  - Nasal oxygen: administer at 2 to 4 L/min.
- Prompt myocardial reperfusion can be accomplished with percutaneous coronary intervention (PCI), fibrinolytic therapy, or coronary artery bypass graft (CABG) surgery. If readily available without delay, PCI is superior to thrombolytic therapy for treating patients with STEMI. It is effective and generally results in more favorable outcomes than thrombolytic therapy. If PCI is planned, use of parental anticoagulation is recommended with either unfractionated heparin, enoxaparin, fondaparinux, or bivalirudin. In patients at high risk of bleeding, use of bivalirudin, is reasonable. Aspirin and a thienopyridine (e.g., clopidogrel) should be loaded before PCI and continued for at least 12 mo in patients who receive a stent. Continuation beyond 15 months may be considered in patients who receive a drug-eluting stent. Thienopyridines can be discontinued early if there is a high risk for bleeding. If coronary artery bypass grafting is planned, the drug should be withheld for at least 5 days unless the urgency of revascularization outweighs the risk of bleeding. Neither facilitation of PCI with reteplase plus abciximab nor facilitation with abciximab alone significantly improves the clinical outcomes compared with abciximab given at the time of PCI in patients with STEMI. Coronary stents after PCI are useful to decrease ischemia, improve long-term patency, and lower the rate of restenosis of the infarct-related artery. In patients with acute MI, treatment with drug-eluting stents is associated with decreased 2-yr mortality rates and a

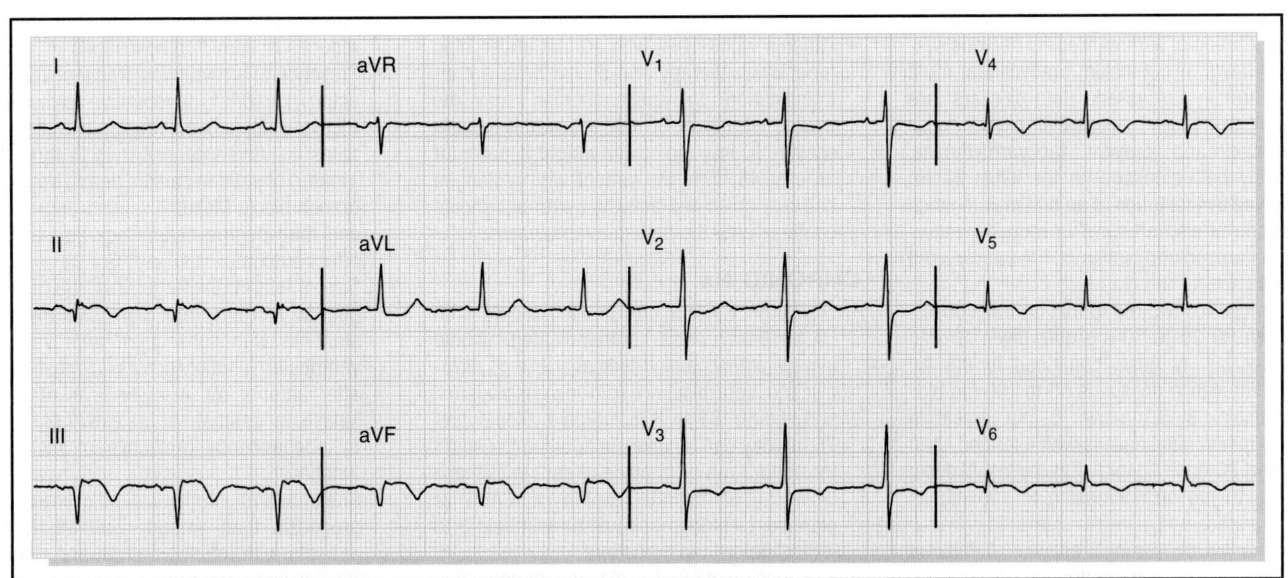

FIGURE 1-205 Evolving inferoposterolateral infarction. Note the prominent Q waves in leads II, III, and aV1, along with ST elevation and T-wave inversion in these leads, as well as V3 through V6. ST depression in I, aV1, V1, and V2 is consistent with a reciprocal change. Relatively tall R waves are also present in V1 and V2. (From Zipes DP et al [eds]: *Braunwald's heart disease,* ed 7, Philadelphia, 2005, Elsevier.)

reduction in the need for repeat revascularization procedures compared with treatment with bare-metal stents.

- Thrombolytic therapy: if the duration of pain has been <6 hr and primary angioplasty is not readily available, recanalization of the occluded arteries should be attempted with thrombolytic agents, possibly in combination with glycoprotein IIb/IIIa inhibition. Because the effectiveness of thrombolytics is time dependent, these agents should ideally be administered either in the field or within 30 min of the patient's arrival in the emergency department. When tissue plasminogen activator (tPA) or reteplase is used, heparin is given to increase the likelihood of patency in the infarct-related artery. In patients receiving fibrinolysis for STEMI, treatment with enoxaparin is superior to treatment with unfractionated heparin for 48 hr but is associated with an increase in major bleeding episodes. In patients receiving streptokinase or APSAC, heparin is not indicated because it does not offer any additional benefit and can result in increased bleeding complications. Tenecteplase and reteplase are comparable with accelerated infusion recombinant tPA in terms of efficacy and safety but are more convenient because they are administered by bolus injection. Lanoplase and heparin bolus plus infusion are as effective as tPA with regard to mortality rate, but the rate of intracranial hemorrhage is significantly higher. Absolute contraindications to thrombolytic therapy include active internal bleeding, intracranial neoplasm or arteriovenous malformation, intracranial surgery in past 6 mo, stroke in past year, head trauma with loss of consciousness in past 6 mo, surgery in noncompressible location in past 6 wk, alteration in mental status, and infectious endocarditis.
- Beta-adrenergic blocking agents should generally be given to all patients with evolving acute MI. Before using beta-blockers, some of the contraindications and side effects (i.e., exacerbation of asthma, central nervous system effects, hypotension, bradycardia) must be carefully assessed. Beta-blockers are useful to reduce myocardial oxygen consumption and prevent tachyarrhythmias. Early IV beta-blockage (in the initial 24 hr) followed by institution of an oral maintenance regimen is also effective in reducing recurrent infarction and ischemia. Frequently used agents are:
  - Metoprolol: IV 5 mg q2min for three doses, then PO 25 to 50 mg q6h, given 15 min after last IV dose, continued for 48 hr; maintenance dosage is 50 to 100 mg bid.
  - Atenolol: IV 5 mg over 5 min, repeat in 10 min if initial dose is well tolerated, then start PO dose 10 min after the last IV dose; PO 50 mg qd, increasing to 100 mg as tolerated.
- Angiotensin-converting enzyme inhibitors (ACEIs) reduce left ventricular dysfunction and dilation and slow the progression of CHF during and after acute MI. They should be initiated within hours of hospitalization, provided the patient does not have hypotension or a contraindication (bilateral renal stenosis, renal failure, or history of angioedema caused by previous treatment with ACEIs). Angiotensin receptor blockers offer no advantage over ACEIs and should be considered only in patients who have a contraindication to the use of ACEIs or cannot tolerate them.
  - Commonly used ACEIs are ramipril 2.5 mg qd, captopril 12.5 mg PO bid, enalapril 2.5 mg bid, or lisinopril 2.5 to 5 mg qd initially, with subsequent titration as needed. Ramipril is associated with lower mortality rate than most ACEIs.
  - ACEIs may be stopped in patients without complications and no evidence of left ventricular dysfunction after 6 to 8 wk.
  - ACEIs should be continued indefinitely in patients with impaired left ventricular function (ejection fraction <40%) or clinical CHF.
- Glycoprotein IIb receptor inhibitors (tirofiban, eptifibatide), when administered with heparin and aspirin, further reduce the incidence of ischemic events in high-risk patients with NSTEMI. The use of IV glycoprotein IIb/IIIa inhibitors (e.g., abciximab) during PCI also reduces the risk of closure after angioplasty. However, the usefulness of initiating therapy for PCI prior to arrival to the cardiac catheterization laboratory is uncertain.
- Assess fasting lipid profile preferably within 24 hr of MI, and initiate statin therapy before hospital discharge to keep low-density lipoprotein cholesterol <70 mg/dl. Consider addition of fenofibrate or niacin if triglycerides are significantly elevated or high-density lipoprotein cholesterol is very low.
- Long-term aldosterone blockade should be prescribed for post-STEMI patients without significant renal dysfunction (Cr ≤2.5 mg/dl in men and ≤2.0 mg/dl in women) or hyperkalemia who are already taking an ACEI and have left ventricular ejection fraction <0.40, and have symptomatic heart failure or diabetes.
- Patients with STEMI who are not undergoing reperfusion therapy and do not have a contraindication to anticoagulation may be treated with IV or SC unfractionated heparin or with SC low-molecular-weight heparin for at least 48 hr. In the patient with prolonged bed rest or limited activity, treatment should continue until the patient is ambulatory.

CHRONIC Rx

- Discharge medications in all patients with UA/NSTEMI (unless contraindicated) should include antiischemic medications (e.g., nitroglycerin, beta-blocker), lipid-lowering agents, and aspirin (81 to 325 mg/day). Clopidogrel 75 mg/day can be given in addition to aspirin for up to 9 mo or in place of aspirin in those who cannot tolerate aspirin. If CABG is planned, clopidogrel should be withheld 5 to 7 days before the procedure.
- The addition of ACEIs is also recommended in all patients with diabetes, CHF, and in those with ejection fraction <40%.
- Evaluation of post-MI patients:
  - Submaximal (low level) treadmill test (can be done 1 to 3 wk after MI) in stable patients without any clinical evidence of significant left ventricular dysfunction or post-MI angina.
    1. Useful to assess the patient's functional capacity and formulate an at-home exercise program
    2. Helpful to determine the patient's prognosis
  - Radionuclide angiography or two-dimensional echocardiography:
    1. To evaluate patient's left ventricular ejection fraction
    2. To evaluate ventricular size and segmental wall motion
    3. Echocardiography to rule out presence of mural thrombi in patients with anterior wall infarction; transesophageal echo is preferred if mural thrombosis is suspected
  - A 24-hr Holter monitor study to evaluate patients who have demonstrated significant arrhythmias during their hospital stay. Selected patients with complex ventricular ectopy may be candidates for programmed electrical stimulation studies and antiarrhythmic therapy or implanted defibrillator, depending on the results of these studies.

DISPOSITION

The prognosis after MI depends on multiple factors:

- Use of beta-blockers: the mortality rate of patients on a regular regimen of beta-blockers is significantly decreased compared with that of control groups. Discharge medication in patients with UA/NSTEMI should include a beta-blocker in all patients without contraindications.
- In patients ≤75 yr who have STEMI and receive aspirin and a standard fibrinolytic regimen, the addition of clopidogrel improves the patency rate of the infarct-related artery and reduces ischemic complications.
- Presence of arrhythmias, frequent ventricular ectopy (≥10/hr), or repetitive forms of ventricular ectopic beats (couplets, triplets) indicates an increased risk (two to three times greater) of sudden cardiac death. New bundle branch block, Mobitz II second-degree block, and third-degree heart block also adversely affect outcome.
- Size of infarct: the larger it is, the higher the post-MI mortality rate. Significant myocardial stunning with subsequent improvement of ventricular function occurs in most patients after anterior MI. A lower level of creatine kinase, an estimate of the extent of necrosis, is independently predictive of recovery of function.
- Site of infarct: inferior wall MI carries a better prognosis than anterior wall MI; however, patients with inferior wall MI and right ventricular involvement have a high risk for arrhythmic complications and cardiac shock.
- Ejection fraction after MI: the lower the left ventricular ejection fraction, the higher the

mortality rate after MI. The risk of sudden death is highest in the first 30 days after MI among patients with left ventricular dysfunction, heart failure, or both.

- Presence of post-MI angina indicates a high mortality rate.
- Performance on low-level exercise test: the presence of ST-segment changes during the test is a predictor of high mortality rate during the first year.
- Presence of pericarditis during the acute phase of MI increases mortality rate at 1 yr.
- Type A behavior (competitive drive, ambitiousness, hostility) is associated with a lower mortality rate after symptomatic MI.
- The Killip classification is an independent predictor of all-cause mortality in patients with non–ST elevation acute coronary syndromes.
- Self-reported moderate alcohol consumption in the year before acute MI is associated with reduced 1-yr mortality rate.
- Discharge medication in patients with UA/NSTEMI should include lipid-lowering agents in patients with hyperlipidemia unresponsive to exercise and dietary restrictions and is beneficial. Statins may also lower vascular inflammation and damage by mechanisms other than reduction of low-density lipoprotein cholesterol. Early initiation of statin treatment in patients with acute MI is associated with reduced 1-yr mortality rate.
- Additional poor prognostic factors include cigarette smoking, history of hypertension or prior MI, presence of ST-segment depression in acute MI, increasing age, diabetes mellitus, and female sex (especially women >50 yr).
- Renal disease, even mild, as assessed by the estimated glomerular filtration rate, is a major risk factor for cardiovascular complications after MI.
- Although black patients with MI have worse outcomes than white patients, these differences did not persist after adjustment for patient factors and site of care.

PEARLS & CONSIDERATIONS

COMMENTS

- Current guidelines recommend an early invasive strategy for patients who have acute coronary syndromes without ST-segment elevation and with an elevated cTnT level. However, a recent trial (ICTUS) comparing early invasive and selectively invasive management for acute coronary syndromes failed to show that, given optimized medical therapy, an early invasive strategy is superior to a selective invasive strategy in patients with acute coronary syndromes without ST-segment elevation and with an elevated cTnT level. All 1200 patients in this trial received aggressive medical therapy, including aspirin, clopidogrel, enoxaparin for 48 hr, abciximab during PCI, and intensive lipid-lowering therapy. The mortality rate was the same in the two groups (2.5%); MI was significantly more frequent in the group assigned to early invasive management (15% vs. 10%), but rehospitalization rate was less frequent in that group (7.4% vs. 10.9%).
- Persons who survive a myocardial infarction for at least 4 weeks are at increased risk for sudden death from cardiac causes mainly due to ventricular tachyarrhythmias. Patients who may be considered for implantable cardioverter-defibrillators post MI are those with EF ≤30%. For patients with EF 30% to 35%, modifying factors include symptomatic heart failure of New York Heart Association class 2 or 3 and with a life expectancy of at least a year. The elderly (>80 yr), those with borderline cognition, and those with systemic immunosuppression or poorly controlled bleeding diatheses should be considered on an individual basis.

EBM EVIDENCE

Please note: Complete text of EBM for this topic is available online.

Key trials and commentary:

This study sought to best estimate the benefits and risks associated with rescue percutaneous coronary intervention (PCI) and repeat fibrinolytic therapy as compared with conservative management in patients with failed fibrinolytic therapy for ST-segment elevation myocardial infarction (STEMI).

This study showed that rescue PCI is associated with improved clinical outcomes for STEMI patients after failed fibrinolytic therapy, but these benefits must be interpreted in the context of potential risks. On the other hand, repeat fibrinolytic therapy is not associated with significant clinical improvement and may be associated with increased harm.

Randomized trials have established that three fibrinolytic agents—SK, anisolylated plasminogen streptokinase activator complex (APSAC), and tissue plasminogen activator (tPA)—each reduced the short-term and long-term mortality rates in patients with acute ST elevation myocardial infarction (STEMI). Nevertheless, angiographic trials have demonstrated that there is suboptimal patency of the infarct-related artery (IRA) in 40% to 50% of patients 90 minutes after administration of fibrin-specific fibrinolytic drugs (tPA, reteplase, tenecteplase). Persistent occlusion of the IRA after acute MI is associated with left ventricular remodeling, resulting in increased left ventricular end-systolic volume, which is a major predictor of survival after acute MI. PCI of an occluded IRA 3 to 28 days after acute MI did not reduce the occurrence of death, reinfarction, or congestive heart failure. The benefit of rescue PCI that is performed within hours after unsuccessful fibrinolytic therapy is the subject of the study performed by Wijeysundera et al.[1]

The Thrombolysis in Myocardial Infarction (TIMI) Study Group formulated angiographic definitions to grade the patency of the IRA in patients with acute MI. Studies that examined the relationship between the TIMI grade flow and clinical outcome concluded that TIMI grade 3 flow, but not TIMI grade 2 flow, improves both in-hospital and long-term mortality rates after acute MI.

Although coronary angiography is the gold standard for assessment of the response to fibrinolytic therapy, resolution of ST-segment elevation also has been used as a noninvasive alternative method of judging the response to fibrinolytic therapy. Compared with complete resolution of ST-segment elevation, incomplete resolution of ST-segment elevation after fibrinolytic therapy is associated with larger infarct size and greater short-term and long-term mortality rates.

Unsuccessful fibrinolytic therapy can be managed in one of three ways: conservative therapy, readministration of a fibrinolytic drug, and "rescue" PCI. The randomized trials that compared rescue PCI with conservative therapy have used a variety of criteria to define unsuccessful fibrinolysis and rescue PCI. The Middlesbrough Early Revascularization to Limit Infarction (MERLIN) trial defined failed fibrinolytic therapy as failure of the ST-segment elevation in the worst lead to have resolved by 50% 60 minutes after the onset of fibrinolytic therapy. The Rescue Angioplasty vs. Conservative Treatment or Repeat Thrombolysis (REACT) trial's definition of rescue PCI was PCI performed within 12 hours after failed fibrinolytic therapy, defined as an electrocardiogram obtained 90 minutes after the start of fibrinolytic therapy that showed <50% resolution of the ST segment in the lead with the greatest ST-segment elevation. Thus, many of the patients who underwent PCI in the REACT trial would meet the TIMI group's definition of either adjunctive PCI, defined as PCI for patients with TIMI 2 or 3 flow, or delayed PCI, defined as PCI >150 minutes after fibrinolytic therapy, rather than rescue PCI as defined by the TIMI group and other investigators.

The randomized trials that compared rescue PCI with conservative therapy were insufficiently powered to detect an effect on the mortality rate. Although differences in trial design and the definition of rescue PCI make it somewhat difficult to compare the results of various trials, at least two meta-analyses of the randomized trials have been published. A pooled analysis of the short-term mortality rate (in-hospital or 30-day) among 942 patients who were enrolled in five randomized trials revealed that the risk of death was 36% lower among patients who were randomized to PCI (RR, 0.64; 95% CI, 0.41 to 1.00; $P = 0.048$). The meta-analysis performed by Wijeysundera et al included six trials that randomized 908 patients to rescue PCI or conservative therapy. Four trials used the angiographic TIMI perfusion grade to define unsuccessful fibrinolysis, and the MERLIN and REACT trials used the electrocardiographic criteria described above. Rescue PCI was not associated with a reduction in the all-cause mortality rate at 6 months (RR, 0.69; 95% CI, 0.46-01.05), but it was associated with significant reductions in the risk of heart failure and reinfarction, and an increased risk of stroke and minor bleeding.

Wijeysundera et al also performed a meta-analysis of three clinical trials that randomized 410 patients to repeat fibrinolysis or conservative therapy. Repeat fibrinolytic therapy was not associated with a significant risk reduction in the all-cause mortality rate (RR, 0.68; 95% CI, 0.41-1.14; $P = 0.14$) or reinfarction (RR, 1.79; 95% CI, 0.92-3.48; $P = 0.09$).

The results of this meta-analysis provide support for the current practice guidelines regarding the management of patients with acute ST-segment elevation MI who undergo unsuccessful fibrinolytic therapy. The class I recommendations for rescue PCI are:

1. Rescue PCI should be performed in patients <75 years old with ST-segment elevation or left bundle branch block in whom shock develops within 36 hours.
2. Rescue PCI should be performed in patients with severe congestive heart failure and/or pulmonary edema and onset of symptoms within 12 hours.

The guidelines include two class IIa recommendations for rescue PCI:

1. Rescue PCI is reasonable for selected patients >75 years old with ST elevation or left bundle branch block in whom shock develops within 36 hours.
2. It is reasonable to perform rescue PCI for patients with 1 or more of the following: (a) hemodynamic or electrical instability, (b) persistent ischemic symptoms[1] **A**

At least one quarter of STEMI patients do not receive reperfusion therapy, and these patients are at high risk for new ischemic events. A separate study evaluated fondaparinux treatment vs. usual care (i.e., placebo or unfractionated (UF) heparin) in a pre-specified subgroup of 2867 (out of 12 092) patients not receiving reperfusion treatment in the OASIS-6 trial.

This study showed that in STEMI patients not receiving reperfusion treatment, fondaparinux reduces the composite of death or myocardial reinfarction without an increase in severe bleedings or strokes as compared to placebo or UF heparin.

Patients with STEMI who have contraindications to fibrinolytic therapy may undergo PCI or may not receive reperfusion therapy. Among 10,954 patients with ST-segment elevation or left bundle-branch block who presented within 12 hours of symptom onset and were enrolled in an international registry, 33% of patients who were eligible to receive reperfusion therapy did not receive a fibrinolytic agent or undergo PCI.

The rationale for anticoagulant therapy in patients with STEMI includes promotion of infarct artery patency, prevention of deep vein thrombosis, pulmonary embolism, left ventricular mural thrombus, and cerebral embolism. Relatively few clinical trials have evaluated the efficacy of anticoagulant agents in patients with STEMI who did not undergo reperfusion therapy.

OASIS-6 was a randomized, double-blind trial that compared usual care (UFH or placebo) with subcutaneous fondaparinux, a synthetic pentasaccharide that binds antithrombin and inhibits factor Xa, in patients with STEMI. Among the total enrollment of 12,092 patients, 2867 patients who did not receive reperfusion therapy were randomized to fondaparinux or usual care (control). Compared with the usual care group, treatment with fondaparinux was associated with a 20% reduction in the composite end point of death or reinfarction at 30 days.[2]

Based on the results of the OASIS-6 study, the 2007 update of the American College of Cardiology/American Heart Association 2004 Guidelines for the Management of Patients with STEMI include a class IIa recommendation (level of evidence B) for administration of fondaparinux to patients with STEMI who do not undergo reperfusion therapy.[2] **A**

Depression following MI is associated with an increased risk of cardiac events, but attempts to alter cardiovascular prognosis by providing antidepressive treatment have not been successful. This may be because of the limited effects of antidepressive treatment on depression itself. A study assessed whether nonresponse to treatment of post-MI depression is associated with new cardiac events.[3]

This study provides further preliminary evidence that nonresponse to treatment of post-MI depression may be associated with cardiac events. Efforts should be dedicated to developing more effective treatments for depressed patients with MI.

We have followed the issue of depression following MI in recent years and of course it has been shown to be associated with significantly increased mortality. However, what to do about it is less clear. In this trial, the authors enrolled patients in a double-blind placebo-controlled trial with mirtazapine, and if they did not respond gave them further open treatment with citalopram. In fact, they found that the rates for recurrent cardiac events were 7.4% if people responded, but 25.6% among nonresponders. Interestingly, the rate among untreated control subjects was 11.2%. This is a definitive trial in this area and should change patient care.[3] **A**

Recurrent ventricular tachycardia (VT) is an important cause of mortality and morbidity late after MI. With frequent use of implantable cardioverter-defibrillators, these VTs are often poorly defined and not tolerated for mapping, factors previously viewed as relative contraindications to ablation. This observational multicenter study assessed the outcome of VT ablation with a saline-irrigated catheter combined with an electroanatomic mapping system.[4]

This study showed that catheter ablation is a reasonable option to reduce episodes of recurrent VT in patients with prior MI, even when multiple and/or unmappable VTs are present. This population remains at high risk for death, warranting surveillance and further study.[4] **A**

For one editor, this study emphasizes that there is still a useful, in fact important, role for ablation techniques to minimize or cure VT in patients with underlying coronary artery disease and previous MI, and even in the presence of an implantable cardioverter defibrillator (ICD), it may be used to minimize shocks and even to reduce the need for medications, some of which can have some very undesirable adverse effects.

The identification and assessment of MI are important for therapeutic and prognostic purposes, yet current recommended diagnostic strategies have significant limitations. This study prospectively tested the performance of delayed-enhancement MRI with gadolinium-based contrast for the detection of MI in an international, multicenter trial.

This study showed that Gadoversetamide-enhanced MRI using doses of ≥0.2 mmol/kg is effective in the detection and assessment of both acute and chronic MI. This study represents the first multicenter trial designed to evaluate an imaging approach for detecting MI.[5]

This article is included because it is the first multicenter, blinded, randomized, dose-finding trial for gadolinium-based contrast agent and a cardiac application. Both cardiac CT and cardiac MRI have commonly used contrast agents for CTA and MRA; however, these have been considered off-label applications. This trial has provided the highest attainable quality of data that allow us to judge the accuracies that result from various doses of the contrast agent. The diagnostic sensitivity of MRI for detecting MI is given according to four different gadoversetamide doses, and the two delay time points (10 min and 30 min). Doses of ≥0.2 mmol/kg result in appropriate accuracies for detection of myocardial infarction. Although the results in this trial are not surprising, and many of us have been acquiring MRI with similar doses and time points, the fact that we now have a multicenter trial, rather than multiple single-center trials and expert opinions, constitutes a remarkable advancement in cardiac MR imaging.[5] **A**

One prospective randomized trial evaluates the impact of early abciximab administration on angiographic and left ventricular function parameters.[6]

This study showed that in patients with AMI treated with primary PCI, early abciximab administration improves pre-PCI angiographic findings, post-PCI tissue perfusion, and 1-month left ventricular function recovery, possibly by starting early recanalization of the infarct-related artery.

Based on current guidelines, the European Society of Cardiology, the American College of Cardiology, and the American Heart Association recommend the use of abciximab in those patients receiving PCI in setting of STEMI. Important to the emergency physician, the authors of this Italian project set out to determine if initiation of abciximab would be more beneficial if initiated in the emergency department (ED) or the cardiac catheterization laboratory (CCL). Although this study was prospectively randomized, patients and their physicians may determine whether or not the patient receives the anticoagulant in the ED or CCL, that is, the patient who is rapidly taken to the laboratory before the medication is available for ED use. The appropriate governing boards and numerous studies advocate rapid treatment and decreased door-to-balloon times. Referencing this study's statistically significant improved outcomes in the early group, the emergency medicine and cardiology leadership can justify storage and use of these anticoagulants in the ED.[6] Ⓐ

Evidence-Based References

1. Wijeysundera HC et al: Rescue angioplasty or repeat fibrinolysis after failed fibrinolytic therapy for ST-segment myocardial infarction: a meta-analysis of randomized trials, *J Am Coll Cardiol* 49:422-430, 2007. Commentary by S.W. Werns, M.D. Ⓐ

2. Oldgren J et al: Effects of fondaparinux in patients with ST-segment elevation acute myocardial infarction not receiving reperfusion treatment, *Eur Heart J* 29:315-323, 2008. Commentary by S.W. Werns, M.D. Ⓐ

3. De Jonge P, MIND-IT Investigators: Nonresponse to treatment for depression following myocardial infarction: association with subsequent cardiac events, *Am J Psychiatry* 164:1371-1378, 2007. Commentary by J.C. Ballenger, M.D. Ⓐ

4. Stevenson WG et al: Irrigated radiofrequency catheter ablation guided by electroanatomic mapping for recurrent ventricular tachycardia after myocardial infarction: the Multicenter Thermocool Ventricular Tachycardia Ablation Trial, *Circulation* 188:2773-2782, 2008. Commentary by A.L. Waldo, M.D. Ⓐ

5. Kim RJ, for the Gadoversetamide Myocardial Infarction Imaging Investigators: Performance of delayed-enhancement magnetic resonance imaging with gadoversetamide contrast for the detection and assessment of myocardial infarction: an international, multicenter, double-blinded, randomized trial, *Circulation* 117:629-637, 2008. Commentary by S. Abbara, M.D. Ⓐ

6. Maioli M et al: Randomized early versus late abciximab in acute myocardial infarction treated with primary coronary intervention (RELAx-AMI Trial), *J Am Coll Cardiol* 49:1517-1524, 2007. Commentary by E.C. Bruno, M.D. Ⓐ

SUGGESTED READINGS

2007 focused update of the ACC/AHA guidelines for the management of patients with ST-elevation myocardial infarction, *J Am Coll Cardiol* 51:210-247, 2008.

2009 focused updates: ACC/AHA guidelines for the management of patients with ST-elevation myocardial infarction (updating the 2004. guideline and 2007. focused update) and ACC/AHA/SCAI guidelines on percutaneous coronary intervention (updating the 2005. guideline and 2007. focused update), *J Am Coll Cardiol* 54:2205-2241, 2009.

Antman EM et al: The TIMI risk score for unstable angina/non-ST elevation MI: a method for prognostication and therapeutic decision making, *JAMA* 284:835-842, 2000.

Becker RC: Antithrombotic therapy after myocardial infarction, *N Engl J Med* 347:1019, 2002.

Cannon CP et al: Intensive versus moderate lipid lowering with statins after acute coronary syndromes, *N Engl J Med* 350:1495, 2004.

Jeremias A, Gibson M: Narrative review: alternative causes for elevated cardiac troponin levels when acute coronary syndromes are excluded, *Ann Intern Med* 142:786-791, 2005.

Mauri L et al: Drug-eluting or bare-metal stents for acute myocardial infarction, *N Engl J Med* 359: 1330-1342, 2008.

Meier MA et al: The new definition of myocardial infarction, *Arch Intern Med* 162:1585, 2002.

Myerburg RJ: Implantable cardioverter-defibrillators after myocardial infarction, *N Engl J Med* 359:2245-2253, 2008.

Newby LK et al: Early statin initiation and outcomes in patients with acute coronary syndromes, *JAMA* 287:3087, 2002.

Sabatine MS et al: Addition of clopidogrel to aspirin and fibrinolytic therapy for MI with ST-segment elevation, *N Engl J Med* 352:1179-1189, 2005.

Thygesen K, Alpert JS, White HD; on behalf of the Joint ESC/ACCF/AHA/WHF Task Force for the Redefinition of Myocardial Infarction: Universal definition of myocardial infarction, *J Am Coll Cardiol* 50:2173-2195, 2007.

AUTHORS: **VICTOR SHIN, M.D.,** and **FRED F. FERRI, M.D.**

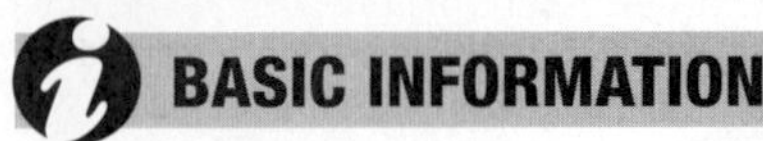

BASIC INFORMATION

DEFINITION

Myocarditis is an inflammatory condition of the myocardium.

ICD-9CM CODES

429.0	Myocarditis, nonspecific
391.2	Myocarditis, rheumatic
422.91	Myocarditis, viral (except Coxsackie)
074.23	Myocarditis, Coxsackie
422.92	Myocarditis, bacterial

EPIDEMIOLOGY & DEMOGRAPHICS

- The incidence of focal myocarditis reported at autopsy is 1% to 7% in asymptomatic patients and ≥50% in patients infected with HIV.
- Myocarditis is a major cause of sudden unexpected death (15% to 20% of cases) in adults <40 yr.

PHYSICAL FINDINGS & CLINICAL PRESENTATION

- Persistent tachycardia out of proportion to fever
- Faint S_1, S_4 sound on auscultation
- Murmur of mitral regurgitation
- Pericardial friction rub if associated with pericarditis
- Signs of biventricular failure (hypotension, hepatomegaly, peripheral edema, distention of neck veins, S_3)
- Patients may present with a history of recent flulike syndrome (fever, arthralgias, malaise); children often have a more fulminant presentation
- Most common presentations are dyspnea (72% of patients), chest pain (32%), arrhythmias (18%)

ETIOLOGY

- Infection
  1. Viral (Coxsackie B virus, cytomegalovirus, echovirus, polio virus, adenovirus, mumps, HIV, Epstein-Barr virus)
  2. Bacterial *(Staphylococcus aureus, Clostridium perfringens,* diphtheria, and any severe bacterial infection)
  3. Mycoplasma
  4. Mycotic *(Candida, Mucor, Aspergillus)*
  5. Parasitic (*Trypanosoma cruzi, Trichinella, Echinococcus,* amoeba, *Toxoplasma*)
  6. *Rickettsia rickettsii*
  7. Spirochetal *(Borrelia burgdorferi*–Lyme carditis)
- Rheumatic fever
- Secondary to drugs (e.g., cocaine, emetine, doxorubicin, sulfonamides, isoniazid, methyldopa, amphotericin B, tetracycline, phenylbutazone, lithium, 5-fluoruracil, phenothiazines, interferon-alfa, tricyclic antidepressants, cyclophosphamides)
- Toxins (carbon monoxide, ethanol, diphtheria toxin, lead, arsenicals)
- Collagen-vascular disease (systemic lupus erythematosus, scleroderma, sarcoidosis, Kawasaki syndrome)
- Sarcoidosis
- Radiation
- Postpartum status

DIAGNOSIS

DIFFERENTIAL DIAGNOSIS

- Cardiomyopathy
- Acute myocardial infarction
- Valvulopathies

The differential diagnosis of chest pain is described in Section II.

WORKUP

- Medical history: the clinical presentation of myocarditis is nonspecific and can consist of fatigue, palpitations, dyspnea, precordial discomfort, and myalgias.
- Diagnostic workup includes chest x-ray examination, ECG, laboratory evaluation, echocardiogram, cardiac catheterization, and endomyocardial biopsy (in selected patients on the basis of the likelihood of finding specific treatable disorders) (Fig. 1-206).

LABORATORY TESTS

- Elevated cardiac troponin T is suggestive of myocarditis in patients with clinically suspected myocarditis. Troponin I specificity is 89%; sensitivity is 34%. A normal level does not rule out the diagnosis.
- Increased creatine kinase (with elevated MB fraction, lactate dehydrogenase), and aspartate aminotransferase from myocardial necrosis.
- Increased erythrocyte sedimentation rate (nonspecific but may be of value in following the progress of the disease and the response to therapy).
- Increased white blood cell count (increased eosinophils if parasitic infection).
- Viral titers (acute and convalescent).
- Cold agglutinin titer, antistreptolysin O titer, blood cultures.
- Lyme disease antibody titer.

IMAGING STUDIES

- Chest radiograph: enlargement of cardiac silhouette

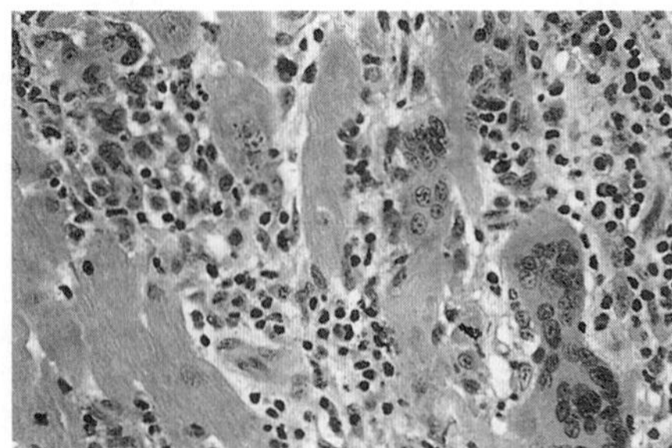

FIGURE 1-206 Giant cell myocarditis. A mixed inflammatory infiltrate, multinucleated giant cells, and extensive myocyte damage. (From Winters GL, McManus BM: Myocarditis. In Silver MD et al [eds]: *Cardiovascular pathology,* ed 3, New York, 2001, Churchill Livingstone, p 269.)

- ECG: sinus tachycardia with nonspecific ST-T wave changes; interventricular conduction defects and bundle branch block may be present
  1. Lyme disease and diphtheria cause all degrees of heart block.
  2. Changes of acute myocardial infarction can occur with focal necrosis.
- Echocardiogram:
  1. Dilated and hypokinetic chambers
  2. Segmental wall motion abnormalities
- Cardiac catheterization and angiography:
  1. To rule out coronary artery disease and valvular disease.
  2. A right ventricular endomyocardial biopsy can confirm the diagnosis, although a negative biopsy result does not exclude myocarditis. Recent studies have shown that myocardial biopsy may be unnecessary because immunosuppression therapy based on biopsy results is generally ineffective.
- Cardiac MRI is a newer promising modality in suspected myocarditis. Regions of myocarditis are reported to correlate closely with regions of abnormal signal on cardiac MRI.

TREATMENT

NONPHARMACOLOGIC THERAPY

- Supportive care is the first line of therapy for patients with myocarditis.
- Restrict physical activity (to decrease cardiac work). Bed rest is advisable during viremia.

ACUTE GENERAL Rx

- Treat underlying cause (e.g., use specific antibiotics for bacterial infection).
- Treat congestive heart failure (CHF) with diuretics, angiotensin-converting enzyme inhibitors, and salt restriction. A beta-blocker may be added once clinical stability has been achieved. Digoxin should be used with caution and only at low doses.
- If ventricular arrhythmias are present, treat with quinidine or procainamide.
- Provide anticoagulation to prevent thromboembolism.
- Use preload and afterload reducing agents for treating cardiac decompensation.
- Corticosteroid use is contraindicated in early infectious myocarditis; it may be justified in only selected patients with intractable CHF, severe systemic toxicity, and severe life-threatening arrhythmias.
- Immunosuppressive drugs (prednisone with cyclosporine or azathioprine) do not have any significant effect on the prognosis of myocarditis and should not be used in the routine treatment of patients with myocarditis. Immunosuppression may have a role in the treatment of myocarditis from systemic autoimmune disease (e.g., lupus, scleroderma) and in patients with idiopathic giant cell myocarditis.

DISPOSITION

Nearly 50% of patients with myocarditis will die within 5 yr of diagnosis. Prognosis is best for patients with fulminant lymphocytic myocarditis (severe hemodynamic compromise, rapid onset of symptoms, or high fever). These patients tend to have complete recovery with total resolution of myocarditis on repeat biopsy.

REFERRAL

Consider heart transplant if patient develops intractable CHF.

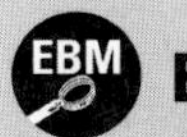

EVIDENCE

Several confounding variables limit the quality of clinical trials conducted in patients with myocarditis and should be considered when interpreting trial findings.

Human studies are limited because of the low incidence of recognized symptomatic myocarditis.

Clinical presentation is highly variable; consequently it is difficult to generalize a treatment response to the whole spectrum of the disease.

Patients of all ages are affected, and disease and treatment response may vary between children and adults.

History, physical examination, and routine investigations have poor specificity for myocarditis. Standardized microscopic criteria exist but are not always used. The validity of these criteria, however, has also been questioned.

Consequently, many of the current treatment strategies for myocarditis are based on clinical experience rather than randomized trials. Furthermore, the evidence for therapies used in the treatment of heart failure is derived from trials in subjects whose heart failure was not necessarily caused by myocarditis. This should be kept in mind when this evidence is used to inform treatment decisions for patients with myocarditis. For more detailed evidence of therapies used in heart failure, see the entry on "Congestive Heart Failure."

IV immunoglobulin has not been found to be superior to placebo in the treatment of adult patients with presumed viral myocarditis. The incidence of death, requirement for cardiac transplant or placement of a left ventricular assist device, and improvement in left ventricular ejection fraction and functional capacity at 12 mo are similar for both treatments.[1] Ⓑ

Evidence-Based Reference

1. Robinson J et al: Intravenous immunoglobulin for presumed viral myocarditis in children and adults, *Cochrane Rev* 1, 2005. Ⓑ

SUGGESTED READINGS

Cooper LT: Myocarditis, *N Engl J Med* 360:1526-1538, 2009.

Wu LA et al: Current role of endomyocardial biopsy in the management of dilated cardiomyopathy and myocarditis, *Mayo Clin Proc* 76:1030, 2001.

AUTHOR: **FRED F. FERRI, M.D.**

Myoclonus

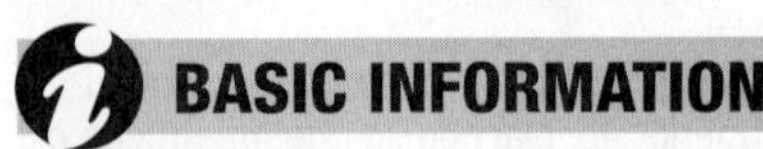

BASIC INFORMATION

DEFINITION

Myoclonus is defined as sudden, brief, jerky, "shocklike" involuntary movements that can involve the muscles of the extremities, face, or trunk. Positive myoclonus is caused by muscle contraction, whereas negative myoclonus is caused by inhibition of active (such as postural) muscles. Myoclonus is a symptom that can be seen in a number of different neurologic disorders.

ICD-9CM CODES
333.2 Myoclonus

EPIDEMIOLOGY & DEMOGRAPHICS

INCIDENCE: 1.3/100,000 persons
PREVALENCE: 8.6/100,000 persons
PREDOMINANT SEX AND AGE: No gender preference; age of onset varies by the etiology of the myoclonus.
GENETICS: Varies by etiology, can be hereditary or sporadic

PHYSICAL FINDINGS & CLINICAL PRESENTATION

- Clinically, myoclonus can be classified by its distribution: focal (only one body part involved), multifocal, segmental (spread to adjacent body parts), axial (muscles innervated by one or several spinal levels), or generalized. It can be stimulus-induced or occur at rest.
- Myoclonus can be seen with involvement or lesions of the cerebral cortex, brainstem, spinal cord, or peripheral nerve. The location of the lesion may not always influence the characteristics of the myoclonus.
- Negative myoclonus is typically seen in postural muscles of the legs, causing a "bobbing" while walking. Asterixis is another form of negative myoclonus.

ETIOLOGY

- The causes of myoclonus are numerous and can be grouped into the categories of physiologic, essential, epileptic, and symptomatic.
- Physiologic myoclonus ranges from sleep (hypnic) jerks to exercise-induced myoclonus and can be seen in normal subjects.
- Essential myoclonus occurs in the absence of other neurologic symptoms and is usually autosomal dominant. When dystonia is present it is called myoclonus-dystonia. The myoclonus is often responsive to alcohol in this condition.
- In epileptic myoclonus, seizures dominate the clinical picture. Syndromes include infantile spasms and juvenile myoclonic epilepsy among others.
- Symptomatic or secondary myoclonus comprises myoclonus in the setting of an underlying neurologic disorder or other precipitant. The number of prevents giving a full list, but common causes include neurodegenerative diseases (Alzheimer's, atypical forms of parkinsonism), CNS infections (Creutzfeldt-Jakob disease, viral encephalitis), metabolic derangements (uremia, hepatic failure), drug-induced (selective serotonin reuptake inhibitors [SSRIs], tricyclics, lithium), and posthypoxic etiologies.

Dx DIAGNOSIS

DIFFERENTIAL DIAGNOSIS

- Tremor: a rhythmic oscillation around a point; slower than myoclonus
- Tic: complex patterned movements that can be suppressed voluntarily for a short time unlike myoclonus, which is simple jerks that are persistent
- Dystonia: patterned contractions of agonist/antagonist muscles causing twisting or pulling; slower than myoclonus
- Chorea: typically slower, writhing, patterned movements
- Psychogenic myoclonus: variable in duration and location, distractible, or entrainable

LABORATORY TESTS

- Evaluate for metabolic precipitants (renal and hepatic function, Mg, Ca, thyroid studies)
- Toxicology screen
- Lumbar puncture if encephalitis is suspected
- Electroencephalography (EEG) to evaluate for epileptic myoclonus

IMAGING STUDIES

MRI of the brain can evaluate for a seizure focus if the myoclonus is epileptic. Creutzfeldt-Jakob disease shows diffusion weighted abnormalities in the basal ganglia.

Rx TREATMENT

NONPHARMACOLOGIC THERAPY

- Treatment should be directed toward correcting the underlying cause if it is reversible (e.g. hepatic or renal failure).
- Carefully remove or decrease potentially causative medications.

ACUTE GENERAL Rx

For acute treatment of epileptic myoclonus, antiepileptic drugs such as valproic acid, levetiracetam, or clonazepam are helpful.

CHRONIC Rx

- Clonazepam, valproic acid, levetiracetam are typically used for all forms of myoclonus, and often combinations of several medications seem to be more effective.
- If dystonia is present (myoclonus-dystonia), a trial of levodopa is worthwhile although only rarely responsive. Anticholinergics may also help dystonia. Botulinum toxin injections are used for focal dystonias.
- Peripheral focal myoclonus can also be helped by botulinum toxin injections.

DISPOSITION

The ultimate prognosis depends on the etiology of the myoclonus.

REFERRAL

Referral to a general neurologist or movement disorders center is appropriate.

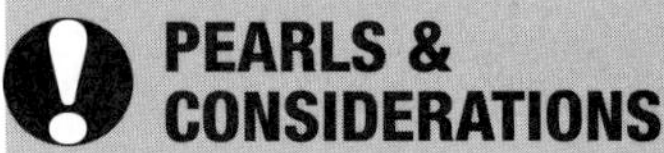

PEARLS & CONSIDERATIONS

COMMENTS

- When myoclonus is seen with parkinsonism, atypical forms of parkinsonism should be high on the differential such as dementia with Lewy bodies, corticobasal degeneration, and multiple system atrophy. Myoclonus is only rarely seen in idiopathic Parkinson's disease.
- Symptomatic palatal myoclonus is a specific syndrome that is often associated with a focal brainstem lesion. In essential palatal myoclonus (no lesion), ear "clicking" is an additional symptom, which is not seen in the symptomatic form.

SUGGESTED READINGS

Borg M: Symptomatic myoclonus, *Clin Neurophys* 36:309-318, 2006.

Caviness JN: Pathophysiology and treatment of myoclonus, *Neurol Clin* 27:757-777, 2009.

Chang VC, Frucht SJ: Myoclonus, *Curr Treat Options Neurol* 10:222–229, 2008.

Vercueil I: Myoclonus and movement disorders, *Clin Neurophys* 36:327-331, 2006.

AUTHOR: **ANDREW DUKER, M.D.**

BASIC INFORMATION

DEFINITION

Inflammatory myopathies are idiopathic diseases of muscle characterized clinically by muscle weakness and pathologically by inflammation and muscle fiber breakdown. The three most common are dermatomyositis (DM), polymyositis (PM), and inclusion body myositis (IBM). See "Inclusion Body Myositis" entry for details regarding the latter.

SYNONYMS

See "Definition."

ICD-9CM CODES
710.3 Dermatomyositis
710.4 Polymyositis

EPIDEMIOLOGY & DEMOGRAPHICS

DM:
- Occurs in children and in adults (bimodal age peak)
- Average age at diagnosis is 40 in adults. Age range in children: 5 to 14 yr.
- More common in females than in males (2:1)
- Incidence 1:100,000
- Prevalence 1 to 10 cases/million in adults and 1 to 3.2 cases/million in children
- Up to one third of patients older than 50 with DM have an associated malignancy

PM:
- Occurs mostly in adults, very rare in children
- Average age at diagnosis >20 yr
- More common in females
- Least common inflammatory myopathy
- Exact incidence unknown

PHYSICAL FINDINGS & CLINICAL PRESENTATION

DM and PM:
- Most patients have a subacute onset over weeks to months.
- Pattern is typically symmetric proximal muscle weakness involving the proximal limbs (shoulder and pelvic girdles).
- Weakness of neck flexion and extension is common.
- Difficulty getting up from a chair, climbing stairs, reaching for objects above head, or combing hair.
- Distal muscle and ocular involvement is uncommon.
- Sensation is preserved.
- Reflexes may be preserved or diminished.
- Dysphagia and dysphonia result from involvement of striated muscle of the pharynx and proximal esophagus.
- Esophageal dysmotility is common in DM.
- Respiratory failure from associated pulmonary fibrosis.
- Cardiac conduction abnormalities can be seen with DM.
- Systemic autoimmune disease occurs frequently in PM, and rarely in DM.
- Skin findings in DM:
    - Heliotrope rash on the upper eyelids (Fig. 1-207)
    - Erythematous rash on the face (see Fig. 1-207)
    - May also involve the back and shoulders (shawl sign), neck and chest (V-shape), knees, and elbows
    - Photosensitivity
    - Gottron's papules (violaceous papules overlying dorsal interphalangeal or metacarpophalangeal areas, elbow or knee joints—Fig. 1-208)
    - Nail cracking, thickening, and irregularity with periungual telangiectasia (see Fig. 1-208)
    - Mechanic's hand: fissured, hyperpigmented, scaly, and hyperkeratotic; also associated with increased risk of interstitial lung disease

ETIOLOGY

DM: complex, immune-mediated microangiopathy. Adaptive immune response via humorally mediated complement attack

PM: unknown:
- Cell-mediated immune major histocompatibility-I (MHC-1) process directed against muscle fibers is likely, given biopsy features.
- A viral etiology has been proposed secondary to the presence of autoantibodies to histidyl transferase, anti-Jo-1, and signal recognition particle.

DIAGNOSIS

- Myopathic pattern of muscle weakness
- Characteristic rash in DM
- EMG shows myopathic (small-amplitude, short-duration, polyphasic) motor potentials with early recruitment
- Majority of patients have "irritable" features (fibrillations and positive sharp waves) on EMG
- See "Laboratory Tests."

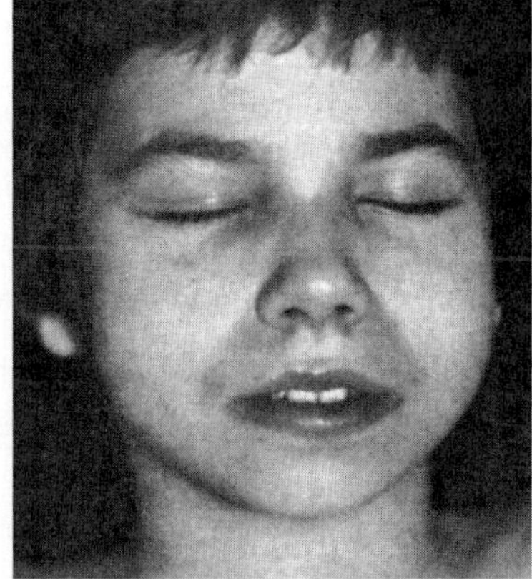

FIGURE 1-207 The facial rash of juvenile dermatomyositis. There is erythema over the bridge of the nose and malar areas, with violaceous (heliotropic) discoloration of the upper eyelids. (From Behrman RE: *Nelson textbook of pediatrics,* ed 17, Philadelphia, 2004, WB Saunders.)

- Biopsy is required for diagnosis and should confirm inflammation before treatment is started: myopathic features (variation in fiber size, fiber splitting, fatty replacement of muscle tissue, and increased endomysial connective tissue) should be seen in addition to the following:
    - DM: perifascicular atrophy, MAC deposition along capillaries
    - PM: endomysial infiltrates composed of CD8+ T cells and macrophages invading nonnecrotic muscle fibers that express MHC-I antigen

DIFFERENTIAL DIAGNOSIS

- IBM
- Muscular dystrophies
- Amyloid myoneuropathy
- Amyotrophic lateral sclerosis
- Myasthenia gravis
- Eaton-Lambert syndrome
- Drug-induced myopathies (e.g., quinidine, NSAIDs, penicillamine, HMG CoA-reductase inhibitors)
- Diabetic amyotrophy
- Guillain-Barré syndrome
- Hyperthyroidism or hypothyroidism
- Lichen planus
- Amyopathic DM (rash without weakness)
- Dermatomyositis siné rash (weakness with characteristic biopsy, but no rash)
- Systemic lupus erythematosus (SLE)
- Contact atopic or seborrheic dermatitis
- Psoriasis

LABORATORY TESTS

- Creatine kinase (CK) is the most sensitive muscle enzyme test for muscle breakdown. It should be checked at onset, and serially monitored several times during treatment.
- CK is typically elevated (5-50x normal) in active PM.
- CK may be normal or only slightly elevated in DM.
- Aldolase, AST, ALT, alkaline phosphatase, and LDH may be elevated.

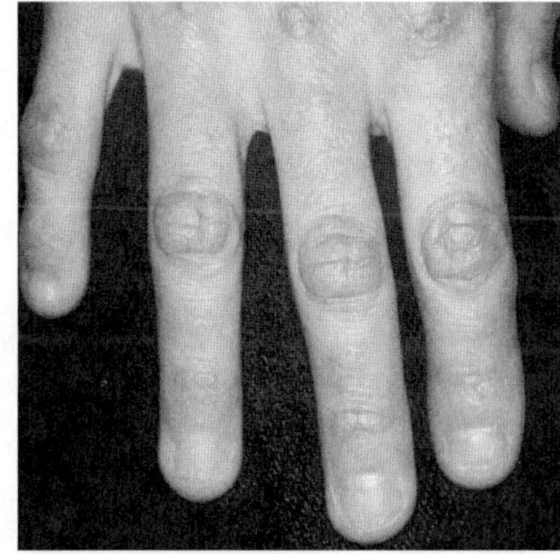

FIGURE 1-208 Dermatomyositis (Gottron's papules). Note erythematous papules over joints and periungual telangiectasias. (From Noble J [ed]: *Textbook of primary care medicine,* ed 2, St Louis, 1996, Mosby.)

- Anti-Jo-1 antibodies are seen in myositis with associated interstitial lung disease but are not specific for either DM or PM.
- Electrolytes, thyroid-stimulating hormone (TSH), Ca, and Mg should be evaluated to exclude other causes of weakness.
- Check ECG for cardiac involvement.

IMAGING STUDIES

- Chest x-ray is used to rule out pulmonary involvement. If suspicious for pulmonary interstitial disease, a high-resolution CT scan of the chest may be helpful.
- Video fluoroscopy or barium swallow study to look for upper esophageal dysfunction in patients with dysphagia and DM.

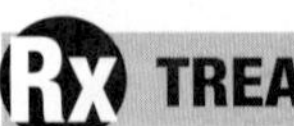

TREATMENT

Goal: maintain function, minimize disease/iatrogenic sequelae

NONPHARMACOLOGIC THERAPY

- Sun-blocking agents with SPF 15 or greater for skin protection in patients with DM
- Physical therapy beneficial for gait training and increasing muscle tone and strength
- Occupational therapy assists with activities of daily living
- Speech therapy to monitor patients with swallowing dysfunction

ACUTE GENERAL Rx

- Corticosteroids are the mainstay of therapy. Start prednisone 1 to 2 mg/kg per day, up to a maximum dose of 100 mg/day. Continue until muscle strength improves or muscle enzymes have normalized for at least 4 wk. Begin tapering by 10 mg/mo until 60 mg/day, then slowly taper by 5 mg/mo. Consider every-other-day prednisone treatment at same dose (may decrease side effects).
- Consider IV immunoglobulin (IVIG) if patient fails to improve on prednisone, or muscle enzymes begin rising when tapering off prednisone. See "Chronic Rx" for specific dosage.
- Hydroxychloroquine can be used to treat the cutaneous lesions of DM.

CHRONIC Rx

- Chronic prednisone therapy may be needed for years, but other immunosuppressive ("steroid-sparing") agents may be added early to decrease long-term steroid side effects.
- Azathioprine 2 to 3 mg/kg per day tapered to 1 mg/kg per day once steroid is tapered to 15 mg/day. Reduce dosage monthly by 25-mg intervals. Maintenance dosage is 50 mg/day.
- Methotrexate 7.5 to 10 mg PO/wk, increased by 2.5 mg/wk to total of 25 mg/wk; consider IM dosing if PO is ineffective.
- IV immunoglobulin 2 g/kg total dose over 2 to 5 days
- IV cyclophosphamide 1 g/M^2 monthly for 6 mo is preferred to oral dosing for refractory cases. However, oral dosing of cyclophosphamide is 1 to 3 mg/kg per day PO or 2 to 4 mg/kg per day in conjunction with prednisone.
- Cyclosporin A: initial dose 2.0 to 2.5 mg/kg bid; long-term maintenance is lowest effective dose.
- Mycophenolate mofetil 500 mg PO bid, titrate to 1500 mg PO bid over 1 to 2 mo.
- Hydroxychloroquine 200 mg PO daily; monitor for visual changes.

DISPOSITION

- 30% to 40% of patients achieve clinical remission with treatment.
- In patients with residual weakness, deficits typically remain stable over long-term follow-up.
- 10% experience recurrent disease.
- Serum CK often returns to normal before symptoms improve.
- During exacerbations, enzymes may rise before clinical symptoms appear.
- Poor prognostic indicators include delay in diagnosis, older age, recalcitrant disease, malignancy, interstitial pulmonary fibrosis, dysphagia, leukocytosis, fever, and anorexia.
- Infection, malignancy, and cardiac and pulmonary dysfunction are the most common causes of death.
- With early treatment, 5- and 8-yr survival rates of 80% and 73%, respectively, have been reported.

REFERRAL

Neurology or rheumatology referral should be made to help establish the diagnosis and implement treatment.

PEARLS & CONSIDERATIONS

- Do not implement treatment before muscle biopsy.
- When assessing response to treatment, clinical muscle strength is more important than muscle enzyme tests.
- The concern for malignancies (ovary, lung, breast, GI) associated with DM is legitimate and merits screening in patients older than age 40 at time of diagnosis and every 2 to 3 yr thereafter.
- There does not appear to be any association between juvenile DM and malignancy.
- Overlap syndrome refers to patients with DM who also meet criteria for a connective tissue disorder (e.g., rheumatoid arthritis, scleroderma, SLE).
- In any patient taking steroids, closely monitor for:
  - Diabetes or glucose intolerance (2-hour oral glucose tolerance test)
  - Osteopenia/osteoporosis (DEXA scan q6mo)
  - Cataracts (yearly ophthalmologic appointment)
  - Hypertension
  - Psychiatric side effects including depression or psychosis
  - Poor sleep
  - Peptic ulcer disease (prescribe H+ antagonist or proton pump inhibitor)

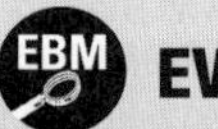

EVIDENCE

Conducting high-quality randomized controlled trials in rare diseases such as the inflammatory myopathies is extremely difficult. Individual clinicians rarely have sufficient numbers of patients; therefore multicenter trials are the only way to study such diseases. But even these are lacking and, coupled with the lack of international consensus on outcome measures, it is easy to see why pooling of data on the inflammatory myopathies, by meta-analysis, is limited.

Immunosuppressants, such as azathioprine and methotrexate, may be used as steroid-sparing agents or in patients who are becoming steroid resistant. Used either singly or in combination, immunosuppressants can increase muscle strength.

A systematic review found that daily azathioprine given with weekly oral methotrexate increased muscle strength over a 6-mo period.[1] Ⓐ

It also found that, compared with placebo, muscle strength increased with azathioprine, though the difference was not statistically significant.[1] Ⓐ

Hand grip strength after 1 yr, however, did not show more improvement with azathioprine than with methotrexate.[1] Ⓐ

Furthermore, it found that there was a slightly greater increase in muscle strength after 6 months of methotrexate plus azathioprine (oral combination), compared with intravenous methotrexate. The difference between the two groups, however, was not statistically significant.[1] Ⓐ

Intravenous immune globulin (IVIG) in high doses is an effective treatment for refractory DM.

A systematic review included a randomized controlled trial on patients with biopsy-proven, treatment-resistant DM. Patients assigned to receive immune globulin had a significant improvement in scores of muscle strength and neuromuscular symptoms, whereas those assigned to placebo did not. Repeat muscle biopsies in patients whose strength improved to almost normal showed an increase in muscle-fiber diameter, amongst other things.[1] Ⓐ

Evidence-Based Reference

1. Dalakas M, Hohlfeld R: Polymyositis and dermatomyositis, *Lancet* 362:971-982, 2003.

AUTHORS: **GAVIN BROWN, M.D.** and **GREGORY J. ESPER, M.D.**

BASIC INFORMATION

DEFINITION

Myotonia is a type of muscular dystrophy in which relaxation of a muscle after contraction is delayed or prolonged. The most common type of muscular dystrophy with myotonia is myotonic dystrophy.

SYNONYMS

Myotonic dystrophy

ICD-9CM CODES
359.2 Myotonic disorders
728.85 Muscle spasm

EPIDEMIOLOGY & DEMOGRAPHICS

- Three to five cases/100,000 persons.
- Genetic disorder inherited as an autosomal-dominant illness.
- Symptoms usually manifest during adolescence or early adulthood. Cases of infantile myotonic dystrophy have been described.

PHYSICAL FINDINGS & CLINICAL PRESENTATION

- Usual first symptom is distal extremity weakness sometimes associated with muscle stiffness, cramps, or difficulty relaxing grasp.
- Weakness spreads to eventually involve all muscle groups. Flexor neck muscle weakness and masseter and temporal wasting are often prominent features, as is dysarthria.
- Percussion of a muscle produces a slow contraction followed by prolonged relaxation. The myotonic reflex is best tested by percussing the thenar muscles and observing a slow flexion followed by slow relaxation of the thumb.
- As the disease progresses, generalized weakness becomes more pronounced and myotonia becomes less evident.
- Extramuscular involvement:
  - Mental retardation of variable severity (may be absent)
  - Frontal baldness (Fig. 1-209)
  - Cataracts
  - Diabetes mellitus
  - Hypogonadism
  - Adrenal failure
  - Cardiomyopathy
- Infantile myotonic dystrophy presents as neonatal extreme hypotonia with "shark mouth" deformity (upper lip forming an inverted V).

ETIOLOGY & PATHOGENESIS

Genetic disorder encoded on chromosome 19 leading to sustained firing of the muscle membrane, causing prolonged muscle contraction. Myotonic dystrophy 1 (the more common form) is caused by an expanded CTG repeat within the noncoding 3′ untranslated region of the myotonic dystrophy protein kinase *(DMPK)* gene. The less common form (myotonic dystrophy 2) is caused by an expanded CCTG repeat in the first intron of the zinc finger protein 9 *(ZNF9)* gene.

Dx DIAGNOSIS

DIFFERENTIAL DIAGNOSIS

The disease is limited to muscles and causes hypertrophy and stiffness after rest. Muscle function normalizes with exercise. There is no weakness. Symptoms are exacerbated by exposure to cold.

- Myotonia congenita (Thomsen's disease)
- May be autosomal dominant or recessive (two distinct varieties)
- Paramyotonia congenita (autosomal-dominant disease): weakness and stiffness of facial muscles and distal upper extremities, especially or exclusively on cold exposure
- Muscular dystrophies
- Inflammatory myopathies (polymyositis)
- Metabolic muscle diseases
- Myasthenic syndromes
- Motor neuron disease

WORKUP

- History and physical examination usually sufficient
- Muscle enzymes usually abnormal (creatine phosphokinase, aldolase, aspartate aminotransferase)
- Electromyography: typical myotonic "dive bomber" bursts
- Muscle biopsy: type I fiber atrophy, ring fibers, increased central nucleation

Rx TREATMENT

- Phenytoin
- Quinine
- Quinidine
- Procainamide
- Acetazolamide
- Genetic counseling
- Assistive devices, orthotics

DISPOSITION

In myotonic dystrophy, death is usually caused by the wasting of skeletal muscle and defects in cardiac function.

REFERRAL

To neurologist

SUGGESTED READINGS

Cooper TA: A reversal of misfortune for myotonic dystrophy, *N Engl J Med* 355:17, 2006.

Kanadia RN et al: Reversal of RNA missplicing and myotonia after muscle blind overexpression in a mouse poly (CUG) model for myotonic dystrophy, *Proc Natl Acad Sci U S A* 103:11748, 2006.

AUTHOR: **FRED F. FERRI, M.D.**

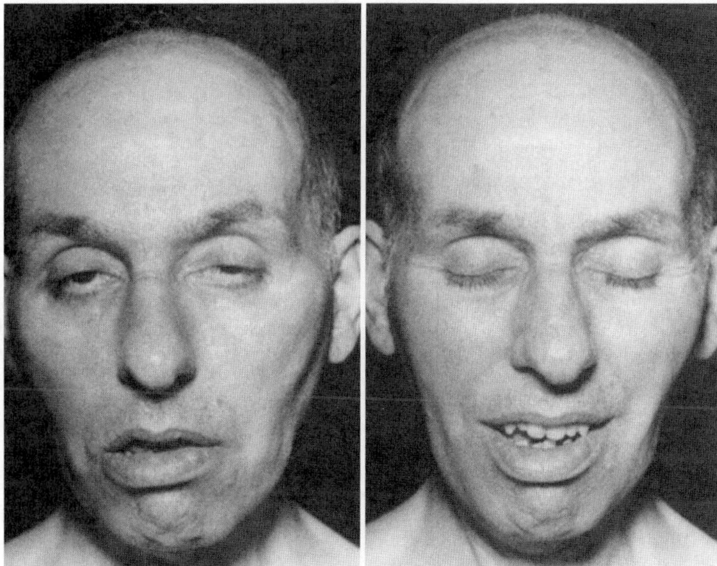

FIGURE 1-209 Myotonic dystrophy with typical myopathic facies, frontal balding, and sunken cheeks. (From Dubowitz V: *Muscle disorders in childhood,* London, 1995, WB Saunders.)

Myxedema Coma

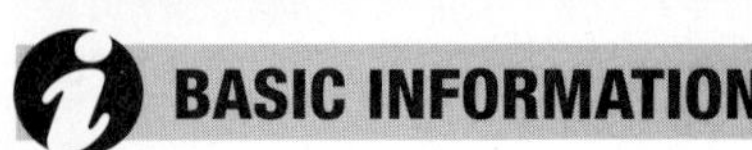

BASIC INFORMATION

DEFINITION

Myxedema coma is a life-threatening complication of hypothyroidism characterized by profound lethargy or coma and usually accompanied by hypothermia.

ICD-9CM CODES
244.8 Myxedema, pituitary
244.1 Myxedema, primary

PHYSICAL FINDINGS & CLINICAL PRESENTATION

- Profound lethargy or coma
- Hypothermia (rectal temperature <35° C [95° F]); often missed by using ordinary thermometers graduated only to 34.5° C or because the mercury is not shaken below 36° C
- Bradycardia, hypotension (attributable to circulatory collapse)
- Delayed relaxation phase of deep tendon reflexes, areflexia
- Myxedema facies (Fig. 1-210)
- Alopecia, macroglossia, ptosis, periorbital edema, nonpitting edema, doughy skin
- Bladder dystonia and distention

ETIOLOGY

Decompensation of hypothyroidism from:

- Sepsis
- Exposure to cold weather
- Central nervous system depressants (sedatives, narcotics, antidepressants)
- Trauma, surgery

Dx DIAGNOSIS

DIFFERENTIAL DIAGNOSIS

- Severe depression, primary psychosis
- Drug overdose
- Cerebrovascular accident, liver failure, renal failure
- Hypoglycemia, CO_2 narcosis, encephalitis

WORKUP

Diagnosis of hypothyroidism and exclusion of contributing factors (e.g., sepsis, cerebrovascular accident) with laboratory and radiographic studies (see "Laboratory Tests")

LABORATORY TESTS

- Markedly increased thyroid-stimulating hormone (if primary hypothyroidism), decreased serum free T_4
- Complete blood count with differential, urine and blood cultures to rule out infectious process
- Electrolytes, blood urea nitrogen, creatinine, liver function tests, calcium, glucose
- Arterial blood gases to rule out hypoxemia and carbon dioxide retention
- Cortisol level to rule out adrenal insufficiency
- Elevated CPK
- Hyperlipidemia

IMAGING STUDIES

- CT scan of head in suspected cerebrovascular accident
- Chest radiograph to rule out infectious process

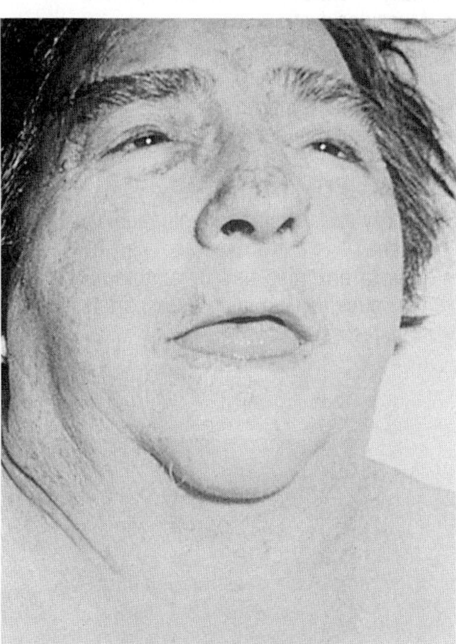

FIGURE 1-210 Myxedema facies. Note dull, puffy, yellowed skin; coarse, sparse hair; temporal loss of eyebrows; periorbital edema; prominent tongue. (Courtesy Paul W. Ladenson, MD, The Johns Hopkins University and Hospital, Baltimore. In Seidel HM [ed]: *Mosby's guide to physical examination,* ed 5, St Louis, 2004, Mosby.)

Rx TREATMENT

NONPHARMACOLOGIC THERAPY

- Prevent further heat loss; cover the patient but avoid external rewarming because it may produce vascular collapse.
- Support respiratory function; intubation and mechanical ventilation may be required.
- Monitor patients in the intensive care unit.

ACUTE GENERAL Rx

- Give levothyroxine 5 to 8 mcg/kg (300 to 500 mcg) IV infused over 15 min, then 100 mcg IV q24h.
- Glucocorticoids should also be administered until coexistent adrenal insufficiency can be ruled out. Hydrocortisone hemisuccinate 100 mg IV bolus is initially given, followed by 50 mg IV q12h or 25 mg IV q6h until initial plasma cortisol level is confirmed normal.
- IV hydration with D_5NS is used to correct hypotension and hypoglycemia (if present); avoid overhydration and possible water intoxication because clearance of free water is impaired in these patients.
- Rule out and treat precipitating factors (e.g., antibiotics in suspected sepsis).

CHRONIC Rx

Refer to "Hypothyroidism" in Section I.

DISPOSITION

Mortality rate in myxedema coma is 20% to 50%.

REFERRAL

Endocrinology consultation

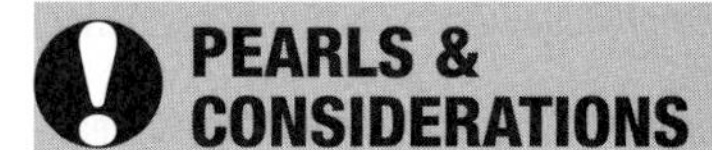

PEARLS & CONSIDERATIONS

COMMENTS

If the diagnosis is suspected, initiate treatment immediately without waiting for confirming laboratory results.

AUTHOR: **FRED F. FERRI, M.D.**

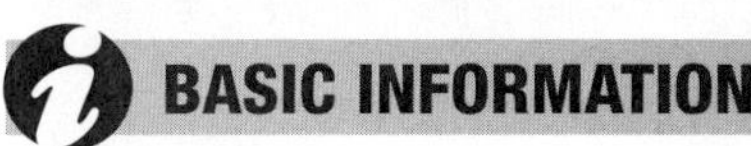

BASIC INFORMATION

DEFINITION

Narcissistic personality disorder (NPD) is characterized by a pattern of grandiosity, need for admiration, and lack of empathy that begins by early adulthood and causes significant distress or impairment in multiple domains of functioning. The individual must meet five or more of the following criteria:

1. Grandiose sense of self-importance. For example, the person may exaggerate achievements and talents or expect recognition as superior without commensurate achievements.
2. Preoccupied with fantasies of unlimited success, power, brilliance, beauty, or ideal love.
3. Views self as "special" and unique and should only associate with other special or highly regarded people and institutions.
4. Requires excessive admiration.
5. Sense of entitlement. For example, unreasonable expectations of especially favorable treatment or automatic compliance with his or her expectations.
6. Interpersonally exploitative.
7. Lacks empathy—unwilling to recognize or identify with the feelings or needs of others.
8. Often envious of others or believes others envious of him or her.
9. Shows arrogant or haughty behaviors.

SYNONYMS

None

ICD-9CM CODES
301.81

EPIDEMIOLOGY & DEMOGRAPHICS

PREVALENCE: Less than 1% of the general population; estimates range from 2% to 16% in the clinical population

PREDOMINANT SEX: More commonly diagnosed in males (up to 3:1)

PREDOMINANT AGE: 20s and 30s

CLINICAL PRESENTATION

- Patients have an underlying sense of inferiority and inadequacy.
- Often related to the failure of parents or parental surrogates to impart a sense of self-worth.
- To avoid these beliefs and their associated painful effects, patients seek to convince self and others that they are special, the best, or unusually talented.
- Astutely aware of status, pecking order.
- Vulnerability in self-esteem makes these patients exquisitely sensitive to criticism, defeat, or perceived weakness, which in turn can lead to feeling humiliated, degraded, and empty.
- These patients react to perceived slights with either more intense grandiosity and admiration seeking or with disdain and rage. Either approach seeks to bolster their sense of self often by devaluing or criticizing the other person.
- Experiences of self-deflation lead to social withdrawal or depressed mood or to feigned humility that protects grandiosity.
- Interpersonal relationships are typically shallow and limited.
- Although ambition and confidence may lead to high achievement, vocational functioning may be disrupted by intolerance for criticism.

ETIOLOGY

- Limited knowledge about role of genetic loading and neurobiologic vulnerability.
- Prevailing hypotheses focus on impaired development of self as "worthy" because of insufficient affirmation and warmth from parents.

Dx DIAGNOSIS

DIFFERENTIAL DIAGNOSIS

- Mania and hypomania
- Dysthymia and major depressive episode
- Substance-induced euphoria, especially cocaine abuse
- Histrionic, borderline, antisocial, and paranoid personality disorders share common features and are often comorbid
- Personality changes from a general medical condition, including central nervous system processes in the frontal-temporal regions of the brain

WORKUP

- History: collateral information essential to establishing presence of longstanding interpersonal pattern in multiple domains of the patient's life
- Physical examination
- Mental status examination

LABORATORY TESTS

Tests necessary to rule out medical causes of personality changes

IMAGING STUDIES

Those necessary to rule out medical causes of personality changes

Rx TREATMENT

NONPHARMACOLOGIC THERAPY

- Cognitive-behavioral therapy to help patients control rage, manage perceived criticism, and develop social skills
- Psychodynamic psychotherapy to help develop improved self-concept, affect tolerance, and interpersonal functioning

ACUTE GENERAL Rx

Benzodiazepines or low-dose antipsychotics to control rage

CHRONIC Rx

- Selective serotonin reuptake inhibitors for impulsivity or comorbid depression
- Mood stabilizers if comorbid bipolar or to improve impulse control

DISPOSITION

- Severity is variable and course is chronic. The majority of patients obtain greater functioning in fifth decade and beyond when pessimism replaces grandiosity. Often lifelong difficulty maintaining intimate relationships.
- At increased risk for major depressive disorder and substance abuse or dependence (especially cocaine).

REFERRAL

If pharmacotherapy is contemplated

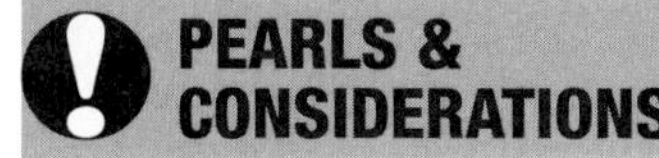

PEARLS & CONSIDERATIONS

COMMENTS

- Illness threatens these patients' image of superiority.
- To defend against this threat, patients may minimize symptoms or deny presence of illness.
- Patients will commonly demand special treatment from senior and well-known physicians.
- Patients may devalue, criticize, or question the behavior or credentials of the treating physician.
- Management guidelines:
  1. Be respectful and nonconfrontational.
  2. Help patient use self-perceived talents in service of treatment.
  3. Do not personalize patient's devaluation, but understand their criticalness as an attempt to manage their own intense insecurity.
  4. Appeal to the patient's narcissism. In other words, agree with the patient that he or she is "entitled" to appropriate care.

SUGGESTED READINGS

Grant BF et al: Prevalence, correlates, and disability of personality disorders in the United States: results from the national epidemiologic survey on alcohol and related conditions, *J Clin Psychiatry* 65(7):948-958, 2004.

Morana HC, Camara FP: International guidelines for the management of personality disorders, *Curr Opin Psychiatry* 19(5):539, 2006.

Ward RK: Assessment and management of personality disorders, *Am Fam Physician* 70(8):1505-1512, 2004.

AUTHOR: **JOHN Q. YOUNG, M.D., M.P.P.**

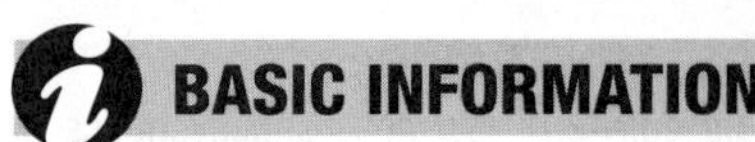

BASIC INFORMATION

DEFINITION

Narcolepsy is a chronic neurological sleep disorder characterized by excessive daytime sleepiness and dysregulation of rapid eye movement (REM) sleep. It is the second most common cause of disabling daytime sleepiness after obstructive sleep apnea. Symptoms of REM sleep dysregulation include cataplexy, sleep paralysis, and hallucinations during transition between wake and sleep.

SYNONYMS

Hypersomnia of central origin
Narcolepsy with cataplexy
Narcolepsy-cataplexy syndrome
Narcolepsy with hypocretin deficiency
Gelineau syndrome

ICD-9CM CODES
347.00 Narcolepsy without cataplexy
347.01 Narcolepsy with cataplexy

EPIDEMIOLOGY & DEMOGRAPHICS

INCIDENCE: 0.74/100,000 person/yr
PREVALENCE: 5 to 50/100,000 people
PREDOMINANT SEX: Males and females are equally affected.
AGE OF ONSET: Peak 15 to 30 yr (range, 10-55 yr)
GENETICS:
- Associated with specific human leukocyte antigen (HLA) subtypes (e.g., DQB1*0602)
- Risk of narcolepsy increases 20 to 40 times if a family member is affected.
- Monozygotic concordance rate is 17% to 36%, thus indicating an incomplete penetrance and suggesting an environmental factor in the disease process.

PHYSICAL FINDINGS & CLINICAL PRESENTATION

- Overwhelming urge to sleep with chronic hypersomnia may occur during the day.
- Cataplexy occurs in 60% to 100% of patients with narcolepsy and is reported as a partial or complete loss of voluntary muscle control with preserved consciousness that is precipitated by a strong emotion, more commonly with laughter. This is the most specific symptom and is considered pathognomonic for narcolepsy.
- Hypnagogic (wake to sleep) or hypnopompic (sleep to wake) hallucinations have been reported in 60% to 80% of patients with narcolepsy.
- Sleep paralysis, defined as loss of muscle tone during the transition between sleep and wakefulness, occurs in 60% to 80% of patients with narcolepsy. It may occur with hallucinations and can be interrupted by sensory stimuli.
- Fragmented sleep is seen in 60% to 80% of narcolepsy patients and can often be mistaken for insomnia or other intrinsic sleep disorder.
- Other symptoms that have been reported in narcolepsy include automatic behavior or semipurposeful movements in 40% of patients and memory disturbance in 50% of patients.

ETIOLOGY

The loss of hypocretin/orexin signaling, genetic factors, and rare brain lesions are presently identified factors in the development of narcolepsy.

HYPOCRETIN/OREXIN:
- Loss of hypocretin-1 and hypocretin-2 (also known as orexin-A and orexin-B) producing neurons in the lateral hypothalamus
- Human cerebrospinal fluid (CSF) levels of hypocretin-1 are low to undetectable in narcoleptics with cataplexy.
- Narcolepsy without cataplexy may have a different cause because CSF hypocretin levels are usually normal in these patients, so there may be a completely separate mechanism in these patients, or it may result from less extensive loss of hypocretin neurons or impaired signaling.

SECONDARY ETIOLOGIES:
- Tumors, vascular malformations, and strokes have all been reported to cause secondary narcolepsy.
- Direct injury to the hypocretin neurons or their projections is the most likely cause of secondary narcolepsy due to central nervous system lesions.
- Narcolepsy has been reported in genetic syndromes, including Prader-Willi syndrome and Niemann-Pick disease type C, as well as paraneoplastic syndromes.

Dx DIAGNOSIS

DIFFERENTIAL DIAGNOSIS

Excessive daytime somnolence:
- Autism
- Autosomal dominant cerebellar ataxia, deafness, and narcolepsy
- Behaviorally induced insufficient sleep syndrome
- Central or obstructive sleep apnea (sleep-disordered breathing)
- Circadian rhythm disorder
- Depression
- Diencephalic lesions
- Drug or alcohol abuse
- Hypothyroidism
- Idiopathic hypersomnia with long or short sleep time
- Inadequate sleep hygiene
- Increased intracranial pressure
- Insomnia
- Kleine-Levin syndrome
- Medication effect
- Menstrual-related hypersomnia
- Posttraumatic narcolepsy
- Seizures
- Sleep fragmentation (multiple causes)

Cataplexy:
- Seizures
- Periodic paralysis
- Cardiovascular insufficiency
- Psychogenic (multiple causes)

WORKUP

- Narcolepsy is often diagnosed by clinical history. The Epworth Sleepiness Scale is very useful in determining the degree of excessive daytime sleepiness.
- The diagnosis of narcolepsy can be made if there is a clear history of cataplexy in the setting of excessive daytime somnolence, without need for further diagnostic testing. Sleep laboratory testing or possibly laboratory testing is required if these symptoms do not exist.
- The medical history should include questions regarding severity of daytime hypersomnia while also evaluating for sleep-disordered breathing, transient muscle weakness triggered by emotion, hallucinations while falling asleep or upon awakening, and inability to move after awakening. The clinical evaluation should also address symptoms of seizures and paraneoplastic disorders while also asking about previous stroke or genetic disorders. A detailed family history is imperative. Hypothalamic dysfunction such as unexplained weight gain, endocrine abnormalities, circadian dysrhythmias, and autonomic nervous system problems may provide useful insight.
- A thorough examination including a detailed neurological examination should be performed.
- Nocturnal polysomnography followed by a multiple sleep latency test remains to be the gold standard for the diagnosis of narcolepsy. A drug screen should also be performed to rule our pharmacological modulations of sleep.

LABORATORY TESTS

HLA subtyping and CSF hypocretin/orexin levels may be attempted in suspected cases of narcolepsy. CSF hypocretin/orexin analysis is primarily a research tool. CSF hypocretin levels below 110 pg/ml are indicative of narcolepsy, but high CSF hypocretin levels do not exclude the diagnosis.

Rx TREATMENT

NONPHARMACOLOGIC THERAPY

Avoidance of over-the-counter drugs and illicit drugs, optimal sleep hygiene and scheduled daily naps, and psychosocial support can be used for symptoms of excessive daytime somnolence. However, nonpharmacologic therapy is typically not sufficient for treatment of narcolepsy alone but is often used as adjunct therapy with medications.

PHARMACOLOGIC THERAPY

For excessive daytime somnolence:

- Sodium oxybate (Xyrem): a central nervous system depressant that can be used for the treatment cataplexy and REM-related symptoms
- Modafinil (Provigil) 200 to 600 mg PO every morning or divided bid
- Armodafinil (Nuvigil) 150 or 250 mg PO as a single dose in the morning
- Methylphenidate (Ritalin) 5 to 15 mg PO bid to tid
- Methylphenidate SR (Concerta) 18 to 54 mg PO every morning or divided bid
- Dextroamphetamine (Dexedrine) 10 to 60 mg PO qd
- Eldepryl (Selegiline HCl) 5 mg PO bid

For cataplexy:

- Sodium oxybate (Xyrem): a central nervous system depressant that can be used for the treatment of cataplexy and REM-related symptoms
- Fluoxetine (Prozac) 20 mg PO qd initially
- Sertraline (Zoloft) 25 mg PO qd initially
- Venlafaxine (Effexor) 25 mg PO qd initially
- Clomipramine (Anafranil) 25 mg/day initially
- Protriptyline (Vivactil) 5 mg tid initially
- Imipramine (Tofranil) 25 to 50 mg/day initially
- Desipramine (Norpramin) 10 mg bid initially

DISPOSITION

This is a chronic sleep disorder that may worsen for the first few years and then persist for life.

REFERRAL

Because the complexity of this disorder and its ever-changing management and treatment, patients should be referred to centers or programs with highly trained sleep specialists with expertise caring for these patients, especially if sodium oxybate (Xyrem) therapy is needed.

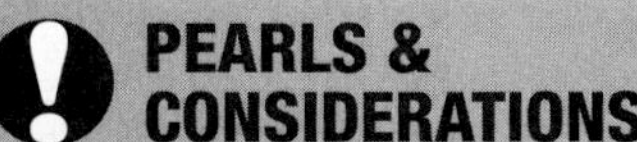

PEARLS & CONSIDERATIONS

Many narcoleptics report the onset of symptoms beginning in childhood to early adulthood with a long delay of actual diagnosis on the order of 10 to 15 yr. Typically, excessive daytime sleepiness is the initial symptom followed by REM dysregulation (e.g., cataplexy, sleep paralysis, hypnagogic hallucinations). Patients with narcolepsy also have higher than expected incidence of other sleep disorders, including obstructive sleep apnea, periodic limb movements of sleep, and REM sleep behavior disorder.

COMMENTS

Narcolepsy is a rare disorder that is underdiagnosed. Cataplexy is specific for narcolepsy, but other symptoms of REM dysregulation, including sleep paralysis and hypnagogic or hypnopompic hallucinations can occur even in normal patients. Sleep-onset REM or REM periods on a MSLT study may occur as a result of sleep deprivation or withdrawal from REM suppressing drugs.

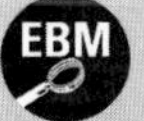

EVIDENCE

The medications, approved by the Food and Drug Administration (FDA) for the treatment of narcolepsy, include sodium oxybate (Xyrem), modafinil (Provigil), and armodafinil (Nuvigil). There is evidence that all three medications are effective in treating daytime hypersomnia while sodium oxybate (Xyrem) is also effective in treating cataplexy.[1-6]

Evidence-Based References

1. Black J et al: Sodium oxybate improves excessive daytime sleepiness in narcolepsy, *Sleep* 29(7):939-946, 2006.
2. Xyrem International Study Group: A double-blind, placebo-controlled study demonstrates sodium oxybate is effective for the treatment of excessive daytime sleepiness in narcolepsy, *J Clin Sleep Med* 1(4):391-397, 2005.
3. A 12-month, open-label, multicenter extension trial of orally administered sodium oxybate for the treatment of narcolepsy, *Sleep* 26:31-35, 2003.
4. Xyrem International Study Group: Further evidence supporting the use of sodium oxybate for the treatment of cataplexy: a double-blind, placebo-controlled study in 228 patients, *Sleep Med* 6(5):415-421, 2005.
5. Randomized trial of modafinil as a treatment for the excessive daytime somnolence of narcolepsy: US Modafinil in Narcolepsy Multicenter Study Group, *Neurology* 54(5):1166-1175, 2000.
6. Garnock-Jones KP et al: Armodafinil, *CNS Drugs* 23(9):793-803, 2009.

SUGGESTED READINGS

Amira SA et al: Diagnosis of narcolepsy using the multiple sleep latency test: analysis of current laboratory criteria, *Sleep* 8(4):325-331, 1985.

Baumann CR et al: Hypocretins (orexins) and sleep-wake disorders, *Lancet Neurol* 4(10):673-682, 2005.

Chervin RD et al: Comparison of the results of the Epworth Sleepiness Scale and the Multiple Sleep Latency Test. *J Psychosom Res* 42(2):145-155, 1997.

Dauvilliers Y et al: Narcolepsy with cataplexy, *Lancet* 369(9560):499-511, 2007.

Longstreth WT Jr et al: The epidemiology of narcolepsy, *Sleep* 30(1):13-26, 2007.

Morgenthaler TI et al: Practice parameters for the treatment of narcolepsy and other hypersomnias of central origin, *Sleep* 30(12):1705-1711, 2007.

Scammell TE: The neurobiology, diagnosis, and treatment of narcolepsy, *Ann Neurol* 53(2):154-166, 2003.

Wise MS et al: Treatment of narcolepsy and other hypersomnias of central origin, *Sleep* 30(12):1712-1727, 2007.

Zeman A et al: Narcolepsy and excessive daytime sleepiness, *BMJ* 329(7468):724-728, 2004.

AUTHOR: **DON HAYES, JR., M.D.**

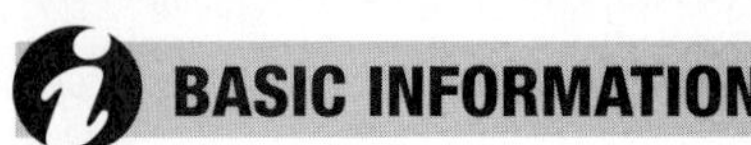

BASIC INFORMATION

DEFINITION

Malignant renal tumor derived from primitive metanephric blastoma. Most tumors are unicentric, but some are multifocal in one or both kidneys. Associated anomalies may be present.

SYNONYMS

Wilms' tumor

ICD-9CM CODES
189.0 Nephroblastoma

EPIDEMIOLOGY & DEMOGRAPHICS

- Pediatric malignancy mean presentation is at 41.5 mo in boys and 46.9 mo in girls
- Slightly more frequent in girls
- Incidence rate is 7.9 cases per year per 1 million white children <15 yr (a little over 500 new cases annually in the U.S.); the incidence is double in black children
- Associated syndromes:
  1. Cryptorchidism
  2. Hypospadias
  3. Hemihypertrophy with or without the Beckwith-Wiedemann syndrome, aniridia
  4. Denys-Drash syndrome (nephroblastoma, pseudohermaphrodism, glomerulonephritis)
  5. WAGR syndrome (***W***ilms' tumor, ***a***niridia, ***g***enitourinary malformations, and mental ***r***etardation)
- Familial nephroblastoma occurs in 1.5% (with younger age at diagnosis and more frequent multifocal tumors)

PHYSICAL FINDINGS & CLINICAL PRESENTATION

- Nephroblastoma often is discovered when a parent notices a mass while bathing or dressing a child, most commonly a child who is approximately age 3 yr, or during a routine physical examination. The mass is unilateral, firm, and nontender and below the costal margin.
- Abdominal swelling and/or pain
- Nausea
- Vomiting
- Constipation
- Loss of appetite
- Fever of unknown origin
- Night sweats
- Hematuria (less common than in adult renal malignancies)
- Malaise
- High blood pressure that is triggered when the tumor obstructs the renal artery
- Varicocele
- Signs of associated syndromes

ETIOLOGY & PATHOGENESIS

- Three cell types: blastomal, stromal, and epithelial may be present. Structural diversity is characteristic.
- Anaplasia is evidenced by the presence of gigantic polyploid nuclei. The term *focal anaplasia* is used to describe such findings when it is confined within the primary tumor in the kidney.
- Staging:

  Stage I: Tumor limited to the kidney whose capsule is intact. The tumor is completely excised.

  Stage II: Tumor extends beyond the kidney but is completely excised. No peritoneal involvement.

  Stage III: Residual tumor confined to the abdomen after surgery. No hematogenous metastases.

  Stage IV: Hematogenous metastases present.

  Stage V: Bilateral renal involvement at time of initial diagnosis.

Dx DIAGNOSIS

DIFFERENTIAL DIAGNOSIS

- Other renal malignancies
  1. Hypernephroma
  2. Transitional cell carcinoma
  3. Lymphoma
  4. Clear cell sarcoma
  5. Rhabdoid tumor of the kidney
- Renal cyst
- Other intraabdominal or retroperitoneal tumors

LABORATORY TESTS

- Complete blood count
- Transaminases (alanine aminotransferase, aspartate aminotransferase)
- Alkaline phosphatase
- Blood urea nitrogen and creatinine
- Serum calcium
- Urinalysis

IMAGING STUDIES

- Renal ultrasound to confirm existence of a solid mass in a kidney
- Abdominal CT scan with contrast (Fig. 1-211)
- Chest radiograph or CT scan

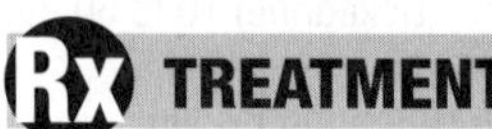

TREATMENT

- Surgical resection and surgical staging:
  1. Stages I and II: surgery followed by chemotherapy
  2. Stages III and IV: surgery followed by radiation and chemotherapy
- Chemotherapeutic agents used in the treatment of nephroblastoma include vincristine, dactinomycin, and doxorubicin

PROGNOSIS

- Stage I: 95% survival
- Stage II: 91% survival
- Stage III: 91% survival
- Stage IV: 81% survival
- Prognosis is better for patients <2 yr

AUTHOR: **FRED F. FERRI, M.D.**

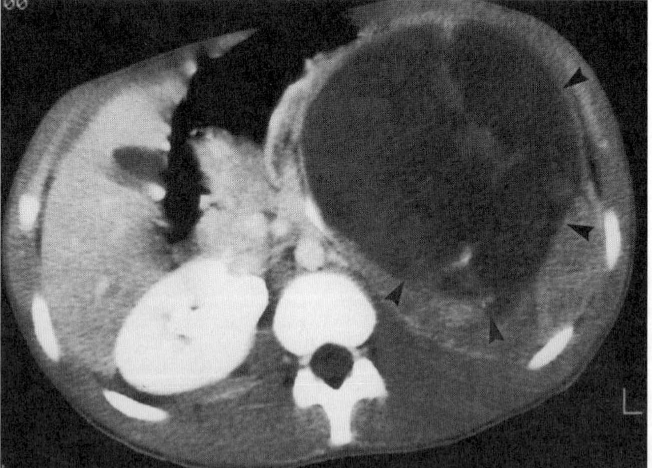

FIGURE 1-211 Transverse computed tomographic image of a nephroblastoma (Wilms' tumor) shows a large intrarenal mass. (From Abeloff MD [ed]: *Clinical oncology,* ed 3, Philadelphia, 2004, Elsevier.)

BASIC INFORMATION

DEFINITION

Nephrotic syndrome is characterized by high urine protein excretion (>3.5 g/1.73 m^3/24 hr), peripheral edema, and metabolic abnormalities (hypoalbuminemia, hypercholesterolemia).

ICD-9CM CODES
581.9 Nephrotic syndrome

EPIDEMIOLOGY & DEMOGRAPHICS

- Nephrotic syndrome occurs predominantly in children ages 2 to 6 yr (2 new cases/100,000 persons/yr) and in adults of all ages (3 to 4 new cases/100,000 persons/yr).
- Membranous glomerulonephritis is the most common cause of nephrotic syndrome.

PHYSICAL FINDINGS & CLINICAL PRESENTATION

- Peripheral edema, eyelid edema (Fig. 1-212)
- Ascites, anasarca
- Hypertension
- Pleural effusion
- Typically patients present with severe peripheral edema, exertional dyspnea, and abdominal fullness secondary to ascites. There is a significant amount of weight gain in most patients

ETIOLOGY

- Idiopathic (may be secondary to the following glomerular diseases: minimal change disease [nil disease, lipoid nephrosis], focal segmental glomerular sclerosis, membranous nephropathy, membranoproliferative glomerular nephropathy) PLA 2 R is a major antigen in the majority of patients with idiopathic membranous nephropathy.
- Associated with systemic diseases (diabetes mellitus, SLE, amyloidosis). Amyloidosis and dysproteinemias should be considered in patients older than 40 yr
- Majority of children with nephrotic syndrome have minimal change disease (this form also associated with allergy, nonsteroidals, and Hodgkin's disease)
- Focal glomerular disease: can be associated with HIV infection, heroin abuse. A more severe form of nephrotic syndrome associated with rapid progression to end-stage renal failure within months can also occur in HIV seropositive patients and is known as "collapsing glomerulopathy"
- Membranous nephropathy: can occur with Hodgkin's lymphoma, carcinomas, SLE, gold therapy
- Membranoproliferative glomerulonephropathy: often associated with upper respiratory infections

Dx DIAGNOSIS

DIFFERENTIAL DIAGNOSIS

- Other edema states (CHF, cirrhosis)
- Primary renal disease (e.g., focal glomerulonephritis, membranoproliferative glomerulonephritis). Table 1-54 summarizes primary renal diseases that present as idiopathic nephrotic syndrome
- Carcinoma, infections
- Malignant hypertension
- Polyarteritis nodosa
- Serum sickness
- Toxemia of pregnancy

WORKUP

Diagnostic workup consists of family history and history of drug use or toxin exposure and laboratory evaluation. Renal biopsy is generally performed in individuals with persistent proteinuria in whom the etiology of the proteinuria is unclear.

LABORATORY TESTS

- Urinalysis reveals proteinuria. The presence of hematuria, cellular casts, and pyuria is suggestive of nephritic syndrome. Oval fat bodies (tubular epithelial cells with cholesterol esters) are also found in the urine in patients with nephrotic syndrome.

TABLE 1-54 Summary of Primary Renal Diseases That Present as Idiopathic Nephrotic Syndrome

	Minimal-Change Nephropathy Syndrome (MCNS)	Focal Segmental Sclerosis	Membranous Nephrotic	MEMBRANOPROLIFERATIVE GLOMERULONEPHRITIS (MPGN)	
				Type I	Type II
Frequency*					
Children	75%	10%	<5%	10%	10%
Adults	15%	15%	50%	10%	10%
Clinical Manifestations					
Age (yr)	2-6	2-10	40-50	5-15	5-15
Sex	2:1	1.3:1	2:1 male	Male-female	Male-female
Nephrotic syndrome	100%	90%	80%	60%	60%
Asymptomatic proteinuria	0	10%	20%	40%	40%
Hematuria	10%-20%	60%-80%	60%	80%	80%
Hypertension	10%	20% early	Infrequent	35%	35%
Rate of progression to renal failure	Does not progress	10 years	50% in 10-20 yr	10-20 yr	5-15 yr
Associated conditions	Allergy? Hodgkin's disease, usually none	None			
Laboratory Findings	Manifestations of nephrotic syndrome	Manifestations of nephrotic syndrome	Renal vein thrombosis, cancer, SLE, hepatitis B	None	Partial lipodystrophy
	↑ BUN in 15%-30%	↑ BUN in 20%-40%	Manifestations of nephrotic syndrome	Low C1, C4, C3–C9	Normal C1, C4, low C3–C9
Immunogenetics	HLA-B8, B12 (3.5)†	Not established	HLA-DRW3 (12–32)†	Not established	C3 nephritic factor
Renal Pathology					Not established
Light microscopy	Normal	Focal	Thickened	Thickened	Lobulation
Immunofluorescence	Negative	IgM	Fine	Granular	C3 only
Electron microscopy	Foot process fusion	Foot	Subepithelial	Mesangial	Dense deposits
Response of Steroids	90%	15%-20%	May slow progression	Not established	Not established

Modified from Goldman L, Ausiello D (eds): *Cecil textbook of medicine,* ed 22, Philadelphia, 2004, WB Saunders.
*Approximate frequency as a cause of idiopathic nephrotic syndrome. About 10% of adult nephrotic syndrome is due to various diseases that usually present with acute glomerulonephritis.
†Relative risk.
↑, Elevated; *BUN,* blood urea nitrogen; *C,* complement; *GBM,* glomerular basement membrane; *hepatitis B,* hepatitis B virus; *HLA,* human leukocyte antigen; *Ig,* immunoglobulin; *SLE,* systemic lupus erythematosus.

- 24-hr urine protein excretion is >3.5 g/ 1.73 m^3/24 hr.
- Abnormalities of blood chemistries include serum albumin <3 g/dl, decreased total protein, elevated serum cholesterol, glucose, azotemia.
- Additional tests in patients with nephrotic syndromes depending on the history and physical examination are ANA, serum and urine immunoelectrophoresis, C3, C4, CH-50, LDH, liver enzymes, alkaline phosphatase, hepatitis B and C screening, and HIV.

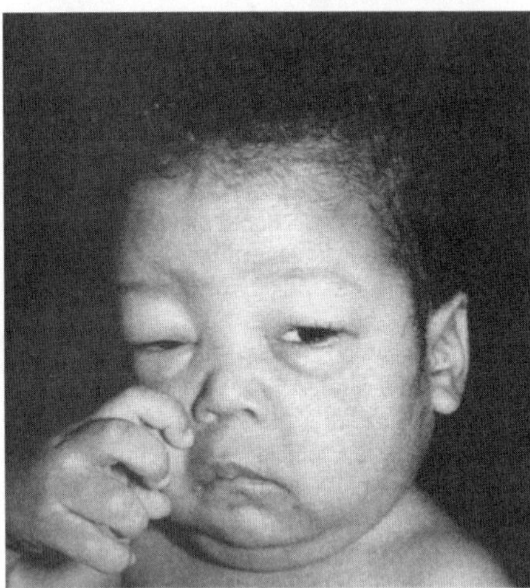

FIGURE 1-212 Marked eyelid edema in a 2-year-old boy with minimal change disease and nephrotic syndrome. Eyelid edema in any child should prompt the performance of urinalysis rather than the presumption of allergy. (From Zitelli BJ, Davis HW: *Atlas of pediatric physical diagnosis,* ed 5, Philadelphia, 2007, Mosby.)

IMAGING STUDIES

- Ultrasound of kidneys
- Chest radiograph

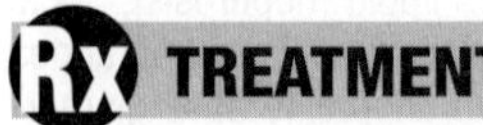

Rx TREATMENT

NONPHARMACOLOGIC THERAPY

- Bed rest as tolerated, avoidance of nephrotoxic drugs, low-fat diet, fluid restriction in hyponatremic patients; normal protein intake unless urinary protein loss exceeds 10 g/24 hr (some patients may require additional dietary protein to prevent negative nitrogen balance and significant protein malnutrition)
- Improved urinary protein excretion and serum lipid changes have been observed with a low-fat soy protein diet providing 0.7 g of protein/kg/day. However, because of increased risk of malnutrition, many nephrologists recommend normal protein intake
- Strict sodium restriction to help manage peripheral edema
- Close monitoring of patients for development of peripheral venous thrombosis and renal vein thrombosis because of hypercoagulable state secondary to loss of antithrombin III and other proteins involved in the clotting mechanism

ACUTE GENERAL Rx

- Furosemide is useful for severe edema.
- Use of ACE inhibitors to reduce proteinuria is generally indicated even in normotensive patients.
- Anticoagulant therapy should be administered as long as patients have nephrotic proteinuria, an albumin level <20 g/L, or both.

The mainstay of therapy is treatment of the underlying disorder:

- Minimal change disease generally responds to prednisone 1 mg/kg/day. Relapses can occur when steroids are discontinued. In these individuals, cyclophosphamide and chlorambucil may be useful.
- Focal and segmental glomerulosclerosis: steroid therapy is also recommended. However, response rate is approximately 35% to 40%, and most patients progress to end-stage renal disease within 3 yr.
- Membranous glomerulonephritis: prednisone 2 mg/kg/day may be useful in inducing remission. Cytotoxic agents can be added if there is poor response to prednisone.
- Membranoproliferative glomerulonephritis: most patients are treated with steroid therapy and antiplatelet drugs. Despite treatment, the majority of patients will progress to end-stage renal disease within 5 yr.

CHRONIC Rx

- Patients should be monitored for azotemia and should be aggressively treated for hypertension and hyperlipidemia. Furosemide is useful for severe edema. Anticoagulants may be necessary for thromboembolic events. Prophylactic anticoagulation should be considered in patients with membranous glomerulonephritis.
- Oral vitamin D is useful in the treatment of hypocalcemia (because of vitamin D loss).

REFERRAL

Nephrology consultation is recommended in all cases of nephrotic syndrome.

AUTHOR: **FRED F. FERRI, M.D.**

BASIC INFORMATION

DEFINITION

Neuroblastomas are tumors of postganglionic sympathetic neurons that typically originate in the adrenal medulla or the sympathetic chain/ganglion. Often present at birth, but not diagnosed until later, when the child shows symptoms of the disease. They are almost exclusively a disease of childhood.

ICD-9CM CODES
194.0 Neuroblastoma, unspecified site

EPIDEMIOLOGY & DEMOGRAPHICS

INCIDENCE (IN U.S.): 8%-10% of all solid tumors of childhood (third most common childhood cancer, after leukemia and brain tumors); 1/10,000 children <15 yr.

PREDOMINANT SEX: Male:female ratio of 1:1.3

PEAK AGE: Early childhood. Mean age of onset is 18 mo; 33% onset by 1 year; 75% onset by 5 year; 97% by 10 year. In rare cases, neuroblastoma can be discovered by fetal ultrasound.

GENETICS: Chromosomal deletions (loss of heterozygosity) found in nearly half of tumors, most commonly localized to chromosomes 1p, 11q, and 14q. Deletion of 1p36 (leading to amplification and overexpression of *N-MYC* protooncogene) associated with poor prognosis. There is a small subset with an autosomal dominant pattern of inheritance.

PHYSICAL FINDINGS & CLINICAL PRESENTATION

- Mass in abdomen, neck, or chest. Approximately two thirds of tumors arise in the abdomen; of these, two thirds arise in the adrenal glands. 70% to 80% of children have regional lymph node involvement or distant metastases at time of presentation.
- Spinal cord/paraspinal: can present with back pain, signs of compression—paraplegia, stool/urine retention.
- Horner's syndrome (ptosis, miosis, anhidrosis).
- Thoracic: difficulty breathing, dysphagia, infections, chronic cough.
- Secondary symptoms referable to metastatic disease: fatigue, chronic pain (typically bony pain), pancytopenia, periorbital ecchymosis, proptosis, anorexia, weight loss, unexplained fever, multiple subcutaneous bluish nodules, irritability.
- Paraneoplastic syndromes: opsoclonus-myoclonus syndrome is described as "dancing eyes, dancing feet," which manifest as myoclonic jerks and chaotic eye movements in all directions. This may be initial presentation before tumor diagnosis; present in 1% to 3% of patients with neuroblastoma; of all patients with opsoclonus-myoclonus, 20% to 50% have an underlying neuroblastoma. Patients who present with this syndrome often have neuroblastomas with more favorable biologic features.
- Progressive cerebellar ataxia.
- Abnormal secretion of vasoactive intestinal peptide by the tumor, leading to distention of the abdomen and secretory diarrhea.

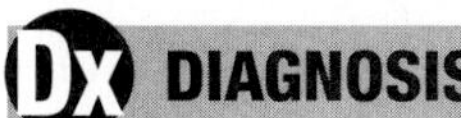

DIAGNOSIS

WORKUP

- Careful general physical examination
- Biopsy and resection of tumor when possible

LABORATORY TESTS

- Complete blood count, coagulation studies, erythrocyte sedimentation rate.
- 24-hour urine for catecholamines: homovanillic acid (HVA) and vanillylmandelic acid (VMA) are secreted by up to 90% of tumors.
- Nonspecific serum markers such as neuron-specific enolase, lactate dehydrogenase, and ferritin.
- Bone marrow biopsy and aspirate: karyotype, DNA index, *N-MYC* copy number.
- Minimum criteria for diagnosis is based on one of the following: (1) unequivocal pathologic diagnosis made from tumor tissue or (2) combination of bone marrow aspirate with unequivocal tumor cells and increased levels of serum or urinary catecholamine metabolites, as described above.
- Genetic/biologic variables have been studied in children with neuroblastoma, in particular the histology, aneuploidy of tumor DNA, and amplification of the *N-MYC* oncogene within tumor tissue, because treatment decisions may be based on these factors.
  - Hyperdiploid DNA is associated with favorable prognosis, especially in infants.
  - *N-MYC* amplification is associated with poor prognosis, regardless of patient age, likely due to association with deletion of chromosome 1p and gain of chromosome 17q.
  - Other biologic factors studied include profile of GABAergic receptors, expression of neurotrophin receptors, level of telomerase RNA and serum ferritin and lactate dehydrogenase.

IMAGING STUDIES

- Chest radiograph, abdominal radiograph, skeletal survey, abdominal ultrasound
- Renal/bladder ultrasound
- CT scan or MRI of the chest and abdomen to provide information about regional lymph nodes, vessel invasion, and distant metastases (Fig. 1-213)
- Body scan with ^{131}I-MIBG (meta-iodobenzylguanidine), which is taken up by neuroblasts and is sensitive to metastases in the bone and soft tissue
- Bone scan with Tc-99 MDP to visualize lytic bone lesions and metastases
- STAGING (International Neuroblastoma Staging System)
  - I. Confined to single organ
  - IIA. Localized tumor with incomplete gross resection; lymph nodes negative
  - IIB. Localized tumor with incomplete gross resection; ipsilateral lymph nodes positive
  - III. Extension across midline, with or without lymph node involvement
  - IV. Distant metastases to lymph nodes, bone, bone marrow, liver, skin
  - IVs. Localized primary tumor with dissemination limited to skin, liver, or bone marrow; limited to infants

DIFFERENTIAL DIAGNOSIS

- Other small, round, blue-cell childhood tumors, such as lymphoma, rhabdomyosarcoma, soft tissue sarcoma, and primitive neuroectodermal tumors (PNETs)
- Wilms' tumor
- Hepatoblastoma

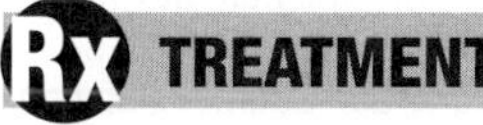

TREATMENT

- Assure patient and family that there is hope for recovery with aggressive treatment.
- Overall, treatment will be determined by several factors, including age at diagnosis, stage of disease, site of primary tumor and metastases, and tumor histology.
- Surgery, particularly for low-risk tumors.

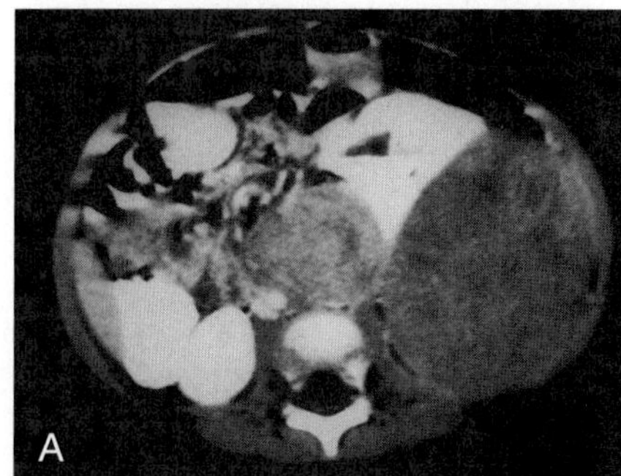

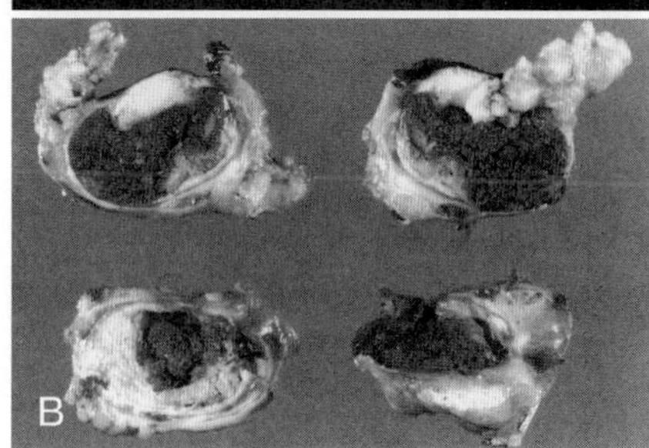

FIGURE 1-213 Computed tomographic scan **(A)** shows adrenal neuroblastoma at diagnosis. Serial sections through adrenal neuroblastoma **(B)** show tumor with large areas of diffuse hemorrhage and calcification. (From Abeloff MD [ed]: *Clinical oncology,* ed 3, Philadelphia, 2004, Elsevier.)

- Radiation therapy may be tried for unresectable tumors or tumors that are not responsive to chemotherapy.
- Multiagent chemotherapy is mainstay of treatment (e.g., cisplatinum, etoposide, Adriamycin, cyclophosphamide, carboplatin).
- Autologous bone marrow transplantation following aggressive chemotherapy for stage IV disease or patients who are at highest risk based on presence of disseminated disease or unfavorable markers such as *N-MYC* amplification.
- Novel therapies include immunotherapy using monoclonal antibodies and vaccines that attempt to initiate an immune reaction against the disease and targeting of tumor cells with drugs that induce apoptosis or have antiangiogenic effect.
- Adrenocorticotropic hormone (ACTH) treatment is thought to be effective for patients with opsoclonus/myoclonus syndrome.

DISPOSITION

- Overall survival is >40%. Children under the age of 1 yr have a cure rate as high as 90%.
- Approximately 70% of patients with neuroblastoma have metastases at diagnoses.
- Prognosis is related to age at time of diagnosis, clinical stage, and regional lymph node involvement. Children with localized disease and infants <1 year at diagnosis and favorable disease characteristics have better prognosis whereas poorer prognosis is noted in older children with stage IV disease (20% survival compared with >95% in stage I), age >1 year at diagnosis, increased number of *N-MYC* copies, adrenal tumor, and chronic 1p deletion.
- Children treated for neuroblastoma may be at risk for second malignancies, including renal cell carcinoma.

REFERRAL

Multidisciplinary oncology team with experience in treating cancers of childhood and adolescence.

PEARLS & CONSIDERATIONS

- Predominantly a tumor of early childhood that originates in the sites where the sympathetic nervous system tissue is present.
- Most common symptoms due to tumor mass or bone pain from metastases.
- Children can present with classic paraneoplastic neurologic symptoms including cerebellar ataxia and opsoclonus/myoclonus.

EVIDENCE

For patients with high-risk neuroblastoma, myoablative chemotherapy with hematopoietic stem-cell transplant is an effective treatment strategy. A large randomized controlled trial evaluated the role of conventional chemotherapy or myoablative therapy with stem-cell transplant. Event free survival was greater in those who received myoablative therapy plus hematopoietic cell transplantation (HCT) (34% vs. 22%).[1] Ⓐ

In most cases of stage IV, neuroblastoma is a favorable disease with minimal therapy achieving an excellent outcome. Infants <2 months of age may require more intensive treatment.[2] Ⓑ

Evidence-Based References

1. Matthay KK et al: Treatment of high-risk neuroblastoma with intensive chemotherapy, radiotherapy, autologous bone marrow transplantation, and 13-*cis*-retinoic acid: Children's Cancer Group, *N Engl J Med* 341:1165, 1999.
2. Nickerson HJ et al: Favorable biology and outcome of stage IV-S neuroblastoma with supportive care or minimal therapy: a Children's Cancer Group study, *J Clin Oncol* 18:477, 2000.

SUGGESTED READINGS

Marcus K et al: Primary tumor control in patients with stage 3/4 unfavorable neuroblastoma treated with tandem double autologous stem cell transplants, *J Pediatr Hematol Oncol* 25:934, 2003.

Maris JM: The biologic basis for neuroblastoma heterogeneity and risk stratification, *Curr Opin Pediatr* 17(1):7-13, 2005.

Pranzatelli MR et al: Screening for autoantibodies in children with opsoclonus-myoclonus-ataxia, *Pediatr Neurol* 27:384, 2002.

Riley RD et al: A systematic review of molecular and biological tumor markers in neuroblastoma, *Clin Cancer Res* 10(1 Pt 1):4-12, 2004.

Roberts SS et al: GABAergic system gene expression predicts clinical outcome in patients with neuroblastoma, *J Clin Oncol* 22(20):4127-4134, 2004.

Rudnick E et al: Opsoclonus-myoclonus-ataxia syndrome in neuroblastoma: clinical outcome and antineuronal antibodies—a report from the Children's Cancer Group Study, *Med Pediatr Oncol* 36(6):612-622, 2001.

Schilling FH et al: Neuroblastoma screening at one year of age, *N Engl J Med* 346:1047, 2002.

Shimada H: International neuroblastoma pathology classification for prognostic evaluation of patients with peripheral neuroblastic tumors: a report from the Children's Cancer Group, *Cancer* 92:2451, 2001.

Woods WG et al: Screening of infants and mortality due to neuroblastoma, *N Engl J Med* 346:1041, 2002.

AUTHOR: **NICOLE J. ULLRICH, M.D., PH.D.**

BASIC INFORMATION

DEFINITION

Neurofibromatosis (NF) is an autosomal-dominant disorder affecting bone, the nervous system, soft tissue, and skin. There are three major subtypes of neurofibromatosis disorders: NF type 1 (NF1), NF type 2 (NF2), and schwannomatosis. Schwannomatosis has only recently been recognized as a distinct disorder; currently very little is known about it.

SYNONYMS

NF1: von Recklinghausen disease, peripheral NF
NF2: bilateral acoustic neurofibromatosis, central NF

ICD-9CM CODES
237.70 Neurofibromatosis, unspecified
237.71 Type 1, von Recklinghausen's
237.72 Type 2, acoustic

EPIDEMIOLOGY & DEMOGRAPHICS

- Incidence of NF1 (one case/3000 live births), NF2 (one case/25,000 live births).
- Prevalence of NF1 (one case/5000 persons), NF2 (one case/210,000 persons).
- NF1 and NF2 are autosomal dominant; approximately 50% of cases have no family history.
- The two disorders affect approximately 100,000 people in the U.S.
- Affects males and females equally.
- NF1 may be associated with optic gliomas, astrocytomas, spinal neurofibromas, pheochromocytomas, and chronic myeloid leukemia.
- NF2 may be associated with meningiomas, spinal schwannomas, and cataracts.
- For schwannomatosis, the incidence is one per 30,000 persons, and the disease is mostly sporadic in nature.

PHYSICAL FINDINGS & CLINICAL PRESENTATION

- Common features of NF1 include:
  1. Café-au-lait macules (100% of children by age 2 yr)
     a. Hyperpigmented skin lesions occurring anywhere on the body except the face, palms, and soles
     b. Appear early in life and increase in size and number during puberty
     c. Are focal or diffuse
  2. Axillary and inguinal freckling (70%).
  3. Multiple neurofibromas (Figs. 1-214 and 1-215) can be soft or firm; three subtypes:
     a. Cutaneous: circumscribed, not specific for NF1
     b. Subcutaneous: circumscribed, not specific for NF1
     c. Plexiform: noncircumscribed, thick and irregular; can cause disfigurement of supportive structures and specific for NF1
  4. Lisch nodule (small hamartoma of the iris) found in >90% of adult cases.
  5. Visual defects possibly related to optic gliomas (2% to 5%).
  6. Neurodevelopment problems such as learning disability and mental retardation (30% to 40%).
  7. Skeletal disorders, including long bone dysplasia, pseudoarthrosis, scoliosis, short stature, and decreased bone mineral density.
- Common features of NF2 include:
  1. Hearing loss and tinnitus related to bilateral acoustic neuromas (>90% of adults)
  2. Cataracts (81%)
  3. Headache
  4. Unsteady gait
  5. Cutaneous and subcutaneous neurofibromas, but less than NF1
  6. Café-au-lait macules (1%)
- Common features of schwannomatosis include painful multiple schwannomas of the spinal, peripheral, or cranial nerves *except* the vestibular nerve.

ETIOLOGY

- NF1 is caused by DNA mutations located on the long arm of chromosome 17 responsible for encoding the protein neurofibromin.
- NF2 is caused by DNA mutations located in the middle of the long arm of chromosome 22 responsible for encoding the protein merlin, which is a potent inhibitor of glioma growth.
- Both proteins are speculated to act as tumor suppressors.
- The etiology of schwannomatosis remains unclear; however, biallelic NF2 mutations are found in the schwannomas but nowhere else, suggesting that they are secondary mutations.

Dx DIAGNOSIS

- NF1 is diagnosed if the person has two or more of the following features:
  1. Six or more café-au-lait macules >5 mm in prepubertal patients and >15 mm in postpubertal patients
  2. Two or more neurofibromas of any type or one plexiform neurofibroma
  3. Axillary or inguinal freckling
  4. Optic glioma
  5. Two or more Lisch nodules (iris hamartomas)
  6. Sphenoid wing dysplasia or cortical thinning of long bones, with or without pseudoarthrosis
  7. A first-degree relative (parent, sibling, or child) with NF1 based on the previous criteria
- NF2 is diagnosed if the person has either of the following two criteria:
  1. Bilateral eighth nerve masses seen by appropriate imaging studies (e.g., CT, MRI)
  2. A first-degree relative with NF2 and either a unilateral eighth nerve mass or two of the following: neurofibroma, meningioma, glioma, schwannoma, or juvenile posterior subcapsular lenticular opacity

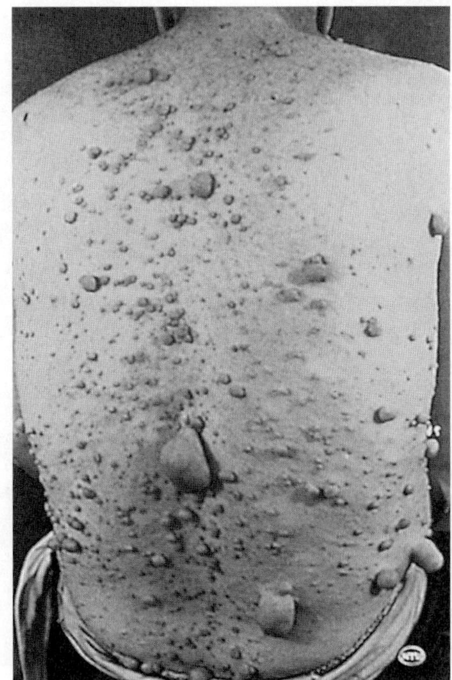

FIGURE 1-214 Nodules. Solid, large (>1 cm), deep-seated mass in dermal or subcutaneous tissues. These nodules are neurofibromas in a patient with neurofibromatosis. (From Goldman L, Ausiello D [eds]: *Cecil textbook of medicine,* ed 22, Philadelphia, 2004, WB Saunders.)

- Schwannomatosis is diagnosed in an individual >30 yr having either of the following two criteria:
  1. Two nonintradermal schwannomas, no vestibular tumor found on MRI scan, no NF2 mutation
  2. One nonvestibular schwannoma and a first-degree relative fitting the above criteria

DIFFERENTIAL DIAGNOSIS

- Abdominal neurofibromatosis
- Myxoid lipoma
- Nodular fasciitis
- Fibrous histiocytoma
- Segmental NF

WORKUP

The diagnosis of NF is usually self-evident. Workup is dictated by clinical symptoms in NF1 and usually includes MRI evaluation of the head and spine in NF2 and schwannomatosis. In fact, if NF2 is suspected but no vestibular nerve schwannomas are found, the diagnosis points to schwannomatosis.

LABORATORY TESTS

- Genetic testing is possible in individuals who desire prenatal diagnosis for NF1. There is no single standard test and multiple tests are required. Results can only tell if an individual is affected but cannot predict the severity of the disease due to variable expression.
- In NF2, linkage analysis testing provides a >99% certainty the individual has NF2.

IMAGING STUDIES

- MRI with gadolinium is the imaging study of choice in both NF1 and NF2 patients. MRI increases detection of optic gliomas, tumors of the spine, acoustic neuromas, and "bright spots" believed to represent hamartomas.
- MRI of the spine is recommended in all patients diagnosed with NF2 to exclude intramedullary tumors.

OTHER TESTS

- Wood lamp examination may be useful in patients with very pale skin for visualizing café-au-lait spots.
- Slit-lamp examination is recommended for children >6 yr to confirm the presence of Lisch nodules and subcapsular opacity.

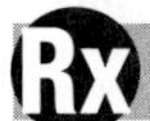 TREATMENT

Treatment is directed primarily at symptoms and complications of NF1 and NF2. As for schwannomatosis, resection should be reserved for tumors that are symptomatic or threaten to cause spinal cord compression.

NONPHARMACOLOGIC THERAPY

- Counseling addressing prognosis and genetic, psychologic, and social issues
- Hearing testing and speech pathology evaluation

ACUTE GENERAL Rx

- Surgery is usually not done on skin tumors unless cosmetically requested or if suspicion of malignant transformation exists.
- Surgery may be indicated for spinal or cranial neurofibromas, gliomas, or meningiomas.
- Acoustic neuromas can be treated by surgical excision.

CHRONIC Rx

- Radiation may be indicated in optic nerve gliomas and patients whose central nervous system tumors show image progression.
- Stereotactic radiosurgery with a gamma knife may be an alternative approach to surgery for acoustic neuromas.

DISPOSITION

- Prognosis varies according to the severity of involvement.
- There is no cure for neurofibromatosis.

REFERRAL

A multidisciplinary team of consultants is needed in patients with neurofibromatosis, including neurosurgeon, otolaryngologist, dermatologist, neurologist, audiologist, speech pathologist, geneticist, and neuropsychologist.

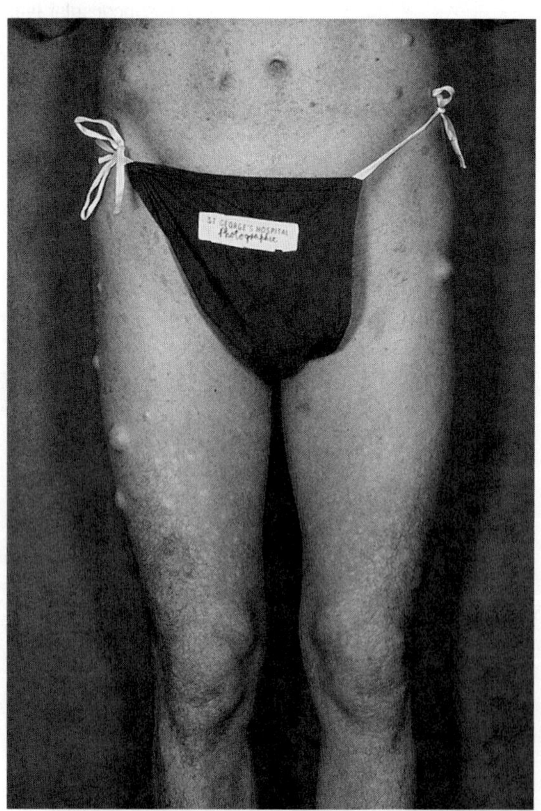

FIGURE 1-215 Type 1 neurofibromatosis: widespread cutaneous neurofibromata are a prominent feature of the classical variant. Courtesy of R.A. Marsden, M.D., St George's Hospital, London. (From McKee PH, Calonje E, Granter SR [eds]: *Pathology of the skin with clinical correlations,* ed 3, St Louis, 2005, Mosby.)

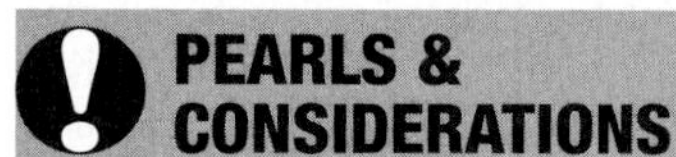 PEARLS & CONSIDERATIONS

- Friedrich Daniel von Recklinghausen first reported his cases in 1882, although there had been similar accounts dating back to the 1600s.
- The first report in the literature of NF2 was by Wishart in 1822.
- A high SPRED1 mutation detection rate has been identified in NF1 mutation-negative families with an autosomal dominant phenotype of CALMs with or without freckling and no other NF1 features.

COMMENTS

For additional information and patient resources, refer to the National Neurofibromatosis Foundation (www.nf.org) or Neurofibromatosis Inc. (www.nfinc.org).

SUGGESTED READINGS

Asthagiri et al: Neurofibromatosis type 2, *Lancet* 373(9679):1974, 2009.

Messiaen L et al: Clinical and mutational spectrum of neurofibromatosis type 1-like syndrome, *JAMA* 302(19):2111-2118, 2009.

Williams VC et al: Neurofibromatosis type 1 revisited, *Pediatrics* 123(1):124, 2009.

AUTHORS: **MARK F. BRADY, M.D., M.P.H.,** and **WEN Y. WU-CHEN, M.D.**

BASIC INFORMATION

DEFINITION

Neuroleptic malignant syndrome (NMS) is a disorder characterized by hyperthermia, muscular rigidity, autonomic dysfunction, and depressed/fluctuating levels of arousal that evolve over 24 to 72 hr. This occurs as an idiosyncratic adverse reaction most commonly to dopamine-receptor antagonists (especially the D2/4 receptor) or sudden withdrawal from a dopaminergic agent or agonist, such as antiparkinsonian medications.

SYNONYMS

None

ICD-9CM CODES
333.92 Neuroleptic malignant syndrome

EPIDEMIOLOGY & DEMOGRAPHICS

INCIDENCE (IN U.S.): 0.07% to 0.15% annual incidence in psychiatric population.
PREDOMINANT SEX: More than two thirds of patients are male.
PREDOMINANT AGE: Young and middle-aged adults
PREDISPOSING FACTORS:
- High-potency dopamine antagonists
- Long-acting depot preparations or multiple agents

PHYSICAL FINDINGS & CLINICAL PRESENTATION

- Muscle rigidity (hypertonia, cogwheeling, or "lead pipe" rigidity)
- Hyperthermia (38.6° to 42.3° C, usually $<$40° C)
- Autonomic symptoms: diaphoresis, sialorrhea, skin pallor, urinary incontinence
- Tachycardia, tachypnea
- Labile blood pressure (hypertension or postural hypotension)
- Agitation, catatonia, fluctuating consciousness, obtundation

ETIOLOGY

- Unknown. Impaired thermoregulation in hypothalamus and limbic cortex may occur as a result of relative lack of dopamine activity (central dopamine-blockade hypothesis: most accepted).
- Neuroleptic drugs have different potencies for inducing NMS:
  1. Typical neuroleptics: high potency, haloperidol; medium potency, chlorpromazine, fluphenazine; low potency, levomepromazine, loxapine
  2. Atypical neuroleptics: low potency, risperidone, olanzapine, clozapine, quetiapine

Dx DIAGNOSIS

DIFFERENTIAL DIAGNOSIS

- Heatstroke, drug-induced states and overdose (ecstasy abuse, phencyclidine), thyrotoxicosis, pheochromocytoma, serotonin syndrome
- Malignant hyperthermia, catatonia, acute psychosis with agitation
- CNS or systemic infections, including sepsis

WORKUP

Careful drug history

LABORATORY TESTS

- Elevated creatine phosphokinase (CPK) (sensitivity 0.71)
- Urinary myoglobin
- Leukocytosis, usually 10,000 to 40,000/mm^3
- Electrolytes and renal function
- Blood gases
- Drug levels

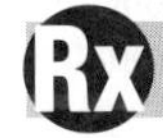

TREATMENT

NONPHARMACOLOGIC THERAPY

- Stop all neuroleptic agents and reinstitute any recently discontinued dopaminergic agents.
- Respiratory support; nutritional support in cases with dysphagia or comatose.
- Careful fluid balance monitoring with adequate hydration (intravenous in severe cases).
- Active cooling (cooling blanket and antipyretics).
- Skilled nursing care is necessary to prevent decubitus ulcers in bed-confined patients.

ACUTE GENERAL Rx

- IV benzodiazepines (e.g., diazepam 2 to 10 mg, with total daily dose of 10 to 60 mg) to relax muscles and control agitation.
- Bromocriptine, a dopamine receptor agonist, is the mainstay of therapy for patients with neuroleptic malignant syndrome. Initial doses of 2.5 to 10 mg are given IV q8h and are increased by 5 mg/day until clinical improvement is seen. The drug should be continued for at least 10 days after the syndrome has been controlled and then tapered slowly.
- Amantadine, an NMDA receptor antagonist with possible dopaminergic properties, administered orally at doses of 100 to 200 mg PO bid, has been shown to reduce mortality in comparison to supportive therapy alone.
- Dantrolene therapy is also effective. Initially, patients can be given 0.25 mg/kg IV q6-12h, followed by a maintenance dose up to 3 mg/kg/day. After 2 to 3 days, patients may be given the drug orally (25 to 600 mg/day in divided doses). Oral dantrolene therapy (50 to 600 mg/day) may be continued for several days afterward.
- Electroconvulsive therapy with neuromuscular blockage in pharmacologically refractory cases. Succinylcholine should not be used because it may cause hyperkalemia and cardiac arrhythmias in patients with rhabdomyolysis or dysautonomia.

CHRONIC Rx

- Respiratory care, nutritional support, and physical therapy may be required in more severe cases.
- Appropriate therapy would be required in patients with persistent neuropsychiatric sequelae of NMS (e.g., antidepressants for depression, cognitive behavioral therapy for cognitive deficits, rehabilitation for contractures).

DISPOSITION

- Mortality rate is currently 5% to 10% despite therapeutic measures. Serious sequelae may occur in a further 20%. Complete recovery occurs in $>$70% of patients. Causes of death include cardiac arrhythmias, myocardial infarction, renal failure secondary to rhabdomyolysis, seizures, pulmonary edema, and bronchopneumonia.
- Factors adversely affecting mortality are development of renal failure and core temperature $>$104°F (40° C).
- Late neuropsychiatric sequelae.
- Monitor closely for future complications of pharmacologic therapy.

REFERRAL

If the patient's condition is critical, it is preferable to treat the patient in a medical/neurologic ICU.

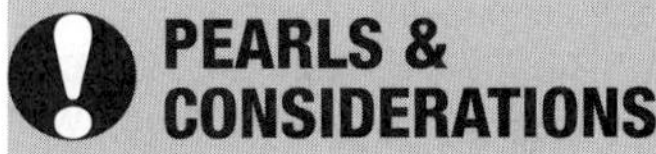

PEARLS & CONSIDERATIONS

COMMENTS

Early detection and diagnosis lead to a more favorable outcome. Treatment is a medical emergency.

SUGGESTED READINGS

Adityanjee, Sajatovic M, Munshi KR: Neuropsychiatric sequelae of neuroleptic malignant syndrome, *Clin Neuropharmacol* 28:197-204, 2005.

Chandran GJ et al: Neuroleptic malignant syndrome: case report and discussion, *CMAJ* 169:439, 2003.

Kipps CM et al: Movement disorder emergencies, *Mov Disord* 20:322-334, 2005.

Sueman VL: Clinical management of neuroleptic malignant syndrome, *Psychiatr Q* 72(4):825, 2001.

Ty EB, Rothner AD: Neuroleptic malignant syndrome in children and adolescents, *J Child Neurol* 16(3):157, 2001.

AUTHOR: **EROBOGHENE E. UBOGU, M.B.B.S. (HONS.)**

Neuropathic Pain 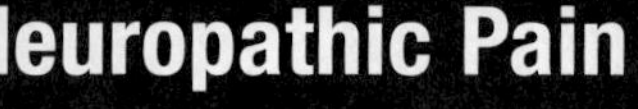

BASIC INFORMATION

DEFINITION

Neuropathic pain is not itself a disease, but rather a symptom that is associated with multiple different diseases. Thus it is not enough to define its presence without searching for a cause. It is defined as the sensation derived from the abnormal discharges of impaired or injured neural structures in either the peripheral or central nervous system. Descriptors include:

- Hyperesthesia: heightened sensitivity to nonpainful stimuli (e.g., light touch)
- Hyperalgesia: heightened sensitivity to painful stimuli (e.g., pinprick), or reduced threshold to feel pain
- Allodynia: pain provoked by a stimulus that is not normally painful

SYNONYMS

Neuralgia

ICD-9CM CODES

782.0 Numbness, paresthesias
729.1 Myositis/myalgia, not otherwise specified
729.2 Neuralgia, neuritis, or radiculitis, not otherwise specified

EPIDEMIOLOGY & DEMOGRAPHICS

- Estimates of the prevalence of neuropathic pain in the general population range from 1.6% to 8.2%.
- Demographics vary widely depending on etiology, for example:
  - Postherpetic neuralgia: affects elderly, pain seen in almost 100% of cases
  - AIDS: 30% of patients affected
  - Diabetes mellitus: 20% to 24% affected (prevalence rates vary, increasing with longer disease duration)
  - Fabry disease: affects mostly children, pain in 81% to 90% of patients

PHYSICAL FINDINGS & CLINICAL PRESENATION

- History: localize the disease with questions
  - Quality (description) of neuropathic pain: burning, hot or cold, "icy hot," "pins and needles," stinging, lancinating, sharp, shooting
  - Distribution of symptoms may aid in localization (i.e., "stocking-glove" symptoms in generalized neuropathy, numbness in a peripheral nerve territory in focal neuropathy)
  - Generalized small fiber neuropathy: dysesthesias without numbness common, but many etiologies (e.g., diabetes) cause both small and large fiber dysfunction
  - Large fiber neuropathy: coexisting numbness, hyporeflexia, or weakness may be seen, usually worse distally
  - Nerve root: coexisting neck or low back pain that radiates along a specific dermatome; most common cause is structural compression
  - Spinal cord symptoms: coexisting spasticity, bowel or bladder involvement, sensory level
  - Prior history of thalamic stroke in central thalamic pain syndrome (Dejerine-Roussy syndrome)
  - Family history may suggest a genetic cause
- Examination: see Table 1-55 and Section III, "Neuropathic Pain."

ETIOLOGY & LABORATORY EVALUATION (Table 1-56)

- Metabolic: diabetes mellitus; malnutrition and alcoholism; vitamin B_{12} deficiency; thiamine deficiency; porphyria; Fabry's disease
- Inflammatory: immune vasculitides (lupus, Sjögren's syndrome, polyarteritis nodosa, etc.), acute inflammatory demyelinating polyneuropathy (classically presents with ascending weakness and numbness, though pain is also a common feature), chronic inflammatory demyelinating polyneuropathy, sarcoid, multiple sclerosis
- Infiltrative: amyloidosis, paraproteinemias (e.g., monoclonal gammopathy of uncertain significance [MGUS])
- Infectious: postviral (brachial neuritis), HIV/AIDS, HSV, varicella-zoster virus (VZV; postherpetic neuralgia), Lyme disease, leprosy (thickened nerves and skin lesions), syphilis
- Neoplastic and paraneoplastic-carcinomatous infiltration of nerve/nerve root, anti-Hu
- Drugs/toxins: history of exposure to alcohol, chemotherapeutic agents (paclitaxel, vincristine), isoniazid, metronidazole, or heavy metals (thallium, arsenic)

Dx DIAGNOSIS

LABORATORY TESTS

- Fasting blood glucose (FBG)
- 2-hour oral glucose tolerance test (OGTT)
- Vitamin B_1 level
- If B_{12} level normal: serum methylmalonic acid and homocysteine levels
- Serum erythrocyte sedimentation rate (ESR), ANA, SS-A and SS-B, c-ANCA, p-ANCA
- RPR or FTA-ABS
- Serum ACE level (sarcoid)
- HIV antibody
- SPEP, UPEP, immunofixation
- Urine and stool protoporphyrins, if porphyria is suspected clinically
- Hu antibody: can be seen in both small cell and non–small cell lung cancers, may be positive without evidence of lung cancer
- Lumbar puncture: protein elevation, oligoclonal bands, CSF/serum IgG index, herpes simplex virus (HSV), VZV, Lyme polymerase chain reaction (PCR), VDRL

ELECTROPHYSIOLOGY STUDIES

- Electrophysiologic testing (electromyography with nerve conduction studies): may be normal in small fiber neuropathies or CNS lesion, but often abnormal in large fiber neuropathies
- Quantitative sensory testing: abnormal in small and large fiber neuropathy
- Evoked potentials (only if suspicion for spinal cord lesion)

PATHOLOGY STUDIES

- Nerve biopsy is occasionally useful in selected cases, particularly when vasculitis, sarcoid, or amyloid neuropathy are in the differential.

TABLE 1-55 Examination

Exam Finding	Localization
Pinprick/temperature loss alone	Small fibers only
Pinprick/temperature loss + vibratory/proprioceptive loss	Small and large fibers
Sensory loss and motor dysfunction worse distally than proximal	Large fiber neuropathy
Sensory loss and motor dysfunction along single nerve distribution	Single nerve
Sensory loss and motor dysfunction along multiple single nerves	Multiple mononeuropathies (i.e., mononeuropathy multiplex)
Motor and sensory loss involving multiple nerves belonging to specific region of brachial or lumbar plexus	Plexopathy
Sensory loss along dermatome with multiple myotomal muscles affected	Nerve root lesion
Asymmetric sensory loss without weakness and pseudoathetosis	Dorsal root ganglion
Vibratory/proprioceptive loss without pinprick/temperature loss	Dorsal column dysfunction (from compressive lesion, B_{12} deficiency, or tabes dorsalis from neurosyphilis)
Sensory level with weakness below the level of lesion and long tract signs (spasticity/Babinski's sign)	Spinal cord lesion
Hemisensory hyperalgesia	Contralateral thalamus

- Skin biopsy for intraepidermal nerve fiber (IENF) density may be useful for small fiber neuropathy when other studies are normal.
- Rectal or abdominal fat pad biopsy may show amyloid deposition in systemic amyloidosis.

IMAGING STUDIES

- MRI (with and without contrast):
  - Of the brain to exclude thalamic pathology if symptoms and signs are consistent with thalamic lesion
  - Of the spinal cord and nerve roots to exclude structural, inflammatory, neoplastic, or infectious causes
  - Of the lumbar spine to evaluate for arachnoiditis
- If MRI cannot be performed, consider:
  - CT of the brain for thalamic pathology
  - CT myelography of the spinal cord to evaluate for structural/neoplastic disease, but only if clinical signs of spinal or nerve root compromise are present

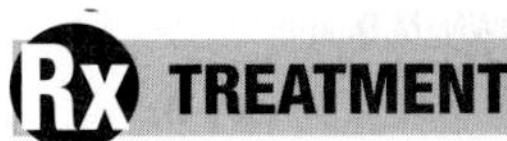

TREATMENT

NONPHARMACOLOGIC THERAPY

- Counseling should be initiated at the beginning of therapy to address psychologic issues exacerbating physiologic pain
- Physical therapy: especially in cases of chronic neck and low back pain

ACUTE GENERAL Rx

- Antidepressants:
  - Tricyclic antidepressants (TCAs): nortriptyline preferred over amitriptyline (fewer anticholinergic side effects with nortriptyline). Begin 25 mg PO qd in adults, or 10 mg qd in elderly. Increase dose by 25 mg every week as tolerated until usual maximal effective dose of 150 mg/day.
  - Paroxetine: begin 10 mg PO qd, increase by 10 mg/wk to a max dose of 60 mg qd.
  - Duloxetine: begin 30 mg daily, increase to 60 to 120 mg daily, qd or bid.
- Antiepileptics:
  - Gabapentin: begin 300 mg PO qd, advance to 300 mg PO tid by the end of the first week. Effective dose: higher than 1600 mg/day. Max dose: 1500 mg PO tid.
  - Carbamazepine: for trigeminal neuralgia. Begin 400 mg PO bid, increase to tid if necessary. Side effects and drug levels help to determine optimal dosing. Risk of aplastic anemia and hyponatremia (monitor CBC and chemistries).
  - Oxcarbazepine: better tolerated than carbamazepine. Start 150 mg PO bid and gradually increase to a maximal dose of 600 mg bid.
  - Lamotrigine: begin 25 mg PO bid, increase slowly (by 100 mg biweekly) until maximum effective dose of 200 to 300 mg PO bid. Risk: Stevens-Johnson syndrome.
  - Pregabalin: begin 50 mg PO tid, increase slowly to 100 to 200 mg PO tid.
- Analgesics:
  - Tramadol: 150 mg/day (50 mg tid), increase by 50 mg/wk, max 200 to 400 mg/day.
  - Morphine (oral): 15 to 30 mg q8h, max 90 to 360 mg/day.
  - Oxycodone: 20 mg q12h, increase by 10 mg/wk, max 40 to 160 mg/day.
  - Fentanyl patch: 25 to 100 mcg transdermally q3 days.
- Topical anesthetics:
  - 5% lidocaine patch, apply to area of pain, max three patches every 12 hr.
  - Capsaicin is inconsistent in its ability to relieve pain and may exacerbate it. Use not recommended.
- Procedural/surgical: this option is considered mostly when the patient suffers from pain secondary to spinal cord or cauda equina injury. Studies are limited and benefit is not completely established. Procedures should

TABLE 1-56 Clinical Presentation and Laboratory Findings

Neuropathy Type	Predisposition	Examination Findings	EMG/NCS	Laboratory Analysis
Idiopathic small fiber PN	Age >50	Strength: normal Reflexes: normal Pos/Vib: normal Pain/Temp: decreased distally	Normal	Serum studies: normal Skin biopsy: abnormal Sudomotor studies: abnormal
Diabetic PN	Longstanding disease Family history	Strength normal to reduced, sensation reduced distally	Abnormal	Abnormal glucose tolerance High fasting glucose
Inherited PN	Family history	Pes cavus, hammer toes, reduced reflexes, sensation reduced distally	Abnormal	Genetic studies may be abnormal, other studies normal
Familial amyloid PN	Family history	Pain/temp loss Reduced reflexes Orthostasis	Abnormal if large fibers affected; also carpal tunnel syndrome	Transthyretin genetic study
Acquired amyloid PN	Monoclonal gammopathy	Pain/temp loss Reduced reflexes Orthostasis	Abnormal if large fibers affected; also carpal tunnel syndrome	SPEP, UPEP, immunofixation abnormal
Fabry's disease	Age <20 Renal failure Strokes	Normal; possible reduced pain/temp sensation	Normal	α-galactosidase levels in cultured fibroblasts
PN + mixed connective tissue disease	History of lupus, rheumatoid arthritis, Sjögren's syndrome	Reduced reflexes and distal sensation	Abnormal	ANA, RF, SS-A/SS-B may be abnormal
Peripheral nerve vasculitis	Asymmetric disease	Multiple peripheral nerves involved	Abnormal	ANA, RF, SS-A/SS-B, ANCA, cryoglobulins may be abnormal
Paraneoplastic neuropathy	Lung cancer risk factors, chemical exposures	Asymmetric sensory loss, pseudoathetosis, relatively preserved strength	Abnormal	Anti-Hu
Sarcoidosis	Pulmonary sarcoid	Multiple mononeuropathies	Abnormal	Abnormal biopsy, elevated serum ACE, CXR abnormal
Arsenic	Pesticides, copper smelting	Reduced reflexes and distal sensation	Abnormal	Elevated arsenic in plasma, urine, and hair
HIV	Promiscuity, unprotected sex, IV drug abuse, blood transfusion	Variable, but most often reduced reflexes and distal sensation	Abnormal if large fibers involved	HIV antibody

ACE, Angiotensin-converting enzyme; *ANA,* antibody to nuclear antigens; *ANCA,* antineutrophil cytoplasmic antibodies; *CXR,* chest x-ray; *EMG,* electromyography; *HbA1C,* glycosylated hemoglobin; *HIV,* human immunodeficiency virus; *IV,* intravenous; *NCS,* nerve conduction studies; *PN,* polyneuropathy; *Pos,* position sensation; *RF,* rheumatoid factor; *SPEP,* serum protein electrophoresis; *SS-A,* Sjögren syndrome A; *SS-B,* Sjögren syndrome B; *Temp,* temperature sensation; *UPEP,* urine protein electrophoresis; *Vib,* vibration sensation.
(Adapted from Mendell JR, Sahenk Z: Painful sensory neuropathy, *N Engl J Med* 348(13):1243, 2003.)

be considered only when all other therapeutic modalities have failed. In addition, the patient should be cautioned that surgical procedures may not result in pain relief and may be associated with significant morbidity and even mortality.
- Dorsal root rhizotomy
- Nerve blocks
- Spinal cord stimulator

DISPOSITION

Prognosis depends on multiple factors including:
- Etiology of pain
- Treatment of any underlying condition
- Initiation of appropriate (often multiple) therapeutic modalities
- Patient compliance with prescribed regimen

Most care is accomplished in the outpatient setting, except when surgery is required.

REFERRAL

- Pain clinic
- Neurology
- Psychiatry
- Psychology
- Physiatry
- Anesthesiology (nerve blocks)
- Neurosurgery if considering surgical management

PEARLS & CONSIDERATIONS

Factitious disorder and malingering frequently manifest with pain complaints. These are diagnoses of exclusion, and require negative evaluation for organic etiologies before diagnosis is made.

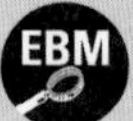

EVIDENCE

Please note: Complete text of EBM for this topic is available online.

Key trials and commentary:

Botulinum toxin type A (BTX-A) has been reported to have analgesic effects independent of its action on muscle tone, possibly by acting on neurogenic inflammation. Such a mechanism may be involved in peripheral neuropathic pain.

These results indicate for the first time that BTX-A may induce direct analgesic effects in patients with chronic neuropathic pain independent of its effects on muscle tone and suggest novel indications for BTX-A in analgesia.[1] Ⓐ

As with many studies comparing the effect of an active treatment vs. placebo in patients with neuropathic pain, BTX-A (Botox) infiltration was significantly better than placebo, but the degree of pain reduction was not impressive. The study does, however, confirm that there may be some pain-relieving effects independent of the drug's effect on muscle tone. Botox is expensive, but if it provides many weeks of pain reduction, its cost may be competitive with many oral medications.

Evidence-Based Reference

1. Ranoux D et al: Botulinum toxin type A induces direct analgesic effects in chronic neuropathic pain, *Ann Neurol* 64:274-283, 2008. Commentary by S. Abram, M.D. Ⓐ

SUGGESTED READING

Mendell JR, Sahenk Z: Painful sensory neuropathy, *N Engl J Med* 348(13):1243, 2003.

AUTHORS: **GAVIN BROWN, M.D.** and **GREGORY J. ESPER, M.D.**

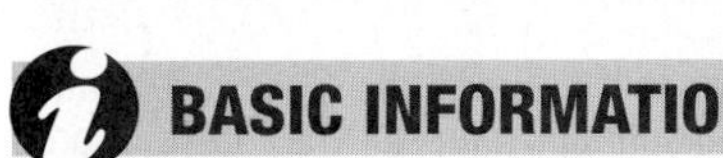

BASIC INFORMATION

DEFINITION

Any disorder affecting the peripheral nervous system, including nerve roots, plexuses, and individual peripheral nerves, that has a genetic basis of inheritance and has been or is capable of being transmitted along generations.

There are many different types of hereditary peripheral neuropathies, including Dejerine-Sottas disease, inherited metabolic neuropathies, hereditary sensory and autonomic neuropathies (HSANs), and hereditary motor neuropathies such as spinal muscular atrophy (SMA). Most disorders are diagnosed in infancy or childhood; as such, adult clinicians rarely see these patients. For this reason, this chapter discusses only the hereditary motor and sensory neuropathies that an adult clinician might encounter.

SYNONYMS

Charcot-Marie-Tooth (CMT) disease, a.k.a. hereditary motor-sensory neuropathy (HMSN)
Hereditary neuropathy with liability to pressure-sensitive palsies (HNPP)

ICD-9CM CODES
CMT: 356.1
HNPP: 689

EPIDEMIOLOGY & DEMOGRAPHICS

All CMT: approximately 30 per 100,000
- CMT type 1 (demyelinating pathophysiology): 1 in 2500
- CMT type 2 (axonal pathophysiology): 7 in 1000
- CMT type 4 and CMT-X: rare (either axonal or demyelinating pathophysiology)

HNPP: 2 to 5 per 100,000

PHYSICAL FINDINGS & CLINICAL PRESENATION

CMT: Highly variable
- Age at onset earlier for CMT-1 than CMT-2, but both may present from childhood to old age.
- Severely affected patients have severe distal weakness and muscle atrophy with hand (prominently affecting interossei) and foot deformities (pes cavus, high arched feet, hammer toes).
- Mildly affected patients may have only foot deformity (pes cavus) with little or no weakness/sensory loss.
- Legs can be affected greater than arms, and patients will complain of gait abnormalities (steppage), which cause them to trip and fall.
- Sensory complaints (paresthesias, numbness, dysesthesia) are uncommon despite physical findings of impaired sensation.
- Decreased or absent reflexes.
- Some patients may have postural tremor of the upper limbs.

HNPP (a.k.a. tomaculous neuropathy):
- Age at onset is commonly adolescence.
- Disorder is characterized by recurrent entrapment of peripheral nerves with accompanying signs and symptoms (paresthesias and/or weakness in anatomical distributions). Most common are:
  1. Median nerve at the wrist (carpal tunnel syndrome)
  2. Ulnar nerve at the elbow (cubital tunnel syndrome)
  3. Painless brachial plexopathies
  4. Lateral femoral cutaneous nerve (meralgia paresthetica)
  5. Peroneal nerve at the fibular head
- May be associated with a generalized polyneuropathy.

ETIOLOGY

CMT: more than 30 subgroups have been identified and have various chromosomal abnormalities.
- Most common mutation is PMP-22 duplication, giving rise to CMT 1A demyelinating phenotype.
- Other mutations include P0 (demyelinating) and neurofilament light chain mutations (demyelinating or axonal phenotype)—see the following.
- Updated information may be available at http://www.neuro.wustl.edu/neuromuscular.

HNPP: deletion of chromosome 17p11.2–12.

DIAGNOSIS

DIFFERENTIAL DIAGNOSIS

CMT: other genetic, metabolic, and multisystem disorders including:
- Spinocerebellar ataxias
- Friedreich's ataxia
- Leukodystrophies
- Refsum's disease (elevated serum phytanic acid)
- Distal spinal muscular atrophies and distal myopathies, which can present with pes cavus and other foot deformities
- Chronic inflammatory demyelinating polyneuropathy (CIDP)

HNPP:
- Hereditary neuralgic amyotrophy (HNA), which typically is painful rather than painless. In addition, in HNA, there is no evidence of generalized polyneuropathy.
- Multifocal motor neuropathy with conduction block (MMNCB)—autoimmune-mediated pure motor neuropathy
- Neuropathy associated with renal failure
- Lead neuropathy
- Neuropathy relating to paraproteinemia (demyelinating pathophysiology)

EVALUATION

CMT
- History of gradual onset symptoms is important to distinguish CMT from other forms of neuropathy.
- Detailed family history with *pedigree* is essential. Consider examination of multiple family members.
- History should evaluate for potential heavy metal exposure.
- History of dysesthesias is uncommon and should prompt search for acquired neuropathy or other inherited neuropathies (e.g., Fabry's disease).

HNPP: genetic testing after identification of multiple entrapment neuropathies on EMG and nerve conduction studies

LABORATORY TESTS

- Neurophysiology: electromyography (EMG) and nerve conduction studies (NCSs) must be done first to determine type of pathophysiology: demyelinating or axonal. This will guide genetic testing.
- NCSs in CMT-1 will reveal demyelinating physiology characterized by very slow conduction velocities (around 15 to 30 m/s) with prolonged distal latencies. Inherited demyelinating disorders can be distinguished from acquired demyelinating disorders (e.g., chronic inflammatory demyelinating polyneuropathy or CIDP) by the presence of conduction block in the latter.
- In HNPP, diffusely prolonged distal latencies with superimposed entrapment neuropathies at common sites will be seen on NCSs.
- EMG will reveal reinnervation characterized by long-duration, large-amplitude, polyphasic motor unit potentials (MUPs) with decreased MUP recruitment.
- Genetic tests are available for some CMT subtypes:
  1. CMT-1A: chromosome 17p11-PMP-22 duplication
  2. CMT-1B: chromosome 1q22-P0 mutation
  3. CMT-2E: chromosome 8p21-neurofilament light chain (NF-L) point mutation
  4. CMT-X: connexin 32 mutations
  5. HNPP: chromosome 17p11 deletion, which includes the PMP-22 gene
- Serum and 24-hour urine levels of heavy metals (arsenic, lead, etc.)
- SPEP, UPEP, immunofixation (for paraprotein).
- Anti-GM1 antibody (positive in ~50% of patients with MMNCB).
- Lumbar puncture may reveal elevated CSF protein in CIDP.
- Peripheral nerve biopsy:
  1. Demyelination with "onion bulb formation." Tomaculae, or focal thickening of myelin sheaths, seen in HNPP
  2. Generally not indicated unless diagnosis is uncertain

IMAGING STUDIES

- Spine plain films: for evaluation of scoliosis.
- MRI: indicated if dissociative sensory loss (dorsal column dysfunction with intact spinothalamic tract function) or if upper motor neuron findings (spasticity, Babinski's sign, clonus, increased tendon reflexes) are present.
- Exclusion of involvement of brain or spinal cord compressive lesions causing arm or leg weakness.
- Some inherited peripheral demyelinating disorders (i.e., CMT-X) are associated with intracerebral white matter abnormalities on MRI.
- Exclusion of structural, infectious, or inflammatory nerve root pathology.

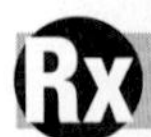

TREATMENT

There is no known cure for any of these disorders. Management is supportive.

NONPHARMACOLOGIC THERAPY

- Physical therapy (PT) and occupational therapy (OT) to provide assistance with gait and coordination.
- PT and OT might provide walking aid such as ankle foot orthosis (AFO), cane, walker, or wheelchair depending on the severity of the neuropathy.
- Wrist splints for superimposed carpal tunnel syndrome.
- Elbow pads (Heelbo Pads) to cushion the ulnar nerve at the elbow.
- Heel-cord strengthening.
- Stretching exercises.
- Analgesics for pain associated with foot deformity.
- Surgical correction of foot deformities by orthopedic surgeons if indicated.

Vincristine may worsen existing neuropathy (important for oncologist to know if patient develops cancer requiring chemotherapy).

SURGICAL TREATMENT

- Patients with HNPP should probably not undergo surgical decompression of the median nerve at the wrist or the ulnar nerve at the elbow; these nerves are sensitive to manipulation. Poor results have been reported with ulnar nerve transposition.
- Anesthesiologists should be aware of HNPP diagnosis in patients undergoing surgery to prevent compression neuropathies from occurring during surgical procedures.

GENETIC COUNSELING

Must be routinely done for patient and family when diagnosis is established. Many aspects of the patient and family's life are affected including:

- Future progeny of patient and/or patient's parents or children
- Psychosocial aspects including social functioning, marriage, employment
- Financial needs
- Medical and life insurability

PROGNOSIS

- CMT: slowly progressive, and patients often remain ambulatory until late in life. Life expectancy is normal. Patients with respiratory involvement (i.e., phrenic nerve involvement with diaphragm paresis) may have shorter life expectancy.
- HNPP: benign prognosis.

DISPOSITION

Outpatient care. Routine follow-up appointments should be done initially every 6 mo, and then every 1 to 2 yr.

REFERRAL

- Neurology and/or neuromuscular disease specialist
- Podiatry for recurrent foot problems, including appropriate arches

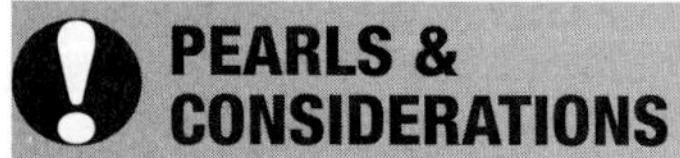

PEARLS & CONSIDERATIONS

PATIENT & FAMILY EDUCATION

Patients can benefit from use of Muscular Dystrophy Association (MDA) resources.

SUGGESTED READINGS

Chance PF: Genetic evaluation of inherited motor/sensory neuropathy, *Suppl Clin Neurophysiol* 57:228, 2004.

Scott KR, Kothari MJ: Hereditary neuropathies, *Semin Neurol* 25(2):174, 2005.

Washington University Neuromuscular Disease Center: http://www.neuro.wustl.edu/neuromuscular.

AUTHORS: **GREGORY J. ESPER, M.D.,** and **GAVIN BROWN, M.D.**

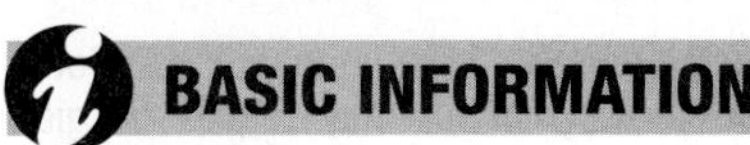

BASIC INFORMATION

DEFINITION

Nocardiosis is an infection caused by aerobic actinomycetes found in soil and characterized by lung, soft tissue, or central nervous system (CNS) involvement.

SYNONYMS

Mycetoma
Nocardia

ICD-9CM CODES
039 Actinomycotic infections
039.9 Nocardiosis NOS, of unspecified site

EPIDEMIOLOGY & DEMOGRAPHICS

- *Nocardia* species are found worldwide in the soil.
- Nocardiosis is found most commonly in patients who are immunocompromised (e.g., those receiving steroids or immunosuppressive therapy; those with lymphoma, leukemia, or lung cancer; transplant recipients; and those with pulmonary infections).
- Other underlying conditions associated with nocardiosis are pemphigus vulgaris, Whipple's disease, Goodpasture's syndrome, Cushing's disease, cirrhosis, ulcerative colitis, and rheumatoid arthritis.
- Use of steroids is an independent risk factor for developing nocardiosis.
- Between 500 and 1000 new cases are diagnosed each year in the U.S.
- Approximately 2% of patients with AIDS develop nocardiosis.
- Occurs more commonly in men than in women (2:1).
- Adults are affected more often than children.

PHYSICAL FINDINGS & CLINICAL PRESENTATION

- Inhalation of *Nocardia* organisms is the most common mode of entry, and pneumonia is the most common presentation, with 75% manifesting with fever, chills, dyspnea, and a productive cough (Fig. 1-216).
  1. Presentation can be acute, subacute, or chronic.
  2. Nocardiosis should be suspected if soft tissue abscesses or CNS tumors or abscesses form in conjunction with the pulmonary infection.
  3. Pulmonary infection may spread into the pericardium, mediastinum, and superior vena cava.
- Cutaneous disease usually occurs by direct inoculation of the organism as a result of skin puncture by a thorn or splinter, surgery, IV catheter use, or animal scratches or bites manifesting in:
  1. Cellulitis
  2. Lymphocutaneous nodules appearing along lymphatic sites draining the infected puncture wound
  3. Mycetoma (Madura foot), a chronic deep nodular infection usually involving the hands or feet that can cause skin breakdown or fistula formation and that spreads along the fascial planes to infect surrounding skin, subcutaneous tissue, and bone
- The CNS system is infected in approximately one third of all cases. Brain abscess is the most common pathologic finding.
- Dissemination of nocardiosis may infect other tissues and organs, including the kidney, heart, skin, and bone.

ETIOLOGY

- The most common *Nocardia* species leading to infection in human beings are:
  1. *N. asteroides* (causing more than 80% of the cases of pulmonary nocardiosis)
  2. *N. brasiliensis* (most common cause of mycetoma)
  3. *N. otitidiscaviarum*
- *N. asteroides* has two subgroups:
  1. *N. farcinica*
  2. *N. nova*

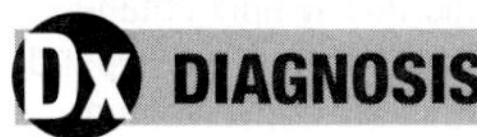

DIAGNOSIS

The diagnosis of nocardiosis requires a high index of suspicion in the proper clinical setting and is confirmed by bacteriologic staining and growth of the organism in culture.

DIFFERENTIAL DIAGNOSIS

There are no pathognomonic findings separating nocardiosis pneumonia from other infectious etiologies of the lung. Diagnoses presenting in a similar manner and often confused for nocardiosis include:

1. Tuberculosis
2. Lung abscess
3. Lung tumor
4. Other causes of pneumonia
5. Actinomycosis
6. Mycosis
7. Cellulitis
8. Coccidioidomycosis
9. Histoplasmosis
10. Aspergillosis
11. Kaposi's sarcoma

WORKUP

All patients with suspected nocardiosis need laboratory identification of the microorganism by obtaining sputum in the case of pneumonia, cultures of the infected skin lesions in mycetoma or lymphocutaneous disease, or the sampling of any purulent material (e.g., brain abscess, lung abscess, or pleural effusion).

LABORATORY TESTS

- Blood tests are not very sensitive in the diagnosis of nocardiosis.
- Gram stain shows gram-positive beaded filaments with multiple branches (Fig.1-217).
- Gomori methenamine silver staining may detect the organism.
- *Nocardia* species are acid-fast on a modified Ziehl-Neelsen stain.
- *Nocardia* are slow-growing organisms; colony growth in cultures may take up to 2 to 3 wk.

IMAGING STUDIES

- Chest radiograph may demonstrate infiltrates, densities, nodules, cavitary masses, or multiple abscesses.
- CT scan of the brain is indicated in the appropriate clinical setting to exclude CNS brain abscesses.

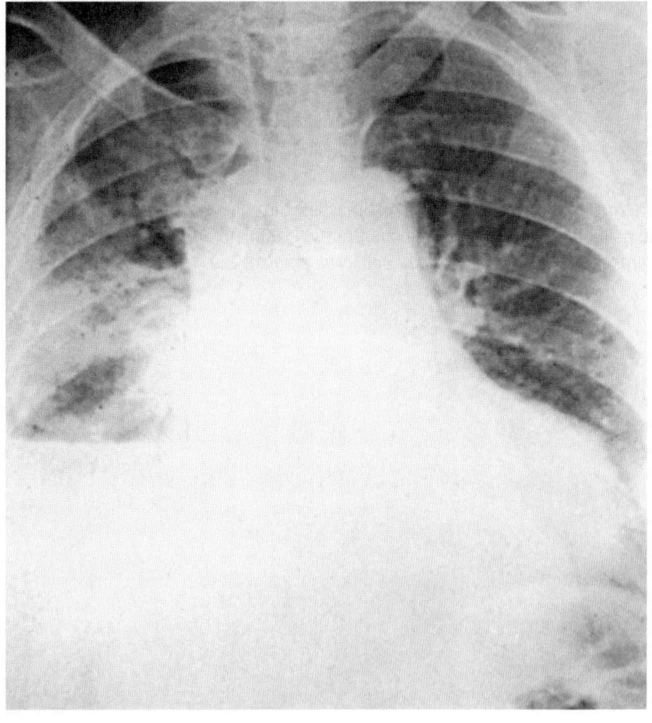

FIGURE 1-216 Right lower lobe *Nocardia* pneumonia in a kidney transplant recipient. (From Gorbach SL: *Infectious diseases,* ed 2, Philadelphia, 1998, WB Saunders.)

Rx TREATMENT

NONPHARMACOLOGIC THERAPY

- Supportive therapy with oxygen in patients with pneumonia
- Chest physiotherapy
- For any abscess formation, surgical drainage is indicated (e.g., skin, lung, or brain)

ACUTE GENERAL Rx

- There are no prospective, randomized trials to date highlighting the most effective treatment of nocardiosis. Nevertheless, sulfonamides are considered the treatment of choice. Sulfadiazine 6 to 10 g is given in 4 to 6 divided oral doses.
- For cutaneous infection, trimethoprim-sulfamethoxazole (TMX-SMX) (5 mg/kg/day divided in 2 doses)
- Severe infection: life-threatening pulmonary or disseminated disease; immunocompromised patients with severe disease should receive two-drug therapy: TMP-SMX 15 mg/kg/day divided into 4 to 6 doses and amikacin 7.5 mg/kg/IV q12h.
- In patients with CNS disease, ceftriaxone 2 g/IV q12h or cefotaxime 2 g q8h or imipenem 500 mg q6h is substituted for amikacin.
- Sulfonamide-resistant disease: any of the following two-drug regimens: amikacin plus one of the following: ampicillin/sulbactam, imipenem, meropenem, ceftriaxone, or cefotaxime.
- Alternative drug treatment includes:
  1. Imipenem
  2. Third-generation cephalosporin
  3. Minocycline 100 to 200 mg bid
  4. Extended-spectrum fluoroquinolones (moxifloxacin)
  5. Linezolid (use of linezolid >4 wk is associated with hematologic toxicity)

CHRONIC Rx

- Although the optimal duration of therapy has not been determined, long-term therapy is generally recommended for all infections caused by *Nocardia.*
- Patients with cellulitis and lymphocutaneous syndrome are treated for 2 to 4 mo depending on whether there is bone involvement.
- Mycetomas are best treated with antibiotics for 6 to 12 mo but may require surgical drainage.
- Pulmonary and systemic nocardiosis excluding the CNS is treated for 6 to 12 mo.
- CNS involvement is treated with drainage and antibiotics for 12 mo.
- All immunosuppressed patients should receive 12 mo of antibiotic therapy.

DISPOSITION

- Patients with pulmonary nocardiosis have a mortality rate of 15% to 30%.
- CNS involvement carries a >40% mortality rate.
- Isolated skin lesions have a low mortality rate.

REFERRAL

Whenever the diagnosis of nocardiosis is suspected, consultation with infectious disease is indicated. Pulmonary evaluation and assistance may be needed in pulmonary nocardiosis. Neurosurgery consultation is indicated in patients with single or multiple brain abscesses.

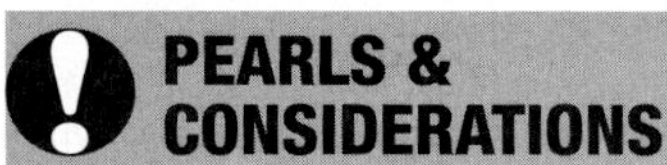

PEARLS & CONSIDERATIONS

- Nocardiosis does not spread from animal to animal.
- Nocardiosis is not transmitted from person to person.
- Nocardiosis is distinguished by its ability to disseminate to any organ and its tendency to relapse despite appropriate antibiotic therapy.

COMMENTS

Tuberculosis and nocardiosis may coexist in the same patient.

SUGGESTED READINGS

Chapman S: Diagnosis and treatment of nocardiosis, *UpToDate,* 15:2, 2007. www.uptodateonline.com.

Corti ME, Villafane-Fioti MF: Nocardiosis: a review, *Int J Infect Dis* 7(4):243, 2003.

Torres HA et al: Nocardiosis in cancer patients, *Medicine* 81(5):388, 2002.

AUTHOR: **TANYA ALI, M.D.**

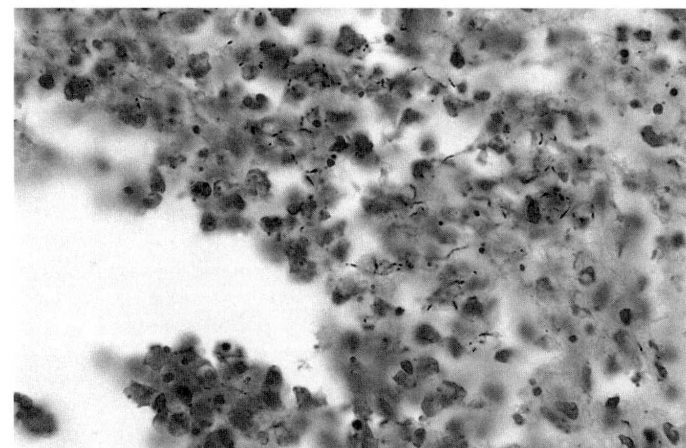

FIGURE 1-217 *Nocardia* pneumonia. Thin, branching, irregularly staining Gram-positive bacilli course through necrotic pulmonary tissue (Brown-Hopps Gram, ×1000). (From Silverberg SG et al [eds]: *Silverberg's principles and practice of surgical pathology and cytopathology,* ed 4, Philadelphia, 2006, Churchill Livingstone.)

BASIC INFORMATION

DEFINITION

Spectrum of diseases based on histiopathologic findings and representing a morphologic rather than a clinical diagnosis. It is liver disease occurring in patients who do not abuse alcohol and manifesting histologically by mononuclear cells and/or polymorphonuclear cells, hepatocyte ballooning, and spotty necrosis.

SYNONYMS

Nonalcoholic steatohepatitis (NASH)
NAFLD
Fatty liver hepatitis
Diabetes hepatitis
Alcohol-like liver disease
Laënnec's disease

ICD-9CM CODES
571.8 Fatty liver

EPIDEMIOLOGY & DEMOGRAPHICS

- Nonalcoholic fatty liver disease (NAFLD) affects 10% to 24% of the general population
- Increased prevalence in obese persons (57% to 74%), type 2 diabetes mellitus, and hyperlipidemia (primarily hypertriglyceridemia)
- Most common cause of abnormal liver test results in adults in the U.S. (accounts for up to 90% of cases of asymptomatic ALT elevations)
- 30 million obese adults have steatosis, 8.6 million may have steatohepatitis
- There is a 3:1 female-to-male predominance

PHYSICAL FINDINGS & CLINICAL PRESENTATION

- Most patients are asymptomatic
- Patients may report a sensation of fullness or discomfort on the right side of the upper abdomen
- Nonspecific complaints of fatigue or malaise may be reported
- Hepatomegaly is generally the only positive finding on physical examination
- Acanthosis nigricans may be found in children

ETIOLOGY

- Insulin resistance is the most reproducible factor in the development of nonalcoholic fatty liver disease
- Risk factors are obesity (especially truncal obesity), diabetes mellitus, hyperlipidemia

DIAGNOSIS

DIFFERENTIAL DIAGNOSIS

- Alcohol-induced liver disease (a daily alcohol intake of 20 g in females and 30 g in males [three 12-oz beers or 12 oz of wine] may be enough to cause alcohol-induced liver disease)
- Viral hepatitis
- Autoimmune hepatitis
- Toxin or drug-induced liver disease

WORKUP

Diagnosis is usually suspected on the basis of hepatomegaly, asymptomatic elevations of transaminases, or "fatty liver" on sonogram of abdomen in obese patients with little or no alcohol use. Liver biopsy will confirm diagnosis and provide prognostic information. It should be considered in patients with suspected advanced liver fibrosis (presence of obesity or type 2 diabetes, AST/ALT ratio 1, age 45 yr).

LABORATORY TESTS

- Elevated ALT, AST: AST/ALT ratio is usually <1, but can increase as fibrosis advances
- Negative serology for infectious hepatitis; generally normal GGTP and serum alkaline phosphatase
- Hyperlipidemia (primarily hypertriglyceridemia) may be present
- Elevated glucose levels may be present
- Prolonged prothrombin time, hypoalbuminuria, and elevated bilirubin may be present in advanced stages
- Elevated serum ferritin and increased transferrin saturation may be found in up to 10% of patients; however, hepatic iron index and hepatic iron level are normal
- Liver biopsy may show a wide spectrum of liver damage, ranging from simple steatosis to advanced fibrosis and cirrhosis

IMAGING STUDIES

- Ultrasound generally reveals diffuse increase in echogenicity as compared with that of the kidneys; CT scan reveals diffuse low-density hepatic parenchyma.
- Occasionally patients may have focal rather than diffuse steatosis, which may be misinterpreted as a liver mass on ultrasound or CT; use of MRI in these cases will identify focal fatty infiltration.

TREATMENT

NONPHARMACOLOGIC THERAPY

- Weight reduction in all obese patients (500 g per week in children and 1600 g per week in adults is preferred)
- Increase physical activity

GENERAL Rx

- No medications have been proved to directly improve liver damage from nonalcoholic fatty liver disease.
- Medications to control hyperlipidemia (e.g., fenofibrates for elevated triglycerides) and hyperglycemia (e.g., metformin) can lead to improvement in abnormal liver test results.
- In a recent trial of pioglitazone therapy in NASH it was associated with several favorable histologic and metabolic outcomes.

DISPOSITION

- Patients with pure steatosis on liver biopsy generally have a relatively benign course.
- The presence of steatohepatitis or advanced fibrosis on liver biopsy is associated with a worse prognosis.

REFERRAL

- Liver transplantation should be considered in patients with decompensated, end-stage disease; however, in these patients there may be a recurrence of nonalcoholic fatty liver disease post-transplantation.

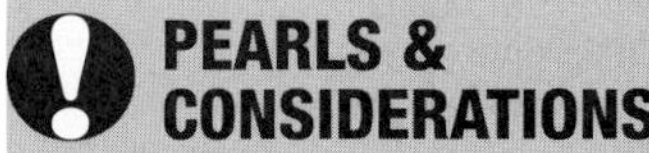

PEARLS & CONSIDERATIONS

COMMENTS

- Nonalcoholic fatty liver disease is closely associated with metabolic disorders, even in nonobese, nondiabetic subjects. It can be considered an early predictor of metabolic disorders, particularly in the normal-weight population. The presence of metabolic syndrome is a strong predictor of nonalcoholic fatty liver disease.
- A diagnosis of nonalcoholic fatty liver disease is contingent on the following factors:
  1. Alcohol consumption in amounts less than those considered hepatotoxic
  2. Absence of serologic evidence of other hepatic diseases or disorders
  3. Liver biopsy showing predominant macrovesicular steatosis or steatohepatitis

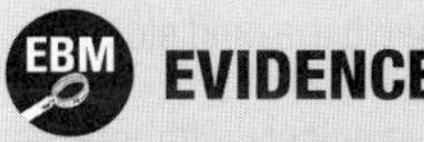

EVIDENCE

Please note: Complete text of EBM for this topic is available online.

SUGGESTED READINGS

Angulo P: Nonalcoholic fatty liver disease, *N Engl J Med* 346:1221, 2002.

Bayard M et al: Nonalcoholic fatty liver disease, *Am Fam Physician* 73:1961, 2006.

Belfort R et al: A placebo-controlled trial of pioglitazone in subjects with nonalcoholic steatohepatitis, *N Engl J Med* 355:2297, 2006.

Clark JM: Nonalcoholic fatty liver disease, *JAMA* 289:3000, 2003.

Ekstedt M et al: Long-term follow-up of patients with NAFLD and elevated liver enzymes, *Hepatology* 44: 865, 2006.

Hamaguchi M et al: The metabolic syndrome as a predictor of nonalcoholic fatty liver disease, *Ann Intern Med* 143:722, 2005.

Kim HJ et al: Metabolic significance of nonalcoholic fatty liver disease in nonobese, nondiabetic adults, *Arch Intern Med* 164:2169, 2004.

AUTHOR: **FRED F. FERRI, M.D.**

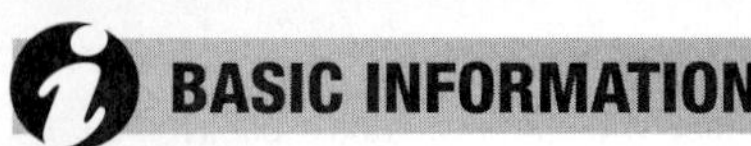

DEFINITION

Nosocomial infections are infections associated with health care, generally occurring over 48 hr after admission to a hospital.

SYNONYMS

Health care-associated infections (HAIs)

ICD-9CM CODES
008.45 Clostridium difficile
041.12 MRSA
482.42 MRSA pneumonia
038.12 MRSA septicemia
998.59 Other postoperative infection
999.31 Infection due to central venous catheter
997.31 Ventilator-assisted pneumonia
996.31 Due to urethral [indwelling] catheter

EPIDEMIOLOGY & DEMOGRAPHICS

INCIDENCE (IN U.S.):
- Develop in at least 5% of hospitalized patients
- In 2002 these HAIs accounted for more than 98,000 deaths
- In 2002 the annual cost of HAIs in the U.S. was estimated as >$5 to 10 billion; adjusts to >$35 billion in 2007 values

PREVALENCE (IN U.S.): 2 to 4 million cases/yr
PREDOMINANT SEX:
- Overall, approximately equal
- Elderly women: predominantly nosocomial urinary tract infections

PREDOMINANT AGE: Newborns and elderly patients (>60 yr) at highest risk
PEAK INCIDENCE: Varies widely with infection site
RISK FACTORS: Patients with the following conditions can develop HAI at any age:
- ICU
- Intubation
- Chronic lung disease
- Renal disease
- Comatose
- Chronic urethral or vascular catheterization
- Malnutrition
- Postoperative state
- Diabetic

PHYSICAL FINDINGS & CLINICAL PRESENTATION

Vary with specific HAIs
ETIOLOGY
- Bacteria
- Fungi
- Viruses

SOURCES AND MODES OF TRANSMISSION:
- Patient's own flora
  - Comprises resistant organisms associated with hospitalization
  - Frequently maintained thereafter by persistent GI colonization
- Unwashed hands of staff
  - Physicians
  - Nurses
- Invasion of protective defenses (intact skin, respiratory cilia, urinary sphincters, and mucosa)
  - IV lines/central lines
  - Catheters
  - Respiratory equipment
  - Surgical wounds
  - Scopes and other imaging devices
- Failure to provide adequate negative pressure, high-volume air flow chambers for airborne infection isolation of patients with TB or disseminated herpes zoster/chickenpox
- Failure to rapidly identify and provide appropriate care (with isolation or precautions) for patients with communicable diseases
- Inanimate environment
- Food
- Fomites

RISKS AMPLIFIED:
- Use of broad-spectrum antibiotics
  - Select highly resistant bacteria
  - Establish highly resistant bacteria as endemic flora in microenvironments within the hospital
- Highly vulnerable patients with specific risk factors
  - Immunosuppression (as a result of therapy, transplantation, AIDS)
  - Old age
  - Postsurgery
  - Prolonged surgery
  - Chronic lung disease
  - Ventilator dependence
  - Antacid therapy
  - Vascular lines
  - Hyperalimentation
  - ICU stay
  - Recent antibiotic therapy
- Clustering of seriously ill patients
  - Often with wounds or drainage of contaminated materials
  - Intensifying probability of cross-infection

PREVENTION STRATEGIES: Hand washing/hand hygiene between all patient contacts is the single most important method of decreasing HAI
- Regular soap and water for at least 15 seconds
- Chlorhexidine (particularly good for gram-positive organisms like methicillin-resistant *Staphylococcus aureus* [MRSA]), alcohol handrub or other antiseptic for resistant organisms
- Purpose of soap and water handwash
  - Degrease hand surfaces
  - Wash away oils and associated bacteria, removal of visible dirt or body fluids
- Procedure
  - Lukewarm water
  - Must include all surfaces
  - Special attention to areas between fingers and to the dirtier dominant hand (most people reflexively wash the cleaner, nondominant hand more vigorously)
- The widespread availability of alcohol-based hand hygiene solutions throughout hospital settings has been shown to improve handwashing frequency (less drying to hands, faster, and no need for wash basin and towels for drying) and to significantly reduce hospital-associated infections; now recommended in essentially all routine health care settings

VANCOMYCIN-RESISTANT *ENTEROCOCCUS FAECIUM* (VREF):
- The percentage of HAIs caused by VREF increased more than twentyfold between 1989 and 1993, rising from 0%, to 3%, to 7%, to 9%. By 2005, VREF, vancomycin-resistant *E. faecalis,* and other vancomycin-resistant species of enterococci had become common and endemic nosocomial pathogens accounting for 15% to 40% of all enterococci isolated in the hospital setting.
- A high percentage of VREF isolated, 80%, are also ampicillin resistant.
- Factors predisposing to VREF colonization or infection include a high percentage of hospital days receiving antibiotic therapy, use of IV, underlying disease, immunosuppression, and abdominal surgery.
- Evidence suggests that vehicle is the hands of medical personnel.
- Control measures:
  - Aggressive isolation of colonized or infected patients
  - Restraint in using broad-spectrum antibiotics

CLOSTRIDIUM DIFFICILE:
- Causes diarrhea as a result of pseudomembranous colitis
- May be transmitted among hospitalized patients
- Warrants contact precautions and bleach for terminal disinfection
- Alcohol-based hand rub may not eliminate spores of this organism so can use soap and water to wash hands at sink

SURVEILLANCE:
- Crucial for early identification of infections:
  - Enables immediate intervention
  - Education
- Prospective, concurrent, hospital surveillance:
  - Electronic data mining provides accurate review
  - Feasible with sophisticated computerized data collection and analysis
- Targeted surveillance address high-risk procedures and patient populations
- Routine rate calculations and statistical analyses:
  - Uses device-specific days or patient-days as denominators
  - Enhances early recognition of microclusters of infections by body site and by organism
  - Facilitates proper early control of potential outbreaks
- Active surveillance cultures for multi-drug resistant organisms (MDROs); for example, high-risk populations for MRSA

DIAGNOSIS

MOST COMMON HAI:
- Urinary tract infections (UTIs) (32%)
- Surgical wound and other soft tissue infections (22%)
- Pneumonia (15%)
- Bloodstream infections (14%)

HOSPITAL-ASSOCIATED UTIs:
- General associations:
  - Foley catheters
  - Inappropriate catheter care (including opening catheter junctions)
  - Female sex
  - Absence of systemic antibiotics
- Physical findings:
  - Fever
  - Dysuria
  - Leukocytosis
  - Pyuria
  - Flank or costovertebral angle tenderness
- Usual organisms:
  - *E. coli*
  - *Klebsiella*
  - *Enterobacter*
  - *Pseudomonas*
  - *Enterococcus*
- Sepsis in 1% to 3% of hospital-associated UTIs
- Prevention:
  - Meticulous technique during insertion and daily perineal care
  - Never open the catheter-collection tubing junction
  - Obtain all specimens using sterile syringe
  - Substitute intermittent catheterization for Foley catheters

HOSPITAL-ASSOCIATED BLOODSTREAM INFECTIONS:
- General associations:
  - IV lines
  - Arterial lines
  - CVP lines: leads to catheter-associated bloodstream infection (CLABSI)
  - Phlebitis
  - Hyperalimentation
- Fever possibly only presenting sign
- Exit site of all vascular lines carefully evaluated for:
  - Erythema
  - Induration
  - Tenderness
  - Purulent drainage
- Usual organism for device-associated bacteremia
  - *S. aureus* (including MRSA)
  - *Staphylococcus epidermidis* for long-term IV lines
  - *Enterobacter*
  - *Klebsiella*
  - *Candida* spp.
  - *Pseudomonas aeruginosa* may come from a water source or reflect cutaneous bacteria
- Phlebitis in 1.3 million patients yearly
- Approximately 10,000 annual deaths from IV sepsis
- Prevention:
  - Meticulous sterile technique during IV insertion.
  - Emphasis should be placed on attention to detail, including hand washing, adherence to guidelines for catheter insertion and maintenance, appropriate use of antiseptic solutions such as chlorhexidine (CHG) for CVPs or chlorhexidine or iodine to prepare the skin around the catheter insertion site, and use of sterile technique for central catheter insertion.
  - Modified catheter may reduce risk for endoluminal colonization and catheter-related sepsis in subclavian lines.
  - Decrease use of routine IVs (patients would rather drink).
  - Avoid using a femoral insertion site. Subclavian site is associated with lower infection rate than jugular.

HOSPITAL-ASSOCIATED PNEUMONIAS:
- More common in ICUs
- General associations:
  - Aspiration
  - Intubation: leads to ventilator-associated pneumonia (VAP)
  - Altered consciousness
  - Old age
  - Chronic lung disease
  - Postsurgery
  - Antacids
  - Head of bed not elevated
- Signs of pneumonia common among patients on general wards:
  - Cough
  - Sputum
  - Fever
  - Leukocytosis
  - New infiltrate on chest x-ray examination
- Signs more subtle in ICUs, because many patients have purulent sputum because of chronic intubation
  - Change in sputum character or volume
  - Small changes on chest x-ray examination
- Usual organisms:
  - *Klebsiella*
  - *Acinetobacter*
  - *Enterobacter*
  - *Pseudomonas aeruginosa*
  - *S. aureus* (including MRSA)
- Less common organisms:
  - *Stenotrophomonas* spp.
  - *Legionella, Flavobacterium*
  - Respiratory syncytial virus (infants)
  - Adenovirus
- 1% of hospitalized patients affected
- Mortality rate high (40%)
- Prevention:
  - Use meticulous sterile technique during suctioning and handling airway.
  - Do not routinely change ventilator breathing circuits and components. For heat and moisture exchangers, no more frequently than q48h.
  - Drain respirator tubing without allowing fluid to return to respirator.
  - Wash hands routinely to prevent colonization of patients and transfer of organisms among patients.

NOSOCOMIAL SOFT TISSUE INFECTIONS:
- Associations:
  - Decubitus ulcers
  - Surgical wound classification (contaminated or dirty-infected)
  - Abdominal surgery
  - Presence of drain
  - Preoperative length of stay
  - Duration of surgery >2 hr
  - Surgeon
  - Presence of other infection
- Physical findings:
  - Decubitus ulcer with fluctuance at margin or under firm eschar
  - Erythema extending >2 cm beyond margin of surgical wound
  - Tenderness
  - Induration
  - Erythema
  - Fluctuance
  - Purulent drainage
  - Dehiscence of sutures
- Usual organisms:
  - *S. aureus* (including MRSA)
  - *Enterococcus*
  - *Enterobacter*
  - *Acinetobacter*
  - *E. coli*
- Prevention:
  - Use careful skin care and frequent, proper positioning of patient to prevent decubitus ulcer.
  - Use meticulous sterile surgical technique.
  - Wash hands to decrease colonization when handling postoperative wound.
  - Limit prophylactic antibiotics to 24 hr perioperatively.
  - Double-wrap contaminated dressings (hold in gloved hand and evert gloves over dressings) before disposal.

LABORATORY TESTS

- Appropriate to specific HAI and specific patient's condition
- Cultures generally indicated for proper confirmation of responsible pathogens:
  - Urine
  - Blood
  - Sputum
  - Soft tissue
- Molecular analysis of nosocomial epidemics:
  - Plasmid fingerprinting
  - Restriction endonuclease digestion (plasmid and genomic DNA)
  - Peptide analysis
  - Immunoblotting
  - Ribosomal RNA (rRNA) typing
  - DNA probes
  - Multilocus enzyme electrophoresis
  - Restriction fragment length polymorphism (RFLP)
  - Polymerase chain reaction (PCR)
  - Provide confirmation of point-source or common strains and corroboration of hypotheses reached utilizing classic epidemiology

IMAGING STUDIES

Rarely needed for diagnosis of HAI

Rx TREATMENT

ACUTE GENERAL Rx

- Appropriate to etiologic organism:
  - Antibiotic
  - Antifungal
  - Antiviral
- Specific therapy determined after careful consideration of resident flora within the microenvironment in which the patient was hospitalized
  - Empiric therapy
    1. Frequently difficult to fashion accurately
    2. Often undesirable, unless the patient's clinical condition requires urgent treatment
  - Consultation for expert advice regarding antibiotic selection in view of known epidemiologic risks within the hospital
    1. Infection preventionist
    2. Hospital epidemiologist
- Avoid unnecessary treatment for organisms that are colonizing but not infecting patients
- Prevention of spread of communicable diseases often requiring isolation or precautions
  - Classic schema (Strict, Respiratory Isolation and Contact [Skin and Wound] Precautions) being replaced by more streamlined Revised Guidelines (Airborne, Droplet, Contact Isolation Precautions, and combinations thereof)
  - Less careful response to some diseases (e.g., hemorrhagic fevers) inadvertently induced by removal of strict isolation category
  - Universal/Standard Precautions and Body Substance Isolation continue within a new Standard Isolation Precautions Guideline
  - Tracking patients of roommates with communicable disease, for example, Norovirus, influenza
- Universal Precautions used for all patients during all contacts with blood, body fluids, or secretions
  - Gloves
  - Goggles/eye shield
  - Impermeable gowns if aerosol or splash is likely
- Consider aggressive isolation to restrict spread of resistant organisms and their plasmids
  - MRSA
  - VREF
  - Highly resistant gram-negative organisms, including extended spectrum β-lactamases (ESBL) gram-negative rods and carbapenem-resistant Enterobacteriaceae (CRE)

DISPOSITION

The infection prevention and control service and/or hospital epidemiologist should be notified when infectious complications occur in the hospital setting; most, but not all, HAIs are potentially avoidable, and every effort should be taken to minimize the risk of infections associated with health care.

REFERRAL

- To infection preventionist
- To hospital epidemiologist

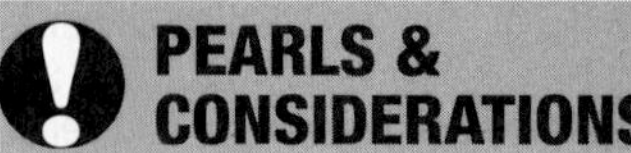

PEARLS & CONSIDERATIONS

COMMENTS

- Sharp and splash injuries to staff are relatively rare, but nearly all are preventable.
  - Nurses incur most injuries.
  - Usual causes:
    1. Needle sticks
    2. Scalpel and surgical needle injuries
    3. Blood splashes
  - Prevention:
    1. Never recap needles.
    2. Dispose of needles only in rigid, impermeable plastic containers.
    3. Clearly announce instrument passes in the operating room or during procedures and use passing trays.
    4. Use needleless systems for vascular access and connectors whenever possible to limit health care workers' use of sharp medical devices.
    5. Use gloves, mask, and goggles/eye shield if aerosol or splash is likely.
    6. Never leave needles or other sharp items in beds.
    7. Never dispose of sharp items in regular trash bags.
  - Infection prevention and control staff should be consulted immediately after exposure to determine need for prophylaxis for hepatitis B or HIV.
  - All clinical staff should be immune to hepatitis B (natural or vaccine).
- Fungi previously considered to be contaminants are now risks for patients with cancer and organ transplantation.
  - *Candida* spp.
    1. *C. guilliermondii*
    2. *C. krusei*
    3. *C. parapsilosis*
    4. *C. tropicalis*
  - *Aspergillus* spp.
  - *Curvularia* spp.
  - *Bipolaris* spp.
  - *Exserohilum* spp.
  - *Alternaria* spp.
  - *Fusarium* spp.
  - *Scopulariopsis* spp.
  - *Pseudallescheria boydii*
  - *Trichosporon beigelii*
  - *Malassezia furfur*
  - *Hansenula* spp.
  - *Microsporum canis*
- Focused, committed efforts by the entire health care staff continuously directed toward prevention.
  - Each HAI addressed as an opportunity to improve the organization and delivery of care
  - Essential that individual staff members understand that small risks applied to large populations result in a large number of total events (i.e., HAI)
- The number of surgical-site *S. aureus* infections acquired in the hospital can be reduced by rapid screening and decolonizing of nasal carriers of *S. aureus* on admission.

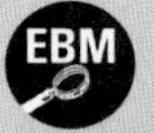

EVIDENCE

Please note: Complete text of EBM for this topic is available online.

Key trials and commentary:

This study sought to determine the effect of an early MRSA detection strategy on nosocomial MRSA infection rates in surgical patients.

This study showed that a universal, rapid MRSA admission screening strategy did not reduce nosocomial MRSA infection in a surgical department with endemic MRSA prevalence but relatively low rates of MRSA infection.[1] Ⓐ

Universal screening for MRSA colonization, early identification of patients colonized with MRSA, and targeted implementation of infection control measures have been recommended by experts and policymakers in an attempt to control MRSA. However, no controlled trial has evaluated the impact of MRSA screening on patient outcome. The strategy of early detection and intervention has been successfully implemented in countries with low prevalence, but reduction of endemic MRSA through universal surveillance has remained controversial. Targeted active surveillance has proven useful in high-risk populations and during outbreaks. This prospective, interventional cohort study is the largest controlled evaluation of the effect of MRSA screening on admission in patients undergoing surgery. The use of a rapid molecular test in this large-scale screening campaign identified 337 previously unknown MRSA carriers. However, the incidence of nosocomial MRSA infections did not decrease during the intervening period (July 2004-May 2006). The trial did not show an added benefit for widespread rapid screening on admission compared with standard MRSA control in preventing nosocomial MRSA infections in a large surgical department. This finding suggests that infection control teams should consider local MRSA epidemiology and patient profiles before embarking on universal MRSA screening.

In this study, the screening was not beneficial to surgical patients because one third of the patients went to surgery before their positive MRSA screening results were known; these patients were not decolonized or given chlorhexidine baths. Initial MRSA screening of surgical patients should be timed whenever possible to allow for consideration of actions to control that MRSA, namely decolonization with mupirocin for five days, daily chlorhexidine baths for five days, and consideration of vancomycin when antibiotic prophylaxis is recommended.

Expansion of active surveillance screening cultures should be done in conjunction with bundled interventions such as hand hygiene, isolation attire usage, and disinfection of both equipment and environment.

Evidence-Based Reference

1. Harbarth S et al: Universal screening for methicillin-resistant Staphylococcus aureus at hospital admission and nosocomial infection in surgical patients, *JAMA* 299:1149-1157, 2008. Commentary by N. Khardori, M.D. Ⓐ

2. Diekema DJ, Climo M: Preventing MRSA infections: finding it is not enough, *JAMA* 299: 1190-1192, 2008.

3. Calfee DP et al: Strategies to prevent transmission of methicillin-resistant Staphylococcus aureus in acute care hospitals, *Infect Control Hosp Epidemiol* 29(Suppl 1): S62-S80, 2008.

SUGGESTED READINGS

Bode LG et al: Preventing surgical-site infections in nasal carriers of Staphylococcus aureus, *N Engl J Med* 362:9-17, 2010.

Centers for Disease Control and Prevention (CDC): Guidelines for hand hygiene in health-care settings. 2002. Available at http://www.cdc.gov/mmwr/PDF/rr/rr5116.pdf. Accessed August 17, 2009.

CDC: Management of multidrug-resistant organisms in healthcare settings, 2006. Available at http://www.cdc.gov/ncidod/dhqp/guidelines.html. Accessed August 26, 2009.

CDC: Guidance for control of infections with carbapenem-resistant or carbapenemase-producing enterobacteriaceae in acute care facilities. Available at http://www.cdc.gov/mmwr/preview/mmwrhtml/mm5810a4.htm. Accessed August 26, 2009.

Darouiche RO et al: Chlorhexidine-alcohol versus povidone-iodine for surgical-site antisepsis, *N Engl J Med* 362:18-26, 2010.

Eriksen HM et al: Prevalence of nosocomial infections and use of antibiotics in long-term care facilities in Norway, 2002 and 2003, *J Hosp Infect* 57(4):316, 2004.

Gastmeier P: Nosocomial infection surveillance and control policies, *Curr Opin Infect Dis* 17(4):295, 2004.

Merle V et al: Knowledge and opinions of surgical patients regarding nosocomial infection, *J Hosp Infect* 60(2): 169, 2005

Scott RD: The direct medical costs of healthcare-associated infection in U.S. hospitals and the benefits of prevention 2009. Available at http://www.cdc.gov/ncidod/dhqp/hai.html. Accessed August 17, 2009.

Society for Healthcare Epidemiology of America (SHEA): Compendium of strategies to prevent HAIs. Available at http://www.shea-online.org/about/compendium.cfm. Accessed August 17, 2009.

Won SP et al: Handwashing program for the prevention of nosocomial infections in a neonatal intensive care unit, *Infect Control Hosp Epidemiol* 25(9):742, 2004.

AUTHORS: **MARLENE FISHMAN, M.P.H., C.I.C., GLENN G. FORT, M.D., M.P.H.,** and **DENNIS J. MIKOLICH, M.D.**

Obesity (PTG) (ALG)

BASIC INFORMATION

DEFINITION

Obesity refers to having an excess amount of body fat in relation to lean body mass, or a body mass index (BMI) of ≥30 kg/m^2. Overweight is defined as BMI of 25 to 29.9 kg/m^2. BMI is used as a surrogate measure of fatness. These conditions result from an imbalance between energy intake and expenditure. Morbid obesity refers to adults with a BMI ≥40 kg/m^2.

SYNONYMS

Overweight

ICD-9CM CODES

278.0 Obesity

EPIDEMIOLOGY & DEMOGRAPHICS

- Obesity has become an epidemic in the U.S. and worldwide; 66% of U.S. adults are overweight.
- Based on data from the 2003-2004 U.S. National Health and Nutrition Examination Survey (NHANES), approximately 66 million American adults (30 million men and 36 million women) are obese and an additional 74 million (42 million men and 32 million women) are overweight.
- The prevalence of individuals who are overweight and obese increases with advancing age until the sixth decade, after which it begins to decline.
- By 2015, it is estimated that two in every five adults and one in every four children in the U.S. will be obese.
- The present cost of obesity in the U.S. population is estimated at $100 billion annually.
- According to the World Health Organization (WHO), in some European countries the prevalence of obesity is as high as 30%.
- For persons with a BMI ≥30 kg/m^2, all-cause mortality is increased by 50% to 100% above that of persons with BMI in the range of 20 to 25 kg/m^2.
- Obesity is associated with cardiac hypertrophy, diastolic dysfunction, and increased aortic stiffness, which are independent predictors of cardiovascular risk.
- Obesity is an independent risk factor for cardiovascular disease (CVD) and CVD risks associated with obesity have also been documented in children.
- Obese individuals are at increased risk of morbidity and death from type 2 diabetes, hypertension, coronary heart disease (CHD), cancer (particularly colon, prostate, and breast cancer), sleep apnea, degenerative joint disease, thromboembolic disorders, digestive tract diseases (gallstones), and dermatologic disorders.
- Significant morbidity and risk of death are projected to begin in young adulthood, resulting in more than 100,000 excess cases of CHD by 2035, even with the most modest projection of future obesity.
- Obesity is a major potentially preventable cause of death and disability in the United States (the other is tobacco).
- Extensive data indicate that weight loss can reverse or arrest the harmful effects of obesity.

PHYSICAL FINDINGS & CLINICAL PRESENTATION

- Physical examination should assess the degree and distribution of body fat and signs of secondary causes of obesity.
- Increased waist circumference is apparent. Excess abdominal fat is clinically defined as a waist circumference >40 inches (>102 cm) in men and >35 inches (>88 cm) in women (in Asian men and women, >36 inches and >33 inches, respectively).
- Symptoms associated with hypertension, coronary artery disease (CAD), and diabetes (e.g., polyuria, polydipsia, retinopathy, and neuropathy) may be present.
- Joint pain and swelling are associated with degenerative joint disease and obesity.
- The physical exam and ECG often underestimate the presence and extent of cardiac dysfunction in obese patient. Jugular venous distention and hepatojugular reflux may not be seen and heart sounds are distant. Obesity is associated with the changes in the ECG such as microvoltage and non specific ST-T changes that may affect the diagnosis of left ventricular hypertrophy (LVH) or CAD.
- A large quantity of fluid is present in the interstitial space of adipose tissue, as the interstitial space is ~10% of the tissue wet weight. Excess fluid in this compartment may have important repercussions in obese individuals with heart failure if this extra volume is redistributed into the circulation. Obese individuals have higher cardiac output and a lower total peripheral resistance than do lean individuals and obesity is associated with persistence of elevated cardiac filling pressure during exercise,
- Cardiomyopathy of obesity (adipositas cordis): excessive epicardial fat and fatty infiltration of the myocardium in the hearts of obese subjects. Thus obesity predisposes to heart failure through different mechanisms, increased total blood volume, increased cardiac output, LVH, left ventricular diastolic dysfunction, and adipositas cordis.

ETIOLOGY

- The pathophysiology of obesity is complex and poorly understood, but includes social, nutritional, physiologic, psychological, and genetic factors.
- Environmental factors such as a sedentary lifestyle and chronic ingestion of excess calories can cause obesity.
- Most human obesity may be related to genetic factors. It is believed that obesity may be polygenic. Genetic studies with adopted children have demonstrated that they have similar BMIs to their biologic parents but not their adoptive parents. Twin studies also demonstrate a genetic influence on BMI.
- Current data also suggest that obesity may spread in social networks in a quantifiable and discernible pattern that depends on the nature of social ties. Moreover, social distance appears to be more important than geographic distance within these networks.

Dx DIAGNOSIS

- BMI will establish the diagnosis of obesity. BMI is a measure of an adult's weight in relation to his or her height—more specifically, the adult's weight in kilograms divided by the square of his or her height—and is closely correlated with total body fat content.
- BMI values can categorize patients into three classes of obesity:
  - Class I (mild): BMI of 30.0 to 34.9 kg/m^2
  - Class II (moderate): BMI of 35.0 to 39.9 kg/m^2
  - Class III (severe): BMI of ≥40 kg/m^2
- Although BMI is commonly used to define obesity, it is not a highly accurate indicator of body fat composition in children, who are undergoing rapid changes in height, or in bodybuilders or athletes who have large amounts of muscle tissue.
- Waist circumference or waist-hip ratio is indicative of visceral adipose tissue, or intraabdominal fat, which may be more deleterious than overall overweight or obesity.

DIFFERENTIAL DIAGNOSIS

It is important to rule out specific causative medical disorders in obese patients. Metabolic syndrome, hypothalamic disorders, hypothyroidism, Cushing's syndrome, insulinoma, depression, diabetes mellitus, and drugs (corticosteroids, antidepressants, second generation antipsychotics, antihistamine agents, antihypertensive agents, and HIV protease inhibitors) can cause obesity.

WORKUP

History should be obtained regarding weight change, family history of obesity, social circles, and eating and exercise behavior. Assessment for eating disorders and depression should be made. Attention should be directed to the use of nutritional supplements, over-the-counter medications, hormones, diuretics, and laxatives. The workup of an obese patient typically requires laboratory work to assess for risks and complications as well as to rule out underlying causative medical conditions.

LABORATORY TESTS

- Obese patients should be assessed for medical consequences of their obesity by screening for metabolic syndrome (measure high density lipoprotein, triglycerides, blood pressure, fasting glucose, and waist circumference).
- In the proper clinical setting, thyroid function studies, dexamethasone suppression testing, morning cortisol level, and insulin level with C-peptide measurements will exclude hypothyroidism, Cushing's syndrome, and insulinoma as underlying causes of obesity.

IMAGING STUDIES

- Several methods are available for determining or calculating total body fat but offer no significant advantage over the BMI. These include measurement of total body water, total body potassium, bioelectrical impedance, and dual-energy x-ray absorptiometry.
- Buoyancy testing is an accurate method for determining total body fat composition.

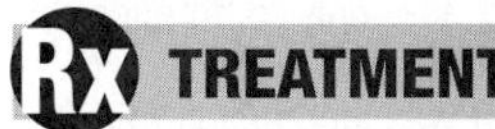

TREATMENT

The National Heart, Lung, and Blood Institute (NHLBI) developed guidelines for selecting treatment strategies for overweight and obese patients based on BMI and comorbidities. They recommend a combination of dietary management, physical activity management, and behavior therapy for anyone with a BMI ≥25. Pharmacotherapy should also be considered for patients with a BMI between 27 and 29.9 with comorbidities and for any patient with a BMI ≥30.

Surgery is indicated for patients with a BMI between 35 and 39.9 with comorbidities and for any patient with a BMI ≥40 (Table 1-57).

NONPHARMACOLOGIC THERAPY

- The cornerstones for weight management and reduction are calorie restriction, exercise, and behavioral modification.
- The NHLBI guidelines recommend an initial diet to produce a calorie deficit of 500 to 1000 kcal/day. This has been shown to reduce total body weight by an average of 8% over 3 to 12 mo.
- These guidelines recommend the use of a food diary to focus on dietary substitutes.
- Thirty minutes of moderate-intensity activity on 5 or more days of the week results in health benefits for obese individuals. Several studies also indicate that 60 to 80 min of moderate to vigorous physical activity can be more beneficial.
- Increased physical activity without caloric restriction (minimal or no weight loss) can reduce abdominal (visceral) adipose tissue and improve insulin resistance.
- The key features of the standard behavioral-modification program include goal setting, self-monitoring, stimulus control (modification of one's environment to enhance behaviors that will support weight management), cognitive restructuring (increased awareness of perceptions of oneself and one's weight), and prevention of relapse (weight regain).

ACUTE GENERAL Rx

- According to the NHLBI *Guidelines on the Identification, Evaluation, and Treatment of Overweight and Obesity in Adults* and the U.S. Food and Drug Administration (FDA), pharmacotherapy is indicated for:
  - Obese patients with a BMI ≥30 *or*
  - Overweight patients with a BMI of ≥27 and concomitant obesity-related risk factors or diseases, such as hypertension, diabetes, or dyslipidemia
- Three general classes of medications are currently approved by the FDA for treating obesity:
  - Sympathomimetic medications approved for long-term use: sibutramine (Meridia) acts as a serotonin norepinephrine reuptake inhibitor and suppresses appetite primarily by increasing satiation.
  - Gastrointestinal lipase inhibitors: orlistat (Xenical) blocks the digestion and absorption of ingested dietary fat. It is a reversible inhibitor of pancreatic, gastric, and carboxyl ester lipases and phospholipase A2, which are required for the hydrolysis of dietary fat in the gastrointestinal tract.
  - Sympathomimetic medications approved for short-term use: phentermine is an amphetamine derivative that increases the amount of norepinephrine in the neuronal cleft, resulting in appetite suppression. Similar drugs include diethylpropion, benzphetamine, and phendimetrazine. In 1997 both dexfenfluramine and fenfluramine were withdrawn from the market because of side effects of valvular heart lesions and pulmonary hypertension.
- Other medications in clinical trials include bupropion (Wellbutrin), topiramate (Topamax), and metformin (Glucophage).

CHRONIC Rx

- According to the NHLBI guidelines, surgical intervention is an option for selected patients with clinically severe obesity (a BMI ≥40 or a BMI ≥35 with comorbid conditions), when patients are at high risk for obesity-associated morbidity or death, and when less invasive methods of weight loss have failed.
- Bariatric surgery for weight loss falls into one of two categories:
  - Restrictive surgeries that limit the amount of food the stomach can hold and slow the rate of gastric emptying. These include vertical banded gastroplasty and laparoscopic adjustable silicone gastric banding (lap banding).
  - Restrictive malabsorptive bypass procedures combine the elements of gastric restriction and selective malabsorption. These include Roux-en-Y gastric bypass (considered the gold standard because of its high level of effectiveness and durability) and biliopancreatic diversion.
- A study on bariatric surgery patients demonstrated a significant reduction in long-term cardiovascular events. Ten-year follow-up estimated relative risk reductions ranging from 18% to 79% according to the Framingham risk score and 8% to 62% with the PROCAM risk score.

DISPOSITION

- The incidence of venous thromboembolism in the upper tertile of BMI was 2.42 times that of the lowest BMI tertile. Obese patients have a higher incidence of postoperative thromboembolic disease in noncardiac surgery.
- Venous insufficiency: in the absence of right heart failure, surgically induced weight loss is effective in correcting the venous stasis disease in the large majority of the patients.
- Perioperative obesity (>140% ideal body weight) may increase morbidity and mortality rates after heart transplantation.
- Weight stable obese subjects have an increased risk of arrhythmias and sudden death even in the absence of cardiac dysfunction in both genders.
- Obesity and the cardiac autonomic nervous system are intrinsically related. A 10% increase in body weight is associated with a decline in parasympathetic tone accompanied by a rise in mean heart rate, and conversely, heart rate declines during weight reduction.
- A 10% weight loss in severely obese patients is associated with significant improvement in autonomic nervous system cardiac modulation. This translates into decreased heart rate and increased heart rate variability (HRV); decreased HRV is associated with increased

TABLE 1-57 Weight-Loss Treatment Guidelines from the National Heart, Lung, and Blood Institute*

	BMI				
Treatment	**25.0-26.9**	**27.0-29.9**	**30.0-34.9**	**35.0-39.9**	**>40.0**
Diet, physical activity, behavioral therapy, or all three	Yes	Yes	Yes	Yes	Yes
Pharmacotherapy†		In patients with obesity-related diseases	Yes	Yes	Yes
Surgery‡				In patients with obesity-related diseases	Yes

*Data are from www.nhlbi.nih.gov/guidelines/obesity/ob_home.htm. These guidelines are generally consistent with those from the American Heart Association, the American Medical Association, the American Diabetic Association, the Obesity Society (Practical Guide), the American Diabetes Association, the American Academy of Family Physicians, the American College of Sports Medicine, and the American Cancer Society. *BMI* denotes body mass index, calculated as the weight in kilograms divided by the square of the height in meters.

†Pharmacotherapy should be considered only in patients who are not able to achieve adequate weight loss with available conventional lifestyle modifications and who have no absolute contraindications for drug therapy.

‡Bariatric surgery should be considered only in patients who are unable to lose weight with available conventional therapy and who have no absolute contraindications for surgery.

 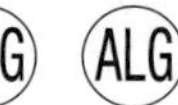

cardiac mortality, independent of ejection fraction.

- Postmortem Determinants of Atherosclerosis in Youth (PDAY) study data provided convincing evidence that obesity in adolescents and young adults accelerates the progression of atherosclerosis decades before the appearance of clinical manifestations.
- Obesity accelerates the progression of native coronary atherosclerosis and after coronary artery bypass grafting.
- In older adults, obesity is associated with protection against hip fracture, but this protective effect on bone status does not offset the extensive array of potential adverse effects on conditions common in the older population.

REFERRAL

- Obesity is commonly seen in the primary care setting. If pharmacologic therapy is considered, consultation with physicians specializing in obesity and experienced with the use of the drug is recommended. In addition, consultation with nutritionists and behavioral therapists is also helpful. A consultation with general surgery is indicated in patients being considered for surgical intervention.
- Recent trials have shown that among adolescents, use of gastric banding compared with lifestyle intervention results in a greater percentage achieving a loss of 50% of excess weight corrected for age. There were associated benefits to health and quality of life.

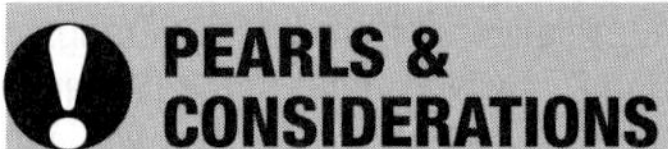

PEARLS & CONSIDERATIONS

COMMENTS

- The NHLBI launched the Obesity Education Initiative in January 1991. The overall purpose of the initiative is to help reduce the prevalence of overweight along with the prevalence of physical inactivity to reduce the risk of CHD and overall morbidity and mortality rates from CHD.
- The American Medical Association produced, with support from the Robert Wood Johnson Foundation, and developed, in collaboration with the U.S. Department of Health and Human Services, a primer for the assessment and management of adult obesity. The primer consists of 10 booklets that offer practical recommendations for addressing adult obesity in the primary care setting.
- Recent research indicates that brown adipose tissue represents a natural target for the modulation of energy expenditure. The presence of brown adipose tissue in humans may be quantified with the use of ^{18}F-FDG PET-CT. The amount of brown adipose tissue is inversely correlated with body mass index, suggesting a potential role of brown adipose tissue in adult human metabolism.
- Obesity, glucose intolerance, and hypertension in childhood are strongly associated with increased rates of premature death from endogenous causes in this population.

PREVENTION

- Prevention of overweight and obesity involves both increasing physical activity and dietary modification to reduce caloric intake.
- There is compelling evidence that prevention of weight regain in formerly obese individuals requires 60 to 90 min of moderate intensity activity or lesser amounts of vigorous intensity activity.
- Moderate intensity activity of approximately 45 to 60 min per day, or 1.7 physical activity level (PAL) is required to prevent the transition to overweight or obesity. For children, even more activity time is recommended.
- Clinicians can help guide patients to develop personalized eating plans and help them recognize the contributions of fat, concentrated carbohydrates, and large portion sizes.
- Clinicians must work with patients to modify other risk factors such as tobacco use, high glycemic intake, and elevated blood pressure to prevent the long-term chronic disease sequelae of obesity.
- Regular screening of body weight and BMI measurements at routine office visits can help identify early weight gain.

PATIENT & FAMILY EDUCATION

Information can be obtained on the American Obesity Association website (http://www.obesity.org) and the American Medical Association website (http://www.ama-assn.org).

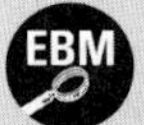

EVIDENCE

Please note: Complete text of EBM for this topic is available online.

Key trials and commentary:

Pulmonary complications following injury significantly contribute to subsequent mortality. Obese patients have preexisting risk factors for pulmonary complications, and are at risk for these complications following elective surgery. Whether or not obesity contributes to pulmonary complications after critical injury is poorly understood.

This study showed that obesity does not appear to be an independent risk factor for increased pulmonary complications after critical injury, but severely obese patients are likely to require longer ICU stays.[1] Ⓐ

One would suspect that obesity would affect outcome during critical illness, but an independent effect of obesity on outcome from critical illness has never been conclusively demonstrated. Early reports suggested that obesity played a large role in determining outcomes in the ICU and after trauma, but more recent reports have suggested no relationship. The conclusions from the literature are limited by mostly retrospective studies and by varying definitions of obesity. The authors of this selection describe the relationship of obesity to pulmonary complications in a large, prospective population of trauma patients with a prevalence of obesity that mirrors the general population. Despite the underlying risk factors for pulmonary complications, the investigators did not detect a difference in pulmonary complications that was related to a patient's body weight. The authors speculate that improvements in the care of the obese patient both in the inpatient and outpatient settings may account for this observation.[1] Ⓐ

This study sought to analyze the influence of severe obesity on mortality and morbidity in mechanically ventilated ICU patients. This study showed that the only difference in morbidity of obese patients who were mechanically ventilated was increased difficulty with tracheal intubation and a higher frequency of postextubation stridor. Obesity was not associated either with increased ICU mortality or with hospital mortality.[2] Ⓐ

Morbid obesity is frequently associated with comorbidities, including cardiovascular, metabolic, and respiratory disorders, which may impair patients' abilities to compensate for the stress associated with critical illness. Many previous studies have shown increased morbidity and mortality in obese patients in the ICU. However, the results derived from many of these studies were retrospective in nature and are extracted from databases. Therefore, the authors prospectively evaluated the influence of morbid obesity on ICU mortality. Their results show that ICU courses were similar in morbidly obese and nonobese patients. However, in obese patients, greater difficulties were encountered during airway management and there was increased frequency of postextubation stridor. The difficulties associated with airway management could be attributed to the anatomic peculiarities associated with obesity such as short neck, large tongue, excessive palatal and pharyngeal soft tissue, a high anterior larynx, and restricted ability to open the mouth. The most surprising finding of this study was that the authors did not find any difference in nosocomial infection rate in obese and nonobese patients from either ventilator-associated pneumonia or catheter-related infection. The explanation for such a "protective" effect of obesity is not clear and does not seem to be related to the underlying disease state, especially when experimental data suggest that obesity is considered as a chronic inflammatory state. In vitro data have suggested that adipose tissue can produce mediators that can modulate inflammatory response.[2] Ⓐ

This study aimed to investigate the effects of calcium supplementation on markers of fat metabolism. This study showed that dairy calcium supplementation in overweight subjects with habitually low calcium intakes failed to alter fat metabolism and energy expenditure under resting conditions and during acute stimulation by caffeine or epinephrine.[3] Ⓐ

The etiology of obesity is multifactorial and involves genetic, environmental, and psychosocial factors. There is good epidemiological evidence linking low calcium intake to increased adiposity. In the first National Health and Nutrition Examination Survey (NHANES I) an inverse relationship was found between dietary calcium intake and body weight. Several other studies supported this finding. Dairy products and calcium supplements both were linked to reduced adiposity, but the effect of calcium supplement on weight is less than that observed with dairy products. Whether decreased adiposity is due to increased calcium intake or to the effect of other nutrients contained in dairy products such as protein, or even due to mild fat malabsorption because of saponification with increased fat excretion, is not clear.

Bortolotti et al investigated the effect of calcium supplementation on fat metabolism in subjects given a low calcium intake (<800 mg/day). They designed a placebo-controlled, crossover experiment in 10 overweight/obese subjects, given 800 mg dairy Ca/placebo for 5 weeks and crossed over after a 10-week washout period. Energy expenditure and fat oxidation were measured by indirect calorimetry, lipolysis was assessed by microdialysis, and gene expression studies were conducted from adipose tissue obtained percutaneously from abdominal subcutaneous stores. Calcium supplementation increased urinary calcium excretion but there was no change in parathyroid hormone levels, resting energy expenditure, fat oxidation, plasma free fatty acid concentrations, or glycerol turnover with calcium supplementation. There was no difference is glycerol turnover after stimulation with caffeine or epinephrine, which would explain a role of calcium in accentuating physiological conditions. The expression of genes involved in lipid metabolism such as hormone-sensitive lipase were not affected by calcium supplementation.

This very elegant study challenges the theory that the observed effect of a low-calcium diet on adiposity is through lipid oxidation. Further studies should be conducted in humans in order to evaluate calcium effect on lipid metabolism in adipocytes and whether its effect is similar in various adipocyte depots (visceral vs. subcutaneous) .[3] Ⓐ

Gastric bypass (GBP) is the most common operation performed in the U.S. for morbid obesity. However, weight loss is poor in 10% to 15% of patients. This study sought to determine the independent factors associated with poor weight loss after GBP. This study showed that gastric bypass results in substantial weight loss in most patients. Diabetes and larger pouch size are independently associated with poor weight loss after GBP.[4] Ⓐ

The beneficial effects of a substantial weight loss through bariatric surgery includes improved metabolic profile, better quality of life, and an increased life span compared to matched obese individuals. Roux-en-Y gastric bypass (RYBG) is the most common bariatric surgery performed in North America. RYBG combines a restrictive and malabsorptive procedure in which a small pouch is created at the proximal part of the stomach and it is anastomosed to the proximal jejunum therefore bypassing part of the stomach, duodenum, and part of the jejunum. The weight loss achieved with RYBG is greater compared to pure gastric restrictive procedures. In spite of the fact that there is an expected weight loss of more that 40% of excess body weight, some patients will lose substantially less weight. Factors associated with a lower weight loss include older age, male sex, greater initial weight and BMI, and the presence of diabetes among others.[4] Ⓐ

Campos et al designed a prospective study in which they investigated whether age, sex, race, marital and insurance status, initial body weight and BMI, comorbidities, surgical procedure (laparoscopic vs. open surgery, pouch area (assessed by swallow studies of the upper gastrointestinal tract on post operative day 1), gastrojejunostomy technique, and alimentary limb length are related to poor weight loss. The authors defined "poor weight loss" as <+40% excess weight loss within 1 year. From the 361 patients recruited, the data from 310 were available for analysis. The mean excess weight loss was 60% (range 8%-117%), and 12.3% of patients had poor weight loss. On univariate analysis, just diabetes and larger pouch size were independently associated with poor weight loss after RYGB.[4] Ⓐ

The relation between pouch size and subsequent weight loss is clear. The problem is standardizing the desired pouch size during surgery, because the pouch size depends on the patient's body habitus and to the surgeon's technique. The reason why diabetic patients lose less weight is less clear. Some plausible explanations are the use of medications that promote weight gain (such as insulin, sulfonylureas, and glitazones), hypoglycemia, and improved glucose control with less glycosuria. On the other hand, a drastic reduction in the need for diabetes medications is seen immediately after surgery, even before any weight loss is achieved. We need more prospective studies to evaluate whether the connection between poor weight loss and diabetes is related to specific medical therapy or hormonal/metabolic factors as shown in the study by Somma et al, in which the authors found that patients with GH and IGF-1 deficiency lose less fat mass after gastric banding.

Weight loss through bariatric surgery reduces overall mortality and induces remission of type 2 diabetes.[5,6] Whether such improvements can also be achieved by pharmacologically induced weight loss with sibutramine [Sibutramine cardiovascular outcome Trial (SCOUT)] or rimonabant[Comprehensive Rimonabant Evaluation Study of Cardiovascular ENDpoints and Outcomes (CRESCENDO)] is under investigation in large outcome trials.

Exercise-induced quality of life improvements is dose dependent and independent of weight loss.[8]

Data support recommendations to limit liquid caloric intake as a mean to accomplish weight loss or avoid excess weight gain.[7]

Evidence-Based References

1. Dossett LA et al: Obesity and pulmonary complications in critically injured adults, *Chest* 134:974-980, 2008. Commentary by D.W. Mozingo, M.D. Ⓐ
2. Frat J-P et al: Impact of obesity in mechanically ventilated patients: a prospective study, *Intensive Care Med* 34:1991-1998, 2008. Commentary by M. Mathru, M.D., F.C.C.P. Ⓐ
3. Bortolotti M et al: Dairy calcium supplementation in overweight or obese persons: its effect on markers of fat metabolism, *Am J Clin Nutr* 88:877-885, 2008. Commentary by R. Ness-Abramof, M.D. Ⓐ
4. Campos GM et al: Factors associated with weight loss after gastric bypass, *Arch Surg* 143: 877-884, 2008. Commentary by R. Ness-Abramof, M.D. Ⓐ
5. Dixon et al: Adjustable gastric banding and conventional therapy for type 2 diabetes; a randomized controlled trial, *JAMA* 299:1547-1560, 2008.
6. Sjostrom et al: Effects of bariatric surgery on mortality in Swedish obese subjects, *N Engl J Med* 357:741-752, 2007.
7. Chen et al: Reduction in consumption of sugar-sweetened beverages is associated with weight loss: the PREMIER trial, *Am J Clin Nutr* 89:1299-306, 2009.
8. Martin et al: Exercise dose and quality of life. A randomized controlled trial, *Arch Intern Med* 169(3): 269, 2009.

SUGGESTED READINGS

DeMaria EJ: Bariatric surgery for morbidly obese, *N Engl J Med* 356:2176, 2008.

Eckel RH: Nonsurgical management of obesity in adults, *N Engl J Med* 358:1941, 2008

Franks PW et al: Childhood obesity, other cardiovascular risk factors, and premature death, *N Engl J Med* 362:485-493, 2010.

Kumanyika SK et al: Population-based prevention of obesity: the need for comprehensive promotion of healthful eating, physical activity, and energy balance. A Scientific Statement from American Heart Association Council on Epidemiology and Prevention, Interdisciplinary Committee for Prevention (Formerly the Expert Panel on Population and Prevention Science), *Circulation* 118:428-464, 2008.

Ludwig DS: Childhood obesity—the shape of things to come, *N Engl J Med* 357:2325, 2007.

Markus P et al; European Society of Hypertension Working Group on Obesity: Obesity-induced hypertension and target organ damage: current knowledge and future directions, *J Hypertens* 27:207-211, 2009.

O'Brien PE et al: Laparoscopic adjustable gastric binding in severely obese adolescents, *JAMA* 303(6): 519-526, 2010.

Poirier P et al: Obesity and cardiovascular disease: pathophysiology, evaluation, and effect of weight loss: an update of the 1997. American Heart Association Scientific Statement on Obesity and Heart Disease from the Obesity Committee of the Council on Nutriition, Physical Activity, and Metabolism, *Circulation* 113:898-918. 2006.

AUTHORS: **SHAHNAZ PUNJANI, M.D.,** and **WEN-CHIH WU, M.D.**

Obsessive-Compulsive Disorder (OCD) (PTG)

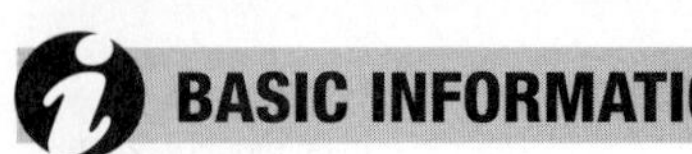

BASIC INFORMATION

DEFINITION

Obsessive-compulsive disorder (OCD) involves recurrent obsessions (intrusive and inappropriate thoughts, impulses, or images) and/or compulsions (behaviors or mental acts performed in response to obsessions or rigid application of rules) that consume >1 hr/day or cause marked impairment or distress. The symptoms are perceived as excessive and unreasonable.

SYNONYMS

Compulsive hoarding, washing, list-making
Intrusive thoughts with ritualized and repetitive behaviors

ICD-9CM CODES
F42.8 Obsessive-compulsive disorder (DSM-IV 300.3)

EPIDEMIOLOGY & DEMOGRAPHICS

PEAK INCIDENCE: Mean age at onset is 19.6 yr.
LIFETIME PREVALENCE (IN U.S.): 2.5% of adults
PREDOMINANT SEX: Approximately equal distribution between sexes
PREDOMINANT AGE:

- Modal age of onset for females is between 20 and 29 yr.
- Modal age of onset for males is between 6 and 15 yr.

DISEASE COURSE:

- Condition is chronic with waxing and waning.
- Symptoms typically worsen with stress.
- 15% show progressive deterioration, whereas 5% show an episodic course with little impairment between episodes.

GENETICS:

- There is no clear genetic pattern.
- Rate of concordance is higher in monozygotic (33%) compared with dizygotic (7%) twins.
- Rate of disorder is also higher in first-degree relatives of individuals with OCD and Tourette's disorder than in the general population.

PHYSICAL FINDINGS & CLINICAL PRESENTATION

- Persistent and recurrent intrusive and egodystonic obsessive ideas, thoughts, impulses, or images that are perceived as alien and beyond one's control.
- Frequent experiencing of obsessions related to contamination (e.g., when using the telephone), excessive doubt (e.g., was the door locked?), organization (the need for a particular order), violent impulses (e.g., to yell obscenities in church), or intrusive sexual imagery.
- Obsessions possibly leading to compulsive behaviors meant to temporarily ameliorate the anxiety caused by obsessions (e.g., repeated hand washing, checking, rearranging), or mental tasks (e.g., counting, repeating phrases).
- Obsessions and compulsions almost always accompanied by high anxiety and subjective distress. Both are seen as excessive and unreasonable.

ETIOLOGY

- Strong evidence of neurobiologic etiology.
- OCD may have onset after infectious illness of central nervous system (e.g., Von Economo's encephalitis, Sydenham's chorea).
- OCD may follow head trauma or other premorbid neurologic condition, including birth hypoxia and Tourette's syndrome.
- Serotonergic pathways believed important in some ritualistic instinctual behaviors, with dysfunction of these pathways possibly giving rise to OCD.

Dx DIAGNOSIS

DIFFERENTIAL DIAGNOSIS

- Obsessive-compulsive personality disorder (OCPD) is a maladaptive personality style defined by excessive rigidity, need for order and control, preoccupation with details, and excessive perfectionism. Unlike OCD, OCPD is ego syntonic.
- Other psychiatric disorders in which obsessive or intrusive thoughts occur (e.g., body dysmorphic disorder, phobias, posttraumatic stress disorder).
- Other conditions in which compulsive or impulse control behaviors are seen (e.g., trichotillomania, gambling, paraphilias).
- Major depression, hypochondriasis, and several anxiety disorders with predominant obsessions or compulsions; however, in these disorders the thoughts are not anxiety provoking or extremes of normal concern.
- Delusions or psychosis, which may be mistaken for obsessive thoughts; unlike OCD, these individuals do not believe their obsessions are unreal and may likely meet criteria for another psychotic spectrum disorder that fully accounts for the obsessions (e.g., schizophrenia).

WORKUP

- Careful history leading to diagnosis
- Typically long delay between symptom onset and treatment
- Neurologic examination to rule out concomitant Tourette's or other tic disorder
- In adolescents and children: psychological testing to reveal learning disabilities

LABORATORY TESTS

No specific tests are indicated.

IMAGING STUDIES

No specific studies are indicated.

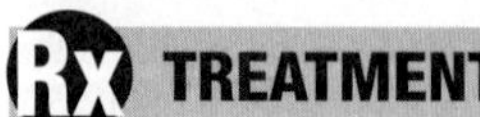

TREATMENT

NONPHARMACOLOGIC THERAPY

- Treatment will help approximately 50% of patients achieve partial remission within the first 6 mo.
- Cognitive-behavioral therapy (especially exposure with response prevention) is successful in up to 70% of patients, but nearly 25% drop out of treatment because of the initial anxiety the exposures create. Best results are found for contamination obsessions and washing compulsions.

ACUTE GENERAL Rx

Clonazepam may be helpful in patients with extreme anxiety or those with a history of seizure disorder.

CHRONIC Rx

- Antidepressants with serotonergic reuptake blockade, including fluoxetine, clomipramine, fluvoxamine, paroxetine, sertraline, venlafaxine, escitalopram, and citalopram; optimal dosages are typically at the high end of the prescription range.
- No response in 15% of patients.
- Indefinite treatment.
- Recent studies suggest that combination cognitive-behavioral therapy and pharmacotherapy yields superior outcomes. More severe symptoms warrant combination therapy.
- Patients with comorbid psychosis and/or tic disorders may benefit from the addition of a neuroleptic.
- Surgical intervention (e.g., cingulotomy) is an option for the most extreme, refractory cases.

DISPOSITION

- Course is chronic with waxing and waning. Symptoms tend to worsen with stress.
- Most mild to moderate cases can be managed on a regular outpatient basis. Treatment should typically start with selective serotonin reuptake inhibitor (SSRI) monotherapy with regular follow-up to assess treatment response and side-effect management. Dose should be increased to maximum tolerated.
- Patient and family education may help improve medical adherence and support.

REFERRAL

- If distinction from other psychiatric conditions, particularly delusional disorder, is not clear
- If patient is refractory to drug treatment and/or requests cognitive-behavioral therapy

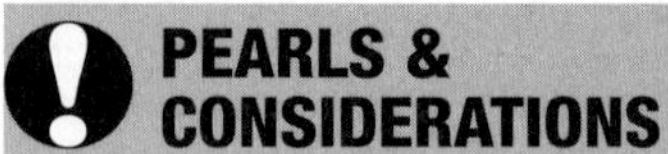

PEARLS & CONSIDERATIONS

Patients with OCD typically have insight regarding the irrationality of their obsessions and compulsions but lack the ability to control them. This may cause intense shame and avoidance of medical care unless patient education and support are provided.

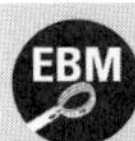

EVIDENCE

SSRIs have been found to be more effective than placebo at reducing symptoms of OCD.[1,2] A

Systematic reviews have also found clomipramine to be more effective than SSRIs (paroxetine, fluoxetine, fluvoxamine, sertraline) in the management of OCD in children and adolescents and more effective than desipramine, imipramine, or nortriptyline. All of the SSRIs were equally effective.[1,3] A

A randomized, controlled trial (RCT) compared fluvoxamine and clomipramine and found no significant difference in symptom severity after 10 wk. Fluvoxamine was better tolerated.[4]

An RCT found no significant difference in symptoms between treatment with venlafaxine and clomipramine at 12 wk. This trial may have been underpowered.[5] B

Both behavioral therapy and cognitive therapy have been found to be significantly more effective than relaxation therapy for the reduction of symptoms in patients with OCD.[6] A

It is unclear if the addition of fluvoxamine to behavioral or cognitive therapy produces superior outcomes.[7,8] However, a recent randomized controlled trial of 108 patients on SSRIs showed that adjunctive cognitive therapy produced significant reductions in OCD symptoms compared with an adjunctive stress reduction intervention.[9]

Evidence-Based References

1. Math SB, Janardhan Reddy YC: Issues in the pharmacological treatment of obsessive-compulsive disorder, *Int J Clin Pract* 61:1188, 2007. A

2. Ackerman DL, Greenland S: Multivariate meta-analysis of controlled drug studies for obsessive-compulsive disorder, *J Clin Psychopharmacol* 22: 309, 2002. A

3. Geller DA et al: Which SSRI? A meta-analysis of pharmacotherapy trials in pediatric obsessive-compulsive disorder, *Am J Psychiatry* 160:1919, 2003. A

4. Mundo E et al: Fluvoxamine in obsessive-compulsive disorder: similar efficacy but superior tolerability in comparison with clomipramine, *Hum Psychopharmacol* 16:461, 2001.

5. Albert U et al: Venlafaxine versus clomipramine in the treatment of obsessive-compulsive disorder: a preliminary single-blind, 12-week, controlled study, *J Clin Psychiatry* 63:1004, 2002. B

6. Abramowitz JS: Effectiveness of psychological and pharmacological treatments for obsessive compulsive disorder: a quantitative review, *J Consult Clin Psychol* 65:44, 1997. A

7. van Balkom AJ et al: Cognitive and behavioral therapies alone versus in combination with fluvoxamine in the treatment of obsessive compulsive disorder, *J Nerv Ment Dis* 186:492, 1998.

8. Hohagen F et al: Combination of behaviour therapy with fluvoxamine in comparison with behaviour therapy and placebo: results of a multicentre study, *Br J Psychiatry* 35(suppl):718, 1998.

9. Simpson HB et al: A randomized, controlled trial of cognitive-behavioral therapy for augmenting pharmacotherapy in obsessive-compulsive disorder, *Am J Psychiatry* 165:621, 2008.

SUGGESTED READINGS

Fineberg NA, Gale TM: Evidence-based pharmacotherapy of obsessive-compulsive disorder, *Int J Neuropsychopharmacol* 8(1):107, 2005.

Harrington P: Obsessive compulsive disorder with associated hypochondriasis, *BMJ* 336(7652):1070-1071, 2008.

Simpson HB et al: A randomized, controlled trial of cognitive-behavioral therapy for augmenting pharmacotherapy in obsessive-compulsive disorder, *Am J Psychiatry* 165(5):621-630, 2008.

AUTHORS: **JASON M. SATTERFIELD, PH.D.,** and **MITCHELL D. FELDMAN, M.D., M.PHIL.**

Ocular Foreign Body

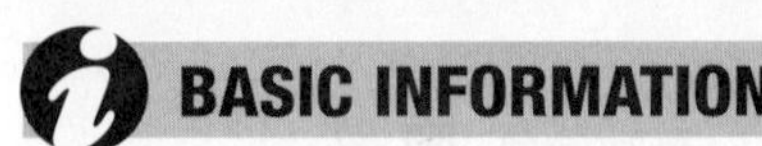

BASIC INFORMATION

DEFINITION

The term *ocular foreign body* refers to a foreign body on the surface of the corneal epithelium.

ICD-9CM CODES
930 Foreign body in external eye

EPIDEMIOLOGY & DEMOGRAPHICS

INCIDENCE (IN U.S.): Universal, with a predominance in active people

PEAK INCIDENCE: Childhood through active adult years

PREDOMINANT SEX: Perhaps slightly more common in men

PREDOMINANT AGE: Childhood through active adult years

PHYSICAL FINDINGS & CLINICAL PRESENTATION

- Pain is most common symptom.
- Causes of most common foreign bodies:
  - Grinding (Fig. 1-218)
  - Drilling
  - Auto repair
  - Working beneath cars
  - Airborne particles, such as blown by fans

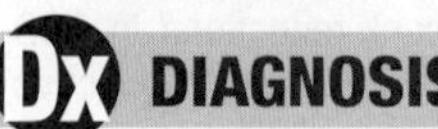

DIAGNOSIS

DIFFERENTIAL DIAGNOSIS

- History of corneal foreign body seen
- Hemorrhage, loss of vision
- Distorted anterior chamber, soft eye
- Corneal abrasion
- Corneal ulceration or laceration
- Glaucoma
- Herpes ulcers
- Infection
- Other keratitis
- Intraocular foreign body

WORKUP

- Fluorescein stain, slit-lamp examination if no foreign body is found
- Ultrasound examination
- Plain radiographs

LABORATORY TESTS

Intraocular pressure to make certain that eye has not been penetrated

IMAGING STUDIES

Occasionally, MRI of the orbits to identify foreign bodies not found by other means. Do not perform MRI if suspect metallic foreign body. Plain radiographs and ultrasound are sufficient.

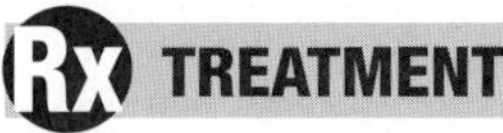

TREATMENT

NONPHARMACOLOGIC THERAPY

- Remove foreign body
- Treat infection
- Repair eye if ruptured
- Treat corneal abrasion or injury

ACUTE GENERAL Rx

- Saline irrigation
- Removal of foreign body with moist cotton-tipped applicator after instillation of topical anesthetic drops
- Use Burr or more aggressive treatment if needed
- Cycloplegics, antibiotics, and pressure dressing after removal of foreign body
- Repair corneal laceration or damaged eye

DISPOSITION

If symptoms persist 24 hr after examination, refer to an ophthalmologist.

REFERRAL

To ophthalmology within 24 hr if patient not completely comfortable

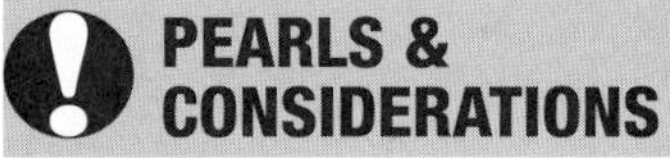

PEARLS & CONSIDERATIONS

COMMENTS

- Make sure foreign body is not intraocular (inside eye).
- Alkaline or acidic chemical foreign bodies can be dangerous; pH test must be performed if either of these is suspected (for all chemical foreign bodies).

SUGGESTED READINGS

Pokhrel P, Loftus SA: Ocular emergencies, *Am Fam Physician* 76:829-836, 2007.

Ta CN, Bowman RW: Hyphema caused by a metallic intraocular foreign body during magnetic resonance imaging, *Am J Ophthalmol* 129(4):533, 2000.

AUTHOR: **MELVYN KOBY, M.D.**

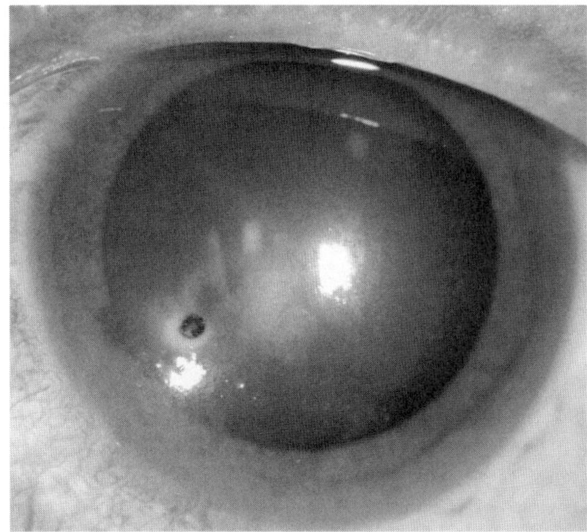

FIGURE 1-218 A small iron foreign body may be seen on external examination. (Courtesy Department of Dermatology, University of North Carolina at Chapel Hill. In Goldstein GB, Goldstein AO: *Practical dermatology,* ed 2, St Louis, 1997, Mosby.)

BASIC INFORMATION

DEFINITION

Onychomycosis is defined as a persistent fungal infection affecting the toenails and fingernails.

SYNONYMS

Tinea unguium
Ringworm of the nails

ICD-9CM CODES
110.1 Onychomycosis

EPIDEMIOLOGY & DEMOGRAPHICS

- Onychomycosis is most commonly found in people between the ages of 40 and 60 yr.
- Onychomycosis rarely occurs before puberty.
- Incidence: 20 to 100 cases/1000 population.
- Toenail infection is 4 to 6 times more common than fingernail infection.
- Onychomycosis affects men more often than women.
- Occurs more frequently in patients with diabetes, peripheral vascular disease, and any conditions resulting in the suppression of the immune system.
- Occlusive footwear, physical exercise followed by communal showering, and incompletely drying the feet predisposes the individual to developing onychomycosis.

PHYSICAL FINDINGS & CLINICAL PRESENTATION

- Onychomycosis causes nails to become thick, brittle, hard, distorted, and discolored (yellow to brown color). Eventually, the nail may loosen, separate from the nail bed, and fall off (Fig. 1-219).
- Onychomycosis is frequently associated with tinea pedis (athlete's foot).

ETIOLOGY

- The most common causes of onychomycosis are dermatophyte, yeast, and nondermatophyte molds.
- The dermatophyte *Trichophyton rubrum* accounts for 80% of all nail infections caused by fungus.
- *Trichophyton interdigitale* and *Trichophyton mentagrophytes* are other fungi causing onychomycosis.
- The yeast *Candida albicans* is responsible for 5% of the cases of onychomycosis.
- Nondermatophyte molds *Scopulariopsis brevicaulis* and *Aspergillus niger,* although rare, can also cause onychomycosis.
- Onychomycosis is classified according to the clinical pattern of nail bed involvement. The main types are:
  1. Distal and lateral subungual onychomycosis (DLSO)
  2. Superficial onychomycosis
  3. Proximal subungual onychomycosis
  4. Endonyx onychomycosis
  5. Total dystrophic onychomycosis

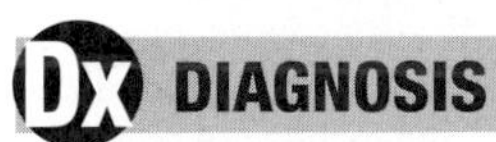

DIAGNOSIS

The diagnosis of onychomycosis is based on the clinical nail findings and confirmed by direct microscopy and culture.

DIFFERENTIAL DIAGNOSIS

- Psoriasis
- Contact dermatitis
- Lichen planus
- Subungual keratosis
- Paronychia
- Infection (e.g., *Pseudomonas*)
- Trauma
- Peripheral vascular disease
- Yellow nail syndrome

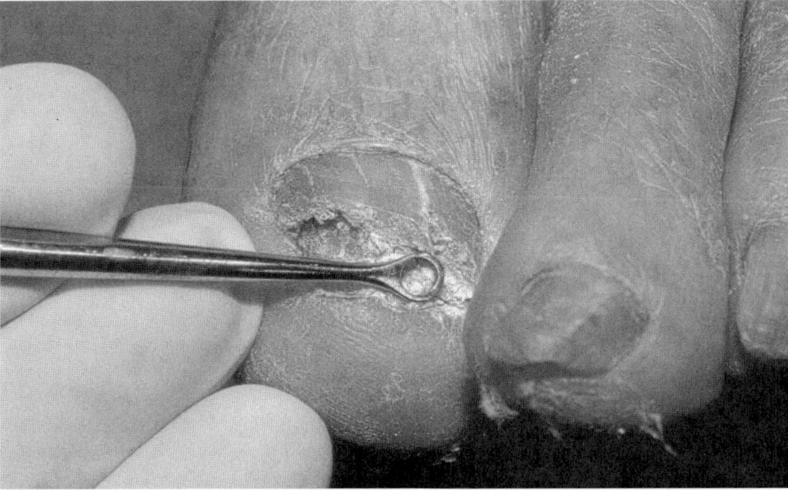

FIGURE 1-219 Collection of nail for culture. The subungual debris is the most valuable material for culture. After cutting back the nail, a curette may be used. Clippings of the nail may be added to the culture. (From White GM, Cox NH [eds]: *Diseases of the skin, a color atlas and text,* ed 2, St Louis, 2006, Mosby.)

WORKUP

The workup of suspected onychomycosis is directed at confirming the diagnosis of onychomycosis by visualizing hyphae under the microscope or by culturing the organism. Although the standard for the diagnosis of fungal nail disease is a positive result on microscopical examination and culture of nail clippings with subungal debris or from surface debris in superficial white onychomycosis, treatment is often prescribed in absence of confirmatory findings.

LABORATORY TESTS

- KOH prep
- Fungal cultures on Sabouraud medium
- Blood tests are not specific in the diagnosis of onychomycosis and therefore not useful

IMAGING STUDIES

- Imaging studies are not very specific in making the diagnosis of onychomycosis and not useful.
- If an infection is present and osteomyelitis is a consideration, an x-ray of the specific area and a bone scan may help establish the diagnosis.

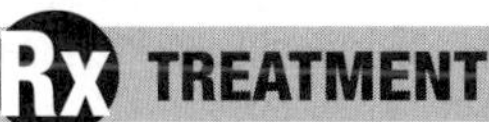

TREATMENT

NONPHARMACOLOGIC THERAPY

- Surgical removal of the nail plate is a treatment option; however, the relapse rate is high.
- Prevention of reinfection by wearing properly fitted shoes, avoiding public showers, and keeping feet and nails clean and dry.

ACUTE GENERAL Rx

- Topical antifungal creams are used for early superficial nail infections.
  1. Miconazole 2% cream applied over the nail plate bid
  2. Clotrimazole 1% cream bid
- Oral agents.
  1. Terbinafine
     a. For toenails: 250 mg/day for 3 mo
     b. For fingernails: 250 mg/day for 6 wk
  2. Itraconazole
     a. For toenails: 200 mg qid for 3 mo
     b. For fingernails: 200 mg PO bid for 7 days, followed by 3 wk of no medicine, for 2 pulses
  3. Fluconazole
     a. For toenails: 150 to 300 mg once weekly, until infection clears
     b. For fingernails: 150 to 300 mg once weekly until infection clears
- All oral agents used for onychomycosis require periodic monitoring of liver function blood tests. Patients should be advised to watch for symptoms of drug-induced hepatitis (anorexia, fatigue, nausea, right upper quadrant pain) while taking these oral antifungal agents. They should stop their medication and contact their physician immediately if symptoms occur.

- Itraconazole is contraindicated in patients taking cisapride, astemizole, triazolam, midazolam, and terfenadine. Statins should be discontinued during itraconazole therapy. Itraconazole requires gastric acidity for absorption; patients should be advised not to take oral antacids, H_2 blockers, or proton pump inhibitors while taking itraconazole.
- Fluconazole is contraindicated in patients taking cisapride and terfenadine.
- Oral antifungal agents should not be initiated during pregnancy.
- Ciclopirox, a topical nail lacquer antifungal agent, is FDA approved for treatment of mild to moderate disease not involving the lunula.

DISPOSITION

- Spontaneous remission of onychomycosis is rare.
- A disease-free toenail is reported to occur in approximately 25% to 50% of patients treated with the oral antifungal agents mentioned previously.

REFERRAL

- Podiatry consultation is indicated in diabetic patients for proper instruction in foot care, footwear, and nail debridement or surgical removal of the toenail.
- Dermatology consultation is indicated in patients refractory to treatment or if another diagnosis is considered (e.g., psoriasis).

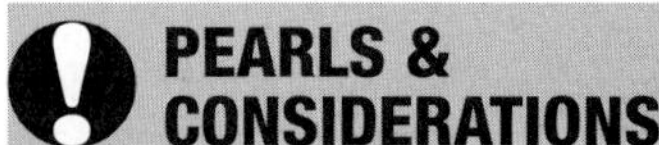

PEARLS & CONSIDERATIONS

COMMENTS

- The growth of fungus on an infected nail typically begins at the end of the nail and spreads under the nail plate to infect the nail bed as well.
- Carefully consider the informational insert regarding drug-drug interactions and contraindications before initiating oral antifungal agents.

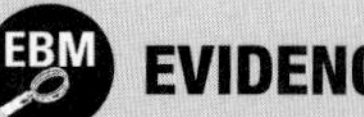

EVIDENCE

Please note: Complete text of EBM for this topic is available online.

Key trials and commentary:

This study estimated the absolute risks of treatment termination and incidence of adverse liver outcomes among all commonly used oral antifungal treatments for superficial dermatophytosis and onychomycosis.

This study showed that oral antifungal therapy against superficial dermatophytosis and onychomycosis, including intermittent and continuous terbinafine, itraconazole, and fluconazole, was associated with a low incidence of adverse events in an immunocompetent population.[1] Ⓐ

I was somewhat surprised (and disappointed) that this article appeared not in a dermatology journal but in a general medical journal. Nevertheless, the results are reassuring. Dermatologists know that oral antifungal agents, specifically oral terbinafine, itraconazole, and fluconazole, are associated with a low incidence of adverse events when used in the treatment of dermatophytosis and onychomycosis. In this study, Chang et al found that pulse therapy was associated with a lower risk of discontinuation because of adverse reactions than was continuous therapy. Overall, fluconazole seemed to have a lower risk of treatment discontinuation because of adverse events. In general, as the dosage of antifungal agents is increased, the incidence of adverse events is increased as well. The overall risk of adverse events was, however, quite low.

Evidence-Based Reference

1. Chang C-H et al: The safety of oral antifungal treatments for superficial dermatophytosis and onychomycosis: a meta-analysis, *Am J Med* 120:791-798, 2007. Commentary by B.H. Thiers, M.D. Ⓐ

SUGGESTED READINGS

Baran R, Kaoukhov A: Topical antifungal drugs for the treatment of onychomycosis: an overview of current strategies for monotherapy and combination therapy, *J Eur Acad Dermatol Venereol* 19(1):21, 2005.

DeBerker D: Fungal nail disease, *N Engl J Med* 360:2108-2116, 2009.

Gupta AK et al: The use of terbinafine in the treatment of onychomycosis in adults and special populations: a review of the evidence, *J Drugs Dermatol* 4(3):302, 2005.

Kulac M et al: Venous insufficiency in patients with toenail onychomycosis, *J Ultrasound Med* 24(8): 1085, 2005.

Romano C, Gianni C, Difonzo EM: Retrospective study of onychomycosis in Italy: 1985-2000, *Mycoses* 48(1):42, 2005.

Sigurgeirsson B, Steingrimsson O: Risk factors associated with onychomycosis, *J Eur Acad Dermatol Venereol* 18(1):48, 2004.

AUTHORS: **GLENN G. FORT, M.D., M.P.H.,** and **DENNIS J. MIKOLICH, M.D.**

BASIC INFORMATION

DEFINITION

- Opioid addiction/dependence is defined as a cluster of cognitive, behavioral, and physiologic symptoms in which the individual continues use of opiates despite significant opiate-induced problems. Opiate dependence is a chronic, relapsing disorder characterized by repeated self-administration that usually results in opiate tolerance, withdrawal, and compulsive drug use. Dependence may occur with or without the physiologic symptoms of tolerance and withdrawal.
- There are four stages of addiction:
  1. Stage I, acute drug effects: rewarding effects of drug result from neurobiologic changes in response to the acute drug use. Duration varies from hours to days.
  2. Stage II, transformation to addiction: associated with changes in neuronal function that accumulate with repeated administration and diminish over days or weeks after discontinuation of drug use.
  3. Stage III, relapse after extended periods of abstinence: precipitated by an incubation of cue-induced craving (people, places, and things as triggers) and priming (relapse precipitated by drug exposure).
  4. Stage IV, end-stage addiction: vulnerability to relapse endures for years and results from prolonged changes at the cellular level.
- Pseudoaddiction: undertreatment of pain resulting in "opiate-seeking" behaviors such as "doctor shopping" and multiple emergency department visits. These behaviors disappear with adequate treatment of pain.

SYNONYMS

Opiate addiction
Opiate abuse
Narcotic addiction
Narcotic abuse

ICD-9CM CODES
304.7X/304.8X Opioid dependence

EPIDEMIOLOGY & DEMOGRAPHICS

INCIDENCE: There are 980,000 opiate addicts in the U.S.; less than one third are in treatment.

PREVALENCE:

- Approximately 6 million persons age ≥12 yr used psychotherapeutic drugs for nonmedical purposes in 2004, which represents 2.5% of the population. Most of them reported abusing opiate pain relievers.
- In 2004, 2.4 million persons age ≥12 yr initiated nonmedical use of prescription pain relievers, surpassing for the first time those who initiated abuse of marijuana (2.1 million).
- Opiate addiction is becoming an adolescent disease. Among twelfth-graders, in 2005, 9.5% reported past-year nonmedical use of oxycodone (Vicodin) and 5.5% reported past-year nonmedical use of oxycodone slow-release tablets (OxyContin).
- The percentage of eighth-, tenth-, and twelfth-graders who have used heroin has more than doubled since the late 1990s. This increase has largely been attributed to decreased price and increased purity in the last decade.

PREDOMINANT SEX: Males abuse opiates more commonly than females, with a male/female ratio of 3:1 for heroin and 1.5:1 for prescription opiates.

PEAK INCIDENCE: The majority of new abusers of opiates are <26 yr.

RISK FACTORS:

- Family history
- Prior history of addiction
- Psychiatric disorders

GENETICS:

- Genetic epidemiologic studies suggest a high degree of heritable vulnerability for opiate dependence.
- Gene polymorphism for dopamine receptor/transporters, opioid receptors, serotonin receptors/transporters, proenkephalin, and catechol-*o*-methyltransferase all appear to be associated with vulnerability to opiate dependence. Future interventions for opiate dependence may include medications identified through genetic research.

PHYSICAL FINDINGS & CLINICAL PRESENTATION

- Physical examination is often noncontributory.
- Small-sized pupils may be the only observable sign of use because only mild tolerance develops for miosis.
- Scars or tracks from chronic IV use may be visible over the veins of the arms, hands, ankles, neck, and breasts.
- Inflamed nasal mucosa or respiratory wheezing may be apparent in patients who are snorting heroin or OxyContin.
- Patients in withdrawal may have more dramatic findings such as tachycardia, hypertension, fever, piloerection (goose flesh), mydriasis, lacrimation, central nervous system (CNS) arousal, irritability, and repeated yawning. In patients with sympathetic overactivity and panic attacks, use of CNS stimulants, such as amphetamines or cocaine, should also be ruled out.
- Although gastrointestinal symptoms of nausea, vomiting, and abdominal pain are common in opiate withdrawal, other causes such as gastroenteritis, pancreatitis, peptic ulcer disease, and intestinal obstruction need to be ruled out.
- The history may provide relevant information in making the diagnosis. Significant findings may include:
  1. A long history of opiate self-administration, typically by the IV or intranasal route but sometimes through smoking as well.
  2. Polysubstance use. Intoxication by drugs other than narcotics (e.g., benzodiazepines, barbiturates) should be ruled out in unconscious patients.
  3. A high incidence of non-opiate-related psychiatric disorders (>80%).
  4. History of problems at work, school, or relationships associated with drug use.
  5. History of legal problems associated with drug use, such as arrest for possession, robbery, or prostitution.
  6. History of interpersonal violence (as perpetrator or victim).
  7. History of physical problems such as skin infections, phlebitis, endocarditis, or liver diseases attributable to acetaminophen toxicity (Vicodin/Percocet) or viral hepatitis. Hepatitis C is the most prevalent blood-borne pathogen. It is present in approximately 90% of opiate-dependent people and is often spread by sharing IV drug paraphernalia or snorting devices. There is also a higher incidence of HIV infection.

ETIOLOGY

Opioid dependence is a biopsychosocial disorder. Pharmacologic, social, genetic, and psychodynamic factors interact to influence abusive behaviors. Pharmacologic factors are especially prominent in opiate addiction because these drugs are strong reinforcing agents because of their euphoric effects and their ability to reduce anxiety and increase self-esteem and the patient's subjective feelings of improved ability to cope with daily challenges.

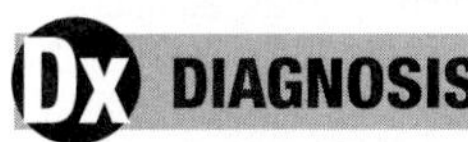

DIAGNOSIS

DIFFERENTIAL DIAGNOSIS

- Psychiatric disorders (e.g., anxiety, depression, bipolar disorder).
- Acute medical illness (e.g., hypoglycemia, seizure disorder, sepsis, renal or hepatic insufficiency) may mimic opiate withdrawal symptoms.

WORKUP

- The history is the most important part of the workup.
- Observation of opiate withdrawal is indicative of opiate addiction.
- Observation of purposeful behaviors such as complaints and manipulations directed at getting more drugs and anxiety during withdrawal is suggestive of opiate addiction.
- Screen blood and urine for opiate metabolites.
- Screen for communicable diseases: HIV, hepatitis B and hepatitis C, tuberculosis.
- Screen for endocarditis in patients with newly diagnosed murmurs.

LABORATORY TESTS

- Urine and serum toxicology screen
- Complete blood count
- Chemistries (alanine aminotransferase, aspartate aminotransferase, serum creatinine): elevated liver function test (LFT) results may be from viral hepatitis or acetaminophen toxicity

 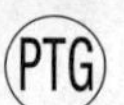

- Hepatitis screen: if hepatitis C antibody positive, follow up with hepatitis C polymerase chain reaction (viral load) even in patients with normal LFTs
- HIV
- PPD

IMAGING STUDIES

Generally not helpful in routine diagnosis and treatment. Consider echocardiography in patients with heart murmurs and liver sonography or CT scan in patients with elevated LFTs or who are positive for hepatitis C or B (increased risk of hepatocellular carcinoma).

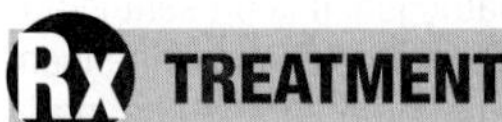

TREATMENT

NONPHARMACOLOGIC THERAPY

- Brief counseling interventions during a visit with their primary care physician or OB/GYN have proven efficacious in motivating patients for treatment.
- Therapeutic communities (residential).
- 12-step or other self-help groups (e.g., Alcoholics Anonymous, Narcotics Anonymous).
- Relapse prevention (counseling).

ACUTE Rx

- Medical withdrawal (not overdosed).
- Short- (30 days) or long-term (30 to 180 days) protocols.
- Buprenorphine (opioid partial agonist) or methadone (opioid agonist) is initiated in tapering doses.
- Clonidine 0.1 mg bid to tid can be used to minimize autonomic symptoms (sweating) and craving.
- Nonsteroidal antiinflammatory drugs for body and muscle aches.
- The anticholinergic dicyclomine can be used to minimize gastrointestinal hyperactivity.
- Nonbenzodiazepine hypnotics, low-dose atypical antipsychotics (e.g., Quetiapine), or low-dose tricyclic antidepressants are effective for promoting adequate sleep.

CHRONIC Rx

Opioid antagonist treatment:

- Naltrexone: does not stabilize neuronal circuitry like partial or full opioid agonists and generally results in poor outcomes, much like Antabuse for alcohol.
- Opioid partial agonist therapy: buprenorphine.
- Opioid agonist therapy: methadone.

NOTE: Buprenorphine and methadone are both metabolized by the cytochrome P450 3a4 and 2d6 I isoenzyme pathways. Prescribers should be aware of multiple possible drug interactions.

PATIENT SELECTION FOR BUPRENORPHINE OR METHADONE

- Appropriate patients for buprenorphine office-based treatment:
  - Patients interested (highly motivated) in treatment
  - Have no major contraindications (see following)
  - Can be expected to be reasonably compliant with treatment
  - Understand the benefits and risks of buprenorphine treatment
  - Willing to follow safety precautions
- Less likely to be appropriate for office-based treatment:
  - Have comorbid dependence on benzodiazepines or other CNS depressants (including ethylene alcohol)
  - Have significant untreated psychiatric comorbidities
  - Have active or chronic suicidal or homicidal ideation or attempts
  - Have multiple previous treatments with frequent relapses
  - Have poor response to previous treatment with buprenorphine
  - Have significant medical complications (e.g., hepatic insufficiency, bacterial endocarditis, active tuberculosis)
- Methadone maintenance: narcotic treatment program (clinic setting) indications
- Evidence of opiate addiction >1 yr
- Two failed previous treatment attempts
- Patients not appropriate for office-based treatment
- Eligible without active "use" if prior methadone maintenance patient within previous 2 mo
- Pregnancy

DISPOSITION

- Opioid addiction is a chronic, relapsing disease.
- High rate of relapse after "detox."
- Relapse potential after medically supervised withdrawal from methadone:
  - 90% after 1 yr stable in treatment
  - 80% after 3 yr stable in treatment
  - 70% after 5 yr stable in treatment

REFERRAL

Refer to addiction medicine specialist or narcotic treatment program when the neurobiologic disease of opioid addiction is identified.

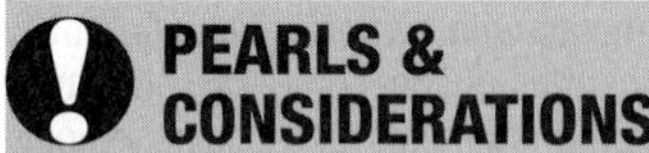

PEARLS & CONSIDERATIONS

COMMENTS

- Methadone maintenance is the gold standard for the pregnant opiate-addicted patient regardless of the duration of the addiction or prior treatment attempts. Detoxification is contraindicated during pregnancy.
- Breastfeeding is encouraged in mothers on methadone maintenance. The American Academy of Pediatrics statement regarding "Transfer of Drugs and Other Chemicals into Human Milk" has placed methadone into the "usually compatible with breastfeeding" group based on the assumption that maternal urine is monitored to detect use of illicit drugs. The U.S. Department of Health and Human Services also recommends that mothers on methadone be encouraged to breastfeed.
- When a physician identifies a patient as a "drug seeker," it is imperative that the physician avoids abruptly stopping the opiate prescription because this will often result in the patient buying the drugs illegally. These patients should be counseled and referred for treatment.
- Patients on methadone or buprenorphine who have pain resulting from an acute injury will need pain medication in addition to their daily dose of methadone or buprenorphine. They will require higher than usual doses of pain medications because of opiate receptor blockade attributable to their methadone or buprenorphine use.
- Opiate-dependent patients have a lower pain threshold resulting from hyperalgesia caused by the long-term use of opiates.

PREVENTION

Education is the hallmark of prevention.

- School drug prevention education programs.
- Educate children about their family medical history, including diseases of addiction.
- Address childhood psychiatric disorders to prevent self-medicating.

PATIENT & FAMILY EDUCATION

- Stigma of addictions and treatment often interferes with good treatment.
- Family needs to be educated so they can support the patient's efforts.
- Encourage family meeting with addiction specialist, counselor.
- Recommend support groups for family members.

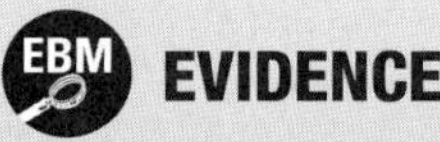

EVIDENCE

Maintenance Treatment

The evidence for the use of naltrexone as a maintenance therapy in people with opioid dependence has been limited because of the small number of trials.[1] B

The evidence for psychosocial interventions in maintenance therapy has been limited by trial sizes and differences. However, systematic reviews have found promising results with some forms of psychosocial therapy used alone or in combination with methadone maintenance therapy.[2,3] B

Treatment of Withdrawal

When tapered methadone was compared with other forms of pharmacologic therapy for opioid withdrawal, a systematic review found that there was no significant difference between treatment methods but that symptoms experienced by subjects differed according to the medication and program used.[4] B

Buprenorphine, when used to manage symptoms of opioid withdrawal, has been found to result in fewer adverse effects and less severe withdrawal symptoms compared with clonidine and a similar effect in terms of completion of therapy to methadone. There is some evidence that withdrawal symptoms resolve faster with buprenorphine than with methadone.[5] Ⓐ

There is some evidence that when naltrexone is used with minimal sedation to initiate withdrawal in people with opioid dependency in combination with an adrenergic agonist, there are more intense but overall less severe withdrawal symptoms than with clonidine or lofexidine alone, but no significant difference in rates of completion of treatment.[6] Ⓐ

There is evidence that clonidine or lofexidine have similar efficacy to reducing doses of methadone when used to manage symptoms of opioid withdrawal, but clonidine may be associated with more adverse effects.[7] Ⓐ

A systematic review found some benefit for the addition of psychosocial therapy to pharmacologic treatment for opioid withdrawal compared with pharmacologic treatment alone. This evidence is limited by the heterogeneity of outcome assessment in the included trials.[8] Ⓑ

Evidence-Based References

1. Minozzi S et al: Oral naltrexone maintenance treatment for opioid dependence, *Cochrane Database Rev* 1, 2006.
2. Amato L et al: Psychosocial combined with agonist maintenance treatments versus agonist maintenance treatments alone for treatment of opioid dependence, *Cochrane Database Rev* 4, 2004.
3. Mayet S et al: Psychosocial treatment for opiate abuse and dependence, *Cochrane Database Rev* 4, 2004.
4. Amato L et al: Methadone at tapered doses for the management of opioid withdrawal, *Cochrane Database Rev* 3, 2005.
5. Gowing L et al: Buprenorphine for the management of opioid withdrawal, *Cochrane Database Rev* 4, 2004.
6. Gowing L et al: Opioid antagonists with minimal sedation for opioid withdrawal, *Cochrane Database Rev* 1, 2006.
7. Gowing L et al: Alpha2 adrenergic agonists for the management of opioid withdrawal, *Cochrane Database Rev* 4, 2004.
8. Amato L et al: Psychosocial and pharmacological treatments versus pharmacological treatments for opioid detoxification, *Cochrane Database Rev* 4, 2004.

SUGGESTED READINGS

Daniel A: Acute pain management for patients receiving methadone or buprenorphine therapy, *Ann Intern Med* 144:127, 2006.

Kalinas PW, Volkow ND: The neural basis of addiction: a pathology of motivation and choice, *Am J Psych* 162:1403, 2005.

Olsen Y, Alford D: Chronic pain management in patients with substance use disorders, *Johns Hopkins Advanced Studies in Medicine* 6:110, 2006.

Sullivan L, Fiellin DA: Narrative review: buprenorphine for opioid-dependent patients in office practice, *Ann Intern Med* 148:662-670, 2008.

Wilford B: *Principles of addiction medicine,* ed 3, Chevy Chase, MD, 2003, American Society of Addiction Medicine.

Woody GE et al: Extended vs short-term buprenorphine-naloxone for treatment of opioid-addicted youth, *JAMA* 300(17):2003-2011, 2008.

AUTHOR: **STEVEN PELIGIAN, D.O.**

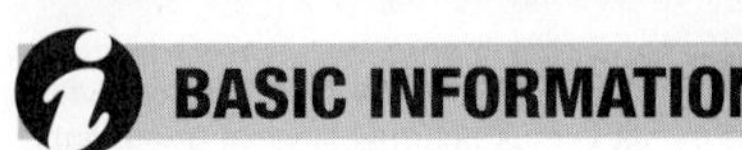

BASIC INFORMATION

DEFINITION

- Optic atrophy refers to the degeneration of the axons of the optic nerve.
- It is a symptom rather than a disease.

SYNONYMS

Unilateral/bilateral optic atrophy

ICD-9CM CODES
377.10 Atrophy, optic nerve

EPIDEMIOLOGY & DEMOGRAPHICS

PREDOMINANT SEX: Unilateral optic atrophy in women is most commonly multiple sclerosis (MS); may also occur after head injury (more commonly in men)
PREDOMINANT AGE: 21 to 40 yr
PEAK INCIDENCE: Varies depending on cause

PHYSICAL FINDINGS & CLINICAL PRESENTATION

- Asymmetry of disc color is often first subtle finding.
- Temporal part of optic disc is pale initially (Fig. 1-220); later the entire disc becomes pale/white.
- Optic disc pallor occurs 4 to 6 wk after optic nerve injury.
- Unilateral lesion produces a relative afferent pupillary defect (RAPD): swing flashlight eye to eye; abnormal pupil dilates to direct light.
- Decreased visual acuity, blurred vision, visual field deficits (e.g., central scotoma), abnormal color vision (e.g., red desaturation).

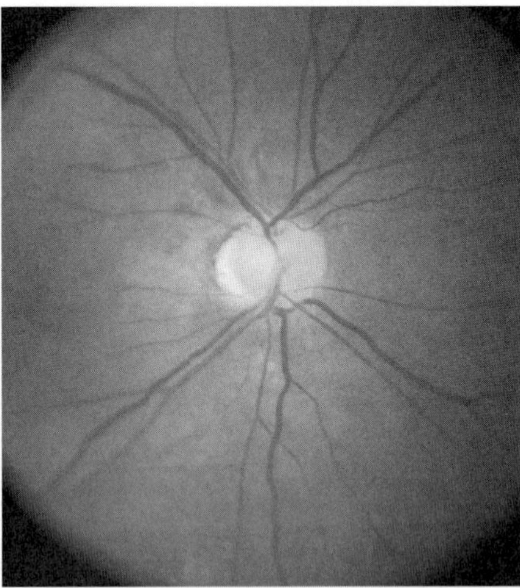

FIGURE 1-220 Optic atrophy. Patient's right eye shows atrophy. (Courtesy John W. Payne, M.D., The Wilmer Ophthalmological Institute, The Johns Hopkins University and Hospital, Baltimore. From Seidel HM [ed]: *Mosby's guide to physical examination,* ed 4, St Louis, 1999, Mosby.)

ETIOLOGY

- Optic neuritis—MS, sarcoidosis, infections (syphilis, CMV, HIV, Lyme disease)
- Vascular—ischemic optic neuropathy, central retinal artery occlusion, temporal arteritis
- Compression—glaucoma, pituitary tumor, meningioma, thyroid eye disease
- Hereditary—Leber's hereditary optic neuropathy
- Nutritional, toxic, and metabolic—Amiodarone, Isoniazid, B_{12} deficiency, tobacco, alcohol
- Trauma

DIAGNOSIS

DIFFERENTIAL DIAGNOSIS

- Nutritional, toxic, and hereditary causes are usually bilateral.
- Unilateral optic atrophy in a young person is more commonly MS.
- Postviral atrophy may be seen in childhood.

WORKUP

- Depends on suspected cause/clinical presentation. History including age of onset, risk factors, acuity of onset of symptoms, trauma, presence of pain, family history, toxic/nutritional factors, and other associated neurologic findings should be considered.
- Visual field testing may help identify cause (e.g., centrocecal field defects may occur with nutritional/toxic causes), but specificity is low.
- To differentiate between optic nerve and macular disease an Amsler chart and/or visual evoked responses may be helpful.
- If high clinical suspicion for MS, consider MRI of brain with contrast, evoked potentials, and LP with oligoclonal bands.
- Measure intraocular pressure (glaucoma).

LABORATORY TESTS

- Depends on suspected cause: none for trauma, tumor, or MS
- Serum B_{12}
- Autoimmune diseases: ESR, ANA, ACE

IMAGING STUDIES

- MRI of the brain with contrast, fat suppression and special (thin) cuts through orbits are necessary to identify compressive lesions in all patients with unexplained optic atrophy; especially important in patients with positive predictive factors for abnormal imaging (e.g., young age, progression, bilateral findings).
- If sarcoid is suspected, order chest x-ray.

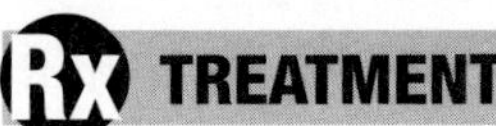

TREATMENT

ACUTE GENERAL Rx

Treat the underlying cause—discontinue identifiable toxins, use B_{12} replacement, neurosurgical intervention is necessary if tumor is found; consider IV steroids if there is evidence for active demyelinating disease.

CHRONIC Rx

The optic nerve does not regenerate, although symptoms often improve.

DISPOSITION

- Visual loss usually occurs over weeks to months.
- Appointment with neurologist or ophthalmologist.

REFERRAL

If tumor or demyelinating lesions are found or if etiology is unknown

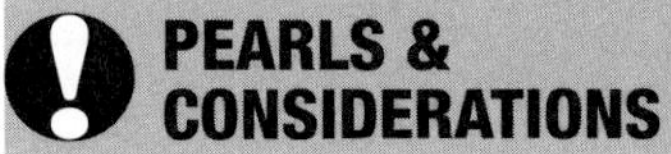

PEARLS & CONSIDERATIONS

COMMENTS

- An experienced clinician should be able to identify pale optic discs and a relative afferent pupillary defect.
- Pupillary dilation with mydriatic agents (e.g., Pilocarpine) may be necessary to optimize funduscopic examination.
- Patient education material can be obtained from the National Eye Institute, Department of Health and Human Services, 9000 Rockville Pike, Bethesda, MD 20892.

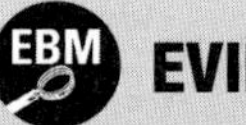

EVIDENCE

Optic atrophy is a syndrome with multiple potential causes, rather than a single disorder, and there are no randomized, controlled clinical trials for the diagnosis or treatment of this syndrome.

SUGGESTED READINGS

Lee AG et al: The diagnostic yield of the evaluation for isolated unexplained optic atrophy, *Ophthalmol* 112(5):757, 2005.

Newman NJ, Biousse V: Hereditary optic neuropathies, *Eye* 18(11):1144, 2004.

Van Stavern GP, Newman NJ: Optic neuropathies. An overview, *Ophthalmol Clin North Am* 14(1):61, 2001.

AUTHOR: **RICHARD S. ISAACSON, M.D.**

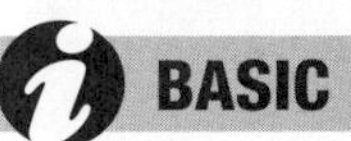

BASIC INFORMATION

DEFINITION

Optic neuritis is an inflammation of the optic nerve resulting in impaired visual function.

SYNONYMS

Optic papillitis
Retrobulbar neuritis

ICD-9CM CODES
377.3 Optic neuritis

EPIDEMIOLOGY & DEMOGRAPHICS

INCIDENCE (IN U.S.): 1 to 5/100,000 person(s) per year; rates vary according to incidence of multiple sclerosis (MS).
PREVALENCE (IN U.S.): Common in patients with MS.
PREDOMINANT SEX: Female/male ratio: 1.8:1
PEAK INCIDENCE: 20 to 49 yr, mean 30.
GENETICS: MS is more common in patients with certain HLA blood types and in monozygotic twins of affected siblings. See topic "Multiple Sclerosis."

PHYSICAL FINDINGS & CLINICAL PRESENTATION

- Presents with acute or subacute (days) visual loss and most often tenderness with movement of affected eye.
- Marcus Gunn pupil (relative afferent pupillary defect [RAPD]): direct and consensual response is normal; however, when swinging flashlight from eye to eye, the affected eye's pupil dilates to direct light.
- Decreased visual acuity.
- Unilateral visual field abnormalities—often a central scotoma.
- Color desaturation, red is most often affected.
- Normal orbit and fundus; occasionally there is disc edema acutely (Fig. 1-221), uveitis, or periphlebitis.

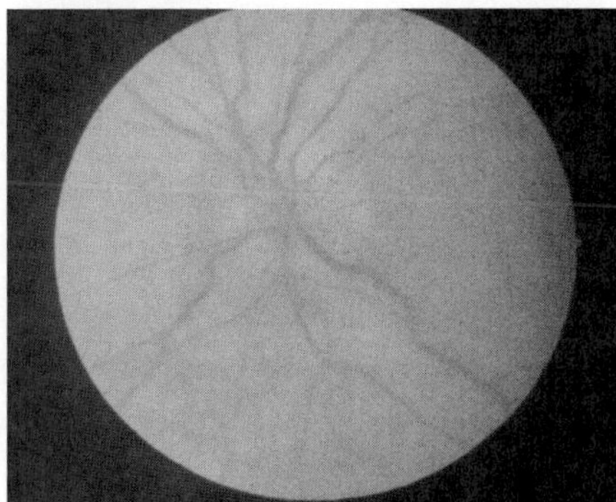

FIGURE 1-221 A case of optic neuritis. The optic disc edema seen here is often not present. Note the otherwise normal fundus. (Courtesy of J. Barton, M.D., Beth Israel Deaconess Medical Center, Boston.)

- May have movement or light-induced phosphenes (flashes of light lasting 1 to 2 sec).
- Uhthoff's phenomenon (benign exercise- or heat-induced deterioration of vision) is seen in some. Vision may also worsen in bright sunlight.
- Over time the optic disc may atrophy and become pale.

ETIOLOGY

An inflammatory response associated with an infection, autoimmune disease (such as MS), or, rarely, a mitochondrial disorder.

DIAGNOSIS

Consistent clinical presentation and exclusion of alternate ocular pathology, infection, and CNS mass lesions. Classic triad includes loss of vision, pain, and dyschromatopsia. 70% unilateral and 30% bilateral.

DIFFERENTIAL DIAGNOSIS

- Inflammatory: MS, neuromyelitis optica, sarcoidosis, lupus, Sjögren's, Behçet's, postinfectious, postvaccination
- Infectious: syphilis, TB, Lyme disease, Bartonella, HIV, CMV, herpes
- Ischemic: giant cell arteritis, anterior and posterior ischemic optic neuropathies, diabetic papillopathy, branch or central retinal artery or vein occlusion
- Mitochondrial: Leber's hereditary optic neuropathy
- Mass lesion: pituitary tumor, aneurysm, meningioma, glioma, metastases, sinus mucocele
- Ocular: optic drusen, retinal detachment, vitreous hemorrhage, uveitis, posterior scleritis, neuroretinitis, maculopathies and retinopathies
- Toxic: B_{12} deficiency, tobacco-ethanol amblyopia, methanol or ethambutol intoxication (painless, most bilateral, typically slowly progressive)
- Other: acute papilledema, retinal migraine, factitious visual loss

WORKUP

A thorough neurologic examination; recommend dilated ophthalmoscopy.

LABORATORY TESTS

- Recommend CBC, ANA, ESR.
- Consider HIV Ab, Lyme titer, ACE, RPR, LHON mtDNA mutations.

IMAGING STUDIES

MRI of the brain and orbits (thin section fat-suppressed T_2-weighted) with gadolinium is needed to look for compressive and infiltrative causes. Often enhancement of the optic nerve is seen. The risk to develop MS can also be assessed.

TREATMENT

NONPHARMACOLOGIC THERAPY

Assure patient that in most cases there is near complete recovery of vision.

ACUTE GENERAL Rx

Not all ophthalmologists and neurologists recommend treatment, but treat if the visual loss is severe or if there is an abnormal MRI (higher risk of MS). Consider methylprednisolone (MP) 250 mg IV every 6 hr for 3 days followed by an oral prednisone taper of 11 days. MP 1 g IV every day for 3 days followed by a prednisone taper is an alternative.

CHRONIC Rx

None, unless at high risk to develop MS. See topic "Multiple Sclerosis."

DISPOSITION

Most often vision is worst at the end of week 1, followed by recovery over several months. In the Optic Neuritis Treatment Trial (ONTT), 90% had 20/40 or better vision at 1 yr and 3% had 20/200 or worse. Of initial 20/200 or worse cases, only 5% remained in that group at 6 mo.

REFERRAL

- To neurologist if patient has other neurologic signs; urgently needed if proptosis or ophthalmoplegia present.
- To ophthalmologist when atypical features or slowly progressive, and urgently when other ocular pathology is present.
- To ophthalmologist if vision worsens or does not improve after several wk, severe or persistent pain, or deteriorates as steroids are tapered.

PEARLS & CONSIDERATIONS

- Bilateral optic neuritis, especially with poor recovery, suggests possible Leber's hereditary optic neuropathy or toxic optic neuropathies.
- Acute bilateral loss with a severe headache or diplopia should raise concern for pituitary apoplexy.

SUGGESTED READINGS

Beck R et al: High and low risk profiles for the development of MS within 10 years after optic neuritis, *Arch Ophthalmol* 121(7):944, 2003.
Beck R et al: Visual function more than 10 years after optic neuritis, *Am J Ophthalmol* 137:77, 2004.
Hickman S et al: Management of acute optic neuritis, *Lancet* 360:1953, 2002.

AUTHOR: **ALEXANDRA DEGENHARDT, M.D.**

Orchitis (PTG)

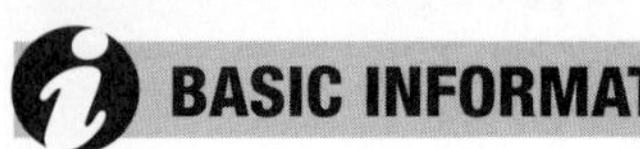

DEFINITION

Orchitis is an inflammatory process (usually infectious) involving the testicles. Infection may be viral or bacterial and can be associated with infection of other male sex organs (prostate, epididymis, or bladder) or lower urogenital tract or sexually transmitted diseases often via hematogenous spread. Common causes are:

- Viral: Mumps—20% postpubertal; coxsackie B virus
- Bacterial: Pyogenic via spread from involving epididymis; bacteria include *Escherichia coli, Klebsiella pneumoniae, P. aeruginosa, Staphylococcus, Streptococcus* or *Rickettsia, Brucella* spp.
- Other:
  - Viral—HIV-associated, CMV
  - Fungi
    1. Cryptococcosis
    2. Histoplasmosis
    3. *Candida*
    4. Blastomycosis
  - *Mycobacterium tuberculosis* and *M. leprae*
  - Parasitic causes: toxoplasmosis, filiariasis, schistosomiasis

SYNONYMS

Epididymoorchitis
Testicular infection
Testicular inflammation

ICD-9CM CODES	
0.72	Mumps
098.13	Acute gonococcal orchitis
095.8	Syphilitic orchitis
016.50	Tuberculous orchitis, unspecified

EPIDEMIOLOGY & DEMOGRAPHICS

PREDOMINANT SEX: Male

PREDOMINANT ORGANISM: The leading cause of viral orchitis is mumps. The mumps virus rarely causes orchitis in prepubertal males but involves one or both testicles in nearly 30% of postpubertal males.

PHYSICAL FINDINGS & CLINICAL PRESENTATION

- Testicular pain, unilateral or bilateral swelling
- May have associated epididymitis, prostatitis, fever, scrotal edema, erythema cellulitis
- Inguinal lymphadenopathy
- Acute hydrocele (bacterial)
- Rare development: abscess formation, pyocele of scrotum, testicular infarction
- Spermatic cord tenderness may be present

Dx DIAGNOSIS

Clinical presentation as described previously with possible history of acute viral illness or concomitant epididymitis.

DIFFERENTIAL DIAGNOSIS

- Epididymoorchitis-gonococcal
- Autoimmune disease
- Vasculitis
- Epididymyosis
- Mumps, with or without parotitis
- Neoplasm
- Hematoma
- Spermatic cord torsion

LABORATORY TESTS

- CBC with differential
- Urinalysis
- Viral titer—mumps
- Urine culture
- Ultrasound of testicle to rule out abscess

IMAGING STUDIES

Ultrasound if abscess suspected

Rx TREATMENT

- Dependent on cause
- Viral (mumps): observation; bed rest, ice packs, analgesics, and a scrotal sling for support may provide some relief of discomfort that accompanies mumps orchitis
- Bacterial: empiric antibiotic treatment with parenteral antibiotic treatment until pathogen identified: ceftriaxone (250 mg IM once) plus doxycycline (100 mg PO bid for 10 days), ofloxacin (300 mg PO bid for 10 days), ciprofloxacin (500 mg PO bid or 400 mg IV bid)
- Surgery for abscess, pyogenic process

DISPOSITION

Follow-up for evidence of recurrence, hypogonadism, and infertility may be needed with bilateral orchitis.

REFERRAL

- To a urologist if surgical drainage is needed
- To an endocrinologist if hypogonadism develops
- To a fertility specialist if infertility develops

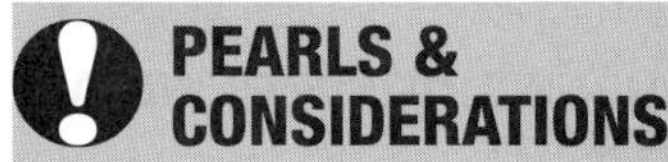

Consider tuberculous orchitis if symptoms fail to respond to standard antibacterial therapy, even in the absence of chest radiographic evidence of pulmonary tuberculosis.

SUGGESTED READINGS

Niizuma T et al: Elevated serum C-reactive protein in mumps orchitis, *Pediatr Infect Dis J* 23(10):971, 2004.

Rajagopal AS: Pseudomonas orchitis in puberty, *Int J STD AIDS* 15(10):707, 2004.

AUTHORS: **GLENN G. FORT, M.D., M.P.H.,** and **DENNIS J. MIKOLICH, M.D.**

BASIC INFORMATION

DEFINITION

Orthostatic hypotension (OH) is defined as the presence of at least one of the following: a decrease in systolic blood pressure by ≥20 mm Hg or a decrease in diastolic blood pressure by ≥10 mm Hg within 3 min of standing. It is a physical sign that requires further investigation to discern its underlying etiology.

SYNONYMS

Postural hypotension

ICD-9CM CODES

458.0 Orthostatic hypotension

EPIDEMIOLOGY & DEMOGRAPHICS

- The incidence of OH is increased in older people.
- OH may cause up to 30% of all syncopal events in the elderly, and OH is associated with an increased risk of cardiovascular disease and all-cause mortality among those aged 55 yr and older.

PHYSICAL FINDINGS & CLINICAL PRESENTATION

- Symptoms may include dizziness, lightheadedness, syncope, visual and auditory disturbances, weakness, diaphoresis, pallor, and nausea. OH may also be asymptomatic, especially in older hypertensive patients.
- Associated with increased autonomic activity during meals (from increased splanchnic blood flow), exercise, and hot weather.
- Supine and nocturnal hypertension in patients with OH may indicate an underlying autonomic dysfunction.

ETIOLOGY

- The assumption of an upright posture results in the pooling of approximately 500 ml of blood in the lower extremities due to gravity and leads to decreased venous return, decreased cardiac output, and decreased arterial pressure. The consequent increase in sympathetic tone due to increased carotid baroreceptor activity causes arterial and venous constriction as well as positive inotropic and chronotropic effects, thereby limiting the fall in blood pressure in the upright position. Peripheral vasoconstriction is also mediated by increased activity of the renin-angiotensin system and decreased activity of atrial natriuretic factor.
- Impairment of the baroreceptor reflex, as in central or peripheral autonomic dysfunction and aging, may cause OH because decreased blood pressure cannot be counteracted by the aforementioned regulatory mechanisms.

Dx DIAGNOSIS

DIFFERENTIAL DIAGNOSIS

Common:

- Medications: antihypertensives, antidepressants (tricyclics), antipsychotics (phenothiazines), alcohol, narcotics, barbiturates, insulin, nitrates, PDE-5 inhibitors, alpha-adrenergic antagonists
- Reduced intravascular volume (hemorrhage, dehydration, hyperglycemia, hypoalbuminemia)
- Postprandial effect (especially in the elderly)
- Vasovagal syncope
- Deconditioning
- Central autonomic dysfunction (Parkinson's disease)
- Peripheral autonomic dysfunction (diabetes mellitus, Guillain-Barré syndrome)

Uncommon:

- Central autonomic dysfunction (Shy-Drager syndrome)
- Postganglionic autonomic dysfunction: impaired norepinephrine release
- Autoimmune autonomic dysfunction: nicotinic acetylcholine receptor autoantibodies
- Paraneoplastic autonomic dysfunction: anti-Hu antibodies (in small cell lung cancer)
- Postural tachycardia syndrome (POTS): usually occurs in young women; an abnormally large increase in heart rate is observed in the upright position caused by increased venous pooling from autonomic dysfunction of the lower extremities, but blood pressure is not affected because of an excess of plasma norepinephrine
- Impaired cardiac output (myocardial infarction, aortic stenosis, arrhythmias)
- Cerebrovascular accident
- Adrenal insufficiency
- Deconditioning
- Carotid sinus hypersensitivity
- Anxiety, panic attacks
- Seizures
- Sepsis
- Idiopathic

WORKUP

- Measure supine blood pressure after the patient has been resting comfortably to ensure stability of the supine blood pressure measurement, stand for 3 min, then measure upright blood pressure. The blood pressure cuff must be held at the level of the right atrium; holding the cuff below this level will result in a 5 to 10 mm Hg underestimation of blood pressure.
- Thorough neurologic examination should be performed.
- Rule out treatable causes (e.g., medications, volume depletion).

LABORATORY TESTS

- Hemoglobin and hematocrit
- Consider when treatable causes of OH have been ruled out:
  - Blood pressure and heart rate monitoring with a tilt table test
  - Plasma norepinephrine measurements (to distinguish postganglionic from preganglionic autonomic dysfunction)
  - Other methods, which use the Valsalva maneuver or measure sweating as indirect means of evaluating the autonomic nervous system

IMAGING STUDIES

None

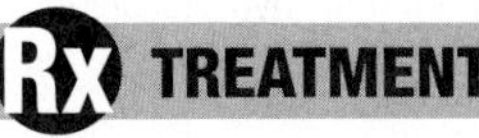

Rx TREATMENT

NONPHARMACOLOGIC THERAPY

- Patient education (leg crossing, prolonged sitting before first standing in the morning, avoid excessive straining and hot baths)
- High-salt diet (e.g., bouillon cubes); caution if history of heart failure
- Liberal fluid intake
- Take needed antihypertensive medications at different times of the day
- Raise the head of the bed at night
- Compression stockings (to include splanchnic circulation)
- Multiple low-carbohydrate meals to avoid postprandial orthostatic hypotension
- Avoid large carbohydrate loads and excess alcohol consumption

ACUTE GENERAL Rx

- Correction of volume status
- Review medication list and attempt to eliminate medications potentially contributing to OH

CHRONIC Rx

- Fludrocortisone: 0.1 mg/day (may combine with an alpha-1 agonist to lower the dose of each); monitor for electrolyte disturbances and supine hypertension
- Midodrine (alpha-1 agonist): 10 mg three times a day; monitor for supine hypertension
- Erythropoietin (consider if anemic)
- Caffeine (for postprandial hypotension)

OTHER TREATMENTS

- Pyridostigmine (enhances renal sodium reabsorption): 0.2 to 0.6 mg/day (not FDA approved for this indication)
- Octreotide: 300 to 600 mg/day (not FDA-approved for this indication)
- Indomethacin (prostaglandin inhibitor)
- DDAVP (experimental)

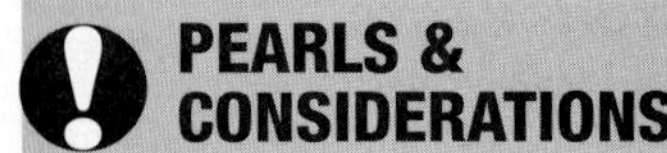

PEARLS & CONSIDERATIONS

COMMENTS

- The presence of OH should always trigger a search for an underlying etiology.
- OH is diagnosed by observing changes in blood pressure, not by observing changes in heart rate.
- Volume depletion should cause an increased heart rate on standing; a lack of heart rate response in this setting suggests autonomic dysfunction.
- Pharmacotherapy with mineralocorticoids may require concomitant potassium replenishment and monitoring for hypertension.
- The etiology of OH is often multifactorial in older patients, but increased susceptibility to volume depletion due to decreased baroreceptor reflexes frequently contributes.
- The physical examination of patients with dizziness, gait disturbance, and/or falls should include an assessment for OH.
- Because OH may be asymptomatic, physical examination of those at risk must include assessment of blood pressure in both the supine and upright positions.

SUGGESTED READINGS

Bradley J, Davis K: Orthostatic hypotension, *Am Fam Physician* 68:2393-2398, 2003.

Bush D: Syncope. In Pompei P, Murphy J (eds): Geriatrics review syllabus: a core curriculum in geriatric medicine, ed 6, New York, 2006, American Geriatrics Society, pp. 168-173.

Freeman R: Neurogenic orthostatic hypotension, *N Engl J Med* 358:615-624, 2008.

Gupta V, Lipsitz LA: Orthostatic hypotension in the elderly: diagnosis and treatment, *Am J Med* 120:841-847, 2007.

Jacob G et al: The neuropathic postural tachycardia syndrome, *N Engl J Med* 343:1008, 2000.

Verwoert G et al: Orthostatic hypotension and risk of cardiovascular disease in elderly people: the Rotterdam study, *JAGS* 56:1816-1820, 2008.

Wieling W, Schatz I. The consensus statement on the definition of orthostatic hypotension: a revisit after 13 years, *J Hypertens* 27: 935-938, 2009.

AUTHOR: **TIMOTHY W. FARRELL, M.D.**

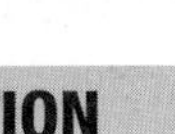

BASIC INFORMATION

DEFINITION

Osgood-Schlatter disease is a painful swelling of the tibial tuberosity that occurs in adolescence.

ICD-9CM CODES
732.4 Osgood-Schlatter disease

EPIDEMIOLOGY & DEMOGRAPHICS

PREVALENCE: Four cases per 100 adolescents
PREDOMINANT SEX: Male/female ratio of 3:1
PREDOMINANT AGE: 11 to 15 yr (bilateral in 20%)

PHYSICAL FINDINGS & CLINICAL PRESENTATION

- Pain at the tibial tubercle aggravated by activity, especially stair-walking and squatting
- Tender swelling and enlargement of the tibial tubercle
- Increased pain with knee extension against resistance

ETIOLOGY

- Unknown
- May be traumatically induced inflammation

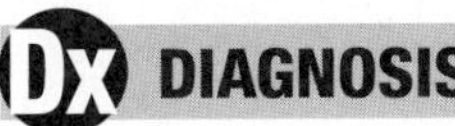

DIAGNOSIS

DIFFERENTIAL DIAGNOSIS

- Referred hip pain (any child with hip pain should have a thorough clinical hip examination)
- Patellar tendinitis

WORKUP

In most cases, the diagnosis is obvious on a clinical basis.

IMAGING STUDIES

- Lateral roentgenogram of the upper portion of the tibia with the leg slightly internally rotated may reveal variable degrees of separation and fragmentation of the upper tibial epiphysis (Fig. 1-222).
- Fragmented area occasionally fails to unite to the tibia and persists into adulthood.

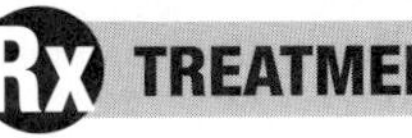
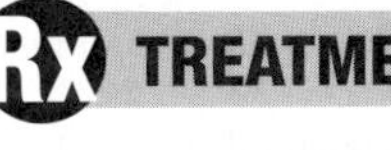

TREATMENT

ACUTE GENERAL Rx

- Ice, especially after exercise
- Nonsteroidal antiinflammatory drugs
- Gentle hamstring and quadriceps stretching exercises
- Abstinence from physical activity
- Temporary immobilization in a knee splint for 2 to 4 wk in resistant cases

DISPOSITION

- Prognosis for complete restoration of function and relief from pain is excellent.
- Condition usually heals when the epiphysis closes.
- Complications are rare.
- Symptoms in the adult:
  1. Although unusual, prominence of the tibial tubercle is usually permanent
  2. May be more susceptible to local irritation, especially when kneeling
  3. Rarely, nonunion of the epiphyseal fragment, but it is usually asymptomatic
  4. Surgery rarely required

REFERRAL

For orthopedic consultation when diagnosis is uncertain or when symptoms persist.

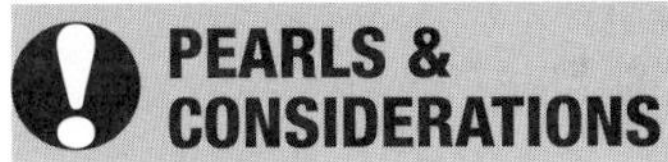

PEARLS & CONSIDERATIONS

COMMENTS

Larsen-Johansson disease is a similar disorder that can develop where either the quadriceps or patellar tendon inserts into the patella. Treatment and prognosis are the same as with Osgood-Schlatter disease.

SUGGESTED READINGS

Bloom OJ et al: What is the best treatment for Osgood-Schlatter disease? *J Fam Pract* 53(2):153, 2004.

Cohen DA, Hinton RY: Bilateral tibial tubercle avulsion fractures associated with Osgood-Schlatter's disease, *Am J Orthop* 37:92, 2008.

Dupuis CS et al: Injuries and conditions of the extensor mechanism of the pediatric knee, *Radiographics* 29:877, 2009.

Duri ZA et al: The immature athlete, *Clin Sports Med* 21(3):461, 2002.

Frank JB et al: Lower extremity injuries in the skeletally immature athlete, *J Am Acad Orthop Surg* 15(6):356, 2007.

Gholve PA et al: Osgood Schlatter syndrome, *Curr Opin Pediatr* 19(1):44, 2007.

Hirano A et al: Magnetic resonance imaging of Osgood-Schlatter disease: the course of the disease, *Skeletal Radiol* 31(6):334, 2002.

Ross MD, Villard D: Disability levels of college-aged men with history of Osgood-Schlatter disease, *J Strength Cond Res* 17(4):659, 2003.

AUTHOR: **LONNIE R. MERCIER, M.D.**

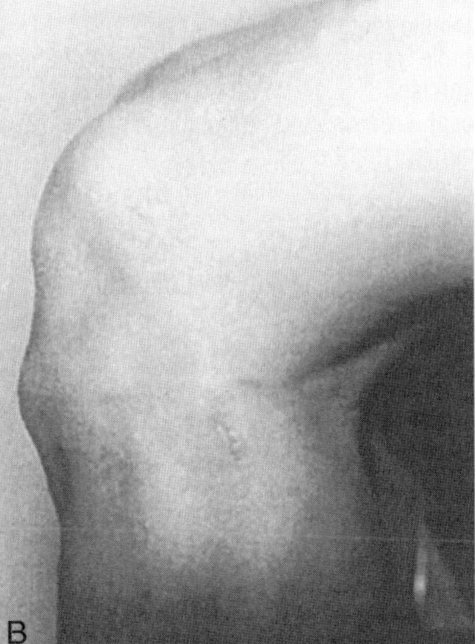

FIGURE 1-222 **A,** Radiograph of Osgood-Schlatter disease demonstrating thickening of patella tendon, fragmentation of the tibial tubercle, and soft tissue swelling. **B,** Clinical picture of bony prominence anteriorly at the tibial tubercle. (From Scuderi G [ed]: *Sports medicine: principles of primary care,* St Louis, 1997, Mosby.)

O

Diseases and Disorders I

Osteoarthritis

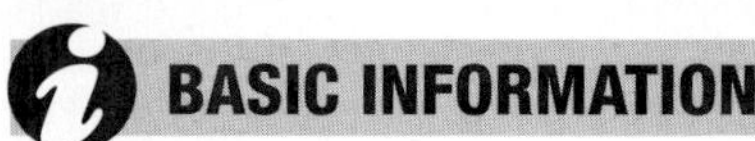

BASIC INFORMATION

DEFINITION

Osteoarthritis is a joint condition in which degeneration and loss of articular cartilage occur, leading to pain and deformity. Two forms are usually recognized: primary (idiopathic) and secondary. The primary form may be localized or generalized.

SYNONYMS

Degenerative joint disease
Osteoarthrosis
Arthrosis

ICD-9CM CODES
715.0 Osteoarthrosis and allied disorders

EPIDEMIOLOGY & DEMOGRAPHICS

PREVALENCE: 2% to 6% of general population
PREDOMINANT SEX: Females and males affected equally
PREDOMINANT AGE: >50 yr

PHYSICAL FINDINGS & CLINICAL PRESENTATION

- Similar symptoms in most forms: stiffness, pain, crepitus
- Joint tenderness, swelling
- Decreased range of motion
- Crepitus with motion
- Bony hypertrophy
- Pain with range of motion
- Distal interphalangeal joint involvement, possibly leading to development of nodular swellings called Heberden's nodes (Fig. 1-223)
- Proximal interphalangeal joint involvement, possibly leading to development of nodular swellings called Bouchard's nodes

ETIOLOGY

Primary osteoarthritis is of unknown cause. Secondary osteoarthritis may result from a number of disorders, including trauma, metabolic conditions, and other forms of arthritis.

DIAGNOSIS

DIFFERENTIAL DIAGNOSIS

- Bursitis, tendinitis
- Radicular spine pain
- Inflammatory arthritides
- Infectious arthritis

WORKUP

- No diagnostic test exists for degenerative joint disease.
- Laboratory evaluation is normal.
- Rheumatoid factor, erythrocyte sedimentation rate, complete blood count, and antinuclear antibody tests may be required if inflammatory component is present.
- Synovial fluid examination is generally normal.

IMAGING STUDIES

- When knee is involved with pain, radiographs should always be taken with the patient standing.
- Roentgenographic evaluation (Fig. 1-224) reveals:
  1. Joint space narrowing
  2. Subchondral sclerosis
  3. New bone formation in the form of osteophytes

TREATMENT

- Rest, restricted use or weight bearing, heat
- Walking aids such as a cane (often helpful for weight-bearing joints)
- Suitable footwear
- Gentle range of motion and strengthening exercise
- Local creams and liniments to provide a counterirritant effect
- Education, reassurance
- Arthroscopic surgery for osteoarthritis of the knee provides no additional benefit to optimized physical and medical therapy.

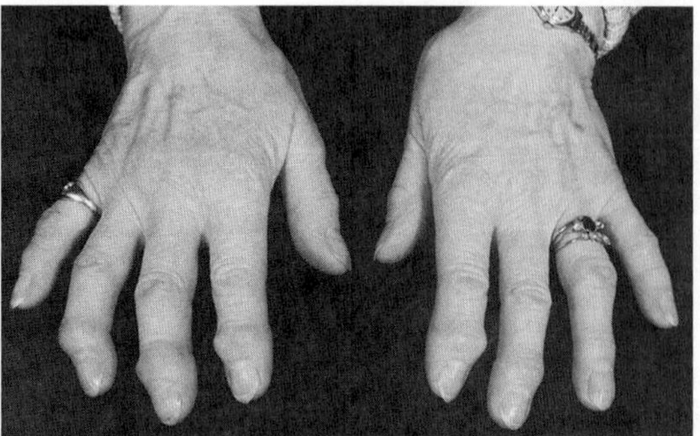

FIGURE 1-223 Osteoarthritis of the distal interphalangeal (DIP) joints. This patient has the typical clinical findings of advanced osteoarthritis of the DIP joints, including large, firm swellings (Heberden's nodes), some of which are tender and red because of associated inflammation of the periarticular tissues and the joint. (From Klippel J et al [eds]: *Primary care rheumatology,* London, 1999, Mosby.)

ACUTE GENERAL Rx

- Mild analgesics for joint pain
- Nonsteroidal anti-inflammatory drugs (NSAIDs) if inflammation is present
- Occasional local corticosteroid injections
- Mild antidepressants, especially at night, if depression is present
- Viscosupplementation (injection of hyaluronic acid products into the degenerative joint) is of uncertain benefit
- Nutritional supplements (glucosamine and chondroitin) are unproven

DISPOSITION

Progression is not always inevitable, and the prognosis is variable depending on the site and extent of the disease.

REFERRAL

Surgical consultation for patients not responding to medical management

PEARLS & CONSIDERATIONS

COMMENTS

Surgical intervention is generally helpful in degenerative joint disease. Arthroplasty, arthrodesis, and realignment osteotomy are the most common procedures performed. Arthroscopic debridement (of the knee) appears to be of questionable value.

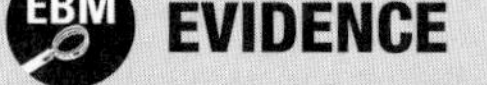

EVIDENCE

Evidence for pharmacological therapy.
There is some evidence for the effectiveness of acetaminophen compared with placebo in the treatment of pain caused by osteoarthritis, although NSAIDs may be slightly more effective.[1,2] Ⓐ

There is limited evidence for the efficacy of intraarticular corticosteroid injections in the short-term treatment of osteoarthritic knee pain.[3-5] Ⓑ

Evidence for surgical treatment.
There is good evidence for the effectiveness of joint replacement as a treatment in osteoarthritis.[6] Ⓐ Ⓑ

Evidence for complementary therapies.
A recent RCT found that acupuncture as a complementary therapy to pharmacologic treatment of osteoarthritis of the knee was more effective than pharmacologic treatment alone, in terms of reducing pain and rigidity, and improving physical functioning and health related quality of life. More evidence is needed.[7] Ⓑ

Evidence-Based References

1. Zhang W et al: Does paracetamol (acetaminophen) reduce the pain of osteoarthritis?: a meta-analysis of randomised controlled trials, *Ann Rheum Dis* 63:901-907, 2004. Ⓐ

2. Wegman A et al: Nonsteroidal anti-inflammatory drugs or acetaminophen for osteoarthritis of hip or

knee? A systematic review of evidence and guidelines, *J Rheumatol* 31:344-354, 2004. Ⓐ

3. Godwin M, Dawes M: Intra-articular steroid injections for painful knees: systematic review with meta-analysis, *Can Fam Physician* 50:241-248, 2004. Ⓑ

4. Arroll B, Goodyear-Smith F: Corticosteroid injections for osteoarthritis of the knee: meta-analysis, *BMJ* 328:869-870, 2004. Ⓑ

5. Steroid injections for OA knee, *Bandolier Journal* 123, 2004. Ⓑ

6. How good is a joint replacement? *Bandolier Journal* 122, 2004. Ⓐ Ⓑ Article

7. Vas J, Mendez C et al: Acupuncture as a complementary therapy to the pharmacological treatment of osteoarthritis of the knee: randomised controlled trial, *BMJ* 329:1216, 2004. Ⓑ

SUGGESTED READINGS

Bedson J, Croft PR: The discordance between clinical and radiographic knee osteoarthritis: a systematic search and summary of the literature, *BMC Musculoskeletal Disord* 9:116, 2008.

Bijsterbosch et al: Illness perceptions in patients with osteoarthritis: Change over time and association with disability, *Arthritis Rheum* 61:1054, 2009.

Callahan JJ et al: Results of Charnley total hip arthroplasty at a minimum of thirty years, *J Bone Joint Surg Am* 86A:690, 2004.

Hartofilakidis G, Karachalios T: Idiopathic osteoarthritis of the hip: incidence, classification and natural history of 272 cases, *Orthopedics* 26:161, 2003.

Kelly MA et al: Osteoarthritis and beyond: a consensus on the past, present and future of hyaluronans in orthopedics, *Orthopedics* 26:1064, 2003.

Kirkley A et al: A randomized trial of arthroscopic surgery for osteoarthritis of the knee, *N Engl J Med* 359:1097, 2008.

Leopold S et al: Corticosteroid compared with hyaluronic acid injections for the treatment of osteoarthritis of the knee, *J Bone Joint Surg* 85:1197, 2003.

Lo HG: Intra-articular hyaluronic acid in treatment of knee osteoarthritis, *JAMA* 290:3115, 2003.

O'Connor MI: Sex differences in osteoarthritis of the hip and knee, *J Am Acad Orthop Surg* 15(suppl 1):S22, 2007.

Ottaviani RA et al: Inflammatory and immunological responses to hyaluronan preparations: study of a murine biocompatibility model, *J Bone Joint Surg Am* 89A:148, 2007.

Pollo FE, Jackson RW: Knee bracing for unicompartmental osteoarthritis, *J Am Acad Orthop Surg* 14:5, 2006.

Ramsey DK et al: A mechanical theory for the effectiveness of bracing for medial compartment osteoarthritis of the knee, *J Bone Joint Surg Am* 89:2398, 2007.

Reichenbach S et al: Meta-analysis: chondroitin for osteoarthritis of the knee or hip, *Ann Intern Med* 146:580, 2007.

Rozendaal RM et al: Effect of glucosamine sulfate on hip osteoarthritis, *Ann Intern Med* 148:268, 2008.

Salk RS et al: Sodium hyaluronate in the treatment of osteoarthritis of the ankle: a controlled, randomized double-blind study, *J Bone Joint Surg Am* 88A: 295, 2006.

Saltzman CL et al: Impact of comorbidities on the measurement of health in patients with ankle osteoarthritis, *J Bone Joint Surg Am* 88A:2366, 2006.

Schimizu M et al: Clinical and biochemical characteristics after intra-articular injection for the treatment of osteoarthritis of the knee: prospective randomized study of sodium hyaluronate and corticosteroid, *J Orthop Sci* 15:51, 2010.

Wang C et al: Therapeutic effects of hyaluronic acid in osteoarthritis of the knee, *J Bone Joint Surg Am* 86A:538, 2004.

Wegman A et al: Nonsteroidal antiinflammatory drugs or acetaminophen for osteoarthritis of the hip or knee? A systematic review of evidence and guidelines, *J Rheumatol* 31:344, 2004.

AUTHOR: **LONNIE R. MERCIER, M.D.**

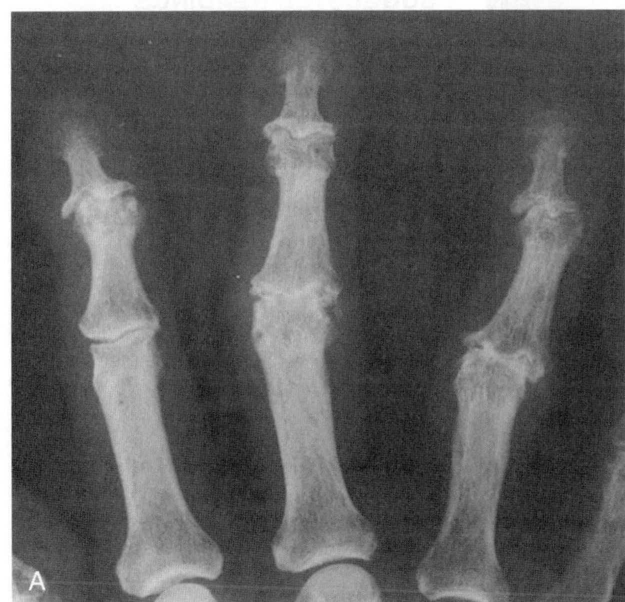

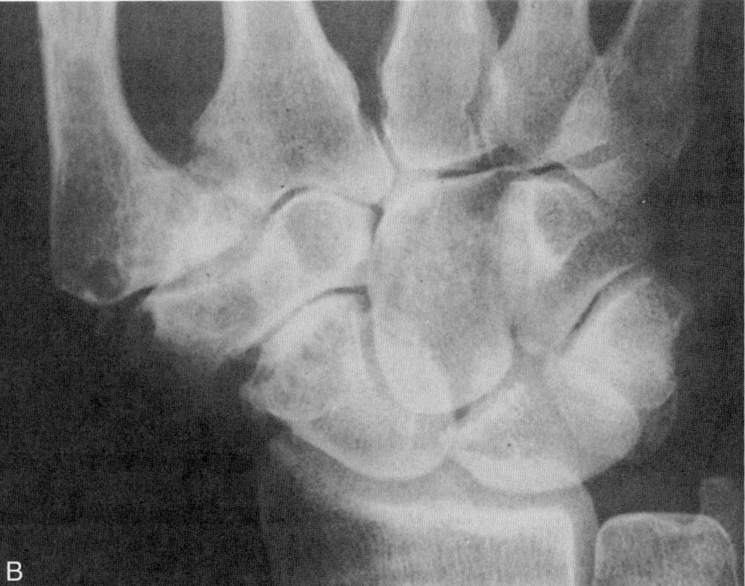

FIGURE 1-224 Osteoarthritis (degenerative joint disease). A, Primary osteoarthritis of the fingers with characteristic cartilage loss, deviations, and spurs of the proximal (Bouchard's nodes) and distal (Heberden's nodes) interphalangeal joints. **B,** Primary osteoarthritis of the carpus showing characteristic involvement of the radial side with cartilage loss, subchondral sclerosis, and small spur formation from the base of the first metacarpal to the distal articular surface of the scaphoid. (From Grainger RG, Allison D: *Grainger & Allison's diagnostic radiology, a textbook of medical imaging,* ed 4, 2001, Churchill Livingstone.)

Osteochondritis Dissecans 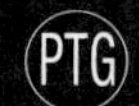

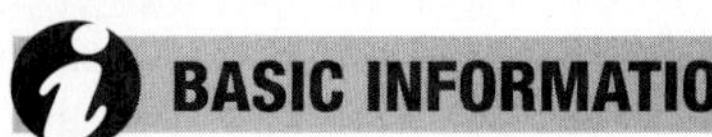

BASIC INFORMATION

DEFINITION

Osteochondritis dissecans is a disorder in which a portion of cartilage and underlying subchondral bone separates from a joint surface and may even become detached.

SYNONYMS

Osteochondrosis
Talar dome fracture: commonly used in describing the lesion of the talus
Panner's disease (capitellum)

ICD-9CM CODES
732.7 Osteochondritis dissecans

EPIDEMIOLOGY & DEMOGRAPHICS

PREVALENCE: 0.3 cases per 1000 persons
PREDOMINANT SEX: Male/female ratio of 3:1
PREDOMINANT AGE: Onset at 10 to 30 yr
The most common joint affected is the knee, with the lateral surface of the medial femoral condyle the most frequent area involved. The capitellum of the humerus, dome of the talus, shoulder, and hip may also be affected.

PHYSICAL FINDINGS & CLINICAL PRESENTATION

- Pain, stiffness, and swelling
- Intermittent locking if the fragment becomes detached
- Occasionally palpable loose body
- Tenderness at the site of the lesion
- When the knee is involved, positive Wilson's sign (pain with knee extension and internal rotation)
- Some asymptomatic cases

ETIOLOGY

Unknown

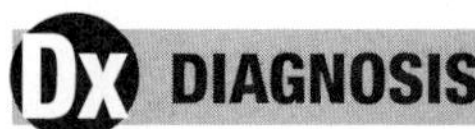

DIAGNOSIS

DIFFERENTIAL DIAGNOSIS

- Acute fracture
- Neoplasm

IMAGING STUDIES

- Plain roentgenography to confirm the diagnosis (Fig. 1-225)
- "Tunnel view" helpful in knee cases
- Typical finding: radiolucent, semilunar line outlining the oval fragment of bone (but findings variable depending on the amount of healing and stability)
- MRI or bone scanning usually not necessary in establishing diagnosis but helpful in determining prognosis and management, especially regarding stability of the lesion

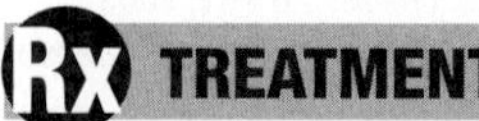

TREATMENT

ACUTE GENERAL Rx

- Observation every 4 to 6 mo for patients in whom the lesion is asymptomatic
- Symptomatic patients who are skeletally immature:
  1. Observation with an initial period of non–weight bearing for 6 to 8 wk (in knee cases)
  2. When symptoms subside, gradual resumption of activities

DISPOSITION

- Juvenile cases with open epiphyses have a favorable prognosis.
- Cases developing after skeletal maturity are more likely to develop osteoarthritis.
- Large fragments, especially those in weight-bearing areas, have a more unfavorable prognosis, especially if they involve the lateral femoral condyle.

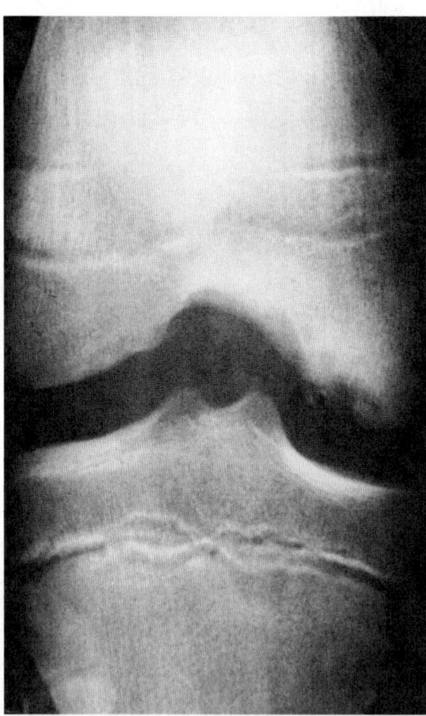

FIGURE 1-225 Osteochondritis dissecans of the knee. The "tunnel" view is often helpful in visualizing the defect. This fragment may become detached and form a loose body. This area should not be confused with the normal irregularity of the distal femoral epiphysis in young children.

- Loose body formation and degenerative joint disease are more common when condition develops after age 20 yr.

REFERRAL

For orthopedic consultation:
- For most adults with unstable lesions
- If a loose body is present
- If symptomatic care has failed

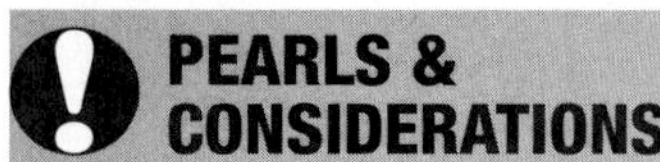

PEARLS & CONSIDERATIONS

COMMENTS

- Although inflammation is suggested by the name, it has not been shown to be of significance in this disorder. *Osteochondral lesion* or *osteochondrosis dissecans* may be more appropriate terms to describe these disorders.
- Repetitive trauma with ischemic necrosis is the most likely cause.
- The condition is often bilateral, especially in the knee, which could suggest the possibility of an endocrine or genetic basis.
- This condition should always be considered in the patient whose "sprained ankle" does not improve over the usual course of treatment.

SUGGESTED READINGS

Bramer JA et al: Increased external tibial torsion and osteochondritis dissecans of the knee, *Clin Orthop* 422:175, 2004.

Crawford DC, Safran MR: Osteochondritis dissecans of the knee, *J Am Acad Orthop Surg* 14:90, 2006.

Frank JB et al: Lower extremity injuries in the skeletally immature athlete, *J Am Acad Orthop Surg* 15: 356, 2007.

Hanna SA et al: Bicondylar osteochondritis dissecans in the knee: a report of two cases, *J Bone Joint Surg* 90:232, 2008.

Kobaynsh K et al: Lateral compression injuries in the pediatric elbow. Panner's disease and osteochondritis dissecans of the capitellum, *J Am Acad Orthop Surg* 12:246, 2004.

Maffulli N et al: Long-term health outcomes of youth sports opportunities, *Br J Sports Med* 44:21, 2010.

Peh WC: Osteochondritis dissecans, *Am J Orthop* 33(1): 46, 2004.

Perumal V et al: Juvenile osteochondritis dissecans of the talus, *J Pediatr Orthop* 27:821, 2007.

Takahara M et al: Classification, treatment and outcome of osteochondritis dissecans of the humeral capitellum, *J Bone Joint Surg Am* 89A:1205, 2007.

Wall EJ et al: The healing potential of stable juvenile osteochondritis dissecans knee lesions, *J Bone Joint Surg Am* 90:2655, 2008.

AUTHOR: **LONNIE R. MERCIER, M.D.**

BASIC INFORMATION

DEFINITION

Osteomyelitis is an acute or chronic infection of the bone secondary to the hematogenous or contiguous source of infection or direct traumatic inoculation, which is usually bacterial.

SYNONYMS

Bone infection

ICD-9CM CODES
730.1 Chronic osteomyelitis
730.2 Acute or subacute osteomyelitis

EPIDEMIOLOGY & DEMOGRAPHICS

PREDOMINANT SEX: Male > female
PREDOMINANT AGE: All ages

PHYSICAL FINDINGS & CLINICAL PRESENTATION

HEMATOGENOUS OSTEOMYELITIS:

- Usually occurs in tibia/fibula (children)
- Localized inflammation: often secondary to trauma with accompanying hematoma or cellulitis
- Abrupt fever
- Lethargy
- Irritability
- Pain in involved bone

VERTEBRAL OSTEOMYELITIS:

- Usually hematogenous.
- Fever: 50%
- Localized pain/tenderness
- Neurologic defects: motor/sensory

CONTIGUOUS OSTEOMYELITIS:

- Direct inoculation.
- Associated with trauma, fractures, surgical fixation
- Chronic infection of skin/soft tissue
- Fever, drainage from surgical site

CHRONIC OSTEOMYELITIS:

- Bone pain
- Sinus tract drainage, nonhealing ulcer
- Chronic low-grade fever
- Chronic localized pain

ETIOLOGY

- *Staphylococcus aureus*
- *S. aureus* (methicillin-resistant)
- *Pseudomonas aeruginosa*
- *Enterobacteriaceae*
- *Streptococcus pyogenes*
- *Enterococcus*
- Mycobacteria
- Fungi
- Coagulase-negative *staphylococci*
- Salmonella (in sickle cell disease)

DIAGNOSIS

DIFFERENTIAL DIAGNOSIS

- Gaucher's disease
- Bone infarction
- Charcot's joint
- Fracture

WORKUP

- ESR, C-reactive protein
- Blood culturing
- Bone culture
- Pathologic evaluation of bone biopsy for acute/chronic changes consistent with necrosis or acute inflammation

IMAGING STUDIES

- Bone radiograph examination
- Triple-phase bone scan (Fig. 1-226)
- Gallium scan
- Indium scan
- CT or MRI (most accurate imaging study)

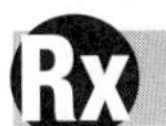

TREATMENT

- Surgical debridement in biopsy-positive cases will guide direction for antibiotic therapy. This will vary with type of osteomyelitis. Duration of therapy is usually 6 wk for acute osteomyelitis; chronic osteomyelitis may need a longer course of medication.
- *S. aureus:* cefazolin IV, nafcillin IV, vancomycin IV (in patient allergic to penicillin)
- *S. aureus* (methicillin resistant): vancomycin IV, linezolid, daptomycin, or tigecycline
- *Streptococcus* spp.: cefazolin or ceftriaxone
- *P. aeruginosa:* piperacillin plus aminoglycoside or cefepime plus aminoglycoside
- Enterobacteriaceae: ceftriaxone or fluoroquinolone
- Hyperbaric oxygen therapy: may be useful in chronic osteomyelitis
- Surgical debridement of all devitalized bone and tissue
- Immobilization of affected bone (plaster, traction) if bone is unstable

DISPOSITION

Acute hematogenous osteomyelitis usually resolves without recurrence or long-term complications, but contiguous focus osteomyelitis, bone infections from open fractures, or osteomyelitis frequently recur.

REFERRAL

- To an orthopedic surgeon if chronic osteomyelitis with need for bone debridement, bone grafting, or stabilization of infected tissue adjacent to a bone fracture
- To an infectious disease specialist for appropriate treatment for difficult-to-treat or recalcitrant infections
- To an hyperbaric oxygen chamber service for nonhealing, chronic osteomyelitis

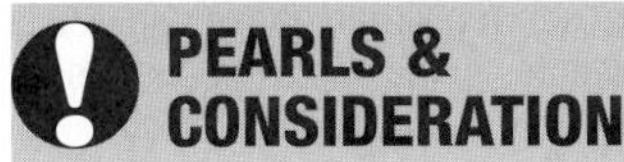

PEARLS & CONSIDERATIONS

Chronic osteomyelitis is one of the most challenging infections to treat; the high failure rate is a consequence of poor vascular supply, nondistensible bone tissue, and limited penetration of bone tissue.

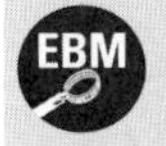

EVIDENCE

Please note: Complete text of EBM for this topic is available online.

SUGGESTED READINGS

Joosten U et al: Effectiveness of hydroxyapatite-vancomycin bone cement in the treatment of Staphylococcus aureus induced chronic osteomyelitis, *Biomaterials* 26(25):5251, 2005.

Schinabeck MK, Johnson JL: Osteomyelitis in diabetic foot ulcers. Prompt diagnosis can avert amputation, *Postgrad Med* 118(1):11, 2005.

Yin LY et al: Comparative evaluation of tigecycline and vancomycin, with and without rifampicin, in the treatment of methicillin-resistant Staphylococcus aureus experimental osteomyelitis in a rabbit model, *J Antimicrob Chemother* 55(6):995, 2005.

AUTHORS: **GLENN G. FORT, M.D., M.P.H.,** and **DENNIS J. MIKOLICH, M.D.**

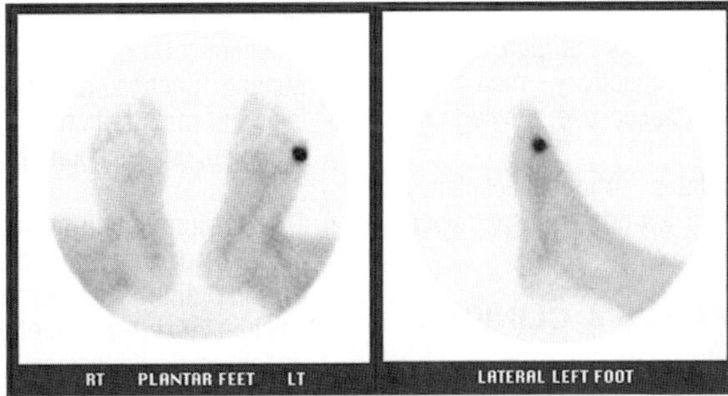

FIGURE 1-226 Osteomyelitis. Intense accumulation of Tc-99m WBC in proximal phalanx of fifth digit of left foot at 4 hr after injection (From Specht N [ed]: *Practical guide to diagnostic imaging,* St Louis, 1998, Mosby.)

Osteoporosis 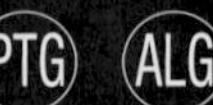

BASIC INFORMATION

DEFINITION

Osteoporosis is characterized by a progressive decrease in bone mass that results in increased bone fragility and a higher fracture risk. The various types are as follows:

PRIMARY OSTEOPOROSIS: Affects 80% of women and 60% of men with osteoporosis.

- Idiopathic osteoporosis: unknown pathogenesis; may occur in children and young adults
- Type I osteoporosis: may occur in postmenopausal women (age range, 51 to 75 yr); characterized by accelerated and disproportionate trabecular bone loss and associated with vertebral body and distal forearm fractures (estrogen withdrawal effect)
- Type II osteoporosis (involutional): occurs in both men and women >70 yr; characterized by both trabecular and cortical bone loss and associated with fractures of the proximal humerus and tibia, femoral neck, and pelvis

SECONDARY OSTEOPOROSIS: Affects 20% of women and 40% of men with osteoporosis; osteoporosis that exists as a common feature of another disease process, heritable disorder of connective tissue, or drug side effect (see "Differential Diagnosis")

ICD-9CM CODES
733.0 Osteoporosis

EPIDEMIOLOGY & DEMOGRAPHICS

PREVALENCE (IN U.S.):

- Approximately 25 million men and women
- Twice as common in women
- Results in 1.5 million fractures annually (70% women)
- Osteoporosis-related fractures in 50% women and 20% men >65 yr
- Results: institutionalization, death, and costs in excess of $10 billion annually

RISK FACTORS:

- Age: each decade after 40 yr associated with a fivefold increase risk
- Genetics:
  1. Ethnicity (white/Asian are affected more often than blacks, with Polynesians affected the least)
  2. Gender (females affected more often than males)
  3. Family history
- Environmental factors: poor nutrition, calcium deficiency, physical inactivity, medication (steroids/heparin), tobacco use, ethylene alcohol use, traumatic injury
- Chronic disease states: estrogen deficiency, androgen deficiency, hyperthyroidism, hypercortisolism, cirrhosis, gastrectomy

PHYSICAL FINDINGS & CLINICAL PRESENTATION

- Most commonly silent with no signs and symptoms
- Insidious and progressive development of dorsal kyphosis (dowager's hump), loss of height, and skeletal pain typically associated with fracture; other physical findings related to other conditions with associated increased risk for osteoporosis (see "Risk Factors")

ETIOLOGY

- Primary osteoporosis: multifactorial, resulting from a combination of factors including nutrition, peak bone mass, genetics, level of physical activity, age of menopause (spontaneous vs. surgical), and estrogen status
- Secondary osteoporosis: associated decrease in bone mass resulting from an identified cause, including endocrinopathies, hypogonadism, hyperthyroidism, hyperparathyroidism, Cushing's syndrome, hyperprolactinemia, acromegaly, diabetes mellitus, gastrointestinal disease, malabsorption, primary biliary cirrhosis, gastrectomy, malnutrition (including anorexia nervosa), and medications (corticosteroids, PPIs, rosiglitazone, pioglitazone)

DIAGNOSIS

DIFFERENTIAL DIAGNOSIS

- Malignancy (multiple myeloma, lymphoma, leukemia, metastatic carcinoma)
- Primary hyperparathyroidism
- Osteomalacia
- Paget's disease
- Osteogenesis imperfecta: types I, III, and IV (see also "Epidemiology and Demographics" and "Etiology")

WORKUP

- History and physical examination (20% of women with type I osteoporosis have associated secondary cause), with appropriate evaluation for identified risk factors and secondary causes
- Diagnosis of osteoporosis made by bone mineral density (BMD) determination (BMD should ideally evaluate the hip, spine, and wrist):
  1. Dual-energy x-ray absorptiometry
  2. Single-energy x-ray
  3. Peripheral dual-energy x-ray
  4. Single-photon absorptiometry
  5. Dual-photon absorptiometry
  6. Quantitative CT scan
  7. Radiographic absorptiometry

LABORATORY TESTS

- Biochemical profile to evaluate renal and hepatic function, primary hyperparathyroidism, and malnutrition
- Complete blood count for nutritional status and myeloma
- Thyroid-stimulating hormone to rule out the presence of hyperthyroidism
- Consideration of 24-hr urine collection for calcium (excess skeletal loss, vitamin D malabsorption/deficiency), creatinine, sodium, and free cortisol (to detect occult Cushing's disease); no need to measure calcitropic hormones (parathyroid hormone, calcitriol, calcitonin) unless specifically indicated
- Biochemical markers of bone remodeling; may be useful to predict rate of bone loss and/or follow therapy response; specific biochemical markers followed (e.g., 3-mo interval) to document normalization as a response to therapy
  1. High-turnover osteoporosis: high levels of resorption markers (lysyl pyridinoline, deoxy lysyl pyridinoline, n-telopeptide of collagen cross-links, C-telopeptide of collagen cross-links) and formation markers (osteocalcin, bone-specific alkaline phosphatase, carboxy-terminal extension peptide of type I procollagen); accelerated bone loss responding best to antiresorptive therapy
  2. Low-normal-turnover osteoporosis: normal or low levels of the markers of resorption and formation (see "high turnover osteoporosis" listed previously); no accelerated bone loss; responds best to drugs that enhance bone formation

IMAGING STUDIES

- BMD determination (see "Workup") should be performed on all women with determined risk factors and/or associated secondary causes; accepted screening criteria are currently being investigated.
  1. Normal: BMD <1 SD of the young adult reference mean
  2. Osteopenia: BMD 1 to 2.5 SD below the young adult reference mean
  3. Osteoporosis: BMD >2.5 SD below the young adult reference mean
- For patient undergoing treatment: annual BMD to follow response to therapy
- X-ray examination of appropriate part of skeleton to evaluate clinical osteoporotic fracture only (Fig. 1-227)

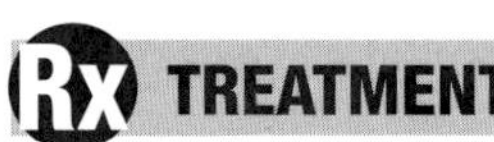

TREATMENT

NONPHARMACOLOGIC THERAPY

Prevention:

- Identification and minimization of risk factors
- Appropriate diagnosis and treatment of secondary causes
- Behavioral modification: proper nutrition (dietary calcium >800 mg/day, vitamin D 400 to 800 U/day), physical activity, fracture prevention strategies

ACUTE GENERAL Rx

- Vitamin D supplement: 400 U/day.
- Calcium supplement: 1000 to 1500 mg/day.
- Estrogen (conjugated equine estrogen or equivalent): 0.3 to 0.625 mg/day.
- Progestin: continuous (e.g., 2.5 mg medroxyprogesterone acetate/day or equivalent) or cyclic (e.g., 10 mg medroxyprogesterone acetate days 16 to 25 each month or equivalent) coadministered in nonhysterectomized women.
- Ibandronate 150 mg once monthly, swallow whole with 8 oz water on empty stomach, with no oral intake for at least 60 min. Do not lie down for 60 min after dose.

- Alendronate (10 mg/day) or risedronate (5 mg/day) on awakening with 8 oz water on empty stomach with no oral intake for at least 30 min.
- Alendronate 70 mg once weekly on awakening, with 8 oz water on empty stomach, with no oral intake for at least 30 min. Use 70-mg dose for treatment of postmenopausal osteoporosis and a 35-mg tablet for the prevention of osteoporosis in postmenopausal women.
- Risedronate: 35 mg once weekly or 75 mg taken on 2 consecutive days per month on awakening, with 8 oz water on empty stomach, with no oral intake for at least 30 min.
- Synthetic salmon calcitonin: 100 U/day SC or 200 U/day intranasally.
- Raloxifene: 60 mg qd.
- Zoledronic acid: a bisphosphonate given by IV infusion over at least 15 min, 5 mg once/year
- Teriparatide is a recombinant human parathyroid hormone used for postmenopausal women with osteoporosis who are at high risk for fracture. It is also used in men with primary or hypogonadal osteoporosis who are at high risk of fracture. It is administered by injection 20 mcg qd SQ into the thigh or abdominal wall. Use for >2 yr not recommended. It reduces the risk of fracture but may increase the risk of stroke in older women with osteoporosis.
- Other FDA-approved drugs (without osteoporosis indication) used to treat osteoporosis:
  1. Calcitriol
  2. Etidronate
  3. Thiazide
- Combination estrogen/alendronate or estrogen-progestin/alendronate may be considered in individualized patients on hormone replacement therapy with identified osteoporosis. BMD baseline obtained before onset of therapy and at 1 yr; decrease of 2% or greater results in dosage adjustment or medication change.
- A recent trial on the effects of lasofoxifene on the risk of fractures showed that in postmenopausal women with osteoporosis, lasofoxifene (0.5 mg/day) decreased risk of vertebral and non-vertebral fractures. It also lowered the risk of ER-positive breast cancer, coronary heart disease, and stroke but it increased the risk of venous thromboembolic events.
- Baseline biochemical markers of remodeling baseline considered; identified high-turnover osteoporosis patients rescreened at 3 mo to document marker return to normal.

CHRONIC Rx

- Lifelong disorder requiring lifelong attention to behavior modification issues (nutrition, physical activity, fracture prevention strategies) and compliance with pharmacologic intervention
- Continuing need to eliminate high-risk factors when possible and to diagnose and optimally manage secondary causes of osteoporosis

DISPOSITION

Goal for diagnosis and treatment: identification of women at risk; initiation of preventive measures for all women lifelong; institution of treatment modalities that will result in a decrease in fracture risk; and reduction of morbidity, mortality, and unnecessary institutionalization, thereby improving quality of independent life and productivity.

REFERRAL

- To reproductive endocrinologist, endocrinologist, gynecologist, or rheumatologist if unfamiliar with diagnosis and management of osteoporosis
- If multidisciplinary management is required, to other specialties depending on presence of acute fracture and/or secondary associated disorders

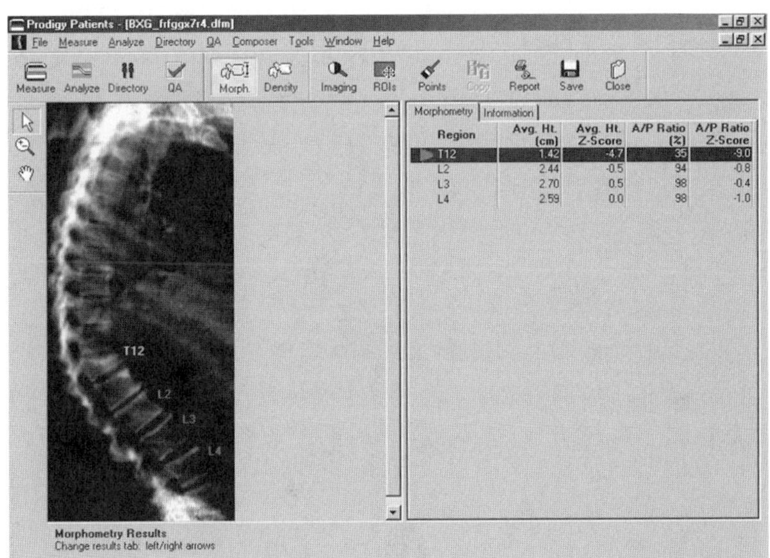

FIGURE 1-227 Vertebral fracture assessment from a dual x-ray absorptiometry image of the spine. Use of dual energy images facilitates the visualization of the lumbar and thoracic spine in a single image. In this example, a fracture has been identified at T12. (From Hochberg MC et al [eds]: *Rheumatology,* ed 3, St Louis, 2003, Mosby.)

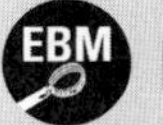

EVIDENCE

Please note: Complete text of EBM for this topic is available online.

Key trials and commentary:

A single infusion of intravenous zoledronic acid decreases bone turnover and improves bone density at 12 months in postmenopausal women with osteoporosis. This study assessed the effects of annual infusions of zoledronic acid on fracture risk during a 3-year period.

This study showed that a once-yearly infusion of zoledronic acid, during a 3-year period, significantly reduced the risk of vertebral, hip, and other fractures.

Osteoporosis is estimated to cost in excess of $18 billion annually in the U.S. Currently, the standard of care treatment includes calcium plus vitamin D supplementation and a biphosphonate (alendronate, risedronate, and ibandronate). Because bisphosphonates are poorly absorbed enterally and cause significant esophageal irritation, patient compliance represents a significant impediment to optimal response, as measured by improved bone density measurements and decreased bone fractures.

In response to this observation, two intravenous antiresorption medications were produced. The use of these medications, ibandronate and zoledronic acid, attempts to improve patient adherence.

In this current study, the authors performed a multicenter, double-blind, randomized, placebo-controlled trial investigating the treatment response to, and adverse effects from, zoledronic acid.

This study serves two major roles—to document that a yearly osteoporosis medication is effective, and to further reinforce the concept that an intravenous medication is a reasonable approach to ensuring patient compliance. Several concerns, which are relatively minor, include the presumption that all of the patients had pure postmenopausal osteoporosis. The authors do not indicate whether the patients had other causes of low BMD, such as medication-induced, inflammatory, or malabsorption disease or family history. A subgroup analysis of response to therapy, based on underlying causes of osteoporosis, would be interesting. Regarding toxicities, the most important adverse event was serious atrial fibrillation. Unfortunately, the authors did not define what this meant; therefore, it is impossible to interpret its clinical relevance. Additionally, zoledronic acid does not appear to increase the incidence of osteonecrosis of the jaw in this study.[1] Ⓐ

Bisphosphonate therapy is the current standard of care for the prevention and treatment of glucocorticoid-induced osteoporosis. Studies of anabolic therapy in patients who are receiving long-term glucocorticoids and are at high risk for fracture are lacking.

One study showed that among patients with osteoporosis who were at high risk for fracture, BMD increased more in patients receiving teriparatide than in those receiving alendronate.

The most common cause of secondary osteoporosis is glucocorticoid induced. Corticosteroids contribute to this condition through several mechanisms, including stimulating osteoblast apoptosis and inhibiting osteoblastogenesis. The current standard of care for osteoporosis treatment is a bisphosphonate. However, because recombinant human parathyroid hormone (teriparatide [Forteo]) directly stimulates osteoblastogenesis and inhibits osteoblast apoptosis, it represents a more rational treatment. Because no randomized controlled trials exist that compare teriparatide with a bisphosphonate in patients with glucocorticoid-induced osteoporosis, the authors performed and report the first 18 months of their prospective 36-month investigation.

This is a randomized double-blind clinical trial investigating the effect of 20 mg of daily subcutaneous teriparatide with 10 mg of daily oral alendronate in patients with established glucocorticoid-induced osteoporosis. The primary outcome was the change in the lumbar spine BMD from baseline to 18 months.

This study is important because it suggests that teriparatide is superior to the bisphosphonates in the treatment of glucocorticoid-induced osteoporosis. Because osteoporosis is so prevalent and costly, aggressive therapy is necessary; however, only an actuarial analysis will determine the cost effectiveness of teriparatide over a bisphosphonante. Despite the lack of a cost effectiveness evaluation, teriparatide appears to be a reasonable choice for treating patients at risk for developing, or who already have, glucocorticoid-induced osteoporosis and are at particularly high risk for fracture.[2] Ⓐ

Evidence-Based References

1. Black DM, for the HORIZON Pivotal Fracture Trial: Once-yearly zoledronic acid for treatment of postmenopausal osteoporosis, *N Engl J Med* 356:1809-1822, 2007. Commentary by S.M. Berney, M.D. Ⓐ

2. Saag KG et al: Teriparatide or alendronate in glucocorticoid-induced osteoporosis, *N Engl J Med* 357:2028-2039, 2007. Commentary by S.M. Berney, M.D. Ⓐ

SUGGESTED READINGS

Black DM et al: Once-yearly zoledronic acid for treatment of postmenopausal osteoporosis, *N Engl J Med* 356:1809, 2007.

Cadarette SM et al: Relative effectiveness of osteoporosis drugs for preventing nonvertebral fracture, *Ann Intern Med* 148:637-646, 2008.

Cummings SR et al: The effects of tibolone in older postmenopausal women, *N Engl J Med* 359:697, 2008.

Cummings SR et al: Lasofoxifene in postmenopausal women with osteoporosis, *N Engl J Med* 362:686-696, 2010.

Liu H et al: Screening for osteoporosis in men: a systematic review for an American College of Physicians Guideline, *Ann Intern Med* 148:685, 2008.

Saag KG et al: Teriparatide or alendronate in glucocorticoid-induced osteoporosis, *N Engl J Med* 357: 2028, 2007.

Sweet MG et al: Diagnosis and treatment of osteoporosis, *Am Fam Physician* 79(3):193-200, 2009.

AUTHORS: **DENNIS M. WEPPNER, M.D.,**
and **RUBEN ALVERO, M.D.**

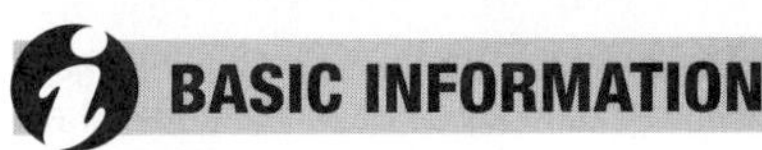

BASIC INFORMATION

DEFINITION

Otitis externa is a term encompassing a variety of conditions causing inflammation and/or infection of the external auditory canal (and/or auricle and tympanic membrane). There are six subgroups of otitis externa:

1. Acute localized otitis externa (furunculosis)
2. Acute diffuse bacterial otitis externa (swimmer's ear)
3. Chronic otitis externa
4. Eczematous otitis externa
5. Fungal otitis externa (otomycosis)
6. Invasive or necrotizing (malignant) otitis externa (Fig. 1-228)

SYNONYMS

See "Definition."

ICD-9CM CODES
38.10 Otitis externa

EPIDEMIOLOGY & DEMOGRAPHICS

INCIDENCE (IN U.S.):

- Among the most common disorders
- Affects 3% to 10% of patients seeking otologic care

PREVALENCE (IN U.S.):

- Diffuse otitis externa (swimmer's ear) is most often seen in swimmers and in hot, humid climates, conditions that lead to water retention in the ear canal.
- Necrotizing otitis externa is more common in elderly, diabetics, and immunocompromised patients.

PREDOMINANT SEX: None

PREDOMINANT AGE:

- Occurs at all ages
- Necrotizing otitis externa: typically occurs in elderly: mean age >65 yr

PHYSICAL FINDINGS & CLINICAL PRESENTATION

The two most common symptoms are otalgia, ranging from pruritus to severe pain exacerbated by motion (e.g., chewing), and otorrhea. Patients may also experience aural fullness and hearing loss as a result of swelling with occlusion of the canal. More intense symptoms may occur with bacterial otitis externa, with or without fever, and lymphadenopathy (anterior to tragus). There are also findings unique to the various forms of the infection:

- Acute localized otitis externa (furunculosis):
  1. Occurs from infected hair follicles, usually in the outer third of the ear canal, forming pustules and furuncles
  2. Furuncles are superficial and pointing or deep and diffuse
- Impetigo:
  1. In contrast to furunculosis, this is a superficial spreading infection of the ear canal that may also involve the concha and the auricle
  2. Begins as a small blister that ruptures, releasing straw-colored fluid that dries as a golden crust
- Erysipelas:
  1. Caused by group A streptococcus
  2. May involve the concha and canal
  3. May involve the dermis and deeper tissues
  4. Area of cellulitis, often with severe pain
  5. Fever, chills, malaise
  6. Regional adenopathy
- Eczematous otitis externa:
  1. Stems from a variety of dermatologic problems that can involve the external auditory canal
  2. Severe itching, erythema, scaling, crusting, and fissuring possible
- Acute diffuse otitis externa (swimmer's ear):
  1. Begins with itching and a feeling of pressure and fullness in the ear that becomes increasingly tender and painful
  2. Mild erythema and edema of the external auditory canal, which may cause narrowing and occlusion of the canal, leading to hearing loss
  3. Minimal serous secretions, which may become profuse and purulent
  4. Tympanic membrane may appear dull and infected
  5. Usually absence of systemic symptoms such as fever, chills
- Otomycosis:
  1. Chronic superficial infection of the ear canal and tympanic membrane
  2. In primary fungal infection, major symptom is intense itching
  3. In secondary infection (fungal infection superimposed on bacterial infection), major symptom is pain
  4. Fungal growth of variety of colors
- Chronic otitis externa:
  1. Dry and atrophic canal
  2. Typically lack of cerumen
  3. Itching, often severe, and mild discomfort rather than pain
  4. Occasionally mucopurulent discharge
  5. With time, thickening of the walls of the canal, causing narrowing of the lumen
- Necrotizing otitis externa (also known as malignant otitis externa). Typically seen in older patients with diabetes or in patients who are immunocompromised.
  1. Redness, swelling, and tenderness of the ear canal
  2. Classic finding of granulation tissue on the floor of the canal and the bone–cartilage junction
  3. Small ulceration of necrotic soft tissue at bone–cartilage junction
  4. Most common symptoms: pain (often severe) and otorrhea
  5. Lessening of purulent drainage as infection advances
  6. Facial nerve palsy often the first and only cranial nerve defect
  7. Possible involvement of other cranial nerves

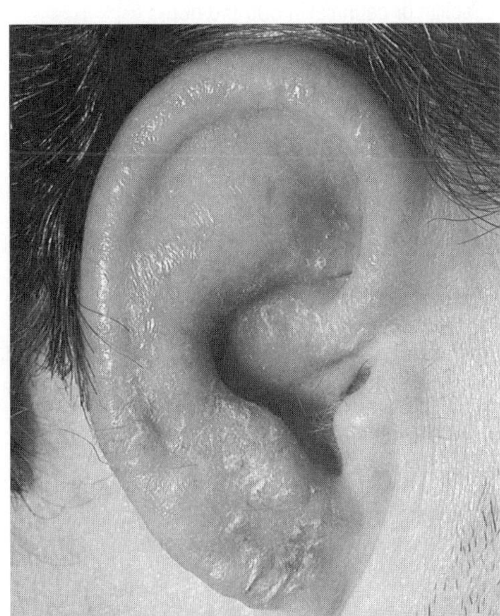

FIGURE 1-228 Malignant external otitis. Severe infection of the ear has occurred after months of chronic inflammation of the pinna. (From Habif TP: *Clinical dermatology: a color guide to diagnosis and therapy,* ed 3, St Louis, 1996, Mosby.)

ETIOLOGY

- Acute localized otitis externa: *Staphylococcus aureus*
- Impetigo:
  1. *S. aureus*
  2. *Streptococcus pyogenes*
- Erysipelas: *S. pyogenes*
- Eczematous otitis externa:
  1. Seborrheic dermatitis
  2. Atopic dermatitis
  3. Psoriasis
  4. Neurodermatitis
  5. Lupus erythematosus
- Acute diffuse otitis externa:
  1. Swimming
  2. Hot, humid climates
  3. Tightly fitting hearing aids
  4. Use of ear plugs
  5. *Pseudomonas aeruginosa*
  6. *S. aureus*
- Otomycosis:
  1. Prolonged use of topical antibiotics and steroid preparations

 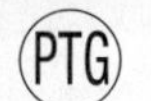

2. *Aspergillus* (80% to 90%)
3. *Candida*

- Chronic otitis externa: persistent low-grade infection and inflammation
- Necrotizing otitis externa (NOE):
  1. Complication of persistent otitis externa
  2. Extends through Santorini's fissures, small apertures at the bone–cartilage junction of the canal, into the mastoid and along the base of the skull
  3. *P. aeruginosa*

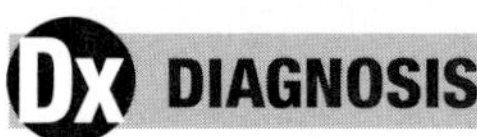

DIAGNOSIS

DIFFERENTIAL DIAGNOSIS

- Acute otitis media
- Bullous myringitis
- Mastoiditis
- Foreign bodies
- Neoplasms

WORKUP

Thorough history and physical examination

LABORATORY TESTS

- Cultures from the canal are usually not necessary unless the condition does not respond to treatment.
- Leukocyte count normal or mildly elevated.
- Erythrocyte sedimentation rate is often quite elevated in malignant otitis externa.

IMAGING STUDIES

- CT scan is the best technique for defining bone involvement and extent of disease in malignant otitis externa.
- MRI is slightly more sensitive in evaluation of soft tissue changes.
- Gallium scans are more specific than bone scans in diagnosing NOE.
- Follow-up scans are helpful in determining efficacy of treatment.

NOTE: Expert opinion supports history and physical examination as the best means of diagnosis. Persistent pain that is constant and severe should raise the question of NOE (particularly in the elderly, diabetics, and immunocompromised patients).

Rx TREATMENT

NONPHARMACOLOGIC THERAPY

- Cleansing and debridement of the ear canal with cotton swabs and hydrogen peroxide or other antiseptic solution allows a more thorough examination of the ear.
- If the canal lumen is edematous and too narrow to allow adequate cleansing, a cotton wick or gauze strip inserted into the canal serves as a conduit for topical medications to be drawn into the canal. Usually remove wick after 2 days.
- Local heat is useful in treating deep furunculosis.
- Incision and drainage is indicated in treatment of superficial pointing furunculosis.

ACUTE GENERAL Rx

Topical medications:

- An acidifying agent, such as 2% acetic acid, inhibits growth of bacteria and fungi
- Topical antibiotics (in the form of otic or ophthalmic solutions) or antifungals, often in combination with an acidifying agent and a steroid preparation
- The following are some of the available preparations:
  1. Neomycin otic solutions and suspensions:
     a. With polymyxin-B-hydrocortisone (Cortisporin)
     b. With hydrocortisone-thonzonium (Coly-Mycin S)
  2. Polymyxin-B-hydrocortisone (Otobiotic)
  3. Quinolone otic solutions:
     a. Ofloxacin 0.3% solution (Floxin Otic)
     b. Ciprofloxacin 0.3% with hydrocortisone (Cipro HC)
  4. Quinolone ophthalmic solutions:
     a. Ofloxacin 0.3% (Ocuflox)
     b. Ciprofloxacin 0.3% (Ciloxan)
  5. Aminoglycoside ophthalmic solutions:
     a. Gentamicin sulfate 0.3% (Garamycin)
     b. Tobramycin sulfate 0.3% (Tobrex)
     c. Tobramycin 0.3% and dexamethasone 0.1% (TobraDex)
  6. Chloramphenicol 0.5% otic solution or 0.25% ophthalmic solution (Chloromycetin)
  7. Gentian violet (methylrosaniline chloride 1%, 2%)
  8. Antifungals:
     a. Amphotericin B 3% (Fungizone lotion)
     b. Clotrimazole 1% solution (Lotrimin)
     c. Tolnaftate 1% (Tinactin)
- Topical preparations should be applied qid (bid for quinolones, antifungals), generally for 3 days after cessation of symptoms (average 10 to 14 days total)

Systemic antibiotics:

- Reserved for severe cases, most often infections with *P. aeruginosa* or *S. aureus*
- Treatment usually for 10 days with ciprofloxacin 750 mg q12h or ofloxacin 400 mg q12h, or with antistaphylococcal agent (e.g., dicloxacillin or cephalexin 500 mg q6h)

Treatment for NOE:

- Requires prolonged therapy up to 3 mo; whether to use oral parenteral therapy based on clinical judgment
- Oral quinolones, ciprofloxacin 750 mg q12h or ofloxacin 400 mg q12h may be appropriate initial therapy or used to shorten the course of IV therapy
- Intravenous antipseudomonals with or without aminoglycosides are also appropriate
- Local debridement

Pain control:

- May require NSAIDs or opioids
- Topical corticosteroids to reduce swelling and inflammation

CHRONIC Rx

- Patients prone to recurrent infections should try to identify and avoid precipitants to infection.
- Swimmers should try tight-fitting ear plugs or tight-fitting bathing caps and remove all excess water from the ears after swimming.
- Treat underlying systemic diseases and dermatologic conditions that predispose to infection.

DISPOSITION

Inadequate treatment of otitis externa may lead to NOE and mastoiditis.

REFERRAL

To an otolaryngologist:

- NOE
- Treatment failure
- Severe pain

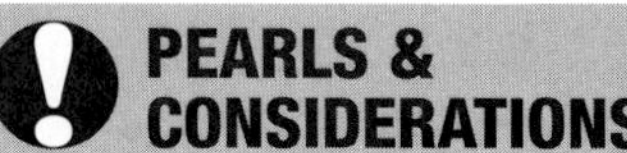

PEARLS & CONSIDERATIONS

Otitis externa varies in severity from a mild irritation of the external acoustic canal (swimmer's ear) that resolves spontaneously by simply removing the offending agent (stay out of fresh water or wear ear plugs) to a life-threatening infection with the risk of intracranial extension, gram-negative bacterial meningitis, and severe neurologic impairment with multiple cranial neuropathy. Do not miss severe malignant otitis externa in patients who are diabetic or immunocompromised.

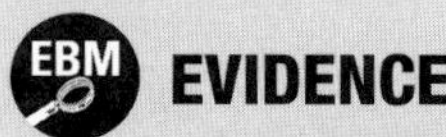

EVIDENCE

A recent systematic review of RCTs comparing topical antimicrobial therapy versus placebo in the treatment of otitis externa found that treatment with topical antimicrobials significantly increased the clinical cure rate (by 46%) and microbial cure rate (by 61%).[1] A

Evidence-Based Reference

1. Rosenfeld RM et al: Systematic review of topical antimicrobial therapy for acute otitis externa, *Otolaryngol Head Neck Surg* 134(4 Suppl):S24-48, 2006. A

SUGGESTED READINGS

Block SL: Otitis externa: providing relief while avoiding complications, *J Fam Pract* 54(8):669, 2005.

Cantrell HF et al: Declining susceptibility to neomycin and polymyxin B of pathogens recovered in otitis externa clinical trials, *South Med J* 97(5):465, 2004.

Hajioff D: Otitis externa, *Clin Evid* (12):755, 2004.

McCoy SI et al: Antimicrobial prescribing for otitis externa in children, *Pediatr Infect Dis J* 23(2):181, 2004.

Osguthorpe JD, Nielsen DR: Otitis externa: review and clinical update, *Am Fam Physician* 74:1510, 2006.

Rutka J: Acute otitis externa: treatment perspectives, *Ear Nose Throat J* 83(9 Suppl 4):20, 2004.

AUTHORS: **GLENN G. FORT, M.D., M.P.H.**, and **DENNIS J. MIKOLICH, M.D.**

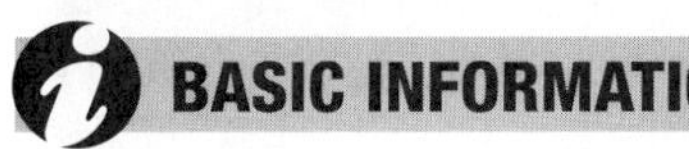

BASIC INFORMATION

DEFINITION

Otitis media is the presence of fluid in the middle ear accompanied by signs and symptoms of infection.

SYNONYMS

Acute suppurative otitis media
Purulent otitis media

ICD-9CM CODES
382.9 Acute or chronic otitis media
382.10 381.00 Otitis media with effusion

EPIDEMIOLOGY & DEMOGRAPHICS

INCIDENCE (IN U.S.):
- Affects patients of all ages but is largely a disease of infants and young children
- Occurs once in approximately 75% of all children
- Occurs three or more times in one third of all children by age 3 yr
- The diagnosis of acute otitis media increased from 9.9 million in 1975 to 25.5 million in 1990
- From 1975 to 1990, office visits for acute otitis media increased threefold for children <2 yr, doubled for children ages 2 to 5 yr, and almost doubled for children ages 6 to 10 yr

PEAK INCIDENCE:
- Between 6 and 36 mo
- Second peak between ages 4 and 6 yr
- Fall, winter, early spring

PREDOMINANT SEX: Males
PREDOMINANT AGE:
- 47% to 60% of all children have their first episode of otitis media during their first year of life and 60% to 70% by their fourth birthday
- Incidence of infection declines with age; seen infrequently in adults

GENETICS:
Familial disposition:
- Native Americans
- Eskimos
- Australian aborigines
- Those with a strong family history

Congenital infection: high incidence in children born with cleft palates and other craniofacial abnormalities

PHYSICAL FINDINGS & CLINICAL PRESENTATION

- Fluid in the middle ear along with signs and symptoms of local inflammation (Figs. 1-229 and 1-230).
    1. Erythema with diminished light reflex
- Erythema of the tympanic membrane without other abnormalities is not a diagnostic criterion for acute otitis media because it may occur with any inflammation of the upper respiratory tract, crying, or nose blowing.
- As infection progresses, middle ear exudation occurs (exudative phase); the exudate rapidly changes from serous to purulent (suppurative phase).
    1. Retraction and poor motility of the tympanic membrane, which then becomes bulging and convex
- At any time during the suppurative phase the tympanic membrane may rupture, releasing the middle ear contents.
- Symptoms:
    1. Otalgia, ranging from slight discomfort to severe, spreading to the temporal region
    2. Ear stuffiness and hearing loss may precede or follow otalgia
    3. Otorrhea
    4. Vertigo, nystagmus, tinnitus, fever, lethargy, irritability, nausea, vomiting, anorexia
- After an episode of acute otitis media:
    1. Persistence of effusion for weeks or months (called secretory, serous, or nonsuppurative otitis media)
    2. Fever and otalgia usually absent
    3. Hearing loss possible (10 to 50 dB, with predominant involvement of the low frequencies)

ETIOLOGY

- Most common etiologic factor is an upper respiratory tract infection (often viral), which causes inflammation and obstruction of the eustachian tube. Bacterial colonization of the nasopharynx in conjunction with eustachian tube dysfunction leads to infection.
- May occasionally develop as a result of hematogenous spread or by direct invasion from the nasopharynx.
- Most common bacterial pathogens:
    1. *Streptococcus pneumoniae* causes 40% to 50% of cases and is the least likely of the major pathogens to resolve without treatment
    2. *Haemophilus influenzae* causes 20% to 30% of cases
    3. *Moraxella catarrhalis* causes 10% to 15% of cases
    4. Of increasing importance, infection caused by penicillin-nonsusceptible *S. pneumoniae* (MIC >0.1 μg/ml), ranging from 8% to 34%. About 50% of PNSSP isolates are penicillin-intermediate (MIC 0.1 to 2.0 μg/ml)
- Viral pathogens:
    1. Respiratory syncytial virus
    2. Rhinovirus
    3. Adenovirus
    4. Influenza
- Others:
    1. *Mycoplasma pneumoniae*
    2. *Chlamydia trachomatis*

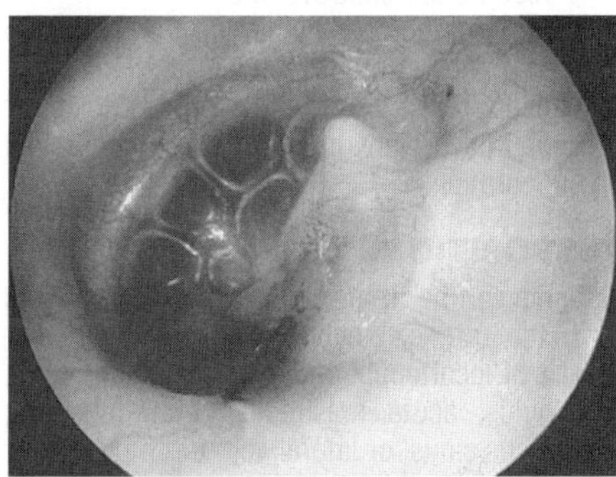

FIGURE 1-229 Otitis media with effusion of left ear. Retracted eardrum, prominent short process of malleus, and air bubbles seen anteriorly through the tympanic membrane. (From Behrman RE: *Nelson textbook of pediatrics,* ed 16, Philadelphia, 1996, WB Saunders.)

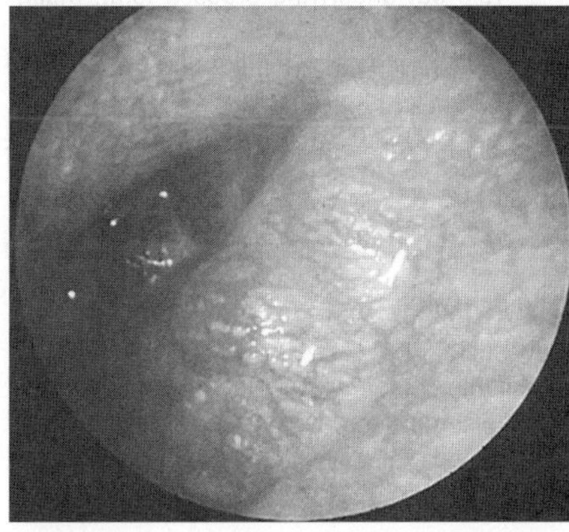

FIGURE 1-230 Acute left otitis media. (From Behrman RE: *Nelson textbook of pediatrics,* ed 16, Philadelphia, 1996, WB Saunders.)

Dx DIAGNOSIS

DIFFERENTIAL DIAGNOSIS

- Otitis externa
- Referred pain
    1. Mouth
    2. Nasopharynx
    3. Tonsils
    4. Other parts of the upper respiratory tract
- Section II describes the differential diagnosis of earache

WORKUP

Thorough otoscopic examination. Adequate visualization of the tympanic membrane requires removal of cerumen and debris.
- Tympanometry
    1. Measures compliance of the tympanic membrane and middle ear pressure
    2. Detects the presence of fluid
- Acoustic reflectometry
    1. Measures sound waves reflected from the middle ear
    2. Useful in infants >3 mo
    3. Increased reflected sound correlated with the presence of effusion

LABORATORY TESTS

- Tympanocentesis
    1. Not necessary in most cases because the microbiology of middle ear effusions has been shown to be quite consistent
    2. May be indicated in:
        a. Highly toxic patients
        b. Patients who do not respond to treatment in 48 to 72 hr
        c. Immunocompromised patients

- Cultures of the nasopharynx: sensitive but not specific
- Blood counts: usually show a leukocytosis with polymorphonuclear elevation
- Plain mastoid radiographs: generally not indicated; will reveal haziness in the periantral cells that may extend to entire mastoid
- CT or MRI may be indicated if serious complications suspected (meningitis, brain abscess)

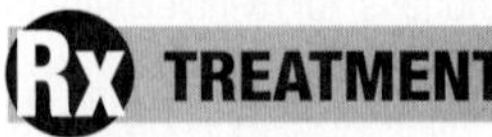

TREATMENT

ACUTE GENERAL Rx

Hydration, avoidance of irritants (e.g., tobacco smoke), nasal systemic decongestants, cool mist humidifier

Antimicrobials:

NOTE: Most uncomplicated cases of acute otitis media resolve spontaneously, without complications. Studies have demonstrated limited therapeutic benefit from antibiotic therapy. However, when opting to use antibiotic therapy:

- Amoxicillin remains the drug of choice for first-line treatment of uncomplicated acute otitis media despite increasing prevalence of drug-resistant *S. pneumoniae.*
- Treatment failure is defined by lack of clinical improvement of signs or symptoms after 3 days of therapy.
- With treatment failure, in the absence of an identified etiologic pathogen, therapy should be redirected to cover:
  1. Drug-resistant *S. pneumoniae*
  2. β-lactamase–producing strains of *H. influenzae* and *M. catarrhalis*
- Agents fulfilling these criteria include amoxicillin/clavulanate, second-generation cephalosporins (e.g., cefuroxime axetil, cefaclor), and ceftriaxone (given IM). Cefaclor, cefixime, loracarbef, and ceftibuten are active against *H. influenzae* and *M. catarrhalis* but less active against pneumococci, especially drug-resistant strains, than the agents listed previously.
- TMP/SMX and macrolides have been used as first- and second-line agents, but pneumococcal resistance to these agents is rising (up to 25% resistance to TMP/SMX and up to 10% resistance to erythromycin).
- Cross-resistance between these drugs and the β-lactams exists; therefore patients who do not respond to amoxicillin are more likely to have infections resistant to TMP/SMX and macrolides.
- Newer fluoroquinolones (grepafloxacin, levofloxacin, moxifloxacin) have enhanced activity against pneumococci compared with older agents (ciprofloxacin, ofloxacin).
- Treatment should be modified according to cultures and sensitivities.
- Generally treatment course is 10 to 14 days.
- Follow up approximately 4 wk after discontinuation of therapy to verify resolution of all symptoms, return to normal otoscopic findings, and restoration of normal hearing.

NOTE: Effusions may persist for 2 to 6 wk or longer in many cases of adequately treated otitis media.

SURGICAL Rx

- No evidence to support the routine of myringotomy, but in severe cases it provides prompt pain relief and accelerates resolution of infection.
- Purulent secretions retained in the middle ear lead to increased pressure that may lead to spread of infection to contiguous areas. Myringotomy to decompress the middle ear is necessary to avoid complications.
- Complications include mastoiditis, facial nerve paralysis, labyrinthitis, meningitis, and brain abscess.
- Other procedures used for drainage of the middle ear include insertion of a ventilation tube and/or simple mastoidectomy.

CHRONIC Rx

- Myringotomy and tympanostomy tube placement for persistent middle ear effusion unresponsive to medical therapy for ≥3 mo if bilateral or ≥6 mo if unilateral.
- Adenoidectomy, with or without tonsillectomy, often advocated for treatment of recurrent otitis media, although indications for this procedure are controversial.
- Long-term complications include tympanic membrane perforations, cholesteatoma, tympanosclerosis, ossicular necrosis, toxic or suppurative labyrinthitis, and intracranial suppuration.

DISPOSITION

Patients can be treated at home as outpatients with the rare exception of patients with evidence of local suppurative complications (e.g., meningitis, acute mastoiditis, brain abscess, cavernous sinus, or lateral vein thrombosis).

REFERRAL

- To otorhinolaryngologist if:
  1. Medical treatment failure
  2. Diagnosis uncertain: adults with one or more episodes of otitis media should be referred for ear-nose-throat evaluation to rule out underlying process (e.g., malignancy)
  3. Any of the above mentioned acute and chronic complications

PEARLS & CONSIDERATIONS

COMMENTS

Prevention:

- Multiple component conjugate vaccines hold promise for decreasing recurrent episodes of acute otitis media
- Breastfeed and bottle-feed infants in an upright position
- Avoidance of irritants (e.g., tobacco smoke)

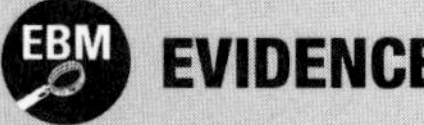

EVIDENCE

Antibiotics appear to have a modest role in the management of acute otitis media.

In acute otitis media in children, a short course of an appropriate antibiotic is modestly effective.[1] (A)

There is limited evidence supporting the effectiveness of tympanostomy tubes in the management of otitis media with effusion.

The insertion of tympanostomy tubes in children with otitis media with effusion has been found to result in hearing improvement, although the improvements are not sustained in the long term.[2] (A)

There is some evidence about the efficacy of adenoidectomy in the treatment of otitis media with effusion but not in the treatment of recurrent acute otitis media.

A recent randomized controlled trial in children aged 10 mo to 2 yr failed to show a significant difference in treatment of recurrent acute otitis media with adenoidectomy versus sulfafurazole given once a day for 6 mo versus placebo in terms of the number of episodes of acute otitis media, visits to a doctor, antibiotic prescriptions, and days with symptoms of respiratory infection.[3] (B)

Evidence-Based References

1. Glasziou PP et al: Antibiotics for acute otitis media in children, *Cochrane Database Rev* 1, 2004. (A)
2. Lous J et al: Grommets (ventilation tubes) for hearing loss associated with otitis media with effusion in children, *Cochrane Database Rev* 1, 2005. (A)
3. Koivunen P et al: Adenoidectomy versus chemoprophylaxis and placebo for recurrent acute otitis media in children aged under 2 years: randomised controlled trial, *BMJ* 328:487, 2004. (B)

SUGGESTED READINGS

Damoiseaux RA et al: Long-term prognosis of acute otitis media in infancy: determinants of recurrent acute otitis media and persistent middle ear effusion, *Fam Pract* 23(1):40, 2006.

Plasschaert AL et al: Trends in doctor consultations, antibiotic prescription, and specialist referrals for otitis media in children: 1995-2003, *Pediatrics* 117(6):1879, 2006.

Ramakrishnan K et al: Diagnosis and treatment of otitis media, *Am Fam Physician* 76:1650, 2007.

AUTHORS: **GLENN G. FORT, M.D., M.P.H.,** and **DENNIS J. MIKOLICH, M.D.**

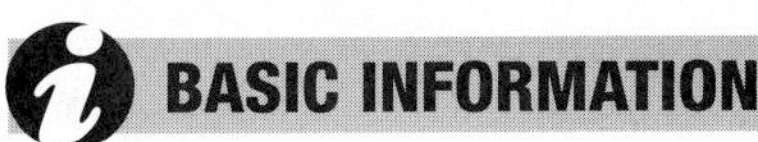

BASIC INFORMATION

DEFINITION

Otosclerosis is conductive hearing loss caused by fixation of the stapes, resulting in gradual hearing loss. Approximately 15% of cases affect only one ear.

ICD-9CM CODES

387.9 Otosclerosis

EPIDEMIOLOGY & DEMOGRAPHICS

INCIDENCE (IN U.S.): Most common cause of hearing loss in young adults
PEAK INCIDENCE: Middle age
PREVALENCE (IN U.S.): Five cases per 1000 persons
PREDOMINANT SEX: Male/female ratio of 2:1
PREDOMINANT AGE: Symptoms start between ages 15 and 30 yr, with slowly progressive hearing loss.
GENETICS: Half of cases are dominantly inherited.

PHYSICAL FINDINGS & CLINICAL PRESENTATION

- Tympanic membrane is normal in most cases (tested with tuning fork).
- Bone conduction is greater than air conduction.
- Weber test localizes to affected ear.

ETIOLOGY

- A disease in which a vascular type of spongy bone is laid down
- Unknown

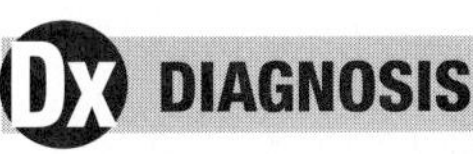

DIAGNOSIS

DIFFERENTIAL DIAGNOSIS

- Hearing loss from any cause: cochlear otosclerosis, polyps, granulomas, tumors, osteogenesis imperfecta, chronic ear infections, trauma.
- A clinical algorithm for evaluation of hearing loss is described in Section III.
- Table 1-58 describes common types of conductive and sensorineural hearing loss.

WORKUP

Audiometry

LABORATORY TESTS

None, unless infection suspected

IMAGING STUDIES

MRI or CT with specific cuts through inner ear (Fig. 1-231)

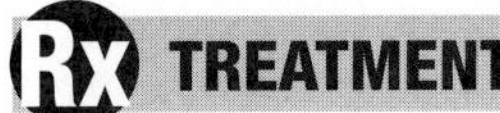

TREATMENT

NONPHARMACOLOGIC THERAPY

Hearing aid only of temporary use

CHRONIC Rx

Progresses to deafness without surgical intervention

DISPOSITION

Referral to ear-nose-throat (ENT) specialist

REFERRAL

To ENT specialist for surgery if moderate hearing loss suspected

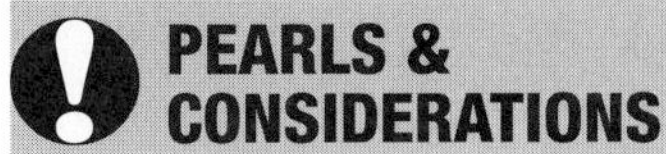

PEARLS & CONSIDERATIONS

COMMENTS

A full ENT evaluation in a young or middle-aged person with hearing loss is mandatory unless the cause is obvious (such as trauma or repeated infection).

SUGGESTED READING

Chole RA, McKenna M: Pathophysiology of otosclerosis, *Otol Neurotol* 22(2):249, 2001.

AUTHOR: **FRED F. FERRI, M.D.**

TABLE 1-58 Common Types of Conductive and Sensorineural Hearing Loss

Conductive Hearing Loss	Sensorineural Hearing Loss
Otitis media with effusion	Presbycusis (hearing loss with aging)
TM perforation	Ototoxicity
Tympanosclerosis	Ménière's disease
Retracted TM (eustachian tube dysfunction)	Idiopathic loss
Ossicular problems	Noise-induced loss
Otosclerosis	Perilymphatic fistula
Foreign body in ear canal	Hereditary (congenital) loss
Cerumen impaction	Multiple sclerosis
Tumor of the ear canal or middle ear	Diabetes
Cholesteatoma	Syphilis, acoustic neuroma

From Rakel RE (ed): *Principles of family practice,* ed 6, Philadelphia, 2002, WB Saunders.
TM, Tympanic membrane.

FIGURE 1-231 A patient with conductive hearing loss. By comparing the normal **(A)** and abnormal **(B)** sides on CT scan, the narrowing of the oval window can be clearly appreciated. This results in fixation of the stapes footplate and conductive hearing loss. (From Grainger RG et al [eds]: *Grainger & Allison's diagnostic radiology,* ed 4, Philadelphia, 2001, Churchill Livingstone.)

Ovarian Cancer (PTG)

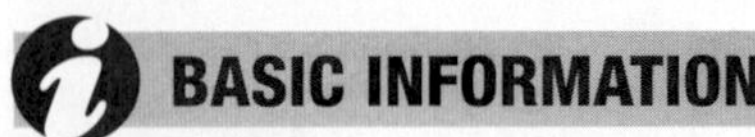

BASIC INFORMATION

DEFINITION

Ovarian tumors can be benign, requiring operative intervention but not recurring or metastasizing; malignant, recurring, metastasizing, and having decreased survival; or borderline, having a small risk of recurrence or metastases but generally having a good prognosis.

SYNONYMS

Epithelial ovarian cancer
Germ cell tumor
Sex cord stromal tumor
Ovarian tumor of low malignant potential

ICD-9CM CODES
183.0 Malignant neoplasm of ovary

EPIDEMIOLOGY & DEMOGRAPHICS

INCIDENCE: 12.9 to 15.1 cases/100,000 persons; approximately 25,000 new cases annually
PREVALENCE: Median age of 61 yr; peaks at age 75 to 79 yr (54/100,000)
RISK FACTORS: Low parity, delayed childbearing, use of talc on the perineum (unlikely), high-fat diet, fertility drugs (unlikely), Lynch II syndrome (nonpolyposis colon cancer, endometrial cancer, breast cancer, and ovarian cancer clusters in first- and second-degree relatives), breast-ovarian familial cancer syndrome, site-specific familial ovarian cancer. Hormone therapy is associated with an increased risk of ovarian cancer regardless of the duration of use, the formulation, estrogen dose, regimen, progestin type, and route of administration.
GENETICS: The greatest risk factors of ovarian cancer are a family history and associated genetic syndromes. Familial susceptibility has been shown with the *BRCA1* gene located on 17q12 to 21. This correlates with breast-ovarian cancer syndrome.

PHYSICAL FINDINGS & CLINICAL PRESENTATION

- 60% present with advanced disease
- Abdominal fullness, early satiety, dyspepsia
- Pelvic pain, back pain, constipation
- Pelvic or abdominal mass
- Lymphadenopathy (inguinal)
- Sister Mary Joseph nodule (umbilical mass)

ETIOLOGY

- Can be inherited as site-specific familial ovarian cancer (two or more first-degree relatives have ovarian cancer)
- Breast-ovarian cancer syndrome (clusters of breast and ovarian cancer among first- and second-degree relatives)
- Lynch syndrome
- No family history and unknown etiology in the majority of ovarian cancer cases

DIAGNOSIS

DIFFERENTIAL DIAGNOSIS

- Primary peritoneal cancer mesothelioma
- Benign ovarian tumor
- Functional ovarian cyst
- Endometriosis
- Ovarian torsion
- Pelvic kidney
- Pedunculated uterine fibroid
- Primary cancer from breast, gastrointestinal tract, or other pelvic organ metastasized to the ovary

WORKUP

- Definitive diagnosis made at laparotomy; epithelial ovarian cancer most common type of ovarian cancer
- Careful physical and history, including family history
- Exclusion of nongynecologic etiologies
- Observation of small cystic masses in premenopausal women for regression for 2 mo

LABORATORY TESTS

- Complete blood count
- Chemistry profile
- CA-125 or lysophosphatidic acid level
- Consider: human chorionic gonadotropin, inhibin, alpha-fetoprotein, neuron-specific enolase, and lactate dehydrogenase in patients at risk for germ cell tumors

IMAGING STUDIES

- Ultrasound
- Chest x-ray examination
- Mammogram
- CT scan to help evaluate extent of disease (Fig. 1-232)
- Other studies (barium enema, MRI, intravenous pyelogram, etc.) as clinically indicated

TREATMENT

NONPHARMACOLOGIC THERAPY

Virtually all cases of ovarian cancer involve surgical exploration. This includes:

- Abdominal cytology
- Total abdominal hysterectomy and bilateral salpingo-oophorectomy (except in early stages in which fertility is an issue)
- Omentectomy
- Diaphragm sampling
- Selective lymphadenectomy (pelvis and para-aortic)
- Primary cytoreduction with a goal of residual tumor diameter <2 cm
- Bowel surgery, splenectomy if needed to obtain optimal (<2 cm) cytoreduction
- Conventional treatment includes surgical debulking followed by chemotherapy

ACUTE GENERAL Rx

- Optimal cytoreduction is generally followed by chemotherapy (except in some early-stage disease).

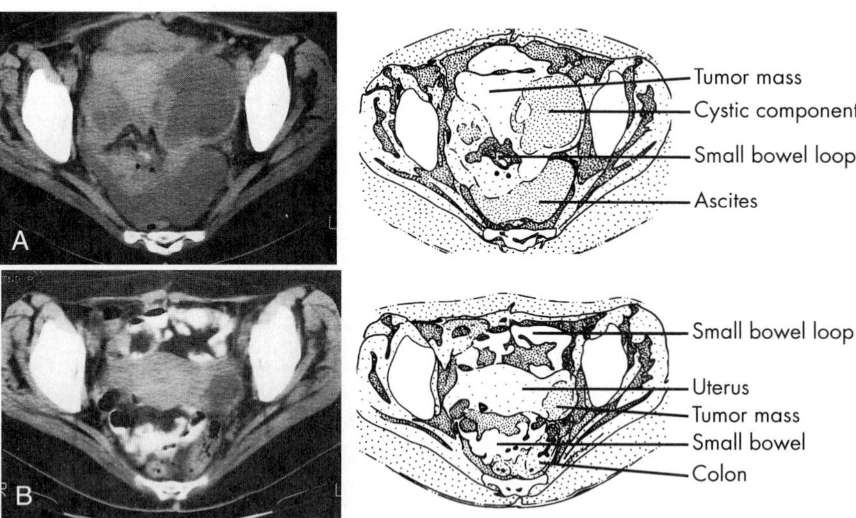

FIGURE 1-232 Response to chemotherapy. A 51-year-old woman presented with a rapid increase in abdominal girth. **A,** On CT scan, she was found to have a 12 x 8 cm ovarian mass with a cystic component; peritoneal involvement was extensive and 6 L of ascites were removed. Pathologic examination showed a poorly differentiated tumor. The tumor was not resectable, and she was treated with combination chemotherapy. After one cycle of therapy, her abdomen returned to normal size. **B,** A CT scan reveals only a small residual ovarian mass. Surgery after four cycles of chemotherapy showed no gross or microscopic tumor. She received four more cycles of chemotherapy but relapsed 1 year later with abdominal metastases. (From Skarin AT: *Atlas of diagnostic oncology,* ed 3, St Louis, 2003, Mosby.)

- Cisplatin-based combination chemotherapy is used for stage II or greater, 6-mo treatment. Compared with IV paclitaxel plus cisplatin, IV paclitaxel plus intraperitoneal cisplatin and paclitaxel improves survival rates in patients with optimally debulked stage III ovarian cancer.
- Chemotherapy regimens continue to change as research continues.
- Consider second-look surgery when chemotherapy is complete.

CHRONIC Rx

- If CA-125 elevated, may have recurrent disease
- Physical and pelvic examinations every 3 mo for 2 yr, every 4 mo during third year, then every 6 mo
- CA-125 every visit
- Yearly Pap smear

DISPOSITION

- Overall 5-yr survival rates remain low because of the preponderance of late-stage disease:
  - Stage I and II: 80% to 100%
  - Stage III: 15% to 20%
  - Stage IV: 5%
- Younger patients (<50 yr) in all stages have a considerably better 5-yr survival than older patients (40% vs. 15%).

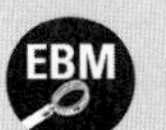

EVIDENCE

Please note: Complete text of EBM for this topic is available online.

Key trials and commentary:

Ovarian cancer (OC) patients experiencing progressive disease (PD) within 6 months of platinum-based therapy in the primary setting are considered platinum resistant (Pt-R). Currently, pegylated liposomal doxorubicin (PLD) is a standard of care for treatment of recurrent Pt-R disease. On the basis of promising phase II results, gemcitabine was compared with PLD for efficacy and safety in taxane-pretreated Pt-R OC patients. Although this was not designed as an equivalency study, gemcitabine and PLD seem to have a comparable therapeutic index in this population of Pt-R taxane-pretreated OC patients. Single-agent gemcitabine may be an acceptable alternative to PLD for patients with Pt-R OC.

This article by Mutch et al focuses on the treatment of patients with recurrent ovarian carcinoma. Mutch et al report the results of a randomized phase III trial comparing gemcitabine with PLD. The study showed that both agents are active in Pt-R disease with no significant differences in level of efficacy. Patients reported better quality of life on PLD as compared with gemcitabine.

The message from this article may be summarized as follows. First, there are a number of active agents in ovarian carcinoma. Despite this, the platinum drugs remain the most active agents in the disease, and patients should be conclusively platinum resistant before nonplatinum regimens are used in the treatment of the disease. Platinum-resistant patients do benefit from further therapy with active nonplatinum agents. The number of lines of therapy ultimately used in the platinum-resistant setting should be the joint decision of the patient and his or her physician after a thorough discussion of expected benefit vs. toxicity of treatment.[1] Ⓐ

A Gynecologic Oncology Group (GOG) randomized phase III trial (GOG 172) in optimal stage III epithelial ovarian cancer showed that intravenous (IV) paclitaxel plus intraperitoneal (IP) cisplatin and paclitaxel significantly lengthened progression-free survival and overall survival compared with IV paclitaxel and cisplatin. The purpose of this report was to comprehensively evaluate the patient-reported outcomes associated with IP vs. IV therapy.

This study showed that during active treatment, patients on the IP arm experienced more health-related quality-of-life disruption, AD, and Ntx compared with patients receiving conventional IV therapy. However, only Ntx remained significantly greater for IP patients 12 months after treatment. This trade-off should be included when discussing treatment options with patients. Future studies to mitigate the added burden associated with IP therapy are planned.

This article focuses on IP chemotherapy for small-volume–residual advanced ovarian carcinoma. Wenzel et al report the results of the quality-of-life component of a randomized phase III GOG study (GOG Protocol 172). The investigators report that quality of life was significantly impaired in patients receiving IP chemotherapy and that this impairment persisted for up to 12 months following completion of the IP therapy. The recommendations focus on standards for the delivery of IP chemotherapy, which is important to the minimizing of adverse effects associated with this method of delivery. Anyone planning the use of IP chemotherapy outside of clinical trials would do well to review these recommendations.[2] Ⓐ

Evidence-Based References

1. Mutch DG et al: Randomized phase III trial of gemcitabine compared with pegylated liposomal doxorubicin in patients with platinum-resistant ovarian cancer, *J Clin Oncol* 25:2811-2818, 2007. Commentary by J.T. Thigpen, M.D. Ⓐ

2. Wenzel LB et al: Health-related quality of life during and after intraperitoneal versus intravenous chemotherapy for optimally debulked ovarian cancer: a Gynecologic Oncology Group Study, *J Clin Oncol* 25:437-443, 2007. Commentary by J.T. Thigpen, M.D. Ⓐ

SUGGESTED READINGS

Armstrong D et al: Intraperitoneal cisplatin and paclitaxel in ovarian cancer, *N Engl J Med* 354:34, 2006.

Clarke-Pearson DL: Screening for ovarian cancer, *N Engl J Med* 361:170-177, 2009.

Roett MA, Evans, P: Ovarian cancer, an overview, *Am Fam Physician* 80(6):609-616, 2009.

Steinrud L et al: Hormone therapy and ovarian cancer, *JAMA* 302(3):298-305, 2009.

AUTHORS: **GIL M. FARKASH, M.D.,** and **RUBEN ALVERO, M.D.**

Ovarian Neoplasm, Benign (PTG)

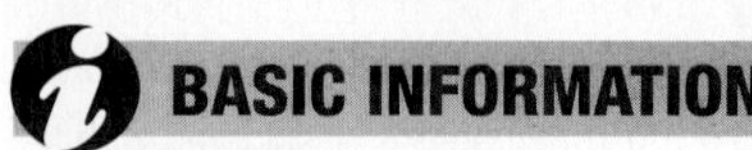

BASIC INFORMATION

DEFINITION

Benign ovarian neoplasms are often clinically indistinguishable from their malignant counterparts. Therefore all persistent adnexal masses must be considered malignant until proven otherwise. Nonneoplastic tumors include:

- Germinal inclusion cyst
- Follicle cyst
- Corpus luteum cyst
- Pregnancy luteoma
- Theca lutein cysts
- Sclerocystic ovaries
- Endometrioma

Neoplastic tumors derived from coelomic epithelium include:

- Cystic tumors: serous cystoma, mucinous cystoma, mixed forms
- Tumors with stromal overgrowth: fibroma, adenofibroma, Brenner tumor

Tumors derived from germ cells are dermoids (benign cystic teratomas).

ICD-9CM CODES
220 Benign neoplasm of ovary

EPIDEMIOLOGY & DEMOGRAPHICS

- Reproductive years:
  1. Most common benign ovarian neoplasms: serous cystadenoma and benign cystic teratoma
  2. Most common adnexal mass: functional cyst
- Risk of malignancy increases after age 40 yr.
- Infants: adnexal masses are usually follicular cysts attributable to maternal hormone stimulation that regress during first few months of life.
- Childhood:
  1. Adnexal masses are rare
  2. 8% malignant
  3. Almost always dysgerminomas or teratomas (germ cell origin)
  4. Frequency of malignancy inversely correlated with age
- Adolescence:
  1. Most common adnexal mass is a functional cyst.
  2. Most common neoplastic ovarian tumor is a benign cystic teratoma.
  3. Solid/cystic adnexal tumors are rare and almost always dysgerminomas or malignant teratomas.

PHYSICAL FINDINGS & CLINICAL PRESENTATION

- Usually asymptomatic
- Pelvic pain or pressure
- Dyspareunia
- Abdominal pain ranging from mild to severe peritoneal irritation
- Increasing abdominal girth or distention
- Adnexal mass of pelvic examination
- Children: abdominal or rectal mass

ETIOLOGY

- Physiologic
- Endometriosis
- Unknown

Dx DIAGNOSIS

DIFFERENTIAL DIAGNOSIS

- Ovarian torsion
- Malignancy: ovary, fallopian tube, colon
- Uterine fibroid
- Diverticular abscess, diverticulitis
- Appendiceal abscess, appendicitis (especially in children)
- Tubo-ovarian abscess
- Paraovarian cyst
- Distended bladder
- Pelvic kidney
- Ectopic pregnancy
- Retroperitoneal cyst or neoplasm

WORKUP

- Complete history and physical examination
- Pelvic or rectovaginal examination to reveal firm, irregular, mobile mass
- Laparoscopy or laparotomy to establish diagnosis

LABORATORY TESTS

- Pregnancy test
- Serum tumor markers:
  1. Cancer antigen 125 (CA 125)
  2. Alpha-fetoprotein (endodermal sinus tumor, immature teratoma)
  3. Beta-human chorionic gonadotropin
  4. Lactate dehydrogenase (dysgerminoma)

IMAGING STUDIES

Ultrasound:

- May differentiate adnexal mass from other pelvic masses
- Features that increase risk of malignancy include solid component, papillae, multiple septations or solitary thick septa, ascites, matted bowel, bilaterality, irregular borders
- CT scan with contrast
- Colonoscopy or barium enema, if symptomatic

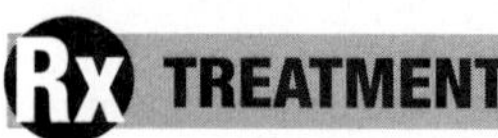

TREATMENT

NONPHARMACOLOGIC THERAPY

Repeat pelvic examination for premenopausal women in 4 to 6 wk

ACUTE GENERAL Rx

Indications for surgery:

- Postmenopausal or premenarcheal palpable adnexal mass
- Adnexal mass with suspicious ultrasound features
- Premenopausal woman with persistent cyst >5 cm
- Any adnexal mass >10 cm
- Suspected torsion or rupture

CHRONIC Rx

- Depends on diagnosis
- Possible suppression of formation of new cysts by oral contraceptives

DISPOSITION

Depends on diagnosis

REFERRAL

- If malignancy suspected
- If surgery required

SUGGESTED READINGS

Dayal M, Barnhart KT: Noncontraceptive benefits and therapeutic uses of the oral contraceptive pill, *Semin Reprod Med* 19(4):295, 2001.

Doret M, Raudrant D: Functional ovarian cysts and the need to remove them, *Euro J Obstet Gynecol Reprod Biol* 100(1):1, 2001.

Kurjak A et al: Ultrasonic assessment of the peri- and postmenopausal ovary, *Maturitas* 41(4):245, 2002.

AUTHORS: **GEORGE T. DANAKAS, M.D.,** and **RUBEN ALVERO, M.D.**

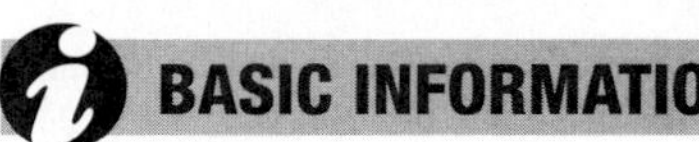

BASIC INFORMATION

DEFINITION

Paget's disease of the bone is a nonmetabolic disease of bone characterized by repeated episodes of osteolysis and excessive attempts at repair that result in a weakened bone of increased mass. Monostotic (solitary lesion) and polyostotic (numerous lesions) disease are both described.

SYNONYMS

Osteitis deformans

ICD-9CM CODES
731.0 Paget's disease (osteitis deformans)

EPIDEMIOLOGY & DEMOGRAPHICS

PREVALENCE: Localized lesions in 3% of patients >50 yr
PREDOMINANT SEX: Male/female ratio of 2:1
PREDOMINANT AGE: Rare before 40 yr

PHYSICAL FINDINGS & CLINICAL PRESENTATION

- Many lesions are asymptomatic.
- Onset is variable.
- Symptoms result mainly from the effects of complications:
  1. Skeletal pain, especially hip and pelvis
  2. Bowing of long bones, sometimes leading to pathologic fracture
  3. Increased heat of extremity (resulting from increased vascularity)
  4. Skull enlargement and spinal involvement caused by characteristic bone enlargement, which can produce neurologic complications (vision and hearing loss, radicular pain, and cord compression)
  5. Thoracic kyphoscoliosis
  6. Secondary osteoarthritis, especially of hip
  7. Heart failure as a result of chest and spine deformity and blood shunting

ETIOLOGY

Unknown

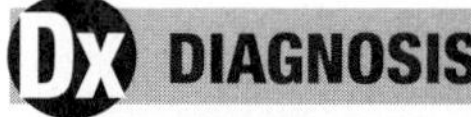

DIAGNOSIS

DIFFERENTIAL DIAGNOSIS

- Fibrous dysplasia
- Skeletal neoplasm (primary or metastatic)
- Osteomyelitis
- Hyperparathyroidism
- Vertebral hemangioma

LABORATORY TESTS

- Increased serum alkaline phosphatase (SAP)
- Normal serum calcium and phosphorus levels
- Increased urinary excretion of pyridinoline cross-links, although test is expensive and not usually required in routine cases
- Other: bone biopsy only in uncertain cases or if sarcomatous degeneration is suspected

IMAGING STUDIES

- Appropriate radiographs reflect the characteristic radiolucency and opacity (Fig. 1-233).
- Bone scanning usually reflects the activity and extent of the disease.

Rx TREATMENT

NONPHARMACOLOGIC THERAPY

- Counseling regarding home environment to prevent falls
- Cane for balance and weight-bearing pain

ACUTE GENERAL Rx

- Bisphosphonates: Can be given by PO or IV.
- Calcitonin: The use of salmon calcitonin has been largely supplanted by the use of bisphosphonates. It is used primarily when bisphosphonates are not tolerated or contraindicated.
- Nonsteroidal anti-inflammatory drugs for pain relief
- General indications for treatment:
  1. All symptomatic patients
  2. Asymptomatic patients with high level of metabolic activity or those at risk for deformity
  3. Preoperative, if surgery involves pagetic site

DISPOSITION

- Many monostotic lesions probably remain asymptomatic.
- Progression of the disease is common.
- Malignant degeneration occurs in <1% of patients and should be considered when there is a sudden increase in pain.
- Sarcomatous change carries a grave prognosis.

REFERRAL

- For dental evaluation if there is involvement of the mandible or maxilla
- For ENT evaluation if there is hearing loss
- For ophthalmologic evaluation if there is impaired vision
- For orthopedic consultation for assessment of pain in bone or joint

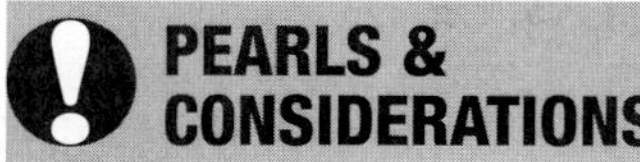

PEARLS & CONSIDERATIONS

COMMENTS

Surgical intervention is often required for neurologic complications or joint symptoms
- Often associated with profuse blood loss
- Elective cases: benefit from preoperative treatment to suppress bone activity and vascularity

SUGGESTED READINGS

Bone HG: Nonmalignant complications of Paget's disease, *J Bone Mineral Res* 21(suppl 2):64, 2006.

Brown JP: Metabolic bone diseases: treating Paget disease: when matters more than how, *Nat Rev Rheumatol* 5:663, 2009.

Haddaway MJ et al: Effect of age and gender on the number and distribution of sites in Paget's disease of bone, *Br J Radiol* 80:532, 2007.

Keating GM, Scott LJ: Zoledronic acid: a review of its use in the treatment of Paget's disease of bone, *Drugs* 67:793, 2007.

Langston AL, Ralston SH: Management of Paget's disease of bone, *Rheumatology* 43(8):955, 2004.

Silverman SL: Paget disease of bone: therapeutic options, *J Clin Rheumatol* 14L:299, 2008.

Singer FR: Paget disease: when to treat and when not to treat, *Nat Rev Rheumatol* 5:483, 2009.

Whyte MP: Paget's disease of bone, *N Engl J Med* 355: 593, 2006.

AUTHOR: **LONNIE R. MERCIER, M.D.**

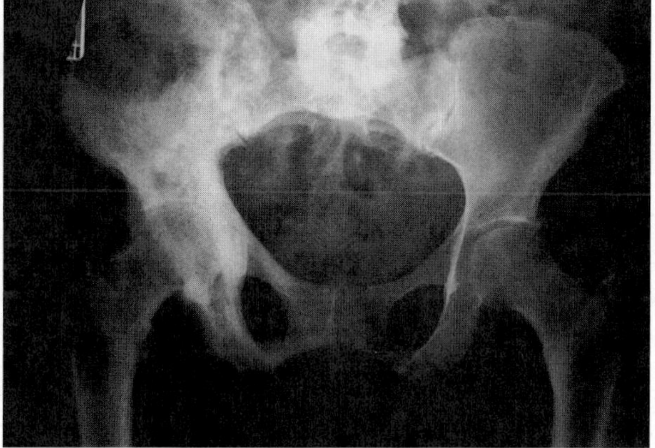

FIGURE 1-233 Frontal radiograph of the pelvis shows marked prominence to the trabeculae in the right ilium, ischium, and pubic bones, with small lytic areas identified as compatible with the later stages of Paget's disease. (From Specht N [ed]: *Practical guide to diagnostic imaging,* St Louis, 1998, Mosby.)

Paget's Disease of the Breast 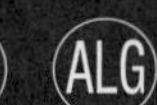

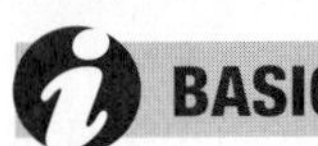

BASIC INFORMATION

DEFINITION

Paget's disease of the breast is a malignant disease that presents itself as a scaly, sore, eroding, bleeding ulcer of the nipple. Microscopically, typical large clear cells (Paget's cells) with pale and abundant cytoplasm and hyperchromatic nuclei with prominent nucleoli are found in the epidermal layer. Paget's disease is more often associated with primary invasive or in situ carcinoma of the breast.

ICD-9CM CODES

174.0 Malignant neoplasm of female breast, nipple, and areola

EPIDEMIOLOGY & DEMOGRAPHICS

- Not common
- Found in one in 100 to 200 breast cancer patients

PHYSICAL FINDINGS & CLINICAL PRESENTATION

- Variable
- Itching or burning nipple and/or reported lump
- Very minimal scaly lesion that may bleed when scales are lifted
- Typical ulcer located on nipple with serous fluid weeping or small amount of bleeding coming from it (Fig. 1-234)
- Palpable carcinoma in the breast of some patients

ETIOLOGY

- Exact origin unknown
- Possibly migration of either in situ or invasive carcinoma cells in breast to nipple skin to produce Paget's disease

DIAGNOSIS

DIFFERENTIAL DIAGNOSIS

- Chronic dermatitis
- Florid papillomatosis of the nipple or nipple adenoma
- Eczema

WORKUP

- Clinically apparent
- Careful breast examination with diagnosis in mind
- Palpable mass or mammographic lesions in 60% to 70% of patients

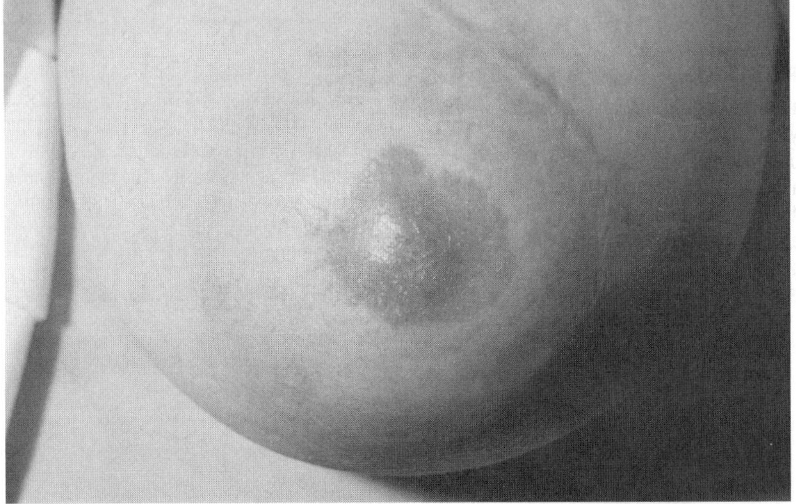

FIGURE 1-234 Paget's disease of the breast. The lesion has insidiously spread for 1 year to infiltrate the areola and surrounding skin. (From Habif TP: *Clinical dermatology: a color guide to diagnosis and therapy,* ed 3, St Louis, 1996, Mosby.)

A clinical algorithm for the evaluation of nipple discharge is described in Section III, "Breast, Nipple Discharge Evaluation."

LABORATORY TESTS

Biopsy of nipple lesion

IMAGING STUDIES

Mammograms to search for possible primary carcinoma

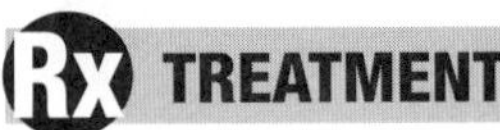

TREATMENT

NONPHARMACOLOGIC THERAPY

- Fewer patients:
  1. Paget's disease of nipple only finding when mammographically negative breast
  2. Consideration of wide excision of nipple with or without radiation
- Other patients: additional invasive or in situ carcinoma recognized
- Either modified mastectomy or breast conservation treatment
- Presence of underlying in situ or invasive carcinoma in mastectomy specimen of majority of patients

ACUTE GENERAL Rx

Systemic adjuvant therapy depending on extent of invasive carcinoma found

DISPOSITION

- Parallel prognosis to that of breast cancer patient without Paget's disease
- Regular follow-up as in other invasive or in situ carcinoma patients

REFERRAL

At outset, all suspicious nipple lesions should be referred for evaluation and treatment.

SUGGESTED READINGS

Sakoratias GH et al: Paget's disease of the breast, *Canc Treat Rev* 27(1):9, 2001.

Sakoratias GH et al: Paget's disease of the breast: a clinical perspective, *Langenbecks Arch Surg* 386(6): 444, 2001.

AUTHORS: **TAKUMA NEMOTO, M.D.,** and **RUBEN ALVERO, M.D.**

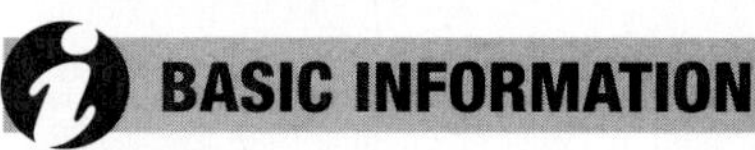

BASIC INFORMATION

DEFINITION

Pancreatic cancer is an adenocarcinoma derived from the epithelium of the pancreatic duct.

ICD-9CM CODES
157.9 Pancreatic cancer
157.0 (head)
157.1 (body)
157.2 (tail)
157.3 (duct)
230.9 (in situ)

EPIDEMIOLOGY & DEMOGRAPHICS

INCIDENCE: One case in 10,000 persons annually. In the U.S. there are >35,000 patients diagnosed with pancreatic cancer and >30,000 deaths yearly.
PREDOMINANT SEX: Male/female ratio of 2:1
PREDOMINANT AGE: Seventh and eighth decades of life

PHYSICAL FINDINGS & CLINICAL PRESENTATION

Presenting symptoms:
- Jaundice
- Abdominal pain
- Weight loss
- Anorexia/change in taste
- Nausea
- Uncommonly: depression, gastrointestinal bleeding, acute pancreatitis, back pain

Physical findings:
- Icterus
- Cachexia
- Excoriations from scratching pruritic skin

ETIOLOGY

Unknown, but several conditions have been associated with pancreatic cancer:
- Smoking
- Alcoholism
- Gallstones
- Diabetes mellitus
- Chronic pancreatitis
- Diet rich in animal fat
- Occupational exposures: oil refining, paper manufacturing, chemical industry
- Overweight or obesity during early adulthood is associated with a greater risk of pancreatic cancer and a younger age of disease onset. Obesity at an older age is associated with a lower overall survival in patients with pancreatic cancer.

Dx DIAGNOSIS

DIFFERENTIAL DIAGNOSIS

- Common duct cholelithiasis
- Cholangiocarcinoma
- Common duct stricture
- Sclerosing cholangitis
- Primary biliary cirrhosis
- Autoimmune pancreatitis
- Drug-induced cholestasis (e.g., phenothiazines)
- Chronic hepatitis
- Sarcoidosis
- Other pancreatic tumors (islet cell tumor, cystadenocarcinoma, epidermoid carcinoma, sarcomas, lymphomas)

WORKUP

Routine Laboratory Tests	*% Abnormal*
Alkaline phosphatase	80
Bilirubin	55
Total protein	15
Amylase	15
Hematocrit	60

IMAGING STUDIES

There is no evidence-based consensus on the optimal preoperative imaging assessment of patients with suspected pancreatic cancer. Helical CT is often the initial study. Multidetector CT and endoscopic ultrasonography represent newer modalities. Compared with multidetector CT, endoscopic ultrasonography is superior for tumor detection and staging but similar for nodal staging and respectability of preoperatively suspected, nonmetastatic pancreatic cancer. Fine-needle aspiration biopsy combined with endoscopic ultrasonography is the preferred modality for evaluation of cystic or mass lesions to determine malignancy.

Noninvasive Imaging	*% Abnormal*
Abdominal ultrasonography	60
Abdominal CT scan (Fig. 1-235) (with or without contrast [IV or oral])	90
Abdominal MRI scan	90
Invasive Imaging	
Endoscopic retrograde cholangiopancreatography	90
CT scan or ultrasonography-guided needle aspiration cytology	90-95

STAGING FOR PANCREATIC CANCER

PRIMARY TUMOR (T):

TX	Primary tumor cannot be assessed
T0	No evidence of primary tumor
T1	Tumor <2 cm
T2	Tumor >2 cm, confined to the pancreas
T3	Tumor extends locally beyond the pancreas
T4	Tumor involves celiac or superior mesenteric arteries

LYMPH NODES (N):

NX	Regional lymph nodes cannot be assessed
N0	No regional lymph node metastasis
N1	Regional lymph node metastasis

DISTANT METASTASES (M):

MX	Presence of distant metastasis cannot be assessed
M0	No distant metastasis
M1	Distant metastasis

STAGING GROUP:

IA	T1, N0, M0
IB	T2, N0, M0
IIA	T3, N0, M0
IIB	T1-3, N1, M0
III	T4, N0-1, M0
IV	T1-4, N0-1, M1

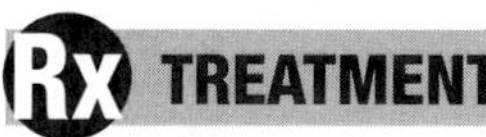

TREATMENT

SURGERY

Curative pancreatectomy (Whipple's procedure) is appropriate for only 10% to 20% of patients whose lesion is <5 cm, solitary, and without metastases. Surgical mortality rate is 5%. Adjuvant chemotherapy may improve postoperative survival. The addition of gemcitabine to adjuvant fluorouracil-based chemotherapy has been reported to have a survival benefit for patients with resected pancreatic cancer, although this

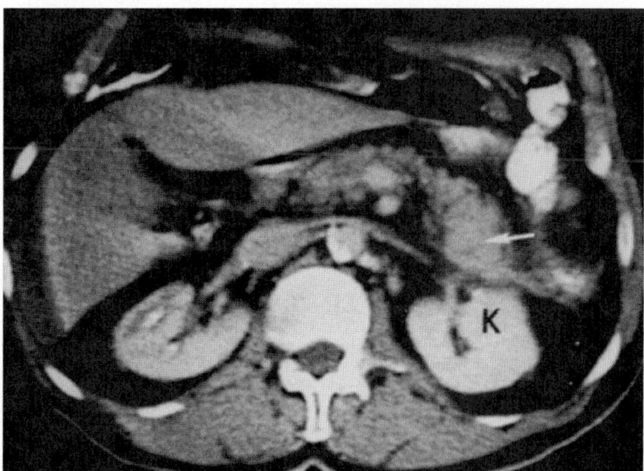

FIGURE 1-235 CT scan of a patient with adenocarcinoma of the body and tail of the pancreas. The tumor *(arrow)* is seen anterior and adjacent to the left kidney *(K)*. At operation, the tumor was invading Gerota's fascia. (From Sabiston D: *Textbook of surgery,* ed 17, Philadelphia, 2005, WB Saunders.)

improvement was not shown to be statistically significant.

PALLIATIVE SURGERY (FOR BILIARY DECOMPRESSION/ DIVERSION)

Palliative therapeutic endoscopic retrograde cholangiopancreatography with stents

CHEMOTHERAPY

The best combination chemotherapy using streptozotocin, mitomycin C, and 5-fluouracil provides only a 19-wk median survival.

RADIATION

- External-beam radiation for palliation of pain.
- Combined chemotherapy and radiation provides a median survival of 11 mo.
- Celiac plexus block by an experienced anesthesiologist provides pain relief in 80% to 90% of cases.

DISPOSITION

- Adjunct chemotherapy has a significant survival benefit in patients with resected pancreatic cancer.
- Recent trials have shown that adjuvant postoperative chemotherapy with gemcitabine significantly delays the development of recurrent disease after complete resection of pancreatic cancer.

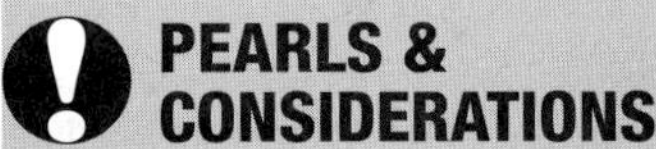

PEARLS & CONSIDERATIONS

COMMENTS

- The U.S. Preventive Services Task Force (USPSTF) recommends against routine screening for pancreatic cancer in asymptomatic adults by abdominal palpation, ultrasonography, or serologic markers. The USPSTF found no evidence that screening for pancreatic cancer is effective in reducing mortality rates. There is potential for significant harm because of the low prevalence of pancreatic cancer, limited accuracy of available screening tests, invasive nature of diagnostic tests, and poor outcome of treatment. As a result, the USPSTF concluded that the harms of screening for pancreatic cancer exceed any potential benefits.
- Recent trials indicate that pancreatic cancer may have a distinct microRNA (miRNA) expression pattern that may differentiate it from normal pancreas and chronic pancreatitis. Current research is aimed at using miRNA expression patterns to distinguish between long- and short-term survivors.

EBM EVIDENCE

Surgical treatment.

Randomized trials comparing surgery with no surgery in people with pancreatic tumors considered suitable for resection would be considered unethical.[1]

A systematic review found that endoscopic insertion of a plastic stent for people with obstructive jaundice secondary to inoperable pancreatic cancer was associated with a reduced rate of complications but higher risk of recurrent biliary obstruction before death compared with surgery.[2] Ⓐ

There is some evidence that metal biliary stents have a lower risk of recurrent biliary obstruction compared with plastic stents.[2] Ⓐ

A recent small multicenter, phase III trial revealed potential benefit for 5-fluouracil–based combination regimens in the setting of advanced inoperable pancreatic cancer.[3] Ⓑ

Erlotinib has been found to provide a small but significant benefit when added to gemcitabine for first-line therapy in patients with advanced inoperable disease.[4] Ⓑ

Evidence-Based References

1. Bazian Ltd: Pancreatic cancer, *Clin Evid* 14:623, 2005. Ⓐ
2. Moss A et al: Palliative biliary stents for obstructing pancreatic carcinoma, *Cochrane Rev* 2, 2006. Ⓐ
3. Oettle H et al: Oxaliplatin/folinic acid/5-fluorouracil plus best supportive care versus supportive care alone in second-line therapy of gemcitabine-refractory advanced pancreatic cancer, *J Clin Oncol* 23:4031, 2005. Ⓑ
4. Moore MJ et al: Erlotinib plus gemcitabine compared to gemcitabine alone in patients with advanced pancreatic cancer: a phase III trial of the National Cancer Institute of Canada Clinical Trials Group, *J Clin Oncol* 23:1, 2005. Ⓑ

SUGGESTED READINGS

Abbruzzese JL: Adjuvant therapy for surgically resected pancreatic adenocarcinoma, *JAMA* 299: 1066, 2008.

Bloomston M et al: MicroRNA expression patterns to differentiate pancreatic adenocarcinoma from normal pancreas and chronic pancreatitis, *JAMA* 297: 1901, 2007.

Freelove R, Walling AD: Pancreatic cancer: diagnosis and management, *Am Fam Physician* 73:485, 2006.

Li D et al: Body mass index and risk, age of onset, and survival in patients with pancreatic cancer, *JAMA* 301(24):2553-2562, 2009.

Oettle H et al: Adjuvant chemotherapy with gemcitabine vs observation in patients undergoing curative-intent resection of pancreatic cancer, *JAMA* 297:267, 2007.

Regine WF et al: Fluorouracil vs gemcitabine chemotherapy before and after fluorouracil-based chemoradiation following resection of pancreatic adenocarcinoma, *JAMA* 299(9):1019-1026, 2008.

U.S. Preventive Task Force: *Screening for pancreatic cancer: a brief evidence update for the USPTS.* Available at http://ahrq.gov/clinic/uspstf/uspspanc.htm.

AUTHOR: **FRED F. FERRI, M.D.**

BASIC INFORMATION

DEFINITION

- Acute pancreatitis is an inflammatory process of the pancreas with intrapancreatic activation of enzymes that may also involve peripancreatic tissue and/or remote organ systems.
- Severe acute pancreatitis (SAP) is diagnosed by the presence of any of the following four criteria:
  1. Organ failure with one or more of the following: shock (systolic blood pressure <90 mm Hg), pulmonary insufficiency (Pa_{O_2} ≤60 mm Hg), renal failure (serum creatinine >2 mg/dl after rehydration), and gastrointestinal bleeding (>500 ml/24 hr)
  2. Local complications such as necrosis, pseudocyst, or abscess
  3. At least three of Ranson's criteria (see below) *or*
  4. At least eight of the Acute Physiology and Chronic Health Evaluation II (APACHE II) criteria

ICD-9CM CODES
577.0 Acute pancreatitis

EPIDEMIOLOGY & DEMOGRAPHICS

- Acute pancreatitis is most often secondary to biliary tract disease and alcohol.
- Incidence in urban areas is twice that of rural areas (20/100,000 persons in urban areas).
- 20% of patients have necrotizing pancreatitis; the remainder have interstitial, or edematous, pancreatitis.
- Acute pancreatitis accounts for >220,000 hospital admissions in the U.S. each year.

PHYSICAL FINDINGS & CLINICAL PRESENTATION

- Epigastric tenderness and guarding; pain usually developing suddenly, reaching peak intensity within 10 to 30 min, severe and lasting several hours without relief
- Hypoactive bowel sounds (from ileus)
- Tachycardia, shock (from decreased intravascular volume)
- Confusion (from metabolic disturbances)
- Fever
- Tachycardia, decreased breath sounds (atelectasis, pleural effusions, acute respiratory distress syndrome [ARDS])
- Jaundice (from obstruction or compression of biliary tract)
- Ascites (from tear in pancreatic duct, leaking pseudocyst)
- Palpable abdominal mass (pseudocyst, phlegmon, abscess, carcinoma)
- Evidence of hypocalcemia ***(Chvostek's sign, Trousseau's sign)***
- Evidence of intraabdominal bleeding (hemorrhagic pancreatitis):
  1. Gray-blue discoloration around the umbilicus ***(Cullen's sign)***
  2. Bluish discoloration involving the flanks ***(Grey Turner's sign)***
- Tender subcutaneous nodules (caused by subcutaneous fat necrosis)

ETIOLOGY

- In >90% of cases: biliary tract disease (calculi or sludge) or alcohol
- Drugs (e.g., thiazides, furosemide, corticosteroids, tetracycline, estrogens, valproic acid, metronidazole, azathioprine, methyldopa, pentamidine, ethacrynic acid, procainamide, sulindac, nitrofurantoin, angiotensin-converting enzyme inhibitors, danazol, cimetidine, piroxicam, gold, ranitidine, sulfasalazine, isoniazid, acetaminophen, cisplatin, opiates, erythromycin, metformin, sitagliptin)
- Abdominal trauma
- Surgery
- Endoscopic retrograde cholangiopancreatography (ERCP)
- Infections (predominantly viral infections)
- Peptic ulcer (penetrating duodenal ulcer)
- Pancreas divisum (congenital failure to fuse of dorsal or ventral pancreas)
- Idiopathic
- Pregnancy
- Vascular (vasculitis, ischemic)
- Hypolipoproteinemia (types I, IV, and V)
- Hypercalcemia
- Pancreatic carcinoma (primary or metastatic)
- Renal failure
- Hereditary pancreatitis
- Occupational exposure to chemicals: methanol, cobalt, zinc, mercuric chloride, creosol, lead, organophosphates, chlorinated naphthalenes
- Others: scorpion bite, obstruction at ampulla region (neoplasm, duodenal diverticula, Crohn's disease), hypotensive shock, autoimmune pancreatitis

Dx DIAGNOSIS

DIFFERENTIAL DIAGNOSIS

- PUD
- Acute cholangitis, biliary colic
- High intestinal obstruction
- Early acute appendicitis
- Mesenteric vascular obstruction
- DKA
- Pneumonia (basilar)
- Myocardial infarction (inferior wall)
- Renal colic
- Ruptured or dissecting aortic aneurysm
- Mesenteric ischemia

LABORATORY TESTS

Pancreatic enzymes:

- Amylase is increased, usually elevated in the initial 3 to 5 days of acute pancreatitis. Isoamylase determinations (separation of pancreatic cell isoenzyme components of amylase) are useful in excluding occasional cases of salivary hyperamylasemia. The use of isoamylase rather than total serum amylase reduces the risk of erroneously diagnosing pancreatitis and is preferred by some as initial biochemical test in patients suspected of having acute pancreatitis.
- Urinary amylase determinations are useful to diagnose acute pancreatitis in patients with lipemic serum, to rule out elevated serum amylase caused by macroamylasemia, and to diagnose acute pancreatitis in patients whose serum amylase is normal.
- Serum lipase levels are elevated in acute pancreatitis; the elevation is less transient than serum amylase; concomitant evaluation of serum amylase and lipase increases diagnostic accuracy of acute pancreatitis. An elevated lipase/amylase ratio is suggestive of alcoholic pancreatitis.
- Elevated serum trypsin levels are diagnostic of pancreatitis (in absence of renal failure); measurement is made by radioimmunoassay. Although not routinely available, the serum trypsin level is the most accurate laboratory indicator for pancreatitis.
- Rapid measurement of urinary trypsinogen-2 (if available) is useful in the emergency department as a screening test for acute pancreatitis in patients with abdominal pain; a negative dipstick test for urinary trypsinogen-2 rules out acute pancreatitis with a high degree of probability, whereas a positive test indicates need for further evaluation.

Additional tests:

- Complete blood count: reveals leukocytosis; hematocrit (Hct) may be initially increased as a result of hemoconcentration; decreased Hct may indicate hemorrhage or hemolysis.
- Blood urea nitrogen (BUN) is increased because of dehydration.
- Elevation of serum glucose in a previously normal patient correlates with the degree of pancreatic malfunction and may be related to increased release of glycogen, catecholamines, and glucocorticoid release and decreased insulin release.
- Liver profile: aspartate aminotransferase (AST) and lactate dehydrogenase (LDH) are increased as a result of tissue necrosis; bilirubin and alkaline phosphatase may be increased from common bile duct obstruction. A threefold or greater rise in serum alanine aminotransferase concentrations is an excellent indicator (95% probability) of biliary pancreatitis.
- Serum calcium is decreased as a result of saponification, precipitation, and decreased parathyroid hormone response.
- Arterial blood gases: Pa_{O_2} may be decreased as a result of ARDS, pleural effusion(s); pH may be decreased as a result of lactic acidosis, respiratory acidosis, and renal insufficiency.
- Serum electrolytes: potassium may be increased from acidosis or renal insufficiency; sodium may be increased from dehydration.

IMAGING STUDIES

- Abdominal plain films are useful initially to distinguish other conditions that may mimic pancreatitis (perforated viscus). They may reveal localized ileus (sentinel loop), pancreatic calcifications (chronic pancreatitis), blurring of left psoas shadow, dilation of transverse colon, calcified gallstones.

- Chest radiographs may reveal elevation of one or both diaphragms, pleural effusions, basilar infiltrates, or platelike atelectasis.
- Abdominal ultrasonography is useful in detecting gallstones (sensitivity of 60% to 70% for detecting stones associated with pancreatitis). It is also useful for detecting pancreatic pseudocysts; its major limitation is the presence of distended bowel loops overlying the pancreas.
- CT scan is superior to ultrasonography in identifying pancreatitis and defining its extent, and it also plays a role in diagnosing pseudocysts (they appear as a well-defined area surrounded by a high-density capsule); gastrointestinal fistulation or infection of a pseudocyst can also be identified by the presence of gas within the pseudocyst. Sequential contrast-enhanced CT is useful for detection of pancreatic necrosis (Fig. 1-236). The severity of pancreatitis can also be graded by CT scan. (A = normal pancreas, B = enlarged pancreas [1 point], C = pancreatic and/or peripancreatic inflammation [2 points], D = single peripancreatic collection [3 points], E = at least two peripancreatic collections and/or retroperitoneal air [4 points]. Percentage of pancreatic necrosis <30% [2 points], 30% to 50% [4 points], >50% [6 points]. The CT severity index is calculated by adding grade points to points assigned for percentage of necrosis.)
- Magnetic resonance cholangiopancreatography is also a useful diagnostic modality if a surgical procedure is not anticipated.
- ERCP should not be performed during the acute stage of disease unless it is necessary to remove an impacted stone in the ampulla of Vater; patients with severe or worsening pancreatitis but without obstructive jaundice (biliary obstruction) do not benefit from early ERCP and papillotomy. ERCP can be deferred as long as no evidence of cholestasis or cholangitis is present.

Rx TREATMENT

NONPHARMACOLOGIC THERAPY

- Bowel rest with avoidance of liquids or solids during the acute illness
- Avoidance of alcohol and any drugs associated with pancreatitis

ACUTE GENERAL Rx

General measures:

- Maintain adequate intravascular volume with vigorous IV hydration.
- Patient should remain NPO until clinically improved, stable, and hungry. Enteral feedings are preferred over total parenteral nutrition. Parenteral nutrition may be necessary in patients who do not tolerate enteral feeding or in whom an adequate infusion rate cannot be reached within 2 to 4 days.
- Nasogastric suction is useful only in severe pancreatitis to decompress the abdomen in patients with ileus.
- Control pain: IV morphine or fentanyl
- Correct metabolic abnormalities (e.g., replace calcium and magnesium as necessary).

Specific measures:

- Pancreatic or peripancreatic infection develops in 40% to 70% of patients with pancreatic necrosis. However, IV antibiotics should not be used prophylactically for all cases of pancreatitis; their use is justified if the patient has evidence of septicemia, pancreatic abscess, or pancreatitis caused by biliary calculi. Their use should generally be limited to 5 to 7 days to prevent development of fungal superinfection. Appropriate empiric antibiotic therapy should cover:
  1. *Bacteroides fragilis* and other anaerobes (cefotetan, cefoxitin, metronidazole, or clindamycin plus aminoglycoside)
  2. *Enterococcus* (ampicillin)
- Surgical therapy has a limited role in acute pancreatitis; it is indicated in the following:
  1. Gallstone-induced pancreatitis: cholecystectomy when acute pancreatitis subsides.
  2. Perforated peptic ulcer.
  3. Excision or drainage of necrotic or infected foci. Necronectomy (debridement) with placement of wide-bore drains for continuous postoperative irrigation is the preferred surgical procedure. Surgery is not indicated for patients with sterile necrosis unless there is clinical deterioration despite intensive medical care.
- Identification and treatment of complications:
  1. Pseudocyst: round or spheroid collection of fluid, tissue, pancreatic enzymes, and blood.
     a. Diagnosed by CT scan or sonography
     b. Treatment: CT scan or ultrasound-guided percutaneous drainage (with a pigtail catheter left in place for continuous drainage) can be used, but the recurrence rate is high; the conservative approach is to reevaluate the pseudocyst (with CT scan or sonography) after 6 to 7 wk and surgically drain it if the pseudocyst has not decreased in size. Generally pseudocysts <5 cm in diameter are reabsorbed without intervention, whereas those >5 cm require surgical intervention after the wall has matured.
  2. Phlegmon: represents pancreatic edema. It can be diagnosed by CT scan or sonography. Treatment is supportive because it usually resolves spontaneously.
  3. Pancreatic abscess: diagnosed by CT scan (presence of bubbles in the retroperitoneum); Gram staining and cultures of fluid obtained from guided percutaneous aspiration usually identify bacterial organism. Therapy is surgical (or catheter) drainage and IV antibiotics (imipenem-cilastatin [Primaxin] is the drug of choice).
  4. Pancreatic ascites: usually caused by leaking of pseudocyst or tear in pancreatic duct. Paracentesis reveals very high amylase and lipase levels in the pancreatic fluid; ERCP may demonstrate the lesion. Treatment is surgical correction if exudative ascites from severe pancreatitis does not resolve spontaneously.
  5. Gastrointestinal bleeding: caused by alcoholic gastritis, bleeding varices, stress ulceration, or disseminated intravascular coagulation (DIC).
  6. Renal failure: caused by hypovolemia, resulting in oliguria or anuria, cortical or tubular necrosis (shock, DIC), or thrombosis of renal artery or vein.
  7. Hypoxia: caused by ARDS, pleural effusion, or atelectasis.

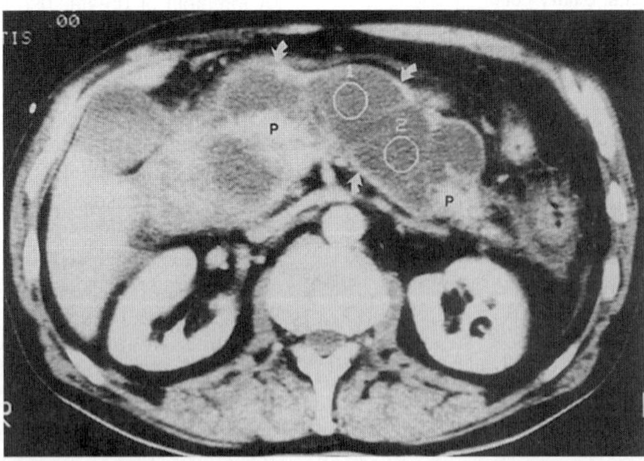

FIGURE 1-236 Acute necrotizing pancreatitis. Dynamic CT shows enlargement of the pancreas, a thin rim of contrast-enhancement *(arrows),* and lack of enhancement of the pancreatic parenchyma, indicating almost complete gland necrosis (cursors 1 and 2 measure soft tissue density: 25 to 30 Hounsfield units). Small islands of normally enhancing parenchyma are seen *(P).* Patient died despite surgery. (From Grainger RG et al [eds]: *Grainger & Allison's diagnostic radiology,* ed 4, Philadelphia, 2001, Churchill Livingstone.)

DISPOSITION

Prognosis varies with the severity of pancreatitis; overall mortality rate in acute pancreatitis is 5% to 10%; poor prognostic signs according to the Ranson criteria are as follows:

- Age >55 yr
- Fluid sequestration >6000 ml
- Laboratory abnormalities on admission: white blood cell count >16,000, blood glucose >200 mg/dl, serum LDH >350 IU/L, AST >250 IU/L

- Laboratory abnormalities during the initial 48 hr: decreased Hct >10% with hydration or Hct <30%, BUN rise >5 mg/dl, serum calcium <8 mg/dl, arterial Po_2 <60 mm Hg, and base deficit >4 mEq/L

REFERRAL

- Hospitalization is indicated in moderate to severe cases of pancreatitis.
- Surgical consultation is needed in suspected gallstone pancreatitis, perforated peptic ulcer, or presence of necrotic or infected foci.

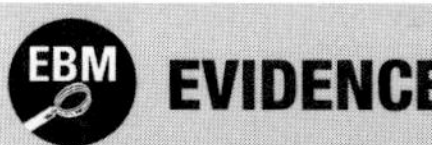

EVIDENCE

Please note: Complete text of EBM for this topic is available online.

Key trials and commentary:

In patients with severe, necrotizing pancreatitis, it is common to administer early, broad-spectrum antibiotics, often a carbapenem, in the hope of reducing the incidence of pancreatic and peripancreatic infections, although the benefits of doing so have not been proved. This study demonstrated no statistically significant difference between the treatment groups for pancreatic or peripancreatic infection, mortality, or requirement for surgical intervention, and did not support early prophylactic antimicrobial use in patients with severe acute necrotizing pancreatitis.

In recent years, the practice of administering broad-spectrum prophylactic antibiotics to patients with severe necrotizing pancreatitis has become common. This approach is based on several small, randomized studies that suggested a decreased risk of pancreatic infection and meta-analyses that suggested an improved survival rate. However, the only published randomized, double-blind trial of antibiotic prophylaxis in this condition showed no advantage over placebo.[4] This is an important question for intensivists because patients with severe necrotizing pancreatitis are routinely admitted to the intensive care unit for supportive care and monitoring.

In this randomized, double-blind, placebo-controlled study, prophylaxis with meropenem was found to have no impact on infection rates, the requirement for surgical intervention, or the mortality rate. Although the study was limited by the relatively small sample size (50 in each group), it is actually comparable in size to the largest studies to address this question. These results strongly call into question the practice of using antimicrobial prophylaxis in patients with this condition.[1] Ⓐ

Evidence-Based Reference

1. Dellinger EP et al: Early antibiotic treatment for severe acute necrotizing pancreatitis: A randomized, double-blind, placebo-controlled study, *Ann Surg* 245:674-683, 2007. Commentary by A. Kumar, M.D. Ⓐ

SUGGESTED READINGS

Balthazar EJ: Acute pancreatitis: assessment of severity with clinical and CT evaluation, *Radiology* 223: 603, 2002.

Bosmann M et al: Coexistence of Cullen's and Grey Turner's signs in acute pancreatitis, *Am J Med* 122: 333-334, 2009.

Finkelberg D et al: Autoimmune pancreatitis, *N Engl J Med* 355:2670, 2006.

Knaus WA et al: APACHE II: a severity of disease classification system, *Crit Care Med* 13:818, 1984.

Swaroop VS et al: Severe acute pancreatitis, *JAMA* 291:2865, 2004.

Vitale GC: Early management of acute gallstone pancreatitis, *Ann Surg* 245:18, 2007.

Whitcomb DC: Acute pancreatitis, *N Engl J Med* 354: 2142, 2006.

AUTHOR: **FRED F. FERRI, M.D.**

Pancreatitis, Chronic (PTG) (ALG)

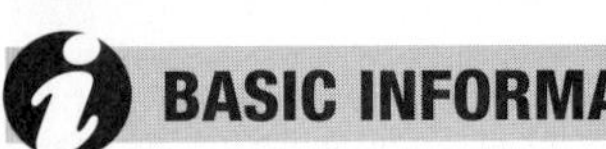

BASIC INFORMATION

DEFINITION

Chronic pancreatitis is a recurrent or persistent inflammatory process of the pancreas characterized by chronic pain and by pancreatic exocrine and/or endocrine insufficiency.

ICD-9CM CODES
577.1 Chronic pancreatitis

EPIDEMIOLOGY & DEMOGRAPHICS

- Chronic pancreatitis occurs in approximately five to 10 per 100,000 persons in industrialized countries.
- Average age at diagnosis is 35 to 55 yr; male/female ratio is 5:1.

PHYSICAL FINDINGS & CLINICAL PRESENTATION

- Persistent or recurrent epigastric and left upper quadrant pain that may radiate to the back
- Tenderness over the pancreas, muscle guarding
- Significant weight loss
- Bulky, foul-smelling stools, greasy in appearance
- Epigastric mass (10% of patients)
- Jaundice (5% to 10% of patients)

ETIOLOGY

- Chronic alcoholism.
- Obstruction (ampullary stenosis, tumor, trauma, pancreas divisum, annular pancreas).
- Hereditary pancreatitis.
- Severe malnutrition.
- Idiopathic.
- Untreated hyperparathyroidism (hypercalcemia).
- Mutations of the cystic fibrosis transmembrane conductance regulator *(CFTR)* gene and the TF genotype.
- Autoimmune pancreatitis (5% of chronic pancreatitis cases): presents clinically with jaundice (63% of patients) and abdominal pain (35%). CT may reveal diffusely enlarged pancreas, enhanced peripheral rim of hypoattenuation "halo," and low-attenuation mass in head of pancreas. Laboratory values reveal elevated serum immunoglobulin (Ig) G4, elevated serum Ig or gamma-globulin level, presence of antilactoferrin antibody (ALA), anticarbonic anhydrase (ACA) II level, anti-smooth-muscle antibody (ASMA), or antinuclear antibody (ANA).
- Sclerosing pancreatitis: a form of chronic pancreatitis characterized by infrequent attacks of abdominal pain, irregular narrowing of the pancreatic duct, and swelling of the pancreatic parenchyma; patients have high levels of serum immunoglobulins (IgG4). Chronic sclerosing pancreatitis is also known as *autoimmune pancreatitis.*

Dx DIAGNOSIS

DIFFERENTIAL DIAGNOSIS

- Pancreatic cancer
- Peptic ulcer disease
- Cholelithiasis with biliary obstruction
- Malabsorption from other etiologies
- Recurrent acute pancreatitis
- Renal insufficiency
- Intestinal ischemia or infarction
- Other: Crohn's disease, gastroparesis, inflammatory bowel disease

WORKUP

Medical history with focus on alcohol use, laboratory tests, diagnostic imaging

LABORATORY TESTS

- Serum amylase and lipase may be elevated (normal amylase levels, however, do not exclude the diagnosis).
- Hyperglycemia, glycosuria, hyperbilirubinemia, and elevated serum alkaline phosphatase may also be present.
- 72-hr fecal fat determination (rarely performed) reveals excess fecal fat. Fecal elastase test requires only 20 g of stool.
- Secretin stimulation test is the best test for diagnosing pancreatic exocrine insufficiency.
- Lipid panel: significantly elevated triglycerides can cause pancreatitis.
- Serum calcium: hyperparathyroidism is a rare cause of chronic pancreatitis.
- Elevated levels of serum IgG4 are found in sclerosing pancreatitis and autoimmune pancreatitis.
- Elevated serum Ig or gamma globulin level, presence of ALA, ACA II level, ASMA, or ANA in autoimmune pancreatitis.

IMAGING STUDIES

- Plain abdominal radiographs may reveal pancreatic calcifications (95% specific for chronic pancreatitis).
- Ultrasound of abdomen may reveal duct dilation, pseudocyst, calcification, and presence of ascites.
- Contrast-enhanced CT scan of abdomen is the initial modality of choice. It is useful to detect calcifications, evaluate for ductal dilation, and rule out pancreatic cancer.
- Endoscopic retrograde cholangiopancreatography (ERCP) has been traditionally used to evaluate for the presence of dilated ducts, strictures, pseudocysts, and intraductal stones. However, for the evaluation of pancreatic parenchyma and duct system newer, less invasive modalities such as magnetic resonance cholangiopancreatography (MRCP) and endoscopic ultrasonography (EUS) may be preferred. EUS has a sensitivity of 97% and a specificity of 60% for chronic pancreatitis and a very low complication rate. Fine-needle aspiration biopsy (FNAB) combined with EUS is the preferred modality for evaluation of cystic or mass lesions to determine malignancy.

Rx TREATMENT

NONPHARMACOLOGIC THERAPY

- Avoidance of alcohol and tobacco
- Frequent, small-volume, low-fat meals

ACUTE GENERAL Rx

- Avoidance of narcotics if possible (simple analgesics or nonsteroidal anti-inflammatory drugs can be used).
- Treatment of steatorrhea with pancreatic supplements (e.g., Pancrease, Creon, Pancrelipase titrated prn based on the amount of steatorrhea and patient's weight loss). Proton pump inhibitors and H_2 blockers reduce inactivation of the enzymes from gastric acid.
- Treatment of complications (e.g., type 1 diabetes mellitus).
- Glucocorticoid therapy in patients with autoimmune pancreatitis and sclerosing pancreatitis can induce clinical remission and significantly decrease serum concentrations of IgG4, immune complexes, and the IgG4 subclass of immune complexes.

CHRONIC Rx

- Surgical intervention may be necessary to eliminate biliary tract disease and improve flow of bile into the duodenum by eliminating obstruction of pancreatic duct.
- ERCP with endoscopic sphincterectomy and stone extraction is useful in selected patients.
- Transduodenal sphincteroplasty or pancreaticojejunostomy in selected patients. Surgery should also be considered in patients with intractable pain.

DISPOSITION

- Long-term survival is poor (50% of patients die within 10 yr from chronic pancreatitis or malignancy).
- Prognosis is best in patients with recurrent acute pancreatitis resulting from cholelithiasis, hyperparathyroidism, or stenosis of the sphincter of Oddi.

REFERRAL

Gastrointestinal referral for ERCP, surgical referral in selected patients (see "Chronic Rx").

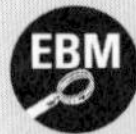

EVIDENCE

Please note: Complete text of EBM for this topic is available online.

Key trials and commentary:

For patients with chronic pancreatitis and a dilated pancreatic duct, ductal decompression is recommended. This study conducted a randomized trial to compare endoscopic and surgical drainage of the pancreatic duct.

This study showed that surgical drainage of the pancreatic duct was more effective than endoscopic treatment in patients with obstruction of the pancreatic duct caused by chronic pancreatitis.

The development of chronic pancreatitis from acute pancreatitis should be viewed from the hepatology spectrum, because it is similar to the relationship of acute hepatitis to cirrhosis. Unfortunately, both tracts are predisposed to development of cancer. With chronic pancreatitis it is pancreatic cancer, whereas with cirrhosis it is hepatocellular cancer. The most common symptom of chronic pancreatitis is abdominal pain that interferes with the quality of life, and it often leads to drug addiction. Chronic pancreatitis is thought to originate from the multitude of causes including ductal obstruction, ischemia, inflammatory damage to pancreatic nerves, and other complications, that is, duodenal obstruction, pseudocyst, etc. Medical management is supportive and includes avoidance of alcohol, pancreatic enzyme replacement, and non-narcotic pain medication. Our attention usually focuses on the reversible causes, that is, pseudocysts, duodenal obstruction, and lastly, pancreatic ductal decompression. The latter can be accomplished either surgically, with a longitudinal pancreaticojejunostomy, or endoscopically, with dilation of pancreatic duct strictures, use of extracorporeal shock wave lithotripsy when needed to fracture stones, and then use of endoscopy for removal of the stones. This study, and other previous studies, reaches the conclusion that surgical drainage provides better pain relief in patients with strictures from chronic pancreatitis.[1] Ⓐ

Evidence-Based Reference

1. Cahen DL et al: Endoscopic versus surgical drainage of the pancreatic duct in chronic pancreatitis, *N Engl J Med* 356:676-684, 2007. Commentary by J.S. Barkin, M.D. Ⓐ

SUGGESTED READINGS

Finkelberg DL et al: Autoimmune pancreatitis, *N Engl J Med* 355:2670, 2006.

Hamano H et al: High serum IgG4 concentrations in patients with sclerosing pancreatitis, *N Engl J Med* 344:732, 2001.

Hollerbach S et al: Endoscopic ultrasonography and fine needle aspiration cytology for diagnosis of chronic pancreatitis, *Endoscopy* 33:824, 2001.

Nair R et al: Chronic pancreatitis, *Am Fam Physician* 76:1679-1688, 2007.

AUTHOR: **FRED F. FERRI, M.D.**

Panic Disorder, with or without Agoraphobia

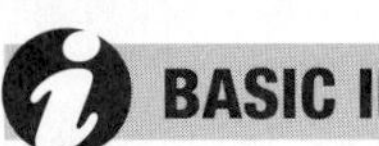

BASIC INFORMATION

DEFINITION

A panic attack is a relatively brief, sudden episode of intense fear or apprehension, often associated with a sense of impending doom and various uncomfortable and disquieting physical symptoms. Panic attacks may be uncued ("out of the blue") or cued (i.e., triggered by a particular object or situation). Panic attacks may be present in a variety of different anxiety-related disorders (e.g., phobias, social anxiety, obsessive-compulsive disorder). Panic disorder is diagnosed after two uncued panic attacks have occurred followed by at least 1 mo (or more) of significant concern about future attacks, worry about their implications, or a major change in behavior related to these attacks. Agoraphobia is anxiety about, and avoidance of, places or situations in which the ability to escape is limited or embarrassing or in which help might not be available in the event of having a panic attack.

SYNONYMS

Anxiety attacks
Fear attacks
Ataque de nervios

ICD-9CM CODES
F41.0 Panic disorder without agoraphobia (DSM-IV 300.01)
F40.01 Panic disorder with agoraphobia (DSM-IV 300.21)

EPIDEMIOLOGY & DEMOGRAPHICS

INCIDENCE (IN U.S.): 1% 1-mo incidence of panic attacks.

PREVALENCE (IN U.S.):
- 15% to 20% lifetime prevalence of one or more panic attacks.
- Panic disorder much more uncommon, with a lifetime prevalence of 1.5% to 3.5%; chronicity of condition reflected by a similar 1-yr prevalence rate of 1% to 2%.
- Agoraphobia relatively rare; 0.3% to 1% lifetime prevalence; 30% to 50% of patients diagnosed with panic disorder also have agoraphobia.

PEAK INCIDENCE:
- Chronic condition with a waxing and waning course.
- Bimodal incidence peaks noted, with the first peak between ages 15 and 24 yr and second peak between ages 35 and 44 yr.

PREDOMINANT SEX:
- Women more commonly affected (>85% of clinical population).
- Panic disorder twice as common in women.
- Panic disorder with agoraphobia three times as common in women.

PREDOMINANT AGE:
- Age of onset is typically late adolescence to mid-30s. Onset earlier in males (24 yr) than females (28 yr).
- Onset after age 45 yr is rare and should raise suspicion of different etiology.

GENETICS:
- Risk of developing panic disorder in first-degree relatives of individuals with panic disorder is four to seven times that of general population.
- Findings in twin studies: approximately 60% of contributing factors to panic are genetic.

PHYSICAL FINDINGS & CLINICAL PRESENTATION

Panic disorder:
- Present either with a panic attack or with fear and anxiety related to anticipation of a future panic attack or its implications.
- Typical presentation: unexpected, untriggered periods of intense anxiety and fear with associated physiologic changes (e.g., palpitations, sweating, tremulousness, shortness of breath, chest pain, gastrointestinal distress, faintness, derealization, paresthesia). Panic attacks are often described as "the most terrifying" episode an individual has experienced.
- Emergency or physician visits often occasioned by physical symptoms such as chest pain, dizziness, or difficulty breathing.

Agoraphobia:
- Rare complaints to physician. May manifest in missed office visits or tardiness. Patients may request home visits or telephone care.
- Activities usually self-limited by avoiding public situations where the patient might experience a panic attack and would be unable to exit readily, such as the following:
  1. Crowded public areas (stores, public transportation, flying, church)
  2. Individual interactions (hairdresser, neighborhood meetings)
  3. Driving (especially if alone, over bridges, or on isolated roads)
- On exposure to or anticipation of exposure to such situations, significant anxiety occurs. Anxiety may generate somatic symptoms that trigger a full-blown panic attack, further reinforcing avoidance of such situations.

ETIOLOGY

Hypotheses (NOTE: There are sufficient data to support each model. Models are not mutually exclusive.)
1. Central dyscontrol of autonomic arousal (typically localized to the locus ceruleus); similar symptoms may be chemically induced with yohimbine, caffeine, or cholecystokinin.
2. Cognitive overreaction (i.e., "catastrophic misinterpretation") to relatively mild or benign physiologic cues that then triggers a genuine autonomic cascade and further misinterpretations.
3. Dysfunction of a central suffocation alarm mechanism; some signs of compensated respiratory alkalosis. Can be experimentally induced with sodium lactate or carbon dioxide.

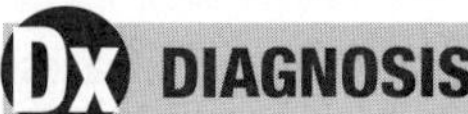

DIAGNOSIS

DIFFERENTIAL DIAGNOSIS

Medical conditions:
- Endocrinopathies:
  1. Hyperthyroidism
  2. Hyperparathyroidism
  3. Pheochromocytoma
  4. Carcinoid tumor
- Cardiac and respiratory diseases:
  1. Arrhythmias
  2. Myocardial infarction
  3. Chronic obstructive pulmonary disease
  4. Asthma
- Metabolic:
  1. Hypoglycemia
  2. Electrolyte imbalances
  3. Porphyria
- Seizure disorders
- Psychiatric disorders (NOTE: Panic attacks are common in a variety of psychiatric disorders. Panic disorder could be conceptualized as a phobia of the somatic sensations or situations that have become paired with panic attacks.)
  1. Phobias (e.g., specific phobia or social phobia)
  2. Obsessive-compulsive disorder (cued by exposure to the object of the obsession)
  3. Posttraumatic stress disorder (cued by recall of a stressor)
- Therapeutic (theophylline, steroids) and recreational (cocaine, amphetamine, caffeine, diet pills) drugs and drug withdrawal (alcohol, barbiturates, benzodiazepines)

WORKUP

- Emergency presentation: cardiac, respiratory, or neurologic symptoms
- History and physical examination to rule out a concomitant medical or substance-related condition

NOTE: Panic disorder and agoraphobia are not diagnoses of exclusion, but exclusion of other conditions is usually required.

LABORATORY TESTS

- Thyroid profile
- Electrolyte measures, including calcium
- Toxicology screen
- ECG
- Acute cases: possible monitoring and cardiac enzymes to rule out arrhythmia or ischemia

IMAGING STUDIES

- For temporal lobe dysfunction (e.g., temporal lesions or as ictal or interictal manifestation of temporal lobe seizures): brain CT scan or MRI or an electroencephalogram in some patients
- Holter monitor to rule out occult or episodic arrhythmias
- Chest x-ray examination, arterial blood gases, or pulmonary function tests if respiratory compromise suspected

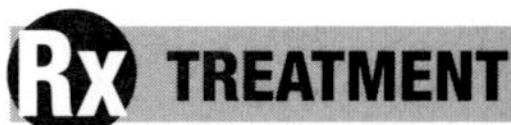

NONPHARMACOLOGIC THERAPY

Cognitive-behavioral therapy (CBT) is generally very effective, with strongest results for cognitive restructuring (i.e., challenging catastrophic misinterpretations of somatic symptoms) and interoceptive exposures (i.e., recreation and management of feared somatic sensations). CBT effect sizes are equal to or larger than for pharmacotherapy, attrition rates are lower, and relapse rates are lower.

ACUTE GENERAL Rx

- Benzodiazepines, particularly alprazolam: highly effective in the acute setting.
- Low-dose alprazolam for patients with rare panic attacks and asymptomatic periods (0.25 to 0.5 mg PO or sublingually prn).
- Start patient on selective serotonin reuptake inhibitor (SSRI) or similar agent and taper patient off of benzodiazepine by wk 2 to 3.

CHRONIC Rx

- Preferred pharmacologic agents: antidepressants with a significant serotonin reuptake inhibitory action. Generally start at low dose and titrate upward. Minimum treatment duration is 6 to 8 mo, but many patients need to take medications indefinitely.
  1. SSRIs: paroxetine (10 to 60 mg/day), sertraline (50 to 200 mg/day), citalopram (20 to 60 mg/day), escitalopram (5 to 30 mg/day), and fluoxetine (5 to 60 mg/day)
  2. Imipramine (100 to 300 mg/day)
  3. Venlafaxine (75 to 225 mg/day)
- Combination CBT plus SSRI has shown good long-term effects and is somewhat better than antidepressants or CBT alone. Combination CBT plus benzodiazepine does not provide any added benefit and may undermine CBT (interoceptive exposures are less effective if patient is taking a benzodiazepine).

DISPOSITION

- Typical course is chronic but with significant waxing and waning (common to have long periods of remission).
- Presence of agoraphobia associated with a more chronic course.
- Findings with long-term follow-up studies: 6 to 10 yr after treatment some 30% are in remission, 40% to 50% have improved with residual symptoms, and the remainder either are unchanged or worse.

REFERRAL

- If patients do not respond to an SSRI.
- Cognitive-behavioral therapy is the preferred treatment.

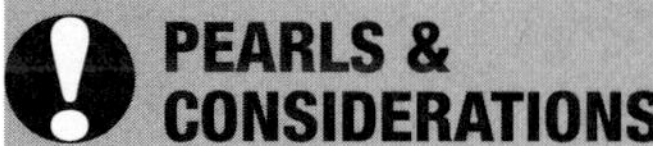

- Patient and family education is an important first step in the management of panic disorder. Education provides more adaptive explanations for the benign somatic sensations paired with panic.
- Resumption of avoided activities or situations is a positive prognostic sign and may promote further therapeutic gains.

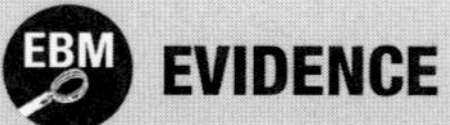

Please note: Complete text of EBM for this topic is available online.

Key trials and commentary:

Study sought to compare the long-term efficacy of venlafaxine extended release (ER) with placebo in preventing panic disorder relapse in outpatient treatment responders.

This study showed that venlafaxine ER was safe, well tolerated, and effective in preventing relapse in outpatients with panic disorder.

It has been somewhat unclear in the research history of venlafaxine how effective it is in panic disorder. Early on, I designed and conducted a large trial that failed to demonstrate efficacy. However, this large definitive trial demonstrates clear efficacy of the extended release venlafaxine. In this study, venlafaxine ER was well tolerated and effective in a relapse prevention design.[1] Ⓐ

Evidence-Based Reference

1. Ferguson JM et al: Relapse prevention of panic disorder in adult outpatient responders to treatment with venlafaxine extended release, *J Clin Psychiatry* 68:58-68, 2007. Commentary by J.C. Ballenger, M.D. Ⓐ

SUGGESTED READINGS

Katon WJ: Clinical practice: panic disorder, *N Engl J Med* 354(22):2360, 2006.

Raffa SD et al: Relapse following combined treatment discontinuation in a placebo-controlled trial for panic disorder, *J Nerv Ment Dis* 196(7):548-555, 2008.

AUTHORS: **JASON M. SATTERFIELD, PH.D.,** and **MITCHELL D. FELDMAN, M.D., M.PHIL.**

Paranoid Personality Disorder (PTG)

BASIC INFORMATION

DEFINITION

Paranoid personality disorder (PPD) is characterized by a pattern of pervasive distrust and suspiciousness of others that leads the person to assign malevolence to the motives of others. PPD begins by early adulthood and causes significant distress or impairment in multiple domains of functioning. Individuals must meet four or more of the following criteria:

1. Suspect, without justification, that others are exploiting, harming, or deceiving them.
2. Preoccupied with unwarranted doubts about the loyalty or trustworthiness of friends or associates.
3. Reluctant to confide in others because of unjustified fear that the information will be used against them in a malicious fashion.
4. Infer demeaning or threatening statements from benign remarks or events.
5. Bear grudges for extended periods. For example, PPD patients are unforgiving of perceived or real insults and slights.
6. Perceive attacks on their character that are not apparent to others. Quick to react angrily or to counterattack.
7. Recurrent suspicions, without justification, regarding fidelity of spouse or partner.

SYNONYMS

None

ICD-9CM CODES
301.0

EPIDEMIOLOGY & DEMOGRAPHICS

PREVALENCE: From 0.5% to 4.4% in the general population, 10% to 30% in inpatient psychiatric settings, and 2% to 10% in outpatient mental health clinics.

PREDOMINANT SEX: More commonly diagnosed in males in clinical samples.

GENETICS: Increased prevalence of PPD in relatives of probands with schizophrenia and delusional disorder, paranoid type.

CLINICAL PRESENTATION

- Signs of PPD in childhood include solitariness, poor peer relationships, social anxiety, underachievement in school, hypersensitivity, peculiar thoughts and language, and idiosyncratic fantasies.
- As children, these patients may have appeared "odd" or "eccentric" and attracted teasing.
- Their excessive suspiciousness often leads to either overt argumentativeness and recurrent complaining or quiet, hostile aloofness.
- These patients maintain interpersonal distance and may refuse to answer personal questions, saying the information is "nobody's business."
- Misinterpret benign actions by others as malicious assaults. PPD patients may, for example, interpret an honest mistake as a deliberate attempt to harm, a casual humorous remark as a serious character attack, a compliment as a veiled criticism, and an offer of help as a judgment of failure.
- Close relationships are impaired by hypervigilance for threats and associated guardedness. May appear as "cold." Suspiciousness can lead to pathologic jealousy where they gather circumstantial evidence to support contention of betrayal.
- To protect themselves from the perceived malice of others, these patients often maintain a high degree of control of relationships and interactions, constantly questioning the whereabouts, intentions, or actions of the other.
- Often rigid and critical of others but have great difficulty accepting criticism themselves.
- Given their lack of trust of others, PPD patients have an excessive need for self-sufficiency and autonomy.
- Quick to counterattack and may be litigious.
- May join "cults" or groups that share their paranoid belief system.
- In response to stress, may experience very brief psychotic episodes (minutes to hours).

ETIOLOGY

- At this point, limited knowledge about role of genetic loading and neurobiologic vulnerability.
- However, increased prevalence in families of probands with schizophrenia and delusional disorder, paranoid type, suggests possible genetic role.

Dx DIAGNOSIS

DIFFERENTIAL DIAGNOSIS

- Schizophrenia, paranoid type, delusional disorder, paranoid type, and mood disorder with psychotic symptoms: require presence of persistent positive psychotic symptoms such as delusions and hallucinations. To give an additional diagnosis of PPD, the personality disorder must be present before the onset of psychotic symptoms and must persist when the psychotic symptoms are in remission.
- Substance-induced paranoia, especially in the context of cocaine or methamphetamine abuse or dependence.
- Personality changes caused by a general medical condition that affects the central nervous system.
- Paranoid traits associated with a sensory disability. For example, hearing impairment.
- Increased risk for major depressive disorder, obsessive-compulsive disorder, agoraphobia, and substance abuse or dependence.
- The most common co-occurring personality disorders are schizotypal, schizoid, narcissistic, avoidant, and borderline:
  1. Schizotypal personality disorder includes magical thinking and unusual perceptual experiences.
  2. Schizoid and borderline personality disorders do not have prominent paranoid ideation.
  3. Avoidant personality disorder includes fear of embarrassment.
  4. Narcissistic personality disorder includes the fear that hidden "flaws" or "inferiority" may be revealed.

WORKUP

- History: collateral information is essential to establishing the presence of longstanding interpersonal pattern in multiple domains of the patient's life.
- Physical examination.
- Mental status examination.

LABORATORY TESTS

Those necessary to rule out medical causes of personality changes

IMAGING STUDIES

Those necessary to rule out medical causes of personality changes

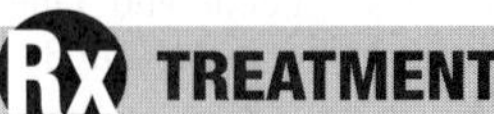

TREATMENT

NONPHARMACOLOGIC THERAPY

- Cognitive-behavioral therapy to help patients control rage, manage perceived criticism, and develop social skills.
- Psychodynamic psychotherapy to help patient develop capacity to trust and improved interpersonal functioning.

ACUTE GENERAL Rx

Benzodiazepines or low-dose antipsychotics to control hostility and paranoia

CHRONIC Rx

- Low-dose antipsychotic medication. Increase dose in small increments to minimize risk of side effects.
- Selective serotonin reuptake inhibitors if comorbid depression, obsessive-compulsive disorder, or agoraphobia.
- Substance abuse treatment if comorbid dependence.

COMPLEMENTARY & ALTERNATIVE MEDICINE

No evidence of efficacy in PPD.

DISPOSITION

- Severity is variable and course is chronic. Often lifelong difficulty maintaining intimate relationships.
- At increased risk for major depressive disorder, obsessive-compulsive disorder, agoraphobia, and substance abuse or dependence.
- In some cases, PPD is a prepsychotic antecedent of delusional disorder, paranoid type.

REFERRAL

- If pharmacotherapy or psychotherapy is contemplated
- If patient's social or occupational functioning is impaired

PEARLS & CONSIDERATIONS

COMMENTS

- Illness exacerbates these patients' sense of vulnerability.
- Communicating personal information to the physician challenges the guarded, self-protective approach to others and will often heighten PPD patients' fear that the physician will harm them.
- The encounter with the physician intensifies hypervigilance. As a result, innocuous or even overtly helpful behaviors by the physician may be perceived as threatening.
- With the perceived threat, these patients will often confront and challenge the physician on their motives and their rationale for diagnosis and treatment. Conflict and argument are not uncommon.
- Thus establishing an alliance with the patient can be challenging.
- Faced with such a patient, physicians may understandably react defensively to unfounded suspicion or distance and not respond to the patient's concerns. Both responses increase the patient's anxiety and paranoia.
- Management guidelines:
  1. Convey intent "to do no harm."
  2. Address the patient's fears and concerns, no matter how irrational, in a clear, direct, and detailed manner.
  3. Remember that behind the patient's hostility lie fears that are real to him or her.
  4. Maintain a professional and neutral stance.
  5. Responding with too much warmth and friendliness will intensify paranoia.
  6. Give patient detailed and factual information about treatment plan.
  7. Give patient as much control as possible, including maximum participation at each decision node.
  8. Do not personalize patient's hostility and suspicion, but understand his or her distrust as an attempt to manage intense fear.
  9. Validate patient's concerns about the diagnosis or treatment plan.

SUGGESTED READINGS

Gomez-Benyto M et al: Posttraumatic stress disorder in primary care with special reference to personality disorder comorbidity, *Br J Gen Pract* 56(526): 349, 2006.

Grant BF et al: Prevalence, correlates, and disability of personality disorders in the United States: results from the national epidemiologic survey on alcohol and related conditions, *J Clin Psychiatry* 65(7):948, 2004.

Lynch TR, Cheavens JS: Dialectical behavior therapy for comorbid personality disorders, *J Clin Psychol* 64(2):154-167, 2008.

Ward RK: Assessment and management of personality disorders, *Am Fam Physician* 70(8):1505, 2004.

AUTHOR: **JOHN Q. YOUNG, M.D., M.P.P.**

Parkinson's Disease (PTG) (ALG)

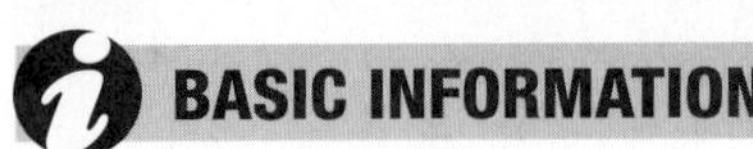

BASIC INFORMATION

DEFINITION

Idiopathic Parkinson's disease (PD) is a progressive neurodegenerative disorder characterized clinically by rigidity, tremor, postural instability, and bradykinesia.

SYNONYMS

Paralysis agitans

ICD-9CM CODES
332.0 Idiopathic Parkinson's disease, primary
332.1 Parkinson's disease, secondary

EPIDEMIOLOGY & DEMOGRAPHICS

PREVALENCE:
- Affects over 1 million people in North America.
- In age group <40 yr, <5/100,000 are affected.
- In those aged >70 yr, 700/100,000 are affected.
- Highest incidence in whites, lowest incidence in Asians and African Americans.

PHYSICAL FINDINGS & CLINICAL PRESENTATION

- Tremor—typically a resting tremor with a frequency of 4 to 6 Hz that is often first noted in the hand as a pill-rolling tremor (thumb and forefinger). Can also involve the leg and lip. Tremor improves with purposeful movement. Usually starts asymmetrically.
- Rigidity—increased muscle tone that persists throughout the range of passive movement of a joint. This, too, is usually asymmetric in onset.
- Akinesia/bradykinesia—slowness in initiating movement.
- Postural instability—tested by "pull test." Ask patient to stand in place with back to examiner. Examiner pulls patient back by the shoulders, and proper response would be to take no steps back or very few steps back without falling. Retropulsion is a positive test as is falling straight back. This is not usually severe early on. If falls and postural reflexes are greatly impaired early on, then consider other disorders.
- Masked facies—face seems expressionless, giving the appearance of depression. Decreased blink; often there is excess drooling.
- Gait disturbance.
- Stooped posture, decreased arm swing.
- Difficulty initiating the first step; small shuffling steps that increase in speed (festinating gait). Steps become progressively faster and shorter while the trunk inclines further forward.
- Other complaints and findings early on include micrographia—handwriting becomes smaller, and hypophonia—voice becomes softer and often "gruffer."

ETIOLOGY

- Unknown.
- Most cases are sporadic, with age being the most common risk factor, although there is probably a combination of both environmental and genetic factors contributing to disease expression. There are rare familial forms with at least seven different genes identified; these include the parkin gene, which is a significant cause of early-onset autosomal recessive PD and LRRK2, which is the most common cause of familial and sporadic parkinsonism.

Dx DIAGNOSIS

A clinical diagnosis can be made based on a comprehensive history and physical examination. The four cardinal signs used to diagnose Prakinson's disease are (mnemonic = TRAP):

1. **T**remor (resting, typically 4-6Hz)
2. **R**igidity, of the Cogwheel type
3. Bradykinesia/**a**kinesia—slowness of movement
4. **P**ostural instability—failure of postural "righting" reflexes leading to poor balance and falls

One need not show all four cardinal signs to make a presumptive diagnosis of PD and begin treatment.

DIFFERENTIAL DIAGNOSIS

- Multiple system atrophy—distinguishing features include autonomic dysfunction (including urinary incontinence, orthostatic hypotension, and erectile dysfunction), parkinsonism, cerebellar signs, and normal cognition.
- Diffuse Lewy body disease—parkinsonism with concomitant dementia. Patients often have early hallucinations and fluctuations in level of alertness and mental status.
- Corticobasal degeneration—often begins asymmetrically with apraxia, cortical sensory loss in one limb, and sometimes alien limb phenomenon.
- Progressive supranuclear palsy—tends to have axial rigidity greater than appendicular (limb) rigidity. These patients have early and severe postural instability. Hallmark is supranuclear gaze palsy that usually involves vertical gaze (especially downward) before horizontal.
- Essential tremor—bilateral postural and action tremor.
- Secondary (acquired) parkinsonism.
  1. Iatrogenic—any of the neuroleptics and antipsychotics. The high potency D_2-blocker neuroleptics are most likely to cause parkinsonism. Quetiapine is an atypical antipsychotic with lower risk of causing parkinsonism. Metoclopramide can also cause parkinsonism.
  2. Postinfectious parkinsonism—von Economo's encephalitis.
  3. Parkinson's pugilistica—after repeated head trauma.
  4. Toxins (e.g., MPTP, manganese, carbon monoxide).
  5. Cerebrovascular disease "vascular parkinsonism" (basal ganglia infarcts); often lower limbs (especially gait) affected more than upper extremities.

WORKUP

Identification of clinical signs and symptoms associated with PD (see "Physical Findings") and elimination of conditions that may mimic it with a comprehensive history and physical examination.

Routine genetic testing is not recommended.

IMAGING STUDIES

Computed tomographic (CT) scan has almost no role in investigations. Magnetic resonance imaging (MRI) of the head may sometimes distinguish between idiopathic PD and other conditions that present with signs of parkinsonism (see "Differential Diagnosis").

Rx TREATMENT

NONPHARMACOLOGIC THERAPY

- Physical therapy, patient education and reassurance, treatment of associated conditions (e.g., depression)
- Avoidance of drugs that can induce or worsen parkinsonism: neuroleptics (especially high potency), certain antiemetics (prochlorperazine, trimethobenzamide), metoclopramide, nonselective MAO inhibitors (may induce hypertensive crisis), reserpine, methyldopa

ACUTE GENERAL Rx

- There is persistent controversy whether levodopa or dopamine agonists should be the initial treatment. In younger patients, agonists are usually the drug of choice; in patients >70 yrs, levodopa is typically the drug of choice.
- It is appropriate to initiate pharmacotherapy when required by symptoms; prior practice of waiting for limitation of ADLs is now outdated.
- Motor complications do develop during the course of the disease and likely reflect the combination of disease progression together with the side effects of dopaminergic medications.

CHRONIC Rx

- Levodopa therapy
  1. Cornerstone of symptomatic therapy—should be used with a peripheral dopa decarboxylase inhibitor (carbidopa) to minimize side effects (nausea, lightheadedness, postural hypotension). The combination of the two drugs is marketed under the trade name Sinemet. Levodopa therapy has been found to reduce morbidity and mortality in PD patients.
  2. Usual starting dose is 25/100 mg (carbidopa/levodopa) tid 1 hr before meals.
  3. Controlled-release preparations (Sinemet CR) are available, but their use should be deferred to a neurologist.

4. Stalevo (combination Sinemet and entacapone, a COMT inhibitor). Useful for patients with motor fluctuations (wearing off). Has no role in treating early patients with PD.

- Dopamine receptor agonists (Ropinirole and Pramipexole) are not as potent as levodopa, but they are often used as initial treatment in younger patients to attempt to delay the onset of complications (dyskinesias, motor fluctuations) associated with levodopa therapy. These medications are more expensive than levodopa. In general they cause more side effects than levodopa, including nausea, vomiting, lightheadedness, peripheral edema, confusion, and somnolence. They can also cause impulse control behaviors such as hypersexuality, binge eating, and compulsive shopping and gambling. Presence of these must be assessed at each visit.
  1. Ropinirole (Requip): initial dose is 0.25 mg tid
  2. Pramipexole (Mirapex): initial dose is 0.125 mg tid
- MAO-B inhibitors can be used as monotherapy early in the disease or as adjunctive therapy in later stages. Milder symptomatic benefit than dopamine agonists or levodopa. Well tolerated and easy to titrate. Concurrent use of stimulants and sympathomimetics should be avoided. Certain food restrictions may apply.
  1. Rasagiline (Azilect): initial dose is 0.5 mg qd, then 1 mg daily. A recent study, ADAGIO, suggests that 1 mg Rasagiline may have disease-modifying benefits, but results must be interpreted with caution.
  2. Selegiline: Usual dose, 5 mg bid with breakfast and lunch. Has amphetamine byproduct so has mild stimulant-like effects, which can be beneficial in some patients.
  3. Amantadine (Symmetrel) can be used alone early in the disease. It is especially useful in the treatment of dyskinesias. Dosage is 100 mg tid (titrate q week from 100 mg qd). Must adjust for elderly and renal impairment. The most notable side effect, especially in the elderly, is confusion.
- Anticholinergic agents are only helpful in treating tremor and drooling in patients with PD. Potential side effects include constipation, urinary retention, memory impairment, and hallucinations. They should be avoided in the elderly.
  1. Trihexyphenidyl (Artane): initial dose, 1 mg PO tid
  2. Benztropine (Cogentin): usual dose, 0.5 to 1 mg qd or bid

SURGICAL OPTIONS

- Pallidal (globus pallidus interna) and subthalamic deep-brain stimulation are currently the surgical options of choice; thalamic DBS may be useful for refractory tremor.
- Surgery is limited to patients with disabling, medically refractory problems, and patients must still have a good response to L-dopa to undergo surgery. DBS results in decreased dyskinesias, fluctuations, rigidity, and tremor.

DISPOSITION

Parkinson's disease usually follows a slowly progressive course leading to disability over the course of several years. However, every patient will progress individually, and patients should be reassured that this diagnosis does not, by definition, result in being either wheelchair- or bed-bound.

REFERRAL

- Neurology consultation is recommended on initial diagnosis of PD.
- Exercise is important for all patients with PD.
- Participation in outpatient physical therapy program is recommended for patients with moderate to advanced disease.

PEARLS & CONSIDERATIONS

- Asymmetry of symptoms at onset is very useful in distinguishing PD from other causes of parkinsonism.
- Although resting tremor is a common presenting symptom, up to 25% of patients with idiopathic PD do not have classic resting tremor.

COMMENTS

Additional patient information on PD can be obtained from the Internet at www.parkinson.org and from the National Parkinson Foundation, Inc., 1501 Ninth Avenue NW, Miami, FL 33136; phone: (800) 327-4545.

EBM EVIDENCE

Please note: Complete text of EBM for this topic is available online.

Key trials and commentary:

After 20 years follow-up of newly diagnosed patients with Parkinson's disease (PD), 100 of 136 (74%) have died. The mortality rate fell in the first 3 years of treatment, then rose compared to the general population, the standardized mortality ratio from 15 to 20 years reaching 3.1. Drug-induced dyskinesia and end of dose failure were experienced by most patients, but the main current problems relate to the non-levodopa responsive features of the disease. Dementia is present in 83% of 20-year survivors. Dementia correlates with increasing age and probably reflects an interplay of multiple pathologies. 17 people with dementia had postmortems. 8 had diffuse Lewy bodies as the only cause of dementia, whereas others had mixed neuropathology. Only one person lives independently and 48% are in nursing homes. Excessive daytime sleepiness is noted in 70%, falls have occurred in 87%, freezing in 81%, fractures in 35%, symptomatic postural hypotension in 48%, urinary incontinence in 71%, moderate dysarthria in 81%, choking in 48%, and hallucinations in 74%. The challenge is to understand the cellular mechanisms underlying the diverse features of advanced PD that go far beyond a lack of dopamine.[1] Ⓐ

This longitudinal study provides rather grim statistics bearing on the long-term outcome of patients with PD. By 20 years follow-up, 74% of the initial cohort of 136 patients had died. Dementia was noted in 83% of 20-year survivors, correlating with increasing age. Moreover, long-term complications were prevalent, including falls, gait freezing, autonomic dysfunction, hallucinations, dysarthria, and dysphagia. In contrast, levodopa motor complications (dyskinesias and motor fluctuations) were relatively low on the list of problems affecting this cohort in the long term. Notable was that these patients were followed and tabulated by a single group of clinician-investigators over the course of 20 years.

These results again bring to forefront the controversy regarding best initial therapy in patients with PD. Some clinicians tend to defer using levodopa until later stages of the disease, arguing that the best responses can be saved for later. The Sydney multicenter study suggests that this may be futile. Thus, many of the disease features that cause major morbidity in the later stages are not levodopa complications, but rather manifestations of nondopaminergic aspects of the disease: dementia, dysautonomia, levodopa-refractory gait, and other motor problems. Deferring use of the most effective treatment (levodopa) for anticipated later gain appears to be a futile strategy.[2] Ⓐ

10-year follow-up results from the Parkinson's Disease Research Group of the U.K. trial demonstrated that there were no long-term advantages to initiating treatment with bromocriptine compared with levodopa in early PD. Increased mortality in patients on selegiline combined with levodopa led to premature termination of this arm after 6 years.

This study showed that initial treatment with the dopamine agonist bromocriptine did not reduce mortality or motor disability and the initially reduced frequency in motor complications was not sustained. We found no evidence of a long-term benefit or clinically relevant disease-modifying effect with initial dopamine agonist treatment.

This study reports the final follow-up (14 years) of the Parkinson's Disease Research Group of the United Kingdom (PDRG-UK) drug trial. This was an open, randomized, multicenter study of three initial treatment options: (1) levodopa, (2) levodopa plus selegiline, and (3) the dopamine agonist bromocriptine. The selegiline plus levodopa arm was discontinued after 6 years because of increased mortality in this group. The 14-year analysis showed that disability and physical functioning scores were better in the group started on levodopa, compared with the group started on bromocriptine; other parameters were not significantly different (mortality rates, dyskinesia prevalence, motor fluctuations, dementia). The initially reduced frequency of motor complication seen in the bromocriptine group was not sustained at 14 years. The authors found no evidence of a long-term advantage or clinically relevant disease-modifying effect with initial dopamine agonist therapy. One limitation of this study is that the final analysis represented only 21% of the original patients.

These findings add to the evidence that early dopamine agonist treatment of PD does not provide long-term advantage over initial levodopa treatment. This seems relevant to current practices because there is no compelling evidence that newer dopamine agonists work substantially better than bromocriptine. The long-term morbidity in PD results from manifestations unrelated to dopaminergic deficiency (dysautonomia, dysphagia, dementia, falls), none of which are influenced by whether the initial treatment is levodopa or an agonist. Even though dyskinesias are commonly seen with long-term levodopa use, the dyskinesias are frequently nondisabling, and can be addressed by medication adjustment or deep brain stimulation. Further, most patients find some dyskinesias more acceptable than an akinetic state.

The optimal treatment of patients with early PD is a controversial topic. Most studies show that patients initially treated with dopamine agonists rather than levodopa show fewer motor complications (dyskinesias and motor fluctuations) but worse motor function after 5 years of follow-up. The most compelling argument for initial dopamine agonist administration is among patients with young-onset PD (e.g., before age 40), where the incidence of dyskinesia and motor fluctuations are high. On the other hand, dopamine agonists are more expensive, and are associated with a higher incidence of nonmotor side effects like hypersomnolence and hallucinations. Of particular concern with dopamine agonists are behavioral syndromes, most notably, pathological gambling or hypersexuality.

Many patients and physicians are under the impression that the initial treatment of PD should be with an agonist, and that levodopa treatment should be delayed. This has been taken to the extreme and the term "levodopa phobia" has been coined. However, this can have very unfortunate consequences where undertreatment during the early years of PD may compromise the lives of PD patients at a time when these medications are most likely to have a meaningful impact on quality of life. Further, even in patients who are initially placed on a dopamine agonist, levodopa is required, as the motor disability related to PD becomes worse.

Several randomized controlled trials (RCTs) have found that dopamine agonists (when used alone or in combination with levodopa rescue therapy) reduce dyskinesias and long-term motor complications compared with levodopa alone in people with early PD. Adding dopamine agonists in later-stage PD reduces required levodopa doses and "off" time, and improves motor impairment; however, this is often at the expense of an increase in dopaminergic adverse effects.[3-7]

There is little convincing evidence that one dopamine agonist is better than another with respect to control of parkinsonian symptoms.[4,5,7]

There are no large randomized controlled trials regarding the use of levodopa; however, experts agree that it is the most potent symptomatic treatment for PD.

Controversy still exists as to whether treatment should be initiated with levodopa or dopamine agonists.

There is evidence from RCTs that rasagiline is useful as monotherapy and adjunctive therapy in Parkinson's disease.[8]

There is evidence that suggests a possible benefit of the early use of rasagiline at 1 mg day. This may be due to disease modifying benefits, but this cannot be definitively concluded based on the existing evidence.[9]

There is evidence from RCTs that selegiline delays the need for levodopa in early Parkinson's disease; however, there is no convincing evidence either for the neuroprotective benefit of or increased mortality with selegiline.[10]

Two RCTs compared modified-release with immediate-release levodopa in patients with early Parkinson's disease. There was no significant difference in motor complications or disease control at 5 years.[11,12]

A systematic review of double-blind crossover trials found that anticholinergics used in de novo or advanced Parkinson's disease are superior to placebo in at least one outcome measure, although reporting of methods and results was incomplete and outcome measures were often heterogenous.[13]

A systematic review of the efficacy of amantadine in the treatment of dyskinesias found insufficient data due to poor design of studies to comment on its utility; however, subsequent studies and clinical experience suggest that it is an effective drug in the treatment of dyskinesias.[14]

Evidence-Based References

1. Hely MA, Reid WGJ, Adena MA: The Sydney Multicenter Study of Parkinson's Disease: The inevitability of dementia at 20 years, *Mov Disord* 23:837-844, 2008. Commentary by N. Kumar, M.D. Ⓐ
2. Katzenschlager R, Parkinson's Disease Research Group of the United Kingdom: Fourteen-year final report of the randomized PDRG-UK trial comparing three initial treatments in PD, *Neurology* 71:474-480, 2008. Commentary by N. Kumar, M.D. Ⓐ
3. Clarke CE et al: Ropinirole for levodopa-induced complications in Parkinson's disease. Cochrane Movement Disorders Group, *Cochrane Database Syst Rev* 3:2005.
4. Clarke CE et al: Ropinirole versus bromocriptine for levodopa-induced complications in Parkinson's disease. Cochrane Movement Disorders Group, *Cochrane Database Syst Rev* 3:2005.
5. Clarke JA: Pramipexole versus bromocriptine for levodopa-induced complications in Parkinson's disease. Cochrane Movement Disorders Group, *Cochrane Database Syst Rev* 3:2005.
6. Holloway RG et al: Pramipexole vs levodopa as initial treatment for Parkinson disease: a 4-year randomized controlled trial, *Arch Neurol* 61:1044, 2004.
7. Navan P et al: Randomized, double-blind, 3-month parallel study of the effects of pramipexole, pergolide and placebo on parkinsonian tremor, *Mov Disord* 18(11):1324, 2003.
8. Parkinson Study Group: A controlled trial of rasagiline in early Parkinson disease: The TEMPO Study, *Arch Neurol* 59:1937-1943, 2002.
9. Olanow CW et al: A double-blind, delayed-start trial of rasagiline in Parkinson's disease, *N Engl J Med* 361:1268-1278, 2009.
10. Macleod AD et al: Monoamine oxidase B inhibitors for early Parkinson's disease. Cochrane Movement Disorders Group, *Cochrane Database Syst Rev* 3:2005.
11. Dupont E et al: Sustained-release Madopar HBS compared with standard Madopar in the long-term treatment of de novo Parkinsonian patients, *Acta Neurol Scand* 93:14, 1996. Reviewed in: *Clin Evid* 11:1736, 2004.
12. Block G et al: Comparison of immediate release and controlled release carbidopa/levodopa in Parkinson's disease, *Eur Neurol* 37:23, 1997. Reviewed in: *Clin Evid* 11:1736, 2004.
13. Katzenschlager R et al: Anticholinergics for symptomatic management of Parkinson's disease. Cochrane Movement Disorders Group, *Cochrane Database Syst Rev* 3:2005.
14. Crosby NJ et al: Amantadine for dyskinesia in Parkinson's disease. Cochrane Movement Disorders Group, *Cochrane Database Syst Rev* 3:2005.

SUGGESTED READINGS

Goetz C et al: Evidence-based medical review update: Pharmacological and surgical treatments of Parkinson's disease: 2001 to 2004, *Mov Disord* 20:523, 2005. Review.

Miyasaki J et al: Practice parameter: Initiation of treatment for Parkinson's disease: An evidence-based review. Report of the Quality Standards Subcommittee of the American Academy of Neurology, *Neurology* 58:11-17, 2002.

Samii A et al: Parkinson's disease, *Lancet* 363(9423):1783, 2004. Review.

Suchowersky O et al: Practice parameter: Neuroprotective strategies and alternative therapies for Parkinson disease (an evidence-based review): Report of the Quality Standards Subcommittee of the American Academy of Neurology, *Neurology* 66:976-982, 2006.

Tetrud J et al: Treatment challenges in early stage Parkinson's disease, *Neurol Clin* 22:S19, 2004.

AUTHOR: **CINDY ZADIKOFF, M.D.**

BASIC INFORMATION

DEFINITION

Paronychia is a localized superficial infection or abscess of the lateral and proximal nail fold. Paronychia may be acute or chronic.

SYNONYMS

Nail bed infection
Nail bed abscess

ICD-9CM CODES
681.9 Paronychia

EPIDEMIOLOGY & DEMOGRAPHICS

- Acute paronychia affects males and females equally.
- Chronic paronychia is more common in females than males (9:1).
- Acute paronychia most often occurs in children.
- Chronic paronychia usually presents in the fifth or sixth decade of life.
- Paronychia is the most common infection of the hand.

PHYSICAL FINDINGS & CLINICAL PRESENTATION

- Acute paronychia usually presents with the sudden onset of redness, swelling, and pain with abscess or cellulitis formation in the nail fold. Fluid with purulence is often present.
- Chronic paronychia is insidious, presenting with mild swelling and erythema of the nail folds.
- Acute paronychia usually involves only one finger.
- Chronic paronychia may involve more than one finger.
- Acute paronychia usually involves the thumb.
- Chronic paronychia commonly involves the middle finger.

ETIOLOGY

- Any disruption of the seal between the proximal nail fold and the nail plate can cause paronychial infections.
- Acute paronychia is almost always bacterial in origin (e.g., *Staphylococcus aureus* [most common], *Streptococcus pyogenes, Enterococcus faecalis, Proteus* and *Pseudomonas* species, and anaerobes).
- Chronic paronychia is commonly caused by *Candida albicans* (70%), with bacterial organisms accounting for the remaining 30%.
- Trauma, nail biting, hangnails, diabetes, and long-term exposure to water are common predisposing features of paronychia.

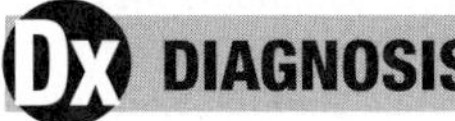

DIAGNOSIS

The diagnosis of paronychia is self-evident on physical examination.

DIFFERENTIAL DIAGNOSIS

- Herpetic whitlow
- Pyogenic granuloma
- Viral warts
- Ganglions
- Squamous cell carcinoma

WORKUP

A workup is usually not pursued unless there is treatment failure.

LABORATORY TESTS

- Gram stain and culture any purulent drainage.
- Potassium hydroxide mount may show pseudohyphae.

IMAGING STUDIES

Radiographs of the digit if concerned about osteomyelitis.

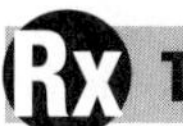

TREATMENT

NONPHARMACOLOGIC THERAPY

- For acute paronychia without purulent drainage, warm soaks tid or qid are helpful. If pus is present, surgical drainage is required.
- For chronic paronychia, avoid frequent immersion in water or exposure to moisture.

ACUTE GENERAL Rx

- First-generation cephalosporin (e.g., cephalexin 250 to 500 mg qid) or penicillinase-resistant penicillin (e.g., dicloxacillin 250 to 500 mg qid) are usually the antibiotics of choice for acute paronychia.
- Alternative antibiotic choices include clindamycin and amoxicillin-clavulanate potassium.
- Surgical drainage is indicated if purulent discharge is noted.
- A No. 11 blade scalpel is used to lift the lateral perionychium and proximal eponychium off the nail, facilitating drainage.
- If the pus is located beneath the nail, the lateral edge of the nail can be lifted off the nail bed and excised.

CHRONIC Rx

- If no fungal organism is found, tincture of iodine (2 drops bid) helps keep the nail and skin dry.
- Chronic paronychia caused by *Candida albicans* is treated with topical antifungal agents (e.g., miconazole or ketoconazole applied tid).
- Unresponsive cases may be treated with itraconazole or fluconazole but should be done in consultation with dermatology and/or infectious disease.
- Surgery may be needed in refractory cases.

DISPOSITION

- Most acute paronychias with appropriate treatment resolve within 7 to 10 days.
- Osteomyelitis is a potential complication of paronychia.
- Untreated chronic paronychia leads to thickening and discoloration with eventual nail loss.

REFERRAL

Chronic paronychia refractory to topical medical therapy is best referred to dermatology and/or infectious disease. A hand surgeon is consulted if abscess drainage or surgery is being considered.

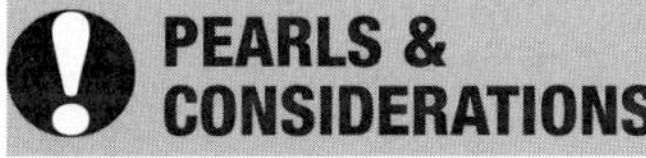

PEARLS & CONSIDERATIONS

COMMENTS

The gastrointestinal tract, including the mouth and bowel, and the genitourinary tract in women are the usual sources of *C. albicans* in chronic paronychia.

SUGGESTED READINGS

Daniel CR et al: Managing simple chronic paronychia and onycholysis with ciclopirox 0.77% and an irritant-avoidance regimen, *Cutis* 73(1):81, 2004.

Griffiths G et al: Paronychia or an abscess: early diagnosis, *Hosp Med* 65(11):696, 2004.

AUTHORS: **GLENN G. FORT, M.D., M.P.H.,** and **DENNIS J. MIKOLICH, M.D.**

Paroxysmal Cold Hemoglobinuria

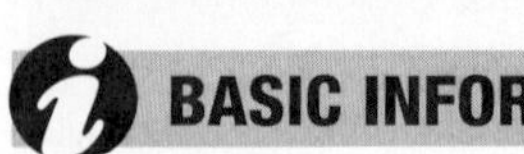

BASIC INFORMATION

DEFINITION

Paroxysmal cold hemoglobinuria (PCH) is a rare disease characterized by episodic massive intravascular hemolysis after exposure to cold temperatures. Hemolysis may occur in an idiopathic form in adults or, more commonly, after a viral infection in children. It was first described in patients with secondary or tertiary syphilis.

SYNONYMS

PCH
Donath-Landsteiner hemoglobinuria

ICD-9CM CODES
283.2 Hemoglobinuria caused by hemolysis from external causes

EPIDEMIOLOGY & DEMOGRAPHICS

- No race or sex predilection
- Accounts for up to 5% of adult cases of autoimmune hemolytic anemia
- Accounts for nearly 30% of childhood cases of autoimmune hemolytic anemia

PHYSICAL FINDINGS & CLINICAL PRESENTATION

- After cold exposure, red to brown urination begins within minutes to hours.
- Associated symptoms include back, leg, and abdominal pain.
- Headaches, nausea, vomiting, and diarrhea are common.
- May be associated with Raynaud's phenomenon.
- Associated with cold urticaria.
- Transient splenomegaly and jaundice may occur.
- Symptoms and gross hemoglobinuria usually resolve within hours.
- Symptoms believed to be mediated by smooth muscle dysfunction as a result of nitric oxide toxicity associated with hemoglobinemia.

ETIOLOGY & PATHOGENESIS

- Polyclonal immunoglobulin (Ig) G (Donath-Landsteiner antibody) binds to P antigen on red blood cell (RBC) membranes when blood is exposed to cold temperatures. As blood warms to body temperature, complement-mediated hemolysis ensues.
- In children, the appearance of the antibody usually follows the onset of a viral respiratory illness by 7 to 10 days. Symptoms may persist for several weeks.
- PCH has been associated with multiple infectious pathogens, including syphilis, *Haemophilus influenzae,* Epstein-Barr virus (EBV), cytomegalovirus (CMV), influenza A, varicella, measles, mumps, and adenovirus.

Dx DIAGNOSIS

DIFFERENTIAL DIAGNOSIS

- Cold agglutinin disease associated with hemoglobinuria, paroxysmal nocturnal hemoglobinuria, rhabdomyolysis.
- Other causes of acute massive intravascular hemolysis.

LABORATORY TESTS

- The presence of IgG that reacts with the RBC at reduced temperatures but not at body temperature. In the Donath-Landsteiner test, a patient's serum is incubated with donated RBCs and complement at 4° C then warmed to 37° C. Lysis is observed in a positive test.
- A more sensitive test involves using radiolabelled monoclonal anti-IgG. This is incubated at 4° C with the patient's serum and donor RBCs. The degree of radioactivity on the separated RBCs will be elevated in PCH compared with a control run at 37° C.
- Elevated bilirubin and lactate dehydrogenase.
- Abnormal RBC forms such as poikilocytosis, spherocytosis, and anisocytosis.
- Erythrophagocytosis by neutrophils and monocytes may be seen.

Rx TREATMENT

NONPHARMACOLOGIC THERAPY

The mainstay of treatment is the avoidance of exposure to cold.

ACUTE GENERAL Rx

- In children in particular, transfusion may be necessary because the anemia may become life threatening and hemolysis may be ongoing for several weeks.
- Testing and treatment for syphilis if present.
- Steroids generally are not be helpful.
- Splenectomy is not indicated.
- Treatment with rituximab has resulted in termination of hemolysis in a case report.

DISPOSITION

- Postinfectious varieties are self-limited.
- There have been a few case reports of recurrent episodes of PCH.
- Adult idiopathic form is generally manageable by avoiding environmental exposure.

REFERRAL

To hematologist to aid in diagnosis

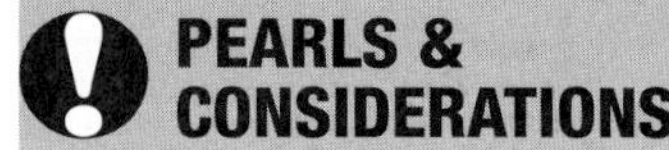

PEARLS & CONSIDERATIONS

- PCH is associated with brown or red discoloration of urine after cold exposure in adults or after a viral infection in children.
- PCH can be associated with viral or bacterial infections, including syphilis, *H. influenzae,* EBV, CMV, influenza A, varicella, measles, mumps, and adenovirus.
- PCH can cause life-threatening hemolysis in children.

SUGGESTED READINGS

Koppel A et al: Rituximab as successful therapy in a patient with refractory paroxysmal cold hemoglobinuria, *Transfusion,* 47(10):1902-1904, 2007.

Ogose T et al: A case of recurrent paroxysmal cold hemoglobinuria with the different temperature thresholds of Donath-Landsteiner antibodies. *J of Ped Hematology/Oncology,* 29(10):716-719, 2007.

AUTHOR: **MICHAEL MAHER, M.D.**

BASIC INFORMATION

DEFINITION

Paroxysmal nocturnal hemoglobinuria (PNH) is a rare disease characterized by episodes of intravascular hemolysis and hemoglobinuria usually occurring at night. Thrombocytopenia, leukopenia, and recurrent venous thrombosis are also associated with PNH.

SYNONYMS

PNH

ICD-9CM CODES

283.2 Paroxysmal nocturnal hemoglobinuria

EPIDEMIOLOGY & DEMOGRAPHICS

- Affects patients of any age (reported spectrum 6 to 82 yr) but most common in patients aged 30 to 50 yr
- Affects both sexes (slight female predominance) and all races

PHYSICAL FINDINGS & CLINICAL PRESENTATION

1. Initial manifestations
   - Anemia symptoms (35%)
   - Hemoglobinuria (25%)
   - Bleeding (20%)
   - Aplastic anemia (15%)
   - Gastrointestinal symptoms (10%)
   - Hemolytic anemia (10%)
   - Iron-deficiency anemia (5%)
   - Venous thrombosis (5%)
   - Infections (5%)
   - Neurologic symptoms
2. Hemoglobinuria
   - Typically the first morning void reveals dark urine with progressive clearing during the day. The cause for the circadian rhythm is unknown.
3. Hemolysis
   - In addition to the circadian hemolysis and resulting hemoglobinuria, episodes of hemolytic exacerbations can accompany infections, menstruation, transfusion, surgery, iron therapy, and vaccinations. Symptoms of severe hemolysis include chest, back, or abdominal pain, headache, fever, malaise, and fatigue.
4. Aplastic anemia
   - Aplastic anemia may be the presenting manifestation of PNH (therefore PNH must be in the differential diagnosis of aplastic anemia) or may develop as a later complication of PNH.
5. Thrombosis (leading cause of death in PNH; occurs in 40% of patients)
   - Lower extremity deep vein thrombosis (DVT)
   - Subclavian thrombosis
   - Portal or mesenteric vein thrombosis
   - Hepatic vein thrombosis (Budd-Chiari syndrome)
   - Cerebrovascular thromboses
6. Renal failure
   - Acute renal failure associated with massive hemoglobinuria (acute tubular necrosis)
   - Progressive renal failure associated with thrombosis within renal small veins
7. Dysphagia
8. Infections (associated with leukopenia or steroid treatment)
9. Physical findings include:
   - Pallor (anemia)
   - Jaundice (hemolysis)
   - Splenomegaly
   - Unilateral extremity swelling (DVT)
   - Ascites (Budd-Chiari syndrome)

ETIOLOGY & PATHOGENESIS

- Complement-mediated hemolysis; the erythrocytes are abnormally sensitive to acidified serum.
- Patients have two populations of red blood cells (RBCs): some sensitive to hemolysis (PNH III cells) and others not (PNH I cells), in variable proportions (10% to 75% PNH III cells). Approximately 20% PNH III are required for hemoglobinuria to be detectable.
- The RBC defects in PNH are in the membrane proteins as follows:
  - Decay-accelerating factor deficiency
  - Membrane inhibitor of reactive lysis deficiency
  - C-8 binding protein deficiency
- These protein deficiencies are the result of an acquired mutation located in the X chromosome, which regulates glycosyl phosphatidyl inositol (GPI). GPI anchors the above-mentioned proteins in the RBC membrane; GPI-deficient RBCs proliferate as an abnormal clone. Because women are affected at least as frequently as men are, the mutation must be expressed as dominant gene. The mechanism by which the mutant stem cells can dominate hematopoiesis in PNH is unknown.
- The pathophysiology of the relation of PNH and aplastic anemia is unknown.

DIAGNOSIS

Clinical situations:
- Intravascular hemolysis
- Hemoglobinuria
- Pancytopenia associated with hemolysis
- Iron deficiency associated with hemolysis
- Recurrent venous thrombosis
- Recurrent episodes of abdominal pain, headache, or back pain associated with hemolysis

DIFFERENTIAL DIAGNOSIS

- See "Hemolytic Anemia" in Section I.
- See "Aplastic Anemia" in Section I.
- See "Anemia" algorithm in Section III.

LABORATORY TESTS

- Complete blood count: anemia, leukopenia, thrombocytopenia
- Reticulocytosis
- RBC smear: spherocytes
- Negative Coombs test
- Low leukocyte alkaline phosphatase
- Elevated lactate dehydrogenase
- Low serum haptoglobin
- Low serum iron saturation, low ferritin
- Elevated urine hemoglobin, urine urobilinogen, urine hemosiderin
- Positive Ham test (acidified serum RBC lysis)
- Normoblastic hyperplasia on bone marrow aspirate or biopsy
- Identification of GPI-anchored protein deficiency on hematopoietic cells by using monoclonal antibodies or flow cytometry; flow cytometric analysis of granulocytes is the best way to diagnose PNH
- Cytogenetic studies are not diagnostic

TREATMENT

- Prednisone (15 to 40 mg qod) helpful, but prolonged use should be avoided
- Eculizumab, a humanized antibody that inhibits the activation of terminal complement components, is an effective therapy for PNH; it reduces intravascular hemolysis, hemoglobinuria, and need for transfusion in patients with PNH. It is very expensive and requires lifelong administration.
- Iron replacement, folic acid supplementation
- Transfusions
- Treatment and prevention of thrombosis (heparin, Coumadin)
- Avoidance of oral contraceptives
- Bone marrow transplantation

REFERRAL

To hematologist

PROGNOSIS

- 50% survival to 10 to 15 yr
- 25% survival to 25 yr
- If thrombosis at presentation, only 40% survival to 4 yr
- 1% incidence of leukemia
- 5% incidence of myelodysplastic syndrome

SUGGESTED READINGS

Brodsky RA: Narrative review: paroxysmal nocturnal hemoglobinuria: the physiology of complement-related hemolytic anemia, *Ann Intern Med* 148:587-595, 2008.

Hillmen P et al: The complement inhibitor eculizumab in paroxysmal nocturnal hemoglobinuria, *N Engl J Med* 355:1233, 2006.

AUTHOR: **FRED F. FERRI, M.D.**

Paroxysmal Supraventricular Tachycardia

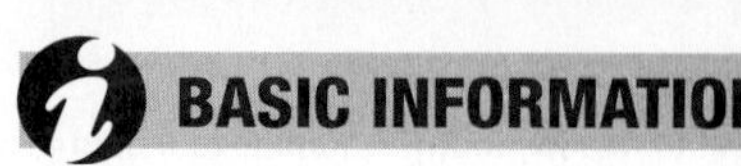

BASIC INFORMATION

DEFINITION

Paroxysmal supraventricular tachycardia (SVT) is a group of tachyarrhythmias that originate from within or above the atrioventricular (AV) node and are characterized by sudden onset and abrupt termination. The most common types include AV nodal reentrant tachycardia (AVNRT), AV reentrant tachycardia (AVRT), and paroxysmal atrial tachycardia (PAT).

SYNONYMS

PAT (old terminology for SVT)
PSVT
Supraventricular tachycardia

ICD-9CM CODES

427.0 Paroxysmal atrial tachycardia

PHYSICAL FINDINGS & CLINICAL PRESENTATION

- Patient is usually asymptomatic.
- Patient may be aware of "fast" heartbeat (palpitations) or have presyncope, syncope, or chest pain.
- Hemodynamic status during arrhythmia may vary and can depend on the patient's comorbidities and presence of underlying structural heart disease.

ETIOLOGY

- AVNRT—Dual electrical pathways within or near the AV node
- AVRT—Accessory pathway (concealed [not evident on ECG], only retrograde ventriculoatrial conduction without antegrade atrioventricular conduction)
- Pre-excitation [Wolff-Parkinson-White] syndrome, evident on ECG as described below)
- Paroxysmal atrial tachycardia—abnormal automaticity of atrial tissue or triggered activity

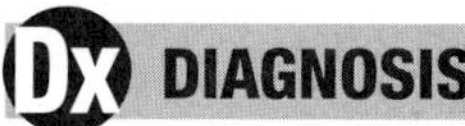

DIAGNOSIS

WORKUP

- Regular rhythm at rate of >100 beats/min is present.
- P waves may or may not be seen (the presence of P waves depends on the relation of atrial to ventricular depolarization).
- Wide QRS complex (>0.12 sec) with initial slurring (delta wave) during sinus rhythm and short PR (<0.12 sec) is characteristic of WPW syndrome.
- QRS complex during supraventricular tachycardia is usually narrow; however, may be widened because of intrinsic conduction disease, myocardial disease, or rate-related bundle branch block. It may also be widened if the patient has pre-excitation syndrome.
- Echocardiography is appropriate to assess for the presence of underlying structural heart disease.

TREATMENT

NONPHARMACOLOGIC THERAPY

- Valsalva maneuver in the supine position is the most effective way to terminate SVT; carotid sinus massage (after excluding occlusive carotid disease) is also commonly used to elicit vagal efferent impulses.
- Synchronized DC shock is used if patient shows signs of hemodynamic instability.

ACUTE GENERAL Rx

- Adenosine is useful for treatment of AVRT and AVNRT, and can uncover the underlying rhythm in paroxysmal atrial tachycardia; it is the first choice of therapy for treatment of almost all episodes of SVT unresponsive to vagal maneuvers. The dose is 6 mg given as a rapid IV bolus; tachycardia is usually terminated within a few seconds. If necessary, may repeat with 12-mg IV bolus. Contraindications are second- or third-degree atrioventricular block, sick sinus syndrome, and atrial fibrillation. Adenosine may cause bronchospasm in asthmatics.
- Verapamil 5 to 10 mg IV is given over 5 min; if no effect, may repeat in 30 min.
  1. Verapamil should be used cautiously in patients with SVT associated with hypotension.
  2. Slow injection of calcium chloride (10 ml of a 10% solution given over 5 to 8 min before verapamil administration) decreases the hypotensive effect without compromising its antiarrhythmic effect.
- Repeat carotid massage after IV verapamil if SVT persists.
- Metoprolol (IV 5 mg/2 min up to 15 mg) or esmolol (500 μg/kg IV bolus, then 50 μg/kg/min) may be effective in the treatment of SVT.
- IV digitalization (0.75 to 1 mg slow IV loading) if other agents are not effective.
  1. Repeat carotid massage 30 min later; if not successful, give additional 0.25 mg IV digoxin and repeat carotid sinus massage 1 hr later.
  2. Digoxin, beta-blockers, and calcium-channel blockers should be avoided in patients with pre-excitation syndrome to avoid increased conduction through the accessory pathway.

DISPOSITION

Most patients respond well with resolution of the paroxysmal atrial tachycardia upon treatment (see "Acute General Rx"). Some patients may need chronic AV blocking agents for recurrence.

REFERRAL

Radiofrequency ablation is the procedure of choice in symptomatic patients who are refractory to medical therapy.

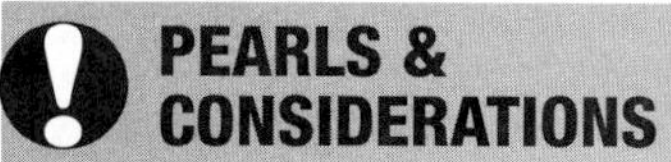

PEARLS & CONSIDERATIONS

COMMENTS

Accessory pathways occur in 0.1% to 0.3% of the general population.

SUGGESTED READINGS

Fox DJ et al: Supraventricular tachycardia: diagnosis and management, *Mayo Clin Proc* 83(12):1400-1411, 2008.

Marine JE: Catheter ablation therapy for supraventricular arrhythmias, *JAMA* 298(3):2768-2778, 2007.

AUTHORS: **SCOTT BRANCATO, M.D., FRED F. FERRI, M.D.,** and **WEN-CHIH WU, M.D.**

BASIC INFORMATION

DEFINITION

Overuse or overload of the patellofemoral region leading to anterior knee pain

SYNONYMS

Retropatellar pain syndrome
Runner's knee
Lateral facet compression syndrome
Idiopathic anterior knee pain

ICD-9CM CODES
719.46 Patellofemoral pain syndrome

EPIDEMIOLOGY & DEMOGRAPHICS

PREVALENCE: Estimated >20% of adolescents
PREDOMINANT SEX AND AGE: Nearly 2:1 female predominance; disproportionately affects active adolescents and adults in the second and third decades of life
RISK FACTORS: Increase in physical activity intensity or duration, overuse, joint overload, trauma

PHYSICAL FINDINGS & CLINICAL PRESENTATION

- Gradual or acute onset of anterior knee pain
- Sometimes localized under or around the patella
- Also described as a catching sensation under the patella
- Worsened pain with squatting, running, prolonged sitting, or ascending or descending steps
- Effusion implies intraarticular pathology not explained by PFPS
- Pain may be elicited by compression of the patella into the trochlear groove while the leg is extended

ETIOLOGY

- No clear consensus; likely multifactorial, including muscle overuse or joint overload with malalignment and/or trauma potentially contributing

DIAGNOSIS

DIFFERENTIAL DIAGNOSIS

- Patellofemoral arthritis, patellar instability, prepatellar bursitis, iliotibial band syndrome, synovitis, chondromalacia, bony abnormalities

WORKUP

- PFPS is a clinical diagnosis of exclusion; evaluate and rule out other possibilities on the differential
- Physical exam findings consistent with PFPS include eliciting pain by compression of the patella into the trochlear groove while the leg is extended.

LABORATORY TESTS

- None

IMAGING STUDIES

- No imaging is necessary in the initial workup.
- Consider plain films if symptoms do not improve after 1 to 2 mo of therapy.

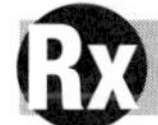

TREATMENT

There is a general lack of consensus.

NONPHARMACOLOGIC THERAPY

- Physical therapy; quadriceps, hamstring, iliotibial band, and calf-stretching exercises; quadriceps and hip abductor strengthening

ACUTE GENERAL Rx

- Short term (2 to 3 wk) NSAIDs for pain relief; activity modification; ice for 10 to 20 min after activity

CHRONIC Rx

- Physical therapy; strengthening and flexibility exercises; consider arch supports or evaluation for custom orthotics.
- Spontaneous resolution may occur in some cases.

DISPOSITION

- Outpatient management

REFERRAL

- Consider referral to orthopedics for surgical evaluation as a last resort if conservative therapies fail.

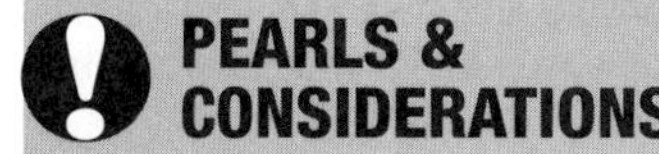

PEARLS & CONSIDERATIONS

COMMENTS

Treatment is most successful when the patient has a disciplined approach.

PATIENT/FAMILY EDUCATION

The American Academy of Family Practice website www.familydoctor.org contains frequently asked questions, patient information, and example stretching and strengthening exercises.

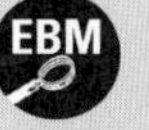

EVIDENCE

Studies indicate that the majority of patients with PFPS will improve with physical therapy (average length is 8 wk).

Physical therapy typically will include strengthening and stretching the muscles of the lower limb, particularly the quadriceps.

Patients who do not experience pain during their rehabilitation program have a greater success of recovery. The use of NSAIDs, ice, and patellar taping are helpful in decreasing pain and increasing exercise tolerance.

Evidence-Based Reference

1. Post WR: Patellofemoral pain: Results of nonoperative treatment, *Clin Orthop* 436:55-59, 2005.

SUGGESTED READING

Juhn MS: Patellofemoral pain syndrome: a review and guidelines for treatment, *Am Fam Physician* 60: 2012-2022, 1999.

AUTHOR: **KATE MAVRICH, M.D.**

Patent Foramen Ovale

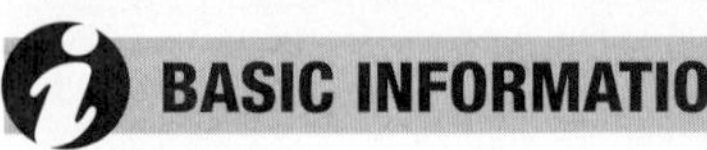

BASIC INFORMATION

DEFINITION

- Patent foramen ovale (PFO) is a vestige of the fetal circulation, and results from failure of the primum and secundum septa to fuse postnatally. Persistence of the one-way flap valve overlying this foramen ovale allows right to left blood flow when right atrial pressure exceeds that of the left.
- Foramen ovale remains open during intrauterine life, in a valve like manner, to allow highly oxygenated blood to reach the left atrium from the inferior vena cava. High right atrial pressure in the fetus keeps it open.
- Soon after birth, as the pulmonary circulation fills, the left atrial pressure rises higher than that of the right atrium. This pushes the septum primum against septum secondum, closing the right-to-left pathway through the foramen ovale.

ICD-9CM CODES

745.5 Patent foramen ovale

EPIDEMIOLOGY & DEMOGRAPHICS

- PFO fails to close in as many as a fourth of the population.
- PFO has similar frequency among males and females.

PHYSICAL FINDINGS & CLINICAL PRESENTATION

- Most patients with isolated PFO are asymptomatic.
- It cannot be detected on clinical examination.

COMPLICATIONS

- Cryptogenic stroke (particularly <55 yr).
- The proposed mechanism of stroke with PFO includes paradoxical embolization, in situ thrombosis within the canal of the PFO, associated atrial arrhythmia and concomitant hypercoagulable state.
- Migraine with aura.
- Decompression sickness and air embolism.
- Increases risk of hypoxemia during sleep in patients with obstructive sleep apnea.
- Platypnea-orthodeoxia syndrome (characterized by both dyspnea and arterial desaturation in the upright position with improvement in supine position).
- Increased risk of postoperative atrial fibrillation and hypoxemia, in off-pump coronary artery bypass surgery.

ETIOLOGY

- Unknown

DIAGNOSIS

- Testing for PFO is primarily performed in patients with a cerebral ischemic event of uncertain origin.
- A variety of echocardiography modalities have been used to diagnose PFO. These include:
  1. Transthoracic echocardiography (TTE)
  2. Transesophageal echocardiogram (TEE)
  3. Transmitral Doppler (TMD)
  4. Transcranial Doppler (TCD) of middle cerebral artery after injection of agitated saline peripherally
- TEE, especially when performed with contrast injected during a cough or valsalva, is the most sensitive and preferred test for diagnosing PFO.
- Essentially, a PFO is suggested by the presence of echo dropout in the atrial septum visualized in more than one plane during echocardiography. The appearance of microbubbles in the left atrium within three to five cardiac cycles after injection of agitated saline peripherally is considered diagnostic of PFO with associated with right-to-left shunt (RLS).
- The diagnosis of PFO is enhanced with multiple intravenous contrast injections with maneuvers that cause transient elevations of right atrial pressure (cough or valsalva) to enhance RLS.
- TCD has the advantage of being noninvasive and easy to perform at bedside. But it can only detect a right-to-left shunt, not the location of the shunt or other cardiac structural anomalies.

TREATMENT

- Management guidelines from professional societies are shown in Table 1-59.
- Most patients with a PFO as an isolated finding receive no special treatment. This is because the yearly risk of cryptogenic stroke in healthy persons with PFO may be as low as 0.1%.
- As it is not associated with increased risk for endocarditis, antibiotic prophylaxis is not indicated.

PHARMACOLOGICAL TREATMENT

When PFO is associated with an otherwise unexplained neurological event, traditional treatment has been antiplatelet treatment (e.g., aspirin) therapy alone in low-risk patients and combined with therapeutic anticoagulants (e.g., warfarin) in high-risk patients.

Risk factors associated with a higher risk of complications, particularly stroke include:

- Coexisting atrial septal aneurysm
- Large PFO
- Spontaneous right-to-left shunting
- Major shunt (>50 bubbles)
- Valsalva provoking activity preceding the onset of stroke
- Presence of Chiari network (a congenital remnant of the right valve of the sinus venosus)
- Eustachian valves
- Younger age (<55 yr)
- Multiple clinical events or infarcts
- Pulmonary hypertension
- Failure or contraindications to anticoagulants
- High risk for recurrent deep venous thrombosis
- Pulmonary embolism at time of initial event
- Hypercoagulable state

PERCUTANEOUS TRANSCATHETER CLOSURE OF PFO

Percutaneous method of closure is usually preferred over open surgical closure because of invasiveness, procedure time, and patient convenience.

- Indications:
  1. Recurrent cryptogenic stroke due to presumed paradoxical embolism through PFO while on adequate medical treatment with antiplatelets or anticoagulants
  2. In presence of contraindications to anticoagulants
- Contraindications:
  1. Presence of thrombus on the implant site or in the venous system used for access
  2. Active endocarditis or bacteremia
  3. Inadequate size of femoral vein for access

TABLE 1-59 Management Guidelines from Professional Societies

	American Academy of Neurology	American College of Chest Physicians
PFO	1. Evidence is insufficient to determine whether warfarin or aspirin is superior in preventing recurrent strokes or death, but minor bleeding is more frequent with warfarin. 2. There is insufficient evidence to evaluate the efficacy of surgical or endovascular closure.	
PFO alone		1. Antiplatelet therapy recommended over no therapy 2. Antiplatelet therapy suggested over warfarin
PFO with other risk factors		Inadequate data available to allow recommendation of optimal medical therapy vs. endovascular or surgical closure
PFO with concomitant deep vein thrombosis or pulmonary embolism	At least 3 months of anticoagulation	Anticoagulation recommended

4. Atrial septal anatomy without an adequate rim to hold the device
5. Atrial septal anatomy that may result in the occlude obstructing an intracardiac structure
6. Known hypercoagulable state
7. Presence of an intracardiac mass or vegetation

- The Food and Drug Administration (FDA) has approved CardioSEAL Septal Occlusion System and Amplatzer PFO Occluder devices for percutaneous PFO closure.
- Requires SBE prophylaxis and antiplatelets (aspirin and clopidogrel for first 3 mo, followed by aspirin for another 3 mo) for 6 mo postprocedure. During this period of endothelialization, the risk of recurrent stroke is highest.
- The 1-yr rate of recurrent neurological events ranged from 0% to 5% with percutaneous closure group vs. 4% to 12% with medical therapy group.
- MRI or metal detectors do not affect these implants, as they are not metallic in nature.

SURGICAL CLOSURE (OPEN THORACOTOMY)

- Indications:
  1. PFO >25 mm in size
  2. Inadequate rim of tissue around the defect
  3. Percutaneous device failure
  4. In presence of other indication for open heart surgery

SUGGESTED READINGS

Aslam F et al: Patent foramen ovale: assessment, clinical significance and therapeutic options, *South Med J* 19(12):1367-1372, 2006.

Horton SC, Bunch TJ: Patent foramen ovale and stroke, *Mayo Clin Proc* 79:79-88, 2004.

Kizer JR, Devereux RB: Patent foramen ovale in young adults with unexplained stroke, *N Engl J Med* 353: 2361-2372, 2005.

Maissel WH, Laskey WK: Patent foramen closure devices: moving beyond equipoise, *JAMA* 294(3):366-369, 2005.

AUTHOR: **HEMANT K. SATPATHY, M.D.**

Pediatric Medication Errors

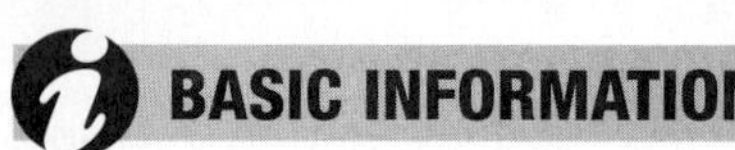

BASIC INFORMATION

DEFINITION

Medication errors represent failure of intended prescription, dispensation, or administration of desired drug therapy. Medication errors may result in inappropriate medication use or an adverse drug event (ADE) (i.e., direct harm or injury to the patient).

SYNONYMS

Dosing errors or mistakes. Medication errors are not synonymous with ADEs because not all cause harm (a requirement of ADEs).

ICD-9CM CODES
Not applicable

EPIDEMIOLOGY & DEMOGRAPHICS

INCIDENCE:

- 15% of pediatric outpatient prescriptions are either underdosed (7%) or overdosed (8%).
- Nearly 6% of medication orders for a hospitalized child contain an error. One percent of medication orders for a child will result in a potential ADE (i.e., an error that would have caused harm but was intercepted before reaching the patient). Less than 1% of medication orders for a child will contain an error that ultimately results in harm or injury.

PEAK INCIDENCE: Among outpatient prescriptions, medication errors occur more frequently in children <4 yr compared with older children (20% vs. 13%)

PREVALENCE: Not applicable

PREDOMINANT SEX AND AGE: Children <4 yr

GENETICS: Not applicable

RISK FACTORS:

- Patient age <4 yr, particularly with prescriptions for asthma and allergy medications or antibiotics
- Off-label (non-FDA approved) medication use
- Prescriptions for analgesics (most commonly written for potential overdose)
- Lack of computerized prescriber order entry (CPOE), standardized order sets, or alert systems
- Prescriptions for antiseizure medications (most commonly written for potential underdose)
- Infants or children with multiple health care needs or those in intensive care

PHYSICAL FINDINGS & CLINICAL PRESENTATION

- Signs and symptoms of toxicity specific to the current drug regimen
- Lack of clinical efficacy of the current drug regimen

ETIOLOGY

Common sources of pediatric medication errors include:

- Prescribing errors: lack of knowledge of medication; lack of recognition of the impact growth and development may have on the pharmacokinetics of a specific drug; use of medical abbreviations within the prescription or medication order
- Calculation errors: mg/kg/*dose* versus mg/kg/*day* dosing recommendations; "tenfold" decimal mistakes such as the use of trailing zeros (1 vs. 1.0) and naked decimals (0.1 vs. 1); patient weight in pounds versus kilograms
- Administration errors: incomplete education provided to patient or caregiver; lack of appropriate drug administration tools such as graduated oral syringes or medication spoons; deviation from the "five rights," (i.e., the *right* drug at the *right* dose for the *right* patient by the *right* route at the *right* time)
- Dispensing errors: inappropriate formulation recommended, prescribed, or dispensed; use of adult formulations for children

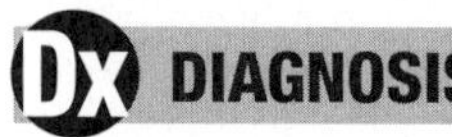

DIAGNOSIS

DIFFERENTIAL DIAGNOSIS

- Iatrogenic adverse drug reaction (unpreventable ADEs)
- Patient nonadherence (may be considered a medication error if appropriate instructions and/or education is not provided to the patient or caregiver)

WORKUP

Alert from CPOE systems, deviation from standardized order set, or detection on review of prescription or medication order by pharmacist or nurse:

- Immediately discontinue medication order or prescription
- Determine if suspected error has reached the patient
- Assess harm to patient and intervene if necessary (if ADE has occurred)
- Determine source of error if possible
- Resume correct drug therapy with appropriate monitoring of efficacy and toxicity
- Report error to institution or facility for tracking and quality improvement purposes
- Report sentinel events (an adverse event that led to death, serious physical or psychologic injury, or the risk of such injury) to the Joint Commission

LABORATORY TESTS

Supratherapeutic or subtherapeutic serum drug concentrations (if applicable)

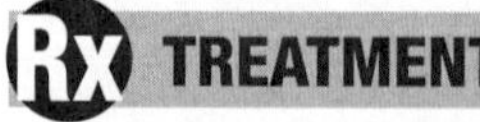

TREATMENT

Management of a medication error resulting in harm to the patient may include acute treatment of a toxic ADE or long-term management of a suboptimally treated condition. It should always include the workup described above.

ACUTE GENERAL Rx

If the medication error has reached the patient and resulted in an ADE, immediate intervention may be required. Disclosure to the patient or caregiver of an error resulting in harm to the patient is necessary.

CHRONIC Rx

Long-term management of injury or harm resulting from a medication error may be necessary.

DISPOSITION

- Prescribers may need to reestablish trust with the patient or caregiver after an error that resulted in harm to ensure optimal care in the future.
- The reporting of medication errors should be nonpunitive in nature and intent on individual education and correction of health systems–related flaws.

REFERRAL

Consultation with a pharmacist trained in pediatric pharmacotherapy may improve individual drug therapy and ensure age-specific drug dosing. Interpreters may be necessary to ensure drug information is accurately relayed to non-English-speaking patients or caregivers.

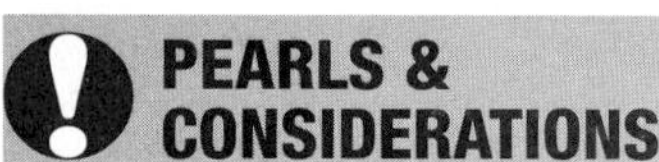

PEARLS & CONSIDERATIONS

COMMENTS

- 20% of ADEs occurring in hospitalized children are preventable.
- Medication errors must be reported for health systems–related flaws to be identified and corrected.
- Careful attention must always be focused on the impact growth and development has on the pharmacokinetic characteristics of drugs used in children. From birth through adolescence, the absorption, distribution, metabolism, and elimination of a particular drug must not be assumed constant, and age-specific dosing recommendations should be used. A child's dose should not exceed that of an adult. Equations that calculate proportionate doses based on body weight or body surface area do not take into consideration these age-related changes.

PREVENTION

- Health systems management: double-checking of calculations and verification of medication orders by pharmacists and nurses reduce preventable ADEs. Eliminate the use of medical abbreviations within medication orders and prescriptions. The use of CPOE, standardized order sets, and electronic prescription filing can provide a prompt at the time of prescribing or ordering and will reduce medication errors resulting from illegible handwriting.
- Communication: open lines of communication between the prescriber, nurse, and pharmacist will help ensure medication errors do not occur. Drug information must be presented and reinforced at a level and in a

language understandable to patients or caregivers.
- Education: health care professionals must remain knowledgeable of current standards of care as well as new drug therapy options.
- Review of drug therapy: reassessment of prescriptions for accurate age-appropriate dosing and the indication for drug therapy, monitoring of efficacy and toxicity, and reconfirming a patient or caregiver's understanding of the drug regimen will limit medication errors and potential harm in chronic medication use.

PATIENT & FAMILY EDUCATION

- Caregivers should always remind a child's doctor of any drug allergies or side effects the child has had in the past.
- Do not use over-the-counter cough and cold medicines for children less than 4 yr.
- A list of all the medicines a child uses should be kept and shared with all the doctors the child sees. Remember to include over-the-counter medicines such as cough medicine and analgesics.
- Caregivers should ask a child's doctor or pharmacist as many questions as needed so that they understand how to correctly use the child's medicine.

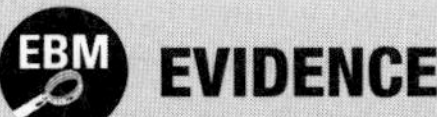

EVIDENCE

The most common sources of error in overdoses involving children within the home include tenfold dosing errors, errors regarding formulation or units of measure, increased frequency of administration, and use of adult dosing.[1] In January 2008, the U.S. Food & Drug Administration recommended that over-the-counter cough and cold medications should not be used in children less than 2 years of age; in October 2008, the Consumer Healthcare Products Association, an organization representing manufacturers of OTC medications, voluntarily removed dosing information for children less than 4 years of age from cough and cold medications.[2] Most medication errors in hospitalized infants and children involve antimicrobial drugs, analgesics and antipyretics, and intravenous electrolyte solutions.[3] Pediatric clinical pharmacy services coupled with computerized physician order entry can reduce medication errors in pediatric inpatient practices.[4]

Evidence-Based References

1. Tzimenatos L et al: Severe injury or death in young children from therapeutic errors: a summary of 238 cases from the American Association of Poison Control Centers, *Clin Toxicol* 47:348, 2009.
2. U.S. Food and Drug Administration Press Announcement: FDA statement following CHPS's announcement on nonprescription over-the-counter cough and cold medicines in children, 2008. Available at: http://www.fda.gov/NewsEvents/Newsroom/PressAnnouncements/2008/ucm116964.htm.
3. Takata G et al: Characteristics of medication errors and adverse drug events in hospitals participating in the California Pediatric Patient Safety Initiative, *Am J Health Syst Pharm* 65:2036, 2008.
4. Wang JK et al: Prevention of pediatric medication errors by hospital pharmacists and the potential benefit of computerized physician order entry, *Pediatrics* 119:e77, 2007.

SUGGESTED READINGS

Kozer E et al: Medication errors in children, *Pediatr Clin North Am* 53:1155, 2006.

Sharek PJ, Classen D: The incidence of adverse events and medical error in pediatrics, *Pediatr Clin North Am* 53:1067, 2006.

Wong ICK et al: Minimising medication errors in children, *Arch Dis Child* 94:161, 2009.

AUTHOR: **BRIAN J. COWLES, PHARM.D.**

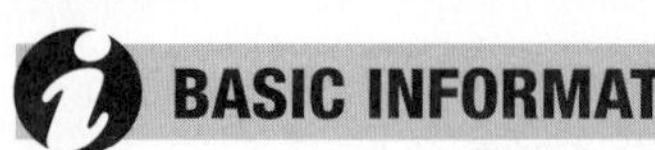

DEFINITION

Pediculosis is lice infestation. Human beings can be infested with three kinds of lice: *Pediculus capitis* (head louse [Fig. 1-237]), *Pediculus corporis* (body louse), and *Phthirus pubis* (pubic, or crab, louse). Lice feed on human blood and deposit their eggs (nits) on the hair shafts (head lice and pubic lice) and along the seams of clothing (body lice). Nits generally hatch within 7 to 10 days. Lice are obligate human parasites and cannot survive away from their hosts for longer than 7 to 10 days.

SYNONYMS

Lice

ICD-9CM CODES
132.9 Pediculosis

EPIDEMIOLOGY & DEMOGRAPHICS

- There are 6 million to 12 million cases of head lice in the U.S. yearly.
- Lice infestation of the scalp is most common in children (girls affected more often than boys).
- Infestation of the eyelashes is most frequently seen in children and may indicate sexual abuse.
- The chance of acquiring pubic lice from one sexual exposure with an infested partner is >90% (most contagious STD known).
- Body lice is most common in conditions of poor hygiene.

PHYSICAL FINDINGS & CLINICAL PRESENTATION

- Pruritus with excoriation may be caused by hypersensitivity reaction, inflammation from saliva, and fecal material from the lice.
- Nits can be identified by examining hair shafts.
- The presence of nits on clothes is indicative of body lice.
- Lymphadenopathy may be present (cervical adenopathy with head lice, inguinal lymphadenopathy with pubic lice).
- Head lice is most frequently found in the back of the head and neck, behind the ears.
- Scratching can result in pustules and crusting.
- Pubic lice may affect the hair around the anus.

ETIOLOGY

Lice are transmitted by close personal contact or use of contaminated objects (e.g., combs, clothing, bed linen, hats).

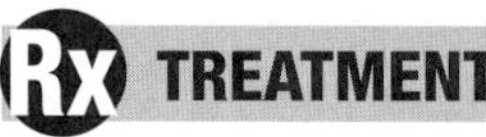

DIFFERENTIAL DIAGNOSIS

- Seborrheic dermatitis
- Scabies
- Eczema
- Other: pilar casts, trichonodosis (knotted hair), monilethrix

WORKUP

Diagnosis is made by seeing the lice or their nits. Combing hair with a fine-toothed comb is recommended because visual inspection of the hair and scalp may miss more than 50% of infestations.

LABORATORY TESTS

Wood's light examination is useful to screen a large number of children: live nits fluoresce, empty nits have a gray fluorescence, nits with unborn louse reveal white fluorescence.

Rx TREATMENT

NONPHARMACOLOGIC THERAPY

- Patients with body lice should discard infested clothes and improve their hygiene.
- Combing out nits is a widely recommended but unproven adjunctive therapy.
- Personal items such as combs and brushes should be soaked in hot water for 15 to 30 min.
- Close contacts and household members should also be examined for the presence of lice.

ACUTE GENERAL Rx

The following products are available for treatment of lice:

- Benzyl alcohol lotion, 5% (Ulesfia) can be used for treatment of head lice in patients >6 mo old. The lotion is applied to dry hair and left on for 10 min. Treatment must be repeated after 7 days because the drug is not ovicidal.
- Permethrin: available over the counter (1% permethrin [Nix]) or by prescription (5% permethrin [Elimite]); should be applied to the hair and scalp and rinsed out after 10 min. A repeat application is generally not necessary in patients with head lice. It can be applied to clean, dry hair and left on overnight (8 to 14 hours) under a shower cap.
- Eyelash infestation can be treated with the application of petroleum jelly rubbed into the eyelashes three times a day for 5 to 7 days. The application of baby shampoo to the eyelashes and brows three or four times a day for 5 days is also effective. The use of fluorescein drops applied to the lids and eyelashes is also toxic to lice.
- In patients who have previously not responded to treatment or in whom resistance with 1% permethrin cream rinse occurs, a 10-day course of trimethoprim-sulfamethoxazole (TMP-SMX) 8 mg/kg/day in divided doses is an effective treatment for head lice infestation, especially for eyelash infestations with *Phthirus pubis*.
- Ivermectin (Mectizan), an antiparasitic drug, given in a single oral dose of 200 mcg/kg is effective for head lice resistant to other treatments (currently not FDA approved for pediculosis).
- Malathion (Ovide), an organophosphate, is effective in head lice. It is available by prescription. Use should be avoided in children ≤2 yr. It is not commonly used because of its objectionable odor, fear of flammability, and prolonged application time (8 to 12 hr).

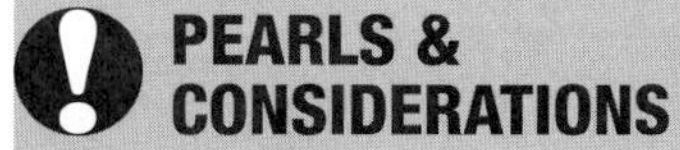

COMMENTS

- Patients with pubic lice should notify their sexual contacts. Sex partners within the last month should be treated.
- Parents of patients should also be educated that head lice infestation (unlike body lice) does not indicate poor hygiene.

SUGGESTED READINGS

Flinders DC, DeSchweinitz P: Pediculosis and scabies, *Am Fam Physician* 69:341, 2004.
Roberts RJ: Head lice, *N Engl J Med* 346:1645, 2002.

AUTHOR: **FRED F. FERRI, M.D.**

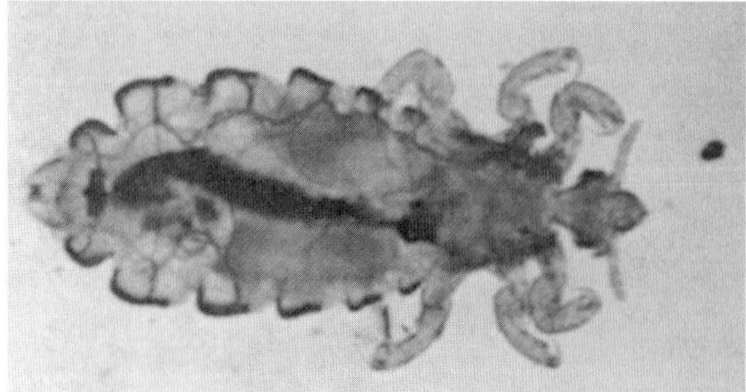

FIGURE 1-237 *Pediculus humanus* var. *capitis* (head louse). (From Mandell GL [ed]: *Mandell, Douglas, and Bennett's principles and practice of infectious diseases,* ed 6, New York, 2005, Churchill Livingstone.)

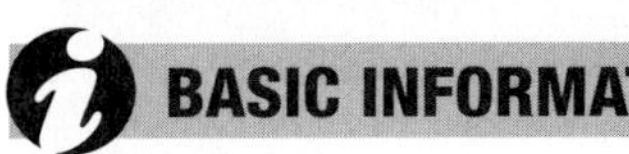

BASIC INFORMATION

DEFINITION

Pedophilia is a sexual disorder that involves recurrent, intense, distressing sexual urges and/or fantasies involving prepubescent children. A person must be at least 16 yr of age and at least 5 yr older than the child affected. The behavior may range from looking, to fondling, masturbation, and various degrees of penetration and coercion.

SYNONYMS

Pedophilia erotica

Acts referred to as child sexual abuse or child molestation

ICD-9CM CODES

302.2 Pedophilia

EPIDEMIOLOGY & DEMOGRAPHICS

PEAK INCIDENCE: Onset in adolescence

PREVALENCE (IN U.S.): 2% of men and 17% of women report being sexually touched by an older person when they were children.

PREDOMINANT SEX:

- Majority of perpetrators are men: 75% attracted to females exclusively; 25% attracted to males exclusively
- Girls sexually abused three times more often than boys; children from the lowest income families are 18 times more likely to be sexually abused.

PREDOMINANT AGE: One of every seven sexual assaults of juveniles occurs in children <6 yr and one third are <12 yr.

GENETICS: None identified

PHYSICAL FINDINGS & CLINICAL PRESENTATION

- Often shy, passive, and with social and interpersonal difficulties
- Frequently has experienced early abuse himself or herself
- May occasionally seek help before any sexual acts with children
- "Belief" among some of those who molest children that their behavior is good for or welcomed by the child

ETIOLOGY

- Personal experience with early molestation may be important, though only a minority of molested children develop pedophilia.
- Influence of personality factors is cited by some experts (i.e., inadequate attachment style rooted in a dysfunctional family).
- Neurodevelopmental perturbations increase the risk of pedophilia in males.

DIAGNOSIS

DIFFERENTIAL DIAGNOSIS

- Psychosis: may present with unusual ideas or statements that may rarely be confused with pedophilia.
- Incest: not necessarily based in pedophilia, but may instead reflect a dysfunctional family unit.
- Paraphilic sexual behavior in the setting of another condition such as mental retardation, brain injury, or drug intoxication.

WORKUP

- History is essential for diagnosis; however, most pedophiles are less than forthcoming even to direct questions by a physician.
- Children who have been sexually abused may display depression and aggressive behaviors, have an increased frequency of anxiety disorders, and have problems with age-appropriate sex roles and sexual functioning.
- Collateral information should be obtained from family members, suspected victims, or legal and social organizations; but even experienced interviewers may be unable to diagnose pedophilia consistently.

LABORATORY TESTS

Hormone profile is sometimes recommended.

IMAGING STUDIES

Useful only if pedophilic behavior is believed to be a consequence of central nervous system damage.

TREATMENT

NONPHARMACOLOGIC THERAPY

- Usually obtain treatment under legal coercion after child molestation charge.
- Behavioral approaches are centered on aversion conditioning, in which an aversive stimulus is paired with the pedophilic fantasy.
- Outpatient group therapy sometimes combined with the administration of antiandrogenic medications.
- For incestuous adult-child relationships not based in pedophilia, intensive family systems investigation and therapy are needed.
- Pedophilia is considered a chronic disorder. Therefore treatment should focus on achieving long-term behavioral change in the community.
- Treat comorbid conditions, such as alcoholism and affective illness.

ACUTE GENERAL Rx & CHRONIC Rx

- Brief periods of inpatient hospitalization may be required as a precaution during periods of heightened stress.
- Chemical castration with antiandrogen compounds; they are generally believed to be safe, effective, and reversible.
- Medroxyprogesterone acetate (Provera) can be administered PO (60 mg/day) or in a depot IM form (200 to 400 mg IM once weekly).
- Testosterone-lowering medications. Although these drugs suppress the intensity of libidinal drive, they generally allow erectile function.
- Serotonin reuptake inhibitors to suppress sexual drive.

DISPOSITION

If untreated, child molesters are highly likely to be repeat offenders.

REFERRAL

Refer to specialty mental health.

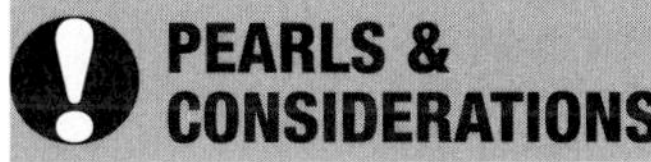

PEARLS & CONSIDERATIONS

Physicians should be aware of reporting requirements in their jurisdiction.

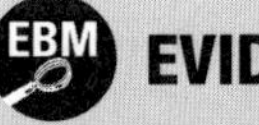

EVIDENCE

A systematic review studied randomized, controlled trials of psychological treatments for children who had been sexually abused. It found that cognitive-behavioral therapy, particularly for young children, had the strongest evidence for improving psychological symptoms.[1] B

Evidence-Based Reference

1. Ramchandani P, Jones DP: Treating psychological symptoms in sexually abused children: from research findings to service provision, *Br J Psychiatry* 183:484, 2003. B

SUGGESTED READINGS

Fagan PJ et al: Pedophilia, *JAMA* 288(19):2458, 2002.

Hughes JR: Review of medical reports on pedophilia, *Clin Pediatr (Phila)* 46(8):667-682, 2007.

Kenworthy T et al: Psychological interventions for those who have sexually offended or are at risk of offending, *Cochrane Rev* 3:CD004858, 2004.

Seto MC: Pedophilia, *Ann Rev Clin Psychol* 5:391-407, 2009.

AUTHOR: **MITCHELL D. FELDMAN, M.D., M.PHIL.**

BASIC INFORMATION

DEFINITION

Pelvic inflammatory disease (PID) is a spectrum of inflammatory disorders of the upper genital tract, including a combination of any of the following:

- Endometritis, salpingitis, tubo-ovarian abscess, or pelvic peritonitis
- Resulting from an ascending lower genital tract infection
- Not related to obstetric or surgical intervention

SYNONYMS

Adnexitis
Pyosalpinx
Salpingitis
Tubo-ovarian abscess

ICD-9CM CODES
614.9 Unspecified inflammatory disease of female pelvic organs and tissue

EPIDEMIOLOGY & DEMOGRAPHICS

INCIDENCE/PREVALENCE:

- Estimated 600,000 to 1 million cases annually (U.S.)
- Diagnosed in 2% to 5% of women seen in sexually transmitted disease clinics
- Most common cause of female infertility and ectopic pregnancy

RISK FACTORS:

- Adolescent sexually active females $<$20 yr (1:8)
- Previous episode of gonococcal PID
- Multiple sexual partners
- Vaginal douching

PHYSICAL FINDINGS & CLINICAL PRESENTATION

- Lower abdominal pain
- Abnormal vaginal discharge
- Abnormal uterine bleeding
- Dysuria
- Dyspareunia
- Nausea and vomiting (suggestive of peritonitis)
- Fever
- Right upper quadrant tenderness (perihepatitis): 5% of PID cases
- Cervical motion tenderness and adnexal tenderness
- Adnexal mass

ETIOLOGY

- *Chlamydia trachomatis*
- *Neisseria gonorrhoeae*
- Polymicrobial infection: *Bacteroides fragilis, Escherichia coli, Gardnerella vaginalis, Haemophilus influenzae, Mycoplasma hominis, Ureaplasma urealyticum*
- *Mycobacterium tuberculosis* (an important cause in developing countries)
- Cytomegalovirus (CMV)

Dx DIAGNOSIS

DIFFERENTIAL DIAGNOSIS

- Ectopic pregnancy
- Appendicitis
- Ruptured ovarian cyst
- Endometriosis
- Urinary tract infection (cystitis or pyelonephritis)
- Renal calculus
- Adnexal torsion
- Proctocolitis

WORKUP

Diagnostic considerations:

- Clinical diagnosis is difficult and imprecise. A clinical algorithm for the evaluation of pelvic pain is described in Section III, "Pelvic Pain, Reproductive-Age Woman"; evaluation of vaginal discharge is described in Section III, "Vaginal Discharge."
- Clinical diagnosis of symptomatic PID has a positive predictive value of 65% to 90% compared with laparoscopy as the standard.
- No single historical, physical, or laboratory finding is both sensitive and specific for the diagnosis of PID.

2002 CDC diagnostic criteria for PID:

- Empiric treatment is based on the presence of all of the following minimum criteria:
  1. Uterine tenderness
  2. Adnexal tenderness
  3. Cervical motion tenderness
- Additional criteria to increase the specificity of the diagnosis of PID in women with severe clinical signs:
  1. Oral temperature $>$38.3° C (101° F)
  2. Abnormal cervical or vaginal discharge
  3. Elevated erythrocyte sedimentation rate (ESR)
  4. Elevated C-reactive protein
  5. Laboratory documentation of cervical infection with *N. gonorrhoeae* or *C. trachomatis*
- Definitive criteria for diagnosing PID warranted in selected cases:
  1. Laparoscopic abnormalities consistent with PID
  2. Histopathologic evidence of endometritis on biopsy
  3. Transvaginal sonography or other imaging techniques showing thickened fluid-filled tubes with or without free pelvic fluid or tubo-ovarian complex

LABORATORY TESTS

- Leukocytosis
- Elevated acute phase reactants: ESR $>$15 mm/hr, C-reactive protein
- Gram stain of endocervical exudate: $>$30 polymorphonuclear cells per high-power field correlates with chlamydial or gonococcal infection
- Endocervical cultures for *N. gonorrhoeae* and *C. trachomatis*
- Fallopian tube aspirate or peritoneal exudate culture if laparoscopy performed
- Human chorionic gonadotropin to rule out ectopic pregnancy

IMAGING STUDIES

- Transvaginal ultrasound to look for adnexal mass has sensitivity for PID of 81%, specificity of 78%, and accuracy of 80%.
- MRI has sensitivity for PID of 95%, specificity of 89%, and accuracy of 93%. It is useful for establishing the diagnosis of PID and detecting other processes responsible for the symptoms. Disadvantages are its higher cost and unavailability in certain areas.

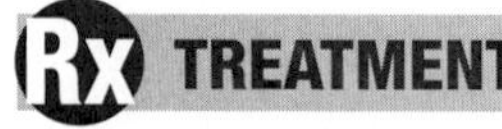

TREATMENT

NONPHARMACOLOGIC THERAPY

- Most patients are treated as outpatients.
- Criteria for hospitalization (CDC, 2006) as follows:
  1. Surgical emergencies such as appendicitis cannot be excluded
  2. Tubo-ovarian abscess
  3. Pregnant patient
  4. Patient is immunodeficient
  5. Severe illness, nausea, or vomiting precluding outpatient management
  6. Patient unable to follow or tolerate outpatient regimens
  7. No clinical response to outpatient therapy

ACUTE GENERAL Rx

Regimens for treatment of PID recommended by the CDC, 2006:

- Outpatient treatment, regimen A:
  1. Ofloxacin 400 mg PO bid × 14 days or levofloxacin 500 mg PO × 14 days with or without metronidazole 500 mg PO bid × 14 days
- Outpatient treatment, regimen B:
  1. Cefoxitin 2 g IM plus probenecid 1 g PO single dose plus doxycycline 100 mg PO bid × 14 days with or without metronidazole 500 mg PO bid × 14 days *or*
  2. Ceftriaxone 250 mg IM once single dose plus doxycycline 100 mg PO bid × 14 days with or without metronidazole 500 mg PO bid × 14 days
- Inpatient treatment, regimen A:
  1. Cefoxitin 2 g IV q6h or cefotetan 2 g IV q12h plus doxycycline 100 mg IV or PO q12h
  2. Continuation of regimen for at least 24 hr after substantial clinical improvement, after which doxycycline 100 mg PO bid is continued for a total of 14 days
- Inpatient treatment, regimen B:
  1. Clindamycin 900 mg IV q8h plus gentamicin loading dose IV or IM (2 mg/kg of body weight), followed by a maintenance dose (1.5 mg/kg) q8h
  2. Continuation of regimen for at least 24 hr after substantial clinical improvement, followed by doxycycline 100 mg PO bid or clindamycin 450 mg PO qid to complete a total of 14 days of therapy

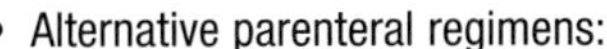

- Alternative parenteral regimens:
  1. Ofloxacin 400 mg IV q12h *or*
  2. Levofloxacin 500 mg IV once daily with or without metronidazole 500 mg IV q8h *or*
  3. Ampicillin/sulbactam 3 g IV q6h plus doxycycline 100 mg PO or IV q12h

CHRONIC Rx

Hospitalized patients receiving IV therapy:

1. Significant clinical improvement is characterized by defervescence, decreased abdominal tenderness, and decreased uterine, adnexal, and cervical motion tenderness within 3 to 5 days.
2. If no clinical improvement occurs, further diagnostic workup is necessary, including possible surgical intervention.

DISPOSITION

- Long-term sequelae of PID: recurrent PID, chronic pelvic pain, ectopic pregnancy, infertility, Fitz-Hugh-Curtis syndrome (Fig. 1-238)
- Risk of tubal infertility related to episodes of PID: first episode, 8%; second episode, 20%; third episode, 40%
- Essential to evaluate and treat male sex partners

REFERRAL

If there is no clinical improvement with outpatient therapy observed within 72 hr, patient should be hospitalized and gynecology consult requested.

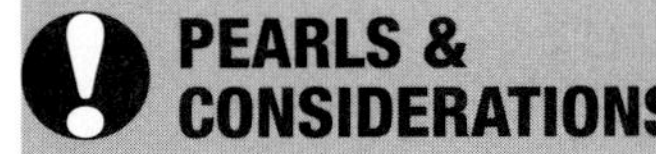

PEARLS & CONSIDERATIONS

COMMENTS

Maintain a low threshold for the diagnosis of PID.

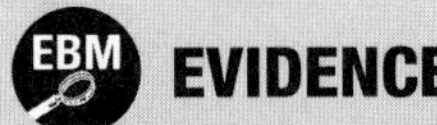

EVIDENCE

Please note: Complete text of EBM for this topic is available online.

Key trials and commentary:

This study sought to evaluate the equivalence of ceftriaxone plus doxycycline or azithromycin for cases of mild pelvic inflammatory disease (PID). It showed that when combined with ceftriaxone, 1 g of azithromycin weekly for 2 weeks is equivalent to ceftriaxone plus a 14-day course of doxycycline for treating mild PID.

Treatment guidelines for STDs were recently reissued by the CDC (2006). In general, ambulatory management of PID requires coverage for *Gonococcus* and *Chlamydia* as well as suggestions that prolonged wide-spectrum coverage, particularly for anaerobes, is prudent. One hurdle for ambulatory management is patient compliance. These researchers investigate what is essentially a 2-dose/2-week regimen substituting azithromycin for the typical 14-day course of doxycycline that is part of recommended treatments. The idea is that compliance will be enhanced by reducing the number of pills the patient needs to take. The fact that the two regimens compared here perform equally well indicates that azithromycin could be a suitable substitute for many outpatients with mild-moderate PID. Because this was performed in a study setting with fairly small sample sizes, it is not easy to assess whether compliance truly will be better with use of azithromycin in a real-world setting. Additionally, although not part of the analysis in this study, the cost for PO azithromycin is considerably higher than 14 days of doxycycline. This fact will temper its widespread implementation in certain settings.[1] Ⓐ

Evidence-Based Reference

1. Savaris RF et al: Comparing ceftriaxone plus azithromycin or doxycycline for pelvic inflammatory disease: a randomized controlled trial, *Obstet Gynecol* 110:53-60, 2007. Commentary by J.S. Dungan, M.D. Ⓐ

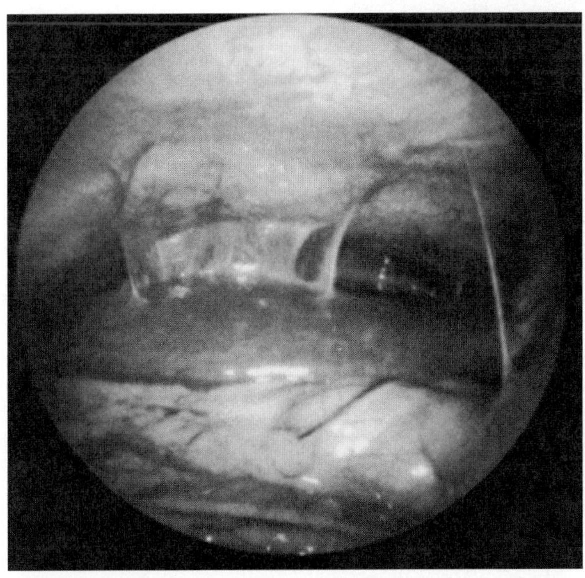

FIGURE 1-238 "Violin string" adhesions are visualized in this patient with Fitz-Hugh-Curtis syndrome. (From Copeland LJ: *Textbook of gynecology,* ed 2, Philadelphia, 2000, WB Saunders.)

SUGGESTED READING

Centers for Disease Control and Prevention: 2006: sexually transmitted diseases treatment guidelines, *MMWR* 55(RR-11):1, 2006.

AUTHORS: **GEORGE T. DANAKAS, M.D.,** and **RUBEN ALVERO, M.D.**

Pemphigus Vulgaris (PTG)

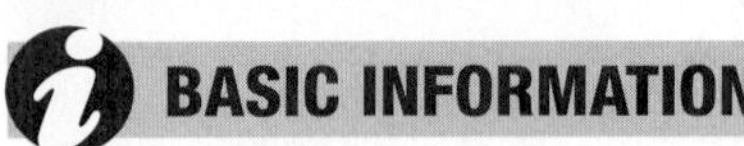

BASIC INFORMATION

DEFINITION

- Pemphigus refers to a group of rare, potentially fatal, chronic, autoimmune blistering diseases of the skin and mucous membranes
- Pemphigus has four main subtypes:
  1. Pemphigus vulgaris (PV) (most common) (Fig. 1-239)
     - Pemphigus vegetans, a rare clinical variant of PV
  2. Pemphigus foliaceus (PF)
     - Pemphigus erythematosus, a variant of PF
  3. Paraneoplastic pemphigus
  4. Immunoglobulin (Ig) A pemphigus

SYNONYMS

Pemphigus

Fogo selvagem: endemic pemphigus foliaceus

Senear-Usher syndrome: pemphigus erythematosus

ICD-9CM CODES

694.4 Pemphigus

EPIDEMIOLOGY & DEMOGRAPHICS

- Incidence is approximately one case per 100,000 persons and varies substantially by geographic region.
- More common in Ashkenazi Jews and people of Middle Eastern descent.
- Typically occurs in the fourth and fifth decades of life, though range of ages affected is broad and may occur in the very young or elderly.
- No gender predilection.

PHYSICAL FINDINGS & CLINICAL PRESENTATION

- History:
  1. Multiple oropharyngeal ulcerations and erosions typically occur first, which can be followed by a more generalized bullous eruption involving the skin within several weeks or months
  2. Blisters are fragile and rupture easily, leaving painful erosions and ulcerations that may be the predominant clinical finding
  3. Pain associated with oral mucosal blistering often results in dysphagia and hoarseness
  4. Not commonly pruritic
- Physical findings:
  1. Anatomic distribution
     a. Oral mucosa
     b. Can also involve the pharynx, larynx, vagina, penis, anus, and conjunctival mucosa
     c. Generalized cutaneous involvement (Figs. 1-240 and 1-241)
  2. Lesion configuration
     a. Any stratified squamous epithelial surfaces can become involved
  3. Lesion morphology
     a. Flaccid bullae and vesicles
     b. Erosion with crusting commonly occurs

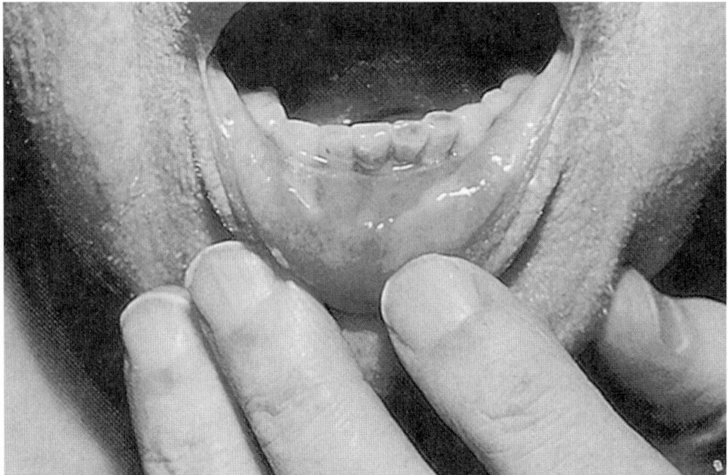

FIGURE 1-239 Pemphigus vulgaris with oral lesions and no intact bullae. (Courtesy Department of Dermatology, University of North Carolina at Chapel Hill. From Goldstein BG, Goldstein AO: *Practical dermatology,* ed 2, St Louis, 1997, Mosby.)

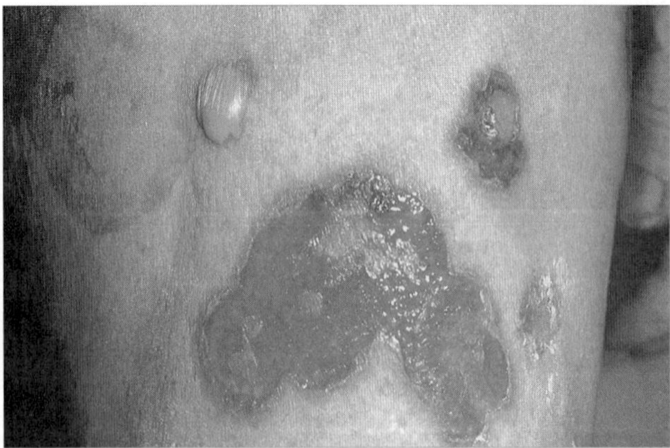

FIGURE 1-240 Pemphigus vulgaris; extensive erosions and blisters are present on the shin. (Courtesy R. A. Marsden, M.D., St. George's Hospital, London. From McKee PH et al [eds]: *Pathology of the skin with clinical correlations,* ed 3, St Louis, 2005, Mosby.)

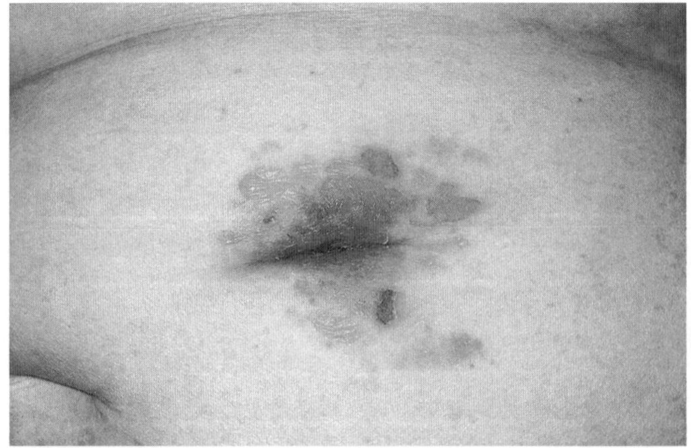

FIGURE 1-241 Pemphigus vulgaris: umbilical lesions showing intact blisters as well as raw erosions. (Courtesy R. A. Marsden, M.D., St. George's Hospital, London. From McKee PH et al [eds]: *Pathology of the skin with clinical correlations,* ed 3, St Louis, 2005, Mosby.)

4. Positive Nikolsky sign: when the clinician applies lateral pressure to normal-appearing skin at the periphery of active lesions, separation of the superficial epidermis occurs

ETIOLOGY

Autoimmune disease caused by autoantibodies against the cell surface of keratinocytes. The predominant antibody in PV is directed against desmoglein 3; in PF it is directed against desmoglein 1.

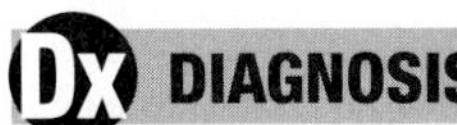

DIAGNOSIS

The diagnosis of pemphigus vulgaris should be suspected in patients with painful oral erosions and flaccid bullae or erosions on the skin.

DIFFERENTIAL DIAGNOSIS

- Bullous pemphigoid (Table 1-60)
- Cicatricial pemphigoid
- Behçet's syndrome
- Erythema multiforme
- Hailey-Hailey disease
- Aphthous stomatitis
- Bullous lupus erythematosus
- Drug eruptions

WORKUP

Skin biopsy is diagnostic; specimens should be sent for routine histochemical staining and direct immunofluorescence. Certain laboratory values may also be useful in establishing the diagnosis of pemphigus.

LABORATORY TESTS

- Indirect immunofluorescence may detect circulating autoantibodies.
- Skin biopsy reveals intraepidermal vesicles, also called *acantholysis* (loss of cell adhesion between the epidermal cells).
- Direct immunofluorescence studies of perilesional skin demonstrate IgG directed against keratinocyte surfaces in the epidermis.

Rx TREATMENT

NONPHARMACOLOGIC THERAPY

- Mild soaps and emollients to skin
- Burow's solution may be useful for weeping erosions
- Soft diet and viscous lidocaine can be used in patients with oral lesions

ACUTE GENERAL Rx

- For localized disease, topical steroids may be effective.
- For generalized disease, systemic corticosteroids (prednisone) are the mainstay of therapy and often work rapidly to halt blistering.
  - Initial dose of prednisone is usually 1 mg/kg/day, then tapered over weeks as blistering decreases
  - Steroid-sparing immunosuppressive therapies are often initiated simultaneously with prednisone to minimize the side effects of prolonged corticosteroid therapy

CHRONIC Rx

- Adjuvant therapy such as immunosuppressants, antiinflammatories, chemotherapeutic agents, and biologics are useful for disease control and to shorten the length of treatment with oral steroids; treatment duration and dosing are determined by clinical response:
  1. Azathioprine 50 to 100 mg/day
  2. Cyclophosphamide 1 to 3 mg/kg/day
  3. Mycophenolate mofetil 500 mg to 2 g daily
- Refractory disease:
  1. IV Ig
  2. Rituximab (anti-CD20 monoclonal antibody)
  3. Plasmapheresis

DISPOSITION

- Before the use of oral corticosteroids, pemphigus was usually a fatal disease with most patients dying within 5 yr of diagnosis.
- Combined corticosteroids and adjuvant therapy has decreased mortality rates to <10%.
- Death generally occurs from sepsis or complications related to medical therapy.

REFERRAL

Dermatology
Otolaryngology

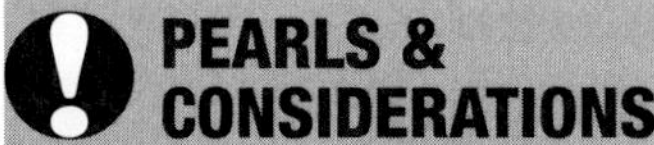

PEARLS & CONSIDERATIONS

COMMENTS

- PV, unlike bullous pemphigoid, is a disease of middle-aged persons.
- Early diagnosis of pemphigus is important to initiate prompt treatment.
- Oral corticosteroids have many substantial side effects, and patients should be monitored for osteoporosis, hypertension, and diabetes.

SUGGESTED READINGS

Bickle K et al: Autoimmune bullous dermatoses: a review, *Am Fam Physician* 65(9):1861, 2002.

Dick SE, Werth V: Pemphigus: a treatment update, *Autoimmunity* 39(7):591-599, 2006.

Joly P et al: A single cycle of rituximab for the treatment of severe pemphigus, *N Engl J Med* 357: 545-552, 2007.

Yeh SW et al: Treatment of pemphigus vulgaris: current and emerging options, *Am J Clin Dermatol* 6(5): 327, 2005.

AUTHORS: **JESSICA RISSER, M.D., M.P.H.,** and **KACHIU LEE, B.A.**

TABLE 1-60 Differentiation of Pemphigus Vulgaris and Bullous Pemphigoid

Characteristics	Pemphigus Vulgaris	Bullous Pemphigoid
Age	Usually occurs in middle aged persons	>60 yr
Site	Oral mucosa, face, chest, groin	Flexural areas, groin, axilla; less often involving mucosal surfaces
Findings	Flaccid bullae and erosions, intraepidermal blisters, IgG autoantibodies against keratinocyte surfaces	Intact bullae, subepidermal blisters, IgG autoantibodies against hemidesmosomal antigens
Treatment	Prednisone 1 mg/kg/day with adjuvant immunosuppressant agents; refractory disease may require IV Ig, plasmapheresis or rituximab	Prednisone 1 mg/kg/day with adjuvant immunosuppressant therapy; localized disease may be controlled with topical steroids
Prognosis	>90% respond; steroid side effects significant	>90% respond; remissions and recurrences common

Ig, Immunoglobulin; *IV,* intravenous.

P

Diseases and Disorders I

Peptic Ulcer Disease (PTG)

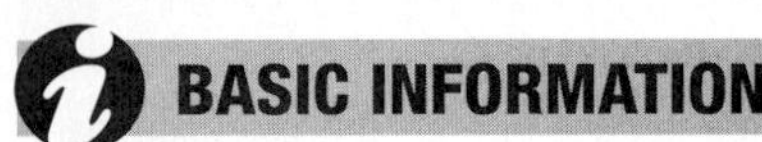

BASIC INFORMATION

DEFINITION

Peptic ulcer disease (PUD) is an ulceration in the stomach or duodenum resulting from an imbalance between mucosal protective factors and various mucosal damaging mechanisms (see "Etiology").

SYNONYMS

PUD
Duodenal ulcer (DU)
Gastric ulcer (GU)

ICD-9CM CODES	
536.8	Peptic ulcer disease
531.3	Peptic ulcer, stomach, acute
531.7	Peptic ulcer, stomach, chronic
532.3	Peptic ulcer, duodenum, acute
532.7	Peptic ulcer, duodenum, chronic

EPIDEMIOLOGY & DEMOGRAPHICS

- Incidence: 250,000 to 500,000 (200,000 to 400,000 duodenal; 50,000 to 100,000 gastric) annually; duodenal ulcer/gastric ulcer ratio is 4:1.
- Anatomic location: $>$90% of duodenal ulcers occur in the first portion of the duodenum; gastric ulcers occur most frequently in the lesser curvature near the incisura angularis.

PHYSICAL FINDINGS & CLINICAL PRESENTATION

- Physical examination is often unremarkable.
- Patient may have epigastric tenderness, tachycardia, pallor, hypotension (from acute or chronic blood loss), nausea and vomiting (if pyloric channel is obstructed), boardlike abdomen and rebound tenderness (if perforated), and hematemesis or melena (with a bleeding ulcer).

ETIOLOGY

Often multifactorial. The following are common mucosal damaging factors:

- *Helicobacter pylori* infection. *H. pylori* is the major cause of peptic ulcer disease. It is found in more than 70% of patients with duodenal ulcers and gastric ulcers in the U.S. Rates are much higher ($>$90%) in other parts of the world. Eradication of *H. pylori* markedly reduces peptic ulcer recurrence.
- Medications (nonsteroidal anti-inflammatory drugs [NSAIDs], glucocorticoids)
- Incompetent pylorus or lower esophageal sphincter
- Bile acids
- Impaired proximal duodenal bicarbonate secretion
- Decreased blood flow to gastric mucosa
- Acid secreted by parietal cells and pepsin secreted as pepsinogen by chief cells
- Cigarette smoking
- Alcohol

Dx DIAGNOSIS

DIFFERENTIAL DIAGNOSIS

- Gastroesophageal reflux disease
- Cholelithiasis syndrome
- Pancreatitis
- Gastritis
- Nonulcer dyspepsia
- Neoplasm (gastric carcinoma, lymphoma, pancreatic carcinoma)
- Angina pectoris, myocardial infarction, pericarditis
- Dissecting aneurysm
- Other: high small-bowel obstruction, pneumonia, subphrenic abscess, early appendicitis

WORKUP

Comprehensive history and physical examination to exclude other diagnoses. Diagnostic modalities include endoscopy or upper gastrointestinal (GI) series. Endoscopy is preferred.

LABORATORY TESTS

- Routine laboratory evaluation is usually unremarkable.
- Anemia may be present in patients with significant GI bleeding.
- *H. pylori* testing by endoscopic biopsy, urea breath test, stool antigen test (*H. pylori* stool antigen), or specific antibody test is recommended:
  1. Serologic testing for antibodies to *H. pylori* is easy and inexpensive; however, the presence of antibodies demonstrates previous but not necessarily current infection. Antibodies to *H. pylori* can remain elevated for months to years after infection has cleared; therefore antibody levels must be interpreted in light of the patient's symptoms and other test results (e.g., PUD seen on upper GI series).
  2. The urea breath test documents active infection (sensitivity and specificity $>$90%). The patient ingests a small amount of urea labeled with carbon 13 or carbon 14. If urease is present (produced by the organism), the urea is hydrolyzed and the patient exhales labeled carbon dioxide that is then collected and measured. This test is more expensive and not as readily available. Use of proton pump inhibitors (PPI) within 2 wk of the urea breath test may interfere with test results. Recently a new card test for ^{14}C urea has been developed, providing a testing option in primary care settings. It uses a flat breath card that is read by a small analyzer.
  3. Histologic evaluation of endoscopic biopsy samples is considered by many the gold standard for accurate diagnosis of *H. pylori* infection. However, detection of *H. pylori* depends on the site and number of biopsy samples, the method of staining, and experience of the pathologist.
  4. Stool antigen test is an enzyme-linked immunosorbent assay (ELISA) that identifies *H. pylori* antigen in a stool specimen through a polyclonal anti–*H. pylori* antibody. It is as accurate as the urea breath test for diagnosis of active infection and follow-up evaluation of patients treated for *H. pylori.* A negative result on the stool antigen test 8 wk after completion of therapy identifies patients in whom eradication of *H. pylori* was unsuccessful.
- Additional laboratory evaluation is indicated only in specific cases (e.g., amylase level in suspected pancreatitis, serum gastrin level in suspected Zollinger-Ellison [ZE] syndrome).

IMAGING STUDIES

Conventional upper GI barium studies identify approximately 70% to 80% of PUD; accuracy can be increased to approximately 90% by using double contrast.

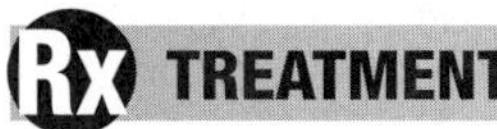

TREATMENT

NONPHARMACOLOGIC THERAPY

- Stop smoking; smoking increases the risk of PUD, decreases the healing rate, and increases the frequency of recurrence.
- Avoid NSAIDs and alcohol.
- Special diets have been proved unrelated to ulcer development and healing; however, avoid foods that cause symptoms.

ACUTE GENERAL Rx

Eradication of *H. pylori,* when present, can be accomplished with various regimens:

1. PPI (e.g., omeprazole 20 mg bid or lansoprazole 30 mg bid, esomeprazole 40 mg qd) *plus* clarithromycin 500 mg bid *and* amoxicillin 1000 mg bid for 10 days. This regimen achieves an eradication rate of 80% to 90% and can be used as first-line therapy for patients not allergic to penicillin.
2. PPI bid *plus* amoxicillin 500 mg bid *plus* metronidazole 500 mg bid for 10 days.
3. PPI bid *plus* clarithromycin 500 mg bid *and* metronidazole 500 mg bid for 10 days. This regimen is useful in those with penicillin allergy.
4. A 1-day quadruple therapy may be as effective as a 7-day triple-therapy regimen. The 1-day quadruple-therapy regimen consists of 2 tablets of 262-mg bismuth subsalicylate qid, 1 500-mg metronidazole tablet qid, 2 g of amoxicillin suspension qid, and 2 capsules of 30 mg of lansoprazole.
5. Bismuth compound qid *plus* tetracycline 500 mg qid *and* metronidazole 500 mg qid for 14 days.
6. A combination of levofloxacin 250 mg bid, amoxicillin 1000 mg bid, and a PPI bid for 10 to 14 days can be used as salvage therapy after unsuccessful attempts to eradicate *H. pylori* using other regimens.

A 10-day sequential therapy has been reported to be superior to standard triple therapy for eradication of *H. pylori.* It consists of 5 days of treatment with a PPI and one antibiotic (usually amoxicillin) followed by 5-day treatment with the PPI and two other antibiotics (usually clarithromycin and metronidazole).

PUD patients testing negative for *H. pylori* should be treated with antisecretory agents:
- H_2 receptor antagonists (H_2RAs): cimetidine, ranitidine, famotidine, and nizatidine are all effective; they are usually given in split dose or at nighttime.
- PPIs: can also induce rapid healing; they are usually given 30 min before meals.

Antacids and sucralfate are also effective agents for the treatment and prevention of PUD.

CHRONIC Rx

Maintenance therapy in duodenal ulcer patients is indicated in the following situations:
- Persistent smokers
- Recurrent ulcerations
- Long-term treatment with NSAIDs, glucocorticoids
- Elderly or debilitated patients
- Aggressive or complicated ulcer disease (e.g., perforation, hemorrhage)
- Asymptomatic bleeders

Misoprostol therapy (100 μg qid with food, increased to 200 μg qid if well tolerated) is useful for the prevention of NSAID-induced gastric ulcers in all patients on long-term NSAID therapy; it is contraindicated in women of childbearing age because of its abortifacient properties. PPIs are also effective at healing ulcers and maintaining remission in patients on long-term NSAIDs.

DISPOSITION

- The recurrence rate for untreated PUD is approximately 60% (>70% in smokers). Treatment decreases the recurrence rate by nearly 30%.
- Patients with recurrent ulcers should be retreated for an additional 8 wk and then placed on maintenance therapy with H_2RAs, PPIs, sucralfate, or antacids.
- An ulcer is considered refractory to treatment if healing is not evident after 8 wk for duodenal ulcers and 12 wk for gastric ulcers. In these patients maximum acid inhibition (e.g., esomeprazole 40 mg bid) is preferred over continued therapy with standard antiulcer therapy.
- Eradication of *H. pylori* (when present) is indicated in all patients. A negative stool antigen test for *H. pylori* 6 wk after treatment accurately confirms cure of *H. pylori* infection with reasonable sensitivity in initially seropositive healthy subjects.
- Screening for ZE syndrome should also be considered in patients with multiple recurrent ulcers; in patients with ZE, the serum gastrin level is >1000 pg/ml and the basal acid output is usually >15 mEq/hr.
- Surgery for refractory ulcers is now only rarely performed; it consists of highly selective vagotomy for duodenal ulcers or ulcer removal with antrectomy or hemigastrectomy without vagotomy for gastric ulcers.

REFERRAL

- GI referral for patients requiring endoscopy
- Surgical referral for patients with nonhealing ulcers despite appropriate medical therapy

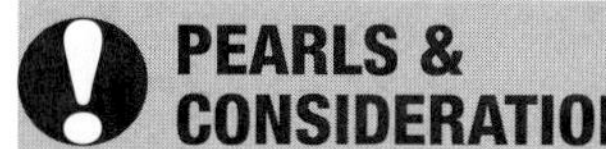

PEARLS & CONSIDERATIONS

COMMENTS

- Patients with gastric ulcers should have repeat endoscopy after 4 to 6 wk of therapy to document healing and test exfoliative cytology for gastric carcinoma.
- After endoscopic treatment of bleeding peptic ulcers, bleeding recurs in up to 20% of patients. PPI administration intravenously by continuous infusion substantially reduces the risk of recurrent bleeding. High dose IV esomeprazole (80 mg IV bolus followed by 8 mg/hr infusion over 72 hr) given after successful endoscopic therapy to patients with high-risk peptic ulcer bleeding has been reported to reduce recurrent bleeding at 72 hr and to maintain sustained clinical benefits for up to 30 days.
- Among low-dose aspirin recipients who had peptic ulcer bleeding, continuous aspirin therapy may increase the risk for recurrent bleeding.

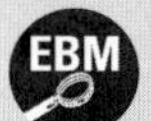

EVIDENCE

Please note: Complete text of EBM for this topic is available online.

Key trials and commentary:

This study sought to compare pantoprazole and somatostatin continuous infusion after endoscopic hemostasis in patients with bleeding peptic ulcers.

This study showed that in patients with a bleeding ulcer, after successful endoscopic hemostasis, despite equipotent acid suppression, pantoprazole continuous infusion was superior to somatostatin to prevent bleeding recurrence and quick disappearance of the endoscopic stigmata. Nevertheless, no differences were seen in the need for surgery, or in mortality.

Despite effective endoscopic therapy, up to 20% of patients with peptic ulcer bleeding have recurrent bleeding. IV continuous infusion of pantoprazole is the current standard of care after endoscopic therapy for peptic ulcer bleeding. However, somatostatin is also effective in this setting, and studies comparing the two modalities in a randomized fashion are lacking. This randomized Greek study including 164 consecutive patients with peptic ulcer bleeding found that pantoprazole was four times more efficacious than somatostatin for the prevention of rebleeding and disappearance of endoscopic stigmata of bleeding at 48 hours despite similar effects on acid suppression, need for surgery, and mortality. Thus there is no evidence for a shift in paradigm from proton pump inhibitor therapy to somatostatin for peptic ulcer bleeding.[1] Ⓐ

A neutral gastric pH is critical for the stability of clots over bleeding arteries. This study investigated the effect of preemptive infusion of omeprazole before endoscopy on the need for endoscopic therapy.

This study showed that infusion of high-dose omeprazole before endoscopy accelerated the resolution of signs of bleeding in ulcers and reduced the need for endoscopic therapy.

The morbidity and mortality of upper GI bleeding from peptic ulcer is based upon its physiological effects (i.e., hypotension, renal failure, etc.) and its endoscopic appearance. The latter ranges from a clean-based ulcer to the presence of a nonbleeding, visible vessel within the ulcer base to a bleeding vessel within the ulcer. Our endoscopic goal is to visualize the source of bleeding and characterize its likelihood of rebleeding, which is almost nil in clear-based ulcers and very high in the bleeding ulcer. Endoscopic therapy of bleeding ulcers reduces their chance of rebleeding. High-dose proton pump inhibitor (PPI) therapy after endoscopic hemostasis has been achieved, which reduces recurrent ulcer bleeding and improves clinical outcome. This effect is likely a result of its beneficial effect on stabilizing clot formation over the bleeding vessel. Lau et al, in a double-blind placebo-controlled, randomized trial, answered the question of whether early initiation of PPI before endoscopy would have a therapeutic effect on bleeding ulcers, reduce the need for endoscopic therapy, and/or improve clinical outcome. Patients received either placebo or 80 mg intravenous injection of omeprazole, followed by infusion of 8 mg per hour until the endoscopic examination. Patients with refractory shock were excluded from the study, and they underwent urgent endoscopy. Patients who were found to have gastroduodenal ulcers with spurting or oozing hemorrhages or who had nonbleeding visible vessels underwent epinephrine injection and coaptive thermocoagulation. Omeprazole was infused for 72 hours after endoscopic therapy and then 40 mg omeprazole was given orally per day for 8 weeks. The patients in the omeprazole group received therapy for 14.7±6.3 hours before the endoscopic procedure. The patients in the omeprazole group required significantly less endoscopic therapy (19.1% vs. 28.4%). Actively bleeding peptic ulcers were seen significantly less frequently in patients given omeprazole before endoscopy than placebo (6.4% vs. 14.7%; $P = 0.01$). The hospital stay was significantly shorter in the omeprazole group. Optimal acid suppression, via PPI infusion, improves clot formation over arteries in bleeding peptic ulcers and reduces the need for endoscopic therapy. In addition, it increases the resolution of signs of bleeding and permits earlier discharge. Therefore, patients awaiting endoscopy should be started on high-dose intravenous omeprazole.[2] Ⓐ

Evidence-Based References

1. Tsibouris P et al: High-dose pantoprazole continuous infusion is superior to somatostatin after endoscopic hemostasis in patients with peptic ulcer bleeding, *Am J Gastroenterol* 102:1192-1199, 2007. Commentary by M.T. Osterman, M.D. Ⓐ
2. Lau JY, Leung WK, Wu JCY: Omeprazole before endoscopy in patients with gastrointestinal bleeding. *N Engl J Med* 356:1631-1640, 2007. Commentary by J.S. Barkin, M.D. Ⓐ

SUGGESTED READINGS

Jafri N et al: Meta-analysis: sequential therapy appears superior to standard therapy for *Helicobacter pylori* infection in patients naive to treatment, *Ann Intern Med* 148:923-931, 2008.

Sung J et al: Intravenous esomeprazole for prevention of recurrent peptic ulcer bleeding, *Ann Intern Med* 150:455, 2009.

Sung J et al: Continuation of low-dose aspirin therapy in peptic ulcer bleeding, *Ann Intern Med* 152:1-9, 2010.

AUTHOR: **FRED F. FERRI, M.D.**

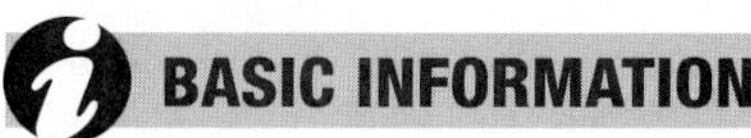

BASIC INFORMATION

DEFINITION

Pericarditis is the inflammation (or infiltration) of the pericardium associated with a wide variety of causes (see “Etiology”).

ICD-9CM CODES
420.91 Pericarditis

EPIDEMIOLOGY & DEMOGRAPHICS

- The incidence of acute pericarditis is 2% to 6%.
- Increased incidence found in male and in adults compared with children.
- The use of thrombolytic agents and early revascularization have greatly reduced the incidence of both early postinfarction pericarditis and Dressler’s syndrome.

PHYSICAL FINDINGS & CLINICAL PRESENTATION

- Severe, constant pain that localizes over the anterior chest and may radiate to arms and back; it can be differentiated from myocardial ischemia because the pain intensifies with inspiration and is relieved by sitting up and leaning forward (the pain of myocardial ischemia is not pleuritic).
- Pericardial friction rub is best heard with the patient upright and leaning forward and by pressing the stethoscope firmly against the chest. It is often confused with the pleural rub. The pericardial friction rub corresponds temporally to movement of the heart within the pericardial sac. Typically the rub is a high-pitched scratchy or squeaky sound heard best at the left sternal border at end expiration. It consists classically of three short, scratchy sounds:
  1. Systolic component
  2. Diastolic component
  3. Late diastolic component (associated with atrial contraction)

  However, in reality, the rub is reported to be triphasic in approximately half of patients, biphasic in a third, and monophasic in the remainder.
- Cardiac tamponade may occur as a complication if the following are observed:
  1. Tachycardia
  2. Low blood pressure and pulse pressure
  3. Distended neck veins
  4. Paradoxic pulse (pulsus paradoxus)

ETIOLOGY

- Most common cause (>40%) of pericarditis is idiopathic
- Infectious (viral, bacterial [1% to 2%], tuberculous [4%], fungal, amebic, toxoplasmosis)
- Collagen-vascular disease (systemic lupus erythematosus, rheumatoid arthritis, scleroderma, vasculitis, dermatomyositis): 3% to 5% of cases
- Drug-induced lupus syndrome (procainamide, hydralazine, phenytoin, isoniazid, rifampin, doxorubicin, mesalamine)
- Acute myocardial infarction (MI) (transmural MI)
- Trauma or posttraumatic
- After MI (Dressler’s syndrome)
- After pericardiotomy
- After mediastinal radiation (e.g., patients with Hodgkin’s disease)
- Uremia
- Sarcoidosis
- Neoplasm (primary or metastatic [breast, lung, leukemia, lymphoma]): 7% of cases
- Leakage of aortic aneurysm into pericardial sac
- Familial Mediterranean fever
- Rheumatic fever
- Other: anticoagulants, amyloidosis, idiopathic thrombocytopenia purpura

Dx DIAGNOSIS

DIFFERENTIAL DIAGNOSIS

- Angina pectoris
- Pulmonary infarction
- Dissecting aneurysm
- Gastrointestinal abnormalities (e.g., hiatal hernia, esophageal rupture)
- Pneumothorax
- Hepatitis
- Cholecystitis
- Pneumonia with pleurisy

WORKUP

Diagnosis is clinical, based on history and physical examination. ECG may help confirm the diagnosis if typical changes are found. Laboratory tests may help on elucidating the potential cause, and an ECG may assist in ruling out significant pericardial effusion.

LABORATORY TESTS

Laboratory tests are generally not clinically helpful, and the clinical presentation should guide any ordering. Initial blood work should be limited to the following tests:

- Complete blood count with differential
- Erythrocyte sedimentation rate (not specific but may be of value in following the course of the disease and the response to therapy)
- Blood urea nitrogen, creatinine, alanine aminotransferase
- Troponin I (plasma troponins are elevated in 35% to 50% of patients with pericarditis, which would indicate myopericarditis)

The following tests may be useful in the absence of an obvious cause:

- Viral titers (acute and convalescent)
- Antinuclear antibody, rheumatoid factor
- Purified protein derivative (PPD), antistreptolysin O titers
- Blood cultures
- Pericardiocentesis is indicated in patients with pericardial tamponade and in those with known or suspected purulent or neoplastic pericarditis. The fluid should be analyzed for red and white blood cell counts, cytology, glucose, lactate dehydrogenase, protein, pH, triglyceride level, and cultured. Polymerase chain reaction assays or elevated levels of adenosine deaminase activity (>30 U/L) are useful when suspecting tuberculous pericarditis.
- Pericardial biopsy may be helpful in recurrent tamponade.

IMAGING STUDIES

- ECG to detect and determine amount of pericardial effusion; absence of effusion does not rule out the diagnosis of pericarditis. Variation in atrioventricular valve inflow with respiration is present in cardiac tamponade and constrictive pericarditis.
- ECG: varies with the evolutionary stage of pericarditis:
  1. Acute phase: PR-segment depression and diffuse ST-segment elevations (particularly evident in the precordial leads), which can be distinguished from acute MI by:
     a. Absence of reciprocal ST-segment depression in oppositely oriented leads. Elevated ST segments concave upward
     c. Absence of Q waves
     d. Reciprocal PR elevation may be seen in aVR and V1
  2. Intermediate phase: return of PR and ST segments to baseline, and T-wave inversion in leads previously showing ST-segment elevation (Fig. 1-242)
  3. Late phase: resolution of the T-wave changes
- Chest radiograph: done primarily to rule out abnormalities of the mediastinum or lung fields that may be responsible for the pericarditis
  1. Cardiac silhouette appears enlarged if more than 250 ml of fluid has accumulated.
  2. Calcifications around the heart may be seen with constrictive pericarditis.

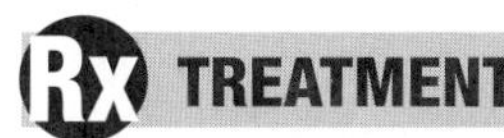

TREATMENT

NONPHARMACOLOGIC THERAPY

- Limitation of activity until the pain abates
- Patient education regarding potential complications (e.g., cardiac tamponade, constrictive pericarditis)

ACUTE GENERAL Rx

- NSAID therapy (e.g., ibuprofen 800 mg tid, naproxen 500 mg bid). Aspirin is preferred in patients with recent MI.
- Colchicine 0.6 mg bid may be used in combination or as an alternative to NSAIDs. Long-term colchicine can also be used for recurrent pericarditis.
- Use of corticosteroids is controversial. Prednisone up to 1.5 mg/kg of body weight daily for up to 4 wk may be added in patients with severe symptoms of acute pericarditis and suspected connective tissue disease. Steroids have also been studied in recurrent pericarditis. They are associated with increased recurrence, side effects, and hospitalizations. One study found that using a lower dose (0.2 to 0.5mg/kg per day) main-

 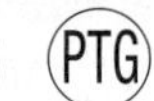

tained for 4 weeks, and then a slow taper had few adverse effects.

- Close observation of patients when there is suspicion for cardiac tamponade.
- Avoidance of anticoagulants (increased risk of hemopericardium).

TREATMENT OF UNDERLYING CAUSE:

- Bacterial pericarditis: systemic antibiotics and surgical drainage of pericardium
- Collagen vascular disease and idiopathic: NSAIDs, prednisone
- Uremic: dialysis

POTENTIAL COMPLICATIONS FROM PERICARDITIS:

1. *Pericardial effusion*: the time required for pericardial effusion to develop is of critical importance. If the rate of accumulation is slow, the pericardium can gradually stretch and accommodate a large effusion (>1000 ml), whereas rapid accumulation can cause tamponade with as little as 200 ml of fluid.
2. Chronic constrictive pericarditis:
   a. Physical examination reveals jugular venous distention, Kussmaul's sign (increase in jugular venous distention during inspiration as a result of increased venous pressure), pericardial knock (early diastolic filling sound heard 0.06 to 0.1 sec after S2), clear lungs, tender hepatomegaly, pedal edema, ascites, scrotal edema, and possible anasarca.
   b. Chest radiograph: clear lung fields, normal or slightly enlarged heart, pericardial calcification.
   c. ECG: low-voltage QRS complex.
   d. Echocardiography: may show respiratory inflow variation over the mitral and tricuspid valves (due to variations in the diastolic ventricular pressure gradients with respiration), pericardial thickening or may be normal.
   e. Cardiac catheterization to confirm elevation of right-sided filling pressures: shows a prominent y descent in the right atrial tracing, a "dip and plateau" tracing of the right ventricular pressure and discordance of right ventricular and left ventricular systolic pressures during respiration.
   f. Therapy: surgical stripping or removal of both layers of the constricting pericardium.
3. *Cardiac tamponade*: occurs in 15% of patients with idiopathic pericarditis but in nearly 60% of those with neoplastic, tuberculous, or purulent pericarditis.
   a. Signs and symptoms: dyspnea, orthopnea, interscapular pain.
   b. Physical examination: distended neck veins, distant heart sounds, decreased apical impulse, diaphoresis, tachypnea, tachycardia, *Ewart's sign* (an area of dullness at the angle of the left scapula caused by compression of the lungs by the pericardial effusion), pulsus paradoxus (decrease in systolic blood pressure >10 mm Hg during inspiration), hypotension, narrowed pulse pressure. Of all the clinical signs, a pulsus paradoxus >10 mm Hg in patients with pericardial effusion is the most specific for tamponade.
   c. Chest radiograph: cardiomegaly ("water-bottle" configuration of the cardiac silhouette may be seen) with clear lungs; the chest x-ray film may be normal when acute tamponade occurs rapidly in the absence of prior pericardial effusion.
   d. ECG reveals decreased amplitude of the QRS complex, variation of the R-wave amplitude from beat to beat (electrical alternans). This results from the heart's oscillating motion in the pericardial sac from beat to beat and frequently occurs with neoplastic effusions.
   e. Echocardiography: may show diastolic collapse of the right ventricle and/or the right atrium, respiratory inflow variation over the mitral valve and tricuspid valve (due to transmission of respiratory changes in intrathoracic pressure to the ventricles), and a paradoxic wall motion may also be seen.
   f. Cardiac catheterization: equalization of pressures within chambers of the heart, elevation of right atrial pressure with a prominent x but no significant y descent.
   g. MRI can also be used to diagnose pericardial effusions.
   h. Therapy for pericardial tamponade consists of immediate pericardiocentesis, preferably by needle paracentesis with the use of echocardiography, fluoroscopy, or CT; in patients with recurrent effusions (e.g., neoplasms), placement of a percutaneous drainage catheter or pericardial window draining in the pleural cavity may be necessary.
4. Effusive-constrictive pericarditis:
   a. Uncommon pericardial syndrome characterized by concomitant tamponade caused by tense pericardial effusion and constriction caused by the visceral pericardium.
   b. Extensive epicardiectomy is the procedure of choice in symptomatic patients.

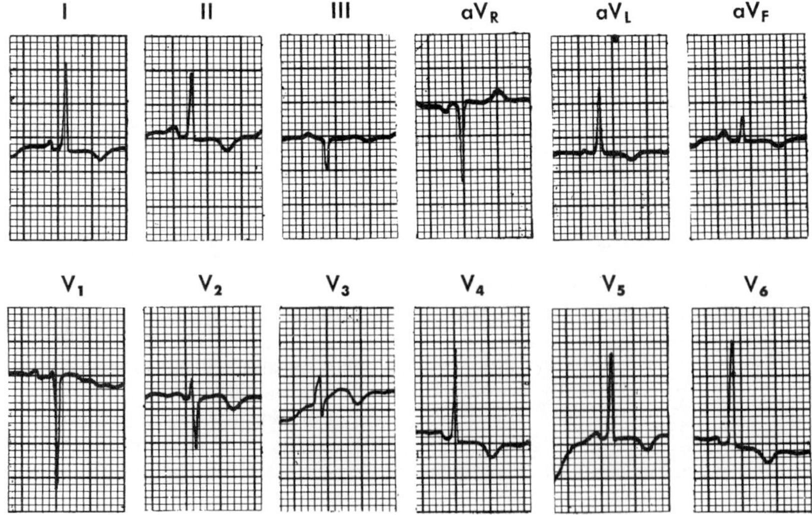

FIGURE 1-242 Note the diffuse T-wave inversions in leads I, II, III, aVL, aVF, and V2 to V6. (From Goldberg AL [ed]: *Clinical electrocardiography,* ed 5, St Louis, 1994, Mosby.)

DISPOSITION

- Complete resolution of pain and other signs and symptoms during the initial 3 wk of therapy.
- Recurrence in 10% to 15% of patients within the initial 12 mo.
- Recurrent pericarditis in 28% of patients.
- Recurrence of large effusion after pericardiocentesis is common in patients with idiopathic chronic pericardial effusion. Pericardiectomy should be considered in these patients.
- Most cases of pericarditis can be treated in the outpatient setting. Indications for hospitalization are fever >38° C, immunosuppressed state, history of trauma, subacute onset, oral anticoagulant therapy, presence of myocarditis, large pericardial effusion, or tamponade.
- In patients with pericardial effusion after cardiac surgery, use of NSAIDs is not recommended because they have not been shown to reduce the size of the effusions or prevent late cardiac tamponade.

SUGGESTED READING

Mevrin P et al: NSAID treatment for postoperative pericardial effusion, *Ann Intern Med* 152:137-143, 2010.

AUTHORS: **SCOTT COHEN, M.D., FRED F. FERRI, M.D.,** and **WEN-CHIH WU, M.D.**

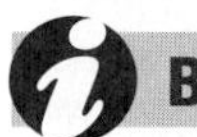

BASIC INFORMATION

DEFINITION

Peripheral arterial disease (PAD) refers to stenotic, occlusive, and aneurysmal diseases of the aorta and its branch arteries, exclusive of the cerebral and coronary arteries. This chapter deals specifically with the arteries of the lower extremities.

SYNONYMS

Peripheral vascular disease (PVD)
Arteriosclerosis obliterans
Atherosclerotic occlusive disease
Atherosclerosis of the extremities
Peripheral arterial stenosis
Vaso-occlusive disease of the legs
Chronic critical limb ischemia

ICD-9CM CODES
443.9 Peripheral vascular disease

EPIDEMIOLOGY & DEMOGRAPHICS

- The prevalence of PAD increases with age. Based on ABI (ankle-brachial index) recordings, the general population prevalence of PAD for individuals ages 40 to 59 yr is 2.5%, ages 60 to 69 yr is 8.3%, and ages 70 to 79 yr is 18.8%.
- Studies have shown a prevalence of up to 29% in patients aged 50 to 69 yr with a history of diabetes and smoking.
- Cigarette smoking and diabetes mellitus are the strongest risk factors.
- More than 80% of patients with PAD are current or former smokers.
- PAD affects men and women equally.
- African Americans and Hispanics with diabetes have a higher prevalence of PAD than whites.
- Cardiovascular disease is the major cause of death in patients with intermittent claudication.
- Patients with newly diagnosed PAD are 6 times more likely to die within the next 10 years when compared with patients without PAD.
- Risk factors associated with PAD are similar to coronary artery disease, including tobacco use, diabetes, hyperlipidemia, hypertension, and advanced age.
- An inverse relationship has been suggested between PAD and alcohol consumption.
- In 2006, the American College of Cardiology/American Heart Association (ACC/AHA) suggested that the following individuals would be at risk from lower-extremity PAD:
  - Age <50 yr, with diabetes and one other atherosclerosis risk factor (smoking, dyslipidemia, hypertension, or hyperhomocysteinemia)
  - Ages 50 to 69 yr and history of smoking or diabetes
  - Age 70 yr or older
  - Symptoms with exertion involving the lower extremities (suggestive of claudication) or ischemic rest pain
  - Abnormal lower extremity pulse examination
  - Known atherosclerotic coronary, carotid, or renal artery disease

PHYSICAL FINDINGS & CLINICAL PRESENTATION

Nearly 50% of patients with PAD are asymptomatic, making PAD an underdiagnosed and undertreated condition. Approximately one-third of patients with PAD present with intermittent claudication described as an aching or cramping leg pain brought on by exertion and relieved with rest, and it can progress with time. However, relying on the classic history of claudication alone will miss the majority of patients with PAD.

Individuals who present with symptoms associated with PAD often present with one or more of the following complaints or findings:

- Painful cramping in buttocks, hip, or leg that occurs while walking but goes away while resting
- Diminished pedal pulses
- Bruits heard over the distal aorta, iliac, or femoral arteries
- Changes in skin color, especially on feet (rubor with prolonged capillary refill on dependency or delayed pallor)
- Cool skin temperature
- Trophic changes of hair loss, brittle nails, and muscle atrophy
- Nonhealing ulcers (Fig. 1-243), necrotic tissue, and gangrene
- Weakness, numbness, or a feeling of heaviness in legs
- Aching or burning in toes and feet during rest and especially while lying flat, which may be a sign of ischemia and more serious PAD

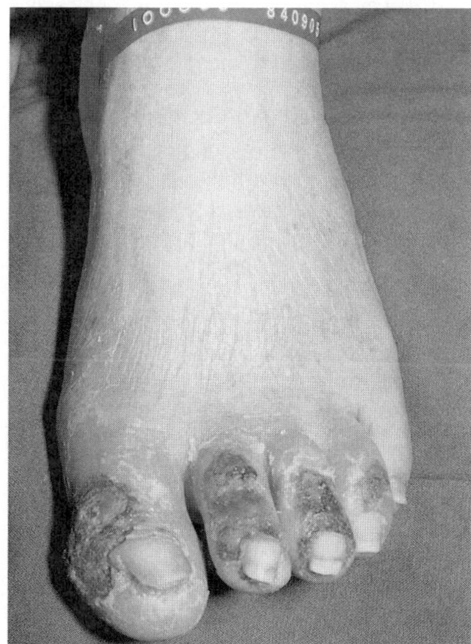

FIGURE 1-243 Ischemic skin ulcer induced by trauma from shoes. This patient with peripheral arterial occlusive disease suffered severe superficial skin necrosis of several toes because of shoes that were too tight. (From Crawford MH et al [eds]: *Cardiology,* ed 2, St Louis, 2004, Mosby.)

ETIOLOGY

The primary cause of PAD is atherosclerosis: atherosclerotic lesions lead to varying percentages of luminal stenosis of peripheral vessels and inability to supply oxygenated blood to meet the demand of limb muscles.

Dx DIAGNOSIS

DIFFERENTIAL DIAGNOSIS

- Spinal stenosis
- Musculoskeletal disorder
- Lumbar spinal stenosis or nerve root compression (neurogenic or pseudoclaudication)
- Peripheral neuropathy
- Reflex sympathetic dystrophy
- Raynaud's disease
- Compartment syndrome

WORKUP

A thorough history and physical examination are critical for evaluating and diagnosing the etiology of lower-extremity pain. Since the differential of lower-extremity pain is relatively broad, careful questioning of symptom onset, duration, and intensity is critical to obtaining an accurate diagnosis. Physical examination for identification of PAD should include assessment of all the major arterial trees in each extremity:

- Measurement of blood pressure in both arms and notation of asymmetry.
- Palpation and recording of carotid pulses, upstroke, amplitude, and presence of bruits.
- Auscultation and palpation of abdomen for bruits, aortic pulsation, and diameter.
- Palpation of brachial, radial, ulnar, femoral, popliteal, dorsalis pedis, and posterior tibial pulses. Pulse intensity should be recorded as follows: 0, absent; 1, diminished; 2, normal; 3, bounding.
- Auscultation of femoral arteries for the presence of bruits.
- Feet should be inspected for color, temperature, and integrity of the skin.
- Findings suggestive of severe PAD—hair loss, trophic skin changes, and hypertrophic nails—should be sought and recorded.
- Measurement of resting ankle-brachial index (ABI) to establish the diagnosis of PAD is appropriate in people aged 70 yr or older presenting with symptoms of exertional leg pain or nonhealing wounds; or in people 50 yr or older with a history of diabetes mellitus or smoking. Once the presence of PAD is identified by an abnormal ABI, exercise treadmill testing is recommended. Comparison of resting and exercise ABI measurements can be helpful for objectively characterizing the severity of the individual's claudication symptoms.
- ABI also subjectively measures the severity of functional limitations related to the claudication. Postexercise ABI measurements can be especially useful in individuals with symptoms of intermittent claudication who have a normal resting ABI.
- Individuals with asymptomatic lower extremity PAD should be identified by examination

and/or measurement of the ABI so that therapeutic interventions known to diminish their risk of cardiovascular disease, myocardial infarction, or stroke may be initiated.

- The ABI is calculated by dividing the highest ankle systolic pressure using either the dorsalis pedis or posterior tibial artery by the highest systolic pressure from either arm.
- A diagnosis of PAD is based on the presence of limb symptoms or a low ABI.
- The lower the ABI the worse the prognosis.
- The severity of PAD is based on the ABI at rest and during treadmill exercise (1 to 2 mph, 5 min, or symptom limited). It is classified as follows:
  - Mild: ABI at rest 0.71 to 0.90 or ABI during exercise 0.50 to 0.90
  - Moderate: ABI at rest 0.41 to 0.70 or ABI during exercise 0.20 to 0.50
  - Severe: ABI at rest <0.40 or ABI during exercise <0.20
- An ABI >1.30 is an indication of vessel calcification. If the ABI is >1, then obtain a toe brachial index since there is no medial calcification of the digital vessels. If the toe brachial index is <0.7, then this is an indication of PAD.

LABORATORY TESTS

Currently there is no laboratory test that can diagnose PAD; however, measurement of lipid profile, hemoglobin A1C, homocysteine levels, fibrinogen, D-dimer, and CRP can be useful in the initiation of treatment for systemic atherosclerotic disease.

IMAGING STUDIES

- The diagnosis of PAD can be confirmed by measuring the ABI or toe-brachial index (determined according to the return of pulsatile flow on deflation of a small blood pressure cuff on the great or second toe with a plethysmographic device).
- Rest or exercise pulse volume recordings (PVRs) and segmental limb pressures are also useful. PVRs measure volume of limb flow per pulse in different segments of the limb (e.g., thigh, calf, ankle, metatarsal, and toes). They help to assess the location and severity of the lesion.
- Duplex ultrasound can be used to diagnose PAD and assess occlusion severity and location. It is also an appropriate modality for surveillance evaluation after femoral popliteal or femoral tibial or pedal surgical bypass with a venous graft.
- Magnetic resonance angiography (MRA) can be used as a noninvasive approach to visualize the aorta and peripheral lower-extremity arteries.
- Contrast CT is an accurate modality to assess presence and severity of PAD in patients with intermittent claudication.
- Angiography remains the gold standard for visualizing the arterial anatomy before revascularization.

Rx TREATMENT

NONPHARMACOLOGIC THERAPY

The mainstays of treatment for PAD include risk factor modification, exercise, antiplatelet therapy, additional pharmacologic therapy (if symptoms warrant), and revascularization (endovascular or surgical).

Aggressive management of risk factors for PAD includes:

- Smoking-cessation programs, diet counseling, and weight-loss programs.
- Smoking goal: complete cessation and no exposure to environmental tobacco smoke.
- Physical activity: 30 to 60 min/day at about 2 miles/hr to near maximal pain every day for 6 months, and resistance training, is encouraged in patients with PAD. Studies have shown that a rigorous exercise-training program may be as beneficial as lower-extremity bypass surgery in symptomatic improvement. Supervised treadmill training and resistance training improve functional performance measured by treadmill walking and quality of life.
- Weight management: goal body mass index, 18.5 to 24.9 kg/m^2. Waist circumference: men <40 inches, women <35 inches.
- Management of hypertension with goal <140/90 or <130/80 if the patient has diabetes or chronic renal disease.
- Tight glycemic control (A1C <7%) in diabetic patients with PAD results in prevention of microvascular complications.
- Control of dyslipidemia with goal for LDL cholesterol of <100 mg/dl or <70 in very high-risk patients. Alternatively, reduction of LDL-cholesterol levels by 50% in patients with high-baseline LDL cholesterol if levels <70 could not be achieved. If triglycerides are >200 mg/dl, non-HDL cholesterol should be lowered to <130 mg/dl.

ACUTE GENERAL Rx

Most individuals will respond fairly well to risk factor modification and exercise. If symptoms become severe, endovascular or surgical therapy is performed for symptom relief.

CHRONIC Rx

- Aspirin 75 to 325 mg daily is recommended for secondary prevention.
- The thienopyridines (ticlopidine and clopidogrel) may be considered as alternatives to aspirin, particularly in patients who cannot tolerate aspirin.
- Pentoxyphylline (Trental, Pentoxil) 400 mg tid provides a small benefit in walking distance when compared with placebo.
- Cilostazol (Pletal) 100 mg bid has been shown to increase maximal walking distance by 40% to 60% in symptomatic patients with infrainguinal PAD after 12 to 24 wk of therapy. It also improves patient quality of life. It should not be given to patients with congestive heart failure and an ejection fraction <40%. Cilostazol may be used in patients with aspirin and/or clopidogrel.

The American College of Cardiology/American Heart Association have suggested the following guidelines for revascularization therapy:

- A revascularization procedure is indicated in less than 10% of people with PAD.
- Revascularization (surgery or percutaneous transluminal angioplasty) is indicated for relief in patients with claudication that limits their lifestyle and is refractory to exercise and pharmacologic therapy, or if there is a very favorable risk-benefit ratio (e.g., focal aortoiliac occlusive disease).
- Endovascular intervention is recommended for TransAtlantic Inter-Society Consensus type A iliac and femoro-popliteal arterial lesions.
- Endovascular therapy is preferred in patients aged 50 yr or younger, because they have a higher risk of graft failure after surgical therapy than older patients.
- Endovascular intervention is not indicated as prophylactic therapy in an asymptomatic patient with lower-extremity PAD, or if there is no significant pressure gradient across a stenosis even after augmentation of flow with vasodilators.
- Primary stent placement is not recommended in the femoral, popliteal, or tibial arteries.
- Surgical intervention is not indicated to prevent progression to limb-threatening ischemia in patients with intermittent claudication.
- Surgical interventions are indicated for individuals with claudication symptoms who have lifestyle-limiting disability, who are unresponsive to exercise or pharmacotherapy, and who have a reasonable chance of symptomatic improvement. Prior to any surgical therapy, patients should have a preoperative cardiovascular risk evaluation.

DISPOSITION

Risk factors for atherosclerosis should be assessed, and appropriate modification instituted. Focus should be placed on smoking cessation, dietary adjustment, and pharmacotherapy for dyslipidemia, hyperglycemia, and hypertension. All patients with PAD should receive aspirin therapy (75 to 325 mg/day) unless contraindicated. Revascularization is performed if the symptoms of PAD do not improve with conservative therapy.

REFERRAL

Consultation with vascular medicine, vascular surgery, or other physicians with expertise in PAD is recommended in patients with rest pain, functional disability from pain, ABI <0.50 at rest, or any physical signs of limb ischemia or gangrene.

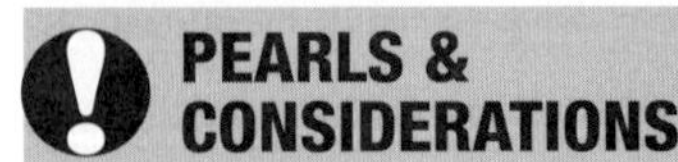

PEARLS & CONSIDERATIONS

COMMENTS

- Although the prevalence of PAD in Europe and North America is estimated at approximately 27 million people, PAD remains underdiagnosed and undertreated.

- Studies of the natural history of claudication show the relative safety of initial conservative treatment of PAD in the absence of critical limb ischemia.
- When PAD limits a patient's ability to walk and exercise, percutaneous revascularization can be considered. Data reveal excellent outcomes with angioplasty and stenting in selected patients. Outcomes will likely be better as peripheral interventional technology and skills improve.
- In patients with peripheral arterial disease, the combination of an oral anticoagulant and antiplatelet therapy was not more effective than antiplatelet therapy alone in preventing major cardiovascular complications and was associated with an increase in life-threatening bleeding.
- Increasing levels of D-dimer and inflammatory biomarkers (CRP) are independently associated with higher mortality in persons with PAD.

PREVENTION

Cardiovascular disease is the major cause of death in patients with intermittent claudication. Therefore, the treatment of claudication is directed not only at improving walking distance but also at reducing cardiovascular risk.

PATIENT & FAMILY EDUCATION

The following organizations offer more information about PAD:

- American College of Cardiology (http://www.acc.org)
- Vascular Disease Foundation (http://www.vdf.org)

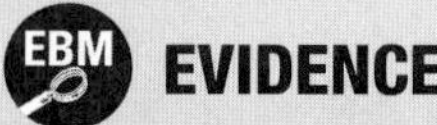

EVIDENCE

Please note: Complete text of EBM for this topic is available online.

Key trials and commentary:

The purpose of this study was to determine the possible benefit of dual antiplatelet therapy in patients with prior myocardial infarction (MI), ischemic stroke, or symptomatic peripheral arterial disease (PAD).

In this analysis of the CHARISMA trial, the large number of patients with documented prior MI, ischemic stroke, or symptomatic PAD appeared to derive significant benefit from dual antiplatelet therapy with clopidogrel plus aspirin. Such patients may benefit from intensification of antithrombotic therapy beyond aspirin alone, a concept that future trials will need to validate. (Clopidogrel for High Atherothrombotic Risk and Ischemic Stabilization, Management, and Avoidance [CHARISMA]; http://clinicaltrials.gov/ct/show/NCT00050817?order51;NCT00050817).

This new analysis of the data from CHARISMA deserves to be read and interpreted with caution. CHARISMA was a trial comparing dual antiplatelet therapy (aspirin plus clopidogrel) with aspirin alone in patients with established atherothrombotic disease (ie, previous coronary events, TIA/strokes, or symptomatic peripheral vascular disease) or multiple vascular risk factors for the prevention of ischemic events. The results did not demonstrate superiority of dual therapy over aspirin for the primary endpoint (cardiovascular death, myocardial infarction, or stroke). This post hoc analysis only included patients enrolled with prior documented myocardial infarction, ischemic stroke, or symptomatic peripheral vascular disease, thus transforming the original trial that assessed primary and secondary prevention into a study exclusively evaluating the value of the dual therapy for secondary prevention. These criteria used to select the population to be considered for this analysis were essentially the same that were used for the CAPRIE trial, which compared clopidogrel with aspirin for secondary prevention of atherothrombotic events. Slightly over a third of the patients included had a previous ischemic stroke.

Although the results of this analysis showed a benefit for the dual therapy in the primary endpoint, some caveats should be kept in mind. The combination of clopidogrel and aspirin for the specific indication of secondary stroke prevention was not superior to clopidogrel alone in the MATCH trial, which additionally found that the risk of hemorrhage was increased in patients receiving both antiplatelet agents. In this post hoc analysis of CHARISMA, the rate of ischemic stroke was not significantly decreased in patients taking clopidogrel plus aspirin and the risk of moderate, albeit not severe or fatal, bleeding was increased in these patients. The rate of hemorrhage in patients enrolled with previous stroke was not reported.

Based on current evidence, the combination of clopidogrel and aspirin cannot be recommended for the indication of secondary stroke prevention. Combining these 2 antiplatelet agents is reasonable in patients with documented vascular disease in multiple locations (the group that benefited most significantly in this analysis), but the risk of hemorrhage should be factored in the decision. Dual antiplatelet therapy might also be beneficial in the acute phase after a TIA or minor stroke, but the effectiveness and safety in these situations still needs to be confirmed.[1] Ⓐ

Atherosclerotic PAD is associated with an increased risk of myocardial infarction, stroke, and death from cardiovascular causes. Antiplatelet drugs reduce this risk, but the role of oral anticoagulant agents in the prevention of cardiovascular complications in patients with PAD is unclear.

This study showed that in patients with PAD, the combination of an oral anticoagulant and antiplatelet therapy was not more effective than antiplatelet therapy alone in preventing major cardiovascular complications and was associated with an increase in life-threatening bleeding.

The results of this multicenter trial of 2161 patients are a mixture of good and bad news. The bad news is that the combined regimen of warfarin and an antiplatelet agent did not result in improved cardiovascular complications and was associated with an increase in life-threatening bleeding. The good news is that a simple regimen of antiplatelet therapy alone was equally effective. The results do, however, come as somewhat of a disappointment. Patients with PAD have a risk of myocardial infarction and death that is three times as high as that in patients without peripheral vascular disease. Moreover, several studies have shown that oral anticoagulants do reduce the incidence of major cardiovascular events in patients with coronary artery disease, and current American College of Cardiology (ACC)/American Heart Association (AHA) guidelines consider oral anticoagulation in combination with aspirin to be an appropriate alternative to aspirin alone in patients with ST-elevation acute myocardial infarction.

Nonetheless, there is a paucity of data on the safety and efficacy of combined therapy, particularly in patients with PAD, and this trial fills in some of the pieces and is consistent with the only other large randomized trial comparing these therapies in patients with PAD. It appears that patients with PAD who are older and have extensive systemic atherosclerosis and probably cerebral vascular disease are at a higher risk of bleeding complications with oral anticoagulants.

It is interesting that the relative risk of myocardial infarction, stroke, or death was increased among patients in this trial from China. Although this may be a chance finding, as often occurs with multiple post hoc analyses, prior studies have questioned whether the target international normalized ratio should be lower for Chinese patients. Moreover, a recent study in patients with atrial fibrillation treated with warfarin demonstrated that the risk of intracranial hemorrhage was highest in Asians, and blacks and Hispanics still had a higher rate than whites. Whether this reflects a greater sensitivity for warfarin, which may have a genetic basis, or a function of greater baseline risk of intracranial hemorrhage regardless of warfarin therapy (and if so, is this a result of underlying intracranial pathology or vascular disease), remains to be clarified.

This trial generates many interesting questions that require answers, but the routine management of patients with PAD with a simple regimen of antiplatelet therapy alone will suffice. In addition, if patients with PAD require warfarin anticoagulation for other reasons, for example, atrial fibrillation, one needs to be very much aware of what appears to be an increased risk of serious bleeding.[2] Ⓐ

This study sought to compare the safety and effectiveness of the Viabahn endoprosthesis with that of percutaneous transluminal angioplasty (PTA) alone in the treatment of symptomatic PAD affecting the superficial femoral artery (SFA).

In this multicenter study, the patency, technical success, and clinical status results obtained with stent-grafts were superior to those obtained with PTA alone.

PTA has been used as the endovascular "standard therapy" to treat femoropopliteal artery (FPA) lesions in patients with chronic limb ischemia, although results have been variable and somewhat disappointing, with 1-year restenosis rates that have ranged from 25% to 80%. The results of endovascular treatment, supplementing PTA with implantation of metallic stents, have also been variable. Metallic stents covered with polyester or expanded polytetrafluoroethylene (ePTFE) were developed with the aim of improving long-term patency and reducing complications, but initial results with early stent-grafts in the SFA were poor with respect to both patency and complications, especially for devices covered with polyester. However, several subsequent nonrandomized studies showed that substantially better results could be achieved in the SFA or FPA with self-expanding nitinol stents covered with ePTFE (Viabahn [formerly Hemobahn]; W.L. Gore, Flagstaff, Arizona). 1-year primary patency rates in these investigations ranged from 58% to 93%.

Although this study addresses the very relevant issue of PTA vs. stent-graft placement, SFA treatment algorithms have changed substantially today, almost 10 years after initiation of this trial. Surgical bypass, nitinol stents and stent-grafts (with varying mechanical characteristics), and PTA are now augmented with subintimal angioplasty, cutting balloon angioplasty, directional atherectomy, laser atherectomy, and cryoplasty. Drug-eluting and biodegradable stents for the SFA are also under development. As the authors note, most of these treatment modalities may have a place in SFA treatment; the question is what place do they have and how do they compare? Although the results of this study showed that SFA stent-graft placement with the Viabahn endoprosthesis was safe and provided significantly better results than PTA alone, further randomized clinical trials comparing stent-grafts and new bioactive stent-grafts with other newer endovascular techniques or with bypass surgery are warranted.[3] Ⓐ

This study sought to determine whether supervised treadmill exercise or lower extremity resistance training improve functional performance of patients with PAD with or without claudication.

This study showed that supervised treadmill training improved 6-minute walk performance, treadmill walking performance, brachial artery flow-mediated dilation, and quality of life but did not improve the short physical performance battery scores of PAD participants with and without intermittent claudication. Lower extremity resistance training improved functional performance measured by treadmill walking, quality of life, and stair climbing ability.

It is known that treadmill exercise training under supervised conditions improves walking performance in patients with PAD and intermittent claudication. The effect of treadmill training on patients with PAD who do not have symptoms of claudication is unknown. Also, it is unknown whether lower extremity resistance (strength) training in patients with PAD provides additional benefits. It is known that adults with PAD have smaller calf muscle area and diminished strength of their legs than those patients without PAD, and that these muscle characteristics are associated with greater functional impairment. This randomized trial was designed to address two questions. The first was to determine whether supervised exercise training on a treadmill improved functional performance in patients with PAD with and without classic symptoms of claudication. The second objective was to determine whether lower extremity strength training improved functional performance in patients with PAD with and without symptoms of claudication.

The study indicated that patients with PAD without symptoms of claudication should be treated with supervised treadmill exercise to improve function and, as suggested by improvements in brachial artery flow-mediated dilatation, improve underlying endothelial dysfunction that may contribute to atherosclerosis. Supervised treadmill exercise produces greater increases in 6-minute walk performance than resistance training. Resistance training, however, also produced potentially clinical improvements on quality of life measures and stair climbing ability. In effect, it is becoming increasingly clear that patients with PAD, whether or not they are symptomatic, should be treated essentially as low-level, deconditioned athletes. Benefits can be measured from both resistance and nonresistance training that may, over time, reduce the accelerated functional decline associated with PAD.[4] Ⓐ

Evidence-Based References

1. Bhatt DL: Patients with prior myocardial infarction, stroke, or symptomatic peripheral arterial disease in the CHARISMA trial, *J Am Coll Cardiol* 49:1982-1988, 2007. Commentary by A.A. Rabinstein, M.D. Ⓐ

2. Anand S, the Warfarin Antiplatelet Vascular Evaluation Trial Investigators: Oral anticoagulant and antiplatelet therapy and peripheral arterial disease, *N Engl J Med* 357:217-227, 2007. Commentary by B.J. Gersh, M.B., Ch.B., D.Phil., F.R.C.P. Ⓐ

3. Saxon RR et al: Randomized, multicenter study comparing expanded polytetrafluoroethylene-covered endoprosthesis placement with percutaneous transluminal angioplasty in the treatment of superficial femoral artery occlusive disease, *J Vasc Interv Radiol* 19:823-832, 2008. Commentary by T.G. Walker, M.D. Ⓐ

4. McDermott MM et al: Treadmill exercise and resistance training in patients with peripheral arterial disease with and without intermittent claudication: a randomized controlled trial, *JAMA* 301:165-174, 2009. Commentary by G.L. Moneta, M.D. Ⓐ

SUGGESTED READINGS

ACC/AHA Guidelines for Secondary Prevention for Patients with Coronary and Other Atherosclerotic Vascular Disease: 2006 update: endorsed by the National Heart, Lung, and Blood Institute, *Circulation* 113:2363-2372, 2006.

Hankey G et al: Medical treatment of peripheral arterial disease, *JAMA* 295:547, 2006.

Hirsch AT et al: ACC/AHA Guidelines for the management of patients with peripheral arterial disease (lower extremity, renal, mesenteric, and abdominal aortic): a collaborative report from the American Association for Vascular Surgery/Society for Vascular Surgery, Society for Cardiovascular Angiography and Interventions, Society of Interventional Radiology, Society for Vascular Medicine and Biology, and the American College of Cardiology/American Heart Association Task Force on Practice Guidelines (Writing Committee to Develop Guidelines for the Management of Patients with Peripheral Arterial Disease), *J Am Coll Cardiol* 47:1239-1312, 2006. Available at http://www.acc.org/clinical/guidelines/pad/index.pdf.

McDermott MM et al: Treadmill exercise and resistance training in patients with peripheral arterial disease with and without intermittent claudication: a randomized controlled trial, *JAMA* 301:165, 2009.

Met R et al: Diagnostic performance of computed tomography angiography in peripheral arterial disease, *JAMA* 301(4):415-424, 2009.

Norgren L et al: Inter-society consensus for the management of peripheral arterial disease (TASC II), *J Vasc Surg* (45):S5, 2007.

Vidula H et al: Biomarkers of inflammation and thrombosis as predictors of near-term mortality in patients with peripheral arterial disease: a cohort study, *Ann Intern Med* 148:85-93, 2008.

The Warfarin Antiplatelet Vascular Evaluation Trial Investigators: Oral anticoagulant and antiplatelet therapy and peripheral arterial disease, *N Engl J Med* 357:217, 2007.

White C: Intermittent claudication, *N Engl J Med* 356:1241-1250, 2007.

AUTHORS: **GARY S. MAK, M.D.** and **PRANAV M. PATEL, M.D.**

BASIC INFORMATION

DEFINITION

Peritonitis refers to the acute onset of severe abdominal pain caused by peritoneal inflammation.

Secondary peritonitis is a localized (abscess) or diffuse peritonitis originating from a defect in abdominal viscus.

SYNONYMS

Acute abdomen
Surgical abdomen

ICD-9CM CODES
567.2 Peritonitis

EPIDEMIOLOGY & DEMOGRAPHICS

Common presentation as a result of diverse etiologies; for example, 5% to 10% of the population has acute appendicitis at some point in their lives.

PHYSICAL FINDINGS & CLINICAL PRESENTATION

- Acute abdominal pain
- Abdominal distention and ascites
- Abdominal rigidity, rebound, and guarding
- Fever, chills
- Exacerbation with movement
- Anorexia, nausea, and vomiting
- Constipation
- Decreased bowel sounds
- Hypotension and tachycardia
- Tachypnea, dyspnea

ETIOLOGY

- Microbiology: most common is gram-negative bacteria (*Escherichia coli, Enterobacter, Klebsiella, Proteus*), gram-positive bacteria (enterococci, streptococci, staphylococci), anaerobic bacteria (*Bacteroides, Clostridium*), and fungi
- Acute perforation peritonitis: gastrointestinal perforation, intestinal ischemia, pelvic peritonitis and other forms
- Postoperative peritonitis: anastomotic leak, accidental perforation, and devascularization
- Posttraumatic peritonitis: after blunt or penetrating abdominal trauma

Dx DIAGNOSIS

DIFFERENTIAL DIAGNOSIS

- Postoperative: abscess, sepsis, bowel obstruction, injury to internal organs
- Gastrointestinal: perforated viscus, appendicitis, inflammatory bowel disease, infectious colitis, diverticulitis, acute cholecystitis, peptic ulcer perforation, pancreatitis, bowel obstruction
- Gynecologic: ruptured ectopic pregnancy, pelvic inflammatory disease, ruptured hemorrhagic ovarian cyst, ovarian torsion, degenerating leiomyoma
- Urologic: nephrolithiasis, interstitial cystitis
- Miscellaneous: abdominal trauma, penetrating wounds, infections caused by intraperitoneal dialysis

WORKUP

- Acute peritonitis is mainly a clinical diagnosis based on patient history and physical examination.
- Laboratory and imaging studies (see "Laboratory Tests") assist in determining the need for and type of intervention.
- If patient is hemodynamically unstable, immediate diagnostic laparotomy should be performed in lieu of adjuvant diagnostic studies.

LABORATORY TESTS

- Complete blood count: leukocytosis, left shift, anemia
- SMA7: electrolyte imbalances, kidney dysfunction
- Liver function tests: ascites from liver disease, cholelithiasis
- Amylase: pancreatitis
- Blood cultures: bacteremia, sepsis
- Peritoneal cultures: infectious etiology
- Blood gas: respiratory versus metabolic acidosis
- Ascitic fluid analysis: exudate versus transudate
- Urinalysis and culture: urinary tract infection
- Cervical cultures for gonorrhea and *Chlamydia*
- Urine/serum human chorionic gonadotropin

IMAGING STUDIES

- Abdominal series: free air from perforation, small or large bowel dilation from obstruction, identification of fecalith
- Chest x-ray examination: elevated diaphragm, pneumonia
- Pelvic/abdominal ultrasound: abscess formation, abdominal mass, intrauterine versus ectopic pregnancy, identify free fluid suggestive of hemorrhage or ascites
- CT: mass, ascites

Rx TREATMENT

NONPHARMACOLOGIC THERAPY

- IV hydration to correct dehydration, hypovolemia
- Blood transfusion to correct anemia from hemorrhage
- Nasogastric decompression, especially if obstruction is present
- Oxygen: intubation if necessary
- Bed rest

ACUTE GENERAL Rx

- Surgery to correct underlying pathology, such as controlling hemorrhage, correcting perforation, draining abscess
- Broad-spectrum antibiotics:
  1. Single agent: ceftriaxone 1 to 2 g IV q24h, cefotaxime 1 to 2 g IV q4-6h
  2. Multiple agents:
     a. Ampicillin 2 g IV q4-6h; gentamicin 1.5 mg/kg/day; clindamycin 600 to 900 mg IV q8h
     b. Ampicillin 2 g IV q4-6h; gentamicin 1.5 mg/kg/day; metronidazole 500 mg IV q6-8h
- Pain control: morphine or meperidine as needed (hold until diagnosis confirmed)

DISPOSITION

Depends on etiology of peritonitis, age of patient, coexisting medical disease, and duration of process before presentation

REFERRAL

Surgical consultation is required in all cases of acute peritonitis.

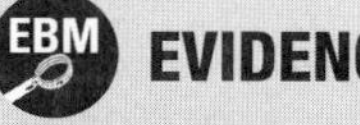

EVIDENCE

A systematic review that aimed to ascertain the efficacy and adverse effects of different antibiotic regimens in treating intraabdominal infections in adults found that no specific recommendations can be made for first-line antibiotics for secondary peritonitis, as all regimens showed similar efficacy, although the reviewers noted that within the limited and small studies available for meta-analysis, the combination of uoroquinolones/antianaerobes and cephalosporins/beta-lactamase inhibitors appear to be statistically more effective clinically.[1] Ⓐ

The reviewers further noted, however, that factors such as local guidelines and preferences, ease of administration, cost, and availability must be used when deciding on the antibiotic regimen and that in acute life-threatening surgical infections requiring immediate therapy, choice of antibiotic treatment must be empirical, taking into account microbial factors such as the presumed spectrum of the bacterial contamination, as well as their pathogenicity and synergism.[1] Ⓐ

Evidence-Based Reference

1. Wong PF et al: Antibiotic regimens for secondary peritonitis of gastrointestinal origin in adults, *Cochrane Database Rev* 2, 2005. Ⓐ

SUGGESTED READINGS

Bosscha K et al: Surgical management of severe secondary peritonitis, *Br J Surg* 86(11):1371, 1999.
Marshall JC, Innes M: Intensive care management of intra-abdominal infection, *Crit Care Med* 31(8):2228, 2003.
Wittmann DH et al: Management of secondary peritonitis, *Ann Surg* 224(1):10, 1996.

AUTHORS: **ARUNDATHI G. PRASAD, M.D.,** and **RUBEN ALVERO, M.D.**

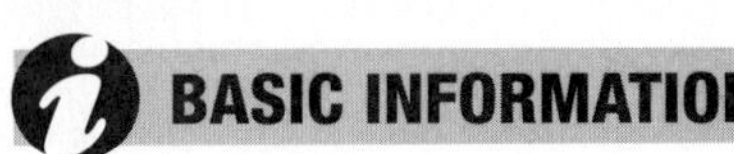

BASIC INFORMATION

DEFINITION

Spontaneous bacterial peritonitis (SBP) is an inflammatory reaction of the peritoneum secondary to the presence of bacteria or other microorganisms. More specifically, SBP is defined as an ascitic fluid infection without an evident intra-abdominal surgically treatable source occurring primarily in patients with advanced cirrhosis of the liver.

SYNONYMS

Primary peritonitis
SBP

ICD-9CM CODES
567.2 Peritonitis

EPIDEMIOLOGY & DEMOGRAPHICS

PREDOMINANT SEX: Males affected more often than females

PHYSICAL FINDINGS & CLINICAL PRESENTATION

- Acute fever with accompanying abdominal pain/ascites, nausea, vomiting, diarrhea
- In cirrhotic patients, presentation may be subtle with a low-grade temperature (100° F) with or without abdominal abnormalities
- In patients with ascites, a heightened degree of awareness is necessary for detection
- Jaundice and encephalopathy
- Deterioration of mental status and/or renal function

ETIOLOGY

- *Escherichia coli*
- *Klebsiella pneumoniae*
- *Streptococcus pneumoniae*
- *Streptococcus and Enterococcus* spp.
- *Staphylococcus aureus*
- Anaerobic pathogens: *Bacteroides, Clostridium* organisms
- Other: fungal, mycobacterial, viral

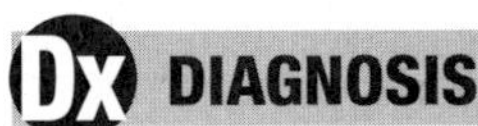

DIAGNOSIS

The diagnosis of SBP is established by a positive ascitic fluid bacterial culture and an elevated ascitic fluid absolute polymorphonuclear leukocyte count ($\geq$250 cells/mm^3).

DIFFERENTIAL DIAGNOSIS

- Appendicitis (in children)
- Perforated peptic ulcer
- Secondary peritonitis
- Peritoneal abscess
- Splenic, hepatic, or pancreatic abscess
- Cholecystitis
- Cholangitis

WORKUP

Paracentesis and ascitic fluid analysis will confirm diagnosis (see "Laboratory Tests").

LABORATORY TESTS

Ascitic fluid analysis reveals the following:

- Polymorphonuclear cell count >250/mm^3
- Presence of bacteria on Gram stain
- pH <7.31
- Lactic acid >32 mg/dl
- Protein <1 g/dl
- Glucose >50 mg/dl
- Lactate dehydrogenase <225 mU/ml
- Positive culture of peritoneal fluid
- Measurement of the serum/ascites/albumin gradient: The serum/ascites/albumin gradient indirectly measures portal pressure. The albumin concentration of ascitic fluid and serum must be obtained on the same day. The ascitic fluid value is subtracted from the serum value to obtain the gradient. If the difference (not a ratio) is >1.1 g/dl, the patient has portal hypertension, with 97% accuracy. If the difference is <1.1 g/dl, portal hypertension is not present. The majority of patients with SBP have portal hypertension as a result of cirrhosis.

IMAGING STUDIES

- Abdominal ultrasound: if there is clinical difficulty in performing paracentesis
- CT scan: to rule out secondary peritonitis (if indicated) and to exclude abscess, mass

Rx TREATMENT

ACUTE GENERAL Rx

Cefotaxime 1 to 2 g IV q8h or ceftriaxone 2 g IV q24h in patients with normal renal function; duration of treatment is generally 7 to 10 days. Oral quinolone therapy (ofloxacin 400 to 800 mg/day) or ciprofloxacin may be an acceptable alternative in selected patients.

PROPHYLAXIS

Give double-strength trimethoprim/sulfamethoxazole qd 5 days/wk or ciprofloxacin 750 mg/wk PO. Both have been shown to decrease occurrence of SBP in patients with cirrhosis.

DISPOSITION

- If possible, the initial management of SBP should be undertaken in the hospital setting; this permits careful follow-up for treatment-related complications, management of underlying portal hypertension, and workup for concomitant diseases.
- Once the diagnosis is confirmed and the patient is stabilized, oral antibiotic therapy can be continued in an outpatient setting if careful follow-up of the patient is ensured.

REFERRAL

- To a gastroenterologist for management of ascites and prevention of recurrent SBP
- To an infectious disease specialist for management of difficult-to-treat infections, antibiotic-resistant bacterial infections, or antibiotic drug intolerance

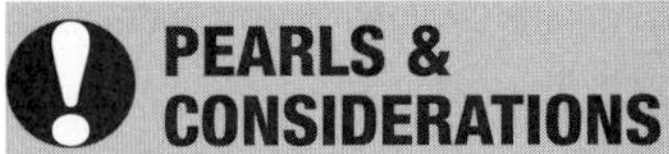

PEARLS & CONSIDERATIONS

COMMENTS

- Renal failure is a major cause of morbidity in cirrhotic patients with SBP. The use of IV albumin (1.5 g/kg at the time of diagnosis and 1 g/kg on day 3) may lower the rate of renal failure and mortality in patients with SBP.
- The criteria for the diagnosis of SBP require that abdominal paracentesis be performed and ascitic fluid be analyzed before a diagnosis of SBP can be made.
- Culturing ascitic fluid as if it were blood (with bedside inoculation of ascitic fluid into blood culture bottles) has been shown to significantly increase the culture positivity of the ascitic fluid.
- Laparotomy may be life threatening in end-stage cirrhosis.
- Positive blood cultures in an individual with ascites require exclusion of a peritoneal source by paracentesis.

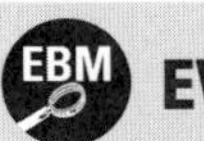

EVIDENCE

Please note: Complete text of EBM for this topic is available online.

SUGGESTED READINGS

Cholongitas E et al: Spontaneous bacterial peritonitis in cirrhotic patients: is prophylactic propranolol therapy beneficial? *J Gastroenterol Hepatol* 21(3):581, 2006.

Gonzalez-Suarez B et al: Pharmacologic treatment of portal hypertension in the prevention of community-acquired spontaneous bacterial peritonitis, *Eur J Gastroenterol Hepatol* 18(1):49, 2006.

Runyon BA: Early events in spontaneous bacterial peritonitis, *Gut* 53(6):782, 2004.

Shaw E et al: Clinical features and outcome of spontaneous bacterial peritonitis in HIV-infected cirrhotic patients: a case control study, *Eur J Clin Microbiol Infect Dis* 25(5):291, 2006.

Wong CL et al: Does this patient have bacterial peritonitis or portal hypertension? How do I perform a paracentesis and analyze the results? *JAMA* 299(10):1166, 2008

AUTHORS: **GLENN G. FORT, M.D., M.P.H.,** and **DENNIS J. MIKOLICH, M.D.**

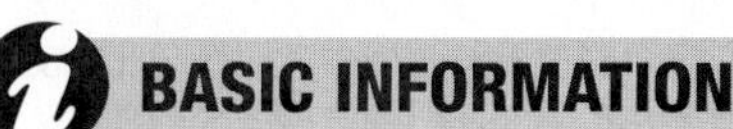

BASIC INFORMATION

DEFINITION

Peritonsillar abscess is an acute infection located between the capsule of the palatine tonsil and the superior constrictor muscle of the pharynx.

SYNONYMS

Quinsy

ICD-9CM CODES
475.0 Peritonsillar abscess

EPIDEMIOLOGY & DEMOGRAPHICS

INCIDENCE (IN U.S.): 30:100,000/yr. It is the most common deep infection of the head and neck
FREQUENCY: There is a bimodal frequency during the year, with highest occurrence from November to December and April to May.
PREDOMINANT SEX: Male = female
PREDOMINANT AGE: Common during adolescence and 20s. Young children may be affected if immunocompromised.

CLINICAL PRESENTATION

- Sore throat, which may be severe
- Dysphagia and odynophagia
- Otalgia
- Foul-smelling breath
- Facial swelling
- Drooling
- Headache
- Fever
- Trismus
- Hoarseness, muffled voice (also called "hot potato voice")
- Tender submandibular and anterior cervical lymph nodes
- Tonsillar hypertrophy
- Contralateral deflection of the uvula
- Stridor

ETIOLOGY

- Peritonsillar abscess is a complication of tonsillitis.
- Group A β-hemolytic Streptococcus is the most common bacterial cause, accounting for 15% to 30% of cases in children and 5% to 10% of cases in adults.
- Less common aerobic causes are *Staphylococcus aureus, Haemophilus influenzae, Neisseria* species.
- The most common anaerobic organism is *Fusobacterium*.

DIAGNOSIS

DIFFERENTIAL DIAGNOSIS

- Tonsillitis
- Infectious mononucleosis
- Peritonsillar cellulitis
- Retropharyngeal abscess
- Epiglottitis
- Dental abscess
- Lymphoma

WORKUP

Thorough history and physical exam

LABORATORY TESTS

- Rapid strep antigen detecting testing and throat swab culture and sensitivity
- Aspiration of the abscess for culture and sensitivity

IMAGING STUDIES

Ultrasound and CT scan can be considered to help differentiate mass from abscess, but the gold standard still remains a culture of the abscess.

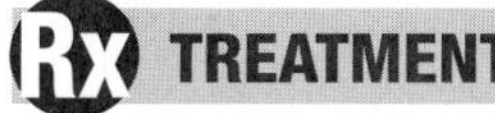

TREATMENT

NONPHARMACOLOGIC THERAPY

- Surgical drainage of the abscess by needle aspiration or by incision and drainage
- Possible subsequent surgery for tonsillectomy

ACUTE GENERAL Rx

- Several methods of initial surgical drainage are equally effective.
- Appropriate selection of antibiotic guided by culture and sensitivity of the organism. After performing aspiration or drainage, appropriate antibiotic therapy, possibly including penicillin, clindamycin, cephalosporins, or metronidazole, must be started.

CHRONIC Rx

- Tonsillectomy usually occurs 3 to 6 mo after diagnosis of abscess or recurrent tonsillitis.
- Though rare, in adults and children with peritonsillar abscess and a history of recurrent pharyngitis or previous peritonsillar abscess, the specialist may proceed with removal of the tonsils directly after placing the patient on IV antibiotics. This is known as a quinsy or hot tonsillectomy.

REFERRAL

Patients may be able to be treated as outpatients, but emergently consider hospitalization or consultation with an otolaryngologist if the patient's airway has the potential to become obstructed or if stridor is appreciated.

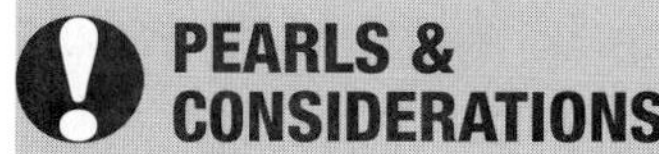

PEARLS & CONSIDERATIONS

COMMENTS

- Any person who has had a peritonsillar abscess is at risk for a recurrence, both immediately (within 4 days) and long term (2 to 3 yr).
- Most recurrences occur shortly after the initial presentation, suggesting continued infection rather than recurrence.
- Regardless of treatment modality, the overall recurrence rate is from 6% to 36%.

PREVENTION

- Strongly encourage completion of the full course of antibiotic treatment for acute pharyngitis (10 to 14 days) to prevent incomplete treatment of infection leading to abscess formation.
- Tonsillectomy is recommended in the event of recurrent peritonsillar abscess or tonsillitis in both children and adults.

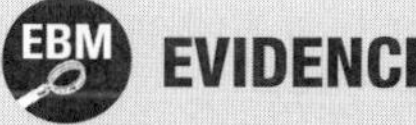

EVIDENCE

There is limited evidence for the use of antibiotic therapy in the management of sore throats without complications.

A systematic review of randomized controlled trials found that, in the management of patients with sore throat, antibiotic therapy reduces the incidence of peritonsillar abscess and other complications compared with placebo, but the overall benefit of antibiotic therapy is small in modern, Westernized societies in that large numbers of patients must be treated for a few to benefit. The reviewers note that the situation may be different in developing economies, where complication rates may be higher.[1] Ⓐ

Evidence-Based Reference

1. Del Mar CB et al: Antibiotics for sore throat, *Cochrane Database Rev* 2, 2006.

SUGGESTED READINGS

Al Yaghchi C et al: Out-patient management of patients with a peritonsillar abscess, *Clin Otolaryngol* 33(1):52-55, 2008.

Johnson RF et al: An evidence-based review of the treatment of peritonsillar abscess, *Otolaryngol Head Neck Surg* 128(3):332-343, 2003.

Steyer TE: Peritonsillar abscess: diagnosis and treatment, *Am Fam Physician* 65:93-96, 2002.

AUTHOR: **CHRISTINE HEALY, D.O.**

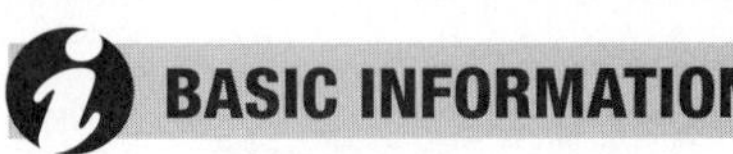

BASIC INFORMATION

DEFINITION

Pertussis is a prolonged bacterial infection of the upper respiratory tract characterized by paroxysms of an intense cough.

SYNONYMS

Whooping cough

ICD-9CM CODES
033.9 Pertussis

EPIDEMIOLOGY

INCIDENCE (IN U.S.): Approximately 5000 new cases annually (Fig. 1-244)

PEAK INCIDENCE:
- Childhood
- Usually affects children aged <1 yr

PREDOMINANT AGE:
- 50% in children aged <1 yr
- 20% in children aged >15 yr

PHYSICAL FINDINGS & CLINICAL PRESENTATION

- Usually begins with a 1- to 2-wk prodrome that resembles a common cold
- After this initial phase, increased production of mucus is noted
- Increased mucus production is followed by an intense, paroxysmal cough, ending with gasps and an inspiratory whoop
- In some children, cyanosis and anoxia are noted
- When prolonged, frank exhaustion and even apnea occur
- Pertussis is characterized by the finding of intense cough with a marked lymphocytosis; posttussive gagging and vomiting are characteristic of pertussis

ETIOLOGY

Gram-negative rod *Bordetella pertussis,* which adheres to human cilia

DIAGNOSIS

DIFFERENTIAL DIAGNOSIS

- Croup
- Epiglottitis
- Foreign body aspiration
- Bacterial pneumonia

WORKUP

- Blood cultures
- Chest radiograph examination
- Culture of bacteria, usually from nasopharynx
- Immunofluorescent staining of nasopharyngeal secretions
- Enzyme-linked immunosorbent assay for detection of antibody to pertussis

LABORATORY TESTS

Complete blood count, which usually demonstrates marked lymphocytosis:
- Up to 18,000 white blood cells
- 70% to 80% lymphocytes

IMAGING STUDIES

Chest x-ray examination is of value if secondary bacterial pneumonia is suspected.

TREATMENT

ACUTE GENERAL Rx

- Intensive supportive care:
  1. Adequate hydration
  2. Control of secretions
  3. Maintenance of airway
- Antibiotics are indicated even though their ability to alter the course of the disease is controversial.
  1. Erythromycin 50 mg/kg/day for 14 days. Recent literature reports indicate that a 7-day treatment regimen may be as effective as a 14-day course of erythromycin. Azithromycin 500 mg on day 1, followed by 250 mg for days 2 to 5. TMP/SMX 320/1600 mg per day in divided doses can be used in patients with allergy or intolerance to macrolides.
  2. Although unproved, dexamethasone 1 mg/kg/day in four doses for severe, life-threatening paroxysms.
  3. Ceftriaxone 75 mg/kg/day in two doses for broad coverage of secondary bacterial pneumonias.
- Vaccination is successful in preventing the disease: universal vaccination is advised for all children aged <7 yr.
- Erythromycin is recommended for all close contacts in the household: TMP/SMX in two oral doses per day for those intolerant to erythromycin.

DISPOSITION

Close attention to accepted vaccination schedules is the best prevention.

REFERRAL

To intensive care setting for life-threatening infections:
- Pulmonologist
- Infectious disease specialist

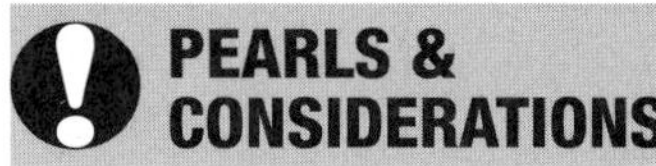

PEARLS & CONSIDERATIONS

- The diagnosis of pertussis in a young child is easily recognized, but in adults pertussis can be a subtle diagnosis and is often missed. The tip-off is often a persistent, hacking, and productive cough with minor or no fever in a previously healthy person that lasts >2 wk.
- Approximately 11% of pertussis cases in the pediatric population are attributable to vaccine refusal, dispelling the myth that herd immunity protects children whose parents refuse pertussis vaccine.

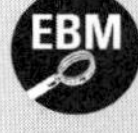

EVIDENCE

Multicomponent acellular pertussis vaccines are effective and have fewer systemic and local adverse effects than whole cell pertussis vaccines.[1] Ⓐ

Evidence-Based Reference

1. Tinnion ON, Hanlon M: Acellular vaccines for preventing whooping cough in children, *Cochrane Rev* 3, 2004.

SUGGESTED READINGS

Glanz JM et al: Parental refusal of pertussis vaccination is associated with an increased risk of pertussis infection in children, *Pediatrics* 123:1446, 2009.

Gregory DS: Pertusssis: a disease affecting all ages, *Am Fam Physician* 74:420, 2006.

Heininger U, Cherry JD: Pertussis immunization in adolescents and adults—*Bordetella pertussis* epidemiology should guide vaccination recommendations, *Expert Opin Biol Ther* 6(7):685, 2006.

Schafer S et al: A community-wide pertussis outbreak, *Arch Intern Med* 166:1317, 2006.

AUTHORS: **GLENN G. FORT, M.D., M.P.H.,** and **DENNIS J. MIKOLICH, M.D.**

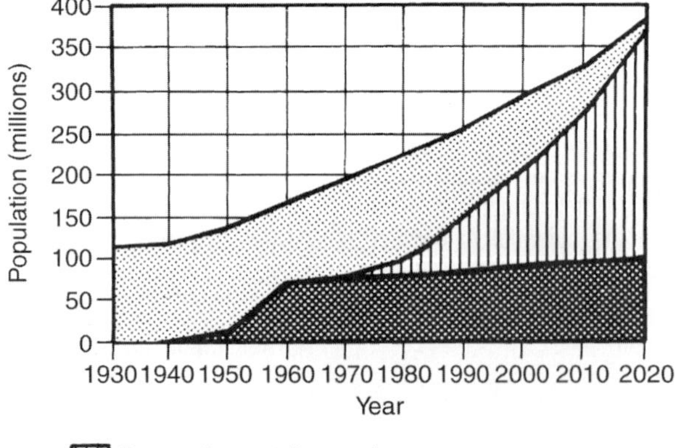

FIGURE 1-244 Projected pertussis epidemiology in the United States through the year 2020 with continued use of present-day whole-cell pertussis vaccines. (Modified from Bass JW, Stephenson SR: The return of pertussis, *Pediatr Infect Dis J* 6:141, 1987.)

BASIC INFORMATION

DEFINITION

- A hamartomatous polyp is a benign intestinal growth that may contain all components of the intestinal mucosa. In gastrointestinal polyposis, multiple such polyps coexist within the intestinal tract, and associated manifestations are usually also present.
- Juvenile polyps are benign polyps composed of cystic dilatations of glandular structures within the fibroblastic stroma of the lamina propria. They may cause bleeding or intussusception.
- Commonly recognized syndromes are Peutz-Jeghers syndrome, juvenile polyposis syndrome, Cowden's disease, Bannagan-Ruvalcaba-Riley syndrome, and Cronkhite-Canada syndrome. Other lesser known inherited hamartomatous polyposis syndromes are hereditary mixed polyposis syndrome, intestinal ganglioneuromatosis and neurofibromatosis (variant of von Recklinghausen's syndrome), Devon family syndrome, basal cell nevus syndrome, and tuberous sclerosis (may involve gastrointestinal tract).

ICD-9CM CODES
759.6 (Peutz-Jeghers syndrome)
211.3 (Cronkhite-Canada syndrome)

EPIDEMIOLOGY

- Colonic adenomas, the precursors of nearly all colorectal cancers, are found in nearly 40% of patients by age 60 yr.
- 25% of men and 15% of women who undergo colonoscopy are found to have one or more adenomas.
- Detection of any adenoma in patients <60 yr confers an increased risk of colorectal cancer (by a factor of 2.6) in their first-degree relatives.

PHYSICAL FINDINGS & CLINICAL PRESENTATION

PEUTZ-JEGHERS SYNDROME:

- Transmission: autosomal dominant with incomplete penetrance
- Disease expression:
  - Stomach, small and large intestinal hamartomas with bands of smooth muscle in the lamina propria
  - Pigmented lesions around mouth (lips and buccal mucosa), nose, hands, feet, genital, and perineal areas
  - Ovarian tumors
  - Sertoli cell testicular tumors
  - Airway polyps
  - Pancreatic cancer
  - Breast cancer
  - Urinary tract polyps
- Cumulative lifetime cancer risk
  - Colon cancer: 39%
  - Stomach cancer: 29%
  - Small intestine cancer: 13%
  - Pancreatic cancer: 36%
  - Breast cancer: 54%
  - Ovarian cancer: 10%
  - Sertoli cell tumor: 9%
  - Overall cancer risk: 93%
- Clinical manifestation:
  - Gastrointestinal, small-bowel obstruction, intussusception, gastrointestinal bleeding
  - See chapters on relevant malignancies for their signs and symptoms

JUVENILE POLYPOSIS SYNDROME:

- Transmission: autosomal dominant
- Disease expression
  - Solitary juvenile polyps numbering 10 or more in the rectum or throughout the gastrointestinal tract; the polyps are smooth and covered with normal epithelium
  - Various congenital abnormalities coexist in 20%
- Cumulative cancer risk is increased (may be as high as 50%)
- Clinical manifestation
  - Intestinal obstruction
  - Intussusception
  - Gastrointestinal bleeding

COWDEN'S DISEASE:

- Transmission: autosomal dominant, rare
- Disease expression
  - Juvenile intestinal polyposis
  - Orocutaneous hamartomas
  - Fibrocystic breast disease and breast cancer
  - Goiter and thyroid cancer
  - Facial tricholemmomas (papules) in 83%
- Cumulative cancer risk
  - Gastrointestinal: same as general population
  - Thyroid: 3% to 10%
  - Breast: 25% to 50%

BANNAGAN-RUVALCABA-RILEY SYNDROME:

- Transmission: autosomal dominant, rare
- Disease expression
  - Juvenile intestinal polyposis
  - Macrocephaly
  - Developmental delay
  - Penile pigmented spots
  - Cumulative cancer risk unknown

CRONKHITE-CANADA SYNDROME:

- Transmission: acquired
- Age of onset: midlife
- Disease expression
  - Diffuse gastrointestinal juvenile polyposis (50% to 95% of cases)
  - Chronic diarrhea and protein-losing enteropathy (the entire intestinal mucosa may be inflamed), which leads to abdominal pain, weight loss, and various complications of malnutrition
  - Dystrophic nails
  - Alopecia
  - Hyperpigmentation
- Cumulative cancer risk: same as the average population

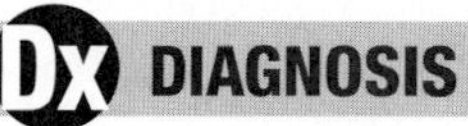

DIAGNOSIS

Diagnosis is suggested in many cases by family history and confirmed by colonoscopy and physical findings described previously.

TREATMENT

GENERAL Rx

Peutz-Jeghers syndrome:
- Colonoscopies with polypectomies
- Screening for breast cancer, testicular cancer, possibly ovarian cancer

Juvenile polyposis syndrome:
- Colonoscopies with polypectomies if few colon polyps
- Total colectomy if numerous polyps
- Esophagogastroscopies and polypectomies

Cowden's disease:
- Rigorous breast cancer screening or prophylactic simple bilateral mastectomy with reconstruction.

Cronkhite-Canada syndrome:
- Progressive malabsorption syndrome is the hallmark of this syndrome, and no specific treatment exists. Enteral or parenteral feeding is the cornerstone of management and can result in remission.

DISPOSITION

- The screening of first-degree relatives of patients with colonic adenomas detected before 60 yr of age is controversial. Some recommend beginning colonoscopic screening at age 40 yr or 10 yr younger than the age at diagnosis of the youngest person in the family with an adenoma.
- Recommended interval between colonoscopies from the U.S. Consensus Guidelines for Colonoscopic Surveillance after Polypectomy are as follows:
  - 10 yr for small, rectal hyperplastic polyps
  - 5 to 10 yr for one to two low-risk adenomas (tubular adenomas <1 cm)
  - 3 yr for low-risk adenomas or any high-risk adenoma (large [≥1 cm] or histologically advanced adenomas [tubulovillous or villous adenomas or villous adenomas and those with high-grade dysplasia)]
  - <3 yr for presence of >10 adenomas
  - 2 to 6 mo for inadequately removed adenomas

SUGGESTED READING

Levine JS, Ahnen DJ: Adenomatous polyps of the colon, *N Engl J Med* 355:2551-2557, 2006.

AUTHOR: **FRED F. FERRI, M.D.**

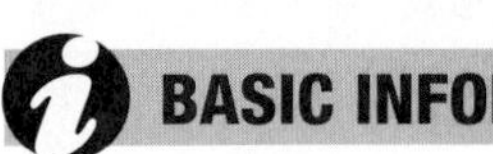

BASIC INFORMATION

DEFINITION

Peyronie's disease is an abnormal curvature and shortening of the penis during an erection. This is caused by scarring of the tunica albuginea of the corpora cavernosa.

SYNONYMS

Plastic induration of the penis
Penile fibromatosis

ICD-9CM CODES
607.89 Peyronie's disease

EPIDEMIOLOGY & DEMOGRAPHICS

- Peyronie's disease occurs in approximately 1% of men.
- It is commonly seen between the ages of 45 and 60 yr.
- A genetic predisposition has been suggested.
- There are no incidence and prevalence data available in the literature.

PHYSICAL FINDINGS & CLINICAL PRESENTATION

- Painful erections
- Tenderness over the scar tissue area
- Erectile dysfunction
- Curvature of the erected penis interfering with penetration
- Dupuytren's contracture is a commonly associated finding in patients with Peyronie's disease

ETIOLOGY

- Specific cause is unknown. It is believed that scar tissue forms on either the dorsal or ventral midline surface of the penile shaft. The scar restricts expansion at the involved site, causing the penis to bend or curve in one direction.
- The precipitating factor appears to be trauma either from repetitive microvascular injury caused by vigorous sexual intercourse, accidents, or prior surgeries (e.g., transurethral or radical prostatectomy, cystoscopy).

Dx DIAGNOSIS

Diagnosis is based on the clinical findings.

DIFFERENTIAL DIAGNOSIS

- The history differentiates congenital from acquired curvatures of the penis.
- Other causes of erectile dysfunction must be excluded, including metabolic, diabetic, thyroid, and renal causes, in addition to hypogonadism and hyperprolactinemia.

WORKUP

History and physical examination alone will usually establish the diagnosis of Peyronie's disease.

LABORATORY TESTS

There are no specific blood tests to diagnose Peyronie's disease. Electrolytes, blood urea nitrogen, creatinine, glucose, thyroid function tests (thyroid-stimulating hormone, T_3U, T_4), testosterone, and prolactin levels are blood tests to exclude other medical causes of erectile dysfunction.

IMAGING STUDIES

Imaging studies are not specific.

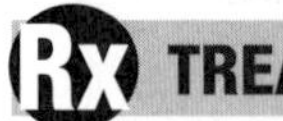

TREATMENT

NONPHARMACOLOGIC THERAPY

A conservative approach of reassurance and observation is taken at first because the disease process may be self-limiting.

ACUTE GENERAL Rx

Although not substantiated by direct randomized, controlled clinical trials, the following treatment modalities have been tried:

- Vitamin E 400 mg bid.
- Paraaminobenzoic acid 12 g/day.
- Colchicine 0.6 mg bid for 2 to 3 wk.
- Fexofenadine 60 mg bid for 3 mo.
- Steroid injection into the scar tissue.
- Collagenase injection into the scar tissue.
- Radiation to the scar tissue area.
- Extracorporeal shockwave therapy (ESWT): Current evidence on the safety, but not the efficacy, of ESWT appears adequate. From comparative studies, the main benefits of ESWT were the alleviation of pain and reduction of angulation of the penis. In one comparative study, 10 of 20 patients receiving ESWT had a decrease in the curvature of at least 30%. Case series evidence also suggested some improvement of sexual performance.
- Other medications that can be helpful include verapamil, tamoxifen, and interferon.

CHRONIC Rx

In patients who have progressed to intractable pain with erection or erectile dysfunction, surgical treatment with excision of the plaque and skin grafting may be indicated.

DISPOSITION

Peyronie's disease evolves slowly and in some cases can resolve on its own. Waiting for 1 yr before proceeding with surgical attempts is recommended.

REFERRAL

A urologic consultation is recommended in patients with progressive symptoms and erectile dysfunction.

PEARLS & CONSIDERATIONS

COMMENTS

- Peyronie's disease is not commonly seen in younger patients because they are able to sustain intracorporeal pressures high enough to stretch the scar tissue, preventing it from deforming the penis during erection.
- Trauma from buckling of the erected penis is thought to be the precipitant cause of scar formation and Peyronie's disease. It is found more often in men who are sexually very active and vigorous, having sexual intercourse daily or almost daily.
- Sexual positions with the women being on top or thrusting the penis into the anterior vaginal wall is thought to increase the chances of developing Peyronie's disease.

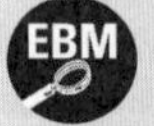

EVIDENCE

Most of the therapies and interventions for the treatment of Peyronie's disease are lacking high quality evidence to support their use. However, there is limited evidence to support the use of some therapies:

A small RCT found no evidence to support the use of Vitamin E, either alone or in combination with interferon-alpha 2b.

A small RCT involving 30 patients randomized patients to receive intralesional interferon-alpha 2b combined with oral vitamin E or intralesional interferon-alpha 2b alone or oral vitamin E alone. A total of 5.0 x 10(6) U of interferon-alpha 2b was given once per week directly into the plaque for a period of 12 wk. Patients received 400 IU of vitamin E orally twice daily for 6 mo. The study found that at 6 mo follow-up, there were no significant changes in the objective parameters (plaque size, location, and presence of calcification) when compared with the initial findings in each group or among the three groups. We did not observe any clinically significant improvement in the subjective parameters (penile pain and quality of sexual intercourse) among the three groups.[1] B

There is some evidence from an RCT to suggest that aminobenzoate potassium is more beneficial than placebo in the stabilization of Peyronie's disease.

A double blind RCT involving 103 patients with Peyronie's disease and a history of $<$12 mo, noncalcified plaques and no previous treatment compared potassium paraaminobenzoate versus placebo, on a regimen of 4 x 3 g/day for 12 mo. Response was defined as regression in plaque-size and/or reduction in penile curvature of at least 30%. It should be noted that analysis was based on 75 patients who completed the study. Response rates were significantly greater on potassium paraaminobenzoate (74.3%) than on placebo (50.0%). Mean plaque size decreased from 259 mm^2 to 142 mm^2 in the treatment arm. In the placebo group, plaque size increased from 259 mm^2 to 303 mm^2 after 6 mo but improved slightly to 233 mm^2 after 12 mo. Differences between the groups were significant. There was no significant improvement in preexisting curvature in the treatment arm, but development of new curvature or deterioration of preexisting curvature remained stable. In contrast, in the placebo group penile curvature deteriorated significantly in 32.5% of the cases. No significant differences in decrease of pain were observed between the two groups.[2] B

One small RCT found that tamoxifen was no more effective than placebo in the treatment of Peyronie's disease; another RCT found tamoxifen was less effective than acetyl-L-carnitine.

A randomized controlled trial (RCT) involving 48 patients with Peyronie's disease compared tamoxifen 20 mg twice daily for 3 mo versus acetyl-L-carnitine 1 g twice daily for 3 mo. The study found acetyl-L-carnitine was significantly more effective than tamoxifen in reducing pain and in inhibiting disease progression. Furthermore, it found acetyl-L-carnitine reduced penile curvature significantly, while tamoxifen did not. Both drugs produced significant reductions in plaque size. B

An RCT involving 25 patients with Peyronie's disease, but without calcified plaques, compared 20 mg tamoxifen twice daily for 3 mo versus placebo. At 4 mo follow-up, no significant differences were found between the treatment and placebo arms for pain, curvature, or plaque size. B

An RCT found that colchicine was no more effective than placebo in the treatment of Peyronie's disease and noted significant drug-related adverse effects.

A randomized controlled trial involving 84 patients with Peyronie's disease, but without calcified plaque, compared 4 mo treatment with colchicine 0.5 to 2.5 mg versus placebo. The study found no significant differences between the two groups in terms of pain resolution, reduction in penile deformity, or decrease in plaque size. Significant drug-related adverse effects occurred in colchicine group and in two cases treatment was discontinued.[3] B

There is evidence from two RCTs that intralesional injections of interferon are more effective than placebo injections in the treatment of Peyronie's disease; another smaller RCT found no benefit from intralesional interferon compared with Vitamin E.

A systematic evidence-based analysis of plaque injection therapy identified seven studies evaluating intralesional interferon injections. Six were assessed as being low-level evidence (case series or poor-quality cohort or case-control studies) and one was assessed as being a good quality randomized controlled trial. Five studies showed benefit from treatment and two showed no significant benefit from treatment. The single-blinded, randomized, placebo-controlled trial involved 117 patients who had at least a 12-mo history of Peyronie's disease and a minimum penile curvature of 30 degrees. It compared intralesional interferon alpha-2b vs saline, administered biweekly for 12 wk. The study found significantly greater improvement in penile curvature, plaque size and density, and erectile pain resolution in patients treated with interferon alpha-2b compared with placebo. However, increase in mean International Index of Erectile Function score was not significantly different between the two arms.[4] A

An RCT involving 39 patients compared 10 ml of saline versus 5 x 10(6) units of IFN alpha-2b intralesional injections every other week for a total of six injections. Increase in penile blood flow was significantly greater in IFN alpha-2b-treated patients compared with those in the placebo group. The number with the nonvascular classification increased significantly in the IFN alpha-2b arm from 31.5% to 57.8%. Improvements in penile curvature, plaque size and density, and pain on erection were also significantly better in the IFN alpha-2b group compared with placebo.[5] B

A small RCT found a straightening-reinforcing (S-R) plication technique was not better than the Nesbit procedure, but the authors suggested the technique may be useful in some situations.

A randomized study of surgery for congenital curvature and Peyronie's disease compared two different plication techniques. Between 1995 and 1998, 50 patients were randomized to straightening-reinforcing (S-R) plication (20 congenital and 5 PD) or Nesbit procedure (20 congenital and 5 PD). S-R plication involved a modified Ebbehoj-Metz technique using a 'straightening-reinforcing' (S-R) double stitch: the first stitch performing the plication, with the second tightening it, thus preventing tension during erection. A further 28 patients, between 1998 and 2000, were assigned exclusively to S-R plication. The study found no patient reported a decrease in erectile function and all reported easy vaginal penetration within 3 mo. In 60% of the patients undergoing the Nesbit technique, restoration of fully satisfactory coital activity was delayed because of pain during erection; 35% of all patients had some problems with the coronal suture which disappeared 1 mo after the operation, and 15% reported decreased sensibility of the glans. Overall, the authors concluded that S-R plication is not better than the Nesbit procedure. However, they suggested for low degrees of penile bending modified plication may be a minimally invasive and effective treatment suitable for most curvatures treated in day clinics and under local anesthesia.[6] B

Two RCTs provide some evidence that iontophoresis with verapamil or verapamil plus dexamethasone is more effective than placebo.

A randomized, double blind, placebo controlled trial involving 42 patients with Peyronie's disease compared 10 mg verapamil in 4 ml of saline versus 4 ml saline alone via electromotive drug administration, given 2 times a wk for 3 mo. No significant differences in change in curvature were found between the treatment and control arms.[7] B

An RCT involving 98 patients with Peyronie's disease compared intraplaque electromotive verapamil/dexamethasone versus electromotive lidocaine. Treatment was with either 5 mg verapamil and 8 mg dexamethasone or 2% lidocaine as control. Treatments were scheduled for 4 sessions per week for 6 weeks. 37 patients in the study group and 36 in the control group completed the treatment course. The study reported significant decreases in median plaque volume and in penile curvature in the study group, whereas there were no significant changes in median volume and curvature in the control group. Significant pain relief occurred in both treatment and control groups, though this was reported as transient in the control group and permanent in the study group.[8] B

Evidence-Based References

1. Inal T et al: Effect of intralesional interferon-alpha 2b combined with oral vitamin E for treatment of early stage Peyronie's disease: a randomized and prospective study, *Urology* 67:1038-1042, 2006. B
2. Weidner W et al; Peyronie's Disease Study Group of Andrological Group of German Urologists: Potassium paraaminobenzoate (POTABA) in the treatment of Peyronie's disease: a prospective, placebo-controlled, randomized study, *Eur Urol* 47:530-535, 2005. B
3. Safarinejad MR: Therapeutic effects of colchicine in the management of Peyronie's disease: a randomized double-blind, placebo-controlled study, *Int J Impot Res* 16:238-243, 2004. B
4. Russell S et al: Systematic evidence-based analysis of plaque injection therapy for Peyronie's disease, *Eur Urol* 51:640-647, 2007. A
5. Kendirci M et al: The impact of intralesional interferon alpha-2b injection therapy on penile hemodynamics in men with Peyronie's disease, *J Sex Med* 2:709-715, 2005. B
6. Mantovani F et al: 'Straightening-reinforcing' technique for congenital curvature and Peyronie's disease, *Urol Int* 75:201-203, 2005. B
7. Greenfield JM et al: Verapamil versus saline in electromotive drug administration for Peyronie's disease: a double-blind, placebo controlled trial, *J Urol* 177:972-975, 2007. B
8. Di Stasi SM et al: A prospective, randomized study using transdermal electromotive administration of verapamil and dexamethasone for Peyronie's disease, *J Urol* 171:1605-1608, 2004. B

SUGGESTED READINGS

Ralph DJ, Minhas S: The management of Peyronie's disease, *BJU Int* 93(2):208, 2004.

Smith CJ et al: Peyronie's disease: the epidemiology, aetiology and clinical evaluation of deformity, *BJU Int* 95(6):729, 2005.

AUTHOR: **TANYA ALI, M.D.**

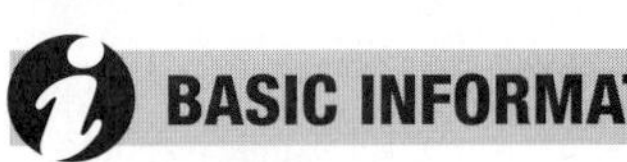

BASIC INFORMATION

DEFINITION

Pharyngitis/tonsillitis is inflammation of the pharynx or tonsils.

SYNONYMS

Sore throat

ICD-9CM CODES
462 Pharyngitis

EPIDEMIOLOGY & DEMOGRAPHICS

PEAK INCIDENCE: Late winter/early spring (group A streptococcal infections)

PREDOMINANT SEX: Females and males affected equally

PREDOMINANT AGE:
- All ages affected
- Streptococcal pharyngitis most common among school-age children

GENETICS: Neonatal infection: pharyngitis at age <3 yr is almost always of viral etiology.

PHYSICAL FINDINGS & CLINICAL PRESENTATION

- Pharynx:
  1. May appear normal to severely erythematous
  2. Tonsillar hypertrophy and exudates commonly seen but do not indicate etiology
- Viral infection:
  1. Rhinorrhea
  2. Conjunctivitis
  3. Cough
- Bacterial infection, especially group A streptococci:
  1. High fever
  2. Systemic signs of infection
- Herpes simplex or enterovirus infection: vesicles
- Streptococcal infection:
  1. Rare complications:
     a. Scarlet fever
     b. Rheumatic fever
     c. Acute glomerulonephritis
  2. Extension of infection: tonsillar, parapharyngeal, or retropharyngeal abscess presenting with severe pain, high fever, trismus

ETIOLOGY

- Viruses:
  1. Respiratory syncytial virus
  2. Influenza A and B
  3. Epstein-Barr virus
  4. Adenovirus
  5. Herpes simplex
- Bacteria:
  1. *Streptococcus pyogenes*
  2. *Neisseria gonorrhoeae*
  3. *Arcanobacterium haemolyticum*
- Other organisms:
  1. *Mycoplasma pneumoniae*
  2. *Chlamydophila pneumoniae*

DIAGNOSIS

DIFFERENTIAL DIAGNOSIS

- Sore throat associated with granulocytopenia, thyroiditis.
- Tonsillar hypertrophy associated with lymphoma.
- Section II describes the differential diagnosis of sore throat.

WORKUP

- Throat swab for culture to exclude *S. pyogenes, N. gonorrhoeae* (requires specific transport medium)
- Rapid streptococcal antigen test (culture should be performed if rapid test negative)
- Monospot

LABORATORY TESTS

- Complete blood count with differential
  1. May help support diagnosis of bacterial infection
  2. Streptococcal infection suggested by leukocytosis >15,000/mm^3
- Viral cultures, serologic studies rarely needed

IMAGING STUDIES

Seldom indicated

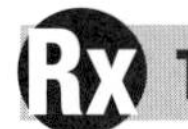

TREATMENT

NONPHARMACOLOGIC THERAPY

- Fluids
- Salt water gargles

ACUTE GENERAL Rx

- Aspirin (acetaminophen culture)
- If streptococcal infection proven or suspected:
  1. Penicillin V 500 mg PO bid for 10 days or benzathine penicillin 1.2 million U IM once (adults)
  2. Erythromycin 500 mg PO bid or 250 mg qid for 10 days if penicillin allergic
- If gonococcal infection proven or suspected: ceftriaxone 125 mg IM once

CHRONIC Rx

- Recurrent streptococcal infections are common and may represent reinfection from other household.
- There is no conclusive evidence from randomized clinical trials that tonsillectomy is superior to antibiotic therapy for recurrent tonsillitis in adults.
- Tonsillopharyngitis is generally managed in an outpatient setting with follow-up arranged in 1 to 2 wk. Admission to the hospital is indicated for local suppurative complications (peritonsillar abscess; lateral pharyngeal or posterior pharyngeal abscess; impending airway closure; or inability to swallow food, medications, or water).

REFERRAL

- To otolaryngologist:
  1. If peritonsillar or other abscess is suspected
  2. If tonsillar hypertrophy persists
- To infectious disease expert if unusual pathogen is suspected

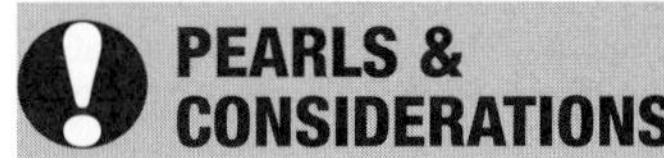

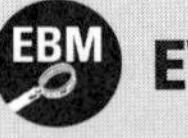

PEARLS & CONSIDERATIONS

COMMENTS

Antibiotic therapy should be avoided unless bacterial etiology is suspected or proven, especially in adults.

The major problem in the diagnosis and treatment of pharyngitis is not which guideline to follow to avoid testing and antibiotic prescribing to patients at low risk for streptococcal pharyngitis but that most physicians fail to follow any guidelines.

EVIDENCE

A systematic review found that antibiotics confer relative benefits in the treatment of sore throat, shortening the duration of symptoms by a mean of one day about half way through the illness (the time of maximal effect), and by about 16 hr overall, and preventing nonsuppurative complications of beta-hemolytic streptococcal pharyngitis. However, the absolute benefits are modest in modern Western societies given the rarity of suppurative and nonsuppurative complications.[1] Ⓐ

Evidence-Based Reference

1. Del Mar CB et al: Antibiotics for sore throat, *Cochrane Database Rev* 4, 2006. Ⓐ

SUGGESTED READINGS

Brook I, Gober AE: Treatment of non-streptococcal tonsillitis with metronidazole, *Int J Pediatr Otorhinolaryngol* 69(1):65, 2005.

Choby BA: Diagnosis and treatment of streptococcal pharyngitis, *Am Fam Phys* 79(5):383-390, 2009.

Frohna JG: Effectiveness of adenotonsillectomy in children with mild symptoms of throat infections or adenotonsillar hypertrophy: open, randomised controlled trial, *J Pediatr* 146(3):435, 2005.

Linder JA et al: Evaluation and treatment of pharyngitis in primary care practice, *Arch Intern Med* 166:1374-1379, 2006.

Patel NN, Patel DN: Acute exudative tonsillitis, *Am J Med* 122:17-20, 2009.

Tewfik TL, Al Garni M: Tonsillopharyngitis: clinical highlights, *J Otolaryngol* 34(suppl 1):S45, 2005.

AUTHORS: **GLENN G. FORT, M.D., M.P.H.,** and **DENNIS J. MIKOLICH, M.D.**

BASIC INFORMATION

DEFINITION

Pheochromocytomas are catecholamine-producing tumors that originate from chromaffin cells of the adrenergic system. They generally secrete both norepinephrine and epinephrine, but norepinephrine is usually the predominant amine.

SYNONYMS

Paraganglioma

ICD-9CM CODES
194.0 Pheochromocytoma
255.6 Medulloadrenal hyperfunction

EPIDEMIOLOGY & DEMOGRAPHICS

- Incidence: 0.05% of population; peak incidence in 30s and 40s.
- "Rough" rule of 10: 10% are extraadrenal, 10% are malignant, 10% are familial, 10% occur in children, 10% involve both adrenals, 10% are multiple (other than bilateral adrenal).
- Approximately 25% of patients with apparently sporadic pheochromocytoma may be carriers of mutations.
- Pheochromocytoma is a feature of two disorders with autosomal-dominant pattern of inheritance:
  1. Multiple endocrine neoplasia (MEN) type 2
  2. Von Hippel-Lindau disease: angioma of the retina, hemangioblastoma of the central nervous system, renal cell carcinoma, pancreatic cysts, and epididymal cystoadenoma
- Pheochromocytomas occur in 5% of patients with neurofibromatosis type 1.

PHYSICAL FINDINGS & CLINICAL PRESENTATION

- Hypertension: can be sustained (55%) or paroxysmal (45%).
- Headache (80%): usually paroxysmal in nature and described as "pounding" and severe.
- Palpitations (70%): can be present with or without tachycardia.
- Hyperhidrosis (60%): most evident during paroxysmal attacks of hypertension.
- Physical examination may be entirely normal if done in a symptom-free interval; during a paroxysm the patient may demonstrate marked increase in both systolic and diastolic pressure, profuse sweating, visual disturbances (caused by hypertensive retinopathy), dilated pupils (from catecholamine excess), paresthesias in the lower extremities (caused by severe vasoconstriction), tremor, tachycardia.

ETIOLOGY

- Catecholamine-producing tumors that are usually located in the adrenal medulla.
- Specific mutations of the RET protooncogene cause familial predisposition to pheochromocytoma in MEN 2.
- Mutations in the von Hippel-Lindau tumor suppressor gene (*VHL* gene) cause familial disposition to pheochromocytoma in von Hippel-Lindau disease.
- Recently identified genes for succinate dehydrogenase subunit D *(SDHD)* and succinate dehydrogenase subunit B *(SDHB)* predispose carriers to pheochromocytoma and globus tumors.

DIAGNOSIS

DIFFERENTIAL DIAGNOSIS

- Anxiety disorder
- Thyrotoxicosis
- Amphetamine or cocaine abuse
- Carcinoid
- Essential hypertension

WORKUP

Laboratory evaluation and imaging studies to locate the neoplasm.

LABORATORY TESTS

- Although there is no consensus on the best test, plasma-free metanephrines have been suggested as the test of first choice for excluding or confirming the tumor. Plasma concentrations of normetanephrines >2.5 pmol/ml or metanephrine levels >1.4 pmol/ml indicate a pheochromocytoma with 100% specificity.
- 24-hr urine collection for metanephrines (up to 100% sensitive) will also show increased metanephrines; the accuracy of the 24-hr urinary levels for metanephrines can be improved by indexing urinary metanephrine levels by urine creatinine levels.
- The clonidine suppression test is useful for distinguishing between high levels of plasma norepinephrine from sympathetic nerves and those from a pheochromocytoma. A decrease <50% in plasma norepinephrine levels after clonidine administration is normal, whereas persistent elevations are indicative of pheochromocytoma.

IMAGING STUDIES (Fig. 1-245)

- Abdominal CT scan (88% sensitivity) is useful in locating pheochromocytomas >0.5 inch in diameter (90% to 95% accurate). There have been concerns that IV contrast may induce a hypertensive crisis. However, studies have shown that IV low-osmolar, contrast-enhanced CT can safely be used in patients with pheochromocytoma who are not receiving alpha or beta blockers.
- MRI: pheochromocytomas demonstrate a distinctive MRI appearance (up to 100% sensitivity); MRI may become the diagnostic imaging modality of choice.
- Scintigraphy with 131 or 1-123 I-MIBG (up to 100% sensitivity): this norepinephrine analog localizes in adrenergic tissue; it is particularly useful in locating extraadrenal pheochromocytomas.
- 6 [^{18}F] Fluorodopamine positron emission tomography is reserved for cases in which clinical symptoms and signs suggest pheochromocytoma and results of biochemical tests are positive but conventional imaging studies cannot locate the tumor. An alternative approach is to use vena caval sampling for plasma catecholamines and metanephrines.

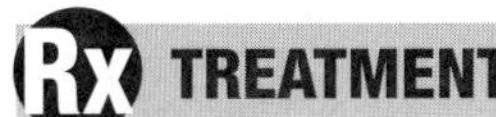

TREATMENT

GENERAL Rx

Laparoscopic removal of the tumor (surgical resection for both benign and malignant disease):

1. Preoperative stabilization with combination of phenoxybenzamine, beta-blocker, metyrosine, and liberal fluid and salt intake starting 10 to 14 days before surgery.
2. Hypertensive crisis preoperatively and intraoperatively can be controlled with phentolamine (Regitine) 2 to 5 mg IV q1-2h prn or nitroprusside used in combination with beta-adrenergic blockers.

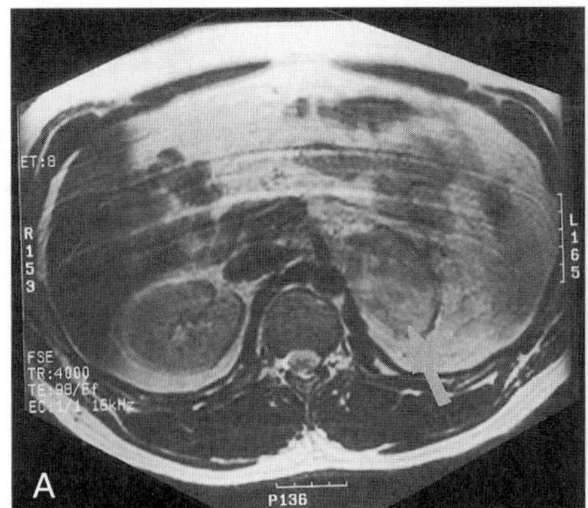

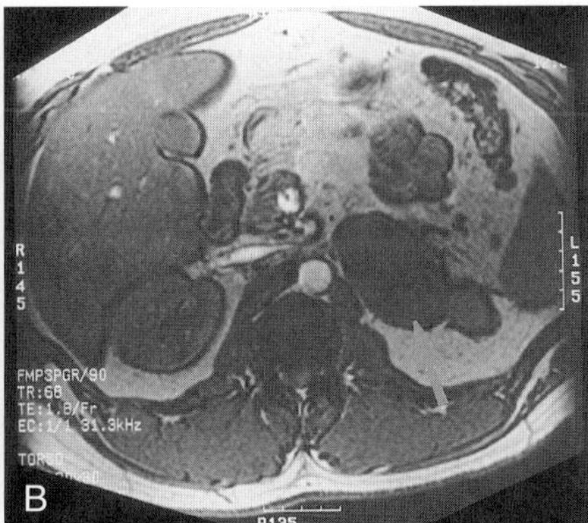

FIGURE 1-245 A, Axial in-phase gradient-echo image demonstrates left adrenal mass *(arrow)*. **B,** Axial image from the out-of-phase gradient-echo sequence demonstrates the left adrenal mass. In comparison to the in-phase image, no suppression of the adrenal mass is present. Suppression is the rule in lipid-containing cortical adenomas. (From Larson PR et al: *William's textbook of Endocrinology,* ed 10, Philadelphia, 2003, Saunders.)

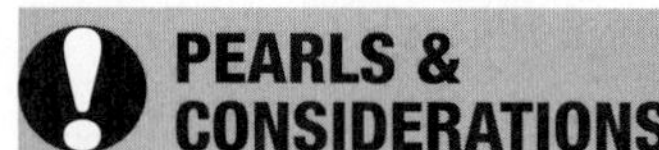

PEARLS & CONSIDERATIONS

COMMENTS

- Obtaining a detailed family history is important because 10% of pheochromocytomas are familial.
- Screening for pheochromocytoma should be considered in patients with any of the following:
  1. Malignant hypertension
  2. Poor response to antihypertensive therapy
  3. Paradoxical hypertensive response
  4. Hypertension during induction of anesthesia, parturition, surgery, or thyrotropin-releasing hormone testing
  5. Hypertension associated with imipramine or desipramine
  6. Neurofibromatosis (increased incidence of pheochromocytoma)
- All patients with pheochromocytoma should be screened for MEN-2 and von Hippel-Lindau disease with pentagastrin test, serum parathyroid hormone, ophthalmoscopy, MRI of the brain, CT scan of the kidneys and pancreas, and ultrasonography of the testes.
- In patients with pheochromocytoma, routine analysis for mutations of *RET, VHL, SDHD,* and *SDHB* is indicated to identify pheochromocytoma-associated syndromes.

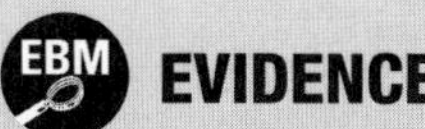

EVIDENCE

There is a lack of randomized, controlled trials evaluating the treatments for and management of pheochromocytoma. Much of the data to support such therapies are derived from case series and retrospective studies. However, recommendations from professional bodies provide some general guidance.

Guidelines from the National Comprehensive Cancer Network Neuroendocrine tumors panel note that surgical resection is the mainstay of treatment. Further notations are that a laparoscopic approach is the preferred treatment for adrenal medullary tumors, including pheochromocytomas. If possible, surgical resection is also recommended for the treatment of isolated distant metastases. Tumor debulking, if possible, with or without radiation therapy is recommended for locally unresectable disease.[1] Ⓒ

Guidelines from the American Association of Clinical Endocrinologists note that whenever possible, surgical excision or maximal debulking of accessible tumor is the preferred treatment of pheochromocytoma.[2] Ⓒ

The perioperative management of blood pressure by alpha- or beta-blockade and selective other agents is important. Guidelines from the National Comprehensive Cancer Network Neuroendocrine tumors panel make the following remarks regarding perioperative management. Before surgery, the patient should have a symptom-free period, which can be accomplished through treatment with alpha-adrenergic blockade (such as phenoxybenzamine) and forced hydration for at least 7 days. Beta-adrenergic blockade may be used after initiation of alpha-adrenergic blockade and 10 days before surgery to prevent tachyarrhythmias after correction of hypovolemia. Alpha-methyltyrosine is also used preoperatively by some clinicians. Tumor debulking, if possible, with or without radiation therapy is recommended for locally unresectable disease. Symptoms can be controlled by using alpha-blockade with or without alpha-methyltyrosine and with or without beta-blockade for locally unresectable or distant metastases.[1] Ⓒ

Guidelines from the American Association of Clinical Endocrinologists note that preoperative management or control of residual disease should involve primarily alpha-adrenergic blocking agents, particularly phenoxybenzamine or prazosin hydrochloride, and allowance of adequate time for vascular volume expansion. Beta-blockers should be added, as needed, to control tachycardia and arrhythmia. Calcium channel blockers are also advantageous as secondary or tertiary agents because they attenuate the pressor response to norepinephrine and can prevent catecholamine-induced coronary spasm.[2] Ⓒ

Management of advanced disease may involve novel therapeutic approaches. Guidelines from the National Comprehensive Cancer Network Neuroendocrine tumors panel make the following remarks regarding distant metastases. Additional treatment options include (1) high-dose iodine-131-MIBG therapy on a compassionate investigational new drug trial; (2) clinical trial; or (3) systemic chemotherapy with cyclophosphamide, vincristine, and dacarbazine.[1] Ⓒ

Evidence-Based References

1. National Comprehensive Cancer Network: NCCN Clinical Practice Guidelines in Oncology. Neuroendocrine tumors 2009. Ⓒ

2. AACE Hypertension Task Force: American Association of Clinical Endocrinologists medical guidelines for clinical practice for the diagnosis and treatment of hypertension, *Endocr Pract* 12:193, 2006. Ⓒ

SUGGESTED READING

Baid SK et al: Brief communication: radiographic contrast infusion and catecholamine release in patients with pheochromocytoma, *Ann Intern Med* 150:27-32, 2009.

AUTHORS: **MARK F. BRADY,** and **FRED F. FERRI, M.D.**

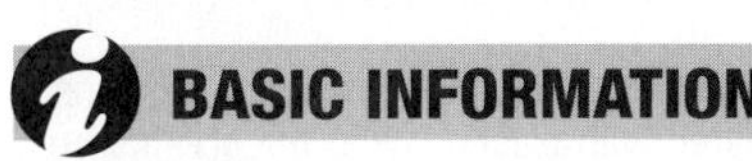

BASIC INFORMATION

DEFINITION

Specific phobias are anxiety disorders characterized by an excessive, persistent fear elicited by a specific object or situation that is then avoided or tolerated with intense distress. The provoking stimulus may be a specific object, such as an animal or insect; natural environments, such as heights or water; or a specific situation, such as the sight of blood, the receiving of an injection, or being in a tunnel or on a bridge. Social phobia is a specific disorder characterized by a fear of being in social or performance situations. Also, those with panic disorder may also have agoraphobia, characterized by an intense anxiety about being in a place or situation from which they would not be able to escape in the event of a panic attack.

SYNONYMS

Simple phobia (obsolete name for specific phobia)
Phobias named for the provoking stimulus, such as arachnophobia (fear of spiders) and acrophobia (fear of heights)
Social anxiety disorder (social phobia)

ICD-9CM CODES
F40.2 Specific phobia (DSM-IV: 300.29)
F40.1 Social phobia (DSM-IV: 300.23), Agoraphobia (DSM-IV: 300.21 [with panic disorder], 300.22 [without panic disorder])

EPIDEMIOLOGY & DEMOGRAPHICS

PEAK INCIDENCE: Specific phobias are often lifelong conditions, but some of those with childhood onset (e.g., some animal phobias) tend to remit spontaneously.

PREVALENCE (IN U.S.):
- Specific phobias are prevalent in 5% to 10% of the general population.
- Social phobia is prevalent in approximately 13% of the general population.

PREDOMINANT SEX AND AGE:
- Females with specific phobias outnumber males, though rates vary according to the phobia.
- More women than men (16% vs. 11%) are affected with social phobia.
- Agoraphobia is also more prevalent in women than in men.
- Childhood is time of onset for most specific phobias.
- Situational phobias have two peaks—the first in childhood and the second in the mid-20s.
- Onset of social phobia usually occurs in the mid-teens, with onset after age 25 being unusual; this disorder is generally lifelong.

GENETICS: Both specific phobias and social phobias are more common in first-degree relatives than in the general population.

PHYSICAL FINDINGS & CLINICAL PRESENTATION

- When approaching the phobic stimulus, the experience of extreme anxiety is often accompanied by autonomic symptoms such as tachycardia, tremor, and diaphoresis; depersonalization may occur in some cases. In blood or injection phobias, these symptoms are often followed by a parasympathetic response that can cause vasovagal syncope.
- Specific phobias frequently occur with other anxiety disorders.
- Social phobias are distinguished from specific phobias in that what is feared is humiliation or embarrassment rather than a specific object or environment.

ETIOLOGY

There is no clear etiology.

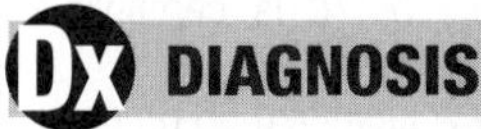

DIAGNOSIS

DIFFERENTIAL DIAGNOSIS

- Panic attacks (with or without agoraphobia): anxiety symptoms seen in specific phobia may resemble symptoms of panic attacks, but the stimulus in the specific or social phobia is clear, whereas panic attacks do not have a clearly associated provoking stimulus.
- Posttraumatic stress disorder (PTSD): anxiety and physiological arousal associated with specific cues from the traumatic event defining the PTSD may resemble the symptoms induced by a phobia.
- Generalized anxiety disorder (GAD): may be difficult to distinguish from social phobia, but in social phobia the focus is fear of embarrassment or humiliation from other people, whereas GAD has no specific focus for the worry.
- Avoidant personality disorder is often comorbid with social phobia.
- Psychotic disorders can present with a fear of being in public that arises from delusions.

WORKUP

- History: usually diagnostic. This should include information about other medical disorders, medications, any history of past trauma, and substance abuse.
- Physical examination: to confirm absence of cardiovascular abnormalities (e.g., a chronic sinus arrhythmia).

LABORATORY TESTS

No specific laboratory tests are indicated.

IMAGING STUDIES

No specific imaging studies are recommended.

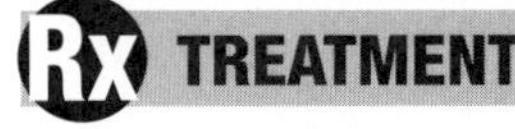

TREATMENT

NONPHARMACOLOGIC THERAPY

- Cognitive-behavioral therapy (CBT) and exposure-based treatments have been found to be effective in treating social phobia in controlled trials.
- Behavioral treatments can involve relaxation training, often paired with visualization and progressive desensitization.
- Success rates in treating specific phobias are higher when the phobia is not complicated by other anxiety disorders.

ACUTE GENERAL Rx

- Benzodiazepines provide rapid relief of anxiety associated with exposure to provoking stimuli.
- Lorazepam or alprazolam can be administered sublingually to increase the rate of absorption.
- Beta-blockers (e.g., propranolol) have been used to decrease autonomic hyperarousal and tremor associated with performance situations (e.g., before public speaking).

CHRONIC Rx

- If the phobic stimulus is rarely encountered, benzodiazepines on an as-needed basis can be an appropriate long-term treatment.
- Selective serotonin reuptake inhibitors are the most effective pharmacologic treatment in reducing symptoms and improving function for people with social phobia.
- Monoamine oxidase inhibitors also have demonstrated efficacy in the treatment of social phobia.

COMPLEMENTARY & ALTERNATIVE MEDICINE

No definitive evidence exists for complementary and alternative medicines in the treatment of phobic disorders.

DISPOSITION

Phobic disorders are generally present for life, though outpatient-based treatment may effectively reduce symptoms.

REFERRAL

Recommended for confirmation of diagnosis and for evaluation for psychotherapy and other treatment modalities.

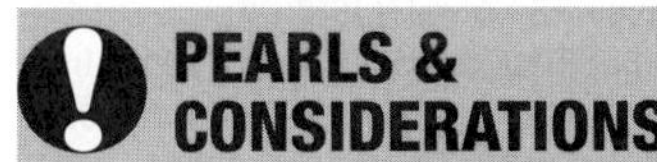

PEARLS & CONSIDERATIONS

People with social phobia often have low self-esteem and fear being scrutinized by others such that they avoid or are fearful of any situation in which others may assess or evaluate them directly or indirectly. More than half are concurrently affected by another anxiety disorder, and alcohol and other substance dependence is common because these patients often use substances to mask their anxiety.

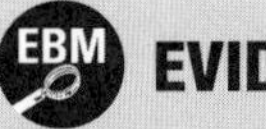

EVIDENCE

Please note: Complete text of EBM for this topic is available online.

Key trials and commentary:

Previous studies examining the relationship between specific phobia and major depression have reported mixed findings. The results of some studies have suggested that specific phobia is associated with a higher prevalence of comorbid depression, whereas others have found no association. The purpose of this study was to further examine whether specific phobia is an independent contributor to major depression by using data from the National Comorbidity Survey, a household probability sample of adults (N = 5877) aged 15 to 54 years in the U.S. After adjusting for demographic differences and comorbid mental disorders, multiple logistic regression analyses confirmed that specific phobia remains positively associated with comorbid depression (odds ratio, 1.9; 95% confidence interval, 1.6-2.4). Additional analysis found this relationship to be specific to individuals with a fear of heights, animals, and closed spaces, as well as those endorsing at least two irrational fears. These results suggest that the types and number of fears play an important role in the probability of lifetime depression.

Most of us were surprised and frankly incredulous at the finding from the National Comorbidity Study that "simple" specific phobias were associated with a significant increase in depression in later life. It just seemed that these specific phobias, which we all considered to be minor problems that could be ignored, could not be the specific risk factor that they appear to be for major depression. However, this recent reanalysis suggests that this relationship is there for people with a fear of heights, animals, and closed spaces, and for those who have two or more irrational fears. Like the article by Widom et al, this is a clear childhood identifier for future depressive problems and one that should command more of our attention.[1] Ⓐ

This study investigated whether anxiety characteristics independently predicted the onset of myocardial infarction (MI) over an average of 12.4 years and whether this relationship was independent of other psychologic variables and risk factors.

This study showed that anxiety-prone dispositions appear to be a robust and independent risk factor of MI among older men.

We have previously and continue to follow the relationship of depression to MI. However, independent factors of anxiety have not been studied. Using 735 older men without a history of coronary disease or diabetes, they were able to demonstrate that anxiety independently and prospectively predicted MI incidence. The anxiety factors they followed were psychasthenia, social introversion, phobia, and manifest anxiety. All of these increased MI incidence. The anxiety effect was separate from other variables of depression, anger, hostility, negative emotion, type A behavior, etc., and health behaviors such as smoking, drinking, etc. The findings of this article dovetail the previous trial of panic disorder seemingly being associated with increased cardiac events in women. However, we do not know if treating anxiety reduces cardiovascular events but it is certainly a question we need answered.[2] Ⓐ

A systematic review identified 36 randomized controlled trials (RCTs) that compared antidepressants with placebo in the treatment of social phobia. The review found that in 26 of the studies short-term treatment with antidepressant therapy of all classes produced significant response when compared with placebo, and that there appears to be benefit in continuing pharmacotherapy in medication responders over the longer-term.

The review found that the response to SSRIs was significantly greater compared with other classes of antidepressant.[3] Ⓐ

CBT is of benefit in the management of social phobia.

An RCT compared phenelzine (a monoamine oxidase inhibitor) to CBT group therapy, a pill placebo, and an attention placebo over a 12-week period in adults with social phobia. At 12 weeks both CBT and phenelzine were equally effective in significantly improving patient responses compared with either placebo.[4] Ⓐ

Evidence shows that exposure therapy is effective in the treatment of social phobia.

An RCT including 375 adults with social phobia compared sertraline with placebo with or without exposure therapy for 24 weeks. At the end of the trial all patients receiving active treatment showed an improved response compared with placebo, with the greatest response seen in patients receiving sertraline alone. Patients were followed up for a further 28 weeks, at which point patients receiving exposure therapy showed continued improvement, whereas some deterioration occurred in patients receiving sertraline. The study suggests that better long-term outcomes may be achieved with exposure therapy.[5] Ⓐ

A meta-analysis of 33 randomized treatment studies demonstrated the efficacy of exposure-based therapies as compared to placebo and to no treatment, and there was similar effect sizes for the variety of specific phobias that were included. Interestingly, placebo treatments were also significantly more effective than no treatment.[6] Ⓐ

Evidence-Based References

1. Choy Y et al: Specific phobia and comorbid depression: a closer look at the National Comorbidity Survey data, *Compr Psychiatry* 48:132-136, 2007. Commentary by J.C. Ballenger, M.D. Ⓐ
2. Shen B-J et al: Anxiety characteristics independently and prospectively predict myocardial infarction in men: the unique contribution of anxiety among psychologic factors. *J Am Coll Cardiol* 51:113-119, 2008. Commentary by J.C. Ballenger, M.D. Ⓐ
3. Stein DJ, et al: Pharmacotherapy for social phobia, *Cochrane Database Rev* (4), 2004.
4. Heimberg RG, et al: Cognitive behavioural group therapy vs phenelzine therapy for social phobia: 12 week outcome, *Arch Gen Psychiatry* 55:1131, 1998.
5. Haug TT et al: Exposure therapy and sertraline in social phobia: 1-year follow-up of a randomised control trial, *Br J Psychiatry* 182:312, 2003.
6. Wolitzky-Taylor KB et al: Psychological approaches in the treatment of specific phobias: a meta-analysis, *Clin Psychol Rev.* 28(6):1021, 2008. Ⓐ

SUGGESTED READINGS

Anxiety Disorders Association of America: http://www.adaa.org

Schneir FR: Clinical practice: social anxiety disorder, *N Engl J Med* 355(10):1029, 2006.

AUTHOR: **ILJIE KIM FITZGERALD, M.D., M.S.**

BASIC INFORMATION

DEFINITION

From the Latin words *pilus,* meaning hair, and *nidus,* meaning nest.

A *pilonidal sinus* is a short tract that extends from the skin surface and most likely represents a distended hair follicle. It is most commonly found in the intergluteal fold sacrococcygeal region, but it can also occur in the interdigital area, umbilicus, chest wall, and scalp. An *acute pilonidal abscess,* which consists of pus and a wall of edematous fat, results from rupture of an infected follicle into fat. A *chronic pilonidal abscess* results when an infected follicle ruptures directly into surrounding tissues; the wall of a chronic pilonidal abscess consists of fibrous tissue. A *pilonidal cyst* develops from a chronic abscess of long duration as a thin and flat lining of epithelium grows into the cavity from the skin surface.

SYNONYMS

Jeep disease

ICD-9CM CODES
685.1 Pilonidal cyst

EPIDEMIOLOGY & DEMOGRAPHICS

INCIDENCE: 26 cases per 100,000 persons
PREDOMINANT SEX: Males are more commonly affected than females (2.2:1)
AVERAGE AGE OF PRESENTATION: 21 yr
RISK FACTORS:
- Male sex
- Caucasian race
- Family predisposition
- Obesity
- Sedentary lifestyle
- Occupation requiring prolonged sitting
- Local hirsutism
- Poor hygiene
- Increased sweat activity

PHYSICAL FINDINGS & CLINICAL PRESENTATION

- May manifest as asymptomatic pits or pores in the natal cleft
- Tenderness after physical activity or prolonged sitting
- Acute pilonidal abscess in 20% of patients with pilonidal disease
- Presents as a hot, tender, fluctuant swelling just lateral to the midline over the sacrum that may exude pus through the midline pit
- Chronic pilonidal abscess in 80% of patients with pilonidal disease
- Acute suppuration, tenderness, swelling, and heat
- Infrequently, systemic reaction: occasionally fever, leukocytosis, and malaise

ETIOLOGY

- Currently believed to be acquired rather than congenital.
- Drilling of hair shed from the perineum or the head into sebaceous or hair follicles in the natal cleft.
- Drilling is facilitated by the friction of the natal cleft.
- Subsequent infection by skin organisms leads to pilonidal abscess.

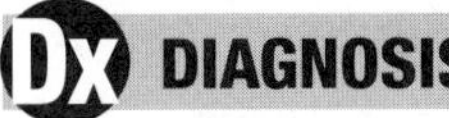

DIAGNOSIS

DIFFERENTIAL DIAGNOSIS

- Perianal abscess arising from the posterior midline crypt
- Hidradenitis suppurativa
- Carbuncle
- Furuncle
- Osteomyelitis
- Anal fistula
- Coccygeal sinus

WORKUP

- Diagnosis is based on history and physical examination.
- Midline pits present behind the anus overlying the sacrum and coccyx.
- Broken hairs are often seen extruding from the midline pits.
- Insert probe in pilonidal sinus in path away from the anus.
- Complicated anal fistula may be angulating posteriorly before passing into a retrorectal abscess, but thorough examination of the anal cavity usually discloses point of origin.

LABORATORY TESTS

Complete blood count

IMAGING STUDIES

CT scan in advanced, recurrent cases

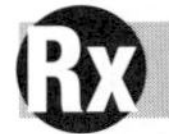

TREATMENT

NONPHARMACOLOGIC THERAPY

Prevention of exacerbations:
1. Local hygiene
2. Avoidance of prolonged sitting position
3. Weight reduction

ACUTE GENERAL Rx

- Procedure of choice for first-episode acute abscess: simple incision and drainage in an outpatient setting
- Cure rate of 76% after 18 mo
- Antibiotics: generally not indicated unless the patient has a medical condition such as rheumatic heart disease or is immunosuppressed

CHRONIC Rx

Elective treatment of pilonidal disease:
1. Minimal surgery:
   a. Remove hair from midline pits and shave buttocks.
   b. May use a fine wire brush with local anesthesia to clear the pits and any lateral openings of granulation tissue and hair.
   c. Keep area clean.
2. Fistulotomy and curettage:
   a. Used when minimal surgery does not control episodes of suppuration
   b. Pass probe to outline the pilonidal sinus and open tract surgically
   c. Curette granulation tissue at the base of the sinus and excise edges of the skin
   d. Keep open granulating wound meticulously clean and allow to heal
   e. If complete healing does not take place, use a skin graft or advancement flap to close the defect
3. Marsupialization:
   a. This is the treatment of choice for chronic pilonidal disease.
   b. Wide excision of the pilonidal area is performed, including all affected skin and subcutaneous tissues down to the presacral fascia.
   c. Wound is left open, allowed to marsupialize, or closed as a primary procedure.
   d. Give antibiotics for 24 hr (particularly those directed against *Staphylococcus* and *Bacteroides* species).
4. Other procedures:
   a. Excision and closure
   b. Excision and skin grafting
   c. Bascom procedure (follicle removal and lateral drainage)
   d. Flaps: *Z*-plasty, V-Y advancement flap, rhomboid flap, gluteus maximus myocutaneous flap

DISPOSITION

- Recurrence rate for excision (most definitive procedure): 1% to 6%
- Incidence of squamous cell carcinoma in a chronic, recurrent pilonidal sinus is rare <1%

REFERRAL

- Emergency department for incision and drainage for an acute abscess
- To a surgeon for elective treatment or management of chronic or recurrent disease

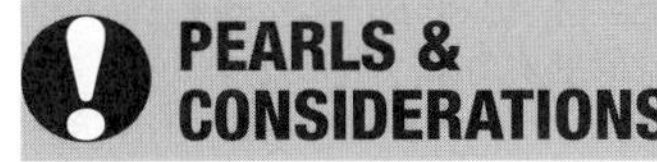

PEARLS & CONSIDERATIONS

COMMENTS

Because of significant associated morbidity, the elective surgical procedures outlined are performed only after the potential risks versus benefits are carefully weighed.

SUGGESTED READINGS

Church JM: Pilonidal cyst: cause and treatment, *Dis Colon Rectum* 43(8):1146, 2000.

Hull TL, Wu J: Pilonidal disease, *Surg Clin North Am* 82(6):1169, 2002.

AUTHORS: **ARUNDATHI G. PRASAD, M.D.,** and **RUBEN ALVERO, M.D.**

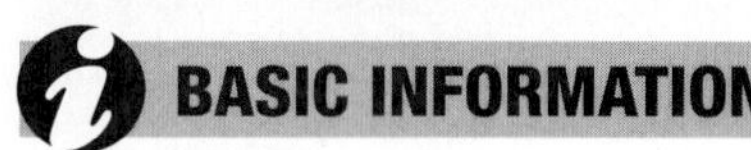

BASIC INFORMATION

DEFINITION

Pinworms are a noninvasive infestation of the intestinal tract by *Enterobius vermicularis,* a helminth of the nematode family.

SYNONYMS

Enterobiasis

ICD-9CM CODES
127.4 Enterobiasis

EPIDEMIOLOGY & DEMOGRAPHICS

- Most common intestinal nematode; approximately 30,000 cases annually in the U.S.
- Worldwide distribution, but most common in temperate climates.
- The prevalence of pinworm infection is lowest in infants and reaches highest infection rate in school-age children (ages 5 to 14 yr).
- Eggs are infective within 6 hr of oviposition and may remain so for 20 days.
- Clusters are found in families, institutionalized persons, and homosexual men.

PHYSICAL FINDINGS & CLINICAL PRESENTATION

- Most infested persons are asymptomatic.
- Perianal itching is the most common reported symptom, with scratching leading to excoriation and sometimes secondary infection.
- Rarely insomnia, irritability, anorexia, and weight loss are described.
- Granulomas have been described in various organs resulting from worms wandering outside the intestines and dying there.

ETIOLOGY & PATHOGENESIS

- *E. vermicularis* is highly prevalent throughout the world, particularly in countries of the temperate zone. Human beings are the only host for this worm. Infestation is by fecal–oral route; ingested eggs hatch in the stomach and the larvae migrate to the colon, where they mature. Gravid female worms containing an average of 10,000 ova migrate to the perianal skin at night, lay their eggs there, and die. The eggs embryonate within 6 hr and cause itching; scratching causes egg deposition under fingernails, from which they can contaminate food or lead to autoreinfection.
- *E. vermicularis* may be transmitted between sexual partners, especially those engaging in oral–anal sex.

Dx DIAGNOSIS

DIFFERENTIAL DIAGNOSIS

- Perianal itching related to poor hygiene
- Hemorrhoidal disease and anal fissures
- Perineal yeast/fungal infections

Section II describes the causes of pruritus ani.

WORKUP

Identification of adult worms or eggs. *E. vermicularis* ova are ovoid but flattened on one side and measure approximately 56 × 27 micrometers (Fig. 1-246). The eggs can be identified on transparent tape placed on the perianal skin on awakening. (NOTE: Five consecutive negative tests rule out the diagnosis.) A single examination detects 50% of infections, three examinations detect 90%, and five examinations detect 99%.

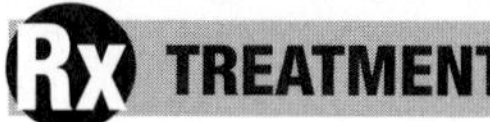

Rx TREATMENT

- Single dose of mebendazole (100 mg) with a repeat dose given after 2 wk.
- Single dose of albendazole (400 mg) with a second dose given 2 wk later is also highly effective.
- Pyrantel pamoate (11 mg/kg up to 1 g) can prevent against *E. vermicularis.* It is available as a suspension and has minimal toxicity (mild transient gastrointestinal symptoms, headache, drowsiness). A repeat dose after 2 wk is recommended because of the frequency of reinfection and autoinfection.
- Other infected family members, classmates, or residents of long-term care facilities should be treated at the same time as the index case.

SUGGESTED READING

Lohiya GS et al: Epidemiology and control of enterobiasis in a developmental center, *West J Med* 172: 305-308, 2000.

AUTHOR: **FRED F. FERRI, M.D.**

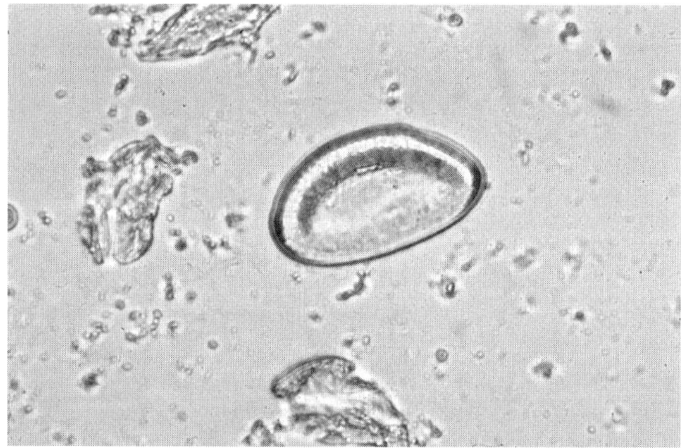

FIGURE 1-246 Enterobius vermicularis embryonated egg. Note larva inside (40 × 10 μm). (From Gorbach SL et al [eds]: *Infectious diseases,* ed 2, Philadelphia, 1998, WB Saunders.)

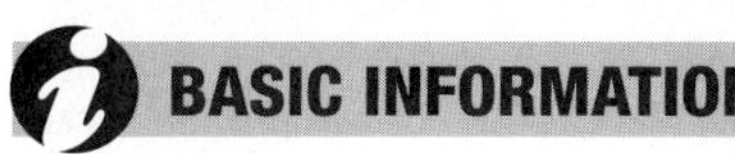

DEFINITION

Pituitary adenoma is a benign neoplasm of the anterior lobe of the pituitary that causes symptoms, either by excess secretion of hormones or by a local mass effect as the tumor impinges on other, nearby structures (e.g., optic chiasm, hypothalamus, pituitary stalk). Pituitary adenomas are classified by their size, function, and features that characterize their appearance. Microadenomas are <10 mm in size, and macroadenomas are ≥10 mm in size.

- *Acromegaly* is the disease state characterized by a pituitary adenoma that secretes growth hormone (GH).
- A *prolactinoma* secretes prolactin (PRL).
- *Cushing's disease* is a disease state of hypersecretion of adrenocorticotropic hormone (ACTH).
- *Thyrotropin-secreting pituitary adenomas* secrete primarily thyroid-stimulating hormone (TSH).
- *Nonsecretory pituitary adenomas* are those in which the neoplasm is a space-occupying lesion whose secretory products do not cause a specific disease state.

ICD-9CM CODES
253 Pituitary adenoma
253.0 Acromegaly
253.1 Prolactinoma

EPIDEMIOLOGY & DEMOGRAPHICS

CLASSIFICATION (BY HORMONE SECRETED):
- PRL only: 35%
- No hormone: 30%
- GH only: 20%
- PRL and GH: 7%
- ACTH: 7%
- Luteinizing hormone (LH), follicle-stimulating hormone (FSH), TSH: 1%

PREVALENCE/INCIDENCE:
- Pituitary adenomas: up to 10% to 15% of all intracranial neoplasms; 3% to 27% at autopsy series
- Prolactinomas: up to 20% in women with unexplained primary or secondary amenorrhea
- GH-secreting pituitary adenoma: 50 to 60 cases per 1 million persons
- Thyrotropin-secreting pituitary adenoma: 2.8% of pituitary adenomas with a slight female/male predominance of 1.7:1
- Corticotropin-secreting pituitary adenomas: female/male predominance of 8:1

PHYSICAL FINDINGS & CLINICAL PRESENTATION

PROLACTINOMAS:
- Females:
  1. Galactorrhea
  2. Amenorrhea
  3. Oligomenorrhea with anovulation
  4. Infertility
  5. Estrogen deficiency leading to hirsutism
  6. Decreased vaginal lubrication
  7. Osteopenia
- Males:
  1. Large tumors more common as a result of delayed diagnosis
  2. Possible impotence, decreased libido, or hypogonadism
  3. Galactorrhea rare because males lack the estrogen-dependent breast growth and differentiation

GH-SECRETING PITUITARY ADENOMA: ACROMEGALY
- Coarse facial features
- Oily skin
- Prognathism
- Carpal tunnel syndrome
- Osteoarthritis
- History of increased hat, glove, or shoe size
- Decreased exercise capacity
- Visual field deficits
- Diabetes mellitus

CORTICOTROPIN-SECRETING PITUITARY ADENOMA: CUSHING'S DISEASE
- Usually present when the tumor is small (1 to 2 mm)
- 50% of the tumors <5 mm
- Other symptoms:
  1. Truncal obesity
  2. Round facies (moon face)
  3. Dorsocervical fat accumulation (buffalo hump)
  4. Hirsutism
  5. Acne
  6. Menstrual disorders
  7. Hypertension
  8. Striae
  9. Bruising
  10. Thin skin
  11. Hyperglycemia

THYROTROPIN-SECRETING PITUITARY ADENOMA:
- In males, larger, more invasive, and more rapidly growing tumors that present later in life
- Other symptoms: thyrotoxicosis, goiter, visual impairment

NONSECRETORY PITUITARY ADENOMAS (ENDOCRINE INACTIVE PITUITARY ADENOMA):
- Usually large at the time of diagnosis
- Symptoms:
  1. Bitemporal hemianopsia as a result of compression of the optic chiasm
  2. Hypopituitarism from compression of the pituitary gland
  3. Hypogonadism in men and in premenopausal women
  4. Cranial nerve deficits caused by extension into the cavernous sinus
  5. Hydrocephalus from extension into the third ventricle, compressing the foramen of Monro
  6. Diabetes insipidus resulting from compression of the hypothalamus or pituitary stalk (a rare complication)

ETIOLOGY

Benign neoplasms of epithelial origin

Dx DIAGNOSIS

DIFFERENTIAL DIAGNOSIS

PROLACTINOMA:
- Pregnancy
- Postpartum puerperium
- Primary hypothyroidism
- Breast disease
- Breast stimulation
- Drug ingestion (especially phenothiazines, antidepressants, haloperidol, methyldopa, reserpine, opiates, amphetamines, and cimetidine)
- Chronic renal failure
- Liver disease
- Polycystic ovarian disease
- Chest wall disorders
- Spinal cord lesions
- Previous cranial irradiation

ACROMEGALY: Ectopic production of GH-releasing hormone from a carcinoid or other neuroendocrine tumor

CUSHING'S DISEASE:
- Diseases that cause ectopic sources of ACTH overproduction (including small-cell carcinoma of the lung, bronchial carcinoid, intestinal carcinoid, pancreatic islet cell tumor, medullary thyroid carcinoma, or pheochromocytoma)
- Adrenal adenomas, adrenal carcinoma
- Nelson's syndrome

THYROTROPIN-SECRETNG PITUITARY ADENOMAS: Primary hypothyroidism

NONSECRETORY PITUITARY ADENOMA: Nonneoplastic mass lesions of various etiologies (e.g., infectious, granulomatous)

WORKUP

See Section III, "Pituitary Tumor".

PROLACTINOMA:
First step: measurement of basal PRL levels
- Elevated PRL levels are correlated with tumor size.
- Level >200 ng/ml is diagnostic, with levels of 100 to 200 ng/ml being equivocal.
- Basal PRL levels between 20 and 100 suggest a microadenoma as well as other conditions such as psychotropic drug ingestion, recent breast examination, and even a recent meal.
- Basal level <20 ng/ml is usually considered normal.
- Prolactin normative data should be developed by each institution for its population.
- Threshold level for obtaining imaging such as MRI should be developed by individual providers depending on the level of specificity and sensitivity desired.

ACROMEGALY:
- First screening tests are the measurement of the serum insulin-like growth factor I level, postprandial serum GH, and TRH stimulation test.
- Follow with an oral glucose tolerance test.
- Failure to suppress serum GH to <2 ng/ml with an oral load of 100 g glucose is considered conclusive.
- A GH-releasing hormone level >300 ng/ml is indicative of an ectopic source of GH.

CUSHING'S DISEASE:
- Normal or slightly elevated corticotropin levels ranging from 20 to 200 pg/ml; normal is 10 to 50 pg/ml (normative data should be developed by each institution for its population).
- Level <10 pg/ml usually indicates an autonomously secreting adrenal tumor.
- Level >200 pg/ml suggests an ectopic corticotropin-secreting neoplasm.
- Cushing's disease is confirmed by demonstration of low-dose dexamethasone, which shows presence of abnormal cortisol suppressibility.
- 24-hr urine collection should demonstrate an increased level of cortisol excretion.

THYROTROPIN-SECRETING PITUITARY ADENOMA:
- Highly sensitive thyrotropin assays, which evaluate the presence of thyrotoxicosis, are one way to detect a thyrotropin-secreting tumor.
- Free alpha subunit is secreted by >80% of tumors, with the ratio of the alpha subunit to thyrotropin <1.
- With central resistance to thyroid hormone, ratio is <1 and the sella is normal.
- Laboratory tests show elevated serum levels of both T_3 and T_4.

NONSECRETORY PITUITARY ADENOMA:
- Visual field testing
- Assessment of the pituitary and organ function to determine if there is hypopituitarism or hypersecretion of hormones (even if the effects of hypersecretion are subclinical)
- TRH to provoke secretion of FSH, LH, and LH-beta-subunit; will not elicit response in normal persons
- Exclusion of Klinefelter's syndrome in patient with longstanding primary hypogonadism, elevated gonadotropin levels, and enlargement of the sella

IMAGING STUDIES

Study of choice: MRI of the pituitary and hypothalamus
- When evaluating Cushing's disease, small size at the onset of symptoms noted
- MRI, in this case, only 60% sensitive at best and may yield false-positive results
- CT scan only when MRI is unavailable or is otherwise contraindicated

Rx TREATMENT

NONPHARMACOLOGIC THERAPY

SURGERY:
- Selective transsphenoidal resection of the adenoma is the treatment of choice for acromegaly, Cushing's disease, and thyrotropin-secreting pituitary adenomas, all of which tend to be microadenomas at the time of onset of symptoms.
- Macroadenomas, such as the nonsecretory pituitary adenoma, may also be surgically removed, but risk of recurrence is greater with these tumors and adjunctive therapy such as irradiation may also be necessary.
- Radiotherapy is reserved for patients who have not responded to surgical treatment and who still have symptoms of the adenoma.
- Bilateral adrenalectomy has been performed in patients with Cushing's disease after failure of other therapies; complications requiring lifelong hormone replacement or Nelson's syndrome may occur.

RADIOTHERAPY:
- Generally reserved for patients who have not responded to surgical treatment
- Used with varying degrees of success in all the different pituitary adenomas

ACUTE GENERAL Rx

PROLACTINOMA:
- Bromocriptine, a dopamine analog, is generally given orally in divided doses of 1.5 to 10 mg.
- Side effects include orthostatic hypotension, nausea, and dizziness; avoided by beginning with low-dose therapy.
- Other compounds include pergolide mesylate, a long-acting ergot derivative with dopaminergic properties, as well as other nonergot derivatives.

ACROMEGALY:
- Octreotide, a somatostatin analog, 100 mcg SC, is the medical therapy of choice but is limited by side effects such as biliary sludge and gallstones, nausea, cramps, steatorrhea, and its parenteral administration.
- Bromocriptine 10 to 20 mg PO tid to qid is less effective than octreotide but has the advantage of oral administration.

CUSHING'S DISEASE:
- Ketoconazole, which inhibits the cytochrome P-450 enzymes involved in steroid biosynthesis, is effective in managing mild to moderate disease in daily oral doses of 600 to 1200 mg.
- Metyrapone and aminoglutethimide can be used to control hypersecretion of cortisol but are generally used when preparing a patient for surgery or while waiting for a response to radiotherapy.

THYROTROPIN-SECRETING PITUITARY ADENOMA:
- Ablative therapy with either radioactive iodide or surgery is indicated.
- Treatment directed to the thyroid alone may accelerate growth of the pituitary adenoma.
- Octreotide has been shown to be effective in doses similar to those used for acromegaly.

NONSECRETORY PITUITARY ADENOMA:
- There is no role for medical therapy at this time.
- Surgery and radiotherapy are indicated.

CHRONIC Rx

For all pituitary adenomas:
- Careful follow-up is important. Patients undergoing transsphenoidal microsurgical resection should be seen in 4 to 6 wk to ensure that the adenoma has been completely removed and that the endocrine hypersecretion is resolved.
- If there is good clinical response, patient should be monitored yearly for recurrence and to follow the level of the hypersecreted hormone.
- Patients who have undergone irradiation should have close follow-up with backup medical therapy because response to radiotherapy may be delayed; incidence of hypopituitarism also increases with time.

EBM EVIDENCE

Please note: Complete text of EBM for this topic is available online.

Key trials and commentary:

The objective of this study was to evaluate the short-term efficacy of the novel multireceptor ligand somatostatin analog pasireotide in patients with de novo, persistent, or recurrent Cushing's disease.

This study showed that Pasireotide produced a decrease in UFC levels in 76% of patients with Cushing's disease during the treatment period of 15 days, with direct effects on ACTH release. These results suggest that pasireotide holds promise as an effective medical treatment for this disorder.

Pituitary surgery is typically the first-line treatment for Cushing's disease. There is currently no effective medical treatment that acts centrally to modulate ACTH overproduction from these pituitary tumors. Using pasireotide (SOM230), a novel, nonspecific somatostatin receptor agonist, these authors participated in a phase II trial looking at the safety and efficacy of treating Cushing's disease patients with 600 μg sq bid for 15 days. 76% of the patients showed a reduction in the UFC levels, with 17% resulting in normalization of their UFC level within the 2 weeks of treatment. It is interesting to note that patients needed to have UFCs twice the upper limit of normal to be included in this study. The rigorous entry criteria may have resulted in a decreased number of patients that completely normalized their UFCs, because the initial UFC was quite elevated. This drug particularly may have a potential role in treating patients with recurrence of Cushing's disease (who often present with low-grade disease) rather than de novo disease. This study suggests that pasireotide (SOM230) may ultimately play an important role in the treatment algorithm of Cushing's disease.[1] Ⓐ

Evidence-Based Reference

1. Boscaro M et al: Treatment of pituitary-dependent Cushing's Disease with the multireceptor ligand somatostatin analog pasireotide (SOM230): a multicenter, phase II trial, *J Clin Endocrinol Metab* 94:115-122, 2009. Commentary by W.H. Ludlam, M.D., Ph.D. Ⓐ

SUGGESTED READINGS

Davis AK et al: Pituitary tumors, *Reproduction* 121(3):363, 2001.

Kovacs K et al: Classification of pituitary adenomas, *J Neurooncol* 54(2):121, 2001.

AUTHORS: **BETH J. WUTZ, M.D.**, and **RUBEN ALVERO, M.D.**

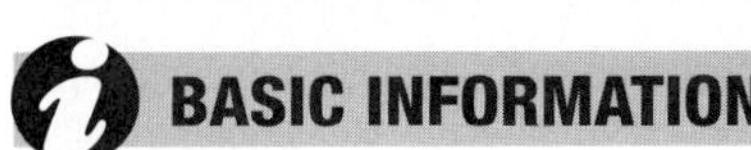

BASIC INFORMATION

DEFINITION

Pityriasis is a common self-limiting skin eruption of unknown etiology.

ICD-9CM CODES
696.3 Pityriasis rosea

EPIDEMIOLOGY & DEMOGRAPHICS

- Most cases of pityriasis rosea occur between ages 10 and 35 yr; mean age is 23 yr.
- The incidence of disease is highest in the fall and spring.
- Female/male ratio is 1.5:1.

PHYSICAL FINDINGS & CLINICAL PRESENTATION

- Initial lesion (herald patch) precedes the eruption by approximately 1 to 2 wk; typically measures 3 to 6 cm; it is round to oval in appearance and most frequently located on the trunk.
- Eruptive phase follows within 2 wk and peaks after 7 to 14 days.
- Lesions are most frequently located in the lower abdominal area. They have a salmon-pink appearance in whites and a hyperpigmented appearance in blacks.
- Most lesions are 4 to 5 mm in diameter; center has a "cigarette paper" appearance; border has a characteristic ring of scale (collarette).
- Lesions occur in a symmetric distribution and follow the cleavage lines of the trunk (Christmas tree pattern [Fig. 1-247]).
- The number of lesions varies from a few to hundreds.
- Most patients are asymptomatic; pruritus is the most common symptom.
- History of recent fatigue, headache, sore throat, and low-grade fever is present in approximately 25% of cases.

ETIOLOGY

Unknown, possibly viral (picornavirus)

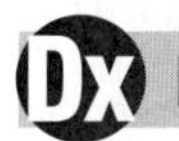

DIAGNOSIS

DIFFERENTIAL DIAGNOSIS

- Tinea corporis (can be ruled out by potassium hydroxide examination)
- Secondary syphilis (absence of herald patch, positive serologic test for syphilis)
- Psoriasis
- Nummular eczema
- Drug eruption: medications that may cause rashes similar to pityriasis rosea include clonidine, captopril, interferon, bismuth, barbiturates, gold, hepatitis B vaccine, and imatinib mesylate
- Viral exanthem
- Eczema
- Lichen planus
- Tinea versicolor (the lesions are more brown and the borders are not as ovoid)

WORKUP

Presence of herald lesion and characteristic rash are diagnostic. Skin biopsy is generally reserved for atypical cases.

LABORATORY TESTS

Generally not necessary; serologic test for syphilis if clinically indicated

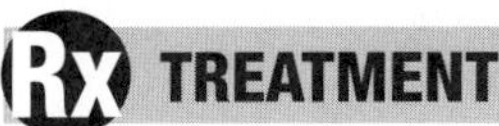

TREATMENT

NONPHARMACOLOGIC THERAPY

The disease is self-limited and generally does not require any therapeutic intervention.

ACUTE GENERAL Rx

- Use calamine lotion or oral antihistamines in patients with significant pruritus.
- Use prednisone tapered over 2 wk in patients with severe pruritus.
- Direct sun exposure or use of ultraviolet light within the first week of eruption is beneficial in decreasing the severity of disease.

DISPOSITION

- Spontaneous complete resolution of the rash within 4 to 8 wk
- Recurrence rare (<2% of cases)

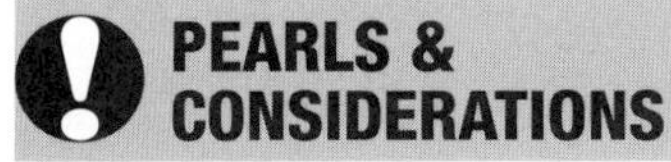

PEARLS & CONSIDERATIONS

COMMENTS

Reassure patient that the disease is not contagious and its course is benign.

SUGGESTED READING

Stulberg D, Wolfrey J: Pityriasis rosea, *Am Fam Physician* 69:87, 2004.

AUTHOR: **FRED F. FERRI, M.D.**

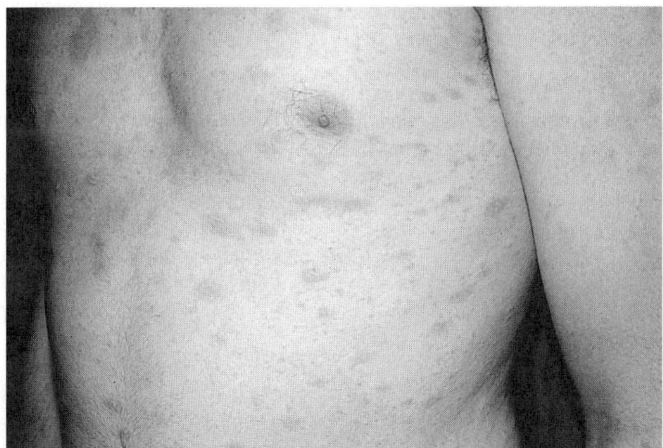

FIGURE 1-247 Scale (pityriasis rosea). Shows example of how unique scaling (collarette of fine scale within several lesions), distribution and shape of lesions (oval lesions with long axis paralleling natural skin cleavage lines), and color (salmon-pink) help in diagnosing skin disease. (From Noble J [ed]: *Textbook of primary care medicine,* ed 3, St Louis, 2001, Mosby.)

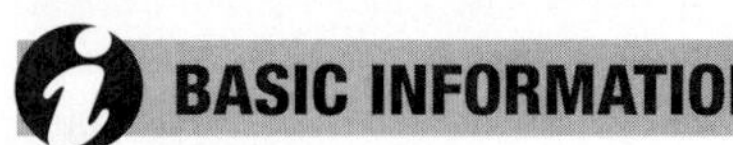

BASIC INFORMATION

DEFINITION

Placenta previa is the implantation of the placenta over the internal os. Four degrees of this abnormality have been defined:

1. Total placenta previa: the internal os is covered completely.
2. Partial placenta previa: the internal os is partially covered.
3. Marginal placenta previa: the edge of the placenta is at the margin of the internal os.
4. Low-lying placenta: the placenta is implanted in the lower uterine segment and, although its edge does not reach the internal os, is in close proximity to it (Fig. 1-248).

ICD-9CM CODES
641.1 Placenta previa

EPIDEMIOLOGY & DEMOGRAPHICS

INCIDENCE: 0.26% to 0.7% of pregnancies

RISK FACTORS:

- Previous cesarean delivery (after one cesarean delivery, the risk is 1% to 4%; after four or more, the risk approaches 10%).
- Multiparity has also been associated with placenta previa.

PHYSICAL FINDINGS & CLINICAL PRESENTATION

The classic presentation of placenta previa is painless vaginal bleeding, usually in the second or third trimester. Uterine contractions may or may not be present. On physical examination, the uterus is soft and pain free. The fetus is often in breech, transverse lie, or high. Fetal distress is usually not present.

ETIOLOGY

Uncertain

DIAGNOSIS

DIFFERENTIAL DIAGNOSIS

- Placenta accreta
- Placenta percreta
- Placenta increta
- Vasa previa
- Abruptio placentae
- Vaginal or cervical trauma
- Labor
- Local malignancy

WORKUP

- Do *not* perform a digital vaginal examination.
- The diagnosis of placenta previa can seldom be firmly established by physical examination alone. A speculum examination in a hospital setting to exclude any local bleeding may be performed.
- This diagnosis should not be dismissed until thorough evaluation, including sonography, has completely excluded its presence.

LABORATORY TESTS

- A complete blood count can be used to monitor hemoglobin and hematocrit
- A Kleihauer-Betke preparation of maternal blood in all Rh-negative women and Rh-immune globulin when indicated

IMAGING STUDIES

- The simplest, most precise, and safest method of placental localization is transabdominal sonography with confirmatory imaging by transvaginal ultrasonography. Transperineal sonography has also proven effective in detection. A distance of $\leq$20 mm from placental edge to interior cervical os is becoming a new criterion for performing term cesarean delivery in women with placenta previa.
- MRI has also been effective in detecting placenta previa, although sonography remains the preferred method.

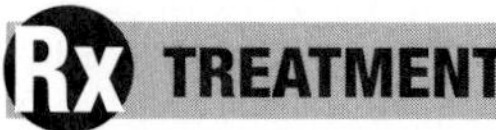

TREATMENT

NONPHARMACOLOGIC THERAPY

- In preterm pregnancies with no active bleeding, close observation and expectant management are indicated. In those with active bleeding, conservative management, including blood transfusions for severe bleeds, is appropriate. The woman should stay in the hospital for at least 48 hr after the bleeding has stopped.
- Bed rest, preferably in a hospital setting, should be prescribed.

ACUTE GENERAL Rx

- Initial assessment for signs of maternal hemodynamic compromise or hemorrhagic shock; large-bore IV access with crystalloid fluid resuscitation
- Assess fetal status and gestational age by sonogram and continuous fetal heart rate monitoring
- Cross-matched blood should be made available during bleeding episodes; if the hemorrhage is severe, cesarean delivery is indicated despite fetal immaturity
- Tocolytic therapy may be considered in those women in preterm labor, as well as the administration of corticosteroids to enhance fetal lung maturity

CHRONIC Rx

- Cesarean delivery is necessary in nearly all cases of placenta previa.
- Uncontrollable hemorrhage after placental removal should be anticipated as a result of the poorly contractile nature of the lower uterine segment. The need for hysterectomy to control bleeding should be discussed with the patient before delivery, if possible.

DISPOSITION

Because of the unpredictable nature of placenta previa, not all women with placenta previa can be treated expectantly.

REFERRAL

Affected women and their families should be aware of all signs and symptoms that would necessitate immediate transport to the hospital. The possibility of hysterectomy should also be discussed early during pregnancy.

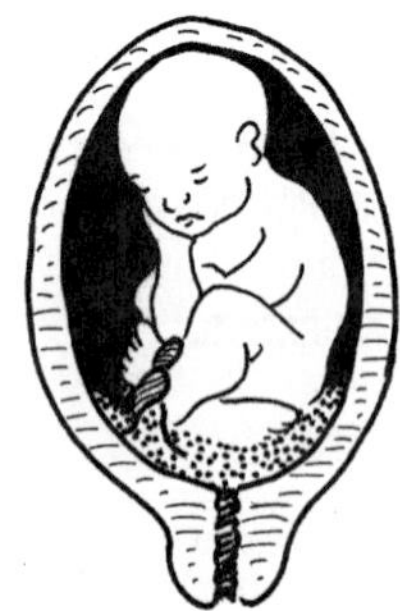

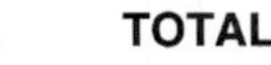

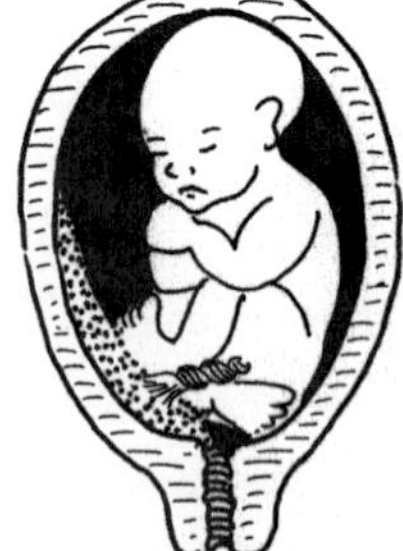

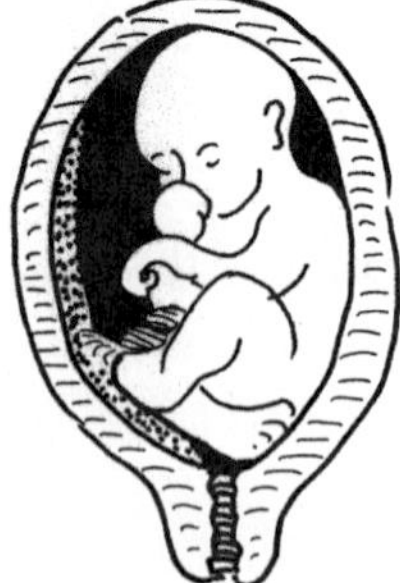

FIGURE 1-248 Various types of placenta previa. A, The cervical os is completely covered by placenta. **B,** The cervical os is partially covered by placenta. **C,** The placenta extends to the edge of the cervical os. (From Rakel RE: *Textbook of family practice*, ed 6, Philadelphia, 2002, WB Saunders.)

SUGGESTED READING

Vergani P et al: Placenta previa: distance to interval os and mode of delivery, *Am J Obstet Gynecol* 201:266, 2009.

AUTHORS: **SONYA S. ABDEL-RAZEQ, M.D.,** and **RUBEN ALVERO, M.D.**

BASIC INFORMATION

DEFINITION

Plantar fasciitis is a common, painful inflammation or degeneration of the plantar fascia, a tissue that extends from the calcaneus to the proximal phalanges of each toe.

SYNONYMS

Painful heel syndrome
Painful heel spur

ICD-9CM CODES
728.71 Plantar fasciitis
726.73 Calcaneal spur

EPIDEMIOLOGY & DEMOGRAPHICS

PREDOMINANT SEX: Males and females affected equally

PREDOMINANT AGE:

- Middle age
- Bilateral in 10% to 20% of cases
- The condition is more likely to occur in persons who are obese and in those who are on their feet most of the day

PHYSICAL FINDINGS & CLINICAL PRESENTATION

- Pain is characteristically worse on arising and after periods of rest; warming up often lessens the pain
- Local tenderness at site involvement, usually the medial tubercle of the calcaneus, sometimes in the midfascia
- Pain sometimes elicited by passive dorsiflexion of toes and ankle, which stretches the plantar fascia
- A tight heel cord may be present

ETIOLOGY

- Uncertain.
- Inflammation, microscopic tears, and/or degeneration.
- The role of the calcaneal traction osteophyte (spur) is unclear. The rate of plantar fascial pain appears unrelated to the occurrence or presence of a calcaneal osteophyte.
- May be associated with tight heel cord.

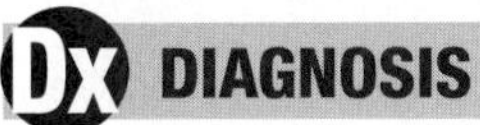

DIAGNOSIS

DIFFERENTIAL DIAGNOSIS

- Other regional tendonitis
- Stress fracture
- Tarsal tunnel syndrome
- Tumor, infection

IMAGING STUDIES

Traction osteophyte or minor soft tissue calcification may be present on plain radiography. Other studies are usually not required.

TREATMENT

- Sensible activity restriction
- Gentle stretching exercises
- NSAIDs
- Local steroid or lidocaine injections (Fig. 1-249)
- Heel lift. Foot orthoses produce small short-term benefits in function and may also produce small reductions in pain for people with plantar fasciitis, but they do not have long-term beneficial effects.
- Extracorporeal shock wave therapy may effectively treat runners with chronic heel pain but is ineffective in other patients
- Night brace, daytime cast brace

DISPOSITION

Disorder is usually self-limited, although full recovery may take 1 to 2 yr.

REFERRAL

- If symptoms fail to respond to medical management
- For surgical consideration (plantar fascia release, excision of osteophyte)

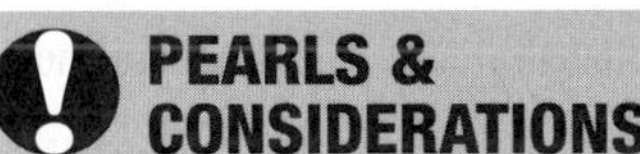

PEARLS & CONSIDERATIONS

Fasciitis may be a misnomer. Inflammation is usually not present on pathologic evaluation of tissue samples in most cases. Tendinosis may be a more proper term. Involvement of the plantar fascia and/or heel cord insertion in the spondyloarthropathies (enthesitis, enthesopathy) is a common association.

COMMENTS

- Various cushions and heel cups are generally ineffective because stretching, not heel strikes, is probably the cause of the disorder.
- Surgical intervention is rarely necessary.
- Shock wave therapy is of unproven benefit.

SUGGESTED READINGS

Aldridge J: Diagnosing heel pain in adults, *Am Fam Physician* 70:332, 2004.

Bachbinder R: Plantar fasciitis, *N Engl J Med* 350:2159, 2004.

Chinn L, Hertel J: Rehabilitation of ankle and foot injuries in athletes, *Clin Sports Med* 29:157, 2010.

Cole C, Seto C, Gazewood J: Plantar fasciitis: evidence-based review of diagnosis and therapy, *Am Fam Physician* 72:2237, 2005.

Cosca DD, Navazio F: Common problems in endurance athletes, *Am Fam Physician* 76:237, 2007.

Flanigan RM et al: The influence of foot position on stretching of the plantar fascia, *Foot Ankle Int* 28(7):815, 2007.

Fredericson M, Misra AK: Epidemiology and aetiology of marathon running injuries, *Sports Med* 37:437, 2007.

Furia JP: The safety and efficacy of high energy extracorporeal shock wave therapy in active, moderately active and sedentary patients with chronic plantar fasciitis, *Orthopedics* 28:685, 2005.

Khoury V et al: Ultrasound of ankle and foot: overuse and sports injuries, *Semin Musculoskeletal Radiol* 11:149, 2007.

Landorf KB et al: Effectiveness of foot orthoses to treat plantar fasciitis, *Arch Intern Med* 166:1305, 2006.

Neufeld SK, Cerrato R: Plantar fasciitis: evaluation the treatment. *J Am Acad Orthop Surg* 16:338, 2008.

Walls RJ et al: Overuse ankle injuries in professional Irish dancers, *Foot Ankle Surg* 16:45, 2010.

AUTHOR: **LONNIE R. MERCIER, M.D.**

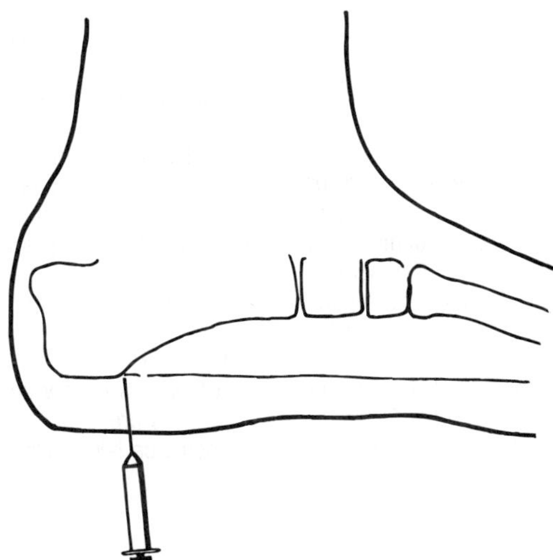

FIGURE 1-249 Injection site for plantar fasciitis. Injection should be through the sole into the area of maximum tenderness. A 25- or 27-gauge needle should be used and the medication injected slowly because some pain may occur. The total volume should be no greater than 1.5 ml. (From Mercier L: *Practical orthopedics*, ed 5, St Louis, 2002, Mosby.)

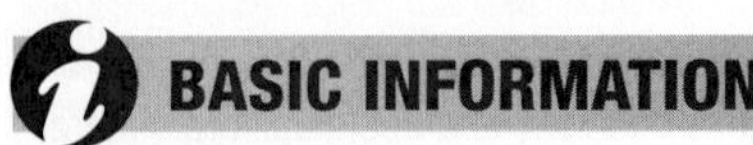

BASIC INFORMATION

DEFINITION

Pleurisy refers to the inflammation of the parietal pleural. This inflammation results in pleuritic chest pain which is characteristically worsened with respiration or movement.

SYNONYMS

Pleuritis

ICD-9CM CODES

511.0 Pleurisy

EPIDEMIOLOGY & DEMOGRAPHICS

INCIDENCE: There are a variety of disorders that may result in pleurisy. Infectious diseases, rheumatologic disorders, thromboembolic events, and trauma may all lead to pleural inflammation. Therefore, the incidence of pleurisy varies in accordance with the underlying etiology.

PHYSICAL FINDINGS & CLINICAL PRESENTATION

- The defining characteristic of pleurisy is chest pain that worsens with respiration, coughing, or sneezing.
- Chest pain is typically described as sharp or stabbing. However, pleurisy may be described as dull pain, burning pain, or a "catch" while breathing.
- Movements of the trunk or chest wall typically exacerbate pain. Many patients may locate the position of minimal discomfort and remain still in that position.
- Dyspnea may be associated with pleurisy.
- Physical exam may be remarkable for a pleural friction rub.
- Decreased breath sounds, rales, or egophony may be appreciated if pneumonia is the underlying etiology of the patient's pleurisy.

ETIOLOGY

- Pleurisy is caused by inflammation of the parietal pleura. The visceral pleura is not innervated by nociceptors. However, injury or inflammation at the periphery of the lung parenchyma often results in inflammation of the overlying parietal pleura. The parietal pleura, which lines the rib cage and the lateral portion of each hemidiaphragm, is innervated by intercostal nerves; therefore pain is localized to the cutaneous distribution of those nerves (over the chest wall). The parietal pleural of the central diaphragm is innervated by fibers that travel with the phrenic nerve; therefore pain associated with inflammation in this area is referred to the ipsilateral shoulder or neck.
- Various underlying etiologies may result in pleurisy, including:
  1. Thromboembolism (pulmonary embolism)
  2. Viral infection (coxsackie viruses, RSV, CMV, adenovirus, EBV, parainfluenza, influenza)
  3. Bacterial infection (pneumonia or tuberculous pleuritis)
  4. Fungal infection (coccidioidomycosis, histoplasmosis)
  5. Rheumatologic disease (rheumatoid arthritis, SLE)
  6. Medications (drug-induced lupus)
  7. Malignancy of the lung or pleura
  8. Trauma (rib fracture)
  9. Hereditary (familial Mediterranean fever, sickle cell disease)

Dx DIAGNOSIS

DIFFERENTIAL DIAGNOSIS

- Cardiac: myocardial infarction, ischemia, pericarditis.
- Intraabdominal process: pancreatitis, cholecystitis.
- Thromboembolic: pulmonary embolism, infarction of lung parenchyma.
- Traumatic/mechanical: rib fracture or pneumothorax.
- Viral infection: viral infections may lead to epidemic pleurodynia (also known as Bornholm's disease). Implicated viruses include coxsackie viruses, RSV, CMV, adenovirus, EBV, parainfluenza, influenza. Of note, viral pleurisy is a diagnosis of exclusion.
- Bacterial infection: pneumonia or tuberculous pleurisy.
- Fungal infection: coccidioidomycosis, histoplasmosis.
- Rheumatologic disease: rheumatoid arthritis, SLE.
- Medications: drug-induced lupus.
- Hereditary causes: familial Mediterranean fever, sickle cell disease.
- Malignancy: malignancy affecting the lung or pleura.
- Uremia.

WORKUP

- A thorough history and physical exam of all patients presenting with pleuritic chest pain should be taken. The time course of the patient's symptoms can provide valuable diagnostic clues. Acute onset of symptoms is suggestive of traumatic injuries, spontaneous pneumothorax, pulmonary embolism, or myocardial infarction. Subacute onset of symptoms suggests a potential infectious, rheumatologic, or medication-induced cause. Viral pleurisy is often associated with prodromal symptoms of upper respiratory infection. Chronic or recurrent symptoms suggest a potential malignant, tuberculous, or hereditary cause.
- Chest x-ray to evaluate for pneumonia, pneumothorax, or pleural effusion.
- EKG to evaluate for infarction, ischemia, or pericarditis.
- Evaluation for pulmonary embolism should be undertaken if clinical suspicion exists.

LABORATORY TESTS

- Laboratory testing varies based on suspected underlying etiology.
- If a pleural effusion is present, diagnostic thoracentesis may provide valuable diagnostic clues to the underlying etiology.

IMAGING STUDIES

- Chest x-ray
- EKG

Rx TREATMENT

- Treatment of pleurisy consists of pain control as well as treating the underlying condition.
- NSAIDs are the preferred first-line agent to control pain associated with pleurisy. Human studies have been limited to trials using indomethacin for pain control, although an NSAID class effect is presumed.
- Indomethacin 50 mg orally up to three times a day has been found to be effective in relieving pain and is associated with an improvement in mechanical lung function.

SUGGESTED READINGS

Jones K et al: Investigation and management of patients with pleuritic chest pain presenting to the accident and emergency department, *J Accid Emerg Med* 16(1):55-59, 1999.

Kass, SM et al: Pleurisy, *Am Fam Physician* 75(9):1357-1364, 2007.

Murray JF, Gebhardt GF: Chest pain. In Mason RJ et al (eds): *Murray and Nadel's textbook of respiratory medicine.* Philadelphia, 2005, Elsevier.

AUTHOR: **MARISA VAN POZNAK, M.D.**

BASIC INFORMATION

DEFINITION

Aspiration pneumonia is a lung infection caused by bacterial organisms aspirated from the nasopharyngeal space.

ICD-9CM CODES
507.0 Aspiration pneumonia

EPIDEMIOLOGY & DEMOGRAPHICS

INCIDENCE (IN U.S.):
- Few reliable data
- 20% to 35% of all pneumonias
- 5% to 15% of all community acquired pneumonias

PEAK INCIDENCE: Elderly patients in hospitals or nursing homes

PREVALENCE (IN U.S.): Unknown (unreliable data)

PREDOMINANT SEX: Males and females affected equally

PREDOMINANT AGE: Elderly

PHYSICAL FINDINGS & CLINICAL PRESENTATION

- Shortness of breath, tachypnea, cough, sputum, fever after vomiting, or difficulty swallowing
- Rales, rhonchi, often diffusely throughout lung

ETIOLOGY

Complex interaction of etiologies, ranging from chemical (often acid) pneumonitis after aspiration of sterile gastric contents (generally not requiring antibiotic treatment) to bacterial aspiration

COMMUNITY-ACQUIRED ASPIRATION PNEUMONIA:
- Generally results from predominantly anaerobic mouth bacteria (anaerobic and microaerophilic streptococci, fusobacteria, gram-positive anaerobic non–spore-forming rods), *Bacteroides* species *(melaninogenicus, intermedius, oralis, ureolyticus), Haemophilus influenzae,* and *Streptococcus pneumoniae*
- Rarely caused by *Bacteroides fragilis* (of uncertain validity in published studies) or *Eikenella corrodens*
- High-risk groups: the elderly; alcoholics; IV drug users; patients who are obtunded; stroke victims; and those with esophageal disorders, seizures, poor dentition, or recent dental manipulations.

HOSPITAL-ACQUIRED ASPIRATION PNEUMONIA:
- Often occurs among elderly patients and others with diminished gag reflex; those with nasogastric tubes, intestinal obstruction, or ventilator support; and especially those exposed to contaminated nebulizers or unsterile suctioning.
- High-risk groups: seriously ill hospitalized patients (especially patients with coma, acidosis, alcoholism, uremia, diabetes mellitus, nasogastric intubation, or recent antimicrobial therapy, who are frequently colonized with aerobic gram-negative rods); patients undergoing anesthesia; those with strokes, dementia, or swallowing disorders; the elderly; and those receiving antacids or H_2 blockers (but not sucralfate).
- Hypoxic patients receiving concentrated O_2 have diminished ciliary activity, encouraging aspiration.
- Causative organisms:
  1. Anaerobes listed above, although in many studies gram-negative aerobes (60%) and gram-positive aerobes (20%) predominate.
  2. *E. coli, P. aeruginosa, S. aureus, Klebsiella, Enterobacter, Serratia, Proteus* spp. *H. influenzae, S. pneumoniae, Legionella,* and *Acinetobacter* spp. (sporadic pneumonias) in two thirds of cases.
  3. Fungi, including *Candida albicans,* in fewer than 1%.

DIAGNOSIS

DIFFERENTIAL DIAGNOSIS

- Other necrotizing or cavitary pneumonias (especially tuberculosis, gram-negative pneumonias)
- See "Pulmonary Tuberculosis"

WORKUP

- Chest x-ray examination
- Complete blood count (CBC), blood cultures
- Sputum Gram stain and culture
- Consideration of tracheal aspirate

LABORATORY TESTS

- CBC: leukocytosis often present
- Sputum Gram stain
  1. Often useful when carefully prepared immediately after obtaining suctioned or expectorated specimen, examined by experienced observer.
  2. Only specimens with multiple white blood cells and rare or absent epithelial cells should be examined.
  3. Unlike nonaspiration pneumonias (e.g., pneumococcal), multiple organisms may be present.
  4. Long, slender rods suggest anaerobes.
  5. Sputum from pneumonia caused by acid aspiration may be devoid of organisms.
  6. Cultures should be interpreted in light of morphology of visualized organisms.

IMAGING STUDIES

- Chest x-ray examination often reveals bilateral, diffuse, patchy infiltrates and posterior segment upper lobes.
- Aspiration pneumonia of several days' or longer duration may reveal necrosis (especially community-acquired anaerobic pneumonias) and even cavitation with air-fluid levels, indicating lung abscess.

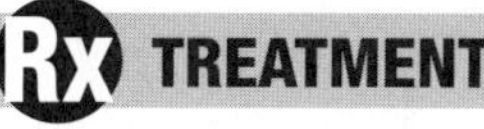

TREATMENT

NONPHARMACOLOGIC THERAPY

- Airway management to prevent repeated aspiration
- Ventilatory support if necessary

ACUTE GENERAL Rx

Acute aspiration of acidic gastric contents without bacteria may not require antibiotic therapy; consult infectious disease or pulmonary expert.

- Community-acquired anaerobic aspiration pneumonia: levofloxacin 500 mg qd or ceftriaxone 1 to 2 g/day
- Nursing home aspirations: levofloxacin 500 mg qd or piperacillin-tazobactam 3.375 g q6h or ceftazidime 2 g q8h
- Hospital-acquired aspiration pneumonia:
  - Piperacillin-tazobactam 3.375 g IV q6h, or clindamycin 450 to 900 mg IV q8h, or cefoxitin 2 g IV q8h.
  - Knowledge of resident flora in the microenvironment of the aspiration within the hospital is crucial to intelligent antibiotic selection; consult infection control nurses or hospital epidemiologist.
  - Confirmed *Pseudomonas* pneumonia should be treated with antipseudomonal beta-lactam agent plus an aminoglycoside until antimicrobial sensitivities confirm that less toxic agents may replace the aminoglycoside.
  - Do not use metronidazole alone for anaerobes.

DISPOSITION

Repeat chest x-ray examination in 6 to 8 wk.

REFERRAL

For consultation with infectious disease and/or pulmonary experts for patients with respiratory distress, hypoxia, ventilatory support, pneumonia in more than one lobe, or necrosis or cavitation on x-ray examination or for those not responding to antibiotic therapy within 2 to 3 days.

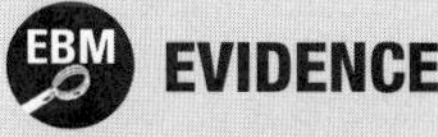

EVIDENCE

Please note: Complete text of EBM for this topic is available online.

SUGGESTED READING

Marik PE: Aspiration pneumonitis and aspiration pneumonia, *N Engl J Med* 344:665, 2001.

AUTHORS: **BETH J. WUTZ, M.D.,** and **RUBEN ALVERO, M.D.**

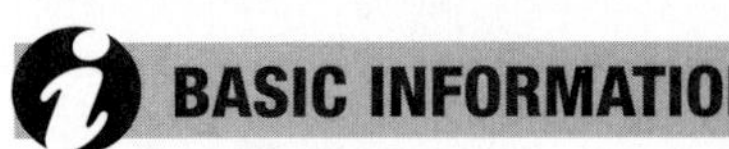

BASIC INFORMATION

DEFINITION

Bacterial pneumonia is an infection involving the lung parenchyma.

ICD-9CM CODES
486.0 Pneumonia, acute
507.0 Pneumonia, aspiration
482.9 Pneumonia, bacterial
481 Pneumonia, pneumococcal
482.1 Pneumonia, Pseudomonas
482.4 Pneumonia, staphylococcal
482.0 Pneumonia, Klebsiella
482.2 Pneumonia, Haemophilus influenzae

EPIDEMIOLOGY & DEMOGRAPHICS

- The incidence of community-acquired pneumonia is 1 in 100 persons.
- The incidence of nosocomial pneumonia is 8 cases per 1000 persons annually.
- Primary care physicians see an average of 10 cases of pneumonia annually.
- Hospitalization rate for pneumonia is 15% to 20%.
- Most cases of pneumonia occur in the winter and in elderly patients.

PHYSICAL FINDINGS & CLINICAL PRESENTATION

- Fever, tachypnea, chills, tachycardia, cough
- Presentation varies with the cause of pneumonia, the patient's age, and the clinical situation:
  1. Patients with streptococcal pneumonia usually present with high fever, shaking chills, pleuritic chest pain, cough, and copious production of purulent sputum.
  2. Mycoplasma pneumoniae*:* insidious onset; headache; dry, paroxysmal cough that is worse at night; myalgias; malaise; sore throat; extrapulmonary manifestations (e.g., erythema multiforme, aseptic meningitis, urticaria, erythema nodosum) may be present.
  3. *Chlamydia pneumoniae:* persistent, nonproductive cough, low-grade fever, headache, sore throat.
  4. *Legionella pneumophila:* fever, mild cough, mental status change, myalgias, diarrhea, respiratory failure.
  5. Elderly or immunocompromised hosts with pneumonia may initially present with only minimal symptoms (e.g., low-grade fever, confusion); respiratory and nonrespiratory symptoms are less commonly reported by older patients with pneumonia.
  6. In general, auscultation of patients with pneumonia reveals crackles and diminished breath sounds.
  7. Percussion dullness is present if the patient has pleural effusion.
  8. The clinical impression of pneumonia has an overall sensitivity of 70% to 90%; specificity ranges from 40% to 70%.

ETIOLOGY

- *Streptococcus pneumoniae*
- *Haemophilus influenzae*
- *L. pneumophila* (1% to 5% of adult pneumonias)
- *Klebsiella, Pseudomonas, Escherichia coli*
- *Staphylococcus aureus*
- Atypical organisms such as *M. pneumoniae, C. pneumoniae,* and *L. pneumophila* implicated in up to 40% of cases of community-acquired pneumonia
- Pneumococcal infection responsible for 50% to 75% of community-acquired pneumonias; gram-negative organisms cause >80% of nosocomial pneumonias
- Predisposing factors:
  1. Chronic obstructive pulmonary disease: *H. influenzae, S. pneumoniae, Legionella*
  2. Seizures: aspiration pneumonia
  3. Compromised hosts: *Legionella,* gram-negative organisms
  4. Alcoholism: *Klebsiella, S. pneumoniae, H. influenzae*
  5. HIV: *S. pneumoniae*
  6. IV drug addicts with right-sided bacterial endocarditis: *S. aureus*
  7. Older patient with comorbid diseases: *C. pneumoniae*

Dx DIAGNOSIS

DIFFERENTIAL DIAGNOSIS

- Exacerbation of chronic bronchitis
- Pulmonary embolism or infarction
- Lung neoplasm
- Bronchiolitis
- Sarcoidosis
- Hypersensitivity pneumonitis
- Pulmonary edema
- Drug-induced lung injury
- Viral pneumonias
- Fungal pneumonias
- Parasitic pneumonias
- Atypical pneumonia
- Tuberculosis

WORKUP

Laboratory evaluation and chest x-ray

LABORATORY TESTS

- Complete blood count with differential; white blood cell count is elevated, usually with left shift.
- Blood cultures (hospitalized patients only): positive in approximately 20% of cases of pneumococcal pneumonia.
- Pulse oximetry or arterial blood gases: hypoxemia with partial pressure of oxygen <60 mm Hg while the patient is breathing room air, a standard criterion for hospital admission.
- Direct immunofluorescent examination of sputum when suspecting *Legionella* (e.g., direct fluorescent antibody stain is a highly specific and rapid test for detecting legionellae in clinical specimen) or urine *Legionella* antigen test.
- Serologic testing for HIV in selected patients.
- Serum electrolytes (hyponatremia in suspected *Legionella* pneumonia), BUN, creatinine.

IMAGING STUDIES

Chest x-ray: findings vary with the stage and type of pneumonia and the hydration of the patient (Fig. 1-250).
- Classically, pneumococcal pneumonia presents with a segmental lobe infiltrate.
- Diffuse infiltrates on chest radiograph can be seen with *L. pneumophila, M. pneumoniae,* viral pneumonias, *P. jirovecii (carinii),* miliary tuberculosis, aspiration, aspergillosis.
- An initial chest radiograph is also useful to rule out the presence of any complications (pneumothorax, empyema, abscesses).

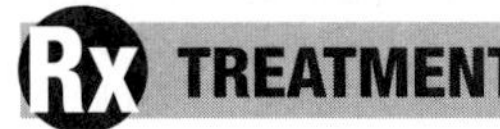

TREATMENT

NONPHARMACOLOGIC THERAPY

- Avoidance of tobacco use
- Oxygen to maintain partial oxygen pressure in arterial blood >60 mm Hg
- IV hydration, correction of dehydration
- Assisted ventilation in patients with significant respiratory failure

ACUTE GENERAL Rx

- Initial antibiotic therapy should be based on clinical, radiographic, and laboratory evaluation.
- Macrolides (azithromycin or clarithromycin) or levofloxacin is recommended for empirical outpatient treatment of community-acquired pneumonia. Cefotaxime or a beta-lactam/beta-lactamase inhibitor can be added in patients with more severe presentation who insist on outpatient therapy. Duration of treatment ranges from 7 to 14 days. The treatment of choice in suspected *Legionella* pneumonia is either a quinolone (e.g. moxifloxaxin) or a macrolide (e.g., azithromycin) antibiotic.
- In the hospital setting, patients admitted to the general ward can be treated empirically with a second- or third-generation cephalosporin (ceftriaxone, ceftizoxime, cefotaxime, or cefuroxime) plus a macrolide (azithromycin or clarithromycin) or doxycycline. An antipseudomonal quinolone (levofloxacin or moxifloxacin) can be substituted in place of the macrolide or doxycycline.
- Empiric therapy in ICU patients: IV beta-lactam (ceftriaxone, cefotaxime, ampicillin-sulbactam) plus an IV quinolone (levofloxacin, moxifloxacin) or IV azithromycin.
- In hospitalized patients at risk for *P. aeruginosa* infection, empirical treatment should consist of an antipseudomonal beta-lactam (cefepime or piperacillin-tazobactam) plus an aminoglycoside plus an antipseudomonal quinolone or macrolide.
- In patients with suspected methicillin-resistant *S. aureus,* vancomycin or linezolid is effective.

CHRONIC Rx

Parapneumonic effusion empyema can be managed with chest tube placement for drainage. Instillation of fibrinolytic agents (streptokinase, urokinase) by chest tube may be necessary in resistant cases.

DISPOSITION

- Most patients respond well to antibiotic therapy.
- Indications for hospital admission are:
  1. Hypoxemia (oxygen saturation <90% while patient is breathing room air)
  2. Hemodynamic instability
  3. Inability to tolerate medications
  4. Active coexisting condition requiring hospitalization

  A criterion often used to determine hospital admission is known as the "CURB-65": **Con**fusion, B**UN** >19.6 mg/dl, **R**espiratory rate >30 breaths/min, Systolic **B**P <90 mg Hg, and diastolic BP ≤60 mm Hg, age ≥**65**. Patients are generally admitted to the hospital if they fulfill 2 or more criteria and to the ICU if they have 3 or more criteria.

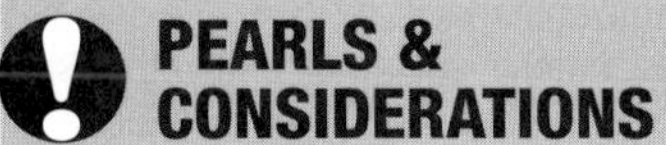

PEARLS & CONSIDERATIONS

COMMENTS

- Use of gastric acid suppressive therapy (H_2 receptor antagonists, proton pump inhibitors [PPIs]) has been associated with an increased risk of community-acquired pneumonia. It appears that PPI therapy started within the previous 30 days is associated with an increased risk for community-acquired pneumonia, whereas longer-term current use is not.
- Causes of slowly resolving or nonresolving pneumonia:
  1. Difficult to treat infections: viral pneumonia, *Legionella,* pneumococci or staphylococci with impaired host response, tuberculosis, fungi
  2. Neoplasm: lung, lymphoma, metastasis
  3. Congestive heart failure
  4. Pulmonary embolism
  5. Immunologic or idiopathic: Wegener's granulomatosis, pulmonary eosinophilic syndromes, systemic lupus erythema-tosus
  6. Drug toxicity (e.g., amiodarone)
- In patients with pneumonia, repeat films should be taken promptly in those who are not doing well. In those with complete clinical recovery, it is reasonable to wait 6 to 8 wk before repeating the radiograph to document clearing of the infiltrate.

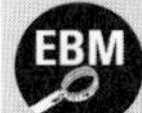

EVIDENCE

Please note: Complete text of EBM for this topic is available online.

Key trials and commentary:

Ventilator-associated pneumonia (VAP) causes substantial morbidity. A silver-coated endotracheal tube has been designed to reduce VAP incidence by preventing bacterial colonization and biofilm formation.

This study showed that patients receiving a silver-coated endotracheal tube had a statistically significant reduction in the incidence of VAP and delayed time to VAP occurrence compared with those receiving a similar, uncoated tube.

VAP is one of the major preventable causes of morbidity and mortality in the ICU. The pathogenesis is thought to be related to colonization of the oropharynx with bacterial pathogens followed by migration of these pathogens into the lung through microaspiration of pooled secretions around the endotracheal cuff. Biofilm formation on the surface of the endotracheal tube may contribute to VAP by shielding pathogens from direct contact with antimicrobials and effectively providing a protected reservoir for the pathogen. The use of antimicrobial/antiseptic-impregnated central venous catheters has shown a high degree of efficacy in reducing the risk of infusion-related sepsis. Similarly, silver-coated urinary catheters substantially reduce the risk of nosocomial urinary tract infections.

This study demonstrates that a similar approach can reduce the risk of VAP by as much as a third. As such, it is an important demonstration of how technological innovation can be harnessed to optimize patient care. Although no formal recommendations recommend use of antiseptic/antimicrobial-impregnated catheters yet, it seems likely that use of these devices will become the standard of practice in the near future, at least for select patients likely to be intubated for more than short periods of time.[1] Ⓐ

Evidence-Based Reference

1. Kollef MH et al: Silver-coated endotracheal tubes and incidence of ventilator-associated pneumonia: the Nascent Randomized Trial, *JAMA* 300:805-813, 2008. Commentary by A. Kumar, M.D. Ⓐ

SUGGESTED READINGS

Aujesky D et al: Prospective comparison of three validated prediction rules for prognosis in community-acquired pneumonia, *Am J Med* 118:384-392, 2005.

Bruns AHW et al: Patterns of resolution of chest radiograph abnormalities in adults hospitalized with severe community-acquired pneumonia, *Clin Infect Dis* 45:983, 2007.

Carratala J et al: Outpatient care compared with hospitalization for community-acquired pneumonia, *Ann Intern Med* 142:165, 2005.

Davidson R et al: Resistance to levofloxacin and failure of treatment of pneumococcal pneumonia, *N Engl J Med* 346:747, 2002.

Halm EA, Teirstein AS: Management of community-acquired pneumonia, *N Engl J Med* 347:2039, 2002.

Sarkar M et al: Proton-pump inhibitor use and the risk for community-acquired pneumonia, *Ann Intern Med* 149:391-398, 2008.

Thibodeau K, Viera AJ: Atypical pathogens and challenges in community-acquired pneumonia, *Am Fam Physician* 69:1699, 2004.

AUTHOR: **FRED F. FERRI, M.D.**

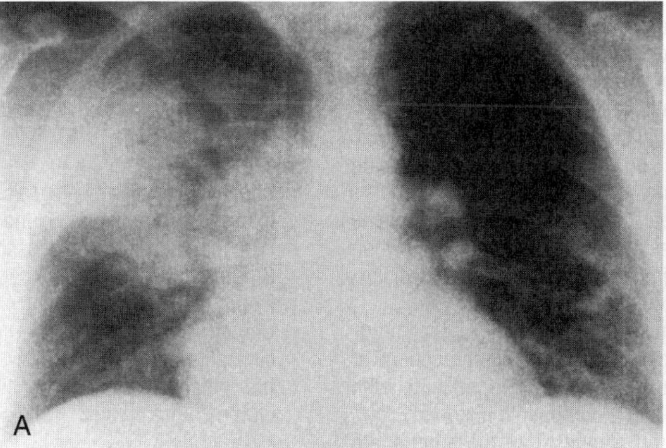

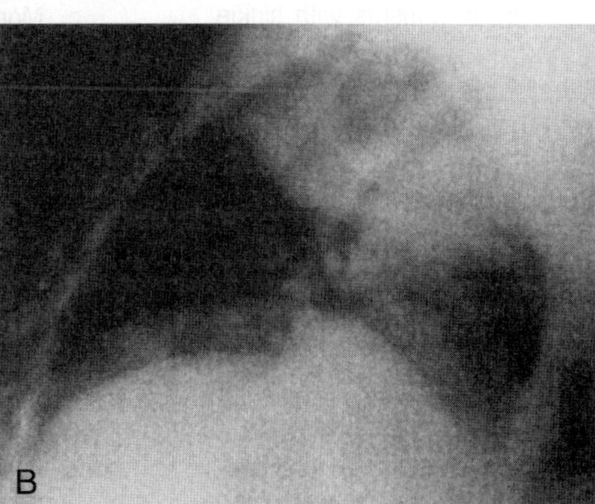

FIGURE 1-250 A, PA and, **B,** lateral chest radiographs reveal right upper-lobe pneumonia and patchy left lower-lobe infiltrate. A variety of organisms can produce this pattern, including *S. pneumoniae* and *H. influenzae.* (From Marx J [ed]: *Rosen's emergency medicine,* ed 5, St Louis, 2003, Mosby.)

Pneumonia, *Mycoplasma* (PTG)

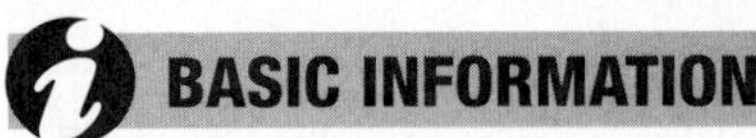

BASIC INFORMATION

DEFINITION

Mycoplasma pneumonia is an infection of the lung parenchyma caused by *Mycoplasma pneumoniae.*

SYNONYMS

Primary atypical pneumonia
Eaton's pneumonia
Walking pneumonia

ICD-9CM CODES
483 *Mycoplasma* pneumonia

EPIDEMIOLOGY & DEMOGRAPHICS

INCIDENCE (IN U.S.):
- Hard to determine incidence precisely because of difficulty in making the diagnosis, but it is a frequent cause of community-acquired pneumonia.
- Many cases probably resolve without coming to medical attention.
- Incidence is estimated at one case per 1000 persons annually.
- Incidence is estimated to at least triple every (approximately) 5 yr during epidemics.

PEAK INCIDENCE:
- Some increased incidence in fall to early winter
- Seems more prevalent in temperate climates

PREVALENCE (IN U.S.):
- Estimated to be present in one in every five patients hospitalized for pneumonia (generally a self-limited disease, so its true prevalence is unknown)
- Estimated to cause 7% of all cases of pneumonia and approximately half the cases in those aged 5 to 20 yr

PREDOMINANT SEX: Equal distribution

PREDOMINANT AGE:
- Most commonly affected: school-age children and young adults (ages 5 to 20 yr)
- Occurs in older adults as well, especially with household exposure to a young child
- More severe infections in affected elderly patients

GENETICS: Familial disposition:
- None known
- May be more severe in patients with sickle cell anemia

Neonatal infection: severe respiratory distress, sometimes requiring intubation, attributed to this disease in infants.

PHYSICAL FINDINGS & CLINICAL PRESENTATION

- Nonexudative pharyngitis (common)
- Headache, otalgia common
- Fever may be mild or not present
- Rhonchi or rales without evidence of consolidation (common) in lower lung zones
- Associated with bullous myringitis (nonspecific finding; perhaps no more frequently than in other pneumonias)
- Skin rashes in up to one fourth of patients
  1. Morbilliform
  2. Urticaria
  3. Erythema nodosum (unusual)
  4. Erythema multiforme (unusual)
  5. Stevens-Johnson syndrome (rare)
- Muscle tenderness (<50% of the patients)
- On examination (and confirmed with testing):
  1. Mononeuritis or polyneuritis
  2. Transverse myelitis
  3. Cranial nerve palsies
  4. Meningoencephalitis
- Lymphadenopathy and splenomegaly
- Conjunctivitis

ETIOLOGY

Infection is spread by droplet infection from respiratory tract secretions.

Dx DIAGNOSIS

DIFFERENTIAL DIAGNOSIS

- *Chlamydia* (now known as *Chlamydophila*) pneumoniae
- *Chlamydophila psittaci*
- *Legionella* spp.
- *Coxiella burnetii*
- Several viral agents
- Q fever
- *Streptococcus pneumoniae*
- Pulmonary embolism or infarction

WORKUP

- Chest x-ray examination
- Thorough history and physical examination
- Laboratory tests
- Evaluation guided by symptoms and findings

LABORATORY TESTS

- White blood cells (WBC):
  1. WBC count >10,000/mm^3 in approximately one fourth of patients
  2. Differential count nonspecific
  3. Leukopenia rare
- Cold agglutinins:
  1. Detected in approximately half of the patients
  2. Also may be found in:
     a. Lymphoproliferative diseases
     b. Influenza
     c. Mononucleosis
     d. Adenovirus infections
     e. Occasionally, Legionnaires' disease
  3. Titers typically >1:64
     a. May be detectable with bedside testing
     b. Appear between days 5 and 10 of the illness (so may be demonstrable when patient is first examined) and disappear within 1 mo
- Complement fixation testing or other immunoassays specific for mycoplasm antigens of paired sera (fourfold rise) in patients with pneumonia and a compatible history:
  1. Considered diagnostic in the appropriate clinical setting
- Culture of the organism from specimens
  1. Only truly specific test for infection
  2. Technically difficult and done reliably by few laboratories
  3. May require weeks to get results
- Sputum
  1. Often no sputum produced for laboratory testing
  2. When present, gram-stained specimens show polymorphonuclear cells without organisms
- Infection occasionally complicated by pancreatitis or glomerulitis
- Disseminated intravascular coagulation is a rare complication
- Electrocardiographic evidence of pericarditis or myocarditis may be present

IMAGING STUDIES

- Predilection for lower lobe involvement (upper lobes involved in less than a fourth), with radiographic abnormalities frequently out of proportion to those on physical examination (Fig. 1-251)
- Small pleural effusions in approximately 30% of patients
- Large effusions: rare
- Infiltrates: patchy, unilateral, and with a segmental distribution, although multilobar involvement may be seen
- Evidence of hilar adenopathy on chest radiographs in 20% to 25%
- Rare cases reported:
  1. Associated lung abscess
  2. Residual pneumatoceles
  3. Lobar collapse
  4. Hyperlucent lung syndrome

Rx TREATMENT

ACUTE GENERAL Rx

- Therapy (10 to 14 days) with erythromycin (500 mg qid), azithromycin (500 mg initially, then 250 mg daily for 4 days), or clarithromycin (500 mg bid) is preferred to tetracycline, especially in young children or women of childbearing age. Respiratory fluoroquinolones such as Levaquin or moxifloxacin are alternative agents for treatment but should not be used in young children.
- Therapy shortens the duration and severity of symptoms and may hasten radiographic clearing, but the disease is self-limiting.

CHRONIC Rx

- Effective antimicrobial therapy does not eliminate the organism from the respiratory secretions, which may be positive for weeks.
- Serum antibody response does not necessarily provide lifelong immunity.
- Chronic symptoms do not occur, although clinical relapses may occur 7 to 10 days after the initial response and may be associated with new areas of infiltration.

DISPOSITION

- Clinical improvement is almost universal within 10 days.

- Infiltrates generally clear within 5 to 8 wk.
- Rare deaths are likely attributable to underlying medical diseases.
- Person-to-person spread can be minimized by avoiding open coughing, especially in enclosed areas.

REFERRAL

- Not responding to treatment
- Severe infection
- Severe extrapulmonary manifestations
- Multilobe involvement accompanied by respiratory embarrassment (very rare)

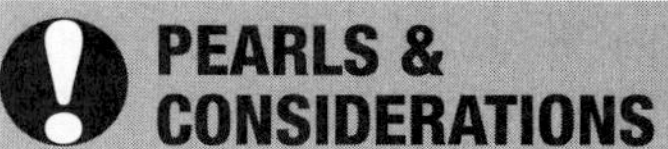

PEARLS & CONSIDERATIONS

COMMENTS

X-ray resolution complete by 8 wk in approximately 90% of patients.

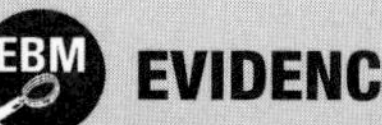

EVIDENCE

Much of the data on treatment of atypical pneumonia have been taken from studies on patients with community-acquired pneumonia, which include a large number of patients with atypical pneumonia.[1]

Oral antibiotic therapy results in a 90% rate of clinical cure or improvement in outpatients with community-acquired pneumonia.[2] Ⓐ

Little evidence exists suggesting superior clinical efficacy of one oral antibiotic over another. Oral azithromycin may be more effective than other macrolides, penicillins, and cephalosporins in the treatment of community-acquired pneumonia, but further study is required in this area to confirm this finding. Beta-lactam agents are ineffective against *M. pneumoniae*.[1,3] Ⓐ Ⓑ

In hospitalized and nonhospitalized patients with community-acquired pneumonia, clinical outcome at 5 to 7 days is significantly better when treated with levofloxacin (oral or IV) compared with IV ceftriaxone or oral cefuroxime axetil.[4] Ⓑ

Monotherapy with levofloxacin is as effective as combination therapy with IV azithromycin plus ceftriaxone in patients hospitalized with community-acquired pneumonia.[5] Ⓑ

Evidence-Based References

1. Loeb M: Community acquired pneumonia, *Clin Evid* (15):2015-2024, 2006.
2. Pomilla PV, Brown RB: Outpatient treatment of community-acquired pneumonia in adults, *Arch Intern Med* 154:1793, 1994. Ⓐ
3. Contopoulos-Ioannidis DG et al: Meta-analysis of randomized controlled trials on the comparative efficacy and safety of azithromycin against other antibiotics for lower respiratory tract infections, *J Antimicrob Chemother* 48:691, 2001. Ⓑ
4. File TM et al: A multicenter, randomized study comparing the efficacy and safety of intravenous and/or oral levofloxacin versus ceftriaxone and/or cefuroxime axetil in treatment of adults with community-acquired pneumonia, *Antimicrob Agents Chemother* 41:1965, 1997. Ⓑ
5. Frank E et al: A multicenter, open-label, randomized comparison of levofloxacin and azithromycin plus ceftriaxone in hospitalized adults with moderate to severe community-acquired pneumonia, *Clin Ther* 24:1292, 2002. Ⓑ

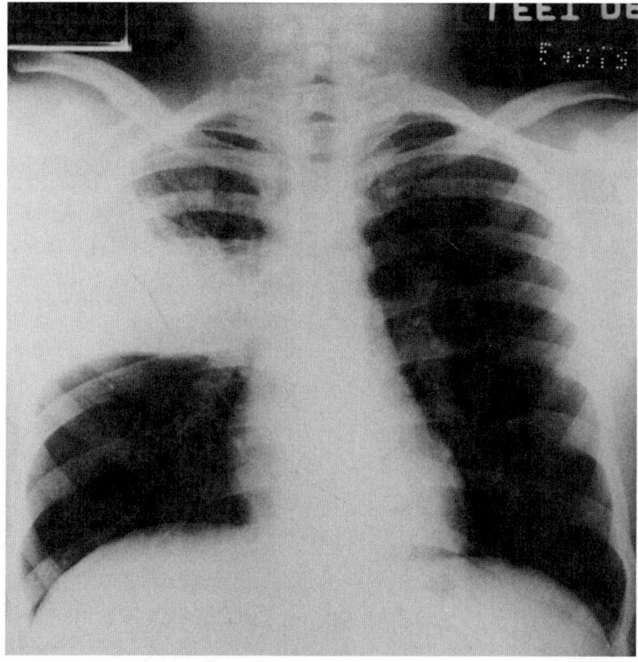

FIGURE 1-251 Localized airspace opacification resulting from *Mycoplasma pneumoniae.* (From Specht N [ed]: *Practical guide to diagnostic imaging,* St Louis, 1998, Mosby.)

SUGGESTED READINGS

La Scola B et al: *Mycoplasma pneumoniae:* a rarely diagnosed agent in ventilator-acquired pneumonia, *J Hosp Infect* 59(1):74, 2005.

Meloni F et al: Acute *Chlamydia pneumoniae* and *Mycoplasma pneumoniae* infections in community-acquired pneumonia and exacerbations of COPD or asthma: therapeutic considerations, *J Chemother* 16(1):70, 2004.

Michelow IC et al: Diagnostic utility and clinical significance of naso- and oropharyngeal samples used in a PCR assay to diagnose *Mycoplasma pneumoniae* infection in children with community-acquired pneumonia, *J Clin Microbiol* 42(7):3339, 2004.

Waites KG, Talkington DF: *Mycoplasma pneumoniae* and its role as a human pathogen, *Clin Microbiol Rev* 17(4):697, 2004.

AUTHORS: **GLENN G. FORT, M.D., M.P.H.,** and **DENNIS J. MIKOLICH, M.D.**

Pneumonia, *Pneumocystis jirovecii (carinii)* (PTG)

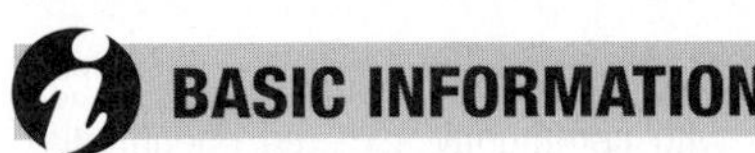

BASIC INFORMATION

DEFINITION

Pneumocystis jirovecii pneumonia (PJP) is a serious respiratory infection caused by the fungal or protozoal organism *P. jirovecii* (formerly known as *P. carinii*).

SYNONYMS

PCP
PJP

ICD-9CM CODES
136.3 *Pneumocystis jirovecii (P. carinii)* pneumonia

EPIDEMIOLOGY & DEMOGRAPHICS

INCIDENCE (IN U.S.):
- Seen primarily in the setting of AIDS
- Approximately 11 cases per 100 patient-years among HIV-infected patients with CD4 lymphocyte counts $<100/\text{mm}^3$
- Also seen in other immunocompromised patients with severe cell-mediated immune deficiency (congenital T-cell deficiency, acute leukemia, lymphoma, bone marrow or organ transplant deficiency)

PEAK INCIDENCE: Age 20 to 40 yr (parallel to AIDS epidemic)

PREDOMINANT SEX: Equal incidence when corrected for HIV status

PREDOMINANT AGE:
- <2 yr
- 20 to 40 yr

GENETICS: Neonatal infection:
- Most frequent opportunistic infection among HIV-infected children, occurring in approximately 30%
- Neonatal occurrence unusual

PHYSICAL FINDINGS & CLINICAL PRESENTATION

- Fever, cough, shortness of breath present in almost all cases
- Lungs frequently clear to auscultation, although rales occasionally present
- Cyanosis and pronounced tachypnea in severe cases
- Hemoptysis unusual
- Spontaneous pneumothorax

ETIOLOGY

- *P. jirovecii* (formerly *P. carinii*) recently reclassified as a fungal organism
- Reactivation of dormant infection
- Extrapulmonary involvement rare

Dx DIAGNOSIS

DIFFERENTIAL DIAGNOSIS

- Other opportunistic respiratory infections:
  1. Tuberculosis
  2. Histoplasmosis
  3. Cryptococcosis
- Nonopportunistic infections:
  1. Bacterial pneumonia
  2. Viral pneumonia
  3. Mycoplasmal pneumonia
  4. Legionellosis
- Occurs virtually exclusively in the setting of profound depression of cellular immunity

WORKUP

- Chest x-ray.
- Arterial blood gases.
- Because *Pneumocystis* cannot be cultured, diagnosis relies on detection of the organism by colorimetric or immunofluorescent stains or PCR.
- Sputum examination for cysts of PJP and to exclude other pathogens.
- Bronchoscopy with bronchoalveolar lavage or lung biopsy for diagnosis if sputum examination is negative or equivocal. Stains such as Gomori methenamine silver stain or toluidine blue O are used to identify the organism.

LABORATORY TESTS

- Arterial blood gas monitoring
- Elevated lactate dehydrogenase in majority of cases
- HIV antibody test if cause of underlying immune deficiency state is unclear

IMAGING STUDIES

Diffuse uptake on gallium scanning of the lungs is suggestive but not diagnostic.

Rx TREATMENT

NONPHARMACOLOGIC THERAPY

- Supplemental oxygen
- Ventilatory support if needed
- Prompt thoracotomy if pneumothorax develops

ACUTE GENERAL Rx

For confirmed or suspected PJP:
- Trimethoprim-sulfamethoxazole (15 to 20 mg/kg trimethoprim and 75 to 100 mg/kg sulfamethoxazole qd) PO or IV per day divided and given q6-8h
- Pentamidine (4 mg/kg IV qd)
- Either regimen with prednisone (40 mg PO bid):
  1. If arterial oxygen pressure <70 mm Hg
  2. If arterial-alveolar oxygen pressure difference >35 mm Hg
  3. Dose tapered to 20 mg bid after 5 days and 20 mg qd after 10 days
- Therapy continued for 3 wk
- Alternative therapies available for patients unable to tolerate conventional therapy:
  1. Dapsone/trimethoprim
  2. Clindamycin/primaquine
  3. Atovaquone

CHRONIC Rx

- After completion of therapy, lifelong prophylaxis should be maintained with trimethoprim-sulfamethoxazole (one single-strength tablet PO qd or double-strength three times weekly).
- Patients intolerant of this therapy should be treated with dapsone (50 mg PO qd) plus pyrimethamine (50 mg PO weekly) plus leucovorin (25 mg PO weekly).
- Inhaled pentamidine (300 mg monthly by standardized nebulizer) is less effective and is reserved for patients intolerant to other forms of prophylaxis.
- Same approach taken to all HIV-infected patients with CD4 lymphocyte counts <200 to $250/\text{mm}^3$ or <20% of the total lymphocyte count because of their high risk of PJP.

DISPOSITION

After completion of therapy, long-term ambulatory follow-up is mandatory to provide secondary prevention of PJP (see "Chronic Rx" above) and management of the underlying immunodeficiency syndrome.

REFERRAL

- To pulmonologist for bronchoscopy if diagnosis cannot be confirmed by sputum examination
- To an infectious disease specialist if case is severe or difficult to manage

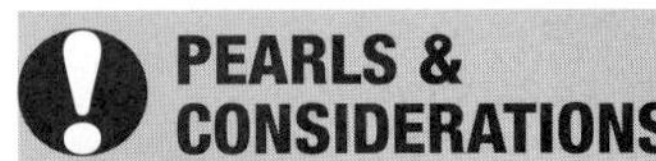

PEARLS & CONSIDERATIONS

COMMENTS

All patients, especially those with severe infection or intolerant of conventional therapy, should be followed by a physician experienced in the management of PJP and, if appropriate, in the long-term management of HIV infection or other underlying disease.

Severe and life-threatening hypoglycemia may occur after 1 or 2 wk after start of IV pentamidine. Monitor closely and advise the patient of symptoms of hypoglycemia.

SUGGESTED READINGS

Kovacs JA, Masur H: Evolving health effects of pneumocystis, *JAMA* 301(24):2578-2585, 2009.

Torres HA et al: Influence of type of cancer and hematopoietic stem cell transplantation on clinical presentation of *Pneumocystis jirovecii* pneumonia in cancer patients, *Eur J Clin Microbiol Infect Dis* 25(6): 382, 2006.

AUTHORS: **GLENN G. FORT, M.D., M.P.H.,** and **DENNIS J. MIKOLICH, M.D.**

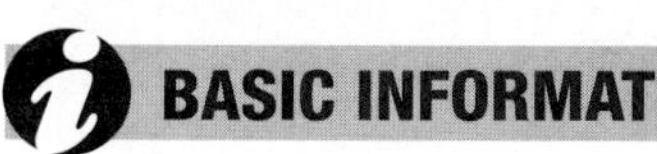

BASIC INFORMATION

DEFINITION

Viral pneumonia is infection of the pulmonary parenchyma caused by any of a large number of viral agents. The most important viruses are discussed.

SYNONYMS

Nonbacterial pneumonia
Atypical pneumonia

ICD-9CM CODES
480.9 Viral pneumonia

EPIDEMIOLOGY & DEMOGRAPHICS

INCIDENCE (IN U.S.):

- Influenza virus:
    1. 10% to 20% of population in temperate zones infected during 1- to 2-mo epidemics occurring yearly during winter months.
    2. Up to 50% infected during pandemics.
    3. Pneumonia develops in small percentage of infected persons.
- Incidence of other important viral pneumonias is not known precisely.

PEAK INCIDENCE:

1. Influenza:
    - Winter months for influenza A
    - Year round for influenza B
    - Peak of pneumonia seen weeks into the outbreak of infection
2. Respiratory syncytial virus (RSV) and parainfluenza virus:
    - Winter and spring
3. Adenovirus:
    - Endemic (military)
4. Varicella:
    - Spring in temperate zones
5. Measles:
    - Year round
6. Cytomegalovirus (CMV):
    - Year round

PREVALENCE (IN U.S.):

- Often related to immune status of the population or presence of an epidemic
- Normal hosts (estimates):
    1. 86% of cases of pneumonia resulting in hospitalization in American adults
    2. 16% of pediatric pneumonias managed as outpatients
    3. 49% of hospitalized infants with pneumonia
- Important problem in hosts with impaired immunity

PREDOMINANT SEX:

- None generally
- Male sex may predispose to more severe respiratory disease in RSV infection

PREDOMINANT AGE:

1. Influenza:
    - Overall incidence greatest at age 5 yr
    - Falls with increasing age
    - The most serious sequelae in those with chronic medical illnesses, especially cardiopulmonary disease
    - Hospitalizations greatest in infants and adults aged >64 yr
2. RSV and parainfluenza virus:
    - Young children (as the major cause of pneumonia)
    - Occurs throughout life
3. Adenoviruses:
    - Young children
    - Adults, primarily military recruits
4. Varicella:
    - Approximately 16% of adults (not infected in childhood) who contract chickenpox
    - Acute varicella during pregnancy more likely to be complicated by severe pneumonia
    - 90% of reported varicella pneumonia cases are in adults (highest incidence ages 20 to 60 yr)
5. Measles:
    - Young adults and older children who received a single vaccination (5% failure rate)
    - Measles during pregnancy more likely to be complicated by pneumonia
    - Underlying cardiopulmonary diseases and immunosuppression predispose to serious pneumonia complicating measles
    - Before availability of measles vaccine, 90% of pneumonias in those <10 yr
    - Currently more than one third of U.S. patients >14 yr
    - 3% to 50% of measles cases are complicated by pneumonia
6. CMV:
    - Neonatal through adult
    - Immunosuppression is key predisposing factor

GENETICS:

Familial disposition:

- Close contact, not genetics, is important in acquisition
- Congenital anomalies and immunosuppression worsen course of RSV pneumonia

Congenital infection:

- CMV is the most common intrauterine infection in the U.S.
- Pneumonia occurs occasionally in infants with symptomatic congenital infection.

Neonatal infection:

- Severe RSV pneumonia
- Adenovirus pneumonia
    1. 5% to 20% mortality rate
    2. Can lead to residual restrictive or obstructive functional abnormalities
- "Varicella neonatorum"
    1. Disseminated visceral disease including pneumonia
    2. May develop in neonates whose mothers develop peripartum chickenpox
- CMV pneumonia
    1. Generally fatal
    2. Associated with severe cerebral damage in this population

PHYSICAL FINDINGS & CLINICAL PRESENTATION

1. Influenza:
    - Fever
    - Uncomfortable or lethargic appearance
    - Prominent dry cough (rarely hemoptysis)
    - Flushed integument and erythematous mucous membranes
    - Rales or rhonchi
2. RSV and parainfluenza:
    - Fever
    - Tachypnea
    - Prolonged expiration
    - Wheezes and rales
3. Adenoviruses:
    - Hoarseness
    - Pharyngitis
    - Tachypnea
    - Cervical adenitis
4. Measles:
    - Conjunctivitis
    - Rhinorrhea
    - Koplik's spots
    - Exanthem
    - Pneumonitis
        a. May occur as a complication in 3% to 4% of adolescents and young adults
        b. Coincident with rash
        c. May also develop after apparent recovery from measles
    - Fever
    - Dry cough
5. Varicella:
    - Fever
    - Maculopapular or vesicular rash
        a. Becomes encrusted
        b. Pneumonia typical 1 to 6 days after rash appears
        c. Pneumonia accompanied by cough and occasionally hemoptysis
    - Few auscultatory abnormalities noted on examination of the lungs
6. CMV:
    - Fever
    - Paroxysmal cough
    - Occasional hemoptysis
    - Diffuse adenopathy when pneumonia occurs after transfusion

ETIOLOGY

Viral infection can lead to pneumonia in both immunocompetent and immunocompromised hosts.

Dx DIAGNOSIS

DIFFERENTIAL DIAGNOSIS

- Bacterial pneumonia, which frequently complicates (i.e., can follow or be simultaneous with) viral (especially influenza) pneumonia
- Other causes of atypical pneumonia:
    1. *Mycoplasma* spp.
    2. *Chlamydia* spp.
    3. *Coxiella* spp.
    4. Legionnaires' disease
- Acute respiratory distress syndrome (ARDS)
- Physical findings and associated hypoxemia confused with pulmonary emboli

WORKUP

- Information about the current prevalent strain of influenza virus can be obtained from local

health departments or from the Centers for Disease Control and Prevention.
- Viral diagnostic tests are usually not necessary once an outbreak has been defined.
- Influenza and other viruses can be cultured from respiratory secretions during the initial few days of the illness (special media and techniques necessary).
- Paired sera antibody titers are also useful.
- Monoclonal antibody tests are available for influenza and other respiratory viruses.
- Measles and adenovirus pneumonia are usually diagnosed clinically.
- Polymerase chain reaction may be able to rapidly detect and identify viral nucleic acid.
- Open lung biopsy is required for definite diagnosis of CMV pneumonia.

LABORATORY TESTS

- Sputum Gram stain (usually produced in scanty amounts) typically shows few polymorphonuclear leukocytes and few bacteria.
- White blood cell count may vary from leukopenic to modest elevation, usually without a leftward shift.
- Disseminated intravascular coagulation occasionally complicates adenovirus type 7 pneumonia.
- Multinucleated giant cells on Tzanck preparation of an unroofed vesicular lesion are useful in diagnosing varicella in a patient with an infiltrate (also found in herpes simplex).
- Severe immunosuppression is associated with symptomatic CMV pneumonia (usually reactivation of latent infection or in previously seronegative recipients from the donor).
- Hypoxemia may be profound.
- Cultures may be helpful in identifying superinfecting bacterial pathogens.
- When they occur, parapneumonic pleural effusions are exudative.

IMAGING STUDIES

- Chest x-ray examination may demonstrate a spectrum of findings from ill-defined, patchy, or generalized interstitial infiltrates, which can be associated with ARDS.
- A localized dense alveolar infiltrate suggests a superimposed bacterial pneumonia.
- Small calcified nodules may develop as a radiographic residual of varicella pneumonia (Fig. 1-252).

Rx TREATMENT

NONPHARMACOLOGIC THERAPY

General:
- Measures to diminish person-to-person transmission
- Modified bed rest
- Maintenance of adequate hydration
- Possible ventilatory support for severe pneumonia or ARDS

Influenza:
- Yearly prophylactic strain-specific influenza vaccination (only subvirion vaccine should be used in children <13 yr) can be given to prevent infection.
- Live, attenuated influenza vaccines administered by nose drops as effective as injected inactivated viral vaccines.

RSV:
- Isolation techniques are important in limiting spread of RSV infections.
- Immunoglobulins with a high RSV-neutralizing antibody titer are beneficial in treatment.

Adenoviruses:
- Intestinal inoculation of respiratory adenoviruses has been used to successfully immunize military recruits.
- Although they produce no disease in recipients, the viruses may be shed chronically and may infect others at a later date.
- These vaccines are not available for civilian populations.

Varicella:
- Live, attenuated varicella vaccine has been successfully used in clinical trials.
- Varicella-zoster immune globulin should be administered within 4 days of exposure to prevent or modify the disease in susceptible persons.
- Nonimmunized persons exposed to varicella are potentially infectious between 10 and 21 days after exposure.

Measles:
- Effective measles vaccine is available:
  - The vaccine should be administered at age 15 mo.
  - A second dose should be administered at the time of school entry.
- Live, attenuated vaccine or gamma-globulin can prevent measles in unvaccinated persons if administered early after exposure.
- Vitamin A given PO for 2 days reduces morbidity and mortality rates from measles in exposed children.

Severe acute respiratory syndrome (SARS) = associated coronaviruses:
- No vaccine currently available.
- Supportive care: ribavirin ineffective, use of steroids or interferon-alpha of unclear value.

ACUTE GENERAL Rx

- **General:** Administer appropriate antibiotics for bacterial superinfections.
- **Influenza:**
  - Amantadine and rimantadine for influenza A (not active against influenza B). Early use can speed recovery from small airways dysfunction, but whether it influences the development or course of pneumonia is uncertain.
  - The neuraminidase inhibitors oseltamivir and zanamivir are effective if given in the first 48 hours of symptoms of influenza; their efficacy in established influenza pneumonia is unclear.
  - Aerosolized ribavirin or amantadine may have a role in severe influenza pneumonia but have not been approved for this indication.
- **RSV and parainfluenza:**
  - Ribavirin aerosol is effective for severe RSV pneumonia.
  - There is no approved antiviral therapy for parainfluenza virus pneumonia.
- **Adenoviruses:** no effective agent; some case reports of cidofovir use but unproved.
- **Varicella:**
  - Varicella pneumonia can be treated with IV acyclovir.
  - Adults who develop chickenpox should be considered for acyclovir treatment, which may prevent the development of pneumonia.
- **Measles:** no effective antimeasles agent.
- **CMV:**
  - Acyclovir can prevent CMV infection in renal transplant recipients.
  - Ganciclovir and foscarnet, with or without CMV hyperimmune globulin, show promise in the treatment of serious CMV infection, including pneumonia, in compromised hosts.

DISPOSITION

- Supportive therapy is useful.
- Death arise possible during acute illness.

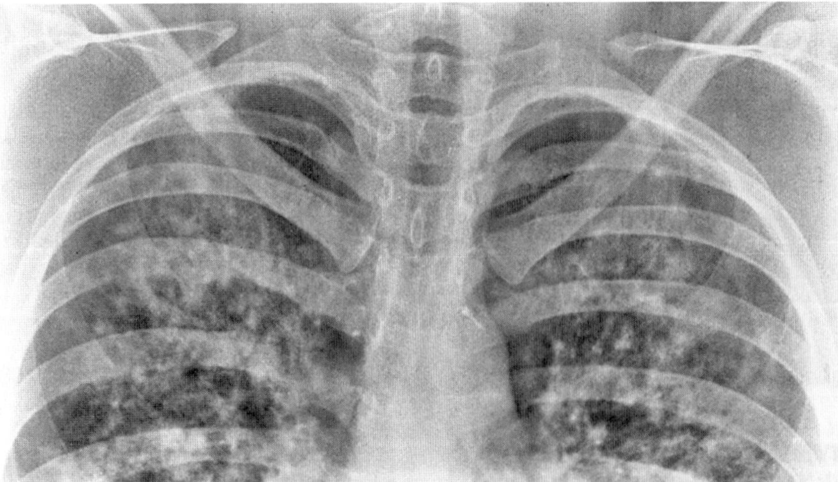

FIGURE 1-252 Chickenpox-varicella pneumonia. Coned-down view of the upper lobes shows multiple ill-defined nodules in both upper lobes. (From McLoud TC: *Thoracic radiology: the requisites,* St Louis, 1998, Mosby.)

- Residual functional abnormalities may be persistent, develop into, or predispose to chronic respiratory diseases in later life.
- Morbidity and mortality rates after most viral pneumonias are increased by bacterial superinfection.

REFERRAL

- Uncertainty about the diagnosis in a compromised host
- Symptoms or findings progressive
- Severe respiratory compromise, diffuse infiltrates, or the development of ARDS

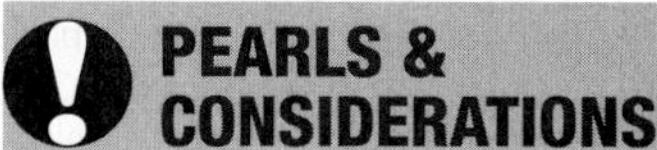

PEARLS & CONSIDERATIONS

COMMENTS

- Influenza spreads by close contact and by small droplets transmitted by cough.
- RSV is effectively transmitted by fomites and by direct contact (little by aerosol).
- Varicella is transmitted by direct contact or by aerosol.
- Of the three major forms of parainfluenza viruses (types 1 to 3), type 3 is the most common cause of viral pneumonia; types 1 and 2 primarily cause laryngotracheitis.
- Recent evidence indicates that a newly discovered virus known as metapneumovirus is a common cause of upper respiratory infections worldwide; this virus can cause pneumonia.

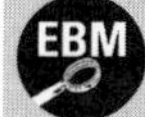

EVIDENCE

Although there is evidence that many antiviral agents reduce the duration of influenza, there is no evidence that these drugs are effective in preventing pneumonia.[1]

A systematic review found limited evidence on the efficacy of ribavirin in the management of hospitalized infants with RSV infection of the lower respiratory tract. Mortality rate and respiratory deterioration were not significantly reduced with ribavirin compared with placebo. Cumulative results from three small trials showed that ribavirin reduced the duration of mechanical ventilator support and may reduce the duration of hospitalization.[2] Ⓐ

Evidence-Based References

1. Hansen L: Influenza, *Clin Evid* 10:867, 2003.
2. Ventre K, Randolph AG: Ribavirin for respiratory syncytial virus infection of the lower respiratory tract in infants and young children, *Cochrane Rev* 4, 2004. Ⓐ

SUGGESTED READINGS

Cheng VC et al: Medical treatment of viral pneumonia including SARS in immunocompetent adults, *J Infect* 49(4):262, 2004.

Falsey AR, Walsh EE: Viral pneumonia in older adults, *Clin Infect Dis* 42(4):518, 2006.

Hohenthal U et al: Measurement of complement receptor 1 on neutrophils in bacterial and viral pneumonia, *BMC Infect Dis* 6:11, 2006.

Luyt, CE, et al: Viral infections in the ICU, *Curr Opin Care* 14(5):605, 2008.

Michelow IC et al: Epidemiology and clinical characteristics of community-acquired pneumonia in hospitalized children, *Pediatrics* 113(4):701, 2004.

Moreno L et al: Development and validation of a clinical prediction rule to distinguish bacterial from viral pneumonia in children, *Pediatr Pulmonol* 41(4):331, 2006.

Tsolia MN et al: Etiology of community-acquired pneumonia in hospitalized school-age children: evidence for high prevalence of viral infections, *Clin Infect Dis* 39(5):681, 2004.

Werno AM et al: Human metapneumovirus in children with bronchiolitis or pneumonia in New Zealand, *J Paediatr Child Health* 40(9-10):549, 2004.

AUTHORS: **DENNIS J. MIKOLICH, M.D.,** and **GLENN G. FORT, M.D., M.P.H.**

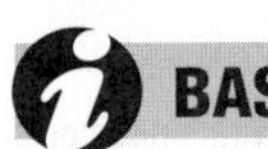

BASIC INFORMATION

DEFINITION

A spontaneous pneumothorax (SP) is defined as the accumulation of air into the pleural space, collapsing the lung (Fig. 1-253). This can be primary SP (without any obvious underlying lung disease) or secondary SP (with underlying lung disease).

SYNONYMS

Primary spontaneous pneumothorax
Secondary spontaneous pneumothorax

ICD-9CM CODES
512.0S **Spontaneous** tension pneumothorax
512.8 Other spontaneous pneumothorax

EPIDEMIOLOGY & DEMOGRAPHICS

- Approximately 20,000 new cases of SP occur each year in the U.S.
- SP is more common in men than women (6:1).
- Incidence of primary SP is 7.4 per 100,000 in men and 1.2 per 100,000 in women.
- Incidence of secondary SP is 6.3 per 100,000 in men and 2.0 per 100,000 in women.
- SP is commonly seen in tall, thin young men aged 20 to 40 yr.
- Tobacco use increases the risk of SP.

PHYSICAL FINDINGS & CLINICAL PRESENTATION

- Sudden onset of pleuritic chest pain (90%), which often becomes dull after a few hours
- Pain is usually unilateral and can be sharp and agonizing and associated with considerable apprehension
- Dyspnea (80%), which often resolves within 24 hr, despite persistence of pneumothorax
- Cough (10%)
- Asymptomatic (5%); may take up to 7 days to come to medical attention
- Tachycardia
- Diminished breath sounds
- Subcutaneous emphysema may be present
- Hyperresonance on percussion

ETIOLOGY

- In primary SP, rupture of small blebs, usually located near the apex of the upper lobes, is a common cause. The check-valve mechanism

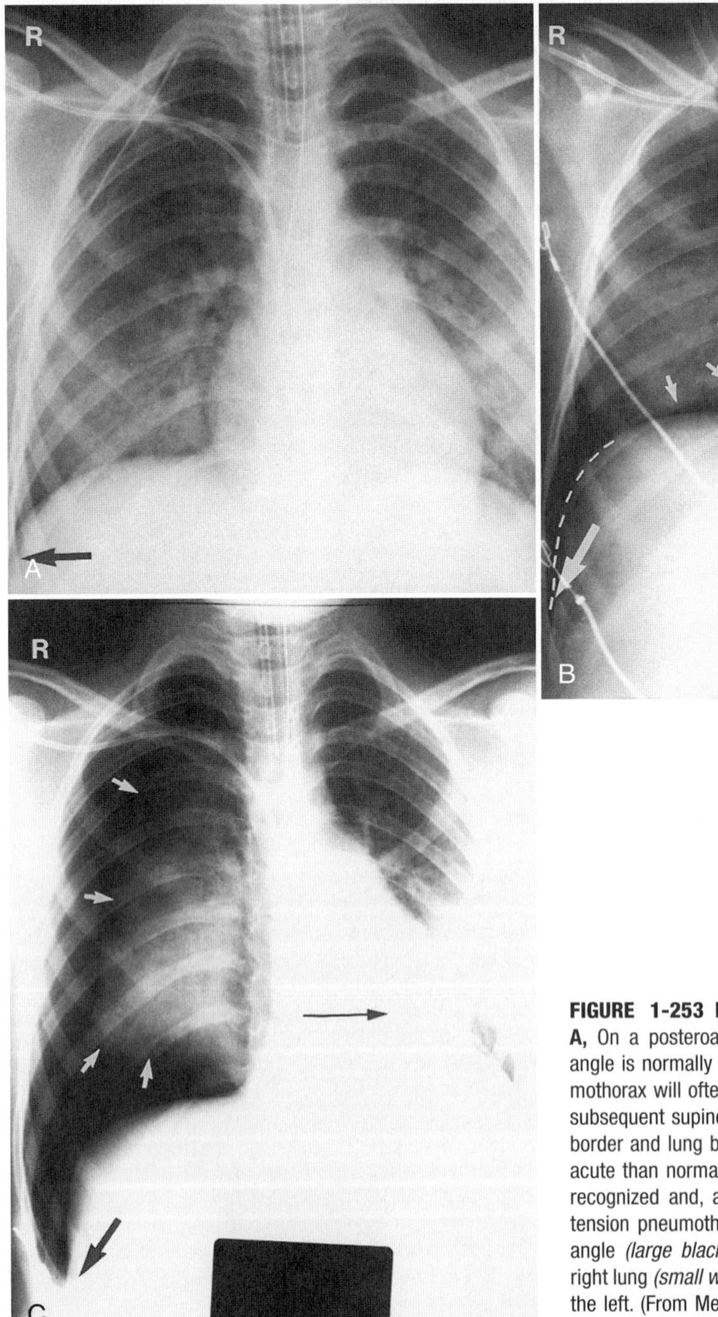

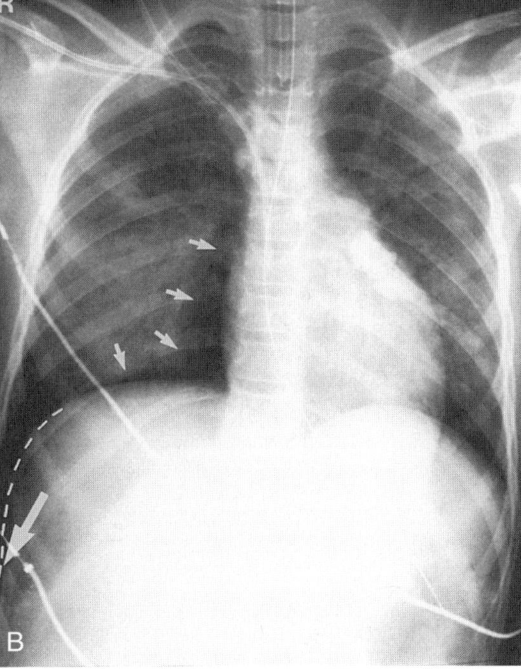

FIGURE 1-253 Deep sulcus sign of pneumothorax. A, On a posteroanterior chest radiograph the costophrenic angle is normally acute *(arrow).* In a supine patient, a pneumothorax will often be anterior, medical, and basilar. **B,** On a subsequent supine film the dark area along the right cardiac border and lung base angle became much deeper and more acute than normal *(large arrow).* **C,** These findings were not recognized and, as a result, the same patient developed a tension pneumothorax with an extremely deep costophrenic angle *(large black arrow)* and almost completely collapsed right lung *(small white arrows)* and shift of the mediastinum to the left. (From Mettler FA [ed]: *Primary care radiology,* Philadelphia, 2000, WB Saunders.)

is uncommon in this case; therefore, tension pneumothorax rarely occurs.

- In secondary SP, chronic obstructive pulmonary disease is the most common cause, but it can also be associated with pneumonia, bronchogenic carcinoma, mesothelioma, sarcoidosis, tuberculosis, cystic fibrosis, and many other lung diseases (Fig. 1-254).

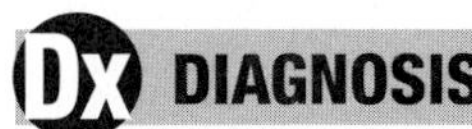

DIAGNOSIS

Established by the chest radiograph (CXR) or CT

DIFFERENTIAL DIAGNOSIS

- Pleurisy
- Pulmonary embolism
- Myocardial infarction
- Pericarditis
- Asthma
- Pneumonia

WORKUP

Includes CXR and, in some cases, CT scan of the chest

LABORATORY TESTS

Arterial blood gases may show hypoxemia and hypocapnia as a result of hyperventilation.

IMAGING STUDIES

- Spontaneous pneumothorax is usually confirmed by upright CXR:
    1. A white visceral pleural line. The absence of vessel markings peripheral to this line helps differentiate from mimicking conditions such as an overlying skin fold. A lateral width of 1 cm corresponds to 10% pneumothorax.
    2. The left lateral decubitus position is the most sensitive and supine position the least sensitive. The increased sensitivity of expiratory films in detecting pneumothorax has never been demonstrated in studies.
    3. As little as 50 ml of air can be detected on upright film.
- Tension pneumothorax is a medical emergency and should be suspected when the patient is hemodynamically unstable or with contralateral tracheal and mediastinal deviation and ipsilateral flattening or inversion of the diaphragm on the CXR.
- CT scan can be done in suspected but difficult-to-visualize pneumothoraces, to differentiate from large subpleural bullae or to evaluate for underlying lung pathology, especially in patients with secondary pneumothorax.

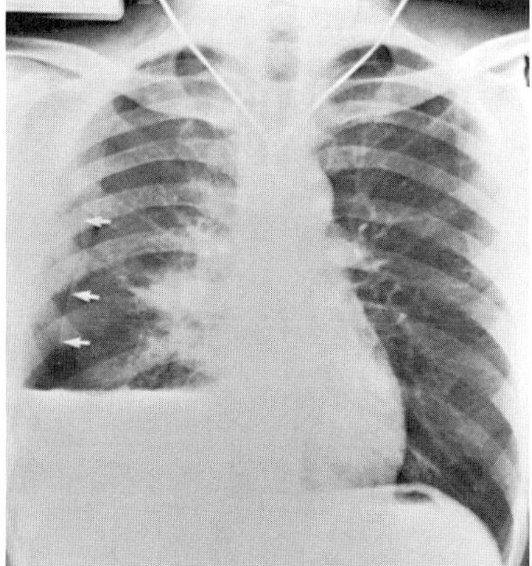

FIGURE 1-254 Chest radiograph shows right hydropneumothorax. Horizontal line in lower right hemithorax is interface between air and liquid in pleural space. *Arrows* point to visceral pleura above level of effusion. There is air in pleural space between visceral pleura and chest wall. (From Weinberg SE et al: *Principles of pulmonary medicine,* ed 5, Philadelphia, 2008, Saunders.)

Rx TREATMENT

NONPHARMACOLOGIC THERAPY

- 100% oxygen administration reduces the partial pressure of nitrogen in pleural capillaries, consequently quadrupling the rate of pneumothorax absorption, and should be administered to all patients with pneumothorax.
- Observation alone is acceptable in the asymptomatic patient with a small (<3 cm between lung and chest wall on CXR) pneumothorax. However, a repeat CXR is necessary to demonstrate the stability of the condition, which requires close monitoring.

ACUTE GENERAL Rx

- Initial management is directed at removing air from the pleural space, with subsequent management directed at preventing recurrence.
- Needle aspiration is performed emergently in unstable patients with a tension pneumothorax as a bridge to allow adequate time for chest tube placement.
- Needle aspiration technique or chest tube placement should be considered for stable patients with large primary spontaneous pneumothorax (>3 cm between the lung and chest wall on a CXR).
- There is no firm conclusion on the initial optimal treatment (simple aspiration versus chest tube insertion) for a first episode of primary SP. Studies suggest that shorter hospital stay can be achieved with the aspiration technique, but there is a potential risk of lung laceration.
- Needle aspiration can be done at the bedside using a large-bore angiocatheter needle or commercially available needle thoracotomy kit. The needle is introduced in the second intercostal space midclavicular line. The catheter is left in place and attached to a three-way stopcock and a large syringe. Air is aspirated until resistance is met or the patient experiences significant coughing. Repeat CXR is done immediately after aspiration and again in 4 to 24 hr to document reexpansion of the lung. If the pneumothorax fails to resolve with aspiration, a chest tube should be placed.
- If there is improvement but not complete resolution of pneumothorax after the aspiration, the catheter can be attached to a Heimlich (one-way) valve to allow further lung expansion. Some stable patients can be discharged home with this device in place if close follow-up monitoring can be obtained.
- Chest tube insertion has been recommended for patients with primary SP who do not respond to simple aspiration and for all patients with secondary SP, recurrent pneumothorax, or tension pneumothorax.

PREVENTION

- Multiple techniques have been used to prevent recurrence, including pleurectomy, laser abrasion of parietal pleural, intrapleural instillation of sclerosing agents, and pleural abrasion with dry gauze. The overall recurrence rate is estimated at <5%.
- The current recommended approach is the use of video-assisted thoracoscopy (VATS) with an aim to excise the associated bullae or perform guided pleurodesis or treatment. Most pulmonologists recommend definitive management after the first recurrence. However, high-risk occupations such as divers or pilots should be considered for surgery after their first pneumothorax. Similarly, complex conditions such as patients with persistent bronchopleural fistula suggested by a persistent air leak from the chest tube should also be considered for VATS and early surgical intervention.
- The recurrence rates for the instillation of sclerosing agents (minocycline 5 mg/kg in 50 ml of normal saline or doxycycline 500 mg in 50 ml of normal saline) are higher than VATS-guided therapy. Therefore this mode of therapy should be reserved for patients who are poor surgical candidates.
- Talc has also been used as a sclerosing agent; however, there are case reports of acute respiratory distress syndrome and pleural calcification occurring after use.
- Open thoracotomy is performed in patients who do not respond to VATS or when VATS is not available.

DISPOSITION

- Approximately 25% of patients with primary SP will have recurrence within 2 yr.
- Smoking cessation should be advised.
- The rates of recurrence after the second and third episode of SP are 60% and 80%, respectively, with the majority of recurrences occurring on the same side as the first pneumothorax.
- Death from primary SP is uncommon. In patients with secondary SP and chronic obstructive pulmonary disease, mortality rates range from 1% to 16%.

REFERRAL

A pulmonary specialist and surgical consultation are recommended.

PEARLS & CONSIDERATIONS

- The rate of pleural air absorption is approximately 1.25% of the volume of the hemithorax per day. Therefore the interval for complete resolution of pneumothorax with observation can be estimated.
- Catamenial pneumothorax is a rare condition characterized by recurrent spontaneous pneumothorax coinciding with the onset of menses. It usually affects the right lung and is believed to be caused by endometriosis with involvement of the diaphragm and/or pleura. It is believed to be hormonally related, and treatment is aimed at endometrial suppression.

COMMENTS

- Patients with AIDS and *Pneumocystis carinii* infection have a high incidence of SP. Treatment typically requires chest tube placement and either thoracoscopy or open thoracotomy.

SUGGESTED READINGS

Baumann MH et al: Management of spontaneous pneumothorax: an American College of Chest Physicians Delphi consensus statement, *Chest* 119(2):590, 2001.

Baumann MH et al: Pneumothorax, *Respirology* 9(2):137, 2004.

Chen F et al: Position of a chest tube at video-assisted thoracoscopic surgery for spontaneous pneumothorax, *Respiration* 73(3):329, 2006.

Deavanand A et al: Simple aspiration versus chest tube insertion in the management of primary spontaneous pneumothorax: a systematic review, *Respir Med* 98(7):579, 2004.

Morimoto T et al: Effects of timing of thoracoscopic surgery for primary spontaneous pneumothorax on prognosis and cost, *Am J Surg* 187(6):767, 2004.

Noppen M et al: Music: a new cause of primary spontaneous pneumothorax, *Thorax* 59(8):722, 2004.

Wakai A: Spontaneous pneumothorax, *Clin Evid* 13:1884, 2005.

AUTHORS: **RICHARD REGNANTE, M.D.,** and **KENNETH KORR, M.D.**

P

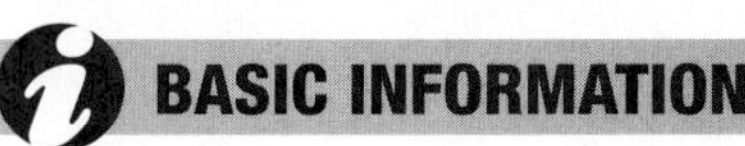

BASIC INFORMATION

DEFINITION

Contact dermatitis caused by exposure to urushiol, the oil of plants of the genus *Toxicodendron,* which includes poison ivy, poison oak, and poison sumac.

SYNONYMS

Rhus dermatitis
Toxicodendron dermatitis

ICD-9CM CODES
ICD 692.6

EPIDEMIOLOGY & DEMOGRAPHICS

INCIDENCE: Affects 10 to 40 million Americans annually

PEAK INCIDENCE: More frequent in months when outdoor activity is more common.

PREVALENCE: From 50% to 75% of the adult population is clinically sensitive to these plants. Sensitivity rates are lower in urban areas. (Tolerance is found in 10% to 15% of the population.)

PREDOMINANT SEX AND AGE: Sensitization occurs most commonly between ages 8 and 14 yr. Sensitivity wanes with age, especially with limited exposure and prior mild reactions.

GENETICS: There is believed to be a genetic susceptibility to sensitivity; however, the rash occurs in all ethnicities and skin types.

RISK FACTORS: Firefighters, forestry workers, farmers, and outdoor workers in general as well as those who participate in outdoor recreation. These plants are indigenous to the United States, Canada, and Mexico, and cases are most common in these areas.

PHYSICAL FINDINGS & CLINICAL PRESENTATION

- Patients typically present with intense pruritus and rash. The patient may not be aware of exposure to the plant.
- Symptoms typically peak from 1 to 14 days after exposure depending on the degree of exposure and thickness of affected skin.
- Dermatitis may initially present as erythema and may develop into papules, vesicles, and bullae.
- Lesions may be found in the classic linear configuration, typically in exposed areas likely to have been in contact with plants. Atypical appearance or location of dermatitis is more common with secondary exposure, such as through pets or infected tools or clothing.
- Face and genital involvement may present with significant edema.
- Inhalation of urushiol aerosolized by fire can cause significant respiratory tract inflammation. This can be a particular occupational hazard of forest firefighters.

ETIOLOGY

- Initial contact with oil of plants in this genus, which is released with damage to plant parts, causes a classic T-lymphocyte–mediated delayed-type allergic reaction.
- Subsequent exposures cause a cell-mediated cytotoxic immune response.

Dx DIAGNOSIS

DIFFERENTIAL DIAGNOSIS

- Allergic contact dermatitis from other plants or nonplant substances
- Irritant contact dermatitis
- Nummular dermatitis
- Arthropod reactions, including scabies and bedbug bites

WORKUP

- Typically not needed. Diagnosis is based on characteristic rash and possibly history of exposure.

Rx TREATMENT

Prevention is the most effective treatment.

NONPHARMACOLOGIC THERAPY

- After known exposure, patients should remove contaminated clothing and wash the skin gently with soap and water. Washing after appearance of dermatitis does not prevent further lesions.
- Calamine lotion, cool compresses, baking soda, or colloidal oatmeal baths may provide symptomatic relief.
- Keep nails short and clean to help prevent secondary bacterial infection.
- Exposed clothing, as well as tools, pets, and equipment, should be washed with soap and water to prevent secondary exposure.

ACUTE GENERAL Rx

- Topical steroids generally should be avoided, although they may be effective in mild, early cases with erythema and pruritus but no vesiculation.
- Topical antibiotics should be avoided.
- Use of antihistamines for associated pruritus may be effective, but this has not been extensively studied.
- Systemic corticosteroids offer significant relief in moderate to severe rhus dermatitis, including generalized rash or severe facial or genital involvement.
- Effective dosing of oral prednisone is 1 mg/kg/day over 7 to 10 days (maximum 60 mg initial dose), with tapering over an additional 7 to 10 days.
- Inadequate doses or too-rapid tapering of systemic steroids may cause symptom rebound.

CHRONIC Rx

- Recurrence may be caused by repeated exposure to fomites, including contaminated clothing, equipment, or pets.
- Secondary bacterial infection of the skin is the most common complication of rhus dermatitis.

DISPOSITION

Untreated rhus dermatitis will resolve in 1 to 3 weeks.

REFERRAL

To dermatology if there is diagnostic confusion

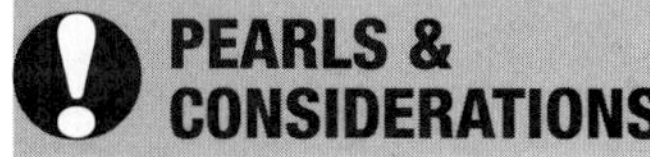

PEARLS & CONSIDERATIONS

PREVENTION

- Patients should be educated regarding identification and avoidance as well as washing to remove the oil after exposure.
- Total avoidance of the plants may not be practical.
- The use of barrier creams applied before exposure to prevent dermatitis may be of some benefit.
- Products available for postexposure prophylaxis are effective; however, equal efficacy may be obtained from less expensive liquid dishwashing soap.
- Desensitization has not been found to be effective.

PATIENT & FAMILY EDUCATION

- "Leaves of three, let it be," is a helpful reminder for patients.
- Patient education material, including access to photographs of the leaves of these plants in a variety of seasons and conditions, may be useful.

SUGGESTED READINGS

Gladman AC: Toxicodendron dermatitis: poison ivy, oak, and sumac, *Wilderness Environ Med* 17(2):120, 2006.

McGovern TW et al: Is it, or isn't it? Poison ivy look-alikes, *Am J Contact Dermat* 11(2):104, 2000.

AUTHOR: **MARGARET TRYFOROS, M.D.**

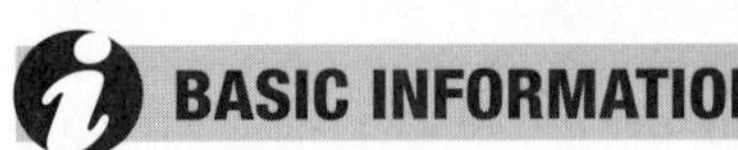

BASIC INFORMATION

DEFINITION

Poliomyelitis is a symptomatic infection caused by poliovirus, which (on rare occasions) may result in paralysis.

SYNONYMS

Polio
Infantile paralysis

ICD-9CM CODES
045.9 Poliomyelitis

EPIDEMIOLOGY & DEMOGRAPHICS

INCIDENCE (IN U.S.):

- Approximately 8 cases/yr.
- All cases in the U.S. and Western Hemisphere are now vaccine associated (because of oral polio vaccine [OPV]).

PREDOMINANT AGE: Almost always infants or young children

GENETICS:

Neonatal Infection: Most cases occur in otherwise healthy infants who receive OPV, or their contacts.

PHYSICAL FINDINGS & CLINICAL PRESENTATION

- Exposure of a nonimmune host to poliovirus usually results in asymptomatic infection.
- A small percentage of individuals may have one of three presentations:
  1. Abortive poliomyelitis: a flulike illness
     a. Fever
     b. Malaise
     c. Headache
     d. Sore throat
  2. Nonparalytic poliomyelitis: an aseptic meningitis that correlates with invasion of the CNS
     a. Headache
     b. Neck stiffness
     c. Change in mental status
  3. Paralytic poliomyelitis
     a. Most commonly affects the lumbar or bulbar regions
     b. Following paralysis, a period of variable degrees of recovery, the majority of which occurs in 2 to 6 mo
     c. Paralysis from involvement of motor neurons in the spinal cord
     d. Flaccid paralysis without sensory defects
     e. Postpolio syndrome late sequela, which may occur many years after the acute illness
     f. Functional deterioration of muscle groups that had recovered from initial paralysis thought to result from failure of reinnervation, which initially was able to restore function to weakened or paralyzed areas

ETIOLOGY

- Virus of genus *Enterovirus* (3 serotypes of polio virus [types 1 to 3])
- Classic endemic and epidemic disease caused by wild-type poliovirus
- All cases in the U.S. currently caused by a live, attenuated virus in the OPV
  1. Extremely rare complication that occurs in vaccine recipients or their contacts
  2. Paralysis from lower motor neuron damage caused by viral infection

Dx DIAGNOSIS

DIFFERENTIAL DIAGNOSIS

- Guillain-Barré syndrome
- CVA
- Botulism food poisoning
- Spinal cord compression
- Other enteroviruses:
  1. Aseptic meningitis
  2. Paralysis (rare)

WORKUP

- Isolation of virus:
  1. Stool or a rectal swab
  2. Throat swabs
  3. Rarely CSF
- Paired sera for antibody titer determinations

LABORATORY TESTS

CSF:

- Aseptic meningitis
- Elevated WBCs
- Elevated protein
- Normal glucose

IMAGING STUDIES

MRI may show involvement of anterior horn of the spinal cord.

Rx TREATMENT

NONPHARMACOLOGIC THERAPY

- Maintenance of respiration and hydration
- Early mobilization and exercise once fever subsides

ACUTE GENERAL Rx

- Aimed at reduction of pain and muscle spasm
- No agent to alter the course of disease

CHRONIC Rx

Physical therapy

DISPOSITION

- In the abortive and nonparalytic forms, complete recovery
- Paralytic disease:
  1. Variable degrees of recovery
  2. 80% usually in the first 6 mo following illness

REFERRAL

Always refer to an infectious disease consultant. Cases should be reported to public health agencies.

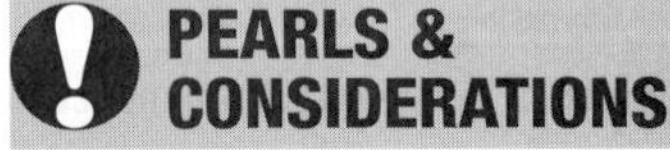

PEARLS & CONSIDERATIONS

COMMENTS

- Risk of disease in recipients of OPV is approximately 1 in 2.5 million.
- Use of inactivated polio vaccine (IPV) is not associated with disease:
  1. Does not confer local (mucosal) immunity
  2. Will not immunize nonvaccinated contacts
  3. Requires boosters
  4. Is given by injection
- To decrease the incidence of vaccine-associated polio, the routine childhood vaccination schedule has been changed. A recent recommendation for use of a sequential IPV-OPV schedule has again been modified. Exclusive use of IPV is now recommended. OPV use is limited to unvaccinated persons with plans for imminent ($<$4 wk) travel to polio-endemic areas.

SUGGESTED READINGS

Alexander LN et al: Vaccine policy changes and epidemiology of poliomyelitis in the United States, *JAMA* 292(14):1696, 2004.

Howard RS: Poliomyelitis and the postpolio syndrome, *BMJ* 330(7503):1314, 2005.

Progress towards poliomyelitis eradication in India, January 2004 to May 2005, *Wkly Epidemiol Rec* 80(27):235, 2005.

Senior K et al: Polio eradication within our grasp? *Lancet Infect Dis* 8(10):591-592, 2008.

Wiysonge CS et al: Eradication of poliomyelitis, *Lancet* 366(9492):1163, 2005.

AUTHORS: **DENNIS J. MIKOLICH, M.D.,** and **GLENN G. FORT, M.D., M.P.H.**

BASIC INFORMATION

DEFINITION

Polyarteritis nodosa is a vasculitic syndrome involving medium-sized to small arteries, characterized histologically by necrotizing inflammation of the arterial media and inflammatory cell infiltration.

SYNONYMS

Periarteritis nodosa
PAN
Necrotizing arteritis

ICD-9CM CODES
446.0 Polyarteritis nodosa

EPIDEMIOLOGY & DEMOGRAPHICS

INCIDENCE: One per 100,000 persons annually. Increased incidence in patients with hepatitis B surface antigen or hepatitis C virus.
PREDOMINANT SEX: Male/female ratio is 2:1.

PHYSICAL FINDINGS & CLINICAL PRESENTATION

- Typical presentation is subacute, with the onset of constitutional symptoms over weeks to months
- Weight loss, nausea, vomiting
- Testicular pain or tenderness
- Myalgias, weakness, or leg tenderness
- Neuropathy (mononeuritis multiplex), foot drop
- Livedo reticularis, ulceration of digits, abdominal pain after meals, hematemesis, hematochezia, hypertension, asymmetric polyarthritis (tending to involve large joints of lower extremities); true synovitis occurs only in a minority of patients
- Fever may be present (polyarteritis nodosa is often a cause of fever of unknown origin) and can range from intermittent, low-grade fevers to high fevers with chills
- Tachycardia is common and often striking

ETIOLOGY

- Unknown.
- Hepatitis B virus–associated polyarteritis nodosa appears to be an immune complex–mediated disease.

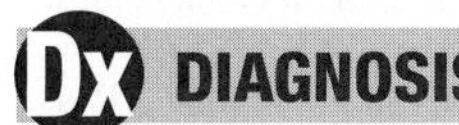

DIAGNOSIS

DIFFERENTIAL DIAGNOSIS

Cryoglobulinemia, systemic lupus erythematosus, infections (e.g., subacute bacterial endocarditis, trichinosis, *Rickettsia*), lymphoma

WORKUP

- Laboratory evaluation, arteriography, and biopsy of small or medium-sized arteries can confirm diagnosis. Clinical manifestations are variable and depend on the arteries involved and the organs affected (e.g., kidney involvement occurs in >80% of cases).
- The presence of any three of the following 10 items allows the diagnosis of polyarteritis nodosa with a sensitivity of 82% and a specificity of 86%:
  1. Weight loss >4 kg
  2. Livedo reticularis
  3. Testicular pain or tenderness
  4. Myalgias, weakness, or leg tenderness
  5. Neuropathy
  6. Diastolic blood pressure >90 mm Hg
  7. Elevated blood urea nitrogen (BUN) or creatinine
  8. Positive test for hepatitis B virus
  9. Arteriography revealing small or large aneurysms and focal constrictions between dilated segments
  10. Biopsy of small or medium-sized artery containing white blood cells

LABORATORY TESTS

- Elevated BUN or creatinine, positive test for hepatitis B virus or hepatitis C.
- Elevated erythrocyte sedimentation rate and C-reactive protein, anemia, elevated platelets, eosinophilia, proteinuria, hematuria.
- Biopsy of small or medium-sized artery of symptomatic sites (muscle, nerve) is >90% specific. Biopsy of the gastrocnemius muscle and sural nerve are commonly performed.
- Assays for antinuclear antibody and rheumatoid factor are negative; however, low, nonspecific titers may be detected.

IMAGING STUDIES

Arteriography can be done in patients with negative biopsies or if there are no symptomatic sites. Visceral angiography will reveal aneurysmal dilation of the renal, mesenteric, or hepatic arteries.

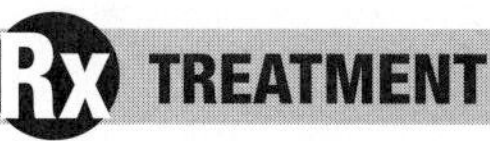

TREATMENT

NONPHARMACOLOGIC THERAPY

Low-sodium diet in hypertensive patients

ACUTE GENERAL Rx

Prednisone 1 to 2 mg/kg/day; cyclophosphamide in refractory cases

CHRONIC Rx

Monitoring for infections and potential complications such as thrombosis, infarction, or organ necrosis

DISPOSITION

The 5-yr survival is <20% in untreated patients. Treatment with corticosteroids increases survival to approximately 50%. Use of both corticosteroids and immunosuppressive drugs may increase 5-yr survival to >80%. Poor prognostic signs are severe renal or gastrointestinal involvement.

REFERRAL

Surgical referral for biopsy

SUGGESTED READING

Stone JH: Polyarteritis nodosa, *JAMA* 288:1632, 2002.

AUTHOR: **FRED F. FERRI, M.D.**

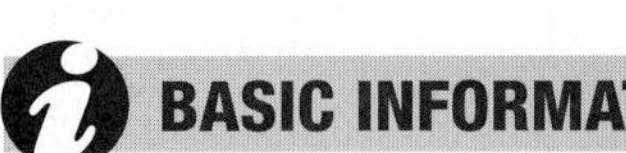

BASIC INFORMATION

DEFINITION

Polycystic kidney disease (PKD) refers to a systemic hereditary disorder characterized by the formation of cysts in the cortex and medulla of both kidneys (Figs. 1-255 and 1-256).

SYNONYMS

Autosomal-dominant polycystic kidney disease (ADPKD)

ICD-9CM CODES

753.1 Polycystic kidney, unspecified type
753.13 Polycystic kidney, autosomal dominant

EPIDEMIOLOGY & DEMOGRAPHICS

- The most common Mendelian disorder of the kidneys
- Affects all racial groups worldwide
- Results in kidney failure in the majority of individuals by the fifth to sixth decade
- PKD occurs in one in 700 to 1000 persons
- Usually presents in the third to fourth decades of life

PHYSICAL FINDINGS & CLINICAL PRESENTATION

- Characterized by focal development of renal and extrarenal cysts in an age-dependent manner, resulting in a slow, gradual, and massive kidney enlargement.

Symptoms:

- Pain (60%): acute pain can be associated renal hemorrhage, passage of stones (20% patients; usually uric acid or calcium oxalate), and urinary tract infections
- Palpable flank mass
- Hypertension: >60% of patients; usually develops before the loss of renal function
- Headache
- Nocturia, hematuria

Renal manifestations:

- Kidney and cyst volumes and renal blood flow (or vascular resistance) are the strongest predictors of renal function decline. Kidney function does not decline in individuals with PKD until kidney size is at least five times greater than normal.
- Morphometric analysis of sequential CT was shown to be sufficiently accurate to monitor rates of renal enlargement in PKD, and MRI-based methods have been developed. Two general groups of kidney volume increase: those with rapid rates (>5% increase in total kidney volume per year) and those with rates of progression <5% per year. Intervals between measurements as short as 6 mo may be adequate to determine an effect of treatment that reduces the rates of volume progression >50% in those with rapidly progressive disease.
- All cysts develop from preexisting renal tubule segments, and only a small portion of the nephrons (1%) undergoes cystic formation.
- Renal failure: in most patients renal function is maintained within normal range, despite relentless growth of cysts, until the fourth to sixth decades of life.
- Nephrolithiasis (20%)
- Urinary tract infection

Extrarenal manifestations:

- Associated with liver cysts (50% to 70%), pancreatic cysts (10%), splenic cysts (5%), central nervous system arachnoid cysts (5%), and cerebral aneurysms (20%)
- Polycystic liver disease: most common extrarenal manifestation-associated with both *PKD1* and non-*PKD1* genotypes
- Vascular manifestations: intracranial aneurysms (occur in approximately 6% of patients with a negative family history of aneurysms and 16% of those with a positive history), thoracic aortic and cervicocephalic artery dissection, and coronary artery aneurysms
- Increased incidence of diverticular disease and mitral valve prolapse

ETIOLOGY

- Dominantly inherited heterogenic systemic disease: mutations in *PKD1* (chromosome region 16p13.3; 85% of cases) or *PKD2* (4q21; approximately 15% of cases).
- Polycystin 1 and polycystin 2 are the protein products of PKD1 and PKD2, which interact and coassemble and seem to function together to regulate the morphologic configuration of epithelial cells. Although individuals with PKD1 are clinically indistinguishable from individuals with PKD2, patients with PKD2 have a less severe course of disease with a later mean age of diagnosis, hypertension, and end-stage renal disease (ESRD).
- Disease penetrance is 100%.

Dx DIAGNOSIS

Sonographic imaging or CT scan:

1. In an individual with a family history for the disease, including:
   - Age <30 yr: at least two unilateral or bilateral cysts
   - 30 to 59 yr: two cysts in each kidney
   - ≥60 yr: four cysts in each kidney
2. In the absence of a family history: bilateral renal enlargement or cysts or the presence of multiple bilateral cysts with hepatic cysts together and in the absence of other manifestations suggesting a different renal cyst disease
   - Genetic testing can be used when the imaging results are equivocal and when a definitive diagnosis is required in a younger individual, such as a potential living related kidney donor.

DIFFERENTIAL DIAGNOSIS

- Simple cysts
- Autosomal-recessive polycystic kidney disease in children
- Tuberous sclerosis
- von Hippel Lindau syndrome
- Acquired cystic kidney disease

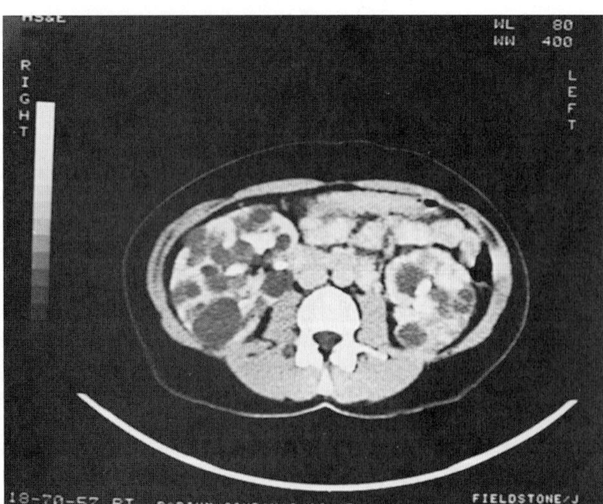

FIGURE 1-255 Tomogram of autosomal-dominant polycystic kidney disease. Kidney cysts. (From Stein JH [ed]: *Internal medicine,* ed 5, St Louis, 1998, Mosby.)

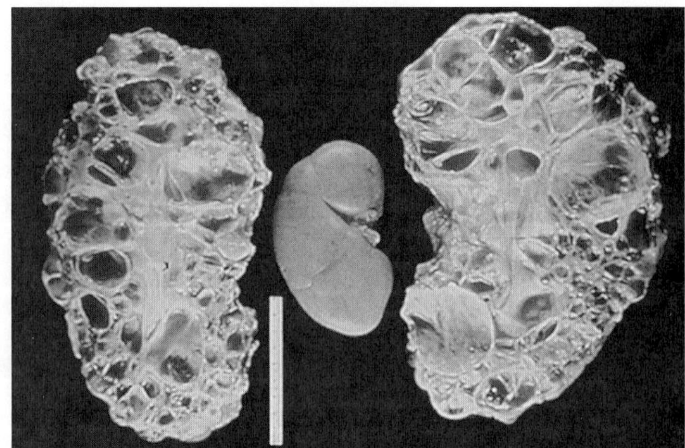

FIGURE 1-256 Markedly enlarged polycystic kidneys from a patient with autosomal-dominant polycystic kidney disease compared with a normal kidney *(middle).* (From Johnson RJ, Feehally J: *Comprehensive clinical nephrology*, ed 2, St Louis, 2000, Mosby.)

LABORATORY TESTS

- Hemoglobin and hematocrit are elevated because of increased secretion of erythropoietin from functioning renal cysts.
- Electrolyte abnormalities commonly seen in any patients with renal insufficiency.
- Blood urea nitrogen and creatinine can be elevated.
- Urinalysis can show microscopic hematuria and proteinuria (seldom >1 g/24 hr). Proteinuria >2 g/day is unusual and suggests the presence of another kidney disease.

IMAGING STUDIES

- A cyst is considered to be present if it measures >2 mm in diameter.
- Abdominal renal ultrasound is the easiest and more cost-efficient test for renal cysts. Renal ultrasound can detect cysts from 1 to 1.5 cm.
- Abdominal CT scan is more sensitive than ultrasound and can detect cysts as small as 0.5 cm.
- Both studies can detect associated hepatic, splenic, and pancreatic cysts.
- MRI is more sensitive than ultrasound and may help distinguish renal cell carcinomas from simple cysts.

Rx TREATMENT

NONPHARMACOLOGIC THERAPY

- Treatment consists of the standard therapies for chronic renal disease, including good blood pressure control and control of hyperlipidemia.
- When conservative measures fail to control the pain, infection, or bleeding, surgical interventions such as cystic decompression by aspiration under ultrasound or CT guidance or laparoscopic or surgical cyst fenestration through lumbotomy or flank incision may be of benefit.
- When above measures fail, nephrectomy should be undertaken in ESRD.
- Combined percutaneous cyst drainage and antibiotic treatment provide the best treatment results for hepatic cyst infection.

ACUTE GENERAL Rx

- Kidney infections should be treated with antibiotics known to penetrate the cyst (e.g., trimethoprim-sulfamethoxazole 1 tablet PO bid or ciprofloxacin 250 mg PO bid).
- Early detection and treatment of hypertension is important because cardiovascular disease is the main cause of death.

CHRONIC Rx

- Dialysis for end-stage renal failure.
- Pretransplant nephrectomy is reserved for patients with a history of infected cyst or frequent bleeding.
- Renal transplantation is the treatment of choice for ESRD.
- Cyst infections are often difficult to treat. Lipophilic agents penetrate the cysts consistently. If fever persists after 1 to 2 wk of appropriate antimicrobial treatment, percutaneous or surgical drainage of the cysts may be needed. Several months of antibiotic treatment may be needed to eradicate the infection.
- Most cases of polycystic liver disease do not need treatment; patients should avoid estrogens and compounds that promote cyclic adenosine monophosphate accumulation (e.g., caffeine).

DISPOSITION

- Most patients with PKD will progress to renal failure.
- Gross hematuria is usually self-limited.

REFERRAL

- Nephrology consultation.
- Urology can also be consulted in patients with nephrolithiasis, for recurrent episodes of gross hematuria, or for consideration for nephrectomy before transplantation.
- Counseling should be done before PKD genetic testing. Benefits include certainty of diagnosis that could affect family planning, early detection and treatment of disease complications, and selection of genetically unaffected family members for living related donor transplantation. Potential discrimination in terms of insurability and employment associated with a positive diagnosis should be discussed.

PEARLS & CONSIDERATIONS

- ESRD patients with PKD do better on dialysis than do patients with other causes of ESRD.
- There is no difference in patient survival after transplantation between patients with PKD and other ESRD populations.
- Widespread screening is not indicated. Indications for screening include family history of aneurysm, subarachnoid hemorrhage, previous aneurysm rupture, preparation for major elective surgery, high-risk occupations (airplane pilots), and patient anxiety despite adequate information.
- Kidney and cyst volumes are the strongest predictors of renal function decline.

COMMENTS

- Conservative management is recommended for patients with a small (<7 mm) cerebral aneurysm, particularly in the anterior circulation. Rescreening of patients with a family history of intracranial aneurysm after 5 to 10 yr seems reasonable.
- Studies with treatment protocols involving vasopressin antagonists, somatostatin, and rapamycin are underway to slow the progression of PKD.

EBM EVIDENCE

There is evidence that antihypertensives are effective in the management of patients with chronic renal disease.

There have been no clinical trials evaluating the efficacy of antihypertensive therapy in patients with polycystic kidney disease. Most information is derived from studies involving patients with chronic renal disease. The following statements are based upon evidence-based consensus:

Multiple antihypertensive agents are usually required to reach target blood pressure.[1] ©

ACE inhibitors are more effective than other antihypertensive agents in slowing the progression of most nondiabetic kidney diseases.[1] ©

ACE inhibitors, ARBs, and nondihydropyridine calcium-channel blockers have a greater antiproteinuric effect than other antihypertensive classes in nondiabetic kidney disease.[1] ©

Diuretics may potentiate the beneficial effects of ACE inhibitors and ARBs in nondiabetic kidney disease.[1] ©

Evidence-Based Reference

1. Kidney Disease Outcomes Quality Initiative (K/DOQI): K/DOQI clinical practice guidelines on hypertension and antihypertensive agents in chronic kidney disease, *Am J Kidney Dis* 43:S1-29, 2004. ©

SUGGESTED READINGS

Chapman AB: Autosomal dominant polycystic kidney disease: time for a change? *J Am Soc Nephrol* 18(5):1399, 2007.

Grantham J: Volume progression in autosomal dominant polycystic kidney disease: the major factor determining clinical outcomes, *Clin J Am Soc Nephrol* 1(1):148, 2006.

Pei Y: Diagnostic approach in autosomal dominant polycystic kidney disease, *Clin J Am Soc Nephrol* 1(5):1108, 2006.

Rapoport J: Autosomal dominant polycystic kidney disease: path physiology and treatment, *Q J Med* 100:1, 2007.

Torres VE et al: Autosomal dominant polycystic kidney disease, *Lancet* 369(9569):1287, 2007.

AUTHOR: **SHAHNAZ PUNJANI, M.D.**

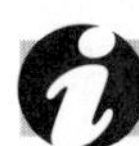

BASIC INFORMATION

DEFINITION

Polycystic ovary syndrome (PCOS) is characterized by an accumulation of incompletely developed follicles in the ovaries due to anovulation and associated with ovarian androgen production. In its complete form it associates polycystic ovaries, amenorrhea, hirsutism, and obesity.

SYNONYMS

Stein-Leventhal syndrome
PCOS

ICD-9CM CODES
256.4 Polycystic ovary syndrome

EPIDEMIOLOGY & DEMOGRAPHICS

- 6% to 7% of reproductive-age women (most common endocrine disorder in this population).
- Symptoms usually begin around the time of menarche, and the diagnosis is often made during adolescence or young adulthood.
- Increased risk of endometrial and ovarian cancers.

PHYSICAL FINDINGS & CLINICAL PRESENTATION

- Oligomenorrhea or amenorrhea
- Dysfunctional uterine bleeding
- Infertility
- Hirsutism
- Acne
- Obesity (40% only)
- Insulin resistance (type 2 diabetes mellitus)

ETIOLOGY & PATHOGENESIS

Elevated serum luteinizing hormone (LH) concentrations and an increased serum LH/follicle-stimulating hormone (FSH) ratio result either from an increased gonadotropin-releasing hormone hypothalamic secretion or less likely from a primary pituitary abnormality. This results in dysregulation of androgen secretion and increased intraovarian androgen, the effect of which in the ovary is follicular atresia, maturation arrest, polycystic ovaries, and anovulation. Hyperinsulinemia is a contributing factor to ovarian hyperandrogenism, independent of LH excess. A role for insulin growth factor (IGF) receptors has been postulated for the association of PCOS and diabetes.

DIAGNOSIS

The diagnosis of PCOS excludes secondary causes (androgen-producing neoplasm, hyperprolactinemia, adult-onset congenital adrenal hyperplasia).

Clinical:

- PCOS is the most common cause of chronic anovulation with estrogen present. A positive progesterone withdrawal test establishes the presence of estrogen. Medroxyprogesterone (Provera) 10 mg qd is administered for 5 days and bleeding occurs if estrogen is present.
- The presence of oligomenorrhea, hirsutism, obesity, and documented polycystic ovaries establishes the diagnosis.

DIFFERENTIAL DIAGNOSIS

Causes of amenorrhea:

- Primary (unusual in PCOS)
  1. Genetic disorder (Turner's syndrome)
  2. Anatomic abnormality (e.g., imperforate hymen)
- Secondary
  1. Pregnancy
  2. Functional (cause unknown, anorexia nervosa, stress, excessive exercise, hyperthyroidism, less commonly hypothyroidism, adrenal dysfunction, pituitary dysfunction, severe systemic illness, drugs such as oral contraceptives, estrogens, or dopamine agonists)
  3. Abnormalities of the genital tract (uterine tumor, endometrial scarring, ovarian tumor)

LABORATORY TESTS

- Glucose tolerance test at the initial presentation and every 2 yr thereafter (rule out diabetes mellitus)
- Fasting lipid panel (rule out dyslipidemia), alanine aminotransferase, aspartate aminotransferase (rule out hepatic steatosis)
- Elevated LH/FSH ratio >2.5
- Prolactin level elevation in 25%
- Elevated androgens (testosterone, DHEA-S) (rule out androgen-secreting tumor)
- Other: thyroid-stimulating hormone (rule out hypothyroidism), 17-hydroxyprogesterone (rule out congenital adrenal hyperplasia), 24-h urine for cortisol and creatinine (rule out Cushing's syndrome)

IMAGING STUDIES

Pelvic ultrasound (or CT scan) reveals the presence of twofold to fivefold ovarian enlargement with a thickened tunica albuginea, thecal hyperplasia, and 20 or more subcapsular follicles from 1 to 15 mm in diameter (Fig. 1-257).

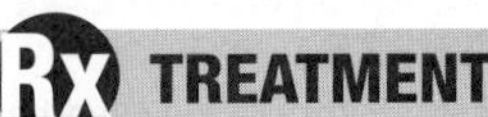

TREATMENT

The goal is to interrupt the self-perpetuating abnormal hormone cycle:

- Reduction of ovarian androgen secretion by laparoscopic ovarian wedge resection
- Reduction of ovarian androgen secretion by using oral contraceptives or LH-releasing hormone (LHRH) analogs
- Weight reduction for all obese women with PCOS
- FSH stimulation with clomiphene HMG or pulsatile LHRH
- Urofollitropin (pure FSH) administration
- Glitazones (rosiglitazone, pioglitazone) may improve ovulation and hirsutism in PCOS
- Metformin improves ovulation, insulin sensitivity, and possibly hyperandrogenemia

Choice of treatment:

- The management of hirsutism without risking pregnancy includes oral contraceptives, glucocorticoids, LHRH analogs, or spironolactone (an antiandrogen). Finasteride and flutamide may be similarly effective in reducing hirsutism as spironolactone.
- Pregnancy can be achieved with clomiphene (alone or with glucocorticoids, human chorionic gonadotropin, or bromocriptine), HMG, urofollitropin, pulsatile LHRH, or ovarian wedge resection. (Metformin may induce ovulation.)

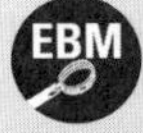

EVIDENCE

Please note: Complete text of EBM for this topic is available online.

Key trials and commentary:

Clomiphene citrate (CC) and metformin are two effective drugs used to induce ovulation in patients with polycystic ovary syndrome (PCOS), even if it is still unclear which compound between them should be initially administered.

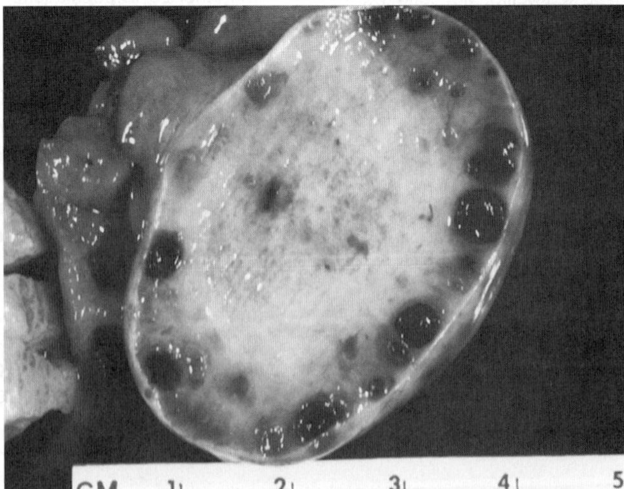

FIGURE 1-257 Sagittal section of a polycystic ovary illustrating large number of follicular cysts and thickened stroma. (From Mishell DR: *Comprehensive gynecology*, ed 3, St Louis, 1997, Mosby.)

The aim of the study was to compare in a clinical setting the efficacy of CC and metformin as first-line approaches for treating anovulation in infertile PCOS patients.

This study showed that a 6-month course of 1700 mg/day metformin treatment and CC administered in an escalation protocol are two effective first-line approaches for improving fertility in anovulatory PCOS women.

The treatment of anovulation in patients with PCOS is often needed for fertility success. CC has been used extensively to induce ovulation and treat infertility in women with PCOS. Because many patients with PCOS have insulin resistance, treatment with metformin has also been effective in improving ovulation. Palomba et al compared the results of 6 months of treatment with CC vs. metformin in inducing ovulatory cycles, pregnancy, and abortion rates. They observed no significant differences between the groups for these parameters. The patients in the current study were not selected for BMI or degree of obesity. Thus, in previous studies, nonobese patients with PCOS responded better to metformin than CC in terms of pregnancy and abortion rates. Although there may be modest differences in ovulation success with metformin or CC, the study confirms that both agents may be used as first-line therapy for treating anovulation in women with PCOS. CC has a higher risk of multiple births than metformin. It is reassuring to be able to offer a selection based on the individual characteristics of the patient with PCOS.

Weight loss and metformin therapy are reported to be beneficial in improving the biochemical hyperandrogenaemia and insulin resistance of PCOS. Rimonabant has been found to reduce weight and improve the metabolic profile in patients with obesity, type 2 diabetes, and metabolic syndrome.

This study sought to compare the effects of insulin sensitization with metformin to weight reduction by rimonabant on biochemical hyperandrogenemia and insulin resistance in patients with PCOS.

This study suggests that the weight loss through rimonabant therapy may be of use in patients with PCOS and appears superior to insulin sensitization by metformin in reducing the FAI and insulin resistance in obese PCOS patients treated over a 12-week period.

PCOS is a common disorder in women of the reproductive age and is characterized by insulin resistance, the metabolic syndrome, oligomenorrhea, and androgen excess. Metformin is commonly used to improve insulin resistance, body weight, and hyperandrogenemia. Rimonabant, a cannabinoid receptor 1 blocker, has been reported to improve the metabolic syndrome, lipid parameters, and insulin resistance in obese persons. This study compared the effects of 12 weeks of treatment with metformin or rimonabant in women with PCOS. Rimonabant but not metformin significantly improved characteristics of the metabolic syndrome and free testosterone index and total testosterone during the therapy. Rimonabant treatment did not significantly affect triglycerides or high-density lipoprotein (HDL) cholesterol. The reduction in weight loss but not in insulin resistance correlated well with androgen reduction in the rimonabant-treated group. Although the lack of benefit with metformin is not consistent with other studies, rimonabant has promise in the treatment of PCOS, and long-term studies are needed to determine safety and efficacy.

Evidence-Based References

1. Palomba S et al: Clomiphene citrate versus metformin as first-line approach for the treatment of anovulation in infertile patients with polycystic ovary syndrome, *J Clin Endocrinol Metab* 92:3498-3503, 2007. Commentary by A.W. Meikle, M.D. Ⓐ

2. Sathyapalan T et al: A comparison between rimonabant and metformin in reducing biochemical hyperandrogenaemia and insulin resistance in patients with polycystic ovary syndrome (PCOS): a randomized open-label parallel study. *Clin Endocrinol* 69:931-935. 2008. Commentary by A.W. Meikle, M.D. Ⓐ

SUGGESTED READINGS

Nestler JE: Metformin for the treatment of polycystic ovary syndrome, *N Engl J Med* 358:47-54, 2008.

Radosh L: Drug treatment for polycystic ovary syndrome, *Am Fam Phys* 79(8):671-676, 2009.

AUTHOR: **FRED F. FERRI, M.D.**

BASIC INFORMATION

DEFINITION

Polycythemia vera is a chronic myeloproliferative disorder characterized mainly by erythrocytosis (increase in red blood cell [RBC] mass).

SYNONYMS

Primary polycythemia
Vaquez disease

ICD-9CM CODES
238.4 Polycythemia vera

EPIDEMIOLOGY & DEMOGRAPHICS

Incidence of 0.5 cases per 100,000 persons; mean age at onset is 60 yr; men are affected more often than are women.

PHYSICAL FINDINGS & CLINICAL PRESENTATION

The patient generally comes to medical attention because of symptoms associated with increased blood volume and viscosity or impaired platelet function:

- Impaired cerebral circulation resulting in headache, vertigo, blurred vision, dizziness, transient ischemic attack, cerebrovascular accident
- Fatigue, poor exercise tolerance
- Pruritus, particularly after bathing (caused by overproduction of histamine)
- Bleeding: epistaxis, upper gastrointestinal bleeding (increased incidence of peptic ulcer disease)
- Abdominal discomfort from splenomegaly; hepatomegaly may be present
- Hyperuricemia may result in nephrolithiasis and gouty arthritis

The physical examination may reveal:

- Facial plethora, congestion of oral mucosa, ruddy complexion
- Enlargement and tortuosity of retinal veins
- Splenomegaly (found in >75% of patients)

Dx DIAGNOSIS

DIFFERENTIAL DIAGNOSIS

Smoking:

- Polycythemia is caused by increased carboxyhemoglobin, resulting in left shift in the hemoglobin (Hgb) dissociation curve.
- Laboratory evaluation shows increased hematocrit (Hct), RBC mass, erythropoietin level, and carboxyhemoglobin.
- Splenomegaly is not present on physical examination.

Hypoxemia (secondary polycythemia):

- Living for prolonged periods at high altitudes, pulmonary fibrosis, congenital cardiac lesions with right-to-left shunts.
- Laboratory evaluation shows decreased arterial oxygen saturation and elevated erythropoietin level.
- Splenomegaly is not present on physical examination.

Erythropoietin-producing states:

- Renal cell carcinoma, hepatoma, cerebral hemangioma, uterine fibroids, polycystic kidneys.
- The erythropoietin level is elevated in these patients, and the arterial oxygen saturation is normal.
- Splenomegaly may be present with metastatic neoplasms.

Stress polycythemia (Gaisböck's syndrome, relative polycythemia):

- Laboratory evaluation demonstrates normal RBC mass, arterial oxygen saturation, and erythropoietin level; plasma volume is decreased.
- Splenomegaly is not present on physical examination.

Hemoglobinopathies associated with high oxygen affinity:

- An abnormal oxyhemoglobin-dissociation curve (P50) is present.

WORKUP

Recent developments in molecular biology have identified a single, acquired point mutation in the Janus kinase 2 *(JAK2)* gene in the majority of patients with polycythemia vera and other pH-negative myeloproliferative disorders. The *JAK2* mutation is found in >95% of patients with polycythemia vera and can be used for diagnostic purposes. Testing for the *JAK2 V617F* mutation with polymerase chain reaction assay is now available. In patients with high hematocrit (>52% in men or >48% in women) and in the absence of coexisting secondary erythrocytosis, the presence of the *JAK2* mutation is sufficient for the diagnosis of polycythemia vera.

The diagnosis of polycythemia vera, using standards from the classic Polycythemia Vera Study Group, generally requires the following three major criteria or the first two major criteria plus two minor criteria:

- Major criteria:
  1. Increased RBC mass (>36 ml/kg in men, >32 ml/kg in women)
  2. Normal arterial oxygen saturation (>92%)
  3. Splenomegaly
- Minor criteria:
  1. Thrombocytosis (>400,000/mm^3)
  2. Leukocytosis (>12,000/mm^3)
  3. Elevated leukocyte alkaline phosphatase (>100)
  4. Elevated serum vitamin B_{12} (>900 pg/ml) or vitamin B_{12} binding protein (>2200 pg/ml)

Serum erythropoietin level is the best initial test for the diagnosis of polycythemia vera. A low serum erythropoietin level is highly suggestive of polycythemia vera. A normal level does not exclude the diagnosis. If the erythropoietin level is elevated, obtain abdominal and pelvic CT to rule out renal cercal carcinoma and other causes of polycythemia.

In patients with elevated erythropoietin level, evaluate for secondary erythrocytosis:

- Measure RBC mass by isotope dilution using ^{51}Cr-labeled autologous RBCs (expensive test); a high value eliminates stress polycythemia.
- Measure arterial saturation; a normal value eliminates polycythemia caused by smoking.
- The diagnosis of hemoglobinopathy with high affinity is ruled out by a normal oxyhemoglobin dissociation curve.
- A diagnostic algorithm for polycythemia is described in Section III.

LABORATORY TESTS

- Elevated RBC count (>6 million/mm^3), elevated Hgb (>18 g/dl in men, >16 g/dl in women), elevated Hct (>54% in men, >49% in women)
- Increased white blood cell count (often with basophilia); thrombocytosis in the majority of patients
- Elevated leukocyte alkaline phosphatase, serum vitamin B_{12}, and uric acid levels
- Low serum erythropoietin level
- Bone marrow aspiration revealing RBC hyperplasia and absent iron stores

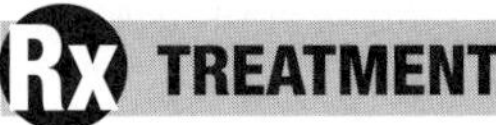

TREATMENT

NONPHARMACOLOGIC THERAPY

Phlebotomy to keep Hct <45% in men and <42% in women is the mainstay of therapy.

ACUTE GENERAL Rx

- Hydroxyurea can be used in conjunction with phlebotomy to decrease the incidence of thrombotic events.
- Interferon-alpha-2b is also effective in controlling RBC values without significant side effects.
- Myelosuppressive therapy with chlorambucil is effective but not routinely used because of its leukemogenic potential.
- Box 1-13 describes an algorithm for management of patients with PV.

CHRONIC Rx

- Patient education regarding need for lifelong monitoring and treatment.
- Adjunctive therapy: treatment of pruritus with antihistamines, control of significant hyperuricemia with allopurinol, reduction of gastric hyperacidity with antacids of H_2 blockers, low-dose aspirin to treat vasomotor symptoms in patients without bleeding diathesis. Low-dose aspirin can safely prevent thrombotic complications in patients with polycythemia vera.

DISPOSITION

- The median survival time without treatment is 6 to 18 mo after diagnosis; phlebotomy extends the average survival time to 12 yr.
- Prognosis is worse in patients >60 yr and those with a history of thrombosis.

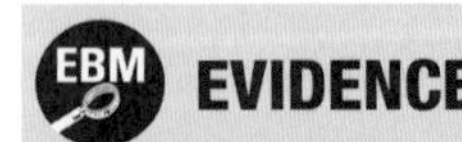

EVIDENCE

Randomized trials have demonstrated the efficacy of regular phlebotomy in increasing overall survival rates in patients with polycythemia vera. Its use is endorsed by expert opinion.

Evidence-based guidelines from the British Society for Haematology (BSH) recommend phlebotomy to maintain the Hct to <0.45.[1] C

Although initial studies were controversial, a recent randomized, controlled trial (RCT) has demonstrated that treatment with low-dose aspirin significantly reduces thrombosis in patients with polycythemia vera. The use of low-dose aspirin is endorsed by expert opinion.

A subsequent RCT compared low-dose aspirin (100 mg/day) and placebo in 518 patients with polycythemia vera. This study found that treatment with aspirin significantly reduced the combined risk of thrombotic events (cardiovascular death, nonfatal myocardial infarction, nonfatal stroke, and major venous thromboembolism) and the rate of thrombotic events. There was no effect on overall mortality rate. Bleeding was not increased with aspirin therapy.[2] A

BOX 1-13 Algorithm for Management of Patients with PV

Low-risk young patients (<60 years) and no prior history of thrombosis, platelet count $<1.5 \times 10^6$ mm^{-3}

Phlebotomy + low-dose aspirin (81 mg/d) to maintain Hct <45% in males and <42% in females. Aspirin should not be used in patients with histories of hemorrhagic episode or with extreme thrombocytosis ($>1.5 \times 10^6$ mm^{-3}) or acquired von Willebrand syndrome.

↓

Thrombosis or hemorrhage
Systemic symptoms
Severe pruritus refractory to histamine antagonists
Painful splenomegaly

↓

Pegylated interferon 90-180 μg/wk or interferon α (3×10^6 units three times/wk; alter dose depending on response and toxicity). Consider the use of pegylated interferon, which can be administered once/wk.

↓

If platelet control is inadequate or patient cannot tolerate interferon, one option could be the use of anagrelide. However, the use of this drug is controversial. In this case, supplemental phlebotomy is required to maintain Hct <45% in males and <42% in females, and the use of hydroxyurea should be considered, especially if patient continues to have thrombotic episodes.

↓

If the patient has increasing splenomegaly, systemic symptoms, or repeated thromboses in spite of adequate dose of hydroxyurea (2-3 g/d) start busulphan 4-6 mg/d PO for 4-8 wk. It should be mentioned that the sequential use of hydroxyurea and busulphan may be associated with an increased risk of leukemia. Supplemental phlebotomy may be required.

↓

Painful splenomegaly
Splenectomy + continued systemic therapy
High-risk patients (>60 years), previous thrombosis, platelet count $>1.5 \times 10^6$ mm^{-3}
Phlebotomy to Hct <42% in females and <45% in males
Aspirin (81 mg/d) to be given only in patients with platelet counts $<1.5 \times 10^6$ mm^{-2}
Myelosuppressive therapy with hydroxyurea 30 mg/kg PO for 1 wk

↓

Then 15-20 mg/kg

If patient continues to have thrombotic episodes and has extreme thrombocytosis or cannot tolerate hydroxyurea, consider pegylated interferon 90-180 μg/wk or add busulphan 4-6 mg/d PO for 4-8 wk.

Stop when blood counts are normalized or platelet count is <300,000 mm^{-3}.

Occasional supplemental phlebotomy if Hct is >42% in females and >45% in males; when patient relapses (patient is symptomatic), initiate busulphan therapy again at same dose.

↓

If patient is poorly compliant, consider ^{32}P: 2.3 mCi/m^2 IV every 12 weeks as needed (limit 5 mCi per dose).

Increase dose by 25% if no response
Patient age >70 years
Phlebotomy + low-dose aspirin + hydroxyurea

↓

No response or poor compliance

Busulphan 4-6 mg/d PO for 4-8 wk. Stop when blood counts are normalized or platelet count is >300,000 mm^{-3}.

↓

No response ^{32}P

(From Hoffmann R et al: *Hematology: basic principles and practice,* ed 5, Philadelphia, 2009, Churchill Livingstone.)

Evidence-based guidelines from BSH recommend aspirin 75 mg/day unless contraindicated.[1] C

The role of hydroxyurea as cytoreductive therapy to reduce thrombosis in polycythemia vera is supported by data from studies evaluating its use in essential thrombocythemia.

A recent RCT compared anagrelide and hydroxyurea in 809 patients with essential thrombocythemia who were at high risk for vascular events. All patients received low-dose aspirin. After median follow-up of 39 mo, this study reported that treatment with hydroxyurea was associated with lower rates of arterial thrombosis, serious hemorrhage, and transformation to myelofibrosis compared with anagrelide. Equivalent long-term control of the platelet count was achieved in both groups.[3] A

The role of cytoreductive therapy for polycythemia vera is endorsed by expert opinion. Evidence-based guidelines from BSH recommend that cytoreduction should be considered in the presence of poor tolerance of venesection; symptomatic or progressive splenomegaly; other evidence of disease progression, such as weight loss, night sweats; or thrombocytosis.[1] C

Recommendations regarding choice of cytoreductive therapy, if indicated, include hydroxyurea, interferon, and anagrelide.[1] C

There is conflicting evidence for the role of hydroxyurea in leukemic transformation in patients with a chronic myeloproliferative disorder. However, recent data suggest no such association.

However, other studies have shown no such increased risk for transformation in this patient group above that expected for all patients with a chronic myeloproliferative disorder.[4] B

A recent large prospective, observational study involving 1638 patients with polycythemia vera used multivariate analysis to assess the risk of leukemic transformation. This study found that treatment with hydroxyurea was not associated with an increased risk for acute leukemia. In this study alternative treatments (including Busulphan and chlorambucil) were independent risk factors for leukemic transformation.[4] B

Retrospective data from case studies suggest that interferon (IFN)-alpha is an alternative agent to hydroxyurea as cytoreductive therapy for patients with polycythemia vera.

Another more recent review of recombinant IFN-alpha in 55 patients with polycythemia vera previously treated with phlebotomy alone or with phlebotomy plus hydroxyurea reported that recombinant IFN-alpha effectively reduced phlebotomy requirements, thrombocythemia, splenomegaly, and thrombohemorrhagic events.[5] B

Evidence-Based References

1. McMullin MF et al: General Haematology Task Force of the British Committee for Standards in Haematology. Guidelines for the diagnosis, inves-

tigation and management of polycythaemia/erythrocytosis, *Br J Haematol* 130:174, 2005. C

2. Landolfi R et al: Efficacy and safety of low-dose aspirin in polycythemia vera, *N Engl J Med* 350:114, 2004. A

3. Harrison CN et al: Hydroxyurea compared with anagrelide in high-risk essential thrombocythemia, *N Engl J Med* 353:33, 2005. A

4. Finazzi G et al: Acute leukemia in polycythemia vera: an analysis of 1638 patients enrolled in a prospective observational study, *Blood* 105:2664, 2005. B

5. Silver RT: Long-term effects of the treatment of polycythemia vera with recombinant interferon-alpha, *Cancer* 107:451, 2006. B

SUGGESTED READINGS

Campbell PJ, Green AR: The myeloproliferative disorders, *N Engl J Med* 355:2452, 2006.

Spivak JL: Narrative review: thrombocytosis, polycythemia vera, and JAK2 mutations: the phenotypic mimicry of chronic myeloproliferation, *Ann Intern Med* 152:300-306, 2010.

Stuart BJ, Vieira AJ: Polycythemia vera, *Am Fam Physician* 69:2139, 2004.

AUTHOR: **FRED F. FERRI, M.D.**

BASIC INFORMATION

DEFINITION

Polymyalgia rheumatica is a disorder of unknown cause that affects older patients. It is characterized by shoulder and hip stiffness and an elevated erythrocyte sedimentation rate (ESR).

SYNONYMS

Anarthritic rheumatoid syndrome

ICD-9CM CODES

725.0 Polymyalgia rheumatica

EPIDEMIOLOGY & DEMOGRAPHICS

PREVALENCE:
One case per 135 persons aged >50 yr
PREDOMINANT SEX: Female/male ratio of 2:1
PREDOMINANT AGE: Rare <50 yr; average age at onset, 70 yr

PHYSICAL FINDINGS & CLINICAL PRESENTATION

- Symptoms are frequently of sudden onset but are often present for months before the diagnosis is made.
- Neck, shoulder, low back, and thigh pain are common complaints.
- Morning stiffness lasting 2 to 3 hr is typical, and patients often have difficulty getting out of bed.
- Malaise, weight loss, depression, and a low-grade fever are common constitutional symptoms and may suggest systemic inflammation.
- Physical findings are usually limited. Synovitis may be present in peripheral joints and may also be responsible for the proximal girdle symptoms despite the fact that they appear to be "muscular" in nature.
- Mild soft tissue tenderness may be present.
- Distal extremity manifestations (knee, wrist, metacarpophalangeal joints) may occur in 25% to 45% of patients.
- The temporal arteries should be carefully examined because of the strong relation of polymyalgia rheumatica with temporal or giant cell arteritis.

ETIOLOGY

Unknown

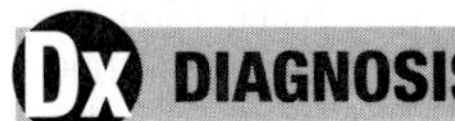

DIAGNOSIS

DIFFERENTIAL DIAGNOSIS

(Table 1-61)

- Rheumatoid arthritis: rheumatoid factor is negative in polymyalgia.
- Polymyositis: enzyme studies are negative in polymyalgia.
- Fibromyalgia.

WORKUP

The diagnosis of polymyalgia rheumatica is suggested by the following findings:

- Pain and stiffness of pectoral and pelvic musculature
- Patient >50 yr
- Morning stiffness >1 hr
- Normal motor strength
- Symptoms for at least 4 to 6 wk
- Elevated ESR (>45)
- Rapid clinical response to low-dose corticosteroid therapy

LABORATORY TESTS

- Complete blood count, ESR, and rheumatoid factor should be measured.
- Mild anemia may be present.

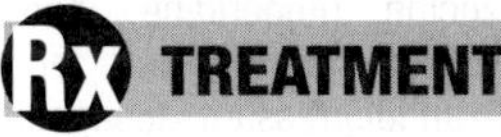

TREATMENT

ACUTE GENERAL Rx

- Prednisone 10 to 20 mg/day is given. The response is often so dramatic that it can be used to confirm the diagnosis. Improvement is usually noted within 24 to 48 hr. Generally, if the initial prednisone dose is 20 mg/day, reduce by 2.5 mg every week to 10 mg/day, then by 1 mg/day every month if tolerated.
- Steroids are gradually tapered over the next few weeks as soon as symptoms permit, but small doses (5 mg/day) may be needed for 2 yr.
- Nonsteroidal antiinflammatory drugs may be tried in mild cases.
- Physical therapy is usually unnecessary.

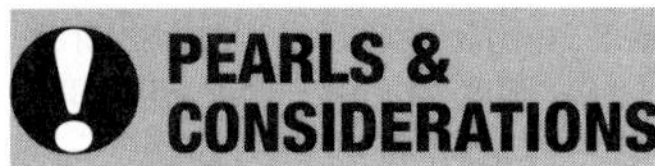

PEARLS & CONSIDERATIONS

COMMENTS

The prognosis is generally favorable. Relapse occasionally occurs in several years, but again responds well to prednisone.

SUGGESTED READINGS

Bird HA: Criteria for polymyalgia rheumatica: tale without end, *J Rheumatol* 35:188, 2008.

Cimmino MA et al: Pulse steroid treatment of polymyalgia rheumatica, *Clin Exp Rheumatol* 22(3):381, 2004.

Clough JD: Polymyalgia rheumatica: not well understood, but important to consider, *Cleve Clin J Med* 71(6):446, 2004.

Dasgupta B et al: Management guidelines and outcome measures in polymyalgia rheumatica (PMR), *Clin Exp Rheumatol* 25(suppl 47):130, 2007.

Hennell S et al: Evidence-based management for polymyalgia rheumatica for rheumatology practitioners, nurses and physiotherapists, *Musculoskeletal Care* 5(2):65, 2007.

Hutchings A et al: Clinical outcomes, quality of life and diagnostic uncertainty in the first year of polymyalgia rheumatica, *Arthritis Rheum* 57(5):803, 2007.

Mandell BF: Polymyalgia rheumatica: clinical presentation is key to diagnosis and treatment, *Cleve Clin J Med* 71(6):489, 2004.

Ntatsaki E, Watts RA: Management of polymyalgia rheumatica, *BMJ* 340:620, 2010.

Salvarani C et al: Polymyalgia rheumatica and giant-cell arteritis, *Lancet* 372:234, 2008.

AUTHOR: **LONNIE R. MERCIER, M.D.**

TABLE 1-61 Differential Features in Polymyalgia Rheumatica and Similar Disorders

Signs/Symptoms	Polymyalgia Rheumatoid	Giant Cell Arteritis	Rheumatica Arthritis	Dermatomyositis	Fibromyalgia
Morning stiffness >30 min	+	±	+*	±	Variable
Headache and/or scalp tenderness	0	+	0	0	Variable
Pain with active joint movement	+	0	+*	0	Inconstant
Tender joints	±	0	+*	0	Tender spots
Swollen joints	±	±	+	0	0
Muscle weakness	±†	0	+*	+	0
Normochromic anemia	+	+	+	0	0
Elevated erythrocyte sedimentation rate	+	+	+	±	0
Elevated serum creatine kinase	0	0	0	+	0
Serum rheumatoid factor	0	0	70%	0	0
Distinct electromyographic abnormality	0	0	0	+	0
Response to nonsteroidal antiinflammatory drug	±	0	+	0	0

From Goldman L, Ausiello D (eds): *Cecil textbook of medicine*, ed 22, Philadelphia, 2004, WB Saunders.
0, Absent; +, present; ±, present in minority of cases.
*Associated with affected joints.
†Pain inhibits movement. Disuse atrophy may occur.

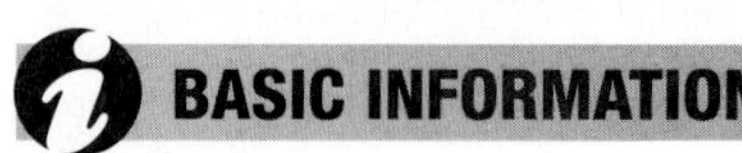

BASIC INFORMATION

DEFINITION

Polypharmacy is the concomitant use of more drugs than are clinically necessary. Older definitions have emphasized specific numbers of medications, commonly five or more drugs per day. The primary issue is that the drugs are inappropriate and increase the risk of medication errors, adverse drug reactions, drug interactions, hospitalizations, and/or cost without a clear benefit to the patient.

SYNONYMS

Potentially inappropriate medications (PIMs)

ICD-9CM CODES
Not applicable

EPIDEMIOLOGY & DEMOGRAPHICS

PEAK INCIDENCE: Estimates vary, but incidence appears to increase between age 70 and 84 yr.

PREVALENCE: One in five Americans receives potentially inappropriate drug therapy, although prevalence may be substantially higher in specific clinical settings.

PREDOMINANT SEX AND AGE:
- Adults aged 65 and older
- Women

RISK FACTORS:
- Multiple chronic diseases
- Frequent hospitalizations with incomplete reconciliation of medications upon admission and medications upon discharge
- Multiple providers such as primary care physician and specialists using electronic health record who do not communicate
- Multiple pharmacies such as one pharmacy for inexpensive generics, one for free antibiotics, mail order for 90-day supply

PHYSICAL FINDINGS & CLINICAL PRESENTATION

- Presence of one or more drugs without a clearly defined purpose
- Presence of therapeutic duplication such as multiple proton pump inhibitors
- Presence of prescriptions for both generic and brand-name version of the same drug
- Unexpected response to drug therapy ranging from lack of efficacy to exaggerated responses
- Failure to use appropriate drugs (aspirin, calcium, etc.) in patients who would clearly benefit
- Expanding list of new medications for a patient late in life or at the end of life
- Decreased patient adherence
- Common unnecessary drugs in polypharmacy such as gastrointestinal and CNS agents
- Presence of a "geriatric syndrome" such as falling, excessive sedation and confusion, urinary retention or incontinence, reduced oral intake, and general failure to thrive

ETIOLOGY

- Inadequate communication between physicians, pharmacists, patients, and their families
- Lack of coordination of medical care
- Extensive use of self-care with OTC drugs by patients
- Prescribing cascade (not recognizing new problem as a drug side effect and prescribing a second drug)
- Increasing number of available medications and intensive marketing to physicians and patients

DIAGNOSIS

DIFFERENTIAL DIAGNOSIS

- Misuse, overuse, or underuse of drug therapy

WORKUP

- Obtain a thorough medication history including prescription and OTC drugs and dietary supplements.
- "Brown bag" approach: visually verify all medication bottles for actual ingredients.
- Although the presence of many drugs does not necessarily identify inappropriate prescribing, the likelihood of at least one or more problem drugs being present increases if at least seven drugs are prescribed.
- Use standard tools to evaluate drug regimens:
  1. Beers criteria drugs to recognize potentially dangerous or ineffective drugs
     Some of these drugs include propoxyphene, pentazocine, meperidine, indomethacin, ketorolac, amitriptyline, and imipramine (in antidepressant dosages); long-acting benzodiazepines, muscle relaxants, and antispasmodic agents; short-acting dipyridamole, ticlopidine, disopyramide, chlorpropamide, and drugs with strong anticholinergic properties.
  2. Zhan Criteria: Potentially inappropriate medication use in the community-dwelling elderly
  3. Classification by Expert Panel of 1997 Beers Criteria medications into three categories: always avoid, rarely appropriate, and appropriate for some indications.
  4. Medication Appropriateness Index evaluates key elements of appropriate prescribing
     - Is there an indication for the drug?
     - Is the medication effective for the condition?
     - Are the directions correct?
     - Are the directions practical?
     - Are there clinically significant drug–drug interactions?
     - Are there clinically significant drug–disease interactions?
     - Is there unnecessary duplication with other drugs?
     - Is the duration of therapy appropriate?
     - Is this drug the least expensive alternative compared with others of equal utility?
  5. The NCQA Healthcare Effectiveness Data and Information Set (HEDIS) 2009 measures include potentially harmful drug–disease interactions in the elderly and use of high-risk medications in the elderly.

TREATMENT

The most important consideration in "treating" polypharmacy is to establish which conditions have the greatest priority for drug treatment, especially from the patient's perspective.

NONPHARMACOLOGIC THERAPY

As drugs are identified to be discontinued, ask patient about his or her interest in non-drug therapies.

ACUTE GENERAL Rx

If acute drug-related problems are identified, establish priorities for safely withdrawing/tapering the offending drugs (as appropriate for the specific agents).

CHRONIC Rx

- A key issue is whether the individual is likely to receive a benefit from a specific medication, especially if multiple comorbid conditions exist and/or their life expectancy is limited.
- Consideration should be given to the incremental benefit from each drug added to a complex drug regimen. For example, what would be the benefit to an individual in his or her 90s from the addition of spironolactone to a regimen consisting of lisinopril, candesartan, and carvedilol for heart failure?
- The goal of therapy for each new medication should be clearly listed by the prescriber.

DISPOSITION

Safe discontinuation of inappropriate medications from a regimen may take at least several months depending on the specific drugs.

REFERRAL

Referral to a clinical pharmacist for a comprehensive drug regimen review and potentially to a geriatrician, especially for frail older adults.

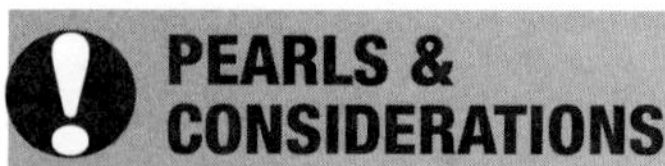

PEARLS & CONSIDERATIONS

COMMENTS

The prevention and/or identification of polypharmacy should focus on the appropriateness of the medications for the *individual* person and not simply the number of medications. The decision regarding what is "appropriate" for an individual should first consider the patient's own priorities and expected risk and benefit to that individual before focusing on clinical practice guidelines that may or may not be applicable to a specific patient.

PREVENTION

- Polypharmacy is prevented by considering whether a drug is needed for a new symptom and whether a new symptom is actually an unrecognized adverse drug reaction.

- Use of technology such as electronic health records in which the medication history is updated regularly may help to prevent polypharmacy.
- OTC drugs and dietary supplements should always be identified when taking a medication history. Although manufacturers make slight changes to common brand names in order to introduce new OTC products, actual ingredients have been completely altered.
- Certain points in the continuum of care are high risk for polypharmacy and inappropriate prescribing. Discharge from the hospital to home (or to a nursing home) is a common time when patients may become confused about the intended drug regimen.
- Consistent use of generic drug names can decrease the risk of polypharmacy. Duplicate prescriptions for the same drug (furosemide and Lasix) commonly occur.
- Medication reconciliation: perform a complete review of medications for the appropriateness of their continued use at least every 6 mo (for older adults), after discharge from the hospital, and whenever new drugs are added.
- Regular evaluation of how frequently "as needed" medications are being used by the patient. For example, the "Rule of 2" for short-acting beta-agonists may identify a need for a change in maintenance therapy.
- Drug use evaluations in hospitals to identify trends in inappropriate prescribing.
- Drug–drug interaction alerts in institutional record systems.
- Geriatric Evaluation and Management (GEM) Program: specialized program of services for both inpatient and outpatient settings. GEM uses an interdisciplinary approach to treatment, rehabilitation, health promotion and social service interventions in older adults. It aims to optimize drug prescribing and reduce unnecessary drug use.
- Use of positive Beers criteria for preferred CNS drugs in older adults can help prescribers select medications preferred for dementia, depression, Parkinson's disease, and psychosis, based on efficacy and safety.

PATIENT/FAMILY EDUCATION

- An up-to-date list of all drugs taken on a regular or as needed basis must be maintained. The list should include all prescription and OTC drugs including eye drops, inhalers, and skin creams. Dietary supplements such as vitamins and herbals should also be on the list. The National Transitions of Care Coalition's "My Medicine List" is an excellent tool for patients (http://www.ntocc.org/Portals/0/My_Medicine_List.pdf), as well as My Medication Action Plan (MAP) from the American Pharmacists Association. Patient should ask physician or pharmacist to review all drugs at least once a year.
- After being discharged from the hospital, compare newly prescribed drugs to your existing drugs. Ask which drugs should be continued and which should be stopped.
- If enrolled in Medicare Part D, determine eligibility for Medication Therapy Management Programs (MTMP). MTMP may be available for beneficiaries who have multiple chronic diseases and Part D drugs, and who are likely to incur significant costs.

SUGGESTED READINGS

Buck MD et al: Potentially inappropriate medication prescribing in outpatient practices: prevalence and patient characteristics based on electronic health records, *Am J Geriatr Pharmacother* 7:84, 2009.

Fick DM et al: Updating the Beers criteria for potentially inappropriate medication use in older adults: results of a US consensus panel of experts. *Arch Intern Med* 163:2716, 2003.

Gallagher PF et al: Inappropriate prescribing in an acutely ill population of elderly patients as determined by Beers' Criteria, *Age Aging* 37:96, 2008.

Hajjar ER, Cafiero AC, Hanlon JR: Polypharmacy in elderly patients, *Am J Geriatr Pharmacother* 5:345-351, 2007.

Hanlon JT et al: A method for assessing drug therapy appropriateness. *J Clin Epidemiol* 45:1045, 1992.

Holmes HM et al: Reconsidering medication appropriateness for patients late in life, *Arch Intern Med* 166:605-609, 2006.

Stefanacci RG et al: Developing explicit positive Beers criteria for preferred central nervous system medications in older adults, *Consult Pharm* 24:601-610, 2009.

Zhan C et al: Potentially inappropriate medication use in the community-dwelling elderly, *JAMA* 286:2823, 2001.

AUTHORS: **ANNE L. HUME, PHARM.D.** and **CHRISTINE EISENHOWER, PHARM.D.**

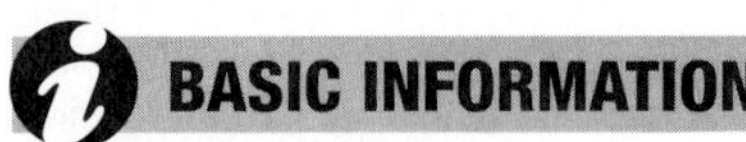

BASIC INFORMATION

DEFINITION

Clinically significant portal hypertension is defined as a portal vein pressure >10 mm Hg, most commonly attributable to liver disease.

SYNONYMS

None

ICD-9CM CODES
572.3 Portal hypertension

EPIDEMIOLOGY & DEMOGRAPHICS

- Incidence of portal hypertension is not known.
- Cirrhosis is the most common cause of portal hypertension in the U.S.
- More than 90% of patients with cirrhosis develop portal hypertension.
- Alcoholic and viral liver diseases are the most common causes of cirrhosis and portal hypertension in the U.S.
- Schistosomiasis is the main cause of portal hypertension outside the U.S.
- Esophageal varices may appear when portal vein pressure rises to >10 mm Hg.
- Variceal hemorrhage is the most serious complication of portal hypertension and may occur when portal pressures rise >12 mm Hg.

PHYSICAL FINDINGS & CLINICAL PRESENTATION

- Jaundice
- Ascites (Figs. 1-258 and 1-259)
- Spider angiomata
- Testicular atrophy
- Gynecomastia
- Palmar erythema
- Dupuytren's contracture
- Asterixis (with advanced liver failure)
- Irritability, encephalopathy
- Splenomegaly
- Dilated veins in the anterior abdominal wall
- Venous pattern on the flanks
- Caput medusae (tortuous collateral veins around the umbilicus)
- Hemorrhoids
- Hematemesis
- Melena
- Pruritus

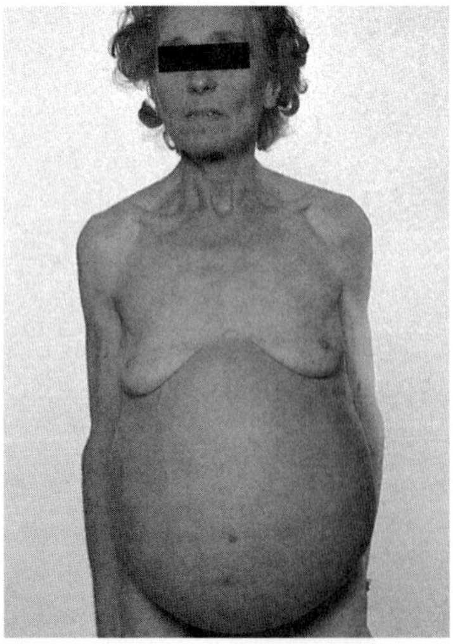

FIGURE 1-258 Ascites secondary to portal hypertension. Note the dilated collateral vein running up the right side of the abdomen. (From Forbes A, Misiewicz JJ, Crompton CC, Levine M et al [eds]: *Atlas of clinical gastroenterology,* ed 3, Oxford, 2005, Mosby.)

ETIOLOGY

Pathophysiologically caused by:

1. Conditions resulting in an increased resistance to flow
   - Prehepatic (e.g., portal vein thrombosis, splenic vein thrombosis, congenital stenosis)
   - Hepatic (e.g., cirrhosis, alcoholic liver disease, primary biliary cirrhosis, schistosomiasis)
   - Posthepatic (e.g., Budd-Chiari syndrome, constrictive pericarditis, inferior vena cava obstruction, cor pulmonale, tricuspid regurgitation)
2. Conditions leading to increase in portal blood flow
   - Splanchnic arterial vasodilation accompanying portal hypertension, mediated by local release of nitric oxide
   - Arterial-portal venous fistulae

DIAGNOSIS

- The diagnosis of portal hypertension is made on clinical grounds after a comprehensive history and physical examination.
- Noninvasive and invasive procedures confirm diagnosis and determine the severity of portal hypertension.

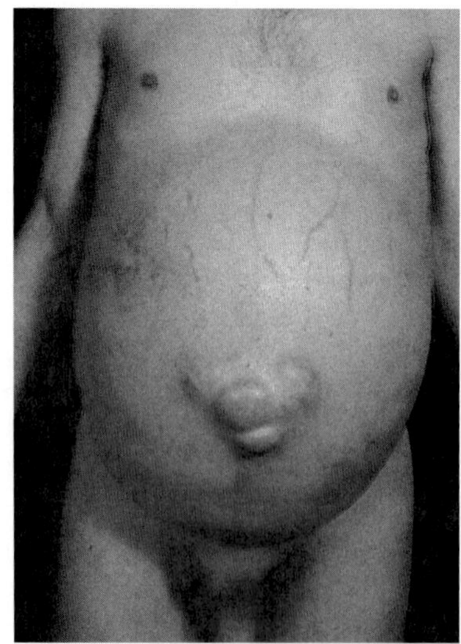

FIGURE 1-259 Ascites in a patient with alcoholic cirrhosis showing distended abdomen; dilated superficial collateral veins; hemorrhagic scratch marks due to pruritus and coagulopathy; umbilical varices; plaster in left iliac fossa indicating diagnostic paracentesis. (From Forbes A, Misiewicz JJ, Crompton CC, Levine M et al [eds]: *Atlas of clinical gastroenterology,* ed 3, Oxford, 2005, Mosby.)

DIFFERENTIAL DIAGNOSIS

- Ascites from infection, neoplasm, or other inflammatory processes
- Obesity
- Abdominal organomegaly

WORKUP

The workup of portal hypertension includes blood tests and noninvasive imaging studies to determine if the cause of portal hypertension is prehepatic, hepatic, or posthepatic. Ascitic fluid analysis is a key part of the diagnosis.

LABORATORY TESTS

- Complete blood count with platelets
- Liver function tests with serum albumin
- Prothrombin and partial thromboplastin times
- Hepatitis B surface antigen and antibody
- Hepatitis C antibody
- In selected cases: iron, total iron-binding capacity, and ferritin; antinuclear antibody, anti–smooth muscle antibodies, antimitochondrial antibody, ceruloplasmin, alpha-1 antitrypsin.
- Ascitic fluid analysis: a serum-ascites albumin gradient ≥1.1 mg/dl suggests portal hypertension. Polymorphonuclear cells ≥250 cells/ml or positive Gram stain or culture suggest complicating spontaneous bacterial peritonitis (SBP).

IMAGING STUDIES

- Duplex-Doppler ultrasound is effective in screening for portal hypertension.
- Less commonly, CT/MRI scanning or liver-spleen nuclear medicine scanning can be used if the results from ultrasound are equivocal.
- Upper endoscopy is the most reliable test documenting the presence of esophageal varices.

TREATMENT

The treatment of portal hypertension is complex and involves measures to reduce the hypertension directly, minimize volume overload, correct underlying disorders, and prevent complications (most notably SBP and variceal bleeding).

NONPHARMACOLOGIC THERAPY

Dietary sodium restriction to generally 2000 mg/day forms the basis of therapy to limit fluid overload.

ACUTE GENERAL Rx

- For tense ascites, serial large volume paracentesis (LVP) is generally recommended. The use of albumin infusion (8 to 10 g/L of ascites fluid removed) during LVP >5 L has been shown to reduce the incidence of postparacentesis circulatory dysfunction, although its use remains somewhat controversial.

- IV diuretics, typically furosemide and spironolactone, are used to achieve natriuresis and net negative salt and water balance. Renal function and serum electrolytes are monitored frequently, with transition to an oral regimen for long-term therapy.
- SBP is treated with IV antibiotics directed against enteric bacteria.
- Acute variceal hemorrhage is treated with crystalloid and blood product resuscitation, IV octreotide, terlipressin/vasopressin or somatostatin, and urgent upper endoscopy, often with sclerotherapy or band ligation. Patients with acute variceal hemorrhage should receive antibiotic prophylaxis against SBP.
- For patients not responding to the above measures, a transjugular intrahepatic portosystemic shunt (TIPS) or surgical shunt placement may be considered.

CHRONIC Rx

- Dietary sodium restriction in combination with diuretics: the typical ratio of furosemide 40 mg to spironolactone 100 mg retains normal serum potassium levels in most patients.
- Nonselective beta-blockers (propranolol and nadolol) in dosages sufficient to reduce the resting heart rate by 25% have been shown to be effective in primary prophylaxis for first-time variceal bleeding and for preventing recurrent variceal bleeding. Dosages are usually given bid and decreased if heart rate falls to <55 beats/min or systolic blood pressure drops to <90 mm Hg. The addition of a long-acting nitrate (e.g., isosorbide-5-mononitrate) has been shown to improve portal hemodynamics. Findings of a prospective trial of beta-blockers to prevent the formation of varices were negative. The combination of beta-blockade plus endoscopic esophageal variceal banding is superior to either intervention alone.
- Intermittent LVP may be needed in "diuretic resistant" patients.
- Patients with prior SBP merit lifelong antibiotics for secondary prevention.
- Abstinence from alcohol or treatment for hepatitis B or hepatitis C. Vaccination for hepatitis A and B as appropriate.
- Hepatic transplantation is an option in selected patients.

DISPOSITION

- The most common complication associated with portal hypertension is variceal bleeding. The risk of bleeding from varices is approximately 15% at 1 yr.
- Development of the hepatorenal syndrome (HRS) is associated with high near-term mortality. In particular, HRS may complicate SBP, which emphasizes the importance of making the diagnosis of SBP and instituting appropriate prophylaxis.

REFERRAL

Consultation with a gastroenterologist is recommended in all patients with portal hypertension to screen for esophageal varices.

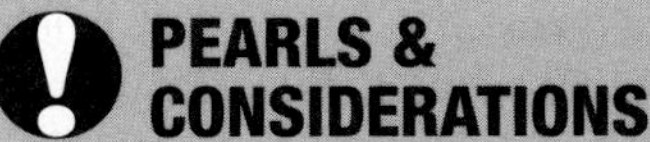

PEARLS & CONSIDERATIONS

Splanchnic arterial vasodilation is increasingly recognized as an important component of the pathophysiology of portal hypertension and ascites. There may be vasodilation in other capillary beds as well; of note, pulmonary arteriolar vasodilation can create a significant shunt fraction and resultant hypoxemia in the absence of chest radiograph or CT chest evidence of parenchymal disease. The diagnosis is suspected when otherwise unexplained hypoxia arises in a patient with cirrhosis, along with platypnea (dyspnea worse when sitting upright) and orthodeoxia (desaturation with upright posture). The diagnosis is confirmed by echocardiography with agitated saline, in which there is delayed appearance of bubbles in the left heart after injection into a peripheral vein.

COMMENTS

Portal hypertension and its complications carry significant morbidity and mortality rates. Emphasize ethanol abstinence, provide vaccinations and prophylactic therapy where indicated, and consider early referral to a specialist for assistance with management and consideration for hepatic transplantation.

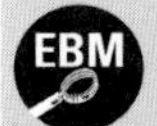

EVIDENCE

Please note: Complete text of EBM for this topic is available online.

Key trials and commentary:

The aim of this study was to identify predictors of clinical decompensation (defined as the development of ascites, variceal hemorrhage [VH], or hepatic encephalopathy [HE]) in patients with compensated cirrhosis and with portal hypertension as determined by the hepatic venous pressure gradient (HVPG).

This study showed that HVPG, MELD, and albumin independently predict clinical decompensation in patients with compensated cirrhosis. Patients with an HVPG <10 mm Hg have a 90% probability of not developing clinical decompensation in a median follow-up of 4 years.

Patients with cirrhosis have different survival rates depending on whether they have compensated cirrhosis with lack of ascites, complication ascites, VH, and encephalopathy or decompensated cirrhosis, with the presence of one or more of these complications that are related to portal hypertension. If there is a linear relation between portal hypertension and complications, then use of portal pressure would be a marker of severity. Ripoll et al evaluated the predictors of clinical decompensation in patients with compensated cirrhosis. The authors previously found that the strongest predictor for development of varices was the presence of HVPG >10 mm Hg. Therefore, there are two stages of compensated cirrhosis—early, or stage 1, which is without varices, and the more advanced compensated stage II with varices. Decompensation occurred in 29% of patients over a 51-month follow-up, which was predicted by HVPG, albumin level, and MELD score, which are related to severity of portal hypertension and liver insufficiency. The higher the HVPG, the more likely it is clinical decompensation; conversely, patients with levels <10 mm Hg had only a 10% risk of clinical decompensation. This study shows the importance of response to medical therapy, because the authors found an independent role of a decrease in HVPG in prediction of clinical decompensation. If our medical therapy is effective, and if taken in the long term by patients who are relatively symptomatic, then we should be able to delay decompensation and improve survival.[1] Ⓐ

The use of the HVPG to assess the efficacy of the pharmacological treatment of portal hypertension in cirrhosis is controversial. The aim of this study was to establish whether target HVPG reduction predicts variceal bleeding in cirrhotic patients receiving variceal bleeding prophylaxis.

Current evidence supports the validity of HVPG end points to monitor drug therapy efficacy for variceal bleeding prophylaxis. HVPG monitoring also provides valuable prognostic information.

Increase in hepatic vein portal vein gradient pressure is associated with increased risk of variceal bleeding. The methods that are available to decrease HVPG include medical therapy with nonselective beta adregenic blockers, alone or combined, with organic nitrates and radiological (transjugular) or surgical shunting. Endoscopic band ligation of varices can decrease bleeding. This requires the esophageal varices to be of a moderate size. Medical therapy results in a 50% reduction in risk of initial bleed. Its therapeutic aim is to reduce portal venous pressure, which is estimated by the HVPG. HVPG can be measured by a reliable, well-tolerated balloon catheter technique done through the internal jugular vein. Albillos et al presented a meta-analysis to assess the validity of the use of target HVPG reduction to predict variceal bleeding prophylaxis. Clinically, this will lead us to determine if we should recommend the use of HVPG measurement to assess the efficacy of drug therapy. The authors found that the risk of first or recurrent variceal bleeding is reduced when drug therapy achieved the reduction in HVPG (<12 mm Hg or ≥20%), which is better if an early hemodynamic response is obtained. Therefore, because most variceal bleeding occurs within the first 24 days of the index bleed, our clinical goal should be to rapidly initiate and reach a clinically appropriate dose of medical therapy and measure HVPG, a clinical practice not routinely performed outside of trials. This meta-analysis showed that HVPG reduction ≤12 mm Hg confers significant protection against bleeding. This occurred in 30% of nonbleeders and 18% of rebleeders. In addition to this bleeding benefit, achieving a response of HVPG reduced liver-related mortality. Will this article change our clinical practice, or will we continue to use the crude measurement of heart rate as the end point of medical therapy? In my opinion, we need to place an objective end point to our medical therapy that will be allowed by measurement.[2] Ⓐ

Evidence-Based References

1. Ripoll C: Hepatic venous pressure gradient predicts clinical decompensation in patients with compensated cirrhosis, *Gastroenterology* 133:481-488, 2007. Commentary by J.S. Barkin, M.D. Ⓐ

2. Albillos A, Bañares R, González M: Value of the hepatic venous pressure gradient to monitor drug therapy for portal hypertension: a meta-analysis, *Am J Gastroenterol* 102:1116-1126, 2007. Commentary by J.S. Barkin, M.D. Ⓐ

SUGGESTED READINGS

Blei AT: Portal hypertension and its complications, *Curr Opin Gastroenterol* 23(3):275, 2007.

Bosch J et al: The management of portal hypertension: rational basis, available treatments and future options, *J Hepatol* 48(suppl 1):S68, 2008.

De Francis R: Evolving consensus in portal hypertension. Report of the Baveno IV consensus workshop on methodology of diagnosis and therapy in portal hypertension, *J Hepatol* 43(1):167, 2005.

Gines P et al: Current concepts: management of cirrhosis and ascites, *N Engl J Med* 350:1646, 2004.

Runyon B: Practice Guidelines Committee, American Association for the Study of Liver Diseases (AASLD): management of adult patients with ascites due to cirrhosis, *Hepatology* 39:841, 2004.

Wong CL et al: Does this patient have bacterial peritonitis or portal hypertension? How do I perform a paracentesis and analyze the results? *JAMA* 299(10):1166, 2008.

AUTHOR: **MEL L. ANDERSON, M.D.**

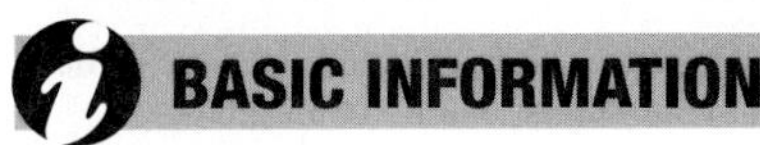

BASIC INFORMATION

DEFINITION

Portal vein thrombosis is thrombotic occlusion of the portal vein.

SYNONYMS

Pylethrombosis

ICD-9CM CODES
452 Portal vein thrombosis
572.1 Septic portal vein thrombosis

EPIDEMIOLOGY & DEMOGRAPHICS

Occurs with equal frequency in children (peak age: 6 yr) and adults (peak age: 40 yr)

PHYSICAL FINDINGS & CLINICAL PRESENTATION

Upper gastrointestinal hemorrhage (hematemesis and/or melena) caused by esophageal varices. If abdominal pain is present, mesenteric venous thrombosis should be suspected (see Mesenteric Venous Thrombosis in Section I).

ETIOLOGY & PATHOPHYSIOLOGY

In children: umbilical sepsis (pathophysiology unknown) In adults:

1. Hypercoagulable states
   - Antiphospholipid syndrome
   - Neoplasm (common cause)
   - Paroxysmal nocturnal hemoglobinuria
   - Myeloproliferative diseases
   - Oral contraceptives
   - Polycythemia vera
   - Pregnancy
   - Protein S or C deficiency
   - Sickle cell disease
   - Thrombocytosis
2. Inflammatory diseases
   - Crohn's disease
   - Pancreatitis
   - Ulcerative colitis
3. Complications of medical intervention
   - Ambulatory dialysis
   - Chemoembolization
   - Liver transplantation
   - Partial hepatectomy
   - Sclerotherapy
   - Splenectomy
   - Transjugular intrahepatic portosystemic shunt
4. Infections
   - Appendicitis
   - Diverticulitis
   - Cholecystitis
5. Miscellaneous
   - Cirrhosis (common cause)
   - Bladder cancer

Pathophysiology: portal vein thrombosis results in portal hypertension, leading to esophageal and gastrointestinal varices. The liver sustained by the hepatic artery maintains normal function.

Dx DIAGNOSIS

DIFFERENTIAL DIAGNOSIS

Causes of upper gastrointestinal hemorrhage are covered in Section II.

WORKUP

- Determination of underlying cirrhosis of the liver should be the foremost step.
- Esophagogastroscopy shows esophageal varices.
- Abdominal ultrasound (Fig. 1-260) or MRI may show the portal vein thrombosis. Abdominal ultrasound color Doppler imaging has a 98% negative predictive value and is considered the imaging modality of choice in diagnosing portal vein thrombosis.

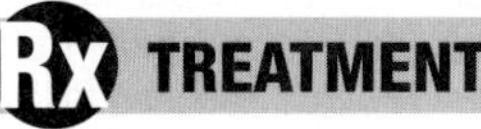

TREATMENT

- Oral anticoagulation if risks of bleeding are low. In patients with concomitant cirrhosis, long-term anticoagulation generally not recommended
- Variceal sclerotherapy or banding
- Surgical mesocaval or splenorenal shunt
- The roles of thrombolysis and transjugular intrahepatic portosystemic shunt continuing to evolve

REFERRAL

To gastroenterologist, surgeon, or both

SUGGESTED READING

Parikh S, Shah R, Kapoor P: Portal vein thrombosis, *Am J Med* 123:111-119, 2010.

AUTHOR: **FRED F. FERRI, M.D.**

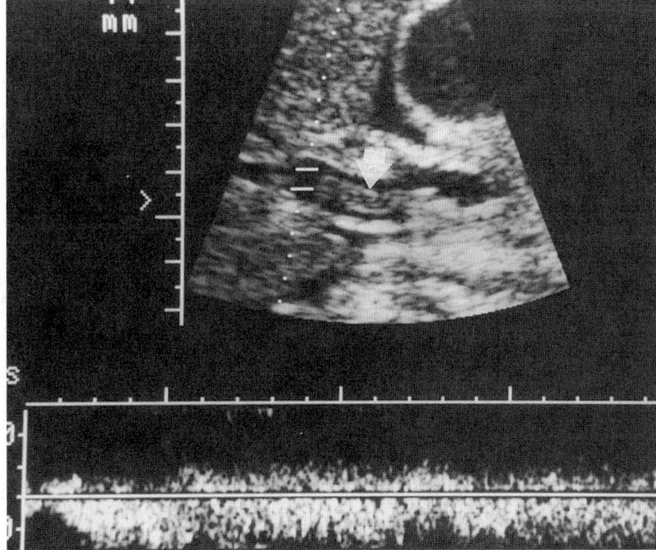

FIGURE 1-260 Thrombus in portal vein evident on pulsed Doppler ultrasonography. An echogenic thrombus *(arrow)* is within the lumen of the portal vein. Doppler tracing indicates flow within portal vein. (From Sabiston D: *Textbook of surgery,* ed 17, Philadelphia, 2005, WB Saunders.)

Postconcussive Syndrome 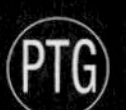

BASIC INFORMATION

DEFINITION

Postconcussive syndrome (PCS) refers to persistent neurologic symptoms that result from traumatic brain injury (TBI) PCS can also follow moderate and severe brain injury, although it is more commonly associated with mild brain injury or concussion. Concussion is an acute trauma-induced alteration of mental function lasting <24 hr, with or without preceding loss of consciousness.

SYNONYMS

Posttraumatic nervous instability or brain injury
Postcontusion syndrome or encephalopathy status post comotio cerebri

ICD-9CM CODES

310.2 Postconcussion syndrome

EPIDEMIOLOGY & DEMOGRAPHICS

- Incidence is approximately 27 cases per 100,000 persons/year.
- From 30% to 80% of patients with mild to moderate brain injury will experience some symptoms of PCS.
- Female gender and increasing age are risk factors for PCS.
- Usually seen in the young, ages 20 to 30 yr.

PHYSICAL FINDINGS & CLINICAL PRESENTATION

- Usually present without focal neurologic deficits on examination.
- Symptoms start within a few days after the head injury and usually persist after 3 mo.
- Can be divided into early and late or persistent (>6 mo).
- 15% of patients will have persistent symptoms 1 yr later.
- Symptoms include (at least three of the following after traumatic brain injury to meet ICD-10 criteria):
  1. Headache (usually of fronto-occipital location and showing characteristics of tension or migraine headache). The International Headache Society suggests that coding and attribution of headaches with characteristics of primary headaches but in the setting of an inticing event should be attributed to the event, unless there was a known history of the headache and the inticing event was seen as aggravating/initiating the preexisting migraine/tension headache.
  2. Fatigue
  3. Dizziness and/or vertigo
  4. Impaired memory
  5. Difficulty in concentrating
  6. Insomnia
  7. Irritability
  8. Lowered tolerance of stress, emotion, or alcohol
- Other associated symptoms: noise sensitivity, neck pain, non-dermatomal paresthesias, interference with social role functioning.

ETIOLOGY

- Caused by TBI from events such as falls, motor vehicle accidents, contact sports.
- Postmortem findings reveal diffuse axonal injury as the primary pathologic finding along with small petechial hemorrhages and local edema.
- Diffuse axon injury is believed to lead to altered neurotransmission and possibly to clinical manifestations.
- A psychogenic origin has been suggested by a number of empiric and clinical observations; however, limitations in methodology and differing definitions preclude firm conclusions.

Dx DIAGNOSIS

A careful history, a nonfocal neurologic examination, and a normal neurologic test will usually establish the diagnosis.

DIFFERENTIAL DIAGNOSIS

- Headache (dissection of the vertebral artery, occipital neuralgia)
- Epidural hematoma
- Subdural hematoma
- Skull fracture
- Cervical spine disk disease
- Whiplash
- Cerebrovascular accident
- Depression
- Anxiety

WORKUP

To exclude other causes of neurologic symptoms after TBI:

- Electroencephalography is normal.
- Evoked potentials are normal.
- Neuropsychologic testing is useful because it reveals difficulties in concentration, memory, language, and executive function.

LABORATORY TESTS

Blood tests are not specific.

IMAGING STUDIES

- 10% of CT scans of the head following mild TBI are abnormal, showing mild subarachnoid hemorrhage, subdural hemorrhage, or contusions.
- MRI of the head is abnormal in 30% of patients with normal CT scans and may show irregular brain contours or old cerebral contusions.

Rx TREATMENT

Must be recognized as a physiologic and psychologic problem and treated accordingly.

GENERAL Rx

- Must be individualized to the patient's particular symptoms.
- Simple reassurance is often the major treatment.
- Supportive care may include the use of nonnarcotic analgesics and antiemetics.
- Pain management.
- Amitriptyline has been widely used for posttraumatic tension-type headaches as well as for nonspecific symptoms such as irritability, dizziness, insomnia, and depression.
- Posttraumatic migraine-type headaches can be treated with a trial of propranolol or amitriptyline alone or in combination.
- Depression can be treated with selective serotonin reuptake inhibitors but may not respond as well when compared with patients without PCS who have depression.
- Some patients may be admitted for severe symptoms; most can be managed as an outpatient.

NONPHARMACOLOGIC THERAPY

- Early psychological intervention and cognitive rehabilitation are key for full recovery.
- Physical and occupational therapy.
- Avoidance of alcohol, narcotics, and sleep deprivation.
- Explanation of symptoms and expectations, combined with early follow-up with reassurance, may hasten resolution of symptoms.

DISPOSITION

- Most patients improve after mild TBI without any residual deficits within 3 months.
- Predictors for the development of persistent PCS include:
  - Female sex
  - Ongoing litigation (conflicting studies)
  - Low socioeconomic status
  - Prior headaches
  - Prior TBI
  - Prior psychiatric illnesses

REFERRAL

Early consultations with psychologists, psychiatrists, neurologists, and rehabilitation specialists in an outpatient setting would be beneficial.

PEARLS & CONSIDERATIONS

- PCS starts within a few days after the injury.
- Recognizing depression and treating pain symptoms early in the course may help prevent the development of persistent PCS (>1 yr).
- The severity of the trauma does not clearly predict the risk of PCS.
- The severity of the brain injury is usually documented by the initial Glasgow coma scale, the length of unconsciousness, and the duration of amnesia; however, the field may be moving towards more subtle tests of function, such as neuropsychological testing.

COMMENTS

- Attempts to determine how much of a role psychological and/or neurologic factors play in the PCS are important but very difficult.

- No medication at hospital discharge has been proven to change the natural course of the disease.

SUGGESTED READINGS

Evans RW: Postconcussion syndrome. Available at http://www.uptodate.com, accessed Aug 28, 2009.

Legome E et al: Postconcussive syndrome, *eMedicine Journal.* Available at http://www.emedicine.com, accessed Aug 28, 2009.

McAllister TW, Arciniegas D: Evaluation and treatment of postconcussive symptoms, *Neuro Rehabil* 17(4): 265, 2002.

McConnell A, Shubrook J: Concussion care: simple strategies, big payoffs, *J Fam Pract* 58(8):410, 2009.

Wood RL: Post concussional syndrome: all in the minds eye! *J Neurol Neurosurg Psychiatry*, 78:552, 2007.

AUTHORS: **WEN Y. WU-CHEN, M.D.,** and **MARK F. BRADY, M.D., M.P.H.**

Postpoliomyelitis Syndrome

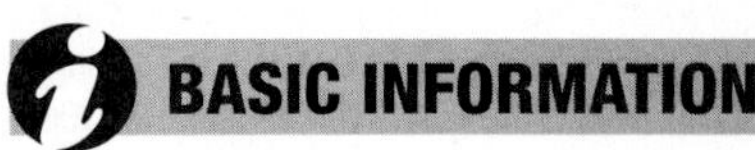

BASIC INFORMATION

DEFINITION

Postpoliomyelitis syndrome (PPS) is a lower motor neuron disease characterized by late-onset chronic progressive weakness, muscle cramps, joint pain, and fatigue (focal muscles or generalized) occurring several years after recovering from an acute poliomyelitis infection.

SYNONYMS

Progressive postpoliomyelitis muscular atrophy

ICD-9CM CODES
138 Late effects of acute poliomyelitis

EPIDEMIOLOGY & DEMOGRAPHICS

INCIDENCE (IN U.S.): 250,000 to 640,000 people survived acute poliomyelitis from the 1940 and 1950 epidemics; of those, 28.5% to 64% will develop PPS.

PEAK INCIDENCE: Occurs 8 to 71 yr (mean 36 yr) from the time of the acute poliomyelitis infection.

RISK FACTORS:
- Severe acute poliomyelitis infection
- Older age of onset of the acute infection
- Less recovery and greater physical activity during the intervening years
- Longer interval since the acute illness
- Recent weight gain
- Muscle and joint pain

PHYSICAL FINDINGS & CLINICAL PRESENTATION

- Polio "wall": generalized fatigue occurring with minimal activity
- A slow, progressive, asymmetric, proximal, distal, or patchy weakness and atrophy, predominately involving muscles previously affected by the acute infection
- Focal muscle fatigue (decreased endurance)
- Muscle tenderness on palpation, pain (aches and soreness), fasciculations, cramps, arthralgia, and joint deformities
- Bulbar muscle dysfunction (dysphasia, dysarthria, aphonia and, less commonly, facial weakness)
- Cold intolerance and vasomotor instability
- Respiratory dysfunction
- Sleep apnea and sleep disturbances
- Diagnostic criteria (set by the PostPolio Task Force in 1997):
  1. A confirmed episode of acute polio myelitis infection with residual motor neuron loss documented by a typical history, neurologic examination, or electromyographic studies
  2. Neurologic and functional stability after recovery from the acute episode for several decades (median, 25 yr)
  3. Insidious onset (can be acute) of new muscle weakness, atrophy, or fatigue (focal muscle fatigability or generalized)
  4. Exclusion of other conditions that can present like PPS

ETIOLOGY

- Controversial.
- The overuse of a weak muscle (most widely held hypothesis): many years of muscle overuse causes excessive metabolic stress on the remaining motor neurons that already have branched out to innervate denervated muscle fibers from the acute infection. This results in the gradual degeneration of those nerve terminals (and eventually the motor neurons) that supply the denervated muscles.
- Vulnerability of the anterior horns: from an earlier acute infection or preexistent since birth.
- Scar tissue forming in the anterior horn: forms "a locus resistentiae minoris" (an area of little resistance) or "a latent inflammatory focus" that could produce new symptoms at any time.
- Chronic persistent polio virus infection.
- Persistent immune-mediated mechanism: supported by the presence of oligoclonal bands in the cerebrospinal fluid (CSF) and lymphocytic infiltration of muscles and spinal cord of some patients.

Dx DIAGNOSIS

DIFFERENTIAL DIAGNOSIS

- Amyotrophic lateral sclerosis
- Cervical and lumbosacral radiculopathy
- Adult spinal muscular atrophy
- Diabetic amyotrophy
- Multifocal motor neuropathy with conduction block
- Chronic inflammatory demyelinating polyneuropathy
- Entrapment neuropathies
- Inflammatory and metabolic myopathies
- Vasculitis
- Connective tissue disease–associated myopathies

WORKUP

- A good history and physical examination demonstrating the characteristic pattern of weakness in an individual who has a history of a documented acute poliomyelitis illness.
- Electromyography (EMG): ongoing denervation and chronic reinnervation. Fibrillation potentials and fasciculations may be present in symptomatic muscles. Single-fiber EMG may show increased jitter and blocking. However, those findings cannot separate PPS from asymptomatic patients with previous poliomyelitis.
- Nerve conduction studies: decreased compound muscle action potential amplitudes with normal distal latencies and conduction velocities. Sensory nerve action potentials are normal.
- Muscle biopsy: fiber-type grouping (remote denervation), isolated angular atrophic fibers (recent localized denervation), and neural cell adhesion molecule–positive myofibers (denervation).
- Lumbar puncture: CSF might show a nonspecific protein elevation and oligoclonal bands.
- Imaging studies (MRI, CT, radiography): to rule out spine disease, such as spondylosis, spinal stenosis, or radiculopathy.
- Pulmonary function test: to assess respiratory muscle strength.
- Sleep study: if there is a suggestion of obstructive sleep apnea.
- Swallow evaluation: using dynamic imaging.
- Cardiac evaluation: check for conduction abnormalities.

LABORATORY TESTS

- Creatine kinase: mildly elevated in many patients.
- Thyroid function test to rule out thyroid disease causing myopathy.
- Antinuclear antigen, rheumatoid factor, double-stranded DNA, erythrocyte sedimentation rate, C-reactive protein, scl-70, and anti-Ro and anti-La to rule out other autoimmune diseases.
- Heavy metal screening should be considered.
- Standard serum studies (complete blood count and electrolytes).

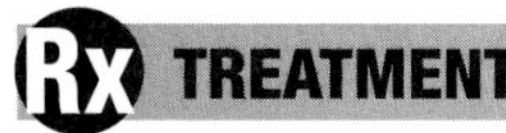

Rx TREATMENT

NONPHARMACOLOGIC THERAPY

- Treatment is supportive and focused on reducing physical exhaustion.
- Generalized fatigue: energy conservation (pacing of physical activities, frequent rest periods and daytime naps), weight loss, and assistive devices (orthoses, canes, intermittent use of wheelchairs).
- New weakness: nonfatiguing aerobic exercise and isometric or isokinetic exercise (short intervals, frequent rest, performed on alternate days). A physical therapist should be involved.
- Respiratory insufficiency: nighttime noninvasive positive-pressure ventilation. Some patients might require tracheostomy and permanent ventilation.
- Dysphagia: speech therapist to teach proper food and swallowing techniques.
- Musculoskeletal pain (joint or muscle pain) and joint instability: pacing activities, lifestyle changes, decreased mechanical stress, bracing, and wheelchairs. Heat and massage might be used.
- Pneumonia and influenza vaccines should be given.
- Smoking cessation.
- Avoid certain medications: beta-blockers, benzodiazepines, neuromuscular blockers, tetracycline, aminoglycosides, phenytoin, lithium, phenothiazines, and barbiturates.
- Social support for psychosocial difficulties.

GENERAL Rx

- Weakness and fatigue:
  - Anticholinesterases (pyridostigmine): an open trial reported improvement of fatigue

with pyridostigmine. Preliminary data from a double-blind, placebo-controlled crossover trial suggested subjective improvement of fatigue and strength in the upper extremities with the same drug.
  - Amantadine, modafinil, amitriptyline, bromocriptine, fluoxetine, and pemoline might be considered.
- Postpolio tinnitus: botulinum toxin A
- Depression: selective serotonin reuptake inhibitors

DISPOSITION

Slow progression, with an average decline in strength of approximately 1% to 2% per year

REFERRAL

- Surgical evaluation for muscle biopsy
- A neurologist or a neuromuscular specialist for neurophysiologic testing
- Physical and occupational therapists

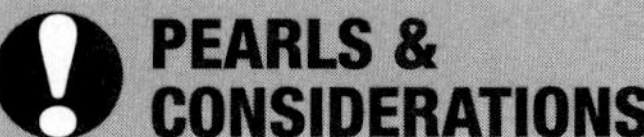

PEARLS & CONSIDERATIONS

COMMENTS

- Risk of falls should be assessed by a physical therapist.
- Interdisciplinary approach should be used in the management of those patients, including primary care physician; physiatrist; neurologist; pulmonologist; psychiatrist; physical, occupational, and respiratory therapists; nurse; and social worker.

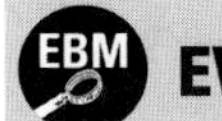

EVIDENCE

Pyridostigmine provided improvement of fatigue[1] and subjective improvement of fatigue and strength in the upper extremities.[2] Moderate-intensity strength training exercise is safe and effective in PPS patients.[3]

Evidence-Based References

1. Trojan DA, Cashman NR: An open trial of pyridostigmine in post-poliomyelitis syndrome, *Can J Neurol Sci* 22(3):223-237, 1995.
2. Seizert BP et al: Pyridostigmine effect on strength, endurance, and fatigue in post-polio patients [abstract], *Arch Phys Med Rehabil* 75:1049, 1994.
3. Chan KM et al: Randomized controlled trial of strength training in post-polio patients, *Muscle Nerve* 27(3):332-338, 2003.

SUGGESTED READINGS

Katirji B et al: *Neuromuscular disorders in clinical practice,* Boston, 2002, Butterworth-Heinemann, pp 403-415.

Nollet F, de Visser M: Postpolio syndrome, *Arch Neurol* 61(7):1142-1144, 2004.

Scolozzi P et al: Successful treatment of a postpolio tinnitus with type A botulinum toxin, *Laryngoscope* 115(7):1288-1290, 2005.

Trojan DA, Cashman NR: Post-poliomyelitis syndrome, *Muscle Nerve* 31(1):6-19, 2005.

AUTHOR: **MUSTAFA A. HAMMAD, M.D.**

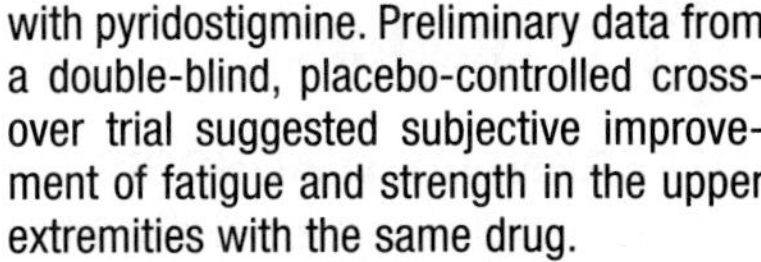

Posttraumatic Stress Disorder (PTG)

BASIC INFORMATION

DEFINITION

Posttraumatic stress disorder (PTSD) is an anxiety disorder that may arise when an individual has witnessed or experienced a potentially fatal or serious injury during which he or she felt helpless or horrified. The individual continues to experience the event in the form of flashbacks (reliving the trauma), intrusive recollections, dreams, or physiologic reactivity. These responses are associated with persistent hyperarousal (e.g., hypervigilance, exaggerated startle response, sleep disturbance, irritability, and difficulty concentrating) and avoidance (both physically and cognitively) of stimuli associated with the traumatic event. In children, the horror may be expressed by disorganized or agitated behavior. Currently, there is controversy regarding the criteria for PTSD to be included in DSM-V. The diagnosis of "complex PTSD" has been suggested for people with multiple traumas, particularly childhood traumas, that are believed to contribute to a predisposition to acute PTSD as well as different trajectories of treatment and recovery. "Developmental trauma disorder" has been suggested for children and adolescents.

SYNONYMS

Soldier's heart
Effort syndrome
Shell shock
Irritable heart
Traumatic necrosis
Survivor syndrome
Concentration camp syndrome
Gross stress reaction (DSM-I, published in 1952)

ICD-9CM CODES
308.3 Posttraumatic stress syndrome, acute (duration of symptoms <3 mo)
309.8 Posttraumatic stress syndrome, chronic (duration of symptoms >3 mo)

EPIDEMIOLOGY & DEMOGRAPHICS

INCIDENCE: Less than 10% of individuals who have experienced a traumatic event will develop PTSD.

PREVALENCE (IN U.S.):
- PTSD is one of the most common psychiatric disorders, with an estimated lifetime prevalence of 7.8% to 12.3%.
- Prevalence estimates among high-risk populations (e.g., combat veterans or victims of violent crimes) range up to 58%.
- PTSD is associated with high rates of depression, anxiety disorders, and substance use. Overall, approximately 80% of persons with PTSD also have a comorbid psychiatric disorder.
- Posttraumatic factors most associated with the development of PTSD are subsequent life stress and perceived lack of social support.

PREDOMINANT SEX: Twice as many women as men are affected, with prevalence rates of 10% to 14% of women and 5% to 6% of men; more than 50% of cases in women are related to sexual assault.

PREDOMINANT AGE: No predisposing age factors have been identified.

GENETICS: Twin studies have demonstrated the important role of genetic vulnerability in the development of PTSD related to combat. No comparable studies exist for civilian trauma.

PHYSICAL FINDINGS & CLINICAL PRESENTATION

- A life-threatening event evoking intense fear or horror (criterion A).
- Reexperiencing of traumatic events in the form of dreams, flashbacks, and intrusive memories (criterion B).
- Depersonalization, detachment, emotional numbing, and dissociation, with avoidance of physical or cognitive reminders of the event (criterion C).
- Hyperarousal, hypervigilance and exaggerated startle response, irritability, anxiety, and difficulty concentrating (criterion D).
- To meet DSM-IV criteria for PTSD, one must meet criterion A plus symptoms from each of the three symptoms clusters A, B, C, and D. A fifth criterion concerns duration of symptoms (>1 mo) and a sixth assesses function (must be impaired).
- Mneumonic: TRAUMA
  *T*raumatic event (criterion A)
  *R*e-experiencing (criterion B)
  *A*voidance (criterion C)
  *U*nable to function (criterion F)
  *M*onth at least (criterion E)
  *A*rousal (criterion D)

ETIOLOGY

- Events that involve interpersonal violence are more likely to give rise to PTSD than are events such as motor vehicle accidents and natural disasters.
- The severity of the physical injury is a weaker predictor of the likelihood of developing PTSD than the psychological distress; the duration of the stress is the most important factor.
- Symptoms are mediated, in part, by the autonomic nervous system and the hypothalamic-pituitary-adrenal (HPA) system. Studies have proposed mechanisms, including an excessive release of norepinephrine that consolidates the memory on the amygdala, an exaggerated negative feedback inhibition of the HPA axis by glucocorticoids, and enhanced postsynaptic alpha-1 response in the central nervous system to norepinephrine.
- Hippocampal volumes in adults with PTSD are smaller than normal. Whether this is a result of PTSD or a predisposing factor is unknown. This finding is theorized as possibly the result of damage caused by glucocorticoids. Hippocampal damage can facilitate consolidation of traumatic memories and prevent laying down of new memories. SSRIs induce neurogenesis of the hippocampus, although the significance of this requires ongoing research.

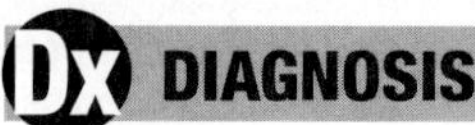

DIAGNOSIS

DIFFERENTIAL DIAGNOSIS

- Adjustment disorders are distinguished from PTSD in that the precipitating stress is less catastrophic and the psychological reaction less specific.
- Acute stress disorder, if symptoms last between 48 hr and 4 wk after trauma.
- Delayed-onset PTSD, if symptoms develop >6 mo after the event.
- Major depression; up to 30% of primary care patients with depression also have PTSD.

WORKUP

- After a traumatic event, the presence of the following symptoms for >1 mo: at least one reexperiencing symptom, at least three avoidance/numbing symptoms, and at least one hypervigilance symptom meet DSM-IV criteria for diagnosis of PTSD.
  Symptoms 1 to 3 mo = acute PTSD
  Symptoms >3 mo = chronic PTSD
  Development of symptoms years after the event = delayed-onset PTSD
- There are numerous self-report questionnaires and structured diagnostic instruments; the best validated tool is the Posttraumatic Diagnostic Scale.
- Laboratory and imaging are not sufficiently validated or replicated to be clinically useful, although other medical conditions that can exacerbate symptoms should be ruled out with studies such as TSH, CBC, urine toxicology, and glucose.
- Primary care PTSD (PC-PTSD) screen recommended by the Veterans Administration:
  In your life, have you ever had any experience that was so frightening, horrible, or upsetting that, in the past month, you:
  1. Have had nightmares about it or thought about it when you did not want to?
     YES NO
  2. Tried hard not to think about it or went out of your way to avoid situations that reminded you of it?
     YES NO
  3. Were constantly on guard, watchful, or easily startled?
     YES NO
  4. Felt numb or detached from others, activities, or your surroundings?
     YES NO

  Current research suggests that the results of the PC-PTSD should be considered positive for PTSD if a patient answers "yes" to any three items.

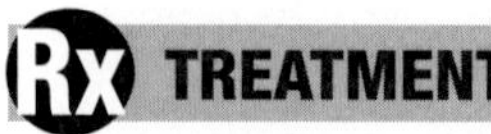

TREATMENT

NONPHARMACOLOGIC THERAPY

- Gold standard treatment is cognitive-behavioral therapy (CBT), particularly with a trauma focus (may include mental imagery and other forms of exposure). Prolonged exposure (PE), a type of CBT that includes education on stress response, breathing training, and prolonged mental recounting of the event to decrease the emotional response, was found to be more effective than standard CBT in female veterans. However, there is some controversy regarding the long-term efficacy of brief therapies and the potential role for long-term psychodynamic psychotherapy.

- Group therapy is helpful for many PTSD victims, particularly combat veterans.
- Eye movement desensitization reprocessing (EMDR) has been shown to be effective in controlled trials.

ACUTE GENERAL Rx

- Studies have shown that immediate postincident debriefing may worsen outcome.
- A brief course of benzodiazepines may be helpful acutely for reducing anxiety but has not been shown to decrease development of core symptoms.
- Increasing evidence exists that beta-adrenergic blockers may be helpful if given within hours after the trauma to disrupt the physiologic stress response.
- Sedating antidepressants or sleep aids such as trazodone may be helpful to treat initial insomnia.

CHRONIC Rx

- SSRIs are the pharmacologic treatment of choice for PTSD.
- Other antidepressants such as TCAs are also helpful in reducing symptoms.
- Beta-adrenergic blockers such as propranolol and alpha-2-adrenergic agonists such as clonidine, and less so, guanfacine, may be helpful in treating arousal symptoms.
- Prazosin, a central α1-adrenergic antagonist, may decrease distressing dreams and improve sleep quality.
- Mood stabilizers and antipsychotics may be needed for severe symptoms such as paranoia, extreme anxiety, or angry outbursts.

COMPLEMENTARY & ALTERNATIVE APPROACHES

Acupuncture was shown to be as effective as CBT in decreasing symptoms of PTSD.

DISPOSITION

- Recovery rates are highest in the first 12 mo after onset of symptoms.
- Average duration of symptoms is 36 mo for those who undergo treatment and 64 mo for those never treated.
- There is a 50% chance of remission at 2 yr, but up to half of patients have chronic symptoms.
- Predictors of chronic course include previous trauma, premorbid psychiatric function, panic reaction at time of event, prolonged terror, or dissociation at time of event.

REFERRAL

Because early intervention improves outcome, refer to psychiatry as soon as diagnosis made.

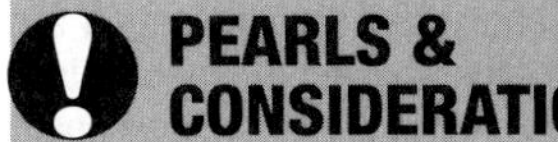

PEARLS & CONSIDERATIONS

- Screen for comorbid substance abuse. Substance use may start or increase as an attempt to manage distressing symptoms.
- Treatment can be effective even if it begins years after the traumatic event occurred.
- As a result of emerging findings regarding disturbances of the limbic system in PTSD, it is increasingly being conceived of as a stress-induced fear-circuitry disorder.

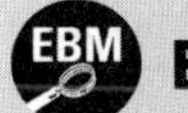

EVIDENCE

Please note: Complete text of EBM for this topic is available online.

Key trials and commentary:

In addition to trauma exposure, other factors contribute to risk for development of posttraumatic stress disorder (PTSD) in adulthood. Both genetic and environmental factors are contributory, with child abuse providing significant risk liability.

The aim of this study was to increase understanding of genetic and environmental risk factors as well as their interaction in the development of PTSD by gene–environment interactions of child abuse, level of non–child abuse trauma exposure, and genetic polymorphisms at the stress-related gene *FKBP5*.

This study showed that four SNPs of the *FKBP5* gene interacted with severity of child abuse as a predictor of adult PTSD symptoms. There were no main effects of the SNPs on PTSD symptoms and no significant genetic interactions with level of non–child abuse trauma as predictor of adult PTSD symptoms, suggesting a potential gene–childhood environment interaction for adult PTSD.

This is an important study illustrating the powerful effects of gene–environment interactions in childhood upon adult psychopathology. The study was meticulous in its design. Gene effects on PTSD risk do not appear to be confounded by the usual suspect, that is, comorbid depression and familial risk for PTSD. What is perhaps most powerful in this study is the extent of the "signal" from the trauma of childhood abuse. The effect is distinct and independent from other trauma experienced in this sample of patients with PTSD. This is an extremely important article in that it illustrates gene–early environment interactions for psychiatric illness in genes. It is also important because of the strength of the "signal" from childhood abuse as a risk factor for the later development of PTSD in adult life.[1] Ⓐ

Evidence-Based Reference

1. Binder EB et al: Association of *FKBP5* polymorphisms and childhood abuse with risk of posttraumatic stress disorder symptoms in adults, *JAMA* 299:1291-1305, 2008. Commentary by P. Buckley, M.D. Ⓐ

SUGGESTED READINGS

Bisson JI: Post-traumatic stress disorder, *BMJ* 334: 789-793, 2007.

Forbes D et al: Australian guidelines for the treatment of adults with acute stress disorder and posttraumatic stress disorder, *Aust N Z J Psychiatry* 41(8):637-648, 2007.

Heim C, Nemeroff CB: Neurobiology of posttraumatic stress disorder. *CNS Spectr* 14(1) Suppl 1:13-24, 2009.

Kubzansky LD et al: Prospective study of posttraumatic stress disorder symptoms and coronary heart disease in the normative aging study, *Arch Gen Psychiatry* 64:109-116, 2007.

National Center for PTSD (NCPTSD), United States Department of Veterans Affairs: Available at http://www.ncptsd.va.gov. Accessed March 2010.

Schottenbauer MA et al: Contributions of psychodynamic approaches to treatment of PTSD and trauma: a review of the empirical treatment and psychopathology literature, *Psychiatry* 71(1):13-34, 2008.

AUTHORS: **ALISON C. MAY, M.D., KAILA COMPTON, M.D., PH.D.**, and **RADHIKA RAMANAN, M.D., M.P.H.**

P

Diseases and Disorders

Precocious Puberty (ALG)

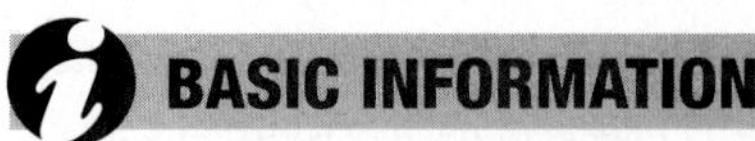

BASIC INFORMATION

DEFINITION

Precocious puberty is defined as sexual development occurring before age 8 yr in females and 9 yr in males.

SYNONYMS

Pubertas praecox

ICD-9CM CODES
259.1 Precocious puberty

EPIDEMIOLOGY & DEMOGRAPHICS

INCIDENCE: Estimated to be between one in 5000 to 10,000.

PREDOMINANT SEX: Females are affected more often than males for the idiopathic variant; for other causes, dependent on the underlying etiology.

GENETICS: The genetics for some of the etiologies of precocious puberty are known.

PHYSICAL FINDINGS & CLINICAL PRESENTATION

- In females: breast development, pubic hair development, accelerated growth, menarche
- In males: increase in testicular volume and penile length, pubic hair development, accelerated growth, muscular development, acne, change in voice, penile erections

ETIOLOGY

- Idiopathic or true: diagnosis of exclusion
- Central nervous system (CNS) pathology: tumors, hydrocephalus, ventricular cysts, benign lesions
- Severe hypothyroidism
- Posttraumatic head injury
- Genetic disorders: neurofibromatosis, tuberous sclerosis, McCune-Albright syndrome, congenital adrenal hyperplasia
- Gonadal tumors
- Nongonadal tumors: hepatoblastoma
- Exposure to exogenous sex steroids

Dx DIAGNOSIS

DIFFERENTIAL DIAGNOSIS

- Most common diagnoses to consider: premature thelarche and premature adrenarche
- Gonadotropin hormone-releasing hormone (GnRH)-dependent precocious puberty: idiopathic, CNS tumors, hypothalamic hamartomas, neurofibromatosis, tuberous sclerosis, hydrocephalus, status after acute head injury, ventricular cysts, status after CNS infection
- GnRH-independent precocious puberty: congenital adrenal hyperplasia, adrenocortical tumors (males), McCune-Albright syndrome (females), gonadal tumors, ectopic human chorionic gonadotropin (hCG)-secreting tumors (chorioblastoma, hepatoblastoma), exposure to exogenous sex steroids, severe hypothyroidism

WORKUP

Thorough history and physical examination are essential to determine if the patient has true precocious puberty. Particular attention should be paid to growth, development, order of appearance of the secondary sexual characteristics, pubertal development in family members, medications, neurologic symptoms, Tanner staging, abdominal and neurologic examination. Section III, "Puberty, Precocious" describes a clinical approach to precocious puberty.

LABORATORY TESTS

- GnRH testing will help determine if dependent or independent cause
- Sex hormone studies: luteinizing hormone, follicle-stimulating hormone, hCG, testosterone (males), estrogen (females). Levels of sex steroids should be determined in the morning, with use of assays that have detection limits adapted to pediatric values. In girls, serum estradiol levels are highly variable and have a rather low sensitivity for the diagnosis of precocious puberty.
- T_4, thyroid-stimulating hormone

IMAGING STUDIES

- CT scan or MRI of the brain to evaluate for CNS pathology
- Consideration of pelvic ultrasound in female patients to evaluate for cysts or tumors
- Abdominal imaging with CT scan if intra-abdominal pathology suspected

Rx TREATMENT

NONPHARMACOLOGIC THERAPY

- Good communication with the parents is essential to care.
- Psychologic support for the child may be needed with regard to self-image and problems with peer acceptance.

ACUTE GENERAL Rx

There is no acute therapy for precocious puberty.

CHRONIC Rx

Therapy depends on the etiology of precocious puberty. For the treatment of central or gonadotropin-dependent precocious puberty depot GnRH agonists (leuprorelin, leuprolide, triptorelin, goserelin, histrelin, buserelin) are effective.

- Leuprolide is given 0.25 to 0.3 mg/kg with a 7.5 mg minimum IM every 4 wk. Local side effects include pain, erythema, and inflammatory reactions. Other side effects include headaches and menopausal-like symptoms (asthenia, hot flashes).
- For other CNS lesions and extragonadal tumors, therapy is dependent on the type of lesion, location of the lesion, and the overall prognosis of the underlying problem.
- For severe hypothyroidism, treatment with thyroid hormone will result in regression of the sexual development. The child will subsequently undergo appropriate pubertal development later in life.
- For familial male gonadotropin-independent precocious puberty, the androgen-synthesis inhibitor ketoconazole can be used at doses of 600 mg/day divided tid, or a combination of the aromatase inhibitor testolactone and spironolactone can be used.

DISPOSITION

- For true precocious puberty and some CNS lesions, long-term outcome is usually very good. When drug therapy is instituted, it is continued until a time when further pubertal development is appropriate. It is then discontinued, allowing the child to progress through puberty.
- For other cases, long-term outcomes depend on the prognosis of the underlying cause.

REFERRAL

- Initial workup can be instituted by the primary care provider.
- Referral to an endocrinologist is indicated for most children because they will need long-term management, monitoring, and treatment.
- Attention to the emotional needs of the child is important.

SUGGESTED READING

Carel JC, Leger J: Precocious puberty, *N Engl J Med* 358:2366, 2008.

AUTHORS: **BETH J. WUTZ, M.D.,** and **RUBEN ALVERO, M.D.**

BASIC INFORMATION

DEFINITION

Preeclampsia involves the triad of hypertension, proteinuria, and edema that develops after the twentieth week of gestation. Mild preeclampsia is defined as a blood pressure of <140/90 mm Hg. Severe preeclampsia is associated with a blood pressure >160/110 mm Hg, proteinuria >5 g in a 24-hr urine collection, oliguria (<400 ml/24 hr), cerebral or visual disturbances, epigastric pain, pulmonary edema, thrombocytopenia, hepatic dysfunction, or severe intrauterine growth restriction.

SYNONYMS

Pregnancy-induced hypertension
Toxemia of pregnancy

ICD-9CM CODES
642.6 Preeclampsia

EPIDEMIOLOGY & DEMOGRAPHICS

INCIDENCE: 0% to 14% in primigravidas, 5.7% to 7.3% in multigravidas
RISK FACTORS: Increased incidence and severity with multiple gestations or renal or collagen-vascular diseases. Extremes of reproductive age, <20 or >35 yr, obesity, African American race, thrombophilia, previous preeclampsia.
GENETICS: Positive correlation with maternal and paternal family history.

PHYSICAL FINDINGS & CLINICAL PRESENTATION

- Generalized swelling or nondependent edema, possibly manifested by rapid weight gain (>4 lb/wk) even in the absence of edema
- Auscultation of pulmonary rales
- Right upper quadrant pain (HELLP syndrome [hemolysis, elevated liver enzymes, and low platelet count] or subcapsular liver hematoma)
- Hyperreflexia or clonus
- Vaginal bleeding (placental abruption)
- Acute or chronic fetal compromise manifested by intrauterine growth restriction or fetal tachycardia with late decelerations, respectively
- Wide range of symptoms attributable to multiorgan system dysfunction, involving hepatic, hematologic, renal, pulmonary, and central nervous systems
- Possibility of severe disease despite "normal" blood pressure readings, so a high index of suspicion must be maintained in high-risk situations

ETIOLOGY

- Exact etiology or toxic substance is unknown
- Theories:
  1. Imbalance between thromboxane A_2 (vasoconstrictor and platelet aggregator) and prostacyclin (vasodilator)
  2. Abnormal trophoblastic invasion of spiral arteries
  3. Increased sensitivity to angiotensin II by the muscular walls of the arteries
  4. Excess circulating soluble fms-like tyrosine kinase 1 (SFIT-1), which binds placental growth factor (PIGF) and vascular endothelial growth factor (VEGF), may have a pathogenic role

DIAGNOSIS

DIFFERENTIAL DIAGNOSIS

- Acute fatty liver of pregnancy
- Appendicitis
- Diabetic ketoacidosis
- Gallbladder disease
- Gastroenteritis
- Glomerulonephritis
- Hemolytic-uremic syndrome
- Hepatic encephalopathy
- Hyperemesis gravidarum
- Idiopathic thrombocytopenia
- Thrombotic thrombocytopenic purpura
- Nephrolithiasis
- Pyelonephritis
- Peptic ulcer disease
- Systemic lupus erythematosus
- Viral hepatitis

WORKUP

- Two blood pressure measurements with the patient in lateral recumbent position 6 hr apart, with an absolute pressure >140/90 mm Hg or an increase of 30 mm Hg systolic or 15 mm Hg diastolic from baseline, an increase in the mean arterial pressure (MAP) of 20 mm Hg, or an absolute MAP >105 mm Hg
- Evaluation for proteinuria as defined by >0.1 g/L on urine dipstick or >300 mg protein on a 24-hr urine collection
- Evaluation of fetal status for evidence of intrauterine growth restriction, oligohydramnios, alteration in umbilical or uterine artery Doppler flow, or acute compromise, such as abruption
- Because of the insidious nature of the disease with potential for multiple organ involvement, complete evaluation for preeclampsia in any pregnant patient presenting with central nervous system derangement or gastrointestinal symptoms after 20 wk of gestation
- Evaluation for associated conditions such as disseminated intravascular coagulation, hepatic dysfunction, or subcapsular hematoma

LABORATORY TESTS

- High-risk patients: baseline assessment of renal function (24-hr urine collection for protein and creatinine clearance), platelets, blood urea nitrogen, creatinine, liver function tests (LFTs), and uric acid should be obtained at the first prenatal visit.
- Complete blood count (hemoglobin, hematocrit, platelets) may show signs of volume contraction or HELLP syndrome.
- LFTs (aspartate aminotransferase, alanine aminotransferase, lactate dehydrogenase) are useful in evaluation for HELLP syndrome or to exclude important differentials.
- Hyperuricemia or increased creatinine may indicate decreasing renal function.
- Prothrombin time, partial thromboplastin time, and fibrinogen should be checked to rule out disseminated intravascular coagulation.
- Peripheral smear may demonstrate microangiopathic hemolytic anemia.
- Complement levels can be used to differentiate from an acute exacerbation of a collagen-vascular disease.
- Increased levels of SFIT-1 and reduced levels of PIGF predict subsequent development of preeclampsia.

IMAGING STUDIES

- CT scan of head if atypical presentation of eclampsia, possibility of intracerebral bleed, or prolonged postictal state
- Sonogram of fetus to evaluate for intrauterine growth restriction, amniotic fluid, placenta
- Sonogram of maternal liver if suspect subcapsular hematoma

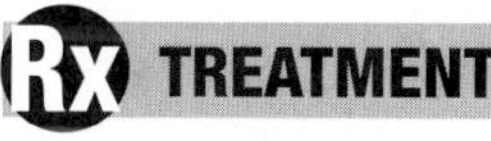

TREATMENT

NONPHARMACOLOGIC THERAPY

Bed rest in left lateral decubitus position

ACUTE GENERAL Rx

Delivery is the treatment of choice and the only cure for the disease. This must be taken in the context of the gestational age of the fetus, severity of the preeclampsia, and the likelihood of a successful induction and reliability of patient.

- Administer magnesium sulfate 6 g IV loading dose, with 2 to 3 g maintenance or phenytoin at 10 to 15 mg/kg loading dose, then 200 mg IV q8h starting 12 hr after loading dose.
- Hydralazine 10 mg IV, labetalol hydrochloride 20 to 40 mg IV, nifedipine 20 mg SL can be used for acute blood pressure control.
- Continuous fetal monitoring is needed.
- Epidural is anesthesia of choice for pain management in labor or cesarean section.
- All patients undergoing induction of labor should receive antiseizure medications regardless of severity of disease.

CHRONIC Rx

- Mild preeclampsia <37 wk: close observation for worsening maternal or fetal condition, with delivery at >37 wk with favorable cervix or at 40 wk regardless of cervical status.
- Severe preeclampsia: delivery in the presence of maternal or fetal compromise, labor, or >34 wk; at 28 to 34 wk consider steroids with close monitoring, and at <24 wk consider termination of pregnancy.
- Methyldopa is drug of choice for long-term blood pressure control during pregnancy.

DISPOSITION

Preeclampsia is a progressive and unpredictable disease process; a course of expectancy should be managed with caution. Up to 20% of patients who have seizures are normotensive.

REFERRAL

Obstetric management is indicated because of the insidious nature of the disease, with transfer of all cases <34 wk to a facility with a level three nursery.

PEARLS & CONSIDERATIONS

COMMENTS

- Low-dose aspirin 81 mg qd and calcium supplementation 1500 mg qd can be considered in high-risk patients to decrease the risk of recurrence.
- Begin after first trimester.
- Although the absolute risk of ESRD in women who have had preeclampsia is low, preeclampsia is a marker for an increased risk of subsequent ESRD.

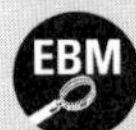

EVIDENCE

In pregnant women with mild-to-moderate hypertension, antihypertensive drug therapy reduces the risk of severe hypertension.

Antihypertensive drug therapy for mild-to-moderate hypertension in pregnancy is associated with a significant reduction in the risk of developing severe hypertension, but there is little evidence of a difference in the risk of developing pre-eclampsia or in the rate of fetal death or small-for-date babies.[1] Ⓐ

The question of whether the reduction in the risk of severe hypertension should be considered sufficient to warrant treatment is a decision to be made by patients in consultation with their clinician.[1]

There is no evidence to favor one agent over another, but methyldopa is often the agent of first choice for clinicians; beta-blockers are as effective, although they are associated with small-for-date babies.

There is insufficient evidence to conclude that one antihypertensive agent is better than another.[1] Ⓐ

In pregnant patients with very high blood pressure, there is no evidence that one antihypertensive is preferable to others in terms of improving outcomes.

Analysis of multiple reviews found no clear evidence that one drug therapy is to be preferred over another.[2] Ⓐ

Antenatal corticosteroids are beneficial to the fetus in women at risk of preterm delivery.

A systematic review found that treatment with antenatal corticosteroids (betamethasone, dexamethasone, or hydrocortisone) versus placebo in women at risk of preterm delivery, including those with pregnancy-related hypertension, is associated with a reduced rate of neonatal death, respiratory distress syndrome, cerebroventricular hemorrhage, necrotizing enterocolitis, and systemic infections, as well as a reduced need for respiratory support and intensive care. There was no evidence of increased risk of maternal death, chorioamnionitis, or puerperal sepsis.[3] Ⓐ

There is insufficient evidence to assess the effects of hospital admission, bed rest, or day care compared with outpatient care.

Systematic reviews have compared hospital admission versus outpatient management, bed rest in hospital versus normal ambulation in hospital, and antenatal day care units versus hospital admission in women who develop hypertension during pregnancy, but the trials are too small for any reliable conclusions to be drawn.[4]

Evidence-Based References

1. Abalos E: Antihypertensive drug therapy for mild to moderate hypertension during pregnancy, *Cochrane Database Rev* 1, 2007. Ⓐ

2. Duley L et al: Drugs for treatment of very high blood pressure during pregnancy, *Cochrane Database Rev* 3, 2006. Ⓐ

3. Roberts D, Dalziel S: Antenatal corticosteroids for accelerating fetal lung maturation for women at risk of preterm birth, *Cochrane Database Rev* 3, 2006. Ⓐ

4. Duley L: Pre-eclampsia and hypertension, *Clin Evid* 14:1776-1790, 2005.

SUGGESTED READINGS

Lain KY, Roberts JM: Contemporary concepts of the pathogenesis and management of preeclampsia, *JAMA* 287:3183, 2002.

Levine RJ et al: Circulating angiogenic factors and risk of preeclampsia, *N Engl J Med* 350:672, 2004.

AUTHORS: **SCOTT J. ZUCCALA, D.O.,** and **RUBEN ALVERO, M.D.**

BASIC INFORMATION

DEFINITION

The *Diagnostic and Statistical Manual of Mental Disorders,* 4th edition, classifies premenstrual dysphoric disorder (PMDD) as a "depressive disorder not otherwise specified" and requires as criteria for definition the presence of five or more of the following symptoms in most menstrual cycles for the past year.

- The symptoms should be present most of the time during the last week of the luteal phase, with remission beginning within a few days after the onset of the follicular phase, and absent during the week after menses, with at least one of the symptoms being either 1, 2, 3, or 4:
    1. Marked depressed mood, feeling of hopelessness, or self-deprecating thoughts
    2. Marked anxiety, tension, feeling of being "keyed up" or "on edge"
    3. Marked affective lability (e.g., feeling suddenly sad or tearful or increased sensitivity to rejection)
    4. Persistent and marked anger or irritability or increased interpersonal conflicts
    5. Decreased interest in usual activities (e.g., work, school, friends, hobbies)
    6. Subjective sense of difficulty in concentrating
    7. Lethargy, easy fatigability, or marked lack of energy
    8. Marked change in appetite, overeating, or specific food cravings
    9. Hypersomnia or insomnia
    10. A subjective sense of being overwhelmed or out of control
    11. Other physical symptoms, such as breast tenderness or swelling, headaches, joint or muscle pain, a sensation of "bloating," or weight gain
- The disturbance markedly interferes with work or school or with usual social activities and relationships with others (e.g., avoidance of social activities, decreased production and efficiency at work or school).
- The disturbance is not merely an exacerbation of the symptoms of another disorder, such as major depressive disorder, panic disorder, dysthymic disorder, or a personality disorder (although it may be superimposed on any of these disorders).
- The first three criteria must be confirmed by prospective daily ratings during at least two consecutive symptomatic cycles (diagnosis may be made provisionally before such confirmation).

NOTE: In menstruating women, the luteal phase corresponds to the period between ovulation and the onset of menses, and the follicular phase begins with menses. In nonmenstruating women (e.g., women who have had a hysterectomy), determination of the timing of the luteal and follicular phases may require measurement of circulating reproductive hormones.

ICD-9CM CODES

625.4 Premenstrual dysphoric syndrome

EPIDEMIOLOGY & DEMOGRAPHICS

- PMDD affects 3% to 10% of women of reproductive age.
- Genetic factors play a significant role (increased incidence in monozygotic twins and in women whose mothers had PMDD).
- 30% to 76% of women with PMDD have a lifetime history of depression.

PHYSICAL FINDINGS & CLINICAL PRESENTATION

- Physical examination may be completely normal.
- Depressed mood, tachycardia, sweating from comorbid disorders (e.g., panic disorder, major depression) may be present.
- Symptoms occur during the last half of the menstrual cycle (the luteal phase) and are absent from the first day of menstruation until ovulation (follicular phase).

ETIOLOGY

Unknown. Serotonin deficiency and altered sensitivity in serotoninergic system in response to phasic hormone fluctuations in the menstrual cycle are believed to play a role.

Dx DIAGNOSIS

DIFFERENTIAL DIAGNOSIS

- Premenstrual syndrome
- Dysthymic syndrome
- Personality disorder
- Panic disorder
- Major depressive disorder
- Hyperthyroidism
- Polycystic ovarian syndrome
- Drug or alcohol abuse
- Irritable bowel syndrome
- Endometriosis

WORKUP

- Diagnosis is based on obtaining a detailed history and ruling out the presence of physical or psychiatric disorders. No objective diagnostic tests exist.
- The diagnosis should be confirmed by using a symptom checklist prospectively for two consecutive menstrual cycles. Commonly used diagnostic instruments include the Calendar of Premenstrual Experiences and the Premenstrual Syndrome Diary.

LABORATORY TESTS

- None are usually necessary.
- A serum thyroid-stimulating hormone test to exclude thyroid problems, complete blood count to rule out anemia, and a chemistry profile to assess electrolytes may be ordered if diagnosis is unclear.

Rx TREATMENT

NONPHARMACOLOGIC THERAPY

- Reduction in intake of caffeine, refined sugars, or sodium may be helpful in some patients.
- Increased aerobic exercise, smoking cessation, alcohol restriction, and regular sleep are often beneficial.
- Stress reduction and management will decrease severity of symptoms.

GENERAL Rx

- Selective serotonin reuptake inhibitors are first-line agents for the treatment of PMDD. Commonly used agents and initial doses are fluoxetine 10 mg qd, sertraline 50 mg qd, paroxetine 10 mg qd, and citalopram 20 mg qd. Many patients will require titration to significantly higher doses to achieve therapeutic benefit. These medications can be administered continuously during the menstrual cycle or only when the patients experience symptoms. Luteal phase or intermittent administration involves initiating medication at the time of ovulation and stopping it at the beginning of menses.
- Second-line agents are benzodiazepines (alprazolam 0.25 mg tid prn) and the tricyclic antidepressant clomipramine (25 mg qd as starting dose).
- Hormonal intervention with monthly intramuscular injections of leuprolide has been reported effective in some patients; however, it should be reserved only for patients unresponsive to first- and second-line agents.
- Nutritional supplementation (vitamin B_6 up to 100 mg/day, vitamin E up to 600 IU/day, calcium carbonate up to 1200 mg/day, and magnesium up to 500 mg/day) are also commonly used and effective in symptom reduction in some patients.
- Ovariectomy may be considered in severe refractory cases.

AUTHOR: **FRED F. FERRI, M.D.**

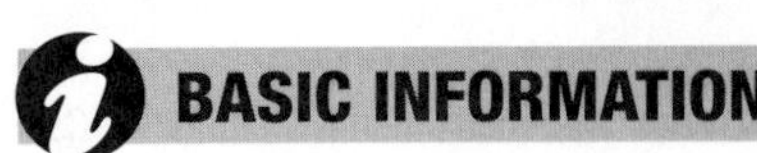

BASIC INFORMATION

DEFINITION

Premenstrual syndrome (PMS) is a cyclic recurrence during the luteal phase of the menstrual cycle of somatic, affective, and behavioral disturbances that are of sufficient severity to affect interpersonal relationships adversely or interfere with normal activities.

SYNONYMS

PMS
PMDD

ICD-9CM CODES
625.4 Premenstrual tension syndromes

EPIDEMIOLOGY & DEMOGRAPHICS

- PMS is believed to be extremely prevalent, intermittently affecting approximately one third of all premenopausal women.
- Severe cases occur in approximately 2% to 10% of women with PMS.
- Those seeking treatment for PMS are usually in their 30s or 40s.
- The natural history of PMS has not been clearly elucidated.

PHYSICAL FINDINGS & CLINICAL PRESENTATION

- Diverse and potentially disabling symptoms
- Associated with >150 psychological, physical, and behavioral symptoms
- Most frequent reason for seeking treatment: emotional symptoms
- Most common emotional symptoms: depression, irritability, anxiety, labile moods, anger, crying easily, sadness, extreme sensitivity, nervous tension
- Most common physical symptoms: headache, bloating, cramps, breast tenderness, migraines, fatigue, weight gain, aches and pains, palpitations
- Most common behavior symptom: food cravings
- Other behavioral symptoms: increased appetite, increased alcohol intake, decreased motivation, decreased efficiency, avoidance of activities, staying home, sleep changes, libido changes, forgetfulness, decreased concentration

ETIOLOGY

- Etiology remains obscure.
- Because of the multifactorial, multiorgan nature of PMS, a single etiologic cause is unlikely.

Dx DIAGNOSIS

DIFFERENTIAL DIAGNOSIS

- A diagnosis of exclusion, so other medical or psychologic disorders should be ruled out.
- Most common disorders: depression or anxiety, thyroid disease.

WORKUP

- History
- Physical examination
- Laboratory studies to rule out alternative diagnosis
- If no alternative diagnosis confirms diagnosis of PMS, basal body temperature charting is used to determine if the patient is ovulating:
  1. If she is not ovulating, it is not PMS.
  2. If she is ovulating, symptoms should be charted for at least two cycles to determine if the symptoms occur in the luteal phase.
  3. If symptoms are not occurring in the luteal phase, it is not PMS and further investigation is needed.
     a. If symptoms occur in the follicular phase, patient has premenstrual exacerbation of another condition.
     b. If symptoms do not occur in the follicular phase, diagnosis of PMS is confirmed.

LABORATORY TESTS

- None available to specifically confirm the diagnosis of PMS
- Thyroid function tests to rule out thyroid disease

Rx TREATMENT

NONPHARMACOLOGIC THERAPY

- Individualization of the treatment plan to maximize therapeutic response
- Psychosocial intervention:
  1. Education
  2. Stress management
  3. Environmental changes
  4. Adequate rest and sleep
  5. Regular exercise
- Nutritional recommendations:
  1. Regularly eaten, well-balanced meals
  2. Adequate amounts of protein, fiber, and complex carbohydrates; low fat
  3. Avoidance of foods that are high in salt and simple sugars; may promote water retention, weight gain, and physical discomfort
  4. Avoidance of caffeine-containing beverages; stimulant effects of caffeine may worsen tension, irritability, and insomnia
  5. Avoidance of alcohol and illicit drugs; may worsen emotional lability
  6. Calcium supplementation (1000 mg/day for women 19 to 50 yr, 1300 mg/day for girls 14 to 18 yr) to reduce the physical and emotional symptoms
  7. Magnesium (360 mg/day) to reduce water retention and the negative effect associated with PMS
  8. Pyridoxine (vitamin B_6) 50 mg bid to improve depression, fatigue, irritability, and natural diuretic ability; neurotoxicity observed at higher dosages

ACUTE GENERAL Rx

Suppression of ovulation:

- Oral contraceptives: one pill per day
- Progestin-only oral contraceptive: one pill per day
- Oral micronized progesterone: 100 mg every morning and 200 mg every evening on days 17 through 28 of menstrual cycle
- Progestin suppository: 200 to 400 mg bid on days 17 through 28 of menstrual cycle
- Oral contraceptive containing drosperinone/ethinyl estradiol: very effective in decreasing physical symptoms
- Medroxyprogesterone: 150 mg IM q3mo
- Levonorgestrel implants: surgical insertion every 5 yr
- Transdermal estradiol: one or two 100-μg patches every 3 days
- Danazol: 100 to 200 mg/day (ovulation not suppressed at this dose)
- Gonadotropin-releasing hormone (GnRH) agonists: daily by intranasal spray or monthly by depot injection

Suppression of physical symptoms:

- Spironolactone: 25 to 50 mg bid on days 14 through 28 of menstrual cycle
- Mefenamic acid
  1. For fluid retention: 250 mg tid on days 24 through 28 of cycle
  2. For pain: 500 mg tid on days 19 through 28 of cycle
- Bromocriptine: 5 mg/day on days 10 through 26 of cycle
- Danazol: 200 mg/day on days 19 through 28 of cycle
- Naproxen: 550 mg bid on days 17 through 28 of cycle, Naprosyn-500 mg bid on days 17 through 28 of cycle

Suppression of psychological symptoms:

- Nortriptyline: 50 to 125 mg/day
- Fluoxetine: 20 mg/day or 90 mg weekly (this medication has indications for premenstrual dysphoric disorder)
- Buspirone: 10 mg bid or tid on days 16 through 28 of cycle, then taper drug
- Alprazolam: 25 mg tid on days 16 through 28 of cycle, then taper drug
- Clonidine: 0.1 mg bid
- Naltrexone: 0.25 mg/day on days 9 through 18 of cycle
- Atenolol: 50 mg/day
- Paroxetine: 20 mg/day
- Sertraline (Zoloft): 50 to 100 mg/day
- Nefazodone (Serzone): initial dosage 100 mg bid; after 1 wk increase to 150 mg bid
- Propranolol: 20 to 40 mg bid
- Verapamil: 100 to 320 mg qd

CHRONIC Rx

- Therapy is largely trial and error, with the goal of providing effective treatment with the safest and most simple therapy.
- For severe intractable PMS: hysterectomy with bilateral oophorectomy; give trial of GnRH therapy or danazol before surgery (hysterectomy and bilateral oophorectomy should be exceedingly rare).

- Estrogen replacement therapy recommended postoperatively to reduce the risk of osteoporosis, heart disease, and genitourinary atrophy.

DISPOSITION

Improved symptoms in 90% of women over time.

REFERRAL

- For counseling with a psychologist or psychiatrist if underlying psychiatric disorder is discovered (cognitive-behavioral therapy)
- To a gynecologist if surgical therapy is contemplated

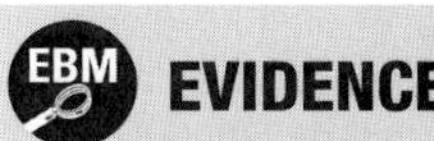

EVIDENCE

A systematic review showed inconsistent results for the benefit of magnesium supplements.[1] B

The same systematic review found calcium to be more effective than placebo in reducing overall PMS symptoms. However, the reviewers concluded that the evidence was not compelling because of methodologic limitations of the trial.[1] B

The review also included trials using herbal medicine, homeopathy, dietary supplementation, relaxation, massage, reflexology, chiropractic, and biofeedback. The authors concluded that on the basis of the current evidence, no complementary or alternative therapy could be recommended as a treatment for PMS.[1] B

There is a small but significant improvement in symptoms with progesterone treatment, but the clinical significance of this is uncertain and the preferred route and timing of delivery remain unclear.[2] B

Three randomized, controlled trials (RCTs) have found that spironolactone is effective in improving irritability, breast tenderness, and bloating; one trial failed to find it superior to placebo.[3-6] B

Treatments for which there is good evidence often have significant side effects or potential harms. GnRH analogs are effective in reducing premenstrual symptoms. Evidence suggests that the use of add-back estrogen and progesterone therapy is less effective than the use of GnRH analogs alone, but more effective than placebo, and the addition of tibolone to GnRH analogs provides no benefit.[7-9] A B

Alprazolam in daily doses of ≥0.75 mg are significantly more effective than placebo in reducing premenstrual symptoms. There is a risk of significant side effects with long-term use.[10] B

There is good evidence to support the use of selective serotonin reuptake inhibitors in the management of severe PMS. A systematic review has confirmed that selective serotonin reuptake inhibitors are significantly better at relieving premenstrual symptoms than placebo in women with severe PMS. However, their long-term use in this chronic condition has not been extensively studied as yet.[11] A

Evidence-Based References

1. Stevinson C, Ernst E: Complementary/alternative therapies for premenstrual syndrome: a systematic review of randomized controlled trials, *Am J Obstet Gynecol* 185:227, 2001. B
2. Wyatt K et al: Efficacy of progesterone and progestogens in management of premenstrual syndrome: systematic review, *BMJ* 323:776, 2001. B
3. Hellberg D et al: Premenstrual tension: a placebo-controlled efficacy study with spironolactone and medroxyprogesterone acetate, *Int J Gynecol Obstet* 34:243, 1991. A
4. Vellacott ID et al: A double-blind, placebo-controlled evaluation of spironolactone in the premenstrual syndrome, *Curr Med Res Opin* 10:450, 1987. A
5. Wang M et al: Treatment of premenstrual syndrome by spironolactone: a double-blind, placebo-controlled study, *Acta Obstet Gynecol Scand* 74:803, 1995. A
6. Burnet RB et al: Premenstrual syndrome and spironolactone, *Aust NZ J Obstet Gynaecol* 31:366, 1991. A
7. Mortola JF et al: Successful treatment of severe premenstrual syndrome by combined use of gonadotrophin-releasing hormone agonist and estrogen/progestin, *J Clin Endocrinol Metab* 72:252A, 1991. B
8. Mezrow G et al: Depot leuprolide acetate with estrogen and progestin add-back for long-term treatment of premenstrual syndrome, *Fertil Steril* 62:932, 1994. B
9. Wyatt K: Premenstrual syndrome, *Clin Evid* 11: 2507, 2004. A
10. Di Carlo C et al: Use of leuprolide acetate plus tibolone in the treatment of severe premenstrual syndrome, *Fertil Steril* 75:380, 2001. A
11. Wyatt KM et al: Selective serotonin reuptake inhibitors for premenstrual syndrome, *Cochrane Rev* 3, 2004. A

SUGGESTED READINGS

Brown C: A new monophasic oral contraceptive containing drospirenone: effect on premenstrual symptoms, *J Reprod Med* 47(1):14, 2002.

Miner C, Brown E: Weekly luteal-phase dosing with enteric-coated fluoxetine 90 mg in premenstrual dysphoric disorder: a randomized, double blind, placebo-controlled clinical trial, *Clin Ther* 24(3): 417, 2002.

Pearlstein T: Selective serotonin reuptake inhibitors for premenstrual dysphoric disorder: the emerging gold standard? *Drugs* 62(13):1869, 2002.

Wyatt K: Premenstrual syndrome, *Clin Evid* 7:338, 2002.

AUTHORS: **GEORGE T. DANAKAS, M.D.,** and **RUBEN ALVERO, M.D.**

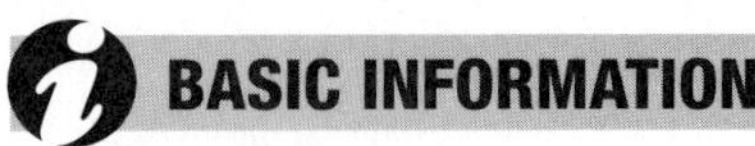

DEFINITION

Priapism is the persistent, usually painful erection associated or unassociated with sexual stimulation. There are two major forms: low-flow (veno-occlusive) priapism and high-flow priapism (associated with increased arterial inflow without increased venous outflow resistance).

ICD-9CM CODES
607.3 Priapism

EPIDEMIOLOGY & DEMOGRAPHICS

- Peak incidence is seen from ages 5 to 10 yr and 20 to 50 yr.
- In the younger group, priapism is often associated with sickle cell disease or neoplasm. In the older group it is often caused by pharmacologic agents.
- Low-flow (veno-occlusive priapism [type I]) is much more common than high-flow (type II).

PHYSICAL FINDINGS & CLINICAL PRESENTATION

- In idiopathic priapism the initial erection is associated with prolonged sexual excitement. Previous transient episodes are frequently reported. The erection involves the corpora cavernosa alone. Detumescence does not occur spontaneously.
- In secondary priapism, sexual excitement need not be involved. Otherwise the clinical picture is the same as in idiopathic priapism.
- Table 1-62 compares normal erection and priapism.

ETIOLOGY

Idiopathic: prolonged sexual arousal
Secondary or associated causes:
- Sickle cell disease
- Diabetes
- Leukemia (especially chronic myelogenous leukemia)
- Solid tumor (malignant) penile infiltration
- Spinal cord injury
- Perineal or penile trauma
- Iatrogenic
- Total parenteral nutrition, which includes a fat emulsion
- Hyperosmolar IV contrast
- Spinal or general anesthesia
- Anticoagulant therapy
- Phenothiazines
- Trazodone
- Intracorporeal injection therapy for impotence
- Phosphodiesterase type 5 inhibitors (e.g., sildenafil [Viagra], tadalafil [Cialis], vardenafil [Levitra])

PATHOPHYSIOLOGY

- Low-flow priapism: prolonged erection leads to edema of the cavernosal trabeculae, resulting in a sequence of statis, thrombosis, venous occlusion, fibrosis, scarring, and possibly impotence.
- High-flow priapism: cavernosal artery rupture leading to an arteriocavernous fistula.

Dx DIAGNOSIS

WORKUP

None if the associated underlying causes are known to be present. Otherwise they should be ruled out. Low-flow priapism can be distinguished from high-flow priapism by obtaining a corporeal blood gas value. A $Po_2 <30$ mm Hg, $Pco_2 >60$ mm Hg, and a pH <7.25 are consistent with low-flow priapism. High-flow priapism can be confirmed by a perineal Doppler ultrasound or arteriography (useful to identify arterial-lacunar fistula).

Rx TREATMENT

Goal: achieve detumescence with preservation of potency.

1. Medical therapies:
   - Ice packs
   - Ice water enemas
   - Hot water enemas
   - Pressure dressing
   - Sedatives
   - Analgesics
   - Antispasmodic/anticholinergic drugs
   - Estrogens
   - Anticoagulants
   - Procaine
   - Amyl nitrite
   - Local or general anesthesia
   - Ketamine (1 mg/lb)
2. In the patient with sickle cell disease: intravenous hydration, alkalinization, transfusion or exchange transfusion, oxygen.
3. Corporeal irrigation with normal saline may be used for low-flow priapism. The midshaft of the penis can be injected with a small-gauge butterfly needle and irrigated with 10 to 20 ml of normal saline, followed by an intracorporeal injection of an alpha-adrenergic agonist every 5 min until detumescence. Commonly used intracavernous vasoconstrictor agents are epinephrine (10 to 20 mcg), phenylephrine (250 to 500 mcg), and ephedrine (50 to 100 mg). It is mandatory to monitor the patient's blood pressure and pulse when using alpha-adrenergic agonists.
4. Surgery:
   - Cavernospongiosum shunt
   - Glans-cavernosum shunt
   - Cavernosaphenous shunt
   - In the less common situation of high-flow priapism (diagnosed by the finding of bright red arterial blood on aspiration), arterial embolization or surgical ligation is recommended.

PROGNOSIS

Impotence is associated with the duration of priapism, with 36 hr being an important threshold.

REFERRAL

To urologist

AUTHOR: **FRED F. FERRI, M.D.**

TABLE 1-62 Comparison of Normal Erection and Priapism

Factor	Normal Erection	Priapism
Portion of penis involved	Corpora cavernosa and corpus spongiosum and glans	Corpora cavernosa
Cause	Vasodilatation of penile arteries	Obstruction of venous outflow Disturbance of neuroarterial mechanism (imbalance between it and adrenergic activity) Increased viscosity
Sexual desire	Present	Absent
Pain	Absent	Present
Duration	Minutes to hours	Hours to days

From Nseyo UO (ed): *Urology for primary care physicians,* Philadelphia, 1999, WB Saunders.

BASIC INFORMATION

DEFINITION

Glaucoma is a chronic degenerative optic neuropathy in which the neuro-retinal rim of the optic nerve becomes progressively thinner, thereby enlarging the optic-nerve cup. The classification of glaucomas is based on the appearance of the iridocorneal angle (open angle vs. closed angle) and is further subdivided into primary and secondary types. Primary open-angle glaucoma can occur with or without elevated intraocular pressure. Normal tension glaucoma refers to primary open-angle glaucoma without elevated intraocular pressure.

SYNONYMS

Chronic simple glaucoma
Chronic open-angle glaucoma (POAG)

ICD-9CM CODES
365.1 Open-angle glaucoma

EPIDEMIOLOGY & DEMOGRAPHICS

INCIDENCE (IN U.S.): Third most common cause of vision loss (75% to 95% of all forms of glaucoma are open angle)

PEAK INCIDENCE:
- Increases after age 40 yr
- Three million cases expected by 2020 because of the rapid increase in aging population

PREVALENCE (IN U.S.):
- Overall prevalence in U.S. population aged >40 yr is estimated to be 1.86%, with 1.57 million white and 398,000 black patients affected.
- 150,000 patients have bilateral blindness.
- Disease occurs in 2% of people >40 yr.
- Prevalence is higher in diabetics, those with high myopia, and older persons.
- More common in blacks (three times the age-adjusted prevalence than whites).

PREDOMINANT AGE:
- Persons >50 yr
- Can occur in 30s and 40s

GENETICS:
- Four to six times higher incidence in blacks than whites
- No clear-cut hereditary patterns but a strong hereditary tendency

PHYSICAL FINDINGS & CLINICAL PRESENTATION

- High intraocular pressures and large optic nerve cup (Ocular Hypertension Treatment Study results very important)
- Corneal edema causes vision loss and blurring
- Abnormal visual fields
- Open-angle gonioscopy
- Red eye
- Restricted vision and field

ETIOLOGY

- Uncertain hereditary tendency
- Topical steroids
- Trauma
- Inflammatory
- High-dose oral corticosteroids taken for prolonged periods

DIAGNOSIS

DIFFERENTIAL DIAGNOSIS

- Other optic neuropathies
- Secondary glaucoma from inflammation and steroid therapy
- Red eye differential
- Trauma
- Contact lens injury

WORKUP

- Intraocular pressure
- Slit lamp examination
- Visual fields
- Gonioscopy
- Nerve fiber analysis (e.g., GDx analyzer, Zeiss, Jena, Germany)
- Corneal thickness—very important in prognosis

LABORATORY TESTS

Blood sugar

IMAGING STUDIES

- Optic nerve photography—stereo photographs
- Visual field testing
- Laser scan of nerve fiber layer, OCT, HRT

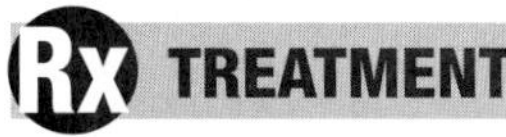

TREATMENT

ACUTE GENERAL Rx

- β-blockers (e.g., Timolol) qd to bid depending on individual response to drug
- Diamox 250 mg qid or 500 mg bid
- Hyperosmotic agents (mannitol) in acute treatment (IV)
- Prostaglandins commonly used as first-line treatment
- Laser trabeculoplasty (SLT) as needed
- Pilocarpine qid

CHRONIC Rx

- At least biannual checks of intraocular pressure and adjustment of medication
- Poor control = frequent examinations; good control = drugs
- Trabeculectomy
- Filter valves

DISPOSITION

Must be followed by ophthalmologist

REFERRAL

Immediately to ophthalmologist

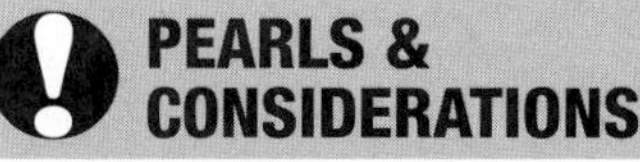

PEARLS & CONSIDERATIONS

COMMENTS

- Glaucoma is a serious blinding disease that must be monitored professionally by an ophthalmologist.
- Early diagnosis and treatment may minimize visual loss.
- Glaucoma is not solely caused by increased intraocular pressure because approximately 20% of patients with glaucoma have normal intraocular pressure. However, high pressure is definitely a risk factor to be considered. Potential sites of increased resistance to aqueous flow are described in Fig. 1-261.

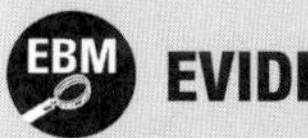

EVIDENCE

The use of adjunctive medications increases the success rate for surgical interventions.

Systematic reviews have found that the use of intraoperative mitomycin C and post-

POTENTIAL SITES OF INCREASED RESISTANCE TO AQUEOUS FLOW

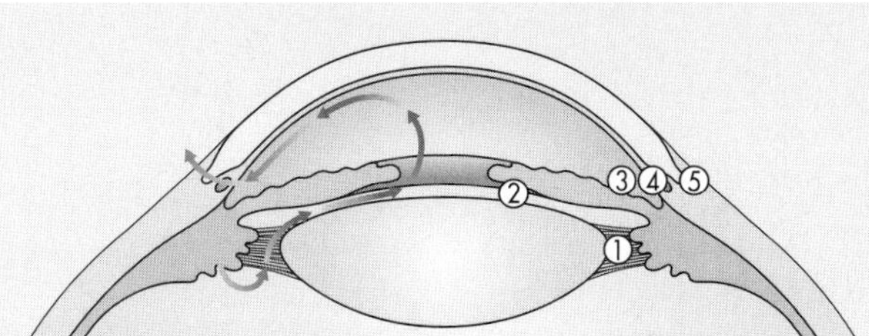

FIGURE 1-261 Potential sites of increased resistance to aqueous flow. (From Yanoff M, Duker JS: *Ophthalmology,* ed 2, St Louis, 2004, Mosby.)

operative 5-fluorouracil reduces the risk of surgical failure in eyes that have undergone no previous surgery and in eyes at high risk of failure.[1] Ⓐ

Evidence-Based Reference

1. Wilkins M et al: Intra-operative mitomycin C for glaucoma surgery, *Cochrane Rev* 4, 2005. Ⓐ

SUGGESTED READINGS

Gordon MO et al: Baseline factors that predict the onset of primary open-angle glaucoma, *Arch Ophthalmol* 120:714, 2002.

Heijl A et al: Reduction of intraocular pressure and glaucoma progression: results from the early manifest glaucoma trial, *Arch Ophthalmol* 120:1268, 2002.

Higginbotham EJ et al: The Ocular Hypertension Treatment Study: topical medication delays or prevents primary open-angle glaucoma in African American individuals, *Arch Ophthalmol* 122(6):813, 2004.

Kwon YH et al: Primary open-angle glaucoma, *N Engl J Med* 360:1113-1124, 2009.

Rezaie T et al: Adult-onset primary open-angle glaucoma caused by mutations in optineurin, *Science* 295:1077, 2002.

AUTHOR: **MELVYN KOBY, M.D.**

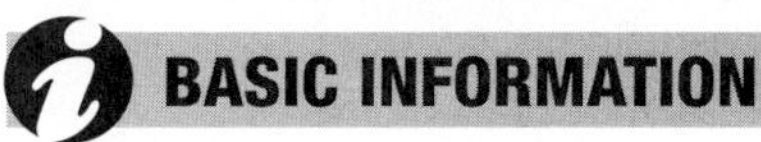

BASIC INFORMATION

DEFINITION

Progressive supranuclear palsy (PSP) is an atypical parkinsonian syndrome characterized by supranuclear gaze impairment, prominent and early postural instability with falls, axial greater than appendicular rigidity, and poor or absent response to levodopa.

SYNONYMS

Steele-Richardson-Olszewski syndrome
Progressive supranuclear ophthalmoplegia

ICD-9CM CODES
333.0 Other degenerative diseases of the basal ganglia

EPIDEMIOLOGY & DEMOGRAPHICS

INCIDENCE: 1.1 per 100,000 (5.3 per 100,000 over age 50)
PREVALENCE: 4.9 per 100,000 (6.4 per 100,000 age-adjusted)
PREDOMINANT SEX AND AGE: Slight male predominance; mean age onset 63 yr, very uncommon for onset <50 yr
GENETICS: Familial cases have been reported only rarely. The vast majority of cases are sporadic.

PHYSICAL FINDINGS & CLINICAL PRESENTATION

Tremorless parkinsonism is the general clinical presentation, and differentiation from idiopathic Parkinson's disease can be challenging early in the disease course. However, there are certain symptoms that can serve as "red flags" to consider PSP:

- Early postural instability and retropulsion leads to frequent falls; falls within the first year of onset of symptoms is typically the rule.
- Supranuclear gaze palsy is often preceded by slowing of vertical saccades; square wave jerks can be present; blepharospasm is common.
- Dystonia of the frontalis and procerus muscles gives the PSP patient a "surprised" or "frightened" expression as opposed to the hypomimia of Parkinson's disease (see Fig. 1-262).
- Speech is typically strained, spastic, hypernasal, with a low-pitched dysarthria.
- Pseudobulbar affect and "emotional incontinence" can be seen, with easy crying or laughter.
- Early cognitive impairment, most commonly with apathy, disinhibition, and anxiety.

ETIOLOGY

PSP is caused by neuronal degeneration of nuclei in the midbrain and basal ganglia, as a result of abnormal tau protein accumulation, most commonly in astrocyte inclusions and neurofibrillary tangles.

DIAGNOSIS

DIFFERENTIAL DIAGNOSIS

- Parkinson's disease: responds more robustly to levodopa, progression much slower, and lacks "red flag" symptoms above
- Corticobasal degeneration: also a tauopathy like PSP, but characterized by parkinsonism with prominent asymmetric dystonia, cortical sensory signs such as astereognosis, typically progressing to apraxia and sometimes an "alien hand" syndrome
- Multiple system atrophy: distinguished by autonomic involvement such as orthostatic hypotension, cerebellar ataxia, and inspiratory stridor
- Dementia with Lewy bodies: dementia coincident with parkinsonism, fluctuating mental status, visual hallucinations often preceding onset of dopaminergic treatment

WORKUP

- PSP is a clinical diagnosis, best made by a neurologist familiar with the disorder such as a movement disorders specialist.
- A robust response to a trial of levodopa may help to lead consideration away from PSP.
- MRI scan (see below) can be helpful.

LABORATORY TESTS

There are no diagnostic laboratory tests.

IMAGING STUDIES

- Dorsal midbrain atrophy is commonly seen on MRI.
- MRI regional apparent diffusion coefficients (rADC) in specific nuclei on diffusion-weighted imaging can reliably differentiate PSP from Parkinson's disease, although not from multiple system atrophy.

TREATMENT

NONPHARMACOLOGIC THERAPY

- Physical therapy, in particular focusing on fall prevention, is essential for avoiding the morbidity associated with frequent falls. Assistive devices such as a walker or wheelchair should be encouraged.
- Dysphagia is a common finding and should be monitored for closely in conjunction with a speech therapist.
- Prisms can be helpful in some patients for the eye movement abnormalities that can result in misalignment and diplopia.

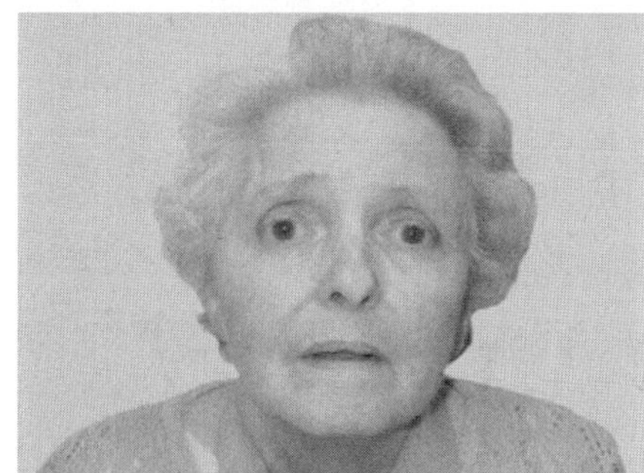

FIGURE 1-262 A patient with progressive supranuclear palsy with staring expression, frontalis overactivity, and retrocolitis. She is wearing a neck sling for a fractured wrist sustained in a fall. (From Burn D, Lees A: Progressive supranuclear palsy: where are we now? *Lancet Neurol* 1:359, 2002.)

CHRONIC Rx

- Although classically felt to be unresponsive to levodopa, there is often a transient response to this medication and it can be useful. The poor response to levodopa is most likely due to the loss of postsynaptic dopamine receptors.
- Anticholinergic medications should be avoided.
- Blepharospasm can be effectively treated with botulinum toxin injections.

DISPOSITION

- Median latency from symptom onset to wheelchair-bound state is 5 yr and to death is 7 yr.

REFERRAL

Referral to a general neurologist or movement disorders center is appropriate.

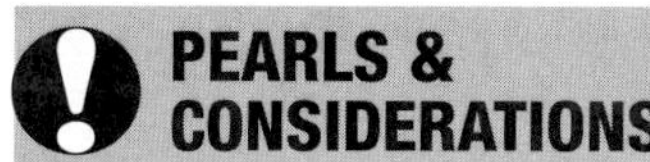

PEARLS & CONSIDERATIONS

COMMENTS

Consider PSP in a parkinsonian patient with the onset of falls within 1 yr of diagnosis, vertical eye movement abnormalities, early cognitive impairment, pseudobulbar affect, frontonasal dystonia, or poor response to levodopa.

PATIENT & FAMILY EDUCATION

Patient and caregiver information and resources can be found at www.wemove.org (a comprehensive movement disorders website) as well as the Society for Progressive Supranuclear Palsy at www.curepsp.org.

SUGGESTED READINGS

Houghton DL, Litvan I: Unraveling progressive supranuclear palsy: from the bedside back to the bench, *Parkinsonism Relat Disord* 13:S341-S346, 2007.

Litvan I et al: Clinical research criteria for the diagnosis of progressive supranuclear palsy (Steele-Richardson-Olszewski syndrome), *Neurology* 47: 1-9, 2003.

Seppi K et al: Diffusion-weighted imaging discriminates progressive supranuclear palsy from PD, but not from the parkinson variant of multiple system atrophy, *Neurology* 60:922-927, 2003.

Williams DR et al: Characteristics of two distinct clinical phenotypes in pathologically proven progressive supranuclear palsy: Richardson's syndrome and PSP-parkinsonism, *Brain* 128:1247-1258, 2005.

AUTHOR: **ANDREW DUKER, M.D.**

Prolactinoma (PTG) (ALG)

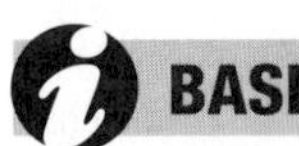

BASIC INFORMATION

DEFINITION

Prolactinomas are monoclonal tumors that secrete prolactin.

ICD-9CM CODES
253.1 Forbes-Albright syndrome

EPIDEMIOLOGY & DEMOGRAPHICS

INCIDENCE: Most common pituitary tumor; nearly 30% of all pituitary adenomas secrete enough prolactin to cause hyperprolactinemia.
PREDOMINANT SEX: Microadenomas are more common in women; macroadenomas are found more frequently in men.

PHYSICAL FINDINGS & CLINICAL PRESENTATION

- Men: decreased facial and body hair, small testicles; may also have decreased libido, impotence, and delayed puberty (caused by decreased testosterone as a result of inhibition of gonadotropin secretion).
- Women: physical examination may be normal; history may reveal amenorrhea, galactorrhea, oligomenorrhea, and anovulation.
- Both sexes: visual field defects and headache may occur depending on size of tumor and its expansion.

ETIOLOGY

Prolactin-secreting pituitary adenomas: microadenomas (<10 mm diameter) or macroadenomas (>10 mm diameter)

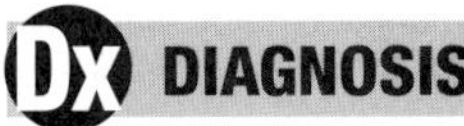

DIAGNOSIS

DIFFERENTIAL DIAGNOSIS

Hyperprolactinemia may be caused by the following:

- Drugs: phenothiazines, methyldopa, reserpine, monoamine oxidase inhibitors, androgens, progesterone, cimetidine, tricyclic antidepressants, haloperidol, meprobamate, chlordiazepoxide, estrogens, narcotics, metoclopramide, verapamil, amoxapine, cocaine, oral contraceptives
- Hepatic cirrhosis, renal failure, primary hypothyroidism
- Ectopic prolactin-secreting tumors (hypernephroma, bronchogenic carcinoma)
- Infiltrating diseases of the pituitary (sarcoidosis, histiocytosis)
- Head trauma, chest wall injury, spinal cord injury
- Polycystic ovary disease, pregnancy, nipple stimulation
- Idiopathic hyperprolactinemia, stress, exercise

WORKUP

- The diagnosis of prolactinoma is established by demonstration of an elevated serum prolactin level (after exclusion of other causes of hyperprolactinemia) and radiographic evidence of a pituitary adenoma.
  1. Normal mean prolactin levels are 8 ng/ml in women and 5 ng/ml in men.
  2. Levels >300 ng/ml are virtually diagnostic of prolactinomas.
  3. Prolactin levels can vary with time of day, stress, sleep cycle, and meals. More accurate measurements can be obtained 2 to 3 hr after awakening, preprandially, and when patient is not distressed.
  4. Serial measurements are recommended in patients with mild prolactin elevations.
- Thyroid-releasing hormone stimulation test may be useful in equivocal cases. The normal response is an increase in serum prolactin levels by 100% within 1 hr of TRH infusion; failure to demonstrate an increase in prolactin level is suggestive of pituitary lesion.
- All patients with prolactinomas should undergo visual field testing. Serial evaluation is recommended, particularly during pregnancy in patients with macroadenomas.

IMAGING STUDIES

- MRI with gadolinium enhancement (Fig. 1-263) is the procedure of choice in the radiographic evaluation of pituitary disease.
- In absence of MRI, a radiographic diagnosis is best accomplished with a high-resolution CT scanner and special coronal cuts through the pituitary region.

Rx TREATMENT

NONPHARMACOLOGIC THERAPY

Pregnancy and breastfeeding should be avoided because they can encourage tumor growth.

ACUTE GENERAL Rx

- Management of prolactinomas depends on their size and encroachment on the optic chiasm and other vital structures, the presence or absence of gonadal dysfunction, and the patient's desires regarding fertility.
- Medical therapy is preferred when fertility is an important consideration.
  1. Bromocriptine (Parlodel): initial dose is 0.625 at bedtime for the first week. After 1 wk, add morning dose of 1.25 mg. Gradually increase dose by 1.25 mg/wk until dose of 5 to 10 mg/day is achieved. Bromocriptine decreases size of the tumor and generally lowers the prolactin level into the normal range when the initial serum prolactin is <500 ng/ml. Side effects of bromocriptine are nausea, constipation, dizziness, and nasal stuffiness. Bromocriptine appears to be safe during pregnancy.
  2. Cabergoline is a longer acting dopamine agonist that is more expensive but may be more effective and better tolerated than bromocriptine; initial dose is 0.25 mg twice weekly.
- Transsphenoidal resection: option in an infertile patient who cannot tolerate bromocriptine or cabergoline or when medical therapy is ineffective. The success rate depends on the location of the tumor (entirely intrasellar), experience of the neurosurgeon, and size of the tumor (<10 mm in diameter); the recurrence rate may reach 80% within 5 yr. Possible complications of transsphenoidal surgery include transient diabetes insipidus, hypopituitarism, cerebrospinal fluid rhinorrhea, and infections (meningitis, wound infection).
- Pituitary irradiation is useful as adjunctive therapy of macroadenomas (>10 mm in diameter) and in patients with persistent hypersecretion after surgery. Potential complications include cranial nerve damage, radionecrosis, and cognitive abnormalities.
- Stereotactic radiosurgery (gamma knife) has become popular as a modality in the treatment of prolactinomas. A high dose of ionizing radiation is delivered to the tumor through multiple ports. Its advantage is minimal irradiation to surrounding tissues. Proximity of the tumor to the optic chiasm limits this therapeutic modality.

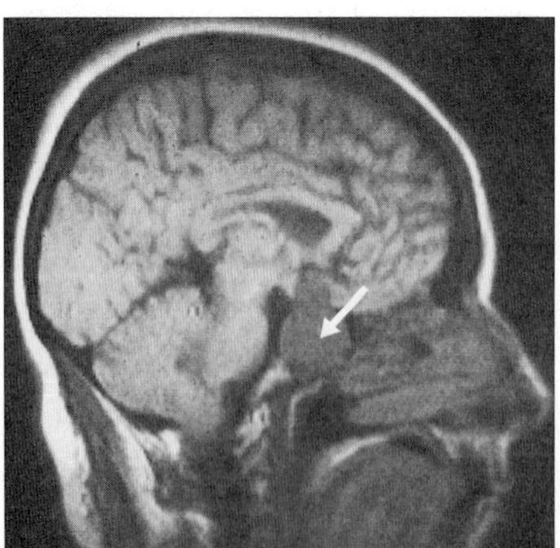

FIGURE 1-263 T1 sagittal MRI depicting a large pituitary prolactinoma *(arrow)* in a 13-year-old girl presenting with headaches and galactorrhea. (From Grainger RG et al [eds]: *Grainger & Allison's diagnostic radiology*, ed 4, Philadelphia, 2001, Churchill Livingstone.)

CHRONIC Rx

- Patients on medical therapy require periodic measurement of prolactin levels. An attempt to reduce the dose of bromocriptine or cabergoline can be made after the prolactin level has been normal for 2 yr. An MRI scan of the pituitary should be obtained to rule out tumor enlargement within 6 mo of initiation of tapering regimen.
- Evaluation and monitoring of pituitary function are recommended after transsphenoidal surgery.

DISPOSITION

- Transsphenoidal surgery will result in a cure in nearly 50% to 75% of patients with microadenomas and 10% to 20% of patients with macroadenomas.

- Nearly 20% of microprolactinomas resolve during long-term dopamine agonist treatment.

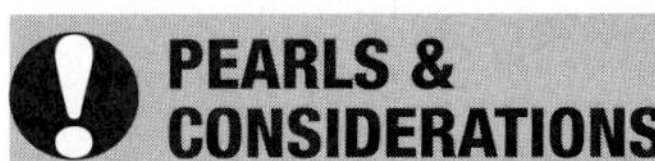

PEARLS & CONSIDERATIONS

COMMENTS

Patients must be monitored for several years after surgery because up to 50% of microadenomas and nearly 90% of macroadenomas can recur.

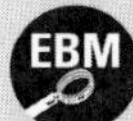

EVIDENCE

Evidence for the treatment of prolactinoma is limited. High-quality trials for the main therapies mentioned are lacking, although some small or nonrandomized trials exist.

One study evaluated the outcome of cabergoline treatment in 52 male patients with prolactinomas. It found that after 24 mo of treatment with cabergoline, serum prolactin levels had normalized in 75% of patients and no patients had galactorrhea. Restoration of normal adrenocorticotropin-releasing hormone, growth hormone, and testosterone levels were achieved in approximately 60% of patients.[1] Ⓐ

Evidence-Based Reference

1. Colao A et al: Outcome of cabergoline treatment in men with prolactinoma: effects of a 24-month treatment on prolactin levels, tumor mass, recovery of pituitary function, and semen analysis, *J Clin Endocrinol Metab* 89:1704, 2004.

SUGGESTED READINGS

Leung A, Pacaud D: Diagnosis and management of galactorrhea, *Am Fam Physician* 70:543, 2004.

Schlechte JA: Prolactinoma, *N Engl J Med* 349:2035, 2003.

AUTHOR: **FRED F. FERRI, M.D.**

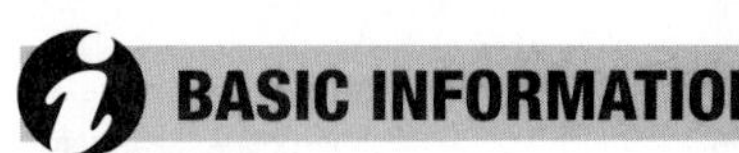

BASIC INFORMATION

DEFINITION

A form of compression neuropathy of the median nerve in the proximal forearm caused primarily by the pronator teres muscle (Fig. 1-264). Occasionally, only the anterior interosseus motor branch is affected, sometimes causing a specific separate clinical presentation.

SYNONYMS

Kiloh-Nevin syndrome (anterior interosseus syndrome)

ICD-9CM CODES
354.1 Median nerve entrapment
354.9 Mononeuritis of upper limb

EPIDEMIOLOGY & DEMOGRAPHICS

PREDOMINANT SEX: Males are affected more often than females.

INCIDENCE: Rare (comprises <1% of median nerve entrapment disorders); most common in dominant arm.

PHYSICAL FINDINGS & CLINICAL PRESENTATION

- Forearm discomfort and fatigue, often resulting from repetitive pronation.
- Insidious onset.
- Nocturnal paresthesias are not typical.
- Vague numbness in hand, primarily in thumb and index finger, may be present.
- Tenderness and enlargement of the pronator teres may be present.
- Tinel's sign may be positive at the site of compression.
- Although there are no reliable provocative tests, painful paresthesias may occasionally be elicited with forced pronation of the forearm against resistance.
- Motor impairment is rare.

Anterior interosseus nerve syndrome:

- Forearm pain and weakness.
- Patient may be unable to form a circle when trying to pinch the index finger and thumb because of the inability to flex distal phalanges of thumb and index finger.
- Sensation to the hand is not affected.

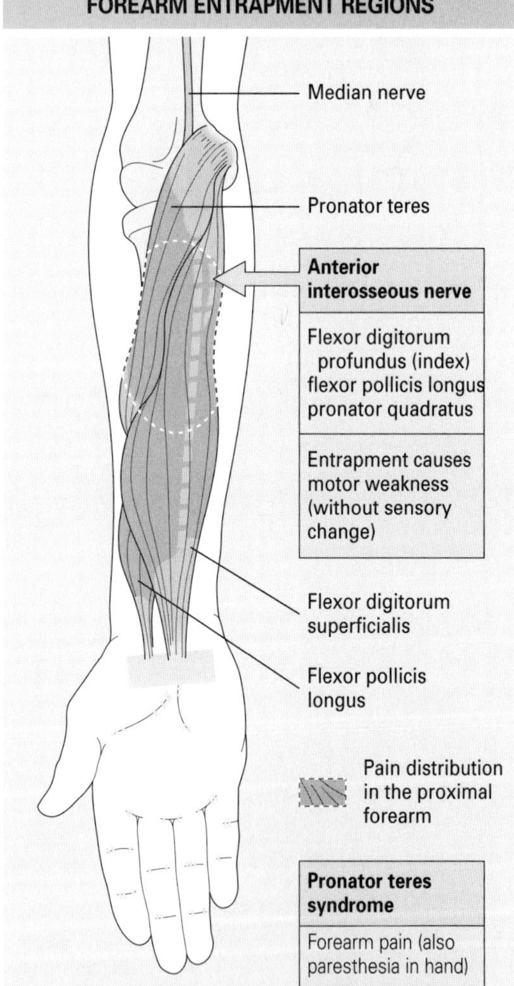

FIGURE 1-264 Forearm entrapment regions. The median nerve may be compressed at several locations in the forearm, most commonly as it traverses the pronator teres muscle. The anterior interosseous branch of the median nerve is solely motor, thus entrapment produces no sensory deficit. (From Hochberg MC et al [eds]: *Rheumatology,* 3rd ed, St Louis, 2003, Mosby.)

ETIOLOGY

- Localized anatomic compression
- Trauma
- Traumatic cut down or phlebotomy

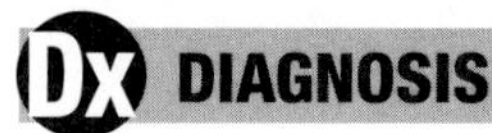

DIAGNOSIS

DIFFERENTIAL DIAGNOSIS

- Carpal tunnel syndrome
- Cervical disc syndrome with radiculopathy
- Tendon rupture
- Tendinitis

WORKUP

- Electrodiagnostic studies may be helpful; they are indicated if symptoms persist >4 to 6 wk or if motor weakness is suspected
- Plain radiography to rule out bony abnormalities causing compression

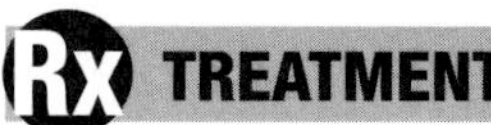

TREATMENT

- Rest, bracing of forearm, sling
- Stretching exercises, physical therapy
- Nonsteroidal antiinflammatory drugs

DISPOSITION

Patients whose symptoms are mainly subjective often respond to nonsurgical management. Motor deficits may not be reversible despite surgery.

REFERRAL

Surgical referral in cases of failed medical management or when motor weakness is present

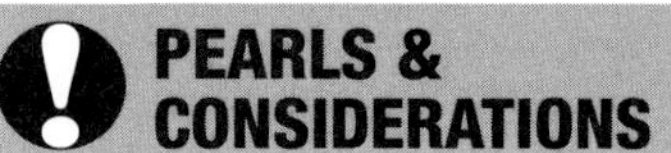

PEARLS & CONSIDERATIONS

COMMENTS

Prognosis for recovery is good. When indicated, surgical intervention is most effective if the diagnosis can be firmly established by objective testing.

SUGGESTED READINGS

Bridgeman C et al: Clinical and electrophysiological presentation of pronator syndrome, *Electromyogr Clin Neurophysiol* 47(2):89, 2007.

Cain EL et al: Elbow injuries in throwing athletes: a current concepts review, *Am J Sports Med* 31(4): 621, 2003.

Neal S, Fields KB: Peripheral nerve entrapment and injury in the upper extremity, *Am Fam Physician* 81(2):147, 2010.

Rehak DC: Pronator syndrome, *Clin Sports Med* 20(3): 531, 2001.

Sellards R, Kuebrich C: The elbow: diagnosis and treatment of common injuries, *Prim Care* 32(1):1, 2005.

Tsai P, Steinberg DR: Median and radial nerve compression about the elbow, *Instr Course Lect* 57:177, 2008.

AUTHOR: **LONNIE R. MERCIER, M.D.**

BASIC INFORMATION

DEFINITION & CLASSIFICATION

Prostate cancer is a neoplasm involving the prostate. Various classifications have been developed to evaluate malignancy potential and prognosis.

- The degree of malignancy varies with the stage:
    1. Stage A: Confined to the prostate, no nodule palpable
    2. Stage B: Palpable nodule confined to the gland
    3. Stage C: Local extension
    4. Stage D: Regional lymph nodes or distant metastases
- In the Gleason classification, two histologic patterns are independently assigned numbers 1 to 5 (best to least differentiated). These numbers are added to give a total tumor score between 2 and 10. Prognosis is best for highly differentiated tumors (e.g., Gleason score 2 to 4) compared with most poorly differentiated tumors (Gleason score 7 to 10).
- Another commonly used classification is the Tumor-Node-Metastasis (TNM) classification of prostate cancer.

ICD-9CM CODES
185 Malignant neoplasm of prostate

EPIDEMIOLOGY & DEMOGRAPHICS

- Prostate cancer has surpassed lung cancer as the most common nonskin cancer in men.
- More than 180,000 cases are diagnosed yearly, and nearly 30,000 males die from prostate cancer each year (second leading cause of death from cancer in U.S. men).
- Incidence of prostate cancer increases with age: uncommon <50 yr; 80% of new cases are diagnosed in patients aged ≥65 yr.
- Average age at time of diagnosis is 72 yr.
- Blacks in the U.S. have the highest incidence of prostate cancer in the world (one in every nine males).
- Incidence is low in Asians.
- Approximately 9% of all prostate cancers may be familial. Obesity is a risk factor for prostate cancer. High insulin levels may also increase the risk of prostate cancer.
- Mortality rates of prostate cancer have declined substantially in the past 15 yr from 34% in 1990 to <20% currently.

PHYSICAL FINDINGS & CLINICAL PRESENTATION

- Generally silent disease until it reaches advanced stages.
- Bone pain and pathologic fractures may be initial symptoms of prostate cancer.
- Local growth can cause symptoms of outflow obstruction.
- Digital rectal examination (DRE) may reveal an area of increased firmness; 10% of patients will have a negative DRE.
- Prostate may be hard, fixed, with extension of tumor to the seminal vesicles in advanced stages.

DIAGNOSIS

DIFFERENTIAL DIAGNOSIS

- Benign prostatic hypertrophy
- Prostatitis
- Prostate stones

LABORATORY TESTS

- Measurement of prostate-specific antigen (PSA) is controversial in early diagnosis of prostate cancer. PSA screening is associated with psychological harm, and its potential benefits remain uncertain. Normal PSA is found in >20% of patients with prostate cancer, whereas only 20% of men with PSA levels between 4 ng/ml and 10 ng/ml have prostate cancer. The American Cancer Society recommends offering the PSA test and DRE yearly to men aged ≥50 yr who have a life expectancy of at least 10 yr. Earlier testing, starting at age 45 yr, is recommended for men at high risk (e.g., blacks, men with family history of prostate cancer). An isolated elevation in PSA level should be confirmed several weeks later before proceeding with further testing, including prostate biopsy. Screening for prostate cancer in men aged ≥75 yr is controversial and generally not recommended.
- Free PSA: the use of serum-free PSA for prostate screening has been proposed by some urologists as a means to decrease unwarranted biopsies without missing a significant number of prostate cancers. This approach is based on the higher free PSA in men with benign prostatic hyperplasia and the higher protein-bound PSA levels in men with prostate cancer. For example, in men with total PSA levels of 4 to 10 ng/ml, the cancer probability is 0.25, but if the percentage of free PSA is ≤17%, the probability of cancer increases to 0.45.
- PSA velocity: the rate of increase of serum PSA (PSA velocity) can aid in the diagnosis of prostate cancer. A yearly PSA velocity >0.75 ng/ml increases the likelihood of later malignancy when total PSA is still within normal range. Proper interpretation of PSA velocity requires at least three PSA measurements over an 18-month period because most PSA variations are physiologic.
- Age-adjusted PSA: there is evidence that the current threshold of 4.0 ng/ml is inadequate for younger men, because in a recent study 22% of men with PSA levels between 2.6 and 4.0 were found to have prostate cancer. The concept of age-related cutoffs remains controversial. Lowering the upper limit of normal for PSA would improve sensitivity but decrease specificity.
- Prostatic acid phosphatase can be used for evaluation of nonlocalized disease.
- Transrectal biopsy and fine-needle aspiration of prostate can confirm the diagnosis. Indications for biopsy include an abnormal PSA level, an abnormal DRE, or a previous biopsy specimen that showed prostatic intraepithelial neoplasia or prostatic atypia. The number of cores taken is patient specific, typically including a minimum of 10 cores. Prostate volume negatively affects cancer detection rate (23% in glands >50 cm^3, 38% in glands <50 cm^3).

IMAGING STUDIES

- Bone scan is useful to evaluate bone metastasis (present or eventually develops in almost 80% of patients). However, according to the American Urological Association (AUA), the routine use of bone scanning is not required for staging of prostate cancer in asymptomatic men with clinically localized cancer if the PSA level is ≤20 ng/ml.
- CT scan, MRI, and transrectal ultrasonography may be useful in selected patients to assess extent of prostate cancer. High-resolution MRI with magnetic nanoparticles has been used for the detection of small and otherwise undetectable lymph node metastases in patients with prostate cancer. However, according to the AUA, transrectal ultrasonography adds little to the combination of PSA and DRE. Similarly, CT and MRI imaging are generally not indicated for cancer staging in men with clinically localized cancer and PSA <25 ng/ml. With regard to pelvic lymph node dissection in staging, the AUA states that it may not be required in patients with PSA levels <10 ng/ml and when PSA level is <20 ng/ml and the Gleason score is <6.

TREATMENT

NONPHARMACOLOGIC THERAPY

Watchful waiting is reasonable in selected patients with early-stage (T-IA) and projected life expectancy <10 yr or in patients with focal and moderately differentiated carcinoma.

ACUTE GENERAL Rx

- Therapeutic approach varies with the following:
    1. Stage of the tumor
    2. Patient's life expectancy
    3. General medical condition
    4. Patient's treatment preference (e.g., patient may be opposed to orchiectomy)
- The optimal treatment of clinically localized prostate cancer is unclear.
    1. Radical prostatectomy is generally performed in patients with localized prostate cancer and life expectancy >10 yr. Radical prostatectomy reduces disease-specific mortality, overall mortality, and the risks of metastasis and local progression. The absolute reduction in the risk of death after 10 yr is small, but the reductions in the risks of metastasis and local tumor progression are substantial. Postoperative complications of radical prostatectomy include urinary incontinence (10% to 20% depending on degree of neurovascular

bundle and urethral preservation, patient age, and correct mucosal apposition) and erectile dysfunction (percentage exceeds 50% and varies with patient age, preoperative erectile dysfunction, stage of tumor at time of surgery, and preservation of neurovascular bundle). Lower complication rates occur in hospitals that perform a large number of prostatectomies. Fewer men will have postsurgical erectile dysfunction after unilateral or bilateral nerve-sparing surgery. Men undergoing minimally invasive prostatectomy (MIRP) experience shorter length of stay and fewer respiratory and miscellaneous surgical complications and strictures but experience more genitourinary complications, erectile dysfunction, and incontinence when compared with open retropubic radical prostatectomy (RPP).

2. Radiation therapy (external-beam irradiation or brachytherapy with implantation of radioactive pellets [iodine-125 or palladium-103 seeds] into the prostate gland) represents an alternative in patients with localized prostate cancer, especially poor surgical candidates or patients with a high-grade malignancy. The efficacy of brachytherapy is comparable to external radiation. In patients receiving external-beam radiation, a total dose of 79.2 Gy (high dose) compared with a total dose of 70.2 Gy (conventional dose) has been reported to lower the risk of recurrence without increased risk of morbidity and mortality. Patients with localized prostate cancer and high risk for extraprostatic disease and disease recurrence (e.g., Gleason score ≤7 with multiple positive biopsy cores and clinical stage T1b-T2b) may benefit (increased overall survival) with the addition of 6 mo of androgen suppression therapy to radiation therapy.
3. Watchful waiting is reasonable in patients who are too old or too ill to survive longer than 10 yr. If the cancer progresses to the point where it becomes symptomatic, palliation can be attempted with several methods. Conservative management is also reasonable for patients with Gleason score of 2 to 4 because these patients do not have a shortened life expectancy and treatment is associated with long-term side effects.

- Patients with advanced disease and projected life expectancy <10 yr are candidates for radiation therapy and hormonal therapy (diethylstilbestrol, luteinizing hormone–releasing hormone analogs, antiandrogens, bilateral orchiectomy).
- Recommended treatment of patients with regional metastatic prostate cancer with projected life expectancy ≥10 yr includes radiation therapy and hormonal therapy.
- Androgen deprivation therapy (ADT) is the mainstay of treatment for metastatic prostate cancer. Adverse effects of ADT include decreased libido, impotence, hot flashes, osteopenia with increased fracture risk, metabolic alterations, and changes in mood and cognition. Adjuvant treatment with luteinizing hormone-releasing hormone (LHRH) agonists (goserelin leuprolide, or triptorelin) plus antiandrogens (flutamide, bicalutamide, or nilutamide), when started simultaneously with external-beam radiation, improves local control and survival in patients with locally advanced prostate cancer. Pamidronate inhibits osteoclast-mediated bone resorption and prevents bone loss in the hip and lumbar spine in men receiving treatment for prostate cancer. Gonadotropin-releasing hormone (GmRH) receptor antagonists can be used for rapid medical castration of men with advanced prostate cancer. Degarelix is an injectable GnRH agonist useful to suppress testosterone in patients with prostate cancer who are not good candidates for LHRH agonists and refuse surgical castration. Assessment of bone density and treatment with once-weekly oral alendronate can prevent and improve the bone loss that occurs in men receiving ADT for prostate cancer.
- Docetaxel plus prednisone or docetaxel plus estramustine can be used in metastatic hormone-refractory prostate cancer.

CHRONIC Rx

- Patients should be monitored at 3- to 6-mo intervals with clinical examination and PSA for the first year, then every 6 mo for the second year, then yearly if stable. For patients who have undergone radical prostatectomy, a rising PSA level suggests evidence of residual or recurrent prostate cancer. Salvage radiotherapy may potentially cure patients with disease recurrence after radical prostatectomy.
- Chest radiography and bone scan should be performed yearly or sooner if patient develops symptoms.

DISPOSITION

- Prognosis varies with the stage of the disease and the Gleason classification (see "Definition"). For patients between ages 65 and 69 yr at diagnosis and a Gleason score of 2 to 4, the probability of dying from prostate cancer 15 yr after diagnosis is 0.06 and that of dying from other causes is 0.56. If the Gleason score is 7 to 10, the probability of dying from prostate cancer increases to 0.72 and from other causes varies from 0.25 to 0.36.
- The ploidy of the tumor also has prognostic value; prognosis is better with diploid tumor cells and worse with aneuploid tumor cells.
- For grade 1 tumors, the extended 10-yr, disease-specific survival is similar for patients with prostatectomy (94%), radiotherapy (90%), and conservative management (93%); survival rate is better with surgery than with radiotherapy or conservative management in patients with grade 2 or 3 localized prostate cancer.
- Expression of the gene *EZH2* has been identified as an important factor in the determination of the aggressiveness of prostate cancer. A recent study revealed that expression of the *EZH2* gene may be a better predictor of clinical failure than Gleason score, tumor stage, or surgical margin status. Testing for *EZH2* protein in prostate cancer tissue may be useful to determine prognosis and direct treatment.
- Preoperative PSA level and PSA velocity have prognostic significance. Men whose PSA level increases by >2.0 mcg/ml during the year before the diagnosis of cancer may have a relatively high risk of death from prostate cancer despite undergoing radical prostatectomy.
- Extraprostatic disease is detected at radical prostatectomy in 38% to 52% of patients and is associated with a risk of disease recurrence, progression, and death. In these patients, adjuvant radiotherapy results in significantly reduced risk of PSA relapse and disease recurrence; however, the improvements in metastases-free survival and overall survival are not statistically significant.

EBM EVIDENCE

Please note: Complete text of EBM for this topic is available online.

Key trials and commentary:

The European Randomized Study of Screening for Prostate Cancer was initiated in the early 1990s to evaluate the effect of screening with prostate-specific antigen (PSA) testing on death rates from prostate cancer.

This study showed that PSA-based screening reduced the rate of death from prostate cancer by 20% but was associated with a high risk of overdiagnosis.

This study and the study by Andriole et al[3] attempt to put the question of PSA testing to rest. Unfortunately, things are just more confusing than ever. Schröder et al examined 182000 men between the ages of 50 and 74 from seven different European studies who were randomized to either be screened or not be screened for prostate cancer. The end point of this study was overall mortality, and this study demonstrated an improvement in overall survival, which was statistically significant with a rate ratio for death from prostate cancer 0.73 (95% CI, 0.56-0.90). Andriole et al randomized roughly 76,000 patients in the U.S. to either annual PSA screening or standard of care. At a median follow-up of 7 years, there was not a demonstrated improvement in overall survival with a risk ratio of death of 1.13 (95% CI, 0.75-1.70).

Why the different results? Both studies have a large sample size, although this abstracted study from Europe had more than twice the number of patients. Perhaps there was possibly contamination in the control arm. In Andriole et al, a significant percentage of the patients in the control arm were actually undergoing PSA screening (roughly 50%). This may have been enough to alter the results. In contrast, in this European study there was relatively little crossover between the patients who received screening and those who did not.

The main problem with this European study (and possibly PSA screening) is that at the relatively short follow-up of approximately 9 years, there were not a lot of deaths from prostate cancer. The authors' estimates were that to prevent one prostate cancer death, 1410 men would have to be screened and 48 men would have to be treated. Clearly, this is a lot of men requiring screening and treatment to save one life. Although I am sure that the man saved benefited, there continues to be concern that we are over treating a significant number of patients.

What does this all mean? Well, the PSA screening debate will continue. I think there are those in the camp that believe that PSA screening benefits all patients, and there are those who are convinced that PSA screening benefits none. I believe there is a middle ground where there are some patients who benefit and some patients who do not. My hope is that in the coming years we identify this cohort of patients. It may simply be on the basis of age or family history or genetic testing. Only the future will tell us.[1] Ⓐ

Several studies have shown the efficacy of endocrine therapy in combination with radiotherapy in high-risk prostate cancer. This study sought o assess the effect of radiotherapy, we did an open phase III study comparing endocrine therapy with and without local radiotherapy, followed by castration on progression.

This study showed that in patients with locally advanced or high-risk local prostate cancer, addition of local radiotherapy to endocrine treatment halved the 10-year prostate-cancer-specific mortality, and substantially decreased overall mortality with fully acceptable risk of side effects compared with endocrine treatment alone. In the light of these data, endocrine treatment plus radiotherapy should be the new standard.

Does local control improve survival of patients with high-risk localized prostate cancer, or should we just be looking to systemic treatment? In other words, should we use radiation therapy or surgery on these patients or just go straight to hormone therapy? Once again, the Swedes have succeeded in answering this question. This multicenter study examines 875 patients with locally advanced prostate cancer. Half of the men received androgen deprivation plus radiation therapy and the other half just androgen deprivation. The authors found that PSA recurrence, prostate-cancer-specific mortality, and overall mortality were all improved in the group of patients who received the radiation therapy in addition to the androgen depravation therapy. This provided strong level I evidence that local control improves the outcomes of patients with locally advanced disease.

This study has the potential to profoundly alter our management of patients with high-risk localized disease. It provides a strong rationale for not simply treating patients with hormone therapy alone but taking patients with advanced T3 and T4 disease and giving them radiation therapy, and possibly taking patients with less advanced T3 disease and high PSAs and treating them with radical prostatectomy. Although the decision to proceed with radical prostatectomy is an extrapolation from the article, I personally believe that radical prostatectomy does a better job of providing local control and, therefore, has the potential to actually do a better job than radiation therapy in this high-risk patient population.[2] Ⓐ

The effect of screening with PSA testing and digital rectal examination on the rate of death from prostate cancer is unknown. This is the first report from the Prostate, Lung, Colorectal, and Ovarian (PLCO) Cancer Screening Trial on prostate-cancer mortality. After 7 to 10 years of follow-up, the rate of death from prostate cancer was very low and did not differ significantly between the two study groups.

This study attempts to put the question of PSA testing to rest. Unfortunately, things are just more confusing than ever. Schröder et al[1] examined 182,000 men between the ages of 50 and 74 from seven different European studies who were randomized to either be screened or not be screened for prostate cancer. The endpoint of this study was overall mortality, and this study demonstrated an improvement in overall survival, which was statistically significant with a rate ratio for death from prostate cancer 0.73 (95% CI, 0.56-0.90). This study by Andriole et al randomized roughly 76,000 patients in the U.S. to either annual PSA screening or standard of care. At a median follow-up of 7 years, there was not a demonstrated improvement in overall survival with a risk ratio of death of 1.13 (95% CI, 0.75-1.70).

Why the different results? Both studies have a large sample size, although impressively the study from Europe had more than twice the number of patients. Perhaps there was possibly contamination in the control arm. In this study by Andriole et al, a significant percentage of the patients in the control arm were actually undergoing PSA screening (roughly 50%). This may have been enough to alter the results. In contrast, in the European study there was relatively little crossover between the patients who received screening and those who did not.

The main problem with the European study (and possibly PSA screening) is that at the relatively short follow-up of approximately 9 years, there were not a lot of deaths from prostate cancer. The authors' estimates were that to prevent one prostate cancer death, 1410 men would have to be screened and 48 men would have to be treated. Clearly, this is a lot of men requiring screening and treatment to save one life. Although I am sure that the man saved benefited, there continues to be concern that we are over treating a significant number of patients.

What does this all mean? Well, the PSA screening debate will continue. I think there are those in the camp that believe that PSA screening benefits all patients, and there are those who are convinced that PSA screening benefits none. I believe there is a middle ground where there are some patients who benefit and some patients who do not. My hope is that in the coming years we identify this cohort of patients. It may simply be on the basis of age or family history or genetic testing. Only the future will tell us.[3] Ⓐ

Secondary analyses of two randomized controlled trials and supportive epidemiologic and preclinical data indicated the potential of selenium and vitamin E for preventing prostate cancer.

This study sought to determine whether selenium, vitamin E, or both could prevent prostate cancer and other diseases with little or no toxicity in relatively healthy men.

This study showed that selenium or vitamin E, alone or in combination at the doses and formulations used, did not prevent prostate cancer in this population of relatively healthy men.

This long-awaited article failed to demonstrate that selenium or vitamin E prevents prostate cancer or any cancer for that matter. For years, when asked by patients what they could do to prevent disease, I told them to give these a shot based on strong, epidemiologic evidence that they worked as well as phase III trials in other diseases that demonstrated a hint that they were protective. This study proved that I was wrong.

So which is correct, the earlier epidemiologic data, or the current randomized trial? Maybe (but not certainly) both. Treatment with a mineral or vitamin for a relatively short time in an older population probably stacks the deck against the treatment. If nutrients are going to work, they probably will have to be ingested early in life, for a prolonged period of time, and as foods not as isolated minerals/vitamins. In other words, there is no substitute for taking care of yourself when you are young by eating nutritious foods. Although this message may not always resonate with the American public, it is probably close to the truth.[4] Ⓐ

Evidence-Based References

1. Schröder FH, for the ERSPC Investigators: Screening and prostate-cancer mortality in a randomized European study, *N Engl J Med* 360:1320-1328, 2009. Commentary by A.S. Kibel, M.D. Ⓐ

2. Widmark A et al: Endocrine treatment, with or without radiotherapy, in locally advanced prostate cancer (SPCG-7/SFUO-3): an open randomised phase III trial, *Lancet* 373:301-308, 2009. Commentary by A.S. Kibel, M.D. Ⓐ

3. Andriole GL, for the PLCO Project Team: Mortality results from a randomized prostate-cancer screening trial, *N Engl J Med* 360:1310-1319, 2009. Commentary by A.S. Kibel, M.D. Ⓐ

4. Lippman SM et al: Effect of selenium and vitamin E on risk of prostate cancer and other cancers: the Selenium and Vitamin E Cancer Prevention Trial (SELECT), *JAMA* 301:39-51, 2009. Commentary by A.S. Kibel, M.D. Ⓐ

SUGGESTED READINGS

D'Amico AV et al: Androgen suppression and radiation vs radiation alone for prostate cancer, *JAMA* 299(3): 289, 2008.

Gittleman M et al: A 1-year, open label, randomized phase II dose finding study of degarelix for the treatment of prostate cancer in North America, *J Urol* 18:1986, 2008.

Greenspan S et al: Effect of once-weekly oral alendronate on bone loss in men receiving androgen deprivation therapy for prostate cancer, *Ann Intern Med* 146:416, 2007.

Hoffman RM et al: Health outcomes in older men with localized prostate cancer: results from the prostate cancer outcomes study, *Am J Med* 119:418, 2006.

Hu JC et al: Comparative effectiveness of minimally invasive vs. open radical prostatectomy, *JAMA* 302(14):1557-1564, 2009.

Lin K et al: Benefits and harms of prostate-specific antigen screening for prostate cancer: an evidence update from the US Preventive Services Task Force, *Ann Intern Med* 149:192-199, 2008.

Sanda MG et al: Quality of life and satisfaction with outcome among prostate cancer survivors, *N Engl J Med* 358:1250-1261, 2008.

Sharifi N et al: Androgen deprivation therapy for prostate cancer, *JAMA* 294:238-244, 2005.

Smith MR et al: Denosumab in men receiving androgen-deprivation therapy for prostate cancer, *N Engl J Med* 361:745-755, 2009.

Thompson IM et al: Adjuvant radiotherapy for pathologically advanced prostate cancer, *JAMA* 296: 2329, 2006.

Walczak J, Carducci M: Prostate cancer: a practical approach to current management of recurrent disease, *Mayo Clin Proc* 82(2):243, 2007.

Walsh PC et al: Localized prostate cancer, *N Engl J Med* 357:26, 2007.

Wilt TS et al: Systematic review: comparative effectiveness and harms of treatments for clinically localized prostate cancer, *Ann Intern Med* 148:435-448, 2008.

AUTHOR: **FRED F. FERRI, M.D.**

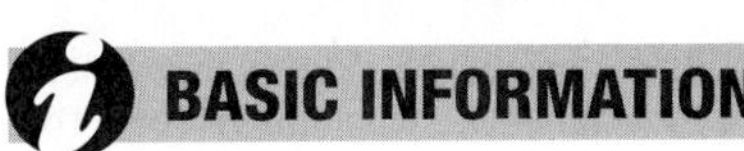

BASIC INFORMATION

DEFINITION

Benign prostatic hyperplasia (BPH) is the benign growth of the prostate, generally originating in the periureteral and transition zones, with subsequent obstructive and irritative voiding symptoms.

SYNONYMS

BPH
Prostatic hypertrophy

ICD-9CM CODES
600 Benign prostatic hyperplasia

EPIDEMIOLOGY & DEMOGRAPHICS

- 80% of men have evidence of BPH by age 80 yr.
- Medical and surgical intervention for problems caused by BPH is required in >20% of males by age 75 yr.
- Transurethral resection of the prostate (TURP) is the tenth most common operative procedure (>400,000/yr in U.S.).
- 10% to 30% of men with BPH have occult prostate cancer.

PHYSICAL FINDINGS & CLINICAL PRESENTATION

- Digital rectal examination (DRE) reveals enlargement of the prostate.
- Focal enlargement may be indicative of malignancy.
- There is poor correlation between size of prostate and symptoms (BPH may be asymptomatic if it does not encroach on the urethral lumen).
- Most patients with BPH report difficulty in initiating urination (hesitancy), decrease in caliber and force of stream, incomplete emptying of bladder often resulting in double voiding (need to urinate again a few minutes after voiding), postvoid "dribbling," and nocturia.

ETIOLOGY

Multifactorial; a functioning testicle is necessary for development of BPH (as evidenced by the absence in males who were castrated before puberty).

Dx DIAGNOSIS

DIFFERENTIAL DIAGNOSIS

- Prostatitis
- Prostate cancer
- Strictures (urethral)
- Medications interfering with the muscle fibers in the prostate and also with bladder function
  - Opiates: impaired autonomic function
  - Decongestants: increased sphincter tone
  - Antihistamines: decreased parasympathetic tone
  - Tricyclic antidepressants: anticholinergic effects
- Neurogenic bladder
- Bladder cancer

WORKUP

Symptom assessment (use of American Urological Association [AUA] Symptom Index for BPH [Table 1-63]), laboratory tests, and imaging studies

LABORATORY TESTS

- Prostate-specific antigen (PSA): protease secreted by epithelial cells of the prostate; elevated in 30% to 50% of patients with BPH. Testing for PSA increases detection rate for prostate cancer and tends to detect cancer at an earlier stage. However, the PSA test does not discriminate well between patients with symptomatic BPH and those with prostate cancer, particularly if the cancer is pathologically localized and curable. The test may also trigger additional evaluation, including ultrasound biopsy of the prostate. Asymptomatic men with PSA levels <2 ng/ml do not need annual testing. According to the AUA, PSA testing and DRE should be offered to any asymptomatic man >50 yr with a life expectancy of 10 yr. PSA testing can also be offered at an earlier age in men at higher risk of prostatic cancer (e.g., first-degree relatives with prostate cancer; African American race).
- Measurement of "free" PSA is useful to assess the probability of prostate cancer in

TABLE 1-63 International Prostate Symptom Score (I-PSS)

	SCORE						
Symptom	**Not at All**	**Less than 1 Time in 5**	**Less than Half the Time**	**About Half the Time**	**More than Half the Time**	**Almost Always**	**Total Score**
Incomplete emptying: Over the past month, how often have you had a sensation of not emptying your bladder completely after you finished urinating?	0	1	2	3	4	5	
Frequency: Over the past month, how often have you had to urinate again <2 hr after you finished urinating?	0	1	2	3	4	5	
Intermittency: Over the past month, how often have you found you stopped and started again several times when you urinated?	0	1	2	3	4	5	
Urgency: Over the past month, how often have you found it difficult to postpone urination?	0	1	2	3	4	5	
Weak stream: Over the past month, how often have you had a weak urinary stream?	0	1	2	3	4	5	
Straining: Over the past month, how often have you had to push or strain to begin urination?	0	1	2	3	4	5	
	None	**1 Time**	**2 Times**	**3 Times**	**4 Times**	**5 or More Times**	
Nocturia: Over the past month, how many times did you most typically get up to urinate from the time you went to bed at night until the time you got up in the morning?	0	1	2	3	4	5	
Total I-PSS score =							

patients with normal DRE and total PSA between 4 and 10 ng/ml. In these patients the global risk of prostate cancer is 25%. However, if the free PSA is >25%, the risk of prostate cancer decreases to 8%, whereas if the free PSA is <10%, the risk of cancer increases to 56%. Free PSA is also useful to evaluate the aggressiveness of prostate cancer. A low free PSA percentage generally indicates a high-grade cancer, whereas a high free PSA percentage is generally associated with a slower growing tumor.
- Urinalysis, urine culture, and sensitivity to rule out infection (if suspected).
- Blood urea nitrogen and creatinine to rule out postrenal insufficiency.

IMAGING STUDIES

- Transrectal ultrasound may be indicated in patients with palpable nodules or significant elevation of PSA. It is also useful to estimate prostate size. BPH may also be evident in suprapubic ultrasound and MRI (Fig. 1-265).
- Uroflowmetry may be used to determine relative impact of obstruction on urine flow. Urethral pressure profile is useful to predict prostatic hypertrophy within the urethral lumen.
- Pressure flow studies, although invasive, are particularly helpful in patients whose history and/or examination suggest primary bladder dysfunction as a cause of symptoms of prostatism. They are also useful in patients for whom a distinction between prostatic obstruction and impaired detrusor contractility may affect the choice of therapy. However, pressure flow studies may not be useful in the workup of the usual patient with symptoms of prostatism.
- Postvoid residual urine measurement has not been proved useful in predicting the need for or response to treatment; it may be useful in monitoring the course of the disease in patients who elect nonsurgical treatment.
- Urethral cystoscopy is an option during later evaluation if invasive treatment is being planned.

Rx TREATMENT

NONPHARMACOLOGIC THERAPY

- Avoidance of caffeine or any other foods that may exacerbate symptoms
- Avoidance of medications that may exacerbate symptoms (e.g., most cold and allergy remedies)

GENERAL Rx

- Asymptomatic patients with prostate enlargement caused by BPH generally do not require treatment. Patients with mild to moderate symptoms are candidates for pharmacologic treatment (see below). For patients who have specific complications from BPH, prostate surgery is usually the most appropriate form of treatment. However, surgery may result in significant complications (e.g., incontinence, infection).
- Alpha-blockers (e.g., tamsulosin, alfuzosin, doxazosin, prazosin, terazosin) relax smooth muscle of the bladder neck and prostate and can increase peak urinary flow rate. They have no effect on the size of the prostate. Alpha-1 blockers are useful in symptomatic patients to relieve symptoms of obstruction by causing relaxation of smooth muscle tone in the prostatic capsule, urethra, and bladder neck.
- Hormonal manipulation with finasteride, a 5-alpha-reductase inhibitor that blocks conversion of testosterone to dihydrotestosterone, can reduce the size of the prostate. Usual dose is 5 mg qd. Treatment requires ≥6 mo for maximal effect.
- Dutasteride is also a 5-alpha-reductase inhibitor useful to decrease prostate size and improve urinary flow. In addition to inhibiting the isoform of 5-alpha-reductase located in the prostate, the medication also inhibits a second isoform and reduces dihydrotestosterone formation in the skin and liver. Usual dose is 0.5 mg qd.
- The dietary supplement saw palmetto is commonly used for relief of symptoms of BPH. Recent trials using 160 mg of saw palmetto bid did not improve symptoms of BPH. This contrasts with the positive findings of many previous studies. Trials with higher dose-ranging protocols are currently in progress.
- TURP is the most commonly used surgical procedure for BPH. Transurethral incision of the prostate (TUIP), a procedure almost equivalent in efficacy, is limited to patients whose estimated resection tissue weight would be 30 g or less. TUIP can be performed in an ambulatory setting or during a 1-day hospitalization. Open prostatectomy is typically performed on patients with very large prostates.
- Laser therapy for BPH is a less invasive alternative to TURP; YAG laser enucleation has minimal effect on potency, libido, or patient satisfaction with his sex life and is associated with retrograde ejaculation. However, recent studies indicate that at least in the initial 7 mo after surgery, TURP is moderately more effective than laser therapy in relieving symptoms of BPH.
- Transurethral needle ablation with radiofrequency to remove periurethral prostate tissue is being increasingly used in patients with prostate volume <60 ml and moderate symptoms. It has a low morbidity rate, but treatment failure is approximately 25% at 5 yr and >80% at 10 yr.
- Balloon dilation of the prostatic urethra is less effective than surgery for relieving symptoms but is associated with fewer complications. It is a reasonable treatment option for patients with smaller prostates and no middle lobe enlargement.
- Surgery need not be the treatment of last resort for most patients; that is, patients need not undergo other treatments for BPH before they can have surgery. However, recommending surgery on the grounds that a patient's surgical risk will "only increase with age" is generally inappropriate.

CHRONIC Rx

- Avoid medications and foods that exacerbate symptoms.
- Symptomatic improvement occurs in >70% of patients with proper treatment.

DISPOSITION

With appropriate therapy, symptoms improve or stabilize in >70% of patients with BPH.

REFERRAL

Urology referral for patients with severe or intolerable symptoms and for any patient suspected of having prostate cancer (10% to 30% of men with BPH).

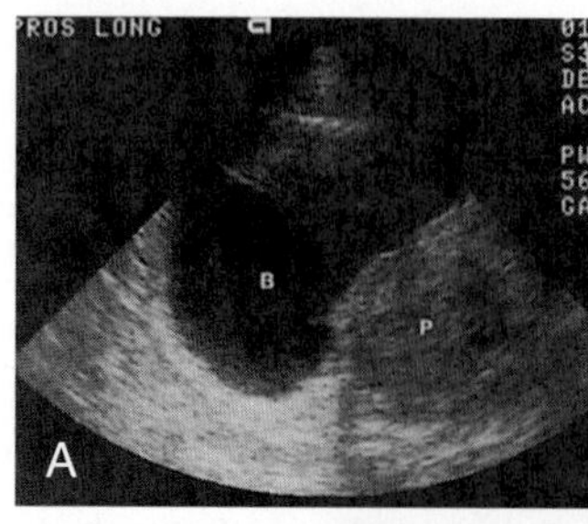

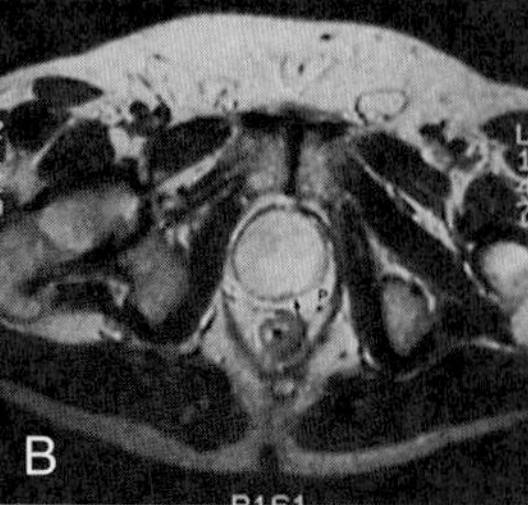

FIGURE 1-265 Benign prostatic nodular hyperplasia. Ultrasound (suprapubic abdominal approach) **(A)** and T2-weighted MRI **(B).** On ultrasound the prostate *(P)* demonstrates uniform low-level acoustic reflectivity, whereas on the MRI the adenomatous enlargement of the prostate and the peripheral zone *(P)* can be distinguished. The two are separated by a low-intensity surgical pseudocapsule *(arrow).* (From Grainger RG et al [eds]: *Grainger & Allison's diagnostic radiology,* ed 4, Philadelphia, 2001, Churchill Livingstone.)

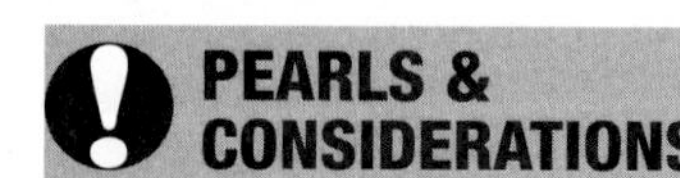

PEARLS & CONSIDERATIONS

COMMENTS

- Emerging technologies for treating BPH include lasers, coils, stents, thermal therapy, and hyperthermia. Laser prostatectomy appears promising; however, long-term effectiveness has not yet been demonstrated.

- The increase in the use of pharmacologic management has resulted in >30% reduction in the total number of TURP procedures.
- Combined drug therapy for BPH with an alpha-blocker and a 5-alpha-reductase inhibitor is superior to monotherapy with either agent.

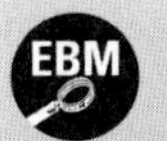 EVIDENCE

Please note: Complete text of EBM for this topic is available online.

Key trials and commentary:

Clinical benign prostatic hyperplasia (BPH) is primarily diagnosed based on a diverse array of progressive lower urinary tract symptoms and is likely distinct from histologic BPH, which is detected by the presence of nonmalignant proliferation of prostate cells but may or may not be associated with symptoms. Pharmacologic management of lower urinary tract symptoms has emerged as an effective initial treatment for clinical BPH because of the introduction of new drug therapies shown to be effective in recent large clinical trials. Despite advances in symptom management and research into disease pathology, diagnostic strategies for the prediction of BPH progression and response to drug modalities are lacking, and questions remain as to the molecular differences underlying clinical (symptomatic) vs. histologic (nonsymptomatic) BPH.

These findings and ongoing Consortium discovery efforts have the potential to provide a greater understanding of the defects underlying disease pathology, and may lead to the development of early and more effective pharmacological treatment strategies for BPH.

As one of them, I believe I'm free to say that there are days when we aging males feel strongly that BPH is too much with us—one of the great downsides of the human condition. BHP is one of the most common diseases in aging men in the U.S. Pathologically diagnosed BPH is characterized by the nonmalignant proliferation of the epithelial and stromal components of the prostate. Such histologic BPH may or may not be associated with clinical BPH, which is defined by the progressive development of lower urinary tract symptoms (LUTS). LUTS primarily result from constriction of the urethra and resulting resistance to urinary flow, and may take the form of urgency, frequency, nocturia, and a weak urine stream with incomplete emptying. If left untreated, LUTS can result in acute urinary retention, urinary incontinence, recurrent urinary tract infection, and/or obstructive uropathy. Interestingly, some men with a significantly enlarged prostate do not present with LUTS, whereas some with a normal-sized prostate experience severe LUTS. BPH is a chronic condition that increases in prevalence and severity with increasing age. Given all this, easily usable and reliable serum markers for BPH would certainly be expected to stand in line as potentially very heavily used tests. The current report details efforts to apply the powerful tools of proteomics to the age-old problem of BPH. To further investigate the efficacy of individual and combination drug therapy for medical management of clinical BPH, National Institute of Diabetes and Digestive and Kidney Diseases (NIDDK) conducted a long-term, randomized trial known as the Medical Therapy of Prostatic Symptoms (MTOPS) study. Importantly, as a component of the study protocol, serum samples were collected from MTOPS patients before randomization, and at yearly intervals during the trial and at the end of the study. Prostate biopsy samples were also collected from a patient subgroup at baseline, year 1, and at the end of the study. These biosamples were banked in anticipation of analyses of potential molecular changes associated with patient responses to the MTOPS clinical protocol.[1] Ⓐ

This study sought to compare the efficacy and safety of transurethral microwave thermotherapy (TUMT) with ProstaLund Feedback Treatment, using the CoreTherm device, with transurethral resection of the prostate (TURP) 5 years after treatment.

The clinical outcome 5 years after TUMT using the CoreTherm device was comparable to the results seen after TURP. The safety of TUMT using the CoreTherm device compared favorably with that of TURP.

TUMT has stood the test of time, and several devices have been thoroughly tested and subjected to randomized trials with long-term follow-up. This is also true for the ProstaLund feedback treatment using the CoreTherm device, which is a high-energy microwave thermotherapy device without water cooling. This device was tested in a randomized, prospective, multicenter trial in the U.S. and Scandinavia, enrolling 154 patients who were randomized to either TUMT or TURP in a 2:1 ratio. 66% of the patients had completed 60 months of follow-up, and the data demonstrate that both symptom score and quality of life are comparable between the TURP and the TUMT groups. Peak urinary flow rate improvements were not as dramatic in the TUMT group compared to the TURP group. However, even in the TURP group, the maximum urinary flow rate was not as good as in some other recent TURP studies. Prostate volume was assessed by ultrasound, and interestingly enough, from an average prostate volume of approximately 50 cm^3, a reduction to ~35 cm^3 was observed at 12 months, but at 60 months those patients available for follow-up had an increase in prostate volume to 45 cm^3, suggesting that the reduction in size is temporary, and that the natural growth tendency of the gland resumes after treatment. The same trend was *not* seen in the TURP group, suggesting that the more complete removal of the transition zone—also evidenced by a more substantial reduction in serum PSA—after a TURP prevents the regrowth of tissue, and thus likely reduces long-term need for retreatment. I like to add that the lack of water cooling in the CoreTherm device requires insertion of a catheter, because patients experience sloughing of tissue, among other side effects, which is somewhat detrimental when using it in a busy private practice setting. The trade-off between the absence of anesthesia during TUMT compared to a TURP, vs. prolonged catheterization may dissuade some patients from choosing this minimally invasive treatment.[2] Ⓐ

Evidence-Based References

1. Mullins C, Lucia MS, Hayward SW: A comprehensive approach toward novel serum biomarkers for benign prostatic hyperplasia: the MPSA consortium, *J Urol* 179:1243-1256, 2008. Commentary by M.G. Bissell, M.D., Ph.D., M.P.H. Ⓐ
2. Mattiasson A, Wagrell L, Schelin S: Five-year follow-up of feedback microwave thermotherapy versus TURP for clinical BPH: a prospective randomized multicenter study, *Urology* 69:91-97, 2007. Commentary by C.G. Roehrborn, M.D. Ⓐ

SUGGESTED READINGS

AUA Practice Guidelines Committee: AUA guideline on management of benign prostatic hyperplasia, *J Urol* 170:2003.

Bent S et al: Saw palmetto for benign prostatic hyperplasia, *N Engl J Med* 354:557, 2006.

Edwards JL: Diagnosis and management of benign prostatic hyperplasia, *Am Fam Physician* 77(10): 1403-1410, 2008.

Lepor H: Insights into the natural history and treatment of benign prostatic hyperplasia, *J Urol* 175: 815, 2006.

AUTHOR: **FRED F. FERRI, M.D.**

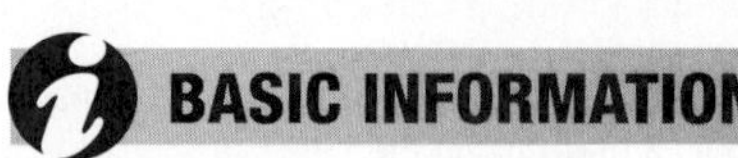

BASIC INFORMATION

DEFINITION

Prostatitis refers to inflammation of the prostate gland. There are four major categories:

1. Acute bacterial prostatitis (type I)
2. Chronic bacterial prostatitis (type II)
3. Chronic prostatitis/pelvic pain syndrome (CP/CPPS) (type III): subdivided in type IIIA (inflammatory) and IIIB (noninflammatory)
4. Asymptomatic inflammatory prostatitis (type IV)

ICD-9CM CODES

601.0	Prostatitis (acute)
601.1	Prostatitis (chronic)
099.54	Prostatitis (chlamydial)

EPIDEMIOLOGY & DEMOGRAPHICS

- 50% of men will have symptoms of prostatitis in their lifetime.
- Acute bacterial prostatitis is uncommon.
- The prevalence of chronic bacterial prostatitis is 5% to 10%.
- CP/CPPS is the most common of the clinically defined prostatitis syndromes, with the prevalence of the syndrome ranging from 9% to 12% of men.

PHYSICAL FINDINGS & CLINICAL PRESENTATION

1. Acute bacterial prostatitis:
   - Sudden or rapidly progressive onset of:
     - Dysuria
     - Frequency
     - Urgency
     - Nocturia
     - Perineal pain that may radiate to the back, rectum, or penis
   - Hematuria or a purulent urethral discharge may occur.
   - Occasionally urinary retention complicates the course.
   - Fever, chills, and signs of sepsis can also be part of the clinical picture.
   - On rectal examination the prostate is typically tender.
2. Chronic bacterial prostatitis:
   - Characterized by positive culture of expressed prostatic secretions. May cause symptoms such as suprapubic, low back, or perineal pain; mild urgency, frequency, and dysuria with urination; and possibly recurrent urinary tract infections.
   - May be asymptomatic when the infection is confined to the prostate.
   - May present as an increase in severity of baseline symptoms of benign prostatic hypertrophy.
   - When cystitis is also present, urinary frequency, urgency, and burning may be reported.
   - Hematuria may be a presenting complaint.
   - In elderly men, new onset of urinary incontinence may be noted.
3. CP/CPPS:
   - Presents similarly with pain in the pelvic region lasting more than 3 mo. Symptoms also can include pain in the suprapubic region, low back, penis, testes, or scrotum.
   - The symptoms can be of variable severity and may include lower urinary tract symptoms, sexual dysfunction, and reduced quality of life.

ETIOLOGY

1. Acute bacterial prostatitis:
   - Acute, usually gram-negative infection of the prostate gland.
     - Generally associated with cystitis
     - Results from the ascent of bacteria into the urethra
   - Occasionally the route of infection is hematogenous or a lymphatogenous spread of rectal bacteria.
   - The condition is seen in young or middle-aged men.
2. Chronic bacterial prostatitis:
   - Often asymptomatic.
   - Exacerbation of symptoms of benign prostatic hypertrophy caused by the same mechanism as in acute bacterial prostatitis.
3. CP/CPPS:
   - Type IIIA: refers to symptoms of prostatic inflammation associated with the presence of white blood cells in prostatic secretions with no identifiable bacterial organism.
   - Chlamydia infection may be etiologically implicated in some cases.
   - Type IIIB: refers to symptoms of prostatic inflammation with no or few white blood cells in the prostatic secretion.
   - Its cause is unknown. Spasm in the bladder neck or urethra may be responsible for the symptoms.

Dx DIAGNOSIS

DIFFERENTIAL DIAGNOSIS

- Benign prostatic hypertrophy with lower urinary tract symptoms
- Prostate cancer
- Also see differential diagnosis of "Hematuria" entry

WORKUP

- Rectal examination:
  1. Tender prostate most suggestive of acute bacterial prostatitis.
  2. Enlarged prostate common in chronic bacterial prostatitis.
  3. Normal prostate is consistent with chronic bacterial prostatitis and CP/CPPS.
- Expression of prostatic secretions by prostate massage is contraindicated in acute bacterial prostatitis but is appropriate in the other three situations.

LABORATORY TESTS

- Urinalysis.
- Urine culture and sensitivity.
- Bacterial localization studies can be performed but are cumbersome and impractical in most clinical settings.
- Cell count and culture of expressed prostatic secretions.
- The yield of a urine culture may be increased if the specimen is obtained after a prostatic massage.
- Prostate-specific antigen (PSA) is not used to diagnose prostatitis and is not recommended unless a nodule is present on digital examination. A rapid rise over baseline should raise the possibility of prostatitis even in the absence of symptoms. In such cases, a follow-up PSA after treatment of prostatitis is appropriate.
- Complete blood count and blood cultures if fever, chills, or signs of sepsis exist.
- If hematuria is present, a workup to rule out a urologic malignancy should be considered if the hematuria does not clear after treatment of prostatitis.

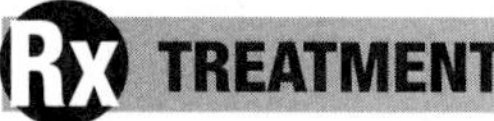

TREATMENT

1. Acute bacterial prostatitis:
   - Culture-guided antibiotic therapy for 4 wk (beginning with a few days of IV antibiotics if the infection is serious or if the patient is bacteremic)
2. Chronic bacterial prostatitis:
   - Trimethoprim-sulfamethoxazole (TMP-SMX) is first line choice for 4 wk if the organism is sensitive.
   - Second line choice for treatment failure or organisms resistant to TMP-SMX is with a quinolone.
   - Patient with refractory infection or with multiple relapses may be offered long-term suppressive therapy.
3. CP/CPPS:
   - No specific treatment. A brief course of nonsteroidal antiinflammatory drugs may be tried until urine localization cultures are completed. Alfzosin may reduce symptoms in men who have not received prior therapy with an alpha-blocker (*N Engl J Med* 359:2663, 2008).
   - Antibiotics are not effective and should be avoided in patients who are afebrile and have normal urinalysis results.
   - A trial of treatment with an alpha-adrenergic blocker (terazosin, doxazosin, or tamsulosin) may be considered, but recent trials failed to show a significant reduction in symptoms.
   - Contributing factors (e.g., stress, neuromuscular factors) should be addressed.
   - Any underlying bladder pathology should be ruled out by cystoscopy and treated if identified.

AUTHORS: **FRED F. FERRI, M.D.**, and **TOM J. WACHTEL, M.D.**

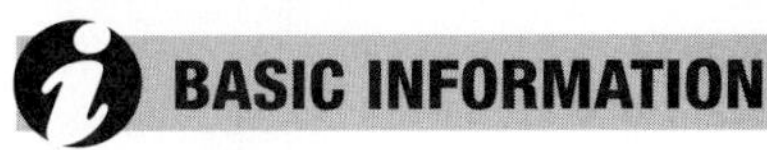

DEFINITION

Pruritus ani refers to an intense chronic itching of the anus and perianal skin.

ICD-9CM CODES
698.0 Pruritus ani

EPIDEMIOLOGY & DEMOGRAPHICS

- Any age can be affected.
- Occurs in 1% to 5% of the population.
- Male/female predominance of 4:1.

PHYSICAL FINDINGS & CLINICAL PRESENTATION

- Anal itching
- Anal fissures
- Hemorrhoids
- Excoriations
- Pinworms
- Fecal incontinence

ETIOLOGY

Anorectal diseases and fecal contamination:
- Diarrhea
- Anal incontinence
- Hemorrhoids
- Fissures
- Fistulae
- Rectal prolapse
- Malignancy: Bowen's disease, epidermoid cancer, perianal Paget's disease

Infections:
- Fungal: candidiasis, dermatophytes
- Parasitic: pinworms, scabies
- Bacterial: *Staphylococcus aureus,* erythrasma
- Lymphogranuloma venereum
- Granuloma inguinale
- Chancroid
- Molluscum contagiosa
- Trichomoniasis
- Venereal: herpes, gonococcal syphilis, human papillomavirus

Local irritants:
- Moisture, obesity, excessive perspiration
- Soaps, hygiene products
- Toilet paper: perfumed, dyed
- Underwear: irritating fabrics, detergents
- Anal creams, suppositories
- Dietary: coffee, beer, acidic foods
- Drugs: mineral oil, ascorbic acid, hydrocortisone sodium succinate, quinine, colchicine

Dermatologic diseases:
- Psoriasis
- Atopic dermatitis
- Seborrheic dermatitis

Section II also describes the various causes of pruritus ani.

Dx DIAGNOSIS

DIFFERENTIAL DIAGNOSIS

- Allergies
- Anxiety
- Dermatologic conditions
- Infections
- Parasites
- Diabetes mellitus
- Chronic liver disease
- Neoplasia
- Proctalgia fugax

WORKUP

- Detailed history regarding bowel habits, hygiene, use of perfumed products, and medical history
- Inspection of perianal area
- Possible biopsy to exclude neoplasia
- Microscopic inspection of scrapings
- Colposcopy of perineum

LABORATORY TESTS

- Chemistry profile
- Urinalysis
- Cultures
- Stool for ova and parasites
- Tape test
- Glucose tolerance test, if necessary

Rx TREATMENT

NONPHARMACOLOGIC THERAPY

- Avoidance of tight, nonbreathable clothing and underclothing
- Discontinuation or curtailment of coffee, beer, citrus fruits, tomatoes, chocolate, and tea
- Cleansing of anal area after bowel movements with a premoistened pad or tissue and avoidance of perfumes and dyes present in toilet paper and soaps
- Avoidance of excessive perspiration
- Aggressive management of fecal leakage or incontinence to avoid soiling of perianal skin

ACUTE GENERAL Rx

- Minimization of frequent loose stools with antidiarrheals and fiber agents if appropriate
- Use of a 1% hydrocortisone cream sparingly bid during the acute phase of pruritus ani but not for >2 wk to avoid atrophy
- Treatment of predisposing factors, such as parasites, diabetes, liver disease, hemorrhoids, and other infections

CHRONIC Rx

- Possible complications: excoriation and secondary bacterial infection; must be treated aggressively
- Longstanding, intractable pruritus ani: good response to intracutaneous injections of methylene blue and other agents, steroid injection

DISPOSITION

- Usually good results with total resolution of symptoms
- In some, persistent and recurrent symptoms

REFERRAL

To colorectal specialist if conservative measures fail

SUGGESTED READING

Heard S: Pruritus ani, *Aust Fam Physician* 33(7):511, 2004.

AUTHORS: **MARIA A. CORIGLIANO, M.D.,** and **RUBEN ALVERO, M.D.**

Pruritus Vulvae (ALG)

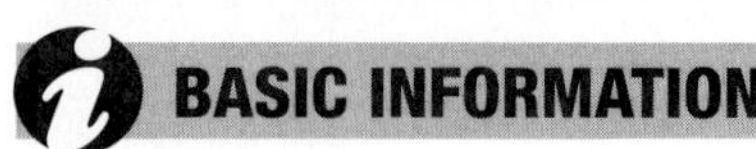

BASIC INFORMATION

DEFINITION

Pruritus vulvae refers to intense itching of the female external genitalia.

SYNONYMS

Vulvodynia

ICD-9CM CODES
698.1 Pruritus of genital organs

EPIDEMIOLOGY & DEMOGRAPHICS

- A female disorder that can affect women at any age
- Young girls: infection is usually causative
- Postmenopausal women: frequently affected because of hypoestrogenic state

PHYSICAL FINDINGS & CLINICAL PRESENTATION

Constant, intense itching or burning of the vulva

ETIOLOGY

- Approximately 50% are caused by monilial infection or trichomoniasis.
- Other infectious causes are herpes simplex, condylomata acuminata, and molluscum contagiosum.
- Other causes:
  1. Infestations with scabies, pediculosis pubis, and pinworms
  2. Dermatoses such as hypertrophic dystrophy, lichen sclerosus, lichen planus, and psoriasis
  3. Neoplasms such as Bowen's disease, Paget's disease, and squamous cell carcinoma
  4. Allergic or chemical dermatitis caused by dyes in clothing or toilet paper, detergents, contraceptive gels, vaginal medications, douches, or soaps
  5. Vulvar or vaginal atrophy
- Severe pruritus is probably caused by degeneration and inflammation of terminal nerve fibers.
- Most intense itching occurs with hyperplastic lesions.
- Children typically (75%) have nonspecific pruritus, lichen sclerosus, bacterial infections, yeast infection, or pinworm infestation.

Dx DIAGNOSIS

DIFFERENTIAL DIAGNOSIS

- Vulvitis
- Vaginitis
- Lichen sclerosus
- Squamous cell hyperplasia
- Pinworms
- Vulvar cancer
- Syringoma of the vulva

WORKUP

- Inspection of vulva, vagina, and perianal area for infection, fissures, ulcerations, induration, or thick plaques
- Must rule out trichomoniasis, candidiasis, bacterial vaginosis, allergy, vitamin deficiencies, diabetes

LABORATORY TESTS

- Wet prep of saline and potassium hydroxide of vaginal discharge
- Tape test to look for pinworms
- Vaginal cultures
- Biopsy when needed

Rx TREATMENT

NONPHARMACOLOGIC THERAPY

- Keep vulva clean and dry.
- Wear white cotton panties.
- Avoid perfumes and body creams over vulvar area because they can cause irritation.
- Reduce stress.
- Apply wet dressings with aluminum acetate (Burow's) solution frequently.
- Avoid coffee and caffeine-containing beverages, chocolate, and tomatoes.
- Sitz baths may be helpful.

ACUTE GENERAL Rx

Need to treat underlying problem:

- Yeast infection: any of the vaginal creams or Diflucan 150-mg one-time dose
- Trichomoniasis or *Gardnerella vaginalis:* Flagyl 500 mg or 375 mg PO bid for 7 days
- Urinary tract infection: treatment of specific organism
- Estrogen replacement therapy if atrophy is the cause of pruritus
- Pinworms: mebendazole (Vermox) 100 mg 1 tablet at diagnosis and repeated in 1 to 2 wk; also treat other members in family aged >2 yr
- Squamous cell hyperplasia: local application of corticosteroids
  1. One of the high- or medium-potency corticosteroids (0.025% or 0.01% fluocinolone acetonide or 0.01% triamcinolone acetonide) can be used to relieve itching.
  2. Rub into vulva bid or tid for 4 to 6 wk.
  3. Once itching is controlled, fluorinated steroid can be discontinued and patient can be switched to hydrocortisone preparation.
- Lichen sclerosus: topical 2% testosterone in petrolatum massaged into the vulvar tissue bid or tid; Temovate (clobetasol propionate gel 0.05%) cream tid for 5 days is effective
- Treatment with immune response modifiers

CHRONIC Rx

- If not relieved by topical measures: intradermal injection of triamcinolone (10 mg/ml diluted 2:1 saline); 0.1 ml of the suspension injected at 1-cm intervals and tissue gently massaged
- If symptoms still uncontrollable: SC injection of absolute alcohol 0.1 ml at 1-cm intervals

DISPOSITION

Usually controlled with conservative measures and topical steroids

REFERRAL

To a gynecologist for further workup if conservative measures do not give relief

SUGGESTED READINGS

Boardman LA et al: Recurrent vulvar itching, *Obstet Gynecol* 105(6):1451, 2005.

Welch B et al: Vulval itch, *Aust Fam Physician* 33(7):505, 2004.

AUTHORS: **MARIA A. CORIGLIANO, M.D.,** and **RUBEN ALVERO, M.D.**

BASIC INFORMATION

DEFINITION

Pseudogout is one of the clinical patterns associated with a crystal-induced synovitis resulting from the deposition of calcium pyrophosphate dehydrate (CPPD) crystals in joint hyaline and fibrocartilage. The cartilage deposition is termed *chondrocalcinosis.*

SYNONYMS

Calcium pyrophosphate dehydrate crystal deposition disease (CPDD)
Chondrocalcinosis
Pyrophosphate arthropathy

ICD-9CM CODES
275.4 Chondrocalcinosis

EPIDEMIOLOGY & DEMOGRAPHICS

PREVALENCE:

- Uncertain
- Probably similar to gout (three per 1000 persons)
- Chondrocalcinosis is present in >20% of all people at age 80 yr, but most are asymptomatic

PREDOMINANT SEX: Female/male ratio of approximately 1.5:1

PREDOMINANT AGE: 0 to 70 yr at onset

PHYSICAL FINDINGS & CLINICAL PRESENTATION

- Symptoms are similar to those of gouty arthritis with acute attacks and chronic arthritis
- Knee joint is most commonly affected
- Swelling, stiffness, and increased heat in affected joint

ETIOLOGY

- Unknown
- Often associated with various medical conditions, including hyperparathyroidism and amyloidosis

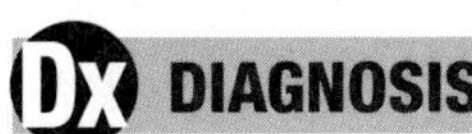

DIAGNOSIS

DIFFERENTIAL DIAGNOSIS

- Gouty arthritis
- Rheumatoid arthritis
- Osteoarthritis
- Neuropathic joint

Section II describes the differential diagnosis of acute monoarticular and oligoarticular arthritis and crystal-induced arthritides. An algorithm for evaluation of arthralgia is described in Section III, "Arthralgia Limited to One or Few Joints."

WORKUP

- Variable clinical presentation
- Diagnosis dependent on the identification of CPPD crystals
- The American Rheumatism Association revised diagnostic criteria for CPPD crystal deposition disease (pseudogout) are often used:
  1. Criteria
     - I. Demonstration of CPPD crystals (obtained by biopsy, arthroscopy, or aspirated synovial fluid) by definitive means (e.g., characteristic "fingerprint" by x-ray diffraction powder pattern or by chemical analysis)
     - II. (a) Identification of monoclinic and/or triclinic crystals showing either no or only a weakly positive birefringence by compensated polarized light microscopy
       (b) Presence of typical calcifications in roentgenograms
     - III. (a) Acute arthritis, especially of knees or other large joints, with or without concomitant hyperuricemia
       (b) Chronic arthritis, especially of knees, hips, wrists, carpus, elbow, shoulder, and metacarpophalangeal joints, especially if accompanied by acute exacerbations; the following features are helpful in differentiating chronic arthritis from osteoarthritis:
         1. Uncommon site: for example, wrist, metacarpophalangeal joint, elbow, shoulder
         2. Appearance of lesion radiologically: for example, radiocarpal or patellofemoral joint space narrowing, especially if isolated (patella "wrapped around" the femur)
         3. Subchondral cyst formation
         4. Severity of degeneration: progressive, with subchondral bony collapse (microfractures) and fragmentation, with formation of intraarticular radiodense bodies
         5. Osteophyte formation: variable and inconstant
         6. Tendon calcifications, especially Achilles, triceps, obturators
  2. Categories
     - Definite: criterion I or II (a) plus (b) must be fulfilled.
     - Probable: criterion II (a) or II (b) must be fulfilled.
     - Possible: criterion III (a) or (b) should alert the clinician to the possibility of underlying CPPD deposition.

LABORATORY TESTS

Crystal analysis of the synovial fluid aspirate to reveal rhomboid calcium pyrophosphate crystals

IMAGING STUDIES

Plain radiographs to reveal the following:

- Stippled calcification in bands running parallel to the subchondral bone margins
- Crystal deposition in menisci, synovium, and ligament tissue; triangular wrist cartilage and symphysis pubis often affected

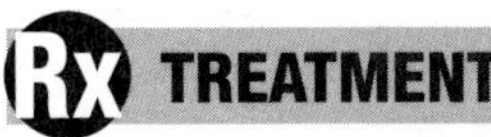

TREATMENT

NONPHARMACOLOGIC THERAPY

General measures such as heat, rest, and elevation as needed

ACUTE GENERAL Rx

- Nonsteroidal antiinflammatory drugs (as for gout)
- Colchicine
- Aspiration or steroid injection

DISPOSITION

Structural joint damage may occasionally occur, requiring arthroplasty in rare cases.

REFERRAL

For orthopedic consultation for destructive joint changes

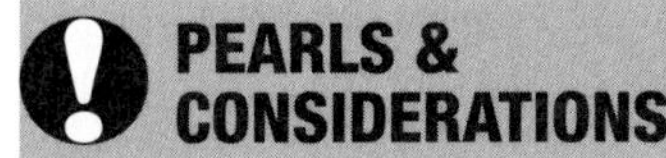

PEARLS & CONSIDERATIONS

COMMENTS

As with gout, acute attacks may be triggered by various surgical or medical events.

SUGGESTED READINGS

Announ N, Guerne PA: Treating difficult crystal pyrophosphate dehydrate deposition disease, *Curr Rheumatol Rep* 10:228, 2008.

Ea HK, Liote F: Advances in understanding calcium-containing crystal disease, *Curr Opin Rheumatol* 21(2):150, 2009.

Liote F, Ea HK: Recent developments in crystal-induced inflammation pathogenesis and management, *Curr Rheumatol Rep* 9(3):243, 2007.

Mader B: Calcium pyrophosphate dihydrate deposition disease of the wrist, *Clin Rheumatol* 23(1):95, 2004.

McGonagle D et al: Successful treatment of resistant pseudogout with anakinra, *Arthritis Rheum* 58:631, 2008.

Rosenthal AK: Crystal arthropathies and other unpopular rheumatic diseases, *Curr Opin Rheumatol* 16(3): 262, 2004.

Wise CM: Crystal-associated arthritis in the elderly, *Rheum Dis Clin North Am* 33(1):33, 2007.

AUTHOR: **LONNIE R. MERCIER, M.D.**

BASIC INFORMATION

DEFINITION

Pseudomembranous colitis is the occurrence of diarrhea and bowel inflammation associated with antibiotic use.

SYNONYMS

Antibiotic-induced colitis

ICD-9CM CODES
008.45 *Clostridium difficile,* pseudomembranous colitis

EPIDEMIOLOGY & DEMOGRAPHICS

- Cephalosporins are the most frequent offending agent in pseudomembranous colitis because of their high rates of use.
- The antibiotic with the highest incidence is clindamycin (10% incidence of pseudomembranous colitis with its use).
- *Clostridium difficile* is responsible for approximately 3 million cases of diarrhea and colitis in the U.S. every year.

PHYSICAL FINDINGS & CLINICAL PRESENTATION

- Abdominal tenderness (generalized or lower abdominal)
- Fever
- In patients with prolonged diarrhea, poor skin turgor, dry mucous membranes, and other signs of dehydration may be present

ETIOLOGY

Risk factors for *C. difficile* (the major identifiable agent of antibiotic-induced diarrhea and colitis):
- Administration of antibiotics: can occur with any antibiotic, but occurs most frequently with clindamycin, ampicillin, and cephalosporins
- Prolonged hospitalization
- Advanced age
- Abdominal surgery
- Hospitalized, tube-fed patients are at risk for *C. difficile*–associated diarrhea. Clinicians should consider testing for *C. difficile* in tube-fed patients with diarrhea unrelated to the feeding solution.

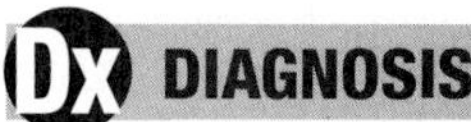

DIAGNOSIS

The clinical signs of pseudomembranous colitis generally include diarrhea, fever, and abdominal cramps after use of antibiotics.

DIFFERENTIAL DIAGNOSIS

- Gastrointestinal bacterial infections (e.g., *Salmonella, Shigella, Campylobacter, Yersinia*)
- Enteric parasites (e.g., *Cryptosporidium, Entamoeba histolytica*)
- Inflammatory bowel disease
- Celiac sprue
- Irritable bowel syndrome
- Ischemic colitis
- Antibiotic intolerance

WORKUP

- All patients with diarrhea accompanied by current or recent antibiotic use should be tested for *C. difficile* (see below).
- Sigmoidoscopy (without cleansing enema) may be necessary when the clinical and laboratory diagnosis is inconclusive and the diarrhea persists.
- In antibiotic-induced pseudomembranous colitis, the sigmoidoscopy often reveals raised white-yellow exudative plaques adherent to the colonic mucosa (Fig. 1-266).

LABORATORY TESTS

- *C. difficile* toxin can be detected by cytotoxin tissue-culture assay (gold standard for identifying *C. difficile* toxin in stool specimen). This test is difficult to perform and results are not available for 24 to 48 hr. A more useful test is the enzyme-linked immunosorbent assay for *C. difficile* toxins A and B. The latter is used most widely in the clinical setting. It has a sensitivity of 85% and a specificity of 100%.
- Fecal leukocytes (assessed by microscopy or lactoferrin assay) are generally present in stool samples.
- Complete blood count usually reveals leukocytosis. A sudden increase in white blood cells to >30,000/mm^3 may be indicative of fulminant colitis.

IMAGING STUDIES

Abdominal film (flat plate and upright) is useful in patients with abdominal pain or evidence of obstruction on physical examination.

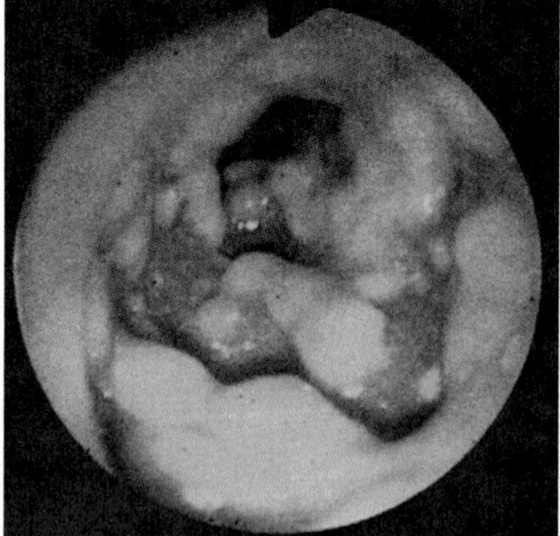

FIGURE 1-266 Pseudomembranous plaques seen with colonoscopy in a patient with *Clostridium difficile*–associated pseudomembranous colitis. (From Gorbach SL: *Infectious diseases,* ed 2, Philadelphia, 1998, WB Saunders.)

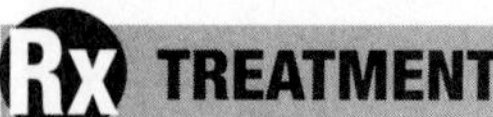

TREATMENT

NONPHARMACOLOGIC THERAPY

- Discontinue offending antibiotic
- Fluid hydration and correction of electrolyte abnormalities

ACUTE GENERAL Rx

- Metronidazole 500 mg PO qid for 10 to 14 days.
- Vancomycin 125 mg PO qid for 10 to 14 days in cases resistant to metronidazole. However, vancomycin may be considered as first-line therapy in hospitalized patients who are seriously ill.
- Cholestyramine 4 g PO qid for 10 days in addition to metronidazole to control severe diarrhea (avoid use with vancomycin).
- When parenteral therapy is necessary (e.g., patient with paralytic ileus), IV metronidazole 500 mg qid can be used. It can also be supplemented with vancomycin 500 mg by nasogastric tube with intermittent clamping or retention enema.
- IV tigecycline (a broad-spectrum antibiotic used for skin or soft-tissue infection) can be used as adjunctive or alternative therapy for severe refractory *C. difficile* toxin infection.
- The addition of monoclonal antibodies against *C. difficile* toxins to antibiotic agents has been shown to reduce the recurrence of *C. difficile* infection.

CHRONIC Rx

Judicious future use of antibiotics to prevent recurrences (e.g., avoid prolonged antibiotic therapy)

DISPOSITION

Most patients recover completely with appropriate therapy. Fever resolves within 48 hr and diarrhea within 4 to 5 days. Overall mortality rate is 1% to 2.5% but exceeds 10% in untreated patients.

REFERRAL

Hospital admission and IV hydration in severe cases

SUGGESTED READINGS

Herpers BL et al: IV tigecycline as adjunctive or alternative therapy for severe refractory *C. difficile* infection, *Clin Infect Dis* 48:1732, 2009.

Kelly CP, La Mont JT: *Clostridium difficile,* more difficult than ever, *N Engl J Med* 359:1932-1940, 2008.

Lowry I et al: Treatment with monoclonal antibodies against *C. difficile* toxins, *N Engl J Med* 362:197-205, 2010.

AUTHOR: **FRED F. FERRI, M.D.**

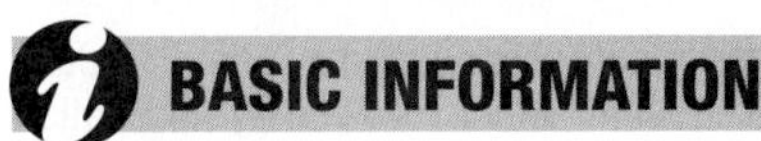

BASIC INFORMATION

DEFINITION

Psittacosis is a systemic infection caused by *Chlamydophila psittaci* (formerly known as *Chlamydia psittaci*).

SYNONYMS

Ornithosis
Parrot pneumonia

ICD-9CM CODES
073.9 Psittacosis

EPIDEMIOLOGY & DEMOGRAPHICS

INCIDENCE (IN U.S.):
- 21 cases reported in 2005
- True incidence possibly higher because infections may be subclinical
- Highest incidence among pet owners and people working with birds

PEAK INCIDENCE: Age 30 to 60 yr
PREVALENCE (IN U.S.):
- Low among human beings
- Organism carried by 5% to 8% of birds

PREDOMINANT SEX: Equal sex distribution
PREDOMINANT AGE: More common in adults

PHYSICAL FINDINGS & CLINICAL PRESENTATION

- Incubation period of 5 to 15 days
- Subclinical infection
- Onset abrupt or insidious
- Most common symptoms:
  1. Fever
  2. Myalgias
  3. Chills
  4. Cough
- Most common clinical syndrome: atypical pneumonia with fever, headache, dry cough, and a chest radiograph more dramatically abnormal than the physical examination
- Ranges from mild disease to respiratory failure and death, although this is extremely unusual
- Other clinical presentations:
  1. Mononucleosis-like syndrome
  2. Typhoidal form
- Most frequent physical findings:
  1. Fever
  2. Pharyngeal erythema
  3. Rales
  4. Hepatomegaly
- Less common findings:
  1. Somnolence
  2. Confusion
  3. Relative bradycardia
  4. Pleural rub
  5. Adenopathy
  6. Splenomegaly
  7. Horder's spots (pink blanching maculopapular rash)
- Besides the lungs, other specific end-organ involvement:
  1. Pericarditis
  2. Myocarditis
  3. Endocarditis
  4. Hepatitis
  5. Joints
  6. Kidneys (glomerulonephritis)
  7. Central nervous system

ETIOLOGY

- *C. psittaci* is an obligate intracellular bacterium.
- Infection is usually spread by the respiratory route from infected birds.
- There is a history of exposure to birds in 85% of patients.
- Strains from turkeys and psittacine birds are most virulent for human beings.
- Cows, goats, and sheep are occasionally implicated.

Dx DIAGNOSIS

DIFFERENTIAL DIAGNOSIS

- Legionella
- Mycoplasma
- *Chlamydophila pneumoniae* (Taiwan acute respiratory strain)
- Viral respiratory infections
- Typhoid fever
- Viral hepatitis
- Aseptic meningitis
- Mononucleosis

WORKUP

- Complete blood count, renal and liver function tests
- *Chlamydophila* serology
- Chest x-ray examination
- Special immunostaining of respiratory secretions

LABORATORY TESTS

- White blood count is normal or slightly elevated.
- Mild liver function abnormalities are common (50%).
- Blood cultures are almost always negative.
- Studies on respiratory secretions:
  1. Direct immunofluorescent antibody of respiratory secretions with monoclonal antibodies to chlamydial antigens
  2. *Chlamydophila* lipopolysaccharide antigen by enzyme immunoassay
  3. Polymerase chain reaction
- Serologic studies:
  1. Complement-fixing antibodies
  2. Microimmunofluorescence
  3. Possible false-negative results and cross-reaction with other chlamydial species with both techniques

IMAGING STUDIES

- Chest x-ray examination is abnormal in 50% to 90% with a variety of patterns.
- Pleural effusions are common.

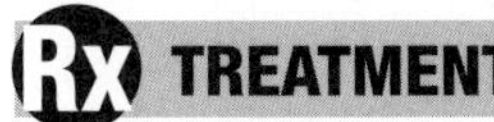

TREATMENT

NONPHARMACOLOGIC THERAPY

Oxygen supplementation as needed

ACUTE GENERAL Rx

- Tetracycline (500 mg PO qid) *or*
- Doxycycline (100 mg PO bid) *or*
- Erythromycin (500 mg PO qid): less effective

CHRONIC Rx

In the rare cases of endocarditis, combination of heart valve replacement and prolonged antibiotic course may be the treatment of choice.

DISPOSITION

- Mortality rate is low (0.7%)
- Poor prognostic factors:
  1. Advanced age
  2. Leukopenia
  3. Severe hypoxemia
  4. Renal failure
  5. Confusion
  6. Multilobe pulmonary involvement
- Possible reinfection

REFERRAL

- To infectious disease expert:
  1. Complicated atypical pneumonia or other end-organ involvement
  2. Suspicion of an outbreak
- To pulmonologist for diagnostic bronchoscopy

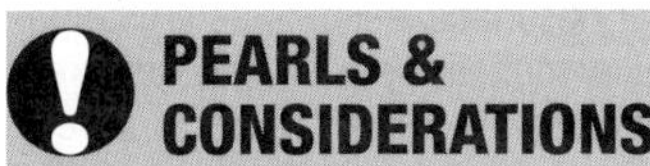

PEARLS & CONSIDERATIONS

COMMENTS

- Hospitalized patients do not require specific isolation precautions.
- Any confirmed or suspected case of psittacosis should be reported to public health authorities.
- Recent evidence indicates that *C. psittaci* may be associated with induction of a rare form of lymphoma found in the ocular adnexa; case reports have described regression of ocular lymphoma with antibiotic treatment for *C. psittaci*.

SUGGESTED READINGS

Cunha BA: The atypical pneumonias: clinical diagnosis and importance, *Clin Microbiol Infect* 3:12, 2006.

Ferreri AJ et al: Evidence for an association between *Chlamydia psittaci* and ocular adnexal lymphomas, *J Natl Cancer Inst* 96(8):586, 2004.

Ferreri AJ et al: Regression of ocular adnexal lymphoma after *Chlamydia psittaci*-eradicating antibiotic therapy, *J Clin Oncol* 23(22):5067, 2005.

Smith KA et al: Compendium of measures to control *Chlamydophila psittaci* (formerly *Chlamydia psittaci*) infection among humans (psittacosis) and pet birds, 2005, *J Am Vet Med Assoc* 226(4):532, 2005.

Vargas RL et al: Is there an association between ocular adnexal lymphoma and infection with *Chlamydia psittaci?* The University of Rochester experience, *Leuk Res* 30(5)547, 2006.

AUTHORS: **GLENN G. FORT, M.D., M.P.H.,** and **DENNIS J. MIKOLICH, M.D.**

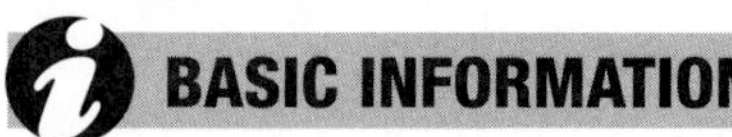

BASIC INFORMATION

DEFINITION

Psoriasis is a chronic skin disorder characterized by excessive proliferation of keratinocytes, resulting in the formation of thickened scaly plaques, itching, and inflammatory changes of the epidermis and dermis. The various forms of psoriasis include guttate, pustular, and arthritis variants.

ICD-9CM CODES
696.0 Psoriasis, arthritis, arthropathic
696.1 Psoriasis, any type except arthropathic

EPIDEMIOLOGY & DEMOGRAPHICS

- Psoriasis affects 1% to 3% of the world's population. Most patients have limited psoriasis involving <5% of their body surface.
- There is a strong association between psoriasis and human leukocyte antigens (HLAs) B13, B17, and B27 (pustular psoriasis).
- Peak age of onset is bimodal (adolescents and at age 60 yr).
- Men and women are affected equally.

PHYSICAL FINDINGS & CLINICAL PRESENTATION

- The primary psoriatic lesion is an erythematous papule topped by a loosely adherent scale. Scraping the scale results in several bleeding points (Auspitz sign).
- Chronic plaque psoriasis generally manifests with symmetric, sharply demarcated, erythematous, silver-scaled patches affecting primarily the intergluteal folds, elbows, scalp, fingernails, toenails, and knees (Fig. 1-267, *A*). This form accounts for 80% of psoriasis cases.
- Psoriasis can also develop at the site of any physical trauma (sunburn, scratching). This is known as Koebner's phenomenon.
- Nail involvement is common (pitting of the nail plate), resulting in hyperkeratosis, onychodystrophy with onycholysis (Fig. 1-267, *B*).
- Pruritus is variable; soreness and bleeding may occur.
- Joint involvement can result in sacroiliitis and spondylitis.
- Guttate psoriasis is generally preceded by streptococcal pharyngitis and manifests with multiple droplike lesions on the extremities and the trunk (Fig. 1-267, *C*).
- Adverse effect on psychological and social functioning, with affected persons often feeling stigmatized.

ETIOLOGY

- Unknown, but there is a strong genetic component and high heritability. There are at least nine chromosomal loci with liinkage to psoriasis. These loci are called psoriasis susceptibility 1 through 9 (PSORS1-PSORS9). PSORS1 locus in the major histocompatibility complex (MHC) region on chromosome 6 is considered the most important susceptibility locus and is believed to account for 35% to 50% of the heritability of the disease.
- Familial clustering (genetic transmission with a dominant mode with variable penetrants).
- One third of persons affected have a positive family history.

DIAGNOSIS

DIFFERENTIAL DIAGNOSIS

- Contact dermatitis
- Atopic dermatitis
- Stasis dermatitis
- Tinea
- Nummular dermatitis
- Candidiasis
- Mycosis fungoides
- Cutaneous systemic lupus erythematosus
- Secondary and tertiary syphilis
- Drug eruption

WORKUP

- Diagnosis is clinical.
- Skin biopsy is rarely necessary.

LABORATORY TESTS

Generally not necessary for diagnosis

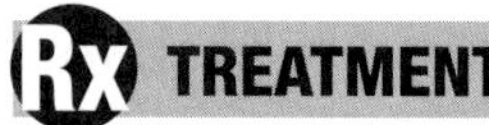

TREATMENT

NONPHARMACOLOGIC THERAPY

- Sunbathing generally leads to improvement.
- Eliminate triggering factors (e.g., stress, certain medications [e.g., lithium, beta-blockers, antimalarials]).
- Patients with psoriasis benefit from a daily bath in warm water followed by application of a cream or ointment moisturizer. Regular use or an emollient moisturizer limits evaporation of water from the skin and allows the stratum corneum to rehydrate itself.

GENERAL Rx

Therapeutic options vary according to the extent of disease. Approximately 70% to 80% of all patients can be treated adequately with topical therapy.

- Patients with limited disease (<20% of the body) can be treated with the following:
  1. Topical steroids: disadvantages are brief remissions, expense, and decreased effect with continued use. Salicylic acid can be compounded by pharmacist in concentrations of 2% to 10% and used in combination with a corticosteroid to decrease the amount of scale.
  2. Calcipotriene (Dovonex): a vitamin D analogue effective for moderate plaque psoriasis. Adults should comb the hair, apply solution to the lesions, and rub it in, avoiding uninvolved skin. Disadvantages include its cost and potential burning and skin irritation. It should not be used concurrently with salicylic acid because calcipotriene is inactivated by the acidic nature of salicylic acid. Taclonex ointment is a combination of calcipotriene and the high-potency corticosteroid betamethasone dipropionate. It is well tolerated and more effective than either agent used alone but also much more expensive.
  3. Tar products (Estar, LCD, psorigel) can be used overnight and are most effective when combined with ultraviolet B (UVB) light (Goeckerman regimen).
  4. Anthralin (Drithocreme): useful for chronic plaques; can result in purple-brown staining; best used with UVB light.
  5. Retinoids such as tazarotene 0.05%, 0.1% cream or gel, are effective in thinning plaques but are expensive and can cause irritation.
  6. Other useful measures include tape or occlusive dressing, UVB and lubricating agents, and interlesional steroids.
- Therapeutic options for persons with generalized disease (affecting >20% of the body) and for those with inadequate response to topical agents:
  1. UVB light exposure three times a week: this therapy does not require administration of a systemic drug (unlike psoralen plus ultraviolet A [PUVA]), but to be effective, it requires removal of scale with keratolytic agents and emollients.
  2. Oral PUVA administered two to three times weekly is effective for generalized disease. It is often considered in patients for whom narrow-band UVB therapy is ineffective. However, many PUVA treatments are required, necessitating frequent office visits, and it may be associated with phototoxicity, such as erythema and blistering, and increased risk of skin cancer.

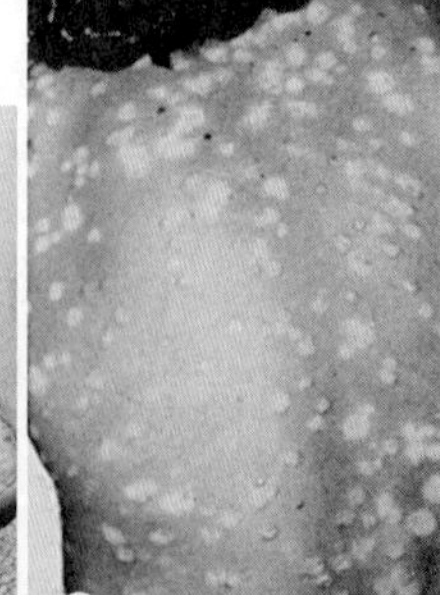

FIGURE 1-267 **A,** Chronic psoriatic plaques on the knee. **B,** Psoriatic nail changes of pitting and dystrophy. **C,** Guttate psoriasis in widespread distribution over the trunk. (From Behrman RE: *Nelson textbook of pediatrics,* ed 17, Philadelphia, 2004, WB Saunders.)

- Systemic treatments include methotrexate 25 mg/wk for severe psoriasis. Etretinate (Tegison) (a synthetic retinoid) is most effective for palmar-plantar pustular psoriasis. Dose is 0.5 to 1 mg/kg/day. It can cause liver enzyme and lipid abnormalities and is teratogenic.
- Cyclosporine is also effective in severe psoriasis; however, relapses are common.
- Chronic plaque psoriasis may be treated with alefacept, a recombinant protein that selectively targets T lymphocytes. Treatment with alefacept for 12 wk (0.025, 0.075, or 0.150 mg/kg of body weight IV weekly) may result in significant improvement. Some patients also demonstrate a sustained clinical response after the cessation of treatment. This medication is very expensive (a 12-wk course costs >$8000).
- TNF inhibitors: Treatment with etanercept, a tumor necrosis factor (TNF) antagonist, for 24 wk can also lead to a reduction in severity of plaque psoriasis. Efalizumab, a humanized monoclonal antibody that inhibits the activation of T cells, has also been reported to produce significant improvement in plaque psoriasis over a 24-wk treatment period. Adalimumab—a fully human, anti-TNF-alpha monoclonal antibody—has been reported to be effective for joint and skin manifestations of psoriasis.
- A newer biologic agent in patients with psoriasis is ustekinumab (an interleukin-12 and interleukin-23 blocker). A recent trial showed that it was more effective than etanercept for the treatment of moderate-to-severe psoriasis.

DISPOSITION

The course of psoriasis is chronic, and the disease may be refractory to treatment.

REFERRAL

- Dermatology referral is recommended in all patients with generalized disease.
- Hospital admission may be necessary for severe diffuse or poorly responsive psoriasis. The Goeckerman regimen combines daily application of tar with UVB exposure and can result in prolonged remissions.

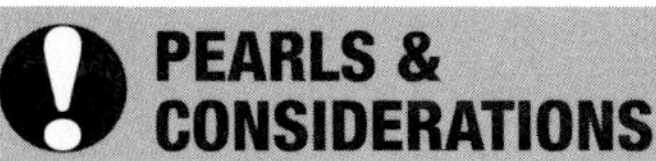

PEARLS & CONSIDERATIONS

COMMENTS

Psoriasis is more emotionally than physically disabling for most patients. Counseling may be indicated, particularly when it affects younger patients.

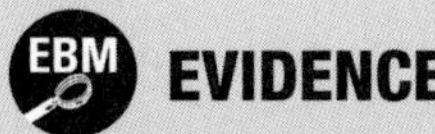

EVIDENCE

Please note: Complete text of EBM for this topic is available online.

Key trials and commentary:

This study sought to determine the risk of mortality in patients with psoriasis. It revealed that severe, but not mild, psoriasis is associated with an increased risk of death.

This article examines the risk of systemic disease in patients with psoriasis. Gelfand et al expanded on previous studies showing a possible increase in mortality in patients with psoriasis, especially in individuals with severe disease requiring hospitalization. They performed a population-based cohort study in the U.K. to determine the risk of mortality in patients with psoriasis. They found a 50% increased risk of mortality in patients with severe psoriasis, whereas patients with milder psoriasis had no increased risk. The cause of the excess mortality in patients with severe psoriasis could not be determined, nor could assessment be made of how the extensive skin disease affected mortality risk, or whether the mortality risk was altered by the various systemic therapies prescribed for these individuals. The authors of this study suggest that the management of patients with psoriasis should address not only their skin disease, but also other risk factors that can increase mortality.[1] Ⓐ

Psoriasis is a common, chronic, inflammatory skin disorder. Smoking may increase the risk of psoriasis, but no prospective data are available on this relation. In this prospective analysis, current and past smoking, and cumulative measures of smoking were associated with the incidence of psoriasis. The risk of incident psoriasis among former smokers decreases nearly to that of never smokers 20 years after cessation.

A link between cigarette smoking and psoriasis has been suggested by previous cross-sectional and case-controlled studies, although no prospective data have been presented. Moreover, an association between the intensity and duration of smoking and the clinical severity of the skin disease has also been reported. In this article, Setty et al prospectively evaluated the relationship between smoking status, duration, intensity, cessation, and exposure to secondhand smoke and incident psoriasis in a large cohort of women without a history of the disease. They found that increasing duration and intensity of cigarette smoking increased the risk of psoriasis in women. Women with more than 10 pack-years of smoking were found to have a risk of psoriasis that increased in a dose-dependent manner. Although the risk of psoriasis returned to that of never smokers after smoking cessation, this did not occur until 20 years later.[2] Ⓐ

Ustekinumab, a human monoclonal antibody against interleukins 12 and 23, has shown therapeutic potential for psoriasis. This study assessed the efficacy and safety of ustekinumab in psoriasis patients and assessed dosing intensification in partial responders.

This study showed that although treatment with ustekinumab every 12 weeks is effective for most patients with moderate-to-severe psoriasis, intensification of dosing to once every 8 weeks with ustekinumab 90mg might be necessary to elicit a full response in patients who only partially respond to the initial regimen.

Ustekinumab will clearly be a welcome addition to our therapeutic armamentarium for patients with severe psoriasis. The benefits are obvious. It is given infrequently (every 3 months) by subcutaneous injection, and therefore can, at least theoretically, be self-administered by the patient. It yields response rates at least as good and in most cases better than currently available therapies. In the current study, adverse events differed little between the active drug and placebo groups. The real question is: are we being lulled into a false sense of security? In Leonardi et al's study, the patients were followed for up to 76 weeks. We all know that psoriasis is a chronic disease, and many patients must be treated for a lifetime. Is 76 weeks really enough to judge the potential for long-term side effects of any drug? Interleukin 12 and interleukin 23 played an important role in immune surveillance. Can an analogy be drawn with cyclosporine, the most potent of the oral agents for psoriasis? Will long-term use of ustekinumab be associated with an increased risk of skin cancer or, even worse, systemic malignancy? These questions cannot be answered with a short-term study. Long-term surveillance is needed and a registry of patients receiving ustekinumab must be created. That will be more difficult to attain if the drug is approved for self-administration. An FDA Advisory Committee recommended, at its June 2008 meeting, that the drug be approved only for administration in a physician's office. Whether the full FDA follows this recommendation should be known by the time this commentary is published.[3] Ⓐ

Etanercept, a soluble tumor necrosis factor (TNF) receptor, has been shown to lessen disease severity in adult patients with psoriasis. This study assessed the efficacy and safety of etanercept in children and adolescents with moderate-to-severe plaque psoriasis.

This study showed that Etanercept significantly reduced disease severity in children and adolescents with moderate-to-severe plaque psoriasis.

Unfortunately, most pediatricians do not tend to think of psoriasis as a pediatric disease. It certainly is. One third of adults with psoriasis have onset at or before 16 years of age. In most cases, this presents as plaque psoriasis. Anyone with psoriasis knows how physically disfiguring it can be, leading to social stigmatization and psychological difficulties. Data also show that psoriasis is associated with other conditions, such as depression, obesity, myocardial infarction, and the metabolic syndrome. The FDA has not approved any systemic therapy for psoriasis for use in children and adolescents. Systemic therapies and phototherapies used in adults have limited application in children because of low tolerability, cumulative adverse effects, and teratogenicity. Part of the problem with systemic therapy in children is the lack of controlled trials of agents done in childhood age groups. This is why this report is so important.

Etanercept is a soluble TNF receptor fusion protein that antagonizes the effects of endogenous TNF. It is widely used to treat adult patients who have moderate-to-severe plaque psoriasis and is indicated for patients as young as 4 years of age with polyarticular juvenile rheumatoid arthritis. Adults treated with etanercept have shown benefits with respect to reduced disease severity, fatigue, and symptoms of depression. Overall, health-related quality of life in adult patients so treated seems to be significantly improved.

In the report of Paller et al, patients with plaque psoriasis who were aged 7 to 17 years were randomly assigned to a double-blind trial of 12 once-weekly subcutaneous injections of placebo or 0.8 mg of etanercept per kilogram of body weight, followed by 24 weeks of once-weekly open-label etanercept. At week 36, 138 patients underwent a second randomization to placebo or etanercept to investigate the effects of withdrawal and retreatment. At all phases of the study, significant improvement was seen with etanercept. Although there were four serious adverse events, mostly infections, all resolved without sequelae.

This randomized, placebo-controlled trial demonstrated that etanercept was effective in children and adolescents with moderate-to-severe plaque psoriasis. This commentary closes with a fast fact regarding a noted individual and his dermatologic disorder. Karl Marx was afflicted with a skin disorder that he claimed limited his productivity. He made no secret of having recurrent boils. According to a paper in the *British Journal of Dermatology* the underlying condition was hidradenitis suppurativa, in which the large sweat glands under the arms and in the groin become blocked and inflamed, and the skin eventually becomes thickened and scarred. Marx often complained in his letters that his skin affected the output and quality of his work. Hidradenitis suppurativa probably contributed to his poverty and to his frankly admitted low self-esteem and self-loathing.[4] Ⓐ

Adalimumab is a fully human monoclonal antibody that binds TNF, a key proinflammatory cytokine involved in the pathogenesis of psoriasis.

This study sought to evaluate clinical efficacy and safety of adalimumab for moderate to severe psoriasis and investigate continuous vs. interrupted therapy.

It showed that Adalimumab is efficacious and well-tolerated in the treatment of chronic plaque psoriasis.

Many articles have been published in recent years to study the efficacy of the new biologic agents in the treatment of psoriasis. Most of these have shown varying degrees of efficacy in trials in which the active drug was compared with an inactive placebo. Sadly lacking are comparative trials in which two active drugs are pitted against one another. Menter et al reports the results of a pivotal phase III clinical trial of adalimumab treatment in patients with moderate-to-severe psoriasis. The results were quite striking, with 71% of individuals treated with the standard dosing regimen achieving $\geq$75% improvement in the PASI score. These numbers are more impressive than have been reported with other self-administered biologic agents, though it is inappropriate to compare results in different studies, because clinical trials differ in key factors including inclusion and exclusion criteria, severity of disease, evaluator producibility, etc. However, comparative studies are not without their inherent faults. For example, I remember a study published several years ago in which oral fluconazole was shown to be as effective as griseofulvin in the treatment of tinea capitis. Unfortunately, the dose of griseofulvin in that study was significantly lower than I would personally use in clinical practice. Nevertheless, more such comparison studies will be welcome to demonstrate the superiority, safety, and cost effectiveness of the newer biologic agents against older, more traditional oral therapies for psoriasis.[5] Ⓐ

Previous studies of infliximab in psoriasis have demonstrated rapid improvement with induction therapy and sustained response with regularly administered maintenance therapy.

In this study the efficacy and safety of continuous (every-8-week) and intermittent (as-needed) maintenance regimens were compared.

This study showed that through week 50, response was best maintained with continuous infliximab therapy. Infliximab was generally well-tolerated in most patients.

This article by Menter et al confirms the high degree of efficacy of infliximab infusions in patients with moderate-to-severe psoriasis. Menter et al demonstrate that for sustained remission, every-8-week continuous maintenance therapy is superior to intermittent as-needed therapy.[6] Ⓐ

Evidence-Based References

1. Gelfand JM, Troxel AB, Lewis JD: The risk of mortality in patients with psoriasis: results from a population-based study, *Arch Dermatol* 143:1493-1499, 2007. Commentary by B.H. Thiers, M.D. Ⓐ
2. Setty AR, Curhan G, Choi HK: Smoking and the risk of psoriasis in women: Nurses' Health Study II, *Am J Med* 120:953-959, 2007. Commentary by B.H. Thiers, M.D. Ⓐ
3. Papp KA, Langley RG, Lebwohl M. Efficacy and safety of ustekinumab, a human interleukin-12/23 monoclonal antibody, in patients with psoriasis: 52-week results from a randomised, double-blind, placebo-controlled trial (PHOENIX 2), *Lancet* 371: 1675-1684, 2008. Commentary by B.H. Thiers, M.D. Ⓐ
4. Paller AS, for the Etanercept Pediatric Psoriasis Study Group: Etanercept treatment for children and adolescents with plaque psoriasis, *N Engl J Med* 358:241-251, 2008. Commentary by J.A. Stockman III, M.D. Ⓐ
5. Menter A, Tyring SK, Gordon K: Adalimumab therapy for moderate to severe psoriasis: A randomized, controlled phase III trial, *J Am Acad Dermatol* 58: 106-115, 2008. Commentary by B.H. Thiers, M.D. Ⓐ
6. Menter A, Feldman SR, Weinstein GD: A randomized comparison of continuous vs. intermittent infliximab maintenance regimens over 1 year in the treatment of moderate-to-severe plaque psoriasis, *J Am Acad Dermatol* 56:31-44, 2007. Commentary by B.H. Thiers, M.D. Ⓐ

SUGGESTED READINGS

Griffiths C, Barker J: Pathogenesis and clinical features of psoriasis, *Lancet* 370:263, 2007.

Griffiths C et al: Comparison of ustekinumab and etanercept for moderate-to-severe psoriasis, *N Engl J Med* 362:118-128, 2010.

Luba KM, Stulberg DL: Chronic plaque psoriasis, *Am Fam Physician* 73:636, 2006.

Menter A, Griffiths C: Current and future management of psoriasis, *Lancet* 370:272, 2007.

Paller AS et al: Etanercept treatment for children and adolescents with plaque psoriasis, *N Engl J Med* 358:3, 2008.

Schon MP, Boehncke WH: Psoriasis, *N Engl J Med* 353:1899, 2005.

Stern RS: Psoralen and ultraviolet A light therapy for psoriasis, *N Engl J Med* 357:682, 2007.

AUTHOR: **FRED F. FERRI, M.D.**

BASIC INFORMATION

DEFINITION

A state in which external reality is distorted by delusions and/or hallucinations (a delusion is a fixed false belief, and a hallucination is a false auditory, visual, olfactory, tactile, or taste perception).

SYNONYMS

Psychosis is a key finding in many mental illnesses, such as brief psychotic disorder, delusional disorder, schizoaffective disorder, schizophrenia, schizophreniform disorder, or shared psychotic disorder.

EPIDEMIOLOGY & DEMOGRAPHICS

One-year prevalence: 4.5 per 1000. The demographics of psychosis depend on the underlying disorder.

PHYSICAL FINDINGS & CLINICAL PRESENTATION

History
- Past medical history of any of the etiologies
- Use of possible offending medications
- Use of illicit substances
- Impaired function
- Intensive care unit stay >5 days

Physical examination
- If associated with a mood disorder, delusions or hallucinations are usually consistent with mood (e.g., auditory hallucinations in a depressed patient may tell the patient what a terrible person he is).
- Altered, disorganized thought pattern, which is usually reflected in disorganized speech (including word salad, thought blocking, rhyming, clang).
- Lack of insight into problems.
- Behavior is odd or unpredictable; patient may clearly be responding to internal stimuli.
- Signs of Parkinson's disease, dementia.

ETIOLOGY

- Pathophysiologically, an interaction among:
  1. Dopaminergic overactivity (particularly in the mesolimbic, nigrostriatal, and mesocortical systems)
  2. Environmental, social, or childhood factors
  3. Genetic predisposition
- Underlying mental disorder: schizophrenia, major depression, brief psychotic disorder, delusional disorder, schizoaffective disorder, schizophreniform disorder, shared psychotic disorder
- Underlying personality disorder: borderline, paranoid, schizoid, schizotypal
- Underlying medical condition: HIV/AIDS, Parkinson's disease, Huntington's disease, leprosy, malaria, sarcoidosis, systemic lupus erythematosus, prion disease, hypoglycemia, postpartum state, cerebrovascular event, temporal lobe epilepsy, brain neoplasm
- Medications: systemic steroids, anticonvulsants, antiparkinsonian medications, some chemotherapy, scopolamine
- Underlying dementia: Alzheimer's disease, Lewy body dementia
- Illicit drugs (usually with chronic use; can be with intoxication or withdrawal): LSD, PCP, cocaine, gamma-hydroxybutyrate (GHB; withdrawal), alcohol, amphetamines, marijuana
- Traumatic brain injury
- Intensive care unit stay: hypoxia, decreased cardiac output, infection, medications, sleep deprivation, alteration of diurnal cycle, sensory deprivation or overload, pain
- Emotional stress

DIAGNOSIS

WORKUP

Any workup would be to better assess etiology and would depend on the clinical situation.

LABORATORY TESTS

Consider checking chemistry panel (calcium), complete blood count, liver function tests, cortisol, HIV, rapid plasma reagin, thyroid-stimulating hormone, toxicology screen, lumbar puncture (LP).

IMAGING STUDIES

Consider chest x-ray examination (sarcoid), electroencephalography, head CT or MRI

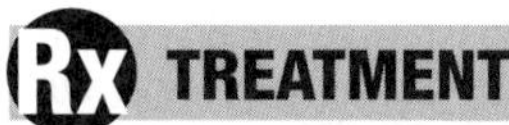

TREATMENT

NONPHARMACOLOGIC THERAPY

- Cognitive-behavioral therapy.
- Social and behavioral skills training.
- Training for self-management of disease.
- Aforementioned strategies favored over psychoanalytic techniques given the relative inability for abstract thought and lack of insight in psychotic patients.
- Family intervention, including education and strategies to reduce emotional expression.
- Counseling for substance abuse.

ACUTE GENERAL Rx

- Antipsychotics, such as haloperidol combined with promethazine, an antihistamine to reduce side effects; low doses should control first episode. Use with caution in elderly patients because adverse effects limit effectiveness.
- Benzodiazepines if agitation is severe.
- Discontinue offending medication if present.

CHRONIC Rx

Second-generation antipsychotics may reduce the incidence of tardive dyskinesia but may increase incidence of metabolic disorders compared with first-generation antipsychotics.

DISPOSITION

Prognosis varies according to etiology of psychosis. In general, the more severe and longer the psychotic episode, the worse the prognosis.

REFERRAL

Patient should be admitted for acute stabilization if actively psychotic to prevent harm to self and others as well as ensure administration of medications.

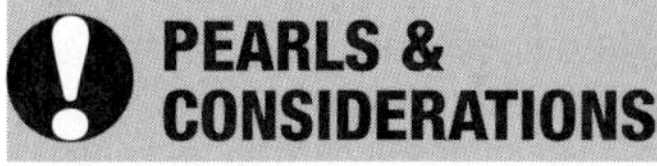

PEARLS & CONSIDERATIONS

- Delusions and/or hallucinations are hallmarks of psychosis.
- Rule out medical or drug causes of psychosis.
- Antipsychotics are the mainstay of acute and chronic treatment.
- Consider alternatives to antipsychotics in elderly or intellectually disabled patients.

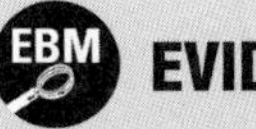

EVIDENCE

Please note: Complete text of EBM for this topic is available online.

Key trials and commentary:

The combination of haloperidol plus promethazine was compared with benzodiazepines (midazolam and lorazepam), olanzapine, and haloperidol alone. All treatments were effective at inducing sleep or tranquil states. However, the side effect profile of benzodiazepines or haloperidol alone, and the short duration of olanzapine, suggests the use of the combination of haloperidol plus promethazine.

Members of the general public often lack the knowledge and skills to intervene effectively to help someone who may be developing a psychotic illness before appropriate professional help is accessed.

These recommendations will improve the provision of first aid to individuals who are developing a psychotic disorder by informing the content of training courses.

This is an incredibly interesting, clever, and innovative study that came up with a comprehensive table that summarizes the three Delphi passes made by 51 clinicians, 45 consumers, and 61 caregivers. When I read the abstract I thought the results would be of immense practical help to family members and the public and, through them, to the ultimate targets—the patients. After all, knowledge about the Heimlich maneuver has been so widely disseminated that at least one patron and/or waiter in every restaurant knows how to do it. The problem here though is that the list is so long and detailed that it's unlikely that any trainer of potential first-responders would ever recall them all, far less be able to communicate them to others; there are simply too many methods that are too diverse. What is needed is a boiled-down version; perhaps using a mnemonic no longer than 10 letters or numbers to convey the essence of what constitutes first aid for persons suffering from a psychotic episode; nonetheless, it is a great first step, however impractical at present.[2] Ⓐ

The ACE project involved 62 participants with a first episode of psychosis randomly assigned to either a cognitive-behavioral therapy (CBT) intervention known as Active Cognitive Therapy for Early Psychosis (ACE) or a control condition known as Befriending. The study hypotheses were that: (1) treating participants with ACE in the acute phase would lead to faster reductions in positive and negative symptoms and more rapid improvement in functioning than Befriending; (2) these improvements in symptoms and functioning would be sustained at a 1-year follow-up; and (3) ACE would lead to fewer hospitalizations than Befriending as assessed at the 1-year follow-up.

This study showed that there is some preliminary evidence that ACE promotes better early recovery in functioning and this finding needs to be replicated in other independent research centers with larger samples.

Psychological treatments for early psychosis are important because they might either reduce the amount of medication used or they might enhance the effect on relapse. Here, this premier Australian center studied CBT against a simple supportive therapy (Befriending therapy). The CBT was not that much better than the less complex and targeted approach. Although a cynic could claim this as a negative study (again) of CBT, perhaps the more encouraging perspective is that both therapies worked and were helpful. So the real message here is that people benefit from psychological treatment—and not just medication— when they experience their first psychotic episode. This makes sense, because the episode is such a challenging experience.[3] Ⓐ

Compared with nonpsychotic depression, psychotic depression is associated with poor prognosis, increased mortality, and severe symptomatology. Although the incidence of psychotic depression is similar to that of schizophrenia, little is known about presentation, course, costs, and effects of treatment.

This study showed that psychotic depression is a common and costly condition, but with no accepted best practice guidance for its management. More attention needs to be focused on this largely under-researched group.

It is hard to believe that (1) no comparison of persons suffering first-break schizophrenia and depression has been undertaken to date and that (2) there is "no accepted best practice guidance" for management of the latter. I recall a statement made by the famous European psychiatrist Luc Ciompi, decades ago, saying that in Europe they treated first-episode psychosis of whatever type with antipsychotics and only after its resolution was antidepressive or antischizophrenic treatment decided on. This, of course, was completely at odds with our American belief that we could differentiate between the two immediately and target treatment accordingly. A finding that is startling in this contribution to the literature is that all who received ECT did well; why do the authors not see that as a "best practice" and why is there such continuing resistance to its use worldwide? In addition, although it is not surprising that those suffering depression had more attempts at self-harm, the authors and I are not clear why they had more "physical health problems." Also, I was not aware either that hospitalizations for psychotic depression were as lengthy and costly as those for schizophrenia. There is much to chew on here.[4] Ⓐ

The authors sought to compare the effects of olanzapine, quetiapine, and risperidone on neurocognitive function in patients with early psychosis.

This study showed that olanzapine, quetiapine, and risperidone all produced significant improvements in neurocognition in early-psychosis patients. Although cognitive improvements were modest, their clinical importance was suggested by relationships with improvements in functional outcome.

The putative advantages of the atypical antipsychotics over traditional antipsychotics have included the suggestion of greater improvement of neurocognitive function. In this trial, there were significant improvements in neurocognition in these early-psychosis patients studied with olanzapine, quetiapine, and risperidone. Improvements were associated with functional improvement also. The results could have been associated with improvement with their overall psychosis, but improvement in the CATIE trial was less than seen previously compared with traditional antipsychotics.

In another report, also from the CATIE trial, the authors compared neurocognitive improvements for the atypicals compared with the traditional antipsychotic perphenazine. In fact, after 18 months of treatment, neurocognitive improvement was greatest in the perphenazine group. The authors suggest that previous studies suggesting greater neurocognitive response to the atypicals may not translate to the type of everyday clinical practice in the CATIE trial, which should temper our enthusiasm for this type of putative advantage of the atypicals. However, they do caution that perphenazine was perhaps the most "atypical" of the traditional antipsychotics and this type of finding might not generalize to other traditional antipsychotics.[5] Ⓐ

Intensive early treatment for first-episode psychosis has been shown to be effective. It is unknown if the positive effects are sustained for 5 years.

This study sought to determine the long-term effects of an intensive early-intervention program (OPUS) for first-episode psychotic patients.

It showed that the intensive early-intervention program improved clinical outcome after 2 years, but the effects were not sustainable up to 5 years later. Secondary outcome measures showed differences in the proportion of patients living in supported housing and days in hospital at the 5-year follow-up in favor of the intensive early-intervention program.

This could be seen as a very discouraging study showing how bad a disease schizophrenia is. And it is, without a doubt. However, maybe there are some things to be learned here that are more positive. For instance, if patients who were treated early on and are now living in the community are better off, maybe we can find out why and apply that across the board to all, including those without early intervention. And maybe if we better understand what makes early-treated patients better for the first 2 years, we can transfer that to the next 3 or 5 or 10 years. Finally, the investigators did not look at the "unusual" individuals who did better, only the group in the aggregate; maybe seeing what worked for some would be transferable to the others. Maybe not, too, but I think given the power of the disease, it's worth a try.[6] Ⓐ

Cannabis use may be a risk factor for schizophrenia. Part of this association may be explained by genotype–environment interaction, and part of it by genotype–environment correlation. The latter issue has not been explored. We investigated whether cannabis use is associated with schizophrenia, and whether gene–environment correlation contributes to this association, by examining the prevalence of cannabis use in groups with different levels of genetic predisposition for schizophrenia.

This study showed that cannabis use was associated with schizophrenia but there was no evidence for genotype–environment correlation.

This study explores the relationship between cannabis use and genetic liability for schizophrenia. It is often considered that drugs of abuse bring on schizophrenia in people who are already vulnerable to develop psychosis. Several years ago another (Australian) group showed evidence for a gene-environment interaction in schizophrenia. This study refutes that proposition. Nevertheless, the higher rates of cannabis abuse in the schizophrenia sample compared with normal subjects again confirm the robust association between cannabis abuse and schizophrenia.[7] Ⓐ

Evidence-Based References

1. Huf G et al: Haloperidol plus promethazine for psychosis-induced aggression, *Cochrane Database Rev* 1, 2008. Commentary by J.A. Talbott, M.D. Ⓐ

2. Langlands RL, Jorm AF, Kelly CM. First Aid Recommendations for Psychosis: Using the Delphi Method to Gain Consensus Between Mental Health Consumers, Carers, and Clinicians. *Schizophr Bull* 2008; 34:435-443. Commentary by J.A. Talbott, M.D. Ⓐ

3. Jackson HJ, McGorry PD, Killackey E: Acute-phase and 1-year follow-up results of a randomized controlled trial of CBT versus Befriending for first-episode psychosis: the ACE project, *Psychol Med* 38:725-735, 2008. Commentary by P. Buckley, M.D. Ⓐ

4. Crebbin K, Mitford E, Paxton R: First-episode psychosis: an epidemiological survey comparing psychotic depression with schizophrenia, *J Affective*

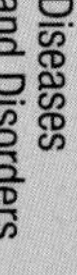

Disord 105:117-124, 2008. Commentary by J.A. Talbott, M.D. Ⓐ

5. Keefe RSE, Sweeney JA, Gu H: Effects of olanzapine, quetiapine, and risperidone on neurocognitive function in early psychosis: a randomized, double-blind 52-week comparison, *Am J Psychiatry* 164:1061-1071, 2007. Commentary by J.C. Ballenger, M.D. Ⓐ

6. Bertelsen M, Jeppesen P, Petersen L: Five-year follow-up of a randomized multicenter trial of intensive early intervention vs standard treatment for patients with a first episode of psychotic illness: the OPUS trial, *Arch Gen Psychiatry* 65:762-771, 2008. Commentary by J.A. Talbott, M.D. Ⓐ

7. Veling W, MacKenbach JP, Van Os J: Cannabis use and genetic predisposition for schizophrenia: a case–control study, *Psychol Med* 38:1251-1256, 2008. Commentary by P. Buckley, M.D. Ⓐ

SUGGESTED READINGS

Bertelsen M et al: Five-year follow-up of a randomized multicenter trial of intensive early intervention vs standard treatment for patients with a first episode of psychotic illness: the OPUS trial, *Gen Psychiatry* 65(7):762, 2008.

Byrne P: Managing the acute psychotic episode, *BMJ* 334(7595):686, 2007.

Cannon T et al: Prediction of psychosis in youth at high clinical risk: A multisite logitudinal study in North America, *Arch Gen Psychiatry* 65(1):28, 2008.

Schneider LS et al: Effectiveness of atypical antipsychotic drugs in patients with Alzheimer's disease, *N Engl J Med* 355(15):1525, 2006.

Tyrer P et al: Risperidone, haloperidol, and placebo in the treatment of aggressive challenging behaviour in patients with intellectual disability: a randomised controlled trial, *Lancet* 371:57, 2008.

AUTHOR: **MICHAEL K. ONG, M.D., PH.D.**

Pubertal Delay (ALG)

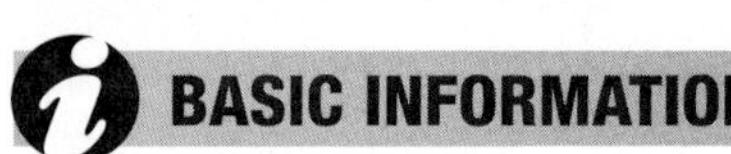

BASIC INFORMATION

DEFINITION

Pubertal delay refers to delayed development and maturation of the reproductive system. The diagnostic criterion is a delay of more than 2 to 3 standard deviations from the mean age of pubertal onset (see Figure 3-248 in Section III).

ICD-9CM CODES
259.0 Delay in sexual development and puberty, not elsewhere classified

EPIDEMIOLOGY & DEMOGRAPHICS

PREVALENCE: 2.5% of healthy adolescents have a diagnosis of pubertal delay using the statistical diagnostic criteria

GENETICS: Constitutional delay of puberty often runs in families. Pubertal delay occurs with some congenital syndromes, such as Prader-Willi syndrome and Noonan syndrome, and in patients with enzyme defects in sex steroid synthesis, as well as others.

PHYSICAL FINDINGS & CLINICAL PRESENTATION

Puberty is clinically delayed for girls if there is no evidence of breast development by 13 yr of age, absence of menarche by age 16 yr, or absence of menarche within 5 yr of pubertal onset. Puberty is clinically delayed for boys if there is no evidence of testicular enlargement by 14 yr of age, or >5 yr between start and completion of growth of genitalia.

ETIOLOGY

Puberty begins with increased pulsatile secretion of gonadotropin-releasing hormone (GnRH) from the hypothalamus, increased pituitary responsiveness to GnRH, secretion of gonadotropins, gonadal maturation, and increasing production of sex steroids. Increased concentration of sex steroids induces the development of secondary sexual characteristics, acceleration of growth, and fertility. Numerous causes can lead to pubertal delay, including chronic disease, normal variation, abnormal chromosomes, or other factors.

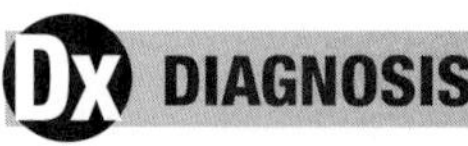

DIAGNOSIS

DIFFERENTIAL DIAGNOSIS

Normal or low serum gonadotropins
- Constitutional delay
- Hypothalamic dysfunction
  - Malnutrition or eating disorder
  - Strenuous exercise
  - Chronic illness
  - Severe obesity
  - Central nervous system tumors
- Hypopituitarism
  - Panhypopituitarism
  - Isolated gonadotropin deficiency
  - Kallman syndrome (associated with anosmia)
  - Growth hormone deficiency
- Hypothyroidism
- Hyperprolactinemia
  - Pituitary adenoma
  - Drug-associated (cannabis, cocaine)

Increased serum gonadotropins
- Turner syndrome (gonadal dysgenesis)
- Klinefelter syndrome
- Bilateral gonadal failure
  - Primary testicular failure
  - Anorchia
  - Premature ovarian failure
  - Resistant ovary syndrome
  - Irradiation, cytotoxic therapy
  - Trauma
  - Infections (e.g., mumps, orchitis)

Other conditions
- Anatomic abnormalities
- Prader-Willi syndrome
- Noonan syndrome
- Androgen resistance
- Steroidogenic enzyme defects

WORKUP

- Given the extensive differential diagnosis for pubertal delay, a systematic and focused approach is necessary. A careful history, including family history and social history, can identify eating and exercise habits, chronic illnesses, and parental history of pubertal delay.
- Growth measurement should include height and weight, a growth chart to assess rate of growth, and calculation of the sex-adjusted midparental height that represents the statistically most probable adult height for the child.
  - For boys add 2.5 inches (6.5 cm) from the mean of the parents' heights. For girls, subtract 2.5 inches (6.5 cm) from the mean of the parents' heights.
  - Physical exam can reveal signs of sexual maturation, stigmata of congenital syndromes, and nutritional status. Include neurologic exam (visual fields, ophthalmologic), thyroid, chest, heart, abdomen, and Tanner staging.

LABORATORY TESTS

- Serum gonadotropin levels (luteinizing hormone, follicle-stimulating hormone) distinguish disorders of congenital or acquired gonadal failure from other causes. By bone age 10 to 12 yr gonadal failure produces elevated levels of serum gonadotropins. If levels are low or normal, constitutional delay is the most frequent diagnosis.
- Chromosomal analysis if there is a suspicion of gonadal dysgenesis or Klinefelter syndrome.
- Screening studies include complete blood count, erythrocyte sedimentation rate, serum prolactin, serum thyroid-stimulating hormone.
- Endocrinologist may do further studies, including growth hormone testing, GnRH stimulation testing, and human chorionic gonadotropin stimulation with testosterone levels.

IMAGING STUDIES

Consider bone age (left hand and wrist film), which is delayed in constitutional delay and GnRH deficiency; CT or MRI of head to evaluate for tumors of pituitary or hypothalamus and absence of olfactory bulb and tract, which occurs in Kallman syndrome (absence of GnRH); and pelvic ultrasound.

TREATMENT

- Treat underlying cause if it is identified.
- Constitutional delay can be managed with reassurance that the delay will have no effect on final adult height or development. Short-term hormonal therapy can be used to hasten puberty if the delay is causing severe psychosocial difficulties. Monthly testosterone injections are used for boys who have begun pubertal development, while oral oxandrolone is used for boys who have not yet begun puberty. Potential side effects include premature epiphyseal closure and hepatic peliosis. Treatment is discontinued when endogenous hormone production has begun.
- Gonadotropin deficiency or hypogonadism requires lifelong sex steroid replacement.
- Psychosocial evaluation, support, and treatment as needed.

REFERRAL

Pediatric endocrinology

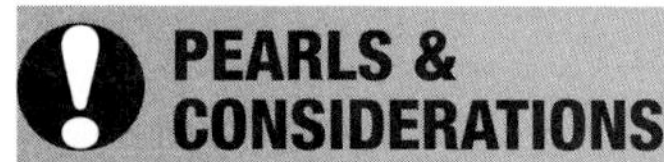

PEARLS & CONSIDERATIONS

COMMENTS

- Constitutional delay is the most common cause of pubertal delay and is often associated with a positive family history in parents and/or siblings, but other causes, such as Turner syndrome and systemic disorders, should be excluded.
- No studies reliably distinguish constitutional delay from gonadotropin deficiency.

PATIENT & FAMILY EDUCATION

- The Magic Foundation, a support group for patients and their families (http://www.magicfoundation.org)
- The American Academy of Family Physicians (http://www.aafp.org)
- American Academy of Pediatrics (http://www.aap.org)

SUGGESTED READINGS

Blondell RD et al: Disorders of puberty, *Am Fam Physician.* Available at http://www.aafp.org/afp/990700ap/209.html. Accessed July 2, 2007.

Master-Hunter T, Heiman D: Amenorrhea: evaluation and treatment, *Am Fam Physician* 73:1376-1382, 2006.

Rosen D, Foster C: Delayed puberty, *Pediatr Rev* 27:9, 2001.

Sedlmeyer IL, Palmort MR: Delayed puberty: analysis of a large case series from an academic center, *J Clin Endocrinol Metab* 87:1613-1620, 2002.

AUTHOR: **NIRALI BORA, M.D.**

BASIC INFORMATION

DEFINITION

Cardiogenic pulmonary edema is a life-threatening condition caused by severe left ventricular decompensation.

SYNONYMS

Cardiogenic pulmonary edema

ICD-9CM CODES

428.1 Acute pulmonary edema with heart disease

PHYSICAL FINDINGS & CLINICAL PRESENTATION

- Dyspnea with rapid, shallow breathing
- Diaphoresis, perioral and peripheral cyanosis
- Pink, frothy sputum
- Moist, bilateral pulmonary rales
- Increased pulmonary second sound, S_3 gallop (in association with tachycardia)
- Hypertension (unless in cardiogenic shock and hypotensive)
- Bulging neck veins

ETIOLOGY

Increased pulmonary capillary pressure attributable to:

- Acute myocardial infarction
- Exacerbation of chronic congestive heart failure
- Valvular regurgitation (e.g., mitral regurgitation)
- Ventricular septal defect
- Severe myocardial ischemia
- Mitral stenosis
- Other: cardiac tamponade, endocarditis, myocarditis, arrhythmias, cardiomyopathy, hypertensive crisis

Dx DIAGNOSIS

DIFFERENTIAL DIAGNOSIS

- Noncardiogenic pulmonary edema
- Pulmonary embolism
- Exacerbation of asthma
- Exacerbation of chronic obstructive pulmonary disease
- Sarcoidosis
- Pulmonary fibrosis
- Viral pneumonitis and other pulmonary infections

LABORATORY TESTS

- Arterial blood gases (ABGs): respiratory and metabolic acidosis, decreased Pao_2, increased Pco_2, low pH. (NOTE: The patient may initially show respiratory alkalosis as a result of hyperventilation in attempts to maintain Pao_2.)
- Measurement of plasma brain natriuretic peptide (elevated).

IMAGING STUDIES

- Chest radiograph:
  1. Pulmonary congestion with Kerley B lines; fluffy perihilar infiltrates in the early stages; bilateral interstitial alveolar infiltrates
  2. Pleural effusions
- Echocardiogram:
  1. Useful to evaluate valvular abnormalities, diastolic versus systolic dysfunction
  2. Can help differentiate cardiogenic versus noncardiogenic pulmonary edema
  3. Can also estimate pulmonary capillary wedge pressure and rule out presence of myxoma or atrial thrombus
- Right heart catheterization (selected patients): cardiac pressures and cardiogenic pulmonary edema reveal increased pulmonary artery diastolic pressure and pulmonary capillary wedge pressure (PCWP) $\geq$25 mm Hg

Rx TREATMENT

ACUTE GENERAL Rx

All the following steps can be performed concomitantly:

- 100% oxygen by face mask. Noninvasive ventilation (continuous positive airway pressure [CPAP]) or noninvasive intermittent positive-pressure ventilation induces a more rapid improvement in respiratory distress and metabolic disturbance than does standard oxygen therapy but has no effect on short-term mortality rate. Both CPAP and bilevel PAP systems can improve oxygenation and lower carbon dioxide tensions. Monitor ABGs; if marked hypoxemia or severe respiratory acidosis, intubate the patient and place on a ventilator. Positive end-expiratory pressure increases functional capacity and improves oxygenation.
- Furosemide: 1 mg/kg IV bolus (typically 40 to 100 mg) to rapidly establish diuresis and decrease venous return through its venodilator action; may double the dose in 30 min if no effect.
- Vasodilator therapy:
  1. Nitrates: particularly useful if the patient has concomitant chest pain.
     a. Nitroglycerin: 150 to 600 mcg SL or nitroglycerin spray may be given immediately on arrival and repeated multiple times if the patient remains symptomatic and blood pressure remains stable.
     b. 2% nitroglycerin ointment: 1 to 3 inches out of the tube applied continuously; absorption may be erratic.
     c. IV nitroglycerin: 100 mg in 500 ml of D_5W solution; start at 6 mcg/min (2 ml/hr).
  2. Nitroprusside: useful for afterload reduction in hypertensive patients with decreased cardiac index (CI).
     a. Increases the CI and decreases left ventricular filling pressure.
     b. Vasodilator and diuretic therapy should be tailored to achieve PCWP $\leq$18 mm Hg, right arterial pressure $\leq$8 mm Hg, and systolic blood pressure $>$90 mm Hg, systemic vascular resistance $>$1200 dynes/sec/cm^{-5}. The use of nitroprusside in patients with acute myocardial infarction is controversial because it may intensify ischemia by decreasing the blood flow to the ischemic left ventricular myocardium.
  3. Morphine: 2 to 4 mg IV, SC, or IM; may repeat q15min prn. It decreases venous return, anxiety, and systemic vascular resistance (naloxone should be available at bedside to reverse the effects of morphine if respiratory depression occurs). Morphine may induce hypotension in volume-depleted patients.
  4. Afterload reduction with angiotensin-converting enzyme (ACE) inhibitors. Captopril 25 mg PO tablet can be used for SL administration (placing a drop or two of water on the tablet and placing it under the tongue helps dissolve it); onset of action is $<$10 min, peak effect can be reached in 30 min. ACE inhibitors can also be given IV (e.g., enalaprilat 1 mg IV given q2h prn).
  5. Dobutamine: parenteral inotropic agent of choice in severe cases of cardiogenic pulmonary edema. It can be administered at a dosage of 2.5 to 10 mcg/kg/min IV. IV phosphodiesterase inhibitors (amrinone, milrinone) may be useful in refractory cases.

EBM EVIDENCE

Please note: Complete text of EBM for this topic is available online.

Key trials and commentary:

This study sought to compare continuous positive airway pressure (CPAP) and proportional assist ventilation (PAV) as modes of noninvasive ventilatory support in patients with severe cardiogenic pulmonary edema.

This study showed that in the present study PAV was not superior to CPAP for noninvasive ventilation in severe cardiogenic pulmonary edema with regard to either efficacy or tolerance.

The use of noninvasive ventilation has been shown to help reverse the oxygenation abnormalities of acute cardiogenic pulmonary edema faster than standard medical therapy and has been shown to produce similar improvements in short-term mortality rates. The best form of noninvasive ventilatory support is still under evaluation. This study compared the use of PAV with the more commonly used masked CPAP in the management of acute cardiogenic pulmonary edema. CPAP is certainly easier to use and most physicians are knowledgeable and comfortable with its use. For now, this noninvasive ventilatory support mode should be the preferred method of support, until there are data that another form of support yields better outcomes.[1] Ⓐ

Noninvasive ventilation (CPAP or noninvasive intermittent positive-pressure ventilation [NIPPV]) appears to be of benefit in the immediate treatment of patients with acute cardiogenic pulmonary edema and may reduce mortality. This study was conducted to determine whether noninvasive ventilation reduces mortality and whether there are important differences in outcome associated with the method of treatment (CPAP or NIPPV).

This study showed that in patients with acute cardiogenic pulmonary edema, noninvasive ventilation induces a more rapid improvement in respiratory distress and metabolic disturbance than does standard oxygen therapy but has no effect on short-term mortality.

This well-designed, multicenter, prospective, randomized trial evaluated standard medical therapy against two forms of positive pressure CPAP and NIPPV in the management of acute cardiogenic pulmonary edema. There has been some concern that the use of NIPPV might lead to more myocardial injury than standard medical management. These results found similar short-term mortality results, despite a more rapid improvement in oxygenation and metabolic improvement with NIPPV. There were no differences in adverse events supporting the safety of the two ventilatory strategies compared with the standard treatment. Based on this study, intensivists should feel comfortable using either CPAP or NIPPV to rapidly improve oxygenation parameters, reduce dyspnea, and improve gas exchange in patients with acute cardiogenic pulmonary edema.[2] Ⓐ

Evidence-Based References

1. Rusterholtz T, Bollaert P-E, Feissel M: Continuous positive airway pressure vs. proportional assist ventilation for noninvasive ventilation in acute cardiogenic pulmonary edema, *Intensive Care Med* 34: 840-846, 2008. Commentary by R.A. Balk, M.D. Ⓐ

2. Gray A, Goodacre S, Newby DE: Noninvasive ventilation in acute cardiogenic pulmonary edema. *N Engl J Med* 359:142-151, 2008. Commentary by R.A. Balk, M.D. Ⓐ

SUGGESTED READINGS

Gray A et al: Non-invasive ventilation in acute cardiogenic pulmonary edema, *N Engl J Med* 359:142, 2008.

Ware LB, Matthay MA: Acute pulmonary edema, *N Engl J Med* 353:2788, 2005.

AUTHORS: **DOUGLAS W. MARTIN, M.D., GAURAV CHOUDHARY, M.D.,** and **FRED F. FERRI, M.D.**

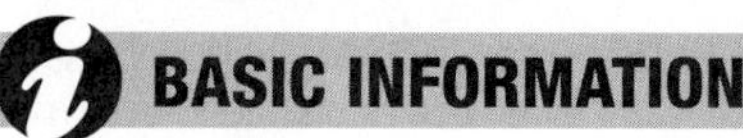

BASIC INFORMATION

DEFINITION

Pulmonary embolism (PE) refers to the lodging of a thrombus or other embolic material from a distant site in the pulmonary circulation.

SYNONYMS

Pulmonary thromboembolism
PE

ICD-9CM CODES

415.1 Pulmonary embolism and infarction

EPIDEMIOLOGY & DEMOGRAPHICS

- 650,000 cases of PE occur in the U.S. each year (increased incidence in women and with advanced age); annually, as many as 300,000 people in the U.S. die from acute PE, and the diagnosis is often not made until after autopsy. The incidence of PE is increasing with the increasing use of spiral CT scans, with a lower severity of illness and lower mortality, suggesting the increase is caused by earlier diagnosis.
- More than 90% of pulmonary emboli originate in the deep venous system of the lower extremities.
- Pulmonary thromboembolism is associated with >200,000 hospitalizations each yr in the U.S.
- 8% to 10% of victims of PE die within the first hr.

PHYSICAL FINDINGS & CLINICAL PRESENTATION

- Most common symptom: dyspnea (85%)
- Tachypnea (30%)
- Chest pain: may be nonpleuritic or pleuritic (infarction) (40%)
- Syncope (massive PE) (10%)
- Fever, diaphoresis, apprehension
- Hemoptysis (2%)
- Evidence of DVT may be present (e.g., swelling and tenderness of extremities)
- Cardiac examination: may reveal tachycardia (23%), increased pulmonic component of S_2, murmur of tricuspid insufficiency, right ventricular heave, right-sided S_3
- Pulmonary examination: may demonstrate rales, localized wheezing, friction rub

ETIOLOGY

- Thrombus, fat, or other foreign material
- Risk factors for PE:
  1. Prolonged immobilization, reduced mobility
  2. Postoperative state, major surgery
  3. Trauma to lower extremities, immobilizer or cast
  4. Estrogen-containing birth control pills, hormone replacement therapy
  5. Prior history of DVT or PE
  6. CHF
  7. Pregnancy and early puerperium
  8. Visceral cancer (lung, pancreas, alimentary and genitourinary tracts)
  9. Spinal cord injury
  10. Advanced age
  11. Obesity
  12. Hematologic disease (e.g., factor V Leiden mutation, antithrombin III deficiency, protein C deficiency, protein S deficiency, lupus anticoagulant, polycythemia vera, dysfibrinogenemia, paroxysmal nocturnal hemoglobinuria, acquired protein C resistance without factor V Leiden, G20210A prothrombin mutation)
  13. COPD, diabetes mellitus, acute medical illness
  14. Prolonged air travel
  15. Central venous catheterization

DIAGNOSIS

DIFFERENTIAL DIAGNOSIS

- Myocardial infarction
- Pericarditis
- Pneumonia
- Pneumothorax
- Chest wall pain
- GI abnormalities (e.g., peptic ulcer, esophageal rupture, gastritis)
- CHF
- Pleuritis
- Anxiety disorder with hyperventilation
- Pericardial tamponade
- Dissection of aorta
- Asthma

WORKUP

- Clinical assessment alone is insufficient to diagnose or rule out PE. It is also important to remember that no single noninvasive test has both high sensitivity and high specificity for PE. Consequently, in addition to clinical assessment, most patients would require an imaging test to diagnose PE. The Wells prediction rules can be used to estimate the probability of PE. Each of the following findings is assigned a score:
  1. Clinical signs/symptoms of deep vein thrombosis (score = 3.0)
  2. No alternate diagnosis likely or more likely than PE (score = 3.0)
  3. Heart rate >100/min (score = 1.5)
  4. Immobilization or surgery in last 4 weeks (score = 1.5)
  5. Previous history of DVT or PE (score = 1.5)
  6. Hemoptysis (score = 1.0)
  7. Cancer actively treated within last 6 months (score = 1.0)
- The probability of PE is high if total score is >6, moderate if 2-6; and low if <2.
- CT angiography is the most commonly used imaging modality.
- V/Q scan is reserved for patients with clinically significant contrast allergies or renal insufficiency.
- Pulmonary angiogram (when indicated) will confirm the diagnosis.
- Serial compressive duplex ultrasonography of lower extremities can be used in patients with "low-probability" lung scan and high clinical suspicion (see "Imaging Studies"). It is useful if positive, negative results do not exclude pulmonary embolism.
- A diagnostic approach to PE is described in Section III.

LABORATORY TESTS

- ABGs may reveal hypoxemia and respiratory alkalosis (decreased PaCO2 and PaCO2 and increased pH); normal results do not rule out PE.
- Alveolar-arteriolar (A-a) oxygen gradient, a measure of the difference in oxygen concentration between alveoli and arterial blood may be elevated. However, a normal A-a gradient does not rule out PE.
- Plasma D-dimer measurement: D-dimer assays by ELISA detect the presence of plasmin-mediated degradation products of fibrin that contain cross-linked D fragments in the whole blood or plasma. A normal plasma D-dimer level is useful to exclude PE in patients with a nondiagnostic lung scan and a low pretest probability of PE. However, it cannot be used to "rule in" the diagnosis because it increases with many other disorders (e.g., metastatic cancer, trauma, sepsis, postoperative state). Plasma D-dimer can also be used in conjunction with lower-extremity compression ultrasonography in patients with indeterminate V/Q and spiral CT scans. Absence of DVT and presence of a normal D-dimer level in these settings generally rules out clinically significant PE.
- Elevated cardiac troponin levels also occur in patients with PE because of right ventricular dilation and myocardial injury; therefore, PE should be considered in the differential diagnosis of all patients presenting with chest pain or dyspnea and elevated cardiac troponin levels.
- Elevated serum BNP levels in patients with acute PE may reflect RV overload.
- ECG is abnormal in 85% of patients with acute PE. Frequent abnormalities are sinus tachycardia; nonspecific ST-segment or T-wave changes; S-1, Q-3, T-3 pattern (10% of patients); S-1, S-2, S-3 pattern; T-wave inversion in V_1 to V_6; acute RBBB; new-onset atrial fibrillation; ST segment depression in lead II; right ventricular strain. A right ventricular strain pattern on ECG in patients with PG and normal blood pressure is associated with adverse short-term outcome and adds incremental prognostic value to echocardiographic evidence of right ventricular function.

IMAGING STUDIES

- Chest x-ray may be normal; suggestive findings include elevated diaphragm, pleural effusion, dilation of pulmonary artery, infiltrate or consolidation, abrupt vessel cut-off, oligemia distal to the PE (Westermark sign) or atelectasis. A wedge-shaped consolidation in the middle and lower lobes is suggestive of a pulmonary infarction and is known as "Hampton's hump."

- Lung scan (in patient with normal chest x-ray examination):
  1. A normal lung scan rules out PE.
  2. A ventilation-perfusion mismatch is suggestive of PE, and a lung scan interpretation of high probability is confirmatory (Fig. 1-268).
  3. If the clinical suspicion of PE is high and the lung scan is interpreted as low probability, moderate probability, or indeterminate, a pulmonary arteriogram is diagnostic; a positive arteriogram confirms diagnosis; a positive compressive duplex ultrasonography for DVT obviates the need for an arteriogram, because treatment with IV anticoagulants is indicated in these patients; the overall sensitivity of compressive ultrasonography for DVT in patients with PE is 29%, specificity 97%; adding ultrasonography in patients with a nondiagnostic lung scan prevents 9% of angiographies; however, this improvement in efficacy is achieved at the cost of unnecessary anticoagulant therapy in 26% of patients who have false-positive ultrasonography results.
- Angiography: pulmonary angiography is the gold standard; however, it is invasive, expensive, and not readily available in some clinical settings. False-positive pulmonary angiograms may result from mediastinal disorders such as radiation fibrosis and tumors.
- CT angiography is an accurate, noninvasive tool in the diagnosis of PE at the main, lobar, and segmental pulmonary artery levels. A major advantage of CT angiography over standard pulmonary angiography is its ability to diagnose intrathoracic disease other than PE that may account for the patient's clinical picture. It is also less invasive, less costly, and more widely available. Its major shortcoming is its poor sensitivity for subsegmental emboli. Gadolinium-enhanced magnetic resonance angiography (MRA) of the pulmonary arteries has a moderate sensitivity and high specificity for the diagnosis of PE; MRA is best reserved for selected patients when CT scan and/or lung scan are inconclusive and the risk of pulmonary angiography is high.
- ECG: Useful for identifying patients with PE who may have poor prognosis. Moderate or severe hypokinesis, persistent pulmonary hypertension, patent foramen ovale, and free-floating right heart thrombus are markers for increased risk of death or recurrent thrombosis. Such patients should be considered for thrombolysis or embolectomy.

Rx TREATMENT

NONPHARMACOLOGIC THERAPY

Correction of risk factors (see "Etiology") to prevent future PE

ACUTE GENERAL Rx

- Unfractionated heparin (UFH) by continuous infusion for at least 5 days or low-molecular-weight heparin (LMWH); many experts recommend a larger initial IV heparin bolus (15,000 to 20,000 U) to block platelet aggregation and thrombi and subsequent release of vasoconstrictive substances.
- Thrombolytic agents (urokinase, tPA, streptokinase): provide rapid resolution of clots; thrombolytic agents are the treatment of choice in patients with massive PE who are hemodynamically unstable and with no contraindication to their use. The use of thrombolytic agents in the treatment of hemodynamically stable patients with acute submassive PE remains controversial. Use of the thrombolytic agents alteplase (100 mg IV over 2-hr period) in normotensive patients with moderate or severe right ventricular dysfunction identified by ECG has been advocated by some physicians. Use of alteplase in conjunction with heparin has been shown to improve the clinical course of stable patients who have acute submassive PE without internal bleeding. Additional studies are needed to confirm these findings before recommending routine use of this therapeutic approach.
- Long-term treatment is generally carried out with warfarin therapy started on day 1 or 2 and given in a dose to maintain the INR at 2 to 3. Preliminary trials reveal that idraparinux, a long-acting inhibitor of activated factor X, given once weekly SC as a fixed dose for 3 or 6 mo has efficacy similar to that of heparin plus a vitamin-K antagonist in the treatment of DVT and causes less bleeding. However, in patients with PE, idraparinux was less efficacious than standard therapy.
- If thrombolytics and anticoagulants are contraindicated (e.g., GI bleeding, recent CNS surgery, recent trauma) or if the patient continues to have recurrent PE despite anticoagulation therapy, vena caval interruption is indicated by transvenous placement of a Greenfield vena caval filter.
- IVC filter may also be considered as an adjunct to anticoagulation in massive PE when thrombolytics cannot be used.
- Acute pulmonary artery embolectomy may be indicated in a patient with massive pulmonary emboli and refractory hypotension.

CHRONIC Rx

Elimination of risk factors (see "Etiology") and monitoring of warfarin dose with INR on a routine basis

DISPOSITION

- Mortality can be reduced to <10% by rapid and effective treatment.
- Mortality from recurrent pulmonary emboli is 8% with effective treatment and >30% in patients with untreated pulmonary emboli.

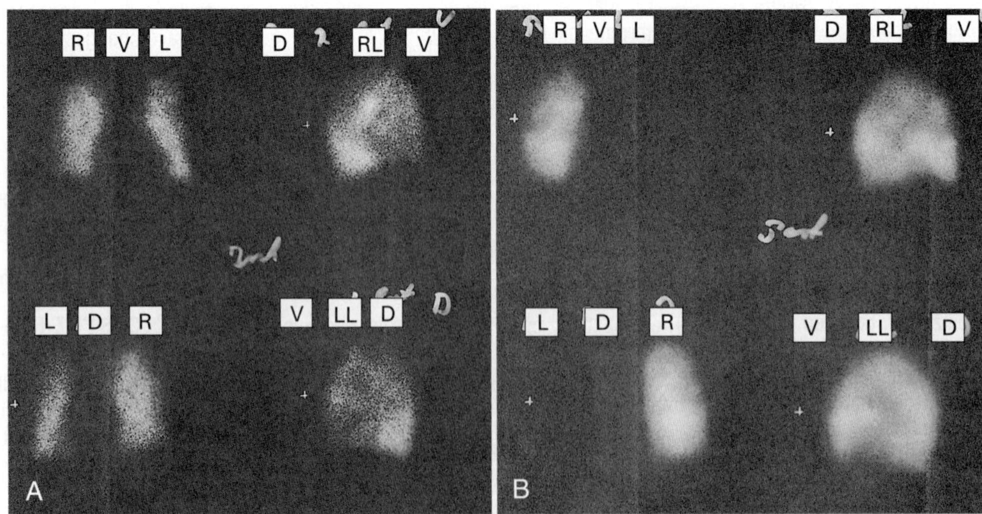

FIGURE 1-268 Ventilation-perfusion lung scan in massive pulmonary embolism. A, A normal pattern on the ventilation scan. **B,** The complete disappearance of the entire left lung from the perfusion scan indicates proximal occlusion of the left pulmonary artery. D, Dorsal; L, left; LL, left lobe; R, right; RL, right lobe; V, ventral. (From Crawford MH et al [eds]: *Cardiology,* ed 2, St Louis, 2004, Mosby.)

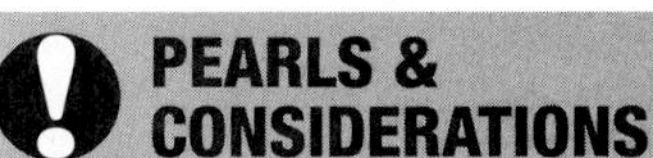

PEARLS & CONSIDERATIONS

COMMENTS

- In hemodynamically stable patients with pulmonary embolism, initial treatment with once-daily SC administration of the synthetic antithrombotic agent fondaparinux without monitoring has been reported to be at least as safe and as effective as adjusted-dose IV UFH. Several other trials have also demonstrated fixed-dose LMWH to be as effective and safe as dose-adjusted IV UFH for the initial treatment of nonmassive PE.
- For cancer-related venous thromboembolism, LMWH is preferred.
- The duration of oral anticoagulant treatment is 6 mo in patients with reversible risk factors and indefinitely in patients with persistence of risk factors that caused the initial PE.
- The risk for fatal PE is 0.19 to 0.49 events per 100 person-years for patients who have finished a course of anticoagulant therapy for a first episode of symptomatic venous thromboembolism. The case fatality rate for death from recurrent PE is 4% to 9%.

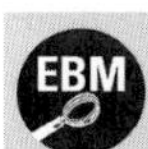

EVIDENCE

Please note: Complete text of EBM for this topic is available online.

Key trials and commentary:

Acute pulmonary embolism (APE) patients with right ventricular dysfunction (RVD) have a worse prognosis. This study assessed RVD, deciding the indexes correlating best with prognosis.

It showed that RVD was a discriminator for a poor prognosis in normotensive patients. Early detection of RVD (especially combination of RV dilation and IVC broadening, RVED/LVED >0.67 and/or SPAP >60 mm Hg) was beneficial for identifying high-risk patients. Hemodynamic instability, 14-day clinical outcomes, and SPAP independently predicted 3-month clinical outcomes.

Right ventricular dysfunction is a poor prognostic factor in APE. In this multicenter trial from China, RVD had double the mortality in normotensive patients with APE than no RVD. The ratio of RV and LV diastolic dimensions >67 and systolic pulmonary artery pressure (SPAP) >60 mm Hg on echo were independent risk factors for increased mortality. RV dilatation and IVC broadening were also found to be associated with a worse prognosis after 2 weeks of APE. These markers were better than worse RV systolic function as markers for a poor prognosis. At 3 months, SPAP elevation was still associated with poor outcome. The findings in Cochrane reviews do not see any evidence to support the practice of giving thrombolytics to patients with even massive PE, but improved outcome is seen in patients who got IVC filters placed when a residual deep venous thrombosis (DVT) was seen.[1] Ⓐ

Evidence-Based Reference

1. Zhu L, Yang Y, Wu Y: Value of right ventricular dysfunction for prognosis in pulmonary embolism, *Int J Cardiol* 127:40-45, 2008. Commentary by M. Ali Raza, M.D. Ⓐ

SUGGESTED READINGS

Chagnon I et al: Comparison of two clinical prediction rules and implicit assessment among patients with suspected pulmonary embolism, *Am J Med* 113(4): 269-275, 2002.

DeMonaco NA et al: Pulmonary embolism incidence is increasing with use of spiral computed tomography, *Am J Med* 121:611-617, 2008.

Douketis JD et al: The risk for fatal pulmonary embolism after discontinuing anticoagulant therapy for venous thromboembolism, *N Engl J Med* 147:766-774, 2008.

Konstantinides S: Acute pulmonary embolism, *N Engl J Med* 359:2806, 2008.

Qaseem A et al: Current diagnosis of venous thromboembolism in primary care: a clinical practice guideline from the American Academy of Family Physicians and the American College of Physicians, *Ann Intern Med* 146:454, 2007.

Stein PD et al: Challenges in the diagnosis acute pulmonary embolism, *Am J Med* 121:565-571, 2008.

Tapson VF: Acute pulmononary embolism, *N Engl J Med* 358:1037-1052, 2008.

Torbicki A, et al: Guidelines on the diagnosis and management of acute pulmonary embolism: the Task Force for the Diagnosis and Management of Acute Pulmonary Embolism of the European Society of Cardiology. *Eur Heart J* 29(18):2276-2315, 2008.

The van Gogh Investigators: Idraparinux versus standard therapy for venous thromboembolic disease, *N Engl J Med* 357:1094, 2007.

Vanni S et al: Prognostic value of ECG among patients with acute pulmonary embolism and normal blood pressure, *Am J Med* 122:257-264, 2009.

AUTHORS: **FREDERICK D. TRONCALES, M.D.**, **FRED F. FERRI, M.D.**, and **GAUGAV CHOUDHARY, M.D.**

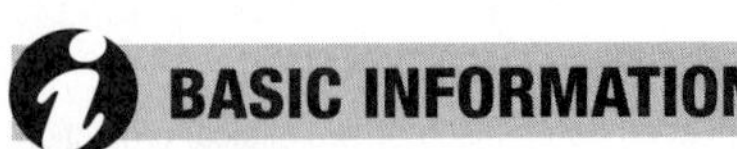

DEFINITION

Pulmonary hypertension (PH) is defined as mean pulmonary artery pressure (PAP) >25 mm Hg at rest or >30 mm Hg with exercise. Sustained elevation in PAP from increased pulmonary venous pressure, hypoxic pulmonary vasoconstriction, or increased flow is often referred to as *secondary pulmonary hypertension.*

SYNONYMS

Idiopathic pulmonary arterial hypertension (IPAH)
Secondary pulmonary hypertension

ICD-9CM CODES
416.0 Primary pulmonary hypertension
416.8 Secondary pulmonary hypertension

EPIDEMIOLOGY & DEMOGRAPHICS

- Idiopathic pulmonary arterial hypertension (IPAH) is rare, occurring in one to two cases per 1 million people per year, with an overall prevalence estimated at 1300 per 1 million.
- IPAH is more common in women than men (1.7:1), usually presenting in the third to fourth decades of life.
- Secondary pulmonary hypertension is more common than IPAH.
- Secondary pulmonary hypertension is the common pathophysiologic mechanism leading to cor pulmonale in patients with underlying pulmonary disease (e.g., chronic obstructive pulmonary disease [COPD], pulmonary embolism).

PHYSICAL FINDINGS & CLINICAL PRESENTATION

IPAH:
- Insidious, may go undetected for years
- Exertional dyspnea most common presenting symptom (60%)
- Fatigue and weakness
- Syncope, classically exertion related or after a warm shower with peripheral vasodilation
- Chest pain
- Hoarse voice from compression of recurrent laryngeal nerve by an enlarged pulmonary artery (Ortner's syndrome)
- Loud P2 component of the second heart sound and paradoxical splitting of second heart sound
- Right-sided S4
- Jugular venous distention
- Abdominal distention and ascites
- Prominent parasternal (right ventricular [RV]) impulse
- Holosystolic tricuspid regurgitation murmur heard best along the left fourth parasternal line that increases in intensity with inspiration
- Peripheral edema

SECONDARY PH: Similar to IPAH but from an underlying cause (e.g., left-sided congestive heart failure, mitral stenosis, COPD)

ETIOLOGY

- The etiology of IPAH is unknown. Most cases are sporadic, but there is a 6% to 12% familial incidence.
- PH is associated with several known risk factors: portal hypertension and liver cirrhosis, appetite-suppressant drugs (fenfluramine), hemoglobinopathies, and HIV disease. It is estimated that 10% of patients with hemoglobinopathies and 0.5% of patients with HIV infection develop moderate to severe pulmonary hypertension. Sickle cell disease and HIV disease may be the most common causes of pulmonary hypertension worldwide.
- Several genetic abnormalities have been associated with the familial form of IPAH, many of which are mutations in the genes that code for members of the tumor growth factor-beta family of receptors (BMPR-II, ALK-1) on chromosome 2q33.
- Familial pulmonary arterial hypertension (PAH) is an autosomal-dominant disease with variable penetrance, affecting only about 10% to 20% of carriers.
- Several factors play a role in the pathogenesis of PAH, including a genetic predisposition, endothelial cell dysfunction, abnormalities in vasomotor control, thrombotic obliteration of the vascular lumen, and vascular remodeling through cell proliferation and matrix production.
- New World Health Organization (WHO) grouping of PH (based on common clinical features)
  1. PAH
     - Idiopathic
     - Familial
     - Associated with collagen vascular diseases, congenital systemic to pulmonary shunts, HIV, portal hypertension, drugs, and toxins
     - Associated with significant venous or capillary involvement: pulmonary veno-occlusive disease, pulmonary capillary hemangiomatosis
     - Persistent PH of the newborn
  2. PH with left heart disease
     - Left-sided atrial, ventricular, or valvular heart disease
  3. PH associated with lung disease and/or hypoxemia
     - COPD, interstitial lung disease, sleep-disordered breathing, alveolar hypoventilation syndromes, long-term exposure to high altitude, neonatal lung disease, alveolar capillary dysplasia
  4. PH from chronic thrombotic and/or embolic disease
     - Pulmonary embolus (thrombus, tumor, parasites, foreign material)
  5. Miscellaneous: schistosomiasis, sarcoidosis, other

Dx DIAGNOSIS

- PAH is a hemodynamic diagnosis involving the detection of elevated pressure in the pulmonary arteries; characterization of this abnormality determines its etiology.
- Right-sided heart catheterization must be performed in all patients suspected of having PAH to establish the diagnosis and to assess pulmonary hemodynamics and acute vasoreactivity response testing.
- Idiopathic PAH is a diagnosis of exclusion.

DIFFERENTIAL DIAGNOSIS

The differential diagnosis is as listed under "Etiology."

EVALUATION

- Consists of establishing the diagnosis and etiology.
- ECG with Doppler technique is a noninvasive measure of systolic PAP. Common findings include tricuspid regurgitation, right heart enlargement, abnormal movement of septum and, rarely, pericardial effusion.
- ECG shows RV enlargement, strain pattern, and right axis deviation.
- Chest radiograph (Fig. 1-269) shows enlarged central pulmonary arteries and right heart enlargement.
- Pulmonary function tests may show obstructive (airway disease) or restrictive disease (parenchymal disease) depending on etiology. Diffusion capacity of carbon monoxide in the lung is reduced, which suggests diffusion defect.
- Right heart catheterization is required to assess pulmonary hemodynamics, exclude shunts and left heart disease, and perform acute vasoreactivity response testing.
- Screening for the presence of PAH with Doppler echocardiography is warranted in individuals with a known predisposing genetic mutation or first-degree relative with IPAH, connective tissue diseases (especially scleroderma), congenital heart disease with left-to-right shunt, or portal hypertension undergoing evaluation for orthotopic liver transplantation.
- Determining the degree of functional impairment, as assessed by the WHO functional classification system (Classes I-IV) and the 6-min walk test (6MWT), is a useful way to monitor disease progression and assess response to treatment.

LABORATORY TESTS

- Complete blood count is usually normal in PAH but may show secondary polycythemia.
- Arterial blood gases show low PO_2 and oxygen saturation.
- Overnight oximetry and sleep study to rule out sleep apnea or hypopnea.
- Other blood tests: antinuclear antibody (ANA), antineutrophil cytoplasmic antibodies (ANCA), and rheumatoid factor (RF) to screen for underlying connective tissue disease, HIV serology, liver function tests, and antiphospholipid antibodies.
- Ventilation perfusion lung scan has high sensitivity for chronic thromboembolic PAH. The diagnosis should be confirmed by pulmonary angiography, which has high specificity.

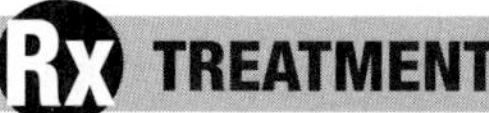

TREATMENT

- Most of the evidence in management of PAH is limited to IPAH. There is some evidence in treatment of PAH associated with connective tissue disease, especially scleroderma, and congenital heart disease. The recommendations for treating PAH associated with other causes are limited to case studies and expert opinions.
- There is some evidence for the use of advanced therapies for sarcoidosis-associated PH. The heterogeneity of sarcoid-associated PH complicates the interpretation.

NONPHARMACOLOGIC THERAPY

- Oxygen therapy to improve alveolar oxygen flow in both idiopathic and secondary PH.
- Avoidance of vigorous exercise and pregnancy.

GENERAL TREATMENT:

1. Diuretics (e.g., furosemide 40 to 80 mg qd) improve dyspnea by reducing afterload and peripheral edema.
2. Digoxin 0.25 mg qd has been used in patients with IPAH with inconclusive benefits.
3. Oral anticoagulation with warfarin B for IPAH, C for other PAH. Recommended INR is 1.5 to 2.5.

CHRONIC Rx

- Acute vasoreactivity response testing should be done in all patients at the time of right heart catheterization. Epoprostenol, adenosine, or nitric oxide is generally used to assess the response. A positive response is a fall in mean PAP of >10 mm Hg to a value of <40 mm Hg, with increased or unchanged cardiac output. Fewer than 10% of patients are responders.
- The positive responders may benefit from treatment with calcium channel blockers (diltiazem, amlodipine, or nifedipine). Verapamil is not recommended because of its negative inotropic effects. All patients should be reassessed in 6 to 8 wk to demonstrate sustained benefit from the calcium channel blocker.
- Nonresponders or nonsustained responders are eligible for selective pulmonary vasodilators.
- Prostanoids (epoprostenol, treprostinil, iloprost, and beraprost) act as potent vasodilators of pulmonary arteries and inhibitors of platelet aggregation. Ideal for class IV patients.
  1. Epoprostenol: IV formulation with very short half-life. Requires long-term IV access with associated risks of infection and thrombosis. Rapid tachyphylaxis, and therefore dose escalation, is seen. Common side effects include jaw pain, abdominal cramping, and diarrhea. Limited evidence exists for use in secondary PAH patients.
  2. Treprostinil: IV and SQ formulation with longer half-life. Main disadvantage is pain at SQ pump site (no long-term evidence for IV formulation).
  3. Iloprost: aerosolized formulation with short half-life requiring 6 to 8 treatments/day.
  4. Beraprost: PO formulation. Not approved in U.S.
- Endothelin receptor antagonists:
  1. Bosentan (nonselective endothelin A and B receptor blocker): oral pulmonary vasodilator, requires monthly liver function tests, often response delay by weeks. Thus, it is not an ideal starting therapy for WHO class IV patients. They are effective in class II and III patients.
  2. Sitaxsentan and ambrisentan (selective endothelin A receptor blockers): both with limited long-term evidence.
- Phosphodiesterase inhibitors: (sildenafil and tadalafil): act by increasing concentration of nitric oxide. Sildenafil is administered as 20 mg PO tid up to 80 mg PO tid. Tadalafil dose is 40 mg once daily. Highly effective in WHO class II patients, both in IPAH and scleroderma-associated PAH.
- Combination therapies: considered when there is no improvement or deterioration on monotherapy.
- Bosentan + inhaled iloprost (STEP trial) showed some benefit over monotherapy.
- IV epoprostenol + oral bosentan (BREATH-2 trial) did not show much difference.
- IV epoprostenol + oral sildenafil (PACES trial) showed benefit over monotherapy.
- Lung transplantation and heart-lung transplantation are other options in patients with end-stage class IV disease. Atrial septostomy may be performed as a bridge to transplant. The defect can be closed at the time of transplantation.
- Atrial septostomy is recommended for individuals with a room air SaO_2 >90% who have severe right-sided heart failure (with refractory ascites) despite maximal diuretic therapy, or who have signs of impaired systemic blood flow (such as syncope) from reduced left heart filling.
- Lung transplant recipients with IPAH had survival rates of 73% at 1 yr, 55% at 3 yr, and 45% at 5 yr.

TREATMENT OF SECONDARY PAH:

- Directed toward cause. At present the guidelines for treatment of PAH do not differentiate between IPAH and secondary PAH. The level of difference varies. Some situations merit mention.
- PAH with congenital heart disease: Eisenmenger's syndrome. Medical treatment generally ineffective. Heart-lung transplantation required in most patients.
- PAH with lung disease or hypoxia: oxygen therapy, control of primary disease process.
- PAH with scleroderma: selective pulmonary vasodilators are effective.
- PAH with HIV: control of viral load by highly active antiretroviral therapy.

FOLLOW-UP

Regular follow-up at 3-mo intervals with clinical assessment: WHO class and 6MWT, 6- to 12-mo objective assessment of RV function by ECG and cardiac catheterization studies.

DISPOSITION

- The 6MWT is predictive of survival in patients with idiopathic PAH. Drop in O_2 saturation >10% during the test increases mortality risk 2.9 times over a median follow-up of 26 mo.
- WHO class II and III patients with PAH have a mean survival of 3.5 yr.
- WHO class IV patients have a mean survival of 6 mo.

REFERRAL

If the diagnosis of IPAH is suspected, a consultation with a pulmonary specialist is recommended. Secondary causes of PH may require disease-specific consultations.

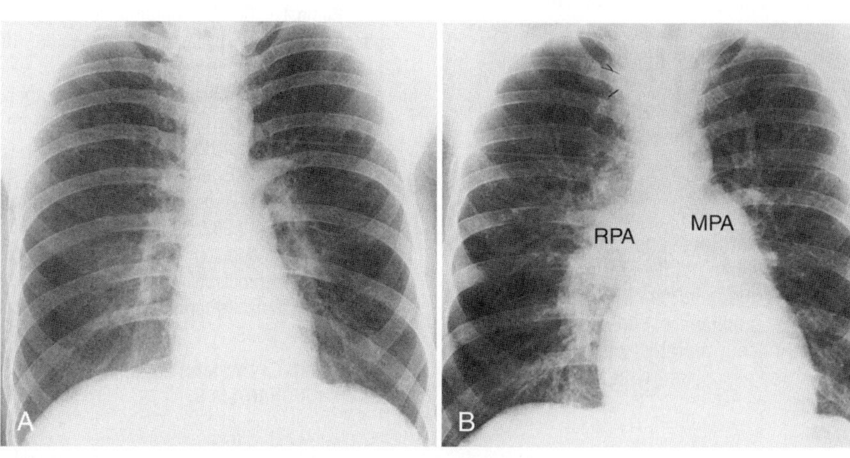

FIGURE 1-269 Progressive pulmonary arterial hypertension. This patient initially presented with a relatively normal chest radiograph **(A).** However, several years later **(B)** there is increasing heart size and marked dilation of the main pulmonary artery (MPA) and right pulmonary artery (RPA). Rapid tapering of the arteries as they proceed peripherally is suggestive of pulmonary hypertension and is sometimes referred to as pruning. (From Mettler FA [ed]: *Primary care radiology,* Philadelphia, 2000, WB Saunders.)

PEARLS & CONSIDERATIONS

- The exertional dyspnea of PAH is typically described by patients as being relentlessly progressive over several months to a year, often out of proportion to, or in the absence of, underlying heart or lung disease.
- Chest radiograph may reveal evidence of interstitial fluid within the lungs in cases of secondary PH. IPAH is not associated with infiltrates on chest radiograph.

COMMENTS

- RV systolic pressure (RVSP) as estimated by echocardiography is not a good indicator of the presence of PAH because RVSP increases with age and body mass index. Athletically conditioned men also have a higher resting RVSP. Thus, these measurements can be misleading.
- Abrupt development of pulmonary edema during acute vasodilator testing suggests pulmonary veno-occlusive disease or pulmonary capillary hemangiomatosis and is a contraindication to long-term vasodilator treatment.

FUTURE TREATMENTS

- Serotonin receptor modulators, platelet-derived growth factor, Rho kinase inhibitors
- Potential of cardiac MRI in assessment of RV function

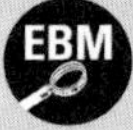

EVIDENCE

Please note: Complete text of EBM for this topic is available online.

Key trials and commentary:

Oral sildenafil and intravenous epoprostenol have independently been shown to be effective in patients with pulmonary arterial hypertension.

This study sought to investigate the effect of adding oral sildenafil to long-term intravenous epoprostenol in patients with pulmonary arterial hypertension.

It showed that in some patients with pulmonary arterial hypertension, the addition of sildenafil to long-term intravenous epoprostenol therapy improves exercise capacity, hemodynamic measurements, time to clinical worsening, and quality of life, but not Borg dyspnea score. Increased rates of headache and dyspepsia occurred with the addition of sildenafil.

Pulmonary arterial hypertension is a chronic debilitating disease without a cure. Current therapies include prostacyclines, endothelin receptor antagonists, and phosphodiesterase 5 inhibitors. Monotherapy with these drugs is effective in increasing exercise capacity and improving hemodynamics, but is still far from being satisfactory. There have been a number of small studies and two randomized trials with two drugs, neither with sildenafil. Although there have been a number of small trials with sildenafil as the single agent or as added to another drug, this trial is the first, large, randomized, placebo-controlled trial where sildenafil is added as a second drug in patients stabilized on an optimal dose of epoprostenol. The patients were symptomatic with 72% being New York Heart Association (NYHA) class III-IV. The dose of sildenafil was gradually increased over the 16-week course and showed, consistent with smaller, nonrandomized studies, that exercise capacity was increased but only in those whose baseline 6-minute walk distance was >325 m. In those whose baseline exercise capacity was <325 m, there was no improvement when sildenafil was added. The hemodynamic benefits in lowering pulmonary artery pressure and vascular resistance, and increasing cardiac output were small but significant. Even though the 6-minute distance was longer, the Borg dyspnea score was the same, suggesting that patients on both drugs could walk farther than those on epoprostenol alone but had the same degree of perceived exertion. One of the most important findings in this study is that the time to clinical worsening events in the group taking both drugs was increased. Because this was only a 16-week trial, certain etiologies of pulmonary artery hypertension such as HIV and unoperated congenital heart disease were not included, and sildenafil was added to stabilized patients already on epoprostenol, these findings should be confined to the population included in this study.[1] Ⓐ

Treprostinil, a long-acting prostacyclin analog, diminished the symptoms of pulmonary arterial hypertension (PAH) in controlled 12-week clinical efficacy studies. This retrospective, single-center, open-label study was designed to assess the efficacy of long-term, subcutaneously administered, treprostinil-based therapy alone or in combination with bosentan for the treatment of moderate-to-severe PAH.

This study showed that long-term treatment with subcutaneous treprostinil-based therapy improved functional parameters and hemodynamics in patients with moderate-to-severe PAH. In patients requiring combination therapy, the addition of oral bosentan to treprostinil-based therapy was safe, well-tolerated, and associated with further clinical improvements.

This study from Dr Benza's group in Alabama gives us more information about the long-term outcome of subcutaneous treprostinil therapy and combination therapy with bosentan.

There have not been many trials looking at long-term data with subcutaneous prostanoids in the U.S. Combination therapy data is also scant and even though most of the pulmonary hypertension centers are treating their New York Heart Association (NYHA) class II-IV patients with a combination of drugs, it is extremely important to have evidence supporting the practice and ensuring safety.[2] Ⓐ

Evidence-Based References

1. Simonneau G, for the PACES Study Group: Addition of sildenafil to long-term intravenous epoprostenol therapy in patients with pulmonary arterial hypertension: a randomized trial, *Ann Intern Med* 149:521-530, 2008. Commentary by M.D. Cheitlin, M.D., M.A.C.C. Ⓐ

2. Benza RL, Rayburn BK, Tallaj JA: Treprostinil-based therapy in the treatment of moderate-to-severe pulmonary arterial hypertension, *Chest* 134:139-145, 2008. Commentary by M. Ali Raza, M.D. Ⓐ

SUGGESTED READINGS

Archer S, Michelakis E: Phosphodiesterase type 5 inhibitors for pulmonary arterial hypertension, *N Engl J Med* 361:1864-1871, 2009.

Barnett CF et al: Pulmonary hypertension, an increasingly recognized complication of hereditary hemolytic anemias and HIV infection, *JAMA* 299(3):324-331, 2008

Chin K, Rubin J: Pulmonary artery hypertension, *J Am Coll Cardiol* 51:1527, 2008.

Ghofrani HA et al. Future perspectives for the treatment of pulmonary arterial hypertension, *J Am Coll Cardiol* 54(1 suppl): S108, 2009.

Hoeper MM et al. Diagnosis, assessment, and treatment of non- pulmonary arterial hypertension pulmonary hypertension, *J Am Coll Cardiol* 54(1 suppl): S85, 2009.

Lee SH, Rubin LJ: Current treatment strategies for pulmonary arterial hypertension, *J Intern Med* 258(3):199, 2005.

McLaughlin VV et al: Prognosis of pulmonary arterial hypertension: ACCP evidence-based clinical practice guidelines, *Chest* 126(suppl 1):S78, 2004.

Rubin LJ, Badesch DB: Evaluation and management of the patient with pulmonary arterial hypertension, *Ann Intern Med* 143:282, 2005.

Simonneau G et al: Addition of sildenafil to long-term intravenous epoprostenol therapy in patients with pulmonary arterial hypertension, *Ann Intern Med* 149:521-530, 2008.

AUTHORS: **DOUGLAS W. MARTIN, M.D.**, and **GAURAV CHOUDHARY, M.D.**

BASIC INFORMATION

DEFINITION

Pulseless electrical activity (PEA) is the absence of cardiac output in the presence of organized electrical activity.

SYNONYMS

Electromechanical dissociation (EMD)

ICD-9CM CODES
427.5 Cardiac arrest

EPIDEMIOLOGY & DEMOGRAPHICS

- Accounts for about 30% of cardiac arrest cases.
- Increasingly recognized as the cause of sudden cardiac death in patients with implantable cardioverter-defibrillators.

PHYSICAL FINDINGS & CLINICAL PRESENTATION

PRIMARY PEA:
- Organized electrical activity (not VT/VF)
- No detectable pulse

SECONDARY PEA: As in primary PEA and may also have:
- Bradycardia: drug overdose
- Tachycardia: hypovolemia, massive PE
- Decreased jugular venous pressure (JVP): hypovolemia
- Elevated JVP and no pulse with CPR: cardiac tamponade, massive PE, tension pneumothorax
- Absent unilateral breath sounds and tracheal deviation: tension pneumothorax
- Cyanosis: hypoxia

ETIOLOGY

PRIMARY PEA: Myocardial excitation and contraction uncoupling secondary to advanced heart muscle disease

SECONDARY PEA: Because of changes in the loading conditions of the heart, ischemia, myocardial depressants
- Massive MI
- Massive PE
- Hypovolemia
- Cardiac tamponade
- Tension pneumothorax
- Hypothermia, hypoxia, acidosis
- Hyperkalemia/hypokalemia
- Hypomagnesemia
- Drug overdose: β-blockers, calcium channel blockers, digoxin, tricyclic antidepressants

DIAGNOSIS

DIFFERENTIAL DIAGNOSIS

- Pseudo-PEA: weak ventricular contractions that do not produce a palpable pulse
- Idioventricular rhythm
- Postdefibrillation idioventricular rhythm
- Ventricular escape rhythm
- Bradyasystolic rhythm

WORKUP

- Stabilizing patient and workup to establish etiology should proceed simultaneously
- History, physical examination, laboratory tests, imaging studies

LABORATORY TESTS

- CBC
- Potassium, magnesium
- Arterial blood gas
- ECG (Fig. 1-270):
  Low voltage: tamponade
  Right heart strain: PE, pneumothorax
  Arrhythmias: MI, metabolic abnormalities, drug effects
  ST changes, Q waves: MI

IMAGING STUDIES

- Chest radiograph: rule out pneumothorax.
- Chest CT/pulmonary arteriogram: rule out PE.
- Echocardiogram: rule out pseudo-EMD, tamponade, valve dysfunction, and atrial myxoma.
- Abdominal radiograph: rule out rupture of abdominal aortic aneurysm.

Rx TREATMENT

Identifying and treating a reversible cause is critical.

NONPHARMACOLOGIC THERAPY

- Activate emergency medical service.
- Begin CPR.
- Intubate and ventilate.
- Obtain IV access.
- Fluid resuscitation.
- Continuous cardiac monitor.
- Confirm absence of blood flow with Doppler ultrasound, arterial line, or bedside echocardiogram.

ACUTE GENERAL Rx

- Treat specific cause if known.
- Epinephrine 1 mg IV push, q3 to 5 min, or vasopressin 40 U IV given once may be used to replace the first or second dose of epinephrine.
- If bradycardic: atropine 1 mg IV q3 to 5 min to a maximum of 3 mg.
- Normal saline (10 to 20 ml) should be given after the drug to improve distribution.
- Alternate routes of medication delivery for epinephrine, vasopressin, and atropine. May take 2 min for medication to reach the heart via these routes:
  1. Intraosseous: safe and effective, use same dose
  2. Tracheal tube: least preferred as plasma concentrations are variable. Epinephrine and atropine given at 2 to 2.5 × the IV dose in 10 ml of sterile water

PROBABLY HELPFUL: Sodium bicarbonate 1 mEq/kg in:
- Severe hyperkalemia
- Tricyclic antidepressant overdose
- Preexisting metabolic acidosis

DISPOSITION

Of hospitalized patients who develop PEA, <15% survive to discharge. Survival rates much lower in patients with prehospital PEA. Survivors often have poor neurologic outcomes.

REFERRAL

As needed for underlying condition

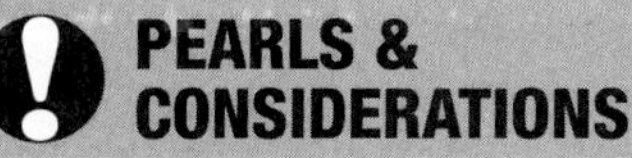

PEARLS & CONSIDERATIONS

- Some support the use of vasopressin instead of or in addition to epinephrine during resuscitation. Randomized trials show no benefit of vasopressin over epinephrine in survival to hospital discharge and suggest it may worsen neurological outcomes.
- Therapeutic hypothermia (32° to 34° C for 12 to 24 hr) may improve neurological outcomes and reduce mortality in unconscious cardiac arrest survivors.
- Prognosis may be guided by median nerve somatosensory-evoked potentials (72 hr) or EEG (24 to 48 hr) after cardiac arrest.

SUGGESTED READINGS

Arrich J, European Resuscitation Council Hypothermia After Cardiac Arrest Registry Study Group: clinical application of mild therapeutic hypothermia after cardiac arrest, *Crit Care Med* 35(4):1041, 2007

Gueugniaud P et al: Vasopressin and epinephrine vs. epinephrine alone in cardiopulmonary resuscitation, *N Engl J Med* 359(1):21, 2008.

Nadkarni VM et al. for the National Registry of Cardiopulmonary Resuscitation Investigators: First documented rhythm and clinical outcome from in-hospital cardiac arrest among children and adults, *JAMA* 295(1):50, 2006.

2005 International Consensus on Cardiopulmonary Resuscitation and Emergency Cardiovascular Care Science with Treatment Recommendations, Part 4: Advanced life support, *Circulation* 112(22 suppl): III-25, 2005.

AUTHOR: **S.K. AULAKH, M.D.**

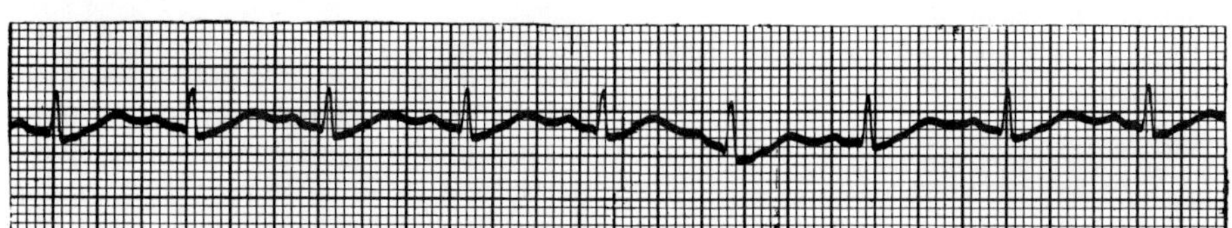

FIGURE 1-270 Sinus rhythm with electromechanical dissociation (EMD). Although the ECG showed sinus rhythm, the patient had no pulse or blood pressure. In this case the EMD was a result of depressed myocardial function after a cardiac arrest. (From Goldberg AL: *Clinical electrocardiography,* ed 5, St Louis, 1994, Mosby.)

Pyelonephritis (PTG)

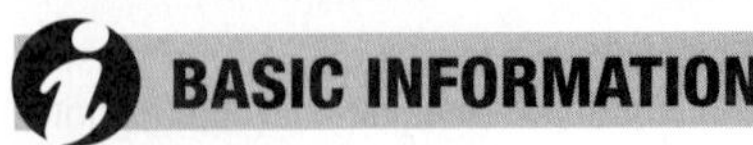

BASIC INFORMATION

DEFINITION

Pyelonephritis is an infection, usually bacterial in origin, of the upper urinary tract.

SYNONYMS

Acute pyelonephritis
Pyonephrosis
Renal carbuncle
Lobar nephronia
Acute bacterial nephritis

ICD-9CM CODES	
590.81	Pyelonephritis
599.0	Urinary tract infection
595.9	Cystitis

EPIDEMIOLOGY & DEMOGRAPHICS

INCIDENCE (IN U.S.): Extremely common
PREDOMINANT SEX: Female
PREDOMINANT AGE:

- Sexually active years in women
- Usually age >50 yr in men

GENETICS: Congenital urologic structural disorders may predispose to infections at an early age.

PHYSICAL FINDINGS & CLINICAL PRESENTATION

- Fever, rigors, chills
- Flank pain
- Dysuria
- Polyuria
- Hematuria
- Toxic feeling and appearance
- Nausea and vomiting
- Headache
- Diarrhea
- Physical examination notable
  1. Costovertebral angle tenderness
  2. Exquisite flank pain

ETIOLOGY

- Gram-negative bacilli such as *Escherichia coli* and *Klebsiella* spp. in more than 95% of cases
- Other, more unusual gram-negative organisms, especially if instrumentation of the urinary system has occurred
- Resistant gram-negative organisms or even fungi in hospitalized patients with indwelling catheters
- Gram-positive organisms such as enterococci
- *Staphylococcus aureus:* presence in urine indicates hematogenous origin
- Viruses: rarely, but these are usually limited to the lower tract

Dx DIAGNOSIS

DIFFERENTIAL DIAGNOSIS

- Nephrolithiasis
- Appendicitis
- Ovarian cyst torsion or rupture
- Acute glomerulonephritis
- Pelvic inflammatory disease
- Endometritis
- Other causes of acute abdomen
- Perinephric abscess
- Hydronephrosis

WORKUP

- No workup usually indicated in sexually active women
- Poorly responding infections, especially with azotemia and frank bacteremia
- Renal sonogram or CT scan to assess for underlying urologic pathology such as hydronephrosis (Fig. 1-271)
- Urologic imaging studies in all young men and boys
- Prostate assessment in older men

LABORATORY TESTS

- Complete blood count with differential
- Renal panel
- Blood cultures
- Gram stain of urine, urinalysis, and urine cultures
- Urgent renal sonography if obstruction or closed space infection suspected
- CT scans may better define the extent of collections of pus
- Helical CT scans excellent to detect calculi

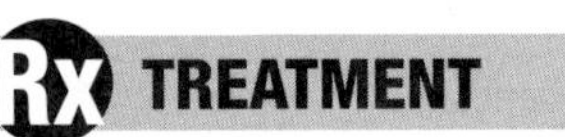

TREATMENT

ACUTE GENERAL Rx

- Hospitalization for:
  1. Toxic patients
  2. Complicated infections
  3. Diabetes
  4. Suspected bacteremia
- Keep patients well hydrated.
- IV fluids are indicated for those unable to take adequate amounts of liquids.
- Give antipyretics such as acetaminophen when necessary.

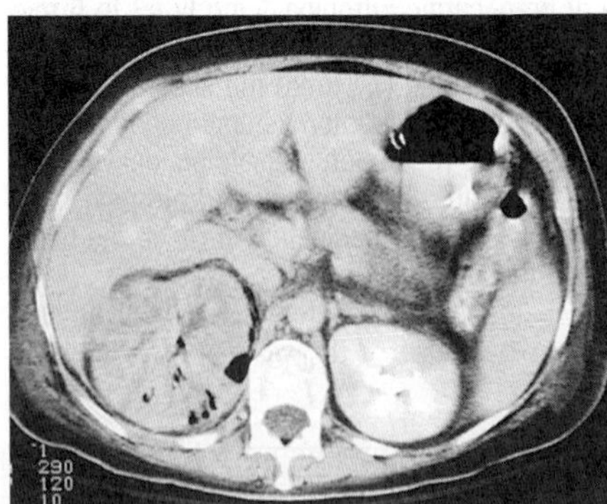

FIGURE 1-271 Emphysematous pyelonephritis in a patient with diabetes. The computed tomographic scan shows an enlarged, inflamed right kidney with air in the parenchyma and subcapsular space. (Courtesy of M. Bergeron, M.D. From Mandell GL et al: Principles and practice of infectious diseases, ed 7, Philadelphia, 2010, Elsevier.)

- Antibiotic therapy should be initiated after cultures are obtained and guided by the results of culture and sensitivity testing.
  1. Oral TMP-SMX DS (bid for 10 days) or ciprofloxacin (500 mg PO bid for 10 days): adequate for stable patients who can tolerate oral medications with sensitive pathogens
  2. TMP-SMX or ciprofloxacin IV for more toxic patients
  3. Ceftazidime 1 g IV q6-8h
  4. Aminoglycosides such as gentamicin (2 mg/kg IV load followed by 1 mg/kg IV q8h adjusted for renal function) added, but nephrotoxicity possible, especially in diabetics with azotemia
  5. Vancomycin 1 g IV q12h or linezolid to cover gram-positive cocci such as enterococci or staphylococci
  6. Ampicillin 1 to 2 g IV q4-6h to cover enterococci with an aminoglycoside for synergy
  7. Oral ampicillin or amoxicillin: no longer adequate for therapy of gram-negative infections because of resistance
- Prompt drainage with nephrostomy tube placement for obstruction.
- Surgical drainage of large collections of pus to control infection.
- Diabetic patients, as well as those with indwelling catheters, are especially prone to complicated infections and abscess formation.

CHRONIC Rx

- Repair underlying structural problems, especially when renal function is compromised.
  1. Reflux
  2. Obstruction
  3. Nephrolithiasis should be considered
- Patients with diabetes mellitus and indwelling urinary catheters are at particular risk of severe and complicated infections.
- When possible, remove catheters.

DISPOSITION

Most patients with uncomplicated pyelonephritis are now treated as outpatients or in short hospitalizations. Indications to admit a patient with pyelonephritis include pregnancy, suspected urinary obstruction, suspected renal abscess or perinephric abscess, bacterial sepsis, diabetes or other immunocompromised states, recurrent or refractory pyelonephritis, or infection with an unusual or antibiotic-resistant microorganism.

REFERRAL

- To a surgeon for correction of underlying urologic problems (e.g., reflux and hydronephrosis)
- To a pediatrician for detection of reflux to avoid recurrent urinary tract infection and loss of renal function
- To an internist for aggressive metabolic and urologic evaluation for patients with nephrolithiasis

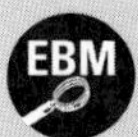

PEARLS & CONSIDERATIONS

Pyelonephritis is a systemic illness and may be a source of bacteremia and sepsis, especially if accompanied by urinary obstruction. Workup for abscess, obstruction, papillary necrosis, and other local complications of pyelonephritis should be initiated if the patient is septic, if patient does not respond to antibiotic therapy after 72 hr of treatment, or if infection is accompanied by worsening renal function.

EBM EVIDENCE

Please note: Complete text of EBM for this topic is available online.

Key trials and commentary:

This study sought to compare the efficacy of oral antibiotic treatment alone with treatment started parenterally and completed orally in children with a first episode of acute pyelonephritis.

It showed that treatment with oral antibiotics is as effective as parenteral then oral treatment in the management of the first episode of clinical pyelonephritis in children.

Historically, infants and children with febrile urinary tract infections were treated with parenteral antibiotics. The authors compare this therapy with oral antibiotics in the treatment of infants and children with pyelonephritis (confirmed by acute phase dimercaptosuccinic acid [DMSA] scan). The incidence of reflux in the study group was 21%, and 60% of the population was female. Even though 20% of the subjects were lost to follow-up, the table in the original article shows that treatment with oral antibiotics is not inferior to parenteral treatment. In those patients without dehydration and vomiting that preclude oral therapy, this approach could reduce costs and the stress associated with hospitalization.[1] Ⓐ

Evidence-Based Reference

1. Montini G, Toffolo A, Zucchetta P: Antibiotic treatment for pyelonephritis in children: multicentre randomised controlled non-inferiority trial. *BMJ* 335:386-388, 2007. Commentary by D.E. Coplen, M.D. Ⓐ

SUGGESTED READINGS

Bloomfield P et al: Antibiotics for acute pyelonephritis in children, *Cochrane Rev* 1:CD003772, 2005.

Hill JB et al: Acute pyelonephritis in pregnancy, *Obstet Gynecol* 105(1):18, 2005.

Pitukkijronnakorn S et al: Maternal and perinatal outcomes in pregnancy with acute pyelonephritis, *Int J Gynaecol Obstet* 89(3):286, 2005.

Scholes D et al: Risk factors associated with acute pyelonephritis in healthy women, *Ann Intern Med* 142(1):20, 2005.

Taskinen S, Ronnholm K: Post-pyelonephritic renal scars are not associated with vesicoureteral reflux in children, *J Urol* 173(4):1345, 2005.

AUTHORS: **GLENN G. FORT, M.D., M.P.H.,** and **DENNIS J. MIKOLICH, M.D.**

Pyoderma Gangrenosum

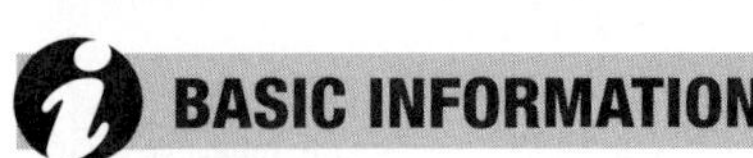

DEFINITION

Pyoderma Gangrenosum (PG) is a rare, noninfectious inflammatory skin disease that is characterized by a pustule that progresses to an ulcer or deep erosion with violaceous overhanging or undermined borders.

SYNONYMS

Classic Pyoderma Gangrenosum
Atypical Pyoderma Gangrenosum
Peristomal Pyoderma Gangrenosum

ICD-9CM CODES
686.01

EPIDEMIOLOGY & DEMOGRAPHICS

INCIDENCE: Unknown
PEAK INCIDENCE: Unknown
PREVALENCE: Between 3 and 10 per million cases or 1 in 100,000
PREDOMINANT AGE: Most common in ages 40 to 60 yr. Infants and adolescents are affected in 3% to 4% of cases.
PREDOMINANT SEX: Prevalence is roughly equal between the genders.
GENETICS: Unknown
RISK FACTORS: Autoimmune diseases particularly ulcerative colitis, Crohn's disease, and rheumatoid arthritis.

PHYSICAL FINDINGS & CLINICAL PRESENTATION

- Typically presents first as a pustule that rapidly and painfully progresses to an ulcer or erosion with tissue necrosis and enlargement of the area. The ulcer or erosion is surrounded by a violaceous or bluish border with erythema extending beyond that.
- Classic PG is commonly found on the legs. Atypical PG occurs more frequently in the upper extremities, head, and neck. Atypical PG lesions begin as pustules and become plaques that may be studded with pustules. Peristomal PG lesions appear similarly to classic PG lesions; however, they occur around surgically created stomas such as in Crohn's disease surgery.
- As many as 30% of lesions occur via pathergy. Pathergy is the development of skin lesions at the sites of injury, including minor injuries. Pathergy-induced PG lesions can be misdiagnosed as cellulitis. Surgery can also induce pathergy.
- Some patients only present with a single episode of PG, while others can have multiple episodes or a chronic relapsing course.
- Approximately 50% of PG sufferers have another underlying systemic disease, including inflammatory bowel disease, myeloproliferative diseases, or inflammatory arthritis.

ETIOLOGY

Exact etiology is unknown. However, neutrophilic infiltration causing cutaneous damage seems to be one part of the injury mechanism.

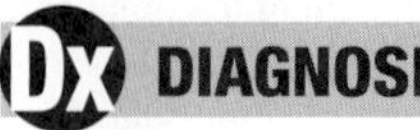

DIFFERENTIAL DIAGNOSIS

- Wegener's Granulomatosis
- Cellulitis
- Fungal infection
- Brown recluse spider bite
- Systemic vasculitis such as polyarteritis nodosa
- Malignancies such as squamous cell carcinoma, cutaneous lymphoma, and metastatic carcinoma
- Sporotrichosis
- Antiphospholipid syndrome
- Erythema nodosum

WORKUP

PG is a diagnosis of exclusion. In particular, workup should include biopsy of lesions and evaluation for associated underlying illness such as inflammatory bowel disease, arthritis, or malignancy. History, particularly as to the timing and progression of the lesions and inciting injury, is particularly important, as well as the physical appearance of the lesions.

LABORATORY TESTS

Skin biopsy is not diagnostic in itself because the findings are nonspecific. However, it may be helpful in excluding other diseases. Histopathologic findings show sterile dermal neutrophilia with or without mixed inflammation or lymphocytic vasculitis. Other appropriate testing could include rheumatologic lab work or colonoscopy to evaluate for inflammatory arthritis or IBD. Tissue cultures should also be performed to rule out bacterial or fungal causes.

IMAGING STUDIES

Consider colonoscopy and/or CT to evaluate for IBD.

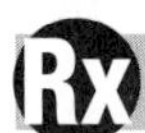 TREATMENT

The major treatment modalities revolve around wound care for the ulcers themselves, as well as either topical or systemic therapy.

NONPHARMACOLOGIC THERAPY

Surgery or aggressive debridement should be avoided in PG lesions because the surgery can cause pathergy and worsen the lesions . When needed, grafting should be performed concurrently with systemic immune-modulating therapy to prevent worsening of the lesions.

ACUTE GENERAL Rx

Care may include one or more of the following:

- Topical wound care and moist healing
- Topical high potency steroids (e.g., clobetasone)
- Topical immune modulators (e.g., tacrolimus)
- Systemic glucocorticoids (e.g., prednisone)
- Systemic immune modulators (e.g., cyclosporine)
- Antibiotics—only in cases of super-infection and if used with one of above
- Infliximab in patients with Crohn's disease
- Thalidomide

CHRONIC Rx

Similar to above except for longer durations or in pulse therapy

COMPLEMENTARY & ALTERNATIVE MEDICINE

Not relevant

DISPOSITION

Can be treated in both inpatient and outpatient settings depending on severity and therapeutic modalities

REFERRAL

- Dermatology
- Rheumatology
- Gastroenterology, especially in cases of IBD-related PG

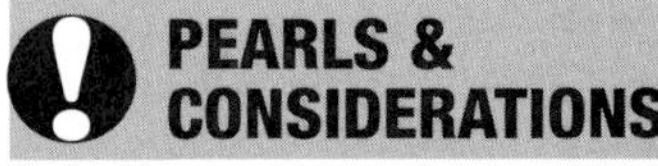

COMMENTS

PG is a diagnosis of exclusion and should only be made after other diseases in the differential have been ruled out and the patient has been evaluated for the associated diseases seen in more than 50% of cases.

PATIENT/FAMILY EDUCATION

Support for PG can often be found in the support groups for associated diseases, particularly Crohn's disease, Ulcerative colitis, and Erythema nodosum.

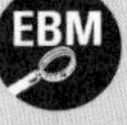 EVIDENCE

Reichrath et al in their recent systematic review suggest that combination treatment with systemic corticosteroids and cyclosporine in combination is effective and has the best evidence for treatment (grade B). Either systemic corticosteroids or cyclosporine used alone were also effective (grade B.) Infliximab as a first line, experimental, therapy was effective in patients who had associated Crohn's disease (grade B). Topical therapy (high potency steroids or tacrolimus) was appropriate in patients with early local disease (grade B). Other modalities such as thalidomide or intravenous immunoglobin therapy were also effective (in patients with no associated disease) (grade C). While surgical intervention should be avoided, when necessary it should be done in conjunction with systemic therapy (grade D).[1,2]

Evidence-Based References

1. Reichrath J et al: Treatment recommendations for pyoderma gangrenosum: an evidence-based review of the literature base on more than 350 patients, *J Am Acad Dermatol* 53:273-83, 2005.

2. Wollina U: Pyoderma gangrenosum—a review, *Orphanet J Rare Dis* 2(19), 2007.

SUGGESTED READINGS

Callen JP, Jackson JM: Pyoderma gangrenosum: an update, *Rheumatic Disease Clinics of North America* 33(4), 2007.

Ephgrave K: Extra-intestinal manifestations of Crohn's disease, *Surgical Clinics of North America* 87(3), 2007.

Habif T: Pyoderma Gangrenosum In Habif T: *Clinical Dermatology.* Edinburg, Mosby, 2004.

AUTHOR: **MICHAEL KLEIN, M.D.**

Pyogenic Granuloma (ALG)

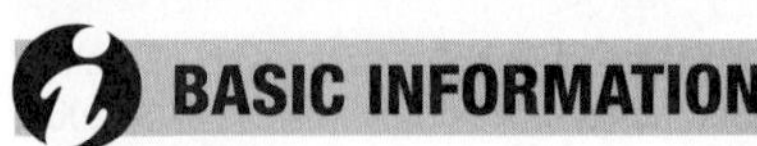

BASIC INFORMATION

DEFINITION

Pyogenic granuloma is a benign vascular lesion of the skin and mucous membranes. The lesions are caused by capillary proliferation, generally the result of trauma.

SYNONYMS

Granuloma pyogenicum
Tumor of pregnancy
Eruptive hemangioma
Lobular capillary hemangioma
Granulation tissue-type hemangioma

ICD-9CM CODES
686.1 Pyogenic granuloma

EPIDEMIOLOGY & DEMOGRAPHICS

- Common in children and young adults.
- Equally prevalent in males and females, with no racial or familial predisposition.
- Caused by trauma or surgery.
- Gingival lesions occur more frequently during pregnancy.

PHYSICAL FINDINGS & CLINICAL PRESENTATION

- Small (<1 cm), yellow to red, dome-shaped lesions (Fig. 1-272)
- May have surrounding scale at base
- Most commonly found on the head, neck, and extremities
- Often found on the gingiva during pregnancy (called *epulis*)
- Extremely friable, can easily ulcerate, and may bleed profusely with minor trauma

ETIOLOGY

Trauma causing focal capillary growth. These lesions are neither infectious in etiology nor granulomatous in histology.

DIAGNOSIS

DIFFERENTIAL DIAGNOSIS

- Amelanotic melanoma
- Bacillary angiomatosis
- Glomus tumor
- Hemangioma
- Irritated nevus
- Wart
- Kaposi's sarcoma

WORKUP

Diagnosis is based on clinical history and appearance. Generally begins with trauma followed by the development of an erythematous papule. The lesion tends to bleed easily and develops over several days to weeks.

LABORATORY TESTS

Pathologic examination should be performed after excision to rule out melanoma.

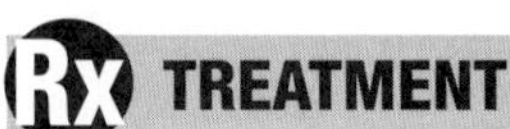

TREATMENT

ACUTE GENERAL Rx

- Excision: using 1% lidocaine for anesthesia, shave or curette at base and border. Follow with electrocauterization or cryotherapy.
- Pulsed-dye laser is also a safe and effective treatment modality.
- Pregnancy epulis generally resolve spontaneously after childbirth.

REFERRAL

Dermatology referral recommended if lesion recurs or multiple satellite lesions occur after excision.

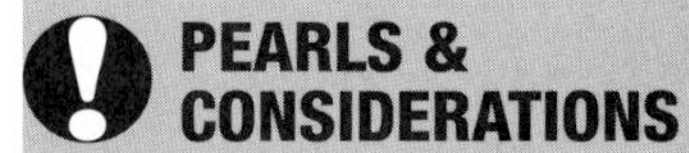

PEARLS & CONSIDERATIONS

COMMENTS

- Removal of entire lesion is essential because lesions may recur at the site of residual tissue.
- Patients and parents should be alerted to the possibility of recurrence after removal.
- Multiple satellite lesions occasionally develop near a primary pyogenic granuloma, usually after destruction of that lesion.

AUTHOR: **JENNIFER R. SOUTHER, M.D.**

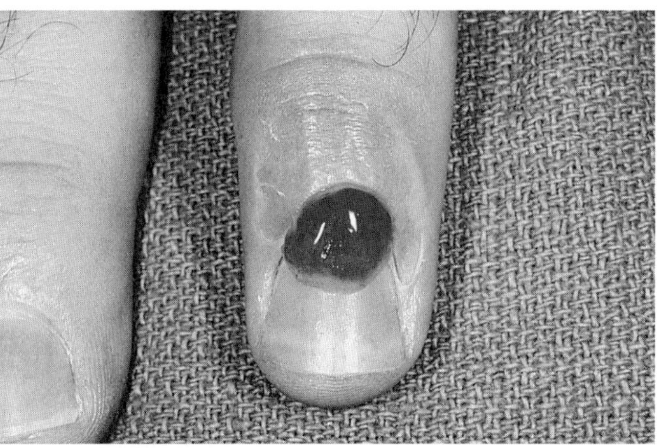

FIGURE 1-272 Pyogenic granuloma. Often the lesions have a collar or moat. (From Callen JP [ed]: *Color atlas of dermatology,* ed 2, Philadelphia, 2000, WB Saunders.)

BASIC INFORMATION

DEFINITION

Q fever is a systemic febrile illness caused by *Coxiella burnetii* that may be acute or chronic.

SYNONYMS

C. burnetii infection

ICD-9CM CODES

083.0 Q fever

EPIDEMIOLOGY & DEMOGRAPHICS

- *C. burnetii* is found worldwide.
- Common animal reservoirs are cattle, sheep, and goats.
- Pets such as cats, rabbits, pigeons are also reservoirs (169 cases were reported in the U.S. in 2006).
- A parturient cat caused an outbreak in Nova Scotia just by delivering in the same room as a card game.
- Most cases are found in individuals who have direct contact with infected animals (e.g., farmers, veterinarians) or who are exposed to contaminated animal urine, feces, milk, or placental tissues.
- Q fever is seen more often in men than in women (ratio of 3:1).
- Its incidence in the U.S. is increasing, with more than 30 cases recently reported in U.S. military personnel recently deployed to Iraq and Afghanistan.

PHYSICAL FINDINGS & CLINICAL PRESENTATION

- Acute Q fever presentation:
  Fever
  Pneumonia
  Hepatitis
  Meningoencephalitis
- Chronic Q fever presentation:
  Endocarditis
  Hepatitis
- Most common clinical symptoms:
  Chills
  Sweats
  Nausea
  Vomiting
  Cough, nonproductive
  Headache
  Fatigue
- Most frequent physical findings:
  Fever
  Inspiratory rales
  Purpuric rash
  Hepatomegaly
  Splenomegaly

ETIOLOGY

- Q fever is caused by the proteobacterium *C. burnetii.*
- *C. burnetii* is a gram-negative coccobacillus transmitted from arthropods to animals to human beings.
- The disease is acquired most often by inhalation of aerosols. In the lungs, it proliferates in macrophages and then gains access to the blood, producing a transient bacteremia. Thereafter it can invade many organs, most commonly the lungs and liver.
- There is an incubation period of 3 to 30 days before systemic symptoms manifest.
- Persons with abnormal heart valves, prosthetic valves, and endovascular grafts are at high risk of progression to chronic Q fever. This includes individuals with bicuspid aortic valves.

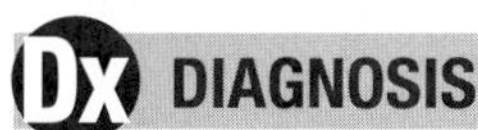

DIAGNOSIS

DIFFERENTIAL DIAGNOSIS

Q fever can have various presentations and must be in the differential diagnosis of fever, hepatitis, pneumonia, endocarditis, and meningitis.

WORKUP

- Complete blood count (CBC), erythrocyte sedimentation rate (ESR), and liver function tests
- Urinalysis
- Serology
- Chest radiograph

LABORATORY TESTS

In acute Q fever:

- CBC and white blood cell count are usually normal.
- Thrombocytopenia can occur (25%).
- Elevation of hepatic transaminases (two to three times the abnormal range) may be seen.
- Antibody detection by immunofluorescence assay is the most commonly used method because of its high sensitivity and specificity. Complement fixation (CF) shows a fourfold rise in titer between acute and convalescent samples.
- Polymerase chain reaction is a promising test for early detection of *C. burnetii* but test availability is limited to reference laboratories and research studies

In chronic Q fever (almost always endocarditis):

- ESR is elevated
- Anemia is present
- Microscopic hematuria
- Blood cultures are almost always negative
- MIF (microimmunofluorescence) titer of >1:800 to phase I antigen is diagnostic

IMAGING STUDIES

- Chest x-ray examination is abnormal, showing segmental lobe consolidation
- Pleural effusions (35%)

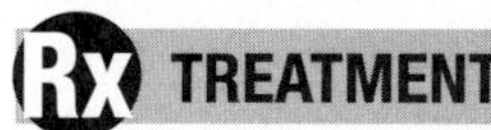

TREATMENT

NONPHARMACOLOGIC THERAPY

Oxygen as needed in patients with pneumonia

ACUTE GENERAL Rx

- Acute Q fever can be treated with doxycycline (100 mg bid) for 14 to 21 days *or*
- Erythromycin (500 mg qid) for 14 days *or*
- Ofloxacin 200 mg PO q8h for 14 to 21 days
- Hydroxychloroquine plus doxycycline for endocarditis associated with Q fever
- Fluoroquinolones are recommended for suspected meningoencephalitis

CHRONIC Rx

- Chronic Q fever is treated with a combination of two antibiotics, doxycycline 100 mg bid and rifampin 300 mg qd *or*
- Doxycycline 100 mg bid and ofloxacin 200 mg PO q8h *or*
- Doxycycline 100 mg bid and hydroxychloroquine 200 mg PO tid
- Duration of treatment: 2 to 3 yr

DISPOSITION

- Patients with acute Q fever respond well with antibiotics, with deaths rarely reported.
- Mortality rate in chronic Q fever endocarditis is high (24%). Most patients will need valve replacement surgery.

REFERRAL

Referral to an infectious disease expert is recommended in any cases of suspected acute or chronic Q fever.

REPORTING

Q fever has been a reportable disease in the U.S. since 1999. The CDC must be notified of cases.

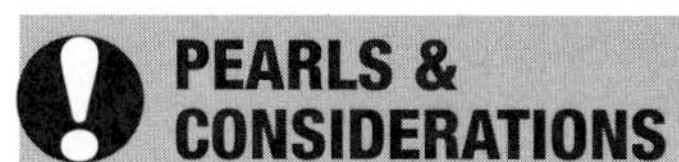

PEARLS & CONSIDERATIONS

COMMENTS

- An acellular (CMR) vaccine is available in the U.S. However, vaccines that are available in other countries such as Australia have been more thoroughly studied.
- Infected patients do not require specific isolation precautions.
- Q fever derived its name in 1935 from Derrick, who was suspicious of a new disease during a series of acute febrile illnesses in abattoir workers of Queensland, Australia, justifying the name of Q fever (for "query").

SUGGESTED READINGS

Carcopino X et al: Managing Q fever during pregnancy: the benefits of long-term cotrimoxazole therapy, *Clin Infect Dis* 45:548, 2007.

Hartzell JD et al: Q fever: epidemiology, diagnosis, and treatment, *Mayo Clin Proc* 83(5):574, 2008.

Healy B et al: The value of follow-up after acute Q fever infection, *J Infect* 52(4):e109, 2006.

Karakousis PC et al: Chronic Q fever in the US, *J Clin Microbiol* 44:2283, 2006.

McQuiston JH et al: National surveillance and the epidemiology of human Q-fever in the United States, 1978. 2004, *Am J Trop Med Hyg* 75(1): 2006.

Milazzo A et al: Q fever vaccine uptake in South Australian meat processors prior to the introduction of the National Q Fever Management Program, *Commun Dis Intell* 29(4):400, 2005.

Oren I et al: An outbreak of Q fever in an urban area in Israel, *Eur J Clin Microbiol Infect Dis* 24(5):338, 2005.

Raoult D et al: Natural history and pathophysiology of Q fever, *Lancet Infect Dis* 5(4):219, 2005.

Rolain JM, Raoult D: Molecular detection of *Coxiella burnetii* in blood and sera during Q fever, *QJM* 98(8):615, 2005.

Tissot-Dupont H et al: Role of sex, age, previous valve lesion, and pregnancy in the clinical expression and outcome of Q fever after a large outbreak, *Clin Infect Dis* 44:232, 2007.

Wagner-Wiening C et al: Serological diagnosis and follow-up of asymptomatic and acute Q fever infections, *Int J Med Microbiol* 40:294, 2006.

AUTHORS: **PATRICIA CRISTOFARO, M.D., GLENN G. FORT, M.D., M.P.H.**, and **DENNIS J. MIKOLICH, M.D.**

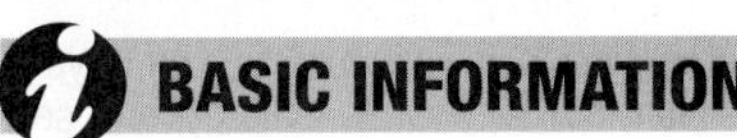

BASIC INFORMATION

DEFINITION

Rabies is a fatal illness caused by the rabies virus and transmitted to human beings by the bite of an infected animal.

SYNONYMS

Hydrophobia

ICD-9CM CODES
071 Rabies

EPIDEMIOLOGY & DEMOGRAPHICS

INCIDENCE (IN U.S.): Approximately two cases annually
PREDOMINANT SEX: Men are more commonly affected (70% of cases)
PREDOMINANT AGE: <16 yr and <55 yr

PHYSICAL FINDINGS & CLINICAL PRESENTATION

- Incubation period of 10 to 90 days
  1. Shorter with bites on the face
  2. Longer if extremities involved
- Prodrome
  1. Fever
  2. Headache
  3. Malaise
  4. Pain or anesthesia at exposure site
  5. Sore throat
  6. Gastrointestinal symptoms
  7. Psychiatric symptoms
- Acute neurologic period, with objective evidence of central nervous system involvement
  1. Extreme hyperactivity and bizarre behavior alternating with periods of relative calm
  2. Hallucinations, disorientation
  3. Seizures
  4. Paralysis
  5. Fear, pain, and spasm of the pharynx and larynx caused by drinking
  6. Coma, death

ETIOLOGY

- Rabies virus
- Cases in U.S. are associated with:
  1. Bats
  2. Raccoons
  3. Foxes
  4. Skunks
- In eight of the 32 cases occurring in the U.S. since 1980, there was a history of exposure to bats without a clinically evident bite or scratch.
- Imported cases are usually associated with dogs.
- Unusual acquisition:
  1. By organ transplantation
  2. By aerosol transmission in laboratory workers and spelunkers

Dx DIAGNOSIS

DIFFERENTIAL DIAGNOSIS

- Delirium tremens
- Tetanus
- Hysteria
- Psychiatric disorders
- Other viral encephalitides
- Guillain-Barré syndrome
- Poliomyelitis

WORKUP

- Rabies antibody
  1. Serum
  2. Cerebrospinal fluid (CSF)
- Viral isolation
  1. Saliva
  2. CSF
  3. Serum
- Rabies fluorescent antibody: skin biopsy from the hair-covered area of the neck
- Characteristic eosinophilic inclusions (Negri bodies) in infected neurons

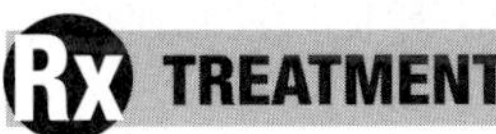

Rx TREATMENT

NONPHARMACOLOGIC THERAPY

- Isolation of the patient to prevent transmission to others
- Supportive therapy

ACUTE GENERAL Rx

- No known beneficial therapy. A recent report describes a 15-yr-old girl who survived rabies and had been treated with a combination of ketamine, midazolam, ribavirin, and amantadine. This therapy is worth trying despite the fact this is a single case report.
- Emphasis is placed on prophylaxis of potentially exposed individuals after an exposure:
  1. Thorough wound cleansing and irrigation of the wound as soon as possible
  2. Active and passive immunization most effective when used within 72 hr of exposure
- Vaccinations:
  1. Human diploid cell vaccine (HDCV) or rhesus monkey diploid cell vaccine (RVA), 1 ml IM (deltoid) on days 0, 3, 7, 14, and 28.
  2. Human rabies hyperimmune globulin (RIG) 20 IU/kg to persons not previously vaccinated. If anatomically feasible, the full dose should be infiltrated into the wound; any remaining volume should be given IM at a site separate from vaccine administration.
- Preexposure prophylaxis with HDCV or RVA (1 ml IM on days 0, 7, and 21 or 28) in individuals at high risk for acquisition:
  1. Veterinarians
  2. Laboratory workers working with rabies virus
  3. Spelunkers
  4. Visitors to endemic areas

DISPOSITION

Virtually always fatal

REFERRAL

- To infectious disease consultant
- To local health authorities

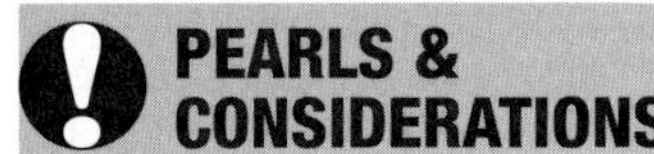

PEARLS & CONSIDERATIONS

COMMENTS

- Most cases in the U.S. are caused by:
  1. Bat bites, often after minimal contact and inapparent exposure to infected bat saliva
  2. Dog bites occurring outside the U.S.
- Rare cases can be transmitted by mucous membrane contact of aerosolized virus (caves, laboratory-acquired cases).

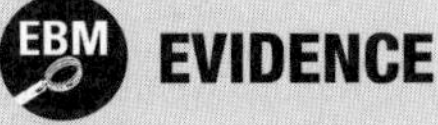

EVIDENCE

Studies conducted in the U.S. by the Centers for Disease Control and Prevention have documented that a regimen of one dose of RIG and five doses of HDCV over a 28-day period was safe and induced an excellent antibody response in all recipients.[1]

Rabies vaccines induce an active immune response with neutralizing antibodies. This antibody response requires 7 to 10 days to develop and usually persists for ≥2 yr.[2]

RIG provides a rapid, passive, short-lived immunity (half-life of approximately 21 days).[1]

Evidence-Based References

1. Centers for Disease Control and Prevention: Human rabies prevention—United States, 1999: recommendations of the Advisory Committee on Immunization Practices (ACIP), *MMWR Recomm Rep* 48:RR-1, 1999.
2. Dreesen DW et al: Two-year comparative trial on the immunogenicity and adverse effects of purified chick embryo cell rabies vaccine for pre-exposure immunization, *Vaccine* 7:397, 1989.

SUGGESTED READINGS

Hemachudha T, Wilde H: Survival after treatment of rabies, *N Engl J Med* 353(10):1068, 2005.

Rupprecht CE, Gibbons RV: Prophylaxis against rabies, *N Engl J Med* 351:2626, 2004.

Srinivasan A et al: Transmission of rabies virus from an organ donor to four transplant recipients, *N Engl J Med* 352:1103, 2005.

Willoughby RE et al: Survival after treatment of rabies with induction of coma, *N Engl J Med* 352:2508-2514, 2005

AUTHORS: **GLENN G. FORT, M.D., M.P.H.,** and **DENNIS J. MIKOLICH, M.D.**

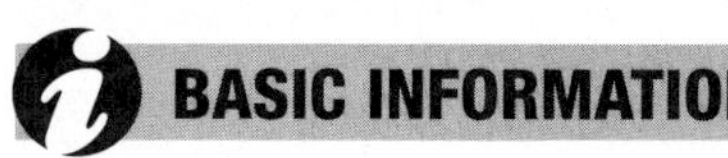

DEFINITION

Radiation that has the potential for injury is called ionizing radiation. Ionizing radiation is a form of radiant energy strong enough to penetrate the body and eject electrons from atoms that form our tissues, creating ions. The biological effects of ionizing radiation depends on the dose of exposure and may produce direct cell damage and death, or changes in the DNA without killing the cell, but these changes may result in neoplasm, and/or heritable DNA changes in reproductive cells.

TYPES OF RADIATION EXPOSURE:
- External irradiation: exposure to ionizing radiation from an external source.
- Contamination: radioactive materials in the form of gases, liquids, or solids are released into the environment and contaminate people through inhalation, ingestion, or skin exposure.
- Incorporation: uptake of radioactive materials by body cells, tissues, and target organs after contamination.

STOCHASTIC EFFECTS OF IONIZING RADIATION: These effects are related to the probability of a biologic effect caused by radiation and not a particular dose of radiation. The scientific community conservatively assumes that any amount of radiation may pose some risk for causing cancer and that the risk is higher for higher radiation exposures. A linear dose–response relationship is used to describe the relationship between radiation dose and the occurrence of cancer. Based on this assumption, any dose of ionizing radiation can alter DNA, causing mutations or carcinogenic changes that may take years to be expressed; hence, there is no safe dose per se and the risk is cumulative. This is mostly a concern with small, but prolonged or repetitive exposure to radiation, such as exposure from medical procedures.

DETERMINISTIC EFFECTS OF IONIZING RADIATION: These effects are dose related, where there is no effect from the exposure below a certain threshold, but there is a dose-dependent effect above it. The higher the dose, the more severe the effects, such as skin erythema, desquamation, and necrosis. The deterministic effects of radiation are consequence of a large exposure, such as the explosion from an atomic bomb or nuclear reactor.

UNITS OF RADIATION:
- Exposure is the measurement of the ionization produced in air by x or gamma rays, the most common form of human-related exposure. It indirectly measures a radiation field by its effect on air. The unit is the *Roentgen* (R), where 1 R = 2.58x10^{-4} Coulombs/kg of air.
- Absorbed dose is the concentration of energy absorbed by a particular tissue. The special unit is *gray* (Gy), where 1 Gy = 1 joule of energy concentrated in 1 kg of tissue. The older unit used was *rad*; 1 Gy = 100 rad.
- Equivalent dose is the estimate of the biologic potency a particular absorbed dose might have. It varies according to the type and energy of the ionizing radiation used. It is typically used for radiation protection purposes. The special unit is the *sievert* (Sv). For x and gamma rays, 1 Sv = 1 Gy. The older unit was *rem*; 1 Sv = 100 rem.
- Effective dose is a hypothetic uniform whole-body dose used to describe the risk of a nonuniform exposure. This allows for risk assessment and comparison between different exposures to particular areas of the body.
- To put things in perspective, the average person in the U.S. receives an effective dose of 3 mSv per year from naturally occurring sources such as radon gas and cosmic radiation.

SYNONYMS

For large exposures (deterministic effects of radiation):
Acute radiation syndrome
Radiation sickness
None, for chronic low-dose exposures (stochastic effects)

ICD-9CM CODES
990 Radiation exposure

PHYSICAL FINDINGS & CLINICAL PRESENTATION

Most of the data linking radiation to cancer comes from studies of the survivors of the atomic bombs. This data relates to a single, large exposure to radiation (>150 mSv). There is much less data on low exposures (<100 mSv) such as medical diagnostic imaging.

ACUTE RADIATION SYNDROME: This syndrome follows a large whole-body exposure of greater than 1 Gy in a very short period of time. The mean lethal dose of radiation required to kill 50% of human beings at 60 days (lethal dose 50/60) of whole-body radiation is between 3.25 and 4 Gy in persons managed without supportive care and 6 to 7 Gy when antibiotics and transfusion support are provided.

The sequence of events has four stages:
1. Stage 1 (prodromal phase): nausea, vomiting, and diarrhea usually occur in the first 48 hr, but may develop up to 6 days after exposure.
2. Stage 2 (latent phase): short period characterized by improvement of symptoms as the person appears to have recovered. Unfortunately this effect is transient, lasting for several days to 1 mo.
3. Stage 3 (manifest illness phase): third to fifth week after exposure. This stage is characterized by recurrence of prodromal symptoms along with additional features such as intense immunosuppression. It is the most difficult to manage. If the person survives this stage, recovery is likely. Signs and symptoms consist of abdominal pain, diarrhea, hair loss, bleeding, and infection. During this stage, several subsyndromes may coexist, overlap, or occur in sequence.
   - Cerebrovascular syndrome: fever, hypotension, ataxia, apathy, lethargy, and seizures. These symptoms may be observed in those receiving more than 20 to 30 Gy of radiation. The prodromal phase is characterized by disorientation, confusion, and prostration. The physical examination may show papilledema, ataxia, decreased or absent deep tendon reflexes, and corneal reflexes.
   - Cutaneous syndrome: caused by thermal or radiation burns and characterized by loss of epidermis, local edema, and increased risk for a compartmental syndrome.
   - Gastrointestinal syndrome: radiation induces loss of intestinal crypts and breakdown of mucosal barrier. These changes result in abdominal pain, anorexia, nausea, vomiting, diarrhea, and dehydration, and predispose patients to superinfection and sepsis.
   - Hematopoietic syndrome: lymphopenia is common and occurs before the onset of other cytopenias; pancytopenia with bleeding diathesis, and sepsis often follow. A predictable decline in lymphocytes occurs after irradiation. A potentially lethal exposure is characterized by a 50% decline in absolute lymphocyte count within the first 24 hr after exposure, followed by a further, more severe decline within 48 hr. The onset of cytopenias varies depending on the dose and dose rate. Granulocyte counts may transiently increase before decreasing in patients with exposure to <5 Gy. This transient increase before decline is known as an *abortive rise* and may indicate a survivable exposure.
4. Stage 4: recovery, lasting weeks to months.

The prognosis of the patient depends on the dose absorbed by the body and the availability of medical care. When expressed in grays:
- Exposure <1 Gy: almost certain survival, even without medical care
- Exposure 1 to 2 Gy: 90% survival with medical care
- Exposure 2 to 3.5 Gy: probable survival with medical care: At a dose of <3 Sv received, a lymphocyte count >1200/mm^3 at 48 hr confers a favorable prognosis; if the count is <1200/mm^3, a fatal dose is possible and more aggressive medical management is warranted. A drop in the number of granulocytes or platelets also portends a severe exposure.
- Exposure 3.5 to 5.5 Gy: 50% survival with medical care
- Exposure 5.5 to 10 Gy: probable death
- Exposure >10 Gy: certain death

CHRONIC LOW-DOSE EXPOSURE: In controlled conditions, an excess of cancers has never been detected in animals or humans for exposures below 100 mSv. However, there is some epidemiologic data from the survivors of the atomic bomb, of a small but significant risk at low exposures (5-100 mSv). Although the evidence is scant, the National Academies' Biological Effects of Ionizing Radiation 7th Report (BEIR VII Phase 2) stated that cancer risk decreases with age and is the highest in children and young adults. This is because children have more years of life during which a potential cancer can be expressed and they are inherently more radiosensitive, since they have a larger proportion of dividing cells (more DNA material). There is usually a long latent period between the exposure and the appearance of a neoplasm, from 2 yr to several decades.

Radiation exposure to the eye can damage the cells covering the posterior surface of the crystalline lens. Symptoms, which range from cloudy vision to severe impairment, can appear as soon as 1 to 2 yr after exposure. The exposure threshold is thought to be somewhere between 0 and 0.8 Gy[2].

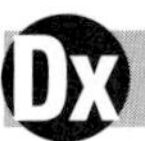

DIAGNOSIS

The key to making the diagnosis of acute radiation exposure and its associated injuries lies in a complete history including the timing of any radiation exposure, and if possible, the dose to which the patient was subjected.

For low-dose chronic exposures, it is currently impossible to determine whether a cancer is radiation induced. Cancers associated with high-dose exposure include leukemia, breast, bladder, colon, liver, lung, esophagus, ovarian, multiple myeloma, and stomach cancers. There is also a possible association between ionizing radiation exposure and prostate, nasal cavity/sinuses, pharyngeal and laryngeal, and pancreatic cancer.

The diagnosis of the lens and skin lesions will also rely on the history of exposure and the physical findings noted above.

ETIOLOGY

SOURCE OF RADIATION:

- Natural
  1. Radon (domestic and mining industry)
  2. Cosmic
  3. Terrestrial
- Ingested (accidentally from contaminated food)Industrial
  1. Medical imaging procedures (nuclear medicine and radiologic procedures). It is estimated that nearly 4 million Americans receive cumulative effective doses that exceed 20 mSv per year. The most common source is CT scans followed by nuclear imaging. A chest X-ray usually provides an effective dose of 0.04 mSv; this is in contrast to 0.7 mSv from a mammogram, 2-10 mSv from computed tomography, 7.5-57 mSv from coronary angioplasty and 14 mSv from a PET scan. Physicians should use these procedures appropriately and adequately inform patients of the risks of exposure to radiation.
  2. Consumer products
  3. Occupational (e.g., nuclear energy)
  4. Weapons

Rx TREATMENT

- For all accidental radiation contamination, the following decontamination steps are considered mandatory:
  1. Perform at site of exposure unless there is continued radiation exposure.
  2. Remove all clothing (and treat as radioactive waste). Providers should use strict isolation precautions, including donning of gown, mask, cap, double gloves, and shoe covers, when evaluating and treating contaminated patients.
  3. Wash patient with soap and water. Dispose of the used water as radioactive waste.
  4. Scrub any open wound.
  5. Depending on the situation, the regional emergency response system should be called for additional measures such as evacuation.
- Management of acute radiation syndrome:
  1. Establish IV access.
  2. Manage the airway if needed.
  3. Manage burns.
  4. Identify and treat other injuries.
  5. Provide analgesia.
  6. Give antiemetics (e.g., ondansetron).
  7. Manage bleeding and transfuse if necessary.
  8. Diagnose and treat sepsis. Administration of antibiotics reduces the mortality rate. In nonneutropenic patients, antibiotic therapy should be directed toward foci of infection and the most likely pathogens. Fluoroquinolones are useful for prophylaxis in neutropenic patients.
  9. Consider colony-stimulating factors (CSFs). In any adult with whole-body or significant partial body exposure $>$3 Gy, treatment with CSFs should be rapidly initiated (e.g., G-CSF or filgrastim, 5 mcg/kg of body weight per day). CSFs may be withdrawn when the absolute neutrophil count reaches a level greater than 1.0×10^9 after recovery from the nadir.
  10. Consider stem cell transplantation in people with exposure dose of 7 to 10 Gy who do not have significant burns or other major organ toxicity and who have an appropriate donor.
  11. Provide counseling; 75% of individuals exposed to nuclear weapon denotations exhibit some form of psychological symptoms, ranging from insomnia to difficulty concentrating and social withdrawal.
- Chronic low-dose exposures: Treatment of radiation-induced organ damages would not differ significantly from non–radiation-induced cancers, cataracts, or skin lesions. Prevention of radiation-induced injuries is paramount, carefully assessing the risks and benefits of each medical imaging procedure, especially in patients who have had these procedures repeatedly. Special attention should be placed in minimizing the dose of radiation utilized for each study.

PEARLS & CONSIDERATIONS

COMMENTS

- The three most useful elements for calculating the acute exposure dose are time to onset of vomiting, lymphocyte depletion kinetics, and the presence of chromosome dicentrics.
- A radiation casualty management software program (biologic assessment tool) is available at the Armed Forces' Radiobiology Research Institute website (http://www.afrri.usuhs.mil).
- Monitoring of lymphocyte count requires obtaining a CBC with leukocyte differential immediately after exposure, three times per day for the next 3 days, then twice per day for the following 6 days. CBC with differential should then be obtained weekly until a nadir in neutrophil count is defined.
- The chromosome aberration cytogenetic bioassay should be obtained from a qualified radiation cytogenetic biodosimetry laboratory.
- Ionizing radiation from medical imaging procedures is not negligible. Since the early 1980s, the per capita dose of radiation from medical imaging has increased by a factor of nearly 6.

EBM EVIDENCE

Please note: Complete text of EBM for this topic is available online.

Key trials and commentary:

Cardiac computed tomography (CT) angiography (CCTA) has emerged as a useful diagnostic imaging modality in the assessment of coronary artery disease. However, the potential risks of exposure to ionizing radiation associated with CCTA have raised concerns.

This study sought to estimate the radiation dose of CCTA in routine clinical practice as well as the association of currently available strategies with dose reduction and to identify the independent factors contributing to radiation dose.

This study showed that median doses of CCTA differ significantly between study sites and CT systems. Effective strategies to reduce radiation dose are available but some strategies are not frequently used. The comparable diagnostic image quality may support an increased use of dose-saving strategies in adequately selected patients.

This large multicenter study that included sites in Europe, North America, South America, the Middle East, Asia, and Australia, recorded and compared radiation doses in a large unselected group of patients. The median dose length product (DLP) of 885 mGy $\times$ cm, which results in an estimated effective radiation dose of 12 mSv, is comparable with that received from technetium-99m myocardial nuclear stress scans (11 mSv) and compares favorably with the 22 mSv received in thallium–201-based scans, but is more than twice the dose typically reported from uncomplicated diagnostic invasive angiography (5 mSv).

What is most remarkable (and has been picked up by the lay press) is that the median DLP per site ranged widely (sixfold!) between sites (from 331 to 2146 mGy × cm) largely because of variability in CT protocols, and differences in the CT units. This article serves to remind us to tailor the scan protocols to the individual patient (minimize scan length to the anatomy of interest, use tube modulation and prospective triggering acquisitions, and down-adjust kVp where appropriate, etc.).[1] Ⓐ

Evidence-Based Reference

1. Hausleiter J, Meyer T, Hermann F: Estimated radiation dose associated with cardiac CT angiography, *JAMA* 301:500-507, 2009. Commentary by S. Abbara, M.D. Ⓐ

SUGGESTED READINGS

Fazel R et al: Exposure to low-dose ionizing radiation from medical imaging procedures, *N Eng J Med* 361:849, 2009.

Health Physics Society: Health Physics Society fact sheet, http://www.hps.org/documents/meddiagimaging.pdf, accessed on September 28, 2009.

National Research Council: *Health risks from exposure to low level ionizing radiation*, BEIR VII. Washington, DC, 2005, National Academies Press.

Neriishi K et al: Postoperative cataract cases among atomic bomb survivors: radiation dose response and threshold, *Radiation Res* 168:404, 2007.

Wagner LK et al: Potential biological effects following high x-ray dose interventional procedures, *J Vas Interv Rad* 5:71, 1994.

Waselenko JK et al: Medical management of the acute radiation syndrome, *Ann Intern Med* 140:1037, 2004.

AUTHORS: **ROBERTO PACHECO, M.D.**, **FRED F. FERRI, M.D.**, and **WEN-CHIH WU, M.D.**

BASIC INFORMATION

DEFINITION

Ramsay Hunt syndrome is a localized herpes zoster infection involving the seventh nerve and geniculate ganglia, resulting in hearing loss, vertigo, and facial nerve palsy.

SYNONYMS

Herpes zoster oticus
Geniculate herpes
Herpetic geniculate ganglionitis

ICD-9CM CODES
053.11 Ramsay Hunt syndrome

EPIDEMIOLOGY & DEMOGRAPHICS

PREDOMINANT SEX: Equal sex distribution
PREDOMINANT AGE:
- Increasingly common with advancing age
- Rare in childhood

PHYSICAL FINDINGS & CLINICAL PRESENTATION

- Characteristic vesicles:
  1. On pinna
  2. In external auditory canal
  3. In distribution of the facial nerve and, occasionally, adjacent cranial nerves
- Facial paralysis on the involved side

ETIOLOGY

Reactivation of dormant infection with varicella-zoster virus after primary varicella

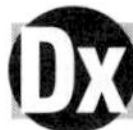

DIAGNOSIS

- Usually made by recognition of the clinical features detailed previously
- Viral culture and/or microscopic examination of specimens taken from active vesicles

DIFFERENTIAL DIAGNOSIS

- Herpes simplex
- External otitis
- Impetigo
- Enteroviral infection
- Bell's palsy of other etiologies
- Acoustic neuroma (before appearance of skin lesions)

The differential diagnosis of headache and facial pain is described in Section II.

WORKUP

If the diagnosis is in doubt, confirm varicella-zoster virus infection.

LABORATORY TESTS

- Viral culture of specimens of vesicular fluid and scrapings of the vesicle base
- Tzanck preparation, which may reveal multinucleated giant cells
- Direct immunofluorescent staining of scrapings

IMAGING STUDIES

MRI may demonstrate enhancement of the facial and vestibulocochlear nerves before appearance of vesicles.

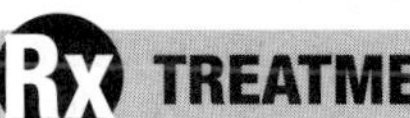

TREATMENT

ACUTE GENERAL Rx

- Prednisone (40 mg PO for 2 days, 30 mg for 7 days, followed by tapering course) is recommended by some authors.
- Acyclovir (800 mg PO five times qd for 10 days), famciclovir (500 mg tid for 7 days), or valacyclovir (1 g q8h for 7 days) may hasten healing.
- Analgesics should be used as indicated.

CHRONIC Rx

- Amitriptyline is effective in some cases of postherpetic pain.
- Other agents for postherpetic pain include gabapentin (Neurontin) and pregabalin (Lyrica).
- Narcotic analgesics may occasionally be necessary.

DISPOSITION

Recurrences are unusual.

REFERRAL

To otolaryngologist: patients with persistent facial paralysis for potential surgical decompression of the facial nerve

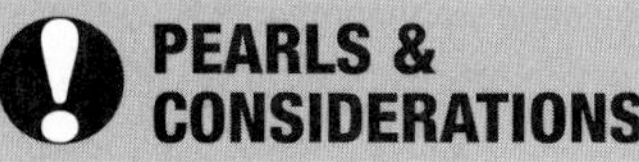

PEARLS & CONSIDERATIONS

COMMENTS

Immunodeficiency states, particularly HIV infection, should be considered in:
- Younger patients
- Severe cases
- Patients with a history of specific risk behavior

SUGGESTED READINGS

Diaz GA et al: A case of Ramsay Hunt-like syndrome caused by herpes simplex virus type 2, *Clin Infect Dis* 40(10):1545, 2005.

Kinishi M et al: Acyclovir improves recovery rate of facial nerve palsy in Ramsay Hunt syndrome, *Auris Nasus Larynx* 28(3):223, 2001.

Verm AM et al: Necrotizing herpetic retinopathy associated with Ramsay Hunt syndrome, *Arch Ophthalmol* 120(7):989, 2002.

AUTHORS: **GLENN G. FORT, M.D., M.P.H.,** and **DENNIS J. MIKOLICH, M.D.**

 BASIC INFORMATION

DEFINITION

Raynaud's phenomenon (RP) is a vasospastic disorder that produces an exaggerated response to cold temperatures and/or emotional stress, resulting in transient digital ischemia. It is characteristically manifest as a cold-induced, symmetric, sharply demarcated white or blue discoloration of the distal fingers or toes, followed by erythema at a variable time after rewarming.

SYNONYMS

Primary Raynaud's phenomenon or Raynaud's disease
Secondary Raynaud's phenomenon

ICD-9CM CODES
443.0 Raynaud's syndrome, Raynaud's disease, Raynaud's phenomenon (secondary)
785.4 If gangrene present

EPIDEMIOLOGY & DEMOGRAPHICS

- RP is classified clinically into primary or secondary forms and affects approximately 3% to 5% of the general population.
- Primary RP usually occurs between the ages of 15 and 25 yr. It is more likely to affect women than men (4:1) and appears to be more common in colder climates.
- 5% to 15% of patients with primary Raynaud's phenomenon develop a secondary cause later in the course of the disease (mostly a connective tissue disorder).
- Secondary RP tends to begin after age 35 to 40 yr.
- Secondary RP occurs in more than 90% of patients with scleroderma and in approximately 30% of patients with systemic lupus erythematosus or Sjögren's syndrome.
- There is also some suggestion that secondary RP may be associated with drugs (nicotine, caffeine, ergotamine, vinyl chloride) or trauma to the hands from vibrating tools such as jack hammers.

PHYSICAL FINDINGS & CLINICAL PRESENTATION

- The typical manifestation of RP is the biphasic color response of the digits to cold exposure and rewarming, which may or may not be accompanied by pain. RP most often affects the hand (Fig. 1-273).
  1. White (pallor) or blue (cyanotic) discoloration of the digit(s) resulting from vasospasm on cold or vibration exposure.
  2. Red (rubor) with or without pain and paresthesia when vasospasm resolves and blood returns to the digit.
- Color changes can sometimes be induced by placing the hand in an ice bath, although this is not recommended as a diagnostic maneuver because responses may be inconsistent even in patients with definite RP.
- Color changes are well delineated, symmetric, and usually bilateral, involving the fingers and toes. The index, middle, and ring fingers are commonly involved and the thumb is usually not.
- Fingertips are most often involved, but feet, ears, nose, tongue, and nipples can also be affected.
- Duration of attacks can range from seconds to hours and average 15 to 20 min.
- Chronic skin changes resulting from repeated attacks may include skin thickening and brittle nails. Ulcerations and, rarely, gangrene may occur.
- Physical examination should also include examination for symptoms associated with autoimmune disease, such as fever, rash, arthritis, dry eyes, dry mouth, myalgias, or cardiopulmonary abnormalities.

ETIOLOGY

- Primary RP can also be called idiopathic Raynaud's phenomenon, primary Raynaud's syndrome, or Raynaud's disease. It occurs in the absence of any associated disease.
- With primary RP, the possibility that another first-degree family member is affected is reported as approximately 25%.
- Secondary RP is associated with an underlying pathologic condition or disorder, use of certain drugs, or related occupation. Secondary RP is associated with:
  1. CREST syndrome (calcinosis, RP, esophageal involvement, sclerodactyly, and telangiectasia)
  2. Scleroderma, Sjögren's syndrome
  3. Mixed connective tissue disease, polymyositis, and dermatomyositis
  4. Systemic lupus erythematosus, arteritis
  5. Rheumatoid arthritis
  6. Thromboangiitis obliterans (Buerger's disease)
  7. Drugs (beta-blockers, ergotamine, methysergide, vinblastine, bleomycin, oral contraceptives, nicotine, clonidine, cocaine, caffeine, vinyl chloride)
  8. Hematologic disorders (polycythemia, cryoglobulinemia, cold agglutinins, paraproteinemia)
  9. Carpal tunnel syndrome
  10. Use of tools that vibrate
  11. Endocrine disorders (hypothyroidism, carcinoid syndrome, metabolic syndrome)
  12. Estrogen replacement therapy without progesterone
  13. Hypercoagulable states, protein C, protein S, antithrombin III deficiency, factor V Leiden deficiency, and anti-phospholipid syndrome
  14. Poliomyelitis is a rare cause
  15. Primary biliary cirrhosis

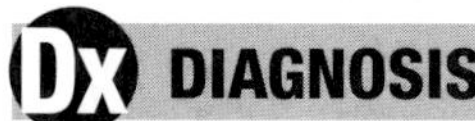

Clinical criteria:
- Definite RP: repeated episodes of biphasic color change on cold exposure
- Possible RP: Uniphasic color changes plus numbness or paresthesia on cold exposure
- No RP: No color change on cold exposure

The suggested criteria for primary RP are:
- Symmetric attacks
- Absence of tissue necrosis, ulceration, or gangrene
- Absence of a secondary cause on the basis of a patient's history and general physical examination
- Negative test for antinuclear antibody (ANA)
- Normal erythrocyte sedimentation rate (ESR)

Secondary RP is suggested by the following findings:
- Onset of symptoms after age 30 yr
- Episodes that are painful, asymmetric, or associated with ischemic skin lesions

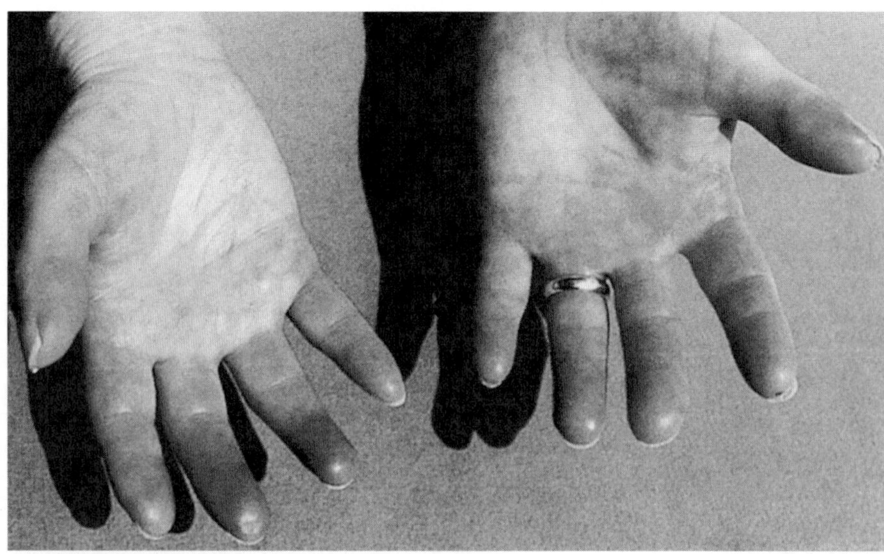

FIGURE 1-273 Raynaud's phenomenon. Sharply demarcated cyanosis of the fingers with proximal venular congestion (livedo reticularis) is seen. (From Klippel J et al [eds]: *Primary care rheumatology,* London, 1999, Mosby.)

- Clinical features suggestive of a connective-tissue disease
- Elevated specific autoantibody tests and ESR
- Evidence of microvascular disease on microscopy of nail-fold capillaries

DIFFERENTIAL DIAGNOSIS

- Neurogenic thoracic outlet syndrome or carpal tunnel syndrome
- Frostbite or cold weather injury
- Medication reaction (ergotamine, chemotherapeutic agents)
- Atherosclerosis, thromboembolic disease
- Buerger's disease, embolic disease
- Acrocyanosis
- Livedo reticularis
- Injury from repetitive motion

WORKUP

- Once the diagnosis of RP is established, differentiating primary from secondary is helpful in treatment and prognosis.
- Patients who are younger when their symptoms occur, have a normal history and physical examination and normal nail-fold capillaries, and have no history of digital ischemic lesions can be considered as having primary RP. These patients can be monitored clinically without any further testing.
- If a secondary cause of RP is suspected, appropriate laboratory testing is recommended (see "Laboratory Tests"). Secondary RP has associated abnormal nail-fold microscopy.

LABORATORY TESTS

- CBC, serum electrolytes, blood urea nitrogen, creatinine, ESR, ANAs, VDRL antibody test, rheumatoid factor, and urinalysis should be included in the initial evaluation.
- If the history, physical examination, and initial laboratory tests suggest a possible secondary cause, specific serologic testing (e.g., anticentromere antibodies, anti-Scl 70, cryoglobulins, complement testing, and serum protein electrophoresis) may be indicated.
- Noninvasive vascular testing includes finger systolic blood pressures, segmental blood pressure measurements, cold recovery time (measure vasoconstrictor and vasodilator responses of finger to cold), fingertip thermography, and laser Doppler with thermal challenge (measures relative change in skin blood flow with ambient warming).

IMAGING STUDIES

- The diagnosis of RP should not be made on the basis of laboratory tests, and imaging studies should not replace a good history and physical examination.
- Duplex ultrasound can image the palmar arch and digital arteries for patency.
- Magnetic resonance angiography is useful for imaging larger arteries.
- Contrast angiography is the gold standard for arterial imaging.
- Nail-fold capillary microscopy can differentiate primary from secondary RP.

Rx TREATMENT

NONPHARMACOLOGIC THERAPY

- Avoid drugs that may precipitate RP (see "Etiology").
- Avoid cold exposure. Use warm gloves, hats, and garments during the winter months or before going into cold environments (e.g., air-conditioned rooms). Sudden shifts in temperature are more likely to precipitate RP.
- Avoid stressful situations, and use relaxation techniques in preventing RP attacks.

ACUTE GENERAL Rx

- Acute measures to terminate an attack include rotating the arms in a windmill pattern, placing the hands under warm water or in a warm body fold such as the axilla, and the swing-arm maneuver. The swing-arm maneuver involves the patient raising both arms over the shoulders in one direction and forcefully swinging them across the body.
- Medications are indicated in the treatment of RP if there are signs of critical ischemia or if the quality of life of the patient is affected to the degree that activities of normal living are no longer possible and preventive techniques do not work.

CHRONIC Rx

- Dihydropyridine calcium channel blockers (e.g., nifedipine, amlodipine, felodipine, nisoldipine, isradipine) are the most effective pharmacologic treatment for RP and are the drugs of choice.
- Nifedipine is most often prescribed at a dose of 10 to 20 mg 30 min before cold exposure. If symptoms occur with long duration, nifedipine XL 30 to 180 mg PO qd is often effective.
- Patients who do not tolerate or do not respond to calcium channel blocker therapy can sometimes benefit from other drugs that directly or indirectly cause vasodilation, either alone or in combination, although data for these therapies are less robust. Some potential therapeutic options include direct vasodilators such as nitroprusside, hydralazine, papaverine, minoxidil, niacin, and griseofulvin. Topical 1% nitroglycerine or topical L-arginine may also be useful, particularly if low blood pressure is a concern.
- Phosphodiesterase inhibitors (cilostazol, pentoxifylline, and sildenafil), angiotensin 2 receptor antagonists (losartan), and selective serotonin reuptake inhibitors (Flouxetine) have been used with some limited success.
- Alpha receptor antagonists such as prazosin and phenoxybenzamine have shown some effectiveness in treating RP.
- The prostaglandins, including inhaled iloprost, IV epoprostenol, and alprostadil, may be promising in severe RP. However, additional experience and controlled studies are needed.
- Anticoagulation with IV unfractionated heparin or subcutaneous low-molecular-weight heparin and addition of aspirin can be considered during the acute phase of a severe ischemic event. Aspirin (81 mg/day) therapy can be considered in all patients with secondary RP with a history of ischemic ulcers or thrombotic events; however, caution should be exercised because aspirin can theoretically worsen vasospasm by the inhibition of prostacyclin. Long-term anticoagulation with heparin or warfarin is not recommended unless there is evidence of a hypercoagulable state.
- Bypass surgery can be performed for severe RP associated with reconstructible arterial occlusive disease.
- Sympathectomy is available for unreconstructible occlusive disease or pure vasospastic disease refractory to medical treatment.
- Ischemic digital lesions should be treated with topical antibiotics and daily cleansing with soap and water. Digits that progress to dry gangrene should be permitted to undergo autoamputation. Surgical amputation is limited for intractable pain or deep tissue infection.

DISPOSITION

The prognosis of patients with RP depends on the etiology.

- Primary RP is fairly benign, usually remaining stable and controlled with nonpharmacologic medical treatment.
- Patients with secondary RP, specifically those with scleroderma, CREST syndrome, or thromboangiitis obliterans, may develop severe ischemic digits with ulceration, gangrene, and autoamputation.

REFERRAL

- Rheumatology consult is indicated if secondary collagen vascular disease is diagnosed.
- Vascular surgery consult is indicated if ulcers, gangrene, or threatened digit loss is noted.

PEARLS & CONSIDERATIONS

- Most patients with RP can be managed by a primary care provider.
- It is important to differentiate primary from secondary forms. Secondary forms may become manifest as far out as 10 yr from the diagnosis of RP. It is important to take immediate action during an attack and patients are encouraged to:
  1. Keep warm
  2. Not use tobacco products
  3. Avoid aggravating medications
  4. Control stress
  5. Exercise
  6. Follow up with a physician

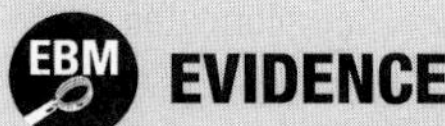

EVIDENCE

Lifestyle measures: There is a lack of evidence from medical research for the standard lifestyle measures often recommended first-line to people with Raynaud's, although most would agree that it is common-sense to suggest to avoid cold.[1]

Medical therapies: Although various medical therapies have been studied the trials can be difficult to interpret because of heterogeneity in terms of diagnostic criteria, combined study of subjects with primary and secondary conditions, and the small numbers of subjects often included.

Calcium channel blockers: When considered as a group, calcium channel blockers significantly reduce the frequency and severity of attacks of primary Raynaud's vs. placebo.[2]

Out of all the calcium channel blockers, the evidence for nifedipine is most convincing since it has been studied most frequently.[2]

Likewise, two small RCTs (included in a systematic review) were unable to find a significant reduction in severity or frequency of attacks when nisoldipine was compared with placebo.[2]

Calcium channel blockers may cause adverse effects such as palpitations, flushing, ankle swelling.[2]

Other medical therapies: A crossover randomized controlled trail (RCT) comparing prazosin 1 mg twice daily vs. placebo in 24 people (14 with the primary disease) found that prazosin significantly reduced the mean number and duration of attacks vs. placebo but not the severity of attacks.[3]

Topical nitrates have been shown to reduce severity and frequency of attacks but side effects are not unusual.[4]

Intravenous iloprost has been found to reduce the frequency and severity of Raynaud's attacks significantly in patients suffering from systemic sclerosis and to prevent and heal digital ulcers.[5]

There was no evidence of an effect on the frequency, severity or duration of attacks for captopril, beraprost, dazoxiben, and ketanserin.[6]

Localized digital sympathectomy has produced promising results in terms of improvement of quality of life and avoidance of digital amputation in people with severe Raynaud's often with nonhealing digital ulcers. This evidence comes from a few retrospective trials of surgery in small numbers of people with severe disease. These trials are too small to produce firm conclusions.[7]

Evidence-Based References

1. Pope J: Raynaud's phenomenon (primary), *Clin Evid* (13):1546, 2005.

2. Thompson AE, Pope JE: Calcium channel blockers for primary Raynaud's phenomenon: a meta-analysis, *Rheumatology* 44:145-150, 2005.

3. Wollersheim H et al: Double-blind, placebo-controlled study of prazosin in Raynaud's phenomenon, *Clin Pharmacol Ther* 40:219, 1986. Reviewed in: *Clin Evid* 11:1603, 2004.

4. Teh LS et al: Sustained-release transdermal glyceral trinitrate patches as treatment for primary and secondary Raynaud's phenomenon, *Br J Rheumatol* 34:636, 1995.

5. Pope J et al: Iloprost and cisaprost for Raynaud's phenomenon in progressive systemic sclerosis, *Cochrane Database Syst Rev* (2):CD000953, 1998.

6. Vinjar B, Stewart M: Oral vasodilaters for primary Raynaud's phenomenon. *Cochrane Database Syst Rev* 16(2):CD006687, 2008.

7. Wang WH et al: Peripheral sympathectomy for Raynaud's phenomenon: a salvage procedure, *Kaohsiung J Med Sci* 22:491-499, 2006.

SUGGESTED READINGS

Bakst R et al: Raynaud's phenomenon: pathogenesis and management, *J Am Acad Dermatol* 59(4):633-53, 2008.

Cook JP et al: Mechanisms of Raynaud's disease, *Vasc Med* 10:297-307, 2005.

Wigley FM: Raynaud's phenomenon, *N Engl J Med* 347:1001-1008, 2002.

AUTHORS: **SYEDA M. SAYEED, M.D.**, and **WEN-CHIH WU, M.D.**

BASIC INFORMATION

DEFINITION

Reflex sympathetic dystrophy (RSD) or complex regional pain syndrome (CRPS) type 1 is a pain disorder characterized by constant and intense limb pain associated with vasomotor and sudomotor abnormalities that occurs without a definable nerve lesion. RSD or CRPS type 1 should be distinguished from CRPS type 2, which refers to pain disorders in which a definable nerve lesion exists.

SYNONYMS

CRPS type 1
Causalgia (or CRPS type 2)
Shoulder-hand syndrome
Sudeck's atrophy
Posttraumatic pain syndrome
RSD

ICD-9CM CODES
337.20 Dystrophy sympathetic (posttraumatic) (reflex)

EPIDEMIOLOGY & DEMOGRAPHICS

- First described by Mitchell et al during the American Civil War.
- The incidence and prevalence is not known.
- Usually initiated by trauma, mostly after orthopedic procedures, especially those on the extremities.
- Can occur in adults or children.
- Often associated with psychiatric and emotional lability, anxiety, and depression.

PHYSICAL FINDINGS & CLINICAL PRESENTATION

RSD is divided into three stages:

- Acute stage (occurring within hr to days after the injury)
  1. Burning or aching pain occurring over the injured extremity
  2. Hyperalgesia (exquisitely sensitive to touch)
  3. Edema
  4. Dysthermia
  5. Increased hair and nail growth
- Dystrophic stage (3 to 6 mo after the injury)
  1. Burning pain radiating both distally and proximally from the site of injury
  2. Brawny edema
  3. Hyperhidrosis
  4. Hypothermia and cyanosis
  5. Muscle tremors and spasms
  6. Increased muscle tone and reflexes
- Atrophic stage (6 mo after injury)
  1. Spread of pain proximally
  2. Cold, pale cyanotic skin
  3. Trophic skin changes with subcutaneous atrophy
  4. Fixed joints
  5. Contractures

ETIOLOGY

- The cause is unknown. It is thought to represent dysfunction of the sympathetic nervous system.
- Any injury can precipitate RSD, including:
  1. Crush blunt trauma, burns, frostbite
  2. Surgery
  3. Parkinson's disease
  4. Cerebrovascular accident
  5. Myocardial infarction
  6. Osteoarthritis, cervical and lumbar disk disease
  7. Carpal tunnel and tarsal tunnel syndrome
  8. Diabetes
  9. Hyperthyroidism
  10. Isoniazid therapy

Dx DIAGNOSIS

The diagnosis is primarily clinical, based on the patient's history and physical presentation.

DIFFERENTIAL DIAGNOSIS

The differential diagnosis includes all the causes mentioned under "Etiology."

WORKUP

- No workup is needed because there are no specific diagnostic tests establishing the diagnosis.
- Electrophysiologic testing is useful to identify patients with type 2 CRPS.
- Long-term skin temperature measurements can be used as a diagnostic test.

LABORATORY TESTS

Blood tests are not specific.

IMAGING STUDIES

- No imaging studies are diagnostic. Three-phase bone imaging may be helpful.
- Autonomic testing, although not commonly done, has been proposed.
  1. Measuring resting sweat output
  2. Measuring resting skin temperature
  3. Quantitative sudomotor axon reflex test
- Radiograph studies of the affected limb may show osteoporosis from disuse.

Rx TREATMENT

Treatment is aimed at relieving the pain and improving disuse atrophy with physical therapy.

NONPHARMACOLOGIC THERAPY

- Physical therapy
- Transcutaneous nerve stimulation

ACUTE GENERAL Rx

- The following has been tried for neuropathic pain relief:
  1. Amitriptyline 10 mg to 150 mg qid
  2. Phenytoin 300 mg qid
  3. Carbamazepine 100 mg bid
  4. Calcium channel blockers, nifedipine extended release 30 to 60 mg qid
  5. Prednisone 60 to 80 mg qid for 2 wk and then tapered over 1 to 2 wk to a maintenance dose of 5 mg qid for 2 to 3 mo
  6. Vitamin C 500 mg daily for 50 days after wrist fracture can decrease the occurrence of CRPS
  7. Gabapentin 300 mg daily up to 3 times a day
- Regional nerve block that provides a perioperative sympathectomy may be advantageous for patients with a history of CRPS who require orthopedic surgery.
- Because CRPS type 2 is the result of a definable nerve lesion, using a surgical technique that minimizes the risk of nerve damage is important.

CHRONIC Rx

- Stellate ganglion and lumbar sympathetic blocks can be tried.
- Intravenous alpha-adrenergic blockade with phentolamine may predict response to subsequent sympatholytic treatment.
- Surgical sympathectomy.
- Surgical correction can be performed for severe foot and ankle contracture.
- Recent trials have shown that intravenous immunoglobulin (IVIG 0.5 gram/mg) can reduce pain in refractory complex regional pain syndrome.

DISPOSITION

Spontaneous remission can occur after several weeks to months.

REFERRAL

RSD is a very difficult diagnosis to make and referral to either rheumatology, neurology, orthopedic, or psychiatry specialists is recommended.

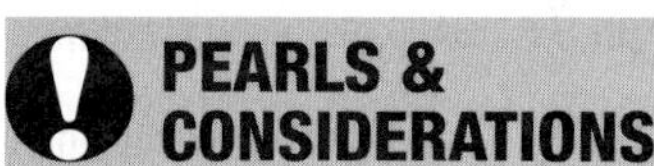

PEARLS & CONSIDERATIONS

COMMENTS

- RSD is a common clinical entity without clear definition, pathophysiologic features, or treatment.
- Pain is the most disabling symptom for most patients and is usually out of proportion to the extent of the injury.

SUGGESTED READINGS

Dowd GSE et al: Complex regional pain syndrome with special emphasis on the knee, *J Bone Joint Surg* 89-B(3):285-290, 2007.

Goebel A et al: Intravenous immunoglobulin treatment of the complex regional pain syndrome, *Ann Intern Med* 152:152-158, 2010.

Krumova EK et al: Long-term skin temperature measurements—a practical diagnostic tool in complex regional pain syndrome, *Pain* 140(1):8-22, Epub 2008.

Low AK et al: Pediatric complex regional pain syndrome, *J Pediatr Orthop* 27(5):567-572, 2007.

Mendicino, RW et al: Correction of severe foot and ankle contracture due to CRPS using external fixation and pain management: report of a pediatric case. *J Foot Ankle Surg* 47(5):434-440, 2008.

Reuben SS, Buvanendran A: Preventing the development of chronic pain after orthopaedic surgery with preventive multimodal analgesic techniques, *J Bone Joint Surg [Am]* 89(6):1343-1358, 2007.

Teasdall RD et al: Complex regional pain syndrome (reflex sympathetic dystrophy), *Clin Sports Med* 23(1):145, 2004.

AUTHOR: **JORGE A. VILLAFUERTE, M.D.**

Reiter's Syndrome (Reactive Arthritis)

BASIC INFORMATION

DEFINITION

Reiter's syndrome is one of the seronegative spondyloarthropathies, so called because serum rheumatoid factor is not present in these forms of inflammatory arthritis. There is an international consensus that the term *reactive arthritis* should replace the name "Reiter's syndrome" to describe this constellation of signs and symptoms. Unfortunately, the original name is still associated with the syndrome. Reiter's syndrome is an asymmetric polyarthritis that affects mainly the lower extremities and is associated with one or more of the following:

- Urethritis
- Cervicitis
- Dysentery
- Inflammatory eye disease
- Mucocutaneous lesions

SYNONYMS

Reiter's disease
Reactive arthritis
Seronegative spondyloarthropathy

ICD-9CM CODES
099.3 Reiter's syndrome

EPIDEMIOLOGY & DEMOGRAPHICS

INCIDENCE (IN U.S.): 0.0035% annually of men ≤50 yr
PEAK INCIDENCE: Most common in the third decade
PREDOMINANT SEX: Male
PREDOMINANT AGE: 20 to 40 yr
GENETICS: Familial disposition: strongly associated with HLA-B27 (63% to 96%)

PHYSICAL FINDINGS & CLINICAL PRESENTATION

- Polyarthritis
  1. Affecting the knee and ankle
  2. Commonly asymmetric
- Heel pain and Achilles tendinitis, especially at the insertion of the Achilles tendon
- Plantar fasciitis
- Large effusions
- Dactylitis, or "sausage toe"
- Urethritis
- Uveitis or conjunctivitis; uveitis can progress to blindness without treatment
- Keratoderma blennorrhagicum, circinate balanitis
  1. Hyperkeratotic lesions on soles of the feet, toes, penis, hands
  2. Closely resembles psoriasis
- Aortic regurgitation similar to that seen in ankylosing spondylitis

ETIOLOGY

- Epidemic Reiter's syndrome after outbreaks of dysentery has been well described.
- Genetically susceptible HLA-B27 individuals are at risk for developing Reiter's syndrome after infection with certain pathogens:
  1. *Salmonella*
  2. *Shigella*
  3. *Yersinia enterocolitica*
  4. *Chlamydia trachomatis*
  5. Molecular mimicry mechanism suspected
- Symptom complex indistinguishable from Reiter's syndrome has been described in association with HIV infection.

Dx DIAGNOSIS

DIFFERENTIAL DIAGNOSIS

- Ankylosing spondylitis
- Psoriatic arthritis
- Rheumatoid arthritis
- Gonococcal arthritis-tenosynovitis
- Rheumatic fever

WORKUP

- X-ray examination of affected joints
- Synovial fluid examination and culture
- Careful examination of eyes and skin
- Cultures for gonococcus (urethral, cervical, stool)

LABORATORY TESTS

- Elevated but nonspecific erythrocyte sedimentation rate
- No specific laboratory tests to diagnose Reiter's syndrome

IMAGING STUDIES

Plain radiographs:

- Juxtaarticular osteopenia of affected joints
- Erosions and joint space narrowing in more advanced disease
- Periostitis and reactive new bone formation at the insertions of the Achilles tendon and the plantar fascia
- Sacroiliitis:
  1. Unilateral or bilateral
  2. Indistinguishable from ankylosing spondylitis
- Vertebral bridging osteophytes

Rx TREATMENT

NONPHARMACOLOGIC THERAPY

Physical therapy to maintain range of motion of the spine and other joints

ACUTE GENERAL Rx

- Flares treated with nonsteroidal anti-inflammatory drugs such as indomethacin (25 to 50 mg PO tid).
- Enteric or urethral infection should be treated with appropriate antibiotic coverage.
- Uveitis should be treated with steroid eye drops in consultation with an ophthalmologist.
- Achilles tendinitis and plantar fasciitis should be treated with injections of methylprednisolone (40 to 80 mg).
- Sulfasalazine (2 to 3 g PO tid) may be effective.
- Careful monitoring for the following is essential:
  1. Gastrointestinal toxicity
  2. Hypersensitivity
  3. Bone marrow suppression
- Persistent and uncontrolled disease should be managed with cytotoxic drugs (methotrexate, azathioprine) in consultation with a rheumatologist.

CHRONIC Rx

Chronic disease is best managed by a team approach with the collaboration of a rheumatologist or other experienced physician and physical therapist.

DISPOSITION

- Recurrences are frequent, even with treatment.
- Long-term sequelae:
  1. Persistent polyarthritis
  2. Chronic back pain
  3. Heel pain
  4. Progressive iridocyclitis
  5. Aortic regurgitation

REFERRAL

- To ophthalmologist if uveitis is suspected
- To rheumatologist if arthritis and tendinitis fail to improve rapidly after a course of nonsteroidal anti-inflammatory drugs

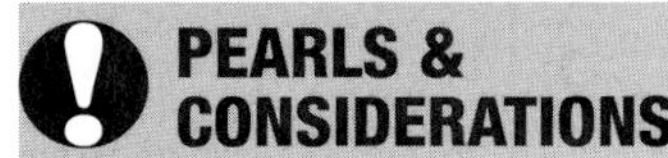

PEARLS & CONSIDERATIONS

COMMENTS

- Infection with HIV is associated with particularly severe cases of Reiter's syndrome.
- HIV testing is recommended, especially if risk factors such as unprotected sexual activity or IV drug use are identified.

SUGGESTED READINGS

Eapen BR: A new insight into the pathogenesis of Reiter's syndrome using bioinformatics tools, *Int J Dermatol* 42(3):242, 2003.

Klecker RJ, Weissman BN: Imaging features of psoriatic arthritis and Reiter's syndrome, *Semin Musculoskelet Radiol* 7(2):115, 2003.

Neumann S et al: Reiter's syndrome as a manifestation of an immune reconstitution syndrome in an HIV-infected patient: successful treatment with doxycycline, *Clin Infect Dis* 36(12):1628, 2003.

Schneider JM et al: Reiter's syndrome, *Cutis* 71(3):198, 2003.

AUTHORS: **GLENN G. FORT, M.D., M.P.H.,** and **DENNIS J. MIKOLICH, M.D.**

BASIC INFORMATION

DEFINITION

Renal artery stenosis (RAS) is the progressive narrowing of the renal artery, most often caused by atherosclerosis or fibromuscular dysplasia. Acute RAS can occur via thrombosis or embolism and can lead to renal infarction. RAS can cause renovascular hypertension and/or lead to ischemic nephropathy.

SYNONYMS

Acute:
  Renal artery thrombosis
  Renal artery embolism
Chronic:
  Renovascular hypertension

ICD-9CM CODES

593.81	Renal artery occlusion
440.1	Renal artery stenosis
405.01	Renovascular hypertension, secondary
447.9	Renal artery hyperplasia

EPIDEMIOLOGY & DEMOGRAPHICS

- In acute renal artery occlusion, the epidemiology depends on the underlying cause (see below).
- Renovascular hypertension:
  1. Prevalence of 0.2% to 5% of all hypertensive patients. RAS is the most common cause of secondary hypertension.
  2. The prevalence is higher in patients with severe hypertension, reaching 43% of white patients and 7% of black patients with malignant hypertension.
- Approximately one in six patients with end-stage renal disease has ischemic nephropathy, and survival of patients with end-stage renal disease associated with ischemic nephropathy is half that of patients with end-stage renal disease from other causes.
- The demographics of atheromatous RAS mirrors the pattern seen in other arteriosclerotic conditions (coronary artery disease, cerebrovascular disease, peripheral vascular disease) and is influenced by the usual risk factors (smoking, family history, diabetes, hyperlipidemia). For example, the prevalence of RAS among hypertensive patients undergoing coronary catheterization is high (47%), with 19% having a stenosis of 50% or more.
- Fibromuscular dysplasia is most likely seen in young adult women, and in approximately 10% of patients with progressive RAS (atherosclerotic RAS is seen in approximately 90%).
- Takayasu's arteritis can involve the renal arteries and is also seen in young to middle-aged women.

PHYSICAL FINDINGS & CLINICAL PRESENTATION

Acute renal artery occlusion:
- Flank or abdominal pain
- Fever
- Nausea or vomiting
- Leukocytosis
- Hematuria (microscopic or gross)
- Elevated aspartate aminotransferase, lactate dehydrogenase, and alkaline phosphatase
- Oliguric renal failure if occlusion is bilateral; normal or near-normal renal function in unilateral occlusion

Cholesterol emboli:
- Multisystem manifestations resembling vasculitis (visual disturbance, painful distal extremities, abdominal pain, signs of organ or limb ischemia). Laboratory findings include eosinophiluria, proteinuria, renal failure, elevated erythrocyte sedimentation rate.

Progressive renal artery stenosis:
- Hypertension in young, white woman without a family history of such (fibromuscular dysplasia), new onset hypertension at age <30 or >55 yr, uncontrolled hypertension refractory to three or more medications, hypertension in any patient without family history or risk factors
- Hypertension in middle-aged man with other evidence of atheromatous disease
- Abdominal bruit (40% of cases)
- Renal failure
- Hypertensive retinopathy
- Pulmonary edema in a hypertensive patient
- Hypokalemia
- Renal failure after the administration of an ACE inhibitor (ACEI) (if bilateral RAS)

ETIOLOGY & PATHOGENESIS

Renal artery thrombosis:
- Atherosclerosis: the most common etiology of RAS (seen in approximately 90% of cases of RAS)
- Fibromuscular dysplasia: second most common etiology of RAS. It is classified into three categories based on the layer of arterial wall affected: intimal, medial (3 subtypes), adventitial
- Extrinsic compression (e.g., neoplasms)
- Neurofibromatosis and fibrous bands
- Arteritis
- Renal artery aneurysm
- Syphilis
- Hypercoagulable state
- Complication of renal transplantation (role of cyclosporine)

Renal artery embolism (cardiac conditions [90%]):
- Myocardial infarction
- Atrial fibrillation
- Cardiomyopathy
- Endocarditis
- Paradoxical emboli from deep vein thrombosis in patient with cardiac septal defect
- Atheromatous plaques (cholesterol emboli)

PATHOGENESIS

The macula densa of the kidney senses a decreased systemic blood pressure owing to the reduced blood flow through the narrowed artery. The decreased perfusion pressure (caused by the stenosis) leads to decreased blood flow (hypoperfusion) to the kidney and a decrease in the glomerular filtration rate. Renal hypoperfusion or ischemia produces an increase in plasma renin that stimulates the conversion of angiotensin I to angiotensin II, causing vasoconstriction and aldosterone secretion, sodium retention, and potassium wasting. Hypertension results and can be self-sustaining after some time, even in the case of unilateral RAS, because of hypertensive damage to the other kidney.

Dx DIAGNOSIS

SCREENING:

American College of Cardiology and American Heart Association (ACC/AHA) guidelines for identifying patients who should be screened for RAS:
- Onset of hypertension at age <30 yr or severe hypertension at age >55 yr
- Malignant hypertension: hypertension with coexistent evidence of acute end-organ damage (acute renal failure, acute decompensated heart failure, new visual or neurologic disturbance, and/or retinopathy)
- Accelerated hypertension: sudden and persistent worsening
- Resistant hypertension: full doses of a three-drug regimen that includes a diuretic
- Sudden unexpected pulmonary edema (especially in azotemic patients)
- New azotemia or worsening renal function after ACEIsand angiotensin receptor blockers (ARBs)

LABORATORY TESTS

- Creatinine
- Glomerular filtration rate
- Potassium level
- Urinalysis
- Peripheral plasma renin activity
- Captopril test (stimulation of excessive renin secretion)

IMAGING STUDIES

- Duplex ultrasound, CT angiography, and magnetic resonance angiography (MRA) are effective diagnostic screening methods. The choice of imaging modality will depend on the availability of the diagnostic tool, the experience and local accuracy of each modality, and patient characteristics, including body size, renal function, contrast allergy, and presence of prior stents.

- Duplex ultrasound is safe and inexpensive. When compared with angiography, duplex ultrasound has a sensitivity of 84% to 98% and a specificity of 62% to 99% for detecting RAS. However, it is highly operator dependent and provides poor visualization of accessory renal arteries. An end-diastolic velocity of >150 cm/sec predicts severe RAS. Duplex ultrasonography may be used to measure the renal artery resistive index, a potentially useful method to identify severe parenchymal disease, which has been shown to limit value of renal revascularization. A renal artery to aortic systolic blood pressure ratio >3.5 is consistent with significant RAS. When ultrasound examination indicates significant asymmetry of kidney size (i.e., size discrepancy >1.5 cm), this suggests significant RAS involving the smaller kidney.
- MRA provides good visualization of both main and accessory renal arteries. Limitations include need to infuse gadolinium (limits use in renal insufficiency due to the possibility of systemic nephrogenic fibrosis), high cost, inability to image within a previously placed metallic stent, and lack of widespread availability.
- CT angiography is fast and effective but requires infusion of iodinated contrast (limits use in renal insufficiency) and involves significant radiation exposure.
- IV digital subtraction catheter angiography (88% sensitivity and 90% specificity) is the reference standard for anatomic diagnosis of RAS. It is not a first-line screening tool but is recommended, if noninvasive tests are inconclusive but clinical suspicion is high. Renal fractional flow reserve (FFR) at the time of catheter angiography can be used to assess severity of RAS using maximal vasodilation with papaverine. One study found that an FFR of <0.9 corresponds to an approximate systolic gradient of 25 mm Hg and is associated with a significant increase in renin production.
- Section III describes an algorithm for the diagnosis of RAS.

Rx TREATMENT

Acute renal artery thrombosis or embolism:
- Thrombolytic therapy.
- Anticoagulation.
- Revascularization (endovascular therapy or surgery). Endovascular renal artery stenting is favored over surgery, and has shown better clinical results when compared with balloon angioplasty (without stenting).
- Blood pressure control.

Cholesterol emboli:
- No treatment

RAS:
- ACEIs, ARBs, and calcium-channel blockers are recommended for the treatment of hypertension in unilateral RAS. Beta-blockers are recommended for the treatment of hypertension in patients with RAS of all types. ACEIs and ARBs should be used with careful supervision in bilateral RAS or unilateral stenosis with solitary kidney to avoid precipitating acute renal failure.
- Angioplasty/stent or surgical revascularization should be reserved for patients whose blood pressure control with medication is difficult and for patients with progressive disease. The ACC/AHA guidelines for clinical indications of renal artery revascularization in the presence of significant stenosis include:
  1. Accelerated, resistant, or malignant hypertension
  2. Hypertension with unilateral small kidney
  3. Hypertension with intolerance to medication
  4. Treatment of cardiac destabilization syndromes such as unexplained heart failure exacerbations, episodes of flash pulmonary edema, and refractory or unstable angina
  5. Progressive chronic kidney disease with bilateral RAS or RAS associated with a solitary functioning kidney

NATURAL HISTORY

- RAS caused by fibromuscular dysplasia generally does not progress. Fibromuscular dysplasia RAS responds well to angioplasty with long-term patency of the lesion typically observed.
- RAS associated with atherosclerosis is progressive. Of patients with >60% stenosis, 5% progress to total occlusion in 1 yr and 11% progress in 2 yr.

EBM EVIDENCE

Please note: Complete text of EBM for this topic is available online.

The degree of renal artery stenosis that would justify any attempt at either surgical intervention or radiologic intervention is not known. A recent study suggested that a ratio of pressure, measured distal to renal artery stenosis, less than 90% relative to aortic pressure, was found to be associated with significant renin release from the affected kidney, renin being measured in the ipsilateral renal vein.[1] This might be useful as a functional measurement of significant renovascular stenosis leading to hypertension and, thus, a marker of those individuals more likely to benefit from angioplasty and stenting.[1]

While the incidence of atherosclerotic RAS is independent of sex, one study showed that female sex (as well as older age, elevated serum creatinine level, coronary artery disease, peripheral vascular disease, hypertension, and cerebrovascular disease) is an independent predictor of RAS progression.[2]

In a study reported in the *New England Journal of Medicine*, the use of a renal resistance index is of value to predict the outcome of therapy in patients aggressively treated for renal artery stenosis.[3] Specifically, an index of greater than 80, indicating small vessel and large vessel disease, was indicative of a poor response to either angioplasty or surgery with respect to improvement in hypertension, renal function, or kidney survival.

A study compared the accuracy of CT angiography and MRA to digital subtraction angiography for diagnosing RAS, and concluded that digital subtraction angiography remains the method of choice to establish a diagnosis.[4]

A surgical bypass study for RAS suggested an operative mortality rate of only 6% and immediate improvement in the serum creatinine level of 32% of surgical bypass procedures in 35 patients with solitary kidneys.[5]

A multicenter trial evaluated the relative benefit of angioplasty versus medical therapy for hypertension associated with RAS.[6] They found that both groups had similar decreases in blood pressure, although the patients who underwent angioplasty used one fewer hypertensive medication. While renal function was improved at 3 mo in those undergoing angioplasty, the function at 12 mo was similar. They concluded that restricting angioplasty to those with atherosclerotic renovascular hypertension persisting despite use of 3 or more antihypertensive medications was prudent. Note that the patients in this trial did not undergo angioplasty with stent placement. In addition, 9% of patients in the medical therapy–only group experienced total occlusion of the affected renal artery on 12-month follow-up angiography.

A randomized study that compared percutaneous transluminal angioplasty (PTA) alone for ostial RAS versus PTA and stenting (PTAS) showed that PTAS is a better technique compared to PTA to achieve vessel patency in ostial atherosclerotic renal artery stenosis.[7] The primary success rate was 57% for PTA alone compared with 88% for PTAS. The restenosis rate after a successful primary procedure was 48% for PTA compared to 14% for PTAS. In the last few years, the use of PTAS in patients with ostial stenosis or early restenosis has led to a considerable reduction in the restenosis rate.

Controversy still surrounds the best approach to patients with atherosclerotic renovascular disease, Large prospective clinical trials are still ongoing and the results from these trials are still pending.[8-10]

Evidence-Based References

1. De Bruyne B et al: Assessment of renal artery stenosis severity by pressure gradient measurements, *J Am Coll Cardiol* 48(9):1851-1855, 2006. A

2. Crowley JJ et al: Progression of renal artery stenosis in patients undergoing cardiac catheterization, *Am Heart J* 136(5):913-918, 1998. A

3. Radermacher J et al: Use of Doppler ultrasonography to predict the outcome of therapy for renal-artery stenosis, *N Engl J Med* 344(6):410-417, 2001. B

4. Vasbinder GB et al: Accuracy of computed tomographic angiography and magnetic resonance angiography for diagnosing renal artery stenosis, *Ann Intern Med* 141(9):674-682, 2004; discussion, 682. B

5. Reilly JM et al: Revascularization of the solitary kidney: a challenging problem in a high risk population, *Surgery* 120(4):732-736, 1996; discussion, 736-737 B

6. van Jaarsveld BC et al: The effect of balloon angioplasty on hypertension in atherosclerotic renal-artery stenosis. Dutch Renal Artery Stenosis Intervention Cooperative Study Group, *N Engl J Med* 342(14):1007-1014, 2000. A

7. van de Ven PJ et al: Arterial stenting and balloon angioplasty in ostial atherosclerotic renovascular disease: a randomised trial, *Lancet* 353(9149):282-286, 1999. B

8. Ives NJ et al: Continuing uncertainty about the value of percutaneous revascularization in atherosclerotic renovascular disease: a meta-analysis of randomized trials, *Nephrol Dial Transplant* 18(2):298-304, 2003. A

9. Textor SC: Ischemic nephropathy: where are we now? *J Am Soc Nephrol* 15(8):1974-1982, 2004. B

10. Plouin PF: Stable patients with atherosclerotic renal artery stenosis should be treated first with medical management, *Am J Kidney Dis* 42(5):851-857, 2003 B

SUGGESTED READINGS

Astral Investigators: Revascularization versus medical therapy for renal-artery stenosis, *N Engl J Med* 361:1953-1962, 2009.

Dworkin LD, Cooper CJ: Renal artery stenosis, *N Engl J Med* 361:1972-1978, 2009.

Regnante RA et al: Renal artery stenosis: clinical and therapeutic implications, *Med Health Rhode Island* 91(10):315, 2008.

Slovut DP, Olin JW: Fibromuscular dysplasia, *N Engl J Med* 350:1862, 2004.

AUTHORS: **KHIET C HOANG, M.D.**, **FRED F. FERRI, M.D.**, and **PRANAV M. PATEL, M.D.**

Renal Cell Adenocarcinoma 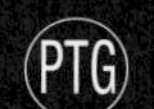

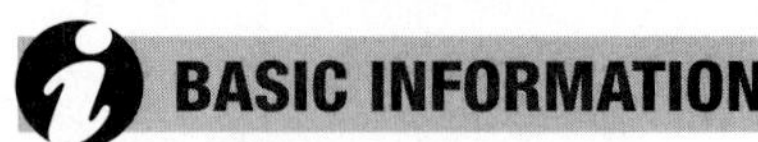

BASIC INFORMATION

DEFINITION

Renal cell adenocarcinoma (RCA) is a primary adenocarcinoma originating in the renal parenchyma from the malignant transformation of proximal renal tubular epithelial cells.

SYNONYMS

Hypernephroma
Clear cell carcinoma of the kidney
Grawitz tumor

ICD-9CM CODES
189.0 Adenocarcinoma of kidney
189.1 (Renal pelvis)

EPIDEMIOLOGY & DEMOGRAPHICS

INCIDENCE: Approximately one in 10,000 persons annually (3% of all adult malignancies). In the U.S., renal cancer is the seventh leading malignant condition among men and twelfth among women. Two percent of cases of renal cancer are associated with inherited syndromes.
PREDOMINANT SEX: Male/female ratio of 2:1
PREDOMINANT AGE: Peaks at age 50 to 70 yr

PHYSICAL FINDINGS & CLINICAL PRESENTATION

The classic presentation of RCA includes the triad of flank pain, hematuria, and a palpable abdominal mass. This now represents an unusual presentation. Current presenting findings in RCA patients now include:

Hematuria	50% to 60%
Elevated erythrocyte sedimentation rate	50% to 60%
Abdominal mass	25% to 45%
Anemia	20% to 40%
Flank pain	35% to 40%
Hypertension	20% to 40%
Weight loss	30% to 35%
Fever	5% to 15%
Hepatic dysfunction	10% to 15%
Classic triad (hematuria, abdominal mass, flank pain)	5% to 10%
Hypercalcemia	3% to 6%
Erythrocytosis	3% to 4%
Varicocele	2% to 3%

ETIOLOGY

Hereditary forms:
- Familial renal carcinoma
- Renal carcinoma associated with von Hippel-Lindau disease
- Hereditary papillary renal cell carcinoma

Risk factors:
- Cigarette smoking
- Obesity
- Use of diuretics
- Phenacetin-containing analgesics
- Asbestos exposure
- Gasoline and other petroleum products
- Lead
- Cadmium
- Thorotrast
- Role of the *VHL* gene on chromosome 3

DIAGNOSIS

DIFFERENTIAL DIAGNOSIS

- Transitional cell carcinomas of the renal pelvis (8% of all renal cancers)
- Wilms' tumor
- Other rare primary renal carcinomas and sarcomas
- Renal cysts
- All causes of hematuria (see Section II)
- Retroperitoneal tumors

WORKUP

- Laboratory tests and imaging studies.
- Section III, "Renal Mass," describes patient evaluation.

LABORATORY TESTS

- Complete blood count: anemia or erythrocytosis
- Elevated sedimentation rate
- Nonmetastatic hepatic dysfunction with elevated alkaline phosphatase, prolonged prothrombin time, and hypoalbuminemia
- Hypercalcemia (caused by parathyroid-related protein)
- Other: elevated ferritin, elevated insulin and glucagon levels, elevated alpha-fetoprotein, and elevated beta–human chorionic gonadotropin

IMAGING STUDIES

Nearly 50% of renal cancers are now detected because a renal mass is incidentally detected on radiographic evaluation.
- Renal ultrasound
- Abdominal CT scan with contrast (Fig. 1-274)
- MRI
- Renal arteriogram
- Intravenous pyelography

STAGING

See Table 1-64.

COMMON SITES OF METASTASES

Lung	50% to 60%
Bone	30% to 40%
Regional nodes	15% to 30%
Main renal vein	15% to 20%
Perirenal fat	10% to 20%
Adrenal (ipsilateral)	10% to 15%
Vena cava	10% to 15%
Brain	10% to 15%
Adjacent organs (colon, pancreas)	10%
Kidney (contralateral)	2%

TREATMENT

- Surgery
  - Surgical nephrectomy is the only effective management for stages I, II, and some stage III tumors.
  - Various forms of partial nephrectomy may be available for patients with bilateral cancers or with a solitary kidney.
  - The role of nephrectomy in patients with metastatic renal cell carcinoma is controversial and should probably be reserved for patients who have a solitary metastasis amenable to surgical resection.
- Angioinfarction (for palliation)
- Radiotherapy (for palliation)
- Chemotherapy (only 5% response rate)
- Hormonal therapy (high-dose progesterone may achieve a 15% to 20% response rate)
- Immunotherapy (interleukin-2 may achieve a 15% to 30% response rate; alpha-, beta-, and gamma-interferons are somewhat less effective; for example, interferon alfa-2b increased postnephrectomy median survival by 30% in one recent trial)
- Antivascular endothelial growth factor antibody Bevacizumab slows disease progression in metastatic renal cancer.
- Sunitinib and sorafenib are oral tyrosine kinase inhibitors useful for therapy of advanced renal cell carcinoma (as first-line therapy) or in patients not responding to or intolerant of cytokine therapy.

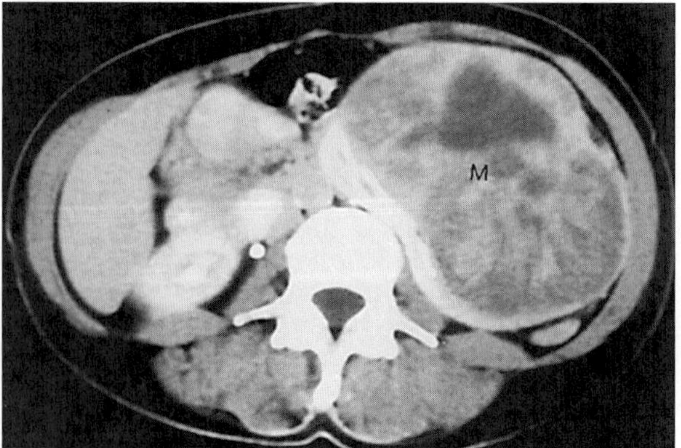

FIGURE 1-274 Large renal cell carcioma. Large mass *(M)* containing areas of high enhancement, low enhancement, and necrosis. (From Stein JH [ed]: *Internal medicine,* ed 5, St Louis, 1998, Mosby.)

- Recent trials with temsirolimus, a specific inhibitor of the mammalian target of rapamycin kinase, have shown promising results. Compared with interferon-alpha, temsirolimus improved overall survival rate among patients with metastatic renal cell carcinoma and a poor prognosis. The addition of temsirolimus to interferon did not improve survival rate.

PROGNOSIS

Prognosis of surgically treated patients:

TNM Stage	*5-yr Survival (%)*
I	95
II	88
III (renal vein or vena cava)	50 to 60
III (nodal involvement)	15 to 25
IV	5 to 20

REFERRAL

To urologist

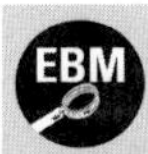

EVIDENCE

Although not supported by data from randomized trials, the role of surgery (nephrectomy) as the primary treatment for stages I to III RCA is supported by expert opinion. In addition, opinion is that selected patients with stage IV disease may benefit from resection of the clinical metastasis.

Guidelines from the National Comprehensive Cancer Network Panel on kidney cancer state that surgical resection is the only effective therapy for clinically localized RCA.[1] Ⓒ

The Guidelines also state that surgery is advised for patients with stage I or II tumors as well as patients with stage III disease.[1] Ⓒ

In addition, candidates for resection of metastases include patients who present with the primary tumor and a solitary extrarenal metastasis and patients who develop a solitary recurrence after nephrectomy for the primary tumor.[1] Ⓒ

There is some evidence that debulking nephrectomy (cytoreductive nephrectomy) is of benefit for selected patients with metastatic RCA who are undergoing immunotherapy.

Data from randomized, controlled trials (RCTs) that compared radical nephrectomy followed by treatment with interferon (IFN)-alpha compared with treatment with IFN-alpha alone has shown that the use of cytoreductive nephrectomy before immunotherapy is associated with improved survival rate compared with treatment with IFN-alpha alone.[2] Ⓐ Ⓑ

Guidelines from the National Comprehensive Cancer Network Panel on kidney cancer state consider that patients most likely to benefit from cytoreductive nephrectomy before immunotherapy are those with lung-only metastases, good prognostic features, and good performance status.[1] Ⓒ

Treatment with immunotherapy (interleukin-2 (IL-2), alone or in combination with IFN) may benefit patients with advanced (metastatic, recurrent, or unresectable) RCA. Limited data suggest that higher doses of IL-2 are more effective. However, its use is associated with high toxicity. Use is supported by expert opinion.

RCTs have shown that treatment with IL-2 induces a clinical response and improves progression-free survival in patients with metastatic renal cell cancer. Data suggest that higher dose treatment with IL-2 is more effective than IFN either alone or in combination with low-dose IL-2, although toxicity may limit its use.[3] Ⓐ

Systematic reviews and meta-analyses have found that treatment with IFN-alpha is associated with a consistent and significant reduction in mortality rate compared with alternative regimens.[4] Ⓐ

Recommendations from the National Comprehensive Cancer Network Panel on kidney cancer are that high-dose IL-2 is considered a category 2A recommendation as first-line therapy in select patients with advanced (relapsed, stage IV, or unresectable) clear cell renal cell carcinoma.[1] Ⓒ

As subsequent or second-line therapy, these guidelines consider high-dose IL-2 or low-dose IL-2 in combination with IFN as category 2B recommendations.[1] Ⓒ

There is limited evidence that targeted therapy with sorafenib or sunitinib may benefit patients with advanced clear cell renal carcinoma. Their use is supported by expert opinion.

A recent large RCT compared sorafenib and placebo in 903 patients with refractory RCA that was resistant to standard therapy. This study found that treatment with sorafenib resulted in significantly improved progression-free survival.[5] Ⓐ

Another recent RCT compared sunitinib and IFN-alpha in 750 patients with previously untreated, metastatic RCA. This study found that treatment with sunitinib resulted in significantly longer progression-free survival compared with IFN. Sunitinib was also associated with a higher objective response rate, and patients reported a significantly better quality of life.[6] Ⓐ

Recommendations from the National Comprehensive Cancer Network Panel on kidney cancer are that use of sorafenib or sunitinib is considered a category 2B recommendation as first-line therapy in select patients with advanced (relapsed, stage IV, or unresectable) clear cell renal cell carcinoma.[1] Ⓒ

As subsequent or second-line therapy, these guidelines consider use of sorafenib or sunitinib as a category 1 recommendation in patients previously treated with IFN or IL-2.[1] Ⓒ

Evidence-Based References

1. National Comprehensive Cancer Network: Clinical practice guidelines in oncology, *Kidney Cancer* 2007.

2. Flanigan RC et al: Cytoreductive nephrectomy in patients with metastatic renal cancer: a combined analysis, *J Urol* 171:1071, 2004.

TABLE 1-64 Comparison of Conventional and TNM Staging Classification of RCAs

Robson Stage	T	N	M
I: Tumor confined by capsule	T_1 (tumor $\le$2.5 cm) T_2 (tumor >2.5 cm, limited to kidney)		
II: Tumor extension to perirenal fat or ipsilateral adrenal but confined by Gerota's fascia	T_3a (tumor invades adrenal gland or perinephric fat but not beyond Gerota's fascia)		
IIIa: Renal vein or inferior vena caval involvement	T_3b (renal vein or caval involvement below diaphragm)	N_0 (nodes negative)	M_0 (no distant metastases)
IIIb: Lymphatic involvement	T_{1-4}	N_1 (single lymph node $\le$2 cm) N_2 (single node 2 to 5 cm, or multiple N_3 (single or multiple nodes >5 cm)	T_3c (caval involvement above nodes <5 cm)
IIIc: Combination of IIIa and IIIb	$T_{3,4}$		
IVa: Spread to contiguous	T_4 (tumor extends beyond organs except ipsilateral adrenal Gerota's fascia)		
IVb: Distant metastases	T_{1-4}		M_1 (distant metastases)

RCC, Renal cell carcinoma.

3. McDermott DF et al: Randomized phase III trial of high-dose interleukin-2 versus subcutaneous interleukin-2 and interferon in patients with metastatic renal cell carcinoma, *J Clin Oncol* 23:133, 2005. Erratum in *J Clin Oncol* 23:2877, 2005.

4. Coppin C et al: Immunotherapy for advanced renal cell cancer, *Cochrane Rev* 3, 2004.

5. Escudier B et al: TARGET Study Group. Sorafenib in advanced clear-cell renal-cell carcinoma, *N Engl J Med* 356:125, 2007.

6. Motzer RJ et al: Sunitinib versus interferon alpha in metastatic renal-cell carcinoma, *N Engl J Med* 356:115-124, 2007.

SUGGESTED READINGS

Cohen HT, McGovern FJ: Renal cell carcinoma, *N Engl J Med* 353:2477, 2005.

Curti BD: Renal cell carcinoma, *JAMA* 292:97, 2004.

Flanigan RC et al: Nephrectomy followed by interferon alpha-2b compared with interferon alfa-2b alone for metastatic renal-cell cancer, *N Engl J Med* 345: 1655, 2002.

Hudes G et al: Temsirolimus, interferon alfa, or both for advanced renal-cell carcinoma, *N Engl J Med* 356: 2271, 2007.

Motzer RJ et al: Sunitinib in patients with metastatic renal cell carcinoma, *JAMA* 295:2516, 2006.

Motzer RJ et al: Sunitinib versus interferon alfa in metastatic renal-cell carcinoma, *N Engl J Med* 356: 115, 2007.

Yang CJ: A randomized trial of Bevacizumab, an anti-vascular endothelial growth factor antibody, for metastatic renal cancer, *N Engl J Med* 349:427, 2003.

AUTHOR: **FRED F. FERRI, M.D.**

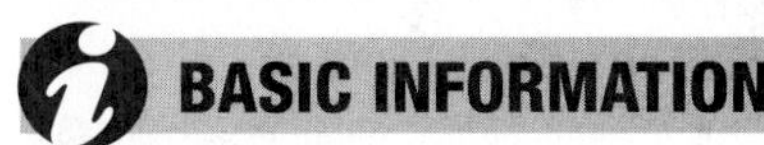

BASIC INFORMATION

DEFINITION

Acute renal failure (ARF) is the rapid impairment in renal function resulting in retention of products in the blood that are normally excreted by the kidneys.

SYNONYMS

ARF

ICD-9CM CODES

584.9 Acute renal failure, unspecified

EPIDEMIOLOGY & DEMOGRAPHICS

- ARF requiring dialysis develops in five in 100,000 persons annually.
- >10% of intensive care unit patients develop ARF.
- >40% of hospital ARF is iatrogenic.
- The most common cause of ARF in hospitalized patients is intrinsic renal failure caused by acute tubular necrosis.
- Acute renal failure occurs in 20% of patients with moderate sepsis and more than 50% of patients with septic shock and positive blood cultures.

PHYSICAL FINDINGS & CLINICAL PRESENTATION

- The physical examination should focus on volume status. The physical findings noted below vary with the duration and rapidity of onset of renal failure.
- Peripheral edema
- Skin pallor, ecchymoses
- Oliguria (however, patients can have nonoliguric renal failure), anuria
- Delirium, lethargy, myoclonus, seizures
- Back pain, fasciculations, muscle cramps
- Tachypnea, tachycardia
- Weakness, anorexia, generalized malaise, nausea

ETIOLOGY

- Prerenal: inadequate perfusion caused by hypovolemia, congestive heart failure, cirrhosis, sepsis. Sixty percent of community-acquired cases of ARF are from prerenal conditions.
- Postrenal: outlet obstruction from prostatic enlargement, ureteral obstruction (stones), bilateral renal vein occlusion. Postrenal causes account for 5% to 15% of community-acquired ARF.
- Intrinsic renal: glomerulonephritis, acute tubular necrosis, drug toxicity, contrast nephropathy. Contrast-induced nephropathy (increase in serum creatinine > 25% within 3 days of intravascular contrast administration in absence of an alternative cause) is the third most common cause of new ARF in hospitalized patients.
- Causes of acute renal failure are described in Section II.

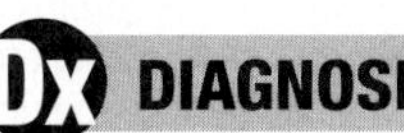

DIAGNOSIS

DIFFERENTIAL DIAGNOSIS

Refer to "Etiology."

LABORATORY TESTS

- Elevated serum creatinine: the rate of rise is approximately 1 mg/dl/day in complete renal failure.
- Elevated blood urea nitrogen (BUN): BUN/creatinine ratio is >20:1 in prerenal azotemia, postrenal azotemia, and acute glomerulonephritis; it is <20:1 in acute interstitial nephritis and acute tubular necrosis (Table 1-65).
- Electrolytes (potassium, phosphate) are elevated; bicarbonate level and calcium are decreased.
- Complete blood count may reveal anemia because of decreased erythropoietin production, hemoconcentration, or hemolysis.
- Urinalysis may reveal the presence of hematuria (glomerulonephritis), proteinuria (nephrotic syndrome), casts (e.g., granular casts in acute tubular necrosis, red blood cell casts in acute GN, white blood cell casts in acute interstitial nephritis), eosinophiluria (acute interstitial nephritis).
- Urinary sodium and urinary creatinine should also be obtained to calculate the fractional excretion of sodium (FE_{Na}) (FE_{Na} = Urine sodium/Plasma sodium × Plasma creatinine/Urine creatinine × 100). FE_{Na} is <1 in prerenal failure and >1 in intrinsic renal failure in patients with urine output <400 ml/day.
- Urinary osmolarity is 250 to 300 mOsm/kg in ATN, <400 mOsm/kg in postrenal azotemia, and >500 mOsm/kg in prerenal azotemia and acute glomerulonephritis (Table 1-66).
- Additional useful studies are blood cultures for patients suspected of sepsis, liver function tests, immunoglobulins, and protein electrophoresis in patients suspected of myeloma; and creatinine kinase in patients with suspected rhabdomyolysis.
- Renal biopsy may be indicated in patients with intrinsic renal failure when considering specific therapy; major uses of renal biopsy are differential diagnosis of nephrotic syndrome, separation of lupus vasculitis from other vasculitis and lupus membranous from idiopathic membranous, confirmation of hereditary nephropathies on the basis of the ultrastructure, diagnosis of rapidly progressing glomerulonephritis, separation of allergic interstitial nephritis from ATN, separation of primary glomerulonephritis syndromes. The biopsy may be performed percutaneously or by open method. The percutaneous approach is favored and generally yields adequate tissue in >90% of cases. Open biopsy is generally reserved for uncooperative patients, those with solitary kidney, and patients at risk for uncontrolled bleeding.

IMAGING STUDIES

- Chest radiograph is useful to evaluate for congestive heart failure and for pulmonary renal syndromes (Goodpasture's syndrome, Wegener's granulomatosis).
- Ultrasound of kidneys is used to evaluate kidney size (useful to distinguish acute from

TABLE 1-65 Serum and Radiographic Abnormalities in Renal Failure

	Prerenal	Postrenal (Acute)	Intrinsic Renal (Acute)	Intrinsic Renal (Chronic)
BUN	↑ 10:1 > Cr	↑ 20-40/day	↑ 20-40/day	Stable; ↑ varies with protein intake
Serum creatinine	N/moderate ↑	↑ 2-4/day	↑ 2-4/day	Stable ↑ (production equals excretion)
Serum potassium	N/moderate ↑	↑ varies with urinary volume	↑↑ (particularly when patient is oliguric)	Normal until end stage, unless tubular dysfunction (type 4 RTA)
			↑↑↑ with rhabdomyolysis	
Serum phosphorus	N/moderate ↑	Moderate ↑	↑	Becomes significantly elevated when serum creatinine surpasses 3 mg/dl
		↑↑ with rhabdomyolysis	Poor correlation with duration of renal disease	
Serum calcium	N	N/↓ with PO_4^{-3} retention	↓ (poor correlation with duration of renal failure)	Usually ↓
Renal size				
By ultrasonography	N/↑	↑ and dilated calyces	N/↑	↓ and with ↑ echogenicity
FE_{Na}*	<1	<1 → >1	>1†	>1

From Kiss B: Renal failure. In Ferri FF (ed): *Practical guide to the care of the medical patient,* ed 8, St Louis, 2011, Mosby.

↑, Increase; ↓, decrease; ↑↑, large increase; ↑↑↑, very high increase; *BUN,* blood urea nitrogen; *Cr,* creatinine; *N,* normal; *Na,* sodium; *P,* plasma; *RTA,* renal tubular acidosis; *U,* urine.

$$*FE_{Na} = \left[\frac{U/P_{Na^+}}{U/P_{Cr}} \times 100\right]$$ (useful only in oliguric patient).

†May be ≤1 in radiocontrast-induced myoglobinuric acute tubular necrosis and in early sepsis.

chronic renal failure), evaluate for the presence of obstruction, and evaluate renal vascular status (with Doppler evaluation).

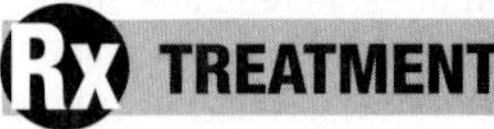

TREATMENT

NONPHARMACOLOGIC THERAPY

- Stop all nephrotoxic medications.
- Dietary modification to supply adequate calories while minimizing accumulation of toxins; appropriate control of fluid balance. Physicians should recommend a nutrition program with an energy prescription of 120 to 150 KJ/kg/day and restriction of potassium (60 mEq/day), sodium (90 mEq/day), and phosphorus (800 mg/day). Ideal protein supplementation ranges from 0.6 to 1.4 g/kg depending on whether dialysis is required.
- Daily weight.
- Modifications of dosage of renally excreted drugs.

ACUTE GENERAL Rx

Treatment is variable with etiology of ARF:

- Prerenal: IV volume expansion in hypovolemic patients.
- Intrinsic renal: discontinuation of any potential toxins and treatment of condition causing the renal failure.
  1. Low-dose dopamine is at times used to influence renal dysfunction and may offer transient improvement in renal physiology; however, there is lack of evidence that it offers significant clinical benefits to patients with or at risk for acute renal failure.
  2. Fenoldopam, a dopamine alpha-1 receptor agonist currently approved for inpatient management of severe hypertension, has been reported to be beneficial in patients at risk for renal failure related to reduced renal blood flow.
  3. Although furosemide is used frequently to convert oliguric to nonoliguric renal failure in patients with early ARF, it has no effect on mortality rate, dialysis requirement, or proportion of patients with persistent oliguria. Its use in a high dose is also associated with increased risk of tinnitus and temporary deafness.
- Postrenal: removal of obstruction.

CHRONIC Rx

- Monitoring of renal function and electrolytes.
- Prevention of further insults to the kidneys with proper hydration, especially before contrast studies, and avoidance of nephrotoxic agents. Hydration with sodium bicarbonate (addition of 154 ml of 1000 mEq/L sodium bicarbonate to 846 ml of 5% dextrose in water) before contrast exposure is more effective than hydration with sodium chloride for prophylaxis of contrast-induced renal failure. Administration of *N*-acetylcysteine prophylaxis has been shown to reduce the risk of contrast-induced nephropathy.
- See "Chronic Renal Failure" entry for indications for initiation of dialysis. Daily hemodialysis is superior to every-other-day hemodialysis in patients with acute tubular necrosis and ARF.

DISPOSITION

- General indications for initiation of dialysis are:
  1. Florid symptoms of uremia (encephalopathy, pericarditis)
  2. Severe volume overload
  3. Severe acid–base imbalance
  4. Significant derangement in electrolyte concentrations (e.g., hyperkalemia, hyponatremia)
- Intermittent hemodialysis and continuous renal replacement therapy have similar outcomes for patients with ARF.
- Renal function recovery (ability to discontinue dialysis) varies from 50% to 75% in survivors of ARF.
- Overall mortality rate in ARF is nearly 50%, varying from 60% in patients with ATN to 35% in patients with prerenal or postrenal ARF.
- The combination of ARF and sepsis is associated with a 70% mortality rate.

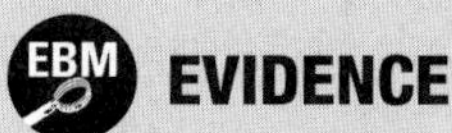

EVIDENCE

Please note: Complete text of EBM for this topic is available online.

SUGGESTED READINGS

Abuelo G: Normotensive ischemic acute renal failure, *N Engl J Med* 357:797, 2007.

Kelly A et al: Meta-analysis: effectiveness of drugs for preventing contrast-induced nephropathy, *Ann Intern Med* 148:284-294, 2008.

Pannu N et al: Renal replacement therapy in patients with acute renal failure, *JAMA* 299(7):793-805, 2008.

AUTHOR: **FRED F. FERRI, M.D.**

TABLE 1-66 Urinary Abnormalities in Renal Failure

	Prerenal	Postrenal (Acute)	Intrinsic Renal (Acute)	Intrinsic Renal (Chronic)
Urinary volume	$\downarrow$	Absent-to-wide fluctuation	Oliguric or nonoliguric	1000 ml + until end stage
Urinary creatinine	$\uparrow$ (U/P Cr $\pm$40)	$\downarrow$ (U/P Cr $\pm$20)	$\downarrow$ (U/P Cr $<$20)	$\downarrow$ (U/P Cr $<$20)
Osmolarity	$\uparrow$ ($\pm$400 mOsm/kg)	($<$350 mOsm/kg)	($<$350 mOsm/kg)	($<$350 mOsm/kg)
Degree of proteinuria	Minimum	Absent	Varies with cause of renal failure: Modest with ATN; Nephrotic range common with acute glomerulopathies, usually $<$2 g/24 hr with interstitial disease*	Varies with cause of renal disease (from 1-2 g/day to nephrotic range)
Urinary sediment	Negative, or occasional hyaline cast	Negative or hematuria with stones or papillary necrosis; Pyuria with infectious prostatic disease	ATN: muddy brown casts; Interstitial nephritis: lymphocytes, eosinophils (in stained preparations), and WBC casts; RPGN: RBC casts; Nephrosis: oval fat bodies	Broad casts with variable renal "residual" acute findings

From Kiss B: Renal failure. In Ferri FF (ed): *Practical guide to the care of the medical patient,* ed 8, St Louis, 2011, Mosby.

$\uparrow$, Increased; $\downarrow$, decreased; *ATN,* acute tubular necrosis; clearance = $\frac{\text{urinary concentration} \times \text{urinary volume}}{\text{plasma concentration}}$; *Cr,* creatinine; *RBC,* red blood cell; *RPGN,* rapidly progressive glomerulonephritis; *U/P,* urine/plasma; *WBC,* white blood cell.

*Except nonsteroidal anti-inflammatory drug-induced allergic interstitial nephritis with concomitant "nil disease."

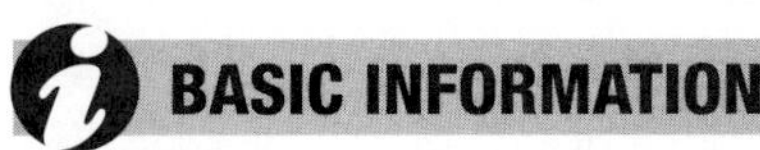

DEFINITION

Chronic renal failure (CRF) is a progressive decrease in renal function (glomerular filtration rate [GFR] <60 ml/min for >3 mo) with subsequent accumulation of waste products in the blood, electrolyte abnormalities, and anemia.

SYNONYMS

CRF
Chronic kidney disease
CKD
End-stage renal disease

ICD-9CM CODES
585 Chronic renal failure

EPIDEMIOLOGY & DEMOGRAPHICS

- The prevalence of patients with chronic kidney disease in the U.S. is approximately 11%.
- The number of patients with end-stage renal disease (ESRD) is increasing at the rate of 7% to 9% per year in the U.S. Each year two in 10,000 persons develop end-stage CRF.
- In the U.S., >250,000 people per year receive dialysis treatment for ESRD.

PHYSICAL FINDINGS & CLINICAL PRESENTATION

- Skin pallor, ecchymoses.
- Edema, leg cramps, restless legs, peripheral neuropathy.
- Hypertension.
- Emotional lability and depression, decreased mental acuity.
- The clinical presentation varies with the degree of renal failure and its underlying etiology. Common symptoms are generalized fatigue, nausea, anorexia, pruritus, sleep disturbances, smell and taste disturbances, hiccups, and seizures.

ETIOLOGY

- Diabetes (37%), hypertension (30%), chronic glomerulonephritis (12%)
- Polycystic kidney disease
- Tubular interstitial nephritis (e.g., drug hypersensitivity, analgesic nephropathy), obstructive nephropathies (e.g., nephrolithiasis, prostatic disease)
- Vascular diseases (renal artery stenosis, hypertensive nephrosclerosis)

Dx DIAGNOSIS

- CRF is primarily distinguished from acute RF by the duration (progression over several months).
- Sonographic evaluation of the kidneys reveals smaller kidneys with increased echogenicity in CRF.

WORKUP

- Laboratory evaluation and imaging studies should be aimed at identifying reversible causes of acute decrements in GFR (e.g., volume depletion, urinary tract obstruction, congestive heart failure [CHF]) superimposed on chronic renal disease.
- Kidney biopsy: generally not performed in patients with small kidneys or with advanced disease.
- GFR is the best overall indicator of kidney function. It can be estimated by using prediction equations that take into account the serum creatinine level and some or all specific variables (body size, age, sex, race). GFR calculators are available on the National Kidney Foundation website (http://www.kidney.org/kls/professionals/gfr_calculator.cfm).

LABORATORY TESTS

- Elevated blood urea nitrogen (BUN), creatinine, creatinine clearance.
- Urinalysis: may reveal proteinuria, red blood cell casts.
- Serum chemistry: elevated BUN and creatinine, hyperkalemia, hyperuricemia, hypocalcemia, hyperphosphatemia, hyperglycemia, decreased bicarbonate.
- Measure urinary protein excretion. The finding of a protein/creatinine ratio of >1000 mg/g suggests the presence of glomerular disease.
- Special studies: serum and urine immunoelectrophoresis (in suspected multiple myeloma), antinuclear antibody (in suspected systemic lupus erythematosus).
- Cystatin C is a cysteine proteinase inhibitor produced by all nucleated cells, freely filtered at the glomerulus but not secreted by tubular cells. Given these characteristics, it may be superior to creatinine concentration both in kidney disease and as a marker of acute kidney injury. It is a better index of kidney function in elderly patients and a better predictor of outcomes than creatinine. The association of cystatin C is stronger than the association of measured GFR with all-cause and cardiovascular mortality in patients with advanced chronic kidney disease.

IMAGING STUDIES

Ultrasound of kidneys to measure kidney size and rule out obstruction

Rx TREATMENT

NONPHARMACOLOGIC THERAPY

- Provide adequate nutrition and calories (147 to 168 kJ/kg/day in energy intake, chiefly from carbohydrate and polyunsaturated fats). Referral to a dietician for nutritional therapy for patients with GFR <50 ml/1.73 m^2 is recommended and is now a covered service by Medicare.
- Restrict sodium (approximately 100 mmol/day), potassium (≤60 mmol/day), and phosphate (<800 mg/day).
- Adjust drug doses to correct for prolonged half-lives.
- Restrict fluid if significant edema is present.
- Protein restriction (≤0.8 g/kg/day) may slow deterioration of renal function; however, recent studies have not confirmed this benefit. There is insufficient evidence to recommend or advise against routine restriction of protein intake.
- Resistance exercise training can preserve lean body mass, nutritional status, and muscle function in patients with moderate chronic kidney disease.
- Avoid radiocontrast agents. Hydration with sodium bicarbonate before contrast exposure is more effective than hydration with sodium chloride for prophylaxis of contrast-induced renal failure.
- Smoking cessation.
- Initiate hemodialysis or peritoneal dialysis (see "Acute General Rx").
- Prompt referral to nephrologist is essential. Late evaluation of patients with chronic renal disease is associated with greater burden and severity of comorbid disease and shorter survival.
- Kidney transplantation in selected patients.

ACUTE GENERAL Rx

- Angiotensin-converting enzyme (ACE) inhibitors and angiotensin receptor blockers (ARBs) are useful in reducing proteinuria and slowing the progression of chronic renal disease, especially in hypertensive diabetic patients. The combination of ACEi and ARBs should be used with great caution in patients with chronic kidney disease due to increased risk of hyperkalemia, hypotension, and worsening renal failure. A systolic blood pressure between 110 and 129 mm Hg may be beneficial in patients with urine protein excretion >1.0 g/day. Systolic blood pressure <110 mm Hg may be associated with a higher risk for kidney disease progression.
- Initiation of dialysis:
  1. Urgent indications: uremic pericarditis, neuropathy, neuromuscular abnormalities, CHF, hyperkalemia, seizures.
  2. Judgmental indications: creatinine clearance 10 to 15 ml/min; progressive anorexia, weight loss, reversal of sleep pattern, pruritus, uncontrolled fluid gain with hypertension and signs of CHF.
- Erythropoiesis-stimulating agents epoetin-alpha and darbepoetin-alpha can be used to reduce the need for transfusions in patients with anemia. Anemia should not be fully corrected in patients with chronic kidney disease. Maintaining a target hemoglobin of 10 g/dl or hematocrit 30% to 33% is satisfactory.
- Diuretics for significant fluid overload (loop diuretics are preferred).
- Correction of hypertension to at least 130/85 mm Hg with ACE inhibitors (avoid in patients with significant hyperkalemia), ARBs, and/or nondihydropyridene calcium channel blockers (verapamil, diltiazem) can be used in patients intolerant to ACE inhibitors or when other agents are needed to control blood pressure.
- Correction of electrolyte abnormalities (e.g., calcium chloride, glucose, sodium polystyrene sulfonate for hyperkalemia), sodium bicarbonate in patients with severe metabolic acidosis.
- Lipid-lowering agents in patients with dyslipidemia; target low-density lipoprotein cholesterol is <100 mg/dl.

- Control of renal osteodystrophy with calcium supplementation and vitamin D. Starting dose of calcium carbonate is 0.5 g with each meal, increased until the serum phosphorus concentration is normalized (most patients require 5 to 10 g/day). Calcitriol 0.125 to 0.25 mcg/day PO is effective in increasing serum calcium concentration. Paricalcitol, a new vitamin D analogue, has been reported to be more effective than calcitriol in lessening the elevations in serum calcium and phosphorus levels.
- Sevelamer is a useful phosphate binder to reduce serum phosphate levels.

DISPOSITION

- Prognosis is influenced by comorbidity of multisystem diseases. Late referral of patients to a nephrologist is associated with higher mortality and morbidity rates and higher costs. Despite recommendations for early referral, up to 64% of patients with CRF are still referred late.
- Apolipoprotein E variation predicts chronic kidney disease progression, independent of diabetes, race, lipid, and nonlipid factors. The e2 allele moderately increases risk of kidney disease progression, whereas allele e4 decreases the risk.
- Kidney transplantation in selected patients improves survival. The 2-yr kidney graft survival rate for living related donor transplantations is >80%, whereas the 2-yr graft survival rate for cadaveric donor transplantation is approximately 70%.

EBM EVIDENCE

Please note: Complete text of EBM for this topic is available online.

Key trials and commentary:

Sodium bicarbonate has been suggested as a possible strategy for prevention of contrast medium–induced nephropathy (CIN), a common cause of renal failure associated with prolonged hospitalization, increased health care costs, and substantial morbidity and mortality.

This study sought to determine if sodium bicarbonate is superior to sodium chloride for preventing CIN in patients with moderate to severe chronic kidney dysfunction who are undergoing coronary angiography.

The results of this study do not suggest that hydration with sodium bicarbonate is superior to hydration with sodium chloride for the prevention of CIN in patients with moderate-to-severe chronic kidney disease who are undergoing coronary angiography.

CIN is a relevant patient care issue, occurring in up to 15% of patients with chronic renal impairment who undergo diagnostic or therapeutic radiographic procedures. A small but significant fraction of these patients (on the order of 1%-10%) may require dialysis and/or prolonged hospitalization; some have persistent decline in renal function over several weeks, evolving toward end-stage renal failure. A higher risk of death has also been reported.

A wide range of preventive strategies have been recommended, including pre-, post-, and peri-procedural hydration with isotonic or hypotonic saline, antioxidant compounds such as N-acetylcysteine or ascorbic acid, and hemofiltration dialysis.

The results of many such studies have been inconclusive or suggest only minimal beneficial therapeutic effects, with intravenous volume expansion the only measure of undisputed efficacy.

However, other randomized studies have recently reported the beneficial effects of administering sodium bicarbonate in reducing the incidence of CIN.

This article, a large-multicenter study in 353 patients undergoing cardiac catheterization, found no benefit to sodium bicarbonate in addition to hydration and N-acetylcysteine, thus reopening the issue once again. This article was especially well done in that patients were tracked not just in the acute phase (i.e., after the first few days) but several weeks to several months after contrast administration.[1] Ⓐ

This study sought to define the role of sodium bicarbonate in preventing CIN in clinical settings.

This study showed that the use of intravenous sodium bicarbonate was associated with increased incidence of CIN. Use of sodium bicarbonate to prevent CIN should be evaluated further rather than adopted into clinical practice.

CIN is one of the leading causes of acute renal failure. The incidence in the general population is only about 1% to 2%. However, in certain high-risk populations with diabetes, anemia, congestive heart failure, and chronic kidney disease, the incidence can exceed 50%. Strategies for the prevention of CIN have included pretreatment with acetylcysteine and several different hydration strategies. The suggestion that hydration with sodium bicarbonate ($NaHCO_3$) containing fluids could reduce the incidence of CIN was demonstrated by the study of Merten et al in 2004, which compared normal saline vs. $NaHCO_3$ hydration strategies. The current article, which is a retrospective review of over 11,000 patients suggests that, despite better baseline renal parameters in the sodium bicarbonate group, $NaHCO_3$ therapy may actually significantly increase the incidence of CIN ($P < 0.0001$). Thus, the role of sodium bicarbonate administration as a protective strategy for CIN remains uncertain and a large, appropriately powered, randomized controlled trial will be required to fully evaluate its risks and benefits. In the meantime, saline-based hydration strategies continue to be the standard choice.[2] Ⓐ

Evidence-Based References

1. Brar SS, Shen AY-J, Jorgensen MB: Sodium bicarbonate vs. sodium chloride for the prevention of contrast medium–induced nephropathy in patients undergoing coronary angiography: a randomized trial, *JAMA* 300:1038-1046, 2008. Commentary by A.D. Elster, M.D. Ⓐ
2. From AM, Bartholmai BJ, Williams AW: Sodium bicarbonate is associated with an increased incidence of contrast nephropathy: a retrospective cohort study of 7977 patients at Mayo Clinic, *Clin J Am Soc Nephrol* 3:10-18, 2008. Commentary by R. Garrick, M.D. Ⓐ

SUGGESTED READINGS

Herget-Rosenthal S et al: Early detection of acute renal failure by serum cystatin C, *Kidney Int* 66:1115, 2004.

Hsu CC et al: Apolipoprotein E and progression of chronic kidney disease, *JAMA* 293:2892, 2005.

Jafar TH et al: Progression of chronic kidney disease: the role of blood pressure control, proteinuria, and angiotensin-converting enzyme inhibition, *Ann Intern Med* 139:244, 2003.

Johnson CA et al: Clinical practice guidelines for chronic kidney disease in adults, *Am Fam Physician* 70:869, 2004.

Kinchen KS et al: The timing of specialist evaluation in chronic kidney disease and mortality, *Ann Intern Med* 137:479, 2003.

Ku E et al: The hazards of dual renin-angiotensin blockade in chronic kidney disease, *Arch Intern Med* 169(11):1015-1018, 2009.

Kunz R et al: Meta-analysis: effect of monotherapy and combination therapy with inhibitors of the renin-angiotensin system on proteinuria in renal disease, *Ann Intern Med* 148:30-48, 2008.

Levey AS et al: National Kidney Foundation practice guidelines for chronic kidney disease: evaluation, classification, and stratification, *Ann Intern Med* 139:137, 2003.

Levey AS: A new equation to estimate glomerular filtration rate, *Ann Intern Med* 150:604-612, 2009.

Mann JFE et al: Effect of telmisartan on renal outcomes, *Ann Intern Med* 151:1-10, 2009.

Menon V et al: Cystatin C as a risk factor for outcomes in chronic kidney disease, *Ann Intern Med* 147:19, 2007.

Merten GJ et al: Prevention of contrast-induced nephropathy with sodium bicarbonate, *JAMA* 291: 2328, 2004.

Meyer TW, Hostetter TH: Uremia, *N Engl J Med* 357: 1316-1325, 2007.

Singh AK et al: Correction of anemia with epoetin alfa in chronic kidney disease, *N Engl J Med* 355:2085, 2006.

Snively C, Gutierrez C: Chronic kidney disease: prevention and treatment of common complications, *Am Fam Physician* 70:1921, 2004.

Sprangers B et al: Late referral of patients with chronic kidney disease: no time to waste, *Mayo Clin Proc* 81:1487, 2006.

AUTHOR: **FRED F. FERRI, M.D.**

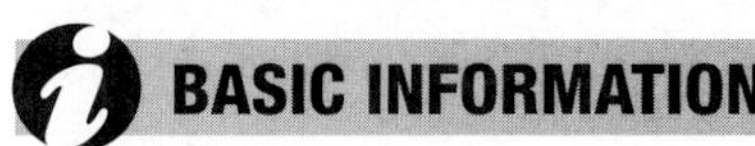

BASIC INFORMATION

DEFINITION

Renal tubular acidosis (RTA) is a disorder characterized by inability to excrete H^+ or inadequate generation of new HCO_3^-. There are four types of renal tubular acidosis:

- Type I (classic, distal RTA): abnormality in distal hydrogen secretion, resulting in hypokalemic hyperchloremic metabolic acidosis.
- Type II (proximal RTA): decreased proximal bicarbonate reabsorption, resulting in hypokalemic hyperchloremic metabolic acidosis.
- Type III (RTA of glomerular insufficiency): normokalemic hyperchloremic metabolic acidosis as a result of impaired ability to generate sufficient NH_3 in the setting of decreased glomerular filtration rate ($<$30 ml/min). This type of RTA is described in older textbooks and is considered by many not to be a distinct entity.
- Type IV (hyporeninemic hypoaldosteronemic RTA): aldosterone deficiency or antagonism, resulting in decreased distal acidification and decreased distal sodium reabsorption with subsequent hyperkalemic hyperchloremic acidosis.

SYNONYMS

RTA

ICD-9CM CODES
588.8 Renal tubular acidosis

EPIDEMIOLOGY & DEMOGRAPHICS

RTA type IV affects mostly adults, whereas RTA types I and II are more frequent in children.

PHYSICAL FINDINGS & CLINICAL PRESENTATION

- Examination may be normal.
- Poor skin turgor may be present from dehydration.
- Muscle weakness and muscle aches from hypokalemia may occur.
- Low back pain and bone pain may be present in patients with abnormalities of calcium metabolism (RTA II).
- There is failure to thrive in children (RTA II).

ETIOLOGY

- Type I RTA: autoimmune disorders, primary biliary cirrhosis and other liver diseases, medications (amphotericin, nonsteroidals), systemic lupus erythematosus, Sjögren's syndrome, genetic disorders (Ehlers-Danlos syndrome, Marfan syndrome, hereditary elliptocytosis), toxins (toluene), disorders with nephrocalcinosis (hyperparathyroidism, vitamin D intoxication, idiopathic hypercalciuria), tubulointerstitial disease (obstructive uropathy, renal transplantation)
- Type II RTA: Fanconi's syndrome, primary hyperparathyroidism, multiple myeloma, medications (acetazolamide)
- Type IV RTA: diabetes mellitus, sickle cell disease, Addison's disease, urinary obstruction

DIAGNOSIS

DIFFERENTIAL DIAGNOSIS

- Diarrhea with significant bicarbonate loss
- Other causes of metabolic acidosis
- Respiratory acidosis

WORKUP

Detection of hyperchloremic metabolic acidosis with arterial blood gases (ABGs) and serum electrolytes and evaluation of potential causes (see "Etiology")

LABORATORY TESTS

- ABGs reveal metabolic acidosis; serum potassium is low in RTA types I and II, normal in type III, and high in type IV.
- Minimal urine pH is $>$5.5 in RTA type I and $<$5.5 in types II, III, and IV.
- Urinary anion gap is 0 or positive in all types of RTA.
- Additional useful studies include serum calcium level and urine calcium.
- Anion gap is normal.
- Parathyroid hormone measurement is useful in patients suspected of primary hyperparathyroidism (may be associated with type II RTA).

IMAGING STUDIES

- Plain abdominal radiography is useful to evaluate for nephrocalcinosis.
- Renal sonogram can be used to evaluate renal size or presence of stones.
- Intravenous pyelogram in patients with nephrocalcinosis or nephrolithiasis.

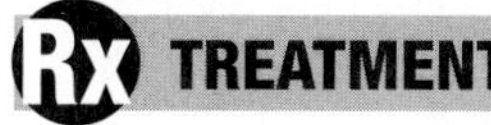

TREATMENT

ACUTE GENERAL Rx

- Types I and II are treated with oral sodium bicarbonate (1 to 2 mEq/kg/day in RTA I, 2 to 4 mEq/kg/day in RTA type II) titrated to correct acidosis.
- Potassium supplementation is needed in hypokalemic patients.
- Type IV RTA can be treated with furosemide to lower elevated potassium levels and sodium bicarbonate to correct significant acidosis. Fludrocortisone 100 to 300 μg/day can be used to correct mineralocorticoid deficiency.

CHRONIC Rx

- Frequent monitoring of potassium levels in RTA type IV
- Monitoring for bone disease in RTA type II
- Monitoring for nephrocalcinosis and nephrolithiasis in RTA type I

DISPOSITION

- Prognosis varies with the presence of associated conditions (see "Etiology").
- Untreated distal RTA may result in hypercalcemia, hyperphosphaturia, nephrolithiasis, and nephrocalcinosis.

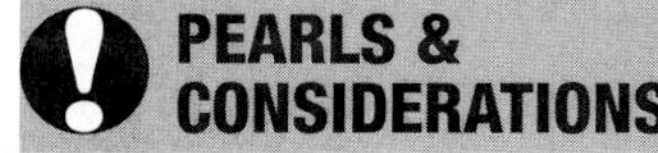

PEARLS & CONSIDERATIONS

COMMENTS

Patient education material can be obtained from the National Kidney and Urologic Diseases Information Clearinghouse, Box NKUDIC, Bethesda, MD 20893.

AUTHOR: **FRED F. FERRI, M.D.**

Renal Vein Thrombosis

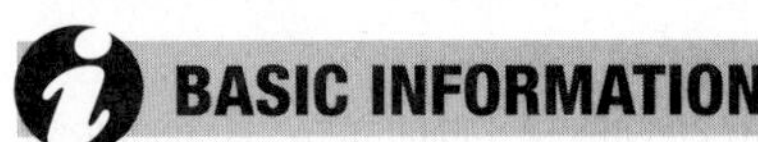

BASIC INFORMATION

DEFINITION

Renal vein thrombosis is the thrombotic occlusion of one or both renal veins.

ICD-9CM CODES
453.3 Renal vein thrombosis

EPIDEMIOLOGY & DEMOGRAPHICS

- Incidence unknown; probably an underdiagnosed condition
- May occur at any age with no gender preference
- Epidemiology tied to the underlying cause

PHYSICAL FINDINGS & CLINICAL PRESENTATION

Acute bilateral renal vein thrombosis:
- Back and bilateral flank pain
- Acute renal failure

Acute unilateral renal vein thrombosis:
- Flank pain
- Decline in renal function
- Hematuria
- Increase in the amount of proteinuria if associated with nephrotic syndrome

Chronic unilateral renal vein thrombosis:
- May be silent
- Pulmonary emboli and hemolysis
- Back pain
- Deep vein thrombosis in lower extremities
- Edema
- Glycosuria
- Hyperchloremic acidosis
- Left varicocele (if the left renal vein is thrombosed)
- Dilated abdominal veins

ETIOLOGY & PATHOGENESIS

- Extrinsic compression by a tumor or retroperitoneal mass
- Invasion of the renal vein or inferior vena cava by tumor (almost always renal cell cancer)
- Trauma
- Hypercoagulable states
- Dehydration
- Glomerulopathies (membranous glomerulonephritis, crescenting glomerulonephritis, systemic lupus erythematosus, amyloidosis) especially in the presence of nephrotic syndrome when the serum albumin is <2 g/dl
- NOTE: For unknown reasons, diabetic nephropathy is not commonly associated with renal vein thrombosis even if the nephrotic syndrome is present

A controversy has existed regarding whether the renal vein thrombosis association with nephrotic syndrome is a complication of nephrotic syndrome or whether renal vein thrombosis occurring in the setting of increased renal vein pressure (e.g., with congestive heart failure, constrictive pericarditis, or extrinsic compression) can independently cause proteinuria. Current evidence is that renal vein thrombosis does not cause nephrotic syndrome.

Dx DIAGNOSIS

DIFFERENTIAL DIAGNOSIS

The diagnosis of renal vein thrombosis does not include any differential consideration. The differential diagnosis is that of proteinuria. Renal vein thrombosis should be considered if proteinuria worsens or if renal function worsens in a patient with glomerulonephritis. Renal vein thrombosis should also be considered in patients with pulmonary emboli and no lower-extremity deep vein thrombosis.

WORKUP

Clinical suspicion (see "Differential Diagnosis") and imaging studies

IMAGING STUDIES

- Abdominal ultrasound
- Abdominal MRI or CT with contrast (Fig. 1-275)
- Renal arteriography (delayed films during venous phase)
- Selective renal vein venography (inferior venacavogram images should be obtained before advancing the catheter in the vena cava because clots, if present, could be dislodged)
- Renal biopsy may be indicated if evidence of nephritis is present (e.g., active urinary sediment)

Rx TREATMENT

- Anticoagulation in acute renal vein thrombosis to prevent pulmonary emboli and in attempt to improve renal function and decrease proteinuria
- Thrombolytic therapy or surgical thrombectomy has also been reported to be effective
- The value of anticoagulation in chronic renal vein thrombosis is dubious except in nephrotic patients with membranous glomerulonephritis with profound hypoalbuminemia where prolonged prophylactic anticoagulation may be of benefit even if renal vein thrombosis has not been documented

PROGNOSIS

Probable worsening of the underlying glomerulonephritis by acute renal vein thrombosis; the effect of chronic renal vein thrombosis is unclear.

AUTHOR: **FRED F. FERRI, M.D.**

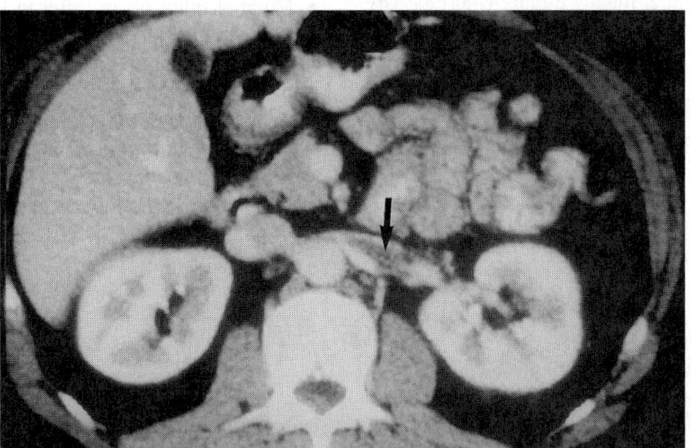

FIGURE 1-275 Renal vein thrombus in a patient with nephritic syndrome. Contrast medium–enhanced CT at the level of the renal vein shows thrombus in the left renal vein *(arrow).* (From Grainger RG et al [eds]: *Grainger & Allison's diagnostic radiology,* ed 4, Philadelphia, 2001, Churchill Livingstone.)

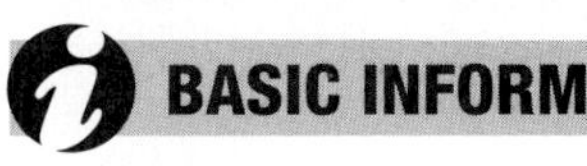

BASIC INFORMATION

DEFINITION

Respiratory syncytial virus (RSV) is an RNA virus that tends to form syncytia in tissue culture. RSV causes repeated acute respiratory tract infections in people of all ages. It is the leading cause of severe lower respiratory tract infections in infants and young children, while it usually manifests as an upper respiratory infection or tracheobronchitis in older children and adults.

ICD-9CM CODES
ICD-079.6

EPIDEMIOLOGY & DEMOGRAPHICS

INCIDENCE: 64 million infections worldwide annually, resulting in 160,000 deaths; it is associated with 120,000 U.S. pediatric hospitalizations annually.
PEAK INCIDENCE: In nontropical areas of the northern hemisphere, seasonal outbreaks usually occur November to April, with a peak in January or February; in nontropical areas of the southern hemisphere, May to September, with a peak in May, June, or July. In the tropics, seasonal outbreaks usually occur during the rainy season.
PREVALENCE: Nearly everyone is infected by age 2 yr, with reinfections occurring throughout life.
PREDOMINANT SEX AND AGE: None generally, but male sex may predispose to more severe respiratory disease in RSV infection. Occurs at all ages but is more likely to be severe in infants, young children, and the elderly.
GENETICS: Severe disease is associated with polymorphisms in various interleukins and CCR5.
RISK FACTORS: For children, risk factors include attending daycare or school and inpatient hospitalization. Severe disease is seen primarily in infants and young children (especially those born before 35 wk of gestation); the elderly; and in patients with cardiac, pulmonary, or immune system dysfunction.

PHYSICAL FINDINGS & CLINICAL PRESENTATION

Physical findings include fever, tachypnea, prolonged expiration, wheezes and rales, cough, rhinorrhea, coryza, conjunctivitis, and otitis media. Clinical presentation can include pneumonia and bronchiolitis.

ETIOLOGY

Humans are the only known reservoir. Transmission is by large respiratory droplets from close contact or contaminated surfaces, where it can survive for several hours. The Centers for Disease Control and Prevention (CDC) recommends handwashing, gowns, and gloves to prevent nosocomial infection, which is especially common on pediatric wards. However, the CDC does not recommend excluding children with respiratory illnesses who are well enough to attend school or daycare as RSV is often spread during early stages of illness.

Dx DIAGNOSIS

DIFFERENTIAL DIAGNOSIS

- Influenza
- Parainfluenza
- Adenovirus

WORKUP

- History with a focus on upper and lower respiratory symptoms, fever, and apnea in infants.
- Focused physical examination, including temperature and pulse oximetry as well as lung and head, eyes, ears, nose, and throat examination.

LABORATORY TESTS

Analysis of respiratory secretions (especially nasal washings) for virus isolation (the standard for definitive diagnosis), viral antigens (most laboratories use this rapid assay), or viral RNA. Other tests include serum antibodies, but this is of dubious usefulness; in infants it is confounded by maternal antibodies and in other patients antibodies are almost universally present due to repeated infections.

IMAGING STUDIES

Chest x-ray for suspected pneumonia, but not routinely in suspected bronchiolitis

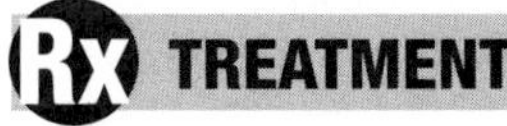

Rx TREATMENT

NONPHARMACOLOGIC THERAPY

Isolation techniques are important in limiting spread of RSV infections.

ACUTE GENERAL Rx

- Mild disease: symptomatic treatment.
- Severe disease may require oxygen therapy, mechanical ventilation, bronchodilators, and corticosteroids.
- Ribavirin aerosol is effective for severe RSV pneumonia.

REFERRAL

To pulmonology for severe disease

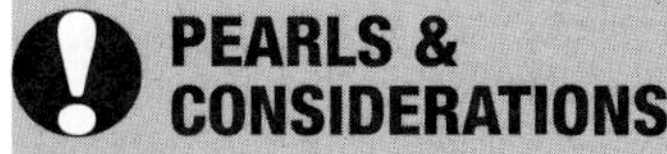

PEARLS & CONSIDERATIONS

PREVENTION

For infants and children with chronic lung disease, prematurity, or otherwise at high risk for RSV complications, preventive treatment may include RSV prophylaxis intravenous immune globulin 750 mg/kg and/or RSV immune globulin (IG) monoclonal antibody (Synagis) 15 mg/kg IM. Updated eligibility criteria for prophylaxis are too detailed to be summarized here, but can be found in the American Academy of Pediatrics Red Book 2009.

PATIENT & FAMILY EDUCATION

Communicate the importance of hand washing.

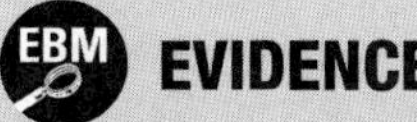

EVIDENCE

Limited evidence suggests that ribavirin may be effective in the management of hospitalized children and infants with RSV bronchiolitis, reducing the duration of mechanical ventilator support and the duration of hospitalization.[1] Ⓐ

Limited evidence suggests that epinephrine may be favorable to albuterol and placebo in outpatients with bronchiolitis, but it has not been shown to be more effective in the inpatient setting.[2] Ⓐ

Evidence on the effects of corticosteroids in bronchiolitis is limited. Corticosteroids do not shorten the duration of hospital admission with acute bronchiolitis, and interpretation of their effect on clinical outcomes has been limited by the diversity of clinical outcome scales used amongst the trials.[3] Ⓐ

Evidence-Based References

1. Ventre K, Randolph AG: Ribavirin for respiratory syncytial virus infection of the lower respiratory tract in infants and young children, *Cochrane Database Rev* 4, 2004. Ⓐ
2. Hartling L et al: Epinephrine for bronchiolitis, *Cochrane Database Rev* 1, 2004. Ⓐ
3. Patel H et al: Glucocorticoids for acute viral bronchiolitis in infants and young children, *Cochrane Database Rev* 3, 2004. Ⓐ

SUGGESTED READINGS

American Academy of Pediatrics, Committee on Infectious Diseases and Committee on Fetus and Newborn: Policy statement: revised indications for the use of palivizumab and respiratory syncytial virus immune globulin intravenous for the prevention of respiratory syncytial virus infections, *Pediatrics* 112: 1442-1446, 2003.

American Academy of Pediatrics Subcommittee on Diagnosis and Management of Bronchiolitis: Diagnosis and management of bronchiolitis, *Pediatrics* 118:1774-1793, 2006.

Centers for Disease Control: www.cdc.gov

Meissner HC et al: Revised indications for the use of palivizumab and respiratory syncytial virus immune globulin intravenous for the prevention of respiratory syncytial virus infections, *Pediatrics* 112:1447-1452, 2003.

Red Book 2009:560-569

WHO: www.who.int

AUTHOR: **STEVEN BUSSELEN, M.D.**

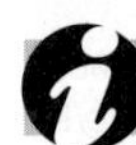

BASIC INFORMATION

DEFINITION

Restless legs syndrome is a sensory-motor disorder with four cardinal features: (1) an uncomfortable sensation or urge to move the legs, (2) discomfort worse in the evening or night, (3) discomfort worse at rest, and (4) discomfort better with movement of the affected leg(s). There are two forms of RLS: primary (familial) and secondary (acquired). Most RLS sufferers (>85%) have periodic leg movements in sleep (PLMS), which also may disrupt sleep.

SYNONYMS

Restless limb syndrome

ICD-9CM CODES
333.99 Restless legs syndrome

EPIDEMIOLOGY & DEMOGRAPHICS

PREVALENCE: 8% to 12%
DEMOGRAPHICS:

- Age <18 yr: unknown
- Ages 18 to 29 yr: 3%
- Ages 30 to 79 yr: 10%
- Ages ≥80 yr: 20%
- Prevalence increases with age (likely because of increases in secondary RLS, which affects males and females equally).
- Symptoms may worsen with age and may spread to the arms or other body areas.
- Prevalence data incomplete for ethnic or racial groups other than whites.
- Primary RLS follows an autosomal-dominant mode of inheritance, shows genetic anticipation, and has a female/male ratio of 3:2.

PHYSICAL FINDINGS & CLINICAL PRESENTATION

- Sensory complaints usually affecting one or both lower extremities during rest:
  1. "Worms" or "bugs" under the skin
  2. Sense of pressure under the skin
  3. Throbbing muscular ache or pain
  4. "Growing pains"
  5. Irresistible urge to move the symptomatic leg(s)
- Many other words used by patients to describe the leg symptoms: creeping, burning, searing, tugging, pulling, drawing, like water flowing, restless, and very often "indescribable."
- Temporary symptomatic relief or improvement with leg movement, rubbing, pressure, walking, or added warmth (bath or heating pad).
- Sleep disruption resulting from leg discomfort, PLMS, and urges to move or walk.
- Leg movements during sleep almost always occur and may be reported by a spouse or parent as kicking or constant movement during the night. These movements are stereotypic, and rhythmic ankle and leg shaking lasting <5 sec can cause arousals during sleep.
- Physical examination is normal in primary RLS but may reveal subtle neuropathy, radiculopathy, or myelopathy in secondary RLS.
- Excessive daytime somnolence, insomnia, and occasional leg symptoms during the day while sedentary are common complaints.

ETIOLOGY

- The most likely mechanism is related to dopaminergic dysregulation at the level of the spinal cord or higher in the central nervous system.
- Primary RLS (50% to 60%) may include iron deficiency.
- Secondary RLS associated with iron deficiency, pregnancy, renal failure, repetitive blood donation, neuropathy, radiculopathy, myelopathy, and rheumatologic conditions.
- Symptoms may be precipitated by medications (selective serotonin reuptake inhibitors [SSRIs] and tricyclic antidepressants [TCAs]), caffeine, alcohol, and sleep deprivation.

Dx DIAGNOSIS

DIFFERENTIAL DIAGNOSIS

- Periodic limb movement disorder (PLMD): repetitive limb movements (lower extremities more than upper extremities) occurring during sleep; no sensory complaints or urges to move the limbs for comfort during periods of rest; associated with arousals in sleep and excessive daytime sleepiness; patient is typically unaware but bed partner may report restlessness or kicking during sleep.
- Peripheral neuropathy, radiculopathy, myelopathy, or other central nervous system injury (e.g., stroke).
- Anxiety and mood disorders.
- Narcolepsy.
- REM sleep behavior disorder.
- Parasomnias (e.g., sleepwalking, confusional arousals, head banging).
- Obstructive sleep apnea.
- Iron deficiency.
- Neuroleptic-induced akathisia.
- Dyskinesias while awake.
- Nocturnal leg cramps with or without peripheral arterial disease.

WORKUP

- History is typically diagnostic, with sensitivity and specificity both >90%.
- Family history of RLS, growing pains, or "night walking."
- Polysomnography with arm and leg leads.
- Ambulatory recording of leg activity over several nights with sleep logs.
- Serum iron studies including total iron-binding capacity, ferritin, and complete blood count.
- Serum vitamin B_{12}, folate, and magnesium.
- Electromyography for neuropathy, radiculopathy, or myelopathy, if suspected.
- Central nervous system MRI for myelopathy or stroke, if suspected.

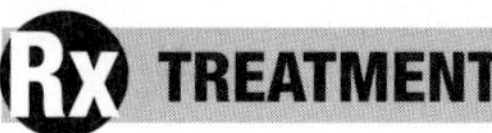

Rx TREATMENT

NONPHARMACOLOGIC THERAPY

- Avoid RLS triggers, which include sleep deprivation, alcohol, caffeine, many antidepressants (most often SSRIs and TCAs), antinausea medications, antihistamines, antipsychotics, and calcium channel blockers.
- Maintain a regular sleep schedule and good sleep hygiene (e.g., use the bed only for sleep, no alerting or light-related activities before bed, avoid daytime cues such as clocks).

CHRONIC Rx

- Dopaminergic medications are first line of treatment (may divide dose bid or tid as needed):
  1. Requip (ropinirole): start 0.25 mg; average dose 2 mg; maximum 12 mg/day
  2. Mirapex (pramipexole): start 0.125 mg; average dose 0.375 mg; maximum 5 mg/day
  3. Permax (pergolide): start 0.05 mg; average dose 0.5 mg; maximum 3 mg/day
  4. Sinemet (levodopa/carbidopa): start 25/100; maximum 3 to 4 doses/day
  5. Sinemet CR (continuous release): start 25/100; maximum 50/200
- Antiepileptics:
  1. Neurontin (gabapentin): start 300 mg; maximum 3600 mg/day
  2. Carbatrol (carbamazepine): start 200 mg; maximum 1200 mg/day
  3. Keppra (levetiracetam): start 250 mg; maximum 2000 mg/day
  4. Topamax (topiramate): start 25 mg; maximum 200 mg/day
- Opiates:
  1. Ultram (tramadol): start 25 mg; maximum 400 mg/day
  2. Dilaudid (hydromorphone): start 2 mg; maximum 24 mg/day
  3. Darvon (propoxyphene HCl): start 65 mg; maximum 195 mg/day
  4. OxyContin (oxycodone-XR): start 10 mg; maximum 30 mg/day
  5. Roxicodone (oxycodone): start 5 mg; maximum 120 mg/day
- Opiate/analgesic combinations:
  1. Vicodin/Lortab (hydrocodone/acetaminophen): start 5/500 mg; maximum 6 doses/day
  2. Percocet (oxycodone/acetaminophen): start 10/325 mg; maximum 6 doses/day
- Benzodiazepines:
  1. Restoril (temazepam): start 15 mg; maximum 30 mg/dose
  2. Klonopin (clonazepam): start 0.25 mg; maximum 3 mg/dose
- Iron supplementation:
  1. Hemocyte (oral ferrous fumarate): 324 mg qd (add vitamin C to enhance absorption)
  2. Ferrlecit (ferrous gluconate) (IV iron): follow published protocols

R

DISPOSITION

This is a chronic condition with periods of variable sensory and motor symptoms that tends to progress in time and may spread to other body areas, including arms, trunk, neck, and head.

REFERRAL

Because of intense investigation concerning phenotype/genotype relations in RLS, familial cases may be referred to university sleep medicine programs for inclusion in research protocols. Pediatric and adolescent cases requiring medical therapy should be referred to a pediatric sleep specialist or university sleep medicine program. Treatment with IV iron therapy is currently under investigation in RLS and may be available at a university sleep medicine program.

PROGNOSIS

Chronic and progressive

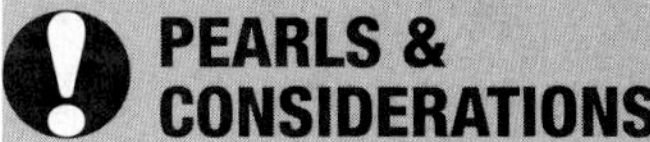

PEARLS & CONSIDERATIONS

- Up to 40% of adults with RLS report the onset of symptoms in childhood.
- In children with attention deficit–hyperactivity syndrome, up to 40% may have undetected RLS and PLMS.
- Some patients may have more sensory symptoms than motor findings (PLMS) or vice versa.
- Because of the night-to-night variability of PLMS, a single night of polysomnography may not be adequate to capture the motor findings related to RLS. Ambulatory accelerometry, or acetometry, over several nights has been shown to be an effective diagnostic tool.
- All dopaminergic medications can cause augmentation (symptoms become more intense) or rebound (symptoms appear later at night or in the morning). This may require discontinuation of the medication or additional therapies.

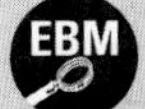

EVIDENCE

Please note: Complete text of EBM for this topic is available online.

Key trials and commentary:

Restless legs syndrome (RLS) is a common neurologic disorder characterized by an irresistible urge to move the legs. It is a major cause of sleep disruption. Periodic limb movements in sleep are detectable in most patients with RLS and represent an objective physiologic metric.

This study revealed a variant associated with susceptibility to periodic limb movements in sleep. The inverse correlation of the variant with iron stores is consistent with the suspected involvement of iron depletion in the pathogenesis of the disease.

RLS as an entity has never been without controversy. Experts and sufferers of RLS describe it as a common and miserably impairing disorder. Critics do not regard RLS as a disease but, rather, as a glorified fabrication of a physiologic aberration by the pharmaceutical industry. Once asleep, most (but not all) patients with RLS have periodic limb movements (PLM) in sleep, which can be objectively recorded and quantified. PLM (and by extension RLS) is linked to frequent sleep arousal, impaired sleep quality, and cardiovascular abnormality.

Since its description over 3 centuries ago, RLS is reported to cluster among family members. The current report showing an association between PLS and a genomic sequence variant, as well as two SNPs, in German and Canadian cohorts with PLS makes the genetic linkage of PLS more secure. But demonstration of genetic linkage does not necessarily validate RLS as a "genuine" disorder. Many physiologic features that vary otherwise in the normal population (e.g., height, weight, and eye color) have genetic bases. The genetic finding reported by the authors, nevertheless, offers hope to patients with RLS and PLS that the syndrome's pathophysiology will be better understood and such knowledge, it is hoped, would lead to more effective treatment.[1] Ⓐ

Evidence-Based Reference

1. Stefansson H, Rye DB, Hicks A: A genetic risk factor for periodic limb movements in sleep, *N Engl J Med* 357:639-647, 2007. Commentary by A. Verma, M.D., D.M. Ⓐ

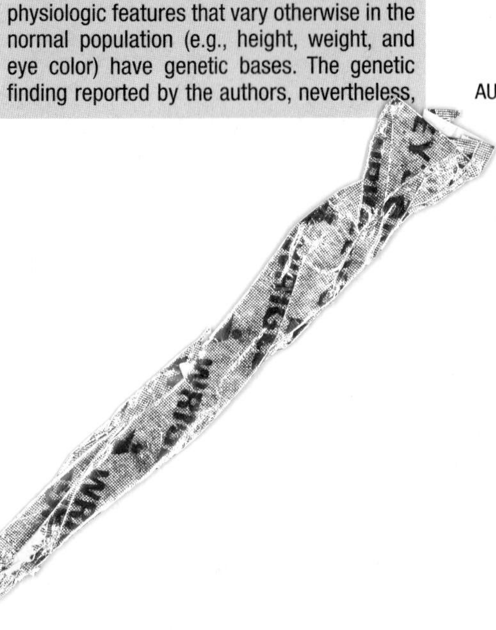

SUGGESTED READINGS

Allen RP et al: Restless legs syndrome prevalence and impact: REST general population study, *Arch Intern Med* 165(11):1286-1292, 2005.

Bayard M, Avonda T, Wadzinski J: Restless legs syndrome, *Am Fam Physician* 78(2):235-240, 2008.

Cortese S et al: Restless legs syndrome and attention-deficit/hyperactivity disorder: a review of the literature, *Sleep* 28(8):1007-1013, 2005.

Earley CJ: Restless legs syndrome, *N Engl J Med* 348: 2103, 2003.

Earley CJ et al: Repeated IV doses of iron provides effective supplemental treatment of restless legs syndrome, *Sleep Med* 6(4):301, 2005.

Happe S, Trenkwalder C: Role of dopamine receptor agonists in the treatment of restless legs syndrome, *CNS Drugs* 18:27, 2004.

Hening W et al: Impact, diagnosis and treatment of restless legs syndrome (RLS) in a primary care population: the REST (RLS epidemiology, symptoms, and treatment) primary care study, *Sleep Med* 5(3):237-246, 2004.

Silber MH et al: An algorithm for the management of restless legs syndrome, *Mayo Clin Proc* 79(7):916-922, 2004. Erratum 79(10):1341, 2004.

Stefansson H et al: A genetic risk factor for periodic limb movements in sleep, *N Engl J Med* 357:639, 2007.

Winkelmann J et al: Complex segregation analysis of restless legs syndrome provides evidence for an autosomal dominant mode of inheritance in early age at onset families, *Ann Neurol* 52:297, 2002.

AUTHOR: **JEFFREY S. DURMER, M.D., PH.D.**

Diseases and Disorders

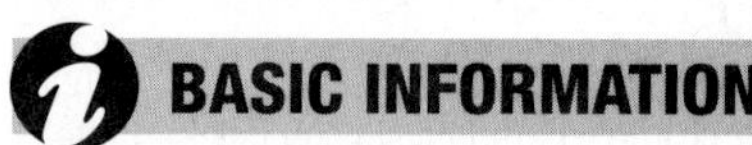

BASIC INFORMATION

DEFINITION

Retinal detachment is a retinal separation in which the inner or neural layer of the retina separates from the pigment epithelial layer. It results from numerous causes.

SYNONYMS

Inflammatory lesions of choroid
Uveitis
Tumor
Vascular lesions
Congenital disorders

ICD-9CM CODES

361 Retinal detachment and defects

EPIDEMIOLOGY & DEMOGRAPHICS

INCIDENCE (IN U.S.):
- 0.02% of the population
- Particularly common in patients with high myopia of 5 diopters or more

PEAK INCIDENCE: Incidence increases with increasing age or increasing myopia.

PREVALENCE (IN U.S.): Busy ophthalmologists may see one or two acute retinal detachments per month.

PREDOMINANT AGE:
- Congenital in younger patients
- Usually trauma in patients aged 30 to 40 yr and older
- High myopia a predisposition

PHYSICAL FINDINGS & CLINICAL PRESENTATION

- Elevation of retina and vessels associated with tears in the retina, fluid, and/or hemorrhage beneath the retina and changes in the vitreous (Fig. 1-276).
- Reports of flashing lights and floaters.

ETIOLOGY

- Trauma
- Tears in the retina
- Uveitis
- Fluid accumulation beneath the retina
- Tumors
- Scleritis
- Inflammatory disease
- Diabetes
- Collagen-vascular disease
- Vascular abnormalities

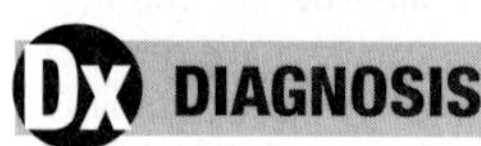

DIAGNOSIS

DIFFERENTIAL DIAGNOSIS

- Detachment
- Hemorrhage
- Tumors

FIGURE 1-276 Retinal detachment. (From Scuderi G [ed]: *Sports medicine: principles of primary care,* St Louis, 1997, Mosby.)

WORKUP

- Full eye examination
- Fluorescein angiography
- Visual fields
- Ultrasonography to show the retinal detachment or tumors beneath it
- Medical workup only when inflammation or systemic disease considered

LABORATORY TESTS

Usually not necessary

IMAGING STUDIES

B scan of the eye

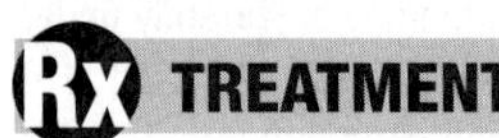

TREATMENT

NONPHARMACOLOGIC THERAPY

Immediate surgery. The three principal methods for reattachment of the retina in patients with primary retinal detachment are scleral buckling, vitrectomy, and pneumatic retinopexy. There is a paucity of randomized trials comparing these procedures and the choice remains subjective. Some data suggests that vitrectomy may be preferable for detachment in pseudophakic eyes, whereas primary detachment in phakic eyes with complexity exceeding the original indications for rheumatic retinopexy may be treated with scleral buckling or vitrectomy.

ACUTE GENERAL Rx

- Early surgery to repair the detachment
- Treatment of the underlying disorder

CHRONIC Rx

Occasionally, steroids or other treatment of underlying disease is indicated.

DISPOSITION

- Immediately refer to an ophthalmologist.
- Early intervention improves outcomes.

REFERRAL

Immediately

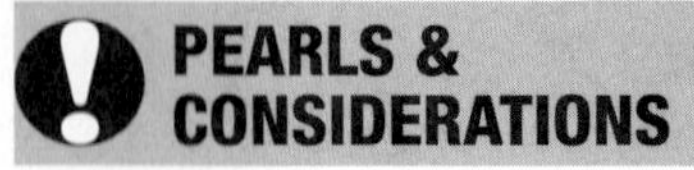

PEARLS & CONSIDERATIONS

COMMENTS

If treated early, most patients will recover a substantial portion of their vision.

SUGGESTED READINGS

Carpineto P et al: Retinal detachment prophylaxis, *Ophthalmology* 109(2):217, 2002.

D'amico DJ: Primary retinal detachment, *N Engl J Med* 359:2346-2354, 2008.

Yazici B et al: Prediction of visual outcome after retinal detachment surgery using the Lotmar visometer, *Br J Ophthalmol* 86(3):278, 2002.

AUTHOR: **MELVYN KOBY, M.D.**

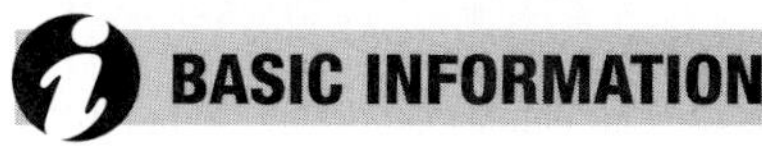

BASIC INFORMATION

DEFINITION

In a retinal hemorrhage, blood accumulates in the retinal and subretinal areas as a result of multiple causes.

SYNONYMS

Pseudoxanthoma elasticum
Coats' disease
Retinal trauma
High-altitude retinopathy

ICD-9CM CODES
362.81 Retinal hemorrhage

EPIDEMIOLOGY & DEMOGRAPHICS

INCIDENCE (IN U.S.): Busy ophthalmologists see one or two cases a month.

PEAK INCIDENCE:

- In children: associated primarily with trauma and hematologic disorders (must consider shaken baby syndrome)
- Associated with trauma, diabetes, vascular disease, macular degeneration, altitude changes (mountain climbing)

PREDOMINANT AGE: Degenerative disease in older patients

PHYSICAL FINDINGS & CLINICAL PRESENTATION

- Hemorrhage within the retina or subretinal area (Fig. 1-277)
- Evidence of retinal tears, tumors, and inflammation; macular degeneration, drugs, diabetes

ETIOLOGY

- Diabetes
- Hypertension
- Trauma
- Inflammation
- Tumors
- Subretinal neovascularization
- Associated with diabetes and aging
- Rapid changes in altitude (mountain climbing or scuba diving)

DIAGNOSIS

DIFFERENTIAL DIAGNOSIS

- Evaluate patients for local and systemic diseases.
- Trauma in children or adults.
- Venous or arterial occlusion associated with atherosclerotic or heart disease may cause retinal hemorrhage.
- Rule out malignant melanoma, trauma, hypertensive cardiovascular disease.

Section II describes the differential diagnosis of acute painless loss of vision.

WORKUP

Complete general physical examination, evaluate for trauma; look for systemic diseases and medication etiologies.

LABORATORY TESTS

- Minimum: complete blood count, erythrocyte sedimentation rate, complete blood chemistries
- Fluorescein
- Angiography
- Visual field testing

IMAGING STUDIES

- Usually not necessary
- Trauma: skull radiographs or head CT
- Ultrasound
- Fluorescein angiography

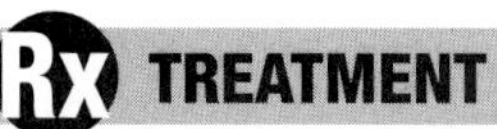

TREATMENT

NONPHARMACOLOGIC THERAPY

- Laser or treatment of underlying disorder
- Treat medical problems (age-related macular degeneration, etc.)

ACUTE GENERAL Rx

- Laser treatment is often indicated.
- Steroids may be indicated with macular degeneration (intravitreal injection).
- Treat underlying disease.
- Repair any damage from trauma.

CHRONIC Rx

- Laser treatment if hemorrhage is recurrent
- Vitamin therapy: high in zinc and antioxidants

DISPOSITION

Consider this condition an emergency.

REFERRAL

Immediate referral to an ophthalmologist; early treatment significantly affects outcome

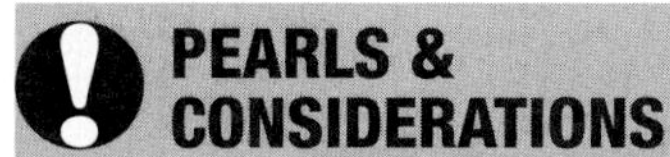

PEARLS & CONSIDERATIONS

COMMENTS

- Vision may return substantially.
- Complete recovery depends on amount of scar tissue formed.
- Chronic situations have poor prognosis.

SUGGESTED READINGS

Duncan BB et al: Hypertensive retinopathy and incident coronary heart disease in high risk men, *Br J Ophthalmol* 86(9):1002, 2002.

Gardner HB: Retinal hemorrhages in children, *Ophthalmology* 110(9):1863, 2003.

Lauritzen DB, Weiter JJ: Management of subretinal hemorrhage, *Int Ophthalmol Clin* 42(3):87, 2002.

Schloff S et al: Retinal findings in children with intracranial hemorrhage, *Ophthalmology* 109(8):1472, 2002.

AUTHOR: **MELVYN KOBY, M.D.**

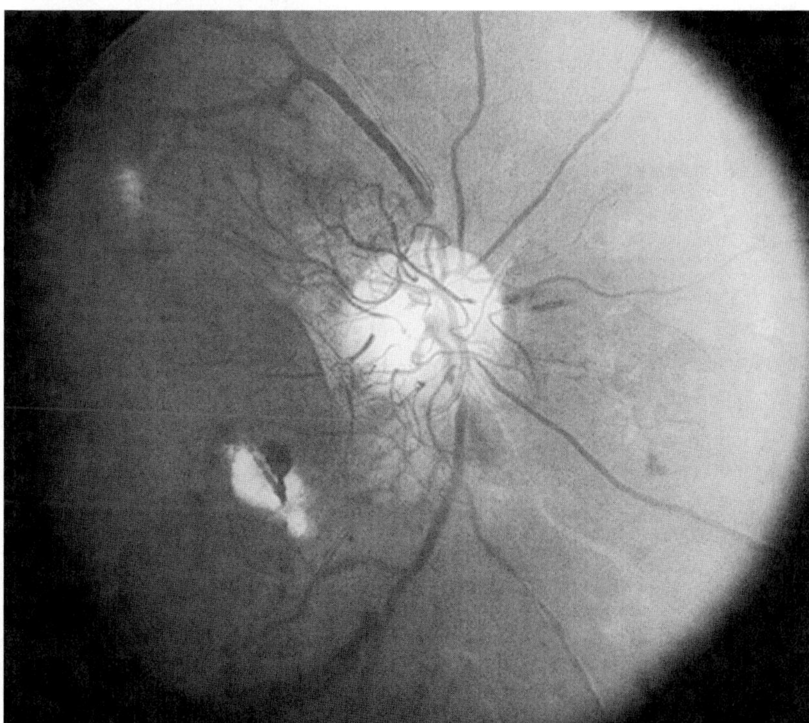

FIGURE 1-277 Fronds of neovascularization on the disc are present in this right eye. Temporally, two cotton-wool spots have adjacent intraretinal hemorrhage and preretinal hemorrhage. Native retinal arteries are narrowed and show evidence of sclerosis. (From Palay D [ed]: *Ophthalmology for the primary care physician*, St Louis, 1997, Mosby.)

Retinitis Pigmentosa

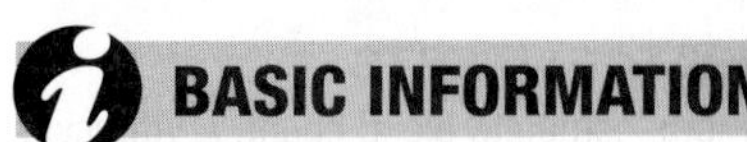

BASIC INFORMATION

DEFINITION

Retinitis pigmentosa is a generalized retinal pigment degeneration associated with a variety of inheritance patterns resulting in decreased vision. A simple recessive pattern is most severe. It may be associated with some rare neurologic syndromes.

ICD-9CM CODES
362.74 Retinitis pigmentosa, pigmentary retinal dystrophy

EPIDEMIOLOGY & DEMOGRAPHICS

PEAK INCIDENCE:
- Recessive incidence: in the 20s
- Dominant form: in the 40s

PREVALENCE (IN U.S.): One in 4000 persons
PREDOMINANT SEX: Depends on inheritance
PREDOMINANT AGE: 60 yr
GENETICS:
- 19% dominant
- 19% recessive
- 8% X-linked
- 46% not known to be genetically related (mutations)
- 8% undetermined cause

PHYSICAL FINDINGS & CLINICAL PRESENTATION

- Deposition of retinal pigment in midperiphery and centrally in the retina with a pale optic nerve and narrowing of blood vessels (Fig. 1-278)
- Possible cataracts and macular edema
- Decrease in night vision and peripheral vision

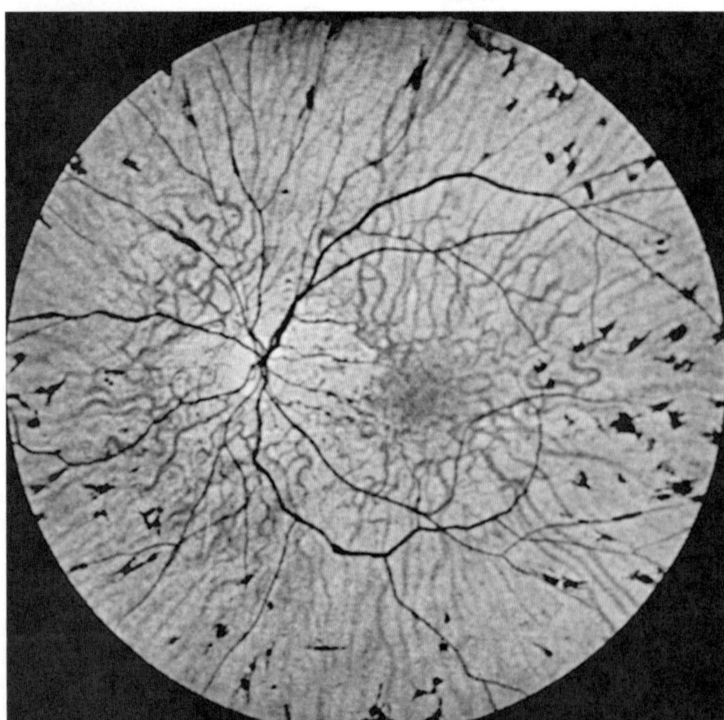

FIGURE 1-278 Retinitis pigmentosa. (From Behrman RE [ed]: *Nelson textbook of pediatrics,* Philadelphia, 2005, WB Saunders.)

ETIOLOGY

Usually hereditary

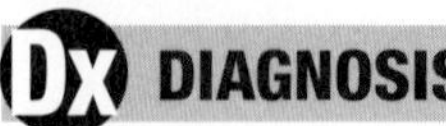

DIAGNOSIS

DIFFERENTIAL DIAGNOSIS

- Syphilis
- Old inflammatory scars
- Old hemorrhage
- Diabetes
- Toxic retinopathies (phenothiazines, chloroquine)

WORKUP

- Electrophysiologic studies
- Dark adaptation studies
- Visual fields

LABORATORY TESTS

- Usually not necessary
- VDRL (syphilis), glucose (selected patients)

IMAGING STUDIES

- Usually not necessary
- Rate of decline of vision for different groups cannot be accurately determined; decline rates are fastest with patients with mutations

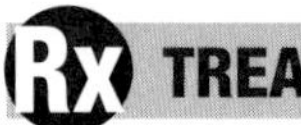

TREATMENT

CHRONIC Rx

- No proven effective therapy
- Sometimes vitamin E or vitamin A may be helpful

DISPOSITION

Disease may be either mild or severe, but if the patient is expected to progress to total blindness, counseling and early education are important.

REFERRAL

To ophthalmologist to confirm diagnosis

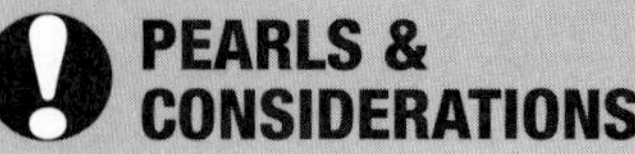

PEARLS & CONSIDERATIONS

COMMENTS

- The spider web–like appearance of macular degeneration should not be confused with the extra pigments sometimes seen in dark-skinned individuals.
- Patient education material can be obtained from the Retinitis Pigmentosa Foundation Fighting Blindness, 1401 Mt. Royal Avenue, 4th Floor, Baltimore, MD 21217.
- Research in fetal retinal pigment transplantation and computer chip implantation is ongoing.

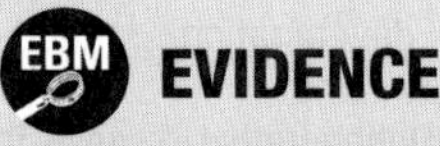

EVIDENCE

Vitamin A

Vitamin A palmitate given at 15,000 IU daily administered to 600 patients with typical retinitis pigmentosa showed a modest but positive slowing of visual loss. Visual loss slowed to a decline of 8.3% per year compared with 10% per year in control subjects.[1]

Some studies have shown that acetazolamide may be of benefit (as measured by improved visual acuity or decreased cystoid macular edema on fluorescein angiogram).[2] For those with cystoid macular edema: initial dose 250 mg daily increased to 500 mg daily if no effect apparent. A trial of several weeks is given.

Docosahexaenoic acid

Trials of docosahexaenoic acid are currently underway.

Evidence-Based References

1. Berson EL et al: A randomized trial of vitamin A and vitamin E supplementation for retinitis pigmentosa, *Arch Ophthalmol* 111:761, 1993.
2. Steinmertz RL et al: Treatment of cystoid macular edema with acetazolamide in a patient with serpiginous choroidopathy, *Retina* 11:412, 1991.

SUGGESTED READINGS

Chow AY et al: The artificial silicon retina microchip for the treatment of vision loss from retinitis pigmentosa, *Arch Ophthalmol* 122(4):460, 2004.

Radtke ND et al: Vision change after sheet transplant of fetal retina with retinal pigment epithelium to a patient with retinitis pigmentosa, *Arch Ophthalmol* 122(8):1159, 2004.

AUTHOR: **MELVYN KOBY, M.D.**

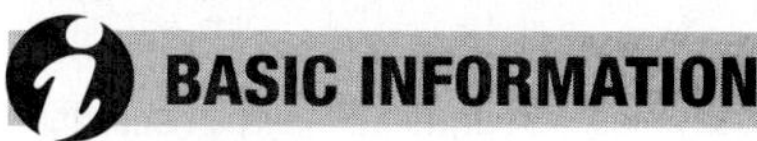

BASIC INFORMATION

DEFINITION

Retinoblastoma is an inherited, highly malignant congenital neoplasm arising from the neural layers of the retina.

ICD-9CM CODES
190.5 Retinoblastoma, malignant neoplasm of eyes, retina

EPIDEMIOLOGY & DEMOGRAPHICS

INCIDENCE (IN U.S.): One in every 23,000 to 34,000 births. It is the most common primary intraocular malignancy of childhood.

PEAK INCIDENCE:

- 6 to 13 mo. Mean age at diagnosis is 12 mo for bilateral tumors and 24 mo for unilateral tumors.
- 72% diagnosed by age 3 yr
- 90% diagnosed by age 4 yr

PREDOMINANT AGE: 8 mo

GENETICS:

- Gene mutation or an autosomal-dominant gene with 80% to 95% penetration
- 5% mutations

PHYSICAL FINDINGS & CLINICAL PRESENTATION

- Leukokoria (white reflex or white pupil) (Fig. 1-279)
- White elevated retinal masses
- Strabismus
- Glaucoma
- Uveitis
- Vitreous masses and opacity

ETIOLOGY

The retinoblastoma gene is a tumor suppressor gene located on the long arm of chromosome 13 at region 14 that codes for the RB protein. Approximately 60% of retinoblastomas are attributable to somatic, nonhereditary mutations.

DIAGNOSIS

DIFFERENTIAL DIAGNOSIS

Examination of eye

- Strabismus
- Retinal detachment
- Uveitis
- Other tumors
- Glaucoma
- Coats' disease (pathologic telangiectatic retinal vessels that leak and lead to accumulation of subretinal fluid and lipid)
- Endophthalmitis
- Cataract
- Infectious

WORKUP

Diagnosis is by ophthalmologic examination with studies including ultrasonography of the eye and MRI of the orbits and brain.

IMAGING STUDIES

- MRI: may show calcifications in retina
- Ultrasonography: good delineation of mass

TREATMENT

NONPHARMACOLOGIC THERAPY

Treatment depends on location and stage of tumor when diagnosed:

- Enucleation of single eye
- External-beam radiation
- Chemotherapy with local vitreous injections
- Radioactive plaque brachytherapy and cryotherapy
- Surgical enucleation of the eye
- Radiation and chemotherapy

DISPOSITION

Usually treated by an ophthalmologist and oncologist; high cure rate (93% 5-yr survival in the U.S.)

REFERRAL

- To ophthalmologist and oncologist
- Prospective parents with a family history of retinoblastoma should be referred for genetic counseling

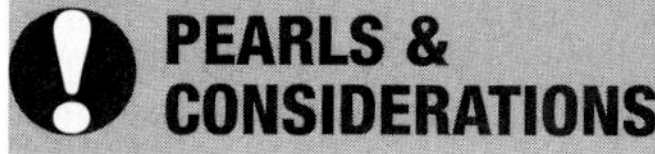

PEARLS & CONSIDERATIONS

COMMENTS

- With early aggressive treatment, many patients may survive.
- High incidence of second tumor in survivors compared with general population.
- High incidence of lung cancer, bladder, and other epithelial cancers.

SUGGESTED READINGS

Brichand B et al: Combined chemotherapy and local treatment in the management of intraocular retinoblastoma, *Med Pediatr Oncol* 38(6):411, 2002.

Butros LJ et al: Delayed diagnosis of retinoblastoma analysis of degree, cause, and potential consequences, *Pediatric* 109(3):E45, 2002.

De Potter P: Current treatment of retinoblastoma, *Curr Opin Ophthalmol* 13(5):331, 2002.

Lee V et al: Globe conserving treatment of the only eye in bilateral retinoblastoma, *Br J Ophthalmol* 87(11):1374, 2003.

Melamud A et al: Retinoblastoma, *Am Fam Physician* 73:1039-1044, 2006.

Schouten-Van Meeteren AY et al: Overview: chemotherapy for retinoblastoma: an expanding area of clinical research, *Med Pediatr Oncol* 38(6):428, 2002.

Sussman DA et al: Comparison of retinoblastoma reduction for chemotherapy vs external beam radiotherapy, *Arch Ophthalmol* 121(7):979, 2003.

AUTHOR: **MELVYN KOBY, M.D.**

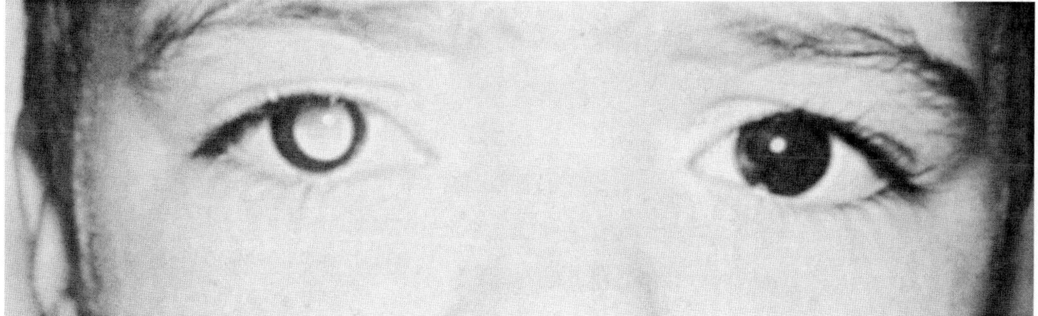

FIGURE 1-279 Leukocoria. White papillary reflex in a child with retinoblastoma. (From Behrman RE [ed]: *Nelson textbook of pediatrics,* Philadelphia, 2005, WB Saunders.)

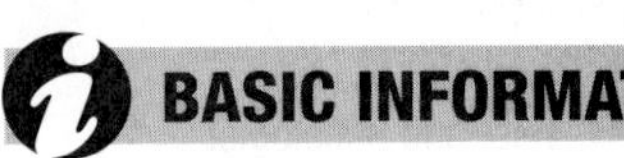

BASIC INFORMATION

DEFINITION

Diabetic retinopathy is an eye abnormality of the retina associated with diabetes and consisting of microaneurysms, punctate hemorrhages, white and yellow exudates, flame hemorrhages, and neovascular vessel growth and can ultimately end in blindness. Diabetic retinopathy can be classified into two stages: nonproliferative and proliferative (Fig. 1-280).

SYNONYMS

Nonproliferative diabetic retinopathy (NPDR)
Proliferative (advanced) diabetic retinopathy (PDR)
Diabetic retinopathy (DR)

ICD-9CM CODES

250.5	Diabetes with ophthalmic manifestations
362.1	Retinopathy, diabetic, background
362.02	Retinopathy, diabetic, proliferative

EPIDEMIOLOGY & DEMOGRAPHICS

INCIDENCE (IN U.S.):
- Affects 11 million persons
- A leading cause of blindness in people ages 20 to 70 yr
- 5000 new cases annually

PEAK INCIDENCE: Begins 10 yr after onset of diabetes

PREVALENCE (IN U.S.): Prevalence of retinopathy increases with duration of diabetes. Found in 18% of people diagnosed with diabetes for 3- to 4-yr duration and in up to 80% of diabetics with a diagnosis of ≥15 yr.

PREDOMINANT SEX: Males and females affected equally

PREDOMINANT AGE: ≥30 yr

GENETICS: Type 1 diabetes: 80% have retinopathy before 30 yr, with 30% having vision-threatening retinopathy.

PHYSICAL FINDINGS & CLINICAL PRESENTATION

- Microaneurysms
- Hemorrhages
- Exudates
- Macular edema
- Neovascularization
- Retinal detachment
- Hemorrhages in the vitreous
- In early cases, patient may not report a visual disturbance

ETIOLOGY

Vascular endothelial growth factor and erythropoietin have been identified as factors involved in angiogenesis in proliferative diabetic retinopathy. Risk factors for diabetic retinopathy are duration of diabetes, hyperglycemia/glycated hemoglobin value, hypertension, hyperlipidemia, pregnancy, and nephropathy or renal disease.

Dx DIAGNOSIS

DIFFERENTIAL DIAGNOSIS

- Retinal examination: look for background retinopathy, microaneurysms, exudate, macular edema, retinal hemorrhage, proliferative neovascular growth on surface of retina
- Retinal inflammatory diseases
- Tumor
- Trauma
- Arteriosclerotic vascular disease
- Hypertension
- Vein or artery occlusion

WORKUP

- Fluorescein angiogram
- Frequent retinal examinations

Rx TREATMENT

NONPHARMACOLOGIC THERAPY

- Tight glycemic and blood pressure control remains the cornerstone in the primary prevention of diabetic retinopathy
- Laser treatment when indicated
- Laser treatment with proliferative disease or macular edema
- Photo coagulation of neovascular areas
- Exercise, diet, sugar control, and blood pressure control can slow progression of background retinopathy but have no effect on proliferative retinopathy

ACUTE GENERAL Rx

- Laser therapy: pan-retinal and focal retinal laser photocoagulation reduces the risk of visual loss in patients with severe diabetic retinopathy and macular edema
- Vitrectomy
- Repair of retinal detachment
- Medical control of disease and complications and associated diseases (e.g., hypertension)

CHRONIC Rx

- Repeated laser treatments may be necessary
- Diet and exercise; good medical control of disease

DISPOSITION

- Retinal examination should be performed on all routine medical visits. Referral if abnormality seen.
- Routine annual eye examination in all patients with diabetes.
- Prognosis is improved with early diagnosis and treatment.

REFERRAL

Refer to ophthalmologist immediately on finding retinal abnormality to institute early treatment.

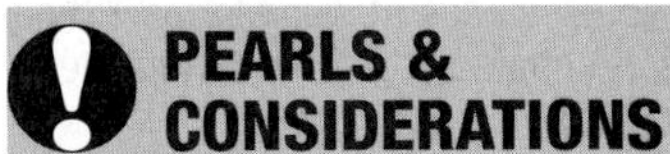

PEARLS & CONSIDERATIONS

COMMENTS

Early laser treatment of severe, nonproliferative, and proliferative retinopathy may minimize complications and visual loss.

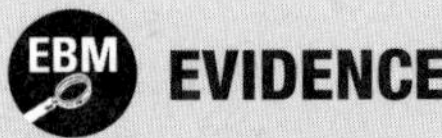

EVIDENCE

Please note: Complete text of EBM for this topic is available online.

SUGGESTED READINGS

Frank RN: Diabetic retinopathy, *N Engl J Med* 350:48, 2004.

Mohamed Q et al: Management of diabetic retinopathy, *JAMA* 298(8):902-916, 2007.

Sjolie AK, Moller F: Medical management of diabetic retinopathy, *Diabetes Med* 21(7):666, 2004.

Watanabe D et al: Erythropoietin as a retinal angiogenic factor in proliferative diabetic retinopathy, *N Engl J Med* 353:782, 2005.

AUTHOR: **MELVYN KOBY, M.D.**

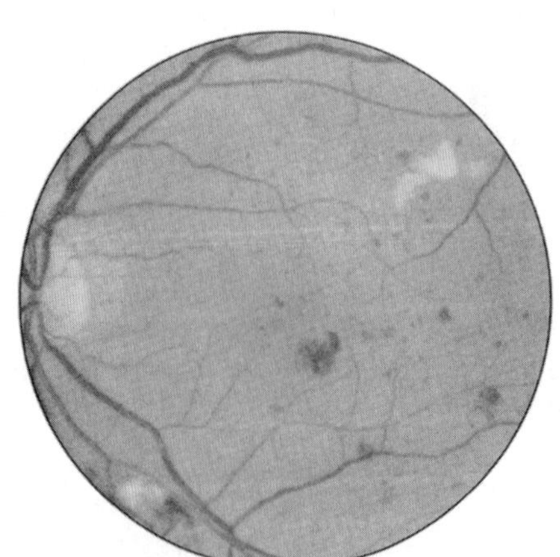

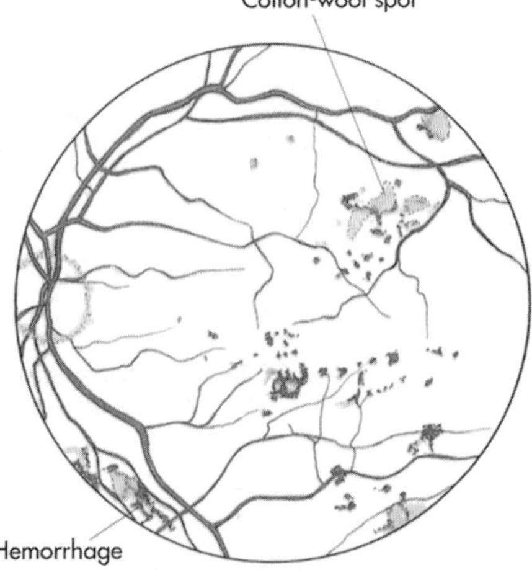

FIGURE 1-280 Background diabetic retinopathy. Note flame-shaped and dot-blot hemorrhages, cotton-wool spots, and microaneurysms. (From Barkaukas VH et al: *Health and physical assessment,* ed 2, St Louis, 1998, Mosby.)

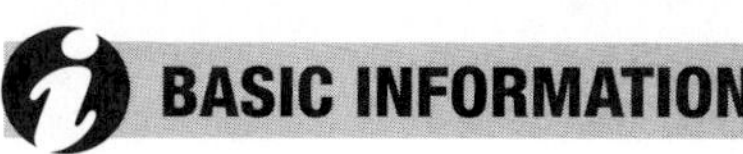

BASIC INFORMATION

DEFINITION

Retropharyngeal abscess is a soft tissue infection of the throat involving retropharyngeal space. The anatomic boundaries of the retropharyngeal space are the middle layer of the deep cervical fascia (abutting the posterior esophageal wall) anteriorly and the deep layer of the deep cervical fascia posteriorly (Fig. 1-281). These two fasciae fuse inferiorly at the level between the first and second thoracic vertebra.

ICD-9CM CODES
478.79

EPIDEMIOLOGY & DEMOGRAPHICS

Retropharyngeal abscess occurs most commonly in children between the ages of 2 and 4 yr, analogous to suppurative cervical adenitis. This represents the peak age group for numerous viral upper respiratory tract infections and their attendant complications, acute otitis media and sinusitis. Retropharyngeal space infection is less common in older children and adults because the lymph nodes atrophy by the age of 3 or 4 yr.

PHYSICAL FINDINGS & CLINICAL PRESENTATION

- The onset of a retropharyngeal infection may be insidious, with little more than fever, irritability, drooling, a muffled voice (dysphonia), or possibly nuchal rigidity.
- The acute symptoms relate to pressure and inflammation produced by the abscess on either the airway or the upper digestive tract and pharynx. The patient may have intense dysphagia, drooling, and odynophagia, or there may be some element of respiratory distress from edema and inflammation of the airway (stridor, tachypnea, or both).
- Unwillingness to move the neck because of discomfort is often a prominent presenting feature and should lead to consideration of retropharyngeal abscess if the child is febrile and irritable.
- Extension of the neck is usually affected more than flexion. This causes the patient to hold his or her neck stiffly or to present with torticollis.
- Trismus is unusual.
- On physical examination it may be possible to appreciate midline or unilateral swelling of the posterior pharyngeal wall. The mass may be fluctuant to the examining finger, and care must be taken to avoid rupture of the abscess into the upper airway.

Complications are numerous and could be fatal; these include airway obstruction, septicemia, thrombosis of the internal jugular vein, carotid artery rupture, and acute necrotizing mediastinitis. Aspiration with resultant pneumonia may complicate retropharyngeal abscess if rupture of the abscess occurs and empties into the airway. Infection can spread from one space in the neck to another.

The most dreaded complication is jugular vein suppurative thrombophlebitis (Lemierre's syndrome), in which the vessels of the carotid sheath become infected, leading to bacteremia and metastatic spread of infection to the lungs, brain, and mediastinum.

ETIOLOGY

- The retropharyngeal space comprises two chains of lymph nodes that drain the nasopharynx, adenoids, posterior paranasal sinuses, middle ear, and eustachian tube. Accordingly, suppurative infections in these areas may provide the seeds for infection for retropharyngeal abscess.
- The predominant bacterial species are *Streptococcus pyogenes* (group A *Streptococcus*), *Staphylococcus aureus,* and respiratory anaerobes (including *Fusobacteria, Prevotella,* and *Veillonella* species). *Haemophilus* species are also occasionally found.
- In young children, infection usually reaches this space by lymphatic spread from a septic focus in the pharynx or sinuses.
- In adults, infection may reach the retropharyngeal space from either local or distant sites. Penetrating trauma (e.g., from chicken bones or after instrumentation) is the usual source of local spread. More distant sources of infection include odontogenic sepsis and peritonsillar abscess (now a rare cause).

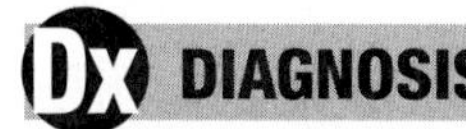

DIAGNOSIS

DIFFERENTIAL DIAGNOSIS

- Cervical osteomyelitis
- Pott's disease
- Meningitis
- Calcific tendonitis of the long muscle of the neck

IMAGING STUDIES

- A lateral neck film may be helpful in delineating the presence of a retropharyngeal abscess and may demonstrate cervical lordosis; the retropharyngeal space is considered widened and pathologic if it is greater than 7 mm at C2 or 14 mm at C6 (Fig. 1-282).
    - There must be attention to technical issues when performing the study, especially in children. The film should be a perfect lateral, and the child must keep the neck in extension during inspiration to avoid a false thickening of the retropharyngeal space. Crying, particularly in infants, may also cause false thickening of the retropharyngeal space.
- A CT scan of the neck is the best tool to identify abscesses in the retropharyngeal area, but it is not perfect. Both the sensitivity and specificity of the CT scan in predicting the presence of drainable purulent material

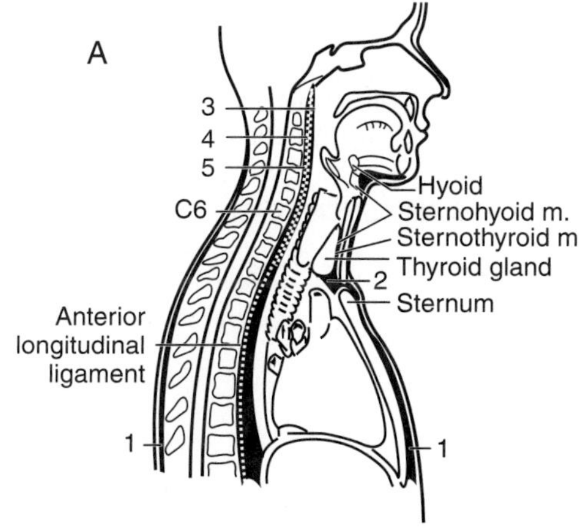

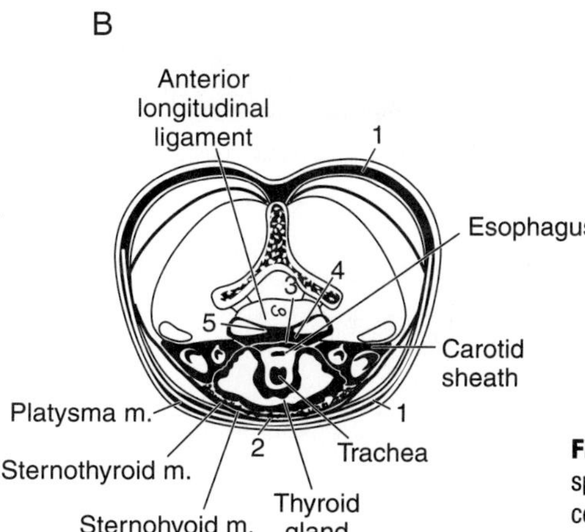

FIGURE 1-281 Relation of various cervical fascial spaces to the superficial and deep layers of the cervical fascia. **A,** Cross-section of the neck at the level of the thyroid isthmus. **B,** Coronal section in the suprahyoid region of the neck. *1,* Superficial space; *2,* pretracheal space; *3,* retropharyngeal space; *4,* "danger" space; *5,* prevertebral space.

are quite variable from study to study, ranging between 68% and 100%.
- The CT scan provides more information than the plain radiograph because it can generally differentiate between retropharyngeal cellulitis and retropharyngeal abscess and can demonstrate extension of the retropharyngeal abscess to contiguous spaces in the neck. Findings on CT common to both cellulitis and abscess are a low-density core, soft tissue swelling, obliterated fat planes, and mass effect. The best differential finding on CT scan is "complete rim enhancement," which is indicative of abscess (Fig. 1-283). The abscess may be seen as a mass impinging on the posterior pharyngeal wall.

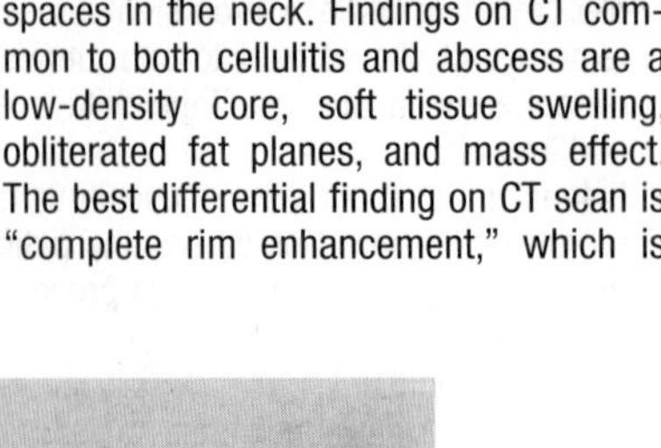

- MRI of the neck is more sensitive than CT, and technetium scanning can be helpful in detecting bone involvement. T2-weighted images may identify and localize areas of pus for drainage or aspiration. Gadolinium enhancement is important to accurately define the soft tissue component. Finally, MRI is useful for imaging vascular lesions, such as jugular thrombophlebitis.

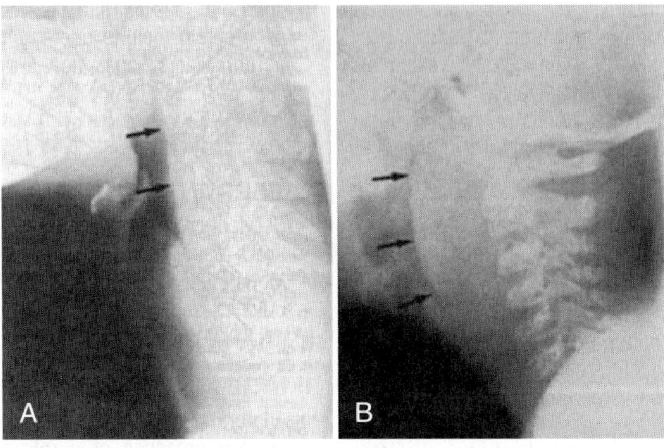

FIGURE 1-282 Lateral radiographs of the neck show normal lateral cervical view **(A)** and expansion of the prevertebral soft tissues by a retropharyngeal abscess **(B).**

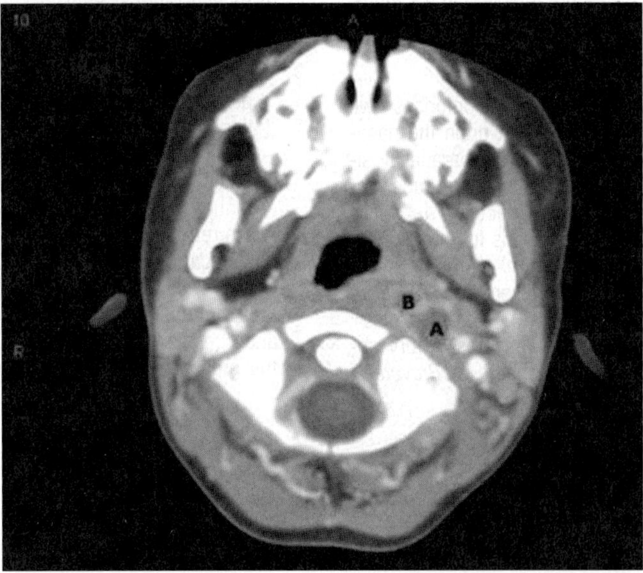

FIGURE 1-283 CT scan of a retropharyngeal abscess (**A** and **B**) demonstrates a low-density core, soft tissue swelling, obliterated fat planes, mass effect, and rim enhancement.

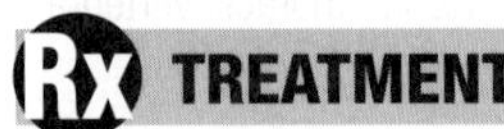

TREATMENT

ACUTE GENERAL & CHRONIC Rx

- High-dose penicillin (2 to 4 million units IV q4h) plus metronidazole (500 mg IV q8h) or ampicillin-sulbactam (50 mg/kg/dose IV q6h) or clindamycin (13 mg/kg/dose IV q8h) are effective antimicrobial selections. Parenteral treatment is maintained until the patient is afebrile and clinically improved. Antibiotics should be adjusted as culture data become available, and oral therapy is continued to complete at least a 14-day course.
- Surgical intervention has historically played a prominent role in the management of retropharyngeal abscess in conjunction with antibiotic therapy. Drainage is indicated when there is a large hypodense area or when a patient has not responded to parenteral therapy alone.
- When the CT does not demonstrate a large hypodense area, a trial of antibiotic therapy without drainage is appropriate. Some investigators also support a trial of IV antibiotic therapy alone when small abscesses are identified by CT scans as long as there is no compromise of the airway.

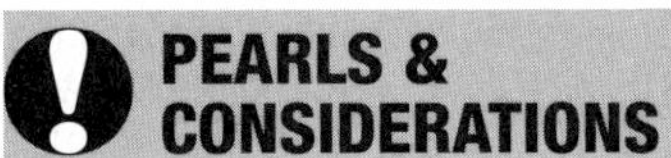

PEARLS & CONSIDERATIONS

PREVENTION

The complications of deep neck infection in any space are numerous and potentially fatal. Early diagnosis, with prompt and appropriate management, is key to avoiding these complications.

AUTHOR: **RUBY SATPATHY, M.D.**

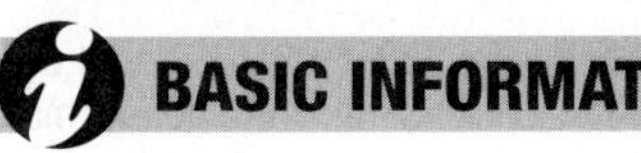

BASIC INFORMATION

DEFINITION

Reye's syndrome is a postinfectious triad consisting of encephalopathy, fatty liver degeneration, and transaminase elevation.

ICD-9CM CODES
331.81 Reye's syndrome

EPIDEMIOLOGY & DEMOGRAPHICS

- During the 1970s, 300 to 600 cases were being reported yearly in the U.S.
- Since the mid-1980s, after the understanding that aspirin is associated with Reye's syndrome, the yearly count has fallen to <20 cases
- Seasonal relation with influenza and varicella outbreaks
- Age: rare in persons aged >18 yr; peak age (in the U.S.) is 6 to 8 yr
- Case fatality rate: 25% to 50%

PHYSICAL FINDINGS & CLINICAL PRESENTATION

Shortly after recovery from a viral infection (flu or chickenpox), an afebrile child begins to vomit intractably. Hepatomegaly is often present. The vomiting can lead to dehydration. Occasionally, symptoms of hypoglycemia are present. After 2 days symptoms of encephalopathy dominate the clinical picture (lethargy, confusion, stupor, coma, seizures, decorticate or decerebrate posture) (Table 1-67).

ETIOLOGY

- Temporal association with influenza and varicella infection
- Epidemiologic association with aspirin or other salicylate use to treat the viral infection
- Possible association with aflatoxin and pesticides
- Pathology
- Liver: no inflammation; the striking finding is panlobular microvesicular hepatocyte infiltration on light microscopy and mitochondrial injury on electron microscopy
- Brain: no inflammation but cerebral edema and anoxic degeneration
- Pathogenesis: not fully understood but mitochondrial dysfunction is clearly center stage

Dx DIAGNOSIS

DIFFERENTIAL DIAGNOSIS

- Inborn errors of metabolism (e.g., carnitine deficiency, ornithine transcarbamylase deficiency)
- Salicylate or amiodarone intoxication
- Jamaican vomiting sickness
- Hepatic encephalopathy of any cause

WORKUP

According to the Centers for Disease Control case definition, the following conditions must be met for consideration as a Reye's syndrome case:

1. Acute noninflammatory encephalopathy documented by:
   - Alteration in the level of consciousness and, if available, a record of cerebrospinal fluid containing ≤8 leukocytes per mm^3 *or*
   - Histologic specimen demonstrating cerebral edema without perivascular or meningeal inflammation
2. Hepatopathy documented either by a liver biopsy or autopsy considered to be diagnostic of Reye's syndrome or by a threefold or greater rise in the levels of serum aspartate aminotransferase, serum alanine aminotransferase, or serum ammonia *and*
3. No more reasonable explanation for the cerebral and hepatic abnormalities

LABORATORY TESTS

- Elevated transaminase (alanine aminotransferase and aspartate aminotransferase)
- Elevated ammonia level
- Occasional elevation of creatine phosphokinase, lactate dehydrogenase, and bilirubin and prolongation of prothrombin time
- Occasional hypoglycemia (in patients <4 yr)
- Cerebrospinal fluid is normal or contains <8 white blood cells per milliliter
- Rarely a liver biopsy is indicated (in infants or in recurrent cases)

Rx TREATMENT

- Supportive
- Mannitol, glycerol, or hyperventilation for cerebral edema if present
- Interferon-alfa (experimental)
- Prevention
  - Influenza vaccine
  - Varicella vaccine
  - Avoidance of aspirin in children, especially during influenza and varicella outbreaks

AUTHOR: **FRED F. FERRI, M.D.**

TABLE 1-67 Clinical Staging of Reye's Syndrome

Grade	Symptoms at Time of Admission
I	Usually quiet, **lethargic** and sleepy, vomiting, laboratory evidence of liver dysfunction
II	Deep lethargy, **confusion,** delirium, combative, hyperventilation, hyperreflexic
III	Obtunded, **light coma,** seizures, decorticate rigidity, intact pupillary light reaction
IV	Seizures, deepening coma, **decerebrate rigidity,** loss of oculocephalic reflexes, fixed pupils
V	Coma, loss of deep tendon reflexes, respiratory arrest, fixed dilated pupils, **flaccidity/decerebrate** intermittent isoelectric electroencephalogram

From Behrman RE: *Nelson textbook of pediatrics,* ed 17, Philadelphia, 2005, WB Saunders.

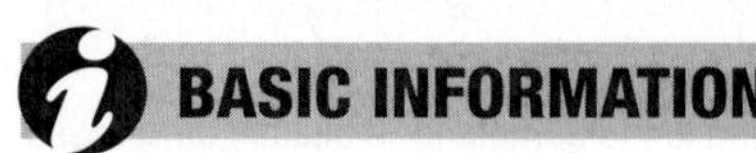

BASIC INFORMATION

DEFINITION

Rh incompatibility occurs when an absence of the D antigen on maternal red blood cells (RBCs) and its presence on fetal RBCs causes risk of isoimmunization.

ICD-9CM CODES
656.1 Rh incompatibility

EPIDEMIOLOGY & DEMOGRAPHICS

INCIDENCE:

- The absence of the D antigen (Rh− blood type) occurs in 15% of whites, 8% of blacks, and virtually no Asians or Native Americans. If the father's blood type is not known, the chance that an Rh− pregnant woman is bearing an Rh+ fetus is approximately 60%.
- Of those pregnancies complicated by Rh incompatibility, the risk of maternal isoimmunization to the D antigen is approximately 8% for each ABO-compatible pregnancy if no prophylaxis is given.
- Maternal-fetal ABO incompatibility is somewhat protective against Rh isoimmunization.

GENETICS: Five major loci determine Rh status: C, D, E, c, e. The presence of the D antigen results in an Rh+ individual. Its absence results in an Rh− individual. Of Rh+ fathers, 45% are homozygotes, and 55% are heterozygotes. For homozygous Rh+ fathers, the probability of an Rh+ offspring is 100%. The probability for heterozygotes is approximately 50%.

RISK FACTORS:

- Antepartum: fetal-to-maternal transfusion
- Intrapartum: fetal-to-maternal transfusion, spontaneous abortion, ectopic pregnancy, abruptio placentae, abdominal trauma, chorionic villus sampling, amniocentesis, percutaneous umbilical blood sampling (PUBS), external cephalic version, manual removal of the placenta, therapeutic abortion, autologous blood product administration

ETIOLOGY

The initial response to D antigen exposure is production of immunoglobulin (Ig) M (molecular weight 900,000) that does not cross the placenta. With a repeated exposure, IgG (MW 160,000) is produced. IgG can cross the placenta and enter the fetal circulation, producing hemolysis in the fetus. This may produce erythroblastosis fetalis or hemolytic disease in the newborn, resulting in antepartum or neonatal death or neurologic damage to the fetus because of hyperbilirubinemia and kernicterus.

DIAGNOSIS

LABORATORY TESTS

ABO and Rh blood type and an antibody screen as part of the initial prenatal profile

- If antibody screen negative:
  1. Repeat antibody screen at 28 wk gestation.
  2. Obtain neonatal blood type after delivery.
  3. If Rh incompatibility is confirmed by the neonatal blood type, a Kleihauer-Betke or rosette test should be performed to determine the amount of fetomaternal transfusion in the following high-risk circumstances: abruptio placentae, placenta previa, cesarean delivery, intrauterine manipulation, manual removal of the placenta.
- If anti-D antibody screen is positive:
  1. Maternal indirect Coombs test is needed to determine antibody titer.
  2. Determine paternal Rh status and zygosity.
  3. If father is heterozygous, PUBS or amniotic fluid is needed to determine fetal Rh status.

IMAGING STUDIES

Ultrasound evaluation can diagnose hydrops fetalis, but it cannot predict it.

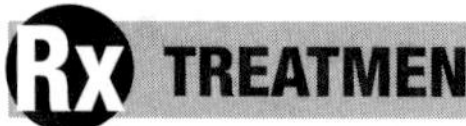

TREATMENT

PREVENTION OF D ISOIMMUNIZATION

- 50 mcg of D immunoglobulin: after spontaneous or induced abortion or ectopic pregnancy <13 wk gestation.
- 300 mcg of D immunoglobulin (protects against 30 ml of fetal blood):
  1. After spontaneous or induced abortion <13 wk gestation, amniocentesis, chorionic villous sampling, PUBS, external cephalic version, or other intrauterine manipulation.
  2. As antepartum prophylaxis at 28 wk gestation. Maternal anti-D prophylaxis does not cause hemolysis in the fetus or newborn.
  3. At delivery if the neonate is D- or Du-positive.
  4. If Kleihauer-Betke or rosette test confirms >30 ml of fetal red blood in maternal circulation, additional D immunoglobulin is indicated. Confirm adequacy of therapy by a maternal indirect Coombs test 48 to 72 hr after Rh immune globulin is given.

MANAGEMENT OF D ISOIMMUNIZED PREGNANCIES

- Serial amniocentesis for assessment of OD_{450} after 25 wk gestation with interpretation of the Delta OD450 according to criteria established by Liley
- PUBS if ultrasonographic evidence of hydrops, rising zone II Delta OD_{450} values on amniocentesis, or maternal history of a severely affected child
- Intrauterine exchange transfusion if severe anemia is documented remote from term
- Initiation of steroids for lung maturation at 28 wk in severely affected pregnancies with delivery at lung maturity
- Delivery as soon as lung maturation is achieved in mild to moderately affected pregnancies

DISPOSITION

Survival of nonhydropic infants is 90%. Of infants with hydrops, 82% survive.

REFERRAL

Refer all Rh isoimmunized pregnancies to a tertiary care center before 18 to 20 wk gestation.

SUGGESTED READING

Maayan-Metzger A et al: Maternal anti-D prophylaxis during pregnancy does not cause neonatal hemolysis, *Arch Dis Child* 84:60, 2001.

AUTHOR: **LAUREL M. WHITE, M.D.**

BASIC INFORMATION

DEFINITION

Rhabdomyolysis is the dissolution or disintegration of muscle, which causes membrane lysis and leakage of muscle constituents, resulting in the excretion of myoglobin in the urine. Renal damage can occur as a result of tubular obstruction by myoglobin as well as hypovolemia.

ICD-9CM CODES
728.89 Rhabdomyolysis

EPIDEMIOLOGY & DEMOGRAPHICS

PREDOMINANT AGE: Rare in children. Increased risk in advanced age (>80 yr).

ONSET: The average length of time on statin therapy before rhabdomyolysis is 1 yr. Average time for onset of rhabdomyolysis after addition of fibrate to statin therapy is 32 days.

PHYSICAL FINDINGS & CLINICAL PRESENTATION

- Variable muscle tenderness. Rhabdomyolysis apart from statin use presents with muscle symptoms only 50% of the time.
- Weakness
- Muscular rigidity
- Fever
- Altered consciousness
- Muscle swelling
- Malaise, fatigue. In statin-induced rhabdomyolysis, fatigue (74%) is nearly as common as muscle pain (88%).
- Dark urine

ETIOLOGY

- Exertion (exercise-induced)
- Electrical injury
- Drug-induced (statins, combination of statins with fibrates, or erythromycin, simvastatin and amiodarone, amphetamines, haloperidol)
- Compartment syndrome
- Multiple trauma
- Malignant hyperthermia
- Limb ischemia
- Reperfusion after revascularization procedures for ischemia
- Extensive surgical (spinal) dissection, bariatric surgery
- Tourniquet ischemia
- Prolonged static positioning during surgery
- Infectious and inflammatory myositis
- Metabolic myopathies
- Hypovolemia and urinary acidification are important precipitating causes in the development of acute renal failure
- Sickle cell trait is a predisposing condition
- Hypothyroidism
- Alcoholism
- Seizures

Dx DIAGNOSIS

DIFFERENTIAL DIAGNOSIS

"Creatine Kinase Elevation" in Section III describes a clinical algorithm for the evaluation of creatine phosphokinase (CPK) elevation.

LABORATORY TESTS

- Screening for myoglobinuria with a simple urine dipstick test using orthotoluidine or benzidine
- Blood urea nitrogen, creatinine
- Increased CK (Fig. 1-284)
- Hyperkalemia
- Hypocalcemia
- Hyperphosphatemia
- Increased urinary myoglobin
- Pigmented granular casts
- Hyperuricemia

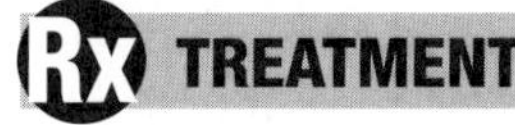

TREATMENT

ACUTE GENERAL Rx

- Early, aggressive, high-volume IV fluid replacement.
- Initiate volume repletion with normal saline at a rate of 200 to 1000 ml/hour depending on the setting and severity. Consider treatment with mannitol (up to 200 g/day and cumulative dose up to 800 g) to induce diuresis to prevent acute renal failure. Check for plasma osmolality and plasma osmolal gap. Discontinue mannitol if diuresis (>20 ml/hr) is not established. Maintain volume repletion until myoglobinuria is cleared (negative urine dipstick for blood).
- Monitor serum potassium frequently. Correct electrolyte imbalances. Correct hypocalcemia only if symptomatic or if severe hyperkalemia occurs.
- Treatment of electrolyte imbalances
- Alkalinization of urine is controversial but appears helpful in research models

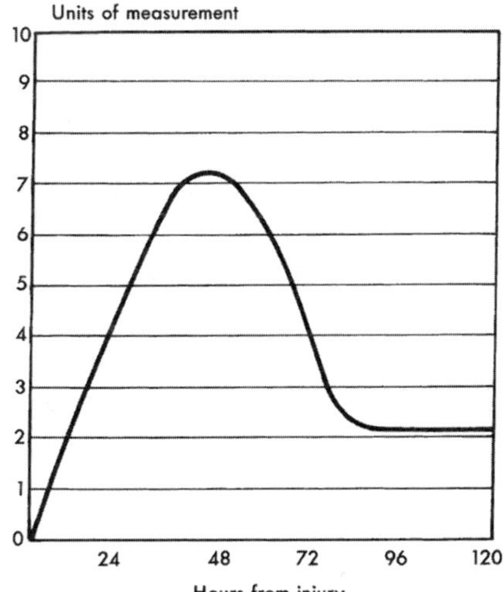

FIGURE 1-284 Typical creatine kinase elimination curve. (From Rosen P [ed]: *Emergency medicine,* ed 4, St Louis, 1998, Mosby.)

DISPOSITION

The condition is easily treatable, but early diagnosis and management are necessary to avoid renal failure, which occurs in 30% of cases.

REFERRAL

Renal consultation

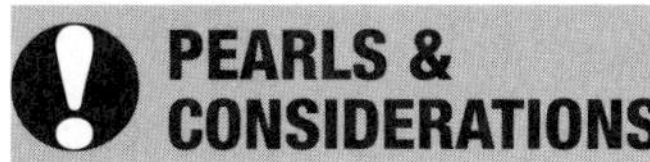

PEARLS & CONSIDERATIONS

COMMENTS

- A clinical algorithm for the evaluation of muscle cramps and aches is described in Fig. 3-216.
- Statin-induced rhabdomyolysis is 12× more frequent when statins are combined with fibrates compared with statin monotherapy.

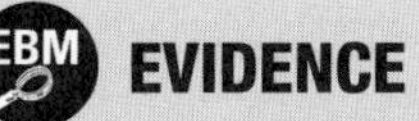

EVIDENCE

There is overwhelming support in the literature for the efficacy of early volume expansion in volume-depleted patients.

Prevention of acute renal failure is imperative with liberal use of IV fluids.

Myoglobin precipitation is prevented with this treatment.

Myoglobinuria usually resolves in 3 to 4 days.

Evidence-Based References

1. Better OS, Stein JH: Early management of shock and prophylaxis of acute renal failure in traumatic rhabdomyolysis, *N Engl J Med* 322:825, 1990.
2. Zager R: Rhabdomyolysis and myohemoglobinuric acute renal failure, *Kidney Int* 49:314, 1996.

SUGGESTED READINGS

Ahn SC: Neuromuscular complications of statins, *Phys Med Rehabil Clin North Am* 19:47, 2008.

Alsheikh-Ali AA et al: Effect of the magnitude of lipid lowering on risk of elevated liver enzymes, rhabdomyolysis, and cancer: insights from large randomized statin trials, *J Am Coll Cardiol* 50(5):409, 2007.

Antons KA et al: Clinical perspectives of statin-induced rhabdomyolysis, *Am J Med* 119:400-409, 2006.

Bosch X et al: Rhabdomyolysis and acute kidney injury, *N Engl J Med* 361:62-72, 2009.

Chatzizisis YS et al: Risk factors and drug interactions predisposing to statin-induced myopathy: implications for risk assessment prevention and treatment, *Drug Saf* 38(3):171, 2010.

Ettinger JE et al: Rhabdomyolysis: diagnosis and treatment in bariatric surgery, *Obes Surg* 17(4):525, 2007.

Finsterer J et al: Severe rhabdomyolysis after excessive bodybuilding, *J Sports Med Phys Fitness* 47:502, 2007.

Joy TR, Hegele RA: Narrative review: statin-related myopathy, *Ann Intern Med* 150:858-868, 2009.

Klopstock T: Drug-induced myopathies, *Curr Opin Neurol* 21:590, 2008.

AUTHOR: **LONNIE R. MERCIER, M.D.**

BASIC INFORMATION

DEFINITION

Rheumatic fever is a multisystem inflammatory disease that occurs in the genetically susceptible host after a pharyngeal infection with group A streptococci.

SYNONYMS

Acute rheumatic fever
Rheumatic carditis

ICD-9CM CODES
390; 716.9 Rheumatic fever

EPIDEMIOLOGY & DEMOGRAPHICS

INCIDENCE (IN U.S.):

- 0.1% to 3% in patients with untreated streptococcal pharyngitis
- Higher incidence of streptococcal pharyngitis with:
  1. Crowding
  2. Poverty
  3. Young age

PREDOMINANT AGE:

- Age 5 to 15 yr for first attack
- Possible relapses later

PEAK INCIDENCE: School-age children

GENETICS: Familial disposition: predisposition to the disease is likely to be genetically determined.

PHYSICAL FINDINGS & CLINICAL PRESENTATION

- Acute streptococcal pharyngitis, which may be subclinical and not reported by the patient
- After latent period of 1 to 5 wk (average, 19 days), acute rheumatic attack
- Patient is febrile, with a migratory polyarthritis of knees, ankles, wrists, elbows; typically severe for 1 wk, remits by 3 to 4 wk
- Carditis
  1. New heart murmur
     a. Mitral regurgitation
     b. Aortic insufficiency
     c. Diastolic mitral murmur
  2. Cardiomegaly
  3. CHF
  4. Pericardial friction rub or effusion
- Rarely, pancarditis is severe and fatal
- Subcutaneous nodules can be palpated over extensor tendon surfaces or bony prominences, such as the skull
- Chorea (Sydenham's chorea) is characterized by rapid involuntary movements affecting all muscles
  1. Muscular weakness
  2. Emotional lability
  3. Rarely seen after adolescence and almost never in adult males
- Erythema marginatum
  1. Evanescent, pink, well-demarcated spreading to trunk and proximal extremities
  2. Not specific
- Arthralgias (joint pain without swelling)
- Abdominal pain

ETIOLOGY

- Group A streptococci not recovered from tissue lesions.
- It does not occur in the absence of a streptococcal antibody response.
- Immunologic cross-reactivity between certain streptococcal antigens and human tissue antigens suggests an autoimmune cause (Fig. 1-285).
- Both initial attacks and recurrences can be completely prevented by prompt treatment of streptococcal pharyngitis with penicillin.

DIAGNOSIS

DIFFERENTIAL DIAGNOSIS

- Rheumatoid arthritis
- Juvenile rheumatoid arthritis (Still's disease)
- Bacterial endocarditis
- Systemic lupus
- Viral infections
- Serum sickness

WORKUP

- "Jones Criteria (revised) for Guidance in the Diagnosis of Rheumatic Fever"
- One major and two minor criteria if supported by evidence of an antecedent group A streptococcal infection
- Major criteria
  1. Carditis
  2. Migratory arthritis
  3. Chorea
  4. Erythema marginatum
  5. Subcutaneous nodules
- Minor criteria
  1. Previous rheumatic fever or rheumatic heart disease
  2. Fever
  3. Arthralgia
  4. Increased acute-phase reactants
     a. ESR
     b. C-reactive protein
     c. Leukocytosis
  5. Prolonged P-R interval

LABORATORY TESTS

- Throat cultures are usually negative.
- Streptococcal antibody tests are more useful in establishing the diagnosis.
  1. Peak at the beginning of the attack
  2. Can document a recent streptococcal infection
- ASO (antistreptolysin O) titers peak:
  1. 4 to 5 wk after a streptococcal throat infection
  2. During the second or third wk of illness
- Anti-DNase B (Streptozyme) is also commonly used but is less reliable.
- High-titer streptococcal antibodies:
  1. Are supportive of diagnosis, but not proof
  2. Should be interpreted in the context of clinical criteria

IMAGING STUDIES

- Chest x-ray to assess heart size
- Echocardiogram:
  1. To evaluate murmurs
  2. To rule out pericardial effusion

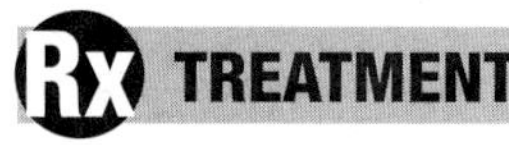

TREATMENT

ACUTE GENERAL Rx

- Course of penicillin to eradicate throat carriage of group A streptococci
- Arthralgia or arthritis without carditis: aspirin 40 mg/lb/day for 2 wk, followed by 20 mg/lb/day for 4 to 6 wk
- Carditis and heart failure:
  1. Prednisone 40 to 60 mg/day
  2. IV corticosteroids, such as methylprednisolone, 10 to 40 mg/day for severe carditis

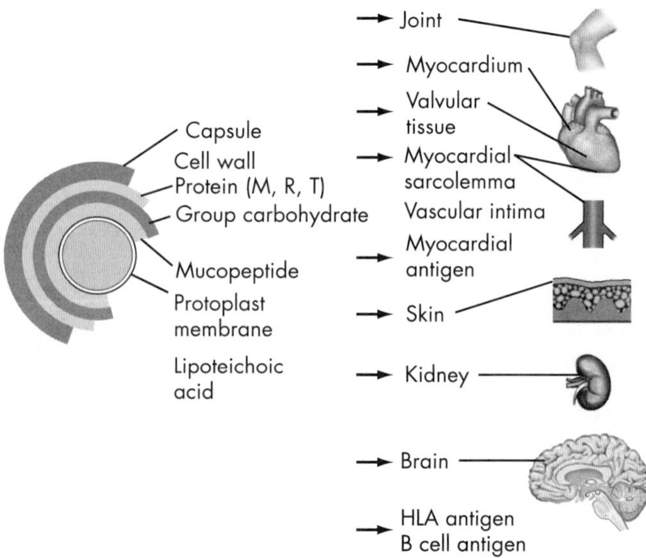

FIGURE 1-285 Structure of the group A streptococcus. Note the wide variety of cross-reactions between its antigens and mammalian tissues. (From Harris ED et al: *Kelley's Textbook of Rheumatology,* ed 8, Saunders, 2009.)

CHRONIC Rx

Secondary prevention (prevention of recurrences):

- Monthly treatment with benzathine penicillin 1.2 million U IM
- Erythromycin in patients with penicillin allergy

DISPOSITION

- Damage of heart valves because of fibrosis
    1. Late sequela of recurrent attacks
    2. Frequent cause of valvular heart disease in developing countries
- May progress to heart failure

REFERRAL

To cardiologist for management of severe carditis

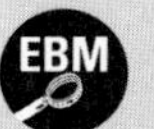

EVIDENCE

There is a lack of information from randomized trials to fully support the use of supportive therapies, such as steroids, aspirin, and bed rest in the management of acute rheumatic fever. The rationale for their use is based on clinical experience and general consensus. However, based on expert opinion, some statements may be made regarding the primary prevention in patients at risk as a result of streptococcal pharyngitis, and for the secondary prevention of recurrent episodes.

Primary prevention:

Recommendations from the American Heart Association are that penicillin is the treatment of choice in the prevention of rheumatic fever in patients with group A beta-hemolytic streptococcal pharyngitis; Penicillin may be administered IM or PO depending on the physician's assessment of the patient's likely adherence to an oral regimen and the risks of rheumatic fever in a particular population.[1] Ⓒ

Recomendations from the American Heart Association are that oral erythromycin is acceptable for patients allergic to penicillin in the prevention of rheumatic fever in patients with group A beta-hemolytic streptococcal pharyngitis.[1] Ⓒ

Secondary prevention:

Recommendations from the American Heart Association are that penicillin is the agent of choice for secondary prophylaxis in patients who have had an attack of rheumatic fever; intramuscular penicillin G is preferred to oral penicillin.[1] Ⓒ

Recommendations from the American Heart Association are that for secondary prophylaxis in patients who have had an attack of rheumatic fever, sulfadiazine may be used in patients allergic to penicillin.[1] Ⓒ

Recommendations from the American Heart Association are that for secondary prophylaxis in patients who have had an attack of rheumatic fever, erythromycin is recommended for the patient who is allergic to penicillin and sulfadiazine.[1] Ⓒ

Evidence-Based Reference

1. American College of Cardiology et al: ACC/AHA 2006 guidelines for the management of patients with valvular heart disease: a report of the American College of Cardiology/American Heart Association Task Force on Practice Guidelines (writing Committee to Revise the 1998 guidelines for the management of patients with valvular heart disease) developed in collaboration with the Society of Cardiovascular Anesthesiologists endorsed by the Society for Cardiovascular Angiography and Interventions and the Society of Thoracic Surgeons. *J Am Coll Cardiol* 48:e1-148, 2006.

SUGGESTED READINGS

Kaplan EL: Pathogenesis of acute rheumatic fever and rheumatic heart disease: evasive after half a century of clinical, epidemiological, and laboratory investigation, *Heart* 91(1):3, 2005.

Robertson KA et al: Antibiotics for the primary prevention of acute rheumatic fever: a meta-analysis, *BMC Cardiovasc Disord* 5(1):11, 2005.

Sharland M et al: Antibiotic prescribing in general practice and hospital admissions for peritonsillar abscess, mastoiditis, and rheumatic fever in children: time trend analysis, *BMJ* 331(7512):328, 2005.

Vijayalakshmi IB et al: The role of echocardiography in diagnosing carditis in the setting of acute rheumatic fever, *Cardiol Young* 15(6):583, 2005.

Walker K, Wilmshurst J: Acute rheumatic fever, *Lancet* 366(9494):1354, 2005.

AUTHORS: **GLENN G. FORT, M.D., M.P.H.,** and **DENNIS J. MIKOLICH, M.D.**

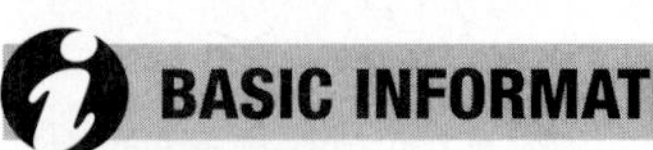

BASIC INFORMATION

DEFINITION

Rheumatoid arthritis (RA) is a systemic disorder characterized by chronic joint inflammation that most commonly affects peripheral joints. This process results in the development of pannus, a destructive tissue that damages cartilage.

ICD-9CM CODES
714.0 Rheumatoid arthritis

EPIDEMIOLOGY & DEMOGRAPHICS

PREVALENCE: 5 to 10 cases/1000 adults. It is the most common autoimmune disease in the world.

PREDOMINANT SEX:

- Female/male ratio of 3:1
- After age 50 yr, sex difference less marked

PREDOMINANT AGE: 35 to 45 yr

PHYSICAL FINDINGS & CLINICAL PRESENTATION

- Usually gradual onset; common prodromal symptoms of weakness, fatigue, and anorexia
- Initial presentation: multiple symmetric joint involvement, most often in the hands and feet, usually metacarpophalangeal, metatarsophalangeal, and proximal interphalangeal joints (Fig. 1-286)
- Joint effusions, tenderness, and restricted motion usually present early in the disease
- Eventual characteristic deformities: subluxations, dislocations, joint contractures
- Extraarticular findings:
    1. Tendon sheaths and bursae frequently affected by chronic inflammation
    2. Possible tendon rupture
    3. Rheumatoid nodules over bony prominences such as the elbow and shaft of the ulna
    4. Splenomegaly, pericarditis, vasculitis
    5. Findings of carpal tunnel syndrome resulting from flexor tenosynovitis

ETIOLOGY

Unknown. There is increasing evidence that the inflammation and destruction of bone and cartilage that occur in many rheumatic diseases are the result of the activation by some unknown mechanism of proinflammatory cells that infiltrate the synovium. These cells, in turn, release various substances, such as cytokines and tumor necrosis factor (TNF)-alpha, which subsequently cause the pathologic changes typical of this group of diseases. Many of the newer therapeutic agents are directed at the suppression of these final mediators of inflammation.

Dx DIAGNOSIS

DIFFERENTIAL DIAGNOSIS

- Systemic lupus erythematosus
- Seronegative spondyloarthropathies
- Polymyalgia rheumatica
- Acute rheumatic fever
- Scleroderma

According to the American College of Rheumatology, rheumatoid arthritis exists when four of seven criteria are present, with criteria 1 to 4 being present for at least 6 wk:

1. Morning stiffness >1 hr
2. Arthritis in three or more joints with swelling
3. Arthritis of hand joints with swelling
4. Symmetric arthritis
5. Rheumatoid nodules
6. Roentgenographic changes typical of RA
7. Positive serum rheumatoid factor

LABORATORY TESTS

- Increase in rheumatoid factor (RF) in 80% of cases (rheumatoid factor also present in the normal population). RF is an antibody directed against the Fc region of the IgG that has been used as a diagnostic marker for rheumatoid arthritis. Patients with rheumatoid arthritis also have autoantibodies against cyclic citrullinated peptide (CCP). Anti-CCp autoantibodies are more specific than RF for diagnosing rheumatoid arthritis and may better predict erosive disease. Sensitivity and specificity of the anti-CCP test for RA is 67% and 95% respectively.
- Possible mild anemia
- Usually, elevated acute phase reactants (erythrocyte sedimentation rate, C-reactive protein)
- Possible mild leukocytosis
- Usually, turbid joint fluid, which forms a poor mucin clot; elevated cell count, with an increase in polymorphonuclear leukocytes

IMAGING STUDIES

Plain radiography:

- Usually reveals soft tissue swelling and osteoporosis early (Fig. 1-287)
- Eventually, joint space narrowing, erosion, and deformity visible as a result of continued inflammation and cartilage destruction

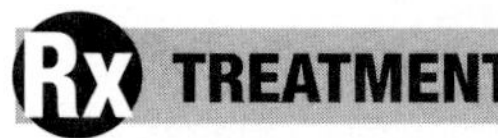

Rx TREATMENT

NONPHARMACOLOGIC THERAPY

Proper management requires close cooperation among primary physician, therapist, rheumatologist, and orthopedist.

- Patient education is important.
- Rest with proper exercise and splinting can prevent or correct joint deformities.
- Maintain proper diet and control obesity.

CHRONIC Rx

- Nonsteroidal anti-inflammatory drugs (NSAIDs): commonly used as the initial treatment to relieve inflammation (drug of choice for most patients is aspirin, but other NSAIDs are also effective)
- Disease-modifying drugs (DMARDs): traditionally begun when NSAIDs are not effective; current recommendations favor early aggressive treatment with DMARDs, seeking to minimize long-term joint damage. Commonly used agents are methotrexate, cyclosporine, hydroxychloroquine, sulfasalazine, leflunomide, and infliximab. Most of these are associated with potential toxicity and require close monitoring. They are also usually slow-acting drugs that require >8 wk to become effective (Table 1-68)
- Oral prednisone
- Intrasynovial steroid injections
- Etanercept, a tumor necrosis factor α-blocker, is useful in moderately to severely active RA in patients who respond inadequately to DMARDs. The combination of etanercept and methotrexate has been reported to be effective and promising in the treatment of RA
- New treatment agents include rituximab (anti-CD 20), abatacept (cytotoxic T-lymphocyte antigen 4 immunoglobulin), and tocilizumab (anti-interleukin 6 receptor)

DISPOSITION

- Remissions and exacerbations are common, but condition is chronically progressive in the majority of cases.
- Joint degeneration and deformity often lead to disability.

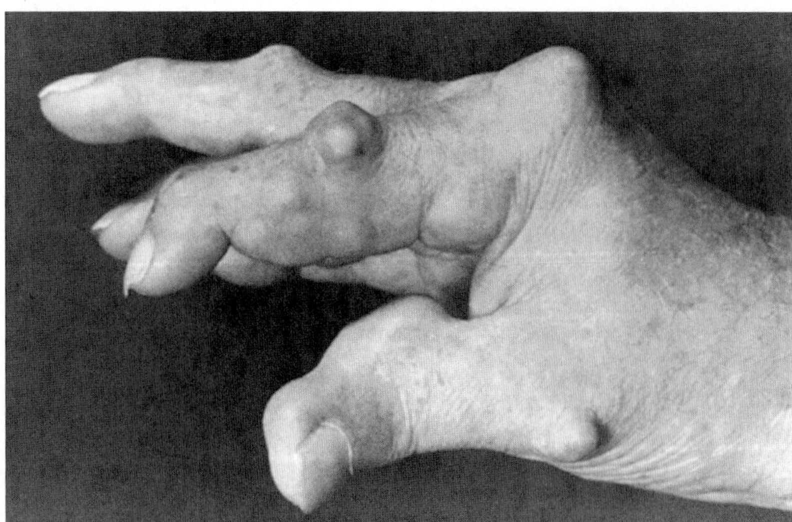

FIGURE 1-286 Rheumatoid arthritis. Hand of a 60-year-old man with seropositive rheumatoid arthritis. There are fixed deformities and gross rheumatoid nodules. (From Canoso JJ: *Rheumatology in primary care,* Philadelphia, 1997, WB Saunders.)

- Early diagnosis and treatment are important and can improve quality of life.

REFERRAL

- Early referral to rheumatologist
- Orthopedic consultation for corrective surgery

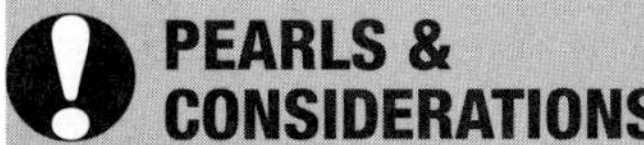

PEARLS & CONSIDERATIONS

- RA often develops acutely in the postpartum patient, a common time for the onset of autoimmune diseases.
- Because of the poor outcomes associated with previous treatment protocols, a much more aggressive approach, often using IV therapies, is presently advocated by many rheumatologists.

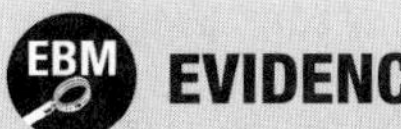

EVIDENCE

Please note: Complete text of EBM for this topic is available online.

Key trials and commentary:

This study sought to investigate intramodality and intermodality agreements of CT and MRI erosion volumes in metacarpophalangeal (MCP) joints in rheumatoid arthritis (RA), and to compare the volumes with erosion scores for CT, MRI, and radiography.

Very high intramodality and high intermodality agreements of CT and MRI erosion volumes were found, encouraging further testing in longitudinal studies. A close correlation with CT and MRI erosion volumes supports the OMERACT RAMRIS erosion score as a valid measure of joint destruction in RA.

RA is a common and debilitating disease process, costing society greatly in reduced productivity and actual medical costs. As more effective drugs are discovered that promise to control disease at an early, nondestructive phase, it is imperative that effective early diagnostic techniques are used to evaluate any changes and validate claims of drug efficacy.

The general radiologist need not be concerned with establishing reliability of assessment techniques for drug studies. However, these studies are important for the general public and add incremental knowledge useful to all radiologists. This study was well conceived, uses adequate numbers of joints for a good statistical analysis, and validates the erosion scoring system currently being used for RA studies. It contains information concerning sources of errors in analysis of erosions.

This article will be useful for the radiologist interested in developing or using a scoring technique for longitudinal studies of RA. **A**

Rheumatoid factor (RF) and autoantibodies against cyclic citrullinated peptide (CCP), are markers that might help physicians diagnose RA.

This study sought to determine whether anti-CCP antibody more accurately identifies patients with RA and better predicts radiographic progression than does RF.

It showed that Anti-CCP antibodies are more specific than RF for diagnosing RA and may better predict erosive disease.

Anti-CCP antibody assays have been developed as a reliable, reproducible, standardized method to detect antibodies, originally described as anti-perinuclear factor and anti-keratin antibodies. Some investigators suggest that anti-CCP antibodies have a pathogenic role in RA because citrullinated fibrin is found in the synovia of patients with RA, and these antibodies appear to be produced locally in inflamed joints. Citrullinated arginyl residues were identified as the epitope, and can be recognized onlinear or cyclic peptides. Both have higher specificity for RA than RF, but CCP assays have higher sensitivity than their linear epitope cousins. Early CCP assays (now called anti-CCP1 assays) had very high specificity (98%) but a lower sensitivity than that of RF. Thus, more sensitive assays (CCP2) were developed, using conformational epitopes selected from libraries of citrullinated peptides. The conclusion from this analysis is that these assays are now equivalent to RF in sensitivity.

Several factors may contribute to the lower specificity of RF. One is that RF occurs in a variety of inflammatory and infectious disorders and is probably best considered a marker for chronic inflammation. Another factor is the varied laboratory techniques used in these studies to measure RF (nephelometry, latex agglutination, ELISA) with different or unspecified lower positive limits. Finally, the specificity may appear higher than it truly is (acquisition bias) because RF positivity is one of the criteria for diagnosing RA, whereas anti-CCP is not. Although the CCP studies may have some heterogeneity in using anti-CCP1 and anti-CCP2 assays, CCP studies may exhibit some publication bias toward positive results.

Other important conclusions that the authors reached from the subset analysis were as follows: the sensitivity and specificity of RF is low when the control patients have other autoimmune diseases associated with RF positivity (e.g., Sjogren syndrome). Additionally, the combination of determining IgM RF with anti-CCP does not significantly improve the diagnostic accuracy of anti-CCP testing alone. Presence of anti-CCP antibody is associated with increased risk of radiographic progression. The anti-CCP2 assay is more sensitive than anti-CCP1 as a marker of RA. Anti-CCP antibody positivity was more specific than IgM RF for early RA, and more predictive of RA development and radiographic progression. As with most tests in medicine, the pretest probability influences the use of the test, and the pretest probability depends on astute clinical judgment.

Effective early treatment appears to be most effective for preventing long-term joint damage; thus, accurate diagnosis is important, especially with the recognition that unnecessary treatment is costly, in terms of health care dollars and risk to the patient.

Thus, to parallel our increasingly aggressive, effective, and costly therapeutic armamentarium, we need equally effective and

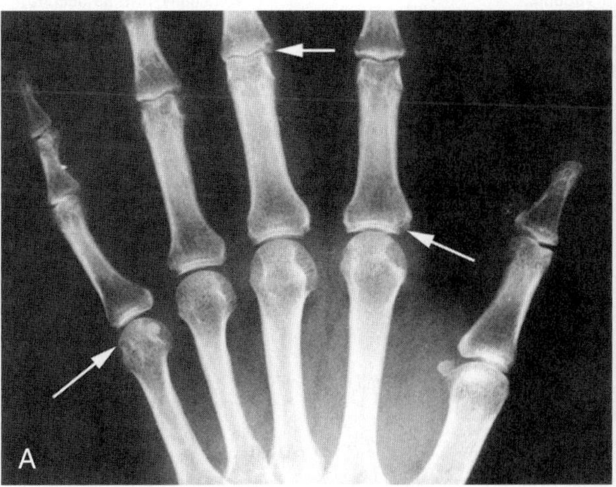

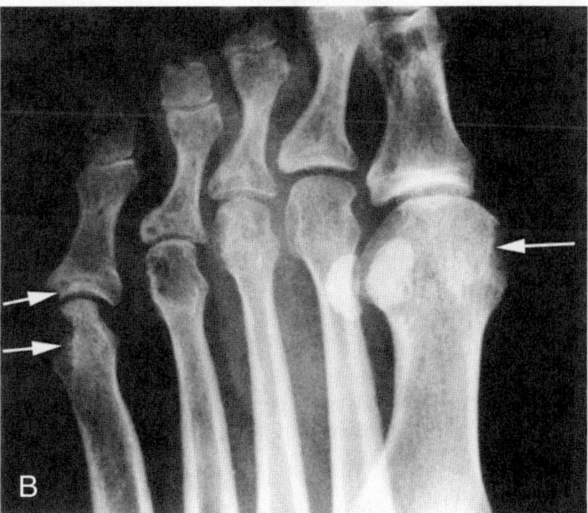

FIGURE 1-287 Rheumatoid arthritis. A, Periarticular osteopenia and marginal erosions in metacarpophalangeal joints and a proximal interphalangeal *(arrows)*. **B,** In the same patient, marginal erosions at metatarsal heads. (From Canoso JJ [ed]: *Rheumatology in primary care.* Philadelphia, 1997, WB Saunders.)

specific diagnostic strategy. This article helps to clarify the use of this test in the context of appropriate clinical judgment.[2] Ⓐ

RANK Ligand (RANKL) is essential for osteoclast development, activation, and survival. Denosumab is a fully human monoclonal IgG2 antibody that binds RANKL, inhibiting its activity. The aim of this multicenter, randomized, double-blind, placebo-controlled, phase II study was to evaluate the effects of denosumab on structural damage in patients with RA receiving methotrexate treatment.

This study showed that addition of twice-yearly injections of denosumab to ongoing methotrexate treatment inhibited structural damage in patients with RA for up to 12 months, with no increase in the rates of adverse events as compared with placebo.

Understanding that osteoclast activity mediated in part by RANKL contributes to erosion formation in RA, the authors of this study set out to determine if the use of denosumab, a fully human monoclonal antibody to RANKL, would slow the progression of structural damage in RA patients receiving methotrexate. This is a multicenter, randomized, double blind, placebo-controlled Phase II clinical trial. 218 patients with rheumatoid arthritis, diagnosed according to ACR 1987 criteria, for >24 months, on a stable dose of methotrexate for >8 weeks and the presence of >6 swollen joints were randomized to receive denosumab 60 mg, denosumab 180 mg or placebo subcutaneously every 6 months in two doses. The patients were evaluated with hand and wrist radiographs and MRIs, DEXA, blood and urine bone and cartilage biomarkers, and clinical assessments at several intervals within a 12-month period. The primary end point was the change in the MRI erosion score from baseline to 6 months. Of the 94% of patients who completed the study, those receiving denosumab 180 mg had statistically significant less change in their MRI erosion score. However, there was no effect

TABLE 1-68 Selected Disease-Modifying Antirheumatic Drugs

Type Generic (Trade) Name	Recommended Dosages	Toxic Effects	Recommended Monitoring
Gold compounds (Myochrysine)	IM: 10 mg followed by 25 mg 1 wk later, then 25-50 mg/wk until there is toxicity, major clinical improvement, or cumulative dose ≥1 g. If effective, interval between doses is increased.	Pruritus, dermatitis (frequent in one third of patients), stomatitis, nephrotoxicity, blood dyscrasias, "nitritoid" reaction: flushing, weakness, nausea, dizziness 30 min after injection.	CBC, platelet count before every other injection
Aurothioglucose (Solganal)	IM: 10 mg; second and third doses 25 mg, fourth and subsequent doses 50 mg. Interval between doses: 1 wk. If improvement and no toxicity, decrease dose to 25 mg or increase interval between doses.	Dermatitis, stomatitis, nephrotoxicity, blood dyscrasias.	CBC, platelet count every 2 wk. Urinalysis before each dose.
Auranofin (Ridaura)	Oral: 3 mg bid or 6 mg qd; may increase to 3 mg tid after 6 mo.	Loose stools, diarrhea (up to 50%), dermatitis.	Baseline CBC, platelet count, U/A, renal, liver function, at onset then CBC with platelet count, U/A 9 mo.
Antimalarial Hydroxychloroquine (Plaquenil)	Oral: 400-600 mg qd with meals then 200-400 mg qd.	Retinopathy, dermatitis, muscle weakness, hypoactive DTRs, CNS.	Ophthalmologic examination every 3 mo (visual acuity, slit lamp, funduscopic, visual field tests), neuromuscular examination.
Penicillamine (Cuprimine, Depen)	Oral: 125-250 mg qd, then increasing at monthly intervals doses to max 750-1000 mg by 125-250 mg.	Pruritus, rash/mouth ulcers, bone marrow depression, proteinuria, hematuria, hypogeusia, myasthenia, myositis, GI distress, pulmonary toxicity, teratogenic.	CBC every 2 wk until dose stable, then every month.
Methotrexate (Rheumatrex)	Oral: 7.5-15 mg/wk.	Pulmonary toxicity, ulcerative stomatitis, leukopenia, thrombocytopenia, GI distress, malaise, fatigue, chills, fever, CNS, elevated LFTs/liver disease, lymphoma, infection.	U/A weekly until dose stable, then every month; hCG as needed.
Azathioprine (Imuran)	Oral: 50-100 mg qd, increase at 4-wk intervals by 0.5 mg/kg/day up to 2.5 mg/kg/day.	Leukopenia, thrombocytopenia, GI, neoplastic if previous Rx with alkylating agents.	CBC with platelet count, LFTs weekly for 6 wk then monthly LFTs, U/A periodically, hCG as needed.
Sulfasalazine (Azulfidine)	Oral: 500 mg/day then increase up to 3 g/day.	GI, skin rash, pruritus, blood dyscrasias, oligospermia.	CBC with platelet count, weekly × 1 mo, 2×/mo. × 2 mo, then monthly, HCG as needed.
Alkylating agents Cyclophosphamide (Cytoxan)	Oral: 50-100 mg/day up to 2.5 mg/kg/day.	Leukopenia, thrombocytopenia, hematuria, GI, alopecia, rash, bladder cancer, non-Hodgkin's lymphoma, infection.	CBC, U/A every 2 wk for 3 mo, then monthly for 9 mo, then every 6 mo.
Chlorambucil (Leukeran)	Oral: 0.1-0.2 mg/kg/day.	Bone marrow suppression, GI, CNS, infection.	CBC with platelet count regularly; hCG as needed.
Cyclosporine (Sandimmune)	Oral 2.5-5 mg/kg/day.	Nephrotoxicity, tremor, hirsutism, hypertension, gum hyperplasia.	CBC with platelet count every week. WBCs 3-4 days after each CBC during first 3-6 wk at therapy; hCG as needed.
Pyrimidine, synthesis inhibitors	Loading dose: 100 mg/day for 3 days.	Hepatotoxicity, carcinogenesis.	Renal function, liver function.
Leflunomide (Arava)	Maintenance therapy: 20 mg/day; if not tolerated, 10 mg/day.	Immunosuppression, long half-life.	LFTs every month, drug levels after discontinuation (after 1 mo therapy, remains in blood for 2 yr without use of cholestyramine).

From Rakel RE (ed): *Principles of family practice,* ed 6, Philadelphia, 2002, WB Saunders.

bid, Twice a day; *CBC,* complete blood count; *CNS,* central nervous system; *DTR,* deep tendon reflex; *GI,* gastrointestinal; *hCG,* human chorionic gonadotropin; *IM,* intramuscular; *LFT,* liver function test; *qd,* every day; *tid,* three times a day; *U/A,* urinalysis; *WBC,* white blood cell count.

of denosumab on the modified Sharp joint space narrowing score or the disease activity as measured by ACR response, HAQ, or DAS28. The denosumab groups also had decreases in the bone turnover markers and an increase in BMD over baseline. The authors concluded that denosumab augmented the methotrexate inhibited structural damage, improved the BMD, and suppressed bone turnover in patients with RA.

The prevention or slowing of structural damage in patients with RA is a goal for all rheumatologists treating this disease. With the introduction of biologic agents, we have had tremendous success in doing so. In this study, denosumab decreased bone destruction in patients taking methotrexate. A large percentage of RA patients are receiving TNF-alpha inhibitors, which appear to slow the progression of erosions. Denosumab may provide an alternative or complementary therapy, recognizing that it does not appear to decrease the synovitis, inflammation, or joint cartilage destruction. A next step in the investigation of denosumab could be to compare this drug to the TNF-alpha inhibitors or even to study its utility in combination with the TNF-alpha inhibitors.[3] Ⓐ

Ocrelizumab, a humanized anti-CD20 monoclonal antibody, was studied in a first-in-human trial in RA patients receiving concomitant methotrexate (MTX).

This study showed that Ocrelizumab therapy in combination with MTX was well tolerated. Doses of 200 mg (two infusions) and higher showed better clinical responses, better reduction of C-reactive protein levels, and very low immunogenicity.

The success of rituximab in the treatment of rheumatoid arthritis has illustrated the importance of B cells in the disease pathogenesis. This is a phase I/II randomized, blinded, placebo-controlled, dose-ranging study of ocrelizumab, a humanized anti-CD20 monoclonal antibody, in the treatment of patients with RA. In phase I of the study, patients received ocrelizumab 10 mg in two infusions to determine its safety. In phase II, 237 patients were randomized to receive placebo or ocrelizumab at doses of 10, 50, 200, 500, or 1000 mg in two infusions 2 weeks apart.

The results of this study show that B-cell depletion was seen in all groups receiving ocrelizumab. Furthermore, more patients in the ocrelizumab groups achieved ACR20, ACR50, or ACR70 responses at week 24 compared with the placebo-treated group. Maximum B-cell depletion seemed to occur at the 200 mg dose, which correlated with the clinical response. Patients receiving ocrelizumab at doses of 200 mg and higher appeared to have a greater clinical benefit than the lower doses.

RA is a complex disease that we do not fully understand, but through investigation of this disease many successful targeted therapies have emerged. B-cell therapy has shown much promise thus far in the form of rituximab, a chimeric monoclonal anti-CD20 antibody. Ocrelizumab is a humanized monoclonal antibody, but the advantages of the humanized antibody over chimeric, such as the development of antichimeric antibodies, are not addressed in this study. Further investigation comparing ocrelizumab with rituximab would be useful.[4] Ⓐ

The aim of this work was to assess the feasibility of using dynamic contrast enhanced (DCE) MRI of bone marrow edema, to compare it with conventional marrow edema scoring systems, and to determine the effects of anti-tumor necrosis factor (TNF)α therapy.

This study showed that dynamic contrast enhanced MRI of bone marrow edema yields additional information to RAMRIS scoring and may be a more sensitive marker of inflammatory activity and response to treatment.

Treatment of RA has entered a new era, and with treatment, the imaging of early RA as well as imaging for early evaluation of the effectiveness of treatment protocols has become increasingly important. An MRI scoring system has been established (Rheumatoid Arthritis MRI Scoring [RAMRIS]), which uses T2-weighted images for this evaluation. It has also been established that dynamic contrast-enhanced MR of the synovium can be used to monitor disease activity and predict progression of erosive disease as well as response to anti-TNF therapy. This article measures dynamic contrast enhancement of bone marrow edema in patients with early RA and following treatment. It shows convincingly that this measurement may prove important in predicting response to treatment earlier than the currently used RAMRIS system. This may prove to save both time and expense in establishing appropriate individual treatment, as well as in drug trials.[5] Ⓐ

Evidence-Based References

1. Døhn UM, Ejbjerg BJ, Hasselquist M: Rheumatoid arthritis bone erosion volumes on CT and MRI: reliability and correlations with erosion scores on CT, MRI and radiography, *Ann Rheum Dis* 66:1388-1392, 2007. Commentary by B.J. Manaster, M.D., Ph.D. Ⓐ

2. Nishimura K, Sigiyama D, Kogata Y: Meta-analysis: diagnostic accuracy of anti-cyclic citrullinated peptide antibody and rheumatoid factor for rheumatoid arthritis, *Ann Intern Med* 146:797-808, 2007. Commentary by D.L. Kimpel, M.D. Ⓐ

3. Cohen SB, Dore RK, Lane NE: Denosumab treatment effects on structural damage, bone mineral density, and bone turnover in rheumatoid arthritis: a twelve-month, multicenter, randomized, double-blind, placebo-controlled, phase II clinical trial, *Arthritis Rheum* 58:1299-1309, 2008. Commentary by S.M. Berney, M.D. Ⓐ

4. Genovese MC, Kaine JL, Lowenstein MB: Ocrelizumab, a humanized anti-CD20 monoclonal antibody, in the treatment of patients with rheumatoid arthritis: a phase I/II randomized, blinded, placebo-controlled, dose-ranging study, *Arthritis Rheum* 58:2652-2661, 2008. Commentary by S.M. Berney, M.D. Ⓐ

5. Hodgson R, Grainger A, O'Connor P: Dynamic contrast enhanced MRI of bone marrow edema in rheumatoid arthritis, *Ann Rheum Dis* 67:270-272, 2008. Commentary by B.J. Manaster, M.D., Ph.D. Ⓐ

SUGGESTED READINGS

Donahue KE et al: Systematic review: comparative effectiveness and harms of disease-modifying medications for rheumatoid arthritis, *Ann Intern Med* 148:124, 2008.

Finckh A et al: Treatment of very early rheumatoid arthritis with symptomatic therapy, disease-modifying antirheumatic drugs, or biologic agents, *Ann Intern Med* 151:612-621, 2009.

Goekoop-Ruiterman JP et al: Comparison of treatment strategies in early rheumatoid arthritis, *Ann Intern Med* 146:406-415, 2007.

Heiberg MS et al: The comparative one-year performance of anti-tumor necrosis factor alpha drugs in patients with rheumatoid arthritis, psoriatic arthritis and ankylosing spondylitis: results from a longitudinal, observational, multicenter study, *Arthritis Rheum* 59:234, 2008.

Nishimura K et al: Meta-analysis: diagnostic accuracy of anti-cyclic citrullinated peptide antibody and rheumatoid factor for rheumatoid arthritis, *Ann Intern Med* 146:797-808, 2007.

Papp SR et al: The rheumatoid wrist, *J Am Acad Orthop Surg* 14:65, 2006.

Sfikakis PP: The first decade of biologic TNF antagonists in practice: lessons learned, unresolved issues, and future directions, *Curr Dir Autoimmun* 11:180, 2010.

Shmerling RH: Testing for anti-cyclic citrullinated peptide antibodies, *Rad Int Med* 169(1):9-14, 2009.

Smolen J et al: New therapies for treatment of rheumatoid arthritis, *Lancet* 370:1861-1874, 2007.

Sokka T: Quantitative assessment of rheumatoid arthritis in standard clinical care: turning clinical care into clinical science, *Best Pract Res Clin Rheumatol* 21(4):653, 2007.

Sokka T et al: Remission and rheumatoid arthritis: data on patients receiving usual care in twenty-four countries, *Arthritis Rheum* 58:2642, 2008.

AUTHOR: **LONNIE R. MERCIER, M.D.**

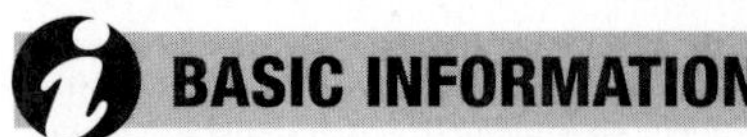

BASIC INFORMATION

DEFINITION

Allergic rhinitis is an IgE-mediated hypersensitivity response to nasally inhaled allergens that causes sneezing, rhinorrhea, nasal pruritus, and congestion. It may be seasonal or perennial.

SYNONYMS

- Hay fever
- IgE-mediated rhinitis

ICD-9CM CODES
477.9 Allergic rhinitis

EPIDEMIOLOGY & DEMOGRAPHICS

- Allergic rhinitis affects approximately 10% to 20% of the U.S. population and 40% of children.
- Mean age of onset is 8 to 12 yr.
- The prevalence of allergic rhinitis in patients presenting to their primary care provider with nasal symptoms is estimated to be 30% to 60%.

PHYSICAL FINDINGS & CLINICAL PRESENTATION

- Pale or violaceous mucosa of the turbinates caused by venous engorgement (this can distinguish it from erythema present in viral rhinitis)
- Nasal polyps
- Lymphoid hyperplasia in the posterior oropharynx with cobblestone appearance
- Erythema of the throat, conjunctival and scleral injection
- Clear nasal discharge
- Clinical presentation: usually consists of sneezing, nasal congestion, cough, postnasal drip, loss of or alteration of smell, and sensation of plugged ears

ETIOLOGY

- Pollens in the springtime, ragweed in fall, grasses in the summer
- Dust, mites, animal allergens
- Smoke or any irritants
- Perfumes, detergents, soaps
- Emotion, changes in atmospheric pressure or temperature
- Fig. 1-288 describes selected mediators present in nasal secretions from allergic rhinitis patients.

Dx DIAGNOSIS

DIFFERENTIAL DIAGNOSIS

- Infections (sinusitis; viral, bacterial, or fungal rhinitis)
- Rhinitis medicamentosa (cocaine, sympathomimetic nasal drops)
- Vasomotor rhinitis (e.g., secondary to air pollutants)
- Septal obstruction (e.g., deviated septum), nasal polyps, nasal neoplasms
- Systemic diseases (e.g., Wegener's granulomatosis, hypothyroidism [rare])

WORKUP

- The initial strategy should be to determine whether patients should undergo diagnostic testing or receive empirical treatment.
- Workup is often unnecessary if the diagnosis is apparent. A detailed medical history is useful in identifying the culprit allergen.
- Selected patients with allergic rhinitis that is not controlled with standard therapy may benefit from allergy testing to target allergen avoidance measures or guide immunotherapy. Allergy testing can be performed using skin testing or radioallergosorbent (RAST) testing. Immunoglobulin E (IgE) testing using newest generation assays is also an excellent tool for diagnosing the cause of symptoms related to rhinitis. Allergy testing should generally be reserved for ambiguous or complicated cases.
- Examination of nasal smears for the presence of neutrophils to rule out infectious causes and the presence of eosinophils (suggestive of allergy) may be useful in selected patients.
- Peripheral blood eosinophil counts are not useful in allergy diagnosis.

Rx TREATMENT

NONPHARMACOLOGIC THERAPY

- Maintain allergen-free environment by covering mattresses and pillows with allergen-proof casings, eliminating carpeting, eliminating animal products, and removing dust-collecting fixtures.
- Use of air purifiers and dust filters is helpful.
- Maintain humidity in the environment below 50% to prevent dust mites and mold.
- Use air conditioners, especially in the bedroom.
- Remove pets from homes of patients with suspected sensitivity to animal allergens.

ACUTE GENERAL Rx

- Determine if the patient is troubled by swollen turbinates (best treated with decongestants) or blockages secondary to mucus (effectively treated by antihistamines).
- Most first-generation antihistamines can cause considerable sedation and anticholinergic symptoms. The second-generation antihistamines (loratadine, fexofenadine, cetirizine, levocetirizine, desloratadine) are preferred because they do not have any significant anticholinergic or sedative effects.
- Montelukast (Singulair), a leukotriene receptor antagonist commonly used for asthma, is also effective for allergic rhinitis. Usual adult dose is 10 mg qd.
- Azelastine (Astelin) is an antihistamine nasal spray effective for seasonal allergic rhinitis. Olopatadine (Patanase) is an intranasal H1-antihistamine alternative to azestaline in mild to moderate seasonal allergic rhinitis.

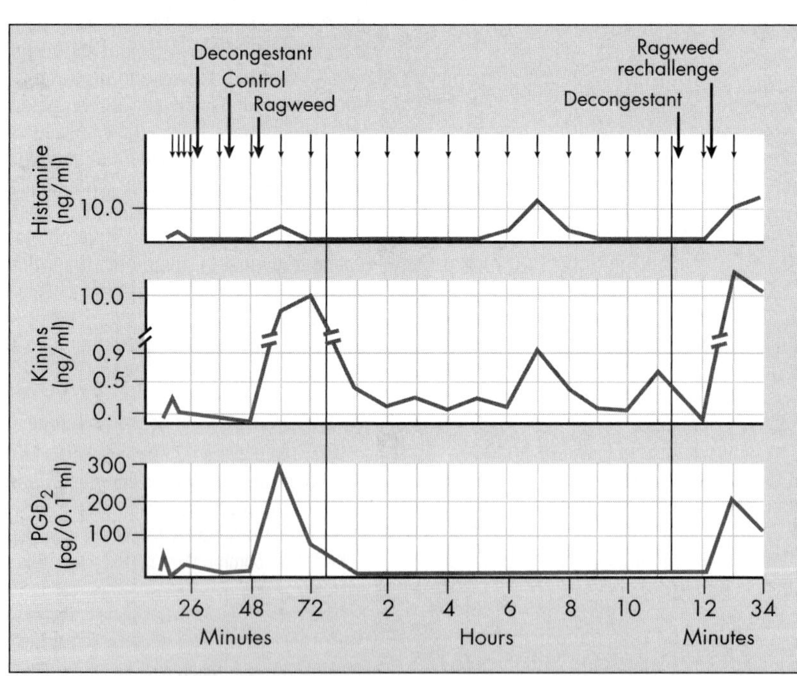

FIGURE 1-288 Profile of selected mediators present in nasal secretions collected by nasal wash from allergic rhinitis patients during early, late, and rechallenge responses to ragweed allergen. The time of each nasal wash is indicated by an *arrow.* Pretreatment with decongestants is necessary, as there are some mediators present in the nasal washes after the initial challenges. Histamine, kinins, tryptase, and prostaglandin D2 (PGD2) are present within minutes (early phase) of challenge with the ragweed allergen. In these experiments, without additional allergen, histamine and kinins reappear in nasal washes 2 to 8 hr after the initial exposure (late phase). Note that PGD2 is not present in secretions during the late-phase reaction. On subsequent reexposure to the allergen during rechallenge, there are prompt increases in these mediators in nasal washes. These data help explain the almost continual (daily) symptoms that many allergic rhinitis patients experience. (From Fireman P: *Atlas of allergies and immunology*, ed 3, St Louis, 2006, Mosby.)

- Topical nasal steroids are very effective and are preferred by many as first-line treatment for allergic rhinitis in adults. Patients should be instructed on proper use and informed that improvement might not occur for at least 1 wk after initiation of therapy. Commonly available inhalers follow:
  1. Beclomethasone dipropionate: one to two sprays in each nostril bid
  2. Fluticasone: initially two sprays in each nostril qd or one spray in each nostril bid, decreasing to one spray in each nostril qd based on response
  3. Flunisolide: initially two sprays in each nostril bid
  4. Budesonide: two sprays in each nostril bid or four sprays in each nostril qam

Table 1-69 compares medications used in relieving allergic and non-allergic rhinitis symptoms.

CHRONIC Rx

- Cromolyn sodium : one spray to each nostril three to four times daily can be used for prophylaxis (mast cell stabilizer).
- Immunotherapy is generally reserved for patients responding poorly to the above treatments.

DISPOSITION

Most patients experience significant relief with avoidance of allergens and proper use of medications.

REFERRAL

Allergy testing in patients with severe symptoms who are unresponsive to therapy or when the diagnosis is uncertain

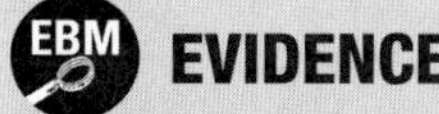

EVIDENCE

Please note: Complete text of EBM for this topic is available online.

Key trials and commentary:

Recent studies have documented the efficacy and safety of sublingual immunotherapy (SLIT) in patients with rhinitis, but the value of this treatment in those with asthma is still debated. This study evaluated the efficacy of SLIT in the treatment of allergic asthma in children by a meta-analysis of randomized, double-blind, and placebo-controlled (DBPC) clinical trials.

SLIT was introduced into the treatment of allergic rhinitis more than 20 years ago and its use is now commonplace in many European countries. There are a variety of reasons why SLIT could be preferable to subcutaneous allergy injections; these include in particular the noninvasive nature of this therapy. The safety profile of SLIT has obvious advantages, also. This meta-analysis of randomized controlled trials of SLIT vs. placebo in allergic asthmatic children showed a statistically significant reduction in the symptoms and medication use of/for asthma. Given the frequent worsening of asthma in the setting of uncontrolled allergic rhinitis, consideration should be given to a randomized, placebo-controlled trial of SLIT in adults with allergic rhinitis and asthma.[1] Ⓐ

This study analyzed the effectiveness of acupuncture in addition to routine care in patients with allergic rhinitis compared with treatment with routine care alone. The results of this trial suggest that treating patients with allergic rhinitis in routine care with additional acupuncture leads to clinically relevant and persistent benefits. In addition, it seems that physician characteristics play a minor role in the effectiveness of acupuncture treatment, although this idea needs further investigation.

This large, randomized, controlled trial compares the effect of acupuncture in addition to routine care with just routine care alone. It contained a nonrandomized arm as well for those patients wishing acupuncture who would not agree to randomization (three out of four eligible patients). It was well-designed using established outcomes instruments (RQLQ and SF-36) and methodology, and provided a reasonable follow-up of 6 months. Of note, all of the patients received their acupuncture from medically trained doctors. Results showed that at 3 months, the RQLQ and SF-36 scores improved significantly more in the acupuncture group compared with the control group ($P < 0.001$ for both). Further, the improvements in both acupuncture groups at 6 months were lower than they had been at 3 months. The glaring issue with this study, as the authors readily admit, is that the patients knew that they were getting "add on" care, and there were no controls (or acupuncture "sham"), which may have been able to mitigate against a considerable placebo effect. It should be noted that several studies in the literature looking at the impact of acupuncture performed with controls ("sham" acupuncture) have yielded inconsistent results. Nevertheless, it is encouraging to see the medical establishment recognizing that alternative (or complementary) approaches exist and are often sought out by patients when conventional techniques are not providing adequate relief. These authors should be applauded for pragmatically and deliberately examining the impact of acupuncture in AR management and resisting the temptation to reflexively dismiss or adopt these presently unsubstantiated approaches. Those on board with traditional remedies (both M.D.s and non-M.D.s alike) might argue that even if the improvement noted in this study is because of placebo effect, that's okay; the important thing is that the patients got better. This flawed line of reasoning may be acceptable to the layperson, but it is a major breach of the scientific method and would undermine the evidence-based thinking that is the foundation of modern-day medicine.[2] Ⓐ

This study analyzed the effect of nasal allergen challenge on the maxillary sinus and the effect of premedication with loratadine. The findings suggest that a neural reflex or systemic allergic inflammation is responsible for the sinus inflammatory response and that this inflammatory response might play a role in the development of rhinosinusitis in allergic subjects.

There has been a long-standing question as to the role of allergic rhinitis (AR) in chronic rhinosinusitis (CRS), given that most patients with CRS also have positive skin tests to common allergens. Both conditions are characterized by chronic inflammation and have similar symptomatology. This interesting study investigated the effect of nasal allergen challenge on the maxillary sinus and studied the effect of premedication with loratadine.

TABLE 1-69 Comparison of Medications in Relieving Allergic and Nonallergic Rhinitis Symptoms

	Oral Antihistamine	Intranasal Antihistamine	Oral or Nasal Decongestant	Nasal Steroid	LT Receptor Antagonist	Intranasal Anticholinergic	Intranasal Cromolyn	Allergen Immunotherapy
Sneezing	+	+	−	+	+	−	−	+
Itching	+	+	−	+	−	−	+	+
Rhinorrhea	+	+	+	+	+	+	+	+
Congestion	−	−	+	+	+	−	−	+
Conjunctivitis	+	−	−	−	+	−	−	+
Vasomotor rhinitis	−	−	+	+	−	+	−	−
Infectious rhinitis	−	−	+	−	−	+	−	−

LT, leukotriene.
From Fireman P: *Atlas of allergies and immunology*, ed 3, St Louis, 2006, Mosby.

These were on operated patients in which a maxillary catheterization technique was used to lavage and collect samples from the maxillary sinus. The design was that of a double-blind, crossover, randomized, placebo-controlled study in 20 allergic subjects out of season. After treatment with either placebo or loratadine (10 mg PO daily) for 1 week, a catheter was inserted into one maxillary sinus and used to lavage the cavity. The subjects then underwent nasal challenge with diluent for the allergen. Nasal and ipsilateral sinus lavages were performed after each challenge and then hourly for 8 hours. Symptoms were recorded and the lavage specimens were evaluated. A control with lactated Ringer's solution was used. The group found that compared with the LR allergen challenge resulted in significant increases in most early- and late-phase nasal parameters. Allergen challenge of the nose also led to a significant increase compared with control values in maxillary sinus eosinophils and the levels of albumin, eosinophil cationic protein, and histamine during the late response. Loratadine resulted in significant inhibition of the nasal early response compared with placebo. Accepting potential problems with catheterization of an unoperated maxillary sinus (in which case, levels measured would be more reflective of the nasal or middle meatal microenvironment and not necessarily that within the maxillary sinus proper), this study had some very intriguing results. In a very direct way, it demonstrated a significant effect of allergen exposure to inflammation within the maxillary sinus. The implications of this are not entirely clear. As the authors discuss, this may suggest a systemic allergic inflammatory response that includes the paranasal (maxillary) sinuses and/or a neurogenic response. Whether or not this response might play a role in the development of rhinosinusitis in allergic subjects is unknown.[3] Ⓐ

Evidence-Based References

1. Penagos M, Passalacqua G, Compalati E: Meta-analysis of the efficacy of sublingual immunotherapy in the treatment of allergic asthma in pediatric patients, 3 to 18 years of age, *Chest* 133:599-609, 2008. Commentary by S.K. Willsie, D.O. Ⓐ
2. Brinkhaus B, Witt CM, Jena S: Acupuncture in patients with allergic rhinitis: a pragmatic randomized trial. *Ann Allergy Asthma Immunol* 101:535-543, 2008. Commentary by R. Sindwani, M.D., FACS, FRCS Ⓐ
3. Baroody FM, Mucha SM, deTineo M: Nasal challenge with allergen leads to maxillary sinus inflammation, *J Allergy Clin Immunol* 121:1126-1132, 2008. Commentary by R. Sindwani, M.D. Ⓐ

SUGGESTED READINGS

Quillen DM, Feller DB: Diagnosing rhinitis: allergic vs. nonallergic, *Am Fam Physician* 73:1583, 2006.

Wallace DV et al: The diagnosis and management of rhinitis: an updated practice parameter, *J Allergy Clin Immunol* 122(2 suppl):S21, 2008.

AUTHOR: **FRED F. FERRI, M.D.**

BASIC INFORMATION

DEFINITION

Rickets is a systemic disease of infancy and childhood in which mineralization of growing bone is deficient as a result of abnormal calcium, phosphorus, or vitamin D metabolism. Osteomalacia is the same condition in the adult. *Renal osteodystrophy* is a term used to describe a similar condition in patients with chronic kidney disease. Certain forms of the disorder may respond only to high doses of vitamin D and are referred to as vitamin D–resistant rickets (VDRR).

ICD-9CM CODES
268.0 Active rickets
275.3 Vitamin D–resistant rickets
588.0 Renal rickets (renal osteodystrophy)
268.2 Osteomalacia

PHYSICAL FINDINGS & CLINICAL PRESENTATION

The child with classic rickets usually develops a number of specific abnormalities:

- Softening of the skull bones (craniotabes) early in the disorder
- Enlargement of the ribs at the costochondral junctions, producing the "rachitic rosary"
- Limb deformities and epiphyseal swelling (Fig. 1-289)
- Height below normal range
- Irritability and easy fatigability
- Pigeon breast deformity and an indentation of the lower ribcage at the insertion of the diaphragm, sometimes referred to as *Harrison's groove;* possible decrease in thoracic volume, resulting in diminished pulmonary ventilation

Physical findings in the adult with osteomalacia are more subtle:

- Possible malaise and bone pain
- Many patients presumed to have osteoporosis but may also have osteomalacia

ETIOLOGY

- Deficiency states
  1. True classic VDRR is rare in Western society.
  2. Absorption of vitamin D, however, may be blocked in several gastrointestinal disorders.
  3. Similar disorders may also prevent absorption of calcium and phosphorus, but in the absence of these other diseases deficiencies of calcium and phosphorus are also rare.
- VDRR, type I results from abnormalities in the gene coding for 25 (OH)D3-1-alpha-hydroxylase, and type II results from defective vitamin D receptors.
- Acquired or inherited renal tubular abnormalities that cause resorptive defects and result in rickets and osteomalacia; syndromes include classical VDRR (probably the most common form of rickets seen in general practice). VDRR are familial hypophosphatemic rickets and hereditary hypophosphatemic rickets with hypercalciuria.
- Chronic renal failure:
  1. Can produce renal rickets or renal osteodystrophy
  2. Results in the retention of phosphate

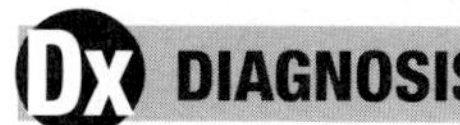

DIAGNOSIS

DIFFERENTIAL DIAGNOSIS

- Osteoporosis
- Hyperparathyroidism
- Hyperthyroidism

LABORATORY TESTS

- Requires a high degree of interest because many of the conditions are so similar that only a complicated laboratory evaluation may establish the diagnosis
- Blood urea nitrogen, creatinine, alkaline phosphatase, calcium, and phosphorus levels in any patient suspected of having metabolic bone disease

IMAGING STUDIES

- In rickets:
  1. Characteristic radiographic changes in the ends of growing long bones caused by the lack of calcification of the cartilage matrix
  2. Widening and irregularity of the epiphyseal plate
- Radiographs in the adult with osteomalacia:
  1. More subtle and often confused with osteoporosis
  2. Possible pseudofractures (Looser's zones) where major arteries cross bone
  3. Insufficiency compression deformities in the vertebral bodies

Rx TREATMENT

- VDRR, type I is treated with vitamin D. Various vitamin D (oral or intramuscular) are available. The earliest biochemical change after initiation of treatment is an increase in the level of phosphorus followed by a rise in calcium level. Serum calcium, phosphorus, alkaline phosphatase and calcidiol levels and urine calcium and phosphorus levels should be obtained within 2 wk of initiation of therapy and periodically. The treatment of type II is more complex and requires consultations with an endocrinologist and nephrologists.
- Familial hypophosphatemic rickets is treated with calcitriol and oral phosphorus.
- Oral phosphorus alone is the treatment of choice for hereditary hypophosphatemic rickets with hypercalciuria.

REFERRAL

- Because of the complex nature of many of these disorders, a qualified endocrinologist and nephrologist should be consulted for treatment.
- The need for orthopedic intervention is rare.
- Surgical care is indicated for slipped capital femoral epiphysis, which is fairly common in renal rickets.
- Deformity may require bracing.

SUGGESTED READINGS

Goodman SB et al: The effects of medications on bone, *J Am Acad Orthop Surg* 15(8):450, 2007.

McKay CP, Portale A: Emerging topics in pediatric bone and mineral disorders 2008, *Semin Nephrol* 29:370, 2009.

Nield LS et al: Rickets: not a disease of the past, *Am Fam Phys* 74:619 2006.

AUTHOR: **LONNIE R. MERCIER, M.D.**

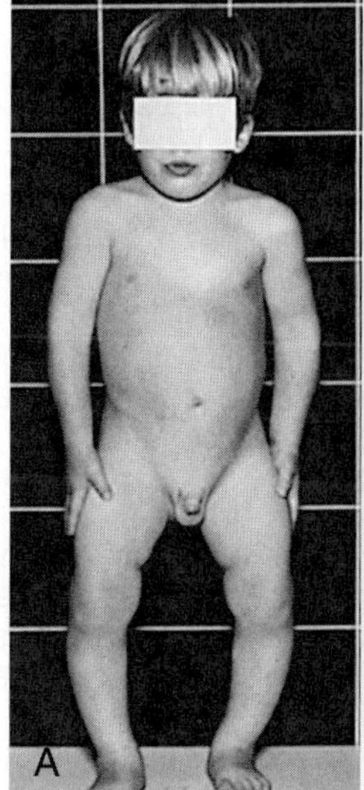

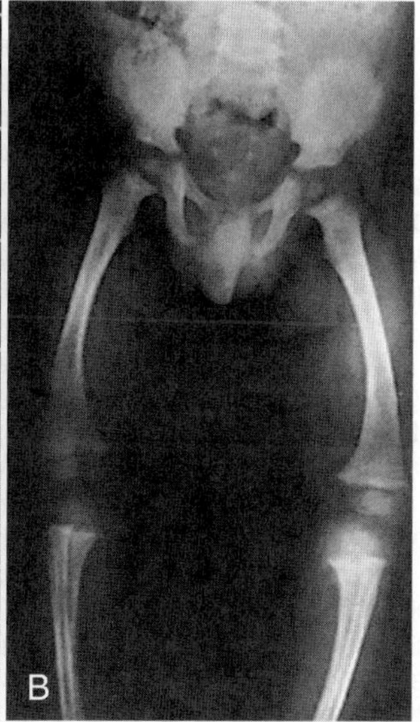

FIGURE 1-289 Clinical **(A)** and radiographic **(B)** appearance of a young boy with X-linked hypophosphatemic rickets. Note the striking bowing of the legs, apparent in both femora and tibiae, with flaring of the ends of the bones at the knee. (Courtesy Dr. Sara B. Arnaud. From Bikle DB: Osteomalacia and rickets. In Wyngaarden JB et al [eds]: *Cecil textbook of medicine,* ed 19, Philadelphia, 1992, WB Saunders.)

Rocky Mountain Spotted Fever

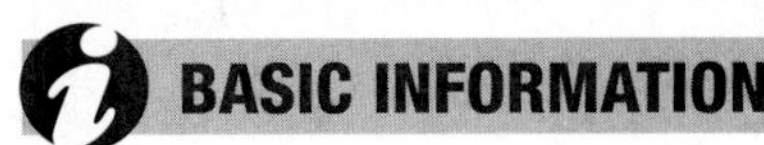

BASIC INFORMATION

DEFINITION

Rocky Mountain spotted fever (RMSF) is a life-threatening, tick-borne febrile illness caused by infection with *Rickettsia rickettsii.* The infection occurs when *R. rickettsii* in the salivary glands of a vector tick is transmitted into the dermis, spreading and replicating in the cytoplasm of endothelial cells and eliciting widespread vasculitis and end-organ damage.

ICD-9CM CODES
082.0 Rocky Mountain spotted fever

EPIDEMIOLOGY & DEMOGRAPHICS

INCIDENCE: 0.18 to 0.32 cases per 100,000 person-years

PREVALENCE: Most prevalent in the Southeast, followed by the South Central states, but seen anywhere. It has recently been reported in eastern Arizona, with common brown dog ticks *(Rhipicephalus sanguineus)* implicated as a vector of *R. rickettsii.*

PREDOMINANT SEX: Affects both genders equally

PREDOMINANT AGE: Occurs at any age, but more likely in children ages 5 to 14 yr

PHYSICAL FINDINGS & CLINICAL PRESENTATION

- Incubation: 3 to 12 days
- First symptoms: fever, headache, malaise, myalgias

Common History, Signs, or Symptoms	%
Tick bite	65
Fever	100
Rash	90
Rash on palms and soles	80
Headache	90
Myalgia	75
Nausea or vomiting	60
Abdominal pain	40
Conjunctivitis	30
Edema	20
Pneumonitis	15
Any severe neurologic complication (including stupor, delirium, seizures, ataxia, papilledema, focal neurologic deficits, and coma)	30

- Rash:
  - Appears during first 3 days in 50%; by day 5, 80% have it. No rash in 10%.
  - Initial appearance: blanching erythematous macules on wrists and ankles that then spread to trunk, palms, and soles.
  - Lesions may evolve into papules and eventually become nonblanching (petechiae or palpable purpura).
- Gastrointestinal symptoms:
  - Nausea, vomiting, and abdominal pain are common
  - Occasionally may mimic an "acute abdomen" (e.g., appendicitis, cholecystitis)
  - Mild hepatitis
- Cardiopulmonary involvement:
  - Interstitial pneumonitis
  - Myocarditis
- Renal problems:
  - Prerenal azotemia
  - Interstitial nephritis
  - Glomerulonephritis
- Neurologic involvement:
  - Encephalitis (confusion, lethargy, delirium)
  - Ataxia
  - Convulsion
  - Cranial nerve palsy
  - Speech impediment
  - Hemiparesis or paraparesis
  - Spasticity
- Fulminant Rocky Mountain spotted fever
  - Early, widespread vascular necrosis leading to multisystem illness and death

ETIOLOGY & PATHOGENESIS

- Infectious agent: *R. rickettsii* (an intracellular bacterium).
- Vector: dog tick and wood tick (vertical transmission exists in ticks, but horizontal transmission involving rodents represents an important reservoir for the agent). In the United States *R. rickettsii* is transmitted mainly by the American dog tick *(Dermacentor variabilis)* and the Rocky Mountain wood tick *(D. andersoni).*
- Pathogenesis: the spread of *R. rickettsii* is hematogenous with attachment to the vascular endothelium, causing a vasculitis. The manifestations of this illness are caused by increased vascular permeability.

Dx DIAGNOSIS

DIFFERENTIAL DIAGNOSIS

Influenza A, enteroviral infection, typhoid fever, leptospirosis, infectious mononucleosis, viral hepatitis, sepsis, ehrlichiosis, gastroenteritis, acute abdomen, bronchitis, pneumonia, meningococcemia, disseminated gonococcal infection, secondary syphilis, bacterial endocarditis, toxic shock syndrome, scarlet fever, rheumatic fever, measles, rubella, typhus, rickettsialpox, Lyme disease, drug hypersensitivity reactions, idiopathic thrombocytopenic purpura, thrombotic thrombocytopenic purpura, Kawasaki disease, immune complex vasculitis, connective tissue disorders

WORKUP

Consider RMSF in any patient with an acute febrile illness with headache and myalgia, especially with an associated history of tick exposure. Absence of rash does not rule out the diagnosis.

LABORATORY TESTS

Routine Tests	%
White cell count	
$<$10,000/mm^3	72
$>$10% bands	69
Platelet count	
$<$150,000/mm^3	52
$<$99,000/mm^3	32
Serum sodium value $<$132 mEq/L	56
Aspartate aminotransferase $\geq$2$\times$ normal	62
Alanine aminotransferase $\geq$2$\times$ normal	39
Bilirubin value $>$1.4 mg/dl	30
Cerebrospinal fluid	
Opening pressure $\geq$250 mm H_2O	14
Glucose value $\leq$50 mg/dl	8
Protein value $\geq$50 mg/dl	35
White cell count $\geq$5/mm^3	38
Mononuclear cell predominance	46
Polymorphonuclear cell predominance	50

- Etiologic tests:
  - Antibody titers to *R. rickettsii* (by indirect fluorescent antibody test). The diagnosis of RMSF requires a fourfold increase 2 wk apart and thus is not helpful in the care of the patients despite a sensitivity and specificity of near 100%.
  - The only test that can provide a timely diagnosis is the immunohistologic demonstration of *R. rickettsii* in skin biopsy specimens.

Rx TREATMENT

- Oral or IV doxycycline, 200 mg/day in 2 divided doses
- Oral tetracycline, 25 to 50 mg/kg/day in 4 divided doses
- Chloramphenicol, 50 to 75 mg/kg/day in 4 divided doses; chloramphenicol may be preferred during pregnancy because of the effects of tetracycline on fetal bones and teeth; therapy continued for at least 2 days after defervescence

PROGNOSIS

Fatality rate: 1% to 4% (five times greater if treatment is initiated after day 5 of illness, which is more likely in the absence of rash and during seasonal nonpeak tick activity). Long-term sequelae seen in patients who recover from severe RMSF: paraparesis, hearing loss; peripheral neuropathy; bladder and bowel incontinence; cerebellar, vestibular, and motor dysfunction; language disorders; limb amputation; and scrotal pain after cutaneous necrosis.

SUGGESTED READINGS

Demma LJ et al: Rocky Mountain spotted fever from an unexpected tick vector in Arizona, *N Engl J Med* 353:587, 2005.

Masters EJ: Rocky Mountain spotted fever, *Arch Intern Med* 163:769, 2003.

AUTHOR: **FRED F. FERRI, M.D.**

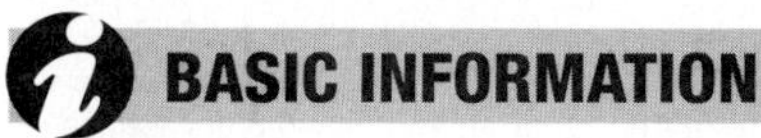

BASIC INFORMATION

DEFINITION

Rosacea is a chronic skin disorder characterized by papules and pustules affecting the face and often associated with flushing and erythema.

SYNONYMS

Acne rosacea

ICD-9CM CODES

695.3 Rosacea

EPIDEMIOLOGY & DEMOGRAPHICS

- Rosacea occurs in one in 20 Americans
- Onset often between ages 30 and 50 yr
- More common in people of Celtic origin; however, this disease may be overlooked in nonwhites because skin pigmentation results in atypical presentation
- Female/male ratio of 3:1

PHYSICAL FINDINGS & CLINICAL PRESENTATION

- Facial erythema, presence of papules, pustules, and telangiectasia.
- Excessive facial warmth and redness is the predominant presenting symptom.
- Itching is generally absent.
- Comedones are absent (unlike acne).
- Women are more likely to show symptoms on the chin and cheeks, whereas in men the nose is commonly involved.
- Ocular findings (mild dryness and irritation with blepharitis, conjunctival injection, burning, stinging, tearing, eyelid inflammation, swelling, and redness) are present in 50% of patients.

Rosacea can be classified into four major subtypes:

1. Erythematotelengiectatic: erythema in central part of face, telangiectasia, flushing
2. Papulopustular: presence of dome-shaped erythematous papules and small pustules, in addition to facial erythema, flushing, and telangiectasia
3. Phymatosis: presence of thickened skin with prominent pores that may affect the nose (rhinophyma), chin (gnathophyma), forehead (metophyma), eyelids (blepharophyma), and ears (otophyma)
4. Ocular: conjunctival injection, sensation of foreign body in the eye, telangiectasia and erythema of lid margins, scaling.

ETIOLOGY

- Unknown.
- Hot drinks, alcohol, and sun exposure may accentuate the erythema by causing vasodilation of the skin.
- Flare-ups may also result from reactions to medications (e.g., simvastatin, angiotensin-converting enzyme inhibitors, vasodilators, fluorinated corticosteroids), stress, extreme heat or cold, wind, humidity, strenuous exercise, spicy drinks, menstruation.

Dx DIAGNOSIS

DIFFERENTIAL DIAGNOSIS

- Drug eruption
- Acne vulgaris
- Contact dermatitis
- Systemic lupus erythematosus
- Carcinoid flush
- Idiopathic facial flushing
- Seborrheic dermatitis
- Facial sarcoidosis
- Photodermatitis
- Mastocytosis
- Perioral dermatitis
- Granulomas of the skin

WORKUP

Diagnosis is based on clinical findings. Distinguishing features between acne and rosacea are the presence of telangiectasia and deep diffuse erythema and absence of comedones in rosacea.

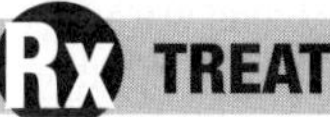

TREATMENT

NONPHARMACOLOGIC THERAPY

- Avoid alcohol, excessive sun exposure, and hot drinks of any type.
- Use of mild, nondrying soap is recommended; local skin irritants should be avoided.
- Reassure patient that rosacea is completely unrelated to poor hygiene.

GENERAL Rx

- Several classes of drugs are used in treatment of rosacea, including the metronidazole family, the tetracycline family, and azelaic acid.
- Topical therapy with metronidazole aqueous gel (MetroGel) applied bid is effective as initial therapy for mild cases or after the use of oral antibiotics. A new 1% formulation of metronidazole (Noritate) applied daily may improve patient compliance. Clindamycin lotion (Cleocin), sulfacetamide, or erythromycin 2% solution may also be effective.
- Systemic antibiotics: Doxycycline 100 mg qd tetracycline 250 mg qid until symptoms diminish, then taper off; doxycycline 100 mg bid is also effective.
- Minocycline 50 to 100 mg qd should be used only in resistant cases because this medication is expensive.
- Oral metronidazole (200 mg qd to bid) for 4 to 6 wk is also effective.
- Isotretinoin (Accutane) 0.5 to 1 mg/kg/day in two divided doses for 15 to 20 wk can be used for refractory papular and pustular rosacea; use of retinoids may, however, worsen erythema and telangiectasis.
- Laser treatment is an option for progressive telangiectasias or rhinophyma.
- Erythema and flushing may respond to low-dose clonidine (0.05 mg bid).
- Treatment of phymatous rosacea: oral tetracyclines, oral isotretinoin, ablative/pulsed dye laser therapy, electrosurgery.
- Treatment of ocular rosacea: topical or oral tetracyclines, artificial tears, and/or lid cleansing for eyelid hygiene.

DISPOSITION

- Rosacea is often resistant to initial treatment and recurrent. Periods of remission and relapse are common.
- The progression of rosacea is variable. Typical stages include:
  1. Facial flushing
  2. Erythema and/or edema and ocular symptoms
  3. Papules and pustules
  4. Rhinophyma

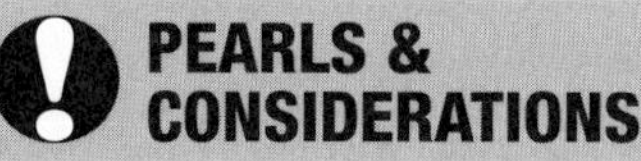

PEARLS & CONSIDERATIONS

COMMENTS

- The course of the disease is typically chronic, with remissions and relapses.
- Patients with resistant cases may have *Demodex folliculorum* mite infestation or tinea infection (diagnosis can be confirmed with potassium hydroxide examination); the role of *D. folliculorum* in rosacea is unclear. These mites can sometimes be found in large numbers in the lesions; however, their numbers do not generally decline with treatment.
- Rosacea can result in emotional and social stigmas, especially because many people associate rosacea and rhinophyma with alcohol abuse.
- Early consultation with an ophthalmologist is recommended in patients with suspected ocular involvement.

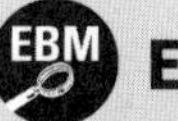

EBM EVIDENCE

Topical metronidazole is effective for treating, and maintaining remission in, patients with moderate to severe rosacea.

A systematic review analyzed the efficacy of treatments for rosacea. It found that the quality of studies was generally poor, but there is evidence that topical metronidazole and azelaic acid are effective. There is some evidence that oral metronidazole and tetracycline are effective as well. There is insufficient evidence, however, concerning the effectiveness of other treatments, thus concluding that good randomized, controlled trials (RCTs) looking at these treatments are urgently needed.[1] A

Another RCT analyzed the efficacy of twice-daily application of metronidazole topical gel 0.75% to the affected areas of the face in patients with mild to moderately severe papulopustular rosacea, of various etiologies and locations, and tried to identify subgroups particularly responsive to it. It found that it was effective in all patient subgroups, and in a variety of climates, and concluded that the findings expand the collected data on the efficacy of this gel beyond that demonstrated in controlled clinical trials. Furthermore, they confirm the utility of this therapy in the community setting.[2] Ⓑ

A further study compared the once-daily application of metronidazole 1% gel with twice-daily applications of azelaic acid 15% gel for the treatment of patients with moderate rosacea. It found that both treatments showed similar reductions in inflammatory lesion counts and concluded that, on average, the efficacy of the once-daily application of metronidazole 1% gel and twice-daily applications of azelaic acid 15% gel were similar.[3]

Azelaic acid appears to have similar efficacy to topical metronidazole in the treatment of patients with moderate rosacea, including the papulopustular variety.

A systematic review analyzed the efficacy of topical 20% azelaic acid cream and 15% azelaic acid gel, compared with their respective vehicles, and metronidazole gel in the treatment of patients with papulopustular rosacea. It concluded that azelaic acid in 20% cream and 15% gel formulations appears to be effective, particularly in regard to decreases in mean inflammatory lesion count and erythema severity. Compared with metronidazole, azelaic acid appears to be an equally effective, if not better, treatment option.[4] Ⓑ

A further study compared the once-daily application of metronidazole 1% gel with twice-daily applications of azelaic acid 15% gel for the treatment of patients with moderate rosacea. It found that both treatments showed similar reductions in inflammatory lesion counts and concluded that, on average, the efficacy of the once-daily application of metronidazole 1% gel and twice-daily applications of azelaic acid 15% gel were similar.[3] Ⓑ

Tetracycline antibiotics are effective for the treatment of moderate to severe rosacea, especially when combined with benzoyl peroxide.

An RCT review analyzed the efficacy of a fixed combination of 5% benzoyl peroxide and 1% clindamycin in a topical gel for the treatment of patients with rosacea. It concluded that the once-daily combined topical application is effective and well tolerated in patients with moderate to severe rosacea.[5] Ⓑ

Erythromycin, especially when combined with benzoyl peroxide, may be a suitable alternative to metronidazole treatment for rosacea.

An RCT analyzed the efficacy of benzoyl peroxide-erythromycin gel compared with metronidazole gel in the treatment of patients with rosacea. The intensities of erythema, telangiectasia, papules/pustules, and nodules were evaluated before, during, and after the treatment. It found that both drugs were significantly effective, especially in treating the papular component of rosacea. Benzoyl peroxide-erythromycin gel was superior to metronidazole gel in decreasing *Demodex folliculorum* by the first examination, but the effect of the two drugs on *D. folliculorum* was similar by the second examination. As a result, it concluded that topically applied combined benzoyl peroxide-erythromycin gel may be an alternative choice of treatment for rosacea.[6] Ⓑ

Evidence-Based References

1. van Zuuren EJ et al: Interventions for rosacea, *Cochrane Rev* 3, 2005.
2. Wolf JE Jr, Del Rosso JQ: The CLEAR trial: results of a large community-based study of metronidazole gel in rosacea, *Cutis* 79:73, 2007.
3. Wolf JE Jr et al: Efficacy and safety of once-daily metronidazole 1% gel compared with twice-daily azelaic acid 15% gel in the treatment of rosacea, *Cutis* 77(4):3, 2006.
4. Liu RH et al: Azelaic acid in the treatment of papulopustular rosacea: a systematic review of randomized controlled trials, *Arch Dermatol* 142: 1047, 2006.
5. Breneman D et al: Double-blind, randomized, vehicle-controlled clinical trial of once-daily benzoyl peroxide/clindamycin topical gel in the treatment of moderate to severe rosacea, *Int J Dermatol* 43:381, 2004.
6. Öztürkcan S et al: Efficiency of benzoyl peroxide-erythromycin gel in comparison with metronidazole gel in the treatment of acne rosacea, *J Dermatol* 31:610, 2004.

SUGGESTED READINGS

Goldgar C, Keahey DJ, Houchins J: Treatment options for acne rosacea, *Am Fam Physician* 80(5):461-468, 2009.

Powell FC: Rosacea, *N Engl J Med* 352:793, 2005.

AUTHOR: **FRED F. FERRI, M.D.**

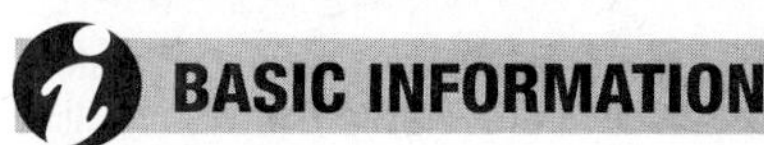

BASIC INFORMATION

DEFINITION

Roseola is a benign viral illness found in infants and characterized by high fevers, followed by a rash.

SYNONYMS

Exanthem subitum
Sixth disease
Roseola infantum

ICD-9CM CODES
057.8 Roseola

EPIDEMIOLOGY & DEMOGRAPHICS

- Nearly one third of all infants develop roseola before the age of 2 yr.
- More than 90% of children older than 2 yr of age are seropositive for the virus causing roseola.
- Roseola is spread from person to person. It is not known how it is spread, but it must be very efficiently spread and presumably via the respiratory tract.
- There is no predilection for gender or time of year.

PHYSICAL FINDINGS & CLINICAL PRESENTATION

- Typically the child develops a high fever, usually up to 104° F (40° C), that lasts for 3 to 5 days
- Fever may be associated with a runny nose, irritability, and fatigue
- A rash appears within 48 hr of defervescence, mainly on the face, neck, trunk, arms, and legs
- The rash is a faint pink maculopapular rash that blanches when palpated
- The rash usually fades away within 48 hr
- Anorexia
- Seizures
- Cervical adenopathy

ETIOLOGY

- Roseola is caused by human herpesvirus-6 (HHV-6).
- The incubation period is between 5 and 15 days.

Dx DIAGNOSIS

The diagnosis of roseola is usually made by the clinical presentation as stated previously.

DIFFERENTIAL DIAGNOSIS

- Measles
- Rubella
- Fifth disease
- Drug eruption
- Mononucleosis
- All causes of fever (e.g., otitis media, pneumonia, and urinary tract infection)
- Meningitis

WORKUP

- If unsure of the diagnosis of roseola in a febrile infant, a fever workup is done to rule out other infectious causes.
- The decision to proceed with a fever workup is a clinical judgment call.

LABORATORY TESTS

- CBC with differential, erythrocyte sedimentation rate (ESR), blood cultures as indicated
- Urinalysis and urine cultures
- Stool cultures if diarrhea is present
- Lumbar puncture if needed to rule out meningitis
- Commercial assays can be used to detect HHV-6-specific IgG antibody responses but IgM assays are not always reliable for acute infection

IMAGING STUDIES

Chest x-ray to rule out pneumonia

Rx TREATMENT

NONPHARMACOLOGIC THERAPY

- Supportive care
- Maintain hydration by drinking clear fluids: water, fruit juice, lemonade, and so forth
- Sponge bathe with lukewarm water if febrile

ACUTE GENERAL Rx

- Acetaminophen 10 to 15 mg/kg per dose at 4-hr intervals for fever
- Ibuprofen 5 to 10 mg/kg per dose at 6-hr intervals (maximal dose 600 mg)

CHRONIC Rx

Roseola is a viral disease that is short lasting; chronic treatment is usually not an issue.

DISPOSITION

- Roseola is generally a benign, self-limited disease that usually lasts approximately 1 wk.
- Complications, although rare, can occur and include:
  1. Febrile seizures
  2. Meningitis
  3. Encephalitis
  4. Pneumonitis
  5. Hepatitis

REFERRAL

Subspecialty consultation is made with the appropriate discipline if any of the previously mentioned complications occur (e.g., neurology for seizures).

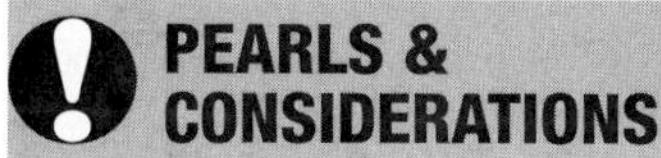

PEARLS & CONSIDERATIONS

COMMENTS

- A child with fever and rash should be excluded from day care.
- HHV-6 is named accordingly because it is the sixth herpesvirus discovered after herpes simplex 1 (HSV-1), HSV-2, cytomegalovirus (CMV), Epstein-Barr virus (EBV), and varicella-zoster virus (VZV).
- Roseola is called sixth disease because it represents the sixth childhood "exanthem"; the other five are measles, scarlet fever, rubella, Dukes disease, and erythema infectiosum.

SUGGESTED READINGS

Caserta MT et al: Human herpesvirus 6, *Clin Infect Dis* 33(6):829, 2001.

Ward KN: The natural history and laboratory diagnosis of human herpesviruses-6 and -7 infections in the immunocompetent, *J Clin Virol* 32(3):183, 2005.

Zerr DM et al: A population-based study of primary human herpesvirus 6 infection, *N Engl J Med* 352(8):768, 2005.

AUTHORS: **GLENN G. FORT, M.D., M.P.H.,** and **DENNIS J. MIKOLICH, M.D.**

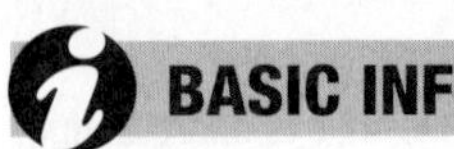

BASIC INFORMATION

DEFINITION

Rotator cuff syndrome refers to a spectrum of afflictions involving the tendons of the rotator cuff (primarily the supraspinatus), ranging from simple strains and tendinitis to complete, massive rupture with cuff-tear arthropathy.

SYNONYMS

Impingement syndrome
Painful arc syndrome
Internal derangement of the subacromial joint
Supraspinatus syndrome
Bursitis of shoulder

ICD-9CM CODES
726.10 Rotator cuff syndrome
727.61 Rotator cuff rupture

EPIDEMIOLOGY & DEMOGRAPHICS

PREVALENCE: 5% to 10% of the general population

PREDOMINANT SEX: More common in males than females

PREDOMINANT AGE: Uncommon <20 yr of age

PHYSICAL FINDINGS & CLINICAL PRESENTATION

- Pain, often at night
- Rotator cuff tenderness
- Referred pain down deltoid, especially with abduction between 70 and 120 degrees ("the painful arc") (Fig. 1-290)
- Weakness in abduction or forward flexion
- Increased pain with overhead activities
- Atrophy in longstanding cases of complete tear
- Positive "drop-arm" test (weakness of abduction against downward pressure at 90 degrees)

ETIOLOGY

- Microtrauma from repetitive use
- Abnormally shaped acromion
- Shoulder instability
- Worsening of process by the overhead throwing motion
- Microcirculatory changes at the musculotendinous junction

DIAGNOSIS

DIFFERENTIAL DIAGNOSIS

- Shoulder instability
- Degenerative arthritis
- Cervical radiculopathy
- Avascular necrosis
- Suprascapular nerve entrapment

WORKUP

- In chronic tendinitis, clinical findings similar to those seen in partial rupture
- Even with complete rupture, may have full, active range of motion in shoulder

IMAGING STUDIES

- Plain radiography
- Ultrasonography may be useful but only in diagnosing moderately large tears
- MRI to evaluate full- or partial-thickness tears, chronic tendinitis, and other causes of shoulder pain
- Since MRI, arthrography is rarely used

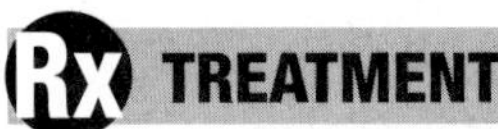

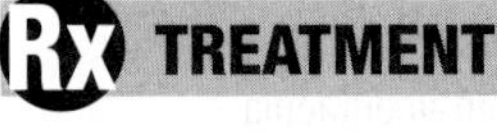

TREATMENT

ACUTE GENERAL Rx

- Rest to avoid overhead activity
- Ice or heat for comfort
- Carefully supervised program of stretching and strengthening
- Medication: nonsteroidal antiinflammatory drugs, subacromial corticosteroid injection (once or twice at 2-wk intervals)

DISPOSITION

- All forms are likely to respond to nonsurgical management.
- Even many complete rotator cuff tears have minimal pain and little loss of function.

REFERRAL

For orthopedic consultation in patients who do not respond to medical management or in whom rotator cuff tear is suspected

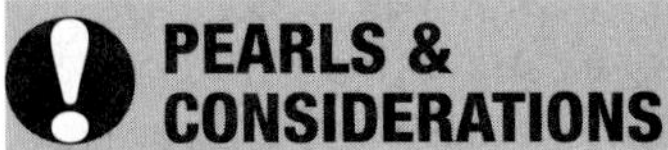

PEARLS & CONSIDERATIONS

COMMENTS

- There is considerable disagreement regarding the likelihood of recovery once a significant rotator cuff rupture has developed.
- Indications for surgery vary among surgeons.
- Injection is contraindicated in the presence of local infection.
- As with other similar musculoskeletal disorders, the underlying pathology involved may be more degenerative (tendinopathy, tendinosis) than inflammatory.
- Once a separation ("tear") develops, there is no way to predict whether it will ever become worse or not.

SUGGESTED READINGS

Cools AM et al: Screening the athlete's shoulder for impingement symptoms: a clinical reasoning algorithm for early detection of shoulder pathology, *Br J Sports Med* 42:628, 2008.

Kim HM et al: Shoulder strength in asymptomatic individuals with intact compared with torn rotator cuffs, *J Bone Joint Surg Am* 91:289, 2009.

Koester MC et al: The efficacy of subacromial corticosteroid injection in the treatment of rotator cuff disease: a systematic review, *J Am Acad Orthop Surg* 15:3, 2007.

Maman E et al: Outcome of nonoperative treatment of symptomatic rotator cuff tears monitored by magnetic resonance imaging, *J Bone Joint Surg* 91:1898, 2009.

Matsen FA: Rotator cuff failure, *N Engl J Med* 358: 2138, 2008.

Mcfarland EG et al: Clinical evaluation of impingement: what to do and what works, *J Bone Joint Surg Am* 88A:432, 2006.

Tashjian RZ et al: Effect of medical comorbidity on self-assessed pain, function, and general health status after rotator cuff repair, *J Bone Joint Surg Am* 88A:536, 2006.

Wolff AB et al: Partial-thickness rotator cuff tears, *J Am Acad Orthop Surg* 14:715, 2006.

Zing PO et al: Clinical and structural outcomes of nonoperative management of massive rotator cuff tears, *J Bone Joint Surg Am* 89A:1928, 2008.

AUTHOR: **LONNIE R. MERCIER, M.D.**

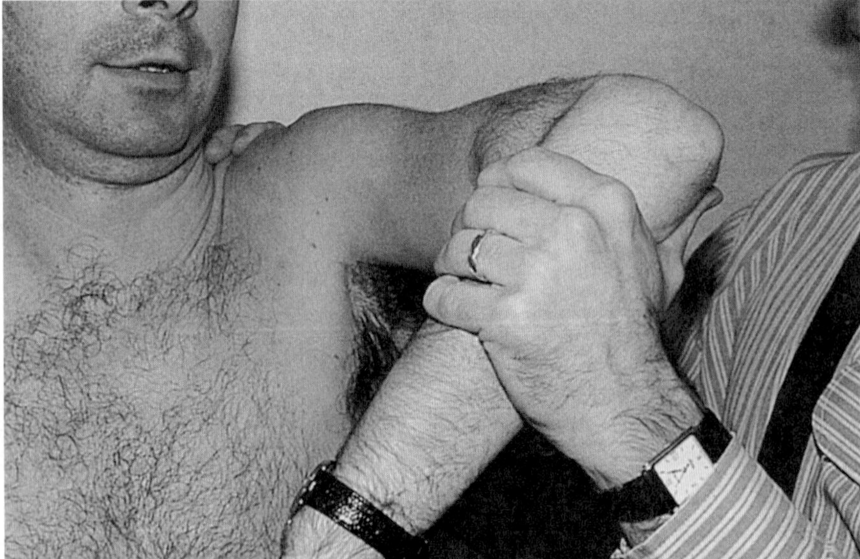

FIGURE 1-290 Rotator cuff lesions are often accompanied by painful impingement of the upwardly subluxating humerus onto the acromion. Evidence for this as a cause of pain is elicited by impingement tests—for example, by forced, passive, internal rotation, and abduction of the shoulder, as shown here. (From Klippel J et al [eds]: *Primary care rheumatology,* London, 1999, Mosby.)

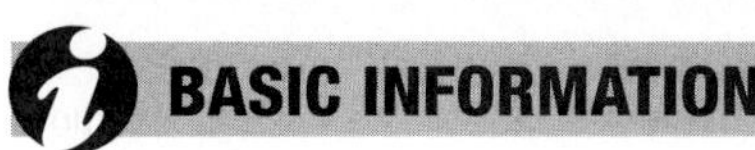

BASIC INFORMATION

DEFINITION

Rubella is a mild illness caused by the rubella virus that can cause severe congenital problems by in vitro transmission to a fetus when a pregnant woman becomes infected.

SYNONYMS

German measles

ICD-9CM CODES
056.9 Rubella
771.0 (Congenital)
V04.3 (Vaccination)

EPIDEMIOLOGY & DEMOGRAPHICS

- Before vaccination (i.e., before 1969):
  - 28 reported cases per 100,000 person-years, eight of which were in persons >15 yr
  - Four cases of congenital rubella syndrome per 100,000 live births
- After mass vaccination (i.e., after 1980) most cases have occurred in unimmunized people, with fewer than one case per 100,000 person-years (acquired and congenital).
- Currently, 10% to 20% of childbearing-age women are susceptible.
- The highest risk of developing long-term complications of congenital infection exists during the first trimester of gestation; both risk of congenital infection and long-term complications drop during the second trimester, and although the risk of congenital infection increases during the third trimester, there is no risk of long-term complication at that point.

PHYSICAL FINDINGS & CLINICAL PRESENTATION

1. Acquired infection:
   - Incubation: 14 to 21 days
   - Prodrome: 1 to 5 days; low-grade fever, headache, malaise, anorexia, mild conjunctivitis, coryza, pharyngitis, cough, and cervical, suboccipital, and postauricular lymphadenopathy
   - Rash: 1 to 5 days
2. Enanthema: palatal macules
3. Exanthema (rash): blotchy eruption beginning on face and neck and then spreading to trunk and limbs
   - Occasional splenomegaly and hepatitis (during rash)
   - Complications: arthritis (15%, mostly in adult women), thrombocytopenia, myocarditis, optic neuritis, encephalitis (all <0.1%)
4. Congenital infection:
   - Deafness: 85%
   - Intrauterine growth retardation: 70%
   - Cataracts: 35%
   - Retinopathy: 35%
   - Patent ductus arteriosus: 30%
   - Pulmonary artery hypoplasia: 25%
   - In utero death: 20%
   - Mental retardation: 10% to 20%
   - Meningoencephalitis: 10% to 20%
   - Behavior disorder: 10% to 20%
   - Hepatosplenomegaly: 10% to 20%
   - Bone radiolucencies: 10% to 20%
   - Diabetes mellitus (type 1): 10% to 20% by age 35 yr
   - Other congenital heart defects: 2% to 5%

ETIOLOGY & PATHOGENESIS

1. Acquired infection:
   - Viral portal of entry is upper respiratory tract.
   - Viral replication occurs in lymph nodes, then hematogenous dissemination occurs to many organs, including placenta if present.
   - Immune complexes may be cause of rash and arthritis.
2. Congenital infection:
   - Fetus is infected by the placenta during maternal acquired infection.
   - Cellular damage in the fetus results from cytolysis of fetal cells, mostly by fetal vasculitis or from immune-mediated inflammation and damage.

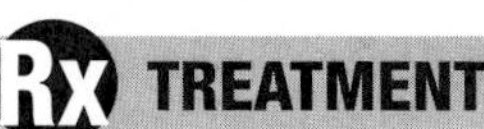

DIAGNOSIS

DIFFERENTIAL DIAGNOSIS

1. Acquired rubella syndrome:
   - Other viral infections by enteroviruses, adenoviruses, human parvovirus B-19, measles
   - Scarlet fever
   - Allergic reaction
   - Kawasaki disease
2. Congenital rubella syndrome:
   - Congenital syphilis, toxoplasmosis, herpes simplex, cytomegalovirus, and enterovirus can cause a similar set of problems.

WORKUP

1. Acquired infection:
   - Serologic test (hemagglutination inhibition, neutralization tests, complement fixation tests, passive agglutination, enzyme immunoassay [EIA], enzyme-linked immunosorbent assay [ELISA])
   - Immunoglobulin (Ig) M antibodies (by EIA) are detected early: second to fourth week
   - IgG antibodies (by ELISA) can be measured as acute phase (7 days after rash onset) and convalescent phase (14 days later)
2. Congenital infection:
   - Viral culture (from nasopharynx)
   - Serologic studies: IgM antirubella virus detection by EIA is the method of choice (after the newborn is age 5 mo)

IMMUNIZATION

- Four existing vaccines provide persisting immunity in 92% of vaccines. Indications:
  - All children ≥12 mo (as part of the measles-mumps-rubella [MMR] vaccine)
  - Postpubertal women
- Vaccinate if not known to be immunized (advise not to become pregnant within 3 mo of vaccination)
- Premarital serologic screening for rubella immunity
- Prenatal or antepartum serologic screening for rubella
- Vaccinate susceptible women postpartum
- Serologic screening for female workers likely to be exposed to rubella (e.g., teachers, child care employees, health care workers)

Contraindications:
- Pregnancy
- Recent receipt of immune globulin or blood transfusion (2 wk before to 3 mo after)
- Immunodeficiency (except AIDS)

Adverse reactions:
- Fever, rash, or lymphadenopathy: 5% to 15%
- Arthralgias: 0.5% in children; 25% in adult women
- Transient peripheral neuropathy (rare)

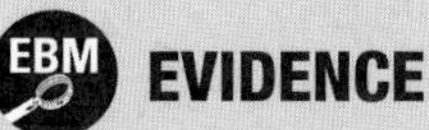

TREATMENT

- No known effective antiviral therapy
- Management of specific congenital problems as appropriate

EBM EVIDENCE

The following statements concern the evidence for the MMR vaccine.

There is evidence that both monovalent rubella and combined MMR vaccines are effective in protecting against rubella infection.[1] A

There are no systematic reviews or RCTs that compare the clinical effects of combined MMR vaccines with the monovalent rubella vaccine in children, although seroconversion rates have been shown to be similar for both.[1] A

A large proportion of the literature on adverse events after immunization is based on passive reporting, which has major limitations such as underreporting events or reporting events that are unassociated with the intervention.[1]

Existing evidence has failed to confirm the much-publicized possible association between MMR vaccines and any autistic disorder, ulcerative colitis, Crohn's disease, or inflammatory bowel disease.[2] A

Evidence-Based References

1. Booy R et al: Measles, mumps and rubella: prevention, *Clinical evidence,* London, 2007, BMJ Publishing Group. A
2. Demicheli V et al: Vaccines for measles, mumps and rubella in children, *Cochrane Rev* 4, 2005.

SUGGESTED READINGS

Madsen KM et al: A population-based study of measles, mumps, and rubella vaccination and autism, *New Engl J Med* 347(19):1477, 2002.

U.S. Department of Health: Control and prevention of rubella: evaluation and management of suspected outbreaks, rubella in pregnant women, and surveillance for congenital rubella syndrome, *MMWR* 50(RR-12):1, 2001.

AUTHOR: **FRED F. FERRI, M.D.**

Salivary Gland Neoplasms (PTG)

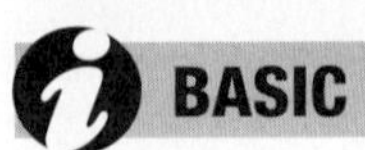

BASIC INFORMATION

DEFINITION

Salivary gland neoplasms are benign or malignant tumors of a salivary gland (parotid, submandibular, or sublingual).

SYNONYMS

These tumors are often named according to their histologic type (see "Diagnosis").

ICD-9CM CODES
142.9 Salivary gland neoplasm
142.0 (Parotid)
142.1 (Submandibular)
142.2 (Sublingual)

EPIDEMIOLOGY & DEMOGRAPHICS

INCIDENCE: One to two cases per 100,000 person-years (1% of all head and neck tumors)

DISTRIBUTION:
- Parotid gland, 85% (80% are benign)
- Submandibular gland, 10% (55% are benign)
- Sublingual and minor glands, 5% (35% are benign)

PHYSICAL FINDINGS & CLINICAL PRESENTATION

- Parotid gland:
  1. Painless swelling overlying the masseter muscle (under the temporomandibular joint)
  2. Pain
  3. Facial nerve palsy
  4. Cervical lymph nodes
  5. Mass in oral cavity
- Submandibular gland: swelling under anterior portion of the mandible
- Sublingual gland: intraoral swelling under the tongue, medial to the mandible

DIAGNOSIS

PATHOLOGY

HISTORY:

Benign Tumors:
- Mixed tumor (usually parotid)
- Adenolymphoma (Warthin's tumor)
- Pleomorphic adenoma
- Capillary hemangioma, lymphangioma (in children)
- Intraductal papilloma
- Other (e.g., myoepithelioma, canalicular adenoma, basal cell adenoma)

Malignant Tumors:
- Mucoepidermoid carcinoma (most common malignant tumor of the parotid gland)
- Adenoid cystic carcinoma
- Adenocarcinoma
- Malignant mixed tumor
- Squamous cell carcinoma
- Other

STAGE (TNM):

T_0 No evidence of primary tumor
T_1 Tumor <2 cm
T_2 Tumor 2 to 4 cm
T_3 Tumor 4 to 6 cm
T_4 Tumor >6 cm
All subdivided into
- Without local extension
- With local extension

N_0 No lymph node metastasis
N_1 Single ipsilateral node <3 cm
N_2 Ipsilateral, contralateral, or bilateral node <6 cm
N_3 Any node >6 cm
M_0 No distant metastasis
M_1 Distant metastasis
Stage I T_{1a} or ${}_{2a}N_0M_0$
Stage II $T_{1b,2b,3a}$ N_0M_0
Stage III $T_{3b,4a}$ N_0M_0 or any T except ${}_{4b}N_1M_0$
Stage IV T_{4b} any N any M or any T $N_{2,3}M_0$ or any T, any N_1M_1

WORKUP

- Fine-needle aspiration. The sensitivity, specificity, and accuracy of parotid gland aspirates is approximately 92%, 100%, and 98%, respectively
- Imaging by CT scan or MRI
- Open biopsy (rarely indicated)

TREATMENT

Malignant tumors:
- Surgery is the mainstay of treatment; gland resection and neck dissection if lymph nodes are involved.
- A lateral lobectomy with preservation of facial nerve should be considered for tumors confined to the superficial lobe of the parotid gland. Gross tumor should not be left in situ, but if the facial nerve is able to be preserved by "peeling" tumor off the nerve, it should be attempted, followed by radiation therapy for microscopic disease.
- Postoperative radiation is indicated for high-grade malignancies demonstrating extraglandular disease, perineural invasion, direct invasion of surrounding tissues, or regional metastases.
- Chemotherapy.

Benign tumors: surgery for tumor resection

PROGNOSIS OF MALIGNANT TUMORS

Five-year survival rates:
- Mucoepidermoid carcinoma: 75% to 95%
- Adenoid cystic carcinoma: 40% to 80%
- Adenocarcinoma: 20% to 75%
- Malignant mixed tumor: 35% to 75%
- Squamous cell carcinoma: 25% to 60%

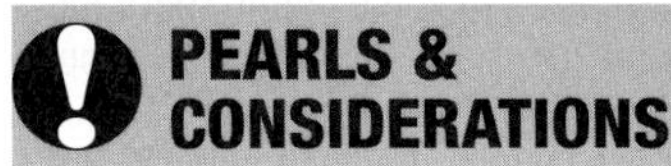

PEARLS & CONSIDERATIONS

COMMENTS

Salivary gland neoplasms most often present as slow-growing, well-circumscribed masses. Pain, rapid growth, nerve weakness, fixation to skin or underlying muscle, and paresthesias usually are indicative of malignancy.

SUGGESTED READING

Stewart CJ et al: Fine needle aspiration cytology of salivary gland: a review of 341 cases, *Diagn Cytopathol* 22:139, 2000.

AUTHOR: **FRED F. FERRI, M.D.**

BASIC INFORMATION

DEFINITION

Salmonellosis is an infection caused by one of several serotypes of *Salmonella.*

SYNONYMS

Typhoid fever
Paratyphoid fever
Enteric fever

ICD-9CM CODES
003.0 Salmonellosis

EPIDEMIOLOGY & DEMOGRAPHICS

INCIDENCE (IN U.S.):

- Estimated 1 million cases/yr of nontyphoidal salmonellosis
- Approximately 500 cases of *Salmonella typhi* infection reported each yr
- Largest outbreak: 200,000 people who ingested contaminated milk

PEAK INCIDENCE: Summer and fall

PREDOMINANT AGE:

- <20 yr old
- >70 yr old
- Highest rates of infection in infants, especially neonates

GENETICS:

Neonatal infection:

- Highly susceptible to infection with nontyphoidal *Salmonella*

PHYSICAL FINDINGS & CLINICAL PRESENTATION

- Infections
  1. Localized to GI tract (gastroenteritis)
  2. Systemic (typhoid fever)
  3. Localized outside of GI tract
- Gastroenteritis
  1. Incubation period: 12 to 48 hr
  2. Nausea, vomiting
  3. Diarrhea, abdominal cramps
  4. Fever
  5. Bacteremia: Occurs mostly in the immunocompromised host or those with underlying conditions, including HIV infection
  6. Self-limited illness lasting 3 or 4 days
  7. Colonization of GI tract persistent for months, especially in those treated with antibiotics
- Typhoid fever
  1. Incubation period of few days to several wk
  2. Prolonged fever, often with a stepwise-increasing temperature pattern
  3. Myalgias
  4. Headache, cough, sore throat
  5. Malaise, anorexia
  6. Abdominal pain
  7. Hepatosplenomegaly
  8. Diarrhea or constipation early in the course of illness
  9. Rose spots (faint, maculopapular, blanching lesions) sometimes seen on chest or abdomen
- Untreated disease
  1. Fever lasting 1 to 2 mo
  2. Main complication: GI bleeding caused by perforation from ulceration of Peyer's patches in the ileum (Fig. 1-291)
  3. Rare complications:
     a. Mental status changes
     b. Shock
  4. Relapse rate of approximately 10%
- Infections outside GI tract
  1. Can occur in virtually any location
  2. Usually occur in patients with underlying diseases
  3. Endocarditis, endovascular infections are caused by seeding of atherosclerotic plaques or aneurysms
  4. Hepatic or splenic abscesses in patients with underlying disease in these organs
  5. Urinary tract infections in patients with renal TB or schistosomiasis
  6. Salmonellae are a frequent cause of gram-negative meningitis in neonates
  7. Osteomyelitis in children with hemoglobinopathies (particularly sickle cell disease)

ETIOLOGY

- More than 2000 serotypes of *Salmonella* exist, but only a few cause disease in humans.
- Some found only in humans are the cause of enteric fever.
  1. *S. typhi*
  2. *S. paratyphi*
- Some responsible for gastroenteritis and frequently isolated from raw meat and poultry and uncooked or undercooked eggs.
  1. *S. typhimurium*
  2. *S. enteritidis*
- *S. choleraesius* is a prototype organism that causes extraintestinal nontyphoidal disease.
- Transmission generally via ingestion of contaminated food or drink.
- Outbreaks of gastroenteritis related to contaminated poultry, meat, and dairy products.
- Typhoid fever is a systemic illness caused by serotypes exclusive to humans.
  1. Acquisition by ingestion of food or water contaminated by other humans
  2. Most cases in the U.S. are:
     a. Acquired during foreign travel
     b. Acquired by ingestion of food prepared by chronic carriers, many of whom have acquired the organism outside of the U.S.

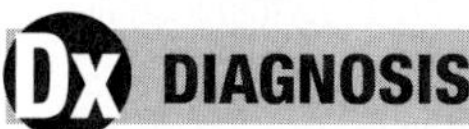

DIAGNOSIS

DIFFERENTIAL DIAGNOSIS

- Other causes of prolonged fever:
  1. Malaria
  2. TB
  3. Brucellosis
  4. Amebic liver abscess

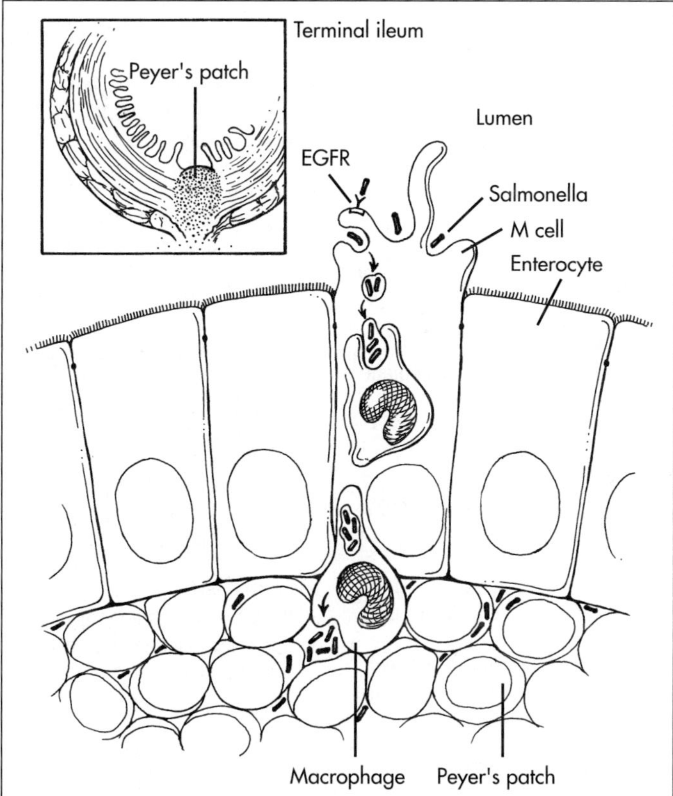

FIGURE 1-291 *Salmonella typhi* invade M cells through membrane ruffling and EGF receptor-dependent pathways. Macrophages originating from Peyer's patch take up *S. typhi* in close association with M cells. *S. typhi* replicate from Peyer's patches and then enter the lymphatic system, leading to bacteremia. Replication in Peyer's patches causes hypertrophy followed by necrosis, which can cause intestinal perforation. (From Stein JH [ed]: *Internal medicine,* ed 5, St Louis, 1998, Mosby.)

 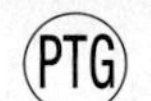

- Other causes of gastroenteritis:
  1. Bacterial: *Shigella, Yersinia, Campylobacter* spp.
  2. Viral: Norwalk virus, rotavirus
  3. Parasitic: *Entamoeba histolytica, Giardia lamblia*
  4. Toxic: enterotoxigenic *E. coli, Clostridium difficile*

WORKUP

- Typhoid fever
  1. Cultures of blood, stool, urine; repeat if initially negative.
  2. Blood cultures are more likely to be positive early in the course of illness.
  3. Stool and urine cultures are more commonly positive in the second and third wk of illness.
  4. Highest yield with bone marrow biopsy cultures: 90% positive
  5. Serology using Widal's test is helpful in retrospect, showing a fourfold increase in convalescent titers.
- Gastroenteritis: stool cultures
- Extraintestinal localized infection:
  1. Blood cultures
  2. Cultures from the site of infection

LABORATORY TESTS

- Neutropenia is common
- Transaminitis is possible
- Culture to grow organism: blood, body fluids, biopsy specimens

IMAGING STUDIES

- Radiographs of bone may be suggestive of osteomyelitis (particularly in patients with sickle cell disease and bone infarctions).
- CT scan or sonogram of abdomen:
  1. May reveal hepatic or splenic abscesses or pleural involvement
  2. May reveal aortic aneurysm

Rx TREATMENT

NONPHARMACOLOGIC THERAPY

Adequate hydration and electrolyte replacement in people with diarrhea

ACUTE GENERAL Rx

- Typhoid fever:
  1. Ciprofloxacin 500 mg PO bid or 400 mg IV bid for 14 days
  2. Ceftriaxone 2 g IV qd for 14 days
  3. If sensitive, may switch therapy to TMP/SMX 1 to 2 DS tabs PO bid or amoxicillin 2 g PO q8h to complete 14 days
  4. Dexamethasone 3 mg IV initially, followed by 1 mg IV q6h for eight doses for patients with shock or mental status changes
- Gastroenteritis:
  1. Usually not indicated for gastroenteritis alone because this illness usually self-limited
  2. May prolong the carrier state
  3. Prophylactic treatment for patients who are at high risk of developing complications from bacteremia
     a. Neonates
     b. Patients with hemoglobinopathies
     c. Patients with atherosclerosis
     d. Patients with aneurysms
     e. Patients with prosthetic devices
     f. Immunocompromised patients
  4. Treatment can be oral or parenteral, with the same regimens used for typhoid, but only for 48 to 72 hr
- Intravascular infections require 6 wk of parenteral therapy.

CHRONIC Rx

- Carrier states are possible in those with typhoid fever.
- More common in people >60 yr of age and in people with gallstones.
- Usual site of colonization is the gallbladder.
- Treatment should be considered for those with persistently positive stool cultures and for food handlers.
- Suggested regimens for eradication of carrier state:
  1. Ciprofloxacin 500 mg PO bid for 4 wk
  2. SMX/TMP 1 to 2 DS tabs PO bid for 6 wk (if susceptible)
  3. Amoxicillin 2 g PO q8h for 6 wk (if susceptible)
- Cholecystectomy may be required in carriers with gallstones who fail medical therapy, but this is rarely indicated for nontyphoidal salmonellosis currently.
- Prolonged course of oral therapy or lifetime suppression for patients with AIDS who have chronic infection.

DISPOSITION

- Typhoid fever
  1. Treated patients usually respond to therapy; small percentage of chronic carriers.
  2. Untreated patients may have serious complications.
- Gastroenteritis
  1. Usually self-limited
  2. May be recurrent or persistent in AIDS patients

REFERRAL

- If gastroenteritis is persistent or recurrent
- If there is evidence of extraintestinal infection, typhoid fever, or chronic carriers

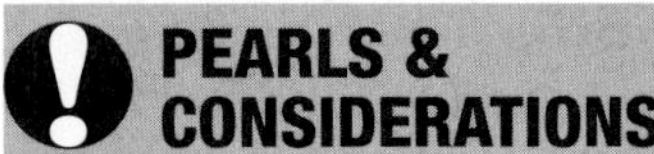

PEARLS & CONSIDERATIONS

COMMENTS

- Quinolones should not be used in children or pregnant women.
- Infections should be reported to local health departments.
- Recent outbreaks in the U.S. have been traced back to raw tomatoes, peanut butter, and frozen pot pies.

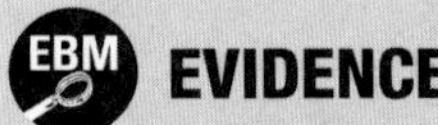

EVIDENCE

Antibiotic therapy has not been shown to have any positive clinical effect in healthy children and adults with mild diarrhea caused by *Salmonella* spp.[1] Ⓐ

Oral rehydration fluids are as effective as IV rehydration fluids in children with mild or moderate dehydration caused by gastroenteritis.[2,3] Ⓐ

Oral rehydration fluid has been shown to be associated with significant reductions in the duration of diarrhea and with increased weight gain at discharge compared with IV rehydration fluid, in a randomized controlled trial conducted in a developing country.[4] Ⓐ

Evidence-Based References

1. Sirinavin S, Garner P: Antibiotics for treating salmonella gut infections, *Cochrane Database Rev* 1, 1999.
2. Gavin N, Merrick N, Davidson B: Efficacy of glucose-based oral rehydration therapy, *Pediatrics* 98:45, 1996. Reviewed in: *Clin Evid* 10:86, 2003.
3. Singh M et al: Controlled trial of oral versus intravenous rehydration in the management of acute gastroenteritis, *Indian J Med Res* 75:691, 1982. Reviewed in: *Clin Evid* 9:367, 2003.
4. Sharifi J et al: Oral versus intravenous rehydration therapy in severe gastroenteritis, *Arch Dis Child* 60:856, 1985. Reviewed in: *Clin Evid* 9:367, 2003.

SUGGESTED READINGS

CDC: Salmonellosis associated with pet turtles—Wisconsin and Wyoming, 2004, *MMWR Morb Mortal Wkly Rep* 54(9):223, 2005.

DuPont HL: Bacterial diarrhea, *N Engl J Med* 361:1560, 2009.

Wells EV et al: Reptile-associated salmonellosis in pre-school aged children in Michigan, January 2001–June 2003, *Clin Infect Dis* 39(5):687, 2004.

AUTHORS: **GLENN G. FORT, M.D., M.P.H.,** and **DENNIS J. MIKOLICH, M.D.**

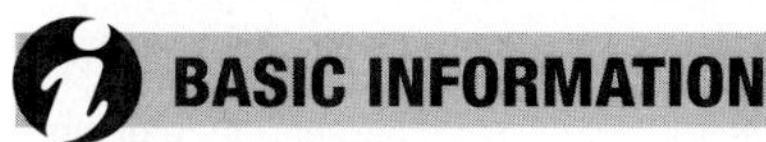

BASIC INFORMATION

DEFINITION

Sarcoidosis is a chronic systemic granulomatous disease characterized histologically by the presence of nonspecific, noncaseating granulomas.

SYNONYMS

Boeck's sarcoid

ICD-9CM CODES
135.0 Sarcoidosis

EPIDEMIOLOGY & DEMOGRAPHICS

INCIDENCE (IN U.S.): 11 in 100,000 whites and 35 in 100,000 blacks; presents most commonly in the winter and early spring
PREDOMINANT SEX: Increased incidence in females
PREDOMINANT AGE: 20 to 40 yr

PHYSICAL FINDINGS & CLINICAL PRESENTATION

- Clinical manifestations often vary with the stage of the disease and degree of organ involvement. Patients may be asymptomatic, but a chest radiograph may demonstrate findings consistent with sarcoidosis (see "Imaging Studies" in next column). Nearly 50% of patients with sarcoidosis are diagnosed by incidental findings on chest radiograph.
- Frequent manifestations:
  1. Pulmonary manifestations: dry, nonproductive cough; dyspnea; chest discomfort
  2. Constitutional symptoms: fatigue, weight loss, anorexia, malaise
  3. Visual disturbances: blurred vision, ocular discomfort, conjunctivitis, iritis, uveitis (65% of patients)
  4. Dermatologic manifestations: erythema nodosum (10% of patients), macules, papules, subcutaneous nodules, hyperpigmentation, lupus pernio (indurated violaceous lesions on the nose, lips, ears, and cheeks that can erode into underlying cartilage and bone)
  5. Myocardial disturbances (5% of patients): arrhythmias, cardiomyopathy
  6. Splenomegaly, hepatomegaly
  7. Rheumatologic manifestations: arthralgias have been reported in up to 40% of patients
  8. Neurologic and other manifestations: cranial nerve palsies, diabetes insipidus, meningeal involvement, parotid enlargement, hypothalamic and pituitary lesions, peripheral adenopathy

ETIOLOGY

Unknown. A cardinal feature of sarcoidosis is the presence of CD4+ T cells that interact with antigen-presenting cells to initiate the formation and maintenance of granulomas. Multiple lines of evidence suggest that sarcoidosis may result from the interaction of multiple genes with environmental exposures or infection.

Dx DIAGNOSIS

DIFFERENTIAL DIAGNOSIS

- Tuberculosis
- Lymphoma
- Hodgkin's disease
- Metastases
- Pneumoconioses
- Enlarged pulmonary arteries
- Infectious mononucleosis
- Lymphangitic carcinomatosis
- Idiopathic hemosiderosis
- Alveolar cell carcinoma
- Pulmonary eosinophilia
- Hypersensitivity pneumonitis
- Fibrosing alveolitis
- Collagen disorders
- Parasitic infection

Section II describes the differential diagnosis of granulomatous lung disease and a classification of granulomatous disorders.

WORKUP

- Workup is aimed at excluding critical organ involvement, determining extent and severity of disease, and excluding other disease. A complete neurologic and ophthalmologic examination is mandatory. A complete occupational and environmental exposure history is recommended.
- Initial laboratory evaluation should include complete blood count, serum chemistries (alanine aminotransferase, aspartate aminotransferase, alkaline phosphatase, electrolytes, blood urea nitrogen, creatinine, serum calcium), urinalysis, and 24-hour urinary excretion of calcium.
- Chest radiograph and ECG should also be obtained in all patients with sarcoidosis.
- Pulmonary function testing; spirometry, diffusion capacity of carbon monoxide–single breath.
- Biopsy should be done on accessible tissues suspected of sarcoid involvement (conjunctiva, skin, lymph nodes); bronchoscopy with transbronchial biopsy is the procedure of choice in patients without any readily accessible site.

LABORATORY TESTS

Laboratory abnormalities:

- Hypergammaglobulinemia, anemia, leukopenia
- Liver function test abnormalities
- Hypercalcemia (11% of patients), hypercalciuria (40% of patients; attributable to increased gastrointestinal absorption, abnormal vitamin D metabolism, and increased calcitriol production by sarcoid granuloma)
- Angiotensin-converting enzyme: elevated in approximately 60% of patients with sarcoidosis; nonspecific and generally not useful as a diagnostic tool and in following the course of the disease

IMAGING STUDIES

- Chest radiograph (Fig. 1-292): adenopathy of the hilar and paratracheal nodes is a frequent finding. Parenchymal changes may also be present, depending on the stage of the disease (stage 0, normal radiograph; stage I, bilateral hilar adenopathy; stage II, stage I plus pulmonary infiltrate; stage III, pulmonary infiltrate without adenopathy; stage IV, advanced fibrosis with evidence of "honeycombing," hilar retraction, bullae, cysts, and emphysema).
- Pulmonary function tests (spirometry and diffusing capacity of the lung for carbon dioxide): may be normal or may reveal a restrictive pattern and/or obstructive pattern.
- For patients without apparent lung involvement, ^{18}F-fluorodeoxyglucose positron emission tomography (FDG-PET) is useful in identifying sites for diagnostic biopsy.
- CT imaging is generally unnecessary for most patients with sarcoidosis. It is indicated when the chest radiograph is atypical for sarcoidosis or if the patient has hemoptysis.
- FDG-PET and MRI with gadolinium are useful in patients with suspected cardiac and neurologic involvement.
- Gallium-67 scan: represents an older testing modality. It will localize in areas of granulomatous infiltrates; however, it is not specific and not necessary. The "panda" sign (localization in the lacrimal and salivary glands, giving a "panda" appearance to the face) is suggestive of sarcoidosis.

Rx TREATMENT

GENERAL Rx

- Many patients with sarcoidosis will not require any treatment. In general, treatment should be instituted when organ function is threatened. Corticosteroids (Table 1-70) are the mainstay of therapy when treatment is required (e.g., prednisone 40 mg qd for 8 to 12 wk with gradual tapering of the dose to 10 mg qod over 8 to 12 mo); corticosteroids should be considered in patients with severe symptoms (e.g., dyspnea, chest pain); hypercalcemia; ocular, central nervous system, or cardiac involvement; or progressive pulmonary disease. Patients with interstitial lung disease benefit from oral steroid therapy for 6 to 24 mo.
- Patients with progressive disease refractory to corticosteroids may be treated with methotrexate 7.5 to 15 mg once per week.
- Hydroxychloroquine is effective for chronic disfiguring skin lesions, hypercalcemia, and neurologic involvement.
- Nonsteroidal anti-inflammatory drugs are useful for musculoskeletal symptoms and erythema nodosum.
- Pulmonary rehabilitation in patients with significant respiratory insufficiency. Consider liver and lung transplantation in patients unresponsive to conventional treatment.

DISPOSITION

- The majority of patients with sarcoidosis have spontaneous remission within 2 yr and do not require treatment. Their course can be followed by periodic clinical evaluation, chest radiographs, and pulmonary function tests.

 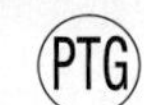

- Blacks have increased rates of pulmonary involvement, a worse long-term prognosis, and more frequent relapses.
- Up to one third of patients have unrelenting disease, leading to clinically significant organ impairment. Adverse prognostic factors in sarcoidosis include age of onset >40 yr, cardiac involvement, neurosarcoidosis, progressive pulmonary fibrosis, chronic hypercalcemia, chronic uveitis, involvement of nasal mucosa, nephrocalcinosis, and presence of cystic bone lesions and lupus pernio.

REFERRAL

Ophthalmologic examination is indicated in all patients with suspected sarcoidosis because ocular findings (iridocyclitis, uveitis, conjunctivitis, and keratopathy) are found in ≥25% of documented cases.

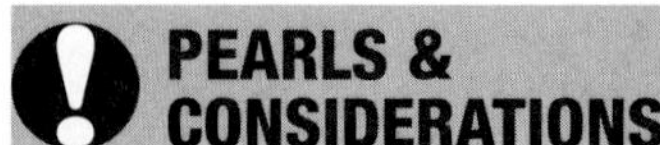

PEARLS & CONSIDERATIONS

COMMENTS

Approximately 15% to 20% of patients with lung involvement advance to irreversible lung impairment (bronchiectasis, cavitation, progressive fibrosis, pneumothorax, and respiratory failure). Death from pulmonary failure occurs in 5% to 7% of patients with sarcoidosis.

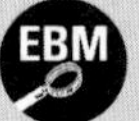

EVIDENCE

Oral corticosteroids improve chest radiographic findings over 3 to 24 mo, and they improve global scores (a combination of symptoms, chest radiograph changes, and lung function) in patients with stage II and III pulmonary sarcoidosis but not in patients with stage I disease. A systematic review found little evidence of an improvement in lung function, and there were insufficient data on the effects of corticosteroids on long-term disease progression.[1] Ⓐ

This review also found limited evidence from one randomized controlled trial that inhaled corticosteroids improved symptoms associated with pulmonary sarcoidosis in the short-term.[1] Ⓑ

Evidence-Based Reference

1. Paramothayan NS et al: Corticosteroids for pulmonary sarcoidosis, *Cochrane Rev* 2, 2005.

SUGGESTED READINGS

Judson MA: The management of sarcoidosis by the primary care physician, *Am J Med* 120:403, 2007.

Iannuzzi MC et al: Sarcoidosis, *N Engl J Med* 357:2153, 2007.

AUTHOR: **FRED F. FERRI, M.D.**

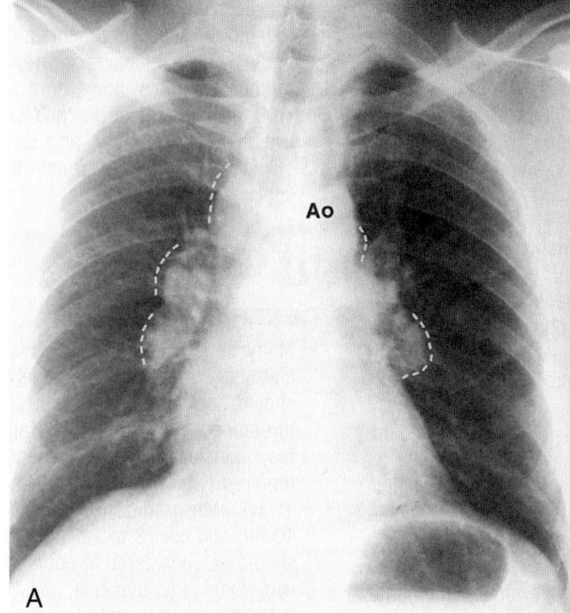

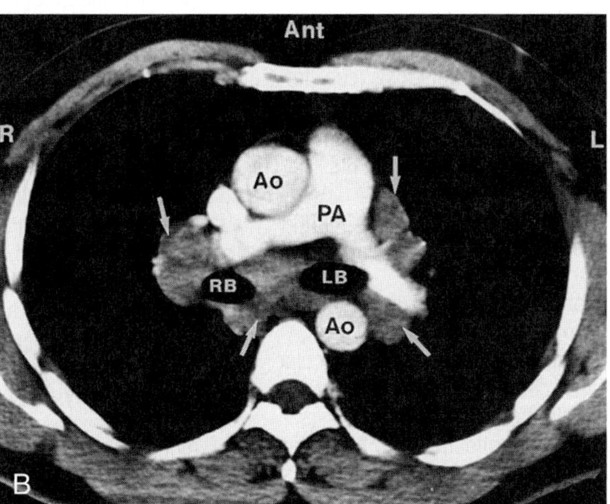

FIGURE 1-292 Sarcoid. Marked lymphadenopathy *(dotted lines)* is seen in the region of both hila in the right paratracheal region **(A).** The transverse contrast-enhanced CT scan of the upper chest **(B)** clearly shows the ascending and descending aorta *(Ao)* as well as the pulmonary artery *(PA)* and superior vena cava. The right and left mainstem bronchus area is also seen. The arrows indicate the extensive lymphadenopathy. *LB,* Left bronchus; *RB,* right bronchus. (From Mettler FA [ed]: *Primary care radiology,* Philadelphia, 2000, WB Saunders.)

TABLE 1-70 Indications for Use of Corticosteroids in Sarcoidosis

Disorder	Treatment
Iridocyclitis	Corticosteroid eye drops; local subconjunctival deposit of cortisone
Posterior uveitis	Oral prednisone
Pulmonary involvement	Steroids rarely recommended for stage I; typically used if infiltrate remains static or worsens over 3-mo period or the patient is symptomatic
Upper airway obstruction	Rare indication for intravenous steroids
Lupus pernio	Oral prednisone shrinks the disfiguring lesions
Hypercalcemia	Responds well to corticosteroids
Cardiac involvement	Corticosteroids usually recommended if patient has arrhythmias or conduction disturbances
CNS involvement	Response is best in patients with acute symptoms
Lacrimal/salivary gland involvement	Corticosteroids recommended for disordered function, not gland swelling
Bone cysts	Corticosteroids recommended if symptomatic

From Andreoli TE (ed): *Cecil essentials of medicine,* ed 5, Philadelphia, 2001, WB Saunders.
CNS, Central nervous system.

BASIC INFORMATION

DEFINITION

Scabies is a contagious disease caused by the mite *Sarcoptes scabiei.*

ICD-9CM CODES
133.0 Scabies

EPIDEMIOLOGY & DEMOGRAPHICS

- Scabies is generally acquired by sleeping with or in the bedding of infested individuals.
- It is generally associated with poor living conditions and is also common in hospitals and nursing homes.

PHYSICAL FINDINGS & CLINICAL PRESENTATION

- Primary lesions are caused when the female mite burrows within the stratum corneum, laying eggs within the tract she leaves behind; burrows (linear or serpiginous tracts) end with a minute papule or vesicle.
- Primary lesions are most commonly found in the web spaces of the hands, wrists, buttocks, scrotum, penis, breasts, axillae, and knees.
- Secondary lesions result from scratching or infection.
- Intense pruritus, especially nocturnal, is common; it is caused by an acquired sensitivity to the mite or fecal pellets and is usually noted 1 to 4 wk after the primary infestation.
- Examination of the skin may reveal burrows, tiny vesicles, excoriations, inflammatory papules.
- Widespread and crusted lesions (Norwegian or crusted scabies) may be seen in elderly and immunocompromised patients.

ETIOLOGY

Human scabies is caused by the mite *S. scabiei,* var. *hominis* (Fig. 1-293).

DIAGNOSIS

DIFFERENTIAL DIAGNOSIS

- Pediculosis
- Atopic dermatitis
- Flea bites
- Seborrheic dermatitis
- Dermatitis herpetiformis
- Contact dermatitis
- Nummular eczema
- Syphilis
- Other insect infestation

WORKUP

Diagnosis is made on the clinical presentation and on the demonstration of mites, eggs, or mite feces.

LABORATORY TESTS

- Microscopic demonstration of the organism, feces, or eggs: a drop of mineral oil may be placed over the suspected lesion before removal; the scrapings are transferred directly to a glass slide; a drop of potassium hydroxide is added and a cover slip is applied.
- Skin biopsy is rarely necessary to make the diagnosis.

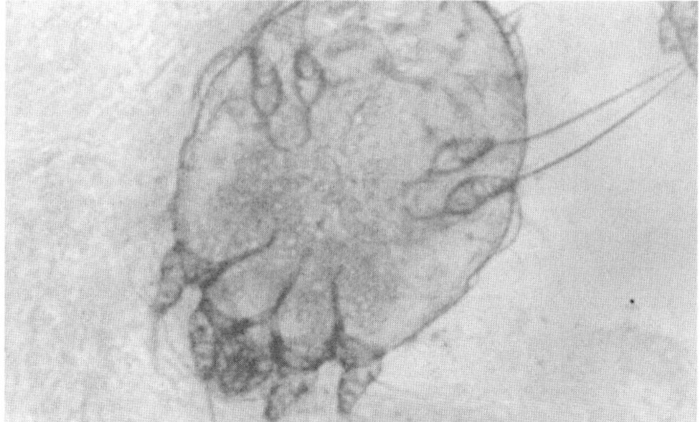

FIGURE 1-293 Scabies organism in a wet mount preparation. (From Mandell GL: *Mandell, Douglas, and Bennett's principles and practice of infectious diseases*, ed 5, New York, 2000, Churchill Livingstone.)

TREATMENT

NONPHARMACOLOGIC THERAPY

Clothing, underwear, and towels used in the 48 hr before treatment must be laundered.

ACUTE GENERAL Rx

- Permethrin 5% cream (Elimite) is usually effective with one treatment; it should be massaged into the skin from head to soles of feet; remove 8 to 14 hr later by washing. If living mites are present after 14 days, treat again.
- A single dose (150 to 200 micrograms/kg in 6-mg tablets) of ivermectin, an antihelmintic agent, is also effective for the treatment of scabies. It is the best treatment for generalized crusted scabies.
- Pruritus generally abates 24 to 48 hr after treatment but can last up to 2 wk; oral antihistamines are effective in decreasing postscabietic pruritus.
- Topical corticosteroid creams may hasten the resolution of secondary eczematous dermatitis.
- If the patient is a resident of an extended care facility, it is important to educate the patients, staff, family, and frequent visitors about scabies and the need to have full cooperation in treatment. Scabicide should be applied to all patients, staff, and frequent visitors, whether symptomatic or not; symptomatic family members of staff and visitors should also receive treatment.

DISPOSITION

Refractory cases usually are seen with immunocompromised hosts or patients with underlying skin diseases.

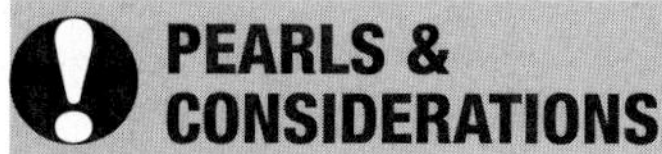

PEARLS & CONSIDERATIONS

COMMENTS

- Lindane is potentially neurotoxic and should not be used on infants or pregnant women (permethrin is safe and effective in these situations).
- Sexual partners should be notified and treated.

SUGGESTED READING

Currie BJ, McCarthy JS: Permethrin and ivermectin for scabies, *N Engl J Med* 362:717, 2010.

AUTHOR: **FRED F. FERRI, M.D.**

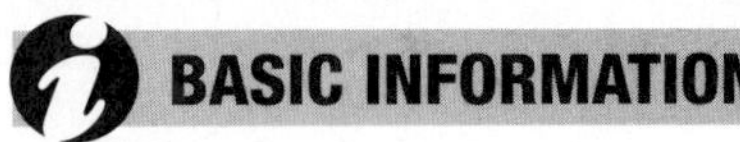

BASIC INFORMATION

DEFINITION

Scarlet fever is a rash involving the skin and tongue and complicating streptococcal group A pharyngitis.

SYNONYMS

Scarlatina
SF

ICD-9CM CODES

034.1 Scarlet fever

EPIDEMIOLOGY & DEMOGRAPHICS

- Same as streptococcal pharyngitis; namely, children ages 5 to 15 yr. May also complicate impetigo.
- Most common in cooler climates during the late fall, winter, and early spring.
- Most cases follow tonsillitis or pharyngitis; however, it has also been reported after wounds ("surgical scarlet fever"), burns, and pelvic or puerperal infections.

PHYSICAL FINDINGS & CLINICAL PRESENTATION

- Diffuse erythema, beginning on face and spreading to neck, back, chest, rest of trunk, and extremities. Most intense on inner aspects of arms and thighs.
- Erythema blanches, but nonblanching petechiae may be present or produced by a tourniquet.
- Strawberry or raspberry tongue.
- Rash lasts approximately 1 wk and then desquamates.
- Febrile illness with headache, malaise, anorexia, and pharyngitis begins after a 2- to 4-day incubation period.
- Scarlatinal rash begins 1 or 2 days after the onset of pharyngitis (Fig. 1-294).

ETIOLOGY

Caused by group A beta-hemolytic *Streptococcus* infection, which produces one of three erythrogenic toxins (NOTE: *Some streptococcal species have the ability to cause both scarlet fever and rheumatic fever).*

DIAGNOSIS

DIFFERENTIAL DIAGNOSIS

- Viral exanthems (covered in Section II)
- Kawasaki disease
- Toxic shock syndrome
- Drug rashes

See differential diagnosis of "Pharyngitis" in Section I.

WORKUP

- Identification of group A *Streptococcus* by throat culture
- Streptolysin O antibody titers

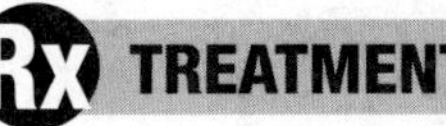

TREATMENT

- Penicillin 250 mg PO qid for 10 days or erythromycin 250 mg PO qid for 10 days in penicillin-allergic patients. A clinical response can be expected in 24 to 48 hr.
- Benzathine penicillin 1 to 2 million U IM once; may be used for a patient who cannot swallow pills.

COMPLICATIONS (RARE)

- Peritonsillar abscess
- Mastoiditis
- Otitis media
- Pneumonia
- Sepsis and distant foci of infection
- Acute rheumatic fever
- Inability to swallow liquids or upper airway obstruction requiring hospitalization

NOTE: Failure to respond to penicillin should raise doubt about the diagnosis because *Streptococcus* may be carried in the pharynx without causing infection.

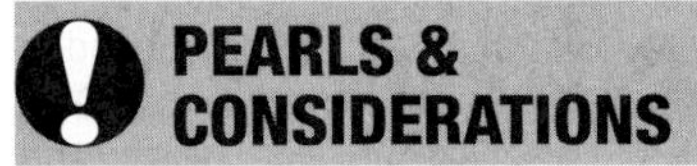

PEARLS & CONSIDERATIONS

COMMENTS

Patients with antibodies against the toxin are spared the rash but still develop other symptoms of the infection (e.g., sore throat).

AUTHOR: **FRED F. FERRI, M.D.**

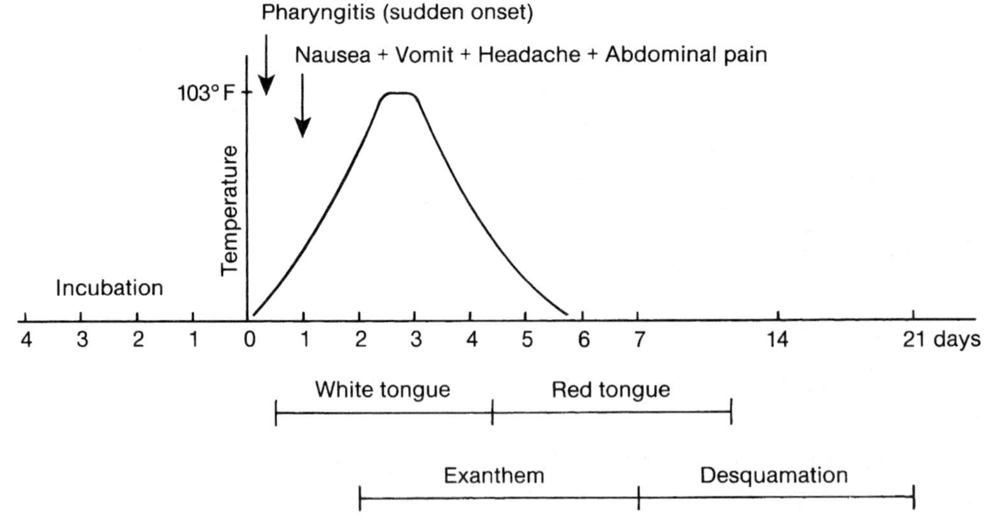

FIGURE 1-294 Scarlet fever. Evolution of signs and symptoms. (From Habif TP: *Clinical dermatology: a color guide to diagnosis and therapy*, ed 3, St Louis, 1996, Mosby.)

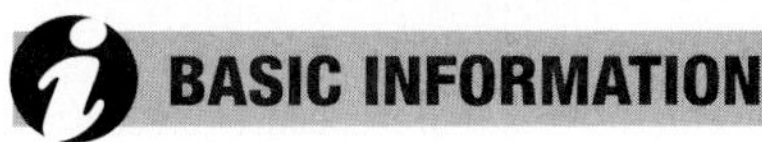

BASIC INFORMATION

DEFINITION

Schistosomiasis is caused by infection with parasite blood flukes known as schistosomes.

SYNONYMS

Bilharziasis
Urinary schistosomiasis
Hepatosplenic schistosomiasis
Swimmers itch
Katayama fever

ICD-9CM CODES
120.9 Schistosomiasis

EPIDEMIOLOGY & DEMOGRAPHICS

INCIDENCE:
- More than 200 million people worldwide and more than 200,000 deaths annually. In U.S., estimated to exceed 400,000 people.
- Geographic distribution of schistosomiasis is confined to an area between 36° north and 34° south latitude, where fresh water temperatures average 25° to 30° C.

PREVALENCE: The greatest cercarial exposure usually occurs in boys ages 5 to 10 yr

DISTRIBUTION:
- *S. mansoni* in tropical and subtropical areas of sub-Saharan Africa, the Middle East, South America, and the Caribbean
- *S. haematobium* in North Africa, sub-Saharan Africa, the Middle East, and India
- *S. japonicum* in Asia, particularly in China, the Philippines, Thailand, and Indonesia
- *S. intercalatum* in central and west Africa
- *S. mekongi* in Cambodia

ETIOLOGY & PATHOGENESIS

- Human infections are caused by *S. mansoni, S. haematobium, S. japonicum, S. mekongi,* and *S. intercalatum.*
- Acquisition of disease via contact with fresh water containing infectious free-living cercarial larvae.
- In U.S., most cases are acquired during foreign travel.
- Human disease is primarily associated with the host's granulomatous response to eggs retained in the tissue.

PHYSICAL FINDINGS & CLINICAL PRESENTATION

ACUTE SYMPTOMS:
- Swimmers itch
- Katayama fever

CHRONIC SYMPTOMS:
- Intestinal schistosomiasis
  1. Abdominal pain
  2. Bloody diarrhea
  3. Iron-deficiency anemia
  4. Intestinal polyp
  5. Bowel ulcer and strictures
- Hepatic schistosomiasis
  1. Hepatomegaly
  2. Splenomegaly
  3. Portal hypertension
  4. Esophageal varices
- Urinary schistosomiasis
  1. Hematuria
  2. Dysuria
  3. Urinary frequency
  4. Fibrosis of bladder and ureters
  5. Squamous cell ca of bladder
  6. Proteinuria
  7. Nephrotic syndrome

COMPLICATIONS:
- Neurologic complication
  1. Granuloma of spinal cord or brain
  2. Transverse myelitis
  3. Epilepsy or focal neurologic deficit
- Pulmonary complication
  1. Granulomatous pulmonary endarteritis
  2. Pulmonary hypertension
  3. Cor pulmonale
- Other complications include tubal obstruction and infertility
- Recurrent bacteremia and recurrent UTI

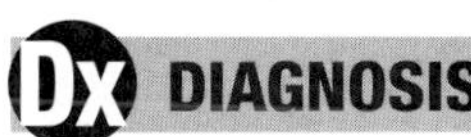

DIAGNOSIS

DIFFERENTIAL DIAGNOSIS

- Amebiasis
- Bacillary dysentery
- Bowel polyp
- Prostatic disease
- Genitourinary tract cancer
- Bacterial infections of the urinary tract

WORKUP

- Microscopy in urine or stool
- Tissue biopsy
- Serology
- CBC
- LFT
- US of abdomen
- CT scan of abdomen

LABORATORY TESTS

- CBC shows eosinophilia, anemia, thrombocytopenia
- LFT with mild increase in alkaline phosphatase and GGT
- Microscopy: stool and urine
- Serology: ELISA for detecting both schistosomal antibodies and antigen
- Rectal biopsy or bladder mucosal biopsy

IMAGING STUDIES

- X-ray of abdomen shows "fetal head" calcification.
- Sonography also documents a thickened bladder wall, hydronephrosis and hydroureter, and bladder polyps or calcification. It also demonstrates the thickened fibrosed portal tracts.
- Esophagoscopy documents esophageal varices.
- Liver biopsy may also demonstrate granuloma and clay pipestem fibrosis.

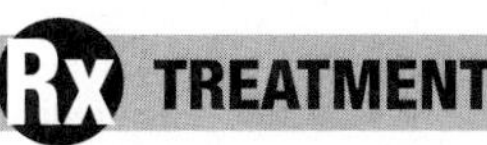

TREATMENT

- Praziquantel 40 mg/kg of body weight PO in one or two doses
- Oxamniquine 15 mg/kg PO once or 20 mg/kg PO daily for 3 days for recalcitrant infections
- Metrifonate 7.5 to 10 mg/kg of body weight given PO in three doses at 2-wk intervals

DISPOSITION

Treated patients usually respond to therapy. Definitive cure has occurred only when there is total disappearance of viable eggs from the excreta for a total of 6 mo after treatment.

REFERRAL

- To an infectious disease specialist knowledgeable in parasitology and geographic medicine for treatment and follow-up
- To a gastroenterologist for sclerotherapy of bleeding esophageal varices, if needed in advanced hepatosplenic schistosomiasis
- To a urologist for management and follow-up of urinary complications of *S. haematobium* infection of the genitourinary tract

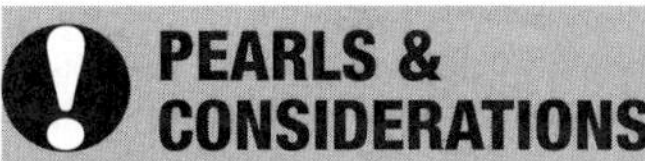

PEARLS & CONSIDERATIONS

COMMENTS

Prevention:
- Chemotherapy
  1. Mass
  2. Targeted population
- Snail control
  1. Molluscicidng
  2. Environmental modification
  3. Biologic control
- Reduction of water contact and contamination
  1. Provision of domestic water supplies
  2. Provision for sanitary disposal of excreta
- Vaccination
- Improved living standards

SUGGESTED READINGS

Steinmann P et al: Schistosomiasis and water resources development: systematic review, meta-analysis, and estimates of people at risk, *Lancet Infect Dis* 6(7):411, 2006.

Swai B et al: Female genital schistosomiasis as an evidence of a neglected cause for reproductive ill-health: a retrospective histopathological study from Tanzania, *BMC Infect Dis* 6:134, 2006.

Vennervald BJ et al: Morbidity in schistosomiasis: an update, *Curr Opin Infect Dis* 17(5):439, 2004.

Wang LD et al: A strategy to control transmission of schistosoma japonicum in China, *N Engl J Med* 360:121-128, 2009.

AUTHORS: **GLENN G. FORT, M.D., M.P.H.,** and **DENNIS J. MIKOLICH, M.D.**

BASIC INFORMATION

DEFINITION

Schizophrenia is a disorder that causes significant distortions in thinking, perception, speech, and behavior. Characteristics include psychosis, apathy, social withdrawal, and cognitive impairment, which result in significant social impairment.

SYNONYMS

Dementia praecox

ICD-9CM CODES

295.9 Schizophrenia

EPIDEMIOLOGY & DEMOGRAPHICS

INCIDENCE: 0.2 per 1000

PREVALENCE: 0.5%; lifetime prevalence risk, 0.4%

PREDOMINANT SEX: Males have a more severe illness with earlier onset; however, distribution is probably equal.

PREDOMINANT AGE:

- The age of onset of psychotic symptoms is the early 20s for males and the late 20s for females.
- The age of onset of negative symptoms is usually earlier (i.e., the mid-teenage years).

PEAK INCIDENCE: Between the ages of 16 and 30 yr

GENETICS:

- Genetics account for 70% of risk; the remaining 30% is associated with urban environments, migration, and cannabis use.
- First-degree relatives of schizophrenic patients have a 10 times greater chance of becoming schizophrenic than the general population.
- Discordant rates among identical twins are higher than expected with the simple inheritance pattern.
- Associations with several chromosomes have been described, but none have been replicated.
- Evidence exists that triplet nucleotide repeat expansion (e.g., such as that seen with Huntington's disease) may play a role in the inheritance of the disease.

PHYSICAL FINDINGS & CLINICAL PRESENTATION

- Schizophrenia is best defined as a dementing illness that begins early in life and that progresses slowly throughout the lifetime.
- Frequent structural brain imaging findings include the enlargement of the ventricular system, a loss of brain volume and cortical gray matter, and an alteration of the white matter tracts.
- The initial "negative" symptoms of adolescence—cognitive decline, social withdrawal and awkwardness, loss of motivation and pleasure, and loss of emotional expressiveness—begin after a period of normal development.
- During early adulthood, positive symptoms of psychosis and thought disturbance occur; psychotic symptoms then wax and wane throughout life. Treatment ameliorates positive symptoms but generally does little for negative ones.
- The condition is also accompanied by cognitive impairment, including problems with attention and concentration, psychomotor speed, learning, memory, and executive functions (e.g., abstract thinking, problem solving).
- Social and occupational dysfunction can be profound.

ETIOLOGY

- The basic determination of whether this is a degenerative or developmental condition has not made.
- The major hypothesis is that the generation of the mesocortical pathways produces the hypofrontality and the negative symptoms. This occurs along with a compensatory hyperactivation of the mesolimbic pathways, which produces the positive symptoms of psychosis.

DIAGNOSIS

DIFFERENTIAL DIAGNOSIS

- Schizophrenia is diagnosed when an individual has experienced at least 1 month of hallucinations, delusions, thought disorders, catatonia, or negative symptoms (e.g., avolition, anhedonia, social isolation, affective flattening).
- Any medical condition, medicine, or substance of abuse that can affect brain homeostasis can cause psychosis; this is distinguished from schizophrenia by a relatively brief course and an alteration in mental status that suggests an underlying delirium.
- Other neurologic conditions that have psychosis as the initial presentation (e.g., Huntington's disease) need to be ruled out.
- Other psychiatric disorders are the source of greatest confusion.
- Mood disorders with psychosis: These are indistinguishable from schizophrenia cross-sectionally but have a longitudinal course that includes full recovery.
- Delusional disorder: This condition involves nonbizarre delusions and lacks the thought disturbance, hallucinations, and negative symptoms of schizophrenia.
- Autism in the adult: This has an early age of onset and lacks significant hallucinations or delusions.

WORKUP

- History and physical examination to help determine whether the psychosis is primary or secondary
- Neurologic examination to uncover the soft neurologic signs (e.g., clumsiness, cortical thumb, loss of fine motor movements) that are common with schizophrenia

LABORATORY TESTS

- No laboratory tests are specific for schizophrenia.
- Laboratory examinations (e.g., chemistry profile, blood count, sedimentation rate, toxicology screen, urinalysis) are geared toward excluding a primary medical condition.

IMAGING STUDIES

- Computed tomography scan or MRI of the brain during the initial workup; repeated if the course of the illness varies from what is expected
- Sometimes electroencephalography to reveal slowing when the psychosis is the result of an encephalopathy
- Chest radiograph during the initial workup to rule out a primary medical condition

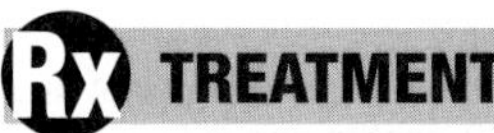

TREATMENT

NONPHARMACOLOGIC THERAPY

- Significant social support is required by most schizophrenic patients, but available support services are grossly inadequate. Schizophrenic patients constitute nearly one third of all homeless individuals. They usually require help with basic social, occupational, and interactive skills.
- For schizophrenic patients who continue to live with their families, family stress can precipitate relapse and rehospitalization. Family interventions can reduce morbidity.
- Cognitive behavioral therapy can reduce the severity of both psychotic and negative symptoms.
- Illness management training for patients can increase medication adherence and reduce distress that results from symptoms.
- Integrated treatment that includes assertive community treatment, family involvement programs, and social skills training reduces the severity of both psychotic and negative symptoms, reduces comorbid substance misuse, reduces hospital days, increases adherence to treatment, and increases satisfaction with treatment.

ACUTE GENERAL Rx

- Acute psychosis is usually adequately controlled with antipsychotic agents.
- Few differences in effectiveness exist between first-generation antipsychotics (e.g., haloperidol, perphenazine, fluphenazine, chlorpromazine) and second-generation antipsychotics (e.g., risperidone, olanzapine, quetiapine, ziprasidone, aripiprazole, clozapine) for nonrefractory patients. First-generation antipsychotics are slightly more likely than second-generation antipsychotics to cause a parkinsonian state and eventual tardive dyskinesia (rate of tardive dyskinesia, 15% to 30%). Antiparkinsonian drugs (e.g., benztropine, amantadine) are used to ameliorate the parkinsonism. Risperidone has been shown to be superior to haloperidol for the prevention of acute psychotic relapse.

- Sedatives (i.e., benzodiazepines and, to a lesser degree, barbiturates) can be used transiently if a patient is in an agitated state.

CHRONIC RX

- Relapse prevention is a major goal of treatment. Noncompliance is common and leads to high relapse rates. Antipsychotic agents usually must be continued at the same doses that controlled psychosis. For noncompliant patients, depot preparations given biweekly or monthly can be used.
- Most patients frequently switch among antipsychotics; there is considerable individual variability with regard to antipsychotic response and vulnerability to specific adverse effects.
- Clozapine is more effective than other agents for treatment-refractory patients.
- Neurocognitive improvement associated with antipsychotic treatment among patients with schizophrenia is small and does not differ between first-generation and second-generation antipsychotics.
- Antiparkinsonian agents may also need to be continued for the long term.
- Tardive dyskinesia (i.e., choreoathetoid movements of the muscles of tongue and face and occasionally of other muscle groups) can occur in as many as 30% of patients with the long-term use of neuroleptics.
- The negative symptoms of schizophrenia can resemble depression. In addition, depressive disorders may occur in schizophrenic patients. Antidepressant treatment of the negative symptoms is usually not effective. However, antidepressants can improve the symptoms of a discrete comorbid depressive episode.
- Mood stabilizers (e.g., lithium, valproate, carbamazepine) are of little use unless the patient has a comorbid impulse control disorder.
- Substance abuse is a major problem for more than a third of schizophrenic patients. More than half of these patients smoke cigarettes. Unfortunately, these individuals do poorly in traditional substance abuse treatment programs. Specialized "dual-diagnosis" programs with highly structured aftercare are required.
- Specific antipsychotic medications have been associated with weight gain (i.e., olanzapine and clozapine) and QT prolongation. Hyperlipidemia and diabetes mellitus are associated with second-generation antipsychotics, and hyperprolactinemia is associated with first-generation antipsychotics. Clozapine is associated with agranulocytosis.

DISPOSITION

- The positive symptoms of as many as 20% to 30% of schizophrenic patients do not respond to available treatments. A much higher fraction of patients experience relapse as a result of poor compliance.
- Negative symptoms are responsible for the 50% to 70% of patients in whom deterioration in occupational and social function continues.
- Approximately 10% of schizophrenic patients will complete suicide.
- The course of the illness most strongly predicted by level of social development attained at the onset of psychosis.
- Schizophrenic patients die 12 to 15 years sooner than the average population, mostly as a result of physical causes related to a lack of access to health care or as a result of health risk factors (e.g., smoking, obesity).

REFERRAL

- If hospitalization is required
- If patient is noncompliant
- If patient is resistant to treatment

PEARLS & CONSIDERATIONS

- Rule out delirium caused by medical conditions, medications, or substance abuse before diagnosing an individual's psychotic behavior as schizophrenia.
- All antipsychotic medications have high discontinuation rates in chronic schizophrenia treatment. Olanzapine and clozapine may be more effective than other antipsychotics for chronic treatment, but they have significant side effects.
- Significant social support is required for most patients with schizophrenia. Nonpharmacologic therapy should be used in conjunction with pharmacotherapy.

EBM EVIDENCE

Please note: Complete text of EBM for this topic is available online.

Key trials and commentary:

Clozapine is more effective than typical antipsychotics for individuals with schizophrenia, particularly those who do not improve with typical antipsychotics. Clozapine is associated with less movement adverse effects than typical antipsychotic drugs, but it may cause serious blood related adverse effects and white blood cell monitoring is mandatory for all individuals taking clozapine.[1]

Cannabis use may be a risk factor for schizophrenia. Part of this association may be explained by genotype–environment interaction, and part of it by genotype–environment correlation. The latter issue has not been explored. This study investigated whether cannabis use is associated with schizophrenia, and whether gene–environment correlation contributes to this association, by examining the prevalence of cannabis use in groups with different levels of genetic predisposition for schizophrenia.

This study shows that cannabis use was associated with schizophrenia, but there was no evidence for genotype–environment correlation.

This study explores the relationship between cannabis use and genetic liability for schizophrenia. It is often considered that drugs of abuse bring on schizophrenia in people who are already vulnerable to develop psychosis. Several years ago another (Australian) group showed evidence for a gene–environment interaction in schizophrenia. This study refutes that proposition. Nevertheless, the higher rates of cannabis abuse in the schizophrenia sample compared with normal subjects again confirm the robust association between cannabis abuse and schizophrenia.[2] Ⓐ

Brain glutathione levels are decreased in schizophrenia, a disorder that often is chronic and refractory to treatment. N-acetyl-cysteine (NAC) increases brain glutathione in rodents. This study was conducted to evaluate the safety and effectiveness of oral NAC (1 g orally twice daily [bid]) as an add-on to maintenance medication for the treatment of chronic schizophrenia over a 24-week period.

Oxidative stress has long been proposed as a mechanism to understand how schizophrenia occurs and how the disease has such a broad constellation of effects. It is proposed that, through vulnerability to oxidative damage, there are free radical effects that impact cellular processes, especially mitochondrial, prostaglandin, and cell membrane functioning. This hypothesis has been elaborated through investigations with plasma and cerebrospinal fluid assays for breakdown products of oxidative stress, brain imaging of neurochemistry using magnetic resonance spectroscopy, and treatment studies using vitamin E and/or fish oil products. Most recently, an Australian group has come up with another approach of giving N-acetyl-cysteine in addition to antipsychotic medications. N-acetyl-cysteine is a precursor of glutathione, a key element in the phospholipid pathway. In this study, Berk et al show how N-acetyl-cysteine (given under placebo-controlled, double-blinded conditions for 24 weeks) could produce at least some (but not dramatic) benefit in overall symptoms. The compound was well tolerated. This is an interesting avenue of research, now taking practical observations into the treatment arena. We are likely to see more of this type of work over time.[3] Ⓐ

Compared with nonpsychotic depression, psychotic depression is associated with poor prognosis, increased mortality, and severe symptomatology. Although the incidence of psychotic depression is similar to that of schizophrenia, little is known about presentation, course, costs, and effects of treatment.

This study showed that psychotic depression is a common and costly condition, but with no accepted best practice guidance for its management. More attention needs to be focused on this largely under-researched group.

It is hard to believe that (1) no comparison of persons suffering first-break schizophrenia and depression has been undertaken to date and that (2) there is "no accepted best practice guidance" for management of the latter. I recall a statement made by the famous European psychiatrist, Luc Ciompi, decades ago, saying that in Europe they treated first-episode psychosis of whatever type with antipsychotics and only after its resolution was antidepressive or antischizophrenic treatment decided on. This, of course, was completely at odds with our American belief that we could differentiate between the two immediately and target treatment accordingly. A finding that is startling in this contribution to the literature is that all who received ECT did well; why do the authors not see that as a "best practice" and why is there such continuing resistance to its use worldwide? In addition, although it is not surprising that those suffering depression had more attempts at self-harm, the authors and I are not clear why they had more "physical health problems." Also, I was not aware either that hospitalizations for psychotic depression were as lengthy and costly as those for schizophrenia. There is much to chew on here.[4] Ⓐ

Major mental disorders are associated with an increased risk for obesity-related cardiovascular mortality, leading to interest in risk-reduction approaches that target weight and risk-related plasma lipids, including use of antipsychotic agents with low metabolic risk. This multicenter, randomized, double-blind study compared the metabolic effects of aripiprazole vs. olanzapine in overweight persons with schizophrenia or schizoaffective disorder who were previously on olanzapine treatment.

Significant improvements in weight and lipids observed during discontinuation of olanzapine and switch to aripiprazole treatment occurred with limited evidence of negative psychiatric effects, relative to uninterrupted continuation of olanzapine treatment. The results suggest that the potential value of therapeutic substitutions involving specific antipsychotic medications should be considered in overall efforts to reduce cardiovascular risk in this population.

Since 2003, the FDA stance toward the second-generation atypical antipsychotics has been that there is not sufficient evidence to differentiate among the six of them for metabolic effects. However, there is a fairly large amount of literature suggesting there are clinically important differences. This trial is another one finding the same issues in a trial of 173 schizophrenic patients that were randomly assigned to receive either aripiprazole or olanzapine. At week 16, there were clear differences. Weight had decreased significantly with aripiprazole (−1.8 kg vs. +1.41 kg). Significantly more patients on aripiprazole had clinically relevant (≥7%) weight loss vs. olanzapine (11.1% vs. 2.6%) and a similar advantage for clinically relevant weight gain (2.5% vs. 9.1%). Although there were no differences on glycemic lab measures, there were again advantages in total cholesterol and high-density lipoprotein cholesterol favoring aripiprazole. In patients with weight gain and metabolic changes on olanzapine who have been switched to aripiprazole, quetiapine, ziprasidone, or risperidone, reduction in weight and other metabolic changes have also been observed. It would appear to be that we do have growing evidence of differences between the second-generation atypical antipsychotics at least for potential metabolic issues.[5] Ⓐ

Psychoeducation programs have been demonstrated to reduce relapse and be cost-effective for schizophrenia in academic settings, although this has not been examined in private care inpatient settings.

This controlled study demonstrated subsequent reduction of costly rehospitalization among patients randomly assigned to STEPS, although study attrition of 46% over 6 months may diminish the confidence in the findings. This is the first study to demonstrate effectiveness of inpatient-initiated psychoeducation in private-sector care. Larger, more comprehensive studies are needed to replicate these findings and identify the active components of the intervention yielding these apparent gains.

I've chosen this article for many reasons. First, I realized there are far too few articles on psychoeducation that I have had abstracted for review. Second, there are far too few articles on psychoeducation published on the subject at all. Third, I'm always looking for studies from "real life" situations using "dirty" patient populations rather than rarefied populations most doctors never see and/or treat. And last, it's always interesting to see if private sector programs are as effective as those conducted in academic settings. The study's principal result—a 20% vs. 56% reduction in rehospitalization in the first 6 months is impressive. A caution, of course, is that we know from other studies that such striking changes tend to be less powerful over time (i.e., after 6 months), but still, as the authors kept pointing out, quoting McFarlane et al's work, every "dollar spent on the program yielded an overall savings of $34 in other treatment costs."[6] Ⓐ

Evidence-Based References

1. Essali A et al: Clozapine versus typical neuroleptic medication for schizophrenia, *Cochrane Database Rev* 2, 2007.
2. Veling W et al: Cannabis use and genetic predisposition for schizophrenia: a case-control study, *Psychol Med* 38:1251-1256, 2008. Commentary by P. Buckley, M.D. Ⓐ
3. Berk M et al: N-acetyl cysteine as a glutathione precursor for schizophrenia—a double-blind, randomized, placebo-controlled trial, *Biol Psychiatry* 64: 361-368, 2008. Commentary by P. Buckley, M.D. Ⓐ
4. Crebbin K et al: First-episode psychosis: an epidemiological survey comparing psychotic depression with schizophrenia, *J Affective Disord* 105:117-124, 2008. Commentary by J.A. Talbott, M.D. Ⓐ
5. Newcomer JW et al: A multicenter, randomized, double-blind study of the effects of aripiprazole in overweight subjects with schizophrenia or schizoaffective disorder switched from olanzapine, *J Clin Psychiatry* 69:1046-1056, 2008. Commentary by J.C. Ballenger, M.D. Ⓐ
6. Vickar GM et al: A randomized controlled trial of a private-sector inpatient-initiated psychoeducation program for schizophrenia, *Psychiatr Serv* 60:117-120, 2009. Commentary by J.A. Talbott, M.D. Ⓐ

SUGGESTED READINGS

Jones PB et al: Randomized controlled trial of the effect on quality of life of second- vs first-generation antipsychotic drugs in schizophrenia: Cost Utility of the Latest Antipsychotic Drugs in Schizophrenia Study (CUtLASS 1), *Arch Gen Psychiatry* 63(10): 1079-1087, 2006.

Lieberman JA et al: Effectiveness of antipsychotic drugs in patients with chronic schizophrenia, *N Engl J Med* 353:1209, 2005.

Picchioni MM, Murray RM: Schizophrenia, *BMJ* 335: 91, 2007.

Ray WA et al: Atypical antipsychotic drugs and the risk of sudden cardiac death, *N Engl J Med* 360:225-235, 2009.

van Os J, Kapur S: Schizophrenia, *Lancet* 374:635, 2009.

AUTHOR: **MICHAEL K. ONG, M.D., PH.D.**

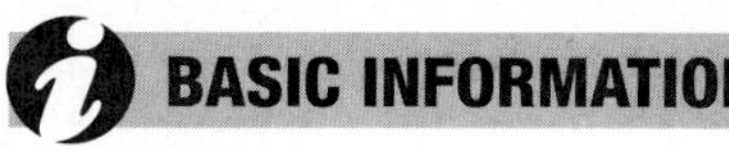

BASIC INFORMATION

DEFINITION

Scleritis is inflammation of the sclera.

SYNONYMS

Anterior scleritis
Diffuse nodular, necrotizing scleritis
Scleromalacia perforans
Scleral melt syndrome

ICD-9CM CODES
379.0 Scleritis and episcleritis

EPIDEMIOLOGY & DEMOGRAPHICS

PEAK INCIDENCE: Increases with increasing age
INCIDENCE (IN U.S.): Busy ophthalmologists may see one or two cases a year
PREVALENCE (IN U.S.): Relatively rare
PREDOMINANT SEX: 61% women
PREDOMINANT AGE: 52 yr

PHYSICAL FINDINGS & CLINICAL PRESENTATION

- Deep, boring eye pain
- Photophobia
- Tearing
- Conjunctival injection (Fig. 1-295)
- Thinning of the sclera
- 44% of patients have associated medical conditions: 7% infections, 37% rheumatic disease. Most common infection is Herpes zoster. Most common rheumatic problem is rheumatoid arthritis; 4% have systemic vasculitis. Most patients with systemic disease are diagnosed before development of scleritis.

ETIOLOGY

- Inflammatory
- Allergic
- Toxic

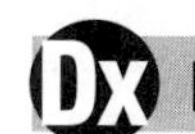

DIAGNOSIS

DIFFERENTIAL DIAGNOSIS

- Most common causes are rheumatoid arthritis and other collagen-vascular diseases.
- Occasionally there are allergic, infectious, or traumatic causes.
- Conjunctivitis, iritis, and episcleritis should be considered in the differential diagnosis.

WORKUP

- Fluorescein angiography
- Eye examination
- Visual field examination
- Workup for autoimmune disease
- Workup for vasculitis
- Collagen vascular workup

LABORATORY TESTS

Rheumatoid factor, antinuclear antibody, erythrocyte sedimentation rate may be useful for underlying etiology

IMAGING STUDIES

Usually not necessary; CT scan of orbit may be useful in selected patients for collagen vascular disease or vasculitis

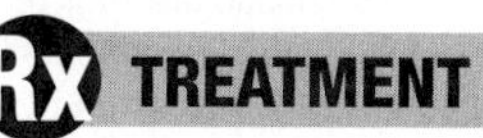

TREATMENT

NONPHARMACOLOGIC THERAPY

- Bandage lenses
- Surgery if thinning of the sclera is severe to prevent eye rupture

ACUTE GENERAL Rx

Immunotherapy (with steroids and Imuran, etc.):

- Steroids (topical, periocular, and systemic)
- Cycloplegic drops
- Nonsteroidal anti-inflammatory drugs (topical and systemic); systemic more effective than topical
- Other immunosuppressive drugs

CHRONIC Rx

- Systemic steroids can be given for the underlying disease.
- Local steroids may be helpful.
- Control underlying disease.

DISPOSITION

Urgent referral to ophthalmologist

REFERRAL

If not referred to an ophthalmologist early, patients may develop uveitis and other complications.

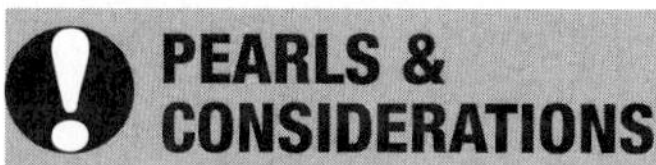

PEARLS & CONSIDERATIONS

COMMENTS

An ominous diagnosis because these patients often have other severe underlying debilitating disease processes.

SUGGESTED READINGS

Akpek EK et al: Evaluation of patients with scleritis for systemic disease, *Ophthalmology* 111(3):501, 2004.

Paresio CG et al: Systemic disorders associated with episcleritis and scleritis, *Curr Opin Ophthalmol* 12(6):471, 2001.

Sainz de la Maza M et al: Ocular characteristics and disease associations in scleritis: associated peripheral keratopathy, *Arch Ophthalmol* 120(1):15, 2002.

Thorne JE et al: Severe scleritis and urticarial lesions, *Am J Ophthalmol* 134(6):932, 2002.

AUTHOR: **MELVYN KOBY, M.D.**

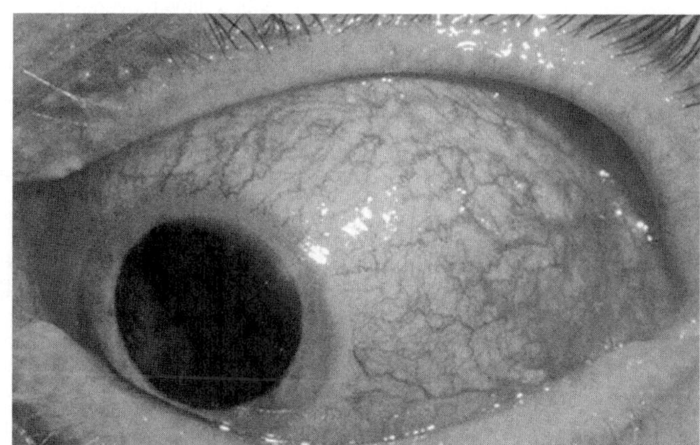

FIGURE 1-295 In diffuse anterior scleritis, widespread injection of the conjunctival and deep episcleral vessels occurs. (From Palay D [ed]: *Ophthalmology for the primary care physician,* St Louis, 1997, Mosby.)

Scleroderma (Progressive Systemic Sclerosis) 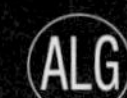 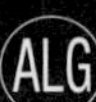

BASIC INFORMATION

DEFINITION

Scleroderma is a connective tissue disorder that is characterized by the thickening and fibrosis of the skin and the variably severe involvement of diverse internal organs. It can be subdivided into two major subgroups: (1) limited cutaneous scleroderma, which involves mainly the face, arms, and hands; and (2) diffuse scleroderma, which affects the skin and one or more internal organs.

SYNONYMS

Systemic sclerosis

Morphea applies to localized scleroderma that affects only the skin

Scleredema is a disease of the skin that is distinct from scleroderma.

ICD-9CM CODES

710.1 Scleroderma

701.0 Morphea

EPIDEMIOLOGY & DEMOGRAPHICS

INCIDENCE: There are 2.3 to 22.8 cases per million persons per yr, but many mild cases go unrecognized.

PREVALENCE: 50 to 300 cases per million persons

PREDOMINANT SEX: Female/male ratio of 4:1

PREDOMINANT AGE: 30 to 50 yr

DISTRIBUTION: Worldwide

PHYSICAL FINDINGS & CLINICAL PRESENTATION

PHYSICAL FINDINGS:

1. Skin
    - Begins on the hands and then moves to the face; the skin is shiny, taut, and sometimes red, with a loss of creases and hair
    - Later skin tightening may limit movement
    - Pigmentary changes occur
    - Skin atrophy occurs during later stages
    - Musculoskeletal symptoms
    - Symmetric inflammatory arthritis
    - Myopathy
2. Gastrointestinal involvement
    - Esophageal dysmotility with heartburn, dysphagia, and odynophagia
    - Delayed gastric emptying
    - Small-bowel dysmotility with abdominal cramps and diarrhea
    - Colon dysmotility with constipation
    - Primary biliary cirrhosis (see "Cirrhosis, Primary Biliary" in Section I)
3. Pulmonary manifestations
    - Pulmonary fibrosis with symptoms of dyspnea and nonproductive cough as well as fine inspiratory crackles on examination
    - Pulmonary hypertension
4. Cardiac involvement
    - Myocardial fibrosis that leads to congestive heart failure
5. Renal involvement
    - Malignant hypertension
    - Rapidly progressive renal failure
6. Other organ involvement
    - Hypothyroidism
    - Erectile dysfunction
    - Sjögren's syndrome
    - Entrapment neuropathies
7. CREST syndrome
    - *C*alcinosis, *R*aynaud's syndrome, *E*sophageal dysmotility, *S*clerodactyly, *T*elangiectasias. With CREST syndrome, scleroderma is limited to the distal extremities. This acronym is now considered obsolete by many because it does not accurately reflect the burden of internal organ involvement.

CLINICAL PRESENTATION:

- Raynaud's phenomenon: initial complaint in 70% of patients (Note: The prevalence of Raynaud's phenomenon is 5% to 10% in the general population; most cases do not progress to scleroderma.)
- Finger or hand swelling that is sometimes associated with carpal tunnel syndrome
- Arthralgias/arthritis
- Internal organ involvement

ETIOLOGY

The etiology of this condition is unknown. Stimulatory autoantibodies against platelet-derived growth factor appear to be a specific hallmark of scleroderma. Their biologic activity on fibroblasts suggests that they have a causal role in the pathogenesis of the disease. In scleroderma, unifying features exist despite heterogenous patterns of organ involvement and disease progression:

- Extracellular connective tissue activation
- Frequent immunologic abnormalities
- Inflammation
- Vasoconstriction

DIAGNOSIS

DIFFERENTIAL DIAGNOSIS

DERMATOLOGIC:

- Mycosis fungoides
- Amyloidosis
- Porphyria cutanea tarda
- Eosinophilic fasciitis
- Reflex sympathetic dystrophy

SYSTEMIC:

- Idiopathic pulmonary fibrosis
- Primary pulmonary hypertension
- Primary biliary cirrhosis
- Cardiomyopathies
- Gastrointestinal dysmotility problems
- Systemic lupus erythematosus and overlap syndromes

WORKUP

Laboratory tests and imaging studies

LABORATORY TESTS

- Antinuclear antibodies (homogeneous, speckled, or nucleolar patterns)
- Negative antibody to native DNA
- Negative anti-smooth muscle antibody
- Autoantibodies against ribonucleoprotein positive in 20% of patients
- Rheumatoid factor positive in 30% of patients
- Anticentromere antibodies in <10% of patients with systemic illness and in 50% to 95% of patients with limited scleroderma (i.e., good prognosis if positive)
- Positive extractable nuclear antibody to SCL 70 in 30% of patients
- Routine biochemistry tests may indicate specific organ involvement (e.g., liver, kidney, muscle)

IMAGING AND OTHER STUDIES

1. Arthritis: joint radiographs
2. Gastrointestinal
    - Barium swallow
    - Cine-esophagography
    - Endoscopy
    - Esophageal manometry
3. Pulmonary
    - Chest x-ray
    - Pulmonary function test
    - Chest computed tomographic scan
    - Bronchoscopy with biopsy
    - Gallium lung scan
    - Bronchoalveolar lavage
4. Heart
    - ECG
    - Ambulatory (Holter) ECG monitoring
    - Echocardiography
    - Cardiac catheterization
5. Kidney: renal biopsy
6. Skin: skin biopsy

TREATMENT

1. D-penicillamine, recombinant human relaxin, and supportive therapies
2. Raynaud's syndrome:
    - Calcium channel blockers (i.e., long-acting dihydropyridines)
    - Peripheral alpha$_1$-adrenergic blockers
    - Angiotensin-II receptor blockers
    - Pentoxifylline
    - Stellate ganglionic blockades
    - Digital sympathectomy
3. Arthralgias: nonsteroidal anti-inflammatory drugs
4. Skin: moisturizing agents (For skin fibrosis, immunomodulatory drugs are used [e.g., D-penicillamine, mycophenolate, cyclophosphamide].)
5. Esophageal reflux
    - H_2-receptor blockers
    - Proton pump inhibitors
6. Pulmonary hypertension and fibrosis
    - Oxygen
    - Diuretics
    - Endothelin-1 receptor inhibitors (Bosentan)
    - Sildenafil
    - Prostacyclin analogues (Epoprostenol)
    - Lung transplant
    - Cyclophosphamide chemotherapy for symptomatic scleroderma-related interstitial lung disease
7. Renal involvement
    - Angiotensin-converting enzyme inhibitors
    - Dialysis
    - Renal transplantation

REFERRAL

Rheumatology consultation

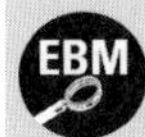

EVIDENCE

Please note: Complete text of EBM for this topic is available online.

Key trials and commentary:

Lung disease has become the leading cause of mortality and morbidity in scleroderma (SSc) patients. The frequency, nature, and progression of interstitial lung disease seen on high-resolution CT (HRCT) scans in patients with diffuse SSc (dcSSc) compared with those with limited SSc (lcSSc) has not been well characterized.

This study showed that PF and GGO were the most common HRCT scan findings in symptomatic SSc patients. HCs were seen in more than one third of cases, being more common in lcSSc vs. dcSSc. There was no relationship between progression and baseline PF extent in lcSSc vs. dcSSc.

This study was completed by members of the Scleroderma Lung Study Research Group with participants in various academic institutions throughout the U.S. The authors explain that the Scleroderma Lung Study (SLS) was a prospective, randomized, double-blind controlled clinical trial to evaluate the effectiveness of oral cyclophosphamide vs. placebo therapy in the treatment of active, symptomatic pulmonary alveolitis inflammation secondary to systemic scleroderma (SSc). The study was limited to symptomatic patients, all of whom had dyspnea, 67.9% with cough and 46.1% with sputum production. Every participant in the study underwent a baseline HRCT scan with prone imaging when possible. Patients were classified as having lcSSc if skin thickening was limited to areas of the extremities below elbows and knees and above the clavicles. Patients with dcSSc were those who had skin thickening involving proximal extremities and/or torso.

The authors state that pulmonary involvement is a significant cause of morbidity and mortality in up to 95% of autopsy cases of patients with SSc. The typical HRCT pulmonary abnormality reported in patients with SSc is GGO in a distribution similar to that seen in patients with nonspecific interstitial pneumonia (NSIP). NSIP can be cellular or fibrotic. Fibrotic NSIP typically manifests with peripheral basilar predominant architectural distortion characterized by reticular opacities and traction bronchiectasis/bronchiolectasis. A less frequent HRCT abnormality is that of peripheral honeycomb cysts, findings associated with usual interstitial pneumonia (UIP) histology. The HRCT findings in the study population are listed in the abstract. However, the authors point out that lung biopsies and histologic correlations were not performed.

Interestingly, although pulmonary function was similar in patients with lcSSc and those with dcSSc, patients with lcSSc had more extensive pulmonary fibrosis. The extent of pulmonary fibrosis was negatively correlated with measurements of forced vital capacity (FVC) and diffusing capacity of the lung for CO (DLCO).[1] Ⓐ

Evidence-Based Reference

1. Goldin JG et al: High-resolution CT scan findings in patients with symptomatic scleroderma-related interstitial lung disease, *Chest* 134:358-367, 2008. Commentary by M.L. Rosado de Christenson, M.D., FACR Ⓐ

SUGGESTED READINGS

Baron SS et al: Stimulatory autoantibodies to the PDGF receptor in systemic sclerosis, *N Engl J Med* 354:2667, 2006.

Gabrielli A et al: Scleroderma, *N Engl J Med* 360:1989-2003, 2009.

Hinchcliff M, Varga J: Systemic sclerosis/scleroderma: a treatable multisystem disease, *Am Fam Physician* 78(8):961-968, 2008.

Tashkin DP et al: Cyclophosphamide versus placebo in scleroderma lung disease, *N Engl J Med* 354:2655, 2006.

AUTHOR: **FRED F. FERRI, M.D.**

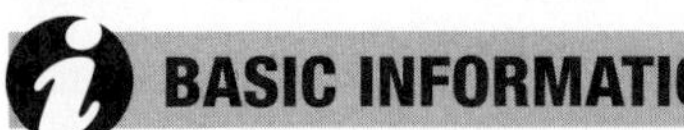

BASIC INFORMATION

DEFINITION

Scoliosis is a lateral curvature of the spine in the upright position, usually 10 degrees or greater. Scoliosis may be classified as either structural (fixed, nonflexible) or nonstructural (flexible, correctable).

ICD-9CM CODES
737.30 Idiopathic scoliosis
737.39 Paralytic scoliosis
754.2 Congenital scoliosis
724.3 Sciatic scoliosis
737.43 Associated with neurofibromatosis

EPIDEMIOLOGY & DEMOGRAPHICS (IDIOPATHIC FORM)

PREDOMINANT SEX: Females are affected more often than males (7:1)
PREVALENCE: Four cases per 1000 persons
PREDOMINANT AGE:
- Onset variable
- Most curves found in adolescents (age ≥11 yr)

PHYSICAL FINDINGS & CLINICAL PRESENTATION

- Record patient age (in years plus months) and height.
- Perform neurologic examination to rule out neuromuscular disease.
- Inspect the shoulders and iliac crests to determine if they are level.
- Palpate the spinous processes to determine their alignment.
- Have the patient bend forward symmetrically at the waist with the arms hanging free (Adams' position); observe from the back or front to detect abnormal spine rotation (Fig. 1-296).

ETIOLOGY

- 90% unknown, usually referred to as *idiopathic* (genetic)
- Congenital spine deformity
- Neuromuscular disease
- Leg-length inequality
- Local inflammation or infection
- Acute pain (disk disease)
- Chronic degenerative disk disease with asymmetric disk narrowing

Curves of an idiopathic nature or those accompanying congenital deformity or neuromuscular disease are associated with structural changes. The nonstructural types (leg-length discrepancy, inflammation, or acute pain) disappear when the offending disorder is corrected.

DIAGNOSIS

WORKUP

- Curvatures associated with congenital spine abnormalities, neuromuscular disease, and other less common forms of scoliosis can usually be identified by history or associated radiographic or physical findings.
- Section III, "Scoliosis," describes an approach to scoliosis screening.

IMAGING STUDIES

- Diagnosis of idiopathic scoliosis is confirmed by a standing roentgenogram of the spine.
- Severity of the curve is measured in degrees, usually by the Cobb method.
- MRI is usually not indicated unless there is pain, a neurologic deficit, or a left thoracic curve (which is often associated with an underlying spinal disorder).

TREATMENT

ACUTE GENERAL Rx

- Treatment or correction of cause if curve is nonstructural
- Early detection is key in treating genetic curve
- Regular observation for curves <20 degrees
- Bracing for idiopathic curves of 20 to 40 degrees to prevent progression
- Surgery for idiopathic curves >40 to 50 degrees in immature patient

DISPOSITION

- The larger the curve at detection, the greater the chance of progression.
- Progression is more common in young children who are beginning their growth spurt.
- Curves in females are more likely to progress.
- Curves <20 degrees will improve spontaneously >50% of the time.
- Failure to diagnose and treat these curves may allow progressive deformity, pain, and cardiopulmonary compromise to develop.
- Spinal deformities >50 degrees in adults may progress and eventually become painful.
- There is no difference in the rate of back pain in the general population and patients with adolescent idiopathic scoliosis.

REFERRAL

For orthopedic consultation if structural curve is present

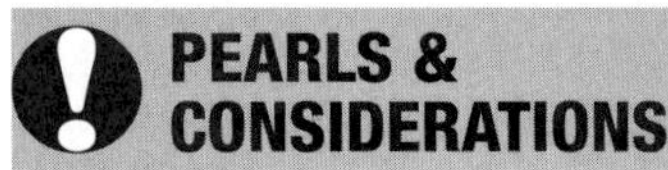

PEARLS & CONSIDERATIONS

COMMENTS

- Congenital scoliosis has a high incidence of cardiac and urinary tract abnormalities.
- Bracing is not intended to completely straighten the idiopathic curve. It may improve the curvature but is mainly used to stabilize and prevent progression.

SUGGESTED READINGS

Davids JR et al: Indications for magnetic resonance imaging in presumed adolescent idiopathic scoliosis, *J Bone Joint Surg Am* 86A:2187, 2004.

Fernandes P, Weinstein SL: Natural history of early onset scoliosis, *J Bone Joint Surg Am* 89A(suppl 1): 21, 2007.

Gillingham BL et al: Early onset idiopathic scoliosis, *J Am Acad Orthop Surg* 14:101, 2006.

Helenius I et al: Long-term health-related quality of life after surgery for adolescent idiopathic scoliosis and spondylolisthesis, *J Bone Joint Surg Am* 90A: 1231, 2008.

Lenke LG, Dobbs MB: Management of juvenile idiopathic scoliosis, *J Bone Joint Surg Am* 89A(suppl 1): 55, 2007.

Richards BS, Vitale MG: Screening for idiopathic scoliosis in adolescents, *J Bone Joint Surg Am* 90A:195, 2008.

Sanders JO et al: Predicting scoliosis progression from skeletal maturity: a simplified classification during adolescence, *J Bone Joint Surg Am* 90A:540, 2008.

Sengupta DK, Webb JK: Scoliosis, the current concepts, *Indian J Orthop* 44(1):5, 2010.

Ugwonali OF et al: Effect of bracing on the quality of life of adolescents with idiopathic scoliosis, *Spine J* 4:254, 2004.

AUTHOR: **LONNIE R. MERCIER, M.D.**

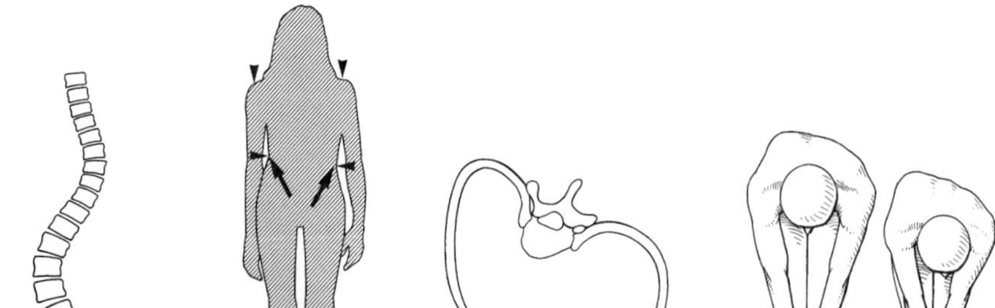

FIGURE 1-296 Structural changes in idiopathic scoliosis. A, As curvature increases, alterations in body configuration develop in both the primary and compensatory curve regions. **B,** Asymmetry of shoulder height, waistline, and the elbow-to-flank distance are common findings. **C,** Vertebral rotation and associated posterior displacement of the ribs on the convex side of the curve are responsible for the characteristic deformity of the chest wall in scoliosis patients. **D,** In the school screening examination for scoliosis, the patient bends forward at the waist. Rib asymmetry of even a small degree is obvious. (From Scoles PV: Spinal deformity in childhood and adolescence. In Behrman RE, Vaughn VC III [eds]: *Nelson textbook of pediatrics*, ed 5, Philadelphia, 1989, WB Saunders.)

BASIC INFORMATION

DEFINITION

Recurrent depressive episodes during autumn and winter alternating with nondepressive episodes during spring and summer. Patients with seasonal affective disorder (SAD) have experienced two episodes of major depression in the last 2 yr that demonstrate the temporal seasonal relations and have had no nonseasonal episodes over this period.

SYNONYMS

Seasonal depression
Winter depression
Wintertime blues

ICD-9CM CODES
296.30 Seasonal affective disorder

EPIDEMIOLOGY & DEMOGRAPHICS

- Climate, genetic vulnerability, and sociocultural factors all play a role. The risk of seasonal mood swings is clearly associated with northern latitudes. The prevalence of SAD is estimated to be 0.5% to 1.5% in northern European populations, but up to 10% to 20% of these populations report milder, recurrent episodes consistent with subsyndromal SAD.
- As with other depressive disorders, women are affected disproportionately compared with men.

PHYSICAL FINDINGS & CLINICAL PRESENTATION

- The symptoms of SAD can be identical to those of other depressive episodes but tend to include features associated with atypical major depression, including low energy, irritability, weight gain, and overeating.
- The average duration of symptoms is 5 mo, generally beginning in November.

ETIOLOGY

- Explanations for the phenomenon of SAD tend to focus on biologic models. The shorter photoperiod and decrease in sunlight exposure experienced by people living in temperate and higher latitudes during the winter are hypothesized to be the main triggers for SAD.
- Several neurotransmitters have been implicated in SAD, including dopamine, serotonin, and norepinephrine. Much current research is focused on the role of serotonin in the mediation of seasonal affective changes.

Dx DIAGNOSIS

Diagnostic workup similar to that for major depression but with a focus on the seasonal nature of the symptoms.

DIFFERENTIAL DIAGNOSIS

- Major depressive disorder
- Minor depression or adjustment disorder
- Bipolar affective disorder
- Evaluate for substance use (especially alcohol)
- Medical illness or medications that may contribute to depression (e.g., endocrine disorders, neurologic disease)

WORKUP

- As with major depression, consider medical etiologies and rule out as indicated by the presenting signs and symptoms. Consider endocrine evaluation, especially thyroid function; sleep studies and a toxicology screen might be considered.
- Structured Interview Guide for the Hamilton Depression Rating Scale-Seasonal Affective Disorders Version (SIGH-SAD) used in research settings.

LABORATORY TESTS

As directed by presenting symptoms

IMAGING STUDIES

Generally not indicated

Rx TREATMENT

NONPHARMACOLOGIC THERAPY

- Phototherapy is based on the principle that the presentation of artificial light at a similar strength to natural sunlight will prevent the biologic changes that mediate SAD during the winter.
- There have been at least 20 randomized trials comparing light treatment with placebo in the treatment of SAD. Some of these trials have found a benefit; others have been unable to demonstrate a benefit over placebo.
- Phototherapy for SAD tends to use 2500 to 10,000 lux delivered by a commercial light box or a portable head-mounted unit. Phototherapy is recommended to begin within 2 wk of the start of symptoms and continue through the winter months. Patients are instructed to sit approximately 18 inches away from the light box for 30 min up to several hours once or twice per day for a minimum of 1 wk.

ACUTE GENERAL Rx

None necessary unless patient is suicidal; immediate hospitalization may be necessary if suicidal ideation and intent are present.

CHRONIC Rx

There is no conclusive evidence from randomized trials to support the use of selective serotonin reuptake inhibitors in the treatment of SAD.

DISPOSITION

Psychiatric referral may be helpful to confirm diagnosis. Recommended for high-risk and suicidal patients.

REFERRAL

For active suicidal ideation, psychosis, symptoms suggestive of bipolar disorder

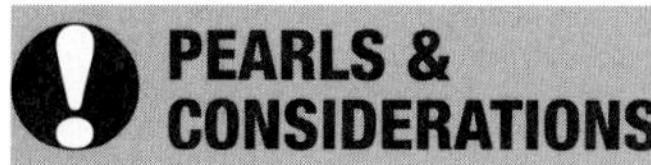

Patients with SAD may present with a complaint of overeating, particularly food high in carbohydrates.

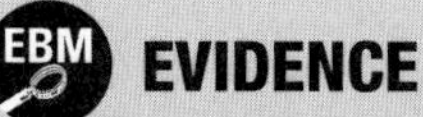

A small randomized, controlled trial (RCT) compared light-box treatment with dawn simulation in patients with winter depression. Improvement in symptoms was noted in both groups, but there was significantly greater improvement in the light-box group. The majority of patients in both treatment groups maintained improvement at 9-wk follow-up.[1] Ⓑ

An RCT compared fluoxetine with placebo over 5 wk in patients with SAD. The rate of clinical response ($\geq$50% reduction in depression score between baseline and study termination) was greater in the fluoxetine group.[2] Ⓑ

Evidence-Based References

1. Lingjaerde O et al: Dawn simulation vs. lightbox treatment in winter depression: a comparative study, *Acta Psychiatr Scand* 98:73, 1998. Ⓑ

2. Lam RW et al: Multicenter, placebo-controlled study of fluoxetine in seasonal affective disorder, *Am J Psychiatry* 152:1765, 1995. Ⓑ

SUGGESTED READINGS

Golden RN et al: The efficacy of light therapy in the treatment of mood disorders: a review and meta-analysis of the evidence, *Am J Psychiatry* 162(4):656, 2005.

Lurie SJ et al: Seasonal affective disorder, *Am Fam Physician* 74(9):1521-1524, 2006.

Rohan KJ et al: A randomized controlled trial of cognitive-behavioral therapy, light therapy, and their combination for seasonal affective disorder, *J Consult Clin Psychol* 75(3):489, 2007.

Westrin A, Lam RW: Seasonal affective disorder: a clinical update, *Ann Clin Psychiatry* 19(4):239, 2007.

AUTHOR: **MITCHELL D. FELDMAN, M.D., M.PHIL.**

Seborrheic Dermatitis (SD) (PTG)

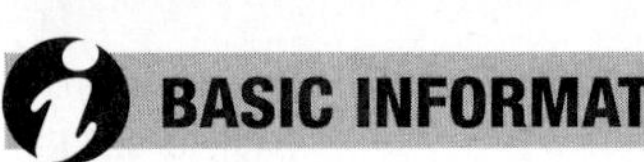

BASIC INFORMATION

DEFINITION

Mild to severe rash characterized by scaling and erythema that occurs in areas of the skin rich in sebaceous glands.

SYNONYMS

Dandruff
Cradle cap
Sebopsoriasis
Seborrheic eczema
Pityriasis capitis

ICD-9CM CODES
690.10 Seborrheic dermatitis

EPIDEMIOLOGY & DEMOGRAPHICS

PREVALENCE: Affects between 1% and 3% of otherwise healthy adults.
PREDOMINANT SEX AND AGE: Can occur from infancy through old age, with peak incidence in adolescents and young adults and increasing again after age 50 yr. More common in men than women.
RISK FACTORS: More common in patients with HIV/AIDS, Parkinson's disease, other neurologic disorders, mood disorders, chronic alcoholic pancreatitis, hepatitis, cancer, and genetic disorders (e.g., Down syndrome). Occurs more often during winter season.

PHYSICAL FINDINGS & CLINICAL PRESENTATION

Mild, greasy scaling of the scalp and nasolabial folds, postauricular skin, beard area, eyebrows, trunk and sometimes the central face. Blepharitis, otitis externa and coexisting acne vulgaris or pityriasis may also be present. Itching and stinging of lesions can occur. Increased occurrence during times of stress or sleep deprivation.

ETIOLOGY

Actual etiology is unknown but has been linked to hormone levels, fungal infections, altered immune function, nutritional deficits, and neurogenic factors. Fungal infections of the *Malassezia* species have been associated with SD.

DIAGNOSIS

DIFFERENTIAL DIAGNOSIS

- Atopic dermatitis
- Candidiasis
- Dermatophytosis
- Langerhans cell histiocytosis
- Psoriasis
- Rosacea
- Systemic lupus erythematosus
- Tinea infection

WORKUP

- Diagnosis usually based on clinical identification of lesions
- Skin biopsies can be performed, if warranted, to distinguish SD from similar disorders

LABORATORY TESTS

Microscopic examination with special stains can be used to determine if yeast cells are present in keratinocytes

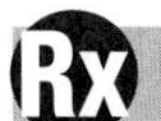

TREATMENT

- Treatment of SD is aimed at resolving lesions but does not prevent recurrence.
- General recommendations: wash skin regularly, soften and remove scales, and apply moisturizing emollients after washing.

ACUTE GENERAL Rx

- Topical steroids: can be in the form of shampoos, creams, or ointments
- Calcineurin inhibitors (e.g., tacrolimus ointment, pimecrolimus cream): good when face and ears are affected
- Keratolytics (e.g., tar, salicylic acid, zinc pyrithione)
- Antifungals (e.g., Nizoral, selenium sulfide, ketoconazole, terbinafine, ciclopirox, fluconazole)

CHRONIC Rx

Recalcitrant seborrheic dermatitis: topical azole combined with desonide regimen (limit use to 2 wk)

COMPLEMENTARY & ALTERNATIVE MEDICINE

Tea tree oil (Melaleuca oil)

REFERRAL

Consider referral to dermatology for recalcitrant cases

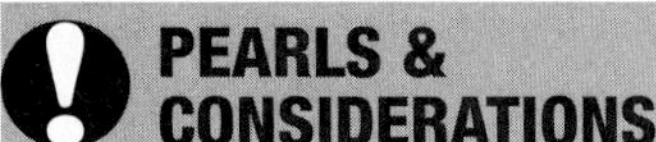

PEARLS & CONSIDERATIONS

- Reserve oral therapy for patients with widespread SD or SD that is refractory to topical therapy. Itraconazole 200 mg/day for 7 days is a sample oral regimen.
- Limit use of steroids to 2-wk course of treatment due to risk of cutaneous atrophy and telangiectasias
- SD of the scalp can be treated with an antifungal (e.g., 2% ketoconazole) or keratolytic shampoo

SUGGESTED READINGS

Finnish Medical Society Duodecim: Seborrhoeic dermatitis. In *EBM Guidelines. Evidence-based medicine,* Helsinki, Finland, 2007, Wiley Interscience.

Gupta AK et al: Seborrheic dermatitis, *J Eur Acad Dermatol Venereol* 18:13-26, 2004.

Naldi L, Rebora A: Seborrheic dermatitis, *N Engl J Med* 360:387-396, 2009.

Schwartz RA et al: Seborrheic dermatitis: an overview, *Am Fam Physician* 74:125-130, 2006.

AUTHOR: **ANNGENE GIUSTOZZI, M.D., M.P.H.**

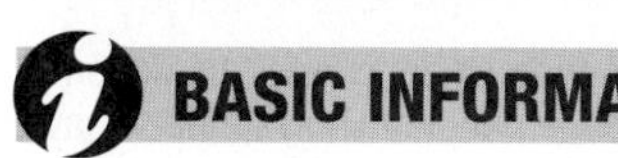

BASIC INFORMATION

DEFINITION

Absence seizures are a type of generalized nonconvulsive seizure characterized by episodes of loss of awareness (typically ≤3 to 15 sec) associated with a 3-Hz generalized spike and slow-wave electroencephalographic (EEG) pattern, followed by abrupt return to full consciousness.

SYNONYMS

Petit mal seizures (obsolete)
Childhood absence epilepsy

ICD-9CM CODES
345.0 Generalized nonconvulsive epilepsy

EPIDEMIOLOGY & DEMOGRAPHICS

INCIDENCE (IN U.S.): Two to 10 cases per 100,000 persons from ages 1 to 10 yr; rare after age 14 yr
PEAK INCIDENCE: Ages 6 to 7 yr
PREVALENCE (IN U.S.): Accounts for 2% to 15% of cases of childhood epilepsy
PREDOMINANT AGE: 4 to 8 yr
PREDOMINANT SEX: Some studies suggest a female predominance
GENETICS: Clear genetic predisposition; undetermined mode of inheritance

PHYSICAL FINDINGS & CLINICAL PRESENTATION

- Findings are normal between seizures in children with typical absence epilepsy.
- During seizure, patient typically appears awake but abruptly ceases ongoing activity and does not respond to or recall stimuli.
- More prolonged episodes may be associated with automatisms and therefore mistaken for complex partial seizures.
- Tonic-clonic seizures can occur in approximately 40% of patients.

ETIOLOGY

- Idiopathic with a presumed genetic cause
- Absence seizures can also be seen with some types of generalized epilepsy syndromes such as juvenile absence epilepsy or juvenile myoclonic epilepsy
- Experimental data: seizures arise from impaired regulation of rhythmic thalamic discharges

Dx DIAGNOSIS

DIFFERENTIAL DIAGNOSIS

- Complex partial seizures
- Daydreaming
- Psychogenic unresponsiveness

WORKUP

- EEG is the most powerful tool for identification of this seizure type.
- In the majority of untreated individuals, vigorous hyperventilation for 3 to 5 min provokes the characteristic EEG finding.

IMAGING STUDIES

None needed for typical presentation

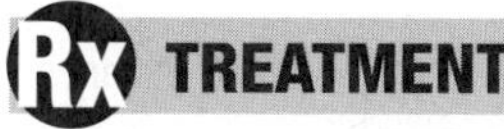

TREATMENT

NONPHARMACOLOGIC THERAPY

Avoid sleep deprivation and hyperventilation.

ACUTE GENERAL Rx

Not indicated for individual typical seizures

CHRONIC Rx

- Drug of choice is ethosuximide or valproate.
- Ethosuximide does not suppress tonic-clonic seizures. Thus valproate is the drug of choice for patients with absence and tonic-clonic seizures.
- In patients with childbearing potential, valproate should be used with caution because of the high risk of adverse fetal effects; lamotrigine may be preferred.
- The initial dose of ethosuximide in children is 10 to 15 mg/kg/day with maintenance dose of 15 to 40 mg/kg/day divided into a bid or tid dosing schedule. Can result in gastrointestinal side effects, so it may be best to take the drug with meals.
- Common pediatric doses for valproate are 15 to 60 mg/kg/day (bid to qid). Can result in hepatotoxicity and blood dyscrasias.
- Lamotrigine is also effective but is not FDA approved for the treatment of absence epilepsy.
- Because most patients will have spontaneous resolution of their seizures, one can consider withdrawing anticonvulsant therapy typically when the patient has been seizure free for at least 2 yr.

DISPOSITION

- Favorable prognosis in typical childhood absence epilepsy without other seizure types
- Excellent response to medication
- Subsidence of seizures with advancing age in 70% to 90% of patients

REFERRAL

If uncertain about diagnosis or treatment

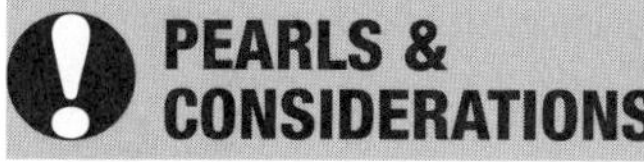

PEARLS & CONSIDERATIONS

COMMENTS

- Absence seizures may be mistakenly diagnosed as complex partial seizures based on clinical descriptions. The EEG is essential for making this distinction.
- Administering other anticonvulsants (particularly carbamazepine or phenytoin) to patients with typical absence epilepsy may exacerbate seizures.
- Patient education information can be obtained from the Epilepsy Foundation, 4351 Garden City Drive, Landover, MD 20785; 800-332-1000; http://www.epilepsyfoundation.org.

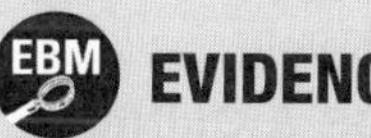

EVIDENCE

A systematic review assessing the efficacy of valproate, ethosuximide, and lamotrigine in the treatment of absence seizures in children and adolescents found insufficient evidence to guide clinical practice because of the poor methodologic quality of the included trials.[1]

Evidence-Based Reference

1. Posner EB et al: Ethosuximide, sodium valproate or lamotrigine for absence seizures in children and adolescents, *Cochrane Rev* 3, 2003.

SUGGESTED READINGS

Bourgeois BF: Chronic management of seizures in the syndromes of idiopathic generalized epilepsy, *Epilepsia* 44(2):27, 2003.

French JA et al: Efficacy and tolerability of the new antiepileptic drugs I: treatment of new onset epilepsy, *Neurology* 62:1252, 2004.

Glauser TA et al: Ethosuximide, valproic acid, and lamotrigine in childhood absence epilepsy, *N Engl J Med* 362:790-799, 2010.

Mattson RH: Overview: idiopathic generalized epilepsies, *Epilepsia* 44(2):2, 2003.

Panayiotopoulos CP: Treatment of typical absence seizures and related epileptic syndromes, *Paediatr Drugs* 3(5):379, 2001.

AUTHORS: **JOHN E. CROOM, M.D., PH.D.,** and **WILLIAM H. HEWITT, M.D.**

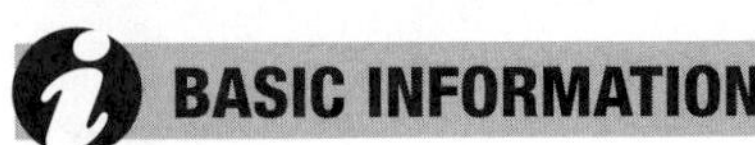

DEFINITION

A febrile seizure is a seizure in infancy or childhood, usually occurring between ages 6 mo and 5 yr, associated with fever but without evidence of intracranial infection or defined cause.

SYNONYMS

Benign febrile seizure
Febrile convulsions

ICD-9CM CODES
780.3 Convulsions

EPIDEMIOLOGY & DEMOGRAPHICS

PREVALENCE (IN U.S.): 2% to 5% in children aged 6 mo to 5 yr
PREDOMINANT SEX: Males are affected more often than females
PREDOMINANT AGE: Most commonly at age 6 mo to 5 yr
GENETICS:
- Family history increases risk
- Mode of inheritance unknown

PHYSICAL FINDINGS & CLINICAL PRESENTATION

- Typically occurs early in the course of an illness when temperature is rising.
- Febrile seizures can be either simple or complex.
- Simple febrile seizures are single events lacking focality and lasting <15 min. The children are neurologically normal and there are no persistent deficits after the seizure.
- Complex febrile seizures have a duration >15 min.
- Symptomatic febrile seizures mean that the child has an underlying neurologic abnormality or acute neurologic illness.
- Children with febrile seizures are at greater than normal risk of later developing epilepsy.

ETIOLOGY

Unknown, though genetics appears to play a role.

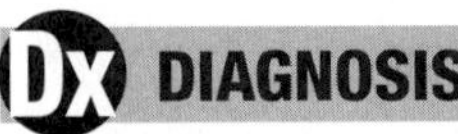

DIFFERENTIAL DIAGNOSIS

- Epilepsy
- Meningitis
- Encephalitis
- Brain abscess

WORKUP

- In children with simple febrile seizures, no further evaluation is usually required.
- In children with complex febrile seizures, investigation is recommended.

LABORATORY TESTS

- Lumbar puncture is indicated in all children <12 mo, in children with complex febrile seizures, or if signs or symptoms of meningitis are present.
- Complex febrile seizures may warrant electroencephalography, toxicology screening, assessment of electrolytes, and neuroimaging depending on history and examination findings.

IMAGING STUDIES

Not needed in simple febrile seizures

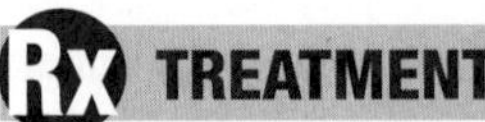

NONPHARMACOLOGIC THERAPY

- Avoid excessive clothing.
- Encourage fluids.
- Apply tepid sponge bath to control fever.

ACUTE GENERAL Rx

- Antipyretics.
- Possibly rectal diazepam in some instances of recurrent febrile seizures.
- For prolonged seizures, can use parenteral diazepam or lorazepam.
- Febrile status epilepticus should be treated as a medical emergency (see "Status Epilepticus" in Section I).

CHRONIC Rx

- Prophylactic treatment with anticonvulsants is not indicated in children with typical simple febrile seizures.
- Phenobarbital and valproate have been shown to prevent recurrence of febrile seizures, but no drug has been shown to alter the subsequent risk of developing afebrile seizures or epilepsy. Because of the high rate of associated adverse drug effects and the generally benign nature of simple febrile seizures, neither drug is indicated for chronic prophylactic therapy.
- May consider anticonvulsant use in children with complex febrile seizures, but risks and benefits must be considered.

DISPOSITION

- Approximately one third of patients will have additional febrile seizures. Less than 6% of patients will have three or more febrile seizures.
- Independent predictors of febrile seizure recurrence include (1) young age at onset (particularly <1 yr), (2) history of first-degree relative with febrile seizures, (3) low degree of fever while in the emergency department, and (4) brief interval between fever onset and seizure presentation.
- Available data show no risk reduction with prophylactic anticonvulsants.

REFERRAL

If uncertain about diagnosis or with atypical presentation

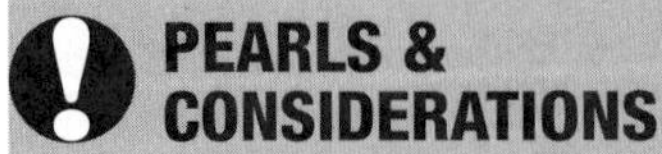

COMMENTS

Febrile seizures typically occur early in the course of a fever. Often the febrile seizure occurs before the fever is noticed by the patient's caregivers, and the patient is only found to have a fever after the seizure has occurred.

CAUTION

A child who presents with a seizure after having been febrile for more than a day should be considered to have encephalitis until proven otherwise and should undergo a workup for meningoencephalitis, including lumbar puncture.

Randomized, controlled trials have found that in children with febrile seizures, diazepam given during febrile illnesses, daily phenobarbital, and daily valproate are each effective at reducing the risk of recurrent febrile seizures. However, phenobarbital was not found to be effective at reducing the incidence of subsequent afebrile seizures or epilepsy in children with febrile seizures.[1-7] Data are lacking for other antiepileptic drugs.

Evidence-Based References

1. Rosman NP et al: A controlled trial of diazepam administered during febrile illnesses to prevent recurrence of febrile seizures, *N Engl J Med* 329(2):79-84, 1993.
2. Camfield PR et al: The first febrile seizure—antipyretic instruction plus either phenobarbital or placebo to prevent recurrence, *J Pediatr* 97(1):16-21, 1980.
3. Bacon CJ et al: Placebo-controlled study of phenobarbitone and phenytoin in the prophylaxis of febrile convulsions, *Lancet* 19;2(8247):600-604, 1981.
4. Mamelle N et al: Prevention of recurrent febrile convulsions—a randomized therapeutic assay: sodium valproate, phenobarbital and placebo, *Neuropediatrics* 15(1):37-42, 1984.
5. Ngwane E, Bower B: Continuous sodium valproate or phenobarbitone in the prevention of 'simple' febrile convulsions. Comparison by a double-blind trial, *Arch Dis Child* 55(3):171-174, 1980.
6. Wolf SM et al: The value of phenobarbital in the child who has had a single febrile seizure: a controlled prospective study, *Pediatrics* 59(3):378-385, 1977.
7. Wolf SM, Forsythe A: Epilepsy and mental retardation following febrile seizures in childhood, *Acta Paediatr Scand* 78(2):291-295, 1989.

SUGGESTED READINGS

Baumann RJ: Prevention and management of febrile seizures, *Paediatr Drugs* 3(8):585, 2001.
Knudsen FU: Febrile seizures: treatment and prognosis, *Epilepsia* 41(1):2, 2000.
Shinnar S, Glauser TA: Febrile seizures, *J Child Neurol* 17(suppl 1):S44, 2002.
Waruiru C, Appleton R: Febrile seizures: an update, *Arch Dis Child* 89(8):751-756, 2004.

AUTHORS: **JOHN E. CROOM, M.D., PH.D.,** and **WILLIAM H. HEWITT, M.D.**

BASIC INFORMATION

DEFINITION

Generalized tonic-clonic seizures (GTCS) are marked by paroxysmal hypersynchronous neuronal activity involving both cerebral hemispheres and resulting in loss of consciousness with tonic muscle contraction followed by rhythmic clonic contractions. The seizure may start focally in one region or hemisphere of the brain with subsequent or secondary generalization.

SYNONYMS

Grand mal seizure (obsolete)

ICD-9CM CODES

345.1 Generalized convulsive epilepsy

EPIDEMIOLOGY & DEMOGRAPHICS

INCIDENCE (IN U.S.): 50 to 70 cases per 100,000 persons annually, with the highest rates during early childhood and in those aged >65 yr. The incidence varies depending on the population reported.

PREVALENCE (IN U.S.): Approximately 6.5 cases per 1000 persons for all types of epilepsy.

PREDOMINANT SEX: Males are affected slightly more often than females.

GENETICS: Genetic predisposition exists for the idiopathic generalized epilepsies; mode of transmission varies with the particular epilepsy syndrome.

PHYSICAL FINDINGS & CLINICAL PRESENTATION

- Generally normal neurologic examination. Focal deficits may be found in patients with an underlying lesion causing the seizures.
- Sequence of motor events during the seizure typically includes widespread tonic muscle contraction evolving to clonic jerking.
- Typically associated with postictal confusion lasting for minutes up to several hours.
- May be associated with tongue, cheek, or lip biting or urinary incontinence.

ETIOLOGY

- Seizures are a symptom of an underlying abnormality affecting the central nervous system (CNS).
- Etiology of GTCS can be divided into idiopathic, symptomatic, or cryptogenic causes.
- With idiopathic GTCS, there is no underlying cause other than a postulated inherited predisposition for the disorder. This includes some epilepsy syndromes such as juvenile myoclonic epilepsy and epilepsy with tonic-clonic seizures on awakening.
- Symptomatic GTCS result from an underlying cause, such as inborn errors of metabolism, acquired metabolic or toxic abnormalities, CNS infection, tumor, or trauma.
- Cryptogenic seizures have an occult underlying cause and are presumed to be symptomatic.

DIAGNOSIS

DIFFERENTIAL DIAGNOSIS

- Syncope
- Psychogenic events

Section II describes the differential diagnosis of epilepsy.

WORKUP

New-onset seizures: a detailed history and physical examination with the goal of determining the underlying etiology

LABORATORY TESTS

- Serum glucose and electrolytes
- Additional blood studies and lumbar puncture as indicated by history and physical examination
- Electroencephalography (EEG): most valuable diagnostic tool for identifying seizure type and predicting the likelihood of recurrence

IMAGING STUDIES

- Generally not necessary in well-documented cases of idiopathic GTCS
- MRI: modality of choice if history, examination, or EEG suggests partial (focal) onset

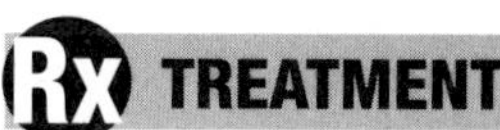

TREATMENT

NONPHARMACOLOGIC THERAPY

Avoid sleep deprivation or environmental precipitants (e.g., photosensitive epilepsy).

ACUTE GENERAL Rx

- Individual seizures lasting <5 min generally require no acute pharmacologic intervention.
- See "Status Epilepticus" in Section I for management of recurrent or prolonged seizures.

CHRONIC Rx

- A single seizure with an identifiable and easily correctable provoking factor (e.g., hyponatremia) does not warrant long-term use of anticonvulsants.
- If there is significant risk of recurrence (Table 1-71) or more than one unprovoked seizure, treatment is indicated.
- Sodium valproate, phenytoin, and carbamazepine are common first-line therapeutic agents in adults but are limited by significant adverse side effects.
- Newer agents such as lamotrigine, topiramate, oxcarbazepine, zonisamide, gabapentin, levetiracetam, and pregabalin may be better tolerated.
- For each patient, anticonvulsant choice is influenced by factors such as effectiveness, cost, adverse effects, ease of administration, and type of epilepsy syndrome if present.

DISPOSITION

- Varies with underlying etiology
- Excellent outcome for most patients with idiopathic GTCS

REFERRAL

If uncertain about diagnosis or seizure type or if the seizures fail to respond to anticonvulsant treatment. Also refer if the patient is considering pregnancy.

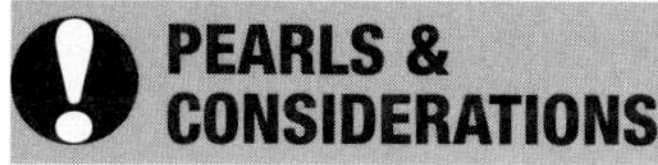

PEARLS & CONSIDERATIONS

CAUTION

EEG is normal in as many as 50% of patients; thus diagnosis is primarily by history. A single seizure is usually not treated with long-term anticonvulsants unless the patient has an epilepsy syndrome in which the seizure recurrence is known to be high.

COMMENTS

Patient education information can be obtained from the Epilepsy Foundation, 4351 Garden City Drive, Landover, MD 20785; 800-332-1000; http://www.epilepsyfoundation.org.

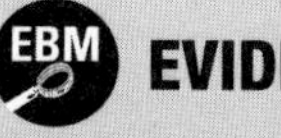

EVIDENCE

Immediate treatment of a single GTCS with antiepileptic drugs reduces the risk of relapse but does not appear to alter the probability of achieving remission from seizures.[1,2]

No placebo-controlled trials have evaluated the classic antiepileptic drugs (phenytoin, valproate, carbamazepine, and phenobarbital) in the treatment of newly diagnosed

TABLE 1-71 Risk of Recurrence After a First Tonic-Clonic Seizure

High	Low
Abnormal neurologic findings	Febrile seizure in a child
Mental retardation	Febrile status epilepticus (child)
Abnormal electroencephalographic findings	Transient metabolic and toxic states
Myoclonic jerks, absences, or atonic seizures	Benign rolandic seizures
Structural brain lesions	Impact seizures in early nonsevere head trauma
Family history of epilepsy	
Elderly individuals	

From Johnson RT, Griffin JW: *Current therapy in neurologic disease,* ed 5, St Louis, 1997, Mosby.

epilepsy, but decades of experience with their use and widespread consensus hold them to be effective. Systematic reviews have found no evidence on which to base the choice of which drug to use.[3]

Lamotrigine, topiramate, and oxcarbazepine have each been found to be as effective as a classic antiepileptic drug in monotherapy for epilepsy with GTCS.[4-10]

Evidence-Based References

1. First Seizure Trial Group (FIRST Group): Randomized clinical trial on the efficacy of antiepileptic drugs in reducing the risk of relapse after a first unprovoked tonic clonic seizure, *Neurology* 43:478-483, 1993.
2. Musicco M et al for the FIRST group: Treatment of first tonic clonic seizure does not improve the prognosis of epilepsy, *Neurology* 49:991-998, 1997.
3. Marson A, Ramaratnam S: Epilepsy, *Clin Evid* 11: 1655-1673, 2004.
4. Brodie MJ et al: Multicentre, double-blind, randomised comparison between lamotrigine and carbamazepine in elderly patients with newly diagnosed epilepsy. The UK Lamotrigine Elderly Study Group, *Epilepsy Res* 37:81-87, 1999.
5. Brodie MJ et al: Double-blind comparison of lamotrigine and carbamazepine in newly diagnosed epilepsy. UK Lamotrigine/Carbamazepine Monotherapy Trial Group, *Lancet* 345:476-479, 1995.
6. Steiner TJ et al: Lamotrigine monotherapy in newly diagnosed untreated epilepsy: a double-blind comparison with phenytoin, *Epilepsia* 40:601-607, 1999.
7. Privitera MD et al: Topiramate, carbamazepine and valproate monotherapy: double-blind comparison in newly diagnosed epilepsy, *Acta Neurol Scand* 107:165-175, 2003.
8. Bill PA et al: A double-blind controlled clinical trial of oxcarbazepine versus phenytoin in adults with previously untreated epilepsy, *Epilepsy Res* 27:195-204, 1997.
9. Christe W et al: A double-blind controlled clinical trial: oxcarbazepine versus sodium valproate in adults with newly diagnosed epilepsy, *Epilepsy Res* 26:451-460, 1997.
10. Dam M et al: A double-blind study comparing oxcarbazepine and carbamazepine in patients with newly diagnosed, previously untreated epilepsy, *Epilepsy Res* 3:70-76, 1989.

SUGGESTED READINGS

Browne TR, Holmes GL: Epilepsy, *N Engl J Med* 344: 1145, 2001.

Chang BS, Lowenstein DH: Mechanisms of disease: epilepsy, *N Engl J Med* 349:1257, 2003.

French JA et al: Efficacy and tolerability of the new antiepileptic drugs I: treatment of new onset epilepsy, *Neurology* 62:1252-1260, 2004.

French JA et al: Efficacy and tolerability of the new antiepileptic drugs II: treatment of refractory epilepsy, *Neurology* 62:1261-1273, 2004.

French JA, Pedley TA: Initial management of epilepsy, *N Engl J Med* 359:166-176, 2008.

AUTHORS: **JOHN E. CROOM, M.D., PH.D.,** and **WILLIAM H. HEWITT, M.D.**

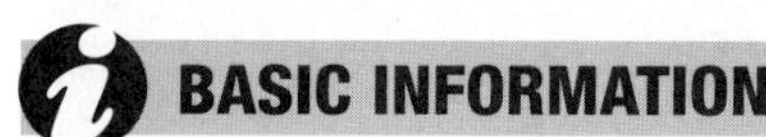

BASIC INFORMATION

DEFINITION

In partial seizures, the onset of abnormal electrical activity originates in a focal region or lobe of the brain. Clinical manifestations may involve sensory, motor, autonomic, or psychic symptoms. Consciousness may be preserved (simple partial seizures) or impaired (complex partial seizures).

SYNONYMS

Localization-related seizures
Focal epilepsy

ICD-9CM CODES
345.4 Partial epilepsy, with impairment of consciousness
345.5 Partial epilepsy, without impairment of consciousness

EPIDEMIOLOGY & DEMOGRAPHICS

INCIDENCE (IN U.S.): 20 cases per 100,000 persons through age 65 yr; incidence then rises sharply.

PREVALENCE (IN U.S.): 6.5 cases per 1000 persons for all types of epilepsy.

PREDOMINANT SEX: Males are affected slightly more often than females.

GENETICS: Most are acquired, but several distinct inherited syndromes have been identified.

PHYSICAL FINDINGS & CLINICAL PRESENTATION

- Range from normal to focal neurologic deficits depending on underlying cause.
- Clinical presentation is varied and depends on the site of origin of the abnormal electrical discharges.
- Symptoms of simple partial seizures can include focal motor or sensory symptoms; language disturbance; olfactory, visual, or auditory hallucinations; visceral sensations; or fear or panic.
- With complex partial seizures, there is a loss or reduction of awareness. This may be preceded by an aura (simple partial seizure). There may be associated automatisms or alterations in behavior.
- There may be a relatively quick "march" or progression of symptoms over seconds to minutes as the ictal focus spreads along the cortex.

ETIOLOGY

- Seizures are a symptom of an underlying abnormality affecting the central nervous system (CNS), not a disease.
- Partial-onset seizures may be caused by underlying disorders, including stroke, tumor, infection, trauma, vascular malformations, or genetic factors.

Dx DIAGNOSIS

DIFFERENTIAL DIAGNOSIS

- Migraine
- Transient ischemic attack
- Presyncope
- Psychogenic phenomena

WORKUP

Because partial seizures are manifestations of an underlying focal CNS disturbance that must be identified if possible, imaging studies, preferably MRI, are essential.

LABORATORY TESTS

Electroencephalography (EEG) is the most powerful tool for localization of the seizure focus (Fig. 1-297).

IMAGING STUDIES

- MRI with contrast: modality of choice because of its high sensitivity for stroke, tumor, abscess, atrophy, and vascular malformations

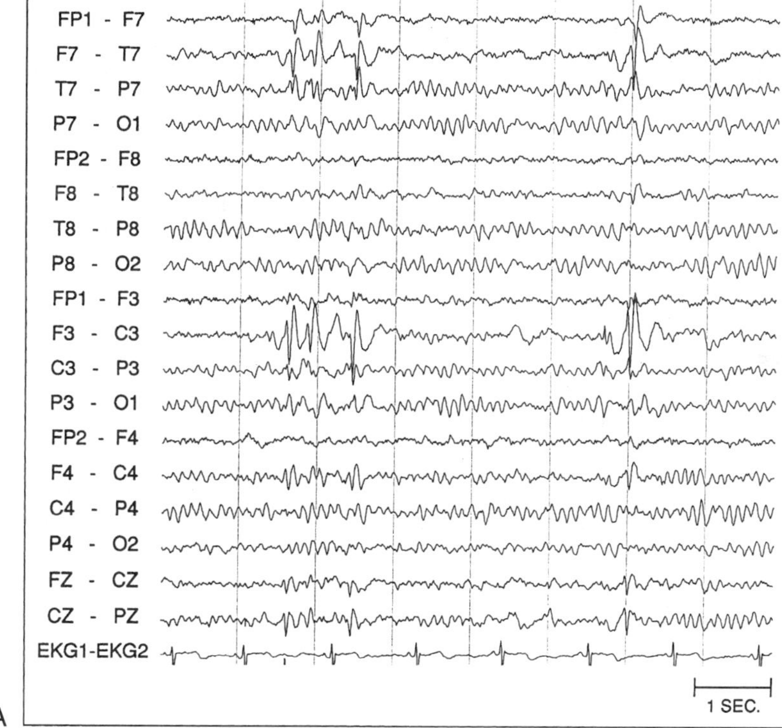

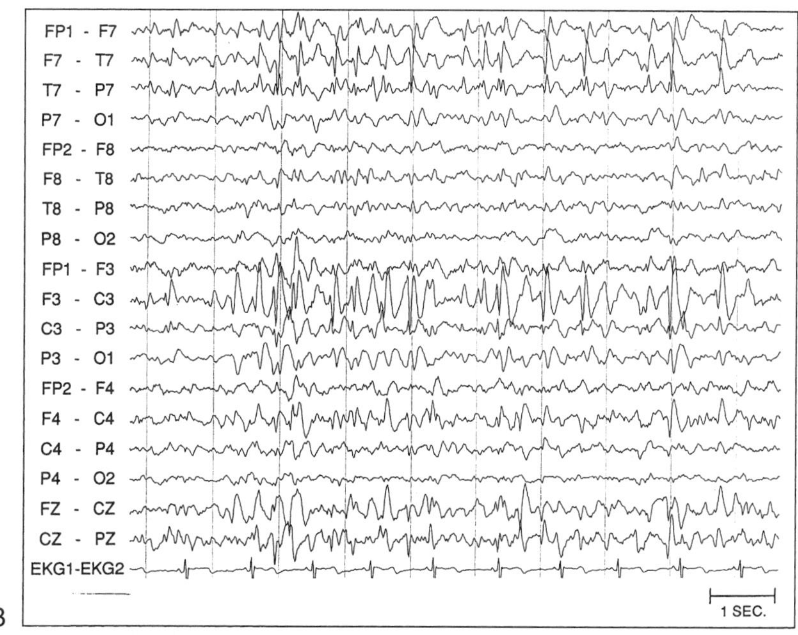

FIGURE 1-297 Benign rolandic epilepsy. Electroencephalograms (EEGs) from a 9-year-old boy with a history of nocturnal generalized tonic-clonic seizures that responded well to antiepileptic drugs. **A,** EEG from the awake background with several sharp waves in the left centrotemporal region. This distribution is typical for benign rolandic epilepsy, but it is not diagnostic for rolandic epilepsy, because other entities such as structural lesions can present with similar spiking. If the clinical history is appropriate, however, the best clinical correlation of these waveforms would be rolandic epilepsy. **B,** There is significant activation of the EEG spiking in sleep. The discharges are often quite continuous. The patients are usually asymptomatic at this time. This fascinating disorder may have a genetic component, and is almost always resolved by the age of 16. If seizures occur they can include simple partial motor seizures of the lower face and generalized tonic-clonic seizures. (From Rosenberg RN: *Atlas of clinical neurology,* Boston, 1998, Butterworth-Heinemann.)

 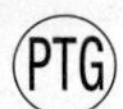

- CT scan without contrast if hemorrhage is suspected

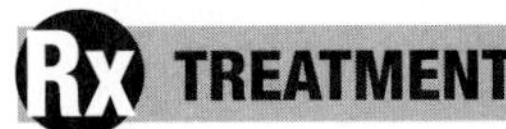

TREATMENT

NONPHARMACOLOGIC THERAPY

Avoid sleep deprivation.

ACUTE GENERAL Rx

Individual seizures lasting <5 min generally require no acute pharmacologic intervention.

CHRONIC Rx

- Sodium valproate, phenytoin, and carbamazepine are common first-line therapeutic agents in adults but are limited by significant adverse side effects.
- Newer agents such as lamotrigine, topiramate, oxcarbazepine, zonisamide, gabapentin, levetiracetam, and pregabalin may be better tolerated.
- For each patient, anticonvulsant choice is influenced by factors such as effectiveness, cost, adverse effects, and ease of administration.

DISPOSITION

- Determined by underlying cause.
- Approximately 70% of patients are controlled with medication.

REFERRAL

If uncertain about diagnosis or patient does not respond to appropriate medication, refer to a neurologist or epilepsy specialist for further evaluation. In addition, some types of partial seizures, particularly temporal lobe epilepsy, are amenable to surgical resection.

PEARLS & CONSIDERATIONS

COMMENTS

- Patient education information can be obtained from the Epilepsy Foundation of America, 4351 Garden City Drive, Landover, MD 20785; 800-332-1000; http://www.epilepsyfoundation.org.
- This is the most underdiagnosed, yet the most common, type of seizure in adults.

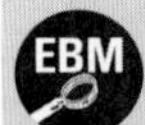

EVIDENCE

No placebo-controlled trials have evaluated the classic antiepileptic drugs (phenytoin, valproate, carbamazepine, and phenobarbital) in the treatment of newly diagnosed epilepsy, but decades of experience with their use and widespread consensus hold them to be effective. Systematic reviews have found no evidence on which to base the choice of which drug to use.[1]

Lamotrigine, topiramate, oxcarbazepine, and gabapentin have each been found to be as effective as a classic antiepileptic drug in monotherapy for epilepsy.[2-9]

Evidence-Based References

1. Marson A, Ramaratnam S: Epilepsy, *Clin Evid* 11: 1655-1673, 2004.

2. Brodie MJ, Overstall PW, Giorgi L: Multicentre, double-blind, randomised comparison between lamotrigine and carbamazepine in elderly patients with newly diagnosed epilepsy. The UK Lamotrigine Elderly Study Group, *Epilepsy Res* 37:81-87, 1999.

3. Brodie MJ, Richens A, Yuen AWC: Double-blind comparison of lamotrigine and carbamazepine in newly diagnosed epilepsy, *Lancet* 345:476-479, 1995.

4. Steiner TJ et al: Lamotrigine monotherapy in newly diagnosed untreated epilepsy: a double-blind comparison with phenytoin, *Epilepsia* 40:601-607, 1999.

5. Privitera MD, Brodie MJ, Mattson RH: Topiramate, carbamazepine and valproate monotherapy: double-blind comparison in newly diagnosed epilepsy, *Acta Neurol Scand* 107:165-175, 2003.

6. Bill PA et al: A double-blind controlled clinical trial of oxcarbazepine versus phenytoin in adults with previously untreated epilepsy, *Epilepsy Res* 27: 195-204, 1997.

7. Christe W et al: A double-blind controlled clinical trial: oxcarbazepine versus sodium valproate in adults with newly diagnosed epilepsy, *Epilepsy Res* 26:451-460, 1997.

8. Dam M et al: A double-blind study comparing oxcarbazepine and carbamazepine in patients with newly diagnosed, previously untreated epilepsy, *Epilepsy Res* 3:70-76, 1989.

9. van Walderveen MAA et al: Histopathologic correlate of hypointense lesions on T1-weighted spin-echo MRI in multiple sclerosis, *Neurology* 51:1282-1288, 1998.

SUGGESTED READINGS

Browne TR, Holmes GL: Epilepsy, *N Engl J Med* 344: 1145, 2001.

Chang BS, Lowenstein DH: Mechanisms of disease: epilepsy, *N Engl J Med* 349:1257, 2003.

French JA et al: Efficacy and tolerability of the new antiepileptic drugs I: treatment of new onset epilepsy, *Neurology* 62:1252-1260, 2004.

French JA et al: Efficacy and tolerability of the new antiepileptic drugs II: treatment of refractory epilepsy, *Neurology* 62:1261-1273, 2004.

AUTHORS: **JOHN E. CROOM, M.D., PH.D.,** and **WILLIAM H. HEWITT, M.D.**

BASIC INFORMATION

DEFINITION

Septicemia is a systemic illness caused by generalized bacterial or fungal infection and characterized by evidence of infection, fever or hypothermia, hypotension, and evidence of end-organ compromise.

SYNONYMS

Sepsis
Sepsis syndrome
Severe sepsis
Systemic inflammatory response syndrome
Septic shock

ICD-9CM CODES
038.9 Sepsis
038.40 Sepsis, gram-negative bacteremia
038.1 Sepsis, *Staphylococcus*

EPIDEMIOLOGY & DEMOGRAPHICS

INCIDENCE (IN U.S.):
- Exact incidence is unknown
- Approximately 750,000 cases of severe sepsis occur among hospitalized patients each year in the U.S.
- Complicates a minority of bacteremia cases and may occur in the absence of documented bacteremia

PREDOMINANT SEX: Males slightly more commonly affected than females

PREDOMINANT AGE:
- Neonatal period
- Patients >65 yr of age account for 60% of all cases of severe sepsis

GENETICS:
- Familial disposition: a great variety of congenital immunodeficiency states and other inherited disorders may predispose to septicemia.
- Neonatal infection: incidence is high in neonatal period.

PHYSICAL FINDINGS & CLINICAL PRESENTATION

- Fever or hypothermia
- Hypotension
- Tachycardia
- Tachypnea
- Altered mental status
- Bleeding diathesis
- Skin rashes
- Symptoms that reflect primary site of infection: urinary tract, GI tract, CNS, respiratory tract

ETIOLOGY

- Disseminated infection with a great variety of bacteria:
  A. Gram-negative bacteria
    1. *E. coli*
    2. *Klebsiella* spp.
    3. *Pseudomonas aeruginosa*
    4. *Proteus* spp.
    5. *Neisseria meningitidis*
  B. Gram-positive bacteria
    1. *Staphylococcus aureus*
    2. *Streptococcus* spp.
    3. *Enterococcus* spp.
- Less common infections:
  1. Fungal
  2. Viral
  3. Rickettsial
  4. Parasitic
- Activation of coagulation, inflammatory cytokines, complement, and kinin cascades with release of a variety of vasoactive endogenous mediators
- Predisposing host factors:
  1. General medical condition
  2. Age
  3. Immunosuppressive therapy
  4. Recent surgery
  5. Granulocytopenia
  6. Hyposplenism
  7. Diabetes
  8. Instrumentation

Dx DIAGNOSIS

DIFFERENTIAL DIAGNOSIS

- Cardiogenic shock
- Acute pancreatitis
- Pulmonary embolism
- Systemic vasculitis
- Toxic ingestion
- Exposure-induced hypothermia
- Fulminant hepatic failure
- Collagen-vascular diseases

WORKUP

- Evaluation should focus on identifying a specific pathogen and localizing the site of primary infection.
- Hemodynamic, metabolic, coagulation disorders should be carefully characterized.
- Intensive monitoring, including the use of central venous or Swan-Ganz catheters, may be necessary.

LABORATORY TESTS

- Cultures of blood and examination and culture of sputum, urine, wound drainage, stool, and CSF
- CBC with differential, coagulation profile
- Routine chemistries, LFTs
- ABGs, lactic acid level; procalcitonin might be useful as a general marker of infection/sepsis
- Urinalysis

IMAGING STUDIES

- Chest x-ray examination
- Other radiographic and radioisotope procedures according to suspected site of primary infection

Rx TREATMENT

NONPHARMACOLOGIC THERAPY

- Tissue oxygenation: mixed venous oxygen saturation maintained >70% if possible; early mechanical ventilation
- Focal infection drained, if possible

ACUTE GENERAL Rx

- Blood pressure support, rapid IV fluid resuscitation and vasopressors, if needed, with the goal of reestablishing a mean arterial blood pressure >65 mm Hg; reduction in blood lactate and mixed venous oxygen saturation >70% within 6 hr of recognition of septic shock is associated with improved survival
  1. IV hydration; crystalloids are as effective as colloids as resuscitation fluids
  2. Therapy with vasopressors (e.g., dopamine, norepinephrine, vasopressin) if mean blood pressure of 70 to 75 mm Hg cannot be maintained by hydration alone. A recent trial comparing low-dose vasopressin with norepinephrine revealed that low-dose vasopressin did not reduce mortality rates as compared with norepinephrine among patients with septic shock who were treated with catecholamine vasopressors.
- Correction of acidosis by improving the tissue perfusion, not by giving bicarbonate
  1. Mechanical ventilation
- Antibiotics
  1. Directed at the most likely sources of infection.
  2. Should generally provide broad coverage of gram-positive and gram-negative bacteria (or fungi if clinically indicated).
  3. Typical regimens:
    a. For hospital-acquired sepsis (pending culture results): vancomycin plus cefepime, imipenem, aztreonam, quinolones, or an aminoglycoside. Monotherapy with appropriate agents appears to be as effective as combination therapy in immunocompetent hosts.
    b. For community-acquired infection in the absence of granulocytopenia: previously listed or single-drug therapy with third-generation cephalosporin.
    c. For infection in the granulocytopenic host: previously listed or dual gram-negative coverage (e.g., cephalosporin and aminoglycoside).
  4. Biological treatment Drotrecogin alfa (Xigris), a genetically engineered form of activated protein C, is approved for use in patients with severe sepsis with multiorgan dysfunction (or APACHE II score >24); when combined with conventional therapy, there may be a reduction in mortality.
  5. The role of corticosteroids in the acute management of septicemia has long been debated. Patients with relative adrenal insufficiency may benefit from low-dose

therapy with hydrocortisone (50 mg IV q6h) and fludrocortisone (50 microgram daily PO) given together for 7 days. Recent trials however revealed that hydrocortisone did not improve survival or reversal of shock, either overall or in patients who did not have a response to corticotropin, although hydrocortisone hastened reversal of shock in patients in whom shock was reversed.

CHRONIC Rx

- Adjust antibiotic therapy on the basis of culture results.
- In general, continue therapy for a minimum of 2 wk.

DISPOSITION

All patients with suspected septicemia should be hospitalized and given access to intensive monitoring and nursing care.

REFERRAL

- To infectious diseases expert
- To physician experienced in critical care

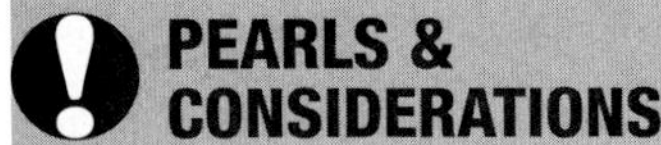

PEARLS & CONSIDERATIONS

COMMENTS

Mortality rises quickly if antibiotic therapy is not instituted promptly and metabolic derangements are not treated aggressively.

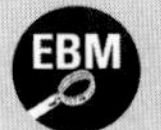

EVIDENCE

Evidence for fluid resuscitation in sepsis:

Evidence-based guidelines recommend that fluid resuscitation in severe sepsis may consist of natural or artificial colloids or crystalloids and that fluid challenge should be administered and repeated based on response (increase in blood pressure and urine output) and tolerance.[1] Ⓒ

Evidence for beta-lactam monotherapy instead of beta-lactam combined with aminoglycoside for sepsis:

A systematic review compared any beta-lactam monotherapy to any combination of one beta-lactam and one aminoglycoside for patients with sepsis. It found that combination therapy was not associated with improved clinical efficacy compared with beta-lactam antibiotic alone and was associated with a higher incidence of nephrotoxicity. The researchers comment that these results may have been limited by deficiencies of the included trials and may not apply to locations in which resistance rates to narrow-spectrum beta-lactams are very low.[2] Ⓐ

Corticosteroids for treating severe sepsis and septic shock:

A systematic review of 15 trials found that overall corticosteroids did not change 28-day all-cause mortality or hospital mortality in patients with severe sepsis and septic shock. However, there was some evidence of reduction in intensive care unit mortality and an increase in the proportion of shock reversal by days 7 and 28.[3] Ⓐ

The researchers highlighted a difference in two groups of trials: the trials performed after 1992 found that a long course of low-dose corticosteroid improved survival in septic shock without causing harm, whereas those with trials performed before 1992 showed no benefit from a short course of high-dose corticosteroids.[3]

Evidence for vasopressors in septic shock:

Existing evidence has not determined whether any particular vasopressor agent has superiority in the management of septic shock.[4] Ⓐ

Treatment for suspected or confirmed neonatal sepsis:

Systematic reviews have been unable to find sufficient evidence to determine the benefit of any one antibiotic regimen over another for the treatment of suspected early (birth to 48 hr of age) neonatal sepsis or late onset (after 48 hr of age) neonatal sepsis.[5,6]

One systematic review was unable to find enough evidence to confirm the effect of the use of granulocyte transfusions in neonates with sepsis and neutropenia. Another review was unable to find any eligible trials studying the effect of recombinant human activated protein C in the management of severe sepsis in newborn infants.[7]

Evidence References

1. Vincent JL, Gerlach H. Fluid resuscitation in severe sepsis and septic shock: an evidence-based review, *Crit Care Med* 2004;32:S451-4.
2. Paul M et al: Beta lactam antibiotic monotherapy versus beta lactam-aminoglycoside antibiotic combination therapy for sepsis, *Cochrane Database Syst Rev* 1: 2006.
3. Annane D et al: Corticosteroids for treating severe sepsis and septic shock, *Cochrane Database Syst Rev* 1: 2004.
4. Müllner M et al: Vasopressors for shock, *Cochrane Database Syst Rev* 2: 2004.
5. Gordon A, Jeffery HE: Antibiotic regimens for suspected late onset sepsis in newborn infants, *Cochrane Database Syst Rev* 3: 2005.
6. Mtitimila EI, Cooke RWI. Antibiotic regimens for suspected early neonatal sepsis, *Cochrane Database Syst Rev* 4: 2004.
7. Kylat RI, Ohlsson A. Recombinant human activated protein C for severe sepsis in neonates, *Cochrane Database Syst Rev* 2: 2006.

SUGGESTED READINGS

De Backer D et al: Comparison of dopamine and norepinephrine in the treatment of shock, *N Engl J Med* 362:779, 2010.

Dellinger RP et al: Surviving Sepsis Campaign: international guidelines for the management of severe sepsis and septic shock, *Crit Care Med* 36(1):296-327, 2008.

The NICE-SUGAR Study Investigators: Intensive versus conventional glucose control in critically ill patients, *N Engl J Med* 360(13):1283-1297, 2009.

O'Brien JM et al: Sepsis, *Am J Med* 120:1012-1022, 2007.

Russell J et al: Vasopressin versus norepinephrine infusion in patients with septic shock, *N Engl J Med* 358:877-887, 2008.

Sprung CL et al: Hydrocortisone therapy for patients with septic shock, *N Engl J Med* 358:111-124, 2008

Toussaint S, Gerlach H: Activated protein C for sepsis, *N Engl J Med* 361:2646, 2009.

AUTHORS: **STEVEN M. OPAL, M.D., GLENN G. FORT, M.D., M.P.H.,** and **DENNIS J. MIKOLICH, M.D.**

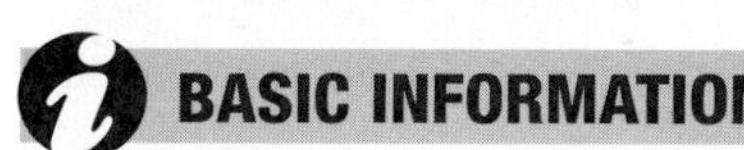

BASIC INFORMATION

DEFINITION

Serotonin syndrome (SS) refers to a group of symptoms resulting from increased activity of serotonin (5-hydroxytryptamine) in the CNS. SS is a drug-induced disorder that is classically characterized by a change in mental status and alteration in neuromuscular activity and autonomic function.

SYNONYMS

SS
Hyperserotonemia
Serotonergic syndrome
Serotonin toxicity

ICD-9CM CODES
333.99 Syndrome serotonin

EPIDEMIOLOGY & DEMOGRAPHICS

- The incidence of SS is not known.
- SS is seen in all age groups, from neonates to elderly.
- SS classically occurs in patients receiving two or more serotonergic drugs, but it can also occur with monotherapy—selective serotonin reuptake inhibitor (SSRI) monotherapy has an incidence of 0.5 to 0.9 cases of SS per 1000 patient-mo.
- Concomitant use of an SSRI with a monoamine oxidase inhibitor (MAOI) poses the greatest risk of developing SS.
- Combination of SSRIs with other serotonergic drugs (e.g., tryptophan, illicit drugs like cocaine and MDMA, "ecstasy") or drugs with serotonin properties (e.g., lithium, meperidine, triptans) may also lead to SS.

PHYSICAL FINDINGS & CLINICAL PRESENTATION

- Findings of clonus with hyperreflexia in the setting of recent (<5 wk) use of serotonergic agents strongly suggests the diagnosis of SS.
- Symptoms can manifest within minutes to hours after starting a new psychopharmacologic treatment, increasing the dose of a serotonergic drug, or after administering a second serotonergic drug.
- Clonus (inducible, spontaneous, and ocular) is the key finding in establishing a diagnosis of SS.
- Other pertinent findings include:
  - Confusion, agitation, hypomania
  - Fever >38° C (100° F), tachycardia, and tachypnea
  - Nausea, vomiting, abdominal pain, and diaphoresis
  - Diarrhea, tremors, shivering, and seizures
  - Hyperreflexia and muscle rigidity

ETIOLOGY

- Hyperstimulation of the brainstem and spinal cord serotonin receptors leading to the neuromuscular and autonomic symptoms.
- Psychopharmacologic drugs—in particular, fluoxetine and sertraline co-administered with MAOI (e.g., tranylcypromine and phenelzine)—have been cited in the literature as a common cause of SS. Triptans (serotonin-receptor agonists used in the treatment of migraines) may also precipitate the SS when used in combination with SSRIs and serotonin-norepinephrine reuptake inhibitors (SNRIs).

Dx DIAGNOSIS

- The diagnosis of SS is made on clinical grounds. There are no specific laboratory tests for SS. A high index of suspicion along with a detailed medication history is the mainstay of diagnosis.
- Diagnostic criteria: most accurate is Hunter Serotonin Toxicity Criteria (sensitivity 84%, specificity 97%, confirmation by toxicologist).
- To fulfill Hunter criteria a patient must have consumed a serotonergic drug and have one of the following:
  1. Spontaneous clonus
  2. Inducible clonus plus agitation or diaphoresis
  3. Ocular clonus plus agitation or diaphoresis
  4. Tremor and hyperreflexia
  5. Temperature greater than 38° C (100° F) plus hypertonia plus ocular clonus or inducible clonus

DIFFERENTIAL DIAGNOSIS

- Neuroleptic malignant syndrome (NMS), substance abuse (e.g., cocaine, amphetamines), anticholinergic toxicity, thyroid storm, infection (e.g., meningitis, encephalitis), alcohol and opioid withdrawal.
- Classic features in differentiation of NMS from SS are that SS develops over 24 hr, involves neuromuscular hyperactivity, and begins to resolve within 24 hr with appropriate therapy, whereas NMS develops gradually over days to weeks, involves sluggish neuromuscular response, and resolves over an average period of 1 wk to 10 days.

WORKUP

- Because SS is a clinical diagnosis, there is no laboratory test that confirms the diagnosis, and serum serotonin concentration does not correlate with clinical picture. Other causes are described in "Differential Diagnosis." Thus, all patients should have blood tests and diagnostic imaging studies to rule out infectious, toxic, and metabolic causes.
- Additional laboratory tests are performed to exclude complicating features of SS (e.g., renal failure secondary to rhabdomyolysis).

LABORATORY TESTS

- CBC with differential to rule out sepsis
- Electrolytes, BUN, and creatinine to rule out acidosis and renal failure
- Blood and urine toxicology screen
- Thyroid function tests
- Creatine-phosphokinase (CPK) with isoenzymes
- Urine and blood cultures
- ECG because ventricular rhythm disturbance is a potentially fatal complication

IMAGING STUDIES

Imaging studies are not very specific in the diagnosis of SS and are only ordered to exclude other causes with similar clinical presentations as SS.

Rx TREATMENT

- Once a diagnosis of SS is established, appropriate consultation with a medical toxicologist, clinical pharmacologist, and/or poison control center should be sought.
- Management includes:
  - Discontinue use of all potential precipitating drugs
  - Provide supportive management
  - Control agitation
  - Administer serotonin antagonists
  - Control autonomic instability
  - Control hyperthermia
  - Reassess the need to resume the use of the serotonergic agent once the symptoms have resolved

NONPHARMACOLOGIC THERAPY

- Discontinuation of the drug is the mainstay of therapy.
- Treatment is supportive: maintaining oxygenation and blood pressure and monitoring respiratory status. Hypotensive patients may require both IV fluids and vasopressor therapy.
- Patients who are severely hyperthermic with temperatures greater than 41° C (106° F) should be given IV sedation, paralyzed, and intubated. Cooling blankets can be used for patients with mild to moderate hyperthermia. There is no role of acetaminophen here.
- Mechanical intubation is recommended for patients unable to protect their airways as a result of mental status changes or seizures.

ACUTE GENERAL Rx

- Benzodiazepines for control of agitation is preferred to physical restraints.
  1. Lorazepam 1 to 2 mg IV every 30 min has been used effectively in treating agitation, muscle rigidity, myoclonus, and seizure complications.
  2. Diazepam is an alternative choice.
- Blood pressure management with short-acting agents such as esmolol and nitroprusside.
- Serotonin antagonists should be titrated to clinical effectiveness in patients for whom nonpharmacologic therapy and benzodiazepines are not achieving adequate response, though substantial and rigorous data is lacking
  1. Cyproheptadine 4-mg tablet or 2 mg/5 ml syrup is given 12 mg initially followed by 2 mg every 2 hr until therapeutic response is achieved in adults (up to 32 mg/day), children ages 7 to 14 should receive 4 mg every 6 hr (up to 16 mg/day), children ages 2 to 6 should receive 2 mg every

6 hr (up to 12 mg/day), and children younger than 2 yr should receive a maximum of 0.25 mg/kg/day as 0.06 mg/kg every 6 hr.
2. Atypical antipsychotic agents with serotonin antagonist properties (e.g., olanzapine 10 mg SL) have been tried with some success.
3. Chlorpromazine 50 to 100 mg IM may be considered in severe cases.

CHRONIC Rx

For patients not requiring hospital admission, cyproheptadine and lorazepam can be given in an oral dose on a prn basis with close follow-up.

DISPOSITION

- SS is a potentially life-threatening condition if not recognized early, though it does exist on a spectrum.
- Prompt diagnosis and withdrawal of the medication results in improvement of symptoms within 24 hr.
- Seizures, rhabdomyolysis, hyperthermia, ventricular arrhythmia, respiratory arrest, and coma are all complicating features of SS.

REFERRAL

All cases of SS secondary to psychotropic medications should be referred to a psychiatrist.

PREVENTION

Modify prescription practices by avoiding multidrug regimens.

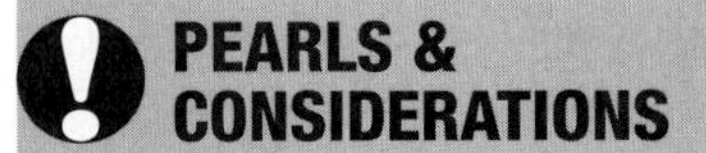

PEARLS & CONSIDERATIONS

The combined use of SSRIs and MAOIs is contraindicated.

COMMENTS

- The use of SSRIs and other serotonergic agents is not an absolute contraindication; however, prompt withdrawal of the medication is recommended if any symptoms suggesting SS occur.
- SS is usually found in patients being treated for depression, bipolar disorders, obsessive-compulsive disorder, attention-deficit disorder, and Parkinson's disease.

SUGGESTED READINGS

Boyer EW, Shannon M: The serotonin syndrome, *N Engl J Med* 352:1112-1120, 2005.

Dunkley EJ et al: The Hunter Serotonin Toxicity Criteria: simple and accurate diagnostic decision rules for serotonin toxicity, *QJM* 96:635, 2003.

Evans RW: The FDA alert on serotonin syndrome with combined use of SSRIs or SNRIs and triptans: an analysis of the 29 case reports, *Med Gen Med* 9(3): 48, 2007.

Sclar DA et al: Concomitant triptan and SSRI or SNRI use: a risk for serotonin syndrome. *Headache* 48: 126-129, 2008.

AUTHOR: **MARK BRADY, M.D., M.P.H., M.M.S.**

BASIC INFORMATION

DEFINITION

Severe acute respiratory syndrome (SARS) is a respiratory illness caused by a coronavirus called SARS-associated coronavirus (SARS-CoV).

CLINICAL CRITERIA:

A. Asymptomatic or mild respiratory illness
B. Moderate respiratory illness
   1. Temperature of >100.4° F (>38° C)* *and*
   2. One or more clinical findings of respiratory illness (e.g., cough, shortness of breath, difficulty breathing, hypoxia)
C. Severe respiratory illness
   1. Temperature of >100.4° F (>38° C)* *and*
   2. One or more clinical findings of respiratory illness (e.g., cough, shortness of breath, difficulty breathing, hypoxia) *and*
      a. Radiographic evidence of pneumonia, *or*
      b. Respiratory distress syndrome, *or*
      c. Autopsy findings consistent with pneumonia or respiratory distress syndrome without an identifiable cause

EPIDEMIOLOGIC CRITERIA:

- Travel (including transit in an airport) within 10 days of onset of symptoms to an area with current or previously documented or suspected community transmission of SARS, *or*
- Close contact† within 10 days of onset of symptoms with a person known or suspected to have SARS.
- The Chinese horseshoe bat, which is a healthy carrier of SARS, has been identified as the reservoir of the virus in nature. The spread of the virus was facilitated by people eating bats or using bat feces in traditional medicine for asthma, kidney ailments, and general malaise.

Laboratory criteria:

- Confirmed:
   1. Detection of antibody to SARS-CoV in a serum sample, *or*
   2. Detection of SARS-CoV RNA by reverse-transcription polymerase chain reaction (PCR) confirmed by a second PCR assay by using a second aliquot of the specimen and a different set of PCR primers, *or*
   3. Isolation of SARS-CoV
- Negative:
   1. Absence of antibody to SARS-CoV in a convalescent-phase serum sample obtained >28 days after symptom onset‡
- Undetermined:
   1. Laboratory testing either not performed or incomplete

Case classification§:

- Probable case: meets the clinical criteria for severe respiratory illness of unknown etiology and epidemiologic criteria for exposure; laboratory criteria confirmed or undetermined.
- Suspect case: meets the clinical criteria for moderate respiratory illness of unknown etiology and epidemiologic criteria for exposure; laboratory criteria confirmed or undetermined.

Exclusion criteria: a case may be excluded as a suspect or probable SARS case if:

- An alternative diagnosis can fully explain the illness.
- The case has a convalescent-phase serum sample (i.e., obtained >28 days after symptom onset) that is negative for antibody to SARS-CoV.‡
- The case was reported on the basis of contact with an index case that was subsequently excluded as a case of SARS, provided other possible epidemiologic exposure criteria are not present.

SYNONYMS

SARS

ICD-9CM CODES
Not available

EPIDEMIOLOGY & DEMOGRAPHICS

- The disease was first recognized in Asia in February 2003 and spread to more than 2 dozen countries in North and South America, Europe, and Asia over the next several months, affecting more than 8000 patients and resulting in more than 750 deaths. In July 2003, cases were no longer being reported, and SARS outbreaks worldwide were considered contained.
- Most reported cases of SARS in the United States were attributed to exposure through foreign travel to countries with community transmission of SARS, with only limited secondary spread to close contacts such as family members and health care workers.
- Incubation period is 2 to 10 days.
- Evidence of airborne transmission of the SARS virus and laboratory-acquired SARS have now been documented.

PHYSICAL FINDINGS & CLINICAL PRESENTATION¶

- Early manifestations: fever, myalgias, and headache. Fever is often high and associated with chills or rigors. Fever may be absent in elderly patients.
- Dry, nonproductive cough occurs within 2 to 4 days of onset of fever.
- Diarrhea may occur in up to 25% of cases.
- Dyspnea and hypoxemia follow the cough and may require intubation in nearly 20% of patients.
- A biphasic course of illness may occur with initial improvement followed by subsequent deterioration in some patients.

ETIOLOGY

SARS-associated coronavirus

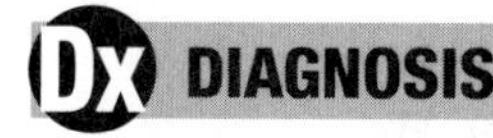

DIAGNOSIS

DIFFERENTIAL DIAGNOSIS

- Legionella pneumonia
- Influenza A and B
- Respiratory syncytial virus
- Acute respiratory distress syndrome (ARDS)

WORKUP

Initial diagnostic testing for suspected SARS patients should include chest radiograph, pulse oximetry, blood cultures, sputum Gram stain and culture, and testing for viral respiratory pathogens, notably influenza A and B and respiratory syncytial virus. A specimen for Legionella and pneumococcal urinary antigen testing should also be considered.

LABORATORY TESTS

When to test for SARS:

- In the absence of documented SARS transmission, diagnostic testing for SARS-

---

*A measured documented temperature of >100.4° F (>38° C) is preferred. However, clinical judgment should be used when evaluating patients for whom a measured temperature of >100.4° F (>38° C) has not been documented. Factors that might be considered include patient self-report of fever, use of antipyretics, presence of immunocompromising conditions or therapies, lack of access to health care, and inability to obtain a measured temperature. Reporting authorities should consider these factors when classifying patients who do not strictly meet the clinical criteria for this case definition.

†Close contact is defined as having cared for or lived with a person known to have SARS or having a high likelihood of direct contact with respiratory secretions and/or body fluids of a patient known to have SARS. Examples of close contact include kissing or embracing, sharing eating or drinking utensils, close conversation (<3 ft), physical examination, and any other direct physical contact between persons. Close contact does not include activities such as walking by a person or sitting across a waiting room or office for a brief period.

‡The World Health Organization has specified that the surveillance period for China should begin on November 1; the first recognized cases in Hong Kong, Singapore, and Hanoi (Vietnam) had onset in February 2003. The date for Toronto is linked to the occurrence of a laboratory confirmed case of SARS in a U.S. resident who had traveled to Toronto; the date for Taiwan is linked to the Centers for Disease Control and Prevention (CDC) issuing travel recommendations.

§The last date for illness onset is 10 days (i.e., one incubation period) after removal of a CDC travel alert. The case patient's travel should have occurred on or before the last date the travel alert was in place.

Assays for the laboratory diagnosis of SARS-CoV infection include enzyme-linked immunosorbent assay, indirect fluorescent-antibody assay, and reverse-transcription PCR assays of appropriately collected clinical specimens (Source: CDC: *Guidelines for collection of specimens from potential cases of SARS.* Available at http://www.cdc.gov/ncidod/sars/specimen_collection_sars2.htm). Absence of SARS-CoV antibody from serum obtained <28 days after illness onset,‡ a negative PCR test, or a negative viral culture does not exclude SARS-CoV infection and is not considered a definitive laboratory result. In these instances a convalescent serum sample obtained >28 days after illness is needed to determine infection with SARS-CoV.

¶Asymptomatic SARS-CoV infection or clinical manifestations other than respiratory illness might be identified as more is learned about SARS-CoV infection.

associated coronavirus (SARS-CoV) should *not* be considered unless the clinician and health department have a high index of suspicion for SARS (e.g., a hospitalized pneumonia patient has a possible SARS exposure during travel and no other explanation for their pneumonia).

- Respiratory specimens should be collected as soon as possible in the course of the illness. The likelihood of recovering most viruses diminishes markedly >72 hours after symptom onset.
- Three types of specimens may be collected for viral or bacterial isolation and PCR. These include (1) nasopharyngeal wash/aspirates, (2) nasopharyngeal swabs, or (3) oropharyngeal swabs. Nasopharyngeal aspirates are the specimen of choice for detection of respiratory viruses and are the preferred collection method among children aged <2 yr.
- Laboratory testing on initial evaluation should also include CBC with differential, platelet count, liver enzymes, LDH, and CPK. Common laboratory abnormalities in SARS include thrombocytopenia, lymphopenia, elevated LDH, and elevated CPK, ALT, AST.

IMAGING STUDIES

- Chest x-ray: patchy focal infiltrates or consolidation with peripheral distribution.
- Chest x-ray may be normal in up to 25% of patients.
- Pleural effusions generally are not present.

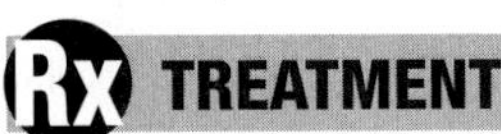

TREATMENT

NONPHARMACOLOGIC THERAPY

- Supportive care.
- Nearly 25% of cases will require ventilator assistance.
- Nutritional support.

ACUTE GENERAL Rx

- There is no specific treatment currently available for SARS.
- Broad-spectrum antibiotics (quinolone or macrolide) are generally started pending laboratory testing.
- Use of corticosteroids (methylprednisolone 40 mg bid or doses up to 2 mg/kg/day) is controversial but may be beneficial in patients with significant hypoxemia and progressive pulmonary infiltrates.
- In a preliminary, uncontrolled study of patients with SARS, use of interferon alfacon-1 plus corticosteroids was beneficial.

DISPOSITION

- Case fatality rate is 3% to 12%.
- Mortality rate is higher in elderly and immunocompromised patients and lower in pediatric age group.

REFERRAL

- Infectious disease consultation and pulmonary consultation is recommended in all cases.
- Notification of state Department of Health is mandatory.

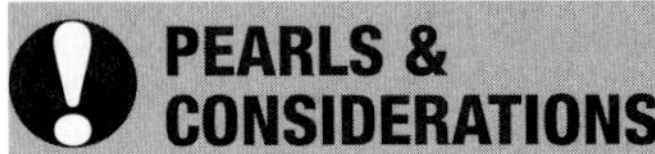

PEARLS & CONSIDERATIONS

COMMENTS

- Persons who may have been exposed to SARS should be vigilant for fever (i.e., measure temperature twice daily) and respiratory symptoms over the 10 days after exposure. During this time, in the absence of both fever and respiratory symptoms, persons who may have been exposed to SARS patients need not limit their activities outside the home and should not be excluded from work, school, out-of-home child care, church, or other public areas.
- Exposed persons should notify their health care provider immediately if fever or respiratory symptoms develop.
- Symptomatic persons exposed to SARS should follow the following infection control precautions:
    1. If fever or respiratory symptoms develop, the person should limit interactions outside the home and not go to work, school, out-of-home child care, church, or other public areas. In addition, the person should use infection control precautions in the home to minimize the risk for transmission, and continue to measure temperature twice daily.
    2. If symptoms improve or resolve within 72 hr after first symptom onset, the person may be allowed, after consultation with local public health authorities, to return to work, school, out-of-home child care, church, or other public areas, and infection control precautions can be discontinued.
    3. For persons who meet or progress to meet the case definition for suspected SARS (e.g., develop fever and respiratory symptoms), infection control precautions should be continued until 10 days after the resolution of fever, provided respiratory symptoms are absent or improving.
    4. If the illness does not progress to meet the case definition, but the individual has persistent fever or unresolving respiratory symptoms, infection control precautions should be continued for an additional 72 hr, at the end of which time a clinical evaluation should be performed. If the illness progresses to meet the case definition, infection control precautions should be continued as described earlier. If case definition criteria are not met, infection control precautions can be discontinued after consultation with local public health authorities and the evaluating clinician.
- Persons who meet or progress to meet the case definition for suspected SARS (e.g., develop fever and respiratory symptoms) or whose illness does not meet the case definition, but who have persistent fever or unresolving respiratory symptoms over the 72 hr after onset of symptoms, should be tested for SARS coronavirus infection.

SUGGESTED READINGS

Lim PL et al: Laboratory-acquired SARS, *N Engl J Med* 350:1740, 2004.

Poutanen SM et al: Identification of severe acute respiratory syndrome in Canada, *N Engl J Med* 348: 20, 2004.

Yu, IT et al: Evidence of airborne transmission of SARS virus, *N Engl J Med* 350:1731, 2004.

AUTHOR: **FRED F. FERRI, M.D.**

BASIC INFORMATION

DEFINITION

A sexual dysfunction in a woman is any disorder that interferes with female sexuality and that causes marked distress to that person. These disorders are generally categorized into four types:

1. Disorders of desire
2. Disorders of arousal
3. Orgasmic disorders
4. Sexual pain disorders (including dyspareunia, vaginismus, and vulvodynia)

SYNONYMS

Female sexual dysfunction

ICD-9CM CODES

302.70 Decreased libido
302.72 Disorders of arousal
302.73 Orgasmic disorders
625.x Sexual pain disorders

EPIDEMIOLOGY & DEMOGRAPHICS

According to the National Health and Social Life Survey, in 1999, approximately 20% to 50% of women reported some form of sexual dysfunction during their lifetimes. One third of women reported a decrease in sexual interest, and one fourth reported an inability to achieve orgasm.

PHYSICAL FINDINGS & CLINICAL PRESENTATION

- History:
  - Important to obtain the patient's definition of the dysfunction, including its onset and duration; to determine whether the dysfunction is situational or global; and to determine whether more than one dysfunction exists and the interrelationship among the dysfunctions
  - Related medical and gynecologic conditions
  - Psychosocial factors, including sexual abuse, sexual orientation, depression, and anxiety
  - Current medications
- Physical examination:
  - External genitalia
  - Vaginal vault
  - Uterus/adnexa
  - Rectovaginal area
  - Other body systems as indicated

ETIOLOGY

- Chronic medical conditions (e.g., diabetes, coronary vascular disease, arthritis, urinary incontinence)
- Medication induced (e.g., antihypertensives, selective serotonin reuptake inhibitors (SSRIs)
- Gynecologic conditions (e.g., cystitis, posthysterectomy, gynecologic cancers, breast cancer [femininity/self-image issues; chemotherapy effects], postpregnancy, postmenopausal)
- Psychosocial (e.g., religion, taboos, identity conflicts, guilt, relationship problems, abuse, rape, life stressors)

DIAGNOSIS

DIFFERENTIAL DIAGNOSIS

- Depression
- Psychosocial stressors
- Medical disease

LABORATORY TESTS

- Cervical cultures and vaginal swabs for infectious disease
- Pap smear
- Appropriate laboratory tests if comorbid or chronic disease is suspected

IMAGING STUDIES

- Appropriate imaging studies if comorbid or chronic disease is suspected

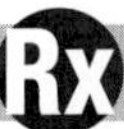

TREATMENT

NONPHARMACOLOGIC THERAPY

- Education
- Activities to enhance stimulation and eliminate routine
- Distraction techniques
- Noncoital behavior
- Position changes (e.g., female astride)
- Lubricants (e.g., non-petroleum based)

ACUTE GENERAL Rx

- NSAIDs before intercourse for sexual pain disorders

CHRONIC Rx

- Treat underlying medical, gynecologic, or psychologic conditions.
- Reduce comorbidities.
- For medication-induced conditions, decrease dose or change medication.
- For postmenopausal women or those with hypoestrogenism, try estrogen replacement therapy with or without progesterone.
- Testosterone therapy (controversial)
- Sildenafil (controversial)
- Behavioral therapy

REFERRAL

- Gynecologic referral for conditions that may be amenable to surgical therapy
- Psychologic referral for conditions (e.g., depression, abuse) that may benefit from counseling or psychotherapy
- Social services referrals for active abuse issues

PEARLS & CONSIDERATIONS

COMMENTS

- Identify the earliest cause in the chain and treat that first.

PATIENT/FAMILY EDUCATION

- When appropriate, involve the patient's partner or significant other in treatment.

EVIDENCE

Please note: Complete text of EBM for this topic is available online.

Key trials and commentary:

Antidepressant-associated sexual dysfunction is a common adverse effect that frequently results in premature medication treatment discontinuation and for which no treatment has demonstrated efficacy in women.

This study sought to evaluate the efficacy of sildenafil for sexual dysfunction associated with selective and nonselective serotonin reuptake inhibitors (SRIs) in women.

In this study population, sildenafil treatment of sexual dysfunction in women taking SRIs was associated with a reduction in adverse sexual effects.

Women are twice as likely to be prescribed antidepressants, most commonly selective serotonin reuptake inhibitors (SSRIs). It is well known that SSRIs may lead to sexual difficulties in both men and women. For this reason, investigation in ways to ameliorate SSRI-induced sexual dysfunction in women is timely and necessary.

Despite similarities in the enzymatic processes involved in both penile erection and vaginal/clitoral engorgement, phosphodiesterase type 5 inhibitors (PDE5Is) such as sildenafil have not shown the same benefit in women that has been observed in men. Several small studies have suggested that women with specific medical problems (such as MS or diabetes) may benefit from PDE5I, but in general this medication class has not proven particularly useful in the management of female sexual dysfunction.

This interesting study suggests another female population in which PDE5I may be useful. In this population of previously sexually healthy women with new onset of sex problems after initiation of SSRI therapy for major depressive disorder, on-demand PDE5Is were found to improve sexual function. Their most significant improvements were noted in ability to attain satisfactory orgasms. This study end point is somewhat analogous to the SEP2 and 3 questions (Were you able to complete sexual intercourse?) used to ascertain PDE5I efficacy in men.[1] Ⓐ

Evidence-Based Reference

1. Nurnberg HG et al: Sildenafil treatment of women with antidepressant-associated sexual dysfunction: a randomized controlled trial, *JAMA* 300:395-404, 2008. Commentary by A. Shindel, M.D. Ⓐ

SUGGESTED READINGS

Basson R et al: Report of the International Consensus Development Conference on Female Sexual Dysfunction: definitions and classifications, *J Urol* 163(3):888-893, 2000.

Laumann EO et al: Sexual dysfunction in the United States: prevalence and predictors, *JAMA* 281:537-544, 1999.

Phillips NA: Female sexual dysfunction: evaluation and treatment, *Am Fam Physician* 62(1):127-136, 2000.

AUTHOR: **ANNGENE A. GIUSTOZZI, M.D., M.P.H.**

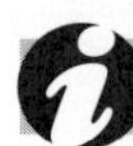

BASIC INFORMATION

DEFINITION

Sheehan's syndrome is a state of hypopituitarism resulting from an infarct of the pituitary secondary to postpartum hemorrhage or shock, causing partial or complete loss of the anterior pituitary hormones (adrenocorticotropic hormone [ACTH], follicle-stimulating hormone [FSH], luteinizing hormone [LH], growth hormone [GH], prolactin [PRL], thyroid-stimulating hormone [TSH]) and their target organ functions.

ICD-9CM CODES
253.2 Sheehan's syndrome

EPIDEMIOLOGY & DEMOGRAPHICS

INCIDENCE: One case in 10,000 deliveries (perhaps more rare in the U.S.)
PREDOMINANT SEX: Affects only females
RISK FACTORS:
- Hypovolemic shock
- Type 1 (insulin-dependent) diabetes mellitus (secondary to microvascular disease)
- Sickle cell anemia (secondary to occlusion of the small vessels in the pituitary)

ONSET OF SYMPTOMS: Average delay of 5 to 7 yr between onset of symptoms and diagnosis of disease.

PHYSICAL FINDINGS & CLINICAL PRESENTATION

- Failure of lactation
- Infertility
- Failure to resume menses after delivery
- Failure to regrow shaved pubic or axillary hair
- Skin depigmentation (including areola)
- Rapid breast involution
- Superinvolution of the uterus
- Hypothyroidism
- Adrenal cortical insufficiency
- Diabetes insipidus (rare)

ETIOLOGY

- Compromise of the blood supply to the low-pressure pituitary sinusoidal system may occur with postpartum hemorrhage or shock, resulting in pituitary infarct and/or necrosis.
- It is hypothesized that locally released factors may mediate vascular spasm of the pituitary blood supply.
- Severity of postpartum hemorrhage does not always correlate with the presence of Sheehan's syndrome.

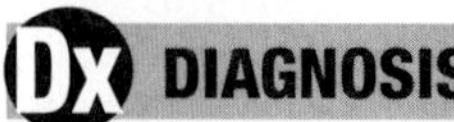

DIAGNOSIS

DIFFERENTIAL DIAGNOSIS

- Chronic infections
- HIV
- Sarcoidosis
- Amyloidosis
- Rheumatoid disease
- Hemochromatosis
- Metastatic carcinoma
- Lymphocytic hypophysitis

WORKUP

- Target gland deficiency should be investigated by measuring levels of ACTH, FSH, LH, TSH (which may be normal or low), and T_4. Cortisol and estradiol (which may be low) should also be measured.
- Provocative testing of pituitary hormone reserves (e.g., metyrapone test, insulin tolerance test, and cosyntropin test): normal, subnormal, or delayed responses may suggest the presence of islands of pituitary cells that no longer have the support of the hypothalamic-portal circulation.
- Measurement of insulin-like growth factor-I to screen for GH deficiency: subnormal levels suggest decreased GH.
- Impaired prolactin response to TRH or dopamine antagonist stimulation is frequently found.
- During pregnancy, adjustments must be made in interpreting both hormone levels and responses to various stimuli because of normal physiologic changes.

IMAGING STUDIES

- Study of choice: MRI of the pituitary
  1. Sella turcica partially or totally empty
  2. Rules out mass lesion
- CT scan of the pituitary when MRI is unavailable or contraindicated

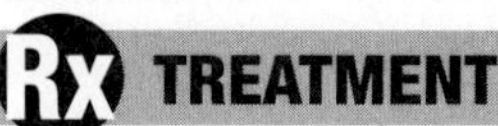

TREATMENT

ACUTE GENERAL Rx

- Acute form can be lethal, presenting with hypotension, tachycardia, failure to lactate, and hypoglycemia.
- A high degree of suspicion is required with any woman who has undergone postpartum hemorrhage and shock.
- IV corticosteroids and fluid replacement should be given initially.
- Diagnosis is confirmed with a full endocrinologic workup, as noted previously.
- Thyroid hormone is replaced as L-thyroxin in doses of 0.1 to 0.2 mg qd.

CHRONIC Rx

- With late-onset disease (symptoms of general hypopituitarism, such as oligomenorrhea or amenorrhea, vaginal atrophic changes, and loss of libido): a full endocrinologic workup and replacement of the appropriate hormones are needed.
- With symptoms of adrenal insufficiency: corticosteroids should be given.
  1. A maintenance dose of cortisone acetate or prednisone may be given.
  2. Because adrenal production of cortisol is not entirely dependent on ACTH, replacement of mineralocorticoids is rarely necessary.
  3. Stress doses of glucocorticoids should be administered during surgery or during labor and delivery.

DISPOSITION

Patients who receive early diagnosis and adequate hormonal replacement may expect favorable outcomes, including subsequent pregnancy.

REFERRAL

Patients should have yearly examinations by an endocrinologist.

SUGGESTED READING

Kovacs K: Sheehan's syndrome, *Lancet* 361(9356): 520, 2003.

AUTHOR: **BETH J. WUTZ, M.D.**

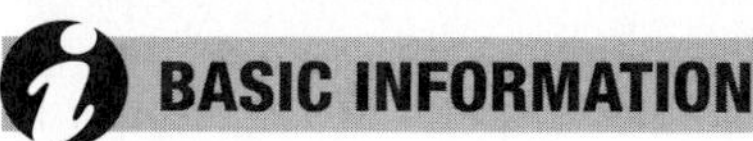

BASIC INFORMATION

DEFINITION

Shigellosis is an inflammatory disease of the bowel caused by one of several species of *Shigella.* It is the most common cause of bacillary dysentery in the U.S.

SYNONYMS

Bacillary dysentery

ICD-9CM CODES
004.9 Shigellosis

EPIDEMIOLOGY & DEMOGRAPHICS

INCIDENCE (IN U.S.): Approximately 15,000 cases/yr
PREDOMINANT SEX: Male homosexuals at increased risk
PREDOMINANT AGE: Young children
PEAK INCIDENCE: Summer
GENETICS: Neonatal infection: rare but severe

PHYSICAL FINDINGS & CLINICAL PRESENTATION

- Possibly asymptomatic, but incubation period can range from 1 to 7 days with an average of 3 days
- Mild illness that is usually self-limited, resolving in a few days
- Fever
- Watery diarrhea
- Bloody diarrhea
- Dysentery (abdominal cramps, tenesmus, and numerous, small-volume stools with blood, mucus, and pus)
- Descending intestinal tract illness, reflecting infection of small bowel first and then the colon
- Severe disease is more common in children and elderly and outside of U.S.
- Complications of severe illness:
    1. Seizures
    2. Megacolon
    3. Intestinal perforation
    4. Death
- Extraintestinal manifestations are rare
- Bacteremia is more common in children; in adults it has been described in patients with AIDS, the elderly, and diabetics
- Hemolytic-uremic syndrome (HUS): usually occurs as the initial illness seems to be resolving
- Reactive arthritis, sometimes as part of Reiter's syndrome

ETIOLOGY

- Shigella
    1. *S. flexneri*
    2. *S. dysenteriae*
    3. *S. sonnei*
    4. *S. boydii*
- *S. sonnei* is the most commonly isolated species in the U.S., and it usually causes a mild watery diarrhea.
- Direct person-to-person transmission is thought to be the most common route. Outbreaks among men who have sex with men have occurred because of direct or indirect oral-anal contact.
- Contaminated food or water may transmit disease.
- A recent outbreak occurred at a community wading pool frequented by toddlers.

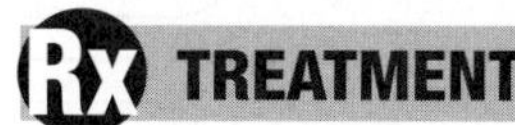

DIAGNOSIS

DIFFERENTIAL DIAGNOSIS

- May mimic any bacterial or viral gastroenteritis
- Dysentery also caused by *Entamoeba histolytica*
- Bloody diarrhea may resemble disease caused by enterotoxigenic *E. coli*

LABORATORY TESTS

- Total WBCs may be low, normal, or high. Leukemoid reactions can occur in children.
- Stool should be cultured from fresh samples, because the yield is increased by processing the specimen soon after passage. The best yield is from the mucoid part of the stool.
- Serology is available but rarely useful.
- Polymerase chain reaction may be diagnostic.
- Fecal leukocyte preparation may show WBCs.

IMAGING STUDIES

Abdominal radiographs may suggest megacolon or perforation in rare, severe cases.

Rx TREATMENT

NONPHARMACOLOGIC THERAPY

- Adequate hydration
- Electrolyte replacement

ACUTE GENERAL Rx

Antibiotics:

- To shorten course of illness.
- To limit transmission of illness.
- For children: IV ceftriaxone (50 mg/kg/day) for severe disease. For oral therapy, can use SMX/TMP or ampicillin for 5 days for susceptible strains. Azithromycin can be used for 5 days when susceptibilities still not known or in areas of high resistance (12 mg/kg for the first day, then 6 mg/kg/day for 4 days).
- For adults: Pending susceptibilities, ciprofloxacin 500 mg PO bid for 5 days should be used. If susceptible, can also use SMX/TMP one DS PO bid for 5 days. Azithromycin is a second alternative.

DISPOSITION

- Most disease is self-limited.
- Severe illness may be fatal.

REFERRAL

For severe illness or complications

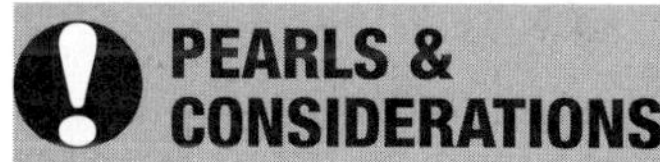

PEARLS & CONSIDERATIONS

COMMENTS

- *Shigella* is one cause of "gay bowel syndrome."
- Illness is worsened by agents that decrease intestinal motility.
- Food handlers, child-care providers, and health care workers should have a negative stool culture documented following treatment.

SUGGESTED READINGS

Ashkenazi S: Shigella infections in children: new insights, *Semin Pediatr Infect Dis* 15(4):246, 2004.
Ekdahl K, Andersson Y: The epidemiology of travel-associated shigellosis-regional risks, seasonality and serogroups, *J Infect* 51(3):222, 2005.
Taylor DN et al: Rifaximin, a nonabsorbed oral antibiotic, prevents shigellosis after experimental challenge, *Clin Infect Dis* 42(9):1283, 2006.

AUTHORS: **GLENN G. FORT, M.D., M.P.H.,** and **DENNIS J. MIKOLICH, M.D.**

Short Body Syndrome

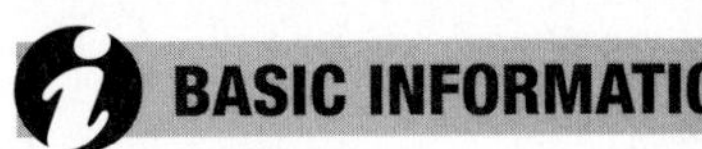

BASIC INFORMATION

DEFINITION

Short bowel syndrome is a malabsorption syndrome that results from extensive small intestinal resection.

SYNONYMS

Short bowel

ICD-9CM CODES

579.3 (postsurgical malabsorption)

EPIDEMIOLOGY & DEMOGRAPHICS

- Parallels Crohn's disease (see "Crohn's Disease" in Section I), which is the most common cause of the syndrome in adults.
- In children, two thirds of short bowels are related to congenital abnormalities (intestinal atresia, gastroschisis, volvulus, aganglionosis) and one third are related to necrotizing enterocolitis.
- Prevalence: 10,000 to 20,000 cases are estimated to exist in the U.S.

PHYSICAL FINDINGS & CLINICAL PRESENTATION

- Diarrhea and steatorrhea
- Weight loss
- Anemia related to iron or vitamin B_{12} absorption
- Bleeding diathesis related to vitamin K malabsorption
- Osteoporosis/osteomalacia related to vitamin D and calcium malabsorption
- Hyponatremia, hypokalemia
- Hypovolemia
- Other macronutrient or micronutrient deficiency states

ETIOLOGY

- Extensive bowel resection for treatment of the conditions mentioned previously (see "Epidemiology").
- Pathogenesis (Fig. 1-298).

The human intestine is 3 to 8 m in length. Removal of up to half of the small intestine produces no disruption in nutrient absorption, and most patients can maintain nutritional balance on oral feeding if they have more than 100 cm (3 ft) of jejunum. Similarly, 100 cm of intact jejunum can maintain a normal water, sodium, and potassium balance under normal circumstances. The presence of an intact colon can compensate for some small intestine loss.

Site-specific functions:

- Calcium, magnesium, phosphorus, iron, and vitamins are absorbed in the duodenum and proximal jejunum.
- Vitamin B_{12} and bile acids are absorbed in the ileum. The resection of more than 60 cm of ileum results in vitamin B_{12} malabsorption. The loss of more than 100 cm results in fat malabsorption (from the loss of bile acids).
- The loss of gastrointestinal endocrine hormones can affect intestinal motility.
- Intestinal bacterial overgrowth may also occur, especially if the ileocecal valve is lost.

DIAGNOSIS

Presence of macronutrient and/or micronutrient loss in a patient with a known history of bowel resection

DIFFERENTIAL DIAGNOSIS

Because the history of significant bowel resection is typically known, there is no differential diagnosis. If that history is not known, all causes of weight loss, malabsorption, and diarrhea must be considered.

TREATMENT

Extensive small bowel resection with colectomy (<100 cm of jejunum)

- Rx: long-term total parenteral nutrition (TPN). Some patients can switch to oral intake after 1 to 2 yr of TPN. In jejunostomy patients, excessive fluid loss can be reduced with H_2 blockers, proton pump inhibitors, or octreotide. Micronutrients are supplemented.

Extensive small bowel resection with partial colectomy (usually patients with Crohn's disease)

- Rx: oral intake alone is possible in all patients with >100 cm of jejunum. In addition to vitamin B_{12} deficiency, these patients often have diarrhea. Consider lactose malabsorption and bacterial overgrowth treated, respectively, with lactose restriction and antibiotics (tetracycline 250 mg tid or metronidazole 500 mg tid for 2 wk). Nonspecific antidiarrheal agents may also be indicated (e.g., Imodium or codeine). The patient must be monitored for micronutrient losses.

COMPLICATIONS

- Oxalate kidney stones
- Cholesterol gallstones
- D-Lactic acidosis

PROGNOSIS

Directly dependent on the extent of the bowel resection and in the case of Crohn's disease by the underlying illness

AUTHOR: **FRED F. FERRI, M.D.**

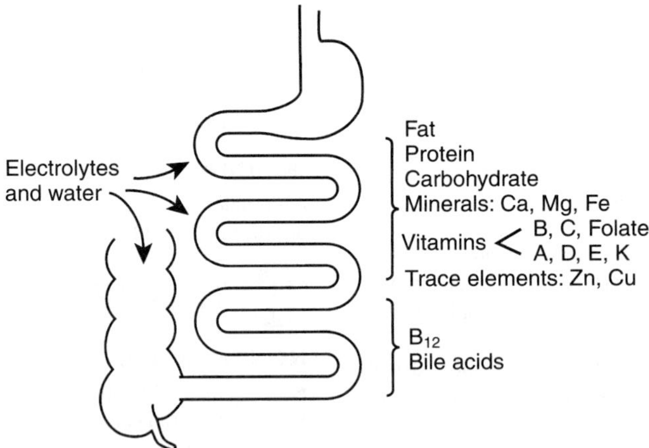

FIGURE 1-298 Specific areas of absorption of constituents of diet and secretions in the gastrointestinal tract. Macronutrients and micronutrients are predominantly absorbed in the proximal jejunum. Bile acids and vitamin B_{12} are only absorbed in the ileum. Electrolytes and water are absorbed in both the small and the large intestine. (From Feldman M et al [eds]: *Sleisenger and Fortran's gastrointestinal and liver disease: pathophysiology, diagnosis, and management,* ed 6, Philadelphia, 1998, WB Saunders.)

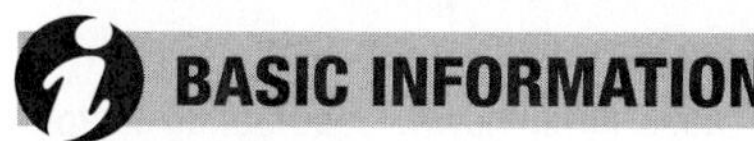

BASIC INFORMATION

DEFINITION

Sialadenitis is an inflammation of the salivary glands.

ICD-9CM CODES
527.2 Sialadenitis

EPIDEMIOLOGY & DEMOGRAPHICS

Parotid or submandibular glands are most frequently affected (Fig. 1-299).

PHYSICAL FINDINGS & CLINICAL PRESENTATION

- Pain and swelling of the affected salivary gland
- Increased pain with meals
- Erythema, tenderness at the duct opening
- Purulent discharge from duct orifice
- Induration and pitting of the skin, with involvement of the masseteric and submandibular spatial planes in severe cases

ETIOLOGY

- Ductal obstruction is generally from a mucus plug caused by stasis of saliva with increased viscosity with subsequent stasis and infection.
- Most frequent infecting organisms are *Staphylococcus aureus, Pseudomonas, Enterobacter, Klebsiella, Enterococcus, Proteus,* and *Candida* spp.
- Sjögren's syndrome, trauma, radiation therapy, chemotherapy, dehydration, and chronic illness are predisposing factors.

Dx DIAGNOSIS

DIFFERENTIAL DIAGNOSIS

- Salivary gland neoplasm
- Ductal stricture
- Sialolithiasis
- Decreased salivary secretion as a result of medications (e.g., amitriptyline, diphenhydramine, anticholinergics)

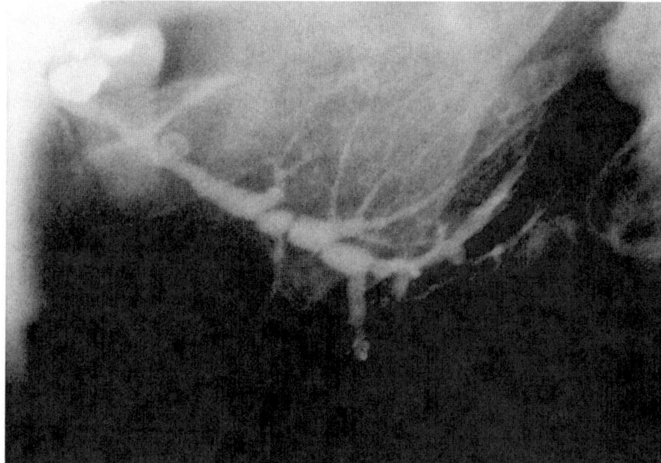

FIGURE 1-299 Sialogram of patient with chronic sialadenitis showing sausage link–like patterns and massive duct dilation. (From Blitzer CE et al: Sialadenitis. In Johnson JT, Yu VL [eds]: *Infectious diseases and antimicrobial therapy of the ears, nose, and throat,* Philadelphia, 1997, WB Saunders.)

WORKUP

- Generally not necessary
- Ultrasound or CT scan in patients not responding to medical treatment

LABORATORY TESTS

- Generally not indicated
- Complete blood count with differential to possibly reveal leukocytosis with left shift

IMAGING STUDIES

- Ultrasound or CT scan may be needed in patients not responding to medical therapy.
- Sialography should not be performed during the acute phase.

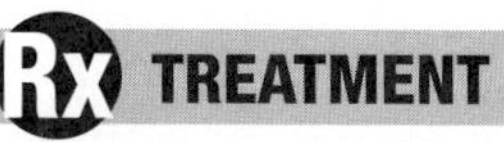

Rx TREATMENT

NONPHARMACOLOGIC THERAPY

- Massage of the gland: may express pus and relieve some of the pressure
- Rehydration
- Warm compresses
- Oral cavity irrigations

ACUTE GENERAL Rx

- Amoxicillin-clavulanate 500 to 875 mg or cefuroxime 250 to 500 mg bid should be given for 10 days. Clindamycin is an alternative choice in patients allergic to penicillin.
- IV antibiotics (e.g., cefoxitin, nafcillin) can be given in severe cases.

DISPOSITION

Complete recovery unless the patient has underlying obstruction (e.g., ductal stricture, tumor, or stone)

REFERRAL

- To ear-nose-throat specialist for nonresolving cases despite appropriate antibiotic therapy
- For salivary gland incision and drainage, which may be necessary in resistant cases

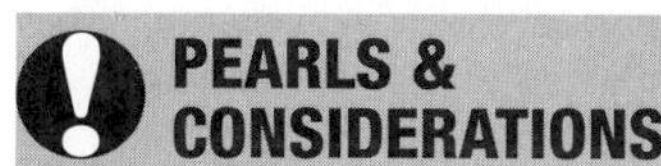

PEARLS & CONSIDERATIONS

COMMENTS

Prevention of dehydration will decrease the risk of sialadenitis.

AUTHOR: **FRED F. FERRI, M.D.**

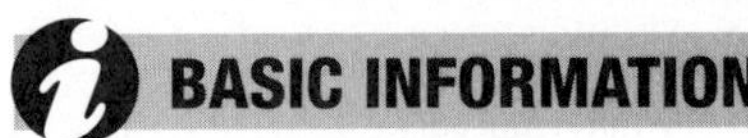

BASIC INFORMATION

DEFINITION

Sialolithiasis is the existence of hardened intraluminal deposits in the ductal system of a salivary gland.

SYNONYMS

Salivary gland stone
Salivary calculus

ICD-9CM CODES

527.5 Sialolithiasis

EPIDEMIOLOGY & DEMOGRAPHICS

Affects patients mostly in the fifth to eighth decades and occurs most commonly in the submandibular gland (80%); only 14% are located in a parotid gland.

PHYSICAL FINDINGS & CLINICAL PRESENTATION

- Symptoms: colicky postprandial pain and swelling of a salivary gland. Tends to have a remitting/relapsing course.
- Signs: swelling and tenderness of a salivary gland. The stone may be felt by palpation of the floor of the mouth (Fig. 1-300).

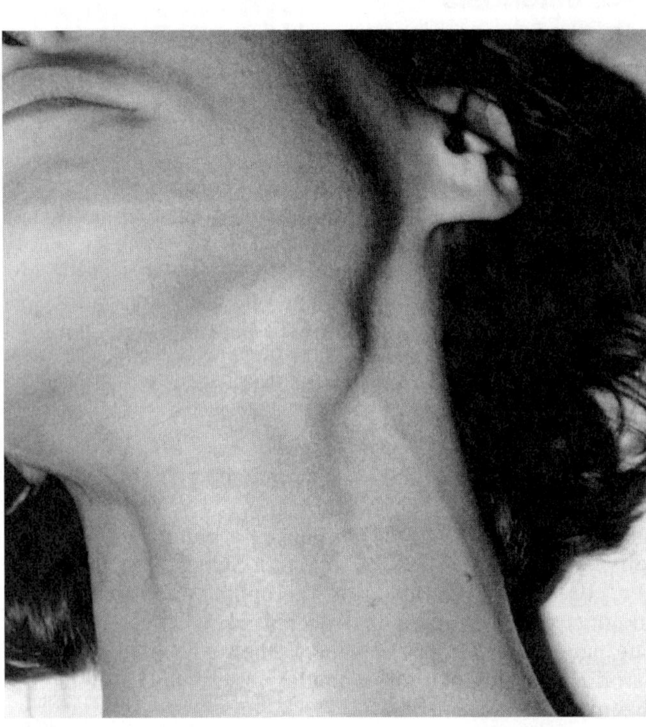

FIGURE 1-300 Patient with large calculus and obstruction of the left submandibular gland. (From Blitzer CE et al: Sialadenitis. In Johnson JT, Yu VL [eds]: *Infectious diseases and antimicrobial therapy of the ears, nose, and throat,* Philadelphia, 1997, WB Saunders.)

ETIOLOGY

- The cause is unknown. Contributing factors include saliva stagnation, sialadenitis (inflammation of a salivary gland), ductal inflammation, or injury.
- Salivary calculus composition is mainly calcium phosphate and carbonate, often combined with small proportions of magnesium, zinc, ammonium salts, and organic materials or debris.

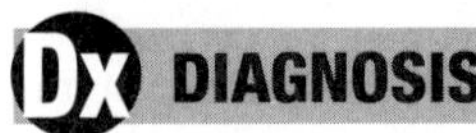

DIAGNOSIS

DIFFERENTIAL DIAGNOSIS

- Lymphadenitis
- Salivary gland tumor
- Salivary gland bacterial (*Staphylococcus* or *Streptococcus*), viral (mumps), or fungal infection (sialadenitis)
- Noninfectious salivary gland inflammation (e.g., Sjögren's syndrome, sarcoidosis, lymphoma)
- Salivary duct stricture
- Dental abscess

IMAGING STUDIES

- Plain radiograph
- Sialography

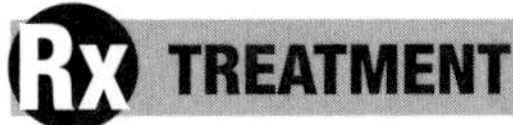

TREATMENT

- Warm soaks to area
- Antibiotics if associated bacterial sialadenitis is present
- Bland diet; avoid citrus fruit and spices
- Manual stone extraction sometimes associated with incisional enlargement of the ductal orifice
- Surgical salivary gland removal for retained hilar calculi

REFERRAL

To otorhinolaryngologist

AUTHOR: **FRED F. FERRI, M.D.**

BASIC INFORMATION

DEFINITION

Sick sinus syndrome is a group of cardiac rhythm disturbances characterized by abnormalities of the sinus node including (1) sinus bradycardia, (2) sinus arrest or exit block, (3) combinations of sinoatrial or atrioventricular conduction defects, and (4) alternating with paroxysmal supraventricular tachyarrhythmias (bradycardia-tachycardia syndrome) that result in atrial rates that are inappropriate for physiologic needs.

SYNONYMS

Bradycardia-tachycardia syndrome

ICD-9CM CODES

427.81 Sick sinus syndrome

EPIDEMIOLOGY & DEMOGRAPHICS

- In children: associated with congenital heart disease
- In adults: primarily a disease of the elderly resulting from degenerative disease of the conduction system. It can also be seen at any age resulting from destruction of the sinus node due to other causes (i.e., ischemia or infarction, infiltrative diseases, endocrinologic abnormalities, etc.).

PHYSICAL FINDINGS & CLINICAL PRESENTATION

- Light-headedness, dizziness, syncope, palpitation
- Physical examination may be normal or reveal abnormalities (e.g., heart murmurs or gallop sounds) associated with the underlying heart disease

ETIOLOGY

- Fibrosis or fatty infiltration involving the sinus node, which may also affect the atrioventricular node, the His bundle, or its branches
- In addition, inflammatory or degenerative changes of the nerves and ganglia surrounding the sinus nodes and other sclerodegenerative changes may be found.

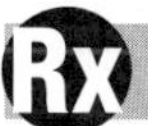

DIAGNOSIS

DIFFERENTIAL DIAGNOSIS

- Bradycardia: atrioventricular block
- Tachycardia: atrial fibrillation
- Atrial flutter
- Paroxysmal atrial tachycardia
- Sinus tachycardia

WORKUP

- ECG
- Ambulatory cardiac rhythm monitoring
- 24-hour ambulatory ECG (Holter) (Fig. 1-301)
- Event recorder
- Electrophysiologic testing including sinus nodal recovery time and sino-atrial conduction time

TREATMENT

- Permanent pacemaker placement if symptoms are present
- In bradycardia-tachycardia syndrome, the drug treatment of the tachycardia (e.g., with digitalis or calcium channel blockers) may worsen or bring out the bradycardia and become the reason for pacemaker requirement

REFERRAL

To cardiologist

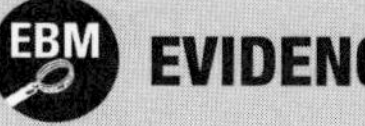

EVIDENCE

Implantation of a permanent pacemaker is the cornerstone of treatment of symptomatic bradycardia in sick sinus syndrome.

A systematic review of dual chamber vs single chamber ventricular pacemakers for sick sinus syndrome and/or atrioventricular block identified five parallel and 26 crossover randomized controlled trials of at least 48 hours duration. Overall, the quality of reporting was found to be poor. Analysis of pooled data from parallel studies showed a statistically nonsignificant preference for physiologic pacing (primarily dual chamber pacing) in terms of the prevention of stroke, heart failure and mortality, and a statistically significant beneficial effect regarding the prevention of atrial fibrillation. With regard to pacemaker syndrome, both parallel and crossover studies favored dual chamber pacing. Analysis of pooled data from crossover studies shows a statistically significant trend toward dual chamber pacing being more favorable in terms of exercise capacity. No individual studies reported a significantly more favorable outcome with single chamber ventricular pacing.[1] Ⓐ

Evidence-Based Reference

1. Dretzke J et al: Dual chamber versus single chamber ventricular pacemakers for sick sinus syndrome and atrioventricular block, *Cochrane Database Rev* 2, 2004. Ⓐ

AUTHORS: **SCOTT BRANCATO, M.D., FRED F. FERRI, M.D.,** and **WEN-CHIH WU, M.D.**

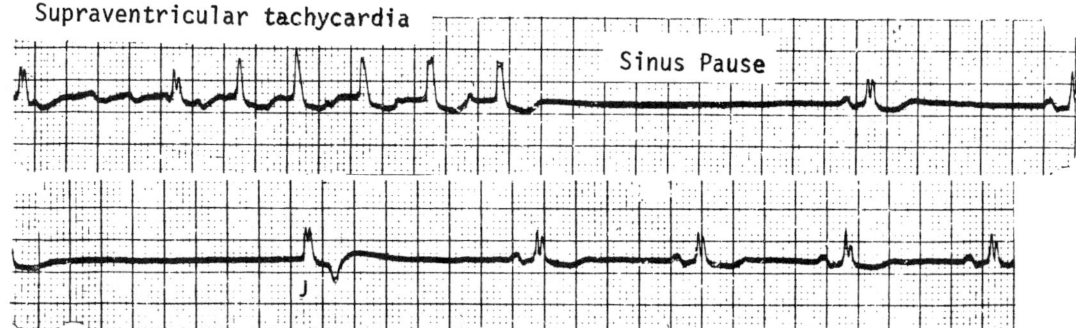

FIGURE 1-301 Brady-tachy (sick sinus) syndrome. This rhythm strip shows a narrow-complex tachycardia (probably atrial flutter) followed by a sinus pause, an AV junctional escape beat *(J),* and then sinus rhythm. (From Goldberger AL: *Clinical electrocardiography,* ed 5, St Louis, 1994, Mosby.)

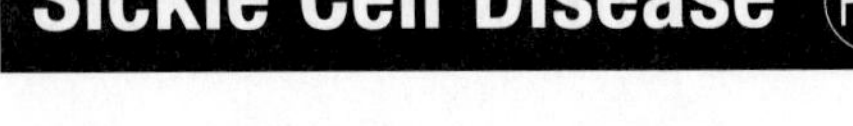

BASIC INFORMATION

DEFINITION

Sickle cell disease is a hemoglobinopathy characterized by the production of hemoglobin S caused by substitution of the amino acid valine for glutamic acid in the sixth position of the gamma-globin chain. When exposed to lower oxygen tension, red blood cells (RBCs) assume a sickle shape, resulting in stasis of RBCs in capillaries. Painful crises are caused by ischemic tissue injury resulting from obstruction of blood flow produced by sickled erythrocytes.

SYNONYMS

Sickle cell anemia
Hemoglobin S disease

ICD-9CM CODES
286.60 Sickle cell anemia

EPIDEMIOLOGY & DEMOGRAPHICS

- Sickle cell hemoglobin S is transmitted by an autosomal-recessive gene. It is found mostly in blacks (one in 400 black Americans).
- Sickle cell trait occurs in nearly 10% of black Americans. It is estimated that 2000 babies are born with sickle cell disease in the U.S. each year.
- There is no predominant sex.

PHYSICAL FINDINGS & CLINICAL PRESENTATION

- Physical examination is variable depending on the degree of anemia and presence of acute vaso-occlusive syndromes or neurologic, cardiovascular, genitourinary, and musculoskeletal complications. Pain in adults with sickle cell disease is the rule rather than the exception and is far more prevalent and severe than reported in older large-scale surveys.
- There is no clinical laboratory finding that is pathognomonic of painful crisis of sickle cell disease. The diagnosis of a painful episode is made solely on the basis of the medical therapy and physical examination.
- Bones are the most common site of pain. Dactylitis, or hand-foot syndrome (acute, painful swelling of the hands and feet), is the first manifestation of sickle cell disease in many infants. Irritability and refusal to walk are other common symptoms. After infancy, musculoskeletal pain can be symmetric, asymmetric, or migratory, and it may or may not be associated with swelling, low-grade fever, redness, or warmth.
- In both children and adults, sickle vaso-occlusive episodes are difficult to distinguish from osteomyelitis, septic arthritis, synovitis, rheumatic fever, or gout.
- When abdominal or visceral pain is present, care should be taken to exclude sequestration syndromes (spleen, liver) or the possibility of an acute condition such as appendicitis, pancreatitis, cholecystitis, urinary tract infection, pelvic inflammatory disease, or malignancy.
- Pneumonia develops during the course of 20% of painful events and can present as chest and abdominal pain. In adults chest pain may be a result of vaso-occlusion in the ribs and often precedes a pulmonary event. The lower back is also a frequent site of painful crisis in adults.
- The acute chest syndrome manifests with chest pain, fever, wheezing, tachypnea, and cough. Chest radiograph reveals pulmonary infiltrates. Common causes include infection (mycoplasma, chlamydia, viruses), infarction, and fat embolism.
- Musculoskeletal and skin abnormalities seen in sickle cell anemia include leg ulcers (particularly on the malleoli) and limb-girdle deformities caused by avascular necrosis of the femoral and humeral heads.
- Endocrine abnormalities include delayed sexual maturation and late physical maturation, especially evident in boys.
- Neurologic abnormalities on examination may include seizures and altered mental status.
- Infections, particularly involving *Salmonella, Mycoplasma,* and *Streptococcus,* are relatively common.
- Severe splenomegaly as a result of sequestration often occurs in children before splenic atrophy.

DIAGNOSIS

DIFFERENTIAL DIAGNOSIS

- Thalassemia
- Iron-deficiency anemia, leukemia
- The differential diagnosis of patients presenting with a painful crisis is discussed in "Physical Findings"

WORKUP

- Screening of all newborns regardless of racial background is recommended. Screening can be performed with sodium metabisulfite reduction test (Sickledex test).
- Hemoglobin electrophoresis will also confirm the diagnosis and is useful to identify hemoglobin variants such as fetal hemoglobin and hemoglobin A2.

LABORATORY TESTS

- Anemia (resulting from chronic hemolysis), reticulocytosis, leukocytosis, and thrombocytosis are common.
- Elevations of bilirubin and lactate dehydrogenase are also common.
- Peripheral blood smear may reveal sickle cells, target cells, poikilocytosis, and hypochromia (Fig. 1-302).
- Elevated blood urea nitrogen and creatinine may be present in patients with progressive renal insufficiency.
- Urinalysis may reveal hematuria and proteinuria.

IMAGING STUDIES

- Chest radiography is useful in patients presenting with chest syndrome. Cardiomegaly may be present on chest x-ray.
- Bone scan is useful to rule out osteomyelitis (usually the result of *Salmonella*). MRI scan is also effective in diagnosing osteomyelitis.
- CT scan or MRI of brain is often needed in patients with neurologic complications such as transient ischemic attack, cerebrovascular accident, seizures, or altered mental status.
- Transcranial Doppler ultrasonograhy (TCD) is a useful commodity to identify children with sickle cell anemia who are at risk for stroke, in adults magnetic resonance angiography (MRA) can be used instead of TCD.
- Doppler echocardiography can be used to diagnose pulmonary hypertension.

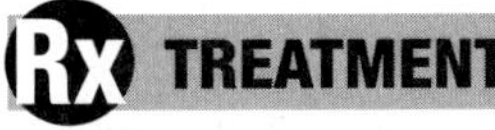

TREATMENT

NONPHARMACOLOGIC THERAPY

- Patients should be instructed to avoid conditions that may precipitate sickling crisis, such as hypoxia, infections, acidosis, and dehydration.
- Maintain adequate hydration (PO or IV).
- Correct hypoxia.

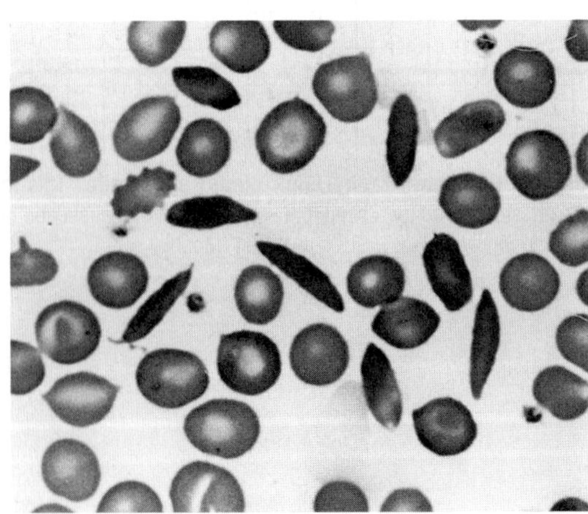

FIGURE 1-302 Photomicrograph of peripheral blood smear with sickle cells, typical of sickle cell anemia. (From Andreoli TE [ed]: *Cecil essentials of medicine,* ed 4, Philadelphia, 1997, WB Saunders.)

S

Diseases and Disorders

ACUTE GENERAL Rx

- Aggressively diagnose and treat suspected infections (*Salmonella* osteomyelitis and pneumococcal infections occur more often in patients with sickle cell anemia because of splenic infarcts and atrophy). Combination therapy with a cephalosporin and erythromycin plus incentive spirometry and bronchodilators is useful in patients with acute chest syndrome.
- Provide pain relief during the vaso-occlusive crisis. The fear of creating or perpetuating addiction or being deceived by patients often causes physicians to prescribe subtherapeutic dosages of opioids. However, available evidence suggests that the prevalence of drug addiction among patients with sickle cell anemia is no higher than in the overall U.S. population. Medications should be administered on a fixed time schedule with a dosing interval that does not extend beyond the duration of the desired pharmacologic effect.
    1. Meperidine is contraindicated in patients with renal dysfunction or central nervous system disease because its metabolite, normeperidine (which is excreted by the kidneys), can cause seizures.
    2. Narcotics (e.g., morphine 0.1 mg/kg IV q3-4h or 0.3 mg/kg PO q4h) should be given on a fixed schedule (not prn for pain), with rescue dosing for breakthrough pain as needed.
    3. Except when contraindications exist, concomitant use of nonsteroidal antiinflammatory drugs should be standard treatment.
    4. Nurses should be instructed not to give narcotics if the patient is heavily sedated or respirations are depressed.
    5. When the patient shows signs of improvement, narcotic drugs should be tapered gradually to prevent withdrawal syndrome. It is advisable to observe the patient on oral pain relief medications for 12 to 24 hr before discharge from the hospital.
    6. Analgesic medications should be used in combination with psychologic, behavioral, and physical modalities in the management of sickle cell disease.
- Aggressively diagnose and treat any potential complications (e.g., septic necrosis of the femoral head, priapism, bony infarcts, and acute chest syndrome).
- Avoid "routine" transfusions but consider early transfusions for patients at high risk for complications. Indications for transfusion include aplastic crises, severe hemolytic crises (particularly during third trimester of pregnancy), acute chest syndrome, and high risk of stroke.
- Hydroxyurea (15 mg/kg body weight per day in patients with normal creatinine clearance) increases hemoglobin F levels and reduces the incidence of vaso-occlusive complications. It is generally well tolerated. Side effects consist primarily of mild, reversible neutropenia. It should be avoided in patients with existing leukopenia, thrombocytopenia, or severe hypoplastic anemia. It is indicated for adults with sickle cell anemia who have moderate to severe disease, typically those with three or more acute painful crises or episodes of the acute chest syndrome in the previous year.
- Replace folic acid (1 mg PO qd) due to loss from increased utilization of folic acid stores due to chronic hemolysis. Sickle cell patients also often have mineral and vitamin deficiencies (calcium, zinc, and vitamins A, C, D, and E) and may need vitamin and nutritional supplementation.

CHRONIC Rx

- Guidelines for prompt management of fever, infections, pain, and specific complications should be reviewed.
- Genetic counseling is recommended in all cases.
- Avoid unnecessary transfusions. Exchange transfusions may be necessary for patients with acute neurologic signs, in aplastic crisis, or undergoing surgery. The target hemoglobin level is 10 to 11 g/dl (hematocrit 30%). Transfusing to a higher Hb/Hct should be avoided due to associated hyperviscosity if there is a substantial portion of HbS in the blood.
- Allogeneic stem cell transplantation can be curative in young patients with symptomatic sickle cell disease; however, the death rate from the procedure is nearly 10%, the marrow recipients are likely to be infertile, and there is an undefined risk of chemotherapy-induced malignancy.
- Penicillin V 125 mg PO bid should be administered by age 2 mo and increased to 250 mg bid by age 3 yr. Penicillin prophylaxis can be discontinued after age 5 yr except in children who have had splenectomy.

REFERRAL

- Hospitalization is generally recommended for most crises and complications.
- Psychosocial counseling and support structures should be developed.

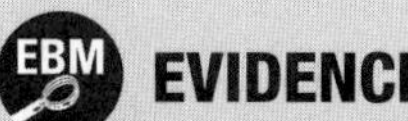

PEARLS & CONSIDERATIONS

COMMENTS

- Pain in adults with sickle cell disease is the rule rather than the exception and needs to be treated appropriately.
- Patients and their families should receive genetic counseling and should be made aware of the difference between sickle cell trait and sickle cell disease.
- Regular immunizations and pneumococcal vaccination are recommended. The prophylactic administration of penicillin soon after birth and the timely administration of pneumococcal and *Haemophilus influenzae* type b vaccines have resulted in a significant decline in the incidence of these infections. The heptavalent conjugated pneumococcal vaccine (Prevan) should be administered from 2 mo of age. The 23-valent unconjugated pneumococcal vaccine is given from age 2 yr and can be boosted once 3 yr later. Influenza vaccination can be given after 6 mo of age.
- Patients should be instructed on a well-balanced diet and appropriate folic acid supplementation.
- The presence of dactylitis, Hb 7, or leukocytosis in the absence of infection during the first 2 yr of life indicates a higher risk of severe sickle cell disease later in life.
- Among patients with sickle cell disease, acute chest syndrome is commonly precipitated by fat embolism and infection, especially community-acquired pneumonia. Among older patients and those with neurologic symptoms, the syndrome often progresses to respiratory failure.
- Poloxamer 188, a nonionic surfactant with hemorrheologic and antithrombotic properties, has been reported to produce a significant but relatively small decrease in the duration of painful episodes and an increase in the proportion of patients who achieved resolution of the symptoms. A more significant effect was observed in patients who received concomitant hydroxyurea.
- Pulmonary hypertension is a complication of chronic hemolysis and is associated with a high risk of death. It can be detected by Doppler echocardiography in more than 30% of adult patients with sickle cell disease. Cardiac catheterization will confirm the diagnosis. It is resistant to hydroxyurea therapy.

EBM EVIDENCE

Please note: Complete text of EBM for this topic is available online.

SUGGESTED READINGS

Brawley OW et al: National Institute of Health Consensus Development Conference Statement: hydroxyurea treatment for sickle cell disease, *Ann Intern Med* 148:932-938, 2008.

Gladwin MT, Vichinski EP: Pulmonary complications of sickle cell disease, *N Engl J Med* 359:2254-2265, 2008.

Lanzkron S et al: Systematic review: hydroxyurea for the treatment of adults with sickle cell disease, *Ann Intern Med* 148:939-955, 2008.

Platt OS: Hydroxyurea for the treatment of sickle cell anemia, *N Engl J Med* 358:1362-1369, 2008.

AUTHOR: **FRED F. FERRI, M.D.**

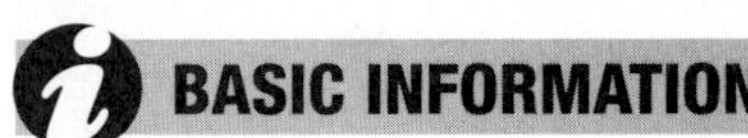

BASIC INFORMATION

DEFINITION

Silicosis is a lung disease attributable to the inhalation of silica (silicon dioxide) in crystalline form (quartz) or in cristobalite or tridymite forms.

SYNONYMS

Pneumoconiosis caused by silica

ICD-9CM CODES
502 Silicosis, occupational
503 Pneumoconiosis caused by other inorganic dust

EPIDEMIOLOGY & DEMOGRAPHICS

- Occupational disease affecting men and women involved in gathering, milling, processing, or using silica-containing rock or sand
- An estimated 1 million Americans are exposed

PHYSICAL FINDINGS & CLINICAL PRESENTATION

- Dyspnea
- Cough
- Wheezing
- Abnormal chest radiograph in an asymptomatic person

ETIOLOGY

- Silica particles are ingested by alveolar macrophages, which in turn release oxidants causing cell injury and cell death, attract fibroblasts, and activate lymphocytes, increasing immunoglobulins in the alveolar space.
- Hyperplasia of alveolar epithelial cells occurs.
- Collagen accumulates in the interstitium.
- Neutrophils also accumulate and secrete proteolytic enzymes, which leads to tissue destruction and emphysema.
- Silica dust may be carcinogenic (not proven).
- Exposure to silicosis predisposes to tuberculosis.
- Some patients develop rheumatoid silicotic pulmonary nodules and may have arthritic symptoms of rheumatoid arthritis (Caplan's syndrome). Scleroderma has also been associated with silicosis.

DIAGNOSIS

DIFFERENTIAL DIAGNOSIS

- Other pneumoconiosis, berylliosis, hard metal disease, asbestosis
- Sarcoidosis
- Tuberculosis
- Interstitial lung disease
- Hypersensitivity pneumonitis
- Lung cancer
- Langerhans' cell granulomatosis (histiocytosis X)
- Granulomatous pulmonary vasculitis

WORKUP

- History of occupational exposure
- Chest radiograph (Fig. 1-303)

Chronic silicosis:
- Characteristic finding: small, rounded lung parenchymal opacities
- Hilar lymphadenopathy with "eggshell" calcifications
- Pleural plaques (uncommon)

Accelerated silicosis (progressive massive fibrosis):
- Large parenchymal lesions resulting from coalesced small nodules

Acute silicosis:
- Ground-glass appearance of the lung fields
- Chest CT scan
- Pulmonary function tests
- Combination of obstructive and restrictive changes with or without reduction in diffusing capacity
- Bronchoscopy with lung biopsy in uncertain cases

COURSE

Chronic silicosis:
- May not progress with absence of further exposure
- Accelerated silicosis: progressive respiratory failure and cor pulmonale

Acute silicosis:
- Fatal course from respiratory failure over several months to a few years

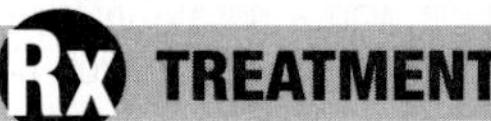

TREATMENT

- Prevention (industrial hygiene)
- Treatment of associated tuberculosis if present
- Supportive measures (oxygen, bronchodilators)
- Lung transplant

AUTHOR: **FRED F. FERRI, M.D.**

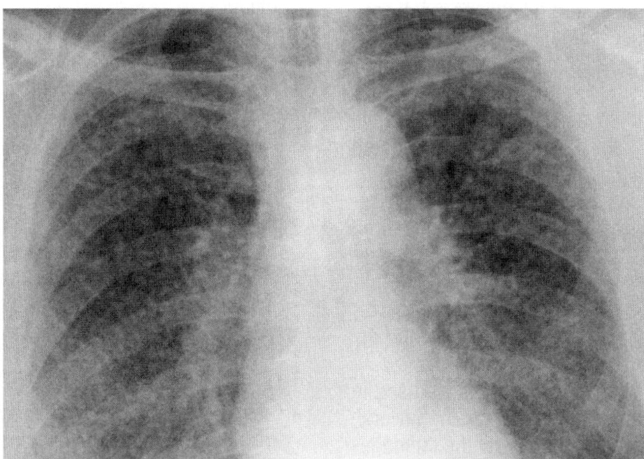

FIGURE 1-303 Simple silicosis. There are multiple small (2- to 4-mm) nodules distributed throughout the lungs, with an upper lobe predominance. (From McLoud TC: *Thoracic radiology: the requisites,* St Louis, 1998, Mosby.)

BASIC INFORMATION

DEFINITION

Sinusitis is inflammation of the mucous membranes lining one or more of the paranasal sinuses. The various presentations are:

- Acute sinusitis: infection lasting <30 days, with complete resolution of symptoms.
- Subacute infection: lasts from 30 to 90 days, with complete resolution of symptoms.
- Recurrent acute infection: episodes of acute infection lasting <30 days, with resolution of symptoms, which recur at intervals at least 10 days apart.
- Chronic sinusitis: inflammation lasting >90 days, with persistent upper respiratory symptoms.
- Acute bacterial sinusitis superimposed on chronic sinusitis: new symptoms that occur in patients with residual symptoms from prior infection(s). With treatment, the new symptoms resolve but the residual ones do not.

SYNONYMS

Rhinosinusitis: sinusitis is almost always accompanied by inflammation of the nasal mucosa; thus it is now the preferred term.

ICD-9CM CODES
473.9 Sinusitis (accessory) (nasal) (hyperplastic) (nonpurulent) (purulent) (chronic)
461.9 Acute sinusitis

EPIDEMIOLOGY & DEMOGRAPHICS

INCIDENCE (IN U.S.): Seems to correlate with the incidence of upper respiratory tract infections

PEAK INCIDENCE: Fall, winter, spring: September through March

PHYSICAL FINDINGS & CLINICAL PRESENTATION

- Patients often give a history of a recent upper respiratory illness with some improvement, then a relapse.
- Mucopurulent secretions in the nasal passage:
  1. Purulent nasal and postnasal discharge lasting 7 to 10 days
  2. Facial tightness, pressure, or pain
  3. Nasal obstruction
  4. Headache
  5. Decreased sense of smell
  6. Purulent pharyngeal secretions, brought up with cough, often worse at night
- Erythema, swelling, and tenderness over the infected sinus in a small proportion of patients:
  1. Diagnosis cannot be excluded by the absence of such findings.
  2. These findings are not common, and do not correlate with number of positive sinus aspirates.
- Intermittent low-grade fever in about half of adults with acute bacterial sinusitis.
- Toothache is a common complaint when the maxillary sinus is involved.
- Periorbital cellulitis and excessive tearing with ethmoid sinusitis:
  1. Orbital extension of infection: chemosis, proptosis, impaired extraocular movements
- Characteristics of acute sinusitis in children with upper respiratory tract infections:
  1. Persistence of symptoms
  2. Cough
  3. Bad breath
- Symptoms of chronic sinusitis (may or may not be present):
  1. Nasal or postnasal discharge
  2. Fever
  3. Facial pain or pressure
  4. Headache
- Nosocomial sinusitis is typically seen in patients with nasogastric tubes or nasotracheal intubation.

ETIOLOGY

- Each of the four paranasal sinuses is connected to the nasal cavity by narrow tubes (ostia), 1 to 3 mm in diameter; these drain directly into the nose through the turbinates. The sinuses are lined with a ciliated mucous membrane (mucoperiosteum).
- Acute viral infection:
  1. Infection with the common cold or influenza
  2. Mucosal edema and sinus inflammation
  3. Decreased drainage of thick secretions/obstruction of the sinus ostia
  4. Subsequent entrapment of bacteria
     a. Multiplication of bacteria
     b. Secondary bacterial infection
- Other predisposing factors:
  1. Tumors
  2. Polyps
  3. Foreign bodies
  4. Congenital choanal atresia
  5. Other entities that cause obstruction of sinus drainage
  6. Allergies
  7. Asthma
- Dental infections lead to maxillary sinusitis.
- Viruses recovered alone or in combination with bacteria (in 16% of cases):
  1. Rhinovirus
  2. Coronavirus
  3. Adenovirus
  4. Parainfluenza virus
  5. Respiratory syncytial virus
- The principal bacterial pathogens in sinusitis are *Streptococcus pneumoniae,* nontypeable *Haemophilus influenzae,* and *Moraxella catarrhalis.*
- In the remainder of cases find *Streptococcus pyogenes, Staphylococcus aureus,* α-hemolytic streptococci, and mixed anaerobic infections (*Peptostreptococcus, Fusobacterium, Bacteroides, Prevotella* spp.).
- Infection is polymicrobial in about one third of cases.
- Anaerobic infections are seen more often in cases of chronic sinusitis and in cases associated with dental infection; anaerobes are unlikely pathogens in sinusitis in children.
- Fungal pathogens are isolated with increasing frequency in immunocompromised patients but remain uncommon pathogens in the paranasal sinuses. Fungal pathogens include: *Phaeohyphomycoses, Aspergillus, Pseudallescheria, Sporothrix,* and *Zygomycetes* spp.
- Nosocomial infections: occur in patients with nasogastric tubes, nasotracheal intubation, cystic fibrosis, and patients who are immunocompromised.
  1. *S. aureus* (including MRSA)
  2. *Pseudomonas aeruginosa*
  3. *Klebsiella pneumoniae*
  4. *Enterobacter* spp.
  5. *Proteus mirabilis*
- Organisms typically isolated in chronic sinusitis:
  1. *S. aureus*
  2. *S. pneumoniae*
  3. *H. influenzae*
  4. *P. aeruginosa*
  5. Anaerobes

Dx DIAGNOSIS

DIFFERENTIAL DIAGNOSIS

- Temporomandibular joint disease
- Migraine headache
- Cluster headache
- Dental infection
- Trigeminal neuralgia

WORKUP

- In the normal healthy host, the paranasal sinuses should be sterile. Although the contiguous structures are colonized with bacteria and likely contaminate the sinuses, the mucociliary lining functions to remove these bacteria.
- Gold standard for diagnosis: recovery of bacteria in high density $\geq 10^4$ colony-forming units/ml from a paranasal sinus, in the setting of a patient with history of upper respiratory infection and symptoms persisting for 7 to 10 days. Sinus aspiration is the best method for obtaining cultures; however, it must be performed by an otorhinolaryngologist and is not practical for the primary care practitioner. Therefore, most diagnoses are based on the clinical history and presentation, possibly supported by radiologic evaluations.
  1. Standard four-view sinus radiographs
     a. Complete opacification and air-fluid levels are most specific findings (average 85% and 80%, respectively)
     b. Mucosal thickening has low specificity (40% to 50%)
     c. Absence of all three of the previous findings has estimated sensitivity of 90%
     d. Overall, standard radiographs are of limited use in diagnosis, although negative films are strong evidence against the diagnosis

2. CT scans:
    a. Much more sensitive than plain radiographs in detecting acute changes and disease in the sinuses
    b. Recommended for patients requiring surgical intervention, including sinus aspiration; it is a useful adjunct to guide therapy
3. Transillumination:
    a. Used for diagnosis of frontal and maxillary sinusitis
    b. Place transilluminator in the mouth or against cheek to assess maxillary sinuses, under medial aspect of the supraorbital ridge to assess frontal sinuses
    c. Absence of light transmission indicates that sinus is filled with fluid
    d. Dullness (decreased light transmission) is less helpful in diagnosing infection
4. Endoscopy:
    a. Used to visualize secretions coming from the ostia of infected sinuses
    b. Culture collection via endoscopy often contaminated by nasal flora; not nearly as good as sinus puncture
5. Sinus puncture:
    a. Gold standard for collecting sinus cultures
    b. Generally reserved for treatment failures, suspected intracranial extension, and nosocomial sinusitis

Rx TREATMENT

NONPHARMACOLOGIC THERAPY

To help promote sinus drainage:

- Air humidification with vaporizers (for steam) or humidifiers (for a cool mist)
- Application of hot, wet towel over the face
- Sipping hot beverages
- Hydration

ACUTE GENERAL Rx

- Sinus drainage:
    1. Nasal vasoconstrictors, such as phenylephrine nose drops, 0.25% or 0.5%
    2. Topical decongestants should not be used for more than a few days because of the risk of rebound congestion
    3. Systemic decongestants
    4. Nasal or systemic corticosteroids, such as nasal beclomethasone, short course oral prednisone
    5. Nasal irrigation, with hypertonic or normal saline (saline may act as a mild vasoconstrictor of nasal blood flow)
    6. Use of antihistamines has no proven benefit, and the drying effect on the mucous membranes may cause crusting, which blocks the ostia, thus interfering with sinus drainage
- Analgesics, antipyretics

Antimicrobial therapy:

- Most cases of acute sinusitis have a viral cause and will resolve within 2 wk without antibiotics.
- Current treatment recommendations favor symptomatic treatment for those with mild symptoms.
- Antibiotics should be reserved for those with moderate to severe symptoms who meet the criteria for diagnosis of sinusitis.
- Antibiotic therapy is usually empiric, targeting the common pathogens:
    1. First-line antibiotics include amoxicillin, erythromycin, TMP/SMX.
    2. Second-line antibiotics include the newer macrolides: clarithromycin, azithromycin, amoxicillin/clavulanate, cefuroxime axetil, cefprozil, cefaclor, loracarbef, ciprofloxacin, levofloxacin, moxifloxacin, clindamycin, metronidazole, and others.
    3. For patients with uncomplicated acute sinusitis, the less expensive first-line agents appear to be as effective as the costlier second-line agents.
- Hospitalization and IV antibiotics may be required for more severe infection and those with suspected intracranial complications. Broader-spectrum antibiotic coverage may be indicated in severe cases, to cover for MRSA, *Pseudomonas,* and fungal pathogens.
- Duration of therapy generally 10 to 14 days, although some have success with much shorter regimens

Surgery:

- Surgical drainage indicated
    1. If intracranial or orbital complications suspected
    2. Many cases of frontal and sphenoid sinusitis
    3. Chronic sinusitis recalcitrant to medical therapy
- Surgical debridement imperative in the treatment of fungal sinusitis

Complications:

- Untreated, sinusitis may lead to a number of serious, life-threatening complications.
- Intracranial complications include meningitis, brain abscess, and epidural and subdural empyema.
- Intracranial sequelae are more common with frontal and ethmoid infections.
- Extracranial complications include orbital cellulitis, blindness, orbital abscess, osteomyelitis.
- Extracranial sequelae are more commonly seen with ethmoid sinusitis.

CHRONIC Rx

- Broad-spectrum antibiotics that cover both aerobes and anaerobes
- Duration of therapy not clearly established: range 3 to 6 wk
- Adjunctive therapy: one or more of the various options listed previously
- Surgical intervention may be necessary in nonresponders

DISPOSITION

Appropriate diagnosis and treatment are necessary to avoid the various sequelae that can occur without proper therapy.

REFERRAL

- To infectious disease specialist if failure to respond to initial therapy
- To otorhinolaryngologist for:
    1. Failure to respond to therapy
    2. Suspected fungal infection
    3. Suspected intracranial or orbital complications

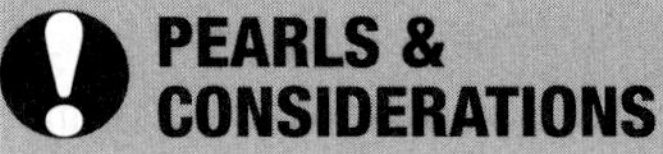

PEARLS & CONSIDERATIONS

- Recurrent sinusitis is usually related to anatomic defects, poor drainage, or immunocompromised states; such patients deserve a thorough workup by an ENT specialist and/or an infectious disease specialist.
- Nosocomial sinusitis from obstruction by nasotracheal or nasogastric tubes is not uncommon and can be difficult to recognize in patients in the critical care units.

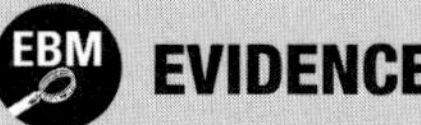

EVIDENCE

Please note: Complete text of EBM for this topic is available online.

SUGGESTED READINGS

Cherry WB, Li J: Chronic rhinosinusitis in adults, *Am J Med* 121:185-189, 2008.

Rosenfeld RM et al: Clinical practice guideline: adult sinusitis. *Otolaryngol Head Neck Surg* 137 (suppl S) S1-31, 2007.

Taxy JB: Paranasal funal sinusitis: contributions of histopathology to diagnosis: a report of 60 cases and literature review, *Am J Surg Pathol* 30(6):713, 2006.

Williamson I et al: Antibiotics and topical nasal steroid for treatment of acute maxillary sinusitis, *JAMA* 298(1):2487-2496, 2007.

AUTHORS: **GLENN G. FORT, M.D., M.P.H.,** and **DENNIS J. MIKOLICH, M.D.**

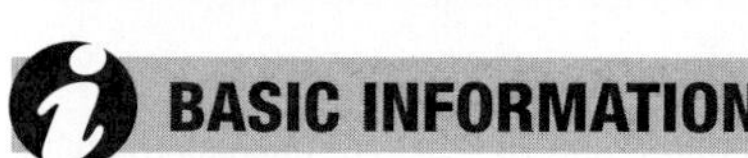

BASIC INFORMATION

DEFINITION

Sjögren's syndrome (SS) is an autoimmune disorder characterized by lymphocytic and plasma cell infiltration and destruction of salivary and lacrimal glands with subsequent diminished lacrimal and salivary gland secretions.

- Primary: dry mouth (xerostomia) and dry eyes (xerophthalmia) develop as isolated entities.
- Secondary: associated with other disorders.

SYNONYMS

SS
Sicca syndrome

ICD-9CM CODES
710.2 Sjögren's syndrome

EPIDEMIOLOGY & DEMOGRAPHICS

INCIDENCE & PREVALENCE: 1-2 million persons in the U.S. are affected. Prevalence is 0.05%-4.8% of population; secondary SS is also common and can affect up to one third of patients with systemic lupus erythematosus (SLE) and nearly 20% of rheumatoid arthritis (RA) patients.
PREDOMINANT SEX: Females are affected much more often than males.
PREDOMINANT AGE: Peak incidence is in the sixth decade.

PHYSICAL FINDINGS & CLINICAL PRESENTATION

- Dry mouth with dry lips (cheilosis), erythema of tongue (Fig. 1-304) and other mucosal surfaces, carious teeth
- Dry eyes (conjunctival injection, decreased luster, and irregularity of the corneal light reflex)
- Possible salivary gland enlargement and dysfunction, with subsequent difficulty in chewing and swallowing food and in speaking without frequent water intake
- Purpura (nonthrombocytopenic, hyperglobulinemic, vasculitic) may be present
- Evidence of associated conditions (e.g., RA or other connective tissue disease, lymphoma, hypothyroidism, chronic obstructive pulmonary disease, trigeminal neuropathy, chronic liver disease, polymyopathy)

ETIOLOGY

Autoimmune disorder

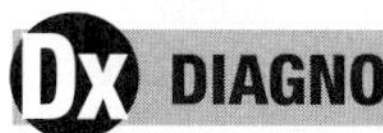

DIAGNOSIS

DIFFERENTIAL DIAGNOSIS

- Medication-related dryness (e.g., anticholinergics)
- Age-related exocrine gland dysfunction
- Mouth breathing
- Anxiety
- Other: sarcoidosis, primary salivary hypofunction, radiation injury, amyloidosis

WORKUP

Workup involves ocular and oral examination and laboratory and radiographic testing to demonstrate the following criteria for diagnosis of primary and secondary SS.

PRIMARY:

- Symptoms and objective signs of ocular dryness:
  1. Schirmer's test: <8 mm wetting per 5 min
  2. Positive rose bengal or fluorescein staining of cornea and conjunctiva to demonstrate keratoconjunctivitis sicca
- Symptoms and objective signs of dry mouth:
  1. Decreased parotid flow using Lashley cups or other methods
  2. Abnormal biopsy result of minor salivary gland (focus score >2 based on average of four assessable lobules)
- Evidence of systemic autoimmune disorder:
  1. Elevated titer of rheumatoid factor $>1{:}320$
  2. Elevated titer of antinuclear antibody (ANA) $>1{:}320$
  3. Presence of anti-SS A (Ro) or anti-SS B (La) antibodies

FIGURE 1-304 "Crocodile tongue" in a patient with Sjögren's syndrome. (From Noble J: *Primary care medicine*, ed 3, St Louis, 2001, Mosby.)

SECONDARY:

- Characteristic signs and symptoms of SS
- Clinical features sufficient to allow a diagnosis of RA, SLE, polymyositis, or scleroderma

LABORATORY TESTS

- Positive ANA ($>60\%$ of patients) with autoantibodies anti-SS A and anti-SS B may be present.
- Additional laboratory abnormalities may include elevated erythrocyte sedimentation rate, anemia (normochromic, normocytic), abnormal liver function studies, elevated serum $beta_2$ microglobulin levels, rheumatoid factor.
- A definite diagnosis of SS can be made with a salivary gland biopsy.

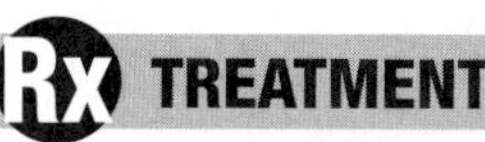

TREATMENT

NONPHARMACOLOGIC THERAPY

- Adequate fluid replacement. Ameliorate skin dryness by gently blotting dry after bathing, leaving a small amount of moisture, and then applying a moisturizer.
- Proper oral hygiene (daily topical fluoride use and antimicrobial mouth rinses) to reduce the incidence of caries. Sugar-free chewing gum and sour lemon lozenges to stimulate salivary secretion.
- Periodic dental and ophthalmology evaluations to screen for complications.

GENERAL Rx

- Use artificial tears frequently.
- Pilocarpine 5 mg PO qid is useful to improve dryness. A cyclosporine 0.05% ophthalmic emulsion (Restasis) may also be useful for dry eyes. Recommended dose is one drop bid in both eyes.
- Cevimeline (Evoxac), a cholinergic agent with muscarinic agonist activity, 30 mg PO tid is effective for the treatment of dry mouth in patients with SS.
- Interferon-alfa, 150 IU tid for 12 wk, has been shown to significantly improve stimulated whole saliva output and decrease reports of xerostomia.
- Hydroxychloroquine may be useful for arthralgias, rituximab for severe inflammatory manifestations.

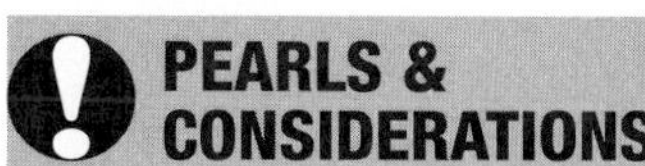

PEARLS & CONSIDERATIONS

COMMENTS

- Unusual presentations of SS may occur in association with polymyalgia rheumatica, chronic fatigue syndrome, fever of unknown origin, and inflammatory myositis.
- The most serious complication of primary SS is the development of non-Hodgkin's lymphoma and other lymphoproliferative disorders.

SUGGESTED READING

Kruszka P, O'Brian RJ: Diagnosis and management of Sjögren syndrome, *Am Fam Phys* 79(6):465-470, 2009.

AUTHOR: **FRED F. FERRI, M.D.**

BASIC INFORMATION

DEFINITION

The *International Classification of Sleep Disorders, Second Edition,* classifies sleep-disordered breathing disorders into three categories: central sleep apnea syndrome, obstructive sleep apnea (OSA), and sleep-related hypoventilation/hypoxic syndromes. The American Academy of Sleep Disorders defines OSA as repetitive episodes of upper airway obstruction that occur during sleep and that are typically associated with oxyhemoglobin desaturations.

SYNONYMS

Sleep apnea syndrome
Sleep-disordered breathing
Obstructive sleep apnea syndrome
Obstructive sleep apnea–hypopnea syndrome

ICD-9CM CODES
327.2 Organic sleep apnea
327.21 Organic sleep apnea, unspecified
327.23 Obstructive sleep apnea (adult) (pediatric)

EPIDEMIOLOGY & DEMOGRAPHICS

OSA is a common disease in the United States. Data from the Wisconsin Cohort Study indicated that the prevalence of OSA in people between the ages of 30 and 60 yr is 9% to 24% for men and 4% to 9% for women. The estimated prevalence of OSA is 4% for men and 2% for women. The prevalence is higher in obese and hypertensive patients. OSA in children most commonly occurs among preschool-aged and early school-aged children, and it is associated with hypertrophy of the adenoids and tonsils.

PHYSICAL FINDINGS & CLINICAL PRESENTATION

- Nocturnal symptoms
- Snoring that can be loud, habitual, and bothersome to others
- Witnessed apneas that often interrupt the snoring and that end with a snort
- Gasping or choking sensations that arouse the patient from sleep
- Restless sleep associated with frequent arousals
- Daytime symptoms:
  - Nonrestorative sleep
  - Not feeling refreshed upon awakening
  - Morning headache
  - Dry mouth or throat upon awakening
  - Excessive daytime sleepiness, typically during quiet activities
  - Daytime fatigue or tiredness
  - Problems with memory, concentration, and cognitive function, especially with executive functioning
  - Easily angered, short tempered, and inattentive
  - Hyperactivity in children
- Systemic hypertension
- Obesity (body mass index >30 kg/m^2)
- Mood swings, anxiety, depression, and decreased libido
- A neck circumference of >43 cm (17 in) in men and of >37 cm (15 in) in women has been associated with an increased risk for OSA.
- The oropharynx may be erythematous as a result of snoring.
- Adenotonsillar hypertrophy, excessive soft tissue, high-arched hard palate, pendulous uvula, prominent tongue, large degree of overjet, and retrognathia or micrognathia can be present.
- A narrowing of the lateral airway walls is an independent predictor of OSA in men but not in women.
- Craniofacial skeletal abnormalities can lead to OSA, particularly among children and nonobese adults.
- A positive family history increases an individual's risk with each additional close family member with OSA.

ETIOLOGY

- Narrowing of upper airway as a result of obesity or increased peripharyngeal fat deposition, retrognathia and/or micrognathia, adenotonsillar hypertrophy, macroglossia, or neuromuscular weakness
- Upper airway muscular weakness as a result of neuromuscular disorders, primary central nervous system disorders (e.g., stroke), or metabolic disorders
- Other diseases associated with the development of OSA (e.g., hypothyroidism, acromegaly)

Dx DIAGNOSIS

DIFFERENTIAL DIAGNOSIS

- Anemia
- Anxiety or panic disorder
- Behaviorally induced insufficient sleep syndrome
- Cardiac or heart disease
- Central sleep apnea
- Circadian rhythm disorder
- Depression
- Drug or alcohol abuse
- Hypothyroidism
- Idiopathic hypersomnia with long or short sleep time
- Inadequate sleep hygiene
- Insomnia
- Medication effect
- Narcolepsy
- Nocturnal asthma
- Nocturnal gastroesophageal reflux
- Obesity–hypoventilation syndrome (i.e., Pickwickian syndrome)
- Parasomnias
- Parkinson's disease
- Periodic limb movement disorder
- Primary snoring
- Pulmonary or lung disease
- Restless legs syndrome
- Sleep fragmentation (multiple causes)

WORKUP

- Evaluation should include questions about snoring, witnessed apneas, gasping or choking episodes, restless sleep, and excessive daytime sleepiness.
- Mood swings and personality changes should be addressed.
- Job performance and difficulty driving or previous motor vehicle accidents related to excessive daytime sleepiness should be discussed
- Additional historic concerns include morning dry mouth or throat, morning headaches, alcohol intake, weight gain, and mood or personality changes.
- A thorough drug history should include muscle relaxants and sedatives.
- A family history should target any family members with OSA.
- The physical examination is frequently normal in patients with OSA except for the presence of obesity, enlarged neck circumference, and hypertension.
- OSA is confirmed by nocturnal polysomnography (PSG), which is the gold standard for diagnosis. The PSG should be performed during the patient's typical sleeping hours; it should all stages of sleep as well as sleep in the supine position.
- The severity of the OSA is determined by the apnea–hypopnea index (AHI), which is derived from the total number of apneas and hypopneas divided by the total sleep time.
- Recommended severity cutoff levels for the AHI are as follows:
  - Mild: 5 to 15 episodes per hour
  - Moderate: 15 to 30 episodes per hour
  - Severe: >30 episodes per hour
- Criteria for the treatment of mild OSA often require symptoms, including excessive daytime sleepiness, cardiovascular disease, hypertension, and mood swings.
- In-home respiratory monitoring is an effective alternative to PSG for the evaluation of OSA.

LABORATORY TESTS

- Arterial blood gas testing should be performed if a patient has suspected pulmonary hypertension or cor pulmonale to rule out daytime hypoxemia or hypercapnia.
- The thyroid-stimulating hormone level should be obtained if hypothyroidism is suspected.
- A CBC is helpful to look for anemia, and iron studies are indicated if anemia is detected.
- Pulmonary function testing is indicated if a pulmonary disorder is suspected or to assess the severity of neuromuscular disease, if present.
- An ECG or possibly an echocardiogram is indicated if a cardiac disorder (e.g., arrhythmia, pulmonary hypertension) is suspected.

IMAGING STUDIES

- Plain radiography of the neck can be helpful to assess the soft tissues of patients with suspected anatomic abnormalities.
- Chest x-ray is indicated if pulmonary disease is suspected.

Rx TREATMENT

NONPHARMACOLOGIC THERAPY

- Behavioral modifications:
  - Weight loss in overweight and obese patients, with consideration of bariatric surgery
  - Avoidance of alcohol for 4 to 6 hours before bedtime
  - Avoidance of muscle relaxants and sedating medications
  - Sleep hygiene training
  - Avoidance or elimination of supine sleeping positions
- Medical treatment:
  - Nasal continuous positive airway pressure (CPAP) is the primary therapy for OSA. It provides a pneumatic splint that relieves the upper airway obstruction.
  - An oral appliance constructed by a reputable and qualified dentist may be effective for the treatment of mild OSA in certain patients, especially those with retrognathia.
  - The optimal treatment of allergic rhinitis is needed; nasal corticosteroids are often helpful.
  - Symptoms of excessive daytime sleepiness may linger and require further investigation or medical therapy.
  - Patients should be considered for surgery if multiple attempts at CPAP therapy have failed and if an oral appliance is not an option. If the patient opts for surgery, ensure that the surgery is performed by a reputable and qualified otolaryngologist and that the surgery is based on the location of airway collapse.
- Surgical treatment:
  - Adenotonsillectomy is often curative for children with OSA.
  - Nasal septoplasty should be considered for patients with nasoseptal deformities.
  - Uvulopalatopharyngoplasty, which involves the resection of the uvula and the soft palate, is effective for approximately 40% of patients. However, predicting which patients will benefit from the procedure is difficult.
  - Tracheostomy is typically reserved for patients with very severe OSA who cannot tolerate CPAP or who have cor pulmonale.

DISPOSITION

- The short-term prognosis for excessive daytime sleepiness and snoring is good to excellent with the regular use of nasal CPAP, but no studies have been performed to address the long-term effects in a large population of patients.
- Residual symptoms of excessive daytime sleepiness can occur in some patients with OSA despite regular CPAP use. This has led the U.S. Food and Drug Administration to approve modafinil (Provigil) for the management of residual sleepiness.

REFERRAL

- Highly trained sleep specialists with expertise in caring for patients with OSA are recommended, especially for complex cases.
- Surgical referral to otolaryngology should be considered for children and for adults who are unresponsive to weight loss and CPAP therapy.
- Referral to a qualified dentist for treatment with an oral appliance may be useful for certain patients with mild OSA.

PEARLS & CONSIDERATIONS

- OSA is a common disorder that is underrecognized and underdiagnosed, so the identification of risk factors is crucial for making the correct diagnosis.
- The prevalence of OSA increases among women after menopause.
- The degree of tonsillar hypertrophy does not correlate with the presence of OSA in children.
- A 10% weight loss can decrease the AHI of a patient with OSA by as much as 50%.
- The single most effective therapy for OSA is nasal CPAP.
- Patients with OSA are more vulnerable than healthy persons to the effects of alcohol consumption and sleep restriction with regard to various driving performance variables.

EBM EVIDENCE

Please note: Complete text of EBM for this topic is available online.

Key trials and commentary:

This study sought to examine the short-term and longer term (6-week) effects of continuous positive airway pressure (CPAP) on myocardial energetics.

Obstructive sleep apnea (OSA) and heart failure (HF) are both states of increased afterload and metabolic demand. This study showed that treatment with CPAP may initially reduce stroke volume but subsequently improves left ventricular function. However, it is not clear whether CPAP therapy favorably affects myocardial energetics and hence improves cardiac efficiency.

In this cohort of patients with HF and OSA, short-term CPAP decreased oxidative metabolism and tended to decrease SVI, but did not alter cardiac efficiency. Longer term CPAP improved cardiac efficiency, indicating an energy-sparing effect. These effects may contribute to the benefits of CPAP therapy.

OSA occurs in more than a third of patients with congestive heart failure (CHF). There are multiple pathophysiologic effects of OSA on the cardiovascular system, including increased left ventricular (LV) transmural pressure because of the periods of increased negative intrathoracic pressures causing increased afterload; increased blood pressure caused by hypoxia; increased sympathetic nervous system activation that increases heart rate and predisposes to arrhythmias; and increased myocardial oxygen demand in the face of decreased myocardial oxygen supply, causing myocardial ischemia. Because heart failure is characterized by an energy-depleted state and high-wall stress increases metabolic demand at the expense of useful kinetic work, OSA, with its repeated apnea-arousal cycles leading to the above cardiovascular effects, aggravates the problem by further increasing myocardial metabolic demand and altering cardiac energetics. In this study, CHF patients with OSA were treated with CPAP and were shown after 6 weeks of therapy to have improved their LV ejection fraction, reduced their oxidative metabolism, and improved their work metabolic index, whereas the heart failure patients without OSA and not on CPAP did not change over the 6 weeks. In CHF patients with OSA, CPAP has been shown to decrease sympathetic nervous system activation[2,4] and improve cardiac efficiency by improving LV function and decreasing oxidative metabolism.[1] Ⓐ

CPAP in patients with obstructive sleep apnea syndrome (OSAS) might lower blood pressure, but evidence from clinical studies is inconsistent, perhaps as a result of small sample size or heterogeneity in study design. This study aimed to assess whether CPAP reduces ambulatory blood pressure in patients with OSAS, to quantify the effect size with precision, and to identify trial characteristics associated with the greatest blood pressure reductions.

This study showed that among patients with OSAS, CPAP reduces 24-hour ambulatory MBP, with greater treatment-related reductions in ambulatory MBP among patients with a more severe degree of OSAS and a better effective nightly use of the CPAP device. These reductions in blood pressure are likely to contribute to a better prognosis in terms of adverse cardiovascular events.

Perhaps the most widely recognized "new" secondary cause of hypertension is sleep apnea; it appears to be particularly common among cases of "resistant" hypertension. Several observational studies have indicated that, if left untreated, sleep apnea is associated with increased cardiovascular risk, and one long-term observational study suggested that long-term CPAP treatment reduces this risk. Some believe that the pathophysiology involves aldosterone, and spironolactone has been successful in reducing blood pressure when given to individuals with resistant hypertension, and to those with obstructive sleep apnea.

This study subjected the existing data from 12 studies about the effects of CPAP on ambulatory blood pressure monitoring to a meta-analysis and finds a small but statistically significant lowering of blood pressure after CPAP was initiated. It is reassuring that their meta-regression analysis showed a larger effect in those with more severe sleep apnea, as assessed by apnea–hypopnea index, arousal index (awakenings per hour of sleep), and effective use of CPAP (in hours/night). It would have been helpful to also observe a larger effect in individuals with higher baseline blood pressures.

These data tend to complete the findings: sleep apnea increases blood pressure, which increases cardiovascular risk, and CPAP not only reduces cardiovascular risk (in a cohort study), but also lowers blood pressure. The stage is now set for a randomized clinical trial comparing blockade of aldosterone (with either spironolactone or eplerenone) with CPAP for both blood pressure lowering and reduction of cardiovascular risk.[2] Ⓐ

The purpose of this study was to corroborate the association between obstructive sleep apnea (OSA) and nocturia in a clinical sample of urogynecologic patients and to explore whether night-time urine concentration predicts the presence of OSA.

This study showed that we should consider a diagnosis of OSA in all patients with nocturia, even those patients with daytime OAB.

Nocturia is a common clinical problem. The differential diagnosis and therapy of nocturia are well established. This article suggests that the prevalence of OSA as a contributing factor to nocturia and nocturnal polyuria is underappreciated and under-reported. If this data can be corroborated, the bigger issue is whether treatment of OSA in affected individuals would satisfactorily improve their nocturia. Currently available treatments for nocturnal polyuria are often ineffective or associated with significant side effects. Perhaps more aggressive case finding for individuals with OSA may lead to improved treatment of this condition.

One prospective cohort study suggests that CPAP reduces mortality in OSA.[4] There is evidence that CPAP is effective treatment in improving daytime sleepiness, mood, and cognitive function in patients with mild and moderate OSA,[5-6] with a *Cochrane Review* article[7] demonstrating these similar effects in severe OSA. Research has demonstrated that CPAP therapy increases quality of life[7-8] and decreases health care costs[9] in OSA. Studies also indicate that CPAP reduces blood pressure, primarily in patients with severe OSA.[10-12] Evidence further reveals that CPAP improves the left ventricular ejection fraction in patients with congestive heart failure and OSA.[3,13] Ⓐ

Evidence-Based References

1. Yoshinaga K et al: The effects of continuous positive airway pressure on myocardial energetics in patients with heart failure and obstructive sleep apnea, *J Am Coll Cardiol* 49:450-458, 2007. Commentary by M.D. Cheitlin, M.D., M.A.C.C. Ⓐ
2. Haentjens P et al: The impact of continuous positive airway pressure on blood pressure in patients with obstructive sleep apnea syndrome: evidence from a meta-analysis of placebo-controlled randomized trials, *Arch Intern Med* 167:757-765, 2007. Commentary by W.J. Elliott, M.D., Ph.D. Ⓐ
3. Lowenstein L et al: The relationship between obstructive sleep apnea, nocturia, and daytime overactive bladder syndrome in women, *Am J Obstet Gynecol* 198:598.e1-598.e5, 2008. Commentary by E.S. Rovner, M.D. Ⓐ
4. Marin JM et al: Long-term cardiovascular outcomes in men with obstructive sleep apnoea-hypopnoea with or without treatment with continuous positive airway pressure: an observational study, *Lancet* 365(9464):1046-1053, 2005.
5. Engleman HM et al: Effect of continuous positive airway pressure treatment on daytime function in sleep apnoea/hypopnoea syndrome, *Lancet* 343(8897):572-575, 1994.
6. Engleman HM et al: Randomized placebo-controlled crossover trial of continuous positive airway pressure for mild sleep apnea/hypopnea syndrome, *Am J Respir Crit Care Med* 159(2):461-467, 1999.
7. Giles TL et al: Continuous positive airways pressure for obstructive sleep apnoea in adults, *Cochrane Database Syst Rev* 3:CD001106, 2006.
8. Bennett LS et al: Health status in obstructive sleep apnea: relationship with sleep fragmentation and daytime sleepiness, and effects of continuous positive airway pressure treatment, *Am J Respir Crit Care Med* 159(6):1884-1890, 1999.
9. Bahammam A et al: Health care utilization in males with obstructive sleep apnea syndrome two years after diagnosis and treatment, *Sleep* 22(6):740-747, 1999.
10. Faccenda JF et al: Randomized placebo-controlled trial of continuous positive airway pressure on blood pressure in the sleep apnea-hypopnea syndrome, *Am J Respir Crit Care Med* 163(2):344-348, 2001.
11. Pepperell JC et al: Ambulatory blood pressure after therapeutic and subtherapeutic nasal continuous positive airway pressure for obstructive sleep apnoea: a randomised parallel trial, *Lancet* 359(9302):204-210, 2002.
12. Becker HF et al: Effect of nasal continuous positive airway pressure treatment on blood pressure in patients with obstructive sleep apnea, *Circulation* 107(1):68-73, 2003.
13. Kaneko Y et al: Cardiovascular effects of continuous positive airway pressure in patients with heart failure and obstructive sleep apnea, *N Engl J Med* 348(13):1233-1241, 2003.

SUGGESTED READINGS

Basner RC: Continuous positive airway pressure for obstructive sleep apnea, *N Engl J Med* 356(17):1751-1758, 2007.

Campos-Rodriguez F et al: Mortality in obstructive sleep apnea-hypopnea patients treated with positive airway pressure, *Chest* 128(2):624-633, 2005.

Capdevila OS et al: Pediatric obstructive sleep apnea: complications, management, and long-term outcomes, *Proc Am Thorac Soc* 5(2):274-282, 2008.

Chan AS et al: Non-positive airway pressure modalities: mandibular advancement devices/positional therapy, *Proc Am Thorac Soc* 5(2):179-184, 2008.

Friedman M et al: Updated systematic review of tonsillectomy and adenoidectomy for treatment of pediatric obstructive sleep apnea/hypopnea syndrome, *Otolaryngol Head Neck Surg* 140(6):800-808, 2009.

Golbin JM et al: Obstructive sleep apnea, cardiovascular disease, and pulmonary hypertension, *Proc Am Thorac Soc* 5(2):200-206, 2008.

Pépin JL et al: Effective compliance during the first 3 months of continuous positive airway pressure. A European prospective study of 121 patients, *Am J Respir Crit Care Med* 160(4):1124-1129, 1999.

Reichmuth KJ et al. Impaired vascular regulation in patients with obstructive sleep apnea: effects of continuous positive airway pressure treatment, *Am J Respir Crit Care Med* 180(11):1143-1150, 2009.

Tonelli de Oliveira AC et al: Diagnosis of obstructive sleep apnea syndrome and its outcomes with home portable monitoring, *Chest* 135(2):330-336, 2009.

Qureshi A et al: Medical treatment of obstructive sleep apnea, *Semin Respir Crit Care Med* 26(1):96-108, 2005.

Vakulin A et al: Effects of alcohol and sleep restriction on simulated driving performance in untreated patients with obstructive sleep apnea, *Ann Intern Med* 151:447-455, 2009.

Won CH et al: Surgical treatment of obstructive sleep apnea: upper airway and maxillomandibular surgery, *Proc Am Thorac Soc* 5(2):193-199, 2008.

Young T et al: Sleep disordered breathing and mortality: eighteen-year follow-up of the Wisconsin sleep cohort, *Sleep* 31(8):1071-1078, 2008.

AUTHOR: **DON HAYES, JR., M.D.**

BASIC INFORMATION

DEFINITION

Smallpox infection is caused by the variola virus, a DNA virus member of the genus *Orthopoxvirus.* It is a human virus with no known nonhuman reservoir of disease. Natural infection occurs after implantation of the virus on the oropharyngeal or respiratory mucosa.

ICD-9CM CODES
050.9 Smallpox NOS
V01.3 Smallpox exposure
050.0 Smallpox, hemorrhagic (pustular)
050.1 Variola minor (alastrim)
050.0 Variola major

EPIDEMIOLOGY & DEMOGRAPHICS

- Smallpox infection was eliminated from the world in 1977. The last cases of smallpox, from laboratory exposure, occurred in 1978. The threat of bioterrorism has brought on renewed interest in the smallpox virus.
- Routine vaccination against smallpox ended in 1972.
- Smallpox is spread from person to person by infected saliva droplets in face-to-face contact with the ill person.
- Persons with smallpox are most infectious during the first week of illness, when the largest amount of virus is present in saliva; however, some risk of transmission lasts until all scabs have fallen off.
- The incubation period is approximately 12 days (range, 7 to 17 days) after exposure.
- Contaminated clothing or bed linens can also spread the virus. Special precautions need to be taken to ensure that all bedding and clothing of patients are cleaned appropriately with bleach and hot water. Disinfectants such as bleach and quaternary ammonia can be used for cleaning contaminated surfaces.

PHYSICAL FINDINGS & CLINICAL PRESENTATION

- Initial symptoms include high fever, fatigue, and headaches and backaches. A characteristic rash, most prominent on the face, arms, and legs, follows in 2 to 3 days (Fig. 1-305).
- The rash starts with flat red lesions that evolve at the same rate. The rash follows a centrifugal pattern.
- Lesions are firm to the touch, domed, or umbilicated. They become pus filled and begin to crust early in the second week.
- Scabs develop and then separate and fall off after approximately 3 to 4 wk. Depigmentation persists at the base of the skin lesions for 3 to 6 mo after illness. Scarring is usually most extensive on the face.
- Associated with the rash may be fever, headache, generalized malaise, vomiting, and colicky abdominal pain.
- Variola major may produce a rapidly fatal toxemia in some patients.
- Complications of smallpox include dehydration, pneumonia, blepharitis, conjunctivitis, and corneal ulcerations.

ETIOLOGY

Smallpox is caused by the variola virus. There are at least two strains of the virus, the most virulent known as *variola major* and a less virulent strain known as *variola minor* (alastrim).

Dx DIAGNOSIS

DIFFERENTIAL DIAGNOSIS

- Rash from other viral illnesses (e.g., hemorrhagic chickenpox, measles, Coxsackie virus)
- Abdominal pain may mimic appendicitis
- Meningococcemia
- Insect bites
- Impetigo
- Dermatitis herpetiformis
- Pemphigus
- Papular urticaria

WORKUP & LABORATORY TESTS

- Laboratory examination requires high-containment (BL-4) facilities.
- Electron microscopy of vesicular scrapings can be used to distinguish poxvirus particles from varicella-zoster virus or herpes simplex. To obtain vesicular or pustular fluid it may be necessary to open lesions with the blunt edge of a scalpel. A cotton swab may be used to collect the fluid.
- In the absence of electron microscopy, light microscopy can be used to visualize variola viral particles (Guarnieri bodies) after Giemsa staining.
- Polymerase chain reaction techniques and restriction fragment-length polymorphisms can rapidly identify variola.

IMAGING STUDIES

Chest radiograph in patients with suspected pneumonia

Rx TREATMENT

NONPHARMACOLOGIC THERAPY

- Supportive therapy
- IV hydration in severe cases
- A suspect case of smallpox should be placed in strict respiratory and contact isolation

ACUTE GENERAL Rx

- There is no proven treatment for smallpox. Vaccination administered within 3 to 4 days may prevent or significantly ameliorate subsequent illness. Vaccinia immune globulin can be used for treatment of vaccine complications and for administration with vaccine to those for whom vaccine is otherwise contraindicated.
- Patients can benefit from supportive therapy (e.g., IV fluids, acetaminophen for pain or fever).
- Antibiotics are indicated only if secondary bacterial infections occur. Penicillinase-resistant antimicrobial agents should be used if smallpox lesions are secondarily infected.
- Topical idoxuridine should be considered for corneal lesions.

DISPOSITION

- The mortality rate for variola major is 20% to 50%. Variola minor has a mortality rate of 1%.
- After severe smallpox, pitted lesions (most commonly on the face) are seen in up to 80% of survivors.
- Panophthalmitis and blindness from viral keratitis or secondary eye infection occur in 1% of patients.
- Arthritis caused by viral infection of the metaphysis of growing bones occurs in 2% of children.

REFERRAL

ID consultation and notification of local health authorities is mandatory in all cases of smallpox.

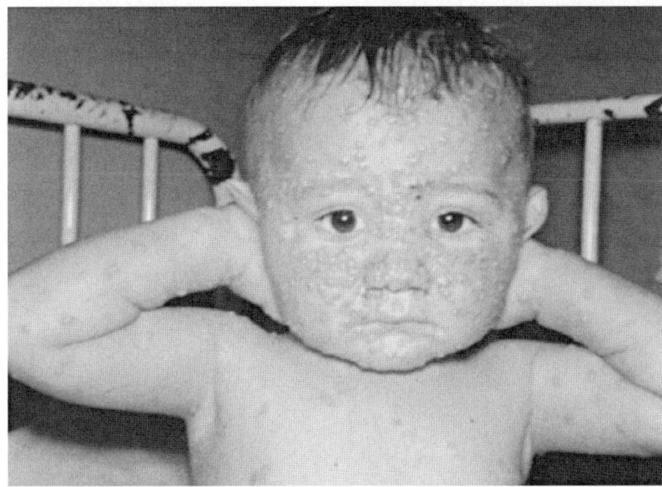

FIGURE 1-305 Appearance of the rash of smallpox on days 6 to 7. All the lesions are in the same stage of development. (From Gorbach SL: *Infectious diseases,* ed 2, Philadelphia, 1998, WB Saunders.)

PEARLS & CONSIDERATIONS

- The smallpox virus is fragile; in the event of an aerosol release, all viruses will be inactivated or dissipated within 1 to 2 days. Buildings exposed to the initial aerosol release of the virus do not need to be decontaminated. By the time the first cases are identified, typically 2 wk after release, the virus in the building will be gone. Infected patients, however, will be capable of spreading the virus and possibly contaminating surfaces while they are sick. Standard hospital-grade disinfectants such as quaternary ammonias are effective in killing the virus on surfaces and should be used for disinfecting hospitalized patients' rooms or other contaminated surfaces. In the hospital setting, patients' linens should be autoclaved or washed in hot water with bleach added. Infectious waste should be placed in biohazard bags and autoclaved before incineration.
- Symptomatic patients with suspected or confirmed smallpox are capable of spreading the virus. Patients should be placed in medical isolation to avoid spread of the virus. In addition, people who have come into close contact with smallpox patients should be vaccinated immediately and closely watched for symptoms of smallpox.

COMMENTS

- In people exposed to smallpox, the vaccine can lessen the severity of or even prevent illness if given within 4 days of exposure.
- The vaccine against smallpox contains another live virus called *vaccinia.* The vaccine does not contain smallpox virus. Smallpox vaccination produces a skin lesion that is infectious. Vaccine virus in the skin lesion can be transferred to others if the skin lesion is touched directly or if the bandage is handled casually with ungloved hands. The vaccination site is infectious until the scab falls off, approximately 21 days after vaccination.
- Primary vaccination confers full immunity to smallpox in more than 95% of persons for up to 10 yr.

SUGGESTED READINGS

Breman JG, Henderson DA: Diagnosis and management of smallpox, *N Engl J Med* 346:1300, 2002.

Frey SE et al: Clinical responses to undiluted and diluted smallpox vaccine, *N Engl J Med* 346:1265, 2002.

Henderson DA et al: Smallpox as a biological weapon, *JAMA* 281:2127, 1999.

AUTHOR: **FRED F. FERRI, M.D.**

BASIC INFORMATION

DEFINITION

Somatization disorder refers to a pattern of recurring multiple somatic complaints that begin before the age of 30 yr and persist over several years. Patients complain of multiple sites of pain (a minimum of four), gastrointestinal symptoms (a minimum of two), a sexual or reproductive symptom, and a pseudoneurologic symptom. These cannot be explained by a medical condition or are in excess of an expected disability from a coexisting medical condition.

SYNONYMS

Briquet's syndrome
Nonorganic physical symptoms
Medically unexplained symptoms
Functional somatic symptoms

ICD-9CM CODES
300.81 Somatization disorder

EPIDEMIOLOGY & DEMOGRAPHICS

PREVALENCE (IN U.S.): Lifetime rates of 0.25% to 2% in women, <0.2% in men
PEAK INCIDENCE: Typically before age 25 yr
PREDOMINANT SEX: Women are more commonly affected in the U.S. (10:1 ratio)
PREDOMINANT AGE: Onset occurs before age 30 yr and usually in adolescence.
GENETICS: In males, there is a high risk of associated substance abuse or antisocial personality disorder.

PHYSICAL FINDINGS & CLINICAL PRESENTATION

- Onset is characteristically in the teens; course is marked by frequent, unexplained, and frequently disabling pain and physical complaints.
- Patient frequently undergoes multiple procedures and seeks treatment from multiple physicians. Symptom focus rotates periodically with new physicians sought for new complaints.
- Patient often has a comorbid psychiatric disorder, most commonly generalized anxiety, panic disorder, or depression.

ETIOLOGY

- Believed to be the physical expression of psychologic distress; there appears to be a biologic predisposition.
- May be more common in individuals without sufficient verbal or intellectual capacity to communicate psychologic distress, individuals with alexithymia (inability to describe emotional states), or individuals from cultural backgrounds that consider emotional distress as an undesirable quality.
- Some aspects of somatization behavior possibly learned from somatizing parents.

DIAGNOSIS

DIFFERENTIAL DIAGNOSIS

- Undifferentiated somatoform disorder (ICD-10 F45.1, DMS-IV 300.81): one or more physical complaints that cannot be explained by a medical condition are present for at least 6 mo (NOTE: Somatization disorder is more severe and less common).
- Conversion disorder: an alteration or loss of voluntary motor or sensory function without demonstrable physical cause and related to a psychologic stress or a conflict (NOTE: With multiple complaints, the diagnosis of conversion is not made).
- Pain disorder: distinguished from somatization disorder by the latter featuring multiple nonpain symptoms.
- Factitious disorder (e.g., Munchausen's syndrome) and malingering: the psychologic basis of the complaints in somatization disorder is not conscious as in factitious disorder, in which the goal is to be in the patient role, and malingering, in which symptoms are also produced consciously but for some secondary gain like a monetary award in litigation or opioids.

WORKUP

- Rule out a general medical condition.
- If somatization is suspected on the basis of a history of repeated, multiple, unexplained complaints, restraint in ordering tests is recommended.

LABORATORY TESTS

No specific laboratory tests are required.

IMAGING STUDIES

No specific imaging studies are required.

TREATMENT

NONPHARMACOLOGIC THERAPY

- Legitimize patient's complaints.
- Minimize diagnostic investigation and symptomatic treatment. Only do invasive testing or procedures when there are clear-cut signs, not just symptom reports.
- Set attainable treatment goals. Patients may benefit from realizing that even though they cannot be cured, that they will be cared for. This may help reassure them that they will continue to have a relationship with the physician.
- Treat coexisting psychiatric conditions such as depression and anxiety.

ACUTE GENERAL Rx

- At each visit do a brief physical examination focusing on the area of complaint.
- Gently praise increased functioning rather than focusing on symptoms.
- Explore recent life events and ask how the patient is handling these.
- Convey empathy with the patient's suffering and psychosocial difficulties.
- No specific pharmacologic therapy has been clearly proven effective, although a number of agents, including gabapentin and St. John's wort, have been useful in some studies.

CHRONIC Rx

- Provide one primary care practitioner to manage care.
- Avoid confronting the patient regarding the psychological origin of symptoms.
- Ensure follow-up visits at regular intervals (e.g., 2- to 4-wk intervals that are not symptom contingent; maintain the regularity even if the symptoms improve so that the patient does not need new symptoms to continue the relationship).
- Avoid invasive or expensive diagnostic procedures unless there are clear signs of new illness, not just symptoms.
- Diagnose and treat mood or anxiety disorders.
- Cognitive behavior therapy groups have been helpful for patients with unexplained somatic symptoms and can dramatically improve functioning.

DISPOSITION

A chronic condition with frequent exacerbations

REFERRAL

If the patient is open to discussing psychological issues, a referral for psychotherapy can be made.

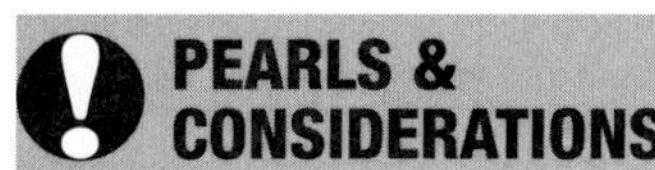

PEARLS & CONSIDERATIONS

Patients with somatization disorder respond best to establishing a regular, working relationship with a primary care provider. Avoiding confrontations about the origins of symptoms, investigating symptoms when related to actual signs of disease, and gently investigating concurrent stressors will help avoid most of the common problems with this population.

Patients with subsyndromal symptoms (i.e., failing to meet the full criteria but having three or more medically unexplained symptoms) may be just as challenging and chronic. They warrant similar approaches as utilized for the full syndrome.

SUGGESTED READINGS

Hatcher S, Arroll B: Assessment and management of medically unexplained symptoms, *BMJ* 17;336(7653):1124-1128, 2008.

Jackson, JL, Kroenke K: Prevalence, impact, and prognosis of multisomatoform disorder in primary care: a 5-year follow-up study. *Psychosom Med* 70(4):430-434, 2008.

olde Hartman TC et al: Medically unexplained symptoms, somatisation disorder and hypochondriasis: course and prognosis. A systematic review, *J Psychosom Res* 66(5)363-377, 2009.

Paras ML et al: Sexual abuse and lifetime diagnosis of somatic disorders: a systematic review and meta-analysis, *JAMA* 302(5):550-561, 2009.

AUTHOR: **STUART J. EISENDRATH, M.D.**

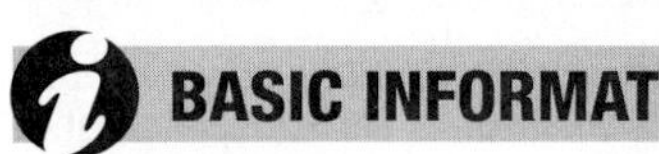

BASIC INFORMATION

DEFINITION

Spina bifida is the term for a group of neural tube disorders that involve the spinal column, including spina bifida occulta and spina bifida cystica. Anencephaly and cranium bifidum (i.e., encephalocele) are also classified as neural tube disorders, but these involve the cranium and brain and thus deserve a separate classification.

Spina bifida occulta is a midline defect that involves the closure of the posterior vertebral arches and laminae and that usually involves the L5-S1 area of the spinal cord.

Spina bifida cystica involves both meningocele and myelomeningocele. Meningocele is a midline defect in which meninges herniate through the posterior vertebral arch defect with a normal spinal cord in a normal position in the spinal canal; this condition makes up about 5% of cases of spina bifida cystica. Myelomeningocele is the most severe form of disease in the spectrum of spina bifida. The meninges, fragments of bone and cartilage, and the spinal cord herniate through the vertebral arches or the skin; this condition makes up about 95% of cases. The majority of these defects (~75%) are located in the lumbosacral area (Figs. 1-306 and 1-307).

SYNONYMS

Dysraphism
Meningomyelocele
Neural tube disorders

ICD-9CM CODES

756.17	Spina bifida occulta
741.9	Meningocele/myelomeningocele (without mention of hydrocephalus)

EPIDEMIOLOGY & DEMOGRAPHICS

INCIDENCE:
- Spina bifida occulta: 10% of the general pediatric population
- Spina bifida cystica: 0.15% of Caucasians, 0.04% of African Americans
- Highest in Ireland and lowest in Japan
- Influenced by season, economic status, maternal age, heat exposure, and a mother who has had other children with neural tube defects

PREVALENCE: About 12 infants are born daily with spina bifida or anencephaly.

PREDOMINANT SEX: Females are affected more frequently than males.

RISK FACTORS:
- Nutritional deficiency (specifically folate)
- Prior children with neural tube defects (risk increases 1.5% to 2%)
- If two prior children had spinal column defects, the risk increases 6% to 10%

GENETICS: Unknown

PHYSICAL FINDINGS & CLINICAL PRESENTATION

- Spina bifida occulta:
  - Most patients are asymptomatic and have a normal neurological examination.
  - In some cases, patients may have a patch of hair, a lipoma, skin discoloration, or a dermal sinus overlying the defect.
  - The condition is occasionally associated with syringomyelia, diastematomyelia, and a tethered cord.
- Meningocele:
  - Patients typically have a normal neurological examination; however, lesions may be accompanied by tethering, syringomyelia, or diastematomyelia.
  - Constipation or bladder dysfunction can develop as a result of an enlargement of the lesion.
- Myelomeningocele:
  - The lesion can be completely exposed, or it may have a skinlike membrane that covers it.
  - The extent of the neurologic deficits depends on the level of the lesion:
    - Thoracolumbar: hypertonic bladder with normal anal tone
    - Below L2: flaccid tone; areflexic paraparesis; sensory loss in L3-L4 dermatomes; bladder and bowel incontinence; and poor anal sphincter tone, which can result in rectal prolapse
    - Below S3: motor deficits are absent; bladder and anal sphincter paralysis with saddle anesthesia
  - Joint deformities include contractures, hip dislocations, scoliosis, clubfoot, and rocker-bottom foot.
  - Hydrocephalus with Chiari type II malformations occurs in up to 90% of lumbosacral myelomeningoceles, and it is seen in more than half of cases at birth.
  - Tethered cord disease manifests with a loss of motor function, spasticity with contractures, a rapid progression of scoliosis with bent posture, back pain, and changes in urodynamics.
  - The condition is associated with disorders of cell migration that cause brain malformations, including heterotopia and schizencephaly.
  - With this disease, there may also be multiorgan developmental disease (e.g., renal agenesis/anomalies, duodenal atresia, cardiac malformations, tracheoesophageal fistulas).

ETIOLOGY

- The posterior neuropore closes at about 26 to 28 days of gestation, which is typically before

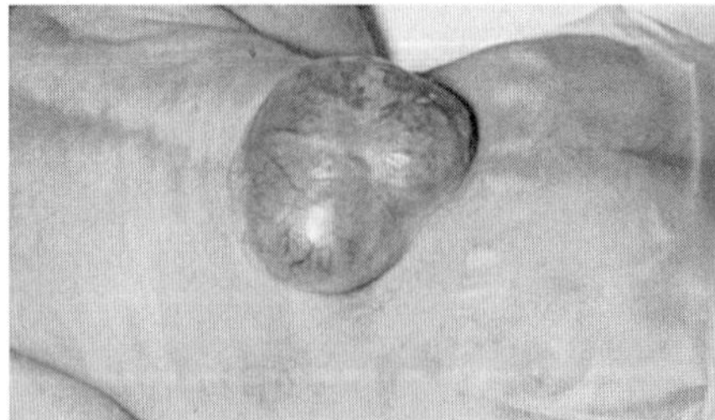

FIGURE 1-306 Lumbosacral myelomeningocele covered by an epithelialized membrane. (From Kliegman RM [ed]: *Nelson textbook of pediatrics,* ed 18, Philadelphia, 2007, Saunders.)

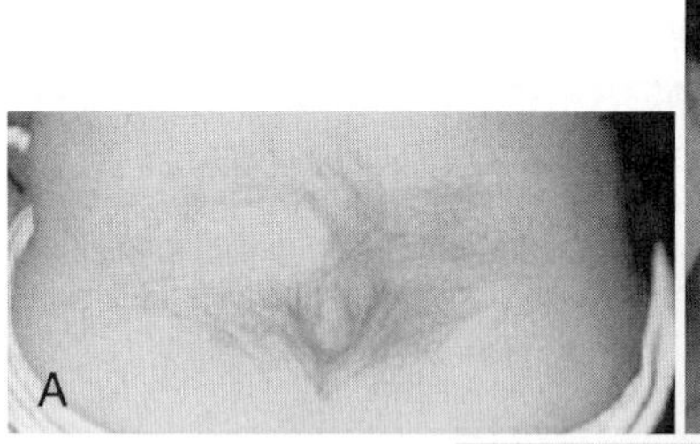

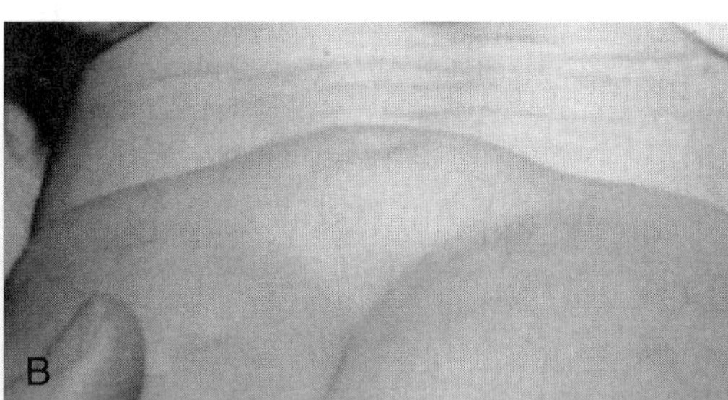

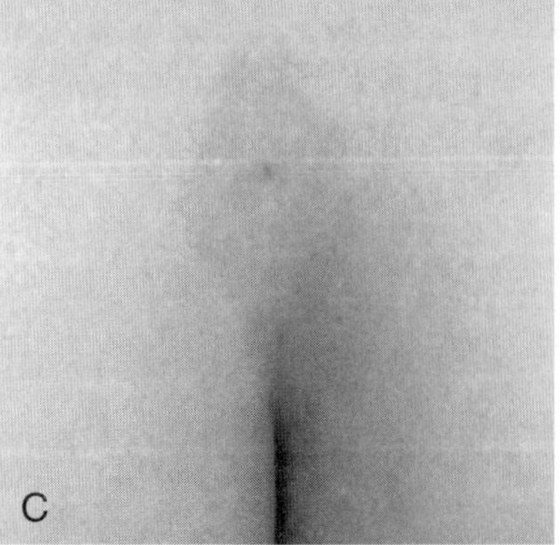

FIGURE 1-307 Examples of cutaneous malformations associated with spina bifida occulta. **A,** Tuft of hair. **B,** Sacral lipoma. **C,** Sinus tract that communicates with a dermoid tumor. (From Zitelli BJ, Davis HW [eds]: *Atlas of pediatric physical diagnosis,* ed 5, Philadelphia, 2007, Saunders.)

the mother has knowledge of the pregnancy. The failure of the closure results in any of the neural tube disorders, with the severity being dependent on the stage of development at closure (i.e., earlier in development results in spina bifida cystica vs. spina bifida occulta).
- The cause of the failure to close is unknown, but it is thought to be multifactorial and to involve genetic defects, environmental toxins, and folate deficiency.

Dx DIAGNOSIS

DIFFERENTIAL DIAGNOSIS

Isolated to this group of disorders

WORKUP

- Spina bifida occulta: none, unless foot deformities, neurogenic bladder, or neurologic deficits develop, which would be concerning for spinal cord pathology
- Spina bifida cystica: mostly includes imaging studies

LABORATORY TESTS

None

IMAGING STUDIES

- Ultrasound
- MRI of head and spine
- Computed tomography is a quicker study and would not require sedation; however, this method exposes the patient to radiation and therefore should be minimized.

Rx TREATMENT

- Spina bifida occulta: if asymptomatic with normal examination, none
- Meningocele: none
- Myelomeningocele: antiepileptic medications, if warranted

NONPHARMACOLOGIC THERAPY

- Spina bifida occulta: These is no nonpharmacologic therapy used for this condition, unless the patient develops neurological disease that is suggestive of underlying spinal cord disease.
- Meningocele: Most of these defects are covered by skin, so there is minimal risk of infection. If the patient has a normal examination with full-thickness skin, surgery can be delayed. However, if cerebrospinal fluid begins to leak or if the skin is thin, then immediate surgical correction is warranted.
- Myelomeningocele: Initial sac closure with a ventriculoperitoneal shunt is usually performed during the first 48 hours of life.
- The in utero closure of spinal lesions has been successful in a few centers, but there is a lack of evidence to support this procedure. The theory is that early closure possibly results in less severe motor disease, joint deformities, and sensory loss.

CHRONIC RX

- Involves a multidisciplinary approach that includes primary care, neurology, urology, orthopedic surgery, neurosurgery, and intense physical and occupational therapy
- Bladder catheterization to ensure the complete emptying of the bladder and the minimization of renal scarring
- Urodynamic evaluations
- Bowel training with stool softeners and enemas (An appendicostomy may be placed for antegrade enemas, if warranted.)
- The goal is to prevent the further loss of function and to maximize ambulation:
  - Close monitoring via physical examination for further worsening of clubfoot, spasticity, sensory loss as a result of possible shunt malfunction, or tethering of cord, which would warrant neurosurgical intervention
  - Orthotics
  - Physical and occupational therapy
- Frequent skin examinations to monitor for decubitus ulcer formation

DISPOSITION

- 70% of patients have normal intelligence; this is affected by episodes of meningitis and encephalitis
- Higher incidence of learning disorders and seizures as compared with the general population, which is likely related to brain malformations

PEARLS & CONSIDERATIONS

PREVENTION

All women of childbearing age should take a daily multivitamin for folate supplementation (0.4 mg/day), because more than half of pregnancies are unplanned, and the greatest benefit is seen when supplements are taken for about 1 month before conception. In addition, women who are taking valproic acid, carbamazepine, methotrexate, sulfamethoxazole/trimethoprim, and other medications that affect folate metabolism probably need a higher dose (e.g., 1 mg/day).

PATIENT/FAMILY EDUCATION

Spina Bifida Family Support and Spina Bifida Central have websites where families can share their experiences and information about their children.

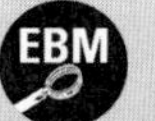

EVIDENCE

Prior to 1991, cereals and grains were not fortified. A nonrandomized trial involving folate supplementation to mothers with history of a prior child with neural tube defect showed an 86% risk reduction for further pregnancy. A randomized clinical trial was then undertaken involving supplementation of 0.4 mg per day of folate periconceptionally to mothers and showed a 72% reduction of incidence in neural tube defects. These studies are what lead to the CDC recommendations of fortified foods and women considering pregnancy to supplement with 0.4 mg/day of folate.

Evidence-Based Reference

Sarwark JF: Common orthopedic problems II: spina bifida, *Pediatr Clin North Am* 43:1151-1158, 1996.

SUGGESTED READINGS

Kliegman: Meningocele. In Kliegman (ed): *Nelson textbook of pediatrics,* ed 18, 2007, Saunders, p. 592.3.

Kliegman: Myelomeningocele. In Kliegman (ed): *Nelson textbook of pediatrics,* ed 18, 2007, Saunders, p. 592.4.

Kliegman: Spina bifida occulta. In Kliegman (ed): *Nelson textbook of pediatrics,* ed 18, 2007, Saunders, p. 592.2.

Menkes JH et al: Neuroembryology, genetic programming, and malformations of the nervous system. In Menkes JH et al (eds): *Child neurology,* ed 7, Philadelphia, 2006, Lippincott Williams & Wilkins, pp. 287-299.

Rowe DE, Jadhav AL: Care of the adolescent with spina bifida, *Pediatr Clin North Am* 55:1359-1374, 2008.

Sarwark JF: Common orthopedic problems II: spina bifida, *Pediatr Clin North Am* 43:1151-1158, 1996.

AUTHOR: **DONITA DILLON LIGHTNER, M.D.**

 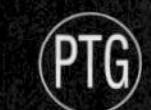

BASIC INFORMATION

DEFINITION

Spinal cord compression is the neurologic loss of spine function. Lesions may be complete or incomplete and develop gradually or acutely. Incomplete lesions often present as distinct syndromes, as follows:

- Central cord syndrome
- Anterior cord syndrome
- Brown-Séquard syndrome
- Conus medullaris syndrome
- Cauda equina syndrome

ICD-9CM CODES
344.89 Brown-Séquard syndrome
344.60 Cauda equina syndrome
336.8 Conus medullaris syndrome
Other lesions listed by site

PHYSICAL FINDINGS & CLINICAL PRESENTATION

Clinical features reflect the amount of spinal cord involvement:

- Motor loss and sensory abnormalities
- Babinski testing usually positive
- Clonus
- Gradual compression, often manifested by progressive difficulty walking, clonus with weight bearing, and involuntary spasm; development of sensory symptoms; bladder dysfunction (late)
- Central cord syndrome: results in a variable quadriparesis with the upper extremities more severely involved than the lower extremities; some sensory sparing
- Anterior cord syndrome: results in motor, pain, and temperature loss below the lesion
- Brown-Séquard syndrome:
  1. Spinal cord syndrome caused by injury to either half of the spinal cord and resulting in the loss of motor function, position, vibration, and light touch on the affected side
  2. Pain and temperature sense loss on the opposite side
- Conus medullaris syndrome: results in variable motor loss in the lower extremities with loss of bowel and bladder function
- Cauda equina syndrome: typical low back pain, weakness in both lower extremities, saddle anesthesia, and loss of voluntary bladder and bowel control

ETIOLOGY

- Trauma
- Tumor
- Infection
- Inflammatory processes
- Degenerative disk conditions with spinal stenosis
- Acute disk herniation
- Cystic abnormalities

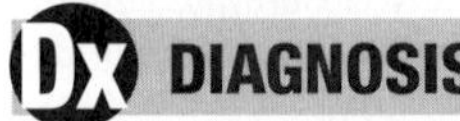

DIAGNOSIS

DIFFERENTIAL DIAGNOSIS

- See "Etiology."
- Section II describes the differential diagnosis of paraplegia.

WORKUP

- Spinal cord compression: requires an immediate referral for radiographic and neurologic assessment
- Laboratory results usually unremarkable unless infectious or inflammatory causes suspected

IMAGING STUDIES

- Depend on the suspected etiology
- MRI usually required

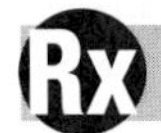

TREATMENT

Urgent surgical decompression is usually indicated as soon as the etiology is established.

DISPOSITION

Important indicators regarding prognosis:

- The greater the distal motor and sensory sparing, the greater the expected recovery.
- When a plateau of recovery is reached, no further improvement is expected.
- The quicker the recovery, the greater the recovery.

REFERRAL

Immediate referral for radiographic and neurologic evaluation and treatment in all suspected cases of spinal cord compression

SUGGESTED READINGS

Baines MJ: Spinal cord compression—a personal and palliative care perspective, *Clin Oncol (R Coll Radiol)* 14(2):135, 2002.

Banerjee R et al: Spinal epidural hematoma induced by leukemia, *Orthopedics* 27:864, 2004.

Benjamin R: Neurologic complications of prostate cancer, *Am Fam Physician* 65(9):1834, 2002.

Berrand T, Samant R: Palliative radiotherapy knowledge among community family physicians and nurses, *J Cancer Educ* 23:156, 2008.

Buchner M, Schiltenwolf M: Cauda equina syndrome caused by intervertebral lumbar disc prolapse: mid-term results of 22 patients and literature review, *Orthopedics* 25:727, 2002.

Carlson GD et al: Sustained spinal cord compression. Part I: time-dependent effect on long-term pathophysiology, *J Bone Joint Surg* 85:86, 2003.

Carlson GD et al: Sustained spinal cord compression. Part II: effect of methylprednisolone on regional blood flow and recovery of somatosensory evoked potentials, *J Bone Joint Surg* 85:95, 2003.

Casey AT et al: Rheumatoid arthritis of the cervical spine: current techniques for management, *Orthop Clin North Am* 33(2):291, 2002.

Jagas M et al: Vertebroplasty with methacrylate bone cement and radiotherapy in the treatment of spinal metastases with epidural spinal cord compression, *Orthop Traumatol Rehabil* 7(5):491, 2005.

Kadanka Z et al: Approaches to spondylotic cervical myelopathy: conservative versus surgical in a 3-year follow-up study, *Spine* 27(20):2205, 2002.

Malcolm GP: Surgical disorders of the cervical spine: presentation and management of common disorders, *J Neurosurg Psychiatry* 73(suppl 1):134, 2002.

Matsunaga S et al: Trauma-induced myelopathy in patients with ossification of the posterior longitudinal ligament, *J Neurosurg* 97(2 suppl):172, 2002.

Mohanty SP, Venkatram N: Does neurological recovery in thoracolumbar and lumbar burst fractures depend on the extent of canal compromise? *Spinal Cord* 40(6):295, 2002.

Nowak DD et al: Central cord syndrome, *J Am Acad Orthop Surg* 17:756, 2009.

Rades D et al: Do bladder cancer patients with metastatic spinal cord compression benefit from radiotherapy alone? *Urology* 69(6):1081, 2007.

Shimomura T et al: Prognostic factors for deterioration of patients with cervical spondylotic myelopathy after nonsurgical treatment, *Spine* 32:2474, 2007.

Sorar M et al: Cervical compression myelopathy: is fusion the main prognostic indicator? *J Neurosurg Spine* 6(6):531, 2007.

Tosteson A et al: Surgical treatment of spinal stenosis with and without degenerative spondylolisthesis: cost-effectiveness after 2 years, *Ann Intern Med* 149:845-853, 2008.

Venkitaraman R et al: Outcome of early detection and radiotherapy for occult spinal cord compression, *Radiother Oncol* 85:469, 2007.

Yagi M et al: Long-term surgical outcome and risk factors in patients with cervical myelopathy and a change in signal intensity of intramedullary spinal cord on magnetic resonance imaging, *J Neurosurg Spine* 12:59, 2010.

AUTHOR: **LONNIE R. MERCIER, M.D.**

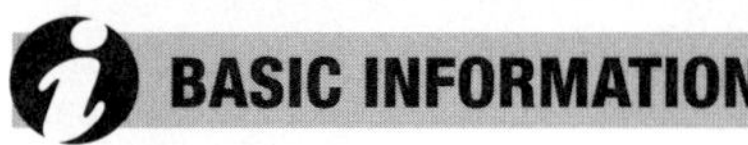

BASIC INFORMATION

DEFINITION

A spinal epidural abscess (SEA) is a focal suppurative infection occurring in the spinal epidural space.

ICD-9CM CODES
324.1 Spinal epidural abscess

EPIDEMIOLOGY & DEMOGRAPHICS

INCIDENCE (IN U.S.):

- 2 to 25 cases/100,000 hospitalized patients/yr
- May be increasing over the past 3 decades

PREDOMINANT AGE:

- Median age of onset approximately 50 yr (35 yr in intravenous drug users)
- Peak incidence in seventh and eighth decades of life

PHYSICAL FINDINGS & CLINICAL PRESENTATION

- The presentation of SEA can be nonspecific.
- Fever, malaise, and back pain are the most consistent early symptoms.
- Pain is often focal. It may initially be mild but can progress to become severe.
- As the disease progresses, root pain can occur, followed by motor weakness, sensory changes, bladder and bowel dysfunction, and paralysis.
- Physical findings may be limited to fever or spinal tenderness.
- The evolution to neurologic deficits can occur as quickly as a few hours, or over weeks to months.
- Once paralysis occurs, it may quickly become irreversible without the appropriate intervention.

ETIOLOGY

- Pyogenic bacteria account for the majority of cases in the U.S. Immigrants from TB-endemic areas may present with tuberculous SEAs. Fungi and parasites can also cause this condition. The most common causative organism is *Staphylococcus aureus.* Most posterior SEAs are thought to originate from distant focus (e.g., skin and soft tissue infections), while anterior SEAs are commonly associated with diskitis or vertebral osteomyelitis. No source was found in approximately one third of cases.
- Associated predisposing conditions include diabetes mellitus, alcoholism, cancer, AIDS, and chronic renal failure, or following epidural anesthesia, spinal surgery or trauma, or IV drug use. No predisposing condition is found in approximately 20% of patients.
- Damage to the spinal cord can be caused by direct compression of the spinal cord, vascular compromise, bacterial toxins, and inflammation.

Dx DIAGNOSIS

DIFFERENTIAL DIAGNOSIS

- Herniated disc
- Vertebral osteomyelitis and diskitis
- Metastic tumors
- Meningitis

LABORATORY TESTS

- WBC may be normal or elevated.
- ESR is usually elevated over 30 mm/hr.
- Blood cultures are positive in approximately 60% of patients with SEA.
- CSF cultures are positive in 19%, but lumbar puncture is unnecessary, and may be contraindicated.
- Once imaging is done, CT-guided aspiration or open biopsy should be done to determine causative organism. Abscess content culture is positive in 90% of patients.

IMAGING STUDIES

- MRI with gadolinium is the imaging modality of choice; CT scan with contrast may show the abscess but is less sensitive than MRI.
- CT with myelography is more sensitive for cord compression.

Rx TREATMENT

NONPHARMACOLOGIC THERAPY

- Surgical decompression is the mainstay of treatment. Decompression within the first 24 hr has been related to an improved prognosis.
- Nonsurgical treatment is effective in some patients, but failure rate may be excessive. This approach should not be considered and should only be attempted in the absence of signs of compressive myelopathy and with very careful follow-up.

ACUTE GENERAL Rx

- In addition to surgery, antibiotics directed at the most likely organism should be initiated.
- If the organism is unknown, broad coverage against staphylococci, streptococci, and gram-negative bacilli should be initiated. The regimen can be adjusted according to culture results. Therapy should continue for at least 4 to 6 wk.

CHRONIC Rx

Neurologic deficits may remain despite aggressive treatment.

DISPOSITION

Irreversible paralysis and death can occur in up to 25% of patients.

REFERRAL

All cases should be referred to a neurosurgeon and an infectious disease specialist.

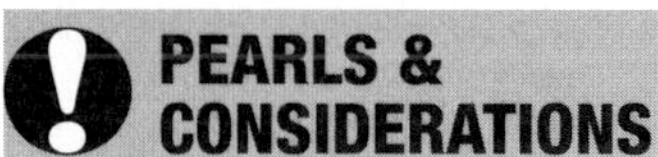

PEARLS & CONSIDERATIONS

It is critically important to recognize this process early; the prognosis is generally excellent if treatment is initiated while symptoms are localized and before evidence of myelopathy develops.

SUGGESTED READINGS

Curry WT et al: Spinal epidural abscess: clinical presentation, management, and outcome, *Surg Neurol* 63(4):364, 2005.

Moriya M et al: Successful management of cervical spinal epidural abscess without surgery, *Intern Med* 44(10):1110, 2005.

Savage K et al: Spinal epidural abscess: early clinical outcome in patients treated medically, *Clin Orthop Relat Res* 439:56, 2005.

Torgovnick J et al: Spinal epidural abscess: clinical presentation, management and outcome, *Surg Neurol* 63:364, 2005.

AUTHORS: **GLENN G. FORT, M.D., M.P.H.,** and **DENNIS J. MIKOLICH, M.D.**

Spinal Stenosis, Lumbar (PTG)

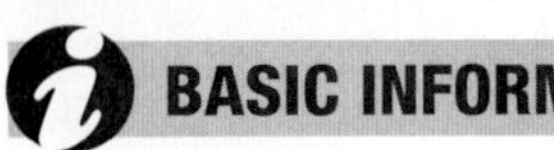

BASIC INFORMATION

DEFINITION

Spinal stenosis is the pathologic condition caused by the compressing or narrowing of the spinal canal, nerve root canal, or intervertebral foramina at the lumbar region.

SYNONYMS

Central spinal stenosis
Lateral spinal stenosis
Spondylosis

ICD-9CM CODES

724.02 Spinal stenosis lumbar, lumbosacral

EPIDEMIOLOGY & DEMOGRAPHICS

More common between 50 and 60 yr of age

PHYSICAL FINDINGS & CLINICAL PRESENTATION

- Symptoms caused by direct mechanical compression or indirect vascular compression of the nerve roots or the cauda equina.
- Neurogenic claudication: leg, buttock, or back pain precipitated by walking and relieved by sitting.
- Pain may radiate down to ankles and is associated with numbness, tingling, and weakness.
- Taking a flexed posture reduces symptoms because it increases the available space in the lumbar spinal canal.
- Decreased lumbar extension.
- Normal peripheral pulses.
- Positive Romberg's sign (decreased proprioception).
- Wide-based gait.
- Reduced knee and ankle reflex.
- Urine incontinence.

ETIOLOGY

Spinal stenosis may be primary or secondary

- Primary stenosis (congenital or developmental narrowing)
  1. Idiopathic
  2. Achondroplasia
  3. Morquio-Ullrich syndrome
- Secondary stenosis (acquired)
  1. Degenerative (hypertrophy of the articular processes, disk degeneration, ligamentum flavum hypertrophy, spondylolisthesis)
  2. Fracture/trauma
  3. Postoperative (postlaminectomy)
  4. Paget's disease
  5. Ankylosing spondylitis
  6. Tumors
  7. Acromegaly

Dx DIAGNOSIS

DIFFERENTIAL DIAGNOSIS

- Osteoarthritis of the knee or hip
- Acute cauda equina syndrome, resulting from compression by epidural abscess or tumors
- Pain and weakness caused by multiple myeloma or osteomyelitis
- Intermittent claudication—peripheral vascular disease
- Peripheral neuropathy such as that caused by a herniated nucleus pulposus
- Scoliosis or spondylolisthesis
- Rheumatoid diseases: ankylosing spondylitis, Reiter's syndrome, fibromyalgia
- Table 1-72 compares clinical features of spinal stenosis, peripheral vascular disease, and disc disease.

WORKUP

History, physical examination, and specific imaging studies

IMAGING STUDIES

- Lumbar spine film sensitivity 66%, specificity 93%.
- Ultrasound of the spinal canal has also been used.
- CT scan of the lumbosacral spine: sensitivity (75% to 85%), specificity (80%).
- MRI of the lumbosacral spine: sensitivity (80% to 90%), specificity (95%).
- Myelogram: sensitivity (77%), specificity (72%). Absolute stenosis is defined as the anterior-posterior (AP) diameter of the spinal canal <10 mm. Relative stenosis: 10 to 12 mm AP diameter.
- Electromyography (EMG) and nerve conduction velocity (NCV) are additional studies particularly useful in differentiating peripheral neuropathy from lumbar spinal stenosis.

Rx TREATMENT

NONPHARMACOLOGIC THERAPY

- Physiotherapy
- Lumbar corsets
- Back exercises
- Abdominal muscle strengthening
- Aquatic exercises

ACUTE GENERAL Rx

- Surgery is indicated in patients with significant compression of nerve roots as determined by MRI or CT and incapacitating symptoms limiting activities of daily living or bladder and bowel incontinence.
- Surgical procedures include decompressive laminectomy, arthrodesis, hemilaminectomy, and medial facetectomy.
- Lumbar interspinous process decompression using X-STOP device: a titanium oval spacer placed between the two adjacent spinous processes of the affected level; provides an unloading distractive force to the stenotic middle column part of the motion segment.

CHRONIC Rx

- Conservative therapy with NSAIDs (ibuprofen 800 mg PO tid, naproxen 500 mg PO bid) may be tried for symptomatic relief in addition to acetaminophen 1 g PO qid.
- Epidural steroid injections may provide temporary relief.

DISPOSITION

- Approximately 20% of patients having surgery require repeat surgery within 10 yr. Nearly one third of these patients continue to experience pain.
- The natural history of spinal stenosis is one of slow progression. Although not very common, cord compression with resultant bowel and bladder incontinence and paresis can occur.
- Operative treatment is more effective in reducing pain and disability than nonoperative treatment.

REFERRAL

- Patients who have spinal stenosis should be referred to an orthopedic surgeon specializing in back surgery or to a neurosurgeon.
- Pain clinic referrals should be made if surgery is contraindicated or if the patient does not want surgery.

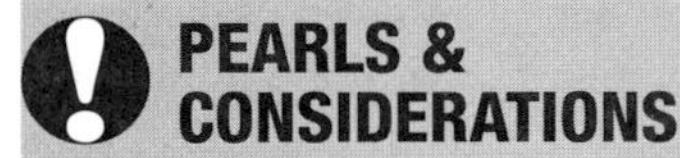

PEARLS & CONSIDERATIONS

COMMENTS

- Approximately one third of patients have coexisting peripheral vascular disease.
- The severity of cauda equina constriction is directly related to the walking ability and the pain intensity in the legs and back.
- Spinal stenosis is also a cause of chronic low back pain in the young.

Table 1-72 Comparative Clinical Features of Spinal Stenosis, Peripheral Vascular Disease, and Disc Disease

Feature	Spinal Stenosis	Disc Prolapse	Peripheral Vascular Disease
Reduced straight leg raise	Rarely	Usually	No
Neurologic deficit	Sometimes	Often	No
Leg pain on walking	Yes	Usually	Yes
Leg pain on sitting	No	Yes	No
Pain relief on standing still	No	No	Yes
Pain relief on sitting	Yes	No	Yes
Numbness/paresthesia	Yes	Yes	Sometimes

(From Carr A, Hamilton W: Orthopedics in primary care, ed 2, Philadelphia, 2005, Elsevier.)

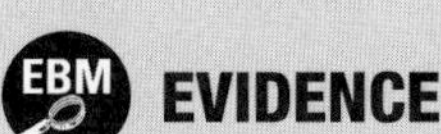

EVIDENCE

There is little evidence that NSAIDs are effective for the treatment of sciatica caused by lumbar disc herniation.

There is limited evidence that diskectomy is superior to epidural steroid injections for the treatment of lumbar disc herniation.

Another RCT compared epidural steroid injections to diskectomy in 100 people with lumbar disc herniation. Diskectomy significantly improved leg pain and function at follow up after 1 to 3 mo compared with epidural injection, although after 2 to 3 yr, there was no significant difference in outcome between either treatment.[1] Ⓐ

There is no clear evidence that arthrodesis is superior to the nonsurgical management of degenerative lumbar disease.

A systematic review identified 31 randomized controlled trials (RCTs) of all forms of surgical treatment for degenerative lumbar spondylosis. Two of the trials evaluated the efficacy of arthrodesis. One of the RCTs found that fusion was superior to physiotherapy. The second trial found that fusion and physical therapy were equally effective.[2] Ⓐ

An additional three RCTs evaluating the efficacy of anterior, posterior, or circumferential fusion showed conflicting results and the authors could not make any conclusions as to which approach was more beneficial.[2] Ⓐ

Evidence-Based References

1. Buttermann GR: Treatment of lumbar disc herniation: epidural steroid injection compared with discectomy. A prospective, randomized study. *J Bone Joint Surg Am* 86-A:670-679, 2004.

2. Gibson JNA, Waddell G: Surgery for degenerative lumbar spondylosis. *Cochrane Database Syst Rev* 4: 2005.

SUGGESTED READINGS

de Graaf I et al: Diagnosis of lumbar spinal stenosis: a systematic review of the accuracy of diagnostic tests, *Spine* 31(10):1168-1176, 2006.

Fu, Yi-Shan MD et al: Long-term outcomes of two different decompressive techniques for lumbar spinal stenosis, *Spine.* 33(5):514-518, March 1, 2008.

Malmivaara A et al (for the Finnish Lumbar Spinal Research Group): Surgical or nonoperative treatment for lumbar spinal stenosis? A randomized controlled trial, *Spine* 32(1):1-8, 2007.

Pua, Yong-Hao et al: Treadmill walking with body weight support is no more effective than cycling when added to an exercise program for lumbar spinal stenosis: a randomised controlled trial, *Austr J Physiother* 53(2):83-89, 2007.

Spengler, DM: Surgery reduced pain at two years but did not differ from nonsurgical treatment for physical function in lumbar spinal stenosis, *J Bone Joint Surgy [Am]* 90(11):2553, 2008.

Tosteson A et al: Surgical treatment of spinal stenosis with and without degenerative spondylolisthesis: cost-effectiveness after 2 years, *Ann Intern Med* 149:845-853, 2008.

Weinstein JN et al: Surgical versus non-surgical therapy for lumbar spinal stenosis, *N Engl J Med* 358: 794-810, 2008.

AUTHOR: **JORGE A. VILLAFUERTE, M.D.**

Spinocerebellar Ataxia

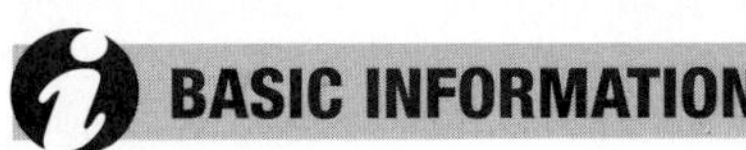

BASIC INFORMATION

DEFINITION

The spinocerebellar ataxias (SCAs) are a heterogeneous group of autosomal dominantly inherited genetic conditions that cause progressive ataxia.

SYNONYMS

Autosomal-dominant cerebellar ataxia (ADCA)
Machado-Joseph disease (eponym for SCA3; this may be the most common SCA)

ICD-9CM CODES

334.2 Primary cerebellar degeneration

EPIDEMIOLOGY & DEMOGRAPHICS

PREVALENCE: The prevalence of the condition is approximately 3 persons per 100,000. The most common SCAs are 1, 2, 3, 6, and 7.

PREDOMINANT SEX: SCA demonstrates no gender preference.

PREDOMINANT AGE: The age of onset is often during the 30s or 40s. However, this can be highly variable, even within family groups; SCAs can occur anytime from childhood to late adulthood.

GENETICS: All SCAs are inherited in an autosomal dominant fashion; however, reduced penetrance can be present.

PHYSICAL FINDINGS & CLINICAL PRESENTATION

- Chronically progressive ataxia is the predominant symptom of all of the SCAs. It typically presents as a combination of balance and gait difficulty, limb incoordination, and dysarthria.
- Previous nomenclature had grouped these conditions into ADCA type I (i.e., ataxia plus other neurologic symptoms, such as pyramidal, extrapyramidal, ophthalmoplegia, dementia, dystonia, or others); ADCA type II (i.e., ataxia with progressive retinopathy); and ADCA type III (i.e., pure cerebellar dysfunction). Current terminology preferentially involves the use of the SCA genetic classification.
- More than 30 different genetic subtypes of SCA have been described to date. Although certain clinical characteristics are common to specific SCA subtypes, there is significant overlap among and variability within these conditions, so making a diagnosis on the basis of the clinical presentation alone can be challenging and sometimes impossible without genetic testing. Some of the more common SCAs and their features include the following:
    - SCA1 can be characterized by ataxia, nystagmus, spasticity, and neuropathy.
    - SCA2 can be characterized by ataxia, slow saccades, gaze palsy, neuropathy, and sometimes parkinsonism or dementia.
    - SCA3, which is also known as *Machado-Joseph disease,* can be characterized by ataxia, neuropathy, amyotrophy, parkinsonism, and dystonia.
    - SCA6 is generally felt to be a pure cerebellar syndrome with ataxia and nystagmus (gaze evoked and downbeat) as well as a frequently later age of onset.
    - SCA7 is characterized by ataxia, vision loss caused by a pigmentary maculopathy, and sometimes ophthalmoplegia.
    - Knowledge in this area is constantly expanding and being updated. Online sources of information (e.g., Online Mendelian Inheritance in Man [http://www.ncbi.nlm.nih.gov/omim]) can be invaluable for tracking new developments.

ETIOLOGY

Several of the SCAs are the result of polyglutamine CAG repeat expansions; this causes the accumulation of mutant proteins inside neurons, which is thought to cause dysfunction and cell death. Higher numbers of repeats are correlated with an earlier onset of symptoms, and anticipation may be present. Other types of repeat expansions and point mutations have been found with several SCAs; for others, the affected gene has not been identified.

Dx DIAGNOSIS

DIFFERENTIAL DIAGNOSIS

- Structural cerebellar abnormality: includes cerebellar tumor, inflammation (e.g., multiple sclerosis), stroke, or hemorrhage; the time course for these causes is typically more acute or subacute than chronic
- Endocrine dysfunction: hypothyroidism or hypoparathyroidism can uncommonly cause ataxia
- Alcoholic cerebellar degeneration: caused by heavy alcohol use; gait ataxia predominates
- Other toxin-induced ataxias: antiepileptic medications, lithium, and chemotherapeutic agents
- Creutzfeldt-Jakob disease: rapidly progressive ataxia, dementia, and myoclonus
- Paraneoplastic cerebellar degeneration: found in association with primary malignancies (e.g., small-cell lung cancer, breast cancer); subacute onset ataxia that progresses rapidly
- Celiac disease: gluten-sensitive enteropathy with malabsorption may be associated with ataxia; autoantibodies such as antigliadin or antiendomysial antibodies are typically present
- Multiple system atrophy: cerebellar variant of this disorder causes ataxia; there is typically associated parkinsonism with some degree of autonomic dysfunction (e.g., orthostatic hypotension, urinary incontinence)
- Friedreich's ataxia: autosomal recessive inheritance, generally younger age of onset (i.e., mean, 15 yr), lower limb areflexia, and posterior column dysfunction
- Ataxia associated with vitamin E deficiency: can be an autosomal recessive disorder or acquired; clinically resembles Friedreich's ataxia, with areflexia and loss of position sense
- Ataxia telangiectasia: autosomal recessive inheritance, childhood onset, oculocutaneous telangiectases, and immunodeficiency
- Wilson's disease: can cause hepatic dysfunction and a variety of movement disorders, including ataxia; particularly important to screen for this in patients who are young at onset because it is treatable
- Dentatorubral pallidoluysian atrophy: autosomal dominant like SCA but typically has ataxia with associated choreoathetosis, myoclonus, epilepsy, and dementia
- Fragile-X–associated tremor–ataxia syndrome: premutation of the fragile X mutation gene; more common among males than females; late onset of ataxia (i.e., >50 yr), tremor, and sometimes parkinsonism; MRI often shows T2 hyperintensity in the middle cerebellar peduncle
- Box 1-14 shows the classification of the various causes of ataxia.

LABORATORY TESTS

- Rule out acquired causes of ataxia, depending on the clinical scenario, with thyroid studies, toxicology screening, and the determination of the vitamin E level and the presence of paraneoplastic antibodies.
- Screen for Wilson's disease with ceruloplasmin and, if indicated, a 24-hour urinary copper determination.
- Genetic testing is commercially available for many but not all of the SCAs.

IMAGING STUDIES

- MRI of the brain should be performed to exclude structural abnormalities.
- Cerebellar or brain stem atrophy can be seen with several of the SCA subtypes

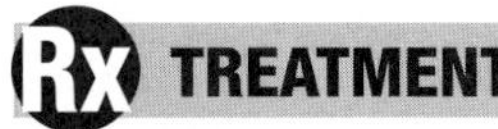

TREATMENT

NONPHARMACOLOGIC THERAPY

- Speech therapy for dysarthria and dysphagia
- Physical therapy
- Occupational therapy

CHRONIC Rx

Treatment is symptomatic and supportive. In some cases, parkinsonism can respond to levodopa. Clonazepam can be helpful if tremor is prominent. Spasticity can be treated with baclofen or tizanidine. Dystonia may benefit from botulinum toxin injections.

DISPOSITION

All SCA disorders are progressive, although the speed is variable from subtype to subtype and from patient to patient. On average, patients become wheelchair bound 15 yr after the onset of ataxia, and death can occur after 20 to 25 yr.

REFERRAL

Referral to a general neurologist or to a movement disorders center is appropriate.

BOX 1-14 Classification of Ataxia

Congenital Ataxias

Hereditary Ataxias

Autosomal Recessive Ataxias
- Friedreich's ataxia
- Ataxia–telangiectasia
- Ataxia with oculomotor apraxia type 1
- Ataxia with oculomotor apraxia type 2
- Autosomal recessive spastic ataxia of Charlevoix-Saguenay
- Abetalipoproteinemia
- Ataxia with isolated vitamin E deficiency
- Refsum's disease
- Cerebrotendinous xanthomatosis
- Marinesco-Sjögren syndrome
- Autosomal recessive ataxia with known gene locus
- Early-onset cerebellar ataxia

X-Linked Ataxias
- Fragile X tremor ataxia syndrome

Autosomal Dominant Ataxias
- Spinocerebellar ataxias
- Dentatorubral–pallidoluysian atrophy
- Episodic ataxias

Nonhereditary Degenerative Ataxias
- Multiple system atrophy, cerebellar type
- Sporadic adult-onset ataxia of unknown etiology

Acquired Ataxias
- Alcoholic cerebellar degeneration
- Ataxia as a result of other toxic causes (e.g., antiepileptic medications, lithium, solvents)
- Paraneoplastic cerebellar degeneration
- Other immune-mediated ataxias (e.g., gluten ataxia, ataxia associated with anti-glutamic acid decarboxylase antibodies)
- Acquired vitamin E deficiency
- Hypothyroidism
- Ataxia as a result of physical causes (e.g., heat stroke, hyperthermia)

(From Goetz CG: *Textbook of clinical neurology*, ed 3, Philadelphia, 2007, Saunders.)

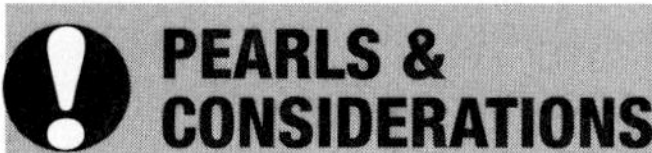

COMMENTS

- Genetic testing can have consequences for both the patient and the family. These issues should be discussed during the informed consent process. Patients who desire asymptomatic testing as a result of a relevant family history should undergo genetic counseling before testing.
- In symptomatic patients with a family history of dominantly inherited ataxia, the diagnostic process is relatively straightforward. Genetic testing that is directed toward likely mutations by phenotype and ethnic origin should be the first step.

PATIENT/FAMILY EDUCATION

Patient educational materials as well as contact information for support and advocacy groups are available on the website of the National Ataxia Foundation: http://www.ataxia.org.

SUGGESTED READINGS

Bird TD: Hereditary ataxia overview. Available at http://www.geneclinics.org/profiles/ataxias/details.html.

Klockgether T: The clinical diagnosis of autosomal dominant spinocerebellar ataxias, *Cerebellum* 7:101-105, 2008.

Neuromuscular Disease Center: Ataxias: classification. Available at http://neuromuscular.wustl.edu/ataxia/aindex.html.

Schols L et al: Autosomal dominant cerebellar ataxias: clinical features, genetics, and pathogenesis, *Lancet Neurol* 3:291, 2004.

AUTHOR: **ANDREW DUKER, M.D.**

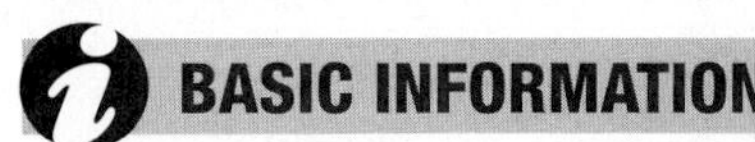

BASIC INFORMATION

DEFINITION

Spontaneous miscarriage is fetal loss before week 20 of pregnancy, calculated from the patient's last menstrual period or the delivery of a fetus weighing <500 g. Early loss is before menstrual week 12, whereas late loss refers to losses from weeks 12 to 20.

Miscarriage can also be classified as incomplete (partial passage of fetal tissue through partially dilated cervix), complete (spontaneous passage of all fetal tissue), threatened (uterine bleeding without cervical dilation or passage of tissue), inevitable (bleeding with cervical dilation without passage of fetal tissue), or missed abortion (intrauterine fetal demise without passage of tissue).

Recurrent miscarriage involves three or more spontaneous pregnancy losses before week 20.

SYNONYMS

Abortion

ICD-9CM CODES
634.0 Spontaneous abortion

EPIDEMIOLOGY & DEMOGRAPHICS

INCIDENCE: 5% to 20% of clinically recognized pregnancies, with 80% of miscarriages occurring in the first trimester

GENETICS:

- Distribution of abnormal karyotypes: autosomal trisomy (50%), monosomy 45,X (20%), triploidy (15%), tetraploidy (10%), structural chromosomal abnormalities (5%).
- With two or more spontaneous miscarriages, a karyotype should be performed to evaluate for balanced translocation, which has 80% risk for abortion, and, if the pregnancy is carried to term, has 3% to 5% risk for unbalanced karyotype.

RISK FACTORS: Prior pregnancy history (risk after live birth, 5%; prior pregnancy aborted, 20% subsequent risk) is the most significant risk factor. Vaginal bleeding, especially >3 days, carries with it a 15% to 20% chance of miscarriage.

PHYSICAL FINDINGS & CLINICAL PRESENTATION

- Profuse bleeding and cramping have a higher association with miscarriage than bleeding without cramping, which is more consistent with a threatened miscarriage.
- Cervical dilation with history or finding of fetal tissue at cervical os may be present.
- In cases of missed abortion, uterine size may be smaller than menstrual dating, in contrast to molar gestation, where size may be greater than dates.

ETIOLOGY

- In a general overview the etiology can be classified in terms of maternal (environmental) and fetal (genetic) factors, with the majority of miscarriages being related to genetic or chromosomal causes.
- Causes: uterine anomalies (unicornuate uterus risk, 50%; bicornuate or septate uterus risk, 25% to 30%); incompetent cervix (iatrogenic or congenital, associated with 20% of mid-trimester losses); diethylstilbestrol exposure in utero (T-shaped uterus); submucous leiomyomas; intrauterine adhesions or synechiae; luteal phase or progesterone deficiency; autoimmune disease such as anticardiolipin antibodies; uncontrolled diabetes mellitus; human leukocyte antigen associations between mother and father; infections such as tuberculosis, *Chlamydia,* and *Ureaplasma;* smoking and alcohol use; irradiation; and environmental toxins.

Dx DIAGNOSIS

DIFFERENTIAL DIAGNOSIS

- Normal pregnancy
- Hydatidiform molar gestation
- Ectopic pregnancy
- Dysfunctional uterine bleeding
- Pathologic endometrial or cervical lesions

WORKUP

- All patients with bleeding in the first trimester should have an evaluation for possible ectopic pregnancy.
- If there are three early, prior pregnancy losses, a workup and treatment for recurrent miscarriage should begin before next conception. If there is a strong history for second-trimester loss, consideration for cerclage should be given, especially if the history is consistent with incompetent cervix (e.g., painless cervical dilation).

LABORATORY TESTS

- Type and antibody screen are used to evaluate the need for Rh immune globulin.
- During the preconception period, hemoglobin A1C, anticardiolipin antibody, lupus anticoagulant, Factor V Leiden, MTHFR, antithrombin III, prothrombin gene 2210A, karyotyping, endometrial biopsy with progesterone level, and cervical cultures or serum antibodies can be checked for suspected disease processes.
- Progesterone level <5 mg/dl indicates nonviable gestation versus >25 mg/dl, which suggests a good prognosis.

IMAGING STUDIES

Transabdominal or transvaginal sonogram (preferably) can be used in combination with menstrual dating and serum quantitative human chorionic gonadotropin to document pregnancy location, fetal heart presence, gestational sac size, and adnexal pathology.

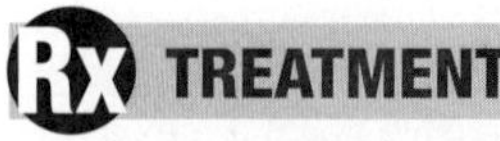

TREATMENT

NONPHARMACOLOGIC THERAPY

Depending on the patient's clinical status, desire to continue the pregnancy, and certainty of the diagnosis, expectant management can be considered. In pregnancies <6 wk or >14 wk, complete expulsion of fetal tissue usually occurs and surgical intervention such as dilation and curettage (D&C) can be avoided.

ACUTE GENERAL Rx

- Incomplete miscarriage between 6 and 14 wk can be associated with large amounts of blood loss; thus these patients should undergo D&C.
- In cases of missed abortion, if fetal demise has occurred >6 wk before or gestational age is >14 wk, there is an increased risk of hypofibrinogenemia with disseminated intravascular coagulation. Thus D&C should be performed early in the disease course. Consider use of misoprostol (Cytotec) 200 mg PO q6h.
- Rh-negative patients should be given Rhogam 300 mcg IM to prevent Rh isoimmunization.

REFERRAL

Refer to obstetrician/gynecologist

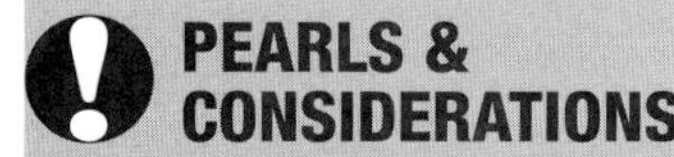

PEARLS & CONSIDERATIONS

Spontaneous pregnancy loss is recommended as a replacement for the term *abortion* and to acknowledge the emotional aspects of losing a pregnancy.

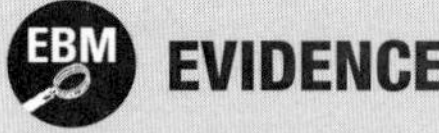

EVIDENCE

Please note: Complete text of EBM for this topic is available online.

SUGGESTED READING

Griebel CP et al: Management of spontaneous abortion, *Am Fam Physician* 72:1243, 2005.

AUTHORS: **SCOTT J. ZUCCALA, D.O.,** and **RUBEN ALVERO, M.D.**

BASIC INFORMATION

DEFINITION

Sporotrichosis is a granulomatous disease caused by the dimorphic fungus *Sporothrix schenckii.*

SYNONYMS

Lymphocutaneous sporotrichosis
Cutaneous sporotrichosis
Pulmonary sporotrichosis

ICD-9CM CODES
117.1 Sporotrichosis

EPIDEMIOLOGY & DEMOGRAPHICS

PREDOMINANT SEX: The most common form, lymphocutaneous sporotrichosis, occurs equally in both sexes. Males predominate in both pulmonary and osteoarticular sporotrichosis.

PREDOMINANT AGE: Generally, lymphocutaneous sporotrichosis occurs in people 35 yr of age or younger, and pulmonary sporotrichosis occurs in people between the ages of 30 and 60 yr.

GENETICS: Neonatal infection: at least one case of transmission from the cheek lesions of the mother to the skin of the infant has been reported.

PHYSICAL FINDINGS & CLINICAL PRESENTATION

- Cutaneous disease
  1. Arises at the site of inoculation
  2. Initial lesion usually located on the distal part of an extremity (Fig. 1-308), although any area may be affected, including the face
  3. Variable incubation period of approximately 3 wk once introduced into the skin
  4. Granulomatous reaction provoked
  5. Lesion becomes papulonodular, erythematous, elastic, variable in size
  6. Subsequently, nodule becomes fluctuant, undergoes central necrosis, breaks down, discharges mucoid pus from which fungus may be isolated
  7. Indolent ulcer with raised erythematous or violaceous borders
  8. Secondary lesions:
     a. Develop along superficial lymphatic channels
     b. Evolve in the same manner as the primary lesion, with subsequent inflammation, induration, and suppuration
- Fixed, or plaque form
  1. Erythematous verrucous, ulcerated, or crusted lesions
  2. Does not spread locally
  3. Does not involve lymphatic vessels
  4. Rarely undergoes spontaneous resolution
  5. More often persists for years without systemic symptoms and within a setting of normal laboratory examinations
- Osteoarticular involvement
  1. Most common extracutaneous form
  2. Usually presents as monoarticular arthritis
  3. Left untreated, may progress to:
     a. Synovitis
     b. Osteitis
     c. Periostitis
     d. All involving elbows, knees, wrists, and ankles
  4. Joint inflamed
     a. Associated with an effusion
     b. Painful on motion
- Early pulmonary disease
  1. Usually associated with a paucity of clinical findings
     a. Low-grade fever
     b. Cough
     c. Fatigue
     d. Malaise
     e. Weight loss
  2. Untreated
     a. Cavitary pulmonary disease
     b. Frank pulmonary dysfunction
  3. Meningitis uncommon
     a. Except perhaps in the immunocompromised patient
     b. Presents with few signs or symptoms of neurologic involvement, usually headache
  4. Few reported cases
     a. Infection of the ocular adnexa
     b. Endophthalmitis without antecedent trauma
     c. Infection of the testes and epididymis

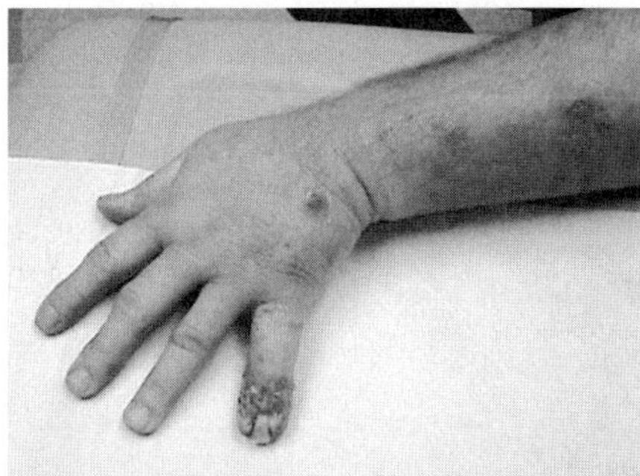

FIGURE 1-308 Sporotrichosis of the fifth finger in a gardener. Three nodular lesions are visible on the hand and arm. (From Mandell GL, Bennett JE, Dolin R: *Principles and practice of infectious diseases,* ed 7, Philadelphia, 2010, Elsevier.)

ETIOLOGY

- *Sporothrix schenckii*
  1. Global in distribution
  2. Often isolated from soil, plants, and plant products
  3. Majority of case reports from tropical and subtropical regions of the Americas
- Occupational or recreational exposure
  1. Hay
  2. Straw
  3. Sphagnum moss
  4. Timber
  5. Thorny plants (e.g., roses and barberry bushes)
- Animal contact
  1. Armadillos
  2. Cats
  3. Squirrels
- Human-to-human transmission
- Tattooing

Dx DIAGNOSIS

DIFFERENTIAL DIAGNOSIS

- Fixed, or plaque, sporotrichosis
  1. Bacterial pyoderma
  2. Foreign body granuloma
  3. Tularemia
  4. Anthrax
  5. Other mycoses: blastomycosis, chromoblastomycosis
- Lymphocutaneous sporotrichosis
  1. *Nocardia brasiliensis*
  2. *Leishmania braziliensis*
  3. Atypical mycobacterial disease: *M. marinum, M. kansasii*
- Pulmonary sporotrichosis
  1. Pulmonary TB
  2. Histoplasmosis
  3. Coccidioidomycosis
- Osteoarticular sporotrichosis
  1. Pigmented villonodular synovitis
  2. Gout
  3. Rheumatoid arthritis
  4. Infection with *M. tuberculosis*
  5. Atypical mycobacteria: *M. marinum, M. kansasii, M. avium-intracellulare*
- Meningitis
  1. Histoplasmosis
  2. Cryptococcosis
  3. TB

WORKUP

- The diagnosis should be considered in individuals who are occupationally exposed to soil, decaying plant matter, and thorny plants (gardeners, horticulturists, farmers) who present with chronic nonhealing ulcers or lesions with or without associated arthritis or pulmonary symptoms.
- Diagnosis is made by culture:
  1. Pus
  2. Joint fluid
  3. Sputum
  4. Blood
  5. Skin biopsy
- Isolation of the fungus from any site is considered diagnostic of infection.
- Saprophytic colonization of the respiratory tract has been described.
- A positive blood culture may indicate infection in an immunocompromised host.
- Increasingly sensitive laboratory culturing systems may detect the fungus in the normal host.
- Biopsy specimens are diagnostic if characteristic cigar-shaped, round, oval, or budding yeast forms are seen.
- Despite special staining, the yeast may remain difficult to detect unless multiple sections are examined.

- No standard method of serologic testing is available.
- Previously described techniques have been hampered by the presence of antibody in the absence of infection.

LABORATORY TESTS

- CBCs and serum chemistries are generally normal.
- Elevated ESR is seen with extracutaneous disease.
- CSF analysis in meningeal disease reveals:
  1. Lymphocytic pleocytosis
  2. Elevated protein
  3. Hypoglycorrhachia
- Nested polymerase chain reaction (PCR) assay represents a future clinical modality to rapidly detect *Sporothrix schenckii.*

IMAGING STUDIES

- Chest x-ray examination: unilateral or bilateral upper lobe cavitary or noncavitary lesions
- Radiographic findings of affected joints:
  1. Loss of articular cartilage
  2. Periosteal reaction
  3. Periarticular osteopenia
  4. Cystic changes

Rx TREATMENT

NONPHARMACOLOGIC THERAPY

Local heat and prevention of bacterial superinfection in cutaneous or plaque form

ACUTE GENERAL Rx

CUTANEOUS AND LYMPHOCUTANEOUS SPOROTRICHOSIS:

- Itraconazole at doses of 100 to 200 mg/day is the drug of choice and should be given for 3 to 6 mo.
- Use saturated solution of potassium iodide (SSKI) 5 to 10 drops PO tid or 1.5 ml PO tid, gradually increasing to 40 to 50 drops PO tid or 3 ml PO tid after meals.
- Maximum tolerated dose should be continued until cutaneous lesions have resolved, approximately 6 to 12 wk.
- Adjunctive therapy with heat is useful and occasionally curative.
- Side effects:
  1. Nausea
  2. Anorexia
  3. Diarrhea
  4. Parotid or lacrimal gland hypertrophy
  5. Acneiform rash

DEEP-SEATED MYCOSES (E.G., OSTEOARTICULAR, NONCAVITARY PULMONARY DISEASE):

- Itraconazole
  1. Appropriate initial chemotherapy
  2. Probably as effective as amphotericin B
  3. Less toxic than amphotericin B
  4. Better tolerated than ketoconazole
  5. 100 to 200 mg bid for 1 to 2 yr with continued lifelong suppressive therapy in selected patients
  6. Absence of relapses from 40 to 68 mo has been documented when at least 200 mg/day administered for 24 mo
  7. Insufficient data for use in disseminated disease (e.g., fungemia and meningitis)
- Parenteral amphotericin B, total course of 2 to 2.5 g or more, results in cure in approximately two thirds of cases
  1. Relapses are common.
  2. Amphotericin B-resistant isolates of *Sporothrix schenckii* have been reported.
  3. Remains the drug of choice for severely ill patients with disseminated disease.
  4. In cavitary pulmonary disease, given perioperatively as an adjunct to surgical resection.
  5. In meningitis, amphotericin B may be used alone or in combination with 5-fluorocytosine.
- Fluconazole
  1. Less effective than itraconazole
  2. Requires daily doses of 400 mg/day for lymphocutaneous disease and 800 mg/day for visceral or osteoarticular disease

CHRONIC Rx

For lymphocutaneous and visceral disease, therapy with itraconazole 200 mg/day for periods of 24 mo or greater. Sporothrix is resistant to voriconazole. It is sensitive *in vitro* to posaconazole, but existing data is very limited at present.

DISPOSITION

- Prognosis for cutaneous disease is good.
- Prognosis is less satisfactory for extracutaneous disease, especially if associated with abnormal immunologic states or other underlying systemic diseases.

REFERRAL

To surgeon; with an established diagnosis of pulmonary sporotrichosis, cavitary lesions require resection of involved tissue

Infectious disease physician

PEARLS & CONSIDERATIONS

COMMENTS

- In patients with underlying immunosuppression (e.g., hematologic malignancy or infection with HIV), progression of the initial infection may develop into multifocal extracutaneous sporotrichosis.
- In this subset of patients, dissemination of cutaneous lesions is accompanied by hematogenous spread to lungs, bone, mucous membranes, CNS.
- Osteoarticular and pulmonary manifestations predominate with the development of polyarticular arthritis and osteolytic bone lesions.
- In the absence of therapy, the infection is ultimately fatal.
- Patients with underlying immunosuppressive states should be carefully evaluated even when presenting with single cutaneous lesions.
- Diagnostic modalities should include:
  1. Radiographic examination of chest
  2. Technetium pyrophosphate bone scan
  3. Culture of synovial fluid, blood, skin lesion(s)
- In patients with AIDS, itraconazole appears to be the drug of choice, although meningitis and pulmonary disease may warrant the use of amphotericin B.
- In patients with AIDS, lifetime suppressive therapy with itraconazole should follow initial therapy because of the potential for relapse and dissemination.

SUGGESTED READINGS

Bernardes-Engermann AR et al: Development of an enzyme-linked immunosorbent assay for the serodiagnosis of several clinical forms of sporotrichosis, *Med Mycol* 43(6):487, 2005.

Da Rosa AC et al: Epidemiology of sporotrichosis; a study of 304 cases in Brazil, *J Am Acad Dermatol* 52(3 Pt 1):451, 2005.

Gottlieb GS et al: Disseminated sporotrichosis associated with treatment with immunosuppressants and tumor necrosis factor-alpha antagonists, *Clin Infect Dis* 37(6):838, 2003.

Kauffman CA et al: Clinical practice guidelines for the management of sporotrichosis: 2007 update by the Infectious Diseases Society of America, *Clin Infect Dis* 45(10):1255, 2007.

Kauffman CA: Sporotrichosis, *Clin Infect Dis* 29(2): 231, 1999.

Neyra E et al: Epidemiology of human sporotrichosis investigated by amplified fragment length polymorphism, *J Clin Microbiol* 43(3):1348, 2005.

Schubach AO, Schubach TM, Barros MB: Epidemic cat-transmitted sporotrichosis, *N Engl J Med* 353(11):1185, 2005.

AUTHORS: **PATRICIA CRISTOFARO, M.D., GLENN G. FORT, M.D., M.P.H.,** and **DENNIS J. MIKOLICH, M.D.**

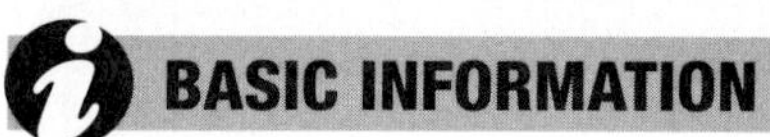

BASIC INFORMATION

DEFINITION

Squamous cell carcinoma (SCC) is a malignant tumor of the skin arising in the epithelium.

SYNONYMS

SCC
Skin cancer

ICD-9CM CODES

173.9 Skin neoplasm, site unspecified

EPIDEMIOLOGY & DEMOGRAPHICS

- SCC is the second most common cutaneous malignancy, comprising 20% of all cases of nonmelanoma skin cancer.
- Incidence is highest in lower latitudes (e.g., southern U.S., Australia).
- Male/female ratio is 2:1.
- Incidence increases with age and sun exposure.
- Average age at diagnosis is 66 yr.

PHYSICAL FINDINGS & CLINICAL PRESENTATION

- SCC commonly affects the scalp, neck region, back of hands, superior surface of the pinna, and the lip.
- The lesion may have a scaly, erythematous macule or plaque.
- Telangiectasia, central ulceration may also be present (Fig. 1-309).
- Most SCCs present as exophytic lesions that grow over a period of months.

ETIOLOGY

Risk factors include ultraviolet B radiation and immunosuppression (kidney transplant recipients have a threefold increased risk).

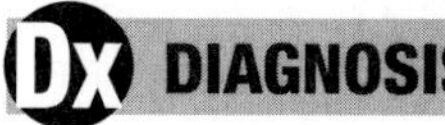

DIAGNOSIS

DIFFERENTIAL DIAGNOSIS

- Keratoacanthomas
- Actinic keratosis
- Amelanotic melanoma
- Basal cell carcinoma
- Benign tumors
- Healing traumatic wounds
- Spindle cell tumors
- Warts

WORKUP

Diagnosis is made by full-thickness skin biopsy (incisional or excisional).

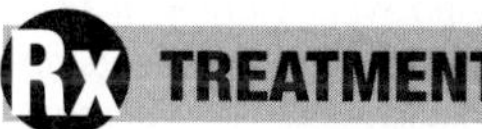

TREATMENT

ACUTE GENERAL Rx

- Electrodesiccation and curettage for small SCCs (<2 cm in diameter), superficial tumors, and lesions located in extremity and trunk.
- Tumors thinner than 4 mm can be managed by simple local removal.
- Lesions between 4 and 8 mm thick or those with deep dermal invasion should be excised.
- Tumors penetrating the dermis can be treated with several modalities, including excision and Mohs' surgery, radiation therapy, and chemotherapy.
- Metastatic SCC can be treated with cryotherapy and combination of chemotherapy using 13-*cis*-retinoic acid and interferon-alpha 2A.

DISPOSITION

- Survival is related to size, location, degree of differentiation, immunologic status of the patient, depth of invasion, and presence of metastases. Risk factors for metastasis include lesions on the lip or ear, increasing lesion depth, and poor cell differentiation.
- Patients whose tumors penetrate through the dermis or exceed 8 mm in thickness are at risk of tumor recurrence.
- The most common metastatic locations are regional lymph nodes, liver, and lung.
- Tumors on the scalp, forehead, ears, nose, and lips also carry a higher risk.
- SCCs originating in the lip and pinna metastasize in 10% to 20% of cases.
- Five-year survival for metastatic squamous cell carcinoma is 34%.

REFERRAL

Oncology referral for metastatic SCC

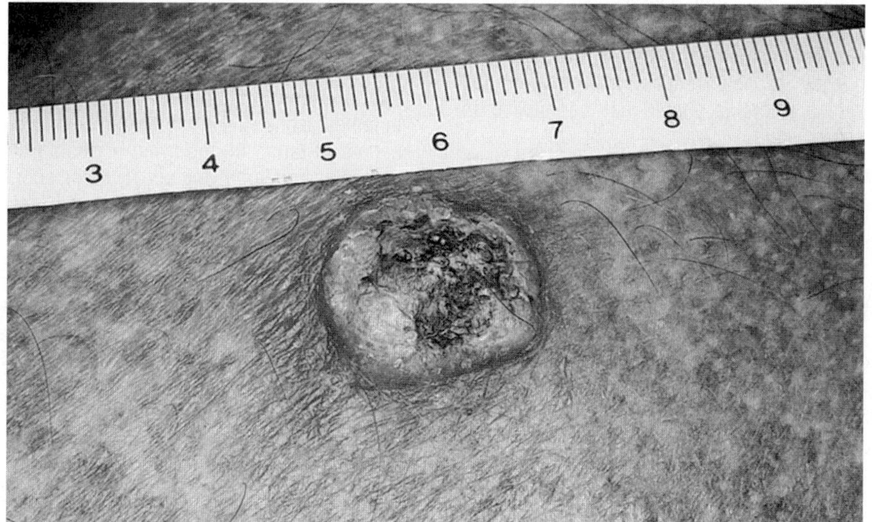

FIGURE 1-309 Squamous cell carcinoma. Nodular hyperkeratotic lesion with central erosion. (From Noble J et al: *Textbook of primary care medicine,* ed 3, St Louis, 2001, Mosby.)

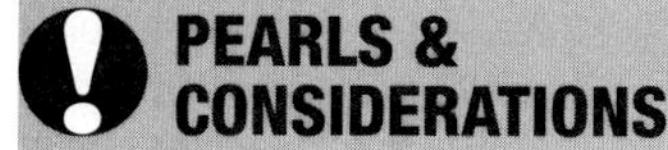

PEARLS & CONSIDERATIONS

COMMENTS

SCC arising in areas of prior radiation, thermal injury, and areas of chronic ulcers or chronic draining sinuses are more aggressive and have a higher frequency of metastasis than those originating in actinic damaged skin.

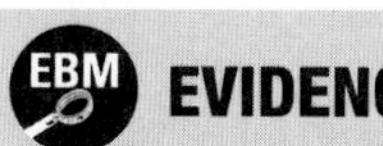

EVIDENCE

Please note: Complete text of EBM for this topic is available online.

SUGGESTED READING

Stulberg DL et al: Diagnosis and treatment of basal cell and squamous cell carcinomas, *Am Fam Physician* 70:1481, 2004.

AUTHOR: **FRED F. FERRI, M.D.**

Stasis Dermatitis (PTG)

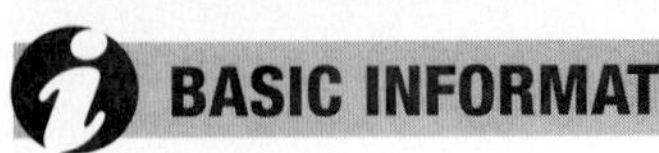

BASIC INFORMATION

DEFINITION

Stasis dermatitis refers to an inflammatory skin disease of the lower extremities, commonly seen in patients with chronic venous insufficiency (Fig. 1-310).

SYNONYMS

Chronic venous insufficiency

ICD-9CM CODES
454.1 Varicose veins of lower extremities with inflammation

EPIDEMIOLOGY & DEMOGRAPHICS

- Prevalence of stasis dermatitis increases with age and obesity
- Rarely seen before age 50 yr
- Twice as common in women than men, although men tend to have more severe disease
- No ethnic predilection for disease

PHYSICAL FINDINGS & CLINICAL PRESENTATION

- Insidious onset
- Pruritus
- Chronic lower extremity edema, sometimes unilateral, often described as "brawny" because of dermal fibrosis
- Ill-defined erythema
- Eczematous patches
- Commonly located over the medial malleolus
- Progressive pigment changes can occur as a result of extravasation of red blood cells and hemosiderin deposition within the cutaneous tissue
- Secondary infections can occur

ETIOLOGY

- Stasis dermatitis is believed to occur as a result of venous incompetence. Common etiologies include:
  1. Deep vein thrombosis
  2. History of lower extremity injury
  3. Pregnancy
  4. Vein stripping or vein harvesting in patients requiring coronary artery bypass grafting
- Venous insufficiency subsequently results in venous hypertension, causing skin inflammation and the aforementioned physical findings and clinical presentation

Dx DIAGNOSIS

The diagnosis of stasis dermatitis is primarily made by a detailed history and physical examination

DIFFERENTIAL DIAGNOSIS

- Contact dermatitis
- Atopic dermatitis
- Cellulitis
- Dermatophyte infection
- Pretibial myxedema
- Nummular eczema
- Lichen simplex chronicus
- Xerosis
- Asteatotic eczema
- Deep vein thrombosis

WORKUP

Directed at excluding potential life-threatening causes (e.g., deep vein thrombosis) and complications (e.g., cellulitis and sepsis).

LABORATORY TESTS

Generally not helpful unless a secondary infection is present

IMAGING STUDIES

- Radiograph, CT scans, and MRIs are generally not necessary for diagnosis
- Doppler studies are indicated in any patient suspected of having deep vein thrombosis

Rx TREATMENT

NONPHARMACOLOGIC THERAPY

- Leg elevation above heart level for 30 min three to four times a day (avoid in arterial occlusive diseases)
- Compression stocking with a gradient of at least 30 to 40 mm Hg; in obese patients, intermittent pneumatic compression pump is recommended
- For weeping skin lesions, wet to dry dressing changes are helpful

ACUTE GENERAL Rx

- The mainstay of treatment of stasis dermatitis is to control leg edema and prevent venous stasis ulcers from developing.
- In patients with acute stasis dermatitis, a compression (Unna) boot can be applied.
- Topical corticosteroid creams or ointments (e.g., triamcinolone 0.1% bid) are used frequently to help reduce inflammation and itching. Steroids should not be applied to stasis ulcers.
- Secondary infections should be treated with appropriate antibiotics. Most secondary infections are the result of *Staphylococcus* or *Streptococcus* organisms.
- Diuretics for controlling edema.

CHRONIC Rx

- Patients with chronic stasis dermatitis can be treated with topical emollients (e.g., white petrolatum, lanolin, Eucerin)
- Surgical therapy:
  - Venous stripping
  - Superficial and deep perforator vein ligation
  - Endovenous stenting

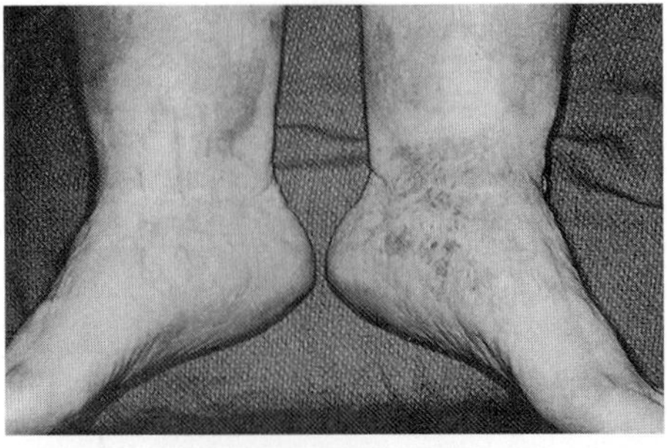

FIGURE 1-310 Moderate stasis dermatitis with hyperpigmentation and bilateral venous insufficiency. (Courtesy Department of Dermatology, University of North Carolina at Chapel Hill. From Goldstein BG, Goldstein AO: *Practical dermatology,* ed 2, St Louis, 1997, Mosby.)

COMPLEMENTARY & ALTERNATIVE MEDICINE

Oral horse chestnut seed extract

REFERRAL

- Dermatology
- Vascular surgery
- Indications for referral:
  - Nonhealing ulcers
  - Uncertainty in the diagnosis
  - Associated arterial insufficiency
  - Persistent stasis dermatitis
  - Suspected contact dermatitis
  - Consideration of superficial venous surgery

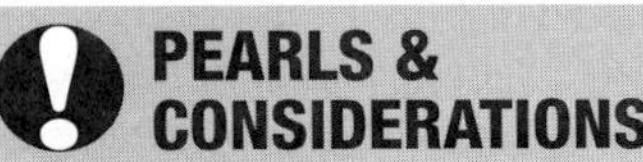

PEARLS & CONSIDERATIONS

COMMENTS

- Inflammatory skin changes from stasis dermatitis are believed to result from poor oxygen perfusion to the lower extremity skin tissue.
- Venous disease is irreversible. Goal of treatment is to alleviate symptoms and prevent progression.
- Stasis ulcers are often associated with stasis dermatitis. Refer to Section I, "Venous Ulcers," for more information.

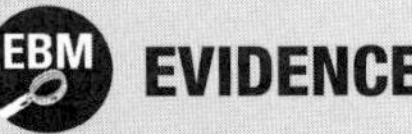

EVIDENCE

Evidence for the treatment of stasis dermatitis is limited, and large, high-quality trials and systematic reviews for the main therapies are lacking. However, there is some limited evidence of benefit for topical corticosteroids.

A small double blind, placebo-controlled trial provides limited evidence that 0.12% betamethasone valerate foam can be of some benefit in terms of improving erythema and petechiae and improving quality of life scores in the treatment of mild to moderate stasis dermatitis.[1] B

Evidence-Based Reference

1. Weiss SC et al: A randomized controlled clinical trial assessing the effect of betamethasone valerate 0.12% foam on the short-term treatment of stasis dermatitis, *J Drugs Dermatol* 4:339-345, 2005. B

SUGGESTED READINGS

Bergan JJ et al: Chronic venous disease, *N Engl J Med* 355(5):488, 2006.

Eberhardt RT: Chronic venous insufficiency, *Circulation* 111:2398, 2005.

AUTHORS: **KACHIU LEE, B.A.,** and **JESSICA RISSER, M.D., M.P.H.**

BASIC INFORMATION

DEFINITION

The term *status epilepticus* refers to continuous seizure activity lasting at least 5 min, or two or more discrete seizures with incomplete recovery of consciousness between them.

SYNONYMS

Generalized convulsive status epilepticus
Nonconvulsive status epilepticus
Complex partial status epilepticus
Absence status epilepticus

ICD-9CM CODES
345.3 Grand mal status

EPIDEMIOLOGY & DEMOGRAPHICS

INCIDENCE (IN U.S.): 100,000 to 152,000 cases per year

PREDOMINANT SEX: Males and females affected equally

PHYSICAL FINDINGS & CLINICAL PRESENTATION

- Patients are typically unresponsive and may have obvious tonic, clonic, or tonic-clonic movements of the extremities (convulsive status epilepticus).
- Some patients are unresponsive or have an altered level of consciousness with no clear observable repetitive motor activity (nonconvulsive status epilepticus).
- Clinical manifestations can evolve and can become subtle with only small-amplitude twitching movements of the face, limbs, or eyes.

ETIOLOGY

- Preexisting epilepsy with breakthrough seizures or low anticonvulsant drug levels
- Central nervous system infection or tumor
- Drug toxicity or metabolic disturbance
- Central nervous system hypoxia
- Head trauma
- Stroke

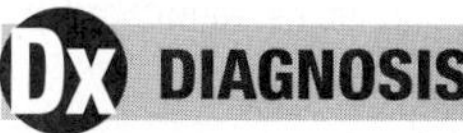

DIAGNOSIS

DIFFERENTIAL DIAGNOSIS

- Coma
- Encephalopathic states
- Psychogenic unresponsiveness

WORKUP

Because convulsive status epilepticus is an emergency with substantial risk of morbidity and mortality if not treated immediately, treatment must be early and aggressive, not postponed until an etiology is determined.

LABORATORY TESTS

- While treatment is being initiated: glucose, electrolytes, blood urea nitrogen, arterial blood gases, drug levels, complete blood count, urinalysis, toxicology screens
- Lumbar puncture in children with fever and in adults suspected to have meningitis or encephalitis

IMAGING STUDIES

Unless the etiology is known, CT or MRI of the brain is recommended as soon as possible after seizures have been controlled.

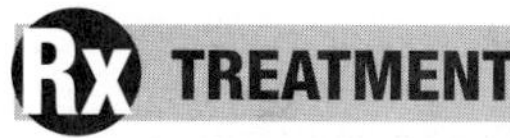

TREATMENT

NONPHARMACOLOGIC THERAPY

- Give oxygen by nasal cannula or nonrebreathing mask.
- Be prepared to intubate the patient.
- Maintain blood pressure.
- Maintain body temperature.
- Monitor ECG.
- Obtain IV access.

ACUTE GENERAL Rx

- Thiamine 100 mg IV and glucose 50 mg D_{50} by IV push (2 ml/kg D_{25} in children) unless hyperglycemic.
- Lorazepam 0.1 mg/kg IV at 2 mg/min.
- If seizures persist, fosphenytoin 20 mg/kg IV at 150 mg/min (if not available, use phenytoin 20 mg/kg IV at up to 50 mg/min as tolerated), followed by an additional 5 to 10 mg/kg IV if needed.
- If seizures persist, phenobarbital 20 mg/kg IV at 50 to 75 mg/min; will likely require intubation.
- If seizures persist, emergency neurologic consultation for management of refractory status epilepticus with additional doses of antiepileptic drugs or general anesthesia with midazolam, propofol, or pentobarbital.
- An electroencephalogram (EEG) should be obtained to evaluate for nonconvulsive status epilepticus in any patient who does not regain consciousness within 1 to 2 hr of cessation of convulsive activity.

CHRONIC Rx

Long-term treatment with anticonvulsants is indicated if there is significant risk of recurrence (e.g., known epilepsy, brain lesion, epileptiform EEG abnormalities).

DISPOSITION

- Generally favorable if treated promptly and there is no underlying acute symptomatic cause such as an underlying central nervous system lesion or systemic metabolic insult.
- Overall mortality rate is 22%; higher in the elderly (38%) and substantially lower in children (2.5%). Difference in mortality rate is mainly because status epilepticus in the elderly is more often the result of an acute symptomatic cause.

REFERRAL

This is an emergency. A neurologist should be involved as soon as possible if seizures do not subside immediately with treatment.

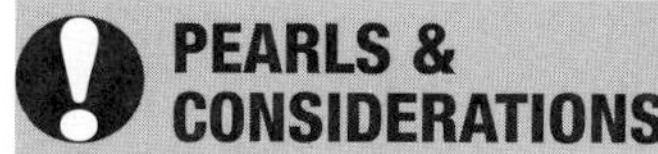

PEARLS & CONSIDERATIONS

COMMENTS

- Because of varied clinical presentations of status epilepticus, without an EEG there is no clinical basis for being certain that seizures have stopped unless the patient regains full consciousness.
- EEG provides definitive information about seizure cessation. If available, use of EEG in the management of status epilepticus is highly recommended.

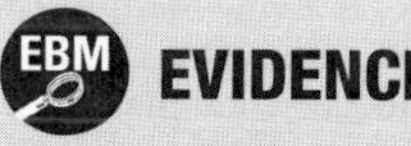

EVIDENCE

Many of the drugs used for the management of status epilepticus have not been fully evaluated for this indication in randomized controlled trials. Treatment regimens used are often influenced by factors such as local protocols, physician preference, and individual patient characteristics such as previous antiepileptic medication

Benzodiazepines

A systematic review of trials in both adult and pediatric patients, published in 2005, included 11 trials and concluded lorazepam was significantly better than diazepam or phenytoin for the immediate control of status epilepticus. For the treatment of premonitory seizures, 30 mg of diazepam as an intrarectal gel was significantly better than 20 mg for cessation of seizures.[1] Ⓐ

Evidence-Based Reference

1. Prasad K et al: Anticonvulsant therapy for status epilepticus, Cochrane Database Rev 2005. Ⓐ

SUGGESTED READINGS

Gaitanis JN, Drislane FW: Status epilepticus: a review of different syndromes, their current evaluation, and treatment, *Neurologist* 9(2):61-76, 2003.

Manno EM: New management strategies in the treatment of status epilepticus, *Mayo Clin Proc* 78(4): 508-518, 2003.

AUTHORS: **JOHN E. CROOM, M.D., PH.D.,** and **WILLIAM H. HEWITT, M.D.**

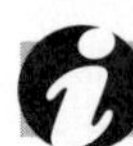

BASIC INFORMATION

DEFINITION

Stevens-Johnson syndrome (SJS) is a rare, severe vesiculobullous form of erythema multiforme affecting the skin, mouth, eyes, and genitalia.

SYNONYMS

SJS
Herpes iris
Febrile mucocutaneous syndrome

ICD-9CM CODES
695.1 Stevens-Johnson syndrome

EPIDEMIOLOGY & DEMOGRAPHICS

- SJS affects predominantly children and young adults.
- Male/female ratio is 2:1.

PHYSICAL FINDINGS & CLINICAL PRESENTATION

- The cutaneous eruption is generally preceded by vague, nonspecific symptoms of low-grade fever and fatigue occurring 1 to 14 days before the skin lesions. Cough is often present. Fever may be high during the active stages.
- Bullae generally occur on the conjunctiva, mucous membranes of the mouth, nares, and genital regions.
- Corneal ulcerations may result in blindness.
- Ulcerative stomatitis results in hemorrhagic crusting.
- Flat, atypical target lesions or purpuric maculae may be distributed on the trunk or be widespread (Fig. 1-311).
- The pain from oral lesions may compromise fluid intake and result in dehydration.
- Thick, mucopurulent sputum and oral lesions may interfere with breathing.

ETIOLOGY

- Drugs (e.g., phenytoin, sulfonamides, lamotrigine, allopurinol, phenobarbitol) are the most common cause.
- Upper respiratory tract infections (e.g., *Mycoplasma pneumoniae*) and herpes simplex viral infections have also been implicated in SJS.

Dx DIAGNOSIS

DIFFERENTIAL DIAGNOSIS

- Toxic erythema (drugs or infection)
- Pemphigus
- Pemphigoid
- Urticaria
- Hemorrhagic fevers
- Serum sickness
- *Staphylococcus* scalded-skin syndrome
- Behçet's syndrome

WORKUP

- Diagnosis is generally based on clinical presentation and characteristic appearance of the lesions.
- Skin biopsy is generally reserved for when classic lesions are absent and diagnosis is uncertain.

LABORATORY TESTS

Complete blood count with differential, cultures in cases of suspected infection

IMAGING STUDIES

Chest radiographs may show patchy changes in patients with pulmonary involvement.

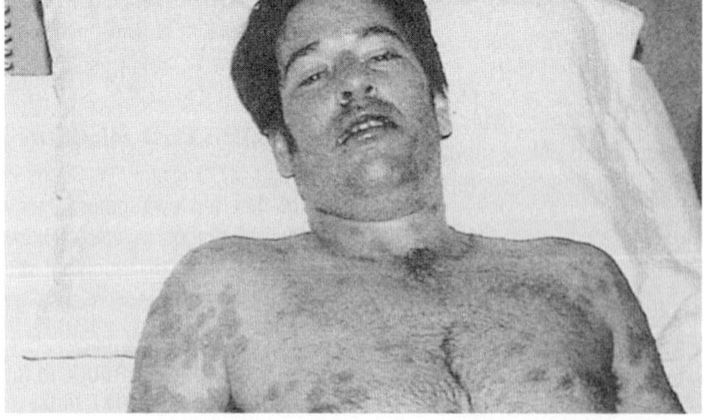

FIGURE 1-311 Stevens-Johnson syndrome. (From Stein JH: *Internal medicine,* ed 5, St Louis, 1998, Mosby.)

Rx TREATMENT

NONPHARMACOLOGIC THERAPY

- Withdrawal of any potential drug precipitants
- Careful skin nursing to prevent secondary infection

ACUTE GENERAL Rx

- Treatment of associated conditions (e.g., acyclovir for herpes simplex virus infection, azithromycin for *Mycoplasma* infection)
- Antihistamines for pruritus
- Treatment of the cutaneous blisters with cool, wet Burow's compresses
- Relief of oral symptoms by frequent rinsing with lidocaine (Xylocaine Viscous)
- Liquid or soft diet with plenty of fluids to ensure proper hydration
- Treatment of secondary infections with antibiotics
- Corticosteroids: use remains controversial and should be used only in severe cases early in the disease; when used, prednisone 20 to 30 mg bid until new lesions no longer appear, then rapidly tapered
- Topical steroids: may use to treat papules and plaques; however, should not be applied to eroded areas
- Vitamin A: may be used for lacrimal hyposecretion
- Consider intravenous immunoglobulins in severe cases

DISPOSITION

- Prognosis varies with severity of disease. It is generally good in patients with limited disease; however, mortality rate may approach 10% in patients with extensive involvement.
- Oral lesions may continue for several months.
- Scarring and corneal abnormalities may occur in 20% of patients.

REFERRAL

- Hospital admission in a unit used for burn care is recommended in severe cases.
- Urethral involvement may necessitate catheterization.
- Ocular involvement should be monitored by an ophthalmologist.

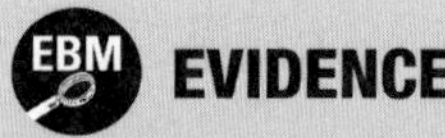

EVIDENCE

Please note: Complete text of EBM for this topic is available online.

SUGGESTED READING

Wetter DA, Camilleri MJ: Clinical, etiologic, and histopathologic features of Stevens-Johnson during an 8-year period at Mayo Clinic, *Mayo Clin Proc* 85(2): 131-138, 2010.

AUTHOR: **FRED F. FERRI, M.D.**

BASIC INFORMATION

DEFINITION

Stomatitis is inflammation involving the oral mucous membranes.

SYNONYMS

Heterogeneous grouping of unrelated illnesses, each with their own designation(s)

ICD-9CM CODES
528.0 Stomatitis
054.2 (herpetic)
528.2 (aphthous)
112.0 (monilial)

PHYSICAL FINDINGS & CLINICAL PRESENTATION

WHITE LESIONS:

- Candidiasis (thrush)
- Caused by yeast infection *(Candida albicans)*
- Examination: white, curdlike material that when wiped off leaves a raw bleeding surface
- Epidemiology: seen in the very young and the very old, those with immunodeficiency (AIDS, cancer), persons with diabetes, and patients treated with antibacterial agents
- Other
  1. Leukoedema: filmy opalescent-appearing mucosa, which can be reverted to normal appearance by stretching. This condition is benign.
  2. White sponge nevus: thick, white corrugated folds involving the buccal mucosa. Appears in childhood as an autosomal dominant trait. Benign condition.
  3. Darier's disease (keratosis follicularis): white papules on the gingivae, alveolar mucosa, and dorsal tongue. Skin lesions also present (erythematous papules). Inherited as an autosomal-dominant trait.
  4. Chemical injury: white sloughing mucosa.
  5. Nicotine stomatitis: whitened palate with red papules.
  6. Lichen planus: linear, reticular, slightly raised striae on buccal mucosa. Skin is involved by pruritic violaceous papules on forearms and inner thighs.
  7. Discoid lupus erythematosus: lesion resembles lichen planus.
  8. Leukoplakia: white lesions that cannot be scraped off; 20% are premalignant epithelial dysplasia or squamous cell carcinoma.
  9. Hairy leukoplakia: shaggy white surface that cannot be wiped off; seen in HIV infection, caused by Epstein-Barr virus.

RED LESIONS:

- Candidiasis may present with red lesions instead of the more frequent white. Median rhomboid glossitis is a chronic variant.
- Benign migratory glossitis (geographic tongue): area of atrophic depapillated mucosa surrounded by a keratotic border. Benign lesion, no treatment required.
- Hemangiomas.
- Histoplasmosis: ill-defined, irregular patch with a granulomatous surface, sometimes ulcerated.
- Allergy.
- Anemia: atrophic reddened glossal mucosa seen with pernicious anemia.
- Erythroplakia: red patch usually caused by epithelial dysplasia or squamous cell carcinoma.
- Burning tongue (glossopyrosis): normal examination; sometimes associated with denture trauma, anemia, diabetes, vitamin B_{12} deficiency, psychogenic problems.

DARK LESIONS (BROWN, BLUE, BLACK):

- Coated tongue: accumulation of keratin; harmless condition that can be treated by scraping
- Melanotic lesions: freckles, lentigines, lentigo, melanoma, Peutz-Jeghers syndrome, Addison's disease
- Varices
- Kaposi's sarcoma: red or purple macules that enlarge to form tumors; seen in patients with AIDS

RAISED LESIONS:

- Papilloma
- Verruca vulgaris
- Condyloma acuminatum
- Fibroma
- Epulis
- Pyogenic granuloma
- Mucocele
- Retention cyst

BLISTERS:

- Primary herpetic gingivostomatitis
- Caused by herpes simplex virus type 1 or, less frequently, type 2
- Course: day 1: malaise, fever, headache, sore throat, cervical lymphadenopathy; days 2 and 3: appearance of vesicles that develop into painful ulcers of 2 to 4 mm in diameter; duration of up to 2 wk
- Recurrent intraoral herpes: rare; recurrences typically involve only the keratinized epithelium (lips)
- Pemphigus and pemphigoid
- Hand-foot-mouth disease: caused by coxsackievirus group A
- Erythema multiforme
- Herpangina: caused by echovirus
- Traumatic ulcer
- Primary syphilis
- Perlèche (or angular cheilitis)
- Recurrent aphthous stomatitis (canker sores)
- Behçet's syndrome (aphthous ulcers, uveitis, genital ulcerations, arthritis, and aseptic meningitis)
- Reiter's syndrome (conjunctivitis, urethritis, and arthritis with occasional oral ulcerations)
- Unknown cause

Course: solitary or multiple painful ulcers may develop simultaneously and heal over 10 to 14 days. The size of the lesions and the frequency of recurrences are variable.

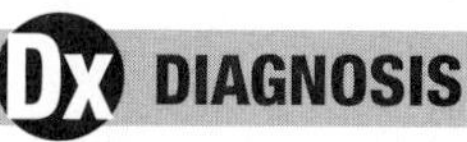

DIAGNOSIS

WORKUP

- White lesions: Candidiasis (thrush) diagnosis: ovoid yeast and hyphae seen in scrapings treated with KOH culture
- Blisters:
  - Exfoliative cytology
  - Viral culture
  - Immunofluorescence for herpes antigen

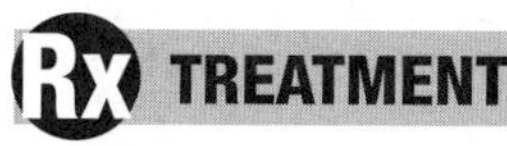

TREATMENT

White lesions: candidiasis (thrush) treatment:

- Topical with nystatin or clotrimazole
- Systemic with ketoconazole or fluconazole

Blisters:

- Supportive
- Consider acyclovir

Recurrent intraoral herpes: topical corticosteroids or systemic steroids for severe cases

SUGGESTED READINGS

Amir J et al: Treatment of herpes simplex gingivostomatitis with acyclovir in children: a randomized double blind placebo controlled study, *BMJ* 314:1800, 1997.

Khandwala A et al: 5% amlexanox oral paste, a new treatment for recurrent minor aphthous ulcers. Clinical demonstration of acceleration of healing and resolution of pain, *Oral Surg Oral Med Oral Pathol* 83:222, 1997.

AUTHOR: **FRED F. FERRI, M.D.**

BASIC INFORMATION

DEFINITION

Strabismus is a condition of the eyes in which the visual axes of the eyes are not straight in the primary position or in which the eyes do not follow each other in the different positions of gaze.

SYNONYMS

Esotropia
Exotropia
Restrictive eye movement

ICD-9CM CODES
378.9 Strabismus

EPIDEMIOLOGY & DEMOGRAPHICS

INCIDENCE (IN U.S.): 2% of all children
PEAK INCIDENCE: Childhood
PREDOMINANT SEX: None
PREDOMINANT AGE: Birth to age 5 yr
GENETICS: None known

PHYSICAL FINDINGS & CLINICAL PRESENTATION

- Conjugate gaze loss in both eyes with the eyes focusing independently (Fig. 1-312).
- Amblyopia (a decrease in best-corrected visual acuity in an otherwise structurally healthy eye) may occur with untreated strabismus.

ETIOLOGY

- Many cases are congenital.
- Accommodative cases occur later with focusing.
- Rarely, there is neurologic disease or severe refractive errors.
- Hereditary form is common, with hyperopia (far-sightedness) the most common.

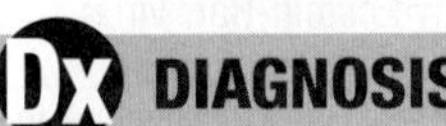

DIAGNOSIS

DIFFERENTIAL DIAGNOSIS

- Measuring eye position and movement
- Vision testing
- Refractive errors
- Central nervous system (CNS) tumors
- Orbital tumors
- Brain and CNS dysfunction

WORKUP

- Eye examination. Strabismus is classified according to the type and magnitude of misalignment. Esotropia refers to an inward deviation of the nonfixing eye and exotropia to the outward deviation of the nonfixing eye. Hypertropia is a vertical deviation in which the nonfixing eye is higher, and hypotropia is a vertical deviation in which the nonfixing eye is lower.
- Visual field
- MRI to rule out tumors that develop later with no apparent cause

LABORATORY TESTS

Generally not needed

IMAGING STUDIES

Necessary only if other neurologic findings are found

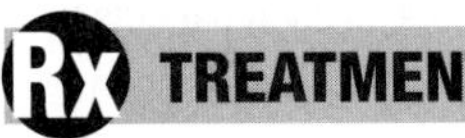

TREATMENT

NONPHARMACOLOGIC THERAPY

- Glasses
- Patching: best between age 3 and 7 yr; vision most improved by 3 to 6 mo
- Prisms
- Atropine: same as patching most of the time, although patching may give better results in resistant cases

CHRONIC Rx

- Glasses
- Alternate eye patching
- Surgery
- Prisms

DISPOSITION

- The earlier the condition is treated, the more likely the child will have normal vision in both eyes.
- After age 7 yr, visual loss is usually permanent from amblyopia.

REFERRAL

- Early for full rehabilitation of eye cosmetically and functionally
- To an ophthalmologist for management (usually)

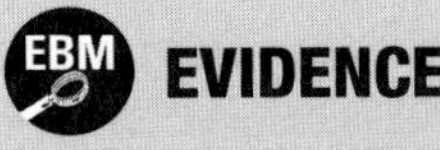

EVIDENCE

Please note: Complete text of EBM for this topic is available online.

SUGGESTED READING

Donahue SP: Pediatric strabismus, *N Engl J Med* 356: 1040, 2007.

AUTHOR: **MELVYN KOBY, M.D.**

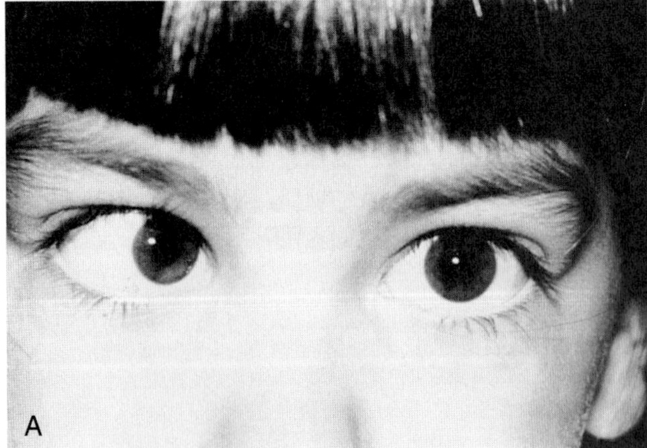

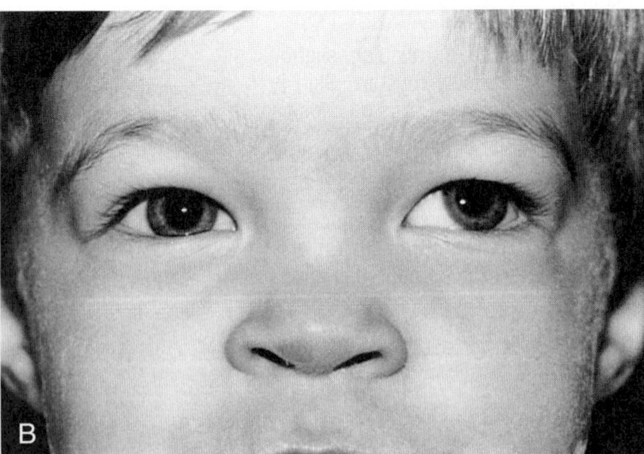

FIGURE 1-312 A, Note the nasal deviation of the right eye with the corneal light reflection temporally displaced on the right eye and centered in the left pupil, indicating an esotropia. **B,** Divergent strabismus of the left eye, defining an exotropia. (From Hodkelman [ed]: *Primary pediatric care*, ed 3, St Louis, 1997, Mosby.)

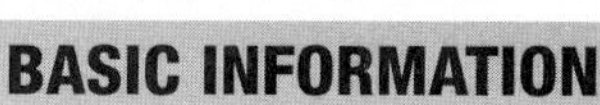

BASIC INFORMATION

DEFINITION

Ischemic stroke is the sudden onset of a focal neurologic deficit as a result of ischemia. Acute ischemic stroke may be defined as relating to the first few days after onset. However, the purpose of this chapter is to help the provider to make decisions regarding the acute stroke patient within the first several hours of symptoms; this is the crucial time for definitive treatment interventions.

SYNONYMS

Stroke
Brain attack
Cerebrovascular attack (This is a nonspecific term and should not be used.)

ICD-9CM CODES
494.31 Ischemic stroke
436 Acute stroke

EPIDEMIOLOGY & DEMOGRAPHICS

INCIDENCE:
- ~750,000 new or recurrent strokes occur each year in the U.S.
- Stroke is the number three cause of death and the leading cause of long-term disability in the U.S.

PREVALENCE: There are ~4.5 million stroke survivors in the U.S.

RISK FACTORS: Hypertension, dyslipidemia, diabetes mellitus, and smoking are the four major risk factors. Other risk factors include atrial fibrillation, mechanical heart valve, patent foramen ovale, recent myocardial infarction, carotid stenosis, hypercoaguable states, and sickle cell disease.

GENETICS: Multifactorial

PHYSICAL FINDINGS & CLINICAL PRESENTATION

The presentation of ischemic stroke varies with the artery involved and the region of the central nervous system affected. Following are some common syndromic presentations. Please note that this list is not comprehensive and that all findings for a particular syndrome may not be listed here.

- Large- to medium-sized arteries:
  - Left middle cerebral artery: right face, arm, and leg weakness and sensory loss with aphasia (expressive, receptive, or both); possible hemianopia
  - Right middle cerebral artery: right face, arm, and leg weakness and sensory loss with hemineglect; possible hemianopia
  - Basilar artery: typically an acute loss of consciousness preceded by vertigo, nausea, vomiting, and diplopia; quadriparesis or quadriplegia may be seen, including the "locked-in" syndrome
  - Posterior cerebral artery: unilateral hemianopia
  - Anterior cerebral artery: unilateral leg weakness and sensory loss
  - Cerebellum: ataxia (typically of the limbs), often with vertigo, nausea, and vomiting
- Small arteries (common lacunar syndromes)
  - Lateral medullary (Wallenberg's) syndrome
  - Posterior limb internal capsule

ETIOLOGY

Etiologies include atherosclerosis, cardioembolism, artery-to-artery embolism, small-vessel lipohyalinosis, arteritis, arterial dissection, and vasospasm.

Dx DIAGNOSIS

DIFFERENTIAL DIAGNOSIS

The differential diagnosis of acute ischemic stroke includes hemorrhagic stroke (primarily intracerebral hemorrhage), seizure with postictal paralysis, migraine with hemiparesis, syncope, hypoglycemia, hypertensive encephalopathy, and conversion disorder.

LABORATORY TESTS

- Immediate (Box 1-15): CBC, metabolic panel that includes blood glucose and renal function, PT/INR, aPTT, cardiac enzymes, troponin I, and urinalysis
- National Institutes of Health Stroke Scale: a brief, focused neurologic examination aimed at providing a numeric estimate of the severity of stroke; can be performed by any provider trained in its use; may increase the likelihood of the correct assessment of stroke
- ECG and telemetry monitoring

IMAGING STUDIES

- Immediate (Fig. 1-313): computed tomography (CT) of the head without contrast or MRI of the brain with stroke protocol to rule out

BOX 1-15 Immediate Diagnostic Studies: Evaluation of a Patient with Suspected Acute Ischemic Stroke

All Patients	Selected Patients
Noncontrast brain computed tomographic scan or magnetic resonance image	Hepatic function tests
Blood glucose level	Toxicology screen
Serum electrolyte and renal function tests	Blood alcohol level
Electrocardiography	Pregnancy test
Markers of cardiac ischemia	Arterial blood gas tests (if hypoxia is suspected)
Complete blood count, including platelet count*	Chest radiography (if lung disease is suspected)
Prothrombin time/international normalized ratio*	Lumbar puncture (if subarachnoid hemorrhage is suspected and computed tomography scan is negative for blood)
Activated partial thromboplastin time*	Electroencephalogram (if seizures are suspected)
Oxygen saturation	

*Although it is desirable to know the results of these tests before giving a patient tissue plasminogen activator, thrombolytic therapy should not be delayed while awaiting the results unless (1) there is clinical suspicion of a bleeding abnormality or thrombocytopenia; (2) the patient has received heparin or warfarin; or (3) the patient's use of anticoagulants is not known.

From Christensen H et al: Abnormalities on ECG and telemetry predict stroke outcome at 3 months, *J Neurol Sci* 234:99-103, 2005.

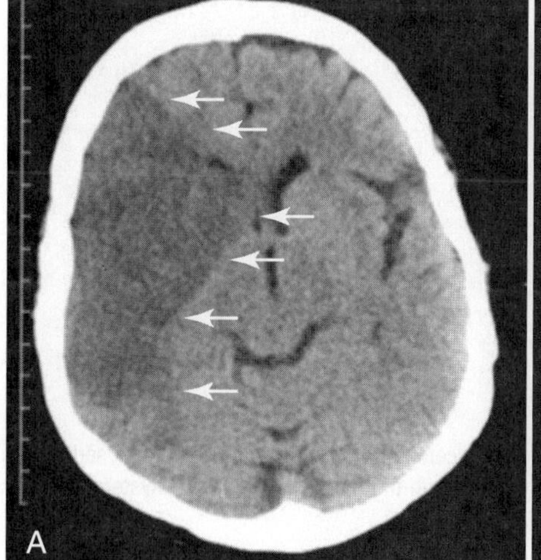

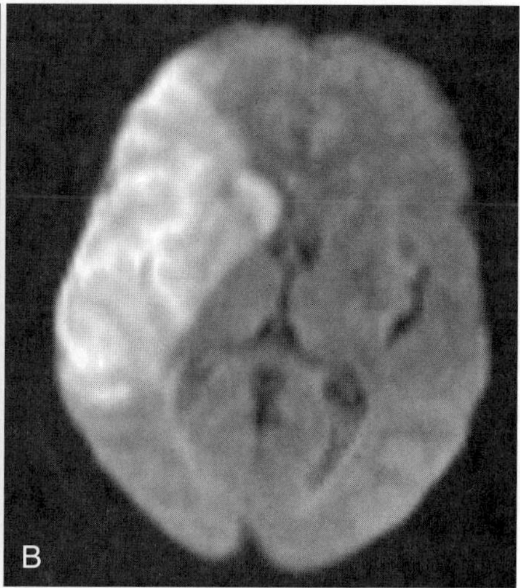

FIGURE 1-313 Large right middle cerebral artery infarct on **A,** an unenhanced computed tomographic scan and **B,** a diffusion-weighted magnetic resonance image. There is a mass effect, and this patient is at risk for cerebral herniation syndromes.

TABLE 1-73 Imaging Modalities for Stroke

Imaging Modality	Advantage	Disadvantage
Cerebral catheter angiography	• Allows for the definitive assessment of cerebral circulation (gold standard) • Allows for the deployment of intra-arterial thrombolysis and thrombectomy devices if a thrombus is found • Allows for the assessment of collateral circulation	• Invasive (significant risks) • High cost • Not available at all facilities
Doppler studies	• Noninvasive • May be performed at the patient's bedside	• Can be limited by the patient's body habitus • Operator dependent
Magnetic resonance angiography	• Excellent view of the large arteries of the neck and brain • No contrast material needed	• Cannot be performed in patients who are critically ill, who are unable to tolerate supine positioning, who have a pacemaker or other ferromagnetic hardware, or who are claustrophobic
Magnetic resonance perfusion	• Assesses cerebral hemodynamics • May show ischemic penumbra (i.e., the area of the brain that may be saved by timely intervention)	• Not commonly available • Not well standardized
CT angiography	• Excellent view of the large arteries of the neck and brain • Similar to magnetic resonance angiography with regard to resolution	• Requires intravenous contrast
CT perfusion	• Assesses cerebral hemodynamics • May show ischemic penumbra (i.e., the area of the brain that may be saved by timely intervention)	• Challenging to interpret in some cases • Not routinely available at many facilities • Requires intravenous contrast

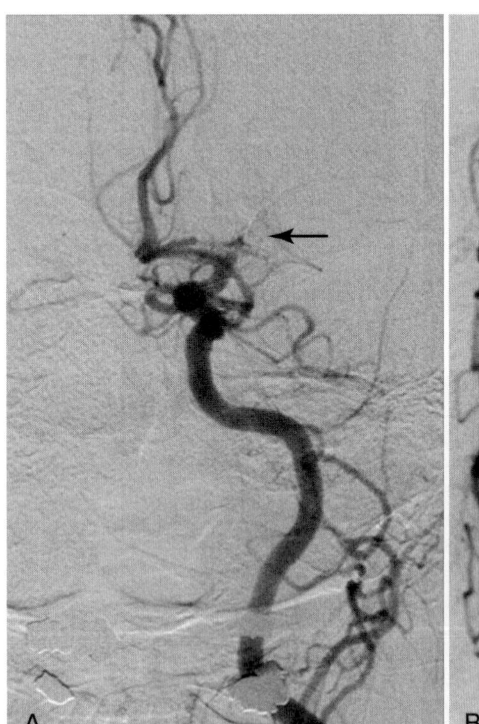

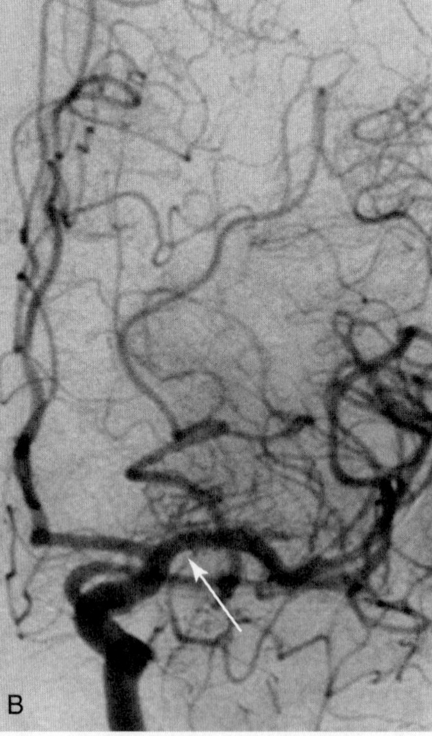

FIGURE 1-314 A, A catheter angiogram showing left middle cerebral artery occlusion, which caused severe stroke symptoms for several hours. **B,** The artery was opened with the Merci® clot retrieval system, and this resulted in normal flow.

hemorrhage and, if possible, to assess the extent of stroke (Because CT typically will not show an ischemic stroke for several hours, it may also be useful to estimating how long ischemia has been present for cases in which the time of onset is unclear.)

- Several other neuroimaging studies are useful during the early stages of acute stroke to assess whether there is a thrombus that is amenable to intervention (Table 1-73).

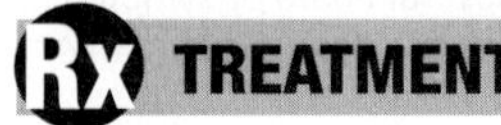

TREATMENT

NONPHARMACOLOGIC THERAPY

GENERAL CONSIDERATIONS:

- Airway and breathing should be maintained.
- Supplemental oxygen should be provided to keep the oxygen saturation at ≥92%.
- Fever is harmful during acute stroke. Ascertaining and addressing the cause while lowering an elevated temperature is strongly advised.
- Pneumatic compression devices or pharmacologic means should be applied to help prevent deep venous thromboses.
- Avoid any and all oral intake until swallowing is clearly unimpaired; this helps to avoid aspiration pneumonia.
- Early mobilization for rehabilitation is desirable.
- Consider neurosurgical intervention for craniectomy in select cases. Typical cases in which craniectomy may be performed include cerebellar ischemia with compression of the brain stem or the fourth ventricle and large right middle cerebral artery ischemia.

IMMEDIATE CATHETER CEREBRAL ANGIOGRAPHY FOR ENDOVASCULAR INTERVENTION (Figs. 1-314 and 1-315): Methods Available:

1. The Merci® clot retrieval system is approved by the U.S. FDA for use up to 8 hr after the onset of symptoms.
2. The Penumbra System is also available at some centers.
3. Intra-arterial tissue plasminogen activator (TPA) is used routinely for up to 6 hr after the onset of symptoms, although it is not approved by the U.S. FDA for this purpose.

Pearls and Caveats:

- Multimodal therapy (i.e., thrombectomy and intra-arterial TPA) is sometimes performed.
- Endovascular treatment may be performed for select cases in which intravenous (IV) TPA has failed to recanalize an occluded artery.
- Endovascular intervention may be an option for cases in which there are systemic contraindications to IV TPA.
- Endovascular intervention is useful only for large, accessible thrombi. Therefore, if a stroke patient is a candidate for IV TPA, then he or she should probably receive IV TPA.
- One can reasonably expect a recanalization rate of 60% in appropriate patients.
- Complications can ensue from the angiogram procedure itself, including an intracerebral hemorrhage rate that is similar to that associated with IV TPA.

- Endovascular intervention is typically available only at select large stroke centers.
- Some practitioners are making use of perfusion imaging (i.e., CT perfusion and magnetic resonance perfusion) to assess whether there is salvageable brain tissue before performing the procedure. In some cases, this may lead to a dramatic expansion of traditional time windows; this practice is currently being studied in clinical trials.

BOX 1-16 Three-Hour Criteria for Tissue Plasminogen Activator (Alteplase [Activase]) Use in Patients with Thromboembolic Stroke

Criteria for considering TPA as a treatment option:
- Noncontrast CT scan without evidence of hemorrhage
- Time since onset of symptoms clearly <3 hr before TPA administration would begin

Criteria for excluding TPA as a treatment option:
- Historic and clinical findings
- Clinical presentation suggestive of subarachnoid hemorrhage, even if CT scan is normal
- Sudden, severe headache, often with a loss of consciousness at onset
- Vomiting common
- Active internal bleeding, increased risk of bleeding, or known bleeding diathesis, including as a result of the following:
  - Recent use of warfarin with an INR of ≥1.7
  - Use of heparin within 48 hr with a prolonged aPTT
  - Platelet count of <100,000/mm^3
  - History of intracranial hemorrhage
  - Known arteriovenous malformation or aneurysm
  - GI or GU bleeding within the past 21 days
  - Arterial puncture within the past 7 days
- Recent lumbar puncture
- Stroke, intracranial surgery, or head trauma within the previous 3 mo
- Major surgery or serious trauma within the preceding 14 days
- Systolic blood pressure >185 mm Hg or diastolic blood pressure >110 mm Hg that does not decrease below that range with treatment
- Seizure at stroke onset
- Rapidly improving neurologic signs
- Isolated mild neurologic deficits
- Acute myocardial infarction
- Post–myocardial infarction pericarditis
- Blood glucose <50 mg/dl or >400 mg/dl
- Patient who is pregnant or lactating
- CT findings
- Evidence of intracranial hemorrhage
- Hypodensity or effacement of the sulci in one third of the territory of the middle cerebral artery

(From Rakel RE [ed]: *Principles of family practice,* ed 6, Philadelphia, 2002, WB Saunders.)

TPA, Tissue plasminogen activator; *CT,* computed tomography; *INR,* international normalized ratio; *aPTT,* activated partial thromboplastin time; *GI,* gastrointestinal; *GU,* genitourinary.

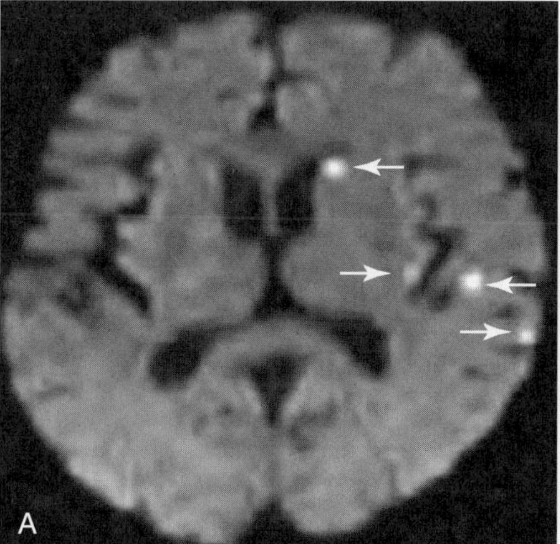

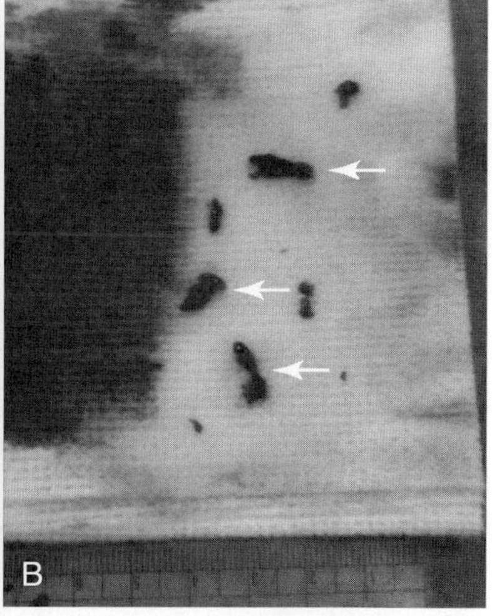

FIGURE 1-315 A, A diffusion-weighted magnetic resonance image of the same patient as shown in previous figure, this time showing only mild left cerebral ischemia after intervention. The patient was clinically normal. **B,** Thrombi removed from the middle cerebral artery with the use of the Merci® clot retrieval system.

ACUTE GENERAL Rx

INTRAVENOUS THROMBOLYSIS:
- IV TPA is the only medical therapy approved by the U.S. FDA for the treatment of ischemic stroke.
- The time window for administration is within 3 hr of symptom onset.
- There are strict criteria for the administration of IV TPA (see Box 1-16).
- The protocol is weight based, with 90 mg being the maximum allowable dose.
- The risk of brain hemorrhage with IV TPA is about 5% in stroke patients.
- Some new data suggest that IV TPA can be administered safely and with benefit in select patients up to 4.5 hours after symptom onset. As of this writing, this should probably not be routine practice. There are additional exclusion criteria if IV TPA is given beyond the 3-hr window.

HYPERTENSION: Elevated blood pressure is common during acute stroke, and it often subsides without specific therapy. In general, hypertension is not treated acutely unless it is extremely high (e.g., >220 mm Hg systolic blood pressure); unless there is evidence of organ damage caused by the hypertension; or unless thrombolysis is being considered, in which case the blood pressure needs to come down (if it can be safely accomplished) to <185/110 mm Hg. It is risky to severely decrease blood pressure in the presence of acute ischemic stroke. A 15% to 25% decrease over the first 24 hours is recommended.

HYPOGLYCEMIA: Hypoglycemia can mimic stroke. The prompt assessment of the serum glucose level and replacement as necessary are important.

HYPERGLYCEMIA: The presence of hyperglycemia worsens ischemic stroke outcome. Hyperglycemia should be managed aggressively.

HYPOTENSION: The presence of systemic hypotension in acute ischemic stroke portends a poor outcome. The cause should be sought, and volume depletion should be corrected with normal saline. Cardiac arrhythmias should be treated. Induced hypertension with vasopressor agents may be useful for select cases with an ischemic penumbra that is at risk, but caution is strongly advised.

ANTIPLATELET THERAPY: Beginning the oral or feeding tube administration of aspirin (325 mg/day) within 48 hours of stroke onset is advised. This will decrease the likelihood of a repeat ischemic stroke. Another oral antiplatelet regimen approved for secondary stroke prophylaxis (e.g., clopidogrel, aspirin plus extended-release dipyridamole) will also suffice and may be superior in the long term.

DISPOSITION

Patients with acute ischemic stroke should be cared for in a stroke unit or an intensive care unit. Nurses with skills in stroke care and telemetry monitoring should be routine. After the patient is stable and the workup is complete, rehabilitation should be arranged.

REFERRAL

Patients with acute ischemic stroke should be transported to a hospital in which providers are skilled with regard to the treatment of stroke. Depending on the severity and duration of symptoms, the patient may qualify for immediate endovascular intervention at a comprehensive stroke center, even if he or she is not a candidate for IV TPA. If complications from brain edema develop, further evaluation by a neurosurgeon may be helpful during the acute phase.

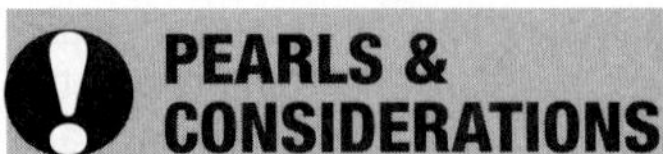

PEARLS & CONSIDERATIONS

PREVENTION

The prevention of acute ischemic stroke depends on the aggressive management of risk factors in individual patients.

PATIENT/FAMILY EDUCATION

Patients and families need to be taught about ways to reduce the risk for recurrent stroke, including lifestyle modifications. Education about rehabilitation goals, when appropriate, should also be accomplished.

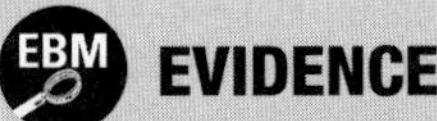

EVIDENCE

Please note: Complete text of EBM for this topic is available online.

SUGGESTED READING

Adams HP Jr et al: Guidelines for the early management of adults with ischemic stroke, *Stroke*, 38(5):1655-1711, 2007.

AUTHOR: **MICHAEL R. DOBBS, M.D.**

BASIC INFORMATION

DEFINITION

Hemorrhagic stroke is the sudden onset of a focal neurologic deficit caused by hemorrhage into or around the brain.

SYNONYMS

Intracerebral hemorrhage
Intracranial hemorrhage
Cerebrovascular attack (This is a nonspecific term and should not be used.)
The term *subarachnoid hemorrhage* refers to a specific location for hemorrhage, which commonly occurs as a result of a ruptured aneurysm. Please see "Subarachnoid Hemorrhage" for additional information.

ICD-9CM CODES

431 Intracerebral hemorrhage
432.9 Unspecified intracranial hemorrhage

EPIDEMIOLOGY & DEMOGRAPHICS

INCIDENCE: There are ~750,000 new or recurrent strokes per year in the U.S., of which ~10% to 15% are hemorrhagic.

RISK FACTORS:
- Hypertension
- Anticoagulant use
- Thrombolysis
- Alcoholism
- Illicit drug use (e.g., cocaine)
- Cerebral amyloid angiopathy

GENETICS: Multifactorial

PHYSICAL FINDINGS & CLINICAL PRESENTATION

The presentation varies with the region of the brain that is affected. The following are common locations for hemorrhage:
- Basal ganglia
- Cerebellum
- Pons
- Lobar (i.e., amyloid angiopathy)

ETIOLOGY

- Rupture of vessels
- Aneurysm
- Arteriovenous malformation
- Brain tumor
- Amyloid angiopathy

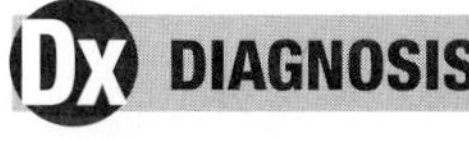

DIAGNOSIS

DIFFERENTIAL DIAGNOSIS

- Ischemic stroke
- Seizure with postictal paralysis
- Migraine with hemiparesis
- Syncope
- Conversion disorder.

LABORATORY TESTS

- CBC, metabolic panel including blood glucose and renal function, PT/INR, aPTT, urinalysis, and toxicology screens
- ECG and telemetry monitoring

IMAGING STUDIES

- Immediate: CT scanning of the head without contrast is highly sensitive for hemorrhage (Fig. 1-316).
- MRI of the brain with a gradient echo sequence is also highly sensitive for hemorrhage, including intracerebral microhemorrhages that may not be visible with computed tomography scanning.

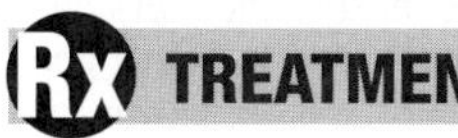

TREATMENT

NONPHARMACOLOGIC THERAPY

- Surgery should be performed promptly for cases of cerebellar hemorrhage of >3 cm when the patient is deteriorating clinically or showing brain stem edema or hydrocephalus.
- Surgery for lobar or deep brain clots may be considered for select cases, although the level of evidence for efficacy is not high.

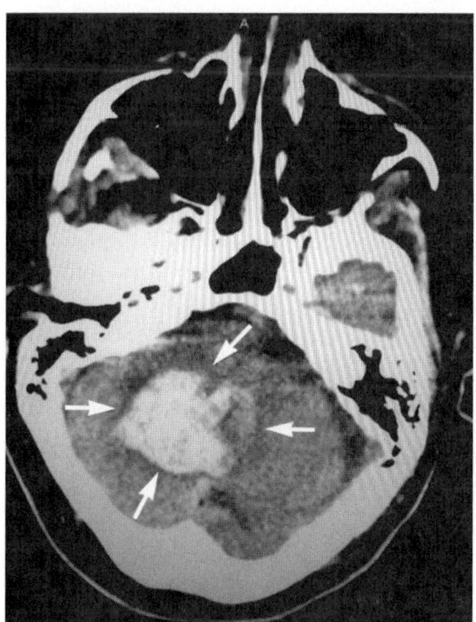

FIGURE 1-316 Nonenhanced computed tomographic scan of a patient with large cerebellar hemorrhage, mass effect, and compression of the fourth ventricle.

- Pneumatic compression devices should be applied to help prevent deep venous thromboses.
- Early mobilization for rehabilitation is desirable.

ACUTE GENERAL Rx

- Hypertension (Box 1-17): Blood pressure should be quickly lowered by 15% and then gradually and safely brought to the individual patient's target range. In theory, this may diminish the expansion of the hematoma.
- Hyperglycemia: A high blood glucose level predicts a worse outcome. Markedly elevated glucose levels should be lowered to <300 mg/dl.
- Seizures: If seizures occur, they should be treated aggressively, including with intravenous medications, if needed.
- Elevated intracranial pressure: This condition should be treated with a graded approach, which may include the elevation of the head of the bed elevation, analgesia/sedation, hyperventilation, and osmotic therapy.
- Antipyretics should be administered for cases that involve fever in addition to searching for a cause of the fever.
- Protamine sulfate is used to treat cases of heparin-induced intracerebral hemorrhage.
- Vitamin K is given for warfarin-associated intracerebral hemorrhage. In addition, recombinant factor VIIa and fresh frozen plasma are sometimes used.
- Recommendations for thrombolytic-associated intracerebral hemorrhage treatment include the consideration of the infusion of platelets and cryoprecipitate.

DISPOSITION

For large hemorrhages or unstable patients, immediate referral to a stroke center

REFERRAL

Patients with hemorrhagic stroke should be transported to a hospital where providers are skilled in the treatment of stroke. Depending on the severity and duration of symptoms, the patient may require neurosurgical intervention.

BOX 1-17 Suggested Recommended Guidelines for the Treatment of Elevated Blood Pressure in Patients with Spontaneous Intracerebral Hemorrhage

1. SBP of >200 mm Hg or MAP of >150 mm Hg: Consider the aggressive reduction of BP with continuous intravenous infusion, with BP monitoring every 5 min.
2. SBP of >180 mm Hg or MAP of >130 mm Hg with evidence or suspicion of elevated ICP: Consider ICP monitor and reducing BP with intermittent or continuous intravenous medications to keep cerebral perfusion pressure >60 to 80 mm Hg.
3. SBP of >180 mm Hg or MAP of >130 mm Hg without evidence or suspicion of elevated ICP: Consider a modest reduction of BP (e.g., MAP of 110 mm Hg or target blood pressure of 160/90 mm Hg) with intermittent or continuous intravenous medications, and clinically reexamine the patient every 15 min.

BP, Blood pressure; *ICP,* intracranial pressure; *MAP,* mean arterial pressure; *SBP,* systolic blood pressure.
Modified from Broderick J et al: Guidelines for the management of spontaneous intracerebral hemorrhage in adults: 2007 update, *Stroke* 38:2001-2023, 2007.

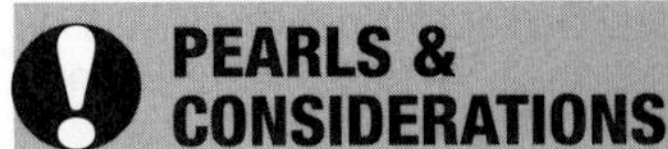

PEARLS & CONSIDERATIONS

- Outcomes are inversely correlated with hemorrhage size.
- Specific reversal agents may be useful for warfarin-, heparin-, or thrombolysis-associated hemorrhage.
- Although they have been investigated in placebo-controlled trials, no procoagulant medications have yet been shown to be safe and effective for the mitigation of spontaneous intracerebral hemorrhage.

PREVENTION

Prevention depends on the aggressive management of risk factors in individual patients, including hypertension, smoking, alcohol use, and cocaine use.

PATIENT/FAMILY EDUCATION

Patients and families need to understand that most patients will not soon achieve functional independence and that rehabilitation will be a long process. Education about avoiding antithrombotic agents should be stressed as appropriate for individual circumstances.

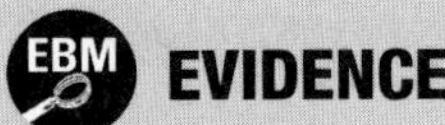

EVIDENCE

Please note: Complete text of EBM for this topic is available online.

SUGGESTED READING

Broderick J et al: Guidelines for the management of spontaneous intracerebral hemorrhage in adults: 2007 update, *Stroke* 38:2001-2023, 2007.

AUTHOR: **MICHAEL R. DOBBS, M.D.**

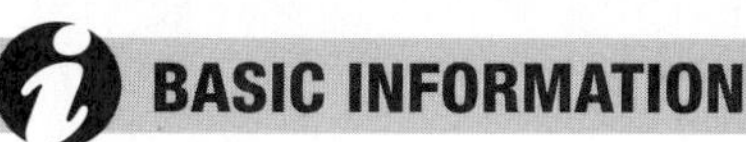

BASIC INFORMATION

DEFINITION

Secondary prevention of stroke involves preventing the recurrence of a cerebral vascular ischemic or hemorrhagic stroke after a primary event.

SYNONYMS

Brain attack
Stroke
Cerebral thrombosis
Cerebral hemorrhage
Brain infarct

ICD-9CM CODES

433 Precerebral vessel occlusion
434 Cerebral vessel thrombosis or occlusion

EPIDEMIOLOGY

Stroke is the third leading cause of death in the U.S. and the leading cause of morbidity. There are a total of 750,000/yr, of which approximately 200,000 are recurrent strokes. Thus, the secondary prevention of ischemic stroke remains the best treatment. Secondary prevention is specifically targeted toward modifiable risk factors.

RISK FACTORS: Age is the most important nonmodifiable risk factor for stroke. Modifiable risk factors include hypertension, hyperlipidemia, cigarette smoking, excessive alcohol consumption, physical inactivity, obesity (i.e., a body mass index of >25 kg/m^2), and diabetes mellitus.

GENETICS: Multifactorial

PHYSICAL FINDINGS & CLINICAL PRESENTATION

- Stroke can present in many ways, and the clinical history and the physical findings can provide the most important clues regarding how to proceed. Typically, the individual has a sudden definable loss of motor, sensory, visual, or cognitive functions that have a clear time of onset and that are noticed by others or by the individual themselves.
- Physical findings such as weakness in one limb or on one side of the body, the sudden loss of a visual field, or the inability to understand or communicate with others raises one's suspicion of a stroke event.
- In addition, there may be eye deviation, facial droop, numbness of the face or extremities, and definable weakness on one side of the body.
- The inability to understand or communicate with others may lead others to classify the person as psychotic or confused; this finding is known as *aphasia.*

ETIOLOGY

- Strokes are broadly divided into ischemic or hemorrhagic (i.e., intraparenchymal or subarachnoid hemorrhage)
- The main causes of ischemic stroke include atherosclerosis; cardioembolic causes (e.g., atrial fibrillation); and lacunar stroke (i.e., small-vessel disease). Rare causes that result from drug use (e.g., cocaine abuse); dissection; and hypercoaguable states need to be considered when ischemic stroke occurs among younger individuals.
- The most common cause of intracerebral hemorrhage is uncontrolled hypertension. Spontaneous rupture of a brain aneurysm causes subarachnoid hemorrhage.

Dx DIAGNOSIS

DIFFERENTIAL DIAGNOSIS

- Seizure and postictal states
- Complicated migraine
- Hypoglycemia
- Brain tumor
- Somatization disorder
- Metabolic disorder

WORKUP

- Blood glucose level at the bedside or in the office
- aPTT, PT/INR, CBC, and CMP
- Fasting lipid panel
- Hypercoagulability tests for young stroke patients with no obvious risk factors

IMAGING STUDIES

- Computed tomography scanning of the head without contrast can differentiate between ischemic and hemorrhagic stroke. MRI of the brain is a more specific test.
- Carotid ultrasound and transcranial Doppler are used to detect large-vessel atherosclerosis. Magnetic resonance and computed tomography angiography are good alternatives.
- Echocardiogram and ECG can be used to detect a cardioembolic source.

Rx TREATMENT

The secondary prevention of stroke is targeted toward modifiable risk factors and toward preventing strokes in specific conditions. Lifestyle modifications, including appropriate diet and exercise, need to be emphasized for every stroke patient. It is important to note that, for all patients with noncardioembolic ischemic stroke or transient ischemic attack (TIA), aspirin (50 to 325 mg/day), the combination of aspirin and extended-release dipyridamole, and clopidogrel are all acceptable options for initial therapy. Both the combination of aspirin and extended-release dipyridamole and clopidogrel were found to be superior to aspirin in comparison trials. A consultation with a neurologist should be considered for young stroke patients and for patients with no obvious cause or with stroke from unusual causes (e.g., hypercoaguable states, dissections).

PREVENTING STROKE IN SPECIFIC CONDITIONS:

1. Cardioembolic strokes as a result of atrial fibrillation: Try to maintain an international normalized ratio between 2.0 and 3.0. For patients who are unable to take oral anticoagulants, aspirin (325 mg/day) is recommended. A recent study suggested that a combination of aspirin and clopidogrel is slightly better than aspirin alone.
2. Cardioembolic strokes as a result of a prosthetic metallic valve: Try to obtain an international normalized ratio between 2.5 and 3.5.
3. Strokes as a result of large-vessel atherosclerois (i.e., symptomatic carotid stenosis): For patients with recent TIA or ischemic stroke within the last 6 months and ipsilateral severe (70% to 99%) carotid artery stenosis, carotid endarterectomy (CEA) performed by a surgeon is recommended and results in a perioperative morbidity and mortality rate of <6%. For patients with recent TIA or ischemic stroke and ipsilateral moderate (50% to 69%) carotid stenosis, CEA is recommended. When the degree of stenosis is <50%, there is no indication for CEA. Carotid stenting is not indicated except for cases in which surgery is high risk.
4. Symptomatic intracranial atherosclerosis: The optimal therapy in these cases is unclear. Warfarin is not superior to aspirin according to the WASID study. Angioplasty/stenting is believed by many to be the treatment of choice, but this remains investigational (Fig. 1-317). Trials are ongoing, but treatment is available at many stroke centers.

RISK FACTOR MODIFICATION:

1. Hypertension: Antihypertensive treatment is recommended for both the prevention of recurrent stroke and the prevention of other vascular events in persons who have had an ischemic stroke or a TIA. An absolute target blood pressure level and reduction are uncertain and should be individualized. Normal blood pressure levels have been defined as <120/80 mm Hg by the JNC-7. Several lifestyle modifications have been associated with blood pressure reduction and should be included as part of a comprehensive antihypertension treatment plan.
2. Diabetes: The goal for the hemoglobin A_{1c} level should be ≤7%.
3. Hyperlipidemia: For patients with ischemic stroke or TIA with elevated cholesterol levels, statin agents are recommended. The target goals for cholesterol lowering are an LDL-C level of <100 mg/dl and an LDL-C level of <70 mg/dl for very high-risk persons with multiple risk factors (e.g., both coronary artery disease and diabetes).
4. Cigarette smoking: Absolute cessation is required.
5. Obesity: Weight reduction may be considered for all overweight ischemic stroke and TIA patients to maintain the goal of a body mass index of between 18.5 and 24.9 kg/m^2 and a waist circumference of <35 in for women and <40 in for men.
6. Excessive alcohol consumption: Patients with ischemic stroke or TIA who are heavy drinkers should eliminate or reduce their consumption of alcohol. Light to moderate levels of no more than two drinks per day for men and one drink per day for nonpregnant women may be considered.

DISPOSITION

Secondary stroke prevention is a multifaceted approach of lifestyle modification and pharmacological intervention that is aimed at preventing or limiting disability.

REFERRAL

- For complicated recurrent strokes, a referral to a neurologist who specializes in stroke is recommended.
- Obtaining previously suggested radiologic studies and laboratory tests before referral is recommended.

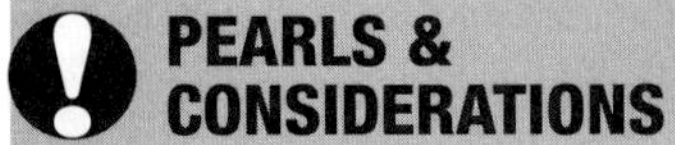

PEARLS & CONSIDERATIONS

The modification of risk factors is the best prevention of stroke. Lifestyle modification is a very important aspect of secondary stroke prevention.

PREVENTION

Prevention is the goal of treatment, and compliance is the most important factor. Review risk factor reduction and pharmacologic therapy as previously discussed.

PATIENT/FAMILY EDUCATION

More information can be obtained from the following sources:

- American Heart Association, National Center, 7272 Greenville Avenue, Dallas, TX 75231
- American Stroke Association, 1-888-4-STROKE or 1-888-478-7653
- H.O.P.E. for Stroke, 250 Duck Pond Drive, Wantagh, NY 11793, 516-804-8495

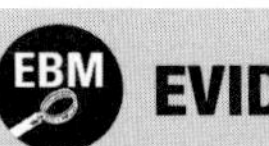

EVIDENCE

Please note: Complete text of EBM for this topic is available online.

SUGGESTED READINGS

Graham GD: Secondary stroke prevention: from guidelines to clinical practice, *J Natl Med Assoc* 100(10):1125-1137, 2008.

Vermeer SE et al: Silent brain infarcts: a systemic review, *Lancet Neurol* 6:611, 2007.

AUTHOR: **NAWAZ HACK, M.D.**

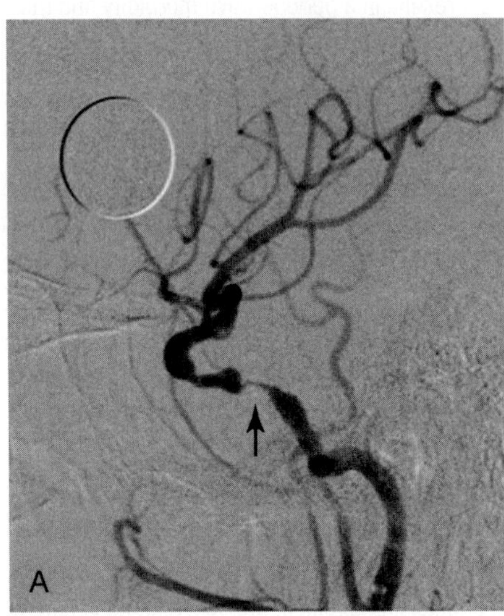

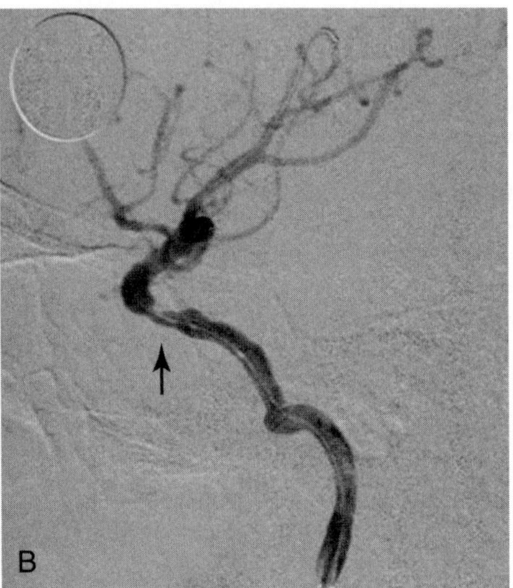

FIGURE 1-317 A, Intracranial high-grade symptomatic stenosis. **B,** This patient failed aggressive medical therapy and responded only to angioplasty and stenting.

BASIC INFORMATION

DEFINITION

Sturge-Weber syndrome (SWS) is a sporadic congenital disorder characterized by a dermal capillary malformation (port-wine stain) occurring in association with vascular malformations of the leptomeninges and the eye.

Sturge first described a patient with epilepsy, a facial capillary malformation, and buphthalmos in 1879. Parkes Weber better characterized the pattern and distribution of the characteristic intracranial calcifications. The complete syndrome generally includes the triad of facial dermal capillary malformation (port-wine stain), ipsilateral central nervous system (CNS) vascular malformation (leptomeningeal angiomatosis), and vascular malformation of the choroid of the eye associated with glaucoma. Partial forms have been reported.

SYNONYMS

Sturge (-Weber) (-Dimitri) disease or syndrome
Encephalocutaneous angiomatosis

ICD-9CM CODES
759.6

EPIDEMIOLOGY & DEMOGRAPHICS

SWS is not a heritable disorder; thus recurrence is unlikely.

PHYSICAL FINDINGS & CLINICAL PRESENTATION

SWS is characterized by a facial angioma (port-wine stain) and an associated leptomeningeal angioma. These vascular malformations are associated with specific ocular and neurologic abnormalities.

CUTANEOUS MANIFESTATIONS:

- Cutaneous port-wine stain is the most common type of vascular malformation, occurring in 0.3% of newborns (Fig. 1-318, *A*). However, only a small number of children with port-wine stains have SWS.
- In SWS, the port-wine stain typically is present on the forehead and upper eyelid, primarily in the distribution of the first or second division of the trigeminal nerve. Extension of the skin lesion to both sides of the face and the trunk and extremities is common.
- The distribution of the cutaneous angioma influences the risk of an associated leptomeningeal angioma. Leptomeningeal angioma occurs in approximately 90% of cases when the port-wine stain involves both the upper and lower eyelids compared with 10% when only one eyelid is affected.
- The skin lesion usually is obvious at birth. However, its appearance changes with age and its size increases as the patient grows. In the newborn, the lesion is flat and usually light pink in color. It typically darkens with age to a deep red, port-wine appearance and vascular ectasias develop (Fig. 1-318, *B*). The vascular ectasias produce nodularity and superficial blebbing, which lead to overgrowth of the underlying soft tissues and sometimes the bone.
- It may extend to mucosal surfaces with concomitant gingival hypertrophy, which may be even further accentuated in patients being treated with phenytoin for seizures. Some patients exhibit accelerated eruption of teeth.

LEPTOMENINGEAL ANGIOMA:

- Leptomeningeal angioma occurs in 10% to 20% of cases when a typical facial lesion is present. The intracerebral lesion usually occurs on the same side as the port-wine stain. Leptomeningeal angiomatosis seldom occurs without an accompanying facial angioma.
- The parietal and occipital areas are affected most commonly, although any portion of the cerebrum can be involved.
- The pathologic appearance of the leptomeninges includes thickening and discoloration caused by the increased vascularity. The angiomatous tissue typically fills the subarachnoid space in the sulci, and large, tortuous venous structures drain superficially or into the deep venous system. The underlying parenchyma may be atrophic and contain multiple calcific granular deposits. The intraparenchymal calcification may result from chronic tissue hypoxia caused by venous stasis.

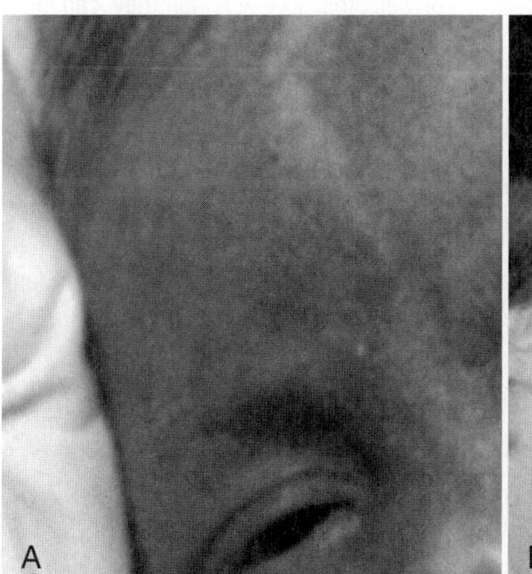

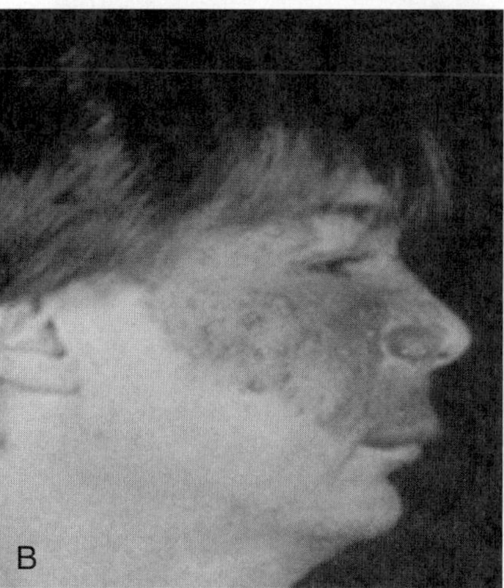

FIGURE 1-318 Port-wine stain at different stages.

OCULAR MANIFESTATIONS:

- Ocular features of SWS include glaucoma and vascular malformations of the conjunctiva, episclera, choroid, and retina.
- The predominant ocular abnormality is glaucoma (increased intraocular pressure), which occurs in 30% to 70% of affected patients. The risk of glaucoma is highest in the first decade. Congenital glaucoma is seen in approximately one half of patients with SWS and presents in newborns with enlargement of the globe *(buphthalmos)*. Patients occasionally develop glaucoma as adults. Thus continued vigilance is needed, even in patients with initially normal intraocular pressure.
- Angioma of the choroid occurs in 30% to 40% of patients with SWS and can lead to increased intraocular pressure. These lesions may be diffuse or localized within the retina.
- Episcleral and conjunctival lesions include anomalous vessels or true angiomata. These may be caused by increased venous pressure in the eye.
- Weber originally noted heterochromia of the iris. The more deeply pigmented iris usually is ipsilateral to the facial angioma. The pigmentation is caused by aggregated melanocytic hamartomata on the anterior surface of the iris.

NEUROLOGIC FEATURES:

- The neurologic features of SWS are progressive and include seizures, focal neurologic deficits, and mental retardation. These disorders occur with variable severity. A small proportion of patients have no neurologic abnormalities.
- The reasons for neurologic progression are uncertain. A possible mechanism is hypoxic-ischemic injury to tissue adjacent to the leptomeningeal angioma. Other proposed mechanisms are venous occlusion and increased venous pressure.

SEIZURES:

1. Seizures occur in 80% of patients with SWS and are more common with bilateral than unilateral port-wine stains. Seizures may develop at any age, although they usually start in early childhood.
2. Seizures are often the first symptom to appear. Initially, seizures are typically focal but often become generalized tonic-clonic. Less often, infantile spasms or myoclonic or atonic seizures are seen. The occurrence of seizures, the age at onset, and the response to treatment affect prognosis. Onset before age 1 yr and poor response to anticonvulsant therapy are associated with a greater likelihood of cognitive impairment.
    - Hemiparesis: often develops acutely in conjunction with the onset of seizures. The deficit occurs contralateral to the facial and intracranial lesions. The affected extremity usually does not grow at a normal rate, resulting in hemiatrophy. Some affected children have progressive loss of motor function or have a series of stroke-like events.
    - Mental retardation: children with SWS typically develop normally for several months after birth, then manifest devel-

opmental delay. However, impairment can be obvious soon after birth, especially in infants with extensive brain involvement. Cognitive function is poorest in patients with bilateral intracerebral lesions. In one report, only 8% of patients with bilateral leptomeningeal angiomata were intellectually normal.

- Behavior problems: are more common in SWS patients than in their unaffected siblings. Higher risk for psychological problems is associated with poorer cognitive function and frequent seizures. However, behavior problems can occur in patients with normal intelligence.
- Other deficits: many patients have visual field defects, typically homonymous hemianopia. This is from the involvement of the leptomeningeal angioma with one or both occipital lobes or optic tracts. Hydrocephalus also may occur. This disorder is believed to result from increased venous pressure caused by thrombosis of the deep venous channels or extensive arteriovenous anastomoses.

ETIOLOGY

The etiology of SWS is unknown. One hypothesis suggests that the capillary angiomata result from somatic mutations in fetal ectodermal tissues that cause inappropriate control or maturation of capillary blood vessel formation.

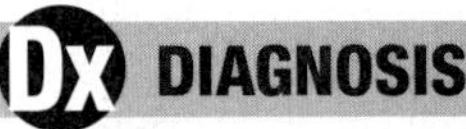

DIAGNOSIS

DIFFERENTIAL DIAGNOSIS

- Klippel-Trenaunay-Weber syndrome (extensive capillary angiomata associated with dysplastic veins involving the limbs and trunk, often with hypertrophy of the affected extremity)
- Von Hippel-Lindau disease (associated with capillary retinal angiomata in contrast to cavernous angiomata seen in SWS)

WORKUP

SWS should be suspected in all patients with facial capillary malformations involving the trigeminal dermatome. At-risk infants should undergo careful physical examination to determine the extent of the malformation.

IMAGING STUDIES

- Most children with facial port-wine stains without an intracranial lesion would be expected to develop normally. Therefore performing neuroimaging studies is helpful to provide prognostic information.
- Plain radiographs of the skull may detect intracranial calcifications, revealing the classic "tram line" appearance, but calcifications are often not present before age 2 yr. Newer radiographic techniques have made plain films obsolete.
- The preferred technique is MRI with gadolinium contrast, which demonstrates the presence of the leptomeningeal angioma and the extent of involvement with brain structures (Fig. 1-319).
- If MRI is not readily available, cranial CT reliably identifies brain calcification and provides some anatomic information.
- In some cases leptomeningeal involvement may not be detected by neuroimaging during infancy and only becomes apparent later. There is no absolute way to exclude intracerebral lesions during the first year after birth.

Rx TREATMENT

No specific treatment exists for SWS. The cutaneous, ocular, and neurologic manifestations are treated with mixed success.

ACUTE GENERAL & CHRONIC Rx

Port-wine stain:

- Port-wine stains can be treated by selective photothermolysis with a pulsed-dye laser. Treatment can be further optimized for individual patients so that blanching of the lesion can be accomplished in the fewest possible sessions.
- The response of facial port-wine stains to laser treatment depends on the location and size of the lesion and the patient's age. The greatest decrease in size occurs in the smallest lesions and in the youngest children (<1 yr). The greater success in the youngest patients may reflect treatment before the development of ectasias.
- Complications of laser therapy include scarring and transient hyperpigmentation. Retinal injury can occur if the eyes are not shielded properly.

Glaucoma:

- The development of new medications has improved the medical management of glaucoma in SWS. However, topical treatment often is ineffective in normalizing intraocular pressure. In these cases, the surgical treatment depends on the etiology of the glaucoma.

Seizures:

- Management of seizures in SWS often is difficult. The success of controlling seizures with anticonvulsant medication is variable and unpredictable. Carbamazepine is the recommended antiepileptic of choice. In refractory cases, hemispherectomy or more limited surgical resection of epileptogenic tissue may be beneficial, although risks often outweigh benefits.

REFERRAL

- Initial ophthalmologic evaluation should be performed in the neonatal period because of the risk of congenital glaucoma.
- If the first complete ophthalmologic evaluation is normal, it should be repeated frequently (some authors have suggested quarterly evaluations) for the first 2 yr of life.
- If the examination results remain normal, the vision should be reevaluated at least annually throughout the patient's lifetime.
- Periodic evaluation by a pediatric neurologist is an essential component of the management of SWS.

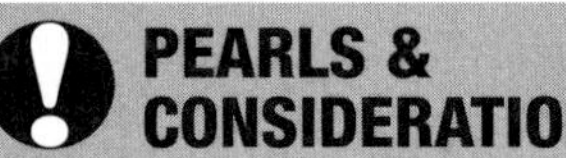

PEARLS & CONSIDERATIONS

COMMENTS

- The prognosis for SWS depends on the extent of the leptomeningeal angioma and its effect on the perfusion of the cerebral cortex as well as the severity of ocular involvement.
- Prognosis also is affected by the age of onset of seizures and whether they can be controlled.
- Neurologic function may deteriorate with age. As a result, approximately half of affected adults are impaired, including those who initially were normal.

PATIENT & FAMILY EDUCATION

- The Sturge-Weber Foundation is an active support group for patients and families (http://www.sturge-weber.com).

SUGGESTED READINGS

Garzon MC et al: Vascular malformations. Part II: associated syndromes, *J Am Acad Dermatol* 56(4):541, 2007.

Nathan N, Thaller SR: Sturge-Weber syndrome and associated congenital vascular disorders: a review, *J Craniofac Surg* 17(4):724, 2006.

AUTHOR: **RUBY SATPATHY, M.D.**

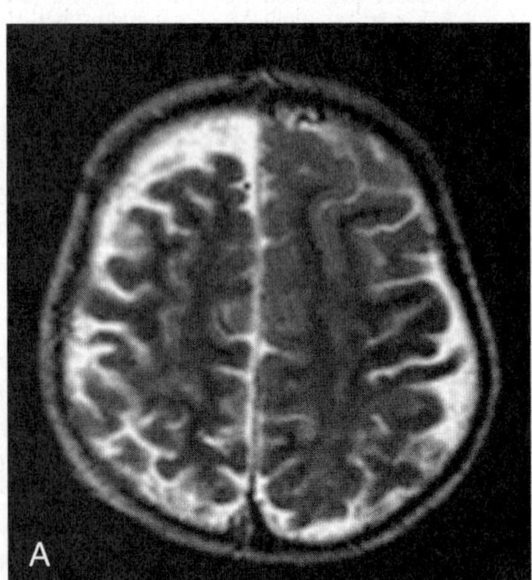

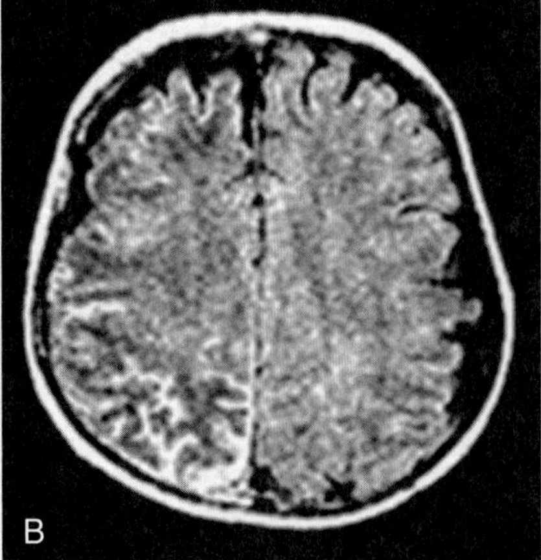

FIGURE 1-319 Axial magnetic resonance image of child with Sturge-Weber syndrome demonstrating atrophy of the left hemisphere and contrast enhancement of the surface of the left hemisphere particularly prominent over the occipital lobe.

BASIC INFORMATION

DEFINITION

Subarachnoid hemorrhage (SAH) is defined as hemorrhage into the subarachnoid space. There are several causes of SAH, with the most common being head trauma and the rupture of an intracerebral aneurysm.

SYNONYMS

Subarachnoid bleed

ICD-9CM CODES

430 Subarachnoid hemorrhage

EPIDEMIOLOGY & DEMOGRAPHICS

INCIDENCE: Approximately 6 to 8 cases/100,000 persons per yr

PREDOMINANT SEX: Women >55 yr old were found to have a 25% greater risk of developing SAH as compared with men of the same age.

PREDOMINANT AGE: The mean age at onset is 55 yr.

PEAK INCIDENCE: Most aneurysmal SAH occurs in people who are between the ages of 55 and 60 yr.

GENETICS:

- First-degree relatives have a 5× to 12× greater risk of developing SAH as compared with the general population.
- If someone has two or more first-degree relatives who have experienced aneurysmal SAH, screening may be worthwhile.
- Autosomal dominant polycystic kidney disease is known to be associated with cerebral aneurysms in 8% of cases; screening is recommended in families with this condition in which one family member has experienced a ruptured aneurysm.

RISK FACTORS: Although genetics seem to play a factor in SAH, lifestyle factors are more important for determining overall risk. These risk factors include smoking, hypertension, oral contraception, pregnancy, and cocaine use.

PHYSICAL FINDINGS & CLINICAL PRESENTATION

- The primary symptom is a sudden, severe headache in 97% of cases. This is classically described as the "worst headache of my life" and also called a *thunderclap headache.*
- 30% to 60% of patients report a history of sentinel bleeds with short last headaches during the weeks before the hemorrhage.
- The onset of the headache may be associated with a brief loss of consciousness, a seizure, nausea or vomiting, and meningismus.
- Altered mental status and coma may result from the direct effect of the SAH causing a mass effect and increased intracranial pressure.
- A posterior communication aneurysm may cause a third cranial nerve palsy.

ETIOLOGY

- Trauma is the most common cause of SAH.
- 75% to 80% of cases of spontaneous SAH are caused by the rupture of a cerebral aneurysm.
- Idiopathic SAH, which is also known as *angiogram-negative SAH,* is found in 15% to 20% of cases of spontaneous SAH. In these cases, no angiographic cause of the hemorrhage is found.
- Other culprits include arteriovenous malformations, bleeding into preexisting tumors, vasculitis, and cerebral artery dissection.
- Cocaine abuse, sickle cell anemia, coagulopathies, and pituitary apoplexy can also result in SAH.

Dx DIAGNOSIS

DIFFERENTIAL DIAGNOSIS

- Intracerebral hemorrhage as a result of trauma, tumors, and stroke with hemorrhagic conversion
- Other causes of headache, including migraines, tension headaches, and cluster headaches

WORKUP

- Look for a history that is suggestive of SAH (e.g., thunderclap headache, "worst headache of my life").
- Computed tomography (CT) will be positive in more than 95% of cases, especially during the acute phase (i.e., 24 to 48 hours) after the onset of bleeding (Fig. 1-320).
- Lumbar puncture is a very important part of the workup, especially because 3% of patients with normal CT scans show evidence of hemorrhage on lumbar puncture. An RBC count of more than 100,000/m^3 is strongly suggestive of SAH. If RBC counts drop between the first and fourth tubes, then the tap is most likely traumatic. The presence of xanthochromia or bilirubin in the cerebrospinal fluid is a sign of SAH.
- A CT angiogram or a cerebral angiogram is imperative for determining the origin of the SAH. Angiography may also be extremely useful, because it may offer a therapeutic benefit via the coiling of the aneurysm.

LABORATORY TESTS

- Basic laboratory values, including CBC, chemistry panel, prothrombin time, partial thromboplastin time, and platelet count
- Troponin and sodium levels also important to guide management

IMAGING STUDIES

- High-resolution CT scanning (Fig. 1-320) correctly identifies more than 95% of SAH cases, with blood appearing hyperdense in the subarachnoid spaces.
- Cerebral angiography is the gold standard for diagnosis and may offer a therapeutic option via coiling.
- MRI is not a good imaging modality during the acute phase; however, its sensitivity increases after 4 to 7 days.

Rx TREATMENT

NONPHARMACOLOGIC THERAPY

- Patients with a depressed level of consciousness may need to be intubated and mechanically ventilated in an intensive care unit setting.
- A lumbar drain or a ventriculostomy is required should the patient develop hydrocephalus and increased intracranial pressure.

ACUTE GENERAL Rx

- Initial management strategies are geared toward stabilizing the patient and preventing rehemorrhage and hydrocephalus.
- Tight blood pressure control is paramount. This can be done with the use of drips (e.g., nipride) or as-needed medications. A systolic blood pressure of 120 to 150 mm Hg is recommended.
- After an aneurysm has been identified, measures to secure it should be undertaken; this can be done by either clipping or coiling the aneurysm. Clipping consists of placing a clip around the neck of the aneurysm and is performed via intra-arterial angiography; it consists of deploying platinum coils inside the aneurysm to cause thrombosis of the aneurysmal sac.
- Pain control is performed with the use of short-acting and less-sedating medications (e.g., codeine, low-dose morphine).
- Seizures occur in about 3% of patients during the acute phase; however, the use of prophylactic antiepileptics is still controversial.
- Vasospasm, which typically begins around day 3 after the hemorrhage and reaches a

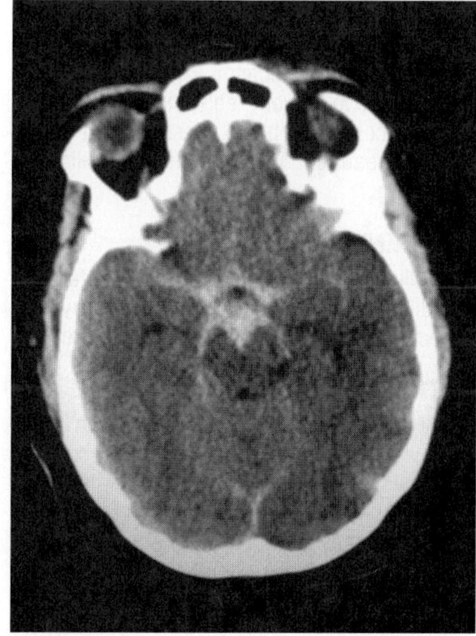

FIGURE 1-320 Non-contrast CT of brain in patient with subarachnoid hemorrhage.

peak on day 6 to e8, is the leading cause of death and disability after aneurysm rupture. Nimodipine has been shown to improve outcomes if it is administered between the days 4 and 21 after the hemorrhage, even if it does not significantly reduce the amount of vasospasm detected on angiography. After vasospasm develops, "triple H" therapy—to achieve *H*ypertension, *H*ypervolemia, and *He*modilution—is used in an attempt to provide adequate cerebral perfusion.

CHRONIC Rx

Chronic treatment usually involves the management of the complications of SAH through means such as intensive physical therapy and rehabilitation.

DISPOSITION

- SAH is often associated with a poor outcome. The death rate associated with SAH is between 40% and 50%, with 10% to 15% of patients dying before they reach the hospital.
- More than 46% of those who survive hospitalization have cognitive impairments that affect their lifestyles.

REFERRAL

Patients should be transferred as soon as possible to a facility with neurosurgical care.

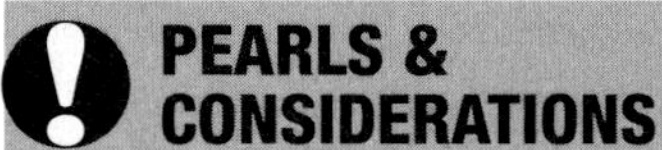

PEARLS & CONSIDERATIONS

COMMENTS

- After the diagnosis of SAH is made, the patient should be transferred to a facility where neurosurgical care in an intensive care unit setting is available.
- All anticoagulation and antiplatelet therapy should be withheld, and coagulopathy should be corrected.
- Patients should be adequately hydrated, and Nimotop should be started to prevent poor outcomes of vasospasm.
- Measures to prevent rebleeding include adequate control of blood pressure and aneurysm treatment with the use of coiling or clipping.

PREVENTION

Controlling some of the modifiable risk factors, including smoking and blood pressure, may help to decrease the risk of aneurysmal rupture.

PATIENT/FAMILY EDUCATION

- SAH is a devastating condition, with most survivors developing significant cognitive deficits. A good support system and an adequate physical and cognitive rehabilitation program may prove useful to survivors.
- Screening may be useful for patients with two or three relatives with SAH.

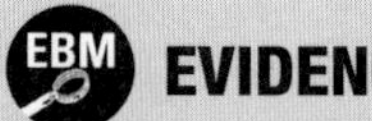

EVIDENCE

Please note: Complete text of EBM for this topic is available online.

Key trials and commentary:

This randomized, double-blind, placebo-controlled, dose-finding study assessed efficacy and safety of 1, 5, and 15 mg/hour intravenous clazosentan, an endothelin receptor antagonist, in preventing vasospasm after aneurysmal subarachnoid hemorrhage.

This study showed that clazosentan significantly decreased moderate and severe vasospasm in a dose-dependent manner and showed a trend for reduction in vasospasm-related morbidity/mortality in patients with aneurysmal subarachnoid hemorrhage when centrally assessed. Overall, the adverse effects were manageable and not considered serious.

Solid experimental data indicates that endothelial dysfunction is a key mechanism in the development of delayed vasospasm after subarachnoid hemorrhage. Endothelin is up-regulated while nitric oxide activity is reduced, thus favoring vasoconstriction. Endothelin receptor antagonists have been shown to reduce vasospasm in animal models. Furthermore, the endothelin receptor A antagonist clazosentan had been previously reported to diminish the incidence and severity of angiographic vasospasm in a pilot study. The multicenter trial CONSCIOUS-1 was designed to confirm these promising results in a much larger population.

In this trial, 413 patients with aneurysmal subarachnoid hemorrhage were randomized to receive placebo or different intravenous doses of clazosentan within 56 hours of aneurysm rupture. The infusion was then continued for up to 14 days. When first presented in abstract, the results of CONSCIOUS-1 were considered mostly disappointing. Although the drug had been very successful in reducing moderate or severe angiographic vasospasm in a convincing dose-dependent manner (for the high-dose vs. placebo comparison the rates were 66% vs. 23% in the intention-to-treat analysis and 67% vs. 31% among actually treated patients), the treatment had failed to improve clinical outcomes. In fact, patients in the placebo group had slightly lower morbidity and mortality than those in the active treatment groups (31% for placebo vs. 38% for the high-dose clazosentan group).

The study is now presented with the addition of a post hoc analysis, which seems to indicate that the medication was actually associated with a trend toward better clinical outcomes when a different definition for morbidity and mortality was used. The original criteria for poor clinical outcome included all new infarcts on repeat CT scan (without requiring that they be related to vasospasm) and relied on the assessment by local investigators at each participating center. The post hoc criteria only included radiologic infarctions deemed because of vasospasm as determined by a central review of the cases with repeat CT scans. On this post hoc analysis, lower rates of vasospasm-related infarctions (5% vs. 19% with placebo) and poor clinical outcome (29% vs. 39% with placebo) were seen in the high-dose arm of clazosentan.

Systemic hypotension, anemia, pulmonary complications (probably related to fluid retention), and death were more common in the treatment arms. However, most fatalities were because of intraoperative complications; hence, they were not thought to be related to the agent under investigation.

The validity of the results of the post hoc analysis of the data is debatable. Nonetheless, the confirmation that clazosentan infusion can substantially decrease the occurrence of angiographic vasospasm merits attention. Two more studies (CONSCIOUS-2 and CONSCIOUS-3 in clipped and coiled patients) evaluating this medication are in different stages of development. Intensive surveillance to prevent systemic hypotension and lung complications from extravascular fluid retention may make the difference between positive or negative clinical results in these upcoming trials.[1]

A Cochrane review identified three randomized controlled trials comparing endovascular coiling to neurosurgical clipping in a total of 2272 patients. The review showed that coiling was associated with a better overall outcome.[2] The International Subarachnoid Aneurysm Trial (ISAT) showed that, the absolute advantage over surgical treatment in the rate of death or dependence was maintained after 1 year, and the early survival advantage was maintained for up to 7 years.[3]

Vasospasm is one of the main causes of morbidity and mortality in SAH. The calcium channel blocker Nimodipine has been shown to significantly reduce the proportion of patients with poor outcome and ischemic neurological deficits after aneurysmal subarachnoid hemorrhage,[4] even though it does not alter radiographic vasospasm[5] or overall mortality.[6]

Evidence-Based References

1. Macdonald RL on behalf of the CONSCIOUS-1 Investigators. Clazosentan to Overcome Neurological Ischemia and Infarction Occurring After Subarachnoid Hemorrhage (CONSCIOUS-1): randomized, double-blind, placebo-controlled phase 2 dose-finding trial, *Stroke* 39:3015-3021, 2008. Ⓐ

2. Molyneux AJ et al and the International Subarachnoid Aneurysm Trial (ISAT) Collaborative Group: International subarachnoid aneurysm trial (ISAT) of neurosurgical clipping versus endovascular coiling in 2143 patients with ruptured intracranial aneurysms: a randomised comparison of effects on survival, dependency, seizures, rebleeding, subgroups, and aneurysm occlusion, *Lancet* 366: 809-817, 2005.

3. Van der Schaaf I et al: Endovascular coiling versus neurosurgical clipping for patients with aneurysmal subarachnoid haemorrhage, *Cochrane Database Rev* 4, 2005.

4. Rinkel GJE et al: Calcium antagonists for aneurysmal subarachnoid haemorrhage, *Cochrane Database Rev* 1, 2005

5. Allen GS et al: Cerebral arterial vasospasm—a controlled trial of nimodipine in patients with subarachnoid hemorrhage, *N Engl J Med* 308:619-624, 1984.

6. Baker FG et al: Efficacy of prophylactic nimodipine for delayed ischemic deficit after subarachnoid hemorrhage: a metaanalysis, *J Neurosurg* 84: 405-414, 1996.

SUGGESTED READINGS

Edlow JA: Diagnosis of subarachnoid hemorrhage, *Neurocrit Care* 2(2):99, 2005.

Rinkel GJE et al: Circulatory volume expansion therapy for aneurysmal subarachnoid haemorrhage, *Cochrane Database Rev* 2, 2004.

Rinkel GJE et al: Calcium antagonists for aneurysmal subarachnoid haemorrhage, *Cochrane Database Rev* 1, 2005.

Van der Schaaf I et al: Endovascular coiling versus neurosurgical clipping for patients with aneurysmal subarachnoid haemorrhage, *Cochrane Database Rev* 4, 2005.

Van Gijn J et al: Subarachnoid hemorrhage, *Lancet* 369:306-318, 2007.

AUTHORS: **WISSAM S. Z. ASFAHANI, M.D.,** and **CHRISTIAN N. RAMSEY, III, M.D.**

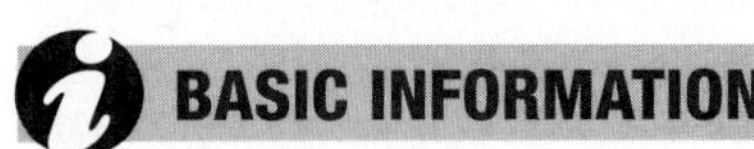

BASIC INFORMATION

DEFINITION

Subclavian steal syndrome is an occlusion or severe stenosis of the proximal subclavian artery leading to decreased antegrade flow or retrograde flow in the ipsilateral vertebral artery and neurologic symptoms referable to the posterior circulation.

SYNONYMS

Proximal subclavian (or innominate) artery stenosis or occlusion

ICD-9CM CODES
435.2 Subclavian steal syndrome

EPIDEMIOLOGY & DEMOGRAPHICS

- Similar to that of other manifestations of atherosclerosis (coronary artery disease, cerebrovascular disease, or peripheral vascular disease)
- Affects middle-aged persons (men somewhat younger than women on average) with arteriosclerotic risk factors, including family history, smoking, diabetes mellitus, hyperlipidemia, hypertension, and sedentary lifestyle

PHYSICAL FINDINGS & CLINICAL PRESENTATION

Symptoms:
- Many patients are asymptomatic.
- Upper extremity ischemic symptoms: fatigue, exercise-related aching, coolness, numbness of the involved upper extremity.
- Neurologic symptoms are reported by 25% of patients with known unilateral subclavian steal. These include brief spells of:
  1. Vertigo
  2. Diplopia
  3. Decreased vision
  4. Oscillopsia
  5. Gait unsteadiness

These spells are only occasionally provoked by exercising the ischemic upper extremity (classic subclavian steal). Left subclavian steal is more common than right, but the latter is more serious.
- Posterior circulation stroke related to subclavian steal is rare.
- Innominate artery stenosis can cause decreased right carotid artery flow and cerebrovascular symptoms of the anterior cerebral circulation, but this is uncommon.

Physical findings:
- Delayed and smaller volume pulse (wrist or antecubital) in the affected upper extremity
- Lower blood pressure in the affected upper extremity
- Supraclavicular bruit

NOTE: Inflating a blood pressure cuff will increase the bruit if it originates from a vertebral artery stenosis and decrease the bruit if it originates from a subclavian artery stenosis.

ETIOLOGY & PATHOGENESIS

Etiology:
- Atherosclerosis
- Arteritis (Takayasu's disease and temporal arteritis)
- Embolism to the subclavian or innominate artery
- Cervical rib
- Long-term use of a crutch
- Occupational (baseball pitchers and cricket bowlers)

Pathogenesis: The vertebral artery originates from the subclavian artery. For subclavian steal to occur, the occlusion must be proximal to the takeoff of the vertebral artery. On the right side, only a small distance separates the bifurcation of the innominate artery and the takeoff of the vertebral artery, explaining why the condition occurs less commonly on the right side. Occlusion of the innominate artery must affect right carotid artery flow.

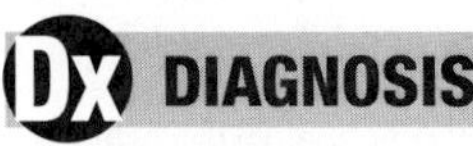

DIAGNOSIS

The carotid arteries should be evaluated at least noninvasively in all cases.

DIFFERENTIAL DIAGNOSIS

- Posterior circulation transient ischemic attack or stroke
- Upper extremity ischemia
  1. Distal subclavian artery stenosis or occlusion
  2. Raynaud's syndrome
  3. Thoracic outlet syndrome

WORKUP

- Noninvasive upper extremity arterial flow studies
- Doppler sonography of the vertebral, subclavian, and innominate arteries
- Arteriography

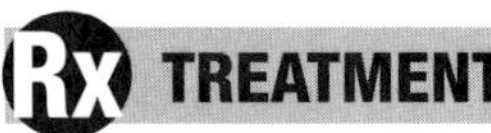

TREATMENT

- In most patients the disease is benign and requires no treatment other than atherosclerosis risk factor modification and aspirin. Symptoms tend to improve over time as collateral circulation develops.
- Vascular surgical reconstruction requires a thoracotomy; it may be indicated in innominate artery stenosis or when upper extremity ischemia is incapacitating.

AUTHOR: **FRED F. FERRI, M.D.**

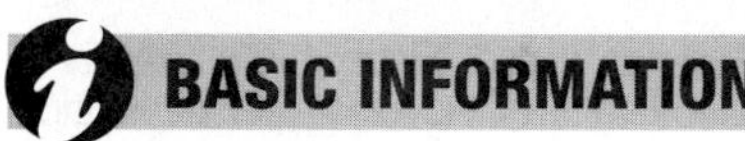

BASIC INFORMATION

DEFINITION

A subdural hematoma (SDH) is a collection of blood or blood products between the arachnoidal (superficial) layer of the brain and the dura or meningeal layer of the brain.

SYNONYMS

Subdural hemorrhage

ICD-9CM CODES

852.10 Subdural hematoma

EPIDEMIOLOGY & DEMOGRAPHICS

INCIDENCE: SDH is a common finding, especially among trauma patients.
PREVALENCE: Unknown
PEAK INCIDENCE: SDH most commonly occurs in the elderly and alcoholic populations as a result of cerebral atrophy and in the infant population (e.g., shaken baby) as a result of the increasing traction on the bridging veins between the brain parenchyma and the dura mater. SDHs are more common than epidural hematomas.
RISK FACTORS: Any conditions that predispose patients to hemorrhage (e.g., anticoagulants, antiplatelet therapy); atrophy of the brain (e.g., dementia, alcoholism); or falls and trauma (e.g., movement disorders, previous stroke)

PHYSICAL FINDINGS & CLINICAL PRESENTATION

Symptoms vary on the basis of acuity, size, and location. Acute traumatic SDHs are often seen in comatose patients. When they are associated with a midline shift (i.e., >5 mm), they can cause signs of cerebral herniation (e.g., ipsilateral pupil dilation, contralateral weakness). Chronic and subacute SDHs present with variable symptoms of headache, mild weakness, slowness of mentation, aphasia, mobility problems, and abulia.

ETIOLOGY

SDH is usually the result of shear and of the tearing of a bridging vein. It can be caused by any source of bleeding into the subdural space (i.e., contusion, extension of parenchymal hemorrhage, rarely other vascular abnormalities [e.g., arteriovenous malformation, aneurysm]).

DIAGNOSIS

DIFFERENTIAL DIAGNOSIS

Other causes of subdural collections, such as hygromas, abscesses, and tumor infiltrations.

WORKUP

- Patient history, including medications with anticoagulant properties, alcohol abuse, trauma, cancer, and recent bacterial infections
- Physical examination, including alertness, pupil and facial symmetry, and motor weakness (i.e., pronator drift)

LABORATORY TESTS

- Prothrombin time (international normalized ratio)
- partial thromboplastin time

IMAGING STUDIES

A noncontrast computed tomographic (CT) scan of the head should be obtained (Fig. 1-321). For comatose and trauma patients, include a cervical spine CT scan. Contrast is only needed if there are concerns about tumor or infection.

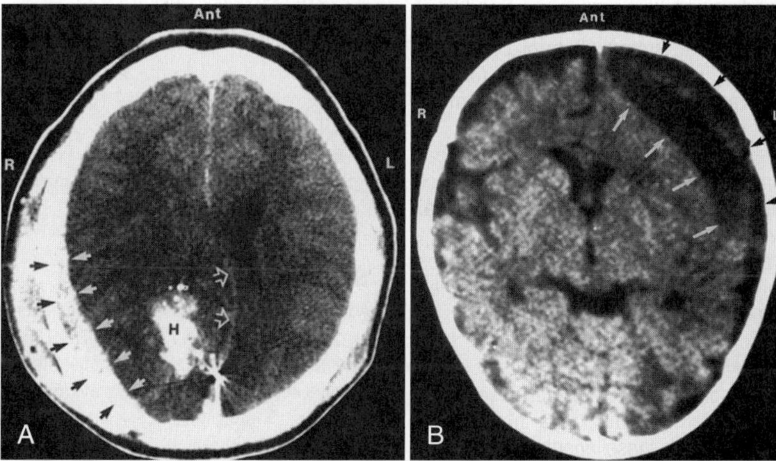

FIGURE 1-321 Subdural hematomas. A, A noncontrast computed tomographic scan of an acute subdural hematoma shows a crescentic area of increased density in the right posterior parietal region between the brain and the skull *(black and white arrows).* An area of intraparenchymal hemorrhage *(H)* is also seen. **B,** A chronic subdural hematoma for a different patient is shown. There is an area of decreased density in the left frontoparietal region *(arrows)* that effaces the sulci, compresses the anterior horn of the left lateral ventricle, and shifts the midline somewhat to the right. (From Mettler FA [ed]: *Primary care radiology,* Philadelphia, 2000, WB Saunders.)

Rx TREATMENT

1. Correction of underlying coagulopathy, if present (e.g., Coumadin reversal)
2. The majority of SDH can be managed without surgery in awake patients with normal neurologic examinations.

NONPHARMACOLOGIC THERAPY

1. For acute SDH with mass effect, midline shift, and clinical effects (e.g., coma, weakness), surgical evacuation is required.
2. For chronic SDH with a mass effect, a change in the clinical examination from the baseline evacuation, or enlargement, evacuation via craniotomy or burr hole should be considered.

COMPLEMENTARY AND ALTERNATIVE MEDICINE

Remember that some herbal and alternative medicines can be associated with coagulopathy.

DISPOSITION

Depending on the size and location of the SDH and the examination of the patient, observation can range from the intensive care unit to outpatient management. When observation of the patient is considered, clinical examinations should be serially performed. Patient baseline and follow-up clinical examinations are more important than CT scan findings.

REFERRAL

Neurosurgical and operative consultation should be made available.

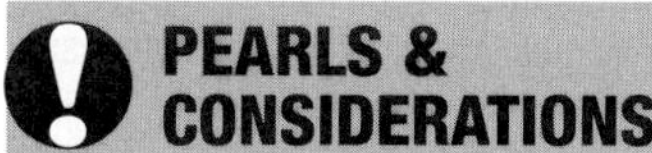

PEARLS & CONSIDERATIONS

COMMENTS

- Many elderly patients have small chronic SDHs or hygromas. Unless these are associated with seizures or clinical or radiographic progression, they are usually not emergent. The important thing is to recognize the cause (e.g., medication, fall risk).
- Recurrence after surgical management for chronic SDH is common.
- SDHs in elderly patients can have a mixed hyperdense and hypodense appearance on noncontrast CT scan; this is suggestive of acute and chronic components.

PREVENTION

Fall risk and prevention, especially among the elderly, are very important when considering anticoagulant medications.

PATIENT/FAMILY EDUCATION

Individuals with SDHs are at higher risk for seizure, so surveillance is important.

AUTHOR: **CHRISTIAN N. RAMSEY, M.D.**

BASIC INFORMATION

DEFINITION

Suicide refers to successful and unsuccessful attempts to kill oneself.

SYNONYMS

Self-murder

ICD-9CM CODES
Categorized by method

EPIDEMIOLOGY & DEMOGRAPHICS

INCIDENCE (IN U.S.):

- Suicide is among the top 10 leading causes of death and the seventh leading cause of years of potential life lost in the U.S.
- U.S. rate of 11.0 cases/100,000 persons
- 18.7/100,000 men; 4.4/100,000 women

PEAK INCIDENCE: Age 65 yr or older for completed suicide

PREDOMINANT AGE:

- Increases with age (13.1 cases/100,000 persons ages 15 to 24 yr, 16.9 cases/100,000 persons ages 65 to 74 yr, and 23.5 cases/100,000 persons ages 75 to 84 yr)
- Third leading cause of death in those ages 15 to 24 yr in United States

GENETICS:

- Family history of suicide is associated with suicidal behavior

PHYSICAL FINDINGS & CLINICAL PRESENTATION

Methods used in attempted suicides differ from those used in completed suicides.

- Overdose used in >70% of attempted suicides.
- Approximately 60% of completed suicides used firearms.
- Several risk factors for completed suicide include psychiatric illness such as depression or anxiety, middle age or advanced age, white race, male gender, a recent divorce or separation, comorbid substance use (particularly when intoxicated), previous history of suicide attempts, fatal plan (e.g., firearms or hanging), history of violence, and family history of suicide. Concurrent chronic physical illness increases the risk for suicide.

ETIOLOGY

- Individuals with a mental disorder or substance use disorder are responsible for >90% of all suicides.
- The concurrence of more than one condition (e.g., depression and alcohol abuse) greatly increases the risk of suicide.
- Hopelessness is a strong predictor of suicide potential.
- Rates are higher in developing countries.
- Rates vary by occupation, ethnicity, and employment status.

DIAGNOSIS

DIFFERENTIAL DIAGNOSIS

- Some disorders are associated with self-injurious behavior that is not suicidal. Borderline personality disorder, for example, manifests with self-mutilation without active suicidal intent. Eating disorders are harmful and may be fatal, but death is rarely the goal.
- Some suicidal behavior is intended as a "call for help." In these situations individuals usually design the suicide so that they will be discovered before significant damage has been done.

WORKUP

- The physician must directly inquire into the presence of suicidal ideation. Approximately one half to two thirds of individuals who commit suicide visit physicians within 1 mo of taking their lives.
- Explicit suicidal intent, hopelessness, and a well-formulated plan indicate high risk. Clinicians can use the mnemonic SAL: Is the method ***s***pecific? Is it ***a***vailable? Is it ***l***ethal?
- The concurrence of multiple psychiatric problems, substance abuse, and multiple physical problems increases the risk.
- Covert suicidal ideation occurs in patients primarily with multiple vague physical complaints, depression, anxiety, or substance abuse.

TREATMENT

NONPHARMACOLOGIC THERAPY

- Major immediate intervention: placement of the patient in a safe environment (usually hospitalization in a psychiatric unit or a medical unit with continuous observation)
- Long-term: psychotherapy aimed at factors that underlie the decision to pursue suicide or at the risk factors contributing to suicidal behavior
- Substance abuse treatment (e.g., Alcoholics Anonymous, Narcotics Anonymous) when substance use disorder is present

ACUTE GENERAL Rx

- Benzodiazepines may be useful in reducing extreme anxiety and dysphoria in a suicidal patient; however, these agents are depressive and should be used only when patient is in a safe environment.
- Antipsychotics can be used if psychosis is present (e.g., voices telling patient to hurt self).
- Mood stabilizers and antidepressants should be started in the acute setting but may have up to a 2-wk latency period.
- "No-harm contracts" supported by expert opinion.

CHRONIC Rx

- Therapy should be aimed at the underlying condition (e.g., antidepressants for depression, anxiolytics or antidepressants for anxiety, substance abuse treatment, or psychotherapy for chronic low self-esteem, hopelessness).
- In elderly, loneliness and medical disability are major reasons for suicide and therefore major targets for intervention.

DISPOSITION

- Prior suicide attempt is the best predictor for completed suicides (i.e., patients who attempt suicide once are at high risk for completing suicide in the future).
- Conditions associated with suicide (e.g., depression, physical ailments) are usually chronic and recurring.

REFERRAL

Patients with active suicidal ideation and intent should be referred to specialty mental health.

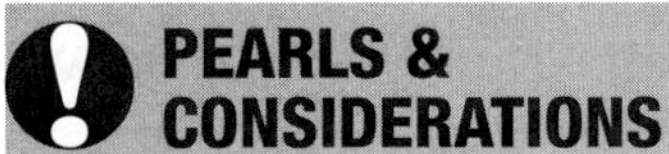

PEARLS & CONSIDERATIONS

- A past episode of suicidal behavior is strongly associated with an increased risk for subsequent suicidal behavior.
- Restriction of access to lethal means is one of the few suicide-prevention policies with proven effectiveness.
- Family history of suicidal behavior is important.

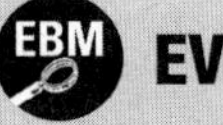

EVIDENCE

Please note: Complete text of EBM for this topic is available online.

SUGGESTED READINGS

Adams SM et al: Pharmacologic management of adult depression, *Am Fam Physician* 77(6):785, 2008.

Feldman MD et al: Let's not talk about it: suicide inquiry in primary care, *Ann Fam Med* 5(5):412, 2007.

Hawton K, van Heeringen K: Suicide, *Lancet* 373(9672):1372-1381, 2009.

AUTHOR: **MITCHELL D. FELDMAN, M.D., M.PHIL.**

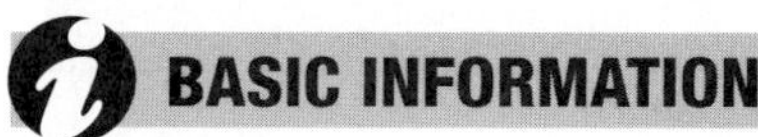

BASIC INFORMATION

DEFINITION

Superior vena cava syndrome is a set of symptoms that results when a mediastinal mass compresses the superior vena cava (SVC) or the veins that drain into it.

ICD-9CM CODES
453.2 Vena cava thrombosis

EPIDEMIOLOGY & DEMOGRAPHICS

- SVC syndrome occurs in 15,000 persons in the U.S. every year.
- Mirrors lung cancer (especially small-cell carcinoma) and lymphoma (see "Lung Neoplasm" and "Lymphoma" in Section I).

PHYSICAL FINDINGS & CLINICAL PRESENTATION

The pathophysiology of the syndrome involves the increased pressure in the venous system draining into the SVC, producing edema of the head, neck, and upper extremities. Symptoms develop over a period of 2 wk in one third of patients and include:

- Shortness of breath
- Chest pain
- Cough
- Dysphagia, hoarseness, stridor
- Headache
- Syncope
- Visual trouble

Signs:

- Chest wall vein distention (Fig. 1-322)
- Neck vein distention
- Facial edema
- Upper extremity swelling
- Cyanosis

ETIOLOGY

- Lung cancer (80% of all cases, of which half are small-cell lung cancer)
- Lymphoma (15%)
- Thymoma
- Tuberculosis
- Goiter
- Aortic aneurysm (arteriosclerotic or syphilitic)
- SVC thrombosis
  1. Primary: associated with a central venous catheter
  2. Secondary: as a complication of SVC syndrome associated with one of the above-mentioned causes
- Inflammatory process, fibrosing mediastinitis

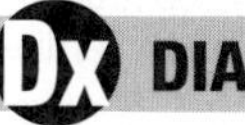

DIAGNOSIS

CT of the chest with contrast is the most useful diagnostic study. MRI is usually adequate to establish the diagnosis of SVC obstruction and to assist in the differential diagnosis of probable cause.

DIFFERENTIAL DIAGNOSIS

The syndrome is characteristic enough to exclude other diagnoses. The differential diagnosis concerns the underlying etiologies listed above.

WORKUP

- Chest radiograph
- Chest CT with contrast or MRI (in patient who cannot tolerate contrast medium)

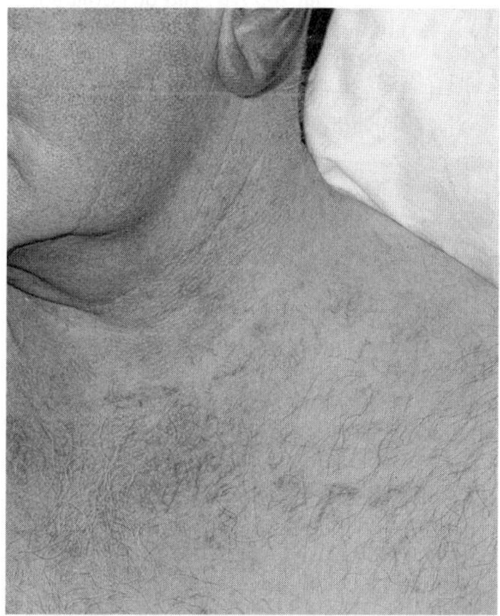

FIGURE 1-322 Superior vena cava obstruction causing dilated veins and plethora of the upper trunk and neck in a patient with bronchial carcinoma. Patients with superior vena cava obstruction are occasionally referred to dermatologists with suspected contact allergy (eyelid swelling) or angioedema (facial or hand swelling). (From White GM, Cox NH [eds]: *Diseases of the skin, a color atlas and text*, ed 2, St Louis, 2006, Mosby.)

- Venography: warranted only when an intervention (e.g., stent or surgery) is planned
- Percutaneous needle biopsy (usually the initial diagnostic modality used to establish a histologic diagnosis)
- Bronchoscopy
- Mediastinoscopy
- Thoracotomy

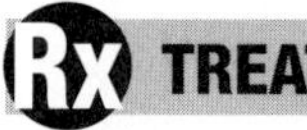

TREATMENT

- Although invasive procedures such as mediastinoscopy or thoracotomy are associated with higher than usual risk of bleeding, a tissue diagnosis is usually needed before commencing therapy.
- Management is guided by the severity of the symptoms and the underlying etiology.
- Emergency empiric radiation is indicated in critical situations such as respiratory failure or central nervous system signs associated with increased intracranial pressure.
- Treatment of the underlying malignancy:
  1. Radiotherapy: the majority of tumors causing SVC syndrome are sensitive to radiotherapy
  2. Systemic chemotherapy
- Anticoagulant or fibrinolytic therapy in patients who do not respond to cancer treatment within a week or if an obstructing thrombus has been documented.
- Loop diuretics are often used, but their effect is limited.
- Upright positioning and fluid restriction until collateral channels develop and allow for clinical regression are useful modalities for SVC syndrome secondary to benign disease.
- Steroids (dexamethasone 4 mg q6h) may be useful in reducing the tumor burden in lymphoma and thymoma.
- Percutaneous self-expandable stents that can be placed under local anesthesia with radiologic manipulation are useful in the treatment of SVC syndrome to bypass the obstruction, especially in cases associated with malignant tumors.
- Surgical bypass grafting is infrequently used to treat SVC syndrome.

REFERRAL

To a thoracic surgeon, pulmonary specialist, or oncologist

AUTHOR: **FRED F. FERRI, M.D.**

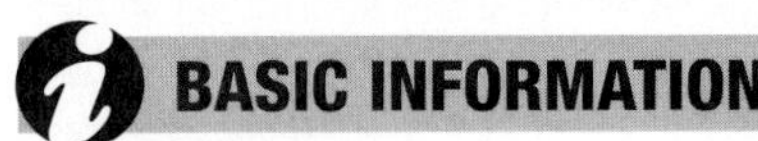

BASIC INFORMATION

DEFINITION

Syncope is the transient loss of consciousness that results from an acute global reduction in cerebral blood flow. Syncope should be distinguished from other causes of transient loss of consciousness.

ICD-9CM CODES
720.2 Syncope

EPIDEMIOLOGY & DEMOGRAPHICS

- Syncope accounts for 3% to 5% of emergency department visits.
- 30% of the adult population will experience at least one syncopal episode during their lifetimes.
- Incidence of syncope is highest in elderly men and young women.

PHYSICAL FINDINGS & CLINICAL PRESENTATION

- Blood pressure: if low, consider orthostatic hypotension; if unequal in both arms (difference >20 mm Hg), consider subclavian steal or dissecting aneurysm. (NOTE: Blood pressure [BP] and heart rate should be recorded in the supine and standing positions.) If there is a drop in BP but no change in heart rate (HR), the patient may be taking a beta-blocker or may have an autonomic neuropathy.
- Pulse: if patient has tachycardia, bradycardia, or irregular rhythm, consider arrhythmia.
- Heart: if there are murmurs present, consider syncope attributable to left ventricular outflow obstruction; if there are jugular venous distension and distal heart sounds, consider cardiac tamponade.
- Carotid sinus pressure: can be diagnostic if it reproduces symptoms and other causes are excluded; a pause >3 sec or a systolic BP drop >50 mm Hg without symptoms or <30 mm Hg with symptoms when sinus pressure is applied separately on each side for <5 sec is considered abnormal. This test should be avoided in patients with carotid bruits or cerebrovascular disease. ECG monitoring, IV access, and bedside atropine should be available when carotid sinus pressure is applied.

ETIOLOGY

- Neurally mediated syncope
  1. Psychophysiologic (emotional upset, panic disorders, hysteria, hyperventilation)
  2. Visceral reflex (micturition, defecation, food ingestion, coughing, ventricular contraction; glossopharyngeal neuralgia)
  3. Carotid sinus pressure
  4. Reduction of venous return caused by Valsalva maneuver
- Orthostatic hypotension
  1. Hypovolemia
  2. Vasodilator medications
  3. Autonomic neuropathy (diabetes, amyloid, Parkinson's disease, multisystem atrophy)
  4. Pheochromocytoma
  5. Carcinoid syndrome
- Cardiac
  1. Reduced cardiac output
     a. Left ventricular outflow obstruction (aortic stenosis, hypertrophic cardiomyopathy)
     b. Obstruction to pulmonary flow (pulmonary embolism, pulmonic stenosis, primary pulmonary hypertension)
     c. Myocardial infarct with pump failure
     d. Cardiac tamponade
     e. Mitral stenosis
     f. Reduction of venous return (atrial myxoma, valve thrombus)
     g. Beta-blocker therapy
  2. Arrhythmias or asystole
     a. Extreme tachycardia (>160 to 180 beats/min)
     b. Severe bradycardia (<30 to 40 beats/min)
     c. Sick sinus syndrome
     d. Atrioventricular block (second or third degree)
     e. Ventricular tachycardia or fibrillation
     f. Long QT syndrome
     g. Pacemaker malfunction
     h. Psychotropic medications and beta-blockers

Dx DIAGNOSIS

DIFFERENTIAL DIAGNOSIS

1. Seizure (see "Workup.")
2. Vertebrobasilar transient ischemic attack (TIA) usually manifests as diplopia, vertigo, or ataxia but not loss of consciousness. Isolated episodes of transient loss of consciousness (TLOC) without accompanying neurologic symptoms are unlikely to be TIAs.
3. Recreational drugs or alcohol.
4. Functional causes, such as stress and somatoform disorders.
5. Sleep disorders, such as sleep attacks and narcolepsy, are also in the differential for TLOC.
6. Head trauma.

WORKUP

The history is crucial to diagnosing the cause of syncope and may suggest a diagnosis that can be evaluated with directed testing. History is also important to determine other etiologies for TLOC, such as seizure.

- Sudden LOC: consider cardiac arrhythmias.
- Gradual LOC: consider orthostatic hypotension, vasodepressor syncope, hypoglycemia.
- History of aura before LOC or prolonged confusion (>1 min), amnesia, or lethargy after LOC suggests seizure rather than syncope.
- Patient's activity at the time of syncope:
  1. Micturition, coughing, defecation: consider syncope caused by decreased venous return.
  2. Turning head or while shaving: consider carotid sinus syndrome.
  3. Physical exertion in a patient with murmur: consider aortic stenosis.
  4. Arm exercise: consider subclavian steal syndrome.
  5. Assuming an upright position: consider orthostatic hypotension.
- Associated events:
  1. Chest pain: consider myocardial infarction, pulmonary embolism.
  2. Palpitations: consider arrhythmias.
  3. Incontinence (urine or fecal) and tongue biting are associated with seizure or syncope.
  4. Brief, transient shaking after LOC may represent myoclonus from global cerebral hypoperfusion and not seizures. However, sustained tonic/clonic muscle action is more suggestive of seizure.
  5. Focal neurologic symptoms or signs point to a neurologic event such as a seizure with residual deficits (e.g., Todd's paralysis) or cerebral ischemic injury.
  6. Psychologic stress: syncope may be vasovagal.
- Review current medications, particularly antihypertensive and psychotropic drugs.

LABORATORY TESTS

Routine blood tests rarely yield diagnostically useful information and should be done only if they are specifically suggested by the results of the history and physical examination. The following are commonly ordered tests:

- Pregnancy test in women of childbearing age
- Complete blood count to look for anemia and signs of infection
- Electrolytes, blood urea nitrogen, creatinine, magnesium, and calcium to look for electrolyte abnormalities and evaluate fluid status
- Serum glucose level
- Cardiac isoenzymes, especially if the patient gives a history of chest pain before the syncopal episode
- Drug and alcohol levels with suspected toxicity

IMAGING STUDIES

- Echocardiography.
- If seizure is suspected, CT scan and/or MRI of the head and electroencephalogram may be useful.
- If head trauma or neurologic signs on examination, CT or MRI may be helpful.
- If arrhythmias are suspected, a 24-hr Holter monitor or admission to a telemetry unit is appropriate. In general, Holter monitoring is rarely useful, revealing a cause for syncope in <3% of cases. Loop recorders that can be activated after syncopal episode to retrieve information about the cardiac rhythm during the preceding 4 min add considerable diagnostic yield in patients with unexplained syncope.
- Implantable cardiac monitors that function as permanent loop recorders or implantable cardioverter-defibrillators, which are placed subcutaneously in the pectoral region with the patient under local anesthesia, are useful in patients with cardiac syncope.

- Electrophysiologic studies may be indicated in patients with structural heart disease and/or recurrent syncope.
- ECG to rule out arrhythmias; may be diagnostic in 5% to 10% of patients.

TILT-TABLE TESTING

- Useful to support a diagnosis of neurally mediated syncope. Patients age >50 yr should have stress testing before tilt-table testing. Positive results would preclude tilt-table testing.
- Indicated in patients with recurrent episodes of unexplained syncope as well as patients in high-risk occupations (e.g., pilots, bus drivers) (Fig. 1-323). The test is also useful for identifying patients with prominent bradycardic response who may benefit from implantation of a permanent pacemaker.
- It is performed by keeping the patient in an upright posture on a tilt table with footboard support. The angle of the tilt table varies from 60 to 80 degrees. The duration of upright posture during tilt-table testing varies from 25 to 45 min.
- The hallmark of neurally mediated syncope is severe hypotension associated with a paradoxic bradycardia triggered by a specific stimulus. The diagnosis of neurally mediated syncope is likely if upright tilt testing reproduces these hemodynamic changes in <15 min and causes presyncope or syncope.

PSYCHIATRIC EVALUATION

- May be indicated in young patients without heart disease who have frequently recurring transient loss of consciousness and other somatic symptoms.
- Generalized anxiety disorder, pain disorder, and major depression predispose patients to neurally mediated reactions and may result in syncope.

Rx TREATMENT

NONPHARMACOLOGIC THERAPY

- Ensure proper hydration; consider thromboembolic stockings and salt tablets in appropriate patients.
- Eliminate medications that may induce hypotension.

ACUTE GENERAL Rx

- Varies with the underlying etiology of syncope (e.g., pacemaker in patients with syncope resulting from complete heart block).
- Syncope caused by orthostatic hypotension is treated with volume replacement in patients with intravascular volume depletion. Also consider midodrine to promote venous return by adrenergic-mediated vasoconstriction and Florinef for its mineralocorticoid effects to increase intravascular volume.

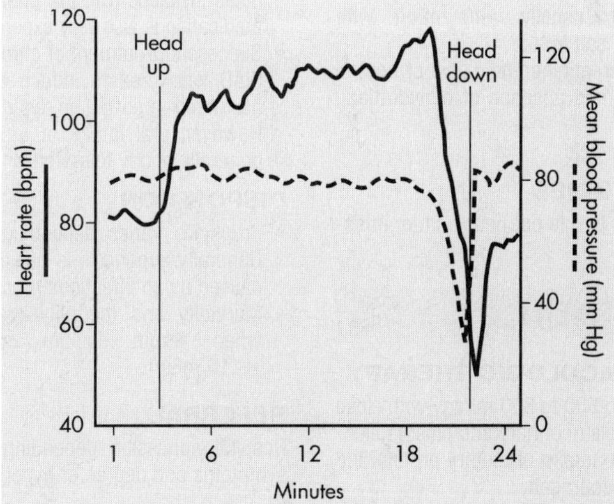

FIGURE 1-323 Head-up tilt test performed on an 18-year-old woman with a history of syncope associated with pain, preceded by a prodrome of dizziness, graying vision, and diaphoresis. A similar prodrome preceded syncope during the test. Note the precipitous and nearly simultaneous decline of heart rate and blood pressure after an initial rise in heart rate. Vital signs returned to normal rapidly after the head was lowered. (Courtesy Robert F. Sprung, University of Utah. In Goldman L, Ausiello D [eds]: *Cecil textbook of medicine,* ed 22, Philadelphia, 2004, WB Saunders.)

DISPOSITION

Prognosis varies with the age of the patient and the etiology of the syncope. In general:

- Benign prognosis (very low 1-yr morbidity rate) in patients:
  1. Age <30 yr and having noncardiac syncope
  2. Age <70 yr and having vasovagal or psychogenic syncope or syncope of unknown cause
- Poor prognosis (high mortality and morbidity rates) in patients with cardiac syncope.
- Patients with the following risk factors have a higher 1-yr mortality rate: abnormal ECG, history of ventricular arrhythmia, history of congestive heart failure.

REFERRAL

Hospital admission in elderly patients without prior history of syncope or unknown etiology of their syncope and in any patients suspected of having cardiac syncope.

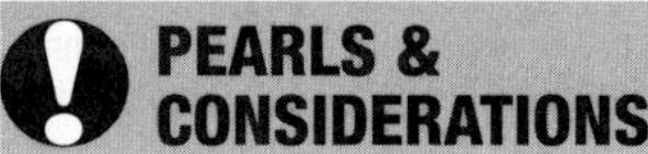

PEARLS & CONSIDERATIONS

COMMENTS

- Section III, "Syncope," describes an algorithmic approach to the patient.
- The etiology of syncope is identified in <50% of cases during the initial evaluation.
- A thorough history and physical examination are the most productive means of establishing a diagnosis in patients with syncope.

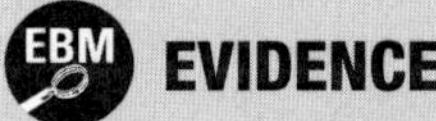

EVIDENCE

Please note: Complete text of EBM for this topic is available online.

SUGGESTED READINGS

Brignole M et al: Guidelines on management (diagnosis and treatment) of syncope 2004, *Europace* 6:467, 2004.

Chen LY et al: Management of syncope in adults: an update, *Mayo Clin Proc* 83(11):1280-1293, 2008.

Fenton AM et al: Vasovagal syncope, *Ann Intern Med* 133:722, 2000.

Grubb BP: Neurocardiogenic syncope, *N Engl J Med* 352:1002-1010, 2005.

Kapoor WN: Syncope, *N Engl J Med* 343:1856, 2000.

Menozzi C et al: Mechanism of syncope in patients with heart disease and negative electrophysiologic test, *Circulation* 105:2741, 2002.

AUTHOR: **SEAN I. SAVITZ, M.D.**

 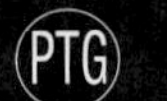

BASIC INFORMATION

DEFINITION

Syndrome of inappropriate antidiuresis (SIAD) is a syndrome characterized by excessive secretion of antidiuretic hormone (ADH) in absence of normal osmotic or physiologic stimuli (increased serum osmolarity, decreased plasma volume, hypotension).

SYNONYMS

SIAD
SIADH
Syndrome of inappropriate antidiuretic hormone secretion
Inappropriate secretion of antidiuretic hormone

ICD-9CM CODES
276.9 Inappropriate secretion of antidiuretic hormone

EPIDEMIOLOGY & DEMOGRAPHICS

The syndrome of inappropriate antidiuresis is the most frequent cause of hyponatremia. Nearly 50% of hyponatremia detected in the hospital setting is caused by SIAD.

PHYSICAL FINDINGS & CLINICAL PRESENTATION

- The patient is generally normovolemic or slightly hypervolemic; edema is absent.
- Delirium, lethargy, and seizures may be present if the hyponatremia is severe or of rapid onset.
- Manifestations of the underlying disease may be evident (e.g., fever from an infectious process or headaches and visual field defects from an intracranial mass).
- Diminished reflexes and extensor plantar responses may occur with severe hyponatremia.

ETIOLOGY

- Neoplasm: lung, oropharynx, stomach, duodenum, pancreas, brain, thymus, bladder, prostate, endometrium, mesothelioma, lymphoma, Ewing's sarcoma
- Pulmonary disorders: pneumonia, aspergillosis, pulmonary abscess, TB, bronchiectasis, emphysema, cystic fibrosis, status asthmaticus, respiratory failure associated with positive-pressure breathing.
- Intracranial pathology: trauma, neoplasms, infections (meningitis, encephalitis, brain abscess), hemorrhage, hydrocephalus, MS, Guillain-Barré syndrome
- Postoperative period: surgical stress, ventilators with positive pressure, anesthetic agents
- Drugs: nicotine, chlorpropamide, thiazide diuretics, vasopressin, desmopressin, oxytocin, chemotherapeutic agents (vincristine, vinblastine, cyclophosphamide), carbamazepine, phenothiazines, MAO inhibitors, tricyclic antidepressants, narcotics, nicotine, clofibrate, haloperidol, SSRIs, NSAIDs
- Other: acute intermittent porphyria, myxedema, psychosis, delirium tremens, ACTH deficiency (hypopituitarism), general anesthesia, endurance exercise

Dx DIAGNOSIS

DIFFERENTIAL DIAGNOSIS

- Hyponatremia associated with hypervolemia (congestive heart failure, cirrhosis, nephrotic syndrome)
- Factitious hyponatremia (hyperglycemia, abnormal proteins, hyperlipidemia)
- Hyponatremia associated with hypovolemia (e.g., burns, GI fluid loss)

WORKUP

- Demonstration through laboratory evaluation (see "Laboratory Tests") of excessive secretion of ADH in absence of appropriate osmotic or physiologic stimuli (abnormal result on test of water load, elevated plasma arginine vasopressin levels despite the presence of hypotonicity and clinical euvolemia)
- Demonstration of normal thyroid, adrenal, and cardiac function
- No recent or concurrent use of diuretics
- Failure to correct hyponatremia after 0.9% saline infusion
- Correction of hyponatremia through fluid restriction

LABORATORY TESTS

- Hyponatremia
- Decreased effective osmolality (<275 mOsm/kg of water)
- Urine osmolality >100 mOsm/kg of water during hypotonicity
- Urinary osmolarity > serum osmolarity
- Urinary sodium usually >40 mEq/L with normal dietary salt intake
- Normal BUN, creatinine (indicative of normal renal function and absence of dehydration), normal TSH
- Decreased uric acid

IMAGING STUDIES

Chest radiograph to rule out neoplasm or infectious process

Rx TREATMENT

NONPHARMACOLOGIC THERAPY

Fluid restriction to 500 to 800 ml/day with close monitoring of levels of urinary and plasma electrolytes. Adequate intake of dietary protein and salt should be encouraged.

ACUTE GENERAL Rx

- In emergency situations (seizures, coma) SIAD can be treated with combination of:
  1. Hypertonic saline solution (slow infusion of 250 ml of 3% NaCl). Infuse 3% saline (513 mmol/L) at a rate of 1 to 2 ml/kg of body weight per hour to increase the serum sodium level by 1 to 2 mmol/L/hr.
  2. Furosemide, 20 to 40 mg IV. This combination increases the serum sodium by causing diuresis of urine that is more dilute than plasma and prevents extracellular fluid volume expansion.
- The rapidity of correction varies depending on the degree of hyponatremia and if the hyponatremia is acute or chronic; generally the serum sodium should be corrected only halfway to normal in the initial 24 hr. A prudent approach is to increase serum sodium by <0.5 mEq/L/hr and limit the total increase to 8 to 12 mmol/L during the first 24 hr.
- Close monitoring of the rate of correction (every 2 to 3 hr) is recommended to avoid overcorrection. In patients with hyponatremia of chronic duration, correction of serum sodium level by >12 mmol/L over a period of 24 hr increases the risk of osmotic demyelination.
- Conivaptan (20 to 40 mg/day IV) or tolvaptan (15 mg/day PO initiative) are selective agrinine vasopressin (AVP) antagonists useful in selected hospitalized patients with moderate-to-severe hyponatremia. Potential problems associated with its use are infusion-site reactions (50% of patients) and risk of osmotic demyelination if serum sodium levels are corrected too rapidly. Oral vasopressin-receptor antagonists (tolvaptan, lixivaptan, satavaptan) are pending FDA approval.

CHRONIC Rx

- Depending on the underlying etiology, fluid restriction may be needed indefinitely. Monthly monitoring of electrolytes is recommended in patients with chronic SIAD.
- Demeclocycline 300 to 600 mg PO bid reduces urinary osmolality and increases serum sodium levels. It may be useful in patients with chronic SIAD (e.g., secondary to neoplasm) but use with caution in patients with hepatic disease; its side effects include nephrogenic diabetes insipidus (DI) and photosensitivity. This medication is also very expensive.
- Successful treatment of chronic nephrogenic SIAD with urea to induce osmotic diuresis has been reported in children and adults. However, oral intake of urea (30 g/day) is generally poorly tolerated.

DISPOSITION

- Prognosis varies depending on the cause. Generally, prognosis is benign when SIAD is caused by an infectious process.
- Morbidity and mortality are high (>40%) when serum sodium concentration is <110 mEq/L.

REFERRAL

Hospital admission depending on severity of symptoms and degree of hyponatremia

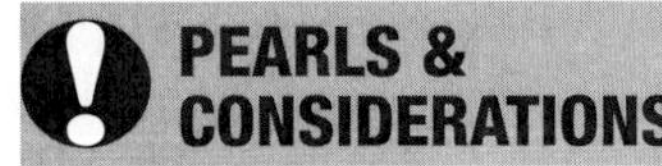

PEARLS & CONSIDERATIONS

COMMENTS

- Use of hypertonic (3%) saline is contraindicated in patients with CHF, nephrotic syndrome, or cirrhosis.
- Too rapid correction of hyponatremia can cause demyelination and permanent central nervous system damage.

SUGGESTED READING

Ellison DH, Berl T: The syndrome of inappropriate antidiuresis, *N Engl J Med* 356:2064-2072, 2007.

AUTHOR: **FRED F. FERRI, M.D.**

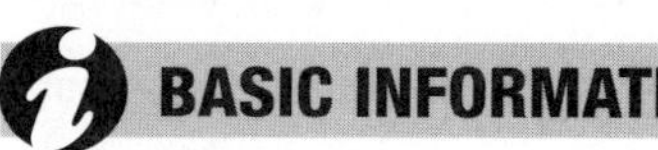

BASIC INFORMATION

DEFINITION

Syphilis is a sexually transmitted treponemal disease, acute and chronic, characterized by primary skin lesions; secondary eruption involving skin and mucous membranes; long periods of latency; and late lesions of the skin, bone, viscera, central nervous system, and cardiovascular system.

SYNONYMS

Lues

ICD-9CM CODES

097.9 Syphilis, acquired unspecified

EPIDEMIOLOGY & DEMOGRAPHICS

- Widespread, primarily involving ages 20 to 35 yr. Racial differences in incidence are related to social factors. Usually more prevalent in urban areas. Estimated annual incidence of 90,000 cases in the U.S. Increase in incidence in the late 1980s to 1990s, likely related to illicit drug use and prostitution. Increase occurred primarily in lower socioeconomic groups.
- Communicability is indefinite and variable. Communicable during primary, secondary, and latent mucocutaneous lesions in up to first 4 yr of latency. Most probable congenital transmission occurs in early maternal syphilis. Adequate penicillin treatment ends infectivity within 24 to 48 hr.

PHYSICAL FINDINGS & CLINICAL PRESENTATION

PRIMARY SYPHILIS: Characteristic lesion is a painless chancre on genitalia, mouth, or anus; atypical primary lesions may occur. Usually appears 3 wk after exposure and may spontaneously involute.

SECONDARY SYPHILIS:

- Localized or diffuse mucocutaneous lesions and generalized lymphadenopathy. Common to have constitutional symptoms, flulike symptoms. May begin approximately 4 to 6 wk after appearance of primary lesion. Manifestations may resolve in 1 wk to 12 mo.
- 60% to 80% of patients have maculopapular lesions on their palms and soles.
- Condylomata lata intertriginous papules form at areas of friction and moisture, such as the vulva.
- 21% to 58% have mucocutaneous or mucosal lesions (pharyngitis, tonsillitis, "mucous patch" lesion on oral and genital mucosa).

EARLY LATENT (≤1 YR): Generally asymptomatic

LATE LATENT (>1 YR):

- Characterized by gummas (nodular, ulcerative lesions) that can involve the skin, mucous membranes, skeletal system, and viscera.
- Manifestations of cardiovascular syphilis include aortitis, aneurysm, or aortic regurgitation.
- Neurosyphilis may be asymptomatic or symptomatic. Tabes dorsalis, meningovascular syphilis, general paralysis, or insanity may occur. Iritis, choroidoretinitis, and leukoplakia may also occur.

ETIOLOGY

- *Treponema pallidum,* a spirochete
- Spread by sexual intercourse or by intrauterine transfer

DIAGNOSIS

DIFFERENTIAL DIAGNOSIS

- Other genitoulcerative diseases such as herpes, chancroid (see Section II)
- See Section III for a clinical algorithm for the evaluation of genital ulcer disease

WORKUP

Confirmation is primarily through laboratory diagnosis.

LABORATORY TESTS

- Dark-field microscopy of fluid from lesion to look for treponeme
- Serologic testing, both nontreponemal (VDRL, RPR) and treponemal (FTA, MHA)
- Lumbar puncture for cerebrospinal fluid VDRL in patients with evidence of latent syphilis

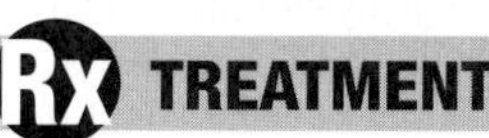

TREATMENT

ACUTE GENERAL Rx

- Early (primary, secondary, early latent): penicillin G benzathine 2.4 million U IM × 1 or doxycycline 100 mg PO bid × 14 days
- Late (late latent, cardiovascular, gumma): penicillin G benzathine 2.4 million U IM qwk × 3 wk or doxycycline 100 mg PO bid × 4 wk
- Neurosyphilis: aqueous crystalline penicillin G 18 to 24 million U/day, administered as 3 to 4 million U IV q4h × 10 to 14 days or procaine penicillin 2.4 million U IM/day plus probenecid 500 mg PO qid, both for 10 to 14 days
- Congenital syphilis: aqueous crystalline penicillin G 50,000 U/kg/dose IV q12h × first 7 days of life and q8h after that for total of 10 days or procaine penicillin G 50,000 U/kg/dose IM/day × 10 days
- Penicillin-allergic patients with primary or secondary syphilis: doxycycline 100 mg PO bid × 14 days, or tetracycline 500 mg PO qid × 14 days, or ceftriaxone 1 g IM or IV × 8 to 10 days, or azithromycin 2 g PO stat (preliminary data only)
- Latent syphilis in penicillin-allergic patient: doxycycline 100 mg PO bid or tetracycline 500 mg qid for 28 days
- Tetracyclines are contraindicated in pregnancy. If pregnant and penicillin allergic, must be desensitized prior to treatment.

DISPOSITION

- Repeat quantitative nontreponemal tests at 3, 6, and 12 mo. Pregnancy requires monthly tests until delivery.
- If a fourfold increase in titer occurs, if initial high titer fails to drop by fourfold within a year, or signs persist retreatment may be indicated. Use treatment regimen for late syphilis.
- Pregnant women without a fourfold drop in titer in a 3-mo period need to be retreated.
- Cases should be reported to local or state health department for referral, follow-up, and partner notification.

REFERRAL

- Pregnant and possible congenital syphilis
- Pregnant and allergic to penicillin, with need to be desensitized
- Late latent syphilis with serious central nervous system, cardiovascular, or other organ system compromise

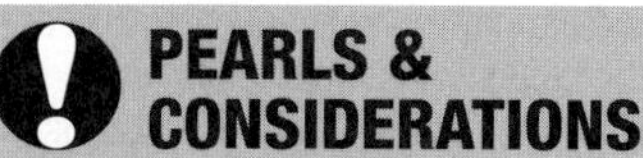

PEARLS & CONSIDERATIONS

- Jarisch-Herxheimer reaction (fever, myalgia, tachycardia, hypotension) may occur within 24 hr of treatment.
- One third of untreated patients develop central nervous system and/or cardiovascular sequelae.
- Up to 80% of those treated during late stages remain seropositive indefinitely.
- Treponemal tests remain positive even after adequate therapy.
- Male circumcision does not decrease the incidence of syphilis (unlike HIV, HSV-2, and HPV infection)

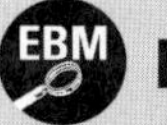

EVIDENCE

Parenteral penicillin-G is the preferred drug for treatment of all stages of syphilis. Evidence for the efficacy of penicillin in the treatment of syphilis is based on expert opinion and is reinforced by case series, clinical trials, and 50 years of clinical experience.[1] Ⓒ

There is little evidence to support the use of alternatives to penicillin in the treatment of early syphilis. Doxycycline and tetracycline are regimens that have been used for many years for nonpregnant penicillin-allergic patients with primary or secondary syphilis.[1] Ⓒ

Evidence-Based Reference

1. Centers for Disease Control and Prevention; Workowski KA, Berman SM: Sexually Transmitted Diseases Treatment Guidelines, 2006, *MMWR Recomm Rep* 55(RR-11):1-94, 2006. Ⓒ

SUGGESTED READINGS

Centers for Disease Control and Prevention: 2006. sexually transmitted diseases treatment guidelines, *MMWR* 55:(RR-11), 2006.

Tobian AA et al: Male circumcision for the prevention of HSV-2 and HPV infections and syphilis, *N Engl J Med* 360:1298-1309, 2009.

AUTHORS: **MARIA A. CORIGLIANO, M.D.,** and **RUBEN ALVERO, M.D.**

BASIC INFORMATION

DEFINITION

Syringomyelia is a disease of the spine characterized by the formation of fluid-filled cavities within the spinal cord, sometimes extending into the brain stem.

ICD-9CM CODES
336.0 Syringomyelia

PHYSICAL FINDINGS & CLINICAL PRESENTATION

- Onset is usually insidious, with symptoms often not beginning until the third or fourth decade.
- Cervical spine is the most commonly affected area.
  1. Intrinsic hand atrophy, weakness, and anesthetic sensory loss may develop.
  2. The latter may lead to unnoticed burns or other injuries in the hand.
  3. Loss of pain and temperature sensation may occur, but tactile sense in the upper extremity is preserved.
  4. Sharp testing elicits no pain, but patient often perceives the sharpness of the object.
  5. A Charcot joint in the shoulder or elbow may develop.
- Reflexes are absent in the upper extremity.
- Spasticity and hyperreflexia are present in the lower extremity.
- Scoliosis is common.
- Nystagmus and Horner's syndrome may also occur.
- Trophic skin changes eventually develop in many cases.

ETIOLOGY

- Cause is unknown, but condition is believed to result from obstruction of the outlet of the fourth ventricle, often associated with a Chiari I malformation, which causes fluid to be diverted down the central cord.
- A history of birth injury often exists.
- Syringes later in life may be the result of trauma or an intramedullary tumor.

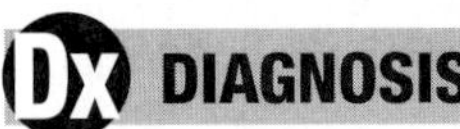

DIAGNOSIS

DIFFERENTIAL DIAGNOSIS

- Amyotrophic lateral sclerosis
- Multiple sclerosis
- Spinal cord tumor
- Tabes dorsalis
- Progressive spinal muscular atrophy

WORKUP

- Plain radiographs usually reveal widening of the bony canal in the region of involvement.
- Bony anomalies are often present at the base of the skull and at the C1-C2 spinal segments.
- Myelography, MRI (Fig. 1-324), and other imaging studies are recommended.

Rx TREATMENT

Drainage and operative repair of any bony anomalies are undertaken, often with decompression laminectomy of C1 and C2.

DISPOSITION

- Condition is slowly progressive in most cases but course may be quite variable, ranging from death in a few months to slow incapacitation over several years; progression may halt at any time.
- Surgical intervention often stops progression but frequently does not lead to improvement in neurologic findings.

REFERRAL

For neurosurgical consultation when diagnosis is suspected

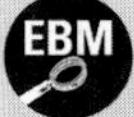

EVIDENCE

Ergun et al. reviewed their surgical results in 18 patients with syringomyelia-Chiari complex who underwent foramen magnum decompression and syringosubarachnoid shunting. Sixteen patients improved and there was no change in two patients.[1]

Di Lorenzo et al. prospectively evaluated 20 patients with syringomyelia-Chiari I complex who underwent surgery. After an average follow-up of 2.4 yr, eight patients were improved and 11 stabilized.[2]

Rauzzino and Oakes reviewed several studies on patients with syringomyelia and Chiari II malformations treated surgically, all showing positive results with favorable outcomes.[3]

Evidence-Based References

1. Ergun R et al: Surgical management of syringomyelia-Chiari complex, *Eur Spine J* 9(6):553, 2000.
2. Di Lorenzo N et al: "Conservative" craniocervical decompression in the treatment of syringomyelia-Chiari I complex. A prospective study of 20 adult cases, *Spine* 20:2479, 1995.
3. Rauzzino M, Oakes WJ: Chiari II malformation and syringomyelia, *Neurosurg Clin N Am* 6:293, 1995.

SUGGESTED READINGS

Akhtar OH, Rowe DE: Syringomyelia-associated scoliosis with and without the Chiari I malformation, *J Am Acad Orthop Surg* 16:407, 2008.

Chu WC et al: A detailed morphologic and functional magnetic resonance imaging study of the craniocervical junction in adolescent idiopathic scoliosis, *Spine* 32(15):1667, 2007.

Fernandez AA et al: Malformations of the craniocervical junction (Chiari type I and syringomyelia: classification, diagnosis, and treatment), *BMC Musculoskelet Disord* 10(Suppl 1):51, 2009.

Klekamp J: The pathophysiology of syringomyelia: historical overview and current concepts, *Acta Neurochir* 144(7):649, 2002.

Mallucci C, Brodbelt A: The enigma of syringomyelia, *Br J Neurosurg* 21:423, 2007.

Riente L et al: Neuropathic shoulder arthropathy associated with syringomyelia and Arnold-Chiari malformation (type I), *J Rheumatol* 29(3):638, 2002.

Wang R et al: Atypical syringomyelia without cavity in a patient with Chiari malformation and hydrocephalus, *Spine* 32(16):467, 2007.

AUTHOR: **LONNIE R. MERCIER, M.D.**

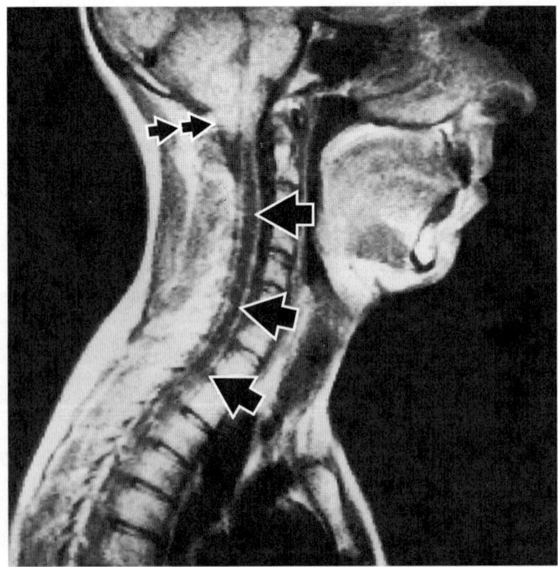

FIGURE 1-324 Midsagittal magnetic resonance image of Arnold-Chiari malformation *(small black arrows)* and syringomyelia *(three large black arrows)* in a 31-yr-old man. Note the cerebellar tonsils extending below the posterior rim of the foramen magnum (*dark structure* immediately above the *black arrow*). The syrinx extends from the medulla well into the thoracic cord. (From Andreoli TE [ed]: *Cecil essentials of medicine,* ed 4, Philadelphia, 1997, WB Saunders.)

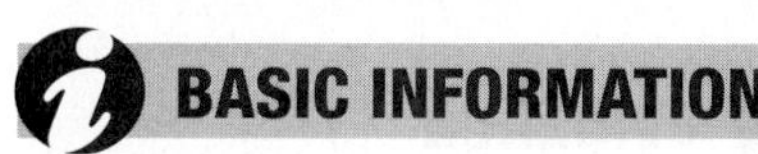

BASIC INFORMATION

DEFINITION

Systemic lupus erythematosus (SLE) is a chronic, multisystemic disease characterized by production of autoantibodies and protean clinical manifestations.

SYNONYMS

SLE

ICD-9CM CODES
710.0 Systemic lupus erythematosus

EPIDEMIOLOGY & DEMOGRAPHICS

PREVALENCE: 20 cases per 100,000 persons. Ethnic groups, such as those of African or Asian ancestry, are at greatest risk of developing the disorder.
PREDOMINANT SEX: Female/male ratio of 9:1
PREDOMINANT AGE: 20 to 45 yr (childbearing years)

PHYSICAL FINDINGS & CLINICAL PRESENTATION

- Skin: erythematous rash over the malar eminences (Fig. 1-325), generally with sparing of the nasolabial folds (butterfly rash); alopecia; raised erythematous patches with subsequent edematous plaques and adherent scales (discoid lupus); leg, nasal, or oropharyngeal ulcerations; livedo reticularis; pallor (from anemia); petechiae (from thrombocytopenia)
- Joints: tenderness, swelling, or effusion, generally involving peripheral joints
- Cardiac: pericardial rub (in patients with pericarditis), heart murmurs (if endocarditis or valvular thickening or dysfunction)
- Other: fever, conjunctivitis, dry eyes, dry mouth (sicca syndrome), oral ulcers, abdominal tenderness, decreased breath sounds (pleural effusions)

ETIOLOGY

Unknown. Autoantibodies are typically present many years before the diagnosis of SLE. A haplotype of STAT4 is associated with increased risk for both rheumatoid arthritis and SLE, suggesting a shared pathway for these illnesses. Genetic susceptibility to lupus is inherited as a complex trait. An interval on the long arm of chromosome 1, 1q23-24 has been linked with SLE in many populations.

Dx DIAGNOSIS

DIFFERENTIAL DIAGNOSIS

- Other connective tissue disorders (e.g., rheumatoid arthritis, mixed connective tissue disease, progressive systemic sclerosis)
- Metastatic neoplasm
- Infection

WORKUP

The diagnosis of SLE can be made by demonstrating the presence of any four or more of the following criteria of the American Rheumatism Association:

1. Butterfly rash
2. Discoid rash
3. Photosensitivity (particularly leg ulcerations)
4. Oral ulcers
5. Arthritis
6. Serositis (pleuritis, pericarditis)
7. Renal disorder (persistent proteinuria >0.5 g/day or 3+ if quantitation not performed, cellular casts)
8. Neurologic disorder (seizures, psychosis [in absence of offending drugs or metabolic derangement])
9. Hematologic disorder:
   a. Hemolytic anemia with reticulocytosis
   b. Leukopenia (<4000/mm^3 total on two or more occasions)
   c. Lymphopenia (<1500/mm^3 on two or more occasions)
   d. Thrombocytopenia (<100,000/mm^3 in the absence of offending drugs)
10. Immunologic disorder:
    a. Positive SLE cell preparation
    b. Anti-DNA (presence of antibody to native DNA in abnormal titer)
    c. Anti-Sm (presence of antibody to Smith nuclear antigen)
    d. False-positive STS known to be positive for at least 6 mo and confirmed by negative TPI or FTA tests
11. Antinuclear antibody (ANA): an abnormal titer of ANA by immunofluorescence or equivalent assay at any time in the absence of drugs known to be associated with "drug-induced lupus" syndrome

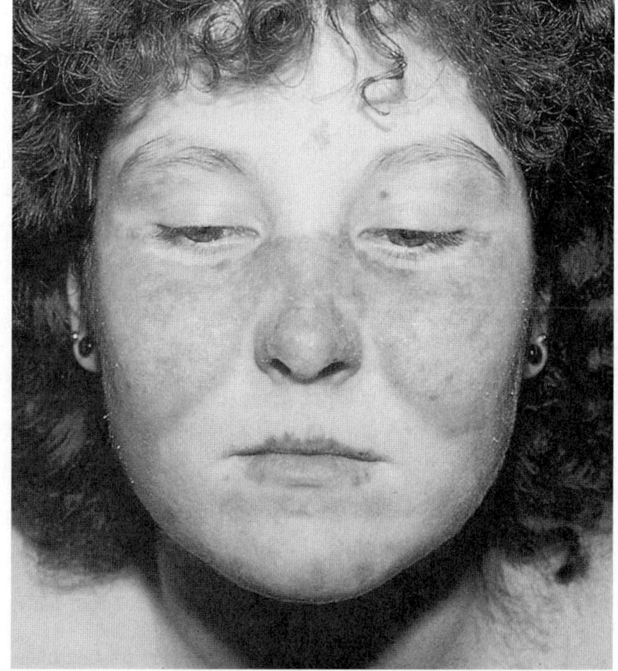

FIGURE 1-325 Acute cutaneous lupus erythematosus (LE) (systemic LE). The classic butterfly rash occurs in 10% to 50% of patients with acute LE. (From Habif TP: *Clinical dermatology: a color guide to diagnosis and therapy,* ed 3, St Louis, 1996, Mosby.)

LABORATORY TESTS

Suggested initial laboratory evaluation of suspected SLE:

- Immunologic evaluation: ANA, anti-DNA antibody, anti-Sm antibody
- Other laboratory tests: complete blood count with differential, platelet count (Coombs test if anemia detected), urinalysis (24-hr urine collection for protein if proteinuria is detected), partial thromboplastin time and anticardiolipin antibodies in patients with thrombotic events, blood urea nitrogen, creatinine to evaluate renal function

IMAGING STUDIES

- Chest radiograph for evaluation of pulmonary involvement (e.g., pleural effusions, pulmonary infiltrates)
- Echocardiogram to screen for significant valvular heart disease (present in 18% of patients with SLE); echocardiography can identify a subset of lesions (valvular thickening and dysfunction) other than verrucous (Libman-Sacks) endocarditis that are prone to hemodynamic deterioration

Rx TREATMENT

NONPHARMACOLOGIC THERAPY

Patients with photosensitivity should avoid sunlight and use high-factor sunscreen.

GENERAL Rx

- Joint pain and mild serositis are generally well controlled with nonsteroidal antiinflammatory drugs; antimalarials are also effective (e.g., hydroxychloroquine [Plaquenil]).
- Cutaneous manifestations are treated with the following:
  1. Topical corticosteroids; intradermal corticosteroids are helpful for individual discoid lesions, especially in the scalp
  2. Antimalarials (e.g., hydroxychloroquine [Plaquenil] and quinacrine)

3. Sunscreens that block ultraviolet (UV) A and UVB radiation
4. Immunosuppressive drugs (methotrexate or azathioprine) are used as steroid-sparing drugs

- Renal disease (lupus nephritis)
  1. The use of high-pulsed doses of cyclophosphamide given at monthly intervals is more effective in preserving renal function than is treatment with glucocorticoids alone. The present standard of care with monthly high-dose IV cyclophosphamide has been challenged on several fronts. Alternative ways of administering cyclophosphamide in much lower doses for shorter periods have emerged. The combination of methylprednisolone and cyclophosphamide is superior to bolus therapy with methylprednisolone or cyclophosphamide alone in patients with lupus nephritis. For patients with proliferative lupus nephritis, short-term therapy with IV cyclophosphamide followed by maintenance therapy with mycophenolate mofetil or azathioprine appears to be more efficacious and safer than long-term therapy with IV cyclophosphamide. In the treatment of severe proliferative lupus nephritis, mycophenolate mofetil represents an excellent alternative to cyclophosphamide.
  2. The use of plasmapheresis in combination with immunosuppressive agents (to prevent the rebound phenomenon of antibody levels after plasmapheresis) is generally reserved for rapidly progressive renal failure or life-threatening systemic vasculitis.
- Central nervous system involvement: treatment generally consists of corticosteroid therapy; however, its efficacy is uncertain, and it is generally reserved for organic brain syndrome. Anticonvulsants and antipsychotics are also indicated in selected cases; headaches are treated symptomatically.
- Hemolytic anemia: treatment of Coombs-positive hemolytic anemia consists of high doses of corticosteroids; nonhemolytic anemia (secondary to chronic disease) does not require specific therapy.
- Thrombocytopenia
  1. Initial treatment consists of corticosteroids.
  2. In patients with poor response to steroids, encouraging results have been reported with the use of danazol, vincristine, and immunoglobulins. Combination chemotherapy with cyclophosphamide and prednisone combined with vincristine, vincristine and procarbazine, or etoposide may be useful in patients with severe refractory idiopathic thrombocytopenic purpura.
  3. Splenectomy generally does not cure the thrombocytopenia of SLE, but it may be necessary as an adjunct in managing selected cases.
- Infections are common because of compromised immune function secondary to SLE and the use of corticosteroid, cytotoxic, and antimetabolite drugs; pneumococcal bacteremia is associated with high mortality rate.
- Close monitoring for exacerbation of the disease and for potential side effects from medications (corticosteroids, cytotoxic agents) with frequent laboratory evaluation and office visits is necessary in all patients with SLE.
- Valvular heart disease is present in 18% of patients with SLE. The prevalence of infective endocarditis is approximately 1% (similar to the prevalence after prosthetic valve surgery, but greater than that after rheumatic valvulitis). Valvular heart disease in patients with SLE frequently changes over time (e.g., vegetations can appear unexpectedly for the first time, resolve, or change in size or appearance). These frequent changes are temporarily unrelated to other clinical features of SLE and can be associated with substantial morbidity and mortality rates.
- Newer treatment modalities include the use of rituximab (a chimeric human-murine monoclonal antibody directed against CD20 on B cells and their precursors) to induce substantial remissions in patients previously unresponsive to conventional agents. Intravenous immunoglobulins are also increasingly being used in the treatment of patients with resistant lupus.

DISPOSITION

- Most patients with SLE experience remissions and exacerbations.
- The leading cause of death in SLE is infection (one third of all deaths); active nephritis causes approximately 18% of deaths, and central nervous system disease causes 7% of deaths; the survival rate is 75% over the first 10 yr. Blacks and Hispanics generally have a worse prognosis.
- Symptomatic pericarditis occurs in one fourth of patients with SLE at some point during the course of the disease. Asymptomatic involvement is estimated to be more than 60% based on autopsy reports.
- Renal histologic studies and evaluation of renal function are useful in determining disease activity and predicting disease outcome (e.g., serum creatinine levels >3 mg/dl or evidence of diffuse proliferative involvement on renal biopsy are poor prognostic factors).
- Atherosclerosis occurs prematurely in patients with SLE and is independent of traditional risk factors for cardiovascular disease.
- Antiphospholipid syndrome with thrombotic manifestations is a major predictor of irreversible organ damage and death in patients with SLE.

REFERRAL

- Rheumatology consultation in all patients with SLE
- Hematology consultation in patients with significant hematologic abnormalities (e.g., severe hemolytic anemia or thrombocytopenia)
- Nephrology consultation in patients with significant renal involvement

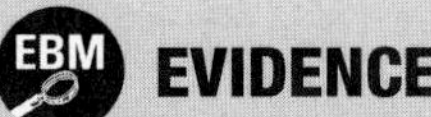

EVIDENCE

Much of the evidence for therapies in people with SLE is the result of a small number of trials with few patients.

Proliferative Lupus Nephritis

There is evidence that cyclophosphamide plus corticosteroids reduces the risk of doubling serum creatinine compared with corticosteroids alone in people with proliferative lupus nephritis.[1] A

From the current evidence, it has been suggested that cyclophosphamide combined with corticosteroids is the best option for preserving renal function but that the smallest effective dose and the shortest duration of treatment should be used.[1]

There is also evidence that azathioprine plus corticosteroids reduces the risk of death from any cause compared with corticosteroids alone, but a systematic review found that it had no impact on renal outcomes.[1] A

Results from a single randomized, controlled trial have indicated that for patients with proliferative lupus nephritis, short-term therapy with IV cyclophosphamide followed by maintenance therapy with mycophenolate mofetil or azathioprine may be more efficacious and safer than long-term therapy with IV cyclophosphamide.[2] B

Neuropsychiatric Involvement of SLE

An randomized, controlled trial of 32 patients with SLE and neuropsychiatric involvement found a significantly higher number of treatment responders with cyclophosphamide compared with methylprednisolone.[3] B

Methotrexate Therapy

The evidence for the benefit of methotrexate in people with SLE and active skin and joint disease is supported by several uncontrolled case series and a single retrospective cohort study.[4]

However, three prospective, randomized trials have reported conflicting results concerning methotrexate therapy in SLE.[4]

Evidence-Based References

1. Flanc RS et al : Treatment for lupus nephritis, *Cochrane Rev* 1, 2004.
2. Contreras G et al: Sequential therapies for proliferative lupus nephritis, *N Engl J Med* 350:971, 2004.
3. Trevisani VFM et al: Cyclophosphamide versus methylprednisolone for treating neuropsychiatric involvement in systemic lupus erythematosus, *Cochrane Rev* 2, 2006.
4. Wong JM, Esdaile JM: Methotrexate in systemic lupus erythematosus, *Lupus* 14:101, 2005.

SUGGESTED READINGS

D'Cruz DP et al: Systemic lupus erythematosus, *Lancet* 369:587, 2007.
Fine DM: Pharmacologic therapy of lupus nephritis, *JAMA* 293:3053, 2005.
Remmers EF et al: STAT4 and the risk of rheumatoid arthritis and systemic lupus erythematosus, *N Engl J Med* 357:977, 2007.

AUTHOR: **FRED F. FERRI, M.D.**

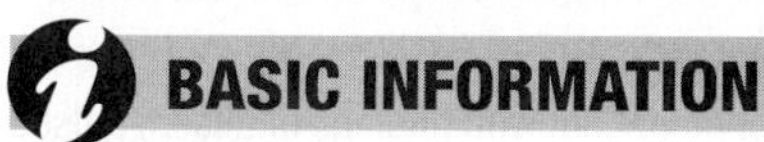

BASIC INFORMATION

DEFINITION

Tabes dorsalis is a form of tertiary neurosyphilis affecting the dorsal columns of the spinal cord and peripheral nerves, characterized by paroxysmal pain, particularly in the abdomen and legs; sensory ataxia; normal strength; autonomic dysfunction; and Argyll-Robertson pupils.

SYNONYMS

Posterior spinal sclerosis
Tabetic neurosyphilis
Syphilitic myeloneuropathy

ICD-9CM CODES
094.0 Tabes dorsalis, ataxia, locomotor

EPIDEMIOLOGY & DEMOGRAPHICS

INCIDENCE (IN U.S.): Rare, but increasing with HIV/AIDS

PEAK INCIDENCE: 15 to 20 yr after initial infection

PREVALENCE (IN U.S.): Rare; more common with HIV/AIDS epidemic. Ten percent of untreated patients with syphilis develop neurosyphilis, 2% to 5% of whom may develop tabes dorsalis. Relative prevalence of tabes dorsalis is reduced compared with the preantibiotic era. This may be the only clinical manifestation of neurosyphilis that has been altered during the antibiotic era.

PREDOMINANT SEX: Male

PHYSICAL FINDINGS & CLINICAL PRESENTATION

- Argyll-Robertson pupils are common (pupil reacts poorly to light but well to accommodation)
- Loss of position and vibration at ankles (wide-based gait, inability to walk in the dark, sensory ataxia)
- Loss of deep pain sensation, resulting in deep foot ulcers
- Degenerative joint disease, especially in knees, caused by severe neuropathy (Charcot joints)
- Normal strength with areflexia in the legs
- Lightning pains in the legs
- Severe intermittent visceral pains, such as gastrointestinal and laryngeal (visceral crises)
- Autonomic dysfunction (urinary and fecal incontinence)

ETIOLOGY

Infectious *(Treponema pallidum)*

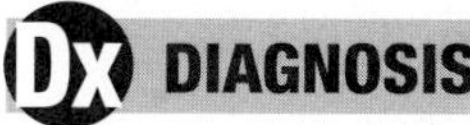

DIAGNOSIS

DIFFERENTIAL DIAGNOSIS

- Vitamin B_{12} deficiency (subacute combined degeneration of the spinal cord)
- Vitamin E deficiency
- Chronic nitrous oxide abuse
- Spinal cord neoplasm (involving conus medullaris)
- Lyme's disease

WORKUP

Thorough neurologic history and examination

LABORATORY TESTS

- Lumbar puncture for elevated Venereal Disease Research Laboratory (VDRL) and Fluorescent Treponemal Antigen-Antibody test (FTA-ABS) titers. False-positive cerebrospinal fluid (CSF) VDRL titers may occur with traumatic tap. CSF mononuclear pleocytosis (>5 white cells/mcL) with increased protein support the diagnosis.
- Serum VDRL test. Results may be normal in 25% to 30% of patients. Serum microhemagglutination-*Treponema pallidum* (MHA-TP) or FTA-ABS is necessary if clinical suspicion high.
- False-positive serum VDRL may occur in Lyme disease, nonvenereal treponematoses, genital herpes simplex, pregnancy, systemic lupus erythematosus, alcoholic cirrhosis, scleroderma, and mixed connective tissue disease.

IMAGING STUDIES

Not necessary if diagnosis confirmed

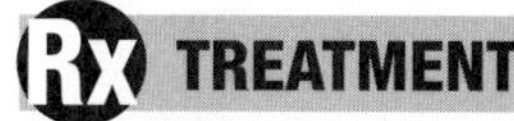

TREATMENT

ACUTE GENERAL Rx

- Procaine penicillin 2 to 4 million U IM qd, along with probenecid 500 mg PO qid, for 14 days or aqueous penicillin G 3 to 4 million U IV q4h for 10 to 14 days.
- If patient is penicillin allergic, doxycycline 200 mg PO bid for 4 wk.
- Many of the symptoms—degenerative neuropathic joint disease, lightning pains—persist after treatment.

CHRONIC Rx

- Physical therapy
- Analgesics, carbamazepine, gabapentin, or steroids may help lightning pain
- Supportive care (wheelchair, toileting issues, etc.)

DISPOSITION

- Close follow-up required. Repeat lumbar puncture is recommended every 6 mo until CSF pleocytosis normalizes. If pleocytosis does not normalize in 6 mo or CSF is still abnormal in 2 yr, repeat treatment.
- Further indication for retreatment: if there is a fourfold increase in titers or a failure of titers >1:32 to decrease at least fourfold by 12 to 24 mo.

REFERRAL

Joint replacement in moderate cases

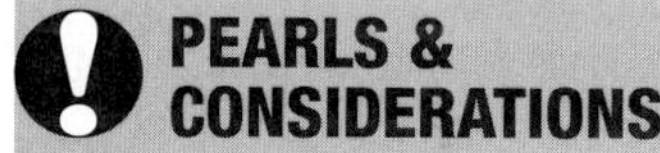

PEARLS & CONSIDERATIONS

COMMENTS

Diagnosis should be considered in all patients with a progressive neuropsychiatric disorder with signs of spinal cord dysfunction and peripheral neuropathy.

SUGGESTED READINGS

Centers for Disease Control and Prevention: 2002 sexually transmitted diseases treatment guidelines, *MMWR* 51:(RR-6), 2002.

Conde-Sendin MA et al: Current clinical spectrum of neurosyphilis in immunocompetent patients, *Eur Neurol* 52:29, 2004.

Timmermans M, Carr J: Neurosyphilis in the modern era, *J Neurol Neurosurg Psychiatry* 75:1727, 2004.

AUTHOR: **EROBOGHENE E. UBOGU, M.D.**

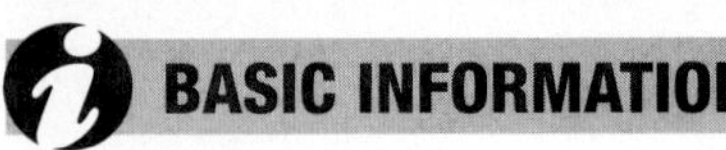

BASIC INFORMATION

DEFINITION

Takayasu's arteritis is a chronic systemic granulomatous vasculitis that primarily affects the aorta and its primary branches. It often presents as a pulseless disease caused by widespread arterial stenosis.

SYNONYMS

Pulseless disease
Aortitis syndrome
Aortic arch arteritis

ICD-9CM CODES
446.7 Takayasu disease or syndrome

EPIDEMIOLOGY & DEMOGRAPHICS

- Most cases have been reported in Japan, China, India, and Mexico.
- The incidence in the U.S. is 2.6/1 million persons.
- The female/male ratio is 9:1.
- The age of onset is usually between 10 and 40 yr.

PHYSICAL FINDINGS & CLINICAL PRESENTATION

- The early phase of Takayasu's arteritis often manifests as constitutional symptoms, including the following:
  1. Low-grade fever
  2. Malaise
  3. Weight loss
  4. Fatigue
  5. Arthralgia and myalgia
- Takayasu's arteritis most frequently involves the aorta and its primary branches. The condition can manifest as follows:
  - Arm or leg claudication, weakness, and numbness
  - Amaurosis fugax, diplopia, headache, orthostasis, vertigo, or syncope
  - Vascular bruits of the carotid artery, subclavian artery, and aorta
  - Discrepancy of blood pressures between the upper extremities, typically of >10 mm Hg
  - Diminished or absent pulses, ischemic ulcerations, or gangrene in advanced disease
  - Hypertension
  - Retinopathy
  - Aortic insufficiency murmur as a result of aortic root dilatation after aortitis and aneurysm formation

ETIOLOGY

- The cause of Takayasu's arteritis is poorly understood. Cell-mediated mechanisms are thought to be important to the pathogenesis.
- The infiltration of inflammatory cells into the vasa vasorum and media of the large elastic arteries leads to thickening and narrowing or obliteration as well as aneurysmal dilation of the affected arteries.

Dx DIAGNOSIS

Diagnostic criteria for Takayasu's arteritis were established by the American College of Rheumatology in 1990 and include the following:

- Age of disease onset <40 yr
- Claudication of extremities
- Decreased brachial artery pulse
- Systolic blood pressure difference >10 mm Hg between left and right arms
- Bruit over subclavian arteries or abdominal aorta
- Abnormal arteriogram

Takayasu's arteritis is diagnosed if at least three of the six criteria are present; this results in a sensitivity of 90% and a specificity of 98%.

DIFFERENTIAL DIAGNOSIS

Other causes of inflammatory aortitis must be excluded:

- Giant cell arteritis
- Syphilis
- Tuberculosis
- Systemic lupus erythematosus
- Rheumatoid arthritis
- Buerger's disease
- Behçet's disease
- Cogan's syndrome
- Kawasaki disease
- Spondyloarthropathies

WORKUP

Any young patient with findings of absent pulses and loud bruits merits a workup for Takayasu's arteritis. The workup generally includes blood testing to look for signs of inflammation as well as imaging studies, with the angiogram being the diagnostic gold standard.

LABORATORY TESTS

- A CBC may reveal a normal or elevated white blood cell count as well as anemia of chronic disease.
- Erythrocyte sedimentation rate (ESR) and serum C-reactive protein levels are usually elevated, which reflects the presence of an inflammatory process

IMAGING STUDIES

- Ultrasound: Carotid, thoracic, and abdominal ultrasound are useful adjunctive imaging studies to diagnose the occlusive disease that results from Takayasu's arteritis (Fig. 1-326).
- Doppler and noninvasive upper and lower extremity studies are helpful to assess blood flow and absent pulses.
- Computed tomographic scanning and MRI may be used to assess the thickness of the large arteries.

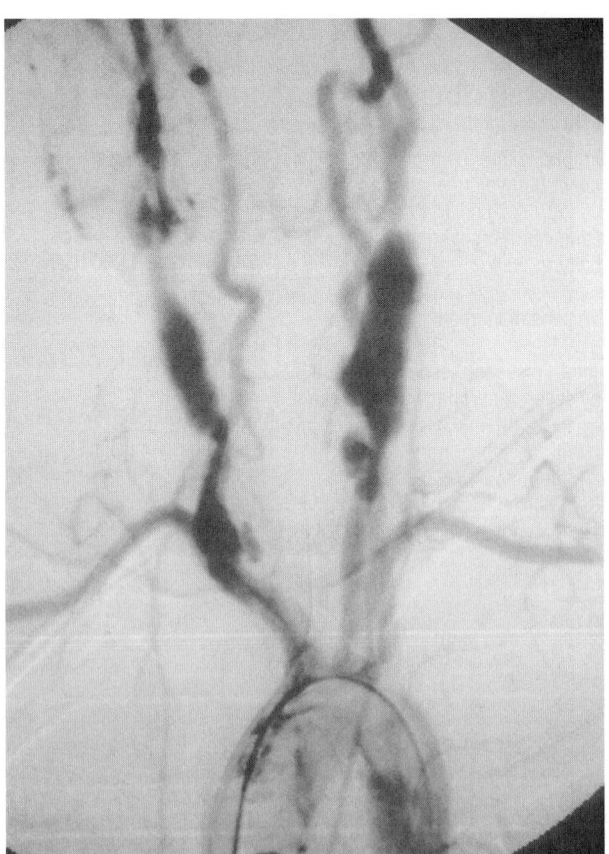

FIGURE 1-326 An angiogram of a child with Takayasu's arteritis that shows massive bilateral carotid dilation, stenosis, and poststenotic dilation. (From Behrman RE: *Nelson textbook of pediatrics,* ed 16, Philadelphia, 2000, WB Saunders.)

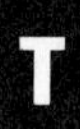

- Angiography can show the narrowing of the aorta and its branches, aneurysm formation, and poststenotic dilation. Collateral circulation may also be visualized. Angiographic findings are classified into four types:
  1. Type I: lesions that involve only the aortic arch and its branches
  2. Type II: lesions that involve only the abdominal aorta and its branches
  3. Type III: lesions that involve the aorta above and below the diaphragm
  4. Type IV: lesions that involve the pulmonary artery

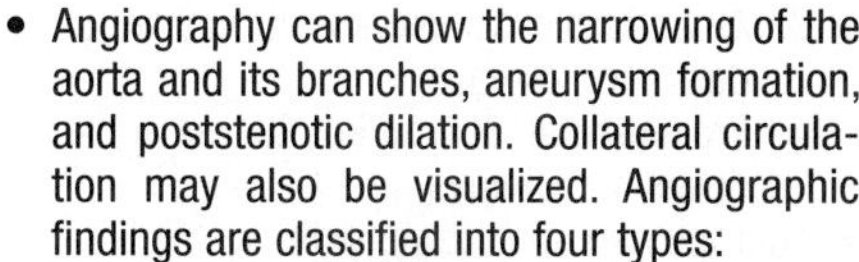

TREATMENT

ACUTE GENERAL RX

- Glucocorticoids are effective to suppress systemic symptoms and to stop the progression of Takayasu's arteritis. Prednisone (40 to 60 mg PO daily or 1 mg/kg/day) can be used for 3 months.
- Patients are monitored for symptoms and ESR. Attempts to taper prednisone can be made in accordance with the resolution of constitutional symptoms and a decrease in ESR and C-reactive protein levels.

CHRONIC RX

- Long-term low-dose prednisone may be necessary to stop the progression of arterial stenoses.
- Methotrexate, azathioprine, or antitumor necrosis factor can be given as adjunctive therapy with glucocorticoids to patients who are in relapse or resistant to other treatments. There is limited experience with cyclophosphamide.
- Percutaneous angioplasty or bypass grafts should be considered for irreversible arterial stenoses with severe ischemia.
- Aortic regurgitation may require valve replacement or repair by surgery.

DISPOSITION

- Treatment improves symptoms within days, with the relief of ischemic claudication, the return of pulses on examination, and the reversal of lumen narrowing on angiograms. However, some patients may continue to have a progression of arterial lesions, despite therapy.
- With the addition of a second agent for patients with treatment resistance or relapse, 50% remission has been seen.
- Quality of life is comparable to that of patients with rheumatoid arthritis or ankylosing spondylitis.
- Mortality results are mixed, with high rates in reports from Asia and lower rates in studies performed in the U.S. (2%).
- Death can occur suddenly from a ruptured aneurysm, a myocardial infarction, or a stroke.

REFERRAL

Whenever the diagnosis of vasculitis is suspected, a rheumatology consultation is appropriate. Vascular surgery and cardiology consultations are recommended for any evidence of carotid, peripheral, or coronary artery disease or if a large abdominal aneurysm is found.

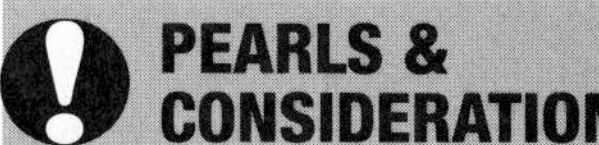

PEARLS & CONSIDERATIONS

With long-term glucocorticoid use, consider measures to protect against bone loss. Bisphosphonates have been studied prospectively with corticosteroid use in this fashion; remember to ensure adequate dietary calcium and vitamin D intake as well.

COMMENTS

The long-term prognosis of patients with treated Takayasu's disease is good, with >90% of patients surviving more than 15 yr.

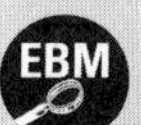

EVIDENCE

A 1991 series involving 26 Mexican children aged 3-15 years, the 5-year survival rate was only 35%. Deaths resulted from rupture of aorta or aneurysms, stroke, cardiac failure, and peritonitis and ventricular fibrillation.[1]

Regimens including weekly methotrexate or daily or monthly intravenous cyclophosphamide have been used in individuals with glucocorticoid-resistant TA. Low-dose weekly methotrexate also has been used as a steroid-sparing agent for patients not tolerating corticosteroid taper. Ozen et al used daily oral cyclophosphamide, which was well tolerated in a small series of children.[2]

Mycophenolate mofetil may be useful to treat individuals with glucocorticoid-resistant disease.[3] Case reports suggest disease control and steroid sparing.

A small series (15 patients) showed that tumor necrosis factor (TNF) inhibition using etanercept or infliximab was successful in inducing clinical remission and permitting corticosteroid taper in patients who are steroid dependent.[4]

Leflunomide has been used in glucocorticoid-resistant and methotrexate-resistant disease.[5]

Of patients with TA who are treated with glucocorticoids, 60% respond; however, as many as 40% relapse on tapering steroids. In the Cleveland Clinic series of 75 patients, 93% achieved remission; only 28% of patients were able to maintain 6 months of remission when steroids were tapered to 10 mg or less.[6]

Evidence-Based References

1. Miller JH et al: Gallium scintigraphic demonstration of arteritis in Takayasu disease, *Clin Nucl Med* 21(11):882-883, 1996 (B)
2. Ozen S et al: Takayasu arteritis in children: preliminary experience with cyclophosphamide induction and corticosteroids followed by methotrexate, *J Pediatr* 150(1):72-76, 2007. (B)
3. Daina E et al: Mycophenolate mofetil for the treatment of Takayasu arteritis: report of three cases, *Ann Intern Med* 130(5):422-426, 1999. (C)
4. Hoffman GS et al: Anti-tumor necrosis factor therapy in patients with difficult to treat Takayasu arteritis, *Arthritis Rheum* 50(7):2296-2304, 2004. (C)
5. Haberhauer G et al: Beneficial effects of leflunomide in glucocorticoid- and methotrexate-resistant Takayasu's arteritis, *Clin Exp Rheumatol* 19(4):477-478, 2001. (C)
6. Maksimowicz-McKinnon K et al: Limitations of therapy and a guarded prognosis in an American cohort of Takayasu arteritis patients, *Arthr Rheum* 56(3):1000-1009, 2007. (C)

SUGGESTED READINGS

Arend WP et al: American College of Rheumatology 1990. criteria for the classification of Takayasu's arteritis, *Arthr Rheum* 33:1129, 1990.

Hahn-Kover K et al: Diagnosis of Takayasu arteritis, *J Clin Rheumatol* 11(3):170, 2005.

Kissin EY et al: Diagnostic imaging in Takayasu arteritis, *Curr Opin Rheumatol* 16:31, 2004.

Maksimowicz-McKinnon K et al: Takayasu arteritis: what is the long term prognosis? *Rheum Dic Clin North Am* 33:777, 2007.

Matsuura K et al: Surgical treatment of aortic regurgitation due to Takayasu arteritis: long-term morbidity and mortality, *Circulation* 112:3707, 2005.

Seko Y: Giant cell and Takayasu arteritis, *Curr Opin Rheumatol* 19:39, 2007.

Weyend CM, Goronzy JJ: Mechanisms of disease: medium and large vessel vasculitis, *N Engl J Med* 349:160, 2003.

AUTHORS: **GARY S. MAK, M.D.,** and **PRANAV M. PATEL, M.D.**

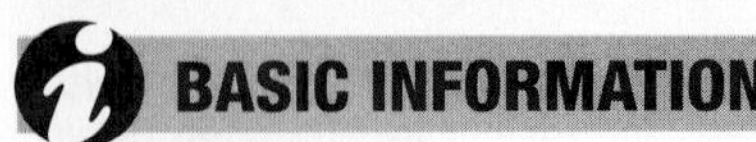

BASIC INFORMATION

DEFINITION

Four species of adult tapeworm may infect humans as the definitive host: *Taenia saginata* (beef tapeworm), *Taenia solium* (pork tapeworm), *Diphyllobothrium latum* (fish tapeworm), and *Hymenolepis nana.* In addition, *T. solium* may infect humans in its larval form (cysticercosis), and several animal tapeworms (see "Echinococcosis" in Section I) may cause infection in an analogous manner.

SYNONYMS

Cysticercosis (larval infection by *T. solium*)

ICD-9CM CODES
123.9 Tapeworm infestation

EPIDEMIOLOGY & DEMOGRAPHICS

INCIDENCE (IN U.S.):
- Diagnosed primarily in immigrants
- Varies widely by country of origin and dietary practices

PREVALENCE (IN U.S.):
- *T. saginata:* <0.1%
- *D. latum:* <0.05%
- *T. solium:* <0.1%
- *H. nana:* sporadic, often in setting of outbreak

PREDOMINANT SEX: Equal sex distribution
PREDOMINANT AGE:
- *T. saginata, T. solium, D. latum:* 20 to 39 yr of age
- *H. nana* in setting of institution outbreaks: children

PHYSICAL FINDINGS & CLINICAL PRESENTATION

Adult worms
1. Attach to bowel mucosa
2. Feed and grow
3. Cause minimal or no symptoms or sequelae

Cysticercosis
1. Mass lesions of brain (neurocysticercosis), soft tissue, viscera
2. Neurocysticercosis may cause seizures, hydrocephalus

Prolonged infection with *D. latum*
1. Vitamin B_{12} deficiency
2. Megaloblastic anemia

ETIOLOGY

TAPEWORM:
- Adult worm resides in small or large bowel; proglottids and eggs are passed in stool.
- Eggs are ingested by the animal intermediate host.
- Eggs hatch into larvae.
- Larvae disseminate largely in skeletal muscle, brain, viscera.
- Humans eat infected beef *(T. saginata),* infected pork *(T. solium),* or infected fish *(D. latum).*
- Larvae mature into adults within the GI lumen.
- *H. nana* infection is acquired by ingesting eggs in human or rodent feces.

CYSTICERCOSIS:
- Humans ingest eggs of *T. solium* in food contaminated with human feces that contain the eggs.
- Eggs hatch into larvae in gut.
- Larvae disseminate widely through tissues (particularly soft tissue and CNS) forming cystic lesions containing either viable or nonviable larvae.

DIAGNOSIS

WORKUP

- Stool examination for eggs or proglottids (tapeworm)
- Cerebral CT scan (neurocysticercosis)
- Serum antibody (neurocysticercosis)

IMAGING STUDIES

- Tapeworm: incidental finding on upper GI series
- Neurocysticercosis:
  1. Cerebral cysts are readily demonstrated by CT scan or MRI.
  2. Calcified lesions are an incidental finding.

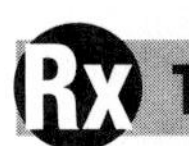

TREATMENT

ACUTE GENERAL Rx

- All patients with intestinal tapeworm infections should be treated with a single oral dose of praziquantel.
  1. *T. solium:* 5 mg/kg
  2. *T. saginata:* 20 mg/kg
  3. *D. latum:* 10 mg/kg
  4. *H. nana:* 25 mg/kg
- An alternative therapy to praziquantel for tapeworm infections is niclosamide, 2 g PO once or 500 mg PO daily for 3 days.
- Therapy that may be considered for symptomatic cysticercosis:
  1. May regress spontaneously
  2. Surgery
  3. Albendazole 15 mg/kg PO qid in three doses for 28 days
  4. Praziquantel 50 mg/kg PO qid in three doses for 15 days
- Therapy contraindicated with:
  1. Ocular infections
  2. Cerebral infections in which local inflammation caused by destruction of the parasite may cause significant damage

CHRONIC Rx

- Retreatment if required
- Avoidance of undercooked pork, meat, or fish
- Cysticercosis: proper hand washing, proper disposal of human waste

DISPOSITION

- Neurologic follow-up for patients with neurocysticercosis
- Ophthalmologic follow-up for patients with ocular involvement

REFERRAL

Patients treated for neurocysticercosis should be evaluated by a physician experienced in managing this infection, if possible.

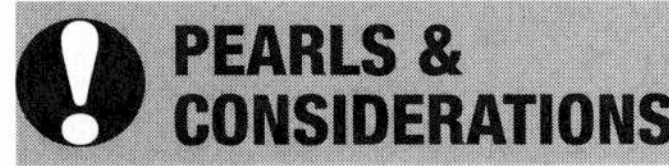

PEARLS & CONSIDERATIONS

COMMENTS

T. solium is the most dangerous of the tapeworms because of the potential for cysticercosis by means of autoinfection.

SUGGESTED READINGS

Buyuk Y et al: Non-ruptured hydatid cyst can lead to death by spread of cyst content into bloodstream: an autopsy case, *Eur J Gastroenterol Hepatol* 17(6): 671, 2005.

DeGiorgio C et al: Sero-prevalence of *Taenia solium* cysticercosis and *Taenia solium* taeniasis in California, USA, *Acta Neurol Scand* 111(2):84, 2005.

Flisser A et al: Short report: evaluation of a self-detection tool for tapeworm carriers for use in public health, *Am J Trop Med Hyg* 72(5):510, 2005.

Infanger M et al: Surgical and medical management of rare echinococcosis of the extremities. Pre- and postoperative long-term chemotherapy, *Scand J Infect Dis* 37(11):954, 2005.

Liu YM et al: Acute pancreatitis cause by tapeworm in the biliary tract, *AM J Trop Med Hyg* 73(2):377, 2005.

AUTHORS: **GLENN G. FORT, M.D., M.P.H.,** and **DENNIS J. MIKOLICH, M.D.**

BASIC INFORMATION

DEFINITION

Tardive dyskinesia (TD) is a syndrome of involuntary movements associated with the long-term use of antipsychotic medication, particularly first-generation antipsychotics. Patients exhibit rapid, repetitive, stereotypic movements that mostly involve the oral, lingual, trunk, and limb areas.

SYNONYMS

Orofacial dyskinesia
Tardive syndrome

ICD-9CM CODES
333.85 Tardive dyskinesia

EPIDEMIOLOGY & DEMOGRAPHICS

- The disorder is caused by dopamine-blocking antipsychotics (e.g., haloperidol).
- The incidence is declining with the use of second-generation antipsychotics. Approximately 0.5% to 1% of all adults develop TD yearly while taking these medications.
- At least 20% of patients treated with first-generation antipsychotic drugs are affected with TD, and approximately 5% are expected to develop TD with each year of antipsychotic treatment.
- Risk increases with the duration of antipsychotic treatment, in elderly patients, and in patients with nonschizophrenia diagnoses.

PHYSICAL FINDINGS & CLINICAL PRESENTATION

- TD is classically described as a chronic condition of insidious onset, but symptoms are variable over time and may even improve despite continued antipsychotic therapy.
- The condition typically appears with the reduction or withdrawal of the antipsychotic medications.
- TD primarily involves stereotypic movements of the mouth and tongue, including lip smacking and puckering, tongue twisting and protrusion, and facial grimacing.
- It may also involve slow, writhing movements of the trunk or choreoathetotic movements of the fingers and toes.
- The involuntary mouth movements associated with TD may be suppressed by voluntary actions (e.g., putting food in the mouth, talking).

ETIOLOGY

TD is generally thought to result from chronic exposure to dopamine-receptor–blocking agents, which are primarily used to treat psychosis. TD has not been reported with dopamine depleters (e.g., reserpine), and it is less common with second-generation antipsychotic drugs. Some drugs used to treat nausea (e.g., metoclopramide, prochlorperazine) and depression (e.g., amoxapine) can also cause TD. TD is believed to be caused by the upregulation and increased sensitivity of dopamine receptors in the basal ganglia and by antipsychotic-induced damage to striatal cholinergic neurons.

DIAGNOSIS

DIFFERENTIAL DIAGNOSIS

- Huntington's disease
- Tourette's syndrome
- Wilson's disease
- Sydenham's chorea
- Hyperthyroidism-induced choreoathetosis
- Edentulous dyskinesias and improperly fitted dentures

WORKUP

TD is a diagnosis of exclusion, with emphasis on a complete neuropsychiatric and medication history and a thorough physical examination.

IMAGING STUDIES

Brain imaging is normal in patients with TD.

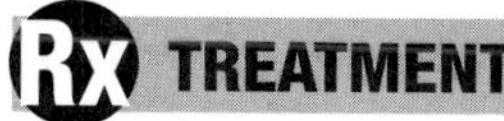

TREATMENT

ACUTE GENERAL RX

- Treatment is predicated on prevention: limit the indications for antipsychotics; use the lowest effective dose; discontinue the drugs, when feasible; and monitor patients frequently.
- Switch to second-generation antipsychotics, if possible.

CHRONIC Rx

- Clozapine has the best evidence for improving the symptoms of TD, although olanzapine and amisulpride may also be of benefit.
- Tetrabenazine, benzodiazepines, vitamin E, vitamin B_6, donepezil, and melatonin may be helpful, although controlled trial evidence is weak.
- Piracetam, which is a gamma-aminobutyric acid derivative, was effective for reducing the symptoms of TD in a randomized clinical trial with short-term follow-up.
- Tetrabenazine, benzodiazepines, vitamin E, vitamin B_6, donepezil, and melatonin may be helpful, although controlled trial evidence is weak.

DISPOSITION

Potentially irreversible long-term adverse effects of treatment with dopamine-receptor–blocking medications

REFERRAL

Movement disorder specialist consultation if symptoms are severe

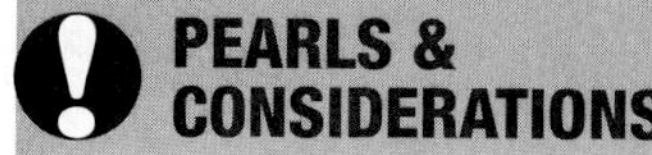

PEARLS & CONSIDERATIONS

- First-generation antipsychotics should be resumed to treat TD in the absence of active psychosis only as a last resort for persistent, disabling, and treatment-resistant TD.
- Avoid the use of anticholinergic medications (e.g., benztropine), which may exacerbate TD symptoms.
- A worsening of the overall psychopathology in patients with schizophrenia is longitudinally associated with the emergence of TD and suggestive of a worse prognosis.
- Recent evidence suggests increased overall mortality among patients with TD, which highlights the need for referral for more aggressive specialized interventions.

T

Diseases and Disorders

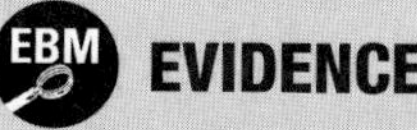

EVIDENCE

Please note: Complete text of EBM for this topic is available online.

Key trials and commentary:

Piracetam is a potent antioxidant, a cerebral neuroprotector, a neuronal metabolic enhancer, and a brain integrative agent. More than 20 years ago, an intravenous preparation of piracetam demonstrated an improvement in the symptoms of tardive dyskinesia. The aim of this study was to reexamine the efficacy of piracetam in the treatment of tardive dyskinesia using an oral preparation.

This study showed that piracetam appears to be effective in reducing symptoms of tardive dyskinesia. The specific mechanism by which piracetam may attenuate symptoms of tardive dyskinesia needs to be further evaluated.

The authors studied piracetam, which is a potent antioxidant and neuroprotective agent. These Israeli authors conducted a 9-week, double-blind, crossover, placebo-controlled trial in tardive dyskinesia. They administered 4 weeks of either piracetam (4800 mg/day) or placebo and then crossed over the patients after a 1-week washout. There was a significant drop, but they observed that piracetam may be effective and certainly needs further study.

In another report, the authors studied another potent antioxidant, vitamin B_6. They conducted a 26-week double-blind trial on 50 inpatients with schizophrenia and tardive dyskinesia. Doses were 1200 mg a day. They also were crossed over after 12 weeks. Vitamin B_6 also appeared to be effective. These two trials need further study but certainly represent exciting treatments for such an awful condition.[1] Ⓐ

The aim of this study was to assess the 1-year risk of second-generation antipsychotics (SGAs) for tardive dyskinesia (TD) in children and adolescents with assumed minimal past exposure to first-generation antipsychotics.

Results across 10 studies suggest relatively low 1-year TD rates in pediatric patients treated with SGAs. However, the available database is limited by the small sample size of studies with SGAs other than risperidone and by the use of relatively low doses, which may have obscured a potentially greater risk for TD in children and adolescents treated with higher total SGA doses and for longer durations. Large, long-term studies of various SGAs, using state-of-the-art methodology, are needed before firm conclusions can be reached about the risk of TD in pediatric patients treated long-term with SGAs.

The occurrence of abnormal movements in adolescents is always of great concern. A promise of the SGA medications was a reduced risk of abnormal movements, particularly TD. Although the risks of metabolic syndrome have been extensively studied, less is known about abnormal movements. But with regard to both metabolic syndrome and abnormal movements, there are risks and they may differ according to the particular medication in question (olanzapine, ziprasidone, risperidone, quetiapine). This study uses as much of the then-extant data to quantify 1-year incidence rates of TD in youth exposed to SGAs. It found, as expected, variations according to the drug. The limited time course of this study makes the authors cautious about making conclusions, but if these data bear out a low risk of TD in this population it will be one source of relief for the many young patients exposed to these medications.[2] Ⓐ

Evidence-Based References

1. Libov I et al: Efficacy of piracetam in the treatment of tardive dyskinesia in schizophrenic patients: a randomized, double-blind, placebo-controlled crossover study, *J Clin Psychiatry* 68:1031-1037, 2007. Commentary by J.C. Ballenger, M.D. Ⓐ

2. Correll CU, Kane JM: One-year incidence rates of tardive dyskinesia in children and adolescents treated with second-generation antipsychotics: a systematic review, *Child Adolesc Psychopharmacol* 17:647-656, 2007. Commentary by A. Mack, M.D. Ⓐ

SUGGESTED READINGS

Dean CE, Thuras PD: Mortality and tardive dyskinesia: long-term study using the US National Death Index, *Br J Psychiatry* 194(4):360, 2009.

Libov I et al: Efficacy of piracetam in the treatment of tardive dyskinesia in schizophrenic patients: a randomized, double-blind, placebo-controlled crossover study, *J Clin Psychiatry* 68(7):1031, 2007.

Margolese HC et al: Tardive dyskinesia in the era of typical and atypical antipsychotics. Part 2: Incidence and management strategies in patients with schizophrenia, *Can J Psychiatry* 50(11):703, 2005.

Soares-Weiser K et al: Tardive dyskinesia, *Semin Neurol* 27:159, 2007.

AUTHOR: **JOHN A. GRAY, M.D., PH.D.**

BASIC INFORMATION

DEFINITION

Tarsal tunnel syndrome is a rare entrapment neuropathy that develops as a result of compression of the posterior tibial nerve in the tunnel formed by the flexor retinaculum behind the medial malleolus of the ankle (Fig. 1-327). This retinaculum arises from the medial malleolus and inserts into the medial aspect of the calcaneus.

SYNONYMS

None

ICD-9CM CODES
355.5 Tarsal tunnel syndrome

EPIDEMIOLOGY & DEMOGRAPHICS

PREVALENCE: Unknown
PREDOMINANT SEX: Females and males affected equally

PHYSICAL FINDINGS & CLINICAL PRESENTATION

- Symptoms are often vague compared with other compression neuropathies such as carpal tunnel syndrome.
- Neuritic symptoms along the course of the posterior tibial nerve in the sole and heel.
- The Valleix phenomenon (proximal radiation of the pain) may occur.
- Swelling over tarsal tunnel.
- Possible positive Tinel's sign.
- Possible reproduction of symptoms with sustained eversion of hindfoot or digital compression of tunnel.
- Sensory loss and motor changes unusual.

ETIOLOGY

- Space-occupying lesions (ganglia, varicosities, lipomas, synovial hypertrophy) or local tendonitis
- Possibly traction on nerve

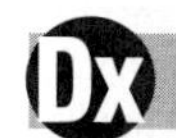

DIAGNOSIS

DIFFERENTIAL DIAGNOSIS

- Plantar fasciitis
- Peripheral neuropathy
- Proximal radiculopathy
- Local tendinitis
- Peripheral vascular disease
- Morton's neuroma

ELECTRICAL STUDIES

Electrodiagnostic testing is often inconclusive. Delayed sensory conduction or increased motor latency may be seen.

Rx TREATMENT

- Nonsteroidal antiinflammatory drugs
- Immobilization for 4 to 6 wk with ankle orthosis or fracture cast boot
- Medial heel wedge or orthotic to minimize heel eversion
- Local steroid injection into tunnel (avoiding the posterior tibial nerve) if symptoms persist

DISPOSITION

Many patients are successfully treated conservatively.

REFERRAL

For surgical decompression if needed. Results of surgery are mixed unless an obvious compressive lesion is found.

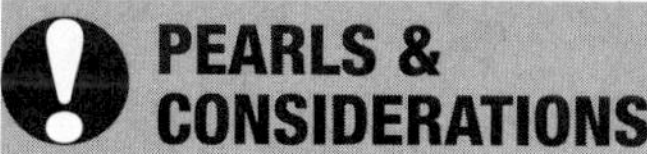

PEARLS & CONSIDERATIONS

- The disorder is controversial and there are many unanswered questions regarding its diagnosis and incidence.
- The condition may be difficult to differentiate from plantar fasciitis, and the two conditions may occur together.

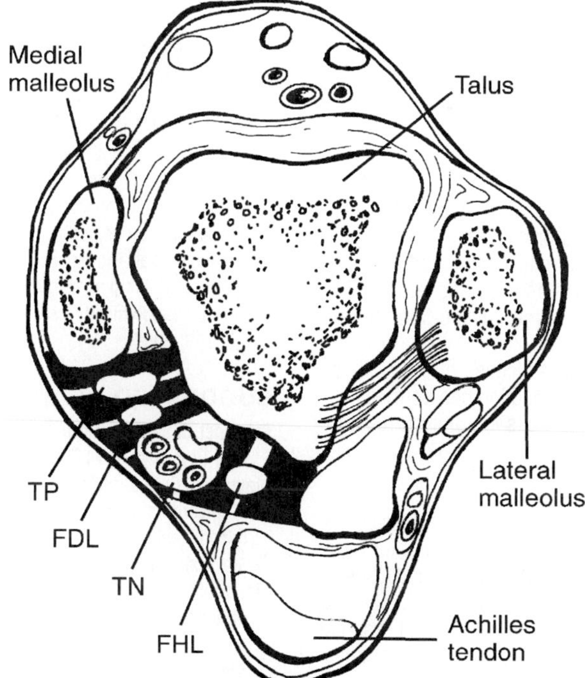

FIGURE 1-327 Anatomy of tarsal tunnel syndrome. Transverse view of ankle. Tendons and neurovascular elements are included in individual fibrous septa that connect periosteum with the deep fascia. *FDL,* Flexor digitorum longus; *FHL,* flexor hallucis longus tendon; *TN,* tibial nerve (single contour), posterior tibial artery, veins; *TP,* tibialis posterior tendon. (From Canoso J: *Rheumatology in primary care,* Philadelphia, 1997, WB Saunders.)

SUGGESTED READINGS

Aldridge T: Diagnosing heel pain in adults, *Am Fam Physician* 70:332, 2004.

Bracilovic A et al: Effect of foot and ankle position on tarsal tunnel compartment volume, *Foot Ankle Int* 27:431, 2006.

Campbell SE: MRI of sports injuries of the ankle, *Clin Sports Med* 25(4):727, 2007.

Campbell WW, Landau ME: Controversial entrapment neuropathies, *Neurosurg Clin N Am* 19:597, 2008.

Kennedy JG, Baxter DE: Nerve disorders in dancers, *Clin Sports Med* 27:329, 2008.

Labib SA et al: Heel pain triad (HPT): the combination of plantar fasciitis, posterior tibial tendon dysfunction and tarsal tunnel syndrome, *Foot Ankle Int* 23(3):212, 2002.

Mizel MS et al: Evaluation and treatment of chronic ankle pain, *Instr Course Lect* 53:311, 2004.

Mondelli M et al: An electrophysiological severity scale in tarsal tunnel syndrome, *Acta Neurol Scand* 109: 284, 2004.

Pecina M: Diagnostic tests for tarsal tunnel syndrome, *J Bone Joint Surg Am* 84A(9):1714, 2002.

Pessis E et al: Nerve and vascular entrapment in athletes, *J Radiol* 88:156, 2007.

Sung KS, Park SJ: Short-term outcome of tarsal tunnel syndrome due to benign space-occupying lesions, *Foot Ankle Int* 30(8):741, 2009.

AUTHOR: **LONNIE R. MERCIER, M.D.**

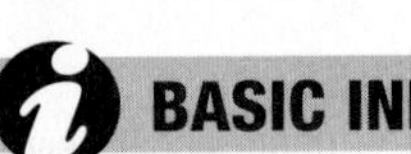

BASIC INFORMATION

DEFINITION

Temporomandibular joint (TMJ) syndrome refers to a group of disorders leading to symptoms of the temporomandibular joint.

SYNONYMS

Temporomandibular dysfunction
Painful temporomandibular joint

ICD-9CM CODES
524.60 Temporomandibular joint pain-dysfunction syndrome

EPIDEMIOLOGY & DEMOGRAPHICS

- 15% of the population have TMJ disorders
- Females are affected more often than males (4:1 ratio)
- Occurs between the second and fourth decades of life
- Usually unilateral, affecting either side with equal frequency

PHYSICAL FINDINGS & CLINICAL PRESENTATION

- Often unilateral pain in the muscles of mastication, usually described as a "dull" ache
- Otalgia
- Odontalgia
- Headaches (frontal, temporal, retro-orbital)
- Tinnitus
- Dizziness
- Clicking or popping sounds with movement of the TMJ
- Joint locking
- Tender to palpation
- Limited range of motion of the TMJ
- Symptoms usually appear in association with a stressful life event

ETIOLOGY

- Multifactorial, encompassing local anatomic anomalies to systemic disease processes.
- Myofascial pain-dysfunction syndrome: the most common cause of TMJ syndrome and results from teeth grinding and clenching the jaw (bruxism)
- Internal TMJ derangement: abnormal connection of the articular disk to the mandibular condyle
- Degenerative joint disease
- Rheumatoid arthritis
- Gouty arthritis
- Pseudogout
- Ankylosing spondylitis
- Trauma
- Prior surgery (orthodontic, intraarticular steroid injection)
- Tumors

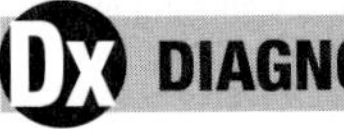

DIAGNOSIS

Can be made based on history and physical examination in most cases.

DIFFERENTIAL DIAGNOSIS

Includes the list provided above. Myofascial pain-dysfunction syndrome, internal TMJ derangement, and degenerative joint disease represent >90% of all causes of TMJ syndrome. Others not mentioned include dental problems such as loss of posterior teeth support and Eagle's syndrome (stylohyoid syndrome, carotidynia, and trigeminal neuralgia).

WORKUP

Radiographic imaging evaluation is used to exclude anatomic or systemic causes of disease when conservative management has failed.

LABORATORY TESTS

Laboratory examination is not very helpful.

IMAGING STUDIES

- Plain radiographs: the most common views are the panoramic, transorbital, and transpharyngeal in both opened and closed positions.
- Arthrography is helpful in looking for meniscus involvement but is seldom performed anymore.
- CT scan is highly accurate in diagnosing meniscal and osseous derangements of the TMJ.
- MRI is the procedure of choice and has replaced arthrography in cases of disabling pain or if locking occurs. It is used to determine disc position and morphology along with degenerative bony changes.

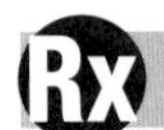

TREATMENT

NONPHARMACOLOGIC THERAPY

- Soft diet to rest the muscles of mastication
- Heat 15 to 20 min four to six times per day
- Massage of the masseter and temporalis muscles
- Formed splints or bite appliances
- Range-of-motion exercises

ACUTE GENERAL Rx

- Nonsteroidal antiinflammatory drugs: ibuprofen 800 PO mg tid prn, naproxen 500 PO mg bid prn, titrated to relieve symptoms
- Muscle relaxants at bedtime: diazepam 2.5 to 5 mg PO tid prn or amitriptyline 5 to 100 mg PO qd prn
- In degenerative joint disease of the TMJ, intraarticular steroid injection can be tried
- Botulism toxin injections into the masticatory muscles

CHRONIC Rx

- Most of the above treatments are used for myofascial pain-dysfunction syndrome; however, they can be applied to other causes of TMJ syndrome. Surgery is usually a measure of last resort in patients who do not respond to nonpharmacologic and acute general treatment.
- Surgical procedures include:
  1. Meniscoplasty
  2. Meniscectomy
  3. Subcondylar osteotomy
  4. TMJ reconstruction

DISPOSITION

The course depends on the underlying etiology; however, a lengthy course with exacerbations of symptoms can be expected.

REFERRAL

All patients with TMJ syndrome refractory to conservative nonpharmacologic and acute therapy should be referred to a periodontist, oral maxillofacial surgeon, or ear-nose-throat surgeon.

PEARLS & CONSIDERATIONS

Patients with rheumatoid arthritis involving the TMJ usually have bilateral involvement.

COMMENTS

Frequently, emotional stress initiates the myofascial pain-dysfunction, which accounts for 85% of all cases of TMJ syndrome.

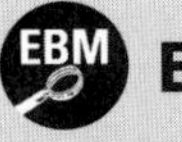

EVIDENCE

A systematic review of occlusal adjustment in the management of TMJ disorders found no difference between occlusal adjustment and control groups (reassurance or no treatment) in terms of symptom-based outcomes.[1] Ⓐ

There is insufficient evidence for or against the use of stabilization splint therapy[2] or low-level laser therapy[3] for the treatment of TMJ pain-dysfunction syndrome. Ⓐ Ⓑ

Acupuncture had a positive influence on the signs and symptoms of TMJ syndrome.[4] Ⓑ

Evidence-Based References

1. Koh H, Robinson PG: Occlusal adjustment for treating and preventing temporomandibular joint disorders, *Cochrane Rev* 1, 2003.
2. Al-Ani MZ et al: Stabilisation splint therapy for temporomandibular pain dysfunction syndrome, *Cochrane Rev* 1:CD002778, 2004.
3. Kulekcioglu S et al: Effectiveness of low-level laser therapy in temporomandibular disorder, *Scand J Rheumatol* 32:114, 2003.
4. Smith P et al: The efficacy of acupuncture in the treatment of temporomandibular joint myofascial pain: a randomised controlled trial. *J Dent* 35(3):259, 2007.

SUGGESTED READINGS

Buescher JJ: Temporomandibular joint disorders, *Am Fam Physician* 76:1477, 2007.

Dimitroulis G: The role of surgery in the management of disorders of the temporomandibular joint: a critical review of the literature. Part 1, *Int J Oral Maxillofac Surg* 34(2):107, 2005.

Dimitroulis G: The role of surgery in the management of disorders of the temporomandibular joint: a critical review of the literature. Part 2, *Int J Oral Maxillofac Surg* 34(3):231, 2005.

Herb K et al: Temporomandibular joint pain and dysfunction, *Curr Pain Headache Rep* 10(6):408, 2006.

Scrivani S et al: Temporomandibular disorders, *N Engl J Med* 359:2693-2705, 2008.

Sommer OJ et al: Cross-sectional and functional imaging of the temporomandibular joint: radiology, pathology, and basic biomechanics of the jaw, *Radiographics* 23(6):e14, 2003.

AUTHORS: **RYAN W. ZUZEK, M.D.,** and **DOUGLAS BURTT, M.D.**

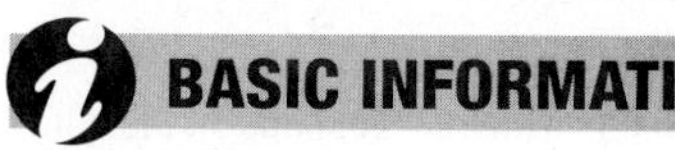

BASIC INFORMATION

DEFINITION

Testicular neoplasms are primary cancers originating in a testis.

SYNONYMS

Testis tumor
Testicular cancer

ICD-9CM CODES

186.9	Testicular neoplasm
M906/3	(seminoma)
M9101/3	(embryonal carcinoma or teratoma)
M9100/3	(choriocarcinoma)

EPIDEMIOLOGY & DEMOGRAPHICS

INCIDENCE: Four cases per 100,000 men annually. Testicular cancer is the most common cancer diagnosis in men between the ages of 15 and 35 yr.
PREVALENCE: 1% to 2% of all cancers in males
PREDOMINANT AGE: Can occur in any age but most common in young adults; average age for embryonal cell carcinoma: 30 yr; average age for seminoma: 36 yr

PHYSICAL FINDINGS & CLINICAL PRESENTATION

- Testicular cancer typically presents as a painless mass in the testis. Any mass within the testicle should be considered cancer until proven otherwise. It may be found by the patient, who brings it to the attention of a physician, or it may be found by a physician on a routine examination.
- Symptoms other than scrotal or testicular swelling are typically absent unless the cancer has metastasized (5% of patients at diagnosis). Occasionally a patient may report scrotal fullness or heaviness. Gynecomastia from tumors that secrete beta-human chorionic gonadotropin (hCG) is found in 1% of men with testicular cancer.
- Testicular palpation should be performed with two hands. Transillumination may distinguish a solid mass (e.g., cancer) and a fluid-filled lesion (e.g., hydrocele or spermatocele). The mass is nontender; indeed, it is less sensitive than a normal testicle.

ETIOLOGY & PATHOLOGY

- Cryptorchidism (undescended testes) is a major risk factor even if corrected by orchiopexy; however, treatment of undescended testis before puberty decreases the risk of testicular cancer from fivefold to twofold. Other risk factors are family history, infertility, tobacco use, and white race.
- Pathology:

Cell Type	*Frequency (%)*
Seminoma	42
Embryonal cell carcinoma	26
Teratocarcinoma	26
Teratoma	5
Choriocarcinoma	1

- Other rare types:
  - Yolk sac carcinoma
  - Mixed germ cell tumors
  - Carcinoid tumor
  - Sertoli cell tumors
  - Leydig cell tumors
  - Lymphoma
  - Metastatic cancer to the testes
- TNM staging system for testicular cancer
  - T_0: No apparent primary
  - T_1: Testis only (excludes rete testis)
  - T_2: Beyond the tunica albuginea
  - T_3: Rete testis or epididymal involvement
  - T_4: Spermatic cord
    1. Spermatic cord
    2. Scrotum
  - N_0: No nodal involvement
  - N_1: Ipsilateral regional nodal involvement
  - N_2: Contralateral or bilateral abdominal or groin nodes
  - N_3: Palpable abdominal nodes or fixed groin nodes
  - N_4: Juxtaregional nodes
  - M_0: No distant metastases
  - M_1: Distant metastases present

The clinical stages consist of stage A, with tumor confined to the testis and cord structures; stage B, with tumor confined to the retroperitoneal lymph nodes; and stage C, with tumor involving the abdominal viscera or disease above the diaphragm.

Dx DIAGNOSIS

DIFFERENTIAL DIAGNOSIS

- Spermatocele
- Varicocele
- Hydrocele
- Epididymitis
- Epidermoid cyst of the testicle
- Epididymis tumors

WORKUP

Physical examination, laboratory tests, and imaging studies (see Section III, "Testicular Mass")

LABORATORY TESTS

- Serum hCG
- Serum alpha-fetoprotein (AFP)

One or both of these tumor markers will be elevated in 70% of cases of testicular cancer.

- Serum lactate dehydrogenase (LDH) level
- Testicular biopsy contraindicated

IMAGING STUDIES

- Ultrasound
- CT scan or MRI of pelvis and abdomen
- Chest radiograph
- CT of the chest in patients with suspected mediastinal, hilar, or lung parenchymal disease; MRI of the brain in patients with neurologic symptoms

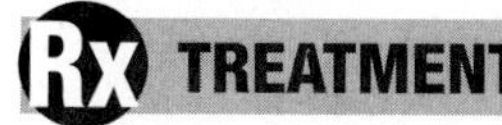

Rx TREATMENT

- Surgical exploration of the testicle through an inguinal incision with a noncrushing clamp placed on the cord before direct testicular examination. If a mass is confined within the body of the testicle, an orchiectomy is performed.
- Retroperitoneal lymph node dissection for clinical stage A and low stage B (lymph nodes <6 cm in greatest diameter) provides cure in 70%.
- Chemotherapy: cisplatin, vinblastine, and bleomycin
  1. Not indicated in clinical stage A
  2. Controversial in low stage B
  3. Cornerstone of treatment in high stage B or stage C
- Radiation therapy for stage A and low stage B seminoma provides cure in 85%
- Posttreatment surveillance for testicular cancer survivors (annually)
  1. General maintenance
  2. Fertility assessment
  3. Sexuality status
  4. Skin examination (increased risk of dysplastic nevi)
  5. Testicular examination (3% to 4% risk of second testicular cancer)
  6. Serum tumor markers (hCG, AFP)
  7. Chest radiograph (for late relapse)
  8. Complications of cisplatin: hypertension, hyperlipidemia, renal failure, hypomagnesemia, hearing loss, tinnitus, peripheral neuropathy, and infertility

DISPOSITION

The overall cure for testicular cancer is >95% (80% for metastatic disease).

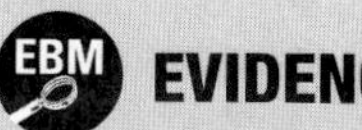

EVIDENCE

A randomized trial of paraaortic (PA) vs. PA plus ipsilateral iliac lymph node radiation for stage I testicular seminoma found low recurrence rates for either treatment and reduced hematologic, gastrointestinal, and gonadal toxicity with adjuvant radiotherapy confined to the PA nodes.[1] B

Evidence-Based Reference

1. Fossa SD et al: Optimal planning target volume for stage I testicular seminoma: a Medical Research Council randomized trial. Medical Research Council Testicular Tumor Working Group, *J Clin Oncol* 17:1146, 1999. B

SUGGESTED READINGS

Feldman DR et al: Medical treatment of advanced testicular cancer, *JAMA* 299(6):672-684, 2008.
Petterson A et al: Age at surgery for undescended testis and risk of testicular cancer, *N Engl J Med* 356:1835, 2007.
Shaw J: Diagnosis and treatment of testicular cancer, *Am Fam Physician* 77(4):469-474, 2008.

AUTHOR: **FRED F. FERRI, M.D.**

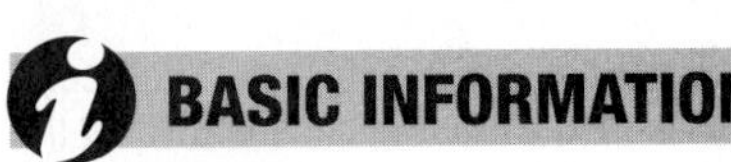

BASIC INFORMATION

DEFINITION

Testicular torsion is a twisting of the spermatic cord leading to cessation of testicular blood flow, ischemia, and infarction if left untreated.

SYNONYMS

Spermatic cord torsion

ICD-9CM CODES
608.2 Testicular torsion

EPIDEMIOLOGY & DEMOGRAPHICS

INCIDENCE: Affects one in 4000 males aged <25 yr
PREDOMINANT AGE: Two thirds of all cases occur between the ages of 12 and 18 yr, but may occur at any age, including antenatally.

PHYSICAL FINDINGS & CLINICAL PRESENTATION

- Typical sequence is sudden onset of hemiscrotal pain, then swelling, nausea, and vomiting without fever or urinary symptoms.
- Physical examination may reveal a tender firm testis, high-riding testis, horizontal lie of testis, absent cremasteric reflex, and no pain with elevation of testis. Absence of the cremasteric reflex (stroking or pinching the medial thigh normally causes contraction of the cremaster muscle and elevation of the testis) is the most sensitive physical finding.
- Painless testicular swelling occurs in 10%.
- One out of three patients reports previous episodes of spontaneously remitting scrotal pain.
- In the neonate, testicular torsion should be presumed in patients with a painless, discolored hemiscrotal swelling.
- In rare cases, torsion may involve an undescended testicle. In such situations an empty hemiscrotum is palpated together with a tender lump in the inguinal area.

ETIOLOGY

- There are two types of testicular torsion: extravaginal, caused by nonadherence of the tunica vaginalis to the dartos layer, and intravaginal, caused by malrotation of the spermatic cord with the tunica vaginalis. Intravaginal torsion accounts for 90% of cases.
- Torsion usually occurs in the absence of any precipitating events. Trauma accounts for <10% of cases.

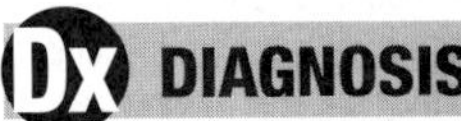

DIAGNOSIS

Diagnosis is made mainly by clinical suspicion. Color Doppler ultrasound evaluation or a nuclear testicular scan (Fig. 1-328) may help with the diagnosis. Ultrasonography will show absent or decreased blood flow; scintigraphy reveals decreased perfusion on symptomatic side.

DIFFERENTIAL DIAGNOSIS

See also Section II.

- Torsion of the testicular appendages (appendix testis)
- Testicular tumor
- Epididymitis
- Incarcerated inguinoscrotal hernia
- Orchitis
- Spermatocele
- Hydrocele, varicocele

WORKUP

The diagnosis is usually based on history and physical examination.

IMAGING STUDIES

- Radionuclide scrotal scanning (technetium-99m): cold testicle
- Doppler ultrasonic stethoscope (Doppler flowmetry)

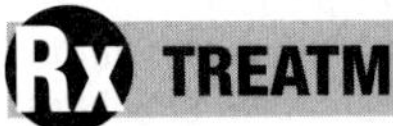

TREATMENT

Surgical derotation of the spermatic cord followed by bilateral testicular fixation with nonabsorbable sutures. If the affected testis is nonviable, orchiectomy of the affected testis and orchiopexy of the contralateral side are performed. Attempts at manual detorsion should not delay surgical consultation.

PROGNOSIS

- The degree of ischemia depends on the duration of torsion and the degree of rotation of the spermatic cord.
- There is an 80% testicular salvage rate if detorsion occurs within 12 hr of onset.
- After 24 hr, irreversible testicular infarction is expected.
- Because the contralateral testes can be affected (immunologic process), when treatment is delayed and return of blood flow does not occur after detorsion, some recommend orchiectomy of the infarcted testicle.

REFERRAL

To urologist

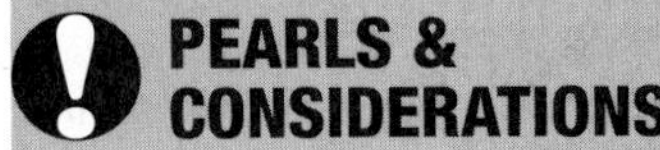

PEARLS & CONSIDERATIONS

- Manual detorsion by external rotation of the testis toward the thigh can be attempted for adolescent intravaginal torsion if an operating facility is not readily available.
- Extravaginal torsion is diagnosed in the newborn. Intravaginal torsion can occur at any age but is usually diagnosed in males ages 12 to 18 yr.

SUGGESTED READING

Ringdahl E, Teague L: Testicular torsion, *Am Fam Physician* 74:1739, 2006.

AUTHOR: **FRED F. FERRI, M.D.**

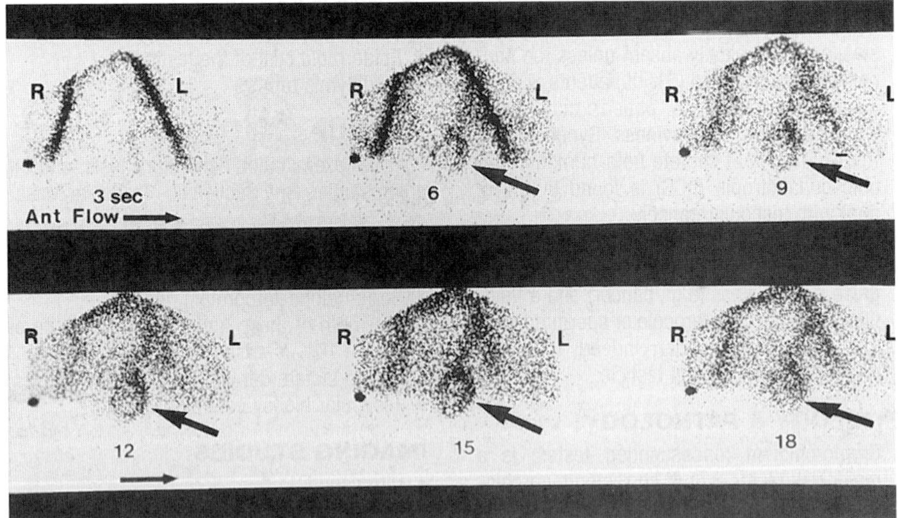

FIGURE 1-328 Testicular torsion. Evaluation of blood flow to the testicle has been done by giving an intravenous bolus of radioactive material. The right and left iliac vessels are clearly identified, and sequential images are obtained every 3 sec. Here, increased flow is seen to the rim of the left testicle *(arrows),* and there is no blood flow centrally. This is the appearance of a testicular torsion in which the torsion has been present for more than approximately 24 hr. (From Mettler FA [ed]: *Primary care radiology,* Philadelphia, 2000, WB Saunders.)

BASIC INFORMATION

DEFINITION

Tetanus is a life-threatening illness manifested by muscle rigidity and spasms; it is caused by a neurotoxin (tetanospasmin) produced by *Clostridium tetani.*

SYNONYMS

Lockjaw
Generalized tetanus
Neonatal tetanus
Cephalic tetanus
Localized tetanus

ICD-9CM CODES
037 Tetanus

EPIDEMIOLOGY & DEMOGRAPHICS

INCIDENCE (IN U.S.): 48 to 64 cases reported annually since 1986
PREDOMINANT AGE: >60 yr of age
GENETICS:
Neonatal infection:
- Rare in U.S.
- Among the leading causes of neonatal mortality in many parts of the world (caused by infection of the umbilical cord stump)

PHYSICAL FINDINGS & CLINICAL PRESENTATION

- Trismus ("lockjaw")
- Risus sardonicus (peculiar grin), characteristic grimace that results from contraction of the facial muscles
- Generalized muscle spasms causing severe pain and, at times, respiratory compromise and death
- Rigid abdominal muscles, flexed arms, and extended legs
- Autonomic dysfunction several days after onset of illness
- Leading cause of death: fluctuations in heart rate and blood pressure
- Usually, absence of fever
- Localized tetanus
  1. Rigidity of muscles near the injury
  2. Weakness as a result of lower motor neuron injury
  3. May be self-limited and resolve spontaneously
  4. More often progresses to generalized tetanus
  5. Cephalic tetanus:
     a. May occur with head injuries or chronic otitis with localized ear or mastoid infection with *C. tetani*
     b. Can manifest as cranial nerve dysfunction

ETIOLOGY

- *C. tetani* is a gram-positive, spore-forming bacillus that resides primarily in the soil.
- Majority of cases are caused by punctures and lacerations.
- Toxin is elaborated from organisms in a contaminated wound.
- Local symptoms are caused by inhibition of neurotransmitter at presynaptic sites.
  1. Over the next 2 to 14 days, the toxin travels up the neurons to the CNS, where it acts on inhibitory neurons to prevent neurotransmitter release.
  2. Unopposed motor activity results in tonic contractions of muscles.

Dx DIAGNOSIS

DIFFERENTIAL DIAGNOSIS

- Strychnine poisoning
- Dystonic reaction caused by neuroleptic agents
- Local infection (dental or masseter muscle) causing trismus
- Severe hypocalcemia
- Hysteria

WORKUP

- Positive wound culture is not helpful in diagnosis.
- Isolation of organism is possible in patients without the illness.

LABORATORY TESTS

- Usually, normal blood counts and chemistries
- Toxicology of serum and urine to rule out strychnine poisoning

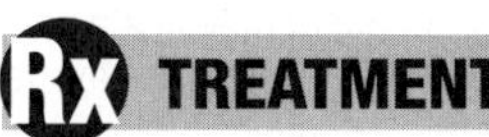

Rx TREATMENT

NONPHARMACOLOGIC THERAPY

- Monitoring in a hospital ICU: keep surroundings dark and quiet
- Intubation or tracheostomy for severe laryngospasm
- Debridement of wound

ACUTE GENERAL Rx

- Human tetanus immunoglobulin (HTIg) 500 U via IM injection
- Tetanus toxoid (Td) 0.5 ml by IM injection at a different site
- Metronidazole 500 mg IV q6h, or penicillin G 1 million U IV q4h for 10 days
- IV diazepam to control muscle spasms
- Neuromuscular blockade if necessary

CHRONIC Rx

- Supportive care
- Possible mechanical ventilation
- Minimal external stimuli
- Control of heart rate and blood pressure:
  1. Labetalol for sympathetic hyperactivity
  2. Pacemaker for sustained bradycardia
- Physical therapy once spasms subside

DISPOSITION

Full recovery over weeks to months if complications can be avoided

REFERRAL

- To emergency department
- To infectious disease specialist

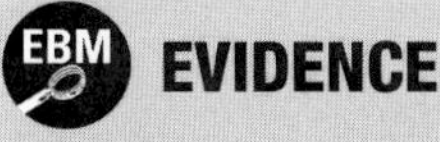

PEARLS & CONSIDERATIONS

COMMENTS

- Illness is preventable.
- Boosters of Td should be given every 10 yr to maintain immune status.
- Passive as well as active immunization (HTIg and Td) should be given for patients with tetanus-prone wounds who have not been adequately immunized in the previous 5 yr.
- A recent U.S. study showed that only 72% of people older than 6 yr had protective levels of antibody.

EBM EVIDENCE

Diazepam
Limited evidence suggests that diazepam is an effective treatment for the muscular spasms and rigidity of tetanus in children. Survival rates are higher when children are treated with diazepam alone, compared with a combination of phenobarbitone and chlorpromazine. Those receiving diazepam (either alone or in conjunction with other anticonvulsants) experience a significantly milder clinical course and shorter duration of hospitalization.[1] B

Magnesium sulfate
A randomized controlled trial involving 256 patients with severe tetanus found that, compared to placebo infusion, a magnesium sulfate infusion significantly reduced the requirement for other drugs to control muscle spasms and the requirement for verapamil to treat cardiovascular instability. However, magnesium sulfate infusion did not significantly reduce the need for mechanical ventilation.[2] B

Evidence-Based References

1. Okoromah CAN, Lesi FEA. Diazepam for treating tetanus, *Cochrane Database Syst Rev* 1, 2004.
2. Thwaites CL et al: Magnesium sulphate for treatment of severe tetanus: a randomised controlled trial, *Lancet* 368:1436-1443, 2006.

SUGGESTED READINGS

Demicheli V et al: Vaccines for women to prevent neonatal tetanus, *Cochrane Database Syst Rev* 4:CD002959, 2005.

Rao KN et al: Structural analysis of the catalytic domain of tetanus neurotoxin, *Toxicon* 45(7):929, 2005.

Rhee P et al: Tetanus and trauma: a review and recommendations, *J Trauma* 58(5):1082, 2005.

Talan DA et al: Tetanus immunity and physician compliance with tetanus prophylaxis practices among emergency department patients presenting with wounds, *Ann Emerg Med* 43(3):305, 2004.

AUTHORS: **GLENN G. FORT, M.D., M.P.H.,** and **DENNIS J. MIKOLICH, M.D.**

BASIC INFORMATION

DEFINITION

Tetralogy of Fallot (TOF) is a congenital heart deformity that consists of the following four features (Fig. 1-329):

1. Ventricular septal defect (VSD)
2. Infundibular stenosis that leads to the obstruction of the right ventricular (RV) outflow tract
3. An aorta that overrides the VSD by <50% of its diameter
4. Concentric RV hypertrophy

ICD-9CM CODES
745.2 Tetralogy of Fallot

EPIDEMIOLOGY & DEMOGRAPHICS

- TOF is the most common cyanotic congenital heart malformation that is diagnosed in patients after the age of 1 yr.
- TOF accounts for nearly 10% of all cases of congenital heart disease.
- TOF occurs in approximately 3000 newborns/yr.

PHYSICAL FINDINGS & CLINICAL PRESENTATION

- Of the four major features of TOF, infundibular stenosis that leads to RV outflow tract obstruction and VSD are the primary defects that result in clinical manifestations. The degree of RV outflow obstruction determines the age and symptoms at presentation. RV outflow tract obstruction and the VSD result in the following:
  - Right-to-left shunting and hypoxemia
  - Altered RV hemodynamics
  - Decreased pulmonary blood flow
- The aforementioned pathophysiologic concepts result in common manifestations of TOF, including the following:
  - Cyanosis of the nail beds and lips as a result of the shunting of deoxygenated blood from the RV through the VSD into the left ventricle, thus bypassing the lungs
  - Dyspnea on exertion
  - Digital clubbing
  - The child assuming a squatting position after exercise to increase systemic vascular resistance, thereby decreasing right-to-left shunting
  - Low birth weight and growth rate
  - Palpable RV impulse
  - Systolic thrill along the left sternal border
  - Single second heart sound with an inaudible P2 component
  - A harsh systolic crescendo/decrescendo murmur that results from RV outflow tract obstruction and that is usually heard along the left mid to upper sternal border with posterior radiation
- After repair, patients may have a low-pitched diastolic murmur at the pulmonic area that is consistent with pulmonary regurgitation or a pansystolic murmur that is consistent with a VSD patch leak. If the patient only has a palliative shunt, a continuous murmur may be heard from the site of the shunt.

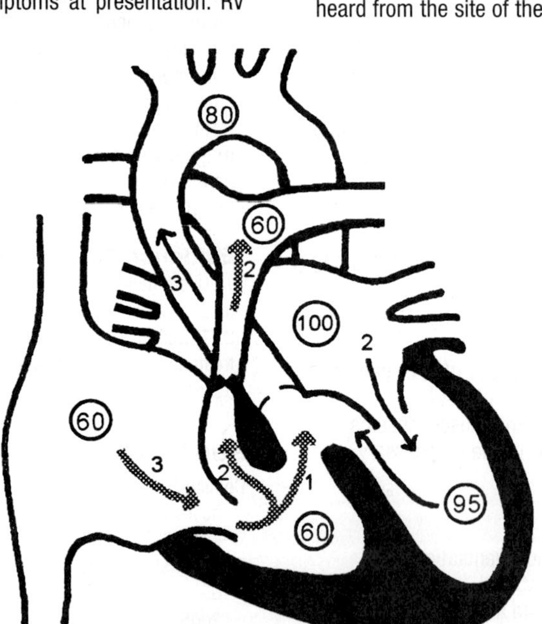

FIGURE 1-329 Physiology of tetralogy of Fallot. The circled numbers represent oxygen saturations. The numbers next to the arrows represent volumes of blood flow (in L/min/m^2). The atrial (mixed venous) oxygen saturation is decreased as a result of the systemic hypoxemia. A total of 3 L/min/m^2 of desaturated blood enters the right atrium and traverses the tricuspid valve: 2 L flow through the right ventricular outflow tract into the lungs, whereas 1 L shunts right to left through the ventricular septal defect *(VSD)* into the ascending aorta. Thus, the pulmonary blood flow is two-thirds normal (Qp:Qs [pulmonary to systemic flow ratio] of 0.7:1). Blood returning to the left atrium is fully saturated. Only 2 L of blood flows across the mitral valve. The oxygen saturation in the left ventricle may be slightly decreased from right-to-left shunting across the VSD. The 2 L of saturated left ventricular blood mixed with 1 L of desaturated right ventricular blood are ejected into the ascending aorta. The aortic saturation is decreased, and the cardiac output is normal. (From Behrman RE: *Nelson textbook of pediatrics,* ed 16, Philadelphia, 2000, WB Saunders.)

ETIOLOGY

TOF likely results from the maldevelopment of the embryologic conotruncus, but the exact mechanism is unknown.

DIAGNOSIS

- The diagnosis of TOF is suspected in any neonate, infant, or child who presents with cyanosis and a heart murmur.
- VSD is associated with other cardiac defects:
  - Persistent foramen ovale/atrial septal defect
  - Pulmonary artery anomalies
  - Right aortic arch
  - Left superior vena cava to coronary sinus
  - Additional VSDs
  - Coronary artery anomalies
- Associated syndromes include the following:
  - DeGeorge
  - DeLange
  - Goldenhar
  - Klippel-Feil
  - VACTERL
  - CHARGE

DIFFERENTIAL DIAGNOSIS

- Asthma
- Isolated VSD
- Pulmonary atresia
- Patent ductus arteriosus
- Aortic stenosis
- Pneumothorax

WORKUP

- Detailed history and physical examination, including pulse oximetry
- Echocardiogram, chest radiograph, 12-lead ECG, and routine laboratory tests

LABORATORY TESTS

- The CBC shows polycythemia from long-standing hypoxemia.
- Arterial blood gas levels show hypoxemia, normal pH, and pCO_2 (carbon dioxide levels).
- ECG commonly demonstrates right axis deviation, RV hypertrophy, and right atrial enlargement. The QRS duration may reflect the degree of RV dilation.
- Exercise testing may help to evaluate functional capacity and exertional arrhythmias.

IMAGING STUDIES

- Chest radiography reveals a boot-shaped heart that is commonly described as *coeur en sabot;* a prominent RV with decreased pulmonary vascularity; and a heart size that is usually normal. Cardiomegaly may reflect important pulmonary or tricuspid regurgitation, and a right-sided aortic arch may be seen.
- Echocardiography demonstrates VSD with a stenotic RV outflow tract and an overriding aorta. After repair, echocardiography can assess the severity of residual RV outflow tract obstruction, pulmonary regurgitation, and any tricuspid regurgitation that may be present. Right ventricular systolic pressures may also be assessed. A residual VSD may be seen, and RV size and function can be determined qualitatively.

- Cardiac catheterization and angiography help to determine hemodynamics, the severity of right-to-left shunting, the localization of the VSD, the flow across a persistent foramen ovale or atrial septal defect, and the severity of the pulmonic regurgitation; it can also be used to anatomically assess the RV outflow tract and the anatomy of the pulmonary artery and the coronary artery. Interventions are also possible, such as the elimination of collateral vessels or systemic–pulmonic artery shunts, dilation or stent implantation for obstructed pulmonary arteries, and possible percutaneous pulmonic valve replacement.
- Cardiac MRI is used for the localization of the VSD, the anatomic assessment of the RV outflow tract, the assessment of RV function, the quantification of pulmonary regurgitation, and the detection of RV myocardial fibrosis. Magnetic resonance angiography can be a noninvasive alternative to cardiac catheterization for the evaluation of pulmonary vascular anatomy and the ascending aorta.
- Multislice spiral computed tomography can be used for diagnosis, and it is extremely important during the planning of the repair procedure. Its use may be limited by the risks associated with radiation exposure in children. It can also be used to make assessments that are similar to those usually made by MRI for patients who are unable to undergo MRI.

Rx TREATMENT

NONPHARMACOLOGIC THERAPY

- Oxygen
- Prostaglandins at time of birth to keep a patent ductus and to maintain ductal flow to the lungs
- Knee–chest position during hypoxemic spells to help reduce venous return and to increase systemic vascular resistance, thereby decreasing right-to-left shunting

ACUTE GENERAL RX

The acute treatment of any infant or child with TOF who is cyanotic with respiratory distress is aimed at increasing systemic vascular resistance and decreasing right-to-left shunting (e.g., phenylephrine 0.1 to 0.5 mcg/kg/min intravenously). Intravenous β-blockers (e.g., propranolol 0.15 to 0.25 mg/kg via slow intravenous push) are used to decrease RV outflow tract contractility, and subcutaneous morphine can be used to decrease venous return.

CHRONIC RX

- Palliative repair includes procedures to increase pulmonary blood flow, thus reducing right-to-left shunting and allowing for pulmonary development. Examples of palliative procedures include the Blalock-Taussig shunt, in which a shunt is made between the subclavian artery and the pulmonary artery; the Waterston shunt, which attaches the ascending aorta to the right pulmonary artery; and the Potts shunt, which attaches the descending aorta to the left pulmonary artery. These are generally performed when the patient is still an infant.
- Complete surgical repair has good success and involves closing the VSD with a Dacron patch and relieving the RV outflow tract obstruction by simple resection of the infundibular stenosis, patch augmentation of the RV outflow, or the placement of a transannular patch). Patients who have the repair before the age of 2 yr are usually symptom free and can generally lead a normal life. If the repair is performed during adulthood, pulmonary valve replacement may be required.
- Postoperative issues include the following:
  - Residual pulmonic regurgitation
  - RV dilation and dysfunction from pulmonary regurgitation
  - Residual RV outflow tract obstruction
  - Branch pulmonary artery stenosis or hypoplasia
  - Sustained ventricular tachycardia
  - Sudden cardiac death
  - Atrioventricular block, atrial flutter, and atrial fibrillation
  - Progressive aortic regurgitation
  - Syndromal associations

DISPOSITION

- Almost all patients with TOF have either palliative or complete surgical repair before they reach adulthood.
- <3% of patients with TOF reach the age of 40 yr without surgery.
- Survival after the complete operative repair of TOF is excellent if the RV outflow tract obstruction has been relieved and the VSD has been closed.
- The 35-yr survival rate for patients after TOF repair is 85%.
- The need for pulmonary valve replacement increases after the second decade of life. It is indicated in symptomatic patients with severe pulmonary regurgitation or asymptomatic patients with severe pulmonary stenosis or regurgitation with signs of progressive or severe RV enlargement or dysfunction.
- A prolonged QRS duration on the preoperative ECG predicts an increased risk of postoperative supraventricular or ventricular arrhythmia. Prolongation of the QRS beyond 180 msec identifies patients who are at increased risk of ventricular tachycardia after surgery.
- Ventricular arrhythmia can lead to sudden cardiac death in 8.3% of surgically repaired patients by the age of 35 yr. Monomorphic ventricular tachycardia is likely the result of a reentry circuit from a scar caused by the surgery.
- Patients with signs or symptoms of arrhythmia should undergo hemodynamic and electrophysiologic testing. Treatment is tailored to the testing results and may include pulmonic valve replacement, residual VSD closure, mapping and ablation of an arrhythmia, antiarrhythmic medication, or the placement of an implantable cardiac defibrillator.
- Reduced exercise capacity is usually the result of chronic pulmonary regurgitation or residual RV outflow tract obstruction.
- Women with repaired TOF should be assessed by a cardiologist before considering pregnancy to determine if pulmonic valve replacement is needed first. The offspring of patients with TOF are more likely to have congenital anomalies than the offspring of the general population.
- Selected patients with normal RV pressures and function without evidence of residual shunt and without atrial or ventricular tachyarrhythmia are eligible to participate in competitive sports.

REFERRAL

- Infants and children with cyanotic heart disease should be referred to a pediatric cardiologist for further diagnostic evaluation. After being diagnosed with TOF, patients should be referred to centers with experience in palliative and complete surgical repair.
- Adult patients with repaired TOF should be comanaged with a cardiologist who specializes in adults with congenital heart disease.

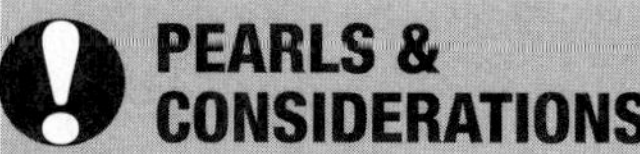

PEARLS & CONSIDERATIONS

- TOF was first described by the French physician Etienne Fallot in 1888.
- The first palliative surgical treatment for TOF was performed by Dr. Alfred Blalock at Johns Hopkins University in 1945 (i.e., the Taussig-Blalock shunt).
- The first surgical repair for TOF was performed by Dr. C. Walton Lillehei at the University of Minnesota in 1954.

COMMENTS

- The severity of RV outflow tract obstruction is the primary determinant of clinical symptoms and outcomes.
- TOF requires subacute bacterial endocarditis prophylaxis before any dental work or nonsterile surgical procedures (e.g., surgery of the bowel or bladder).
- Children with TOF are at risk for neurodevelopmental delay when they reach school age.

SUGGESTED READINGS

Graham TP Jr et al: Task Force 2: congenital heart disease, *J Am Coll Cardiol* 45(8):1326, 2005.

Shinebourne E et al: Tetralogy of Fallot: from fetus to adult, *Heart* 92(9):1353, 2006.

Verheugt C et al: Long-term prognosis of congenital heart defects: a systematic review, *Int J Cardiol* 131(1), 2008.

Warnes CA: The adult with congenital heart disease: born to be bad? *J Am Coll Cardiol* 46(1):1, 2005.

Warnes CA et al: ACC/AHA guidelines for adults with congenital heart disease, *J Am Coll Cardiol* 52(23), 2008.

AUTHORS: **SCOTT COHEN, M.D.,** and **WEN-CHIH WU, M.D.**

T

Diseases and Disorders

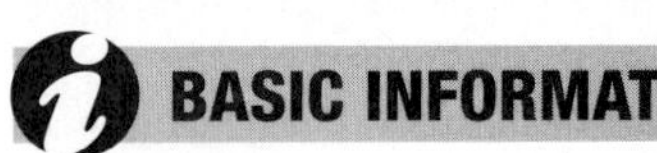

BASIC INFORMATION

DEFINITION

Thalassemias are a heterogeneous group of disorders of hemoglobin synthesis that have in common a deficient synthesis of one or more of the polypeptide chains of the normal human hemoglobin, resulting in a quantitative abnormality of the hemoglobin thus produced. There are no qualitative changes such as those encountered in the hemoglobinopathies (e.g., sickle cell disease).

SYNONYMS

Mediterranean anemia
Cooley's anemia

ICD-9CM CODES

282.4 Thalassemia

EPIDEMIOLOGY & DEMOGRAPHICS

- Thalassemia is among the most common genetic disorders worldwide. Approximately 4.83% of the world's population carry globin variants, including 1.67% of the population that are heterozygous for alpha-thalassemia and beta-thalassemia.
- The highest concentration of alpha-thalassemia is found in Southeast Asia and the African west coast. For example, the prevalence is 5% to 10% in Thailand. It is also common among blacks, with a prevalence of approximately 5%.
- The worldwide prevalence of beta-thalassemia is approximately 3%; in certain regions of Italy and Greece the prevalence reaches 15% to 30%. This high prevalence can be found in Americans of Italian or Greek descent.
- The distribution of thalassemia in Europe and Africa parallels that of malaria, suggesting that thalassemic persons are more resistant to the parasite, thus permitting evolutionary survival advantage.

CLASSIFICATION

Beta-thalassemia:

- Beta (+) thalassemia (suboptimal beta-globin synthesis)
- Beta (o) thalassemia (total absence of beta-globin synthesis)
- Delta-beta-thalassemia (total absence of both delta-globin and beta-globin synthesis)
- Lepore hemoglobin (synthesis of small amounts of fused delta-beta-globin and total absence of delta- and beta-globin)
- Hereditary persistence of fetal hemoglobin (HPHF) (increased hemoglobin F synthesis and reduced or absence of delta- and beta-globin)

Alpha-thalassemia:

- Silent carrier (three alpha-globin genes present)
- Alpha thalassemia trait (two alpha-globin genes present)
- Hemoglobin H disease (one alpha-globin gene present)
- Hydrops fetalis (no alpha-globin gene)
- Hemoglobin constant sprint (elongated alpha-globin chain)

Thalassemic hemoglobinopathies:

- Hb Terre Haute, Hb Quong Sze, HbE, Hb Knossos

PHYSICAL FINDINGS & CLINICAL PRESENTATION

Beta-thalassemia:

- Heterozygous beta-thalassemia (thalassemia minor): no or mild anemia, microcytosis and hypochromia, mild hemolysis manifested by slight reticulocytosis and splenomegaly
- Homozygous beta-thalassemia (thalassemia major): intense hemolytic anemia; transfusion dependency; bone deformities (skull and long bones); hepatomegaly; splenomegaly; iron overload leading to cardiomyopathy, diabetes mellitus, and hypogonadism; growth retardation; pigment gallstones; susceptibility to infection
- Thalassemia intermedia caused by combination of beta- and alpha-thalassemia or beta-thalassemia and Hb Lepore: resembles thalassemia major but is milder

Alpha-thalassemia:

- Silent carrier: no symptoms.
- Alpha-thalassemia trait: microcytosis only.
- Hemoglobin H disease: moderately severe hemolysis with microcytosis and splenomegaly.
- The loss of all four alpha-globin genes is incompatible with life (stillbirth of hydropic fetus). NOTE: Pregnancies with hydrops fetalis are associated with a high incidence of toxemia.

ETIOLOGY

- Beta-thalassemia: it is caused by more than 200 point mutations and, rarely, by deletions. The reduction of beta-globin synthesis results in redundant alpha-globin chains (Heinz bodies), which are cytotoxic and cause intramedullary hemolysis and ineffective erythropoiesis. Fetal hemoglobin may be increased.
- Alpha-thalassemia: several mutations can result in insufficient amounts of alpha-globin available for combination with non–alpha-globins.

DIAGNOSIS

LABORATORY TESTS

Beta-thalassemia:

- Microcytosis (mean cell volume: 55 to 80 FL)
- Normal red blood cell (RBC) distribution width index (RDW)
- Smear: nucleated RBCs, anisocytosis, poikilocytosis, polychromatophilia, Pappenheimer and Howell-Jolly bodies
- Hemoglobin electrophoresis: absent or reduced hemoglobin A, increased fetal hemoglobin, variable increase in the amount of hemoglobin A_2
- Markers of hemolysis: elevated indirect bilirubin and lactate dehydrogenase, decreased haptoglobin

Alpha-thalassemia:

- Microcytosis in the absence of iron deficiency
- Hemoglobin electrophoresis normal except for the presence of hemoglobin H in hemoglobin H disease

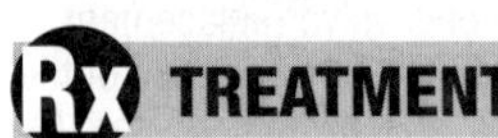

TREATMENT

- Thalassemia minor: no treatment, but avoid iron administration for incorrect diagnosis of iron deficiency.
- Beta-thalassemia major (and hemoglobin H disease):
    1. Transfusion as required together with chelation of iron with desferrioxamine (by IV or subcutaneous administration, 8 to 12 hr nightly, 5 to 6 days a week at a dose of 2 to 6 g/day with a portable infusion pump).
    2. Splenectomy for hypersplenism if present.
    3. Bone marrow transplantation. Although hematopoietic stem cell transplantation is the only curative approach for thalassemia, it has been limited by the high cost and scarcity of human leukocyte antigen–matched donors. Before transplantation, it is necessary to administer myeloablative regimens to eradicate the endogenous thalassemic bone marrow. Commonly used agents are hydroxyurea, azathioprine, fludarabine, busulfan, and cyclophosphamide.
    4. Hydroxyurea may increase the level of hemoglobin F.

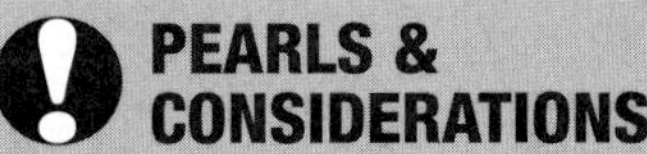

PEARLS & CONSIDERATIONS

- Polymerase chain reaction can be used to detect point mutations or deletions in chorionic villous samples, enabling first-trimester, DNA-based testing for thalassemia.
- Preimplantation genetic diagnosis can be extended to human leukocyte antigen typing on embryonic biopsies, allowing the selection of an embryo that is not affected by thalassemia and that may also serve as a stem cell donor for a previously affected child within the same family.

SUGGESTED READING

Round D, Rachmilewitz E: Beta thalassemia, *N Engl J Med* 353:1135, 2005.

AUTHOR: **FRED F. FERRI, M.D.**

BASIC INFORMATION

DEFINITION

Thoracic outlet syndrome describes a condition producing upper extremity symptoms believed to result from neurovascular compression at the thoracic outlet. Three types are described on the basis of point of compression: (1) cervical rib and scalenus syndrome, in which abnormal scalene muscles or the presence of a cervical rib may cause compression; (2) costoclavicular syndrome, in which compression may occur under the clavicle; and (3) hyperabduction syndrome, in which compression may occur in the subcoracoid area.

ICD-9CM CODES

353.0 Thoracic outlet syndrome

EPIDEMIOLOGY & DEMOGRAPHICS

PREVALENCE: Varies from source to source; presence of cervical ribs in 0.5% to 1% of population (50% bilateral), but most are asymptomatic

PREDOMINANT SEX: Females affected more often than males (ratio of 3.5:1)

PREDOMINANT AGE: Rare in those aged <20 yr

PHYSICAL FINDINGS & CLINICAL PRESENTATION

- Symptoms and signs are related to the degree of involvement of each of the various structures at the level of the first rib.
- True venous or arterial involvement is not common.
- Diagnosis is most often used in the consideration of neural pain affecting the arm, which suggests involvement of the brachial plexus.
  1. Arterial compression: pallor, paresthesias, diminished pulses, coolness, digital gangrene, and a supraclavicular bruit or mass
  2. Venous compression: edema and pain; thrombosis causing superficial venous dilation in the shoulder area
  3. "True" neural compression: lower trunk (C8, T1) findings with intrinsic weakness and diminished sensation to the ring finger and small fingers and ulnar aspect of the forearm
  4. Possible supraclavicular tenderness
  5. Provocative tests (Adson's, Wright's): may reproduce pain but are of disputed usefulness

ETIOLOGY

- Congenital cervical rib or fibrous extension of cervical rib (Fig. 1-330)
- Abnormal scalene muscle insertion
- Drooping of shoulder girdle from generalized hypotonia or trauma
- Narrowed costoclavicular interval as a result of downward and backward pressure on shoulder (sometimes seen in individuals who carry heavy backpacks)
- Acute venous thrombosis with exercise (effort thrombosis)
- Bony abnormalities of first rib
- Abnormal fibromuscular bands
- Malunion of clavicle fracture

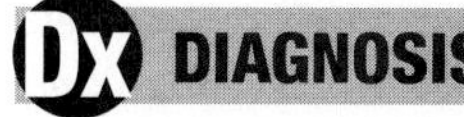

DIAGNOSIS

DIFFERENTIAL DIAGNOSIS

- Carpal tunnel syndrome
- Cervical radiculopathy
- Brachial neuritis
- Ulnar nerve compression
- Reflex sympathetic dystrophy
- Superior sulcus tumor

WORKUP

Except for venous or arterial pathology, no ancillary diagnostic tests are reliable for diagnostic confirmation.

IMAGING STUDIES

- Arteriography or venography when vascular pathology is strongly suspected clinically
- Cervical spine radiographs to rule out cervical disk disease
- Chest radiograph to rule out lung tumor
- Electromyography, nerve conduction velocity studies to rule out carpal tunnel syndrome, cervical radiculopathy

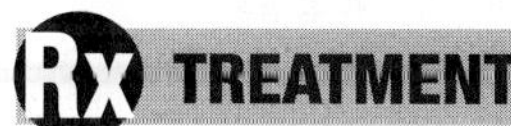

TREATMENT

ACUTE GENERAL Rx

- Sling for pain relief
- Physical therapy modalities plus shoulder girdle–strengthening exercises
- Postural reeducation
- Nonsteroidal anti-inflammatory drugs

DISPOSITION

- Surgery: generally successful for vascular disorders
- Nonsurgical treatment: often successful for patients with pain as the primary symptom

REFERRAL

For vascular surgery consultation when venous or arterial impairment is present

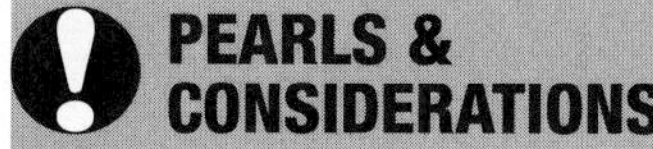

PEARLS & CONSIDERATIONS

COMMENTS

- True thoracic outlet syndrome is probably an uncommon condition.
- Diagnosis is often used to describe a wide variety of clinical symptoms.
- Considerable disagreement exists regarding the frequency of this disorder.

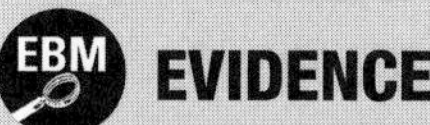

EVIDENCE

Home exercise treatment programs provide relief to patients with thoracic outlet syndrome symptoms.[1]

Evidence-Based Reference

1. Lindgren KA: Conservative treatment of thoracic outlet syndrome: a 2-year follow-up, *Arch Phys Med Rehab* 78:373, 1997.

SUGGESTED READINGS

Arthur LG et al: Pediatric thoracic outlet syndrome: a disorder with serious vascular complications, *J Pediatr Surg* 43:1089, 2008.

Campbell WW, Landau ME: Controversial entrapment neuropathies, *Neurosurg Clin N Am* 19:597, 2008.

Malas FU et al: Etiologic factors in thoracic outlet syndrome, *Orthopedics* 30(6):425, 2007.

Monica JT et al: Thoracic outlet syndrome with subclavian artery thrombosis undetectable by magnetic resonance angiography, *J Bone Joint Surg Am* 89:1589, 2007.

Nichols AW: Diagnosis and management of thoracic outlet syndrome, *Curr Sports Med Rep* 8:240, 2009.

Sadat U et al: Diagnosis of thoracic outlet syndrome: an overview, *Br J Hosp Med* 69:260, 2008.

Sanders RJ et al: Diagnosis of thoracic outlet syndrome, *J Vasc Surg* 46:601, 2007.

Urschel HC, Kourlis H: Thoracic outlet syndrome: a 50-year experience at Baylor University Medical Center, *Proc (Bayl Univ Med Cent)* 20(2):125, 2007.

Wehbe MA, Leinberry CF: Current trends in treatment of thoracic outlet syndrome, *Hand Clin* 20:119, 2004.

AUTHOR: **LONNIE R. MERCIER, M.D.**

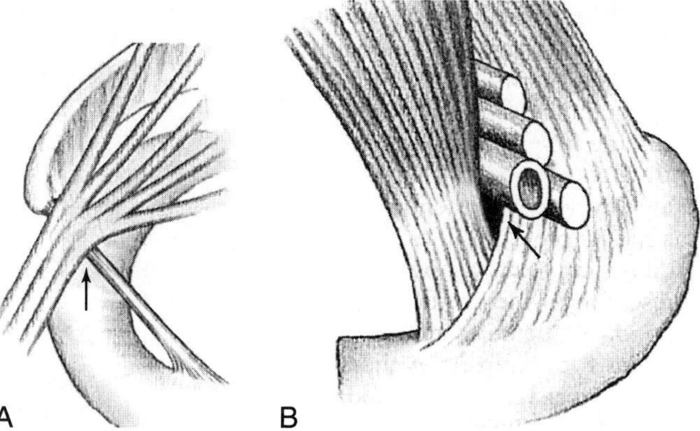

FIGURE 1-330 **A,** Compression caused by a cervical rib *(arrow).* **B,** Abnormal scalene muscle insertions that may cause compression at the cervicobrachial region *(arrow).* (From Mercier LR: *Practical orthopedics,* ed 5, St Louis, 2000, Mosby.)

Thromboangiitis Obliterans

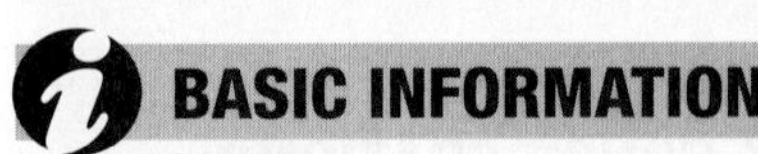

BASIC INFORMATION

DEFINITION

Thromboangiitis obliterans (TAO), or Buerger's disease, is a nonatherosclerotic inflammatory occlusive disease that commonly affects the small and medium-sized arteries, veins, and nerves of the upper and lower extremities.

SYNONYMS

Buerger's disease
Presenile gangrene

ICD-9CM CODES
443.1 Thromboangiitis obliterans (Buerger's disease)

EPIDEMIOLOGY & DEMOGRAPHICS

- TAO is most prevalent in the Middle East, the Far East, and Asia, where the prevalence can be as high as 45% to 63%.
- In the U.S., the prevalence has been estimated at 12.6 to 20 cases/100,000 persons.
- A genetic predisposition has been proposed on the basis of the higher incidence in Israel among Jews of Ashkenazi ancestry with peripheral artery disease.
- The symptoms almost always begin before the age of 40 yr, and almost all patients affected are smokers.
- TAO predominantly affects young men. However, there has been a recent increase in the prevalence of TAO among women; this has been attributed to increased smoking among women.
- Death from TAO is rare, but this disease can shorten the life span.
- Amputation is common, and major amputations (i.e., of limbs rather than of fingers or toes) are almost twice as common among patients who continue to smoke.
- The death rate has not been consistently shown to be higher among patients who do not stop smoking, but, for this and other health concerns, quitting is highly recommended.
- Female patients tend to have much higher longevity rates than men.

PHYSICAL FINDINGS & CLINICAL PRESENTATION

- TAO generally begins with hand or foot ischemia caused by the involvement of the distal small arteries and veins of the limbs.
- In 70% to 80% of cases, rest pain and diminished sensation from ischemic neuropathy are seen. This can sometimes lead to ischemic ulcerations of the toes or feet before the diagnosis of TAO is made.
- Rest pain generally occurs on the forefoot and causes continuous pain; patients may therefore sleep with their legs dangling downward.
- Ischemia of the upper limbs is clinically evident in 40% to 50% of patients, but it may be detected in 63% of patients with the use of Allen's test.
- There is evidence of prolonged capillary refill with dependent rubor and migratory thrombophlebitis.
- Systemic involvement, intestinal involvement, and central nervous system involvement are rare.

ETIOLOGY

- The cause of TAO is not completely known.
- Exposure to tobacco is essential for the initiation and progression of the disease; a small number of cases have been reported to be attributed to the use of chewing tobacco.
- Studies have suggested the presence of impaired endothelium-dependent vasorelaxation in the peripheral vasculature of patients with TAO.
- Pathologic studies have described three phases of thromboangiitis obliterans. The acute phase of the disease is characterized by the formation of occlusive inflammatory thrombi composed of multinucleated giant cells and polymorphonuclear leukocytes that typically involve the distal small vessels of the limbs. The organization of the thrombus takes place during the intermediate phase. The inflammation eventually subsides and leads to the chronic phase, which is characterized by vascular fibrosis and the organized thrombus of the affected vessels.
- There is no evidence to suggest that hypercoagulability abnormalities play a role in the disease mechanism.
- There is no overwhelming evidence to suggest a predominantly genetic or immunologic etiology for TAO.
- A seasonal variation of TAO that occurs with increased incidence during the winter months has been observed.

DIAGNOSIS

DIFFERENTIAL DIAGNOSIS

- Limb ischemia as a result of emboli or atherosclerotic occlusive disease
- Antiphospholipid antibody syndrome
- Autoimmune disorders
- Acrocyanosis
- Carpal tunnel syndrome
- CREST syndrome (i.e., *C*alcinosis cutis, *R*aynaud's phenomenon, *E*sophageal motility disorder, *S*clerodactyly, and *T*elangiectasia)
- Systemic lupus erythematosus
- Diabetes mellitus
- Repetitive vibratory equipment use
- Hypothenar hammer syndrome
- Raynaud's phenomenon
- Ergotamine intoxication
- Polyarteritis nodosa
- Cannabis arteritis
- Peripheral neuropathy

WORKUP

- The diagnosis of TAO is difficult because of the lack of specific clinical, radiologic, and biologic features of the disease. Point scoring systems are available to help with the diagnosis; however, at this time, no criteria have been validated or accepted internationally. The general rule is to suspect TAO in smokers who present with distal ischemia of the hands or feet. A definitive diagnosis is made when the histopathology examination identifies the acute-phase lesion in patients with signs of the disease. Without histopathology, the diagnosis is made by trying to eliminate the differential diagnoses and to search for other signs of the disease:
  1. Peripheral vascular disease occurring predominantly in men <40 yr old
  2. Typically affecting the arms and the legs and not just the lower extremities, as is seen with arteriosclerosis
  3. Found solely in tobacco smokers, with improvement seen among those who abstain
  4. Associated with migratory thrombophlebitis
  5. No other atherosclerotic risk factors (e.g., diabetes, cholesterol, hypertension)
- Angiographic criteria (see "Imaging Studies" later in this topic)
- TAO is an inflammatory disease; however, in contrast with all the major forms of arteritis, fibrinoid necrosis of the arterial wall is not observed, and the vascular wall is preserved. This feature distinguishes TAO from other types of systemic vasculitis and from arteriosclerosis, in which there is usually a disruption of the internal elastic lamina and the media.

LABORATORY TESTS

TAO cannot be diagnosed on the basis of a specific laboratory test. The primary goal of a laboratory workup in patients who are believed to have the disease is to exclude other disease processes from the differential diagnosis. Unlike with other forms of vasculitis, the Westergren sedimentation rate and the serum C-reactive protein level are usually normal in patients with TAO. Common autoantibodies (e.g., antinuclear antibody, rheumatoid factor), circulating immune complexes, complement levels, and cryoglobulins are negative in patients with TAO.

IMAGING STUDIES

- Noninvasive vascular studies help to differentiate proximal occlusive disease characteristic of arterial sclerosis from distal disease typical of TAO.
- Echocardiography should be performed for patients who are believed to have TAO to exclude a proximal source of emboli as the cause of distal vessel occlusion.
- Angiography findings of TAO include the following:
  - Involvement of distal small and medium-sized vessels
  - Occlusions that are segmental, multiple, smooth, and tapered
  - Collateral circulation that gives a "tree root" or "spider leg" appearance
  - Involvement of both the upper and lower extremities

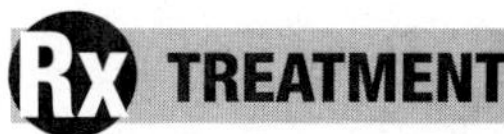

TREATMENT

NONPHARMACOLOGIC THERAPY

Abstaining from smoking is the only way to stop the progression of TAO. Medical and surgical treatments will prove to be futile if the patient continues to smoke. The exacerbation of ischemic ulcers is directly related to tobacco use.

ACUTE GENERAL RX

- The goals of medical treatment are to provide relief from ischemic pain and to heal ischemic ulcers. If the patient does not completely abstain from tobacco, medical measures will not be helpful.
- Treatment with intravenous iloprost, which is a prostaglandin analogue, has been shown to be effective for improving symptoms and reducing the amputation rate among patients with TAO.
- Epidural anesthesia and hyperbaric oxygen have a vasodilator effect and have been shown to provide relief from the pain of ischemic ulcers.
- Dalteparin may be beneficial for patients with associated foot ulcers, because it may help to improve skin oxygenation.
- Intermittent pneumatic compression devices enhance calf blood inflow in patients with limb ischemia and may serve as adjunctive therapy for patients with TAO.

CHRONIC RX

- As with medical treatment, surgical bypass procedures and sympathectomy will not be efficacious unless the patient stops smoking.
- Surgical bypass may be difficult because the occlusions of TAO are distal.
- Sympathectomy leads to increased blood flow by decreasing the vasoconstriction of distal vessels. It has also been shown to help heal and relieve the pain of ischemic ulcers.
- Debridement can be performed on necrotic ulcers, if needed.
- Amputation is frequently required for gangrenous digits.
- There are limited data regarding experimental gene transfer to induce therapeutic angiogenesis in patients with TAO.
- Carperitide (i.e., recombinant human atrial natriuretic peptide) may have therapeutic potential for the treatment of patients with refractory disease.
- The autologous transplantation of bone marrow mononuclear cells and related treatments remain controversial therapeutic options, because they have not been clearly proven to benefit patients with TAO.

DISPOSITION

The course of TAO can be dramatically changed by the cessation of tobacco smoking. If a patient continues to smoke, recurrent exacerbations of ischemic ulcers, necrosis, and gangrene leading to small digit amputations are inevitable.

REFERRAL

Smoking cessation counseling, rheumatology consultation, and vascular surgery consultation are recommended for any young smoker with claudication and ischemic ulcers, especially if both the upper and lower extremities are involved.

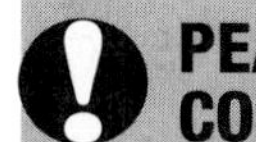

PEARLS & CONSIDERATIONS

COMMENTS

Smoking cessation is mandatory. For individuals who quit smoking, the prognosis is markedly improved.

PATIENT/FAMILY EDUCATION

Patients with TAO must be warned about tobacco use and secondhand smoke. Information for patients can be obtained from the following organizations:

- Vascular Disease Foundation (http://www.vdf.org)
- Mayo Foundation for Medical Education and Research (http://www.mayoclinic.com)

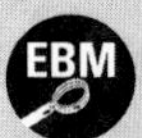

EVIDENCE

- Tobacco cessation is the only definitive therapy for TAO.[1]
- Seasonal variation of TAO, with increase incidence in the winter months, has been observed.[2,3]
- Prostacyclin analogues may help patients with critical limb ischemia seen in TAO.[4]
- Carperitide (recombinant human atrial natriuretic peptide) has therapeutic potential in treatment of refractory disease.[5]
- Recent experimental genetic and cell-based therapeutic approaches have been proposed to help in the treatment of TAO; however, further study is required.[6-8]
- Intermittent pneumatic compression devices enhance calf inflow in patients with limb ischemia and may serve as adjunctive therapy in patients with TAO.[9]
- Dalteparin may be beneficial in patients with associated foot ulcers because it may help improve skin oxygenation.[10]

Evidence-Based References

1. Olin JW et al: Thromboangiitis obliterans (Buerger's disease), *N Engl J Med* 343:864, 2000. Ⓐ
2. Laohapensang K et al: Seasonal variation of Buerger's disease in northern part of Thailand, *Eur J Vasc Endovasc Surg* 28(4):418, 2004. Ⓑ
3. Tavakoli H et al: Buerger's disease: a 10-year experience in Tehran, Iran, *Clin Rheumatol* 27(3):369, 2008. Ⓑ
4. Fiessinger JN et al: Trial of iloprost versus aspirin treatment for critical limb ischemia of thromboangiitis obliterans: the TAO study, *Lancet* 335:555, 1990. Ⓑ
5. Park K et al: Therapeutic potential of atrial natriuretic peptide administration on peripheral arterial diseases, *Endocrinology* 149(2):483, 2008. Ⓒ
6. Kim DI et al: Angiogenesis facilitated by autologous whole bone marrow stem cell transplantation for Buerger's disease, *Stem Cells* 24:1194, 2006. Ⓒ
7. Kim SW et al: Successful stem cell therapy using umbilical cord blood derived multi-potent stem cells for Buerger's disease and ischemic limb disease animal model, *Stem Cells* 24:1620, 2006. Ⓒ
8. De Vriese AS et al: Autologous transplantation of bone marrow mononuclear cells for limb ischemia in a Caucasian population with atherosclerosis obliterans, *J Intern Med* 263(4):395, 2008. Ⓒ
9. Labropoulos N et al: Acute effects of intermittent pneumatic compression on popliteal artery blood flow, *Arch Surg* 133:1072, 1998. Ⓒ
10. Kalani M et al: Effect of dalteparin on healing of chronic foot ulcers in diabetic patients with peripheral arterial occlusive disease: a prospective, randomized, double-blind, placebo-controlled study, *Diabetes Care* 26(9):2689, 2003. Ⓐ

SUGGESTED READINGS

Olin JW et al: Thromboangiitis obliterans (Buerger's disease), *Curr Opin Rheumatol* 18(1):18, 2006.

Puéchal X et al: Thromboangiitis obliterans or Buerger's disease: challenges for the rheumatologist, *Rheumatology* 46(2):192, 2007.

AUTHORS: **KHIET C. HOANG, M.D.,** and **PRANAV M. PATEL, M.D.**

BASIC INFORMATION

DEFINITION

Thrombocytosis is an elevated platelet count (>450,000/μl) in the peripheral blood. It may be caused by the cytokine-driven (reactive) overproduction of platelets or by a clonal expansion of megakaryocytes (i.e., autonomous thrombocytosis). The latter is defined as a chronic myeloproliferative disorder (CMPD) and classified into several subgroups, of which four are well characterized: chronic myelogenous leukemia (CML), polycythemia vera (PV), primary myelofibrosis (PMF), and essential thrombocythemia (ET). Extreme thrombocytosis is defined as a platelet count of >1,000,000/μl.

SYNONYMS

Thrombocythemia

ICD-9CM CODES
289.9 Unspecified diseases of blood and blood-forming organs
238.71 Essential thrombocytosis

EPIDEMIOLOGY & DEMOGRAPHICS

The following information applies to essential thrombocytosis.

INCIDENCE: 2.5 new cases per 100,000 population/yr

PREVALENCE: Estimated at 24 cases per 100,000 population

PREDOMINANT SEX: Female/male ratio is 2:1

PREDOMINANT AGE: The median age at diagnosis is 60 yr.

PHYSICAL FINDINGS & CLINICAL PRESENTATION

- Regardless of the cause, a high platelet count may be associated with vasomotor symptoms such as headache, visual disturbances, dizziness, atypical chest pain, acral dysesthesia, and erythromelalgia.
- Thrombotic and bleeding complications can occur.
- Symptoms and complications are much more likely to occur in association with autonomous thrombocytosis than with reactive thrombocytosis.
- The degree of thrombocytosis cannot predict the likelihood of autonomous thrombocytosis, and it does not generally correlate with the risk of thrombosis.
- Splenomegaly is common with CMPD.
- Coexistent leukocytosis and erythrocytosis are common with CML and PV.
- Disease transformation from ET to PV, PMF, or acute myeloid leukemia is uncommon. The incidences have been reported as 2.7%, 4%, and 1.4%, respectively, after a median follow-up of 9.2 years.

ETIOLOGY

- JAK2 mutation is frequent with CMPD (100% with PV, 50% with ET, and 40% to 60% with PMF).
- MPL mutation is seen in 1% to 4% of ET patients.

DIAGNOSIS

DIFFERENTIAL DIAGNOSIS

- For spurious thrombocytosis:
  - Mixed cryoglobulinemia
  - Circulating cytoplasmic fragments in patients with leukemia, lymphoma, or severe hemolysis or burns counted as platelets
- For reactive thrombocytosis:
  - Acute hemorrhage
  - Iron deficiency anemia
  - Hemolytic anemia
  - Rheumatologic disorders
  - Inflammatory bowel disease
  - Celiac disease
  - Functional and surgical asplenia
  - Trauma
  - Thermal burn
  - Myocardial infarction
  - Acute pancreatitis
  - Recent surgery
  - Chronic infection (e.g., tuberculosis)
  - Renal failure
  - Nephrotic syndrome
  - Exercise
  - Medications (e.g., vincristine, epinephrine)
- For autonomous thrombocytosis:
  - Chronic myelogenous leukemia
  - Polycythemia vera
  - Primary myelofibrosis
  - Myelodysplastic syndrome (i.e., 5q− syndrome)
  - Acute myeloid leukemia with inv(3), t(3; 3)
  - Essential thrombocytosis

WORKUP

- Repeat CBC with peripheral blood smear to exclude spurious thrombocytosis
- Comprehensive history and physical examination to exclude many of the common causes of reactive thrombocytosis; acute blood loss, iron deficiency, acute or chronic infection or inflammation, medication use, asplenia, malignancy, and trauma should be looked for

LABORATORY TESTS

- CBC with peripheral blood smear: Howell-Jolly bodies and target cells are present in patients with asplenia; nucleated RBCs, teardrop RBCs, and WBC precursors are seen in patients with PMF.
- Serum ferritin level: Low ferritin levels suggest iron deficiency.
- Serum C-reactive protein, erythrocyte sedimentation rate, and plasma fibrinogen are nonspecific markers of infection and inflammation.
- Philadelphia chromosome or *BCR-ABL* rearrangement is positive with CML.
- Serum erythropoietin assay is low to normal with PV and ET.
- JAK2 mutation analysis should be done for suspected PV and ET.
- Bone marrow chromosome analysis should be done for suspected 5q− syndrome, other myelodysplastic syndromes, and CML.

TREATMENT

Reactive thrombocytosis has rarely been associated with thrombosis or bleeding and generally does not require specific therapy.

ACUTE GENERAL RX

- Vasomotor symptoms are easily manageable with low-dose aspirin (e.g., 40 to 81 mg/day).
- For bleeding:
  - Discontinue any platelet antiaggregating agents (e.g., aspirin, nonsteroidal anti-inflammatory drugs).
  - Evaluate for disseminated intravascular coagulopathy and coagulation factor deficiency. Acquired factor V deficiency is occasionally present in association with autonomous thrombocytosis. If that is the case, treat the patient with a fresh frozen plasma infusion.
  - In cases of extreme thrombocytosis, acquired von Willebrand's disease may occur. Immediate platelet apheresis with definitive therapy with a platelet-lowering agent is essential for these patients.
- For thrombosis:
  - If the platelet count is >800,000/μl, platelet apheresis coupled with a platelet-lowering agent should be started, with the goal being a platelet count of <400,000/μl.
  - The initial workup should include a search for additional thrombophilic diseases such as protein C and S deficiency, antithrombin deficiency, anticardiolipin antibody, factor V Leiden mutation, prothrombin gene mutation, and plasma homocysteine.
  - Anticoagulant therapy should be continued for 3 to 9 months on the basis of the presence or absence of additional thrombophilic defects.

CHRONIC RX

- Treatment strategies for ET are based on the presence or absence of risk factors for thrombosis. Cytoreductive therapy is indicated for high-risk patients who are 60 yr old or older or who have a history of thrombosis.
- Low-dose aspirin (<81 mg/day) may be safe and possibly effective for the prevention of vascular events.
- Hydroxyurea (HU) vs. anagrelide: HU plus aspirin is thought to be safer and more effective than anagrelide plus aspirin with regard to thrombosis, bleeding, and transformation to PMF at 5 years in a randomized trial.
- The incidence of leukemic conversion in patients with ET treated with HU alone is reported as 0% to 5%.
- Interferon-alpha may be effective for controlling the platelet count of patients for whom treatment with HU is ineffective.

DISPOSITION

Most patients with ET have a normal life expectancy without disease-related complications.

T

REFERRAL

Hematology or oncology consultation when the platelet count is consistently >450,000/μl without known causes of reactive thrombocytosis

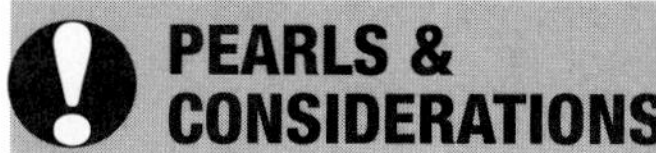

PEARLS & CONSIDERATIONS

COMMENTS

- Some patients with clinically apparent ET have Philadelphia chromosome or *BCR-ABL* rearrangement, even in the absence of other features of CML. It is suggested that these should be looked for in all patients with ET because of the potential therapeutic implications.
- The risk of bleeding with aspirin use among patients with ET is increased when the platelet count is >1,000,000/μl.

PATIENT/FAMILY EDUCATION

Smoking cessation is encouraged in patients with ET and in those with reactive thrombocytosis.

SUGGESTED READINGS

Campbell PJ et al: Definition of subtypes of essential thrombocythemia and relation to polycythemia vera based on JAK2 V617F mutation status: a prospective study, *Lancet* 366:1945, 2005.

Harrison CN et al: Hydroxyurea compared with anagrelide in high-risk essential thrombocythemia, *N Engl J Med* 353:33, 2005.

Schafer AI: Molecular basis of the diagnosis and treatment of polycythemia vera and essential thrombosis, *Blood* 107:4214, 2006.

AUTHOR: **ETSUKO AOKI, M.D., PH.D.**

BASIC INFORMATION

DEFINITION

Superficial thrombophlebitis is inflammatory thrombosis in subcutaneous veins. Superficial suppurative thrombophlebitis is an inflammation of the vein wall caused by the presence of microorganisms and occurring as a complication of either dermal infection or use of an indwelling intravenous catheter.

SYNONYMS

Phlebitis
Superficial suppurative thrombophlebitis

ICD-9CM CODES
451.0 Thrombophlebitis, superficial

EPIDEMIOLOGY & DEMOGRAPHICS

- 20% of superficial thrombophlebitis cases are associated with occult deep vein thrombosis (DVT).
- Catheter-related thrombophlebitis incidence is 100 in 100,000. The disease occurs more frequently when plastic catheters are inserted in the lower extremities. The mean duration of preceding venous cannulation is 4.8 days, and the latent interval from removal of the catheter to development of symptoms ranges from 2 to 10 days.

PHYSICAL FINDINGS & CLINICAL PRESENTATION

- Subcutaneous vein is palpable, tender; tender cord is present with erythema and edema of the overlying skin and subcutaneous tissue.
- Induration, redness, and tenderness are localized along the course of the vein. This linear appearance rather than circular appearance is useful to distinguish thrombophlebitis from other conditions (cellulitis, erythema nodosum).
- There is no significant swelling of the limb (superficial thrombophlebitis generally does not produce swelling of the limb).
- Low-grade fever may be present. High fever and chills are suggestive of septic phlebitis.
- Superficial suppurative thrombophlebitis may be difficult to identify because local findings of inflammation may be absent. Fever is present in >70% of cases but rigors are rare. Local findings (warmth, erythema, tenderness, swelling, lymphangitis) are present in only one third of patients.

ETIOLOGY

- Trauma to preexisting varices.
- Intravenous cannulation of veins (most common cause).
- Abdominal cancer (e.g., carcinoma of pancreas).
- Infection: *Staphylococcus aureus* was the most common pathogen, found in 65% to 78% of the cases of superficial suppurative thrombophlebitis before 1970; now most cases are caused by *Enterobacteriaceae*, especially *Klebsiella-Enterobacter* spp. These agents are acquired nosocomially and are often resistant to multiple antibiotics. Infection with fungi or gram-negative aerobic bacilli is often seen in patients who are receiving broad-spectrum antibiotics at the time of the superficial suppurative phlebitis.
- Hypercoagulable state.
- DVT.

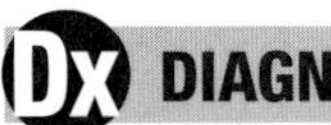

DIAGNOSIS

DIFFERENTIAL DIAGNOSIS

- Lymphangitis
- Cellulitis
- Erythema nodosum
- Panniculitis
- Kaposi's sarcoma

WORKUP

Laboratory evaluation to exclude infectious etiology and imaging studies to rule out DVT in suspected cases

LABORATORY TESTS

- Complete blood count with differential, blood cultures, culture of IV catheter tip (when secondary to intravenous cannulation). Bacteremia occurs in 80% to 90% of the cases of superficial suppurative thrombophlebitis.
- Culture of the catheter may be misleading because even though bacteria are isolated in 60% of the cases, a positive culture does not correlate with inflammation.
- Exploratory venotomy may be necessary in suspected superficial suppurative thrombophlebitis.

IMAGING STUDIES

- Serial compression ultrasound in patients with suspected DVT
- CT scan of abdomen and pelvis in patients with suspected malignancy (Trousseau's syndrome: recurrent migratory thrombophlebitis)

Rx TREATMENT

NONPHARMACOLOGIC THERAPY

- Warm, moist compresses.
- It is not necessary to restrict activity; however, if there is extensive thrombophlebitis, bed rest with the leg elevated will limit the thrombosis and improve symptoms.

ACUTE GENERAL Rx

- Nonsteroidal anti-inflammatory drugs to relieve symptoms
- Treatment of septic thrombophlebitis with antibiotics with adequate coverage of *Enterobacteriaceae* and *Staphylococcus.* Initial empirical treatment with a semisynthetic penicillin (IV nafcillin 2 g q4-6h plus either an aminoglycoside [gentamicin 1 mg/kg IV q8h] or a third-generation cephalosporin [cefotaxime] or a quinolone [ciprofloxacin]).
- Oral dicloxacillin or cephalexin may be adequate for outpatient treatment or mild cases of superficial thrombophlebitis.
- Ligation and division of the superficial vein at the junction to avoid propagation of the clot in the deep venous system when the thrombophlebitis progresses toward the junction of the involved superficial vein with deep veins.
- The role of antifungal therapy for superficial suppurative thrombophlebitis caused by *Candida albicans* is controversial. Most of these infections can be cured by vein excision. Because of the propensity of these infections for hematogenous spread, a 10- to 14-day course of amphotericin B or fluconazole is advisable.

DISPOSITION

Clinical improvement within 7 to 10 days

REFERRAL

Surgical referral in selected cases (see "Acute General Rx")

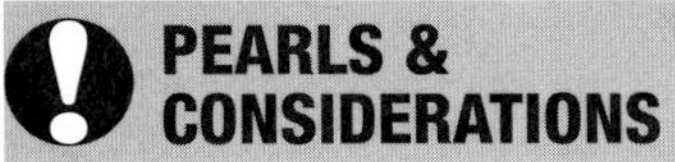

PEARLS & CONSIDERATIONS

COMMENTS

- Patients with positive cultures should be evaluated and treated for endocarditis.
- Suppurative thrombophlebitis is a particular problem in burned patients; it represents a common cause of death from infection.
- Septic thrombophlebitis is more common in IV drug addicts.

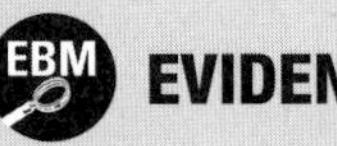

EVIDENCE

A systematic review found that low-molecular-weight heparin is at least as effective as unfractionated heparin in preventing recurrent venous thromboembolism and significantly reduces the occurrence of major hemorrhage during initial treatment and overall mortality rate at follow-up. The reviewers conclude that it can be adopted safely as the standard therapy for DVT.[1] Ⓐ

Evidence-Based Reference

1. van den Belt AGM et al: Fixed dose subcutaneous low molecular weight heparins versus adjusted dose unfractionated heparin for venous thromboembolism, *Cochrane Rev* 4, 2004. Ⓐ

SUGGESTED READING

Gillespie P et al: Cannula related suppurative thrombophlebitis in the burned patient, *Burns* 26:200-204, 2000.

AUTHOR: **FRED F. FERRI, M.D.**

BASIC INFORMATION

DEFINITION

Thrombotic thrombocytopenic purpura (TTP) is a rare disorder characterized by thrombocytopenia (often accompanied by purpura) and microangiopathic hemolytic anemia; neurologic impairment, renal dysfunction, and fever may also be present.

SYNONYMS

TTP

ICD-9CM CODES

446.6 Thrombotic thrombocytopenic purpura

EPIDEMIOLOGY & DEMOGRAPHICS

- TTP primarily affects females between ages 10 and 50 yr.
- Frequency is 11 cases annually per 1 million persons.

PHYSICAL FINDINGS & CLINICAL PRESENTATION

- Most patients present with nonspecific constitutional symptoms (weakness, nausea, abdominal pain, vomiting)
- Purpura (secondary to thrombocytopenia)
- Jaundice, pallor (from hemolysis)
- Mucosal bleeding
- Fever
- Fluctuating levels of consciousness (caused by thrombotic occlusion of the cerebral vessels)
- Renal failure and neurologic events are usually end-stage features

ETIOLOGY

- TTP is caused in some patients by an acquired deficiency of a circulating metalloproteinase. It can also be caused, in very rare cases, by a hereditary deficiency of ADAMTS13.
- Many drugs, including clopidogrel, penicillin, antineoplastic agents, oral contraceptives, quinine, and ticlopidine, have been associated with TTP. Other precipitating causes include infectious agents, pregnancy, malignancies, allogenic bone marrow transplantation, and neurologic disorders.

Dx DIAGNOSIS

DIFFERENTIAL DIAGNOSIS

- Disseminated intravascular coagulation (DIC)
- Malignant hypertension
- Vasculitis
- Eclampsia or preeclampsia
- Hemolytic-uremic syndrome (typically encountered in children, often after a viral infection)
- Gastroenteritis as a result of a serotoxin-producing serotype of *Escherichia coli*
- Medications: clopidogrel, ticlopidine, penicillin, antineoplastic chemotherapeutic agents, oral contraceptives

WORKUP

- A comprehensive history, physical examination, and laboratory evaluation usually confirm the diagnosis.
- The disease often begins as a flulike illness ultimately followed by clinical and laboratory abnormalities.
- An algorithm for the diagnosis of TTP is described in Section III.

LABORATORY TESTS

- Severe anemia and thrombocytopenia (platelet count $<$50,000 or $>$50% reduction from previous counts
- Elevated blood urea nitrogen and creatinine
- Evidence of hemolysis: elevated reticulocyte count, indirect bilirubin, lactate dehydrogenase, decreased haptoglobin
- Urinalysis: hematuria (red blood cells [RBCs] and RBC casts in urine sediment) and proteinuria
- Peripheral smear: severely fragmented RBCs (schistocytes). More than 4% RBC fragments in the peripheral blood.
- No laboratory evidence of DIC (normal fibrin degradation product, fibrinogen)
- The ADAMTS13 level is not necessary and metalloproteinase deficiency need not be proved for diagnosis of TTP

Rx TREATMENT

ACUTE GENERAL Rx

- Discontinue potential offending agents.
- The American Association of Blood Banks, the American Society for Apheresis, and the British Committee for Standards in Haematology recommend daily plasma exchange with replacement of 1.0 to 1.5 times the predicted plasma volume of the patient as standard therapy for TTP. The British guidelines recommend that plasma exchange therapy be continued for a minimum of 2 days after the platelet count returns to normal ($>$150,000 cells/m^3).
- Corticosteroids (prednisone 1 to 2 mg/kg/day) use is controversial. They may be effective alone in patients with mild disease or may be administered concomitantly with plasmapheresis plus plasma exchange with fresh frozen plasma.
- High-dose plasma infusion (25 ml/kg/day) may be useful only if plasma exchange cannot be promptly started and for patients with very severe or refractory disease between plasma exchange sessions. High-dose plasma infusions can cause volume overload in patients with renal insufficiency.
- The monoclonal antibody rituximab has also been used for treatment of TTP.
- Platelet transfusions are contraindicated except in severely thrombocytopenic patients with documented bleeding.
- Use of antiplatelet agents (acetylsalicylic acid, dipyridamole) is controversial.
- Splenectomy is performed in refractory cases.

CHRONIC Rx

- Relapsing TTP may be treated with plasma exchange.
- Remission of chronic TTP that is unresponsive to conventional therapy has been reported after treatment with cyclophosphamide and the monoclonal antibody rituximab.
- Splenectomy done while the patients are in remission has been used in some centers to decrease the frequency of relapse in TTP.

DISPOSITION

- Survival of patients with TTP currently exceeds 80% with plasma exchange therapy.
- Relapse occurs in 20% to 40% of patients who have TTP in remission.

REFERRAL

Surgical referral for splenectomy in selected patients (see "Acute General Rx" and "Chronic Rx.")

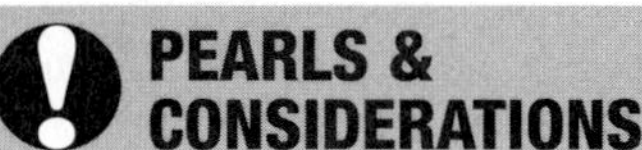

PEARLS & CONSIDERATIONS

COMMENTS

Thrombotic microangiopathy can also be associated with administration of cyclosporine and mitomycin C and with HIV infection.

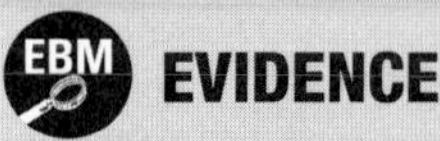

EVIDENCE

Plasma exchange versus plasma infusion with fresh frozen plasma is associated with a significantly higher response rate (increase in platelet count) and lower mortality rate in patients receiving treatment with aspirin and dipyridamole for TTP.[1] B

There is no significant difference in outcome between plasma exchange with fresh frozen plasma compared with exchange with cryoprecipitate-poor plasma as initial treatment for patients with TTP.[2] B

Evidence-Based References

1. Rock GA et al: Comparison of plasma exchange with plasma infusion in the treatment of thrombotic thrombocytopenic purpura. Canadian Apheresis Study Group, *N Engl J Med* 325:393, 1991. B
2. Zeigler ZR et al: Cryoprecipitate poor plasma does not improve early response in primary adult thrombotic thrombocytopenic purpura (TTP), *J Clin Apheresis* 16:19, 2001. B

SUGGESTED READINGS

Crowther MA, George JN: Thrombotic thrombocytopenic purpura: 2008 update, *Cleve Clin J Med* 75:369, 2008.

George JN: Thrombotic thrombocytopenic purpura, *N Engl J Med* 354:1927, 2006.

AUTHOR: **FRED F. FERRI, M.D.**

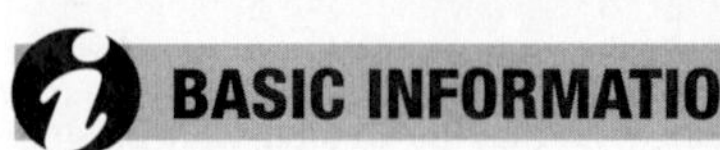

BASIC INFORMATION

DEFINITION

Thyroid carcinoma is a primary neoplasm of the thyroid. There are four major types of thyroid carcinoma: papillary, follicular, anaplastic, and medullary.

SYNONYMS

Papillary carcinoma of thyroid
Follicular carcinoma of thyroid
Anaplastic carcinoma of thyroid
Medullary carcinoma of thyroid

ICD-9CM CODES
193 Malignant neoplasm of thyroid

EPIDEMIOLOGY & DEMOGRAPHICS

- Thyroid cancer is the most common endocrine cancer, with an annual incidence of 14,000 new cases in the U.S. and approximately 1100 deaths.
- Female/male ratio is 3:1.
- Most common type (50% to 60%) is papillary carcinoma.
- Median age at diagnosis: 45 to 50 yr.

PHYSICAL FINDINGS & CLINICAL PRESENTATION

- Presence of thyroid nodule
- Hoarseness and cervical lymphadenopathy
- Painless swelling in the region of the thyroid

ETIOLOGY

- Risk factors: prior neck irradiation
- Multiple endocrine neoplasia II (medullary carcinoma)

DIAGNOSIS

DIFFERENTIAL DIAGNOSIS

- Multinodular goiter
- Lymphocytic thyroiditis
- Ectopic thyroid

WORKUP

The workup of thyroid carcinoma includes laboratory evaluation and diagnostic imaging. However, diagnosis is confirmed with fine-needle aspiration or surgical biopsy. The characteristics of thyroid carcinoma vary with the type:

- Papillary carcinoma:
  1. Most frequently occurs in women during second or third decades
  2. Histologically, psammoma bodies (calcific bodies present in papillary projections) are pathognomonic; found in 35% to 45% of papillary thyroid carcinomas
  3. Majority are not papillary lesions but mixed papillary follicular carcinomas
  4. Spread is by lymphatics and by local invasion
- Follicular carcinoma:
  1. More aggressive than papillary carcinoma
  2. Incidence increases with age
  3. Tends to metastasize hematogenously to bone, producing pathologic fractures
  4. Tends to concentrate iodine (useful for radiation therapy)
- Anaplastic carcinoma:
  1. Very aggressive neoplasm
  2. Two major histologic types: small cell (less aggressive, 5-yr survival approximately 20%) and giant cell (death usually within 6 mo of diagnosis)
- Medullary carcinoma:
  1. Unifocal lesion: found sporadically in elderly patients
  2. Bilateral lesions: associated with pheochromocytoma and hyperparathyroidism; this combination is known as MEN-II and is inherited as an autosomal-dominant disorder

LABORATORY TESTS

- Thyroid function studies are generally normal. Thyroid-stimulating hormone (TSH), T_4, and serum thyroglobulin levels should be obtained before thyroidectomy in patients with confirmed thyroid carcinoma.
- Increased plasma calcitonin assay in patients with medullary carcinoma (tumors produce thyrocalcitonin).

IMAGING STUDIES (Fig. 1-331)

- Thyroid scanning with iodine-123 or technetium-99m can identify hypofunctioning (cold) nodules, which are more likely to be malignant. However, warm nodules can also be malignant.
- Thyroid ultrasound can detect solitary solid nodules that have a high risk of malignancy. However, a negative ultrasound does not exclude diagnosis of thyroid carcinoma.
- Fine-needle aspiration biopsy is the best method to assess a thyroid nodule (see "Thyroid Nodule" in Section I).

TREATMENT

ACUTE GENERAL Rx

- Papillary carcinoma:
  1. Total thyroidectomy is indicated if the patient has:
     a. Extrapyramidal extension of carcinoma
     b. Papillary carcinoma limited to thyroid but a positive history of irradiation to the neck
     c. Lesion >2 cm
  2. Lobectomy with isthmectomy may be considered in patients with intrathyroid papillary carcinoma <2 cm and no history of neck or head irradiation; most follow surgery with suppressive therapy with thyroid hormone because these tumors are TSH responsive. The accepted practice is to suppress serum TSH concentrations to <0.1 mcU/ml.
  3. Radiotherapy with iodine-131 (after total thyroidectomy), followed by thyroid suppression therapy with triiodothyronine, can be used in metastatic papillary carcinoma.
- Follicular carcinoma:
  1. Total thyroidectomy followed by TSH suppression, as previously noted
  2. Radiotherapy with iodine-131 followed by thyroid suppression therapy with triiodothyronine is useful in patients with metastasis
- Anaplastic carcinoma:
  1. At diagnosis, this neoplasm is rarely operable; palliative surgery is indicated for extremely large tumor compressing the trachea.
  2. Management is usually restricted to radiation therapy or chemotherapy (combination of doxorubicin, cisplatin, and other antineoplastic agents); these measures rarely provide significant palliation.

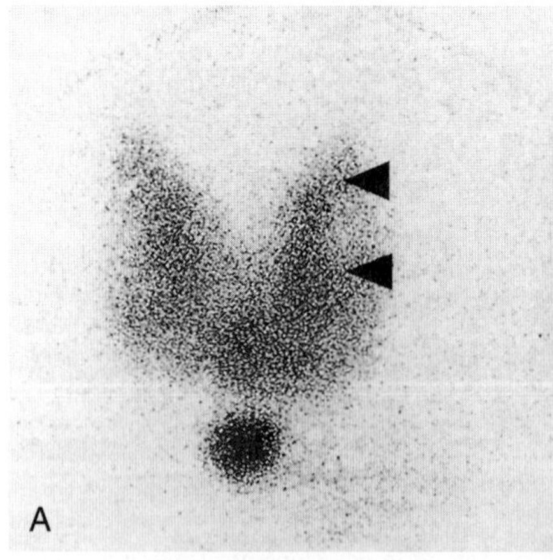

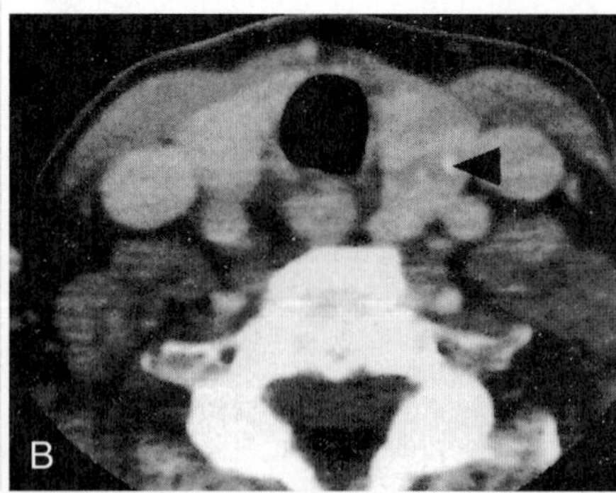

FIGURE 1-331 Papillary adenocarcinoma. A 74-year-old woman presented with a thyroid nodule. **A,** An I123 thyroid scan (anterior view) demonstrates a "cold" nodule *(arrows)* in the upper portion of the left thyroid lobe. The "hot" spot below the thyroid is a suprasternal marker. **B,** An axial CT scan demonstrates an irregular density within the left thyroid lobe at the level of the lesion seen on the radionuclide scan. The lesion contains a single area of calcification *(arrow)* and is not sharply demarcated from normal thyroid tissue. At operation, there proved to be extracapsular extension. (From Skarin AT: *Atlas of diagnostic oncology,* ed 3, St Louis, 2003, Mosby.)

- Medullary carcinoma:
    1. Thyroidectomy should be performed.
    2. Patients and their families should be screened for pheochromocytoma and hyperparathyroidism.

DISPOSITION

Prognosis varies with the type of thyroid carcinoma: 5-yr survival approaches 80% for follicular carcinoma and is approximately 5% with anaplastic carcinoma.

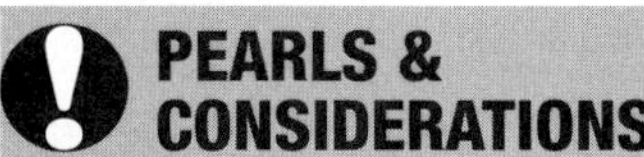

PEARLS & CONSIDERATIONS

COMMENTS

Family members of patients with medullary carcinoma should be screened; DNA analysis for the detection of mutations in the *RET* gene structure permits the identification of *MEN IIA* gene carriers.

Motesanib, an oral inhibitor of vascular endothelial growth factor (VEGF) receptors, has been reported effective in inducing partial responses in patients with advanced or metastatic differentiated thyroid cancer that is progressive.

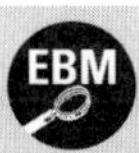

EVIDENCE

A lack of randomized trials has evaluated the use of the primary treatments for differentiated thyroid carcinoma. Their use is governed by clinical experience and supported by consensus opinion.

Guidelines from the American Thyroid Association include the following statements regarding thyroid surgery in the treatment of differentiated thyroid carcinoma:

For most patients with thyroid cancer, the initial surgical procedure should be near-total or total thyroidectomy.[1] C

Thyroid lobectomy alone may be sufficient treatment for small, low-risk, isolated intrathyroidal papillary carcinomas in the absence of cervical nodal metastases.[1] C

Guidelines from the American Thyroid Association include the following statements relating to the role of neck dissection in the treatment of differentiated thyroid carcinoma:

Routine central-compartment (level VI) neck dissection should be considered for patients with papillary thyroid carcinoma and suspected Hürthle carcinoma. Near-total or total thyroidectomy without central node dissection may be appropriate for follicular cancer, and when followed by radioactive iodine therapy may provide an alternative approach for papillary and Hürthle cell cancers.[1] C

Lateral neck compartmental lymph node dissection should be performed for patients with biopsy-proven metastatic cervical lymphadenopathy detected clinically or by imaging, especially when they are likely to be unresponsive to radioactive iodine treatment based on lymph node size, number, or other factors, such as aggressive histology of the primary tumor.[1] C

Patients with persistent or recurrent disease confined to the neck should undergo complete ipsilateral or central compartmental dissection of involved compartments while sparing vital structures.[1] C

Guidelines from the American Thyroid Association include the following recommendation regarding radioablation:

Radioiodine ablation is recommended for patients with TNM stages III and IV disease; all patients with stage II disease <45 yr and most patients with stage II disease ≥45 yr; and selected patients with stage I disease, especially those with multifocal disease, nodal metastases, extrathyroidal or vascular invasion, and/or more aggressive histologies.[1] C

Guidelines from the American Thyroid Association include the following statement relating to the role of external-beam radiation in the treatment of differentiated thyroid carcinoma:

The use of external-beam irradiation should be considered in patients >45 yr with grossly visible extrathyroidal extension at the time of surgery and a high likelihood of microscopic residual disease and for those patients with gross residual tumor in whom further surgery or radioactive iodine would likely be ineffective.[1] C

Guidelines from the American Thyroid Association include the following statements relating to the role of chemotherapy in the treatment of differentiated thyroid carcinoma:

No data support the use of adjunctive chemotherapy in the management of differentiated thyroid cancer, and there is no role for its routine use in this context.[1] C

Doxorubicin (Adriamycin) may act as a radiation sensitizer in some tumors of thyroid origin and could be considered for patients with locally advanced disease undergoing external-beam radiation.[1] C

A lack of randomized trials have evaluated the use of the primary treatments for medullary carcinoma of the thyroid. The use of surgery as the major treatment modality is governed by clinical experience and supported by consensus opinion.

Guidelines from the National Comprehensive Cancer Network panel on thyroid carcinoma include the following statements regarding the treatment of medullary carcinoma:

Surgery is the main treatment for medullary thyroid carcinoma because there is no known curative systemic therapy for medullary carcinoma.[2] C

Total thyroidectomy is indicated in all patients with medullary thyroid carcinoma, especially because of the high frequency of bilateral disease in both sporadic and familial disease.[2] C

If a patient with inherited disease is diagnosed early enough, the recommendation is generally to perform total thyroidectomy by age 5 yr.[2] C

A bilateral central neck dissection (level VI) is preferred for all patients with pathologically demonstrated medullary thyroid carcinoma and for those with MEN2B.[2] C

Postoperative thyroid hormone therapy is indicated; however, TSH suppression is not appropriate because C cells lack TSH receptors.[2] C

Adjuvant radiotherapy can be considered for patients with T4 disease whose tumors are ≥1.0 cm in diameter.[2] C

As for differentiated carcinoma, external-beam radiation therapy can also be given to palliate painful or progressing bone metastases.[2] C

A lack of randomized trials have evaluated the use of the primary treatments for anaplastic carcinoma of the thyroid. The use of surgery as the major treatment modality is governed by clinical experience and supported by consensus opinion.

Guidelines from the National Comprehensive Cancer Network panel on thyroid carcinoma include the following general statements regarding the treatment of anaplastic carcinoma:

If the disease is deemed likely to be resectable, an attempt at total or near-total thyroidectomy should be made, with selective resection of all involved local or regional structures and nodes.[2] C

Patients with tumors that cannot be completely removed should instead receive efforts to protect their airway, including the possibility of a prophylactic tracheostomy.[2] C

All patients, regardless of surgical resection, should then undergo multimodality therapy.[2] C

Evidence-Based References

1. Cooper DS et al: The American Thyroid Association Guidelines Taskforce. Management guidelines for patients with thyroid nodules and differentiated thyroid cancer, *Thyroid* 16:109, 2006.
2. National Comprehensive Cancer Network: NCCN Clinical Practice Guidelines in Oncology, *Thyroid carcinoma,* 2007.

SUGGESTED READING

Sherman SI et al: Motesanib diphosphate in progressive differentiated thyroid cancer, *N Engl J Med* 359:31, 2008.

AUTHOR: **FRED F. FERRI, M.D.**

 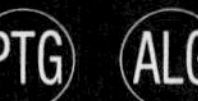

BASIC INFORMATION

DEFINITION

A thyroid nodule is an abnormality found on physical examination of the thyroid gland; nodules can be benign (70%) or malignant.

ICD-9CM CODES
241.0 Nodule, thyroid

EPIDEMIOLOGY & DEMOGRAPHICS

- Palpable thyroid nodules occur in 4% to 7% of the population.
- Thyroid nodules can be found in 50% of autopsies; however, only one in 10 is palpable.
- Malignancy is present in 5% to 30% of palpable nodules.
- Incidence of thyroid nodules increases after age 45 yr. They are found more frequently in women.
- History of prior head and neck irradiation increases the risk of thyroid cancer.
- Increased likelihood that nodule is malignant: nodule increasing in size or >2 cm, regional lymphadenopathy, fixation to adjacent tissues, age <40 yr, symptoms of local invasion (dysphagia, hoarseness, neck pain, male sex, family history of thyroid cancer or polyposis [Gardner syndrome]), rapid growth during levothyroxine therapy.

PHYSICAL FINDINGS & CLINICAL PRESENTATION

- Palpable, firm, and nontender nodule in the thyroid area should prompt suspicion of carcinoma. Signs of metastasis are regional lymphadenopathy and inspiratory stridor.
- Signs and symptoms of thyrotoxicosis can be found in functioning nodules.

ETIOLOGY

- History of prior head and neck irradiation
- Family history of pheochromocytoma, carcinoma of the thyroid, and hyperparathyroidism (medullary carcinoma of the thyroid is a component of MEN-II)

Dx DIAGNOSIS

DIFFERENTIAL DIAGNOSIS

- Thyroid carcinoma
- Multinodular goiter
- Thyroglossal duct cyst
- Epidermoid cyst
- Laryngocele
- Nonthyroid neck neoplasm
- Branchial cleft cyst

WORKUP

- Fine-needle aspiration (FNA) biopsy is the best diagnostic study; the accuracy can be >90%, but it is directly related to the level of experience of the physician and the cytopathologist interpreting the aspirate.
- FNA biopsy is less reliable with thyroid cystic lesions; surgical excision should be considered for most thyroid cysts not abolished by aspiration.
- A diagnostic approach to thyroid nodule is described in Section III.

LABORATORY TESTS

- Thyroid-stimulating hormone (TSH), T_4, and serum thyroglobulin levels should be obtained before thyroidectomy in patients with confirmed thyroid carcinoma on FNA biopsy.
- Serum calcitonin at random or after pentagastrin stimulation is useful when suspecting medullary carcinoma of the thyroid and in anyone with a family history of medullary thyroid carcinoma.
- Serum thyroid autoantibodies (see "Thyroiditis" in Section I) are useful when suspecting thyroiditis.

IMAGING STUDIES

- Thyroid ultrasound is done in some patients to evaluate the size of the thyroid and the number, composition (solid vs. cystic), and dimensions of the thyroid nodule; solid thyroid nodules have a higher incidence of malignancy, but cystic nodules can also be malignant.
- The introduction of high-resolution ultrasonography has made it possible to detect many nonpalpable nodules (incidentalomas) in the thyroid (found at autopsy in 30% to 60% of cadavers). Most of these lesions are benign. For most patients with nonpalpable nodules that are incidentally detected by thyroid imaging, simple follow-up neck palpation is sufficient.
- Thyroid scan can be performed with technetium-99m pertechnetate, iodine-123, or iodine-131. Iodine isotopes are preferred because up to 35% of nodules that appear functioning on pertechnetate scanning (Fig. 1-332) may appear nonfunctioning on radioiodine scanning. A thyroid scan:
  1. Classifies nodules as hyperfunctioning (hot), normally functioning (warm), or nonfunctioning (cold); cold nodules have a higher incidence of malignancy.
  2. Scan has difficulty evaluating nodules near the thyroid isthmus or at the periphery of the gland.
  3. Normal tissue over a nonfunctioning nodule might mask the nodule as "warm" or normally functioning.
- Both thyroid scan and ultrasound provide information about the risk of malignant neoplasia based on the characteristics of the thyroid nodule, but their value in the initial evaluation of a thyroid nodule is limited because neither provides a definite tissue diagnosis.

Rx TREATMENT

GENERAL Rx

- Evaluation of results of FNA:
  1. Normal cells: may repeat biopsy during present evaluation or reevaluate patient after 3 to 6 mo of suppressive therapy (l-thyroxine, prescribed in doses to suppress the TSH level to 0.1 to 0.5)
     a. Failure to regress indicates increased likelihood of malignancy.
     b. Reliance on repeat FNA biopsy is preferable to routine surgery for nodules not responding to thyroxine.
  2. Malignant cells: surgery
  3. Hypercellularity: thyroid scan
     a. Hot nodule: ^{131}I therapy if the patient is hyperthyroid
     b. Warm or cold nodule: surgery (rule out follicular adenoma vs. carcinoma)

DISPOSITION

Variable with results of FNA biopsy

REFERRAL

Surgical referral for FNA biopsy

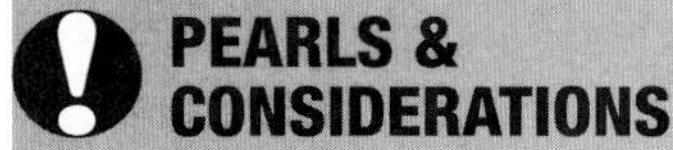

PEARLS & CONSIDERATIONS

COMMENTS

- Most solid, benign nodules grow; therefore an increase in nodule volume alone is not a reliable predictor of malignancy.
- Surgery is indicated in hard or fixed nodule, presence of dysphagia or hoarseness, and rapidly growing solid masses regardless of "benign" results on FNA.
- Suppressive therapy of malignant thyroid nodules postoperatively with thyroxine is indicated. The use of suppressive therapy for benign solitary nodules is controversial.
- The preferred approach when repeated FNA fails to yield an adequate specimen remains a challenge. Immunohistochemical markers (galectin-3, human bone marrow endothelial

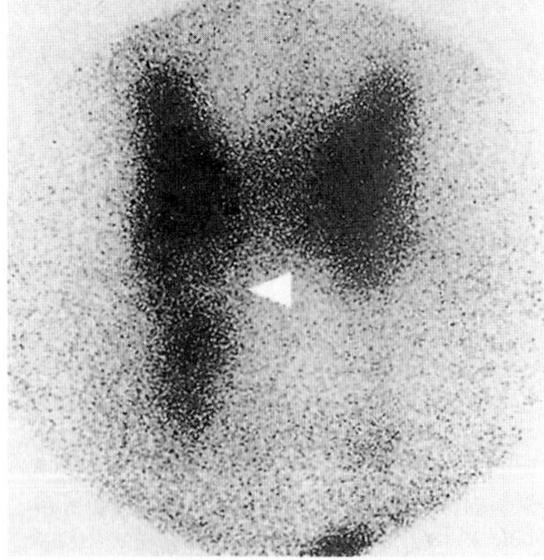

FIGURE 1-332 Follicular adenoma. A 51-year-old woman with a history of previous irradiation of the neck had a thyroid scintiscan as a routine follow-up procedure. A mass could not be palpated. This pertechnetate scan (anterior view) shows a "cold" defect *(arrow)* in the medial aspect of the lower portion of the right thyroid lobe. The left lobe is much smaller than the right. (From Skarin AT: *Atlas of diagnostic oncology,* ed 3, St Louis, 2003, Mosby.)

cell) have shown promise in preliminary studies. Routine calcitonin measurement for early detection of medullary carcinoma remains controversial because of the low frequency of this cancer and the high cost associated with case detection.

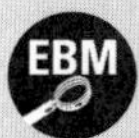

EVIDENCE

The use of surgery in the treatment of benign cystic nodules is endorsed by expert opinion. Guidelines from the American Association of Clinical Endocrinologists (AACE) state that surgical indications in a patient with a thyroid nodule include[1]: C

Associated local symptoms

Hyperthyroidism from a large toxic nodule or hyperthyroidism and concomitant multinodular goiter

Growth of the nodule

Suspicious or malignant FNA results

Recommendations for surgical procedure are[1]: C

For a solitary benign nodule, lobectomy plus isthmectomy is sufficient.

For bilateral nodules, a near-total thyroidectomy is appropriate.

Few randomized controlled trials have evaluated the use of radioablation in the treatment of thyroid nodules. However, based on uncontrolled and observational studies, the AACE make the following recommendations regarding the use of radioiodine[1]: C

Consider radioiodine treatment for small goiters (volume <100 ml), in those without suspected malignant potential, in patients with a history of previous thyroidectomy, and in those at risk for surgical intervention.

Radioiodine treatment is not the first-line therapy if compressive symptoms are present, if patients have large nodules that require high amounts of radioiodine and may be resistant to treatment, or if immediate resolution of thyrotoxicosis is desired.

Radioiodine treatment is effective and safe. Large epidemiologic studies have shown no associated clinically significant increase in the risk of cancers or leukemia.

Give radioiodine therapy cautiously in elderly patients, especially those with heart disease.

Radioiodine is contraindicated in pregnant or lactating women; always perform a pregnancy test before administration of radioiodine in women of childbearing age.

Avoid use of iodine contrast agents or iodinated drugs before administration of radioiodine; withdraw antithyroid drugs at least 3 wk before treatment and resume such regimens 3 to 5 days after radioiodine therapy.

Follow-up of patients should include monitoring of serum levels of TSH, free T4, and free T3; consider repeating treatment in 3 to 6 mo if TSH is still <0.1 mcU/mL.

Consensus opinion is that the routine use of levothyroxine (LT4) is not recommended. Its use in select patients is qualified with certain caveats[1]: C

Recent guidelines from both the AACE and the American Thyroid Association on the management of thyroid nodules do not recommend routine suppression therapy with LT4.[2]

Use of LT4 therapy may be considered in patients from geographic areas with iodine deficiency, young patients with small thyroid nodules, and nodular goiters with no evidence of functional autonomy.

Use of LT4 therapy should be avoided in most cases and especially in the following: large thyroid nodules and goiters, particularly in the presence of symptoms or signs of functional autonomy; clinically suspicious lesions or lesions with an inadequate cytologic sample; postmenopausal women and men >60 yr; patients with osteoporosis or systemic illnesses; and patients with cardiovascular disease.

LT4 treatment induces a clinically significant reduction of thyroid nodule volume in only a minority of patients.

Long-term TSH suppression may be associated with bone loss and arrhythmia in elderly patients and menopausal women.

LT4 treatment should never be fully suppressive (TSH <0.1 mcU/ml).

Nodule regrowth is usually observed after cessation of LT4 therapy.

If nodule size decreases, LT4 therapy should be continued long term.

If thyroid nodule grows during LT4 treatment, reaspiration and possibly surgical treatment should be considered.

The use of percutaneous ethanol injections (PEI) in the treatment of benign cystic nodules is endorsed by expert opinion:

Guidelines from the AACE recommend that PEI should be the first line of treatment for recurrent cystic nodules of the thyroid gland after FNA has ruled out a malignant lesion.[1] C

Limited data from clinical studies supports the use of PEI in benign thyroid nodules:

Nonrandomized studies have shown that ethanol injections reduce nodule size in recurrent cystic nodules and also in autonomously functioning nodules. In autonomously functioning nodules, PEI may reduce TSH levels.[3] B

Evidence-Based References

1. AACE/AME Task Force on Thyroid Nodules: American Association of Clinical Endocrinologists and Associazione Medici Endocrinologi medical guidelines for clinical practice for the diagnosis and management of thyroid nodules, *Endocr Pract* 12: 63-102, 2006.

2. Cooper DS et al: The American Thyroid Association Guidelines Taskforce. Management guidelines for patients with thyroid nodules and differentiated thyroid cancer, *Thyroid* 16:109-142, 2006.

3. Guglielmi R et al: Percutaneous ethanol injection treatment in benign thyroid lesions: role and efficacy, *Thyroid* 14:125-131, 2004.

SUGGESTED READINGS

Castro MR, Gharib H: Continuing controversies in the management of thyroid nodules, *Ann Intern Med* 142:926, 2005.

Shetty SK et al: Significance of incidental thyroid lesions detected on CT: correlation among CT, sonography, and pathology, *Am J Roentgenol* 187:1349, 2006.

AUTHOR: **FRED F. FERRI, M.D.**

Thyroiditis (PTG) (ALG)

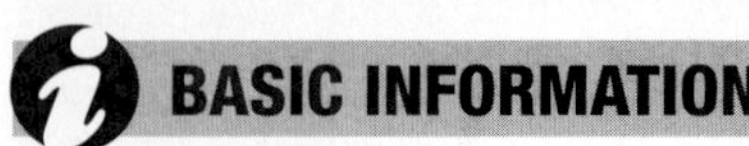

BASIC INFORMATION

DEFINITION

Thyroiditis is an inflammatory disease of the thyroid. It is a multifaceted disease with various etiologies, different clinical characteristics (depending on the stage), and distinct histopathology. Thyroiditis can be subdivided into three common types (Hashimoto's, painful, and painless) and two rare forms (suppurative and Riedel's). To add to the confusion, there are various synonyms for each form, and there is no internationally accepted classification of autoimmune thyroid disease.

SYNONYMS

Hashimoto's thyroiditis: chronic lymphocytic thyroiditis, chronic autoimmune thyroiditis, lymphadenoid goiter

Painful subacute thyroiditis: subacute thyroiditis, giant cell thyroiditis, de Quervain's thyroiditis, subacute granulomatous thyroiditis, pseudogranulomatous thyroiditis

Painless postpartum thyroiditis: subacute lymphocytic thyroiditis, postpartum thyroiditis

Painless sporadic thyroiditis: silent sporadic thyroiditis, subacute lymphocytic thyroiditis

Suppurative thyroiditis: acute suppurative thyroiditis, bacterial thyroiditis, microbial inflammatory thyroiditis, pyogenic thyroiditis

Riedel's thyroiditis: fibrous thyroiditis

ICD-9CM CODES

245.2 Hashimoto's thyroiditis
245.1 Subacute thyroiditis
245.9 Silent thyroiditis
245.0 Suppurative thyroiditis
245.3 Riedel's thyroiditis

PHYSICAL FINDINGS & CLINICAL PRESENTATION

- Hashimoto's: patients may have signs of hyperthyroidism (tachycardia, diaphoresis, palpitations, weight loss) or hypothyroidism (fatigue, weight gain, delayed reflexes) depending on the stage of the disease. Usually there is diffuse, firm enlargement of the thyroid gland; the gland may also be of normal size (atrophic form with clinically manifested hypothyroidism).
- Painful subacute: exquisitely tender, enlarged thyroid, fever; signs of hyperthyroidism are initially present; signs of hypothyroidism can subsequently develop.
- Painless thyroiditis: clinical features are similar to subacute thyroiditis except for the absence of tenderness of the thyroid gland.
- Suppurative: patient is febrile with severe neck pain, focal tenderness of the involved portion of the thyroid, erythema of the overlying skin.
- Riedel's: slowly enlarging hard mass in the anterior neck; often mistaken for thyroid cancer; signs of hypothyroidism occur in advanced stages.

ETIOLOGY

- Hashimoto's: autoimmune disorder that begins with the activation of CD4 (helper) T-lymphocytes specific for thyroid antigens. The etiologic factor for the activation of these cells is unknown.
- Painful subacute: possibly postviral; usually follows a respiratory illness not considered to be a form of autoimmune thyroiditis.
- Painless thyroiditis: frequently occurs postpartum.
- Suppurative: infectious etiology, generally bacterial, although fungi and parasites have also been implicated; often occurs in immunocompromised hosts or after a penetrating neck injury.
- Riedel's: fibrous infiltration of the thyroid; etiology unknown.
- Drug induced: lithium, interferon-alfa, amiodarone, interleukin-2.

Dx DIAGNOSIS

DIFFERENTIAL DIAGNOSIS

- The hyperthyroid phase of Hashimoto's, subacute, and silent thyroiditis can be mistaken for Graves' disease.
- Riedel's thyroiditis can be mistaken for carcinoma of the thyroid.
- Painful subacute thyroiditis can be mistaken for infections of the oropharynx and trachea or for suppurative thyroiditis.
- Factitious hyperthyroidism can mimic silent thyroiditis.

WORKUP

- The diagnostic workup includes laboratory and radiologic evaluation to rule out other conditions that may mimic thyroiditis (see above) and differentiate the various forms of thyroiditis.
- The patient's medical history may be helpful in differentiating the various types of thyroiditis (e.g., presentation after childbirth is suggestive of silent [postpartum, painless] thyroiditis; occurrence after a viral respiratory infection suggests subacute thyroiditis; history of penetrating injury to the neck indicates suppurative thyroiditis).

LABORATORY TESTS

- Thyroid-stimulating hormone, free T_4: may be normal or indicative of hypothyroidism or hyperthyroidism depending on the stage of the thyroiditis.
- White blood cell (WBC) with differential: increased WBC with left shift occurs with subacute and suppurative thyroiditis.
- Antimicrosomal antibodies: detected in $>$90% of patients with Hashimoto's thyroiditis and 50% to 80% of patients with silent thyroiditis.
- Serum thyroglobulin levels are elevated in patients with subacute and silent thyroiditis; this test is nonspecific but may be useful in monitoring the course of subacute thyroiditis and distinguishing silent thyroiditis from factitious hyperthyroidism (low or absent serum thyroglobulin level).

IMAGING STUDIES

Twenty-four-hour radioactive iodine uptake (RAIU) is useful to distinguish Graves' disease (increased RAIU) from thyroiditis (normal or low RAIU).

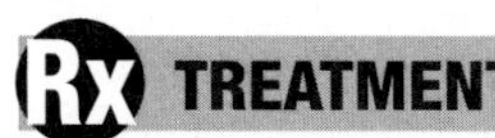

TREATMENT

ACUTE GENERAL Rx

- Treat hypothyroid phase with levothyroxine 25 to 50 mcg/day initially and monitor serum thyroid-stimulating hormone initially every 6 to 8 wk.
- Control symptoms of hyperthyroidism with beta-blockers (e.g., propranolol 20 to 40 mg PO q6h).
- Control pain in patients with subacute thyroiditis with nonsteroidal antiinflammatory drugs. Prednisone 20 to 40 mg qd may be used if nonsteroidals are insufficient, but it should be gradually tapered off over several weeks.
- Use IV antibiotics and drain abscess (if present) in patients with suppurative thyroiditis.

DISPOSITION

- Hashimoto's thyroiditis: long-term prognosis is favorable; most patients recover their thyroid function.
- Painful subacute thyroiditis: permanent hypothyroidism occurs in 10% of patients.
- Painless thyroiditis: 6% of patients have permanent hypothyroidism.
- Suppurative thyroiditis: there is usually full recovery after treatment.
- Riedel's thyroiditis: hypothyroidism occurs when fibrous infiltration involves the entire thyroid.

REFERRAL

Surgical referral in patients with compression of adjacent neck structures and in some patients with suppurative thyroiditis

SUGGESTED READINGS

Bindra A, Braunstein GD: Thyroiditis, *Am Fam Physician* 73:1769, 2006.

Pearce EN et al: Thyroiditis, *N Engl J Med* 348:2646, 2003.

AUTHOR: **FRED F. FERRI, M.D.**

BASIC INFORMATION

DEFINITION

Thyrotoxic storm is the abrupt and severe exacerbation of thyrotoxicosis.

ICD-9CM CODES
242.9 Thyrotoxic storm
242.0 With goiter
242.2 Multinodular
242.3 Adenomatous
242.8 Thyrotoxicosis factitia

PHYSICAL FINDINGS & CLINICAL PRESENTATION

- Goiter
- Tremor, tachycardia, fever
- Warm, moist skin
- Lid lag, lid retraction, proptosis
- Altered mental status (psychosis, coma, seizures)
- Other: evidence of precipitating factors (infection, trauma)

ETIOLOGY

- Major stress (e.g., infection, myocardial infarction [MI], diabetic ketoacidosis) in an undiagnosed hyperthyroid patient
- Inadequate therapy in a hyperthyroid patient

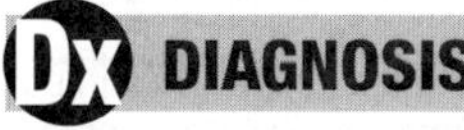

DIAGNOSIS

The clinical presentation is variable. The patient may present with the following signs and symptoms:

- Fever
- Marked anxiety and agitation, psychosis
- Hyperhidrosis, heat intolerance
- Marked weakness and muscle wasting
- Tachyarrhythmias, palpitations
- Diarrhea, nausea, vomiting
- Elderly patients may have a combination of tachycardia, congestive heart failure (CHF), and mental status changes

DIFFERENTIAL DIAGNOSIS

- Psychiatric disorders
- Alcohol or other drug withdrawal
- Pheochromocytoma
- Metastatic neoplasm

WORKUP

- Laboratory evaluation to confirm hyperthyroidism (elevated free T_4, decreased thyroid-stimulating hormone [TSH])
- Evaluation for precipitating factors (e.g., ECG and cardiac enzymes in suspected MI, blood and urine cultures to rule out sepsis)
- Elimination of disorders noted in the differential diagnosis (e.g., psychiatric history, evidence of drug and alcohol abuse)

LABORATORY TESTS

- Free T_4, TSH
- Complete blood count with differential
- Blood and urine cultures
- Glucose
- Liver enzymes
- Blood urea nitrogen, creatinine
- Serum calcium
- Creatine phosphokinase

IMAGING STUDIES

Chest radiograph to exclude infectious process, neoplasm, CHF in suspected cases

Rx TREATMENT

NONPHARMACOLOGIC THERAPY

- Nutritional care: replace fluid deficit aggressively (daily fluid requirement may reach 6 L); use solutions containing glucose and add multivitamins to the hydrating solution.
- Monitor for fluid overload and CHF in the elderly and in those with underlying cardiovascular or renal disease.
- Treat significant hyperthermia with cooling blankets.

ACUTE GENERAL Rx

- Inhibition of thyroid hormone synthesis:
  1. Administer propylthiouracil (PTU) 300 to 600 mg initially (PO or by nasogastric tube), then 150 to 300 mg q6h.
  2. If the patient is allergic to PTU, use methimazole (Tapazole) 80 to 100 mg PO or rectally followed by 30 mg PR q8h.
- Inhibition of stored thyroid hormone:
  1. Iodide can be administered as sodium iodine 250 mg IV q6h, saturated solution of potassium iodide, 5 gtt PO q8h, or Lugol's solution, 10 gtt q8h. It is important to administer PTU or methimazole 1 hr *before* the iodide to prevent the oxidation of iodide to iodine and its incorporation in the synthesis of additional thyroid hormone.
  2. Corticosteroids: dexamethasone 2 mg IV q6h or hydrocortisone 100 mg IV q6h for approximately 48 hr is useful to inhibit thyroid hormone release, impair peripheral conversion of T_3 from T_4, and provide additional adrenocortical hormone to correct deficiency (if present).
- Suppression of peripheral effects of thyroid hormone:
  1. Beta-adrenergic blockers: administer propranolol 80 to 120 mg PO q4-6h. Propranolol may also be given IV 1 mg/min for 2 to 10 min under continuous ECG and blood pressure monitoring. Beta-adrenergic blockers must be used with caution in patients with severe CHF or bronchospasm. Cardioselective beta-blockers (e.g., esmolol or metoprolol) may be more appropriate for patients with bronchospasm, but these patients must be closely monitored for exacerbation of bronchospasm because these agents lose their cardioselectivity at high doses.
- Control of fever with acetaminophen 325 to 650 mg q4h; avoidance of aspirin because it displaces thyroid hormone from its binding protein
- Consider digitalization of patients with CHF and atrial fibrillation (these patients may require higher than usual digoxin doses)
- Treatment of any precipitating factors (e.g., antibiotics if infection is strongly suspected)

DISPOSITION

Patients with thyrotoxic crisis should be treated and appropriately monitored in the ICU.

REFERRAL

Endocrinology referral is appropriate in patients with thyrotoxic crisis.

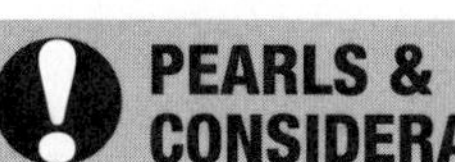

PEARLS & CONSIDERATIONS

COMMENTS

If the diagnosis is strongly suspected, therapy should be started immediately without waiting for laboratory confirmation.

AUTHOR: **FRED F. FERRI, M.D.**

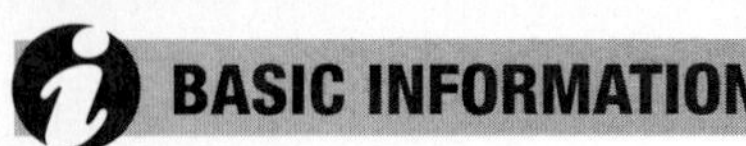

BASIC INFORMATION

DEFINITION

Tinea capitis is a dermatophyte infection of the scalp.

SYNONYMS

Ringworm of the scalp, ringworm of the head, gray patch tinea capitis, black dot tinea capitis, tinea tonsurans, superficial mycosis, dermatophytosis, kerion

ICD-9CM CODES
110.0 Tinea capitis

EPIDEMIOLOGY & DEMOGRAPHICS

Tinea capitis is the most common dermatophytosis of childhood, primarily affecting children between ages 3 and 7 yr. Approximately 3% to 8% of American children are affected, and 34% of household contacts are asymptomatic carriers. African-American children are particularly susceptible. Adult and geriatric populations are less frequently affected, possibly because of the fungistatic effect of the sebum found in older persons. In urban populations, large family size, low socioeconomic status, and crowded living conditions may contribute to an increased incidence of tinea capitis. The predominant etiologic agent of tinea capitis in the U.S. and in Western Europe has changed from *Microsporum audouinii* to *Trichophyton tonsurans* in the past 50 yr.

PHYSICAL FINDINGS & CLINICAL PRESENTATION

- Triad of scalp scaling, alopecia, and cervical adenopathy.
- Primary lesions including plaques, papules, pustules, or nodules on the scalp (usually occipital region).
- Secondary lesions include scales, alopecia (usually reversible), erythema, exudates, and edema.
- Two distinctly different forms:
  1. Gray patch: lesions are scaly and well demarcated. The hairs within the patch break off a few millimeters above the scalp. One or several lesions may be present; sometimes the lesions join to form larger ones.
  2. Black dot: early lesions with erythema and scaling patch are easily overlooked until areas of alopecia develop. Hairs within the patches break at the surface of the scalp, leaving behind a pattern of swollen black dots.
- Scalp pruritus may be present.
- Fever, pain, and lymphadenopathy (commonly postcervical) with inflammatory lesions.
- Kerion: inflamed, exudative, pustular, boggy, tender nodules exhibiting marked edema, and hair loss seen in severe tinea capitis. Caused by immune response to the fungus. May lead to some scarring.
- Favus: production of scutula (hair matted together with dermatophyte hyphae and keratin debris), characterized by yellow cup-shaped crusts around hair shafts. A fetid odor may be present.

ETIOLOGY

Most commonly caused by the *Trichophyton* (>90% of the cases in the U.S.) or *Microsporum* genera (5%). Most common causative species for black dot tinea capitis is *T. tonsurans* and for gray patch tinea capitis are *M. audouinii* and *M. canis*. Transmission occurs by infected persons or asymptomatic carriers, fallen infected hairs, animal vectors, and fomites. *M. audouinii* is commonly spread by dogs and cats. Infectious fungal particles may remain viable for many months.

Dx DIAGNOSIS

DIFFERENTIAL DIAGNOSIS

Alopecia areata, impetigo, pediculosis, trichotillomania, traction alopecia, folliculitis, pseudopelade, seborrhea/atopic dermatitis, psoriasis, carbuncles, pyoderma, lichen ruber planus, lupus erythematosus

WORKUP

- Potassium hydroxide testing of hair shaft extracted from the lesion, not the scale, because the *T. tonsurans* spores attach to or reside inside hair shafts and are rarely found in the scales.
- Wood's ultraviolet light fluoresces blue-green on hair shafts for *Microsporum* infections but will fail to identify *T. tonsurans*.
- Fungal culture of hairs and scales on fungal medium such as Sabouraud's agar may be used to confirm the diagnosis, especially if uncertain.
- Histology of biopsies with fungal staining in cases where mycology tests are negative because of treatment initiation.

Rx TREATMENT

- Griseofulvin: gold standard FDA-approved treatment with less cost and excellent long-term safety profile. Micronized and ultramicronized preparations are absorbed better, and side effects are infrequent, especially when administered with fatty meals. Periodic monitoring of hematologic, liver, and renal function may be indicated, especially in prolonged treatment >8 wk.
  1. Children: 20 mg/kg/day orally (to a maximum of 0.5 to 1.0 g/day) for 6 to 12 wk (until hair regrowth occurs or 2 wk beyond cure to prevent relapse).
  2. Adults: 250 mg orally bid or 500 mg qd (or 250 mg tid for a few cases of black dot type) for 6 to 12 wk.
- New alternative treatments: oral terbinafine, itraconazole, or fluconazole are comparable in efficacy and safety to griseofulvin, with shorter treatment and better patient compliance. Preferred when resistant or allergies to Griseofulvin are of concern. Monitoring of CBC, liver function tests, and renal function may be indicated.
- Terbinafine:
  - 10 to 20 kg: 62.5 mg daily for 4 weeks
  - 20 to 40 kg: 125 mg daily for 4 weeks
  - Above 40 kg: 250 mg daily for 4 weeks
- Itraconazole: 3.5 mg/kg daily for 4 to 6 weeks or pulse therapy of 5 mg/kg daily for one week each month for 2 to 3 months
- Fluconazole: the only oral antifungal agent approved for children younger than 2 years, 6 mg/kg/day for 6 weeks in children (3 to 6 weeks in adults) or 8 mg/kg weekly for 8 to 12 weeks (cap at 150 mg weekly for adults).
- Four wk of terbinafine therapy is as effective as 8 wk of griseofulvin therapy for *Trichophyton* infections; however terbinafine is not very effective against *Microsporum* infections.
- The adjuvant use of antifungal shampoos is recommended for all patients and household contacts. Shampoo like selenium sulfide 2.5% used on scalp for at least 5 min 2 to 3 times/wk can help prevent infection or eradicate asymptomatic carrier state by inhibiting fungal growth.
- Severe inflammatory kerion can be managed with additional prednisone 40 mg daily (1 mg/kg/day in children) and tapering over 2 weeks.

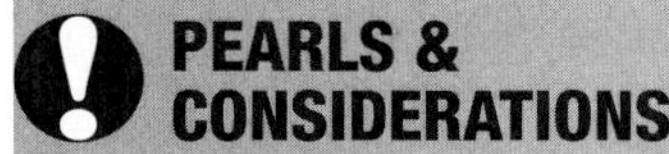

PEARLS & CONSIDERATIONS

COMMENTS

- Confirming the diagnosis of tinea capitis with a laboratory specimen is important because misdiagnosis will result in delay or improper treatment.
- Look for sources of infections and disinfect contaminated objects such as combs, brushes, towels, and headgear. Avoid sharing personal hygiene items.
- Culture of hairs and scalp dander facilitates carrier identification and prevention.
- Pets that are infected or asymptomatic carriers should be treated.
- Recommend follow-up visit every 2 to 4 wk with Wood's light, microscopic study, and fungal culture. A mycologically documented cure is the goal of treatment.

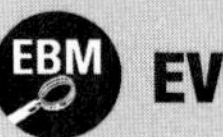

EVIDENCE

Please note: Complete text of EBM for this topic is available online.

SUGGESTED READINGS

Andrews MD, Burns M: Common tinea infections in children, *Am Fam Physician* 77(10):1415-1420, 2008.

Gilbert DN et al: *The Sanford guide to antimicrobial therapy* 2007, Hyde Park, VT, 2007, Antimicrobial Therapy.

Goldstein AO et al: Dermatophyte (tinea) infections, UpToDate Online 17.3, 2009.

Mohrenschlager M et al: Pediatric tinea capitis: recognition and management, *Am J Clin Dermatol* 6(4): 203-213, 2005.

Roberts BJ, Friedlander SF: Tinea capitis: a treatment update, *Pediatr Ann* 34(3):191-200, 2005.

Seebacher C et al: Tinea capitis: ringworm of the scalp, *Mycoses* 50(3):218-226, 2007.

Shy R: Tinea corporis and tinea capitis, *Pediatr Rev* 28(5):164-174, 2007.

Trovato MJ et al: Tinea capitis: current concepts in clinical practice, *Cutis* 77(2):93–99, 2006.

AUTHOR: **MARIE ELIZABETH WONG, M.D.**

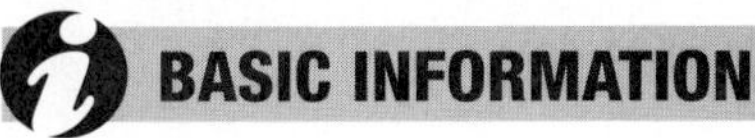

BASIC INFORMATION

DEFINITION

Tinea corporis is a dermatophyte fungal infection caused by the genera *Trichophyton* or *Microsporum.*

SYNONYMS

Ringworm
Body ringworm
Tinea circinata

ICD-9CM CODES

110.5 Tinea corporis

EPIDEMIOLOGY & DEMOGRAPHICS

- The disease is more common in warm climates.
- There is no predominant age or sex.

PHYSICAL FINDINGS & CLINICAL PRESENTATION

- Typically appears as single or multiple annular lesions with an advancing scaly border; the margin is slightly raised, reddened, and may be pustular.
- The central area becomes hypopigmented and less scaly as the active border progresses outward (Fig. 1-333).
- The trunk and legs are primarily involved.
- Pruritus is variable.
- It is important to remember that recent topical corticosteroid use can significantly alter the appearance of the lesions.

ETIOLOGY

Trichophyton rubrum is the most common pathogen.

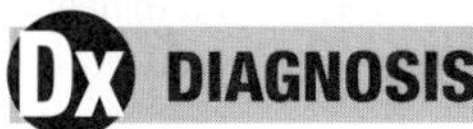

DIAGNOSIS

DIFFERENTIAL DIAGNOSIS

- Pityriasis rosea
- Erythema multiforme
- Psoriasis
- Cutaneous systemic lupus erythematosus
- Secondary syphilis
- Nummular eczema
- Eczema
- Granuloma annulare
- Lyme disease
- Tinea versicolor
- Contact dermatitis

WORKUP

Diagnosis is usually made on clinical grounds. It can be confirmed by direct visualization under the microscope of a small fragment of the scale using wet mount preparation and potassium hydroxide solution; dermatophytes appear as translucent branching filaments (hyphae) with lines of separation appearing at irregular intervals.

LABORATORY TESTS

- Microscopic examination of hyphae
- Mycotic culture is usually not necessary
- Biopsy is indicated only when the diagnosis is uncertain and the patient has not responded to treatment

Rx TREATMENT

NONPHARMACOLOGIC THERAPY

Affected areas should be kept clean and dry.

ACUTE GENERAL Rx

- Various creams are effective; the application area should include normal skin approximately 2 cm beyond the affected area:
  1. Butenafine cream applied qd for 14 days
  2. Terbinafine cream applied bid for 14 days
- Systemic therapy is reserved for severe cases and is usually given up to 4 wk; commonly used agents:
  1. Fluconazole, 200 mg qd
  2. Terbinafine, 250 mg qd

DISPOSITION

Majority of cases resolve without sequelae within 3 to 4 wk of therapy.

REFERRAL

Dermatology referral in patients with persistent or recurrent infections

SUGGESTED READINGS

Andrews MD, Burns M: Common tinea infections in children, *Am Fam Physician* 77(10):1415-1420, 2008.

Hainer BL: Dermatophyte infections, *Am Fam Physician* 67:101, 2003.

Weinstein A, Berman B: Topical treatment of common superficial tinea infections, *Am Fam Physician* 65: 2095, 2002.

AUTHOR: **FRED F. FERRI, M.D.**

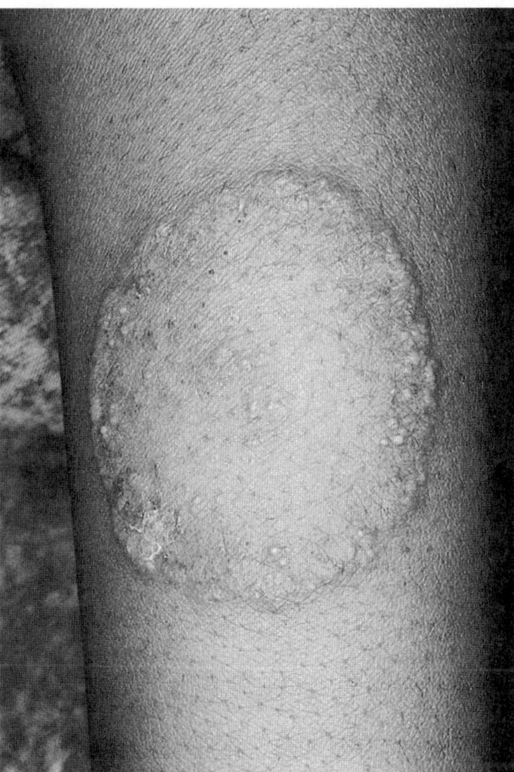

FIGURE 1-333 Annular lesion (tinea corporis). Note raised erythematous, scaling border and central clearing. (From Noble J et al: *Textbook of primary care medicine,* ed 3, St Louis, 2001, Mosby.)

Tinea Cruris (PTG)

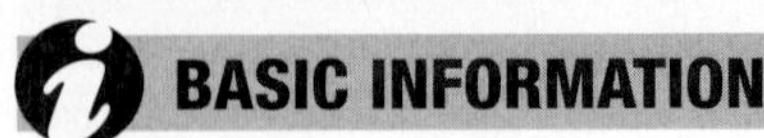

BASIC INFORMATION

DEFINITION

Tinea cruris is a dermatophyte infection of the groin.

SYNONYMS

Jock itch
Ringworm

ICD-9CM CODES
110.3 Tinea cruris

EPIDEMIOLOGY & DEMOGRAPHICS

- Most common during the summer in adolescent and young adult males.
- Males are affected more frequently than females; however, it has become more common in postpubertal females who are overweight or who often wear tight jeans or pantyhose.
- The infection often coexists with tinea pedis.

PHYSICAL FINDINGS & CLINICAL PRESENTATION

- Erythematous plaques have a half-moon shape and a scaling border.
- The acute inflammation tends to move down the inner thigh and usually spares the scrotum; in severe cases the fungus may spread onto the buttocks.
- Itching may be severe.
- Red papules and pustules may be present.
- An important diagnostic sign is the advancing well-defined border with a tendency toward central clearing (Fig. 1-334).

ETIOLOGY

- Dermatophytes of the genera *Trichophyton, Epidermophyton,* and *Microsporum. T. rubrum* and *E. floccosum* are the most common infecting agents.
- Transmission from direct contact (e.g., infected persons, animals). The patient's feet should be evaluated as a source of infection because tinea cruris is often associated with tinea pedis.

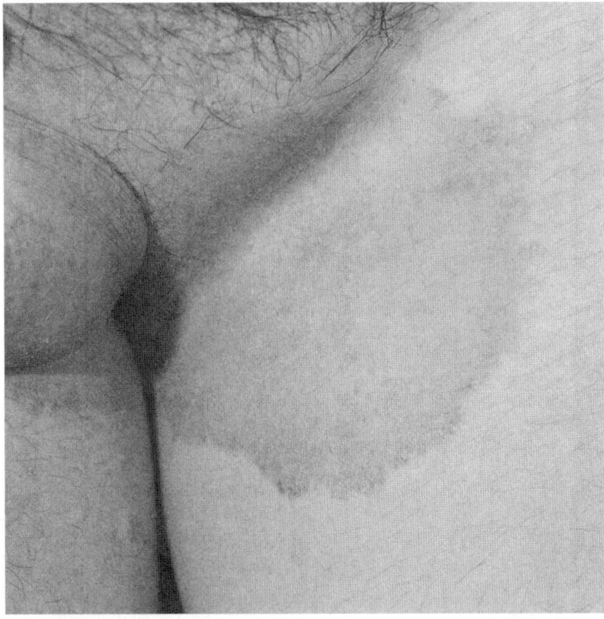

FIGURE 1-334 Tinea cruris. A half-moon–shaped plaque has a well-defined, scaling border. (From Habif TB: *Clinical dermatology: a color guide to diagnosis and therapy,* ed 3, St Louis, 1996, Mosby.)

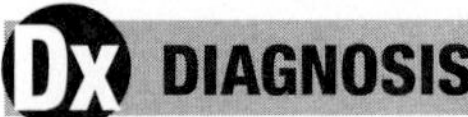

DIAGNOSIS

DIFFERENTIAL DIAGNOSIS

- Candidal intertrigo
- Psoriasis
- Seborrheic dermatitis
- Erythrasma
- Contact dermatitis
- Tinea versicolor

WORKUP

Diagnosis is based on clinical presentation and demonstration of hyphae microscopically using potassium hydroxide.

LABORATORY TESTS

- Microscopic examination
- Cultures are generally not necessary

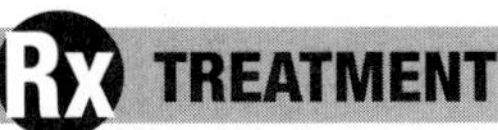

TREATMENT

NONPHARMACOLOGIC THERAPY

- Keep infected area clean and dry.
- Boxer shorts are preferred to regular underwear.

ACUTE GENERAL Rx

- Various topical antifungal agents are available:
  1. Butenafine cream, applied qd × 14 days
  2. Terbinafine cream, applied bid × 14 days
- Drying powders (e.g., Miconazole nitrate) may be useful in patients with excessive perspiration.
- Oral antifungal therapy is generally reserved for cases unresponsive to topical agents or can be used along with topical agents in severe cases. Effective medications are fluconazole 200 mg qd × 10 days and terbinafine 250 mg qd × 30 days.

DISPOSITION

Most cases respond promptly to therapy with complete resolution within 2 to 3 wk.

SUGGESTED READINGS

Andrews MD, Burns M: Common tinea infections in children, *Am Fam Physician* 77(10):1415-1420, 2008.

Hainer BL: Dermatophyte infections, *Am Fam Physician* 67:101, 2003.

AUTHOR: **FRED F. FERRI, M.D.**

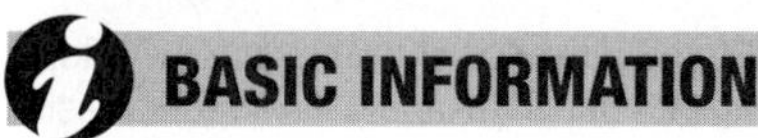

BASIC INFORMATION

DEFINITION

Tinea pedis is a dermatophyte infection of the feet.

SYNONYMS

Athlete's foot

ICD-9CM CODES

110.4 Tinea pedis

EPIDEMIOLOGY & DEMOGRAPHICS

- Most common dermatophyte infection
- Increased incidence in hot humid weather; occlusive footwear is a contributing factor
- Occurrence is rare before adolescence
- More common in adult males

PHYSICAL FINDINGS & CLINICAL PRESENTATION

- Typical presentation is variable and ranges from erythematous scaling plaques (Fig. 1-335) and isolated blisters to interdigital maceration.
- The infection usually starts in the interdigital spaces of the foot. Most infections are found in the toe webs or on the soles.
- Fourth or fifth toes are most commonly involved.
- Pruritus is common and is most intense after removal of shoes and socks.
- Infection with *tinea rubrum* often manifests with a "moccasin" distribution affecting the soles and lateral feet.

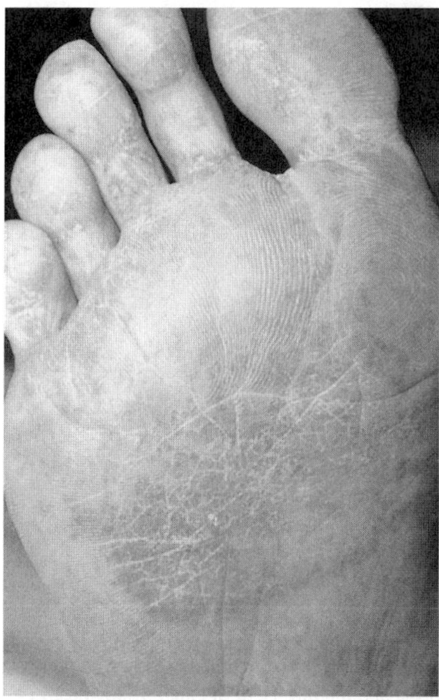

FIGURE 1-335 Tinea pedis. (From Goldstein BG, Goldstein AO: *Practical dermatology,* ed 2, St Louis, 1997, Mosby.)

ETIOLOGY

Dermatophyte infection caused by *T. rubrum, T. mentagrophytes,* or less commonly *E. floccosum*

DIAGNOSIS

DIFFERENTIAL DIAGNOSIS

- Contact dermatitis
- Toe web infection (bacterial or candidal infection)
- Eczema
- Psoriasis
- Keratolysis exfoliativa
- Juvenile plantar dermatosis

WORKUP

- Diagnosis is usually made by clinical observation.
- Laboratory testing, when performed, generally consists of a simple potassium hydroxide preparation with mycologic examination under a light microscope to confirm the presence of dermatophytes.

LABORATORY TESTS

- Microscopic examination of a scale or the roof of a blister with 10% KOH under low or medium power will reveal hyphae.
- Mycologic culture is rarely indicated in the diagnosis of tinea pedis.
- Biopsy is reserved for when the diagnosis remains in question after testing or failure to respond to treatment.

TREATMENT

NONPHARMACOLOGIC THERAPY

- Keep infected area clean and dry. Aerate feet by using sandals when possible.
- Use 100% cotton socks rather than nylon socks to reduce moisture.
- Areas likely to become infected should be dried completely before being covered with clothes.

ACUTE GENERAL Rx

- Butenafine HCL 1% cream applied bid for 1 wk or qd for 4 wk is effective in interdigital tinea pedis.
- Terbinafine cream applied bid × 14 days.
- Ciclopirox 0.77% cream applied bid for 4 wk.
- Clotrimazole 1% cream is an over-the-counter treatment. It should be applied to affected and surrounding area bid for up to 4 wk.
- Naftifine 1% cream applied qd or gel applied bid for 4 wk also produces a significantly high cure rate.
- When using topical preparations, the application area should include normal skin approximately 2 cm beyond the affected area.
- Areas of maceration can be treated with Burow's solution soaks for 10 to 20 min bid followed by foot elevation.
- Oral agents (fluconazole 150 mg once per week for 4 wk) can be used in combination with topical agents in resistant cases.

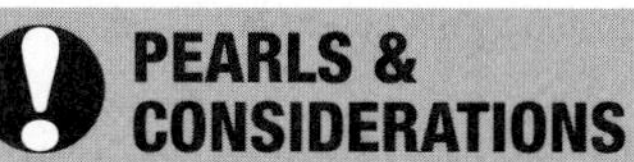

PEARLS & CONSIDERATIONS

Combination therapy of antifungal and corticosteroid (clotrimazole/betamethasone [Lotrisone]) should only be used when the diagnosis of fungal infection is confirmed and inflammation is a significant issue.

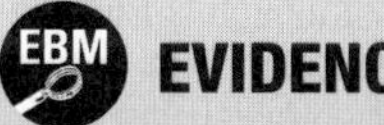

EVIDENCE

There is some evidence from randomized, controlled trials that tea tree oil is more effective than placebo for the treatment of tinea pedis, achieving in one trial a mycologic cure rate at 4 wk of 64% compared with 31% with placebo. However, another trial has shown tea tree oil to be significantly less effective than tolnaftate.[1,2] B

Evidence-Based References

1. Warshaw EM et al: Pulse versus continuous terbinafine for onychomycosis: a randomized, double-blind, controlled trial, *J Am Acad Dermatol* 53:578, 2005.
2. Gupta AK et al: Evaluation of the efficacy of ciclopirox 0.77% gel in the treatment of tinea pedis interdigitalis (dermatophytosis complex) in a randomized, double-blind, placebo-controlled trial, *Int J Dermatol* 44:590, 2005.

SUGGESTED READING

Andrews MD, Burns M: Common tinea infections in children, *Am Fam Physician* 77(10):1415, 2008.

AUTHOR: **FRED F. FERRI, M.D.**

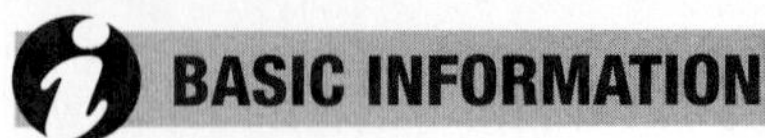

BASIC INFORMATION

DEFINITION

Tinea versicolor is a fungal infection of the skin caused by the yeast *Pityrosporum orbiculare (Malassezia furfur).*

SYNONYMS

Pityriasis versicolor

ICD-9CM CODES
111.0 Tinea versicolor

EPIDEMIOLOGY & DEMOGRAPHICS

- Increased incidence in adolescence and young adulthood
- More common during the summer (hypopigmented lesions are more evident when the skin is tanned)

PHYSICAL FINDINGS & CLINICAL PRESENTATION

- Most lesions begin as multiple small, circular macules of various colors.
- The macules may be darker or lighter than the surrounding normal skin and will scale with scraping.
- Most frequent site of distribution is trunk.
- Facial lesions are more common in children (forehead is most common facial site).
- Eruption is generally of insidious onset and asymptomatic.
- Lesions may be hyperpigmented in blacks.
- Lesions may be inconspicuous in fair-complexioned individuals, especially during the winter.
- Most patients become aware of the eruption when the involved areas do not tan (Fig. 1-336).

ETIOLOGY

The infection is caused by the lipophilic yeast *P. orbiculare* (round form) and *P. ovale* (oval form), which are normal inhabitants of the skin flora. Factors that favor proliferation are pregnancy, malnutrition, immunosuppression, oral contraceptives, and excess heat and humidity.

DIAGNOSIS

DIFFERENTIAL DIAGNOSIS

- Vitiligo
- Pityriasis alba
- Secondary syphilis
- Pityriasis rosea
- Seborrheic dermatitis

WORKUP

Diagnosis is based on clinical appearance; identification of hyphae and budding spores ("spaghetti and meatballs" appearance) with microscopy confirms diagnosis.

LABORATORY TESTS

Microscopic examination with potassium hydroxide confirms diagnosis.

TREATMENT

NONPHARMACOLOGIC THERAPY

Sunlight accelerates repigmentation of hypopigmented areas.

ACUTE GENERAL Rx

- Topical treatment: selenium sulfide 2.5% suspension (Selsun or Exsel) applied daily for 10 min for 7 consecutive days results in a cure rate of 80% to 90%.
- Antifungal topical agents (e.g., miconazole, ciclopirox, clotrimazole) are also effective.
- Oral treatment can be given along with topical agents but is generally reserved for resistant cases. Effective agents are ketoconazole 200 mg qd for 5 days, or single 400-mg dose (cure rate >80%), fluconazole 400 mg given as a single dose (cure rate >70% at 3 wk after treatment), or itraconazole 200 mg/day for 5 days.

DISPOSITION

The prognosis is good, with death of the fungus usually occurring within 3 to 4 wk of treatment; however, recurrence is common.

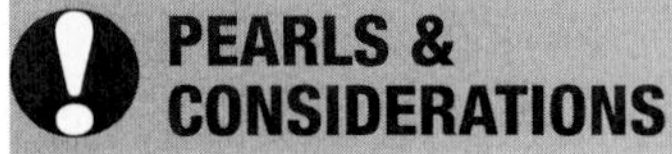

PEARLS & CONSIDERATIONS

COMMENTS

Patients should be informed that the hypopigmented areas will not disappear immediately after treatment and that several months may be necessary for the hypopigmented areas to regain their pigmentation.

AUTHOR: **FRED F. FERRI, M.D.**

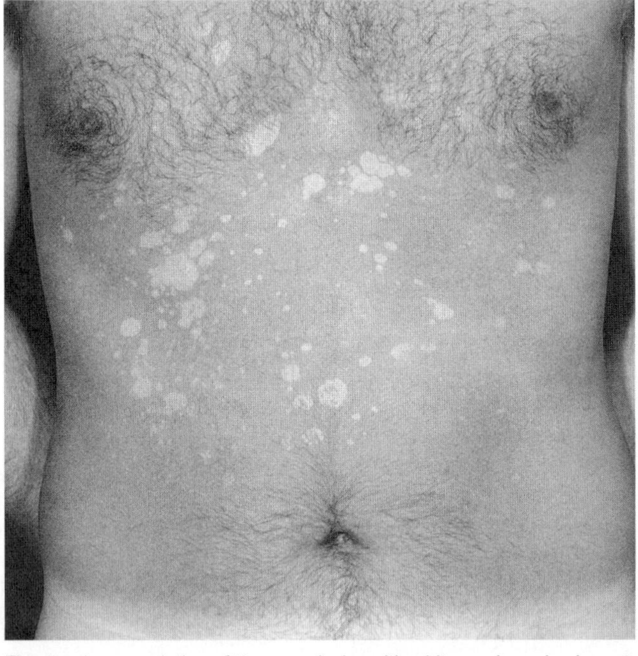

FIGURE 1-336 The classic presentation of tinea versicolor with white, oval, or circular patches on tan skin. (From Habif TB: *Clinical dermatology: a color guide to diagnosis and therapy,* ed 3, St Louis, 1996, Mosby.)

BASIC INFORMATION

DEFINITION

Tinnitus is an unwanted auditory perception of internal origin, usually localized and rarely heard by others. It usually involves a high-pitched sound with a buzzing or ringing quality.

SYNONYMS

Ringing in the ear(s)

ICD-9CM CODES
388.30 Tinnitus

EPIDEMIOLOGY & DEMOGRAPHICS

Tinnitus increases with age. The most recent prevalence statistics from the National Center for Health Statistics (1999) indicate that tinnitus affects approximately 18% of the population. The American Tinnitus Association reports that 50 million Americans have tinnitus. It is slightly more common in men, frequently associated with hearing impairment, and more common in Caucasians than African Americans. The prevalence is double in the southern states compared to the northern states. It is most prevalent at ages 40 to 70 yr.

PHYSICAL FINDINGS & CLINICAL PRESENTATION

- Patient complaints are of sounds in ears. Determine onset, localization, pitch, loudness, duration, and nature: can be pulsatile, or described as ringing, buzzing, cricketlike, hissing, humming, or whistling.
- Objective tinnitus is pulsatile, with bursts of sound energy coinciding with the pulse.

ETIOLOGY

- Mechanism is poorly understood; central in origin, it may originate at any point along the auditory pathway. Theories include injured cochlear hair cells, spontaneous activity in auditory nerve fibers, hyperactivity in the auditory nuclei in the brain stem, or a reduction in suppressive activity of the central auditory cortex.
- Medications implicated in tinnitus are aspirin, NSAIDs, aminoglycosides, chloramphenicol, erythromycin, tetracycline, vancomycin, bleomycin, cisplatin, mechlorethamine, vincristine, bumetanide, ethacrynic acid, furosemide, chloroquine, heavy metals, heterocyclic antidepressants, and quinine.
- Classified as either objective or subjective.
  - Subjective causes: (1) otologic: hearing loss, Meniere's disease, acoustic neuroma, cerumen impaction; (2) ototoxic medications; (3) neurologic: multiple sclerosis, head injury; (4) metabolic: thyroid disorder, hyperlipidemia, vitamin B_{12} deficiency; (5) psychogenic: depression, anxiety, fibromyalgia; and (6) infectious: otitis media, Lyme disease, meningitis, syphilis.
  - Objective causes: (1) vascular: arterial bruit, venous hum, AV malformation, vascular tumors; (2) neurologic: palatomyoclonus, idiopathic stapedial muscle spasm; and (3) patulous (lax) Eustachian tube

DIAGNOSIS

DIFFERENTIAL DIAGNOSIS

Subjective or objective tinnitus

WORKUP

- History of exposure to ototoxic substances or disease processes that predispose to tinnitus
- Association with depression: screen for depression

LABORATORY TESTS

- Audiometry, tympanometry, pitch masking
- Evaluate for metabolic abnormalities: thyroid disease, hyperlipidemia, anemia, B_{12} deficiency, zinc deficiency, CBC, complete blood chemistry
- Electronystagmograph: Meniere's disease

IMAGING STUDIES

- MRI/CT: Consider brain imaging to rule out multiple sclerosis, acoustic neuroma, brain stem tumor
- MRI/MRA for pulsatile tinnitus

TREATMENT

NONPHARMACOLOGIC THERAPY

Unknown effectiveness: psychotherapy, biofeedback, acupuncture, tinnitus-masking devices

ACUTE GENERAL Rx

- No FDA-approved medications; possibly beneficial are tricyclic antidepressants (one randomized controlled trial [RCT])
- Benzodiazepines possibly effective
- Lidocaine not found to be effective

CHRONIC Rx

Tinnitus retraining therapy: education, support, counseling and feedback device, multidisciplinary team. Duration of therapy is >1 yr; success rates of 80%, but no RCTs have been done.

COMPLEMENTARY & ALTERNATIVE MEDICINE

- Possibly effective: acupuncture, relaxation therapy, hypnosis (based on systemic reviews)
- *Ginkgo biloba* not found to be effective (based on one systemic review, one RCT)

DISPOSITION

Evaluate for all treatable causes, careful history to raise awareness of pulsatile tinnitus; determine subjective or objective

REFERRAL

ENT, neurology

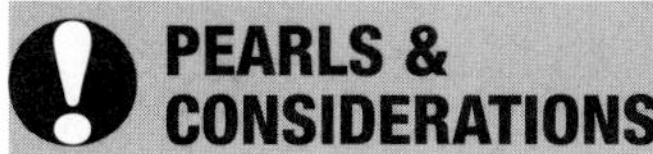

PEARLS & CONSIDERATIONS

COMMENTS

- Up to 18% of population may have tinnitus, with 0.5% severely effected; be aware of high prevalence.
- Be aware of concurrent depression; screen and treat for it. Treat all treatable underlying causes.

PREVENTION

Avoid ototoxic drugs and loud, chronic noise exposure.

PATIENT & FAMILY EDUCATION

- American Tinnitus Association: 800-634-8978, http://www.ata.org
- American Academy of Audiology: 800-AAA-2336, http://www.audiology.org
- Hear USA: http://www.hearusa.org
- Counsel families and patients that tinnitus may be irreversible and that they should be aware of the condition's effect on their lives.

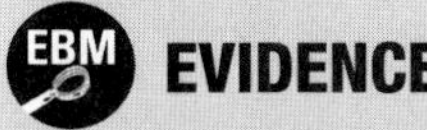

EVIDENCE

Please note: Complete text of EBM for this topic is available online.

SUGGESTED READINGS

Crummer RW: Diagnostic approach to tinnitus, *Am Fam Physician* 69(1):120, 2004.

Lockwood A: Tinnitus, *Neurology Clinics* 23:893, 2005.

Lockwood A: Tinnitus, *N Engl J Med* 347(12):904, 2002.

Waddell A: Tinnitus: clinical evidence concise, *Am Fam Physician* 69(3):591, 2004.

AUTHOR: **JUDITH NUDELMAN, M.D.**

BASIC INFORMATION

DEFINITION

Torticollis is a contraction or contracture of the muscles of the neck that causes the head to be tilted to one side. It is usually accompanied by rotation of the chin to the opposite side with flexion (Fig. 1-337). Usually it is a symptom of some underlying disorder. This term is often used incorrectly in cases when the torticollis may simply be positional.

SYNONYMS

Twisted neck
"Wry neck"

ICD-9CM CODES

723.5	Spastic (intermittent) torticollis
754.1	Congenital muscular (sternocleidomastoid)
300.11	Hysterical
714.0	Rheumatoid
333.83	Spasmodic

PHYSICAL FINDINGS & CLINICAL PRESENTATION

- Congenital muscular torticollis:
  1. Palpable soft tissue "mass" in the sternocleidomastoid shortly after birth
  2. Mass gradually subsides, leaving a shortened, contracted sternocleidomastoid muscle
  3. Head characteristically tilted toward the side of the mass and rotated in the opposite direction
  4. Facial asymmetry and other secondary changes persisting into adulthood
- Spasmodic torticollis:
  1. "Spasms" in the cervical musculature; may be bilateral and uncontrollable
  2. Head often tilted toward the affected side
- Findings in other cases depend on etiology

ETIOLOGY

Torticollis has been found to have more than 50 different causes:

- Localized fibrous shortening of unknown cause involving the sternocleidomastoid, leading to the condition termed *congenital muscular torticollis*
- Spasmodic torticollis: of uncertain etiology, possibly a variant of dystonia musculorum deformans
- Infection, specifically pharyngitis, tonsillitis, retropharyngeal abscess
- Miscellaneous rare causes: congenital musculoskeletal deformities, trauma, inflammation from rheumatoid arthritis, vestibular disturbances, posterior fossa tumor, syringomyelia, neuritis of spinal accessory nerve, and drug reactions

DIAGNOSIS

DIFFERENTIAL DIAGNOSIS

- Usually involves separating each disorder from the others
- Acquired positional disorders (e.g., ocular disturbances, acute disk herniation)

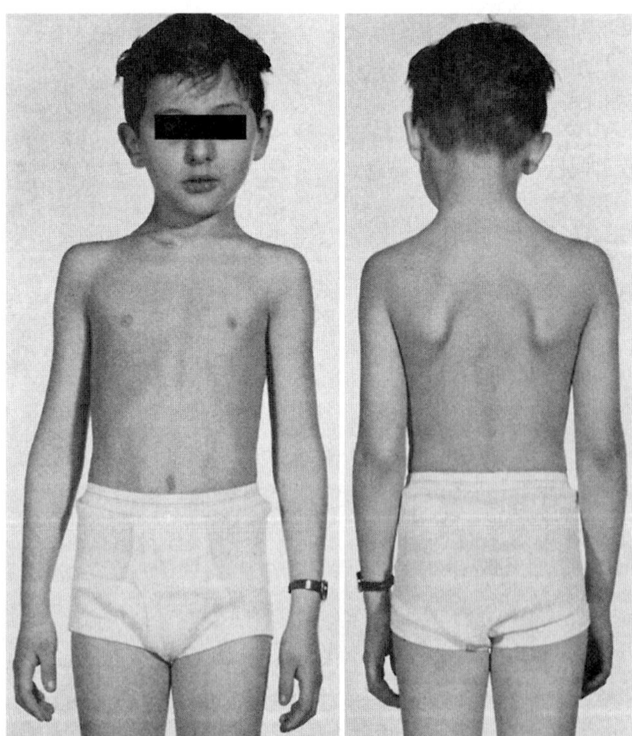

FIGURE 1-337 Torticollis. In this child, the right sternocleidomastoid muscle is contracted. (From Brinker MR, Miller MD: *Fundamentals of orthopaedics,* Philadelphia, 1999, WB Saunders.)

WORKUP

- Workup depends on the clinical situation.
- Laboratory studies are usually not helpful unless infection or rheumatoid disease is suspected.
- Section II describes a differential diagnosis for the evaluation and therapy of neck pain.
- Any child with a gradually increasing torticollis should have a complete eye examination.

IMAGING STUDIES

- Plain radiographs in cases of trauma or to rule out congenital abnormalities
- MRI in appropriate cases
- Electrodiagnostic studies: only rarely indicated to rule out neurologic causes

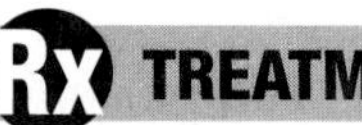

TREATMENT

- Congenital muscular torticollis: gentle stretching exercises carried out by the parent
- Spasmodic torticollis: physical therapy, psychotherapy, cervical braces, biofeedback, and pain control
- Other forms: treated according to etiology

DISPOSITION

- Most patients with congenital muscular torticollis respond well to conservative treatment.
- Spasmodic torticollis is often resistant to normal conservative treatment.
- Prognosis of other forms of torticollis depends on etiology.

REFERRAL

- Torticollis often requires a multidisciplinary approach unless the etiology is obvious.
- Children usually do not require any specific studies; however, an orthopedic consultation is recommended.
- Fixed deformity in the child; may need orthopedic referral for surgical release.

SUGGESTED READINGS

Crowner BE: Cervical dystonia: disease profile and clinical management, *Phys Ther* 87:1511, 2007.

Ferreira JJ et al: The management of cervical dystonia, *Expert Opin Pharmacother* 8(2):129, 2007.

Hosalkar HS et al: Congenital osseous anomalies of the upper cervical spine, *J Bone Joint Surg Am* 90A:337, 2008.

Papadimitriou NG et al: Acute torticollis after isolated stress fracture of the first rib in a child, *J Bone Joint Surg Am* 87A:2537, 2005.

Parikh SN et al: Magnetic resonance imaging in the evaluation of infantile torticollis, *Orthopedics* 27:509, 2004.

Sankar WN et al: Orthopedic conditions in the newborn, *J Am Acad Orthop Surg* 17:112, 2009.

Slawek J et al: Factors affecting the health-related quality of life of patients with cervical dystonia and the impact of botulinum toxin type A injections, *Funct Neurol* 22(2):95, 2007.

AUTHOR: **LONNIE R. MERCIER, M.D.**

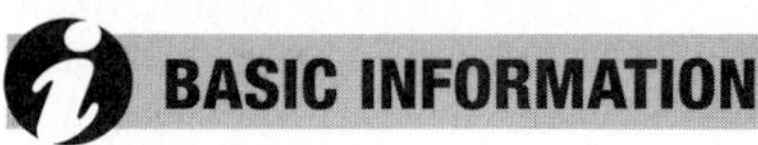

BASIC INFORMATION

DEFINITION

Tics are sudden, brief, intermittent involuntary or semivoluntary movements (motor tics) or sounds (phonic or vocal tics) that mimic fragments of normal behavior.

Tourette's syndrome (TS) is an inherited neuropsychiatric disorder characterized by multiple motor and vocal tics that change during the course of the illness. Onset is typically before age 18 (new-onset tics can occasionally occur after age 18 yr, but for DSM-IV criteria of TS, they must begin before this age).

SYNONYMS

Gilles de la Tourette syndrome

ICD-9CM CODES

307.23 Gilles de la Tourette disorder

EPIDEMIOLOGY & DEMOGRAPHICS

PREVALENCE (IN U.S.): Unknown; estimates range from 0.7% to 5%

PREDOMINANT SEX: Approximate male/female ratio of 3:1

PREDOMINANT AGE: Typical age of onset is between 2 and 15 yr (mean 5 to 7 yr)

PHYSICAL FINDINGS & CLINICAL PRESENTATION

- Neurologic examination is normal.
- Vocal tics (clearing of throat, repetitive short phrases, e.g., "you bet," swearing [coprolalia]).
- Motor tics can be simple (e.g., blinking, grimacing, head jerking) or complex (e.g., gesturing). Tics wax, wane, and change over time. Often they can be suppressed for short periods. Commonly they are preceded by an urge to perform the tic.
- TS is often associated with a variety of behavioral symptoms, most commonly attention deficit hyperactivity disorder (ADHD) and obsessive-compulsive disorder (OCD).

TS can be diagnosed using the DSM-IV-TR criteria as follows:

1. Both multiple motor and one or more vocal tics must be present at some time during the illness.
2. Tics occur many times a day (usually in bouts over >1 year, during which time there must be no tic-free period of >3 consecutive mo.
3. Age at onset is <18 yr.
4. Disturbance is not attributable to the direct physiologic effects of a substance (e.g., stimulants) or a general medical condition (e.g., Huntington's disease or postviral encephalitis).

ETIOLOGY

There is a large genetic contribution to TS. There is a strong family history of OCD or TS in patients with tics, and twin studies provide evidence for the importance of genetic factors. However, although multiple candidate genes have been identified, no simple mutation has been found thus far. Dopamine is believed to be one of the major neurotransmitters involved.

Dx DIAGNOSIS

DIFFERENTIAL DIAGNOSIS

- Sydenham's chorea: occurs after infection with group A streptococcus.
- PANDAS: pediatric autoimmune neuropsychiatric disorder associated with streptococcal infection.
- Sporadic tic disorders: tend to be motor or vocal but not both.
- Head trauma.
- Drug intoxication: many drugs are known to induce or exacerbate tic disorder, including methylphenidate, amphetamines, pemoline, anticholinergics, and antihistamines.
- Postinfectious encephalitis.
- Inherited disorders: Huntington's disease, Hallervorden Spatz, and neuroacanthocytosis. All these conditions should have other observed abnormalities on neurologic examination.

WORKUP

Clinical observation and history to confirm diagnosis

LABORATORY TESTS

No definitive laboratory tests.

IMAGING STUDIES

CT scan and MRI of brain are normal and unnecessary in the absence of abnormal neurologic examination.

Rx TREATMENT

NONPHARMACOLOGIC THERAPY

Multidisciplinary: parents, teachers, psychologists, school nurses

ACUTE GENERAL Rx

Dopamine-blocking agents may be used to reduce severity of tics acutely (e.g., haloperidol 0.25 mg PO qhs initially). There are risks of side effects, such as acute dystonic reactions.

CHRONIC Rx

Tics only require treatment when they interfere with psychosocial, educational, and occupational functioning of a person.

TICS

- Clonidine: many choose this as a first-line agent because of fewer long-term side effects. Start at 0.05 mg and slowly titrate to approximately 0.45 mg daily (needs tid/qid dosing). May also help with symptoms of ADHD.
- Guanfacine (Tenex) is another alpha-agonist similar to clonidine but can be administered once daily. Typical starting dose is 0.5 mg titrating to 1 to 3 mg qd.
- Tetrabenazine: dopamine-depleting agent that recently became available in the U.S. Avoids many of the typical side effects of the neuroleptics; most notably does not cause tardive dyskinesias.
- Atypical antipsychotics such as ziprasidone (Geodon), risperidone (Risperdal), and olanzapine (Zyprexa). These have fewer side effects than typical neuroleptics.
- Dopamine-blocking agents: neuroleptics (pimozide, Haldol, Prolixin). These should be avoided until other options have been exhausted.
- Dopamine agonists: a few small, open-label studies have found that ropinirole and pramipexole in low doses may be effective in reducing tic severity.

ADHD

Stimulants (dextroamphetamine, methylphenidate) are useful for symptoms of ADHD but may exacerbate tics.

OCD

Selective serotonin reuptake inhibitors, such as fluoxetine, are the most effective.

DISPOSITION

- In the later teen years, intensity and frequency of tics typically diminish.
- One third of patients will achieve significant remission, although complete, lifelong remission is rare.
- One third will have mild, persistent, but "non-impairing" tics.

REFERRAL

To a neurologist to confirm initial diagnosis and for treatment in difficult cases

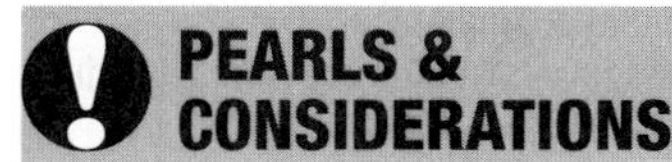

PEARLS & CONSIDERATIONS

Tics do not need treatment unless they interfere with an individual's ability to function.

COMMENTS

Patient education may be obtained from the Tourette's Syndrome Association, 4240 Bell Blvd., Bayside, NY 11361-2864; 800-237-0717 or 718-224-2999; http://www.tsa-usa.org.

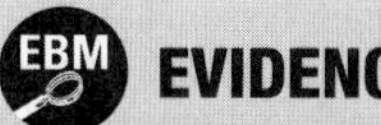

EVIDENCE

Evidence for specific therapies is limited. A recent double-blind, placebo-controlled study showed that methylphenidate (compared with clonidine) does not actually cause a worsening of tics.[1]

Evidence-Based Reference

1. *Neurology* 58:527-536, 2002.

SUGGESTED READINGS

Kenney C, Kuo SH, Jimenez-Shahed J: Tourette's syndrome, *Am Fam Physician* 77(5):651, 2008.

Marcus D, Kurlan R: Tics and its disorders. In Hurtig H, Stern M (eds): *Neurologic clinics: movement disorders,* 19:3, 2001.

Pringsheim T: Tics, *Curr Opin Neurol* 16:523-527, 2003.

Sandor P: Pharmacological management of tics in patients with TS, *J Psychosom Res* 55:41-48, 2003.

AUTHOR: **CINDY ZADIKOFF, M.D.**

Toxic Shock Syndrome (PTG)

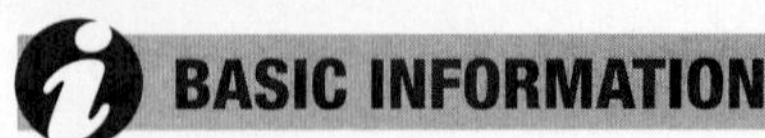

BASIC INFORMATION

DEFINITION

Toxic shock syndrome (TSS) is an acute febrile illness resulting in multiple organ system dysfunction caused most commonly by a bacterial exotoxin. Disease characteristics also include hypotension, vomiting, myalgia, watery diarrhea, vascular collapse, and an erythematous sunburnlike cutaneous rash that desquamates during recovery.

ICD-9CM CODES
040.89 Toxic shock syndrome

EPIDEMIOLOGY & DEMOGRAPHICS

- Case reported incidence peak: 14 cases per 100,000 menstruating women annually in 1980; has since fallen to one case per 100,000 persons
- Occurs most commonly between ages 10 and 30 yr in healthy, young, menstruating white females
- Case fatality ratio of 3%

PHYSICAL FINDINGS & CLINICAL PRESENTATION

- Fever ($>38.0°$ C)
- Diffuse macular erythrodermatous rash that desquamates 1 to 2 wk after disease onset in survivors
- Orthostatic hypotension
- Gastrointestinal symptoms: vomiting, diarrhea, abdominal tenderness
- Constitutional symptoms: myalgia, headache, photophobia, rigors, altered sensorium, conjunctivitis, arthralgia
- Respiratory symptoms: dysphagia, pharyngeal hyperemia, strawberry tongue
- Genitourinary symptoms: vaginal discharge, vaginal hyperemia, adnexal tenderness
- End-organ failure
- Severe hypotension and acute renal failure
- Hepatic failure
- Cardiovascular symptoms: disseminated intravascular coagulation, pulmonary edema, acute respiratory distress syndrome (ARDS), endomyocarditis, heart block

ETIOLOGY

- Menstruation-associated TSS: 45% of cases associated with tampons, diaphragm, or vaginal sponge use
- Non–menstruation-associated TSS: 55% of cases associated with puerperal sepsis, post–cesarean section endometritis, mastitis, wound or skin infection, insect bite, pelvic inflammatory disease, and postoperative fever
- Causative agent: *Staphylococcus aureus* infection of a susceptible individual (10% of population lacking sufficient levels of antitoxin antibodies), which liberates the disease mediator TSST-1 (exotoxin)
- Other causative agents: coagulase-negative streptococci producing enterotoxins B or C, and exotoxin A producing group A beta-hemolytic streptococci

DIAGNOSIS

DIFFERENTIAL DIAGNOSIS

- Staphylococcal food poisoning
- Septic shock
- Mucocutaneous lymph node syndrome
- Scarlet fever
- Rocky Mountain spotted fever
- Meningococcemia
- Toxic epidermal necrolysis
- Kawasaki's syndrome
- Leptospirosis
- Legionnaires' disease
- Hemolytic-uremic syndrome
- Stevens-Johnson syndrome
- Scalded skin syndrome
- Erythema multiforme
- Acute rheumatic fever

WORKUP

Broad-spectrum syndrome with multiorgan system involvement and variable but acute clinical presentation, including the following:

- Fever ($>38.0°$ C)
- Classic desquamating rash (1 to 2 wk)
- Hypotension/orthostatic systolic blood pressure ≤ 90 mm Hg
- Syncope
- Negative throat and cerebrospinal fluid cultures
- Negative serologic test for Rocky Mountain spotted fever, rubeola, and leptospirosis
- Clinical involvement of three or more of the following:
  1. Cardiopulmonary: ARDS, pulmonary edema, endomyocarditis, second- or third-degree atrioventricular block
  2. Central nervous system: altered sensorium without focal neurologic findings
  3. Hematologic: thrombocytopenia (platelets <100 k)
  4. Liver: elevated liver function test results
  5. Renal: >5 cells/high-powered field, negative urine cultures, azotemia, and increased creatinine (double normal)
  6. Mucous membrane involvement: vagina, oropharynx, conjunctiva
  7. Musculoskeletal: myalgia, creatine phosphokinase twice normal
  8. Gastrointestinal: vomiting, diarrhea

LABORATORY TESTS

- Pan culture (cervix and vagina, throat, nasal passages, urine, blood, cerebrospinal fluid, wound) for *Staphylococcus, Streptococcus,* and other pathogenic organisms
- Electrolytes to detect hypokalemia, hyponatremia
- Complete blood count with differential and clotting profile for anemia (normocytic or normochromic), thrombocytopenia, leukocytosis, coagulopathy, and bacteremia
- Chemistry profile to detect decreased protein, increased aspartate aminotransferase, increased alanine aminotransferase, hypocalcemia, elevated blood urea nitrogen and creatinine, hypophosphatemia, increased lactate dehydrogenase, increased creatine phosphokinase
- Urinalysis to detect white blood cells (>5 cells/high-powered field), proteinemia, microhematuria
- Arterial blood gases to assess respiratory function and acid–base status
- Serologic tests considered for Rocky Mountain spotted fever, rubeola, and leptospirosis

IMAGING STUDIES

- Chest x-ray examination to evaluate pulmonary edema
- ECG to evaluate arrhythmia
- Sonography, CT scan, or MRI considered if pelvic abscess or tubo-ovarian abscess suspected

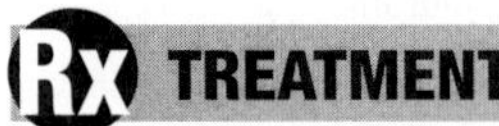

TREATMENT

NONPHARMACOLOGIC THERAPY

- For optimal outcome: high index of suspicion and early and aggressive supportive management in an ICU setting
- Aggressive fluid resuscitation (maintenance of circulating volume, cardiac output, systolic blood pressure)
- Thorough search for a localized infection or nidus: incision and drainage, debridement, removal of tampon or vaginal sponge
- Central hemodynamic monitoring, Swan-Ganz catheter and arterial line for surveillance of hemodynamic status and response to therapy
- Foley catheter to monitor hourly urine output
- Possible military antishock trousers as temporary measure
- Acute ventilator management if severe respiratory compromise
- Renal dialysis for severe renal impairment
- Surgical intervention for indicated conditions (i.e., ruptured tubo-ovarian abscess, wound abscess, mastitis)

ACUTE GENERAL Rx

- Isotonic crystalloid (normal saline solution) for volume replacement following "7–3" rule (refers to the response in mm Hg of the pulmonary artery wedge pressure to volume replacement).
- Electrolyte replacement ($K+$, $Ca+$)
- Packed red blood cells, coagulation factor replacement, fresh frozen plasma to treat anemia or dilation and curettage
- Vasopressor therapy for hypotension refractory to fluid volume replacement (e.g., dopamine beginning at 2 to 5 μg/kg/min)
- Naloxone infusion (0.5 mg/kg/hr) to improve systolic blood pressure by blocking endogenous endorphin effects
- Parenteral antibiotic therapy; β-lactamase–resistant antibiotic (methicillin, nafcillin, oxacillin) initiated early
- Broad-spectrum antibiotic added if concurrent sepsis suspected
- Tetracycline added if considering Rocky Mountain spotted fever

CHRONIC Rx

- Severely ill patient: may require prolonged hospitalization and supportive management with gradual recovery and/or sequelae from severe end-organ involvement (ARDS or renal failure requiring dialysis)
- Majority of patients: complete recovery
- Early late-onset complications (within 2 wk):
  1. Skin desquamation
  2. Impaired digit sensation
  3. Denuded tongue
  4. Vocal cord paralysis
  5. Acute tubular necrosis
  6. ARDS
- Late-onset complications (after 8 wk):
  1. Nail splitting and loss
  2. Alopecia
  3. Central nervous system sequelae
  4. Renal impairment
  5. Cardiac dysfunction
- Recurrent TSS:
  1. More common in menstruation-related cases
  2. Less common in patients treated with beta-lactamase–resistant antistaphylococcal antibiotics
  3. Patients with history of TSS: if suspect signs and symptoms occur, have high index of suspicion and low threshold for evaluation and treatment

PREVENTION

- Avoidance of tampons or use of low-absorbency tampons only (<4 hr in situ) and alternate with napkins
- Education for patients concerning signs and symptoms of TSS
- Avoidance of tampons for patients with history of TSS

DISPOSITION

- Complete recovery for most patients
- Long-term management of early- and late-onset complications for minority of patients

REFERRAL

- For multidisciplinary management, involving primary physician, gynecologist, internist, infectious disease specialist, and other supportive care specialists
- To tertiary-level hospital

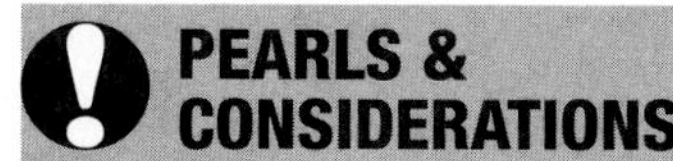

PEARLS & CONSIDERATIONS

COMMENTS

Patient information is available from American College of Gynecologists and Obstetricians.

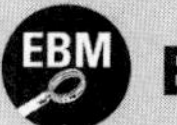

EVIDENCE

In patients with bacterial sepsis or septic shock, treatment with polyclonal intravenous immunoglobulin has been shown to significantly reduce both overall and sepsis-related death, but larger multicenter trials are needed to support these findings.[1,2] Ⓐ

Existing evidence has not determined whether any particular vasopressor agent has superiority in the management of septic shock.[3] Ⓑ

Treatment with a long course of low-dose corticosteroids has been shown to significantly reduce 28-day all-cause mortality rate and intensive care unit and hospital mortality rate in patients with severe sepsis or septic shock compared with control groups.[4] Ⓐ

A randomized, controlled trial has found that early goal-directed therapy, begun in the emergency department before admission to the intensive care unit, provides significant benefits regarding outcome (including in-hospital death) in patients with severe sepsis and septic shock.[5] Ⓑ

Evidence-Based References

1. Alejandria MM et al: Intravenous immunoglobulin for treating sepsis and septic shock, *Cochrane Rev* 1, 2002.

2. Darenberg J et al: Intravenous immunoglobulin G therapy in streptococcal toxic shock syndrome: a European randomized, double-blind, placebo-controlled trial, *Clin Infect Dis* 37:333, 2003. Ⓑ

3. Müllner M et al: Vasopressors for shock, *Cochrane Rev* 2, 2004.

4. Annane D et al: Corticosteroids for treating severe sepsis and septic shock, *Cochrane Rev* 1, 2004.

5. Rivers E et al: Early Goal-Directed Therapy Collaborative Group: early goal-directed therapy in the treatment of severe sepsis and septic shock, *N Engl J Med* 345:1368, 2001. Ⓑ

SUGGESTED READINGS

Issa NC et al: Staphylococcal toxic shock syndrome: suspicion and prevention are keys to control, *Postgrad Med* 110(4):55, 2001.

Miche CA, Shah V: Managing toxic shock syndrome, *Nursing Times* 99(5):26, 2003.

AUTHORS: **DENNIS M. WEPPNER, M.D.,** and **RUBEN ALVERO, M.D.**

T

Diseases and Disorders

Toxoplasmosis (PTG)

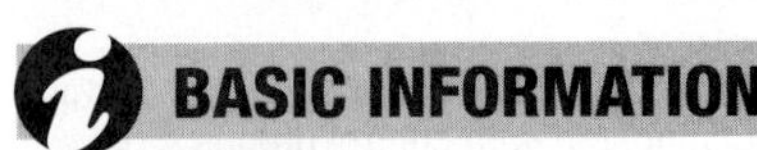

BASIC INFORMATION

DEFINITION

Toxoplasmosis is an infection caused by the protozoal parasite *Toxoplasma gondii.*

ICD-9CM CODES
130.9 Toxoplasmosis

EPIDEMIOLOGY & DEMOGRAPHICS

INCIDENCE (IN U.S.):
- 3% to 70% of healthy adults
- Increases with age
- Increases with certain activities
  1. Slaughterhouse workers
  2. Cat owners
- Increases with certain geographic locations: high prevalence of cats

PREDOMINANT SEX: Equal gender distribution

PREDOMINANT AGE:
- Infancy (congenital infection)
- Prevalence increases with age

PEAK INCIDENCE: Temperate climates

GENETICS: Congenital infection:
- Incidence and severity vary with the trimester of gestation during which the mother acquired infection.
  1. 10% to 25% (first trimester)
  2. 30% to 54% (second trimester)
  3. 60% to 65% (third trimester)
- Congenital infection occurring in the first trimester is the most severe.
- 89% to 100% of infections in the third trimester are asymptomatic.
- Risk to the fetus is not correlated with symptoms in the mother.

PHYSICAL FINDINGS & CLINICAL PRESENTATION

- Acquired (immunocompetent host)
  1. 80% to 90% asymptomatic
  2. Adenopathy (usually cervical)
  3. Fever
  4. Myalgias
  5. Malaise
  6. Sore throat
  7. Maculopapular rash
  8. Hepatosplenomegaly
  9. Chorioretinitis rare
- Acquired (in patients with AIDS)
  1. 89% of symptomatic cases
     a. Encephalitis
     b. Intracerebral mass lesions
  2. Pneumonitis
  3. Chorioretinitis
  4. Other end organ
- Acquired (immunocompromised patients)
  1. Encephalitis
  2. Myocarditis (especially in heart transplant patients)
  3. Pneumonitis
- Ocular infection in the immunocompetent host
  1. Congenital infection
  2. Blurred vision
  3. Photophobia
  4. Pain
  5. Loss of central vision if macula involved
  6. Focal necrotizing retinitis
  7. Typically presents in second or third decade
- Congenital
  1. Results from acute infection acquired by the mother within 6 to 8 wk before conception or during gestation
  2. Usually, asymptomatic mother
  3. No sign of disease
  4. Chorioretinitis
  5. Blindness
  6. Epilepsy
  7. Psychomotor or mental retardation
  8. Intracranial calcifications
  9. Hydrocephalus
  10. Microcephaly
  11. Encephalitis
  12. Anemia
  13. Thrombocytopenia
  14. Hepatosplenomegaly
  15. Lymphadenopathy
  16. Jaundice
  17. Rash
  18. Pneumonitis
  19. Most infected infants are asymptomatic at birth

ETIOLOGY

- *Toxoplasma gondii*
  1. Ubiquitous intracellular protozoan
  2. Present worldwide
  3. Cat is definitive host
- Human infection
  1. Ingestion of oocysts shed by cats
  2. Ingestion of meat containing tissue cysts
  3. Vertical transmission

Dx DIAGNOSIS

DIFFERENTIAL DIAGNOSIS

- Lymphadenopathy
  1. Infectious mononucleosis
  2. CMV mononucleosis
  3. Cat-scratch disease
  4. Sarcoidosis
  5. Tuberculosis
  6. Lymphoma
  7. Metastatic cancer
- Cerebral mass lesions in immunocompromised host
  1. Lymphoma
  2. Tuberculosis
  3. Bacterial abscess
- Pneumonitis in immunocompromised host
  1. *Pneumocystis jirovecii (carinii)* pneumonia
  2. Tuberculosis
  3. Fungal infection
- Chorioretinitis
  1. Syphilis
  2. Tuberculosis
  3. Histoplasmosis (competent host)
  4. CMV
  5. Syphilis
  6. Herpes simplex
  7. Fungal infection
  8. Tuberculosis (AIDS patient)
- Myocarditis
  1. Organ rejection in heart transplant recipients
- Congenital infection
  1. Rubella
  2. CMV
  3. Herpes simplex
  4. Syphilis
  5. Listeriosis
  6. Erythroblastosis fetalis
  7. Sepsis

WORKUP

- Acute infection, immunocompetent host
  1. CBC
  2. *Toxoplasma* serology (IgG, IgM) in serial blood specimens 3 wk apart
  3. Lymph node biopsy if diagnosis uncertain
- Immunocompromised host
  1. CNS symptoms
     a. Cerebral CT scan or MRI if CNS symptoms present
     b. Spinal tap, if safe
     c. Brain biopsy if no response to empiric therapy
  2. Ocular symptoms
     a. Funduscopic examination
     b. Serologic studies
     c. Rarely, vitreous tap
  3. Pulmonary symptoms
     a. Chest x-ray examination
     b. Bronchoalveolar lavage
     c. Transbronchial or open-lung biopsy
  4. Myocarditis
     a. Cardiac enzymes
     b. Electrocardiogram
     c. Endomyocardial biopsy for definitive diagnosis
- Toxoplasmosis in pregnancy
  1. Initial maternal screening with IgM and IgG
     a. If negative, mother at risk of acute infection and should be retested monthly
     b. If both IgG and IgM positive, obtain IgA and IgE ELISA, AC/HS test
     c. IgA and IgE ELISA, AC/HS test elevated in acute infection
     d. Ig high for 1 yr or more
     e. IgG repeated 3 to 4 wk later to determine if titer is stable
  2. Acute maternal infection not excluded or documented
     a. Fetal blood sampling (for culture, Ig, IgA, IgE)
     b. Amniotic fluid polymerase chain reaction (PCR)
  3. Fetal ultrasound every other wk if maternal infection documented
- Congenital toxoplasmosis
  1. Placental histology
  2. Specific IgM or IgA in infant's blood

LABORATORY TESTS

- Antibody studies
  1. More than one test necessary to establish diagnosis of acute toxoplasmosis
  2. IgM antibody
     a. Appears 5 days into infection
     b. Peaks at 2 wk

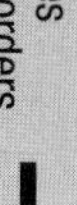

c. Falls to low level or disappears within 2 mo
d. May persist at low levels for 1 yr or more
3. Antibody not measurable
a. Ocular toxoplasmosis
b. Reactivation
c. Immunocompromised hosts
4. IgA ELISA, IgE ELISA, and IgE ASAGA
a. More sensitive tests
b. Disappear more rapidly than Ig, establishing diagnosis of acute infection
5. IgG antibody
a. Appears 1 to 2 wk after infection
b. Peaks at 6 to 8 wk
c. Gradually declines over months to years

IMAGING STUDIES

- Chest x-ray if pulmonary involvement suspected
- Cerebral CT scan (Fig. 1-338) or MRI if encephalitis suspected

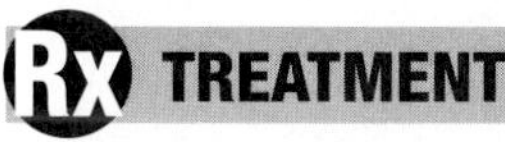

TREATMENT

NONPHARMACOLOGIC THERAPY

- Selected cases of ocular infection
  1. Photocoagulation
  2. Vitrectomy
  3. Lentectomy
- Selected cases of congenital cerebral infection
  1. Ventricular shunting

ACUTE GENERAL Rx

- Acute infection, immunocompetent host
  1. No treatment, unless severe and persistent symptoms or vital organ damage

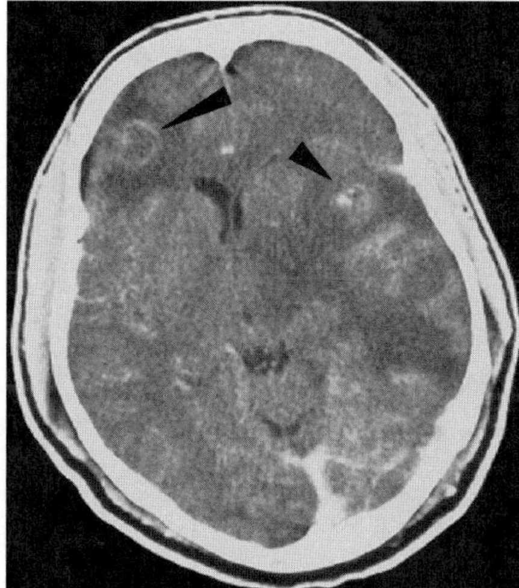

FIGURE 1-338 Toxoplasmic encephalitis in person who has AIDS. A cranial CT scan shows bilateral contrast-enhanced ring lesions with peripheral edema and mass effect. (From Cohen J, Powderly WG: *Infectious diseases,* ed 2, St Louis, 2004, Mosby.)

- Acute infection, immunocompromised host, non-AIDS
  1. Treat even if asymptomatic
  2. Duration
     a. Until 4 to 6 wk after resolution of all signs and symptoms
     b. Usually 6 mo or longer
- Reactivated infection, immunocompromised host, non-AIDS
  1. Treat if symptomatic
- Acute or reactivated infection, AIDS
  1. Treat in all cases
  2. Induction course
     a. 3 to 6 wk.
     b. Maintenance therapy continued for life; consider discontinuation of suppressive therapy if the patient has a good response to highly active antiretroviral therapy and if the CD4 count remains >200 cell/mm^3 for more than 3 mo.
  3. Empiric therapy
     a. AIDS with positive IgG
     b. Multiple ring-enhancing lesions on cerebral CT scan or MRI
     c. Response seen by day 7 in 71% and day 14 in 91%
- Ocular infection
  1. Treat in all cases
  2. Therapy continued for 1 mo or longer if needed
  3. Response seen in 70% within 10 days
  4. Retreat as needed
  5. Steroids may be indicated
  6. Surgical treatment in selected cases
- Treatment regimens
  1. Pyrimethamine 100 to 200 mg loading dose once PO, then 25 mg PO qid (50 to 75 mg in AIDS), plus
  2. Leucovorin 10 to 20 mg PO qid, plus
  3. Sulfadiazine 1 to 1.5 g PO q6h

Other treatment options (if sulfa-hypersensitivity or allergy is present): pyrimethamine 50 to 75 mg/day PO with leucovorin 10 to 20 mg/day PO and either (1) clindamycin 600 mg IV or PO q6h, or (2) clarithromycin 1 gm PO bid, or (3) dapsone 100 mg/day PO, or (4) atovaquone 750 mg PO q6h.

- Acute infection in pregnancy
  1. Treat immediately
  2. Risk of fetal infection reduced by 60% with treatment
     a. First trimester
        i. Spiramycin 3 g PO qid in two to four divided doses
        ii. Sulfadiazine 4 g PO qid in four divided doses
     b. Second and third trimester
        i. Sulfadiazine as previously described, *plus*
        ii. Pyrimethamine 25 mg PO qid, *plus*
        iii. Leucovorin 5 to 15 mg PO qid
        iv. Spiramycin as previously described
- Congenital infection
  1. Sulfadiazine 50 mg/kg PO bid, plus
  2. Pyrimethamine 2 mg/kg PO for 2 days, then 1 mg/kg PO, three times weekly, plus
  3. Leucovorin 5 to 20 mg PO three times weekly
  4. Minimum duration of treatment: 12 mo

CHRONIC Rx

- Maintenance therapy in AIDS patients because of the high risk (80%) of relapse
  1. Pyrimethamine 25 mg PO qid
  2. Sulfadiazine 500 mg PO qid
  3. Leucovorin 10 to 20 mg PO qid

DISPOSITION

- Prognosis
  1. Excellent in the immunocompetent host
  2. Good in ocular infection (although relapses are common)
- Treatment of acute infection in pregnancy
  1. Reduces incidence and severity of congenital toxoplasmosis
- Treatment of congenital infection
  1. Improvement in intellectual function
  2. Regression of retinal lesions
- AIDS
  1. 70% to 95% response to therapy

REFERRAL

- To infectious disease expert:
  1. Immunocompromised hosts
  2. Pregnant women
  3. Difficulty in making a diagnosis or deciding on treatment
- To pediatric infectious disease expert:
  1. Congenital infection
- To obstetrician:
  1. Pregnant seronegative mother
  2. Acute seroconversion
- To ophthalmologist:
  1. Congenital infection
  2. Any case of ocular infection

PEARLS & CONSIDERATIONS

COMMENTS

- Prevention of toxoplasmosis is most important in seronegative pregnant women and immunocompromised hosts.
- Patient instructions:
  1. Cook meat to 66° C.
  2. Cook eggs.
  3. Do not drink unpasteurized milk.
  4. Wash hands thoroughly after handling raw meat.
  5. Wash kitchen surfaces that come in contact with raw meat.
  6. Wash fruits and vegetables.
  7. Avoid contact with materials potentially contaminated with cat feces.

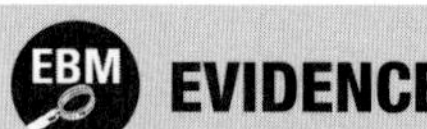

EVIDENCE

Acute infection in immunocompromised patients:

- Recommendations from the CDC, the National Institutes of Health, and the Infectious Diseases Society of America regarding management of toxoplasmosis state that:

- The initial therapy of choice consists of the combination of pyrimethamine plus sulfadiazine plus leucovorin.[1] C
- The preferred alternative regimen for patients unable to tolerate or who fail to respond to first-line therapy is pyrimethamine, plus clindamycin, plus leucovorin.[1] C
- Another alternative in adults is atovaquone (1500 mg orally twice daily, administered with meals), plus pyrimethamine and leucovorin, or atovaquone with sulfadiazine alone, or atovaquone as a single agent among patients intolerant to both pyrimethamine and sulfadiazine.[2] C
- Acute therapy should be continued for at least 6 wk, if there is clinical and radiologic improvement.[1] C
- Patients who have successfully completed a 6-wk course of initial therapy for toxoplasmic encephalitis (TE) should be administered lifelong secondary prophylaxis (i.e., chronic maintenance therapy) unless immune reconstitution occurs because of antiretroviral therapy (ART).[1] C
- HIV-infected children with acquired CNS, ocular, or systemic toxoplasmosis should be treated with pyrimethamine (2 mg/kg/day for 3 days, followed by 1 mg/kg/day) and leucovorin (10 to 25 mg/day) plus sulfadiazine (25 to 50 mg/kg/dose given four times daily).[2] C
- Acute therapy should be continued for 6 wk, assuming clinical and radiological improvement.[2] C

Data suggests that while pyrimethamine plus sulfadiazine (plus folinic acid) remains the standard regimen for toxoplasmic encephalitis, treatment with clindamycin or trimethoprim plus sulfamethoxazole are alternatives for patients unable to tolerate sulfadiazine.

- A Cochrane review of these trials and regimens concluded that the available evidence fails to identify any one superior regimen for the treatment of toxoplasmic encephalitis. The choice of therapy is often directed by available therapy. Given the current evidence, TMP-SMX appears to be an effective alternative therapy for toxoplasmic encephalitis in resource-poor settings where pyrimethamine plus sulfadiazine are not available.[3]

Subsequent maintenance therapy for toxoplasmosis is supported by expert opinion.

Initial therapy and subsequent maintenance treatment of congenital toxoplasmosis is supported by expert opinion.

- Recommendations from the CDC, the National Institutes of Health, and the Infectious Diseases Society of America state that:
  - Pregnant women with suspected or confirmed primary toxoplasmosis and newborns with possible or documented congenital toxoplasmosis should be managed in consultation with an appropriate specialist. If an HIV-infected woman has a symptomatic toxoplasma infection during pregnancy, empiric therapy of the newborn should be strongly considered, whether or not the mother was treated during pregnancy.[2] C
  - The preferred treatment for congenital toxoplasmosis is pyrimethamine (loading dose of 2 mg/kg body weight/day for 2 days, then 1 mg/kg/day for 2 to 6 mo, followed by 1 mg/kg administered three times a wk) combined with sulfadiazine (50 mg/kg/dose twice daily), with supplementary leucovorin (folinic acid) to minimize pyrimethamine-associated hematologic toxicity.[2] C
  - Although the optimal duration of therapy is undefined, the recommended duration of treatment of congenital toxoplasmosis for infants without HIV infection is 12 mo.[2] C
  - HIV-infected children with acquired CNS, ocular, or systemic toxoplasmosis should be treated with pyrimethamine (2 mg/kg/day for 3 days, followed by 1 mg/kg/day) and leucovorin (10 to 25 mg/day) plus sulfadiazine (25 to 50 mg/kg/dose given four times daily).[2] C
  - Acute therapy should be continued for 6 wk, assuming clinical and radiological improvement.[2] C

Data from clinical studies supports the active treatment of congenital toxoplasmosis.

- In a retrospective study of 120 infants with congenital toxoplasmosis treated with pyrimethamine plus sulfadiazine, therapy was initiated shortly after birth and continued for 12 mo. This study reported that treatment of infants without substantial neurologic disease at birth with pyrimethamine and sulfadiazine for 1 yr resulted in normal cognitive, neurologic, and auditory outcomes for all patients. For those patients with moderate or severe neurologic disease, 72% had normal neurologic and/or cognitive outcomes, with all having normal auditory outcomes. In addition, 91% of children without substantial neurologic disease and 64% of those with moderate or severe neurologic disease at birth did not develop new eye lesions.[4] B

Evidence-Based References

1. Benson CA et al: Treating opportunistic infections among HIV-infected adults and adolescents: recommendations from CDC, the National Institutes of Health, and the HIV Medicine Association/Infectious Diseases Society of America, *Clin Infect Dis* 40(Suppl 3):S131-S235, 2005.
2. Mofenson LM et al: Treating opportunistic infections among HIV-exposed and infected children: recommendations from CDC, the National Institutes of Health, and the Infectious Diseases Society of America, *Clin Infect Dis* 40:S1-S84, 2005.
3. Dedicoat M, Livesley N: Management of toxoplasmic encephalitis in HIV-infected adults (with an emphasis on resource-poor settings). *Cochrane Database Syst Rev* 3: 2006.
4. McLeod R et al: Toxoplasmosis study group. Outcome of treatment for congenital toxoplasmosis, 1981-2004: the national collaborative Chicago-based, congenital toxoplasmosis study. *Clin Infect Dis* 42:1383-1394, 2006.

SUGGESTED READINGS

Boyer KM et al: Risk factors for Toxoplasma gondii infection in mothers of infants with congenital toxoplasmosis: implications for prenatal management and screening, *Am J Obstet Gynecol* 192(2): 564, 2005.

Campbell AL et al: First case of toxoplasmosis following small bowel transplantation and systematic review of tissue-invasive toxoplasmosis following noncardiac solid organ transplantation, *Transplantation* 81(3):408, 2006.

Fricker-Hidalgo H et al: Disseminated toxoplasmosis with pulmonary involvement after heart transplantation, *Transpl Infect Dis* 7(1):38, 2005.

Kravetz JD, Federman DG: Prevention of toxoplasmosis in pregnancy: knowledge of risk factors, *Infect Dis Obstet Gynecol* 13(3):161, 2005.

Kravetz JD, Federman DG: Toxoplasmosis in pregnancy, *Am J Med* 118:212, 2005.

Montoya JG, Rosso F: Diagnosis and management of toxoplasmosis, *Clin Perinatol* 32(3):705, 2005.

Soheilian M et al: Prospective randomized trial of trimethoprim/sulfamethoxazole versus pyrimethamine and sulfadiazine in the treatment of ocular toxoplasmosis, *Ophthalmology* 112(11):1876, 2005.

AUTHORS: **GLENN G. FORT, M.D., M.P.H.,** and **DENNIS J. MIKOLICH, M.D.**

BASIC INFORMATION

DEFINITION

Bacterial tracheitis is an acute infectious disease affecting the trachea and large conducting airways. Tracheal inflammation may be caused by a large number of inhaled stimuli, but bacterial infection is a life-threatening illness associated with purulent secretions and subglottic edema.

SYNONYMS

Bacterial tracheobronchitis
Pseudomembranous croup
Membranous laryngotracheobronchitis

ICD-9CM CODES
464.10 Tracheitis

EPIDEMIOLOGY & DEMOGRAPHICS

INCIDENCE (IN U.S.):
- Uncommon
- May be the most common cause of acute upper airway obstruction requiring admission to pediatric ICUs

PEAK INCIDENCE: Three fourths of cases reported in winter
PREDOMINANT SEX: Boys > girls in one series
PREDOMINANT AGE:
- 1 mo to 8 yr
- Almost all <13 yr (most <3 yr)

GENETICS:
- Down syndrome is a possible predisposing factor.
- Congenital infection: Some cases have been found in those with anatomic abnormalities of the upper airways.

PHYSICAL FINDINGS & CLINICAL PRESENTATION

- Croupy or "brassy" cough
- Inspiratory stridor (frequent)
- Wheezing (unusual)
- Fever (often >102° F)
- Thick, purulent secretions expectorated
  1. Minority of patients expectorate "ricelike" pellets.
  2. Most patients are unable to mobilize secretions.
     a. Become inspissated
     b. Form pseudomembranes

ETIOLOGY

- *Staphylococcus aureus*
- *Haemophilus influenzae*
- β-Hemolytic streptococcal infection
- Secondary to viral infections of the respiratory tract
  1. Primary influenza
  2. RSV
  3. Parainfluenza
- Many cases follow measles
  1. Especially when accompanied by chest radiographic infiltrates
  2. Sometimes fatal outcome
  3. Associated with prolonged endotracheal intubation

DIAGNOSIS

DIFFERENTIAL DIAGNOSIS

- Viral croup
- Epiglottitis
- Diphtheria
- Necrotizing herpes simplex infection in the elderly
- CMV in immunocompromised patients
- Invasive aspergillosis in immunocompromised patients

WORKUP

Direct laryngoscopy
1. Typical secretions
   a. May form pseudomembranes
   b. Airway obstruction
2. Normal epiglottis rules out epiglottitis
3. Possible subglottic edema

LABORATORY TESTS

- WBC is sometimes elevated.
- On differential, left shift is almost universal.
- Gram stain and culture of tracheal secretions confirm diagnosis.
- Blood cultures are positive in a minority.

IMAGING STUDIES

- Lateral x-ray examination of neck
  1. Normal epiglottis
  2. Vague density or a "dripping candle" appearance of tracheal mucosa
     a. Secretions
     b. Pseudomembranes
- Chest radiograms
  1. Not diagnostic
  2. Should not be performed on patients in acute respiratory distress, because severe or fatal upper airway obstruction can develop suddenly
- Pneumonic infiltrates frequent
- Atelectasis: unusual but can lead to lobar collapse

TREATMENT

NONPHARMACOLOGIC THERAPY

- Aggressive maintenance of a patent airway
  1. Laryngoscopy or bronchoscopy used diagnostically and therapeutically to strip away pseudomembranes
  2. Voluminous and tenacious secretions suctioned from the underlying friable mucosa
     a. May extend from between the vocal cords to the main carina
     b. Larger channels of rigid instruments for more effective suctioning
- Prevention of complete large airway obstruction
  1. Nasotracheal intubation
  2. Humidification of inspired gas
  3. Frequent saline instillation and suctioning
  4. Intubation with general anesthesia, performed in the operating room, is preferred by some
- Ventilatory support necessary with initial management in ICU

ACUTE GENERAL Rx

- Antibiotic therapy: start immediately, generally continued for 1 to 2 wk
- Initial therapy directed against *H. influenzae* and *S. aureus* (e.g., cefotaxime and vancomycin)
- Oral therapy is usually sufficient after 5 or 6 days of IV administration

DISPOSITION

- Most patients are extubated in 5 to 6 days after initiating antibiotic therapy.
- Anoxic encephalopathy is reported in 7% of survivors.

REFERRAL

Suspected diagnosis

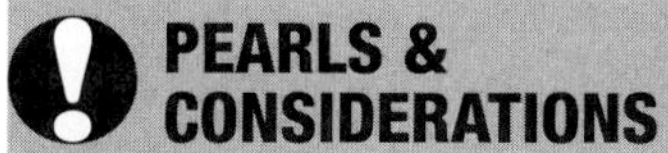

PEARLS & CONSIDERATIONS

COMMENTS

- Infants are at increased risk of airway obstruction because of the small airway dimension.
- Presence of pneumonia and a staphylococcal cause are thought to worsen prognosis.
- Reported complications: toxic shock syndrome, persistent postextubation stridor, pneumothorax, and volutrauma

SUGGESTED READINGS

Gaugler C et al: Neonatal necrotizing tracheobronchitis: three case reports, *J Perinatol* 24(4):259, 2004.
Kinebuchi S et al: Tracheo-bronchitis associated with Crohn's disease improved on inhaled corticotherapy, *Intern Med* 43(9):829, 2004.
Salamone FN et al: Bacterial tracheitis reexamined: is there a less severe manifestation? *Otolaryngol Head Neck Surg* 131(6):871, 2004.

AUTHORS: **GLENN G. FORT, M.D., M.P.H.,** and **DENNIS J. MIKOLICH, M.D.**

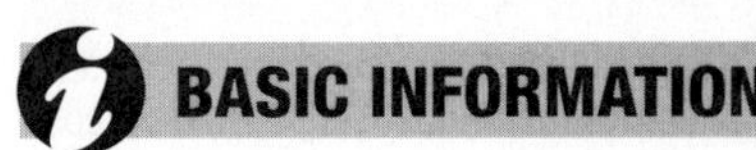

BASIC INFORMATION

DEFINITION

Hemolytic transfusion reaction is acute intravascular hemolysis caused by mismatches in the ABO system. It is caused by complement-fixing immunoglobulin (Ig) and IgG antibodies to group A and B red blood cells. Hemolytic transfusion reactions can also be caused by minor antigen systems; however, they are usually less severe. In delayed serologic transfusion reactions, hemolysis with hemoglobinemia is unusual; in delayed reactions the only manifestations may be the development of a newly positive Coombs test and fever.

ICD-9CM CODES
999.8 Other transfusion reaction

EPIDEMIOLOGY & DEMOGRAPHICS

Acute intravascular hemolysis occurs in fewer than one in 50,000 transfusions.

PHYSICAL FINDINGS & CLINICAL PRESENTATION

- Hypotension
- Pain at the infusion site
- Fever, tachycardia, chest or back pain, dyspnea
- Severe reactions often occur in surgical patients under anesthesia who are unable to give any warning signs

See Table 1-74.

ETIOLOGY

Most fatal hemolytic reactions are caused by clerical errors and mislabeled specimens.

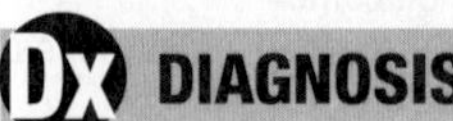

DIAGNOSIS

DIFFERENTIAL DIAGNOSIS

- Bacterial contamination of blood
- Hemoglobinopathies

WORKUP

The transfusion must be stopped immediately. The blood bank must be notified, and the donor transfusion bag must be returned to the blood bank along with a freshly drawn posttransfusion specimen.

LABORATORY TESTS

- Positive Coombs test, elevated blood urea nitrogen, creatinine, bilirubin
- Hemoglobinuria (wine-colored urine), hemoglobinemia (pink plasma)
- Decreased hematocrit and serum haptoglobin

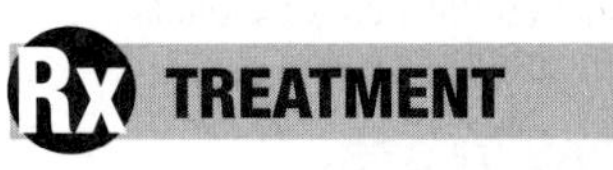

TREATMENT

NONPHARMACOLOGIC THERAPY

- Stop transfusion immediately. Test anticoagulated blood from the recipient for the presence of free hemoglobin in the plasma.
- Monitor vital signs.

ACUTE GENERAL Rx

- Vigorous IV hydration to maintain urine flow at >100 ml/hr until hypotension is corrected and hemoglobinuria clears. IV furosemide may be necessary to maintain adequate renal flow.
- The addition of mannitol may prevent renal damage (controversial).
- Monitor for the presence of disseminated intravascular coagulation.
- Use of IV steroids is controversial.

DISPOSITION

Mortality rate exceeds 50% in severe transfusion reactions.

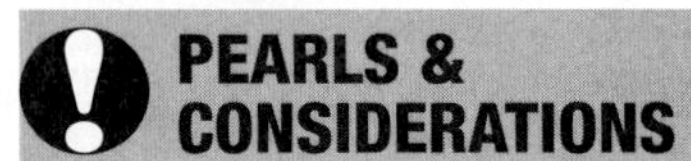

PEARLS & CONSIDERATIONS

COMMENTS

Hemolysis caused by minor antigen systems is generally less severe and may be delayed 5 to 10 days after transfusion.

AUTHOR: **FRED F. FERRI, M.D.**

TABLE 1-74 Signs and Symptoms of Acute Adverse Reactions to Blood Transfusion

Reaction	Fever	Chills/ Rigors	Nausea/ Vomiting	Chest Discomfort/ Pain	Facial Flushing	Wheezing/ Dyspnea	Back/ Lumbar Pain	Discomfort at Infusion Site	Hypotension
Acute hemolytic	X	X	X	X	X	X	X	X	X
Febrile nonhemolytic	X	X		X	X				
Nonimmune hemolysis									
Acute lung injury	X			X		X			X
Allergic									
Massive transfusion complications									
Anaphylaxis	X	X	X	X	X	X	X	X	X
Passive cytokine infusion	X	X	X			X			
Hypervolemia						X			
Bacterial sepsis	X	X	X				X	X	X
Air embolus				X		X			

From Goldman L, Bennett JC (eds): *Cecil textbook of medicine,* ed 22, Philadelphia, 2004, WB Saunders.

BASIC INFORMATION

DEFINITION

Transient ischemic attack (TIA) refers to a transient neurologic dysfunction caused by focal brain or retinal ischemia with symptoms typically lasting <60 min but always <24 hr, followed by a full recovery of function. Acute brain ischemia is a medical emergency requiring prompt neurologic evaluation and potential intervention.

SYNONYMS

TIA

ICD-9CM CODES
435.9 Unspecified transient cerebral ischemia

EPIDEMIOLOGY & DEMOGRAPHICS

INCIDENCE (IN U.S.): 49 cases per 100,000 persons annually
PEAK INCIDENCE: After age 60 yr
PREDOMINANT SEX: Males are affected more often than females

PHYSICAL FINDINGS & CLINICAL PRESENTATION

- During an episode, neurologic abnormalities are confined to a discrete vascular territory.
- Typical carotid territory symptoms are ipsilateral monocular visual disturbance, contralateral homonymous hemianopsia, contralateral motor or sensory dysfunction, and language dysfunction (dominant hemisphere) alone or in combination.
- Typical vertebrobasilar territory symptoms are binocular visual disturbance, vertigo, diplopia, dysphagia, dysarthria, and motor or sensory dysfunction involving the ipsilateral face and contralateral body.

ETIOLOGY

- Embolic
- Large-vessel atherothrombotic disease
- Lacunar disease
- Hypoperfusion with fixed arterial stenosis
- Hypercoagulable states

DIAGNOSIS

DIFFERENTIAL DIAGNOSIS

- Hypoglycemia
- Seizures
- Migraine
- Subdural hemorrhage
- Mass lesions
- Vestibular disease
- Section II describes the differential diagnosis of neurologic deficits, both focal and multifocal.

WORKUP

- Thorough history and physical examination
- Ancillary investigations, including neuroimaging aimed at identifying the etiology quickly

LABORATORY TESTS

- Complete blood count with platelets
- Prothrombin time (INR) and partial thromboplastin time
- Glucose
- Lipid profile
- Erythrocyte sedimentation rate (if clinical suspicion for infectious or inflammatory process)
- Urinalysis
- Chest radiograph
- ECG and consider cycling cardiac enzymes
- Other tests as dictated by suspected etiology

IMAGING STUDIES

- Head CT scan to exclude hemorrhage, including a subdural hemorrhage.
- MRI and MR angiography (MRA). (In several studies, MRI with diffusion-weighted imaging identified early ischemic brain injury in up to 50% of patients with TIA). MRA of the brain and neck can identify large-vessel intracranial and extracranial stenoses, arteriovenous malformations, and aneurysms.
- Carotid Doppler studies identify carotid stenosis; neck ultrasound can also visualize stenoses of the vertebrobasilar arteries.
- CT angiography.
- Echocardiography to look for a cardiac source.
- Telemetry for hospitalized patients for at least 24 hr. May consider 24-hr Holter if patient is being discharged.
- Four-vessel cerebral angiogram in selected cases.

TREATMENT

NONPHARMACOLOGIC THERAPY

- Carotid endarterectomy for carotid territory TIA associated with an ipsilateral symptomatic stenosis of 70% to 99%; should be done by a surgeon who is experienced with and performs this procedure frequently. Carotid stenting is also being performed in patients who are not surgical candidates. Trials comparing stenting versus surgery for carotid disease are ongoing.
- Modification of risk factors, including smoking cessation.

ACUTE GENERAL Rx

- Depends on etiology.
- If the time of the onset of symptoms is clear, there are significant deficits on neurologic examination, and brain hemorrhage has been ruled out, then the patient may be a candidate for thrombolytic therapy; however, this should be discussed with a neurologist or a specialist in cerebrovascular disease.
- Acute anticoagulation: no data supporting benefits in the acute setting. Heparin is considered for new-onset atrial fibrillation and atherothrombotic carotid disease causing recurrent transient neurologic symptoms, especially in the setting before carotid endarterectomy or carotid stenting. Also consider for basilar artery thrombosis given concern for progression to brain stem stroke with high morbidity and mortality rates.
- Section III, "Transient Ischemic Attacks," describes a treatment algorithm.

CHRONIC Rx

- No data supporting the use of long-term anticoagulation in the management of TIA, although stroke patients with atrial fibrillation or demonstrated cardiac thrombi have been shown to benefit from long-term warfarin therapy.
- In the past, treatment for secondary stroke prevention has traditionally been aspirin. No significant benefit of high-dose aspirin (up to 1500 mg/day) has been conclusively found over lower doses (75 mg to 325 mg/day).
- Clopidogrel is superior to aspirin for secondary vascular event prevention (including stroke) and should be strongly considered as first line therapy. Aspirin/dipyridamole extended release capsules (Aggrenox) is also superior to aspirin for stroke prevention. A recent head-to-head clinical trial failed to show any benefit for Aggrenox over clopidogrel in secondary stroke prevention.
- In patients with cerebrovascular disease, HMG-CoA reductase inhibitors (statins) have been shown to provide significant protection against subsequent vascular events such as myocardial infarction and stroke even for low-density lipoprotein (LDL) levels <100 mg/dl. Consider starting a statin agent unless LDL is <70 mg/dl.
- Control of hypertension is paramount, as are diabetic control and smoking cessation.

DISPOSITION

- According to one study, 10% to 20% of patients will have a stroke in the next 90 days, and in 50% of these patients stroke occurs in the first day or two after the TIA.
- Another study showed a stroke risk of 4.4% in the first month and 11.6% in the first year.
- The annual risk of myocardial infarction is 2.4%.
- One-year and 3-yr survival rates are 98% and 94%, respectively.

REFERRAL

Recommend referring all patients with TIA for an urgent neurologic evaluation and management.

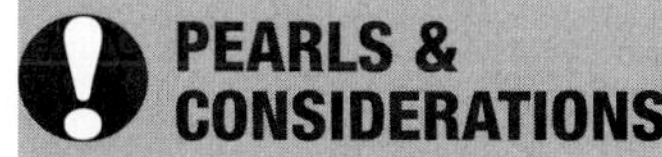

PEARLS & CONSIDERATIONS

CAVEAT

Urgently evaluate all patients who present with symptoms suggestive of acute brain ischemia. Do not wait for symptoms to resolve to differentiate TIA from stroke.

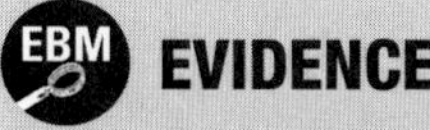

EVIDENCE

Evidence for antiplatelet therapy.
There is no evidence to support the use of dipyridamole alone over aspirin alone in patients with vascular disease.[1] A

Evidence for anticoagulation therapy.

Expert guidelines recommend that patients with atrial fibrillation (AF) who have suffered a recent stroke or TIA commence long-term oral anticoagulation (target INR, 2.5; range, 2.0 to 3.0).[2] Ⓒ

A meta-analysis of two trials has found that anticoagulants are significantly more effective than antiplatelet agents both for preventing all vascular events and for preventing recurrent stroke in people with nonrheumatic AF and recent TIA or minor ischemic stroke. However, major extracranial bleeding complications occur more often in those taking anticoagulants than antiplatelets.[3] Ⓐ

Evidence for surgical treatment.

The evidence for carotid or vertebral percutaneous transluminal angioplasty/stenting versus medical treatment or carotid endarterectomy in people with a recent TIA or minor ischemic stroke who have severe stenosis of the ipsilateral carotid or vertebral artery is limited.[4]

Evidence for antihypertensive therapy in secondary prevention.

Antihypertensive treatment is recommended for both prevention of recurrent stroke and prevention of other vascular events in persons who have had an ischemic stroke or TIA and are beyond the hyperacute period.[5] Ⓒ

Evidence for cholesterol reduction.

A systematic review that included a variety of groups of people including those with and without prior history of stroke, TIA, or coronary artery disease found that statins significantly reduced the risk of stroke compared with placebo or no treatment after a mean of 4.3 yr follow-up.[6] Ⓐ

A randomized controlled trial comparing atorvastatin 80 mg a day with placebo in people who had a history of stroke or TIA, low-density lipoprotein (LDL) cholesterol levels of 100 to 190 mg/dL (2.6 to 4.9 mmol/L), and no known coronary heart disease, found that atorvastatin was associated with a reduced overall incidence of stroke and of cardiovascular events, despite a small increase in the incidence of hemorrhagic stroke compared with placebo. The overall mortality rate was similar in each group.[7] Ⓑ

Evidence-Based References

1. De Schryver EL et al: Dipyridamole for preventing stroke and other vascular events in patients with vascular disease, *Cochrane Database Rev* 2, 2006. Ⓐ
2. Albers GW et al: Antithrombotic and thrombolytic therapy for ischemic stroke: the Seventh ACCP Conference on Antithrombotic and Thrombolytic Therapy, *Chest* 126(3 Suppl):483S-512S, 2004. Ⓒ
3. Saxena R, Koudstaal PJ: Anticoagulants versus antiplatelet therapy for preventing stroke in patients with nonrheumatic atrial fibrillation and a history of stroke or transient ischemic attack, *Cochrane Database Rev* 4, 2004. Ⓐ
4. Lip GYH et al: Stroke prevention, *Clin Evid,* London, 2007, BMJ Publishing Group.
5. Sacco RL et al; American Heart Association; American Stroke Association Council on Stroke; Council on Cardiovascular Radiology and Intervention; American Academy of Neurology: Guidelines for prevention of stroke in patients with ischemic stroke or transient ischemic attack: a statement for healthcare professionals from the American Heart Association/American Stroke Association Council on Stroke: co-sponsored by the Council on Cardiovascular Radiology and Intervention: the American Academy of Neurology affirms the value of this guideline, *Stroke* 37:577-617, 2006. Ⓒ
6. Amarenco P et al: Statins in stroke prevention and carotid atherosclerosis: systematic review and up-to-date meta-analysis, *Stroke* 35:2902-2909, 2004. Ⓐ
7. Amarenco P et al: High-dose atorvastatin after stroke or transient ischemic attack, *N Engl J Med* 355:549-559, 2006. Ⓑ

SUGGESTED READINGS

Albers GW: A review of published TIA treatment recommendations, *Neurology* 62:S26, 2004.

Albers GW et al: Transient ischemic attack—proposal for a new definition, *N Engl J Med* 347:1713, 2002.

Albers GW et al: Antithrombotic and thrombolytic therapy for ischemic stroke, *Chest* 126:483S, 2004.

Algra A et al: Oral anticoagulants versus antiplatelet therapy for preventing further vascular events after transient ischemic attack or minor stroke of presumed arterial origin, *Stroke* 34:234, 2003.

Chaturvedi S et al: Carotid endarterectomy—an evidence-based review: report of the Therapeutics and Technology Assessment Subcommittee of the American Academy of Neurology, *Neurology* 65: 794, 2005.

Diener HC et al: Aspirin and clopidogrel compared with clopidogrel alone after recent ischemic stroke or transient ischaemic attack in high risk patients (MATCH): randomized, double-blind, placebo-controlled trial, *Lancet* 364:331, 2004.

Heart Protection Study Collaborative Group: MRC/BHF heart protection study of cholesterol lowering with simvastatin in 20,536 high-risk individuals: a randomized placebo-controlled trial, *Lancet* 360:7, 2002.

Johnston SC: Clinical practice. Transient ischemic attack, *N Engl J Med* 347:1687, 2002.

Mas JL et al: Endarterectomy versus stenting in patients with symptomatic severe carotid stenosis, *N Engl J Med* 355:1660-1671, 2006.

AUTHOR: **SEAN I. SAVITZ, M.D.**

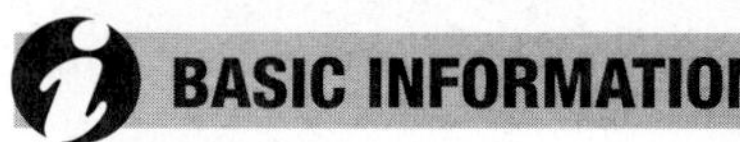

BASIC INFORMATION

DEFINITION

Trichinosis is an infection by one of various species of *Trichinella.*

SYNONYMS

Trichinella spiralis muscle infection

ICD-9CM CODES
124 Trichinosis

EPIDEMIOLOGY & DEMOGRAPHICS

INCIDENCE (IN U.S.): <100 cases/yr
GENETICS: Congenital infection:
- Abrupt delivery of stillbirths in infected pregnant women
- Vertical infection of the fetus

PHYSICAL FINDINGS & CLINICAL PRESENTATION

- Symptoms:
  1. May vary widely depending on the time from ingestion of contaminated meat and on worm burden
  2. Most people asymptomatic
- Enteral phase:
  1. Correlates with penetration of ingested larvae into the intestinal mucosa
  2. May last from 2 to 6 wk
  3. Mild, transient diarrhea and nausea
  4. Abdominal pain
  5. Diarrhea or constipation
  6. Vomiting
  7. Malaise
  8. Low-grade fevers
- Migratory or parenteral phase:
  1. In the intestine, maturation and mating
  2. Newborn larvae
     a. Penetrate into lymphatic and blood vessels
     b. Migrate to muscles, where they penetrate into muscle cells, enlarge, coil, and develop a cyst wall
  3. Patients may present with:
     a. Fever
     b. Myalgias
     c. Periorbital or facial edema
     d. Headache
     e. Skin rash
     f. Other symptoms caused by the penetration of tissues by the newborn migrating larvae
  4. Peak in symptoms 2 to 3 wk after infection, then slowly subside
- Severe complications:
  1. Brain damage by granulomatous inflammation or occlusion of arteries
  2. Cardiac involvement
  3. Can lead to death

ETIOLOGY

- The nematode responsible for this illness is an obligate intracellular parasite belonging to the genus *Trichinella.*
- It is one of the most ubiquitous parasites in the world and may be found in virtually all warm-blooded animals.
- Infection in humans occurs by the ingestion of contaminated animal meat that is raw or partially cooked and contains viable cysts.
- Most cases are now related to the consumption of poorly processed pork or wild game (bear, wild boar, cougar, and walrus).

Dx DIAGNOSIS

DIFFERENTIAL DIAGNOSIS

- Different presentations have different differential diagnoses.
- Early illness may resemble gastroenteritis.
- Later symptoms may be confused with:
  1. Measles
  2. Dermatomyositis
  3. Glomerulonephritis

WORKUP

- Antibody assay of serum is usually positive by approximately 2 wk after infection.
- Muscle biopsy is used to detect the larva in muscle tissue if diagnosis unclear; best done by placing the tissue between two slides.

LABORATORY TESTS

- CBC: leukocytosis with prominent eosinophilia
- ESR: usually normal
- Elevation of muscle enzymes common (i.e., CPK, aldolase)

IMAGING STUDIES

Soft-tissue radiographs may show calcified cyst walls.

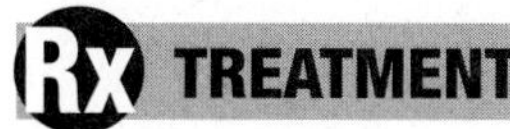

TREATMENT

NONPHARMACOLOGIC THERAPY

Bed rest for myalgias

ACUTE GENERAL Rx

- Albendazole 400 mg PO for 1 to 2 wk.
- Salicylates to decrease muscle discomfort.
- Steroids in critically ill patients.
- Mebendazole 200 mg PO tid for 3 days, followed by mebendazole 400 mg PO tid, is an alternative to albendazole.

DISPOSITION

- Most symptoms subside over time.
- Reports of long-term sequelae:
  1. Myalgias
  2. Headaches
- Occasionally, death occurs.

REFERRAL

Diagnosis uncertain

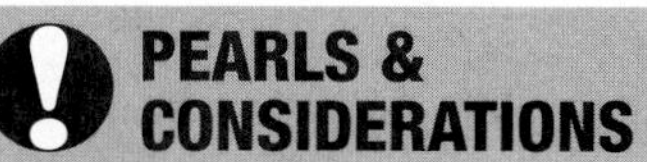

PEARLS & CONSIDERATIONS

COMMENTS

- Prevention by thorough cooking of meats.
- Inadequate to smoke, cure, or dry meats.
- Freezing at specified temperatures kills *T. spiralis* larvae in pork.
- *T. nativa* is a freeze-resistant species that remains viable after freezing, even for months or years; it has been associated with infection from ingestion of bear meat.

SUGGESTED READINGS

Astudillo LM, Arlet PM: Images in clinical medicine. The chemosis of trichinosis, *N Engl J Med* 351(5): 487, 2004.

Awada A, Kojan S: Neurological disorders and travel, *Int J Antimicrob Agents* 21(2):189, 2003.

Centers for Disease Control and Prevention (CDC): Trichinellosis associated with bear meat—New York and Tennessee, *MMWR* 53(27):606, 2004.

Moller LN et al: Outbreak of trichinellosis associated with consumption of game meat in West Greenland, *Vet Parasitol* 132(1-2):131, 2005.

Piergili-Fioretti D et al: Re-evaluation of patients involved in a trichinellosis outbreak caused by *Trichinella britovi* 15 years after infection, *Vet Parasitol* 132(1-2):119, 2005.

Wu Z et al: Tumor necrosis factor receptor-mediated apoptosis in *Trichinella spiralis*-infected muscle cells, *Parasitology* 131(Pt 3):373, 2005.

AUTHORS: **GLENN G. FORT, M.D., M.P.H.,** and **DENNIS J. MIKOLICH, M.D.**

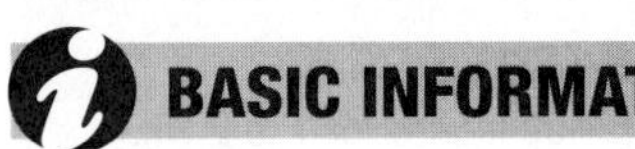

BASIC INFORMATION

DEFINITION

Tricuspid regurgitation (TR) refers to an abnormal flow of blood from the right ventricle to the right atrium (Fig. 1-339).

SYNONYMS

Tricuspid insufficiency
Tricuspid incompetence

ICD-9CM CODES
397.0 Diseases of the tricuspid valve
424.2 Tricuspid valve disorders, specified as non-rheumatic

EPIDEMIOLOGY & DEMOGRAPHICS

- In the adult population, TR is usually functional rather than structural.
- In adolescents and young adults, most cases of TR are the result of congenital cardiac abnormalities.
- In patients with rheumatic heart disease, TR rarely occurs alone; it is usually associated with mitral or aortic valve disease.
- A small degree (i.e., trace to mild) of TR is present in approximately 70% of normal adults. On echocardiography, this "normal" degree of regurgitation is localized to a small region adjacent to valve closure, it often does not extend throughout systole, and it has a low signal strength.

PHYSICAL FINDINGS & CLINICAL PRESENTATION

- Isolated TR can cause nonspecific symptoms (e.g., exercise intolerance).
- Signs and symptoms in the presence of TR are usually the result of an underlying cause.
- Signs and symptoms may be caused by accompanying right-sided heart failure (e.g., jugular venous distension, peripheral edema, ascites, hepatomegaly, right-sided S3).
- A lower-left parasternal holosystolic murmur may be found; the murmur becomes louder during inspiration (Carvallo's sign) and during maneuvers that increase venous return.
- Prominent V waves in the jugular venous waveform can occur (see Fig. 1-339).
- Severe TR may produce systolic propulsion of the eyeballs, pulsatile varicose veins, a venous systolic thrill and murmur in the neck, a mid-diastolic murmur in severe regurgitation, and systolic hepatic pulsation.
- Atrial fibrillation or flutter is common as a result of right atrial enlargement.

ETIOLOGY

- Tricuspid valve dysfunction can occur with structurally normal (functional TR) or abnormal valves (structural TR).
- Functional TR involves conditions that lead to the dilation of the tricuspid annulus or right ventricular enlargement, including the following:
    - Any cause of pulmonary hypertension (e.g., chronic obstructive pulmonary disease, pulmonary embolism, restrictive lung disease, collagen vascular disease, primary pulmonary hypertension)
    - Left-sided heart failure that leads to right-sided heart failure
    - Dilated cardiomyopathy
    - Right ventricular infarction
- Structural TR involves conditions directly affect the tricuspid valve apparatus, including the following:
    - Rheumatic valvulitis
    - Congenital conditions (e.g., Ebstein's anomaly, tricuspid atresia)
    - Endocarditis, either bacterial (particularly related to intravenous drug use) or marantic (e.g., systemic lupus erythematosus, rheumatoid arthritis)
    - Tricuspid valve prolapse or chordae rupture
    - Carcinoid syndrome
    - Marfan's syndrome
    - Iatrogenic damage to the valve (e.g., pacemaker, implantable cardioverter defibrillator, myocardial biopsy, anorectic drugs)
    - External trauma (e.g., deceleration injury)
    - Right atrial myxoma
    - Collagen vascular diseases
    - Radiation injury

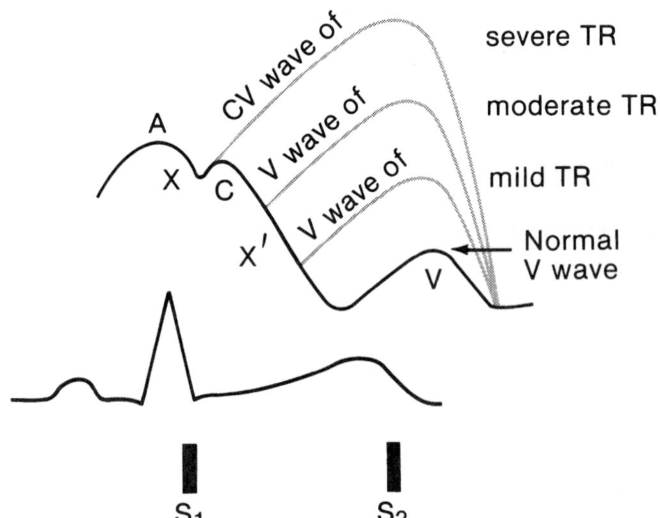

FIGURE 1-339 The jugular venous pulse in tricuspid regurgitation. The jugular venous pulse wave normally drops during ventricular systole. As tricuspid regurgitation becomes more severe, the CV wave becomes more obvious during ventricular systole. (From Conn R: *Current diagnosis,* ed 9, Philadelphia, 1997, WB Saunders.)

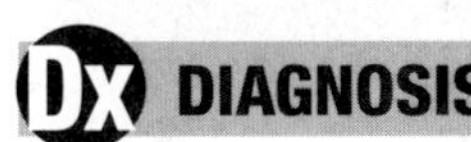

DIAGNOSIS

The diagnosis of TR is made noninvasively by physical examination and imaging techniques (e.g., echocardiography) and invasively by right-sided heart catheterization in selected cases.

DIFFERENTIAL DIAGNOSIS

On the basis of heart auscultation, the diagnosis of TR may be confused with other causes of systolic murmurs, such as mitral regurgitation, aortic stenosis, pulmonary stenosis, ventricular septal defect, and hypertrophic cardiomyopathy.

WORKUP

Any who is patient suspected of having significant TR should undergo the following:
- Chest x-ray
- ECG
- Echocardiogram (confirmatory)
- Right-sided cardiac heart catheterization (in selected cases)

LABORATORY TESTS

ECG may show evidence of the following:
- Right atrial enlargement (e.g., P-wave amplitude in leads II or III or aVF of $>$2.5 mV)
- Right ventricular enlargement or hypertrophy (e.g., R wave $>$ S wave in lead V_1)
- Right axis deviation of $>$100 degrees
- Atrial fibrillation

IMAGING STUDIES

- A chest x-ray may show the following:
    - Evidence of chronic obstructive pulmonary disease (e.g., flattened diaphragms, barrel chest, dilated pulmonary arteries, increased retrosternal air space) or restrictive lung disease
    - Enlarged right atrium
    - Enlarged right ventricle
- An echocardiogram (either transthoracic or transesophageal; Fig. 1-340) will do the following:
    - Assess tricuspid valve structure and motion, measure annular size, and identify other cardiac abnormalities
    - Estimate the severity of TR
    - Estimate the pulmonary artery pressure
    - Exclude vegetation, mass, or prolapse
    - Assess left and right ventricular function
- Right-sided cardiac heart catheterization shows the following:
    - Elevated right atrial and right ventricular systolic and end-diastolic pressures
    - Large V waves

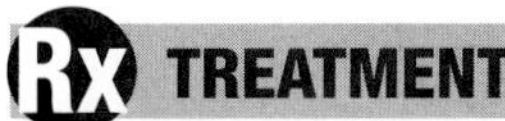

TREATMENT

The treatment of TR is usually directed at the underlying cause.

NONPHARMACOLOGIC THERAPY

Oxygen therapy is beneficial for patients with functional TR caused by underlying pulmonary hypertension provoked by alveolar hypoxia.

ACUTE GENERAL RX

- Functional TR caused by left-sided heart failure is treated in the standard way with preload reduction, afterload reduction, or inotropic therapy (see "Congestive Heart Failure").
- The reversal of pulmonary hypertension with vasodilators or pulmonary thromboendarterectomy has been shown to reverse functional TR.
- Structural TR treatment depends on the underlying cause of heart disease.

CHRONIC RX

- The 2006 American College of Cardiology/American Heart Association Guidelines Pertaining to the Surgical Management of Tricuspid Valve Disease/Regurgitation include the following:
  - Class I: Tricuspid valve repair is beneficial for severe TR in patients with mitral valve (MV) disease that requires MV surgery. B
  - Class IIa: Tricuspid valve replacement or annuloplasty is reasonable for a symptomatic patient with severe primary TR and for severe TR as a result of diseased or abnormal tricuspid valve leaflets that are not amenable to annuloplasty or repair. C
  - Class IIb: Tricuspid annuloplasty may be considered for less-than-severe TR in patients who are undergoing MV surgery when there is pulmonary hypertension or tricuspid annular dilatation (usually >21 mm/m^2 body surface area [BSA]). C
  - Class III: Tricuspid valve replacement or annuloplasty is not indicated for asymptomatic patients with TR whose pulmonary artery pressure is <60 mm Hg in the presence of a normal MV or for those with mild TR. C
- Patients with severe TR of any cause have poor long-term outcomes as a result of right ventricular dysfunction or systemic venous congestion.
- During recent years, annuloplasty has become an established surgical approach to significant TR. A recent study showed that tricuspid valve (TV) repair with an annuloplasty ring results in improved long-term outcomes.
- When the valve leaflets themselves are diseased, abnormal, or destroyed, valve replacement with a low-profile mechanical valve or bioprosthesis is often necessary.
- A biologic prosthesis is preferred because of the high rate of thromboembolic complications that occur with mechanical prostheses in the tricuspid position.

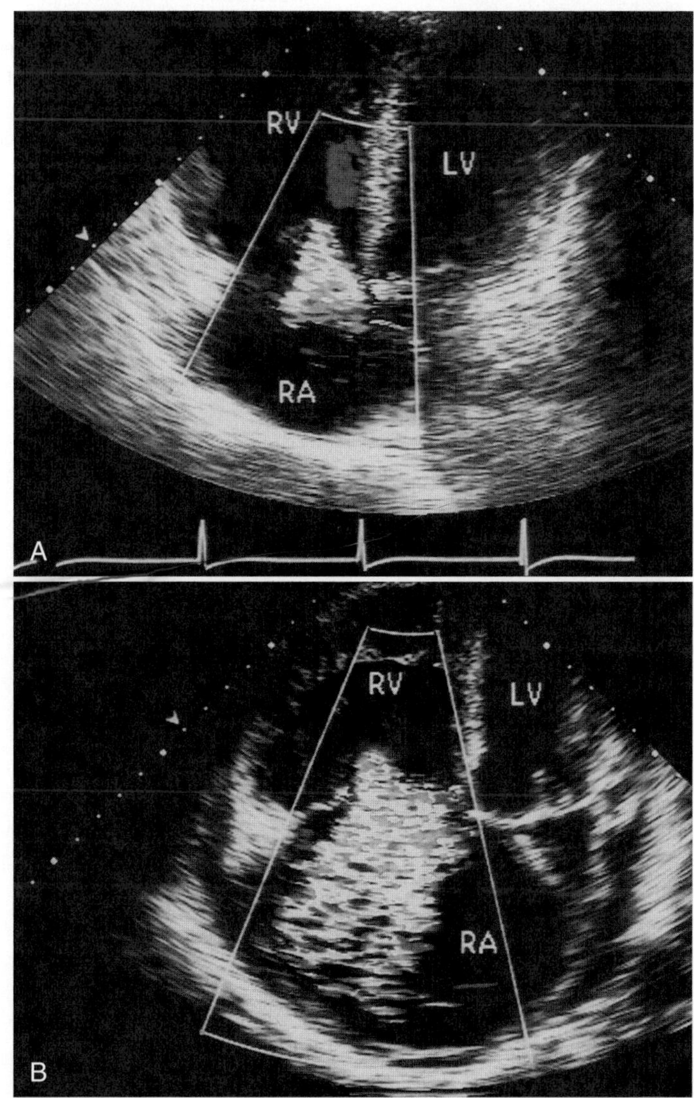

FIGURE 1-340 Two-dimensional echocardiograms with color-flow imaging of patients with tricuspid regurgitation. A, Echocardiogram of a patient with severe tricuspid insufficiency. **B,** Echocardiogram of a patient with severe tricuspid regurgitation. *LV,* Left ventricle; *RA,* right atrium; *RV,* right ventricle. (From Zipes DP et al [eds]: *Braunwald's heart disease,* ed 7, Philadelphia, 2005, Elsevier.)

DISPOSITION

- Regardless of the cause, a greater-than-mild degree of TR is associated with decreased survival.
- Clinically insignificant TR can be detected by color Doppler imaging in many normal people. This is not an indication for either routine follow-up or prophylaxis against bacterial endocarditis.
- Isolated TR should not pose a significant problem during pregnancy, although greater care may be necessary for protection from diuretic-induced hypoperfusion.
- Isolated TR with normal right ventricular function does not preclude an individual's involvement in competitive sports.

REFERRAL

For patients with significant symptomatic TR, a cardiology consultation is recommended.

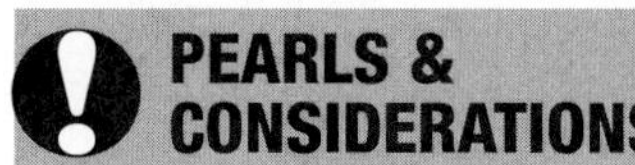

PEARLS & CONSIDERATIONS

- TR that results from tricuspid valve prolapse is often associated with concurrent MV prolapse.
- Secondary TR commonly occurs in combination with left-sided valvular heart disease. It often does not improve, despite correction of the left-sided valve dysfunction.
- Functional tricuspid insufficiency, if left uncorrected, carries serious long-term consequences.

COMMENTS

- Antibiotic prophylaxis for dental, gastrointestinal, or genitourinary procedures is no longer recommended for patients with only structural tricuspid valve abnormalities.

- Tricuspid annuloplasty at the time of MV surgery results in improved functional capacity without any increase in perioperative morbidity or mortality.
- During TR of the donor heart after cardiac transplantation, tricuspid valve replacement with a biologic prosthesis is a safe, durable, and effective method of treating TR after transplantation. This allows for future endomyocardial biopsies to be performed. Mechanical valves should be avoided.

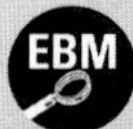

EVIDENCE

Please note: Complete text of EBM for this topic is available online.

Key trials and commentary:

Tricuspid regurgitation (TR) is common in patients undergoing mitral valve surgery, and atrial fibrillation (AF) can cause progression of TR. This study examined the hypothesis that correction of AF with the Maze procedure can prevent the late progression of TR after mitral valve surgery.

This study showed that continued AF after mitral valve surgery can predispose a patient to progression of TR, and this progression is prevented in patients having successful concomitant Maze procedure.

This group from the Mayo Clinic has provided some very interesting data regarding the effect of successful Maze procedures on outcome in patients with AF. They have previously provided data that in patients with heart failure, improvement can be expected following successful Maze procedure in selected patients. This article provides another bit of useful information, namely the fact that the restoration of sinus rhythm by the Maze procedure during mitral valve surgery was associated with significantly decreased progression of late tricuspid regurgitation in comparison with patients who continued to have AF postoperatively, and in their multivariable model, an effective Maze procedure was identified as the only significant predictive factor in halting this progression. The implication clearly is that AF was the most important factor contributing to the progression of tricuspid regurgitation in these patients.[1] Ⓐ

Evidence-Based Reference

1. Stulak JM et al: Restoration of sinus rhythm by the Maze procedure halts progression of tricuspid regurgitation after mitral surgery. *Ann Thorac Surg* 86:40-44, 2008. Commentary by A.L. Waldo, M.D. Ⓐ

SUGGESTED READINGS

Bonow RO et al: 2008 Focused update incorporated into ACC/AHA 2006. guidelines for the management of patients with valvular heart disease: a report of the American College of Cardiology/American Heart Association Task Force on Practice Guidelines (Writing Committee to Revise the 1998. Guidelines for the Management of Patients With Valvular Heart Disease), *Circulation* 118:e523-e661, 2008.

Raman SV et al: Tricuspid valve disease: tricuspid valve complex perspective, *Curr Probl Cardiol* 27:97-144, 2002.

Rogers JH et al: The tricuspid valve: current perspective and evolving management of tricuspid regurgitation, *Circulation* 119:2718-2725, 2009.

Singh SK et al: Midterm outcomes of tricuspid valve repair versus replacement for organic tricuspid disease, *Ann Thorac Surg* 82:1735-1741, 2006.

Song H: Percutaneous mitral valvuloplasty versus surgical treatment in mitral stenosis with severe tricuspid regurgitation, *Circulation* 116:1-246-1-250, 2007.

Trichon BH, O'Connor CM: Secondary mitral and tricuspid regurgitation accompanying left ventricular systolic function: is it important, and how is it treated? *Am Heart J* 144(3):373-376, 2002.

AUTHORS: **FREDERICK D. TRONCALES, M.D.,** and **GAURAV CHOUDHARY, M.D.**

BASIC INFORMATION

DEFINITION

Tricuspid stenosis (TS) is an uncommon valvular pathology that is caused by the narrowing of the tricuspid valve orifice, which results in the restriction of right atrial emptying. TS is most often rheumatic in origin, and it often presents with a combination of regurgitation and stenosis.

SYNONYMS

Tricuspid valve stenosis
TS

ICD-9CM CODES

397.0 Disease of the tricuspid valve

EPIDEMIOLOGY & DEMOGRAPHICS

- TS is most commonly caused by rheumatic heart disease, and it almost always occurs with associated mitral or aortic valve disease.
- Antibiotic therapy has made rheumatic heart disease and TS in the U.S. very rare.
- TS is present at autopsy in 15% of patients with rheumatic heart disease, but it is clinically significant in only 5%.

PHYSICAL FINDINGS & CLINICAL PRESENTATION

- Obstruction to tricuspid flow limits cardiac output.
- Symptoms and physical examination findings usually depend on the presence and severity of concomitant mitral or aortic valve disease.
- Symptoms of right heart failure include fatigue, right upper quadrant abdominal pain (from hepatic congestion), ascites, hepatomegaly, and peripheral edema.
- Jugular venous distention, a prominent a wave, and a palpable hepatic pulsation are noted during the sinus rhythm.
- A right atrial pulsation may be palpated to the right of the sternum, and a diastolic thrill that increases with inspiration may be felt over the left sternal edge.
- An opening snap and a low-frequency diastolic murmur are best heard along the left sternal border of the fourth intercostal space. These are augmented by inspiration (i.e., Carvallo's sign), leg raises, isotonic exercise, and squatting.

ETIOLOGY

- Rheumatic heart disease results in the scarring of the valve leaflets, the shortening of the chordae tendineae, and the fusion of the commissures, thereby leading to the immobility of the valve leaflets and the narrowing of the tricuspid valve orifice.
- Other causes are congenital, infectious (e.g., endocarditis), metabolic, and enzymatic abnormalities (e.g., carcinoid syndrome, Whipple's disease, Fabry's disease); right atrial or metastastic tumors; and, rarely, scarring and adhesions as a result of complications of pacemaker placement.

Dx DIAGNOSIS

DIFFERENTIAL DIAGNOSIS

- Congenital tricuspid atresia
- Right heart diastolic dysfunction: endomyocardial fibrosis or constrictive pericarditis
- Extrinsic compression of the right ventricle: severe pectum excavatum, massive ascites, pleural effusion, pericardial effusion, or tumor
- Obstruction of right atrial emptying: right atrial myxoma, metastatic tumor, right atrial thrombi, or tricuspid valve vegetation (particularly in association with a permanent pacemaker lead)

WORKUP

- ECG is the diagnostic test of choice to look for atrial arrhythmias, atrial fibrillation, or atrial flutter as a result of an enlarged right atrium.
- Chest x-ray
- Right heart catheterization is an option when ECG cannot be used to make a definitive diagnosis.

IMAGING STUDIES

- ECG reveals the thickening and shortening of the tricuspid valve leaflets, the restriction of the movement of the leaflets and the leaflet tips, a reduction in the diameter of the anulus, and diastolic doming of the valve. Evidence of right atrial enlargement is present in most cases.
- Doppler echocardiography or cardiac catheterization demonstrates a reduced tricuspid valve area (severe when <1 cm^2) and a diastolic pressure gradient across the tricuspid valve (normal gradient, <1 mm Hg).
- Chest radiography may reveal an enlarged right atrium and a reduced pulmonary blood volume.

Rx TREATMENT

NONPHARMACOLOGIC THERAPY

Salt and fluid restriction are essential to decrease peripheral edema.

ACUTE GENERAL RX

- Assess and treat the underlying cause of the valvular pathology.
- Treat bacterial endocarditis with antibiotics.
- Manage right atrium volume overload with diuretics.
- Prescribe rate-controlling atrioventricular nodal blockers and anticoagulants, especially for patients with atrial arrhythmia.

CHRONIC RX

- Symptoms of systemic venous hypertension and congestion can be controlled with diuretics and angiotensin-converting inhibitors or angiotensin receptor antagonists.
- Balloon valvuloplasty or dilation of the stenosed tricuspid valve has been shows to be effective. Tricuspid regurgitation that is more than mild is generally considered a contraindication to valvotomy. Tumor masses, vegetations, and thrombi are also contraindications to valvotomy.
- Surgery for TS is usually recommended when the valve is not treatable by balloon valvuloplasty and the valve area is <2 cm^2 with a mean diastolic gradient across the tricuspid valve of >5 mm Hg.
- Isolated tricuspid valve replacement surgery almost never occurs. It is typically performed in the setting of concomitant mitral or aortic valve surgery.
- Surgical procedures for TS include commissurotomy and tricuspid valve replacement.

DISPOSITION

The natural course of severe TS is not well known.

REFERRAL

TS may be difficult to diagnose, so consultation with a cardiologist is recommended.

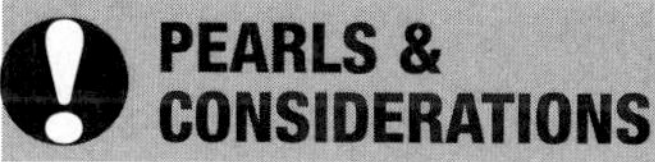

PEARLS & CONSIDERATIONS

- Rheumatic heart disease accounts for $>90\%$ of stenotic tricuspid valves.
- Rheumatic TS almost always occurs in association with mitral valve disease and sometimes with aortic valve disease.
- The majority of cases present with tricuspid regurgitation or a combination of regurgitation and stenosis.

COMMENTS

Tricuspid valve replacement carries a 30-day operative morbidity and mortality rate of 5% to 7% in addition to a high risk of right heart thrombus formation. Therefore, surgical procedures are reserved for patients who are not candidates for balloon dilation techniques. Unlike patients with mitral stenosis, patients with TS typically do not report dyspnea, orthopnea, or paroxysmal nocturnal dyspnea.

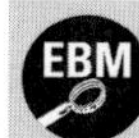

EVIDENCE

No studies have compared balloon valvuloplasty with surgical valvotomy, and only case series on long-term follow-up of these treatments have been published.[1] Limited data support balloon valvuloplasty for severe TS that is not controlled with angiotensin-converting enzyme inhibitors and diuretics.[2]

Evidence-Based References

1. Roguin A et al: Long-term follow-up of patients with severe rheumatic tricuspid stenosis, *Am Heart J* 136:103, 1998.

2. Sancaktar O et al: Late results of combined percutaneous balloon valvuloplasty of mitral and tricuspid valves, *Cathet Cardiovasc Diagn* 45:246, 1998.

SUGGESTED READINGS

AHA/ACC Guidelines for the management of patients with valvular heart disease, *J Am Coll Cardiol* 48:e1-148, 2006.

Block PC, Bonhoeffer P: Percutaneous approaches to valvular heart disease, *Curr Cardiol Rep* 7(2):108-113, 2005.

Mehra MR et al: Difficult cases in heart failure: isolated tricuspid stenosis and heart failure: a focus on carcinoid heart disease, *Congest Heart Fail* 9(5):294, 2003.

Raman SV et al: Tricuspid valve disease: tricuspid valve complex perspective, *Curr Probl Cardiol* 27(3):103, 2002.

Zaibag AM et al Percutaneous balloon valvuloplasty in tricuspid stenosis. *Br Heart J* 57:51-53, 1987.

AUTHORS: **FREDERICK D. TRONCALES, M.D.,** and **GAURAV CHOUDHARY, M.D.**

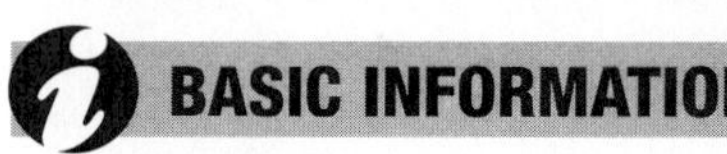

DEFINITION

Tricyclic antidepressants (TCAs) are secondary or tertiary amines that have variable abilities to inhibit reuptake of neurotransmitters (norepinephrine, dopamine, and serotonin) and to be anticholinergic, antihistaminic, and sedating. These properties are important to consider when prescribing these agents and when managing an intentional or accidental overdose.

SYNONYMS

Tricyclic antidepressant intoxication or poisoning
TCA OD

ICD-9CM CODES
969.0

EPIDEMIOLOGY & DEMOGRAPHICS

- TCAs are the most common cause of death from prescription drug overdose in the U.S.
- Available TCAs: amitriptyline, imipramine, desipramine, nortriptyline, doxepin, amoxapine, clomipramine, protriptyline, and others.

PHYSICAL FINDINGS & CLINICAL PRESENTATION

Cardiovascular:

- Intraventricular conduction delay (QRS prolongation)
- Sinus tachycardia
- Atrioventricular block
- Prolongation of the QT interval
- Ventricular tachycardia
- Wide complex tachycardia without P waves
- Refractory hypotension (the most common cause of death from TCA overdose)
- Late arrhythmias or sudden death (in addition to the arrhythmias, which occur during the first 24 to 48 hr; late problems can occur up to 5 days after the overdose)

Central nervous system:

- Coma
- Delirium
- Myoclonus
- Seizures

Other:

- Hyperthermia
- Ileus
- Urinary retention
- Pulmonary complications (e.g., aspiration pneumonitis)
- Life-threatening overdose exists with the ingestion of more than 1 g of a TCA. Among patients who reach a hospital, most deaths occur within the first 24 hr; lack of initial symptoms can be deceptive.

ETIOLOGY & PATHOGENESIS

- Mechanisms of tricyclic antidepressant cardiovascular toxicity (Table 1-75)
- CNS toxicity:
  1. Cholinergic blockade is believed to cause hyperthermia, ileus, urinary retention, pupillary dilation, delirium, and coma.
  2. The mechanism of myoclonus and seizures is not fully understood.

Dx DIAGNOSIS

DIFFERENTIAL DIAGNOSIS

Cardiotoxicity from TCA can be confused with intoxication by drugs that cause QRS prolongation. These include class Ia antiarrhythmic agents (disopyramide, procainamide, quinidine), class Ic antiarrhythmic agents (encainide, flecainide, propafenone), cocaine, propranolol, quinine, chloroquine, neuroleptics, propoxyphene, and digoxin. Other causes of QRS prolongation include hyperkalemia, ischemic heart disease, cardiomyopathy, and cardiac conduction system dysfunction.

WORKUP

- Clinical presentation
- Knowledge of the overdose
- Serum drug levels (TCA concentration >1 mcg/ml is life threatening; TCA concentration >3 mcg/ml is often fatal)
- Baseline complete blood count, prothrombin time, blood urea nitrogen, creatinine, and electrolytes

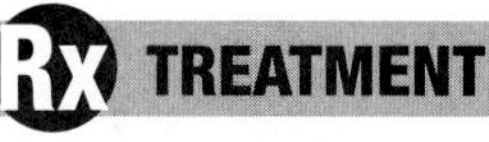

ACUTE GENERAL Rx

1. Initial measures:
   - Hospitalization with cardiac monitoring as well as monitoring of vital signs and temperature
   - Initiate IV access
   - Administer activated charcoal with sorbitol

TABLE 1-75 Mechanism of Tricyclic Antidepressant Cardiovascular Toxicity

Toxic Effect	Mechanism
Conduction Delays, Arrhythmias	
QRS prolongation atrioventricular block	Cardiac sodium channel → slowed depolarization in atrioventricular node, His-Purkinje fibers, and ventricular myocardium
Sinus tachycardia	Cholinergic blockade, inhibition of norepinephrine reuptake
Ventricular tachycardia	
Monomorphic	Cardiac sodium channel inhibition → reentry
Torsades de pointes	Cardiac potassium channel inhibition → prolonged repolarization
Ventricular bradycardia	Impaired cardiac automaticity
Hypotension	
Vasodilation	Vascular alpha-adrenergic receptor blockade
Decreased cardiac contractility	Cardiac sodium channel inhibition → impaired excitation-contraction coupling

- Large-bore tube gastric lavage is of unproven benefit
- Ipecac is contraindicated
- 12-Lead ECG
- If no evidence of cardiotoxicity has been noted during the first 6 hr of observation, further monitoring is not necessary; if there is evidence of cardiotoxicity, monitoring should continue for 24 hr after all signs of toxicity have resolved

2. See Table 1-76 for treatment of specific complications of TCA toxicity.
3. When the patient is medically stable, psychiatric evaluation should be obtained.

SUGGESTED READING

Glauser J: Tricyclic antidepressant poisoning, *Cleve Clin J Med* 67:704, 2000.

AUTHOR: **FRED F. FERRI, M.D.**

TABLE 1-76 Treatment of Complications of Tricyclic Antidepressant Toxicity

Toxic Effect	Treatment
Cardiovascular	
QRS prolongation	Hypertonic $NaHCO_3$ if QRS prolongation is marked or progressing; not clear if treatment is needed in the absence of hypotension or arrhythmias
Hypotension	Intravascular volume expansion, $NaHCO_3$ Vasopressors (norepinephrine) or inotropic agents (dopamine) Correct hyperthermia, acidosis, seizures Consider mechanical support
Ventricular tachycardia	$NaHCO_3$, lidocaine, overdrive, pacing Correct hypotension, hypothermia, acidosis, seizures
Torsades de pointes	Overdrive, pacing
Ventricular bradycardia	Chronotropic agent (epinephrine), pacemaker
Sinus tachycardia	Treatment rarely needed
Atrioventricular block type II second or third degree	Pacemaker
Hypertension	Rapidly titratable antihypertensive agent (nitroprusside)
Central Nervous System	
Delirium	Restraints, benzodiazepine Neuromuscular blockade for hyperthermia, acidosis
Seizures	Benzodiazepine Neuromuscular blockade for hyperthermia, acidosis
Coma	Intubation, ventilation if needed
Other	
Hyperthermia	Control seizures, agitation Cooling measures
Acidosis	$NaHCO_3$ Correct hypotension, hypoventilation

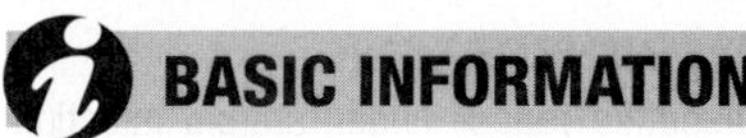

BASIC INFORMATION

DEFINITION

Trigeminal neuralgia is a syndrome characterized by recurrent excruciating paroxysms of lancinating pain in the distribution of one or more divisions of the trigeminal (fifth) nerve.

SYNONYMS

Tic douloureux

ICD-9CM CODES
350.1 Trigeminal neuralgia

EPIDEMIOLOGY & DEMOGRAPHICS

INCIDENCE (IN U.S.): Three to five cases per 100,000 persons
PREVALENCE (IN U.S.): 155 in 1 million persons
PREDOMINANT SEX: Slight predominance of females to males
PEAK INCIDENCE: Median age: 67 yr
GENETICS: Uncommonly familial and possibly caused by underlying genetic etiology (see "Rare causes" under "Etiology")

PHYSICAL FINDINGS & CLINICAL PRESENTATION

- Each attack lasts only seconds but may cluster.
- Attacks often are brought on by mild stimulation of trigger zones located in the affected division of the fifth nerve. These triggers include light touching, eating, drinking, shaving, and drafts.

ETIOLOGY

- Most cases are idiopathic.
- It is believed that many cases are caused by compression of the trigeminal nerve root at the cerebellopontine angle by an aberrant loop of artery or vein, and rarely a saccular aneurysm or arteriovenous malformation.
- Compressive lesions such as schwannomas, epidermoid cysts, and meningiomas also are typically at the cerebellopontine angle.
- Bony compression of the fifth nerve (e.g., from an osteoma or deformity resulting from osteogenesis imperfecta).
- Primary demyelinating disorders: 2% to 4% of patients. In multiple sclerosis, there usually is a plaque of demyelination at the root entry zone of the fifth nerve in the pons.
- Rare causes: (1) infiltrative disorders such as carcinomatous or amyloid deposits in the fifth nerve root, nerve proper, or ganglion; (2) familial occurrence has been reported in Charcot-Marie-Tooth disease.

Dx DIAGNOSIS

DIFFERENTIAL DIAGNOSIS

- Dental pathology.
- The differential diagnosis of headache and facial pain is described in Section II.

WORKUP

MRI scans (CT scan with thin posterior fossa cuts if MRI not available) for all patients to exclude mass lesions or evidence of central demyelination as in multiple sclerosis

Rx TREATMENT

NONPHARMACOLOGIC THERAPY

- In refractory cases, surgical options, including percutaneous radiofrequency gangliolysis and microvascular decompression. Motor cortex stimulation has provided hopeful results; however, this is a new approach, and evidence is largely based on case reports at this stage.
- Gamma-knife radiosurgery is an increasingly popular alternative to conventional surgery for trigeminal neuralgia.

ACUTE GENERAL Rx

None; episodes are too brief

CHRONIC Rx

- Carbamazepine is the treatment of choice, providing relief to at least 75% of patients. Begin with 100 mg bid and increase gradually as tolerated with a tid regimen.
- If carbamazepine is not tolerated or effective, use gabapentin, 400 mg PO tid. Doses as high as 3600 mg/day are easily tolerated. Topiramate 25 mg qhs gradually titrated up to 100 mg bid is also sometimes effective. Other drugs in use include oxcarbazepine and baclofen.

DISPOSITION

Spontaneous remissions may occur after months to years.

REFERRAL

If uncertain about diagnosis or if surgical treatment is necessary

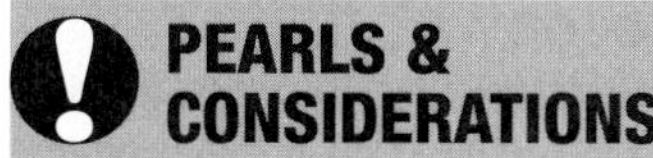

PEARLS & CONSIDERATIONS

Even in patients with multiple sclerosis, vascular compression may be the source of symptoms and thus may benefit from intervention such as surgery.

COMMENTS

Because prolonged remission may occur, drug tapering at yearly intervals is recommended.

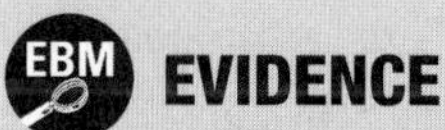

EVIDENCE

There is evidence for increased pain relief with carbamazepine in trigeminal neuralgia.

Carbamazepine has been found to provide better pain relief than placebo by a systematic review that included three relevant randomized controlled trials (RCTs).[1] Ⓐ

Evidence-Based Reference

1. Wiffen PJ et al: Carbamazepine for acute and chronic pain, *Cochrane Database Rev* 3, 2005. Ⓐ

SUGGESTED READINGS

Chesire WP: Trigeminal neuralgia: diagnosis and treatment, *Curr Neurol and Neurosci Rep* 5:79, 2005.
Elias WJ and Burchiel KJ: Trigeminal neuralgia and other neuropathic pain syndromes of the head and face, *Curr Pain Headache Rep* 6(2):115, 2002.
Krafft R: Trigeminal neuralgia, *Am Fam Physician* 77(9): 1291, 2008
Zakrzewska JM, Lopez BC: Trigeminal neuralgia, *Clin Evid* 14(1-2), 2005.

AUTHOR: **U. SHIVRAJ SOHUR, M.D., PH.D.**

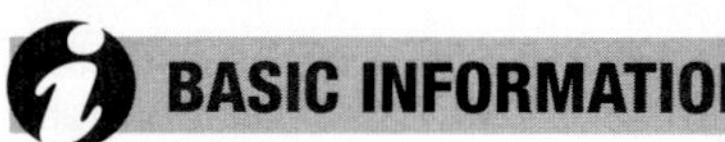

BASIC INFORMATION

DEFINITION

Trigger finger, or digital stenosing tenosynovitis, refers to an inflammatory process of the digital flexor tendon sheath.

SYNONYMS Digital stenosing tenosynovitis

ICD-9CM CODES
727.03 Trigger finger (acquired)

EPIDEMIOLOGY & DEMOGRAPHICS

- Trigger finger can be found in all age groups but is commonly found in patients >45 yr
- More frequently affects females (4:1)
- Repetitive use occupational risk groups: meat cutters, seamstress, tailors, and dentists
- In adults, the middle finger is most often affected (Fig. 1-341)
- In children, the thumb is most often affected

PHYSICAL FINDINGS & CLINICAL PRESENTATION

- Tenosynovitis of the flexor tendon always precedes the mechanical symptoms of triggering
- Painful triggering or snapping with flexion of the affected digit
- Locking or loss of active digital extension is the most common symptom
- The digit is usually fixed in flexion (trapped or incarcerated)
- Usually affects one digit
- If more digits are involved, a systemic cause is most likely present (e.g., diabetes, rheumatoid arthritis)
- A palpable tender nodule is noted at the metacarpophalangeal (MCP) joint of the affected digit
- Pain over the flexor tendon with resisting flexion isometrically
- Pain with passive stretching

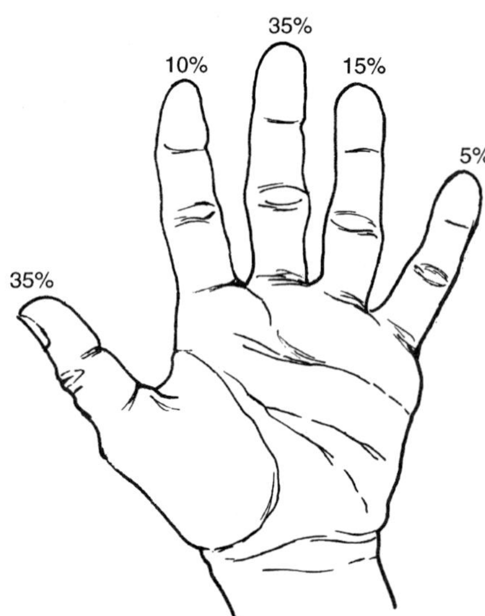

FIGURE 1-341 Trigger finger. Frequency of trigger finger according to digit in adults. In children, virtually all cases occur in the thumb. (From Canoso J: *Rheumatology in primary care,* Philadelphia, 1997, WB Saunders.)

ETIOLOGY

Trigger finger is described as being primary or secondary:

- Primary (idiopathic)
- Secondary
  1. Diabetes
  2. Rheumatoid arthritis
  3. Hypothyroidism
  4. Histiocytosis
  5. Amyloidosis
  6. Gout

Dx DIAGNOSIS

Clinical history and physical examination

DIFFERENTIAL DIAGNOSIS

- Dupuytren's contracture
- De Quervain's tenosynovitis
- Acute digital tenosynovitis
- Proliferative tenosynovitis
- Ulnar collateral ligament injury (gamekeeper's thumb)
- Carpal tunnel syndrome
- Flexion tendon rupture
- Posttraumatic MCP osteoarthritis

WORKUP

Pursued if a secondary cause is suspected.

LABORATORY TESTS

- Complete blood count with differential
- Electrolytes, blood urea nitrogen, creatinine
- Blood glucose
- Thyroid function tests
- Uric acid
- Rheumatoid factor

IMAGING STUDIES

Radiograph studies are not helpful unless a secondary cause has affected other organs (e.g., rheumatoid lung).

Rx TREATMENT

The goals of treatment are to reduce swelling and inflammation in the flexor tendon sheath and allow smooth movement of the tendon under the A-1 pulley of the MCP joint.

NONPHARMACOLOGIC THERAPY

Splinting or buddy taping to the adjacent finger for 4 to 6 wk

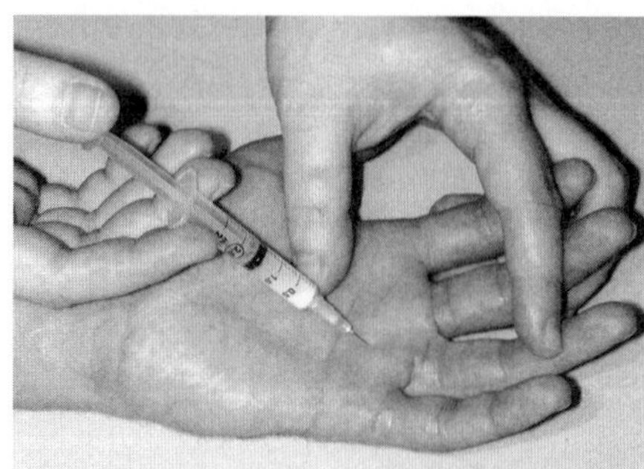

FIGURE 1-342 Injection into the palm for trigger finger. (From Carr A, Hamilton W: *Orthopedics in primary care,* ed 2, Philadelphia, 2005, Elsevier.)

ACUTE GENERAL Rx

- In idiopathic trigger finger, steroid injection with 15 to 20 mg depot methylprenisolone acetate in 1 ml 1% Xylocaine (Fig. 1-342) has been used with success if conservative immobilization has failed.
- Triamcinolone 10 mg with 1 ml 1% Xylocaine is an alternative steroid for patients who do not respond to the first injection.
- If symptoms do not resolve in 6 wk, a repeat injection can be tried.

CHRONIC Rx

- Surgical release is indicated in patients with refractory symptoms (e.g., locked digits) despite nonpharmacologic and acute treatment.
- Surgery is also indicated in patients with recurrent symptoms despite two steroid injections.

DISPOSITION

- After steroid injection, symptoms usually resolve in 3 to 5 days, and locking resolves in 60% of the cases in 2 to 3 wk.
- If symptoms recur, a repeat steroid injection improves the symptoms in ≥80% of patients.
- Diabetic patients do not have the same success rate with steroid injections as the idiopathic group.

REFERRAL

If steroid injection therapy is considered, a rheumatology consult is requested.

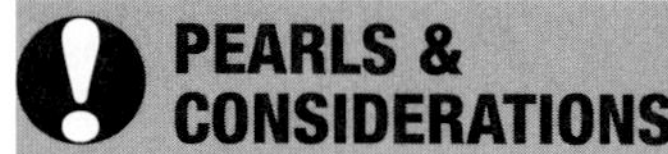

PEARLS & CONSIDERATIONS

COMMENTS

If more than one digit is involved, a workup for a secondary systemic cause is in order.

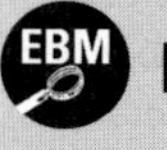

EVIDENCE

There are few randomized controlled trials of the treatment of trigger finger.

In a randomized controlled trial, 24 patients received a steroid and lidocaine or a placebo injection for treatment of primary trigger finger. One injection cured 9 of 14 patients in the intervention group compared with 2 of 10 controls.[1] B

Evidence-Based Reference

1. Murphy D et al: Steroid versus placebo injection for trigger finger, *J Hand Surg Am* 20:628-631, 1995. B

SUGGESTED READINGS

Akhtar S et al: Management and referral for trigger finger/thumb, *BMJ* 331(7507):30, 2005.

Ryzewicz M, Wolf J: Trigger digits: principles, management and complications, *J Hand Surg* 31(1):135, 2006.

Saldana MJ: Trigger digits: diagnosis and treatment, *J Am Acad Orthop Surg* 9(4):246, 2001.

AUTHORS: **RYAN W. ZUZEK, M.D.,** and **PAUL GORDON, M.D.**

BASIC INFORMATION

DEFINITION

Trochanteric bursitis is a presumed inflammation or irritation of the gluteus maximus bursa or the bursa separating the greater trochanter from the gluteus medius and gluteus minimus (Fig. 1-343).

SYNONYMS

Greater trochanteric pain syndrome

ICD-9CM CODES
726.5 Bursitis trochanteric area

EPIDEMIOLOGY & DEMOGRAPHICS

- Trochanteric bursitis is commonly associated with other conditions:
  1. Osteoarthritis of the hip
  2. Lumbar spinal degenerative joint disease
  3. Rheumatoid arthritis
- Incidence peaks between the fourth and sixth decades of life but can occur at any age group
- Occurs in females more often than males (ratio of 4:1)

PHYSICAL FINDINGS & CLINICAL PRESENTATION

- Hip pain is the most common symptom. The pain is chronic, intermittent, and located over the lateral thigh.
- Numbness can be present.
- Pain is precipitated with prolonged lying or standing on the affected side.
- Walking, climbing, and running exacerbate the pain.
- Point tenderness over the greater trochanter is noted.
- Pain is reproduced with resisted hip abduction.

ETIOLOGY

- The specific cause of trochanteric bursitis is not known, although repetitive high-intensity use of the hip joint, trauma, infection (tuberculosis and bacterial), and crystal deposition can precipitate the disease.
- Trochanteric bursitis can occur when other conditions such as osteoarthritis of the knee and hip and bunions of the feet cause changes in the patient's gait, placing varus stress on the hip joint.

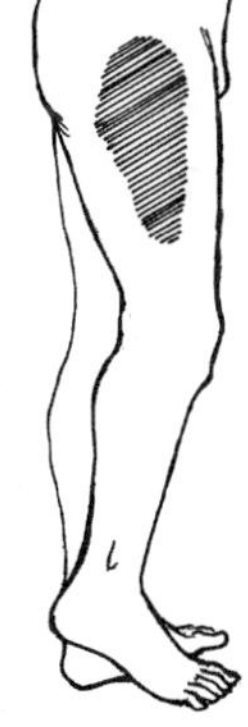

FIGURE 1-343 Typical location of pain in trochanteric bursitis syndrome. This is also a frequent pain radiation site for lumbar spine lesion, various nerve compression syndromes, and hip disease, particularly in osteonecrosis of the femoral head. (From Canoso JJ: *Rheumatology in primary care,* Philadelphia, 1997, WB Saunders.)

Dx DIAGNOSIS

A detailed physical examination and clinical presentation usually make the diagnosis of trochanteric bursitis. Laboratory tests and x-ray images are helpful adjunctive studies used to exclude other conditions either associated with or mimicking trochanteric bursitis.

DIFFERENTIAL DIAGNOSIS

- Osteoarthritis of the hip
- Osteonecrosis of the hip
- Stress fracture of the hip
- Osteoarthritis of the lumbar spine
- Fibromyalgia
- Iliopsoas bursitis
- Trochanteric tendonitis
- Gout
- Pseudogout
- Trauma
- Neuropathy
- Tuberculosis of the greater trochanter
- Metastatic bone disease

WORKUP

A workup is indicated if suspected associated conditions exist; otherwise treatment can be started on clinical grounds alone.

LABORATORY TESTS

- Complete blood count with differential may show elevated white blood cell count if infection is present.
- Erythrocyte sedimentation rate is elevated in an inflammatory process.

IMAGING STUDIES

- Plain radiographs of the hip generally are not helpful in diagnosing trochanteric bursitis. Sometimes calcifications may be seen around the greater trochanter.
- Bone scan can be done but is usually not necessary.
- CT and MRI may show bursitis but are usually not warranted because they will not alter treatment.

Rx TREATMENT

NONPHARMACOLOGIC THERAPY

- Heat 15 to 20 min 4 to 6 times per day
- Ultrasound therapy
- Rest
- Partial weight bearing
- Physical therapy to strengthen back, hip, and knee muscles

ACUTE GENERAL Rx

- Nonsteroidal anti-inflammatory drugs (NSAIDs) for pain relief: ibuprofen 800 mg PO tid or naproxen 500 mg PO bid
- Acetaminophen 500-mg tablet, 1 to 2 tablets PO q6h prn, can be used with NSAIDs or alternating with NSAIDs.
- Corticosteroid injection (30 to 40 mg depot methylprednisolone acetate mixed with 3 ml 1% Xylocaine).

CHRONIC Rx

Although rarely done, surgical removal of the bursa is possible for patients with refractory symptoms or infection.

DISPOSITION

- Most patients respond to NSAIDs and/or nonpharmacologic therapy.
- If steroid injection is used, approximately 70% of patients respond after the first injection and more than 90% respond to two injections.
- 25% of patients receiving steroid injection may develop a relapse.

REFERRAL

A rheumatology or orthopedics referral is made if steroid injection therapy is needed or if the etiology is believed to be infectious.

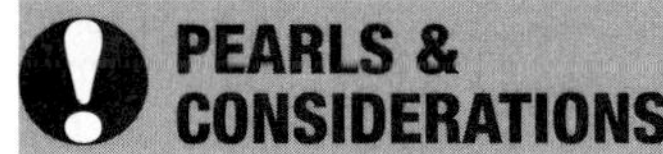

PEARLS & CONSIDERATIONS

Patients with trochanteric bursitis will commonly report "hip" pain. The physical examination readily distinguishes true hip pain from trochanteric bursitis.

COMMENTS

- The absence of pain with flexion and extension differentiates trochanteric bursitis from degenerative joint disease of the hip.
- Localization of pain over the lateral thigh differentiates trochanteric bursitis from pain caused by meralgia paresthetica located over the anterolateral thigh and pain from osteoarthritis located over the inner thigh groin area.

SUGGESTED READINGS

Adkins SB, Figler RA: Hip pain in athletes, *Am Fam Physician* 61(7):2109, 2000.

Canoso JJ: Hip pain. In Canoso JJ, Kersey R (eds): *Rheumatology in primary care,* Philadelphia, 1997, WB Saunders.

Cardone DA, Tallia AF: Diagnostic and therapeutic injection of the hip and knee, *Am Fam Physician* 67: 2147, 2003.

Martin RL, Sekika JK: The interrater reliability of 4 clinical tests used to assess individuals with musculoskeletal hip pain, *J Orthop Sports Phys Ther* 38(2):71, 2008.

Segal NA et al: Multicenter Osteoarthritis Study Group: Greater trochanteric pain syndrome: epidemiology and associated factors, *Arch Phys Med Rehabil* 88(8):988, 2007.

AUTHOR: **MEL L. ANDERSON, M.D.**

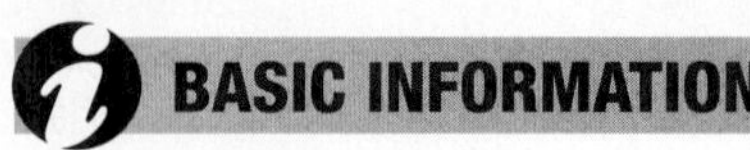

BASIC INFORMATION

DEFINITION

Tropical sprue is a malabsorption syndrome occurring primarily in tropical regions, including Puerto Rico, India, and Southeast Asia.

SYNONYMS

Postinfectious tropical malabsorption
"Tropical enteropathy," referring to a subclinical form of tropical sprue

ICD-9CM CODES

579.1 Tropical sprue

EPIDEMIOLOGY & DEMOGRAPHICS

- Tropical sprue is endemic in tropical regions of Venezuela, Colombia, the Middle East, the Far East, the Caribbean (Puerto Rico, Haiti, Dominican Republic, Cuba), and India.
- The disease affects mainly adults, although it has been reported in all age groups.

PHYSICAL FINDINGS & CLINICAL PRESENTATION

- The classic clinical features of tropical sprue are nonspecific and simply reflect the symptom of malabsorption. Onset is generally not insidious, and most patients can pinpoint when their disorder began.
- Diffuse, nonspecific abdominal tenderness and distention. Abdominal pain is crampy in nature.
- Low-grade fever.
- Glossitis, cheilosis, hyperkeratosis, hyperpigmentation.
- Diarrhea, often with mucus and foul-smelling stools from fat malabsorption.
- Nausea, which leads to decreased appetite and decreased oral intake.
- Lactose intolerance often develops early in the course of tropical sprue.

ETIOLOGY

- Unknown. There is a strong presumption that it is caused by an enteric infection, perhaps in individuals predisposed by some nutritional deficiency.
- Associated with overgrowth of predominantly coliform bacteria in the small intestine.

DIAGNOSIS

The clinical features of tropical sprue include anorexia, diarrhea, weight loss, abdominal pain, and steatorrhea; these symptoms can develop in expatriates even several months after returning to temperate regions.

DIFFERENTIAL DIAGNOSIS

- Celiac disease
- Parasitic infestation
- Inflammatory bowel disease
- Other causes of malabsorption (e.g., Whipple's disease)
- Lymphoma
- Pancreatic tumor
- Intestinal tuberculosis
- Microsporidia-associated HIV enteropathy

WORKUP

Diagnostic workup includes a comprehensive history (especially travel history), physical examination, laboratory evidence of malabsorption (see below), and jejunal biopsy; the biopsy results are nonspecific, with blunting, atrophy, and even disappearance of the villi and subepithelial lymphocytic infiltration. Partial villus atrophy distinguishes tropical sprue histologically from celiac sprue, which reveals flattened mucosa.

LABORATORY TESTS

- Megaloblastic anemia (>50% of cases)
- Vitamin B_{12} deficiency, folate deficiency
- Abnormal D-xylose absorption (72-hr fecal fat determination or serum carotene concentration)
- Stool examination to exclude *Giardia* spp.

IMAGING STUDIES

Gastrointestinal series with small-bowel follow-through may reveal coarsening of the jejunal folds.

TREATMENT

NONPHARMACOLOGIC THERAPY

Monitoring of weight and calorie intake

ACUTE GENERAL Rx

- Folic acid therapy (5 mg bid for 2 wk followed by a maintenance dose of 1 mg tid) will improve anemia and malabsorption in more than two thirds of patients.
- Tetracycline 250 mg qid for 4 to 6 wk in individuals who have returned to temperate zones, up to 6 mo in patients in endemic areas; ampicillin 500 mg bid for at least 4 wk in patients intolerant to tetracycline.
- Correction of vitamin B_{12} deficiency: vitamin B_{12} 1000 mcg IM weekly for 4 wk, then monthly for 3 to 6 mo.
- Correction of other nutritional deficiencies (e.g., calcium, iron).

DISPOSITION

Complete recovery with appropriate therapy

REFERRAL

Gastrointestinal referral for jejunal biopsy

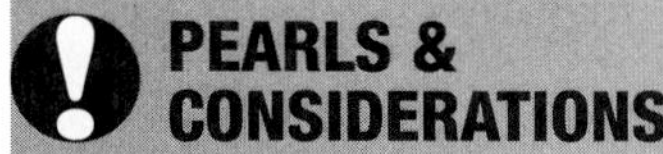

PEARLS & CONSIDERATIONS

COMMENTS

- Tropical sprue should be considered in any patient who presents with chronic diarrhea, weight loss, and malabsorption, especially if there is significant travel and exposure history.
- Important factors in the medical history in addition to travel history are use of medications that may predispose to a small-bowel overgrowth, HIV exposure (increased risk of chronic diarrhea), and any surgical procedure that may predispose to blind loop syndrome.
- Most of the functional changes in tropical sprue may be related to small-bowel mucosal damage; however, there is also dysfunctional hormonal regulation of the gut (increased enteroglucagon, motilin levels, decreased postprandial insulin and gastric inhibitory peptide) and decreased ability of the colon to absorb water.
- Even with prolonged therapy relapses can occur; however, some may be attributable to reexposure to an infecting organism rather than relapsing disease.

AUTHOR: **FRED F. FERRI, M.D.**

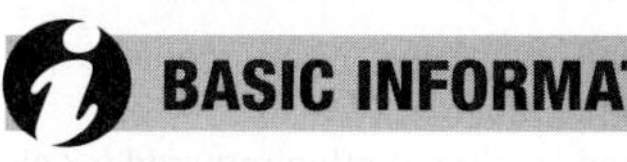

DEFINITION

Miliary tuberculosis (TB) is an infection of disseminated hematogenous disease, caused by the bacterium *Mycobacterium tuberculosis* (Mtb), and is often characterized as resembling millet seeds on examination. Extrapulmonary disease may occur in virtually every organ site.

SYNONYMS

Disseminated TB

ICD-9CM CODES
018.94 Miliary tuberculosis

EPIDEMIOLOGY & DEMOGRAPHICS

INCIDENCE (IN U.S.): >38% of AIDS patients with TB have disseminated disease, often with concurrent pulmonary and extrapulmonary active sites. (See "Pulmonary Tuberculosis" in Section I.)

PREVALENCE (IN U.S.):

- Undetermined
- Highest prevalence
  1. AIDS patients
  2. Minorities
  3. Children
  4. Foreign-born persons
  5. Elderly

PREDOMINANT SEX:

- No specific predilection
- Male predominance in AIDS, shelters, and prisons reflected in disproportionate male TB incidence

PREDOMINANT AGE: Predominantly among 24- to 45-yr-olds

PEAK INCIDENCE: HIV-positive patients, regardless of age

PHYSICAL FINDINGS & CLINICAL PRESENTATION

- See also "Etiology"
- Common symptoms
  1. High intermittent fever
  2. Night sweats
  3. Weight loss
- Symptoms referable to individual organ systems may predominate
  1. Meninges
  2. Pericardium
  3. Liver
  4. Kidney
  5. Bone
  6. GI tract
  7. Lymph nodes
  8. Serous spaces
     a. Pleural
     b. Pericardial
     c. Peritoneal
     d. Joint
  9. Skin
  10. Lung: cough, shortness of breath
- Adrenal insufficiency possible, caused by infection of adrenal gland
- Pancytopenia
  1. With fever and weight loss *or*
  2. Without other localizing symptoms or signs *or*
  3. With only splenomegaly
- TB hepatitis
  1. Tender liver
  2. Obstructive enzymes (alkaline phosphatase) elevated out of proportion to minimal hepatocellular enzymes (SGOT, SGPT) and bilirubin
- TB meningitis
  1. Gradual-onset headache
  2. Minimal meningeal signs
  3. Malaise
  4. Low-grade fever (may be absent)
  5. Sudden stupor or coma
  6. Cranial nerve VI palsy
- TB pericarditis
  1. Effusions resembling TB pleurisy
  2. Cardiac tamponade
- Skeletal TB
  1. Large joint arthritis (with effusions resembling TB pericarditis)
  2. Bone lesions (especially ribs)
  3. Pott's disease
     a. TB spondylitis, especially of lower thoracic spine
     b. Paraspinous TB abscess
     c. Possible psoas abscess
     d. Frequent cord compression (often relieved by steroids)
- Genitourinary TB
  1. Renal TB
     a. Papillary necrosis
     b. Destruction of renal pelvis
     c. Strictures of upper third of ureters
     d. Hematuria
     e. Pyuria with misleading bacterial cultures
     f. Preserved renal function
  2. TB orchitis or epididymitis
     a. Scrotal mass
     b. Draining abscess
  3. Chronic prostatic TB
- GI TB
  1. Diarrhea
  2. Pain
  3. Obstruction
  4. Bleeding
  5. Especially common with AIDS
  6. Bowel lesions
     a. Circumferential ulcers
     b. Short strictures
     c. Calcified granulomas
     d. TB mesenteric caseous adenitis
     e. Abscess, but rare fistula formation
     f. Often difficult to distinguish from granulomatous bowel disease (Crohn's disease)
- TB peritonitis
  1. Fluid resembles TB pleurisy
  2. PPD often negative
  3. Tender abdomen
  4. Doughy peritoneal consistency, often with ascites
  5. Peritoneal biopsy indicated for diagnosis
- TB lymphadenitis (scrofula)
  1. May involve all node groups
  2. Common adenopathies
     a. Cervical
     b. Supraclavicular
     c. Axillary
     d. Retroperitoneal
  3. Biopsy generally needed for diagnosis
  4. Surgical resection of nodes may be necessary
  5. Especially common with AIDS
- Cutaneous TB
  1. Skin infection from autoinoculation or dissemination
  2. Nodules or abscesses
  3. Tuberculids (possibly allergic reactions)
  4. Erythema nodosum
- Miscellaneous presentations
  1. TB laryngitis
  2. TB otitis
  3. Ocular TB
     a. Choroidal tubercles
     b. Iritis
     c. Uveitis
     d. Episcleritis
  4. Adrenal TB
  5. Breast TB

ETIOLOGY

- See also "Pulmonary Tuberculosis" in Section I
- Mtb, a slow-growing, aerobic, non–spore forming, nonmotile bacillus
- Humans are the only reservoir for Mtb
- Pathogenesis:
  1. Acid fast bacilli (AFB) (Mtb) are ingested by macrophages in alveoli, then transported to regional lymph nodes where spread is contained.
  2. Some AFB reach the bloodstream and disseminate widely.
  3. Immediate active disseminated disease may ensue or a latent period may develop.
  4. During latent period, T-cell immune mechanisms contain infection in granulomas until later reactivation occurs as a result of immunosuppression or other undefined factors in conjunction with reactivated pulmonary TB or alone.
- Miliary TB may occur as a consequence of the following:
  1. Primary infection: inability to contain primary infection leads to a hematogenous spread and progressive disseminated disease.
  2. In late chronic TB and in those with advanced age or poor immunity, a continuous seeding of the blood may develop and lead to disseminated disease.

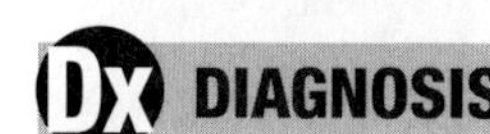

DIFFERENTIAL DIAGNOSIS

Widespread sites of possible dissemination associated with myriad differential diagnostic possibilities:

- Lymphoma
- Typhoid fever

- Brucellosis
- Other tumors
- Collagen-vascular disease

WORKUP

- Prompt evaluation is essential
- Sputum for AFB stain and culture
- Chest x-ray examination
- PPD
- Fluid analysis and culture wherever available
  1. Sputum
  2. Blood: particularly helpful in patients with AIDS
  3. Urine
  4. CSF
  5. Pleural
  6. Pericardial
  7. Peritoneal
  8. Gastric aspirates
- Biopsy of any involved tissue is advisable to make immediate diagnosis
  1. Transbronchial biopsy preferred and easily accessible
  2. Bone marrow
  3. Lymph node
  4. Scrotal mass if present
  5. Any other involved site
  6. Positive granuloma or AFB on biopsy specimen is diagnostic
- Imaging studies as needed

LABORATORY TESTS

- Culture and fluid analysis as described previously
- Smear-negative sputum often is positive weeks later on culture
- CBC is usually normal
- ESR is usually elevated

IMAGING STUDIES

- Chest x-ray examination (may or may not be positive) (see "Pulmonary Tuberculosis" in Section I)
- CT scan or MRI of brain and spinal cord (Fig. 1-344)
  1. Tuberculoma
  2. Basilar arachnoiditis
- Barium studies of bowel

Rx TREATMENT

NONPHARMACOLOGIC THERAPY

- Bed rest during acute phase of treatment
- High-calorie, high-protein diet to reverse malnutrition and enhance immune response to TB
- Isolation in negative-pressure rooms with high-volume air replacement and circulation (with health care provider wearing proper protective 0.5- to 1-micron filter respirators)
  1. Until three consecutive sputum AFB smears are negative, if pulmonary disease coexists
  2. Isolation not required for closed-space TB infections

ACUTE GENERAL Rx

- See "Pulmonary Tuberculosis" in Section I.
- Therapy should be initiated immediately. Do not wait for definitive diagnosis.
- More rapid response to chemotherapy by disseminated TB foci than cavitary pulmonary TB.
- Treatment for 6 mo with INH plus rifampin plus PZA.
  1. Treatment for 12 mo often required for bone and renal TB.
  2. Prolonged treatment often required for CNS and pericardial.
  3. Prolonged treatment often required for all disseminated TB in infants.
- Compliance (rigid adherence to treatment regimen) is the chief determinant of success.
  1. Supervised directly observed therapy (DOT) is recommended for all patients.
  2. Supervised DOT is mandatory for unreliable patients.
- Steroids are often helpful additions in fulminant miliary disease with the hypoxemia and DIC.

CHRONIC Rx

- Generally not indicated beyond treatment described previously
- Prolonged treatment supervised by infectious disease expert required in a few complicated infections caused by resistant organisms

DISPOSITION

- Monthly follow-up by physician experienced in TB treatment
- Confirm sensitivity testing, and alter treatment appropriately (see "Pulmonary Tuberculosis" in Section I)

REFERRAL

- To infectious disease expert for:
  1. HIV-positive patient
  2. Patient with suspected drug-resistant TB
  3. Patient previously treated for TB
  4. Patient whose fever has not decreased and sputum (if positive) has not converted to negative in 2 to 4 wk
  5. Patients with overwhelming pulmonary or extrapulmonary TB

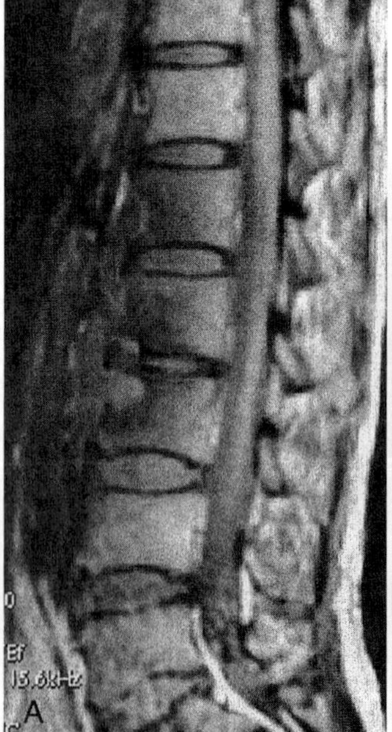

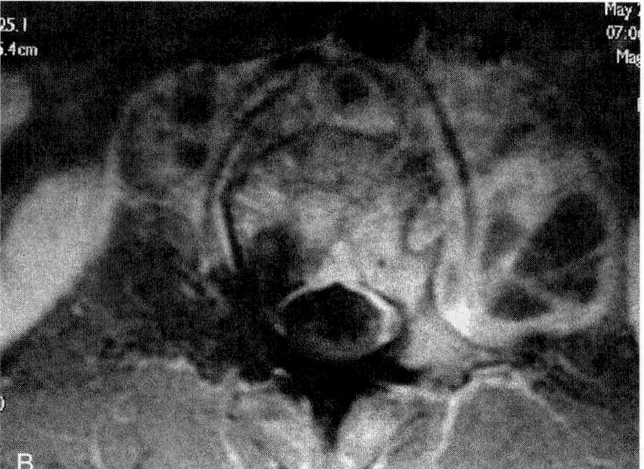

FIGURE 1-344 A, B, MR images of tuberculous spinal osteomyelitis with scalloping of the vertebrae (tuberculous caries) and paraspinal "cold" abscesses. (From Grainger RG, Allison D: *Grainger & Allison's diagnostic radiology, a textbook of medical imaging,* ed 4, 2001, Churchill Livingstone.)

- To pulmonary, orthopedic, or GI physicians for examinations or biopsy

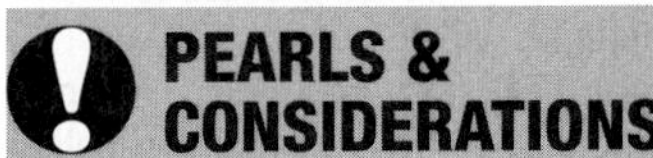

PEARLS & CONSIDERATIONS

COMMENTS

- All contacts (especially close household contacts and infants) should be properly tested for PPD conversions >3 mo following exposure.
- Those with positive PPD should be evaluated for active TB and properly treated or given prophylaxis.

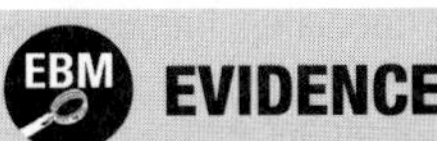

EVIDENCE

Evidence for fluoroquinolones in the treatment of people with newly diagnosed tuberculosis:

- A systematic review found that when ciprofloxacin or ofloxacin was added or substituted into the standard treatment regimen for people with pulmonary TB, there was no significant difference in terms of cure, treatment failure, or clinical or radiological improvement compared with a standard regimen.[1] A
- The authors of the review comment that newer fluoroquinolones may be more effective, but further research is required.[1]

Evidence for the practice of direct observation therapy:

- A systematic review found insufficient evidence from randomized controlled trials (RCTs) demonstrating the efficacy of direct observation of tablet swallowing in the treatment of TB in low-, middle-, and high-income country settings. There was no significant difference between direct observation and self-treatment for cure or treatment completion.[2] A

Treatment and prevention of TB in people with coexistent HIV infection:

- A systematic review of RCTs studied the effectiveness of TB preventive therapy in reducing the risk of active TB and death in patients infected with HIV. Preventive therapy (with any anti-TB regimen) was associated with a significantly lower incidence of active TB compared with placebo, but all-cause mortality rates were similar in both groups. Those with a positive tuberculin skin test were more likely to benefit from treatment than were those with a negative test.[3] A
- Limited evidence from this review suggested that the protective effect of therapy may have declined over the short to medium term. No one regimen was found to be superior, however short-course multidrug regimens were much more likely to be discontinued because of adverse effects, compared to isoniazid monotherapy.[3] A

Evidence-Based References

1. Ziganshina LE et al: Fluoroquinolones for treating tuberculosis, *Cochrane Database Syst Rev* 3, 2005.
2. Volmink J, Garner P: Directly observed therapy for treating tuberculosis, *Cochrane Database Syst Rev* 2, 2006.
3. Woldehanna S, Volmink J: Treatment of latent tuberculosis infection in HIV infected persons, *Cochrane Database Syst Rev* 1, 2004.

SUGGESTED READINGS

American Thoracic Society, CDC and the Infectious Disease Society of America: Controlling tuberculosis in the United States, *MMWR* 54(RR-12):1, 2005.

Golden MP, Vikram HR: Extrapulmonary tuberculosis: an overview, *Am Fam Physician* 72(9):1761, 2005.

Maher D et al: Tuberculosis deaths in countries with high HIV prevalence: what is their use as an indicator in tuberculosis programme monitoring and epidemiological surveillance? *Int J Tuberc Lung Dis* 9(2):123, 2005.

Matsushima T: Miliary tuberculosis or disseminated tuberculosis, *Intern Med* 44(7):687, 2005.

Mitnick CD et al: Comprehensive treatment of extensively drug-resistant tuberculosis, *N Engl J Med* 369:563-574, 2008

Miyoshi I et al: Miliary tuberculosis not affecting the lungs but complicated by acute respiratory distress syndrome, *Intern Med* 44(6):622, 2005.

Sharma SK et al: Miliary tuberculosis: new insights into an old disease, *Lancet Infect Dis* 5(7):415, 2005.

Torgersen J et al: Molecular epidemiology of pleural and other extrapulmonary tuberculosis: a Maryland state review, *Clin Infect Dis* 42(10):1375, 2006.

AUTHORS: **GLENN G. FORT, M.D., M.P.H.,** and **DENNIS J. MIKOLICH, M.D.**

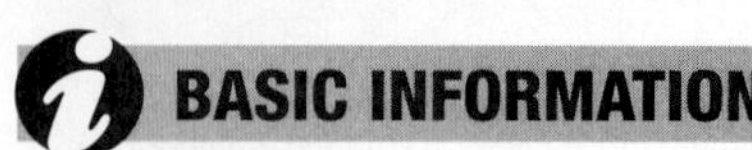

BASIC INFORMATION

DEFINITION

Pulmonary tuberculosis (TB) is an infection of the lung and, occasionally, surrounding structures, caused by the bacterium *Mycobacterium tuberculosis* (Mtb).

SYNONYMS

TB

ICD-9CM CODES
011.9 Pulmonary tuberculosis

EPIDEMIOLOGY & DEMOGRAPHICS

INCIDENCE (IN U.S.):
- Approximately 7 cases/100,000 persons—lowest in reported history
- >90% of new cases each yr from reactivated prior infections
- 9% newly infected
- Only 10% of patients with purified protein derivative (PPD) conversions (higher [8%/yr] in HIV-positive patients) will develop TB, most within 1 to 2 yr
- Two thirds of all new cases in racial and ethnic minorities
- 80% of new cases in children in racial and ethnic minorities
- Occurs most frequently in geographic areas and among populations with highest AIDS prevalence
  1. Urban blacks and Hispanics between 25 and 45 yr old
  2. Poor, crowded urban communities
- Nearly 36% of new cases from new immigrants

PREVALENCE (IN U.S.):
- Estimated 10 million people infected
- Varies widely among population groups

PREDOMINANT SEX:
- No specific predilection
- Male predominance in AIDS, shelters, and prisons reflected in disproportionate male incidence

PREDOMINANT AGE:
- 24 to 45 yr old
- Childhood cases common among minorities
- Nursing home outbreaks among elderly

PEAK INCIDENCE:
- Infancy
- Teenage years
- Pregnancy
- Elderly
- HIV-positive patients, regardless of age, at highest risk

GENETICS:
- Populations with widespread low native resistance have been intensely infected when initially exposed to TB.
- Following elimination of those with least native resistance, incidence and prevalence of TB tend to decline.

PHYSICAL FINDINGS & CLINICAL PRESENTATION

- See "Etiology"
- Primary pulmonary TB infection generally asymptomatic
- Reactivation pulmonary TB
  1. Fever
  2. Night sweats
  3. Cough
  4. Hemoptysis
  5. Scanty nonpurulent sputum
  6. Weight loss
- Progressive primary pulmonary TB disease: same as reactivation pulmonary TB
- TB pleurisy
  1. Pleuritic chest pain
  2. Fever
  3. Shortness of breath
- Rare massive, suffocating, fatal hemoptysis secondary to erosion of pulmonary artery within a cavity (Rasmussen's aneurysm)
- Chest examination
  1. Not specific
  2. Usually underestimates extent of disease
  3. Rales accentuated following a cough (posttussive rales)

ETIOLOGY

- Mtb, a slow-growing, aerobic, non-spore-forming, nonmotile bacillus, with a lipid-rich cell wall:
  1. Lacks pigment
  2. Produces niacin
  3. Reduces nitrate
  4. Produces heat-labile catalase
  5. Mtb staining, acid-fast and acid-alcohol fast by Ziehl-Neelsen method, appearing as red, slightly bent, beaded rods 2 to 4 microns long (acid-fast bacilli [AFB]), against a blue background
  6. Polymerase chain reaction (PCR) to detect <10 organisms/ml in sputum (compared with the requisite 10,000 organisms/ml for AFB smear detection)
  7. Culture
     a. Growth on solid media (Löwenstein-Jensen; Middlebrook 7H11) in 2 to 6 wk
     b. Growth in liquid media (BACTEC, using a radioactive carbon source for early growth detection) often in 9 to 16 days
     c. Enhanced in a 5% to 10% carbon dioxide atmosphere
  8. DNA fingerprinting (based on restriction fragment length polymorphism [RFLP])
     a. Facilitates immediate identification of Mtb strains in early growing cultures
     b. False negatives possible if growth suboptimal
  9. Humans are the only reservoir for Mtb
  10. Transmission
     a. Facilitated by close exposure to high-velocity cough (unprotected by proper mask or respirators) from patient with AFB-positive sputum and cavitary lesions, producing aerosolized droplets containing AFB, which are inhaled directly into alveoli
     b. Occurs within prisons, nursing homes, and hospitals
- Pathogenesis
  1. AFB (Mtb) ingested by macrophages in alveoli, then transported to regional lymph nodes, where spread is contained
  2. Some AFB may reach bloodstream and disseminate widely
  3. Primary TB (asymptomatic, minimal pneumonitis in lower or midlung fields, with hilar lymphadenopathy) essentially an intracellular infection, with multiplication of organisms continuing for 2 to 12 wk after primary exposure, until cell-mediated hypersensitivity (detected by positive skin test reaction to tuberculin PPD) matures, with subsequent containment of infection
  4. Local and disseminated AFB thus contained by T-cell-mediated immune responses
     a. Recruitment of monocytes
     b. Transformation of lymphocytes with secretion of lymphokines
     c. Activation of macrophages and histiocytes
     d. Organization into granulomas, where organisms may survive within macrophages (Langhans' giant cells), but within which multiplication essentially ceases (95%) and from which spread is prohibited
  5. Progressive primary pulmonary disease
     a. May immediately follow the asymptomatic phase
     b. Necrotizing pulmonary infiltrates
     c. Tuberculous bronchopneumonia
     d. Endobronchial TB
     e. Interstitial TB
     f. Widespread miliary lung lesions
  6. Postprimary TB pleurisy with pleural effusion
     a. Develops after early primary infection, although often before conversion to positive PPD
     b. Results from pleural seeding from a peripheral lung lesion or rupture of lymph node into pleural space
     c. May produce a large (sometimes hemorrhagic) exudative effusion (with polymorphonuclear cells early, rapidly replaced by lymphocytes), frequently without pulmonary infiltrates
     d. Generally resolves without treatment
     e. Portends a high risk of subsequent clinical disease, and therefore must be diagnosed and treated early (pleural biopsy and culture) to prevent future catastrophic TB illness
     f. May result in disseminated extrapulmonary infection
  7. Reactivation pulmonary TB
     a. Occurs months to years following primary TB
     b. Preferentially involves the apical posterior segments of the upper lobes and superior segments of the lower lobes
     c. Associated with necrosis and cavitation of involved lung, hemoptysis, chronic fever, night sweats, weight loss
     d. Spread within lung occurs via cough and inhalation

8. Reinfection TB
   a. May mimic reactivation TB
   b. Ruptured caseous foci and cavities, which may produce endobronchial spread
9. Mtb in both progressive primary and reactivation pulmonary TB
   a. Intracellular (macrophage) lesions (undergoing slow multiplication)
   b. Closed caseous lesions (undergoing slow multiplication)
   c. Extracellular, open cavities (undergoing rapid multiplication)
   d. INH and rifampin are cidal in all three sites
   e. Pyrazinamide (PZA) especially active within acidic macrophage environment
   f. Extrapulmonary reactivation disease also possible
10. Rapid local progression and dissemination in infants with devastating illness before PPD conversion occurs
11. Most symptoms (fever, weight loss, anorexia) and tissue destruction (caseous necrosis) from cytokines and cell-mediated immune responses
12. Mtb has no important endotoxins or exotoxins
13. Granuloma formation related to tumor necrosis factor (TNF) secreted by activated macrophages

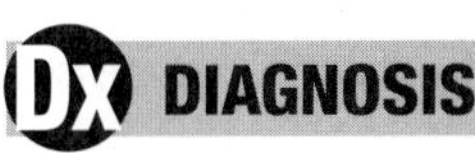

DIAGNOSIS

DIFFERENTIAL DIAGNOSIS

- Necrotizing pneumonia (anaerobic, gram-negative)
- Histoplasmosis
- Coccidioidomycosis
- Melioidosis
- Interstitial lung diseases (rarely)
- Cancer
- Sarcoidosis
- Silicosis
- Rare pneumonias
  1. *Rhodococcus equi* (cavitation)
  2. *Bacillus cereus* (50% hemoptysis)
  3. *Eikenella corrodens* (cavitation)

WORKUP

- Sputum for AFB stains
- Chest x-ray (Fig. 1-345)
- PPD
  1. Recent conversion from negative to positive within 3 mo of exposure is highly suggestive of recent infection.
  2. Single positive PPD is not helpful diagnostically.
  3. Negative PPD never rules out acute TB.
  4. Be certain that positive PPD does not reflect "booster phenomenon" (prior positive PPD may become negative after several yr and return to positive only after second repeated PPD; repeat second PPD within 1 wk), which thus may mimic skin test conversion.
  5. Positive PPD reaction is determined as follows:
     a. Induration after 72 hr of intradermal injection of 0.1 ml of 5 TU-PPD
     b. 5-mm induration if HIV-positive (or other severe immunosuppressed state affecting cellular immune function), close contact of active TB, fibrotic chest lesions
     c. 10-mm induration if in high–medical risk groups (immunosuppressive disease or therapy, renal failure, gastrectomy, silicosis, diabetes), foreign-born high-risk group (Southeast Asia, Latin America, Africa, India), low socioeconomic groups, IV drug addict, prisoner, health care worker
     d. 15-mm induration if low risk
  6. Anergy antigen testing (using mumps, *Candida,* tetanus toxoid) may identify patients who are truly anergic to PPD and these antigens, but results are often confusing. Not recommended.
  7. Patients with TB may be selectively anergic only to PPD.
  8. Positive PPD indicates prior infection but does not itself confirm active disease.
- A new diagnostic test for latent TB infection, known as the quantaferon test (QFT-G), is now available. This is a blood test that measures interferon response to specific Mtb antigens. The test is FDA approved and is available in some large TB centers and state health departments. It may assist in distinguishing true positive reactions, from individuals with latent TB, from PPD reactions related to: nontuberculous mycobacteria; prior BCG vaccination; or difficult-to-interpret skin test results from people with dermatologic conditions or immediate allergic reactions to PPD. The diagnostic utility of the test as a replacement or supplement to the standard PPD is not yet fully determined. The enzyme-linked immunospot assay (Elispot plus) incorporating a novel antigen, RV3879c, when used in combination with tuberculin testing, has been reported to enable rapid exclusion of active infection in patients with moderate to high pretest probability of TB.

LABORATORY TESTS

- Sputum for AFB stains and culture
  1. Induced sputum if patient not coughing productively
- Sputum from bronchoscopy if high suspicion of TB with negative expectorated induced sputum for AFB
  1. Positive AFB smear is essential before or shortly after treatment to ensure subse-

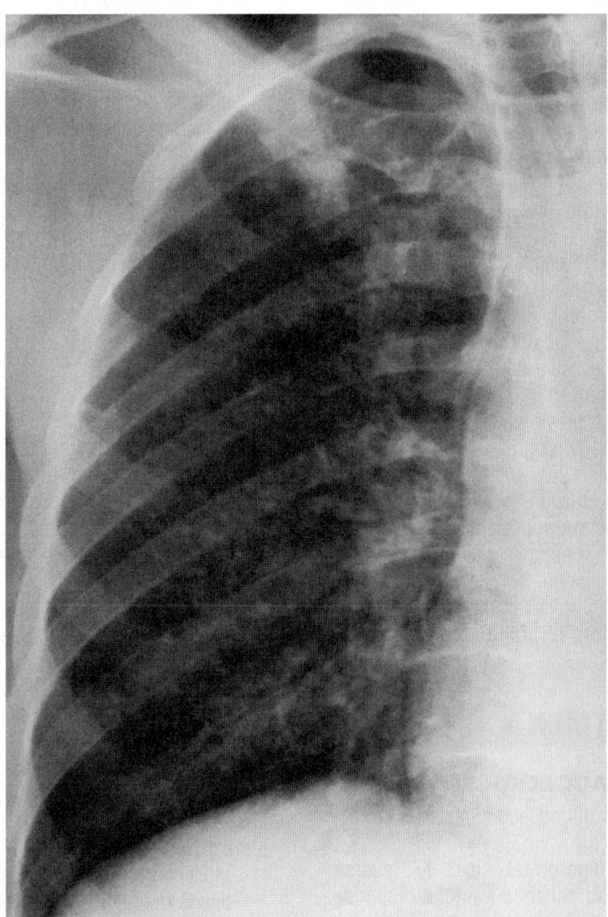

FIGURE 1-345 Miliary pattern in tuberculosis consists of numerous nodules of uniform size. (From Grainger RG et al [eds]: *Grainger & Allison's diagnostic radiology,* ed 4, Philadelphia, 2001, Churchill Livingstone.)

quent growth for definitive diagnosis and sensitivity testing
  2. Consider lung biopsy if sputum negative, especially if infiltrates are predominantly interstitial
- AFB stain-negative sputum may grow Mtb subsequently
- Gastric aspirates reliable, especially in HIV-negative patients
- CBC
  1. Variable values
     a. WBCs: low, normal, or elevated (including leukemoid reaction: >50,000)
     b. Normocytic, normochromic anemia often
  2. Rarely helpful diagnostically
- ESR usually elevated
- Thoracentesis
  1. Exudative effusion
     a. Elevated protein
     b. Decreased glucose
     c. Elevated WBCs (polymorphonuclear leukocytes early, replaced later by lymphocytes)
     d. May be hemorrhagic
  2. Pleural fluid usually AFB-negative
  3. Pleural biopsy often diagnostic—may need to be repeated for diagnosis
  4. Culture pleural biopsy tissue for AFB
- Bone marrow biopsy is often diagnostic in difficult-to-diagnose cases, especially miliary TB

IMAGING STUDIES

- Chest radiograph examination
  1. Primary infection reflected by calcified peripheral lung nodule with calcified hilar lymph node
  2. Reactivation pulmonary TB
     a. Necrosis
     b. Cavitation (especially on apical lordotic views)
     c. Fibrosis and hilar retraction
     d. Bronchopneumonia
     e. Interstitial infiltrates
     f. Miliary pattern
     g. Many of previous findings may also accompany progressive primary TB
  3. TB pleurisy
     a. Pleural effusion, often rapidly accumulating and massive
  4. TB activity not established by single chest x-ray examination
  5. Serial chest x-ray examinations are excellent indicators of progression or regression

Rx TREATMENT

NONPHARMACOLOGIC THERAPY

- Increased rest during acute phase of treatment
- High-calorie, high-protein diet to reverse malnutrition and enhance immune response to TB
- Isolation in negative-pressure rooms with high-volume air replacement and circulation, with health care provider wearing proper protective 0.5- to 1-micron filter respirators, until three consecutive sputum AFB smears are negative

ACUTE GENERAL Rx

- Compliance (rigid adherence to treatment regimen) chief determinant of success.
  1. Supervised directly observed therapy (DOT) recommended for all patients and mandatory for unreliable patients
- Preferred adult regimen: DOT.
  1. Isoniazid (INH) 15 mg/kg (max 900 mg), rifampin 600 mg, ethambutol (EMB) 30 mg/kg (max 2500 mg), and pyrazinamide (PZA) (2 g [<50 kg]; 2.5 g [51 to 74 kg]; 3 g [>75 kg]) thrice weekly for 6 mo
  2. Alternative, more complicated DOT regimens
- Rifapentine, a rifampin derivative with a much longer serum half-life, was shown to be as effective when administered weekly (with weekly isoniazid) as conventional regimens for drug-sensitive pulmonary TB in non–HIV-infected patients.
- Short-course daily therapy: adult.
  1. HIV-negative patient: 6 mo total therapy (2 mo INH 300 mg, rifampin 600 mg, and EMB 15 mg/kg [max 2500 mg]) and PZA (1.5 g [<50 kg]; 2 g [51 to 74 kg]; 2.5 g [>75 kg]) daily and until smear negative and sensitivity confirmed; then INH and rifampin daily for 4 mo
  2. HIV-positive patient: 9 mo total therapy (2 mo INH, rifampin, EMB, and PZA daily until smear negative and sensitivity confirmed; then INH and rifampin qid for 7 mo)
  3. Continue treatment at least 3 mo following conversion to negative cultures
- Drug resistance (often multiple drug resistance TB [MDRTB]) increased by:
  1. Prior treatment
  2. Acquisition of TB in developing countries
  3. Homelessness
  4. AIDS
  5. Prisoners
  6. IV drug addicts
  7. Known contact with MDRTB
- Never add single drug to failing regimen.
- Never treat TB with fewer than two to three drugs or two to three new additional drugs.
- Monitor for clinical toxicity (especially hepatitis).
  1. Patient and physician awareness that anorexia, nausea, right upper quadrant pain, and unexplained malaise require immediate cessation of treatment
  2. Evaluation of liver function testing
     a. Minimal SGOT/SGPT elevations without symptoms generally transient and not clinically significant
- Preventive treatment for PPD conversion only (infection without disease).
  1. Must be certain that chest x-ray examination is negative and patient has no symptoms of TB
  2. INH 300 mg daily for 9 to 12 mo; at least 12 mo if HIV-positive patient
  3. Most important groups:
     a. HIV-positive and other severely immunocompromised patients
     b. Close contact with active TB
     c. Recent converter
     d. Old TB on chest x-ray examination
     e. IV drug addict
     f. Medical risk factor
     g. High-risk foreign country
     h. Homeless
- Infants generally given prophylaxis immediately if recent contact with active TB (even if infant PPD negative), then retested with PPD in 3 mo (continuing INH if PPD becomes positive and stopping INH if PPD remains negative).
- Chronic, stable PPD (several yr) given INH prophylaxis generally only if patient is <35 yr old.
  1. INH toxicity may outweigh benefit
  2. Individualize decision
- Preventive therapy for suspected INH-resistant organisms is unclear.

CHRONIC Rx

- Generally not indicated beyond treatment described previously
- Prolonged treatment, supervised by infectious disease expert, in a few very complicated infections caused by resistant organisms

DISPOSITION

- Monthly follow up by physician experienced in TB treatment
- Confirm sensitivity testing and alter treatment appropriately
- Frequent sputum samples until culture is negative
- Confirm chest x-ray regression at 2 to 3 mo

REFERRAL

- To infectious disease expert for:
  1. HIV-positive patient
  2. Patient with suspected drug-resistant TB
  3. Patients previously treated for TB
  4. Patients whose fever has not decreased and sputum has not converted to negative in 2 to 4 wk
  5. Patients with overwhelming pulmonary or extrapulmonary TB
- To pulmonologist for bronchoscopy or pleural biopsy

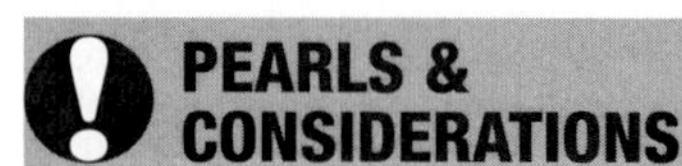

PEARLS & CONSIDERATIONS

COMMENTS

- All contacts (especially close household contacts and infants) should be properly tested for PPD conversions during 3 mo following exposure.
- Those with positive PPD should be evaluated for active TB and properly treated or given prophylaxis.
- Previous treatment is a common risk factor for extensively drug-resistant and multidrug-resistant TB.

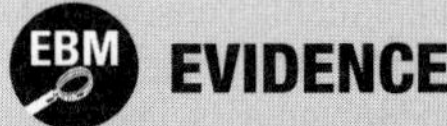

EVIDENCE

Evidence for fluoroquinolones in the treatment of people with newly diagnosed TB:

A systematic review found that when ciprofloxacin or ofloxacin was added or substituted into the standard treatment regimen for people with pulmonary TB there was no significant difference in terms of cure, treatment failure, or clinical or radiological improvement compared with a standard regimen.[1] Ⓐ

The authors of the review comment that newer fluoroquinolones may be more effective, but further research is required.[1]

Evidence for the practice of direct observation therapy:

A systematic review found insufficient evidence from randomized controlled trials (RCTs) demonstrating the efficacy of direct observation of tablet swallowing in the treatment of TB in low-, middle-, and high-income country settings. There was no significant difference between direct observation and self-treatment for cure or treatment completion.[2] Ⓐ

Treatment and prevention of TB in people with coexistent HIV infection:

A systematic review of RCTs studied the effectiveness of TB preventive therapy in reducing the risk of active TB and death in patients infected with HIV. Preventive therapy (with any anti-TB regimen) was associated with a significantly lower incidence of active TB compared with placebo, but all-cause mortality rates were similar in both groups. Those with a positive tuberculin skin test were more likely to benefit from treatment than those with a negative test.[3] Ⓐ

Limited evidence from this review suggested that the protective effect of therapy may have declined over the short to medium term. No one regimen was found to be superior, however short-course multidrug regimens were much more likely to be discontinued because of adverse effects, compared to isoniazid monotherapy.[3] Ⓐ

Evidence-Based References

1. Ziganshina LE et al:. Fluoroquinolones for treating tuberculosis, *Cochrane Database Syst Rev* 3, 2005.
2. Volmink J, Garner P: Directly observed therapy for treating tuberculosis, *Cochrane Database Syst Rev* 2, 2006.
3. Woldehanna S, Volmink J: Treatment of latent tuberculosis infection in HIV infected persons, *Cochrane Database Syst Rev* 1, 2004.

SUGGESTED READINGS

Aderaye G et al: The relationship between disease pattern and disease burden by chest radiography, *M. tuberculosis* load, and HIV status in patients with pulmonary tuberculosis in Addis Ababa, *Infection* 32(6):333, 2004.

American Thoracic Society, CDC, and the Infectious Disease Society of America: Controlling tuberculosis in the United States, *MMWR* 54(RR-12):1, 2005.

Dosanjh D et al: Improved diagnostic evaluation of suspected tuberculosis, *Ann Intern Med* 148:325-336, 2008

Ismail Y: Pulmonary tuberculosis—a review of clinical features and diagnosis in 232 cases, *Med J Malaysia* 59(1):56, 2004.

Jacob JT et al: Acute forms of tuberculosis in adults, *Am J Med* 122:12-17, 2009.

Kliiman K, Altraja A: Predictors of extensively drug-resistant pulmonary tuberculosis, *Ann Intern Med* 150(11):766-775, 2009.

Maartens G: Tuberculosis, *Lancet* 370:2030, 2007.

Rubin EJ: Toward a new therapy for tuberculosis, *N Engl J Med* 352:933, 2005.

van Lettow M et al: Micronutrient malnutrition and wasting in adults with pulmonary tuberculosis with and without HIV co-infection in Malawi, *BMC Infect Dis* 4(1):61, 2004.

Wei CJ et al: Computed tomaography features of acute pulmonary tuberculosis, *Am J Emerg Med* 22(3):171, 2004.

AUTHORS: **GLENN G. FORT, M.D., M.P.H.,** and **DENNIS J. MIKOLICH, M.D.**

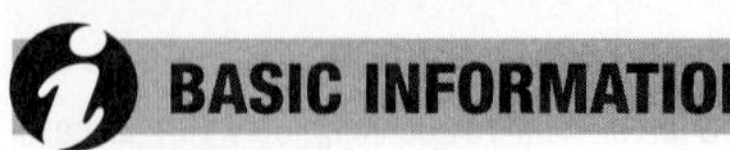

BASIC INFORMATION

DEFINITION

Tuberous sclerosis (TS) is an inherited neurocutaneous disorder that is characterized by pleomorphic features involving many organ systems, including multiple benign neoplasms (hamartomas) of the brain, kidney, and skin.

ICD-9CM CODES
759.5 Tuberous sclerosis

EPIDEMIOLOGY & DEMOGRAPHICS

INCIDENCE: TS has an estimated incidence of 1 case per 6000 live births. Thus, it is the second most common neurocutaneous syndrome after neurofibromatosis.

PREVALENCE: The disorder affects about 1 in 10,000 persons in the general population.

PREDOMINANT SEX: TS has no predilection for gender or race.

GENETICS:

- TS is an autosomal dominant disorder with almost complete penetrance but a wide range of clinical severity. However, only one third of cases are familial. The apparently nonfamilial cases can represent either spontaneous mutations or mosaicism.
- Genetic research has identified two TS genes. One is located on chromosome 9 (*TSC1* gene) and the other on chromosome 16 (*TSC2* gene). About 68% of cases occur as a result of new gene mutations. Because of the genetic transmission and new mutations, antenatal diagnosis is difficult.

PHYSICAL FINDINGS & CLINICAL PRESENTATION

- Dermatologic manifestations may be the only clues the family physician has to the diagnosis of the disorder, which is also marked by childhood seizures and mental retardation (Figs. 1-346 through 1-348).
- The diagnostic criteria for TS were recently revised at a consensus conference. Major and minor features are listed in Table 1-77.
- The classic diagnostic triad of seizures, mental retardation, and facial angiofibromas (Vogt's triad) occurs in fewer than 50% of patients with TS.
- All of the clinical features of TS may not be apparent in the first yr of life. Thus, a child is often initially diagnosed with possible or probable TS and the diagnosis of definite TS is made after additional features are identified.
- Dermatologic manifestations: A careful skin examination of patients at risk for TS continues to be the easiest and most accessible method of establishing the diagnosis (Table 1-78).
- Neurologic manifestations: These are the leading cause of morbidity and mortality in patients with TS. Brain hamartomas in the form of cortical tubers, subependymal nodules, and subependymal giant cell astrocytomas are often responsible for intractable seizures, most commonly as infantile spasms. Approximately 90% to 96% of TS patients suffer from seizures. Approximately 85% of patients have their first epileptic episode in the first 2 yr of life. Behavioral and cognitive dysfunction, including autism and mental retardation, can be seen in 40% to 50% of patients.
- Renal and pulmonary manifestations are strongly associated with TS.
- Angiomyolipoma is the most common renal lesion found in TS patients. Clinically evident pulmonary involvement in TS patients is relatively rare, with an estimated incidence of 1% to 6%. The most common lesion is lymphangiomyomatosis (LAM), a progressive cystic lung disease with progressive dyspnea and spontaneous pneumothorax in a childbearing woman.
- Cardiovascular manifestations: These are often the earliest diagnostic findings in patients with TS. Rhabdomyoma is the most common primary cardiac tumor in infants and children. Its incidence in TS patients ranges between 47% and 60%. In fact, 80% to 95% of patients with cardiac rhabdomyomas have TS.
- The most common ocular findings in TS are retinal hamartomas, appearing in 40% to 50% of patients.

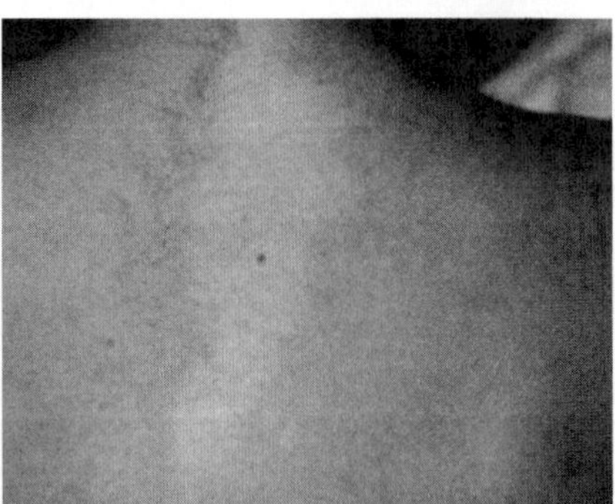

FIGURE 1-346 Hypomelanotic macules ("ash left" spots).

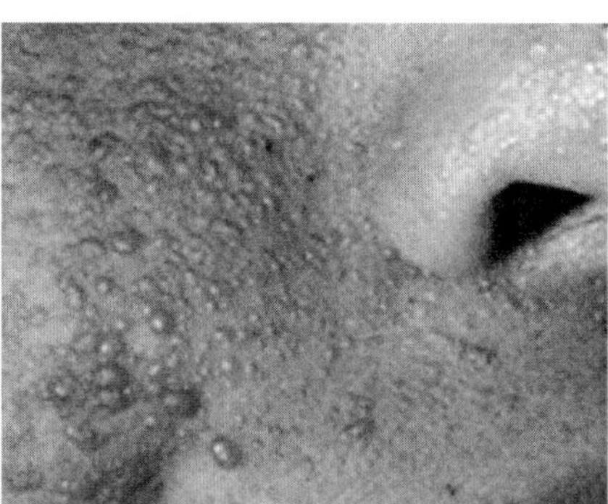

FIGURE 1-347 Facial angiofibromas.

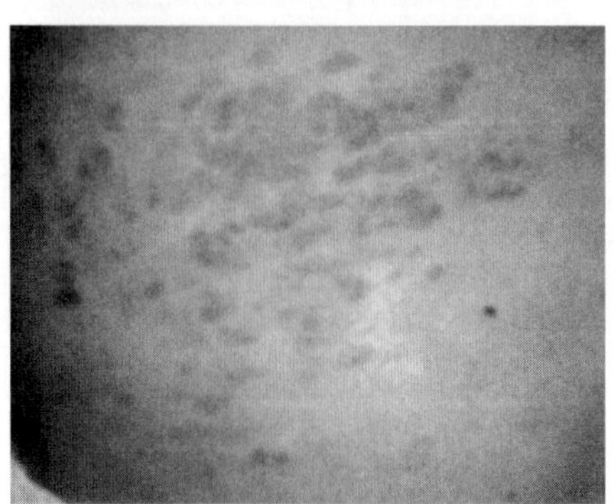

FIGURE 1-348 Shagreen patches.

ETIOLOGY

TS is an autosomal dominant disorder.

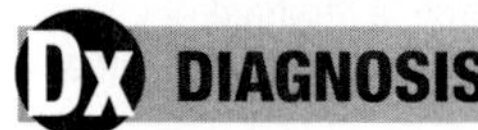

DIAGNOSIS

DIFFERENTIAL DIAGNOSIS

Cutaneous manifestations:

- Nevus anemicus
- Nevus depigmentosus (nevus achromicus)
- Vitiligo

WORKUP

- The dermatologic manifestations of TS are helpful in diagnosing this disorder. When TS has been inherited in the autosomal dominant form, dermatologic signs are almost universally present in one of the patient's parents.

TABLE 1-77 Revised Diagnostic Criteria for Tuberous Sclerosis Complex (TSC)

Major features

1. Facial angiofibromas or forehead plaque
2. Nontraumatic ungual or periungual fibroma
3. Hypomelanotic macule (3 or more)
4. Shagreen patch (connective tissue nevus)
5. Multiple retinal nodular hamartomas
6. Cortical tuber
7. Subependymal nodule
8. Subependymal giant cell astrocytoma
9. Cardiac rhabdomyoma, single or multiple
10. Lymphangiomyomatosis
11. Renal angiomyolipoma

Minor features

1. Multiple, randomly distributed pits in dental enamel
2. Hamartomatous rectal polyps
3. Bone cysts
4. Cerebral white matter radial migration lines
5. Gingival fibromas
6. Nonrenal hamartomas
7. Retinal achromic patch
8. "Confetti" skin lesions
9. Multiple renal cysts

Definite TSC: Either two major features or one major feature plus two minor features. Probable TSC: One major plus one minor feature. Possible TSC: Either one major feature or two or more minor features.

- No specific prenatal laboratory test is available.
- Early recognition of TS is vital because prompt implementation of the recommended diagnostic evaluation (neuroimaging studies, EEG, ECG, renal ultrasonography, and chest CT) may prevent serious clinical consequences.

LABORATORY TESTS

- Molecular genetic testing: In recent years, molecular genetic testing for TS has become clinically available. Such testing identifies mutations in the *TSC1* and *TSC2* genes by one of several methods, most commonly polymerase chain reaction (PCR) amplification of individual exons, followed by DNA sequencing on DNA obtained from a patient's blood sample.
- DNA testing for TS is potentially useful in several settings:
  - First, it can be helpful in confirming a clinical diagnosis of TS, especially in young patients in whom many clinical signs and symptoms have yet to develop.
  - Second, in many families with a history of TS in which there is a sporadic case of TS in a new child, genetic testing can provide reassurance to parents, children, and other family members that they do not carry the TS gene mutation.
  - Third, DNA testing is useful for prenatal diagnosis.

Rx TREATMENT

The management of TS complex (TSC) is presently symptomatic.

NONPHARMACOLOGIC THERAPY

Genetic counseling should be offered to families with affected members, even though accurate counseling remains difficult because of the variability of gene expression.

ACUTE GENERAL Rx & CHRONIC Rx

- Treatment methods currently available for patients with disfiguring facial angiofibromas include cryosurgery, curettage, dermabrasion, chemical peeling, excision, and laser therapy.
- Some patients have been treated successfully with antiepileptic medications; unfortunately, there are multiple cases of intractable seizure in which medical treatment is ineffective. In some cases of intractable epilepsy, neurosurgical intervention becomes a life-saving option.
- In such drug-resistant cases of TS, the early administration of vigabatrin (a-vinyl-gamma aminobutyric acid), a selective irreversible inhibitor of GABA-transaminase, has been proven to result in 80% to 100% cessation rates of infantile spasms. Vigabatrin is marketed in many European countries, but remains unavailable in the U.S. and has not been approved by the FDA.
- Embolization and/or renal sparing surgery are treatment options for renal angiomyolipomas.
- Oopherectomy, medroxyprogesterone, and tamoxifen use have been advocated in patients with LAM, but therapeutic benefit is unclear. Lung transplantation is reserved for patients with end-stage LAM.
- Most rhabdomyomas tend to regress with increasing age, although tumor growth has been documented in some at puberty. Surgery is recommended only for life-threatening situations, such as hemodynamic compromise.
- Oral rapamycin or sirolimus therapy can induce regression of brain astrocytomas associated with TS. Ongoing therapeutic trials with rapamycin in lymphangioleiomyomatosis appear promising.

REFERRAL

A multidisciplinary team including genetics, neurology, ophthalmology, nephrology, dermatology, neurosurgery, and plastic surgery should evaluate children suspected of having TS.

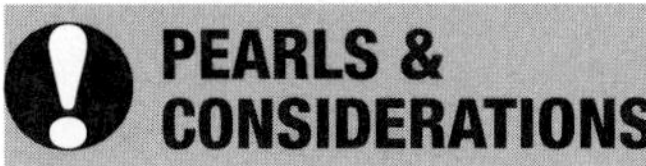

PEARLS & CONSIDERATIONS

PREVENTION

It is speculated that if one could establish the prenatal diagnosis of TS and begin using rapamycin early, one might prevent the development of TS manifestations.

SUGGESTED READINGS

Bissler JJ et al: Sirolimus for angiomyolipoma in tuberous sclerosis complex or lymphangioleiomyomatosis, *N Engl J Med* 358:140-151, 2008.

Crino PB et al: The tuberous sclerosis complex , *N Engl J Med* 355:1345-1356, 2006.

Hurst JS, Wilcoski S: Recognizing an index case of tuberous sclerosis, *Am Fam Physician* 61(3):703-708, 2001.

Schwartz RA: Tuberous sclerosis complex: advances in diagnosis, genetics, and management, *J Am Acad Dermatology,* 57(2):189-202, 2007.

AUTHOR: **RUBY SATPATHY, M.D.**

TABLE 1-78 Cutaneous Manifestations Associated with Tuberous Sclerosis Complex (TSC)

Cutaneous Lesions	Descriptions	Age of Onset	Prevalence	Diagnostic Classification
Hypomelanotic macules ("ash leaf" spots) or Fitzpatrick patches	Leaf-shaped or polygonal white spots enhanced by Wood's lamp examination	Earliest cutaneous lesion; usually present at birth or infancy on buttocks	97.2%	Major
Facial angiofibromas	Red to pink papules with a smooth surface, symmetrically distributed over the centrofacial areas, sparing the upper lips	Second to fifth yr of life; become more prominent with age	74.5%	Major
Shagreen patches	Slightly elevated patch or plaque, usually found on the dorsal body surfaces, especially the lumbosacral area; its rough surface resembles an orange peel; represents a connective tissue nevus, sometimes called collagenoma	Rare during infancy; tend to increase in size and number with age	48.1%	Major
Molluscum pendulum	Multiple soft pedunculated skin growths on neck; rarely in axilla or groin	More common during first decade of life; rare during infancy	22.6%	Minor
Forehead fibrous plaque	Yellowish-brown or skin-colored plaques of variable size and shape, usually located on the forehead or scalp	Common at any age and can be seen at birth or early infancy	18.9%	Major
Periungual fibromas	Skin-colored or reddish nodules seen on the lateral nail groove, nail plate, or along the proximal nail folds; more commonly found on the toes than on the fingers	Present at puberty or soon after; become more common with age	15.1%	Major
"Confetti-like" macules	Multiple 1-2 mm white spots symmetrically distributed over extremities	Second decade or adulthood	2.8%	Minor

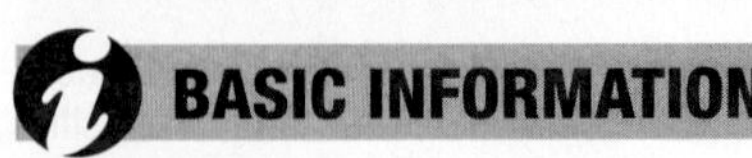

BASIC INFORMATION

DEFINITION

Acute tubular necrosis (ATN) refers to intrinsic tubular damage induced by hypoperfusion to renal parenchymal cells, particularly tubular epithelium, that results in sodium loss and fractional excretion of sodium (FE_{Na}) >1%.

SYNONYMS

Ischemic or nephrotoxic ARF

ICD-9CM CODES

584.5 With lesion of tubular necrosis
Renal failure with (acute) tubular necrosis
Tubular necrosis: NOS, acute

997.5 Urinary complications
Tubular necrosis (acute) specified as resulting from procedure

EPIDEMIOLOGY & DEMOGRAPHICS

- Accounts for 90% of intrinsic renal failure.
- Most common cause of intrinsic renal failure among hospitalized patients, including pediatric and adult, especially on surgical services in patients undergoing major cardiovascular surgery or in intensive care units in patients suffering severe trauma, hemorrhage, sepsis, or volume depletion.

PHYSICAL FINDINGS & CLINICAL PRESENTATION

- No apparent physical findings. Clinical features include recent hemorrhage, hypotension, or surgery, thereby suggesting ischemic ARF. Recent radiocontrast study, nephrotoxic drugs, history suggestive of rhabdomyolysis, hemolysis, or myeloma may suggest toxin-mediated ARF.
- Three phases of ischemic ARF:
  1. Initiation phase (hr to days)—renal hypoperfusion, evolving ischemia.
  2. Maintenance phase (1 to 2 wk)—renal cell injury established, GFR stabilizes at its nadir (5 to 10 ml/min), urine output at its lowest, uremic complications arise.
  3. Recovery phase (>2 wk)—renal parenchymal cell repair and regeneration, gradual return of GFR to premorbid levels; may be complicated by a marked diuretic phase because of excretion of retained salt and water and other solutes, continued use of diuretics, or delayed recovery of epithelial cell function (solute and water reabsorption) relative to glomerular filtration.

PATHOLOGIC FINDINGS

- Ischemic ARF—patchy and focal necrosis of tubule epithelium with detachment from its basement membrane and occlusion of tubule lumens with casts composed of epithelial cells, cellular debris, Tamm-Horsfall mucoprotein (represents the matrix of all urinary casts), and pigments. Also present is leukocyte accumulation in vasa recta (capillaries that return the NaCl and water reabsorbed in the loop of Henle and medullary collecting tubule to the systemic circulation). Morphology of glomeruli and renal vasculature remain normal. Necrosis most severe in pars recta (straight portion of proximal tubule and thick ascending limb of loop of Henle).
- Nephrotoxic ARF-morphologic changes in convoluted and straight portion of proximal tubule. Tubule cell necrosis less pronounced than in ischemic ARF.

ETIOLOGY

Hypotension or shock, prolonged prerenal azotemia, postoperative sepsis syndrome, rhabdomyolysis, hemolysis (hypercalcemia, hemoglobin, urate, oxalate, myeloma light chains), antimicrobial drugs (acyclovir, foscarnet, aminoglycosides, amphotericin B, pentamidine), radiocontrast (contrast nephropathy), chemotherapy (cisplatin, ifosfamide).

DIAGNOSIS

DIFFERENTIAL DIAGNOSIS

Allergic interstitial nephritis, acute bilateral pyelonephritis

LABORATORY TESTS

- Urinalysis for specific gravity (SG), U_{Na}, P_{Cr}, P_{Na}, U_{Cr}
- Calculate $FE_{Na} = [(U_{Na} \times P_{Cr}) / (P_{Na} \times U_{Cr})] \times 100$

LABORATORY FINDINGS

- FE_{Na} >1%
- U_{Na} >20 mmol/L
- SG <1.015

IMAGING STUDIES

Not necessary

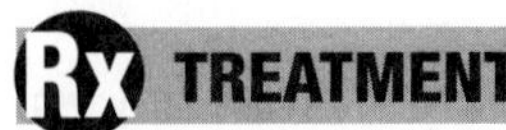

TREATMENT

ACUTE GENERAL Rx

Should focus on providing cause-specific supportive care or correction of primary hemodynamic abnormality. No specific therapies for established ATN. Peritoneal or hemodialysis for replacement of renal function until regeneration and repair restore renal function.

DISPOSITION

Recovery typically takes 1 to 2 wk after normalization of renal perfusion because it requires repair and regeneration of renal cells.

REFERRAL

Renal consultation for severe cases of ATN requiring dialysis.

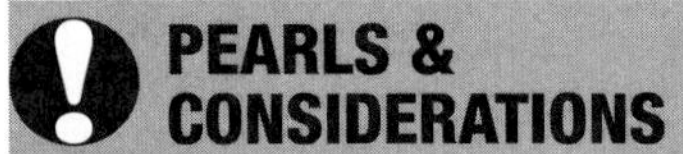

PEARLS & CONSIDERATIONS

COMMENTS

Prevention is paramount.

PREVENTION

Aggressive restoration of intravascular volume in surgical/trauma patients to prevent ischemic ARF. Tailoring dosage of potential nephrotoxins to body size and GFR to limit renal injury.

SUGGESTED READINGS

Barletta et al: Acute renal failure in children and infants, *Curr Opin Crit Care* 10(6):499-504, 2004.

Lameire N et al: Acute renal failure, *Lancet* 365:417-430, 2005.

Lameire N: The pathophysiology of acute renal failure, *Crit Care Clin* 21(2):197-210, 2005.

AUTHOR: **CHAITANYA V. REDDY, D.O.**

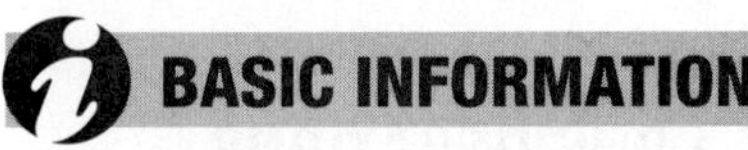

BASIC INFORMATION

DEFINITION

Tularemia is a zoonosis caused by small, facultative gram-negative intracellular coccobacillus *Francisella tularensis.* Clinical manifestations range from asymptomatic illness to septic shock and death.

SYNONYMS

Rabbit fever
Deerfly fever
O'Hara's disease

ICD-9CM CODES
021.9 Tularemia

EPIDEMIOLOGY & DEMOGRAPHICS

INCIDENCE (IN U.S.): Highest overall incidence in Arkansas, Missouri, and Oklahoma. It is also found in Canada, Mexico, European countries, Turkey, Israel, China, and Japan.
PREDOMINANT SEX: Male
PREDOMINANT AGE: Occurs at any age
PEAK INCIDENCE: June through August and in December

PHYSICAL FINDINGS & CLINICAL PRESENTATION

Physical findings:

- Incubation period is 3 to 5 days but may range from 1 to 21 days.
- Most common initial signs and symptoms:
  1. Fever
  2. Chills
  3. Headache
  4. Malaise
  5. Anorexia
  6. Fatigue
  7. Cough
  8. Myalgias
  9. Chest discomfort
  10. Vomiting
  11. Abdominal pain
  12. Diarrhea
  13. Conjunctivitis
  14. Lymphadenitis

Clinical presentation:

- Ulceroglandular and glandular: account for 75% to 80% of cases. Fever and a single erythematous papuloulcerative lesion with a central eschar accompanied by tender lymphadenopathy (Fig. 1-349)
- Oculoglandular: accounts for 1% to 2% of cases. Painful inflamed conjunctiva with numerous yellowish nodules and pinpoint ulcers. Purulent conjunctivitis with regional lymphadenopathy. Corneal perforation may occur.
- Oropharyngeal and gastrointestinal: account for 1% to 4% of cases. Acute exudative membranes pharyngitis associated with cervical lymphadenopathy. Ulcerative intestinal lesion associated with mesenteric lymphadenopathy, diarrhea, abdominal pain, nausea, vomiting, and GI bleeding.
- Pulmonary: occurs often in the elderly and has a higher mortality. Symptoms include nonproductive cough, dyspnea, or pleuritic chest pain.
- Typhoidal: 10% of all cases of tularemia. Rare in U.S. Symptoms include high continuous fever, signs of endotoxemia, and severe headache. Mortality can approach 30%.

COMPLICATIONS

1. Intravascular coagulation
2. Renal failure
3. Rhabdomyolysis
4. Jaundice
5. Hepatitis
6. Meningitis
7. Encephalitis
8. Pericarditis
9. Peritonitis
10. Osteomyelitis
11. Splenic rupture
12. Thrombophlebitis
13. Myositis and septicemia

ETIOLOGY

- Caused by infection with *F. tularensis.*
- Two main biovars of *F. tularensis:* Type A and Type B. Type A produces severe disease in humans. Type B produces milder subclinical infection.
- Transmitted by ticks, tabanid flies, and mosquitoes. Also acquired by inhalation and ingestion.
- Cases also occur after exposure to animals (wild rabbit, squirrels, birds, sheep, beavers, muskrats, and domestic dogs and cats) or animal products.
- Laboratory acquisition is possible.
- Pathogenesis: after inoculation into the skin the organism multiplies locally within 2 to 5 days, then it produces erythematous tender or pruritic papule. The papule rapidly enlarges and forms an ulcer with a black base. The bacteria spread to the regional lymph nodes producing lymphadenopathy, and with bacteremia may spread to distant organs.

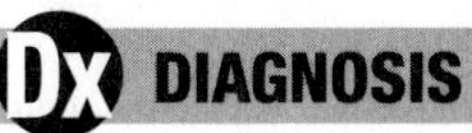

DIAGNOSIS

DIFFERENTIAL DIAGNOSIS

- Rickettsial infections
- Meningococcal infections
- Cat-scratch disease
- Infectious mononucleosis
- Atypical pneumonia
- Group A strep pharyngitis
- Typhoid fever
- Fungal infection—sporotrichosis
- Anthrax
- Plague
- Bacterial skin infections

WORKUP

- CBC
- Chest x-ray examination
- Cultures of blood, lymph node, pleural fluid, wounds, sputum, and gastric aspirate
- Antigen detection in urine
- Polymerase chain reaction (PCR)
- Serology

LABORATORY TESTS

- WBC count and ESR normal or elevated.
- Rarely seen on gram-stained smears or tissue biopsies.
- Antibodies to *F. tularensis* demonstrated by tube agglutination, microagglutination, hemagglutination, and ELISA; definitive serologic diagnosis requires a fourfold or greater rise in titer between acute and convalescent specimens.
- PCR to facilitate early diagnosis.

IMAGING STUDIES

Chest x-ray examination to show bilateral patchy infiltrate, lobar parenchymal infiltrate, cavitary lesion, pleural effusion, or emphysema

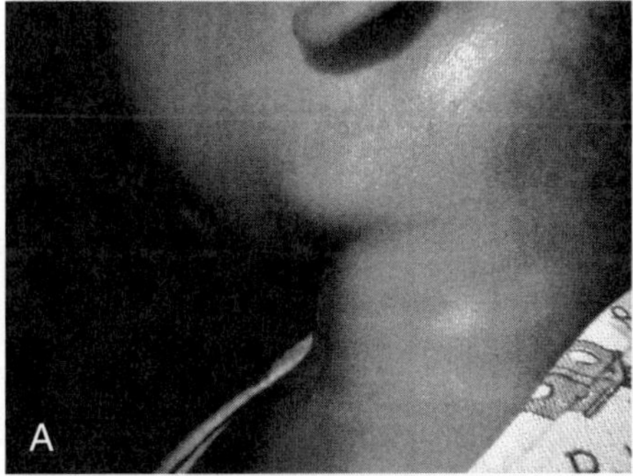

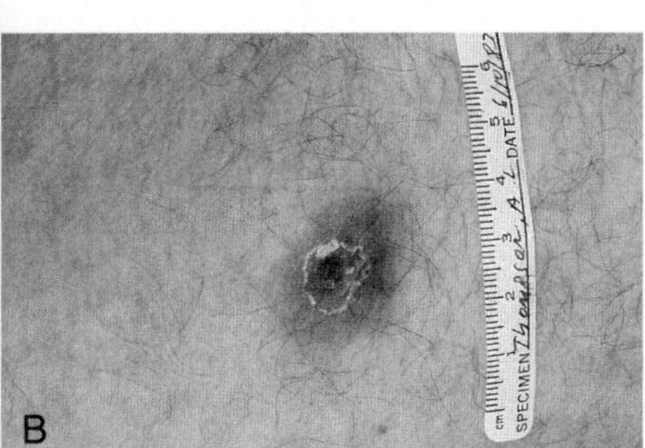

FIGURE 1-349 Examples of primary lesions seen in ulceroglandular tularemia. A, Large cervical and submandibular lymph nodes in a young child; an ulcer was found under the hairline on her forehead at the site of a tick bite. **B,** Papule undergoing central necrosis with desquamation on the thigh of a middle-aged man. (**A** Courtesy of Dr. Joseph A. Bocchini, Louisiana State University Health Sciences Center, Shreveport, LA. **B** From Mandell GL, Bennett JE, Dolin R: *Principles and practice of infectious diseases,* ed 6, Philadelphia, 2005, Elsevier.)

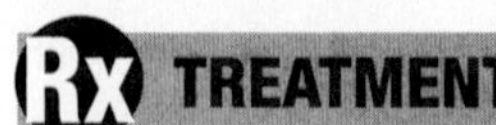

ACUTE GENERAL Rx

- Immediate therapy to limit extent of acute illness and complication
- Streptomycin 10 mg/kg IM q12h (daily dose should not exceed 2 g) or gentamicin 3 to 5 mg/kg/day in 2 or 3 divided doses.
- Tetracycline 500 mg PO qid or doxycycline 100 mg PO bid or chloramphenicol 25 to 50 mg/kg q6h (do not exceed 6 g).
- Quinolones offer new options for the treatment of tularemia.
- Combination antibiotics required for tularemic meningitis—chloramphenicol plus streptomycin.
- Surgical therapies are limited to drainage of abscessed lymph nodes and chest tube drainage of empyemas.

PROGNOSIS

The mortality rate of severe untreated infection (tularemic pneumonia and typhoidal tularemia) can be as high as 30%. Overall mortality associated with tularemia is 2% to 4% with appropriate treatment. Lifelong immunity usually follows tularemia.

DISPOSITION

Follow-up as outpatient

PREVENTION

- Educate the public to prevent sick or dead animals.
- Use insect repellants.
- Remove ticks promptly.
- Drink only potable water.
- Adequately cook wild meats.
- Tularemia vaccine has been developed but is not commercially available in the U.S.; however, it is available from the Centers for Disease Control and Prevention (CDC). Vaccination of high-risk individuals working with large quantities of cultured organism is recommended.
- Avoid skinning wild animals, especially rabbits; wear gloves while handling animal carcasses.
- Do not use wells or other water that is contaminated by dead animals.
- Hospitalized patients with tularemia do not need special isolation (no person to person transmission). Standard universal precautions for contaminated secretion are adequate when handling drainage from wounds.
- Laboratory personnel should be notified of potential danger of growing this organism in the laboratory and generation of an infectious aerosol from dried culture media.

REFERRAL

- For consultation with infectious diseases specialist in suspected cases.
- A cluster of tularemia cases, particularly in an urban area or nonendemic regions, should prompt concern over the possibility of bioterrorism; the local public health authorities should be contacted immediately to investigate the possibility of deliberate release of tularemia as a weapon of terror.

PEARLS & CONSIDERATIONS

- Alert the microbiology laboratory to the possibility of tularemia; this is a major biohazard in the laboratory.
- Do not use doxycycline or tetracycline in children or pregnant women.
- Because of its highly contagious nature with low inoculums, tularemia is considered an agent that could be used by terrorists. It is classified as a category A critical biologic agent by the CDC.

SUGGESTED READINGS

Centers for Disease Control and Prevention: Tularemia transmitted by insect bites—Wyoming, 2001-2003, *MMWR Morb Mortal Wkly Rep* 54(7):170, 2005.

Daya M, Nakamura Y: Pulmonary disease from biological agents: anthrax, plague, Q fever, and tularemia, *Crit Care Clin* 21(4):747-763, 2005.

Feldman KA et al: An outbreak of primary pneumonic tularemia on Martha's Vineyard, *N Engl J Med* 345(22):1601-1606, 2001.

McMurry JA et al: Tularemia vaccines, an overview, Medicine & Health, Rhode Island, 90:311, 2007.

Schmitt P et al: A novel screening ELISA and a confirmatory Western blot useful for diagnosis and epidemiological studies of tularemia, *Epidemiol Infect* 133(4):759-766, 2005.

Staples JE et al: Epidemiologic and molecular analysis of human tularemia, United States, 1964-2004, *Emerg Infect Dis* 12(7):1113, 2006.

AUTHORS: **STEVEN M. OPAL, M.D., GLENN G. FORT, M.D., M.P.H.,** and **DENNIS J. MIKOLICH, M.D.**

BASIC INFORMATION

DEFINITION

Turner's syndrome is a pattern of malformation characterized by short stature, ovarian hypofunction, loose nuchal skin, and cubitus valgus, as described by Turner in 1938. An associated 45,X chromosome constitution was recognized by Ford et al in 1959.

ICD-9CM CODES
758.6 Syndrome, Turner's

EPIDEMIOLOGY & DEMOGRAPHICS

One case in every 2500 to 5000 live female births

PHYSICAL FINDINGS & CLINICAL PRESENTATION

- Turner's phenotype is recognizable at any point on the developmental spectrum.
- In spontaneous abortions it is the most common sex chromosome abnormality detected (45,X chromosome constitution) and accounts for 20% of such cases.
- In fetuses, it is suspected with ultrasonographic manifestations such as thickening of the nuchal folds, frank nuchal cystic hygromas, or mild shortness of the femur at midtrimester.
- In infants:
  1. At birth may display loose nuchal skin (pterygium colli) and edema on the dorsa of hands and feet
  2. Canthal folds reflecting midface hypoplasia and redundant skin in the periorbital region
  3. Nipples appearing widely spaced
  4. Heart and cardiovascular system: murmur of aortic stenosis or bicuspid aortic valve or diminished femoral pulses suggestive of aortic coarctation
  5. Renal ultrasonography: renal ectopia such as pelvic kidney or horseshoe kidneys
- In older children:
  1. Slow linear growth
  2. Short stature: may be improved with growth hormone therapy (Fig. 1-350)
  3. Delayed or absent menses: secondary sex characteristics possibly normalized with estrogen replacement therapy
  4. Intelligence is often normal, but delays in spatial perception or visual-motor integration are commonly observed; frank mental retardation is rare

ETIOLOGY

- Phenotype caused by absence of the second sex chromosome, whether X or Y
- 45,X chromosome constitution in approximately 50% of affected individuals
- Other chromosome aberrations (40% of cases): isochromosome Xq (46,X,i[Xq]) or mosaicism (XX/X)
- With deletions involving the short (or "p") arm of the X chromosome: short stature but little ovarian hypofunction
- Deletions involving Xq13-q27: ovarian failure
- Usually a deficiency of paternal contribution of sex chromosome, reflecting paternal nondisjunction

Dx DIAGNOSIS

DIFFERENTIAL DIAGNOSIS

- Noonan syndrome, an autosomally dominant inherited disorder also characterized by loose nuchal skin, midface hypoplasia, canthal folds, and stenotic cardiac valvular defects and affecting males and females equally; also have normal chromosome constitutions
- Other conditions in the differential diagnosis of loose skin, whether or not associated with edema:
  1. Fetal hydantoin syndrome (loose nuchal skin, midface hypoplasia, distal digital hypoplasia)
  2. Disorders of chromosome constitution (trisomy 21, tetrasomy 12p mosaicism)
  3. Congenital lymphedema (Milroy edema)

WORKUP

- Giemsa banded karyotype to confirm clinical diagnosis
- Once diagnosis is established: cardiologic consultation for evaluation for cardiac valvular abnormalities or aortic coarctation
- Renal ultrasonography
- Endocrine evaluations in older patients with short stature or amenorrhea
- Psychometrics to document known or suspected learning disabilities

LABORATORY TESTS

- As noted, routine Giemsa banded karyotype on peripheral lymphocytes to confirm the clinical impression in all suspected cases of Turner's syndrome
- Important to exclude the presence of Y chromosome in mosaics
- Recognition of associated medical problems, such as hypergonadotropic hypogonadism or autoimmune thyroiditis, prompting periodic evaluation of these potential areas

IMAGING STUDIES

- Echocardiogram
- Renal ultrasonography
- Abdominal ultrasonography for evaluation of ovarian and uterine size and morphology
- MRI of brain (especially in cases with known or suspected neurologic impairment)

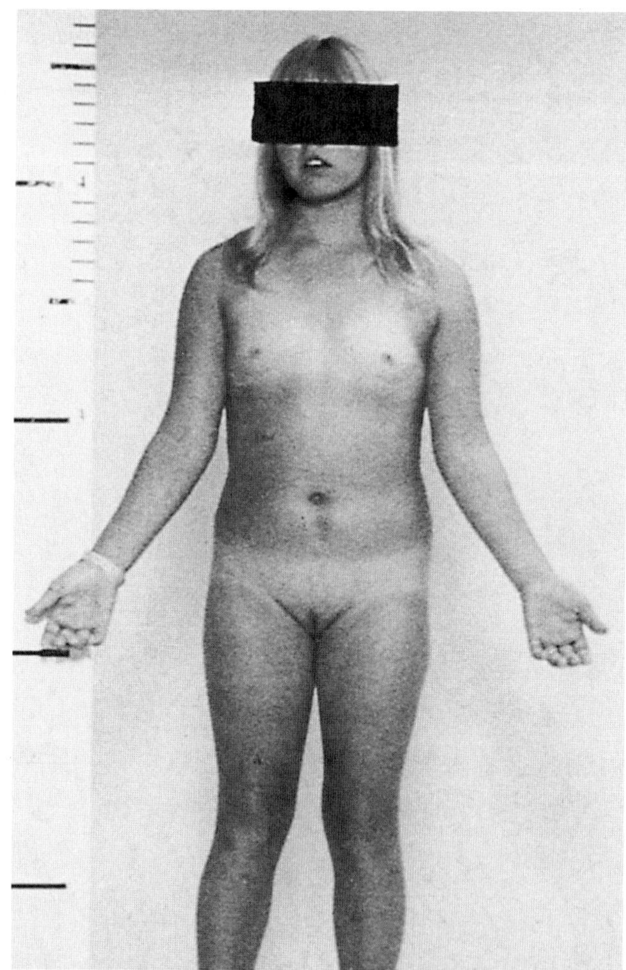

FIGURE 1-350 A 17-year-old patient with Turner's syndrome, demonstrating short stature, poor sexual development, and increased carrying angles at elbows. Patient also has webbing of the neck. (From Mishell D [ed]: *Comprehensive gynecology,* ed 3, St Louis, 1997, Mosby.)

- Radiographs (for evaluation of carpal/metacarpal abnormalities, radioulnar synostosis)
- Bone age (for evaluation of short stature)

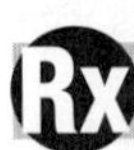

TREATMENT

Recognition of the multisystem involvement of Turner's syndrome necessitates multiple medical specialists working in concert with the primary care provider to maximize and improve outcome while minimizing unnecessary or redundant testing.

NONPHARMACOLOGIC THERAPY

General medical care guided by normal medical standards with special attention paid to identifying such age-related problems as developmental delays, learning disabilities, slow growth, or amenorrhea.

ACUTE GENERAL Rx

Specific treatment geared to the specific medical problem (e.g., cardiac or renal dysfunction)

CHRONIC Rx

- Estrogen-replacement therapy in early adolescence
- Some benefit from recombinant human growth hormone therapy

REFERRAL

- To geneticist: clinical diagnosis, differential diagnosis, recurrence risk counseling, cytogenetic tests
- To endocrinologist (pediatric): evaluation of short stature, estrogen or growth hormone replacement therapy
- To cardiologist: for cardiac valvular abnormalities or aortic coarctation

PEARLS & CONSIDERATIONS

COMMENTS

- Although newer studies are optimistic regarding outcomes, previous reports suffered from retrospective observations, case reports, and ascertainment bias, contributing to a generally poor interaction between physician and patient.
- Affected individuals and families often benefit from the contemporary experiences and expertise of members of genetic support groups. The Turner Syndrome Society of the United States (800-365-9944; http://www.turnersyndrome.org) and the Alliance of Genetic Support Groups (800-336-4363 or 202-966-5557; http://geneticalliance.org) are valuable resources.
- A Turner syndrome diagnosis should be considered in all girls with short stature or primary amenorrhea.
- Almost all women with Turner syndrome are infertile, although some conceive with assisted reproduction.

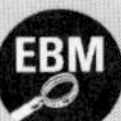

EVIDENCE

Data suggests that treatment with recombinant growth hormone improves short-term growth and final adult height in girls with Turner syndrome.

A Cochrane systematic review identified four RCTs (involving 365 patients) that compared recombinant human growth hormone (hGH) vs placebo/no treatment in children and adolescents with Turner syndrome. In all trials, hGH treatment was initiated prior to the patients reaching final adult height.[1] Ⓐ

The review found that hGH (at doses between 0.3 and 0.375 mg/kg/wk) increases short-term growth in girls with Turner syndrome by approx. 3 cm in the first year of treatment (and by approx. 2 cm/year after 2 yr). However, the treatment group remained substantially shorter, in terms of final adult height, than the comparative normal population.[1] Ⓐ

Evidence-Based Reference

1. Baxter L et al: Recombinant growth hormone for children and adolescents with Turner syndrome, *Cochrane Database Rev* 1, 2007. Ⓐ

SUGGESTED READINGS

Conniff C: Turner's syndrome, *Adolesc Med* 13(2):359, 2002.

Elsheikh M et al: Turner's syndrome in adulthood, *Endocr Rev* 23(1):120, 2002.

AUTHORS: **LUTHER K. ROBINSON, M.D.,** and **RUBEN ALVERO, M.D.**

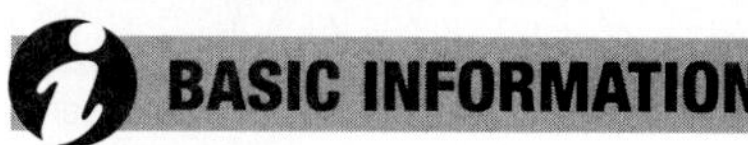

BASIC INFORMATION

DEFINITION

Typhoid fever is a systemic infection caused by *Salmonella typhi.*

SYNONYMS

Typhoid
Enteric fever

ICD-9CM CODES
002.0 Typhoid fever

EPIDEMIOLOGY & DEMOGRAPHICS

INCIDENCE (IN U.S.): Approximately 237 cases of *S. typhi* infections are reported annually in recent surveys. Over three quarters of the cases reported in the U.S. are now associated with foreign travel (most from Asia, Africa, and Central America).

PHYSICAL FINDINGS & CLINICAL PRESENTATION

- Incubation period of a few days to several wk.
- Usual manifestations:
  1. Prolonged fever
  2. Myalgias
  3. Headache
  4. Cough
  5. Sore throat
  6. Malaise
  7. Anorexia, at times with abdominal pain and hepatosplenomegaly
  8. Diarrhea or constipation may occur early in the course of illness
  9. Rose spots, which are faint, maculopapular, blanching lesions, may sometimes be seen on the chest or abdomen
- In the untreated patient, fever may last 1 to 2 mo. The main complication of untreated disease is GI bleeding as a result of perforation from ulceration of Peyer's patches in the ileum. Mental status changes and shock are rare complications. The relapse rate is approximately 10%.

ETIOLOGY

- *Salmonella typhi.*
- *S. paratyphi.*
- *S. typhi* or *S. paratyphi* found only in humans.
- Acquisition of disease by ingestion of food or water contaminated by other humans.
- In the U.S. most cases are acquired either during foreign travel or by ingestion of food prepared by chronic carriers, many of whom acquired the organism outside of the U.S.

Dx DIAGNOSIS

DIFFERENTIAL DIAGNOSIS

- Malaria
- Tuberculosis
- Brucellosis
- Amebic liver abscess

WORKUP

- Blood, stool, and urine cultures are helpful.
- Cultures should be repeated if initially negative.
- Blood cultures are more likely to be positive early in the course of illness.
- Stool and urine cultures are more commonly positive in the second and third wk of illness.
- Bone marrow biopsy cultures are 90% positive, although this procedure is usually not necessary.
- Serology using Widal test is helpful in retrospect, showing a fourfold increase in convalescent titers.

LABORATORY TESTS

- Neutropenia is common.
- Transaminitis is possible.
- Culture:
  1. Blood
  2. Body fluids
  3. Biopsy specimens

Rx TREATMENT

ACUTE GENERAL Rx

- Ciprofloxacin 500 mg PO bid or 400 mg IV bid for 14 days
- Ceftriaxone 2 g IV qd for 14 days
- If organism sensitive
  1. SMX/TMP, 1 to 2 DS tabs PO bid *or*
  2. Amoxicillin, 2 g PO q8h to complete 14 days
- Dexamethasone, 3 mg/kg IV initially, followed by 1 mg/kg IV q6h for 8 doses for patients with septic shock or mental status changes

CHRONIC Rx

- Carrier states possible
- More common in age >60 yr and in people with gallstones
- Usual site of colonization: gallbladder
- Treatment in those with persistently positive stool cultures and in food handlers
- Suggested regimens for eradication of carrier state
  1. Ciprofloxacin 500 mg PO bid for 4 wk
  2. SMX/TMP 1 to 2 tabs PO bid for 6 wk (if susceptible)
  3. Amoxicillin, 2 g PO q8h for 6 wk (if susceptible)
- Cholecystectomy possibly required in carriers with gallstones who fail medical therapy

DISPOSITION

- Treated patients usually respond to therapy, with a small percentage becoming chronic carriers.
- The relapse rate is approximately 10%.
- Untreated patients may have serious complications.

REFERRAL

- Failure of therapy
- Chronic carrier

PEARLS & CONSIDERATIONS

COMMENTS

- Oral and parenteral vaccines are available for travelers to areas of high risk.
- Vaccines are about 70% effective and well tolerated but are infrequently used.
- Immunity wanes after several yr.
- Parenteral preparations are accompanied by frequent side effects:
  1. Pain at injection site
  2. Fever
  3. Malaise
  4. Headaches
- Infection with antimicrobial-resistant *S. typhi* strains among U.S. patients with typhoid fever is associated with travel to the Indian subcontinent, and an increasing proportion of these infections are due to *S. typhi* strains with decreased susceptibility to fluoroquinolones.

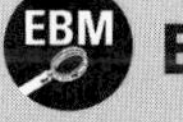

EVIDENCE

Antimicrobial resistance has increased and a quinolone or a third-generation cephalosporin may be the best choice for empiric therapy of typhoid. Regrettably, resistance to the fluoroquinolones is now increasing in *S. typhi* isolates.

In a randomized controlled trial (RCT), 20 patients with blood culture–positive typhoid fever were openly randomized to receive ciprofloxacin and 22 to receive ceftriaxone. Six patients in the ceftriaxone group but none in the ciprofloxacin group had an outcome classed as treatment failure. All six in the ceftriaxone group who experienced treatment failure were switched to ciprofloxacin and became afebrile and asymptomatic within 48 hr.[1] B

In an RCT of a 10-day compared with a 14-day regimen of ciprofloxacin in 69 patients with enteric fever, 52.2% of whom had infection with multidrug-resistant strains of *Salmonella typhi* or *S. paratyphi,* a 100% cure rate was observed for both regimens. Relapse occurred in two patients (on the 14-day regimen).[2] B

In an RCT, 64 patients with positive blood or stool cultures for *Salmonella typhi* or *S. paratyphi* were randomized to receive azithromycin (36) or ciprofloxacin (28). Twenty-one patients had multidrug-resistant infection (to ampicillin, chloramphenicol, and trimethoprim-sulfamethoxazole). All patients in both groups improved and were cured.[3] B

Of 64 children with uncomplicated typhoid fever and blood cultures positive for *S. typhi,* all susceptible to azithromycin and ceftriaxone, 31 of 34 treated with azithromycin and 29 of 30 treated with ceftriaxone were cured.[4] B

Vaccination is recommended when traveling in high-risk endemic areas. The World Health Organization and the CDC recommend vaccination when traveling to areas where typhoid fever is endemic.[5] Ⓒ A systematic review of 17 studies involving nearly 2 million people found that the older whole-cell vaccines produced more prolonged protection than either the Ty21a or Vi vaccine but were associated with higher toxicity.[6] Ⓐ

Evidence-Based References

1. Wallace MR et al: Ciprofloxacin versus ceftriaxone in the treatment of multiresistant typhoid fever, *Eur J Clin Microbiol Infect Dis* 12:907, 1993. Ⓑ
2. Alam MN et al: Efficacy of ciprofloxacin in enteric fever: comparison of treatment duration in sensitive and multidrug-resistant *Salmonella, Am J Trop Med Hyg* 53:306, 1995. Ⓑ
3. Girgis NI et al: Azithromycin versus ciprofloxacin for treatment of uncomplicated typhoid fever in a randomized trial in Egypt that included patients with multidrug resistance, *Antimicrob Agents Chemother* 43:1441, 1999. Ⓑ
4. Frenck RW Jr et al: Azithromycin versus ceftriaxone for the treatment of uncomplicated typhoid fever in children, *Clin Infect Dis* 31:1134, 2000. Ⓑ
5. Centers for Disease Control and Prevention: Typhoid immunization: recommendations of the Advisory Committee on Immunization Practices, *MMWR Recomm Rep* 43(RR-14):1, 1994. Ⓒ
6. Engels EA, Lau J: Vaccines for preventing typhoid fever, *Cochrane Database Syst Rev* 4, 1998. Ⓐ

SUGGESTED READINGS

Bhan MK et al: Typhoid and paratyphoid fever, *Lancet* 366:749, 2005.

Connor BA, Schwartz E: Typhoid and paratyphoid fever in travelers, *Lancet Infect Dis* 5(10):623, 2005.

House D et al: Use of paired serum samples for serodiagnosis of typhoid fever, *J Clin Microbiol* 43(9): 4889, 2005.

Huang DB, DuPont HL: Problem pathogens: extra-intestinal complications of *Salmonella enterica* serotype Typhi infection, *Lancet Infect Dis* 5(6):341, 2005.

Kadhiravan T et al: Clinical outcomes in typhoid fever: adverse impact of infection with nalidixic acid-resistant *Salmonella typhi, BMC Infect Dis* 5(1):37, 2005.

Lynch MF et al: Typhoid fever in the United States, 1999-2006, *JAMA* 302(8):859-865, 2009.

Steinberg EB et al: Typhoid fever in travelers: who should be targeted for prevention? *Clin Infect Dis* 39(2):186, 2004.

Vollaard AM et al: Helicobacter pylori infection and typhoid fever in Jakarta, Indonesia, *Epidemiol Infect* 134(1):163, 2006.

AUTHORS: **STEVEN M. OPAL, M.D., GLENN G. FORT, M.D., M.P.H.,** and **DENNIS J. MIKOLICH, M.D.**

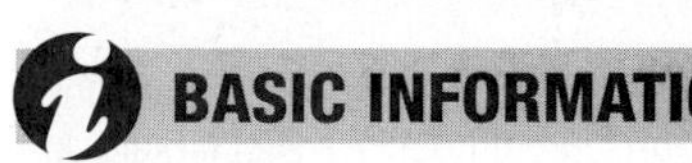

BASIC INFORMATION

DEFINITION

Ulcerative colitis is a chronic inflammatory bowel disease of undetermined etiology.

SYNONYMS

Inflammatory bowel disease (IBD)
Idiopathic proctocolitis

ICD-9CM CODES

556.9 Ulcerative colitis

EPIDEMIOLOGY & DEMOGRAPHICS

INCIDENCE:

- 50 to 150 cases per 100,000 persons; most common between ages 15 and 40 yr, with a second peak between 50 and 80 yr. The disease affects men and women at similar rates.
- Appendectomy for an inflammatory condition (appendicitis or lymphadenitis) but not for nonspecific abdominal pain is associated with a low risk of subsequent ulcerative colitis. This inverse relation is limited to patients who undergo surgery before age 20 yr.

PHYSICAL FINDINGS & CLINICAL PRESENTATION

- Patients with ulcerative colitis often present with bloody diarrhea accompanied by tenesmus, fever, dehydration, weight loss, anorexia, nausea, and abdominal pain.
- Abdominal distention and tenderness.
- Bloody diarrhea.
- Fever, evidence of dehydration.
- Evidence of extraintestinal manifestations may be present in nearly 25% of patients: liver disease, sclerosing cholangitis, iritis, uveitis, episcleritis, arthritis, erythema nodosum, pyoderma gangrenosum, aphthous stomatitis.

Dx DIAGNOSIS

DIFFERENTIAL DIAGNOSIS

- Crohn's disease
- Bacterial infections
  1. Acute: *Campylobacter, Yersinia, Salmonella, Shigella, Chlamydia, Escherichia coli, Clostridium difficile,* gonococcal proctitis
  2. Chronic: Whipple's disease, tuberculosis, enterocolitis
- Irritable bowel syndrome
- Protozoal and parasitic infections (amebiasis, giardiasis, cryptosporidiosis)
- Neoplasm (intestinal lymphoma, carcinoma of colon)
- Ischemic bowel disease
- Diverticulitis
- Celiac sprue, collagenous colitis, radiation enteritis, endometriosis, gay bowel syndrome

WORKUP

Diagnostic workup includes:

- Comprehensive history, physical examination
- Laboratory tests (see below)
- Colonoscopy to establish the presence of mucosal inflammation; typical endoscopic findings in ulcerative colitis are friable mucosa; diffuse, uniform erythema replacing the usual mucosal vascular pattern; and pseudopolyps. Rectal involvement is invariably present if the disease is active.

LABORATORY TESTS

- Anemia and high erythrocyte sedimentation rate (in severe colitis) are common.
- Potassium, magnesium, calcium, and albumin may be decreased.
- Stool examinations for ova and parasites, stool culture, and testing for *Clostridium difficile* toxin may be useful to eliminate other causes of chronic diarrhea.
- Antineutrophil cytoplasmic antibodies (ANCA) with a perinuclear staining pattern (pANCA) can be found in >45% of patients; there is an increased frequency in treatment-resistant left-sided colitis, suggesting a possible association between these antibodies and a relative resistance to medical therapy in patients with ulcerative colitis.

IMAGING STUDIES

Image studies are generally not indicated. A double-contrast barium enema and small-bowel follow-through, when used (in cases in which colonic strictures prevent a thorough evaluation), may reveal continuous involvement (including the rectum), pseudopolyps, decreased mucosal pattern, and fine superficial ulcerations.

Rx TREATMENT

NONPHARMACOLOGIC THERAPY

- Correct nutritional deficiencies; total parenteral nutrition with bowel rest may be necessary in severe cases. Folate supplementation may reduce the incidence of dysplasia and cancer in chronic ulcerative colitis.
- Avoid oral feedings during acute exacerbation to decrease colonic activity; a low-roughage diet may be helpful in *early* relapse.
- Psychotherapy is useful in most patients. Referral to self-help groups is also important because of the chronicity of the disease and the young age of the patients.

ACUTE GENERAL Rx

The therapeutic options vary with the degree of disease (mild, severe, fulminant) and areas of involvement (distal, extensive).

- Mild or moderate disease can be treated with mesalamine. It can be administered as an enema (40 mg once daily at bedtime for 3 to 6 wk) or suppository (500 mg bid) for patients with distal colonic disease. Oral forms in which the 5-acetyl salicylic acid is in a slow-release or pH-dependent matrix (Pentasa 1 g qid, Asacol 800 mg PO tid) can deliver therapeutic concentrations to the more proximal small bowel or distal ileum.
- Olsalazine can be useful for maintenance of remission of ulcerative colitis in patients intolerant to sulfasalazine. Usual dose is 500 mg bid taken with food.
- Balsalazide is indicated for mild to moderately active ulcerative colitis. Usual dose is three 750-mg capsules tid.
- Severe disease usually responds to oral corticosteroids (e.g., prednisone 40 to 60 mg/day); corticosteroid suppositories or enemas are also useful for distal colitis.
- Infliximab, a chimeric monoclonal antibody, has been shown to be effective in patients who have not responded to corticosteroid therapy.
- Fulminant disease generally requires hospital admission and parenteral corticosteroids (e.g., IV hydrocortisone 100 mg q6h). When bowel movements have returned to normal and the patient is able to eat normally, oral prednisone is resumed. IV cyclosporine can also be used in severe refractory cases; renal toxicity is a potential complication.
- Surgery is indicated in patients who do not respond to intensive medical therapy. Colectomy is usually curative in these patients and also eliminates the high risk of developing adenocarcinoma of the colon (10% to 20% of patients develop it after 10 yr with the disease); newer surgical techniques allow preservation of the sphincter.

CHRONIC Rx

- Colonoscopic surveillance and multiple biopsies should be instituted approximately 10 yr after diagnosis because of the increased risk of colon carcinoma.
- Erythropoietin is useful in patients with anemia refractory to treatment with iron and vitamins.
- In patients on long-term steroid therapy, periodic bone density scans are recommended to screen for glucocorticoid-induced osteoporosis.

DISPOSITION

The clinical course is variable. Approximately 66% of patients will achieve clinical remission with medical therapy, and nearly 80% of treatment compliant patients maintain remission. From 15% to 20% of patients eventually require colectomy; >75% of patients treated medically will experience relapse.

REFERRAL

- Gastrointestinal consultation for initial diagnostic sigmoidoscopy/colonoscopy in suspected cases
- Surgical referral for patients with severe disease unresponsive to medical therapy

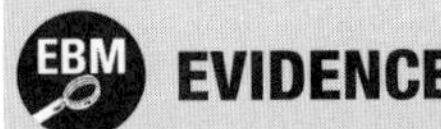

EVIDENCE

Please note: Complete text of EBM for this topic is available online.

Key trials and commentary:

In patients with severe attacks of ulcerative colitis (UC), IV steroids represent the first-line treatment, leading to clinical improvement in approximately 50% to 60% of patients. The aim of this study was to prospectively compare the efficacy and safety of different modalities of steroid administration, and to evaluate predictors of failure to therapy.

This study showed that in severe attacks of UC, 6-methylprednisolone given as a continuous infusion was no better than bolus administration in terms of efficacy and safety.

Approximately 15% of individuals present with a severe attack of UC during the course of their disease. IV corticosteroids represent the mainstay of therapy for this population of patients with severe UC. For severe attacks of UC, the optimal daily dose and route of steroid administration has not been formally investigated; however, most clinicians use an IV bolus of corticosteroids (hydrocortisone, methylprednisolone, and betamethasone). To date, a single controlled trial comparing a dosage of 40 mg of oral prednisone given either once daily or 10 mg four times a day in patients with active ulcerative colitis has been published. Similar rates of adverse events were found in the two groups, with a trend toward a higher frequency of hypertension in the multiple dosing group ($P = 0.059$). There has been no study to date that has evaluated a potential difference in adverse events between intravenously infused steroids delivered in a continuous fashion vs. those delivered in a bolus fashion. The aim of the study was, thus, to prospectively compare efficacy and safety of different modalities of steroid administration and to evaluate predictors of failure to medical therapy. The center was a single-center study treating patients with 6-methylprednisolone, either bolus or continuous infusion, using 1 mg/kg/day. A small number of patients, 36 in total, 15 of whom were in their first attack of UC; 50% of patients in the bolus injection group, and 50% in the continuous infusion group entered remission. 31 patients eventually underwent colectomy, 12 of 32 patients in the bolus injection group, and 9 of 34 patients in the continuous-infusion group. 28 patients had steroid-related adverse events, 15 were in the bolus injection group, and 13 were in the continuous-infusion group. The differences between these groups were not statistically significant. The use of steroids and active smoking did confer an independent prediction of nonresponse in this study. The authors thus concluded that for severe attacks of UC, methylprednisolone given as a continuous infusion was no better than bolus administration in terms of efficacy and safety. It should be pointed out that the size of a study that is attempting to show a difference in treatment with similar treatments as such would likely require several hundred patients; hence, this study is grossly underpowered. The terminology the authors use when stating that one therapy was no better than the other is inaccurate. The overall "take home message" that can be suggested from this particular study is that this represents a pilot study at best.

The authors are to be congratulated, however, on performing the first randomized trial directly comparing bolus vs. continuous infusion of methylprednisolone during a severe phase of the disease; however, from a pharmacokinetic standpoint, it remains uncertain whether this is a necessary study to perform directly given the pharmacokinetics of corticosteroids. The authors do relate that the study was not designed to demonstrate equivalency of the two treatment modalities. A sample size of 2500 subjects would be needed. They do, however, suggest that the easier modality, bolus injection, could be preferable. I would caution that such a conclusion cannot be reached based on this grossly underpowered study and until a prospective study is performed of adequate size, one can use either continuous infusion or bolus infusion. The study does not answer the question as to which is best for the patient.[1] Ⓐ

This study sought to determine the therapeutic equivalence and safety of once daily (OD) versus three times daily (TID) dosing of a total daily dose of 3g Salofalk (mesalazine) granules in patients with active ulcerative colitis.

This study showed that OD 3 g mesalazine granules are as effective and safe as a TID 1g schedule. With respect to the best possible adherence of patients to the treatment, OD dosing of mesalazine should be the preferred application mode in active UC.

This study shows once daily mesalazine (Salofalk) is equivalent to dosing three times daily for the management of acute UC. This is a very well done noninferiority trial that was adequately powered. Although Salofalk is not available in the U.S., the results of this trial are consistent with what has been reported in previous studies of once daily MMX mesalamine confirming efficacy for acute UC. This study did report a better efficacy in the once daily group for distal colitis. It is unclear whether this is clinically important. The once daily regimen was tolerated equally well as the thrice daily. One of the most important considerations of the management of UC is medication compliance. Poor compliance is related to dosing regimen and an important reason for lack of efficacy of mesalamine in UC. Once daily regimens have the best compliance. Current accepted regimens vary from once daily to four times daily therapy. Once daily therapy should be considered in all patients with UC. This will lead to better compliance and better outcomes among patients with UC.[2] Ⓐ

This study was designed to evaluate the accuracy of four different fecal markers in discriminating between irritable bowel syndrome, inflammatory bowel disease, and other forms of colitis and to examine the feasibility of collecting fecal samples in outpatients.

This study showed that IBD-SCAN and PhiCal-Test have the best overall accuracy for detection of colitis, followed by LEUKO-TEST, Hexagon OBTI, C-reactive protein, and blood leukocytes. Accuracy of fecal markers is high even in patients with Crohn's disease in remission. Fecal sampling feasibility was high in outpatients. Because fecal markers are unspecific, endoscopic workup remains crucial to determine the underlying cause of colitis.

Physicians often face difficulty when attempting to differentiate patients who have irritable bowel syndrome from those who have inflammatory bowel disease. The symptoms of these diseases have significant overlap, with frequent occurrence of diarrhea, abdominal pain, and altered bowel function. If a patient is suspected of having irritable bowel syndrome, at least a sigmoidoscopy in younger patients and a colonoscopy for patients over the age of 50 years is suggested. In an effort to avoid these procedures that have been considered somewhat invasive, there has been an attempt to use noninvasive markers that have the potential to differentiate these two gastrointestinal disorders. The standard noninvasive evaluation of intestinal inflammation has been the assessment of a 4-day fecal excretion of indium 111-labelled granulocytes. This, however, is not appropriate to use in clinical practice given that it is an expensive test, exposes the patient to radiation, and mandates sterile handling in a labeling facility.

The authors prospectively evaluated four different tests that evaluate for fecal leukocytes: IBD-SCAN, PhiCal-Test, LEUKO-TEST, and Hexagon OBTI. The accuracy for differentiating irritable bowel syndrome from inflammatory bowel disease was found to be 91%, 89%, 93%, and 92%. Specificity of inflammatory disease, that is, accuracy of differentiating inflammatory bowel disease from other forms of colitis with these fecal markers, was from 43% to 50% and the overall accuracy (in percent) of differentiating Crohn's disease in remission from irritable bowel syndrome was 90%, 90%, 85%, and 77%. When patients were not in remission (CDAI $>$150), the accuracy was $>$95% in all tests.

This study emphasizes that these markers are not specific for inflammatory bowel disease and should thus be used in conjunction with standard diagnostic testing (endoscopy and radiography). Thus, although the goal of the authors was to assess the ability of these noninvasive diagnostic tests to accurately define disease, they were not successful. They did, however, neither assess the accuracy of two or three or even more of these markers

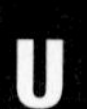

when used together nor the impact of family history on this. Thus, at present we will still need to do endoscopy, radiographic, and microbiologic studies when newly diagnosing a patient with inflammatory bowel disease.[3] Ⓐ

Inflammatory bowel disease (IBD) has a typical onset during the peak reproductive years. Evidence of the risk of adverse pregnancy outcomes in IBD is important for the management of pregnancy to assist in its management.

The aim of this study was to provide a clear assessment of risk of adverse outcomes during pregnancy in women with IBD. The study showed a higher incidence of adverse pregnancy outcomes in patients with IBD. Further studies are required to clarify which women are at higher risk, because this was not determined in the present study. This study's results should affect the management of patients with IBD during pregnancy, who should be treated as a potentially high-risk group.

There is growing concern about adverse pregnancy outcomes in women with IBD. It is uncertain which patients are at risk for adverse outcomes. In an effort to better define risk potential, the Medline literature was searched. In women with IBD, there was a 1.87-fold increase in prematurity compared with controls, a 2.37-fold increased risk of congenital abnormalities, and the incidence of low birth weight was over twice that of normal controls. In this study, women with IBD were more likely to undergo a cesarean section.

The authors of this study are to be congratulated for identifying these increased risks for pregnant women with IBD. However, the study did not identify which patients are likely to develop these problems; this remains to be determined.

It is unlikely that a meta-analysis will help identify which patients with IBD are most at risk for adverse pregnancy outcomes. The authors will need patient level data from studies to identify who will develop these problems. Another approach to this problem is to develop a database, which the Crohn's and Colitis Foundation of America is currently doing.[4] Ⓐ

Evidence-Based References

1. Bossa F et al: Continuous infusion versus bolus administration of steroids in severe attacks of ulcerative colitis: a randomized, double-blind trial, *Am J Gastroenterol* 102:601-608, 2007. Commentary by G.R. Lichtenstein, M.D. Ⓐ
2. Kruis W on behalf of the International Salofalk OD Study Group: Once daily versus three times daily mesalazine granules in active ulcerative colitis: a double-blind, double-dummy, randomised, non-inferiority trial, *Gut* 58:233-240, 2009. Commentary by M.F. Picco, M.D. Ⓐ
3. Schoepfer AM et al: Accuracy of four fecal assays in the diagnosis of colitis, *Dis Colon Rectum* 50:1697-1706, 2007. Commentary by G.R. Lichtenstein, M.D. Ⓐ
4. Cornish J et al: A meta-analysis on the influence of inflammatory bowel disease on pregnancy, *Gut* 56:830-837, 2007. Commentary by G.R. Lichtenstein, M.D. Ⓐ

SUGGESTED READINGS

Abraham C, Cho J: Inflammatory bowel disease, *N Engl J Med* 361:2066-2078, 2009.

Langan RC et al: Ulcerative colitis: diagnosis and treatment, *Am Fam Physician* 76:1323-1330, 2007.

AUTHOR: **FRED F. FERRI, M.D.**

Urethritis, Gonococcal 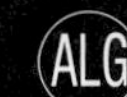

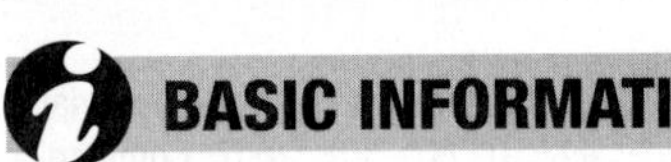

BASIC INFORMATION

DEFINITION

Urethritis is a well-defined clinical syndrome manifested by dysuria, a urethral discharge, or both.

ICD-9CM CODES
597.80 Urethritis, unspecified
098.20 Gonococcal

EPIDEMIOLOGY & DEMOGRAPHICS

- The major single specific etiology of acute urethritis is *Neisseria gonorrhoeae,* producing gonococcal urethritis (GCU). Urethritis of all other etiologies is called *nongonococcal urethritis* (NGU).
- NGU is twice as common as GCU in the U.S. NGU is the most common sexually transmitted disease (STD) syndrome occurring in men, accounting for 6 million office visits annually. NGU is more frequently encountered in higher socioeconomic groups. GCU is more common in homosexual males than heterosexual males with acute urethritis.
- *N. gonorrhoeae* is a gram-negative, kidney-shaped diplococcus with flattened opposed margins. The urethra is the most common site of infection in all men. In heterosexual men, the pharynx is infected in 7%, and in homosexual men the pharynx is infected in 40% and the rectum in 25%. A single episode of intercourse with an infected partner carries a transmission risk of 20% for males; female partners of an infected male will contract the disease 80% of the time.

PHYSICAL FINDINGS & CLINICAL PRESENTATION

- Symptoms of gonococcal urethritis: urethral discharge and dysuria are the most common symptoms. There is complaint of urethral itching. Prostatic involvement can cause frequency, urgency, and nocturia. It can involve the epididymis through spreading down the vas deferens, causing acute epididymitis.
- Incubation period: 3 to 10 days. Without treatment urethritis persists for 3 to 7 wk, with 95% of men becoming asymptomatic after 3 mo. GCU is asymptomatic in up to 60% of contacts.
- Signs of gonococcal urethritis: yellow-brown discharge, meatal edema, urethral tenderness to palpation. Rectal bleeding with pus is seen with gonococcal proctitis. Periurethritis leading to urethral stenosis can occur. Disseminated infection can occur. Tenosynovitis and arthritis can occur. Rarely, hepatitis, myocarditis, endocarditis, and meningitis can occur.

Dx DIAGNOSIS

DIFFERENTIAL DIAGNOSIS

- NGU
- Herpes simplex virus

LABORATORY TESTS

- Calcium alginate or rayon swab on a metal shaft (*not* cotton-tipped swabs, which are bactericidal) of the urethra should be performed anywhere from 2 to 4 hr after voiding to prevent bacterial washout with voiding.
- Cultures of the pharynx and rectum when indicated.
- Gram staining with modified Thayer-Martin media is indicated.
- On examination of the urethral smear, the presence of small numbers of polymorphonuclear cells (PMNs) provides objective evidence of urethritis. The complete absence of PMNs on a urethral smear argues against urethritis. If in addition to the PMNs there are gram-negative, intracellular diplococci, the diagnosis of gonorrhea is established.

Rx TREATMENT

NONPHARMACOLOGIC THERAPY

Behavioral management: avoid intercourse until cure has been attained and sexual partners have been evaluated and treated.

ACUTE GENERAL Rx

- For uncomplicated urethral, cervical, and rectal GCU: Ceftriaxone 125 mg IM + doxycycline 100 mg bid × 7 days. Alternative therapy: ciprofloxacin 500 mg PO × 1 day or ofloxacin 400 mg PO × 1 day (all alternative therapies should be followed by 7 days of doxycycline 100 mg PO bid).
- In uncomplicated gonococcal infections, single-drug regimens using selected fluoroquinolones, selected cephalosporins, or spectinomycin are highly effective and safe.
- Resistance to penicillins, sulfonamides, and tetracyclines is now widespread.
- Dual treatment for gonococcal and chlamydial infections is based on theory and expert opinion rather than evidence from clinical trials.
- For epididymitis: ceftriaxone 250 mg IM followed by doxycycline 100 mg PO bid × 10 days. Alternative therapy: ofloxacin 300 mg PO bid × 10 days.

CHRONIC Rx

Postgonococcal urethritis (PGU): reinfection is the most common cause of recurrence. Repeat swab and culture of the urethra, pharynx, and rectum (where applicable) are mandatory. Persistence of PMNs with the absence of gram-negative intracellular diplococci suggests a diagnosis of postgonococcal urethritis. This occurs when GCU is treated with a regimen that is ineffective against coincident chlamydial infection; it represents NGU after GCU. The syndrome should be treated as NGU. Persistence of *N. gonorrhoeae* by smear or culture requires treatment for *N. gonorrhoeae.*

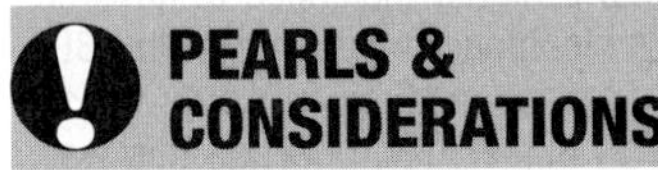

PEARLS & CONSIDERATIONS

COMMENTS

- CAUTION: Tetracyclines and fluoroquinolones are *contraindicated* in pregnancy. *Chlamydia* infection in pregnancy can be treated with amoxicillin 500 mg PO tid for 7 days or with clindamycin 450 mg PO tid for 10 days.
- Posttreatment cultures are required.

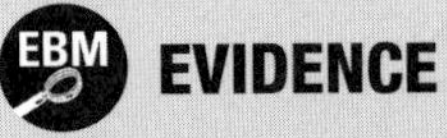

EVIDENCE

A single dose of oral cefixime is as effective as a single intramuscular dose of ceftriaxone in the treatment of genital gonococcal infection.[1] Ⓐ

Single-dose regimens of oral cefuroxime and oral ciprofloxacin are both equally effective in eradicating penicillinase-producing *N. gonorrhea* from males and females with uncomplicated gonorrheal infections.[2] Ⓑ

In the treatment of genital gonococcal infection in pregnancy, amoxicillin plus probenecid, spectinomycin, and ceftriaxone produce similar overall cure rates.[3] Ⓑ

Evidence-Based References

1. Brocklehurst P: Antibiotics for gonorrhoea in pregnancy, *Clin Evid* 11:2104, 2004. Ⓐ
2. Thorpe EM: Comparison of single dose cefuroxime axetil with ciprofloxacin in treatment of uncomplicated gonorrhoea caused by penicillinase producing and non-penicillinase producing *N. gonorrhoeae* strains, *Antimicrob Agents Chemother* 40:2775, 1996. Ⓑ
3. Cavenee M et al: Treatment of gonorrhea in pregnancy, *Am J Obstet Gynecol* 185:629, 2001. Ⓑ

AUTHORS: **PHILIP J. ALIOTTA, M.D., M.S.H.A.,** and **RUBEN ALVERO, M.D.**

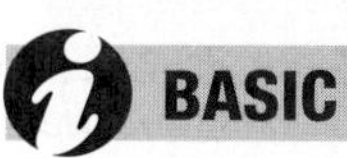

BASIC INFORMATION

DEFINITION

Nongonococcal urethritis (NGU) is urethral inflammation caused by any of several organisms.

SYNONYMS

NGU

ICD-9CM CODES
099.40 Nongonococcal
099.41 Chlamydial

EPIDEMIOLOGY & DEMOGRAPHICS

- Occurrence is 50% in sexually transmitted disease clinics.
- NGU most commonly affects men in a higher socioeconomic class, affecting heterosexual men more frequently than homosexual men.
- NGU carries a greater morbidity rate than gonococcal urethritis (GCU).

PHYSICAL FINDINGS & CLINICAL PRESENTATION

- Incubation period: 2 to 35 days
- Symptoms: dysuria, whitish-clear urethral discharge, and urethral itching. The onset of symptoms in NGU is less acute than GCU.
- Signs: whitish-clear urethral discharge, meatal edema, and erythema. Infected women manifest pyuria, and the disease can present as acute urethral syndrome.

COMPLICATIONS

Epididymitis in heterosexual men may be linked to nonbacterial prostatitis, proctitis in homosexual men, or Reiter's syndrome.

ETIOLOGY

- Most common agent is *Chlamydia* spp., an obligate intracellular parasite possessing both DNA and RNA, which replicates by binary fission. It causes 20% to 50% of NGU cases. Two species exist:
  1. *Chlamydia psittaci*
  2. *Chlamydia trachomatis* with its 15 serotypes
     - Serotypes A through C cause hyperendemic-blinding trachoma.
     - Serotypes D through K cause genital tract infection.
     - Serotypes L1 through L3 cause lymphogranuloma venereum.
- Other causes of NGU: *Ureaplasma urealyticum,* causing 15% to 30% of the cases of NGU; *Trichomonas vaginalis;* and herpes simplex virus. The cause of 20% of the cases of NGU has not been identified.
- Asymptomatic infection occurs in 28% of the contacts of women with chlamydial cervical infection.

Dx DIAGNOSIS

DIFFERENTIAL DIAGNOSIS

- GCU
- Herpes simplex virus
- Trichomoniasis

LABORATORY TESTS

- Requires demonstration of urethritis and exclusion of infection with *N. gonorrhoeae.*
- The appearance of polymorphonuclear cells (PMNs) on urethral smear confirms the diagnosis of urethritis. Because *Chlamydia* is an intracellular parasite of the columnar epithelium, the best specimen for culture is an endourethral swab taken from an area 2 to 4 cm inside the urethra. The organism can only be grown in tissue culture, which is expensive.
- New techniques have been developed and are useful in making the diagnosis: nucleic acid hybridization, enzyme-linked immunosorbent assay, and direct immunofluorescence.
- For culture, a Dacron-tipped swab is used; avoid calcium alginate or cotton swabs.

Rx TREATMENT

Because it is impossible to differentiate among the common etiologies of NGU, the condition is treated syndromically, including in the initial treatment regimen those drugs effective against the common causative agents.

- Recommended: azithromycin 1000 mg as a single dose or doxycycline 100 mg PO bid for 7 days
- Other: tetracycline 500 mg PO qid for 7 days
- Alternative regimens: erythromycin base 500 mg PO qid for 7 days, ofloxacin 300 mg PO bid for 7 days, levofloxacin 500 mg PO daily for 7 days

In pregnant women:

- Both amoxicillin and erythromycin are likely effective in achieving microbiologic cure.
- Clindamycin and erythromycin have a similar effect on cure rates.
- A single dose of azithromycin is more effective in achieving microbiologic cure of *C. trachomatis* than a 7-day course of erythromycin.

In men and nonpregnant women:

- Multiple-dose regimens of tetracyclines and macrolides achieve microbiologic cure in at least 95% of patients.
- Erythromycin daily dose of 2 g is likely beneficial.
- Ciprofloxacin is less effective in the treatment of *C. trachomatis* infection when compared with doxycycline.
- A single dose of azithromycin is as successful at curing *C. trachomatis* as a 7-day course of doxycycline.

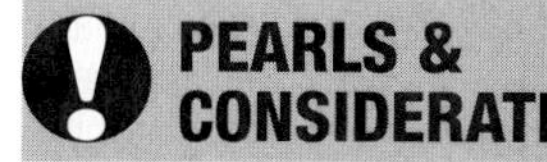

PEARLS & CONSIDERATIONS

COMMENTS

- CAUTION: Tetracyclines and fluoroquinolones are *contraindicated* in pregnancy. *Chlamydia* infection in pregnancy can be treated with amoxicillin 500 mg PO tid for 7 days or with clindamycin 450 mg PO tid for 10 days.
- Posttreatment cultures are required.

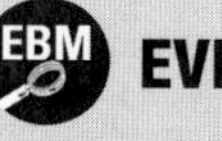

EVIDENCE

Treatment of *Chlamydia trachomatis.*

Both azithromycin 1 g and a 7-day course of doxycycline (100 mg twice daily) produced high clinical cure rates within 2 wk in the treatment of genital chlamydial infection in men and nonpregnant women.[1] Ⓐ

In the treatment of genital chlamydial infection in pregnant women, a single dose of azithromycin 1 g is highly effective and well tolerated, being equally as effective as a 7-day course of amoxicillin and significantly more effective than a 7-day course of erythromycin.[2-4] Ⓐ Ⓑ

Evidence-Based References

1. Lau C-Y, Qureshi AK: Azithromycin versus doxycycline for genital chlamydial infections: a meta-analysis of randomised clinical trials, *Sex Transm Dis* 29:497, 2002. Ⓐ
2. Brocklehurst P, Rooney G: Interventions for treating genital *Chlamydia trachomatis* infection in pregnancy, *Clin Evid* 11:2064, 2004. Ⓑ
3. Jacobson JF et al: A randomized controlled trial comparing amoxicillin and azithromycin for the treatment of *Chlamydia trachomatis* in pregnancy, *Am J Obstet Gynecol* 184:1352, 2001. Ⓐ
4. Kacmar J et al: A randomized trial of azithromycin versus amoxicillin for the treatment of *Chlamydia trachomatis* in pregnancy, *Infect Dis Obstet Gynecol* 9:197, 2001. Ⓐ

AUTHORS: **PHILIP J. ALIOTTA, M.D., M.S.H.A.,** and **RUBEN ALVERO, M.D.**

Urinary Tract Infection (PTG) (ALG)

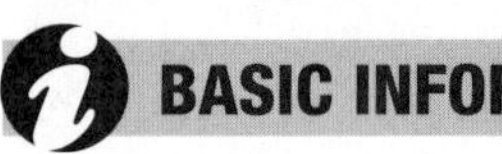

BASIC INFORMATION

DEFINITION

Urinary tract infection (UTI) is a term that encompasses a broad range of clinical entities that have in common a positive urine culture. A conventional threshold is growth of >100,000 colony-forming units per milliliter from a midstream-catch urine sample. In symptomatic patients, a smaller number of bacteria (between 100 and 10,000 colony-forming units per milliliter of midstream urine) is recognized as an infection.

SYNONYMS

UTI

ICD-9CM CODES
595.0 Acute cystitis
595.3 Trigonitis
595.2 Chronic cystitis
590.1 Acute pyelonephritis
590.0 Chronic pyelonephritis
590.8 Nonspecific pyelonephritis

CLASSIFICATION

- First infection: the first documented UTI; tends to be uncomplicated and is easily treated.
- Unresolved bacteriuria: UTI in which the urinary tract is not sterilized during therapy. Main causes are bacterial resistance, patient noncompliance with medication, resistance, mixed bacterial infection, rapid reinfection, azotemia, infected stones, Münchhausen syndrome, and papillary necrosis.
- Bacterial persistence: UTI in which the urine cultures become sterile during therapy, but a persistent source of infection from a site within the urinary tract that was excluded from the high urinary concentrations gives rise to reinfection by the same organism. Causes include infected stone, chronic bacterial prostatitis, atrophic infected kidney, vesicovaginal or enterovesical fistulas, obstructive uropathy, infected pyelocaliceal diverticula, infected ureteral stump after nephrectomy, infected necrotic papillae from papillary necrosis, infected urachal cysts, infected medullary sponge kidney, urethral diverticula, and foreign bodies.
- Reinfection: UTI in which a new infection occurs with new pathogens at variable intervals after a previous infection has been eradicated.
- Relapse: the less common form of recurrent infection; occurs within 2 wk of treatment when the same organism reappears in the same site as the previous infection. Relapsing infections of the urinary tract most commonly occur in pyelonephritis, kidney obstruction from a stone, and prostatitis.

EPIDEMIOLOGY & DEMOGRAPHICS

INCIDENCE:

- In neonates: more common in boys as a result of anatomic abnormalities.
- In preschool children: more common in girls (4.5% vs. 0.5% for boys).
- In adulthood: more common in women, with a 1% to 3% prevalence in nonpregnant women. In pregnancy at 12 wk, the incidence of asymptomatic bacteriuria is similar to nonpregnant women, at 2% to 10%. However, 70% to 80% of women with asymptomatic bacteriuria develop acute pyelonephritis, especially in the second and third trimesters, and have a pyelonephritic recurrence rate of 10%. In adults aged ≥65 yr, at least 10% of men and 20% of women have bacteriuria.

PHYSICAL FINDINGS & CLINICAL PRESENTATION

- UTI presentation is inconsistent and cannot be relied on to diagnose UTI accurately or to localize the site of infection. Patients report:
  1. Urinary frequency, urgency
  2. Dysuria
  3. Urge incontinence
  4. Suprapubic pain
  5. Gross or microscopic hematuria
- When negative cultures are associated with significant pyuria, vaginal discharge, or hematuria, infections with *Chlamydia trachomatis, Neisseria gonorrhoeae,* and *Trichomonas vaginalis* should be considered.
- Acute pyelonephritis presents with fever, flank or abdominal pain, chills, malaise, vomiting, and diarrhea. It is these systemic symptoms that distinguish pyelonephritis from cystitis. Complications of acute pyelonephritis are renal abscess, perinephric abscess, emphysematous pyelonephritis, and pyonephrosis.

ETIOLOGY & PATHOGENESIS

- Four major pathways:
  1. Ascending from the urethra
  2. Lymphatic
  3. Hematogenous
  4. Direct extension from another organ system
- Other risk factors: neurologic diseases, renal failure, diabetes; anatomic abnormalities: bladder outlet obstruction, urethral stricture, vesicoureteral reflux, fistula, urinary diversion, megacystis, infected stones, age, pregnancy, instrumentation, poor patient compliance, poor hygiene, infrequent voiding, diaphragm contraceptives, tampon use, douches, and catheters.
- Catheters: all patients who require a long-term Foley catheter eventually develop significant levels of bacteriuria. Treatment is reserved for individuals who become symptomatic (leukocytosis, fever, chills, malaise, loss of appetite, etc.) Using prophylactic antibiotics to treat patients who have chronic catheters is to be discouraged because of the risk of acquiring bacteria resistant to antibiotic therapy.
- Once bacteria reach the urinary tract, three factors determine whether the infection occurs (Box 1-18). These factors also determine the anatomic level of the UTI:
  1. Virulence of the microorganism
  2. Inoculum size
  3. Adequacy of the host defense mechanisms
- Urinary pathogens: in 95% of UTIs the infecting organism is a member of the Enterobacteriaceae, enterococci, or, in young women, *Staphylococcus saprophyticus.* In contrast, the organisms that commonly colonize the distal urethra and skin of both men and women and the vagina of women are *S. epidermidis,* diphtheroides, lactobacilli, *Gardnerella vaginalis,* and a variety of anaerobes that rarely cause UTI. In general, the isolation of two or more bacterial species from a urine culture signifies a contaminated specimen unless the patient is being managed with an indwelling catheter or urinary diversion or has a chronic complicated infection.
- Defense mechanisms against cystitis: low pH and high osmolarity, mucopolysaccharide glycosaminoglycan protective layer, normal bladder that empties completely and has no incontinence, and the presence of estrogen.

BOX 1-18 Bacterial Factors

1. The size of the inoculum
2. The virulence of the infecting organism:
   a. Virulence factors:
      i. P-fimbriae facilitate the adherence of bacteria to biologic surfaces.
      ii. K-antigens facilitate adherence and protect the organisms from the host-immune response.
      iii. O-antigens are an important source of the systemic reactions, such as fever and shock, that occur with bacterial infections.
      iv. H-antigens are associated with flagella and are related to bacterial locomotion.
      v. Hemolysin may potentiate tissue damage and facilitate local bacterial growth.
      vi. Urease alkalinizes the urine and facilitates stone formation, thus potentiating infection.
   b. Biofilms harbor bacteria on prosthetic devices and may be a source of recurrent infections.
   c. The presence of sialosyl galactosyl globoside on the surface of kidney cells. This compound is a highly powerful receptor for *Escherichia coli* bacteria.
   d. Women with a deficiency in human beta-defensin-1 are at greater risk for urinary tract infection.
3. Adequacy of host defense mechanisms

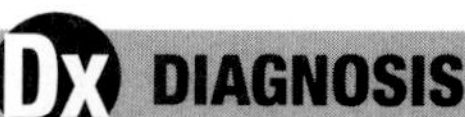

DIAGNOSIS

DIFFERENTIAL DIAGNOSIS

- Interstitial cystitis
- Vaginitis
- Urethritis (gonococcal, nongonococcal, *Trichomonas*)
- Frequency-urgency syndrome, prostatitis (acute and chronic)
- Obstructive uropathy
- Infected stones
- Fistulas
- Papillary necrosis
- Vesicoureteral reflux

LABORATORY TESTS

- Urinalysis with microscopic evaluation of clean-catch urine for bacteria and pyuria
- Urine culture and sensitivity
- Complete blood count with differential (shows leukocytosis)
- Antibody-coated bacteria are seen with pyelonephritis

IMAGING STUDIES

- Warranted only if renal infection or genitourinary abnormality is suspected
- KUB (kidneys, ureter, and bladder); voiding cystourethrogram; renal sonogram; intravenous pyelogram; CT scan; nuclear scan
- Specialty examination: cystoscopy with occasional retrograde pyelography to rule out obstructive uropathy; stenting the obstruction possibly required

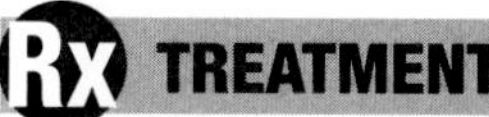

TREATMENT

NONPHARMACOLOGIC THERAPY

- Hot sitz baths, anticholinergics, urinary analgesics
- For pyelonephritis: bed rest, analgesics, antipyretics, and IV hydration

ACUTE GENERAL Rx

- Conventional therapy of 7 days; short-term therapy of 1, 3, or 5 days.
- Agents of choice: amoxicillin/clavulanate, cephalosporins, fluoroquinolones, nitrofurantoin, and trimethoprim plus sulfonamide.
- For pyelonephritis: hospitalization until afebrile and stable, then at home by home care agency with IV antibiotic composed of aminoglycoside plus cephalosporin for 1 wk followed by oral agents (based on sensitivity) for 2 wk. Moderate forms of pyelonephritis have been successfully treated with fluoroquinolone therapy for 21 days without requiring hospitalization. Most important, complicating factors such as obstructive uropathy or infected stones must be identified and treated.
- "Urinary Tract Infection" in Section III describes an approach to the management of UTI.

PEARLS & CONSIDERATIONS

COMMENTS

- Asymptomatic bacteriuria: occurs in both anatomically normal and abnormal urinary tracts. This can clear spontaneously, persist, or lead to symptomatic kidney infection. Treatment is recommended in patients with vesicoureteral reflux, stones, obstructive uropathy, parenchymal renal disease, or diabetes mellitus and in pregnant or immunocompromised patients.
- Pregnancy: 20% to 40% of pregnant women with untreated bacteriuria develop pyelonephritis. This is associated with prematurity and low-birth-weight infants. Confirmed significant bacteriuria should be treated with an aminopenicillin and cephalosporin.
- Recurrent UTI: caused by an unresolved infection, vaginal colonization of the originally infecting organism, or reinfection with a new strain. Management of recurrent UTI includes continuous antibiotic prophylaxis, intermittent self-treatment, and postcoital prophylaxis. Prophylaxis is recommended for women who have two or more symptomatic UTIs over a 6-mo period or three or more episodes over a 12-mo period.
  1. Changes after menopause: lower levels of lactobacilli, decreased estrogen, senile atrophy of the genitalia, and loss of bladder elasticity (compliance).
  2. Biologic factors altering defense systems: the presence of sialosyl galactosyl globoside on the surface of the kidney acts as a powerful receptor for *Escherichia coli* and increases the risk for UTI; the presence of the blood group P1 causes increased binding of *E. coli* that is resistant to normal infection-fighting mechanisms in the body. It is believed that some individuals are deficient in a compound called human beta-defensin-1, a naturally occurring antibiotic that fights *E. coli* within the urinary tract.

RESISTANCE:

- Because of the overuse of antibiotics, organisms once sensitive to a number of antimicrobial agents are now increasingly more resistant, making effective management of UTI and pyelonephritis more difficult and potentially more dangerous. Most important has been the increasing resistance to trimethoprim plus sulfamethoxazole (TMP-SMX), the current primary care provider drug of choice for acute uncomplicated UTI in women.
- When choosing a treatment regimen, physicians should consider such factors as:
  1. In vitro susceptibility
  2. Adverse effects
  3. Cost effectiveness
  4. Resistance rates in their respective communities

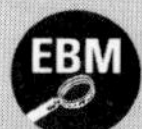

EVIDENCE

There is a general consensus that antibiotics are more effective than placebo in the treatment of active UTI and so it is unlikely that randomized, placebo-controlled trials would now be performed. Most randomized controlled trials that have been carried out are aimed at comparing different antimicrobial agents and different treatment regimens. However, some placebo-controlled trials have been carried out in the context of prophylaxis against recurrent UTI. In problematic cases, choice of antibiotic therapy should be made in consultation with the local microbiology service, which will have knowledge of local organism and resistance patterns.

Adults

Choice and duration of therapy for active UTI:

A systematic review designed to compare the efficacy of 3-day versus 5-day (or longer) courses of antibiotics for the treatment of urinary tract infections in women included 32 trials involving a total of 9605 patients. It found no significant differences in terms of symptomatic failure rates, either in short- or long-term follow-up, between 3-day antibiotic regimens and 5 to 10 day regimens. However, in terms of bacteriological failure rates, 3-day regimens were found to be significantly less effective than 5 to 10 day regimens, particularly at long-term follow-up.[1] Ⓐ

Prophylaxis and prevention of recurrent UTI:

A systematic review found some evidence that, compared with placebo, continuous antibiotic prophylaxis with cephalexin, co-trimoxazole, nitrofurantoin, norfloxacin, or a quinolone for 6 to 12 mo significantly reduced the rate of recurrent urinary tract infection in nonpregnant women during the period of prophylaxis. However, two RCTs identified found no significant difference in recurrence rates at 6 months between placebo and antibiotics after completing prophylaxis. Limited evidence suggested that for sexual intercourse–associated UTI, there was no significant difference between postcoital administration vs continuous daily administration of ciprofloxacin as a means of prophylaxis. The review did not find evidence for any clear benefit of one antibiotic over another for the purpose of prophylaxis.[2] Ⓐ

A systematic review included six trials that evaluated cranberry juice (or cranberry-lingonberry juice) vs. placebo juice or water, and two trials that evaluated cranberry tablets versus placebo. Two of the RCTs, which were of good quality, found cranberry products significantly reduced the incidence of UTIs in adult women at 12 mo, compared to placebo. There was no significant difference in the incidence of UTIs between cranberry juice vs cranberry capsules. Five trials were not included in the meta-analyses due to methodological flaws or lack of available data. Side effects were common in all trials and dropouts from the trials were common.[3] B

Prophylaxis and prevention of recurrent UTI:

A systematic review of long-term antibiotics to reduce recurrent UTI in children included eight studies involving a total of 618 children. Five of the studies, involving a total of 406 children, compared antibiotics versus placebo or no treatment for periods between 10 weeks and 12 mo. Compared to placebo or no treatment, antibiotics significantly reduced the risk of repeat positive urine culture. One study identified reported nitrofurantoin as being significantly more effective than trimethoprim in preventing recurrence over a 6 mo period, although it caused significantly more (mainly gastrointestinal) side effects. Another study reported cefixime as more effective than nitrofurantoin; however, 62% of patients on cefixime experienced an adverse reaction in the first 6 months of treatment, compared with 26% of those on nitrofurantoin.[4] A

Evidence-Based References

1. Milo G et al: Duration of antibacterial treatment for uncomplicated urinary tract infection in women, *Cochrane Database Rev* 2, 2005. A

2. Albert X et al: Antibiotics for preventing recurrent urinary tract infection in non-pregnant women, *Cochrane Database Rev* 3, 2004. B

3. Jepson RG et al: Cranberries for preventing urinary tract infections, *Cochrane Database Rev* 2, 2004. A

4. Williams GJ et al: Long-term antibiotics for preventing recurrent urinary tract infection in children, *Cochrane Database Rev* 3, 2006. A

AUTHORS: **PHILIP J. ALIOTTA, M.D., M.S.H.A.,** and **RUBEN ALVERO, M.D.**

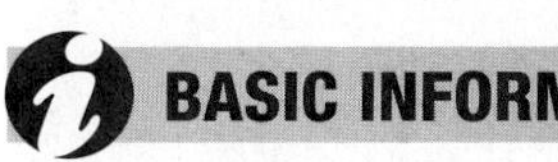

BASIC INFORMATION

DEFINITION

Urolithiasis is the presence of calculi within the urinary tract. The five major types of urinary stones are calcium oxalate (>50%), calcium phosphate (10% to 20%), uric acid (8%), struvite (15%), and cystine (3%).

SYNONYMS

Kidney stones
Renal colic

ICD-9CM CODES

592.9 Urinary calculus

EPIDEMIOLOGY & DEMOGRAPHICS

- Urinary stone disease afflicts 250,000 to 750,000 persons in the U.S. annually.
- The male/female ratio is 4:1; after the sixth decade, it is 1.5:1.
- The incidence of symptomatic nephrolithiasis is greatest during the summer as a result of increased humidity and temperatures with a concomitant increased risk of dehydration and concentrated urine.
- Calcium oxalate or mixed calcium oxalate/calcium phosphate stones account for 70% of uroliths.

PHYSICAL FINDINGS & CLINICAL PRESENTATION

Stones may be asymptomatic, or they may cause the following signs and symptoms as a result of obstruction:

- Sudden onset of flank tenderness
- Nausea and vomiting
- The patient being in constant movement in an attempt to lessen the pain (Patients with an acute abdomen are usually still because movement exacerbates the pain.)
- Pain that is referred to the testes or labium by the progression of stone down the urinary ureter
- Fever and chills that accompany the acute colic if there is superimposed infection
- Pain that may radiate anteriorly over to the abdomen and result in intestinal ileus

ETIOLOGY

- Increased absorption of calcium in the small bowel: type I absorptive hypercalciuria (i.e., independent of calcium intake)
- Idiopathic hypercalciuria nephrolithiasis (This is the most common diagnosis for patients with calcium stones; the diagnosis is made only if there is no hypercalcemia and no known cause of the hypercalciuria.)
- Increased vitamin D synthesis (e.g., as a result of renal phosphate loss: type III absorptive hypercalciuria)
- Renal tubular malfunction with inadequate reabsorption of calcium and resulting hypercalciuria
- Heterozygous mutations in the NPT2a gene that result in hypophosphatemia and urinary phosphate loss
- Hyperparathyroidism with resulting hypercalcemia
- Elevated uric acid level (e.g., metabolic defects, dietary excess)
- Chronic diarrhea (e.g., inflammatory bowel disease) with increased oxalate absorption
- Type I (distal tubule) renal tubular acidosis (<1% of calcium stones)
- Long-term hydrochlorothiazide treatment
- Chronic infections with urease-producing organisms (e.g., *Proteus, Providencia, Pseudomonas, Klebsiella*) (Struvite, or magnesium ammonium phosphate crystals, are produced when the urinary tract is colonized by bacteria, thus producing elevated concentrations of ammonia.)
- Abnormal excretion of cystine
- Chemotherapy for malignancies

Dx DIAGNOSIS

DIFFERENTIAL DIAGNOSIS

- Urinary tract infection
- Pyelonephritis
- Diverticulitis
- Pelvic inflammatory disease
- Ovarian pathology
- Factitious (i.e., in drug addicts)
- Appendicitis
- Small-bowel obstruction
- Ectopic pregnancy

The differential diagnosis of obstructive uropathy is described in Section II.

WORKUP

- Laboratory and imaging studies: Stone analysis should be performed on recovered stones.
- A clinical algorithm for the evaluation of nephrolithiasis is described in Section III.
- Box 1-19 describes events in the medical history that may be significant with regard to urolithiasis.

LABORATORY TESTS

- Urinalysis: Hematuria may be present; however, its absence does not exclude urinary stones. The evaluation of the urinary pH is of value for the identification of the type of stone: a pH of >7.5 is associated with struvite stones, whereas a pH of <5 generally is seen with uric acid or cystine stones). A low serum bicarbonate concentration with a urine pH of ≥6 is suggestive of renal tubular acidosis.
- Urine culture and sensitivity results should be obtained for all patients.
- Serum chemistries should include calcium, electrolytes, phosphate, and uric acid.
- Additional tests: 24-hr urine collection for calcium, uric acid, phosphate, oxalate, and citrate excretion is generally reserved for patients with recurrent stones.

IMAGING STUDIES

- Plain films of the abdomen can identify radiopaque stones (e.g., calcium, uric acid) of ≥5mm in diameter.
- Renal sonogram is generally not sensitive for small stones, but it may be helpful for identifying associated hydronephrosis.
- Unenhanced (noncontrast) helical computed tomography scanning can be used to visualize the calculus, which is identified by the "rim sign" or "halo" that represents the edematous ureteral wall around the stone. The test is fast and accurate (sensitivity, 15% to 100%; specificity, 94% to 96%), and it can be used to readily identify all stone types in all locations. This modality is being used increasingly during the initial assessment of renal colic.
- Intravenous pyelography demonstrates the size and location of the stone as well as the degree of obstruction. However, this modality has largely been replaced by computed tomography.

BOX 1-19 Components of the Medical History That Are Significant for Urolithiasis

- Diseases associated with disturbances of calcium metabolism: primary hyperparathyroidism, Wilson's disease, medullary sponge kidney, osteoporosis, immobilization, sarcoidosis, osteolytic metastases, plasmacytoma, neuroendocrine tumors, Paget's disease
- Dietary history: purine gluttony, calcium excess, milk alkali, oxalate excess, sodium excess, low citrus fruit intake
- Medications: uricosurics, diuretics, analgesics, vitamins C and D, antacids (especially phosphorus-binding agents), acetazolamide, calcium channel blockers, triamterene, theophylline, protease inhibitors (indinavir), sulfonamides
- Diseases associated with disturbances of oxalate metabolism: primary hyperoxaluria types I and II, Crohn's disease, ulcerative colitis, intestinal bypass surgery (especially jejunoileal bypass), ileal resection
- Diseases associated with disturbances of purine metabolism
- Intrinsic metabolic disorders: anemia, neoplastic disorders (especially leukemias), intoxication, myocardial infarction, irradiation, cytotoxic chemotherapy
- Enzyme deficiency: primary gout, Lesch-Nyhan syndrome
- Altered excretion: renal insufficiency, metabolic acidosis
- Infectious history: organisms (particularly *Proteus* and *Klebsiella*), febrile, upper tract involvement, and dates (if hospitalized)

From Nseyo UO (ed): *Urology for primary care physicians,* Philadelphia, 1999, WB Saunders.

TREATMENT

NONPHARMACOLOGIC THERAPY

- An increase in water or other fluid intake is recommended; in fact, a doubling of previous fluid intake should occur unless the patient has a history of congestive heart failure or fluid overload. Generally, patients at increased risk for the development of stones should increase their fluid intake to >2 L/day (68 oz/day) to maintain a urine volume of >2 L/day.
- Normal dietary calcium intake is recommended. If one does not consume enough calcium, less is available to bind to dietary oxalate; as a result, more oxalate reaches the colon, is absorbed into the bloodstream, and excreted as calcium oxalate, thus setting the stage for calcium urolithiasis.
- Sodium restriction to decrease calcium excretion and decreased protein intake to 1 g/kg/day to decrease uric acid, calcium, and oxalate excretion should be considered.
- Increasing the amount of bran in the diet may decrease bowel transit time with an increased binding of calcium and a subsequent decrease in urinary calcium.

ACUTE GENERAL Rx

- Pain control: Ketorolac (60 mg intramuscularly) can be used for moderate pain. However, the use of narcotics is generally indicated because of the severity of pain.
- Specific therapy is tailored to the stone type:
  - Uric acid calculi: control of hyperuricosuria with allopurinol 100 to 300 mg/day; increase urinary pH with potassium citrate 10-mEq tablets tid
  - Calcium stones:
    1. Hydrochlorothiazide 25 to 50 mg qd in patients with type I absorptive hypercalciuria
    2. Decrease bowel absorption of calcium with cellulose phosphate 10 g/day in patients with type I absorptive hypercalciuria
    3. Orthophosphates to inhibit vitamin B synthesis in patients with type III absorptive hypercalciuria
    4. Potassium citrate supplementation for patients with hypocitraturic calcium nephrolithiasis
    5. Purine dietary restrictions or allopurinol for patients with hyperuricosuric calcium nephrolithiasis
  - Struvite stones:
    1. Most of these stones are large and cause obstruction and bleeding.
    2. Extracorporeal shockwave lithotripsy (ESWL) and percutaneous nephrolithotomy are generally necessary.
    3. The prolonged use of antibiotics directed against the predominant urinary tract organism may be beneficial to prevent recurrence.
  - Cystine stones: hydration and alkalization of the urine to pH >6.5; penicillamine and tiopronin can be used to reduce the formation of cystine; captopril is also beneficial and causes fewer side effects
- Possibly useful medications to help with the passage of distal ureteral stones of <10 mm in diameter are tamsulosin (alpha-adrenergic antagonist) and nifedipine (calcium channel blocker used for ureteral dilatation and relaxation). Side effects may include dizziness with tamsulosin and hypotension with nifedipine.
- Administer antibiotics if fever or pyuria (>5 to 20 leukocytes/high-power field) are present.
- Surgical treatment for patients with severe pain that is unresponsive to medication and patients with persistent fever or nausea or significant impediment of urine flow:
  - Ureteroscopic stone extraction
  - ESWL for most renal stones
- In 1997, the American Urological Association issued the following guidelines for the treatment of ureteral stones:
  - Proximal ureteral stones <1 cm in diameter: The options are ESWL, percutaneous nephroureterolithotomy, and ureteroscopy.
  - Proximal ureteral stones >1 cm in diameter: The options are ESWL, percutaneous nephroureterolithotomy, and ureteroscopy. The placement of a ureteral stent should be considered if the stone is causing high-grade obstruction.
  - Distal ureteral stones <1 cm in diameter: Most of these stones pass spontaneously. ESWL and ureteroscopy are two accepted modes of therapy.
  - Distal ureteral stones >1 cm in diameter: The options are watchful waiting, ESWL, and ureteroscopy (after stone fragmentation).

Section III describes an approach to the management of ureteral calculi.

CHRONIC Rx

The maintenance of proper hydration and dietary restrictions (see "Acute General Rx")

DISPOSITION

- >50% of patients will pass the stone within 48 hr.
- Stones will recur in approximately 50% of patients within 5 yr if no medical treatment is provided.

REFERRAL

A urology referral should be undertaken for patients with complicated or recurrent urolithiasis. Most patients with small uncomplicated ureteral or renal calculi can be followed up as outpatients, whereas patients with persistent vomiting, suspected urinary tract infection, pain that is unresponsive to oral analgesics, or obstructing calculus associated with a solitary kidney should be admitted.

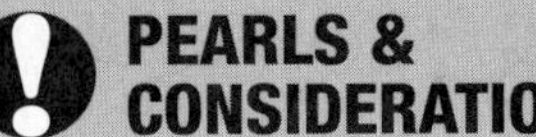

PEARLS & CONSIDERATIONS

COMMENTS

- The early identification and aggressive treatment of urinary tract infections is indicated for all patients with struvite stones.
- The alkalinization of urine (i.e., getting to a pH of >7.5 with the use of penicillamine) is useful for patients with recurrent cystine stones.
- An algorithmic approach to the management of ureteral calculi is described in Section III.

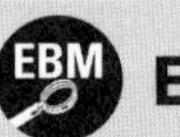

EVIDENCE

There is good evidence that nonsteroidal anti-inflammatory drugs (NSAIDs) and opioids are effective in pain management in patients with renal colic. However, treatment with NSAIDs may be superior to opioids as first-line treatment because these drugs are associated with a lower incidence of vomiting.

A systematic review identified 20 randomized, controlled trials (RCTs) involving 1613 patients comparing NSAIDs and opioids in the treatment of acute renal colic. This review found that both NSAIDs and opioids significantly reduced patient-reported pain scores.[1]

This study also reported that patients treated with NSAIDs were significantly less likely to require rescue medication and had significantly less vomiting than patients treated with opioids (in particular patients treated with pethidine).[1]

There is some evidence that treatment with nifedipine or an alpha-blocker may facilitate stone passage. A meta-analysis of RCTs found that treatment with calcium channel blockers (nifedipine) or alpha-blockers (tamsulosin) significantly increased the passage rate of urinary calculi.[2]

Ureteroscopy is superior to ESWL in achieving ureteric stone removal but is associated with greater morbidity. A systematic review identified six RCTs involving 833 patients that compared ESWL and ureteroscopy with stone retrieval in the treatment of urinary calculi. This review found that although ureteroscopy resulted in a higher stone-free rate, use of ESWL was associated with a lower complication rate and shorter hospital stay.[3]

The use of stenting after ureteroscopy may not benefit clinical outcome and is associated with an increased incidence of urinary tract complications. A systematic review identified nine RCTs involving 832 patients comparing stenting with no stenting after ureteroscopy. Meta-analysis found that use of stenting after ureteroscopy was associated with a significantly higher incidence of subsequent lower urinary tract complications compared with no stenting. In addition, the use of stents did not

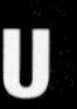

influence need for analgesia, the subsequent stone-free rate, rate of urinary tract infection, or ureteric stricture formation.[4]

Potassium citrate is effective in the prevention of renal calculi recurrence in patients with low rates of urinary citrate excretion. A recent systematic review that identified six RCTs comparing alkali citrate treatment (usually potassium citrate) and control/placebo in patients with nephrolithiasis or urolithiasis found that treatment with alkali citrate resulted in significantly lower rates of stone recurrence and greater rates of stone clearance.[5]

The same review reported on 21 uncontrolled studies involving >1000 patients and reported that treatment with alkali citrate reduced the stone formation rate by 47% to 100%.[5]

Based on consensus opinion, the American Urological Association has made the following recommendations for the management of staghorn calculi of the kidney:

Percutaneous nephrolithotomy should be the first treatment utilized for most patients.

If combination therapy is undertaken, percutaneous nephroscopy should be the last procedure for most patients.

ESWL monotherapy should not be used for most patients; however, if it is undertaken, adequate drainage of the treated renal unit should be established before treatment.

ESWL monotherapy should not be used for patients with staghorn or partial staghorn cystine stones.

ESWL monotherapy or percutaneous-based therapy may be considered for children.

Open surgery (nephrolithotomy by any method) should not be used for most patients.

Nephrectomy should be considered when the involved kidney has negligible function.

Evidence-Based References

1. Holdgate A, Pollock T: Nonsteroidal anti-inflammatory drugs (NSAIDs) versus opioids for acute renal colic, *Cochrane Rev* 1, 2004.

2. Hollingsworth JM et al: Medical therapy to facilitate urinary stone passage: a meta-analysis, *Lancet* 368:1171, 2006.

3. Nabi G et al: Extra-corporeal shock wave lithotripsy (ESWL) versus ureteroscopic management for ureteric calculi, *Cochrane Rev* 1, 2007.

4. Nabi G et al: Outcomes of stenting after uncomplicated ureteroscopy: systematic review and meta-analysis, *BMJ* 334:572, 2007.

5. Mattle D, Hess B: Preventive treatment of nephrolithiasis with alkali citrate: a critical review, *Urol Res* 33:73, 2005.

SUGGESTED READINGS

Borghi L et al: Comparison of two diets for the prevention of recurrent stones in idiopathic hypercalciuria, *N Engl J Med* 346:77, 2002.

Pietrow PK, Karellas ME: Medical management of common urinary calculi, *Am Fam Physician* 74:86, 2006.

Prie D et al: Nephrolithiasis and osteoporosis associated with hypophosphatemia caused by mutations in the type 2a sodium-phosphate cotransporter, *N Engl J Med* 347:983, 2002.

Worster A et al: The accuracy of noncontrast helical computed tomography versus intravenous pyelography in the diagnosis of suspected acute urolithiasis: a meta-analysis, *Ann Intern Med* 40:280, 2002.

AUTHOR: **FRED F. FERRI, M.D.**

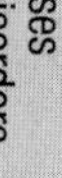

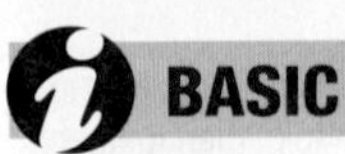

BASIC INFORMATION

DEFINITION

Urticaria is a pruritic rash involving the epidermis and the upper portions of the dermis caused by localized capillary vasodilation and followed by transudation of protein-rich fluid in the surrounding tissue and manifesting clinically with the presence of hives. Urticaria is classified according to its chronicity into acute (<6 wk duration) and chronic (>6 wk duration).

SYNONYMS

Hives
Wheals

ICD-9CM CODES

708.8 Other unspecified urticaria

EPIDEMIOLOGY & DEMOGRAPHICS

- 12% to 24% of the population will have one episode of hives during their lifetime.
- Incidence is increased in atopic patients.
- The etiology of chronic urticaria (hives lasting >6 wk) is determined in only 5% to 20% of cases.

PHYSICAL FINDINGS & CLINICAL PRESENTATION

- Presence of elevated, erythematous, or white nonpitting plaques that change in size and shape over time; they generally last a few hours and disappear without a trace.
- Annular configuration with central pallor (Fig. 1-351).
- Angioedema occurs in approximately 40% of cases of urticaria and is caused by mast cell mediator release in the subcutaneous tissue and deep dermis.

ETIOLOGY

- Foods (e.g., shellfish, eggs, strawberries, nuts)
- Drugs (e.g., penicillin, aspirin, sulfonamides)
- Systemic diseases (e.g., systemic lupus erythematosus, serum sickness, autoimmune thyroid disease, polycythemia vera)
- Food additives (e.g., salicylates, benzoates, sulfites)
- Infections (viral infections, fungal infections, chronic bacterial infections)
- Physical stimuli (e.g., pressure urticaria, exercise-induced, solar urticaria, cold urticaria)
- Inhalants (e.g., mold spores, animal dander, pollens)
- Contact (nonimmunologic) urticaria (e.g., caterpillars, plants)
- Other: hereditary angioedema, urticaria pigmentosa, pregnancy, cryoglobulinemia, hair bleaches, chemicals, saliva, cosmetics, perfumes, pemphigoid, emotional stress, malignancy (lymphomas, endocrine tumors)

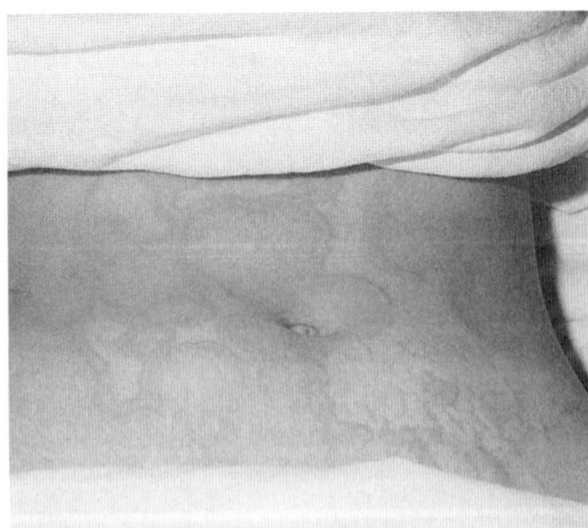

FIGURE 1-351 Wheal (urticaria). Note central cleaning, giving annular configuration. (From Noble J et al: *Textbook of primary care medicine,* ed 3, St Louis, 2001, Mosby.)

DIAGNOSIS

DIFFERENTIAL DIAGNOSIS

- Erythema multiforme
- Erythema marginatum
- Erythema infectiosum
- Urticarial vasculitis
- Herpes gestationis
- Drug eruption
- Multiple insect bites
- Bullous pemphigoid

WORKUP

- It is useful to determine whether hives are acute or chronic; a medical history focused on various etiologic factors is necessary before embarking on extensive laboratory testing.
- Most cases of acute urticaria resolve spontaneously and diagnostic testing is not required.
- A diagnostic approach to chronic urticaria is described in Section III.

LABORATORY TESTS

- Complete blood count with differential.
- Stool for ova and parasites in patients with suspected parasitic infestations.
- Skin testing with allergic extracts and screening for dermatographism by attempting to elicit a wheal after application of linear skin pressure should be performed only after withholding antihistamines for 36 to 72 hr to prevent false-negative results.
- Antinuclear antibody, erythrocyte sedimentation rate, thyroid-stimulating hormone, antithyroid antibodies, *Helicobacter pylori* serology, liver function tests, and eosinophil count are indicated only in patients with chronic urticaria.
- Measurement of C_4 may be helpful in patients who present with angioedema alone.
- Skin biopsy is helpful in patients with fever, arthralgias, and elevated erythrocyte sedimentation rate. Histologic evidence of leukocytoclasia (neutrophilic infiltration with fragmentation of nuclei) is indicative of urticarial vasculitis.
- When suspecting food allergy in acute urticaria, testing can be performed using skin prick, immunoCAP, and radioallergosorbent testing.

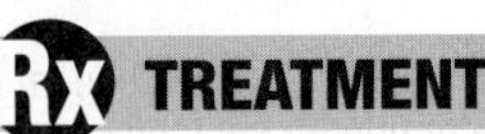

TREATMENT

NONPHARMACOLOGIC THERAPY

- Remove suspected etiologic agents (e.g., stop aspirin and all nonessential drugs), restrict diet (e.g., elimination of tomatoes, nuts, eggs, shellfish).
- Elimination of yeast should be attempted in patients with chronic urticaria (*Candida albicans* sensitivity may be a factor in patients with chronic urticaria).

ACUTE GENERAL Rx

- Oral antihistamines: use of nonsedating antihistamines (e.g., loratadine 10 mg qd, cetirizine 10 mg qd, fexofenadine 180 mg qd, levocetirizine 5 mg qd) is preferred over first-generation antihistamines (e.g., hydroxyzine, diphenhydramine).
- Doxepin (a tricyclic antidepressant) that blocks both H_1 and H_2 receptors 25 to 75 mg qhs may be effective in patients with chronic urticaria.
- Oral corticosteroids should be reserved for refractory cases (e.g., prednisone 20 mg qd or 20 mg bid).
- H_2 receptor antagonists (cimetidine, ranitidine, famotidine) can be added to H_1 antagonists in refractory cases.

CHRONIC Rx

- Use of nonsedating antihistamines, doxepin, and/or oral corticosteroids (see "Acute General Rx")
- Low dose of the immunosuppressant cyclosporine (2.5 to 3 mg/kg body weight/day) has been shown to be effective and corticosteroid sparing in chronic urticaria.
- There are insufficient data to support use of leukotriene antagonists (zafirlukast, montelukast) in patients with chronic urticaria.

DISPOSITION

- Most cases of urticaria resolve within 6 wk.
- Only 25% of patients with a history of chronic urticaria are completely cured after 5 yr.

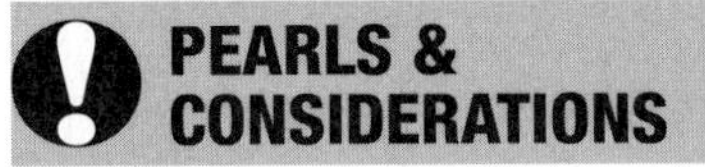

PEARLS & CONSIDERATIONS

COMMENTS

Local treatment (e.g., starch baths or oatmeal baths) may be helpful in selected patients; however, local treatment is generally not rewarding.

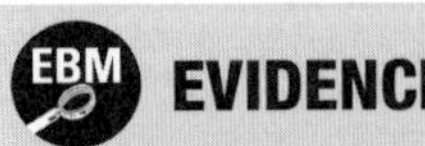

EVIDENCE

Evidence for the treatments used in urticaria and angioedema is limited. Systematic reviews and large, high-quality randomized, controlled trials (RCTs) for the main treatments are lacking, although some smaller RCTs have been published.

Expert opinion and a number of RCTs support H_1 antihistamines as the mainstay of treatment of urticaria and angioedema. Two RCTs found cetirizine significantly better than placebo at relieving the symptoms of chronic idiopathic urticaria. Cetirizine was also found to act more rapidly than hydroxyzine and astemizole.[1] B

A number of RCTs have shown desloratadine to be significantly better than placebo at relieving the signs and symptoms of chronic idiopathic urticaria.[2] B

One of these trials also showed desloratadine alone to be more effective than montelukast (a leukotriene receptor antagonist) alone, and the combination of the drugs did not convey additional benefit over desloratadine alone.[2] B

Evidence-Based References

1. Handa S et al: Comparative efficacy of cetirizine and fexofenadine in the treatment of chronic idiopathic urticaria, *J Dermatolog Treat* 15:55-57, 2004. B

2. Di Lorenzo G et al: Randomized placebo-controlled trial comparing desloratadine and montelukast in monotherapy and desloratadine plus montelukast in combined therapy for chronic idiopathic urticaria, *J Allergy Clin Immunol* 114:619-625, 2004. B

SUGGESTED READING

Komarow HD, Metcalfe DD: Office-based management of urticaria, *Am J Med* 121:379, 2008.

AUTHOR: **FRED F. FERRI, M.D.**

BASIC INFORMATION

DEFINITION

Uterine fibroids are benign tumors of muscle cell origin. They are discrete nodular tumors that vary in size and number and that may be found as subserosal, intramural, or submucosal masses. They can also be located in the cervix, broad ligament, or on a stalk (pedunculated).

SYNONYMS

Leiomyomas, myomas

ICD-9CM CODES
218.9 Leiomyomas, fibroids

EPIDEMIOLOGY & DEMOGRAPHICS

- Estimated prevalence of 20% of reproductive age women
- The most common benign uterine tumor
- More common in black women than white women
- Asymptomatic fibroids may be present in 40% to 50% of women aged >40 yr
- May occur singly but are often multiple
- Fewer than half of all fibroids are estimated to produce symptoms
- Frequently diagnosed incidentally on pelvic examination
- There is increased familial incidence
- Potential to enlarge during pregnancy as well as regress after menopause
- Infrequent primary cause of infertility in <3% of infertile patients
- Symptomatic fibromas are the primary indication for approximately 30% of all hysterectomies

PHYSICAL FINDINGS & CLINICAL PRESENTATION

- Enlarged, irregular uterus on pelvic examination.
- Presenting symptoms:
  1. Menorrhagia (most common)
  2. Chronic pelvic pain (dysmenorrhea, dyspareunia, pelvic pressure)
  3. Acute pain (torsion of pedunculated fibroma, infarction, and degeneration)
  4. Urinary symptoms (frequency from bladder pressure, partial ureteral obstruction, complete ureteral obstruction)
  5. Rectosigmoid compression with constipation or intestinal obstruction
  6. Prolapse through cervix of pedunculated submucosal tumor
  7. Venous stasis of lower extremities
  8. Polycythemia
  9. Ascites

ETIOLOGY

Incompletely understood. It is suggested that fibromas arise from an original single smooth muscle cell in the myometrium. Each individual fibroma is monoclonal (all the cells are derived from one progenitor myocyte). Malignant degeneration of preexisting leiomyoma is extremely uncommon (<0.5%).

Dx DIAGNOSIS

DIFFERENTIAL DIAGNOSIS

Leiomyosarcoma, ovarian mass (neoplastic, nonneoplastic, endometrioma), inflammatory mass, pregnancy

WORKUP

- Complete pelvic examination, rectovaginal examination, Pap test
- Estimation of size of mass in centimeters
- Endometrial sampling may be indicated (biopsy or dilation and curettage) when abnormal bleeding and pelvic mass are present
- If urinary symptoms are prominent, cystometry, cystoscopy to rule out bladder lesions, intravenous pyelogram to rule out impingement on urinary system

LABORATORY TESTS

- Pregnancy test
- Pap smear
- Complete blood count, erythrocyte sedimentation rate
- Fecal occult blood

IMAGING STUDIES

- Pelvic ultrasound (transvaginal may have higher diagnostic accuracy) is useful (Fig. 1-352).
- CT scan is helpful in planning treatment if malignancy is strongly suspected.
- Hysteroscopy may provide direct evidence of intrauterine pathology or submucosal leiomyoma that distorts uterine cavity.

Rx TREATMENT

Management should be based on primary symptoms and may include observation with close follow-up, temporizing surgical therapies, medical management, or definitive surgical procedures. Treatment is generally indicated only when symptoms are present and are severe enough to be unacceptable to the patient.

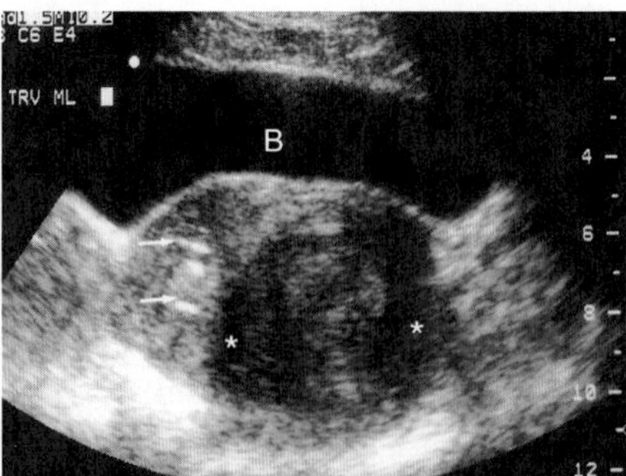

FIGURE 1-352 Transverse real-time ultrasound image through the uterine fundus in a patient with abdominal pain. A large hypoechoic mass is seen to the left of the midline (asterisks) compatible with a uterine fibroid. Note several portions of an IUD (arrows) within the plane of the scan. B, Bladder. (From Skarin AT: *Atlas of diagnostic oncology,* ed 3, St Louis, 2003, Mosby.)

NONSURGICAL Rx

- Patient observation and follow-up with periodic repeat pelvic examinations to ensure that tumors are not growing rapidly.
- Gonadotropin-releasing hormone (GnRH) agonist use results in 40% to 60% reduction in uterine volume. Hypoestrogenism, reversible bone loss, and hot flushes are associated with use. Limit to short-term use and consider low-dose hormonal replacement to minimize hypoestrogenic effects.
- Regrowth occurs in approximately 50% of women treated a few months after cessation.
- Indications for GnRH:
  1. Fertility preservation in women with large myomas before attempting conception or preoperative myectomy treatment
  2. Anemia treatment to normalize hemoglobin before surgery
  3. Women approaching menopause to avoid surgery
  4. Preoperative for large myomas to make vaginal hysterectomy, hysteroscopic resection/ablation, or laparoscopic destruction more feasible
  5. Women with medical contraindications for surgery
  6. Personal or medical indications for delaying surgery
- Progestational agents may also result in decrease in uterine size and amenorrhea, allowing iron therapy to treat anemia with limited success.
- Other drugs used and under investigation:
  1. Danazol: androgen and multienzyme inhibitor of steroidogenesis
  2. Mifepristone: antiprogestogen shown to reduce the fibroid volume by 40% to 50% with amenorrhea
  3. Raloxifene: selective estrogen receptor modulator, either alone or with a GnRHa, shown to reduce the fibroid volume 70% up to 1 yr but only in postmenopausal women
  4. Fadrozole: aromatase inhibitor reported to have produced a 71% reduction in volume

SURGICAL Rx

- Indications
  1. Abnormal uterine bleeding with anemia refractory to hormonal therapy
  2. Chronic pain with severe dysmenorrhea, dyspareunia, or lower abdominal pressure/pain
  3. Acute pain, torsion, or prolapsing submucosal fibroid
  4. Urinary symptoms or signs such as hydronephrosis
  5. Rapid uterine enlargement premenopausal or any growth after menopause
  6. Infertility or recurrent pregnancy loss with submucous leiomyoma as only finding
  7. Enlarged uterus with compression symptoms or discomfort
- Procedures
  1. Hysterectomy (definitive procedure)
  2. Abdominal myomectomy (to preserve fertility)

3. Vaginal myomectomy for prolapsed pedunculated submucous fibroid
4. Hysteroscopic resection
5. Laparoscopic myomectomy
6. Uterine artery embolization

COMPLICATIONS

- Red degeneration
- Leiomyosarcoma (<0.1%)

REFERRAL

Consultation with gynecologic oncologist if suspicion of malignancy

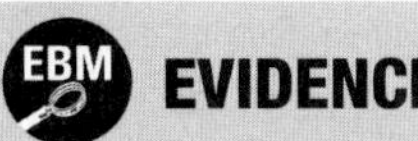

EVIDENCE

Another systematic review, of ten RCTs (two of which were included in the review above), found that the levonorgestrel-releasing intrauterine system (IUS), the most commonly studied progestogen IUS, is more effective than luteal phase oral progestogens in women with primary menorrhagia, and despite the more frequent short-term side effects, women are more satisfied and willing to continue its use compared to those treated with oral progestogens.[1] A

Myolysis, especially when combined with endometrial destructive techniques, can reduce the need for hysterectomy in women with symptomatic fibroids.

A prospective trial examined the efficacy of laparoscopic cryomyolysis for the management of symptomatic fibroids. It found that almost all patients had complete resolution of their complaints after treatment. Myomas regressed up to 80%, and major blood supply to the myomas was eliminated.[2] B

Uterine artery embolization results in a speedier recovery for women with symptomatic fibroids, compared to either hysterectomy or myomectomy.

A systematic review analyzed the efficacy of uterine artery embolization (UAE), compared with either hysterectomy or myomectomy, in women with symptomatic fibroids. UAE involved shorter hospital stays and a speedier return to routine activities, compared with hysterectomy. There was no evidence of benefit of UAE compared to surgery (hysterectomy/myomectomy), however, for levels of satisfaction. It concluded that women with symptomatic fibroids may be offered UAE as a treatment option, but it cautioned that more research with a longer follow-up is still needed.[3] A

Evidence-Based References

1. Lethaby AE et al: Progesterone or progestogen-releasing intrauterine systems for heavy menstrual bleeding, *Cochrane Database Rev* 4, 2005. A

2. Zupi E et al: Directed laparoscopic cryomyolysis: a possible alternative to myomectomy and/or hysterectomy for symptomatic leiomyomas, *Am J Obstet Gynecol* 190:639-643, 2004. B

3. Gupta JK et al: Uterine artery embolization for symptomatic uterine fibroids, *Cochrane Database Rev* 1, 2006. A

SUGGESTED READINGS

DeWaay DJ et al: Natural history of uterine polyps and leiomyomata, *Obstet Gynecol* 100:3, 2002.

Goodwin SC, Spies JB: Uterine fibroid embolization, *N Engl J Med* 361(7):690-697, 2009.

Olive DL et al: Non-surgical management of leiomyoma, *Curr Opin Obstet Gynecol* 16(3):239, 2004.

AUTHORS: **ARUNDATHI G. PRASAD, M.D.,** and **RUBEN ALVERO, M.D.**

BASIC INFORMATION

DEFINITION

Uterine malignancy includes tumors from the endometrium and sarcomas. Uterine sarcoma is an abnormal proliferation of cells originating from the mesenchymal, or connective tissue, elements of the uterine wall.

SYNONYMS

Leiomyosarcomas
Endometrial stromal sarcoma
Malignant mixed Müllerian tumors
Adenosarcomas

ICD-9CM CODES
182.0 Malignant neoplasm of body of uterus (corpus uteri), except isthmus
182.1 Malignant neoplasm of body of uterus, isthmus
182.8 Malignant neoplasm of body of uterus, other specified sites of body of uterus

EPIDEMIOLOGY & DEMOGRAPHICS

INCIDENCE: 17.1 cases per 1 million females. Endometrial cancer remains the most common gynecologic malignancy in the U.S.
PREVALENCE: Uterine sarcoma accounts for 4.3% of all cancers of the uterine corpus and is the most lethal gynecologic malignancy.
MEAN AGE AT DIAGNOSIS: 52 yr
RISK FACTORS: Similar to endometrial carcinoma

PHYSICAL FINDINGS & CLINICAL PRESENTATION

- Abnormal vaginal bleeding is the most common symptom
- May also present as pelvic pain or pressure and pelvic mass on examination
- May appear as tumor protruding through the cervix
- Vaginal discharge may also be a presenting symptom
- Rapidly enlarging uterus

ETIOLOGY

- The exact etiology is unknown.
- Prior pelvic radiation is a risk factor for sarcoma.
- Black women may be at higher risk.

DIAGNOSIS

DIFFERENTIAL DIAGNOSIS

Leiomyoma

WORKUP

Diagnosis is made histologically by biopsy for abnormal bleeding.

LABORATORY TESTS

Chest radiography, CT scans, and MRI are used to evaluate spread.

IMAGING STUDIES

- Chest radiography is usually done as routine preoperative testing.
- CT scans and MRI are good for assessing tumor spread once diagnosis is made.

TREATMENT

NONPHARMACOLOGIC THERAPY

- Surgical excision is the mainstay of treatment.
- Grade and stage of tumor affect prognosis (Fig. 1-353).
- The benefit of adjuvant radiotherapy in stage I endometrial adenocarcinoma to improve pelvic disease control and improve survival remains controversial despite several phase 3 trials.
- Chemotherapeutic agents have produced only partial and short-term responses.

DISPOSITION

- Survival varies with each type of sarcoma but is generally very poor.
- Five-year survival for leiomyosarcoma ranges from 48% for stage I to 0% for stage IV.
- Five-year survival for malignant mixed mesodermal tumor ranges from 36% for stage I to 6% for stage IV.

REFERRAL

Uterine sarcoma should be managed by a gynecologic oncologist and radiation oncologist.

SUGGESTED READINGS

Elima Y et al: Para-aortic lymph node metastasis in relation to serum CA 125 levels and nuclear grade in endometrial carcinoma, *Acta Obstet Gynecol Scand* 81(5):458, 2002.

Lee CM et al: Frequency and effect of adjuvant radiation therapy among women with stage I endometrial adenocarcinoma, *JAMA* 295:389, 2006.

Pitsm G et al: Stage II endometrial carcinoma: prognostic factors and risk classification in 170 patients, *Int J Radiat Oncol Biol Phys* 53(4):862, 2002.

AUTHORS: **GIL M. FARKASH, M.D.,** and **RUBEN ALVERO, M.D.**

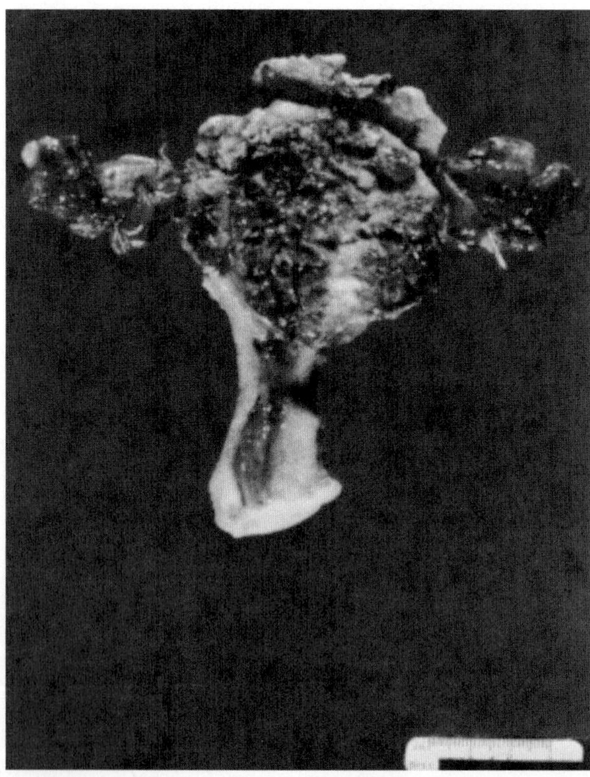

FIGURE 1-353 This grade 3 adenocarcinoma demonstrates extensive myometrial invasion. The tumor has penetrated the uterine serosa and upper left broad ligament. (From Copeland LJ: *Textbook of gynecology,* ed 2, Philadelphia, 2000, WB Saunders.)

BASIC INFORMATION

DEFINITION

Uterine prolapse refers to the protrusion of the uterus into or out of the vaginal canal. In a first-degree uterine prolapse, the cervix is visible when the perineum is depressed. In a second-degree uterine prolapse, the uterine cervix has prolapsed through the vaginal introitus, with the fundus remaining within the pelvis proper. In a third-degree uterine prolapse (i.e., complete uterine prolapse, uterine procidentia), the entire uterus is outside the introitus. Table 1-79 compares the various types of prolapse.

SYNONYMS

Genital prolapse
Uterine descensus
Pelvic organ prolapse

ICD-9CM CODES
618.8 Genital prolapse
618.1 Uterine descensus
618.8 Pelvic organ prolapse

EPIDEMIOLOGY & DEMOGRAPHICS

PREVALENCE: Most prevalent in postmenopausal multiparous women.

RISK FACTORS:
- Pregnancy
- Labor
- Vaginal childbirth
- Obesity
- Chronic coughing
- Constipation
- Pelvic tumors
- Ascites
- Strenuous physical exertion
- Caucasian race

GENETICS: Increased incidence in women with spina bifida occulta.

PHYSICAL FINDINGS & CLINICAL PRESENTATION

- Pelvic pressure
- Bearing-down sensation
- Bilateral groin pain
- Sacral backache
- Coital difficulty
- Protrusion from vagina
- Spotting
- Ulceration
- Bleeding
- Examination of patient in lithotomy, sitting, and standing positions and before, during, and after a maximum Valsalva effort
- Erosion or ulceration of the cervix possible in the most dependent area of the protrusion

ETIOLOGY

- Vaginal childbirth and chronic increases in intraabdominal pressure leading to detachments, lacerations, and denervations of the vaginal support system
- Further weakening of pelvic support system by hypoestrogenic atrophy
- Some cases from congenital or inherited weaknesses within the pelvic support system
- Neonatal uterine prolapse mostly coexistent with congenital spinal defects

Dx DIAGNOSIS

DIFFERENTIAL DIAGNOSIS

- Occasionally, elongated cervix; body of the uterus remains undescended.
- Diagnosis is based on history and physical examination. Currently there is only one genital tract prolapse classification system that has attained international acceptance and recognition: the patient pelvic organ prolapse quantification (POP-Q) (Boxes 1-20 and 1-21).

WORKUP

- If erosion or ulceration of the cervix is present, a Pap smear followed by a cervical biopsy should be performed if indicated.
- If urinary symptoms are significant, further urodynamic workup is indicated, looking for concurrent cystourethrocele, cystocele, enterocele, or rectocele.

LABORATORY TESTS

Urine culture

IMAGING STUDIES

Ultrasound if concurrent fibroids need further evaluation

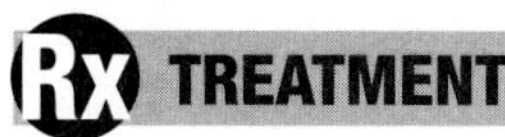

TREATMENT

NONPHARMACOLOGIC THERAPY

- Prophylactic measures
  1. Diagnosis and treatment of chronic respiratory and metabolic disorders
  2. Correction of constipation
  3. Weight control, nutrition, and smoking cessation counseling
  4. Teaching of pelvic muscle exercises

TABLE 1-79 Types of Genital Prolapse

Original Position of Organs	Prolapse	Symptoms (in addition to the general symptoms of discomfort, dragging, the feeling of a 'lump' and, rarely, coital problems)
Anterior	Urethrocele Cystocele	Urinary symptoms (stress incontinence, urinary frequency)
Central	Cervix/uterus: 1st, 2nd and 3rd degree Procidentia	Bleeding and/or discharge from ulceration in association with procidentia
Posterior	Rectocele Enterocele	Bowel symptoms, particularly the feeling of incomplete evacuation and sometimes having to press the posterior wall backwards to pass stool

From Drife J, Magowan B: *Clinical obstetrics and gynaecology,* Philadelphia, 2004, Saunders.

BOX 1-20 Staging of Pelvic Organ Prolapse Based on POP-Q Examination

Stage 0	No prolapse.
Stage I	Most distal prolapse >1 cm above hymenal ring.
Stage II	Most distal point is ≤ 1 cm above hymenal ring.
Stage III	Most distal point is >1 cm below the hymenal ring but not farther than 2 cm less the total vaginal length (TVL) (i.e., ≥ 1 cm but $\leq$ (TVL $-$ 2) cm.
Stage IV	Complete vaginal eversion.

From Pemberton J (ed): *The pelvic floor,* Philadelphia, 2002, WB Saunders.

BOX 1-21 Points of Reference for POP-Q

Point A: 3 cm above the hymen on anterior vaginal wall (Aa) or posterior vaginal wall (Ap). Point Aa roughly corresponds with the urethrovesical junction. These points can range from -3 cm (no prolapse) to $+3$ cm (maximal prolapse).
Point B: The lowest extent of the segment of vagina between point A and the apex of the vagina. Unlike point A, it is not fixed but will be the same as A if point A is the most protruding point. In maximal prolapse it will be the same as point C.
Point C: The most distal part of the cervix or vaginal vault.
Point D: The posterior fornix, which is omitted in women with prior hysterectomy.
Genital hiatus: From midline external urethral meatus to inferior hymenal ring.
Perineal body: From inferior hymenal ring to middle of anal orifice.
Vaginal length: This should be measured without undue stretching of the vagina.

From Pemberton J (ed): *The pelvic floor,* Philadelphia, 2002, WB Saunders.

- Supportive pessary therapy
  1. Ring-type pessary useful for first- or second-degree prolapse
  2. Gellhorn pessary preferred for more advanced prolapse
  3. Use of pessaries in conjunction with continuous hormone replacement therapy, unless contraindicated
  4. Perineorrhaphy under local anesthesia possibly needed to support the pessary if the vaginal outlet is very relaxed

ACUTE GENERAL Rx

- Patients who are only infrequently symptomatic: insertion of a tampon or diaphragm for temporary relief when prolonged standing is anticipated
- Neonatal uterine prolapse: simple digital reduction or the use of a small pessary

CHRONIC Rx

- Hormone replacement therapy at the time of menopause helps preserve tissue strength, maintain elasticity of the vagina, and promote the durability of surgical repairs.
- Gold standard for therapy is vaginal hysterectomy.
- Vaginal apex should be well suspended, but a prophylactic sacrospinous ligament fixation is not routinely required.
- If occult enterocele present, McCall culdoplasty is performed.
- If vaginal approach to hysterectomy is contraindicated, abdominal hysterectomy is performed; vaginal apex likewise well supported.
- Colpocleisis is considered for the elderly patient who is sexually inactive and is a high-risk patient from a surgical point of view; can be done rapidly under local anesthesia with mild sedation if necessary.
- For symptomatic women who desire childbearing: management with pessaries or pelvic muscle exercises is recommended; if surgical correction is required, transvaginal sacrospinous fixation is the preferred method.
- Other surgical options are sling operations and sacral cervicopexy.

DISPOSITION

If untreated, uterine prolapse progressively worsens.

REFERRAL

To a gynecologist/urologist if pessary fitting or surgical intervention is needed

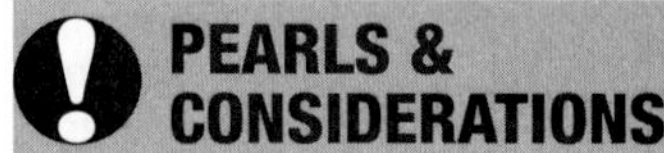

PEARLS & CONSIDERATIONS

COMMENTS

Surgery contraindicated in mild or asymptomatic uterine prolapse because the patient will seldom benefit from the operation although exposed to its risks.

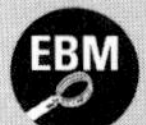

EVIDENCE

Any benefits of hormone replacement therapy (HRT) need to be balanced against the harms associated with its use.

Unopposed estrogen significantly increases the risk of endometrial hyperplasia compared with placebo.[1] A

Hysterectomy is a definitive treatment for uterine prolapse but may not remove all associated symptoms.

A randomized controlled trial compared urogenital function after vaginal hysterectomy (combined with anterior and/or posterior colporrhaphy) and abdominal sacrocolpopexy (with preservation of the uterus) and found discomfort/pain, overactive bladder, and obstructive micturition were significantly higher in the abdominal group than in the vaginal group, and reoperation was more frequent in those who underwent abdominal surgery (9 of 41 compared with 1 of 41).[2] B

There is a lack of evidence concerning the use of pessaries in the treatment of uterine prolapse.

A systematic review found no evidence from randomized controlled trials upon which to base treatment of women with pelvic organ prolapse through the use of mechanical devices/pessaries.[3] A

Although there is evidence for the benefit of pelvic floor exercises in the treatment of urinary incontinence, there is a lack of evidence on their use for treatment of uterine prolapse specifically.

There is no rigorous evidence from randomized controlled trials regarding the use of conservative interventions in the management of pelvic organ prolapse.[4] A

Evidence-Based References

1. Lethaby A et al: Hormone replacement therapy in postmenopausal women: endometrial hyperplasia and irregular bleeding, *Cochrane Database Rev* 3, 2004. A
2. Roovers JP et al: A randomised controlled trial comparing abdominal and vaginal prolapse surgery: effects on urogenital function, *BJOG* 111:50-56, 2004. B
3. Adams E et al: Mechanical devices for pelvic organ prolapse in women, *Cochrane Database Rev* 2, 2004. A
4. Hagan S et al: Conservative management of pelvic organ prolapse in women, *Cochrane Database Rev* 2, 2004. A

SUGGESTED READING

Thaker R: Management of uterine prolapse, *BMJ* 324:1258, 2002.

AUTHORS: **ARUNDATHI G. PRASAD, M.D.,** and **RUBEN ALVERO, M.D.**

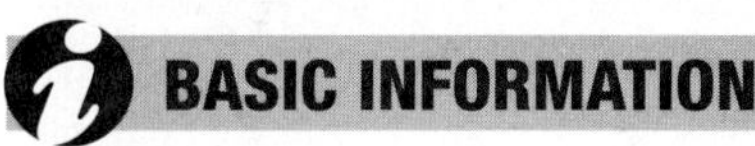

BASIC INFORMATION

DEFINITION

Uveitis is inflammation of the uveal tract, including the iris, ciliary body, and choroid. It may also involve other closed structures such as the sclera, retina, and vitreous humor.

SYNONYMS

Anterior uveitis
Posterior uveitis
Acute or chronic uveitis
Granulomatous or nongranulomatous uveitis
Iritis
Chroroiditis
Pars planitis
Iridocyclitis

ICD-9CM CODES
364.3 Unspecified iridocyclitis, uveitis

EPIDEMIOLOGY & DEMOGRAPHICS

INCIDENCE (IN U.S.): Common; busy ophthalmologist will see two or more cases per week.
PEAK INCIDENCE: Middle age or older; uveitis in childhood rare; equal in boys and girls; 25% idiopathic and 75% related to toxoplasmosis, juvenile rheumatoid arthritis, pars planitis, toxicaris canis, or Behçet's disease
PREVALENCE (IN U.S.): 17 cases per 100,000 persons
PREDOMINANT SEX: None
PREDOMINANT AGE: 38 yr

PHYSICAL FINDINGS & CLINICAL PRESENTATION

- Symptoms of uveitis depend on the site of involvement and whether process is acute or insidious:
  - Acute anterior uveitis: pain and photophobia. Vision may not be affected initially.
  - Posterior uveitis: floaters, hazy vision. Involvement of the retina may produce blind spots or flashing lights.
  - Insidious anterior uveitis: symptoms may not be present until scarring cataracts and loss of vision occur.
- Photophobia
- Blurred visual acuity
- Irregular pupil
- Hazy cornea
- Abnormal cells and flare in anterior chamber or vitreous humor
- Retinal hemorrhage, vascular sheathing
- Conjunctival injection
- Ciliary flush
- Keratitic precipitates (precipitates on the cornea)
- Hazy vitreous
- Retinal inflammation
- Iris nodules
- Glaucoma
- Rheumatoid arthritis
- Scleritis
- Systemic symptoms related to etiology

ETIOLOGY

- Infections: herpes simplex virus, cytomegalovirus, toxoplasmosis, tuberculosis, syphilis, HIV
- Systemic disorders: sarcoidosis, Behçet's syndrome, HLA-B27–associated diseases (e.g., ankylosing spondylitis, reactive arthritis), inflammatory bowel disease, juvenile idiopathic arthritis
- Idiopathic

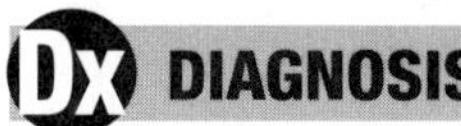

DIAGNOSIS

DIFFERENTIAL DIAGNOSIS

- Glaucoma
- Conjunctivitis
- Retinal detachment
- Retinopathy
- Keratitis
- Scleritis
- Episcleritis
- Masquerading syndromes: lymphoma, uveal melanoma, metastases (breast, lung, renal), leukemia, retinitis pigmentosa, retinoblastoma

WORKUP

- Associated with arthritis, syphilis, tuberculosis, granulomatous disease, collagen-vascular disease, allergies, AIDS, sarcoid, Behçet's disease, histoplasmosis, toxoplasmosis, and toxicaris canis
- Slit lamp examination, indirect ophthalmoscopy

LABORATORY TESTS

- Complete blood count
- Laboratory tests for specific inflammatory causes cited previously in "Workup" (e.g., antinuclear antibody, erythrocyte sedimentation rate, syphilis (VDRL), HLA-B27, purified protein derivative, Lyme titer)
- Visual field testing

IMAGING STUDIES

- Chest radiograph in suspected sarcoidosis, tuberculosis, histoplasmosis
- Sacroiliac radiograph in suspected ankylosing spondylitis

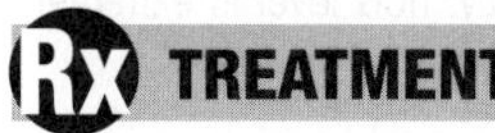

TREATMENT

NONPHARMACOLOGIC THERAPY

- Treat the underlying disease. Treatment is often multidisciplinary (ophthalmologist, internist, rheumatologist, internal disease specialist).
- Treat photophobia and local pain.

ACUTE GENERAL Rx

- Corticosteroids are the mainstay of therapy for noninfectious causes. The route of administration depends on the location of inflammation, the severity, and the presence of systemic disease. Cycloplegic drops (cyclopentolate [Cyclogyl]) or cycloplegic agents (homatropine hydrobromide [Optic] 1 gtt q3-4h while awake) and topical steroids (prednisone acetate 1% 1 gtt qh during day, prn at night until favorable response, then q4-6h); avoid topical corticosteroids in infectious uveitis. Periocular corticosteroid injections can be used for posterior disease; they have the advantage of achieving high intraocular levels of steroids without the systemic side effects of oral corticosteroids.
- Antibiotics for bacterial infections and antiviral agents, when infection is suspected, should be started to prevent retinal damage.
- Systemic steroids if appropriate for the underlying disease. Systemic corticosteroid therapy is generally reserved for patients with systemic disorders and those with bilateral disease that is refractory to local medication or those with major ocular disability or retinitis.
- Antimetabolites when indicated. Immunosuppressive medications used in steroid-dependent or refractory uveitis include methotrexate, sulfasalazine, azathioprine, cyclosporine, and tacrolimus. These medications can have significant toxicity and should be prescribed only by physicians experienced with their use.

CHRONIC Rx

- Topical steroids and cycloplegics
- Treat underlying cause

DISPOSITION

Urgent referral to ophthalmologist for diagnosis and treatment

REFERRAL

- Eye problem should be monitored early on by an ophthalmologist.
- Underlying medical disease should be treated by the primary care physician.

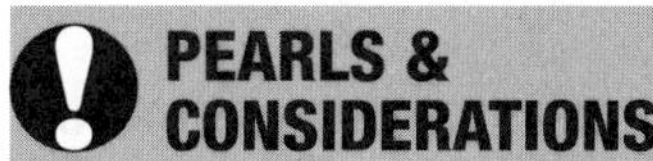

PEARLS & CONSIDERATIONS

COMMENTS

- In 90% of cases the condition is idiopathic.
- Associated causes are found approximately 10% of the time, usually chronic and recurrent.
- Chronic glaucoma, cataracts, retinal degeneration, and other severe eye problems occur with the disease and the treatment.

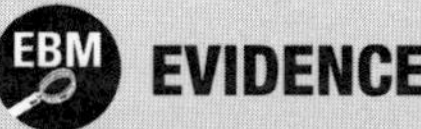

EVIDENCE

Please note: Complete text of EBM for this topic is available online.

SUGGESTED READINGS

Hajj-Ali RA et al: Uveitis in the internist's office: are a patient's eye symptoms serious? *Cleve Clin J Med* 72:329-339, 2005.

Kadayifcilar S et al: Uveitis in childhood, *J Pediatr Ophthalmol Strabismus* 40(6):335, 2003.

AUTHOR: **MELVYN KOBY, M.D.**

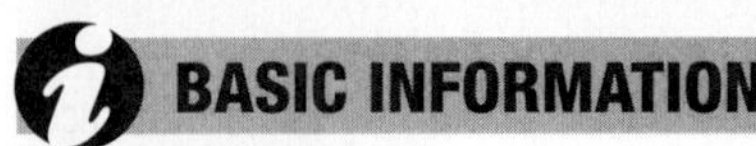

BASIC INFORMATION

DEFINITION

Bleeding per vagina at any time during pregnancy must be regarded as abnormal and is associated with an increased likelihood of pregnancy complications.

SYNONYMS

Hemorrhage

ICD-9CM CODES

634.9	Spontaneous abortion
633.9	Ectopic pregnancy
630/631	Molar pregnancy
622.7	Cervical polyps
180.9/180.0/180.8	Cervical dysplasia/cancer
616.0	Cervicitis
616.10	Vulvovaginitis
184.0	Vaginal cancer
644.2	Premature labor term labor
641.1	Placenta previa
641.2	Placental abruption

EPIDEMIOLOGY & DEMOGRAPHICS

- Common in U.S.; 20% to 25% of patients have vaginal spotting/bleeding in first trimester; of those, miscarriage occurs in 50%.
- Occurs in women of childbearing age.
- Between 1% and 2% of all pregnancies in the U.S. are ectopic.
- After one ectopic pregnancy, the chance of another is 7% to 15%.
- Ectopic pregnancy is the leading cause of maternal mortality in the first trimester.
- Average reported frequency for placental abruption is about 1 in 150 deliveries (0.3%).
- Incidence of placenta previa is <1 in 200 deliveries (0.5%).

PHYSICAL FINDINGS & CLINICAL PRESENTATION

- Bleeding: ranges from scant to life-threatening with hemodynamic instability
- Color: brown to bright red
- Can be painless or painful (cramps, back pain, severe abdominal pain)
- Fetal compromise: ranges from none to fetal demise

ETIOLOGY

- Influenced by gestational age
- Vaginal
- Cervical
- Uterine

Dx DIAGNOSIS

DIFFERENTIAL DIAGNOSIS

- Any gestational age:
  1. Cervical lesions: polyps, decidual reaction, neoplasia
  2. Vaginal trauma
  3. Cervicitis/vulvovaginitis
  4. Postcoital trauma
  5. Bleeding dyscrasias
- Gestation <20 wk:
  1. Spontaneous abortion
  2. Presence of intrauterine device
  3. Ectopic pregnancy
  4. Molar pregnancy
  5. Implantation bleeding
  6. Low-lying placenta
- Gestation >20 wk:
  1. Molar pregnancy
  2. Placenta previa
  3. Placental abruption
  4. Vasa previa
  5. Marginal separation of the placenta
  6. Bloody show at term
  7. Preterm labor
- Section II describes the differential diagnosis of vaginal bleeding in pregnancy.

WORKUP

- Gestation <20 wk (Section III, "Bleeding, Early Pregnancy")
  1. Pelvic examination
  2. Culdocentesis
  3. Laparoscopy
  4. Laparotomy
  5. Ultrasound to verify viable intrauterine pregnancy
- Gestation >20 wk:
  1. Ultrasound to locate placenta before pelvic examination
  2. If placenta previa, no speculum or bimanual examination
  3. If preterm labor, appropriate evaluation done

LABORATORY TESTS

- Urine pregnancy test: if positive, get quantitative β human chorionic gonadotropin (hCG)
  1. Early pregnancy: follow serially every 48 hr
  2. Normal pregnancy: hCG doubles approximately every 48 hr
  3. Spontaneous abortion: hCG level will fall
  4. Ectopic pregnancy: hCG level will rise inappropriately
  5. Molar pregnancy: hCG level is extremely high
- CBC
- Blood type and screen (Rh-negative patients need RhoGAM)
- Coagulation profile (useful in missed abortion and abruption)
- Cervical cultures/wet mount
- Pap smear for cervical malignancy; caution with biopsy, because cervix can bleed extensively

IMAGING STUDIES

Ultrasound:

- 5 to 6 wk: gestational sac (transvaginally); hCG >2500 mIU/ml (third IS) or >1000 mIU/ml (second IS)
- 8 to 9 wk: fetal cardiac activity
- Molar pregnancy: characteristic cluster of cysts
- Location of placenta
- Degree of placental separation: difficult to assess

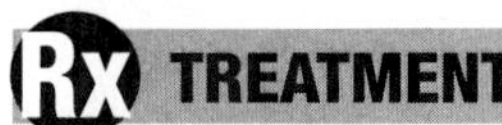

Rx TREATMENT

NONPHARMACOLOGIC THERAPY

- Pelvic rest: no coitus, douching, or tampons
- Bed rest, if >20 wk
- Counseling: genetic, bereavement

ACUTE GENERAL Rx

- Hemodynamic stabilization
- Emergency D&C, laparotomy, or cesarean section as necessary

CHRONIC Rx

Depends on diagnosis

DISPOSITION

Depends on diagnosis

REFERRAL

- If patient is unstable and needs emergency ob/gyn management and/or surgery
- If patient has diagnosis of ectopic or molar pregnancy, because immediate surgical treatment is indicated
- Perinatal consultation for high-risk pregnancy

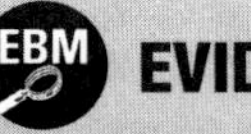

EVIDENCE

Administration of anti-D immunoglobulin to Rhesus-negative women at 24 weeks and 34 weeks gestation during the first pregnancy reduces the risk of Rhesus-D alloimmunization from 1.5% to 0.2%.[1] Ⓐ

Evidence-Based Reference

1. Crowther CA: Anti-D administration in pregnancy for preventing Rhesus alloimmunization. In: *Cochrane Library*, 2, 2004. Ⓐ

SUGGESTED READING

Coppola PT, Coppola M: Vaginal bleeding in the first 20 weeks of pregnancy, *Emerg Med Clin North Am* 21(3):667, 2003.

AUTHORS: **GEORGE T. DANAKAS, M.D.,** and **RUBEN ALVERO, M.D.**

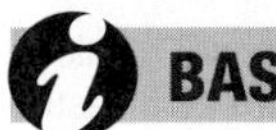

BASIC INFORMATION

DEFINITION

Vaginal malignancy is an abnormal proliferation of vaginal epithelium demonstrating malignant cells below the basement membrane.

SYNONYMS

Squamous cell carcinoma of the vagina
Adenocarcinoma of the vagina
Melanoma of the vagina
Sarcoma of the vagina
Endodermal sinus tumor

ICD-9CM CODES

184.0 Vagina, vaginal neoplasm

EPIDEMIOLOGY & DEMOGRAPHICS

INCIDENCE: 0.42 cases per 100,000 persons
PREVALENCE: Vaginal cancer is the second rarest gynecologic cancer. It comprises 2% of malignancies of the female genital tract.
MEAN AGE AT DIAGNOSIS: Predominantly a disease of menopause. Mean age at diagnosis is 60 yr.

PHYSICAL FINDINGS & CLINICAL PRESENTATION

- Majority of cases are asymptomatic
- Postmenopausal vaginal bleeding and/or vaginal discharge are the most common symptoms
- May also present as pelvic pain or pressure, dyspareunia, dysuria, malodor, or postcoital bleeding
- May present as a vaginal lesion or abnormal Pap smear

ETIOLOGY

- The exact etiology is unknown.
- Vaginal intraepithelial neoplasia is believed to be a precursor for squamous cell carcinoma of the vagina.
- Long-term pessary use has been associated with vaginal malignancy.
- Prior pelvic radiation may be a risk factor.
- Clear-cell adenocarcinoma is related to in utero diethylstilbestrol exposure.

DIAGNOSIS

DIFFERENTIAL DIAGNOSIS

- Extension from other primary carcinoma more common than primary vaginal cancer
- Vaginitis

WORKUP

- Diagnosis is made histologically by biopsy.
- Colposcopy and biopsy should follow suspicious Pap smear.
- Cystoscopy, proctosigmoidoscopy, chest radiography, IV urography, and barium enema may be used for clinical staging.
- CT scan and MRI are used to evaluate spread.
- Staging I to IV (Fig. 1-354).

IMAGING STUDIES

- Chest radiography, IV urography, and barium enema are used for staging.
- CT scan and MRI are good for assessing tumor spread.

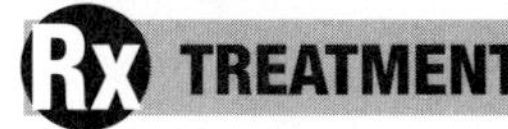

TREATMENT

NONPHARMACOLOGIC THERAPY

- Radiation therapy is the mainstay of treatment.
- Stage I tumors that are small and confined to the posterior, upper third of the vagina may be treated with radical surgery.
- Other stages require a whole-pelvis, interstitial, and/or intracavitary radiation therapy.
- Chemotherapy is used in conjunction with radiotherapy in rare select cases.

DISPOSITION

Five-year survival ranges from 80% for stage I to 17% for stage IV.

REFERRAL

Vaginal cancer should be managed by a gynecologic oncologist and radiation oncologist.

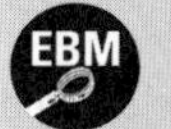

EVIDENCE

A retrospective review of 121 women with vaginal intraepithelial neoplasia found recurrence rates after partial vaginectomy, laser, and 5-fluorouracil of 0%, 38%, and 59%, respectively, after at least 7 mo of follow-up.[1] B

A retrospective review of 71 patients with primary vaginal carcinoma treated with interstitial iridium-192 with or without external-beam radiotherapy found that interstitial irradiation resulted in local control in the majority of patients with primary vaginal carcinoma with acceptable rates of morbidity.[2] B

A retrospective review of 84 patients with primary invasive vaginal cancer managed at one institution over a 25-yr period found that patients with stage I and II squamous cell vaginal carcinoma managed by initial surgery followed by selective radiotherapy had good outcomes in terms of survival and local tumor control.[3] B

Evidence-Based References

1. Dodge JA et al: Clinical features and risk of recurrence among patients with vaginal intraepithelial neoplasia, *Gynecol Oncol* 83:363, 2001. B
2. Tewari KS et al: Primary invasive carcinoma of the vagina: treatment with interstitial brachytherapy, *Cancer* 91:758, 2001. B
3. Tjalma WA et al: The role of surgery in invasive squamous carcinoma of the vagina, *Gynecol Oncol* 81:360, 2001. B

SUGGESTED READING

Kim H et al: Case report: magnetic resonance imaging of vaginal malignant melanoma, *J Comput Assist Tomogr* 27(3):357, 2003.

AUTHORS: **GIL M. FARKASH, M.D.,** and **RUBEN ALVERO, M.D.**

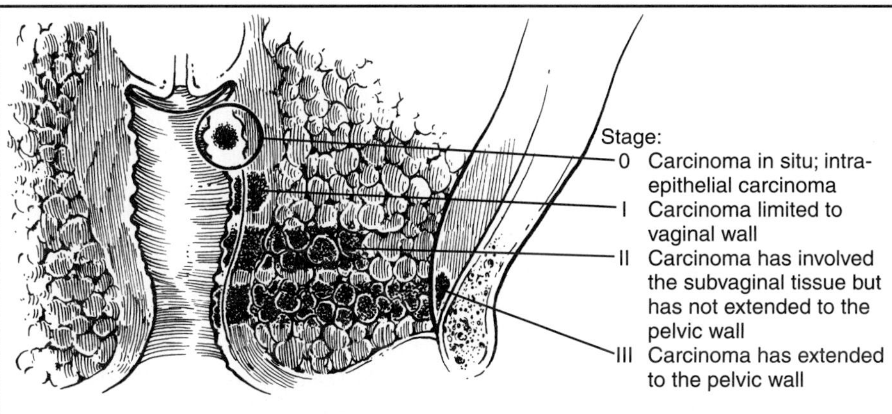

FIGURE 1-354 Staging system for vaginal cancer. Metastatic disease that involves the bladder or rectum is stage IV-a. Metastatic disease beyond the pelvis is stage IV-b. (From Copeland LJ: *Textbook of gynecology,* ed 2, Philadelphia, 2000, WB Saunders.)

Vaginismus

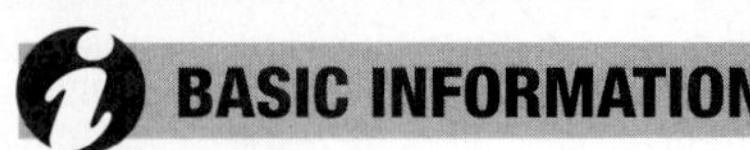

BASIC INFORMATION

DEFINITION

Vaginismus refers to the involuntary spasm of the vaginal, introital, and/or levator ani muscles, preventing penetration or causing painful intercourse.

ICD-9CM CODES

300.11	Hysterical vaginismus
306.51	Psychogenic or functional vaginismus
625.1	Reflex vaginismus

EPIDEMIOLOGY & DEMOGRAPHICS

INCIDENCE: Estimated at 11.7% to 42% of women presenting to sexual dysfunction clinics

PREVALENCE: Affects approximately 1 in 200 women

PREDOMINANT SEX: Affects only females

RISK FACTORS: Any previous sexual trauma, including incest or rape

PHYSICAL FINDINGS & CLINICAL PRESENTATION

- Fear of pain with coitus
- Dyspareunia
- Orgasmic dysfunction

ETIOLOGY

- Learned conditioned response to real or imagined painful vaginal experience (e.g., traumatic speculum examination, incest, rape)
- Vaginitis
- Pelvic inflammatory disease
- Endometriosis
- Anatomic anomalies
- Atrophic vaginitis
- Mucosal tears
- Inadequate lubrication
- Focal vulvitis
- Painful hymenal tags
- Scarring secondary to episiotomy
- Skin disorders
- Topical allergies
- Postherpetic neuralgia

Dx DIAGNOSIS

WORKUP

- Thorough history (including sexual history)
- Careful pelvic examination
- Behavioral therapy

Rx TREATMENT

NONPHARMACOLOGIC THERAPY

- Deconditioning the response by systematic self-administered progressive dilation techniques using fingers or dilators
- Behavioral and/or psychosexual therapy

ACUTE GENERAL Rx

- Botulinum toxin therapy given locally has been shown to relieve the perineal muscle spasms associated with vaginismus, allowing resumption of intercourse.
  1. Acts by preventing neuromuscular transmission, causing muscle weakness
  2. Considered experimental treatment for vaginismus at this time
- Cause should be determined by history and explained to the patient so that she understands the mechanics of the muscle spasms.
- Patient must be motivated to desire painless vaginal insertion for such reasons as pleasurable coitus, tampon insertion, or gynecologic examination.
- Patient (and her partner) must be willing to patiently undergo the process of systematic desensitization and counseling.

DISPOSITION

A high percentage of successfully treated patients

REFERRAL

To a gynecologist or sex therapist

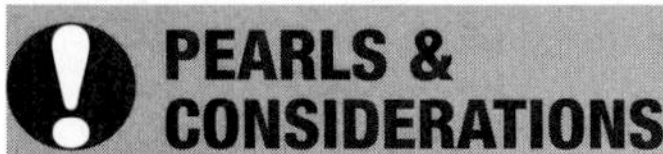

PEARLS & CONSIDERATIONS

COMMENTS

- May uncover early sexual abuse or an aversion to sexuality in general
- American Association of Sex Educators, Counselors and Therapists, 11 Dupont Circle, NW, Washington, DC, 20036.
- Sex Information and Education Council of the U.S. (SIECUS), 85th Avenue, New York, NY 10022.

SUGGESTED READINGS

Heim LJ: Evaluation and differential diagnosis of dyspareunia, *Am Fam Physician* 63(8):1535, 2001.

McGuire H, Hawton K: Interventions for vaginismus, *Cochrane Rev* 1:CD001760, 2003.

AUTHORS: **BETH J. WUTZ, M.D.,** and **RUBEN ALVERO, M.D.**

BASIC INFORMATION

DEFINITION

Bacterial vaginosis (BV) is a thin, gray, homogenous, malodorous vaginal discharge that results from a shift in the vaginal flora from a predominance of lactobacilli to high concentrations of anaerobic bacteria.

SYNONYMS

Before 1955: nonspecific vaginitis
1955: *Haemophilus vaginalis* vaginitis
1963: *Corynebacterium vaginalis* vaginitis
1980: *Gardnerella vaginalis* vaginitis
1990: Bacterial vaginosis

ICD-9CM CODES

616.10 Vaginitis, bacterial

EPIDEMIOLOGY & DEMOGRAPHICS

- Most common vaginal infection
- *Gardnerella, Mycoplasma,* and *Mobiluncus* are harbored in the urethra of male partners; however:
  1. Male partners are asymptomatic.
  2. There is no improved cure rate or lower reinfection rate if the infected patient's male partner is treated.
  3. Abstinence from intercourse or condom use while the patient completes her treatment regimen may improve cure rates and lessen recurrences.

PHYSICAL FINDINGS & CLINICAL PRESENTATION

- 50% of patients are asymptomatic
- A thin, dark, or dull gray homogenous discharge that adheres to the vaginal walls
- An offensive, "fishy" odor that is accentuated after intercourse or menses
- Pruritus (only in 13%)

ETIOLOGY

- *Gardnerella vaginalis* is detected in 40% to 50% of vaginal secretions.
  1. Increase in vaginal pH caused by decrease in hydrogen peroxide–producing lactobacilli
  2. Anaerobes predominate and produce amines
- Amines, when alkalinized by semen, menstrual blood, the use of alkaline douches, or the addition of 10% potassium hydroxide, volatilize and cause the unpleasant "fishy" odor.
- In BV:
  1. *Bacteroides* (anaerobes) species are increased 1000× the usual concentration.
  2. *G. vaginalis* are 100× normal.
  3. *Peptostreptococcus* are 10× normal.
  4. *Mycoplasma hominis* and Enterobacteriaceae members are present in increased concentrations.

DIAGNOSIS

WORKUP

Seattle Group criteria:

- The presence of three of the four following signs will diagnose 90% correctly, with <10% false-positive results:
  1. Thin, gray, homogenous, malodorous discharge that adheres to the vaginal walls
  2. Elevated pH >4.5
  3. Positive potassium hydroxide whiff test
  4. Clue cells present on wet mount
- Cultures are unnecessary.
- Pap smear will not identify *G. vaginalis.*
- Gram stain of vaginal secretions will reveal clue cells and abnormal mixed bacteria (Fig. 1-355).

TREATMENT

ACUTE GENERAL Rx

- Recommended regimens (equal efficacy):
  1. Metronidazole 500 mg PO bid for 7 days
  2. 0.75% metronidazole gel in vagina bid for 5 days
  3. 2% clindamycin cream qd for 7 days
- Alternate regimens (lower efficacy for BV):
  1. Clindamycin ovules 100 g intravaginally qhs for 3 days
  2. Clindamycin 300 mg PO bid for 7 days (increased incidence of diarrhea)
  3. Metronidazole ER 750 mg PO qd for 7 days
  4. Metronidazole 2 g PO single dose (higher relapse rate)
- Patients should be advised to avoid alcohol while taking metronidazole and for 24 hr thereafter.
- Treatment in pregnancy:
  - All pregnant patients proven to have BV should be treated because of its association with preterm labor, chorioamnionitis, and premature rupture of membranes (PROM).
- Recommended regimens:
  1. Metronidazole 250 mg PO tid for 7 days
  2. Clindamycin 300 mg PO bid for 7 days
- Existing data do not support the use of topical agents during pregnancy.
- Multiple studies and meta-analyses have not demonstrated associations between metronidazole use during pregnancy and teratogenic effects in newborns.
  3. Tinidazole, an oral antiprotozoal drug, is now FDA approved for treatment of bacterial vaginosis. Dosage is 2 gm once/day for 2 days or 1 gm qd x 5 days
- Recurrent BV:
  1. Condom use may help reduce the risk of recurrence.
  2. Concurrent treatment of male partner is controversial. Consider treating the male partner if there is recurrent vaginitis or any suspicion of associated upper genital tract infection.

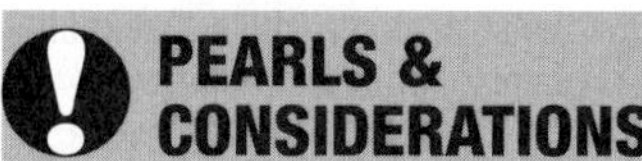

PEARLS & CONSIDERATIONS

- Bacterial vaginosis has been associated with pelvic inflammatory disease, cystitis, posthysterectomy vaginal cuff cellulitis, postabortal infection, preterm delivery, PROM, amnionitis, chorioamnionitis, and postpartum endometritis. New evidence also shows BV increases women's risk of acquiring HIV.
- Higher cumulative cure rates have been found at 3 to 4 wk for a 7-day regimen of metronidazole (500 mg twice daily) than with a single dose (2 g).
- Persistent bacterial vaginosis is associated with several bacteria in the *Clostridiales* order, *Megasphaera* phylotype 2, and *P. lacrimalis*

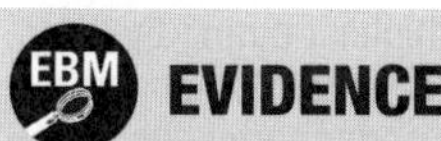

EVIDENCE

Please note: Complete text of EBM for this topic is available online.

SUGGESTED READINGS

Marrazzo JM et al: Relationship of specific vaginal bacteria and bacterial vaginosis treatment failure in women who have sex with women, *Ann Intern Med* 149:130, 2008.

Mitchell H: Vaginal discharge: causes, diagnosis, and treatment, *BMJ* 328(7451):1306, 2004.

AUTHORS: **ARUNDATHI G. PRASAD, M.D.,** and **RUBEN ALVERO, M.D.**

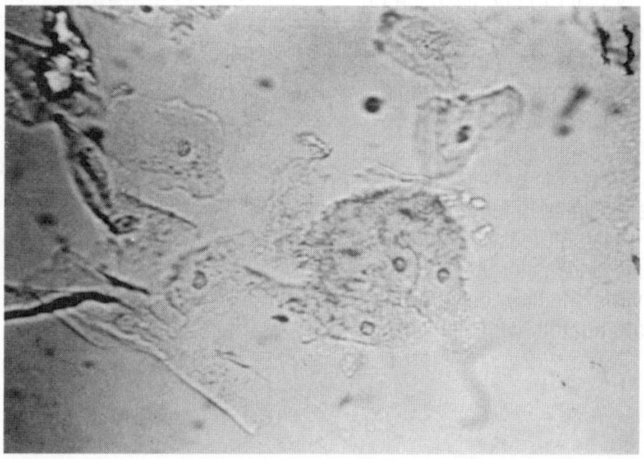

FIGURE 1-355 Clue cells characteristic of bacterial vaginosis, squamous epithelial cells whose borders are obscured by bacteria. (From Carlson K [ed]: *Primary care of women,* St Louis, 1995, Mosby.)

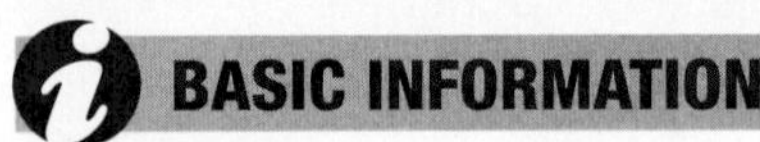

BASIC INFORMATION

DEFINITION

Varicella is a common viral illness that is characterized by the acute onset of a generalized vesicular rash and fever.

SYNONYMS

Chickenpox

ICD-9CM CODES
052.9 Varicella

EPIDEMIOLOGY & DEMOGRAPHICS

- Varicella is extremely contagious. More than 90% of unvaccinated contacts become infected.
- The incubation period of chickenpox ranges from 9 to 21 days.
- The peak incidence is during the springtime.
- The predominant age is 5 to 10 yr.
- The infectious period begins 2 days before the onset of clinical symptoms and lasts until all of the lesions have crusted.
- Most patients will have lifelong immunity after an attack of chickenpox; protection from the virus after a varicella vaccine is approximately 6 yr.

PHYSICAL FINDINGS & CLINICAL PRESENTATION

- Findings vary with the clinical course. Initial symptoms consist of fever, chills, backache, generalized malaise, and headache.
- Symptoms are generally more severe in adults.
- Initial lesions generally occur on the trunk (centripetal distribution) and occasionally on the face; these lesions consist primarily of 3- to 4-mm red papules with an irregular outline and a clear vesicle on the surface (i.e., the appearance of dewdrops on a rose petal).
- Intense pruritus generally accompanies the initial stage.
- New lesion development generally ceases by the fourth day, with subsequent crusting by the sixth day.
- Lesions generally spread to the face and the extremities (i.e., centrifugal spread).
- Patients generally present with lesions that are in different stages at the same time.
- Crusts generally fall off within 5 to 14 days.
- The fever is usually highest during the eruption of the vesicles; the patient's temperature generally returns to normal after the disappearance of vesicles.
- Signs of potential complications (e.g., bacterial skin infections, neurologic complications, pneumonia, hepatitis) may be present on physical examination.
- Mild constitutional symptoms (e.g., anorexia, myalgias, headaches, restlessness) may be present; these are most common among adults.
- Excoriations may be present if scratching is prominent.

ETIOLOGY

Varicella-zoster virus is a human herpes virus III that can manifest with either varicella or herpes zoster (i.e., shingles, which is a reactivation of varicella).

DIAGNOSIS

DIFFERENTIAL DIAGNOSIS

- Other viral infection
- Impetigo
- Scabies
- Drug rash
- Urticaria
- Dermatitis herpetiformis
- Smallpox

WORKUP

The diagnosis is usually made on the basis of the patient's history and clinical presentation.

LABORATORY TESTS

- Laboratory evaluation is generally not necessary.
- The CBC may reveal leukopenia and thrombocytopenia.
- Serum varicella titers (i.e., a significant rise in the serum varicella immunoglobulin G antibody level), skin biopsies, or Tzanck smears are used only when diagnosis is in question.

TREATMENT

NONPHARMACOLOGIC THERAPY

- Use antipruritic lotions for symptomatic relief.
- Avoid scratching to prevent excoriations and superficial skin infections.
- Use a mild soap for bathing.
- Hands should be washed often.

ACUTE GENERAL Rx

- Use acetaminophen for fever and myalgias; aspirin should be avoided because of the associated increased risk for Reye's syndrome.
- Oral acyclovir (20 mg/kg qid for 5 days) initiated at the earliest sign (i.e., within 24 hr of illness) is useful for healthy, nonpregnant individuals 13 yr old or older to decrease the duration and severity of signs and symptoms. Immunocompromised hosts should be treated with intravenous acyclovir 500 mg/m^2 or 10 mg/kg q8h for 7 to 10 days.
- Varicella is most contagious from 2 days before to a few days after the onset of the rash. Varicella vaccine is available for children and adults; protection lasts at least 6 yr. Healthy, nonimmune adults and children exposed to varicella-zoster virus should receive prophylaxis with live attenuated varicella vaccine (Varivax). Patients with HIV or other immunocompromised patients should not receive the live attenuated vaccine.
- Exposed patients with contraindications to varicella vaccine can be treated with varicella-zoster immunoglobulin (VariZIG), which effectively prevents varicella in susceptible individuals. The dose is 12.5 U/kg IM up to a maximum of 625 U. VariZIG must be administered as early as possible after presumed exposure (i.e., within 4 days). If VariZIG cannot be obtained and administered within 4 days, providers should consider the use of intravenous immunoglobulin within 4 days of exposure.
- Pruritus from chickenpox can be controlled with antihistamines (e.g., hydroxyzine 25 mg q6h) and oral antipruritic lotions (e.g., calamine).
- Oral antibiotics are not routinely indicated and should be used only in patients with secondary infection and infected lesions; the most common infective organisms are *Streptococcus* sp. and *Staphylococcus* sp.

DISPOSITION

- The course is generally benign in immunocompetent adults and children.
- Infants who develop chickenpox are incapable of controlling the infection and should be given varicella-zoster immunoglobulin or gamma globulin if VariZIG is not available.

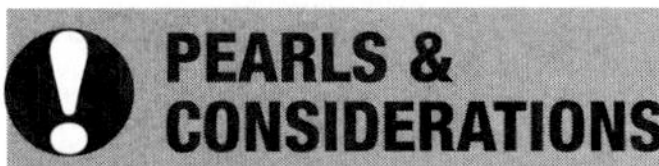

PEARLS & CONSIDERATIONS

COMMENTS

- VariZIG can be obtained from the nearest regional Red Cross Blood Center or the Centers for Disease Control and Prevention in Atlanta.
- Varicella immunization is recommended for all who have not had chickenpox; the dosage for adults and adolescents (>13 yr old) is two 0.5-ml doses 4 to 8 wk apart.

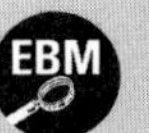

EVIDENCE

There is evidence that oral acyclovir reduces the symptoms of chickenpox in otherwise healthy people if started early, but its clinical importance in this area remains controversial.

The reviewers note that the clinical importance of acyclovir in otherwise healthy children remains controversial.[1] Ⓐ

Evidence-Based Reference

1. Klassen TP et al: Acyclovir for treating varicella in otherwise healthy children and adolescents, *Cochrane Database Syst Rev* 2:CD002980, 2004. Ⓐ

AUTHOR: **FRED F. FERRI, M.D.**

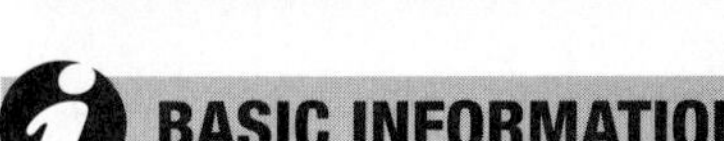

BASIC INFORMATION

DEFINITION

A varicocele is a collection of dilated and tortuous veins in the pampiniform plexus surrounding the spermatic cord in the scrotum.

SYNONYMS

Sometimes referred to as "bag of worms" (Fig. 1-356)

ICD-9CM CODES
456.4

EPIDEMIOLOGY & DEMOGRAPHICS

PREVALENCE: A varicocele is present in up to 20% of all males. It occurs in approximately 30% of infertile men. However, only 10% to 15% of males with varicoceles have fertility problems.

RISK FACTORS: There are no reliable data on epidemiologic risk factors for varicocele, such as a family history or environmental exposures.

PHYSICAL FINDINGS & CLINICAL PRESENTATION

- Patients may report a mass lying posterior to and above the testis. When the patient is supine, dilation of the veins is generally decreased. Dilation and tortuosity of the veins are increased when the patient is upright and when the patient performs a Valsalva maneuver.
- The majority of cases occur more commonly on the left side because the left spermatic vein enters the left renal vein at a 90-degree angle, whereas the right testicular vein drains directly into the vena cava.

ETIOLOGY

Varicoceles are caused by dysfunction of the valves in the spermatic vein, which allows pooling of blood in the pampiniform plexus.

DIAGNOSIS

DIFFERENTIAL DIAGNOSIS

- Hydrocele
- Spermatocele
- Epididymal orchitis
- Testicular tumor

WORKUP

Patient should be examined in an upright position and supine position.

LABORATORY TESTS

Semen analysis if a varicocele is detected and the patient is infertile

IMAGING

High-resolution color-flow Doppler ultrasound or Doppler ultrasound are the most common and least invasive technique to confirm a varicocele and differentiate from other scrotal abnormalities.

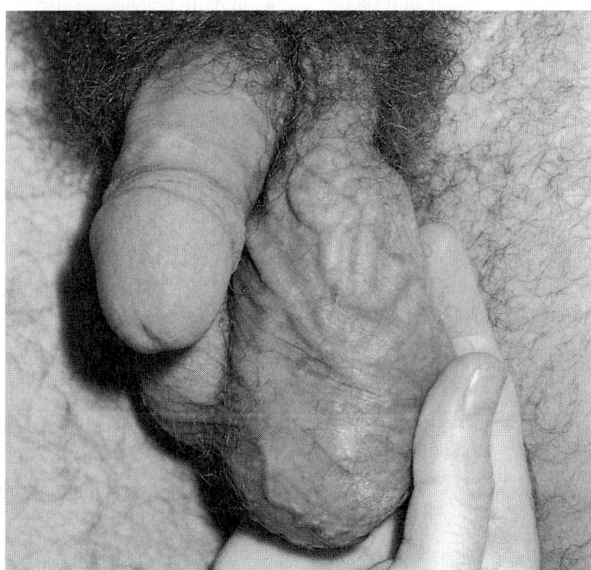

FIGURE 1-356 Varicocele. (From Swartz MH: *Textbook of physical diagnosis,* ed 5, Philadelphia, 2006, Saunders.)

TREATMENT

Once a varicocele is identified, providers must document bilateral testicular size at regular intervals. If the testicle on the affected side is small, spermatogenesis may have been adversely affected.

SURGERY

- Varicocelectomy is performed by ligation of the veins of the pampiniform plexus through an inguinal incision or by ligating the internal spermatic vein in the retroperitoneum. This is generally performed as an ambulatory surgery.
- The goal of varicocelectomy is to maximize chances for fertility.
- Surgical treatment is indicated when there is significant disparity in testicular size or pain. Also, surgery should be performed if the contralateral testis is diseased or absent. Surgery may be considered if the varicocele is large, even without a disparity in testicular size.
- Postoperatively the involved testis typically enlarges and catches up to the uninvolved side in 1 to 2 yr. Semen parameters also improve significantly in 65%.
- The success rate of surgical repair is close to 98%; that of percutaneous repair is significantly lower.

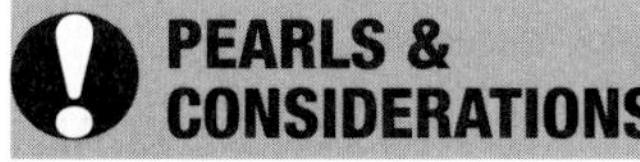

PEARLS & CONSIDERATIONS

- A varicocele in a boy <10 yr or on the right side may be indicative of an abdominal or retroperitoneal mass. Ultrasound should be performed.
- The sudden occurrence of a left-sided varicocele in an older man indicates occlusion of the spermatic vein and should prompt evaluation for a renal tumor.

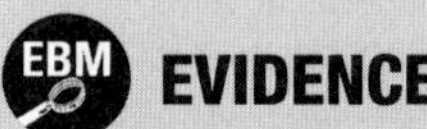

EVIDENCE

Please note: Complete text of EBM for this topic is available online.

SUGGESTED READINGS

Behrman RE et al: *Nelson textbook of pediatrics,* ed 16, Philadelphia, 2000, Saunders, pp 1652-1654.

Diamond DA: Adolescent varicocele, *Curr Opin Urol* 17(4):263, 2007.

Nseyo UO et al: Urology for primary care physicians, Philadelphia, 1999, Saunders, pp 339-346.

AUTHORS: **BETH NOWAK, M.D.,** and **JANICE PATACSIL-TRULL, M.D.**

Varicose Veins (PTG)

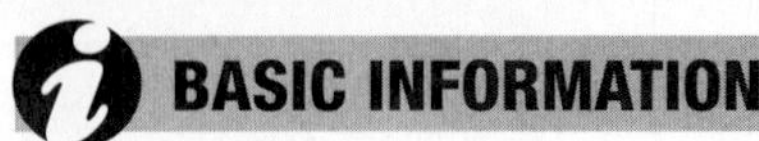

BASIC INFORMATION

DEFINITION

Varicose veins are dilated networks of the subcutaneous venous system that result from valvular incompetence.

SYNONYMS

Chronic venous insufficiency
Stasis skin changes

ICD-9CM CODES
454.9 Varicose veins

EPIDEMIOLOGY & DEMOGRAPHICS

PREVALENCE:

- Approximately 30% of adults, with increasing incidence with age
- Increased incidence during pregnancy, especially with advanced maternal age

PREDOMINANT SEX: Females are more commonly affected

GENETICS:

- Familial tendency
- Evidence for dominant, recessive, and multifactorial types of inheritance

RISK FACTORS:

- Advancing age
- Prolonged standing
- Pregnancy
- Obesity
- Use of oral contraceptives

PHYSICAL FINDINGS & CLINICAL PRESENTATION

- Visible tortuous veins in the territory of either the long saphenous vein (most common), short saphenous vein, or both
- Dull ache, burning, or cramping in leg muscles
- Worsening discomfort with standing, warm temperatures, or menses
- Blowouts: localized dilations
- Tortuous dilation of superficial veins
- Dermatitis, hyperpigmentation or hypopigmentation, edema, eczema
- Varicose ulcer, sometimes with superficial infection

ETIOLOGY

- Normally, blood flow directed from the superficial venous system to the deep venous system by communication of perforating vessels
- Best thought of as "venous hypertension"
- Valvular incompetence in perforator veins of lower extremity leading to reverse flow of fluid from high-pressure deep venous system to low-pressure superficial venous system, resulting in dilation of superficial veins, leg edema, and pain
- Rarely associated with deep vein thrombophlebitis
- Exacerbated by restrictive clothing

Dx DIAGNOSIS

DIFFERENTIAL DIAGNOSIS

Conditions that can lead to superficial venous stasis other than primary valvular insufficiency include:

- Arterial occlusive disease
- Diabetes
- Deep vein thrombophlebitis
- Peripheral neuropathies
- Unusual infections
- Carcinoma

WORKUP

- Mainly a clinical diagnosis: Trendelenburg test
- Arterial studies to rule out arterial insufficiency before initiating therapy for venous insufficiency

LABORATORY TESTS

Not useful

IMAGING STUDIES

Duplex ultrasound:

- Gold standard for evaluation of varicose veins
- Quantitation of flow through venous valves under direct visualization
- Allows precise anatomic identification of source of venous reflux
- Rarely ascending venography and varicography for unusually located varices and recurrence after surgical treatment.

Rx TREATMENT

NONPHARMACOLOGIC THERAPY

- Leg elevation and rest
- Graded compression stockings: used early in morning before edema accumulates and removed before going to bed
- Weight loss
- Avoidance of occlusive clothing

ACUTE GENERAL Rx

- For associated stasis dermatitis: topical corticosteroids
- Treatment of secondary infection with appropriate antibiotics

CHRONIC Rx

- Compression sclerotherapy: injection of 1% to 3% solution of sodium tetradecyl sulfate or 5% ethanolamine oleate
- Surgery: indications include the following:
  1. Persistent varicosities with conservative treatment
  2. Failed sclerotherapy
  3. Previous or impending bleeding from ulcerated varicosities
  4. Disabling pain
  5. Cosmetic concerns
- Surgical methods include (must be combined with compressive therapy):
  1. Saphenous vein ligation
  2. Ligation of incompetent perforating veins
  3. Saphenous vein stripping with or without avulsion of varicosities
  4. Ambulatory "mini-phlebectomies": avulsion of superficial varicosities with saphenous vein stripping
  5. New treatments: endovenous obliteration using radiofrequency (diathermy) or laser as an alternative to traditional stripping of the long saphenous vein and powered phlebectomy for avulsing calf varicosities.

COMPLICATIONS:

- Hemorrhage
- Thrombophlebitis
- Atrophie blanche
- Varicose eczema
- Lipodermatosclerosis
- Venous ulceration

DISPOSITION

A chronic condition in which a combination of compressive and surgical therapy can adequately control varicosities

REFERRAL

- To dermatologist for dermatitis complications
- To surgeon for failed conservative management or varicose veins with complications

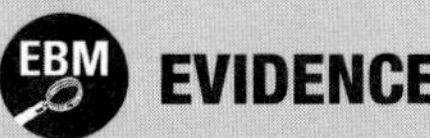

EVIDENCE

Please note: Complete text of EBM for this topic is available online.

SUGGESTED READINGS

Crane J, Cheshire N: Recent developments in vascular surgery, *BMJ* 327(7420):911, 2003.

Hagen MD, Johnson ED: What treatments are effective for varicose veins? *J Fam Pract* 52(4):329, 2003.

Jones RH, Carek PJ: Management of varicose veins, *Am Fam Phys* 78(11):1289-1294, 2008.

AUTHORS: **ARUNDATHI G. PRASAD, M.D.,** and **RUBEN ALVERO, M.D.**

BASIC INFORMATION

DEFINITION

Venous ulcers are shallow wounds with irregular borders that usually occur on the lower extremities between the mid calf and the ankle. These ulcerations develop in patients with venous insufficiency as a result of incompetent valves, obstructed veins, or immobility.

SYNONYMS

Stasis ulcers
Peripheral venous insufficiency
Venous leg ulcers

ICD-9CM CODES

459.3	Chronic venous hypertension, including stasis edema
459.81	Peripheral venous insufficiency
707.1	Ulcer of the lower limb

EPIDEMIOLOGY & DEMOGRAPHICS

PREVALENCE: Venous ulcers primarily occur in patients who are between 60 and 80 yr old, with women being affected more frequently than men.

RISK FACTORS:
- Smoking
- Obesity
- Diabetes mellitus
- Phlebitis
- Increasing age
- Family history of varicose veins
- History of deep vein thrombosis
- Congestive heart failure

PHYSICAL FINDINGS & CLINICAL PRESENTATION

- Patients with venous stasis often have chronic skin changes on their lower limbs, including hyperpigmentation as a result of the deposition of hemosiderin, hyperkeratosis, and dependent edema.
- Venous dermatitis or stasis dermatitis is characterized by pruritic, red, and scaly eczematous changes.
- The smooth white plaques of atrophic sclerosis, which are known as *atrophie blanche,* are a result of chronic fibrosis.
- Venous ulcers are shallow, full-thickness ulcers with irregular borders and areas of granulation tissue; necrosis is extremely rare.
- Patients often report a long history of dependent lower-extremity edema and aching pain in the legs that is often worse after they have stood for a long period.

ETIOLOGY

Venous stasis develops from valvular incompetence or obstruction and results in venous hypertension. Some researchers propose that venous hypertension leads to the malformation of capillaries, which subsequently causes the leakage of fluid and reduced blood flow to the skin. The resultant hypoxic tissue is prone to ulceration after minor trauma, and the underlying vascular deficiency also impedes wound healing.

Dx DIAGNOSIS

DIFFERENTIAL DIAGNOSIS

- Peripheral arterial disease (with ischemia and necrosis)
- Diabetic ulceration (often as a result of neuropathy)
- Decubitus ulceration (caused by pressure over a bony prominence)
- Vasculitis (with erythema and bullae)
- Necrotic ulceration from infection
- Basal cell carcinoma
- Squamous cell carcinoma

WORKUP

- The majority of patients can be diagnosed clinically from the physical examination; however, up to 25% of patients have concomitant arterial disease. In these patients, an ankle–brachial index should be performed. Arterial insufficiency is suggested by an ankle–brachial index of <1.0.
- Patients with lower-extremity ulcers should also be evaluated for diabetes.
- In patients with a known or suspected history of deep venous thrombosis, a thrombophilia workup is indicated.
- If vasculitis is suspected, a biopsy of the edge of the ulcer can confirm the diagnosis.
- Any wound that is present for more than 3 months should be biopsied to rule out malignancy.

IMAGING STUDIES

- Duplex ultrasonography can evaluate for deep and superficial reflux among patients who are considering surgery.
- Venography may be recommended for patients with postthrombotic disease, especially if some type of intervention is considered.
- If the ulcer appears to be infected, consider plain x-ray films to evaluate for osteomyelitis.

Rx TREATMENT

NONPHARMACOLOGIC THERAPY

- The goal of therapy is to improve venous return to the heart, thereby decreasing edema, inflammation, and tissue ischemia.
- The first-line treatment of ulcers includes compression stockings or bandages and the elevation of the leg for at least 30 minutes three to four times per day. Bandages are used under compression stockings to provide a clean, moist environment to promote healing. Highly exudative wounds require absorbent dressings, whereas dry wounds may need a more occlusive dressing. There is no conclusive evidence that supports one type of dressing over another.
- Venous stasis can be treated with the use of compression stockings alone. Knee-high stockings with graded pressure that provide at least 35 to 40 mm Hg of pressure at the ankle and 20 to 25 mm Hg at the knee are most effective. The stockings should be removed at night and replaced every 6 months.
- Compression with either bandages or stockings is to be used only after arterial disease has been excluded, because the compression can cause limb ischemia.
- Surgical intervention is not routine; however, options include sclerotherapy, the replacement of venous valves, ligation, and the stripping of veins. Skin grafts are also an option for wounds that do not heal.

ACUTE GENERAL Rx

- Moist occlusive dressings and certain topical agents can help with the healing of venous ulcers.
- Dressings can be nonadherent (e.g., Telfa), occlusive (e.g., Tegaderm, DuoDERM), or medicated (e.g., unna boot). Occlusive bandages have the advantage of reducing pain, and they can be changed by the patient every 5 to 7 days. These bandages do not increase the rate of wound infection if they are used appropriately.
- Daily aspirin (300 mg) is recommended to accelerate healing.
- Underlying systemic hypertension and diabetes should be aggressively treated.
- Pentoxifylline (800 mg tid) has been shown to be a modestly effective adjuvant to compression therapy. Daflon (micronized purified flavonoid fractions, 1000 mg daily) has been shown to inhibit inflammatory mediators, and it may increase healing rates.
- Antiseptics (e.g., iodine) cause cellular toxicity and should not be used on ulcers. In addition, silver sulfadiazine (e.g., Silvadene), neomycin, and bacitracin are common causes of contact dermatitis and skin irritation; thus, they are not recommended.
- Systemic antibiotics are not indicated unless there are obvious signs of infection (e.g., erythema, heat, purulent drainage, pain).
- The prevention of recurrence is essential and includes the continued use of compression stockings, leg elevation, smoking cessation, and weight loss.

COMPLEMENTARY & ALTERNATIVE MEDICINE

Horse chestnut seed extract (50 mg bid) may reduce the edema associated with venous stasis. It can be used in patients who cannot tolerate compression therapy.

DISPOSITION

The overall prognosis for this condition is poor. Although 50% of ulcers will heal after 4 months, 20% are nonhealing after 2 years of treatment, and 8% are nonhealing after 8 years. Recurrence is common.

REFERRAL

- Referral to a wound clinic should be considered for patients with large ($>5 \times 5$ cm) or longstanding wounds.
- All patients should be evaluated after 1 month of therapy. If the wound shows little to no improvement, then referral is suggested.

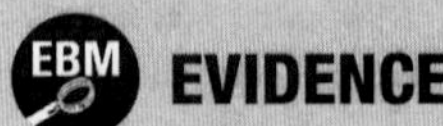

Please note: Complete text of EBM for this topic is available online.

SUGGESTED READINGS

Darmas B: Should incompetent perforating vein surgery be a part of the surgical management of venous ulceration? *Surgeon* 7:238-242, 2009.

Etufugh CN et al: Venous ulcers, *Clin Dermatol* 25:121-130, 2007.

Gohel MS, Davies AH: Pharmacological agents in the treatment of venous disease: an update of the available evidence, *Curr Vasc Pharmacol* 7:303-308, 2009.

Raju S, Neglen P: Chronic venous insufficiency and varicose veins, *N Engl J Med* 360:2319-2327, 2009.

AUTHORS: **KELLY BOSSENBROEK FEDORIW, M.D.,** and **JEFFREY M. BORKAN, M.D., PH.D.**

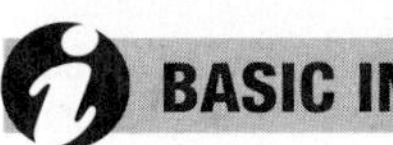

BASIC INFORMATION

DEFINITION

- Ventricular septal defect (VSD) refers to an abnormal communication through the septum that separates the right and left ventricles of the heart.
- VSDs may be large or small and single or multiple.
- VSDs are located at various anatomic regions of the septum and classified as follows:
  - Membranous (75% to 80%): This is the most common type of defect, and it extends into the membranous portion of the interventricular septum. The septal leaflet of the tricuspid valve may become adherent and form a "pouch" of the septum that can limit the left-to-right shunting.
  - Muscular or trabecular (5% to 20%): This defect is entirely surrounded by muscular tissue.
  - Canal or inlet (8%): This defect commonly lies beneath the septal leaflet of the tricuspid valve; it is often seen in patients with Down's syndrome.
  - Subarterial, outlet, infundibular, or supracristal (5% to 7%): This is the least common type of defect. It is usually found beneath the aortic valve, and it may lead to aortic regurgitation.

SYNONYMS

VSD

ICD-9CM CODES
745.4 Ventricular septal defect

EPIDEMIOLOGY & DEMOGRAPHICS

- VSD was first described by Dalrymple in 1847.
- VSDs are one of the most common congenital heart abnormalities, accounting for 30% of all congenital cardiac defects.
- VSD accounts for approximately 25% of all congenital heart defects in children and for approximately 10% of defects in adults (the decrease is a result of spontaneous closure that occurs by adulthood).
- The prevalence of VSD is 1.17/1000 live births and 0.5/1000 adults.
- VSD is found with equal frequency among both males and females.
- VSD may be associated with the following conditions:
  - Atrial septal defect (35%)
  - Patent ductus arteriosus (22%)
  - Coarctation of the aorta (17%)
  - Subvalvular aortic stenosis (4%)
  - Subpulmonic stenosis
- Multiple VSDs are more prevalent among patients with tetralogy of Fallot and double-outlet right ventricular defects.

PHYSICAL FINDINGS & CLINICAL PRESENTATION

- Clinical presentation depends on the direction and volume of the VSD shunt, which is dictated by the size of the defect and the ratio of the pulmonary vascular resistance.
  - Defects of ≤25% of the aortic annulus diameter are small defects that typically involve small left-to-right shunts, no left ventricular volume overload, and no pulmonary artery hypertension.
  - Defects that are 25% to 75% of aortic annulus diameter are considered to be moderate in size, with small to moderate left-to-right shunting, mild to moderate left ventricular volume overload, and mild or no pulmonary artery hypertension. Patients may have symptoms of congestive heart failure that may improve with medical therapy or with age as the defect decreases in size relative to increasing body size.
  - Defects of ≥75% of the aortic annulus diameter usually have moderate to large left-to-right shunting, left ventricular volume overload, and pulmonary artery hypertension. These patients usually have a history of congestive heart failure, or they may possibly develop right-to-left shunting in the setting of Eisenmenger's syndrome during late childhood, adolescence, or young adulthood.
- Infants may be asymptomatic at birth because of elevated pulmonary artery resistance. During the first few weeks of life, pulmonary arterial resistance decreases, thereby allowing for more left-to-right shunting through the VSD. This results in a subsequent increase in flow into the lungs, the left atrium, and the left ventricle, which can potentially cause left ventricular volume overload. Tachypnea, failure to thrive, and congestive heart failure may then ensue.
- In adults with VSD, the shunt is left to right in the absence of pulmonary stenosis and pulmonary hypertension. Patients typically manifest symptoms of left-sided heart failure (e.g., shortness of breath, orthopnea, dyspnea on exertion).
- A spectrum of physical findings may be seen, including the following:
  - Machinelike holosystolic murmur that is heard best along the left sternal border (i.e., shorter duration of the murmur as right ventricular pressure increases)
  - Systolic thrill
  - Mid-diastolic rumble heard at the apex
  - S_3 heart sound
  - Rales
- With the development of pulmonary hypertension, the following occur:
  - An augmented pulmonic component of the S_2 heart sound
  - Cyanosis, clubbing, right ventricular heave, and signs of right heart failure (i.e., as seen with Eisenmenger's complex, with a reversal of the shunt in a right-to-left direction)

ETIOLOGY

- VSD is usually congenital (which is the focus of this review), but it may occur after myocardial infarction.
- After acute myocardial infarction, the rupture of the intraventricular septum typically occurs 1 to 5 days after the event in 0.2% of patients in the current fibrinolytic, primary angioplasty era.

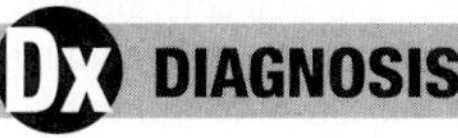

DIAGNOSIS

The diagnosis of VSD can be suspected during a physical examination. Imaging studies—particularly transthoracic echocardiography with color Doppler—establish the diagnosis.

DIFFERENTIAL DIAGNOSIS

On the basis of the physical examination alone, the diagnosis of VSD may be confused with other causes of systolic murmurs, such as mitral regurgitation, tricuspid regurgitation, aortic stenosis, pulmonary stenosis, and hypertrophic cardiomyopathy.

WORKUP

Any person who is suspected of having a VSD should undergo an ECG, a chest radiograph, and an echocardiogram.

LABORATORY TESTS

- Laboratory tests are not specific but may offer insight into the severity of the disease.
- The CBC may show polycythemia, especially in patients with Eisenmenger's complex.
- Arterial blood gas results may demonstrate hypoxemia.

IMAGING STUDIES

- ECG findings vary in accordance with the size of the VSD and depending on whether pulmonary hypertension is present. With large VSDs with pulmonary hypertension, right-axis deviation is seen, along with evidence of right ventricular hypertrophy.
- Chest x-ray findings in patients with VSD include the following:
  - Cardiomegaly that results from left ventricular volume overload that directly relates to the magnitude of the shunt
  - The enlargement of the proximal pulmonary arteries along with the redistribution and pruning of the distal pulmonary vessels as a result of sustained pulmonary hypertension (Fig. 1-357, *A*)
- Echocardiography is the imaging modality of choice for the diagnosis of VSD:
  - Two-dimensional echocardiography and color Doppler display the size and location of the VSD (Fig. 1-357, *B*), the chamber sizes, ventricular function, the presence of aortic valve prolapse or regurgitation, outflow tract obstruction, and the presence of tricuspid regurgitation.
  - Continuous-wave Doppler approximates the gradient between the left and right ventricle and estimates the pulmonary artery pressure.
  - The magnitude of the shunt can be determined by the calculation of the pulmonary-to-systemic flow ratio with the use of echocardiography.

- Right and left heart catheterization may confirm the echocardiography findings of the measurement of right heart pressures and the calculation of the pulmonary-to-systemic flow ratio.
- Ventriculography may help to locate the VSD:
  - MRI and computed tomography scanning can be useful to assess the pulmonary artery, the pulmonary vein, and the aortic anatomy and to confirm the anatomy of unusual VSDs (e.g., inlet or apical defects) that are not seen well with echocardiography.

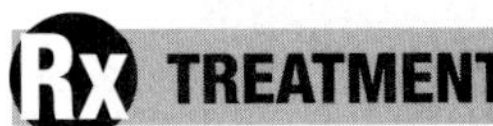

TREATMENT

The decision to close a VSD depends on the type, size, and shunt severity as well as the patient's pulmonary vascular resistance, functional capacity, and associated valvular abnormalities.

NONPHARMACOLOGIC THERAPY

- In young children and adults, a small, asymptomatic VSD with a large left-to-right ventricular pressure gradient, a pulmonary-to-systemic blood flow ratio of less than 1.5:1, and no evidence of pulmonary hypertension can be observed (i.e., restrictive defect).
- Oxygen for hypoxemia and a low-salt diet are recommended for patients with congestive heart failure.

ACUTE GENERAL & CHRONIC RX

Closure is indicated for the following patients:

- Infants with congestive heart failure
- Children between the ages of 1 and 6 yr with persistent VSD and a pulmonary-to-systemic blood flow ratio (Qp/Qs) of $>$2:1
- Adults with a Qp/Qs of $\geq$2 and clinical evidence of left ventricular volume overload (class I):
  - Positive history of infective endocarditis (class I)
  - Adults with a Qp/Qs of $>$1.5 with pulmonary artery pressure that is less than two thirds of the systemic pressure and pulmonary vascular resistance that is less than two thirds of the systemic vascular resistance (class IIa)
  - Adults with a Qp/Qs of $>$1.5 in the presence of left ventricular systolic or diastolic failure (class IIa)

Surgical closure with Dacron or Gore-Tex patches or primary surgical closure has long been the gold standard of therapy. However, with improvements in cardiac imaging and catheter devices, percutaneous transcatheter closure has risen in popularity. Either an Amplatzer or CardioSEAL occluder device can be used for congenital (muscular or perimembranous), postsurgical, and some traumatic VSDs of certain sizes, certain geometry, and certain locations on the septum. There have been studies that have shown similar success rates for both surgical and percutaneous closures, and there are significantly fewer complications, days in the hospital, and blood transfusions after percutaneous closures. Postinfarct VSDs usually carry a high mortality rate, and surgical closure is still the preferred method of treatment for this type.

DISPOSITION

- The natural history of an isolated VSD depends on the type of defect, its size, and any associated abnormalities.
- Approximately 75% to 80% of small VSDs close spontaneously by the time the patient reaches the age of 10 yr.
- Only 10% to 15% of large VSDs will close spontaneously.
- Large VSDs that are left untreated may lead to arrhythmias, congestive heart failure, pulmonary hypertension, and Eisenmenger's complex.
- Eisenmenger's complex carries a poor prognosis, with most patients dying before the age of 40 yr.
- Issues to monitor in adults with unrepaired or repaired and catheter-closed VSDs include the following:
  - The development of aortic regurgitation
  - The assessment of associated coronary artery disease
  - The development of tricuspid regurgitation

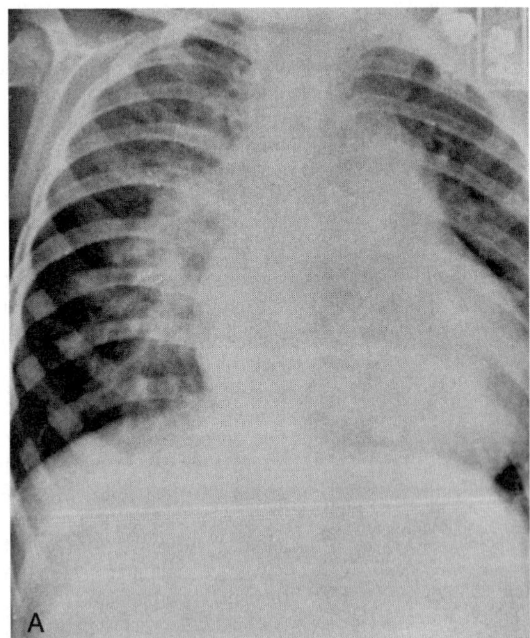

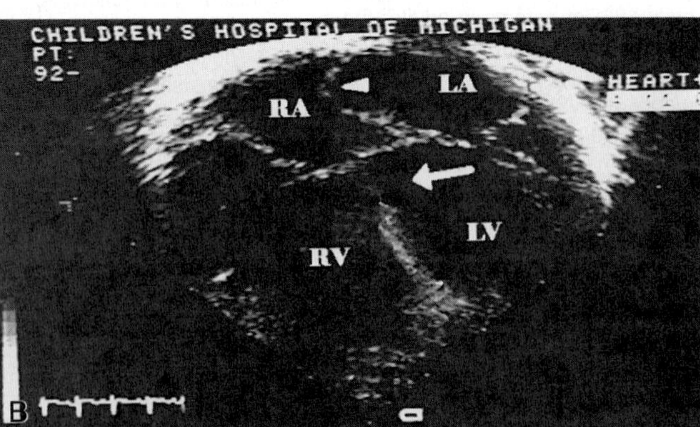

FIGURE 1-357 A, Chest roentgenogram of a child with a large ventricular septal defect, large pulmonary blood flow, and pulmonary hypertension but only mild elevation of peripheral vascular resistance. This is reflected in the evidence of left and right ventricular enlargement, the enlargement of the main pulmonary artery, and a marked increase in pulmonary blood flow. **B,** Apical four-chamber echocardiographic view of ventricular septal defect *(large arrow).* The small arrow points to the interatrial septum. *LA,* Left atrium; *LV,* left ventricle; *RA,* right atrium; *RV,* right ventricle. (**A,** From Pacifico AD et al: Surgical treatment of ventricular septal defect. In Sabiston DC Jr, Spencer FC [eds]: *Surgery of the chest,* ed 5, Philadelphia, 1990, WB Saunders. **B,** Courtesy of Richard Humes, MD, Children's Hospital of Michigan, Detroit.)

- ○ The assessment of the degree of left-to-right shunting (in unrepaired or residual VSD after repair)
- ○ Ventricular dysfunction
- ○ The assessment of pulmonary pressure
- ○ The development of subpulmonary stenosis (usually as a result of a double-chambered right ventricle)
- ○ The development of discrete subaortic stenosis
- ○ The development of arrhythmia or heart block
- ○ Thromboembolic complications
- ○ Infective endocarditis
- After closure, late survival is excellent when ventricular function is normal. Pulmonary artery hypertension may improve, progress, or remain the same. Late operations may be required for tricuspid or aortic regurgitation.

REFERRAL

All infants and children diagnosed with VSD should be referred to a pediatric cardiologist. Adults with VSD should be referred to an adult cardiologist. Cardiothoracic surgeons who have experience with congenital heart disease surgery should be consulted if surgery is indicated.

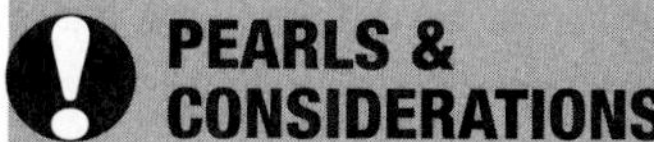

PEARLS & CONSIDERATIONS

COMMENTS

- A loud murmur does not imply a large VSD. Small, hemodynamically insignificant VSDs can cause loud murmurs.
- In patients with Eisenmenger's complex, the right-to-left shunting across the VSD is usually not associated with an audible murmur.
- The risk of patients with unrepaired VSD developing infective endocarditis is 4%. The risk is higher if aortic insufficiency is present.
- For patients with endocarditis, routine antibiotic prophylaxis for dental or surgical procedures is no longer indicated for isolated VSDs, except in the following circumstances:
  - ○ In the presence of complex congenital heart disease with cyanosis
  - ○ In the presence of a residual VSD after surgical closure
  - ○ During the first 6 mo after surgical patch or percutaneous transcatheter closure
- Any patient with a newly diagnosed murmur or hemodynamic compromise after a myocardial infarction should undergo evaluation for possible VSD.
- Pregnancy with a VSD is generally well tolerated in women with small VSDs, no pulmonary artery hypertension, and no associated lesions. Women with large shunts may experience arrhythmias, ventricular dysfunction, and the progression of pulmonary hypertension.
- Women with VSDs and severe pulmonary artery hypertension or Eisenmenger's physiology should be counseled against pregnancy because of associated excessive maternal and fetal mortality.

SUGGESTED READINGS

Butera G et al: Percutaneous closure of ventricular septal defects. State of the art, *J Cardiovasc Med,* 8(1):39-45, 2007.

Minette MS, Sahn DJ: Ventricular septal defects, *Circulation* 114(20):2190, 2006.

Warnes et al: ACC/AHA 2008. Guidelines for Adults with CHD, *J Am Coll Cardiol* 52(23), 2008.

Wilson W et al: Prevention of infective endocarditis. Guidelines from the American Heart Association, *Circulation* 115:739, 2007.

Zheng Q et al: A comparative study: early results and complications of percutaneous and surgical closure of ventricular septal defect, *Cardiology* 114(4): 238-243, 2009.

AUTHORS: **SCOTT COHEN, M.D.,** and **WEN-CHIH WU, M.D.**

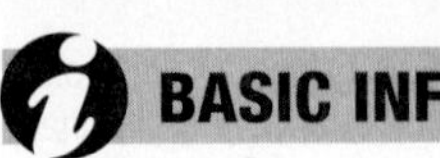

BASIC INFORMATION

DEFINITION

Vertebral compression fractures (VCFs) are defined as fractures of spinal vertebrae in which a bony surface is driven toward another bony surface. These fractures are classified as radiographic reductions in vertebral body height of more than 15% to 20%.

SYNONYMS

Thoracolumbar vertebral compression fractures
Osteoporotic fractures

ICD-9CM CODES	
805.8	Compression fracture, spine
805.4	Compression fracture, lumbar vertebra
805.2	Compression fracture, thoracic vertebra
733.13	Compression fracture, L2 vertebra

EPIDEMIOLOGY & DEMOGRAPHICS

Approximately 700,000 VCFs occur in the U.S. each year, and they affect approximately 25% of postmenopausal women. The prevalence increases with age, reaching a peak of 40% among women who are more than 80 yr old. Compression fractures are also a major concern among men, although their rates of VCF are lower.

RISK FACTORS:

- Modifiable: tobacco or alcohol use, osteoporosis, estrogen deficiency (i.e., early menopause, bilateral ovariectomy, premenopausal amenorrhea for more than 1 yr), frailty, impaired vision, abusive situations, inadequate physical activity, low body mass index, and dietary deficiency of vitamin D or calcium
- Nonmodifiable: advanced age, female gender, dementia, Caucasian, history of fractures in adulthood and among first-degree relatives, and falls

PHYSICAL FINDINGS & CLINICAL PRESENTATION

- Asymptomatic: Most VCFs are asymptomatic, except for height loss or kyphosis (i.e., dowager hump), which is often a sign of multiple VCFs.
- Symptomatic: Many VCFs often present as acute back pain after activity (e.g., bending, lifting) or coughing; neck strain and rib pain may also be present.

ETIOLOGY

- VCFs take place when the combination of bending and the axial load on the spine exceed the strength of the vertebral body.
- The primary etiology of VCF is osteoporosis.

DIAGNOSIS

DIFFERENTIAL DIAGNOSIS

- Hyperparathyroidism
- Osteomalacia
- Granulomatous diseases (e.g., tuberculosis)
- Hematologic/oncologic diseases (e.g., multiple myeloma, malignancy)

WORKUP

- Only one third of VCFs are diagnosed.
- VCF can be clinically suspected from the history and physical alone.
- There may or may not be a specific injury or a remembered event that led to the VCF.

LABORATORY TESTS

Tests to rule out infection or cancer may be helpful, such as a CBC, an erythrocyte sedimentation rate, an alkaline phosphatase level, and a C-reactive protein level; these tests can be reserved for individuals for whom there is a clinical suspicion.

IMAGING STUDIES

- Plain frontal and lateral radiographs (x-rays) are the initial imaging method (Fig. 1-358) and may be sufficient, particularly when no neurologic abnormalities are present. MRI and computed tomography (CT) scans may be uncomfortable or painful for the patient, especially during the acute phase.
- Although CT scans are not routinely necessary, they can be helpful for visualizing fractures that are not seen on plain films, for evaluating the integrity of the posterior vertebral wall, for ruling out other causes of back pain, for detecting spinal canal narrowing, and for assessing instability.
- MRI may be useful when spinal cord compression is suspected, if neurologic symptoms are present, or to distinguish malignancy from osteoporosis (e.g., in patients <55 yr with VCR after minimum or no trauma).
- Bone density studies may be helpful to determine the severity of osteoporosis, which is a key risk factor for future fractures.

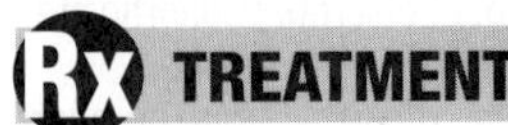

TREATMENT

NONPHARMACOLOGIC THERAPY

- Physical therapy
- External back braces
- Exercise programs: Getting the person active as soon as possible is extremely important for both the short and long term.

ACUTE GENERAL Rx

- Analgesics for pain control, including acetaminophen and opioids (oral or parenteral). The prevention of constipation is important with opioids.
- Nonsteroidal anti-inflammatory drugs are helpful but must be used with caution among elderly patients or when contraindicated.
- Muscle relaxants should be used judiciously.
- Carefully selected patients who do not respond to several weeks of conservative therapy may be considered for percutaneous vertebroplasty. With this procedure, acrylic bone cement is injected into the affected

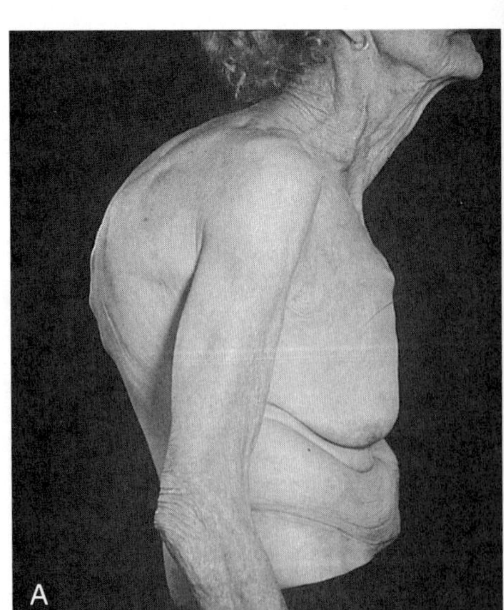

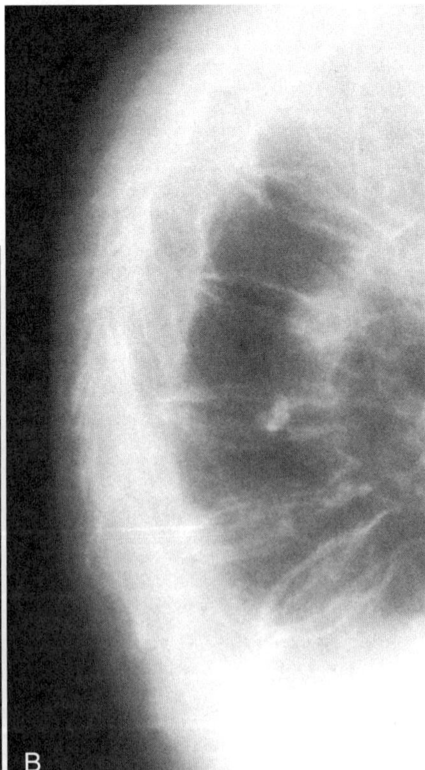

FIGURE 1-358 Dowager's hump. A, Marked thoracic kyphosis due to multiple osteoporotic fractures in an elderly woman with **B,** corresponding radiograph. (From Hochberg MC et al [eds]: *Rheumatology,* ed 3, St Louis, 2003, Mosby.)

vertebral body in an effort to stabilize the fracture and reduce pain. These patients may also be candidates for kyphoplasty, during which a high-pressure inflatable bone tamp or balloon is expanded before the injection of bone cement into the cavity of the fractured vertebral body. Although these are potentially useful procedures for pain relief, there is controversy regarding the amount of time that conservative therapy alone should be pursued. In addition, a recent trial found no beneficial effect of vertebroplasty as compared with a sham procedure in patients with painful osteoporotic vertebral fractures at 1 wk or at 1, 3, or 6 mo after treatment.

CHRONIC Rx

Osteoporosis should be treated with the reduction of risk factors (e.g., smoking, alcohol), diet exercise, calcium and vitamin D supplements, and potentially the use of medications that are more commonly used to treat osteoporosis (e.g., bisphosphonates).

REFERRAL

Referral is indicated for neurologic abnormalities, unremitting pain, instability, continued disability, or when the investigation of the cause of the fracture reveals serious underlying pathology.

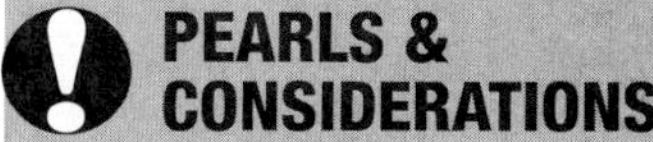

PEARLS & CONSIDERATIONS

COMMENTS

- VCFs should be suspected in anyone >50 yr old with the acute onset of low back pain. There are many opportunities for diagnosis and treatment that are easy to miss, especially for males.
- Solitary vertebral fractures higher than T7 are unusual and may be suspicious for other pathologic causes.
- Diagnosing and treating osteoporosis reduces the incidence of VCFs.
- Getting people with VCF physically active as soon as possible will be efficacious both acutely and in the long term.
- In general, VCF can perhaps be best managed through a partnership of the patient, the primary care physician, an orthopedist, a physical therapist, a dietician, and a social worker.

PREVENTION

Reducing the effects of modifiable risk factors is key.

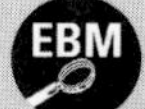

EVIDENCE

Please note: Complete text of EBM for this topic is available online.

Key trials and commentary:

Balloon kyphoplasty is a minimally invasive procedure for the treatment of painful vertebral fractures, which is intended to reduce pain and improve quality of life. This study assessed the efficacy and safety of the procedure. The findings suggest that balloon kyphoplasty is an effective and safe procedure for patients with acute vertebral fractures; the findings will help to inform decisions regarding its use as an early treatment option.

Postmenopausal osteoporosis is effectively prevented or treated with the currently available antiresorptive or anabolic agents in most cases. However, these agents prevent at most only 50% to 70% of the vertebral fractures that would have occurred without therapy. Each year 1.4 million vertebral fractures occur worldwide. Patients occasionally experience vertebral fractures when on therapy. Vertebral fractures cause height loss, kyphosis, reduced pulmonary function, mobility and balance impairment, and increase the risk of subsequent vertebral and other fractures for at least the first year after fracture.

Vertebral fractures that occur with or without therapy for osteoporosis are variably painful, but many patients experience moderate to severe pain that does not improve over time, as expected. Balloon kyphoplasty is a minimally invasive procedure for treatment of painful vertebral fractures that is intended to reduce pain and improve quality of life.[5]

The authors of this study randomized 149 patients with one to three acute vertebral compression fractures to balloon kyphoplasty, and 151 patients to nonsurgical care, including analgesia, bed rest, physiotherapy, and/or back bracing. The primary end point of the study was the difference in change between the two groups in the physical component summary score on the SF-36 short form (scale from 0-100) from baseline to 1 month. Of the randomized subjects, 138 patients in the kyphoplasty group and 128 patients in the nonsurgical care group completed 1 month of follow-up. The SF-36 physical component summary improved by 7.2 points in the kyphoplasty group (from 26.0 at baseline to 33.4 at one month), and by 2.0 points in the nonsurgical treatment group (from 25.5 at baseline to 27.4 at 1 month). Adverse events did not differ significantly between the groups. The authors concluded that balloon kyphoplasty is an effective and safe procedure for patients with acute vertebral compression fractures.

This study is important because it is the first large randomized trial to demonstrate that patients with painful vertebral fractures improve with balloon kyphoplasty compared with nonsurgical care. Other investigators have reported improvement in pain and functional outcome after kyphoplasty treatment, but without nonsurgically treated controls. Other prospective randomized trials comparing kyphoplasty or vertebroplasty, a related procedure, to nonsurgical care are under way. One small, randomized vertebroplasty trial showed short-term improvement in disability and quality of life at 2 weeks after treatment. One uncontrolled study has shown an increased risk of subsequent vertebral compression fracture after kyphoplasty. Information obtained from ongoing randomized controlled clinical trials will help place kyphoplasty and vertebroplasty in their proper perspective for management of osteoporotic vertebral fractures.[1] Ⓐ

Evidence-Based Reference

1. Wardlaw D et al: Efficacy and safety of balloon kyphoplasty compared with non-surgical care for vertebral compression fracture (FREE): a randomised controlled trial, *Lancet* 373:1016–1024, 2009. Commentary by B. Clarke, M.D. Ⓐ

SUGGESTED READINGS

Banerjee S et al: Back stab: percutaneous vertebroplasty in severe back pain, *Can Fam Physician* 53(7):1169, 2007.

Brunton S et al: Vertebral compression fractures in primary care: recommendations from a consensus panel, *J Fam Pract* 54(9):781-788, 2005.

Buchbinder R et al: A randomized trial of vertebroplasty for painful osteoporotic vertebral fractures, *N Engl J Med* 361:557-568, 2009.

Freedman BA et al: Osteoporosis and vertebral compression fractures—continued missed opportunities, *Spine J* 8:756-762, 2008.

Garfin SR, Reilley MA: Minimally invasive treatment of osteoporotic vertebral body compression fractures, *Spine J* 1:76-80, 2002.

Lavelle W et al: Vertebroplasty and kyphoplasty, *Med Clin North Am* 91(2):299-314, 2007.

Old JL, Calvert M: Vertebral compression fractures in the elderly, *Am Fam Physician* 69:111-116, 2004.

AUTHOR: **JEFFREY BORKAN, M.D., PH.D**

Vestibular Neuronitis

BASIC INFORMATION

DEFINITION

Vestibular neuronitis is a syndrome of sudden-onset, often severe, prolonged vertigo of peripheral origin.

SYNONYMS

Labyrinthitis, vestibular neuronitis, acute neuritis

ICD-9CM CODES
078.81 Vestibular neuronitis
386.12 Neuronitis, vestibular

EPIDEMIOLOGY & DEMOGRAPHICS

Viral origin supported by the fact that it occurs in epidemics, may affect several family members, and occurs more commonly in spring and early summer. Male-to-female ratio is similar. Thought to result from selective inflammation of the vestibular nerve; etiology presumed to be viral. There is selective damage to the superior part of the vestibular labyrinth, supplied by the superior division of the vestibular nerve.

PHYSICAL FINDINGS & CLINICAL PRESENTATION

- Course: develops over period of hours, resolves over periods of days, though with frequent long-term sequela; may have viral prodrome.
- Symptoms of vertigo, spontaneous peripheral nystagmus, positive head-thrust test, imbalance. Patient reports intense sensation of rotation, difficulty standing and walking, tends to veer toward affected side, autonomic symptoms with pallor, sweating, nausea and vomiting.

ETIOLOGY

Thought to be viral in origin, thought to possibly be caused by herpes zoster, but trial of valacyclovir with and without methylprednisolone showed no efficacy for valacyclovir but efficacy for the steroid.

DIAGNOSIS

DIFFERENTIAL DIAGNOSIS

Labyrinthitis: similar cause, but includes hearing loss
- Labyrinthine infarction
- Perilymph fistula
- Brain stem and cerebellar infarction
- Migraine-associated vertigo
- Multiple sclerosis

WORKUP

Head-thrust test: grasp patient's head, apply brief small-amplitude rapid head turn, first to one side and then the other; patient fixates on examiner's nose: positive test is lack of corrective eye movement "saccades" on affected side.

LABORATORY TESTS

- ENG: testing of the vestibular apparatus with physical challenges, unilateral lack of caloric response
- Audiogram: normal

IMAGING STUDIES

Brain imaging: CT or MRI—normal

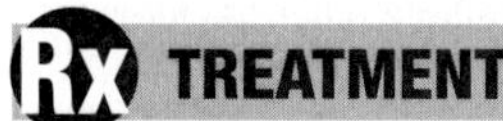

TREATMENT

NONPHARMACOLOGIC THERAPY

Vestibular exercises, when tolerated, will accelerate recovery.

ACUTE GENERAL Rx

- Methylprednisolone: 100 mg days 1 to 3, 80 mg days 4 to 6, 60 mg days 7 to 9, 40 mg days 10 to 12, 20 mg days 13 to 15, 10 mg days 14 to 16, 5 mg days 18 to 20
- Antihistamines: meclizine, dimenhydrinate, promethazine
- Anticholinergics: scopolamine
- Antidopaminergics: droperidol, prochlorperazine
- Anti-GABA agents: diazepam, valium

CHRONIC Rx

- Vestibular rehabilitation exercises
- Anti-GABA agents
- Antihistamines

DISPOSITION

Most patients can be treated as outpatients, but if dehydrated because of severe vomiting, they may require brief parenteral therapy.

REFERRAL

- ENT: if diagnosis is uncertain, these patients are at risk for BPPV subsequently, also symptoms may linger.
- Neurology: if question of central origin or migraine.

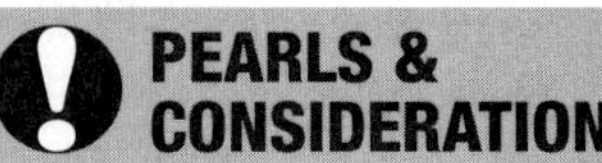

PEARLS & CONSIDERATIONS

COMMENTS

- Utility of steroids questioned until study reported in *NEJM* 7/04 demonstrated steroids improve recovery of vestibular function. Often damage to labyrinth is permanent, but compensated. These patients are at risk to develop BPPV because of damaged vestibular apparatus. Patients recover from dramatic acute symptoms, but subtle vestibular deficits may linger for prolonged period, if not indefinitely.
- Program of vestibular habituation head movement exercises can reduce imbalance symptoms.

PREVENTION

None

PATIENT & FAMILY EDUCATION

Vestibular Disorders Association: http://www.vestibular.org

Timothy Hain, M.D., director of Balance Center at Northwestern University, maintains http://www.tchain.com.

SUGGESTED READINGS

Baloh RW: Vestibular neuritis, *N Eng J Med* 348:1027-1032, 2003.

Cohen HS, Kimball KT: Decreased ataxia and improved balance after vestibular rehabilitation, *Otolaryngol Head Neck Surg* 130(4):418-425, 2004.

Strupp M et al: Methylprednisolone, valacyclovir or the combination for vestibular neuritis, *N Eng J Med* 351(4):354-361, 2004.

AUTHORS: **JUDITH NUDELMAN, M.D.,** and **JEFFREY M. BORKAN, M.D., Ph.D.**

BASIC INFORMATION

DEFINITION Vitiligo is the acquired loss of epidermal pigmentation that is characterized histologically by the absence of epidermal melanocytes. There are two major forms: nonsegmental (generalized) vitiligo, which accounts for >80% of cases, and segmental vitiligo, which accounts for 30% of childhood cases.

ICD-9CM CODES
709.1 Vitiligo

EPIDEMIOLOGY & DEMOGRAPHICS

PREVALENCE: Vitiligo affects 0.5% to 1% of the population; it is the most common depigmenting disorder.

PREDOMINANT AGE: Vitiligo can begin at any age, but the age at onset is <20 yr for half of patients.

GENETICS: A positive family history is present in 25% to 30% of patients, and both sexes are equally affected. There are no differences in the rates of occurrence with regard to skin type or race.

PHYSICAL FINDINGS & CLINICAL PRESENTATION

- Hypopigmented and depigmented lesions (Figure 1-359) favor sun-exposed regions, intertriginous areas, genitalia, and sites over bony prominences (i.e., nonsegmental or type A vitiligo).
- Areas around the body orifices are also frequently involved.
- The lesions tend to be symmetric.
- Occasionally the lesions are linear or pseudodermatomal (i.e., segmental or type B vitiligo).
- Vitiligo lesions may occur at trauma sites (i.e., Koebner's phenomenon).
- The hair in affected areas may be white.
- The margins of the lesions are usually well demarcated; when a ring of hyperpigmentation is seen, the term *trichrome vitiligo* is used.
- The term *marginal inflammatory vitiligo* is used to describe lesions with raised borders.
- Initially the disease is limited, but the lesions tend to become more extensive over time.
- Type B vitiligo is more common among children.
- Vitiligo may begin around pigmented nevi and produce a halo (i.e., Sutton's nevus); in such cases, the central nevus often regresses and disappears over time.

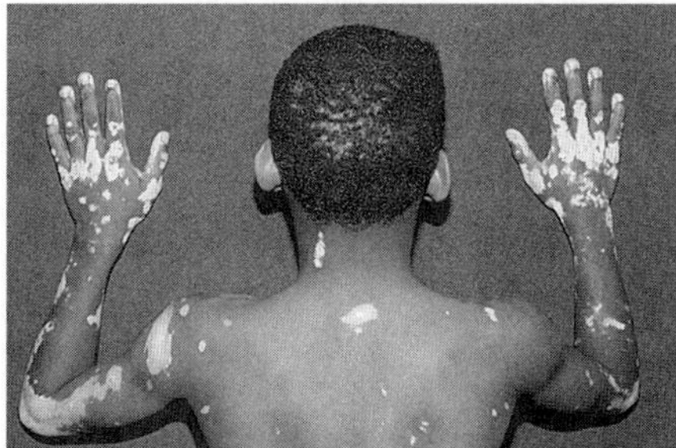

FIGURE 1-359 Multiple, sharply demarcated, symmetric, depigmented areas of vitiligo. (From Behrman RE: *Nelson textbook of pediatrics,* Philadelphia, 2006, WB Saunders.)

ETIOLOGY & PATHOGENESIS

- Three pathophysiologic theories:
  1. Autoimmune theory (i.e., autoantibodies against melanocytes)
  2. Neural theory (i.e., neurochemical mediators selectively destroy melanocytes)
  3. Self-destructive process in which melanocytes fail to protect themselves against cytotoxic melanin precursors
- Although vitiligo is considered to be an acquired disease, 25% to 30% of cases are familial. The mode of transmission is unknown; the condition seems to be polygenic or autosomal dominant with incomplete penetrance and variable expression.
- Associated disorders:
  - Alopecia areata
  - Type 1 diabetes mellitus
  - Adrenal insufficiency
  - Hyperthyroidism and hypothyroidism
  - Mucocutaneous candidiasis
  - Pernicious anemia
  - Polyglandular autoimmune syndromes
  - Melanoma

DIAGNOSIS

DIFFERENTIAL DIAGNOSIS

- Acquired hypopigmentation disorders:
  - Chemical-induced (e.g., chloroquine, imatinib, phenolic-catecholic derivatives [e.g., adhesives, deodorants, latex gloves, lacquer resins, varnish, soap antioxidants, insecticides, printing ink, paints, motor oil additives, disinfectants])
  - Halo nevus
  - Idiopathic guttate hypomelanosis
  - Leprosy
  - Leukoderma associated with melanoma
  - Pityriasis alba
  - Postinflammatory hypopigmentation
  - Tinea versicolor
  - Vogt-Koyanagi syndrome (i.e., vitiligo, uveitis, and deafness)
  - Melasma
  - Mycosis fungoides
- Congenital hypopigmentation disorders:
  - Albinism, partial (piebaldism)
  - Albinism, total
  - Nevus anemicus
  - Nevus depigmentosus
  - Tuberous sclerosis
  - Ito's hypomelanosis

WORKUP

- Inquire about a personal and family history of autoimmune disease.
- Perform a physical examination.
- A Wood's light examination may enhance the lesions of light-skinned individuals.

TREATMENT

Treatment is indicated primarily for cosmetic purposes when depigmentation causes emotional or social distress. Depigmentation is more noticeable among patients with darker complexions.

- Cosmetic masking agents (e.g., Dermablend, Covermark) or stains (e.g., DY-O-Derm, Vitadye)
- Sunless tanning lotions (e.g., dihydroxyacetone)
- Repigmentation (This is achieved by the activation and migration of melanocytes from hair follicles; therefore, skin with little or no hair responds poorly to treatment.)
- Narrow-band ultraviolet B radiation (This is the preferred treatment for nonsegmental vitiligo. It is given twice weekly [not on successive days] during sessions that last from 5 to 10 min. The best results are achieved on the face, trunk, and limbs.)
- Psoralens and sunlight (e.g., PUVAsol)
- Topical mid-potency steroids (e.g., triamcinolone 0.1% or desonide 0.05% cream qd for 3 to 4 mo)
- Topical calcineurin inhibitors for face and neck lesions
- Intralesional steroid injection
- Systemic steroids (e.g., betamethasone 5 mg qd on two consecutive days per week for 2 to 4 mo)
- Total depigmentation in cases of extensive vitiligo with 20% monobenzyl ether or hydroquinone (This is a permanent procedure, and patients will require lifelong protection from sun exposure.)
- Topical immunomodulators (e.g., tacrolimus, pimecrolimus) (These substances can also induce the repigmentation of vitiliginous skin lesions. However, their potential for systemic immunosuppression or for increasing the risk of skin or other malignancies remains to be defined.)
- Calcipotriol, which is a synthetic analog of vitamin D_3 (This has also been used in combination with ultraviolet light or clobetasol, with limited results.)
- Surgical techniques

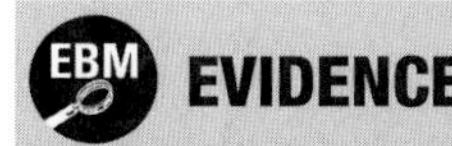

EVIDENCE

Key trial:
A 2006 Cochrane Review found some evidence of short-term benefit to support existing therapies (e.g., topical steroids, light therapies) for vitiligo, but the different designs and outcome measurements, lack of quality-of-life measures, and adverse effect reporting in the studies limit the usefulness of their findings. The reviewers call for high-quality, randomized trials using standardized measures of repigmentation that address relevant clinical outcomes, including quality of life.[1]

Evidence-Based Reference

1. Whitton ME et al: Interventions for vitiligo, *Cochrane Rev* 1, 2006.

SUGGESTED READING

Tareb A, Picardo M: Vitiligo, *N Engl J Med* 360:160-169, 2009.

AUTHOR: **FRED F. FERRI, M.D.**

Von Hippel-Lindau Disease

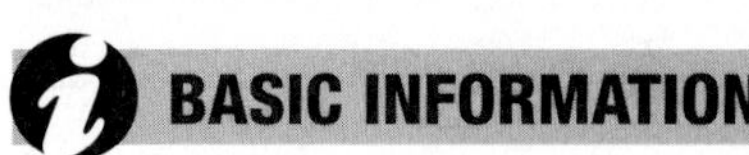

BASIC INFORMATION

DEFINITION

Von Hippel-Lindau disease (VHL) is a rare, autosomal-dominant, inherited disorder that is characterized by the formation of hemangioblastomas, cysts, and malignancies that involve multiple organ systems.

SYNONYMS

Hippel-Lindau syndrome
Cerebelloretinal hemangioblastomatosis
Retinocerebellar angiomatosis

ICD-9CM CODES
759.6 von Hippel-Lindau disease

EPIDEMIOLOGY & DEMOGRAPHICS

- The incidence of VHL is 1 case/36,000 live births.
- The mean age at the onset of clinical manifestations is 26 yr, but the disease can present from infancy until the seventh decade of life.
- In the U.S., approximately 6000 to 7000 people have VHL.
- Affected individuals are at risk for the development of renal cell carcinoma, pheochromocytoma, pancreatic islet cell tumor, endolymphatic sac tumor, and hemangioblastomas of the cerebellum and the retina.

PHYSICAL FINDINGS & CLINICAL PRESENTATION

- There are two clinical types of VHL:
  - Type 1 has no pheochromocytoma
  - Type 2 has pheochromocytoma:
    1. Type 2A: hemangioblastoma in the central nervous system (CNS) with no renal cell carcinoma
    2. Type 2B: renal cell carcinoma and other tumors
    3. Type 2C: only pheochromocytoma; associated with Chuvash polycythemia
- Retinal angiomas (60% prevalence):
  1. Usually occurs by age 25 yr with both VHL type 1 and VHL type 2
  2. Often multifocal and bilateral
  3. Detached retina
  4. Glaucoma
  5. Blindness
- CNS hemangioblastomas (70% prevalence):
  1. Cerebellum and spinal cord are the most common sites, followed by the medulla
  2. Usually multiple; mean age at diagnosis is 25 yr; found with VHL types 1, 2A, and 2B
  3. Headache, ataxia, slurred speech, nystagmus, vertigo, nausea, and vomiting
- Renal cysts (approximately 60% prevalence) and clear cell renal cell carcinoma (RCC; approximately 25% to 45% prevalence):
  1. Usually occur by the age of 40 yr
  2. May be asymptomatic or cause abdominal and flank pain
  3. RCC is bilateral in 75% of patients
- Pancreatic cysts:
  1. Usually asymptomatic
  2. Large cysts can cause biliary obstructive symptoms
  3. Diarrhea and diabetes may develop if enough of the pancreas is replaced by cysts
- Pheochromocytoma (7% to 18% prevalence):
  1. Found with VHL types 2A, 2B, and 2C
  2. Bilateral in 50% to 80% of cases
  3. Hypertension, palpitations, sweating, and headache
  4. Commonly occurs with pancreatic islet cell tumors
- Papillary cystadenoma of the epididymis (25% to 60% of men with VHL):
  1. Palpable scrotal mass
  2. May be unilateral or bilateral
- Papillary cystadenoma of the broad ligaments (unknown prevalence):
  1. Usually asymptomatic
  2. Reported symptoms include pain, dyspareunia, and menorrhagia
- Endolymphatic sac tumors of the middle ear (approximately 15% prevalence):
  1. Vertigo
  2. Hearing loss
  3. Facial paralysis

ETIOLOGY

VHL is primarily caused by a mutation of the von Hippel-Lindau gene, which is located on the short arm of chromosome 3. The VHL gene codes for a cytoplasmic protein that functions in tumor suppression.

Dx DIAGNOSIS

DIFFERENTIAL DIAGNOSIS

Table 1-80 compares genetic diseases associated with the development of pancreatic or gut endocrine tumors.

WORKUP

- A clinical diagnosis is established in the presence of a positive family history plus a single CNS hemangioblastoma or a visceral lesion (e.g., RCC, pheochromocytoma, pancreatic cysts or tumors).
- If no clear family history is present, two or more hemangioblastomas or one hemangioblastoma with a visceral lesion are required to make the diagnosis.
- Genetic screening is up to 100% sensitive and specific, although, in the 20% of patients with de novo VHL mutations, the test may be falsely negative as a result of somatic mosaicism.
- Screening family members is essential for the early detection of VHL disease.

WORKUP

Screening laboratory values and ophthalmoscopic, genetic, and imaging studies to look for sites of involvement

LABORATORY TESTS

- CBC may reveal erythrocytosis that requires periodic phlebotomies
- Electrolytes and renal function tests
- Urine for norepinephrine, epinephrine, and vanillylmandelic acid to look for pheochromocytoma
- Genetic studies: complete sequencing of coding region, Southern blot, and fluorescent in situ hybridization

IMAGING STUDIES

- Indirect and direct ophthalmoscopy, fluorescein angiography, and tonometry are used to screen for retinal angiomas and glaucoma.
- Computed tomographic scanning of the abdomen is used for the screening, detection, and monitoring of patients with renal cysts or tumors, pheochromocytomas, and pancreatic cysts or tumors:
  1. Renal cysts grow an average of 0.5 cm/yr.
  2. Renal tumors grow an average of 1.5 cm/yr.
  3. Computed tomography scans are performed every 6 mo for the first 2 yr and every year for life in patients who have had surgery for RCC.
- MRI with gadolinium is used for the screening and evaluation of CNS and spinal cord hemangioblastomas, endolymphatic sac tumors, and pheochromocytomas.
- Angiography may be performed before CNS surgery.

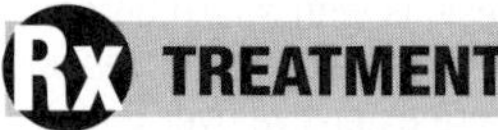

TREATMENT

NONPHARMACOLOGIC THERAPY

Genetic counseling

TABLE 1-80 Genetic Diseases Associated with the Development of Pancreatic or Gut Endocrine Tumors

Gene	Disease	Phenotype
Menin	Multiple endocrine neoplasia type 1	Parathyroid, pituitary, and pancreatic endocrine tumors
VHL	von Hippel-Lindau disease	Pancreatic endocrine tumors, hemangiomas, and multiple neoplasms
NF-1	Neurofibromatosis	Neurofibromas and pheochromocytomas
TSC1/2	Tuberous sclerosis	Pancreatic endocrine tumors and hamartomas

From Larsen PR et al: *Williams textbook of endocrinology*, ed 10, Philadelphia, 2003, WB Saunders.

ACUTE GENERAL RX

- Laser photocoagulation and cryotherapy are used for patients with retinal angiomas to prevent blindness (Table 1-81).
- For cerebellar hemangioblastomas, treatment is surgical. External-beam radiation and stereotactic radiosurgery can also be performed.
- For renal tumors, surgery is delayed until one of the renal tumors reaches 3 cm in diameter. Nephron-sparing surgery is the preferred approach.
- Pancreatic islet cell tumors usually require surgical removal.
- Adrenalectomy is performed for pheochromocytoma.
- Antiangiogenic therapy has been shown to improve the survival of patients with RCC, with studies ongoing to assess combination therapy.

CHRONIC RX

- Dialysis has been delayed for many patients with the use of nephron-sparing surgery.
- Renal transplantation is usually delayed for 1 yr after bilateral nephrectomy for renal tumors to ensure that no metastases have occurred.

DISPOSITION

The median life expectancy of patients with this condition is 49 yr.

REFERRAL

Geneticist, neurosurgeon, urologist, nephrologist, ophthalmologist, otolaryngologist, neurologist, endocrinologist, and radiation oncologist referrals should be considered.

TABLE 1-81 The Management of Different Manifestations of von Hippel-Lindau Disease

Tumor	Treatment	Screening
Retinal angiomas	If small, laser photocoagulation/cryotherapy; in severe cases, the removal of the affected eye	Retinal examinations once per year soon after birth
Central nervous system hemangioblastomas	Surgical resection for symptomatic patients or large tumors; gamma knife if difficult to remove from primary site	MRI for patients >10 yr once per year
Renal cysts/carcinomas	For tumors <3 cm in diameter, observation; for one tumor >3 cm in diameter, remove all tumors by enucleation or partial nephrectomy; percutaneous radiofrequency ablation and cryosurgery are also performed; surgical resection is not recommended for any cyst without a tumor inside of it; nephrectomy is indicated for patients with end-stage renal disease who require dialysis because of the malignancy potential	CT/MRI scan once yearly; if the patient has relatives with the condition, he or she is checked once per year with CT before the age of 20 yr
Pancreatic cysts	Partial resection of the pancreas, depending on the site of the cyst	
Pheochromocytomas	Preferable to remove only the tumor itself and thus to conserve adrenal function	CT scan once per year for patients <10 yr old

CT, Computed tomography; *MRI,* magnetic resonance imaging.

PEARLS & CONSIDERATIONS

- The most common cause of death in patients with VHL is RCC.
- More information for patients can be obtained at from the von Hippel-Lindau Family Alliance (http://vhl.org).

SUGGESTED READINGS

Butman JA et al: Neurologic manifestations of von Hippel-Lindau disease, *JAMA* 300(11):1334-1342, 2008.

Lonser RR et al: von Hippel-Lindau disease, *Lancet* 361:2059, 2003.

Meister M et al: Radiological evaluation, management, and surveillance of renal masses in von Hippel-Lindau disease, *Clin Radiol* 64(6):589, 2009.

Shuin T et al: von Hippel-Lindau disease: molecular pathological basis, clinical criteria, genetic testing, clinical features of tumors and treatment, *Jpn J Clin Oncol* 36(6):337, 2006.

AUTHORS: **MARK F. BRADY, M.D., M.P.H.,** and **WEN-Y. WU-CHEN, M.D.**

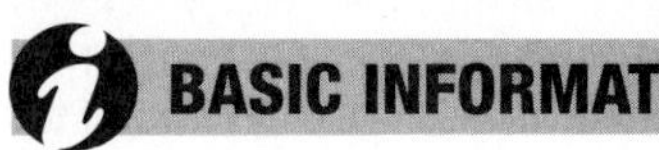

BASIC INFORMATION

DEFINITION

Von Willebrand's disease is a congenital disorder of hemostasis characterized by defective or deficient von Willebrand factor (vWF). There are several subtypes of von Willebrand's disease. The most common type (80% of cases) is type I, which is caused by a quantitative decrease in vWF; type IIA and type IIB are results of qualitative protein abnormalities; and type III is a rare, autosomal recessive disorder characterized by a near-complete quantitative deficiency of vWF. Acquired von Willebrand's disease (AvWD) is a rare disorder that usually occurs in elderly patients and usually presents with mucocutaneous bleeding abnormalities and no clinically meaningful family history. It is often accompanied by a hematoproliferative or autoimmune disorder. Successful treatment of the associated illness can reverse the clinical and laboratory manifestations.

SYNONYMS

Pseudohemophilia

ICD-9CM CODES

286.4 von Willebrand's disease

EPIDEMIOLOGY & DEMOGRAPHICS

- Autosomal-dominant disorder
- Most common inherited bleeding disorder
- Prevalence is 1% to 2% in general population, according to screening studies; estimates based on referral for symptoms of bleeding suggest a prevalence of 30 to 100 cases per million

PHYSICAL FINDINGS & CLINICAL PRESENTATION

- Generally normal physical examination
- Mucosal bleeding (gingival bleeding, epistaxis) and gastrointestinal bleeding may occur
- Easy bruising
- Postpartum bleeding, bleeding after surgery or dental extraction, menorrhagia

ETIOLOGY

Quantitative or qualitative deficiency of vWF (see "Definition")

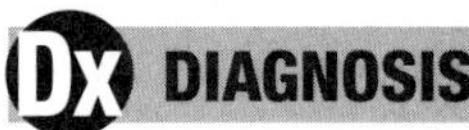

DIAGNOSIS

DIFFERENTIAL DIAGNOSIS

Platelet function disorders, clotting factor deficiencies

WORKUP

- Laboratory evaluation (see "Laboratory Tests")
- Initial testing includes partial thromboplastin time (increased), platelet count (normal), and bleeding time (prolonged)
- Subsequent tests include vWF level (decreased), factor VIII:C (decreased), and ristocetin agglutination (increased in type II B) (Table 1-82)

LABORATORY TESTS

- Normal platelet number and morphology
- Prolonged bleeding time
- Decreased factor VIII coagulant activity
- Decreased vWF antigen or ristocetin cofactor
- Normal platelet aggregation studies
- Type II A von Willebrand disease can be distinguished from type I by absence of ristocetin cofactor activity and abnormal multimer
- Type IIB von Willebrand disease is distinguished from type I by abnormal multimer

Rx TREATMENT

NONPHARMACOLOGIC THERAPY

- Avoidance of aspirin and other nonsteroidal antiinflammatory drugs.
- Evaluation for likelihood of bleeding (with measurement of bleeding time) before surgical procedures. When a patient undergoes surgery or receives repeated therapeutic doses of concentrates, factor VIII activity should be assayed every 12 hr on the day a dose is administered and every 24 hr thereafter.

GENERAL Rx

- The mainstay of treatment in von Willebrand's disease is the replacement of the deficient protein at the time of spontaneous bleeding or before invasive procedures are performed.
- Desmopressin acetate (DDAVP) is useful to release stored vWF from endothelial cells. It is used to cover minor procedures and traumatic bleeding in mild type I von Willebrand's disease. Dose is 0.3 mcg/kg in 100 ml of normal saline solution IV infused >20 min. DDAVP is also available as a nasal spray (dose of 150 mcg spray administered to each nostril) as a preparation for minor surgery and management of minor bleeding episodes. DDAVP is not effective in type IIA von Willebrand's disease and is potentially dangerous in type IIB (increased risk of bleeding and thrombocytopenia).
- In patients with severe disease, replacement therapy in the form of cryoprecipitate is the method of choice. The standard dose is 1 bag of cryoprecipitate per 10 kg of body weight.
- Factor VIII concentrate rich in vWF (Humate-P) is useful to correct bleeding abnormalities in type IIA, IIB, and type III von Willebrand's disease without alloantibodies. Alloantibodies that inactivate vWF and form circulating immune complexes develop in 15% of patients with type III von Willebrand's disease who have received multiple transfusions. In these patients, recombinant factor VIII is preferred because autoantibodies can elicit life-threatening anaphylactic reactions because of complement activation by immune complexes.
- Life-threatening hemorrhage unresponsive to therapy with cryoprecipitate or factor VIII concentrate may require transfusion of normal platelets.

SUGGESTED READING

Mannucci PM: Treatment of von Willebrand's disease, *N Engl J Med* 351:683, 2004.

AUTHOR: **FRED F. FERRI, M.D.**

TABLE 1-82 Genetic and Laboratory Findings in von Willebrand's Disease

Parameter Type	BT	VIII-c	vw-Ag	R-cof	Ripa	Multimer Structure	Mode of Inheritance
I (classic)	P	R	R	R	R	Normal	AD
II							
A	P	N/R	N/R	R	R	Abnormal	AD
B	P	N/R	N/R	N/R	I	Abnormal	AD
III	P	R	R	R	R	Variable	AR

From Behrman RE: *Nelson textbook of pediatrics,* ed 17, Philadelphia, 2004, WB Saunders.

AD, Autosomal dominant; *AR,* autosomal recessive; *BT,* bleeding time; *I,* increased; *N/R,* normal or reduced; *P,* prolonged; *R,* reduced; *R-Cof,* ristocetin cofactor; *RIPA,* ristocetin-induced platelet aggregation (agglutination); *vW-Aq,* von Willebrand antigen (protein); *VIII-C,* factor VIII coagulant activity.

BASIC INFORMATION

DEFINITION

Vulvar cancer is an abnormal cell proliferation arising on the vulva and exhibiting malignant potential. The majority are of squamous cell origin; however, other types include adenocarcinoma, basal cell carcinoma, sarcoma, and melanoma.

SYNONYMS

Squamous cell carcinoma of the vulva (90%)
Basal cell carcinoma of the vulva
Adenocarcinoma of the vulva
Melanoma of the vulva
Bartholin gland carcinoma
Verrucous carcinoma of the vulva
Vulvar sarcoma

ICD-9CM CODES
184.4 Vulvar neoplasm

EPIDEMIOLOGY & DEMOGRAPHICS

INCIDENCE: 1.8 cases per 100,000 persons
PREVALENCE: Vulvar cancer is uncommon. It comprises 4% of malignancies of the female genital tract. It is the fourth most common gynecologic malignancy.
MEAN AGE AT DIAGNOSIS: Predominantly a disease of menopause. Mean age at diagnosis is 65 yr.

PHYSICAL FINDINGS & CLINICAL PRESENTATION

- Vulvar pruritus or pain is present.
- May produce a malodorous discharge or present as bleeding.
- Raised lesion that may have fleshy, ulcerated, leukoplakic, or warty appearance; may have multifocal lesions.
- Lesions are usually located on labia majora but may be seen on labia minora, clitoris, and perineum.
- The lymph nodes of groin may be palpable.

ETIOLOGY

- The exact etiology is unknown.
- Vulvar intraepithelial neoplasia has been reported in 20% to 30% of invasive squamous cell carcinoma of the vulva, but the malignant potential is unknown.
- Human papillomavirus is found in 30% to 50% of vulvar carcinoma, but its exact role is unclear.
- Chronic pruritus, wetness, industrial wastes, arsenicals, hygienic agents, and vulvar dystrophies have been implicated as causative agents.

DIAGNOSIS

DIFFERENTIAL DIAGNOSIS

- Lymphogranuloma inguinale
- Tuberculosis
- Vulvar dystrophies
- Vulvar atrophy
- Paget's disease

WORKUP

- Diagnosis is made histologically by biopsy
- Thorough examination of the lesion and assessment of spread
- Possible colposcopy of adjacent areas
- Cytologic smear of vagina and cervix
- Cystoscopy and proctosigmoidoscopy may be necessary

IMAGING STUDIES

- Chest radiography
- CT scan and MRI for assessing local tumor spread

TREATMENT

NONPHARMACOLOGIC THERAPY

- Treatment is individualized depending on the stage of the tumor.
- Stage I tumors with <1 mm stromal invasion are treated with complete local excision without groin node dissection. Imiquimod 5% cream, a topical immune response modulator, is also effective in the treatment of vulvar intraepithelial neoplasia.
- Stage I tumors with >1 mm stromal invasion are treated with complete local excision with groin node dissection.
- Stage II tumors require radical vulvectomy with bilateral groin node dissection.
- Advanced-stage disease may require the addition of radiation and chemotherapy to the surgical regimen.
- Section III describes a treatment algorithm for management of vulvar cancer.

DISPOSITION

Five-year survival ranges from 90% for stage I to 15% for stage IV.

REFERRAL

Vulvar cancer should be managed by a gynecologic oncologist and radiation oncologist.

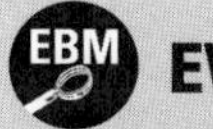

EVIDENCE

Please note: Complete text of EBM for this topic is available online.
Key trials and commentary:
Vulvar and vaginal cancers among younger women are often related to infection with human papillomavirus (HPV). These cancers are preceded by high-grade vulval intraepithelial neoplasia (VIN2-3) and vaginal intraepithelial neoplasia (VaIN2-3). The aim of this study was to do a combined analysis of three randomized clinical trials to assess the effect of a prophylactic quadrivalent HPV vaccine on the incidence of these diseases.

This study showed that prophylactic administration of quadrivalent HPV vaccine was effective in preventing high-grade vulval and vaginal lesions associated with HPV-16 or HPV-18 infection in women who were naive to these types before vaccination. With time, such vaccination could result in reduced rates of HPV-related vulval and vaginal cancers.

This article by Joura et al and an article by the Future II Study Group present additional evidence documenting the efficacy of the Merck vaccine in preventing high-grade vulvar and vaginal lesions associated with HPV-16 or HPV-18. The maximum effect is achieved in girls who are vaccinated in early adolescence, and it is anticipated that widespread use of this vaccine will reduce morbidity, mortality, and health care costs associated with cervical cancer. Nevertheless, a number of important questions about the use of these vaccines remain, and are discussed explicitly in an accompanying commentary on the Future II Study Group article. These questions include the duration of protection from HPV infection after immunization, the best age at which to vaccinate, the possible benefits of vaccinating boys and young men, the need for protection against infection by other virus types that might lead to cervical neoplasia, and the cost barrier to widespread use of the vaccine, especially in the developing world. Other important hurdles include the absence of a health-delivery infrastructure in many countries, the political debate surrounding the issue of voluntary vs. mandatory vaccination, the unsubstantiated claims that HPV vaccination will encourage promiscuity, and the belief by some that vaccination may be unnecessary, given the effectiveness of cervical screening strategies.[1] Ⓐ

Evidence-Based Reference

1. Joura EA et al: Efficacy of a quadrivalent prophylactic human papillomavirus (types 6, 11, 16, and 18) L1 virus-like-particle vaccine against high-grade vulval and vaginal lesions: a combined analysis of three randomised clinical trials, *Lancet* 369: 1693-1702, 2007. Commentary by B.H. Thiers, M.D. Ⓐ

SUGGESTED READING

Van Seters M et al: Treatment of vulvar intraepithelial neoplasia with topical imiquimod, *N Engl J Med* 358:1465-1473, 2008.

AUTHORS: **GIL M. FARKASH, M.D.,** and **RUBEN ALVERO, M.D.**

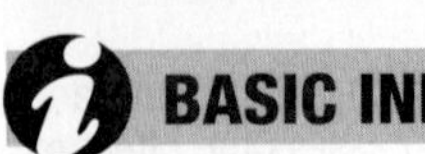

BASIC INFORMATION

DEFINITION

Bacterial vulvovaginitis is inflammation affecting the vagina, only rarely affecting the vulva, caused by anaerobic and aerobic bacteria.

SYNONYMS

Bacterial vaginosis
Gardnerella vaginalis
Haemophilus vaginalis
Corynebacterium vaginalis

ICD-9CM CODES

616.10 Vulvovaginitis

EPIDEMIOLOGY & DEMOGRAPHICS

- Most prevalent form of vaginal infection of reproductive age women in the U.S.
- 32% to 64% in patients visiting STD clinics
- 12% to 25% in other clinic populations
- 10% to 26% in patients visiting obstetric clinics
- May be associated with adverse pregnancy outcomes: premature rupture of membranes, preterm labor, preterm birth
- Organisms frequently found in postpartum or postcesarean endometritis

PHYSICAL FINDINGS & CLINICAL PRESENTATION

- >50% of all women may be without symptoms.
- Unpleasant, fishy, or musty vaginal odor in about 50% to 70% of all patients. Odor exacerbated immediately after intercourse or during menstruation.
- Vaginal discharge is increased.
- Vaginal itching and irritation occur.

ETIOLOGY

- Synergistic polymicrobial infection characterized by an overgrowth of bacteria normally found in the vagina
- Anaerobics: *Bacteroides* spp., *Peptostreptococcus* spp., *Mobiluncus* spp.
- Facultative anaerobes: *G. vaginalis, Mycoplasma hominis*
- Concentration of anaerobic bacteria increased to 100 to 1000 times normal
- Lactobacilli are absent or greatly reduced

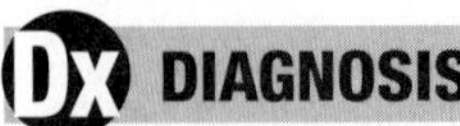

DIAGNOSIS

DIFFERENTIAL DIAGNOSIS

- Fungal vaginitis
- *Trichomonas* vaginitis
- Atrophic vaginitis
- Cervicitis

WORKUP

- Pelvic examination
- Speculum examination
- Normal saline and 10% KOH slide of discharge
- Amsel criteria for diagnosis (three of four should be present):
  1. pH >4.5
  2. Clue cells (epithelial cells covered with bacteria) on saline solution slide
  3. Positive whiff test on 10% KOH
  4. Homogeneous, white, adherent discharge
- Section III, "Vaginal Discharge," describes the evaluation of discharge

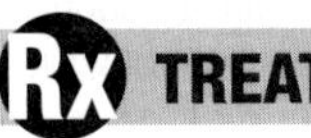

TREATMENT

ACUTE GENERAL Rx

- Metronidazole 500 mg PO bid × 7 days, >90% cure rate
- Metronidazole 2 g PO × 1 day, 67% to 92% cure rate
- Metronidazole gel 5 g, intravaginal bid × 5 days
- Clindamycin 2% cream 5 g, intravaginal qd × 7 days
- Clindamycin 300 mg PO bid × 7 days in pregnancy

CHRONIC Rx

Clindamycin 300 mg PO bid × 7 days; cure rate similar to those achieved with metronidazole
Related to adverse pregnancy outcomes
- Metronidazole 250 mg PO bid × 7 days
- Metronidazole zympoxidase
- Clindamycin 300 mg PO bid × 7 days
- Good hygiene: avoidance of douching, harsh shower gels, bubble baths; cotton underwear

DISPOSITION

- Reevaluate if not cured with treatment
- Recurrence fairly common

REFERRAL

Refer to obstetrician/gynecologist for recurrence or pregnant patient with bacterial vaginosis

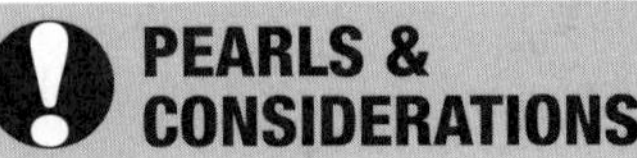

PEARLS & CONSIDERATIONS

COMMENTS

Treating sexual partners has failed to demonstrate a benefit.

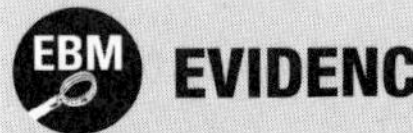

EVIDENCE

The limited evidence comparing oral vs intravaginal treatment and metronidazole versus clindamycin concludes that there is little difference in outcome between the two agents.[1] Ⓐ

Good-quality trials have shown that antibiotic therapy is effective at eradicating bacterial vaginosis during pregnancy. However, evidence does not support treating asymptomatic women to prevent preterm birth, but for women with previous preterm delivery, it may reduce the risk of preterm rupture of membranes and low birth weight.[2] Ⓐ

Evidence-Based References

1. Joesoef MR, Schmid G: Bacterial vaginosis, *Clin Evid* 13:1968-1978, 2007. Ⓐ
2. McDonald HM et al: Antibiotics for treating bacterial vaginosis in pregnancy, *Cochrane Database Rev* 1, 2007. Ⓐ

SUGGESTED READINGS

Eckert LO: Acute vulvovaginitis, *N Engl J Med* 355: 1244-1252, 2006.
Sexually transmitted diseases treatment guidelines, *MMWR* 55(RR-11):49-56, 2006.

AUTHORS: **JULIE ANNE SZUMIGALA, M.D.,** and **RUBEN ALVERO, M.D.**

BASIC INFORMATION

DEFINITION

Estrogen-deficient vulvovaginitis is the irritation and/or inflammation of the vulva and vagina because of progressive thinning and atrophic changes secondary to estrogen deficiency (Fig. 1-360).

SYNONYMS

Atrophic vaginitis

ICD-9CM CODES
616.10 Vulvovaginitis

EPIDEMIOLOGY & DEMOGRAPHICS

- Seen most often in postmenopausal women
- Average age of menopause is 52 yr
- In 1990, there were 36 million women 50 yr of age or older

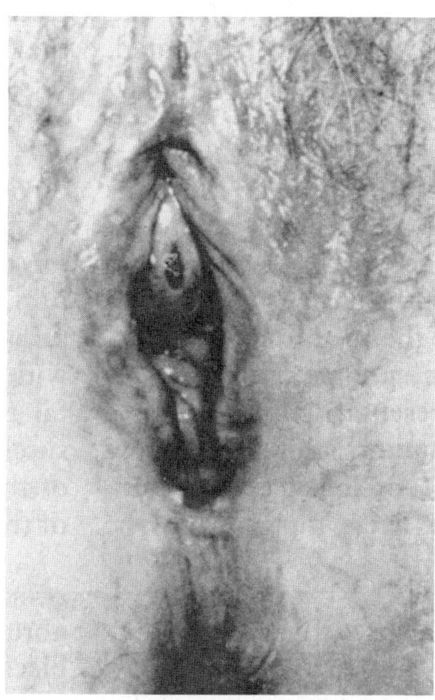

FIGURE 1-360 Advanced postmenopausal atrophy of the vulva in a 72-year-old woman. (From Symonds EM, Macpherson MBA: Color atlas of obstetrics and gynecology, St Louis, 1994, Mosby.)

PHYSICAL FINDINGS & CLINICAL PRESENTATION

- Thinning of pubic hair, labia minora and majora
- Decreased secretions from the vestibular glands, with vaginal dryness
- Regression of subcutaneous fat
- Vulvar and vaginal itching
- Dyspaereunia
- Dysuria and urinary frequency
- Vaginal spotting

ETIOLOGY

Estrogen deficiency

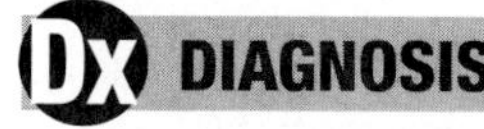

DIAGNOSIS

DIFFERENTIAL DIAGNOSIS

- Infectious vulvovaginitis
- Squamous cell hyperplasia
- Lichen sclerosus
- Vulvar malignancy
- Vaginal malignancy
- Cervical and endometrial malignancy

WORKUP

- Pelvic examination
- Speculum examination
- Pap smear
- Possible endometrial biopsy if bleeding

LABORATORY TESTS

FSH and estradiol: generally after menopause, estradiol $<$15 pg and FSH $>$40 mIU/ml

TREATMENT

ACUTE GENERAL Rx

- Premarin 0.625 mg PO qd.
- Estraderm patch 0.05 mg $\times$ 2 per week.
- If uterus present:
  1. Estrogen + 2.5 mg PO Provera qd *or*
  2. Estrogen + 10 mg PO Provera $\times$ 10 days each mo
- Conjugated estrogen vaginal cream intravaginally. Estradiol vaginal cream 0.01%.
  2 to 4 g/day $\times$ 2 wk then
  1 to 2 g/day $\times$ 2 wk then
  1 to 2 g $\times$ 3 days/wk
- Vagifem (estradiol vaginal tablets) 25 mg inserted intravaginally daily for 2 wk then twice weekly. May take up to 12 wk to feel the full benefits of the medication.
- Conjugated estrogen vaginal cream: 2 to 4 g qd (3 wk on, 1 wk off) for 3 to 5 mo.

CHRONIC Rx

See "Acute General Rx." May discontinue vaginal estrogen cream once symptoms alleviate.

DISPOSITION

The symptoms should be improved with the therapy. Caution for vaginal bleeding if uterus present.

REFERRAL

To obstetrician/gynecologist if vaginal bleeding

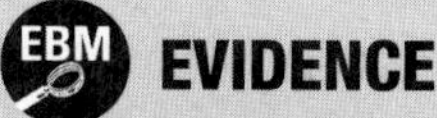

EVIDENCE

Phytoestrogen and plant progestin therapies lack robust evidence of efficacy as treatments for atrophic vaginitis.

A small RCT analyzing the efficacy of a soy-rich diet on urogenital symptoms in peri- and post-menopausal Thai women concluded that it was not effective.[1] Ⓑ

"Botanicals" include an array of foods and supplements derived from any plant part, but robust evidence of efficacy is lacking. Many women, however, report beneficial effects on menopausal signs and symptoms, including atrophic vaginitis.

A double-blind study analyzing the efficacy of a black cohosh preparation on markers vaginal maturity concluded that it had beneficial, weak estrogen-like effects in the vaginal mucosa.[2] Ⓑ

Evidence-Based References

1. Manonai J et al: The effect of a soy-rich diet on urogenital atrophy: a randomized, cross-over trial, *Maturitas* 54:135-140, 2006. Ⓑ

2. Wuttke W et al: Effects of black cohosh (Cimicifuga racemosa) on bone turnover, vaginal mucosa, and various blood parameters in postmenopausal women: a double-blind, placebo-controlled, and conjugated estrogens-controlled study, *Menopause* 13:185-196, 2006. Ⓑ

AUTHORS: **JULIE ANNE SZUMIGALA, M.D.,** and **RUBEN ALVERO, M.D.**

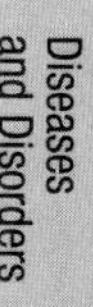

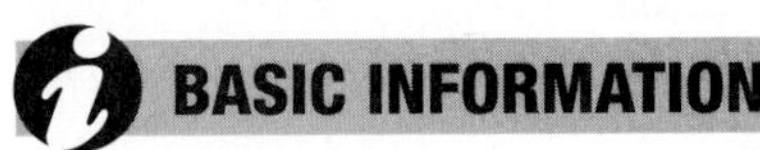

DEFINITION

Fungal vulvovaginitis is the inflammation of vulva and vagina caused by *Candida* spp.

SYNONYMS

Monilial vulvovaginitis
Vulvovaginal candidiasis

ICD-9CM CODES

112.1 Vulvovaginitis, monilial

EPIDEMIOLOGY & DEMOGRAPHICS

- Second most common cause of vaginal infection.
- Approximately 13 million people were affected in 1990.
- 75% of women will have at least one episode during their childbearing years, and approximately 40% to 50% of these will have a second attack.
- No symptoms in 20% to 40% of women who have positive cultures.

PHYSICAL FINDINGS & CLINICAL PRESENTATION

- Intense vulvar and vaginal pruritus
- Edema and erythema of vulva
- Thick, curdlike vaginal discharge
- Adherent, dry, white, curdy patches attached to vaginal mucosa

ETIOLOGY

- *Candida albicans* is responsible for 80% to 95% of vaginal fungal infections.
- *Candida tropicalis* and *Torulopsis glabrata (Candida glabrata)* are the most common nonalbicans *Candida* species that can induce vaginitis.

PREDISPOSING HOST FACTORS

- Pregnancy
- Oral contraceptives (high-estrogen)
- Diabetes mellitus
- Antibiotics
- Immunosuppression (e.g., HIV)
- Tight, poorly ventilated, nylon underclothing, with increased local perineal moisture and temperature

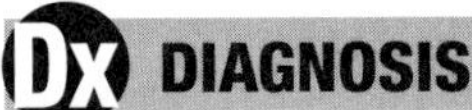

DIFFERENTIAL DIAGNOSIS

- Bacterial vaginosis
- *Trichomonas* vaginitis
- Atrophic vaginitis

Section II describes the differential diagnosis of vaginal discharges and infections.

WORKUP

- Pelvic examination
- Speculum examination
- Hyphae or budding spores on 10% KOH preparation (positive in 50% to 70% of individuals with yeast infection)

Section III, "Vaginal Discharge," describes the evaluation of discharge.

LABORATORY TESTS

Culture, especially recurrence for identification

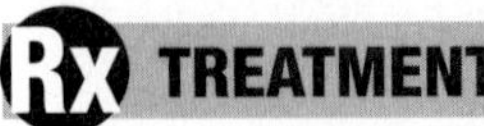

ACUTE GENERAL Rx

- Cure rate of the various azole derivatives 85% to 90%; little evidence of superiority of one azole agent over another
- No significant differences in persistent symptoms with oral or vaginal treatment
- Fluconazole (oral) associated with increased frequency of mild nausea, headache, abdominal pain
- Cure rate of polyene (Nystatin) cream and suppositories: 75% to 80%
- Miconazole 200-mg suppository (Monistat 3), one suppository × 3 days or 2% vaginal cream (Monistat 7), one applicator full intravaginally qhs × 7
- Clotrimazole 200-mg vaginal tablet, one tablet intravaginally qhs × 3 or 100-mg vaginal tablet (Gyne-Lotrimin, Mycelex-G) one tablet intravaginally qhs × 7, or 1% vaginal cream intravaginally qhs × 7
- Butoconazole 2% cream (Femstat) one applicator intravaginally qhs × 3
- Terconazole 80-mg suppository or 0.8% vaginal cream (Terazol 3), one suppository or one applicator intravaginally qhs × 3 or 0.4% vaginal cream (Terazol 7), one applicator intravaginally qhs × 7
- Gynecazole-1 vaginal cream one applicator intravaginally × 1
- Tioconazole 6.5% ointment (Vagi-stat), one applicator intravaginally × 1
- Fluconazole (Diflucan) 150 mg PO × 1

CHRONIC Rx (FOUR OR MORE SYMPTOMATIC EPISODES ANNUALLY)

- Resistance or recurrence
  1. 14- to 21-day course of 7-day regimens mentioned in "Acute General Rx" above
  2. Fluconazole (Diflucan) 150 mg PO × 1
  3. Ketoconazole (Nizoral) 200 mg PO bid × 5 to 14 days
  4. Itraconazole (Sporanox) 200 mg PO qd × 3 days
  5. Boric acid 600-mg capsule intravaginally bid × 14 days
- Prophylactic regimens
  1. Clotrimazole one 500-mg vaginal tablet each month
  2. Ketoconazole 200 mg PO bid × 5 days each month
  3. Fluconazole 150 mg PO × 1 each month
  4. Miconazole 100-mg vaginal tablet × 2 weekly

DISPOSITION

- If symptoms do not resolve completely with treatment, or if they recur within a 2- to 3-mo period, further evaluation is indicated.
- Reexamination and possibly culture are necessary.
- Positive culture in absence of symptoms should not lead to treatment. Approximately 30% of women harbor *Candida* spp. and other species in the vagina.

REFERRAL

To obstetrician/gynecologist for recurrence

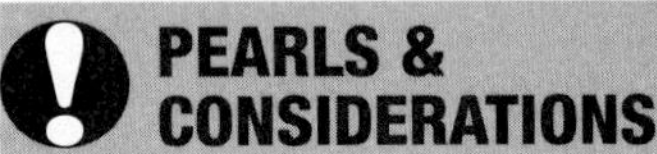

COMMENTS

No evidence that treating a woman's male sexual partner significantly improves woman's infection or reduces their rate of relapse.

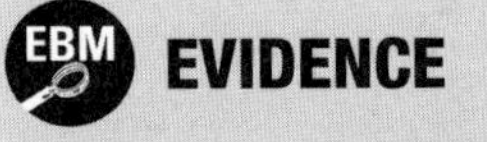

Vulvovaginal Candidiasis

Several randomized controlled trials (RCTs) found that topical imidazoles were more effective than placebo for the treatment of vulvovaginal candidiasis in nonpregnant women.[1] Ⓐ

An RCT compared intravaginal nystatin with placebo in nonpregnant women with symptomatic vulvovaginal candidiasis. Nystatin significantly reduced the number of patients reporting a poor symptomatic response after 2 wk.[2] Ⓑ

A systematic review found that topical imidazole therapy was more effective than nystatin in the management of vaginal candidiasis in pregnancy. Treatment for 7 days may be necessary during pregnancy.[3] Ⓐ

A systematic review compared oral and topical azoles in nonpregnant women with vulvovaginal candidiasis. Both routes of administration were found to be equally effective in terms of clinical and mycologic cure.[4] Ⓐ

Evidence-Based References

1. Spence D: Candidiasis (vulvovaginal), *Clin Evid* 10:2044, 2003. Ⓐ
2. Isaacs JH: Nystatin vaginal cream in monilial vaginitis, *Illinois Med J* 3:240, 1973. Ⓑ
3. Young GL, Jewell D: Topical treatment for vaginal candidiasis (thrush) in pregnancy, *Cochrane Rev* 1, 2004. Ⓐ
4. Watson MC et al: Oral versus intra-vaginal imidazole and triazole anti-fungal treatment of uncomplicated vulvovaginal candidiasis (thrush), *Cochrane Rev* 1, 2004. Ⓐ

AUTHORS: **JULIE ANNE SZUMIGALA, M.D.,** and **RUBEN ALVERO, M.D.**

BASIC INFORMATION

DEFINITION

Prepubescent vulvovaginitis is an inflammatory condition of the vulva and vagina.

ICD-9CM CODES
616.10 Vulvovaginitis

EPIDEMIOLOGY & DEMOGRAPHICS

- Most common gynecologic problem of the premenarcheal female.
- Prepubertal girl is susceptible to irritation and trauma because of the absence of protective hair and labial fat pads and the lack of estrogenization with atrophic vaginal mucosa.
- Symptoms of vulvovaginitis and introital irritation and discharge account for 80% to 90% of gynecologic visits.
- Nonspecific etiology in approximately 75% of children with vulvovaginitis.
- Majority of vulvovaginitis in children involves a primary irritation of the vulva with secondary involvement of the lower third of the vagina.

PHYSICAL FINDINGS & CLINICAL PRESENTATION

- Vulvar pain, dysuria, pruritus
  1. Discharge is not a primary symptom.
  2. If present, vaginal discharge may be foul smelling or bloody.

ETIOLOGY

- Infections
  1. Bacterial
  2. Protozoal
  3. Mycotic
  4. Viral
- Endocrine disorders
- Labial adhesions
- Poor hygiene
- Sexual abuse
- Allergic substance
- Trauma
- Foreign body
- Masturbation
- Constipation

Section II describes the differential diagnosis of vaginal discharge in prepubertal girls.

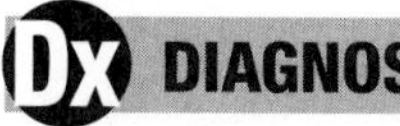

DIAGNOSIS

DIFFERENTIAL DIAGNOSIS

- Physiologic leukorrhea
- Foreign body
- Bacterial vaginosis
- Gonorrhea
- Fungal vulvovaginitis
- *Trichomonas* vulvovaginitis
- Sexual abuse
- Pinworms

WORKUP

- Pelvic, genital examination
- Speculum examination
- Rectal examination
- KOH and normal saline preparation of discharge

Section III, "Vaginal Discharge," describes the evaluation of discharge.

LABORATORY TESTS

- Urinalysis to rule out urinary tract infection and diabetes
- Cultures including sexually transmitted diseases

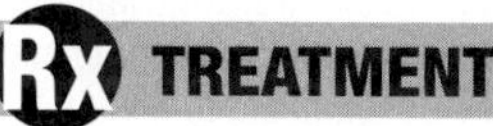

TREATMENT

NONPHARMACOLOGIC THERAPY

- Avoid tight clothing
- Perineal hygiene
- Avoid irritant chemicals
- Reassurance

ACUTE GENERAL Rx

- Group A beta *Streptococcus* and *Streptococcus pneumoniae:* penicillin V potassium 125 to 250 mg PO qid × 10 days
- *Chlamydia trachomatis:* erythromycin 50 mg/kg/day PO × 10 days
  - Children >8 yr, doxycycline 100 mg bid PO × 7 days
- *Neisseria gonorrhoeae:* ceftriaxone 125 mg IM × 1 day
  - Children >8 yr should also be given doxycycline 100 mg bid PO × 7 days
- *Staphylococcus aureus:* amoxicillin-clavulanate 20 to 40 mg/kg/day PO × 7 to 10 days
- *Haemophilus influenzae:* amoxicillin 20 to 40 mg/kg/day PO × 7 days
- *Trichomonas:* metronidazole 125 mg (15 mg/kg/day) tid PO × 7 to 10 days
- Pinworms: mebendazole 100-mg tablet chewable, repeat in 2 wk
- Labial agglutination: spontaneous resolution or topical estrogen cream for 7 to 10 days

CHRONIC Rx

See "Referral."

DISPOSITION

Further education:

- Young child: hygiene
- Adolescent: pregnancy prevention and safe sexual practices

REFERRAL

- To obstetrician/gynecologist
- To pediatrician

SUGGESTED READING

Van Neer PA, Korver CR: Constipation presenting as recurrent vulvovaginitis in prepubertal children, *J Am Acad Dermatol* 43(4):718, 2000.

AUTHORS: **JULIE ANNE SZUMIGALA, M.D.,** and **RUBEN ALVERO, M.D.**

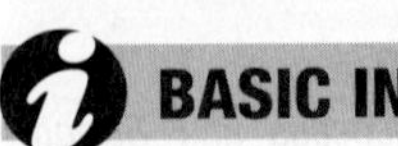

BASIC INFORMATION

DEFINITION

Trichomonas vulvovaginitis is the inflammation of vulva and vagina caused by *Trichomonas* spp.

SYNONYMS

Trichomonas vaginalis
Trichomoniasis

ICD-9CM CODES
131.01 Vulvovaginitis, trichomonal

EPIDEMIOLOGY & DEMOGRAPHICS

- Acquired through sexual contact
- Diagnosed in:
  1. 50% to 75% of prostitutes
  2. 5% to 15% of women visiting gynecology clinics
  3. 7% to 32% of women in sexually transmitted disease (STD) clinics
  4. 5% of women in family planning clinics

PHYSICAL FINDINGS & CLINICAL PRESENTATION

- Profuse, yellow, malodorous vaginal discharge and severe vaginal itching
- Vulvar itching
- Dysuria
- Dyspareunia
- Intense erythema of the vaginal mucosa
- Cervical petechiae ("strawberry cervix")
- Asymptomatic in approximately 50% of women and 90% of men

ETIOLOGY

Single-cell parasite known as trichomonad

RISK FACTORS

- Multiple sexual partners
- History of previous STDs

DIAGNOSIS

DIFFERENTIAL DIAGNOSIS

(Table 1-83)

- Bacterial vaginosis
- Fungal vulvovaginitis
- Cervicitis
- Atrophic vulvovaginitis

WORKUP

- Pelvic examination
- Speculum examination
- Mobile trichomonads seen on normal saline preparation: 70% sensitivity
- Elevated pH (>5) of vaginal discharge
- Culture is most sensitive commercially available method
- A large number of inflammatory cells on normal saline preparation

Section III describes the evaluation of vaginal discharge.

LABORATORY TESTS

- Culture (modified Diamond media): 90% sensitivity
- Direct enzyme immunoassay
- Fluorescein-conjugated monoclonal antibody test
- Pap test 40% detected

TREATMENT

NONPHARMACOLOGIC THERAPY

Condom use

ACUTE GENERAL Rx

Metronidazole (Flagyl) 2 g PO × 1 or 500 mg PO bid × 7 days *or* Tindamax (tinidazole) single 2 g oral dose in both sexes

CHRONIC Rx

- Metronidazole gel: less likely to achieve therapeutic levels; therefore not recommended
- Metronidazole (retreat): 500 mg PO bid × 7 days
- Treatment of future recurrences: metronidazole 2 g PO qd × 3 to 5 days
- Allergy, intolerance, or adverse reactions: alternatives to metronidazole are not available. Patients who are allergic to metronidazole can be managed by desensitization.
- Pregnancy
  1. Associated with adverse outcomes (i.e., premature rupture of membranes)
  2. Metronidazole 2 g PO × 1 day

DISPOSITION

Trichomonas infection is considered an STD; therefore treatment of the sexual partner is necessary.

REFERRAL

To obstetrician/gynecologist for recurrence and pregnancy

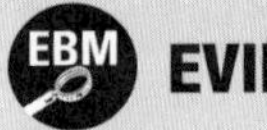

EVIDENCE

A single oral dose of any nitroimidazole is effective in achieving parasitologic cure at short-term follow-up.[1] (A)

Treatment of sexual partners may significantly reduce reinfection rates of *Trichomonas vaginalis*.[2] (A)

The effects of metronidazole treatment on pregnancy outcomes remains uncertain; therefore treatment in pregnancy should be reserved for symptomatic infections only.[3] (A)

Evidence-Based References

1. Forna F, Gülmezoglu AM: Interventions for treating trichomoniasis in women, *Cochrane Rev* 3, 2004.
2. Lyng J, Christensen J: A double-blind study of the value of treatment with a single dose tinidazole of partners to females with trichomoniasis, *Acta Obstet Gynecol Scand* 60:199, 1981.
3. Gülmezoglu AM: Interventions for trichomoniasis in pregnancy, *Cochrane Rev* 3, 2004.

SUGGESTED READING

Workowski KA, Levine WC: Sexually transmitted diseases treatment guidelines, *MMWR* 55:11, 2006.

AUTHORS: **JULIE ANNE SZUMIGALA, M.D.,** and **RUBEN ALVERO, M.D.**

TABLE 1-83 Differential Diagnosis of Vaginitis

Characteristics of Vaginal Discharge	*C. Albicans* Vaginitis	*T. Vaginalis* Vaginitis	Bacterial Vaginosis
pH	4.5	>5.0	>5.0
White curd	Usually	No	No
Odor with KOH	No	Yes	Yes
Clue cells	No	No	Usually
Motile trichomonads	No	Usually	No
Yeast cells3	Yes	No	No

From Goldman L, Ausiello D (eds): *Cecil textbook of medicine,* ed 22, Philadelphia, 2004, WB Saunders.

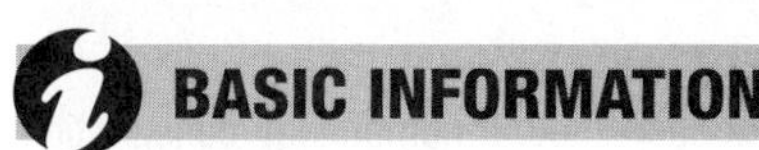

BASIC INFORMATION

DEFINITION

Waldenström's macroglobulinemia (WM) is a plasma cell dyscrasia characterized by the presence of increased blood concentration of monoclonal immunoglobulin (IgM).

SYNONYMS

WM
Monoclonal macroglobulinemia
Lymphoplasmacytic lymphoma

ICD-9CM CODES

273.3 Waldenström's macroglobulinemia

EPIDEMIOLOGY & DEMOGRAPHICS

- Accounts for 2% of all hematologic cancers
- 1500 people diagnosed each yr in the U.S.
- Overall incidence: 3.4 per million person-yr in men, 1.7 per million person-yr in women
- Median age approximately 63 yr
- More common among men than women and among whites than blacks

PHYSICAL FINDINGS & CLINICAL PRESENTATION

- Weakness
- Fatigue
- Weight loss
- Pallor
- Headache, dizziness, vertigo, deafness, and seizures (hyperviscosity syndrome)
- Easy bleeding (e.g., epistaxis)
- Retinal vein link-sausage shaped
- Lymphadenopathy (15%)
- Hepatomegaly (20%)
- Most commonly encountered neurological presentation is symmetric polyneuropathy
- Splenomegaly (15%)
- Purpura
- Symmetric peripheral neuropathy (5%)
- Fever and night sweats

ETIOLOGY

- The exact cause of WM is not known.
- Multiple reports suggest familial clustering, which indicates a genetic predisposition. In one study, chromosomal deletions in 6q21–22.1 were confirmed in 42% of WM patients, regardless of family history. In another study, the strongest evidence of linkage was found on chromosomes 1q and 4q.
- The main risk factor for development of WM is having IgM monoclonal gammopathy of unknown significance (MGUS).
- Radiation exposure, occupational chemicals, viral infection, and chronic inflammatory stimulation have been suggested, but there is insufficient evidence to substantiate these hypotheses.
- There is a twofold to threefold increased risk of of WM in people with a personal history of autoimmune diseases with autoantibodies, There is also increased risk with HIV, hepatitis, and rickettsiosis.

Dx DIAGNOSIS

The diagnosis of WM is usually established by laboratory blood tests and by bone marrow biopsy.

DIFFERENTIAL DIAGNOSIS

- MGUS
- Multiple myeloma
- Chronic lymphocytic leukemia
- Hairy-cell leukemia
- Lymphoma
- Smoldering macroglobulinemia

WORKUP

In any patient suspected of having WM, specific blood tests (CBC, erythrocyte sedimentation rate [ESR], serum or urine protein electrophoresis [SPEP or UPEP, respectively], IgM level, beta 2-microglobulin, serum viscosity) should be ordered. Bone marrow biopsy confirms the diagnosis.

LABORATORY TESTS

- CBC with differential:
  1. Anemia is a common finding, with a median hemoglobin value of approximately 10 g/dl. WBC count is usually normal; thrombocytopenia can occur.
  2. Peripheral smear may reveal "stacked coin" rouleaux formations and malignant lymphoid cells in terminal patients.
- Elevated ESR.
- SPEP: homogeneous M spike (monoclonal gammopathy)
- Immunoelectrophoresis: confirms IgM responsible for the M spike. Table 1-84 describes physiochemical and immunological properties of the monoclonal IgM protein in Waldenström macroglobulinemia.
- Urine immunoelectrophoresis: monoclonal light chains are usually kappa chains. Bence Jones protein can be seen, but is not the typical finding in WM
- IgM levels are high, generally >3 g/dl
- Beta 2-microglobulin: elevated in 55%, high levels are associated with poor prognosis.
- Serum viscosity: symptoms usually occur when the serum viscosity is four times the viscosity of normal serum; classical feature although present in only 15% of cases.
- Cryoglobulins, rheumatoid factor, or cold agglutinins may be present
- Bone marrow biopsy: lymphoplasmacytoid cells are characteristic.

IMAGING STUDIES

Chest radiograph can be obtained to rule out pulmonary involvement.

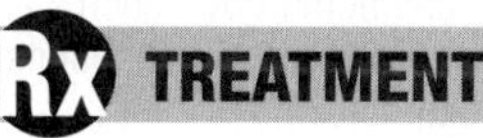

TREATMENT

- Because of the incurable nature of WM, the aim of treatment is to relieve symptoms and reduce the risk of organ damage. Considerations for the initiation of treatment include the following: hemoglobin concentration less than 100×10^9/L, significant adenopathy or organomegaly, symptomatic hyperviscosity, severe neuropathy, amyloidosis, cryoglobu-

TABLE 1-84 Physicochemical and Immunologic Properties of the Monoclonal Immunoglobulin Protein in Waldenström's Macroglobulinemia

Properties of Monoclonal Immunoglobulin Protein	Diagnostic Condition	Clinical Manifestations
Pentameric structure	Hyperviscosity	Headaches, blurred vision, epistaxis, retinal hemorrhages, leg cramps, impaired mentation, and intracranial hemorrhage
Prescription on cooling	Cryoglobulinemia (type I)	Raynaud's phenomenon, acrocyanosis, ulcers, purpura, and cold urticaria
Autoantibody activity to myelin-associated glycoprotein, ganglioside M1, and sulfatide moieties on peripheral nerve sheaths	Peripheral neuropathies	Sensorimotor neuropathies, painful neuropathies, ataxic gait, and bilateral foot drop
Autoantibody activity to immunoglobulin G	Cryoglobulinemia (type II)	Purpura, arthralgias, renal failure, and sensorimotor neuropathies
Autoantibody activity to red blood cell antigens	Cold agglutinins	Hemolytic anemia, Raynaud's phenomenon, acrocyanosis, and livedo reticularis
Tissue deposition as amorphous aggregates	Organ dysfunction	Skin: bullous skin disease, papules, and Schnitzler syndrome Gastrointestinal: diarrhea, malabsorption, and bleeding Kidney: proteinuria and renal failure (light-chain component)
Tissue deposition as amyloid fibrils (Light-chain fibrils are commonly the most component.)	Organ dysfunction	Fatigue, weight loss, edema, periorbital purpura, hepatomegaly, macroglossia, and organ dysfunction of the involved organs: heart, kidney, liver, and peripheral sensory and autonomic nerves.

From Hoffmann R et al: *Hematology, basic principles and practice,* ed 5, Philadelphia, 2009, Churchill Livingstone.

linemia, cold-agglutinin disease, or evidence of disease transformation.

- Treatment is directed at both hyperviscocity and the lymphoproliferative disorder itself.

NONPHARMACOLOGIC THERAPY

Asymptomatic patients do not require treatment, and these patients should be monitored periodically for the onset of symptoms or changes in blood tests (e.g., worsening anemia, thrombocytopenia, rising IgM, and serum viscosity).

ACUTE GENERAL Rx

1. Plasmapharesis is the treatment used to alleviate symptoms of hyperviscocity.
2. Treatment of the lymphoproliferative disorder includes single or combination therapy, though no single or combination of agents has been demonstrated to be superior:
   a. Rituximab, a monoclonal anti-CD 20 antibody, in combination with nucleoside analogs.
   b. Nucleoside analogs and alkylator agents (chlorambucil).
   c. Combination chemotherapy such as CHOP (cyclophosphamide, vincristine, prednisone, doxorubicin).

CHRONIC Rx

- Refractory patients can be retried on original therapy if length of response from initial therapy is greater than 2 yr. If the response from the initial therapy was <2 yr, alternative first-line agents such as fludarabine or cladribine can be used.
- Other treatment options: interferon alpha, thalidomide, and autologous stem cell transplantation.

DISPOSITION

- The onset of WM is slow and insidious. Most patients die from progression of the disease with hyperviscosity, hemorrhage, and infection, or from congestive heart failure.
- Some patients develop acute myelogenous leukemia, immunoblastic sarcoma, or chronic myelogenous leukemia as a preterminal event.
- Median survival in patients with WM is about 4 to 5 yr.
- Approximately 10% of patients will achieve complete remission, with prognosis being more favorable (median survival 11 yr).
- A staging system using serum beta 2-microglobulin concentration, hemoglobin concentration, and serum IgM concentration before treatment provides insight into prognosis and survival.
- Other factors can negatively affect the survival: age >65, male gender, the presence of organomegaly and the presence of cytopenias.

REFERRAL

If WM is suspected, a hematology consultation is helpful in guiding future workup, treatment, and monitoring.

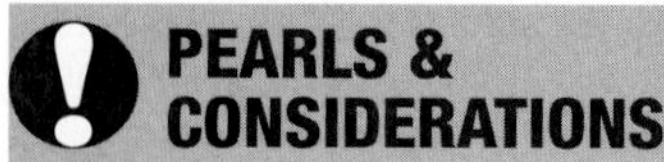

COMMENTS

- WM was first described in 1944 by the Swedish physician Jan Gosta Waldenström.
- Amyloidosis is rare, occurring in 5% of patients with WM.

SUGGESTED READINGS

Dimopoulos MA, Anagnostopoulos A: Waldenström's macroglobulinemia, *Best Pract Res Clin Haematol* 18(4):747, 2005.

Fonseca R, Hayman S: Waldenström macroglobulinaemia, *Br J Haematol* 138:700, 2007.

Gertz MA: Waldenström macroglobulinemia: a review of therapy, *Am J Hematol* 79(2):147, 2005.

Koshiol J et al: Chronic immune stimulation and subsequent Waldenstrom macroglobulinemia, *Arch Intern Med* 168(17):1903-1909, 2008.

Vijay A, Gertz MA: Waldenström macroglobulinemia, *Blood* 109(12):5096, 2007.

AUTHOR: **MARK BRADY, M.D., M.P.H., M.M.S.**

BASIC INFORMATION

DEFINITION

Warts are benign epidermal neoplasms caused by human papillomavirus (HPV).

SYNONYMS

Verruca vulgaris (common warts)
Verruca plana (flat warts)
Condyloma acuminatum (venereal warts)
Verruca plantaris (plantar warts)
Mosaic warts (cluster of many warts)

ICD-9CM CODES
078.10 Viral warts
078.19 Venereal wart (external genital organs)

EPIDEMIOLOGY & DEMOGRAPHICS

- Common warts occur most frequently in children and young adults.
- Anogenital warts are most common in young, sexually active patients. Genital warts are the most common viral sexually transmitted disease in the U.S., with up to 24 million Americans carrying the causative virus.
- Common warts are longer lasting and more frequent in immunocompromised patients (e.g., lymphoma, AIDS, immunosuppressive drugs).
- Plantar warts occur most frequently at points of maximal pressure (over the heads of the metatarsal bones or on the heels).

PHYSICAL FINDINGS & CLINICAL PRESENTATION

- Common warts (Fig. 1-361) have an initial appearance of a flesh-colored papule with a rough surface; they subsequently develop a hyperkeratotic appearance with black dots on the surface (thrombosed capillaries). They may be single or multiple and are most common on the hands.
- Warts obscure normal skin lines (important diagnostic feature). Cylindrical projections from the wart may become fused, forming a mosaic pattern.
- Flat warts generally are pink or light yellow, slightly elevated, and often found on the forehead, back of hands, mouth, and beard area. They often occur in lines corresponding to trauma (e.g., a scratch), are often misdiagnosed (particularly when present on the face), and inappropriately treated with topical corticosteroids.
- Filiform warts have a fingerlike appearance with various projections; they are generally found near the mouth, beard, or periorbital and paranasal regions.
- Plantar warts are slightly raised and have a roughened surface; they may cause pain when walking; as they involute, small hemorrhages (caused by thrombosed capillaries) may be noted.
- Genital warts are generally pale pink with several projections and a broad base. They may coalesce in the perineal area to form masses with a cauliflower-like appearance.
- Genital warts on the cervical epithelium can produce subclinical changes that may be noted on Pap smear or colposcopy.

ETIOLOGY

- HPV infection; >60 types of viral DNA have been identified. Transmission of warts is by direct contact.
- Genital warts are usually caused by HPV types 6 or 11.

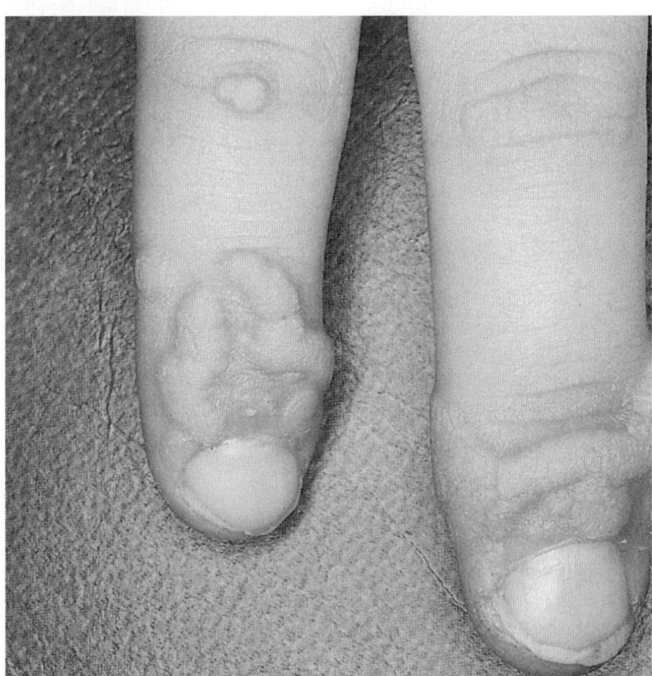

FIGURE 1-361 Verruca vulgaris, or common viral warts. These papules often have verrucous surface changes. (From Callen JP: *Color atlas of dermatology,* ed 2, Philadelphia, 2000, WB Saunders.)

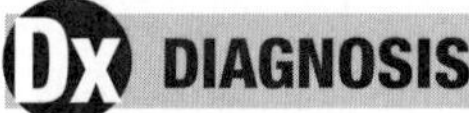

DIAGNOSIS

DIFFERENTIAL DIAGNOSIS

- Molluscum contagiosum
- Condyloma latum
- Acrochordon (skin tags) or seborrheic keratosis
- Epidermal nevi
- Hypertrophic actinic keratosis
- Squamous cell carcinomas
- Acquired digital fibrokeratoma
- Varicella zoster virus in patients with AIDS
- Recurrent infantile digital fibroma
- Plantar corns (may be mistaken for plantar warts)

WORKUP

- Diagnosis is generally based on clinical findings.
- Suspect lesions should be biopsied.

LABORATORY TESTS

Colposcopy with biopsy of patients with cervical squamous cell changes

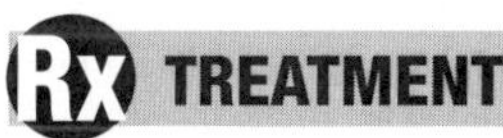

TREATMENT

NONPHARMACOLOGIC THERAPY

- Importance of use of condoms to reduce transmission of genital warts should be emphasized.
- Watchful waiting is an acceptable option in the treatment of warts because many warts will disappear without intervention over time.
- Plantar warts that are not painful do not need treatment.

GENERAL Rx

- Common warts:
  1. Application of topical salicylic acid 17%. Soak area for 5 min in warm water and dry. Apply thin layer once or twice daily for up to 12 wk, avoiding normal skin. Bandage.
  2. Liquid nitrogen and electrocautery are also common methods of removal.
  3. Blunt dissection can be used in large lesions or resistant lesions.
  4. Duct tape occlusion is also effective for treating common warts. It is cut to cover warts and left in place for 6 days. It is removed after 6 days and the warts are soaked in water and then filed with pumice stones. New tape is applied 12 hr later. This treatment can be repeated until warts resolve.
- Filiform warts: surgical removal is necessary.
- Flat warts: generally more difficult to treat.
  1. Tretinoin cream applied at bedtime over the involved area for several weeks may be effective.
  2. Application of liquid nitrogen.
  3. Electrocautery.
  4. 5-Fluorouracil cream applied once or twice a day for 3 to 5 wk is also effective. Persistent hyperpigmentation may occur after Efudex use.

- Plantar warts:
  1. Salicylic acid therapy (e.g., Occlusal-HP). Soak wart in warm water for 5 min, remove loose tissue, dry. Apply to area, allow to dry, reapply. Use once or twice daily; maximum 12 wk. Use of 40% salicylic acid plasters (Mediplast) is also a safe, nonscarring treatment; it is particularly useful in treating mosaic warts covering a large area.
  2. Blunt dissection is also a fast and effective treatment modality.
  3. Laser therapy can be used for plantar warts and recurrent warts; however, it leaves open wounds that require 4 to 6 wk to fill with granulation tissue.
  4. Interlesional bleomycin is also effective but generally used when all other treatments fail.
- Genital warts:
  1. Can be effectively treated with 20% podophyllin resin in compound tincture of benzoin applied with a cotton tip applicator by the treating physician and allowed to air dry. The treatment can be repeated weekly if necessary.
  2. Podofilox (Condylox 0.5% gel) is now available for application by the patient. Local adverse effects include pain, burning, and inflammation at the site.
  3. Cryosurgery with liquid nitrogen delivered with a probe or as a spray is effective for treating smaller genital warts.
  4. Carbon dioxide laser can also be used for treating primary or recurrent genital warts (cure rate >90%).
  5. Imiquimod cream, 5%, is a patient-applied immune response modifier effective in the treatment of external genital and perianal warts (complete clearing of genital warts in >70% of females and >30% of males in 4 to 16 wk). Sexual contact should be avoided while the cream is on the skin. It is applied three times per week before normal sleeping hours and is left on the skin for 6 to 10 hr.
  6. Sinecatechins (Veregen), a botanical drug product, is also effective for treatment of external genital and perianal warts. Formulation is a 15% ointment applied to affected area tid for up to 16 wk.
- Application of trichloroacetic acid or bichloracetic acid 80% to 90% is also effective for external genital warts. A small amount should be applied only to warts and allowed to dry, at which time a white "frosting" develops. This treatment can be repeated weekly if necessary.

DISPOSITION

- Warts can be effectively treated with the previous modalities with complete resolution in the majority of patients; however, recurrence rate is high.
- Cervical carcinomas and precancerous lesions in women are associated with genital papillomavirus infection.
- Squamous cell anal cancer is also associated with a history of genital warts.

REFERRAL

- Dermatology referral for warts resistant to conservative therapy
- Surgical referral in selected cases
- Sexually transmitted disease counseling for patients with anogenital warts

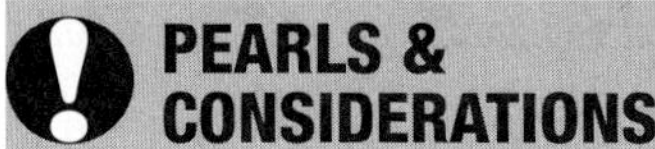

PEARLS & CONSIDERATIONS

COMMENTS

- Subungual and periungual warts are generally more resistant to treatment. Dermatology referral for cryosurgery is recommended in resistant cases.
- Examination of sex partners is not necessary for the management of genital warts because no data indicate that reinfection plays a role.
- HPV vaccination is available for females ages 11 to 26 and males ages 8 to 18.

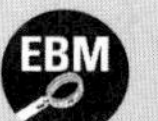

EVIDENCE

Please note: Complete text of EBM for this topic is available online.

Key trials and commentary:

Human papillomavirus types 16 (HPV-16) and 18 (HPV-18) cause ~70% of cervical cancers worldwide. A phase III trial was conducted to evaluate a quadrivalent vaccine against HPV types 6, 11, 16, and 18 (HPV-6/11/16/18) for the prevention of high-grade cervical lesions associated with HPV-16 and HPV-18.

This study showed that in young women who had not been previously infected with HPV-16 or HPV-18, those in the vaccine group had a significantly lower occurrence of high-grade cervical intraepithelial neoplasia related to HPV-16 or HPV-18 than did those in the placebo group (ClinicalTrials.gov number, NCT00092534).

The new quadrivalent vaccine marketed by Merck targets HPV serotypes 6, 11, 16, and 18. Types 6 and 11 are associated with anogenital warts and some low-grade neoplastic lesions, whereas types 16 and 18 cause most cervical cancers. This study shows that the vaccine is highly effective against precancerous cervical lesions and anogenital warts. The vaccine efficacy was 90% to 100% in both trials over 3 years in young women not previously infected with the vaccine serotypes. However, it was considerably less effective in unselected women, some of whom either were already infected or had HPV-related diseases. The question of who should be vaccinated and when they should be vaccinated has been the source of considerable debate, with political, social, and religious factors clouding what should be a purely medical issue. Moreover, the HPV vaccines are probably most needed in the developing world, where 80% of deaths from cervical cancer occur. However, in these countries the cost can be a deterrent. Finally, the efficacy of the vaccine in preventing cervical cancer is limited by at least two factors. First, not all cervical cancer is caused by HPV-16 or HPV-18, and second, for the vaccine to be effective, young women must be vaccinated before they are infected with these two serotypes. Other questions that require answers are the durability of immune protection and whether young men should be vaccinated as well.[1] Ⓐ

Evidence-Based Reference

1. Koutsky LA for the FUTURE II Study Group: Quadrivalent vaccine against human papillomavirus to prevent high-grade cervical lesions, *N Engl J Med* 356:1915-1927, 2007. Commentary by B.H. Thiers, M.D. Ⓐ

SUGGESTED READINGS

Bacelieri R, Johnson SM: Cutaneous warts: an evidence-based approach to therapy, *Am Fam Physician* 72: 647, 2005.

Huang CM: Human papillomavirus and vaccination, *Mayo Clin Proc* 83(6):701, 2008.

AUTHOR: **FRED F. FERRI, M.D.**

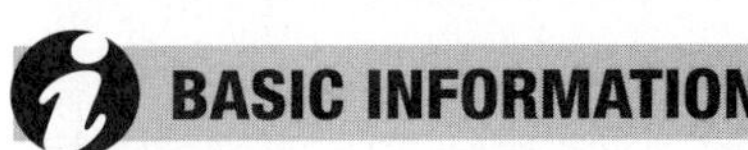

BASIC INFORMATION

DEFINITION

Wegener granulomatosis is a multisystem disease generally consisting of the classic triad of:

1. Necrotizing granulomatous lesions in the upper or lower respiratory tract
2. Generalized focal necrotizing vasculitis involving both arteries and veins
3. Focal glomerulonephritis of the kidneys

"Limited forms" of the disease can also occur and may evolve into the classic triad; Wegener granulomatosis can be classified using the "ELK" classification, which identifies the three major sites of involvement: *E,* ears, nose, and throat or respiratory tract; *L,* lungs; *K,* kidneys.

ICD-9CM CODES
446.4 Wegener's granulomatosis

EPIDEMIOLOGY & DEMOGRAPHICS

INCIDENCE: 3/100,000 persons, equal in men and women

MEAN AGE AT ONSET: 41 yr

PHYSICAL FINDINGS & CLINICAL PRESENTATION

- Clinical manifestations often vary with the stage of the disease and degree of organ involvement. 90% of patients present with symptoms involving the upper or lower airways or both.
- Frequent manifestations are:
  1. Upper respiratory tract: chronic sinusitis, chronic otitis media, mastoiditis, nasal crusting, obstruction and epistaxis, nasal septal perforation, nasal lacrimal duct stenosis, saddle nose deformities (resulting from cartilage destruction)
  2. Lung: hemoptysis, multiple nodules, diffuse alveolar pattern
  3. Kidney: renal insufficiency, glomerulonephritis
  4. Skin: necrotizing skin lesions
  5. Nervous system: mononeuritis multiplex, cranial nerve involvement
  6. Joints: monarthritis or polyarthritis (nondeforming), usually affecting large joints
  7. Mouth: chronic ulcerative lesions of the oral mucosa, "mulberry" gingivitis
  8. Eye: proptosis, uveitis, episcleritis, retinal and optic nerve vasculitis

ETIOLOGY

Unknown

DIAGNOSIS

DIFFERENTIAL DIAGNOSIS

- Other granulomatous lung diseases (e.g., sarcoidosis, lymphomatoid granulomatosis, Churg-Strauss syndrome, necrotizing sarcoid granulomatosis, bronchocentric granulomatosis, sarcoidosis); the differential diagnosis of granulomatous lung disease is described in Section II
- Neoplasms (especially lymphoproliferative disease)
- Goodpasture's syndrome
- Bacterial or fungal sinusitis
- Midline granuloma
- Viral infections
- Other causes of glomerulonephritis (e.g., poststreptococcal nephritis)

WORKUP

- Wegener granulomatosis should be suspected in anyone presenting with sinus disease that does not respond to conventional treatment, pulmonary hemorrhage, glomerulonephritis, mononeuritis multiplex resulting in wrist or foot drop, progressive migratory arthralgias or arthritis, and unexplained multisystem disease.
- Chest x-ray, laboratory evaluation, PFTs, and tissue biopsy.

LABORATORY TESTS

- Positive test for cytoplasmic pattern of ANCA (c-ANCA).
- Anemia, leukocytosis.
- Urinalysis: may reveal hematuria, RBC casts, and proteinuria.
- Elevated serum creatinine, decreased creatinine clearance.
- Increased ESR, positive rheumatoid factor, and elevated C-reactive protein may be found.

IMAGING STUDIES

- Chest x-ray: may reveal bilateral multiple nodules, cavitated mass lesions, pleural effusion (20%). Up to one third of patients without pulmonary signs or symptoms have an abnormal chest x-ray (Fig. 1-362).
- PFTs: useful in detecting stenosis of the airways.

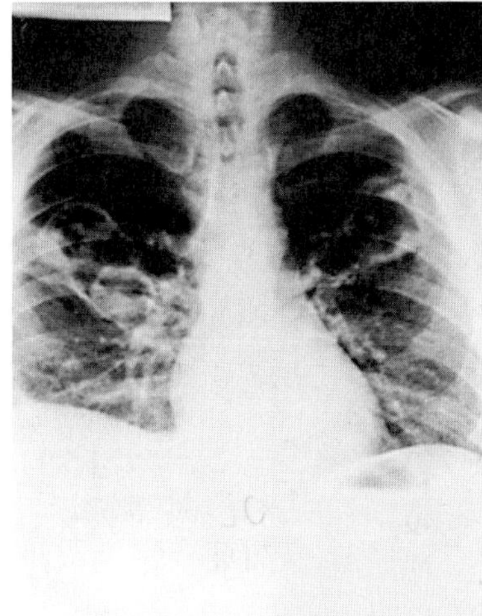

FIGURE 1-362 Chest radiograph shows multiple cavitary pulmonary nodules in patient with Wegener granulomatosis. (From Weinberg SE et al: *Principles of pulmonary medicine,* ed 5, Philadelphia, 2008, Saunders.)

- Biopsy of one or more affected organs should be attempted; the most reliable source for tissue diagnosis is the lung. Lesions in the nasopharynx (if present) can be easily biopsied but biopsy is positive in only 20%. Biopsy of radiographically abnormal pulmonary parenchyma provides the highest yield (>90%).

TREATMENT

NONPHARMACOLOGIC THERAPY

- Ensure proper airway drainage.
- Give nutritional counseling.

ACUTE GENERAL Rx

- Prednisone 60 to 80 mg/day and cyclophosphamide 2 mg/kg are generally effective and are used to control clinical manifestations; once the disease comes under control, prednisone is tapered and cyclophosphamide is continued. Other potentially useful agents in patients intolerant to cyclophosphamide are methotrexate, azathioprine, and mycophenolate mofetil.
- TMP-SMX therapy may represent a useful alternative in patients with lesions limited to the upper or lower respiratory tracts in absence of vasculitis or nephritis. Treatment with TMP-SMX (160 mg/800 mg bid) also reduces the incidence of relapses in patients with Wegener granulomatosis in remission. It is also useful in preventing *Pneumocystis jirovecii* pneumonia, which occurs in 10% of patients receiving induction therapy. When used for prophylaxis, dose of TMP-SMX (160 mg/800 mg) is 1 tablet three times/wk.

DISPOSITION

Five-year survival with aggressive treatment is approximately 80%; without treatment 2-yr survival is <20%.

REFERRAL

Surgical referral for biopsy

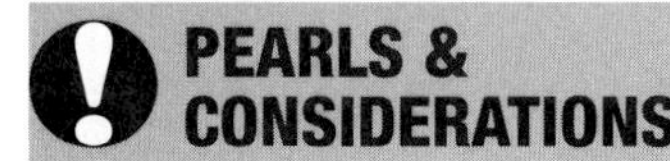

PEARLS & CONSIDERATIONS

COMMENTS

- Methotrexate (20 mg/wk) represents an alternative to cyclophosphamide in patients who do not have immediately life-threatening disease.
- C-ANCA levels should not dictate changes in therapy, because they correlate erratically with disease activity.
- The incidence of venous thrombotic events in Wegener granulomatosis is significantly higher than the general population. Clinicians should maintain a heightened awareness of the risks of venous thrombosis and a lower threshold for evaluating patients for possible DVT or pulmonary embolism.

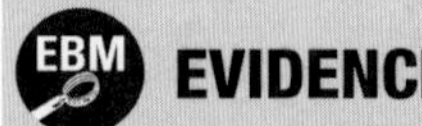

Please note: Complete text of EBM for this topic is available online.

Key trials and commentary:

Immunosuppressive therapies for antineutrophil cytoplasmic antibody (ANCA)–associated vasculitis have greatly advanced patient survival but have turned ANCA-associated vasculitis (AAV) into chronic, relapsing disorders. Long-term treatment and disease-related morbidity are major threats. The last decade has seen a collaborative international effort to determine effective treatment.

This study sought to analyze the reported evidence on AAV therapy in order to provide physicians with a rational approach for dealing with various clinical scenarios.

This study showed that although AAV therapies should be tailored to the patient's specific clinical situation, evidence for treatment of several disease states is lacking. There is a need for safer and more effective drugs

ANCA–associated vasculitis describes a spectrum of disorders that affect small- to medium-sized blood vessels. The diverse clinical manifestations of these life-threatening conditions include signs and symptoms recognized as Wegener's granulomatosis, Churg-Strauss syndrome, and microscopic polyangiitis. The authors propose a model for the pathogenesis of these disorders and review the literature on their treatment. They found a surprising lack of evidence-based data to support the effectiveness of traditional immunosuppressive treatment and suggest that future research efforts explore new immunosuppressive drugs and biologic agents such as rituximab and infliximab that have shown promise in limited early trials.[1] Ⓐ

Evidence-Based Reference

Bosch X et al: Treatment of antineutrophil cytoplasmic antibody–associated vasculitis: a systematic review, *JAMA* 298:655-669, 2007. Commentary by B.H. Thiers, M.D. Ⓐ

SUGGESTED READINGS

Finkielman JD et al: Antiproteinase 3 antineutrophil cytoplasmic antibodies and disease activity in Wegener granulomatosis, *Ann Intern Med* 147(9): 611-619, 2007.

Langford CA: Update on Wegener granulomatosis, *Cleve Clin J Med* 72:689-697, 2005.

Merkel PA et al: Brief communication: high incidence of venous thrombotic events among patients with Wegener granulomatosis: the Wegener's Clinical Occurrence of Thrombosis (WeCLOT) study, *Ann Intern Med* 142:620-626, 2005.

AUTHOR: **FRED F. FERRI, M.D.**

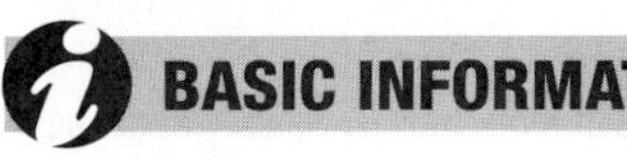

BASIC INFORMATION

DEFINITION

Wernicke's encephalopathy is the syndrome of acute extraocular muscle dysfunction, confusion, and ataxia, resulting from thiamine deficiency.

SYNONYMS

Korsakoff's syndrome
Wernicke-Korsakoff syndrome
Alcoholic polyneuritic psychosis

ICD-9CM CODES

265.1 Wernicke's encephalopathy, disease, or syndrome

EPIDEMIOLOGY & DEMOGRAPHICS

- Most commonly associated with alcohol abuse
- Slightly more common in males
- Age of onset evenly distributed between ages 30 and 70

PHYSICAL FINDINGS & CLINICAL PRESENTATION

- Disturbance of extraocular motility, including nystagmus, abducens nerve palsy, and disorders of conjugate gaze.
- Encephalopathy.
- Ataxia of gait.
- Peripheral neuropathy may be seen in addition to the typical findings described previously.

ETIOLOGY

Thiamine deficiency from alcohol abuse or other malnourished state. It may be iatrogenic from prolonged dextrose infusion without thiamine supplementation.

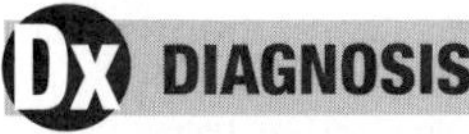

DIAGNOSIS

DIFFERENTIAL DIAGNOSIS

- Thiamine deficiency, including alcohol abuse, malnutrition, or iatrogenic cause
- Stroke, mass lesion, or trauma affecting upper brainstem, thalamus, and associated structures

WORKUP

Patients must be evaluated with a high index of suspicion, and treated rapidly, even in advance of laboratory results.

LABORATORY TESTS

- CBC.
- Serum chemistries.
- Serum pyruvate is elevated.
- Whole-blood or erythrocyte transketolase are decreased; rapid resolution to normal in 24 hr with thiamine repletion.

IMAGING STUDIES

- MRI may show T2 hyperintense diencephalic and mesencephalic lesions acutely, but there is no definitive radiologic study for diagnosis.
- CT scan may show cerebral atrophy from chronic alcoholism.

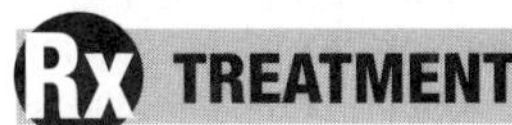

TREATMENT

NONPHARMACOLOGIC THERAPY

Alcoholics Anonymous

ACUTE GENERAL Rx

- 100 mg thiamine IV or IM immediately; typically thiamine IV for 3 to 5 days, then PO.
- Avoid dextrose-containing fluids until thiamine repleted.
- Prophylactic treatment for delirium tremens if alcoholic.

CHRONIC Rx

- Attempt to treat alcoholism or underlying malnourished state.
- Chronic oral thiamine repletion; typical dose 5 mg/day.
- Case reports suggest donepezil may help chronic memory problems.
- Inadequately treated disease may progress to Korsakoff's psychosis (see relevant entry).

DISPOSITION

Enter substance abuse program after acute phase. Long-term care is determined by level of recovery.

REFERRAL

Neurologist should be consulted if symptoms do not resolve after thiamine therapy.

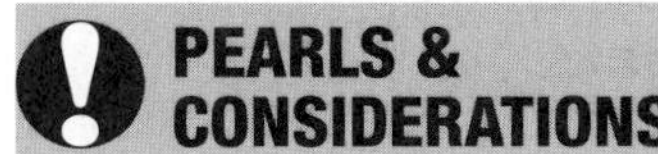

PEARLS & CONSIDERATIONS

COMMENTS

- Give thiamine if the disease is even suspected.
- Prognosis is generally poor, with 10% to 20% mortality even with treatment. Most patients will be left with impaired learning and memory, which may be subtle.
- A preventable cause is prolonged dextrose-containing IV fluids without supplemental thiamine.

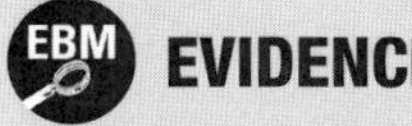

EVIDENCE

The use of thiamine in the management of Korsakoff's psychosis is supported by limited data from randomized studies and endorsed by expert opinion.

A recent Cochrane review identified two RCTs evaluating the use of thiamine in people at risk of Korsakoff's secondary to alcohol excess, of which only one contained sufficient data for quantitative analysis. This review found that although thiamine administration is strongly recommended for alcohol-abusing patients, there is insufficient evidence to make specific recommendations of the dose, frequency, route, or duration of thiamine administration either in the prophylaxis or treatment of Wernicke-Korsakoff syndrome.[1] Ⓐ

Recommendations from the American Society of Addiction Medicine are that parenteral administration of thiamine (100 mg daily for at least 3 days, IV or IM) is recommended to prevent or treat Wernicke-Korsakoff syndrome.[2] Ⓒ

Evidence-Based References

1. Day E et al: Thiamine for Wernicke-Korsakoff Syndrome in people at risk from alcohol abuse. *Cochrane Database Syst Rev* 1, 2004.
2. Mayo-Smith MF et al: Working Group on the Management of Alcohol Withdrawal Delirium, Practice Guidelines Committee, American Society of Addiction Medicine. Management of alcohol withdrawal delirium. An evidence-based practice guideline. *Arch Intern Med* 164:1405-1412, 2004.

SUGGESTED READINGS

Cochrane et al: Acetylcholinesterase inhibitors for the treatment of Wernicke-Korsakoff syndrome—three further cases show response to donepezil, *Alcohol Alcohol* 40(2):151-154, 2005.

Cook CC: Prevention and treatment of Wernicke-Korsakoff syndrome, *Alcohol Alcohol Suppl* 35 (suppl 1):19, 2000.

Martin PR et al: The role of thiamine deficiency in alcoholic brain disease, *Alcohol Res Health* 27(2):134-142, 2003.

Zubaran C et al: Wernicke-Korsakoff syndrome, *Postgrad Med J* 73(855):27, 1997.

AUTHOR: **DANIEL T. MATTSON, M.D., M.SC. (MED.)**

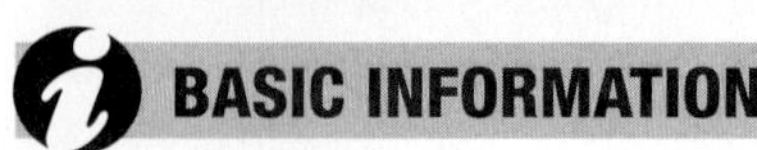

BASIC INFORMATION

DEFINITION

West Nile virus (WNV) infection is an illness affecting the CNS, caused by the mosquito-borne WNV.

SYNONYMS

West Nile virus fever
West Nile virus encephalitis
Neuroinvasive West Nile virus infection
Nonneuroinvasive West Nile virus infection

ICD-9CM CODES
066.4 West Nile virus infection

EPIDEMIOLOGY & DEMOGRAPHICS

- Before 1999, WNV infection was confined to areas in the Middle East, with occasional outbreaks in Europe. The infection began being diagnosed in the Western hemisphere in 1999. First seen in the northeast and mid-Atlantic states, WNV virus infection has spread steadily each year to new regions of the U.S., with a general westward migration pattern. In 2003, a record number of cases were reported from the U.S., with over 7000 cases reported, resulting in several hundred deaths. Most deaths occur in elderly patients with WNV encephalitis. In 2003, Illinois, Ohio, Michigan, and Louisiana were hardest hit. Since 2004 the incidence of WNV infection diminished gradually as it spread to the western states. Human cases of WNV infection have now been reported across all the contiguous continental U.S. (sparing only Hawaii and Alaska). A total of 1400 neuroinvasive and non-neuroinvasive cases were reported in the U.S. in 2008.
- The virus is carried by a number of species of birds, as well as horses and several other animals. It is transmitted to humans through the bite of an infected mosquito. For this reason, WNV infection is seen primarily from mid-summer to mid-autumn, the period of maximum mosquito intensity.
- The majority of severe cases have been reported among individuals >50 yr of age. There is no gender predilection.
- Person-to-person transmission is fortunately rare but has been reported to occur by blood transfusion, organ transplantation, breast-feeding, and perhaps by perinatal transmission; the blood supply is now routinely tested by nucleic acid testing methods to reduce the risk of transmission-acquired WNV in the U.S.

PHYSICAL FINDINGS & CLINICAL PRESENTATION

- Less than 20% of infected individuals develop symptomatic disease. The initial phase of illness is nonspecific, with abrupt onset of fever accompanied by malaise, eye pain, anorexia, headache, and, occasionally, rash and lymphadenopathy. Less commonly, myocarditis, hepatitis, or pancreatitis may occur.
- In approximately 1 in 150 cases, especially among elderly patients, severe neurologic sequelae will occur. Most common among these are ataxia, cranial nerve palsies, optic neuritis, seizures, myelitis, and polyradiculitis.

ETIOLOGY

The WNV is a member of the flavivirus group, along with the yellow fever, dengue, St. Louis, and Japanese encephalitis viruses. It has a large reservoir in nature, infecting many species of birds, as well as certain mammals, and is thought to be spread to humans exclusively by various species of mosquito. Neurologic disease is caused by direct invasion of the CNS.

Dx DIAGNOSIS

DIFFERENTIAL DIAGNOSIS

- Meningitis or encephalitis caused by more common viruses (e.g., enteroviruses, herpes simplex)
- Bacterial meningitis
- Vasculitis
- Fungal meningitis (e.g., cryptococcal infection)
- Tuberculous meningitis

LABORATORY TESTS

- CBC, electrolytes (hyponatremia common)
- Spinal tap and CSF examination: typically demonstrates lymphocytic pleocytosis with normal level of glucose and elevated level of protein
- CSF WNV IgM antibody level: rare false-positive results in people recently vaccinated against Japanese encephalitis or yellow fever viruses

IMAGING STUDIES

CT or MRI studies of the brain to exclude mass lesions and cerebral edema

Rx TREATMENT

NONPHARMACOLOGIC THERAPY

Hospitalization, IV hydration, ventilator support may be necessary.

ACUTE GENERAL Rx

No specific therapy has been established in clinical trials. Ribavirin and interferon alfa-2b have been shown to have in vitro activity against the virus. IV immunoglobulin (IVIG) from convalescent patient plasma is under study but no controlled trials have been reported as yet.

CHRONIC Rx

Chronic rehabilitation therapy usually necessary for patients with severe neurologic impairment. Mental status defects following WNV neuroinvasive disease appear to be more common and severe than initially recognized.

DISPOSITION

Chronic rehabilitation as needed following recovery from acute infection. Physical and mental outcome measures seem to normalize within approximately 1 yr in patients with WNV. The presence of preexisting comorbid conditions is associated with longer recovery.

REFERRAL

- Infectious disease consultant
- Public health authorities

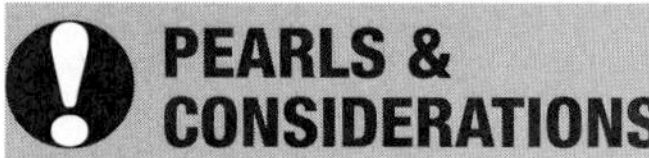

PEARLS & CONSIDERATIONS

COMMENTS

- Diagnosis requires a high index of suspicion, because disease course may be nonspecific and may mimic other, more common disorders.
- Specific laboratory diagnostic studies are available only through public-health laboratories.
- Best means of prevention is reduction in mosquito population by draining of stagnant water deposits and, if necessary, insecticide spraying.
- Individuals may reduce risk by covering arms and legs in areas where mosquitoes are likely to be found and using insect repellent containing DEET.

SUGGESTED READINGS

Carson PJ et al: Long-term clinical and neuropsychological outcomes of West Nile virus infection, *Clin Infect Dis* 43(6):723, 2006.

CDC: Update: West Nile virus activity–United States, 2005, *MMWR* 54(34):851-852, 2005.

Gottfried K et al: Clinical description and follow-up investigation of human West Nile Virus cases, *South Med J* 98(6):603-606, 2005.

Haaland KY et al: Mental status after West Nile virus infection, *Emerg Infect Dis* 12(8):1260, 2006.

Higgs S et al: Nonviremic transmission of West Nile virus, *Proc Natl Acad Sci USA* 102(25):8871-8874, 2005.

Loeb M et al: Prognosis after West Nile virus infection, *Ann Intern Med* 149:232-241, 2008.

Stramer SL et al: West Nile virus among blood donors in the United States, 2003 and 2004, *N Engl J Med* 353(5):451-459, 2005.

AUTHORS: **STEVEN M. OPAL, M.D., GLENN G. FORT, M.D., M.P.H.,** and **DENNIS J. MIKOLICH, M.D.**

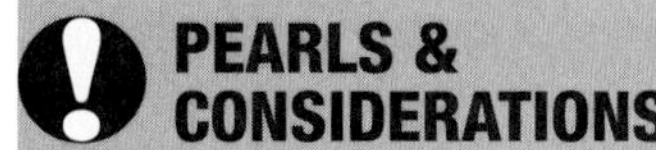

BASIC INFORMATION

DEFINITION

Whiplash refers to a hyperextension injury to the neck, often the result of being struck from behind by a fast-moving vehicle.

SYNONYMS

Acceleration flexion-extension neck injury

ICD-9CM CODES

847.0 Whiplash injury or syndrome

EPIDEMIOLOGY & DEMOGRAPHICS

- Whiplash occurs in more than 1 million people each year.
- Most injuries (40%) are the result of rear-end motor vehicle accidents.
- Whiplash occurs at all ages, in both sexes, and at all socioeconomic levels.
- Incidence is 4 per 1000 persons and is higher in women than men.
- Nearly 50% of patients with whiplash seek legal advice.
- Whiplash is also seen in shaken baby syndrome.

PHYSICAL FINDINGS & CLINICAL PRESENTATION

- Most present with a history of being involved in a motor vehicle accident and being rear-ended by another vehicle
- Pain not present initially but usually develops hr to a few days later
- Neck tightness and stiffness
- Occipital headache
- Shoulder, arm, and back pain
- Numbness in the arms
- Tinnitus
- Temporomandibular jaw (TMJ) pain
- Dysphagia (retropharyngeal hematoma)
- Decreased range of motion of the neck
- Depressive symptoms

ETIOLOGY

- The mechanism of injury is the result of the sudden acceleration of the body forward, forcing the neck to hyperextend backward, causing injury to ligaments, muscles, bone, and/or intervertebral disk. At the end of the accident the head is thrust forward in a flexion position, sometimes causing injury to the cervical spine: C5-C6-C7.
- Motor vehicle accidents, trauma from falls, contact sports, physical abuse, and altercations are all possible causes of whiplash.
- The incidence of whiplash injury following polytrauma is low.
- Low-velocity crashes constitute a major cause of whiplash injury.

DIAGNOSIS

DIFFERENTIAL DIAGNOSIS

- Osteoarthritis
- Cervical disk disease
- Fibrositis
- Neuritis
- Torticollis
- Spinal cord tumor
- TMJ syndrome
- Tension headache
- Migraine headache

WORKUP

Any patient who presents with symptoms of whiplash and musculoskeletal or neurologic signs merits a workup to exclude cervical spine fractures or herniated disk disease.

LABORATORY TESTS

Laboratory studies are not helpful.

IMAGING STUDIES

- Plain C-spine films (antero-posterior, lateral, and odontoid views)
- Flexion/extension x-rays
- CT scan to exclude fracture
- MRI as alternative or in addition to CT in selected cases

TREATMENT

NONPHARMACOLOGIC THERAPY

- Soft cervical collar for no longer than 72 hr
- Moist heat 15 to 20 min four to six times per day.
- Continue with usual activities.

ACUTE GENERAL Rx

- Analgesics
  1. Ibuprofen 800 mg PO tid
  2. Naproxen 500 mg PO bid
  3. Acetaminophen 1 g PO qid
- Muscle relaxants (short-term use)
  1. Cyclobenzaprine 10 mg PO tid
  2. Methocarbamol 1 g PO qid
  3. Carisoprodol 350 mg PO qid

CHRONIC Rx

NSAIDs can be used long term.

DISPOSITION

- Most patients recover from the acute whiplash injury within weeks.
- 20% to 40% may develop chronic whiplash syndrome (symptoms of headache, neck pain, and psychiatric complaints that persist for 6 mo).
- Older age, female gender, lawyer involvement, and at work at entry to the clinic were found to be prognostic factors associated with a negative outcome.

REFERRAL

Orthopedic

PEARLS & CONSIDERATIONS

- Nearly one third of all personal injury cases involve cervical injuries.
- There is no dose-response relationship between trauma severity and incidence of whiplash injury.

COMMENTS

The entity of chronic whiplash syndrome remains elusive. Some authorities argue that financial motivation is a factor leading to persistent neck symptoms. Other studies do not substantiate this, showing a true chronic injury to the soft tissues of the neck.

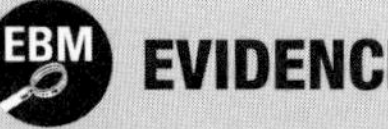

EVIDENCE

Overall, there is a general lack of high-quality evidence for the therapies used in the treatment of cervical hyperextension injuries. There is a trend toward active interventions being more effective than are passive interventions.

There is debate over the evidence supporting the use of corticosteroids in acute spinal injury, with one review suggesting the current evidence does not support the use of methylprednisolone as a standard treatment for acute spinal injury.[1] Ⓐ

Two systematic reviews found a general lack of evidence supporting treatments used in acute whiplash injury.[2]

Evidence-Based References

1. Sayer FT et al: Methylprednisolone treatment in acute spinal cord injury: the myth challenged through a structured analysis of published literature, *Spine J* 6:335-343, 2006.
2. Verhagen AP et al: Conservative treatments for whiplash, *Cochrane Database Syst Rev* 2: 2007.

SUGGESTED READINGS

Carroll LJ et al: Frequency, timing and course of depressive symptomatology after whiplash. *Spine* 31(16):E551-E556, 2006.

Dufton JA et al: Prognostic factors associated with minimal improvement following acute whiplash-associated disorders. *Spine* 31(20):E759-E765, 2006.

Giannoudis PV et al: Incidence and outcome of whiplash injury after multiple trauma. *Spine* 32(7):776-781, 2007.

Rodriquez AA et al: Whiplash: pathophysiology, diagnosis, treatment, and prognosis, *Muscle Nerve* 29(6):768, 2004.

Sterner Y, Gerdle B: Acute and chronic whiplash disorders—a review, *J Rehabil Med* 36(5):193, 2004.

AUTHOR: **JORGE A. VILLAFUERTE, M.D.**

Whipple's Disease

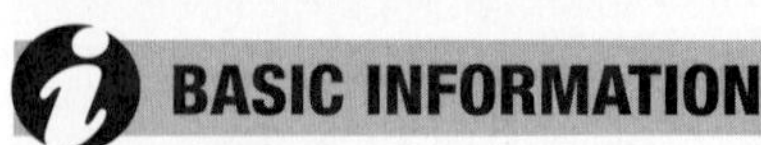

BASIC INFORMATION

DEFINITION

Whipple's disease is a multisystem illness characterized by malabsorption and its consequences, lymphadenopathy, arthritis, cardiac involvement, ocular symptoms, and neurologic problems; it is caused by the gram-positive bacillus *Tropheryma whippelii.*

SYNONYMS

Intestinal lipodystrophy (name used by Whipple in 1907)

ICD-9CM CODES
040.2 Whipple's disease

EPIDEMIOLOGY & DEMOGRAPHICS

- Uncommon illness (only about 1000 cases have been reported to date)
- Peak age: 30 to 60 yr; mean age at diagnosis 50 yr
- More frequent in men than women and in Caucasians
- Specific environmental factors have not been associated with Whipple's disease

PHYSICAL FINDINGS & CLINICAL PRESENTATION

PHYSICAL FINDINGS:
- Abdominal distention, sometimes with tenderness and less commonly fullness or mass, which represents enlarged mesenteric lymph nodes
- Signs of weight loss, cachexia
- Clubbing
- Lymphadenopathy
- Inflamed joints
- Heart murmur or rub
- Sensory loss or motor weakness related to peripheral neuropathy
- Abnormal mental status examination
- Pallor

CLINICAL PRESENTATION: Whipple's disease is characterized by two stages: a prodromal stage and a much later steady-state stage. The prodromal stage is marked by protean symptoms and chronic arthralgias and arthritis. The steady-state stage, which follows the prodromal stage by an average time of 6 yr, is manifested by weight loss, diarrhea, or both. When the disease presents with extraintestinal symptoms (e.g., arthralgia), few clinicians will suspect the diagnosis unless or until gastrointestinal (GI) symptoms are present. Weight loss, diarrhea, and arthropathies are found together in 75% of patients at time of diagnosis. The GI manifestations are those seen in malabsorption of any cause:
- Diarrhea: five to 10 semiformed, malodorous steatorrheic stools per day
- Abdominal bloating and cramps
- Anorexia

Extraintestinal manifestations of malabsorption:
- Weight loss, fatigue
- Anemia
- Bleeding diathesis
- Edema and ascites
- Osteomalacia

Extraintestinal involvement:
- Arthritis (intermittent, migratory; affecting small, large, and axial joints)
- Pleuritic chest pain and cough
- Pericarditis, endocarditis
- Dementia, ophthalmoplegia, myoclonus, and many other symptoms because any portion of the central nervous system may be a disease site
- Fever

ETIOLOGY & PATHOGENESIS

- Infectious disease caused by *Tropheryma whippelii,* an actinobacter.
- The bacillus has never been cultured, nor has direct transmission from patient to patient ever been documented; however, the agent can be seen in tissue samples by electron microscopy and identified by polymerase chain reaction (PCR).
- Predictable response to appropriate antibiotic therapy confirms the pathogenic role of the infection.
- Tissue infiltration by macrophages is believed to be the mechanism of specific organ dysfunction and symptoms.
- Subtle defects of the cell-mediated immunity exist in active and inactive Whipple's disease that may predispose certain individuals to clinical manifestations. HLA-B27 positivity is found in 26% of patients (four times higher than expected).

Dx DIAGNOSIS

DIFFERENTIAL DIAGNOSIS

Malabsorption/maldigestion:
- Celiac disease
- *Mycobacterium avium-intracellulare* intestinal infection in patients with AIDS
- Intestinal lymphoma
- Abetalipoproteinemia
- Amyloidosis
- Systemic mastocytosis
- Radiation enteritis
- Crohn's disease
- Short bowel syndrome
- Pancreatic insufficiency
- Intestinal bacterial overgrowth
- Lactose deficiency
- Postgastrectomy syndrome
- Other cause of diarrhea (see Section III, "Diarrhea, Acute" and "Diarrhea, Chronic")
- Seronegative inflammatory arthritis
- Pericarditis and pleuritis
- Lymphadenitis
- Neurologic disorders

WORKUP

Laboratory tests and imaging studies are useful; however, the diagnosis of Whipple's disease is usually made by upper endoscopy and biopsy. Endoscopic findings reveal a pale yellow, shaggy mucosa alternating with an erythematous, erosive, or friable mucosa in the duodenum or jejunum.

LABORATORY TESTS

- Anemia (iron, folate, or vitamin B_{12} deficiency)
- Hypokalemia
- Hypocalcemia
- Hypomagnesemia
- Hypoalbuminemia
- Prolonged prothrombin time
- Low serum carotene
- Low cholesterol
- Leukocytosis
- Steatorrhea demonstrated by a Sudan fecal fat stain
- 72-hr stool collection demonstrating more than 7 g/24 hr of fat in the stool is impractical to perform, especially in ambulatory patients
- Defective d-xylose absorption

IMAGING STUDIES

Small bowel radiographs after barium ingestion often show thickening of mucosal folds.

BIOPSY

Infiltration of the intestinal lamina propria by PAS-positive macrophages containing gram-positive, acid-fast negative bacilli, associated with lymphatic dilation (diagnostic); PCR of the involved tissue in uncertain cases. If PAS staining of the small-bowel biopsy specimen is positive and the PCR assay is negative, the diagnosis of Whipple's disease must be confirmed; this can be done by immunohistochemical testing with an antibody to *T. whippelii.* If this test is positive, Whipple's disease is confirmed.

Rx TREATMENT

- Antibiotics: TMP/SMX DS bid for 12 to 24 mo, usually preceded by parenteral administration of streptomycin (1 g/day) together with penicillin G (1.2 million U/day) or ceftriaxone (2 g/day) for 2 wk.
- Alternative regimen consists of doxycycline (200 mg/day) plus hydroxychloroquine (200 mg tid).
- Treat specific vitamin, mineral, and nutrient deficiencies.
- Patients with a neurologic recurrence of Whipple's disease have a poor prognosis. Interferon gamma has been proposed for treatment of recurrent central nervous system disease.

SUGGESTED READING

Fenollar F et al: Whipple's disease, *N Engl J Med* 356: 55, 2007.

AUTHOR: **FRED F. FERRI, M.D.**

BASIC INFORMATION

DEFINITION

Wilson's disease is a disorder of copper transport with inadequate biliary copper excretion, leading to an accumulation of the metal in liver, brain, kidneys, and corneas.

SYNONYMS

Progressive hepatolenticular degeneration

ICD-9CM CODES
275.1 Wilson's disease

EPIDEMIOLOGY & DEMOGRAPHICS

PREVALENCE: One case in 30,000
PREDOMINANT SEX: Affects men and women equally (autosomal recessive gene)
ONSET OF SYMPTOMS: Ages 3 to 40 yr

PHYSICAL FINDINGS & CLINICAL PRESENTATION

Hepatic presentation:

- Acute hepatitis with malaise, anorexia, nausea, jaundice, elevated transaminase, prolonged prothrombin time; rarely fulminant hepatic failure
- Chronic active (or autoimmune) hepatitis with fatigue, malaise, rashes, arthralgia, elevated transaminase, elevated serum immunoglobulin G, positive antinuclear antibody and anti-smooth muscle antibody
- Chronic liver disease/cirrhosis with hepatosplenomegaly, ascites, low serum albumin, prolonged prothrombin time, portal hypertension

Neurologic presentation:

- Movement disorder: tremors, ataxia
- Spastic dystonia: masklike facies, rigidity, gait disturbance, dysarthria, drooling, dysphagia

Ophthalmic:

- Kaiser-Fleisher ring
- Sunflower cataracts

Psychiatric presentation:

- Depression, obsessive-compulsive disorder, psychopathic behaviors, neuroses

Other organs:

- Hemolytic anemia
- Renal disease (i.e., Fanconi's syndrome with hematuria, phosphaturia, renal tubular acidosis, vitamin D–resistant rickets)
- Cardiomyopathy
- Arthritis
- Hypoparathyroidism
- Hypogonadism

PHYSICAL FINDINGS:

- Ocular: the Kayser-Fleischer ring is a gold-yellow ring seen at the periphery of the iris (Fig. 1-363); these should be sought with slit-lamp examination by a skilled examiner.
- Stigmata of acute or chronic liver disease.
- Neurologic abnormalities: see previous.

ETIOLOGY & PATHOGENESIS

- Dietary copper is transported from the intestine to the liver, where normally it is metabolized into ceruloplasmin. In Wilson's disease, defective incorporation of copper into ceruloplasmin and a decrease of biliary copper excretion lead to accumulation of this mineral.
- The gene for Wilson's disease is located in chromosome 13.

DIAGNOSIS

DIFFERENTIAL DIAGNOSIS

- Hereditary hypoceruloplasminemia.
- Menkes' disease.
- Consider the diagnosis of Wilson's disease in all cases of acute or chronic liver disease for which another cause has not been established.
- Consider Wilson's disease in patients with movement disorders or dystonia even without symptomatic liver disease.

LABORATORY TESTS

- Abnormal liver function tests (note that aspartate aminotransferase may be higher than alanine aminotransferase)
- Low serum ceruloplasmin level (<200 mg/L)
- Low serum copper (<65 mcg/L)
- 24-hr urinary copper excretion greater than 100 mcg (normal <30 mcg); increases to greater than 1200 mcg/24 hr after 500 mg of d-penicillamine (normal <500 mcg/24 hr)
- Low serum uric acid and phosphorus
- Abnormal urinalysis (hematuria)

BIOPSY

- Early:
  - Steatosis, focal necrosis, glycogenated hepatocyte nuclei
  - May reveal inflammation and piecemeal necrosis
- Late: cirrhosis
- Hepatic copper content (>250 mcg/g of dry weight) (normal is 20 to 50 mcg)
- Histochemical confirmation of excess copper can be helpful in diagnosis, but if absent, does not exclude Wilson's disease. The lack of immunoreactivity to copper-binding protein can occur because of the diffuse presence of copper in the cytoplasm and because of the assay's low sensitivity. Rhodamine and rubeanic acid stains can show dense granular lysosomal copper deposition in hepatocytes at the stage of cirrhotic nodular regeneration.

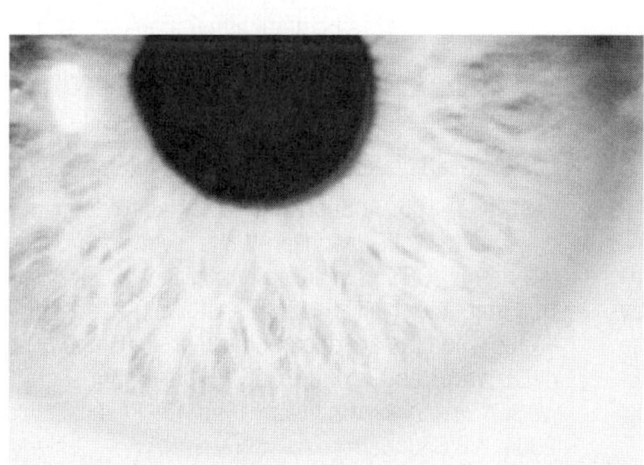

FIGURE 1-363 Wilson's disease. A Kayser-Fleisher ring, which is a gold-yellow ring, extends to the limbus without a clear interval. (From Palay D [ed]: *Ophthalmology for the primary care physician,* St Louis, 1997, Mosby.)

Rx TREATMENT

- Penicillamine: (chelator therapy)
  - 0.75 to 1.5 g/day divided bid (with pyridoxine 25 mg/day)
  - Monitor complete blood count (CBC) and urinalysis weekly
- Trientine: (triethylene tetramine) (chelator therapy)
  - 1 to 2 g/day divided tid
  - Monitor CBC
- Zinc: (inhibits intestinal copper absorption)
  - 50 mg tid
  - Monitor zinc level
- Ammonium tetrathiomolybdate for neurologic symptoms
- Antioxidants
- Liver transplantation (for severe hepatic failure unresponsive to chelation); liver transplantation corrects the underlying pathophysiology and can be lifesaving

PROGNOSIS

Good with early chelation treatment

REFERRAL

To gastroenterologist, neurologist

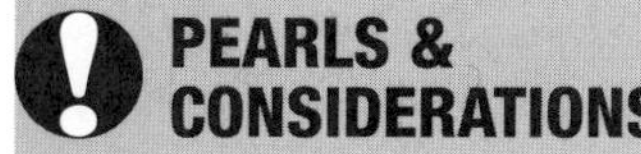

PEARLS & CONSIDERATIONS

COMMENTS

Family screening of first-degree relatives must be undertaken. Genetic diagnosis is also useful in patients with indeterminate clinical and biochemical features.

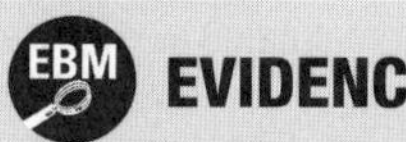

EVIDENCE

Liver transplantation is recommended for patients with decompensated cirrhosis who do not respond to medical therapy and those with fulminant hepatic failure.[1] Ⓒ

Evidence-Based Reference

1. Murray KF, Carithers RL Jr: AASLD practice guidelines: evaluation of the patient for liver transplantation, *Hepatology* 41:1407, 2005. Ⓒ

SUGGESTED READING

Ala A et al: Wilson's disease, *Lancet* 369:397, 2007.

AUTHOR: **FRED F. FERRI, M.D.**

Wolff-Parkinson-White Syndrome

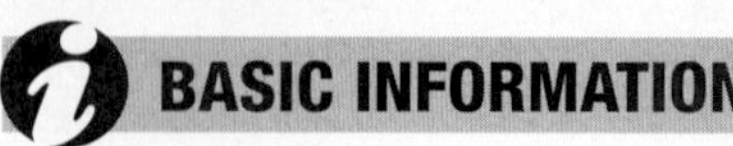

BASIC INFORMATION

DEFINITION

Wolff-Parkinson-White (WPW) syndrome is defined as the presence of preexcitation of the ventricles of the heart due to an abnormal electrical communication from the atria to the ventricles through an accessory pathway. It is typically manifested by a short PR interval (i.e., <120 msec) and the presence of a delta wave in the ECG (WPW pattern).

SYNONYMS

Preexcitation syndrome

ICD-9CM CODES
426.7 Wolff-Parkinson-White syndrome
426.81 Lown-Ganong-Levine syndrome

EPIDEMIOLOGY & DEMOGRAPHICS

- The prevalence of a WPW pattern on the surface ECG is 0.15% to 0.25% in the general population.
- In a study of a presumed healthy population of more than 20,000 patients, the WPW pattern was recognized in 0.25%. Of these patients, only 1.8% had documented arrhythmias that were consistent with the WPW syndrome.
- The prevalence of WPW is higher among males and decreases with age.
- Most patients with WPW syndrome have structurally normal hearts, but associations with mitral valve prolapse, cardiomyopathies, and Ebstein's anomaly have been reported.

PHYSICAL FINDINGS & CLINICAL PRESENTATION

- The physical examination may be entirely normal.
- Symptoms are typically related to tachyarrhythmias, including the following:
  - Palpitations
  - Syncope or near syncope
  - Sudden cardiac death (rarely)
- The type of tachycardia can be one of the following:
  - Supraventricular tachycardia: atrioventricular (AV) reentrant tachycardia (either through the orthodromal pathway [narrow complex] or the antidromal pathway [wide complex]; 80%)
  - Atrial fibrillation (~10% to 30%)
  - Atrial flutter (~5%)
  - Ventricular tachycardia: rare

ETIOLOGY & PATHOGENESIS

- The existence of an accessory pathway allows for conduction from the atria to the ventricles while bypassing the AV node.
- If the accessory pathway is capable of anterograde conduction, two parallel routes of AV conduction are possible: one is subject to delay through the AV node, and the other occurs without delay through the accessory pathway. The resulting QRS complex is a fusion beat, with the delta wave representing rapid ventricular activation through the accessory pathway and the later ventricular activation occurring via conduction through the AV node (Figure 1-364).
- Tachycardias occur when conduction is anterograde in one pathway (usually the normal AV pathway) and retrograde in the other (usually the accessory pathway) as a result of different refractory periods. Some patients (~5% to 10%) with WPW syndrome have multiple accessory pathways.
- In patients with WPW syndrome, the development of atrial fibrillation may be associated with very rapid ventricular rates from AV conduction over the anomalous AV pathway.
- In patients with atrial fibrillation with rapid ventricular response, rapid conduction to the ventricles by way of the accessory pathway may result in degeneration into ventricular fibrillation.

Dx DIAGNOSIS

- Three basic features characterize the ECG abnormalities associated with WPW syndrome (Figure 1-365):
  1. PR interval <120 msec
  2. QRS complex >120 msec with a slurred, slowly rising onset of QRS in some leads (i.e., delta wave)
  3. Secondary ST-T wave changes
- Variants:
  - Lown-Ganong-Levine syndrome: atriohisian pathway with a short PR interval and a normal QRS complex on ECG (i.e., no delta wave)
  - Atriofascicular accessory pathways: duplication of the AV node with normal baseline ECG

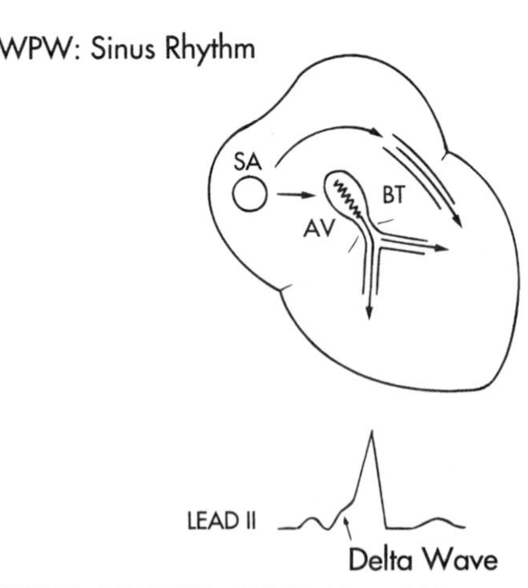

FIGURE 1-364 With Wolff-Parkinson-White syndrome, an abnormal accessory conduction pathway called a *bypass tract (BT)* connects the atria and the ventricles. (From Goldberger AL [ed]: *Clinical electrocardiography: a simplified approach,* ed 6, St Louis, 1999, Mosby.)

Rx TREATMENT

- There is no definitive recommendation for treatment in the absence of tachyarrhythmias. However, there is an American Heart Association/American College of Cardiology class IIa recommendation for radiofrequency ablation for asymptomatic patients whose lifestyles may be adversely affected by a tachyarrhythmia.
- For the acute termination of narrow complex regular tachyarrhythmias, carotid sinus massage or the Valsalva maneuver may be successful. First-line pharmacologic therapy includes adenosine or verapamil for patients without atrial fibrillation or flutter.
- For patients with a rapid ventricular response with hemodynamic compromise, urgent electrical cardioversion is warranted.
- Digitalis should not be used, because it can reduce refractoriness in the accessory pathway and accelerate the tachycardia. Cardioversion should be used in the presence of hemodynamic impairment.
- Drug therapy for the chronic prevention of narrow complex regular tachyarrhythmias includes class IC antiarrhythmics, β-blockers, calcium channel blockers, digoxin, amiodarone, or sotalol. The choice of drug therapy is dictated by the underlying mechanism of the tachyarrhythmia.
- For the treatment of atrial fibrillation in patients with WPW, the administration of AV nodal-blocking agents will not slow the ventricular rate, because the accessory pathways capable of rapid conduction do not respond to AV-blocking agents. Procainamide is the drug of choice for controlling the ventricular rate and restoring the sinus rhythm in patients with WPW who have atrial fibrillation.

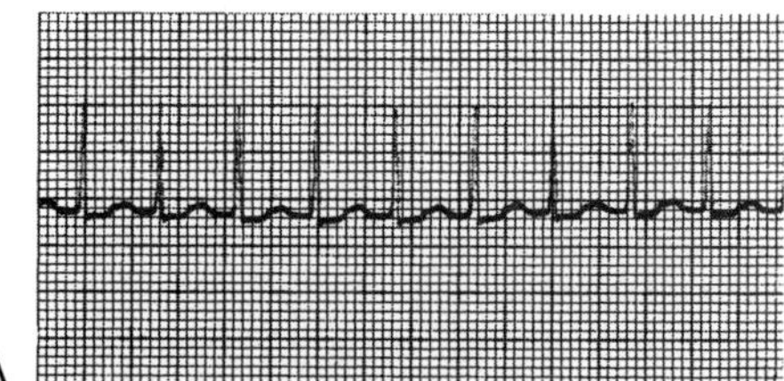

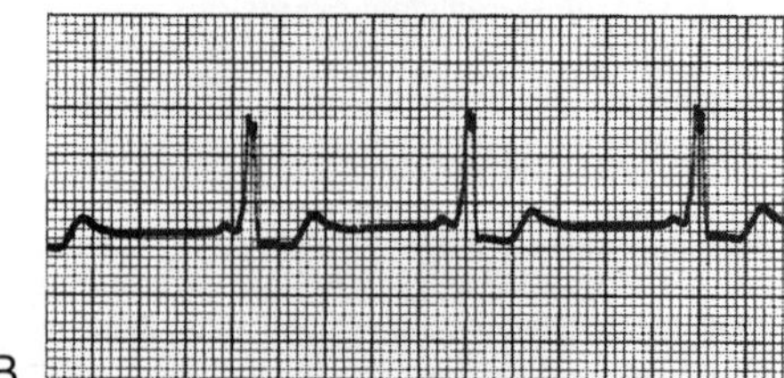

FIGURE 1-365 A, Supraventricular tachycardia in a child with Wolff-Parkinson-White syndrome. Note the normal QRS complexes during the tachycardia. **B,** Later, the typical features of Wolff-Parkinson-White syndrome are apparent: a short P-R interval, a delta wave, and a wide QRS. (From Behrman RE: *Nelson textbook of pediatrics,* ed 17, Philadelphia, 2004, WB Saunders.)

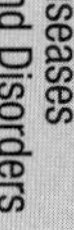

- When medical therapy fails or the patient cannot tolerate it, radiofrequency ablation should be performed (class I indication).

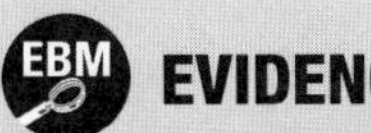

EVIDENCE

In a literature review of studies of children receiving hospital treatment in the U.S. for WPW syndrome, catheter ablation was found to have lower cost, mortality rate, and morbidity rate than either medical management or surgery. The authors concluded that it is the treatment of choice for the child aged ≥5 yr with WPW and supraventricular tachycardia.[1,2]

Evidence-Based References

1. Garson A, Kanter RJ: Management of the child with Wolff-Parkinson-White syndrome and supraventricular tachycardia: model for cost effectiveness, *J Cardiovasc Electrophysiol* 8(11):1320, 1997.
2. Pappone C et al: Radiofrequency ablation in children with asymptomatic WPW, *N Engl J Med* 351:1197, 2004.

SUGGESTED READINGS

Epstein AE et al: ACC/AHA/HRS 2008. Guidelines for Device-Based Therapy of Cardiac Rhythm Abnormalities: a report of the American College of Cardiology/American Heart Association Task Force on Practice Guidelines (Writing Committee to Revise the ACC/AHA/NASPE 2002. Guideline Update for Implantation of Cardiac Pacemakers and Antiarrhythmia Devices): developed in collaboration with the American Association for Thoracic Surgery and Society of Thoracic Surgeons, *Circulation* 117:e350, 2008.

Fitzsimmons PJ et al: The natural history of Wolff-Parkinson-White syndrome in 228 military aviators: a long-term follow-up of 22 years, *Am Heart J* 142(3):530-536, 2001.

Marine JE: Catheter ablation therapy for supraventricular arrhythmias, *JAMA* 298(23):2768, 2007.

AUTHORS: **THOMAS J. EARL, M.D., FRED F. FERRI, M.D.,** and **WEN-CHIH WU, M.D.**

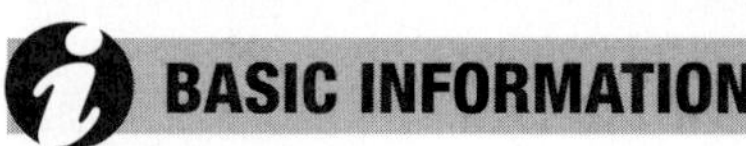

BASIC INFORMATION

DEFINITION

Yellow fever is an infection, primarily of the liver, with systemic manifestations caused by the yellow fever virus (YFV). The clinical spectrum ranges from asymptomatic infection to life-threatening disease with severity and mortality highest in the elderly.

SYNONYMS

Tropical hemorrhagic fever from YFV

ICD-9CM CODES
060.9 Yellow fever

EPIDEMIOLOGY & DEMOGRAPHICS

GEOGRAPHIC DISTRIBUTION:

- South America and Africa, in countries between +15 and −15 degrees latitude.
- The World Health Organization estimates there are more than 200,000 cases a yr with 30,000 deaths per yr. More than 90% of cases occur in Africa.

INCIDENCE: Approximate attack rates of 3% in Africa and Amazon

PREVALENCE: Endemic areas: 20% of population

PREDOMINANT SEX: In Africa and the Amazon, male agricultural workers.

PHYSICAL FINDINGS & CLINICAL PRESENTATION

- Most subclinical.
- The onset of illness appears suddenly 3 to 6 days after the bite of an infected mosquito.
- Viremic (early) phase:
  1. Fever, chills
  2. Severe headache
  3. Lumbosacral pain
  4. Myalgias, nausea, malaise
  5. Conjunctivitis
  6. Relative bradycardia (Faget's sign)
- After brief recovery, toxic phase:
  1. Jaundice
  2. Oliguria
  3. Albuminuria
  4. Hemorrhage
  5. Encephalopathy
  6. Shock
  7. Acidosis
- Case fatality rate 25% to 50%.

ETIOLOGY

- YFV *(L. flavus)*
  1. Flavivirus infects hepatic cells.
  2. Late in infection, cytopathic effects (antibody- and cell-mediated) produce pathology.
- Vector
  1. *Aedes aegypti* (urban).
  2. *Aedes* spp., Haemagogus (especially in Amazon) mosquitos (sylvan).
  3. Primary hosts: humans and simian species.
  4. Exists in two transmission cycles:
     a. Sylvatic or jungle cycle involving mosquitos and nonhuman primates.
     b. Urban cycle involving mosquitos and humans.

PATHOGENESIS & PATHOLOGY

- Virus replication begins at site of mosquito bite, spreading to lymphatic channels and regional lymph nodes. Viremic spread to other organs, especially liver, spleen, and bone marrow.
- Shock and fatal illness result from direct damage to organs and vasoactive cytokines.
- Viral antigen found in hepatocytes, kidneys, and myocardium.
- Midzone of liver lobules primarily affected.
- Hemorrhages of mucosal surfaces of GI tract.

Dx DIAGNOSIS

DIFFERENTIAL DIAGNOSIS

- Viral hepatitis
- Leptospirosis
- Malaria
- Typhoid fever
  1. Typhus
  2. Relapsing fever
- Other hemorrhagic fevers such as Dengue

LABORATORY TESTS

- CBC
  1. Mild leukopenia
  2. Thrombocytopenia
  3. Anemia
- LFTs
  1. AST levels exceed ALT levels.
  2. Alkaline phosphatase normal or slightly elevated.
  3. Elevated bilirubin levels.
- Elevated BUN and creatinine
- Proteinuria
- Coagulation studies
  1. Demonstrate abnormal prothrombin time *or*
  2. Reveal DIC
- Terminal hypoglycemia
- CSF
  1. Pleocytosis
  2. Elevated protein count
- Specific diagnosis confirmed by:
  1. Viral isolation from blood
  2. Viral antigen in serum (ELISA)
  3. Viral RNA by polymerase chain reaction (PCR)
  4. IgM-capture ELISA
     a. Preferred serologic test.
     b. Appears within 5 to 7 days.
     c. Rising Ab confirmed by paired sera.
     d. Cross-reactivity with other flavivirus infections.
  5. Immunohistochemical staining of post-mortem liver biopsy specimens

Rx TREATMENT

ACUTE GENERAL Rx

- Acetaminophen (for headache and fever) and H_2 blockers (GI bleeding); avoid aspirin because of bleeding risk
- Blood transfusion, volume replacement for hemorrhage and shock
- Dialysis for renal failure
- Avoidance of sedatives and drugs dependent on hepatic metabolism

DISPOSITION

Follow up until hepatic, renal, CNS disease resolved

REFERRAL

To infectious diseases expert for accurate diagnosis and management

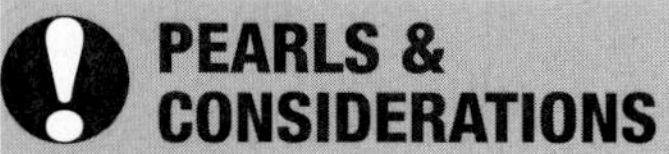

PEARLS & CONSIDERATIONS

PREVENTION

- Yellow fever is preventable.
- Recovery from yellow fever confers lasting immunity.
- Live, attenuated yellow fever vaccine (YF-Vax) provides protective immunity in 95% of vaccinated patients within 10 days of vaccination. Reimmunization at 10-yr intervals for travelers. Vaccine certificate to verify immunization status is required before travel in many tropical countries in South America and Africa.
- Vaccine contraindicated in:
  1. Infants <6 mo (postvaccinal encephalitis)
  2. Immunosuppressed patients
  3. Pregnant women and nursing mothers
  4. Patients with egg hypersensitivity
- Adverse effects of vaccine:
  1. General
     a. Mild headaches, myalgias, low-grade fevers (25% vaccinees in clinical trials).
     b. Immediate hypersensitivity reaction (history of egg allergy).
  2. Vaccine-associated neurotropic disease (postvaccine encephalitis) (1.8 cases per million)
     a. Primarily among infants.
     b. Adult cases only in first-time vaccine recipients.
  3. Vaccine-associated viscerotropic disease (2.2 cases per million)
     a. Disease syndrome resembling wild-type yellow fever, often fatal.
     b. All cases in first-time vaccinees.

SUGGESTED READINGS

Doblas A et al: Yellow fever vaccine-associated viscerotropic disease and death in Spain, *J Clin Virol* 36(2):156, 2006.

Massad E et al: Yellow fever vaccination: how much is enough? *Vaccine* 23(30):3908, 2005.

Monath TP: Dengue and yellow fever—challenges for the development and use of vaccines, *N Engl J Med* 357(22):2222-2225, 2007.

Monath TP: Yellow fever vaccine, *Expert Rev Vaccines* 4(4):553, 2005.

Pugachev KV, Guirakhoo F, Monath TP: New developments in flavivirus vaccines with special attention to yellow fever, *Curr Opin Infect Dis* 18(5):387, 2005.

AUTHORS: **STEVEN M. OPAL, M.D., GLENN G. FORT, M.D., M.P.H.,** and **DENNIS J. MIKOLICH, M.D.**

BASIC INFORMATION

DEFINITION

Zenker's diverticulum (ZD) refers to the acquired physiologic obstruction of the esophageal introitus that results from mucosal herniation posteriorly between the cricopharyngeus muscle and the inferior pharyngeal constrictor muscle (Fig. 1-366).

SYNONYMS

Pharyngoesophageal diverticulum
Pulsion diverticulum

ICD-9CM CODES

530.6 Zenker's diverticulum (esophagus)

EPIDEMIOLOGY & DEMOGRAPHICS

- The most common type of diverticulum of the upper gastrointestinal tract
- Rare disease with annual incidence estimated 1/50,000 per year
- Most commonly presents after the age of 60 yr, more commonly seen in males
- Peak incidence is seventh to ninth decades
- Associated with gastroesophageal reflux disease (GERD) and hiatal hernia

PHYSICAL FINDINGS & CLINICAL PRESENTATION

A small ZD may be asymptomatic. As it becomes larger, symptoms may include:

- Dysphagia to solids and liquids (most common)
- Regurgitation of undigested food
- Sensation of globus or fullness in the neck
- Cough
- Halitosis
- Aspiration pneumonia
- Weight loss
- Voice changes
- Sialorrhea (excessive drooling)

ETIOLOGY

- The specific cause is not known. The leading hypothesis suggests a discoordination of the swallowing muscles (specifically, incomplete relaxation of the cricopharyngeus muscle) that leads to an increased pressure on the mucosa of the hypopharynx, resulting in a progressive distention of that mucosa in its weakest area (posterior wall in "Killian's triangle," the point between the oblique fibers of the inferior pharyngeal muscle and the horizontal fibers of the cricopharyngeus muscle). The end result is the formation of a false diverticulum where food elements and secretions may be lodged, causing the symptoms listed previously.
- ZD may also occur after anterior spinal surgery or cervical spine injury.

DIAGNOSIS

- Clinical presentation and barium swallow typically make the diagnosis of ZD.
- Neck ultrasound can also be used.
- Esophageal manometry can help elucidate the pathogenesis but not required for diagnosis

DIFFERENTIAL DIAGNOSIS

The differential diagnosis is similar to anyone presenting with dysphagia:

- Achalasia
- Esophageal spasm
- Esophageal carcinoma
- Esophageal webs
- Peptic stricture
- Lower esophageal (Schatzki) ring
- Foreign bodies
- Central nervous system disorders (stroke, Parkinson's disease, amyotrophic lateral sclerosis, multiple sclerosis, myasthenia gravis, muscular dystrophies)
- Dermatomyositis
- Infection

WORKUP

Barium swallow is the test of choice. Upper endoscopy runs the risk of perforation.

LABORATORY TESTS

Not specific

IMAGING STUDIES

- Barium swallow: demonstrates a herniated sac with a narrow diverticular neck that typically originates proximal to the cricopharyngeus at the level of C5–C6 (Fig. 1-367).
- Endoscopy is only indicated if barium studies show mucosal irregularities to rule out neoplasia.
- Oropharyngeal-esophageal scintigraphy has recently been shown to be an effective, sensitive, and simple diagnostic study for both qualitative and quantitative analyses.
- A chest x-ray is performed in cases of suspected aspiration pneumonia.

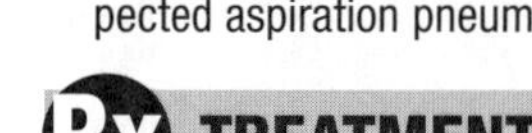

TREATMENT

NONPHARMACOLOGIC THERAPY

- Soft mechanical diet can be tried in patients with symptoms of dysphagia.
- Avoid seeds, skins, and nuts.

ACUTE GENERAL Rx

- Surgical repair is the conventional treatment for symptomatic patients (dysphagia, cough, aspiration) with excellent relief of symptoms in nearly all patients and low procedural mortality (<1.5%). Procedures include:
  1. Cervical diverticulectomy with cricopharyngeal myotomy (most common approach)
  2. Diverticulopexy or diverticular inversion with cricopharyngeal myotomy
  3. Diverticulectomy alone
  4. Cricopharyngeal myotomy alone
- Endoscopic techniques (esophagodiverticulostomy) have largely replaced conventional surgery and include:
  1. Endoscopic stapler diverticulotomy (may be the initial treatment of choice)
  2. Microendoscopic carbon dioxide laser surgical diverticulotomy
  3. Diverticula <3 cm is a contraindication to endosurgical approach
  4. Head-to-head comparison with surgical repairs showed endoscopic techniques to be similar in results, relief of symptoms, and patient satisfaction

CHRONIC Rx

In patients not having surgery, treatment is directed toward any complications that may occur:

- Antibiotics for aspiration pneumonia
- H_2 antagonists for ulcerations that can develop within the diverticulum
- Botulinum toxin for temporary relief of dysphagia

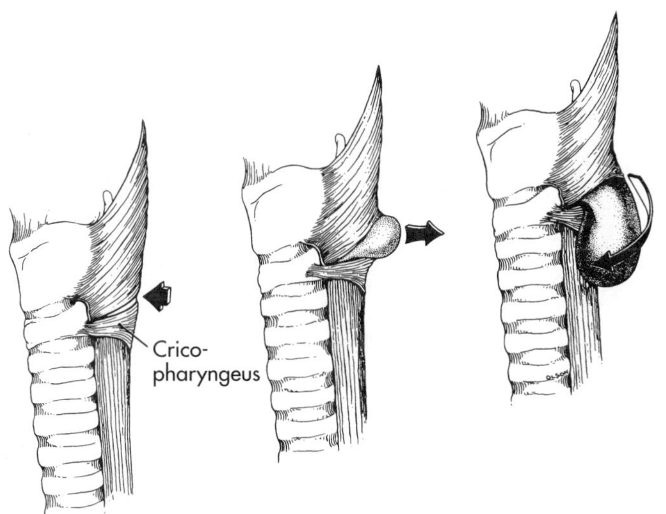

FIGURE 1-366 Formation of pharyngoesophageal (Zenker's) diverticulum. *Left,* Herniation of the pharyngeal mucosa and submucosa occurs at the point of transition *(arrow)* between the oblique fibers of the thyropharyngeus muscle and the more horizontal fibers of the cricopharyngeus muscle. *Center and right,* As the diverticulum enlarges, it dissects toward the left side and downward into the superior mediastinum in the prevertebral space. (From Sabiston D: *Textbook of surgery,* ed 15, Philadelphia, 1997, WB Saunders.)

DISPOSITION

- If left untreated, progressive enlargement of the diverticulum occurs.
- The risk of complications (e.g., aspiration pneumonia) increases with the size of the diverticulum.
- Postsurgical recurrence can occur (4%); however, these are usually asymptomatic.

REFERRAL

Any patient with dysphagia requires a gastroenterology consultation. A thoracic surgical, ENT, or head and neck surgeon may be consulted if surgery is considered.

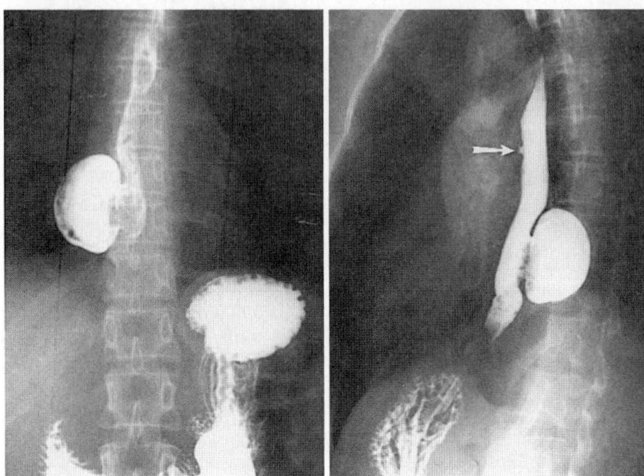

FIGURE 1-367 Posteroanterior *(left)* and oblique *(right)* views from barium esophagogram showing both a typical diverticulum of the junction of the mid-esophagus and distal esophagus and a small traction diverticulum *(arrow)* of the mid-esophagus. (From Sabiston D: *Textbook of surgery,* ed 15, Philadelphia, 1997, Saunders.)

COMMENTS

The association with cancer is rare (0.4%).

SUGGESTED READINGS

Bonavina L et al: Long-term results of endosurgical and open surgical approach for Zenker diverticulum, *World J Gastroenterol* 14;13(18):2586, 2007.

Ferreira LE et al: Zenker's diverticula: pathophysiology, clinical presentation, and flexible endoscopic management, *Dis Esophagus* 21(1):1-8, 2008.

Ruiz-Tovar J et al:. 20 years experience in the management of Zenker's diverticulum in a third-level hospital, *Rev Esp Enferm Dig* 98(6):429, 2006.

Wirth D et al: Outcome and quality of life after open surgery versus endoscopic stapler-assisted esophagodiverticulostomy for Zenker's diverticulum, *Dis Esophagus* 19(4): 294, 2006.

AUTHORS: **ROBERT M. KIRCHNER, M.D.,** and **PAUL GORDON, M.D.**

BASIC INFORMATION

DEFINITION

Zollinger-Ellison (ZE) syndrome is a hypergastrinemic state caused by a pancreatic or extrapancreatic non–beta islet cell tumor (gastrinoma) resulting in peptic acid disease.

SYNONYMS

Gastrinoma

ICD-9CM CODES
251.5 Zollinger-Ellison syndrome

EPIDEMIOLOGY & DEMOGRAPHICS

- Incidence is unknown, but 0.1% of all duodenal ulcers are believed to be caused by ZE.
- Occurs in both genders and at any age (most common in ages 30 to 50 yr).
- Two thirds of gastrinomas are sporadic, and one third are associated with multiple endocrine neoplasia type 1 (MEN-1), an autosomal-dominant genetic disorder that also includes hyperparathyroidism and pituitary tumors.
- Approximately 60% of gastrinomas are malignant.

PHYSICAL FINDINGS & CLINICAL PRESENTATION

- The majority of patients (95%) present with symptoms of peptic ulcer (see Section I, "Peptic Ulcer Disease").
- 60% of patients have symptoms related to gastroesophageal reflux disease (see Section I, "Gastroesophageal Reflux Disease").
- One third of patients with ZE have diarrhea and, less commonly, steatorrhea.

The following circumstances warrant suspicion of ZE syndrome:

- Ulcers distal to the first portion of the duodenum
- Multiple peptic ulcers
- Ineffective treatment for peptic ulcer disease with the usual drug doses and schedules
- Peptic ulcer and diarrhea
- Familial history of peptic ulcer
- Patients with a personal or family history suggesting parathyroid or pituitary tumors of dysfunction
- Peptic ulcer and urinary tract calculi
- Patients with peptic ulcer who are negative for *Helicobacter pylori* and do not have a history of nonsteroidal antiinflammatory drug use

ETIOLOGY

- The pathophysiologic manifestations of ZE syndrome are related to the effects of hypergastrinemia. Gastrin stimulates gastric acid secretion, which in turn is responsible for the development of duodenal ulcers and diarrhea. Gastrin also promotes gastric mucosal epithelial cell growth and resulting parietal cell hyperplasia.
- Gastrinomas are usually small (0.1 to 2 cm) but sometimes large (>20 cm) tumors.
- 60% of gastrinomas are malignant, with liver and regional lymph nodes the most common site of metastases. Histology is not a good predictor of the biology of gastrinomas.
- 60% of patients with MEN-1 have gastrinomas.
- 10% of patients with ZE syndrome have islet cell hyperplasia rather than gastrinomas; in 10% to 20% of patients with gastrinoma the tumors cannot be located because of small size.

DIAGNOSIS

DIFFERENTIAL DIAGNOSIS

- Peptic ulcer disease (see Section I, "Peptic Ulcer Disease")
- Gastroesophageal reflux disease (see Section I, "Gastroesophageal Reflux Disease")
- Diarrhea (see Section III, "Diarrhea, Acute" and "Diarrhea, Chronic")

WORKUP

- Diagnosis of peptic ulcer:
  - Upper gastrointestinal series (may also show prominent gastric rugal folds)
  - Endoscopy
- Gastric acid secretion:
  - Serum gastrin level (fasting) >150 pg/ml (causes of false-positive results: pernicious anemia, renal failure, retained gastric antrum syndrome, diabetes mellitus, rheumatoid arthritis)
- Provocative gastrin level tests:
  - Secretin stimulation
  - Calcium stimulation
  - Standard test meal stimulation
- Gastrinoma localization:
  - Arteriography
  - Abdominal sonography
  - Abdominal CT scan
  - Abdominal MRI
  - Selective portal vein branch gastrin level
  - Octreotide scan

TREATMENT

- Surgical resection of the gastrinoma (NOTE: 90% of gastrinomas can be located, resulting in a 40% overall cure rate)
- Total gastrectomy or vagotomy (palliative in some patients)
- Medical treatment
  - Proton pump inhibitors (e.g., omeprazole, lansoprazole)
  - Somatostatin or octreotide
  - Chemotherapy for metastatic gastrinoma with streptozotocin, 5-fluorouracil, and doxorubicin

PROGNOSIS

Five-yr survival:

- Two thirds of all patients
- 20% with liver metastases
- 90% without liver metastases

REFERRAL

To gastroenterologist and surgeon

SUGGESTED READING

Norten JA et al: Surgery to cure Zollinger-Ellison syndrome, *N Engl J Med* 341:635, 1999.

AUTHOR: **FRED F. FERRI, M.D.**

SECTION II

Differential Diagnosis

ABDOMINAL DISTENTION

ICD-9CM # 787.3

NONMECHANICAL OBSTRUCTION

Excessive intraluminal gas.
Intraabdominal infection.
Trauma.
Retroperitoneal irritation (renal colic, neoplasms, infections, hemorrhage).
Vascular insufficiency (thrombosis, embolism).
Mechanical ventilation.
Extraabdominal infection (sepsis, pneumonia, empyema, osteomyelitis of spine).
Metabolic/toxic abnormalities (hypokalemia, uremia, lead poisoning).
Chemical irritation (perforated ulcer, bile, pancreatitis).
Peritoneal inflammation.
Severe pain, pain medications.

MECHANICAL OBSTRUCTION

Neoplasm (intraluminal, extraluminal).
Adhesions, endometriosis.
Infection (intraabdominal abscess, diverticulitis).
Gallstones.
Foreign body, bezoars.
Pregnancy.
Hernias.
Volvulus.
Stenosis at surgical anastomosis, radiation stenosis.
Fecaliths.
Inflammatory bowel disease.
Gastric outlet obstruction.
Hematoma.
Other: parasites, superior mesenteric artery (SMA) syndrome, pneumatosis intestinalis, annular pancreas, Hirschsprung's disease, intussusception, meconium.

ABDOMINAL PAIN, ADOLESCENCE[26]

ICD-9CM # 789.67

Acute gastroenteritis.
Appendicitis.
Inflammatory bowel disease.
Peptic ulcer disease.
Cholecystitis.
Neoplasm.
Diabetic ketoacidosis.
Functional abdominal pain.
Pelvic inflammatory disease.
Pregnancy.
Pyelonephritis.
Renal stone.
Trauma.

ABDOMINAL PAIN, CHILDHOOD[26]

ICD-9CM # 789.67

Acute gastroenteritis.
Appendicitis.
Constipation.
Cholecystitis, acute.
Intestinal obstruction.
Pancreatitis.
Neoplasm.
Inflammatory bowel disease.
Other:
- Functional abdominal pain.
- Pyelonephritis.
- Pneumonia.
- Diabetic ketoacidosis.
- Heavy metal poisoning.
- Sickle cell crisis.
- Trauma.

ABDOMINAL PAIN, CHRONIC LOWER[38]

ICD-9CM # 789.64 Abdominal Pain Left Lower Quadrant
789.63 Abdominal Pain Right Lower Quadrant
789.85 Abdominal Pain Suprapubic

ORGANIC DISORDERS

Common

Gynecological disease.
Lactase deficiency.
Diverticulitis.
Crohn's disease.
Intestinal obstruction.

Uncommon

Chronic intestinal pseudoobstruction.
Mesenteric ischemia.
Malignancy (e.g., ovarian carcinoma).
Abdominal wall pain.
Spinal disease.
Testicular disease.
Metabolic diseases (e.g., diabetes mellitus, familial Mediterranean fever, C1 esterase deficiency [angioneurotic edema], porphyria, lead poisoning, tabes dorsalis, renal failure).

FUNCTIONAL DISORDERS

Common

Irritable bowel syndrome.
Functional abdominal bloating.

Uncommon

Functional abdominal pain.

ABDOMINAL PAIN, DIFFUSE

ICD-9CM # 789.67

Early appendicitis.
Aortic aneurysm.
Gastroenteritis.
Intestinal obstruction.
Diverticulitis.
Peritonitis.
Mesenteric insufficiency or infarction.
Pancreatitis.
Inflammatory bowel disease.
Irritable bowel.
Mesenteric adenitis.
Metabolic: toxins, lead poisoning, uremia, drug overdose, diabetic ketoacidosis (DKA), heavy metal poisoning.
Sickle cell crisis.
Pneumonia (rare).
Trauma.
Urinary tract infection, pelvic inflammatory disease (PID).
Other: acute intermittent porphyria, tabes dorsalis, periarteritis nodosa, Henoch-Schönlein purpura, adrenal insufficiency.

ABDOMINAL PAIN, EPIGASTRIC

ICD-9CM # 789.66

Gastric: peptic ulcer disease (PUD), gastric outlet obstruction, gastric ulcer.
Duodenal: PUD, duodenitis.
Biliary: cholecystitis, cholangitis.
Hepatic: hepatitis.
Pancreatic: pancreatitis.
Intestinal: high small bowel obstruction, early appendicitis.
Cardiac: angina, MI, pericarditis.
Pulmonary: pneumonia, pleurisy, pneumothorax.
Subphrenic abscess.
Vascular: dissecting aneurysm, mesenteric ischemia.

ABDOMINAL PAIN, INFANCY[26]

ICD-9CM # 789.67

Acute gastroenteritis.
Appendicitis.
Intussusception.
Volvulus.
Meckel diverticulum.
Other: colic, trauma.

ABDOMINAL PAIN, LEFT LOWER QUADRANT

ICD-9CM # 789.64

Intestinal: diverticulitis, intestinal obstruction, perforated ulcer, inflammatory bowel disease, perforated descending colon, inguinal hernia, neoplasm, appendicitis.
Reproductive: ectopic pregnancy, ovarian cyst, torsion of ovarian cyst, tuboovarian abscess, mittelschmerz, endometriosis, seminal vesiculitis.
Renal: renal or ureteral calculi, pyelonephritis, neoplasm.
Vascular: leaking aortic aneurysm.
Psoas abscess.
Trauma.

ABDOMINAL PAIN, LEFT UPPER QUADRANT

ICD-9CM # 789.32

Gastric: PUD, gastritis, pyloric stenosis, hiatal hernia.
Pancreatic: pancreatitis, neoplasm, stone in pancreatic duct or ampulla.
Cardiac: MI, angina pectoris.
Splenic: splenomegaly, ruptured spleen, splenic abscess, splenic infarction.

Renal: calculi, pyelonephritis, neoplasm.
Pulmonary: pneumonia, empyema, pulmonary infarction.
Vascular: ruptured aortic aneurysm.
Cutaneous: herpes zoster.
Trauma.
Intestinal: high fecal impaction, perforated colon, diverticulitis.

ABDOMINAL PAIN, NONSURGICAL CAUSES

ICD-9CM # 789.9

Irritable bowel syndrome.
Urinary tract infection, pyelonephritis, salpingitis, PID.
Gastroenteritis, gastritis, peptic ulcer.
Diverticular spasm.
Hepatitis, mononucleosis.
Pancreatitis.
Inferior wall myocardial infarction.
Basilar pneumonia, pulmonary embolism.
Diabetic ketoacidosis.
Strain or hematoma of rectus muscle.
Ruptured Graafian follicle.
Herpes zoster.
Nerve root compression.
Sickle cell crisis.
Acute adrenal insufficiency.
Other: acute porphyria, familial Mediterranean fever, tabes dorsalis.

ABDOMINAL PAIN, PERIUMBILICAL

ICD-9CM # 789.65

Intestinal: small bowel obstruction or gangrene, early appendicitis.
Vascular: mesenteric thrombosis, dissecting aortic aneurysm.
Pancreatic: pancreatitis.
Metabolic: uremia, DKA.
Trauma.

ABDOMINAL PAIN, POORLY LOCALIZED[26]

ICD-9CM # 789.60

EXTRAABDOMINAL

Metabolic
DKA, acute intermittent porphyria, hyperthyroidism, hypothyroidism, hypercalcemia, hypokalemia, uremia, hyperlipidemia, hyperparathyroidism.
Hematologic
Sickle cell crisis, leukemia or lymphoma, Henoch-Schönlein purpura.
Infectious
Infectious mononucleosis, Rocky Mountain spotted fever, acquired immunodeficiency syndrome (AIDS), streptococcal pharyngitis (in children), herpes zoster.
Drugs and Toxins
Heavy metal poisoning, black widow spider bites, withdrawal syndromes, mushroom ingestion.
Referred Pain
Pulmonary: pneumonia, pulmonary embolism, pneumothorax.
Cardiac: angina, myocardial infarction, pericarditis, myocarditis.
Genitourinary: prostatitis, epididymitis, orchitis, testicular torsion.
Musculoskeletal: rectus sheath hematoma.
Functional
Somatization disorder, malingering, hypochondriasis, Munchausen syndrome.

INTRAABDOMINAL

Early appendicitis, gastroenteritis, peritonitis, pancreatitis, abdominal aortic aneurysm, mesenteric insufficiency or infarction, intestinal obstruction, volvulus, ulcerative colitis.

ABDOMINAL PAIN, PREGNANCY[26]

ICD-9CM # 789.67

GYNECOLOGIC (GESTATIONAL AGE IN PARENTHESES)

Miscarriage	(<20 wk; 80% <12 wk)
Septic abortion	(<20 wk)
Ectopic pregnancy	(<14 wk)
Corpus luteum cyst rupture	(<12 wk)
Ovarian torsion	(especially <24 wk)
Pelvic inflammatory disease	(<12 wk)
Chorioamnionitis	(>16 wk)
Abruptio placentae	(>16 wk)

NONGYNECOLOGIC

Appendicitis	(Throughout)
Cholecystitis	(Throughout)
Hepatitis	(Throughout)
Pyelonephritis	(Throughout)
Preeclampsia	(>20 wk)

ABDOMINAL PAIN, RIGHT LOWER QUADRANT

ICD-9CM # 789.63

Intestinal: acute appendicitis, regional enteritis, incarcerated hernia, cecal diverticulitis, intestinal obstruction, perforated ulcer, perforated cecum, Meckel diverticulitis.
Reproductive: ectopic pregnancy, ovarian cyst, torsion of ovarian cyst, salpingitis, tuboovarian abscess, mittelschmerz, endometriosis, seminal vesiculitis.
Renal: renal and ureteral calculi, neoplasms, pyelonephritis.
Vascular: leaking aortic aneurysm.
Psoas abscess.
Trauma.
Cholecystitis.

ABDOMINAL PAIN, RIGHT UPPER QUADRANT

ICD-9CM # 789.61

Biliary: calculi, infection, inflammation, neoplasm.
Hepatic: hepatitis, abscess, hepatic congestion, neoplasm, trauma.
Gastric: PUD, pyloric stenosis, neoplasm, alcoholic gastritis, hiatal hernia.
Pancreatic: pancreatitis, neoplasm, stone in pancreatic duct or ampulla.
Renal: calculi, infection, inflammation, neoplasm, rupture of kidney.
Pulmonary: pneumonia, pulmonary infarction, right-sided pleurisy.
Intestinal: retrocecal appendicitis, intestinal obstruction, high fecal impaction, diverticulitis.
Cardiac: myocardial ischemia (particularly involving the inferior wall), pericarditis.
Cutaneous: herpes zoster.
Trauma.
Fitz-Hugh-Curtis syndrome (perihepatitis).

ABDOMINAL PAIN, SUPRAPUBIC

ICD-9CM # 789.85

Intestinal: colon obstruction or gangrene, diverticulitis, appendicitis.
Reproductive system: ectopic pregnancy, mittelschmerz, torsion of ovarian cyst, PID, salpingitis, endometriosis, rupture of endometrioma.
Cystitis, rupture of urinary bladder.

ABDOMINAL WALL MASSES[38]

ICD-9CM # varies with specific diagnosis

LUMPS ARISING IN THE SKIN AND SUBCUTANEOUS FAT (THAT COULD OCCUR ANYWHERE ON THE BODY)

Lipoma.
Sebaceous cyst.

LUMPS ARISING IN THE SKIN AND SUBCUTANEOUS FAT (SPECIFIC TO THE ANTERIOR ABDOMINAL WALL)

Tumor nodule of the umbilicus (secondary to the intraperitoneal malignancy, also called Sister Mary Joseph nodule).

LUMPS ARISING IN THE FASCIA AND MUSCLE

Rectus sheath hematoma (usually painful).
Desmoid tumor (associated with Gardner's syndrome).

HERNIA

Incisional	It has an overlying scar. The sac may be very much larger than the neck of the hernia.
Umbilical	The hernia is through the umbilical scar. Those presenting at birth commonly resolve in the first years of life.
Paraumbilical	The neck is just lateral to the umbilical scar. Patients usually present later in life.
Epigastric	It occurs in the midline between the xiphoid process and the umbilicus. They are usually small (<2 cm). They result when a knuckle of extraperitoneal fat extrudes through a small defect in the linea alba. Commonly irreducible and without an expansile cough impulse.
Spigelian	A rare hernia found along the linea semilunaris at the lateral edge of the rectus sheath, most commonly a third of the way between the umbilicus and the pubis.

DIVARICATION OF THE RECTI

Supraumbilical elliptical swelling of the attenuated linea alba (no cough impulse).

ABORTION, RECURRENT

ICD-9CM # 761.8

Congenital anatomic abnormalities.
Adhesions (uterine synechiae).
Uterine fibroids.
Endometriosis.
Endocrine abnormalities (luteal phase insufficiency, hypothyroidism, uncontrolled diabetes mellitus [DM]).
Parenteral chromosome abnormalities.
Maternal infections (cervical mycoplasma, ureaplasma, chlamydia).
DES exposure, heavy metal exposure.
Thrombocytosis.
Allogenic immunity, autoimmunity, lupus anticoagulant.

ACHES AND PAINS, DIFFUSE[24]

ICD-9CM # 719.49

Postviral arthralgias/myalgias.
Bilateral soft tissue rheumatism.
Overuse syndromes.
Fibrositis.
Hypothyroidism.
Metabolic bone disease.
Paraneoplastic syndrome.
Myopathy (polymyositis, dermatomyositis).
Rheumatoid arthritis (RA).
Sjögren's syndrome.
Polymyalgia rheumatica.
Hypermobility.
Benign arthralgias/myalgias.
Chronic fatigue syndrome.
Hypophosphatemia.

ACIDOSIS, LACTIC

ICD-9CM # 276.2

TISSUE HYPOXIA

Shock (hypovolemic, cardiogenic, endotoxic).
Respiratory failure (asphyxia).
Severe CHF.
Severe anemia.
Carbon monoxide or cyanide poisoning.

ASSOCIATED WITH SYSTEMIC DISORDERS

Neoplastic diseases (e.g., leukemia, lymphoma).
Liver or renal failure.
Sepsis.
DM.
Seizure activity.
Abnormal intestinal flora.
Alkalosis.
HIV.

SECONDARY TO DRUGS OR TOXINS

Salicylates.
Ethanol, methanol, ethylene glycol.
Fructose or sorbitol.
Biguanides (phenformin, metformin [usually occurring in patients with renal insufficiency]).
Isoniazid.
Streptozocin.
Nucleoside reverse transcriptase inhibitors (zidovudine, didanosine, stavudine).

HEREDITARY DISORDERS

G6PD deficiency and others.

ACIDOSIS, METABOLIC

ICD-9CM # 276.2

METABOLIC ACIDOSIS WITH INCREASED AG (AG ACIDOSIS)

Lactic acidosis.
Ketoacidosis (DM, alcoholic ketoacidosis).
Uremia (chronic renal failure).
Ingestion of toxins (paraldehyde, methanol, salicylate, ethylene glycol).
High-fat diet (mild acidosis).

METABOLIC ACIDOSIS WITH NORMAL AG (HYPERCHLOREMIC ACIDOSIS)

Renal tubular acidosis (including acidosis of aldosterone deficiency).
Intestinal loss of HCO_3^- (diarrhea, pancreatic fistula).
Carbonic anhydrase inhibitors (e.g., acetazolamide).
Dilutional acidosis (as a result of rapid infusion of bicarbonate-free isotonic saline).
Ingestion of exogenous acids (ammonium chloride, methionine, cystine, calcium chloride).
Ileostomy.
Ureterosigmoidostomy.
Drugs: amiloride, triamterene, spironolactone, β-blockers.

ACIDOSIS, RESPIRATORY

ICD-9CM # 276.2

Pulmonary disease (COPD, severe pneumonia, pulmonary edema, interstitial fibrosis).
Airway obstruction (foreign body, severe bronchospasm, laryngospasm).
Thoracic cage disorders (pneumothorax, flail chest, kyphoscoliosis).
Defects in muscles of respiration (myasthenia gravis, hypokalemia, muscular dystrophy).
Defects in peripheral nervous system (amyotrophic lateral sclerosis, poliomyelitis, Guillain-Barré syndrome, botulism, tetanus, organophosphate poisoning, spinal cord injury).
Depression of respiratory center (anesthesia, narcotics, sedatives, vertebral artery embolism or thrombosis, increased intracranial pressure).
Failure of mechanical ventilator.

ACUTE SCROTUM

ICD-9CM # 608.9

Testicular torsion.
Epididymitis.
Testicular neoplasm.
Orchitis.

ADNEXAL MASS[26]

ICD-9CM # varies with specific disorder

Ovary (neoplasm, endometriosis, functional cyst).
Fallopian tube (ectopic pregnancy, neoplasm, tuboovarian abscess, hydrosalpinx, paratubal cyst).
Uterus (fibroid, neoplasm).
Retroperitoneum (neoplasm, abdominal wall hematoma or abscess).
Urinary tract (pelvic kidney, distended bladder, urachal cyst).
Inflammatory bowel disease.
GI tract neoplasm.
Diverticular disease.
Appendicitis.
Bowel loop with feces.

ADRENAL MASSES[36]

ICD-9CM # 194.0 Adrenocortical Carcinoma
255.8 Adrenal Hyperplasia

UNILATERAL ADRENAL MASSES

Functional Lesions

Adrenal adenoma.
Adrenal carcinoma.
Pheochromocytoma.
Primary aldosteronism, adenomatous type.

Nonfunctional Lesions

Incidentaloma of adrenal.
Ganglioneuroma.
Myelolipoma.
Hematoma.
Adenolipoma.
Metastasis.

BILATERAL ADRENAL MASSES

Functional Lesions

ACTH-dependent Cushing's syndrome.
Congenital adrenal hyperplasia.
Pheochromocytoma.
Conn's syndrome, hyperplastic variety.
Micronodular adrenal disease.
Idiopathic bilateral adrenal hypertrophy.

Nonfunctional Lesions

Infection (tuberculosis, fungi).
Infiltration (leukemia, lymphoma).
Replacement (amyloidosis).
Hemorrhage.
Bilateral metastases.

ADYNAMIC ILEUS[26]

ICD-9CM # 560.1

Abdominal trauma.
Infection (retroperitoneal, pelvic, intrathoracic).
Laparotomy.
Metabolic disease (hypokalemia).
Renal colic.
Skeletal injury (rib fracture, vertebral fracture).
Medications (e.g., narcotics).

AEROPHAGIA (BELCHING, ERUCTATION)

ICD-9CM # 787.3

Anxiety disorders.
Rapid food ingestion.
Carbonated beverages.
Nursing infants (especially when nursing in horizontal position).
Eating or drinking in supine position.
Gum chewing.
Poorly fitting dentures, orthodontic appliances.
Hiatal hernia, gastritis, nonulcer dyspepsia.
Cholelithiasis, cholecystitis.
Ingestion of legumes, onions, peppers.

AIRWAY OBSTRUCTION, PEDIATRIC AGE[19]

ICD-9CM #		
	496	Obstruction Due to Bronchospasm
	934.9	Obstruction Due to Foreign Body
	478.75	Obstruction Due to Laryngospasm
	506.9	Obstruction Due to Inhalation of Fumes or Vapors

CONGENITAL CAUSES

Craniofacial dysmorphism.
Hemangioma.
Laryngeal cleft/web.
Laryngoceles, cysts.
Laryngomalacia.
Macroglossia.
Tracheal stenosis.
Vascular ring.
Vocal cord paralysis.

ACQUIRED INFECTIOUS CAUSES

Acute laryngotracheobronchitis.
Epiglottitis.
Laryngeal papillomatosis.
Membranous croup (bacterial tracheitis).
Mononucleosis.
Retropharyngeal abscess.
Spasmodic croup.
Diphtheria.

ACQUIRED NONINFECTIOUS CAUSES

Anaphylaxis.
Foreign body aspiration.
Supraglottic hypotonia.
Thermal/chemical burn.
Trauma.
Vocal cord paralysis.
Angioneurotic edema.

AKINETIC/RIGID SYNDROME[1]

ICD-9CM # code not available

Parkinsonism (idiopathic, drug-induced).
Catatonia (psychosis).
Progressive supranuclear palsy.
Multisystem atrophy (Shy-Drager syndrome, olivopontocerebellar atrophy).
Diffuse Lewy-body disease.
Toxins (MPTP, manganese, carbon monoxide).
Huntington's disease and other hereditary neurodegenerative disorders.

ALKALOSIS, METABOLIC

ICD-9CM # 276.3

CHLORIDE-RESPONSIVE

Vomiting.
Nasogastric (NG) suction.
Diuretics.
Posthypercapnic alkalosis.
Stool losses (laxative abuse, cystic fibrosis, villous adenoma).
Massive blood transfusion.
Exogenous alkali administration.

CHLORIDE-RESISTANT

Hyperadrenocorticoid states (Cushing's syndrome, primary hyperaldosteronism, secondary mineralocorticoidism [licorice, chewing tobacco]).
Hypomagnesemia.
Hypokalemia.
Bartter's syndrome.

ALKALOSIS, RESPIRATORY

ICD-9CM # 276.3

Hypoxemia (pneumonia, pulmonary embolism, atelectasis, high-altitude living).
Drugs (salicylates, xanthenes, progesterone, epinephrine, thyroxine, nicotine).
Central nervous system (CNS) disorders (tumor, cerebrovascular accident [CVA], trauma, infections).
Psychogenic hyperventilation (anxiety, hysteria).
Hepatic encephalopathy.
Gram-negative sepsis.
Hyponatremia.
Sudden recovery from metabolic acidosis.
Assisted ventilation.

ALOPECIA[14,28]

ICD-9CM #		
	704.00	Alopecia NOS
	704.01	Alopecia, Androgenic
	704.01	Alopecia Areata
	757.4	Alopecia, Congenital
	316	Alopecia, Psychogenic

SCARRING ALOPECIA

Congenital (aplasia cutis).
Tinea capitis with inflammation (kerion).
Bacterial folliculitis.
Discoid lupus erythematosus.
Lichen planopilaris.
Folliculitis decalvans.
Neoplasm.
Trauma.

NONSCARRING ALOPECIA

Cosmetic treatment.
Tinea capitis.
Structural hair shaft disease.
Trichotillomania (hair pulling).
Anagen arrest.
Telogen arrest.
Alopecia areata.
Androgenetic alopecia.

ALVEOLAR CONSOLIDATION

ICD-9CM # 514

Infection.
Neoplasm (bronchoalveolar carcinoma, lymphoma).
Aspiration.
Trauma.
Hemorrhage (Wegener's Goodpasture, bleeding diathesis).
ARDS.
CHF.
Renal failure.
Eosinophilic pneumonia.
Bronchiolitis obliterans.
Pulmonary alveolar proteinosis.

ALVEOLAR HEMORRHAGE[28]

ICD-9CM # 770.3

Hematologic disorders (coagulopathies, thrombocytopenia).
Goodpasture syndrome (anti–basement-membrane antibody disease).
Wegener's vasculitis.
Immune complex–mediated vasculitis.
Idiopathic pulmonary hemosiderosis.
Drugs (penicillamine).
Lymphangiogram contrast.
Mitral stenosis.

AMENORRHEA

ICD-9CM # 626.0

PREGNANCY

EARLY MENOPAUSE

HYPOTHALAMIC DYSFUNCTION: defective synthesis or release of LHRH, anorexia nervosa, stress, exercise.

PITUITARY DYSFUNCTION: neoplasm, postpartum hemorrhage, surgery, radiotherapy.

OVARIAN DYSFUNCTION: gonadal dysgenesis, 17-α-hydroxylase deficiency, premature ovarian failure, polycystic ovarian disease, gonadal stromal tumors.

UTEROVAGINAL ABNORMALITIES

Congenital: imperforate hymen, imperforate cervix, imperforate or absent vagina, Müllerian agenesis.

Acquired: destruction of endometrium with curettage (Asherman's syndrome), closure of cervix or vagina caused by traumatic injury, hysterectomy.

OTHER

Metabolic diseases (liver, kidney), malnutrition, rapid weight loss, exogenous obesity, endocrine abnormalities (Cushing's syndrome, Graves' disease, hypothyroidism).

AMNESIA

ICD-9CM # 292.83 Drug Induced
300.12 Hysterical
780.9 Retrograde
437.7 Transient Global

Degenerative diseases (e.g., Alzheimer's, Huntington's disease).
CVA (especially when involving thalamus, basal forebrain, and hippocampus).
Head trauma.
Postsurgical (e.g., mammillary body surgery, bilateral temporal lobectomy).
Infections (herpes simplex encephalitis, meningitis).
Wernicke-Korsakoff syndrome.
Cerebral hypoxia.
Hypoglycemia.
CNS neoplasms.
Creutzfeldt-Jakob disease.
Medications (e.g., midazolam and other benzodiazepines).
Psychosis.
Malingering.

ANAL ABSCESS AND FISTULA[38]

ICD-9CM # 566

Primary anal gland infection.
Secondary abscess:
Inflammatory bowel disease:
- Crohn's disease.
- Ulcerative colitis.

Infection:
- Tuberculosis.
- Actinomycosis.
- Threadworm.

Trauma.
Leucopenia.
Immunosuppression:
- HIV.
- Drugs.

Rectal cancer.
Diabetes mellitus.

ANAL INCONTINENCE[26]

ICD-9CM # 787.6

TRAUMATIC

Nerve injured in surgery.
Spinal cord injury.
Obstetric trauma.
Sphincter injury.

NEUROLOGIC

Spinal cord lesions.
Dementia.
Autonomic neuropathy (e.g., DM).
Obstetrics: pudendal nerve stretched during surgery.
Hirschsprung's disease.

MASS EFFECT

Carcinoma of anal canal.
Carcinoma of rectum.
Foreign body.
Fecal impaction.
Hemorrhoids.

MEDICAL

Procidentia.
Inflammatory disease.
Diarrhea.
Laxative abuse.

PEDIATRIC

Congenital.
Meningocele.
Myelomeningocele.
Spina bifida.
After corrective surgery for imperforate anus.
Sexual abuse.
Encopresis.

ANAPHYLAXIS[21]

ICD-9CM # 995.0

PULMONARY

Laryngeal edema.
Epiglottitis.
Foreign body aspiration.
Pulmonary embolus.
Asphyxiation.
Hyperventilation.

CARDIOVASCULAR

Myocardial infarction.
Arrhythmia.
Hypovolemic shock.
Cardiac arrest.

CNS

Vasovagal reaction.
CVA.
Seizure disorder.
Drug overdose.

ENDOCRINE

Hypoglycemia.
Pheochromocytoma.
Carcinoid syndrome.
Catamenial (progesterone-induced anaphylaxis).

PSYCHIATRIC

Vocal cord dysfunction syndrome.
Munchausen syndrome.
Panic attack/globus hystericus.

OTHER

Hereditary angioedema.
Cord urticaria.
Idiopathic urticaria.
Mastocytosis.
Serum sickness.
Idiopathic capillary leak syndrome.
Sulfite exposure.
Scombroid poisoning (tuna, blue fish, mackerel).

ANDROGEN EXCESS, REPRODUCTIVE-AGE WOMAN

ICD-9CM # varies with specific disorder

Polycystic ovary syndrome.
Idiopathic.
Medications (e.g., anabolizing agents, testosterone, danazol).
Pregnancy (luteoma, hyperreactio luteinalis).
Sertoli-Leydig ovarian neoplasm.
Adrenal adenoma or hyperplasia.
Cushing's syndrome.
Glucocorticoid resistance.
Hypothyroidism.
Hyperprolactinemia.

ANEMIA, APLASTIC[20]

ICD-9CM # 284

ACQUIRED APLASTIC ANEMIA

Secondary aplastic anemia.
Irradiation.
Drugs and chemicals.
Regular effects.
Cytotoxic agents.
Benzene.
Idiosyncratic reactions.
Chloramphenicol.
Nonsteroidal anti-inflammatory drugs.
Antiepileptics.
Gold.
Other drugs and chemicals.
Viruses.
Epstein-Barr virus (infectious mononucleosis).
Hepatitis virus (non-A, non-B, non-C, non-G hepatitis).
Parvovirus (transient aplastic crisis, some pure red cell aplasia).

Human immunodeficiency virus (acquired immunodeficiency syndrome).
Immune diseases.
Eosinophilic fascitis.
Hyperimmunoglobulinemia.
Thymoma and thymic carcinoma.
Graft-versus-host disease in immunodeficiency.
Paroxysmal nocturnal hemoglobinuria.
Pregnancy.
Idiopathic aplastic anemia.

INHERITED APLASTIC ANEMIA

Fanconi anemia.
Dyskeratosis congenita.
Shwachman-Diamond syndrome.
Reticular dysgenesis.
Amegakaryocytic thrombocytopenia.
Familial aplastic anemias.
Preleukemia (e.g., monosomy 7).
Nonhematologic syndromes (e.g., Down's, Dubowitz, Seckel).

ANEMIA, APLASTIC, DUE TO DRUGS AND CHEMICALS[1]

ICD-9CM # 284.89

Agents that regularly produce marrow depression as a major toxic effect when used in commonly employed doses or normal exposures:
Cytotoxic drugs used in cancer chemotherapy.
Alkylating agents (busulfan, melphalan, cyclophosphamide).
Antimetabolites (antifolic compounds, nucleotide analogs), antimitotics (vincristine, vinblastine, colchicine).
Some antibiotics (daunorubicin, doxorubicin [Adriamycin]).
Benzene (and less often benzene-containing chemicals; kerosene, carbon tetrachloride, Stoddard solvent, chlorophenols).
Agents probably associated with aplastic anemia but with a relatively low probability relative to their use:
Chloramphenicol.
Insecticides.
Antiprotozoals (quinacrine and chloroquine).
Nonsteroidal anti-inflammatory drugs (including phenylbutazone, indomethacin, ibuprofen, sulindac, diclofenac, naproxen, piroxicam, fenoprofen, fenbufen, aspirin).
Anticonvulsants (hydantoins, carbamazepine, phenacemide, ethosuximide).
Gold, arsenic, and other heavy metals such as bismuth and mercury.
Sulfonamides as a class.
Antithyroid medications (methimazole, methylthiouracil, propylthiouracil).
Antidiabetes drugs (tolbutamide, carbutamide, chlorpropamide).
Carbonic anhydrase inhibitors (acetazolamide, methazolamide, mesalazine).
D-Penicillamine.
2-Chlorodeoxyadenosine.
Agents more rarely associated with aplastic anemia:
Antibiotics (streptomycin, tetracycline, methicillin, ampicillin, mebendazole and albendazole, sulfonamides, flucytosine, mefloquine, dapsone).
Antihistamines (cimetidine, ranitidine, chlorpheniramine).
Sedatives and tranquilizers (chlorpromazine, prochlorperazine, piperacetazine, chlordiazepoxide, meprobamate, methyprylon, remoxipride).
Antiarrhythmics (tocainide, amiodarone).
Allopurinol (can potentiate marrow suppression by cytotoxic drugs).
Ticlopidine.
Methyldopa.
Quinidine.
Lithium.
Guanidine.
Canthaxanthin.
Thiocyanate.
Carbimazole.
Cyanamide.
Deferoxamine.
Amphetamines.

ANEMIA, DRUG-INDUCED[17]

ICD-9CM # 283.0

DRUGS THAT MAY INTERFERE WITH RED CELL PRODUCTION BY INDUCING MARROW SUPPRESSION OR APLASIA

Alcohol.
Antineoplastic drugs.
Antithyroid drugs.
Antibiotics.
Oral hypoglycemic agents.
Phenylbutazone.
Azidothymidine (AZT).

DRUGS THAT INTERFERE WITH VITAMIN B_{12}, FOLATE, OR IRON ABSORPTION OR UTILIZATION

Nitrous oxide.
Anticonvulsant drugs.
Antineoplastic drugs.
Isoniazid, cycloserine A.

DRUGS CAPABLE OF PROMOTING HEMOLYSIS

Immune Mediated
Penicillins.
Quinine.
Alpha-methyldopa.
Procainamide.
Mitomycin C.
Oxidative Stress
Antimalarials.
Sulfonamide drugs.
Nalidixic acid.

DRUGS THAT MAY PRODUCE OR PROMOTE BLOOD LOSS

Aspirin.
Alcohol.
Nonsteroidal anti-inflammatory agents.
Corticosteroids.
Anticoagulants.

ANEMIA, HYPOCHROMIC[20]

ICD-9CM # varies with specific diagnosis
280.9 Iron deficiency
285.0 Sideroblastic

DECREASED BODY IRON STORES

Iron-deficiency anemia.

NORMAL OR INCREASED BODY IRON STORES

Impaired iron metabolism.
Anemia of chronic disease.
Defective absorption, transport, or use of iron.
Disorders of globin synthesis:
- Thalassemia.
- Other microcytic hemoglobinopathies.

Disorders of heme synthesis: sideroblastic anemias:
- Hereditary.
- Acquired.

ANEMIA, LOW RETICULOCYTE COUNT[1]

ICD-9CM # 285.9

MICROCYTIC ANEMIA (MCV <80)

Iron deficiency.
Thalassemia minor.
Sideroblastic anemia.
Lead poisoning.

MACROCYTIC ANEMIA (MCV >100)

Megaloblastic anemias.
Folate deficiency.
Vitamin B_{12} deficiency.
Drug-induced megaloblastic anemia.
Nonmegaloblastic macrocytosis.
Liver disease.
Hypothyroidism.

NORMOCYTIC ANEMIA (MCV 80-100)

Early iron deficiency.
Aplastic anemia.
Myelophthisic disorders.
Endocrinopathies.
Anemia of chronic disease.
Uremia.
Mixed nutritional deficiency.

ANEMIA, MEGALOBLASTIC[36]

ICD-9CM # 281.0 Pernicious Anemia
281.1 B_{12} Deficiency
281.2 Folate Deficiency
281.3 B_{12} with Folate Deficiency
281.4 Protein or Amino Acid Deficiency
281.8 Nutritional
281.9 NOS

COBALAMIN (CBL) DEFICIENCY

NUTRITIONAL CBL DEFICIENCY (INSUFFICIENT CBL INTAKE): vegetarians, vegans, breast-fed infants of mothers with pernicious anemia.

ABNORMAL INTRAGASTRIC EVENTS (INADEQUATE PROTEOLYSIS OF FOOD CBL): atrophic gastritis, partial gastrectomy with hypochlorhydria.
LOSS/ATROPHY OF GASTRIC OXYNTIC MUCOSA (DEFICIENT IF MOLECULES): total or partial gastrectomy, pernicious anemia (PA), caustic destruction (lye).
ABNORMAL EVENTS IN SMALL BOWEL LUMEN:
Inadequate pancreatic protease (R-CBL not degraded, CBL not transferred to IF).
- Insufficiency of pancreatic protease—pancreatic insufficiency.
- Inactivation of pancreatic protease—Zollinger-Ellison syndrome.

Usurping of luminal CBL (inadequate CBL binding to IF).
- By bacteria—stasis syndromes (blind loops, pouches of diverticulosis, strictures, fistulas, anastomoses); impaired bowel motility (scleroderma, pseudoobstruction), hypogammaglobulinemia.
- By *Diphyllobothrium latum.*

DISORDERS OF ILEAL MUCOSA/IF RECEPTORS (IF-CBL NOT BOUND TO IF RECEPTORS):
Diminished or absent IF receptors—ileal bypass/resection/fistula.
Abnormal mucosal architecture/function—tropical/nontropical sprue, Crohn's disease, TB ileitis, infiltration by lymphomas, amyloidosis.
IF-/post IF-receptor defects—Imerslund-Graesbeck syndrome, TC II deficiency.
Drug-induced effects (slow K, biguanides, cholestyramine, colchicine, neomycin, PAS).

DISORDERS OF PLASMA CBL TRANSPORT (TC II-CBL NOT DELIVERED TO TC II RECEPTORS)

Congenital TC II deficiency, defective binding of TC II-CBL to TC II receptors (rare).

METABOLIC DISORDERS (CBL NOT UTILIZED BY CELL)

Inborn enzyme errors (rare).
Acquired disorders: (CBL oxidized to cob[III]alamin)—N_2O inhalation.

FOLATE DEFICIENCY

Nutritional Causes
Decreased dietary intake—poverty and famine (associated with kwashiorkor, marasmus), institutionalized individuals (psychiatric/nursing homes), chronic debilitating disease/goats' milk (low in folate), special diets (slimming), cultural/ethnic cooking techniques (food folate destroyed) or habits (folate-rich foods not consumed).
Decreased diet and increased requirements:
- Physiologic: pregnancy and lactation, prematurity, infancy.
- Pathologic: intrinsic hematologic disease (autoimmune hemolytic disease), drugs, malaria; hemoglobinopathies (SS, thalassemia), RBC membrane defects (hereditary spherocytosis, paroxysmal nocturnal hemoglobinopathy); abnormal hematopoiesis (leukemia/lymphoma, myelodysplastic syndrome, agnogenic myeloid metaplasia with myelofibrosis); infiltration with malignant disease; dermatologic (psoriasis).

Folate Malabsorption
With normal intestinal mucosa:
- Some drugs (controversial).
- Congenital folate malabsorption (rare).

With mucosal abnormalities—tropical and nontropical sprue, regional enteritis.
Defective Cellular Folate Uptake—Familial Aplastic Anemia (Rare) Inadequate Cellular Utilization
Folate antagonists (methotrexate).
Hereditary enzyme deficiencies involving folate.
Drugs (Multiple Effects on Folate Metabolism)
Alcohol, sulfasalazine, triamterene, pyrimethamine, trimethoprim-sulfamethoxazole, diphenylhydantoin, barbiturates.

MISCELLANEOUS MEGALOBLASTIC ANEMIAS (NOT CAUSED BY CBL OR FOLATE DEFICIENCY)

Congenital Disorders of DNA Synthesis (Rare)
Orotic aciduria, Lesch-Nyhan syndrome, congenital dyserythropoietic anemia.
Acquired Disorders of DNA Synthesis
Thiamine-responsive megaloblastosis (rare).
Malignancy—erythroleukemia—refractory sideroblastic anemias—all antineoplastic drugs that inhibit DNA synthesis.
Toxic—alcohol.

ANERGY, CUTANEOUS[36]

ICD-9CM # 279.9

IMMUNOLOGIC

Acquired (AIDS, acute leukemia, carcinoma, CLL, Hodgkin's lymphoma, NHL).
Congenital (ataxia-telangiectasia, Di George's syndrome, severe combined immunodeficiency, Wiskott-Aldrich syndrome).

INFECTIONS

Bacterial (bacterial pneumonia, brucellosis).
Disseminated mycotic infections.
Mycobacterial (lepromatous leprosy, TB).
Viral (varicella, hepatitis, influenza, mononucleosis, measles, mumps).

IMMUNOSUPPRESSIVE MEDICATIONS

Systemic corticosteroids.
Methotrexate, cyclophosphamide.
Rifampin.

OTHER

Alcoholic cirrhosis, biliary cirrhosis, sarcoidosis, rheumatic disease.
Diabetes, Crohn's disease, uremia.
Anemia, pyridoxine deficiency, sickle cell anemia.
Burns, malnutrition, pregnancy, old age, surgery.

ANEURYSMS, THORACIC AORTA

ICD-9CM # 441.2

Trauma.
Infection.
Inflammatory (syphilis, Takayasu's disease).
Collagen vascular disease (RA, ankylosing spondylitis).
Annuloaortic ectasia (Marfan's syndrome, Ehlers-Danlos syndrome).
Congenital.
Coarctation.
Cystic medial necrosis.

ANHYDROSIS

ICD-9CM # 705.1

Drugs (anticholinergics).
Dehydration.
Hysteria.
Obstruction of sweat ducts (e.g., inflammation, miliaria).
Local radiant heat or pressure.
CNS lesions (medulla, hypothalamus, pons).
Spinal cord lesions.
Lesions of sympathetic nerves.
Congenital sweat gland disturbances.

ANION GAP INCREASE

ICD-9CM # 276.9

Uremia.
Ketoacidosis (diabetic, starvation, alcoholic).
Lactic acidosis.
Ethylene glycol poisoning.
Salicylate overdose.
Methanol poisoning.

ANISOCORIA

ICD-9CM # 379.41

Mydriatic or miotic drugs.
Prosthetic eye.
Inflammation (keratitis, iridocyclitis).
Infections (herpes zoster, syphilis, meningitis, encephalitis, TB, diphtheria, botulism).
Subdural hemorrhage.
Cavernous sinus thrombosis.
Intracranial neoplasm.
Cerebral aneurysm.
Glaucoma.
CNS degenerative diseases.
Internal carotid ischemia.
Toxic polyneuritis (alcohol, lead).
Adie's syndrome.
Horner's syndrome.
DM.
Trauma.
Congenital.

ANOREXIA[38]

ICD-9CM # 783.0

SELECTED CAUSES OF ANOREXIA

Gastrointestinal tract/liver
Gastric outlet obstruction or small bowel obstruction.
Gastric cancer.
Hepatic metastases.
Acute viral hepatitis.
Metabolic
Addison's disease.
Hypopituitarism.
Hyperparathyroidism.
Functional
Extremely unpleasant sight/smell.
Systemic
Chronic pain.
Renal failure.
Severe congestive heart failure.
Respiratory failure.
Psychiatric
Depression.
Anorexia nervosa.
Medications
Digoxin.
Narcotic analgesics.
Diuretics.
Antihypertensives.
Chemotherapeutic agents.
Amphetamines.
Miscellaneous
Excessive smoking.
Excessive alcohol intake.
Oral cavity disease.
Thiamine deficiency.
Early pregnancy.
Hypogeusia or dysgeusia.

ANOVULATION

ICD-9CM # 628.0

Anorexia and bulimia.
Strenuous exercise.
Weight loss/malnutrition.
Empty sella syndrome.
Pituitary disorders (infarction, infection, trauma, irradiation, surgery, microadenomas, macroadenomas).
Idiopathic hypopituitarism.
Drug induced.
Thyroid dysfunction (hypothyroidism, hyperthyroidism).
Systemic diseases (e.g., liver disease).
Adrenal hyperfunction (Cushing's syndrome, congenital adrenal hyperplasia).
Polycystic ovarian syndrome.
Isolated gonadotropin deficiency.

APPETITE LOSS IN INFANTS AND CHILDREN[19]

ICD-9CM # 783.0 Appetite Loss
307.59 Appetite Loss, Psychogenic Origin

ORGANIC DISEASE

Infection (Acute or Chronic)
Neurologic
Congenital degenerative disease.
Hypothalamic lesion.
Increased intracranial pressure (including a brain tumor).
Swallowing disorders (neuromuscular).
Gastrointestinal
Oral lesions (e.g., thrush or herpes simplex).
Gastroesophageal reflux.
Obstruction (especially with gastric or intestinal distention).
Inflammatory bowel disease.
Celiac disease.
Constipation.
Cardiac
Congestive heart failure (especially associated with cyanotic lesions).
Metabolic
Renal failure and/or renal tubule acidosis.
Liver failure.
Congenital metabolic disease.
Lead poisoning.
Nutritional
Marasmus.
Iron deficiency.
Zinc deficiency.
Fever
RA.
Rheumatic fever.
Drugs
Morphine.
Digitalis.
Antimetabolites.
Methylphenidate.
Amphetamines.
Miscellaneous
Prolonged restriction of oral feedings, beginning in the neonatal period.
Systemic lupus erythematosus (SLE).
Tumor.

PSYCHOLOGIC FACTORS

Anxiety, fear, depression, mania (limbic influence on the hypothalamus).
Avoidance of symptoms associated with meals (abdominal pain, diarrhea, bloating, urgency, dumping syndrome).
Anorexia nervosa.
Excessive weight loss and food aversion in athletes, simulating anorexia nervosa.

ARTERIAL OCCLUSION[15]

ICD-9CM # 444.22 Arterial Occlusion, Lower Extremities
444.21 Arterial Occlusion, Upper Extremities

Thromboembolism (post-MI, mitral stenosis, rheumatic valve disease, atrial fibrillation, atrial myxoma, marantic endocarditis, bacterial endocarditis, Libman-Sacks endocarditis).
Atheroembolism (microemboli composed of cholesterol, calcium, and platelets from proximal atherosclerotic plaques).
Arterial thrombosis (endothelial injury, altered arterial blood flow, trauma, severe atherosclerosis, acute vasculitis).
Vasospasm.
Trauma.
Hypercoagulable states.
Miscellaneous (irradiation, drugs, infections, necrotizing).

ARTHRITIS AND ABDOMINAL PAIN

ICD-9CM # varies with specific disorder

Viral syndrome.
Inflammatory bowel disease.
Celiac disease.
Vasculitis.
SLE.
RA.
Scleroderma.
Amyloidosis.
Chronic hepatitis C.
Whipple's disease.
Polyarteritis nodosa.
Behçet's disease.
Familial Mediterranean fever.
Blind loop syndrome.

ARTHRITIS AND DIARRHEA

ICD-9CM # varies with specific disorder

Viral syndrome.
Inflammatory bowel disease.
Celiac disease.
Whipple's disease.
Enterogenic (bacterial) reactive arthritis.
Collagenous colitis.
Behçet's disease.
Hyperthyroidism.
Spondyloarthropathy.
Blind loop syndrome.

ARTHRITIS AND EYE LESIONS[6]

ICD-9CM # varies with specific diagnosis

SLE.
Sjögren's syndrome.
Behçet's syndrome.

Sarcoidosis.
Subacute bacterial endocarditis (SBE).
Lyme disease.
Wegener's granulomatosis.
Giant cell arteritis.
Takayasu's arteritis.
RA, JRA.
Scleroderma.
Inflammatory bowel disease.
Whipple's disease.
Ankylosing spondylitis.
Reactive arthritis.
Psoriatic arthritis.

ARTHRITIS AND HEART MURMUR[6]

ICD-9CM # varies with specific diagnosis

SBE.
Cardiac myxoma.
Ankylosing spondylitis.
Reactive arthritis.
Acute rheumatic fever.
RA.
SLE with Libman-Sacks endocarditis.
Relapsing polychondritis.

ARTHRITIS AND MUSCLE WEAKNESS[8]

ICD-9CM # varies with specific diagnosis

RA.
Ankylosing spondylitis.
Polymyositis.
Dermatomyositis.
SLE, scleroderma, mixed connective tissue disease.
Sarcoidosis.
HIV-associated arthritis.
Whipple's disease.

ARTHRITIS AND RASH[6]

ICD-9CM # varies with specific diagnosis

Chronic urticaria.
Vasculitic urticaria.
SLE.
Dermatomyositis.
Polymyositis.
Psoriatic arthritis.
Reactive arthritis.
Chronic sarcoidosis.
Serum sickness.
Sweet's syndrome.
Leprosy.

ARTHRITIS AND SUBCUTANEOUS NODULES[6]

ICD-9CM # varies with specific diagnosis

RA.
Gout.
Pseudogout (rare).
Sarcoidosis.
Light chain (LA) amyloidosis (primary, multiple myeloma).
Acute rheumatic fever (ARF).
Hemochromatosis.
Whipple's disease.
Multicentric reticulohistiocytosis.

ARTHRITIS AND WEIGHT LOSS[6]

ICD-9CM # varies with specific diagnosis

Severe RA.
RA with vasculitis.
Reactive arthritis.
RA or psoriatic arthritis or ankylosing spondylitis with amyloidosis.
Cancer.
Enteropathic arthritis (Crohn's, ulcerative colitis).
HIV infection.
Whipple's disease.
Blind loop syndrome.
Scleroderma with intestinal bacterial overgrowth.

ARTHRITIS, AXIAL SKELETON

ICD-9CM # 720.0 Arthritis, Rheumatoid, Spine
696.0 Arthritis, Psoriatic
715.9 Arthritis, Degenerative, NOS
720.0 Ankylosing Spondylitis

RA.
Psoriatic arthritis.
Reiter's syndrome.
Ankylosing spondylitis.
Juvenile RA.
Degenerative disease of the nucleus pulposus.
Spondylosis deformans.
Diffuse idiopathic skeletal hyperostosis (DISH).
Alkaptonuria.
Infection.

ARTHRITIS, FEVER, AND RASH[6]

ICD-9CM # varies with specific diagnosis

Rubella, parvovirus B-19.
Gonococcemia, meningococcemia.
Secondary syphilis, Lyme borreliosis.
Adult acute rheumatic fever, adult Still's disease, adult Kawasaki disease.
Vasculitic urticaria.
Acute sarcoidosis.
Familial Mediterranean fever.
Hyperimmunoglobulinemia D and periodic fever syndrome.

ARTHRITIS, MONOARTICULAR AND OLIGOARTICULAR[2]

ICD-9CM # 715.3 Osteoarthritis, Localized
711.9 Infectious Arthritis
716.6 Monoarticular Arthritis; 5th digit to be added to the above depending on site of arthritis
0. Site Unspecified
1. Shoulder Region
2. Upper Arm
3. Forearm
4. Hand
5. Pelvic Region and Thigh
6. Lower Leg
7. Ankle and/or Foot
8. Other Specified Except Spine

Septic arthritis (*S. aureus, Neisseria gonorrhea, Meningococci, Streptococci, S. pneumoniae,* enteric gram-negative bacilli).
Crystalline-induced arthritis (gout, pseudogout, calcium oxalate, hydroxyapatite and other basic calcium/phosphate crystals).
Traumatic joint injury.
Hemarthrosis.
Monoarticular or oligoarticular flare of an inflammatory polyarticular rheumatic disease (RA, psoriatic arthritis, Reiter's syndrome, SLE).

ARTHRITIS, PEDIATRIC AGE[19]

ICD-9CM # 711.9 Infectious Arthritis
714.30 Juvenile Chronic or Unspecified
714.31 Juvenile Rheumatoid Polyarticular Acute
714.32 Juvenile Rheumatoid Pauciarticular
714.33 Juvenile Rheumatoid Monoarticular

RHEUMATIC DISEASES OF CHILDHOOD

Acute rheumatic fever.
SLE.
Juvenile ankylosing spondylitis.
Polymyositis and dermatomyositis.
Vasculitis.
Scleroderma.
Psoriatic arthritis.
Mixed connective tissue disease and overlap syndromes.
Kawasaki disease.
Behçet's syndrome.
Familial Mediterranean fever.
Reiter's syndrome.
Reflex sympathetic dystrophy.
Fibromyalgia (fibrositis).

INFECTIOUS DISEASES

Bacterial arthritis.
Viral or postviral arthritis.
Fungal arthritis.
Osteomyelitis.
Reactive arthritis.

NEOPLASTIC DISEASES

Leukemia.
Lymphoma.
Neuroblastoma.
Primary bone tumors.

NONINFLAMMATORY DISORDERS

Trauma.
Avascular necrosis syndromes.
Osteochondroses.
Slipped capital femoral epiphysis.
Diskitis.
Patellofemoral dysfunction (chondromalacia patellae).
Toxic synovitis of the hip.
Overuse syndromes.

GENETIC OR CONGENITAL SYNDROMES

Hematologic Disorders

Sickle cell disease.
Hemophilia.

INFLAMMATORY BOWEL DISEASE

Miscellaneous

Growing pains.
Psychogenic arthralgias (conversion reactions).
Hypermobility syndrome.
Villonodular synovitis.
Foreign body arthritis.

ARTHRITIS, POLYARTICULAR

ICD-9CM # 715.09 Generalized Osteoarthritis, Multiple Sites
716.89 Arthritis, Multiple Sites
714.31 Juvenile Rheumatoid, Polyarticular, Acute

RA, juvenile (rheumatoid) polyarthritis.
SLE, other connective tissue diseases, erythema nodosum, palindromic rheumatism, relapsing polychondritis.
Psoriatic arthritis, ankylosing spondylitis.
Sarcoidosis.
Lyme arthritis, bacterial endocarditis, *Neisseria gonorrhoeae* infection, rheumatic fever, Reiter's disease.
Crystal deposition disease.
Hypersensitivity to serum or drugs.
Hepatitis B, HIV, rubella, mumps.
Other: serum sickness, leukemias, lymphomas, enteropathic arthropathy, Whipple's disease, Behçet's syndrome, Henoch-Schönlein purpura, familial Mediterranean fever, hypertrophic pulmonary osteoarthropathy.

ASCITES

ICD-9CM # 789.5 Ascites NOS
197.6 Ascites, Cancerous (Malignant)
457.8 Ascites, Chylous

Hypoalbuminemia: nephrotic syndrome, protein-losing gastroenteropathy, starvation.
Cirrhosis.
Hepatic congestion: CHF, constrictive pericarditis, tricuspid insufficiency, hepatic vein obstruction (Budd-Chiari syndrome), inferior vena cava or portal vein obstruction.
Peritoneal infections: TB and other bacterial infections, fungal diseases, parasites.
Neoplasms: primary hepatic neoplasms, metastases to liver or peritoneum, lymphomas, leukemias, myeloid metaplasia.
Lymphatic obstruction: mediastinal tumors, trauma to the thoracic duct, filariasis.
Ovarian disease: Meigs' syndrome, struma ovarii.
Chronic pancreatitis or pseudocyst: pancreatic ascites.
Leakage of bile: bile ascites.
Urinary obstruction or trauma: urine ascites.
Myxedema.
Chylous ascites.

ASTHENIA

ICD-9CM # 780.79

Depression.
Chronic fatigue syndrome.
Sleep disorders.
Anemia.
Hypothyroidism.
Sedentary lifestyle.
Medications (e.g., narcotics, sedatives).
Infections.
Dehydration/electrolyte disorders.
COPD and other pulmonary disorders.
Renal failure.
CHF.
Diabetes.
Addison's disease.
Paraneoplastic syndrome.

ASTHMA, CHILDHOOD[4]

ICD-9CM # 493.0 use 5th digit
0. Without Mention of Status Asthmaticus
1. With Status Asthmaticus

INFECTIONS

Bronchiolitis (RSV).
Pneumonia.
Croup.
Tuberculosis, histoplasmosis.
Bronchiectasis.
Bronchiolitis obliterans.
Bronchitis.
Sinusitis.

ANATOMIC, CONGENITAL

Cystic fibrosis.
Vascular rings.
Ciliary dyskinesia.
B-lymphocyte immune defect.
Congestive heart failure.
Laryngotracheomalacia.
Tumor, lymphoma.
H-type tracheoesophageal fistula.
Repaired tracheoesophageal fistula.
Gastroesophageal reflux.

VASCULITIS, HYPERSENSITIVITY

Allergic bronchopulmonary aspergillosis.
Allergic alveolitis, hypersensitivity pneumonitis.
Churg-Strauss syndrome.
Periarteritis nodosa.

OTHER

Foreign body aspiration.
Pulmonary thromboembolism.
Psychogenic cough.
Sarcoidosis.
Bronchopulmonary dysplasia.
Vocal cord dysfunction.

ATAXIA

ICD-9CM # 781.3 Ataxia NOS
303.0 Alcoholic, Acute
303.9 Alcoholic, Chronic
334.3 Cerebellar
331.89 Cerebral
334.0 Friedreich's
300.11 Hysterical

Vertebral-basilar artery ischemia.
Diabetic neuropathy.
Tabes dorsalis.
Vitamin B_{12} deficiency.
Multiple sclerosis and other demyelinating diseases.
Meningomyelopathy.
Cerebellar neoplasms, hemorrhage, abscess, infarct.
Nutritional (Wernicke's encephalopathy).
Paraneoplastic syndromes.
Parainfectious: Guillain-Barré syndrome, acute ataxia of childhood and young adults.
Toxins: phenytoin, alcohol, sedatives, organophosphates.
Wilson's disease (hepatolenticular degeneration).
Hypothyroidism.
Myopathy.
Cerebellar and spinocerebellar degeneration: ataxia/telangiectasia, Friedreich's ataxia.
Frontal lobe lesions: tumors, thrombosis of anterior cerebral artery, hydrocephalus.
Labyrinthine destruction: neoplasm, injury, inflammation, compression.
Hysteria.
AIDS.

ATAXIA, ACUTE OR RECURRENT[11]

ICD-9CM # varies with specific diagnosis
781.3 Ataxia NOS
0.94 Locomotor ataxia
334.0 Friedreich's ataxia
334.2 Cerebellar ataxia, primary
334.3 Other cerebellar ataxia
334.8 Ataxia-telangiectasia

Drug ingestion (e.g., phenytoin, carbamazepine, sedatives, hypnotics, and phencyclidine) or intoxication (e.g., alcohol, ethylene glycol, hydrocarbon fumes, lead, mercury, or thallium).
Postinfectious (cerebellitis [e.g., varicella], acute disseminated encephalomyelitis).
Head trauma.
Basilar migraine.
Benign paroxysmal vertigo (migraine equivalent).
Brain tumor or neuroblastoma (if accompanied by opsoclonus or myoclonus [i.e., "dancing eyes, dancing feet"]).
Hydrocephalus.
Infection (e.g., labyrinthitis, abscess).
Seizure (ictal or postictal).
Vascular events (e.g., cerebellar hemorrhage or stroke).
Miller-Fisher variant of Guillain-Barré syndrome (ataxia, ophthalmoplegia, and areflexia). Warning: If bulbar signs present, disease is likely progressive; patient may lose ability to protect airway and/or ability to breathe.
Inherited ataxias.
Inborn errors of metabolism (e.g., mitochondrial disorders, amino-acidopathies, urea cycle defects).
Conversion reaction.
Multiple sclerosis.

ATAXIA, CHRONIC OR PROGRESSIVE[11]

ICD-9CM # varies with specific diagnosis
781.3 Ataxia NOS
0.94 Locomotor ataxia
334.0 Friedreich's ataxia
334.2 Cerebellar ataxia, primary
334.3 Other cerebellar ataxia
334.8 Ataxia-telangiectasia

Hydrocephalus.
Hypothyroidism.
Tumor or paraneoplastic syndrome.
Low vitamin E levels (e.g., cystic fibrosis).
Wilson disease.
Inborn errors of metabolism.
Inherited ataxias (e.g., ataxia-telangiectasia, Friedreich's ataxia).

ATELECTASIS

ICD-9CM # 518.0

Lung neoplasm (primary or metastatic).
Infection (pneumonia, TB, fungal, histoplasmosis).
Postoperative (lower lobes).
Sarcoidosis.
Mucoid impaction.
Foreign body.
Postinflammatory (middle lobe syndrome).
Pneumothorax.
Pleural effusion.
Pneumoconiosis.
Interstitial fibrosis.
Bulla.
Mediastinal or adjacent mass.

ATRIUM ENLARGEMENT, RIGHT ATRIUM

ICD-9CM # varies with specific disorder

Right ventricular failure.
Atrial septal defect.
Tricuspid regurgitation.
Tricuspid stenosis.
Pulmonary hypertension.
Restrictive cardiomyopathy.
Right atrial myxoma.
Ebstein's anomaly.
Anomalous pulmonary venous drainage to the right atrium.
Endomyocardial fibrosis.
Sinus of Valsalva fistula.
Arrhythmogenic right ventricular dysplasia.

AV NODAL BLOCK[15]

ICD-9CM # 426.10 AV Block (Incomplete, Partial)
426.0 AV Block, Complete

Idiopathic fibrosis (Lenègre's disease).
Sclerodegenerative processes (e.g., Lev's disease with calcification of the mitral and aortic annuli).
AV node radiofrequency ablation procedure.
Medications (e.g., digoxin, beta-blockers, calcium channel blockers, class III antiarrhythmics).
Acute inferior wall MI.
Myocarditis.
Infections (endocarditis, Lyme disease).
Infiltrative diseases (e.g., hemochromatosis, sarcoidosis, amyloidosis).
Trauma (including cardiac surgical procedures).
Collagen vascular diseases.
Aortic root diseases (e.g., spondylitis).
Electrolyte abnormalities (e.g., hyperkalemia).

BACK PAIN

ICD-9CM # 724.5 Back Pain (Postural)
724.2 Low Back Pain
307.89 Back Pain Psychogenic
724.8 Stiff Back
847.9 Back Strain
724.6 Backache, Sacroiliac

Trauma: injury to bone, joint, or ligament.
Mechanical: pregnancy, obesity, fatigue, scoliosis.
Degenerative: osteoarthritis.
Infections: osteomyelitis, subarachnoid or spinal abscess, TB, meningitis, basilar pneumonia.
Metabolic: osteoporosis, osteomalacia.
Vascular: leaking aortic aneurysm, subarachnoid or spinal hemorrhage/infarction.
Neoplastic: myeloma, Hodgkin's disease, carcinoma of pancreas, metastatic neoplasm from breast, prostate, lung.
GI: penetrating ulcer, pancreatitis, cholelithiasis, inflammatory bowel disease.
Renal: hydronephrosis, calculus, neoplasm, renal infarction, pyelonephritis.
Hematologic: sickle cell crisis, acute hemolysis.
Gynecologic: neoplasm of uterus or ovary, dysmenorrhea, salpingitis, uterine prolapse.
Inflammatory: ankylosing spondylitis, psoriatic arthritis, Reiter's syndrome.
Lumbosacral strain.
Psychogenic: malingering, hysteria, anxiety.
Endocrine: adrenal hemorrhage or infarction.

BACK PAIN, CHILDREN AND ADOLESCENTS

ICD-9CM # 724.2

Trauma (muscle strain, vertebral fracture).
Idiopathic scoliosis, kyphosis.
Psychological problem.
Infection (pyelonephritis, osteomyelitis).
Inflammatory spondyloarthropathy.
Tumor.
Herniated disc.
Spondylolysis, spondylolisthesis.
Sickle cell crisis.
Syrinx.

BACK PAIN, VISCEROGENIC ORIGIN

ICD-9CM # varies with specific disorder

Urolithiasis.
Aortic aneurysm.
Colorectal carcinoma.
Endometriosis.
Tubal pregnancy.
Prostatitis.
Peptic ulcer.
Pancreatitis.
Diverticular spasm.
Metastatic neoplasm (e.g., bladder, uterus, ovary, kidney).

BACTERIAL OVERGROWTH, SMALL INTESTINE[38]

ICD-9CM # varies with specific diagnosis

Gastric surgery—Billroth II.
Small bowel diverticula.
Small bowel stricture:
- Crohn's disease.
- Radiation enteritis.

Impaired small intestinal motility:
- Scleroderma.
- Diabetes mellitus.
- Chronic intestinal pseudoobstruction.

Miscellaneous/multifactorial
- Elderly.
- Immune deficiency syndrome.
- Chronic pancreatitis.
- Cirrhosis.

BALLISM*

ICD-9CM # 333.5

Cerebral infarction or hemorrhage.
Medications (e.g., dopamine agonists, phenytoin).
CNS neoplasm (primary or metastatic).
Nonketotic hyperosmolar state.

*Violent, flinging, nonpatterned rapid movements

BILE DUCT, DILATED[38]

ICD-9CM # varies with specific diagnosis

Normal variant.
Post-cholecystectomy.
Unsuspected bile duct stone.
Sphincter of Oddi stenosis.
Occult bile duct stricture.
Previous bile duct injury.
Early carcinoma of the pancreas, carcinoma of the bile duct or carcinoma of the ampulla.
Extrinsic compression of the bile duct by a primary or secondary neoplasm.

BLEEDING, LOWER GI

ICD-9CM # 578.9

(ORIGINATING BELOW THE LIGAMENT OF TREITZ)

Small Intestine

Ischemic bowel disease (mesenteric thrombosis, embolism, vasculitis, trauma).
Small bowel neoplasm: leiomyomas, carcinoids.
Hereditary hemorrhagic telangiectasia (Rendu-Osler-Weber syndrome).
Meckel diverticulum and other small intestine diverticula.
Aortoenteric fistula.
Intestinal hemangiomas: blue rubber-bleb nevi, intestinal hemangiomas, cutaneous vascular nevi.
Hamartomatous polyps: Peutz-Jeghers syndrome (intestinal polyps, mucocutaneous pigmentation).
Infections of small bowel: tuberculous enteritis, enteritis necroticans.
Volvulus.
Intussusception.
Lymphoma of small bowel, sarcoma, Kaposi's sarcoma.
Irradiation ileitis.
AV malformation of small intestine.
Inflammatory bowel disease.
Polyarteritis nodosa.
Other: pancreatoenteric fistulas, Henoch-Schönlein purpura, Ehlers-Danlos syndrome, SLE, amyloidosis, metastatic melanoma.

Colon

Carcinoma (particularly left colon).
Diverticular disease.
Inflammatory bowel disease.
Ischemic colitis.
Colonic polyps.
Vascular abnormalities: angiodysplasia, vascular ectasia.
Radiation colitis.
Infectious colitis.
Uremic colitis.
Aortoenteric fistula.
Lymphoma of large bowel.
Hemorrhoids.
Anal fissure.
Trauma, foreign body.
Solitary rectal/cecal ulcers.
Long-distance running.

BLEEDING, LOWER GI, PEDIATRIC[2]

ICD-9CM # 578.9

<3 MO

Swallowed maternal blood.
Infectious colitis.
Milk allergy.
Bleeding diathesis.
Intussusception.
Midgut volvulus.
Meckel diverticulum.
Necrotizing enterocolitis.

<2 YR

Anal fissure.
Infectious colitis.
Milk allergy.
Colitis.
Intussusception.
Meckel diverticulum.
Polyp.
Duplication.
Hemolytic uremic syndrome.
Inflammatory bowel disease.
Pseudomembranous enterocolitis.

<5 YR

Infectious colitis.
Anal fissure.
Polyp.
Intussusception.
Meckel diverticulum.
Henoch-Schönlein purpura.
Hemolytic uremic syndrome.
Inflammatory bowel disease.
Pseudomembranous enterocolitis.

5 TO 18 YR

Infectious colitis.
Inflammatory bowel disease.
Pseudomembranous enterocolitis.
Polyp.
Hemolytic-uremic syndrome.
Hemorrhoid.

BLEEDING, RECTAL[38]

ICD-9CM # 578.9

IN PATIENTS <40 YR

Very common:

Hemorrhoids.
Anal fissure.
Inflammatory bowel disease (mainly proctitis).

Less common:

Polyps (hamartomatous or adenomatous).
Infective colitis.
Meckel's diverticulum.
Intussusception.

Rare:

Colorectal cancer.

IN PATIENTS >40 YR

Hemorrhoids.
Anal fissure.
Colorectal cancer.
Colorectal polyps (mostly adenomas).
Angiodysplasia.
Diverticular disease.
Inflammatory bowel disease.
Ischemic colitis.
Infective colitis.

BLEEDING, UPPER GI

ICD-9CM # 578.9

(ORIGINATING ABOVE THE LIGAMENT OF TREITZ)

Oral or pharyngeal lesions: swallowed blood from nose or oropharynx.

Swallowed Hemoptysis

Esophageal: varices, ulceration, esophagitis, Mallory-Weiss tear, carcinoma, trauma.
Gastric: peptic ulcer (including Cushing and Curling's ulcers), gastritis, angiodysplasia, gastric neoplasms, hiatal hernia, gastric diverticulum, pseudoxanthoma elasticum, Rendu-Osler-Weber syndrome.
Duodenal: peptic ulcer, duodenitis, angiodysplasia, aortoduodenal fistula, duodenal diverticulum, duodenal tumors, carcinoma of ampulla of Vater, parasites (e.g., hookworm), Crohn's disease.
Biliary: hematobilia (e.g., penetrating injury to liver, hepatobiliary malignancy, endoscopic papillotomy).

BLEEDING, UPPER GI, PEDIATRIC[2]

ICD-9CM # 578.9

<3 MO

Swallowed maternal blood.
Gastritis.
Ulcer, stress.
Bleeding diathesis.
Foreign body (NG tube).
Vascular malformation.
Duplication.

<2 YR

Esophagitis.
Gastritis.
Ulcer.
Pyloric stenosis.
Mallory-Weiss syndrome.
Vascular malformation.
Duplication.

<5 YR

Esophagitis.
Gastritis.
Ulcer.
Esophageal varices.
Foreign body.
Mallory-Weiss syndrome.
Hemophilia.
Vascular malformations.

5 TO 18 YR

Esophagitis.
Gastritis.

Ulcer.
Esophageal varices.
Mallory-Weiss syndrome.
Inflammatory bowel disease.
Hemophilia.
Vascular malformation.

BLINDNESS, GERIATRIC AGE

ICD-9CM # 369.4

Cataracts.
Glaucoma.
Diabetic retinopathy.
Macular degeneration.
Trauma.
CVA.
Corneal scarring.
Giant cell arteritis.
Ocular herpes zoster.

BLINDNESS, MONOCULAR, TRANSIENT

ICD-9CM # 369.67

Migraine (vasospasm).
Embolic cerebrovascular disease.
Intermittent angle-closure glaucoma.
Partial retinal vein occlusion.
Hyphema.
Optic disc edema.
Giant cell arteritis.
Psychogenic.
Hypotension.
Hypercoagulopathy disorders.
Multiple sclerosis.

BLINDNESS, PEDIATRIC AGE[23]

ICD-9CM # varies with specific disorder

CONGENITAL

Optic nerve hypoplasia or aplasia.
Optic coloboma.
Congenital hydrocephalus.
Hydranencephaly.
Porencephaly.
Microencephaly.
Encephalocele, particularly occipital type.
Morning glory disc.
Aniridia.
Anterior microphthalmia.
Peter's anomaly.
Persistent pupillary membrane.
Glaucoma.
Cataracts.
Persistent hyperplastic primary vitreous.

PHAKOMATOSES

Tuberous sclerosis.
Neurofibromatosis (special association with optic glioma).
Sturge-Weber syndrome.
von Hippel–Lindau disease.

TUMORS

Retinoblastoma.
Optic glioma.
Perioptic meningioma.
Craniopharyngioma.
Cerebral glioma.
Posterior and intraventricular tumors when complicated by hydrocephalus.
Pseudotumor cerebri.

NEURODEGENERATIVE DISEASES

Cerebral storage disease.
Gangliosidoses, particularly Tay-Sachs disease (infantile amaurotic familial idiocy), Sandhoff's variant, generalized gangliosidosis.
Other lipidoses and ceroid lipofuscinoses, particularly the late-onset amaurotic familial idiocies such as those of Jansky-Bielschowsky and of Batten-Mayou-Spielmeyer-Vogt.
Mucopolysaccharidoses, particularly Hurler's syndrome and Hunter's syndrome.
Leukodystrophies (dysmyelination disorders), particularly metachromatic leukodystrophy and Canavan's disease.
Demyelinating sclerosis (myelinoclastic diseases), especially Schilder's disease and Devic's neuromyelitis optica.
Special types: Dawson's disease, Leigh's disease, Bassen-Kornzweig syndrome, Refsum's disease.
Retinal degenerations: retinitis pigmentosa and its variants, Leber's congenital type.
Optic atrophies: congenital autosomal recessive type, infantile and congenital autosomal dominant types, Leber's disease, and atrophies associated with hereditary ataxias—the types of Behr, of Marie, and of Sanger-Brown.

INFECTIOUS PROCESSES

Encephalitis, especially in the prenatal infection syndromes caused by *Toxoplasma gondii,* cytomegalovirus, rubella virus, *Treponema pallidum,* herpes simplex.
Meningitis, arachnoiditis.
Chorioretinitis.
Endophthalmitis.
Keratitis.

HEMATOLOGIC DISORDERS

Leukemia with central nervous system involvement.

VASCULAR AND CIRCULATORY DISORDERS

Collagen vascular diseases.
Arteriovenous malformations—intracerebral hemorrhage, subarachnoid hemorrhage.
Central retinal occlusion.

TRAUMA

Contusion or avulsion of optic nerves, chiasm, globe, cornea.
Cerebral contusion or laceration.
Intracerebral, subarachnoid, or subdural hemorrhage.

DRUGS AND TOXINS

Other

Retinopathy of prematurity.
Sclerocornea.
Conversion reaction.
Optic neuritis.
Osteopetrosis.

BLISTERS, SUBEPIDERMAL

ICD-9CM # 919.2

Burns.
Porphyria cutanea tarda.
Bullous pemphigoid.
Bullous drug reaction.
Arthropod bite reaction.
Toxic epidermal necrosis.
Dermatitis herpetiformis.
Polymorphous light eruption.
Variegate porphyria.
SLE.
Epidermolysis bullosa.
Pseudoporphyria.
Acute graft-versus-host reaction.
Linear IgA disease.
Leukocytoclastic vasculitis.
Pressure necrosis.
Urticaria pigmentosa.
Amyloidosis.

BONE LESIONS, PREFERENTIAL SITE OF ORIGIN[35]

ICD-9CM # 170.0 Skull and Face
170.1 Mandible
170.2 Vertebral Column
170.3 Ribs, Sternum, Clavicle
170.4 Scapula, Long Bones Upper Limb
170.5 Short Bones and Upper Limb
170.6 Pelvic Bones, Sacrum Coccyx
170.7 Long Bones Lower Limb
170.8 Short Bones Lower Limb
170.9 Bone Cancer NOS
198.5 Bone Cancer, Metastatic

EPIPHYSIS

Chondroblastoma.
Giant-cell tumor—after fusion of growth plate.
Langerhans' cell histiocytosis.
Clear cell chondrosarcoma.
Osteosarcoma.

METAPHYSIS

Parosteal sarcoma.
Chondrosarcoma.
Fibrosarcoma.
Nonossifying fibroma.
Giant-cell tumor—before fusion of growth plate.
Unicameral bone cyst.
Aneurysmal bone cyst.

DIAPHYSIS

Myeloma.
Ewing's tumor.
Reticulum cell sarcoma.

METADIAPHYSEAL

Fibrosarcoma.
Fibrous dysplasia.
Enchondroma.
Osteoid osteoma.
Chondromyofibroma.

BONE MARROW FAILURE SYNDROMES, INHERITED[20]

ICD-9CM # 284

BI-LINEAGE AND TRI-LINEAGE CYTOPENIAS

Fanconi anemia.
Shwachman-Diamond syndrome.
Dyskeratosis congenita.
Amegakaryocytic thrombocytopenia:
- Other inherited thrombocytopenia disorders.

Other genetic syndromes:
- Down's syndrome.
- Dubowitz syndrome.
- Seckel syndrome.
- Reticular dysgenesis.
- Schimke immunoosseous dysplasia.
- Noonan syndrome.
- Cartilage-hair hypoplasia.
- Familial marrow failure (non-Fanconi).

UNI-LINEAGE CYTOPENIA

Diamond-Blackfan anemia.
Kostmann syndrome/Congenital neutropenia:
- *ELA2* mutations.
- *HAX1* mutations.
- *GFI1* mutations.
- *WASP* mutations.
- Constitutive cell surface G-CSF-R mutations.

Other inherited neutropenia syndromes:
- Barth syndrome.
- Glycogen storage disease 1b.
- Miscellaneous.

Thrombocytopenia with absent radii.
Congenital dyserythropoietic anemias (CDAs):
- Types I, II, III, IV.
- Variants.
- Nonclassifiable CDAs.
- Groups IV, V, VI, VII.

BONE MARROW FIBROSIS[14]

ICD-9CM # 289.9

MYELOID DISORDERS

Myelofibrosis with myeloid metaplasia.
Metastatic cancer.
Chronic myeloid leukemia.
Myelodysplastic syndrome.
Atypical myeloid disorder.
Acute megakaryocytic leukemia.
Other acute myeloid leukemias.
Gray platelet syndrome.

LYMPHOID DISORDERS

Hairy cell leukemia.
Multiple myeloma.
Lymphoma.

NONHEMATOLOGIC DISORDERS

Connective tissue disorder.
Infections (tuberculosis, kala-azar).
Vitamin D–deficiency rickets.
Renal osteodystrophy.

BONE MINERAL DENSITY, INCREASED

ICD-9CM # 733.99

Paget's disease of bone.
Skeletal metastases.
DISH.
Osteonecrosis.
Sarcoidosis.
Hypoparathyroidism, pseudohypoparathyroidism.
Milk-alkali syndrome.
Osteopetrosis.
Hypervitaminosis A or D.
Dysplasias (craniodiaphyseal, craniometaphyseal, frontometaphyseal).
Endosteal hyperostosis.
Fluorosis.
Heavy metal poisoning.
Ionizing radiation.
Other: lymphoma, leukemia, mastocytosis, multiple myeloma, polycythemia vera.

BONE PAIN

ICD-9CM # code not available

Trauma.
Neoplasm (primary or metastatic).
Osteoporosis with compression fracture.
Paget's disease of bone.
Infection (osteomyelitis, septic arthritis).
Osteomalacia.
Viral syndrome.
Sickle cell disease.
Anxiety.

BONE RESORPTION[35]

ICD-9CM # 733.90 Bone Disorder

DISTAL CLAVICLE

Hyperparathyroidism.
RA.
Scleroderma.
Posttraumatic osteolysis.
Progeria.
Pycnodysostosis.
Cleidocranial dysplasia.

INFERIOR ASPECT OF RIBS

Vascular impression, associated with but not limited to coarctation of the aorta.
Hyperparathyroidism.
Neurofibromatosis.

TERMINAL PHALANGEAL TUFTS

Scleroderma.
Raynaud's phenomenon.
Vascular disease.
Frostbite, electrical burns.
Psoriasis.
Tabes dorsalis.
Hyperparathyroidism.

GENERALIZED RESORPTION

Paraplegia.
Myositis ossificans.
Osteoporosis.

BRADYCARDIA, SINUS[15]

ICD-9CM # 427.89

Idiopathic.
Degenerative processes (e.g., Lev's disease, Lenègre's disease).
Medications
Beta-blockers.
Some calcium channel blockers (diltiazem, verapamil).
Digoxin (when vagal tone is high).
Class I antiarrhythmic agents (e.g., procainamide).
Class III antiarrhythmic agents (amiodarone, sotalol).
Clonidine.
Lithium carbonate.
Acute Myocardial Ischemia and Infarction
Right or left circumflex coronary artery occlusion or spasm.
High vagal tone (e.g., athletes).

BREAST INFLAMMATORY LESION[12]

ICD-9CM # 611.0 Acute Mastitis
610.1 Chronic Cystic Mastitis
771.5 Neonatal Infective Mastitis
778.7 Neonatal Noninfective Mastitis

Mastitis (*S. aureus,* beta-hemolytic *Streptococcus*).
Trauma.
Foreign body (sutures, breast implants).
Granuloma (TB, fungal).
Fat necrosis post biopsy.
Necrosis or infarction (anticoagulant therapy, pregnancy).
Breast malignancy.

BREAST MASS

ICD-9CM # 611.72

Fibrocystic breasts.
Benign tumors (fibroadenoma, papilloma).
Mastitis (acute bacterial mastitis, chronic mastitis).
Malignant neoplasm.
Fat necrosis.
Hematoma.
Duct ectasia.
Mammary adenosis.

BREATH ODOR[34]

ICD-9CM # 784.9 Halitosis

Sweet, fruity: DKA, starvation ketosis.
Fishy, stale: uremia (trimethylamines).
Ammonia-like: uremia (ammonia).
Musty fish, clover: fetor hepaticus (hepatic failure).
Foul, feculent: intestinal obstruction/diverticulum.

Foul, putrid: nasal/sinus pathology (infection, foreign body, cancer), respiratory infections (empyema, lung abscess, bronchiectasis).
Halitosis: tonsillitis, gingivitis, respiratory infections, Vincent's angina, gastroesophageal reflux, achalasia.
Cinnamon: pulmonary TB.

BREATHING, NOISY[34]

ICD-9CM # 786.09 Breathing, Labored
789.09 Snoring, Wheezing
786.1 Stridor

Infection: upper respiratory infection, peritonsillar abscess, retropharyngeal abscess, epiglottitis, laryngitis, tracheitis, bronchitis, bronchiolitis.
Irritants and allergens: hyperactive airway, asthma (reactive airway disease), rhinitis, angioneurotic edema.
Compression from outside of the airway: esophageal cysts or foreign body, neoplasms, lymphadenopathy.
Congenital malformation and abnormality: vascular rings, laryngeal webs, laryngomalacia, tracheomalacia, hemangiomas within the upper airway, stenoses within the upper airway, cystic fibrosis.
Acquired abnormality (at every level of the airway): nasal polyps, hypertrophied adenoids and/or tonsils, foreign body, intraluminal tumors, bronchiectasis.
Neurogenic disorder: vocal cord paralysis.

BROWN URINE

ICD-9CM # 788.69

Bile pigments.
Myoglobin.
Concentrated urine.
Use of multivitamin supplements.
Medications (antimalarials, metronidazole, nitrofurantoin, levodopa, methyldopa, Phenazopyridine).
Diet rich in fava beans.
Urinary tract infection.

BRUISING

ICD-9CM # 459.89

Medication-induced (warfarin, aspirin, NSAIDs, prednisone).
Alcohol abuse.
Senile purpura.
Purpura simplex.
Physical abuse.
Vasculitis.
Platelet disorders.
Coagulation factor deficiencies.
Cushing's disease.
Vitamin C deficiency.
Marfan's syndrome.
Ehlers-Danlos syndrome.
Disseminated intravascular coagulation.
Leukemia.
Hereditary hemorrhagic telangiectasia.

BULLOUS DISEASES

ICD-9CM # 694.9 Bullous Dermatoses
694.5 Bullous Pemphigoid
694.4 Pemphigus Vulgaris
694.4 Pemphigus Foliaceus

Bullous pemphigoid.
Pemphigus vulgaris.
Pemphigus foliaceus.
Paraneoplastic pemphigus.
Cicatricial pemphigoid.
Erythema multiforme.
Dermatitis herpetiformis.
Herpes gestationis.
Impetigo.
Erosive lichen planus.
Linear IgA bullous dermatosis.
Epidermolysis bullosa acquisita.

CALCIFICATION ON CHEST X-RAY

ICD-9CM # 722.92

Lung neoplasm (primary or metastatic).
Silicosis.
Idiopathic pulmonary fibrosis.
Tuberculosis.
Histoplasmosis.
Disseminated varicella infection.
Mitral stenosis (end-stage).
Secondary hyperparathyroidism.

CALCIFICATIONS, CUTANEOUS

ICD-9CM # 709.3

Calcification, Raynaud's phenomenon, esophageal dysmotility, sclerodactyly, and telangiectasia (CREST) syndrome.
Trauma.
Pancreatitis or pancreatic cancer.
Chronic renal failure.
Sarcoidosis.
Hyperparathyroidism.
Milk-alkali syndrome.
Hypervitaminosis D.
Panniculitis.
Idiopathic.
Iatrogenic (e.g., application of calcium alginate dressing to skin).
Multiple myeloma.
Dermatomyositis.
Parasitic infections.
Leukemia.
Lymphoma.

CALCIUM STONES

ICD-9CM # 592.9

Medications (e.g., antacids, loop diuretics, vitamin D, acetazolamide, glucocorticoids).
Primary hyperparathyroidism.
Hypercalcemia from malignancy.
Sarcoidosis.
Prolonged immobilization.
Hyperoxaluria (e.g., Crohn's disease, celiac disease, chronic pancreatitis).
Hyperuricosuria (e.g., hyperuricemia, excessive dietary purine, allopurinol, probenecid).
Renal tubular acidosis.
Milk-alkali syndrome.
Thyrotoxicosis.
Hypocitraturia (e.g., metabolic acidosis, hypomagnesemia, hypokalemia).

CARDIAC ARREST, NONTRAUMATIC[26]

ICD-9CM # 427.5 Cardiac Arrest NOS

Cardiac (coronary artery disease, cardiomyopathies, structural abnormalities, valve dysfunction, arrhythmias).
Respiratory (upper airway obstruction, hypoventilation, pulmonary embolism, asthma, COPD exacerbation, pulmonary edema).
Circulatory (tension pneumothorax, pericardial tamponade, PE, hemorrhage, sepsis).
Electrolyte abnormalities (hypokalemia or hyperkalemia, hypomagnesemia or hypermagnesemia, hypocalcemia).
Medications (tricyclic antidepressants, digoxin, theophylline, calcium channel blockers).
Drug abuse (cocaine, heroin, amphetamines).
Toxins (carbon monoxide, cyanide).
Environmental (drowning/near-drowning, electrocution, lightning, hypothermia or hyperthermia, venomous snakes).

CARDIAC DEATH, SUDDEN[1]

ICD-9CM # varies with specific disorder

NONCARDIAC

CNS hemorrhage.
Massive pulmonary embolus.
Drug overdose.
Hypoxia secondary to lung disease.
Aortic dissection or rupture.

CARDIAC

Ventricular tachycardia.
Bradyarrhythmia, sick sinus syndrome.
Aortic stenosis.
Tetralogy of Fallot.
Pericardial tamponade.
Cardiac tumors.
Complications of infective endocarditis.
Hypertrophic cardiomyopathy (arrhythmia or obstruction).
Myocardial ischemia.
Atherosclerosis.
Prinzmetal's angina.
Kawasaki's arteritis.

CARDIAC ENLARGEMENT[15]

ICD-9CM # 429.3 Cardiomegaly, Idiopathic
746.89 Cardiomegaly, Congenital
402.0 Cardiomegaly, Malignant
402.1 Cardiomegaly, Benign

CARDIAC CHAMBER ENLARGEMENT

Chronic Volume Overload

Mitral or aortic regurgitation.
Left-to-right shunt (PDA, VSD, AV fistula).

Cardiomyopathy

Ischemic.
Nonischemic.

Decompensated Pressure Overload

Aortic stenosis.
Hypertension.

High-Output States

Severe anemia.
Thyrotoxicosis.

Bradycardia

Severe sinus bradycardia.
Complete heart block.

LEFT ATRIUM

LV failure of any cause.
Mitral valve disease.
Myxoma.

RIGHT VENTRICLE

Chronic volume overload.
Tricuspid or pulmonic regurgitation.
Left-to-right shunt (ASD).
Decompensated pressure overload:
Pulmonic stenosis.
Pulmonary artery hypertension:
- Primary.
- Secondary (PE, COPD).

Pulmonary venoocclusive disease.

RIGHT ATRIUM

RV failure of any cause.
Tricuspid valve disease.
Myxoma.
Ebstein's anomaly.

MULTICHAMBER ENLARGEMENT

Hypertrophic cardiomyopathy.
Acromegaly.
Severe obesity.

PERICARDIAL DISEASE

Pericardial effusion with or without tamponade.
Effusive constrictive disease.
Pericardial cyst, loculated effusion.

PSEUDOCARDIOMEGALY

Epicardial fat.
Chest wall deformity (pectus excavatum, straight back syndrome).
Low lung volumes.
AP chest x-ray.
Mediastinal tumor, cyst.

CARDIAC MURMURS

ICD-9CM # varies with specific disorder

SYSTOLIC

Mitral regurgitation (MR).
Tricuspid regurgitation (TR).
Ventricular septal defect (VSD).
Aortic stenosis (AS).
Idiopathic hypertrophic subaortic stenosis (IHSS).
Pulmonic stenosis (PS).
Innocent murmur of childhood.
Coarctation of aorta.
Mitral valve prolapse (MVP).

DIASTOLIC

Aortic regurgitation (AR).
Atrial myxoma.
Mitral stenosis (MS).
Pulmonary artery branch stenosis.
Tricuspid stenosis (TS).
Graham Steell murmur (diastolic decrescendo murmur heard in severe pulmonary hypertension).
Pulmonic regurgitation (PR).
Severe mitral regurgitation (MR).
Austin Flint murmur (diastolic rumble heard in severe AR).
Severe VSD and patent ductus arteriosus.

CONTINUOUS

Patent ductus arteriosus.
Pulmonary AV fistula.

CARDIOEMBOLISM

ICD-9CM # 410.9

Acute MI.
Atrial fibrillation.
Left ventricular aneurysm.
Valvular heart disease (e.g., rheumatic mitral valve disease, mitral valve prolapse).
Dilated cardiomyopathy.
Atrial septal defect.
Patent foramen ovale.
Cardioversion for atrial fibrillation.
Infective endocarditis.
Atrial septal aneurysm.
Sick sinus syndrome and cardiac arrhythmias.
Nonbacterial thrombotic endocarditis.
Prosthetic heart valves.
Atrial myxoma and other intracardiac tumors.
Cyanotic heart disease.
Balloon angioplasty.
Coronary artery bypass grafting.
Aneurysms of sinus of Valsalva.
Other: VVI pacing, ventricular support devices, heart transplantation, intracardiac defects with paradoxical embolism.

CARDIOGENIC SHOCK

ICD-9CM # 785.51

Myocardial infarction.
Arrhythmias.
Pericardial effusion/tamponade.
Chest trauma.
Valvular heart disease.
Myocarditis.
Cardiomyopathy.
CHF, end-stage.

CAVITARY LESION ON CHEST X-RAY[16]

ICD-9CM # 793.1 Chest X-Ray Lung Shadow

NECROTIZING INFECTIONS

Bacteria: anaerobes, *Staphylococcus aureus,* enteric gram-negative bacteria, *Pseudomonas aeruginosa, Legionella* species, *Haemophilus influenzae, Streptococcus pyogenes, Streptococcus pneumoniae* (?), *Rhodococcus, Actinomyces.*
Mycobacteria: *Mycobacterium tuberculosis, Mycobacterium kansasii,* MAI.
Bacteria-like: *Nocardia* species.
Fungi: *Coccidioides immitis, Histoplasma capsulatum, Blastomyces hominis, Aspergillus* species, *Mucor* species.
Parasitic: *Entamoeba histolytica, Echinococcus, Paragonimus westermani.*

CAVITARY INFARCTION

Bland infarction (with or without superimposed infection).
Lung contusion.

SEPTIC EMBOLISM

S. aureus, anaerobes, others.

VASCULITIS

Wegener's granulomatosis, periarteritis.

NEOPLASMS

Bronchogenic carcinoma, metastatic carcinoma, lymphoma.

MISCELLANEOUS LESIONS

Cysts, blebs, bullae, or pneumatocele with or without fluid collections.
Sequestration.
Empyema with air-fluid level.
Bronchiectasis.

CEREBRAL INFARCTION SECONDARY TO INHERITED DISORDERS

ICD-9CM # 434.91

Homocystinuria.
Marfan's syndrome.
Ehlers-Danlos syndrome.
Rendu-Osler-Weber syndrome.
Pseudoxanthoma elasticum.
Fabry's disease.

CEREBROVASCULAR DISEASE, ISCHEMIC[40]

ICD-9CM # 437.9

VASCULAR DISORDERS

Large-vessel atherothrombotic disease.
Lacunar disease.
Arterial-to-arterial embolization.
Carotid or vertebral artery dissection.

Fibromuscular dysplasia.
Migraine.
Venous thrombosis.
Radiation.
Complications of arteriography.
Multiple, progressive intracranial arterial occlusions.

INFLAMMATORY DISORDERS

Giant cell arteritis.
Polyarteritis nodosa.
SLE.
Granulomatous angiitis.
Takayasu's disease.
Arteritis associated with amphetamine, cocaine, or phenylpropanolamine.
Syphilis, mucormycosis.
Sjögren's syndrome.
Behçet's syndrome.

CARDIAC DISORDERS

Rheumatic heart disease.
Mural thrombus.
Arrhythmias.
Mitral valve prolapse.
Prosthetic heart valve.
Endocarditis.
Myxoma.
Paradoxical embolus.

HEMATOLOGIC DISORDERS

Thrombotic thrombocytopenic purpura.
Sickle cell disease.
Hypercoagulable states.
Polycythemia.
Thrombocytosis.
Leukocytosis.
Lupus anticoagulant.

CHEST PAIN, CHILDREN[4]

ICD-9CM # 786.50 Chest Pain NOS
786.59 Chest Pressure
786.52 Chest Pain, Pleuritic

MUSCULOSKELETAL (COMMON)

Trauma (accidental, abuse).
Exercise, overuse injury (strain, bursitis).
Costochondritis (Tietze's syndrome).
Herpes zoster (cutaneous).
Pleurodynia.
Fibrositis.
Slipping rib.
Sickle cell anemia vasoocclusive crisis.
Osteomyelitis (rare).
Primary or metastatic tumor (rare).

PULMONARY (COMMON)

Pneumonia.
Pleurisy.
Asthma.
Chronic cough.
Pneumothorax.
Infarction (sickle cell anemia).
Foreign body.
Embolism (rare).
Pulmonary hypertension (rare).
Tumor (rare).

GASTROINTESTINAL (LESS COMMON)

Esophagitis (gastroesophageal reflux).
Esophageal foreign body.
Esophageal spasm.
Cholecystitis.
Subdiaphragmatic abscess.
Perihepatitis (Fitz-Hugh-Curtis syndrome).
Peptic ulcer disease.

CARDIAC (LESS COMMON)

Pericarditis.
Postpericardiotomy syndrome.
Endocarditis.
Mitral valve prolapse.
Aortic or subaortic stenosis.
Arrhythmias.
Marfan's syndrome (dissecting aortic aneurysm).
Anomalous coronary artery.
Kawasaki disease.
Cocaine, sympathomimetic ingestion.
Angina (familial hypercholesterolemia).

IDIOPATHIC (COMMON)

Anxiety, hyperventilation.
Panic disorder.

OTHER (LESS COMMON)

Spinal cord or nerve root compression.
Breast-related pathologic condition.
Castleman's disease (lymph node neoplasm).

CHEST PAIN (NONPLEURITIC)[9]

ICD-9CM # 786.50 Chest Pain NOS
786.59 Chest Discomfort

Cardiac: myocardial ischemia/infarction, myocarditis.
Esophageal: spasm, esophagitis, ulceration, neoplasm, achalasia, diverticula, foreign body.
Referred pain from subdiaphragmatic GI structures.
Gastric and duodenal: hiatal hernia, neoplasm, PUD.
Gallbladder and biliary: cholecystitis, cholelithiasis, impacted stone, neoplasm.
Pancreatic: pancreatitis, neoplasm.
Dissecting aortic aneurysm.
Pain originating from skin, breasts, and musculoskeletal structures: herpes zoster, mastitis, cervical spondylosis.
Mediastinal tumors: lymphoma, thymoma.
Pulmonary: neoplasm, pneumonia, pulmonary embolism/infarction.
Psychoneurosis.
Chest pain associated with mitral valve prolapse.

CHEST PAIN (PLEURITIC)

ICD-9CM # 786.52 Chest Pain, Pleuritic

Cardiac: pericarditis, postpericardiotomy/Dressler's syndrome.
Pulmonary: pneumothorax, hemothorax, embolism/infarction, pneumonia, empyema, neoplasm, bronchiectasis, pneumomediastinum, TB, carcinomatous effusion.
GI: liver abscess, pancreatitis, esophageal rupture, Whipple's disease with associated pericarditis or pleuritis.
Subdiaphragmatic abscess.
Pain originating from skin and musculoskeletal tissues: costochondritis, chest wall trauma, fractured rib, interstitial fibrositis, myositis, strain of pectoralis muscle, herpes zoster, soft tissue and bone tumors.
Collagen vascular diseases with pleuritis.
Psychoneurosis.
Familial Mediterranean fever.

CHOLESTASIS[14]

ICD-9CM # 574.71

EXTRAHEPATIC

Choledocholithiasis.
Bile duct stricture.
Cholangiocarcinoma.
Pancreatic carcinoma.
Chronic pancreatitis.
Papillary stenosis.
Ampullary cancer.
Primary sclerosing cholangitis.
Choledochal cysts.
Parasites (e.g., ascaris, clonorchis).
AIDS.
Cholangiography.
Biliary atresia.
Portal lymphadenopathy.
Mirizzi's syndrome.

INTRAHEPATIC

Viral hepatitis.
Alcoholic hepatitis.
Drug induced.
Ductopenia syndromes.
Primary biliary cirrhosis.
Benign recurrent intrahepatic cholestasis.
Byler's disease.
Primary sclerosing cholangitis.
Alagille's syndrome.
Sarcoid.
Lymphoma.
Postoperative.
Total parenteral nutrition.
Alpha-1-antitrypsin deficiency.

CHOREA

ICD-9CM # 333.5

Medications (e.g., neuroleptics, tricyclics, antiparkinsonian drugs).
Cerebral palsy.
Huntington's disease.
Benign hereditary chorea.
Thyroid disorder (hyperthyroidism, hypothyroidism).
Friedreich's ataxia.
Ataxia-telangiectasia.
Hypoglycemia, hyperglycemia.
Electrolyte abnormalities (hyponatremia, hypocalcemia, hypomagnesemia, hypernatremia).
Vitamin B_{12} deficiency.
SLE.
Wilson's disease.
Alcohol.

Cocaine.
Carbon monoxide poisoning.
Mercury poisoning.

CHOREOATHETOSIS[28]

ICD-9CM # 275.1 Choreoathetosis-Agitans Syndrome
33.5 Choreoathetosis Paroxysmal

SYSTEMIC DISEASES

SLE.
Polycythemia.
Thyrotoxicosis.
Rheumatic fever.
Cirrhosis of the liver (acquired hepatocerebral degeneration).
DM.
Wilson's disease.

PRIMARY DEGENERATIVE BRAIN DISEASES

Huntington's chorea.
Olivopontocerebellar atrophies.
Neuroacanthocytosis.

FOCAL BRAIN DISEASES

Hemichorea.
Stroke.
Tumor.
Arteriovenous malformation.

DRUG-INDUCED CHOREOATHETOSIS

Parkinson's Disease Drugs
Levodopa.
Epilepsy Drugs
Phenytoin.
Carbamazepine.
Phenobarbital.
Gabapentin.
Valproate.
Psychostimulant Drugs
Cocaine.
Amphetamine.
Methamphetamine.
Dextroamphetamine.
Methylphenidate.
Pemoline.
Psychotropic Drugs
Lithium.
Tricyclic antidepressant drugs.
Oral Contraceptive Drugs
Cimetidine.

CHYLOTHORAX

ICD-9CM # 457.8

Post lymph node dissection of neck or chest.
Subclavian venous catheterization.
Thoracic aneurysm repair.
Trauma to chest and neck.
Mediastinal tumor resection.
Esophagectomy, pneumonectomy.
Lymphangitis, mediastinitis.
Neoplasms (lymphoma, carcinoma of esophagus, lung, mediastinal malignancies).
Sympathectomy.
Venous thrombosis.
Congenital.

CLOUDY URINE

ICD-9CM # 788.69

Concentrated urine.
Use of multivitamin supplements.
Diet high in purine-rich foods.
Pyuria.
Phosphaturia.
Urinary tract infection.
Lipiduria.
Chyluria.
Hyperoxaluria.

CLUBBING

ICD-9CM # 781.5 Clubbing Finger

Pulmonary neoplasm (lung, pleura).
Other neoplasm (GI, liver, Hodgkin's, thymus, osteogenic sarcoma).
Pulmonary infectious process (empyema, abscess, bronchiectasis, TB, chronic pneumonitis).
Extrapulmonary infectious process (subacute bacterial endocarditis, intestinal TB, bacterial or amebic dysentery, arterial graft sepsis).
Pneumoconiosis.
Cystic fibrosis.
Sarcoidosis.
Cyanotic congenital heart disease.
Endocrine (Graves' disease, hyperparathyroidism).
Inflammatory bowel disease.
Celiac disease.
Chronic liver disease, cirrhosis (particularly biliary and juvenile).
Pulmonary AV malformations.
Idiopathic.
Thyroid acropachy.
Hereditary (pachydermoperiostosis).
Chronic trauma (jackhammer operators, machine workers).

COBALAMIN DEFICIENCY[20]

ICD-9CM # 266.2

ETIOPATHOPHYSIOLOGIC CLASSIFICATION OF COBALAMIN DEFICIENCY

Nutritional cobalamin deficiency (i.e., insufficient cobalamin intake):
  Vegetarians, poverty-imposed near-vegetarians, breast-fed infants of mothers with pernicious anemia.
Abnormal intragastric events (i.e., inadequate proteolysis of food cobalamin):
  Atrophic gastritis, partial gastritis with hypochlorhydria, proton-pump inhibitors, H_2 blockers.
Loss or atrophy of gastric oxyntic mucosa (i.e., deficient intrinsic factor [IF] molecules):
  Total or partial gastrectomy, pernicious anemia, caustic destruction (lye).
Abnormal events in small bowel lumen:
  Inadequate pancreatic protease (e.g., R-cobalamin not degraded, cobalamin not transferred to IF):
  - Insufficient pancreatic protease (i.e., pancreatic insufficiency).
  - Inactivation of pancreatic protease (i.e., Zollinger–Ellison syndrome).

  Usurping of luminal cobalamin (i.e., inadequate cobalamin binding to IF):
  - By bacteria, during stasis syndromes (e.g., blind loops, pouches of diverticulosis, strictures, fistulas, anastomosis), impaired bowel motility (e.g., scleroderma), hypogammaglobulinemia.
  - By *Diphyllobothrium latum* (fish tapeworm).

Disorders of ileal mucosa/IF–cobalamin receptors (i.e., IF–cobalamin not bound to IF–cobalamin receptors):
  Diminished or absent IF–cobalamin receptors (e.g., ileal bypass, resection, fistula).
  Abnormal mucosal architecture/function (e.g., tropical or nontropical sprue, Crohn's disease, tuberculosis ileitis, infiltration by lymphomas, amyloidosis).
  IF-/post-IF–cobalamin receptor defects (e.g., Imerslund–Gräsbeck syndrome, transcobalamin II [TC II] deficiency).
  Drug effects (e.g., slow K, metformin, cholestyramine, colchicine, neomycin).
Disorders of plasma cobalamin transport (i.e., TC II–cobalamin not delivered to TC II receptors):
  Congenital TC II deficiency, defective binding of TC II–cobalamin to TC II receptors (rare).
Metabolic disorders (i.e., cobalamin not used by cells):
  Inborn enzyme errors (rare).
  Acquired disorders (e.g., cobalamin functionally inactivated by irreversible oxidation, N_2O inhalation).

COLIC, ACUTE ABDOMINAL[38]

ICD-9CM # 789.0

Acute gastroenteritis.
Food poisoning.
Non-specific causes.
Constipation.
Gastric outlet obstruction:
- Chronic peptic ulceration.
- Gastric cancer.

Small bowel obstruction:
  Adhesions:
  - Postsurgical.
  - Inflammatory (e.g., diverticular).
  - Radiation.
  - Meckel's diverticulum.
  - Metastatic.

  Stricture:
  - Ischemic.
  - Radiation.
  - Inflammatory (e.g., Crohn's disease).

  Volvulus Intussusception:
  - Tumor (e.g., Peutz-Jegher's syndrome).
  - Superior mesenteric artery syndrome.

Intraluminal bolus:
- Gallstone.
- Bezoar.

Hernia:
- Abdominal wall.
- Internal.

Neoplasm:
- Benign (e.g., leiomyoma).
- Malignant (e.g., carcinoid tumor, adenocarcinoma).

Large bowel obstruction:
- Colon cancer.
- Diverticular disease.
- Volvulus.

Uterine:
- Missed abortion.
- Parturition.
- Period pain.

COLOR CHANGES, CUTANEOUS[34]

ICD-9CM # 709.00 Pigmentation Anomaly

BROWN

Generalized: pituitary, adrenal, liver disease, ACTH-producing tumor (e.g., oat cell lung carcinoma).
Localized: nevi, neurofibromatosis.

WHITE

Generalized: albinism.
Localized: vitiligo, Raynaud's syndrome.

RED (ERYTHEMA)

Generalized: fever, polycythemia, urticaria, viral exanthems.
Localized: inflammation, infection, Raynaud's syndrome.

YELLOW

Generalized: liver disease, chronic renal disease, anemia.
Generalized (except sclera): hypothyroidism, increased intake of vegetables containing carotene.
Localized: resolving hematoma, infection, peripheral vascular insufficiency.

BLUE

Lips, mouth, nail beds: cardiovascular and pulmonary diseases, Raynaud's.

COMA

ICD-9CM # 780.01

Vascular: hemorrhage, thrombosis, embolism.
CNS infections: meningitis, encephalitis, cerebral abscess.
Cerebral neoplasms with herniation.
Head injury: subdural hematoma, cerebral concussion, cerebral contusion.
Drugs: narcotics, sedatives, hypnotics.
Ingestion or inhalation of toxins: CO, alcohol, lead.
Metabolic disturbances.
Hypoxia.
Acid-base disorders.
Hypoglycemia, hyperglycemia.
Hepatic failure.
Electrolyte disorders.
Uremia.
Hypothyroidism.
Hypothermia, hyperthermia.
Hypotension, malignant hypertension.
Postictal.

COMA, NORMAL COMPUTED TOMOGRAPHY[1]

ICD-9CM # 780.01

MENINGEAL DISORDERS

Subarachnoid hemorrhage (uncommon).
Bacterial meningitis.
Encephalitis.
Subdural empyema.

EXOGENOUS TOXINS

Sedative drugs and barbiturates.
Anesthetics and γ-hydroxybutyrate.*
Alcohols.
Stimulants:
  Phencyclidines.†
  Cocaine and amphetamines.‡
Psychotropic drugs:
  Cyclic antidepressants.
  Phenothiazines.
  Lithium.
Anticonvulsants.
Opioids.
Clonidine.§
Penicillins.
Salicylates.
Anticholinergics.
Carbon monoxide, cyanide, and methemoglobinemia.

ENDOGENOUS TOXINS/ DEFICIENCIES/DERANGEMENTS

Hypoxia and ischemia.
Hypoglycemia.
Hypercalcemia.
Osmolar:
  Hyperglycemia.
  Hyponatremia.
  Hypernatremia.
Organ system failure:
  Hepatic encephalopathy.
  Uremic encephalopathy.
  Pulmonary insufficiency (carbon dioxide narcosis).

SEIZURES

Prolonged postictal state.
Spike-wave stupor.

HYPOTHERMIA OR HYPERTHERMIA

Brain stem ischemia.
Basilar artery stroke.
Brain stem or cerebellar hemorrhage.
Conversion or malingering.

---

*General anesthetic, similar to γ-aminobutyric acid; recreational drug and body building aid. Rapid onset, rapid recovery often with myoclonic jerking and confusion. Deep coma (2-3 hr; Glasgow Coma Scale = 3) with maintenance of vital signs.

†Coma associated with cholinergic signs: lacrimation, salivation, bronchorrhea, and hyperthermia.

‡Coma after seizures or status (i.e., a prolonged postictal state).

§An antihypertensive agent active through the opiate receptor system; frequent overdose when used to treat narcotic withdrawal.

COMA, PEDIATRIC POPULATION[31]

ICD-9CM # 780.01

ANOXIA

Birth asphyxia.
Carbon monoxide poisoning.
Croup/epiglottitis.
Meconium aspiration.

INFECTION

Hemolysis.
Blood loss.
Hydrops fetalis.
Infection.
Meningoencephalitis.
Sepsis.
Postimmunization encephalitis.

INCREASED INTRACRANIAL PRESSURE

Anoxia.
Inborn metabolic errors.
Toxic encephalopathy.
Reye's syndrome.
Head trauma/intracranial bleed.
Hydrocephalus.
Posterior fossa tumors.

HYPERTENSIVE ENCEPHALOPATHY

Coarctation of aorta.
Nephritis.
Vasculitis.
Pheochromocytoma.

ISCHEMIA

Hypoplastic left heart.
Shunting lesions.
Aortic stenosis.
Cardiovascular collapse (any cause).

PURPURIC CAUSES

Disseminated intravascular coagulation.
Hemolytic-uremic syndrome.
Leukemia.
Thrombotic purpura.

HYPERCAPNIA

Cystic fibrosis.
Bronchopulmonary dysplasia.
Congenital lung anomalies.

NEOPLASM

Medulloblastoma.
Glioma of brain stem.
Posterior fossa tumors.

DRUGS/TOXINS

Maternal sedation.
Alcohol.
Any drug.
Lead.
Salicylism.
Arsenic.
Pesticides.

ELECTROLYTE ABNORMALITIES

Hypernatremia (diarrhea, dehydration, salt poisoning).
Hyponatremia (SIADH, androgenital syndrome, gastroenteritis).
Hyperkalemia (renal failure, salicylism, androgenitalism).
Hypokalemia (diarrhea, hyperaldosteronism, salicylism, DKA).
Hypocalcemia (vitamin D deficiency, hyperparathyroidism).
Severe acidosis (sepsis, cold injury, salicylism, DKA).

HYPOGLYCEMIA

Birth injury or stress.
Diabetes.
Alcohol.
Salicylism.
Hyperinsulinemia.
Iatrogenic.

POSTSEIZURE

Renal Causes
Nephritis.
Hypoplastic kidneys.
Hepatic Causes
Acute hepatitis.
Fulminant hepatic failure.
Inborn metabolic errors.
Bile duct atresia.

CONJUNCTIVAL NEOPLASM

ICD-9CM # varies with specific disorder

MALIGNANT

Squamous cell carcinoma.
Melanoma.
Sebaceous carcinoma.
Kaposi's sarcoma.
Metastatic neoplasms.

BENIGN

Melanocytic nevus.
Squamous papilloma.
Hemangioma.
Lymphangioma.
Myxoma.

CONSTIPATION

ICD-9CM # 564.0

Intestinal obstruction.
Fecal impaction.
Diverticular disease.
GI neoplasm.
Strangulated femoral hernia.
Gallstone ileus.
Tuberculous stricture.
Adhesions.
Ameboma.
Volvulus.
Intussusception.
Inflammatory bowel disease.
Hematoma of bowel wall, secondary to trauma or anticoagulants.
Poor dietary habits: insufficient bulk in diet, inadequate fluid intake.
Change from daily routine: travel, hospital admission, physical inactivity.
Acute abdominal conditions: renal colic, salpingitis, biliary colic, appendicitis, ischemia.
Hypercalcemia or hypokalemia, uremia.
Irritable bowel syndrome, pregnancy, anorexia nervosa, depression.
Painful anal conditions: hemorrhoids, fissure, stricture.
Decreased intestinal peristalsis: old age, spinal cord injuries, myxedema, diabetes, multiple sclerosis, Parkinsonism and other neurologic diseases.
Drugs: codeine, morphine, antacids with aluminum, verapamil, anticonvulsants, anticholinergics, disopyramide, cholestyramine, alosetron, iron supplements.
Hirschsprung's disease, meconium ileus, congenital atresia in infants.

CONSTIPATION, ADULT PATIENT[38]

ICD-9CM # 564

NO GROSS STRUCTURAL ABNORMALITY

Inadequate fiber intake.
Irritable bowel syndrome (associated with abdominal pain) or functional constipation.
Idiopathic slow-transit constipation.
"Obstructed defecation"—pelvic floor dysfunction (or dyssynergia).

STRUCTURAL DISORDERS

Anal fissure, infection or stenosis.
Colon cancer or stricture.
Aganglionosis and/or abnormal myenteric plexus:
- Hirschsprung's disease.
- Chagas' disease.
- Neuropathic pseudoobstruction.

Abnormal colonic muscle:
- Myopathy.
- Dystrophia myotonica.
- Systemic sclerosis.

Idiopathic megarectum and/or megacolon.
Proximal megacolon.

NEUROLOGIC CAUSES

Diabetic autonomic neuropathy.
Damage to the sacral parasympathetic outflow.
Spinal cord damage or disease (e.g., multiple sclerosis).
Parkinson's disease.
Blunting of consciousness, mental retardation, psychosis.
Pain induced by straining (e.g., sciatic nerve compression).

ENDOCRINE OR METABOLIC CAUSES

Hypothyroidism.
Hypercalcemia.
Porphyria.
Pregnancy.

PSYCHOLOGIC DISORDERS

Depression.
Anorexia nervosa.
Denied bowel habit.

DRUG SIDE EFFECTS

CORNEAL SENSATION, DECREASED

ICD-9CM # 371.89

Herpes (simplex, zoster).
Contact lens wear.
Topical agents (NSAIDs, anesthetics, betablockers).
Diabetes.
Eye trauma.
Postsurgery.

COUGH

ICD-9CM # 786.2

Infectious process (viral, bacterial).
Postinfectious.
"Smoker's cough."
Rhinitis (allergic, vasomotor, postinfectious).
Asthma.
Exposure to irritants (noxious fumes, smoke, cold air).
Drug-induced (especially ACE inhibitors, betablockers).
GERD.
Interstitial lung disease.
Lung neoplasms.
Lymphomas, mediastinal neoplasms.
Bronchiectasis.
Cardiac (CHF, pulmonary edema, mitral stenosis, pericardial inflammation).
Recurrent aspiration.
Inflammation of larynx, pleura, diaphragm, mediastinum.
Cystic fibrosis.
Anxiety.
Other: pulmonary embolism, foreign body inhalation, aortic aneurysm, Zenker's diverticulum, osteophytes, substernal thyroid, thyroiditis, PMR.

CUTANEOUS INFECTIONS, ATHLETES

ICD-9CM # 686.9

Tinea pedis.
Tinea cruris.
Molluscum contagiosum.
Herpes simplex.
Verruca vulgaris.
Folliculitis.
Impetigo.
Furuncles.
Otitis externa.
Erythrasma.

CYANOSIS

ICD-9CM # 782.5 Cyanosis NOS
770.8 Cyanosis, Newborn

Congenital heart disease with right-to-left shunt.
Pulmonary embolism.
Hypoxia.
Pulmonary edema.
Pulmonary disease (oxygen diffusion and alveolar ventilation abnormalities).
Hemoglobinopathies.
Decreased cardiac output.
Vasospasm.
Arterial obstruction.
Pulmonary AV fistulas.
Elevated hemidiaphragm.
Neoplasm (bronchogenic carcinoma, mediastinal neoplasm, intrahepatic lesion).
Substernal thyroid.
Infectious process (pneumonia, empyema, TB, subphrenic abscess, hepatic abscess).
Atelectasis.
Idiopathic.
Eventration.
Phrenic nerve dysfunction (myelitis, myotonia, herpes zoster).
Trauma to phrenic nerve or diaphragm (e.g., surgery).
Aortic aneurysm.
Intraabdominal mass.
Pulmonary infarction.
Pleurisy.
Radiation therapy.
Rib fracture.
Superior vena cava syndrome.

DAYTIME SLEEPINESS

ICD-9CM # varies with specific disorder

Sleep deprivation.
Medication induced (e.g., benzodiazepines, beta-blockers, narcotics, sedative antidepressants, gabapentin).
Depression.
Obstructive sleep apnea.
Medical illness (e.g., severe anemia, hypothyroidism, COPD, hepatic failure, renal insufficiency, CHF, electrolyte disturbances).
Circadian rhythm abnormalities (e.g., jet lag, shift work sleep disorder).
Restless legs syndrome.
Posttrauma.
Narcolepsy.
Neurologic disorders (e.g., neurodegenerative disorders; parkinsonism; multiple sclerosis; lesions affecting thalamus, hypothalamus, or brainstem).

DELIRIUM[26]

ICD-9CM # 780.09 Delirium NOS
293.0 Acute Delirium

PHARMACOLOGIC AGENTS

Anxiolytics (benzodiazepines).
Antidepressants (e.g., amitriptyline, doxepin, imipramine).
Cardiovascular agents (e.g., methyldopa, digitalis, reserpine, propranolol, procainamide, captopril, disopyramide).
Antihistamine.
Cimetidine.
Corticosteroids.
Antineoplastics.
Drugs of abuse (alcohol, cannabis, amphetamines, cocaine, hallucinogens, opioids, sedative-hypnotics, phencyclidine).

METABOLIC DISORDERS

Hypercalcemia.
Hypercarbia.
Hypoglycemia.
Hyponatremia.
Hypoxia.

INFLAMMATORY DISORDERS

Sarcoidosis.
SLE.
Giant cell arteritis.

ORGAN FAILURE

Hepatic encephalopathy.
Uremia.

NEUROLOGIC DISORDERS

Alzheimer's disease.
CVA.
Encephalitis (including HIV).
Encephalopathies.
Epilepsy.
Huntington's disease.
Multiple sclerosis.
Neoplasms.
Normal pressure hydrocephalus.
Parkinson's disease.
Pick's disease.
Wilson's disease.

ENDOCRINE DISORDERS

Addison's disease.
Cushing's disease.
Panhypopituitarism.
Parathyroid disease.
Postpartum psychosis.
Recurrent menstrual psychosis.
Sydenham's chorea.
Thyroid disease.

DEFICIENCY STATES

Niacin.
Thiamine, vitamin B_{12}, and folate.

DELIRIUM, DIALYSIS PATIENT[26]

ICD-9CM # 293.0 Acute Delirium
293.9 Encephalopathy from Dialysis

STRUCTURAL

Cerebrovascular accident (particularly hemorrhage).
Subdural hematoma.
Intracerebral abscess.
Brain tumor.

METABOLIC

Disequilibrium syndrome.
Uremia.
Drug effects.
Meningitis.
Hypertensive encephalopathy.
Hypotension.
Postictal state.
Hypernatremia or hyponatremia.
Hypercalcemia.
Hypermagnesemia.
Hypoglycemia.
Severe hyperglycemia.
Hypoxemia.
Dialysis dementia.

DEMYELINATING DISEASES[40]

ICD-9CM # 341.9

MULTIPLE SCLEROSIS

Relapsing and chronic progressive forms.
Acute multiple sclerosis.
Neuromyelitis optica (Devic's disease).

DIFFUSE CEREBRAL SCLEROSIS

Schilder's encephalitis periaxialis diffusa.
Baló's concentric sclerosis.

ACUTE DISSEMINATED ENCEPHALOMYELITIS

After measles, chickenpox, rubella, influenza, mumps.
After rabies or smallpox vaccination.

NECROTIZING HEMORRHAGIC ENCEPHALITIS

Hemorrhagic leukoencephalitis.

LEUKODYSTROPHIES

Krabbe's globoid leukodystrophy.
Metachromatic leukodystrophy.
Adrenoleukodystrophy.
Adrenomyeloneuropathy.
Pelizaeus-Merzbacher leukodystrophy.
Canavan's disease.
Alexander's disease.

DIARRHEA, ACUTE WATERY AND BLOODY[38]

ICD-9CM # varies with specific diagnosis
009.3 Infectious diarrhea
558.9 Non-infectious diarrhea
564.5 Functional diarrhea
787.91 Diarrhea

ACUTE WATERY DIARRHEA

Gastrointestinal infections:
- Protozoal (e.g., *Giardia*).
- Bacterial (e.g., enterotoxigenic *Escherichia coli,* cholera).
- Viral (e.g., rotavirus, Norwalk virus).

Drugs.
Toxins.
Dietary constituents (e.g., lactose intolerance).
Onset of chronic diarrheal illness.

ACUTE BLOODY DIARRHEA

Infectious colitis:
- Confluent proctocolitis (e.g., *Shigella*, *Campylobacter*, *Salmonella*, *Entamoeba histolytica*).
- Segmental colitis (e.g., *Campylobacter*, *Salmonella*, enteroinvasive *E. coli*, *Aeromonas*, *E. histolytica*).

Drug-induced colitis (e.g., nonsteroidal anti-inflammatory drugs [NSAIDs]).
Inflammatory bowel disease.
Ischemic colitis (usually elderly patient with underlying heart disease or arrhythmias).
Antibiotic-associated colitis.

DIARRHEA, TUBE-FED PATIENT[14]

ICD-9CM # 564.4

COMMON CAUSES UNRELATED TO TUBE FEEDING

Elixir medications containing sorbitol.
Magnesium-containing antacids.
Antibiotic-induced sterile gut.
Pseudomembranous colitis.

POSSIBLE CAUSES RELATED TO TUBE FEEDING

Inadequate fiber to form stool bulk.
High fat content of formula (in the presence of fat malabsorption syndrome).
Bacterial contamination of enteral products and delivery systems (causal association with diarrhea not documented).
Rapid advancement in rate (after the GI tract is unused for prolonged periods).

UNLIKELY CAUSES RELATED TO TUBE FEEDING

Formula hyperosmolality (proven not to be the cause of diarrhea).
Lactose (absent from nearly all enteral feeding formulas).

DIPLOPIA, BINOCULAR

ICD-9CM # 368.2

Cranial nerve palsy (3rd, 4th, 6th).
Thyroid eye disease.
Myasthenia gravis.
Decompensated strabismus.
Orbital trauma with blowout fracture.
Orbital pseudotumor.
Cavernous sinus thrombosis.

DIPLOPIA, MONOCULAR

ICD-9CM # 368.2

Postoperative corrected longstanding tropia.
Defective contact lenses.
Poorly fitting bifocals.
Trauma to iris.
Corneal disorder (e.g., dry eye, astigmatism).
Cataracts.
Lens subluxation.
Nystagmus.
Eyelid twitching.
Foreign body in aqueous or vitreous media.
Migraine.
Lesions of occipital cortex.
Psychogenic.

DIPLOPIA, VERTICAL

ICD-9CM # 368.2

Myasthenia.
Superior oblique palsy.
Myositis or pseudotumor with orbital involvement.
Lymphoma or metastases affecting the orbits.
Brain stem or cerebellar lesions.
Hydrocephalus.
Third nerve palsy.
Botulism.
Wernicke's encephalopathy.
Dysthyroid orbitopathy (muscle infiltration).

DIZZINESS

ICD-9CM # 780.4

Viral syndrome.
Anxiety, hyperventilation.
Benign positional paroxysmal vertigo.
Medications (e.g., sedatives, antihypertensives, analgesics).
Withdrawal from medications (e.g., benzodiazepines, SSRIs).
Alcohol or drug abuse.
Postural hypotension.
Hypoglycemia, hyperglycemia.
Hematologic disorders (e.g., anemia, polycythemia, leukemia).
Head trauma.
Menière's disease.
Vertebrobasilar ischemia.
Cervical osteoarthritis.
Cardiac abnormalities (arrhythmias, cardiomyopathy, CHF, pericarditis).
Multiple sclerosis.
Peripheral vestibulopathy.
Air or sea travel.
Electrolyte abnormalities.
Eye problems (cornea, lens, retina).
Migraine.
Brain stem infarct.
Autonomic neuropathy.
Chronic otomastoiditis.
Complex partial seizures.
Ramsey Hunt syndrome.
Arteritis.
Syncope and presyncope.
Perilymph fistula.
Cerebellopontine tumor.
Hepatic or renal disease.

DRY EYE

ICD-9CM # 375.15

Contacts.
Medications (antihistamines, clonidine, beta-blockers, ibuprofen, scopolamine).
Keratoconjunctivitis sicca.
Trauma.
Environmental causes (air conditioning in patient with contacts).

DYSPAREUNIA[12]

ICD-9CM # 625.0 Dyspareunia
608.89 Dyspareunia, Male
302.76 Dyspareunia, Psychogenic

INTROITAL

Vaginismus.
Intact or rigid hymen.
Clitoral problems.
Vulvovaginitis.
Vaginal atrophy: hypoestrogen.
Vulvar dystrophy.
Bartholin or Skene gland infection.
Inadequate lubrication.
Operative scarring.

MIDVAGINAL

Urethritis.
Trigonitis.
Cystitis.
Short vagina.
Operative scarring.
Inadequate lubrication.

DEEP

Endometriosis.
Pelvic infection.
Uterine retroversion.
Ovarian pathology.
GI.
Orthopedic.
Abnormal penile size or shape.

DYSPHAGIA

ICD-9CM # 787.2

Esophageal obstruction: neoplasm, foreign body, achalasia, stricture, spasm, esophageal web, diverticulum, Schatzki's ring.
Peptic esophagitis with stricture, Barrett's stricture.
External esophageal compression: neoplasms (thyroid neoplasm, lymphoma, mediastinal tumors), thyroid enlargement, aortic aneurysm, vertebral spurs, aberrant right subclavian artery (dysphagia lusoria).
Hiatal hernia, GERD.
Oropharyngeal lesions: pharyngitis, glossitis, stomatitis, neoplasms.
Hysteria: globus hystericus.
Neurologic and/or neuromuscular disturbances: bulbar paralysis, myasthenia gravis, ALS, multiple sclerosis, Parkinsonism, CVA, diabetic neuropathy.
Toxins: poisoning, botulism, tetanus, postdiphtheritic dysphagia.
Systemic diseases: scleroderma, amyloidosis, dermatomyositis.
Candida and herpes esophagitis.
Presbyesophagus.

DYSPHAGIA, OROPHARYNGEAL[38]

ICD-9CM # 787.22

FUNCTIONAL DISORDERS

Central nervous system

Stroke.
Head injury.
Parkinson's disease.
Motor neuron disease.
Multiple sclerosis.
Tumor.
Drugs (e.g., phenothiazines).
Malformations (e.g., syrinx, Arnold Chiari).

Neural

Motor neuron disease.
Myasthenia gravis.
Radiotherapy.
Poliomyelitis.
Familial dysautonomia.

Muscle

Autoimmune myopathy (polymyositis, dermatomyositis, systemic lupus erythematosus).
Thyrotoxic myopathy.
Guillain-Barré motor neuropathy.
Muscular dystrophies.

STRUCTURAL DISORDERS

Head/neck surgery.
Stricture.
Radiotherapy.
Tumor.
Pharyngeal pouch.
Web.
Extrinsic (e.g., osteophytes).

MISCELLANEOUS

Xerostomia.

DYSPNEA

ICD-9CM # 786.00

Upper airway obstruction: trauma, neoplasm, epiglottitis, laryngeal edema, tongue retraction, laryngospasm, abductor paralysis of vocal cords, aspiration of foreign body.
Lower airway obstruction: neoplasm, COPD, asthma, aspiration of foreign body.
Pulmonary infection: pneumonia, abscess, empyema, TB, bronchiectasis.
Pulmonary hypertension.
Pulmonary embolism/infarction.
Parenchymal lung disease.
Pulmonary vascular congestion.
Cardiac disease: ASHD, valvular lesions, cardiac dysrhythmias, cardiomyopathy, pericardial effusion, cardiac shunts.
Space-occupying lesions: neoplasm, large hiatal hernia, pleural effusions.
Disease of chest wall: severe kyphoscoliosis, fractured ribs, sternal compression, morbid obesity.
Neurologic dysfunction: Guillain-Barré syndrome, botulism, polio, spinal cord injury.
Interstitial pulmonary disease: sarcoidosis, collagen vascular diseases, DIP, Hamman-Rich pneumonitis, etc.
Pneumoconioses: silicosis, berylliosis, etc.
Mesothelioma.
Pneumothorax, hemothorax, pleural effusion.
Inhalation of toxins.
Cholinergic drug intoxication.
Carcinoid syndrome.
Hematologic: anemia, polycythemia, hemoglobinopathies.
Thyrotoxicosis, myxedema.
Diaphragmatic compression caused by abdominal distention, subphrenic abscess, ascites.
Lung resection.
Metabolic abnormalities: uremia, hepatic coma, DKA.
Sepsis.
Atelectasis.
Psychoneurosis.
Diaphragmatic paralysis.
Pregnancy.

DYSURIA

ICD-9CM # 788.1 Dysuria
306.53 Dysuria, Psychogenic

Urinary tract infection.
Estrogen deficiency (in postmenopausal female).
Vaginitis.
Genital infection (e.g., herpes, condyloma).
Interstitial cystitis.
Chemical irritation (e.g., deodorant aerosols, douches).
Meatal stenosis or stricture.
Reiter's syndrome.
Bladder neoplasm.
GI etiology (diverticulitis, Crohn's disease).
Impaired bladder or sphincter action.
Urethral carbuncle.
Chronic fibrosis posttrauma.
Radiation therapy.
Prostatitis.
Urethritis (gonococcal, *Chlamydiae*).
Behçet's syndrome.
Stevens-Johnson syndrome.

EARACHE[33]

ICD-9CM # 388.70 Earache
388.72 Ear Pain, Referred

Otitis media.
Serous otitis media.
Eustachitis.
Otitis externa.
Otitic barotrauma.
Mastoiditis.
Foreign body.
Impacted cerumen.
Referred otalgia, as with TMJ dysfunction, dental problems, and tumors.

ECTOPIC ACTH SECRETION[14]

ICD-9CM # 255.0

Small cell carcinoma of lung.
Endocrine tumors of foregut origin.
- Thymic carcinoid.
- Islet cell tumor.
- Medullary carcinoid, thyroid.
- Bronchial carcinoid.

Pheochromocytoma.
Ovarian tumors.

EDEMA, CHILDREN[19]

ICD-9CM # 782.3 Edema NOS

CARDIOVASCULAR

Congestive heart failure.
Acute thrombi or emboli.
Vasculitis of many types.

RENAL

Nephrotic syndrome.
Glomerulonephritis of many types.
End-stage renal failure.

ENDOCRINE OR METABOLIC

Thyroid disease.
Starvation.
Hereditary angioedema.

IATROGENIC

Drugs (diuretics and steroids).
Water or salt overload.

HEMATOLOGIC

Hemolytic disease of the newborn.

GASTROINTESTINAL

Hepatic cirrhosis.
Protein-losing enteritis.
Lymphangiectasis.
Cystic fibrosis.
Celiac disease.
Enteritis of many types.

LYMPHATIC ABNORMALITIES

Congenital (gonadal dysgenesis).
Acquired.

EDEMA, GENERALIZED

ICD-9CM # 782.3 Edema NOS

Congestive heart failure (CHF).
Cirrhosis.
Nephrotic syndrome.
Pregnancy.
Idiopathic.
Acute nephritic syndrome.
Myxedema.
Medications (NSAIDs, estrogens, vasodilators).

EDEMA, LEG, UNILATERAL[26]

ICD-9CM # 782.3

WITH PAIN

DVT.
Postphlebitic syndrome.
Popliteal cyst rupture.
Gastrocnemius rupture.
Cellulitis.
Psoas or other abscess.

WITHOUT PAIN

DVT.
Postphlebitic syndrome.
Other venous insufficiency (after saphenous vein harvest, varicosities).
Lymphatic obstruction/lymphedema (carcinoma, lymphoma, sarcoidosis, filariasis, retroperitoneal fibrosis).

EDEMA OF LOWER EXTREMITIES

ICD-9CM # 782.3

CHF (right-sided).
Hepatic cirrhosis.
Nephrosis.
Myxedema.
Lymphedema.
Pregnancy.
Abdominal mass: neoplasm, cyst.
Venous compression from abdominal aneurysm.
Varicose veins.
Bilateral cellulitis.
Bilateral thrombophlebitis.
Vena cava thrombosis, venous thrombosis.
Retroperitoneal fibrosis.

EJECTION SOUND OR CLICK

ICD-9CM # 785.3

Aortic regurgitation.
Aortic root dilatation.
Systemic hypertension.
Chronic pulmonary hypertension.
Tetralogy of Fallot.
Atrial septal defect.
Pulmonary valve stenosis.
Aortic aneurysm.

ELBOW PAIN

ICD-9CM # 719.42

Trauma.
Infection.
Inflammatory arthritis.
Lateral or medial epicondylitis.
Entrapment neuropathy.
Olecranon bursitis.
Osteoarthritis.
Gout.
Cervical disease (referred pain).
Shoulder disease (referred pain).
Partial subluxation.
Synovial osteochondromatosis.
Loose body.

ELEVATED HEMIDIAPHRAGM

ICD-9CM # 519.4 Diaphragm Disorder
519.4 Diaphragm Paralysis
756.6 Diaphragm Eventration, Congenital

Neoplasm (bronchogenic carcinoma, mediastinal neoplasm, intrahepatic lesion).
Substernal thyroid.
Infectious process (pneumonia, empyema, TB, subphrenic abscess, hepatic abscess).
Atelectasis.
Idiopathic.
Eventration.
Phrenic nerve dysfunction (myelitis, myotonia, herpes zoster).
Trauma to phrenic nerve or diaphragm (e.g., surgery).
Aortic aneurysm.
Intraabdominal mass.
Pulmonary infarction.
Pleurisy.
Radiation therapy.
Rib fracture.

EMBOLI, ARTERIAL[26]

ICD-9CM # 444.22 Embolism, Artery, Lower Extremity
444.21 Embolism, Artery, Upper Extremity

Myocardial infarction with mural thrombi.
Atrial fibrillation.
Cardiomyopathies.
Prosthetic heart valves.
CHF.
Endocarditis.
Left ventricular aneurysm.
Left atrial myxoma.
Sick sinus syndrome.
Paradoxical embolus from venous thrombosis.
Aneurysms of large blood vessels.
Atheromatous ulcers of large blood vessels.

EMESIS, PEDIATRIC AGE[19]

ICD-9CM # 787.03

INFANCY

Gastrointestinal Tract

Congenital:

Regurgitation—chalasia, gastroesophageal reflux.
Atresia—stenosis (tracheoesophageal fistula, prepyloric diaphragm, intestinal atresia).
Duplication.
Volvulus (errors in rotation and fixation, Meckel diverticulum).
Congenital bands.
Hirschsprung's disease.
Meconium ileus (cystic fibrosis), meconium plug.

Acquired:

Acute infectious gastroenteritis, food poisoning (staphylococcal, clostridial).
Pyloric stenosis.
Gastritis, duodenitis.
Intussusception.
Incarcerated hernia—inguinal, internal secondary to old adhesions.
Cow's milk protein intolerance, food allergy, eosinophilic gastroenteritis.
Disaccharidase deficiency.
Celiac disease—presents after introduction of gluten in diet; inherited risk.
Adynamic ileus—the mediator for many nongastrointestinal causes.
Neonatal necrotizing enterocolitis.
Chronic granulomatous disease with gastric outlet obstruction.

Nongastrointestinal Tract

Infectious—otitis, urinary tract infection, pneumonia, upper respiratory tract infection, sepsis, meningitis.
Metabolic—aminoaciduria and organic aciduria, galactosemia, fructosemia, adrenogenital syndrome, renal tubular acidosis, diabetic ketoacidosis, Reye's syndrome.
Central nervous system—trauma, tumor, infection, diencephalic syndrome, rumination, autonomic responses (pain, shock).
Medications—anticholinergics, aspirin, alcohol, idiosyncratic reaction (e.g., codeine).

CHILDHOOD

Gastrointestinal Tract

Peptic ulcer—vomiting is a common presentation in children younger than 6 yr old.
Trauma—duodenal hematoma, traumatic pancreatitis, perforated bowel.
Pancreatitis—mumps, trauma, cystic fibrosis, hyperparathyroidism, hyperlipidemia, organic acidemias.
Crohn's disease.
Idiopathic intestinal pseudoobstruction.
Superior mesenteric artery syndrome.

Nongastrointestinal Tract

Central nervous system—cyclic vomiting, migraine, anorexia nervosa, bulimia.

ENCEPHALOMYELITIS, NONVIRAL CAUSES[25]

ICD-9CM # varies with specific disorder

Subacute bacterial endocarditis.
Rocky Mountain spotted fever.
Typhus.
Ehrlichia.
Q fever.
Chlamydia.
Mycoplasma.
Legionella.
Brucellosis.
Listeria.
Whipple's disease.
Cat-scratch disease.
Syphilis (meningovascular).
Relapsing fever.
Lyme disease.
Leptospirosis.
Nocardia.
Actinomycosis.
Tuberculosis.
Cryptococcus.
Histoplasma.
Toxoplasma.
Plasmodium falciparum.
Trypanosomiasis.
Behçet's disease.
Vasculitis.
Carcinoma.
Drug reactions.

ENCEPHALOPATHY, METABOLIC[36]

ICD-9CM # 291.2 Alcoholic Encephalopathy
572.2 Hepatic Encephalopathy
251.2 Hypoglycemic Encephalopathy
349.82 Toxic Encephalopathy
984.9 Lead Encephalopathy
293.9 Encephalopathy

Substrate deficiency: hypoxia/ischemia, carbon monoxide poisoning, hypoglycemia.
Cofactor deficiency: thiamine, vitamin B_{12}, pyridoxine (INH administration).
Electrolyte disorders: hyponatremia, hypercalcemia, carbon dioxide narcosis, dialysis, hypermagnesemia, disequilibrium syndrome.
Endocrinopathies: DKA, hyperosmolar coma, hypothyroidism, hyperadrenocorticism, hyperparathyroidism.
Endogenous toxins: liver disease, uremia, porphyria.
Exogenous toxins: drug overdose (sedative/hypnotics, ethanol, narcotics, salicylates, tricyclic antidepressants), drug withdrawal, toxicity of therapeutic medications, industrial toxins (e.g., organophosphates, heavy metals), sepsis.
Heat stroke.
Epilepsy (postictal).

ENTHESOPATHY

ICD-9CM # code not available

Viremia or bacteremia.
Ankylosing spondylitis.
Psoriatic arthritis.
Drug-induced (quinolones, etretinate).
Reactive arthritis.
DISH.
Reiter's syndrome.

EPIGASTRIC PAIN[38]

ICD-9CM # 789.66

No specific cause found.
Peptic ulceration (uncomplicated).*
Peptic ulceration (perforated).*
Biliary colic.*
Acute pancreatitis.*
Abdominal aortic aneurysm.

*Conditions that also cause right upper quadrant pain.

EPILEPSY

ICD-9CM # 345.9 Epilepsy NOS

Psychogenic spells.
Transient ischemic attack.
Hypoglycemia.
Syncope.
Narcolepsy.
Migraine.
Paroxysmal vertigo.
Arrhythmias.
Drug reaction.

EPISTAXIS

ICD-9CM # 784.7

Trauma.
Medications (nasal sprays, NSAIDs, anticoagulants, antiplatelets).
Nasal polyps.
Cocaine use.
Coagulopathy (hemophilia, liver disease, DIC, thrombocytopenia).
Systemic disorders (hypertension, uremia).
Infections.
Anatomic malformations.
Rhinitis.
Nasal polyps.
Local neoplasms (benign and malignant).
Desiccation.
Foreign body.

ERECTILE DYSFUNCTION, ORGANIC[31]

ICD-9CM # 607.84

Neurogenic abnormalities: Somatic nerve neuropathy, central nervous system abnormalities.
Psychogenic causes: Depression, performance anxiety, marital conflict.
Endocrine causes: Hyperprolactinemia, hypogonadotropic hypogonadism, testicular failure, estrogen excess.
Trauma: Pelvic fracture, prostate surgery, penile fracture.
Systemic disease: DM, renal failure, hepatic cirrhosis.
Medications: Diuretics, antidepressants, H_2 blockers, exogenous hormones, alcohol, antihypertensives, nicotine abuse, finasteride, etc.
Structural abnormalities: Peyronie's disease.

EROSIONS, GENITALIA

ICD-9CM # 599.84

Candidiasis.
Intraepithelial neoplasia.
Squamous cell carcinoma.
Lichen planus.
Pemphigus vulgaris.
Erythema multiforme.
Lichen sclerosus.
Bullous pemphigoid.
Extramammary Paget's disease.
Impetigo.

ERYTHEMATOUS ANNULAR SKIN LESIONS

ICD-9CM # varies with diagnosis

Tinea corporis.
Warfarin plaques.
Erythema multiforme.
Erythema annulare.
Cutaneous lupus.
Cutaneous sarcoidosis.
Trauma.
Acute febrile neutrophilic dermatosis (Sweet's syndrome).

ERYTHRODERMA

ICD-9CM # 695.9 Secondary
696.2 Maculopapular
696.1 Psoriaticum
695.89 Exfoliative
778.8 Neonatorum

Drug reaction (e.g., allopurinol, ampicillin, phenytoin, vancomycin, dapsone, omeprazole, carbamazepine).
Atopic dermatitis.
Psoriasis.
Contact dermatitis.
Idiopathic.
Pityriasis rubra.
Chronic actinic dermatitis.
Bullous pemphigoid.
Paraneoplastic.
Cutaneous T-cell lymphoma.
Connective tissue disease.
Hypereosinophilia syndrome.

ESOPHAGEAL PERFORATION[26]

ICD-9CM # 530.4 Perforation, Nontraumatic
862.22 Injury, Traumatic

Trauma.
Caustic burns.
Iatrogenic.
Foreign bodies.
Spontaneous rupture (Boerhaave's syndrome).
Postoperative breakdown of anastomosis.

ESOPHAGITIS[25]

ICD-9CM # 530.12

INFECTIOUS

Candidiasis.
Cytomegalovirus.
Herpes simplex virus.
HIV infection, acute.

NONINFECTIOUS

Gastroesophageal reflux.
Mucositis from cancer chemotherapy.
Mucositis from radiation therapy.
Aphthous ulcers.

ESOTROPIA

ICD-9CM # Nonaccommodative 378.00
Accommodative 378.35
Alternating 378.05

Congenital.
Accommodative esotropia.
Myasthenia gravis.
Abducens palsy.
Pseudo-sixth nerve palsy.
Medial rectus entrapment (e.g., blowout fracture).
Posterior internuclear ophthalmoplegia.
Wernicke's encephalopathy.
Thyroid myopathy.
Chiari malformation.

EXANTHEMS[28]

ICD-9CM # 782.1

Measles.
Rubella.
Erythema infectiosum (fifth disease).
Roseola exanthema.
Varicella.
Enterovirus.
Adenovirus.
Epstein-Barr virus.
Kawasaki disease.
Staphylococcal scalded skin.
Scarlet fever.
Meningococcemia.
Rocky Mountain spotted fever.

EYELID NEOPLASM

ICD-9CM # varies with specific disorder

MALIGNANT

Melanoma.
Basal cell carcinoma.
Squamous cell carcinoma.
Bowen's disease.
Sebaceous cell carcinoma.
Metastatic lymphoma/leukemia.

BENIGN

Melanocytic nevus.
Pilar, eccrine, or apocrine tumor.
Neurofibroma.
Keratosis.
Squamous papilloma.
Keratoacanthoma.

EYELID RETRACTION

ICD-9CM # 374.89

Congenital.
Graves' ophthalmopathy.
Myasthenia gravis.
Postsurgical.
Guillain-Barré syndrome.
Cerebellar disease.
Horizontal gaze palsy.
Partial palsy of superior rectus muscle.
Encephalitis.
Closed head injury.
Disseminated sclerosis.
Eye trauma.
Contact lens wear.
Proptosis.
Eyelid neoplasm.
Atopic dermatitis.
Herpes zoster ophthalmicus.
Botulinum toxin injection.
Cyclic oculomotor paralysis.
Spheroid wing meningioma.
Hepatic cirrhosis.
Down's syndrome.
Essential hypertension.
Meningitis.
Paget's disease of bone.

EYE PAIN

ICD-9CM # 379.91

Foreign body.
Herpes zoster.
Trauma.
Conjunctivitis.
Iritis.
Iridocyclitis.
Uveitis.
Blepharitis.
Ingrown lashes.
Orbital or periorbital cellulitis/abscess.
Sinusitis.
Headache.
Glaucoma.
Inflammation of lacrimal gland.
Tic douloureux.
Cerebral aneurysm.
Cerebral neoplasm.
Entropion.
Retrobulbar neuritis.
UV light.
Dry eyes.
Irritation or inflammation from eye drops, dust, cosmetics, etc.

FACIAL PAIN

ICD-9CM # 784.0

Infection, abscess.
Postherpetic neuralgia.
Trauma, posttraumatic neuralgia.
Tic douloureux.
Cluster headache, "lower-half headache."
Geniculate neuralgia.
Anxiety, somatization syndrome.
Glossopharyngeal neuralgia.
Carotidynia.

FACIAL PARALYSIS[28]

ICD-9CM # 351.0 Facial (7th Nerve) Palsy

INFECTION

Bacterial: otitis media, mastoiditis, meningitis, Lyme disease.
Viral: herpes zoster, mononucleosis, varicella, rubella, mumps, Bell's palsy.
Mycobacterial: TB, meningitis, leprosy.
Miscellaneous: syphilis, malaria.

TRAUMA

Temporal bone fracture, facial laceration.
Surgery.

NEOPLASM

Malignant: squamous cell carcinoma, basal cell and adenocystic tumors, leukemia, parotid neoplasms, metastatic tumors.
Benign: facial nerve neuroma, vestibular schwannoma, congenital cholesteatoma.

IMMUNOLOGIC

Guillain-Barré syndrome, periarteritis nodosa.
Reaction to tetanus antiserum.

METABOLIC

Pregnancy.
Hypothyroidism.
DM.

FAILURE TO THRIVE

ICD-9CM # 783.4

MALABSORPTION

Cow's milk protein allergy.
Cystic fibrosis.
Celiac disease.
Biliary atresia.

INSUFFICIENT CALORIC INTAKE

Parental neglect.
Feeding difficulties (CNS lesion, severe reflux, oromotor abnormalities).
Use of diluted formula preparation.
Food shortage (poverty).

INCREASED NEEDS

Hyperthyroidism.
Congenital heart defects.
Malignancy.
Renal or hepatic disease.
HIV.

IMPROPER UTILIZATION

Storage disorders.
Amino acid disorders.
Trisomy 13, 21, 18.

FATIGUE

ICD-9CM # 780.7 Fatigue NOS
300.5 Fatigue Psychogenic
780.7 Chronic Fatigue Syndrome

Depression.
Anxiety, emotional stress.
Inadequate sleep.
Chronic fatigue syndrome.
Prolonged physical activity.
Pregnancy and postpartum period.
Anemia.
Hypothyroidism.
Medications (beta-blockers, anxiolytics, antidepressants, sedating antihistamines, clonidine, methyldopa).
Viral or bacterial infections.
Sleep apnea syndrome.
Dieting.
Renal failure, CHF, COPD, liver disease.

FATTY LIVER

ICD-9CM # 571.8

Obesity.
Alcohol abuse.
DM.
Acute fatty liver of pregnancy.
Medications (tetracycline, valproic acid, glucocorticoids, amiodarone, estrogen, methotrexate).
Reye's syndrome.
Wilson's disease.
Nonalcoholic steatosis.

FEVER AND JAUNDICE

ICD-9CM # 789.6 Fever
782.4 Jaundice

Cholecystitis.
Hepatic abscess (pyogenic, amebic).
Ascending cholangitis.
Pancreatitis.
Malaria.
Neoplasm (hepatic pancreatic, biliary tract, metastatic).
Mononucleosis.
Viral hepatitis.
Sepsis.
Babesiosis.
HIV (cryptosporidium).
Biliary ascariasis.
Toxic shock syndrome.
Yersinia infection, leptospirosis, yellow fever, Dengue fever, relapsing fever.

FEVER AND RASH

ICD-9CM # 782.1 Exanthem
57.9 Exanthem Viral
789.6 Fever

Drug hypersensitivity: penicillin, sulfonamides, thiazides, anticonvulsants, allopurinol.
Viral infection: measles, rubella, varicella, erythema infectiosum, roseola, enterovirus infection, viral hepatitis, infectious mononucleosis, acute HIV.
Other infections: meningococcemia, staphylococcemia, scarlet fever, typhoid fever, *Pseudomonas* bacteremia, Rocky Mountain spotted fever, Lyme disease, secondary syphilis, bacterial endocarditis, babesiosis, brucellosis, listeriosis.
Serum sickness.
Erythema multiforme.
Erythema marginatum.
Erythema nodosum.
SLE.
Dermatomyositis.
Allergic vasculitis.
Pityriasis rosea.
Herpes zoster.

FEVER IN RETURNING TRAVELERS AND IMMIGRANTS[28]

ICD-9CM # varies with specific disorder

Differential diagnosis of some selected systemic febrile illnesses to consider in returned travelers and immigrants.*

COMMON

Acute respiratory tract infection (worldwide).
Gastroenteritis (worldwide) [foodborne, waterborne, fecal-oral].
Enteric fever, including typhoid (worldwide) [food, water].
Urinary tract infection (worldwide) [sexual contact].
Drug reactions [antibiotics, prophylactic agents, other] {rash frequent}.
Malaria (tropics, limited areas of temperate zones) [mosquitoes].
Arboviruses (Africa; tropics) [mosquitoes, ticks, mites].
Dengue (Asia, Caribbean, Africa) [mosquitoes].
Viral hepatitis (worldwide).
Hepatitis A (worldwide) [food, fecal-oral].
Hepatitis B (worldwide, especially Asia, sub-Saharan Africa) [sexual contact] {long incubation period}.
Hepatitis C (worldwide) [blood or sexual contact].
Hepatitis E (Asia, North Africa, Mexico, ?others) [food, water].
Tuberculosis (worldwide) [airborne, milk] {long period to symptomatic infection}.
Sexually transmitted diseases (worldwide) [sexual contact].

LESS COMMON

Filariasis (Asia, Africa, South America) [biting insects] {long incubation period, eosinophilia}.
Measles (developing world) [airborne] {in susceptible individual}.
Amebic abscess (worldwide) [food].
Brucellosis (worldwide) [milk, cheese, food, animal contact].
Listeriosis (worldwide) [foodborne] {meningitis}.
Leptospirosis (worldwide) [animal contact, open fresh water] {jaundice, meningitis}.
Strongyloidiasis (warm and tropical areas) [soil contact] {eosinophilia}.
Toxoplasmosis (worldwide) [undercooked meat].

RARE

Relapsing fever (western Americas, Asia, northern Africa) [ticks, lice].
Hemorrhagic fevers (worldwide) [arthropod and nonarthropod transmitted].
Yellow fever (tropics) [mosquitoes] {hepatitis}.
Hemorrhagic fever with renal syndrome (Europe, Asia, North America) [rodent urine] {renal impairment}.
Hantavirus pulmonary syndrome (western North America, ?other) [rodent urine] {respiratory distress syndrome}.
Lassa fever (Africa) [rodent excreta, person to person] {high mortality rate}
Other—chikungunya, Rift Valley, Ebola-Marburg, etc. (various) [insect bites, rodent excreta, aerosols, person to person] {often severe}.
Rickettsial infections {rashes and eschars}.
Leishmaniasis, visceral (Middle East, Mediterranean, Africa, Asia, South America) [biting flies] {long incubation period}.
Acute schistosomiasis (Africa, Asia, South America, Caribbean) [fresh water].
Chagas' disease (South and Central America) [reduviid bug bites] {often asymptomatic}.
African trypanosomiasis (Africa) [tsetse fly bite] {neurologic syndromes, sleeping sickness}.
Bartonellosis (South America) [sandfly bite; cb] {skin nodules}.
HIV infection/AIDS (worldwide) [sexual and blood contact].
Trichinosis (worldwide) [undercooked meat] {eosinophilia}.
Plague (temperate and tropical plains) [animal exposures and fleas].
Tularemia (worldwide) [animal contact, fleas, aerosols] {ulcers, lymph nodes}.
Anthrax (worldwide) [animal, animal product contact] {ulcers}.
Lyme disease (North America, Europe) [tick bites] {arthritis, meningitis, cardiac abnormalities}.

*Diagnoses for which particular symptoms are indicative are in *italics*. Exposure to regions of the world that are most likely to be significant to the diagnosis are presented in (parentheses). Vectors, risk behaviors, and sources associated with acquisition are presented in [brackets]. Special clinical characteristics are listed within {braces}.

FINGER LESIONS, INFLAMMATORY

ICD-9CM # varies with specific disorder

Paronychia.
Herpes simplex type 1 (herpetic whitlow).
Dyshidrotic eczema (pompholyx).
Herpes zoster.
Bacterial endocarditis (Osler's nodes).
Psoriatic arthritis.

FLATULENCE AND BLOATING[33]

ICD-9CM # 787.3

Ingestion of nonabsorbable carbohydrates.
Ingestion of carbonated beverages.
Malabsorption: pancreatic insufficiency, biliary disease, celiac disease, bacterial overgrowth in small intestine.
Lactase deficiency.
Irritable bowel syndrome.
Anxiety disorders.
Food poisoning, giardiasis.

FLUSHING[27]

ICD-9CM # 782.62

Physiologic flushing: menopause, ingestion of monosodium glutamate (Chinese restaurant syndrome), ingestion of hot drinks.
Drugs: alcohol (with or without disulfiram, metronidazole, or chlorpropamide), nicotinic acid, diltiazem, nifedipine, levodopa, bromocriptine, vancomycin, amyl nitrate.
Neoplastic disorders: carcinoid syndrome, VIPoma syndrome, medullary carcinoma of thyroid, systemic mastocytosis, basophilic chronic myelocytic leukemia, renal cell carcinoma.
Anxiety.
Agnogenic flushing.

FOLATE DEFICIENCY[20]

ICD-9CM # 281.2

ETIOPATHOPHYSIOLOGIC CLASSIFICATION OF FOLATE DEFICIENCY

Nutritional causes:
- Decreased dietary intake:
  - Poverty and famine.
  - Institutionalized individuals (e.g., psychiatric, nursing homes), chronic debilitating disease.
  - Prolonged feeding of infants with goat's milk, special slimming diets or food fads (i.e., folate-rich foods not consumed), cultural or ethnic cooking techniques (i.e., food folate destroyed).
- Decreased diet and increased requirements:
  - Physiologic (e.g., pregnancy and lactation, prematurity, hyperemesis gravidarum, infancy).
  - Pathologic (e.g., intrinsic hematologic diseases involving hemolysis with compensatory erythropoiesis, abnormal hematopoiesis, or bone marrow infiltration with malignant disease and dermatologic disease such as psoriasis).

Folate malabsorption:
- With normal intestinal mucosa:
  - Some drugs (controversial).
  - Congenital folate malabsorption (rare).
- With mucosal abnormalities (e.g., tropical and nontropical sprue, regional enteritis).

Defective cellular folate uptake:
- Familial aplastic anemia (rare).
- Acute cerebral folate deficiency.

Inadequate cellular use:
- Folate antagonists (e.g., methotrexate).
- Hereditary enzyme deficiencies involving folate.

Drugs:
- Multiple effects on folate metabolism (e.g., alcohol, sulfasalazine, triamterene, pyrimethamine, trimethoprim-sulfamethoxazole, diphenylhydantoin, barbiturates).

Acute folate deficiency:
- Intensive care unit setting.
- Uncertain origin.

FOOT AND ANKLE PAIN, IN DIFFERENT AGE GROUPS[8]

ICD-9CM # varies with specific diagnosis

COMMON CAUSES OF FOOT AND ANKLE PAIN IN DIFFERENT AGE GROUPS

Childhood (2-10 yr)
Intraarticular:
Club foot.
Congenital midfoot and forefoot deformities.
Septic arthritis.
Periarticular:
Osteomyelitis.
Adolescence (10-18 yr)
Intraarticular:
Arch disorders (pes cavus, pes planus).
Periarticular:
Osteomyelitis.
Tumors.
Early adulthood (18-30 yr)
Intraarticular:
Metatarsalgia.
Hallux valgus.
Hallux rigidus.
Osteochondritis.
Accessory ossicles.
Periarticular:
Achilles tendonitis.
Achilles tendon rupture.
Fasciitis.
Referred:
Lumbar spine.
Knee.
Adulthood (30-50 yr)
Intraarticular:
Osteoarthritis.
Inflammatory arthritis.
Gout.
Metatarsalgia.
Hallux valgus.
Hallux rigidus.
Osteochondritis.
Accessory ossicles.
Periarticular:
Ischemic foot pain.
Diabetes.
Bursitis.
Tendonitis.
Plantar fasciitis.
Corns.
Referred:
Lumbar spine.
Knee.
Old age (>50 yr)
Intraarticular:
Osteoarthritis.
Inflammatory arthritis.
Gout.
Metatarsalgia.
Hallux valgus.
Hallux rigidus.
Periarticular:
Ischemic foot pain.
Diabetes.
Bursitis.
Tendonitis.
Plantar fasciitis.
Corns.
Referred:
Lumbar spine.
Knee.

FOOT DERMATITIS

ICD-9CM # varies with specific disorder

Tinea pedis.
Dyshidrotic eczema.
Tylosis (mechanically induced hyperkeratosis, fissuring, and dryness).
Allergic contact dermatitis.
Psoriasis.
Peripheral vascular insufficiency.
Neuropathic foot ulcers (DM, poorly fitting shoes).
Acquired plantar keratoderma.
Sézary's syndrome.

FOOTDROP

ICD-9CM # varies with specific disorder

Peripheral neuropathy.
L5 radiculopathy.
Peroneal nerve compression.
Sciatic nerve palsy.
Scapuloperoneal syndromes.
Spasticity.
Peroneal nerve compression.
Myopathy.
Dystonia.

FOOT LESION, ULCERATING

ICD-9CM # 917.9

Cellulitis.
Plantar wart.
Squamous cell carcinoma.
Actinomycosis (Madura foot).
Plantar fibromatosis.
Pseudoepitheliomatous hyperplasia.

FOOT PAIN

ICD-9CM # varies with specific diagnosis

Trauma (fractures, musculoskeletal and ligamentous strain).
Inflammation (plantar fasciitis, Achilles tendonitis or bursitis, calcaneal apophysitis).
Arterial insufficiency, Raynaud's phenomenon, thromboangiitis obliterans.
Gout, pseudogout.
Calcaneal spur.
Infection (cellulitis, abscess, lymphangitis, gangrene).

Decubitus ulcer.
Paronychia, ingrown toenail.
Thrombophlebitis, postphlebitic syndrome.

FOREARM AND HAND PAIN

ICD-9CM # 959.3 Forearm Injury
959.4 Hand Injury

Epicondylitis.
Tenosynovitis.
Osteoarthritis.
Cubital tunnel syndrome.
Carpal tunnel syndrome.
Trauma.
Herpes zoster.
Peripheral vascular insufficiency.
Infection (cellulitis, abscess).

GAIT ABNORMALITY

ICD-9CM # 781.2 Gait Abnormality

Parkinsonism.
Degenerative joint disease (hips, back, knees).
Multiple sclerosis.
Trauma, foot pain.
CVA.
Cerebellar lesions.
Infections (tabes, encephalitis, meningitis).
Sensory ataxia.
Dystonia, cerebral palsy, neuromuscular disorders.
Metabolic abnormalities.

GALACTORRHEA[28]

ICD-9CM # 611.6

Prolonged suckling.
Drugs (INH, phenothiazines, reserpine derivatives, amphetamines, spironolactone and tricyclic antidepressants).
Major stressors (surgery, trauma).
Hypothyroidism.
Pituitary tumors.

GASTRIC EMPTYING, DELAYED[1]

ICD-9CM # 536.8 Gastric Motility Disorder

MECHANICAL OBSTRUCTION

Duodenal or pyloric channel ulcer.
Pyloric stricture.
Tumor of the distal stomach.

FUNCTIONAL OBSTRUCTION (GASTROPARESIS)

Drugs: anticholinergics, beta-adrenergics, opiates.
Electrolyte imbalance: hypokalemia, hypocalcemia, hypomagnesemia.
Metabolic disorders: DM, hypoparathyroidism, hypothyroidism, pregnancy.
Vagotomy.
Viral infections.
Neuromuscular disorders (myotonic dystrophy, autonomic neuropathy, scleroderma, polymyositis).
Gastric pacemaker (i.e., tachygastria).
Brain stem tumors.
GERD.
Psychiatric disorders: anorexia nervosa, psychogenic vomiting.
Idiopathic.

GASTRIC EMPTYING, RAPID

ICD-9CM # 536.8 Gastric Motility Disorder

Pancreatic insufficiency.
Dumping syndrome.
Peptic ulcer.
Celiac disease.
Promotility agents.
Zollinger-Ellison disease.

GENITAL DISCHARGE, FEMALE[12]

ICD-9CM # 629.9

Physiologic discharge: cervical mucus, vaginal transudation, bacteria, squamous epithelial cells.
Individual variation.
Pregnancy.
Sexual response.
Menstrual cycle variation.
Infection.
Foreign body: tampon, cervical cap, other.
Neoplasm.
Fistula.
IUD.
Cervical ectropion.
Spermicide.
Nongenital causes: urinary incontinence, urinary tract fistula, Crohn's disease, rectovaginal fistula.

GENITAL SORES[1]

ICD-9CM # 054.10 Genital Herpes
91.0 Genital Syphilis
078.11 Condyloma Acuminatum
099.0 Chancroid
099.2 Granuloma Inguinale
099.1 Lymphogranuloma Venereum
629.8 Ulcer, Genital Site, Female
608.89 Ulcer, Genital Site, Male

Herpes genitalis.
Syphilis.
Chancroid.
Lymphogranuloma venereum.
Granuloma inguinale.
Condyloma acuminatum.
Neoplastic lesion.
Trauma.

GLOSSODYNIA[38]

ICD-9CM # 529.6

DENTURE-RELATED

Dentures (ill-fitting, monomer from denture base).
Dental plaque.
Oral parafunction.

INFECTIVE/DERMATOLOGICAL

Candidiasis.
Lichen planus.

DEFICIENCY STATES

Iron, B_{12}, folate, B_2 (riboflavin), B_6 (pyridoxine), zinc.

ENDOCRINE

Diabetes.
Myxedema.*
Hormonal changes occurring during menopause.*

NEUROLOGICALLY MEDIATED

Referred from tonsils, teeth.
Lingual nerve neuropathy.
Glossopharyngeal neuralgia.
Esophageal reflux.*

IATROGENIC

Mouthwash.

XEROSTOMIA

PSYCHOGENIC

IDIOPATHIC

*Unproven associations

GLUCOCORTICOID DEFICIENCY[14]

ICD-9CM # 255.4

ACTH-independent causes.
TB.
Autoimmune (idiopathic).
Other rare causes:
- Fungal infection.
- Adrenal hemorrhage.
- Metastases.
- Sarcoidosis.
- Amyloidosis.
- Adrenoleukodystrophy.
- Adrenomyeloneuropathy.
- HIV infection.
- Congenital adrenal hyperplasia.
- Medications (e.g., ketoconazole).

ACTH-dependent causes:
Hypothalamic-pituitary-adrenal suppression.
- Exogenous.
- Glucocorticoid.
- ACTH.
- Endogenous—cure of Cushing's syndrome.

Hypothalamic-pituitary lesions.
- Neoplasm:
  - Primary pituitary tumor.
  - Metastatic tumor.
  - Craniopharyngioma.
- Infection:
  - Tuberculosis.
  - Actinomycosis.
  - Nocardiosis.
- Sarcoid.
- Head trauma.
- Isolated ACTH deficiency.

GOITER

ICD-9CM # 240.9 Goiter, Unspecified
241.9 Goiter, Adenomatous
246.1 Goiter, Congenital
240.9 Goiter, Nontoxic Diffuse
241.1 Goiter, Nontoxic Multinodular
240.0 Simple Goiter
242.1 Thyrotoxic Goiter

Thyroiditis.
Toxic multinodular goiter.
Graves' disease.
Medications (PTU, methimazole, sulfonamides, sulfonylureas, ethionamide, amiodarone, lithium, etc.).
Iodine deficiency.
Sarcoidosis, amyloidosis.
Defective thyroid hormone synthesis.
Resistance to thyroid hormone.

GRANULOMATOUS DERMATITIDES

ICD-9CM # varies with specific disorder

Granuloma annulare.
Sarcoidosis.
Necrobiosis lipoidica diabeticorum.
Cutaneous Crohn's disease.
Rheumatoid nodules.
Annular elastolytic giant cell granuloma (actinic granuloma).
Foreign body granuloma.

GRANULOMATOUS DISORDERS[32]

ICD-9CM # 446.4 Granulomatosis
288.1 Granulomatous Disease

INFECTIONS

Fungi
Histoplasma.
Coccidioides.
Blastomyces.
Sporothrix.
Aspergillus.
Cryptococcus.
Protozoa
Toxoplasma.
Leishmania.
Metazoa
Toxocara.
Schistosoma.
Spirochetes
Treponema pallidum.
T. pertenue.
T. carateum.
Mycobacteria
M. tuberculosis.
M. leprae.
M. kansasii.
M. marinum.
M. avian.
Bacille Calmette-Guérin (BCG) vaccine.
Bacteria
Brucella.
Yersinia.
Other Infections
Cat scratch.
Lymphogranuloma.

NEOPLASIA

Carcinoma.
Reticulosis.
Pinealoma.
Dysgerminoma.
Seminoma.
Reticulum cell sarcoma.
Malignant nasal granuloma.

CHEMICALS

Beryllium.
Zirconium.
Silica.
Starch.

IMMUNOLOGIC ABERRATIONS

Sarcoidosis.
Crohn's disease.
Primary biliary cirrhosis.
Wegener's granulomatosis.
Giant-cell arteritis.
Peyronie's disease.
Hypogammaglobulinemia.
SLE.
Lymphomatoid granulomatosis.
Histiocytosis X.
Hepatic granulomatous disease.
Immune complex disease.
Rosenthal-Melkersson syndrome.
Churg-Strauss allergic granulomatosis.

LEUKOCYTE OXIDASE DEFECT

Chronic granulomatous disease of childhood.

EXTRINSIC ALLERGIC ALVEOLITIS

Farmer's lung.
Bird fancier's.
Mushroom worker's.
Suberosis (cork dust).
Bagassosis.
Maple bark stripper's.
Paprika splitter's.
Coffee bean.
Spatlese lung.

OTHER DISORDERS

Whipple's disease.
Pyrexia of unknown origin.
Radiotherapy.
Cancer chemotherapy.
Panniculitis.
Chalazion.
Sebaceous cyst.
Dermoid.
Sea urchin spine injury.

GRANULOMATOUS LIVER DISEASE

ICD-9CM # 572.8

Sarcoidosis.
Wegener's granulomatosis.
Vasculitis.
Inflammatory bowel disease.
Allergic granulomatosis.
Erythema nodosum.
Infections (fungal, viral, parasitic).
Primary biliary cirrhosis.
Lymphoma.
Hodgkin's disease.
Drugs (e.g., allopurinol, hydralazine, sulfonamides, penicillins).
Toxins (copper sulfate, beryllium).

GREEN OR BLUE URINE

ICD-9CM # 788.69

Pseudomonal urinary tract infection
Medications: triamterene, amitriptyline, IV cimetidine, IV promethazine.
Biliverdin.
Dyes (methylene blue, indigo carmine).

GROIN LUMP[38]

ICD-9CM # varies with specific diagnosis

COMMON CAUSES

Inguinal hernia.
Femoral hernia.
Lymph node.

OTHER CAUSES

Saphena varix.
Femoral artery aneurysm/pseudoaneurysm.
Psoas abscess.
Lipoma of the cord.
Encysted hydrocele of the cord (male).
Testicular maldescent (male).
Hydrocele of canal of Nuck (female).

GROIN MASSES

ICD-9CM # 959.1

Hernia (inguinal, femoral).
Hydrocele.
Varicocele.
Sebaceous cyst.
Hydradenitis of inguinal apocrine glands.
Neoplasm: lymphoma, metastases.
Lipoma.
Hematoma.
Reactive inguinal adenopathy, femoral adenitis.
Folliculitis, psoas abscess.
Epididymitis, testicular torsion, ectopic testes.
Aneurysm or pseudoaneurysm of femoral artery.

GROIN PAIN, ACTIVE PATIENT[37]

ICD-9CM # 959.1 Groin Injury
848.8 Groin Pain

MUSCULOSKELETAL

Avascular necrosis of the femoral head.
Avulsion fracture (lesser trochanter, anterior superior iliac spine, anterior inferior iliac spine).
Bursitis (iliopectineal, trochanteric).
Entrapment of the ilioinguinal or iliofemoral nerve.
Gracilis syndrome.

Muscle tear (adductors, iliopsoas, rectus abdominis, gracilis, sartorius, rectus femoris).
Myositis ossificans of the hip muscles.
Osteitis pubis.
Osteoarthritis of the femoral head.
Slipped capital femoral epiphysis.
Stress fracture of the femoral head or neck and pubis.
Synovitis.

HERNIA-RELATED

Avulsion of the internal oblique muscle in the conjoined tendon.
Defect at the insertion of the rectus abdominis muscle.
Direct inguinal hernia.
Femoral ring hernia.
Indirect inguinal hernia.
Inguinal canal weakness.

UROLOGIC

Epididymitis.
Fracture of the testis.
Hydrocele.
Kidney stone.
Posterior urethritis.
Prostatitis.
Testicular cancer.
Torsion of the testis.
Urinary tract infection.
Varicocele.

GYNECOLOGIC

Ectopic pregnancy.
Ovarian cyst.
Pelvic inflammatory disease.
Torsion of the ovary.
Vaginitis.

LYMPHATIC ENLARGEMENT IN GROIN

GYNECOMASTIA

ICD-9CM # 611.1 Gynecomastia, Nonpuerperal

Physiologic (puberty, newborns, aging).
Drugs (estrogen and estrogen precursors, digitalis, testosterone and exogenous androgens, clomiphene, cimetidine, spironolactone, ketoconazole, amiodarone, ACE inhibitors, isoniazid, phenytoin, methyldopa, metoclopramide, phenothiazine).
Increased prolactin level (prolactinoma).
Liver disease.
Adrenal disease.
Thyrotoxicosis.
Increased estrogen production (hCG-producing tumor, testicular tumor, bronchogenic carcinoma).
Secondary hypogonadism.
Primary gonadal failure (trauma, castration, viral orchitis, granulomatous disease).
Defects in androgen synthesis.
Testosterone deficiency.
Klinefelter's syndrome.

HALITOSIS

ICD-9CM # 784.9

Tobacco use.
Alcohol use.
Dry mouth (mouth breathing, inadequate fluid intake).
Foods (onion, garlic, meats, nuts).
Disease of mouth or nose (infections, cancer, inflammation).
Medications (antihistamines, antidepressants).
Systemic disorders (diabetes, uremia).
GI disorders (esophageal diverticula, hiatal hernia, GERD, achalasia).
Sinusitis.
Pulmonary disorders (bronchiectasis, pneumonia, neoplasms, TB).

HAND PAIN AND SWELLING[6]

ICD-9CM # varies with specific diagnosis

Trauma.
Gout.
Pseudogout.
Cellulitis.
Lymphangitis.
DVT of upper extremity.
Thrombophlebitis.
RA.
Remitting seronegative symmetrical synovitis with pitting edema (RS3PE).
Polymyalgia rheumatica.
Mixed connective tissue disease.
Scleroderma.
Rupture of the olecranon bursa.
Metzger's syndrome (neoplasia).
The puffy hand of drug addiction.
Reflex sympathetic dystrophy.
Eosinophilic fasciitis.
Sickle cell (hand-foot syndrome).
Leprosy.
Factitial (the rubber band syndrome).

HEADACHE[13]

ICD-9CM # 784.0 Headache NOS
307.81 Headache, Tension
346.2 Headache, Cluster
346.9 Headache, Migraine
784.0 Headache, Vascular

Vascular: migraine, cluster headaches, temporal arteritis, hypertension, cavernous sinus thrombosis.
Musculoskeletal: neck and shoulder muscle contraction, strain of extraocular and/or intraocular muscles, cervical spondylosis, temporomandibular arthritis.
Infections: meningitis, encephalitis, brain abscess, sepsis, sinusitis, osteomyelitis, parotitis, mastoiditis.
Cerebral neoplasm.
Subdural hematoma.
Cerebral hemorrhage/infarct.
Pseudotumor cerebri.
Normal pressure hydrocephalus (NPH).
Postlumbar puncture.
Cerebral aneurysm, arteriovenous malformations.
Posttrauma.
Dental problems: abscess, periodontitis, poorly fitting dentures.
Trigeminal neuralgia, glossopharyngeal neuralgia.
Otitis and other ear diseases.
Glaucoma and other eye diseases.
Metabolic: uremia, carbon monoxide inhalation, hypoxia.
Pheochromocytoma, hypoglycemia, hypothyroidism.
Effort induced: benign exertional headache, cough, headache, coital cephalalgia.
Drugs: alcohol, nitrates, histamine antagonists.
Paget's disease of the skull.
Emotional, psychiatric.

HEADACHE, ACUTE[11]

ICD-9CM # 784.0

DIFFERENTIAL DIAGNOSIS OF ACUTE HEADACHE

Evaluation of the first acute headache should exclude pathologic causes listed here before consideration of more common etiologies..
Increased intracranial pressure (ICP): Trauma, hemorrhage, tumor, hydrocephalus, pseudotumor cerebri, abscess, arachnoid cyst, cerebral edema.
Decreased ICP: After ventriculoperitoneal shunt, lumbar puncture, cerebrospinal fluid leak from basilar skull fracture.
Meningeal inflammation: Meningitis, leukemia, subarachnoid or subdural hemorrhage.
Vascular: Vasculitis, arteriovenous malformation, hypertension, cerebrovascular accident.
Bone, soft tissue: Referred pain from scalp, eyes, ears, sinuses, nose, teeth, pharynx, cervical spine, temporomandibular joint.
Infection: Systemic infection, encephalitis, sinusitis, etc.
First migraine.

HEADACHE AND FACIAL PAIN[36]

ICD-9CM # 784.0 Headache NOS
784.0 Facial Pain

VASCULAR HEADACHES

Migraine

Migraine with headaches and inconspicuous neurologic features:

- Migraine without aura ("common migraine").

Migraine with headaches and conspicuous neurologic features:

- With transient neurologic symptoms:
  Migraine with typical aura ("classic migraine").
  Sensory, basilar, and hemiplegic migraine.
- With prolonged or permanent neurologic features ("complicated migraine"):
  Ophthalmoplegic migraine.
  Migrainous infarction.

Migraine without headaches but with conspicuous neurologic features ("migraine equivalents"):

- Abdominal migraine.
- Benign paroxysmal vertigo of childhood.
- Migraine aura without headache ("isolated auras," transient migrainous accompaniments).

Cluster Headaches

Episodic cluster headache ("cyclic cluster headaches").

Chronic cluster headaches.

Chronic paroxysmal hemicrania.

Other Vascular Headaches

Headaches of reactive vasodilation (fever, drug-induced, postictal, hypoglycemia, hypoxia, hypercarbia, hyperthyroidism).

Headaches associated with arterial hypertension:

- Chronic severe hypertension (diastolic 120 mm Hg).
- Paroxysmal severe hypertension (pheochromocytoma, some coital headaches).

Headaches caused by cranial arteritis:

- Giant cell arteritis ("temporal arteritis").
- Other vasculitides.

HEADACHES ASSOCIATED WITH DEMONSTRABLE MUSCLE SPASM

Headache caused by posturally induced or perilesional muscle spasm:

- Headaches of sustained or impaired posture (e.g., prolonged close work, driving).
- Headaches associated with cervical spondylosis and other diseases of cervical spine.
- Myofascial pain dysfunction syndrome (headache or facial pain associated with disorders of teeth, jaws, and related structures, or "TMJ syndrome").

Headaches caused by psychophysiologic muscular contraction ("muscle contraction headaches," or tension-type headache associated with disorder of pericranial muscles).

HEADACHES AND FACIAL PAIN WITHOUT DEMONSTRABLE PHYSICAL SUBSTRATE

Headaches of uncertain etiology:

- "Tension headaches" (tension-type headache unassociated with disorder of pericranial muscles).
- Some forms of posttraumatic headache.

Psychogenic headaches (e.g., hypochondriacal, conversional, delusional, malingered).

Facial pain of uncertain etiology ("atypical facial pain").

COMBINED TENSION-MIGRAINE HEADACHES

Episodic migraine superimposed on chronic tension headaches.

Chronic daily headaches:

- Associated with analgesic and/or ergotamine overuse ("rebound headaches").
- Not associated with drug overuse.

HEADACHES AND HEAD PAINS CAUSED BY DISEASES OF EYES, EARS, NOSE, SINUSES, TEETH, OR SKULL

HEADACHES CAUSED BY MENINGEAL INFLAMMATION

Subarachnoid hemorrhage.

Meningitis and meningoencephalitis.

Others (e.g., meningeal carcinomatosis).

HEADACHES ASSOCIATED WITH ALTERED INTRACRANIAL PRESSURE ("TRACTION HEADACHES")

Increased Intracranial Pressure

Intracranial mass lesions (neoplasm, hematoma, abscess, etc.).

Hydrocephalus.

Benign intracranial hypertension.

Venous sinus thrombosis.

Decreased Intracranial Pressure

Post–lumbar puncture headaches.

Spontaneous hypoliquorrheic headaches.

HEADACHES AND HEAD PAINS CAUSED BY CRANIAL NEURALGIAS

Presumed irritation of superficial nerves

Occipital neuralgia.

Supraorbital neuralgia.

Presumed irritation of intracranial nerves

Trigeminal neuralgia ("tic douloureux").

Glossopharyngeal neuralgia.

HEADACHE, CHRONIC[11]

ICD-9CM # 784.0

DIFFERENTIAL DIAGNOSIS OF RECURRENT OR CHRONIC HEADACHES

Migraine (with or without aura).

Tension.

Analgesic rebound.

Caffeine withdrawal.

Sleep deprivation (e.g., in children with sleep apnea) or chronic hypoxia.

Tumor.

Psychogenic: Conversion disorder, malingering.

Cluster headache.

HEAD AND NECK, SOFT TISSUE MASSES

ICD-9CM # varies with specific diagnosis

Lipoma.

Pilar cyst.

Epidermal inclusion cyst.

Dermoid cyst.

Bone cyst.

Hemangioma.

Eosinophilic granuloma.

Other: facial nerve neuroma, teratoma, rhabdomyoma, rhabdomyosarcoma, branchial cleft cyst.

HEARING LOSS, ACUTE[26]

ICD-9CM # 388.2

Infectious: mumps, measles, influenza, herpes simplex, herpes zoster, CMV, mononucleosis, syphilis.

Vascular: macroglobulinemia, sickle cell disease, Berger's disease, leukemia, polycythemia, fat emboli, hypercoagulable states.

Metabolic: diabetes, pregnancy, hyperlipoproteinemia.

Conductive: cerumen impaction, foreign bodies, otitis media, otitis externa, barotrauma, trauma.

Medications: aminoglycosides, loop diuretics, antineoplastics, salicylates, vancomycin.

Neoplasm: acoustic neuroma, metastatic neoplasm.

HEARTBURN AND INDIGESTION[33]

ICD-9CM # 787.1 Heartburn
536.8 Indigestion

Reflux esophagitis.

Gastritis.

Nonulcer dyspepsia.

Functional GI disorder (anxiety disorder, social/environmental stresses).

Excessive intestinal gas (ingestion of flatulogenic foods, GI stasis, constipation).

Gas entrapment (hepatitis or splenic flexure syndrome).

Neoplasm (adenocarcinoma of stomach or esophagus, lymphoma).

Gallbladder disease.

HEART FAILURE, PREGNANCY

ICD-9CM # 428.90

Congenital valvular heart disease exacerbated by pregnancy.

Peripartum cardiomyopathy.

Untreated thyrotoxicosis.

Hypothyroidism.

Pulmonary hypertension.

Myocardial infarction.

HEEL PAIN

ICD-9CM # varies with specific diagnosis

Achilles tendonitis/tendinopathy (insertional, noninsertional).

Retrocalcaneal bursitis (superficial, deep).

Plantar fasciopathy.

Neuropathy (tarsal tunnel, posterior tibial nerve [medial calcaneal branch], abductor digiti quinti).

Calcaneal stress fracture.

Puncture wound, foreign body.

Cellulitis.

Spondyloarthropathy.

Fat pad atrophy.

Soft tissue tumor.

S1 radiculopathy.

Paget's disease of bone.

Haglund deformity.
Primary or metastatic bone tumor.

HEEL PAIN, PLANTAR[24]

ICD-9CM # 729.5

SKIN

Keratoses.
Verruca.
Ulcer.
Fissure.

CONNECTIVE TISSUE

Fat
Atrophy.
Panniculitis.
Dense Connective Tissue
Inflammatory fasciitis.
Fibromatosis.
Enthesopathy.
Bursitis.
Bone (Calcaneus)
Stress fracture.
Paget's disease.
Benign bone cyst/tumor.
Malignant bone tumor.
Metabolic bone disease (osteopenia).
Nerve
Tarsal tunnel.
Plantar nerve entrapment.
S1 nerve root radiculopathy.
Painful peripheral neuropathy.

INFECTION

Dermatomycoses.
Acute osteomyelitis.
Plantar abscess.

MISCELLANEOUS

Foreign body.
Nonunion calcaneus fracture.
Psychogenic.
Idiopathic.

HEMARTHROSIS

ICD-9CM # 848.9 Hemarthrosis (Sprain) NOS

Trauma.
Anticoagulant therapy.
Thrombocytopenia, thrombocytosis.
Bleeding disorders (e.g., von Willebrand's disease).
Charcot's joint.
Idiopathic.
Other: pigmented villonodular synovitis, hemangioma, synovioma, AV fistula, ruptured aneurysm.

HEMATEMESIS[38]

ICD-9CM # 578.0

CAUSES OF HEMATEMESIS

Very common
Gastric or duodenal ulcer or erosions.
Common
Mallory-Weiss tear (a laceration at the gastroesophageal junction).
Ulcerative esophagitis.
Esophageal varices.
Uncommon
Vascular malformations.
Ulcerated gastrointestinal stromal tumor.
Carcinoma of esophagus or stomach.
Aortoenteric fistula.

HEMATURIA

ICD-9CM # 599.7 Hematuria, Benign (Essential)

Use the mnemonic TICS:

T (trauma): blow to kidney, insertion of Foley catheter or foreign body in urethra, prolonged and severe exercise, very rapid emptying of overdistended bladder.
(tumor): hypernephroma, Wilms' tumor, papillary carcinoma of the bladder, prostatic and urethral neoplasms.
(toxins): turpentine, phenols, sulfonamides and other antibiotics, cyclophosphamide, NSAIDs.
I (infections): glomerulonephritis, TB, cystitis, prostatitis, urethritis, *Schistosoma haematobium,* yellow fever, blackwater fever.
(inflammatory processes): Goodpasture's syndrome, periarteritis, postirradiation.
C (calculi): renal, ureteral, bladder, urethra.
(cysts): simple cysts, polycystic disease.
(congenital anomalies): hemangiomas, aneurysms, AVM.
S (surgery): invasive procedures, prostatic resection, cystoscopy.
(sickle cell disease and other hematologic disturbances): hemophilia, thrombocytopenia, anticoagulants.
(somewhere else): bleeding genitals, factitious (drug addicts).

HEMATURIA, DIFFERENTIAL BASED ON AGE AND SEX

ICD-9CM # 599.7 Hematuria Benign (Essential)
other codes vary with cause

0 TO 20 YR

Acute urinary tract infections.
Acute glomerulonephritis.
Congenital urinary tract anomalies with obstruction.
Trauma to genitals.

20 TO 40 YR

Acute urinary tract infection.
Trauma to genitals.
Urolithiasis.
Bladder cancer.

40 TO 60 YR (WOMEN)

Acute urinary tract infection.
Bladder cancer.
Urolithiasis.

40 TO 60 YR (MEN)

Acute urinary tract infection.
Bladder cancer.
Urolithiasis.

60 YR AND OLDER (WOMEN)

Acute urinary tract infection.
Bladder cancer.
Vaginal trauma or irritation.
Urolithiasis.

60 YR AND OLDER (MEN)

Acute urinary tract infection.
Benign prostatic hyperplasia.
Bladder cancer.
Urolithiasis.
Trauma.

HEMIPARESIS/HEMIPLEGIA

ICD-9CM # 436.0 Acquired Due to Acute CVA, Flaccid
436.1 Acquired Due to CVA, Acute, Spastic

CVA.
Transient ischemic attack.
Cerebral neoplasm.
Multiple sclerosis or other demyelinating disorder.
CNS infection.
Migraine.
Hypoglycemia
Subdural hematoma.
Vasculitis.
Todd's paralysis.
Epidural hematoma.
Metabolic (hyperosmolar state, electrolyte imbalance).
Psychiatric disorders.
Congenital disorders.
Leukodystrophies.

HEMOLYSIS AND HEMOGLOBINURIA

ICD-9CM # 773.2 Hemolysis
791.2 Hemoglobinuria

Erythrocyte trauma (prosthetic cardiac valves, marching and severe trauma, extensive burns).
Infections (malaria, *Bartonella, Clostridium Welchii*).
Brown recluse spider bite.
Incompatible blood transfusions.
Hemolytic uremic syndrome.
Thrombotic thrombocytopenic purpura (TTP).
Paroxysmal nocturnal hemoglobinuria (PNH).
Drugs (penicillins, quinidine, methyldopa, sulfonamides, nitrofurantoin).
Erythrocyte enzyme deficiencies (e.g., exposure to fava beans in patients with glucose-6-phosphate dehydrogenase deficiency).

HEMOLYSIS, INTRAVASCULAR

ICD-9CM # 283.2

Infections.
Exertional hemolysis (e.g., prolonged march).
Valve hemolysis.
Microangiopathic hemolytic anemia.
Osmotic and chemical agents.
Thermal injury.

Cold agglutinins.
Venoms (snakes, spiders).
Paroxysmal nocturnal hemoglobinuria (PNH).

HEMOLYSIS, MECHANICAL

ICD-9CM # 283.19

Prosthetic heart valves.
Aortic stenosis.
Malignant hypertension.
Metastatic adenocarcinoma.
Traumatic exercise.
Renal transplants.
Renal cortical necrosis.
Glomerulonephritis.
Thrombotic thrombocytopenic purpura (TTP), hemolytic-uremic syndrome (HUS).
Renal vasculitis.
Scleroderma.
Diabetes.

HEMOPERITONEUM

ICD-9CM # 568.81

Ruptured Graafian follicle.
Ruptured spleen.
Ectopic pregnancy.
Traumatic laceration of liver.
Ruptured aneurysm.
Ruptured bladder.
Traumatic laceration of bowel, pancreas, uterus.

HEMOPTYSIS

ICD-9CM # 786.3

CARDIOVASCULAR

Pulmonary embolism/infarction.
Left ventricular failure.
Mitral stenosis.
AV fistula.
Severe hypertension.
Erosion of aortic aneurysm.

PULMONARY

Neoplasm (primary or metastatic).
Infection.
Pneumonia: *Streptococcus pneumoniae, Klebsiella pneumoniae, Staphylococcus aureus, Legionella pneumophila.*
Bronchiectasis.
Abscess.
TB.
Bronchitis.
Fungal infections (aspergillosis, coccidioidomycosis).
Parasitic infections (amebiasis, ascariasis, paragonimiasis).
Vasculitis: Wegener's granulomatosis, Churg-Strauss syndrome, Henoch-Schönlein purpura.
Goodpasture's syndrome.
Trauma (needle biopsy, foreign body, right-sided heart catheterization, prolonged and severe cough).
Cystic fibrosis, bullous emphysema.
Pulmonary sequestration.
Pulmonary AV fistula.
SLE.
Idiopathic pulmonary hemosiderosis.
Drugs: aspirin, anticoagulants, penicillamine.
Pulmonary hypertension.
Mediastinal fibrosis.

OTHER

Epistaxis, trauma.
Laryngeal bleeding (laryngitis, laryngeal neoplasm).
Hematologic disorders (clotting abnormalities, DIC, thrombocytopenia).

HEPATIC CYSTS[36]

ICD-9CM # 751.62 Hepatic Cyst, Congenital
122.8 Echinococcus Infection, Liver

CONGENITAL HEPATIC CYSTS

Parenchymal: solitary cyst, polycystic disease.
Ductal: localized dilatation, multiple cystic dilatations of intrahepatic ducts (Caroli's disease).

ACQUIRED HEPATIC CYSTS

Inflammatory cysts: retention cysts, echinococcal cyst, amebic cyst.
Neoplastic cyst.
Peliosis hepatis.

HEPATIC GRANULOMAS[1]

ICD-9CM # 572.8

INFECTIONS

Bacterial, spirochetal: TB and atypical mycobacterial infections, tularemia, brucellosis, leprosy, syphilis, Whipple's disease, listeriosis.
Viral: mononucleosis, CMV.
Rickettsial: Q fever.
Fungal: coccidioidomycosis, histoplasmosis, cryptococcal infections, actinomycosis, aspergillosis, nocardiosis.
Parasitic: schistosomiasis, clonorchiasis, toxocariasis, ascariasis, toxoplasmosis, amebiasis.

HEPATOBILIARY DISORDERS

Primary biliary cirrhosis, granulomatous hepatitis, jejunoileal bypass.

SYSTEMIC DISORDERS

Sarcoidosis, Wegener's granulomatosis, inflammatory bowel disease, Hodgkin's disease, lymphoma.

DRUGS/TOXINS

Beryllium, parenteral foreign material (starch, talc, silicone, etc.), phenylbutazone, α-methyldopa, procainamide, allopurinol, phenytoin, nitrofurantoin, hydralazine.

HEPATITIS, ACUTE[25]

ICD-9CM # varies with specific disorder

Infectious:
- Hepatitis A, B, C, D, G.
- Epstein-Barr virus.
- Cytomegalovirus.
- Herpes simplex virus.
- Yellow fever.
- Leptospirosis.
- Q fever.
- HIV.
- Brucellosis.
- Lyme disease.
- Syphilis.

Noninfectious:
- Drug induced.
- Autoimmune.
- Ischemic.
- Acute fatty liver of pregnancy.
- Acute Budd-Chiari syndrome.
- Wilson's disease.

HEPATITIS, CHRONIC[25]

ICD-9CM # 571.40 Hepatitis, Noninfectious, Chronic
072.22 Hepatitis B, Chronic
070.44 Hepatitis C, Chronic

Chronic viral hepatitis:
- Hepatitis B.
- Hepatitis C.
- Hepatitis D.

Autoimmune hepatitis and variant syndromes.
Hereditary hemochromatosis.
Wilson's disease.
α-Antitrypsin deficiency.
Fatty liver and nonalcoholic steatohepatitis.
Alcoholic liver disease.
Drug-induced liver disease.
Hepatic granulomas:
- Infectious.
- Drug induced.
- Neoplastic.
- Idiopathic.

HEPATOMEGALY

ICD-9CM # 789.1

FREQUENT JAUNDICE

Infectious hepatitis.
Toxic hepatitis.
Carcinoma: liver, pancreas, bile ducts, metastatic neoplasm to liver.
Cirrhosis.
Obstruction of common bile duct.
Alcoholic hepatitis.
Biliary cirrhosis.
Cholangitis.
Hemochromatosis with cirrhosis.

INFREQUENT JAUNDICE

CHF.
Amyloidosis.
Liver abscess.
Sarcoidosis.
Infectious mononucleosis.
Alcoholic fatty infiltration.
Nonalcoholic steatohepatitis.
Lymphoma.
Leukemia.
Budd-Chiari syndrome.
Myelofibrosis with myeloid metaplasia.
Familial hyperlipoproteinemia type 1.

Other: amebiasis, hydatid disease of liver, schistosomiasis, kala-azar *(Leishmania donovani),* Hurler's syndrome, Gaucher's disease, kwashiorkor.

HEPATOMEGALY, BY SHAPE OF LIVER[38]

ICD-9CM # 789.1

DIFFUSELY ENLARGED AND SMOOTH

Massive

Metastatic disease.
Alcoholic liver disease with fatty infiltration.
Myeloproliferative diseases (e.g., polycythemia rubra vera, myelofibrosis).

Moderate

The above causes.
Hemochromatosis.
Hematological disease (e.g., chronic myeloid leukemia, lymphoma).
Fatty liver (e.g., diabetes mellitus, obesity).
Infiltrative disorders (e.g., amyloid).

Mild

The above causes.
Hepatitis (viral, drugs).
Cirrhosis.
Biliary obstruction.
Granulomatous disorders (e.g., sarcoid).
HIV infection.

DIFFUSELY ENLARGED AND IRREGULAR

Metastatic disease.
Cirrhosis.
Hydatid disease.
Polycystic liver disease.

LOCALIZED SWELLINGS

Riedel's lobe (a normal variant—the lobe may be palpable in the right lumbar region).
Metastasis.
Large simple hepatic cyst.
Hydatid cyst.
Hepatoma.
Liver abscess (e.g., amoebic abscess).

HERMAPHRODITISM[4]

ICD-9CM # 752.7 Hermaphroditism, Congenital

FEMALE PSEUDOHERMAPHRODITISM

Androgen exposure:
- Fetal source:
  - 21-Hydroxylase (P450 c21) deficiency.
  - 11β-Hydroxylase (P450 c11) deficiency.
  - 3β-Hydroxysteroid dehydrogenase II (3β-HSD II) deficiency.
  - Aromatase (P450arom) deficiency.
- Maternal source.
- Virilizing ovarian tumor.
- Virilizing adrenal tumor.
- Androgenic drugs.

Undetermined origin:
- Associated with genitourinary and GI tract defects.

MALE PSEUDOHERMAPHRODITISM

Defects in testicular differentiation:
- Denys-Drash syndrome (mutation in WT1 gene).
- WAGR syndrome (*W*ilms tumor, *a*niridia, *g*enitourinary malformation, *r*etardation).
- Deletion of 11p13.
- Camptomelic syndrome (autosomal gene at 17q24.3-q25.1) and SOX 9 mutation.
- XY pure gonadal dysgenesis (Swyer syndrome).
  - Mutation in SRY gene.
  - Unknown cause.
- XY gonadal agenesis.

Deficiency of testicular hormones:
- Leydig cell aplasia.
- Mutation in LH receptor.
- Lipoid adrenal hyperplasia (P450 scc) deficiency; mutation in StAR (steroidogenic acute regulatory protein).
- 3b-HSDII deficiency.
- 17-Hydroxylase/17, 20-lyase (P450 c17) deficiency.
- Persistent Müllerian duct syndrome.
  - Gene mutations, Müllerian-inhibiting substance (MIS).
  - Receptor defects for MIS.

Defect in androgen action:
- 5α-Reductase II mutations.
- Androgen receptor defects:
  - Complete androgen insensitivity syndrome.
  - Partial androgen insensitivity syndrome.
  - Reifenstein and other syndromes.
  - Smith-Lemli-Opitz syndrome.

Defect in conversion of 7-dehydrocholesterol to cholesterol.

TRUE HERMAPHRODITISM

XX.
XY.
XX/XY chimeras.

HICCUPS[21]

ICD-9CM # 786.8

TRANSIENT HICCUPS

Sudden excitement, emotion.
Gastric distention.
Esophageal obstruction.
Alcohol ingestion.
Sudden change in temperature.

PERSISTENT OR CHRONIC HICCUPS

Toxic/metabolic: uremia, DM, hyperventilation, hypocalcemia, hypokalemia, hyponatremia, gout, fever.
Drugs: benzodiazepines, steroids, α-methyldopa, barbiturates.
Surgery/general anesthesia.
Thoracic/diaphragmatic disorders: pneumonia, lung cancer, asthma, pleuritis, pericarditis, myocardial infarction, aortic aneurysm, esophagitis, esophageal obstruction, diaphragmatic hernia or irritation.
Abdominal disorders: gastric ulcer or cancer, hepatobiliary or pancreatic disease, IBD, bowel obstruction, intraabdominal or subphrenic abscess, prostatic infection or cancer.
Central nervous system disorders: traumatic, infectious, vascular, structural.
Ear, nose, and throat disorders: pharyngitis, laryngitis, tumor, irritation of auditory canal.
Psychogenic disorders.
Idiopathic disorders.

HIP PAIN, CHILDREN[26]

ICD-9CM # 959.6 Hip Injury
719.95 Hip Joint Disorder
843.9 Hip Strain

TRAUMA

Hip or pelvis fractures.
Overuse injuries.

INFECTION

Septic arthritis.
Osteomyelitis.

INFLAMMATION

Transient synovitis.
Juvenile RA.
Rheumatic fever.

NEOPLASM

Leukemia.
Osteogenic or Ewing's sarcoma.
Metastatic disease.

HEMATOLOGIC DISORDERS

Hemophilia.
Sickle cell anemia.

MISCELLANEOUS

Legg-Calvé-Perthes disease.
Slipped capital femoral epiphysis.

HIP PAIN, IN DIFFERENT AGE GROUPS[8]

ICD-9CM # 719.45

COMMON CAUSES OF HIP PAIN IN DIFFERENT AGE GROUPS

Childhood (2-10 yr)

Intraarticular:
Developmental dislocation of the hip.
Perthes' disease.
Irritable hip.
Rickets.
Periarticular:
Osteomyelitis.
Referred:
Abdominal.

Adolescence (10-18 yr)

Intraarticular:
Slipped upper femoral epiphysis.
Torn labrum.
Periarticular:
Trochanteric bursitis.
Snapping hip.
Osteomyelitis.
Tumors.

Referred:
Abdominal.
Lumbar spine.
Early adulthood (18-30 yr)
Intraarticular:
Inflammatory arthritis.
Torn labrum.
Periarticular:
Bursitis.
Referred:
Abdominal.
Lumbar spine.
Adulthood (30-50 yr)
Intraarticular:
Osteoarthritis.
Inflammatory arthritis.
Osteonecrosis.
Transient osteoporosis.
Periarticular:
Bursitis.
Referred:
Abdominal.
Lumbar spine.
Old age (>50 yr)
Intraarticular:
Osteoarthritis.
Inflammatory arthritis.
Referred:
Abdominal.
Lumbar spine.

HIRSUTISM

ICD-9CM # 704.1

Idiopathic: familial, possibly increased sensitivity to androgens.
Menopause.
Polycystic ovarian syndrome.
Drugs: androgens, anabolic steroids, methyltestosterone, minoxidil, diazoxide, phenytoin, glucocorticoids, cyclosporine.
Congenital adrenal hyperplasia.
Adrenal virilizing tumor.
Ovarian virilizing tumor: arrhenoblastoma, hilus cell tumor.
Pituitary adenoma.
Cushing's syndrome.
Hypothyroidism (congenital and juvenile).
Acromegaly.
Testicular feminization.

HIV INFECTION, ANORECTAL LESIONS[26]

ICD-9CM # 042 HIV infection, symptomatic
V08 HIV infection, asymptomatic

COMMON CONDITIONS

Anal fissure.
Abscess and fistula.
Hemorrhoids.
Pruritus ani.
Pilonidal disease.

COMMON STDs

Gonorrhea.
Chlamydia.
Herpes.
Chancroid.
Syphilis.
Condylomata acuminata.

ATYPICAL CONDITIONS

Infectious: TB, CMV, actinomycosis, cryptococcus.
Neoplastic: lymphoma, Kaposi's sarcoma, squamous cell carcinoma.
Other: idiopathic and ulcer.

HIV INFECTION, CHEST RADIOGRAPHIC ABNORMALITIES[26]

ICD-9CM # 042 HIV infection, symptomatic
V08 HIV infection, asymptomatic

DIFFUSE INTERSTITIAL INFILTRATION

Pneumocystis carinii.
Cytomegalovirus.
Mycobacterium tuberculosis.
Mycobacterium avium complex.
Histoplasmosis.
Coccidioidomycosis.
Lymphoid interstitial pneumonitis.

FOCAL CONSOLIDATION

Bacterial pneumonia.
Mycoplasma pneumoniae.
Pneumocystis carinii.
Mycobacterium tuberculosis.
Mycobacterium avium complex.

NODULAR LESIONS

Kaposi's sarcoma.
Mycobacterium tuberculosis.
Mycobacterium avium complex.
Fungal lesions.
Toxoplasmosis.

CAVITARY LESIONS

Pneumocystis carinii.
Mycobacterium tuberculosis.
Bacterial infection.

PLEURAL EFFUSION

Kaposi's sarcoma.
(Small effusion may be associated with any infection).

ADENOPATHY

Kaposi's sarcoma.
Lymphoma.
Mycobacterium tuberculosis.
Cryptococcus.

PNEUMOTHORAX

Kaposi's sarcoma.

HIV INFECTION, COGNITIVE IMPAIRMENT[25]

ICD-9CM # 042 HIV Infection, Symptomatic

EARLY TO MID-STAGE HIV DISEASE

Depression.
Alcohol and substance abuse.
Medication-induced cognitive impairment.
Metabolic encephalopathies.
HIV-related cognitive impairment.

ADVANCED HIV DISEASE (CD4+ <100/mm^3)

Opportunistic infection of CNS.
Neurosyphilis.
CNS lymphoma.
Progressive multifocal leukoencephalopathy.
Depression.
Metabolic encephalopathies.
Medication-induced cognitive impairment.
Stroke.
HIV dementia.

HIV INFECTION, CUTANEOUS MANIFESTATIONS[21]

ICD-9CM # 042 HIV Infection, Symptomatic
V08 HIV Infection, Asymptomatic

BACTERIAL INFECTION

Bacillary angiomatosis: Numerous angiomatous nodules associated with fever, chills, weight loss.
Staphylococcus aureus: Folliculitis, ecthyma, impetigo, bullous impetigo, furuncles, carbuncles.
Syphilis: May occur in different forms (primary, secondary, tertiary); chancre may become painful because of secondary infection.

FUNGAL INFECTION

Candidiasis: Mucous membranes (oral, vulvovaginal), less commonly candida intertrigo or paronychia.
Cryptococcoses: Papules or nodules that strongly resemble molluscum contagiosum; other forms include pustules, purpuric papules, and vegetating plaques.
Seborrheic dermatitis: Scaling and erythema in the hair-bearing areas (eyebrows, scalp, chest, and pubic area).

ARTHROPOD INFESTATIONS

Scabies: Pruritus with or without rash, usually generalized but can be limited to a single digit.

VIRAL INFECTION

Herpes simplex: Vesicular lesion in clusters; perianal, genital, orofacial, or digital; can be disseminated.
Herpes zoster: Painful dermatomal vesicles that may ulcerate or disseminate.

HIV: Discrete erythematous macules and papules on the upper trunk, palms, and soles are the most characteristic cutaneous finding of acute HIV infection.
Human papillomavirus: Genital warts (may become unusually extensive).
Kaposi's sarcoma (herpesvirus): Erythematous macules or papules; enlarge at varying rates; violaceous nodules or plaques; occasionally painful.
Molluscum contagiosum: Discrete umbilicated papules commonly on the face, neck, and intertriginous sites (axilla, groin, or buttocks).

NONINFECTIOUS

Drug reactions: More frequent and severe in HIV patients.
Nutritional deficiencies: Mainly seen in children and patients with chronic diarrhea; diffuse skin manifestations, depending upon the deficiency.
Psoriasis: Scaly lesions; diffuse or localized; can be associated with arthritis.
Vasculitis: Palpable purpuric eruption (can resemble septic emboli).

HIV INFECTION, ESOPHAGEAL DISEASE

ICD-9CM # varies with specific diagnosis

Candida infection.
Cytomegalovirus infection.
Aphthous ulcer.
Herpes simplex.

HIV INFECTION, HEPATIC DISEASE[25]

ICD-9CM # 042 HIV Infection, Symptomatic

VIRUSES

Hepatitis A.
Hepatitis B.
Hepatitis C.
Hepatitis D (with HBV).
Epstein-Barr virus.
Cytomegalovirus.
Herpes simplex virus.
Adenovirus.
Varicella-zoster virus.

MYCOBACTERIA

Mycobacterium avium complex.
Mycobacterium tuberculosis.

FUNGI

Histoplasma capsulatum.
Cryptococcus neoformans.
Coccidioides immitis.
Candida albicans.
Pneumocystis carinii.
Penicillium marneffei.

PROTOZOA

Toxoplasma gondii.
Cryptosporidium parvum.
Microsporida spp.
Schistosoma.

BACTERIA

Bartonella henselae (peliosis hepatis).

MALIGNANCY

Kaposi's sarcoma (HHV-8).
Non-Hodgkin's lymphoma.
Hepatocellular carcinoma.

MEDICATIONS

Zidovudine.
Didanosine.
Ritonavir.
Other HIV-1 protease inhibitors.
Fluconazole.
Macrolide antibiotics.
Isoniazid.
Rifampin.
Trimethoprim-sulfamethoxazole.

HIV INFECTION, LOWER GI TRACT DISEASE[25]

ICD-9CM # 042 HIV Infection, Symptomatic

CAUSES OF ENTEROCOLITIS

Bacteria

Campylobacter jejuni and other spp.
Salmonella spp.
Shigella flexneri.
Aeromonas hydrophila.
Plesiomonas shigelloides.
Yersinia enterocolitica.
Vibrio spp.
Mycobacterium avium complex.
Mycobacterium tuberculosis.
Escherichia coli (enterotoxigenic, enteroadherent).
Bacterial overgrowth.
Clostridium difficile (toxin).

Parasites

Cryptosporidium parvum.
Microsporida (*Enterocytozoon bieneusi, Septata intestinalis*).
Isospora belli.
Entamoeba histolytica.
Giardia lamblia.
Cyclospora cayetanensis.

Viruses

Cytomegalovirus.
Adenovirus.
Calicivirus.
Astrovirus.
Picobirnavirus.
Human immunodeficiency virus.

Fungi

Histoplasma capsulatum.

CAUSES OF PROCTITIS

Bacteria

Chlamydia trachomatis.
Neisseria gonorrhoeae.
Treponema pallidum.

Viruses

Herpes simplex.
Cytomegalovirus.

HIV INFECTION, OCULAR MANIFESTATIONS[36]

ICD-9CM # 042 HIV Infection, Symptomatic
V08 HIV Infection, Asymptomatic

EYELIDS

Molluscum contagiosum.
Kaposi's sarcoma.

CORNEA/CONJUNCTIVA

Keratoconjunctivitis sicca.
Bacterial/fungal ulcerative keratitis.
Herpes simplex.
Herpes zoster ophthalmicus.
Conjunctival microvasculopathy.
Kaposi's sarcoma.

RETINA, CHOROID, AND VITREOUS

Microvasculopathy.
Endophthalmitis.
Cytomegalovirus retinitis.
Acute retinal necrosis.
Syphilis.
Toxoplasmosis.
Pneumocystis choroidopathy.
Cryptococcosis.
Mycobacterial infection.
Intraocular lymphoma.
Candidiasis.
Histoplasmosis.

DRUGS ASSOCIATED WITH OCULAR TOXICITY

Rifabutin.
Didanosine.

NEUROOPHTHALMIC

Disc edema.
Primary or secondary optic neuropathy.
Cranial nerve palsies.

ORBITAL

Lymphoma.
Infection.
Pseudotumor.

HIV INFECTION, PULMONARY DISEASE[25]

ICD-9CM # 042 HIV Infection, Symptomatic

MYCOBACTERIAL

M. tuberculosis.
M. kansasii.
M. avium complex.
Other nontuberculous mycobacteria.

OTHER BACTERIAL

Streptococcus pneumoniae.
Staphylococcus aureus.
Haemophilus influenzae.
Enterobacteriaceae.
Pseudomonas aeruginosa.
Moraxella catarrhalis.

Group A *Streptococcus.*
Nocardia spp.
Rhodococcus equi.
Chlamydia pneumoniae.

FUNGAL

Pneumocystis carinii.
Cryptococcus neoformans.
Histoplasma capsulatum.
Coccidioides immitis.
Aspergillus spp.
Blastomyces dermatitidis.
Penicillium marneffei.

VIRAL

Cytomegalovirus.
Herpes simplex virus.
Adenovirus.
Respiratory syncytial virus.
Influenza viruses.
Parainfluenza virus.

OTHER

Toxoplasma gondii.
Strongyloides stercoralis.
Kaposi's sarcoma.
Lymphoma.
Lung cancer.
Lymphocytic interstitial pneumonitis.
Nonspecific interstitial pneumonitis.
Bronchiolitis obliterans with organizing pneumonia.
Pulmonary hypertension.
Emphysema-like or bullous disease.
Pneumothorax.
Congestive heart failure.
Diffuse alveolar damage.
Pulmonary embolus.

HOARSENESS

ICD-9CM # 784.49

Allergic rhinitis.
Infections (laryngitis, epiglottitis, tracheitis, croup).
Vocal cord polyps.
Voice strain.
Irritants (tobacco smoke).
Vocal cord trauma (intubation, surgery).
Neoplastic involvement of vocal cord (primary or metastatic).
Neurologic abnormalities (multiple sclerosis, ALS, parkinsonism).
Endocrine abnormalities (puberty, menopause, hypothyroidism).
Other (laryngeal webs or cysts, psychogenic, muscle tension abnormalities).

HYDROCEPHALUS

ICD-9CM # 331.4

Head trauma.
Brain neoplasm (primary or metastatic).
Spinal cord tumor.
Cerebellar infarction.
Exudative or granulomatous meningitis.
Cerebellar hemorrhage.
Subarachnoid hemorrhage.
Aqueductal stenosis.
Third ventricle colloid cyst.
Hindbrain malformation.
Viral encephalitis.
Metastases to leptomeninges.

HYPERCALCEMIA

ICD-9CM # 275.42 Hypercalcemia Disorder

Malignancy: increased bone resorption via osteoclast-activating factors, secretion of PTH-like substances, prostaglandin E2, direct erosion by tumor cells, transforming growth factors, colony-stimulating activity. Hypercalcemia is common in the following neoplasms:
  Solid tumors: breast, lung, pancreas, kidneys, ovary.
  Hematologic cancers: myeloma, lymphosarcoma, adult T-cell lymphoma, Burkitt's lymphoma.
Hyperparathyroidism: increased bone resorption, GI absorption, and renal absorption; etiology:
  Parathyroid hyperplasia, adenoma.
  Hyperparathyroidism or renal failure with secondary hyperparathyroidism.
Granulomatous disorders: increased GI absorption (e.g., sarcoidosis).
Paget's disease: increased bone resorption, seen only during periods of immobilization.
Vitamin D intoxication, milk-alkali syndrome; increased GI absorption.
Thiazides: increased renal absorption.
Other causes: familial hypocalciuric hypercalcemia, thyrotoxicosis, adrenal insufficiency, prolonged immobilization, vitamin A intoxication, recovery from acute renal failure, lithium administration, pheochromocytoma, disseminated SLE.

HYPERCALCEMIA, MALIGNANCY-INDUCED

ICD-9CM # 275.42

Lung carcinoma	(6% frequency, 35% of hypercalcemic cases)
Breast carcinoma	(10% frequency, 25% of hypercalcemic cases)
Multiple myeloma	(33% frequency, 10% of hypercalcemic cases)
Lymphoma	(4% of hypercalcemic cases)
Genitourinary cancer	(6% of hypercalcemic cases)

HYPERCAPNIA, PERSISTENT[36]

ICD-9CM # 786.09

Hypercapnia with normal lungs: CNS disturbances (CVA, parkinsonism, encephalitis), metabolic alkalosis, myxedema, primary alveolar hypoventilation, spinal cord lesions.
Diseases of the chest wall (e.g., kyphoscoliosis, ankylosing spondylitis).
Neuromuscular disorders (e.g., myasthenia gravis, Guillain-Barré syndrome, amyotrophic lateral sclerosis, muscular dystrophy, poliomyelitis).
COPD.

HYPERCOAGULABLE STATE, ASSOCIATED DISORDERS[20]

ICD-9CM # 289.82

Systemic lupus erythematosus in association with the presence of a lupus anticoagulant or antiphospholipid antibodies.
Malignancy:
  Disease-related: includes migratory superficial thrombophlebitis (Trousseau syndrome), nonbacterial thrombotic endocarditis, thrombosis associated with chronic DIC, thrombotic microangiopathy.
  Treatment-related: associated with the administration of various chemotherapeutic agents (L-asparaginase, mitomycin, some adjuvant chemotherapeutic agents for treatment of breast cancer, thalidomide or lenalidomide in conjunction with high doses of dexamethasone).
Infusion of prothrombin complex concentrates.
Nephrotic syndrome.
Heparin-induced thrombocytopenia.
Myeloproliferative disorders.
Paroxysmal nocturnal hemoglobinuria.

DIC, Disseminated intravascular coagulopathy.

HYPERGASTRINEMIA

ICD-9CM # varies with specific disorder

Decreased gastrin release inhibition from medications (proton pump inhibitors [PPIs], H_2 receptor antagonists), vagotomy.
Chronic renal failure.
Hypochlorhydria due to atrophic gastritis, gastric carcinoma, pernicious anemia.
Gastrinoma (Zollinger-Ellison syndrome).
Pyloric obstruction.
Hyperplasia of antral G cells.
RA.

HYPERHIDROSIS[4]

ICD-9CM # 780.8 hyperhidrosis

CORTICAL

Emotional.
Familial dysautonomia.
Congenital ichthyosiform erythroderma.
Epidermolysis bullosa.
Nail-patella syndrome.
Jadassohn-Lewandowsky syndrome.
Pachyonychia congenita.
Palmoplantar keratoderma.

HYPOTHALAMIC

Drugs

Antipyretics.
Emetics.
Insulin.
Meperidine.

Exercise Infection
Defervescence.
Chronic illness.
Metabolic
Debility.
DM.
Hyperpituitarism.
Hyperthyroidism.
Hypoglycemia.
Obesity.
Porphyria.
Pregnancy.
Rickets.
Infantile scurvy.
Cardiovascular
Heart failure.
Shock.
Vasomotor
Cold injury.
Raynaud phenomenon.
RA.
Neurologic
Abscess.
Familial dysautonomia.
Postencephalitic.
Tumor.
Miscellaneous
Chédiak-Higashi syndrome.
Compensatory.
Phenylketonuria.
Pheochromocytoma.
Vitiligo.
Medullary
Physiologic gustatory sweating.
Encephalitis.
Granulosis rubra nasi.
Syringomyelia.
Thoracic sympathetic trunk injury.
Spinal
Cord transection.
Syringomyelia.
Changes in Blood Flow
Mallucci syndrome.
Arteriovenous fistula.
Klippel-Trenaunay syndrome.
Glomus tumor.
Blue rubber bleb nevus syndrome.

HYPERKALEMIA

ICD-9CM # 276.7

Pseudohyperkalemia.
Hemolyzed specimen.
Severe thrombocytosis (platelet count 0.106 ml).
Severe leukocytosis (white blood cell count 0.105 ml).
Fist clenching during phlebotomy.
Excessive potassium intake (often in setting of impaired excretion).
Potassium replacement therapy.
High-potassium diet.
Salt substitutes with potassium.
Potassium salts of antibiotics.
Decreased renal excretion.
Potassium-sparing diuretics (e.g., spironolactone, triamterene, amiloride).
Renal insufficiency.
Mineralocorticoid deficiency.
Hyporeninemic hypoaldosteronism (DM).
Tubular unresponsiveness to aldosterone (e.g., SLE, multiple myeloma, sickle cell disease).
Type 4 RTA.
ACE inhibitors.
Heparin administration.
NSAIDs.
Trimethoprim-sulfamethoxazole.
Beta-blockers.
Pentamidine.
Redistribution (excessive cellular release).
Acidemia (each 0.1 decrease in pH increases the serum potassium by 0.4 to 0.6 mEq/L). Lactic acidosis and ketoacidosis cause minimal redistribution.
Insulin deficiency.
Drugs (e.g., succinylcholine, markedly increased digitalis level, arginine, beta-adrenergic blockers).
Hypertonicity.
Hemolysis.
Tissue necrosis, rhabdomyolysis, burns.
Hyperkalemic periodic paralysis.

HYPERKINETIC MOVEMENT DISORDERS[30]

ICD-9CM # 314.8 Hyperkinetic Syndrome
275.1 Choreoathetosis
335.5 Hemiballism
333.7 Dystonia Due to Drugs
333.6 Dystonia, Idiopathic

Chorea, choreoathetosis: drug-induced, Huntington's chorea, Sydenham's chorea.
Tardive dyskinesia (e.g., phenothiazines).
Hemiballismus (lacunar CVA near subthalamic nuclei in basal ganglia, metastatic lesions, toxoplasmosis [in AIDS]).
Dystonia (idiopathic, familial, drug-induced [prochlorperazine, metoclopramide]), Wilson's disease.
Liver failure.
Thyrotoxicosis.
SLE, polycythemia.

HYPERMAGNESEMIA

ICD-9CM # 275.2

Renal failure (decreased GFR).
Decreased renal excretion secondary to salt depletion.
Abuse of antacids and laxatives containing magnesium in patients with renal insufficiency.
Endocrinopathies (deficiency of mineralocorticoid or thyroid hormone).
Increased tissue breakdown (rhabdomyolysis).
Redistribution: acute DKA, pheochromocytoma.
Other: lithium, volume depletion, familial hypocalciuric hypercalcemia.

HYPERPHOSPHATEMIA

ICD-9CM # 275.3

Excessive phosphate administration.
Excessive oral intake or IV administration.
Laxatives containing phosphate (phosphate tablets, phosphate enemas).
Decreased renal phosphate excretion.
Acute or chronic renal failure.
Hypoparathyroidism or pseudohypoparathyroidism.
Acromegaly, thyrotoxicosis.
Bisphosphonate therapy.
Tumor calcinosis.
Sickle cell anemia.
Transcellular shift out of cells.
Chemotherapy of lymphoma or leukemia, tumor lysis syndrome, hemolysis.
Acidosis.
Rhabdomyolysis, malignant hyperthermia.
Artifact: in vitro hemolysis.
Pseudohyperphosphatemia: hyperlipidemia, paraproteinemia, hyperbilirubinemia.

HYPERPIGMENTATION[5]

ICD-9CM # 709.00

Addison's disease.*
Arsenic ingestion.
ACTH- or MSH-producing tumors (e.g., oat cell carcinoma of the lung).*
Drug induced (i.e., antimalarials, some cytotoxic agents).
Hemochromatosis ("bronze" diabetes).
Malabsorption syndrome (Whipple's disease and celiac sprue).
Melanoma.
Melanotropic hormone injection.*
Pheochromocytoma.
Porphyrias (porphyria cutanea tarda and variegate porphyria).
Pregnancy.
Progressive systemic sclerosis and related conditions.
PUVA therapy (psoralen administration) for psoriasis and vitiligo.*

ACTH, Adrenocorticotropic hormone; *MSH,* melanocyte-stimulating hormone; *PUVA,* psoralen plus ultraviolet A.
*Accentuation on sun-exposed surfaces.

HYPERSPLENISM, ASSOCIATED CONDITIONS

ICD-9CM # 289.4

Cirrhosis.
Portal vein thrombosis.
Myeloproliferative diseases.
Lymphomas.
Leukemias.
Splenic vein thrombosis.
Autoimmune disease.
Sickle cell disease.
Thalassemias.
Gaucher's disease.
Niemann-Pick disease.

HYPERTRICHOSIS[7]

ICD-9CM # 704.1 Hypertrichosis NOS
757.4 Hypertrichosis, Congenital

DRUGS

Dilantin.
Streptomycin.
Hexachlorobenzene.
Penicillamine.
Diazoxide.
Minoxidil.
Cyclosporine.

SYSTEMIC ILLNESS

Hypothyroidism.
Anorexia nervosa.
Malnutrition.
Porphyria.
Dermatomyositis.

IDIOPATHIC

HYPERTROPHIC OSTEOARTHROPATHY

ICD-9CM # 731.2

Idiopathic.
Pulmonary disease (e.g., pulmonary fibrosis, cystic fibrosis, sarcoidosis).
Bronchogenic carcinoma.
AIDS.
GI neoplasm (e.g., esophagus, colon).
Hepatic neoplasm, cirrhosis.
Cardiovascular diseases, aortic aneurysm, aortic prosthesis.
Congenital cyanotic heart disease, patent ductus arteriosus.
Pulmonary infections, bacterial endocarditis, amebic dysentery.
Inflammatory bowel disease.
Connective tissue diseases.
Lymphomas.
Thyroid acropachy.

HYPERVENTILATION, PERSISTENT[36]

ICD-9CM # 786.01

Fibrotic lung disease.
Metabolic acidosis (e.g., diabetes, uremia).
CNS disorders (midbrain and pontine lesions).
Hepatic coma.
Salicylate intoxication.
Fever.
Sepsis.
Psychogenic (e.g., anxiety).

HYPOCALCEMIA

ICD-9CM # 275.41

Renal insufficiency: hypocalcemia caused by:
- Increased calcium deposits in bone and soft tissue secondary to increased serum PO423 level.
- Decreased production of 1,25-dihydroxyvitamin D.
- Excessive loss of 25-OHD (nephrotic syndrome).

Hypoalbuminemia: each decrease in serum albumin (g/L) will decrease serum calcium by 0.8 mg/dl but will not change free (ionized) calcium.
Vitamin D deficiency:
- Malabsorption (most common cause).
- Inadequate intake.
- Decreased production of 1,25-dihydroxyvitamin D (vitamin D–dependent rickets, renal failure).
- Decreased production of 25-OHD (parenchymal liver disease).
- Accelerated 25-OHD catabolism (phenytoin, phenobarbital).
- End-organ resistance to 1,25-dihydroxyvitamin D.

Hypomagnesemia: hypocalcemia caused by:
- Decreased PTH secretion.
- Inhibition of PTH effect on bone.

Pancreatitis, hyperphosphatemia, osteoblastic metastases: hypocalcemia is secondary to increased calcium deposits (bone, abdomen).
Pseudohypoparathyroidism (PHP): autosomal recessive disorder characterized by short stature, shortening of metacarpal bones, obesity, and mental retardation; the hypocalcemia is secondary to congenital end-organ resistance to PTH.
Idiopathic hypoparathyroidism, surgical removal of parathyroids (e.g., neck surgery).
"Hungry bones syndrome": rapid transfer of calcium from plasma into bones after removal of a parathyroid tumor.
Sepsis.
Massive blood transfusion (as a result of EDTA in blood).

HYPOCAPNIA

ICD-9CM # 786.01

Hyperventilation.
Pneumonia, pneumonitis.
Fever, sepsis.
Medications (salicylates, beta-adrenergic agonists, progesterone, methylxanthines).
Pulmonary disease (asthma, interstitial fibrosis).
Pulmonary embolism.
Hepatic failure.
Metabolic acidosis.
High altitude.
CHF.
Pregnancy.
Pain.
CNS lesions.

HYPOGLYCEMIA

ICD-9CM # 251.2 Spontaneous
250.3 Diabetic
251.0 Due to Insulin
579.3 Postoperative
251.2 Reactive

Oral hypoglycemics (therapeutic, factitious).
Exogenous insulin (therapeutic, factitious).
Postoperative gastric emptying (alimentary hyperinsulinism).
Severe malnutrition.
Liver disease.
Hypermetabolic state (sepsis).
Ketotic hypoglycemia.
Insulinoma.
Antibodies to endogenous insulin.
Hormone deficiencies (glucagon, growth hormone, hypoadrenalism).
Enzyme disorders in metabolism of glycogen, hexose, glycolysis, and Krebs cycle.
Idiopathic.

HYPOGONADISM

ICD-9CM # 256.3 Female
257.2 Male
256.3 Ovarian
253.4 Pituitary
257.2 Testicular

HYPERGONADOTROPIC HYPOGONADISM

Hormone resistance (androgen, LH insensitivity).
Gonadal defects (e.g., Klinefelter's syndrome, myotonic dystrophy).
Drug-induced (e.g., spironolactone, cytotoxins).
Alcoholism, radiation-induced.
Mumps orchitis.
Anatomic defects, castration.

HYPOGONADOTROPIC HYPOGONADISM

Pituitary lesions (neoplasms, granulomas, infarction, hemochromatosis, vasculitis).
Drug-induced (e.g., glucocorticoids).
Hyperprolactinemia.
Genetic disorders (Laurence-Moon-Biedl syndrome, Prader-Willi).
Delayed puberty.
Other: chronic disease, nutritional deficiency, Kallmann's syndrome, idiopathic isolated LH or FSH deficiency.

HYPOKALEMIA

ICD-9CM # 276.8

Cellular shift (redistribution) and undetermined mechanisms.
Alkalosis (each 0.1 increase in pH decreases serum potassium by 0.4 to 0.6 mEq/L).
Insulin administration.
Vitamin B_{12} therapy for megaloblastic anemias, acute leukemias.
Hypokalemic periodic paralysis: rare familial disorder manifested by recurrent attacks of flaccid paralysis and hypokalemia.
Beta-adrenergic agonists (e.g., terbutaline), decongestants, bronchodilators, theophylline, caffeine.
Barium poisoning, toluene intoxication, verapamil intoxication, chloroquine intoxication.
Correction of digoxin intoxication with digoxin antibody fragments (Digibind).
Increased renal excretion.

Drugs:
- Diuretics, including carbonic anhydrase inhibitors (e.g., acetazolamide).
- Amphotericin B.
- High-dose sodium penicillin, nafcillin, ampicillin, or carbenicillin.
- Cisplatin.
- Aminoglycosides.
- Corticosteroids, mineralocorticoids.
- Foscarnet sodium.

RTA: distal (type 1) or proximal (type 2).
Diabetic ketoacidosis (DKA), ureteroenterostomy.
Magnesium deficiency.
Postobstruction diuresis, diuretic phase of ATN.
Osmotic diuresis (e.g., mannitol).
Bartter's syndrome: hyperplasia of juxtaglomerular cells leading to increased renin and aldosterone, metabolic alkalosis, hypokalemia, muscle weakness, and tetany (seen in young adults).
Increased mineralocorticoid activity (primary or secondary aldosteronism), Cushing's syndrome.
Chronic metabolic alkalosis from loss of gastric fluid (increased renal potassium secretion).
GI loss:
- Vomiting, nasogastric suction.
- Diarrhea.
- Laxative abuse.
- Villous adenoma.
- Fistulas.
- Inadequate dietary intake (e.g., anorexia nervosa).
- Cutaneous loss (excessive sweating).
- High dietary sodium intake, excessive use of licorice.

HYPOMAGNESEMIA

ICD-9CM # 275.2

GASTROINTESTINAL AND NUTRITIONAL

Defective GI absorption (malabsorption).
Inadequate dietary intake (e.g., alcoholics).
Parenteral therapy without magnesium.
Chronic diarrhea, villous adenoma, prolonged nasogastric suction, fistulas (small bowel, biliary).

EXCESSIVE RENAL LOSSES

Diuretics.
RTA.
Diuretic phase of ATN.
Endocrine disturbances (DKA, hyperaldosteronism, hyperthyroidism, hyperparathyroidism), SIADH, Bartter's syndrome, hypercalciuria, hypokalemia.
Cisplatin, alcohol, cyclosporine, digoxin, pentamidine, mannitol, amphotericin B, foscarnet, methotrexate.
Antibiotics (gentamicin, ticarcillin, carbenicillin).
Redistribution: hypoalbuminemia, cirrhosis, administration of insulin and glucose, theophylline, epinephrine, acute pancreatitis, cardiopulmonary bypass.
Miscellaneous: sweating, burns, prolonged exercise, lactation, "hungry-bones" syndrome.

HYPONATREMIA

ICD-9CM # 276.1

Renal loss from renal disease, diuretics.
GI loss (diarrhea, vomiting, suction).
Hypertonic hyponatremia (e.g., increased serum osmolality from hyperglycemia).
Transcutaneous loss (extensive burns, excessive sweating).
Fluid sequestration (e.g., ascites).
Osmotic diuresis (e.g., mannitol, glucose).
Dilutional (psychogenic polydipsia, iatrogenic).
Syndrome of inappropriate antidiuretic hormone secretion.
Edema with water and sodium retention.
Artifact (e.g., severe hyperlipidemia).
Laboratory error.
Adrenal insufficiency.

HYPOPHOSPHATEMIA

ICD-9CM # 275.3

Decreased intake (prolonged starvation [alcoholics], hyperalimentation, or IV infusion without phosphate).
Malabsorption.
Phosphate-binding antacids.
Renal loss:
- RTA.
- Fanconi syndrome, vitamin D–resistant rickets.
- ATN (diuretic phase).
- Hyperparathyroidism (primary or secondary).
- Familial hypophosphatemia.
- Hypokalemia, hypomagnesemia.
- Acute volume expansion.
- Glycosuria, idiopathic hypercalciuria.
- Acetazolamide.

Transcellular shift into cells:
- Alcohol withdrawal.
- DKA (recovery phase).
- Glucose-insulin or catecholamine infusion.
- Anabolic steroids.
- Total parenteral nutrition.
- Theophylline overdose.
- Severe hyperthermia; recovery from hypothermia.
- "Hungry bones" syndrome.

HYPOPIGMENTATION

ICD-9CM # 709.00

Vitiligo.
Tinea versicolor.
Atopic dermatitis.
Chemical leukoderma.
Idiopathic hypomelanosis.
Sarcoidosis.
SLE.
Scleroderma.
Oculocutaneous albinism.
Phenylketonuria.
Nevoid hypopigmentation.

HYPOTENSION, POSTURAL

ICD-9CM # 458.0

Antihypertensive medications (especially α-blockers, diuretics, ACE inhibitors).
Volume depletion (hemorrhage, dehydration).
Impaired cardiac output (constrictive pericarditis, aortic stenosis).
Peripheral autonomic dysfunction (DM, Guillain-Barré).
Idiopathic orthostatic hypotension.
Central autonomic dysfunction (Shy-Drager syndrome).
Peripheral venous disease.
Adrenal insufficiency.

ILIAC FOSSA PAIN, LEFT SIDED[38]

ICD-9CM # varies with specific diagnosis

GASTROINTESTINAL CAUSES OF ACUTE LEFT ILIAC FOSSA PAIN

Non-specific left iliac fossa pain including constipation.
Acute gastroenteritis.
Acute diverticulitis.
Colonic carcinoma.
Colonic ischemia.
Localized small bowel perforation.

ILIAC FOSSA PAIN, RIGHT SIDED[38]

ICD-9CM # varies with specific diagnosis

DIFFERENTIAL DIAGNOSIS OF RIGHT ILIAC FOSSA PAIN

Gastrointestinal causes

Non-specific right iliac fossa pain.
Acute appendicitis.
Mesenteric adenitis.
Terminal ileitis.
Acute inflammation of a Meckel's diverticulum.
Crohn's disease of the terminal ileum.
Cecal carcinoma.
Inflammatory cecal lesion (e.g., diverticulitis in a solitary cecal diverticulum).
Inflammatory lesion of the terminal ileum (e.g., foreign body perforation).

Non-gastrointestinal causes

Ruptured ovarian follicle (Mittelschmerz).
Acute salpingitis (pelvic inflammatory disease).
Rupture/torsion or hemorrhage of an ovarian cyst.
Endometriosis.
Ectopic pregnancy.
Urinary tract infection.

IMPOTENCE[27]

ICD-9CM # 302.72 Psychosexual
607.84 Organic
997.99 Organic Postprostatectomy

Psychogenic.
Endocrine: hyperprolactinemia, DM, Cushing's syndrome, hypothyroidism or hyperthyroidism, abnormality of hypothalamic-pituitary-testicular axis.

Vascular: arterial insufficiency, venous leakage, AV malformation, local trauma.
Medications.
Neurogenic: autonomic or sensory neuropathy, spinal cord trauma or tumor, CVA, multiple sclerosis, temporal lobe epilepsy.
Systemic illness: renal failure, COPD, cirrhosis of liver, myotonic dystrophy.
Peyronie's disease.
Prostatectomy.

INCONTINENCE, FECAL[38]

ICD-9CM # 787.6

NORMAL SPHINCTER

Diarrhea.
Anorectal conditions:

- Rectal carcinoma.
- Inflammatory bowel disease.
- Hemorrhoids.
- Mucosal prolapse.
- Fissure-in-ano.
- Abnormal rectal sensation.

ABNORMAL SPHINCTER

Congenital abnormalities.
Anal sepsis.
Neurological conditions.
Rectal prolapse.
Sphincter trauma.
Neurogenic (idiopathic) incontinence.

INFERTILITY, FEMALE[14]

ICD-9CM # 628.9

FALLOPIAN TUBE PATHOLOGY

PID or puerperal infection.
Congenital anomalies.
Endometriosis.
Secondary to past peritonitis of nongenital origin.
Amenorrhea and anovulation.
Minor anovulatory disturbances.

CERVICAL AND UTERINE FACTORS

Leiomyomas and polyps.
Uterine anomalies.
Intrauterine synechiae (Asherman's syndrome).
Destroyed endocervical glands (postsurgery or postinfection).

VAGINAL FACTORS

Congenital absence of vagina.
Imperforate hymen.
Vaginismus.
Vaginitis.

IMMUNOLOGIC FACTORS

Sperm-immobilizing antibodies.
Sperm-agglutinating antibodies.

NUTRITIONAL AND METABOLIC FACTORS

Thyroid disorders.
DM.
Severe nutritional disturbances.

INFERTILITY, MALE[14]

ICD-9CM # 606.9

DECREASED PRODUCTION OF SPERMATOZOA

Varicocele.
Testicular failure.
Endocrine disorders.
Cryptorchidism.
Stress, smoking, caffeine, nicotine, recreational drugs.

DUCTAL OBSTRUCTION

Epididymal (postinfection).
Congenital absence of vas deferens.
Ejaculatory duct (postinfection).
Postvasectomy.

INABILITY TO DELIVER SPERM INTO VAGINA

Ejaculatory disturbances.
Hypospadias.
Sexual problems (i.e., impotence), medical or psychological.

ABNORMAL SEMEN

Infection.
Abnormal volume.
Abnormal viscosity.
Abnormal sperm motion.

IMMUNOLOGIC FACTORS

Sperm-immobilizing antibodies.
Sperm-agglutinating antibodies.

INSOMNIA[33]

ICD-9CM # 780.52 Insomnia NOS
307.42 Insomnia, Chronic Associated with Anxiety or Depression
780.51 Insomnia with Sleep Apnea

Anxiety disorder, psychophysiologic insomnia.
Depression.
Drugs (e.g., caffeine, amphetamines, cocaine), hypnotic-dependent sleep disorder.
Pain, fibromyalgia.
Inadequate sleep hygiene.
Restless leg syndrome.
Obstructive sleep apnea.
Sleep bruxism.
Medical illness (e.g., GERD, sleep-related asthma, parkinsonism and movement disorders).
Narcolepsy.
Other: periodic leg movement of sleep, central sleep apnea, REM behavioral disorder.

INTESTINAL PSEUDOOBSTRUCTION[36]

ICD-9CM # 560.1 Adynamic Intestinal Obstruction
564.9 Intestinal Disorder, Functional

"PRIMARY" (IDIOPATHIC INTESTINAL PSEUDOOBSTRUCTION)

Hollow visceral myopathy:
Familial.
Sporadic.
Neuropathic:
Abnormal myenteric plexus.
Normal myenteric plexus.

SECONDARY

Scleroderma.
Myxedema.
Amyloidosis.
Muscular dystrophy.
Hypokalemia.
Chronic renal failure.
DM.
Drug toxicity caused by:
Anticholinergics.
Opiate narcotics.
Ogilvie's syndrome.

INTRACEREBRAL HEMORRHAGE, NONHYPERTENSIVE CAUSES

ICD-9CM # 431

Trauma.
Anticoagulation.
Intracranial tumors.
Vascular malformations.
Bleeding disorders.
Vasculitides (e.g., polyarteritis nodosa, granulomatous angiitis).
Cocaine and other sympathomimetic agents.
Cerebral amyloid angiopathy.

INTRACRANIAL LESION

ICD-9CM # 348.8

Tumor (primary or metastatic).
Abscess.
Stroke.
Intracranial hemorrhage.
Angioma.
Multiple sclerosis (initial single lesion).
Granuloma.
Herpes encephalitis.
Artifact.

INTRAOCULAR NEOPLASM

ICD-9CM # varies with specific disorder

MALIGNANT

Retinoblastoma.
Melanoma.
Reticulum cell sarcoma.
Metastatic tumor.

BENIGN
Melanocytic nevus.
Hemangioma.
Reactive lymphoid hyperplasia.

IRON OVERLOAD[20]
ICD-9CM # 275.0

HEREDITARY IRON OVERLOAD
Hereditary hemochromatosis:
  HFE-associated (type 1).
  Non–HFE-associated:
  • Transferrin receptor 2–associated (type 3).
Juvenile hemochromatosis (type 2):
  Hemojuvelin-associated (type 2A).
  Hepcidin-associated (type 2B).
Autosomal dominant hemochromatosis:
  Ferroportin-associated (type 4).
DMT1-associated hemochromatosis.
Atransferrinemia.
Aceruloplasminemia.

ACQUIRED IRON OVERLOAD
Iron-loading anemias (refractory anemias with hypercellular erythroid marrow).
Chronic liver disease.
Porphyria cutanea tarda.
Insulin resistance–associated hepatic iron overload.
African dietary iron overload.[a]
Medical iron ingestion.[a]
Parenteral iron overload:
  Transfusional iron overload.
  Inadvertent iron overload from therapeutic injections.

PERINATAL IRON OVERLOAD
Neonatal hemochromatosis.
Trichohepatoenteric syndrome.
Cerebrohepatorenal syndrome.
GRACILE[b] (Fellman) syndrome.

FOCAL SEQUESTRATION OF IRON
Idiopathic pulmonary hemosiderosis.
Renal hemosiderosis.
Associated with neurologic abnormalities:
  Pantothenate kinase–associated neurodegeneration (formerly called Hallervorden-Spatz syndrome).
  Neuroferritinopathy.
  Friedreich's ataxia.

[a]May have a genetic component.
[b]GRACILE, growth retardation, aminoaciduria, cholestasis, iron overload, lactic acidosis, and early death.

ISCHEMIC COLITIS, NONOCCLUSIVE[21]
ICD-9CM # 557.1

ACUTE DIMINUTION OF COLONIC INTRAMURAL BLOOD FLOW
Small Vessel Obstruction
Collagen-vascular disease.
Vasculitis, diabetes.
Oral contraceptives.

Nonocclusive Hypoperfusion
Hemorrhage.
CHF, MI, arrhythmias.
Sepsis.
Vasoconstricting agents: vasopressin, ergot.
Increased viscosity: polycythemia, sickle cell disease, thrombocytosis.

INCREASED DEMAND ON MARGINAL BLOOD FLOW
Increased Motility
Mass lesion, stricture.
Constipation.
Increased Intraluminal Pressure
Bowel obstruction.
Colonoscopy.
Barium enema.

ISCHEMIC NECROSIS OF CARTILAGE AND BONE[14]
ICD-9CM # 733.90

ENDOCRINE/METABOLIC
Ethanol abuse.
Glucocorticoid therapy.
Cushing's disease.
DM.
Hyperuricemia.
Osteomalacia.
Hyperlipidemia.

STORAGE DISEASES (E.G., GAUCHER'S DISEASE)
Hemoglobinopathies (e.g., sickle cell disease).
Trauma (e.g., dislocation, fracture).
HIV infection.
Dysbaric conditions (e.g., caisson disease).
Collagen-vascular disorders.
Irradiation.
Pancreatitis.
Organ transplantation.
Hemodialysis.
Burns.
Intravascular coagulation.
Idiopathic, familial.

JAUNDICE
ICD-9CM # 782.4 Jaundice NOS
576.8 Jaundice, Obstructive
277.4 Bilirubin Excretion Disorders

PREDOMINANCE OF DIRECT (CONJUGATED) BILIRUBIN
Extrahepatic obstruction.
Common duct abnormalities: calculi, neoplasm, stricture, cyst, sclerosing cholangitis.
Metastatic carcinoma.
Pancreatic carcinoma, pseudocyst.
Ampullary carcinoma.
Hepatocellular disease: hepatitis, cirrhosis.
Drugs: estrogens, phenothiazines, captopril, methyltestosterone, labetalol.
Cholestatic jaundice of pregnancy.
Hereditary disorders: Dubin-Johnson syndrome, Rotor's syndrome.
Recurrent benign intrahepatic cholestasis.

PREDOMINANCE OF INDIRECT (UNCONJUGATED) BILIRUBIN
Hemolysis: hereditary and acquired hemolytic anemias.
Inefficient marrow production.
Impaired hepatic conjugation: chloramphenicol.
Neonatal jaundice.
Hereditary disorders: Gilbert's syndrome, Crigler-Najjar syndrome.

JOINT PAIN, ANTERIOR HIP, MEDIAL THIGH, KNEE[28]
ICD-9CM # 719.4 add 5th digit
0 Site NOS
1 Shoulder Region
2 Upper Arm (Elbow, Humerus)
3 Forearm (Radius, Wrist, Ulna)
4 Hand
5 Pelvic Region and Thigh
6 Lower Leg (Fibula, Patella, Tibia)
7 Ankle and/or Foot

ACUTE
Acute rheumatic fever.
Adductor muscle strain.
Avascular necrosis.
Crystal arthritis.
Femoral artery (pseudo) aneurysm.
Fracture (femoral neck or intertrochanteric).
Hemarthrosis.
Hernia.
Herpes zoster.
Iliopectineal bursitis.
Iliopsoas tendinitis.
Inguinal lymphadenitis.
Osteomalacia.
Painful transient osteoporosis of hip.
Septic arthritis.

SUBACUTE AND CHRONIC
Adductory muscle strain.
Amyloidosis.
Acute rheumatic fever.
Femoral artery aneurysm.
Hernia (inguinal or femoral).
Iliopectineal bursitis.
Iliopsoas tendinitis.
Inguinal lymphadenopathy.
Osteochondromatosis.
Osteomyelitis.
Osteitis deformans (Paget's disease).
Osteomalacia (pseudofracture).
Postherpetic neuralgia.
Sterile synovitis (e.g., RA, psoriatic, SLE).

JOINT PAIN, HIP, LATERAL THIGH[28]
ICD-9CM # 959.6 Hip Injury
719.95 Hip Joint Disorder
843.9 Hip Strain

ACUTE
Herpes zoster.
Iliotibial tendinitis.
Impacted fracture of femoral neck.

Lateral femoral cutaneous neuropathy (meralgia paresthetica).
Radiculopathy: L4-5.
Trochanteric avulsion fracture (greater trochanter).
Trochanteric bursitis.
Trochanteric fracture.

SUBACUTE AND CHRONIC

Lateral femoral cutaneous neuropathy (meralgia paresthetica).
Osteomyelitis.
Postherpetic neuralgia.
Radiculopathy: L4-5.
Tumors.

JOINT PAIN, POLYARTICULAR

ICD-9CM # 719.40

Osteoarthritis.
RA.
Fibromyalgia.
Viral syndrome (e.g., human parvovirus B19 infection).
SLE.
Psoriatic arthritis.
Ankylosing spondylitis.

JOINT PAIN, POSTERIOR HIPS, THIGH, BUTTOCKS[28]

ICD-9CM # 719.4 add 5th digit
0 Site NOS
1 Shoulder Region
2 Upper Arm (Elbow, Humerus)
3 Forearm (Radius, Wrist, Ulna)
4 Hand
5 Pelvic Region and Thigh
6 Lower Leg (Fibula, Patella, Tibia)
7 Ankle and/or Foot

ACUTE

Gluteal muscle strain.
Herpes zoster.
Ischial bursitis.
Ischial or sacral fracture.
Osteomalacia (pseudofracture).
Sciatic neuropathy.
Radiculopathy: L5-S1.

SUBACUTE AND CHRONIC

Gluteal muscle strain.
Ischial bursitis.
Lumbar spinal stenosis.
Osteoarthritis of hip.
Osteitis deformans (Paget's disease).
Osteomyelitis.
Osteochondromatosis.
Osteomalacia (pseudofracture).
Postherpetic neuralgia.
Radiculopathy: L5-S1.
Tumors.

JOINT SWELLING

ICD-9CM # 719.0 add 5th digit
0 Site NOS
1 Shoulder Region
2 Upper Arm (Elbow, Humerus)
3 Forearm (Radius, Wrist, Ulna)
4 Hand
5 Pelvic Region and Thigh
6 Lower Leg (Fibula, Patella, Tibia)
7 Ankle and/or Foot

Trauma.
Osteoarthritis.
Gout.
Pyogenic arthritis.
Pseudogout.
RA.
Viral syndrome.

JUGULAR VENOUS DISTENTION

ICD-9CM # 459.89 Increased Venous Pressure

Right-sided heart failure.
Cardiac tamponade.
Constrictive pericarditis.
Goiter.
Tension pneumothorax.
Pulmonary hypertension.
Cardiomyopathy (restrictive).
Superior vena cava syndrome.
Valsalva maneuver.
Right atrial myxoma.
COPD.

KERATITIS, NONINFECTIOUS

ICD-9CM # 370.9

Collagen vascular disease.
Atopic keratoconjunctivitis.
Chemical injury.
Thermal injury.
Ectropion/entropion.
Lid defects.
Exophthalmos.
Keratoconjunctivitis sicca.
Erythema multiforme.
Mucous membrane pemphigoid.
DM (delayed epithelial healing).
Neuroparalytic (cranial nerve VII).
Neurotrophic (diabetes, cranial nerve V).

KIDNEY ENLARGEMENT, UNILATERAL[38]

ICD-9CM # 591

Hydronephrosis (may be bilateral).
Polycystic kidney (may be bilateral).
Simple cyst of kidney.
Renal cell carcinoma.
Pyonephrosis (may be bilateral).
Acute renal vein thrombosis.

KNEE PAIN[28]

ICD-9CM # 844.1 Collateral Ligament Sprain, Medial
844.2 Cruciate Ligament Sprain
716.96 Knee Inflammation
959.7 Knee Injury
718.86 Knee Instability
836.1 Lateral Meniscus Tear
836.0 Medial Meniscus Tear
844.8 Patellar Sprain
719.56 Knee Stiffness
719.06 Knee Swelling

DIFFUSE

Articular.
Anterior.
Prepatellar bursitis.
Patellar tendon enthesopathy.
Chondromalacia patellae.
Patellofemoral osteoarthritis.
Cruciate ligament injury.
Medial plica syndrome.

MEDIAL

Anserine bursitis.
Spontaneous osteonecrosis.
Osteoarthritis.
Medial meniscal tear.
Medial collateral ligament bursitis.
Referred pain from hip and L3.
Fibromyalgia.

LATERAL

Iliotibial band syndrome.
Meniscal cyst.
Lateral meniscal tear.
Collateral ligament.
Peroneal tenosynovitis.

POSTERIOR

Popliteal cyst (Baker's cyst).
Tendinitis.
Aneurysms, ganglions, sarcoma.

KNEE PAIN, IN DIFFERENT AGE GROUPS[8]

ICD-9CM # 719.46

COMMON CAUSES OF KNEE PAIN IN DIFFERENT AGE GROUPS

Childhood (2-10 yr)
Intraarticular:
Juvenile arthritis.
Osteochondritis dissecans.
Infection.
Torn discoid meniscus.
Periarticular:
Osteomyelitis.
Referred:
Perthes' disease.
Irritable hip.
Adolescence (10-18 yr)
Intraarticular:
Osteochondritis dissecans.
Torn meniscus.
Anterior knee pain syndrome.
Patellar instability.
Periarticular:
Osgood–Schlatter disease.
Sinding–Larsen–Johansson syndrome.
Osteomyelitis.
Bone tumors.

Referred:
Slipped upper femoral epiphysis.
Early adulthood (18-30 yr)
Intraarticular:
Torn meniscus.
Patellar instability.
Anterior knee pain syndrome.
Inflammatory arthritis.
Periarticular:
Ligament injuries.
Bursitis.
Adulthood (30-50 yr)
Intraarticular:
Degenerate meniscal tears.
Osteoarthritis.
Inflammatory arthritis.
Periarticular:
Bursitis.
Referred:
Osteoarthritis of hip.
Spinal disorders.
Old age (>50 yr)
Intraarticular:
Osteoarthritis.
Inflammatory arthritis.
Periarticular:
Bursitis.
Referred:
Osteoarthritis of hip.
Spinal disorders.

LEFT AXIS DEVIATION[22]

ICD-9CM # 426.3 Left Bundle Branch Block
426.2 Left Bundle Branch Hemiblock
429.3 Left Ventricular Hypertrophy

Normal variation.
Left anterior fascicular block (hemiblock).
Left bundle branch block.
Left ventricular hypertrophy.
Mechanical shifts causing a horizontal heart, high diaphragm, pregnancy, ascites.
Some forms of ventricular tachycardia.
Endocardial cushion defects and other congenital heart disease.

LEFT BUNDLE BRANCH BLOCK

ICD-9CM # 426.3

Ischemic heart disease.
Electrolyte abnormalities (e.g., hyperkalemia).
Cardiomyopathy.
Idiopathic.
LVH.
Pulmonary embolism.
Cardiac trauma.
Bacterial endocarditis.

LEG CRAMPS, NOCTURNAL

ICD-9CM # 729.82 Muscle Cramps

Diabetic neuropathy.
Medications.
Electrolyte abnormalities (hypokalemia, hyponatremia, hypocalcemia, hyperkalemia, hypophosphatemia).
Respiratory alkalosis.
Uremia.
Hemodialysis.
Peripheral nerve injury.
ALS.
Alcohol use.
Heat cramps.
Vitamin B_{12} deficiency.
Hyperthyroidism.
Contractures.
DVT.
Hypoglycemia.
Peripheral vascular insufficiency.
Baker's cyst.

LEG LENGTH DISCREPANCIES[23]

ICD-9CM # 736.81 Leg Length Discrepancy, Acquired
755.30 Leg Length Discrepancy, Congenital

CONGENITAL

Proximal femoral local deficiency.
Coxa vara.
Hemiatrophy-hemihypertrophy (anisomelia).
Development dysplasia of the hip.

DEVELOPMENTAL

Legg-Calvé-Perthes disease.

NEUROMUSCULAR

Polio.
Cerebral palsy (hemiplegia).

INFECTIOUS

Pyogenic osteomyelitis with physeal damage.

TRAUMA

Physeal injury with premature closure.
Overgrowth.
Malunion (shortening).

TUMOR

Physeal destruction.
Radiation-induced physeal injury.
Overgrowth.

LEG MOVEMENT WHEN STANDING, INVOLUNTARY

ICD-9CM # varies with specific disorder

Benign essential tremor.
Orthostatic tremor.
Spastic ataxia.
Cerebellar truncal tremor.
Postanoxic myoclonus.

LEG PAIN WITH EXERCISE

ICD-9CM # 729.82 Muscle Cramps

Shin splints.
Arteriosclerosis obliterans.
Neurogenic (spinal cord compression or ischemia).
Venous claudication.
Popliteal cyst.
DVT.
Thromboangiitis obliterans.
Adventitial cysts.
Popliteal artery entrapment syndrome.
McArdle syndrome.

LEG ULCERS[28]

ICD-9CM # 440.23 Lower Limb, Arteriosclerotic
707.1 Lower Limb, Chronic
707.1 Lower Limb, Neurogenic
250.70 Lower Limb, Chronic DM Type 2
250.71 Lower Limb, Chronic, DM Type 1

VASCULAR

Arterial: arteriosclerosis, thromboangiitis obliterans, AV malformation, cholesterol emboli.
Venous: superficial varicosities, incompetent perforators, DVT, lymphatic abnormalities.

VASCULITIS HEMATOLOGIC

Sickle cell anemia, thalassemia, polycythemia vera, leukemia, cold agglutinin disease.
Macroglobulinemia, protein C and protein S deficiency, cryoglobulinemia, lupus anticoagulant, antiphospholipid syndrome.

INFECTIOUS

Fungus: Blastomycosis, coccidioidomycosis, histoplasmosis, sporotrichosis.
Bacterial: Furuncle, ecthyma, septic emboli.
Protozoal: leishmaniasis.

METABOLIC

Necrobiosis lipoidica diabeticorum.
Localized bullous pemphigoid.
Gout, calcinosis cutis, Gaucher's disease.

TUMORS

Basal cell carcinoma, squamous cell carcinoma, melanoma.
Mycosis fungoides, Kaposi's sarcoma, metastatic neoplasms.

TRAUMA

Burns, cold injury, radiation dermatitis.
Insect bites.
Factitial, excessive pressure.

NEUROPATHIC

Diabetic trophic ulcers.
Tabes dorsalis, syringomyelia.

DRUGS

Warfarin, IV colchicine extravasation, methotrexate, halogens, ergotism, hydroxyurea.

PANNICULITIS

Weber-Christian disease.
Pancreatic fat necrosis, alpha-antitrypsinase deficiency.

LEPTOMENINGEAL LESIONS

ICD-9CM # varies with specific disorder

Metastases.
Multiple sclerosis.
Bacterial or viral meningitis.
Vasculitis.
Lyme disease.
Tuberculosis.
Fungal infections (e.g., *Cryptococcus*).
Sarcoidosis.
Wegener's granulomatosis.
Neurocysticercosis.
Rheumatoid nodules.
Histiocytosis.

LEUKOCORIA

ICD-9CM # 379.90

Cataract.
Retinal detachment.
Retinoblastoma.
Retinal telangiectasia.
Retrolenticular vascularized membrane.
Familial exudative vitreoretinopathy.

LIMP

ICD-9CM # 781.2 Gait Abnormality
719.75 Gait Disorder Due to Joint Abnormality in Hip, Buttock, or Femur
719.76 Gait Disorder Due to Joint Abnormality in Lower Leg
719.77 Gait Disorder Due to Joint Abnormality in Ankle and/or Foot
300.11 Hysterical Gait Disorder

Degenerative joint disease, osteochondritis dissecans, chondromalacia patellae.
Trauma to extremities, vertebral disc, hips.
Poorly fitting shoes, foreign body in shoe, unequal leg length.
Splinter in foot.
Joint infection (septic arthritis, osteomyelitis), viral arthritis.
Abdominal pain (e.g., appendicitis, incarcerated hernia), testicular torsion.
Polio, neuromuscular disorders, Guillain-Barré syndrome, multiple sclerosis.
Osgood-Schlatter disease.
Legg-Calvé-Perthes disease.
Factitious, somatization syndrome.
Neoplasm (local or metastatic).
Other: diskitis, periostitis, sickle cell disease, hemophilia.

LIMPING, PEDIATRIC AGE[23]

ICD-9CM # 781.2 Gait Abnormality

TODDLER (1-3 YR)

Infection:
- Septic arthritis:
  - Hip.
  - Knee.
- Osteomyelitis.
- Diskitis.

Occult trauma:
- Toddler's fracture.

Neoplasia.

CHILDHOOD (4-10 YR)

Infection:
- Septic arthritis:
  - Hip.
  - Knee.
- Osteomyelitis.
- Diskitis.
- Transient synovitis, hip.

LCPD.
Tarsal coalition.
Rheumatologic disorder:
- JRA.

Trauma.
Neoplasia.

ADOLESCENCE (11+ YR)

SCFE.
Rheumatologic disorder:
- JRA.

Trauma.
Tarsal coalition.
Hip dislocation (DDH).
Neoplasia.

DDH, Developmental dysplasia of the hip; *JRA,* juvenile RA; *LCPD,* Legg-Calvé-Perthes disease; *SCFE,* slipped capital femoral epiphysis.

LIVEDO RETICULITIS

ICD-9CM # code not available

Emboli (SBE, left atrial myxoma, cholesterol emboli).
Thrombocythemia or polycythemia.
Antiphospholipid antibody syndrome.
Cryoglobulinemia, cryofibrinogenemia.
Leukocytoclastic vasculitis.
SLE, RA, dermatomyositis.
Pancreatitis.
Drugs (quinine, quinidine, amantadine, catecholamines).
Physiologic (cutis marmorata).
Congenital.

LIVER DISEASE, PREGNANCY[38]

ICD-9CM # varies with specific diagnosis

INCIDENTAL TO PREGNANCY

Viral hepatitis.
Alcohol related.
Autoimmune chronic active hepatitis.

RELATED TO PREGNANCY (possibly influenced by hormones present in pregnancy)

Complicated gallstone disease.
Hepatic adenoma.
Focal nodular hyperplasia.
Budd-Chiari syndrome.

SPECIFIC TO PREGNANCY

Severe hyperemesis gravidarum.
Benign intrahepatic cholestasis.
Acute fatty liver of pregnancy.
Pre-eclampsia (HELLP).

LIVER LESIONS, BENIGN, OFTEN CONFUSED WITH MALIGNANCY

ICD-9CM # 573.8

Fatty infiltration.
Adenoma.
Hemangioma.
Cysts.
Flow artifacts.
Focal nodular hyperplasia.
Nonenhanced vessels.

LOW-VOLTAGE ECG

ICD-9CM # 794.31

Hypothyroidism.
Obesity.
Pericardial effusion.
Anasarca.
Pleural effusion.
Pneumothorax.
Amyloidosis.
Aortic stenosis.

LYMPHADENOPATHY[14]

ICD-9CM # 785.6

GENERALIZED

AIDS.
Lymphoma: Hodgkin's disease, non-Hodgkin's lymphoma.
Leukemias, reticuloendotheliosis.
Infectious mononucleosis, CMV, and other viral infections.
Diffuse skin infection: generalized furunculosis, multiple tick bites.
Parasitic infections: toxoplasmosis, filariasis, leishmaniasis, Chagas' disease.
Serum sickness.
Collagen vascular diseases (RA, SLE).
Dengue (arbovirus infection).
Sarcoidosis and other granulomatous diseases.
Drugs: INH, hydantoin derivatives, antithyroid and antileprosy drugs.
Secondary syphilis.
Hyperthyroidism, lipid-storage diseases.

LOCALIZED

Cervical Nodes

Infections of the head, neck, ears, sinuses, scalp, pharynx.
Mononucleosis.
Lymphoma.
TB.
Malignancy of head and neck.
Rubella.

Scalene/Supraclavicular Nodes

Lymphoma.
Lung neoplasm.
Bacterial or fungal infection of thorax or retroperitoneum.
GI malignancy.

Axillary Nodes
Infections of hands and arms.
Cat-scratch disease.
Neoplasm (lymphoma, melanoma, breast carcinoma).
Brucellosis.
Epitrochlear Nodes
Infections of the hand.
Lymphoma.
Tularemia.
Sarcoidosis, secondary syphilis (usually bilateral).
Inguinal Nodes
Infections of leg or foot, folliculitis (pubic hair).
LGV, syphilis.
Lymphoma.
Pelvic malignancy.
Pasteurella pestis.
Hilar Nodes
Sarcoidosis.
TB.
Lung carcinoma.
Fungal infections, systemic.
Mediastinal Nodes
Sarcoidosis.
Lymphoma.
Lung neoplasm.
TB.
Mononucleosis.
Histoplasmosis.
Abdominal/Retroperitoneal Nodes
Lymphoma.
TB.
Neoplasm (ovary, testes, prostate, and other malignancies).

LYMPHANGITIS[25]

ICD-9CM # 457.2

Acute:
- Group A streptococci.
- *Staphylococcus aureus.*
- *Pasteurella multocida.*

Chronic:
- *Sporothrix schenckii* (sporotrichosis).
- *Mycobacterium marinum* (swimming pool granuloma).
- *Mycobacterium kansasii.*
- *Nocardia brasiliensis.*
- *W. bancrofti.*

LYMPHOCYTOSIS, ATYPICAL[25]

ICD-9CM # 288.8

Epstein-Barr virus primary infection (infectious mononucleosis).
Cytomegalovirus primary infection (heterophile-negative mono).
Human herpesvirus 6 primary infection (roseola).
Primary HIV infection.
Toxoplasmosis.
Acute viral hepatitis.
Rubella, mumps.
Drug reactions (e.g., phenytoin, sulfa).

MACROTHROMBOCYTOPENIA, INHERITED[20]

ICD-9CM # varies with specific diagnosis

Bernard-Soulier syndrome.
MHY9-related disorders:
- May-Hegglin anomaly.
- Sebastian syndrome.
- Fechtner syndrome.
- Epstein syndrome.

Gray platelet syndrome.
Montreal platelet syndrome.
Mediterranean macrothrombocytopenia.
Mediterranean stomatocytosis/macrothrombocytenia.
GATA1 mutations.
Sialyl-Lewis-S antigen deficiency.
Paris-Trousseau syndrome.
Platelet-type von Willebrand's disease.

MALABSORPTION[38]

ICD-9CM # 579

CAUSES OF MALABSORPTION

More Common
Celiac disease.
Chronic pancreatitis.
Post gastrectomy.
Crohn's disease.
Small bowel resection.
Small intestinal bacterial overgrowth.
Lactase deficiency.
Less Common
AIDS (*Myobacterium avium* intracellulare, AIDS enteropathy).
Whipple's disease.
Intestinal lymphoma.
Immunoproliferative small intestinal disease (alpha heavy chain disease).
Radiation enteritis.
Collagenous sprue.
Tropical sprue.
Non-granulomatous ulcerative jejunoileitis.
Eosinophilic gastroenteritis.
Amyloidosis.
Zollinger-Ellison syndrome.
Intestinal lymphangiectasia.
Systemic mastocytosis.
Chronic mesenteric ischemia.
Abetalipoproteinemia (autosomal recessive).

MEDIASTINAL COMPARTMENTS, ANATOMY AND PATHOLOGY[39]

ICD-9CM # varies with specific diagnosis

Anterior

Normal Structures
Lymph nodes.
Connective tissue.
Thymus (remnant in adults).
Masses
Thymoma.
Germ cell neoplasm.
Lymphoma.
Thyroid enlargement (intrathoracic goiter).
Other tumors.

Middle

Normal Structures
Pericardium.
Heart.
Vessels: Ascending aorta, venae cavae, main pulmonary arteries.
Trachea.
Lymph nodes.
Nerves: Phrenic, upper vagus.
Masses
Carcinoma.
Lymphoma.
Pericardial cyst.
Bronchogenic cyst.
Benign lymph node enlargement (granulomatous disease).

Posterior

Normal Structures
Vessels: Descending aorta.
Esophagus.
Vertebral column.
Nerves: Sympathetic chain, lower vagus.
Lymph nodes.
Connective tissue.
Masses
Neurogenic tumor.
Diaphragmatic hernia.

MEDIASTINAL MASSES OR WIDENING ON CHEST X-RAY

ICD-9CM # 785.6 Adenopathy
519.3 Disease NEC
793.2 Shift (CXR)

Lymphoma: Hodgkin's disease and non-Hodgkin's lymphoma.
Sarcoidosis.
Vascular: aortic aneurysm, ectasia or tortuosity of aorta or bronchocephalic vessels.
Carcinoma: lungs, esophagus.
Esophageal diverticula.
Hiatal hernia.
Achalasia.
Prominent pulmonary outflow tract: pulmonary hypertension, pulmonary embolism, right-to-left shunts.
Trauma: mediastinal hemorrhage.
Pneumomediastinum.
Lymphadenopathy caused by silicosis and other pneumoconioses.
Leukemias.
Infections: TB, viral (rare), *Mycoplasma* (rare), fungal, tularemia.
Substernal thyroid.
Thymoma.
Teratoma.
Bronchogenic cyst.
Pericardial cyst.
Neurofibroma, neurosarcoma, ganglioneuroma.

MEDIASTINITIS, ACUTE[25]

ICD-9CM # 519.2

Esophageal perforation.
Iatrogenic.
EGD, esophageal dilation, esophageal variceal sclerotherapy, nasogastric tube, Sengstaken-Blackmore tube, endotracheal intubation, esophageal surgery, paraesophageal surgery, transesophageal echocardiography, anterior stabilization of cervical vertebral bodies.
Swallowed foreign bodies.
Trauma.
Spontaneous perforation (e.g., emesis, carcinoma).
Head and neck infections (e.g., tonsillitis, pharyngitis, parotitis, epiglottitis, odontogenic).
Infections originating at another site (e.g., TB, pneumonia, pancreatitis, osteomyelitis of sternum, clavicle, ribs).
Cardiothoracic surgery (median sternotomy) (e.g., CABG, valve replacement, other types of cardiothoracic surgery).

MELANONYCHIA

ICD-9CM # varies with specific disorder

Pregnancy.
Trauma.
Medications (e.g., AZT, 5-fluorouracil, doxorubicin, psoralens).
Nail matrix nevus.
HIV infection.
Onychomycosis.
Melanocyte hyperplasia.
Verrucae.
Pustular psoriasis.
Lichen planus.
Basal cell carcinoma.
Nail matrix melanoma.
Subungual keratosis.
Addison's disease.
Bowen's disease.

MEMORY LOSS SYMPTOMS, ELDERLY PATIENTS

ICD-9CM # varies with specific disorder

Age-related mild cognitive impairment.
Depression (pseudodementia).
Medications (e.g., anticholinergics, sedatives).
Hypothyroidism.
Chronic hypoxia.
Cerebrovascular infarcts.
Alzheimer's disease.
Hepatic disease.
Chronic renal failure.
Hyperthyroidism.
Frontotemporal dementia.
Lewy body dementia.

MENINGITIS, CHRONIC[26]

ICD-9CM # 322.2

TB.
Fungal CNS infection.
Tertiary syphilis.
CNS neoplasm.
Metabolic encephalopathies.
Multiple sclerosis.
Chronic subdural hematoma.
SLE cerebritis.
Encephalitides.
Sarcoidosis.
NSAIDs.
Behçet's syndrome.
Anatomic defects (traumatic, congenital, postoperative).
Granulomatous angiitis.

MENINGITIS, RECURRENT[25]

ICD-9CM # varies with specific disorder

Drug induced (with rechallenge).
Parameningeal focus.
 Infection (sinusitis, mastoiditis, osteomyelitis, brain abscess).
 Tumor (epidermoid cyst, craniopharyngioma).
Posttraumatic (bacterial).
Mollaret's meningitis.
SLE.
Herpes simplex virus.

MESENTERIC ISCHEMIA, NONOCCLUSIVE[26]

ICD-9CM # 557.0 Mesenteric Artery Embolism or Infarction
557.1 Mesenteric Artery Insufficiency, Chronic
902.39 Mesenteric Vein Injury

Cardiovascular disease resulting in low-flow states (CHF, cardiogenic shock, post cardiopulmonary bypass, dysrhythmias).
Septic shock.
Drug induced (cocaine, vasopressors, ergot alkaloid poisoning).

MESENTERIC VENOUS THROMBOSIS[26]

ICD-9CM # 557.0

Hypercoagulable states (protein C or S deficiency, antithrombin III deficiency, Factor V Leyden, malignancy, polycythemia vera, sickle cell disease, homocystinemia, lupus anticoagulant, cardiolipin antibody).
Trauma (operative venous injury, abdominal trauma, postsplenectomy).
Inflammatory conditions (pancreatitis, diverticulitis, appendicitis, cholangitis).
Other: CHF, renal failure, portal hypertension, decompression sickness.

METASTATIC NEOPLASMS

ICD-9CM # 198.5 Bone and Bone Marrow
198.3 Brain and Spinal Cord
197.7 Liver
197.0 Lung

To: Bone	*To: Brain*
Breast	Lung
Lung	Breast
Prostate	Melanoma
Thyroid	GU tract
Kidney	Colon
Bladder	Sinuses
Endometrium	Sarcoma
Cervix	Skin
Melanoma	Thyroid
To: Liver	*To: Lung*
Colon	Breast
Stomach	Colon
Pancreas	Kidney
Breast	Testis
Lymphomas	Stomach
Bronchus	Thyroid
Lung	Melanoma
Sarcoma	
Choriocarcinoma	
Kidney	

MICROCEPHALY[4]

ICD-9CM # 742.1 Microcephalus

PRIMARY (GENETIC)

Familial (autosomal recessive).
Autosomal dominant.
Syndromes:
 Down's (21-trisomy).
 Edward (18-trisomy).
 Cri-du-chat (5 p-).
 Cornelia de Lange.
 Rubinstein-Taybi.
 Smith-Lemli-Opitz.

SECONDARY (NONGENETIC)

Radiation.
Congenital infections:
 Cytomegalovirus.
 Rubella.
 Toxoplasmosis.
Drugs:
 Fetal alcohol.
 Fetal hydantoin.
Meningitis/encephalitis.
Malnutrition.
Metabolic.
Hyperthermia.
Hypoxic-ischemic encephalopathy.

MICROPENIS[27]

ICD-9CM # 752.69 Penile Agenesis or Atresia
607.89 Penile Atrophy
752.64 Micropenis (Congenital)

HYPOGONADOTROPIC HYPOGONADISM (HYPOTHALAMIC OR PITUITARY DEFICIENCIES)

Kallmann's syndrome: autosomal dominant; associated with hyposmia.

Prader-Willi syndrome: hypotonia, mental retardation, obesity, small hands and feet.
Rud syndrome: hyposomia, ichthyosis, mental retardation.
De Morsier's syndrome (septooptic dysplasia): hypopituitarism, hypoplastic optic discs, absent septum pellucidum.

HYPERGONADOTROPIC HYPOGONADISM

Primary testicular defect: disorders of testicular differentiation or inborn errors of testosterone synthesis.
Klinefelter syndrome.
Other X polysomies (i.e., XXXXY, XXXY).
Robinow's syndrome: brachymesomelic dwarfism, dysmorphic facies.

PARTIAL ANDROGEN INSENSITIVITY

Idiopathic

Defective morphogenesis of the penis.

MIOSIS

ICD-9CM # 379.42 Miosis, Persistent not Due to Miotics

Medications (e.g., morphine, pilocarpine).
Neurosyphilis.
Congenital.
Iritis.
CNS pontine lesion.
CNS infections.
Cavernous sinus thrombosis.
Inflammation/irritation of cornea or conjunctiva.

MONOARTHRITIS, ACUTE

ICD-9CM # 716.60

Overuse.
Trauma.
Gout.
Pseudogout.
Osteoarthritis.
Infectious arthritis (e.g., gonococcal, Lyme disease, viral, mycobacteria, fungi).
Osteomyelitis.
Avascular necrosis of bone.
Hemarthrosis.
Bowel disease associated arthritis.
Bone malignancy.
Psoriatic arthritis.
Juvenile RA.
Sarcoidosis.
Hemoglobinopathies.
Vasculitic syndromes.
Behçet's syndrome.
Foreign body synovitis.
Hypertrophic pulmonary osteoarthropathy.
Amyloidosis, familial Mediterranean fever.

MONOCYTOSIS[20]

ICD-9CM # 288.63

Inflammatory diseases:
- Infectious diseases:
  - Tuberculosis.
  - Syphilis.
  - Subacute bacterial endocarditis.
  - Fever of unknown origin.
- Autoimmune/granulomatous.
- Systemic lupus erythematosus.
- Rheumatoid arthritis.
- Temporal arteritis.
- Myositis.
- Polyarteritis.
- Ulcerative colitis.
- Regional enteritis.
- Sarcoidosis.

Malignant disorders:
- Preleukemia.
- Nonlymphocytic leukemia.
- Histiocytoses.
- Hodgkin's disease.
- Non-Hodgkin's lymphoma.
- Carcinomas.

Miscellaneous:
- Chronic neutropenia.
- Post splenectomy.

MONONEUROPATHY

ICD-9CM # 355.9

Herpes zoster.
Herpes simplex.
Vasculitis.
Trauma, compression.
Diabetes.
Postinfectious or inflammatory.

MUSCLE WEAKNESS

ICD-9CM # 728.9

Physical deconditioning.
Impaired cardiac output (e.g., mitral stenosis, mitral regurgitation).
Uremia, liver failure.
Electrolyte abnormalities (hypokalemia, hyperkalemia, hypophosphatemia, hypercalcemia), hypoglycemia.
Drug induced (e.g., statin myopathy).
Muscular dystrophies.
Steroid myopathy.
Alcoholic myopathy.
Myasthenia gravis, Lambert-Eaton syndrome.
Infections (polio, botulism, HIV, hepatitis, diphtheria, tick paralysis, neurosyphilis, brucellosis, TB, trichinosis).
Pernicious anemia, other anemias, beriberi.
Psychiatric illness (depression, somatization syndrome).
Organophosphate or arsenic poisoning.
Inflammatory myopathies (e.g., collagen vascular disease, RA, sarcoidosis).
Endocrinopathies (e.g., adrenal insufficiency, hypothyroidism), diabetic neuropathy.
Other: motor neuron disease, mitochondrial myopathy, L-tryptophan (eosinophilia-myalgia), rhabdomyolysis, glycogen storage disease, lipid storage disease.

MUSCLE WEAKNESS, LOWER MOTOR NEURON VERSUS UPPER MOTOR NEURON[40]

ICD-9CM # 728.9

LOWER MOTOR NEURON

Weakness, usually severe.
Marked muscle atrophy.
Fasciculations.
Decreased muscle stretch reflexes.
Clonus not present.
Flaccidity.
No Babinski sign.
Asymmetric and may involve one limb only in the beginning to become generalized as the disease progresses.

UPPER MOTOR NEURON

Weakness, usually less severe.
Minimal disuse muscle atrophy.
No fasciculations.
Increased muscle stretch reflexes.
Clonus may be present.
Spasticity.
Babinski sign.
Often initial impairment of only skilled movements.
In the limbs the following muscles may be the only ones weak or weaker than the others: triceps; wrist and finger extensors; interossei; iliopsoas; hamstrings; and foot dorsiflexors, inverters, and extroverters.

MYDRIASIS

ICD-9CM # 379.43 Mydriasis, Persistent not Due to Mydriatics

Coma.
Medications (cocaine, atropine, epinephrine, etc.).
Glaucoma.
Cerebral aneurysm.
Ocular trauma.
Head trauma.
Optic atrophy.
Cerebral neoplasm.
Iridocyclitis.

MYELIN DISORDERS

ICD-9CM # varies with specific disorder

Multiple sclerosis.
Vitamin B_{12} deficiency.
Radiation.
Hypoxia.
Toxicity from carbon monoxide, alcohol, mercury.
Progressive multifocal encephalopathy.
Acute disseminated encephalomyelitis.
Acute hemorrhagic leukoencephalopathy.
Phenylketonuria.
Adrenoleukodystrophy.
Krabbe's disease.

MYELOPATHY AND MYELITIS[36]

ICD-9CM # 722.70 Myelopathy, Discogenic Intervertebral NOS
336.9 Myelopathy, Nondiscogenic Unspecified

INFLAMMATORY

Infectious: spirochetal TB, zoster, rabies, HIV, polio, rickettsial, fungal, parasitic.
Noninfectious: idiopathic transverse myelitis, multiple sclerosis.

TOXIC/METABOLIC

DM, pernicious anemia, chronic liver disease, pellagra, arsenic.

TRAUMA COMPRESSION

Spinal neoplasm, cervical spondylosis, epidural abscess, epidural hematoma.

VASCULAR

AV malformation, SLE, periarteritis nodosa, dissecting aortic aneurysm.

PHYSICAL AGENTS

Electrical injury, irradiation.

NEOPLASTIC

Spinal cord tumors, paraneoplastic myelopathy.

MYOCARDIAL ISCHEMIA[36]

ICD-9CM # 414.8 Ischemia (Chronic)
411.89 Ischemia, Acute without MI

Atherosclerotic obstructive coronary artery disease.
Nonatherosclerotic coronary artery disease:
Coronary artery spasm.
Congenital coronary artery anomalies:
- Anomalous origin of coronary artery from pulmonary artery.
- Aberrant origin of coronary artery from aorta or another coronary artery.
- Coronary arteriovenous fistula.
- Coronary artery aneurysm.

Acquired disorders of coronary arteries:
- Coronary artery embolism.
- Dissection:
  - Surgical.
  - During percutaneous coronary angioplasty.
  - Aortic dissection.
  - Spontaneous (e.g., during pregnancy).
- Extrinsic compression:
  - Tumors.
  - Granulomas.
  - Amyloidosis.
- Collagen-vascular disease:
  - Polyarteritis nodosa.
  - Temporal arteritis.
  - RA.
  - SLE.
  - Scleroderma.
- Miscellaneous disorders:
  - Irradiation.
  - Trauma.
  - Kawasaki disease.

Syphilis.
Hereditary disorders:
- Pseudoxanthoma elasticum.
- Gargoylism.
- Progeria.
- Homocystinuria.
- Primary oxaluria.

"Functional" causes of myocardial ischemia in absence of anatomic coronary artery disease:
- Syndrome X.
- Hypertrophic cardiomyopathy.
- Dilated cardiomyopathy.
- Muscle bridge.
- Hypertensive heart disease.
- Pulmonary hypertension.
- Valvular heart disease; aortic stenosis, aortic regurgitation.

MYOCLONUS

ICD-9CM # 333.2

Physiologic (e.g., exercise or anxiety induced).
Renal failure.
Hepatic failure.
Hyponatremia.
Hypoglycemia or severe hyperglycemia.
Postdialysis.
Epileptic myoclonus.
Postencephalitis.
CNS lesion (stroke, neoplasm).
CNS trauma.
Parkinson's disease.
Medications (e.g., tricyclics, L-dopa).
Friedreich's ataxia.
Ataxia telangiectasia.
Wilson's disease.
Huntington's disease.
Progressive supranuclear palsy.
Heavy metal poisoning.
Benign familial.

MYOPATHIES, INFECTIOUS

ICD-9CM # 359.8

HIV.
Viral myositis.
Trichinosis.
Toxoplasmosis.
Cysticercosis.

MYOPATHIES, INFLAMMATORY

ICD-9CM # 359.9

SLE, RA.
Sarcoidosis.
Paraneoplastic syndrome.
Polymyositis, dermatomyositis.
Polyarteritis nodosa.
Mixed connective tissue disease.
Scleroderma.
Inclusion body myositis.
Sjögren's syndrome.
Cimetidine, D-penicillamine.

MYOPATHIES, TOXIC[1]

ICD-9CM # 359.4

Inflammatory: cimetidine, D-penicillamine.
Noninflammatory necrotizing or vacuolar: cholesterol-lowering agents, chloroquine, colchicine.
Acute muscle necrosis and myoglobinuria: cholesterol-lowering drugs, alcohol, cocaine.
Malignant hyperthermia: halothane, ethylene, others; succinylcholine.
Mitochondrial: zidovudine.
Myosin loss: nondepolarizing neuromuscular blocking agents; glucocorticoids.

MYOSITIS, INFLAMMATORY[1]

ICD-9CM # 729.1

INFECTIOUS

Viral myositis:
- Retroviruses (HIV, HTLV-I).
- Enteroviruses (echovirus, Coxsackievirus).
- Other viruses (influenza, hepatitis A and B, Epstein-Barr virus).

Bacterial: pyomyositis.
Parasites: trichinosis, cysticercosis.
Fungi: candidiasis.

IDIOPATHIC

Granulomatous myositis (sarcoid, giant cell).
Eosinophilic myositis.
Eosinophilia-myalgia syndrome.

ENDOCRINE/METABOLIC DISORDERS

Hypothyroidism.
Hyperthyroidism.
Hypercortisolism.
Hyperparathyroidism.
Hypoparathyroidism.
Hypocalcemia.
Hypokalemia.

METABOLIC MYOPATHIES

Myophosphorylase deficiency (McArdle's disease).
Phosphofructokinase deficiency.
Myoadenylate deaminase deficiency.
Acid maltase deficiency.
Lipid storage diseases.
Acute rhabdomyolysis.

DRUG-INDUCED MYOPATHIES

Alcohol.
D-Penicillamine.
Zidovudine.
Colchicine.
Chloroquine, hydroxychloroquine.
Lipid-lowering agents.
Cyclosporine.
Cocaine, heroin, barbiturates.
Corticosteroids.

NEUROLOGIC DISORDERS

Muscular dystrophies.
Congenital myopathies.
Motor neuron disease.
Guillain-Barré syndrome.
Myasthenia gravis.

NAIL CLUBBING

ICD-9CM # 703.9

COPD.
Pulmonary malignancy.
Cirrhosis.
Inflammatory bowel disease.
Chronic bronchitis.
Congenital heart disease.
Endocarditis.
AV malformations.
Asbestosis.
Trauma.
Idiopathic.

NAIL, HORIZONTAL WHITE LINES (BEAU'S LINES)

ICD-9CM # 703.8

Malnutrition.
Idiopathic.
Trauma.
Prolonged systemic illnesses.
Pemphigus.
Raynaud's disease.

NAIL KOILONYCHIA

ICD-9CM # 703.8

Trauma.
Iron deficiency.
SLE.
Hemochromatosis.
Raynaud's disease.
Nail-patella syndrome.
Idiopathic.

NAIL ONYCHOLYSIS

ICD-9CM # 703.8

Infection.
Trauma.
Psoriasis.
Connective tissue disorders.
Sarcoidosis.
Hyperthyroidism.
Amyloidosis.
Nutritional deficiencies.

NAIL PITTING

ICD-9CM # 703.8

Psoriasis.
Alopecia areata.
Reiter's syndrome.
Trauma.
Idiopathic.

NAIL SPLINTER HEMORRHAGE

ICD-9CM # 703.8

SBE.
Trauma.
Malignancies.
Oral contraceptives.
Pregnancy.
SLE.
Antiphospholipid syndrome.
Psoriasis.
RA.
Peptic ulcer disease.

NAIL STRIATIONS

ICD-9CM # 703.8

Psoriasis.
Alopecia areata.
Trauma.
Atopic dermatitis.
Vitiligo.

NAIL TELANGIECTASIA

ICD-9CM # 703.8

RA.
Scleroderma.
Trauma.
SLE.
Dermatomyositis.

NAIL WHITENING (TERRY'S NAILS)

ICD-9CM # 703.8

Malnutrition.
Trauma.
Liver disease (cirrhosis, hepatic failure).
DM.
Hyperthyroidism.
Idiopathic.

NAIL YELLOWING

ICD-9CM # 703.8

Tobacco abuse.
Nephrotic syndrome.
Chronic infections (TB, sinusitis).
Bronchiectasis.
Lymphedema.
Raynaud's disease.
RA.
Pleural effusions.
Thyroiditis.
Immunodeficiency.

NAUSEA AND VOMITING

ICD-9CM # 787.01

Infections (viral, bacterial).
Intestinal obstruction.
Metabolic (uremia, electrolyte abnormalities, DKA, acidosis, etc.).
Severe pain.
Anxiety, fear.
Psychiatric disorders (bulimia, anorexia nervosa).
Pregnancy.
Medications (NSAIDs, erythromycin, morphine, codeine, aminophylline, chemotherapeutic agents, etc.).
Withdrawal from substance abuse (drugs, alcohol).
Head trauma.
Vestibular or middle ear disease.
Migraine headache.
CNS neoplasms.
Radiation sickness.
PUD.
Carcinoma of GI tract.
Reye's syndrome.
Eye disorders.
Abdominal trauma.

NECK AND ARM PAIN

ICD-9CM # 723.1 Neck Pain
847.0 Neck Strain
959.09 Neck Injury
959.2 Arm Injury
840.9 Arm Strain

Cervical disc syndrome.
Trauma, musculoskeletal strain.
Rotator cuff syndrome.
Bicipital tendonitis.
Glenohumeral arthritis.
Acromioclavicular arthritis.
Thoracic outlet syndrome.
Pancoast tumor.
Infection (cellulitis, abscess).
Angina pectoris.

NECK MASS[28]

ICD-9CM # 784.2

CONGENITAL ANOMALIES

Thyroglossal duct cyst.
Bronchial apparatus anomalies.
Teratomas.
Ranula.
Dermoid cysts.
Hemangioma.
Laryngoceles.
Cystic hygroma.

NONNEOPLASTIC INFLAMMATORY ETIOLOGIES

Folliculitis.
Adenopathy secondary to peritonsillar abscess.
Retropharyngeal or parapharyngeal abscess.
Salivary gland infections.
Viral infections (mononucleosis, HIV, CMV).
TB.
Cat-scratch disease.
Toxoplasmosis.
Actinomyces.
Atypical mycobacterium.
Jugular vein thrombus.

NEOPLASM (PRIMARY OR METASTATIC)

Lipoma.

NECK PAIN[28]

ICD-9CM # 723.1 Neck Pain (Nondiscogenic)
959.09 Neck Injury

INFLAMMATORY DISEASES

RA.
Spondyloarthropathies.
Juvenile RA.

NONINFLAMMATORY DISEASE

Cervical osteoarthritis.
Diskogenic neck pain.
Diffuse idiopathic skeletal hyperostosis.
Fibromyalgia or myofascial pain.

INFECTIOUS CAUSES

Meningitis.
Osteomyelitis.
Infectious diskitis.

NEOPLASMS

Primary.
Metastatic.

REFERRED PAIN

Temporomandibular joint pain.
Cardiac pain.
Diaphragmatic irritation.
GI sources (gastric ulcer, gallbladder, pancreas).

NEPHRITIC SYNDROME, ACUTE[1]

ICD-9CM # 580.89

LOW SERUM COMPLEMENT LEVEL

Acute postinfectious glomerulonephritis.
Membranoproliferative glomerulonephritis.
SLE.
Subacute bacterial endocarditis.
Visceral abscess "shunt" nephritis.
Cryoglobulinemia.

NORMAL SERUM COMPLEMENT LEVEL

IgA nephropathy.
Idiopathic rapidly progressive glomerulonephritis.
Antiglomerular basement membrane disease.
Polyarteritis nodosa.
Wegener's glomerulonephritis.
Henoch-Schönlein purpura.
Goodpasture's syndrome.

NEPHROCALCINOSIS

ICD-9CM # 275.49

Sarcoidosis.
Hyperparathyroidism.
Chronic glomerulonephritis.
Milk-alkali syndrome.
Distal renal tubular acidosis.
Medullary sponge kidney.
Bartter's syndrome.
Hypervitaminosis D.
Idiopathic hypercalciuria.
Hyperoxaluria.
Cortical necrosis.
Tuberculosis.
Idiopathic hypercalciuria.
Rapidly progressive osteoporosis.

NEUROGENIC BLADDER[29]

ICD-9CM # 396.54

SUPRATENTORIAL

CVA.
Parkinson's disease.
Alzheimer's disease.
Cerebral palsy.

SPINAL CORD

Spinal cord injury.
Spinal stenosis.
Central cord syndrome.
ALS.
Multiple sclerosis.
Myelodysplasia.

PERIPHERAL NEUROPATHY

Diabetes.
Alcohol.
Shingles.
Syphilis.

NEUROLOGIC DEFICIT, FOCAL[26]

ICD-9CM # 436 CVA
435.9 TIA

TRAUMATIC: INTRACRANIAL, INTRASPINAL

Subdural hematoma.
Intraparenchymal hemorrhage.
Epidural hematoma.
Traumatic hemorrhagic necrosis.

INFECTIOUS

Brain abscess.
Epidural and subdural abscesses.
Meningitis.

NEOPLASTIC

Primary central nervous system tumors.
Metastatic tumors.
Syringomyelia.
Vascular.
Thrombosis.
Embolism.
Spontaneous hemorrhage: arteriovenous malformation, aneurysm, hypertensive.

METABOLIC

Hypoglycemia.
B_{12} deficiency.
Postseizure.
Hyperosmolar nonketotic.

OTHER

Migraine.
Bell's palsy.
Psychogenic.

NEUROLOGIC DEFICIT, MULTIFOCAL[26]

ICD-9CM # 436 CVA
435.9 TIA

Acute disseminated encephalomyelitis: postviral or postimmunization.
Infectious encephalomyelitis: poliovirus, enteroviruses, arbovirus, herpes zoster, Epstein-Barr virus.
Granulomatous encephalomyelitis: sarcoid.
Autoimmune: SLE.
Other: Familial spinocerebellar degenerations.

NEUROPATHIC BLADDER

ICD-9CM # 596.59

Diabetes.
Stroke.
Multiple sclerosis.
Parkinson's disease.
Dementia.
Encephalopathy.
Brain trauma.
Spinal cord trauma.
Pelvic surgery.
Spina bifida.

NEUROPATHIES WITH FACIAL NERVE INVOLVEMENT

ICD-9CM # varies with specific disorder

Sarcoidosis.
HIV.
Lyme disease.
Guillain-Barré.
Others: chronic inflammatory polyneuropathy, Tangier disease, amyloidosis.

NEUROPATHIES, PAINFUL[40]

ICD-9CM # 355.9 Neuropathy NOS
357.5 Alcoholic
357.8 Chronic Progressive or Relapsing
356.2 Congenital Sensory
356.0 Dejerine-Sottas
356.60 Diabetic Polyneuropathy, type II
356.61 Diabetic Polyneuropathy type I

MONONEUROPATHIES

Compressive neuropathy (carpal tunnel, meralgia paresthetica).
Trigeminal neuralgia.
Ischemic neuropathy.
Polyarteritis nodosa.
Diabetic mononeuropathy.
Herpes zoster.
Idiopathic and familial brachial plexopathy.

POLYNEUROPATHIES

DM.
Paraneoplastic sensory neuropathy.
Nutritional neuropathy.
Multiple myeloma.

Amyloid.
Dominantly inherited sensory neuropathy.
Toxic (arsenic, thallium, metronidazole).
AIDS-associated neuropathy.
Tangier disease.
Fabry's disease.

NEUTROPENIA WITH DECREASED MARROW RESERVE[20]

ICD-9CM # 288.09

Primary

Severe congenital neutropenia.
Shwachman–Diamond syndrome.
Cyclic neutropenia.

Secondary

Lymphoproliferative disorder of granular lymphocytes.
Chemotherapy.
Drug induced (nonimmune).
Nutritional.
Viral infection (varicella, EBV, measles, CMV, hepatitis, HIV).

NEUTROPENIA WITH NORMAL MARROW RESERVE[20]

ICD-9CM # 288.0

Chronic benign neutropenia of infancy and childhood.
Ethnic or benign familial neutropenia.
Autoimmune neutropenia.
Alloimmune neutropenia.
Drug induced neutropenia.
Infection-related neutropenia.
Hypersplenism.

NEUTROPHILIA[20]

ICD-9CM # 288.60

CLASSIFICATION OF NEUTROPHILIA

Primary (no other evident associated disease)
Hereditary neutrophilia.
Chronic idiopathic neutrophilia.
Chronic myelogenous leukemia (CML) and other myeloproliferative diseases.
Familial myeloproliferative disease.
Congenital anomalies and leukemoid reaction.
Leukocyte adhesion factor deficiency (LAD).
Familial cold urticaria and leukocytosis.
Secondary
Infection.
Stress neutrophilia.
Chronic inflammation.
Drug induced.
Nonhematologic malignancy.
Generalized marrow stimulation as in hemolysis.
Asplenia and hyposplenism.

NIPPLE LESIONS

ICD-9CM # varies with specific disorder

Contact dermatitis.
Trauma.
Paget's disease.
Sebaceous hyperplasia.
Neurofibroma.
Accessory nipple.
Papillary adenoma.
Nevoid hyperkeratosis.
Cellulitis.

NODULAR LESIONS, SKIN

ICD-9CM # 782.2

Lipoma.
Cherry angioma.
Angiokeratoma.
Hemangioma.
Classic Kaposi's sarcoma.
Nodular melanoma.
Pyogenic granuloma.
Angiosarcoma.
Eccrine poroma.

NODULES, PAINFUL

ICD-9CM # varies with specific disorder

Arthropod bite or sting.
Erythema nodosum.
Glomus tumor.
Neuroma.
Leiomyoma.
Angiolipoma.
Dermatofibroma.
Osler's node.
Blue rubber bleb nevus.
Vasculitis.
Sweet's syndrome.

NYSTAGMUS

ICD-9CM # 379.50 Nystagmus NOS
386.11 Benign Positional
386.2 Central Positional
379.59 Congenital

Medications (meperidine, barbiturates, phenytoin, phenothiazines, etc.).
Multiple sclerosis.
Congenital.
Neoplasm (cerebellar, brain stem, cerebral).
Labyrinthine or vestibular lesions.
CNS infections.
Optic atrophy.
Other: Arnold-Chiari malformation, syringobulbia, chorioretinitis, meningeal cysts.

NYSTAGMUS, MONOCULAR

ICD-9CM # 379.50

Amblyopia.
Strabismus.
Multiple sclerosis.
Monocular blindness.
Internuclear ophthalmoplegia.
Lid fasciculations.
Brain stem infarct.

ODYNOPHAGIA[38]

ICD-9CM # varies with specific diagnosis

CAUSES OF ODYNOPHAGIA

Infections
Herpes simplex virus.
Cytomegalovirus.
Candidiasis.
Chemical, inflammatory
Gastroesophageal reflux.
Drug induced (Slow-K, tetracyclines, quinidine).
Radiation.
Graft-versus-host disease.
Crohn's disease.
Dermatological diseases (pemphigus and pemphigoid).

OPHTHALMOPLEGIA[1]

ICD-9CM # 378.9 Ophthalmoplegia NOS
378.52 Cerebellar Ataxia Syndrome
376.22 Exophthalmic

BILATERAL

Botulism.
Myasthenia gravis.
Wernicke's encephalopathy.
Acute cranial polyneuropathy.
Brain stem stroke.

UNILATERAL

Carotid-posterior (3rd cranial nerve, pupil involved communicating aneurysm).
Diabetic-idiopathic (3rd or 6th cranial nerve, pupil spared).
Myasthenia gravis.
Brain stem stroke.

OPSOCLONUS*

ICD-9CM # 379.59

Multiple sclerosis.
Encephalitis.
CNS lymphoma.
Hydrocephalus.
Pontine hemorrhage.
Thalamic disorder (glioma, hemorrhage).
Hyperosmolar coma.
Carcinoma, paraneoplastic.
Cocaine.
Medications (e.g., phenytoin, haloperidol, amitriptyline, diazepam, vidarabine).

*Spontaneous, multivector, chaotic eye movement

ORAL MUCOSA, ERYTHEMATOUS LESIONS[9]

ICD-9CM # 528.3 Oral Abscess
528.9 Oral Disease (Soft Tissue)
528.8 Hyperplasia (Tongue)

Allergy.
Erythroplakia.
Candidiasis.
Geographic tongue.
Stomatitis areata migrans.

Plasma cell gingivitis.
Pemphigus vulgaris.

ORAL MUCOSA, PIGMENTED LESIONS[9]

ICD-9CM # 528.3 Oral Abscess
528.9 Oral Disease (Soft Tissue)
528.8 Hyperplasia (Tongue)

Racial pigmentation.
Oral melanotic macule.
Peutz-Jeghers syndrome.
Neurofibromatosis.
Albright's syndrome.
Addison's disease.
Chloasma.
Drug reaction: quinacrine, Minocin, chlorpromazine, Myleran.
Amalgam tattoo.
Lead line.
Smoker's melanosis.
Nevi.
Melanoma.

ORAL MUCOSA, PUNCTATE EROSIVE LESIONS[9]

ICD-9CM # 528.3 Oral Abscess
528.9 Oral Disease (Soft Tissue)
528.8 Hyperplasia (Tongue)

Viral lesion: Herpes simplex, coxsackievirus (A, B, A16), herpes zoster.
Aphthous stomatitis.
Sutton's disease (giant aphthae).
Behçet's syndrome.
Reiter's syndrome.
Neutropenia.
Acute necrotizing ulcerative gingivostomatitis (ANUG).
Drug reaction.
Inflammatory bowel disease.
Contact allergy.

ORAL MUCOSA, WHITE LESIONS[9]

ICD-9CM # 528.3 Oral Abscess
528.9 Oral Disease (Soft Tissue)
528.8 Hyperplasia (Tongue)

Leukoplakia.
White, hairy leukoplakia.
Squamous cell carcinoma.
Lichen planus.
Stomatitis nicotinica.
Benign intraepithelial dyskeratosis.
White spongy nevus.
Leukoedema.
Darier-White disease.
Pachyonychia congenital.
Candidiasis.
Allergy.
SLE.

ORAL ULCERS, ACUTE

ICD-9CM # varies with diagnosis
528.9 Traumatic Ulcer of Oral Mucosa

Trauma (including thermal trauma).
Aphthous stomatitis.
Syphilis.
Herpes simplex infection.
Herpes zoster.

ORAL VESICLES AND ULCERS[1]

ICD-9CM # 528.9

Aphthous stomatitis.
Primary herpes simplex infection.
Vincent's stomatitis.
Syphilis.
Coxsackievirus A (herpangina).
Fungi (histoplasmosis).
Behçet's syndrome.
SLE.
Reiter's syndrome.
Crohn's disease.
Erythema multiforme.
Pemphigus.
Pemphigoid.

ORBITAL LESIONS, CALCIFIED

ICD-9CM # 376.89

Chronic inflammation.
Phlebolith.
Dermoid cyst.
Mucocele walls.
Tumors (lacrimal gland, fibro-osseous).
Meningioma (optic sheath).
Lymphangioma.
Orbital varix.

ORBITAL LESIONS, CYSTIC

ICD-9CM # 376.9

Sweat gland cyst.
Dermoid cyst.
Lacrimal gland cyst.
Abscess.
Conjunctival cyst.
Lymphangioma.
Schwannoma.

ORGASM DYSFUNCTION[12]

ICD-9CM # 302.73 Orgasm Inhibited, Female Psychosexual
302.74 Orgasm Inhibited, Male Psychosexual

Anorgasmia: inadequate stimulation or learning.
Spinal cord lesion or injury.
Multiple sclerosis.
Alcoholic neuropathy.
Amyotrophic lateral sclerosis.
Spinal cord accident.
Spinal cord trauma.
Peripheral nerve damage.
Radical pelvic surgery.
Herniated lumbar disk.
Hypothyroidism.
Addison's disease.
Cushing's disease.
Acromegaly.
Hypopituitarism.
Pharmacologic agents (e.g., SSRIs, beta-blockers).
Psychogenic.

OROFACIAL PAIN

ICD-9CM # 784.0

Dental abscess.
Sinusitis.
Otitis media.
Otitis externa.
Wisdom tooth eruption.
Sialoadenitis.
Herpes zoster.
Trigeminal neuralgia.
Parotitis.
Anxiety disorder.
Malingering.

OSTEOPOROSIS, SECONDARY CAUSES

ICD-9CM # 733.00

Medication induced (e.g., glucocorticoids, anticonvulsants, heparin, LHRH agonists or antagonists).
Hyperparathyroidism.
Hyperthyroidism.
Prolonged immobilization.
Chronic renal failure.
Sickle cell disease.
Multiple myeloma.
Myeloproliferative diseases.
Leukemias and lymphomas.
Acromegaly.
Prolactinoma.
DM.
Total parenteral nutrition.
Malabsorption.
Chronic hypophosphatemia.
Connective tissue disorders (e.g., osteogenesis imperfecta, Marfan's syndrome, Ehlers-Danlos).
Hepatobiliary disease.
Postgastrectomy.
Aluminum containing antacids.
Systemic mastocytosis.
Homocystinuria.

OVULATORY DYSFUNCTION[21]

ICD-9CM # 628.0 Anovulatory Cycle
626.5 Ovulation Pain

HYPERANDROGENIC ANOVULATION

Polycystic ovarian syndrome.
Late-onset congenital adrenal hyperplasias.
Ovarian hyperthecosis.
Androgen-producing ovarian tumors.
Androgen-producing adrenal tumors.
Cushing's syndrome.

HYPOESTROGENIC ANOVULATION (HYPOTHALAMIC OR PITUITARY ETIOLOGY)

Hypogonadotropic Hypoestrogenic States

Reversible:
- Functional hypothalamic amenorrheas:
  - Eating disorders (anorexia nervosa, excessive weight loss).
  - Excessive athletic training.

Neoplastic:
- Craniopharyngioma.
- Pituitary stalk compression.

Infiltrative diseases:
- Histiocytosis-X.
- Sarcoidosis.

Hypophysitis.
Pituitary adenomas:
- Hyperprolactinemia.
- Euprolactinemic galactorrhea.

Endocrinopathies:
- Hypothyroidism/hyperthyroidism.
- Cushing's disease.

Irreversible:
- Kallmann's syndrome.
- Isolated gonadotropin deficiency (hypothalamic or pituitary origin).
- Panhypopituitarism/pituitary insufficiency:
  - Sheehan's syndrome, pituitary apoplexy.
  - Pituitary irradiation or ablation.

Hypergonadotropic Hypoestrogenic States

Physiologic states:
- Menopause.
- Perimenopause.

Premature ovarian failure.
Immune-related:
- Radiation/chemotherapy-induced.

Ovarian dysgenesis.
Turner's syndrome.
46XX with mutations of X.
Androgen insensitivity syndrome.

MISCELLANEOUS

Endometriosis.
Luteal phase defect.

PAIN, MIDFOOT

ICD-9CM # 719.47

MEDIAL ASPECT

Tendonitis of posterior tibialis.
Tendonitis of flexor digitorum longus.
Tendonitis of flexor hallucis longus.
Infection (osteomyelitis, septic arthritis, cellulitis) of foot.
Peripheral vascular insufficiency.
Fracture.
Osteoarthritis.
Gout, pseudogout.
Neuropathy.
Tumor.

LATERAL ASPECT

Peroneus longus tendonitis.
Peroneus brevis tendonitis.
Infection (osteomyelitis, septic arthritis, cellulitis) of foot.
Peripheral vascular insufficiency.
Fracture.
Osteoarthritis.
Gout, pseudogout.
Neuropathy.
Tumor.

PAIN, PLANTAR ASPECT, HEEL

ICD-9CM # 719.47

Plantar fasciitis.
Tarsal tunnel syndrome.
Neuroma.
Infection (osteomyelitis, septic arthritis, cellulitis) of foot.
Peripheral vascular insufficiency.
Fracture.
Bone cyst.
Osteoarthritis.
Gout, pseudogout.
Neuropathy.
Tumor.
Heel pad atrophy.
Plantar fascia rupture.

PAIN, POSTERIOR HEEL

ICD-9CM # 729.5

Achilles tendonitis.
Retrocalcaneal bursitis.
Retroachilles bursitis.
Infection (osteomyelitis, septic arthritis, cellulitis) of foot.
Peripheral vascular insufficiency.
Fracture.
Osteoarthritis.
Gout, pseudogout.
Neuropathy.
Tumor.

PALINDROMIC RHEUMATISM[6]

ICD-9CM # 719.3 use 5th digit
0. Site Unspecified
1. Shoulder Region
2. Upper Arm (Elbow, Humerus)
3. Forearm (Radius, Wrist, Ulna)
4. Hand (Carpal, Metacarpal, Fingers)
5. Pelvic Region and Thigh
6. Lower Leg
7. Ankle and Foot
8. Other
9. Multiple

Palindromic RA.
Essential palindromic rheumatism.
Crystal synovitis (gout, CPPD, pseudogout, calcific periarthritis).
Lyme borreliosis, stages 2 and 3.
Sarcoidosis.
Whipple's disease.
Acute rheumatic fever.
Reactive arthritis (rare).

PALMOPLANTAR HYPERKERATOSIS

ICD-9CM # 701.1

Superficial skin infection.
Chronic eczema.
Repeated trauma.
Psoriasis.
Reiter's syndrome.
Paraneoplastic acrokeratosis.

PALPITATIONS[33]

ICD-9CM # 785.1 Palpitations

Anxiety.
Electrolyte abnormalities (hypokalemia, hypomagnesemia).
Exercise.
Hyperthyroidism.
Ischemic heart disease.
Ingestion of stimulant drugs (cocaine, amphetamines, caffeine).
Medications (digoxin beta-blockers, calcium channel antagonists, hydralazines, diuretics, minoxidil).
Hypoglycemia in type 1 DM.
Mitral valve prolapse.
Wolff-Parkinson-White (WPW) syndrome.
Sick sinus syndrome.

PANCREATIC CALCIFICATIONS

ICD-9CM # 577.8

Chronic pancreatitis.
Hyperparathyroidism.
Metastatic neoplasm.
Pseudocyst.
Hereditary pancreatitis.
Cystoadenoma.
Cystoadenocarcinoma.
Cavernous lymphangioma.
Hemorrhage.
Acute pancreatitis (saponification).

PANCYTOPENIA[20]

ICD-9CM # 284.1

PANCYTOPENIA WITH HYPOCELLULAR BONE MARROW

Acquired aplastic anemia.
Inherited aplastic anemia (Fanconi anemia and others).
Some myelodysplasia syndromes.
Rare aleukemic leukemia (acute myelogenous leukemia).
Some acute lymphoblastic leukemias.
Some lymphomas of bone marrow.

PANCYTOPENIA WITH CELLULAR BONE MARROW

Primary bone marrow diseases.
Myelodysplasia syndromes.
Paroxysmal nocturnal hemoglobinuria.
Myelofibrosis.
Some aleukemic leukemias.
Myelophthisis.
Bone marrow lymphoma.
Hairy cell leukemia.
Secondary to systemic diseases.
Systemic lupus erythematosus, Sjögren syndrome.
Hypersplenism.
Vitamin B_{12}, folate deficiency (familial defect).
Overwhelming infection.
Alcohol.
Brucellosis.
Ehrlichiosis.
Sarcoidosis.
Tuberculosis and atypical mycobacteria.

HYPOCELLULAR BONE MARROW ± CYTOPENIA

Q fever.
Legionnaires disease.
Mycobacteria.
Tuberculosis.*
Anorexia nervosa, starvation.
Hypothyroidism.

*Pancytopenia in tuberculosis only rarely is associated with a hypocellular bone marrow at biopsy or autopsy. Marrow failure in the setting of tuberculosis is almost always fatal; exceptional patients probably had underlying myelodysplasia or acute leukemia.

PAPILLEDEMA

ICD-9CM # 377.00 Papilledema NOS
377.02 With Decreased Ocular Pressure
377.01 With Increased Intracranial Pressure
377.03 With Retinal Disorder

CNS infections (viral, bacterial, fungal).
Medications (lithium, cisplatin, corticosteroids, tetracycline, etc.).
Head trauma.
CNS neoplasm (primary or metastatic).
Pseudotumor cerebri.
Cavernous sinus thrombosis.
SLE.
Sarcoidosis.
Subarachnoid hemorrhage.
Carbon dioxide retention.
Arnold-Chiari malformation and other developmental or congenital malformations.
Orbital lesions.
Central retinal vein occlusion.
Hypertensive encephalopathy.
Metabolic abnormalities.

PAPULOSQUAMOUS DISEASES[14]

ICD-9CM # 709.8

Psoriasis.
Pityriasis rubra pilaris.
Pityriasis rosea.
Lichen planus.
Lichen nitidus.
Secondary syphilis.
Pityriasis lichenoides.
Parapsoriasis.
Mycosis fungoides.
Dermatophytosis.
Tinea versicolor.

PARANEOPLASTIC NEUROLOGIC SYNDROMES

ICD-9CM # varies with specific disorder

Lambert-Eaton myasthenic syndrome.
Myasthenia gravis.
Guillain-Barré syndrome.
Amyotrophic lateral sclerosis.
Dermatomyositis.
Carcinoid myopathy.
Cerebellar degeneration.
Encephalomyelitis.
Optic neuritis, uveitis, retinopathy.
Stiff-man syndrome.
Autonomic neuropathy.
Brachial neuritis.
Sensory neuropathy.
Progressive multifocal leukoencephalopathy.

PARANEOPLASTIC SYNDROMES, ENDOCRINE[36]

ICD-9CM # varies with specific disorder

Hypercalcemia.
Syndrome of inappropriate secretion of antidiuretic hormone.
Hypoglycemia.
Zollinger-Ellison syndrome.
Ectopic secretion of human chorionic gonadotropin.
Cushing's syndrome.

PARANEOPLASTIC SYNDROMES, NONENDOCRINE[36]

ICD-9CM # varies with specific disorder

CUTANEOUS

Dermatomyositis.
Acanthosis nigricans.
Sweet's syndrome.
Erythema gyratum repens.
Systemic nodular panniculitis (Weber-Christian disease).

RENAL

Nephrotic syndrome.
Nephrogenic diabetes insipidus.

NEUROLOGIC

Subacute cerebellar degeneration.
Progressive multifocal leukoencephalopathy.
Subacute motor neuropathy.
Sensory neuropathy.
Ascending acute polyneuropathy (Guillain-Barré syndrome).
Myasthenic syndrome (Eaton-Lambert syndrome).

HEMATOLOGIC

Microangiopathic hemolytic anemia.
Migratory thrombophlebitis (Trousseau's syndrome).
Anemia of chronic disease.

RHEUMATOLOGIC

Polymyalgia rheumatica.
Hypertrophic pulmonary osteoarthropathy.

PARAPLEGIA

ICD-9CM # 344.1 Paraplegia, Acquired
343.0 Paraplegia, Congenital
438.50 Paraplegia, Late Effect of CVA

Trauma: penetrating wounds to motor cortex, fracture-dislocation of vertebral column with compression of spinal cord or cauda equina, prolapsed disk, electrical injuries.
Neoplasm: parasagittal region, vertebrae, meninges, spinal cord, cauda equina, Hodgkin's disease, NHL, leukemic deposits, pelvic neoplasms.
Multiple sclerosis and other demyelinating disorders.
Mechanical compression of spinal cord, cauda equina, or lumbosacral plexus: Paget's disease, kyphoscoliosis, herniation of intervertebral disk, spondylosis, ankylosing spondylitis, RA, aortic aneurysm.
Infections: spinal abscess, syphilis, TB, poliomyelitis, leprosy.
Thrombosis of superior sagittal sinus.
Polyneuritis: Guillain-Barré syndrome, diabetes, alcohol, beriberi, heavy metals.
Heredofamilial muscular dystrophies.
ALS.
Congenital and familial conditions: syringomyelia, myelomeningocele, myelodysplasia.
Hysteria.

PARESTHESIAS

ICD-9CM # 782.0

Multiple sclerosis.
Nutritional deficiencies (thiamin, vitamin B_{12}, folic acid).
Compression of spinal cord or peripheral nerves.
Medications (e.g., INH, lithium, nitrofurantoin, gold, cisplatin, hydralazine, amitriptyline, sulfonamides, amiodarone, metronidazole, dapsone, disulfiram, chloramphenicol).
Toxic chemicals (e.g., lead, arsenic, cyanide, mercury, organophosphates).
DM.
Myxedema.

Alcohol.
Sarcoidosis.
Neoplasms.
Infections (HIV, Lyme disease, herpes zoster, leprosy, diphtheria).
Charcot-Marie-Tooth syndrome and other hereditary neuropathies.
Guillain-Barré neuropathy.

PARKINSONISM-PLUS SYNDROMES

ICD-9CM # varies with specific disorder

Parkinson's disease.
Shy-Drager syndrome.
Corticobasal degeneration.
Olivo-ponto-cerebellar atrophy.
Dementia with Lewy bodies.
Progressive supranuclear palsy.
Striatonigral degeneration.

PAROTID SWELLING[3]

ICD-9CM # 527.2 Allergic Parotitis
72.9 Infectious Parotitis
527.8 Salivary Gland Obstruction
527.5 Salivary Gland Obstruction with Calculus
527.8 Salivary Gland Stricture
527.3 Salivary Gland Abscess
235.1 Salivary Gland Neoplasm

INFECTIOUS

Mumps.
Parainfluenza.
Influenza.
Cytomegalovirus infection.
Coxsackievirus infection.
Lymphocytic choriomeningitis.
Echovirus infection.
Suppuration (bacterial).
Actinomyces infection.
Mycobacterial infection.
Cat-scratch disease.

NONINFECTIOUS

Drug hypersensitivity (thiouracil, phenothiazines, thiocyanate, iodides, copper, isoprenaline, lead, mercury, phenylbutazone).
Sarcoidosis.
Tumors, mixed.
Hemangioma, lymphangioma.
Sialectasis.
Sjögren's syndrome.
Mikulicz's syndrome (scleroderma, mixed connective tissue disease, SLE).
Recurrent idiopathic parotitis.
Pneumoparotitis.
Trauma.
Sialolithiasis.
Foreign body.
Cystic fibrosis.
Malnutrition (marasmus, alcohol cirrhosis).
Dehydration.
DM.
Waldenström's macroglobulinemia.
Reiter's syndrome.
Amyloidosis.

NONPAROTID SWELLING

Hypertrophy of masseter muscle.
Lymphadenopathy.
Rheumatoid mandibular joint swelling.
Tumors of jaw.
Infantile cortical hyperostosis.

PELVIC MASS

ICD-9CM # 789.39

Hemorrhagic ovarian cyst.
Simple ovarian cyst (follicle or corpus luteum).
Ovarian carcinoma, carcinoma of fallopian tube, colorectal carcinoma, metastatic carcinoma, prostate carcinoma, bladder carcinoma, lymphoma, Hodgkin's disease.
Cystadenoma, teratoma, endometrioma.
Leiomyoma.
Leiomyosarcoma.
Diverticulitis, diverticular abscess.
Appendiceal abscess, tuboovarian abscess.
Ectopic pregnancy, intrauterine pregnancy.
Paraovarian cyst.
Hydrosalpinx.

PELVIC PAIN, CHRONIC[7]

ICD-9CM # 625.9 Pelvic Pain, Female
789.09 Pelvic Pain, Male

GYNECOLOGIC DISORDERS

Primary dysmenorrhea.
Endometriosis.
Adenomyosis.
Adhesions.
Fibroids.
Retained ovary syndrome after hysterectomy.
Previous tubal ligation.
Chronic pelvic infection.

MUSCULOSKELETAL DISORDERS

Myofascial pain syndrome.

GASTROINTESTINAL DISORDERS

Irritable bowel syndrome.
Inflammatory bowel disease.

URINARY TRACT DISORDERS

Interstitial cystitis.
Nonbacterial urethritis.

PELVIC PAIN, GENITAL ORIGIN[26]

ICD-9CM # 625.9 Pelvic Pain, Female
789.09 Pelvic Pain, Male

PERITONEAL IRRITATION

Ruptured ectopic pregnancy.
Ovarian cyst rupture.
Ruptured tuboovarian abscess.
Uterine perforation.

TORSION

Ovarian cyst or tumor.
Pedunculated fibroid.

INTRATUMOR HEMORRHAGE OR INFARCTION

Ovarian cyst.
Solid ovarian tumor.
Uterine leiomyoma.

INFECTION

Endometritis.
Pelvic inflammatory disease.
Trichomonas cervicitis or vaginitis.
Tuboovarian abscess.

PREGNANCY-RELATED

First Trimester

Ectopic pregnancy.
Abortion.
Corpus luteum hematoma.

Late Pregnancy

Placental problems.
Preeclampsia.
Premature labor.

MISCELLANEOUS

Endometriosis.
Foreign objects.
Pelvic adhesions.
Pelvic neoplasm.
Primary dysmenorrhea.

PENILE RASH

ICD-9CM # 782.1

Herpes simplex 2.
Balanitis (candida).
Condyloma acuminata.
Molluscum contagiosum.
Scabies.
Pediculosis pubis.
Pearly penile papules.
Lichen nitidus.
Fox-Forcyte disease (follicular papules).

PERIANAL PAIN[38]

ICD-9CM # 569.42

Fissure-in-ano
Anal sepsis
- Anal abscess
- Anal fistula

Hemorrhoids
- Internal hemorrhoids
- External hemorrhoids

Pruritus ani
Proctalgia fugax
Chronic perianal pain syndromes
- Coccygodynia
- Descending perineum syndrome
- Levator ani syndrome
- Idiopathic perineal pain

PERICARDIAL EFFUSION

ICD-9CM # 420.90

Pericarditis.
Uremia.
Myxedema.
Neoplasm (leukemia, lymphoma, metastatic).

Hemorrhage (trauma, leakage of thoracic aneurysm).
SLE, rheumatoid disease.
Myocardial infarction.

PERIODIC PARALYSIS, HYPERKALEMIC

ICD-9CM # 344.9

Chronic renal failure.
Renal insufficiency with excessive potassium supplementation.
Potassium-sparing diuretics.
Endocrinopathies (hypoaldosteronism, adrenal insufficiency).

PERIODIC PARALYSIS, HYPOKALEMIC

ICD-9CM # 344.9

Chronic diarrhea (laxative abuse, sprue, villous adenoma).
Potassium depleting diuretics.
Medications (amphotericin B, corticosteroids).
Chronic licorice ingestion.
Thyrotoxicosis.
Renal tubular acidosis.
Conn's syndrome.
Barter's syndrome.
Barium intoxication.

PERITONEAL CARCINOMATOSIS[14]

ICD-9CM # 197.6

PRIMARY DISORDERS OF THE PERITONEUM: MESOTHELIOMA

Metastatic spread from:
- Stomach.
- Colon.
- Pancreas.
- Carcinoid.

Other Intraabdominal Organs

Ovary.
Pseudomyxoma peritonei.

Extraabdominal Primary Tumors

Breast.
Lung.

Hematologic Malignancy

Lymphoma.

PERITONEAL EFFUSION[18]

ICD-9CM # 792.9

TRANSUDATES

Increased hydrostatic pressure or decreased plasma oncotic pressure.
Congestive heart failure.
Hepatic cirrhosis.
Hypoproteinemia.

EXUDATES

Increased capillary permeability or decreased lymphatic resorption.
Infections (TB, spontaneous bacterial peritonitis, secondary bacterial peritonitis).
Neoplasms (hepatoma, metastatic carcinoma, lymphoma, mesothelioma).
Trauma.
Pancreatitis.
Bile peritonitis (e.g., ruptured gallbladder).

CHYLOUS EFFUSION

Damage or obstruction to thoracic duct.
Trauma.
Lymphoma.
Carcinoma.
Tuberculosis.
Parasitic infection.

PERIUMBILICAL SWELLING

ICD-9CM # 789.3

Umbilical hernia.
Lipoma.
Epigastric hernia.
Umbilical granuloma.
Omphalocele.
Gastroschisis.
Caput medusae.

PHOTODERMATOSES[14]

ICD-9CM # 692.72

Polymorphous light eruption.
Chronic actinic dermatitis.
Solar urticaria.
Phototoxicity and photoallergy.
Porphyrias.

PHOTOSENSITIVITY

ICD-9CM # 692.72

Solar urticaria.
Photoallergic reaction.
Phototoxic reaction.
Polymorphous light eruption.
Porphyria cutanea tarda.
SLE.
Drug induced (e.g., tetracyclines).

PLEURAL EFFUSIONS

ICD-9CM # 511.9 Pleural Effusion, Unspecified

EXUDATIVE

Neoplasm: bronchogenic carcinoma, breast carcinoma, mesothelioma, lymphoma, ovarian carcinoma, multiple myeloma, leukemia, Meigs' syndrome.
Infections: viral pneumonia, bacterial pneumonia, *Mycoplasma,* TB, fungal and parasitic diseases, extension from subphrenic abscess.
Trauma.
Collagen vascular diseases: SLE, RA, scleroderma, polyarteritis, Wegener's granulomatosis.
Pulmonary infarction.
Pancreatitis.
Postcardiotomy/Dressler's syndrome.
Drug-induced SLE (hydralazine, procainamide).
Postabdominal surgery.
Ruptured esophagus.
Chronic effusion secondary to congestive failure.

TRANSUDATIVE

CHF.
Hepatic cirrhosis.
Nephrotic syndrome.
Hypoproteinemia from any cause.
Meigs' syndrome.

PLEURAL EFFUSIONS, MALIGNANCY-ASSOCIATED

ICD-9CM # 197.2

Lung cancer	(30% to 40%)
Breast cancer	(20% to 25%)
Lymphoma	(10% to 15%)
Leukemia	(5% to 10%)
GI tract	(5%)
GU tract	(5%)
Reproductive	(3%)

PNEUMONIA, RECURRENT

ICD-9CM # 482.9 Bacterial Pneumonia
480.9 Viral Pneumonia
484.1 Fungal Pneumonia
485 Segmental Pneumonia

Mechanical obstruction from neoplasm.
Chronic aspiration (tube feeding, alcoholism, CVA, neuromuscular disorders, seizure disorder, inability to cough).
Bronchiectasis.
Kyphoscoliosis.
COPD, CHF, asthma, silicosis, pulmonary fibrosis, cystic fibrosis.
Pulmonary TB, chronic sinusitis.
Immunosuppression (HIV, corticosteroids, leukemia, chemotherapy, splenectomy).

POLYCYTHEMIA

ICD-9CM # 790.0

Tobacco abuse.
Chronic lung disease.
High altitude.
Sleep apnea.
Right-to-left cardiac shunts.
Erythropoietin administration.
Androgens/anabolic steroids.
Polycystic kidney disease.
Renal cell carcinoma.
Hepatocellular carcinoma.
Polycythemia vera.
Carbon monoxide exposure.
Primary familial and congenital polycythemia.
High-oxygen–affinity hemoglobins.
Uterine leiomyoma, meningioma, pheochromocytoma, parathyroid carcinoma.
Cobalt exposure.

POLYCYTHEMIA, RELATIVE VERSUS ABSOLUTE[20]

ICD-9CM # 790.0

RELATIVE OR SPURIOUS POLYCYTHEMIA

Decreased plasma volume—reduced fluid intake, marked loss of body fluids (diaphoresis, vomiting, diarrhea, "third-spacing").

Gaisböck syndrome.
Overfilling of blood in collection vacuum tubes.

ABSOLUTE POLYCYTHEMIA

Primary Congenital and Familial Polycythemia
Secondary Polycythemia:

Acquired:
- Hypoxia:
  - Pulmonary disease.
  - Cyanotic congenital heart disease.
  - Hypoventilation syndromes—sleep apnea, Pickwickian syndrome.
- High altitude.
- Smokers' polycythemia, carbon monoxide intoxication due to industrial exposure.
- Postrenal transplantation erythrocytosis.
- Aberrant erythropoietin production:
  - Tumors—renal cell carcinoma, Wilms tumor, hepatic carcinoma, uterine leiomyomata, virilizing ovarian tumors, vascular cerebellar tumors.
  - Miscellaneous renal and hepatic disorders—solitary renal cysts, polycystic kidney disease, renal artery stenosis hydronephrosis, viral hepatitis.
- Endocrine disorders—Cushing's syndrome, primary aldosteronism.
- Androgen use.
- Erythropoietin use.

Congenital:
- Abnormal high-affinity hemoglobin variants.
- Bisphosphoglycerate deficiency.
- Congenital methemoglobinemia.
- Chuvash polycythemia (von Hippel–Lindau mutations).
- Prolyl hydroxylase mutations.

Polycythemia Vera

POLYNEUROPATHY[40]

ICD-9CM # 357.9

PREDOMINANTLY MOTOR

Guillain-Barré syndrome.
Porphyria.
Diphtheria.
Lead.
Hereditary sensorimotor neuropathy, types I and II.
Paraneoplastic neuropathy.

PREDOMINANTLY SENSORY

Diabetes.
Amyloidosis.
Leprosy.
Lyme disease.
Paraneoplastic neuropathy.
Vitamin B_{12} deficiency.
Hereditary sensory neuropathy, types I-IV.

PREDOMINANTLY AUTONOMIC

Diabetes.
Amyloidosis.
Alcoholic neuropathy.
Familial dysautonomias.

MIXED SENSORIMOTOR

Systemic diseases: renal failure, hypothyroidism, acromegaly, RA, periarteritis nodosa, SLE, multiple myeloma, macroglobulinemia, remote effect of malignancy.
Medications: isoniazid, nitrofurantoin, ethambutol, chloramphenicol, chloroquine, vincristine, vinblastine, dapsone, disulfiram, diphenylhydantoin, cisplatin, 1-tryptophan.
Environmental toxins: *N*-hexane, methyl *N*-butyl ketone, acrylamide, carbon disulfide, carbon monoxide, hexachlorophene, organophosphates.
Deficiency disorders: malabsorption, alcoholism, vitamin B_1 deficiency, Refsum's disease, metachromatic leukodystrophy.

POLYNEUROPATHY, DRUG-INDUCED[40]

ICD-9CM # 357.6

DRUGS IN ONCOLOGY

Vincristine.
Procarbazine.
Cisplatin.
Misonidazole.
Metronidazole (Flagyl).
Taxol.

DRUGS IN INFECTIOUS DISEASES

Isoniazid.
Nitrofurantoin.
Dapsone.
ddC (dideoxycytidine).
ddI (dideoxyinosine).

DRUGS IN CARDIOLOGY

Hydralazine.
Perhexiline maleate.
Procainamide.
Disopyramide.

DRUGS IN RHEUMATOLOGY

Gold salts.
Chloroquine.

DRUGS IN NEUROLOGY AND PSYCHIATRY

Diphenylhydantoin.
Glutethimide.
Methaqualone.

MISCELLANEOUS

Disulfiram (Antabuse).
Vitamin: pyridoxine (megadoses).

POLYNEUROPATHY, SYMMETRIC[40]

ICD-9CM # 357.9

ACQUIRED NEUROPATHIES

Toxic:
- Drugs.
- Industrial toxins.
- Heavy metals.
- Abused substances.

Metabolic/endocrine:
- Diabetes.
- Chronic renal failure.
- Hypothyroidism.
- Polyneuropathy of critical illness.

Nutritional deficiency:
- Vitamin B_{12} deficiency.
- Alcoholism.
- Vitamin E deficiency.

Paraneoplastic:
- Carcinoma.
- Lymphoma.

Plasma cell dyscrasia:
- Myeloma, typical, atypical, and solitary forms.
- Primary systemic amyloidosis.

Idiopathic chronic inflammatory demyelinating polyneuropathies.
Polyneuropathies associated with peripheral nerve autoantibodies.
Acquired immunodeficiency syndrome.

INHERITED NEUROPATHIES

Neuropathies with Biochemical Markers

Refsum's disease.
Bassen-Kornzweig disease.
Tangier disease.
Metachromatic leukodystrophy.
Krabbe's disease.
Adrenomyeloneuropathy.
Fabry's disease.

Neuropathies without Biochemical Markers or Systemic Involvement

Hereditary motor neuropathy.
Hereditary sensory neuropathy.
Hereditary sensorimotor neuropathy.

POLYURIA

ICD-9CM # 788.42

DM.
Diabetes insipidus.
Primary polydipsia (compulsive water drinking).
Hypercalcemia.
Hypokalemia.
Postobstructive uropathy.
Diuretic phase of renal failure.
Drugs: diuretics, caffeine, alcohol, lithium.
Sickle cell trait or disease, chronic pyelonephritis (failure to concentrate urine).
Anxiety, cold weather.

POPLITEAL SWELLING

ICD-9CM #	
459.2	Venous Obstruction
747.4	Vein Anomaly, Lower Limb Vessel
442.3	Artery Aneurysm
904.41	Artery Injury
447.8	Entrapment Syndrome
727.51	Baker's Cyst
451.2	Phlebitis, Lower Extremity
727.67	Rupture of Achilles Tendon

Phlebitis (superficial).
Lymphadenitis.
Trauma: fractured tibia or fibula, contusion, traumatic neuroma.

DVT.
Ruptured varicose vein.
Baker's cyst.
Popliteal abscess.
Osteomyelitis.
Ruptured tendon.
Aneurysm of popliteal artery.
Neoplasm: lipoma, osteogenic sarcoma, neurofibroma, fibrosarcoma.

PORTAL HYPERTENSION[1]

ICD-9CM # 572.3

INCREASED RESISTANCE TO FLOW

Presinusoidal

Portal or splenic vein occlusion (thrombosis, tumor).
Schistosomiasis.
Congenital hepatic fibrosis.
Sarcoidosis.

Sinusoidal

Cirrhosis (all causes).
Alcoholic hepatitis.

Postsinusoidal

Venoocclusive disease.
Budd-Chiari syndrome.
Constrictive pericarditis.

INCREASED PORTAL BLOOD FLOW

Splenomegaly not caused by liver disease.
Arterioportal fistula.

POSTMENOPAUSAL BLEEDING

ICD-9CM # 627.1

Hormone replacement therapy.
Neoplasm (uterine, ovarian, cervical, vaginal, vulvar).
Atrophic vaginitis.
Vaginal infection.
Polyp.
Extragenital (GI, urinary).
Tamoxifen.
Trauma.

POSTURAL HYPOTENSION, NONNEUROLOGIC CAUSES

ICD-9CM # 458.0

Diuretics and hypertensive agents.
GI hemorrhage.
Alcohol.
Excessive heat.
Rapid volume loss from diarrhea, vomiting.
Hemodialysis.
Extensive burns.
Pyrexia.
Aortic stenosis (impaired output).
Constrictive pericarditis, atrial myxoma (impaired cardiac filling).
Adrenal insufficiency.
Diabetes insipidus.
Vasodilatory agents (e.g., nitrates).

PREMATURE GRAYING, SCALP HAIR

ICD-9CM # varies with specific disorder

Chemical exposure (e.g., phenol/catechol derivatives, sulfhydryls, arsenic).
Physical agents (e.g., ionizing radiation, lasers).
Hyperthyroidism.
Vitamin B_{12} deficiency.
Down's syndrome.
Chronic and severe protein deficiency.
Vitiligo.
Idiopathic.
Myotonic dystrophy.
Ataxia telangiectasia.
Progeria.
Wermer's syndrome.

PROPTOSIS[30]

ICD-9CM # 376.30

Thyrotoxicosis.
Orbital pseudotumor.
Optic nerve tumor.
Cavernous sinus AV fistula, cavernous sinus thrombosis.
Cellulitis.
Metastatic tumor to orbit.

PROPTOSIS AND PALATAL NECROTIC ULCERS

ICD-9CM # 528.9 Ulcer of Palate
376.30 Proptosis

Cavernous sinus thrombosis.
Bacterial orbital cellulitis.
Metastatic neoplasm.
Rhinocerebral mucormycosis.
Ecthyma gangrenosum.
CNS aspergillosis.

PROTEINURIA

ICD-9CM # 791.0

Nephrotic syndrome as a result of primary renal diseases.
Malignant hypertension.
Malignancies: multiple myeloma, leukemias, Hodgkin's disease.
CHF.
DM.
SLE, RA.
Sickle cell disease.
Goodpasture's syndrome.
Malaria.
Amyloidosis, sarcoidosis.
Tubular lesions: cystinosis.
Functional (after heavy exercise).
Pyelonephritis.
Pregnancy.
Constrictive pericarditis.
Renal vein thrombosis.
Toxic nephropathies: heavy metals, drugs.
Radiation nephritis.
Orthostatic (postural) proteinuria.
Benign proteinuria: fever, heat, or cold exposure.

PRURITUS

ICD-9CM # 698.9 Pruritus NOS
697.0 Pruritus Ani
698.1 Pruritus, Genital Organs

Dry skin.
Drug-induced eruption, fiberglass exposure.
Scabies.
Skin diseases.
Myeloproliferative disorders: mycosis fungoides, Hodgkin's lymphoma, multiple myeloma, polycythemia vera.
Cholestatic liver disease.
Endocrine disorders: DM, thyroid disease, carcinoid, pregnancy.
Carcinoma: breast, lung, gastric.
Chronic renal failure.
Iron deficiency.
AIDS.
Neurosis.
Sjögren's syndrome.

PRURITUS ANI[26]

ICD-9CM # 697.0

FECAL IRRITATION

Poor hygiene.
Anorectal conditions (fissure, fistula, hemorrhoids, skin tags, perianal clefts).
Spicy foods, citrus foods, caffeine, colchicine, quinidine.

CONTACT DERMATITIS

Anesthetic agents, topical corticosteroids, perfumed soap.

DERMATOLOGIC DISORDERS

Psoriasis, seborrhea, lichen simplex or sclerosus.

SYSTEMIC DISORDERS

Chronic renal failure, myxedema, DM, thyrotoxicosis, polycythemia vera, Hodgkin's disease.

SEXUALLY TRANSMITTED DISEASES

Syphilis, herpes simplex virus, human papillomavirus.

OTHER INFECTIOUS AGENTS

Pinworms.
Scabies.
Bacterial infection, viral infection.

PSEUDOCYANOSIS, ETIOLOGY

ICD-9CM # varies with etiology

Medications: amiodarone, minocycline, chlorpromazine.
Heavy metals:
Gold (systemic absorption).
Silver (systemic absorption).
Local contact with color dyes, gold, silver.

PSEUDOHERMAPHRODITISM, FEMALE

ICD-9CM # 255.2 Adrenal
752.7 Without Adrenocortical Disorder

Congenital adrenal hyperplasia.
Maternal use of testosterone or related steroids.
Virilizing ovarian or adrenal tumor.
Virilizing luteoma of pregnancy.
Disturbances in differentiation of urogenital structures, non-androgen related.
Maternal virilizing adrenal hyperplasia.
Fetal P450 aromatase deficiency.

PSEUDOHERMAPHRODITISM, MALE

ICD-9CM # 255.2 Adrenal
752.7 Without Adrenocortical Disorder

Maternal ingestion of progestogens.
End-organ resistance to androgenic hormones.
5-Alpha-reductase-2 deficiency.
XY gonadal dysgenesis.
Testicular regression syndrome.
Defects in testosterone metabolism by peripheral tissues.
Testosterone biosynthesis defects.

PSEUDOINFARCTION[22]

ICD-9CM # code not available

Cardiac tumors, primary and secondary.
Cardiomyopathy (particularly hypertrophic and dilated).
Chagas' disease.
Chest deformity.
COPD (particularly emphysema).
HIV infection.
Hyperkalemia.
Left anterior fascicular block.
Left bundle branch block.
Left ventricular hypertrophy.
Myocarditis and pericarditis.
Normal variant.
Pneumothorax.
Poor R wave progression, rotational changes, and lead placement.
Pulmonary embolism.
Trauma to chest (nonpenetrating).
Wolff-Parkinson-White syndrome.
Rare causes: pancreatitis, amyloidosis, sarcoidosis, scleroderma.

PSYCHOSIS[28]

ICD-9CM # 298.9 Psychosis NOS
298.90 Psychosis, Affective
291.0 Psychosis, Alcoholic
290.41 Psychosis, Acute Arteriosclerotic

PRIMARY

Schizophrenia related.*
Major depression.
Dementia.
Bipolar disorder.

SECONDARY

Drug use.†
Drug withdrawal.‡
Drug toxicity.§
Charles Bonnet syndrome.
Infections (pneumonia).
Electrolyte imbalance.
Syphilis.
Congestive heart failure.
Parkinson's disease.
Trauma to temporal lobe.
Postpartum psychosis.
Hypothyroidism/hyperthyroidism.
Hypomagnesemia.
Epilepsy.
Meningitis.
Encephalitis.
Brain abscess.
Herpes encephalopathy.
Hypoxia.
Hypercarbia.
Hypoglycemia.
Thiamine deficiency.
Postoperative states.

*Includes schizophrenia, schizophreniform disorder, brief reactive psychosis.
†Includes hypnotics, glucocorticoids, marijuana, phencyclidine, atropine, dopaminergic agents (e.g., amantadine, bromocriptine, L-dopa), immunosuppressants.
‡Includes alcohol, barbiturates, benzodiazepines.
§Includes digitalis, theophylline, cimetidine, anticholinergics, glucocorticoids, catecholaminergic agents.

PTOSIS

ICD-9CM # 374.30 Ptosis NOS
743.61 Congenital
374.33 Mechanical
374.32 Myogenic
374.31 Paralytic

Third nerve palsy.
Myasthenia gravis.
Horner's syndrome.
Senile ptosis.

PUBERTY, DELAYED[27]

ICD-9CM # 259.0

NORMAL OR LOW SERUM GONADOTROPIN LEVELS

Constitutional delay in growth and development.
Hypothalamic and/or pituitary disorders:
- Isolated deficiency of growth hormone.
- Isolated deficiency on Gn-RH.
- Isolated deficiency of LH and/or FSH.
- Multiple anterior pituitary hormone deficiencies.
- Associated with congenital anomalies: Kallmann's syndrome; Prader-Willi syndrome; Laurence-Moon-Biedl syndrome; Friedreich's ataxia.
- Trauma.
- Postinfection.
- Hyperprolactinemia.
- Postirradiation.
- Infiltrative disease (histiocytosis).
- Tumor.
- Autoimmune hypophysitis.
- Idiopathic.

Functional:
- Chronic endocrinologic or systemic disorders.
- Emotional disorders.
- Drugs: cannabis.

INCREASED SERUM GONADOTROPIN LEVELS

Gonadal abnormalities:
Congenital:
- Gonadal dysgenesis.
- Klinefelter's syndrome.
- Bilateral anorchism.
- Resistant ovary syndrome.
- Myotonic dystrophy in males.
- 17-Hydroxylase deficiency in females.
- Galactosemia.

Acquired:
- Bilateral gonadal failure resulting from trauma or infection or after surgery, irradiation, or chemotherapy.
- Oophoritis: isolated or with other autoimmune disorders.

Uterine or vaginal disorders:
- Absence of uterus and/or vagina.
- Testicular feminization: complete or incomplete androgen insensitivity.

PUBERTY, PRECOCIOUS

ICD-9CM # 255.2

Idiopathic.
Congenital virilizing adrenal hyperplasia.
Hypothalamic tumors.
Head trauma.
Hydrocephalus.
Degenerative CNS disease.
Arachnoid cyst.
Sex chromosome abnormalities (e.g., 47, XXY, 48, XXXY).
Perinatal asphyxia.
CNS infection (e.g., meningitis, encephalitis).

PULMONARY CRACKLES

ICD-9CM # code not available

Pneumonia.
Left ventricular failure.
Asbestosis, silicosis, interstitial lung disease.
Chronic bronchitis.
Alveolitis (allergic, fibrosing).
Neoplasm.

PULMONARY INFILTRATES, IMMUNOCOMPROMISED HOST[39]

ICD-9CM # 518.3

CAUSES OF PULMONARY INFILTRATES IN THE IMMUNOCOMPROMISED HOST

Infections:
- Bacteria:
  - Gram-positive cocci, especially *Staphylococcus.*
  - Gram-negative bacilli.
  - *Mycobacterium tuberculosis.*
  - Nontuberculous mycobacteria.
  - *Nocardia.*
- Viruses:
  - Cytomegalovirus.
  - Herpesvirus.
- Fungi:
  - *Aspergillus.*
  - *Cryptococcus.*
  - *Candida.*
  - *Mucor.*
  - *Pneumocystis jiroveci.*
- Protozoa:
  - *Toxoplasma gondii* (rare).

Pulmonary effects of therapy:
- Chemotherapeutic agents.
- Radiation therapy.

Pulmonary hemorrhage.
Congestive heart failure.
Disseminated malignancy.
Nonspecified interstitial pneumonitis (no defined etiology).

PULMONARY LESIONS

ICD-9CM #	
518.3	Pulmonary Infiltrate
518.89	Pulmonary Nodule
508.9	Pulmonary Disorder Due to Unspecified External Agent
861.20	Pulmonary Injury NOS

TB.
Legionella pneumonia.
Mycoplasma pneumonia.
Viral pneumonia.
Pneumocystis carinii.
Hypersensitivity pneumonitis.
Aspiration pneumonia.
Fungal disease (aspergillosis, histoplasmosis).
ARDS associated with pneumonia.
Psittacosis.
Sarcoidosis.
Septic emboli.
Metastatic cancer.
Multiple pulmonary emboli.
Rheumatoid nodules.

PULMONARY NODULE, SOLITARY

ICD-9CM # 518.89

Bronchogenic carcinoma.
Granuloma from histoplasmosis.
TB granuloma.
Granuloma from coccidioidomycosis.
Metastatic carcinoma.
Bronchial adenoma.
Bronchogenic cyst.
Hamartoma.
AV malformation.
Other: fibroma, intrapulmonary lymph node, sclerosing hemangioma, bronchopulmonary sequestration.

PULSELESS ELECTRICAL ACTIVITY

ICD-9CM # code not available

Hypovolemia.
Hypoxia.
Hyperkalemia.
Acidosis.
Cardiac tamponade.
Tension pneumothorax.
Pulmonary embolus.
Drug overdose.
Hypothermia.

PUPILLARY DILATATION, POOR RESPONSE TO DARKNESS

ICD-9CM # varies with specific disorder

Drugs (narcotics, general anesthetics, cholinergics).
Acute trauma (spasm from prostaglandin release).
Inflammation, infection (interruption of inhibitory fibers to the Edinger-Westphal nucleus).
Old age (loss of inhibition at midbrain from reticular activating formation).
Horner's syndrome (sympathetic neuron interruption).
Adie's syndrome tonic pupil.
Lymphoma.
Congenital miosis.

PURPURA

ICD-9CM #	
287.2	Purpura NOS
287.0	Autoimmune
287.0	Henoch-Schönlein
287.3	Idiopathic thrombocytopenic
446.6	Thrombocytopenic

THROMBOTIC

Trauma.
Septic emboli, atheromatous emboli.
DIC.
Thrombocytopenia.
Meningococcemia.
Rocky Mountain spotted fever.
Hemolytic-uremic syndrome.
Viral infection: echo, coxsackie.
Scurvy.
Other: left atrial myxoma, cryoglobulinemia, vasculitis, hyperglobulinemic purpura.

PURPURA, NONPALPABLE[20]

ICD-9CM # 287.2

INCREASED TRANSMURAL PRESSURE GRADIENT

Acute (Valsalva, coughing, vomiting, high altitude, weight lifting).
Chronic—Venous stasis.

DECREASED MECHANICAL INTEGRITY OF MICROCIRCULATION AND SUPPORTING TISSUES

Age related (infancy and actinic purpura).
Glucocorticoid excess—Cushing syndrome and glucocorticoid therapy.
Vitamin C deficiency (scurvy).
Abnormal connective tissue—Ehlers-Danlos syndrome.
Amyloid infiltration of blood vessels.[a]
Colloid milium.
Hormonal—Female easy bruising syndrome (purpura simplex).
Lorenzo's oil.
MELAS syndrome.

TRAUMA TO BLOOD VESSELS

Physical:
- Injuries.
- Child abuse.
- Factitial purpura.

Ultraviolet purpura:
- Purpuric sunburn.
- Solar purpura.

Infectious:
- Bacteriala.
- Rickettsial.
- Fungala.
- Viral.
- Parasitic.

Embolic:
- Infectious organisms.
- Atheroemboli (cholesterol crystal emboli).
- Fat emboli.

Allergic and/or inflammatory:
- Serum sickness.
- Pigmented purpuric eruptions.
- Pyoderma gangrenosum.
- Contact dermatitis.
- Familial Mediterranean fever.

Neoplastica.
Metabolic:
- Erythropoietic porphyria.
- Calciphylaxis.

Immunoglobulin related (hyperglobulinemic purpura of Waldenström and light-chain vasculitis).
Drug related.

Thrombotic:
- Disseminated intravascular coagulation.
- Warfarin (coumarin)-induced skin necrosis.
- Protein C or protein S deficiency, factor V Leiden, prothrombin G20201A.
- Purpura fulminans.
- Paroxysmal nocturnal hemoglobinuria.
- Antiphospholipid antibody syndrome.
- Hemangioma with thrombocytopenia and consumptive coagulopathy (Kasabach-Merritt syndrome).

UNKNOWN CAUSE—PSYCHOGENIC PURPURA

[a]May also have a palpable purpuric component.

PURPURA, NONPURPURIC DISORDERS SIMULATING PURPURA[1]

ICD-9CM # varies with specific diagnosis

Disorders with telangiectasias:
- Cherry angiomas.
- Hereditary hemorrhagic telangiectasia.
- Chronic actinic telangiectasia.
- Scleroderma.
- CREST syndrome.
- Ataxia-telangiectasia.
- Chronic liver disease.
- Pregnancy-related telangiectasia.

Kaposi sarcoma and other vascular sarcomas.[c]
Fabry disease.
Neonatal extramedullary hematopoiesis.
Angioma serpiginosum.

PURPURA, PALPABLE[20]

ICD-9CM # 287.2

Cutaneous vasculitis:
- Systemic vasculitides.
- Paraneoplastic vasculitis.
- Henoch-Schönlein purpura.
- Acute hemorrhagic edema of infancy.
- Livedoid vasculitis.
- Idiopathic.
- Urticarial.

Cryoglobulinemia.
Cryofibrinogenemia.
Primary cutaneous diseases.

QT INTERVAL PROLONGATION[22]

ICD-9CM # 794.31

Drugs:
- Class I antiarrhythmics (e.g., disopyramide, procainamide, quinidine).
- Class III antiarrhythmics.
- Tricyclic antidepressants.
- Phenothiazines.
- Astemizole.
- Terfenadine.
- Adenosine.
- Antibiotics (e.g., erythromycin and other macrolides).
- Antifungal agents.
- Pentamidine, chloroquine.

Ischemic heart disease.
Cerebrovascular disease.
Rheumatic fever.
Myocarditis.
Mitral valve prolapse.
Electrolyte abnormalities.
Hypocalcemia.
Hypothyroidism.
Liquid protein diets.
Organophosphate insecticides.
Congenital prolonged QT syndrome.

RECTAL MASS, PALPABLE[38]

ICD-9CM # varies with specific diagnosis

Rectal carcinoma.
Rectal polyp.
Hypertrophied anal papilla.
Diverticular phlegmon (prolapsing into the pouch of Douglas).
Sigmoid colon carcinoma (prolapsing into the pouch of Douglas).
Metastatic deposits at the pelvic reflection (Blumer's shelf).
Primary pelvic malignancy (uterine, ovarian, prostatic or cervical).
Mesorectal lymph nodes.
Endometriosis.
Solitary rectal ulcer syndrome.
Foreign body.
Feces (indent).
Presacral cyst.
Amoebic granuloma.
Vaginal tampon and even the pubic bone may be mistaken for a rectal mass.

RECTAL PAIN

ICD-9CM # 569.42

Anal fissure.
Thrombosed hemorrhoid.
Anorectal abscess.
Foreign bodies.
Fecal impaction.
Endometriosis.
Neoplasms (primary or metastatic).
Pelvic inflammatory disease.
Inflammation of sacral nerves.
Compression of sacral nerves.
Prostatitis.
Other: proctalgia fugax, uterine abnormalities, myopathies, coccygodynia.

RED BLOOD CELL APLASIA, ACQUIRED, ETIOLOGY

ICD-9CM # 284.0

Idiopathic (>50% of cases).
Medications (most frequent with phenytoin).
Non-Hodgkin's lymphoma.
Viral infections (parvovirus B-19, EB virus, mumps, hepatitis).
Myelodysplastic syndromes.
Thymoma.
Autoimmune diseases.
Allogenic bone marrow transplant from ABO incompatible donor.
Pregnancy.

RED EYE

ICD-9CM # 379.93

Infectious conjunctivitis (bacterial, viral).
Allergic conjunctivitis.
Acute glaucoma.
Keratitis (bacterial, viral).
Iritis.
Trauma.

RED HOT JOINT

ICD-9CM # varies with specific disorder

Trauma.
Gout.
Infection (septic joint).
Pseudogout (calcium pyrophosphate dehydrate crystal deposition).
Psoriatic arthropathy.
Reactive arthritis.
Palindromic rheumatism.

RED URINE

ICD-9CM # 788.69

Hematuria.
Porphyrins.
Hemoglobinuria.
Myoglobinuria.
Medications (phenazopyridine, aminosalicylic acid, deferoxamine, phenazopyridine, phenolphthalein, NSAIDs, rifampin, phenytoin, methyldopa, doxorubicin, phenacetin).
Foods (beets, berries, maize).
Urate crystalluria.

RENAL ARTERY OCCLUSION, CAUSES

ICD-9CM # 593.81

Atrial fibrillation.
Angiography or stent placement.
Abdominal aortic surgery.
Trauma.
Renal artery aneurysm/dissection.
Vasculitis.
Thrombosis in patient with fibromuscular dysplasia.
Atherosclerosis.
Septic embolism.
Mural thrombus thromboembolism.
Atrial myxoma thromboembolism.
Mitral stenosis thromboembolism.
Prosthetic valve thromboembolism.
Renal cell carcinoma.

RENAL CYSTIC DISORDERS

ICD-9CM # varies with specific disorder

Simple cysts.
Acquired cystic kidney disease.
Autosomal dominant polycystic kidney disease.
Autosomal recessive polycystic kidney disease.
Medullary cystic disease.
Medullary sponge kidney.

RENAL FAILURE, INTRINSIC OR PARENCHYMAL CAUSES[36]

ICD-9CM # 584. Acute, use 4th digit
5. With Acute Tubular Necrosis
6. With Cortical Necrosis
7. With Medullary Necrosis
8. With Other Unspecified Pathologic Condition in Kidney
9. Renal Failure Unspecified
585 Renal Failure, Chronic

ABNORMALITIES OF THE VASCULATURE

Renal arteries: atherosclerosis, thromboembolism, arteritis.
Renal veins: thrombosis.
Microvasculature: vasculitis, thrombotic microangiopathy.

ABNORMALITIES OF GLOMERULI (ACUTE GLOMERULONEPHRITIS)

Antiglomerular membrane disease (Goodpasture's syndrome).
Immune complex glomerulonephritis: SLE, postinfectious, idiopathic, membranoproliferative.

ABNORMALITIES OF INTERSTITIUM (ACUTE INTERSTITIAL NEPHRITIS)

Drugs (e.g., antibiotics, NSAIDs, diuretics, anticonvulsants, allopurinol).
Infectious pyelonephritis.
Infiltrative: lymphoma, leukemia, sarcoidosis.

ABNORMALITIES OF TUBULES

Physical obstruction (uric acid, oxalate, light chains).
Acute tubular necrosis:
- Ischemic.
- Toxic (antibiotics, chemotherapy, immunosuppressives, radiocontrast dyes, heavy metals, myoglobin, hemolysed RBCs).

RENAL FAILURE, POSTRENAL CAUSES[36]

ICD-9CM # 584. Acute, use 4th digit
5. With Acute Tubular Necrosis
6. With Cortical Necrosis
7. With Medullary Necrosis
8. With Other Unspecified Pathologic Condition in Kidney
9. Renal Failure Unspecified
585 Renal Failure, Chronic

URETER AND RENAL PELVIS

Intrinsic obstruction:
- Blood clots.
- Stones.
- Sloughed papillae: diabetes, sickle cell disease, analgesic nephropathy.
- Inflammatory: fungus ball.

Extrinsic obstruction:
- Malignancy.
- Retroperitoneal fibrosis.
- Iatrogenic: inadvertent ligation of ureters.

BLADDER

Prostatic hypertrophy or malignancy.
Neuropathic bladder.
Blood clots.
Bladder cancer.
Stones.

URETHRAL

Strictures.
Congenital valves.

RENAL FAILURE, PRERENAL CAUSES[36]

ICD-9CM # 584. Acute, use 4th digit
5. With Acute Tubular Necrosis
6. With Cortical Necrosis
7. With medullary necrosis
8. With Other Unspecified Pathologic Condition in Kidney
9. Renal Failure Unspecified
585 Renal Failure, Chronic

DECREASED CARDIAC OUTPUT

CHF.
Arrhythmias.
Pericardial constriction or tamponade.
Pulmonary embolism.

HYPOVOLEMIA

GI tract loss (vomiting, diarrhea, nasogastric suction).
Blood losses (trauma, GI tract surgery).
Renal losses (diuretics, mineralocorticoid deficiency, postobstructive diuresis).
Skin losses (burns).

VOLUME REDISTRIBUTION (DECREASE IN EFFECTIVE BLOOD VOLUME)

Hypoalbuminemic states (cirrhosis, nephrosis).
Sequestration of fluid in "third" space (ischemic bowel, peritonitis, pancreatitis).
Peripheral vasodilation (sepsis, vasodilators, anaphylaxis).

ALTERED RENAL VASCULAR RESISTANCE

Increase in afferent vascular resistance (NSAIDs, liver disease, sepsis, hypercalcemia, cyclosporine).
Decrease in efferent arteriolar tone (ACE inhibitors).

RENAL VEIN THROMBOSIS, CAUSES

ICD-9CM # 453.3

Nephrotic syndrome.
Renal cell carcinoma.
Aortic aneurysm causing compression.
Lymphadenopathy.
Retroperitoneal fibrosis.
Estrogen therapy.
Pregnancy.
Renal cell carcinoma with vein invasion.
Severe dehydration.

RESPIRATORY FAILURE, HYPOVENTILATORY[28]

ICD-9CM # 518.81 Respiratory Failure

ABNORMAL RESPIRATORY CAPACITY (NORMAL RESPIRATORY WORKLOADS)

Acute depression of central nervous system:
- Various causes.

Chronic central hypoventilation syndromes:
- Obesity-hypoventilation syndrome.
- Sleep apnea syndrome.
- Hypothyroidism.
- Shy-Drager syndrome (multisystem atrophy syndrome).

Acute toxic paralysis syndromes:
- Botulism.
- Tetanus.
- Toxic ingestion or bites.
- Organophosphate poisoning.

Neuromuscular disorders (acute and chronic):
- Myasthenia gravis.
- Guillain-Barré syndrome.
- Drugs.
- Amyotrophic lateral sclerosis.
- Muscular dystrophies.
- Polymyositis.
- Spinal cord injury.
- Traumatic phrenic nerve paralysis.

ABNORMAL PULMONARY WORKLOADS

Chronic obstructive pulmonary disease:
- Chronic bronchitis.
- Asthmatic bronchitis.
- Emphysema.

Asthma and acute bronchial hyperreactivity syndromes.
Upper airway obstruction.
Interstitial lung diseases.

ABNORMAL EXTRAPULMONARY WORKLOADS

Chronic thoracic cage disorders:
- Severe kyphoscoliosis.
- After thoracoplasty.
- After thoracic cage injury.

Acute thoracic cage trauma and burns.
Pneumothorax.
Pleural fibrosis and effusions.
Abdominal processes.

RETINOPATHY, HYPERTENSIVE

ICD-9CM # 362.11

Retinal venous obstruction.
Diabetic retinopathy.
Ocular ischemic syndrome.
Hyperviscosity.
Tortuosity of retinal artery.

RHINITIS

ICD-9CM # 472.0

Allergic rhinitis.
Infectious rhinitis.
Vasomotor rhinitis.
Exercise-induced rhinitis.
Emotional rhinitis.
Rhinitis medicamentosa.
Hormone-mediated rhinitis (menses, pregnancy, oral contraceptives, hypothyroidism).
GERD.
Chemical- or irritant-induced rhinitis.
Rhinitis mimics:
- Deviated septum.
- Enlarged adenoids.
- Nasal polyps/tumors.
- Foreign bodies.
- CSF rhinorrhea.
- Sarcoidosis.
- Midline granuloma.
- Wegener's granulomatosis.
- SLE.
- Sjögren's syndrome.

RIGHT AXIS DEVIATION[22]

ICD-9CM # varies with specific diagnosis

Normal variation.
Right ventricular hypertrophy.
Left posterior fascicular block.
Lateral myocardial infarction.
Pulmonary embolism.
Dextrocardia.
Mechanical shifts or emphysema causing a vertical heart.

SALIVARY GLAND ENLARGEMENT

ICD-9CM # 527.1

Neoplasm.
Sialolithiasis.
Infection (mumps, bacterial infection, HIV, TB).
Sarcoidosis.
Idiopathic.
Acromegaly.
Anorexia/bulimia.
Chronic pancreatitis.
Medications (e.g., phenylbutazone).
Cirrhosis.
DM.

SALIVARY GLAND SECRETION, DECREASED

ICD-9CM # 527.7

Medications (antihistamines, antidepressants, neuroleptics, antihypertensives).
Dehydration.
Anxiety.
Sjögren's syndrome.
Sarcoidosis.
Mumps.
Amyloidosis.
CNS disorders.
Head and neck radiation.

SCROTAL PAIN[28]

ICD-9CM # 878.2 Scrotal Injury, Traumatic
608.9 Scrotal Disorder NOS
608.4 Scrotal Cellulitis
608.83 Scrotal Hemorrhage, Nontraumatic
608.4 Scrotal Nodule, Inflammatory

Torsion:
- Appendages.
- Spermatic cord.

Infection:
- Orchitis.
- Abscess.
- Epididymitis.

Neoplasia:
- Benign.
- Malignant.

Incarcerated hernia.
Trauma.
Hydrocele.
Spermatocele.
Varicocele.

SCROTAL SWELLING

ICD-9CM # 608.86

Hydrocele.
Varicocele.
Neoplasm.
Acute epididymitis.
Orchitis.
Trauma.
Hernia.
Torsion of spermatic cord.
Torsion of epididymis.
Torsion of testis.
Insect bite.
Folliculitis.
Sebaceous cyst.
Thrombosis of spermatic vein.
Other: lymphedema, dermatitis, fat necrosis, Henoch-Schönlein purpura, idiopathic scrotal edema.

SEIZURE

ICD-9CM # 780.39

Syncope.
Alcohol abuse/withdrawal.
TIA.
Hemiparetic migraine.
Psychiatric disorders.
Carotid sinus hypersensitivity.
Hyperventilation, prolonged breath holding.
Hypoglycemia.
Narcolepsy.
Movement disorders (tics, hemiballismus).
Hyponatremia.
Brain tumor (primary or metastatic).
Tetanus.
Strychnine, phencyclidine poisoning.

SEIZURE, PEDIATRIC[2]

ICD-9CM # 780.39 Infantile Seizures
779.0 Seizures, Newborn

FIRST MONTH OF LIFE

First Day

Hypoxia.
Drugs.
Trauma.
Infection.
Hyperglycemia.
Hypoglycemia.
Pyridoxine deficiency.

Day 2-3

Infection.
Drug withdrawal.
Hypoglycemia.
Hypocalcemia.
Developmental malformation.
Intracranial hemorrhage.
Inborn error of metabolism.
Hyponatremia or hypernatremia.

Day >4

Infection.
Hypocalcemia.
Hyperphosphatemia.
Hyponatremia.
Developmental malformation.
Drug withdrawal.
Inborn error of metabolism.

1 TO 6 MO

As above.

6 MO TO 3 YR

Febrile seizures.
Birth injury.
Infection.
Toxin.
Trauma.
Metabolic disorder.
Cerebral degenerative disease.

>3 YR

Idiopathic.
Infection.
Trauma.
Cerebral degenerative disease.

SEXUALLY TRANSMITTED DISEASES, ANORECTAL REGION[26]

ICD-9CM # 569.49 Infection and Region

ULCERATIVE

Lymphogranuloma venereum.
Herpes simplex virus.
Early (primary) syphilis.
Chancroid *(Haemophilus ducreyi).*
Cytomegalovirus.
Idiopathic (usually HIV positive).

NONULCERATIVE

Condyloma acuminatum.
Gonorrhea.
Chlamydia *(Chlamydia trachomatis).*
Syphilis.

SEXUAL PRECOCITY[41]

ICD-9CM # 259.1

TRUE PRECOCIOUS PUBERTY

Premature reactivation of LHRH pulse generator.

INCOMPLETE SEXUAL PRECOCITY

(Pituitary gonadotropin independent).

Males

Chorionic gonadotropin-secreting tumor.
Leydig cell tumor.
Familial testotoxicosis.
Virilizing congenital adrenal hyperplasia.
Virilizing adrenal tumor.
Premature adrenarche.

Females

Granulosa cell tumor (follicular cysts may be manifested similarly).
Follicular cyst.
Feminizing adrenal tumor.
Premature thelarche.
Premature adrenarche.
Late-onset virilizing congenital adrenal hyperplasia.

In both sexes

McCune-Albright syndrome.
Primary hypothyroidism.

SHOULDER PAIN

ICD-9CM # 952.2 Shoulder Injury
718.81 Shoulder Instability
726.19 Shoulder Ligament or Muscle Instability
840.9 Shoulder Strain, Site Unspecified

WITH LOCAL FINDINGS IN SHOULDER

Trauma: contusion, fracture, muscle strain, trauma to spinal cord.
Arthrosis, arthritis, RA, ankylosing spondylitis.
Bursitis, synovitis, tendinitis, tenosynovitis.
Aseptic (avascular) necrosis.
Local infection: septic arthritis, osteomyelitis, abscess, herpes zoster, TB.

WITHOUT LOCAL FINDINGS IN SHOULDER

Cardiovascular disorders: ischemic heart disease, pericarditis, aortic aneurysm.
Subdiaphragmatic abscess, liver abscess.
Cholelithiasis, cholecystitis.
Pulmonary lesions: apical bronchial carcinoma, pleurisy, pneumothorax, pneumonia.
GI lesions: PUD, gastric neoplasm, peptic esophagitis.
Pancreatic lesions: carcinoma, calculi, pancreatitis.
CNS abnormalities: neoplasm, vascular abnormalities.
Multiple sclerosis.
Syringomyelia.
Polymyositis/dermatomyositis.
Psychogenic.
Polymyalgia rheumatica.
Ectopic pregnancy.

SHOULDER PAIN BY LOCATION

ICD-9CM # 952.2 Shoulder Injury
726.19 Shoulder Ligament or Muscle Instability
840.8 Shoulder Separation

TOP OF SHOULDER (C4)

Cervical source.
Acromioclavicular.
Sternoclavicular.
Diaphragmatic.

SUPEROLATERAL (C5)

Rotator cuff tendinitis.
Impingement.
Adhesive capsulitis.
Glenohumeral arthritis.

ANTERIOR

Bicipital tendinitis and rupture.
Glenoid labral tear.
Adhesive capsulitis.
Glenohumeral arthritis.
Osteonecrosis.

AXILLARY

Neoplasm (Pancoast's, mediastinal).
Herpes zoster.

SHOULDER PAIN, IN DIFFERENT AGE GROUPS[8]

ICD-9CM # 719.41

COMMON CAUSES OF SHOULDER PAIN IN DIFFERENT AGE GROUPS

Childhood (2-10 yr)

Intraarticular:
Instability.
Periarticular:
Osteochondromas.

Adolescence (10-18 yr)

Intraarticular:
Instability.

Early adulthood (18-30 yr)

Intraarticular:
Instability.
Acromioclavicular joint sprain.
Periarticular:
Calcific tendonitis.
Impingement.
Referred:
Cervical.

Adulthood (30-60 yr)

Intraarticular:
Osteochondritis.
Osteoarthritis.
Frozen shoulder.
Inflammatory arthritis.
Periarticular:
Calcific tendonitis.
Impingement.
Rotator cuff tear.
Bicipital tendonitis.
Referred:
Cervical.

Old age (>60 yr)

Intraarticular:
Osteochondritis.
Osteoarthritis.
Frozen shoulder.
Inflammatory arthritis.
Periarticular:
Impingement.
Rotator cuff tear.
Referred:
Cervical.

SMALL BOWEL MASSES[38]

ICD-9CM # varies with specific diagnosis

Cyst:
- Mesenteric cyst.

Tumor:
- Benign.
- Malignant.

Intussusception.
Inflammation:
- Crohn's disease.

SMALL BOWEL OBSTRUCTION[26]

ICD-9CM # 751.1 Small Intestine Obstruction, Congenital
560.81 Small Intestine Obstruction Due to Adhesion

INTRINSIC

Congenital (atresia, stenosis).
Inflammatory (Crohn's, radiation enteritis).
Neoplasms (metastatic or primary).
Intussusception.
Traumatic (hematoma).

EXTRINSIC

Hernias (internal and external).
Adhesions.
Volvulus.
Compressing masses (tumors, abscesses, hematomas).

INTRALUMINAL

Foreign body.
Gallstones.
Bezoars.
Barium.
Ascaris infestation.

SMALL INTESTINE ULCERATION

ICD-9CM # 569.82

Inflammatory bowel disease.
Celiac disease.
Vasculitis, SLE, Behçet's syndrome.
Uremia.
Infections (*Campylobacter,* TB, *Yersinia,* parasites, typhoid, cytomegalovirus [CMV], *Clostridium).*
Mesenteric insufficiency.
Neoplasms.
Radiation.
Drugs (salicylates, potassium, indomethacin, antimetabolites).
Meckel diverticulum.
Zollinger-Ellison syndrome.
Lymphocytic enterocolitis.
Stomal ulceration.

SMELL DISTURBANCE

ICD-9CM # varies with specific disorder

Upper respiratory tract infection.
Nasal or paranasal sinus disease.
Exposure to noxious vapors.
Head trauma.
Idiopathic.
Dental caries, periodontal disease.
Medications.

SORE THROAT[33]

ICD-9CM #	
426	Pharyngitis
075	Mononucleosis
472.1	Chronic Pharyngitis
487.1	Pharyngitis, Influenzal
074.0	Coxsackie Virus Pharyngitis

WITHOUT PHARYNGEAL ULCERS

Viral pharyngitis.
Allergic pharyngitis.
Infectious mononucleosis.
Streptococcal pharyngitis.
Gonococcal pharyngitis.
Sinusitis with postnasal drip.

WITH PHARYNGEAL ULCERS

Herpangina.
Herpes simplex.
Candidiasis.
Fusospirochetal infection (Vincent's angina).

SPASTIC PARAPLEGIAS

ICD-9CM # 344.1

Cervical spondylosis.
Friedreich's ataxia.
Multiple sclerosis.
Spinal cord tumor.
HIV.
Tertiary syphilis.
Vitamin B_{12} deficiency.
Spinocerebellar ataxias.
Syringomyelia.
Spinal cord AV malformations.
Adrenoleukodystrophy.

SPINAL CORD COMPRESSION, EPIDURAL

ICD-9CM # varies with specific disorder

Osteoarthritis.
Meningioma.
Spinal epidural abscess.
Spinal epidural hematoma.
Spinal epidural vascular malformations.
RA.
Metastatic cancer (vertebral, intramedullary, leptomeninges).
Radiation myelopathy.
Neurofibroma.
Sarcoidosis.
Paraneoplastic myelopathy.
Histiocytosis.

SPINAL CORD DYSFUNCTION

ICD-9CM #	
336.9	Spinal Cord Compression
336.9	Spinal Cord Disease NOS
742.9	Spinal Cord Disease, Congenital
281.1	Spinal Cord Degeneration, B_{12} Deficiency Anemia
336.8	Spinal Cord Atrophy, Acute
336.10	Spinal Cord Atrophy, Adult

Trauma.
Multiple sclerosis.
Transverse myelitis.
Neoplasm (primary, metastatic).
Syringomyelia.
Spinal epidural abscess.
HIV myelopathy.
Diskitis.
Spinal epidural hematoma.
Spinal cord infarction.
Spinal AV malformation.
Subarachnoid hemorrhage.

SPINAL CORD ISCHEMIC SYNDROMES

ICD-9CM # varies with specific disorder

Systemic hypotension.
Venous or arterial occlusion.
Arterial dissection.
Thromboembolism.
Endovascular procedures.
Vasculitis.
Fibrocartilaginous embolism.
Regional hemodynamic compromise.

SPINAL TUMORS[14]

ICD-9CM # 299.7

EXTRADURAL

Metastases.
Primary bone tumors arising in spine.

INTRADURAL EXTRAMEDULLARY

Meningiomas.
Neurofibromas.
Schwannomas.
Lipomas.
Arachnoid cysts.
Epidermoid cysts.
Metastasis.

INTRAMEDULLARY

Ependymoma.
Glioma.
Hemangioblastoma.
Lipoma.
Metastases.

SPLENOMEGALY

ICD-9CM #	
789.2	Splenomegaly Unspecified
289.51	Chronic Congestive
759.0	Congenital
789.2	Unknown Origin

Hepatic cirrhosis.
Neoplastic involvement: CML, CLL, lymphoma, multiple myeloma.
Bacterial infections: TB, infectious endocarditis, typhoid fever, splenic abscess.
Viral infections: infectious mononucleosis, viral hepatitis, HIV.
Gaucher's disease and other lipid storage diseases.
Sarcoidosis.
Parasitic infections (malaria, kala-azar, histoplasmosis).
Hereditary and acquired hemolytic anemias.
Idiopathic thrombocytopenic purpura (ITP).
Collagen vascular disorders: SLE, RA (Felty's syndrome), polyarteritis nodosa.
Serum sickness, drug hypersensitivity reaction.
Splenic cysts and benign tumors: hemangioma, lymphangioma.
Thrombosis of splenic or portal vein.
Polycythemia vera, myeloid metaplasia.

SPLENOMEGALY AND HEPATOMEGALY[38]

ICD-9CM #	
789.2	Splenomegaly
789.1	Hepatomegaly

CAUSES OF SPLENOMEGALY AND HEPATOSPLENOMEGALY

Massive Splenomegaly

Hematological disease (e.g., chronic myeloid leukemia, myelofibrosis).

Moderate Splenomegaly

The above causes.
Portal hypertension.
Hematological disease (e.g., lymphoma, leukemia, thalassemia).
Storage disease (e.g., Gaucher's disease).

Small Splenomegaly

The above causes.
Infective (hepatitis, leptospirosis, malaria, bacterial endocarditis).
Hematological disease (e.g., hemolytic anemias, essential thrombocythemia, polycythemia rubra vera).
Connective tissue diseases or vasculitis (e.g., rheumatoid arthritis, systemic lupus erythematosus, polyarteritis nodosa).
Solitary cyst, polycystic syndrome, hydatid cyst.

Infiltration (amyloid, sarcoid).

Hepatosplenomegaly

Chronic liver disease with portal hypertension.
Hematological disease (e.g., myeloproliferative disease, lymphoma).
Infection (e.g., amyloid, sarcoid).
Connective tissue disease (e.g., systemic lupus erythematosus).

SPLENOMEGALY, CHILDREN[20]

ICD-9CM # 782.2

DISORDERS OF THE BLOOD

Hemolytic anemia: congenital/acquired.
Thalassemia.
Sickle cell disease.
Leukemia.
Osteopetrosis.
Myelofibrosis/myeloid metaplasia/thrombocythemia.

INFECTIONS: ACUTE AND CHRONIC

Viral:
- Congenital (e.g., TORCH association).
- Mononucleosis (e.g., EBV, CMV infection).
- Virus associated hemophagocytic syndrome.
- Human immunodeficiency virus.

Bacterial:
- Sepsis/abscess.
- Brucellosis.
- Salmonellosis.
- Tularemia.
- Tuberculosis.
- Subacute bacterial endocarditis.
- Syphilis.
- Lyme disease.

Fungal:
- Histoplasmosis (disseminated).

Rickettsial:
- Rocky Mountain spotted fever.
- Cat scratch disease.

Parasitic:
- Toxoplasmosis.
- Malaria.
- Leishmaniasis (kala-azar).
- Schistosomiasis.
- Echinococcosis.

HEPATIC/PORTAL SYSTEM DISORDERS

Acute/chronic active hepatitis.
Cirrhosis/hepatic fibrosis/biliary atresia.
Portal or splenic venous obstruction (Banti syndrome).

AUTOIMMUNE DISEASE

Juvenile rheumatoid arthritis.
Systemic lupus erythematosus.
Autoimmune lymphoproliferative syndrome (Canale–Smith syndrome).

NEOPLASMS/CYSTS

Lymphomas (Hodgkin and non-Hodgkin).
Hemangiomas/lymphangiomas.
Hamartomas.
Congenital or acquired (posttraumatic) cysts.

STORAGE DISEASES/INBORN ERRORS OF METABOLISM

Lipidoses: Gaucher disease, Niemann–Pick disease, others.
Mucopolysaccharidoses.
Defects in carbohydrate metabolism: galactosemia, fructose intolerance.
Sea-blue histiocyte syndrome.

MISCELLANEOUS DISORDERS

Histiocytoses:
- Reactive.
- Langerhans cell.
- Malignant.

Sarcoidosis.
Congestive heart failure.
Familial Mediterranean fever.

CMV, Cytomegalovirus; *EBV,* Epstein-Barr virus; *TORCH,* toxoplasmosis, other infections, rubella, cytomegalovirus infection, herpes simplex.

STEATOHEPATITIS

ICD-9CM # 571.8

Alcohol abuse.
Obesity.
DM.
Parenteral nutrition.
Medications (high-dose estrogen, amiodarone, corticosteroids, methotrexate, nifedipine).
Jejunoileal bypass.
Abetalipoproteinemia.
Wilson's disease, Weber-Christian disease.

STOMATITIS, BULLOUS

ICD-9CM # 528.0

Erythema multiforme.
Erosive lichen planus.
Bullous pemphigoid.
SLE.
Pemphigus vulgaris.
Mucous membrane pemphigoid.

STRIDOR, PEDIATRIC AGE[4]

ICD-9CM # 786.1 Stridor
748.3 Stridor Laryngeal Congenital

RECURRENT

Allergic (spasmodic) croup.
Respiratory infections in a child with otherwise asymptomatic anatomic narrowing of the large airways.
Laryngomalacia.

PERSISTENT

Laryngeal obstruction:
- Laryngomalacia.
- Papillomas, other tumors.
- Cysts and laryngoceles.
- Laryngeal webs.
- Bilateral abductor paralysis of the cords.
- Foreign body.

Tracheobronchial disease:
- Tracheomalacia.
- Subglottic tracheal webs.
- Endotracheal, endobronchial tumors.
- Subglottic tracheal stenosis.
- Congenital.
- Acquired.

Extrinsic masses.
Mediastinal masses.
Vascular ring.
Lobar emphysema.
Bronchogenic cysts.
Thyroid enlargement.
Esophageal foreign body.
Tracheoesophageal fistulas.
Other.
Gastroesophageal reflux.
Macroglossia, Pierre Robin syndrome.
Cri-du-chat syndrome.
Hysterical stridor.
Hypocalcemia.

STROKE[36]

ICD-9CM # 436 Acute Stroke

Hypoglycemia.
Drug overdose or intoxication.
Hysterical conversion reaction.
Hyperventilation.
Metabolic encephalopathy.
Migraine.
Syncope.
Transient global amnesia.
Seizures.
Vestibular vertigo.

STROKE, PEDIATRIC AGE[23]

ICD-9CM # 436 Stroke, Acute

CARDIAC DISEASE

Congenital:
- Aortic stenosis.
- Mitral stenosis; mitral prolapse.
- Ventricular septal defects.
- Patent ductus arteriosus.
- Cyanotic congenital heart disease involving right-to-left shunt.

Acquired:
- Endocarditis (bacterial, SLE).
- Kawasaki disease.
- Cardiomyopathy.
- Atrial myxoma.
- Arrhythmia.
- Paradoxical emboli through patent foramen ovale.
- Rheumatic fever.
- Prosthetic heart valve.

HEMATOLOGIC ABNORMALITIES

Hemoglobinopathies:
- Sickle cell (SS) disease.
- Sickle (SC) disease.

Polycythemia.
Leukemia/lymphoma.
Thrombocytopenia.
Thrombocytosis.
Disorders of coagulation:
- Protein C deficiency.
- Protein S deficiency.
- Factor V Leiden.

Antithrombin III deficiency.
Lupus anticoagulant.
Oral contraceptive pill use.
Pregnancy and the postpartum state.
Disseminated intravascular coagulation.
Paroxysmal nocturnal hemoglobinuria.
Inflammatory bowel disease (thrombosis).

INFLAMMATORY DISORDERS

Meningitis:
Viral.
Bacterial.
Tuberculosis.
Systemic infection:
Viremia.
Bacteremia.
Local head and neck infections.
Drug-induced inflammation:
Amphetamine.
Cocaine.
Autoimmune disease:
SLE.
Juvenile RA.
Takayasu's arteritis.
Mixed connective tissue disease.
Polyarteritis nodosum.
Primary CNS vasculitis.
Sarcoidosis.
Behçet's syndrome.
Wegener's granulomatosis.

METABOLIC DISEASE ASSOCIATED WITH STROKE

Homocystinuria.
Pseudoxanthoma elasticum.
Fabry's disease.
Sulfite oxidase deficiency.
Mitochondrial disorders:
MELAS.
Leigh syndrome.
Ornithine transcarbamylase deficiency.

INTRACEREBRAL VASCULAR PROCESSES

Ruptured aneurysm.
Arteriovenous malformation.
Fibromuscular dysplasia.
Moyamoya disease.
Migraine headache.
Postsubarachnoid hemorrhage vasospasm.
Hereditary hemorrhagic telangiectasia.
Sturge-Weber syndrome.
Carotid artery dissection.
Postvaricella.

TRAUMA AND OTHER EXTERNAL CAUSES

Child abuse.
Head trauma/neck trauma.
Oral trauma.
Placental embolism.
ECMO therapy.

CNS, Central nervous system; *ECMO,* extracorporeal membrane oxygenation; *MELAS,* mitochondrial encephalomyopathy, lactic acidosis, and stroke.

STROKE, YOUNG ADULT, CAUSES[1]

ICD-9CM # 436

Cardiac factors (ASD, MVP, patent foramen ovale).
Inflammatory factors (SLE, polyarteritis nodosa).
Infections (endocarditis, neurosyphilis).
Drugs (cocaine, heroin, oral contraceptives, decongestants).
Arterial dissection.
Hematolic factors (DIC, TTP, deficiency of protein S, protein C, antithrombin III).
Migraine.
Postpartum angiopathy.
Other: premature atherosclerosis, fibromuscular dysplasia.

ST SEGMENT ELEVATIONS, NONISCHEMIC

ICD-9CM # 794.31

Early repolarization.
Acute pericarditis.
LVH.
Normal pattern variant.
LBBB.
Pulmonary embolism.
Hyperkalemia.
Postcardioversion.

SUDDEN DEATH, PEDIATRIC AGE[4]

ICD-9CM # varies with specific disorder

SIDS AND SIDS "MIMICS"

SIDS.
Long QT syndromes.
Inborn errors of metabolism.
Child abuse.
Myocarditis.
Duct-dependent congenital heart disease.

CORRECTED OR UNOPERATED CONGENITAL HEART DISEASE

Aortic stenosis.
Tetralogy of Fallot.
Transposition of great vessels (postoperative atrial switch).
Mitral valve prolapse.
Hypoplastic left heart syndrome.
Eisenmenger's syndrome.

CORONARY ARTERIAL DISEASE

Anomalous origin.
Anomalous tract.
Kawasaki disease.
Periarteritis.
Arterial dissection.
Marfan's syndrome.
Myocardial infarction.

MYOCARDIAL DISEASE

Myocarditis.
Hypertrophic cardiomyopathy.
Dilated cardiomyopathy.
Arrhythmogenic right ventricular dysplasia.

CONDUCTION SYSTEM ABNORMALITY/ARRHYTHMIA

Long Q-T syndromes.
Proarrhythmic drugs.
Preexcitation syndromes.
Heart block.
Commotio cordis.
Idiopathic ventricular fibrillation.
Heart tumor.

MISCELLANEOUS

Pulmonary hypertension.
Pulmonary embolism.
Heat stroke.
Cocaine.
Anorexia nervosa.
Electrolyte disturbances.

SIDS, Sudden infant death syndrome.

SUDDEN DEATH, YOUNG ATHLETE

ICD-9CM # varies with specific diagnosis

Hypertrophic cardiomyopathy.
Coronary artery anomalies.
Myocarditis.
Ruptured aortic aneurysm (Marfan's syndrome).
Arrhythmias.
Aortic valve stenosis.
Asthma.
Trauma (cerebral, cardiac).
Drug and alcohol abuse.
Heat stroke.
Cardiac sarcoidosis.
Atherosclerotic coronary artery disease.
Dilated cardiomyopathy.

SWOLLEN LIMB

ICD-9CM # 729.81 Swollen Arm or Hand
729.81 Swollen Leg or Foot

Trauma.
Insect bite.
Abscess.
Lymphedema.
Thrombophlebitis.
Lipoma.
Neurofibroma.
Postphlebitic syndrome.
Myositis ossificans.
Nephrosis, cirrhosis, CHF.
Hypoalbuminemia.
Varicose veins.

TALL STATURE[27]

ICD-9CM # 253.0 Growth Hormone Overproduction, Gigantism

Constitutional (familial or genetic)—most common cause

ENDOCRINE CAUSES

Growth hormone excess—gigantism.
Sexual precocity (tall as children, short as adults):
True sexual precocity.
Pseudosexual precocity.
Androgen deficiency:
Klinefelter's syndrome.
Bilateral anorchism.

GENETIC CAUSES

Klinefelter's syndrome.
Syndromes of XYY, XXYY.

MISCELLANEOUS SYNDROMES AND DISORDERS

Cerebral gigantism or Sotos' syndrome: prominent forehead, hypertelorism, high arched palate, dolichocephaly, mental retardation, large hands and feet, and premature eruption of teeth. Large at birth, with most rapid growth in first 4 yr of life.
Marfan's syndrome: disorder of mesodermal tissues, subluxation of the lenses, arachnodactyly, and aortic aneurysm.
Homocystinuria: same phenotype as Marfan's syndrome.
Obesity: tall as infants, children, and adolescents.
Total lipodystrophy: large hands and feet, generalized loss of subcutaneous fat, insulin-resistant DM, and hepatomegaly.
Beckwith-Wiedemann syndrome: neonatal tallness, omphalocele, macroglossia, and neonatal hypoglycemia.
Weaver-Smith syndrome: excessive intrauterine growth, mental retardation, megalocephaly, widened bifrontal diameter, hypertelorism, large ears, micrognathia, camptodactyly, broad thumbs, and limited extension of elbows and knees.
Marshall-Smith syndrome: excessive intrauterine growth, mental retardation, blue sclerae, failure to thrive, and early death.

TARDIVE DYSKINESIA[13]

ICD-9CM # 781.3 Dyskinesia
300.11 Hysterical Dyskinesia
333.82 Orofacial Dyskinesia
307.9 Psychogenic Dyskinesia

DIFFERENTIAL DIAGNOSIS:

Medications (antidepressants, anticholinergics, amphetamines, lithium, L-dopa, phenytoin).
Brain neoplasms.
Ill-fitting dentures.
Huntington's disease.
Idiopathic dystonias (tics, blepharospasm, aging).
Wilson's disease.
Extrapyramidal syndrome (postanoxic or postencephalitic).
Torsion dystonia.

TASTE AND SMELL LOSS[1]

ICD-9CM # 781.1 Smell and Taste Disturbance of Sensation

TASTE

Local: radiation therapy.
Systemic: cancer, renal failure, hepatic failure, nutritional deficiency (vitamin B_{12}, zinc), Cushing's syndrome, hypothyroidism, DM, infection (influenza), drugs (antirheumatic and antiproliferative).
Neurologic: Bell's palsy, familial dysautonomia, multiple sclerosis.

SMELL

Local: allergic rhinitis, sinusitis, nasal polyposis, bronchial asthma.
Systemic: renal failure, hepatic failure, nutritional deficiency (vitamin B_{12}), Cushing's syndrome, hypothyroidism, DM, infection (viral hepatitis, influenza), drugs (nasal sprays, antibiotics).
Neurologic: head trauma, multiple sclerosis, Parkinson's disease, frontal brain tumor.

TELANGIECTASIA

ICD-9CM # 448.9

Oral contraceptive agents.
Pregnancy.
Rosacea.
Varicose veins.
Trauma.
Drug induced (corticosteroids, systemic or topical).
Spider telangiectases.
Hepatic cirrhosis.
Mastocytosis.
SLE, dermatomyositis, systemic sclerosis.

TENDINOPATHY[26]

ICD-9CM # 727.9

INTRINSIC FACTORS

Anatomic Factors
Malalignment.
Muscle weakness or imbalance.
Muscle inflexibility.
Decreased vascularity.
Systemic Factors
Inflammatory conditions (e.g., SLE).
Pregnancy.
Quinolone-induced tendinopathy.
Age-Related Factors
Tendon degeneration.
Increased tendon stiffness.
Tendon calcification.
Decreased vascularity.

EXTRINSIC FACTORS

Repetitive Mechanical Load
Excessive duration.
Excessive frequency.
Excessive intensity.
Poor technique.
Workplace factors.
Equipment Problems
Footwear.
Athletic field surface.
Equipment factors (e.g., racquet size).
Protective gear.

TESTICULAR FAILURE[10]

ICD-9CM # 257.1 Testicular Failure

PRIMARY

Klinefelter's syndrome (XXY).
XYY.
Vanishing testes syndrome (in utero or early postnatal torsion).
Noonan's syndrome.
Varicocele.
Myotonic dystrophy.
Orchitis (mumps, gonorrhea).
Cryptorchidism.
Chemical exposure.
Irradiation to testes.
Spinal cord injury.
Polyglandular failure.
Idiopathic oligospermia or azoospermia.
Germinal cell aplasia (Sertoli cell–only syndrome).
Idiopathic testicular failure.
Testicular torsion.
Testicular trauma.
Diethylstilbestrol (maternal use during pregnancy resulting in in utero estrogen exposure).
Testicular tumor with subsequent irradiation therapy, chemotherapy, or surgery (retroperitoneal lymph node dissection or orchiectomy).

SECONDARY

Delayed puberty.
Kallmann's syndrome.
Isolated gonadotropin deficiency.
Prader-Labhart-Willi syndrome.
Lawrence-Moon-Biedl syndrome.
Central nervous system irradiation.
Prepubertal panhypopituitarism.
Postpubertal panhypopituitarism.
Hypogonadism secondary to hyperprolactinemia.
Adrenogenital syndrome.
Chronic liver disease.
Chronic renal failure/uremia.
Hemochromatosis.
Cushing's syndrome.
Malnutrition.
Massive obesity.
Sickle cell anemia.
Hyper/hypothyroidism.
Anabolic steroid use.

TESTICULAR PAIN

ICD-9CM # 608.9

Testicular torsion.
Trauma.
Epididymitis.
Orchitis.
Neoplasm.

Urolithiasis.
Inguinal hernia.
Infection (cellulitis, abscess, folliculitis).
Anxiety.

TESTICULAR SIZE VARIATIONS[10]

ICD-9CM # 608.3 Testicular Atrophy
608.89 Testicular Mass
257.2 Hypogonadism

SMALL TESTES

Hypothalamic-pituitary dysfunction.
Gonadotropin deficiency.
Growth hormone deficiency.
Normal variant.
Primary hypogonadism.
Autoimmune destruction, chemotherapy, cryptorchidism, irradiation, Klinefelter's syndrome, orchiditis, testicular regression syndrome, torsion, trauma.

LARGE TESTES

Adrenal rest tissue.
Compensatory.
Fragile X syndrome.
Idiopathic.
Tumor.

TETANUS[26]

ICD-9CM # 037

Acute abdomen.
Black widow spider bite.
Dental abscess.
Dislocated mandible.
Dystonic reaction.
Encephalitis.
Head trauma.
Hyperventilation syndrome.
Hypocalcemia.
Meningitis.
Peritonsillar abscess.
Progressive fluctuating muscular rigidity (stiff-man syndrome).
Psychogenic.
Rabies.
Sepsis.
Subarachnoid hemorrhage.
Status epilepticus.
Strychnine poisoning.
Temporomandibular joint syndrome.

THROMBOCYTOPENIA

ICD-9CM # 287.3 Congenital or Primary
287.4 Secondary
287.5 Thrombocytopenia NOS

INCREASED DESTRUCTION

Immunologic

Drugs: quinine, quinidine, digitalis, procainamide, thiazide diuretics, sulfonamides, phenytoin, aspirin, penicillin, heparin, gold, meprobamate, sulfa drugs, phenylbutazone, nonsteroidal anti-inflammatory drugs (NSAIDs), methyldopa, cimetidine, furosemide, INH, cephalosporins, chlorpropamide, organic arsenicals, chloroquine, platelet glycoprotein IIb/IIIa receptor inhibitors, ranitidine, indomethacin, carboplatin, ticlopidine, clopidogrel.
Idiopathic thrombocytopenic purpura (ITP).
Transfusion reaction: transfusion of platelets with plasminogen activator (PLA) in recipients without PLA-1.
Fetal/maternal incompatibility.
Collagen vascular diseases (e.g., SLE).
Autoimmune hemolytic anemia.
Lymphoreticular disorders (e.g., CLL).

Nonimmunologic

Prosthetic heart valves.
Thrombotic thrombocytopenic purpura (TTP).
Sepsis.
DIC.
Hemolytic-uremic syndrome (HUS).
Giant cavernous hemangioma.

DECREASED PRODUCTION

Abnormal marrow.
Marrow infiltration (e.g., leukemia, lymphoma, fibrosis).
Marrow suppression (e.g., chemotherapy, alcohol, radiation).
Hereditary disorders.
Wiskott-Aldrich syndrome: X-linked disorder characterized by thrombocytopenia, eczema, and repeated infections.
May-Hegglin anomaly: increased megakaryocytes but ineffective thrombopoiesis.
Vitamin deficiencies (e.g., vitamin B_{12}, folic acid).

SPLENIC SEQUESTRATION, HYPERSPLENISM

DILUTIONAL, AS A RESULT OF MASSIVE TRANSFUSION

THROMBOCYTOPENIA, IN PREGNANCY[20]

ICD-9CM # 287.4

Incidental thrombocytopenia of pregnancy (gestational thrombocytopenia).
Preeclampsia/eclampsia.*
Disseminated intravascular coagulation (DIC) secondary to:
- Abruptio placentae.
- Endometritis.
- Amniotic fluid embolism.
- Retained fetus.

Preeclampsia/eclampsia:*
- Peripartum/postpartum thrombotic microangiopathy.
- Thrombotic thrombocytopenic purpura.
- Hemolytic uremic syndrome.

*Preeclampsia/eclampsia usually is not associated with overt DIC.

THROMBOCYTOPENIA, INHERITED DISORDERS[1]

ICD-9CM # 287.3

Amegakaryocytic thrombocytopenia.
Thrombocytopenia absent radii.
MYH9-related thrombocytopenia:
- May-Hegglin anomaly.
- Fechtner syndrome.
- Epstein syndrome.
- Sebastian syndrome.

X-linked macrothrombocytopenia.
Wiskott-Aldrich syndrome.
X-linked thrombocytopenia.
Thrombocytopenia and radioulnar synostosis.
Familial platelet disorder—AML.
Familial dominant thrombocytopenia.
Paris-Trousseau thrombocytopenia.
Bernard-Soulier syndrome.
Bernard-Soulier carrier/Mediterranean macrothrombocytopenia.

THROMBOCYTOSIS

ICD-9CM # 289.9 Thrombocytosis, Essential

Iron deficiency.
Posthemorrhage.
Neoplasms (GI tract).
CML.
Polycythemia vera.
Myelofibrosis with myeloid metaplasia.
Infections.
After splenectomy.
Postpartum.
Hemophilia.
Pancreatitis.
Cirrhosis.
Idiopathic.

THROMBOSIS OR THROMBOTIC DIATHESIS[1]

ICD-9CM # 444

DIFFERENTIAL DIAGNOSIS OF THE PATIENT PRESENTING WITH THROMBOSIS OR THROMBOTIC DIATHESIS

Inherited (Primary) Hypercoagulable States

Activated protein C resistance caused by factor V Leiden mutation.
Prothrombin gene mutation (G to A transition at position 20210 in the 3 -untranslated region).
Antithrombin III deficiency.
Protein C deficiency.
Protein S deficiency.
Dysfibrinogenemias (rare).

Acquired (Secondary) Hypercoagulable States

In association with physiologic or thrombogenic stimuli:
- Pregnancy (especially the postpartum period).
- Estrogen use (oral contraceptives, hormone replacement therapy).
- Immobilization.
- Trauma.
- Postoperative state.

Advancing age.
Obesity.
Prolonged air travel.
Lupus anticoagulant or antiphospholipid antibody syndrome.
In association with other clinical disorders .

Mixed/Unknown

Activated protein C resistance in the absence of factor V Leiden.
Elevated factor VIII level.
Elevated factor XI level.
Elevated factor IX level.
Elevated thrombin activatable fibrinolysis inhibitor (TAFI) level.
Decreased free tissue factor pathway inhibitor (TFPI) level.
Decreased plasma fibrinolytic activity.

THYROMEGALY

ICD-9CM # varies with specific diagnosis

Goiter.
Graves' disease.
Thyroiditis (lymphocytic, granulomatous, suppurative).
Toxic adenoma.
Neoplasm (primary, metastatic).

TICK-RELATED INFECTIONS

ICD-9CM # 082.0 Rocky Mountain Spotted Fever
066.1 Colorado Tick Fever
088.82 Babesiosis
082.8 Ehrlichiosis
088.81 Lyme Disease

Lyme disease.
Rocky Mountain spotted fever.
Babesiosis.
Tularemia.
Q fever.
Colorado tick fever.
Ehrlichiosis.
Relapsing fever.

TICS

ICD-9CM # 307.20

Tourette's syndrome.
Physiologic tic.
Anxiety disorder.
Huntington's disease.
Medications (e.g., antipsychotics, carbamazepine, phenytoin, phenobarbital).
Encephalitis.
Head trauma.
Schizophrenia.
Carbon monoxide poisoning.
Stroke.
Sydenham's chorea.
Creutzfeldt-Jakob disease.

TORSADES DE POINTES[22]

ICD-9CM # code not available

Antiarrhythmics known to increase the QT interval (e.g., quinidine, procainamide, amiodarone, disopyramide, sotalol).
Tricyclic antidepressants and phenothiazines.
Histamine (H1) antagonists (e.g., astemizole, terfenadine).
Antiviral and antifungal agents and antibiotics.
Hypokinemia.
Hypomagnesemia.
Insecticide poisoning.
Bradyarrhythmias.
Congenital long QT syndrome.
Subarachnoid hemorrhage.
Chloroquinine, pentamidine.
Cocaine abuse.

TREMOR

ICD-9CM # 781.0 Tremor NOS
333.1 Benign Essential Tremor
333.1 Familial Tremor

REST TREMORS

Parkinson's disease.
Other parkinsonian syndromes (less commonly).
Midbrain (rubral) tremor: rest < postural < kinetic.
Wilson's disease (also acquired hepatocerebral degeneration).
Essential tremor—only if severe: rest < postural and action.

POSTURAL AND ACTION (TERMINAL) TREMORS

Physiological tremor.
Exaggerated physiological tremor (these factors can also aggravate other forms of tremor).
  Stress, fatigue, anxiety, emotion.
  Endocrine: hypoglycemia, thyrotoxicosis, pheochromocytoma, adrenocorticosteroids.
  Drugs and toxins: β-agonists, dopamine agonists, amphetamines, lithium, tricyclic antidepressants, neuroleptics, theophylline, caffeine, valproic acid, alcohol withdrawal, mercury (Hatter's shakes), lead, arsenic, others.
Essential tremor (familial or sporadic) ?subtypes.
Primary writing tremor.
With other CNS disorders.
  Parkinson's disease.
  Other akinetic-rigid syndromes.
  Idiopathic dystonia, including focal dystonias.
With peripheral neuropathy.
  Charcot-Marie-Tooth syndrome (controversial whether to call this the Roussy-Levy syndrome).
  Variety of other peripheral neuropathies (especially dysgammaglobulinemia).
Cerebellar tremor.

KINETIC (INTENTION) TREMOR

Disease of cerebellar outflow (dentate nucleus and superior cerebellar peduncle): multiple sclerosis, trauma, tumor, vascular disease, Wilson's acquired hepatocerebral degeneration, drugs, toxins (e.g., mercury), others.

MISCELLANEOUS RHYTHMICAL MOVEMENT DISORDERS

Psychogenic tremor.
Orthostatic tremor.
Rhythmical movements in dystonia (dystonic tremor).
Rhythmical myoclonus (segmental myoclonus—e.g., palatal or branchial myoclonus, spinal myoclonus, limb myorhythmia).
Oscillatory myoclonus.
Asterixis.
Clonus.
Epilepsia partialis continua.
Hereditary chin quivering.
Spasmus nutans.
Head bobbing with third ventricular cysts.
Nystagmus.

TUBULOINTERSTITIAL DISEASE, ACUTE[14]

ICD-9CM # 584.5

DRUGS

Antibiotics, penicillins, cephalosporins, rifampin.
Sulfonamides: cotrimoxazole, sulfamethoxazole.
NSAIDs: propionic acid derivatives.
Miscellaneous: phenytoin, thiazides, allopurinol, cimetidine, ifosfamide.

INFECTIONS

Invasion of renal parenchyma.
Reaction to systemic infections: streptococcal, diphtheria, hantavirus.

SYSTEMIC DISEASES

Immune mediated: SLE, transplanted kidney, cryoglobulinemias.
Metabolic: Urate, oxalate.
Neoplastic: Lymphoproliferative diseases.

IDIOPATHIC

TUBULOINTERSTITIAL KIDNEY DISEASE[14]

ICD-9CM # 584.5

Ischemic and toxic acute tubular necrosis.
Allergic interstitial nephritis.
Interstitial nephritis secondary to immune complex-related collagen vascular disease (e.g., SLE, Sjögren's).
Granulomatous diseases (sarcoidosis, uveitis).
Pigment-related tubular injury (myoglobinuria, hemoglobinuria).
Hypercalcemia with nephrocalcinosis.
Tubular obstruction (drugs such as indinavir, uric acid in tumor lysis syndrome).
Myeloma kidney or cast nephropathy.
Infection-related interstitial nephritis: *Legionella, Leptospira.*
Infiltrative diseases (e.g., lymphoma).

TUMOR MARKERS ELEVATION[38]

ICD-9CM # 795.8

CAUSES OF ELEVATED LEVELS OF TUMOR MARKERS

Carcinoembryonic Antigen (CEA)

Colonic cancer (higher levels if the tumor is more differentiated or is extensive or has spread to the liver).
Lung or breast cancer; seminoma.
Cigarette smokers.
Cirrhosis, inflammatory bowel disease, rectal polyps, pancreatitis.
Advanced age.

Alpha Fetoprotein

Hepatocellular cancer: very high titers or a rising titer is strongly suggestive, but >10% of patients do not have an elevated level.
Hepatic regeneration (e.g., cirrhosis, alcoholic or viral hepatitis).
Cancer of the stomach, colon, pancreas, or lung.
Teratocarcinoma or embryonal cell carcinoma (testis, ovary, extragonadal).
Pregnancy.
Ataxia telangiectasia.
Normal variant.

Prostate-Specific Antigen

Prostate carcinoma (localized disease).
Prostatic hyperplasia.
Prostatitis.
Prostatic infarction.

Cancer-Associated Antigen (CA-19-9)[1]

Pancreatic carcinoma (80% with advanced, well-differentiated cancer have an elevated level).
Other gastrointestinal cancers: colon, stomach, bile duct.
Acute or chronic pancreatitis.
Chronic liver disease.
Biliary tract disease.

[1]Patients who cannot synthesize Lewis blood group antigens (~5% of the population) do not produce CA-19-9 antigen.

URETHRAL DISCHARGE AND DYSURIA

ICD-9CM # 788.7 Urethral Discharge
599.9 Urethral Discharge Bloody
788.1 Dysuria

Urethritis (gonococcal, chlamydial, trichomonal).
Cystitis.
Prostatitis.
Vaginitis (candidiasis, chemical).
Meatal stenosis.
Interstitial cystitis.
Trauma (foreign body, masturbation, horseback or bike riding).

URIC ACID STONES

ICD-9CM # 792.9

Hyperuricemia.
Excessive dietary purine.
Medications (salicylates, allopurinol, probenecid).
Urine pH <5.5 (e.g., diarrhea, high animal protein diet).
Decreased urine output (dehydration, malabsorption, diarrhea, inadequate fluid intake).
Tumor lysis.
Hemolytic anemia.
Myeloproliferative disorders.

URINARY RETENTION, ACUTE

ICD-9CM # 788.20

Mechanical obstruction: urethral stone, foreign body, urethral stricture, BPH, prostate carcinoma, prostatitis, trauma with hematoma formation.
Neurogenic bladder.
Neurologic disease (MS, parkinsonism, tabes dorsalis, CVA).
Spinal cord injury.
CNS neoplasm (primary or metastatic).
Spinal anesthesia.
Lower urinary tract instrumentation.
Medications (antihistamines, antidepressants, narcotics, anticholinergics).
Abdominal or pelvic surgery.
Alcohol toxicity.
Pregnancy.
Anxiety.
Encephalitis.
Postoperative pain.
Spina bifida occulta.

URINE CASTS

ICD-9CM # 791.7

Normal finding.
Pyelonephritis.
Chronic renal disease.
Nephrotic syndrome.
Acute tubular necrosis.
Interstitial nephritis.
Nephritic syndrome.
Glomerulonephritis.
Eclampsia.
Heavy metal ingestion.
Allograft rejection.
Hypothyroidism.

URINE, RED[29]

ICD-9CM # varies with specific diagnosis

WITH A POSITIVE DIPSTICK

Hematuria.
Hemoglobinuria: negative urinalysis.
Myoglobinuria: negative urinalysis.

WITH A NEGATIVE DIPSTICK

Drugs

Aminosalicylic acid.
Deferoxamine mesylate.
Ibuprofen.
Phenacetin.
Phenolphthalein.
Phensuximide.
Rifampin.
Anthraquinone laxatives.
Doxorubicin.
Methyldopa.
Phenazopyridine.
Phenothiazine.
Phenytoin.

Dyes

Azo dyes.
Eosin.

Foods

Beets, berries, maize.
Rhodamine B.

Metabolic

Porphyrins.
Serratia marcescens (red diaper syndrome).
Urate crystalluria.

UROPATHY, OBSTRUCTIVE[36]

ICD-9CM # 599.6

INTRINSIC CAUSES

Intraluminal

Intratubular deposition of crystals (uric acid, sulfas).
Stones.
Papillary tissue.
Blood clots.

Intramural

Functional.
Ureter (ureteropelvic or ureterovesical dysfunction).
Bladder (neurogenic): spinal cord defect or trauma, diabetes, multiple sclerosis, Parkinson's disease, cerebrovascular accidents.
Bladder neck dysfunction.

Anatomic

Tumors.
Infection, granuloma.
Strictures.

EXTRINSIC CAUSES

Originating in the Reproductive System
Prostate: benign hypertrophy or cancer.
Uterus: pregnancy, tumors, prolapse, endometriosis.
Ovary: abscess, tumor, cysts.

Originating in the Vascular System
Aneurysms (aorta, iliac vessels).
Aberrant arteries (ureteropelvic junction).
Venous (ovarian veins, retrocaval ureter).

Originating in the Gastrointestinal Tract
Crohn's disease.
Pancreatitis.
Appendicitis.
Tumors.

Originating in the Retroperitoneal Space
Inflammations.
Fibrosis.
Tumor, hematomas.

UTERINE BLEEDING, ABNORMAL[12]

ICD-9CM # 626.9

PREGNANCY

Threatened abortion.
Incomplete abortion.
Complete abortion.
Molar pregnancy.
Ectopic pregnancy.
Retained products of conception.

OVULATORY

Vulva: infection, laceration, tumor.
Vagina: infection, laceration, tumor, foreign body.
Cervix: polyps, cervical erosion, cervicitis, carcinoma.
Uterus: fibroids (submucous fibroids most likely to cause abnormal bleeding), polyps, adenomyosis, endometritis, intrauterine device, atrophic endometrium.
Pregnancy complications: ectopic pregnancy; threatened, incomplete, complete abortion; retained products of conception.
Abnormality of clotting system.
Midcycle bleeding.
Halban's disease (persistent corpus luteum).
Menorrhagia.
Pelvic inflammatory disease.

ANOVULATORY

Physiologic causes:
- Puberty.
- Perimenopausal.

Pathologic causes:
- Ovarian failure (FSH over 40 IU/ml).
- Hyperandrogenism.
- Hyperprolactinemia.
- Obesity.
- Hypothalamic dysfunction (polycystic ovaries); LH/FSH ratio greater than 2:1.
- Hyperplasia.
- Endometrial carcinoma.
- Estrogen-producing tumors.
- Hypothyroidism.

VAGINAL BLEEDING, PREGNANCY[7]

ICD-9CM # 626.6 Irregular Vaginal Bleeding

FIRST TRIMESTER

Implantation bleeding.
Abortion.
- Threatened.
- Complete.
- Incomplete.
- Missed.

Ectopic pregnancy.
Neoplasia.
Hydatidiform mole.
Cervix.

THIRD TRIMESTER

Placenta previa.
Placental abruption.
Premature labor.
Choriocarcinoma.

VAGINAL DISCHARGE, PREPUBERTAL GIRLS[19]

ICD-9CM # 623.5 Vaginal Discharge

Irritative (bubble baths, sand).
Poor perineal hygiene.
Foreign body.
Associated systemic illness (group A streptococci, chickenpox).
Infections.
Escherichia coli with foreign body.
Shigella organisms.
Yersinia organisms.
Infections (consider sexual abuse).
- *Chlamydia trachomatis.*
- *Neisseria gonorrhoeae.*
- *Trichomonas vaginalis.*

Tumor (rare).

VASCULITIS, CLASSIFICATION[26]

ICD-9CM # 447.6

LARGE VESSEL DISEASE

Arteritis
Giant cell arteritis.
Takayasu's arteritis.
Arteritis associated with Reiter's syndrome, ankylosing spondylitis.

MEDIUM AND SMALL VESSEL DISEASE

Polyarteritis Nodosa
Primary (idiopathic).
Associated with viruses (Hepatitis B or C, CMV, HIV, herpes zoster).
Associated with malignancy (hairy cell leukemia).
Familial Mediterranean fever.

Granulomatous Vasculitis
Wegener's granulomatosis.
Lymphomatoid granulomatosis.

Behçet's Disease
Kawasaki Disease (Mucocutaneous Lymph Node Syndrome)

PREDOMINANTLY SMALL VESSEL DISEASE

Hypersensitivity Vasculitis (Leukocytoclastic Vasculitis)
Henoch-Schönlein purpura.
Mixed cryoglobulinemia.
Serum sickness.
Vasculitis associated with connective tissue diseases (SLE, Sjögren's syndrome).
Vasculitis associated with specific syndromes:
- Primary biliary cirrhosis.
- Lyme disease.
- Chronic active hepatitis.
- Drug-induced vasculitis.

Churg-Strauss Syndrome
Goodpasture's Syndrome
Erythema Nodosum
Panniculitis
Buerger's Disease (Thrombophlebitis Obliterans)

VASCULITIS (DISEASES THAT MIMIC VASCULITIS)[28]

ICD-9CM # varies with specific disease

EMBOLIC DISEASE

Infectious or marantic endocarditis.
Cardiac mural thrombus.
Atrial myxoma.
Cholesterol embolization syndrome.

NONINFLAMMATORY VESSEL WALL DISRUPTION

Atherosclerosis.
Arterial fibromuscular dysplasia.
Drug effects (vasoconstrictors, anticoagulants).
Radiation.
Genetic disease (neurofibromatosis, Ehlers-Danlos syndrome).
Amyloidosis.
Intravascular malignant lymphoma.

DIFFUSE COAGULATION

Disseminated intravascular coagulation.
Thrombotic thrombocytopenic purpura.
Hemolytic-uremic syndrome.
Protein C and S deficiencies, factor V/Leiden mutation.
Antiphospholipid syndrome.

VENTILATION–PERFUSION MISMATCH ON LUNG SCAN

ICD-9CM # varies with specific disorder

Pulmonary embolism.
Emphysema.
Irradiation.
Pulmonary hypertension.
AV malformations.
Pulmonary thrombosis.
External compression of pulmonary artery (neoplasm, cysts, fibrosing mediastinitis).

Vasculitis.
Tuberculosis.
Pulmonary thrombosis.
Congenital (pulmonary artery hypoplasia, congenital heart disease with upper lobe diversion).
Sequestered segment.
Parasitic lung disease.
Intraluminal obstruction from catheter fragments.

VENTRICULAR FAILURE

ICD-9CM # 429.9 Ventricular Dysfunction

LEFT VENTRICULAR FAILURE

Systemic hypertension.
Valvular heart disease (AS, AR, MR).
Cardiomyopathy, myocarditis.
Bacterial endocarditis.
Myocardial infarction.
Idiopathic hypertrophic subaortic stenosis.

RIGHT VENTRICULAR FAILURE

Valvular heart disease (mitral stenosis).
Pulmonary hypertension.
Bacterial endocarditis (right-sided).
Right ventricular infarction.

BIVENTRICULAR FAILURE

Left ventricular failure.
Cardiomyopathy.
Myocarditis
Arrhythmias.
Anemia.
Thyrotoxicosis.
Arteriovenous fistula.
Paget's disease.
Beriberi.

VERRUCOUS LESIONS

ICD-9CM # varies with specific disorder

Warts.
Seborrheic keratosis.
Lichen simplex.
Acanthosis nigricans.
Scabies (Norwegian, crusted).
Verrucous carcinoma.
Nevus sebaceous.
Deep fungal infection.

VERTIGO

ICD-9CM # 780.4 Vertigo NOS
386.11 Benign Paroxysmal Positional
386.2 Central Origin
386.10 Peripheral
386.12 Vestibular (Neuronitis)

PERIPHERAL

Otitis media.
Acute labyrinthitis.
Vestibular neuronitis.
Benign positional vertigo.
Ménière's disease.
Ototoxic drugs: streptomycin, gentamicin.
Lesions of the eighth nerve: acoustic neuroma, meningioma, mononeuropathy, metastatic carcinoma.
Mastoiditis.

CNS OR SYSTEMIC

Vertebrobasilar artery insufficiency.
Posterior fossa tumor or other brain tumors.
Infarction/hemorrhage of cerebral cortex, cerebellum, or brainstem.
Basilar migraine.
Metabolic: drugs, hypoxia, anemia, fever.
Hypotension/severe hypertension.
Multiple sclerosis.
CNS infections: viral, bacterial.
Temporal lobe epilepsy.
Arnold-Chiari malformation, syringobulbia.
Psychogenic: ventilation, hysteria.

VESICULOBULLOUS DISEASES[14]

ICD-9CM # 709.8

IMMUNOLOGICALLY MEDIATED DISEASES

Bullous pemphigoid.
Herpes gestationis.
Mucous membrane pemphigoid.
Epidermolysis bullosa acquisita.
Dermatitis herpetiformis.
Pemphigus (vulgaris, foliaceus, paraneoplastic).

HYPERSENSITIVITY DISEASES

Erythema multiforme minor.
Erythema multiforme major (Stevens-Johnson syndrome).
Toxic epidermal necrolysis.

METABOLIC DISEASES

Porphyria cutanea tarda.
Pseudoporphyria.
Diabetic blisters.

INHERITED GENETIC DISORDERS

Epidermolysis bullosa.
- Simplex.
- Junctional.
- Dystrophic.

INFECTIOUS DISEASES

Impetigo.
Staphylococcal scalded skin syndrome.
Herpes simplex.
Varicella.
Herpes zoster.

VISION LOSS, ACUTE, PAINFUL

ICD-9CM # 368.11 Vision Loss, Sudden

Acute angle-closure glaucoma.
Corneal ulcer.
Uveitis.
Endophthalmitis.
Factitious.
Somatization syndrome.
Trauma.

VISION LOSS, ACUTE, PAINLESS

ICD-9CM # 368.11 Vision Loss, Sudden

Retinal artery occlusion.
Optic neuritis.
Retinal vein occlusion.
Vitreous hemorrhage.
Retinal detachment.
Exudative macular degeneration.
CVA.
Ischemic optic neuropathy.
Factitious.
Somatization syndrome, anxiety reaction.

VISION LOSS, CHILDREN

ICD-9CM # 368.9

Craniopharyngioma.
Hereditary optic atrophy.
Optic nerve glioma.
Glioma of chiasm.
Albinism.
Optic nerve hypoplasia.

VISION LOSS, CHRONIC, PROGRESSIVE

ICD-9CM # 369.9 Vision Loss NOS

Cataract.
Macular degeneration.
Cerebral neoplasm.
Refractive error.
Open-angle glaucoma.

VISION LOSS, MONOCULAR, TRANSIENT

ICD-9CM # 369.9

Thromboembolism.
Vasculitis.
Migraine (vasospasm).
Anxiety reaction.
CNS tumor.
Temporal arteritis.
Multiple sclerosis.

VOCAL CORD PARALYSIS

ICD-9CM # 478.30 Unspecified
478.31 Unilateral Partial
478.32 Unilateral Complete
478.33 Bilateral Partial
478.34 Bilateral Complete

Neoplasm: primary or metastatic (e.g., lung, thyroid, parathyroid, mediastinum).
Neck surgery (parathyroid, thyroid, carotid endarterectomy, cervical spine).
Idiopathic.
Viral, bacterial, or fungal infection.
Trauma (intubation, penetrating neck injury).
Cardiac surgery.
RA.
Multiple sclerosis.
Parkinsonism.
Toxic neuropathy.
CVA.

CNS abnormalities: hydrocephalus, Arnold-Chiari malformation, meningomyelocele.

VOLUME DEPLETION[1]

ICD-9CM # 276.5

GI losses:
- Upper: bleeding, nasogastric suction, vomiting.
- Lower: bleeding, diarrhea, enteric or pancreatic fistula, tube drainage.

Renal losses:
- Salt and water: diuretics, osmotic diuresis, postobstructive diuresis, acute tubular necrosis (recovery phase), salt-losing nephropathy, adrenal insufficiency, renal tubular acidosis.

Water loss: diabetes insipidus.

Skin and respiratory losses:
- Sweat, burns, insensible losses.

Sequestration without external fluid loss:
- Intestinal obstruction, peritonitis, pancreatitis, rhabdomyolysis, internal bleeding.

VOLUME EXCESS[1]

ICD-9CM # varies with specific diagnosis

PRIMARY RENAL SODIUM RETENTION (INCREASED EFFECTIVE CIRCULATING VOLUME)

Renal failure, nephritic syndrome, acute glomerulonephritis.
Primary hyperaldosteronism.
Cushing's syndrome.
Liver disease.

SECONDARY RENAL SODIUM RETENTION (DECREASED EFFECTIVE CIRCULATING VOLUME)

Heart failure.
Liver disease.
Nephrotic syndrome (minimal change disease).
Pregnancy.

VOMITING

ICD-9CM # 787.03

GI disturbances:
- Obstruction: esophageal, pyloric, intestinal.
- Infections: viral or bacterial enteritis, viral hepatitis, food poisoning, gastroenteritis.
- Pancreatitis.
- Appendicitis.
- Biliary colic.
- Peritonitis.
- Perforated bowel.
- Diabetic gastroparesis.

Other: gastritis, PUD, IBD, GI tract neoplasms.
Drugs: morphine, digitalis, cytotoxic agents, bromocriptine.
Severe pain: MI, renal colic.
Metabolic disorders: uremia, acidosis/alkalosis, hyperglycemia, DKA, thyrotoxicosis.
Trauma: blows to the testicles, epigastrium.
Vertigo.
Reye's syndrome.
Increased intracranial pressure.
CNS disturbances: trauma, hemorrhage, infarction, neoplasm, infection, hypertensive encephalopathy, migraine.
Radiation sickness.
Nausea and vomiting of pregnancy, hyperemesis gravidarum.
Motion sickness.
Bulimia, anorexia nervosa.
Psychogenic: emotional disturbances, offensive sights or smells.
Severe coughing.
Pyelonephritis.
Boerhaave's syndrome.
Carbon monoxide poisoning.

VULVAR LESIONS[12]

ICD-9CM # 625.8 Vulvar Mass
098.0 Vulvar Ulcer, Gonococcal
091.0 Vulvar Ulcer, Syphilitic
616.51 Behçet's
624.0 Leukoplakia
624.8 Dysplasia
233.3 Carcinoma
616.9 Inflammatory Lesion
624.4 Vulvar Scar (Old)
624.1 Vulvar Atrophy

RED LESION

Infection/Infestation

Fung I infection:
- *Candida.*
- *Tinea cruris.*
- Intertrigo.
- *Pityriasis versicolor.*

Sarcoptes scabiei.
Erythrasma: *Corynebacterium minutissimum.*
Granuloma inguinale: Calymmatobacterium granulomatis.
Folliculitis: *Staphylococcus aureus.*
Hidradenitis suppurativa.
Behçet's syndrome.

Inflammation

Reactive vulvitis.
Chemical irritation:
- Detergent.
- Dyes.
- Perfume.
- Spermicide.
- Lubricants.
- Hygiene sprays.
- Podophyllum.
- Topical 5-FU.
- Saliva.
- Gentian violet.
- Semen.

Mechanical trauma: scratching.
Vestibular adenitis.
Essential vulvodynia.
Psoriasis.
Seborrheic dermatitis.

Neoplasm

Vulvar intraepithelial neoplasia (VIN):
- Mild dysplasia.
- Moderate dysplasia.
- Severe dysplasia.
- Carcinoma-in-situ.

Vulvar dystrophy.
Bowen's disease.
Invasive cancer:
- Squamous cell carcinoma.
- Malignant melanoma.
- Sarcoma.
- Basal cell carcinoma.
- Adenocarcinoma.
- Paget's disease.
- Undifferentiated.

WHITE LESION

Vulvar dystrophy:
- Lichen sclerosus.
- Vulvar dystrophy.
- Vulvar hyperplasia.
- Mixed dystrophy.

VIN.
Vitiligo.
Partial albinism.
Intertrigo.
Radiation treatment.

DARK LESION

Lentigo.
Nevi (mole).
Neoplasm (see Neoplasm, Vulvar, below).
Reactive hyperpigmentation.
Seborrheic keratosis.
Pubic lice.

ULCERATIVE LESION

Infection

Herpes simplex.
Vaccinia.
Treponema pallidum.
Granuloma inguinale.
Pyoderma.
Tuberculosis.

Noninfection

Behçet's disease.
Crohn's disease.
Pemphigus.
Pemphigoid.
Hidradenitis suppurativa (see Neoplasm, Vulvar, below).

Neoplasm

Basal cell carcinoma.
Squamous cell carcinoma.
Vulvar tumor <1 cm:
- Condyloma acuminatum.
- Molluscum contagiosum.
- Epidermal inclusion.
- Vestibular cyst.
- Mesonephric duct.
- VIN.
- Hemangioma.
- Hidradenoma.
- Neurofibroma.
- Syringoma.
- Accessory breast tissue.
- Acrochordon.
- Endometriosis.
- Fox-Fordyce disease.
- Pilonidal sinus.

Vulvar tumor >1 cm:
- Bartholin cyst or abscess.
- Lymphogranuloma venereum.
- Fibroma.
- Lipoma.
- Verrucous carcinoma.
- Squamous cell carcinoma.
- Hernia.
- Edema.
- Hematoma.
- Acrochordon.
- Epidermal cysts.
- Neurofibromatosis.
- Accessory breast tissue.

WEAKNESS, ACUTE, EMERGENT[26]

ICD-9CM # 780.7

Demyelinating disorders (Guillain-Barré, chronic inflammatory demyelinating polyneuropathy [CIDP]).
Myasthenia gravis.
Infectious (poliomyelitis, diphtheria).
Toxic (botulism, tick paralysis, paralytic shellfish toxin, puffer fish, newts).
Metabolic (acquired or familial hypokalemia, hypophosphatemia, hypermagnesemia).
Metal poisoning (arsenic, thallium).
Porphyria.

WEAKNESS, GRADUAL ONSET

ICD-9CM # 780.7

Depression.
Malingering.
Anemia.
Hypothyroidism.
Medications (e.g., sedatives, antidepressants, narcotics).
CHF.
Renal failure.
Liver failure.
Respiratory insufficiency.
Alcoholism.
Nutritional deficiencies.
Disorders of motor unit.
Basal ganglia disorders.
Upper motor neuron lesions.

WEAKNESS, NONNEUROMUSCULAR CAUSES

ICD-9CM # 780.79

Anxiety disorder.
Infectious process.
Anemia.
Renal insufficiency.
Hyperventilation.
Malignancy.
Hypothyroidism.
Hypotension.
Hypercapnia.
Hypoglycemia.
Cardiac arrhythmias.
Hepatic insufficiency.
Electrolyte imbalance.
Malnutrition.
Cerebrovascular insufficiency.

WEIGHT GAIN

ICD-9CM # 783.1 Abnormal Weight Gain
278.00 Obesity

Sedentary lifestyle.
Fluid overload.
Discontinuation of tobacco abuse.
Endocrine disorders (hypothyroidism, hyperinsulinism associated with maturity-onset DM, Cushing's syndrome, hypogonadism, insulinoma, hyperprolactinemia, acromegaly).
Medications (nutritional supplements, oral contraceptives, glucocorticoids, etc.).
Anxiety disorders with compulsive eating.
Laurence-Moon-Biedl syndrome, Prader-Willi syndrome, other congenital diseases.
Hypothalamic injury (rare; <100 cases reported in medical literature).

WEIGHT LOSS

ICD-9CM # 783.2 Abnormal Weight Loss

Malignancy.
Psychiatric disorders (depression, anorexia nervosa).
New-onset DM.
Malabsorption.
COPD.
AIDS.
Uremia, liver disease.
Thyrotoxicosis, pheochromocytoma, carcinoid syndrome.
Addison's disease.
Intestinal parasites.
Peptic ulcer disease.
Inflammatory bowel disease.
Food faddism.
Postgastrectomy syndrome.

WHEEZING

ICD-9CM # 786.09

Asthma.
COPD.
Interstitial lung disease.
Infections (pneumonia, bronchitis, bronchiolitis, epiglottitis).
Cardiac asthma.
GERD with aspiration.
Foreign body aspiration.
Pulmonary embolism.
Anaphylaxis.
Obstruction of airway (neoplasm, goiter, edema or hemorrhage from trauma, aneurysm, congenital abnormalities, strictures, spasm).
Carcinoid syndrome.

WHEEZING, PEDIATRIC AGE[4]

ICD-9CM # 786.09 Wheezing

Reactive airways disease.
Atopic asthma.
Infection-associated airway reactivity.
Exercise-induced asthma.
Salicylate-induced asthma and nasal polyposis.
Asthmatic bronchitis.
Other hypersensitivity reactions:
- Hypersensitivity pneumonitis.
- Tropical eosinophilia.
- Visceral larva migrans.
- Allergic bronchopulmonary aspergillosis.

Aspiration:
- Foreign body.
- Food, saliva, gastric contents.
- Laryngotracheoesophageal cleft.
- Tracheoesophageal fistula, H-type.
- Pharyngeal incoordination or neuromuscular weakness.

Cystic fibrosis.
Primary ciliary dyskinesia.
Cardiac failure.
Bronchiolitis obliterans.
Extrinsic compression of airways:
- Vascular ring.
- Enlarged lymph node.
- Mediastinal tumor.
- Lung cysts.

Tracheobronchomalacia.
Endobronchial masses.
Gastroesophageal reflux.
Pulmonary hemosiderosis.
Sequelae of bronchopulmonary dysplasia.
"Hysterical" glottic closure.
Cigarette smoke, other environmental insults.

WRIST AND HAND PAIN, IN DIFFERENT AGE GROUPS[8]

ICD-9CM # 959.3

COMMON CAUSES OF WRIST AND HAND PAIN IN DIFFERENT AGE GROUPS

Childhood (2-10 yr)
Intraarticular:
Infection.
Periarticular:
Fracture.
Osteomyelitis.
Adolescence (10-18 yr)
Intraarticular:
Infection.
Periarticular:
Trauma.
Osteomyelitis.
Tumors.
Ganglion.
Idiopathic wrist pain.
Early adulthood (18-30 yr)
Intraarticular:
Inflammatory arthritis.
Infection.
Osteoarthritis.
Periarticular:
Peripheral nerve entrapment.
Tendonitis.
Referred:
Cervical.
Adulthood (30-50 yr)
Intraarticular:
Inflammatory arthritis.
Infection.

Osteoarthritis.
Periarticular:
Peripheral nerve entrapment.
Tendonitis.
Referred:
Cervical.
Chest.
Cardiac.
Old age (>50 yr)
Intraarticular:
Inflammatory arthritis.
Osteoarthritis.
Periarticular:
Peripheral nerve entrapment.
Tendonitis.
Referred:
Cervical.
Chest.
Cardiac.

WRIST PAIN

ICD-9CM # 959.3

MECHANICAL

Osteoarthritis.
Ligament tear.
Fracture.
Ganglion.
De Quervain's tenosynovitis.
Avascular necrosis (scaphoid, lunate).
Nonunion of scaphoid or lunate.
Neoplasm.

METABOLIC

Pregnancy.
Diabetes.
Gout.
Pseudogout.
Paget's disease.
Acromegaly.
Hypothyroidism.
Hyperparathyroidism.

INFECTIOUS

Osteomyelitis.
Septic arthritis.
Cat-scratch disease.
Tick bite (Lyme disease, babesiosis).
Tuberculosis.

NEUROLOGIC

Peripheral neuropathy.
Nerve injury (median, ulnar, radial nerve).
Thoracic outlet compression syndrome.
Distal posterior interosseous nerve syndrome.

RHEUMATOLOGIC

Psoriasis.
RA.
SLE, mixed connective tissue disorder (MCTD).
Scleroderma.

MISCELLANEOUS

Granulomatous (sarcoidosis).
Amyloidosis.
Multiple myeloma.
Leukemia.

XEROPHTHALMIA[28]

ICD-9CM # 372.53 Xerophthalmia

MEDICATIONS

Tricyclic antidepressants: amitriptyline (Elavil), doxepin (Sinequan).
Antihistamines: diphenhydramine (Benadryl), chlorpheniramine (Chlor-Trimeton), promethazine (Phenergan), and many cold and decongestant preparations.
Anticholinergic agents: antiemetics such as scopolamine, antispasmodic agents such as oxybutynin chloride (Ditropan).

ABNORMALITIES OF EYELID FUNCTION

Neuromuscular disorders.
Aging.
Thyrotoxicosis.

ABNORMALITIES OF TEAR PRODUCTION

Hypovitaminosis A.
Stevens-Johnson syndrome.
Familial diseases affecting sebaceous secretions.

ABNORMALITIES OF CORNEAL SURFACES

Scarring from past injuries and herpes simplex infection.

XEROSTOMIA[28]

ICD-9CM # 527.7

MEDICATIONS

Tricyclic antidepressants: amitriptyline (Elavil), doxepin (Sinequan).
Antihistamines: diphenhydramine (Benadryl), chlorpheniramine (Chlor-Trimeton), promethazine (Phenergan), and many cold and decongestant preparations.
Anticholinergic agents: antiemetics such as scopolamine, antispasmodic agents such as oxybutynin chloride (Ditropan).

DEHYDRATION

Debility.
Fever.

POLYURIA

Alcohol intake.
Arrhythmia.
Diabetes.

PREVIOUS HEAD AND NECK IRRADIATION SYSTEMIC DISEASES

Sjögren's syndrome.
Sarcoidosis.
Amyloidosis.
Human immunodeficiency virus (HIV) infection.
Graft-versus-host disease.

YELLOW URINE

ICD-9CM # 788.69

Normal coloration.
Concentrated urine.
Use of multivitamin supplements.
Diet rich in carrots.
Use of Cascara.
Urinary tract infection.

REFERENCES

1. Andreoli TE (ed): *Cecil essentials of medicine,* ed 5, Philadelphia, 2001, WB Saunders.
2. Barkin RM, Rosen P: *Emergency pediatrics: a guide to ambulatory care,* ed 5, St Louis, 1998, Mosby.
3. Baude AI: *Infectious diseases and medical microbiology,* ed 2, Philadelphia, 1986, WB Saunders.
4. Behrman RE: *Nelson textbook of pediatrics,* ed 16, Philadelphia, 2000, WB Saunders.
5. Callen JP: *Color atlas of dermatology,* ed 2, Philadelphia, 2000, WB Saunders.
6. Canoso J: *Rheumatology in primary care,* Philadelphia, 1997, WB Saunders.
7. Carlson KJ: *Primary care of women,* ed 2, St Louis, 2000, Mosby.
8. Carr A, Hamilton W: *Orthopedics in Primary Care,* ed 2, Philadelphia, 2005, Elsevier.
9. Conn R: *Current diagnosis,* ed 9, Philadelphia, 1997, WB Saunders.
10. Copeland LJ: *Textbook of gynecology,* ed 2, Philadelphia, 2000, WB Saunders.
11. Custer JW, Rau RE: *The Harriet Lane Handbook,* ed 18, St Louis, Mosby, 2009.
12. Danakas G (ed): *Practical guide to the care of the gynecologic/obstetric patient,* St Louis, 1997, Mosby.
13. Goldberg RJ: *The care of the psychiatric patient,* ed 3, St Louis, 2006, Mosby.
14. Goldman L, Ausiello D: *Cecil textbook of medicine,* ed 21, Philadelphia, 2004, WB Saunders.
15. Goldman L, Braunwauld E (eds): *Primary cardiology,* Philadelphia, 1998, WB Saunders.
16. Gorbach SL: *Infectious diseases,* ed 2, Philadelphia, 1998, WB Saunders.

17. Harrington J: *Consultation in internal medicine,* ed 2, St Louis, 1997, Mosby.
18. Henry JB: *Clinical diagnosis and management by laboratory methods,* ed 20, Philadelphia, 2001, WB Saunders.
19. Hoekelman R: *Primary pediatric care,* ed 3, St Louis, 1997, Mosby.
20. Hoffmann R et al: *Hematology, Basic Principles and Practice*, ed 5, Philadelphia, 2009, Churchill Livingstone.
21. Kassirer J (ed): *Current therapy in adult medicine,* ed 4, St Louis, 1998, Mosby.
22. Khan MG: *Rapid ECG interpretation,* Philadelphia, 2003, WB Saunders.
23. Kliegman R: *Practical strategies in pediatric diagnosis and therapy,* Philadelphia, 1996, WB Saunders.
24. Klippel J (ed): *Practical rheumatology,* London, 1995, Mosby.
25. Mandell GL: *Mandell, Douglas, and Bennett's principles and practice of infectious diseases,* ed 6, New York, 2005, Churchill Livingstone.
26. Marx J (ed): *Rosen's emergency medicine: concepts and clinical practice,* ed 5, St Louis, 2002, Mosby.
27. Moore WT, Eastman RC: *Diagnostic endocrinology,* ed 2, St Louis, 1996, Mosby.
28. Noble J (ed): *Primary care medicine,* ed 3, St Louis, 2001, Mosby.
29. Nseyo UO: *Urology for primary care physicians,* Philadelphia, 1999, WB Saunders.
30. Palay D (ed): *Ophthalmology for the primary care physician,* St Louis, 1997, Mosby.
31. Rakel RE: *Principles of family practice,* ed 6, Philadelphia, 2002, WB Saunders.
32. Schwarz MI: *Interstitial lung disease,* ed 2, St Louis, 1993, Mosby.
33. Seller RH: *Differential diagnosis of common complaints,* ed 4, Philadelphia, 2000,WB Saunders.
34. Siedel HM (ed): *Mosby's guide to physical examination,* ed 4, St Louis, 1999, Mosby.
35. Specht N: *Practical guide to diagnostic imaging,* St Louis, 1998, Mosby.
36. Stein JH (ed): *Internal medicine,* ed 5, St Louis, 1998, Mosby.
37. Swain R, Snodgrass: *Phys Sportmed* 23:56, 1995.
38. Talley NJ, Martin CJ: *Clinical gastroenterology*, ed 2, Sydney, 2006, Churchill Livingstone.
39. Weinberg SE et al: *Principles of Pulmonary Medicine*, ed 5, Philadelphia, 2008, Saunders.
40. Wiederholt WC: *Neurology for non-neurologists,* ed 4, Philadelphia, 2000, WB Saunders.
41. Wilson JD: *Williams textbook of endocrinology*, ed 9, Philadelphia, 1998, WB Saunders.

SECTION III

Clinical Algorithms

PLEASE NOTE: These algorithms are designed to assist clinicians in the evaluation and treatment of patients. They may not apply to all patients with a particular disorder and are not intended to replace the clinician's individual judgment.

Additional algorithms available at www.expertconsult.com:

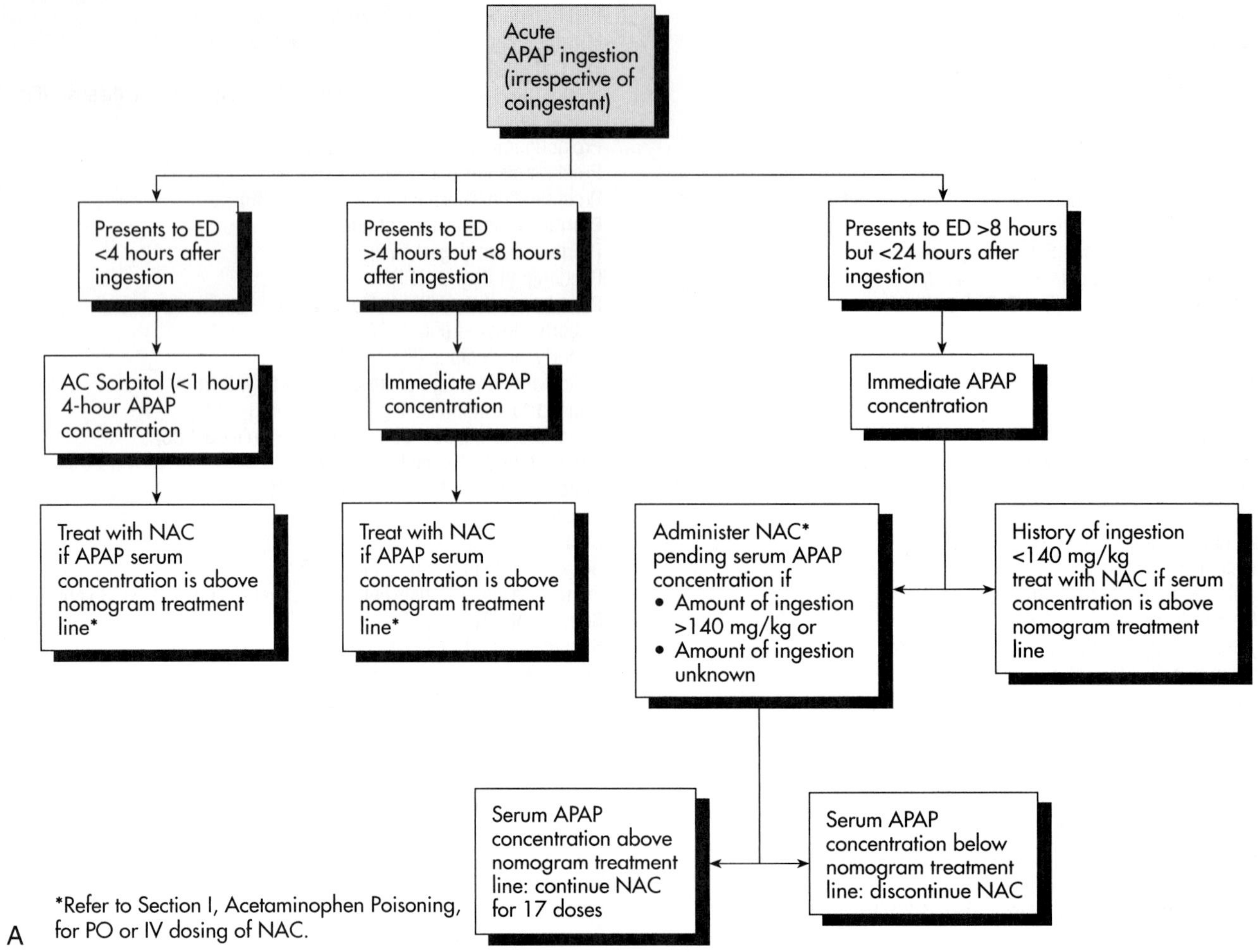

Acute APAP ingestion (irrespective of coingestant)

- Presents to ED <4 hours after ingestion
  - AC Sorbitol (<1 hour) 4-hour APAP concentration
    - Treat with NAC if APAP serum concentration is above nomogram treatment line*
- Presents to ED >4 hours but <8 hours after ingestion
  - Immediate APAP concentration
    - Treat with NAC if APAP serum concentration is above nomogram treatment line*
- Presents to ED >8 hours but <24 hours after ingestion
  - Immediate APAP concentration
    - Administer NAC* pending serum APAP concentration if
      - Amount of ingestion >140 mg/kg or
      - Amount of ingestion unknown
        - Serum APAP concentration above nomogram treatment line: continue NAC for 17 doses
        - Serum APAP concentration below nomogram treatment line: discontinue NAC
    - History of ingestion <140 mg/kg treat with NAC if serum concentration is above nomogram treatment line

*Refer to Section I, Acetaminophen Poisoning, for PO or IV dosing of NAC.

A

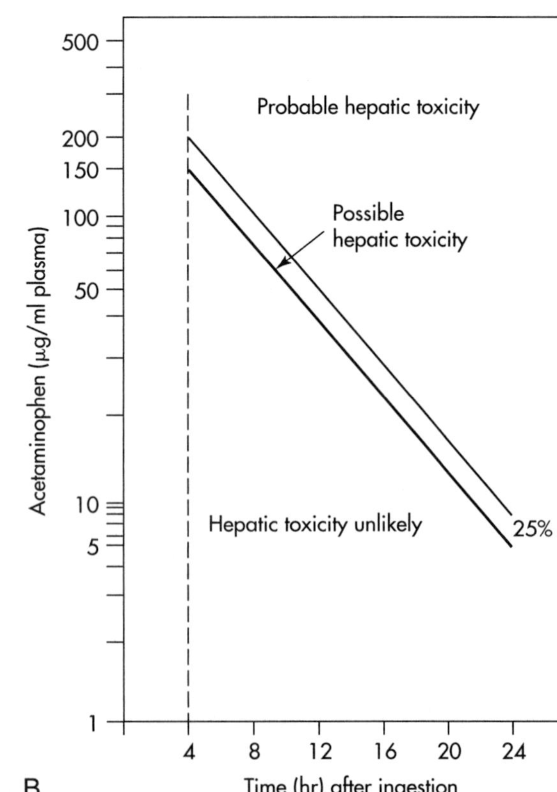

B

FIGURE 3-3 A, Treatment of acetaminophen ingestion. *APAP,* Acetaminophen; *ED,* emergency department; *NAC, N*-acetylcysteine. (From Marx J [ed]: *Rosen's emergency medicine,* ed 5, St Louis, 2002, Mosby.) **B,** Rumack-Matthew nomogram for acetaminophen poisoning. (Modified from Rumack BH, Matthew H: *Pediatrics* 55:871, 1975. In Marx J [ed]: *Rosen's emergency medicine,* ed 6, St Louis, 2006, Mosby.)

ICD-9CM # 276.2 Lactic acidosis
276.2 Metabolic acidosis
276.2 Respiratory acidosis
276.3 Respiratory alkalosis
276.3 Metabolic alkalosis

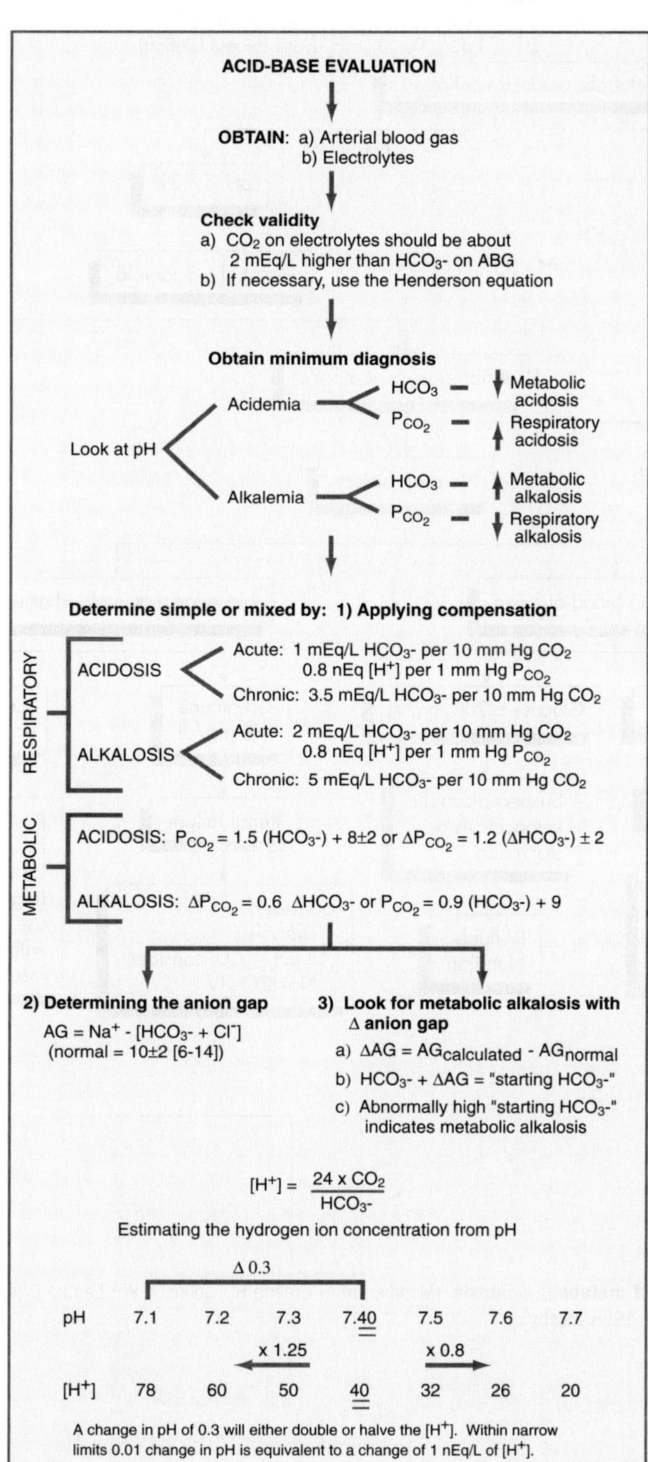

FIGURE 3-4 Scheme for assessing acid-base homeostasis. (From Andreoli TE [ed]: *Cecil essentials of medicine,* ed 7, Philadelphia, 2008, WB Saunders.)

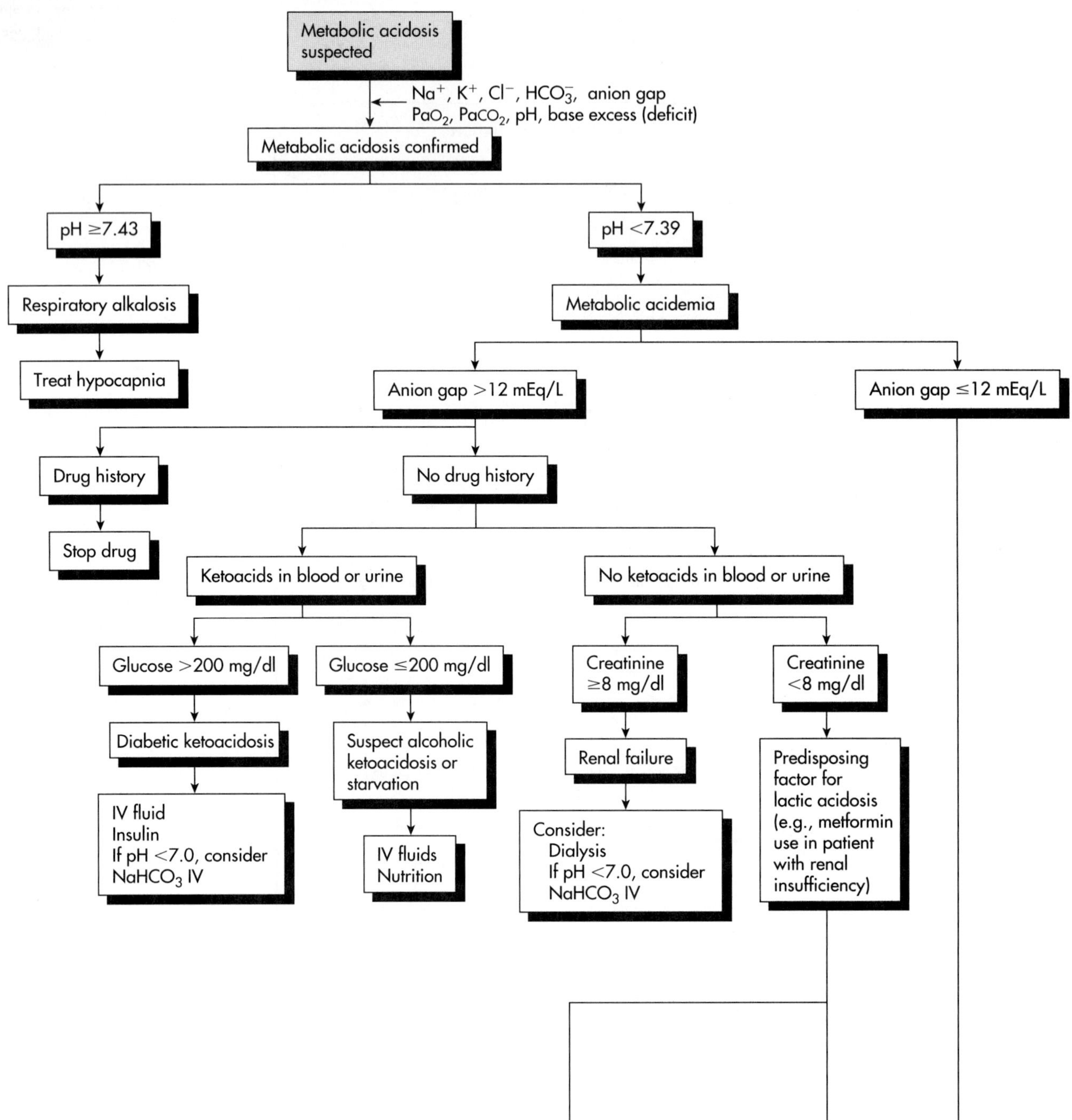

FIGURE 3-5 Suspected metabolic acidosis. (Modified from Greene HL, Johnson WP, Lemke D [eds]: *Decision making in medicine,* ed 2, St Louis, 1998, Mosby.)

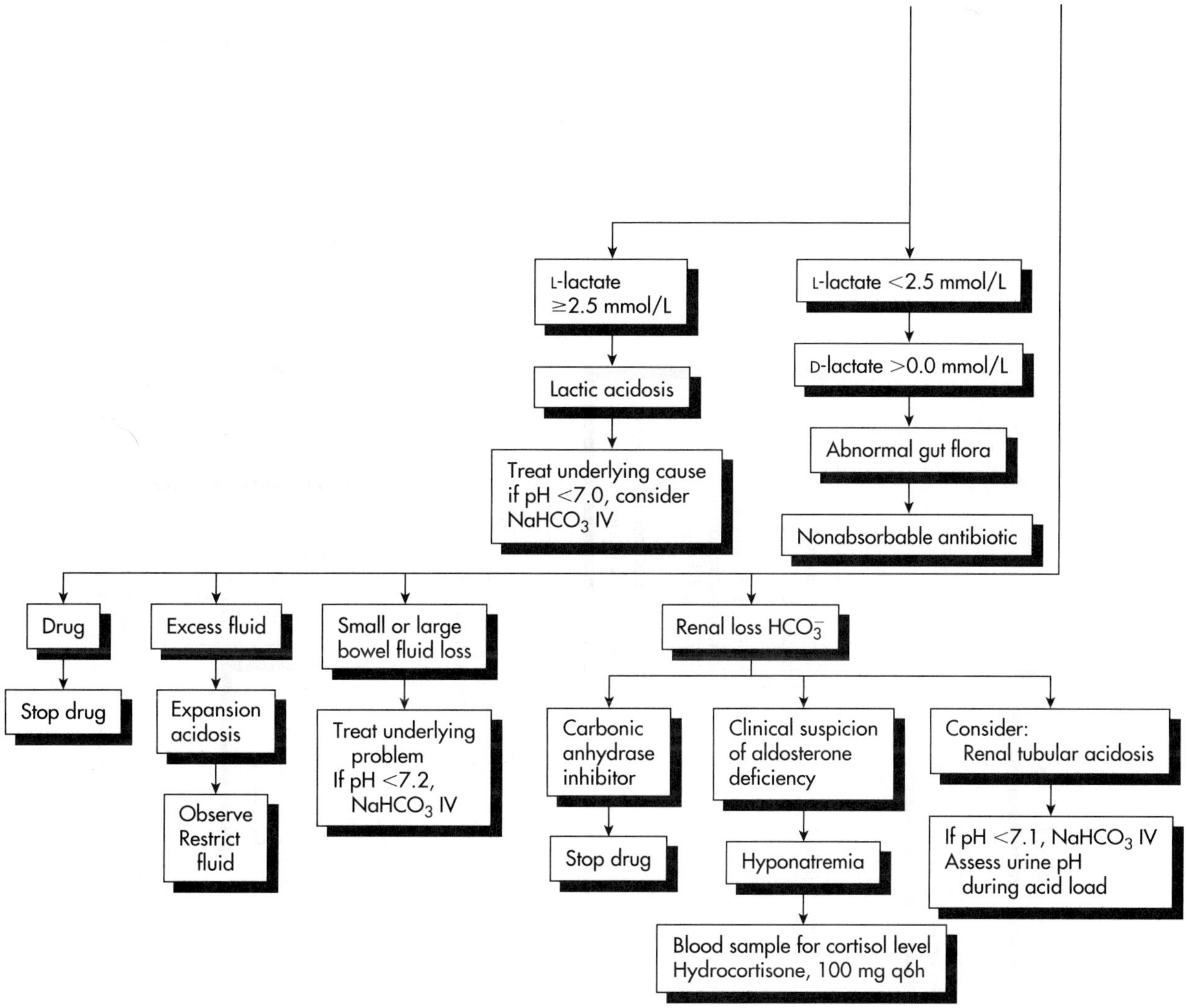

L-lactate ≥2.5 mmol/L

Lactic acidosis

Treat underlying cause if pH <7.0, consider $NaHCO_3$ IV

L-lactate <2.5 mmol/L

D-lactate >0.0 mmol/L

Abnormal gut flora

Nonabsorbable antibiotic

Drug

Stop drug

Excess fluid

Expansion acidosis

Observe Restrict fluid

Small or large bowel fluid loss

Treat underlying problem If pH <7.2, $NaHCO_3$ IV

Renal loss HCO_3^-

Carbonic anhydrase inhibitor

Stop drug

Clinical suspicion of aldosterone deficiency

Hyponatremia

Blood sample for cortisol level Hydrocortisone, 100 mg q6h

Consider: Renal tubular acidosis

If pH <7.1, $NaHCO_3$ IV Assess urine pH during acid load

FIGURE 3-5 (Continued)

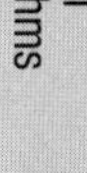

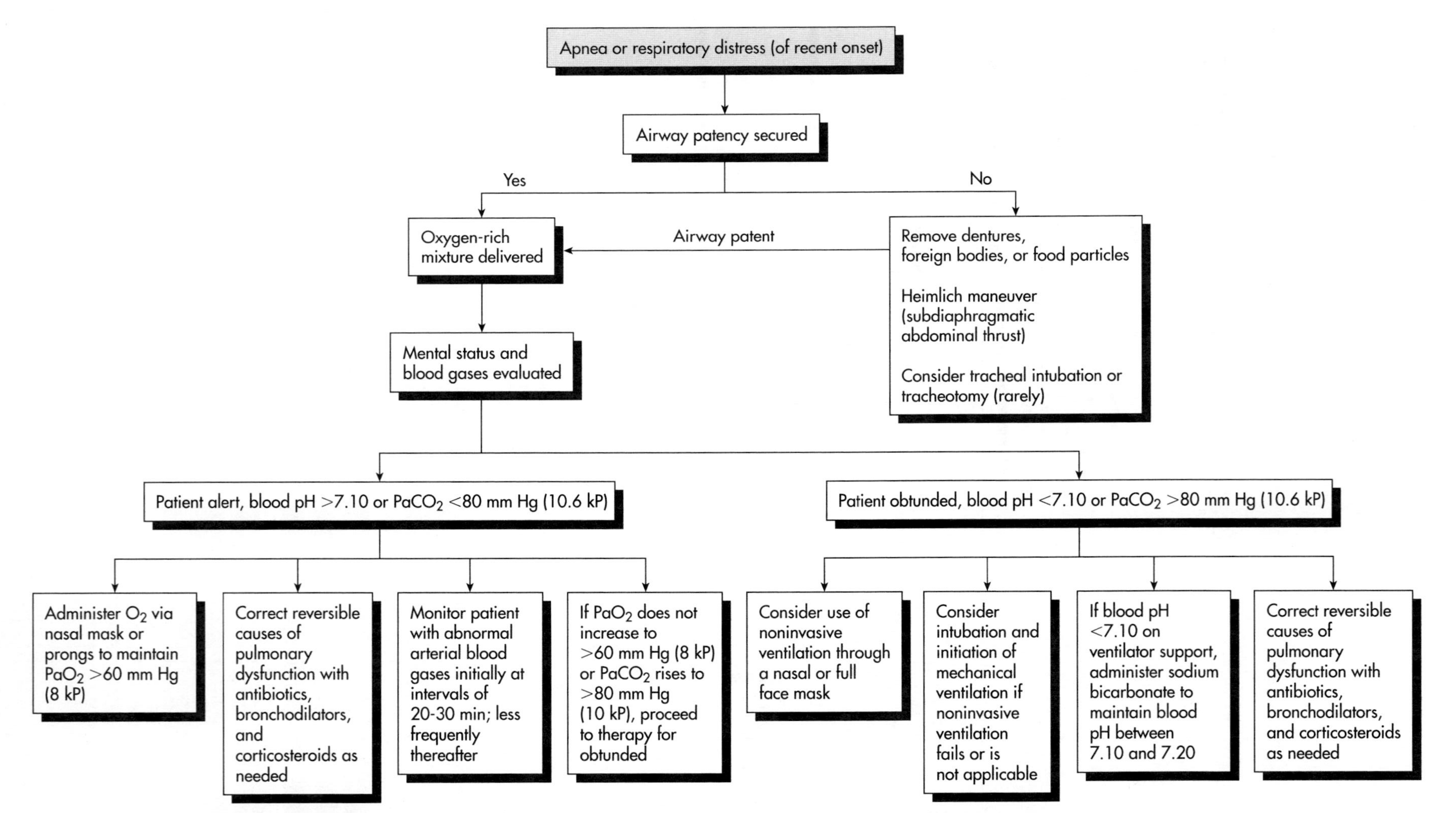

FIGURE 3-6 Algorithm for management of acute respiratory acidosis. (From Feehally J, Floege J, Johnson RJ: *Comprehensive clinical nephrology*, ed 3, St Louis, 2007, Mosby.)

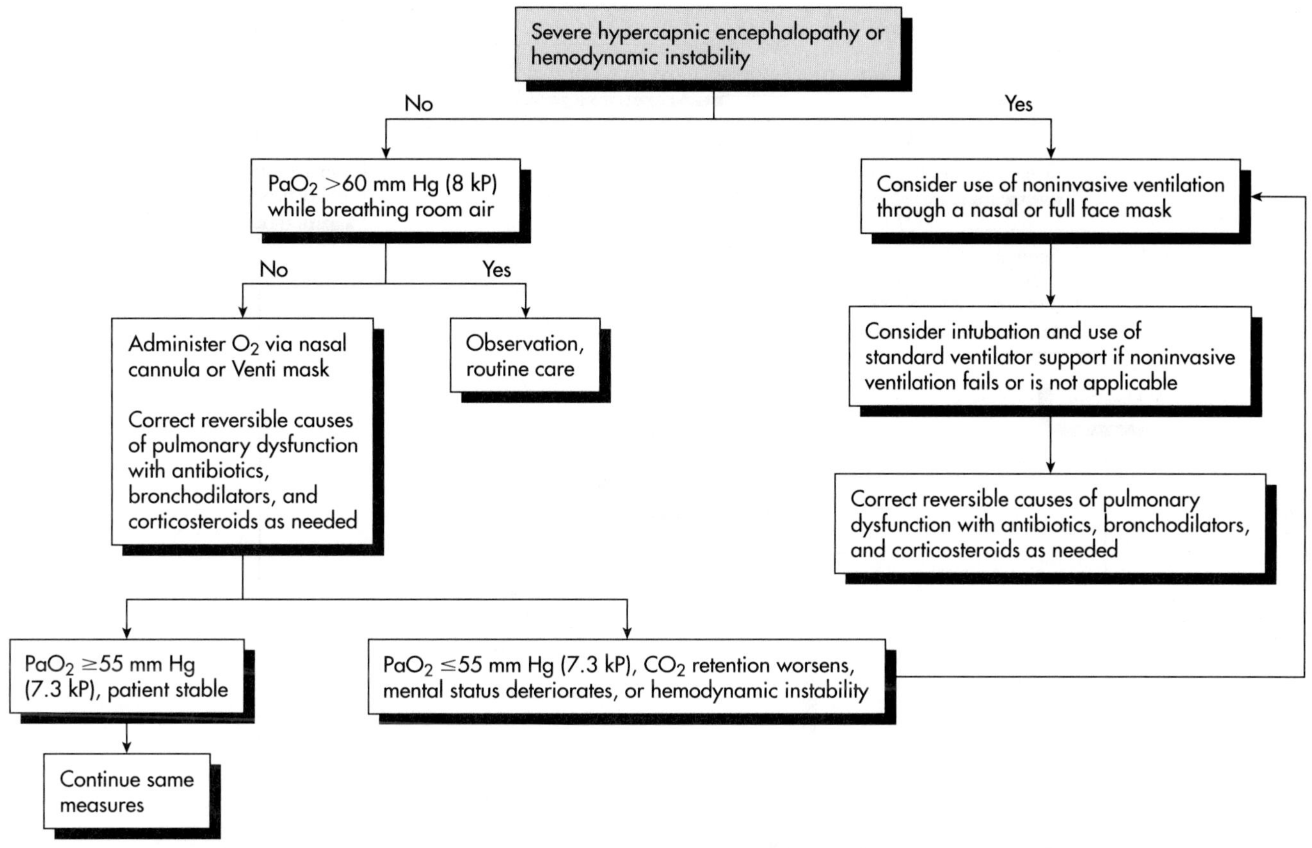

FIGURE 3-7 Algorithm for management of chronic respiratory acidosis. (From Feehally J, Floege J, Johnson RJ: *Comprehensive clinical nephrology*, ed 3, St Louis, 2007, Mosby.)

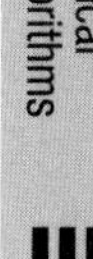

ICD-9CM # 194.0 Adrenal cortical carcinoma site NOS M8370/3
255.8 Adrenal hyperplasia

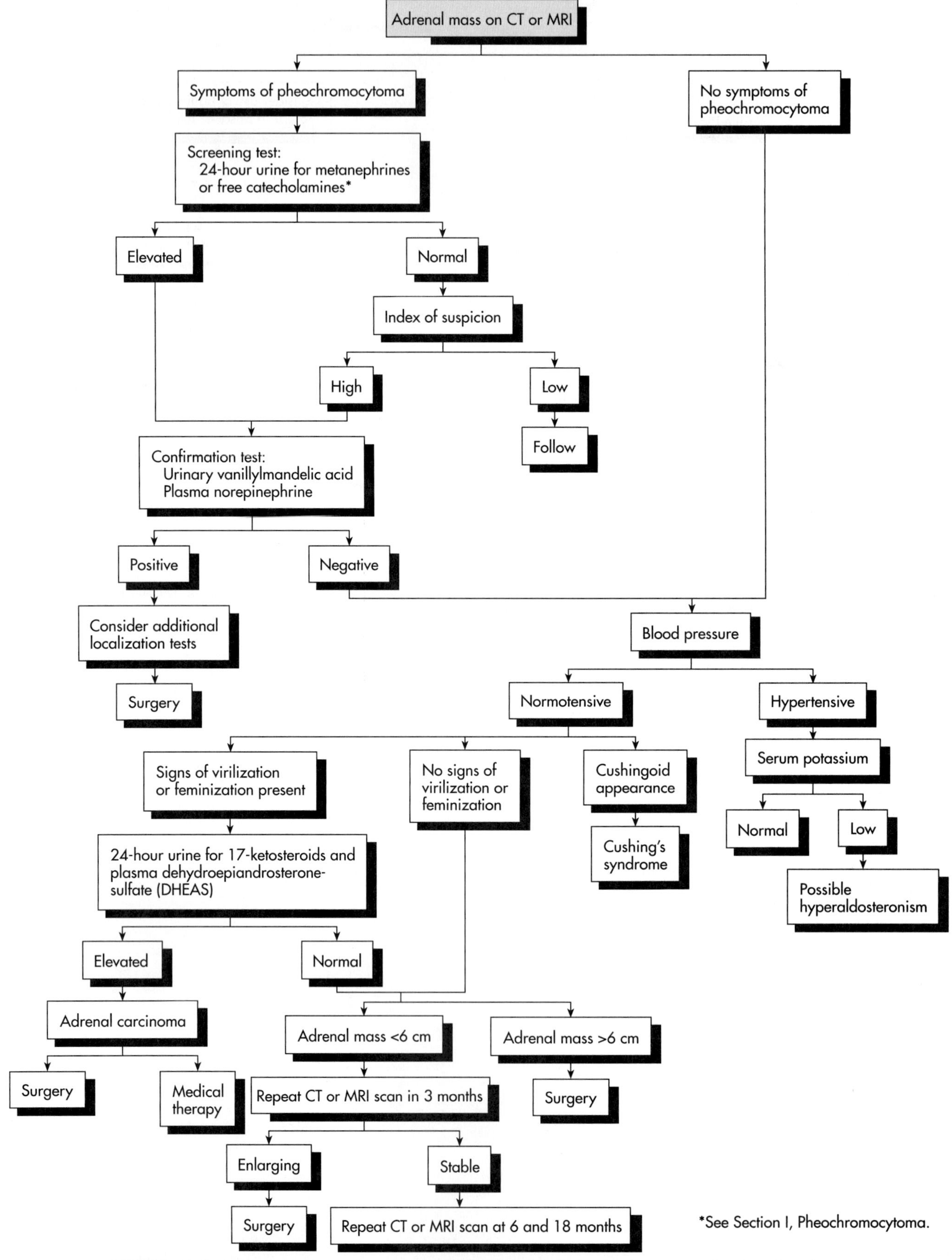

FIGURE 3-11 Evaluation of adrenal mass. *CT,* Computed tomography; *MRI,* magnetic resonance imaging. (From Greene HL, Johnson WP, Lemcke D [eds]: *Decision making in medicine,* ed 2, St Louis, 1998, Mosby.)

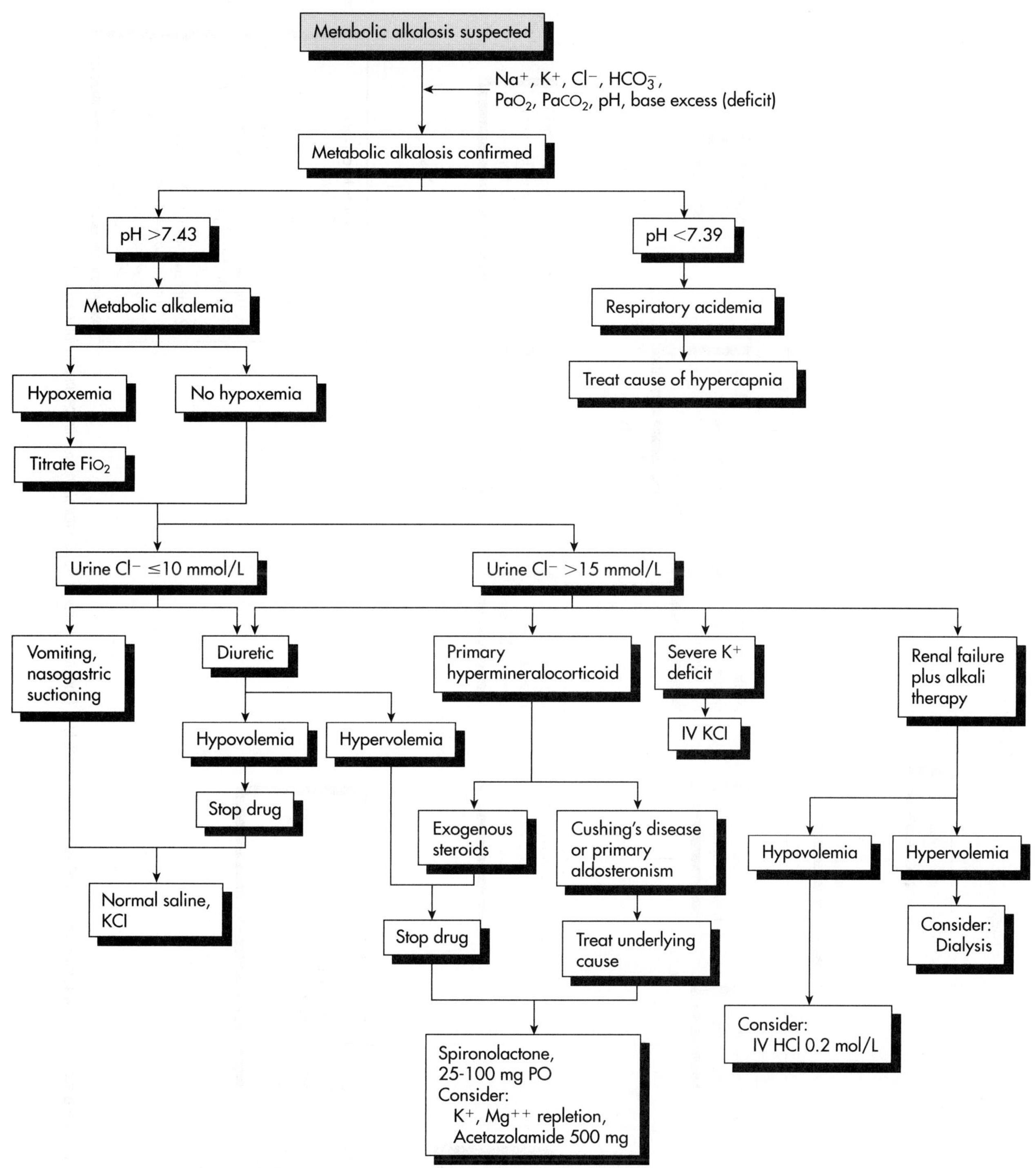

FIGURE 3-15 Suspected metabolic alkalosis. (From Greene HL, Johnson WP, Lemke D [eds]: *Decision making in medicine*, ed 2, St Louis, 1998, Mosby.)

ICD-9CM # 276.3

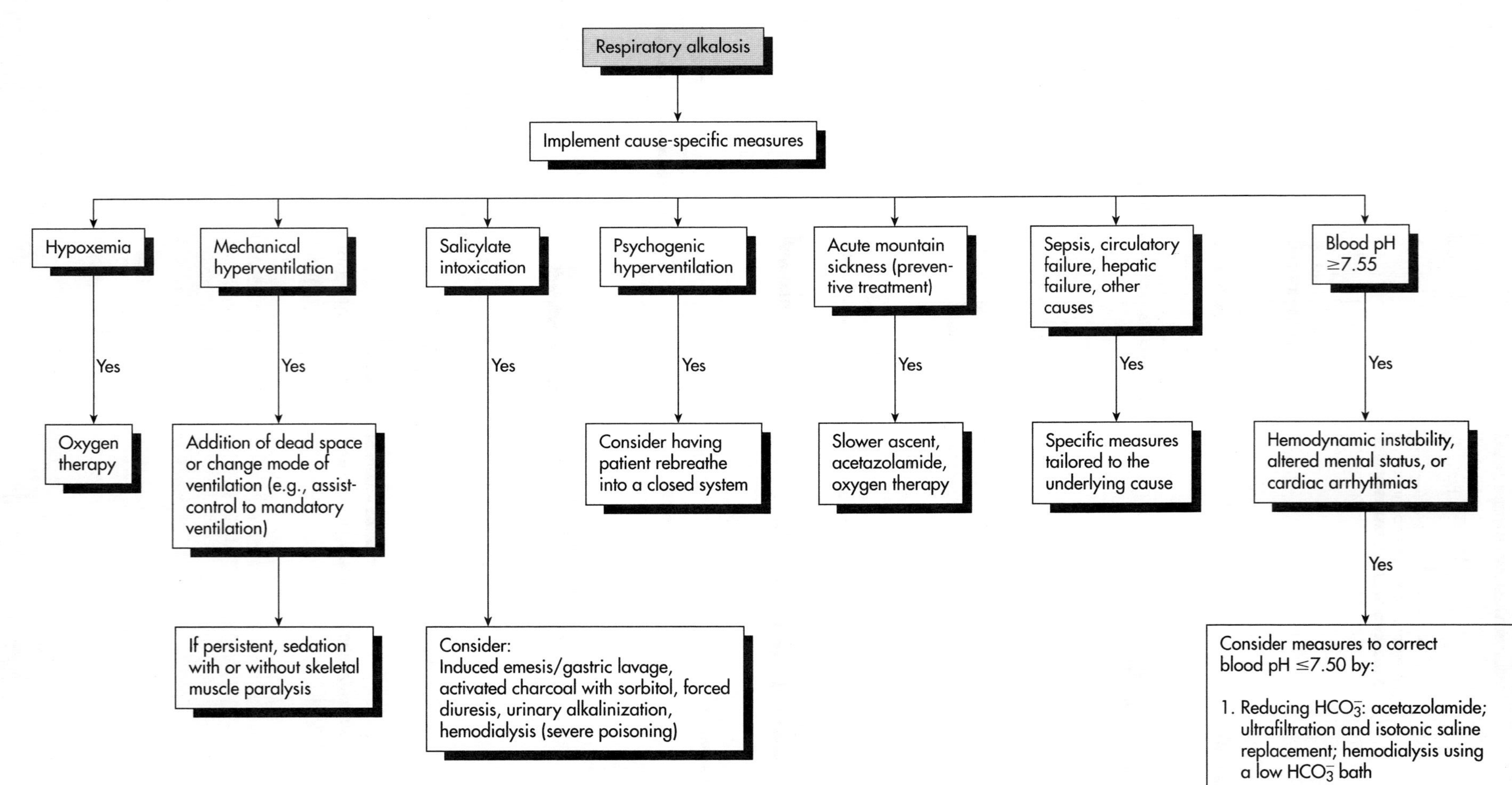

FIGURE 3-16 Recommended treatment of respiratory alkalosis. (From Feehally J, Floege J, Johnson RJ: *Comprehensive clinical nephrology*, ed 3, St Louis, 2007, Mosby.)

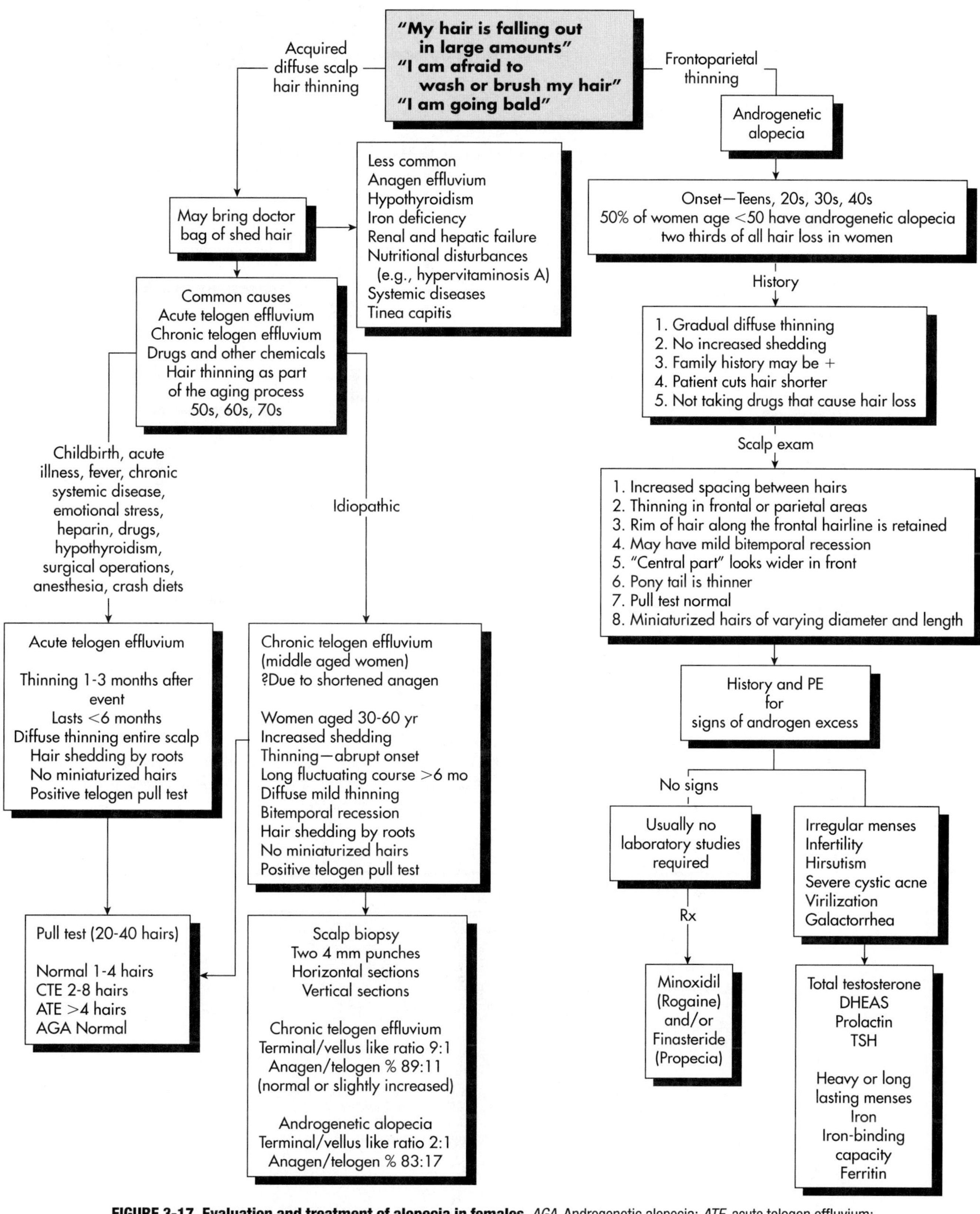

FIGURE 3-17 Evaluation and treatment of alopecia in females. *AGA,* Androgenetic alopecia; *ATE,* acute telogen effluvium; *CTE,* chronic telogen effluvium; *DHEAS,* dehydroepiandrosterone-sulfate; *PE,* physical examination; *TSH,* thyroid-stimulating hormone. (Modified from Habif TA: *Clinical dermatology,* ed 4, St Louis, 2004, Mosby.)

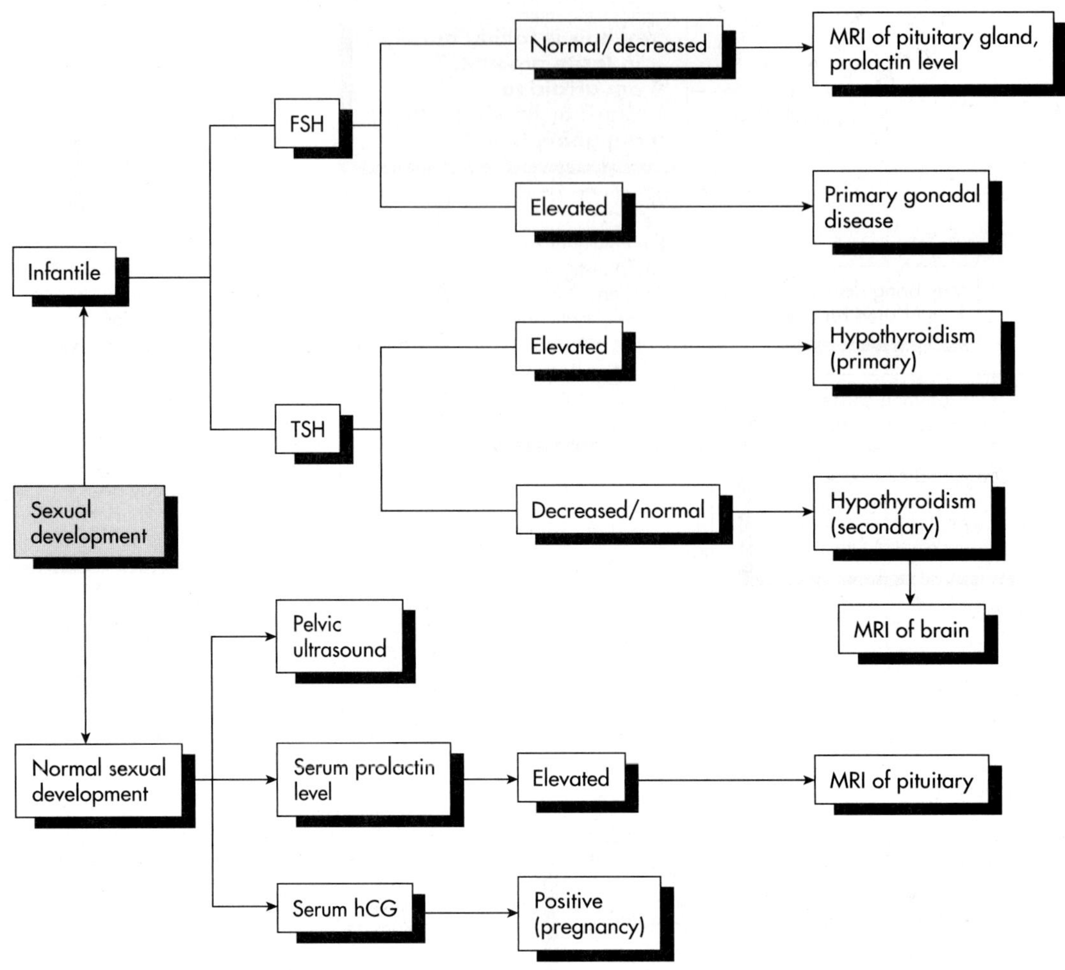

Note: Refer to Section I for additional information on this topic.

FIGURE 3-19 Evaluation of primary amenorrhea. *FSH,* Follicle-stimulating hormone; *hCG,* human chorionic gonadotropin; *MRI,* magnetic resonance imaging; *TSH,* thyroid-stimulating hormone. (From Ferri FF: *Ferri's best test: a practical guide to clinical laboratory medicine and diagnostic imaging,* ed 2, Philadelphia, 2009, Elsevier Mosby.)

BOX 3-1 Amenorrhea, Primary

Diagnostic imaging	**Lab evaluation**
Best test	***Best tests***
MRI of pituitary/hypothalamus with gadolinium when hypothalamic/pituitary lesion is suspected	FSH Prolactin TSH
Ancillary tests	***Ancillary tests***
Pelvic ultrasound	Serum hCG

From Ferri FF: *Ferri's best test: a practical guide to clinical laboratory medicine and diagnostic imaging,* ed 2, Philadelphia, 2009, Elsevier Mosby.

FSH, Follicle-stimulating hormone; *hCG,* human chorionic gonadotropin; *MRI,* magnetic resonance imaging; *TSH,* thyroid-stimulating hormone.

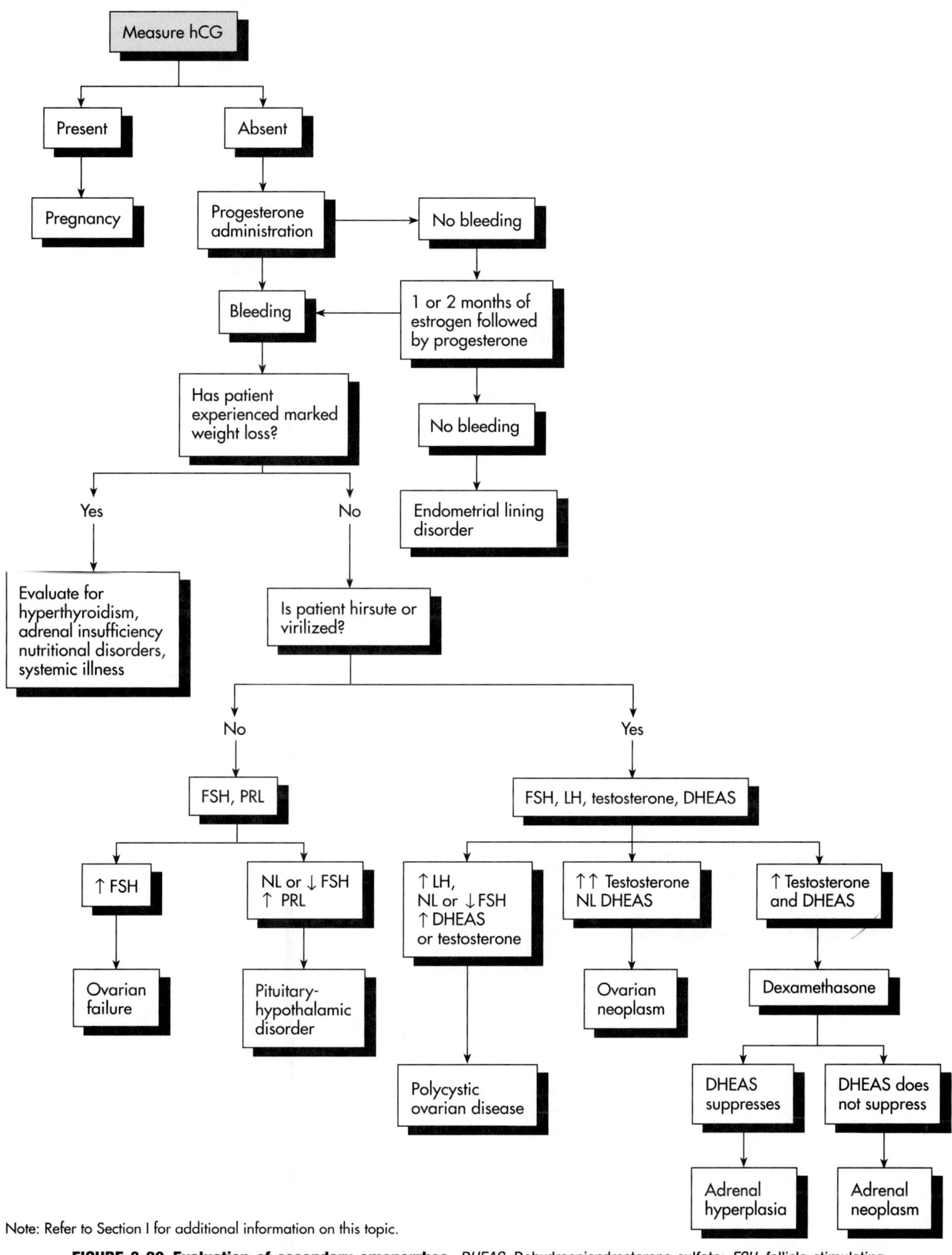

Note: Refer to Section I for additional information on this topic.

FIGURE 3-20 Evaluation of secondary amenorrhea. *DHEAS,* Dehydroepiandrosterone-sulfate; *FSH,* follicle-stimulating hormone; *hCG,* human chorionic gonadotropin; *LH,* luteinizing hormone; *NL,* normal; *PRL,* prolactin; ↑, increased; ↑↑, markedly increased; ↓, decreased. (From Andreoli TE [ed]: *Cecil essentials of medicine,* ed 7, Philadelphia, 2008, WB Saunders.)

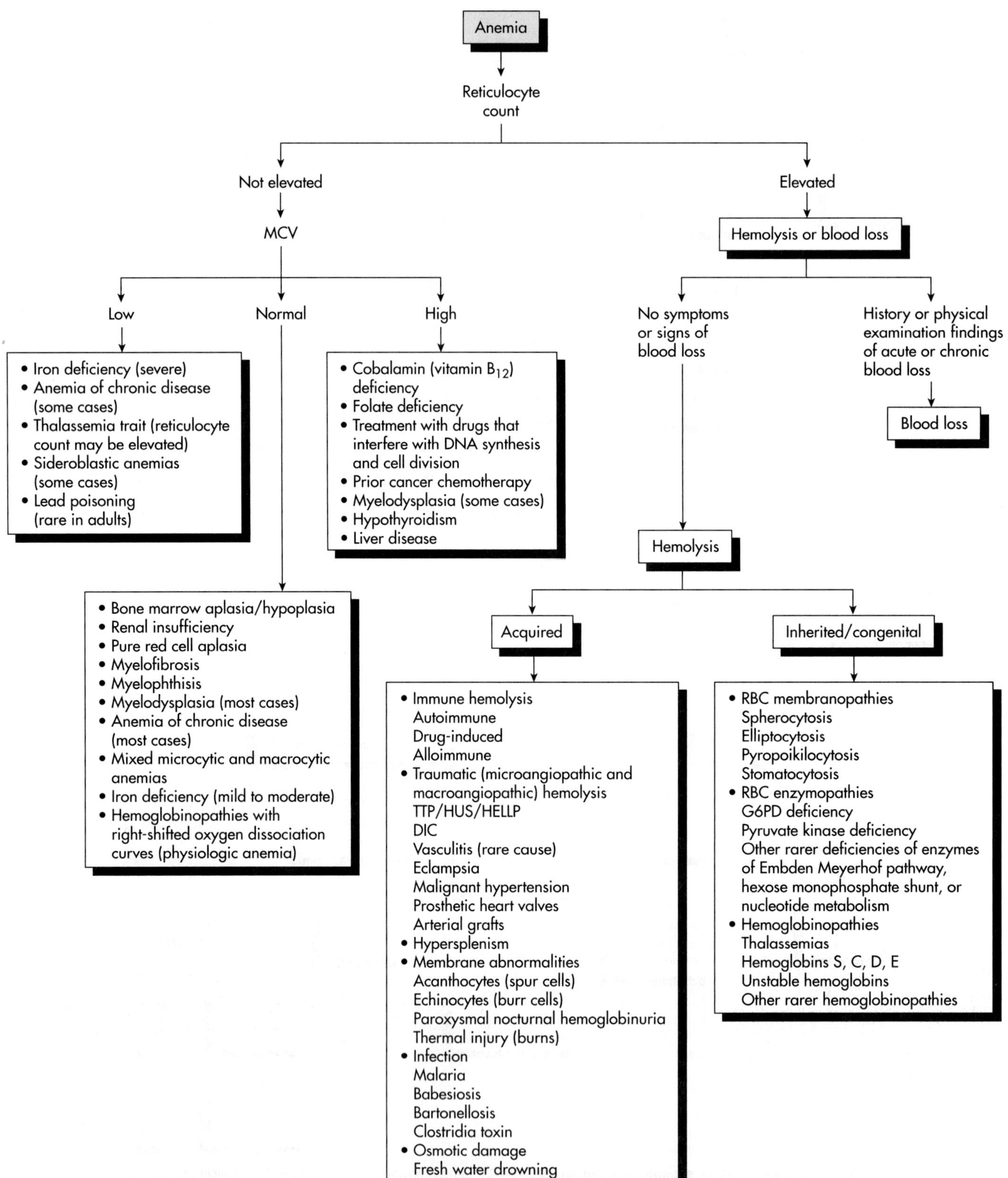

FIGURE 3-22 Algorithm for diagnosis of anemias. *DIC,* Disseminated intravascular coagulation; *G6PD,* glucose-6-phosphate-dehydrogenase; *HELLP, h*epatomegaly-*e*levated *l*iver (function tests)-*l*ow *p*latelets; *HUS,* hemolytic-uremic syndrome; *MCV,* mean corpuscular volume; *RBC,* red blood cell; *TTP,* thrombotic thrombocytopenic purpura. (From Goldman L, Ausiello D [eds]: *Cecil textbook of medicine,* ed 23, Philadelphia, 2008, WB Saunders.)

ANEMIA, MACROCYTIC

ICD-9CM # 281.9

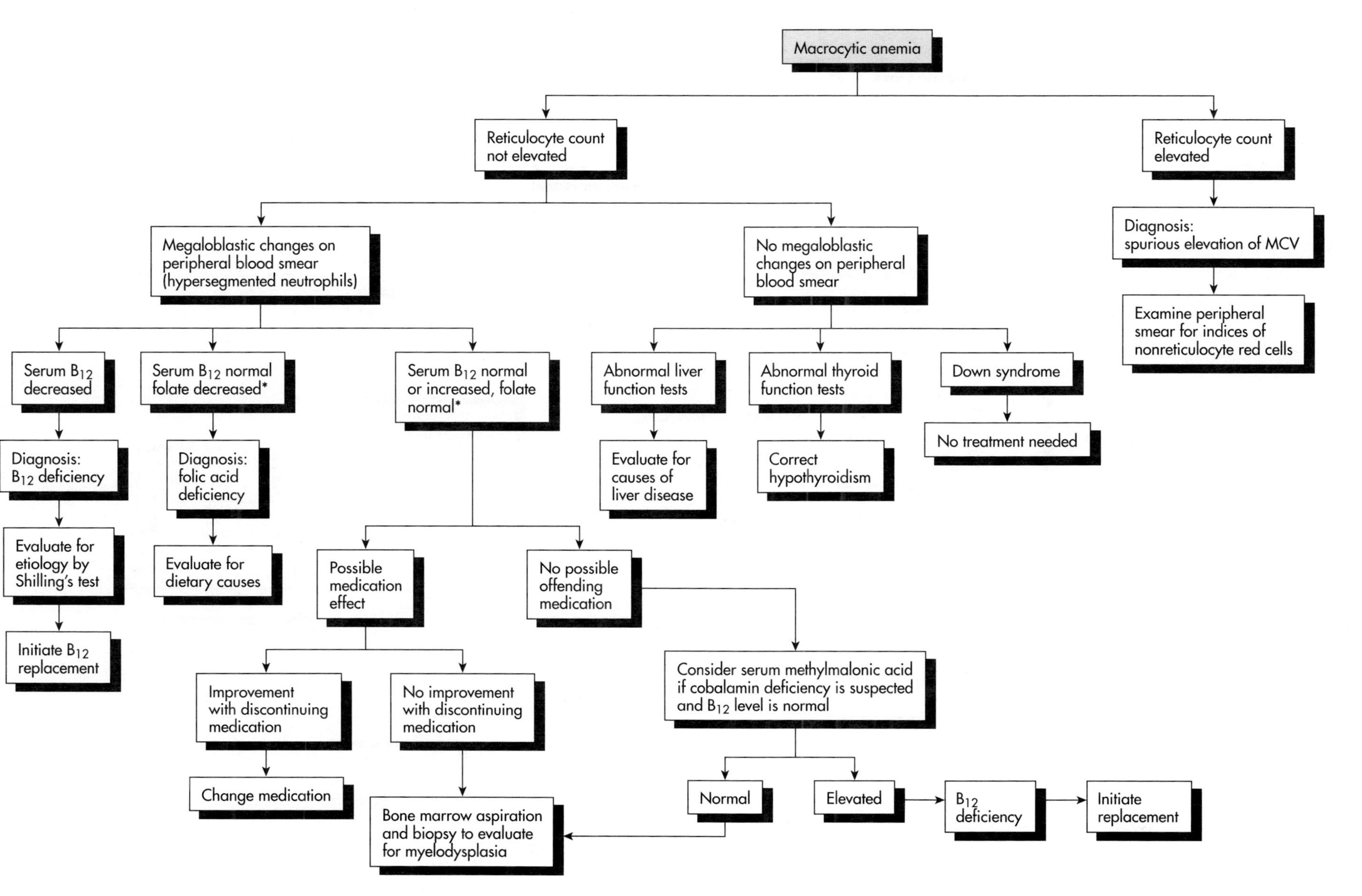

*Measure both serum and RBC folate levels.

FIGURE 3-27 Differential diagnosis of macrocytic anemia. (Modified from Rakel RE [ed]: *Principles of family practice*, ed 7, Philadelphia, 2007, WB Saunders.)

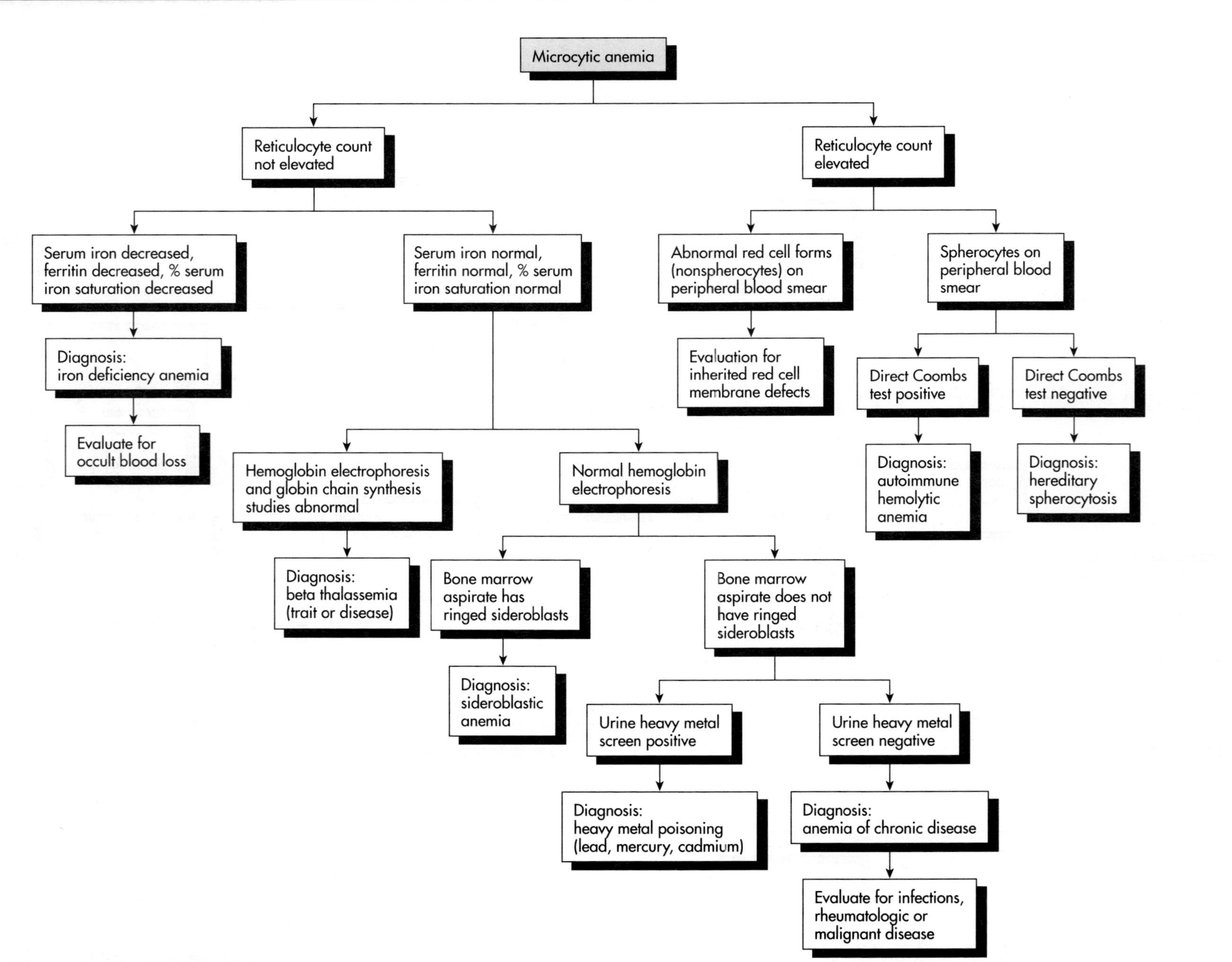

FIGURE 3-28 Differential diagnosis of microcytic anemia. (Modified from Rakel RE [ed]: *Principles of family practice*, ed 7, Philadelphia, 2007, WB Saunders.)

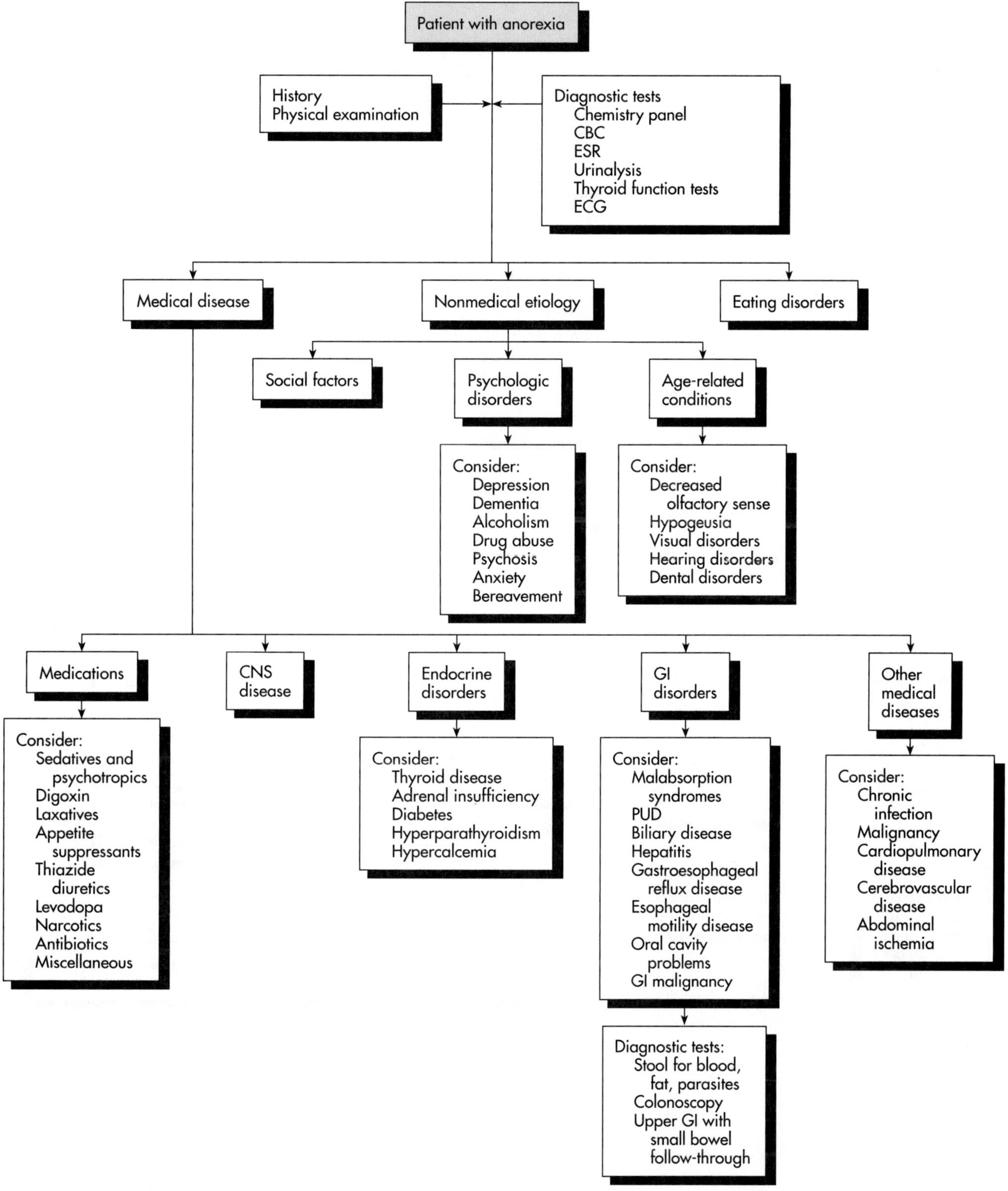

FIGURE 3-33 Evaluation of anorexia. *CBC,* Complete blood count; *CNS,* central nervous system; *ECG,* electrocardiogram; *ESR,* erythrocyte sedimentation rate; *GI,* gastrointestinal; *PUD,* peptic ulcer disease. (Modified from Greene HL, Johnson WP, Lemcke D [eds]: *Decision making in medicine,* ed 2, St Louis, 1998, Mosby.)

ICD-9CM # 719.40 Arthralgia site NOS
719.41 Arthralgia, shoulder region
719.42 Arthralgia, upper arm
719.43 Arthralgia, forearm
719.44 Arthralgia, hand
719.45 Arthralgia, pelvic region and thigh
719.46 Arthralgia, lower leg
719.47 Arthralgia, ankle and/or foot

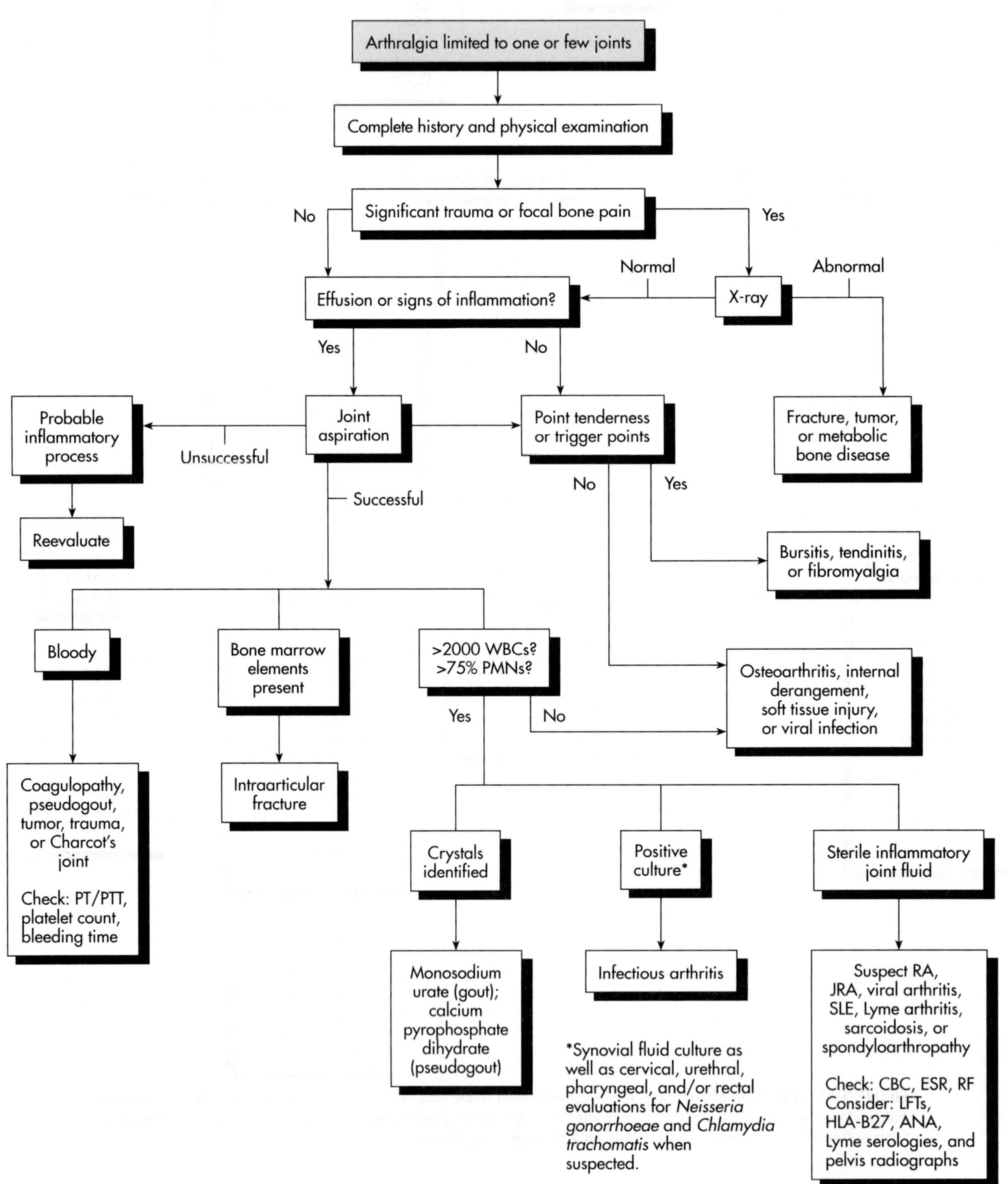

FIGURE 3-39 A diagnostic approach to arthralgia in a few joints. *ANA,* Antinuclear antibodies; *CBC,* complete blood count; *ESR,* erythrocyte sedimentation rate; *JRA,* juvenile rheumatoid arthritis; *LFTs,* liver function tests; *PMNs,* polymorphonuclear neutrophils; *PT,* prothrombin time; *PTT,* partial thromboplastin time; *RA,* rheumatoid arthritis; *RF,* rheumatoid factor; *SLE,* systemic lupus erythematosus; *WBCs,* white blood cells. (Modified from American College of Rheumatology Ad Hoc Committee on Clinical Guidelines: *Arthritis Rheum* 39:1, 1996.)

ASCITES

ICD-9CM # 789.5 Ascites NOS
197.6 Ascites, cancerous (malignant) M8000/6
457.8 Chylous
014.0 Tuberculous

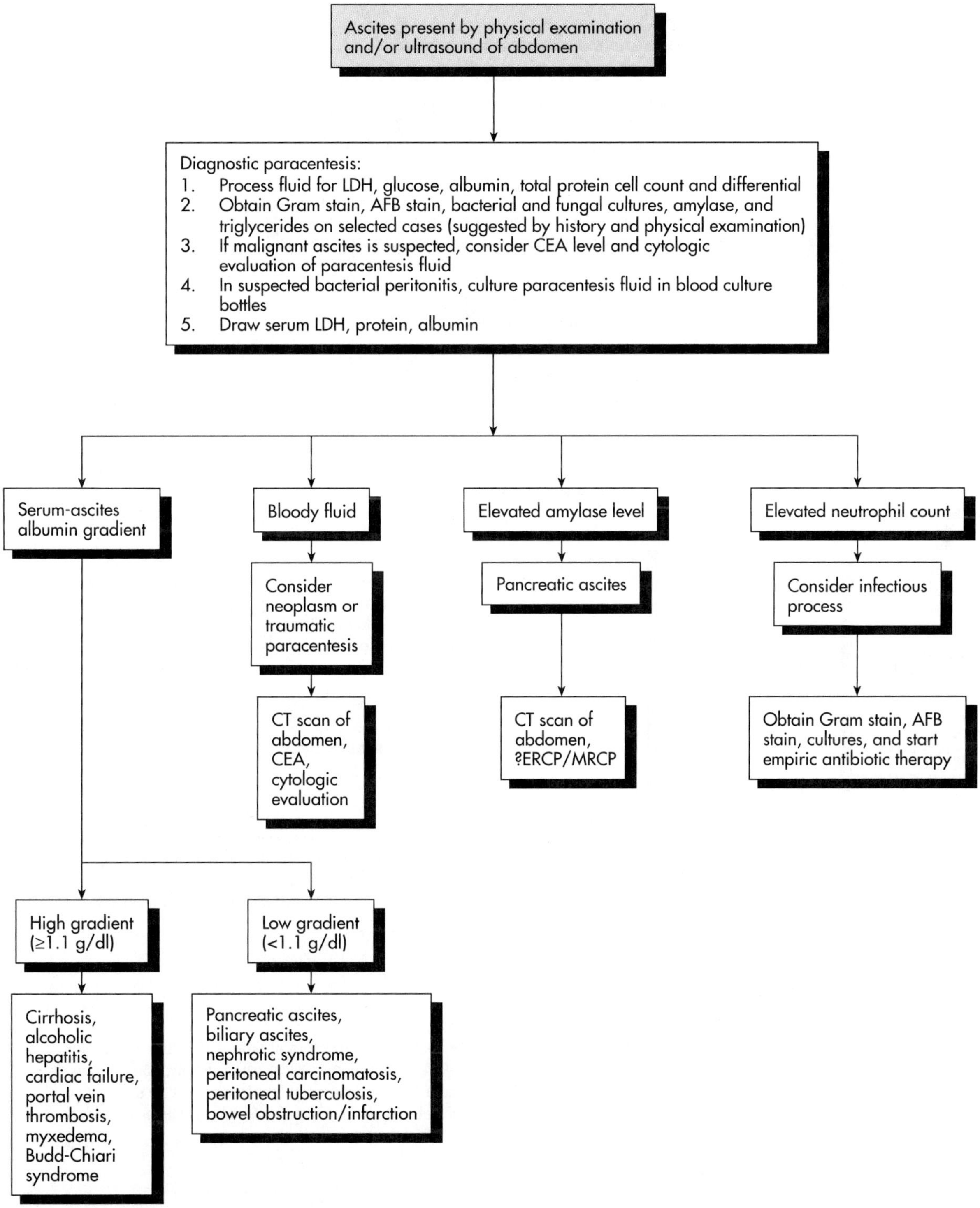

Ascites present by physical examination and/or ultrasound of abdomen

↓

Diagnostic paracentesis:

1. Process fluid for LDH, glucose, albumin, total protein cell count and differential
2. Obtain Gram stain, AFB stain, bacterial and fungal cultures, amylase, and triglycerides on selected cases (suggested by history and physical examination)
3. If malignant ascites is suspected, consider CEA level and cytologic evaluation of paracentesis fluid
4. In suspected bacterial peritonitis, culture paracentesis fluid in blood culture bottles
5. Draw serum LDH, protein, albumin

↓

- Serum-ascites albumin gradient
  - High gradient (≥1.1 g/dl) → Cirrhosis, alcoholic hepatitis, cardiac failure, portal vein thrombosis, myxedema, Budd-Chiari syndrome
  - Low gradient (<1.1 g/dl) → Pancreatic ascites, biliary ascites, nephrotic syndrome, peritoneal carcinomatosis, peritoneal tuberculosis, bowel obstruction/infarction
- Bloody fluid → Consider neoplasm or traumatic paracentesis → CT scan of abdomen, CEA, cytologic evaluation
- Elevated amylase level → Pancreatic ascites → CT scan of abdomen, ?ERCP/MRCP
- Elevated neutrophil count → Consider infectious process → Obtain Gram stain, AFB stain, cultures, and start empiric antibiotic therapy

FIGURE 3-40 Evaluation of ascites. *AFB,* Acid-fast bacillus; *CEA,* carcinoembryonic antigen; *CT,* computed tomography; *ERCP,* endoscopic retrograde cholangiopancreatography; *LDH,* lactate dehydrogenase; *MRCP,* magnetic resonance cholangiopancreatography.

ICD-9CM # 781.3 Ataxia NOS
303.9 Alcoholic, chronic
334.3 Cerebellar
331.89 Cerebral
334.0 Friedreich's

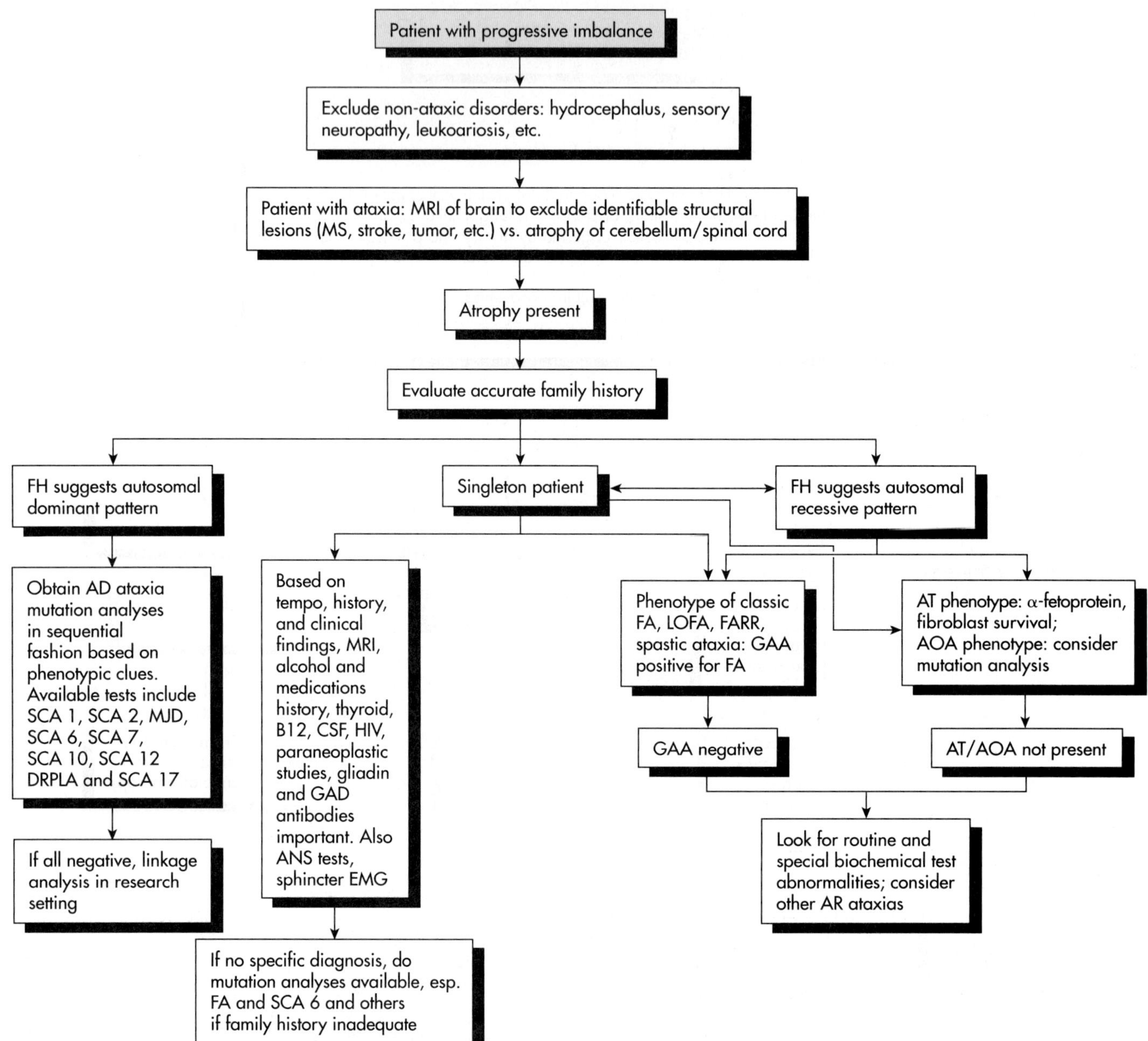

FIGURE 3-47 An algorithm for a diagnostic approach to patients with progressive ataxia. *AOA,* Ataxia with oculomotor apraxia; *AT,* ataxia-telengiectasia; *CSF,* cerebrospinal fluid; *DRPLA,* dentatorubral-pallidoluysian atrophy; *EMG,* electromyelography; *FA,* Friedreich's ataxia; *FH,* family history; *GAD,* glutamate decarboxylase; *HIV,* human immunodeficiency virus; *MRI,* magnetic resonance imaging; *MS,* multiple sclerosis; *SCA,* spinocerebellar ataxia. (From Bradley WG et al [eds]: *Neurology in clinical practice,* ed 4, Philadelphia, 2004, Butterworth Heinemann.)

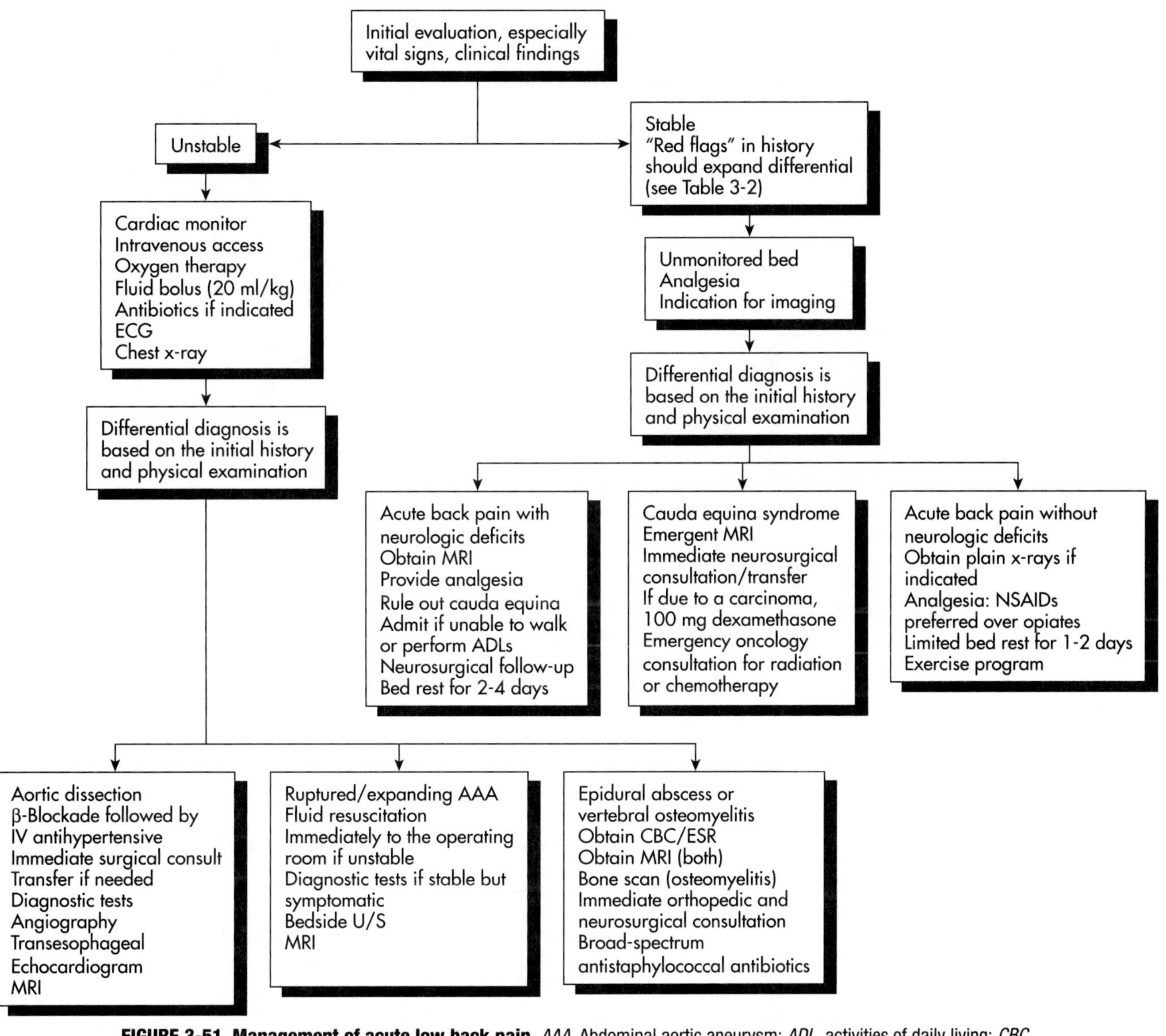

FIGURE 3-51 Management of acute low back pain. *AAA,* Abdominal aortic aneurysm; *ADL,* activities of daily living; *CBC,* complete blood count; *ECG,* electrocardiogram; *ESR,* erythrocyte sedimentation rate; *IV,* intravenous; *MRI,* magnetic resonance imaging; *NSAIDs,* nonsteroidal anti-inflammatory drugs. (From Marx JA [ed]: *Rosen's emergency medicine,* ed 6, St Louis, 2006, Mosby.)

TABLE 3-2 Red Flags for Potentially Serious Conditions

Possible Fracture	Possible Tumor or Infection	Possible Cauda Equina Syndrome
From Medical History		
Major trauma, such as vehicle accident or fall from height Minor trauma or even strenuous lifting (in older or potentially osteoporotic patient)	Age over 50 or under 20 yr History of cancer Constitutional symptoms, such as recent fever or chills or unexplained weight loss Risk factors for spinal infection: recent bacterial infection (e.g., urinary tract infection), intravenous drug abuse, or immune suppression (from steroids, transplant, or human immunodeficiency virus) Pain that worsens when supine; severe nighttime pain	Saddle anesthesia Recent onset of bladder dysfunction, such as urinary retention, increased frequency, or overflow incontinence Severe or progressive neurologic deficit in the lower extremity

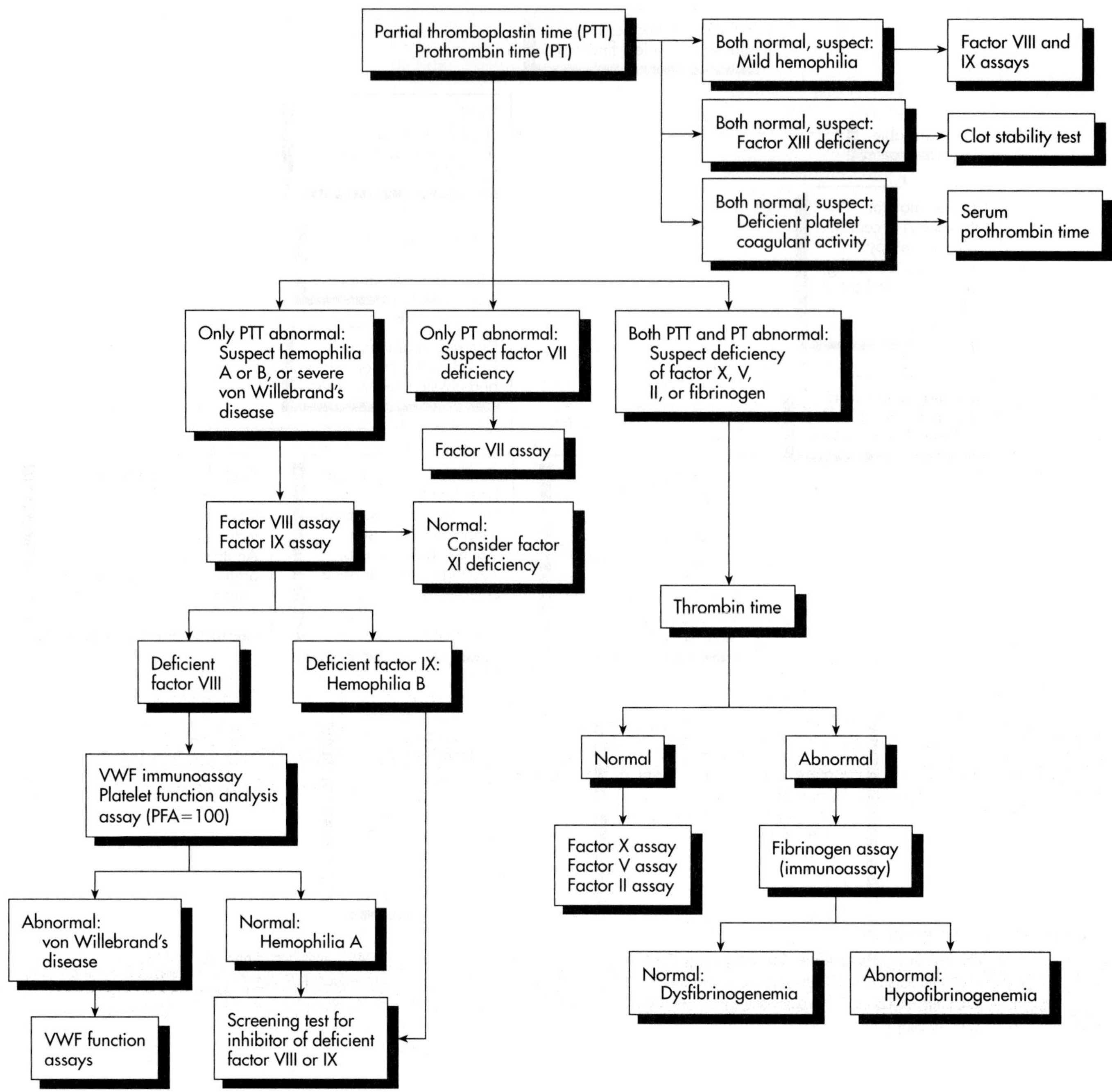

FIGURE 3-53 Laboratory evaluation of a patient with a bleeding disorder in whom the history and physical examination suggest a congenital coagulation disorder. *VWF,* von Willebrand factor. (Modified from Stein JH [ed]: *Internal medicine,* ed 5, St Louis, 1998, Mosby.)

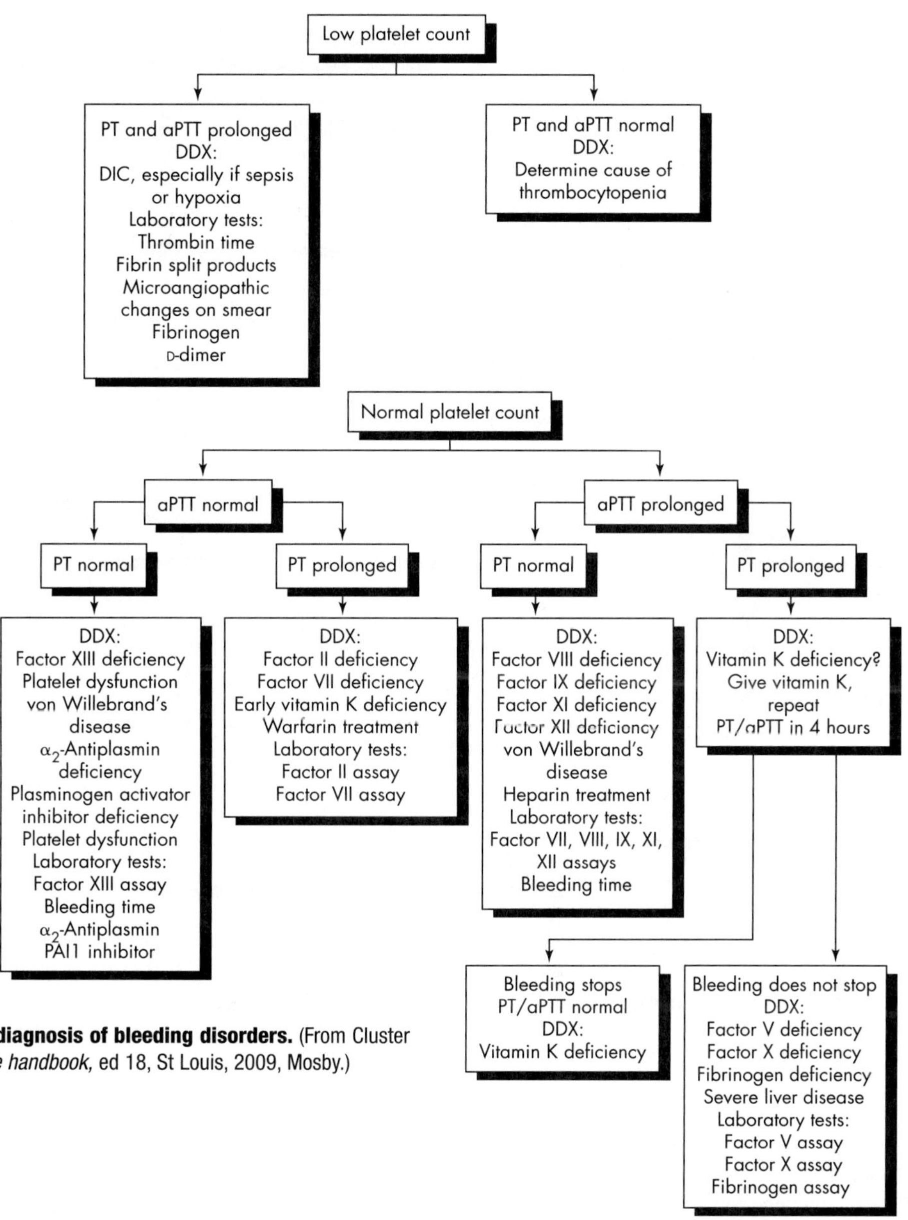

FIGURE 3-54 Differential diagnosis of bleeding disorders. (From Cluster JW, Rau RE: *The Harriet Lane handbook,* ed 18, St Louis, 2009, Mosby.)

Clinical Algorithms III

BOX 3-3 Bleeding Disorders

Congenital	Acquired
Disorder of platelet number or function	**Disseminated intravascular coagulation:** Characterized by prolonged PT and aPTT, decreased fibrinogen and platelets, increased fibrin degradation products, and elevated D-dimers. Treatment includes identifying and treating underlying disorder. Replacement of depleted coagulation factors with FFP may be necessary in severe cases, especially when bleeding is present; 10-15 ml/kg will raise clotting factors 20%. Fibrinogen, if depleted, can be given as cryoprecipitate. Platelet transfusions may also be necessary.
Thrombocytopenia: Secondary to bone marrow disease or defective megakaryocyte maturation	**Liver disease:** The liver is the major site of synthesis of factors V, VII, IX, X, XI, XII, XIII, prothrombin, plasminogen, fibrinogen, protein C and S, and ATIII. Treatment with FFP and platelets may be needed, but this will increase hepatic protein load. Vitamin K should be given to patients with liver disease and clotting abnormalities.
Disorders of platelet function: Bernard-Soulier syndrome, Glanzmann thrombasthenia, storage pool diseases	**Vitamin K deficiency:** Factors II, VII, IX, X, protein C, and protein S are vitamin K dependent. Early vitamin K deficiency may present with isolated prolonged PT because factor VII has the shortest half-life. Fibrinogen should be normal.
Factor VIII deficiency: See text **Factor IX deficiency:** See text **Von Willebrand disease:** See text	**Hemolytic-uremic syndrome/thrombotic thrombocytopenic purpura (HUS/TTP):** Characterized by the triad of microangiopathic hemolytic anemia, uremia, and thrombocytopenia. HUS/TTP is often triggered by bacterial enteritis, especially caused by *Escherichia coli* O157:H7, although there are a variety of causes. HUS does not typically include coagulation abnormalities, such as those seen in DIC. Avoid blood products in patients with HUS thought to be secondary to pneumococcal infection. TTP includes the triad of HUS in addition to fever and CNS changes and is more common in older adolescents and adults.

(From Custer JW, Rau RE: *The Harriet Lane handbook*, ed 18, St Louis, 2009, Mosby.)

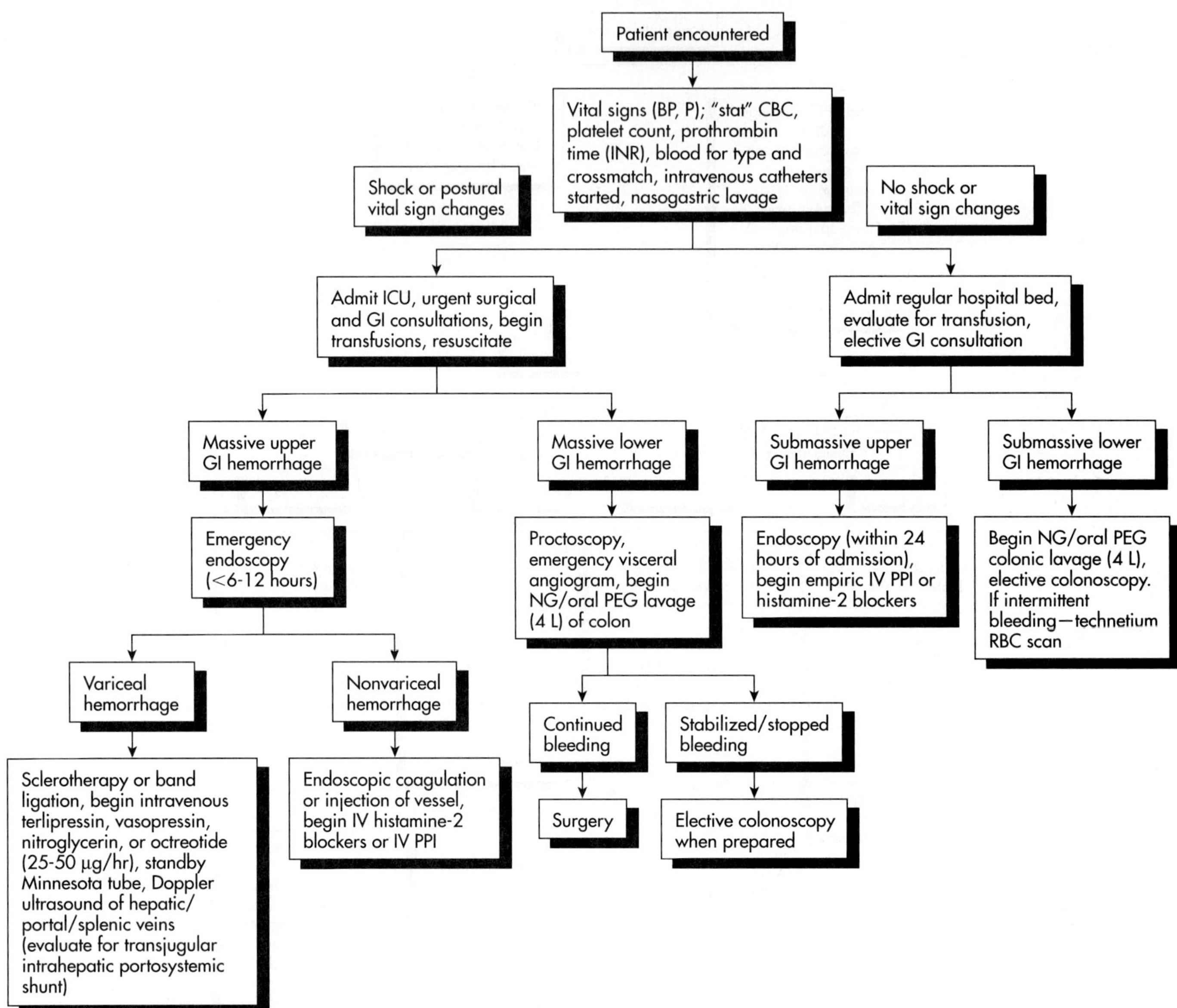

FIGURE 3-56 Approach to the patient with gastrointestinal hemorrhage. *BP,* Blood pressure; *CBC,* complete blood count; *GI,* gastrointestinal; *ICU,* intensive care unit; *IV,* intravenous; *NG,* nasogastric; *P,* weight; *PEG,* percutaneous endoscopic gastrostomy; *PPI,* proton pump inhibitor; *RBC,* red blood cell. (Modified from Goldman L, Ausiello D [eds]: *Cecil textbook of medicine,* ed 23, Philadelphia, 2008, WB Saunders.)

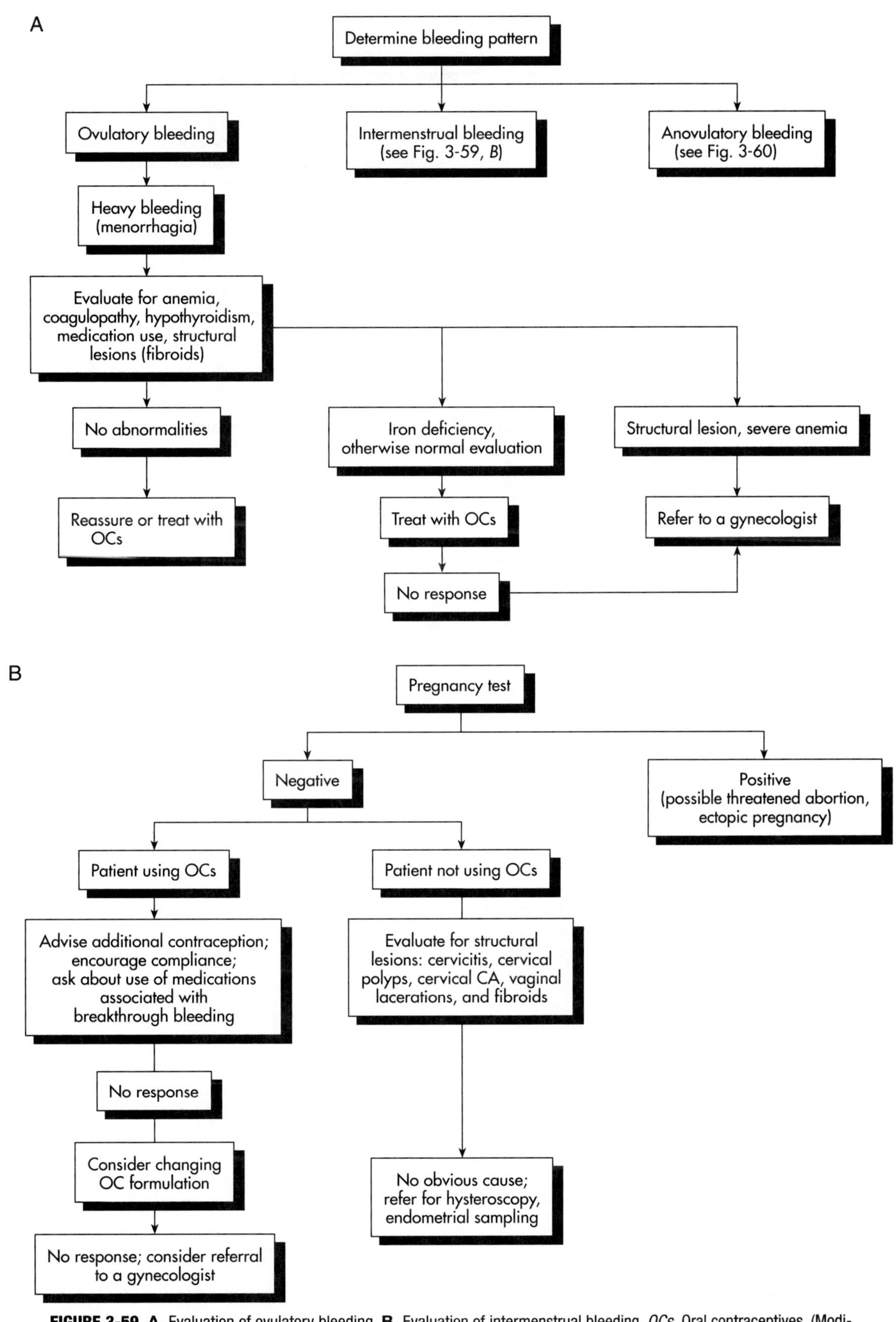

FIGURE 3-59 **A,** Evaluation of ovulatory bleeding. **B,** Evaluation of intermenstrual bleeding. *OCs,* Oral contraceptives. (Modified from Appleby J, Henderson M, Wathen PI: *Intern Med* Sept:17, 1996.)

Clinical Algorithms III

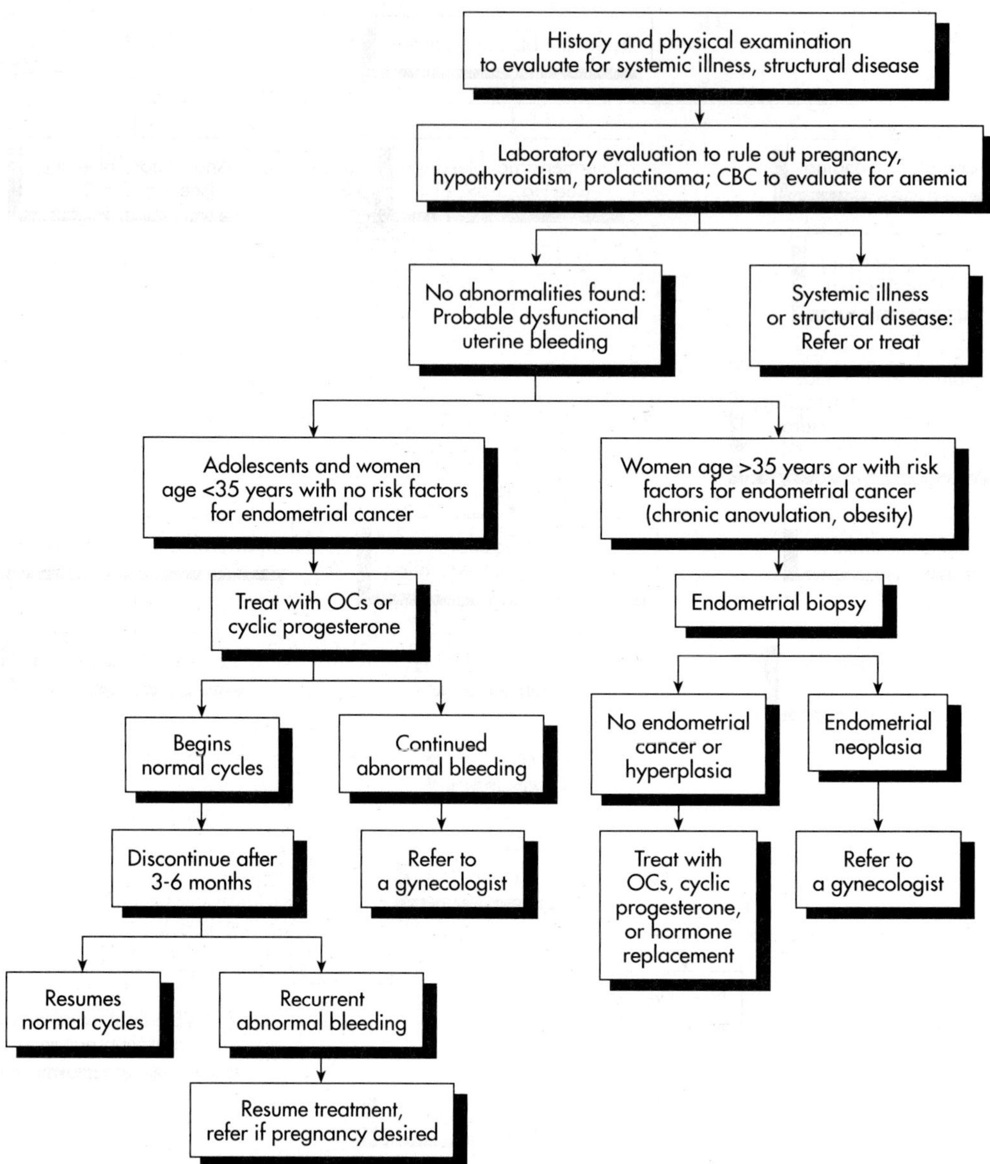

FIGURE 3-60 Evaluation of anovulatory bleeding. *CBC,* Complete blood count; *OCs,* oral contraceptives. (From Appleby J, Henderson M, Wathen PI: *Intern Med,* Sept:17, 1996.)

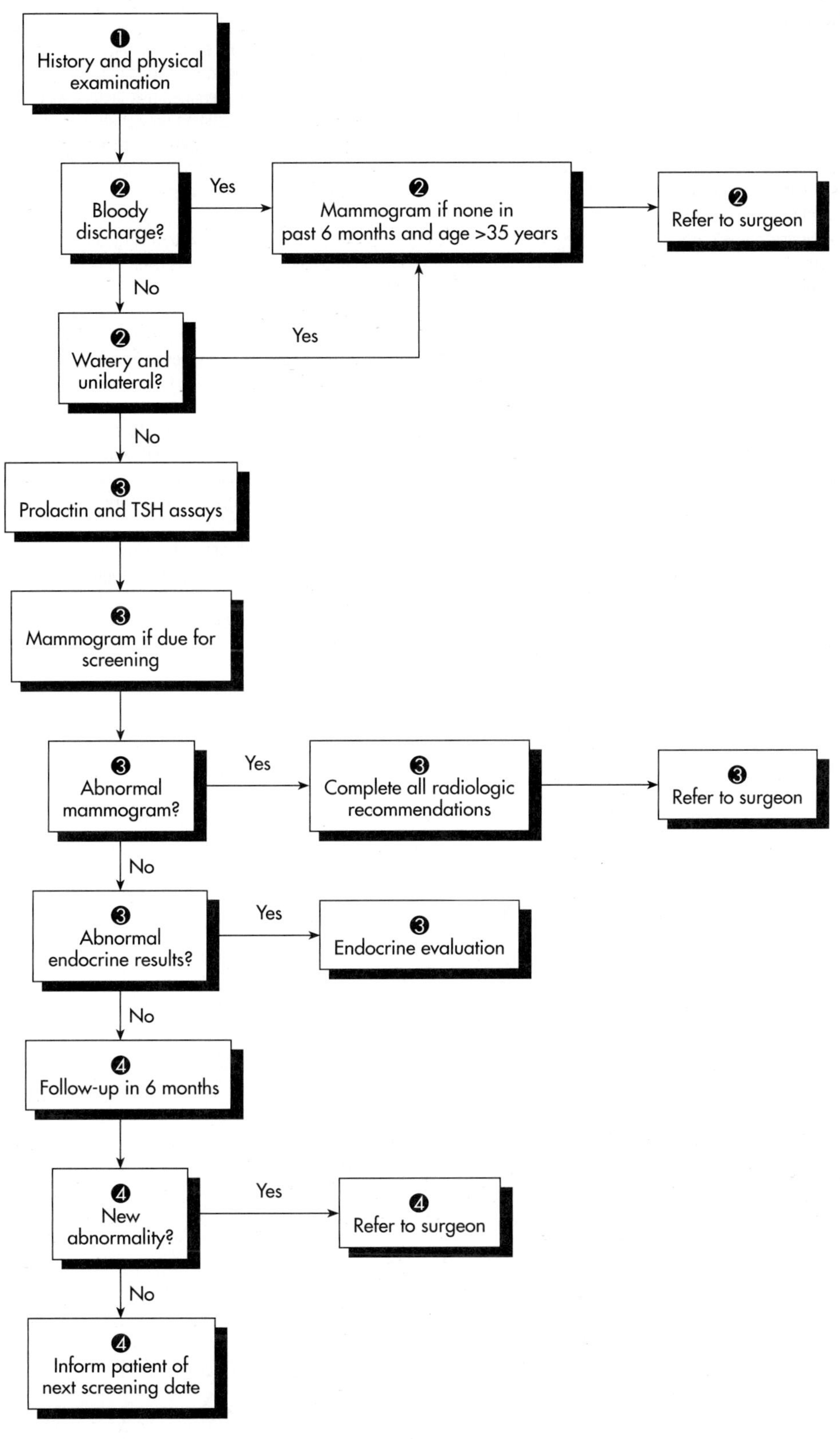

*Without palpable mass.

FIGURE 3-63 Breast cancer screening and evaluation. (From Institute for Clinical Systems Integration, Minneapolis: *Postgrad Med* 100:182, 1996.)

Continued on following page

FIGURE 3-63 (Continued)

1. **History and physical examination.*** Patients who present with a complaint of nipple discharge should be evaluated with breast-related history taking and a physical examination. History taking is aimed at uncovering and characterizing any other breast-related symptom. A risk assessment should also be undertaken for identified risk factors, including patient age over 50 years, any past personal history of breast cancer, history of hyperplasia on previous breast biopsies, and family history of breast cancer in first-degree relatives (mother, sister, daughter). Physical examination should include inspection of the breast for any evidence of ulceration or contour changes and inspection of the nipple for Paget's disease. Palpation should be performed with the patient in both the upright and the supine positions to determine the presence of any palpable mass.
2. **Bloody discharge?** If the discharge appears frankly bloody, the patient should be referred to a surgeon for evaluation. At the time of referral, a mammogram of the involved breast should be obtained if the patient is over 35 years of age and has not had a mammogram within the preceding 6 months. Similarly, patients with a watery, unilateral discharge should be referred to a surgeon for evaluation and possible biopsy.
3. **Endocrine tests. Mammogram.** If the discharge appears frankly milky or is bilateral, serum prolactin and serum thyroid-stimulating hormone *(TSH)* assays should be performed to rule out the presence of an endocrinologic basis for the symptoms. At the time of that visit, a mammogram should also be performed if the patient is due for routine mammographic screening according to the recommended intervals. A patient with an abnormal mammogram should be further evaluated radiologically to better characterize the lesion and then be referred to a surgeon if appropriate. Make certain that all recommended additional views, ultrasound examinations, and follow-up studies have been obtained before referral to a surgeon. Should the mammogram appear normal, results of the assays for TSH and prolactin should be reviewed. If the results are abnormal, the patient should undergo appropriate evaluation for etiology, either by a primary care physician or by an endocrinologist.
4. **Six-month follow-up results.** If results of the mammogram and the endocrinologic screening studies are normal, the patient should return for a follow-up visit in 6 months to ensure that there has been no specific change in the character of the discharge, such as development of frank bleeding or Paget's disease, that would warrant surgical evaluation. If the evaluation at that follow-up visit fails to reveal any palpable or visible abnormalities, the patient should be returned to the routine screening process with studies performed at the recommended intervals.

---

*ICSI health care guidelines are designed to assist clinicians by providing an analytic framework for the evaluation and treatment of patients. They are not intended either to replace a clinician's judgment or to establish a protocol for all patients with a particular condition. A guideline will rarely establish the only approach to a problem. In addition, guidelines are "living documents" that are expected to be imperfect and are subject to annual review and revision.

CARDIOMEGALY ON CHEST X-RAY

ICD-9CM # 429.3 Idiopathic cardiomegaly
746.89 Congenital cardiomegaly
402.0 Hypertensive cardiomegaly, malignant
402.1 Hypertensive cardiomegaly, benign
402.11 Hypertensive cardiomegaly with congestive heart failure

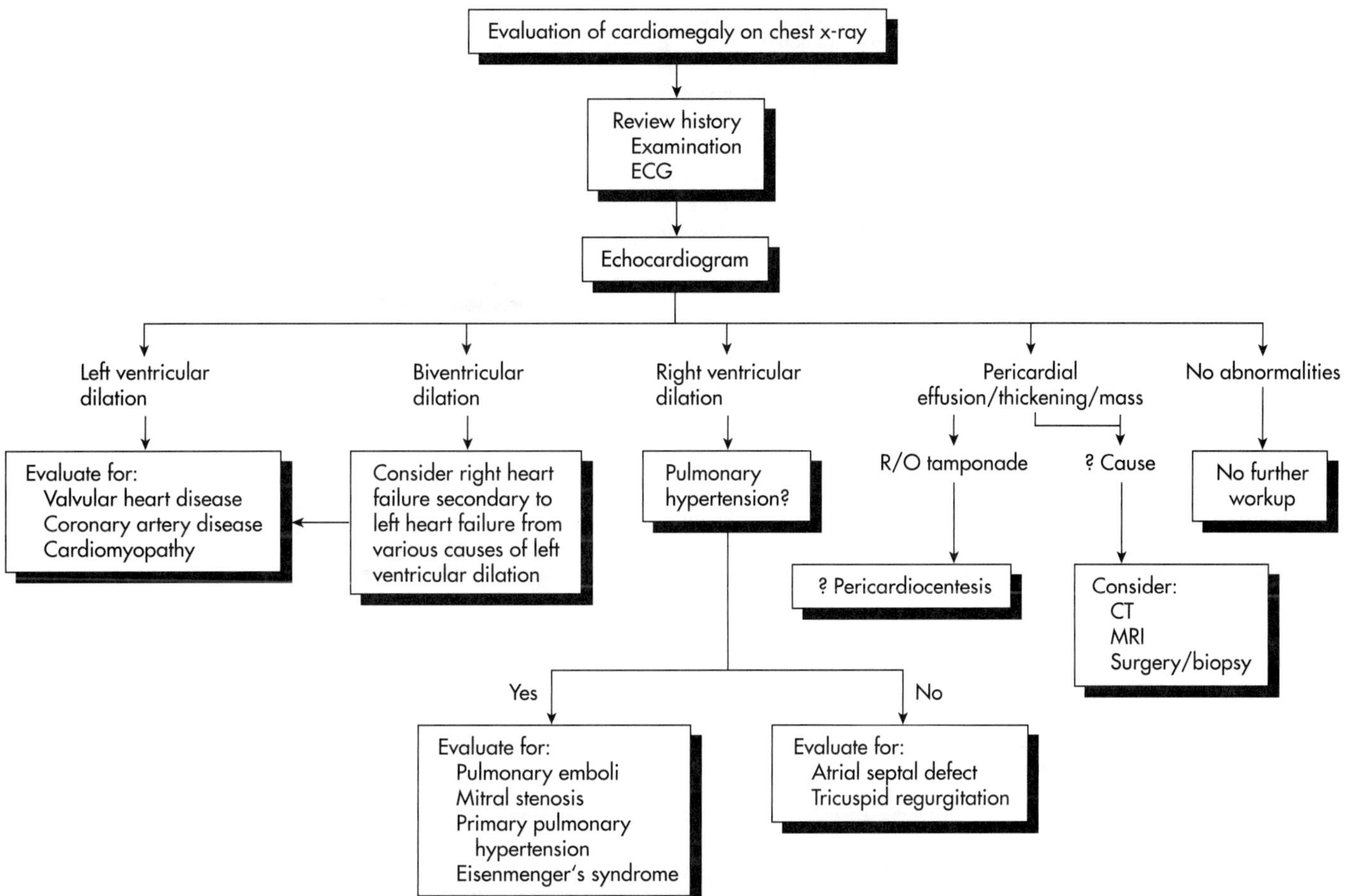

FIGURE 3-69 Approach to the patient with cardiomegaly. When cardiomegaly is found on the chest radiograph, the history and physical examination should be reviewed and an electrocardiogram *(ECG)* performed before obtaining a two-dimensional Doppler echocardiographic study. Cardiomegaly may be explained by left ventricular dilation, biventricular dilation, right ventricular dilation, or pericardial abnormalities, or it may be found to be spurious on the echocardiogram. Rarely, isolated abnormalities of the atrium, particularly the left atrium, may cause abnormalities on the chest radiograph but will not cause true cardiomegaly. Depending on the echocardiographic findings, further tests can help elucidate the cause of echocardiographically confirmed cardiomegaly. *CT,* Computer tomography; *MRI,* magnetic resonance imaging; *R/O,* rule out. (From Goldman L, Braunwald E [eds]: *Primary cardiology,* ed 2, Philadelphia, 2003, WB Saunders.)

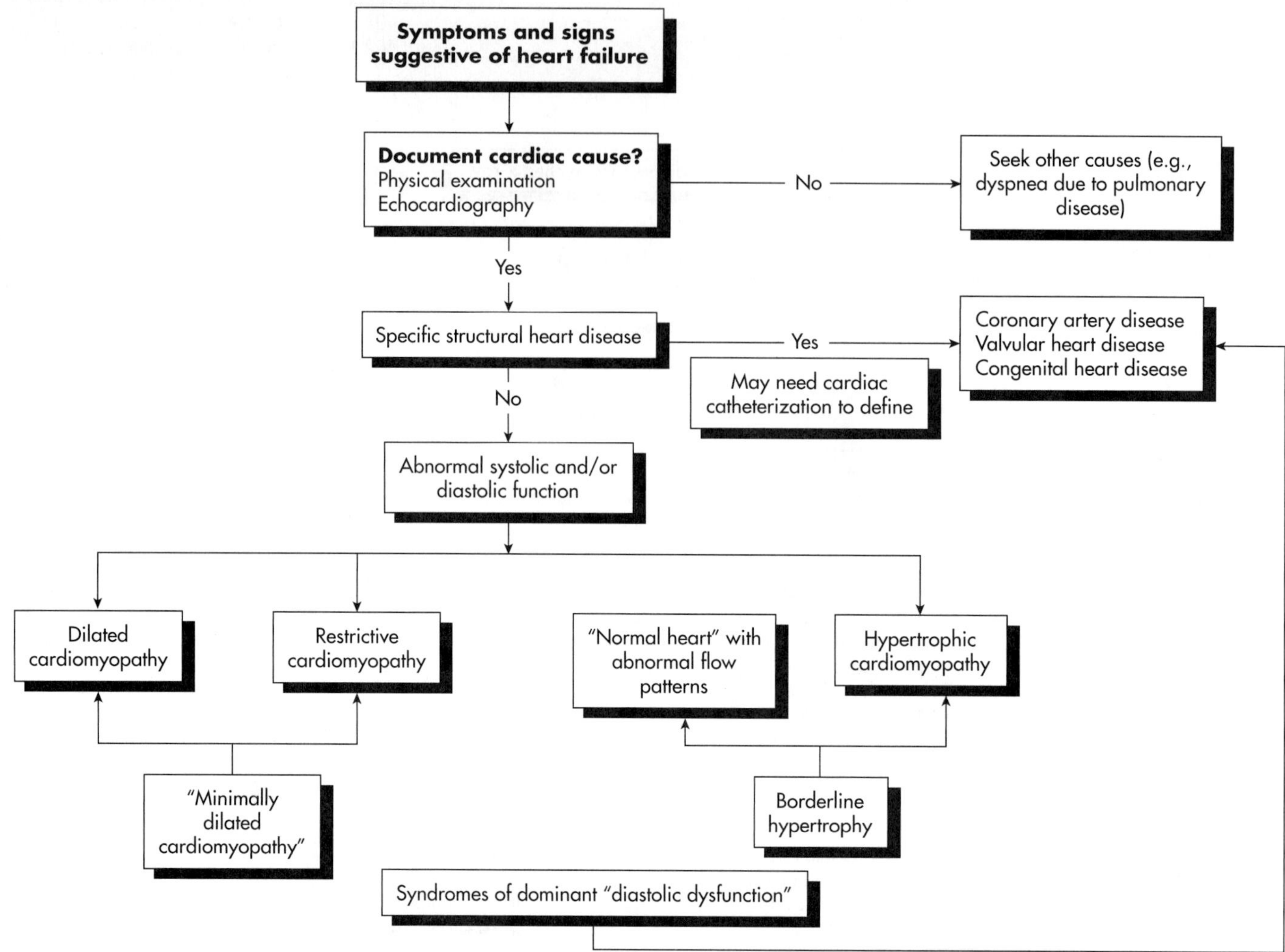

FIGURE 3-70 Initial approach to classification of cardiomyopathy. The evaluation of symptoms or signs consistent with heart failure first includes confirmation that they can be attributed to a cardiac cause. Although this conclusion is often apparent from routine physical examination, echocardiography serves to confirm cardiac disease and provides clues to the presence of other cardiac disease, such as focal abnormalities, suggesting primary valve disease or congenital heart disease. Having excluded these conditions, cardiomyopathy is generally considered to be dilated, restrictive, or hypertrophic. Patients with apparently normal cardiac structure and contraction are occasionally found to demonstrate abnormal intracardiac flow patterns consistent with diastolic dysfunction but should also be evaluated carefully for other causes of their symptoms. Most patients with so-called diastolic dysfunction also demonstrate at least borderline criteria for left ventricular hypertrophy, frequently in the setting of chronic hypertension and diabetes. A moderately decreased ejection fraction without marked dilation or a pattern of restrictive cardiomyopathy is sometimes referred to as "minimally dilated cardiomyopathy," which may represent either a distinct entity or a transition between acute and chronic disease. (From Goldman L, Ausiello D [eds]: *Cecil textbook of medicine,* ed 23, Philadelphia, 2008, WB Saunders.)

TABLE 3-4 Profiles of Symptomatic Cardiomyopathy

	Dilated	Restrictive	Hypertrophic
Ejection fraction (normal >55%)	<30%	25%-50%	>60%
Left ventricular diastolic dimension (normal <55 mm)	≥60 mm	<60 mm	Often decreased
Left ventricular wall thickness	Decreased	Normal or increased	Markedly increased
Atrial size	Increased	Increased; may be massive	Increased
Valvular regurgitation	Mitral first during decompensation; tricuspid regurgitation in late stages	Frequent mitral and tricuspid regurgitation, rarely severe	Mitral regurgitation
Common first symptoms*	Exertional intolerance	Exertional intolerance, fluid retention	Exertional intolerance; may have chest pain
Congestive symptoms*	Left before right, except right prominent in young adults	Right often exceeds left	Primary exertional dyspnea
Risk for arrhythmia	Ventricular tachyarrhythmias; conduction block in Chagas' disease, giant cell myocarditis, and some families; atrial fibrillation	Ventricular tachyarrhythmias uncommon except in sarcoidosis; conduction block in sarcoidosis and amyloidosis, atrial fibrillation	Ventricular tachyarrhythmias, atrial fibrillation

From Goldman L, Ausiello D [eds]: *Cecil textbook of medicine,* ed 23, Philadelphia, 2008, WB Saunders.

*Left-sided symptoms of pulmonary congestion: dyspnea on exertion, orthopnea, paroxysmal nocturnal dyspnea. Right-sided symptoms of systemic venous congestion: discomfort on bending, hepatic and abdominal distention, peripheral edema.

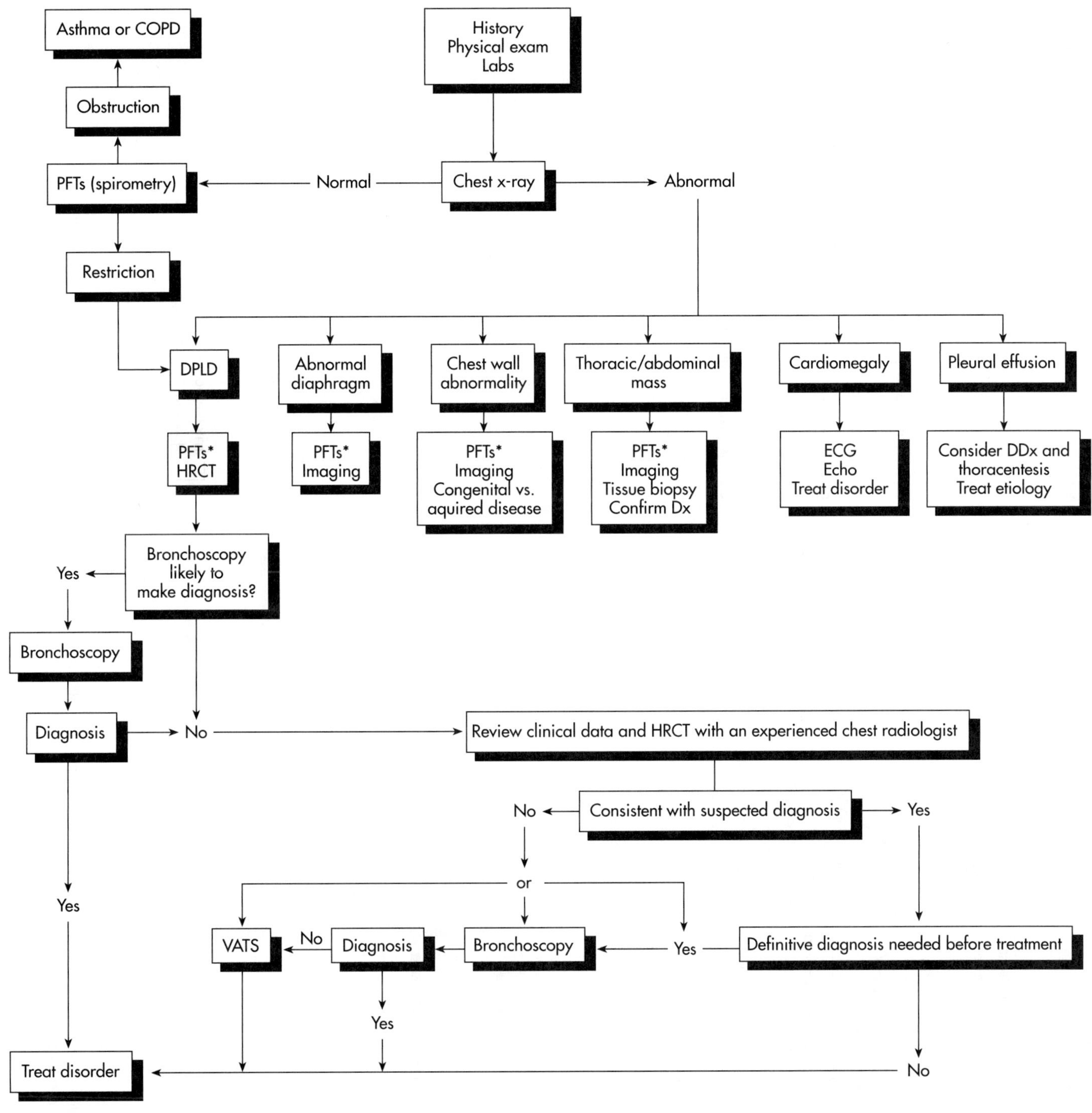

FIGURE 3-75 Diagnostic algorithm. *COPD,* Chronic obstructive pulmonary disease; *DDx,* differential diagnosis; *DLCO,* diffusion capacity; *DPLD,* diffuse parenchymal lung disease; *ECG,* electrocardiogram; *HRCT,* high-resolution computed tomography; *PFTs,* pulmonary function tests; *VATS,* video-assisted thoracoscopic surgery. (From Runge MS, Greganti MA: *Netter's internal medicine,* Philadelphia, 2008, WB Saunders.)

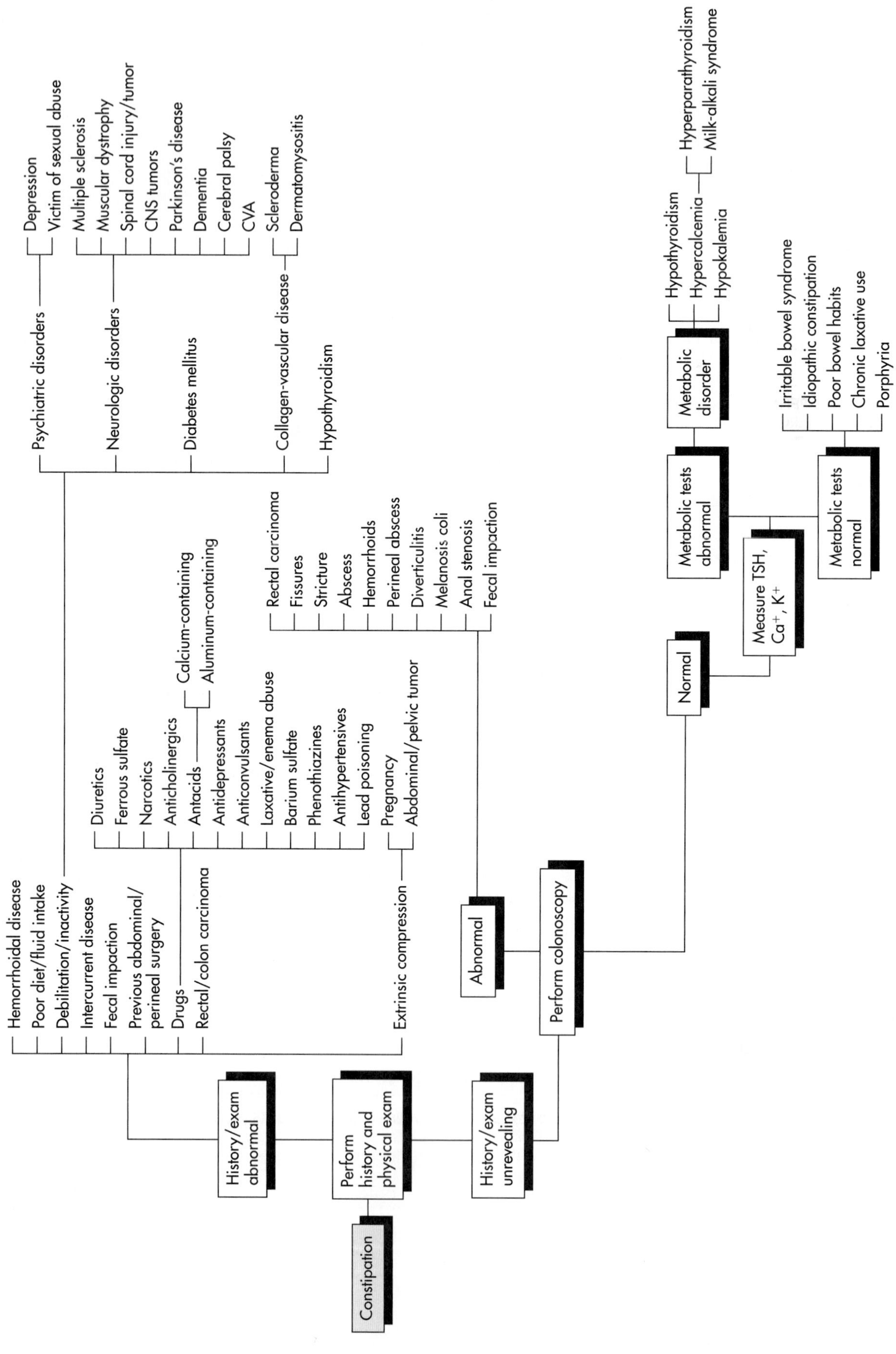

CONSTIPATION

ICD-9CM # 564.0

Constipation

Perform history and physical exam

History/exam abnormal
- Hemorrhoidal disease
- Poor diet/fluid intake
- Debilitation/inactivity
  - Psychiatric disorders
    - Depression
    - Victim of sexual abuse
  - Neurologic disorders
    - Multiple sclerosis
    - Muscular dystrophy
    - Spinal cord injury/tumor
    - CNS tumors
    - Parkinson's disease
    - Dementia
    - Cerebral palsy
    - CVA
  - Diabetes mellitus
  - Collagen-vascular disease
    - Scleroderma
    - Dermatomysositis
  - Hypothyroidism
- Intercurrent disease
- Fecal impaction
- Previous abdominal/perineal surgery
- Drugs
  - Diuretics
  - Ferrous sulfate
  - Narcotics
  - Anticholinergics
  - Antacids
    - Calcium-containing
    - Aluminum-containing
  - Antidepressants
  - Anticonvulsants
  - Laxative/enema abuse
  - Barium sulfate
  - Phenothiazines
  - Antihypertensives
  - Lead poisoning
- Rectal/colon carcinoma
- Extrinsic compression
  - Pregnancy
  - Abdominal/pelvic tumor

History/exam unrevealing
- Perform colonoscopy
  - Abnormal
    - Rectal carcinoma
    - Fissures
    - Stricture
    - Abscess
    - Hemorrhoids
    - Perineal abscess
    - Diverticulitis
    - Melanosis coli
    - Anal stenosis
    - Fecal impaction
  - Normal
    - Measure TSH, Ca^+, K^+
      - Metabolic tests abnormal
        - Metabolic disorder
          - Hypothyroidism
          - Hypercalcemia
            - Hyperparathyroidism
            - Milk-alkali syndrome
          - Hypokalemia
      - Metabolic tests normal
        - Irritable bowel syndrome
        - Idiopathic constipation
        - Poor bowel habits
        - Chronic laxative use
        - Porphyria

FIGURE 3-77 Constipation. *BE,* Barium enema; *CNS,* central nervous system; *CVA,* cerebral vascular accident; *TSH,* thyroid-stimulating hormone. (From Healey PM: *Common medical diagnosis,* ed 3, Philadelphia, 2000, WB Saunders.)

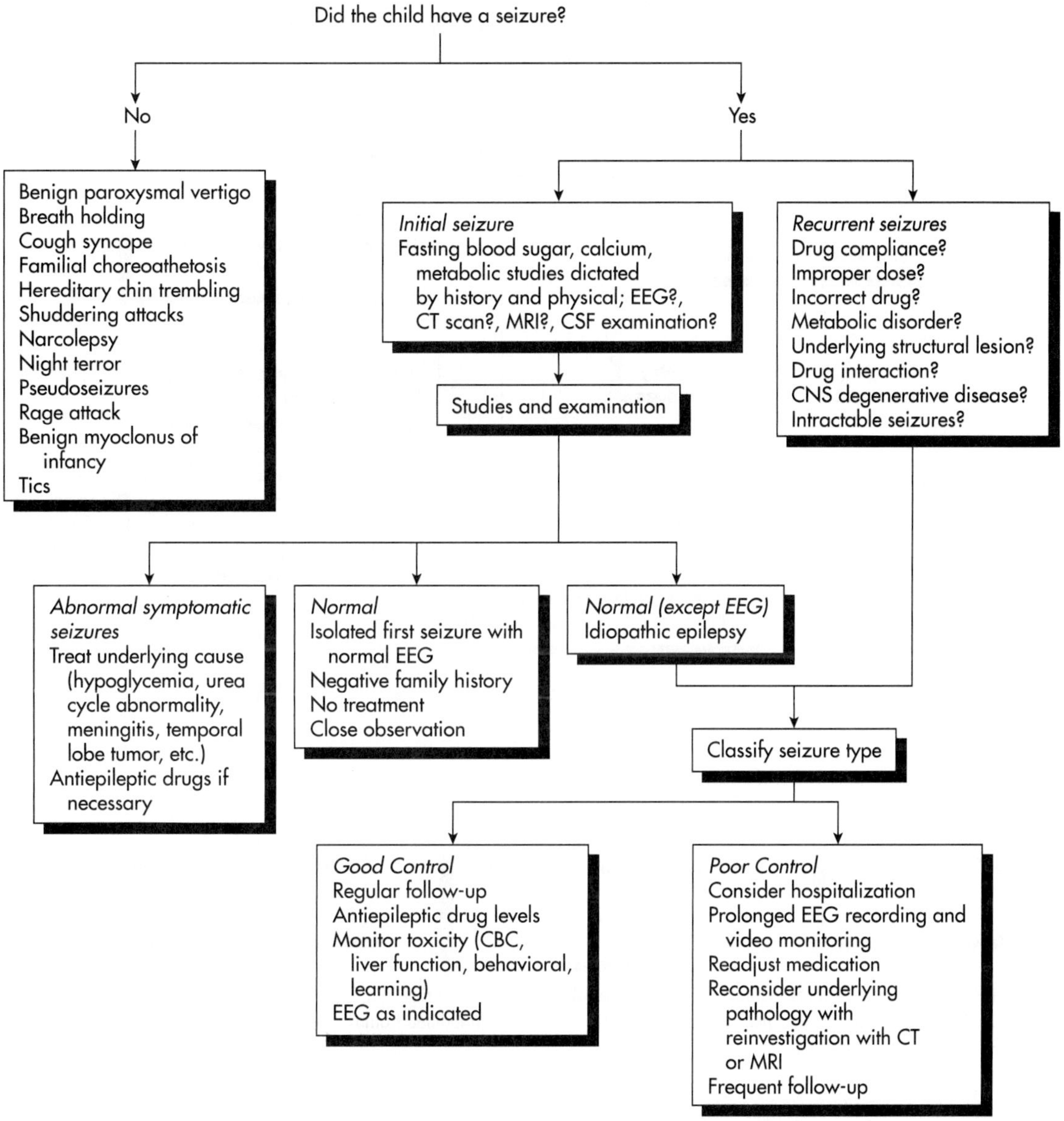

Did the child have a seizure?

No

- Benign paroxysmal vertigo
- Breath holding
- Cough syncope
- Familial choreoathetosis
- Hereditary chin trembling
- Shuddering attacks
- Narcolepsy
- Night terror
- Pseudoseizures
- Rage attack
- Benign myoclonus of infancy
- Tics

Yes

Initial seizure
Fasting blood sugar, calcium, metabolic studies dictated by history and physical; EEG?, CT scan?, MRI?, CSF examination?

→ Studies and examination

Abnormal symptomatic seizures
Treat underlying cause (hypoglycemia, urea cycle abnormality, meningitis, temporal lobe tumor, etc.)
Antiepileptic drugs if necessary

Normal
Isolated first seizure with normal EEG
Negative family history
No treatment
Close observation

Normal (except EEG)
Idiopathic epilepsy

Recurrent seizures
Drug compliance?
Improper dose?
Incorrect drug?
Metabolic disorder?
Underlying structural lesion?
Drug interaction?
CNS degenerative disease?
Intractable seizures?

→ Classify seizure type

Good Control
Regular follow-up
Antiepileptic drug levels
Monitor toxicity (CBC, liver function, behavioral, learning)
EEG as indicated

Poor Control
Consider hospitalization
Prolonged EEG recording and video monitoring
Readjust medication
Reconsider underlying pathology with reinvestigation with CT or MRI
Frequent follow-up

FIGURE 3-80 An approach to the child with a suspected convulsive disorder. *CBC,* Complete blood count; *CNS,* central nervous system; *CSF,* cerebrospinal fluid; *CT,* computed tomography; *EEG,* electroencephalogram; *MRI,* magnetic resonance imaging. (From Behrman RE: *Nelson textbook of pediatrics,* ed 18, Philadelphia, 2007, WB Saunders.)

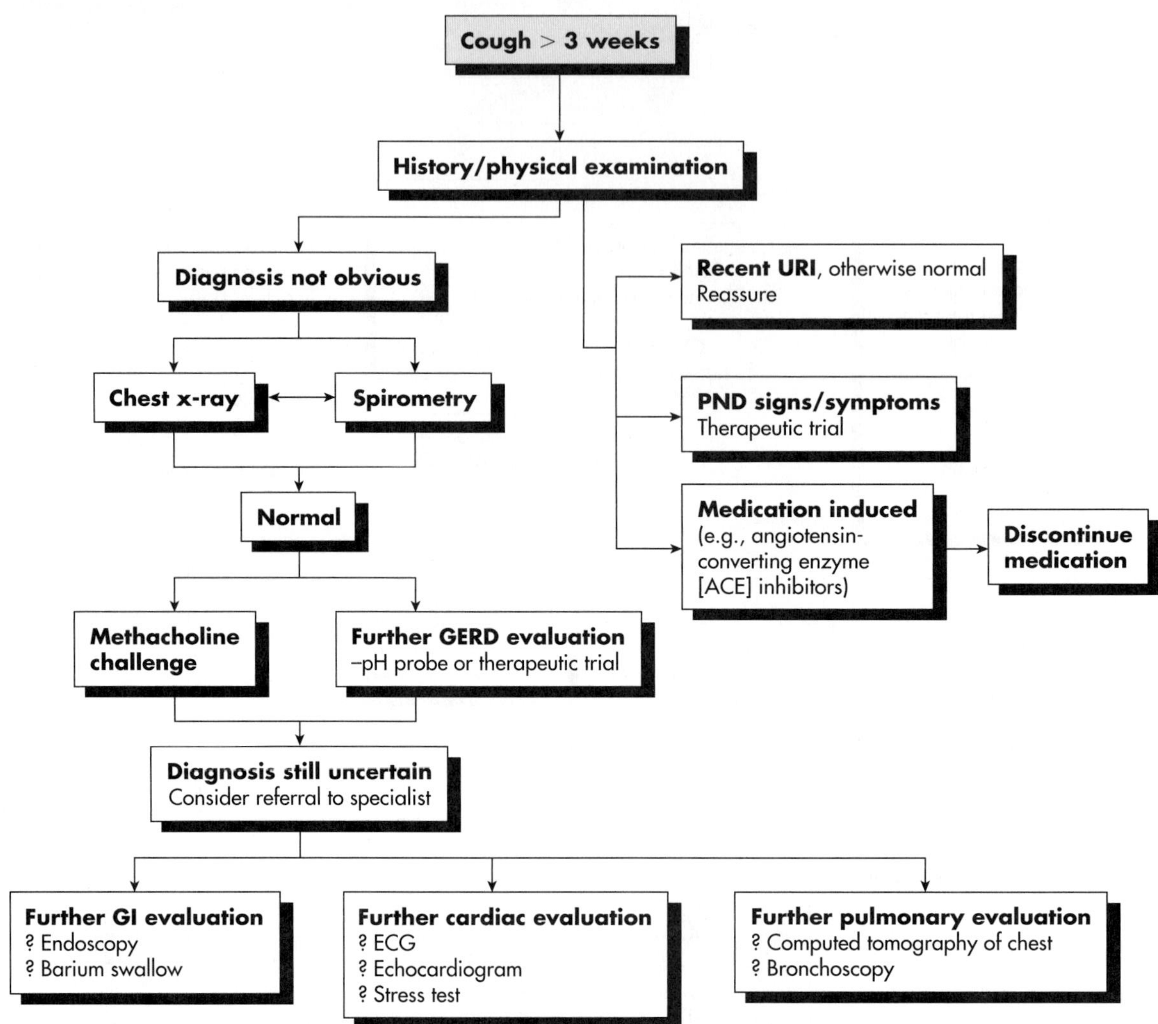

FIGURE 3-83 Diagnostic approach to chronic cough. *ECG,* Electrocardiogram; *GERD,* gastroesophageal reflux disease; *PND,* paroxysmal nocturnal dyspnea; *URI,* upper respiratory infection. (Modified from Carlson KJ et al: *Primary care of women,* ed 2, St Louis, 2002, Mosby.)

CREATINE KINASE ELEVATION

ICD-9CM # V72.6

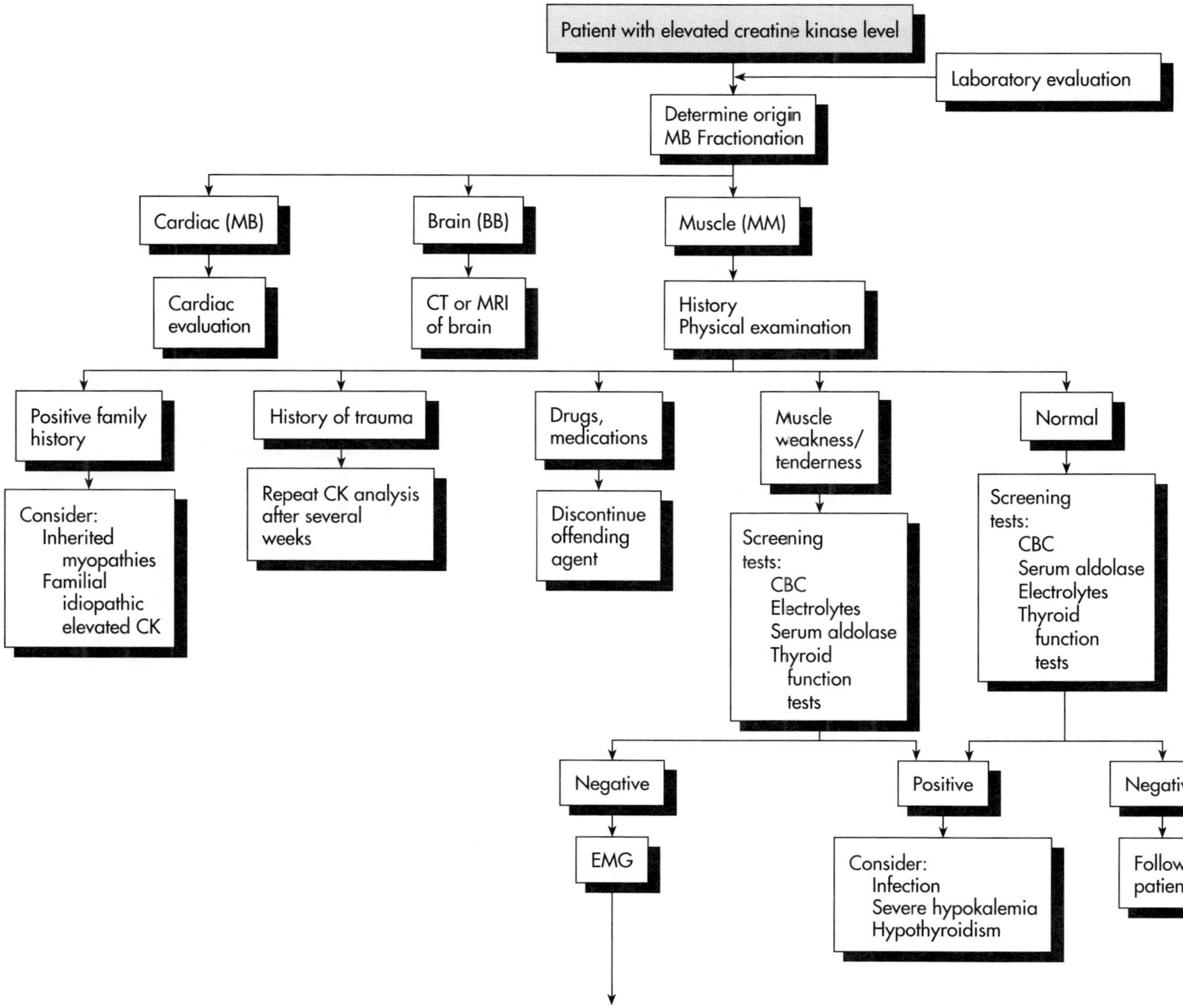

- Patient with elevated creatine kinase level
  - (Laboratory evaluation →) Determine origin MB Fractionation
    - Cardiac (MB) → Cardiac evaluation
    - Brain (BB) → CT or MRI of brain
    - Muscle (MM) → History Physical examination
      - Positive family history → Consider: Inherited myopathies; Familial idiopathic elevated CK
      - History of trauma → Repeat CK analysis after several weeks
      - Drugs, medications → Discontinue offending agent
      - Muscle weakness/tenderness → Screening tests: CBC; Electrolytes; Serum aldolase; Thyroid function tests
        - Negative → EMG
        - Positive → Consider: Infection; Severe hypokalemia; Hypothyroidism
      - Normal → Screening tests: CBC; Serum aldolase; Electrolytes; Thyroid function tests
        - Positive → Consider: Infection; Severe hypokalemia; Hypothyroidism
        - Negative → Follow patient

FIGURE 3-84 Evaluation of creatine kinase elevation. *CBC,* Complete blood count; *CK,* creatine kinase; *CT,* computed tomography; *EMG,* electromyography; *MRI,* magnetic resonance imaging. (Modified from Greene HL, Johnson WP, Lemcke D [eds]: *Decision making in medicine,* ed 2, St Louis, 1998, Mosby.)

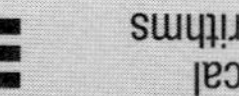

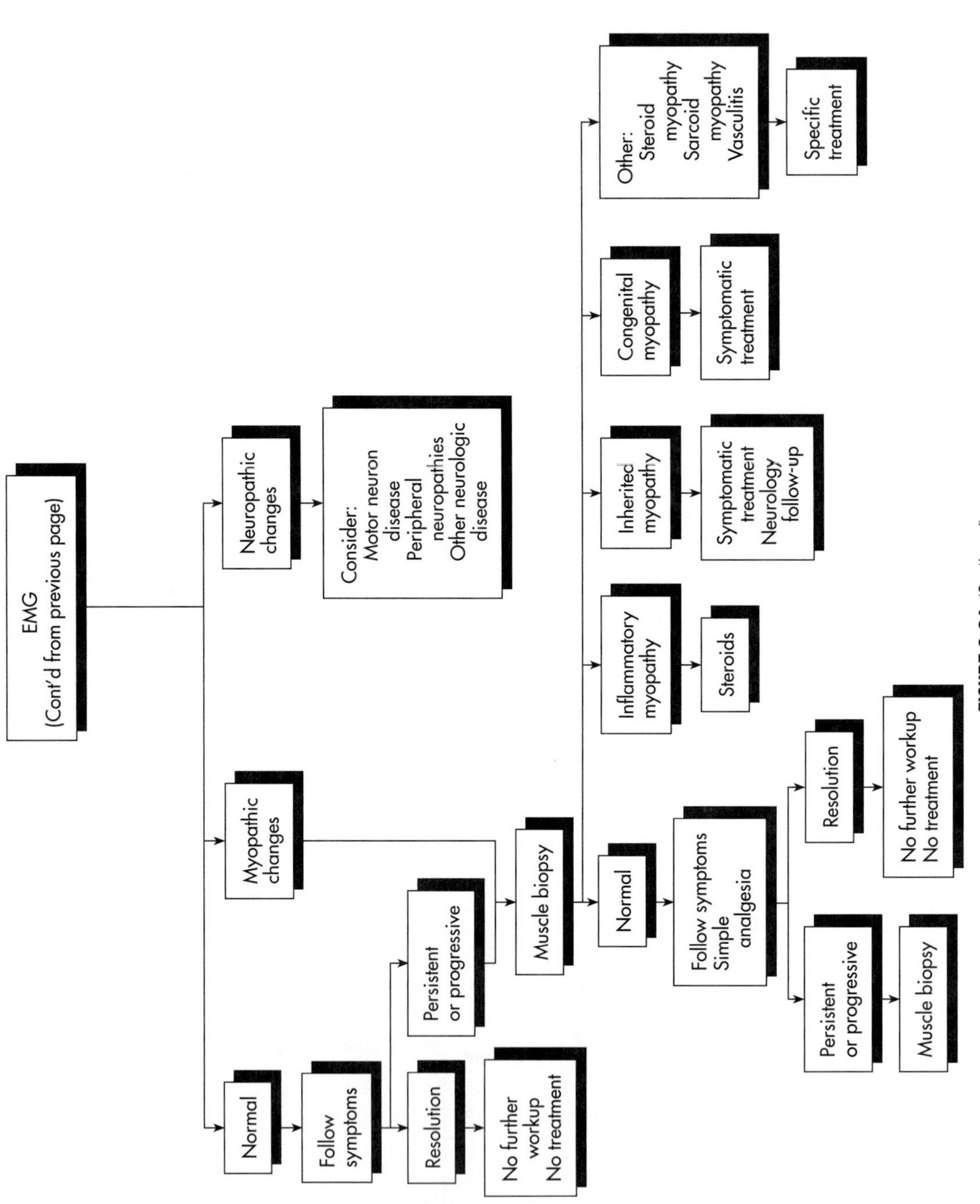

FIGURE 3-84 (Continued)

CYANOSIS

ICD-9CM # 782.5 Cyanosis NOS

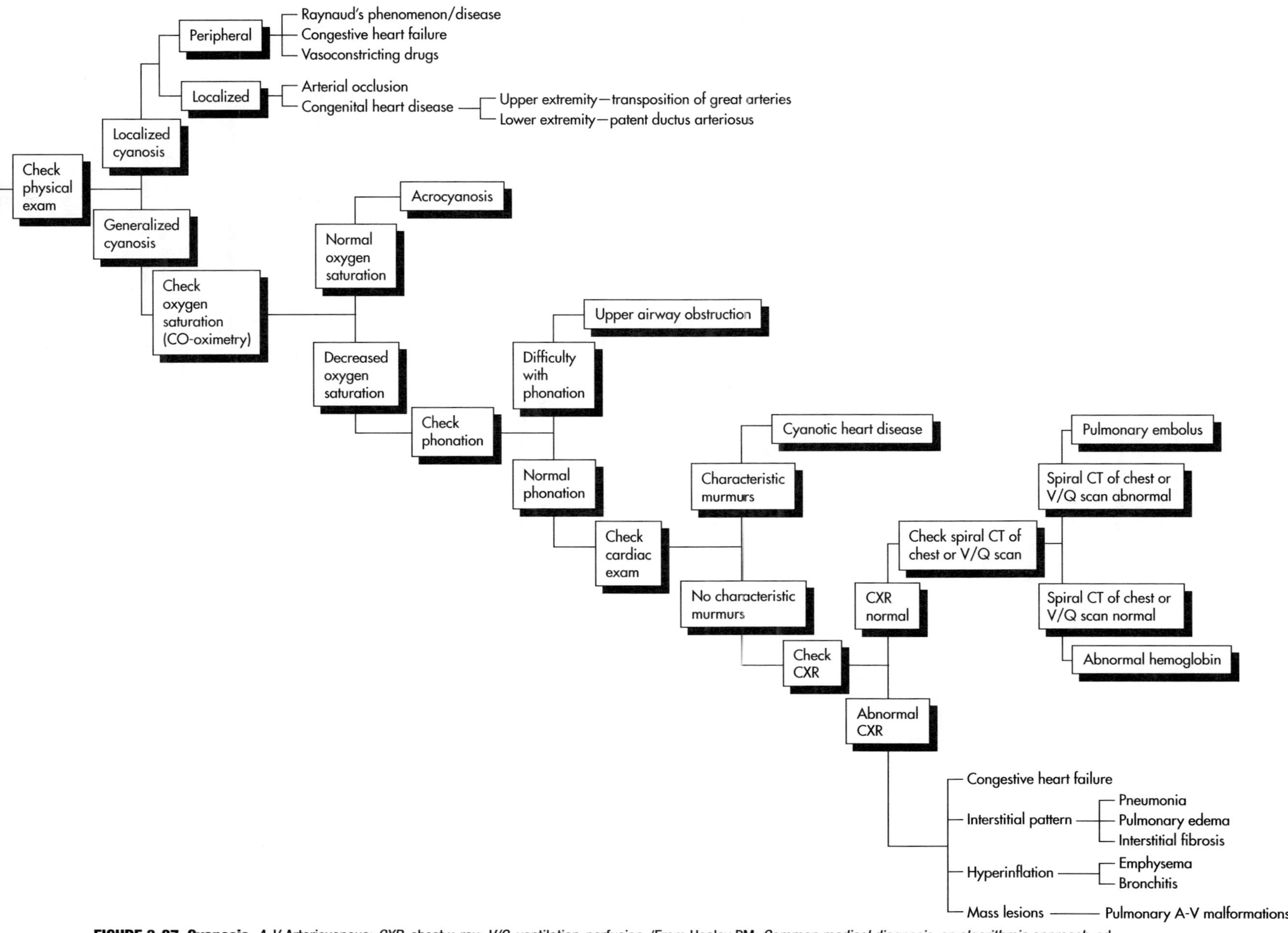

FIGURE 3-87 Cyanosis. *A-V,* Arteriovenous; *CXR,* chest x-ray; *V/Q,* ventilation-perfusion. (From Healey PM: *Common medical diagnosis: an algorithmic approach,* ed 3, Philadelphia, 2000, WB Saunders.)

DELIRIUM, GERIATRIC PATIENT

ICD-9CM # 293.0 Delirium, acute
292.81 Delirium, drug induced
293.1 Delirium, subacute
293.81 Delirium, transient organic with delusions
293.82 Delirium, transient organic with hallucinations

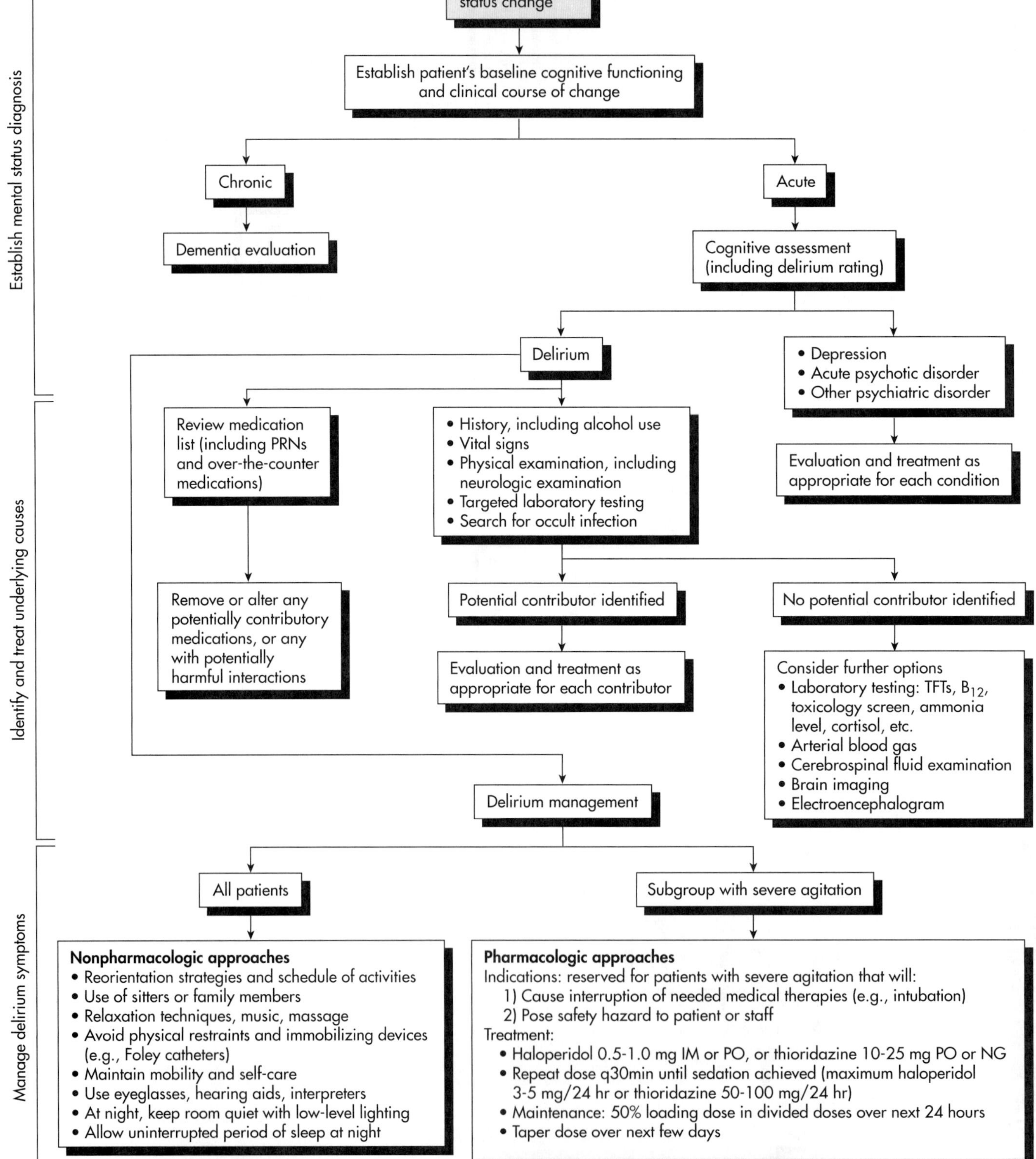

FIGURE 3-94 Algorithm for evaluation of suspected mental status change in an older patient. *IM,* Intramuscular; *NG,* nasogastric; *PO,* by mouth; *PRN,* as needed; *TFTs,* thyroid function tests. (From Goldman L, Ausiello D [eds]: *Cecil textbook of medicine,* ed 23, Philadelphia, 2008, WB Saunders.)

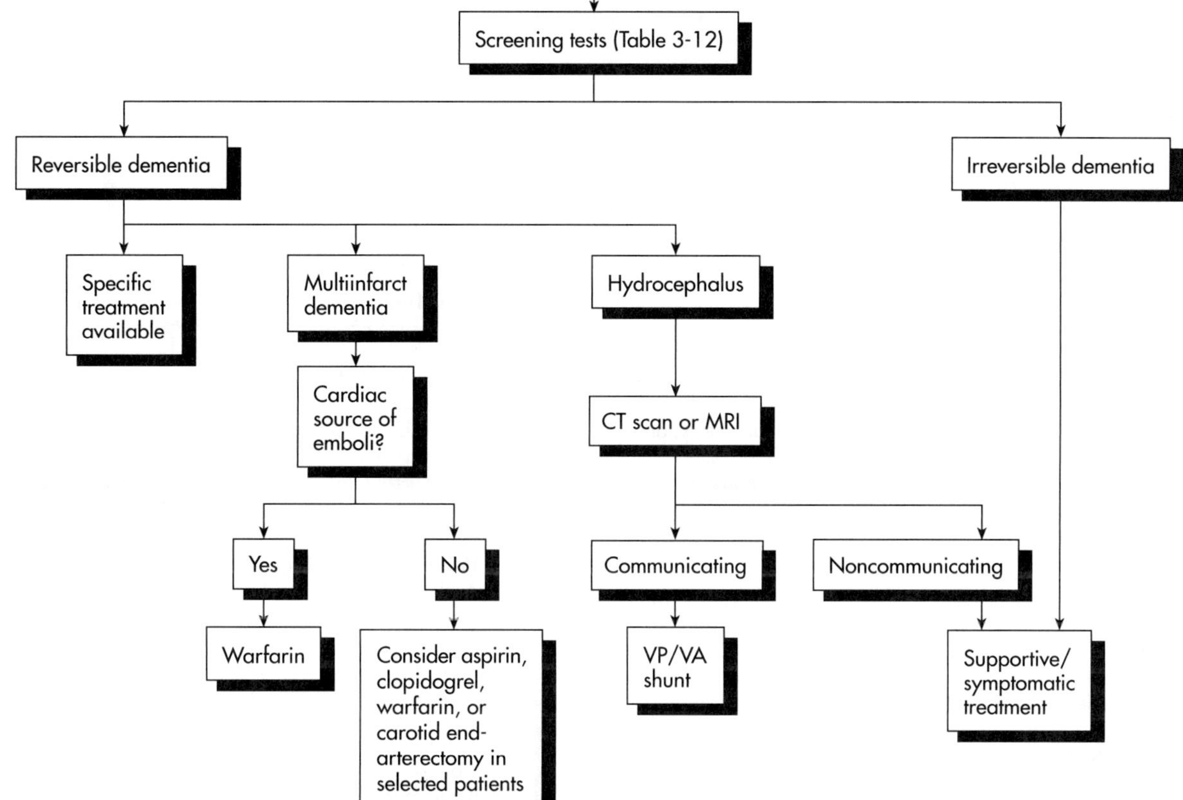

FIGURE 3-95 Management of dementia. *VA,* Ventriculoatrial; *VP,* ventriculoperitoneal.

ICD-9CM # 250.1 Diabetic ketoacidosis
250.2 Hyperosmolar hyperglycemic state

Adult patient with DKA or HHS

Complete initial evaluation, including (but not limited to):
- Medical history and physical examination
- Complete blood count with differential
- Fingerstick blood glucose
- Serum chemistries ("Chem-10" plus serum ketones)
- Urine for urinalysis and ketones
- Cultures as indicated (wound, blood, urine, etc.)
- Chest ± abdominal x-ray
- 12-lead electrocardiogram

Concurrently, begin empiric fluid resuscitation with 0.9% NaCl at 1000 ml/hr
Consider volume expanders if hypovolemic shock is present
Continue fluid resuscitation until volume status and cardiovascular parameters (pulse, blood pressure) have been restored

IV fluids
Based on corrected serum sodium*
If high/normal, use 0.45% NaCl
If low/normal, use 0.9% NaCl
Continue IV fluids at 250-1000 ml/hr, depending on volume status, cardiovascular history, and cardiovascular status (pulse, BP)

Insulin therapy
Regular insulin bolus, 0.15 U/kg
IV infusion, 0.10 U/kg hr
Check serum glucose hourly—should fall by 50-80 mg/dl/hr.
If serum glucose falling too rapidly, back off on insulin infusion
If serum glucose rising or falling too slowly, increase insulin infusion rate by 50%-100%

When serum glucose reaches 250-300 mg/dl:
Add dextrose to IV fluids. Continue IV fluids at 150-250 ml/hr, and adjust insulin infusion to maintain serum glucose of 200-250 mg/dl until metabolic control is achieved:
For DKA, continue until anion gap has closed and acidosis has resolved
For HHS, continue until plasma osmolality drops below 310 mOsm/kg
Begin more exhaustive search for precipitant of metabolic decompensation

Continuing management:
Follow and replete serum electrolytes (including divalent cations) q2-4h until stable
After resolution of hyperglycemic state, follow blood glucose q4h and initiate sliding scale regular insulin coverage
Convert IV insulin to subcutaneous injections (or resumption of prior therapy), ensuring adequate overlap if treating patients without endogenous insulin secretion
Begin clear liquid diet and advance as tolerated. Encourage resumption of ambulation and activity
Review and update diabetes education, with special attention to prevention of further hyperglycemic crises

Potassium (K^+) repletion
Obtain baseline serum potassium
Obtain 12-lead ECG

$[K^+] \geq 5.5$ mEq/L → Hold K^+ therapy → Treat hyperkalemia if ECG changes present → Recheck $[K^+]$ in 2 hr

$[K^+] < 5.5$ mEq/L and adequate urine output → Add K^+ to IV fluids (Use KCl and/or KPhos)
$[K^+] = 4.5$-5.4: add 20 mEq/L IVF
$[K^+] = 3.5$-4.4: add 30 mEq/L IVF
$[K^+] < 3.5$: add 40 mEq/L IVF

Follow serum $[K^+]$ every 2-4 hours until stable: anticipate rapid drop of serum $[K^+]$ during therapy, due to dilution and intracelular shifting
Ensure adequate urine output to avoid over-repletion and hyperkalemia
Continue K^+ repletion until serum $[K^+]$ is stable at between 4-5 mEq/L
If refractory hypokalemia, ensure concurrent magnesium repletion
Repletion may need to be continued for several days, as total body losses may reach up to 500 mEq

Bicarbonate therapy
Obtain ABG
Obtain baseline serum bicarbonate

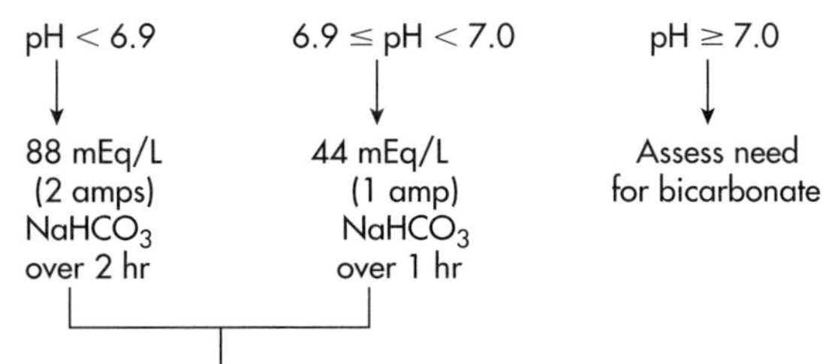

Repeat ABG after bicarbonate administration
Repeat $NaHCO_3$ therapy until pH ≥7.0, then discontinue therapy
Follow serum bicarbonate q4h until stable

*Sodium correction: Serum sodium should be corrected for hyperglycemia. For every 100 mg/dl of glucose elevation above 100 mg/dl, add 1.6 mEq/L to the measured sodium value; this will yield the correction serum sodium concentration.

Note: Refer to Section I for additional information on these topics.

FIGURE 3-100 Management of diabetic ketoacidosis *(DKA)* and hyperosmolar hyperglycemic state *(HHS).* *ABG,* Arterial blood gas; *DKA,* diabetic ketoacidosis; *ECG,* electrocardiograph. (From Goldman L, Ausiello D [eds]: *Cecil textbook of medicine,* ed 23, Philadelphia, 2008, WB Saunders.)

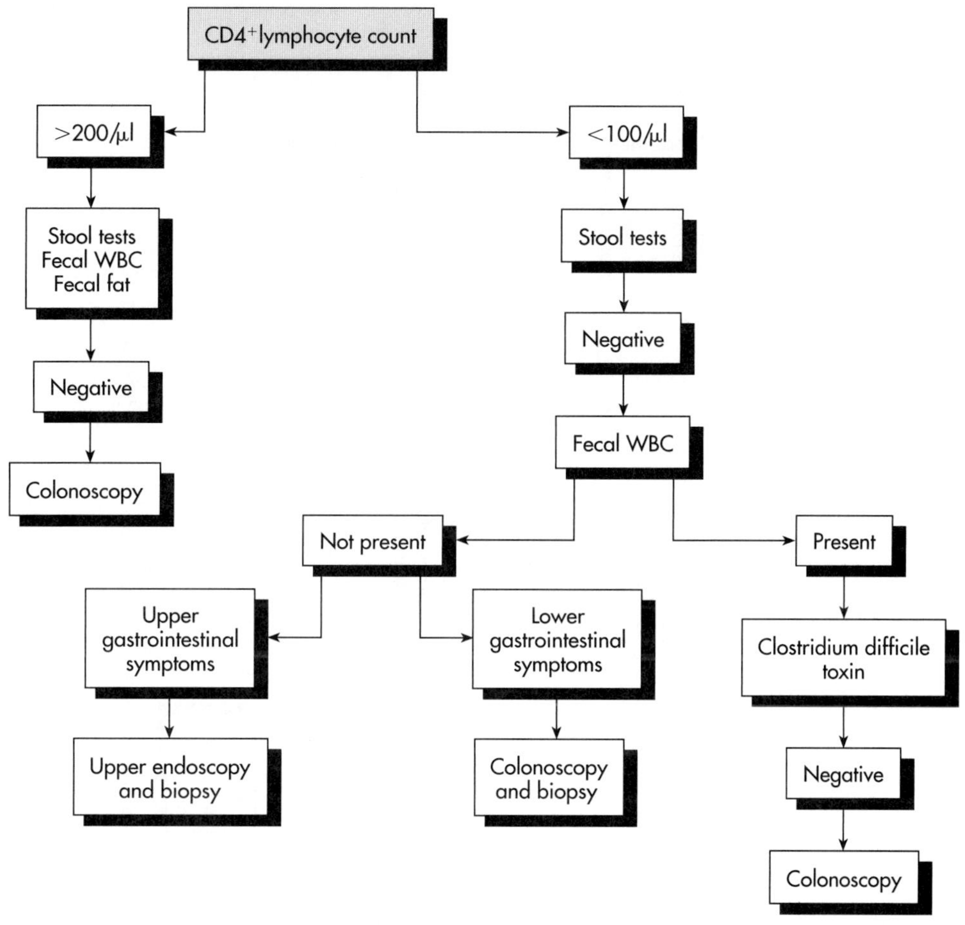

FIGURE 3-103 Approach to evaluating chronic diarrhea in patients with HIV infection. *WBC,* White blood cell count. (Modified from Wilcox CM: *Gastrointest Dis Today* 5:9, 1996.)

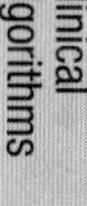

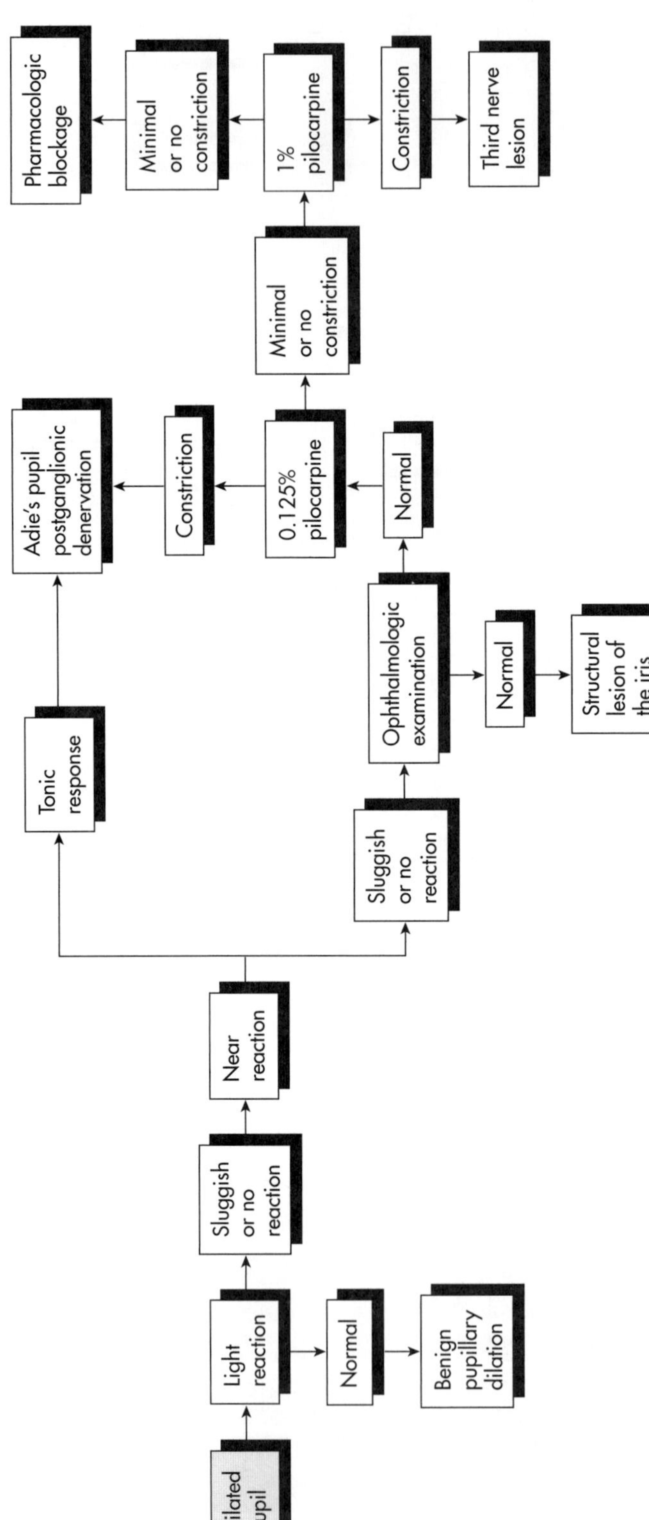

FIGURE 3-104 Use of pilocarpine to help differentiate between different causes of a dilated pupil. (From Goldman L, Ausiello D [eds]: *Cecil textbook of medicine*, ed 23, Philadephia, 2008, WB Saunders.)

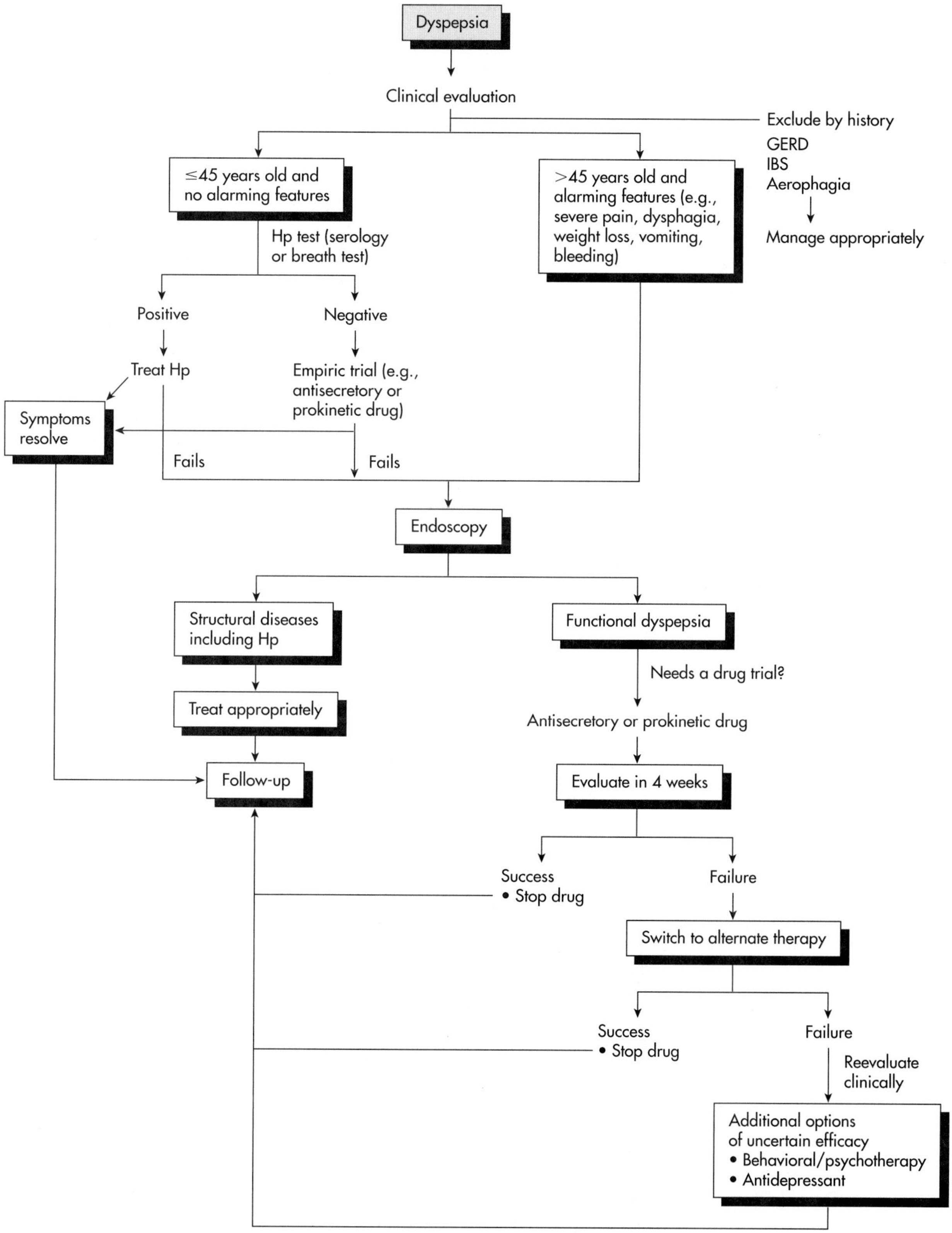

CD-9CM # 563.3 Dyspepsia atonic
536.8 Dyspepsia disorders other unspecified function of stomach
306.4 Dyspepsia, psychogenic

Dyspepsia

Clinical evaluation

Exclude by history
GERD
IBS
Aerophagia

Manage appropriately

≤45 years old and no alarming features

Hp test (serology or breath test)

Positive

Treat Hp

Negative

Empiric trial (e.g., antisecretory or prokinetic drug)

Symptoms resolve

Fails

Fails

>45 years old and alarming features (e.g., severe pain, dysphagia, weight loss, vomiting, bleeding)

Endoscopy

Structural diseases including Hp

Treat appropriately

Follow-up

Functional dyspepsia

Needs a drug trial?

Antisecretory or prokinetic drug

Evaluate in 4 weeks

Success
• Stop drug

Failure

Switch to alternate therapy

Success
• Stop drug

Failure

Reevaluate clinically

Additional options of uncertain efficacy
• Behavioral/psychotherapy
• Antidepressant

FIGURE 3-107 Algorithm for the evaluation of dyspepsia. *GERD,* Symptomatic gastroesophageal reflux disease; *Hp, Helicobacter pylori; IBS,* irritable bowel syndrome. (From Goldman L, Ausiello D [eds]: *Cecil textbook of medicine,* ed 23, Philadelphia, 2008, WB Saunders.)

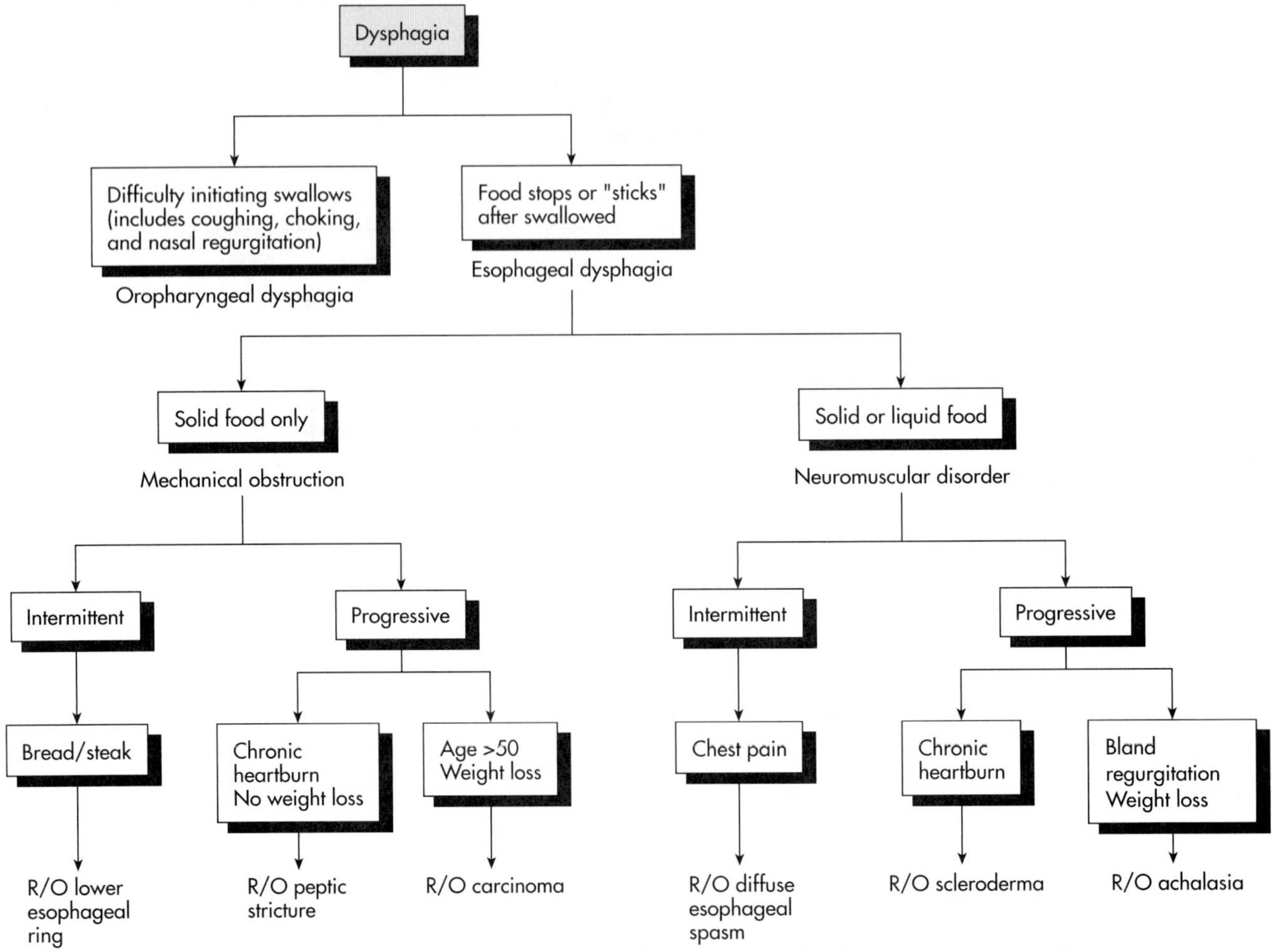

- Dysphagia
  - Difficulty initiating swallows (includes coughing, choking, and nasal regurgitation) — Oropharyngeal dysphagia
  - Food stops or "sticks" after swallowed — Esophageal dysphagia
    - Solid food only — Mechanical obstruction
      - Intermittent
        - Bread/steak → R/O lower esophageal ring
      - Progressive
        - Chronic heartburn, No weight loss → R/O peptic stricture
        - Age >50, Weight loss → R/O carcinoma
    - Solid or liquid food — Neuromuscular disorder
      - Intermittent
        - Chest pain → R/O diffuse esophageal spasm
      - Progressive
        - Chronic heartburn → R/O scleroderma
        - Bland regurgitation, Weight loss → R/O achalasia

FIGURE 3-108 Differential diagnosis of dysphagia. (Modified from Andreoli TE [ed]: *Cecil essentials of medicine,* ed 7, Philadelphia, 2008, WB Saunders.)

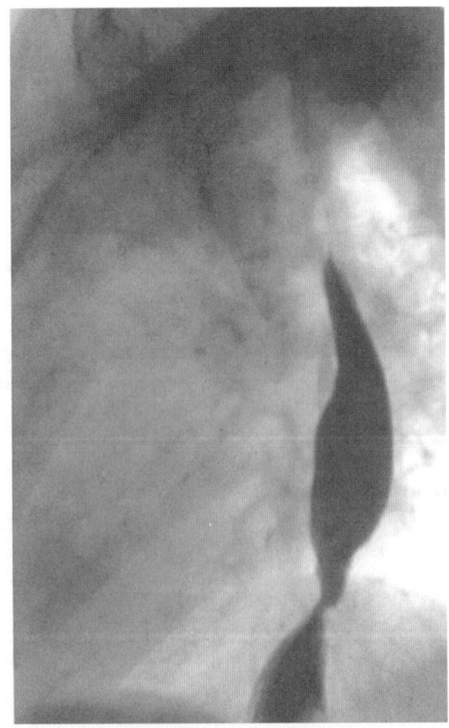

FIGURE 3-109 Barium swallow demonstrating a benign peptic stricture in a patient with gastro-esophageal reflux disease and dysphagia. (From Talley NJ, Martin C: *Clinical gastroenterology: a practical problem-based approach,* ed 2, Sydney, 2006, Elsevier.)

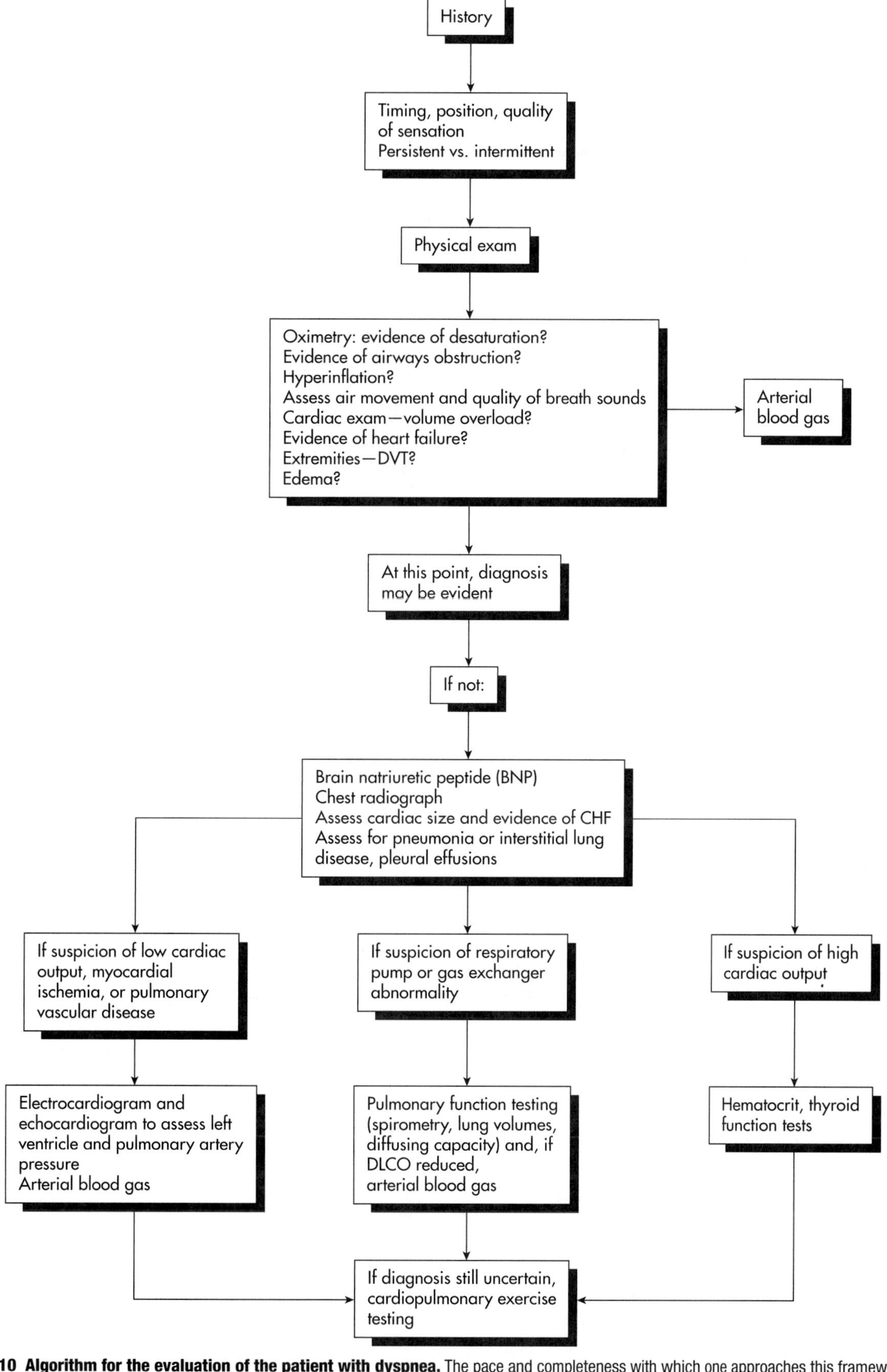

FIGURE 3-110 Algorithm for the evaluation of the patient with dyspnea. The pace and completeness with which one approaches this framework depends on the intensity and acuity of the patient's symptoms. In a patient with severe, acute dyspnea, for example, an arterial blood gas measurement may be one of the first laboratory evaluations, whereas this measurement might not be obtained until much later in the workup in a patient with chronic breathlessness of unclear cause. A therapeutic trial of a medication, for example, a bronchodilator, may be instituted at any point if one is fairly confident of the diagnosis based on the data available at that time. *CHF,* Congestive heart failure; *DLCO,* diffusing capacity of the lung for carbon monoxide; *DVT,* deep venous thrombosis. (From Schwartzstein RM, Feller-Kopman D: Approach to the patient with dyspnea. In Braunwald E, Goldman L [eds]: *Primary cardiology,* ed 2, Philadelphia, 2003, WB Saunders.)

Management of Ear Pain

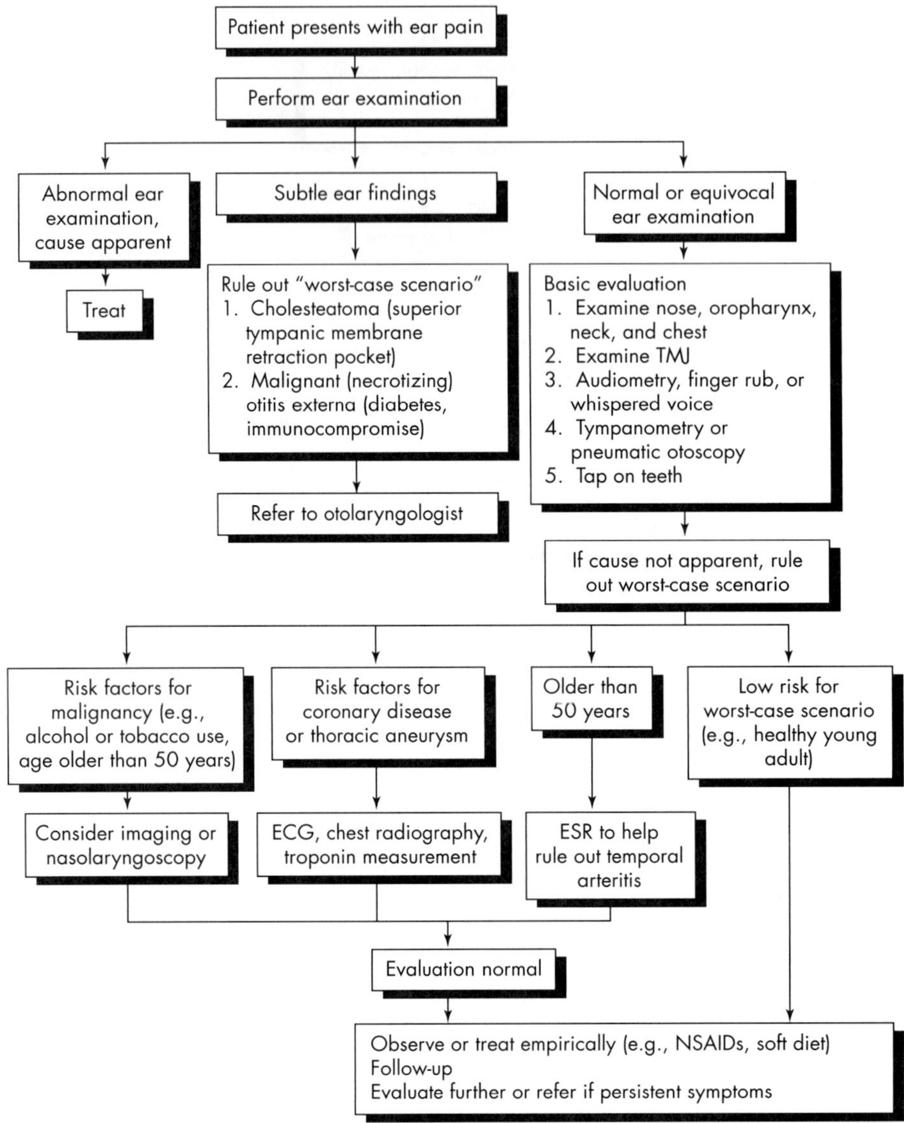

FIGURE 3-112 Management of ear pain. *ECG,* Electrocardiography; *ESR,* erythrocyte sedimentation rate; *NSAIDs,* nonsteroidal anti-inflammatory drugs; *TMJ,* temporomandibular joint. (From Ely JW et al: Diagnosis of ear pain, *Am Fam Physician* 77(5):622, 2008.)

Edema
History
Physical examination
Generalized edema
Regional edema (see Fig. 3-115)
Check JVP, BNP
JVP normal
JVP elevated
BNP elevated
Check serum albumin
Chest radiography
CHF
Cardiomegaly
Normal heart size
Check echocardiogram
Evaluate lung fields
Pericardial effusion
Poor contractibility
Pulmonary hypertension pattern
Clear lung fields
Pericarditis/ tamponade
CHF
Evaluate for cor pulmonale
Evaluate for pericardial constriction
Normal serum albumin
Decreased serum albumin
Normal urinalysis
Abnormal urine sediment
Proteinuria
Normal urinalysis
Check BUN/ creatinine
Check 24-hour urine protein
Check TFTs
Evaluate for renal pathology
>3.5 g protein
<3.5 g protein
Nephrotic syndrome
Check LFTs
Normal TFTs
Decreased TFTs
Abnormal LFTs
Normal LFTs
Myxedema
Evaluate for liver pathology
Check prealbumin
Drug-induced edema
Idiopathic edema
Prealbumin <20 mg/dl
Prealbumin >20 mg/dl
Malnutrition
Capillary leak
Abnormal protein synthesis
Protein-losing enteropathy

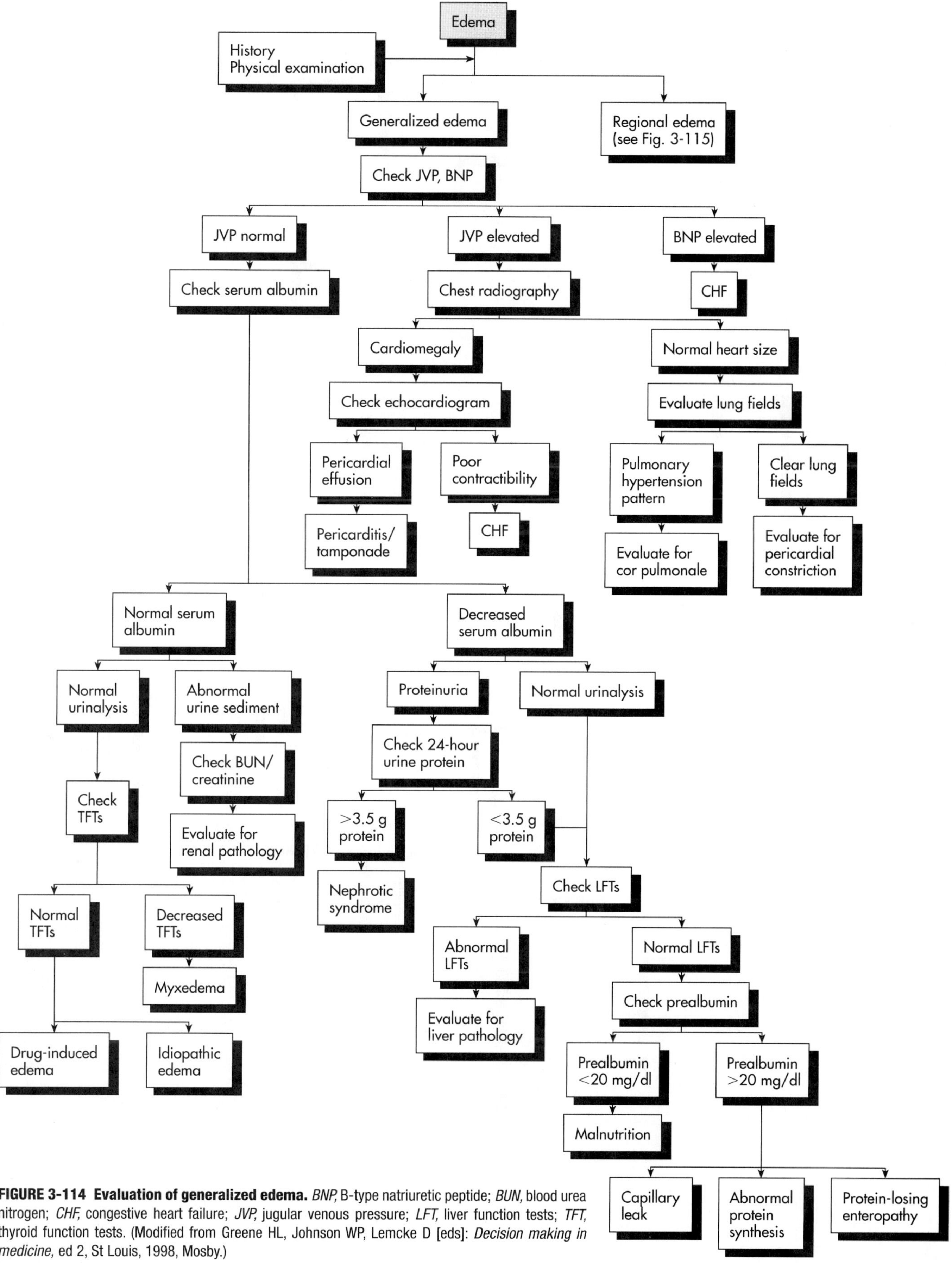

FIGURE 3-114 Evaluation of generalized edema. *BNP,* B-type natriuretic peptide; *BUN,* blood urea nitrogen; *CHF,* congestive heart failure; *JVP,* jugular venous pressure; *LFT,* liver function tests; *TFT,* thyroid function tests. (Modified from Greene HL, Johnson WP, Lemcke D [eds]: *Decision making in medicine,* ed 2, St Louis, 1998, Mosby.)

EDEMA, REGIONAL

ICD-9CM # 250.6

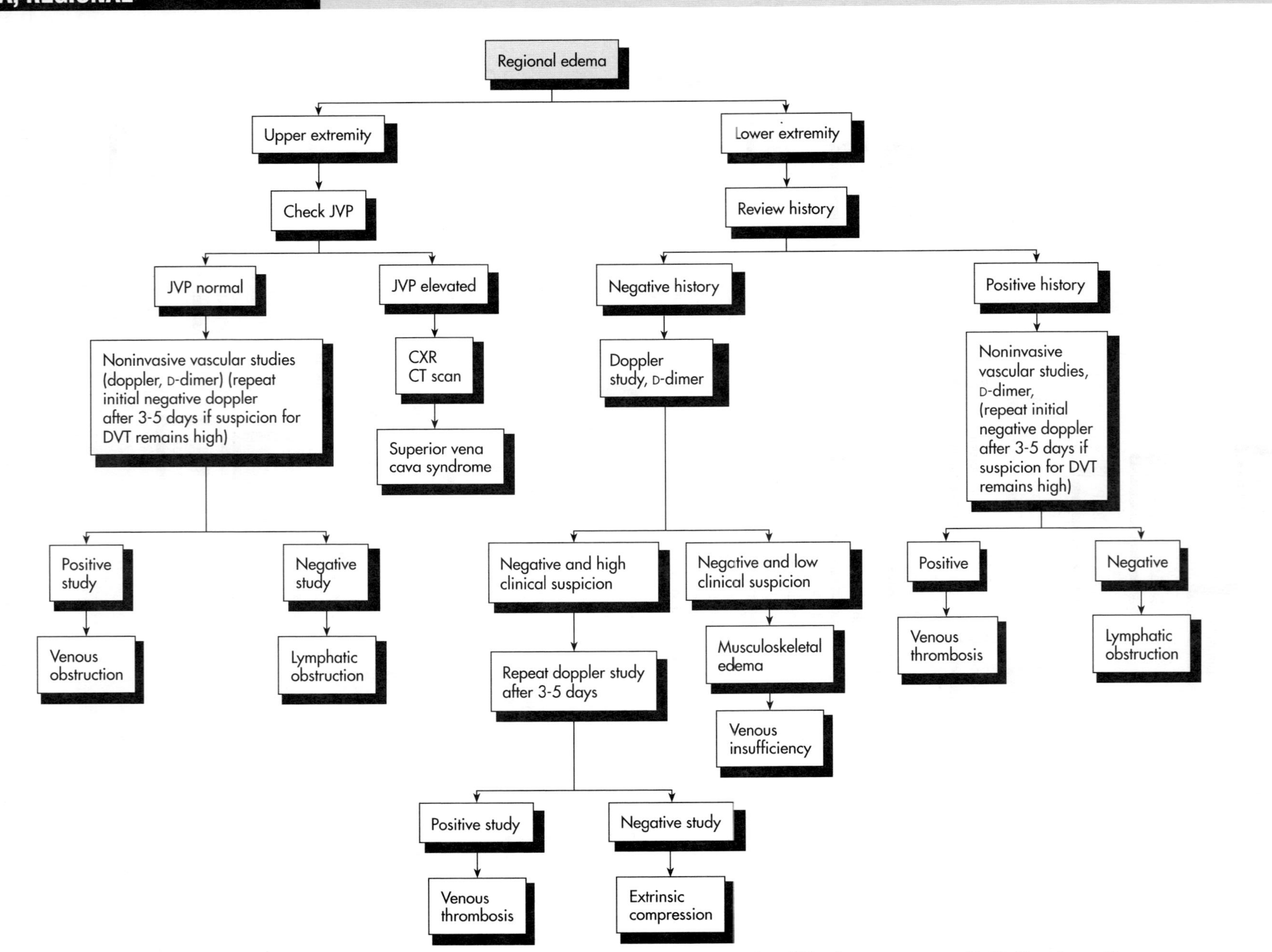

FIGURE 3-115 Evaluation of regional edema. *CT,* Computed tomography; *CXR,* chest x-ray examination; *JVP,* jugular venous pressure. (Modified from Greene HL, Johnson WP, Lemcke D [eds]: *Decision making in medicine,* ed 2, St Louis, 1998, Mosby.)

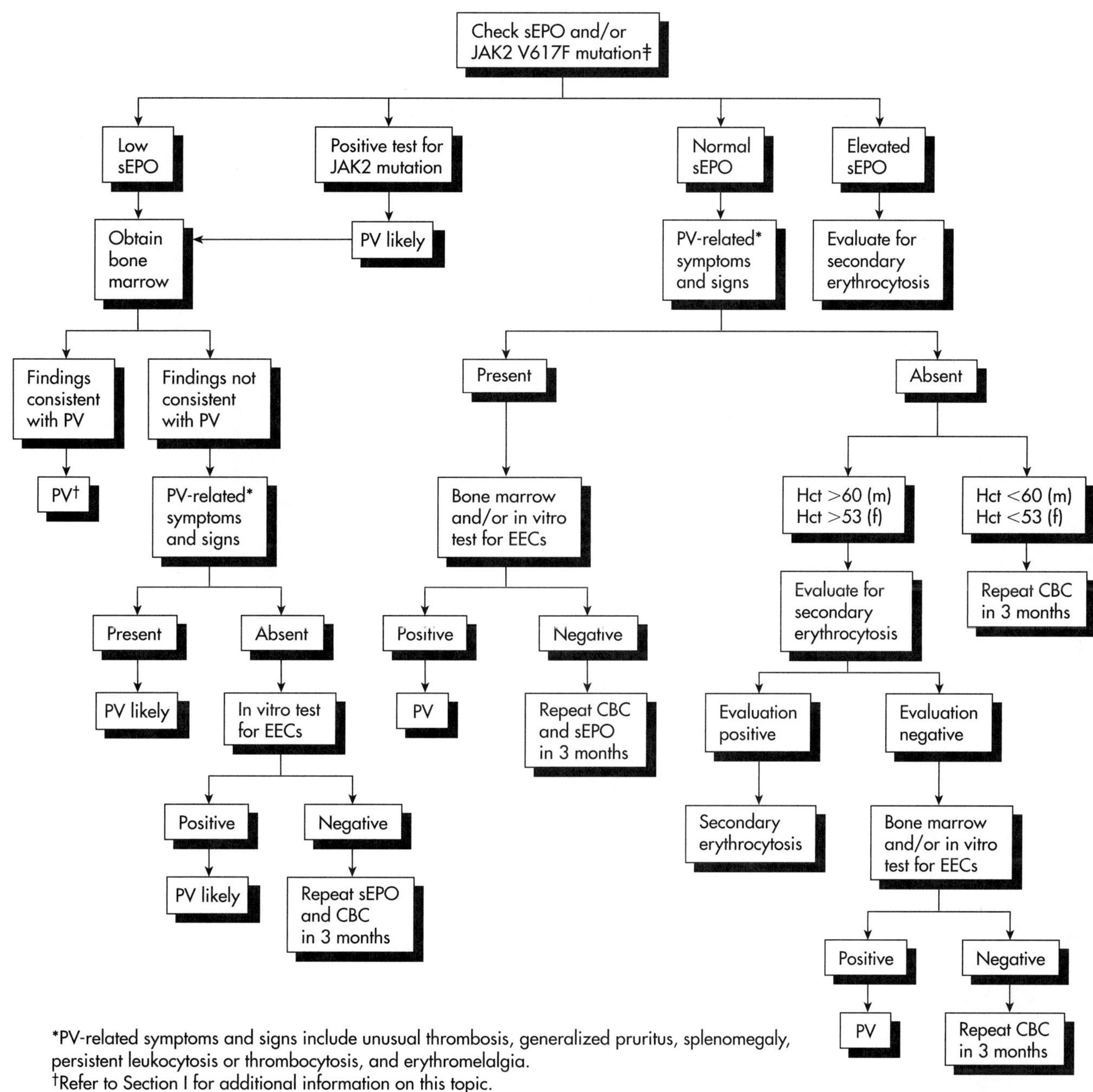

*PV-related symptoms and signs include unusual thrombosis, generalized pruritus, splenomegaly, persistent leukocytosis or thrombocytosis, and erythromelalgia.
†Refer to Section I for additional information on this topic.
‡The JAK2 mutation is found in >95% of patients with PV and can be used for diagnostic purposes.

FIGURE 3-121 A diagnostic approach to acquired erythrocytosis. *CBC,* Complete blood cell count; *EEC,* endogenous (spontaneous) erythroid colonies; *f,* female; *Hct,* hematocrit; *m,* male; *PV,* polycythemia vera; *sEPO,* serum erythropoietin level. (Modified from Goldman L, Ausiello D [eds]: *Cecil textbook of medicine,* ed 23, Philadelphia, 2008, WB Saunders.)

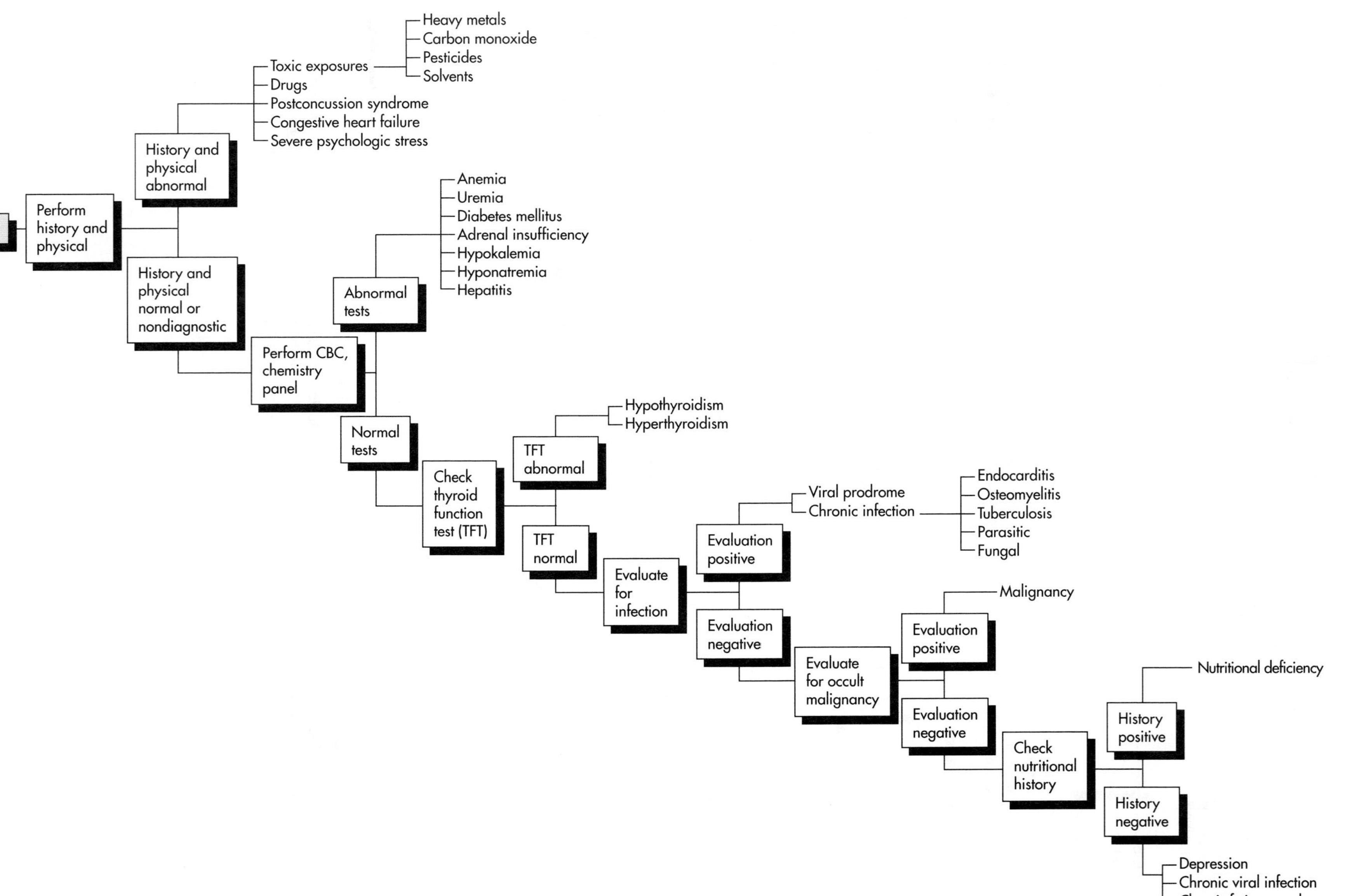

FIGURE 3-123 Evaluation of fatigue. *CBC*, Complete blood count. (From Healey PM: *Common medical diagnosis: an algorithmic approach*, ed 3, Philadelphia, 2000, WB Saunders.)

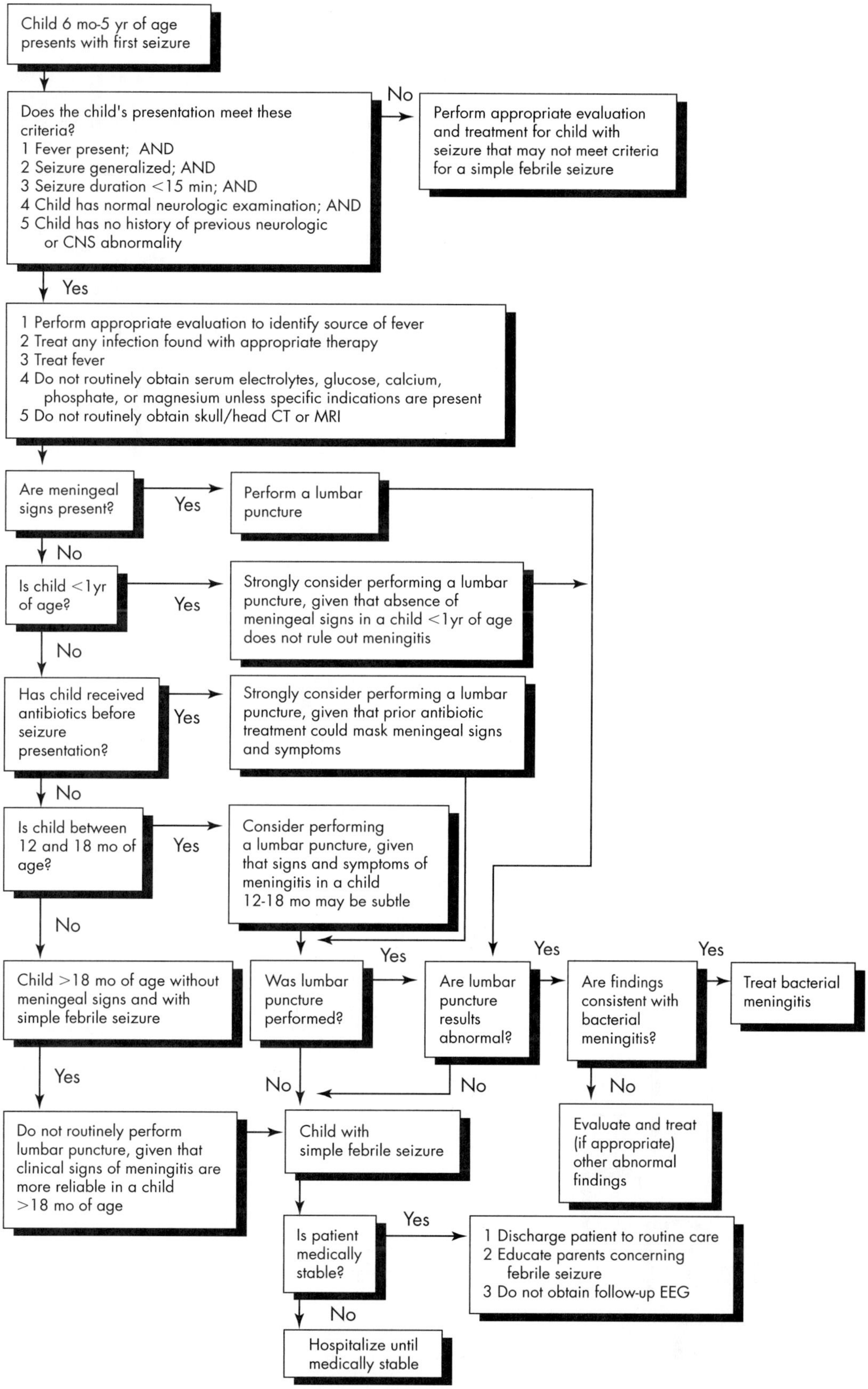

Child 6 mo-5 yr of age presents with first seizure

Does the child's presentation meet these criteria?
1 Fever present; AND
2 Seizure generalized; AND
3 Seizure duration <15 min; AND
4 Child has normal neurologic examination; AND
5 Child has no history of previous neurologic or CNS abnormality

No → Perform appropriate evaluation and treatment for child with seizure that may not meet criteria for a simple febrile seizure

Yes ↓

1 Perform appropriate evaluation to identify source of fever
2 Treat any infection found with appropriate therapy
3 Treat fever
4 Do not routinely obtain serum electrolytes, glucose, calcium, phosphate, or magnesium unless specific indications are present
5 Do not routinely obtain skull/head CT or MRI

Are meningeal signs present? — Yes → Perform a lumbar puncture

No ↓

Is child <1yr of age? — Yes → Strongly consider performing a lumbar puncture, given that absence of meningeal signs in a child <1yr of age does not rule out meningitis

No ↓

Has child received antibiotics before seizure presentation? — Yes → Strongly consider performing a lumbar puncture, given that prior antibiotic treatment could mask meningeal signs and symptoms

No ↓

Is child between 12 and 18 mo of age? — Yes → Consider performing a lumbar puncture, given that signs and symptoms of meningitis in a child 12-18 mo may be subtle

No ↓

Child >18 mo of age without meningeal signs and with simple febrile seizure

Yes ↓

Do not routinely perform lumbar puncture, given that clinical signs of meningitis are more reliable in a child >18 mo of age → Child with simple febrile seizure

Was lumbar puncture performed? — Yes → Are lumbar puncture results abnormal? — Yes → Are findings consistent with bacterial meningitis? — Yes → Treat bacterial meningitis

Was lumbar puncture performed? — No → Child with simple febrile seizure

Are lumbar puncture results abnormal? — No → Child with simple febrile seizure

Are findings consistent with bacterial meningitis? — No → Evaluate and treat (if appropriate) other abnormal findings

Child with simple febrile seizure ↓

Is patient medically stable? — Yes → 1 Discharge patient to routine care
2 Educate parents concerning febrile seizure
3 Do not obtain follow-up EEG

No ↓

Hospitalize until medically stable

FIGURE 3-124 Guidelines for febrile seizure evaluation. (From Custer JW, Rau RE: *The Harriet Lane handbook,* ed 18, St Louis, 2009, Mosby.)

FEVER OF UNDETERMINED ORIGIN

ICD-9CM # 780.6 Pyrexia of undetermined origin

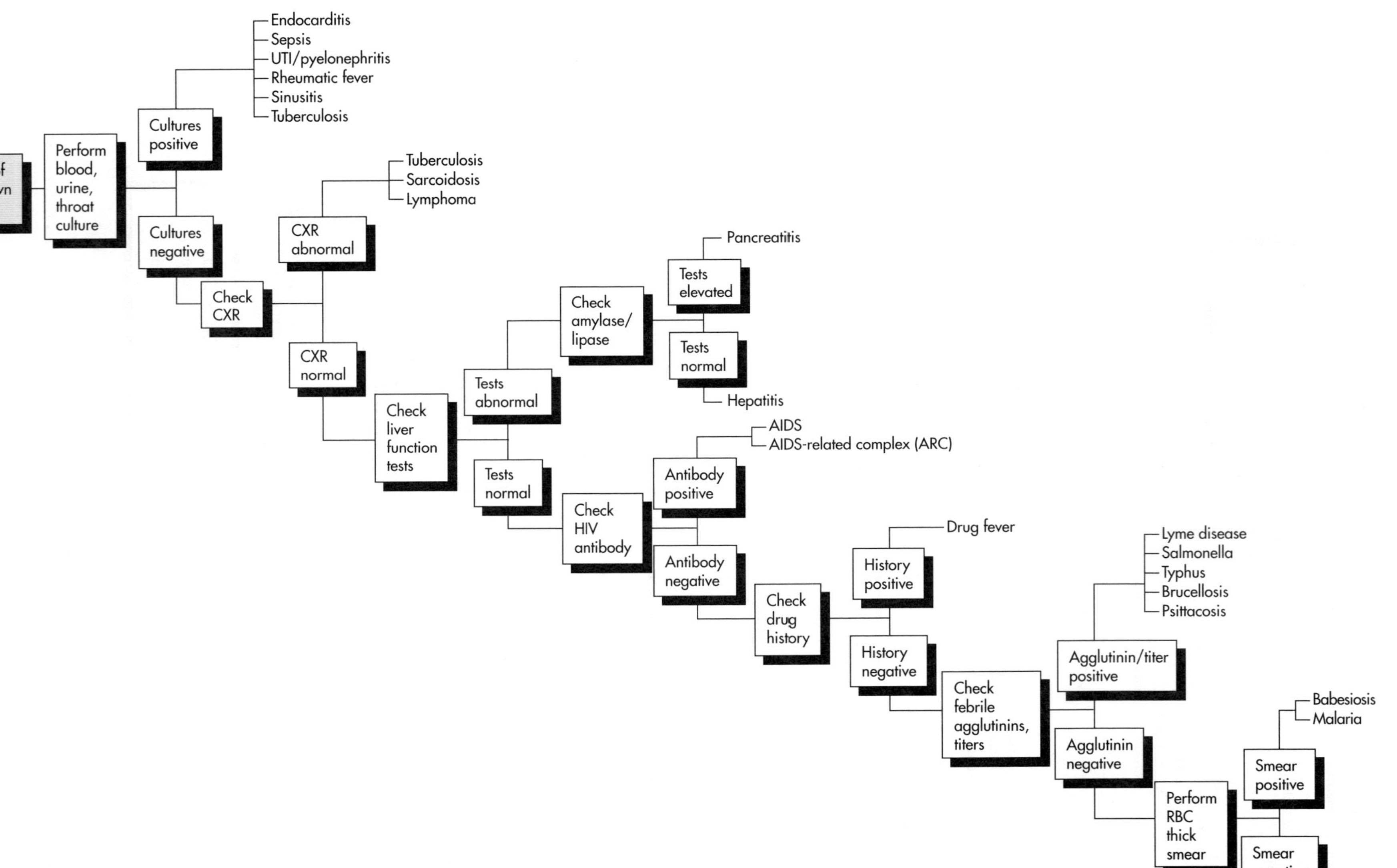

*Refer to Section I for additional information on this topic.

FIGURE 3-128 Approach to the patient with fever of undetermined origin. *AIDS,* Acquired immunodeficiency syndrome; *ANA,* antinuclear antibody; *CT,* computed tomography; *CSR,* chest x-ray; *ESR,* erythrocyte sedimentation rate; *GI,* gastrointestinal; *HIV,* human immunodeficiency virus; *RBC,* red blood cell; *UTI,* urinary tract infection. (Modified from Healey PM: *Common medical diagnosis: an algorithmic approach,* ed 3, Philadelphia, 2000, WB Saunders.)

FEVER OF UNDETERMINED ORIGIN—cont'd

ICD-9CM # 780.6 Pyrexia of undetermined origin

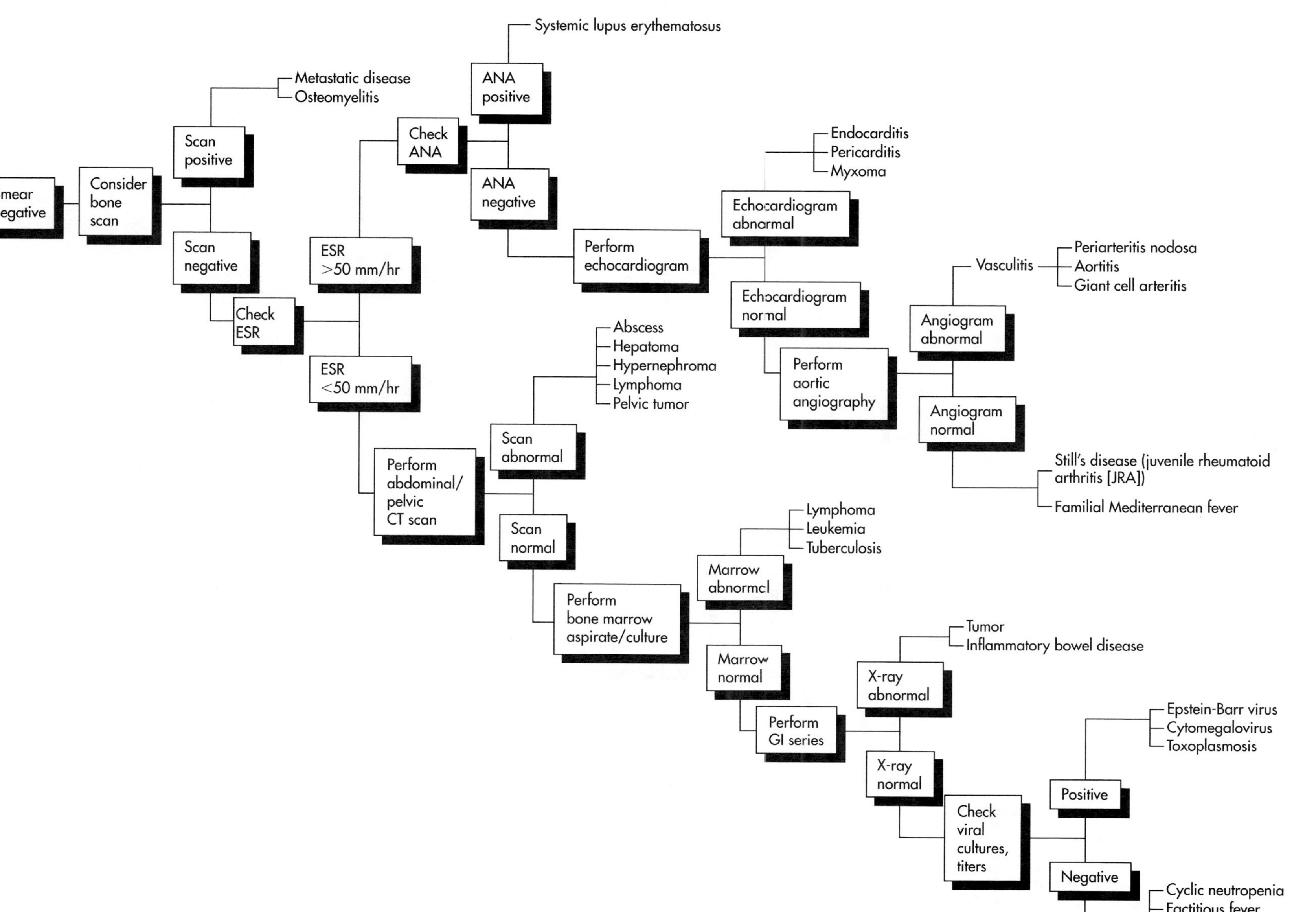

FIGURE 3-128 (Continued)

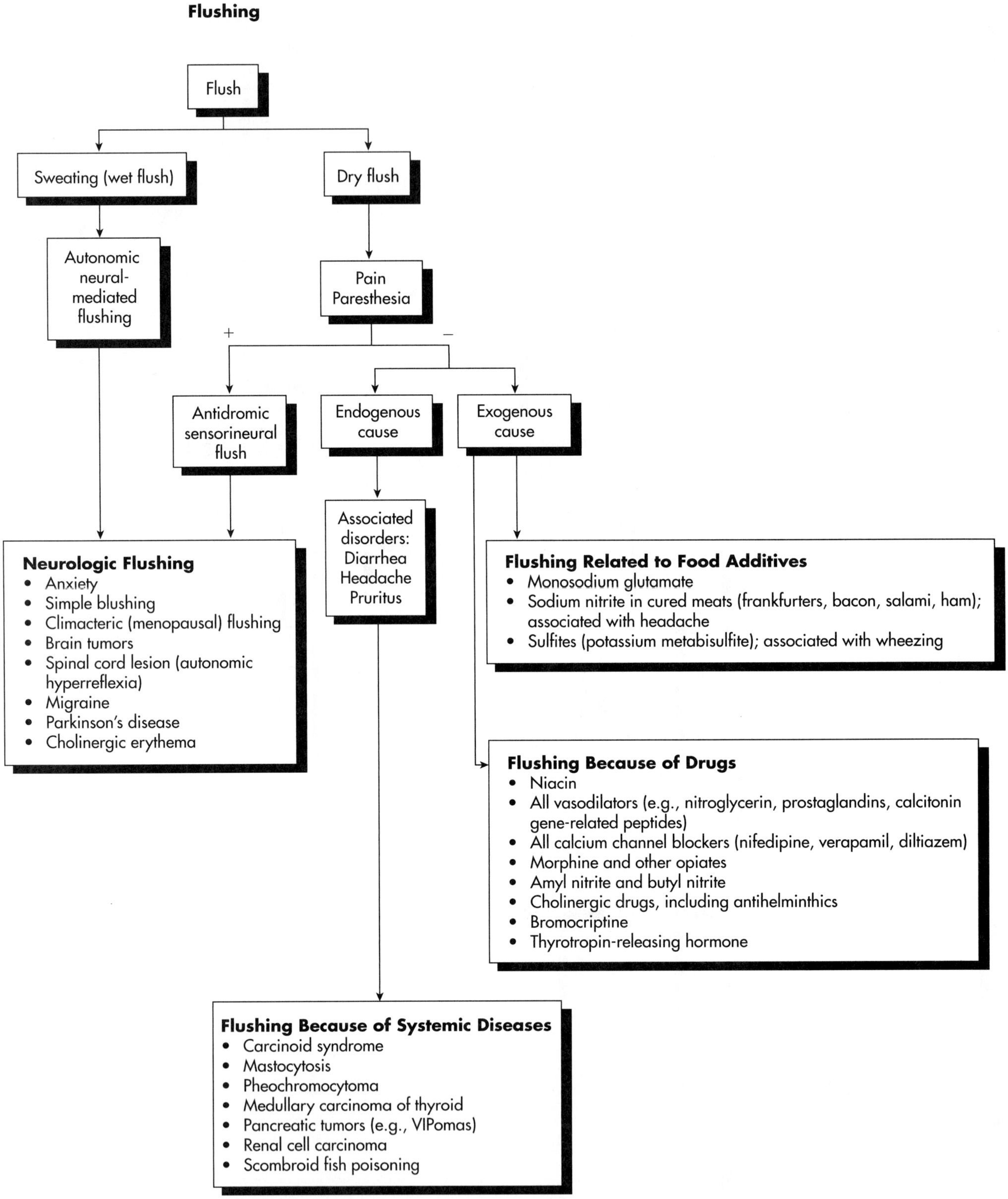

Flushing

Flush

Sweating (wet flush)

Dry flush

Autonomic neural-mediated flushing

Pain Paresthesia

+

−

Antidromic sensorineural flush

Endogenous cause

Exogenous cause

Associated disorders: Diarrhea Headache Pruritus

Neurologic Flushing
- Anxiety
- Simple blushing
- Climacteric (menopausal) flushing
- Brain tumors
- Spinal cord lesion (autonomic hyperreflexia)
- Migraine
- Parkinson's disease
- Cholinergic erythema

Flushing Related to Food Additives
- Monosodium glutamate
- Sodium nitrite in cured meats (frankfurters, bacon, salami, ham); associated with headache
- Sulfites (potassium metabisulfite); associated with wheezing

Flushing Because of Drugs
- Niacin
- All vasodilators (e.g., nitroglycerin, prostaglandins, calcitonin gene-related peptides)
- All calcium channel blockers (nifedipine, verapamil, diltiazem)
- Morphine and other opiates
- Amyl nitrite and butyl nitrite
- Cholinergic drugs, including antihelminthics
- Bromocriptine
- Thyrotropin-releasing hormone

Flushing Because of Systemic Diseases
- Carcinoid syndrome
- Mastocytosis
- Pheochromocytoma
- Medullary carcinoma of thyroid
- Pancreatic tumors (e.g., VIPomas)
- Renal cell carcinoma
- Scombroid fish poisoning

FIGURE 3-130 Evaluation of patients with flushing. (From Bolognia JL et al [eds]: *Dermatology,* ed 2, St Louis, 2008, Mosby.)

ICD-9CM # 054.10 Genital herpes
91.0 Genital syphilis
078.11 Condyloma acuminatum
099.0 Chancroid
099.2 Granuloma inguinale
099.1 Lymphogranuloma venereum
629.8 Ulcer, genital site, female
608.89 Ulcer, genital site, male

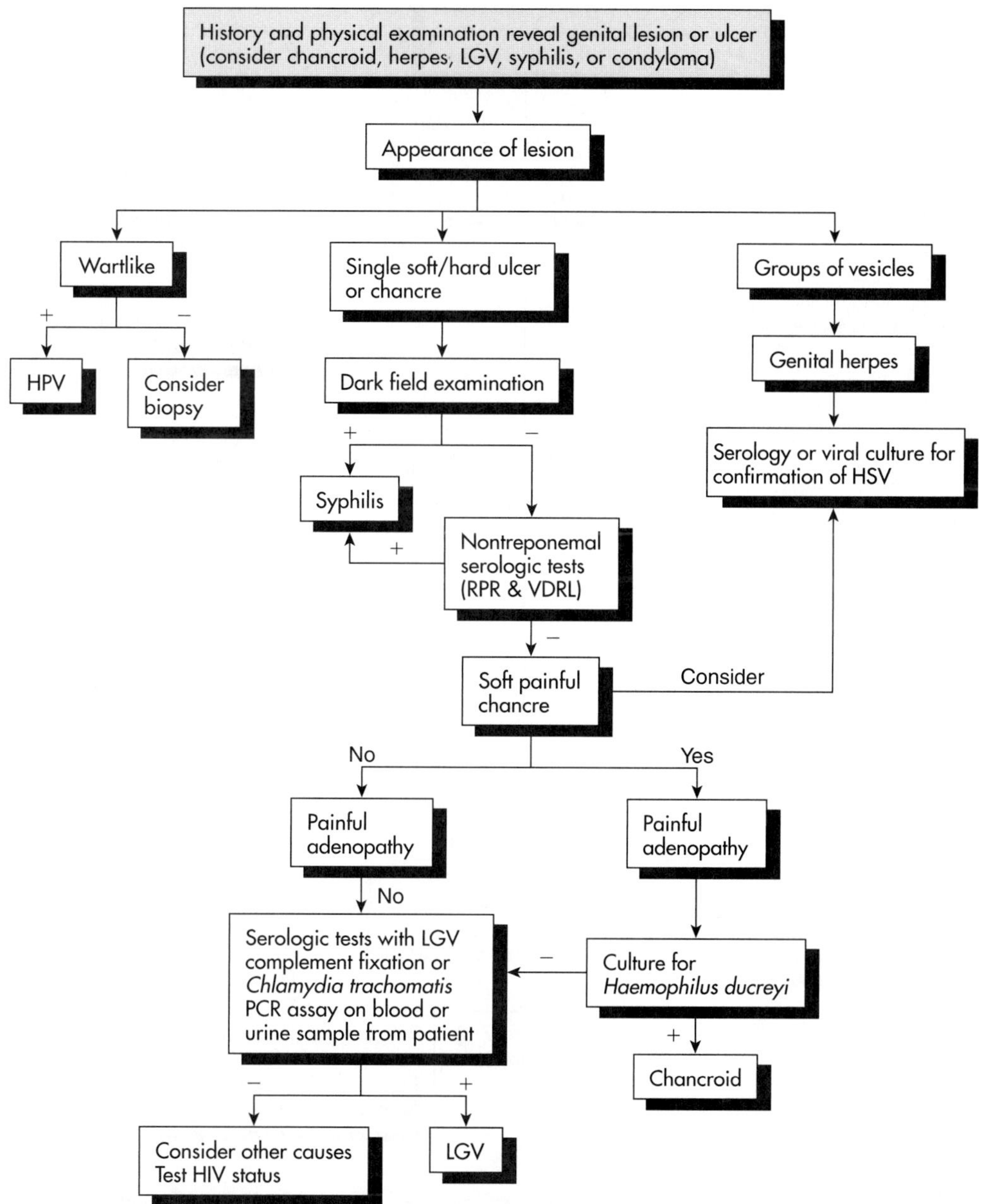

FIGURE 3-132 Evaluation of patients with genital lesions or ulcers. *HIV,* Human immunodeficiency virus; *HPV,* human papillomavirus; *HSV,* herpes simplex virus; *LGV,* lymphogranuloma venereum; *RPR,* rapid plasma reagin; *VDRL,* Venereal Disease Research Laboratory. (Modified from Nseyo UO [ed]: *Urology for primary care physicians,* Philadelphia, 1999, WB Saunders.)

GOITER EVALUATION AND MANAGEMENT

ICD-9CM # 240.9 Goiter, unspecified
240.0 Goiter, simple
241.9 Goiter, adenomatous
246.1 Goiter, congenital
242.1 Goiter, uninodular with thyrotoxicosos
242.2 Goiter, multinodular with thyrotoxicosos

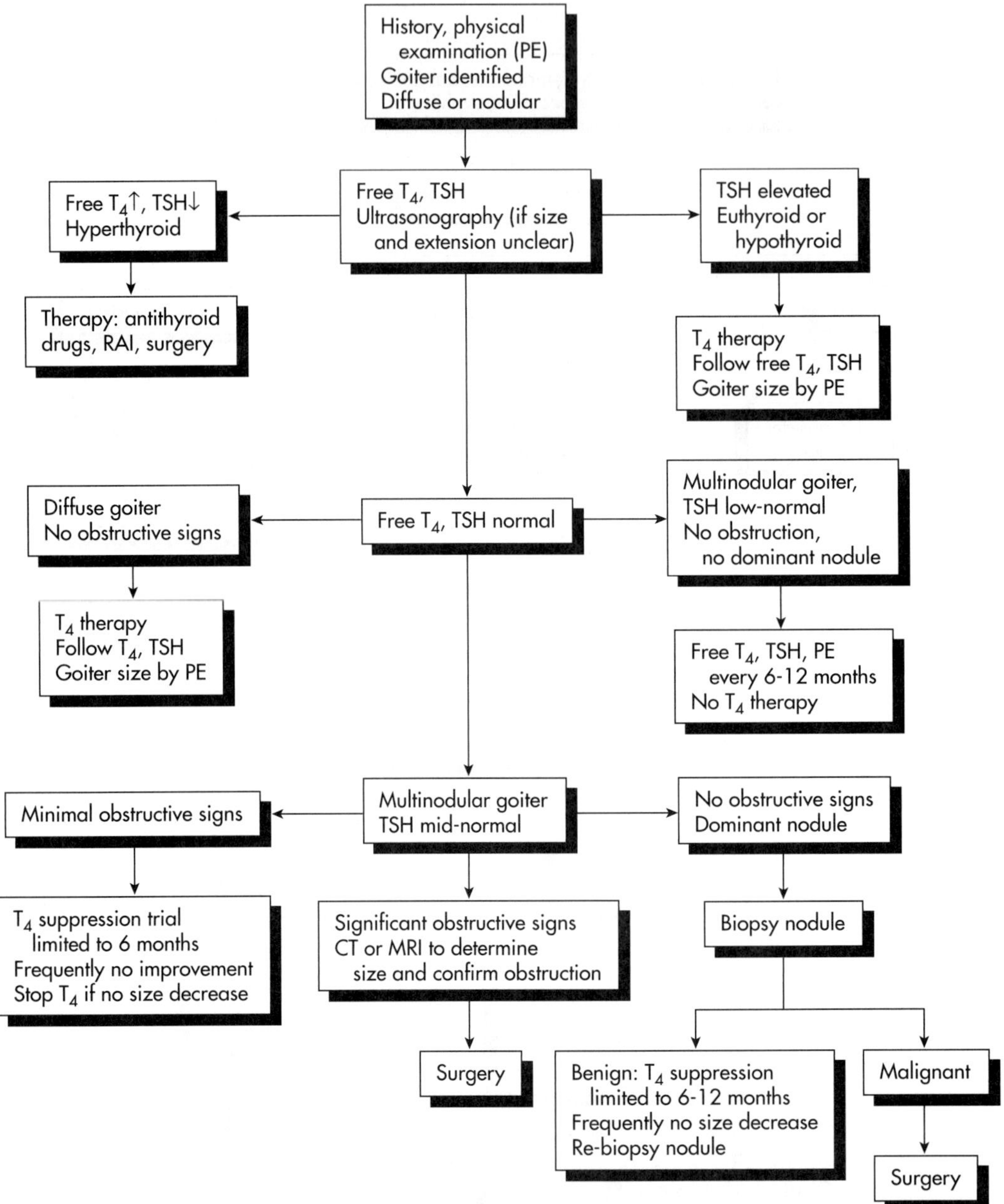

FIGURE 3-135 Evaluation and management of patients with nontoxic diffuse and nodular goiter and undetermined thyroid status. *CT,* Computed tomography; *MRI,* magnetic resonance imaging; *RAI,* radioactive iodine; *TSH,* thyroid-stimulating hormone. (From Goldman L, Ausiello D [eds]: *Cecil textbook of medicine,* ed 23, Philadelphia, 2008, WB Saunders.)

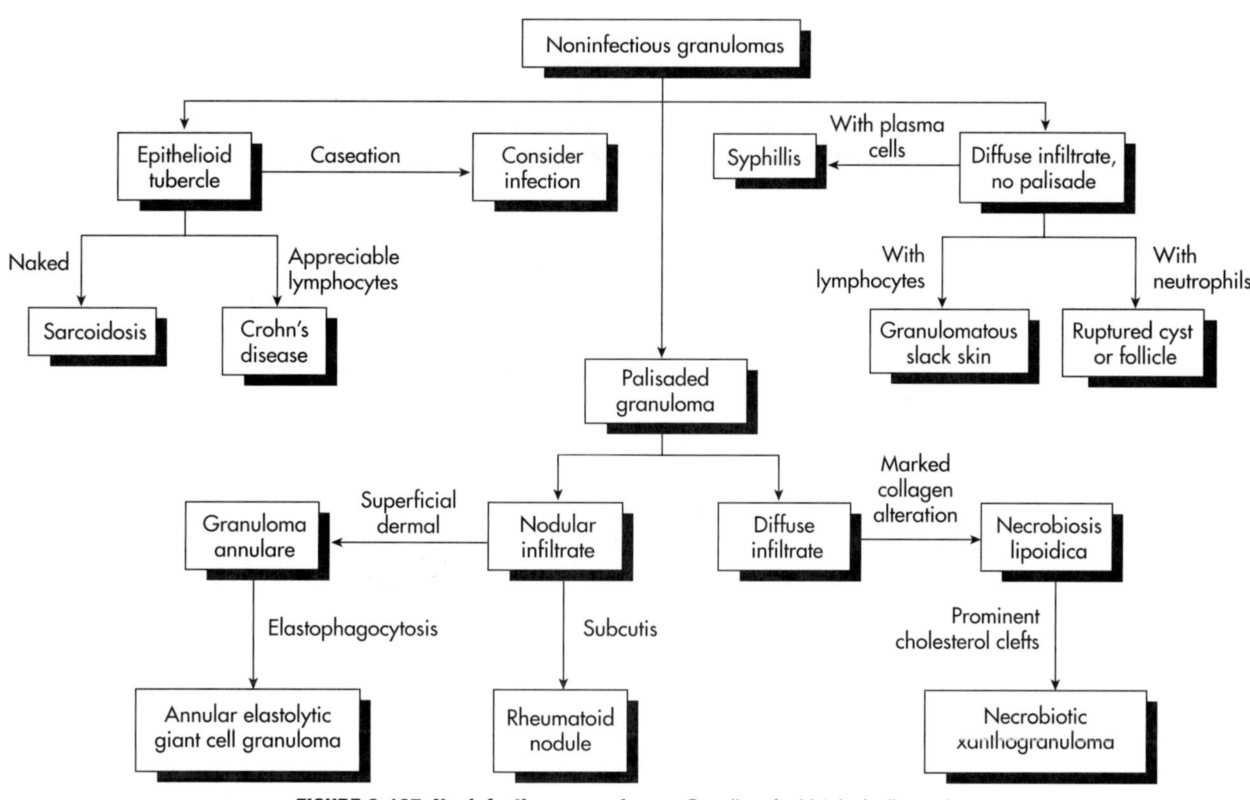

FIGURE 3-137 Noninfectious granulomas. Paradigm for histologic diagnosis.

TABLE 3-15 Clinical Features of the Major Granulomatous Dermatitides

	Sarcoidosis	Classic GA*	NLD	AEGCG	Crohn's Disease	Rheumatoid Nodule
Average age (years)	25-35, 45-65	<30		40	35	30-40
Sex	Female	Female	Female	Female	Female	Female
Racial predilection in United States	African American	None	None	Caucasian	None	None
Site	Symmetric on face, neck, upper trunk, extremities	Hands, feet, extremities	Anterior and lateral distal lower extremities	Face, neck, forearms	Genital areas, lower > upper extremities	Juxtaarticular areas, elbows, hands, ankles, feet
Appearance	Red to red-brown papules and plaques	Papules coalescing into annular plaques	Plaques with elevated borders, telangiectasias centrally	Annular plaques	Dusky erythema and swelling, ulceration	Skin-colored, firm, mobile subcutaneous nodules
Size of lesions	1-5 cm	1-2 mm papules, <5 cm annular plaques	>10 cm	1-6 cm	Variable	1-3 cm
Number of lesions	Variable	1-10	1-10	1-10	1-5	1-10
Associations	Systemic manifestations of sarcoidosis	Rare diabetes mellitus, malignancy	Diabetes mellitus	Actinic damage	Intestinal Crohn's disease	Rheumatoid arthritis
Special clinical characteristics	Occasional central atrophy and hypopigmentation	Central hyperpigmentation	Yellow-brown atrophic centers, ulceration	Central atrophy and hypopigmentation	Draining sinuses and fistulae	Occasional ulceration, especially at site of trauma

From Bolognia JL et al: *Dermatology,* ed 2, St Louis, 2008, Mosby.
AEGCG, Annular elastolytic giant cell granuloma; *GA,* granuloma annulare; *NLD,* necrobiosis lipoidica diabeticorum.
*Clinical variants include generalized, micropapular, nodular, perforating, subcutaneous, and patch GA.

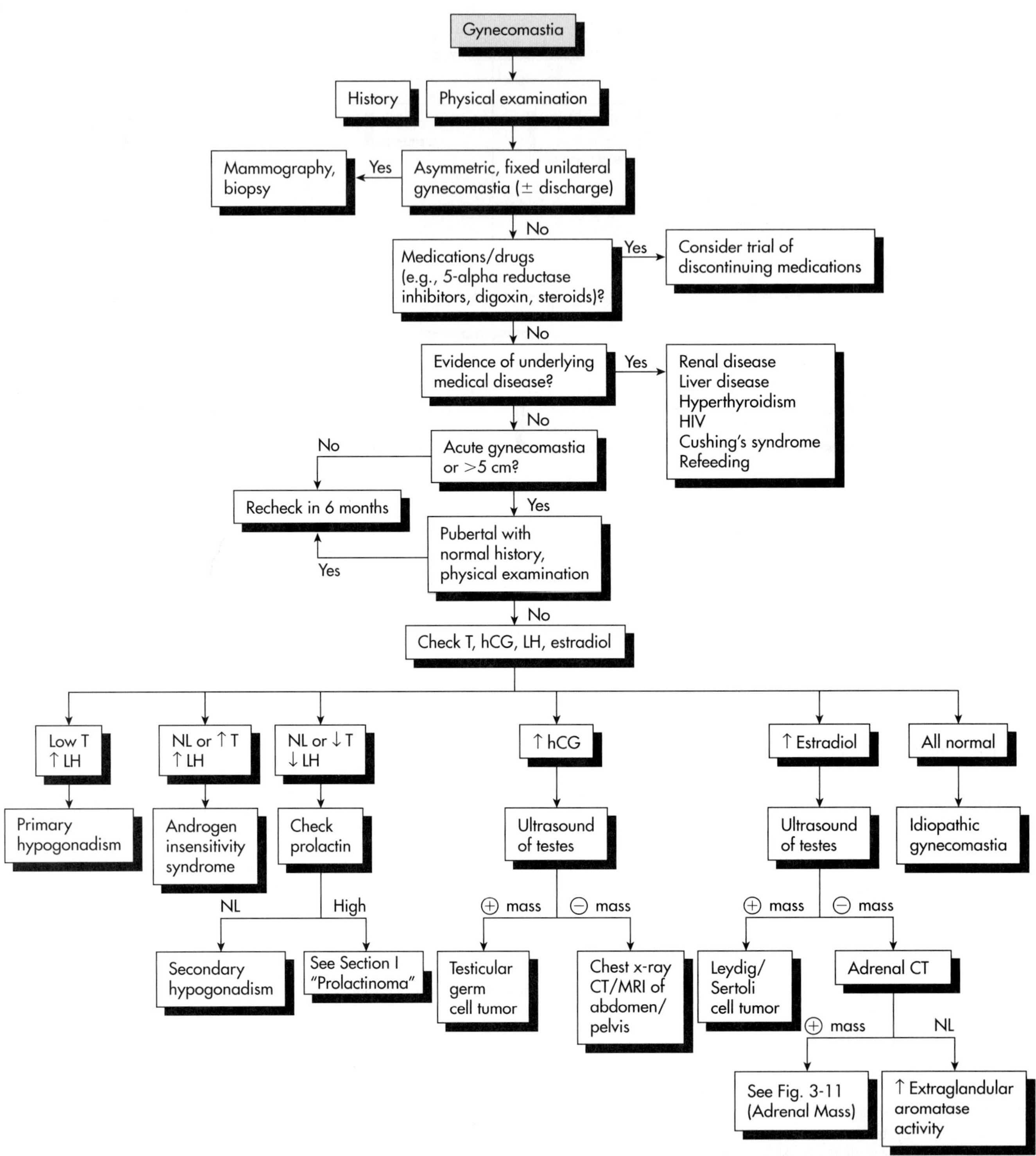

FIGURE 3-138 Evaluation of gynecomastia. *CT,* Computed tomography; *hCG,* human chorionic gonadotropin; *HIV,* human immunodeficiency syndrome; *LH,* luteinizing hormone; *MRI,* magnetic resonance imaging; *NL,* normal limits; *T,* testosterone. (Modified from Noble J: *Primary care medicine,* ed 3, St Louis, 2001, Mosby.)

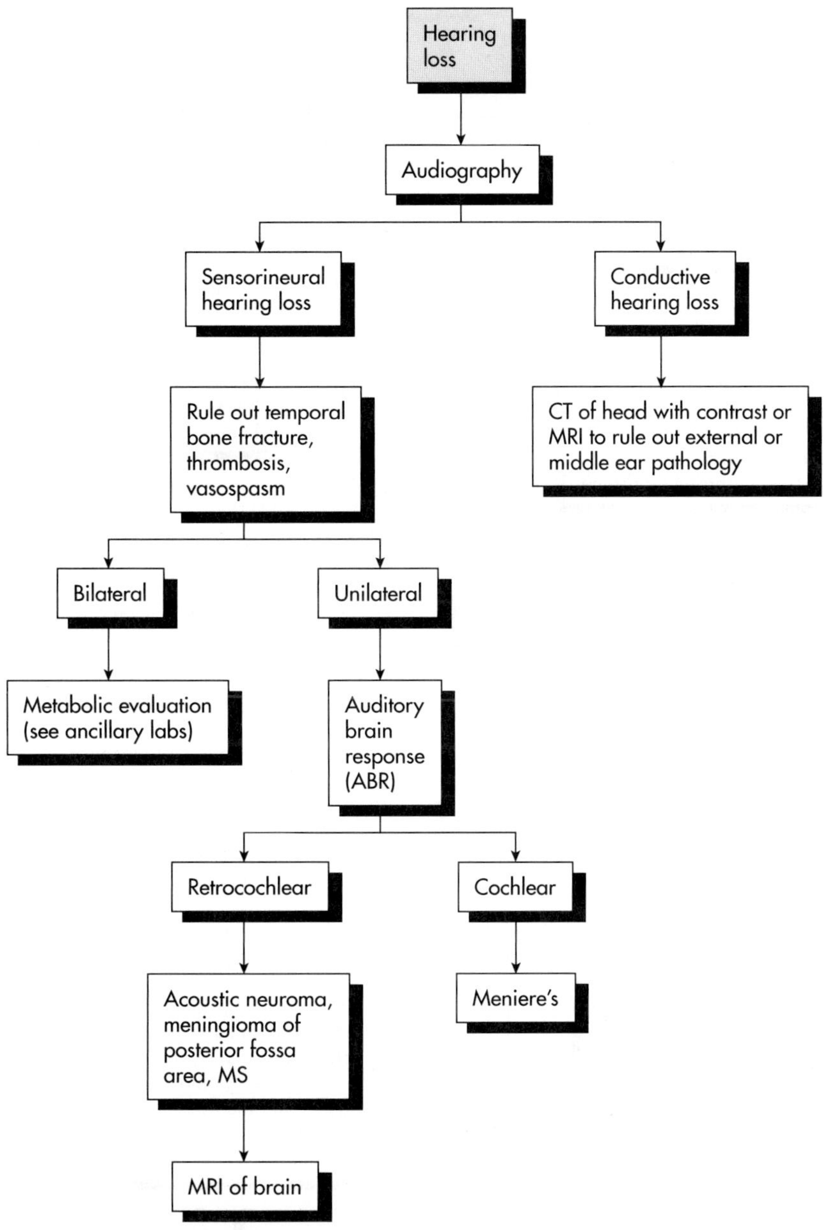

FIGURE 3-139 Evaluation of hearing loss. *CT,* Computed tomography; *MRI,* magnetic resonance imaging. (From Ferri FF: *Ferri's best test: a practical guide to clinical laboratory medicine and diagnostic imaging,* ed 2, Philadelphia, 2009, Elsevier Mosby.)

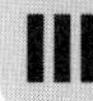

BOX 3-7 Hearing Loss

Diagnostic imaging	Lab evaluation
Best test	***Best test***
None	None
Ancillary tests	***Ancillary tests***
CT of head with contrast or MRI with contrast	CBC
CT of temporal bone without contrast	ALT, AST
	ANA, VDRL
	TSH

From Ferri FF: *Ferri's best test: a practical guide to clinical laboratory medicine and diagnostic imaging,* ed 2, Philadelphia, 2009, Elsevier Mosby.

ALT, Alanine aminotransferase; *ANA,* antibody to nuclear antigens; *AST,* angiotensin sensitivity test; *CBC,* complete blood count; *CT,* computed tomography; *TSH,* thyroid-stimulating hormone; *VDRL,* Venereal Disease Research Laboratory test.

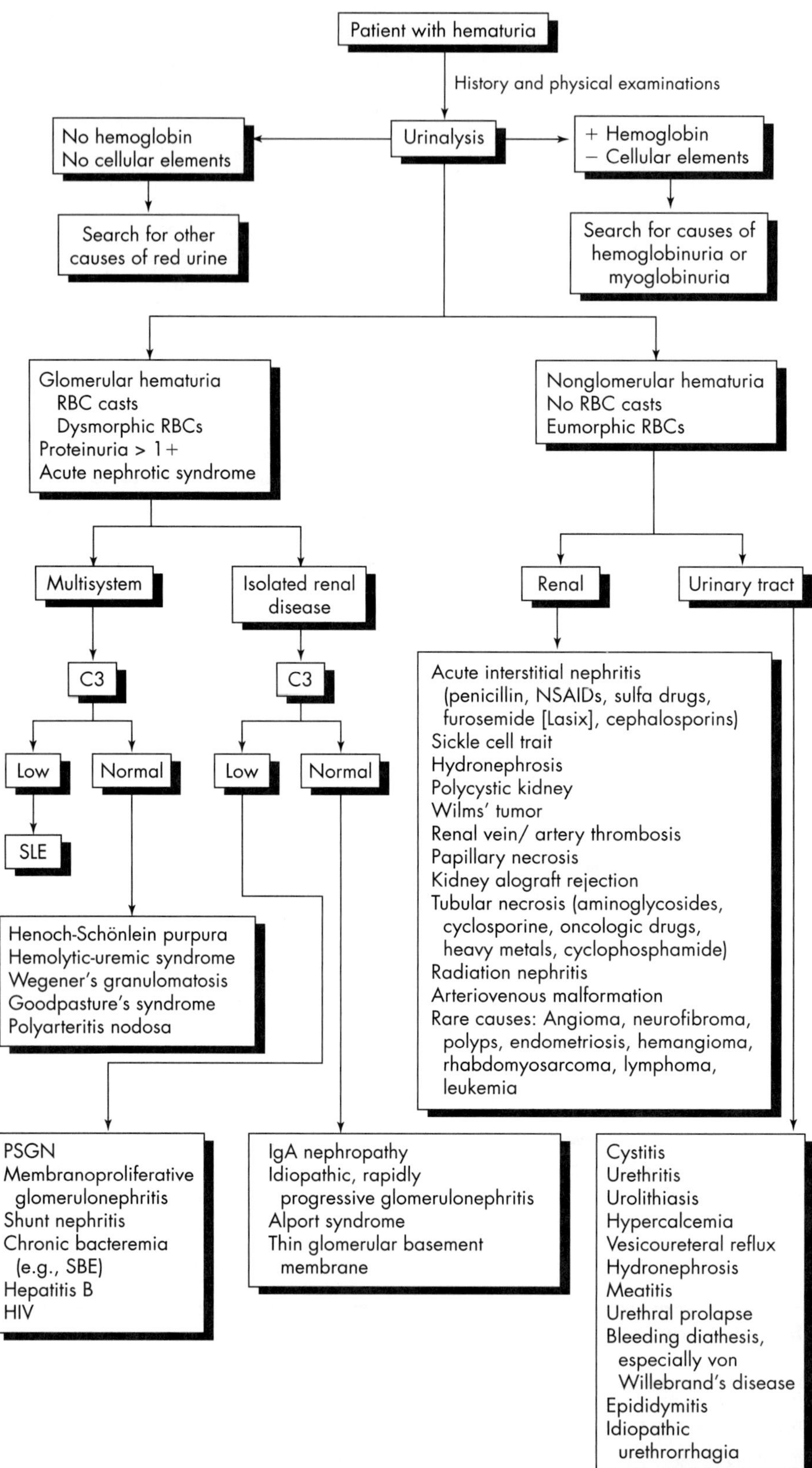

FIGURE 3-142 A diagnostic strategy for hematuria. *HIV,* Human immunodeficiency virus; *NSAIDs,* nonsteroidal anti-inflammatory drugs; *PSGN,* poststreptococcal glomerulonephritis; *RBC,* red blood cell; *SBE,* subacute bacterial endocarditis; *SLE,* systemic lupus erythematosus. (From Custer JW, Rau RE: *The Harriet Lane handbook,* ed 18, St Louis, 2009, Mosby.)

HEMOPTYSIS

ICD-9CM # 786.3

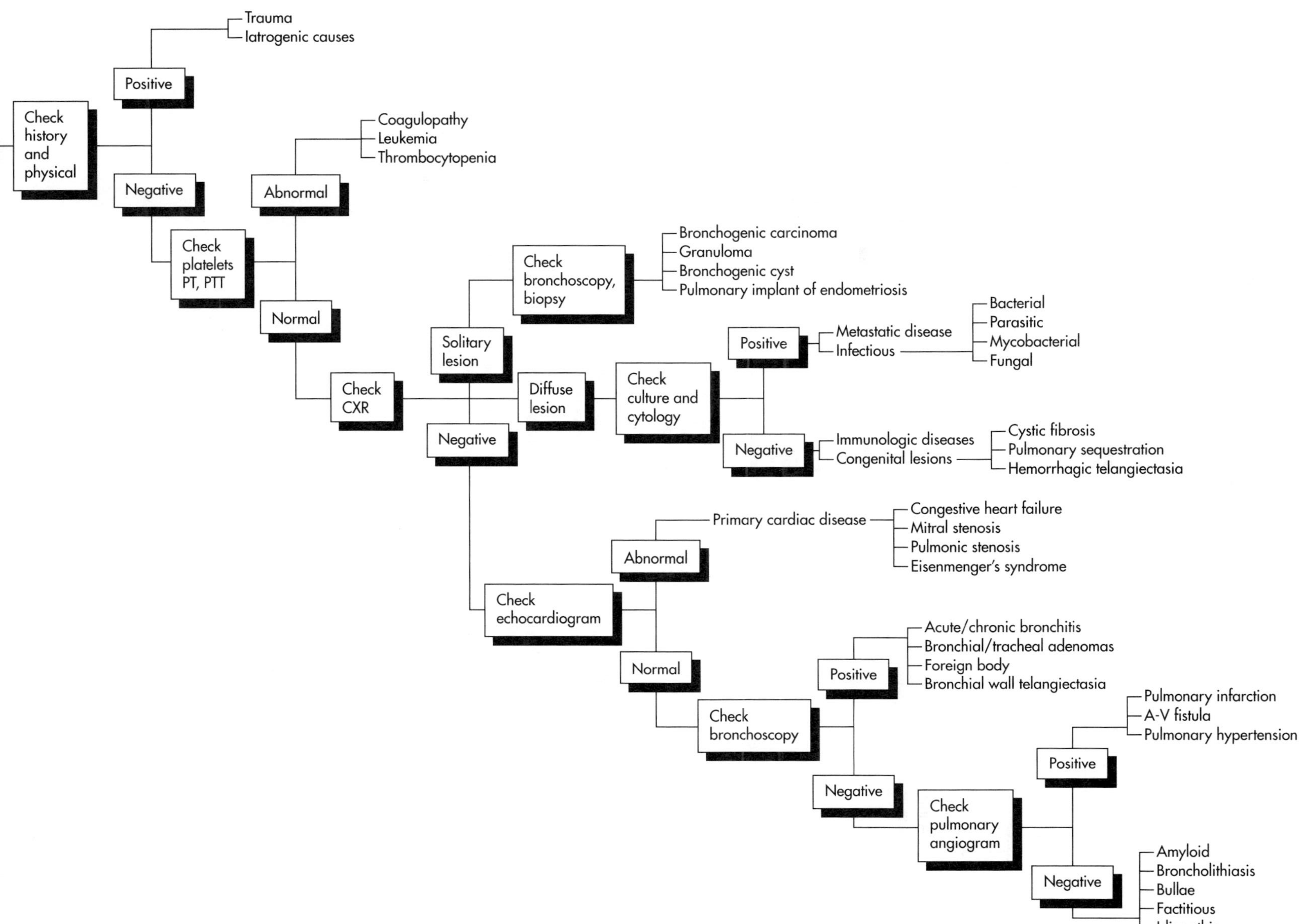

FIGURE 3-144 Evaluation of hemoptysis. *A-V,* Arteriovenous; *CXR,* chest x-ray; *PT,* prothrombin time; *PTT,* partial thromboplastin time. (From Healey PM: *Common medical diagnosis: an algorithmic approach,* ed 3, Philadelphia, 2000, WB Saunders.)

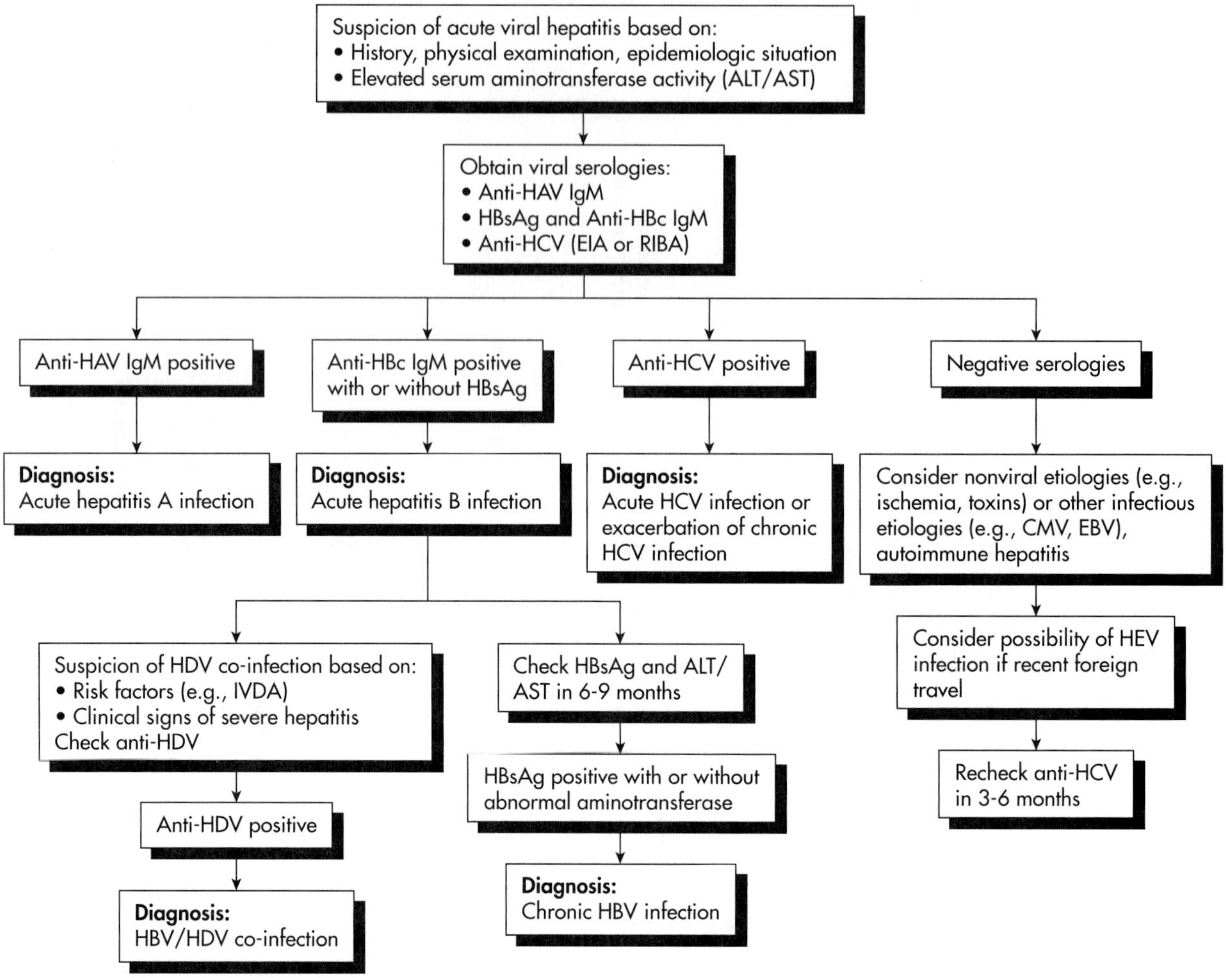

Suspicion of acute viral hepatitis based on:
• History, physical examination, epidemiologic situation
• Elevated serum aminotransferase activity (ALT/AST)

Obtain viral serologies:
• Anti-HAV IgM
• HBsAg and Anti-HBc IgM
• Anti-HCV (EIA or RIBA)

Anti-HAV IgM positive

Diagnosis:
Acute hepatitis A infection

Anti-HBc IgM positive with or without HBsAg

Diagnosis:
Acute hepatitis B infection

Suspicion of HDV co-infection based on:
• Risk factors (e.g., IVDA)
• Clinical signs of severe hepatitis
Check anti-HDV

Anti-HDV positive

Diagnosis:
HBV/HDV co-infection

Check HBsAg and ALT/AST in 6-9 months

HBsAg positive with or without abnormal aminotransferase

Diagnosis:
Chronic HBV infection

Anti-HCV positive

Diagnosis:
Acute HCV infection or exacerbation of chronic HCV infection

Negative serologies

Consider nonviral etiologies (e.g., ischemia, toxins) or other infectious etiologies (e.g., CMV, EBV), autoimmune hepatitis

Consider possibility of HEV infection if recent foreign travel

Recheck anti-HCV in 3-6 months

FIGURE 3-146 A flow diagram showing the use of specific serologic tests for the diagnosis of acute viral hepatitis in relation to the clinical and epidemiologic setting. Co-infections and superinfections of chronic hepatitis B or C patients should always be considered in cases that do not fit well with the clinical or serologic picture. *CMV,* Cytomegalovirus; *EBV,* Epstein-Barr virus; *EIA,* enzyme immunoassay; *HBV,* hepatitis B virus; *HCV,* hepatitis C virus; *HDV,* hepatitis D virus; *HEV,* hepatoencephalomyelitis virus; *IVDA,* intravenous drug abuse; *RIBA,* recombinant immunoblot assay. (Modified from Mandell GL: *Mandell, Douglas, and Bennett's principles and practice of infectious diseases,* ed 6, New York, 2005, Churchill Livingstone.)

HEPATOMEGALY

ICD-9CM # 789.1

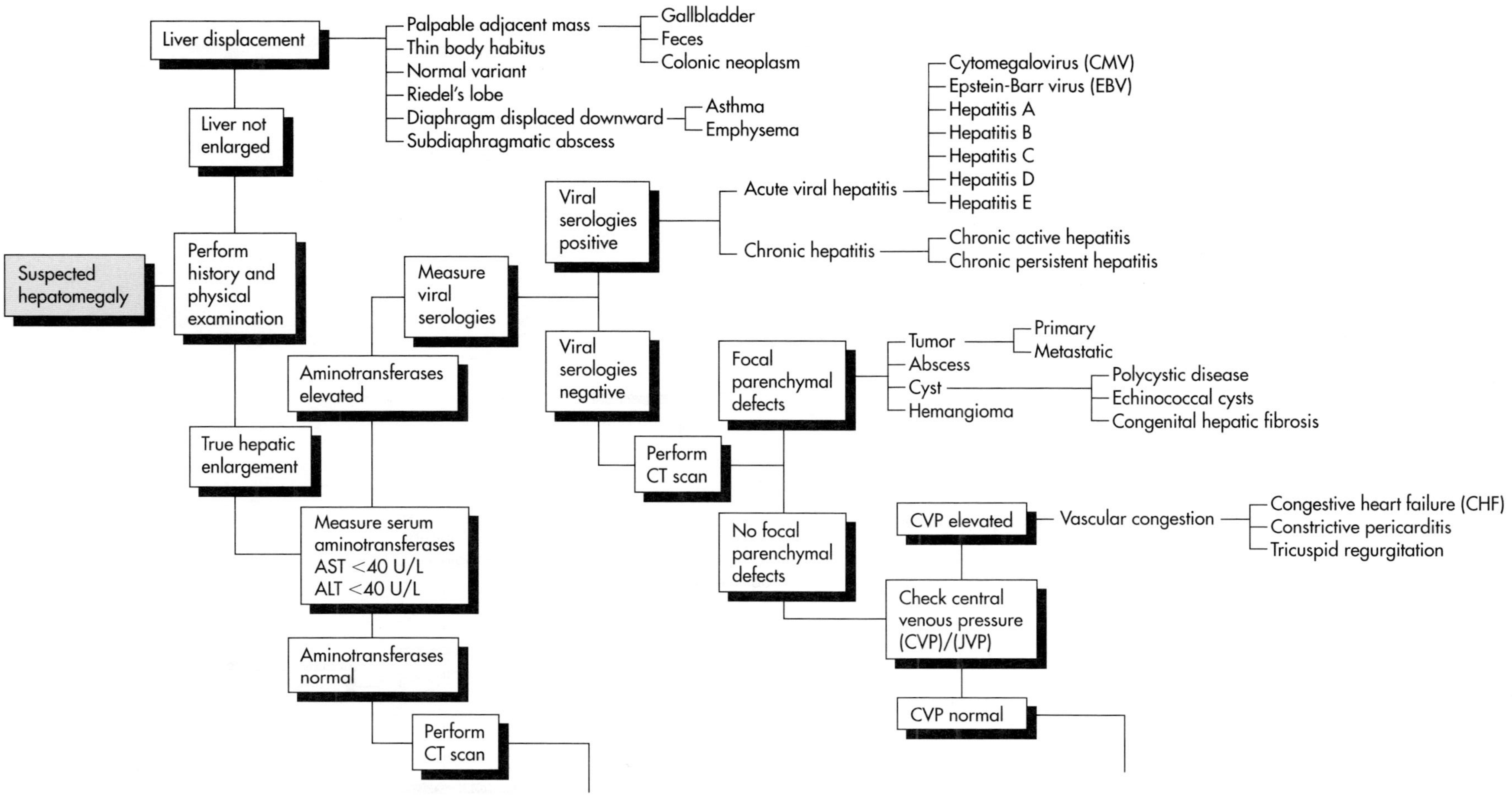

- Suspected hepatomegaly
  - Perform history and physical examination
    - Liver not enlarged
      - Liver displacement
        - Palpable adjacent mass
          - Gallbladder
          - Feces
          - Colonic neoplasm
        - Thin body habitus
        - Normal variant
        - Riedel's lobe
        - Diaphragm displaced downward
          - Asthma
          - Emphysema
        - Subdiaphragmatic abscess
    - True hepatic enlargement
      - Measure serum aminotransferases AST <40 U/L ALT <40 U/L
        - Aminotransferases elevated
          - Measure viral serologies
            - Viral serologies positive
              - Acute viral hepatitis
                - Cytomegalovirus (CMV)
                - Epstein-Barr virus (EBV)
                - Hepatitis A
                - Hepatitis B
                - Hepatitis C
                - Hepatitis D
                - Hepatitis E
              - Chronic hepatitis
                - Chronic active hepatitis
                - Chronic persistent hepatitis
            - Viral serologies negative
              - Perform CT scan
                - Focal parenchymal defects
                  - Tumor
                    - Primary
                    - Metastatic
                  - Abscess
                  - Cyst
                    - Polycystic disease
                    - Echinococcal cysts
                    - Congenital hepatic fibrosis
                  - Hemangioma
                - No focal parenchymal defects
                  - Check central venous pressure (CVP)/(JVP)
                    - CVP elevated
                      - Vascular congestion
                        - Congestive heart failure (CHF)
                        - Constrictive pericarditis
                        - Tricuspid regurgitation
                    - CVP normal
        - Aminotransferases normal
          - Perform CT scan

FIGURE 3-147 Hepatomegaly. *ALT,* Alanine aminotransferase; *AST,* aspartate aminotransferase; *CT,* computed tomography; *JVP,* jugular venous pressure. (Modified from Healey PM: *Common medical diagnosis: an algorithmic approach,* ed 3, Philadelphia, 2000, WB Saunders.)

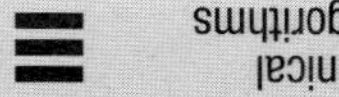

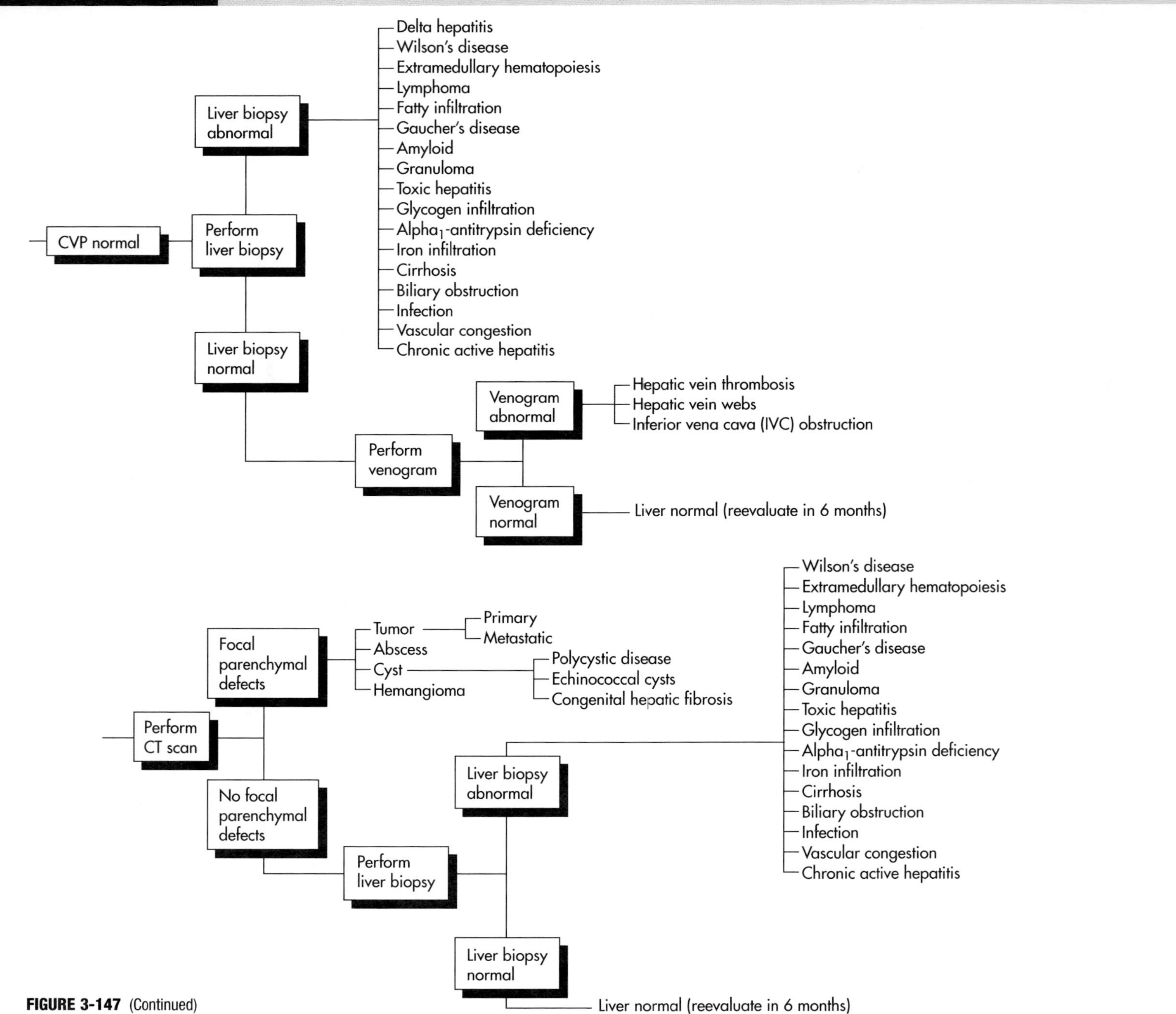

FIGURE 3-147 (Continued)

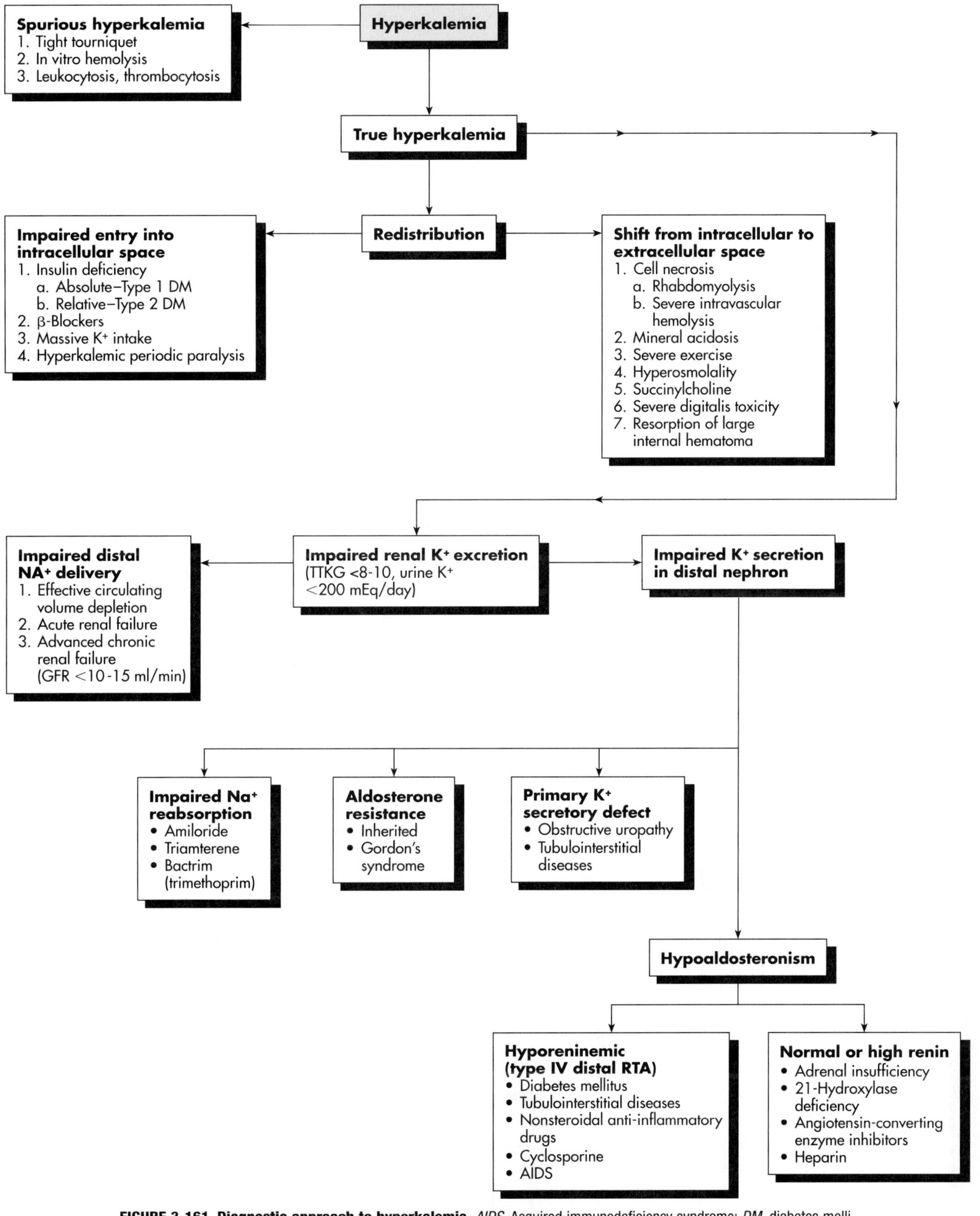

FIGURE 3-161 Diagnostic approach to hyperkalemia. *AIDS,* Acquired immunodeficiency syndrome; *DM,* diabetes mellitus; *GFR,* glomerular filtration rate; *RTA,* renal tubular acidosis; *TTKG,* transtubular potassium gradient. (From Andreoli TE [ed]: *Cecil essentials of medicine,* ed 7, Philadelphia, 2008, WB Saunders.)

HYPERMAGNESEMIA

ICD-9CM # 275.2

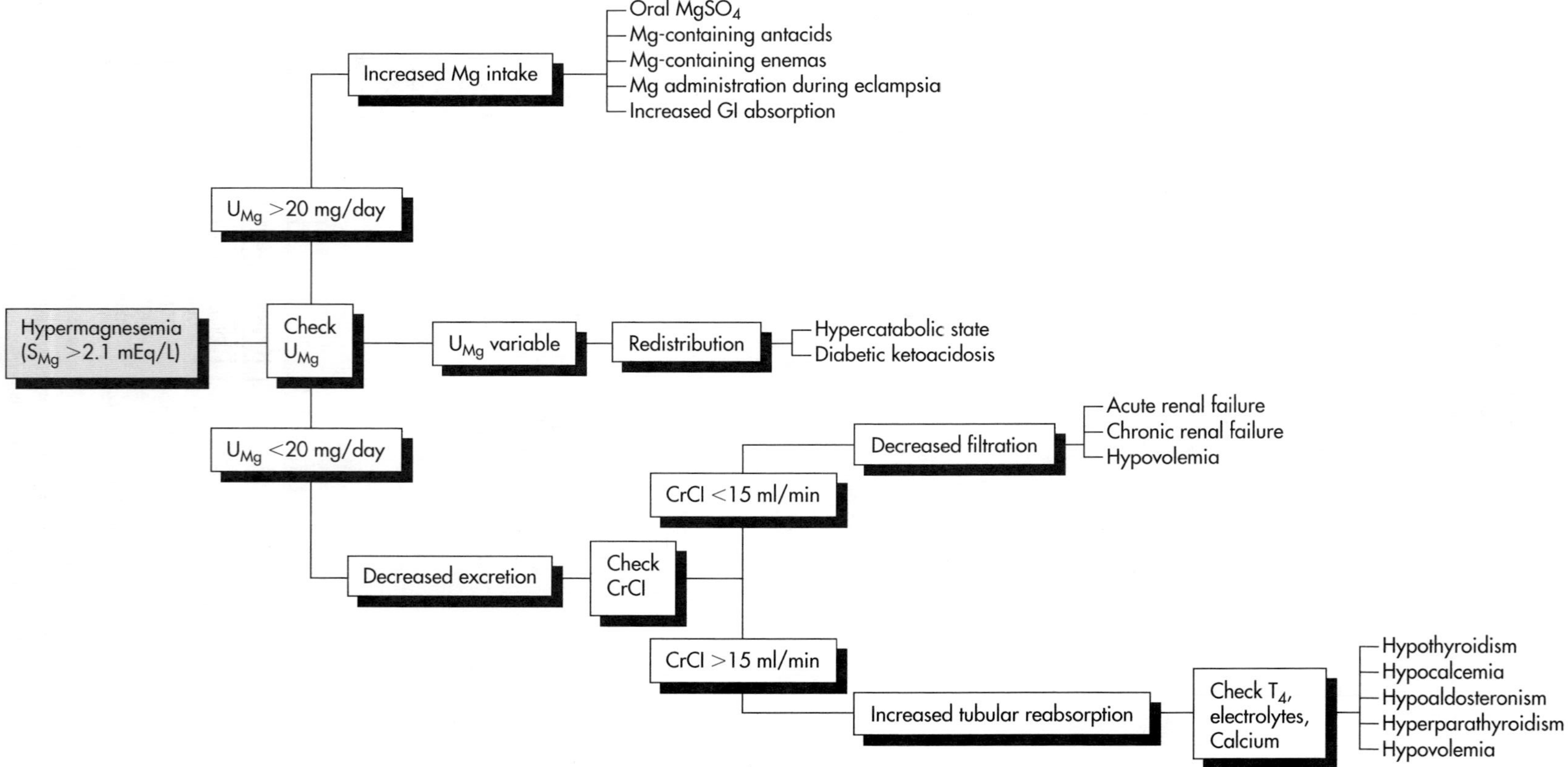

FIGURE 3-164 Hypermagnesemia. *CrCl,* Creatinine clearance; *GI,* gastrointestinal; *MgSO,* magnesium sulfate. (From Healey PM: *Common medical diagnosis: an algorithmic approach,* ed 3, Philadelphia, 2000, WB Saunders.)

HYPERNATREMIA

ICD-9CM # 276.0

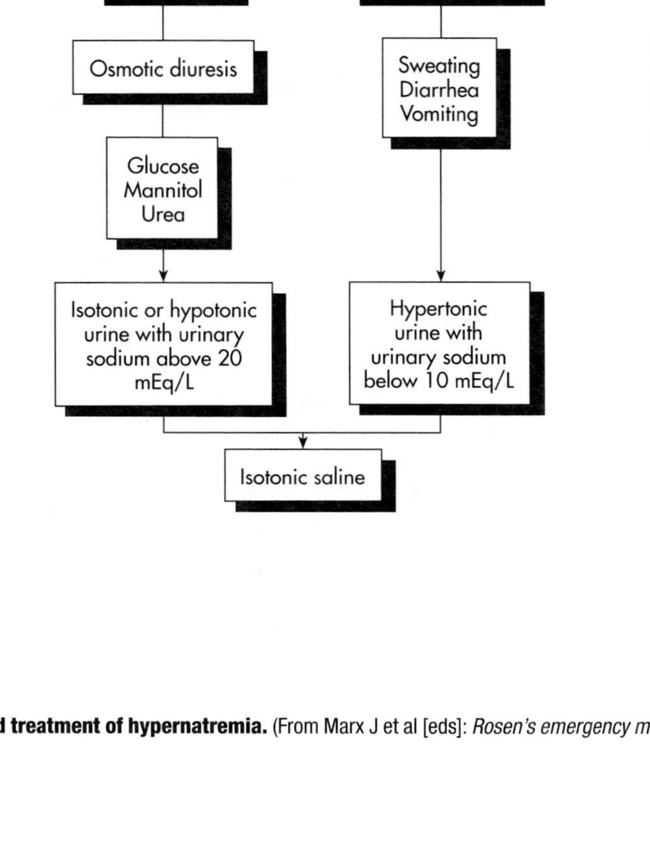

FIGURE 3-165 Evaluation and treatment of hypernatremia. (From Marx J et al [eds]: *Rosen's emergency medicine: concepts and clinical practice,* ed 6, St Louis, 2006, Mosby.)

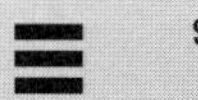
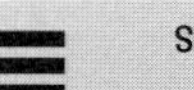

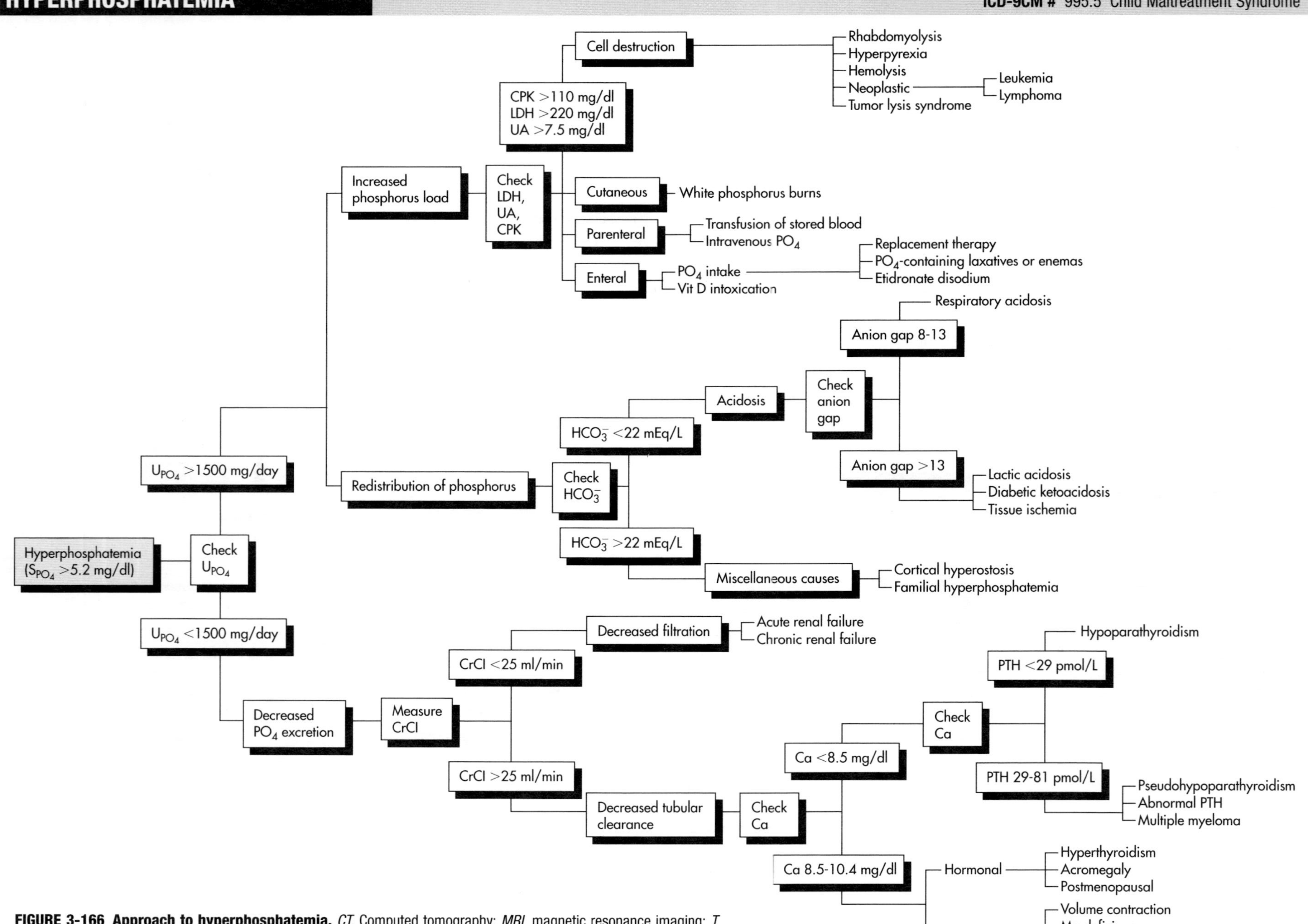

FIGURE 3-166 Approach to hyperphosphatemia. *CT,* Computed tomography; *MRI,* magnetic resonance imaging; *T,* thyroxine; *TSH,* thyroid-stimulating hormone. (From Healey PM: *Common medical diagnosis: an algorithmic approach,* ed 3, Philadelphia, 2000, WB Saunders.)

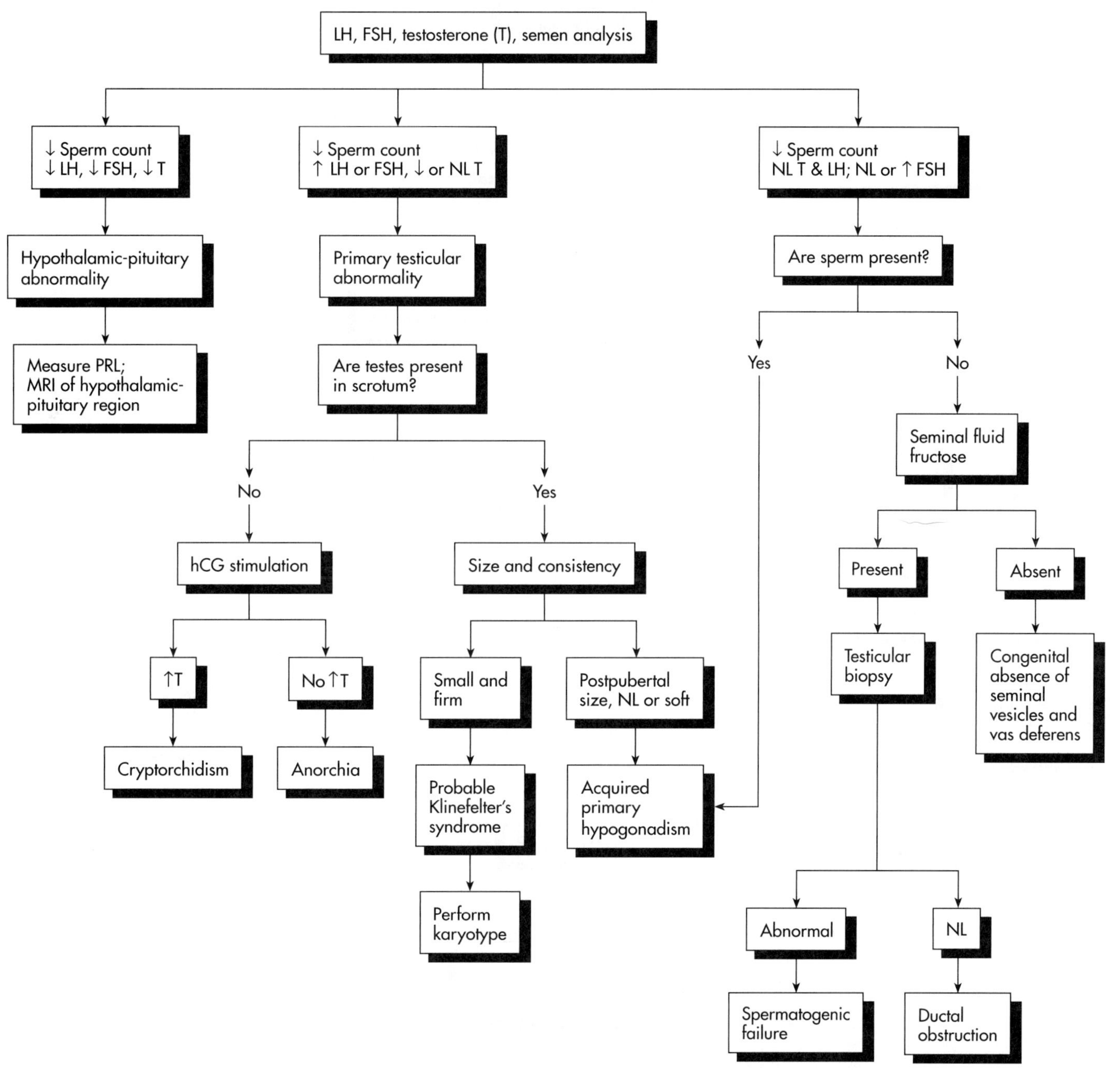

FIGURE 3-177 Laboratory evaluation of hypogonadism. *FSH,* Follicle-stimulating hormone; *hCG,* human chorionic gonadotropin; *LH,* luteinizing hormone; *MRI,* magnetic resonance imaging; *NL,* normal; *PRL,* prolactin; ↑, elevated; ↓, decreased or low. (From Andreoli TE [ed]: *Cecil essentials of medicine*, ed 7, Philadelphia, 2008, WB Saunders.)

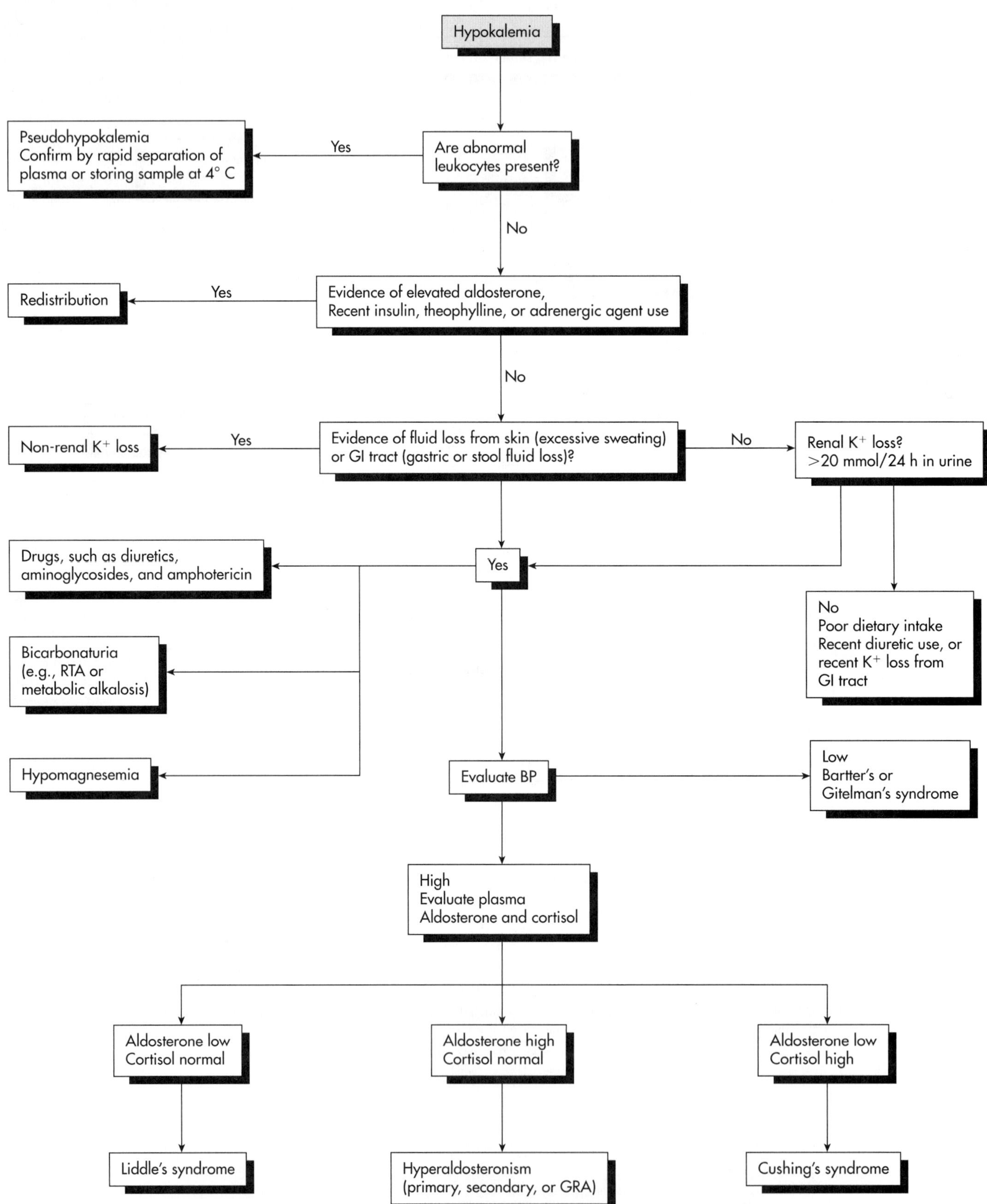

FIGURE 3-178 Diagnostic evaluation of hypokalemia. *BP,* Blood pressure; *GI,* gastrointestinal; *GRA,* glucose remediable aldosteronism; *RTA,* renal tubular acidosis. (From Feehally J, Floege J, Johnson RJ: *Comprehensive clinical nephrology,* ed 3, St Louis, 2007, Mosby.)

HYPOMAGNESEMIA

ICD-9CM # 275.2

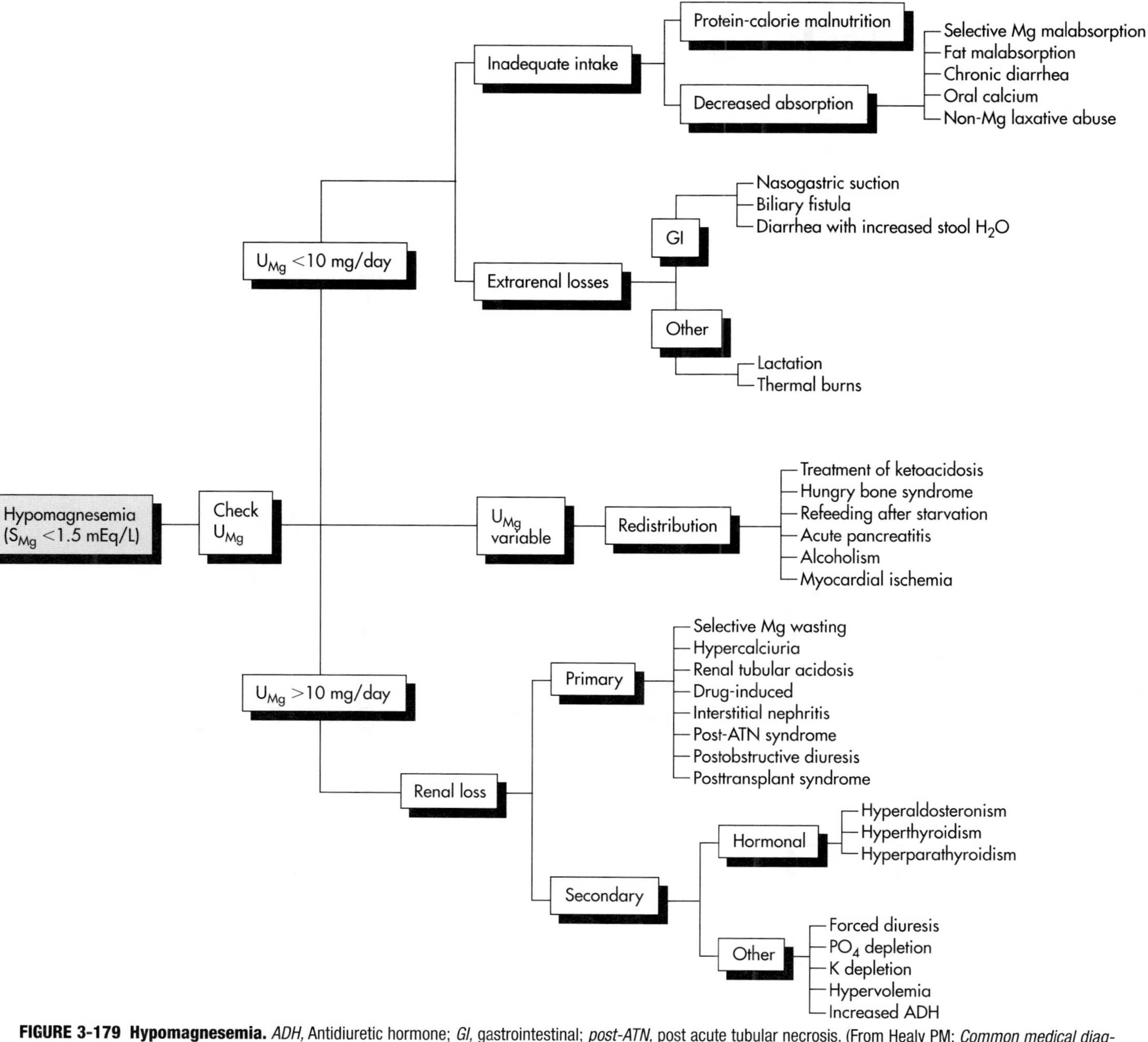

FIGURE 3-179 Hypomagnesemia. *ADH,* Antidiuretic hormone; *GI,* gastrointestinal; *post-ATN,* post acute tubular necrosis. (From Healy PM: *Common medical diagnosis: an algorithmic approach,* ed 3, Philadelphia, 2000, WB Saunders.)

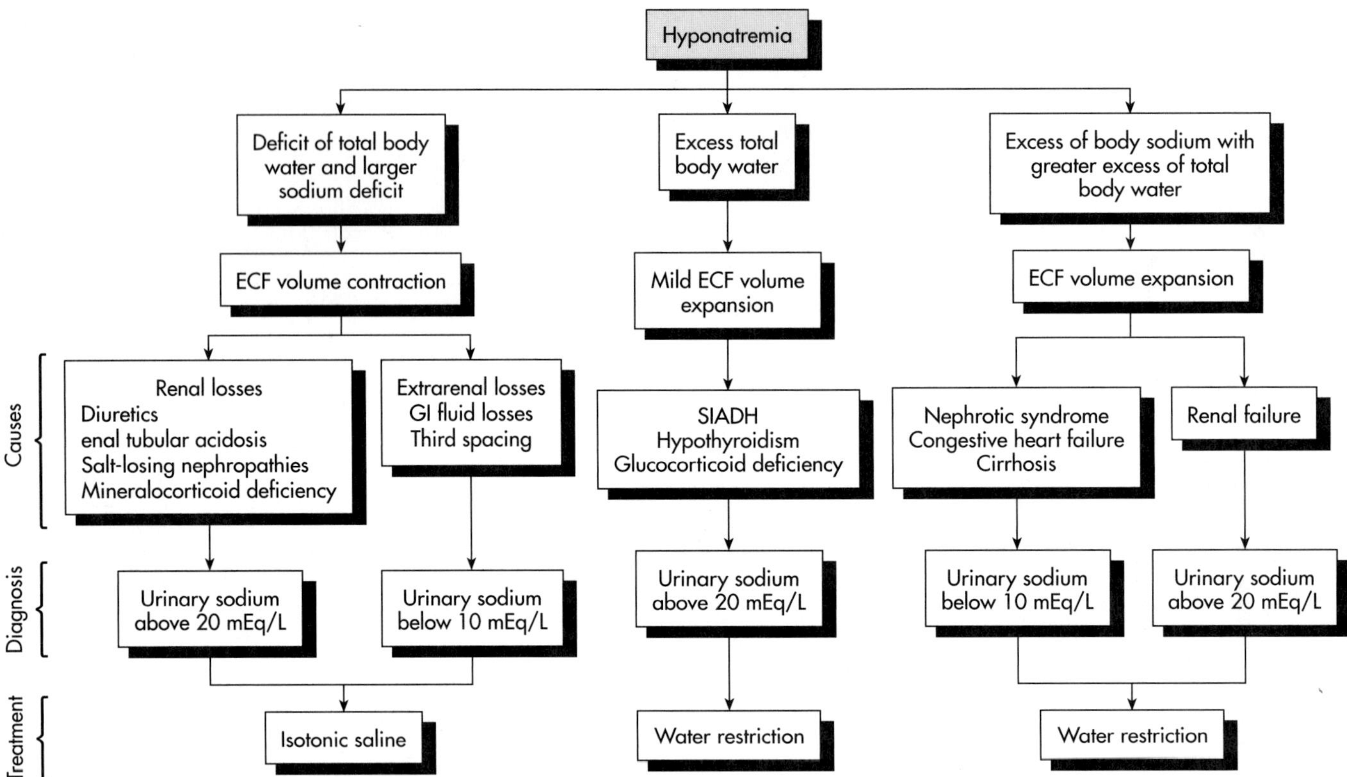

FIGURE 3-180 Evaluation and treatment of asymptomatic, mild hyponatremia. *ECF,* Extracellular fluid; *GI,* gastrointestinal; *SIADH,* syndrome of inappropriate secretion of antidiuretic hormone. (From Marx J et al [eds]: *Rosen's emergency medicine: concepts and clinical practice,* ed 6, St Louis, 2006, Mosby.)

TABLE 3-19 Drugs Associated with Hyponatremia*

Vasopressin Analogs	Drugs that Potentiate Renal Action of Vasopressin
Desmopressin (DDAVP)	Chlorpropamide
Oxytocin	Cyclophosphamide
	Nonsteroidal anti-inflammatory agents
	Acetaminophen (paracetamol)
Drugs that Enhance Vasopressin Release	**Drugs that Cause Hyponatremia by Unknown Mechanisms**
Chlorpropamide	*Haloperidol*
Clofibrate	Fluphenazine
Carbamazepine–oxycarbazepine	Amitriptyline
Vincristine	Thioradazine
Nicotine	Fluoxetine
Narcotics	*Methamphetamine (MDMA or Ecstacy)*
Antipsychotics/antidepressants	Sertraline
Ifosfamide	

(From Johnson RJ, Feehally J: *Comprehensive clinical nephrology,* ed 2, St Louis, 2000, Mosby.)
Italics: The common causes
*Not including diuretics

HYPOTENSION

ICD-9CM # 458.9 Hypotension, NOS
458.1 Hypotension, chronic
458.2 Hypotension, iatrogenic
458.0 Hypotension, orthostatic or postural

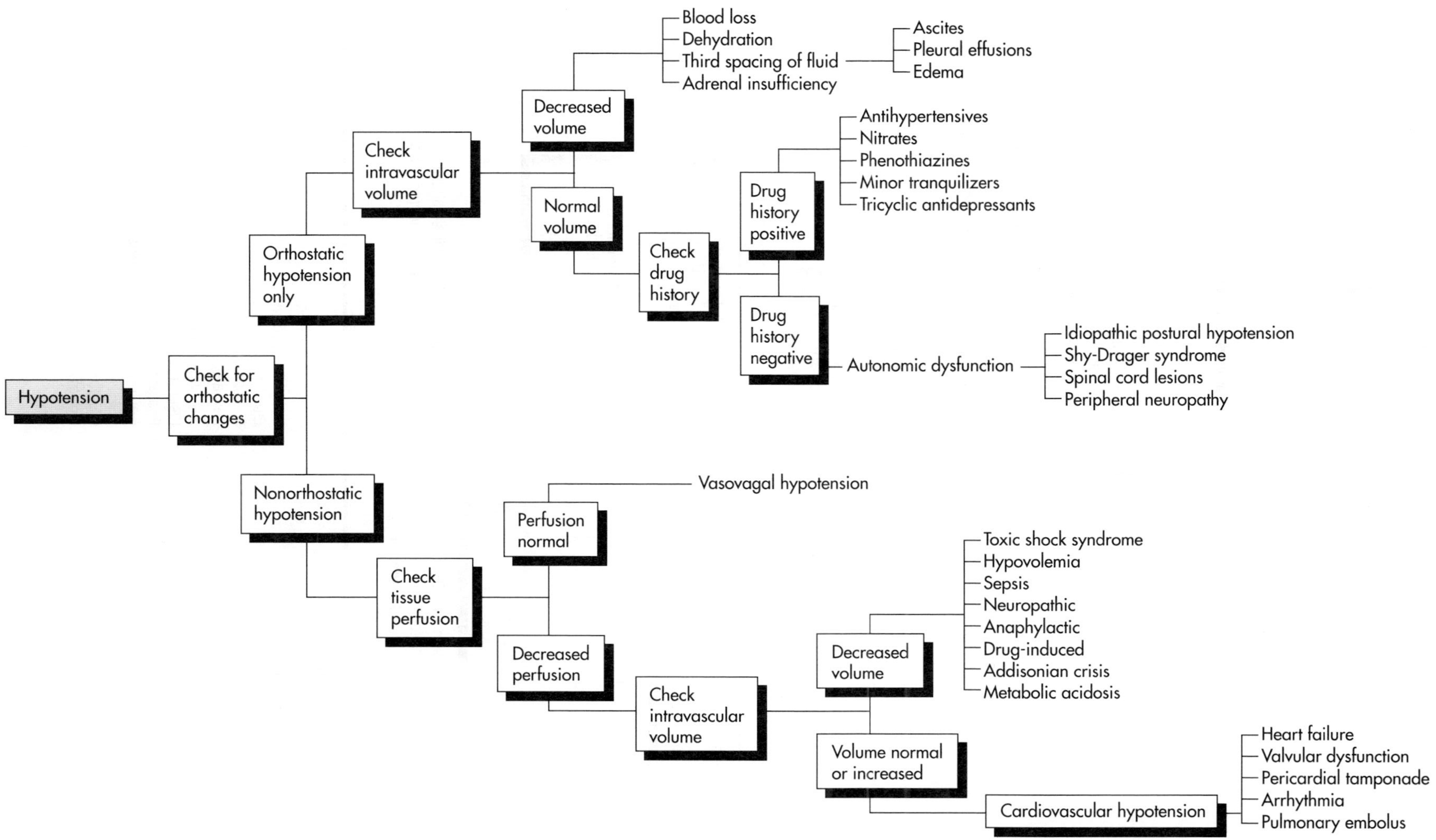

- Hypotension
  - Check for orthostatic changes
    - Orthostatic hypotension only
      - Check intravascular volume
        - Decreased volume
          - Blood loss
          - Dehydration
          - Third spacing of fluid
            - Ascites
            - Pleural effusions
            - Edema
          - Adrenal insufficiency
        - Normal volume
          - Check drug history
            - Drug history positive
              - Antihypertensives
              - Nitrates
              - Phenothiazines
              - Minor tranquilizers
              - Tricyclic antidepressants
            - Drug history negative
              - Autonomic dysfunction
                - Idiopathic postural hypotension
                - Shy-Drager syndrome
                - Spinal cord lesions
                - Peripheral neuropathy
    - Nonorthostatic hypotension
      - Check tissue perfusion
        - Perfusion normal
          - Vasovagal hypotension
        - Decreased perfusion
          - Check intravascular volume
            - Decreased volume
              - Toxic shock syndrome
              - Hypovolemia
              - Sepsis
              - Neuropathic
              - Anaphylactic
              - Drug-induced
              - Addisonian crisis
              - Metabolic acidosis
            - Volume normal or increased
              - Cardiovascular hypotension
                - Heart failure
                - Valvular dysfunction
                - Pericardial tamponade
                - Arrhythmia
                - Pulmonary embolus

FIGURE 3-182 Hypotension. (From Healey PM: *Common medical diagnosis: an algorithmic approach,* ed 3, Philadelphia, 2000, WB Saunders.)

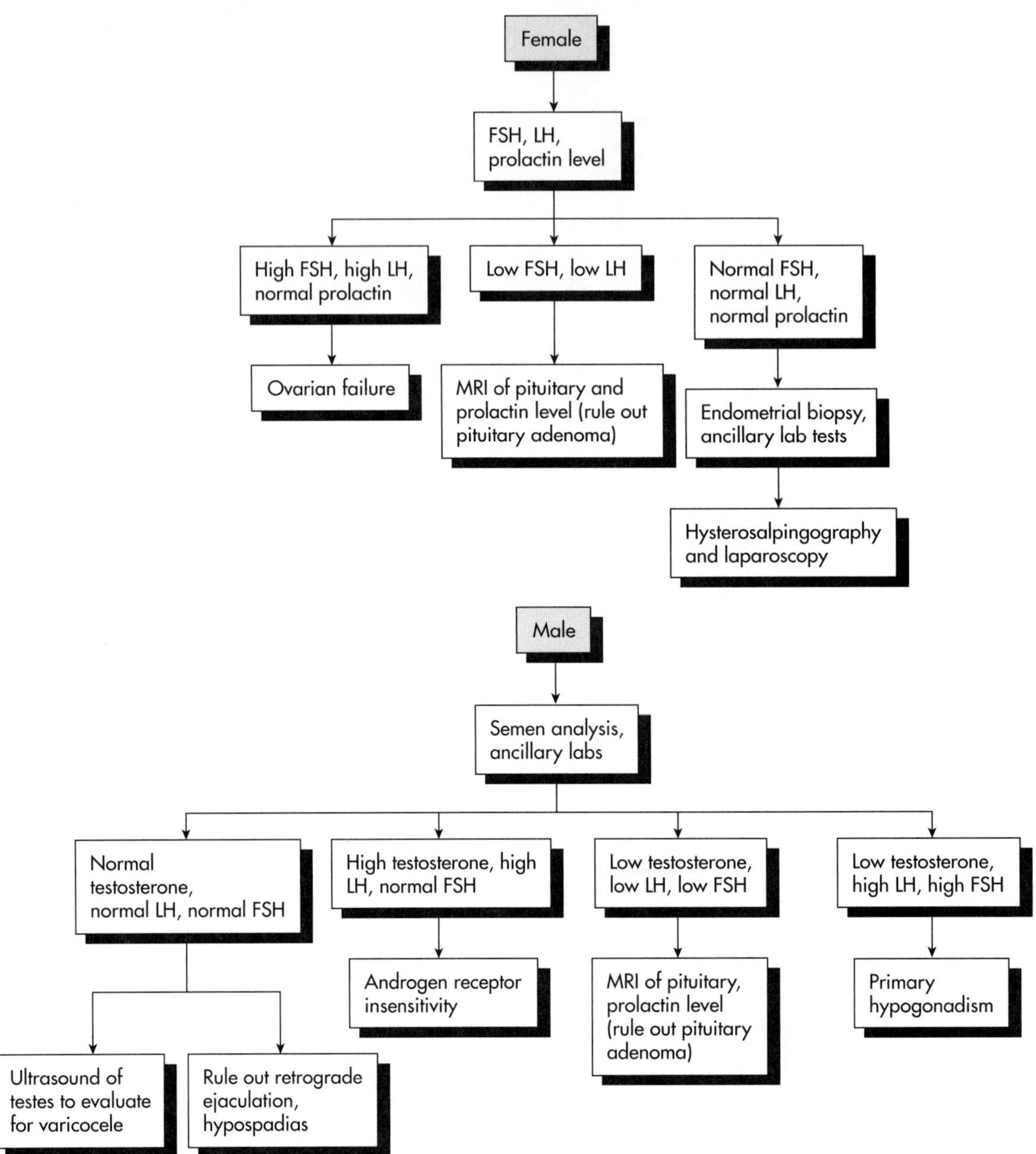

FIGURE 3-186 Approach to infertility diagnosis and management. *FSH,* Follicle-stimulating hormone; *LH,* luteinizing hormone; *MRI,* magnetic resonance imaging. (From Ferri FF: *Ferri's best test: a practical guide to clinical laboratory medicine and diagnostic imaging,* ed 2, Philadelphia, 2009, Elsevier Mosby.)

BOX 3-9 Infertility

Diagnostic imaging
Best test
None

Ancillary tests
MRI of pituitary with contrast
Hysterosalpingography
Testicular ultrasound

Lab evaluation
Best tests
Male: semen analysis
Female: endometrial biopsy

Ancillary tests
FSH, LH
Prolactin
Serum testosterone (male)
TSH
CBC, ESR, FBS
Urinalysis, VDRL, *Mycoplasma* culture, chlamidiae serology

Ferri FF: *Ferri's best test: a practical guide to clinical laboratory medicine and diagnostic imaging,* ed 2, Philadelphia, 2009, Elsevier Mosby.

CBC, Complete blood count; *ESR,* erythrocyte sedimentation rate; *FBS,* fasting blood sugar; *FSH,* follicle-stimulating hormone; *LH,* luteinizing hormone; *MRI,* magnetic resonance imaging; *VDRL,* Venereal Disease Research Laboratory (test).

ICD-9CM # 440.23 Ulcer, lower limb, arteriosclerotic
707.1 Ulcer, lower limb, chronic
707.1 Ulcer, lower limb, neurogenic
707.9 Ulcer, non-healing
707.0 Pressure ulcer

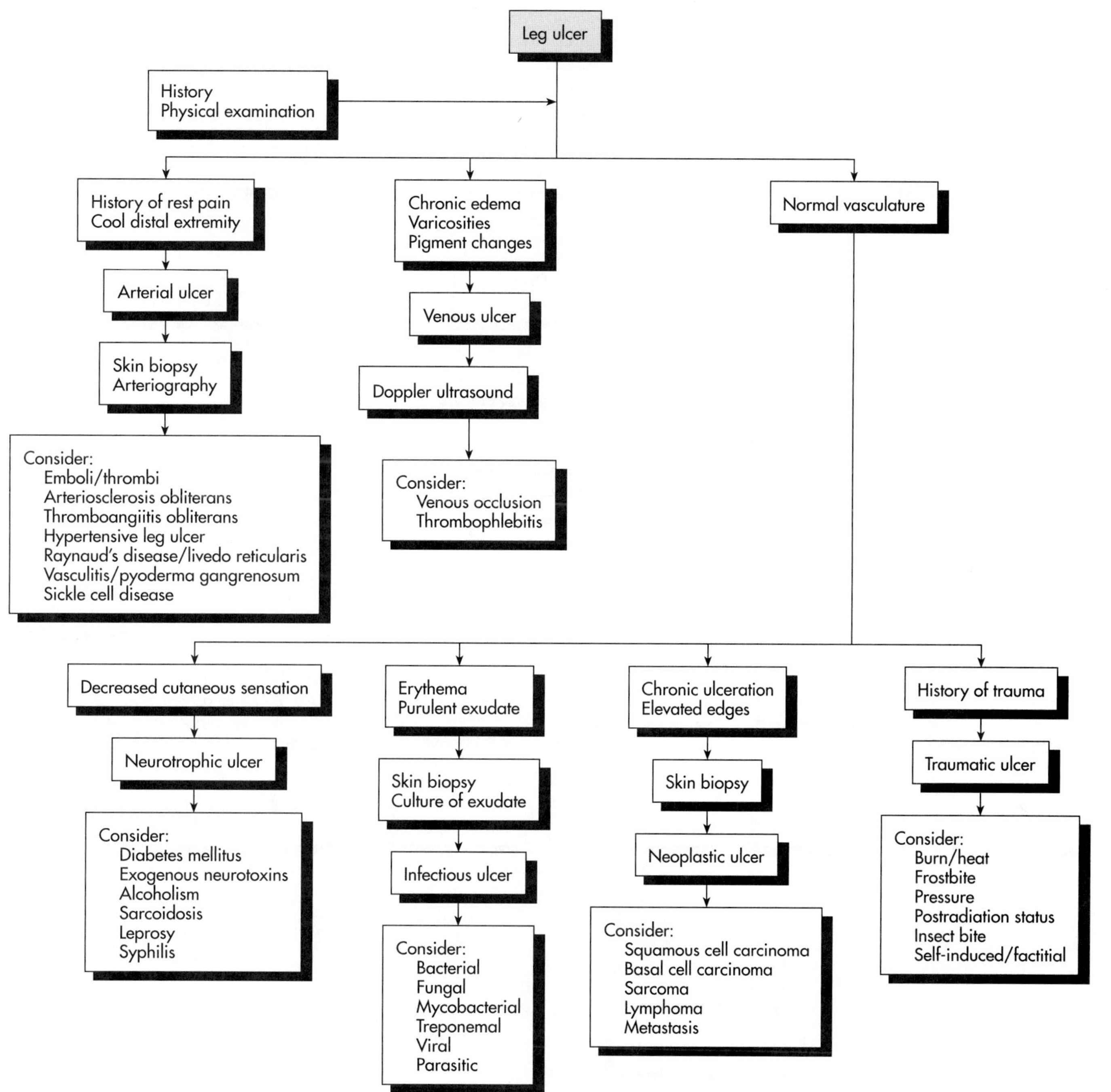

FIGURE 3-197 Leg ulcer. (From Greene HL, Johnson WP, Lemcke D [eds]: *Decision making in medicine*, ed 2, St Louis, 1998, Mosby.)

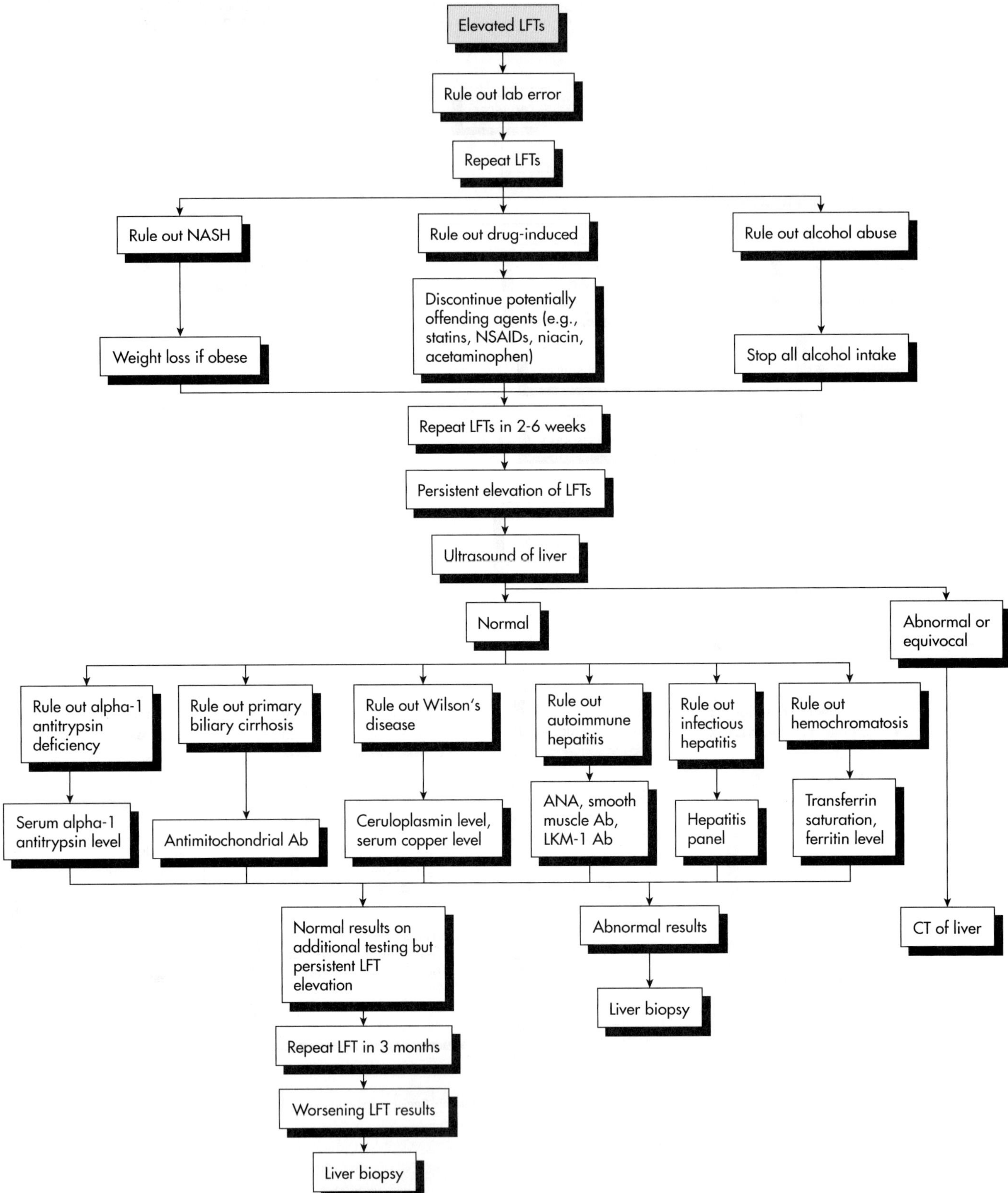

FIGURE 3-199 Liver function test elevations. *Ab,* Antibody; *ANA,* antibody to nuclear antigens; *CT,* computed tomography; *IEP,* immuno-electrophoresis; *LFT,* liver function test; *LKM,* liver-kidney microsome; *NASH,* nonalcoholic steatohepatitis; *NSAIDs,* nonsteroidal anti-inflammatory drugs.

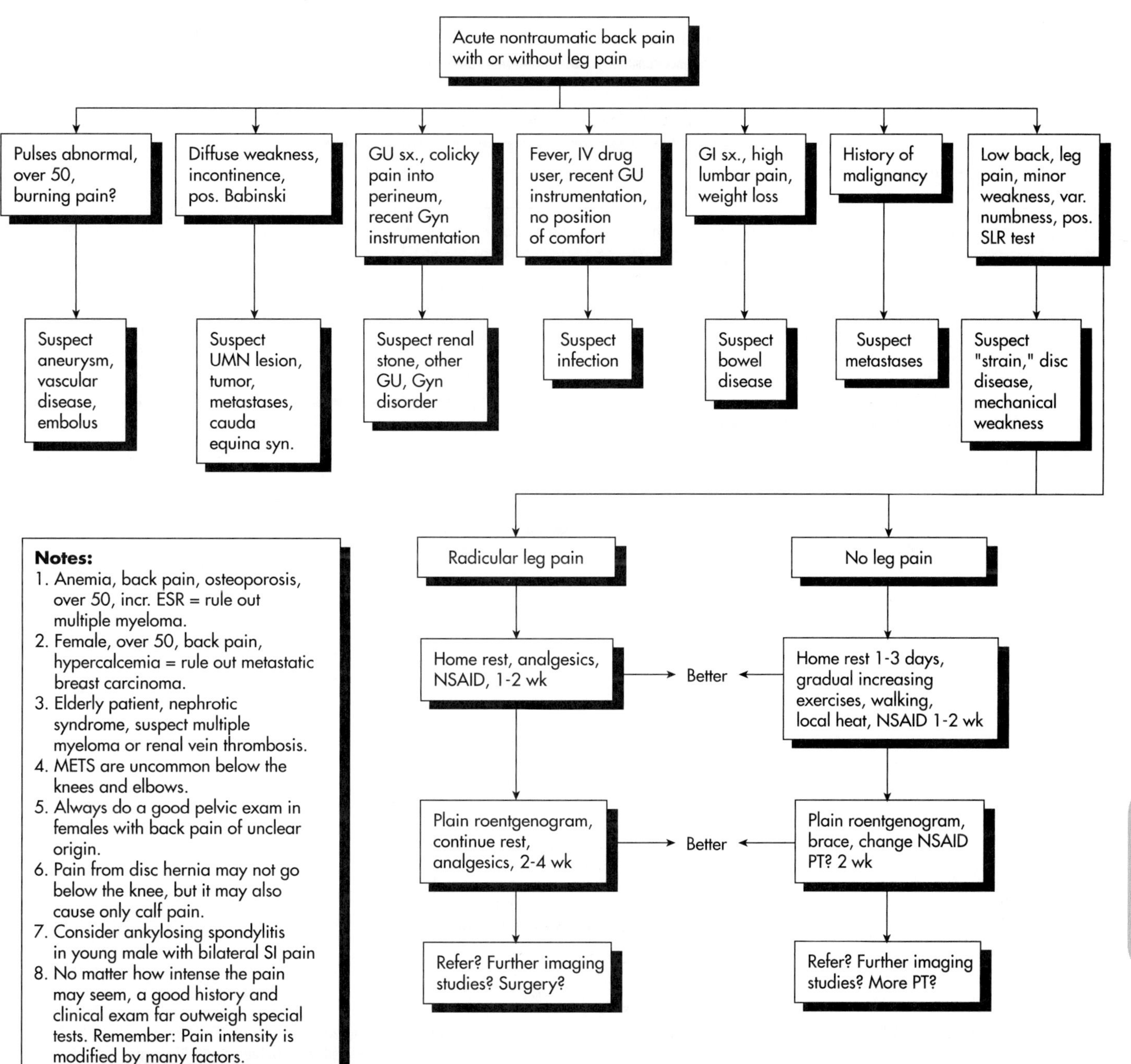

FIGURE 3-200 Algorithm for low back and/or leg pain. *GI*, Gastrointestinal; *GU*, genitourinary; *IV*, intravenous; *METS*, metabolic equivalents; *NSAID*, nonsteroidal anti-inflammatory drug; *PT*, physical therapy; *SLR*, straight-leg raising; *UMN*, upper motor neuron. (From Mercier LR: *Practical orthopedics*, ed 2, St Louis, 2000, Mosby.)

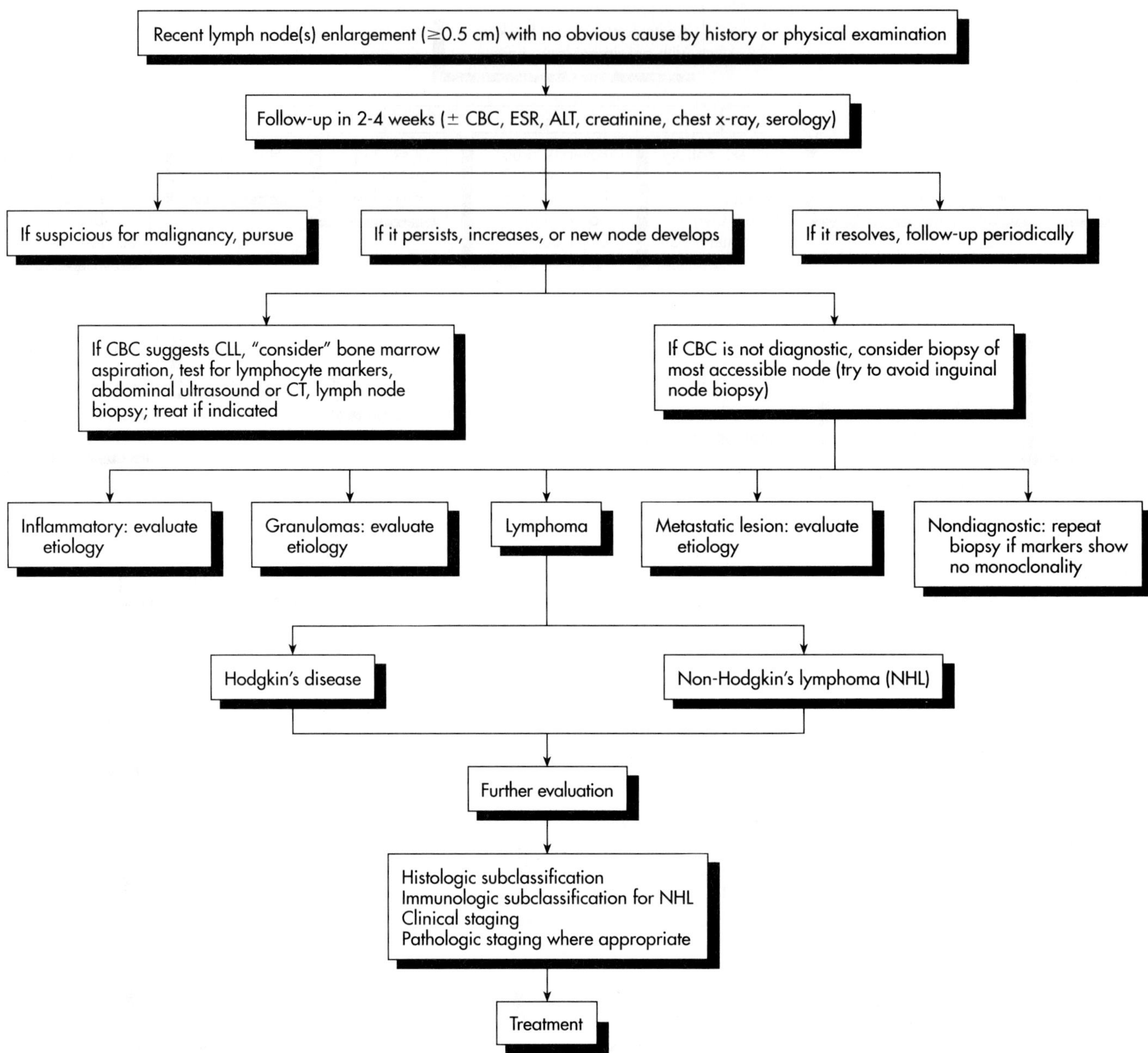

FIGURE 3-204 Workup of lymphadenopathy. *ALT,* Alanine aminotransferase; *CBC,* complete blood count; *CLL,* chronic lymphocytic leukemia; *CT,* computed tomography; *ESR,* erythrocyte sedimentation rate. (Modified from Noble J [ed]: *Primary care medicine*, ed 3, St Louis, 2001, Mosby.)

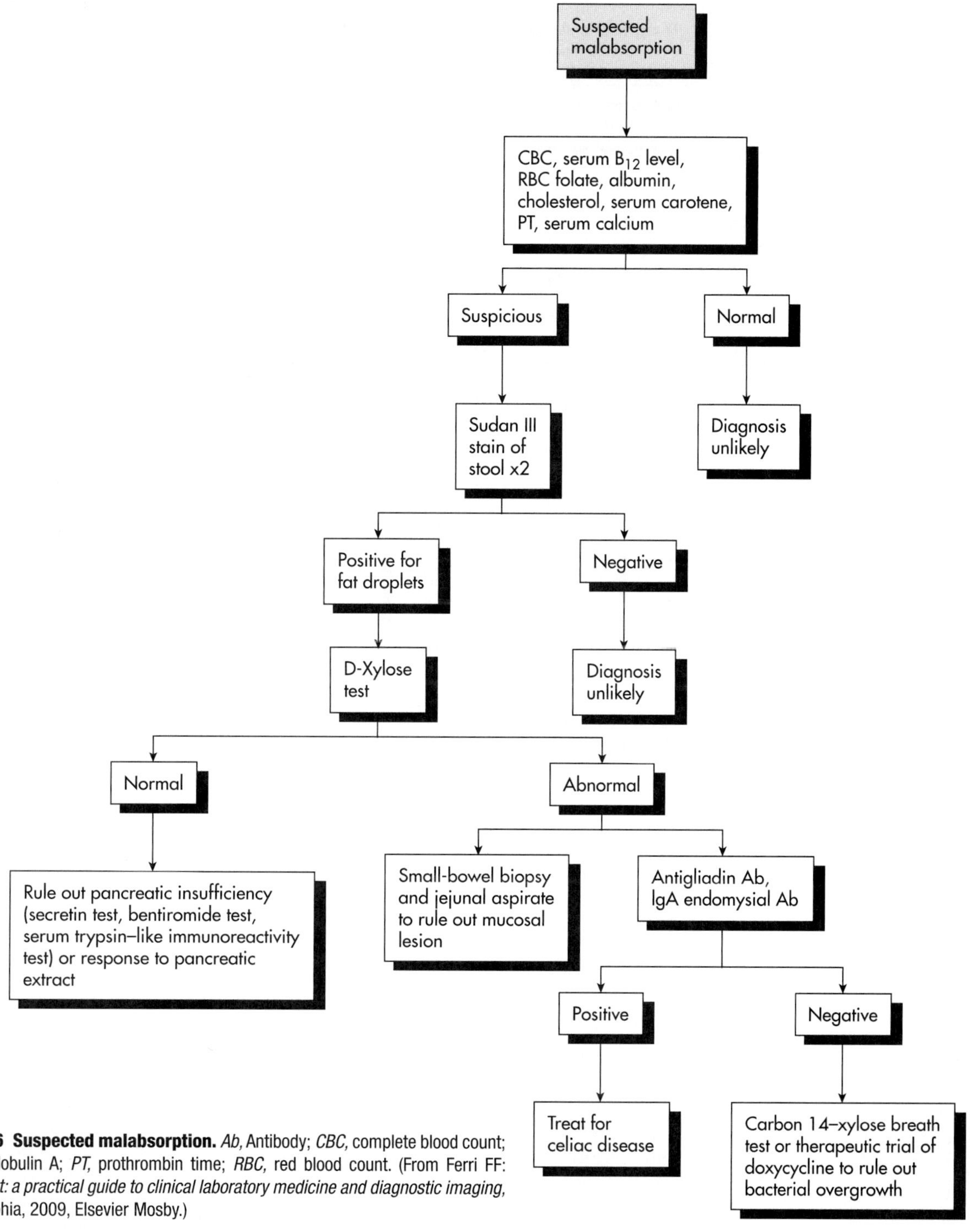

FIGURE 3-206 Suspected malabsorption. *Ab,* Antibody; *CBC,* complete blood count; *IgA,* immunoglobulin A; *PT,* prothrombin time; *RBC,* red blood count. (From Ferri FF: *Ferri's best test: a practical guide to clinical laboratory medicine and diagnostic imaging,* ed 2, Philadelphia, 2009, Elsevier Mosby.)

BOX 3-10 Malabsorption, Suspected

Diagnostic imaging
Best test
Small-bowel series

Ancillary test
CT of pancreas with IV contrast

Lab evaluation
Best test
Biopsy of small bowel

Ancillary tests
Albumin, total protein
ALT, AST, PT
Serum lytes, BUN, creatinine
Sudan III stain of stool for fecal leukocytes
CBC, RBC folate, serum iron, serum carotene, cholesterol, serum calcium
Hydrogen 14-C xylose breath test
D-Xylose test, secretin test
Quantitative fecal test
Antigliadin antibody, IgA endomysial antibody

From Ferri FF: *Ferri's best test: a practical guide to clinical laboratory medicine and diagnostic imaging,* ed 2, Philadelphia, 2009, Elsevier Mosby.
ALT, Alanine aminotransferase; AST, aspartate aminotransferase; BUN, blood urea nitrogen; CBC, complete blood count; CT, computed tomography; IgA, immunoglobulin A; IV, intravenous; PT, prothrombin time; RBC, red blood count.

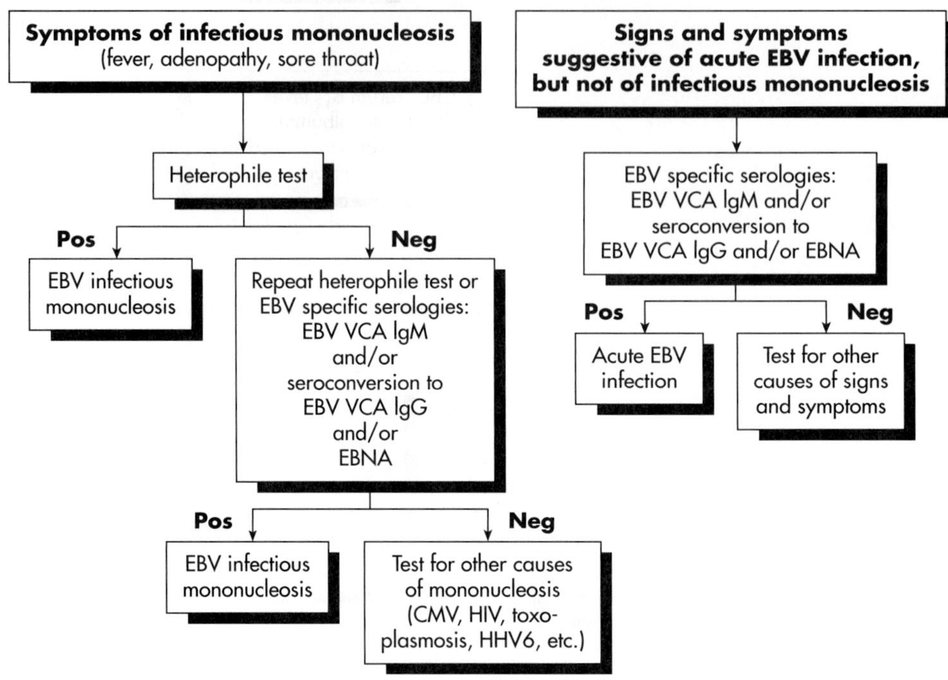

*Refer to Section I for additional information on this topic.

FIGURE 3-210 Diagnostic algorithm for EBV infection and infectious mononucleosis. *CMV,* Cytomegalovirus; *EBV,* Epstein-Barr virus; *HIV,* human immunodeficiency virus. (From Young NS, Gerson SL, High KA [eds]: *Clinical hematology,* St Louis, 2006, Mosby.)

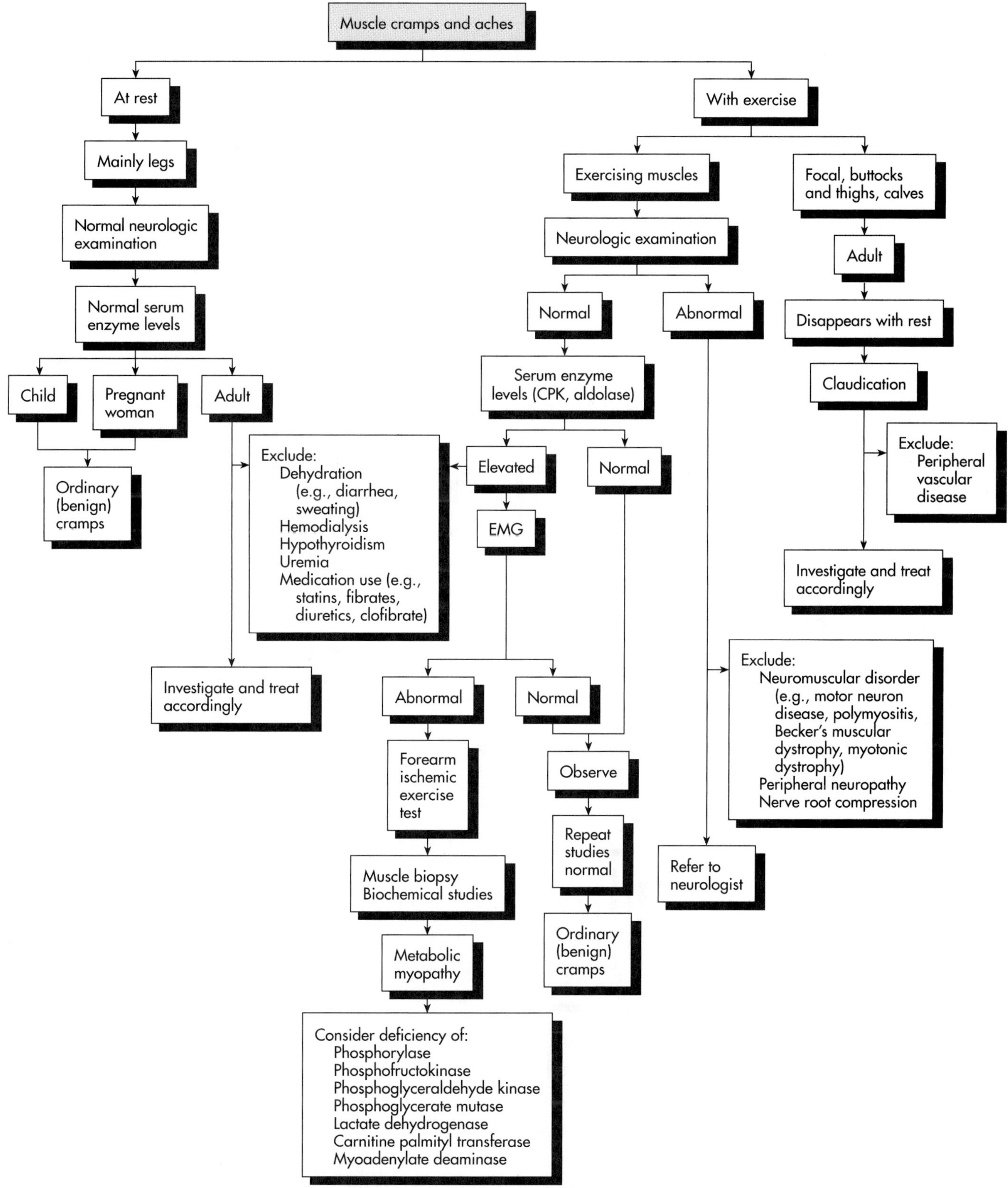

FIGURE 3-216 Evaluation of muscle cramps and aches. *CPK,* Creatine phosphokinase; *EMG,* electromyography. (From Greene HL, Johnson WP, Lemcke D [eds]: *Decision making in medicine,* ed 2, St Louis, 1998, Mosby.)

MUSCLE WEAKNESS

ICD-9CM # 782.9

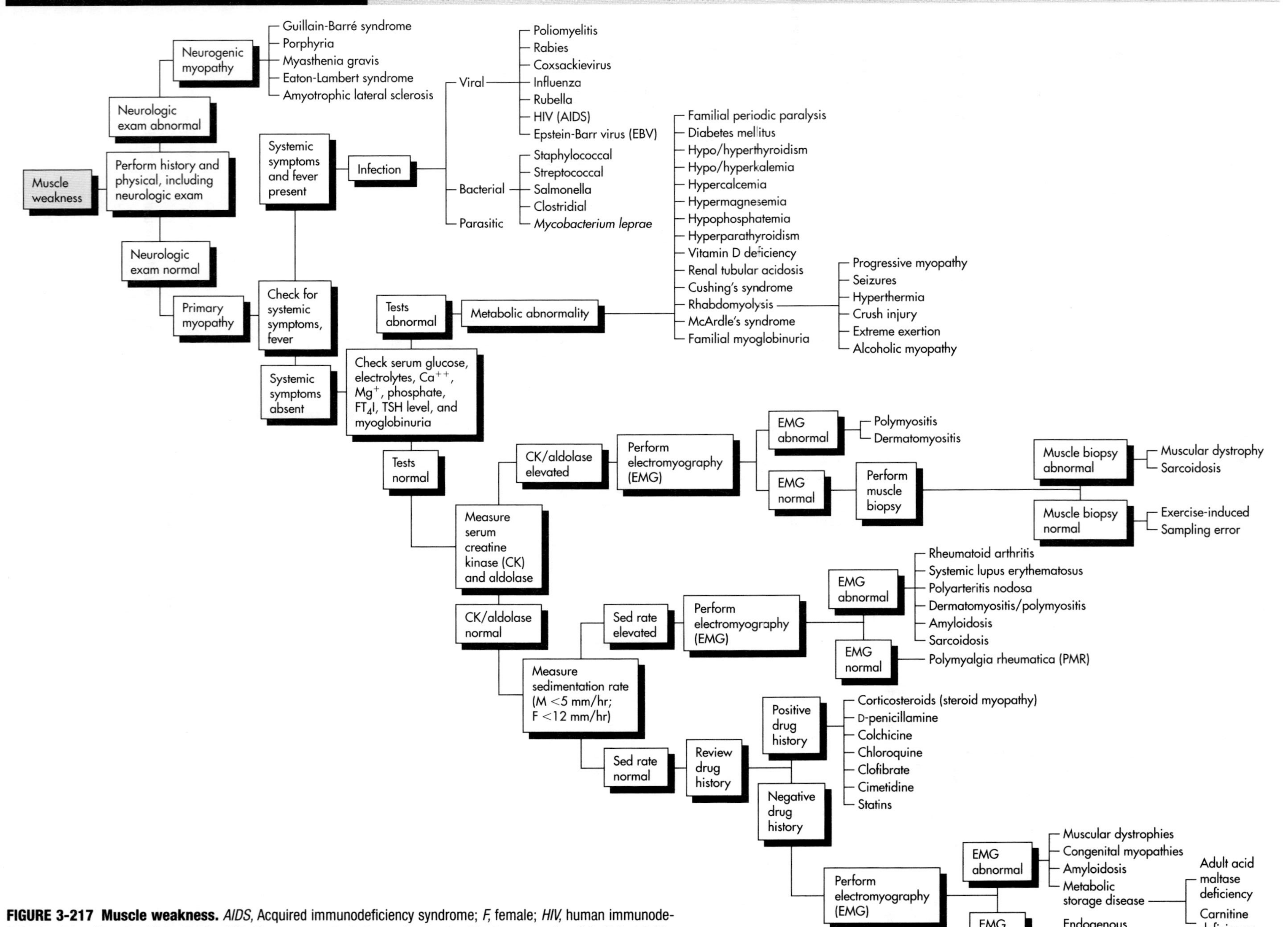

FIGURE 3-217 Muscle weakness. *AIDS,* Acquired immunodeficiency syndrome; *F,* female; *HIV,* human immunodeficiency virus; *M,* male. (From Healey PM: *Common medical diagnosis: an algorithmic approach,* ed 3, Philadelphia, 2000, WB Saunders.)

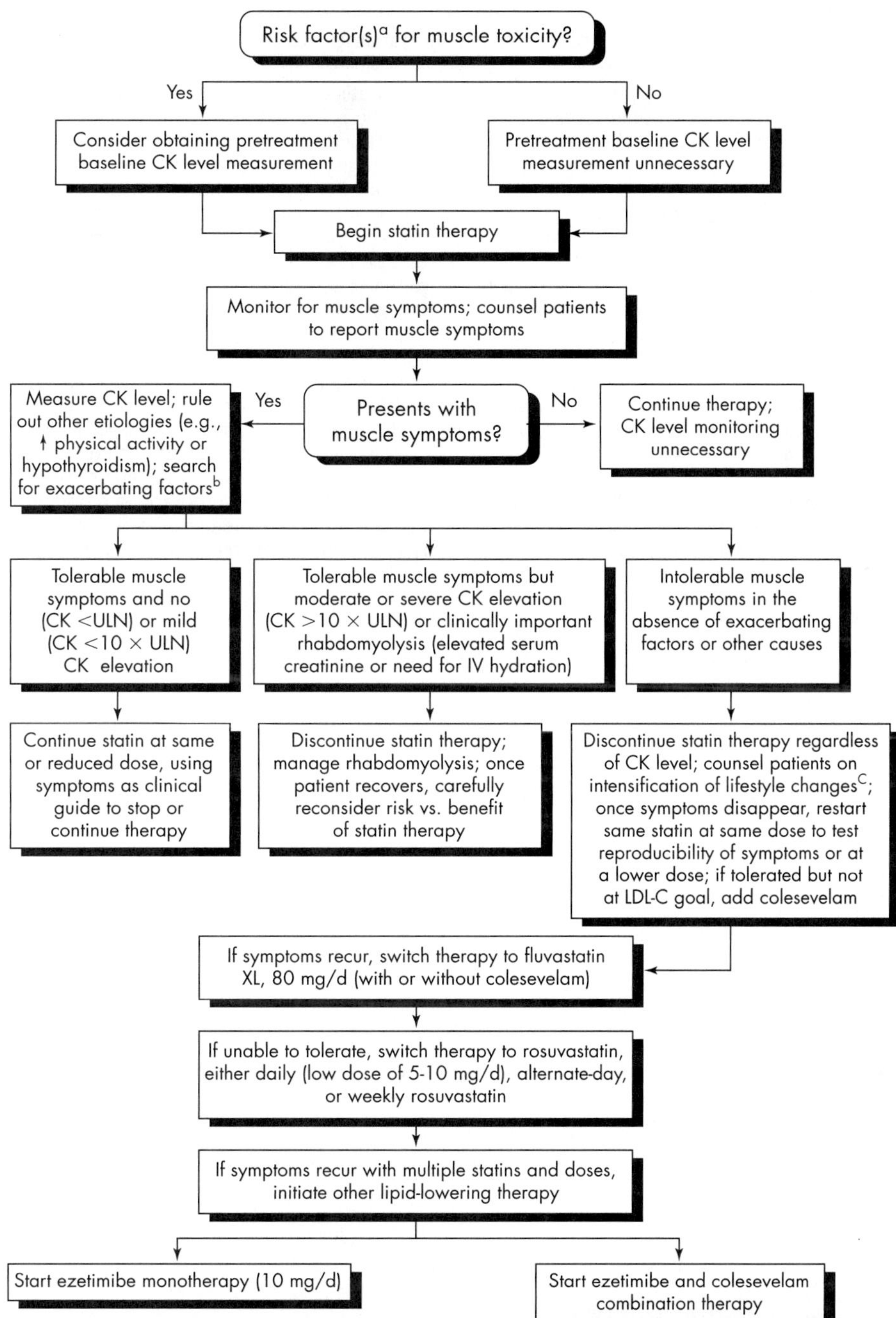

FIGURE 3-221 Algorithm for monitoring and management of suspected statin-associated myopathy. a, Risk factors for muscle toxicity include advanced age and frailty, small body frame, deteriorating renal function, infection, untreated hypothyroidism, interacting drugs, perioperative periods, and alcohol abuse. **b,** Causes for elevated CK levels/muscle toxicity are increased physical activity, trauma, falls, accidents, seizure, shaking chills, hypothyroidism, infections, carbon monoxide poisoning, polymyositis, dermatomyositis, alcohol abuse, and drug abuse (cocaine, amphetamines, heroin, or PCP). **c,** Patient counseling regarding intensification of therapeutic lifestyle changes (reduced intake of saturated fats and cholesterol, increased physical activity, and weight control) should be an integral part of management in all patients with statin-associated intolerable muscle symptoms. *CK,* Creatine kinase; *IV,* intravenous; *LDL-C,* low-density lipoprotein cholesterol; *PCP,* phencyclidine; *ULN,* upper limit of normal; *XL,* extended release. (Modified from Jacobson TA: Toward "pain-free" statin prescribing, *Mayo Clin Proc* 83(60): 696, 2008.)

BOX 3-11 Recommendations to Health Care Professionals Regarding Statin and Muscle Safety

Whenever muscle symptoms or an increased CK level are encountered in patients receiving statin therapy, health professionals should attempt to rule out other causes, because these are most likely to explain the findings. Other comon causes include increased physical activity, trauma, falls, accidents, seizure, shaking chills, hypothyroidism, infections, carbon monoxide poisoning, polymyositis, dermatomyositis, alcohol abuse, and drug abuse (cocaine, amphetamines, heroin, or PCP).

Obtaining a pretreatment, baseline CK level can be considered in patients who are at high risk of experiencing muscle toxicity (e.g., older patients or those combining a statin with an agent known to increase myotoxicity), but this is not routinely necessary in other patients.

It is unnecessary to measure CK levels in asymptomatic patients during the course of statin therapy, because marked, clinically important CK elevations are rare and are usually related to physical exertion or other causes.

Patients receiving statin therapy should be counseled about the increased risk of muscle symptoms, particularly if initiation of vigorous, sustained endurance exercise or a surgical operation is being contemplated; they should be advised to report such muscle symptoms to a health professional.

Creatine kinase measurements should be obtained in symptomatic patients to help gauge the severity of muscle damage and facilitate decision of whether to continue therapy or alter doses.

In patients who develop intolerable muscle symptoms with or without CK elevation and for whom other etiologies have been ruled out, the statin should be discontinued. Once symptoms disappear, the same or different statin at the same or a lower dose can be restarted to test the reproducibility of symptoms. Recurrence of symptoms with multiple statins and doses requires initiation of other lipid-altering therapy.

In patients who develop tolerable muscle symptoms or have no symptoms but have a CK level $<10 \times$ ULN, statin therapy may be continued at the same or reduced doses and symptoms may be used as the clinical guide to stop or continue therapy.

In patients who develop rhabdomyolysis (CK $>$10,000 IU/L or $>10 \times$ ULN with an elevation in serum creatinine or need for intravenous hydration therapy), statin therapy should be stopped. Intravenous hydration therapy in a hospital should be instituted if indicated for patients experiencing rhabdomyolysis. Once patients recover, risk vs benefit of statin therapy should be carefully reconsidered.

(From McKenney JM et al: Final conclusions and recommendations of the National Lipid Association Statin Safety Assessment Task Force, *Am J Cardiol,* 97 (suppl 8A):89C-94C, 2006.)

CK, Creatine kinase; *PCP,* phencyclidine; *ULN,* upper limit of normal.

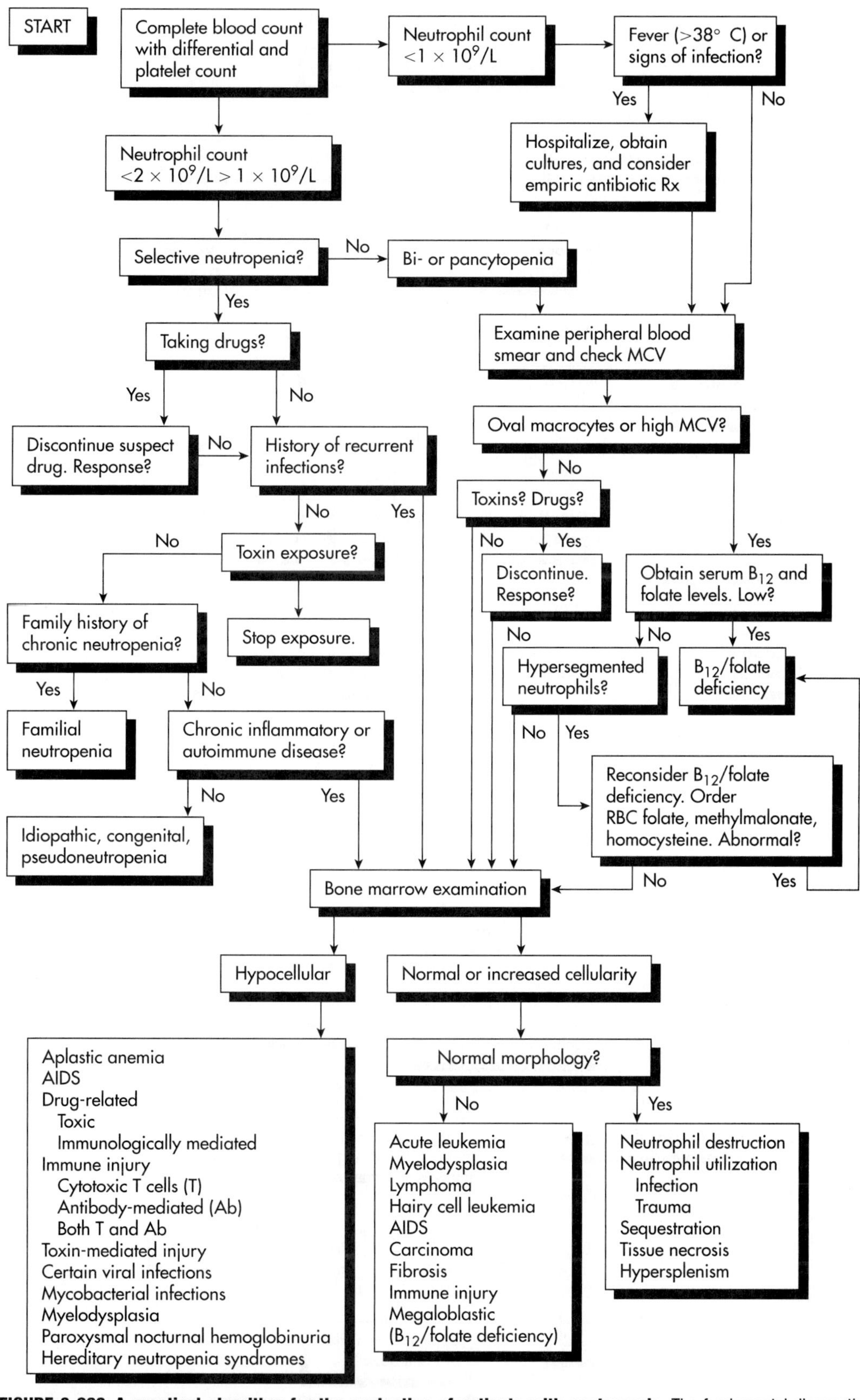

FIGURE 3-228 A practical algorithm for the evaluation of patients with neutropenia. The fundamental diagnostic principle is that for patients with severe neutropenia or for those with bicytopenia or pancytopenia, bone marrow examination will likely be necessary unless the following diagnoses are made: (1) a nutritional (folate or vitamin B_{12}) deficiency or (2) drug- or toxin-induced neutropenia in a patient whose neutropenia resolves after discontinuation of the offending agent. *AIDS,* Acquired immunodeficiency syndrome; *MCV,* mean corpuscular volume; *RBC,* red blood cell. (From Goldman L, Ausiello D [eds]: *Cecil textbook of medicine,* ed 23, Philadelphia, 2008, WB Saunders.)

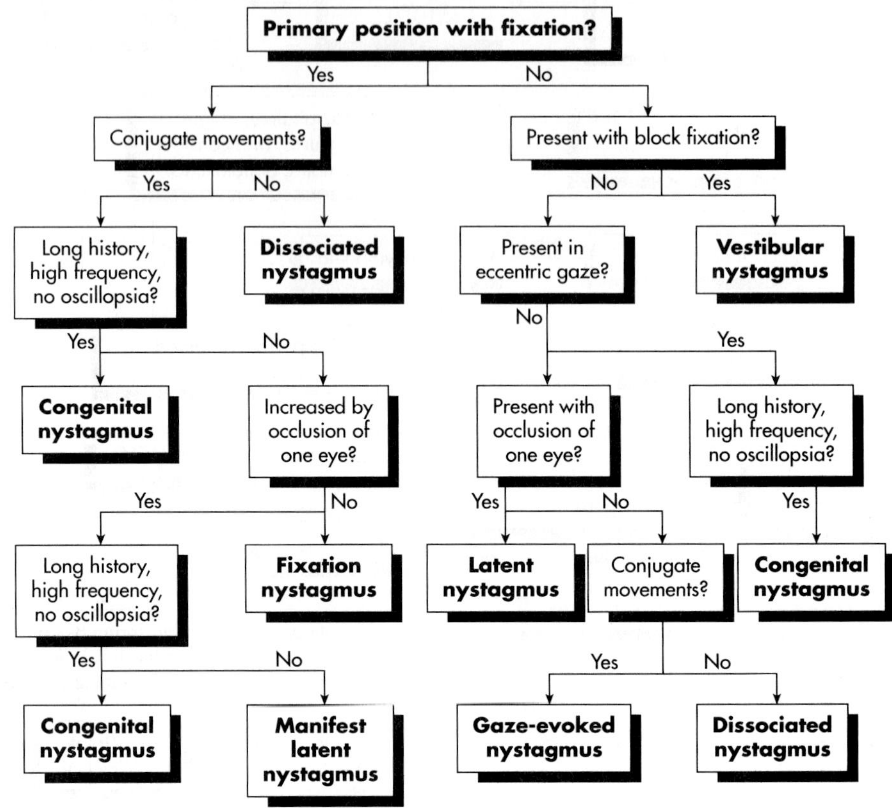

FIGURE 3-232 Identification of types of nystagmus. (From Yanoff M, Duker JS: *Ophthalmology,* ed 2, St Louis, 2004, Mosby.)

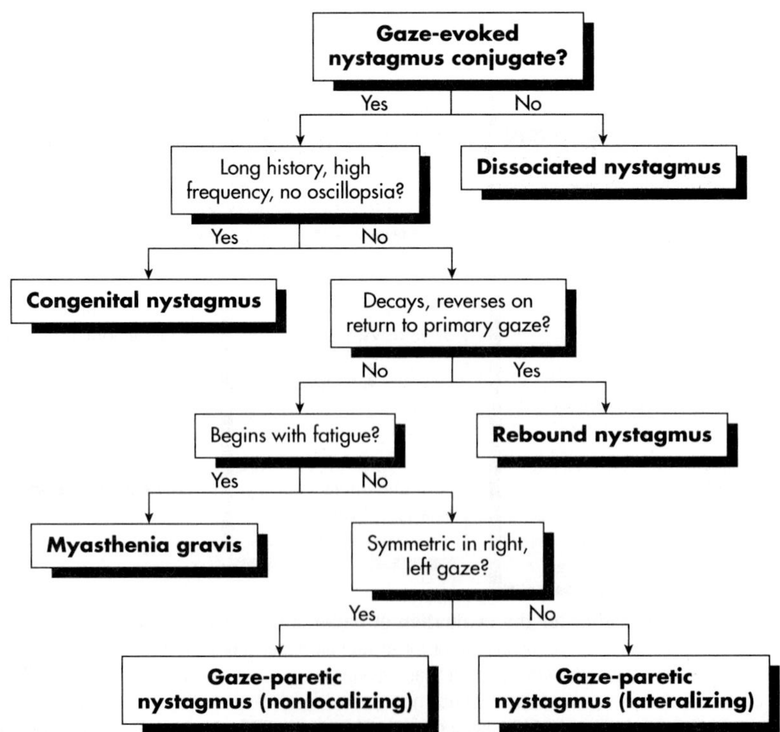

FIGURE 3-234 Identification of types of gaze-evoked nystagmus. (From Yanoff M, Duker JS: *Ophthalmology,* ed 2, St Louis, 2004, Mosby.)

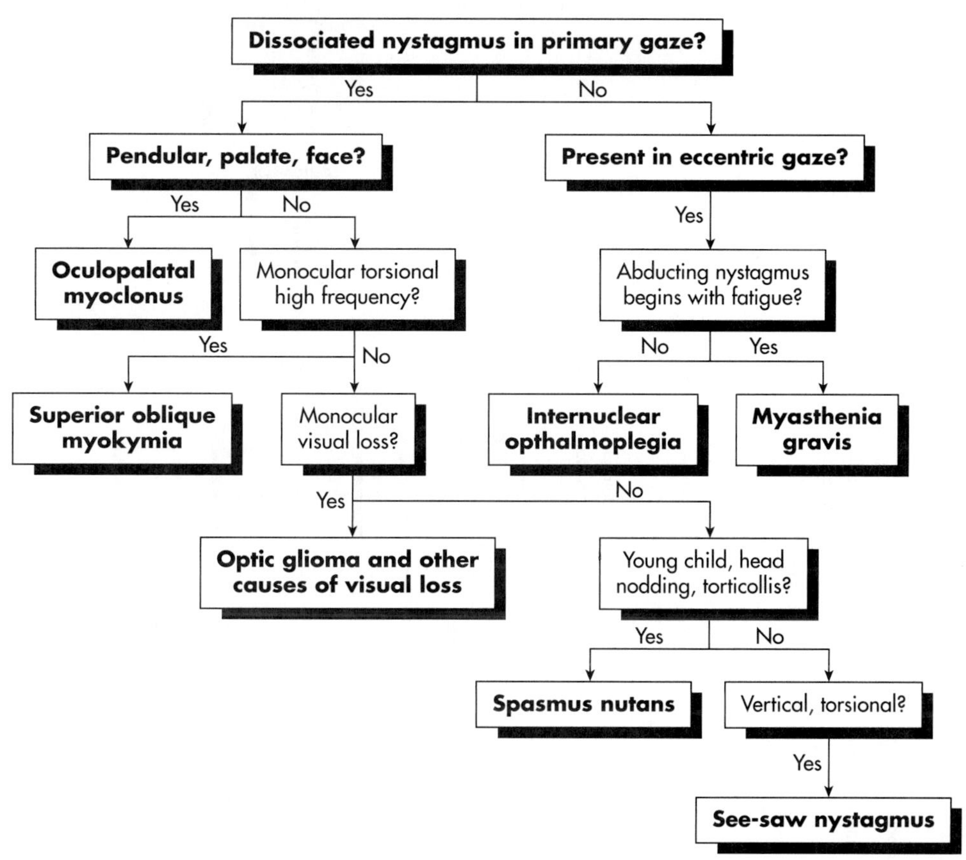

FIGURE 3-235 Identification of types of dissociated nystagmus. (From Yanoff M, Duker JS: *Ophthalmology,* ed 2, St Louis, 2004, Mosby.)

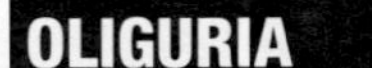

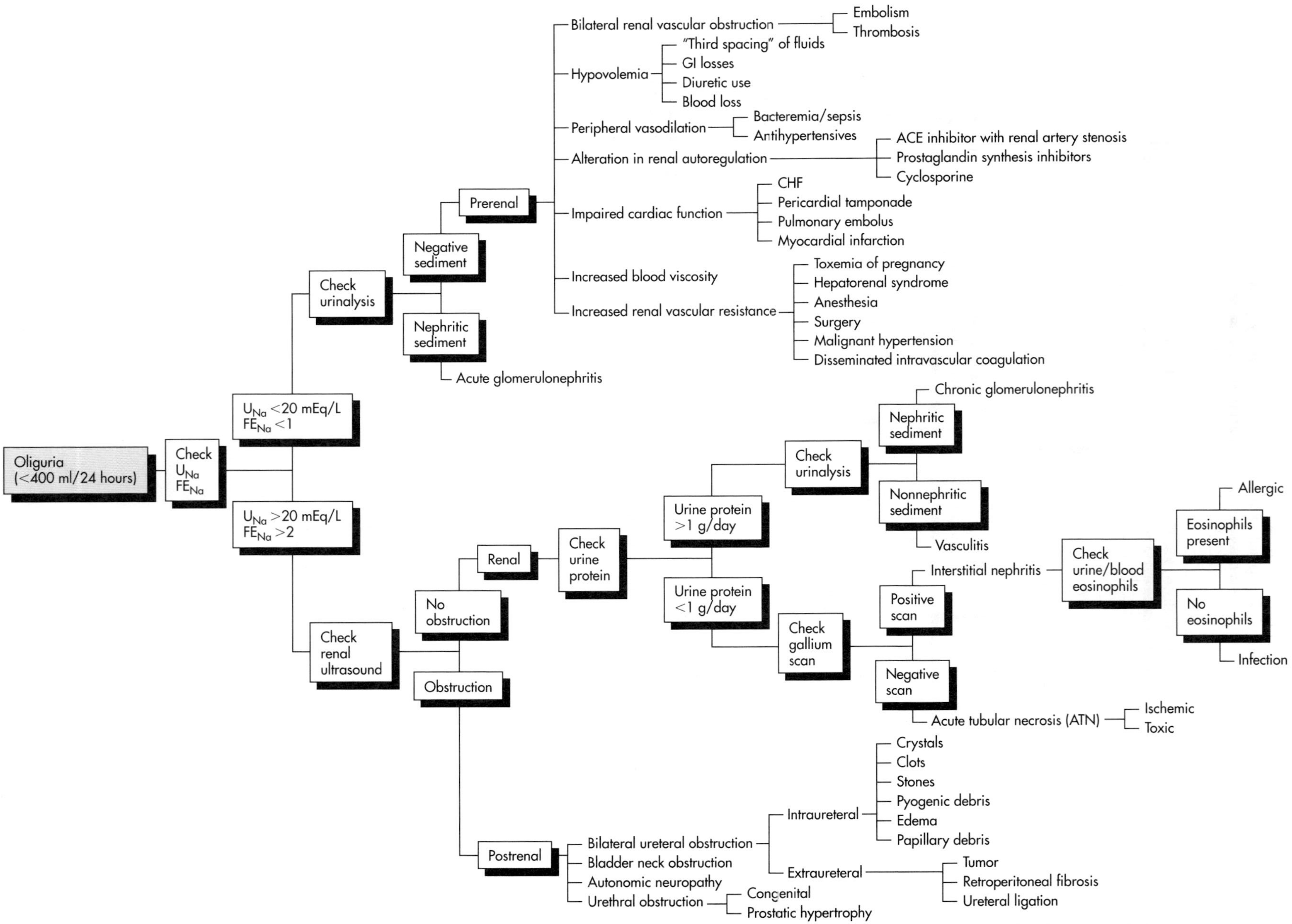

OLIGURIA

ICD-9CM # 788.5

Oliguria (<400 ml/24 hours)

Check U_{Na} FE_{Na}

- U_{Na} <20 mEq/L, FE_{Na} <1
  - Check urinalysis
    - Negative sediment
      - Prerenal
        - Bilateral renal vascular obstruction
          - Embolism
          - Thrombosis
        - Hypovolemia
          - "Third spacing" of fluids
          - GI losses
          - Diuretic use
          - Blood loss
        - Peripheral vasodilation
          - Bacteremia/sepsis
          - Antihypertensives
        - Alteration in renal autoregulation
          - ACE inhibitor with renal artery stenosis
          - Prostaglandin synthesis inhibitors
          - Cyclosporine
        - Impaired cardiac function
          - CHF
          - Pericardial tamponade
          - Pulmonary embolus
          - Myocardial infarction
        - Increased blood viscosity
        - Increased renal vascular resistance
          - Toxemia of pregnancy
          - Hepatorenal syndrome
          - Anesthesia
          - Surgery
          - Malignant hypertension
          - Disseminated intravascular coagulation
    - Nephritic sediment
      - Acute glomerulonephritis
- U_{Na} >20 mEq/L, FE_{Na} >2
  - Check renal ultrasound
    - No obstruction
      - Renal
        - Check urine protein
          - Urine protein >1 g/day
            - Check urinalysis
              - Nephritic sediment
                - Chronic glomerulonephritis
              - Nonnephritic sediment
                - Vasculitis
          - Urine protein <1 g/day
            - Check gallium scan
              - Positive scan
                - Interstitial nephritis
                  - Check urine/blood eosinophils
                    - Eosinophils present
                      - Allergic
                    - No eosinophils
                      - Infection
              - Negative scan
                - Acute tubular necrosis (ATN)
                  - Ischemic
                  - Toxic
    - Obstruction
      - Postrenal
        - Bilateral ureteral obstruction
          - Intraureteral
            - Crystals
            - Clots
            - Stones
            - Pyogenic debris
            - Edema
            - Papillary debris
          - Extraureteral
            - Tumor
            - Retroperitoneal fibrosis
            - Ureteral ligation
        - Bladder neck obstruction
        - Autonomic neuropathy
        - Urethral obstruction
          - Congenital
          - Prostatic hypertrophy

FIGURE 3-238 Evaluation of oliguria. *ACE,* Angiotensin-converting enzyme; *CHF,* congestive heart failure; *GI,* gastrointestinal. (From Healey PM: *Common medical diagnosis: an algorithmic approach,* ed 3, Philadelphia, 2000, WB Saunders.)

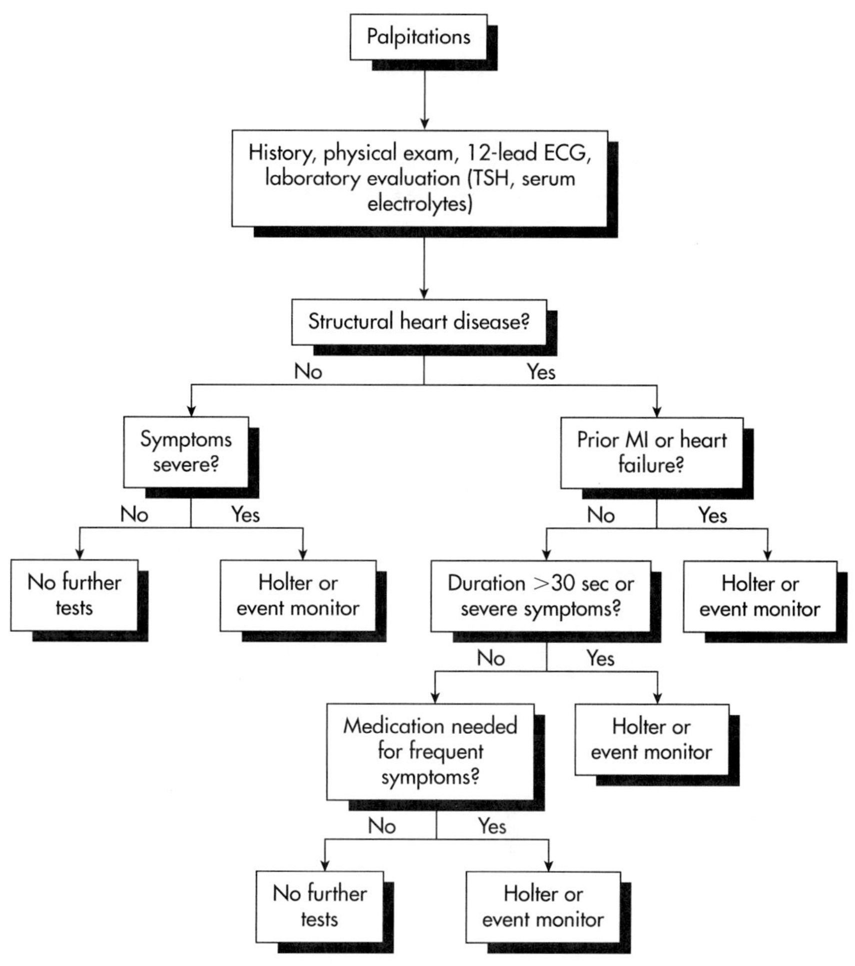

FIGURE 3-243 Diagnostic approach to the patient with palpitations. *ECG,* Electrocardiogram; *MI,* myocardial infarction; *TSH,* thyroid-stimulating hormone. (From Hiatky MA: Approach to the patient with palpitations. In Braunwald E, Goldman L [eds]: *Primary cardiology,* ed 2, Philadelphia, 2003, WB Saunders.)

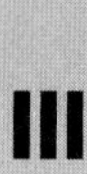

TABLE 3-24 Items to be Covered in History of Patient with Palpitation

Does the Palpitation Occur:	If So, Suspect:
As isolated "jumps" or "skips"?	Extrasystoles
In attacks known to be of abrupt beginning, with a heart rate of 120 beats/min or over, with regular or irregular rhythm?	Paroxysmal rapid heart action
Independent of exercise or excitement adequate to account for the symptom?	Atrial fibrillation, atrial flutter, thyrotoxicosis, anemia, febrile states, hypoglycemia, anxiety state
In attacks developing rapidly though not absolutely abruptly, unrelated to exertion or excitement?	Hemorrhage, hypoglycemia, tumor of the adrenal medulla
In conjunction with the taking of drugs?	Tobacco, coffee, tea, alcohol, epinephrine, ephedrine, aminophylline, atropine, thyroid extract, monoamine oxidase inhibitors
On standing?	Postural hypotension
In middle-aged women, in conjunction with flushes and sweats?	Menopausal syndrome
When the rate is known to be normal and the rhythm regular?	Anxiety state

(From Goldman L, Braunwald E: Chest discomfort and palpitation. In Isselbacher KJ, Braunwald E, et al [eds]: *Harrison's principles of internal medicine,* ed 13, New York, 1994, McGraw-Hill.)

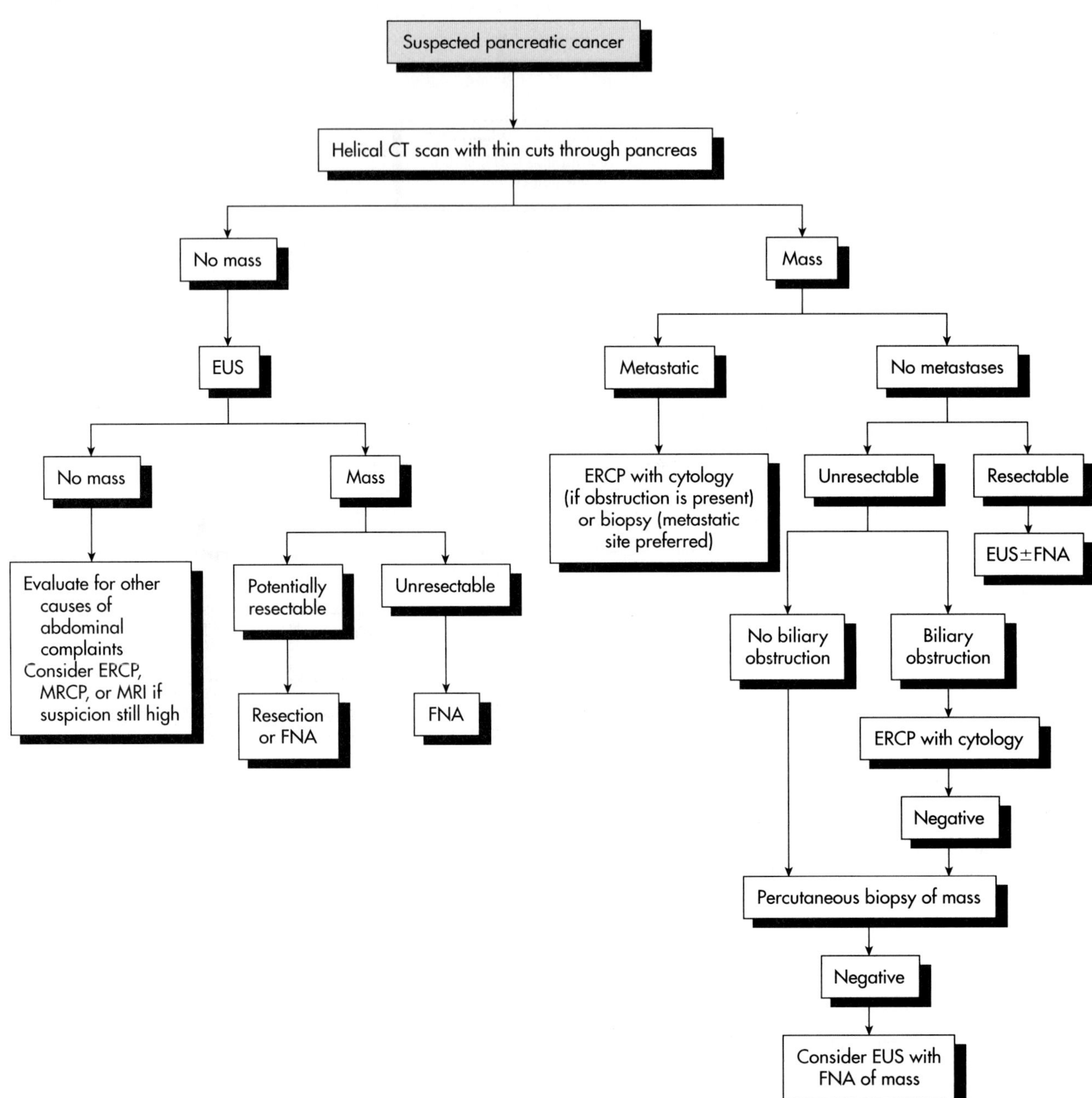

FIGURE 3-245 Diagnostic algorithm for pancreatic cancer. Intraoperative fine-needle aspiration (FNA) if found inoperable during surgery. *CT,* Computed tomography; *ERCP,* endoscopic retrograde cholangiopancreatography; *EUS,* endoscopic ultrasonography; *MRI,* magnetic resonance imaging. (From Goldman L, Ausiello D [eds]: *Cecil textbook of medicine,* ed 23, Philadelphia, 2008, WB Saunders.)

Review medical and psychiatric history
Physical examination
Evidence of major psychiatric disorder
Bizarre complaints or behavior
Sensorium clear
Consider: Acute psychosis Schizophrenia Delusional disorder Psychotic depression
Psychiatric referral
Sensorium confused
Consider: Delirium Dementia
Identify and treat underlying cause
Plausible complaints
Primary depression
Antidepressant medication trial
Psychiatric consultation if no response
Primary anxiety disorder
Stress management Relaxation exercises Judicious use of benzodiazepines, SSRIs, or buspirone trial
No evidence of major psychiatric disorder
Recent stress
Reactive hypochondriasis
Removal from stress Emotional support and reassurance
Conversion disorder
Removal from stress Supportive emotional and physical interventions Positive suggestion
No recent stress
Evidence of deceit
Evidence of secondary gain
Malingering
Confrontation Notification of involved health providers
No obvious secondary gain
Factitious disorder
Avoidance of unnecessary procedures Firm but supportive management Psychiatric consultation
No evidence of deceit
Hypochondriasis or related disorder
Support and reassurance Avoidance of procedures or multiple physician contacts
Undiagnosed physical disorder

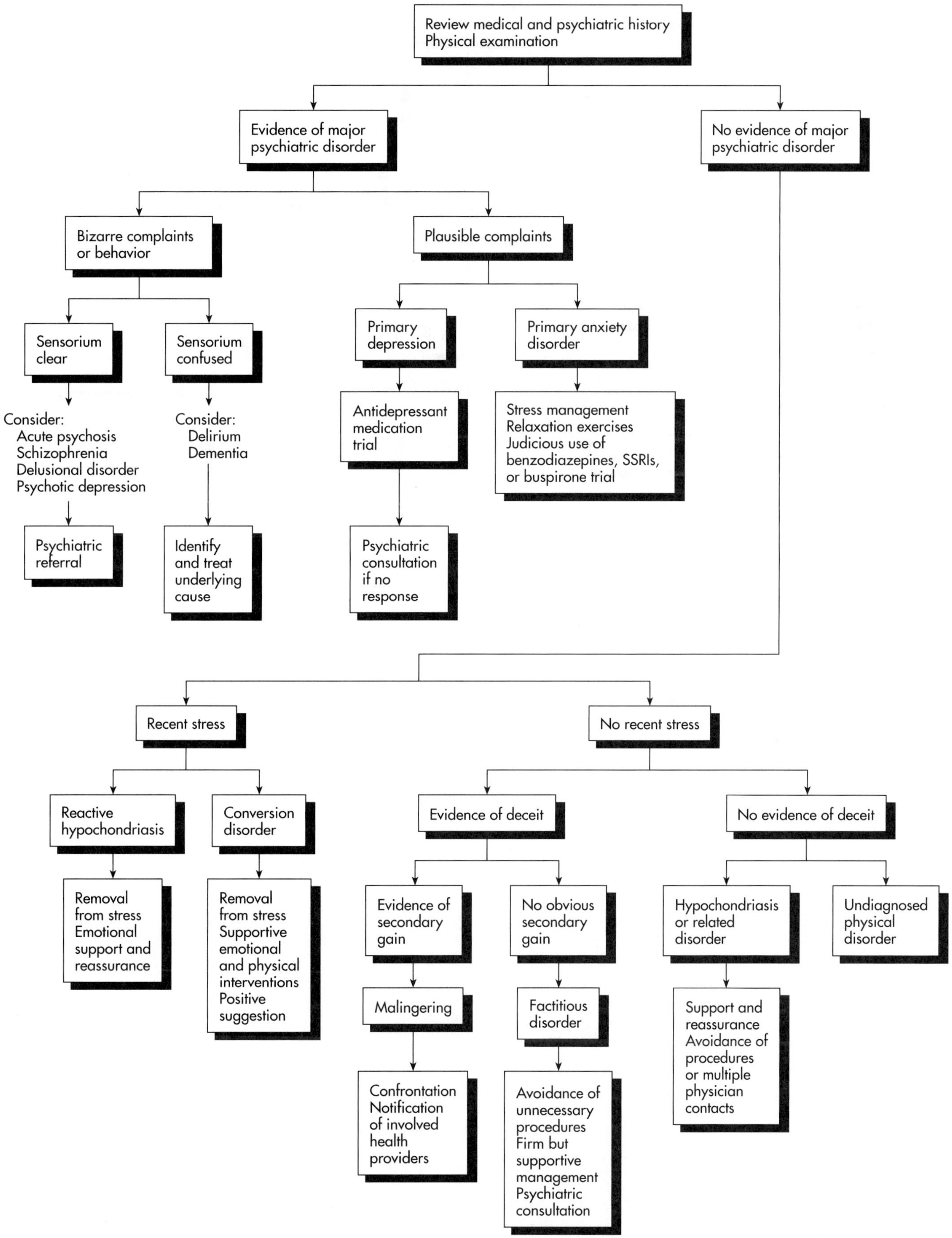

FIGURE 3-250 Patient with ill-defined physical complaints. Previous or recent evaluations are noncontributory. *SSRIs,* Selective serotonin reuptake inhibitors. (From Greene H, Johnson WP, Lemcke D [eds]: *Decision making in medicine,* ed 2, St Louis, 1998, Mosby.)

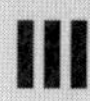

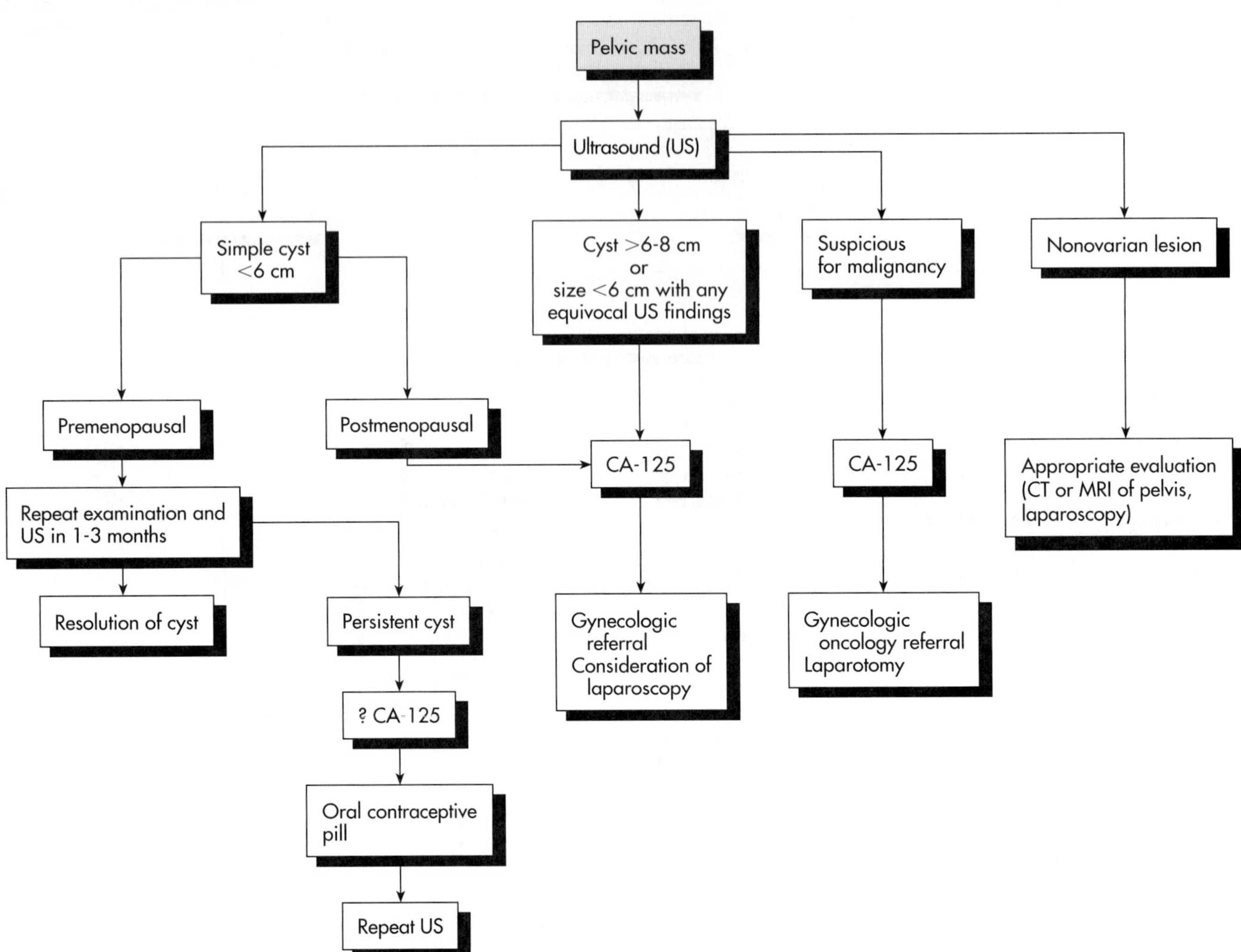

FIGURE 3-251 Approach to the patient with a pelvic mass. *CT,* Computed tomography; *MRI,* magnetic resonance imaging. (Modified from Carlson KJ et al: *Primary care of women,* ed 2, St Louis, 2002, Mosby.)

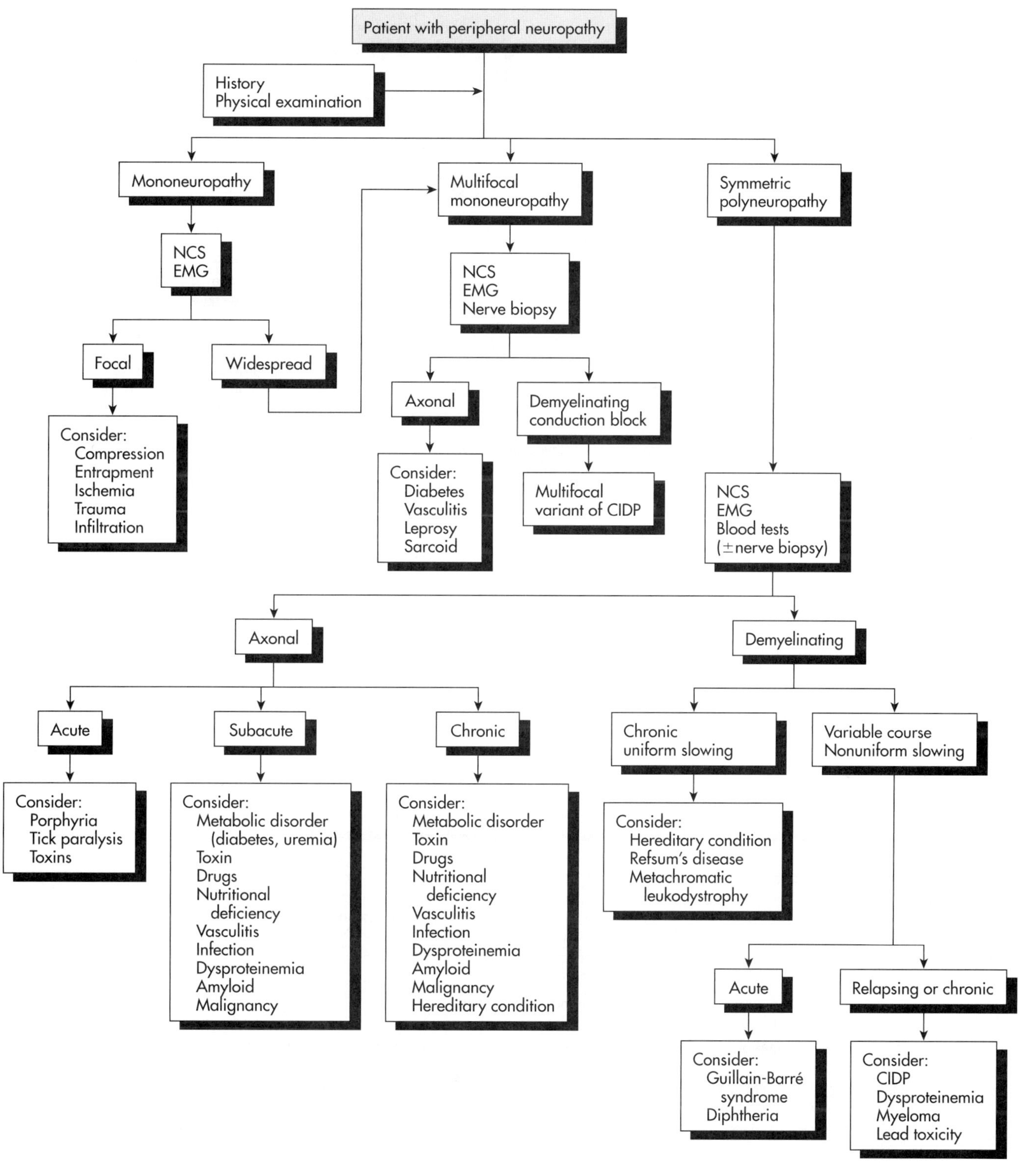

FIGURE 3-255 Approach to the patient with peripheral neuropathy. *CIDP,* Chronic inflammatory demyelinating polyradioneuropathy; *EMG,* electromyogram; *NCS,* nerve conduction studies. (From Greene HL, Johnson WP, Lemcke DL: *Decision making in medicine,* ed 2, St Louis, 1988, Mosby.)

ICD-9CM # 253 Pituitary adenoma
253.0 Acromegaly
253.1 Prolactinoma

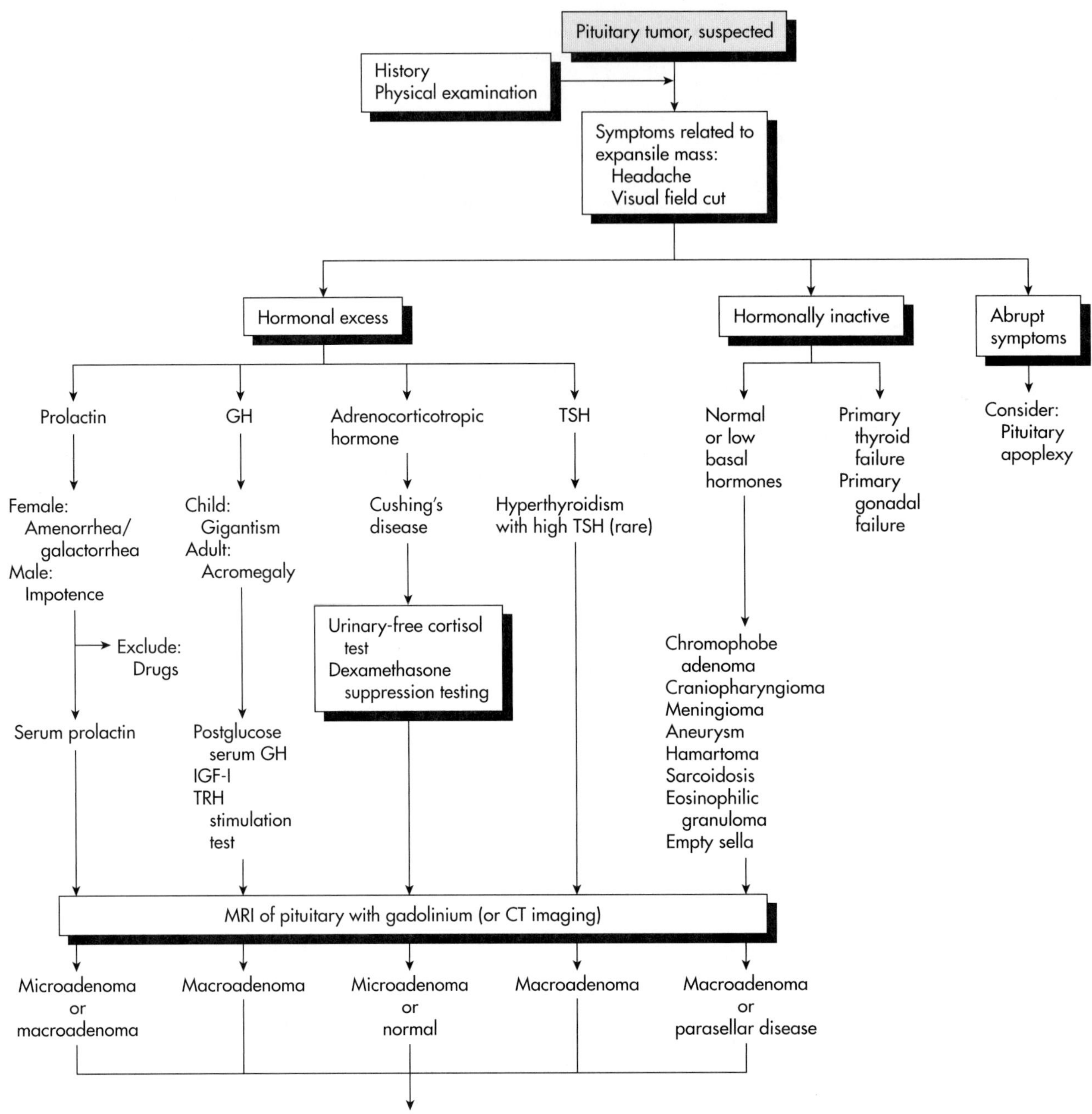

FIGURE 3-258 Evaluation of suspected pituitary tumor. *CT,* Computed tomography; *GH,* growth hormone; *IGF-I,* one of the insulin-like growth factors; *MRI,* magnetic resonance imaging; *TRH,* thyrotropin-releasing hormone; *TSH,* thyroid-stimulating hormone. (From Greene HL, Johnson WP, Lemcke D: *Decision making in medicine,* ed 2, St Louis, 1998, Mosby.)

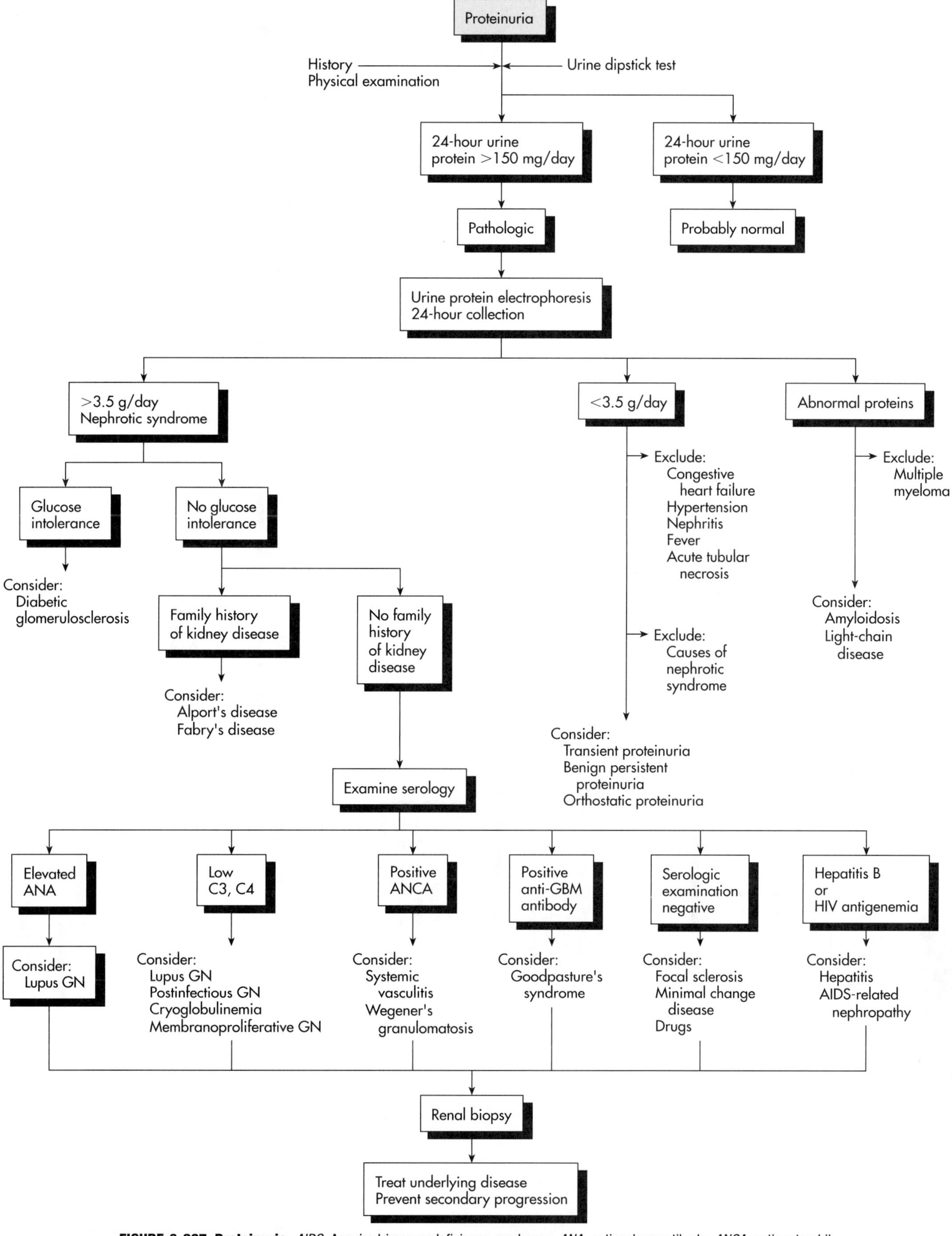

FIGURE 3-267 Proteinuria. *AIDS,* Acquired immunodeficiency syndrome; *ANA,* antinuclear antibody; *ANCA,* antineutrophil cytoplasmic autoantibody; *anti-GBM,* anti–glomerular basement membrane; *GN,* glomerulonephritis. (From Greene HL, Johnson WP, Lemcke D [eds]: *Decision making in medicine,* ed 2, St Louis, 1998, Mosby.)

PRURITUS, GENERALIZED

ICD-9CM # 698.9 Pruritus NOS

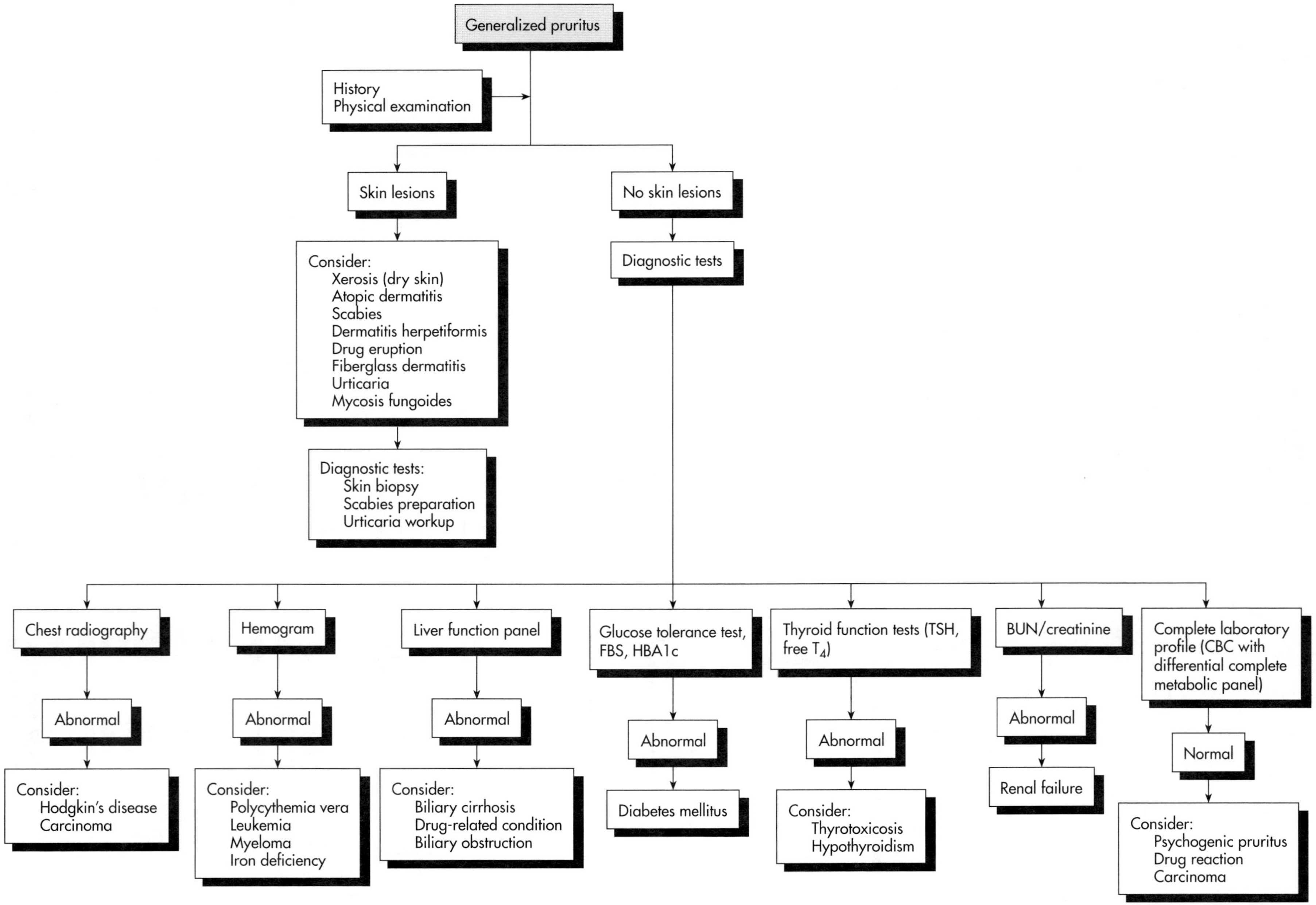

FIGURE 3-268 Evaluation of generalized pruritus. *BUN,* Blood urea nitrogen; *CBC,* complete blood count; *FBS,* fasting blood sugar; *HBA1c,* hemoglobin A1c; T_4, thyroxine; *TSH,* thyroid-stimulating hormone. (From Greene HL, Johnson WP, Lemcke D [eds]: *Decision making in medicine,* ed 2, St Louis, 1998, Mosby.)

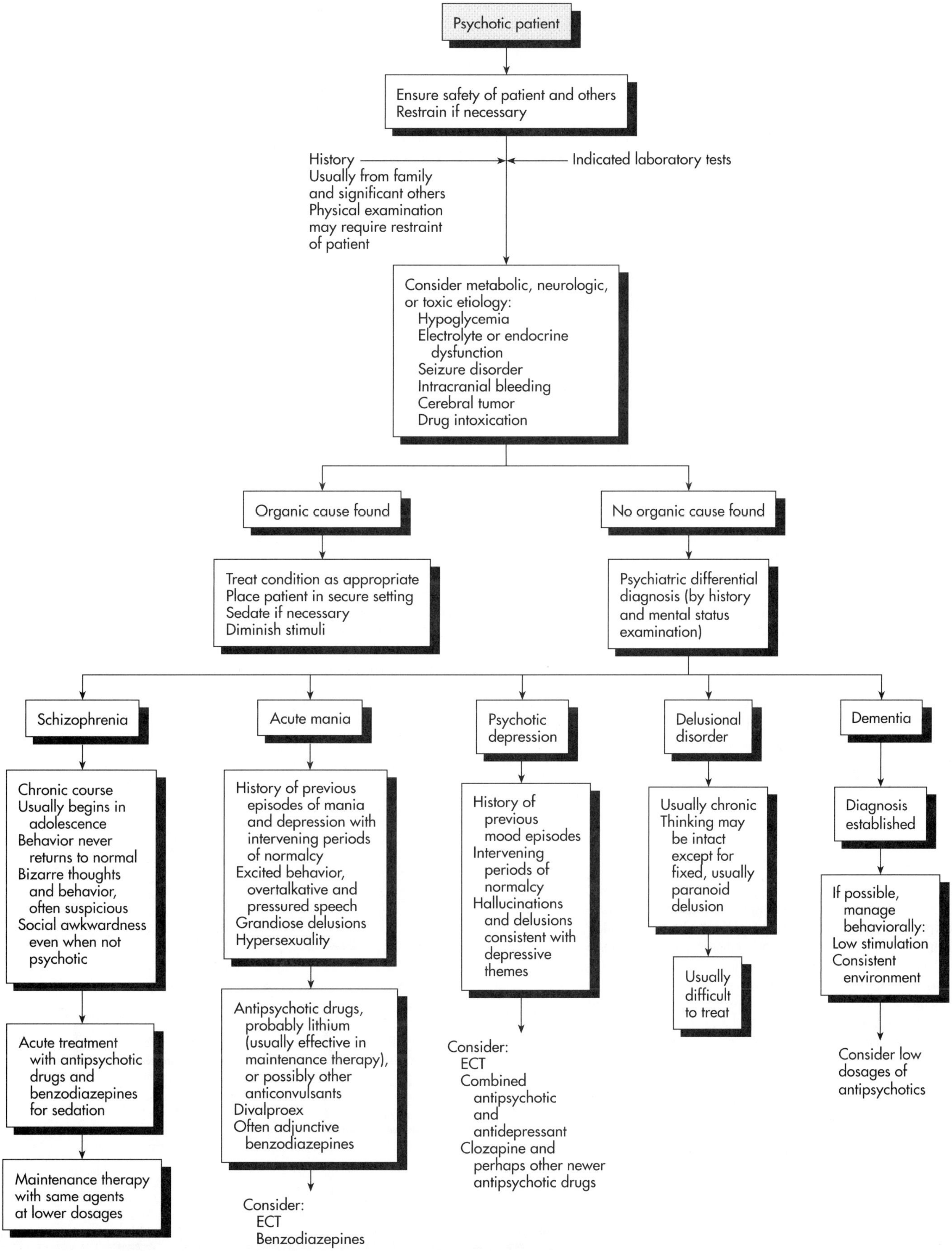

Psychotic patient

Ensure safety of patient and others
Restrain if necessary

History
Usually from family
and significant others
Physical examination
may require restraint
of patient

Indicated laboratory tests

Consider metabolic, neurologic, or toxic etiology:
Hypoglycemia
Electrolyte or endocrine dysfunction
Seizure disorder
Intracranial bleeding
Cerebral tumor
Drug intoxication

Organic cause found

Treat condition as appropriate
Place patient in secure setting
Sedate if necessary
Diminish stimuli

No organic cause found

Psychiatric differential diagnosis (by history and mental status examination)

Schizophrenia

Chronic course
Usually begins in adolescence
Behavior never returns to normal
Bizarre thoughts and behavior, often suspicious
Social awkwardness even when not psychotic

Acute treatment with antipsychotic drugs and benzodiazepines for sedation

Maintenance therapy with same agents at lower dosages

Acute mania

History of previous episodes of mania and depression with intervening periods of normalcy
Excited behavior, overtalkative and pressured speech
Grandiose delusions
Hypersexuality

Antipsychotic drugs, probably lithium (usually effective in maintenance therapy), or possibly other anticonvulsants
Divalproex
Often adjunctive benzodiazepines

Consider:
ECT
Benzodiazepines

Psychotic depression

History of previous mood episodes
Intervening periods of normalcy
Hallucinations and delusions consistent with depressive themes

Consider:
ECT
Combined antipsychotic and antidepressant
Clozapine and perhaps other newer antipsychotic drugs

Delusional disorder

Usually chronic
Thinking may be intact except for fixed, usually paranoid delusion

Usually difficult to treat

Dementia

Diagnosis established

If possible, manage behaviorally:
Low stimulation
Consistent environment

Consider low dosages of antipsychotics

FIGURE 3-273 Evaluation of psychotic patient. *ECT,* Electroconvulsive therapy. (From Greene HL, Johnson WP, Lemcke D [eds]: *Decision making in medicine,* ed 2, St Louis, 1998, Mosby.)

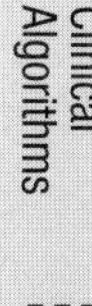

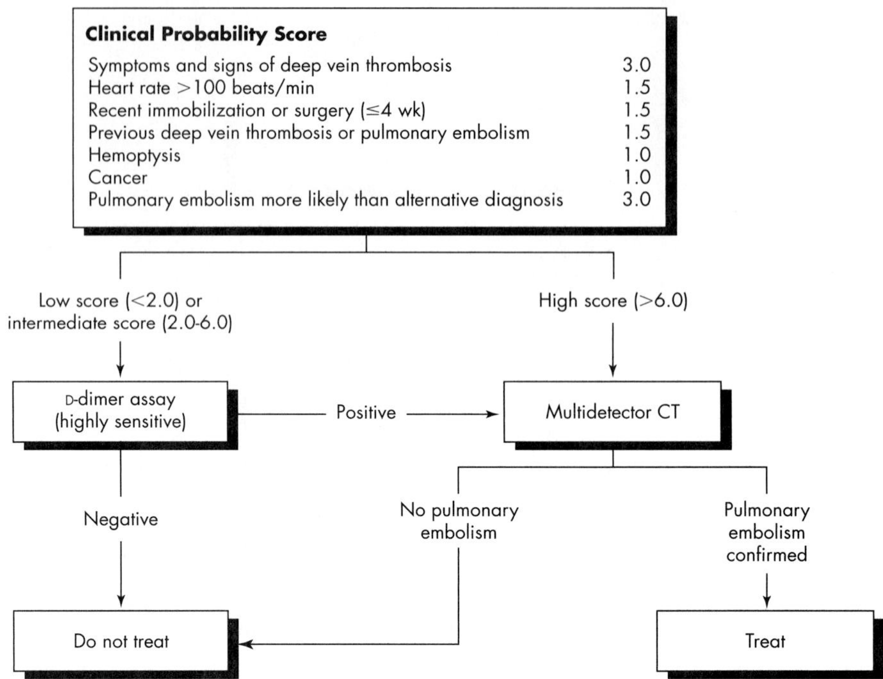

Note: Refer to Section I for additional information on this topic.

FIGURE 3-276 Diagnostic algorithm for suspected pulmonary embolism in a patient without hypotension or shock. This assessment of clinical probability is based on the Wells score (which has a range of 0 to 12.5, with higher scores indicating higher clinical probability). The revised Geneva score may be used as an alternative. If a moderately sensitive latex-derived D-dimer assay is used instead of the highly sensitive enzyme-linked immunosorbent D-dimer assay, pulmonary embolism can be ruled out only in patients with a low clinical probability. Alternatively, the Wells score can be dichotomized, classifying pulmonary embolism as unlikely (≤4.0) or likely (>4.0). For patients in whom pulmonary embolism is considered unlikely, either a highly sensitive or a moderately sensitive D-dimer assay can be used to rule out the diagnosis without need for further testing. If multidetector CT pulmonary angiography, with or without venography, is negative in a patient with a high clinical probability, the possibility of a false negative result should be considered and further testing performed to rule out pulmonary embolism. Options include serial venous ultrasonography, ventilation-perfusion lung scanning, and pulmonary angiography. If a multidetector CT scan shows only subsegmental defects in a patient with a low clinical probability, the possibility of a false positive result should be considered, and further testing (e.g., venous ultrasonography) should be performed to confirm the diagnosis. This may also apply to patients with an intermediate clinical probability, although the need for further tests is less well established for these patients. (From Konstantinides S: Acute pulmonary embolism, *N Engl J Med* 359:2804:2806, 2008.)

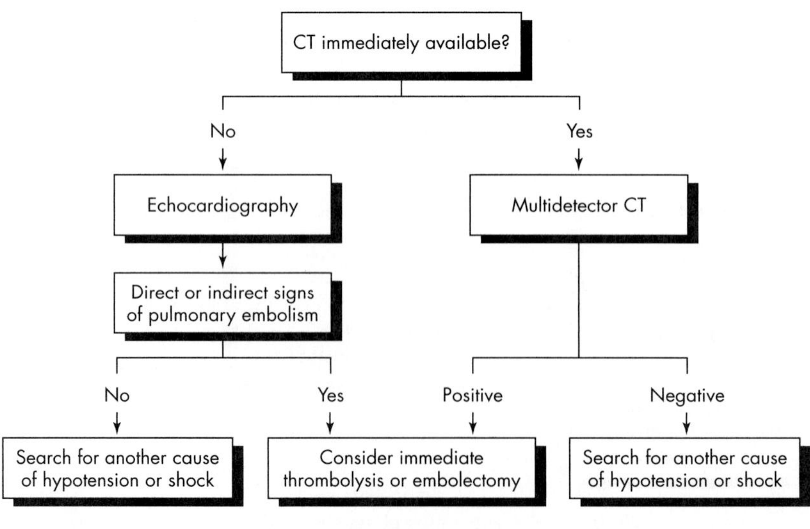

FIGURE 3-277 Emergency diagnostic workup for suspected pulmonary embolism in a patient with hypotension or shock. A direct sign of pulmonary embolism on a transthoracic or transesophageal echocardiogram is the presence of thrombi in the right atrium, right ventricle, or pulmonary artery. Thrombi may protrude into the left atrium through a patent foramen ovale. Indirect signs include right ventricular dysfunction (identified by the finding of dilation, free-wall hypokinesia, or paradoxical septal-wall motion); a systolic pressure gradient between the right ventricle and the right atrium of more than 30 mm Hg; and a pulmonary arterial flow acceleration time of less than 80 msec. When direct or indirect signs of pulmonary embolism are present, immediate treatment (without further diagnostic tests) is justified, particularly if CT angiography is still not available and arterial hypotension or shock persists. Adapted from the 2008 Guidelines on the Diagnosis and Management of Acute Pulmonary Embolism of the European Society of Cardiology. Since validation of diagnostic algorithms in prospective trials excluded hemodynamically unstable patients, these recommendations reflect expert opinion. (From Konstantinides S: Acute pulmonary embolism, *N Engl J Med* 359:2804:2087, 2008.)

TABLE 3-29 Anticoagulant Drugs for Initial Treatment of Pulmonary Embolism.*

Drug	Dose	Remarks
Unfractionated heparin (intravenous infusion)†	80 IU/kg of body weight as an intravenous bolus, followed by continuous infusion at the rate of 18 IU/kg/hr	Adjust infusion rate to maintain aPTT between 1.5 and 2.5 times control, corresponding to therapeutic heparin levels (0.3 to 0.7 IU/ml by factor Xa inhibition)††; monitor platelet count at baseline and every other day from day 4 to day 14 or until heparin is stopped; investigate for heparin-induced thrombocytopenia if platelet count falls by ≥50% or a thrombotic event occurs.
Low-molecular-weight heparins (subcutaneous injection)§		Low-molecular-weight heparins have not been tested in patients with arterial hypotension or shock and thus are not recommended for such patients; monitoring of anti–factor Xa levels may be helpful in patients at increased risk for bleeding, particularly those with moderate or severe renal impairment; the need for monitoring anti–factor Xa levels in pregnant women remains controversial; monitor platelet count at baseline and every 2 to 4 days from day 4 to day 14 or until heparin is stopped.¶
Enoxaparin	1.0 mg/kg every 12 hr or 1.5 mg/kg once daily‖	If creatinine clearance is <30 ml/min, reduce enoxaparin dose to 1 mg/kg once daily; consider unfractionated heparin infusion as an alternative.
Tinzaparin	175 U/kg once daily	
Fondaparinux§	5 mg (body weight, <50 kg); 7.5 mg (body weight, 50-100 kg); or 10 mg (body weight, >100 kg), administered once daily	This drug is contraindicated in patients with severe renal impairment (creatinine clearance, <30 ml/min); no routine platelet monitoring is necessary.

(From Konstantinides S: Acute pulmonary embolism, *N Engl J Med* 359:2804:2808, 2008.)

*The abbreviation aPTT denotes activated partial thromboplastin time.

†Unfractionated heparin is the preferred treatment in patients with severe renal dysfunction (creatinine clearance, <30 ml per minute), since it is not eliminated by the kidneys, and in patients with an increased risk of bleeding (i.e., those with congenital or acquired bleeding diathesis, active ulcerative or angiodysplastic gastrointestinal disease, recent hemorrhagic stroke, recent brain, spinal, or ophthalmologic surgery diabetic retinopathy, or bacterial endocarditis), owing to its short half-life and reversible anticoagulant effects.

††It is recommended that the treatment dose be adjusted on the basis of standardized nomograms such as that proposed by Raschke et al.

§Tinzaparin and fondaparinux are explicitly approved for the treatment of acute pulmonary embolism. Enoxaparin is approved for the treatment of deep vein thrombosis with or without pulmonary embolism.

¶This recommendation applies to postoperative patients and to medical or obstetrical patients who have received unfractionated heparin within the past 100 days. For medical or obstetrical patients who have received only low-molecular-weight heparin, some authorities recommend no routine monitoring of platelet counts.

‖Once-daily injection of enoxaparin at a dose of 1.5 mg per kilogram is approved for inpatient treatment of pulmonary embolism in the United States and in some, but not all, European countries.

TABLE 3-30 Stratification of Risk of Death Associated with Pulmonary Embolism and Severity-Adjusted Treatment.*

Early Risk of Death	Risk Factor			Recommended Treatment
	Shock or Hypotension (on Clinical Examination)	***Right Ventricular Dysfunction (on Echocardiography or Multidetector CT)***	***Myocardial Injury (on Cardiac Troponin Testing)***	
High	Present	Present†	NA††	Unfractionated heparin plus thrombolysis or embolectomy
Non-high				
Intermediate§	Absent	Present	Present	Low-molecular-weight heparin or fondaparinux; as a rule, no early thrombolysis; monitor clinical status and right ventricular function
	Absent	Present	Absent	
	Absent	Absent	Present	
Low	Absent	Absent	Absent	Low-molecular-weight heparin or fondaparnux; consider outpatient treatment

(From Konstantinides S: Acute pulmonary embolism, *N Engl J Med* 359:2804:2810, 2008.)

*Adapted with modifications from the 2008 Guidelines on the Diagnosis and Management of Acute Pulmonary Embolism of the European Society of Cardiology. NA denotes not applicable.

†If RV function is normal on echocardiography, or if a CT scan shows no RV dilatation in a patient with hemodynamic compromise and clinically suspected pulmonary embolism, an alternative diagnosis should be sought.

††Troponin test results do not influence risk assessment or treatment in hemodynamically compromised patients with acute pulmonary embolism.

§Although it has been suggested that normotensive patients with both RV dysfunction and myocardial injury have a higher risk of death than those with only one of these risk factors, there is currently no definitive proof that they should receive more aggressive treatment.

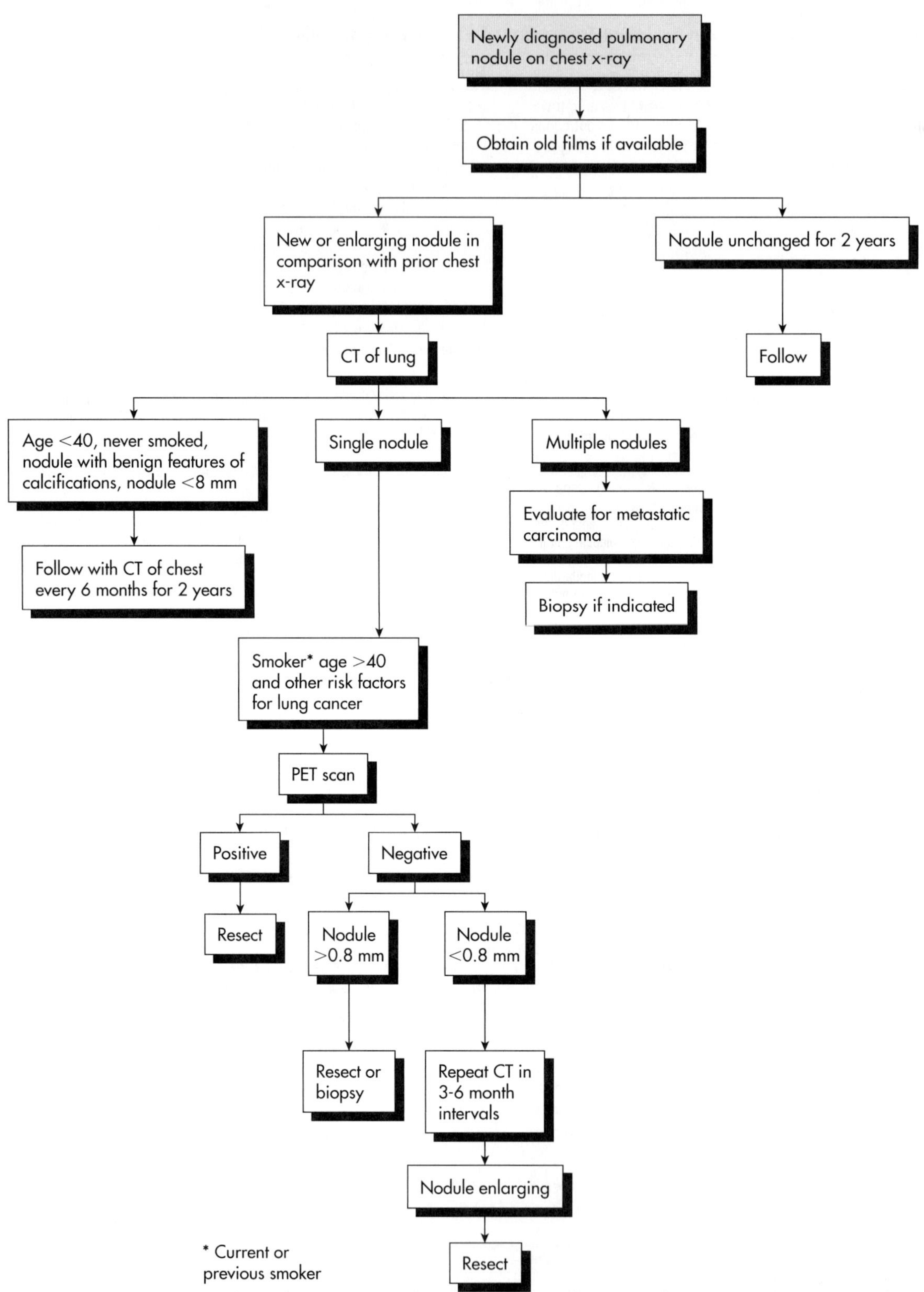

FIGURE 3-278 Pulmonary nodule. *CT,* Computed tomography; *PET,* positron emission tomography.

FIGURE 3-279 Differential diagnosis of purpura. (From Bolognia JL, Jorizzo JL, Rapini RP: *Dermatology,* St Louis, 2003, Mosby.)

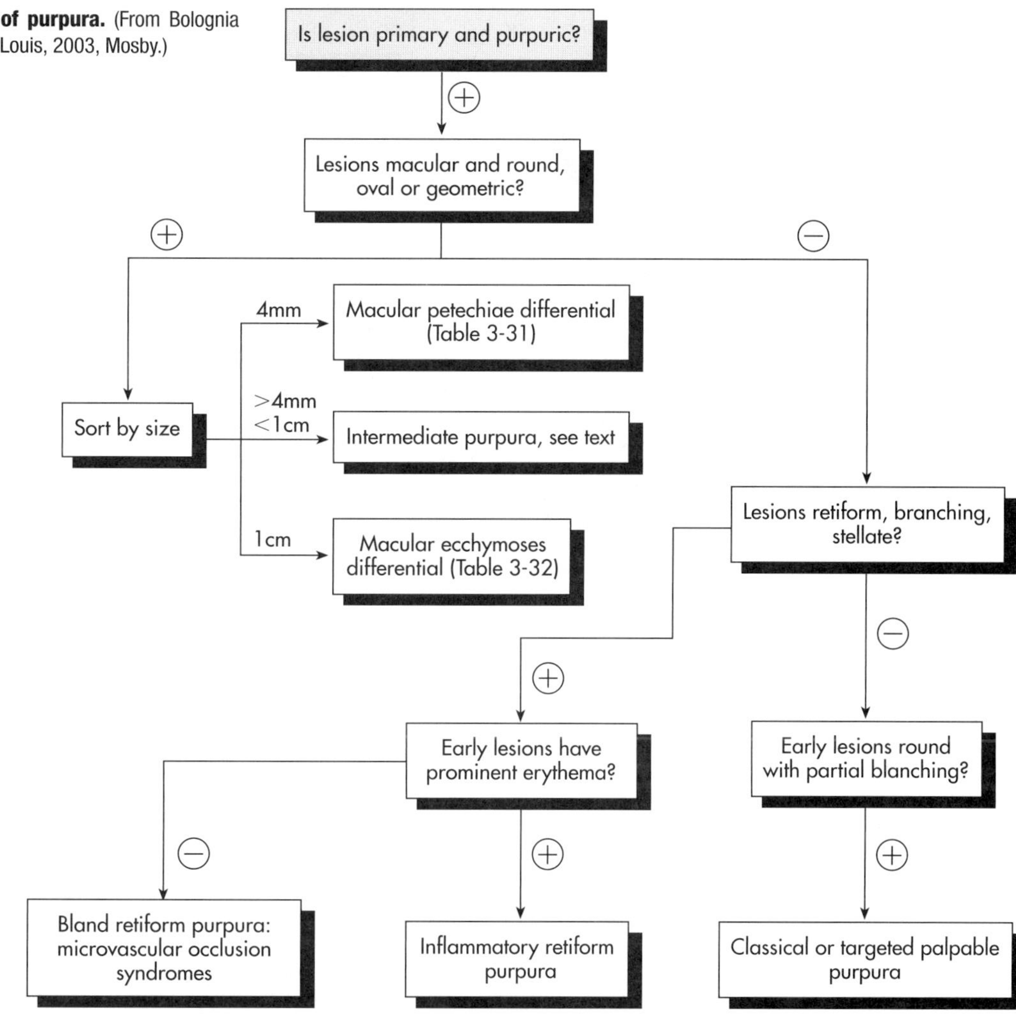

TABLE 3-31 Differential Diagnosis of Petechial Hemorrhage—Non-Palpable, Non-Retiform and ≤4 mm in Diameter

Pathophysiology: hemostatically relevant thrombocytopenia (<50,000/mm³) **

Major etiologies*
1. Idiopathic thrombocytopenic purpura
2. Thrombotic thrombocytopenic purpura
3. Disseminated intravascular coagulation
4. Other acquired thrombocytopenias, including drug-related
   a. Peripheral destruction (e.g., quinine, quinidine)
   b. Decreased production, idiosyncratic or dose-related (e.g., chemotherapy)
   c. Bone marrow infiltration, fibrosis or failure

Pathophysiology: abnormal platelet function

Major etiologies*
1. Congenital or hereditary platelet function defects
2. Acquired platelet function defects
   a. Aspirin, NSAIDs
   b. Renal insufficiency
   c. Monoclonal gammopathy
3. Thrombocytosis in myeloproliferative disease (often >1,000,000/mm³)

Pathophysiology: non-platelet etiologies

Major etiologies*
1. Spiking elevations of intravascular venous pressure (Valsalva maneuver-like, e.g., repetitive vomiting, childbirth, paroxysmal coughing, seizure)
2. Fixed increased pressure (e.g., stasis, ligatures)
3. Trauma (often linear)
4. Perifollicular (vitamin C deficiency)
5. Mildly inflammatory conditions
   a. Chronic pigmented purpura
   b. Hypergammaglobulinemic purpura of Waldenström

TABLE 3-32 Differential Diagnosis for Macular Purpura and Ecchymoses—Non-Palpable and Non-Retiform

Intermediate macular purpura (>4 mm, <1 cm in diameter)

Major etiologies*
1. Hypergammaglobulinemic purpura of Waldenström
2. Infection/inflammation in patients with thrombocytopenia
3. Rarely, minimally inflamed immune complex vasculitis (usually dependent distribution)

Ecchymoses (≥1 cm in diameter)

A. Pathophysiology: procoagulant defect plus minor trauma*
   1. Anticoagulant use
   2. Hepatic insufficiency with poor procoagulant synthesis
   3. Vitamin K deficiency
   4. Disseminated intravascular coagulation (some)
B. Pathophysiology: poor dermal support of vessels plus minor trauma*
   1. Actinic (solar, senile) purpura
   2. Corticosteroid therapy, topical or systemic
   3. Vitamin C deficiency (scurvy)
   4. Systemic amyloidosis (light chain-related, some familial types)
   5. Ehlers-Danlos syndrome (primarily type IV)
C. Pathophysiology: other causes plus minor trauma*
   1. Hypergammaglobulinemic purpura of Waldenström
   2. Platelet function defects, including von Willebrand disease, medications, metabolic diseases
   3. Acquired or congenital thrombocytopenia

*Partial list.
**Most patients do not have petechiae until platelets ≤20,000/mm³.

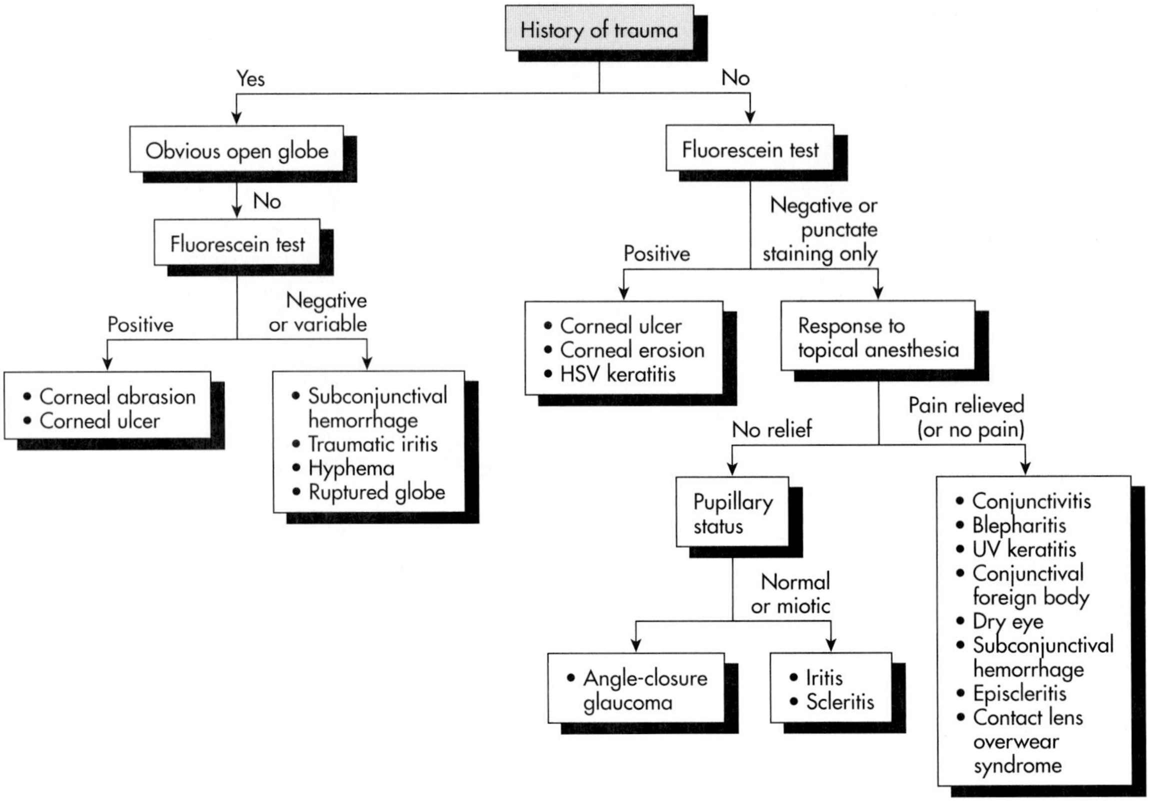

- History of trauma
  - Yes → Obvious open globe
    - No → Fluorescein test
      - Positive → • Corneal abrasion • Corneal ulcer
      - Negative or variable → • Subconjunctival hemorrhage • Traumatic iritis • Hyphema • Ruptured globe
  - No → Fluorescein test
    - Positive → • Corneal ulcer • Corneal erosion • HSV keratitis
    - Negative or punctate staining only → Response to topical anesthesia
      - No relief → Pupillary status
        - → • Angle-closure glaucoma
        - Normal or miotic → • Iritis • Scleritis
      - Pain relieved (or no pain) → • Conjunctivitis • Blepharitis • UV keratitis • Conjunctival foreign body • Dry eye • Subconjunctival hemorrhage • Episcleritis • Contact lens overwear syndrome

FIGURE 3-281 Algorithm showing diagnostic procedure for the acute red eye. *HSV,* Herpes simplex virus; *UV,* ultraviolet. (From Auerbach PS: *Wilderness medicine,* ed 5, St Louis, 2007, Mosby.)

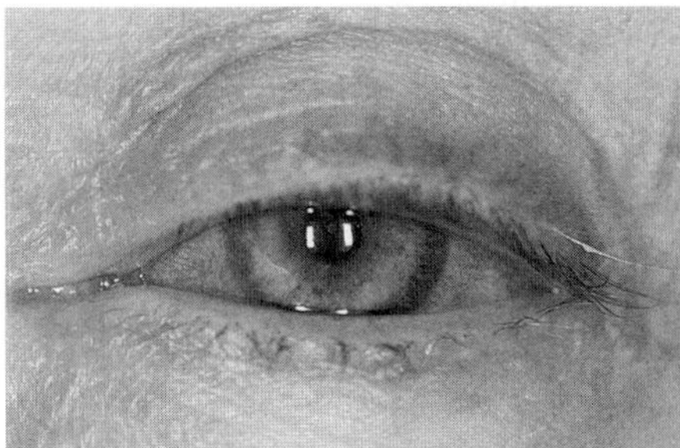

FIGURE 3-282 Contact lens acute red eye. This is often accompanied by pain and photophobia. (From Yanoff M, Duker JS: *Ophthalmology,* ed 2, St Louis, 2004, Mosby.)

Acute renal failure*
Prerenal
1. Absolute decrease in effective blood volume
Hemorrhage
Skin losses (burns, sweating)
Gastrointestinal losses (diarrhea, vomiting)
Renal losses (diuretics, glycosuria)
Fluid pooling (peritonitis, burns)
2. Relative decrease in blood volume (ineffective arterial volume)
Congestive heart failure
Sepsis
Anaphylaxis
Liver failure
3. Arterial occlusion
Bilateral thromboembolism
Thromboembolism of solitary kidney
Intrinsic renal
Vascular
Examples:
vasculitis, malignant hypertension, microscopic polyarteritis
Acute glomerulonephritis
Examples:
postinfectious glomerulonephritis, anti–basement membrane antibody disease
Acute interstitial nephritis
Examples:
drug-associated acute interstitial nephritis (methicillin)
Acute tubular necrosis
Ischemic
Hypotension
Nephrotoxic
Exogenous
Nephrotoxins:
1. Antibiotics (gentamicin, kanamycin, neomycin, amikacin, tobramycin, streptomycin, amphotericin B)
2. Iodinated contrast agents
3. Metals (mercury, cisplatin)
4. Solvents (carbon tetrachloride, ethylene glycol)
Endogenous
1. Intratubular pigments (hemoglobinuria, myoglobinuria)
2. Intratubular proteins (myeloma)
3. Intratubular crystals (uric acid, oxalate)
Postrenal
1. Obstruction of collecting system
Bladder outlet obstruction
Bilateral ureteral obstruction (unusual)
Ureteral obstruction in a solitary kidney

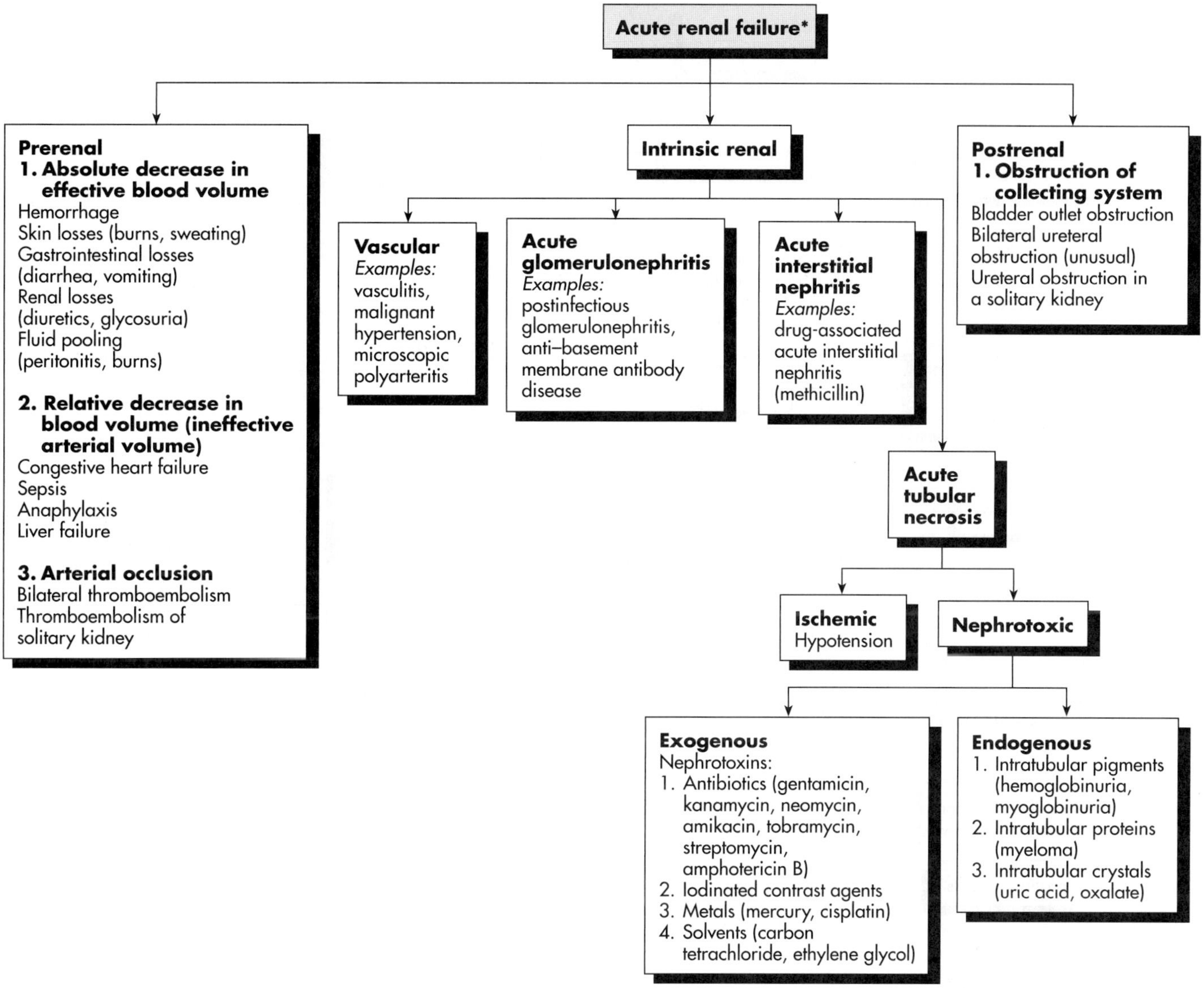

*Refer to Section I for additional information on this topic.

FIGURE 3-286 Causes of acute renal failure. (From Andreoli TE [ed]: *Cecil essentials of medicine,* ed 7, Philadelphia, 2008, WB Saunders.)

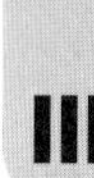

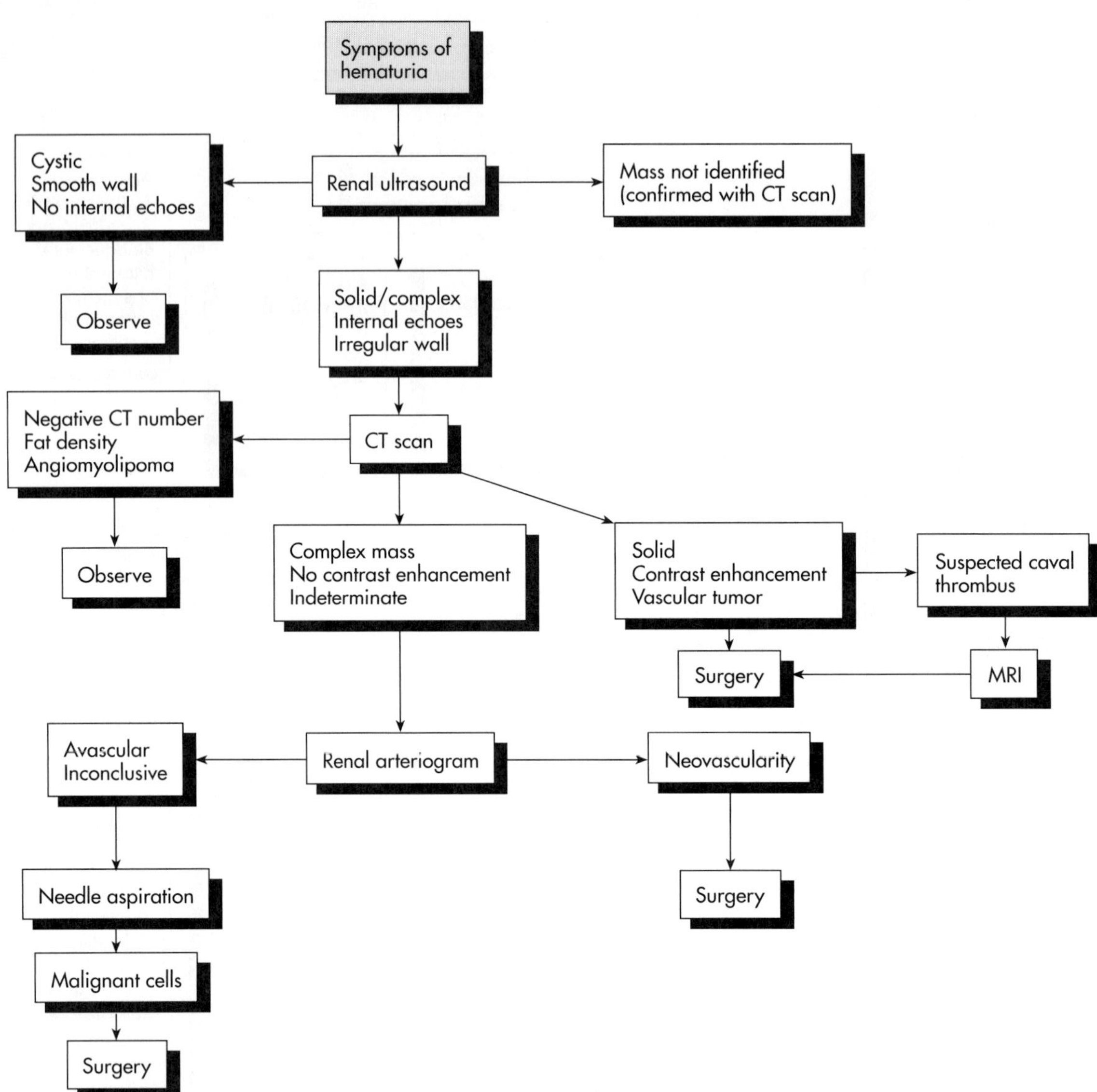

FIGURE 3-287 Evaluation of a patient with a renal mass. *CT,* Computed tomography; *MRI,* magnetic resonance imaging. (Modified from Williams RD: Tumors of the kidney, ureter, and bladder. In Goldman L, Ausiello D [eds]: *Cecil textbook of medicine,* ed 23, Philadelphia, 2008, WB Saunders.)

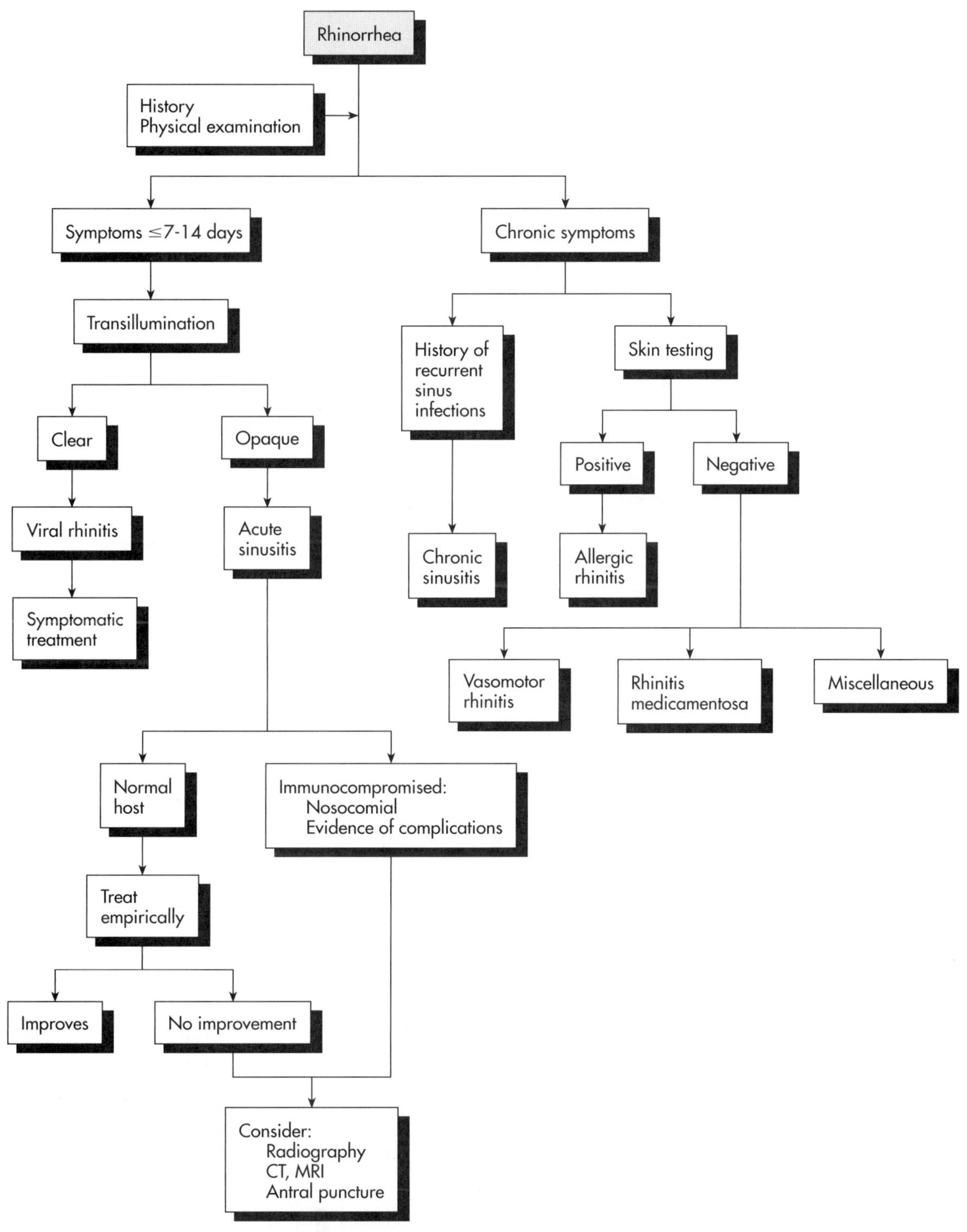

FIGURE 3-290 Approach to a patient with rhinorrhea. *CT,* Computed tomography; *MRI,* magnetic resonance imaging. (From Noble J [ed]: *Primary care medicine,* ed 3, St Louis, 2001, Mosby.)

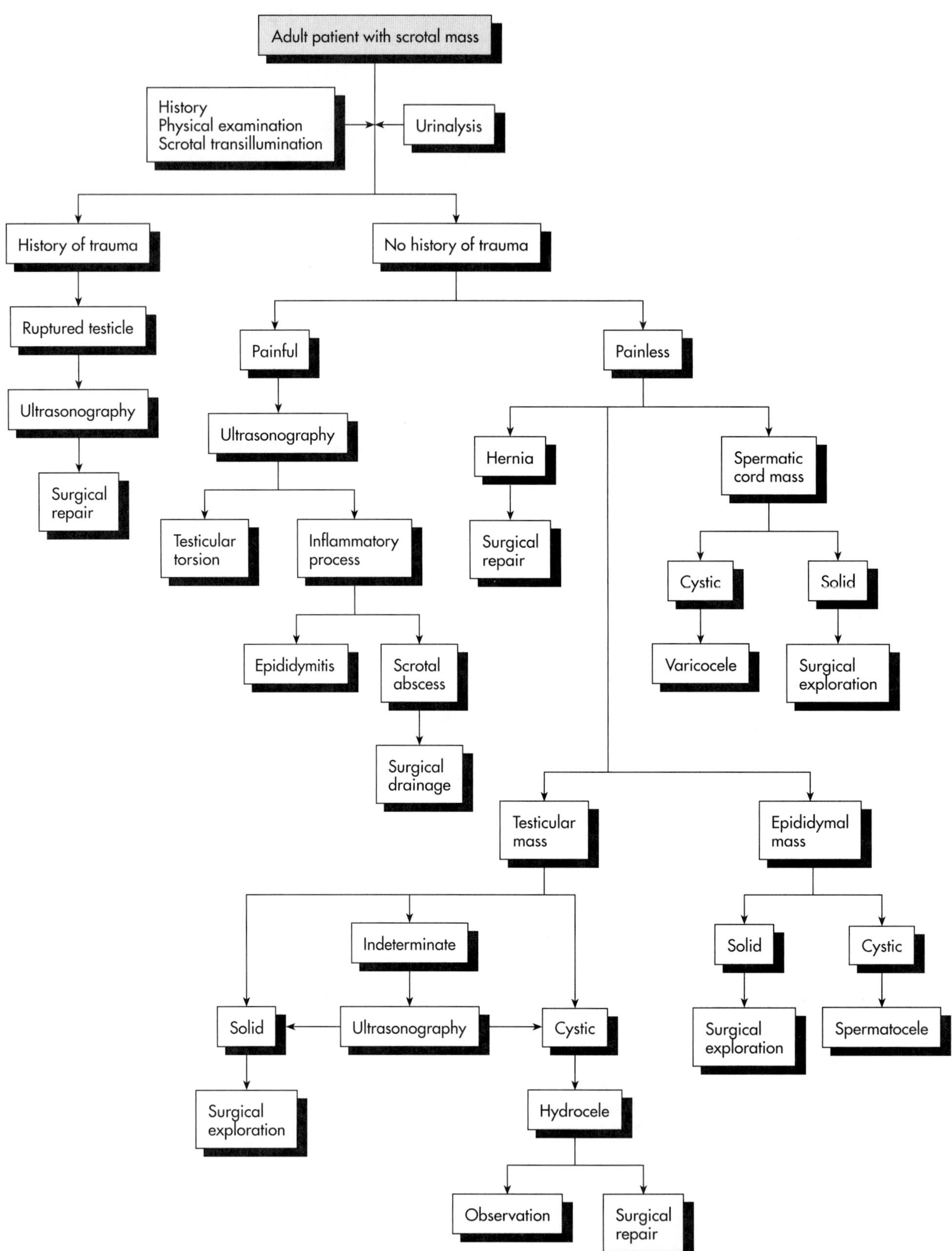

FIGURE 3-293 Evaluation of scrotal mass. (From Greene HL, Johnson WP, Lemcke D [eds]: *Decision making in medicine,* ed 2, St Louis, 1998, Mosby.)

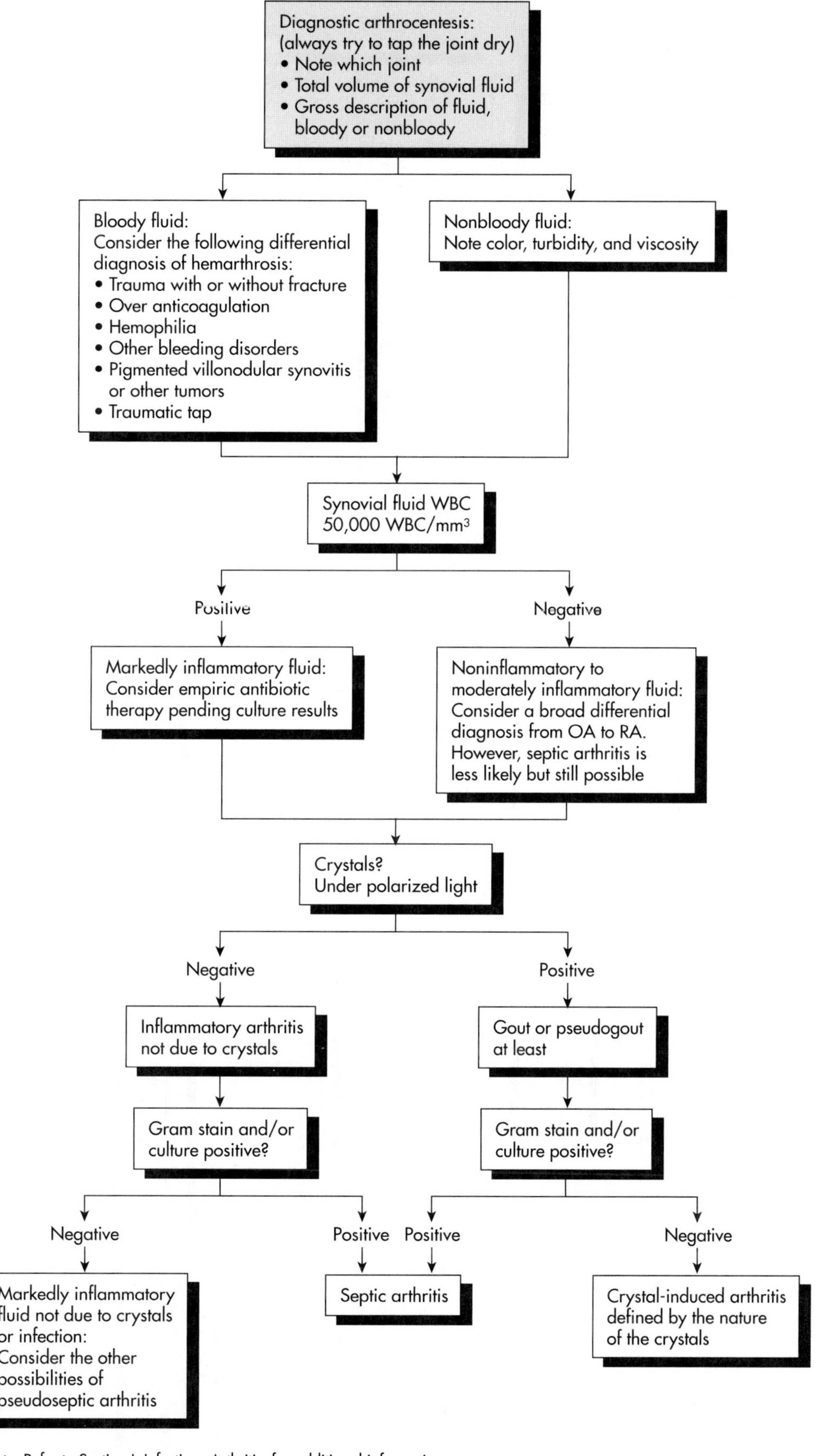

Note: Refer to Section I, Infectious Arthritis, for additional information.

FIGURE 3-295 Algorithm for synovial fluid analysis in septic arthritis. *OA,* Osteoarthritis; *RA,* rheumatoid arthritis. (From Harris ED et al [eds]: *Kelley's textbook of rheumatology,* ed 7, Philadelphia, 2005, Saunders.)

SEXUAL DYSFUNCTION

ICD-9CM # 309.2 Sexual disorder (psychosexual)
V41.7 Sexual function problem

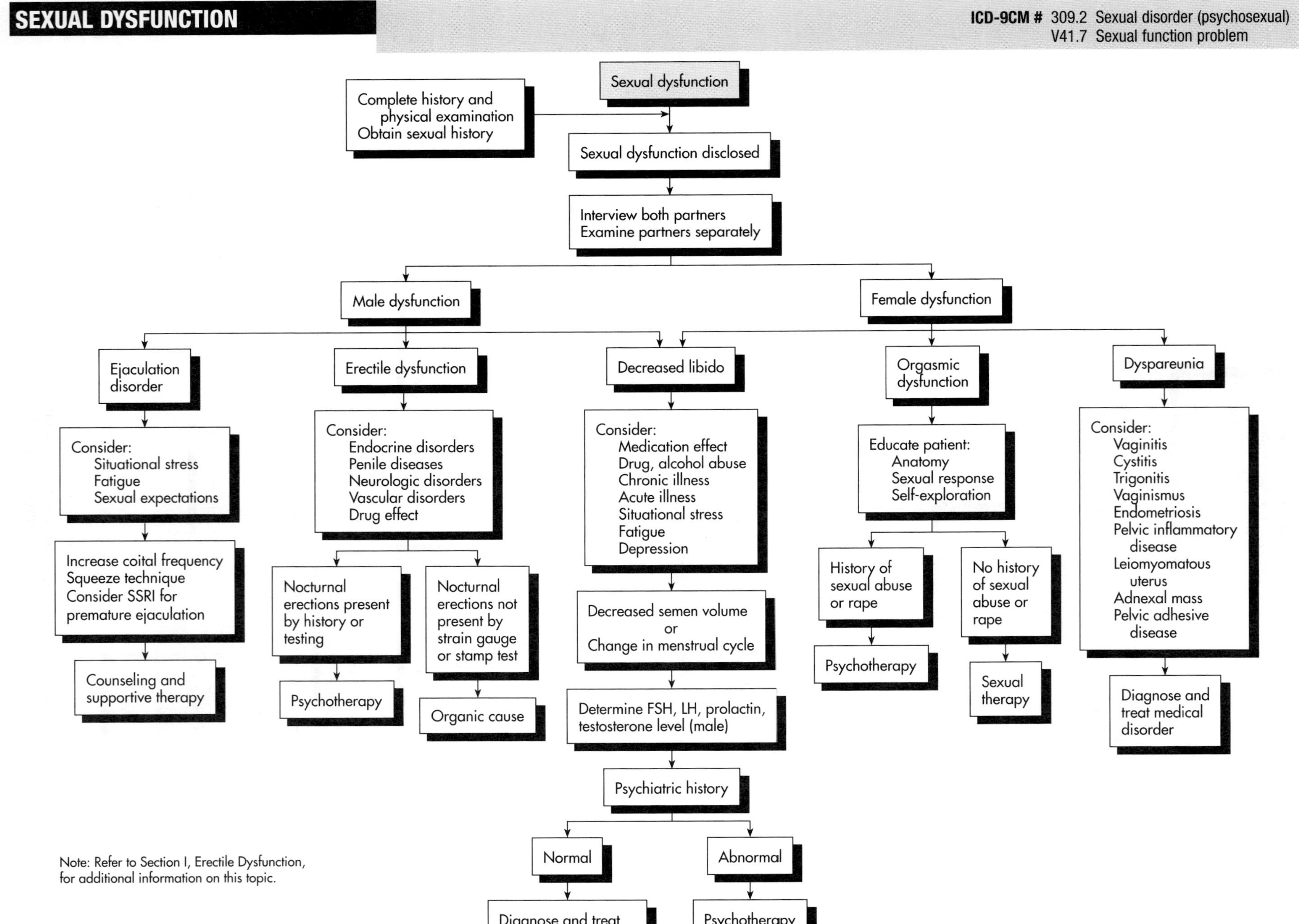

Note: Refer to Section I, Erectile Dysfunction, for additional information on this topic.

FIGURE 3-296 Evaluation of sexual dysfunction. *FSH,* Follicle-stimulating hormone; *LH,* luteinizing hormone; *SSRI,* selective serotonin reuptake inhibitor. (Modified from Greene HL, Johnson WP, Lemcke D [eds]: *Decision making in medicine,* ed 2, St Louis, 1998, Mosby.)

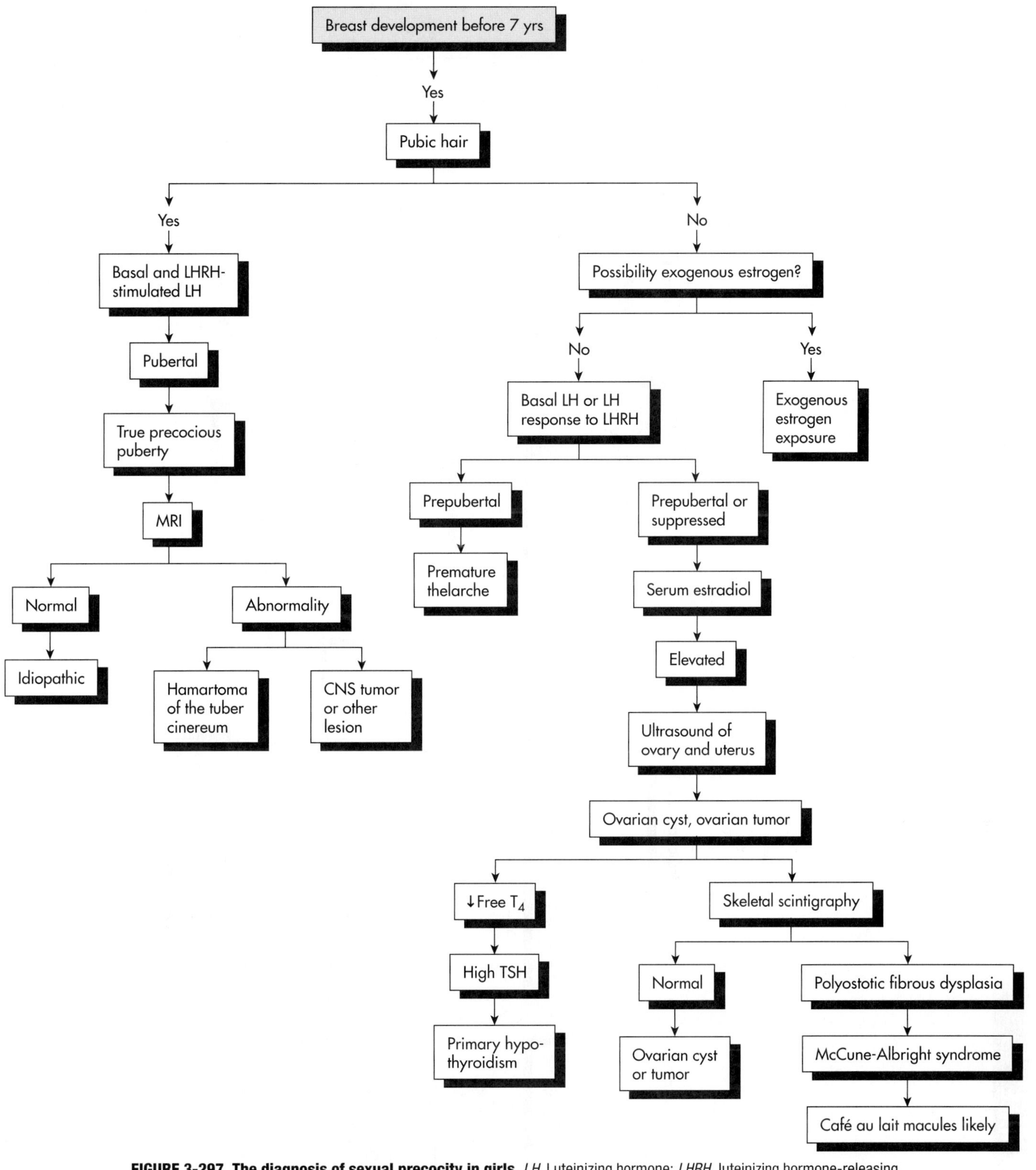

FIGURE 3-297 The diagnosis of sexual precocity in girls. *LH,* Luteinizing hormone; *LHRH,* luteinizing hormone-releasing hormone; *MRI,* magnetic resonance imaging; T_4, thyroxine; *TSH,* thyroid-stimulating hormone; *yrs,* years. (From Larsen PR, Kronenberg HM, Memlmed S, Polansky, KS [eds]: *Williams textbook of endocrinology,* ed 11, Philadelphia, 2008, Saunders.)

SEXUAL PRECOCITY, MALE

ICD-9CM # 259.1

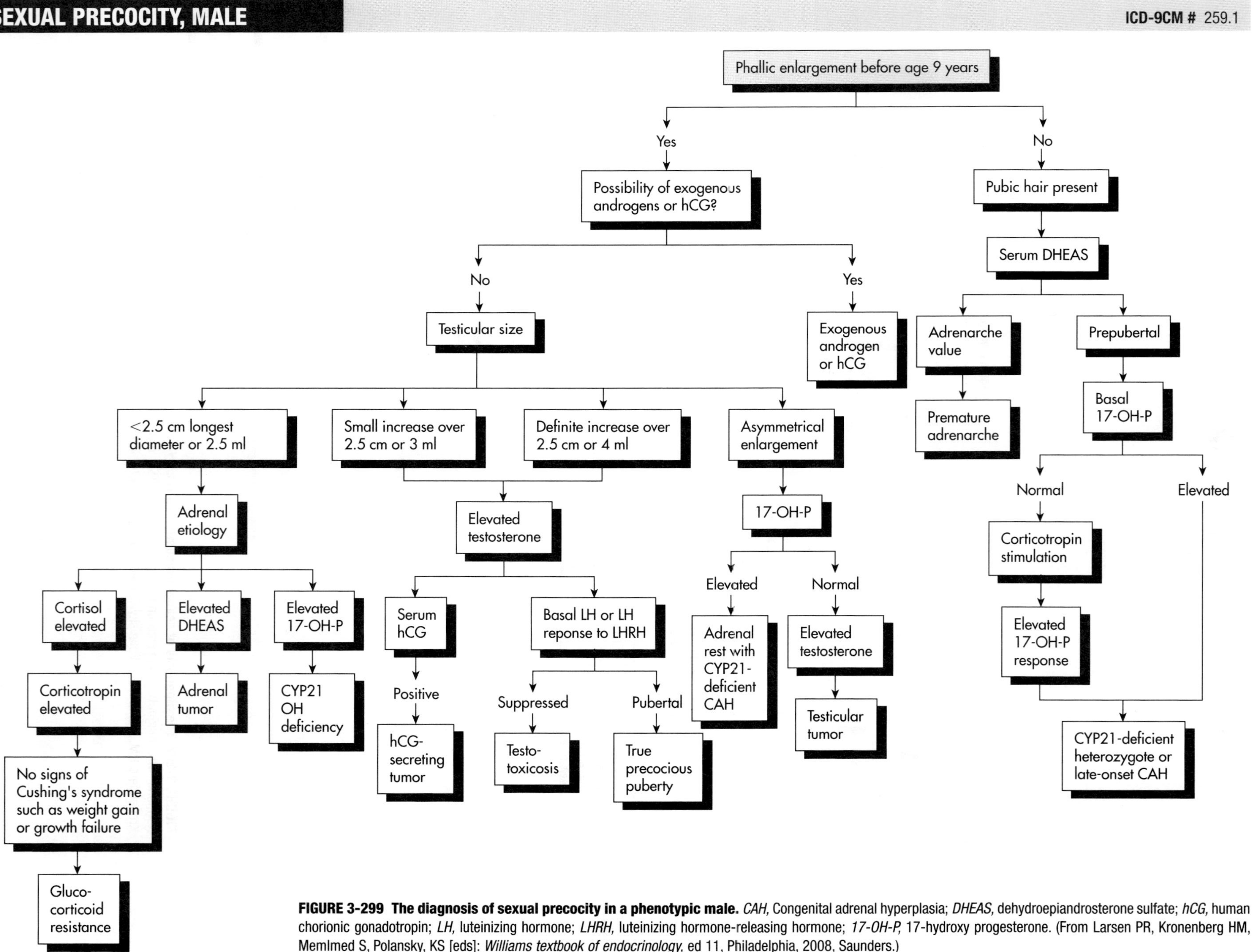

FIGURE 3-299 The diagnosis of sexual precocity in a phenotypic male. *CAH,* Congenital adrenal hyperplasia; *DHEAS,* dehydroepiandrosterone sulfate; *hCG,* human chorionic gonadotropin; *LH,* luteinizing hormone; *LHRH,* luteinizing hormone-releasing hormone; *17-OH-P,* 17-hydroxy progesterone. (From Larsen PR, Kronenberg HM, Memlmed S, Polansky, KS [eds]: *Williams textbook of endocrinology,* ed 11, Philadelphia, 2008, Saunders.)

SEXUAL PRECOCITY, MALE—cont'd

ICD-9CM # 259.1

TABLE 3-34 Differential Diagnosis of Sexual Precocity

	Plasma Gonadotropins	LH Response to LHRH	Serum Sex Steroid Concentration	Gonadal Size	Miscellaneous
True Precocious Puberty (premature reactivation of LHRH pulse generator)	Prominent LH pulses, initially during sleep	Pubertal LH response	Pubertal values of testosterone or estradiol	Normal pubertal testicular enlargement or ovarian and uterine enlargement (by ultrasonography)	MRI of brain to rule out CNS tumor or other abnormality; skeletal survey for McCune-Albright syndrome
Incomplete Sexual Precocity (pituitary gonadotropin-independent)					
Males					
Chorionic gonadotropin-secreting tumor in males	High hCG, low LH	Prepubertal LH response	Pubertal value of testosterone	Slight to moderate uniform enlargement of testes	Hepatomegaly suggests hepatoblastoma; CT scan of brain if chorionic gonadotropin-secreting CNS tumor suspected
Leydig cell tumor in males	Suppressed	No LH response	Very high testosterone	Irregular asymmetrical enlargement of testes	
Familial testotoxicosis	Suppressed	No LH response	Pubertal values of testosterone	Testes symmetrical and larger than 2.5 cm but smaller than expected for pubertal development; spermatogenesis occurs	Familial; probably sex-limited, autosomal dominant trait
Virilizing congenital adrenal hyperplasia	Prepubertal	Prepubertal LH response	Elevated 17-OHP in CYP21 deficiency or elevated 11-deoxycortisol in CYP11B1 deficiency	Testes prepubertal	Autosomal recessive, may be congenital or late-onset form, may have salt loss in CYP21 deficiency or hypertension in CYP11B1 deficiency
Virilizing adrenal tumor	Prepubertal	Prepubertal LH response	High DHEAS and androstenedione values	Testes prepubertal	CT, MRI, or ultrasonography of abdomen
Premature adrenarche	Prepubertal	Prepubertal LH response	Prepubertal testosterone, DHEAS, or urinary 17-ketosteroid values appropriate for pubic hair stage 2	Testes prepubertal	Onset usually after 6 years of age; more frequent in CNS-injured children
In Both Sexes					
McCune-Albright syndrome	Suppressed	Suppressed	Sex steroids pubertal or higher	Ovarian (on ultrasound); slight testicular enlargement	Skeletal survey for polyostotic fibrous dysplasia and skin examination for café au lait spots
Primary hypothyroidism	LH prepubertal; FSH may be slightly elevated	Prepubertal FSH may be increased	Estradiol may be pubertal	Testicular enlargement; ovaries cystic	TSH and prolactin elevated; T_4 low

From Larson PR, Kronenberg HM, Memlmed S, Polansky, KS [eds]: *Williams textbook of endocrinology*, ed 11, Philadelphia, 2008, Saunders.
CNS, Central nervous system; *CT*, computed tomography; *DHEAS*, dehydroepiandrosterone sulfate; *hCG*, human chorionic gonadotropin; *LH*, luteinizing hormone; *MRI*, magnetic resonance imaging; *17-OHP*, 17-hydroxy progesterone; T_4, thyroxine; *TSH*, thyrotropin.

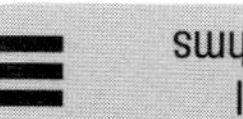
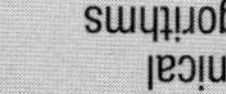

ICD-9CM # 785.50 Shock NOS
995.0 Shock anaphylactic
785.51 Shock cardiogenic
785.59 Shock septic
958.4 Shock traumatic
977.9 Shock due to drug, medicine incorrectly administered

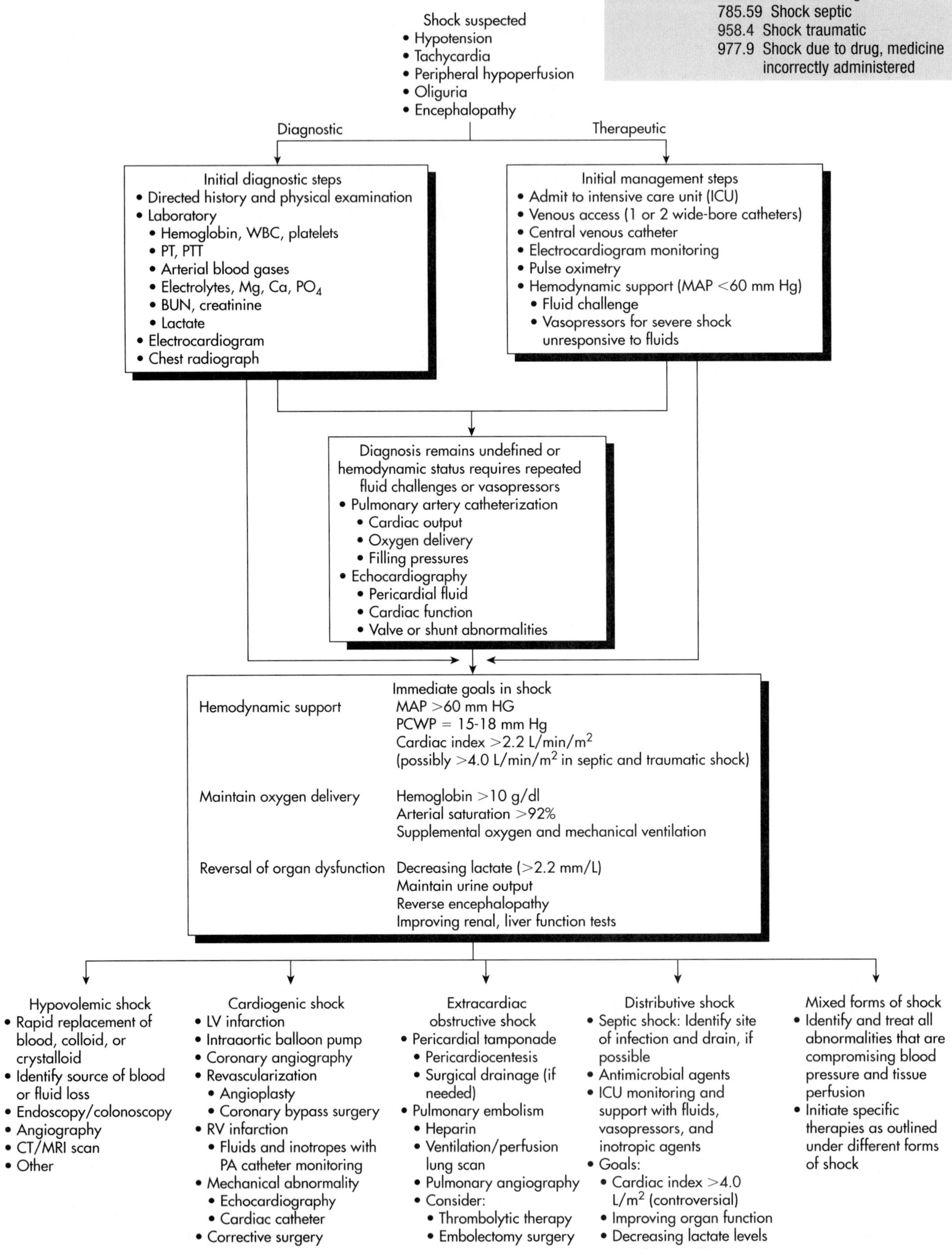

Shock suspected
- Hypotension
- Tachycardia
- Peripheral hypoperfusion
- Oliguria
- Encephalopathy

Diagnostic

Initial diagnostic steps
- Directed history and physical examination
- Laboratory
  - Hemoglobin, WBC, platelets
  - PT, PTT
  - Arterial blood gases
  - Electrolytes, Mg, Ca, PO_4
  - BUN, creatinine
  - Lactate
- Electrocardiogram
- Chest radiograph

Therapeutic

Initial management steps
- Admit to intensive care unit (ICU)
- Venous access (1 or 2 wide-bore catheters)
- Central venous catheter
- Electrocardiogram monitoring
- Pulse oximetry
- Hemodynamic support (MAP <60 mm Hg)
  - Fluid challenge
  - Vasopressors for severe shock unresponsive to fluids

Diagnosis remains undefined or hemodynamic status requires repeated fluid challenges or vasopressors
- Pulmonary artery catheterization
  - Cardiac output
  - Oxygen delivery
  - Filling pressures
- Echocardiography
  - Pericardial fluid
  - Cardiac function
  - Valve or shunt abnormalities

Immediate goals in shock

Hemodynamic support	MAP >60 mm HG PCWP = 15-18 mm Hg Cardiac index >2.2 L/min/m^2 (possibly >4.0 L/min/m^2 in septic and traumatic shock)
Maintain oxygen delivery	Hemoglobin >10 g/dl Arterial saturation >92% Supplemental oxygen and mechanical ventilation
Reversal of organ dysfunction	Decreasing lactate (>2.2 mm/L) Maintain urine output Reverse encephalopathy Improving renal, liver function tests

Hypovolemic shock
- Rapid replacement of blood, colloid, or crystalloid
- Identify source of blood or fluid loss
- Endoscopy/colonoscopy
- Angiography
- CT/MRI scan
- Other

Cardiogenic shock
- LV infarction
- Intraaortic balloon pump
- Coronary angiography
- Revascularization
  - Angioplasty
  - Coronary bypass surgery
- RV infarction
  - Fluids and inotropes with PA catheter monitoring
- Mechanical abnormality
  - Echocardiography
  - Cardiac catheter
- Corrective surgery

Extracardiac obstructive shock
- Pericardial tamponade
  - Pericardiocentesis
  - Surgical drainage (if needed)
- Pulmonary embolism
  - Heparin
  - Ventilation/perfusion lung scan
  - Pulmonary angiography
  - Consider:
    - Thrombolytic therapy
    - Embolectomy surgery

Distributive shock
- Septic shock: Identify site of infection and drain, if possible
- Antimicrobial agents
- ICU monitoring and support with fluids, vasopressors, and inotropic agents
- Goals:
  - Cardiac index >4.0 L/m^2 (controversial)
  - Improving organ function
  - Decreasing lactate levels

Mixed forms of shock
- Identify and treat all abnormalities that are compromising blood pressure and tissue perfusion
- Initiate specific therapies as outlined under different forms of shock

FIGURE 3-301 An approach to the diagnosis and treatment of shock. *BUN,* Blood urea nitrogen; *CT,* computed tomography; *LV,* left ventricular; *MAP,* mean arterial pressure; *MRI,* magnetic resonance imaging; *PA,* pulmonary arterial; *PCWP,* pulmonary capillary wedge pressure; *PT,* prothrombin time; *PTT,* partial thromboplastin time; *RV,* right ventricular; *WBC,* white blood cell count. (From Goldman L, Ausiello D [eds]: *Cecil textbook of medicine,* ed 23, Philadelphia, 2008, WB Saunders.)

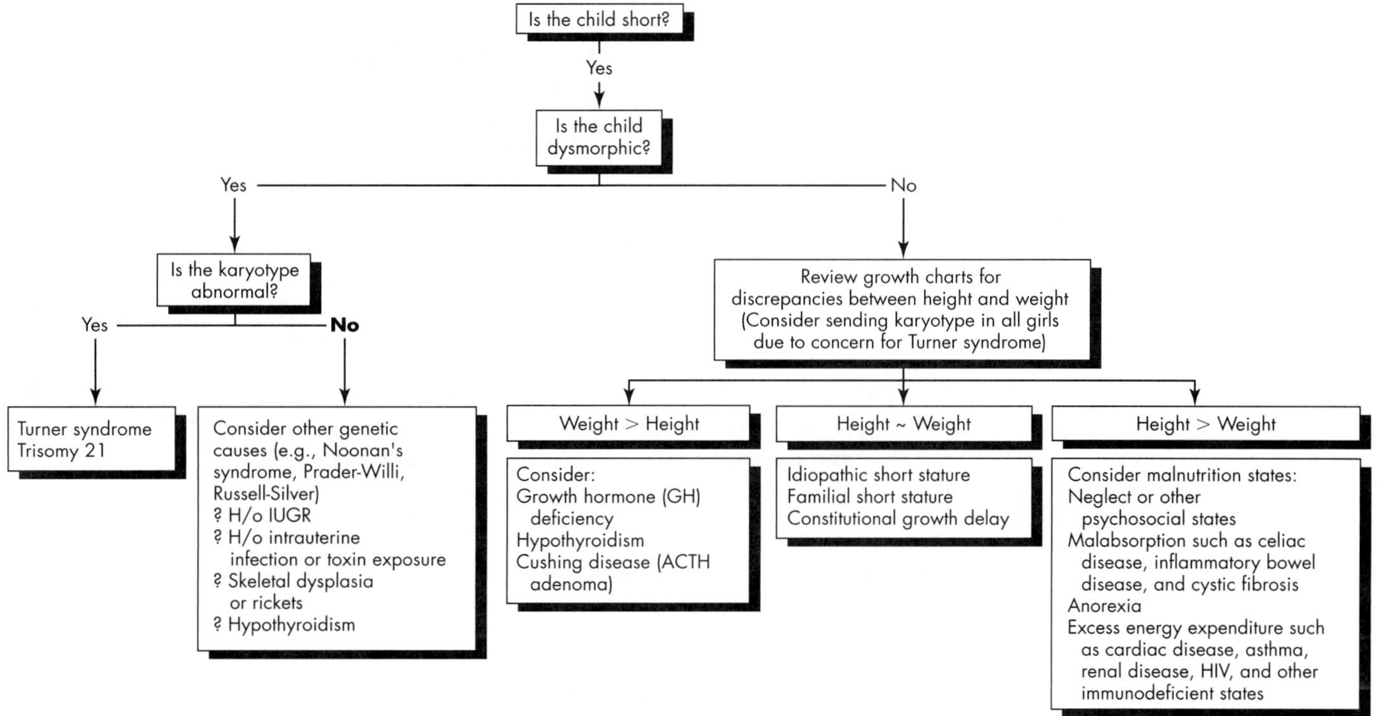

FIGURE 3-302 Differential diagnosis of short stature. (From Custer JW, Rau RE: *The Harriet Lane handbook,* ed 18, St Louis, 2009, Mosby.)

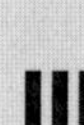

A
Sleep disturbance
History
Insomnia
Hypersomnia
See Algorithm B
Sleep-associated affective and behavioral disturbance
See Algorithm C
Duration >3 weeks
Duration <3 weeks
Consider:
Situational disorder
Work shift change
Jet lag syndrome
Spontaneous resolution
Reassurance
Possible short course of Zolpidem
Normal sleep hygiene
Poor sleep hygiene
Advise on rules of better sleep hygiene
Stress related
Not stress related
Psychiatric
Psychiatric consultation and therapy
Psychophysiologic condition
Alcohol or drug use
Abstention
Counseling
Stress reduction
Relaxation techniques
Stimulus control
Daily exercise
Deconditioning
PSG may reassure and exclude other possibilities
Consider:
Restless legs syndrome
Periodic movements of sleep
Central sleep apnea
Chronic respiratory failure
Alpha delta sleep pattern
PSG to confirm diagnosis
Chronic pain syndrome
Identify source
Treat

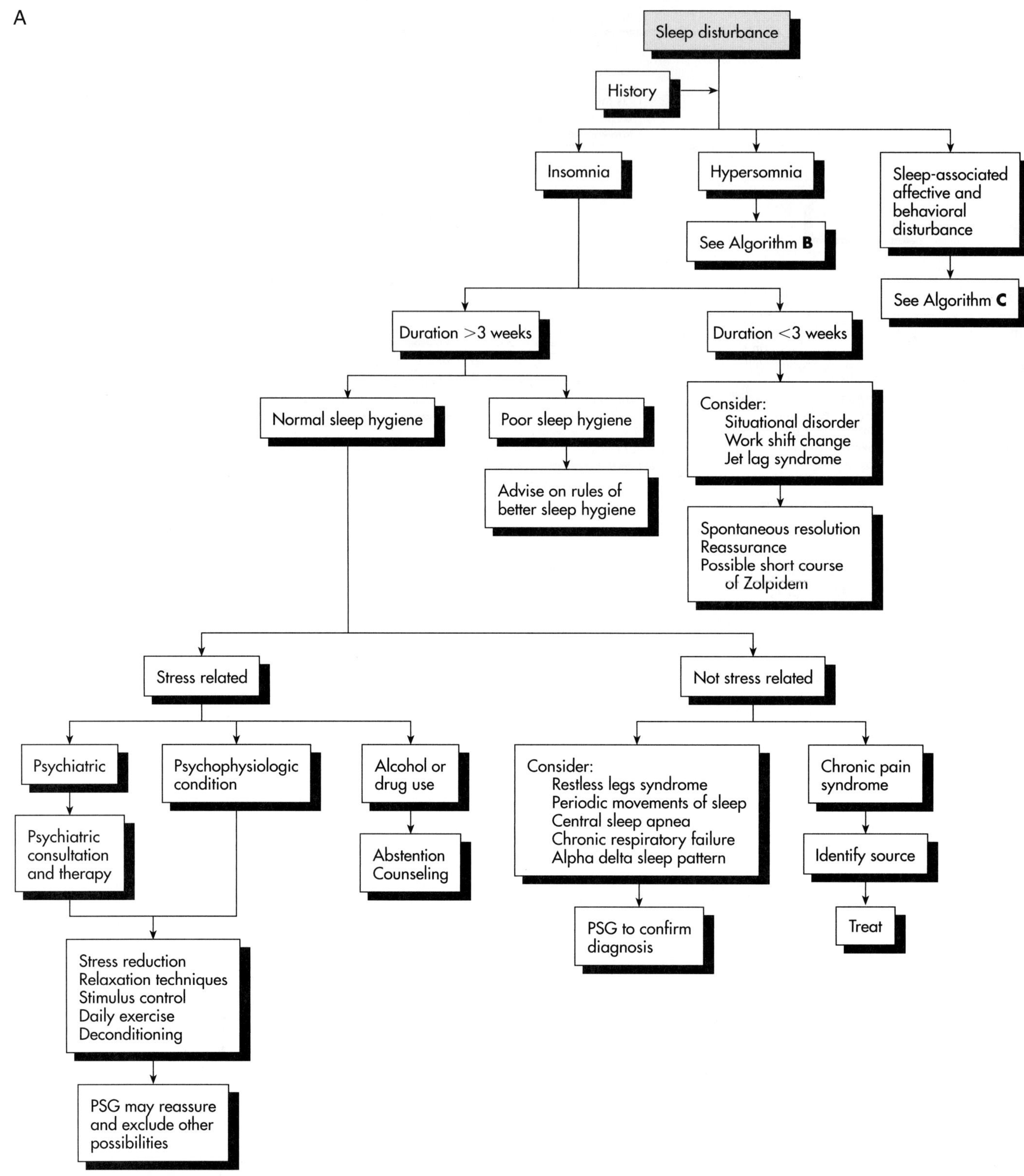

FIGURE 3-306 A, Patient with sleep disturbance. *MSLT,* Multiple sleep latency tests; *PSG,* polysomnography. (Modified from Greene HL, Johnson WP, Lemcke D [eds]: *Decision making in medicine,* ed 2, St Louis, 1998, Mosby.)

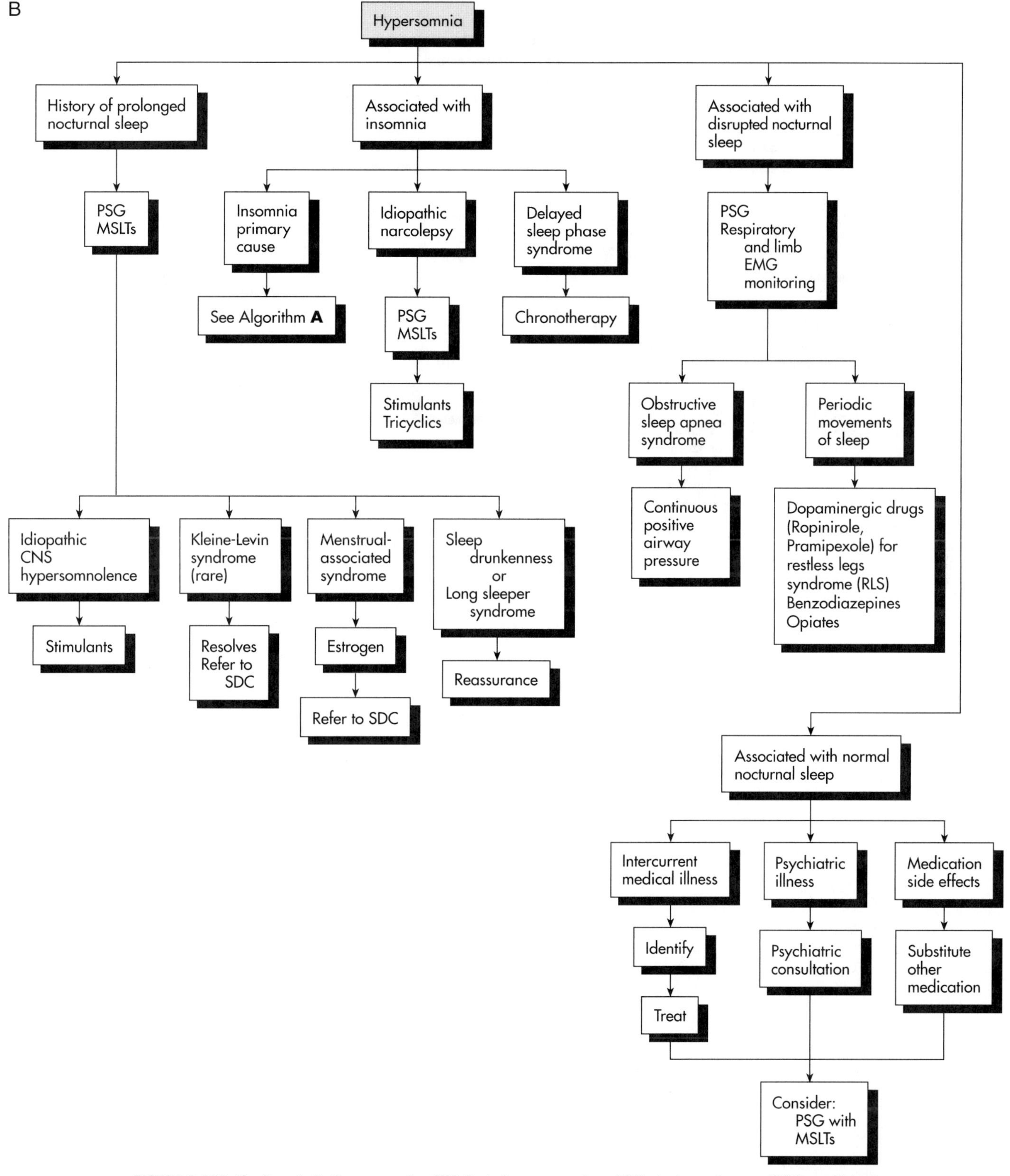

FIGURE 3-306 (Continued) **B, Hypersomnia.** *CNS,* Central nervous system; *EMG,* electromyelogram; *MSLTs,* multiple sleep latency tests; *PSG,* polysomnography; *SDC,* sleep disorders clinic. (Modified from Greene HL, Johnson WP, Lemcke D [eds]: *Decision making in medicine,* ed 2, St Louis, 1998, Mosby.)

Continued on following page

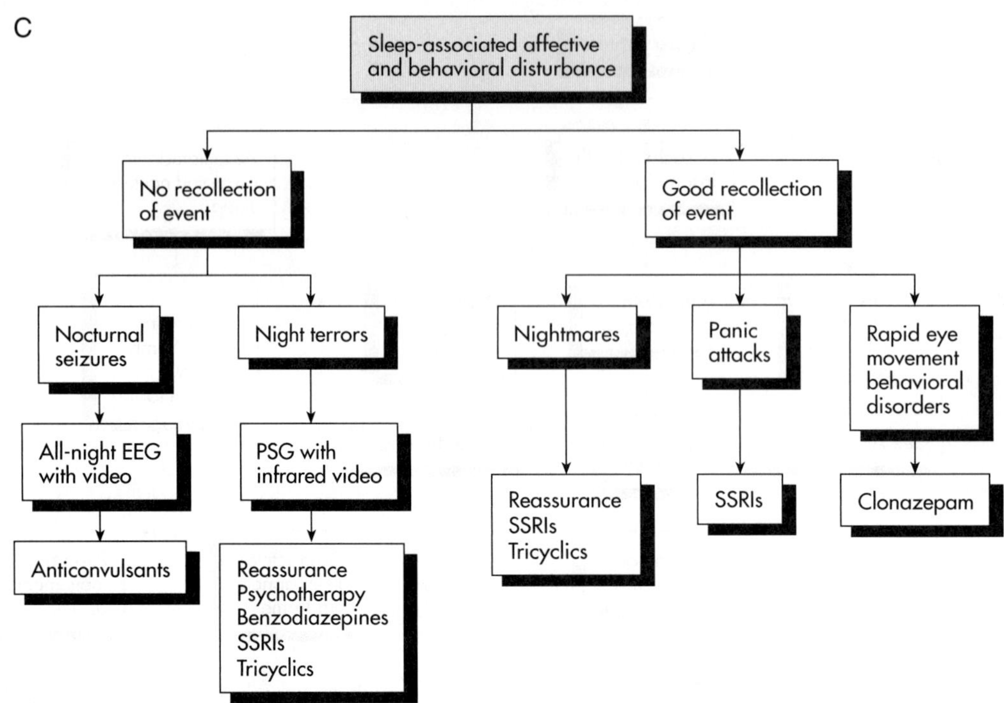

FIGURE 3-306 (Continued) **C, Sleep-associated affective and behavioral disturbance.** *EEG,* Electroencephalogram; *PSG,* polysomnography; *SSRIs,* selective serotonin reuptake inhibitors. (Modified from Greene HL, Johnson WP, Lemcke D [eds]: *Decision making in medicine,* ed 2, St Louis, 1998, Mosby.)

SPLENOMEGALY

ICD-9CM # 789.2 Splenomegaly, unspecified
289.51 Splenomegaly, chronic congestive
759.0 Splenomegaly, congenital
789.2 Splenomegaly, unknown etiology

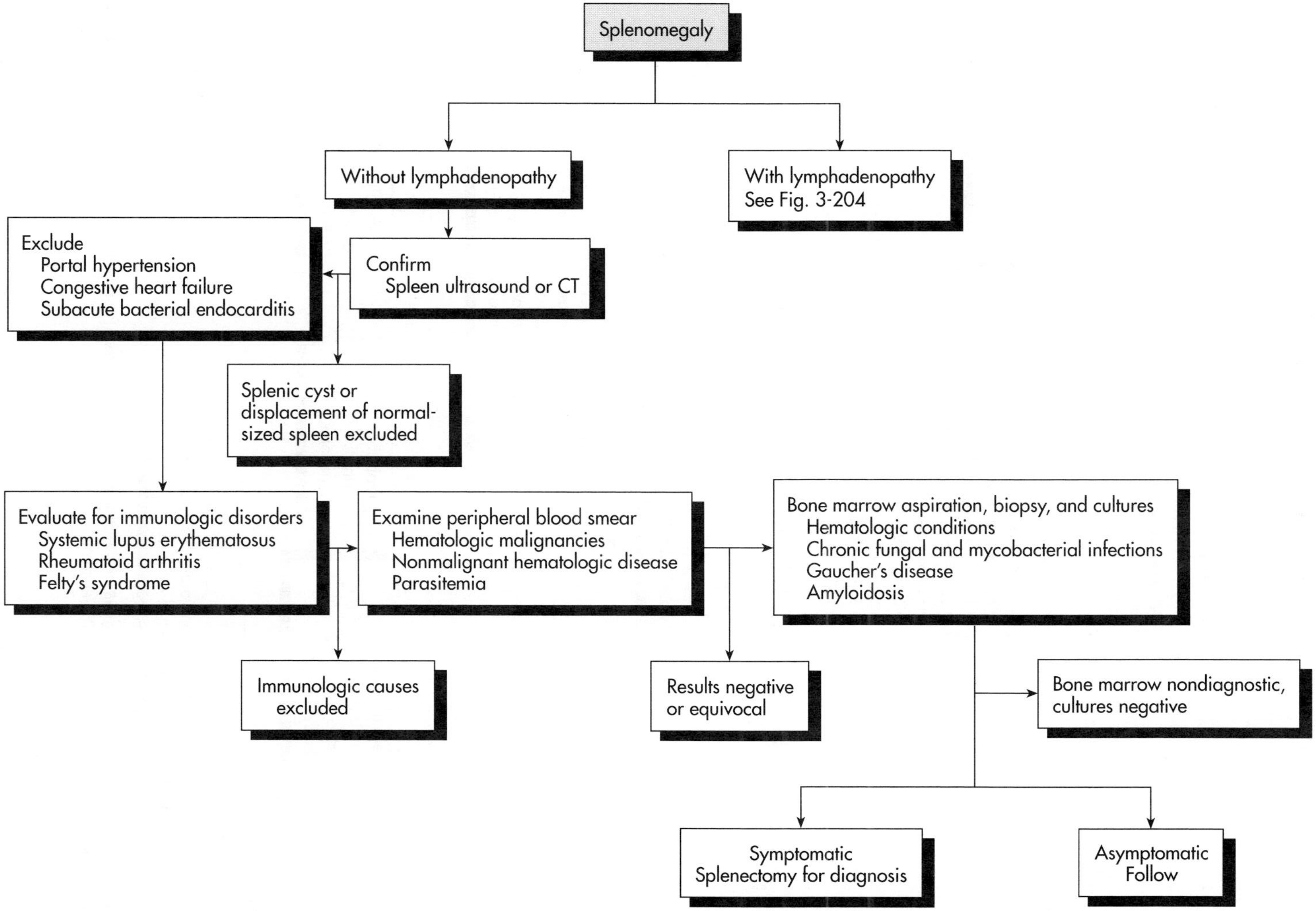

Splenomegaly

Without lymphadenopathy

With lymphadenopathy
See Fig. 3-204

Confirm
Spleen ultrasound or CT

Exclude
Portal hypertension
Congestive heart failure
Subacute bacterial endocarditis

Splenic cyst or displacement of normal-sized spleen excluded

Evaluate for immunologic disorders
Systemic lupus erythematosus
Rheumatoid arthritis
Felty's syndrome

Immunologic causes excluded

Examine peripheral blood smear
Hematologic malignancies
Nonmalignant hematologic disease
Parasitemia

Results negative or equivocal

Bone marrow aspiration, biopsy, and cultures
Hematologic conditions
Chronic fungal and mycobacterial infections
Gaucher's disease
Amyloidosis

Bone marrow nondiagnostic, cultures negative

Symptomatic
Splenectomy for diagnosis

Asymptomatic
Follow

FIGURE 3-308 Clinical approach to patient with splenomegaly. *CT,* Computed tomography. (Modified from Stein JH [ed]: *Internal medicine,* ed 5, St Louis, 1998, Mosby.)

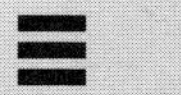
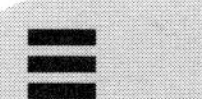

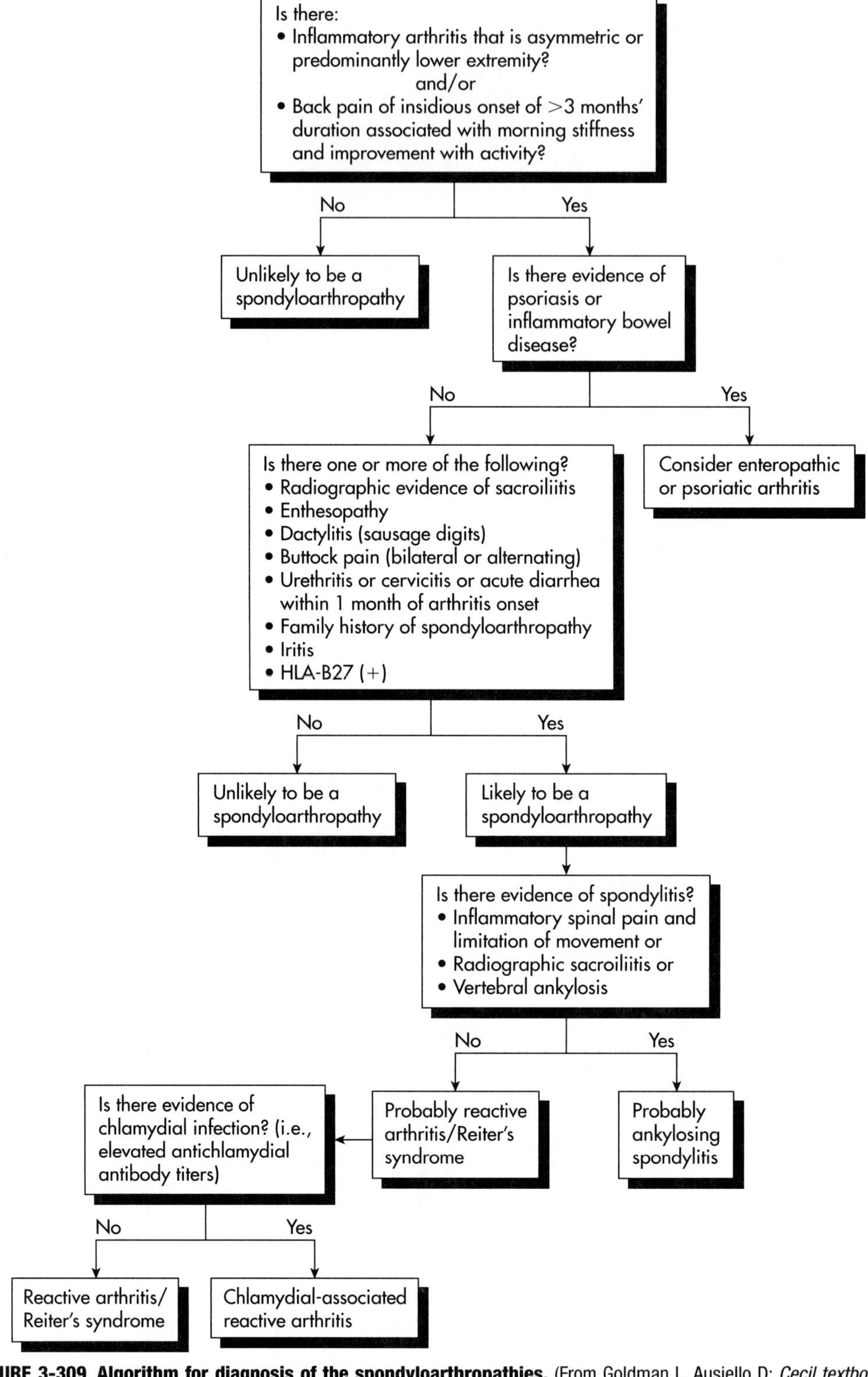

FIGURE 3-309 Algorithm for diagnosis of the spondyloarthropathies. (From Goldman L, Ausiello D: *Cecil textbook of medicine,* ed 23, Philadelphia, 2008, WB Saunders.)

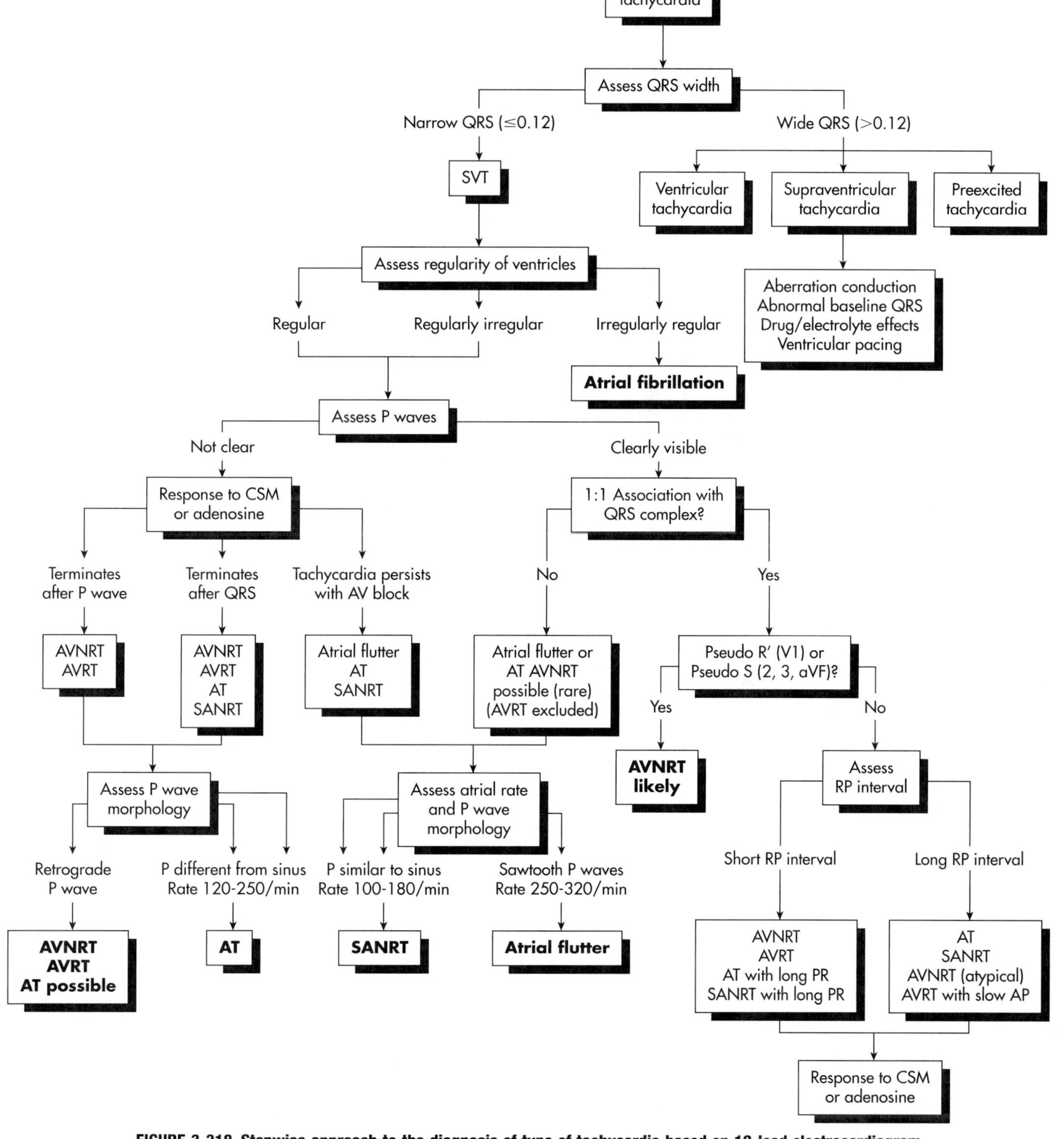

FIGURE 3-318 Stepwise approach to the diagnosis of type of tachycardia based on 12-lead electrocardiogram during the episode. The initial step is to determine whether the tachycardia has a wide or narrow QRS complex (Fig. 3-319). For wide-complex tachycardia, see Figure 3-320; the remainder of the algorithm is helpful in diagnosiing the type of narrow-complex tachycardia. *AP,* Accessory pathway; *AT,* atrial tachycardia; *AV,* atrioventricular; *AVNRT,* AV nodal reentrant tachycardia; *AVRT,* AV reciprocating tachycardia; *CSM,* carotid sinus massage; *SANRT,* sinoatrial nodal reentry tachycardia; *SVT,* supraventricular tachycardia. (From Zipes DP, Libby P, Bonow RO, Braunwald E [eds]: *Braunwald's heart disease,* ed 7, Philadelphia, 2005, Elsevier.)

ICD-9CM # 427.2 Paroxysmal tachycardia
427.0 Supraventricular paroxysmal tachycardia
427.42 Ventricular flutter
427.1 Ventricular paroxysmal tachycardia
427.89 Atrial tachycardia

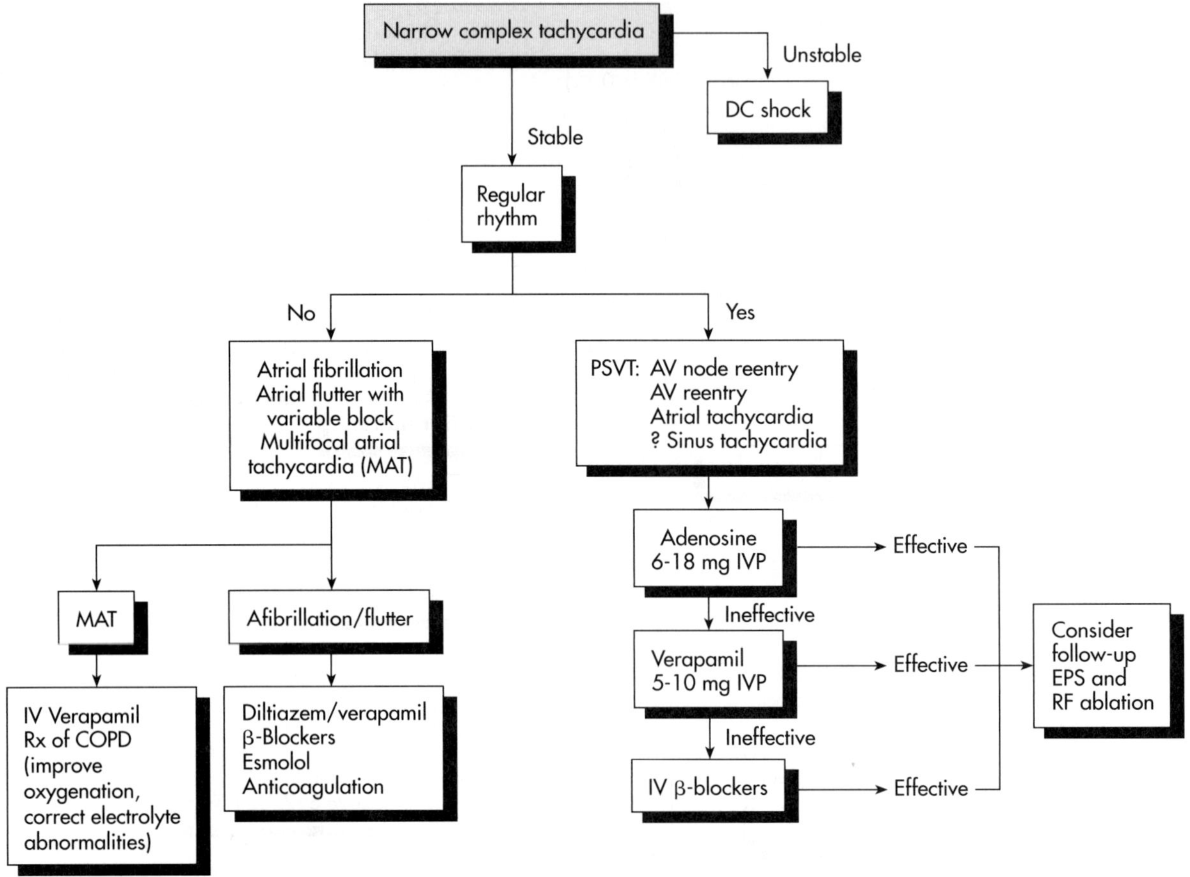

FIGURE 3-319 Evaluation and management of narrow complex tachycardia. *AV,* Atrioventricular; *COPD,* chronic obstructive pulmonary disease; *EPS,* electrophysiologic studies; *IV,* intravenous; *IVP,* intravenous push; *PSVT,* paroxysmal supraventricular tachycardia; *RF,* radiofrequency.

ICD-9CM # 427.2 Paroxysmal tachycardia
427.0 Supraventricular paroxysmal tachycardia
427.42 Ventricular flutter
427.1 Ventricular paroxysmal tachycardia
427.89 Atrial tachycardia

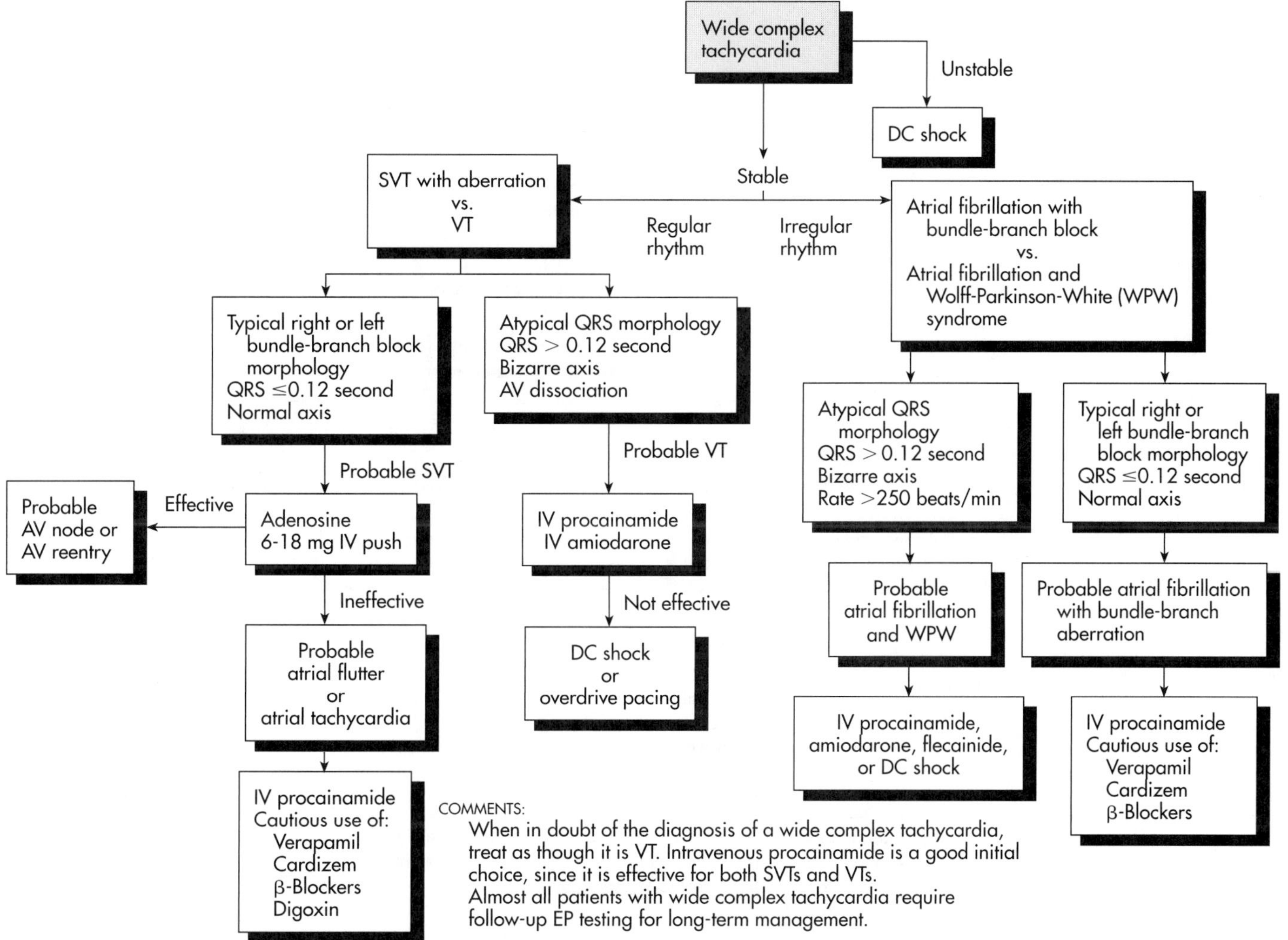

FIGURE 3-320 Evaluation and management of wide complex tachycardia. *AV,* Atrioventricular; *EP,* electrophysiologic; *IV,* intravenous; *SVT,* supraventricular tachycardia; *VT,* ventricular tachycardia. (From Driscoll CE et al: *The family practice desk reference,* ed 3, St Louis, 1996, Mosby.)

TABLE 3-36 Major Features in the Differential Diagnosis of Wide QRS Beats Versus Tachycardia

Supports SVT	Supports VT
Slowing or termination by vagal tone	Fusion beats
Onset with premature P wave	Capture beats
RP interval ≤100 msec	AV dissociation
P and QRS rate and rhythm linked to suggest that ventricular activation depends on atrial discharge, e.g., 2:1 AV block rSR′ V1	P and QRS rate and rhythm linked to suggest that atrial activation depends on ventricular discharge, e.g., 2:1 VA block
Long-short cycle sequence	"Compensatory" pause Left axis deviation; QRS duration >140 msec Specific QRS contours (see text)

(From Zipes DP et al [eds]: *Braunwauld's heart disease,* ed 7, Philadelphia, 2005, Elsevier.)
SVT, Supraventricular tachycardia; *VT,* ventricular tachycardia.

ICD-9CM # 186.9 Testicular neoplasm
M906/3 (seminoma)
M9101/3 (embryonal carcinoma or teratoma)
M9100/3 (choriocarcinoma)

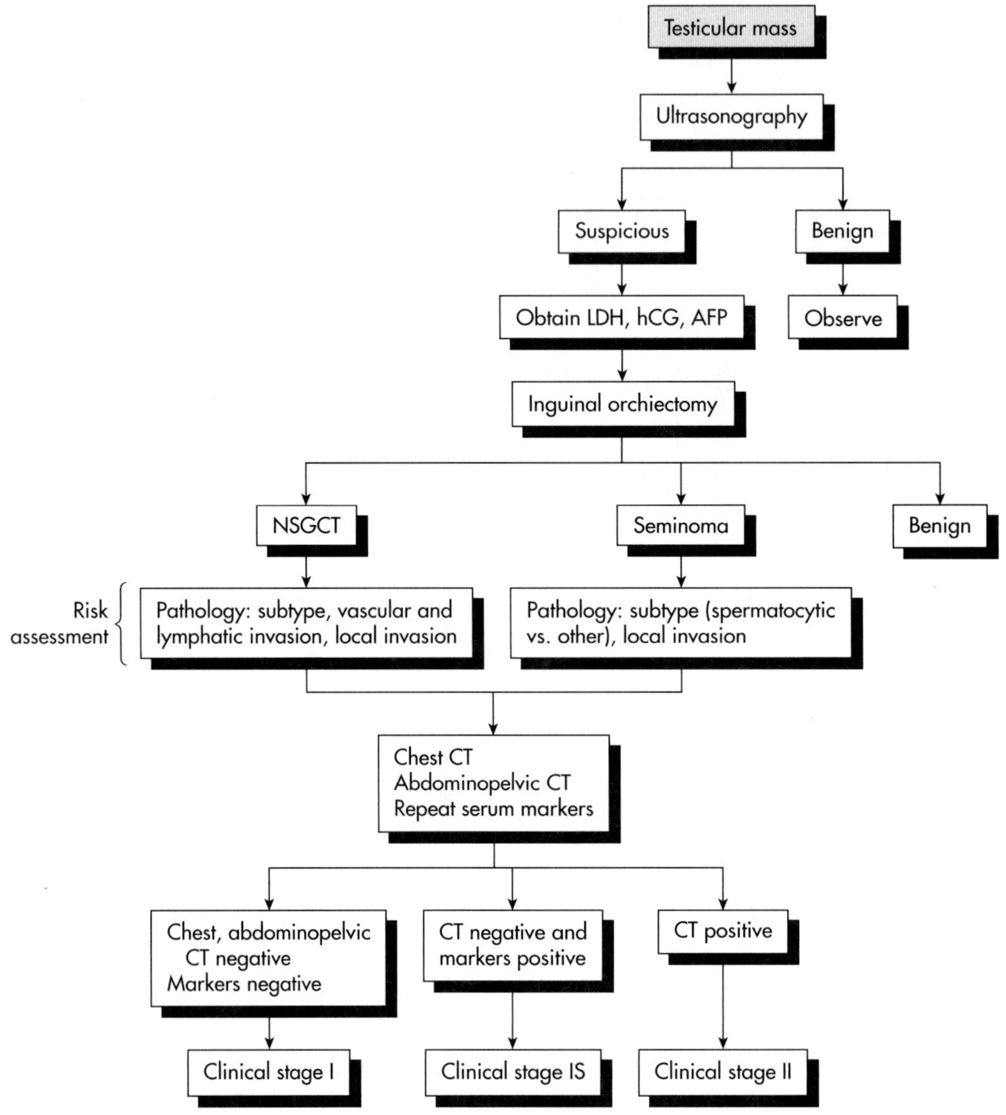

FIGURE 3-321 Diagnosis, staging, and risk assessment of patients with testicular germ cell tumor. *AFP,* α-fetoprotein; *CT,* computed tomography; *hCG,* human chorionic gonadotropin; *LDH,* lactic dehydrogenase; *NSGCT,* nonseminoma germ cell tumor. (From Abeloff MD: *Clinical oncology,* ed 3, New York, 2004, Churchill Livingstone.)

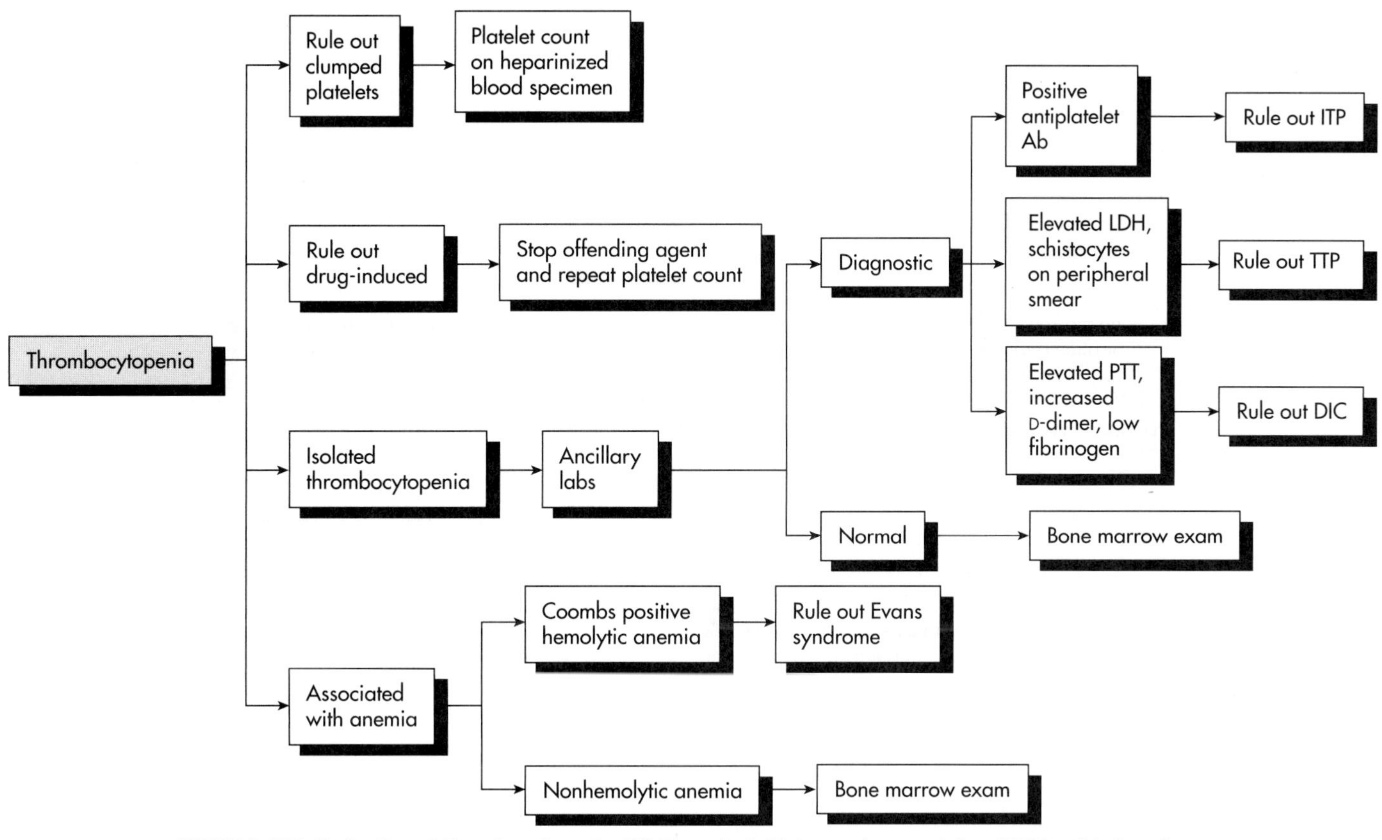

FIGURE 3-323 Evaluation of thrombocytopenia. *DIC,* Disseminated intravascular coagulation; *ITP,* idiopathic thrombocytopenic purpura; *LDH,* lactic dehydrogenase; *PPT,* partial thromboplastin time; *TTP,* thrombotic thrombocytopenic purpura. (From Ferri FF: *Ferri's best test: a practical guide to clinical laboratory medicine and diagnostic imaging,* ed 2, Philadelphia, 2009, Elsevier Mosby.)

BOX 3-15 Thrombocytopenia

Diagnostic imaging	Lab evaluation
Best Test	***Best Test***
None	Bone marrow exam
Ancillary test	***Ancillary tests***
CT of abdomen if splenomegaly is present	CBC, PT, PTT
	LDH
	HIV, ANA
	Antiplatelet Ab
	D-dimer
	Coombs tests

From Ferri FF: *Ferri's best test: a practical guide to clinical laboratory medicine and diagnostic imaging,* ed 2, Philadelphia, 2009, Elsevier Mosby.

ANA, Antibody to nuclear antigens; *CBC,* complete blood count; *CT,* computed tomography; *HIV,* human immunodeficiency virus; *LDH,* lactic dehydrogenase; *PT,* prothrombin time; *PTT,* partial thromboplastin time.

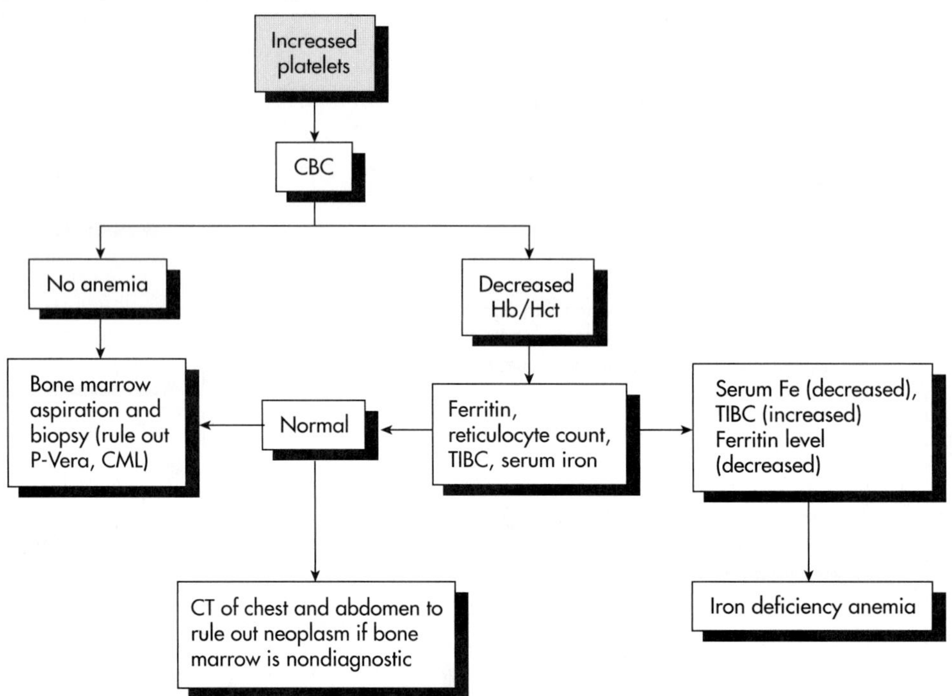

FIGURE 3-324 Thrombocytosis diagnosis. *CBC,* Complete blood count; *CML,* chronic myelogenous leukemia; *CT,* computed tomography; *Fe,* iron; *Hb/Hct,* hemoglobin/hematocrit; *TIBC,* total iron-binding capacity. (From Ferri FF: *Ferri's best test: a practical guide to clinical laboratory medicine and diagnostic imaging,* ed 2, Philadelphia, 2009, Elsevier Mosby.)

BOX 3-16 Thrombocytosis

Diagnostic imaging	Lab evaluation
Best Test	***Best Test***
None	Bone marrow exam
Ancillary test	***Ancillary tests***
CT of chest and abdomen	CBC
	Reticulocyte count
	Stool for OB ×3
	Serum ferritin, TIBC, iron

From Ferri FF: *Ferri's best test: a practical guide to clinical laboratory medicine and diagnostic imaging,* ed 2, Philadelphia, 2009, Elsevier Mosby.

CBC, Complete blood count; *CT,* computed tomography; *OB,* occult blood; *TIBC,* total iron-binding capacity.

THYROID TESTING

ICD-9CM # V77.0

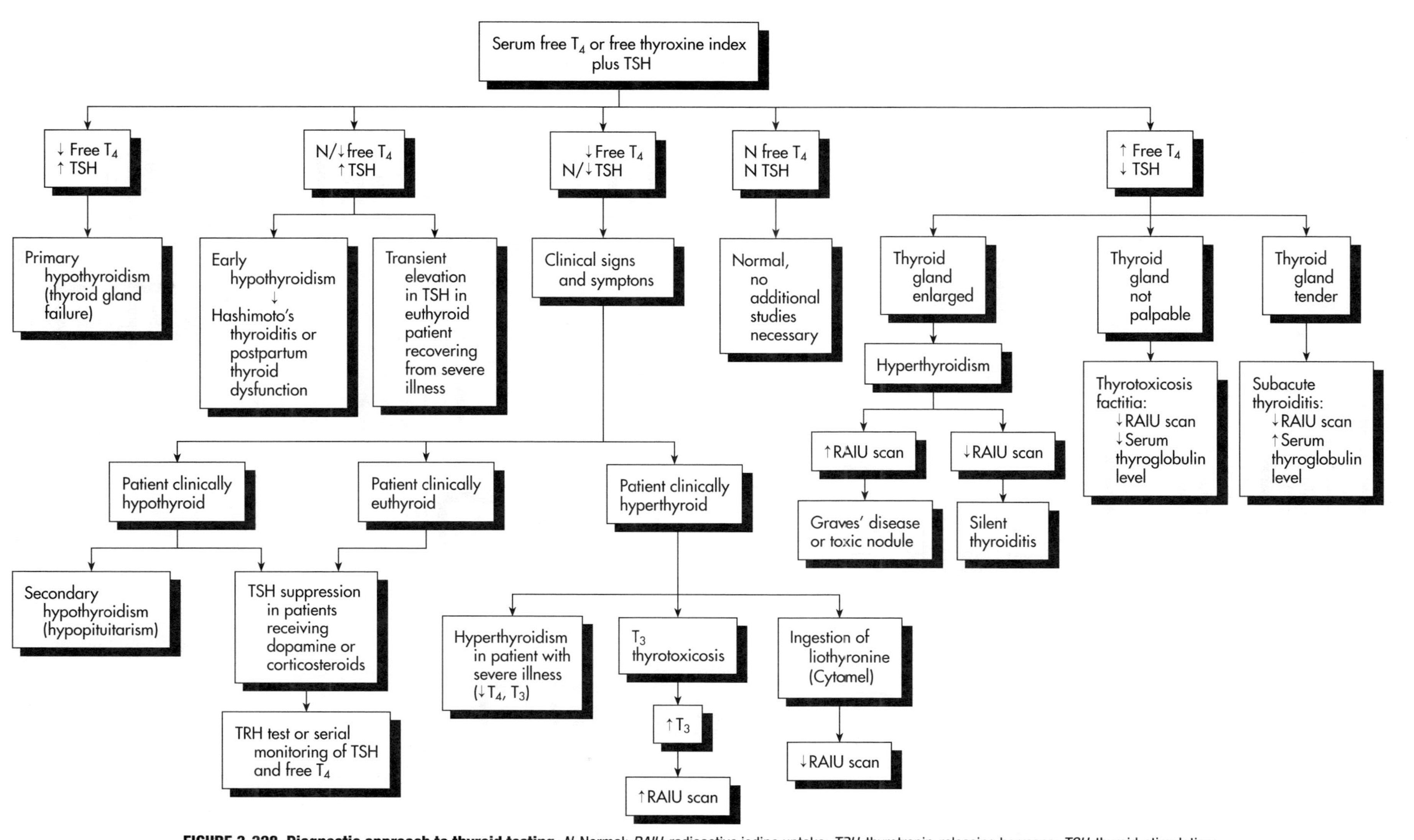

FIGURE 3-328 Diagnostic approach to thyroid testing. *N,* Normal; *RAIU,* radioactive iodine uptake; *TRH,* thyrotropin-releasing hormone; *TSH,* thyroid-stimulating hormone. (From Ferri FF: *Practical guide to the care of the medical patient,* ed 8, St Louis, 2011, Mosby.)

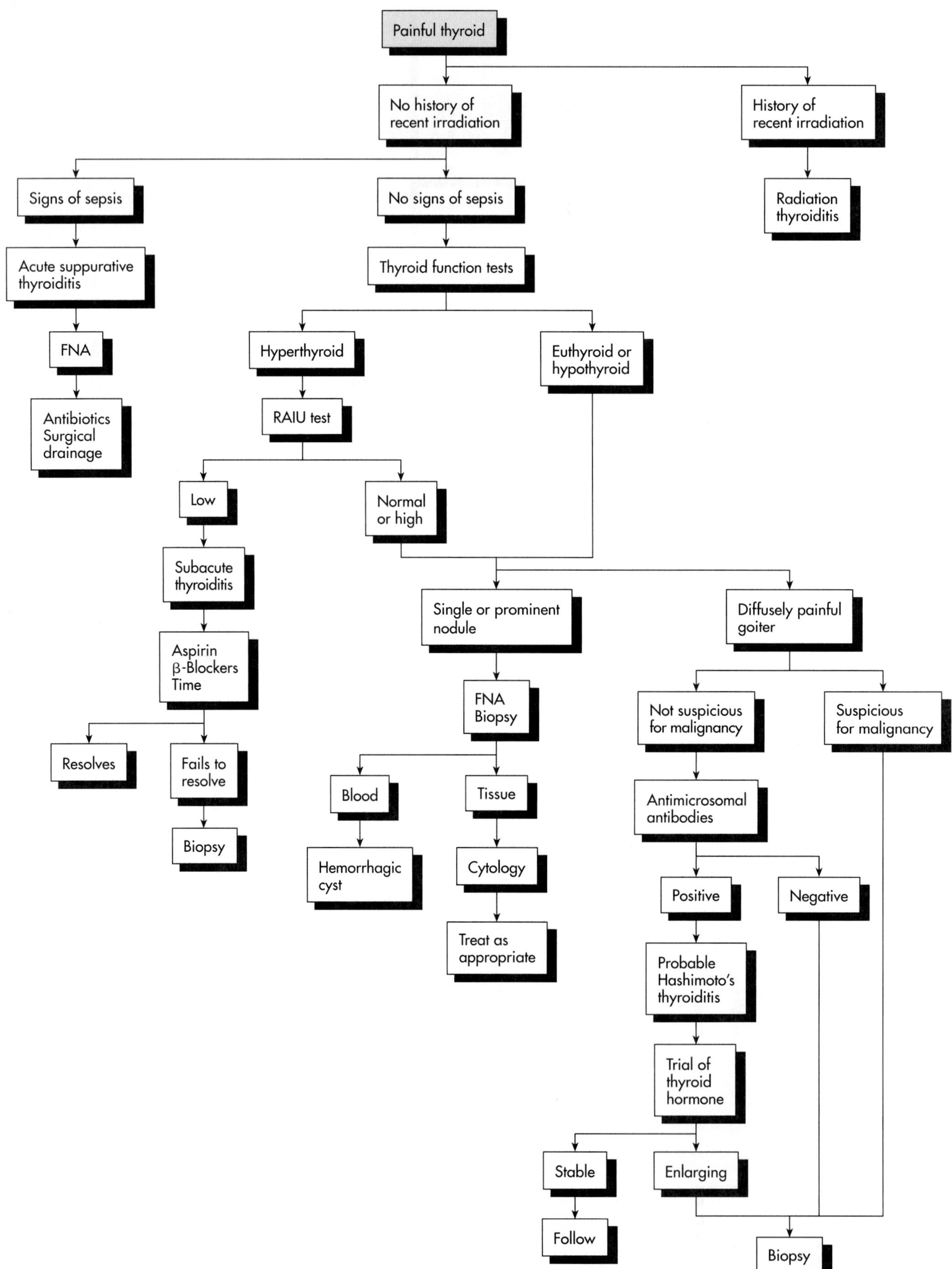

FIGURE 3-329 Painful thyroid. *FNA,* Fine-needle aspiration; *RAIU,* radioactive iodine uptake. (From Greene HL, Johnson WP, Lemcke D [eds]: *Decision making in medicine,* ed 2, St Louis, 1998, Mosby.)

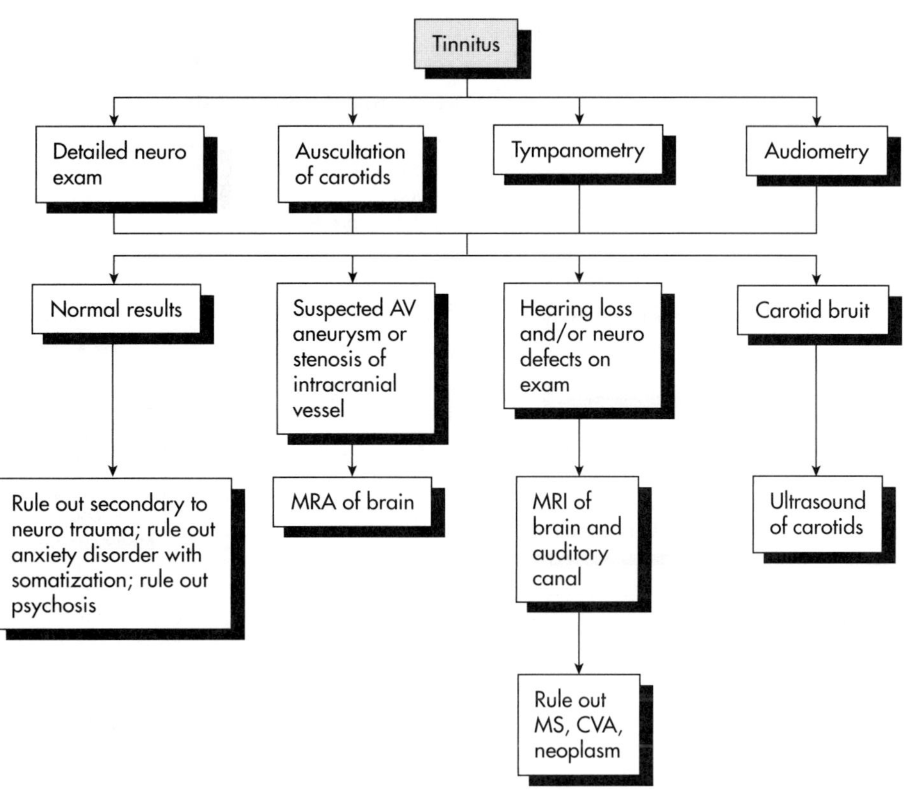

FIGURE 3-330 Tinnitus evaluation. *AV,* Atrioventricular; *CVA,* cerebrovascular accident; *MRA,* magnetic resonance angiography; *MRI,* magnetic resonance imaging; *MS,* multiple sclerosis. (From Ferri FF: *Ferri's best test: a practical guide to clinical laboratory medicine and diagnostic imaging,* ed 2, Philadelphia, 2009, Elsevier Mosby.)

BOX 3-17 Tinnitus

Diagnostic imaging	Lab evaluation
Best Test	***Best Test***
None	None
Ancillary tests	***Ancillary tests***
Carotid Doppler ultrasound	CBC
MRI of brain and auditory canals	Lipid panel
Brain MRA	

From Ferri FF: *Ferri's best test: a practical guide to clinical laboratory medicine and diagnostic imaging,* ed 2, Philadelphia, 2009, Elsevier Mosby.

CBC, Complete blood count; *MRA,* magnetic resonance angiography; *MRI,* magnetic resonance imaging.

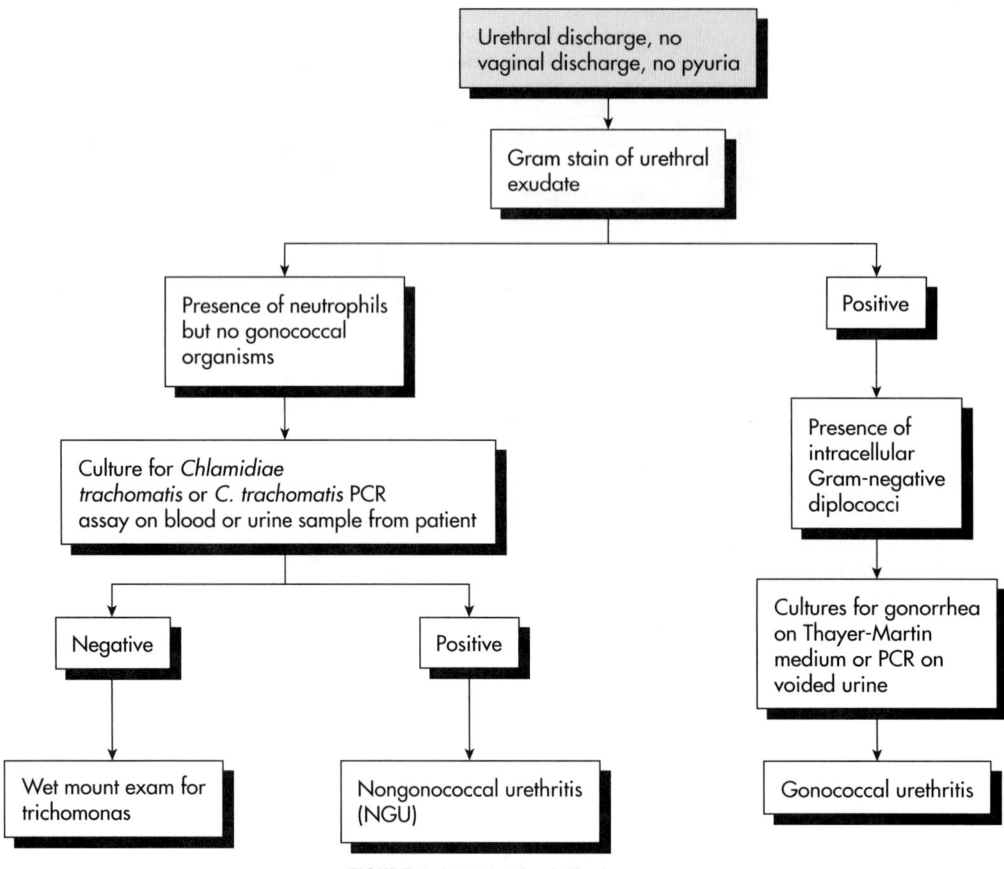

FIGURE 3-334 Urethral discharge.

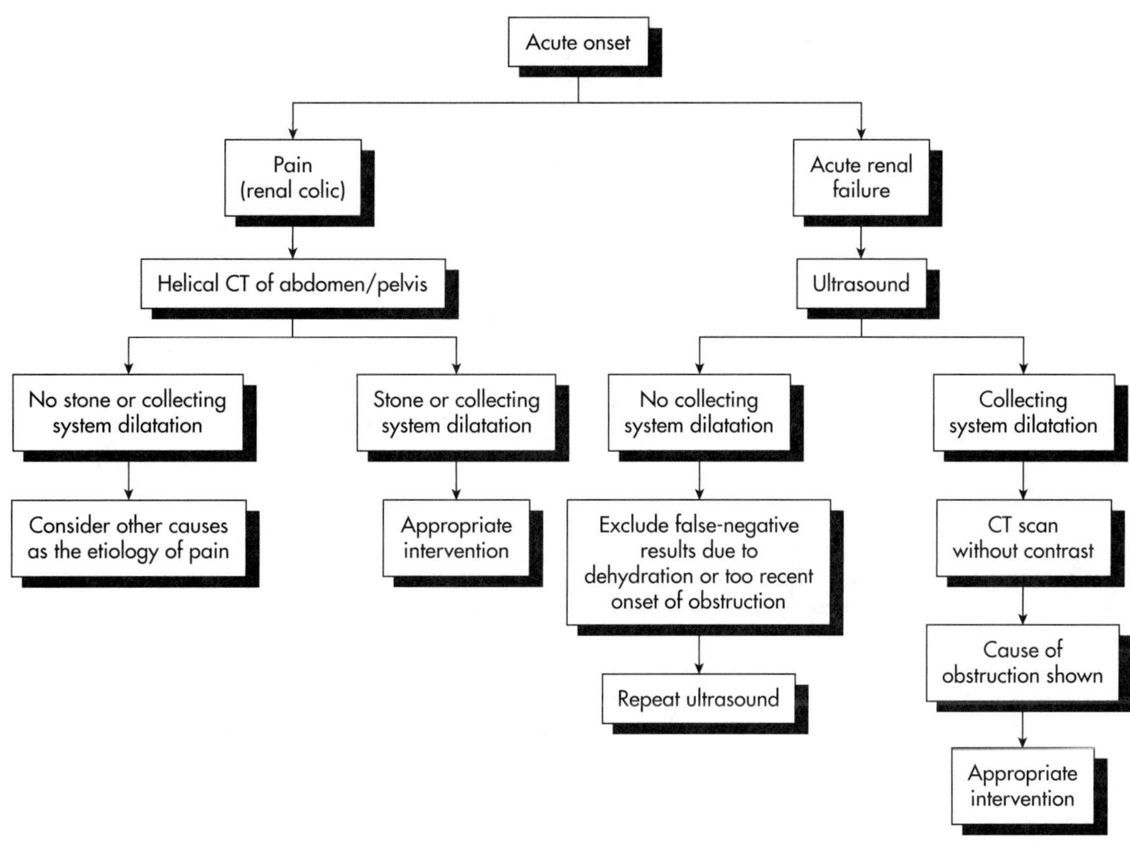

FIGURE 3-336 Scheme of a diagnostic approach to urinary tract obstruction. *CT,* Computed tomography; *IVP,* intravenous pyelography; *KUB,* kidneys, ureter, bladder (a flat film of the abdomen without contrast medium). (Modified from Goldman L, Ausiello D [eds]: *Cecil textbook of medicine,* ed 23, Philadelphia, 2008, WB Saunders.)

BOX 3-18 Diagnostic Tests Used in Obstructive Uropathy

Upper Urinary Tract Obstruction
Sonography (ultrasound)
Plain films of the abdomen (KUB)
Excretory or intravenous pyelography (very rarely needed)
Retrograde pyelography
Isotopic renography
Computed tomography (helical CT)
Magnetic resonance imaging
Pressure flow studies (the Whitaker test)

Lower Urinary Tract Obstruction
Some of the tests listed above
Cystoscopy
Voiding cystourethrogram
Retrograde urethrography
Urodynamic tests
Debimetry
Cystometrography
Electromyography
Urethral pressure profile

KUB, Kidneys, ureter, bladder.

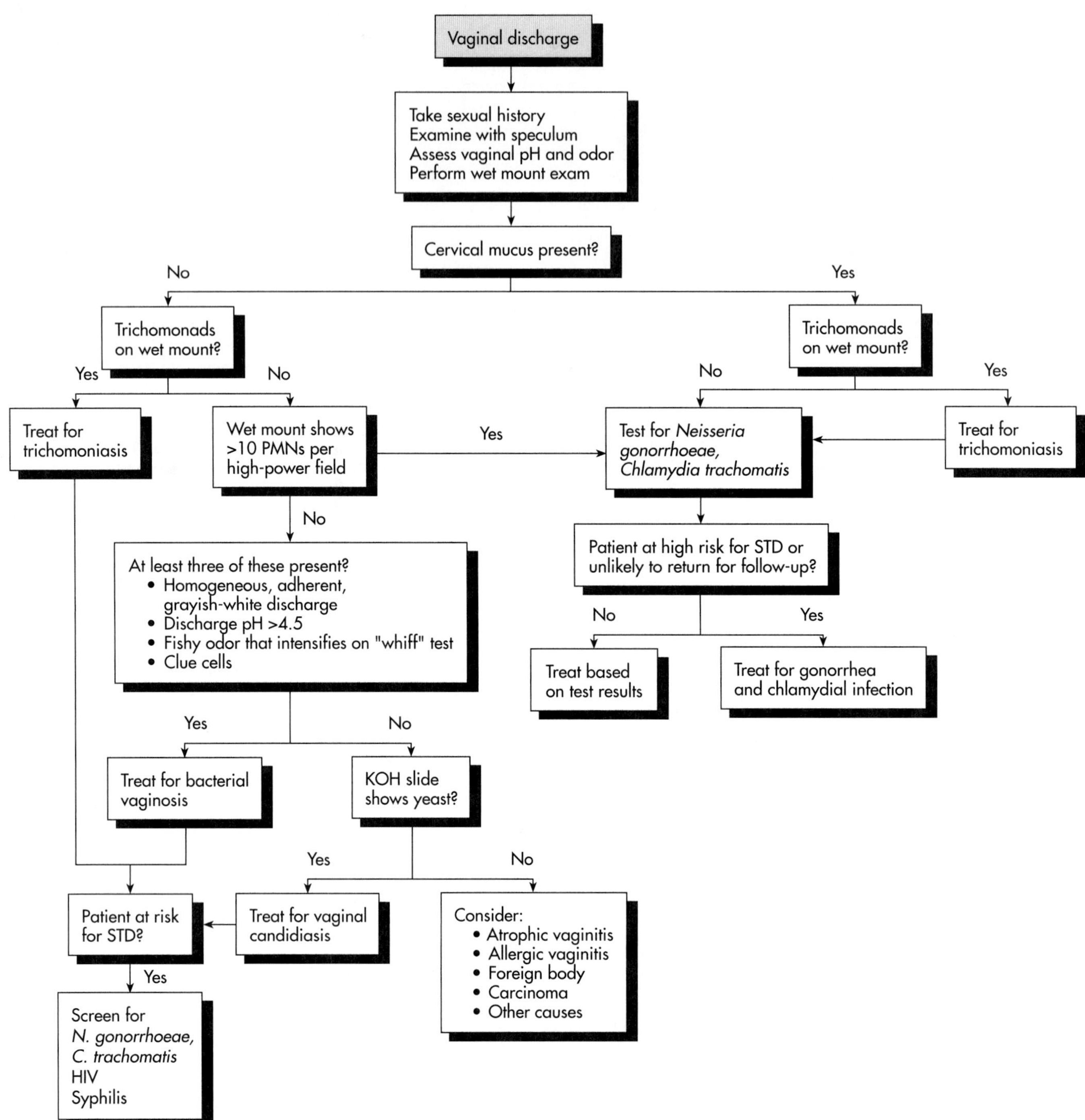

FIGURE 3-340 Evaluation of vaginal discharge. *HIV,* Human immunodeficiency virus; *KOH,* potassium hydroxide; *PMN,* polymorphonuclear leukocyte; *STD,* sexually transmitted disease. (From Fox KK, Behets FMT: *Postgrad Med* 98:87, 1995.)

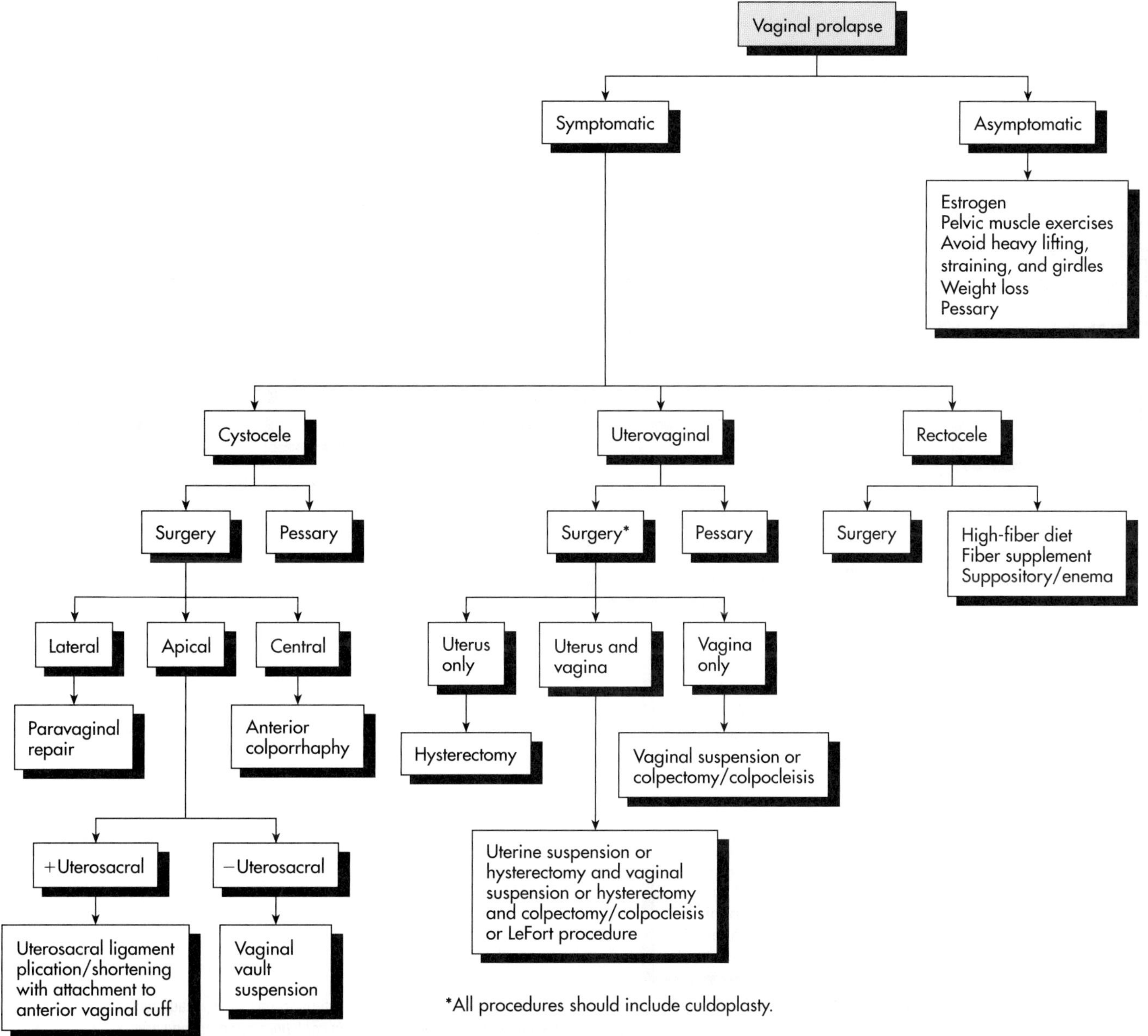

FIGURE 3-341 Management of vaginal prolapse. (From Zuspan FP [ed]: *Handbook of obstetrics, gynecology, and primary care,* St Louis, 1998, Mosby.)

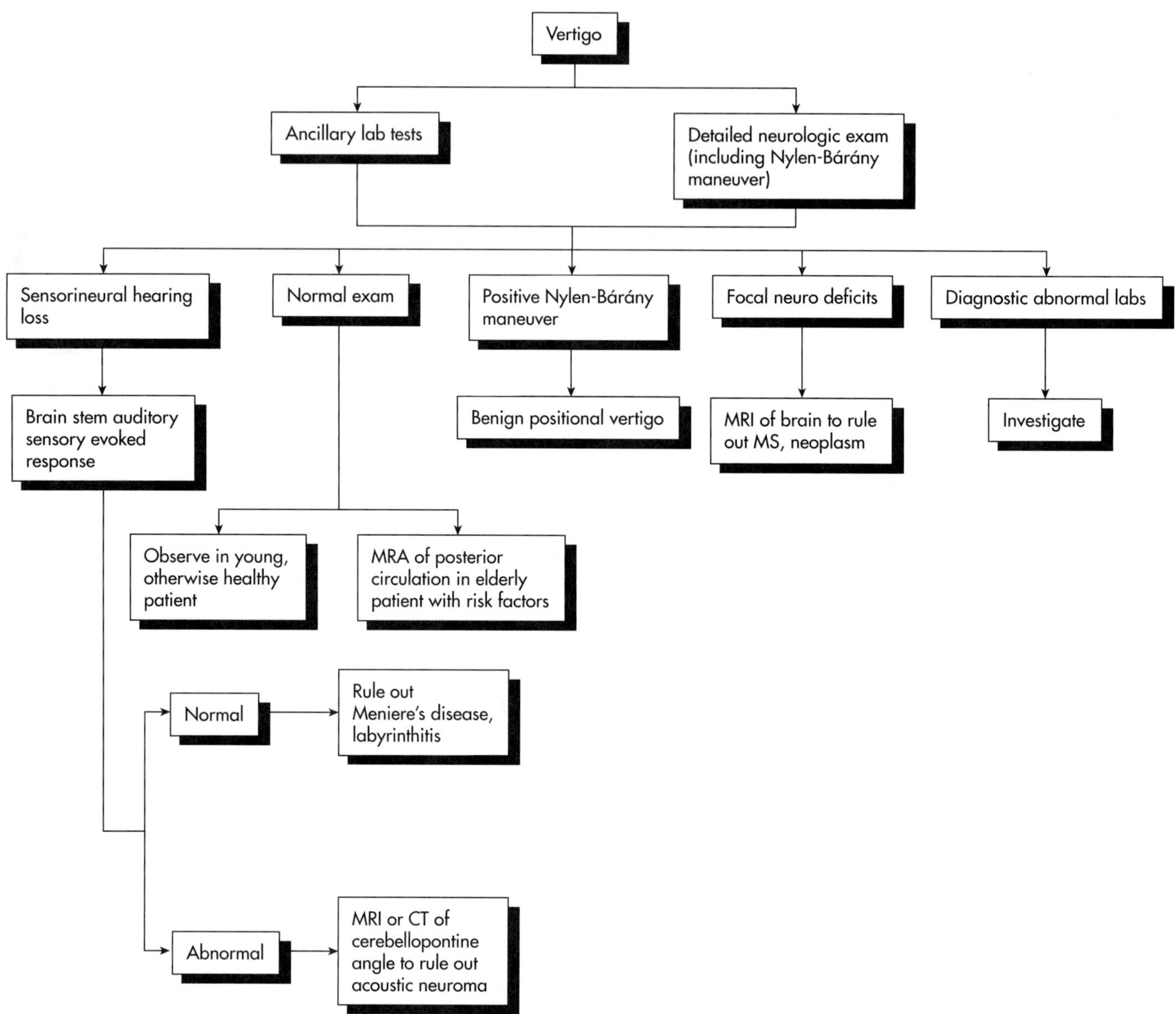

FIGURE 3-342 Vertigo evaluation. *CT,* Computed tomography; *MRA,* magnetic resonance arteriography; *MRI,* magnetic resonance imaging; *MS,* multiple sclerosis. (From Ferri FF: *Ferri's best test: a practical guide to clinical laboratory medicine and diagnostic imaging,* ed 2, Philadelphia, 2009, Elsevier Mosby.)

BOX 3-19 Vertigo

Diagnostic imaging
Best test
MRI of brain
Ancillary tests
MRA of posterior circulation
CT of cerebellopontine region if MRI is contraindicated
Lab evaluation
Best test
None
Ancillary tests
CBC with differential
Serum glucose, creatinine, ALT, electrolytes

From Ferri FF: *Ferri's best test: a practical guide to clinical laboratory medicine and diagnostic imaging,* ed 2, Philadelphia, 2009, Elsevier Mosby.

ALT, Alanine aminotransferase; *CBC,* complete blood count; *CT,* computed tomography; *MRA,* magnetic resonance angiography; *MRI,* magnetic resonance imaging.

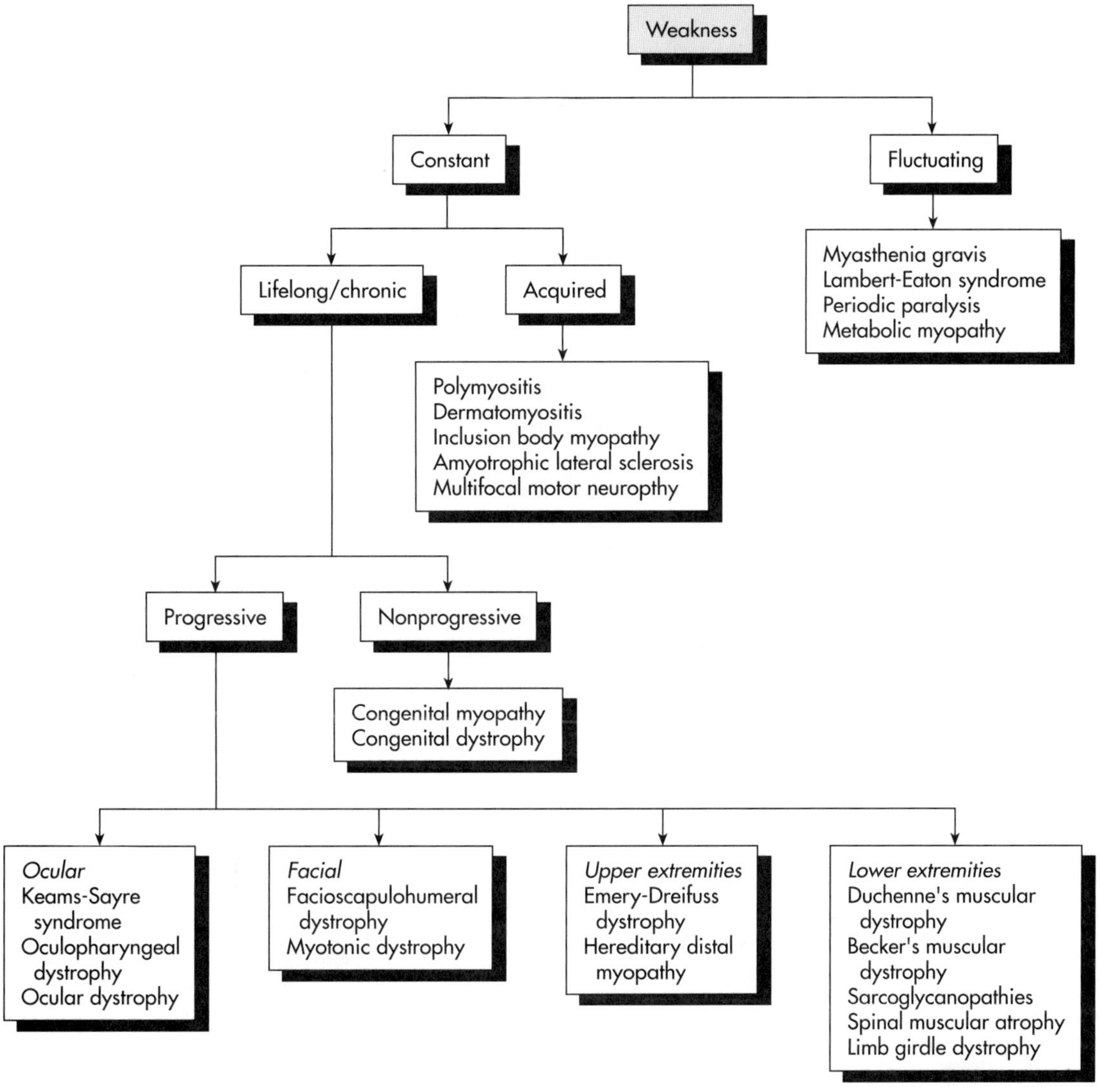

- Weakness
  - Constant
    - Lifelong/chronic
      - Progressive
        - *Ocular*
          - Keams-Sayre syndrome
          - Oculopharyngeal dystrophy
          - Ocular dystrophy
        - *Facial*
          - Facioscapulohumeral dystrophy
          - Myotonic dystrophy
        - *Upper extremities*
          - Emery-Dreifuss dystrophy
          - Hereditary distal myopathy
        - *Lower extremities*
          - Duchenne's muscular dystrophy
          - Becker's muscular dystrophy
          - Sarcoglycanopathies
          - Spinal muscular atrophy
          - Limb girdle dystrophy
      - Nonprogressive
        - Congenital myopathy
        - Congenital dystrophy
    - Acquired
      - Polymyositis
      - Dermatomyositis
      - Inclusion body myopathy
      - Amyotrophic lateral sclerosis
      - Multifocal motor neuropthy
  - Fluctuating
    - Myasthenia gravis
    - Lambert-Eaton syndrome
    - Periodic paralysis
    - Metabolic myopathy

FIGURE 3-344 An algorithm for the approach to the patient with weakness. (From Bradley WG, Daroff RB, Fenichel GM, Jankovic J [eds]: *Neurology in clinical practice,* ed 4, Philadelphia, 2004, Butterworth Heinemann.)

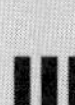

ICD-9CM # 783.1 Abnormal weight gain
278.00 Obesity

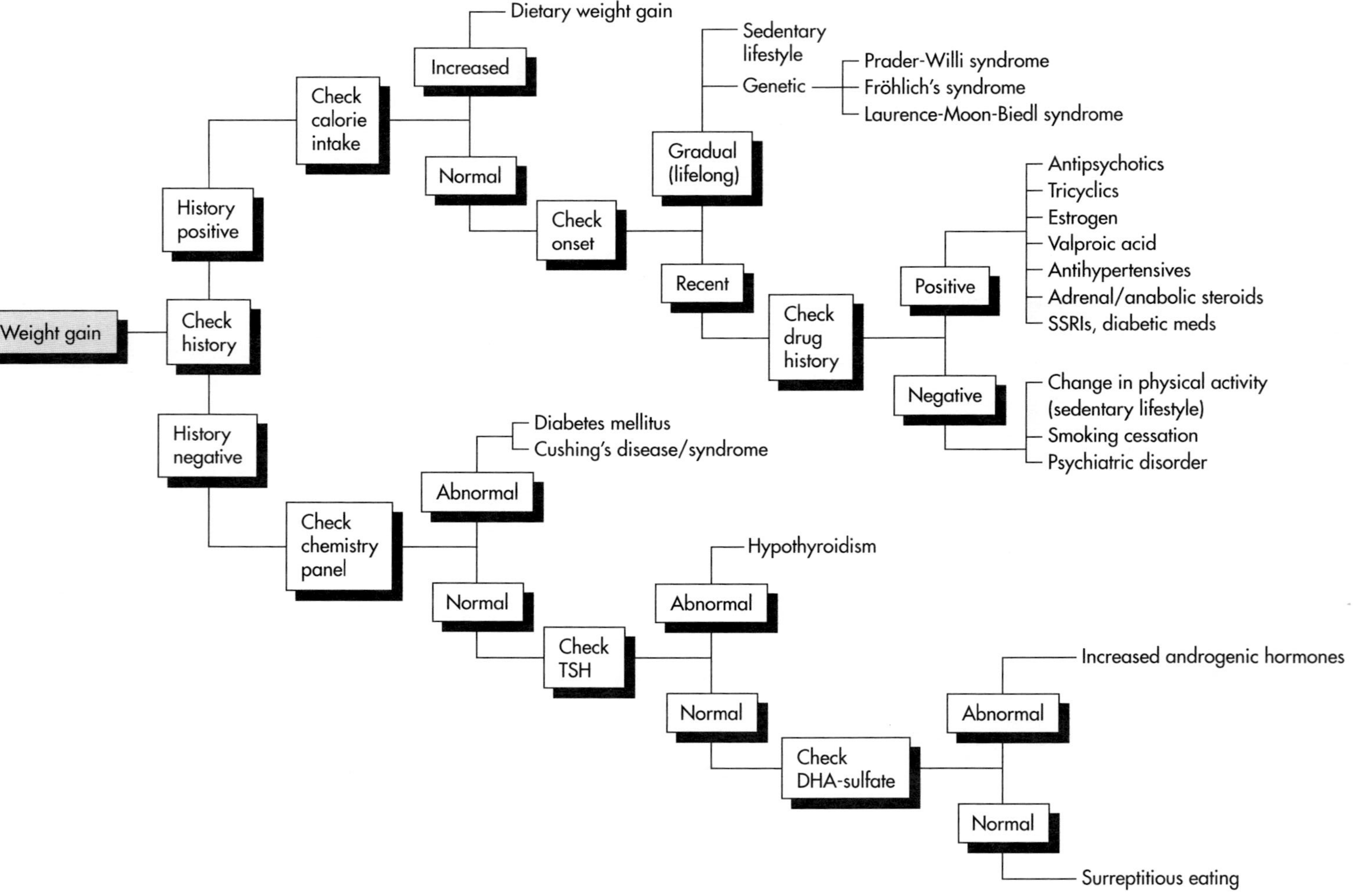

FIGURE 3-345 Weight gain. *DHA,* Dehydroepiandrosterone; *SSRIs,* serotonin reuptake inhibitors; *TSH,* thyroid-stimulating hormone. (Modified from Healey PM: *Common medical diagnosis: an algorithmic approach,* ed 3, Philadelphia, 2000, WB Saunders.)

Documented involuntary weight loss (IWL)
No recent institution of diuretic
Recent institution of diuretic
Observe
Repeat weight at 1-2 months
Documented further IWL
Stable weight
Usual follow-up
Complete history and physical
Review diet and appetite
Update routine indicated cancer screening tests
Preexisting chronic illness known to cause IWL
Review prescription and over-the-counter medications for anorectic side effects
History or examination findings suggestive of illnesses known to cause IWL
No history or examination findings suggestive of cause
Reevaluate and optimize therapy
Eliminate or modify offending medications
Focus evaluation directed by abnormal findings
CBC, SMA 12
Urinalysis
Thyroid-stimulating hormone level
Chest x-ray
Stool guaiacs
Abnormal findings
Normal findings
Follow-up abnormal values
More detailed psychosocial history:
Screen for depression, anxiety, eating disorders
Screen for socioeconomic factors (poverty, lack of transportation, isolation)
Screen for substance abuse
Consider food diary
Probable psychosocial cause detected
No abnormalities detected
Treat appropriately
Unexplained IWL
Follow at close intervals (high risk)

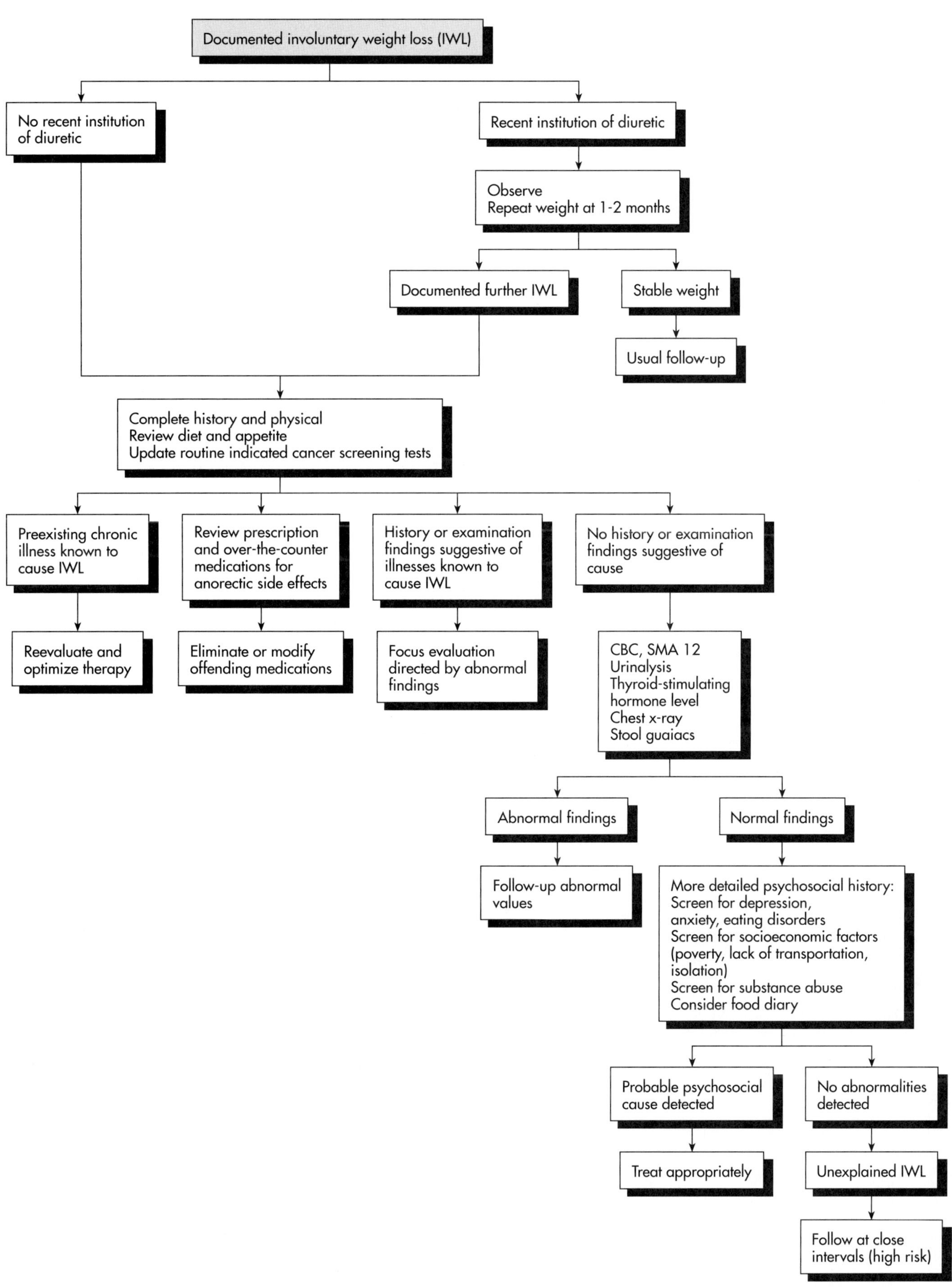

FIGURE 3-346 Involuntary weight loss. *CBC,* Complete blood count. (From Greene HL, Johnson WP, Lemcke D [eds]: *Decision making in medicine,* ed 2, St Louis, 1998, Mosby.)

SECTION IV

Laboratory Tests and Interpretation of Results

This section contains more than 300 commonly performed laboratory tests. In general, the tests are discussed in the following format:

1. Laboratory test.
2. Normal range in adult patients. Normal values are given using the present (traditional) reference interval, followed by the Système Internationale (SI) reference interval, the conversion factor (CF), and the suggested minimum increment (SMI).
3. Common abnormalities, such as positive test, increased or decreased value.
4. Causes of abnormal result.

The normal ranges may differ slightly, depending on the laboratory. The reader should be aware of the "normal range" of the particular laboratory performing the test. Every attempt has been made to present current laboratory test data, with emphasis on practical considerations.

ACE LEVEL

See ANGIOTENSIN-CONVERTING ENZYME

ACETONE (serum or plasma)

Normal: Negative
Elevated in: DKA, starvation, isopropanol ingestion

ACETYLCHOLINE RECEPTOR (AChR) ANTIBODY

Normal: <0.03 nmol/L
Elevated in: Myasthenia gravis. Changes in AChR concentration correlate with the clinical severity of myasthenia gravis following therapy and during therapy with prednisone and immunosuppressants. False-positive AChR antibody results may be found in patients with Eaton-Lambert syndrome.

ACID-BASE REFERENCE VALUES

See Tables 4-1 and 4-2.

ACID PHOSPHATASE (serum)

Normal range: 0-5.5 U/L (0-90 nkat/L [CF: 16.67; SMI: 2 nkat/L])
Elevated in: Carcinoma of prostate, other neoplasms (breast, bone), Paget's disease, osteogenesis imperfecta, malignant invasion of bone, Gaucher's disease, multiple myeloma, myeloproliferative disorders, benign prostatic hypertrophy, prostatic palpation or surgery, hyperparathyroidism, liver disease, chronic renal failure, idiopathic thrombocytopenic purpura, bronchitis

ACID SERUM TEST

See HAM TEST

ACTIVATED CLOTTING TIME (ACT)

Normal: This test is used to determine the dose of protamine sulfate to reverse the effect of heparin as an anticoagulant during angioplasty, cardiac surgery, and hemodialysis. The accepted goal during cardiopulmonary bypass surgery is usually 400-500 sec.

ACTIVATED PARTIAL THROMBOPLASTIN TIME (APTT, aPTT)

See PARTIAL THROMBOPLASTIN TIME

ADRENOCORTICOTROPIC HORMONE

Normal: 9-52 pg/ml
Elevated in: Addison's disease, ectopic ACTH-producing tumors, congenital adrenal hyperplasia, Nelson's syndrome, pituitary-dependent Cushing's disease
Decreased in: Secondary adrenocortical insufficiency, hypopituitarism, adrenal adenoma or adrenal carcinoma

ALANINE AMINOTRANSFERASE (ALT, SGPT)

Normal range: 0-35 U/L (0.058 μkat/L [CF: 0.02 μkat/L])
Elevated in: Liver disease (hepatitis, cirrhosis, Reye's syndrome), hepatic congestion, infectious mononucleosis, myocardial infarction, myocarditis,

TABLE 4-1 Commonly Used Acid-Base Reference Values for Arterial and Venous Plasma or Serum (Averaged from Various Sources)

	ARTERIAL		VENOUS	
	Conventional Units	**SI Units***	**Conventional Units**	**SI Units***
pH	7.40 (7.35-7.45)	7.40 (7.35-7.45)	7.37 (7.32-7.42)	7.37 (7.32-7.42)
Pco_2	40 mm Hg (35-45)	5.33 kPa (4.67-6.10)	45 mm Hg (45-50)	6.10 kPa (5.33-6.67)
Po_2	80-100 mm Hg	10.66-13.33 kPa	40 mm Hg (37-43)	5.33 kPa (4.93-5.73)
HCO_3 (CO_2 combining power)	24 mEq/L (20-28)	24 mmol/L (20-28)	26 mEq/L (22-30)	26 mmol/L (22-30)
CO_2 content	25 mEq/L (22-28)	25 mmol/L (22-28)	27 mEq/L (24-30)	27 mmol/L (24-30)

Reprinted from Ravel R: *Clinical laboratory medicine,* ed 6, St Louis, 1995, Mosby.
*International system.

Laboratory Tests

IV

TABLE 4-2 Summary of Laboratory Findings in Primary Uncomplicated Respiratory and Metabolic Acid-Base Disorders*

Disorder	Pco_2	pH	Base Excess
Acute primary respiratory hypoactivity (respiratory acidosis)	Increase	Decrease	Normal/positive
Acute primary respiratory hyperactivity (respiratory alkalosis)	Decrease	Increase	Normal/negative
Uncompensated metabolic acidosis	Normal	Decrease	Negative
Uncompensated metabolic alkalosis	Normal	Increase	Positive
Partially compensated metabolic acidosis	Decrease	Decrease	Negative
Partially compensated metabolic alkalosis	Increase	Increase	Positive
Chronic primary respiratory hypoactivity (compensated respiratory acidosis)	Increase	Normal	Positive
Fully compensated metabolic alkalosis	Increase	Normal	Positive
Chronic primary respiratory hyperactivity (compensated respiratory alkalosis)	Decrease	Normal	Negative
Fully compensated metabolic acidosis	Decrease	Normal	Negative

Reprinted from Ravel R: *Clinical laboratory medicine,* ed 6, St Louis, 1995, Mosby.
*Base excess results refer to negative (−) values more than 22 and positive (+) values more than 12.

severe muscle trauma, dermatomyositis/polymyositis, muscular dystrophy, drugs (antibiotics, narcotics, antihypertensive agents, heparin, labetalol, statins, NSAIDs, amiodarone, chlorpromazine, phenytoin), malignancy, renal and pulmonary infarction, convulsions, eclampsia, shock liver

ALBUMIN (serum)

Normal range: 4-6 g/dl (40-60 g/L [CF: 10; SMI: 1 g/L])
Elevated in: Dehydration (relative increase)
Decreased in: Liver disease, nephrotic syndrome, poor nutritional status, rapid IV hydration, protein-losing enteropathies (e.g., inflammatory bowel disease), severe burns, neoplasia, chronic inflammatory diseases, pregnancy, oral contraceptives, prolonged immobilization, lymphomas, hypervitaminosis A, chronic glomerulonephritis

ALCOHOL DEHYDROGENASE

Normal: 0-7 U/L
Elevated in: Drug-induced hepatocellular damage, obstructive jaundice, malignancy, inflammation, infection

ALDOLASE (serum)

Normal range: 0-6 U/L (0-100 nkat/L [CF: 16.67; SMI: 20 nkat/L])
Elevated in: Muscular dystrophy, rhabdomyolysis, dermatomyositis/polymyositis, trichinosis, acute hepatitis and other liver diseases, myocardial infarction, prostatic carcinoma, hemorrhagic pancreatitis, gangrene, delirium tremens, burns
Decreased in: Loss of muscle mass, late stages of muscular dystrophy

ALDOSTERONE

Normal range:
Recumbent: 50-150 ng/L
Upright: 150-300 ng/L
(Highest levels in neonates, decreasing over time to adult levels)
Elevated in: Primary aldosteronism, secondary aldosteronism, pseudoprimary aldosteronism
Decreased in:
Patient with hypertension: diabetes mellitus, Turner's syndrome, acute alcohol intoxication, excess secretion of deoxycorticosterone, corticosterone, and 18-hydroxycorticosterone
Patient without hypertension: Addison's disease, hypoaldosteronism resulting from renin deficiency, isolated aldosterone deficiency

ALKALINE PHOSPHATASE (serum)

Normal range: 30-120 U/L (0.5-2 μkat/L [CF: 0.01667; SMI: 0.1 μkat/L])
Elevated in:
LIVER AND BILIARY TRACT ORIGIN
Extrahepatic bile duct obstruction
Intrahepatic biliary obstruction
Liver cell acute injury
Liver passive congestion
Drug-induced liver cell dysfunction
Space-occupying lesions
Primary biliary cirrhosis
Sepsis
BONE ORIGIN (OSTEOBLAST HYPERACTIVITY)
Physiologic (rapid) bone growth (childhood and adolescence)
Metastatic tumor with osteoblastic reaction
Fracture healing
Paget's disease of bone
CAPILLARY ENDOTHELIAL ORIGIN
Granulation tissue formation (active)
PLACENTAL ORIGIN
Pregnancy
Some parenteral albumin preparations
OTHER
Thyrotoxicosis
Benign transient hyperphosphatasemia
Primary hyperparathyroidism
Decreased in: Hypothyroidism, pernicious anemia, hypophosphatemia, hypervitaminosis D, malnutrition

ALPHA-1-ANTITRYPSIN (serum)

Normal range: 110-140 mg/dl
Decreased in: Homozygous or heterozygous deficiency

ALPHA-1-FETOPROTEIN (serum)

See α-1 FETOPROTEIN

ALT

See ALANINE AMINOTRANSFERASE

ALUMINUM (serum)

Normal range: 0-6 ng/ml
Elevated in: Chronic renal failure on dialysis, parenteral nutrition, industrial exposure

AMEBIASIS SEROLOGIC TEST

Test description: Test is used to support diagnosis of amebiasis caused by *Entamoeba histolytica*. Serum acute and convalescent titers are drawn 1-3 weeks apart. A fourfold increase in titer is the most indicative result.

AMINOLEVULIC ACID (d-ALA) (24-h urine collection)

Normal: 1.5-7.5 mg/day
Elevated in: Acute porphyries, lead poisoning, DKA, pregnancy, anticonvulsant drugs, hereditary tyrosinemia
Decreased in: Alcoholic liver disease

AMMONIA (serum)

Normal range: 10-80 μg/dl (5-50 μmol/L [CF: 0.5872; SMI: 5 μmol/L])
Elevated in: Hepatic failure, hepatic encephalopathy, Reye's syndrome, portacaval shunt, drugs (diuretics, polymyxin B, methicillin)
Decreased in: Drugs (neomycin, lactulose, tetracycline), renal failure

AMYLASE (serum)

Normal range: 0-130 U/L (0-2.17 μkat/L [CF: 0.01667; SMI: 0.01 μkat/L])
Elevated in: Acute pancreatitis, pancreatic neoplasm, abscess, pseudocyst, ascites, macroamylasemia, perforated peptic ulcer, intestinal obstruction, intestinal infarction, acute cholecystitis, appendicitis, ruptured ectopic pregnancy, salivary gland inflammation, peritonitis, burns, diabetic ketoacidosis, renal insufficiency, drugs (morphine), carcinomatosis (of lung, esophagus, ovary), acute ethanol ingestion, mumps, prostate tumors, post–endoscopic retrograde cholangiopancreatography, bulimia, anorexia nervosa
Decreased in: Advanced chronic pancreatitis, hepatic necrosis, cystic fibrosis

AMYLASE, URINE

See URINE AMYLASE

AMYLOID A PROTEIN (serum)

Normal: <10 mcg/ml
Elevated in: Inflammatory disorders (acute phase–reacting protein), infections, acute coronary syndrome, malignancies

ANA

See ANTINUCLEAR ANTIBODY

ANCA

See ANTINEUTROPHIL CYTOPLASMIC ANTIBODY

ANDROSTENEDIONE (serum)

Normal:
Male: 75-205 ng/dl
Female: 85-275 ng/dl
Elevated in: Congenital adrenal hyperplasia, polycystic ovary syndrome, ectopic ACTH-producing tumor, Cushing's syndrome, hirsutism, hyperplasia of ovarian stroma, ovarian neoplasm
Decreased in: Ovarian failure, adrenal failure, sickle cell anemia

ANGIOTENSIN II

Normal: 10-60 pg/ml
Elevated in: Hypertension, CHF, cirrhosis, rennin-secreting renal tumor, volume depletion
Decreased in: ACE inhibitor drugs, ARB drugs, primary aldosteronism, Cushing's syndrome

ANGIOTENSIN-CONVERTING ENZYME (ACE level)

Normal range: <40 nmol/ml/min (<670 nkat/L [CF: 16.67; SMI: 10 nkat/L])
Elevated in: Sarcoidosis, primary biliary cirrhosis, alcoholic liver disease, hyperthyroidism, hyperparathyroidism, diabetes mellitus, amyloidosis, multiple myeloma, lung disease (asbestosis, silicosis, berylliosis, allergic alveolitis, coccidioidomycosis), Gaucher's disease, leprosy

ANION GAP

Normal range: 9-14 mEq/L
Elevated in: Lactic acidosis, ketoacidosis (diabetes, alcoholic starvation), uremia (chronic renal failure), ingestion of toxins (paraldehyde, methanol, salicylates, ethylene glycol), hyperosmolar nonketotic coma, antibiotics (carbenicillin)
Decreased in: Hypoalbuminemia, severe hypermagnesemia, IgG myeloma, lithium toxicity, laboratory error (falsely decreased sodium or overestimation of bicarbonate or chloride), hypercalcemia of parathyroid origin, antibiotics (e.g., polymyxin)

ANTICARDIOLIPIN ANTIBODY (ACA)

Normal range: Negative. Test includes detection of IgG, IgM, and IgA antibodies to phospholipid, cardiolipin
Present in: Antiphospholipid antibody syndrome, chronic hepatitis C

ANTICOAGULANT

See CIRCULATING ANTICOAGULANT

ANTIDIURETIC HORMONE

Normal range: mOsm/kg 295-300 4-12 pg/ml[EN4]
Elevated in: SIADH, antipsychotic medications, ectopic ADH from systemic neoplasm, Guillain-Barré syndrome, CNS infections, brain tumors, nephrogenic diabetes insipidus
Decreased in: Central diabetes insipidus, nephritic syndrome, psychogenic polydipsias, demeclocycline, lithium, phenytoin, alcohol

ANTI-DNA

Normal range: Absent
Present in: Systemic lupus erythematosus, chronic active hepatitis, infectious mononucleosis, biliary cirrhosis

ANTI-ds DNA

Normal: <25 U
Elevated in: Systemic lupus erythematosus

ANTIGLOMERULAR BASEMENT ANTIBODY

See GLOMERULAR BASEMENT MEMBRANE ANTIBODY

ANTIHISTONE

Normal: <1 U
Elevated in: Drug-induced lupus erythematosus

ANTIMITOCHONDRIAL ANTIBODY

Normal range: <1:20 titer
Elevated in: Primary biliary cirrhosis (85%-95%), chronic active hepatitis (25%-30%), cryptogenic cirrhosis (25%-30%)

ANTINEUTROPHIL CYTOPLASMIC ANTIBODY (ANCA)

Positive test: Cytoplasmic pattern (cANCA): positive in Wegener's granulomatosis
Perinuclear pattern (pANCA): positive in inflammatory bowel disease, primary biliary cirrhosis, primary sclerosing cholangitis, autoimmune chronic active hepatitis, crescenteric glomerulonephritis

ANTINUCLEAR ANTIBODY (ANA)

Normal range: <1:20 titer
Positive test: Systemic lupus erythematosus (more significant if titer >1:160), drugs (phenytoin, ethosuximide, primidone, methyldopa, hydralazine, carbamazepine, penicillin, procainamide, chlorpromazine, griseofulvin, thiazides), chronic active hepatitis, age over 60 years (particularly age over 80 years), rheumatoid arthritis, scleroderma, mixed connective tissue disease, necrotizing vasculitis, Sjögren's syndrome, tuberculosis, pulmonary interstitial fibrosis. Table 4-3 describes diseases associated with ANA subtypes. Fig. 4-1 illustrates various fluorescent ANA test patterns.

TABLE 4-3 Disease-Associated ANA Subtypes

Nuclear Location	Disease(s)
"Native" DNA (dsDNA, or dsDNA/ssDNA complex)	SLE (60%-70%; range, 35%-75%) Also PSS (5%-55%), MCTD (11%-25%), RA (5%-40%), DM (5%-25%), SS (5%)
sNP	SLE (50%) Also other collagen diseases
DNP (DNA-histone complex)	SLE (52%) Also MCTD (8%), RA (3%)
Histones	Drug-induced SLE (95%) Also SLE (30%), RA (15%-24%)
ENA Sm	SLE (30%-40%; range, 28%-40%) Also MCTD (0%-8%); RNP (U1-RNP) MCTD (in high titer without any other ANA subtype present: 95%-100%) Also SLE (26%-50%), PSS (11%-22%), RA (10%), SS (3%)
SS-A (Ro)*	SS without RA (60%-70%) Also SLE (26%-50%), neonatal SLE (over 95%), PSS (30%), MCTD (50%), SS with RA (9%), PBC (15%-19%)
SS-B (La)	SS without RA (40%-60%) Also SLE (5%-15%), SS with RA (5%)
Scl-70*	PSS (15%-43%)
Centromere*	CREST syndrome (70%-90%; range 57%-96%) Also PSS (4%-20%), PBC (12%)
Nucleolar	PSS (scleroderma) (54%-90%) Also SLE (25%-26%), RA (9%)
RAP (RANA)	SS with RA (60%-76%) Also SS without RA (5%)
Jo-1	Polymyositis (30%)
PM-1	Polymyositis or PMS/PSS overlap syndrome (60%-90%) Also DM (17%)
ssDNA	SLE (60%-70%) Also CAH, infectious mononucleosis, RA, chronic GN, chronic infections, PBC
Cytoplasmic Location	**Disease(s)**
Mitochondrial	Primary biliary cirrhosis (90%-100%) Also CAH (7%-30%), cryptogenic cirrhosis (30%), acute hepatitis, viral hepatitis (3%), other liver diseases (0%-20%), SLE (5%), SS and PSS (8%)
Microsomal†	Chronic active hepatitis (60%-80%), Hashimoto's thyroiditis (97%)
Ribosomal	SLE (5%-12%)
Smooth muscle‡	Chronic active hepatitis (60%-91%) Also cryptogenic cirrhosis (28%), acute hepatitis, viral hepatitis (5%-87%), infectious mononucleosis (81%), MS (40%-50%), malignancy (67%), PBC (10%-50%)

Reprinted from Ravel R: *Clinical laboratory medicine,* ed 6, St Louis, 1995, Mosby.
CAH, Chronic active hepatitis; *DM,* dermatomyositis; *GN,* glomerulonephritis; *MS,* multiple sclerosis; *PBC,* primary biliary cirrhosis; *SS,* Sjögren's syndrome.
*Not detected using rat or mouse liver or kidney tissue method.
†Not detected by cultured cell method.
‡Detected by cultured cells but better with rat or mouse tissue.

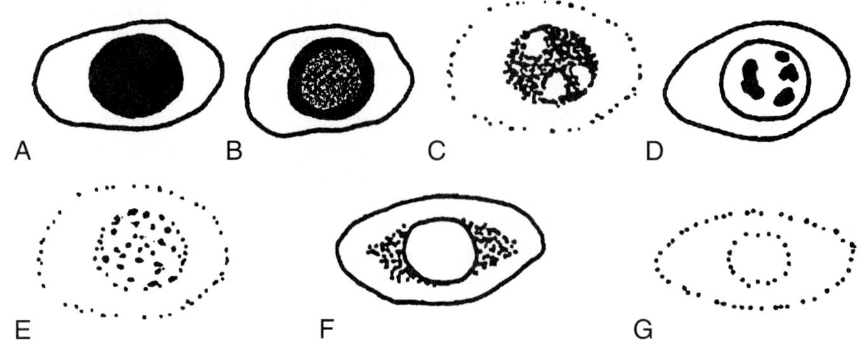

FIGURE 4-1 Fluorescent antinuclear antibody test patterns (HEP-2 cells). A, Solid (homogeneous). **B,** Peripheral (rim). **C,** Speckled. **D,** Nucleolar. **E,** Anticentromere. **F,** Antimitochondrial. **G,** Normal (nonreactive). (Reprinted from Ravel R [ed]: *Clinical laboratory medicine,* ed 6, St Louis, 1995, Mosby.)

ANTI-RNP ANTIBODY

See EXTRACTABLE NUCLEAR ANTIGEN

ANTI-Scl-70

Normal: Absent
Elevated in: Scleroderma

ANTI-Sm (anti-Smith) ANTIBODY

See EXTRACTABLE NUCLEAR ANTIGEN

ANTI-SMOOTH MUSCLE ANTIBODY

See SMOOTH MUSCLE ANTIBODY

ANTISTREPTOLYSIN O TITER (Streptozyme, ASLO titer)

Normal range for adults: <160 Todd units
Elevated in: Streptococcal upper airway infection, acute rheumatic fever, acute glomerulonephritis, increased levels of β-lipoprotein

NOTE: A fourfold increase in titer between acute and convalescent specimens is diagnostic of streptococcal upper airway infection regardless of the initial titer.

ANTITHROMBIN III

Normal range: 81%-120% of normal activity; 17-30 mg/dl
Decreased in: Hereditary deficiency of antithrombin III, disseminated intravascular coagulation, pulmonary embolism, cirrhosis, thrombolytic therapy, chronic liver failure, postsurgery, third trimester of pregnancy, oral contraceptives, nephrotic syndrome, IV heparin >3 days, sepsis, acute leukemia, carcinoma, thrombophlebitis
Elevated in: Warfarin drugs, post–myocardial infarction

APOLIPOPROTEIN A-1 (Apo A-1)

Normal: Recommended >120 mg/dl
Elevated in: Familial hyperalphalipoproteinemia, statins, niacin, estrogens, weight loss, familial cholesteryl ester transfer protein (CETP) deficiency
Decreased in: Familial hypoalphalipoproteinemia, Tangier disease, diuretics, androgens, cigarette smoking, hepatocellular disorders, chronic renal failure, nephritic syndrome, coronary heart disease, cholestasis

APOLIPOPROTEIN B (Apo B)

Normal: Desirable <100 mg/dl; high risk >120 mg/dl
Elevated in: High saturated fat diet, high-cholesterol diet, hyperapobetalipoproteinemia, familial combined hyperlipidemia, anabolic steroids, diuretics, beta-blockers, corticosteroids, progestins, diabetes, hypothyroidism, chronic renal failure, liver disease, Cushing's syndrome, coronary heart disease
Decreased in: Statins, niacin, low-cholesterol diet, malnutrition, abetalipoproteinemia, hypobetalipoproteinemia, hyperthyroidism

ARTERIAL BLOOD GASES

Normal range:
Po_2: 75-100 mm Hg
Pco_2: 35-45 mm Hg
HCO_3: 24-28 mEq/L
pH: 7.35-7.45
Abnormal values: Acid-base disturbances (see the following)

METABOLIC ACIDOSIS
Metabolic acidosis with increased AG (AG acidosis)
Lactic acidosis
Ketoacidosis (diabetes mellitus, alcoholic ketoacidosis)
Uremia (chronic renal failure)
Ingestion of toxins (paraldehyde, methanol, salicylate, ethylene glycol)
High-fat diet (mild acidosis)
Metabolic acidosis with normal AG (hyperchloremic acidosis)
Renal tubular acidosis (including acidosis of aldosterone deficiency)
Intestinal loss of HCO_3^- (diarrhea, pancreatic fistula)
Carbonic anhydrase inhibitors (e.g., acetazolamide)
Dilutional acidosis (as a result of rapid infusion of bicarbonate-free isotonic saline)
Ingestion of exogenous acids (ammonium chloride, methionine, cystine, calcium chloride)
Ileostomy
Ureterosigmoidostomy
Drugs: amiloride, triamterene, spironolactone, β-blockers

RESPIRATORY ACIDOSIS
Pulmonary disease (COPD, severe pneumonia, pulmonary edema, interstitial fibrosis)
Airway obstruction (foreign body, severe bronchospasm, laryngospasm)
Thoracic cage disorders (pneumothorax, flail chest, kyphoscoliosis)
Defects in muscles of respiration (myasthenia gravis, hypokalemia, muscular dystrophy)
Defects in peripheral nervous system (amyotrophic lateral sclerosis, poliomyelitis, Guillain-Barré syndrome, botulism, tetanus, organophosphate poisoning, spinal cord injury)
Depression of respiratory center (anesthesia, narcotics, sedatives, vertebral artery embolism or thrombosis, increased intracranial pressure)
Failure of mechanical ventilator

METABOLIC ALKALOSIS
Divided into chloride-responsive (urinary chloride <15 mEq/L) and chloride-resistant forms (urinary chloride level >15 mEq/L)
Chloride-responsive
Vomiting
Nasogastric (NG) suction
Diuretics
Posthypercapnic alkalosis
Stool losses (laxative abuse, cystic fibrosis, villous adenoma)
Massive blood transfusion
Exogenous alkali administration

Chloride-resistant
Hyperadrenocorticoid states (Cushing's syndrome, primary hyperaldosteronism, secondary mineralocorticoidism [licorice, chewing tobacco])
Hypomagnesemia
Hypokalemia
Bartter's syndrome
RESPIRATORY ALKALOSIS
Hypoxemia (pneumonia, pulmonary embolism, atelectasis, high-altitude living)
Drugs (salicylates, xanthines, progesterone, epinephrine, thyroxine, nicotine)
Central nervous system (CNS) disorders (tumor, cerebrovascular accident [CVA], trauma, infections)
Psychogenic hyperventilation (anxiety, hysteria)
Hepatic encephalopathy
Gram-negative sepsis
Hyponatremia
Sudden recovery from metabolic acidosis
Assisted ventilation

ARTHROCENTESIS FLUID

Interpretation of results:
1. **Color:** Normally it is clear or pale yellow; cloudiness indicates inflammatory process or presence of crystals, cell debris, fibrin, or triglycerides.
2. **Viscosity:** Normally it has a high viscosity because of hyaluronate; when fluid is placed on a slide, it can be stretched to a string >2 cm in length before separating (low viscosity indicates breakdown of hyaluronate [lysosomal enzymes from leukocytes] or the presence of edema fluid).
3. **Mucin clot:** Add 1 ml of fluid to 5 ml of a 5% acetic acid solution and allow 1 minute for the clot to form; a firm clot (does not fragment on shaking) is normal and indicates the presence of large molecules of hyaluronic acid (this test is nonspecific and infrequently done).
4. **Glucose:** Normally it approximately equals serum glucose level; a difference of more than 40 mg/dl is suggestive of infection.
5. **Protein:** Total protein concentration is <2.5 g/dl in the normal synovial fluid; it is elevated in inflammatory and septic arthritis.
6. **Microscopic examination for crystals**
   a. **Gout:** Monosodium urate crystals
   b. **Pseudogout:** Calcium pyrophosphate dihydrate crystals

ASLO TITER

See ANTISTREPTOLYSIN O TITER

ASPARTATE AMINOTRANSFERASE (AST, SGOT)

Normal range: 0-35 U/L (0-0.58 μkat/L [CF: 0.01667, SMI: 0.01 μkat/L])
Elevated in:
HEART
Acute myocardial infarction
Pericarditis (active: some cases)
LIVER
Hepatitis virus, Epstein-Barr, or cytomegalovirus infection
Active cirrhosis
Liver passive congestion or hypoxia
Alcohol- or drug-induced liver dysfunction
Space-occupying lesions (active)
Fatty liver (severe)
Extrahepatic biliary obstruction (early)
Drug-induced
SKELETAL MUSCLE
Acute skeletal muscle injury
Muscle inflammation (infectious or noninfectious)
Muscular dystrophy (active)
Recent surgery
Delirium tremens
KIDNEY
Acute injury or damage
Renal infarct
OTHER
Intestinal infarction
Shock
Cholecystitis
Acute pancreatitis
Hypothyroidism
Heparin therapy (60%-80% of cases)

ATRIAL NATRIURETIC HORMONE (ANH)

Normal: 20-77 pg/ml
Elevated in: CHF, volume overload, cardiovascular disease with high filling pressure
Decreased with: Prazosin

B-TYPE NATRIURETIC PEPTIDE

Normal range: Up to 100 pg/ml
Elevated in: Heart failure. This test is useful in the emergency department setting to differentiate heart failure patients from those with chronic obstructive pulmonary disease presenting with dyspnea.

BASOPHIL COUNT

Normal range: 0.4%-1% of total WBC; 40-100/mm^3
Elevated in: Leukemia, inflammatory processes, polycythemia vera, Hodgkin's lymphoma, hemolytic anemia, after splenectomy, myeloid metaplasia, myxedema
Decreased in: Stress, hypersensitivity reaction, steroids, pregnancy, hyperthyroidism, postirradiation

BICARBONATE

Normal: Arterial: 21-28 mEq/L
Venous: 22-29 mEq/L
Elevated in: Metabolic alkalosis, compensated respiratory acidosis, diuretics, corticosteroids, laxative abuse
Decreased in: Metabolic acidosis, compensated respiratory alkalosis, acetazolamide, cyclosporine, cholestyramine, methanol or ethylene glycol poisoning

BILE ACID BREATH TEST

Normal: The test determines the radioactivity of $_{14}CO_2$ in breath samples at 2 and 4 hr.
  2 hr after dose: 0.11 ± 0.14
  4 hr after dose: 0.52 ± 0.09
Elevated in: GI bacterial overgrowth, cimetidine

BILE, URINE

See URINE BILE

BILIRUBIN, DIRECT (conjugated bilirubin)

Normal range: 0-0.2 mg/dl (0-4 μmol/L [CF: 17.10; SMI: 2 μmol/L])
Elevated in: Hepatocellular disease, biliary obstruction, drug-induced cholestasis, hereditary disorders (Dubin-Johnson syndrome, Rotor's syndrome)

BILIRUBIN, INDIRECT (unconjugated bilirubin)

Normal range: 0-1.0 mg/dl (2-18 μmol/L [CF: 17.10; SMI: 2 μmol/L])
Elevated in:
A. Increased bilirubin production (if normal liver, serum unconjugated bilirubin is usually less than 4 mg/100 ml)
   1. Hemolytic anemia
      a. Acquired
      b. Congenital
   2. Resorption from extravascular sources
      a. Hematomas
      b. Pulmonary infarcts
   3. Excessive ineffective erythropoiesis
      a. Congenital (congenital dyserythropoietic anemias)
      b. Acquired (pernicious anemia, severe lead poisoning; if present, bilirubinemia is usually mild)

B. Defective hepatic unconjugated bilirubin clearance (defective uptake or conjugation)
   1. Severe liver disease
   2. Gilbert's syndrome
   3. Crigler-Najjar type I or II
   4. Drug-induced inhibition
   5. Portacaval shunt
   6. Congestive heart failure
   7. Hyperthyroidism (uncommon)

BILIRUBIN, TOTAL

Normal range: 0-1.0 mg/dl (2-18 μmol/L [CF: 17.10, SMI: 2 μmol/L])
Elevated in: Liver disease (hepatitis, cirrhosis, cholangitis, neoplasm, biliary obstruction, infectious mononucleosis), hereditary disorders (Gilbert's disease, Dubin-Johnson syndrome), drugs (steroids, diphenylhydantoin, phenothiazines, penicillin, erythromycin, clindamycin, captopril, amphotericin B, sulfonamides, azathioprine, isoniazid, 5-aminosalicylic acid, allopurinol, methyldopa, indomethacin, halothane, oral contraceptives, procainamide, tolbutamide, labetalol), hemolysis, pulmonary embolism or infarct, hepatic congestion secondary to congestive heart failure

BILIRUBIN, URINE

See URINE BILE

BLADDER TUMOR ASSOCIATED ANTIGEN

Normal: ≤14 U/ml. Test is used to detect bladder cancer recurrence. Sensitivity 57%-83% and specificity 68%-72%.
Elevated in: Bladder cancer, renal stones, nephritis, UTI, hematuria, renal cancer, cystitis, recent bladder or urinary tract trauma

BLEEDING TIME (modified Ivy method)

Normal range: 2 to 9.5 min
Elevated in: Thrombocytopenia, capillary wall abnormalities, platelet abnormalities (Bernard-Soulier disease, Glanzmann's disease), drugs (aspirin, warfarin, antiinflammatory medications, streptokinase, urokinase, dextran, β-lactam antibiotics, moxalactam), disseminated intravascular coagulation, cirrhosis, uremia, myeloproliferative disorders, von Willebrand's disease

BLOOD VOLUME, TOTAL

Normal: 60-80 ml/kg
Elevated in: Polycythemia vera, pulmonary disease, CHF, renal insufficiency, pregnancy, acidosis, thyrotoxicosis
Decreased in: Anemia, hemorrhage, vomiting, diarrhea, dehydration, burns, starvation

BORDETELLA PERTUSSIS SEROLOGY

Test description: PCR of nasopharyngeal aspirates or secretions is used to identify *Bordetella pertussis*, the organism responsible for whooping cough.

BRCA ANALYSIS

DESCRIPTION OF ANALYSIS

Comprehensive BRCA analysis:

BRCA1: Full sequence determination in both forward and reverse directions of approximately 5500 base pairs comprising 22 coding exons and one noncoding exon (exon 4) and approximately 800 adjacent base pairs in the noncoding intervening sequence (intron). Exon 1, which is noncoding, is not analyzed. The wild-type *BRCA1* gene encodes a protein comprising 1863 amino acids.

BRCA2: Full sequence determination in both forward and reverse directions of approximately 10,200 base pairs comprising 26 coding exons and approximately 900 adjacent base pairs in the noncoding intervening sequence (intron). Exon 1, which is noncoding, is not analyzed. The wild-type *BRCA2* gene encodes a protein comprising 3418 amino acids.

The noncoding intronic regions of *BRCA1* and *BRCA2* that are analyzed do not extend more than 20 base pairs proximal to the 5′ end and 10 base pairs distal to the 3′ end of each exon.

Single-site bracanalysis: DNA sequence analysis for a specified mutation in *BRCA1* and/or *BRCA2.*

Multisite 3 bracanalysis: DNA sequence analysis of specific portions of *BRCA1* exon 2, *BRCA1* exon 20, and *BRCA2* exon 11 designed to detect only mutations 187delAG and 5385insC in *BRCA1* and 6174delT in *BRCA2.*

Interpretive Criteria:

"Positive for a deleterious mutation": Includes all mutations (nonsense, insertions, deletions) that prematurely terminate ("truncate") the protein product of *BRCA1* at least 10 amino acids from the C-terminus, or the protein product of *BRCA2* at least 110 amino acids from the C-terminus (based on documentation of deleterious mutations in *BRCA1* and *BRCA2*).
In addition, specific missense mutations and noncoding intervening sequence (IVS) mutations are recognized as deleterious on the basis of data derived from linkage analysis of high-risk families, functional assays, biochemical evidence, and/or demonstration of abnormal mRNA transcript processing.

"Genetic variant, suspected deleterious": Includes genetic variants for which the available evidence indicates a likelihood, but not proof, that the mutation is deleterious. The specific evidence supporting such an interpretation will be summarized for individual variants on each such report.

"Genetic variant, favor polymorphism": Includes genetic variants for which available evidence indicates that the variant is highly unlikely to contribute substantially to cancer risk. The specific evidence supporting such an interpretation will be summarized for individual variants on each such report.

"Genetic variant of uncertain significance": Includes missense mutations and mutations that occur in analyzed intronic regions whose clinical significance has not yet been determined, as well as chain-terminating mutations that truncate *BRCA1* and *BRCA2* distal to amino acid positions 1853 and 3308, respectively.

"No deleterious mutation detected": Includes nontruncating genetic variants observed at an allele frequency of approximately 1% of a suitable control population (providing that no data suggest clinical significance), as well as all genetic variants for which published data demonstrate absence of substantial clinical significance. Also includes mutations in the protein-coding region that neither alter the amino acid sequence nor are predicted to significantly affect exon splicing, and base pair alterations in noncoding portions of the gene that have been demonstrated to have no deleterious effect on the length or stability of the mRNA transcript.
There may be uncommon genetic abnormalities in *BRCA1* and *BRCA2* that will not be detected by *BRCA* analysis. This analysis, however, is believed to rule out the majority of abnormalities in these genes, which are believed responsible for most hereditary susceptibility to breast and ovarian cancer.

"Specific variant/mutation not identified": Specific and designated deleterious mutations or variants of uncertain clinical significance are not present in the individual being tested. If one (or rarely two) specific deleterious mutations have been identified in a family member, a negative analysis for the specific mutation(s) indicates that the tested individual is at the general population risk of developing breast or ovarian cancer.

BREATH HYDROGEN TEST

Normal: This test is for bacterial overgrowth. H_2 excretion fasting: 4.6 ± 5.1, after lactulose, early increase <12. Lactulose usually results in a colonic response >30 min after ingestion.
Elevated in: A high fasting breath H_2 level and an increase of at least 12 ppm within 30 min after lactulose challenge are indicative of bacterial overgrowth in the small intestine. The increase must precede the colonic response.
Fast positives in: Accelerated gastric emptying, laxative use
Fast negatives in: Use of antibiotics and patients who are nonhydrogen producers

BUN

See UREA NITROGEN, BLOOD

C282Y AND H63D MUTATION ANALYSIS

Procedure: Detection of the C282Y and H63D mutations is accomplished by amplification of exons 2 and 4 of the *HFE* gene on chromosome 6 by polymerase chain reaction (PCR) followed by allele-specific hybridization and chemiluminescent detection of hybridized probes. H63D is viewed by some as a polymorphism rather than a mutation because of its prevalence in the population, because 15% of the individuals affected with hereditary hemochromatosis (HH) are compound heterozygotes for C282Y and H63D and about 1% of patients are H63D homozygotes, which suggests that H63D may be causative in the development of the disorder at reduced penetrance. The test is performed by Quest Diagnostics pursuant to a license agreement with Roche Molecular systems, Inc.

Interpretation: Homozygosity for the C282Y mutation has been associated with an increased risk of being affected with HH compared with the general population. The genotype is observed in 60%-90% of individuals affected with HH and occurs in less than 1% of the general population. However, approximately 25% of asymptomatic individuals with this genotype do not develop the disorder.

C3

See COMPLEMENT

C4

See COMPLEMENT

CALCITONIN (serum)

Normal range: <100 pg/ml (<100 ng/L [CF: 1; SMI: 10 ng/L])
Elevated in: Medullary carcinoma of the thyroid (particularly if level >1500 pg/ml), carcinoma of the breast, apudomas, carcinoids, renal failure, thyroiditis

CALCIUM (serum)

Normal range: 8.8-10.3 mg/dl (2.2-2.58 μmol/L [CF: 0.2495; SMI: 0.02 μmol/L])

ELEVATED

Relatively common:

Neoplasia (noncutaneous)
Bone primary
Myeloma
Acute leukemia
Nonbone solid tumors
Breast
Lung
Squamous nonpulmonary
Kidney
Neoplasm secretion of parathyroid hormone-related protein (PTHrP, "ectopic PTH")
Primary hyperparathyroidism
Thiazide diuretics
Tertiary (renal) hyperparathyroidism
Idiopathic
Spurious (artifactual) hypercalcemia
Dehydration
Serum protein elevation
Laboratory technical problem

Relatively uncommon:

Neoplasia (less common tumors)
Sarcoidosis
Hyperthyroidism
Immobilization (mostly seen in children and adolescents)
Diuretic phase of acute renal tubular necrosis
Vitamin D intoxication
Milk-alkali syndrome
Addison's disease
Lithium therapy
Idiopathic hypercalcemia of infancy
Acromegaly
Theophylline toxicity

Table 4-4 describes the laboratory differential diagnosis of hypercalcemia.

DECREASED

Artifactual
Hypoalbuminemia
Hemodilution
Primary hypoparathyroidism
Pseudohypoparathyroidism
Vitamin D–related
Vitamin D deficiency
Malabsorption
Renal failure

TABLE 4-4 Laboratory Differential Diagnosis of Hypercalcemia

	PLASMA TESTS					URINE TESTS			
Diagnosis	**Ca**	**PO_4**	**PTH**	**25(OH)D**	**$1,25(OH)_2D$**	**cAMP**	**TmP/GFR**	**Ca**	**Comments**
Primary hyperparathyroidism	↑	N/↓	↑	N	N/↑	↑	↓	↑	Parathyroid adenoma most common
MEN I									Parathyroid hyperplasia; also includes pituitary and pancreatic neoplasms
MEN IIa									Parathyroid hyperplasia; also includes medullary thyroid carcinoma and heochromocytoma
MEN IIb									Parathyroid disease uncommon, primarily medullary thyroid carcinoma and pheochromocytoma
FHH	↑	N	N/↑	N	N	N/↑	N/↓	↓↓	Autosomal dominant inheritance; hypercalcemia present within first decade; benign
Malignancy									
Solid tumor, humoral	↑	N/↓	↓	N	N	↑	↓	↑↑	Primarily epidermoid tumors; PTH-related protein(s) is mediator
Solid tumor, osteolytic	↑	N/↑	↓	N	N	↓	↑	↑↑	
Lymphoma	↑	N/↑	↓	N/↓	↑	↓	↑	↑↑	
Granulomatous disease	↑	N/↑	↓	N/↓	↑↑	↓	↑	↑↑	Sarcoid most common etiology
Vitamin D intoxication	↑	N/↑	↓	↑↑	N	↓	↑	↑↑	
Hyperthyroidism	↑	N	↓	N	N	N	N	↑↑	Plasma concentrations of T_4 and/or T_3 are elevated

Reprinted from Moore WT, Eastman RC: *Diagnostic endocrinology,* ed 2, St Louis, 1996, Mosby.

Ca, Calcium; *cAMP,* cyclic adenosine monophosphate; *FHH,* familial hypocalciuric hypercalcemia; *GFR,* glomerular filtration rate; *MEN,* multiple endocrine neoplasia; *25(OH)D,* 25 hydroxyvitamin D; *PO_4,* phosphate; *PTH,* parathyroid hormone; *T_3,* triiodothyronine; *T_4,* thyroxine; *TmP,* renal threshold for phosphorus.

TABLE 4-5 Laboratory Differential Diagnosis of Hypocalcemia

	PLASMA TESTS					URINE TESTS					
Diagnosis	**Ca**	**PO_4**	**PTH**	**25(OH)D**	**1,25$(OH)_2$D**	**cAMP**	**cAMP after PTH**	**TmP/GFR**	**TmP/GFR after PTH**	**Ca**	**Comments**
Hypoparathyroidism	↓	↑	N/↓	N	↓	↓	↑↑	↑	↓↓	N/↓	Deficiency of PTH
Pseudohypoparathyroidism											
Type I	↓	↑	↑↑	N	↓	↓	NC	↑	↑	N/↓	Resistance to PTH; patients may have Albright's hereditary osteodystrophy and resistance to multiple hormones
Type II	↓	N	↑↑	N	↓	↓	↑	↑	↑	N/↓	Renal resistance to cAMP
Vitamin D deficiency	↓	N/↓	↑↑	↓↓	N/↓	↑	↑	↓	↓	↓↓	Deficient supply (e.g., nutrition) or absorption (e.g., pancreatic insufficiency) of vitamin D
Vitamin D–dependent rickets											
Type I	↓	N/↓	↑↑	N	↓	↑		↓		↓↓	Deficient activity of renal 25(OH)D-1a-hydroxylase
Type II	↓	N/↓	↑↑	N	↑↑	↑		↓		↓↓	Resistance to 1,25$(OH)_2$D

Reprinted from Moore WT, Eastman RC: *Diagnostic endocrinology,* ed 2, St Louis, 1996, Mosby.

Ca, Calcium; *cAMP,* cyclic adenosine monophosphate; *FHH,* familial hypocalciuric hypercalcemia; *GFR,* glomerular filtration rate; *MEN,* multiple endocrine neoplasia; *NC,* no change or small increase; *(OH)D,* hydroxycalciferol D; *PO_4,* phosphate; *PTH,* parathyroid hormone; *T_3,* triiodothyronine; *T_4,* thyroxine; *TmP,* renal threshold for phosphorus.

Magnesium deficiency
Sepsis
Chronic alcoholism
Tumor lysis syndrome
Rhabdomyolysis
Alkalosis (respiratory or metabolic)
Acute pancreatitis
Drug-induced hypocalcemia
Large doses of magnesium sulfate
Anticonvulsants
Mithramycin
Gentamicin
Cimetidine

Table 4-5 describes the laboratory differential diagnosis of hypocalcemia.

CALCIUM, URINE

See URINE CALCIUM

CANCER ANTIGEN 15-3 (CA 15-3)

Normal: <30 U/ml

Elevated in: Approximately 80% of women with metastatic breast cancer. Clinical sensitivity is 0.60, specificity 0.87, positive predictive value 0.91. This test is generally used to predict recurrence of breast cancer and evaluate response to therapy. May also be elevated in liver cancer, pancreatic cancer, ovarian cancer, colorectal cancer. Elevations can also occur with benign breast and liver disease.

CANCER ANTIGEN 27-29 (CA 27-29)

Normal: <38 U/ml

Elevated in: Approximately 75% of women with metastatic breast cancer. Clinical sensitivity is 0.57, specificity 0.97, positive predictive value 0.83, negative predictive value 0.92. This test is generally used to predict recurrence of breast cancer and evaluate response to therapy. May also be elevated in liver cancer, pancreatic cancer, ovarian cancer, colorectal cancer. Elevations can also occur with benign breast and liver disease.

CANCER ANTIGEN 72-4 (CA 72-4)

Normal: <4.0 ng/ml

Elevated in: Gastric cancer (elevated in >50% of patients). Often used in combination with CA 72-4, CA 19.9, and CEA to monitor gastric cancer after treatment.

CANCER ANTIGEN 125 (CA 125)

Normal range: <1.4%

This test uses an antibody against antigen from tissue culture of an ovarian tumor cell line. Various published evaluations report sensitivity of about 75%-80% in patients with ovarian carcinoma. There is also an appreciable incidence of elevated values in nonovarian malignancies and in certain benign conditions (see below). Test values may transiently increase during chemotherapy.

MALIGNANT

Epithelial ovarian carcinoma, 75%-80% (range, 25%-92%; better in serous than mucinous cystadenocarcinoma)
Endometrial carcinoma, 25%-48% (2%-90%)
Pancreatic carcinoma, 59%
Colorectal carcinoma, 20% (15%-56%)
Endocervical adenocarcinoma, 83%
Squamous cervical or vaginal carcinoma, 7%-14%
Lung carcinoma, 32%
Breast carcinoma, 12%-40%
Lymphoma, 35%

BENIGN

Cirrhosis, 40%-80%
Acute pancreatitis, 38%
Acute peritonitis, 75%
Endometriosis, 88%
Acute pelvic inflammatory disease, 33%
Pregnancy first trimester, 2%-24%
During menstruation (occasionally)
Renal failure (?frequency)
Normal persons, 0.6%-1.4%

CAPTOPRIL STIMULATION TEST

Normal: Test performed by giving 25 mg captopril orally after overnight fast. Patient should be seated during test. After captopril, aldosterone <15 ng/dl, rennin >2 ng, angiotensin I/ml/hr

Interpretation: In patients with primary aldosteronism, plasma aldosterone remains high and plasma rennin activity remains low after captopril.

CARBAMAZEPINE (Tegretol)

Normal therapeutic range: 4-12 mcg/ml

CARBOHYDRATE ANTIGEN 19-9

Normal: <37.0 U/ml

Elevated in: GI cancer, most frequently pancreatic cancer. Amount of elevation has no relation to tumor mass. Elevations can also occur with cirrhosis, cholangitis, and chronic or acute pancreatitis.

CARBON DIOXIDE, PARTIAL PRESSURE

Normal:
Male: 35-48 mm Hg
Female: 32-45 mm Hg
Elevated in: Respiratory acidosis
Decreased in: Respiratory alkalosis

CARBON MONOXIDE

See CARBOXYHEMOGLOBIN

CARBOXYHEMOGLOBIN

Normal range: Saturation of hemoglobin <2%; smokers <9% (coma: 50%; death: 80%)

Elevated in: Smoking, exposure to smoking, exposure to automobile exhaust fumes, malfunctioning gas-burning appliances

CARCINOEMBRYONIC ANTIGEN (CEA)

Normal range:
Nonsmokers: 0-2.5 ng/ml (0-2.5 μg/L [CF: 1; SMI: 0.1 μg/L])
Smokers: 0-5 ng/ml (0-5 μg/L [CF: 1; SMI: 0.1 μg/L])
Elevated in:
Colorectal carcinomas, pancreatic carcinomas, and metastatic disease (usually produce higher elevations: >20 ng/ml)
Carcinomas of the esophagus, stomach, small intestine, liver, breast, ovary, lung, and thyroid (usually produce lesser elevations)
Benign conditions (smoking, inflammatory bowel disease, hypothyroidism, cirrhosis, pancreatitis, infections) (usually produce levels <10 ng/ml)

CAROTENE (serum)

Normal range: 50-250 μg/dl (0.9-4.6 μmol/L [CF: 0.01863; SMI: 0.1 μmol/L])

Elevated in: Carotenemia, chronic nephritis, diabetes mellitus, hypothyroidism, nephrotic syndrome, hyperlipidemia

Decreased in: Fat malabsorption, steatorrhea, pancreatic insufficiency, lack of carotenoids in diet, high fever, liver disease

CATECHOLAMINES, URINE

See URINE CATECHOLAMINES

CBC

See COMPLETE BLOOD COUNT

CD40 LIGAND

Normal: <5 mcg/L. CD40 ligand is a soluble protein that is shed from activated leukocytes and platelets and used in risk stratification for acute coronary syndrome.

Elevated in: Acute coronary syndrome. Increased CD40 ligand is associated with higher incidence of death or nonfatal MI.

CD4+ T-LYMPHOCYTE COUNT (CD4+ T-cells)

Calculated as total WBC × % lymphocytes × % lymphocytes stained with CD4.

This test is used primarily to evaluate immune dysfunction in HIV infection and should be done every 3-6 months in all HIV-infected persons. It is useful as a prognostic indicator and as a criterion for initiating prophylaxis for several opportunistic infections that are sequelae of HIV infection. Progressive depletion of CD4+ T-lymphocytes is associated with an increased likelihood of clinical complications (Table 4-6). Adolescents and adults with HIV are classified as having AIDS if their CD4+ lymphocyte count is under 200/μL and/or if their CD4+ T-lymphocyte percentage is less than 14%. HIV-infected patients whose CD4+ count is less than 200/μL and who acquire certain infectious diseases or malignancies are also classified as having AIDS. Corticosteroids decrease CD4+ T-cell percentage and absolute number.

TABLE 4-6 Relation of CD4 Lymphocyte Counts to the Onset of Certain HIV-Associated Infections and Neoplasms in North America

CD4 Count (Cells/mm^3)*	Opportunistic Infection or Neoplasm	Frequency (%)†
>500	Herpes zoster, polydermatomal	5-10
200-500	*Mycobacterium tuberculosis* infection, pulmonary and extrapulmonary	2-20
	Oral hairy leukoplakia	40-70
	Candida pharyngitis (thrush)	40-70
	Recurrent *Candida* vaginitis	15-30 (F)
	Kaposi's sarcoma, mucocutaneous	15-30 (M)
	Bacterial pneumonia, recurrent	15-20
	Cervical neoplasia	1-2 (F)
100-200	*Pneumocystis carinii* pneumonia	15-60
	Herpes simplex, chronic, ulcerative	5-10
	Histoplasma capsulatum infection, disseminated	0-20
	Kaposi's sarcoma, visceral	3-8 (M)
	Progressive multifocal leukoencephalopathy	2-3
	Lymphoma, non-Hodgkin's	2-5
<100	*Candida* esophagitis	15-20
	Mycobacterium avium-intracellulare, disseminated	25-40
	Toxoplasma gondii encephalitis	5-25
	Cryptosporidium enteritis	2-10
	CMV retinitis	20-35
	Cryptococcus neoformans encephalitis	2-5
	CMV esophagitis or colitis	6-12
	Lymphoma, central nervous system	4-8

Reprinted from Andreoli TE (ed): *Cecil essentials of medicine,* ed 5, Philadelphia, 2000, WB Saunders.
CMV, Cytomegalovirus; *F,* exclusively in women; *HIV,* human immunodeficiency virus; *M,* almost exclusively in men.
*Table indicates CD4 count at which specific infections or neoplasms generally begin to appear. Each infection may recur or progress during the subsequent course of HIV disease.
†Even within the United States, great regional differences in the incidence of specific opportunistic infections are apparent. For example, disseminated histoplasmosis is common in the Mississippi River drainage area but very rare in individuals who have lived exclusively on the East or West Coast.

CEA

See CARCINOEMBRYONIC ANTIGEN

CEREBROSPINAL FLUID (CSF)

Interpretation of results:

1. Appearance of the fluid
   a. Clear: normal.
   b. Yellow color (xanthochromia) in the supernatant of centrifuged CSF within 1 hour or less after collection is usually the result of previous bleeding (subarachnoid hemorrhage); it may also be caused by increased CSF protein, melanin from meningeal melanosarcomas, or carotenoids.
   c. Pinkish color is usually the result of a bloody tap; the color generally clears progressively from tubes 1 to 4 (the supernatant is usually crystal clear in traumatic taps).
   d. Turbidity usually indicates the presence of leukocytes (bleeding introduces approximately 1 WBC/500 RBCs into the CSF).
2. CSF pressure: elevated pressure can be seen with meningitis, meningoencephalitis, pseudotumor cerebri, mass lesions, and intracerebral bleeding.
3. Cell count: in the adult the CSF is normally free of cells (although up to 5 mononuclear cells/mm^3 is considered normal); the presence of granulocytes is never normal.
   a. Neutrophils: seen in bacterial meningitis, early viral meningoencephalitis, and early tuberculosis (TB) meningitis.

TABLE 4-7 Cerebrospinal Fluid Findings in Central Nervous System Disorders

Condition	Pressure (mm H_2O)	Leukocytes (mm³)	Protein (mg/dl)	Glucose (mg/dl)	Comments
Normal	50-80	<5, ≥75% lymphocytes	20-45	>50 (or 75% serum glucose)	
Common Forms of Meningitis					
Acute bacterial meningitis	Usually elevated (100-300)	100-10,000 or more; usually 300-2000; PMNs predominate	Usually 100-500	Decreased, usually <40 (or <66% serum glucose)	Organisms usually seen on Gram stain and recovered by culture; latex agglutination of CSF usually positive
Partially treated bacterial meningitis	Normal or elevated	5-10,000; PMNs usual but mononuclear cells may predominate if pretreated for extended period	Usually 100-500	Normal or decreased	Organisms may be seen on Gram stain; latex agglutination CSF may be positive; pretreatment may render CSF sterile
Viral meningitis or meningoencephalitis	Normal or slightly elevated (80-150)	Rarely >1000 cells; eastern equine encephalitis and lymphocytic choriomeningitis may have cell counts of several thousand; PMNs early but mononuclear cells predominate through most of the course	Usually 50-200	Generally normal; may be decreased to <40 in some viral diseases, particularly mumps (15%-20% of cases)	HSV encephalitis is suggested by focal seizures or by focal findings on CT or MRI scans or EEG. Enteroviruses and HSV infrequently recovered from CSF. HSV and enteroviruses may be detected by PCR of CSF.
Uncommon Forms of Meningitis					
Tuberculous meningitis	Usually elevated	10-500; PMNs early but lymphocytes predominate through most of the course	100-3000; may be higher in presence of block	<50 in most cases; decreases with time if treatment is not provided	Acid-fast organisms almost never seen on smear; organisms may be recovered in culture of large volumes of CSF; *Mycobacterium tuberculosis* may be detected by PCR of CSF
Fungal meningitis	Usually elevated	5-500; PMNs early but mononuclear cells predominate through most of the course; cryptococcal meningitis may have no cellular inflammatory response	25-500	<50; decreases with time if treatment is not provided	Budding yeast may be seen; organisms may be recovered in culture; cryptococcal antigen (CSF and serum) may be positive in cryptococcal infection
Syphilis (acute) and leptospirosis	Usually elevated	50-500; lymphocytes predominate	50-200	Usually normal	Positive CSF serology; spirochetes not demonstrable by usual techniques of smear or culture; darkfield examination may be positive
Amoebic (Naegleria) meningoencephalitis	Elevated	1000-10,000 or more; PMNs predominate	50-500	Normal or slightly decreased	Mobile amebae may be seen by hanging-drop examination of CSF at room temperature

Reprinted from Behrman RE: *Nelson textbook of pediatrics,* ed 17, Philadelphia, 2004, WB Saunders.

CNS, Central nervous system; *CSF,* cerebrospinal fluid; *CT,* computed tomography; *EEG,* electroencephalogram; *HSV,* herpes simplex virus; *MRI,* magnetic resonance imaging; *PCR,* polymerase chain reaction; *PMN,* polymorphonuclear neutrophils.

b. Increased lymphocytes: TB meningitis, viral meningoencephalitis, syphilitic meningoencephalitis, fungal meningitis.

4. Protein: serum proteins are generally too large to cross the normal blood–CSF barrier; however, increased CSF protein is seen with meningeal inflammation, traumatic tap, increased CNS synthesis, tissue degeneration, obstruction to CSF circulation, and Guillain-Barré syndrome.
5. Glucose
   a. Decreased glucose is seen with bacterial meningitis, TB meningitis, fungal meningitis, subarachnoid hemorrhage, and some cases of viral meningitis.
   b. A mild increase in CSF glucose can be seen in patients with very elevated serum glucose levels.

Table 4-7 describes CSF findings in central nervous system disorders.

CERULOPLASMIN (serum)

Normal range: 20-35 mg/dl (200-350 mg/L [CF: 10; SMI: 10 mg/L])
Elevated in: Pregnancy, estrogens, oral contraceptives, neoplastic diseases (leukemias, Hodgkin's lymphoma, carcinomas), inflammatory states, systemic lupus erythematosus, primary biliary cirrhosis, rheumatoid arthritis
Decreased in: Wilson's disease (values often <10 mg/dl), nephrotic syndrome, advanced liver disease, malabsorption, total parenteral nutrition, Menkes' syndrome

CHLAMYDIA GROUP ANTIBODY SEROLOGIC TEST

Test description: Acute and convalescent sera is drawn 2-4 weeks apart. A fourfold increase in titer between acute and convalescent sera is necessary for confirmation. A single titer ≥1:64 is considered indicative of psittacosis or LGV.

TABLE 4-7 Cerebrospinal Fluid Findings in Central Nervous System Disorders—cont'd

Condition	Pressure (mm H_2O)	Leukocytes (mm^3)	Protein (mg/dl)	Glucose (mg/dl)	Comments
Brain and Parameningeal Abscesses					
Brain abscess	Usually elevated (100-300)	5-200; CSF rarely acellular; lymphocytes predominate; if abscess ruptures into ventricle, PMNs predominate and cell count may reach >100,000	75-500	Normal unless abscess ruptures into ventricular system	No organisms on smear or culture unless abscess ruptures into ventricular system
Subdural empyema	Usually elevated (100-300)	100-5000; PMNs predominate	100-500	Normal	No organisms on smear or culture of CSF unless meningitis also present; organisms found on tap of subdural fluid
Cerebral epidural abscess	Normal to slightly elevated	10-500; lymphocytes predominate	50-200	Normal	No organisms on smear or culture of CSF
Spinal epidural abscess	Usually low, with spinal block	10-100; lymphocytes predominate	50-400	Normal	No organisms on smear or culture of CSF
Chemical (drugs, dermoid cysts, myelography dye)	Usually elevated	100-1000 or more; PMNs predominate	50-100	Normal or slightly decreased	Epithelial cells may be seen within CSF by use of polarized light in some children with dermoids
Noninfectious Causes					
Sarcoidosis	Normal or elevated slightly	0-100; mononuclear	40-100	Normal	No specific findings
Systemic lupus erythematosus with CNS involvement	Slightly elevated	0-500; PMNs usually predominate; lymphocytes may be present	100	Normal or slightly decreased	No organisms on smear or culture; LE preparation may be positive; positive neuronal and ribosomal P protein antibodies in CSF
Tumor, leukemia	Slightly elevated to very high	0-100 or more; mononuclear or blast cells	50-1000	Normal to decreased (20-40)	Cytology may be positive

CHLAMYDIA TRACHOMATIS PCR

Test description: Test is performed on endocervical swab, urine, and intraurethral swab
Normal: Negative

CHLORIDE (serum)

Normal range: 95-105 mEq/L (95-105 mmol/L [CF: 1; SMI: 1 mmol/L])
Elevated in: Dehydration, excessive infusion of normal saline solution, cystic fibrosis (sweat test), hyperparathyroidism, renal tubular disease, metabolic acidosis, prolonged diarrhea, drugs (ammonium chloride administration, acetazolamide, boric acid, triamterene)
Decreased in: Congestive heart failure, syndrome of inappropriate antidiuretic hormone secretion, Addison's disease, vomiting, gastric suction, salt-losing nephritis, continuous infusion of D_5W, thiazide diuretic administration, diaphoresis, diarrhea, burns, diabetic ketoacidosis

CHLORIDE (sweat)

Normal: 0-40 mmol/L
Borderline/indeterminate: 41-60 mmol/L
Consistent with cystic fibrosis: >60 mmol/L
False low results can occur with edema, excessive sweating, and hypoproteinemia.

CHLORIDE, URINE

See URINE CHLORIDE

CHOLECYSTOKININ-PANCREOZYMIN (CCK, CCK-PZ)

Normal: <80 pg/ml
Elevated in: Pancreatic disease, celiac disease, gastric ulcer, postgastrectomy, IBS, fatty food intolerance

CHOLESTEROL, HIGH-DENSITY LIPOPROTEIN

See HIGH-DENSITY LIPOPROTEIN CHOLESTEROL

CHOLESTEROL, LOW-DENSITY LIPOPROTEIN

See LOW-DENSITY LIPOPROTEIN CHOLESTEROL

CHOLESTEROL, TOTAL

Normal range: Varies with age
Generally <200 mg/dl (<5.20 mmol/L [CF: 0.02586; SMI: 0.05 mmol/L])
Elevated in: Primary hypercholesterolemia, biliary obstruction, diabetes mellitus, nephrotic syndrome, hypothyroidism, primary biliary cirrhosis, high-cholesterol diet, pregnancy third trimester, myocardial infarction, drugs (steroids, phenothiazines, oral contraceptives)
Decreased in: Starvation, malabsorption, sideroblastic anemia, thalassemia, abetalipoproteinemia, hyperthyroidism, Cushing's syndrome, hepatic failure, multiple myeloma, polycythemia vera, chronic myelocytic leukemia, myeloid metaplasia, Waldenström's macroglobulinemia, myelofibrosis

CHORIONIC GONADOTROPINS, HUMAN (serum)

Normal range, serum: Female, premenopausal: <0.8 IU/L; postmenopausal <3.3 IU/L
Male: <0.7 IU/L
Elevated in:
Pregnancy, choriocarcinoma, gestational trophoblastic neoplasia (including molar gestations), placental site trophoblastic tumors; human antimouse antibodies (HAMA) can produce false serum assay for hCG.
The principal use of this test is to diagnose pregnancy. The concentration of hCG increases significantly during the initial 6 weeks of pregnancy. Peak values approaching 100,000 IU/L occur 60-70 days following implantation.
hCG levels generally double every 1-3 days. In patients with concentration <2000 IU/L, an increase of serum hCG <66% after 2 days is suggestive of spontaneous abortion or ruptured ectopic gestation.

TABLE 4-8 Characteristics of Coagulation Factors

Factor	Descriptive Name	Source	Approximate Half-Life (hr)	Function
I	Fibrinogen	Liver	120	Substrate for fibrin clot (CP)
II	Prothrombin	Liver (VKD)	60	Serine protease (CP)
V	Proaccelerin, labile factor	Liver	12-36	Cofactor (CP)
VII	Serum prothrombin conversion accelerator, proconvertin	Liver (VKD)	6	(?) Serine protease (EP)
VIII	Antihemophilic factor or globulin	Endothelial cells and (?) elsewhere	12	Cofactor (IP)
IX	Plasma thromboplastin component, Christmas factor	Liver (VKD)	24	Serine protease (IP)
X	Stuart-Prower factor	Liver (VKD)	36	Serine protease (CP)
XI	Plasma thromboplastin antecedent	(?) Liver	40-84	Serine protease (IP)
XII	Hageman factor	(?) Liver	50	Serine protease contact activation (IP)
XIII	Fibrin-stabilizing factor	(?) Liver	96-180	Transglutaminase (CP)
Prekallikrein	Fletcher factor	(?) Liver	?	Serine protease contact activation (IP)
High-molecular-weight kininogen	Fitzgerald factor, Flaujeac or Williams factor	(?) Liver	?	Cofactor, contact activation (IP)

Reprinted from Noble J (ed): *Primary care medicine,* ed 3, St Louis, 2001, Mosby.
CP, Common pathway; *EP,* extrinsic pathway; *IP,* intrinsic pathway; *VKD,* vitamin K dependent.

CHYMOTRYPSIN

Normal: <10 mcg/L
Elevated in: Acute pancreatitis, chronic renal failure, oral enzyme preparations, gastric cancer, pancreatic cancer
Decreased in: Chronic pancreatitis, late cystic fibrosis

CIRCULATING ANTICOAGULANT (lupus anticoagulant)

Normal: Negative
Detected in: Systemic lupus erythematosus, drug-induced lupus, long-term phenothiazine therapy, multiple myeloma, ulcerative colitis, rheumatoid arthritis, postpartum, hemophilia, neoplasms, chronic inflammatory states, AIDS, nephrotic syndrome

NOTE: The name is a misnomer because these patients are prone to hypercoagulability and thrombosis.

CK

See CREATINE KINASE

CLONIDINE SUPPRESSION TEST

Interpretation: Clonidine inhibits neurogenic catecholamine release and will cause a decrease in plasma norepinephrine into the reference interval in hypertensive subjects without pheochromocytoma.Test is performed by giving 4.3 mcg clonidine/kg orally after overnight fast. Norepinephrine is measured at 3 hr. Result should be within established reference range and decrease to <50% of baseline concentration. Lack of decrease in norepinephrine is suggestive of pheochromocytoma.

CLOSTRIDIUM DIFFICILE TOXIN ASSAY (stool)

Normal: Negative
Detected in: Antibiotic-associated diarrhea and pseudomembranous colitis

CO

See CARBOXYHEMOGLOBIN

COAGULATION FACTORS

See Table 4-8 for characteristics of coagulation factors.
Factor reference ranges:
V: >10%
VII: >10%
VIII: 50%-170%
IX: 60%-136%
X: >10%
XI: 50%-150%
XII: >30%

Table 4-9 describes screening laboratory results in coagulation factor deficiencies.

COLD AGGLUTININS TITER

Normal range: <1:32
Elevated in:
Primary atypical pneumonia (mycoplasma pneumonia), infectious mononucleosis, CMV infection
Others: hepatic cirrhosis, acquired hemolytic anemia, frostbite, multiple myeloma, lymphoma, malaria

COMPLEMENT

Normal range:
C3: 70-160 mg/dl (0.7-1.6 g/L [CF: 0.01; SMI: 0.1 g/L])
C4: 20-40 mg/dl (0.2-0.4 g/L [CF: 0.01; SMI: 0.1 g/L])

TABLE 4-9 Screening Laboratory Results in Coagulation Factor Deficiencies

Deficient Factor	Frequency	PT	PTT	TT
I (fibrinogen)	Rare	↑	↑	↑
II (prothrombin)	Very rare	↑	↑	↑
V 1:1,000,000	↑	↑	NL	
VII	1:500,000	↑	NL	NL
VIII	1:5000 (male)	NL	↑	NL
IX	1:30,000 (male)	NL	↑	NL
X 1:500,000	↑	↑	NL	
XI	Rare*	NL	↑	NL
XII or HMWK or PK†	Rare	NL	↑	NL
XIII	Rare	NL	NL	NL

Reprinted from Andreoli TE (ed): *Cecil essentials of medicine,* ed 5, Philadelphia, 2001, WB Saunders.
↑ Increased over normal range; *HMWK,* high-molecular-weight kininogen; *NL,* normal; *PK,* prekallikrein; *PT,* prothrombin time; *PTT,* partial thromboplastin time; *TT,* thrombin time.
*Except in those of Ashkenazi Jewish descent (approximately 4% are heterozygous for factor XI deficiency).
†Not associated with clinical bleeding.

Abnormal values:

Decreased C3: Active SLE, immune complex disease, acute glomerulonephritis, inborn C3 deficiency, membranoproliferative glomerulonephritis, infective endocarditis, serum sickness, autoimmune/chronic active hepatitis

Decreased C4: Immune complex disease, active SLE, infective endocarditis, inborn C4 deficiency, hereditary angioedema, hypergammaglobulinemic states, cryobulinemic vasculitis

Table 4-10 describes complement deficiency states.

COMPLETE BLOOD COUNT (CBC)

White blood cells 3200-9800 mm^3 ($3.2\text{-}9.8 \times 10^9/L$ [CF: 0.001; SMI: $0.1 \times 10^9/L$])

Red blood cells
- Male: $4.3\text{-}5.9 \times 10^6/mm^3$ ($4.3\text{-}5.9 \times 10^{12}/L$ [CF: 0.001; SMI: $0.1 \times 10^{12}/L$])
- Female: $3.5\text{-}5 \times 10^6/mm^3$ ($3.5\text{-}5 \times 10^{12}/L$ [CF: 0.001; SMI: $0.1 \times 10^{12}/L$])

Hemoglobin
- Male: 13.6-17.7 g/dl (136-172 g/L [CF: 10; SMI: 1 g/L])
- Female: 12-15 g/dl (120-150 g/L [CF: 10; SMI: 1 g/L])

Hematocrit
- Male: 39%-49% (0.39-0.49 [CF: 0.01; SMI: 0.01])
- Female: 33%-43% (0.33-0.43 [CF: 0.01; SMI: 0.01])

Mean corpuscular volume (MCV): 76-100 μm^3 (76-100 fL [CF: 1; SMI: 1 fL])

TABLE 4-10 Complement Deficiency States

Component	No. of Reported Patients	Mode of Inheritance	Functional Defects	Disease Associations
Classic Pathway				
C1qrs	31	ACD	Impaired IC handling, delayed C′ activation, impaired immune response	CVD, 48%; infection (encapsulated bacteria), 22%; both, 18%; healthy, 12%
C4	21	ACD	Impaired C′ activation in absence of specific antibody	Infection (meningococcal), 74%; healthy, 26%
C2	109	ACD		
Alternative pathway				
D	3	ACD	Impaired IC handling, opson/phag; granulocytosis, CTX, immune response and absent SBA	CVD, 79%; recurrent infection (encapsulated bacteria), 71%
P	70	XL		
Junction of classic and alternative pathways				
C3	19	ACD	Impaired CTX; absent SBA	Infection (*Neisseria,* primarily meningococcal), 58%; CVD, 4%
Terminal components				
C5	27	ACD	Absent SBA	Both, 1%
C6	77	ACD		Healthy, 25%
C7	73	ACD		
C8	73	ACD		
C9	165	ACD	Impaired SBA	Healthy, 91%; infection, 9%
Plasma proteins regulating C′ activation				
C1-INH	Many	AD	Uncontrolled generation of an inflammatory mediator on C′ activation	Hereditary angioedema
H	13	Acq	Uncontrolled AP activation → low C3	CVD, 40%; CVD plus infection (encapsulated bacteria), 40%; healthy, 20%
I	14	ACD	Uncontrolled AP activation → low C3	Infection (encapsulated bacteria), 100%
Membrane proteins regulating C′ activation	Many	Acq	Impaired regulation of C3b and C8 deposited on host RBCs; PMN, platelets → cell lysis	Paroxysmal nocturnal hemoglobinuria
Decay-accelerating factor				
Homologous restriction factor				
CD59	>20	ACD	Impaired PMN adhesive functions (i.e., margination), CTX, C3bi-mediated opson/phag	Infection (*Staphylococcus aureus, Pseudomonas* spp.), 100%
CR3 autoantibodies				
C3 nephritic factors	>59	Acq	Stabilize AP, convertase → low C3	MPGN, 41%; PLD, 25%; infection (encapsulated bacteria), 16%; MPGN plus PLD, 10%; PLD plus infection, 5%; MPGN plus PLD plus infection, 3%; MPGN plus infection, 2%
C4 nephritic factor		Acq	Stabilize CP, C3 convertase → low C3	Glomerulonephritis, 50%; CVD, 50%

Reprinted from Mandell GL: *Mandell, Douglas, and Bennett's principles and practice of infectious diseases,* ed 6, New York, 2005, Churchill Livingstone.

ACD, Autosomal codominant; *Acq,* acquired; *AD,* autosomal dominant; *AP,* alternative pathway; *C′,* complement; *CP,* classic pathway; *CTX,* chemotaxis; *CVD,* collagen-vascular disease; *IC,* immune complex, *MPGN,* membranoproliferative glomerulonephritis; *PLD,* partial lipodystrophy; *PMN,* polymorphonuclear neutrophil; *RBCs,* red blood cells; *SBA,* serum bactericidal activity; *XL,* X-linked.

Mean corpuscular hemoglobin (MCH): 27-33 pg (27-33 pg [CF: 1; SMI: 1 pg])
Mean corpuscular hemoglobin concentration (MCHC): 33-37 g/dl (330-370 g/L [CF: 10; SMI: 10 g/L])
Red blood cell distribution width index (RDW): 11.5%-14.5%
Platelet count: 130-400 $\times$ 10^3/mm^3 (130-400 $\times$ 10^9/L [CF: 1; SMI: 5 $\times$ 10^9/L])
Differential:
2-6 stabs (bands, early mature neutrophils)
60-70 segs (mature neutrophils)
1-4 eosinophils
0-1 basophils
2-8 monocytes
25-40 lymphocytes

CONJUGATED BILIRUBIN

See BILIRUBIN, DIRECT

COOMBS, DIRECT

Normal: Negative
Positive: Autoimmune hemolytic anemia, erythroblastosis fetalis, transfusion reactions, drugs (α-methyldopa, penicillins, tetracycline, sulfonamides, levodopa, cephalosporins, quinidine, insulin)
False-positive: May be seen with cold agglutinins

COOMBS, INDIRECT

Normal: Negative
Positive: Acquired hemolytic anemia, incompatible cross-matched blood, anti-Rh antibodies, drugs (methyldopa, mefenamic acid, levodopa)

COPPER (serum)

Normal range: 70-140 μg/dl (11-22 μmol/L [CF: 0.1574, SMI: 0.2 μmol/L])
Decreased in: Wilson's disease, Menkes' syndrome, malabsorption, malnutrition, nephrosis, total parenteral nutrition, acute leukemia in remission
Elevated in: Aplastic anemia, biliary cirrhosis, systemic lupus erythematosus, hemochromatosis, hyperthyroidism, hypothyroidism, infection, iron deficiency anemia, leukemia, lymphoma, oral contraceptives, pernicious anemia, rheumatoid arthritis

COPPER, URINE

See URINE COPPER

CORTICOTROPIN RELEASING HORMONE (CRH) STIMULATION TEST

Normal: A dose of 0.5 mg of dexamethasone is given every 6 hours for 2 days; 2 hours after last dose 1 mcg/kg CRH is given IV. Samples are drawn after 15 min. Normally there is a twofold to fourfold increase in mean baseline concentration of ACTH or cortisol. Cortisol >1.4 mcg/L is virtually 100% specific and 100% diagnostic.
Interpretation:
Normal or exaggerated response: Pituitary Cushing's disease
No response: Ectopic ACTH-secreting tumor
A positive response to CRH or a suppressed response to high-dose dexamethasone has a 97% positive predictive value for Cushing's disease. However, a lack of response to either test excludes Cushing's disease in only 64%-78% of patients. When the tests are considered together, negative responses from both have a 100% predictive value for ectopic ACTH secretion.

CORTISOL, PLASMA

Normal range: Varies with time of collection (circadian variation):
8 AM: 4-19 μg/dl (110-520 nmol/L [CF: 27.59; SMI: 10 nmol/L])
4 PM: 2-15 μg/dl (50-410 nmol/L [CF: 27.59; SMI: 10 nmol/L])
Elevated in: Ectopic adrenocorticotropic hormone production (i.e., oat cell carcinoma of lung), loss of normal diurnal variation, pregnancy, chronic renal failure, iatrogenic, stress, adrenal or pituitary hyperplasia, or adenomas
Decreased in: Primary adrenocortical insufficiency, anterior pituitary hypofunction, secondary adrenocortical insufficiency, adrenogenital syndromes

C-PEPTIDE

Elevated in: Insulinoma, sulfonylurea administration
Decreased in: Insulin-dependent diabetes mellitus, factitious insulin administration

CPK

See CREATINE KINASE

C-REACTIVE PROTEIN

Normal range: 6.8-820 μg/dl (68-8200 μg/L [CF: 10; SMI: 10 μg/L])
Elevated in: Rheumatoid arthritis, rheumatic fever, inflammatory bowel disease, bacterial infections, myocardial infarction, oral contraceptives, third trimester of pregnancy (acute phase reactant), inflammatory and neoplastic diseases

C-REACTIVE PROTEIN, HIGH SENSITIVITY (hs-CRP, cardio-CRP)

This is a cardiac risk marker. It is increased in patients with silent atherosclerosis years before a cardiovascular event and is independent of cholesterol level and other lipoproteins. It can be used to help stratify cardiac risk.
INTERPRETATION OF RESULTS:

Cardio-CRP result (mg/L)	*Risk*
0.6	Lowest risk
0.7-1.1	Low risk
1.2-1.9	Moderate risk
2.0-3.8	High risk
3.9-4.9	Highest risk
≥5.0	Results may be confounded by acute inflammatory disease. If clinically indicated, a repeat test should be performed in 2 or more weeks.

CREATINE KINASE (CK, CPK)

Normal range: 0-130 U/L (0-2.16 μkat/L [CF: 0.01667; SMI: 0.01 μkat/L])
Elevated in: Myocardial infarction, myocarditis, rhabdomyolysis, myositis, crush injury/trauma, polymyositis, dermatomyositis, vigorous exercise, muscular dystrophy, myxedema, seizures, malignant hyperthermia syndrome, IM injections, cerebrovascular accident, pulmonary embolism and infarction, acute dissection of aorta
Decreased in: Steroids, decreased muscle mass, connective tissue disorders, alcoholic liver disease, metastatic neoplasms

CREATINE KINASE ISOENZYMES

CK-BB:
Elevated in: Cerebrovascular accident, subarachnoid hemorrhage, neoplasms (prostate, gastrointestinal tract, brain, ovary, breast, lung), severe shock, bowel infarction, hypothermia, meningitis
CK-MB:
Elevated in: Myocardial infarction (MI), myocarditis, pericarditis, muscular dystrophy, cardiac defibrillation, cardiac surgery, extensive rhabdomyolysis, strenuous exercise (marathon runners), mixed connective tissue disease, cardiomyopathy, hypothermia

NOTE: CK-MB exists in the blood in two subforms. MB_2 is released from cardiac cells and converted in the blood to MB_1. Rapid assay of CK-MB subforms can detect MI (CK-MB_2 ≥1.0 U/L, with a ratio of CK-MB_2/CK-MB_1 ≥1.5) within 6 hours of onset of symptoms.

Fig. 4-2 illustrates the time course of CK, AST, troponins, and LDH activity after acute MI.
CK-MM:
Elevated in: Crush injury, seizures, malignant hyperthermia syndrome, rhabdomyolysis, myositis, polymyositis, dermatomyositis, vigorous exercise, muscular dystrophy, IM injections, acute dissection of aorta

CREATININE (serum)

Normal range: 0.6-1.2 mg/dl (50-110 μmol/L [CF: 88.4; SMI: 10 μmol/L])
Elevated in: Renal insufficiency (acute and chronic), decreased renal perfusion (hypotension, dehydration, congestive heart failure), urinary tract infection, rhabdomyolysis, ketonemia

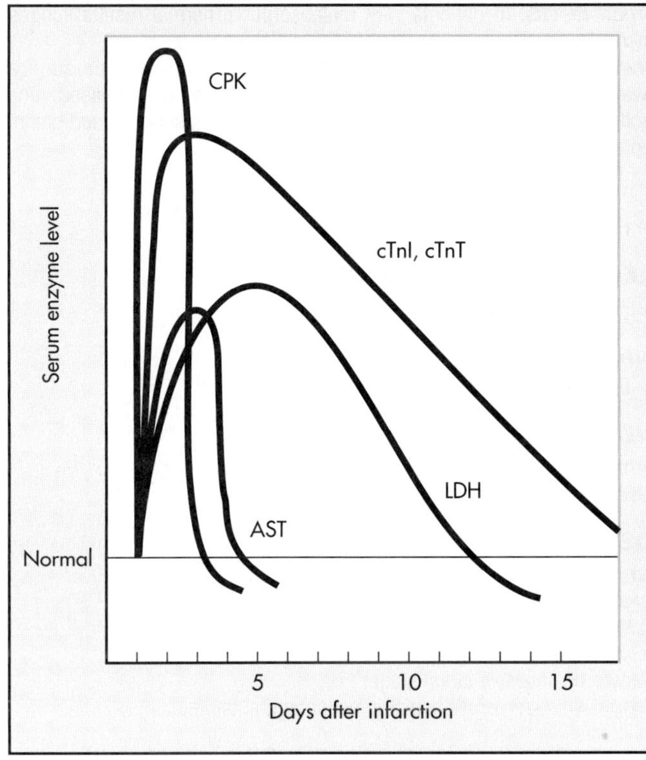

FIGURE 4-2 Evaluation of creatine kinase elevation. *CBC,* Complete blood count; *CK,* creatine kinase; *EMG,* electromyography. (Reprinted from Greene HL, Johnson WP, Lemcke D [eds]: *Decision making in medicine,* ed 2, St Louis, 1998, Mosby.)

Drugs (antibiotics [aminoglycosides, cephalosporins], hydantoin, diuretics, methyldopa)
Falsely elevated in: Diabetic ketoacidosis, administration of some cephalosporins (e.g., cefoxitin, cephalothin)
Decreased in: Decreased muscle mass (including amputees and older persons), pregnancy, prolonged debilitation

CREATININE CLEARANCE

Normal range: 75-124 ml/min (1.24-2.08 ml/sec [CF: 0.01667; SMI: 0.02 ml/sec])

Box 4-1 describes a formula for calculation of creatinine clearance.

The Cockcroft-Gault formula to calculate creatinine clearance is described in Box 4-2.

BOX 4-1 Calculation of the Creatinine Clearance

$C_{cr} = U_{cr} \times V/P_{cr}$
where C_{cr} = clearance of creatinine (ml/min)
U_{cr} = urine creatinine (mg/dl)
V = volume of urine (ml/min) (for 24-hr volume: divide by 1440)
P_{cr} = plasma creatinine (mg/dl)
Normal range: 95 to 105 ml/min/1.75m^2

BOX 4-2 Cockcroft-Gault Formula to Calculate Creatinine Clearance (C_{cr})

$$C_{cr} = \frac{(140 - \text{age in year}) \times (\text{lean body weight in kg})}{S_{cr} \text{ in mg/dl} - 72}$$

Elevated in: Pregnancy, exercise
Decreased in: Renal insufficiency, drugs (cimetidine, procainamide, antibiotics, quinidine)

CREATININE, URINE

See URINE CREATININE

CRYOGLOBULINS (serum)

Normal range: Not detectable
Present in: Collagen vascular diseases, chronic lymphocytic leukemia, hemolytic anemias, multiple myeloma, Waldenström's macroglobulinemia, chronic active hepatitis, Hodgkin's disease

CRYPTOSPORIDIUM ANTIGEN BY EIA (stool)

Normal range: Not detected
Present in: Cryptosporidiosis

CSF

See CEREBROSPINAL FLUID

CYSTATIN C

Normal: Cystatin C is a cysteine protease inhibitor that is produced at a constant rate by all nucleated cells. It is freely filtered by the glomerulus and reabsorbed (but not secreted) by the renal tubules with no extrarenal excretion. Its concentration is not affected by diet, muscle mass, or acute inflammation. Normal range when measured by particle-enhanced nephelometric immunoassay (PENIA) is <0.28 mg/L.
Elevated in: Renal disorders. Good predictor of the severity of acute tubular necrosis. Cystatin C increases more rapidly than creatinine in the early stages of GFR impairment. The cystatin C concentration is an independent risk factor for heart failure in older adults and appears to provide a better measure of risk assessment than the serum creatinine concentration.

CYSTIC FIBROSIS PCR

Test description: Test can be performed on whole blood or tissue. Common mutations in the cystic fibrosis transmembrane regulator (CFTR) gene can be used to detect 75%-80% of mutant alleles.

CYTOMEGALOVIRUS BY PCR

Test description: Test can be performed on whole blood, plasma, or tissue. Qualitative PCR is highly sensitive but may not be able to differentiate between latent and active infection.

D-DIMER

Normal range: <0.5 mcg/ml
Elevated in:

DVT, pulmonary embolism, high levels of rheumatoid factor, activation of coagulation and fibrolytic system from any cause

D-dimer assay by ELISA assists in the diagnosis of DVT and pulmonary embolism. This test has significant limitations because it can be elevated whenever the coagulation and fibrinolytic systems are activated and can also be falsely elevated with high rheumatoid factor levels.

DEHYDROEPIANDROSTERONE SULFATE

Normal:
Males:

Ages 19-30:	125-619 mcg/dl
31-50:	59-452 mcg/dl
51-60:	20-413 mcg/dl
61-83:	10-285 mcg/dl

Females:

Ages 19-30:	29-781 mcg/dl
31-50:	12-379 mcg/dl
Postmenopausal:	30-260 mcg/dl

Elevated in: Hirsutism, congenital adrenal hyperplasia, adrenal carcinomas, adrenal adenomas, polycystic ovary syndrome, ectopic ACTH-producing tumors, Cushing's disease, spironolactone

DEHYDROTESTOSTERONE (serum, urine)

Normal:
Serum: Males: 30-85 ng/dl; females: 4-22 ng/dl
Urine, 24 h: Males: 20-50 mcg/day; females: <8 mcg/day
Elevated in: Hirsutism
Decreased in: 5-α-reductase deficiency, hypogonadism

DEOXYCORTICOSTERONE (11-deoxycorticosterone, DOC) (serum)

Normal: 2-19 ng/dl. Normal secretion depends on ACTH and is suppressible by dexamethasone.
Elevated in: Adrogenital syndromes due to 17- and 11-hydroxylase deficiencies, pregnancy
Decreased in: Preeclampsia

DEXAMETHASONE SUPPRESSION TEST, OVERNIGHT

Normal: Test is performed by giving 1 mg dexamethasone orally at 11 PM and measuring serum cortisol at 8 AM the following morning. Normal response is cortisol suppression to <3 mcg/dl; If dose of 4 mg dexamethasone is given, cortisol suppression will be to <50% of baseline.
Interpretation: Cushing's syndrome (>10 mcg/dl), endogenous depression (half of patients suppress test values >5 mcg/dl). Most patients with pituitary Cushing's disease demonstrate suppression, whereas patients with adrenal adenoma, carcinoma, and ectopic ACTH-producing tumors do not.

DIGOXIN (Lanoxin)

Normal therapeutic range: 0.5-2 ng/ml
Elevated in: Impaired renal function, excessive dosing, concomitant use of quinidine, amiodarone, verapamil, fluoxetine, nifedipine

DILANTIN

See PHENYTOIN

DISACCHARIDE ABSORPTION TESTS

Normal: Test is used to diagnose malabsorption due to disaccharide deficiency. It is performed by giving disaccharide orally 1 g/kg body weight to a total of 25 g. Blood is drawn at 0, 30, 60, 90, and 120 min. Normal response is a change in glucose from fasting value >30 mg/dl, inconclusive when increase is 20-30 mg/dl, abnormal when increase is <20 mg/dl. Test can also be performed by measuring air at 0, 30, 60, 90, and 120 min. Normal is H_2 >20 ppm above baseline level before a colonic response.
Decreased in: Disaccharide deficiency (lactose, fructose, sorbitol), celiac disease, sprue, acute gastroenetetitis

DOC

See DEOXYCORTICOSTERONE

DONATH-LANDSTEINER (D-L) TEST FOR PAROXYSMAL COLD HEMOGLOBINURIA

Normal: No hemolysis
Interpretation: Hemolysis indicates presence of bithermic cold hemolysins or Donath-Landsteiner antibodies (D-L Ab)

DOPAMINE

Normal range: 175 pg/ml
Elevated in: Pheochromocytomas, neuroblastomas, stress, vigorous exercise, certain foods (bananas, chocolate, coffee, tea, vanilla)

D-XYLOSE ABSORPTION

Normal range: 21%-31% excreted in 5 hr (0.21-0.31 [CF: 0.01; SMI: 0.01])
Decreased in: Malabsorption syndrome

D-XYLOSE ABSORPTION TEST

Normal range:
URINE: ≥4 g/5 hours (5-hour urine collection in adults >12 years [25-g dose])
SERUM: ≥25 mg/dl (adult, 1 h, 25-g dose, normal renal function)
Normal results: In patients with malabsorption, normal results suggest pancreatic disease as an etiology of the malabsorption.
Abnormal results: Celiac disease, Crohn's disease, tropical sprue, surgical bowel resection, AIDS. False-positives can occur with decreased renal function, dehydration/hypovolemia, surgical blind loops, decreased gastric emptying, vomiting.

ELECTROPHORESIS, HEMOGLOBIN

See HEMOGLOBIN ELECTROPHORESIS

ELECTROPHORESIS, PROTEIN

See PROTEIN ELECTROPHORESIS

ENA COMPLEX

See EXTRACTABLE NUCLEAR ANTIGEN

ENDOMYSIAL ANTIBODIES

Normal: Not detected
Present in: Celiac disease, dermatitis herpetiformis

EOSINOPHIL COUNT

Normal range: 1%-4% eosinophils (0-440/mm^3)
Elevated in:
HELMINTHIC PARASITES
Ascaris lumbricoides (invasive larval stage)
Hookworms (invasive larval stage)
Strongyloides stercoralis (initial infection and autoinfection)
Trichinosis
Filariasis
Echinococcus granulosus and *E. multilocularis*
Toxocara species
Animal hookworms
Angiostrongylus cantonensis and *A. costaricensis*
Schistosomiasis
Liver flukes
Fasciolopsis buski
Anisakiasis
Capillaria philippinensis
Paragonimus westermani
"Tropical eosinophilia" (unidentified microfilariae)
OTHER INFECTIONS/INFESTATIONS
Pulmonary aspergillosis
Severe scabies
ALLERGIES
Asthma
Hay fever
Drug reactions
Atopic dermatitis
AUTOIMMUNE AND RELATED DISORDERS
Polyarteritis nodosa
Necrotizing vasculitis
Eosinophilic fasciitis
Pemphigus
NEOPLASTIC DISEASES
Hodgkin's disease
Mycosis fungoides
Chronic myelocytic leukemia
Eosinophilic leukemia
Polycythemia vera
Mucin-secreting adenocarcinomas
IMMUNODEFICIENCY STATES
Hyperimmunoglobulin E with recurrent infection
Wiskott-Aldrich syndrome
OTHER
Addison's disease
Inflammatory bowel disease
Dermatitis herpetiformis
Toxic/chemical syndrome

Eosinophilic myalgia syndrome, tryptophan, toxic oil syndrome
Hypereosinophilic syndrome (unknown etiology)

EPINEPHRINE, PLASMA

Normal range: 0-90 pg/ml
Elevated in: Pheochromocytomas, neuroblastomas, stress, vigorous exercise, certain foods (bananas, chocolate, coffee, tea, vanilla), hypoglycemia

EPSTEIN-BARR VIRUS SEROLOGY

Normal range: IgG anti-VCA <1:10 or negative
Abnormal:
IgG anti-VCA >1:10 or positive indicates either current or previous infection
IgM anti-VCA >1:10 or positive indicates current or recent infection
Anti-EBNA ≥1.5 or positive indicates previous infection
Table 4-11 and Fig. 4-3 describe test interpretation.

ERYTHROCYTE SEDIMENTATION RATE (ESR; Westergren)

Normal range:
Male: 0-15 mm/hr
Female: 0-20 mm/hr
Elevated in: Collagen vascular diseases, infections, myocardial infarction, neoplasms, inflammatory states (acute phase reactant), hyperthyroidism, hypothyroidism, rouleaux formation

Decreased in: Sickle cell disease, polycythemia, corticosteroids, spherocytosis, anisocytosis, hypofibrinogenemia, increased serum viscosity

ERYTHROPOIETIN (EP)

Normal: 3.7-16.0 IU/L by radioimmunoassay
Erythropoietin is a glycoprotein secreted by the kidneys that stimulates RBC production by acting on erythroid-committed stem cells.
Increased in:
Extremely high: Generally seen in patients with severe anemia (Hct <25, <7) such as in cases of aplastic anemia, severe hemolytic anemia, hematologic cancers
Very high: Patients with mild to moderate anemia (Hct, 25-35; Hb, 7-10)
High: Patients with mild anemia (e.g., AIDS, myelodysplasia)
Erythropoietin can be inappropriately elevated in patients with malignant neoplasms, renal cysts, postrenal transplant, meningioma, hemangioblastoma, and leiomyoma.
Decreased in: Renal failure, polycythemia vera, autonomic neuropathy

ESTRADIOL (serum)

Normal range:
Female, premenopausal: 30-400 pg/ml, depending on phase of menstrual cycle
Female, postmenopausal: 0-30 pg/ml
Male, adult: 10-50 pg/ml
Decreased in: Ovarian failure
Elevated in: Tumors of ovary, testis, adrenal, or nonendocrine sites (rare)

TABLE 4-11 Antibody Tests in Epstein-Barr Viral Infection

	Appearance	Peak	Disappears
Heterophil Ab	3-5 days after onset of Sx (range, 0-21 days)	During second wk after onset of Sx (1-4 wk)	2-3 mo after onset of Sx (still found at 1 yr in 20% of cases)
VCA-IgM	Beginning of Sx (1 wk before to 1 wk after Sx begin)	During first wk after onset of Sx (0-21 days)	2-3 mo after onset of Sx (1-6 mo)
VCA-IgG	3 days after onset of Sx (0-2 wk)	During second wk after onset of Sx (1-3 wk)	Decline to lower level, then persists for life
EBNA-IgG	3 wk after onset of Sx (1-4 wk)	8 mo after appearance (3-12 mo)	Lifelong
EA-D	5 days after onset of Sx (during first 1-2 wk after onset of Sx)	14-21 days after onset of Sx (1-4 wk)	9 wk after appearance (2-6 mo)
EBNA-IgM	Same as VCA-IgM	Same as VCA-IgM	Same as VCA-IgM

Reprinted from Ravel R: *Clinical laboratory medicine,* ed 6, St Louis, 1995, Mosby.
Ab, Antibody; *EA,* early antigen; *EBNA,* Epstein-Barr virus nuclear antigen; *Sx,* symptoms; *VCA,* viral capsid antigen.

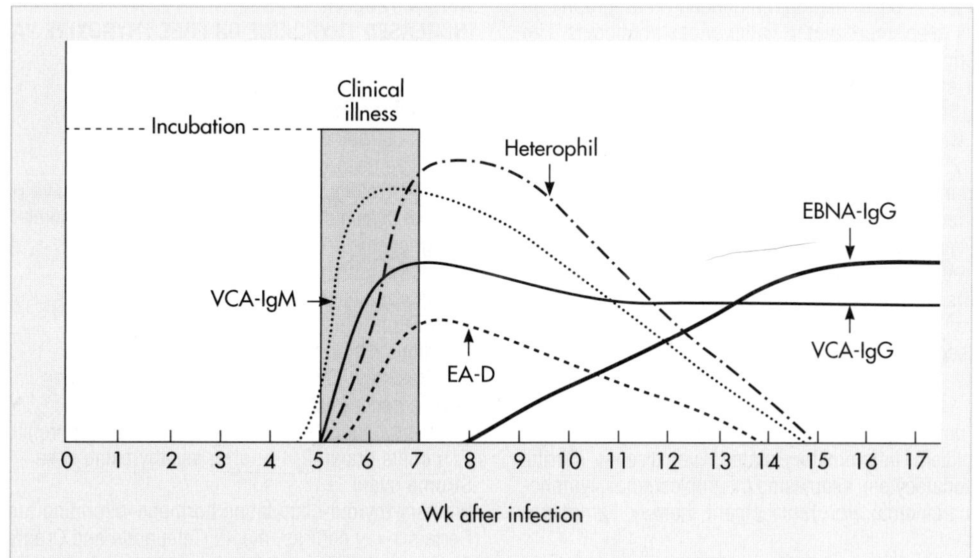

FIGURE 4-3 Tests in Epstein-Barr viral infection. See Table 4-11 for abbreviations. (Reprinted from Ravel R [ed]: *Clinical laboratory medicine,* ed 6, St Louis, 1995, Mosby.)

ESTROGEN

Normal range (serum):
Males: 20-80 pg/ml
Females:
Follicular: 60-200 pg/ml
Luteal: 160-400 pg/ml
Postmenopausal: <130 pg/ml
Normal range (urine):
Males: 4-23 μg/g creatinine
Females:
Follicular: 7-65 μg/g creatinine
Midcycle: 32-104 μg/g creatinine
Luteal: 8-135 μg/g creatinine
Elevated in: Hyperplasia of adrenal cortex, ovarian tumors producing estrogen, granulosa and thecal cell tumors, testicular tumors
Decreased in: Menopause, hypopituitarism, primary ovarian malfunction, anorexia nervosa, hypofunction of adrenal cortex, ovarian agenesis, psychogenic stress, gonadotropin-releasing hormone deficiency

ETHANOL (blood)

Normal range:
Negative (values <10 mg/dl are considered negative)
Ethanol is metabolized at 10-25 mg/dl/hour. Levels ≥80 mg/dl are considered evidence of impairment for driving. Fatal blood concentration is considered to be >400 mg/dl.

EXTRACTABLE NUCLEAR ANTIGEN (ENA complex, anti-RNP antibody, anti-SM, anti-Smith)

Normal: Negative
Present in: Systemic lupus erythematosus, rheumatoid arthritis, Sjögren's syndrome, mixed connective tissue disease

FACTOR V LEIDEN

Test description: PCR test performed on whole blood or tissue. This single mutation, found in 2%-8% of the general Caucasian population, is the single most common cause of hereditary thrombophilia.

FDP

See FIBRIN DEGRADATION PRODUCT

FECAL FAT, QUANTITATIVE (72-hr collection)

Normal range: 2-6 g/24 hr (7-21 mmol/dl [CF: 3.515; SMI: 1 mmol/dl])
Elevated in: Malabsorption syndrome

FECAL GLOBIN IMMUNOCHEMICAL TEST

Normal: Negative. This test is performed by immunochromatography on a cellulose strip that has been impregnated with various antibodies. The test uses a small amount of toilet water as the specimen and is placed onto absorbent pads of card similar to traditional OB card. There is no direct handling of stool. This test is specific for the globin portion of the hemoglobin molecule, which confers lower GI bleeding specificity. It specifically detects blood from the lower GI tract; guaic tests are not lower GI specific. It is more sensitive than typical Hemoccult test (detection limit 50 mcg Hb/g feces versus >500 mcg Hb/g feces for Hemoccult). It has no dietary restrictions and gives no false-positives due to plant peroxidases and red meats. It has no medication restrictions. Iron supplements and NSAIDs do not cause false-positives. Vitamin C does not cause false-negatives.
Positive in: Lower GI bleeding

FERRITIN (serum)

Normal range: 18-300 ng/ml (18-300 μg/L [CF: 1; SMI: 10 μg/L])
Elevated in: Hyperthyroidism, inflammatory states, liver disease (ferritin elevated from necrotic hepatocytes), neoplasms (neuroblastomas, lymphomas, leukemia, breast carcinoma), iron replacement therapy, hemochromatosis, hemosiderosis
Decreased in: Iron deficiency anemia

α-1 FETOPROTEIN

Normal range: 0-20 ng/ml (0-20 μg/L [CF: 1; SMI: 1 μg/L])
Elevated in: Hepatocellular carcinoma (usually values >1000 ng/ml), germinal neoplasms (testis, ovary, mediastinum, retroperitoneum), liver disease (alcoholic cirrhosis, acute hepatitis, chronic active hepatitis), fetal anencephaly, spina bifida, basal cell carcinoma, breast carcinoma, pancreatic carcinoma, gastric carcinoma, retinoblastoma, esophageal atresia

FIBRIN DEGRADATION PRODUCT (FDP)

Normal range: <10 μg/ml
Elevated in: Disseminated intravascular coagulation, primary fibrinolysis, pulmonary embolism, severe liver disease

NOTE: The presence of rheumatoid factor may cause falsely elevated FDP.

FIBRINOGEN

Normal range: 200-400 mg/dl (2-4 g/L [CF: 0.01; SMI: 0.1 g/L])
Elevated in: Tissue inflammation or damage (acute phase protein reactant), oral contraceptives, pregnancy, acute infection, myocardial infarction
Decreased in: Disseminated intravascular coagulation, hereditary afibrinogenemia, liver disease, primary or secondary fibrinolysis, cachexia

FOLATE (folic acid)

Normal range:
Plasma: 2-10 ng/ml (4-22 nmol/L [CF: 2.266; SMI: 2 nmol/L])
Red blood cells: 140-960 ng/ml (550-2200 nmol/L [CF: 2.266; SMI: 10 nmol/L])
Decreased in: Folic acid deficiency (inadequate intake, malabsorption), alcoholism, drugs (methotrexate, trimethoprim, phenytoin, oral contraceptives, Azulfidine), vitamin B_{12} deficiency (defective red cell folate absorption), hemolytic anemia
Elevated in: Folic acid therapy

FOLLICLE-STIMULATING HORMONE (FSH)

Normal range: 5-20 mIU/ml
Elevated in: Menopause, primary gonadal failure, alcoholism, castration, Klinefelter's syndrome, gonadotropin-secreting pituitary hormones
Decreased in: Pregnancy, polycystic ovary disease, anorexia nervosa, anterior pituitary hypofunction

FREE T_4

See T_4, FREE

FREE THYROXINE INDEX

Normal range: 1.1-4.3
INCREASED THYROXINE OR FREE THYROXINE VALUES
Laboratory error
Primary hyperthyroidism (T_4/T_3 type)
Severe thyroxine-binding globulin elevation
Excess therapy of hypothyroidism
Excessive dose of levothyroxine
Active thyroiditis (subacute, painless, early active Hashimoto's disease)
Familial dysalbuminemic hyperthyroxinemia (some FT_4 kits, especially analog types)
Peripheral resistance to T_4 syndrome
Amiodarone or propranolol
Postpartum transient toxicosis
Factitious hyperthyroidism
Jod-Basedow (iodine-induced) hyperthyroidism
Severe nonthyroid illness
Acute psychosis (especially paranoid schizophrenia)
T_4 sample drawn 2-4 hr after levothyroxine dose
Struma ovarii
Pituitary thyroid-stimulating hormone–secreting tumor
Certain x-ray contrast media (Telepaque and Oragrafin)
Acute porphyria
Heparin effect (some T_4 and FT_4 kits)

Amphetamine, heroin, methadone, and phencyclidine abuse
Perphenazine or 5-fluorouracil
Antithyroid or anti-IgG heterophil (HAMA) autoantibodies
"T_4" hyperthyroidism
Hyperemesis gravidarum; about 50% of patients
High altitudes

DECREASED THYROXINE OR FREE THYROXINE VALUES

Laboratory error
Primary hypothyroidism
Severe nonthyroid illness*
Lithium therapy
Severe thyroxine-binding globulin decrease (congenital, disease, or drug-induced) or severe albumin decrease*
Dilantin, Depakene, or high-dose salicylate drugs*
Pituitary insufficiency
Large doses of inorganic iodide (e.g., saturated solution of potassium iodide)
Moderate or severe iodine deficiency
Cushing's syndrome
High-dose glucocorticoid drugs
Pregnancy, third trimester (low normal or small decrease)
Addison's disease; some patients (30%)
Heparin effect (a few FT_4 kits)
Desipramine or amiodarone drugs
Acute psychiatric illness

FTA-ABS (serum)

Normal: Nonreactive
Reactive in: Syphilis, other treponemal diseases (yaws, pinta, bejel), SLE, pregnancy

FUROSEMIDE STIMULATION TEST

Normal: Test is performed by giving 60 mg furosemide orally after overnight fast. Patient should be on a normal diet without medications the week before the test. Normal results: renin 1-6 ng angiotensin I/ml/hr.
Elevated in: Renovascular hypertension, Barrter's syndrome, high-renin essential hypertension, pheochromocytoma
No response in: Primary aldosteronism, low-renin essential hypertension, hyporeninemic hypoaldosteronism

GAMMA-GLUTAMYL TRANSFERASE (gGt)

See γ-GLUTAMYL TRANSFERASE

GASTRIN (serum)

Normal range: 0-180 pg/ml (0-180 ng/L [CF: 1; SMI: 10 ng/L])
Elevated in: Zollinger-Ellison syndrome (gastrinoma), pernicious anemia, hyperparathyroidism, retained gastric antrum, chronic renal failure, gastric ulcer, chronic atrophic gastritis, pyloric obstruction, malignant neoplasms of the stomach, H_2-blockers, omeprazole, calcium therapy, ulcerative colitis, rheumatoid arthritis

GASTRIN STIMULATION TEST

Normal: Gastrin stimulation test after calcium infusion is performed by giving a calcium infusion (15 mg Ca/Kg in 500 ml normal saline over 4 hours). Serum is drawn in fasting state before infusion and at 1, 2, 3, and 4 hr. Normal response is little or no increase over baseline gastrin level.
Elevated in: Gastrinoma (gastrin >400 pg/ml), duodenal ulcer (gastrin level increase <400 ng/L)
Decreased in: Pernicious anemia, atrophic gastritis

GLIADIN ANTIBODIES, IgA AND IgG

Normal: <25 U, equivocal 20-25 U, positive >25 U. Test is useful to monitor compliance with gluten-free diet in patients with celiac disease.
Elevated in: Celiac disease with dietary noncompliance

GLOMERULAR BASEMENT MEMBRANE (gBm) ANTIBODY

Normal: Negative
Present in: Goodpasture's syndrome

GLOMERULAR FILTRATION RATE

Normal:

Ages 20-29	116 ml/min/1.73 m^2
Ages 30-39	107 ml/min/1.73 m^2
Ages 40-49	99 ml/min/1.73 m^2
Ages 50-59	93 ml/min/1.73 m^2
Ages 60-69	85 ml/min/1.73 m^2
Ages >75	75 ml/min/1.73 m^2

Decreased in: Renal insufficiency, decreased renal blood flow

GLUCAGON

Normal: 20-100 pg/ml
Elevated in: Glucagonoma (900-7800 pg/ml), chronic renal failure, diabetes mellitus, glucocorticoids, insulin, nifedipine, danazol, sympathomimetic amines
Decreased in: Hyperlipoproteinemia (types III, IV), beta-blockers, secretin

GLUCOSE, FASTING

Normal range: 70-110 mg/dl (3.9-6.1 mmol/L [CF: 0.05551; SMI: 0.1 mmol/L])
Elevated in: Diabetes mellitus, stress, infections, myocardial infarction, cerebrovascular accident, Cushing's syndrome, acromegaly, acute pancreatitis, glucagonoma, hemochromatosis, drugs (glucocorticoids, diuretics [thiazides, loop diuretics]), glucose intolerance
Decreased in: Sulfonylurea therapy, insulin therapy, reactive hypoglycemia (e.g., s/b subtotal gastrectomy), starvation, insulinoma, glycogen storage disorders, severe liver disease or renal disease, ethanol-induced hypoglycemia, mesenchymal tumors that secrete insulinlike hormones

GLUCOSE, POSTPRANDIAL

Normal range: <140 mg/dl (<7.8 mmol/L [CF: 0.05551; SMI: 0.1 mmol/L])
Elevated in: Diabetes mellitus, glucose intolerance
Decreased in: Post–gastrointestinal resection, reactive hypoglycemia, hereditary fructose intolerance, galactosemia, leucine sensitivity

GLUCOSE TOLERANCE TEST

Normal values above fasting:
30 min: 30-60 mg/dl (1.65-3.3 mmol/L [CF: 0.05551; SMI: 0.1 mmol/L])
60 min: 20-50 mg/dl (1.1-2.75 mmol/L [CF: 0.05551; SMI: 0.1 mmol/L])
120 min: 5-15 mg/dl (0.28-0.83 mmol/L [CF: 0.05551; SMI: 0.1 mmol/L])
180 min: fasting level or below
Abnormal in: Glucose intolerance, diabetes mellitus, Cushing's syndrome, acromegaly, pheochromocytoma, gestational diabetes

GLUCOSE-6-PHOSPHATE DEHYDROGENASE (G6PD) SCREEN (blood)

Normal: G6PD enzyme activity detected
Abnormal: If a deficiency is detected, quantitation of G6PD is necessary; a G6PD screen may be falsely interpreted as "normal" after an episode of hemolysis because most G6PD-deficient cells have been destroyed.

γ-GLUTAMYL TRANSFERASE (GGT)

Normal range: 0-30 U/L (0.050 μkat/L [CF: 0.01667; SMI: 0.01 μkat/L])
Elevated in: Chronic alcoholic liver disease, neoplasms (hepatoma, metastatic disease to the liver, carcinoma of the pancreas), systemic lupus erythematosus, congestive heart failure, trauma, nephrotic syndrome, sepsis, cholestasis, drugs (phenytoin, barbiturates)

GLYCATED (glycosylated) HEMOGLOBIN (HbA_{1c}) (glycohemoglobin)

Normal range: 4.0%-5.9%
Elevated in: Uncontrolled diabetes mellitus (glycated hemoglobin levels reflect the level of glucose control over the preceding 120 days), lead toxicity, alcoholism, iron deficiency anemia, hypertriglyceridemia
Decreased in: Hemolytic anemias, decreased red blood cell survival, pregnancy, acute or chronic blood loss, chronic renal failure, insulinoma, congenital spherocytosis, hemoglobin S, C, and D diseases

GROWTH HORMONE

Normal: Male: 1-9 ng/ml; female: 1-16 ng/ml
Elevated in: Pituitary gigantism, acromegaly, ectopic GH secretion, cirrhosis, renal failure, anorexia nervosa, stress, exercise, prolonged fasting, amphetamines, beta-blockers, insulin, levodopa, metoclopramide, clonidine, vasopressin
Decreased in: Hypopituitarism, pituitary dwarfism, adrenocortical hyperfunction, bromocriptine, corticosteroids, glucose

GROWTH HORMONE RELEASING HORMONE (GHRH)

Normal: <50 pg/ml
Elevated in: Acromegaly caused by GHRH secretion by neoplasms

GROWTH HORMONE SUPPRESSION TEST (after glucose)

Normal: Test is done by giving 1.75 g glucose/kg orally after overnight fast. Blood is drawn at baseline, after 60 min, and after 120 min of glucose load. Normal response is growth hormone suppression to <2 ng/ml or undetectable levels.
Abnormal: There is no or incomplete suppression from the high basal level in gigantism or acromegaly.

HAM TEST (acid serum test)

Normal: Negative
Positive in: Paroxysmal nocturnal hemoglobinuria
False-positive in: Hereditary or acquired spherocytosis, recent transfusion with aged red blood cells, aplastic anemia, myeloproliferative syndromes, leukemia, hereditary dyserythropoietic anemia type II

HAPTOGLOBIN (serum)

Normal range: 50-220 mg/dl (0.50-2.2 g/L [CF: 0.01; SMI: 0.01 g/L])
Elevated in: Inflammation (acute phase reactant), collagen vascular diseases, infections (acute phase reactant), drugs (androgens), obstructive liver disease
Decreased in: Hemolysis (intravascular more than extravascular), megaloblastic anemia, severe liver disease, large tissue hematomas, infectious mononucleosis, drugs (oral contraceptives)

HDL

See HIGH-DENSITY LIPOPROTEIN CHOLESTEROL

HELICOBACTER PYLORI (serology, stool antigen)

Normal range: Not detected
Detected in: *H. pylori* infection. Positive serology can indicate current or past infection. Positive stool antigen test indicates acute infection (sensitivity and specificity >90%). Stool testing should be delayed at least 4 weeks after eradication therapy.

HEMATOCRIT

Normal range:
Male: 39%-49% (0.39-0.49 [CF: 0.01; SMI: 0.01])
Female: 33%-43% (0.33-0.43 [CF: 0.01; SMI: 0.01])
Elevated in: Polycythemia vera, smoking, chronic obstructive pulmonary disease, high altitudes, dehydration, hypovolemia
Decreased in: Blood loss (gastrointestinal, genitourinary) anemia

HEMOGLOBIN

Normal range:
Male: 13.6-17.7 g/dl (136-172 g/L [CF: 10; SMI: 1 g/L])
Female: 12.0-15.0 g/dl (120-150 g/L [CF: 10; SMI: 1 g/L])
Elevated in: Hemoconcentration, dehydration, polycythemia vera, chronic obstructive pulmonary disease, high altitudes, false elevations (hyperlipemic plasma, white blood cells >50,000/mm^3), stress
Decreased in: Hemorrhagic (gastrointestinal, genitourinary) anemia

HEMOGLOBIN A_{1c}

See GLYCATED HEMOGLOBIN

HEMOGLOBIN ELECTROPHORESIS

Normal range:
HbA_1: 95%-98%
HbA_2: 1.5%-3.5%
HbF: <2%
HbC: absent
HbS: absent

HEMOGLOBIN, GLYCATED

See GLYCATED HEMOGLOBIN

HEMOGLOBIN, GLYCOSYLATED

See GLYCATED HEMOGLOBIN

HEMOGLOBIN H

Normal: Negative
Present in: Hemoglobin H disease, alpha-thalassemia trait, unstable hemoglobin disorders

HEMOGLOBIN, URINE

See URINE HEMOGLOBIN

HEMOSIDERIN, URINE

See URINE HEMOGLOBIN

HEPARIN-INDUCED THROMBOCYTOPENIA ANTIBODIES

Normal: Antigen assay: Negative, <0.45; weak, 0.45-1.0; strong, >1.0
Elevated in: Heparin-induced thrombocytopenia

HEPATITIS A ANTIBODY

Normal: Negative
Present in: Viral hepatitis A; can be IgM or IgG (if IgM, acute hepatitis A; if IgG, previous infection with hepatitis A)
See Fig. 4-4 for serologic tests in HAV infection.

HAV-IgM ANTIBODY

Appearance: About the same time as clinical symptoms (3-4 weeks after exposure, range 14-60 days), or just before beginning of AST/ALT elevation (range 10 days before to 7 days after)
Peak: About 3-4 weeks after onset of symptoms (1-6 weeks)
Becomes nondetectable: 3-4 months after onset of symptoms (1-6 months). In a few cases HAV-IgM antibody can persist as long as 12-14 months.

HAV TOTAL ANTIBODY

Appearance: About 3 weeks after IgM becomes detectable (therefore about the middle of clinical symptom period to early convalescence)
Peak: About 1-2 months after onset
Becomes nondetectable: Remains elevated for life but can somewhat slowly fall

HEPATITIS A VIRAL INFECTION

Best all-purpose test(s) to diagnose acute HAV infection = HAV-Ab (IgM)
Best all-purpose test(s) to demonstrate past HAV infection/immunity = HAV-Ab (total)

HEPATITIS B SURFACE ANTIGEN (HBsAg)

Normal: Not detected
Detected in: Acute viral hepatitis type B, chronic hepatitis B
Appearance: 2-6 weeks after exposure (range, 6 days to 6 months); 5%-15% of patients are negative at onset of jaundice
Peak: 1-2 weeks before to 1-2 weeks after onset of symptoms
Becomes nondetectable: 1-3 months after peak (range, 1 week to 5 months)

HEPATITIS B VIRAL INFECTION

Figs. 4-5, 4-6, and 4-7 illustrate antigens and antibodies in hepatitis B infection.

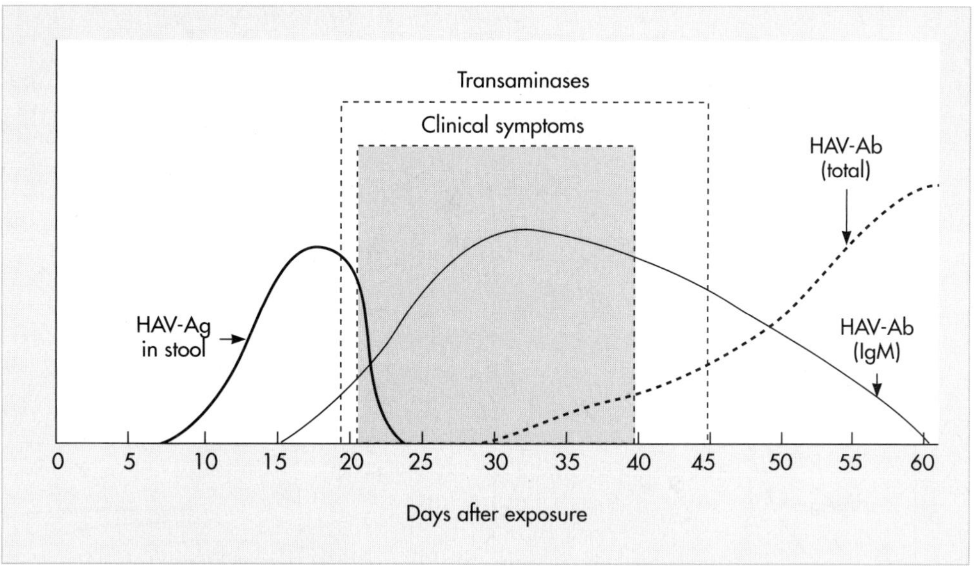

FIGURE 4-4 Serologic tests in HAV infection. (Reprinted from Ravel R [ed]: *Clinical laboratory medicine,* ed 6, St Louis, 1995, Mosby.)

HB_S

-Ag

HB_SAg: shows current active HBV infection.

Persistence over 6 months indicates carrier/chronic HBV infection.

HBV nucleic acid probe: present before and longer than HB_SAg.

More reliable marker for increased infectivity than HB_SAg and/or HB_eAg.

-Ab

HB_SAb-total: shows previous healed HBV infection and evidence of immunity.

HB_C

-Ab

HB_CAb-IgM: shows either acute or very recent infection by HBV.

In convalescent phase of acute HBV, may be elevated when HB_SAg has disappeared (core window).

Negative HB_CAb-IgM with positive HB_SAg suggests either very early acute HBV or carrier/chronic HBV.

HB_CAb-total: only useful to show past HBV infection if HB_SAg and HB_cAb-IgM are both negative.

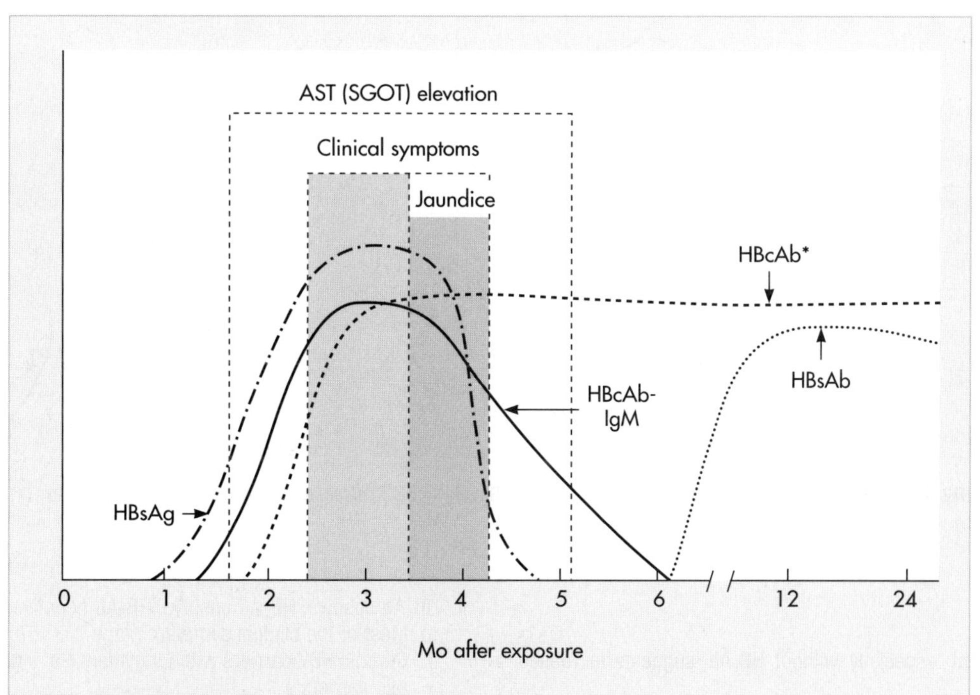

FIGURE 4-5 HBV surface antigen-antibody and core antibodies. Note "core window." *HB_CAb = HB_CAb-IgM + HBCAb-IgG (combined). (Reprinted from Ravel R [ed]: *Clinical laboratory medicine,* ed 6, St Louis, 1995, Mosby.)

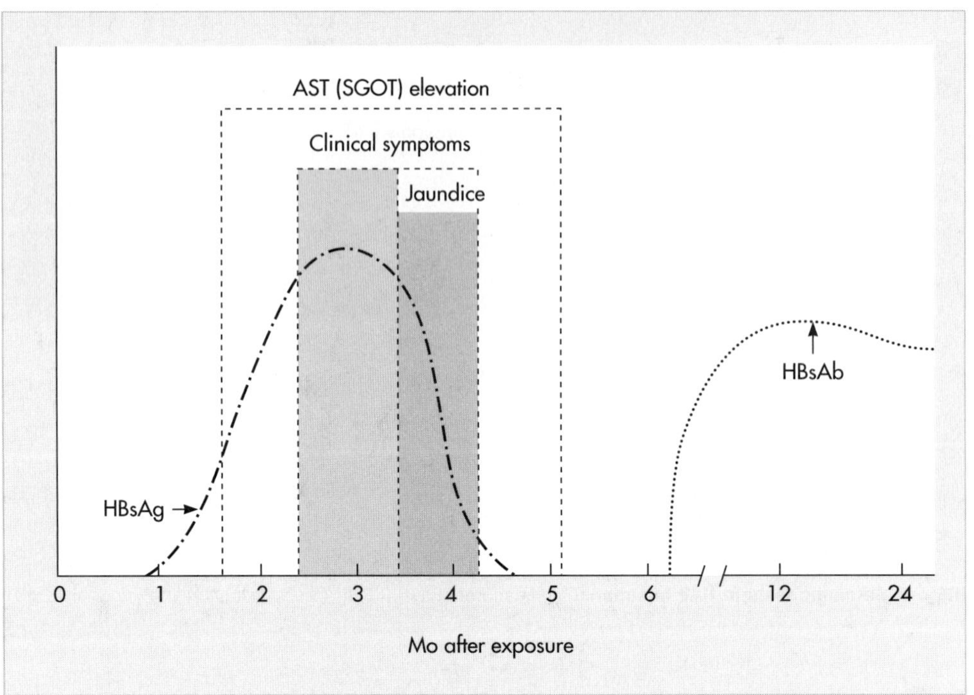

FIGURE 4-6 HBV surface antigen and antibody (HB_SAg and HB_SAb-total). (Reprinted from Ravel R [ed]: *Clinical laboratory medicine,* ed 6, St Louis, 1995, Mosby.)

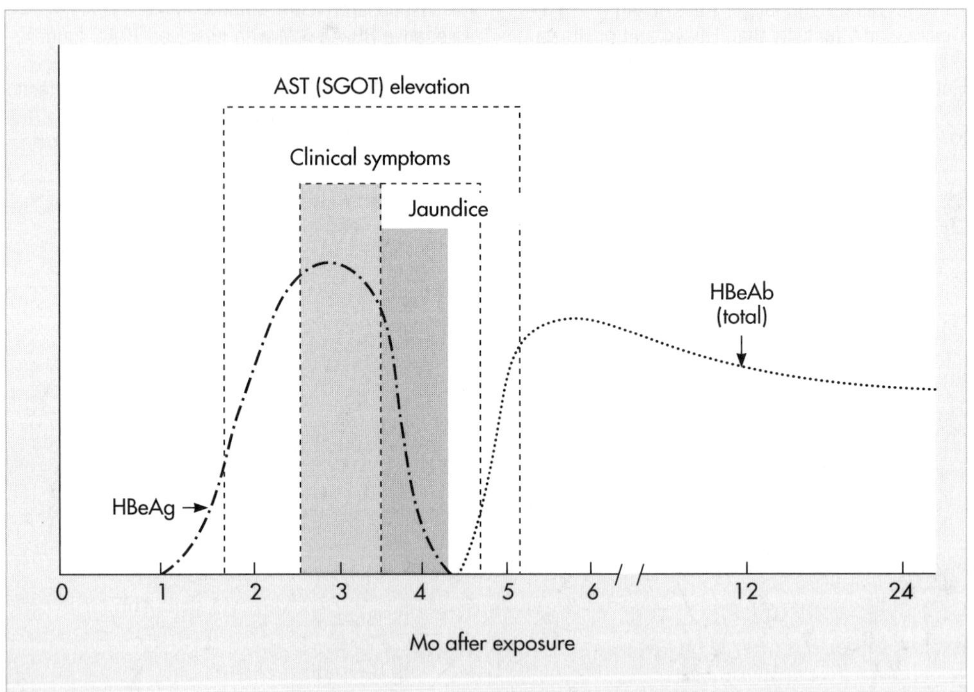

FIGURE 4-7 HBVe antigen and antibody. (Reprinted from Ravel R [ed]: *Clinical laboratory medicine,* ed 6, St Louis, 1995, Mosby.)

HB_e
-Ag

HB_e-AbAg: when present, especially without HB_eAb, suggests increased patient infectivity.

HB_eAb-total: when present, suggests less patient infectivity.

I. HB_SAg positive, HB_CAb negative*
   About 5% (range, 0%-17%) of patients with early-stage HBV acute infection (HB_CAb rises later)

II. HB_SAg positive, HB_CAb positive, HB_SAb negative
   a. Most of the clinical symptom stage
   b. Chronic HBV carriers without evidence of liver disease ("asymptomatic carriers")
   c. Chronic HBV hepatitis (chronic persistent type or chronic active type)

III. HB_SAg negative, HB_CAb positive,* HB_SAb negative
   a. Late clinical symptom stage or early convalescence stage (core window)

b. Chronic HBV infection with HB_SAg below detection levels with current tests
c. Old previous HBV infection

IV. HB_SAg negative, HB_CAb positive, HB_SAb positive
a. Late convalescence to complete recovery
b. Old infection

HEPATITIS C VIRAL INFECTION

Fig. 4-8 illustrates antigens and antibodies in hepatitis C infection.

HEPATITIS C RNA

Normal: Negative
Elevated in: Hepatitis C. Detection of hepatitis C-RNA is used to confirm current infection and to monitor treatment. Quantitative assays (viral load) are needed before treatment to assess response (<2 log decrease after 12-week treatment indicates lack of response).

HCV
-Ag
HCV nucleic acid probe: shows current infection by HCV (especially with PCR amplification).
-Ab
HCV-Ab (IgG): current, convalescent, or old HCV infection.

HAV
-Ag
HAV-Ag by EM: shows presence of virus in stool early in infection.
-Ab
HAV-Ab (IgM): current or recent HAV infection.
HAV-Ab (total): convalescent or old HAV infection.

HEPATITIS D VIRAL INFECTION

Fig. 4-9 illustrates antigens and antibodies in hepatitis D infection.
Best current all-purpose screening test = ADV-Ab (total)
Best test to differentiate acute from chronic infection = HDV-Ab (IgM)

DELTA HEPATITIS COINFECTION (acute HDV1 acute HBV) OR SUPERINFECTION (acute HDV1 chronic HBV)

HDV
-Ag
HDV-Ag: shows current infection (acute or chronic) by HDV.
HDV nucleic acid probe: detects antigen before and longer than HDV-Ag by EIA.
-Ab
HDV-Ab (IgM): high elevation in acute HDV; does not persist.
Low or moderate elevation in convalescent HDV; does not persist.
Low to high persistent elevation in chronic HDV (depends on degree of cell injury and sensitivity of the assay).
HDV-Ab (total): high elevation in acute HDV; does not persist.
High persistent elevation in chronic HDV.

HDV-AG

Detected by DNA probe, less often by immunoassay
Appearance: Prodromal stage (before symptoms); just at or after initial rise in ALT (about a week after appearance of HB_SAg and about the time HB_CAb-IgM level begins to rise)
Peak: 2-3 days after onset
Becomes nondetectable: 1-4 days (may persist until shortly after symptoms appear)

HDV-AB (IgM)

Appearance: About 10 days after symptoms begin (range, 1-28 days)
Peak: About 2 weeks after first detection
Becomes nondetectable: About 35 days (range, 10-80 days) after first detection (most other IgM antibodies take 3-6 months to become nondetectable)

HDV-AB (total)

Appearance: About 50 days after symptoms begin (range, 14-80 days); about 5 weeks after HDV-Ag (range, 3-11 weeks)
Peak: About 2 weeks after first detection
Becomes nondetectable: About 7 months after first detection (range, 4-14 months)

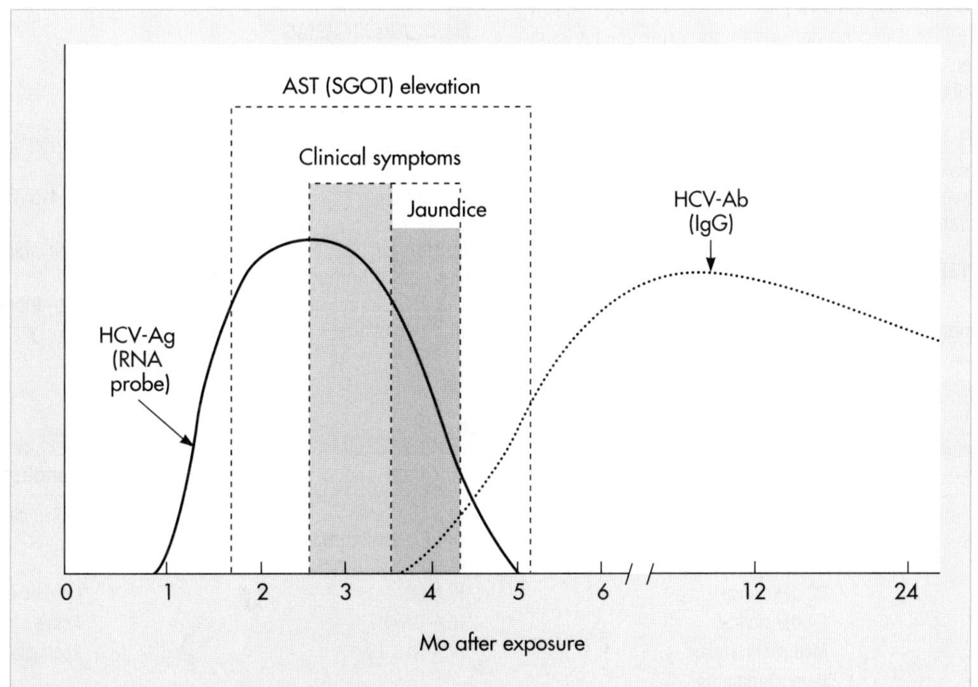

FIGURE 4-8 HCV antigen and antibody. (Reprinted from Ravel R [ed]: *Clinical laboratory medicine,* ed 6, St Louis, 1995, Mosby.)

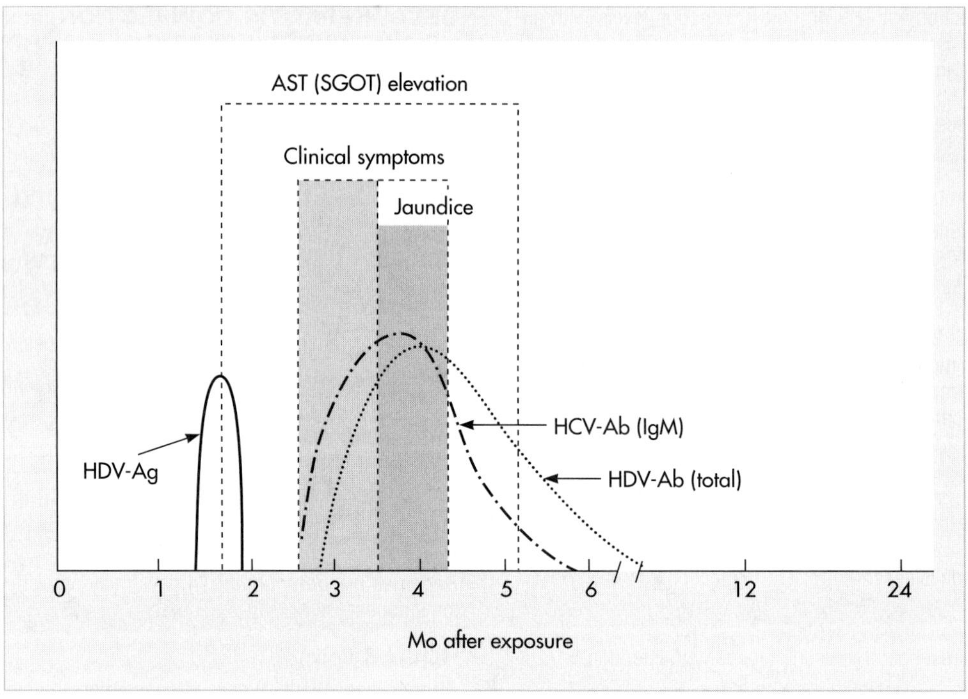

FIGURE 4-9 HDV antigen and antibodies. (Reprinted from Ravel R [ed]: *Clinical laboratory medicine,* ed 6, St Louis, 1995, Mosby.)

HER-2/*NEU*

Normal: Negative
Present in: Present in 25%-30% of primary breast cancers. It can also be found in other epithelial tumors, including lung, hepatocellular, pancreatic, colon, stomach, ovarian, cervical, and bladder cancer. Trastuzumab (Herceptin) is a humanized monoclonal antibody against Her-2/*neu.* This test is useful to identify patients with metastatic; recurrent; and/or treatment refractory, unresectable, locally advanced breast cancer for trastuzumab treatment.

HERPES SIMPLEX VIRUS (HSV)

Test description: The PCR test can be performed on serum biopsy samples, CSF, vitreous humor.

Table 2-3 describes laboratory diagnosis of herpes virus infections.

HFE SCREEN FOR HEREDITARY HEMOCHROMATOSIS

Test description: PCR test can be performed on whole blood or tissue. One mutation (C282Y) and two polymorphisms (H63D, S65C) account for the majority of alleles associated with this disease.

HETEROPHIL ANTIBODY

Normal: Negative
Positive in: Infectious mononucleosis

HIGH-DENSITY LIPOPROTEIN (HDL) CHOLESTEROL

Normal range:
Male: 40-70 mg/dl (0.8-1.8 mmol/L [CF: 0.02586; SMI: 0.05 mmol/L])
Female: 50-90 mg/dl (1.1-2.35 mmol/L [CF: 0.02586; SMI: 0.05 mmol/L])
Increased in: Use of gemfibrozil, statins, fenofibrate, nicotinic acid, estrogens, regular aerobic exercise, small (1 oz) daily alcohol intake
Decreased in: Deficiency of apoproteins, liver disease, probucol ingestion, Tangier disease

NOTE: A cholesterol/HDL ratio >4.0 is associated with increased risk of coronary artery disease.

HLA ANTIGENS

Associated disorders: see Table 4-12.

HOMOCYSTEINE (plasma)

Normal range:
0-30 years: 4.6-8.1 mcmol/L
30-59 years: 6.3-11.2 mcmol/L (males), 4-5-7.9 mcmol/L (females)
>59 years: 5.8-11.9 mcmol/L
Increased: Thrombophilic states, B_6, B_{12}, folic acid, riboflavin deficiency, pregnancy, homocystinuria

NOTE: An increased homocysteine level is an independent risk factor for atherosclerosis.

TABLE 4-12 HLA Antigens Associated with Specific Diseases

Antigen	Condition	Antigen	Condition
HLA-B27	Ankylosing spondylitis	HLA-B8, Dw3	Celiac disease
Reiter's syndrome	HLA-B8, Dw3	Dermatitis herpetiformis	
Psoriatic arthritis	HLA-B8	Myasthenia gravis	
HLA-A10, B18, Dw2	C2 deficiency	HLA-B8	Chronic active hepatitis in children
HLA-A2, B40, Cw3	C4 deficiency	HLA-Drw4	Active chronic hepatitis in adults
HLA-B7, Dw2	Multiple sclerosis	HLA-B13, Bw17	Psoriasis
HLA-A3	Hemochromatosis		

Reprinted from Cerra FB: *Manual of critical care,* St Louis, 1987, Mosby.
HLA, Human leukocyte antigen.

HUMAN HERPES VIRUS 8 (HHV8)

Test description: PCR test can be performed on whole blood, tissue, bone marrow, and urine. HHV8 is found in all forms of Kaposi's sarcoma.

HUMAN CHORIONIC GONADOTROPIN (hCG)

Normal range: Varies with gestational stage:

1 wk:	5-50 mU/ml
1-2 wk:	50-550 mU/ml
2-3 wk:	up to 5000 mU/ml
3-4 wk:	up to 10,000 mU/ml
4-5 wk:	up to 50,000 mU/ml
2-3 mo:	10,000-100,000 mU/ml

Elevated in: Normal pregnancy, hydatidiform mole, choriocarcinoma, germ cell tumors of testicle, some nontrophoblastic neoplasms (e.g., neoplasms of cervix, gastrointestinal tract, ovary, lung, breast)

HUMAN IMMUNODEFICIENCY VIRUS ANTIBODY, TYPE 1 (HIV-1)

Normal range: Not detected

Abnormal result: HIV antibodies usually appear in the blood 1-4 months after infection.

Testing sequence:

1. ELISA is the recommended initial screening test. Sensitivity and specificity are >99%. False-positive ELISA may occur with autoimmune disorders, administration of immune globulin manufactured before 1985, within 6 weeks of testing, in the presence of rheumatoid factor, in the presence of DLA-DR antibodies in multigravida female, with administration of influenza vaccine within 3 months of testing, with hemodialysis, with positive plasma reagin test, and with certain medical disorders (hemophilia, hypergammaglobulinemia, alcoholic hepatitis).
2. A positive ELISA is confirmed with Western blot. False-positive Western blot may result from connective tissue disorders, human leukocyte antigen antibodies, polyclonal gammopathies, hyperbilirubinemia, presence of antibody to another human retrovirus, or cross-reaction with other non-virus-derived proteins in healthy persons. Undetermined Western blot may occur in AIDS patients with advanced immunodeficiency (caused by loss of antibodies) and in recent HIV infections.
3. PCR is used to confirm indeterminate Western blot results or negative results in persons with suspected HIV infection.

Fig. 4-10 describes tests in HIV infection; indications for plasma HIV RNA testing are described in Table 4-13.

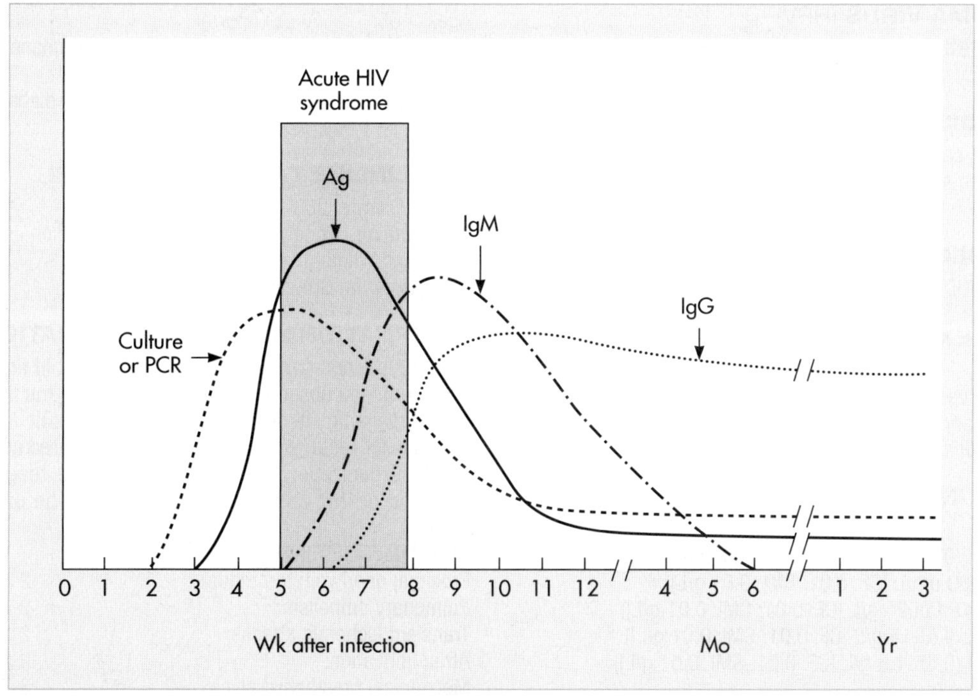

FIGURE 4-10 Tests in HIV-1 infection. (Reprinted from Ravel R [ed]: *Clinical laboratory medicine,* ed 6, St Louis, 1995, Mosby.)

TABLE 4-13 Indications for Plasma HIV RNA Testing*

Clinical Indication	Information	Use
Syndrome consistent with acute HIV infection	Establishes diagnosis when HIV antibody test is negative or indeterminate	Diagnosis†
Initial evaluation of newly diagnosed HIV infection	Baseline viral load set point	Decision to start or defer therapy
Every 3-4 mo in patients not on therapy	Changes in viral load	Decision to start therapy
4-8 wk after initiation of antiretroviral therapy	Initial assessment of drug efficacy	Decision to continue or change therapy
3-4 mo after start of therapy	Maximal effect of therapy	Decision to continue or change therapy
Every 3-4 mo in patients on therapy	Durability of antiretroviral effect	Decision to continue or change therapy
Clinical event or significant decline in CD4+ T cells	Association with changing or stable	Decision to continue, initiate, or change

Reprinted from *MMWR,* 47:RR-5, 1998.

*Acute illness (e.g., bacterial pneumonia, tuberculosis, HSV, PCP) and immunizations can cause increase in plasma HIV RNA for 2-4 wk; viral load testing should not be performed during this time. Plasma HIV RNA results should usually be verified with a repeat determination before starting or making changes in therapy. HIV RNA should be measured using the same laboratory and the same assay.

†Diagnosis of HIV infection determined by HIV RNA testing should be confirmed by standard methods (e.g., Western blot serology) performed 2-4 mo after the initial indeterminate or negative test.

HUMAN IMMUNODEFICIENCY VIRUS TYPE 1 (HIV-1) ANTIGEN (p24), QUALITATIVE (p24 antigen)

Normal range: Negative. This test detects uncomplexed HIV-1 p24 antigen. The core protein p24 is the first detectable protein encoded by the group-specific antigen *(gag)* gene. This protein is a marker for viremia. This test should not be used in place of HIV-1 antibody testing as a screen for HIV-1 infection. HIV-1 p24 may be detectable in the first month of acute HIV-1 infection and generally falls to undetectable levels during the asymptomatic stage of HIV-1 infection. A negative result does not exclude the possibility of infection or exposure to HIV-1. It is recommended that a negative result be followed with repeat testing at least 8 weeks after the original test. This test is used primarily for screening of donated blood and plasma and as an aid for the prognosis of HIV-1 infection.

HUMAN IMMUNODEFICIENCY VIRUS TYPE 1 (HIV-1) VIRAL LOAD

Normal range: HIV-1 RNA, quant. bDNA 3: less than 50 copies/ml or less than 1.7 log copies/ml

This test should be used only in individuals with documented HIV-1 infection for monitoring the progression of infection, response to antiretroviral therapy, and disease prognosis. It is not indicated for diagnosis of HIV infection.

HUMAN PAPILLOMA VIRUS (HPV)

Test description: PCR test can be performed on cervical smears, biopsies, scrapings, liquid cytology specimen, and anogenital tissues.

HUNTINGTON'S DISEASE PCR

Test description: PCR can be performed on whole blood. Huntington's disease is caused by the expansion of the trinucleotide repeat CAG within IT 15 (huntingtin).

5-HYDROXYINDOLE-ACETIC ACID, URINE

See URINE 5-HYDROXYINDOLE-ACETIC ACID

IMMUNE COMPLEX ASSAY

Normal: Negative
Detected in: Collagen vascular disorders, glomerulonephritis, neoplastic diseases, malaria, primary biliary cirrhosis, chronic acute hepatitis, bacterial endocarditis, vasculitis

IMMUNOGLOBULINS

Normal range:

IgA:	50-350 mg/dl (0.5-3.5 g/L [CF: 0.01; SMI: 0.01 g/L])
IgD:	<6 mg/dl (<60 mg/L [CF: 0.01; SMI: 0.01 g/L])
IgE:	<25 μg/dl (<0.00025 g/L [CF: 0.01; SMI: 0.01 g/L])
IgG:	800-1500 mg/dl (8-15 g/L [CF: 0.01; SMI: 0.01 g/L])
IgM:	45-150 mg/dl (0.45-1.5 g/L [CF: 0.01; SMI: 0.01 g/L])

Elevated in:

IgA: Lymphoproliferative disorders, Berger's nephropathy, chronic infections, autoimmune disorders, liver disease
IgE: Allergic disorders, parasitic infections, immunologic disorders, IgE myeloma
IgG: Chronic granulomatous infections, infectious diseases, inflammation, myeloma, liver disease
IgM: Primary biliary cirrhosis, infectious diseases (brucellosis, malaria), Waldenström's macroglobulinemia, liver disease

Decreased in:

IgA: Nephrotic syndrome, protein-losing enteropathy, congenital deficiency, lymphocytic leukemia, ataxia-telangiectasia, chronic sinopulmonary disease
IgE: Hypogammaglobulinemia, neoplasma (breast, bronchial, cervical), ataxia-telangiectasia
IgG: Congenital or acquired deficiency, lymphocytic leukemia, phenytoin, methylprednisolone, nephrotic syndrome, protein-losing enteropathy
IgM: Congenital deficiency, lymphocytic leukemia, nephrotic syndrome

INFLUENZA A AND B TESTS

Test description: PCR can be performed on nasopharyngeal swab, wash, or aspirate
Normal: Negative

INSULIN AUTOANTIBODIES

Normal: Negative
Present in: Exogenous insulin from insulin therapy. The presence of islet cell antibodies indicates ongoing beta cell destruction. This test is useful in the early diagnosis of type 1a diabetes mellitus and in the identification of patients at high risk for type 1a diabetes.

INSULIN, FREE

Normal: <17 mcU/ml
Elevated in: Insulin overdose, insulin resistance syndromes, endogenous hyperinsulinemia
Decreased in: Inadequately treated type 1 DM

INSULINLIKE GROWTH FACTOR-1 (IGF-1) (serum)

Normal range:

Ages 16-24:	182-780 ng/ml
Ages 25-39:	114-492 ng/ml
Ages 40-54:	90-360 ng/ml
Ages >55:	71-290 ng/ml

Elevated in: Adolescence, acromegaly, pregnancy, precocious puberty, obesity
Decreased in: Malnutrition, delayed puberty, diabetes mellitus, hypopituitarism, cirrhosis, old age

INSULINLIKE GROWTH FACTOR-II

Normal range: 288-736 ng/ml
Elevated in: Hypoglycemia associated with non–islet cell tumors, hepatoma, and Wilms' tumor
Decreased in: Growth hormone deficiency

INTERNATIONAL NORMALIZED RATIO (INR)

The INR is a comparative rating of prothrombin time (PT) ratios. The INR represents the observed PT ratio adjusted by the International Reference Thromboplastin. It provides a universal result indicative of what the patient's PT result would have been if measured using the primary World Health Organization International Reference reagent. For proper interpretation of INR values, the patient should be on stable anticoagulant therapy.

RECOMMENDED INR RANGES:

Proximal deep vein thrombosis:	2-3
Pulmonary embolism:	2-3
Transient ischemic attacks:	2-3
Atrial fibrillation:	2-3
Mechanical prosthetic valves:	3-4.5
Recurrent venous thromboembolic disease:	3-4.5

INTRINSIC FACTOR ANTIBODIES

Normal: Negative
Present in: Pernicious anemia (>50% of patients). Cyanocobalamin may give false-positive results.

IRON (serum)

Normal: Male: 65-175 mcg/dl; female: 50-1170 mcg/dl
Elevated in: Hemochromatosis, excessive iron therapy, repeated transfusions, lead poisoning, hemolytic anemia, aplastic anemia, pernicious anemia
Decreased in: Iron deficiency anemia, hypothyroidism, chronic infection

IRON-BINDING CAPACITY, TOTAL (TIBC)

Normal range: 250-460 μg/dl (45-82 μmol/L [CF: 0.1791; SMI: 1 μmol/L])
Elevated in: Iron deficiency anemia, pregnancy, polycythemia, hepatitis, weight loss

TABLE 4-14 Serum Iron and Total Iron-Binding Capacity Patterns

SI↓	TIBC↓	Chronic diseases Uremia
SI↓	TIBC↑	Chronic iron deficiency anemia Pregnancy in third trimester
SI↑	TIBC↓	Hemachromatosis Iron therapy overload (TIBC may be normal) Hemolytic anemia; thalassemia; lead poisoning; megaloblastic anemia; aplastic, pyridoxine deficiency, or other sideroblastic anemias
SI↑	TIBC↑	Oral contraceptives Acute hepatitis (some report TIBC is low normal) Chronic hepatitis (some patients)
SI↑	TIBC NL	B_{12} or folate deficiency
SI↓	TIBC NL	Chronic iron deficiency (some patients) Acute infection, surgery, tissue damage
SI NL	TIBC↑	B_{12}/folate deficiency plus iron deficiency

Reprinted from Ravel R: *Clinical laboratory medicine*, ed 6, St Louis, 1995, Mosby.
NL, Normal; *SI,* serum iron; *TIBC,* total iron-binding capacity.

Decreased in: Anemia of chronic disease, hemochromatosis, chronic liver disease, hemolytic anemias, malnutrition (protein depletion)

Table 4-14 describes TIBC and serum iron abnormalities.

LACTATE (blood)

Normal range: 0.5-2.0 mEq/L
Elevated in: Tissue hypoxia (shock, respiratory failure, severe CHF, severe anemia, carbon monoxide or cyanide poisoning), systemic disorders (liver or renal failure, seizures), abnormal intestinal flora (D-lactic acidosis), drugs or toxins (salicylates, ethanol, methanol, ethylene glycol), G6PD deficiency

LACTATE DEHYDROGENASE (LDH)

Normal range: 50-150 U/L (0.82-2.66 μkat/L [CF: 0.01667; SMI: 0.02 μkat/L])
Elevated in:
Infarction of myocardium, lung, kidney
Diseases of cardiopulmonary system, liver, collagen, central nervous system
Hemolytic anemias, megaloblastic anemias, transfusions, seizures, muscle trauma, muscular dystrophy, acute pancreatitis, hypotension, shock, infectious mononucleosis, inflammation, neoplasia, intestinal obstruction, hypothyroidism

LACTATE DEHYDROGENASE ISOENZYMES

Normal range:
LDH_1: 22%-36% (cardiac, red blood cell) (0.22-0.36 [CF: 0.01, SMI: 0.01])
LDH_2: 35%-46% (cardiac, red blood cell) (0.35-0.46)
LDH_3: 13%-26% (pulmonary) (0.15-0.26)
LDH_4: 3%-10% (striated muscle, liver) (0.03-0.1)
LDH_5: 2%-9% (striated muscle, liver) (0.02-0.09)
Normal ratios:
$LDH_1 < LDH_2$
$LDH_5 < LDH_4$
Abnormal values:
$LDH_1 > LDH_2$: Myocardial infarction (can also be seen with hemolytic anemias, pernicious anemia, folate deficiency, renal infarct)
$LDH_5 > LDH_4$: Liver disease (cirrhosis, hepatitis, hepatic congestion)

LACTOSE TOLERANCE TEST (serum)

Normal: Test is performed by giving 2 g/kg body weight lactose orally and drawing glucose level at 0, 30, 45, 60, and 90 min. Normal response is change in glucose from fasting value to >30 mg/dl. Inconclusive response is increase of 20-30 mg/dl, abnormal response is increase <20 mg/dl.
Abnormal in: Lactase deficiency

LAP SCORE

See LEUKOCYTE ALKALINE PHOSPHATASE

LEAD

Normal: Child, <10 mcg/dl; adult, <25 mcg/dl; acceptable for industrial exposure, <50 mcg/dl
Elevated in: Lead exposure, lead poisoning

LDH

See LACTATE DEHYDROGENASE

LDL

See LOW-DENSITY LIPOPROTEIN CHOLESTEROL

LEGIONELLA TITER

Normal: Negative
Positive in: Legionnaire's disease (presumptive: ≥1:256 titer; definitive: fourfold titer increase to ≥1:128)

LEGIONELLA PNEUMOPHILA PCR

Test description: PCR can be performed on lung tissue, water sputum, bronchoalveolar lavage, and other respiratory fluids.

LEUKOCYTE ALKALINE PHOSPHATASE (LAP)

Normal range: 13-100 (33-188 U)
Elevated in: Leukemoid reactions, neutrophilia secondary to infections (except in sickle cell crisis—no significant increase in LAP score), Hodgkin's disease, polycythemia vera, hairy cell leukemia, aplastic anemia, Down's syndrome, myelofibrosis
Decreased in: Acute and chronic granulocytic leukemia, thrombocytopenic purpura, paroxysmal nocturnal hemoglobinuria, hypophosphatemia, collagen disorders

LEUKOCYTE COUNT

See COMPLETE BLOOD COUNT

LIPASE

Normal range: 0-160 U/L (0-2.66 μkat/L [CF: 0.01667; SMI: 0.02 μkat/L])
Elevated in: Acute pancreatitis, perforated peptic ulcer, carcinoma of pancreas (early stage), pancreatic duct obstruction, bowel infarction, intestinal obstruction

LIPOPROTEIN(a)

Normal: Male: 1.35-19.6 mg/dl; female: 1.24-20.1 mg/dl
Elevated in: Coronary artery disease, uncontrolled diabetes, hypothyroidism, chronic renal failure, pregnancy, tobacco use, infections, nephritic syndrome
Decreased in: Niacin, omega-3 fatty acids, estrogens, tamoxifen

LIPOPROTEIN CHOLESTEROL, HIGH-DENSITY

See HIGH-DENSITY LIPOPROTEIN CHOLESTEROL

LIPOPROTEIN CHOLESTEROL, LOW-DENSITY

See LOW-DENSITY LIPOPROTEIN CHOLESTEROL

LIVER KIDNEY MICROSOME TYPE 1 ANTIBODIES (LKM1)

Normal: <20 U
Elevated in: Autoimmune hepatitis type 2

LOW-DENSITY LIPOPROTEIN (LDL) CHOLESTEROL

Normal range: 50-130 mg/dl (1.30-1.68 mmol/L [CF: 0.02586; SMI: 0.05 mmol/L])

<70	Optimal in diabetics, prior MI, and patients with cardiac risk factors
100-129	Near or above optimal
130-159	Borderline high
160-189	High
≥190	Very high

LUPUS ANTICOAGULANT

See CIRCULATING ANTICOAGULANT

LUTEINIZING HORMONE

Normal range: 5-25 mIU/ml

Elevated in: Postmenopause, pituitary adenoma, primary gonadal dysfunction, polycystic ovary syndrome

Decreased in: Severe illness, anorexia nervosa, malnutrition, pituitary or hypothalamic impairment, severe stress

LYME DISEASE ANTIBODY TITER

Normal range: Negative

Positive result: Fig. 4-11 illustrates the usual serologic response in Lyme disease.

A serologic test is not necessary or helpful for several days after a tick bite because it is only 40%-50% sensitive in this stage, and a negative test does not rule out the diagnosis.

LYMPHOCYTES

Normal range: 15%-40%

Total lymphocyte count = 800-2600/mm^3

Total T lymphocyte: = 800-2200/mm^3

CD4 lymphocytes = $\geq$400/mm^3

CD8 lymphocytes = 200-800/mm^3

Normal CD4/CD8 ratio is 2.0.

Elevated in: Chronic infections, infectious mononucleosis and other viral infections, chronic lymphocytic leukemia, Hodgkin's disease, ulcerative colitis, hypoadrenalism, idiopathic thrombocytopenia

Decreased in:

AIDS, bone marrow suppression from chemotherapeutic agents or chemotherapy, aplastic anemia, neoplasms, steroids, adrenocortical hyperfunction, neurologic disorders (multiple sclerosis, myasthenia gravis, Guillain-Barré syndrome)

CD4 lymphocytes are calculated as total white blood cells $\times$ % lymphocytes $\times$ % lymphocytes stained with CD4. They are decreased in AIDS and other immune dysfunction.

Table 4-15 describes various lymphocyte abnormalities in peripheral blood.

MAGNESIUM (serum)

Normal range: 1.8-3.0 mg/dl (0.80-1.20 mmol/L [CF: 0.4114; SMI: 0.02 mmol/L])

CAUSES OF HYPERMAGNESEMIA

I. Decreased renal excretion
   A. Renal failure—glomerular filtration rate less than 30 ml/min
   B. Hyperparathyroidism
   C. Hypothyroidism
   D. Addison's disease
   E. Lithium intoxication
   F. Familial hypocalciuric hypercalcemia
II. Other causes: usually in association with decrease in glomerular filtration rate
   A. Endogenous loads
      1. Diabetic ketoacidosis
      2. Severe tissue injury—burns
   B. Exogenous loads
      1. Gastrointestinal
         a. Magnesium-containing laxatives and antacids
         b. High-dose vitamin D analogs
      2. Parenteral: management of toxemia of pregnancy

CAUSES OF HYPOMAGNESEMIA

Alcoholic abuse
Diuretic use
Renal losses
Acute and chronic renal failure
Postobstructive diuresis
Acute tubular necrosis
Chronic glomerulonephritis
Chronic pyelonephritis
Interstitial nephropathy
Renal transplantation
Gastrointestinal losses
Chronic diarrhea
Nasogastric suctioning
Short bowel syndrome
Protein calorie malnutrition
Bowel fistula
Total parenteral nutrition
Acute pancreatitis
Endocrine
Diabetes mellitus
Hyperaldosteronism
Hyperthyroidism
Hyperparathyroidism
Acute intermittent porphyria
Pregnancy
Drugs
Aminoglycosides
Amphotericin
β-agonists
Cisplatin
Cyclosporine
Diuretics
Foscarnet

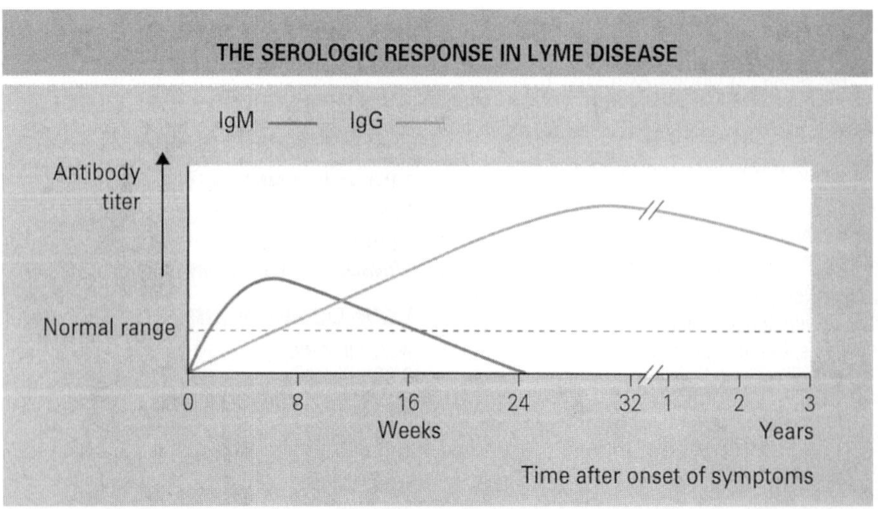

FIGURE 4-11 IgM and IgG response in Lyme disease.

TABLE 4-15 Differential Diagnosis of Abnormal Lymphocytes in Peripheral Blood

Lymphocyte Type	Usual Disease Association	Cytologic Features	Laboratory Features	Clinical Features
Small lymphocyte	Chronic lymphocytic leukemia	B-cell surface markers with low concentration of surface immunoglobulin, CD5 antigen	Hypogammaglobulinemia in 50%; positive direct Coombs' test in 15%; on node biopsy, diffuse, well-differentiated lymphocytic infiltrate	Elderly adults; presentation runs gamut from asymptomatic with lymphocytosis only to bulky disease with adenopathy, splenomegaly, and "packed" bone marrow
Atypical lymphocyte	Infectious mononucleosis, other viral illnesses	Suppressor T-cell markers	Heterophil agglutinin; positive serology for Epstein-Barr virus, cytomegalovirus, toxoplasma, HBsAg	Pharyngitis, fever, adenopathy, rash, splenomegaly, palatal petechiae, jaundice
Plasmacytoid lymphocyte	Waldenström's macroglobulin anemia	Cytoplasmic IgM, periodic acid-Schiff positivity	IgM paraprotein, rouleaux, cryoglobulins	Adenopathy, splenomegaly, absence of bone lesions, hyperviscosity syndrome, cryopathic phenomena
Lymphoblast	ALL	Terminal transferase positivity, common ALL antigen, B- or T-precursor markers	Anemia, granulocytopenia, thrombocytopenia, hyperuricemia, diffuse bone marrow infiltration	Peak incidence in childhood, acute onset, bone pain frequent
Lymphosarcoma cell	Lymphocytic lymphoma	B-cell surface markers with high concentration of monoclonal surface immunoglobulin	Nodular or diffuse, poorly differentiated lymphocytic lymphoma on node biopsy, patchy, peritrabecular bone marrow involvement	Middle-aged to older adults, generalized adenopathy, constitutional symptoms
Sézary cell	Cutaneous lymphomas	T-lymphocyte surface markers	Skin biopsy is diagnostic	Exfoliative erythroderma, cutaneous plaques or tumors
Hairy cell	Hairy cell leukemia	B-lymphocyte markers, cytoplasmic projections, tartrate-resistant acid phosphatase, interleukin-2 receptors, CD11 antigen	Pancytopenia	Middle-aged males, moderate to marked splenomegaly without adenopathy
Prolymphocyte	Prolymphocytic leukemia	B-cell surface markers with high concentration of surface immunoglobulin, CD5 negative	Marked lymphocytosis (frequently $>100 \times 10^9$/L)	Elderly adults, massive splenomegaly, minimum adenopathy, poor response to therapy

Reprinted from Stein JH (ed): *Internal medicine,* ed 5, St Louis, 1998, Mosby.
ALL, Acute lymphoblastic leukemia.

Pentamidine
Theophylline
Congenital disorders
Familial hypomagnesemia
Maternal diabetes
Maternal hypothyroidism
Maternal hyperparathyroidism

MEAN CORPUSCULAR VOLUME (MCV)

Normal range: 76-100 μm³ (76-100 fL) (76-100 fL [CF: 1; SMI: 1 fL])
See Tables 4-16 and 4-17 for descriptions of MCV abnormalities.

METANEPHRINES, URINE

See URINE METANEPHRINES

METHYLMALONIC ACID, SERUM

Normal: <0.2 mcmol/L
Elevated in: Vitamin B_{12} deficiency, pregnancy, methylmalonic acidemia

MITOCHONDRIAL ANTIBODY (AMA)

Normal: Negative
Present in: Primary biliary cirrhosis (>90% of patients)

MONOCYTE COUNT

Normal range: 2%-8%
Elevated in: Viral diseases, parasites, infections, neoplasms, inflammatory bowel disease, monocytic leukemia, lymphomas, myeloma, sarcoidosis
Decreased in: Aplastic anemia, lymphocytic leukemia, glucocorticoid administration

MYCOPLASMA PNEUMONIAE PCR

Test description: PCR can be performed on sputum, bronchoalveolar lavage, nasopharyngeal and throat swabs, other respiratory fluids, and lung tissue

MYELIN BASIC PROTEIN, CEREBROSPINAL FLUID

Normal: <2.5 ng/ml
Elevated in: Multiple sclerosis, CNS trauma, stroke, encephalitis

MYOGLOBIN, URINE

See URINE MYOGLOBIN

NEISSERIA GONORRHOEA PCR

Test description: Test can be performed on endocervical swab, urine, and intraurethral swab
Normal: Negative

NEUTROPHIL COUNT

Normal range: 50%-70%
Subsets:
Stabs (bands, early mature neutrophils): 2%-6%
Segs (mature neutrophils): 60%-70%
Elevated in: Acute bacterial infections, acute myocardial infarction, stress, neoplasms, myelocytic leukemia
Decreased in: Viral infections, aplastic anemias, immunosuppressive drugs, radiation therapy to bone marrow, agranulocytosis, drugs (antibiotics, antithyroidals, clopidogrel), lymphocytic and monocytic leukemias
Table 4-18 describes various drugs that can cause neutropenia.

NOREPINEPHRINE

Normal range: 0-600 pg/ml
Elevated in: Pheochromocytomas, neuroblastomas, stress, vigorous exercise, certain foods (bananas, chocolate, coffee, tea, vanilla)

5′-NUCLEOTIDASE

Normal range: 2-16 IU/L ($3\text{-}27 \times 10^8$ kat/L [CF: 1.67×10^8; SMI: 1×10^8 kat/L])
Elevated in: Biliary obstruction, metastatic neoplasms to liver, primary biliary cirrhosis, renal failure, pancreatic carcinoma, chronic active hepatitis

TABLE 4-16 Some Causes of Increased Mean Corpuscular Volume (Macrocytosis)

Causes	% of all Macrocytosis Patients*	% of Macrocytosis in Each Disease†
Common		
Folate or B_{12} deficiency	20-30 (5-50)‡	80-90 (4-100)
Chronic liver disease	15-20 (6-28)	25-30 (8-65)
Chronic alcoholism	10-12 (3-15)	60 (26-90)
Cytotoxic chemotherapy	10-15 (2-20)	30-40 (13-82)
Cardiorespiratory abnormality	8 (7-9.5)	?
Reticulocytosis	6-7 (0-15)	Depends on severity
Myelodysplastic syndromes	Frequent over age 40 yr	>60 in RAEB and RARS
Unexplained	25 (22.5-27)	—
Normal newborn		
Less Common	**<4%**	
Noncytotoxic drugs		
Zidovudine		
Phenytoin		30 (14-50)
Azathioprine		
Hypothyroidism		20-30 (8-55)
Chronic leukemia/myelofibrosis		
Radiotherapy for malignancy		
Chronic renal disease (occasional patients)		
Distance-runner macrocytosis (some persons)		
Down's syndrome		
Artifactual (e.g., cold agglutinins)		

Reprinted from Ravel R: *Clinical laboratory medicine,* ed 6, St Louis, 1995, Mosby.
RAEB, Refractory anemia with excessive blasts; RARS, refractory anemia with ring sideroblasts (formerly called IASA, or idiopathic acquired sideroblastic anemia).
*Percentage of all patients with macrocytosis.
†Percentage of patients with each condition listed who have macrocytosis.
‡Numbers in parentheses are literature range.

TABLE 4-17 Some Causes of Decreased Mean Corpuscular Volume (Microcytosis)

Common	Less Common
Chronic iron deficiency	Some cases of polycythemia
α- or β-thalassemia (minor)	Some cases of lead poisoning
Anemia of chronic disease	Some cases of congenital spherocytosis
	Some cases of sideroblastic anemia
	Certain abnormal hemoglobins (HbE, Hb Lepore)

Reprinted from Ravel R: *Clinical laboratory medicine,* ed 6, St Louis, 1995, Mosby.

OSMOLALITY (serum)

Normal range: 280-300 mOsm/kg (280-300 mmol/kg [CF: 1; SMI: 1 mmol/kg])

It can also be estimated by the following formula:

$$2([Na] + [K]) + glucose/18 + BUN/2.8$$

Elevated in: Dehydration, hypernatremia, diabetes insipidus, uremia, hyperglycemia, mannitol therapy, ingestion of toxins (ethylene glycol, methanol, ethanol), hypercalcemia, diuretics

Decreased in: Syndrome of inappropriate diuretic hormone secretion, hyponatremia, overhydration, Addison's disease, hypothyroidism

OSMOLALITY, URINE

See URINE OSMOLALITY

OSMOTIC FRAGILITY TEST

Normal: Hemolysis begins at 0.50, w/v [5.0 g/L] and is complete at 0.30, w/v [3.0 g/L] NaCl.

TABLE 4-18 Drugs that Cause Neutropenia

Antiarrhythmics
- Tocainide, procainamide, propranolol, quinidine

Antibiotics
- Chloramphenicol, penicillins, sulfonamides, p-aminosalicylic acid (PAS), rifampin, vancomycin, isoniazid, nitrofurantoin

Antimalarials
- Dapsone, quinine, pyrimethamine

Anticonvulsants
- Phenytoin, mephenytoin, trimethadione, ethosuximide, carbamazepine

Hypoglycemic agents
- Tolbutamide, chlorpropamide

Antihistamines
- Cimetidine, brompheniramine, tripelennamine

Antihypertensives
- Methyldopa, captopril

Antiinflammatory agents
- Aminopyrine, phenylbutazone, gold salts, ibuprofen, indomethacin

Antithyroid agents
- Propylthiouracil, methimazole, thiouracil

Diuretics
- Acetazolamide, hydrochlorothiazide, chlorthalidone

Phenothiazines
- Chlorpromazine, promazine, prochlorperazine

Immunosuppressive agents
- Antimetabolites

Cytotoxic agents
- Alkylating agents, antimetabolites, anthracyclines, Vinca alkaloids, cisplatin, hydroxyurea, dactinomycin

Other agents
- Recombinant interferons, allopurinol, ethanol, levamisole, penicillamine, zidovudine, streptokinase, carbamazepine, clopidogrel, ticlopidine

Modified from Goldman L, Ausiello D (eds): *Cecil textbook of medicine,* ed 22, Philadelphia, 2004, WB Saunders.

Elevated in: Hereditary spherocytosis, hereditary stomatocytosis, spherocytosis associated with acquired immune hemolytic anemia
Decreased in: Iron deficiency anemia, thalassemias, liver disease, leptocytosis associated with asplenia

PARACENTESIS FLUID

Testing and evaluation of results:
1. Process the fluid as follows:
   a. Tube 1: LDH, glucose, albumin
   b. Tube 2: protein, specific gravity
   c. Tube 3: cell count and differential
   d. Tube 4: save until further notice
2. Draw serum LDH, protein, albumin.
3. Gram stain, AFB stain, bacterial and fungal cultures, amylase, and triglycerides should be ordered only when clearly indicated; bedside inoculation of blood-culture bottles with ascitic fluid improves sensitivity in detecting bacterial growth.
4. If malignant ascites is suspected, consider a carcinoembryonic antigen level on the paracentesis fluid and cytologic evaluation.
5. In suspected spontaneous bacterial peritonitis (SBP) the incidence of positive cultures can be increased by injecting 10 to 20 ml of ascitic fluid into blood culture bottles.
6. Peritoneal effusion can be subdivided as exudative or transudative based on its characteristics (see Section II).
7. The serum-ascites albumin gradient (serum albumin level–ascitic fluid albumin level) correlates directly with portal pressure and can also be used to classify ascite. Patients with gradients $\geq$1.1 g/dl have portal hypertension, and those with gradients $\leq$1.1 g/dl do not; the accuracy of this method is $>$95%.
8. For the differential diagnosis of ascites, refer to Section II.
9. An ascitic fluid polymorphonuclear leukocyte count $>500/\mu l$ is suggestive of SBP.
10. A blood-ascitic fluid albumin gradient.

PARIETAL CELL ANTIBODIES

Normal: Negative
Present in: Pernicious anemia ($>$90%), atrophic gastritis (up to 50%), thyroiditis (30%), Addison's disease, myasthenia gravis, Sjögren's syndrome, type 1 DM

PARTIAL THROMBOPLASTIN TIME (PTT), ACTIVATED PARTIAL THROMBOPLASTIN TIME (APTT)

Normal range: 25-41 sec
Elevated in: Heparin therapy, coagulation factor deficiency (I, II, V, VIII, IX, X, XI, XII), liver disease, vitamin K deficiency, disseminated intravascular coagulation, circulating anticoagulant, warfarin therapy, specific factor inhibition (PCN reaction, rheumatoid arthritis), thrombolytic therapy, nephrotic syndrome

NOTE: Useful to evaluate the intrinsic coagulation system.

PEPSINOGEN I

Normal: 124-142 ng/ml
Elevated in: ZE syndrome, duodenal ulcer, acute gastritis
Decreased in: Atrophic gastritis, gastric carcinoma, myxedema, pernicious anemia, Addison's disease

pH, BLOOD

Normal values:
Arterial: 7.35-7.45
Venous: 7.32-7.42

For abnormal values, refer to ARTERIAL BLOOD GASES.

pH, URINE

See URINE pH

PHENOBARBITAL

Normal therapeutic range: 15-30 mcg/ml for epilepsy control

PHENYTOIN (Dilantin)

Normal therapeutic range: 10-20 mcg/ml

PHOSPHATASE, ACID

See ACID PHOSPHATASE

PHOSPHATASE, ALKALINE

See ALKALINE PHOSPHATASE

PHOSPHATE (serum)

Normal range: 2.5-5 mg/dl (0.8-1.6 mmol/L [CF: 0.3229; SMI: 0.05 mmol/L])

DECREASED
Parenteral hyperalimentation
Diabetic acidosis
Alcohol withdrawal
Severe metabolic or respiratory alkalosis
Antacids that bind phosphorus
Malnutrition with refeeding using low-phosphorus nutrients
Renal tubule failure to reabsorb phosphate (Fanconi's syndrome; congenital disorder; vitamin D deficiency)
Glucose administration
Nasogastric suction
Malabsorption
Gram-negative sepsis
Primary hyperthyroidism
Chlorothiazide diuretics
Therapy of acute severe asthma
Acute respiratory failure with mechanical ventilation

INCREASED
Renal failure
Severe muscle injury
Phosphate-containing antacids
Hypoparathyroidism
Tumor lysis syndrome

PLATELET AGGREGATION

Normal: Full aggregation (generally $>$60%) in response to epinephrine, thrombin, ristocetin, ADP, collagen
Elevated in: Heparin, hemolysis, lipemia, nicotine, hereditary and acquired disorders of platelet adhesion, activation, and aggregation
Decreased in: Aspirin, some penicillins, chloroquine, chlorpromazine, clofibrate, captopril, Glanzmann's thrombasthenia, Bernard-Soulier syndrome, Wiskott-Aldrich syndrome, cyclooxygenase deficiency. In von Willebrand's disease there is normal aggregation with ADP, collagen, and epinephrine but abnormal agglutination with ristocetin.

PLATELET ANTIBODIES

Normal: Absent
Present in: ITP ($>$90% of patients with chronic ITP). Patients with nonimmune thrombocytopenias may have false-positive results.

PLATELET COUNT

Normal range: 130-400 $\times$ $10^3/mm^3$ (130-400 $\times$ $10^9/L$ [CF: 1; SMI: 5 $\times$ $10^9/L$])
Elevated in:

REACTIVE THROMBOCYTOSIS
Infections or inflammatory states—vasculitis, allergic reactions, etc.
Surgery and tissue damage—myocardial infarction, pancreatitis, etc.
Postsplenectomy state
Malignancy—solid tumors, lymphoma
Iron deficiency anemia, hemolytic anemia, acute blood loss
Uncertain etiology
Rebound effect after chemotherapy or immune thrombocytopenia
Renal disorders—renal failure, nephrotic syndrome

MYELOPROLIFERATIVE DISORDERS
Chronic myeloid leukemia
Primary thrombocythemia

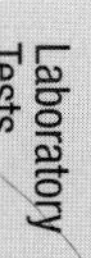

Polycythemia vera
Idiopathic myelofibrosis
Decreased:

A. Increased destruction
  1. Immunologic
    a. Drugs: quinine, quinidine, digitalis, procainamide, thiazide diuretics, sulfonamides, phenytoin, aspirin, penicillin, heparin, gold, meprobamate, sulfa drugs, phenylbutazone, NSAIDs, methyldopa, cimetidine, furosemide, INH, cephalosporins, chlorpropamide, organic arsenicals, chloroquine
    b. Idiopathic thrombocytopenic purpura
    c. Transfusion reaction: transfusion of platelets with platelet antigen HPA-1a (PL^{A1}) in recipients without PL^{A1}
    d. Fetal/maternal incompatibility
    e. Vasculitis (e.g., systemic lupus erythematosus)
    f. Autoimmune hemolytic anemia
    g. Lymphoreticular disorders (e.g., chronic lymphocytic leukemia)
  2. Nonimmunologic
    a. Prosthetic heart valves
    b. Thrombotic thrombocytopenic purpura
    c. Sepsis
    d. Disseminated intravascular coagulation
    e. Hemolytic-uremic syndrome
    f. Giant cavernous hemangioma
B. Decreased production
  1. Abnormal marrow
    a. Marrow infiltration (e.g., leukemia, lymphoma, fibrosis)
    b. Marrow suppression (e.g., chemotherapy, alcohol, radiation)
  2. Hereditary disorders
    a. Wiskott-Aldrich syndrome: X-linked disorder characterized by thrombocytopenia, eczema, and repeated infections
    b. May-Hegglin anomaly: increased megakaryocytes but ineffective thrombopoiesis
  3. Vitamin deficiencies (e.g., vitamin B_{12}, folic acid)
C. Splenic sequestration, hypersplenism
D. Dilutional, secondary to massive transfusion

POTASSIUM (serum)

Normal range: 3.5-5 mEq/L (3.5-5 mmol/L [CF: 1; SMI: 0.1 mmol/L])

CAUSES OF HYPERKALEMIA

I. Pseudohyperkalemia
  A. Hemolysis of sample
  B. Thrombocytosis
  C. Leukocytosis
  D. Laboratory error
II. Increased potassium intake and absorption
  A. Potassium supplements (oral and parenteral)
  B. Dietary—salt substitutes
  C. Stored blood
  D. Potassium-containing medications
III. Impaired renal excretion
  A. Acute renal failure
  B. Chronic renal failure
  C. Tubular defect in potassium secretion
    1. Renal allograft
    2. Analgesic nephropathy
    3. Sickle cell disease
    4. Obstructive uropathy
    5. Interstitial nephritis
    6. Chronic pyelonephritis
    7. Potassium-sparing diuretics
    8. Miscellaneous (lead, systemic lupus erythematosus, pseudohypoaldosteronism)
  D. Hypoaldosteronism
    1. Primary (Addison's disease)
    2. Secondary
      a. Hyporeninemic hypoaldosteronism (type IV RTA)
      b. Congenital adrenal hyperplasia
      c. Drug-induced
        (1) NSAIDs
        (2) ACE inhibitors
        (3) Heparin
        (4) Cyclosporine
IV. Transcellular shifts
  A. Acidosis
  B. Hypertonicity
  C. Insulin deficiency
  D. Drugs
    1. β-blockers
    2. Digitalis toxicity
    3. Succinylcholine
  E. Exercise
  F. Hyperkalemic periodic paralysis
V. Cellular injury
  A. Rhabdomyolysis
  B. Severe intravascular hemolysis
  C. Acute tumor lysis syndrome
  D. Burns and crush injuries

CAUSES OF HYPOKALEMIA

I. Decreased intake
  A. Decreased dietary potassium
  B. Impaired absorption of potassium
  C. Clay ingestion
  D. Kayexalate
II. Increased loss
  A. Renal
    1. Hyperaldosteronism
      a. Primary
        (1) Conn's syndrome
        (2) Adrenal hyperplasia
      b. Secondary
        (1) Congestive heart failure
        (2) Cirrhosis
        (3) Nephrotic syndrome
        (4) Dehydration
      c. Bartter's syndrome
    2. Glycyrrhizic acid (licorice, chewing tobacco)
    3. Excessive adrenal corticosteroids
      a. Cushing's syndrome
      b. Steroid therapy
      c. Adrenogenital syndrome
    4. Renal tubular defects
      a. Renal tubular acidosis
      b. Obstructive uropathy
      c. Salt-wasting nephropathy
    5. Drugs
      a. Diuretics
      b. Aminoglycosides
      c. Mannitol
      d. Amphotericin
      e. Cisplatin
      f. Carbenicillin
  B. Gastrointestinal
    1. Vomiting
    2. Nasogastric suction
    3. Diarrhea
    4. Malabsorption
    5. Ileostomy
    6. Villous adenoma
    7. Laxative abuse
  C. Increased losses from the skin
    1. Excessive sweating
    2. Burns
III. Transcellular shifts
  A. Alkalosis
    1. Vomiting
    2. Diuretics

3. Hyperventilation
4. Bicarbonate therapy
B. Insulin
1. Exogenous
2. Endogenous response to glucose
C. β_2-Agonists (albuterol, terbutaline, epinephrine)
D. Hypokalemia periodic paralysis
1. Familial
2. Thyrotoxic
IV. Miscellaneous
A. Anabolic state
B. Intravenous hyperalimentation
C. Treatment of megaloblastic anemia
D. Acute mountain sickness

POTASSIUM, URINE

See URINE POTASSIUM

PROCAINAMIDE

Normal therapeutic range: 4-10 mcg/ml

PROGESTERONE (serum)

Normal:
Female: Follicular phase: 15-70 ng/dl
Luteal phase: 200-2500 ng/dl
Male: 15-70 ng/dl
Elevated in: Congenital adrenal hyperplasia, clomiphene, corticosterone, 11-deoxycortisol, dihydroprogesterone, molar pregnancy, lipoid ovarian tumor
Decreased in: Primary or secondary hypogonadism, oral contraceptives, ampicillin, threatened abortion

PROLACTIN

Normal range: <20 ng/ml (<20 μg/L [CF: 1; SMI: 1 μg/L])
Elevated in: Prolactinomas (level >200 highly suggestive), drugs (phenothiazines, cimetidine, tricyclic antidepressants, metoclopramide, estrogens, antihypertensives [methyldopa], verapamil, haloperidol), postpartum, stress, hypoglycemia, hypothyroidism

PROSTATE-SPECIFIC ANTIGEN (PSA)

Normal range: 0-4 ng/ml

Table 4-19 describes age-specific reference ranges for PSA.

Elevated in: Benign prostatic hypertrophy, carcinoma of prostate, postrectal examination, prostate trauma.

Factors affecting serum PSA are described in Table 4-20.

NOTE: Measurement of free PSA is useful to assess the probability of prostate cancer in patients with normal digital rectal examination and total PSA between 4 and 10 ng/ml. In these patients, the global risk of prostate cancer is 25%; however, if the free PSA is >25%, the risk of prostate cancer decreases to 8%, whereas if the free PSA is <10%, the risk of cancer increases to 56%. Free PSA is also useful to evaluate the aggressiveness of prostate cancer. A low free PSA percentage generally indicates a high-grade cancer, whereas a high free PSA percentage is generally associated with a slower growing tumor.

Decreased in: Finasteride therapy, dutasteride therapy, saw palmetto use, bedrest, antiandrogens

TABLE 4-19 Age-Specific Reference Ranges for PSA

	Serum PSA (ng/ml)		
Age (yr)	**Whites**	**Japanese**	**African Americans**
40-49	0-2.5	0-2.0	0-2.0
50-59	0-3.5	0-3.0	0-4.0
60-69	0-4.5	0-4.0	0-4.5
70-79	0-6.5	0-5.0	0-5.5

Reprinted from Nseyo UO (ed): *Urology for primary care physicians,* Philadelphia, 1999, WB Saunders.
PSA, Prostate-specific antigen.

TABLE 4-20 Factors Affecting Serum PSA

Factors Affecting Serum PSA	Duration of Effect
Prostate cell number	NA
Prostate size	NA
Recent ejaculation	6-48 hours
Prostate manipulation	
Vigorous massage	1 week
Cystoscopy	1 week
Prostate biopsy	4-6 weeks
Prostatitis	
Acute	3-6 months
Chronic	Unknown
Prostate cancer	NA
Drugs: finasteride (Proscar)*	3-6 months

Reprinted from Nseyo UO (ed): *Urology for primary care physicians,* Philadelphia, 1999, WB Saunders.
NA, Not applicable; *PSA,* prostate-specific antigen.
*Lowers PSA for as long as patient is on the medication.

PROSTATIC ACID PHOSPHATASE

Normal: 0-0.8 U/L
Elevated in: Prostate cancer (especially in metastatic prostate cancer), BPH, prostatitis, post–prostate surgery or manipulation, hemolysis, androgens, clofibrate
Decreased in: Ketoconazole

PROTEIN (SERUM)

Normal range: 6-8 g/dl (60-80 g/L [CF: 10; SMI: 1 g/L])
Elevated in: Dehydration, multiple myeloma, Waldenström's macroglobulinemia, sarcoidosis, collagen vascular diseases
Decreased in: Malnutrition, low-protein diet, overhydration, malabsorption, pregnancy, severe burns, neoplasms, chronic diseases, cirrhosis, nephrosis

PROTEIN C ASSAY

Normal: 70%-140%
Elevated in: Oral contraceptives, stanozol
Decreased in: Congenital protein C deficiency, warfarin therapy, Vitamin K deficiency, renal insufficiency, consumptive coagulopathies

PROTEIN ELECTROPHORESIS (serum)

Normal range:
Albumin: 60%-75% (0.6-0.75 [CF: 0.01; SMI: 0.01])
α-1: 1.7%-5% (0.02-0.05)
α-2: 6.7%-12.5% (0.07-0.13)
β: 8.3%-16.3% (0.08-0.16)
γ: 10.7%-20% (0.11-0.2)
Albumin: 3.6-5.2 g/dl (36-52 g/L [CF: 0.01; SMI: 1 g/L])
α-1: 0.1-0.4 g/dl (1-4 g/L)
α-2: 0.4-1 g/dl (4-10 g/L)
β: 0.5-1.2 g/dl (5-12 g/L)
γ: 0.6-1.6 g/dl (6-16 g/L)
Elevated in:
Albumin: dehydration
α-1: neoplastic diseases, inflammation
α-2: neoplasms, inflammation, infection, nephrotic syndrome

β: hypothyroidism, biliary cirrhosis, diabetes mellitus
γ: See IMMUNOGLOBULINS

Decreased in:

Albumin: malnutrition, chronic liver disease, malabsorption, nephrotic syndrome, burns, systemic lupus erythematosus
α-1: emphysema (α-1 antitrypsin deficiency), nephrosis
α-2: hemolytic anemias (decreased haptoglobin), severe hepatocellular damage
β: hypocholesterolemia, nephrosis
γ: See IMMUNOGLOBULINS

Fig. 4-12 describes serum protein electrophoretic patterns.

PROTEIN S ASSAY

Normal: 65%-140%

Elevated in: Presence of lupus anticoagulant

Decreased in: Hereditary deficiency, acute thrombotic events, DIC, surgery, oral contraceptives, pregnancy, hormone replacement therapy, L-asparaginase treatment

PROTHROMBIN TIME (PT)

Normal range: 10-12 sec

Elevated in: Liver disease, oral anticoagulants (warfarin), heparin, factor deficiency (I, II, V, VII, X), disseminated intravascular coagulation, vitamin K deficiency, afibrinogenemia, dysfibrinogenemia, drugs (salicylate, chloral hydrate, diphenylhydantoin, estrogens, antacids, phenylbutazone, quinidine, antibiotics, allopurinol, anabolic steroids)

Decreased in: Vitamin K supplementation, thrombophlebitis, drugs (glutethimide, estrogens, griseofulvin, diphenhydramine)

PROTOPORPHYRIN (free erythrocyte)

Normal range: 16-36 μg/dl of red blood cells (0.28-0.64 μmol/L [CF: 0.0177; SMI: 0.02 μmol/L])

Elevated in: Iron deficiency, lead poisoning, sideroblastic anemias, anemia of chronic disease, hemolytic anemias, erythropoietic protoporphyria

PSA

See PROSTATE-SPECIFIC ANTIGEN

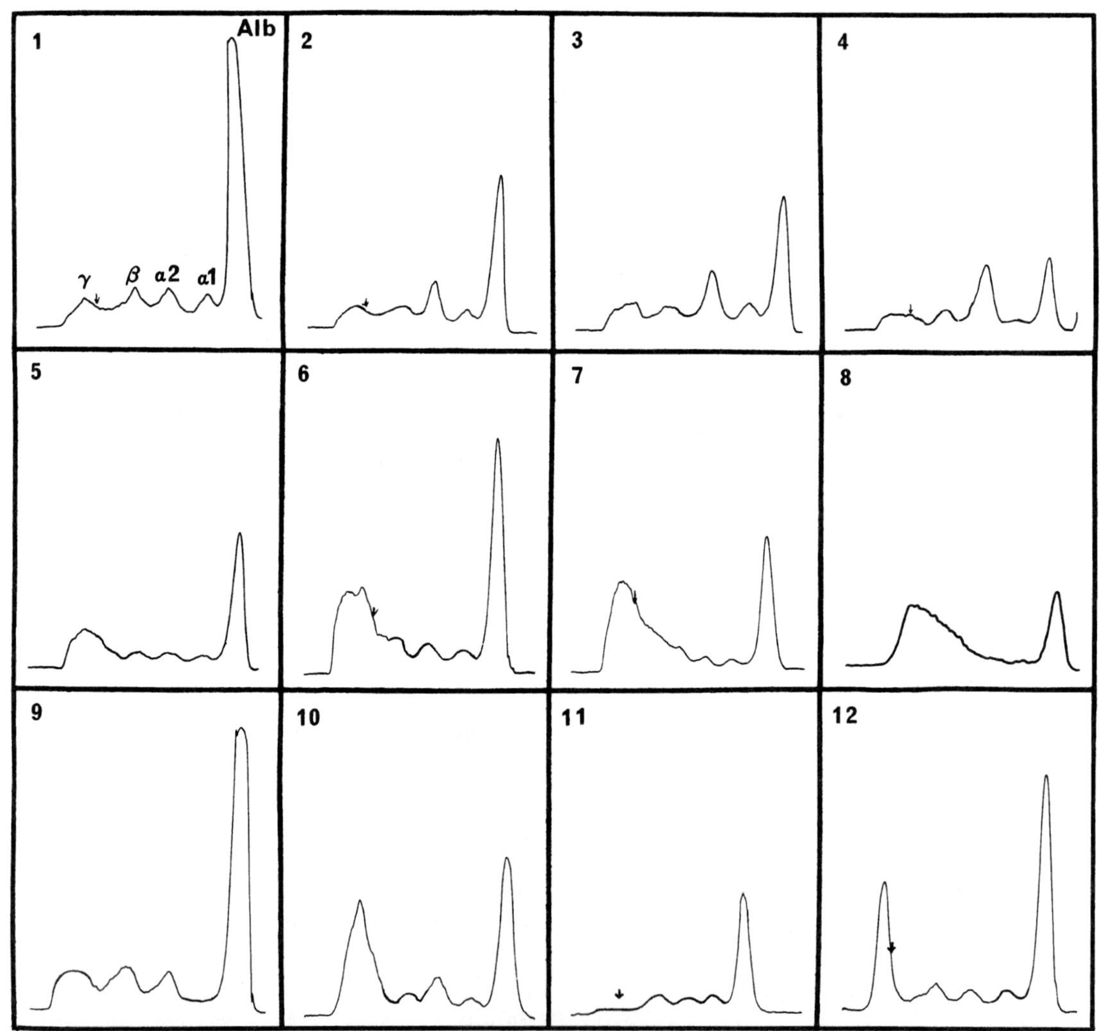

FIGURE 4-12 Typical serum protein electrophoretic patterns. *1,* Normal (*arrow* near γ region indicates serum application point). *2,* Acute reaction pattern. *3,* Acute reaction or nephrotic syndrome. *4,* Nephrotic syndrome. *5,* Chronic inflammation, cirrhosis, granulomatous diseases, rheumatoid-collagen group. *6,* Same as 5, but γ elevation is more pronounced. There is also partial (but not complete) β-γ fusion. *7,* Suggestive of cirrhosis but could be found in the granulomatous diseases or the rheumatoid-collagen group. *8,* Characteristic pattern of cirrhosis. *9,* α-1 Antitrypsin deficiency with mild γ elevation suggesting concurrent chronic disease. *10,* Same as 5, but the γ elevation is marked. The configuration of the γ peak superficially mimics that of myeloma, but is more broad-based. There are superimposed acute reaction changes. *11,* Hypogammaglobulinemia or light-chain myeloma. *12,* Myeloma, Waldenström's macroglobulinemia, idiopathic or secondary monoclonal gammopathy. (Reprinted from Ravel R [ed]: *Clinical laboratory medicine,* ed 6, St Louis, 1995, Mosby.)

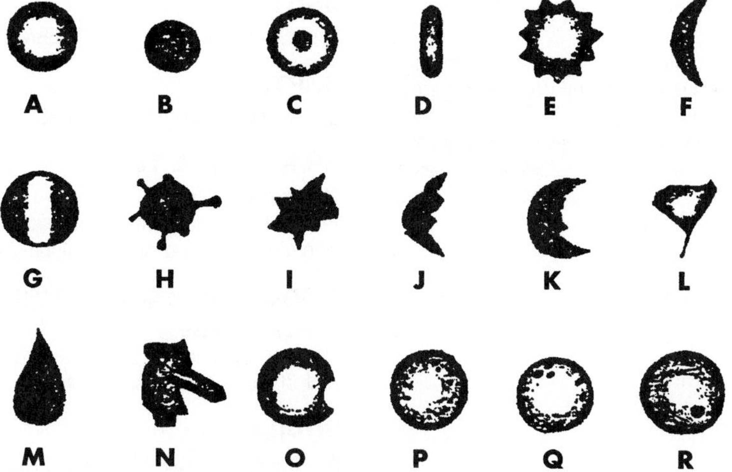

FIGURE 4-13 Abnormal red blood cells (RBCs). A, Normal RBC. **B,** Spherocyte. **C,** Target cell. **D,** Elliptocyte. **E,** Echinocyte. **F,** Sickle cell. **G,** Stomatocyte. **H,** Acanthocyte. **I** to **L,** Schistocytes. **M,** Teardrop RBC. **N,** Distorted RBC with Hb C crystal protruding. **O,** Degmacyte. **P,** Basophilic stippling. **Q,** Pappenheimer bodies. **R,** Howell-Jolly body. (Reprinted from Ravel R [ed]: *Clinical laboratory medicine,* ed 6, St Louis, 1995, Mosby.)

PT
See PROTHROMBIN TIME

PTT
See PARTIAL THROMBOPLASTIN TIME

RDW
See RED BLOOD CELL DISTRIBUTION WIDTH

RED BLOOD CELL (RBC) COUNT
Normal range:
Male: 4.3-5.9 $\times$ 10^6/mm^3 (4.3-5.9 $\times$ 10^{12}/L [CF: 1; SMI: 0.1 $\times$ 10^{12}/L])
Female: 3.5-5 $\times$ 10^6/mm^3 (3.5-5 $\times$ 10^{12}/L [CF: 1; SMI: 0.1 $\times$ 10^{12}/L])
Elevated in: Polycythemia vera, smokers, high altitude, cardiovascular disease, renal cell carcinoma and other erythropoietin-producing neoplasms, stress, hemoconcentration/dehydration
Decreased in: Anemias, hemolysis, chronic renal failure, hemorrhage, failure of marrow production

RED BLOOD CELL DISTRIBUTION WIDTH (RDW)
Measures variability of red cell size (anisocytosis)
Normal range: 11.5-14.5
Normal RDW and elevated mean corpuscular volume (MCV): Aplastic anemia, preleukemia
Normal MCV: Normal, anemia of chronic disease, acute blood loss or hemolysis, chronic lymphocytic leukemia (CLL), chronic myelocytic leukemia, nonanemic enzymopathy or hemoglobinopathy
Decreased MCV: Anemia of chronic disease, heterozygous thalassemia
Elevated RDW and elevated MCV: Vitamin B_{12} deficiency, folate deficiency, immune hemolytic anemia, cold agglutinins, CLL with high count, liver disease
Normal MCV: Early iron deficiency, early vitamin B_{12} deficiency, early folate deficiency, anemic globinopathy
Decreased MCV: Iron deficiency, red blood cell fragmentation, HbH disease, thalassemia intermedia

RED BLOOD CELL FOLATE
See FOLATE

RED BLOOD CELL MASS (volume)
Normal range:
Male: 20-36 ml/kg body weight (1.15-1.21 L/m^2 body surface area)
Female: 19-31 ml/kg body weight (0.95-1.00 L/m^2 body surface area)
Elevated in: Polycythemia vera, hypoxia (smokers, high altitude, cardiovascular disease), hemoglobinopathies with high oxygen affinity, erythropoietin-producing tumors (renal cell carcinoma)
Decreased in: Hemorrhage, chronic disease, failure of marrow production, anemias, hemolysis

RED BLOOD CELL MORPHOLOGY
See Fig. 4-13.

RENIN (serum)
Elevated in: Drugs (thiazides, estrogen, minoxidil), chronic renal failure, Bartter's syndrome, pregnancy (normal), pheochromocytoma, renal hypertension, reduced plasma volume, secondary aldosteronism
Decreased in: Adrenocortical hypertension, increased plasma volume, primary aldosteronism, drugs (propranolol, reserpine, clonidine)

Table 4-21 describes typical renin-aldosterone patterns in various conditions.

TABLE 4-21 Typical Renin-Aldosterone Patterns in Various Conditions

	Plasma Renin	Aldosterone
Primary aldosteronism	Low	High
"Low-renin" essential hypertension	Low	Normal
Cushing's syndrome	Low	Low-normal
Licorice ingestion syndrome	Low	Low
High-salt diet	Low	Low
Oral contraceptives	High	Normal
Cirrhosis	High	High
Malignant hypertension	High	High
Unilateral renal disease	High	High
"High-renin" essential hypertension	High	High
Pregnancy	High	High
Diuretic overuse	High	High
Juxtaglomerular tumor (Bartter's syndrome)	High	High
Low-salt diet	High	High
Addison's disease	High	Low
Hypokalemia	High	Low

Reprinted from Ravel R: *Clinical laboratory medicine,* ed 6, St Louis, 1995, Mosby.

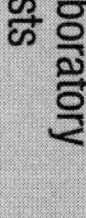

RETICULOCYTE COUNT

Normal range: 0.5%-1.5%
Elevated in: Hemolytic anemia (sickle cell crisis, thalassemia major, autoimmune hemolysis), hemorrhage, postanemia therapy (folic acid, ferrous sulfate, vitamin B_{12}), chronic renal failure
Decreased in: Aplastic anemia, marrow suppression (sepsis, chemotherapeutic agents, radiation), hepatic cirrhosis, blood transfusion, anemias of disordered maturation (iron deficiency anemia, megaloblastic anemia, sideroblastic anemia, anemia of chronic disease)

RHEUMATOID FACTOR

Normal: Negative. Present in titer >1:20
RHEUMATIC DISEASES
Rheumatoid arthritis
Sjögren's syndrome
Systemic lupus erythematosus
Polymyositis/dermatomyositis
Mixed connective tissue disease
Scleroderma
INFECTIOUS DISEASES
Subacute bacterial endocarditis
Tuberculosis
Infectious mononucleosis
Hepatitis
Syphilis
Leprosy
Influenza
MALIGNANCIES
Lymphoma
Multiple myeloma
Waldenström's macroglobulinemia
Postradiation or postchemotherapy
MISCELLANEOUS
Normal adults, especially the elderly
Sarcoidosis
Chronic pulmonary disease (interstitial fibrosis)
Chronic liver disease (chronic active hepatitis, cirrhosis)
Mixed essential cryoglobulinemia
Hypergammaglobulinemic purpura

RNP

See EXTRACTABLE NUCLEAR ANTIGEN

ROTAVIRUS SEROLOGY

Test description: PCR test is performed on stool specimen
Normal: Negative

SEDIMENTATION RATE

See ERYTHROCYTE SEDIMENTATION RATE

SEMEN ANALYSIS

Table 4-22 describes semen analysis reference ranges.

TABLE 4-22 Semen Analysis Reference Ranges

Color	Grayish white
pH	7.3-7.8 (literature range, 7.0-7.8)
Volume	2.0-5.0 ml (literature range, 1.5-6.0 ml)
Sperm count	20-250 million/ml (literature range for upper limit varies from 100-250 million/ml)
Motility	>60% motile <3 hours after specimen is obtained (literature range, >40% to >70%)
% Normal sperm	>60% (literature range, >60% to >70%)
Viscosity	Can be poured from a pipet in droplets rather than a thick strand

From Ravel R (ed): *Clinical laboratory medicine,* ed 6, St Louis, 1995, Mosby.

SGOT

See ASPARTATE AMINOTRANSFERASE

SGPT

See ALANINE AMINOTRANSFERASE

SICKLE CELL TEST

Normal: Negative
Positive in: Sickle cell anemia, sickle cell trait, combination of *Hb S* gene with other disorders such as alpha-thalassemia, beta-thalassemia.

SMOOTH MUSCLE ANTIBODY

Normal: Negative
Present in: Chronic acute hepatitis (≥1:80), primary biliary cirrhosis (≤1:80), infectious mononucleosis

SODIUM (serum)

Normal range: 135-147 mEq/L (135-147 mmol/L [CF: 1; SMI: 1 mmol/L])
HYPONATREMIA
A. Sodium and water depletion (deficit hyponatremia)
  1. Loss of gastrointestinal secretions with replacement of fluid but not electrolytes
     a. Vomiting
     b. Diarrhea
     c. Tube drainage
  2. Loss from skin with replacement of fluids but not electrolytes
     a. Excessive sweating
     b. Extensive burns
  3. Loss from kidney
     a. Diuretics
     b. Chronic renal insufficiency (uremia) with acidosis
  4. Metabolic loss
     a. Starvation with acidosis
     b. Diabetic acidosis
  5. Endocrine loss
     a. Addison's disease
     b. Sudden withdrawal of long-term steroid therapy
  6. Iatrogenic loss from serous cavities
     a. Paracentesis or thoracentesis
B. Excessive water (dilution hyponatremia)
  1. Excessive water administration
  2. Congestive heart failure
  3. Cirrhosis
  4. Nephrotic syndrome
  5. Hypoalbuminemia (severe)
  6. Acute renal failure with oliguria
C. Inappropriate antidiuretic hormone (IADH) syndrome
D. Intracellular loss (reset osmostat syndrome)
E. False hyponatremia (actually a dilutional effect)
  1. Marked hypertriglyceridemia
  2. Marked hyperproteinemia
  3. Severe hyperglycemia

HYPERNATREMIA
Dehydration is the most frequent overall clinical finding in hypernatremia.
1. Deficient water intake (either orally or intravenously)
2. Excess kidney water output (diabetes insipidus, osmotic diuresis)
3. Excess skin water output (excess sweating, loss from burns)
4. Excess gastrointestinal tract output (severe protracted vomiting or diarrhea without fluid therapy)
5. Accidental sodium overdose
6. High-protein tube feedings

STREPTOZYME

See ANTISTREPTOLYSIN O TITER

SUCROSE HEMOLYSIS TEST (sugar water test)

Normal: Absence of hemolysis

Positive in:

Paroxysmal nocturnal hemoglobinuria

False-positive: autoimmune hemolytic anemia, megaloblastic anemias

False-negative: may occur with use of heparin or EDTA

SUDAN III STAIN (qualitative screening for fecal fat)

Normal: Negative. Test should be preceded by diet containing 100-150 g of dietary fat/day for 1 week, avoidance of high-fiber diet, and avoidance of suppositories or oily material before specimen collection.

Positive in: Steatorrhea, use of castor oil or mineral oil droplets

SYNOVIAL FLUID ANALYSIS

Table 4-23 describes the classification and interpretation of synovial fluid analysis.

T_3 (triiodothyronine)

See Table 4-24 for T_3 abnormalities.

Normal range: 75-220 ng/dl (1.2-3.4 nmol/L [CF: 0.01536; SMI: 0.1 nmol/L])

Abnormal values:

A. Elevated in hyperthyroidism (usually earlier and to a greater extent than serum T_4).

B. Useful in diagnosing:
   1. T_3 hyperthyroidism (thyrotoxicosis): increased T_3, normal FTI.
   2. Toxic nodular goiter: increased T_3, normal or increased T_4.
   3. Iodine deficiency: normal T_3, possibly decreased T_4.
   4. Thyroid replacement therapy with liothyronine (Cytomel): normal T_4, increased T_3 if patient is symptomatically hyperthyroid.

Not ordered routinely but indicated when hyperthyroidism is suspected and serum free T_4 or FTI inconclusive.

T_3 RESIN UPTAKE (T_3RU)

Normal range: 25%-35%

Abnormal values: Increased in hyperthyroidism. T_3 resin uptake (T_3RU or RT_3U) measures the percentage of free T_4 (not bound to protein); it does not measure serum T_3 concentration; T_3RU and other tests that reflect thyroid hormone binding to plasma protein are also known as *thyroid hormone-binding ratios* (THBR).

T_4, FREE (free thyroxine)

Normal range: 0.8-2.8 ng/dl

Elevated in:

Graves' disease, toxic multinodular goiter, toxic adenoma, iatrogenic and factitious causes, transient hyperthyroidism

Serum free T_4 directly measures unbound thyroxine. Free T_4 can be measured by equilibrium dialysis (gold standard of free T_4 assays) or by

TABLE 4-23 Classification and Interpretation of Synovial Fluid Analysis

Group	Diseases	Appearance	Viscosity	Mucin Clot	WBC/mm^3	% PMN	Glucose (mg/dl) (Blood-Synovial Fluid)	Protein (g/dl)
Normal	—	Clear	↑	Firm	<200	<25	<10	<2.5
I (noninflammatory)	Osteoarthritis, aseptic necrosis, traumatic arthritis, erythema nodosum, osteochondritis dissecans	Clear, yellow (may be xanthochromic if traumatic arthritis)	↑	Firm	↑ Up to 10,000	<25	<10	<2.5
II (inflammatory)	Crystal-induced arthritis, rheumatoid arthritis, Reiter's syndrome, collagen vascular disease, psoriatic arthritis, serum sickness, rheumatic fever	Clear, yellow, turbid	↓	Friable	↑↑ Up to 100,000	40-90	<40	>2.5
III (septic)	Bacterial (staphylococcal, gonococcal, tuberculosis)	Turbid	↓/↑	Friable	↑↑↑ Up to 5 million	40-100	20-100	>2.5

↑, Elevated; ↑↑, markedly high; ↓, decreased; *PMN*, polymorphonuclear leukocytes. Note that there is considerable overlap in the numbers listed above.

TABLE 4-24 Findings in Thyroid Function Tests in Various Clinical Conditions

TRH Condition	T_4	FT$_4$I	T_3	FT$_3$I	TSH	TSI	Stimulation
Hyperthyroidism							
Graves' disease	↑	↑	↑	↑	↓	+	↓
Toxic nodular goiter	↑	↑	↑	↑	↓	−	↓
Pituitary TSH-secreting tumors	↑	↑	↑	↑	↑	−	↓
T_3 thyrotoxicosis	N	N	↑	↑	↓	+, −	↓
T_4 thyrotoxicosis	↑	↑	N	N	↓	+, −	↓
Hypothyroidism							
Primary	↓	↓	↓	↓	↑	+, −	↑
Secondary	↓	↓	↓	↓	↓ N	−	↓
Tertiary	↓	↓	↓	↓	↓, N	−	N
Peripheral unresponsiveness	↑, N	↑, N	↑, N	↑	↑, N	−	N, ↑

Reprinted from Tilton RC, Barrows A: *Clinical laboratory medicine,* St Louis, 1992, Mosby.
N, Normal; ↑, increased; ↓, decreased; +, − variable.

immunometric techniques (influenced by serum levels of lipids, proteins, and certain drugs). The free thyroxine index (FTI) can also be easily calculated by multiplying T_4 times T_3RU and dividing the result by 100; the FTI corrects for any abnormal T_4 values secondary to protein binding: FTI = $T_4 \times T_3$RU/100.

Normal values equal 1.1 to 4.3.

T_4, SERUM T_4

Normal range: 0.8-2.8 ng/dl (10-36 pmol/L [CF: 12.87; SMI: 1 pmol/L])
Abnormal values: Serum thyroxine (T_4)
Elevated in:

1. Graves' disease
2. Toxic multinodular goiter
3. Toxic adenoma
4. Iatrogenic and factitious
5. Transient hyperthyroidism
   a. Subacute thyroiditis
   b. Hashimoto's thyroiditis
   c. Silent thyroiditis
6. Rare causes: hypersecretion of TSH (e.g., pituitary neoplasms), struma ovarii, ingestion of large amounts of iodine in a patient with preexisting thyroid hyperplasia or adenoma (Jod-Basedow phenomenon), hydatidiform mole, carcinoma of thyroid, amiodarone therapy of arrhythmias.

Serum thyroxine test measures both circulating thyroxine bound to protein (represents >99% of circulating T_4) and unbound (free) thyroxine. Values vary with protein binding; changes in the concentration of T_4 secondary to changes in thyroxine-binding globulin (TBG) can be caused by the following:

Increased TBG (↑ T_4)	*Decreased TBG (↓ T_4)*
Pregnancy	Androgens, glucocorticoids
Estrogens	Nephrotic syndrome, cirrhosis
Acute infectious hepatitis	Acromegaly
	Hypoproteinemia
Oral contraceptives	Familial
Familial	Phenytoin, ASA and other heroin, methadone, NSAIDs, high-dose penicillin, asparaginase
Fluorouracil, clofibrate	
	Chronic debilitating illness

To eliminate the suspected influence of protein binding on thyroxine values, two additional tests are available: T_3 resin uptake and serum free thyroxine.

TEGRETOL

See CARBAMAZEPINE and Table 4-24, under T_3 (Triiodothyronine).

TESTOSTERONE (total testosterone)

Normal range: Variable with age and sex
Serum/plasma
Males: 280-1100 ng/dl Females: 15-70 ng/dl
Urine
Males: 50-135 μg/day Females: 2-12 μg/day
Elevated in: Testicular tumors, ovarian masculinizing tumors
Decreased in: Hypogonadism

THEOPHYLLINE

Normal therapeutic range: 10-20 mcg/ml

THORACENTESIS FLUID

Testing and evaluation of results:

1. Pleural effusion fluid should be differentiated in exudate or transudate. The initial laboratory studies should be aimed only at distinguishing an exudate from a transudate.
   a. Tube 1: protein, LDH, albumin.
   b. Tubes 2, 3, 4: save the fluid until further notice. In selected patients with suspected empyema, a pH level may be useful (generally ≤7.0). See following for proper procedure to obtain a pH level from pleural fluid.

   NOTE: Do not order further tests until the presence of an exudate is confirmed on the basis of protein and LDH determinations (see Section III); however, if the results of protein and LDH determinations cannot be obtained within a reasonable time (resulting in unnecessary delay), additional laboratory tests should be ordered at the time of thoracentesis.
2. A serum/effusion albumin gradient of ≤1.2 g/dl is indicative of exudative effusions, especially in patients with congestive heart failure (CHF) treated with diuretics.
3. Note the appearance of the fluid:
   a. A grossly hemorrhagic effusion can be a result of a traumatic tap, neoplasm, or an embolus with infarction.
   b. A milky appearance indicates either of the following:
      (1) Chylous effusion: caused by trauma or tumor invasion of the thoracic duct; lipoprotein electrophoresis of the effusion reveals chylomicrons and triglyceride levels >115 mg/dl.
      (2) Pseudochylous effusion: often seen with chronic inflammation of the pleural space (e.g., TB, connective tissue diseases).
4. If transudate, consider CHF, cirrhosis, chronic renal failure, and other hypoproteinemic states and perform subsequent workup accordingly.
5. If exudate, consider ordering these tests on the pleural fluid:
   a. Cytologic examination for malignant cells (for suspected neoplasm).
   b. Gram stain, cultures (aerobic and anaerobic), and sensitivities (for suspected infectious process).
   c. AFB stain and cultures (for suspected TB).
   d. pH: a value <7.0 suggests parapneumonic effusion or empyema; a pleural fluid pH must be drawn anaerobically and iced immediately; the syringe should be prerinsed with 0.2 ml of 1:1000 heparin.
   e. Glucose: a low glucose level suggests parapneumonic effusions and rheumatoid arthritis.
   f. Amylase: a high amylase level suggests pancreatitis or ruptured esophagus.
   g. Perplexing pleural effusions are often a result of malignancy (e.g., lymphoma, malignant mesothelioma, ovarian carcinoma), TB, subdiaphragmatic processes, prior asbestos exposure, and postcardiac injury syndrome.

THROMBIN TIME (TT)

Normal range: 11.3-18.5 sec
Elevated in: Thrombolytic and heparin therapy, disseminated intravascular coagulation, hypofibrinogenemia, dysfibrinogenemia

THYROGLOBULIN

Normal: 3-40 ng/ml. Thyroglobulin is a tumor marker for monitoring the status of patients with papillary or follicular thyroid cancer following resection.
Elevated in: Papillary or follicular thyroid cancer, Hashimoto's thyroiditis, Graves' disease, subacute thyroiditis

THYROID MICROSOMAL ANTIBODIES

Normal: Undetectable. Low titers may be present in 5%-10% of normal individuals
Elevated in: Hashimoto's disease, thyroid carcinoma, early hypothyroidism, pernicious anemia

THYROID-STIMULATING HORMONE (TSH)

Normal range: 2-11 μU/ml (2-11 mU/L [CF: 1; SMI: 1 mU/L])
CONDITIONS THAT INCREASE SERUM THYROID-STIMULATING HORMONE VALUES
Laboratory error
Primary hypothyroidism
Synthroid therapy with insufficient dose
Lithium or amiodarone; some patients
Hashimoto's thyroiditis in later stage
Large doses of inorganic iodide (e.g., SSKI)

Severe nonthyroid illness in recovery phase
Iodine deficiency (moderate or severe)
Addison's disease
TSH specimen drawn in evening (peak of diurnal variation)
Pituitary TSH-secreting tumor
Therapy of hypothyroidism (3-6 wk after beginning therapy [range, 1-8 wk]; sometimes longer when pretherapy TSH is over 100 μU/ml)
Acute psychiatric illness
Peripheral resistance to T_4 syndrome
Antibodies (e.g., HAMA) interfering with monoclonal sandwich method of TSH assay
Telepaque (iopanoic acid) and Oragrafin (ipodate) x-ray contrast media
Amphetamines
High altitudes

CONDITIONS THAT DECREASE SERUM THYROID-STIMULATING HORMONE VALUES

Laboratory error
T_4/T_3 toxicosis (diffuse or nodular etiology)
Excessive therapy for hypothyroidism
Active thyroiditis (subacute, painless, or early active Hashimoto's disease)
Multinodular goiter containing areas of autonomy
Severe nonthyroid illness (especially acute trauma, dopamine, or glucocorticoid)
T_3 toxicosis
Pituitary insufficiency
Cushing's syndrome (and some patients on high-dose glucocorticoid)
Jod-Basedow (iodine-induced) hyperthyroidism
Thyroid-stimulating hormone drawn 2-4 hr after levothyroxine dose
Postpartum transient toxicosis
Factitious hyperthyroidism
Struma ovarii
Radioimmunoassay, surgery, or antithyroid drug therapy for hyperthyroidism 4-6 weeks (range, 2 wk to 2 yr) after the treatment
Interleukin-2 drugs (3%-6% of cases) or α-interferon therapy (1% of cases)
Hyperemesis gravidarum
Amiodarone therapy

THYROTROPIN (TSH) RECEPTOR ANTIBODIES

Normal: <130% of basal activity
Elevated in: Values between 1.3 and 2.0 are found in 10% of patients with thyroid disease other than Graves' disease. Values >2.8 have been found only in patients with Graves' disease.

THYROTROPIN RELEASING HORMONE (TRH) STIMULATION TEST

Elevated in: Celiac disease (specificity, 94%-97%; sensitivity, 90%-98%), dermatitis herpetiformis

THYROXINE (T_4)

Normal range: 4-11 μg/dl (51-142 nmol/L [CF: 12.87; SMI: 1 nmol/L])

TIBC

See IRON-BINDING CAPACITY

TISSUE TRANSGLUTAMINASE ANTIBODY

Normal: Negative
Present in: Celiac disease (specificity, 94%-97%, sensitivity, 90%-98%), dermatitis herpetiformis

TRANSFERRIN

Normal range: 170-370 mg/dl (1.7-3.7 g/L [CF: 0.01; SMI: 0.01 g/L])
Elevated in: Iron deficiency anemia, oral contraceptive administration, viral hepatitis, late pregnancy
Decreased in: Nephrotic syndrome, liver disease, hereditary deficiency, protein malnutrition, neoplasms, chronic inflammatory states, chronic illness, thalassemia, hemochromatosis, hemolytic anemia

TRIGLYCERIDES

Normal range: <150 mg/dl (<1.80 mmol/L [CF: 0.01129; SMI: 0.02 mmol/L])
Elevated in: Hyperlipoproteinemias (types I, IIb, III, IV, V), hypothyroidism, pregnancy, estrogens, acute myocardial infarction, pancreatitis, alcohol intake, nephrotic syndrome, diabetes mellitus, glycogen storage disease
Decreased in: Malnutrition, congenital abetalipoproteinemias, drugs (e.g., gemfibrozil, fenofibrate, nicotinic acid, clofibrate)

TRIIODOTHYRONINE

See T_3

TROPONINS, SERUM

Normal range: 0-0.4 ng/ml (negative). If there is clinical suspicion of evolving acute MI or ischemic episode, repeat testing in 5-6 hours is recommended.
Indeterminate: 0.05-0.49 ng/ml. Suggest further tests. In a patient with unstable angina and this troponin I level, there is an increased risk of a cardiac event in the near future.
Strong probability of acute MI:
≥0.05 ng/ml

Cardiac troponin T (CTNT) is a highly sensitive marker for myocardial injury for the first 48 hours after MI and for up to 5-7 days (see Fig. 4-2, under "Creatine Kinase Isoenzymes"). It may also be elevated in renal failure, chronic muscle disease, and trauma.

Cardiac troponin I (CTNI) is highly sensitive and specific for myocardial injury (≥CK-MB) in the initial 8 hours, peaks within 24 hours and lasts up to 7 days. With progressively higher levels of cTnI, the risk of mortality increases because the amount of necrosis increases.

TSH

See THYROID-STIMULATING HORMONE

TT

See THROMBIN TIME

TUBERCULIN TEST (PPD)

Abnormal results: see Boxes 4-3 and 4-4 for interpretation.

BOX 4-3 PPD Reaction Size Considered "Positive" (Intracutaneous 5 TU Mantoux Test at 48 hr)

5 mm or More
- HIV infection or risk factors for HIV
- Close recent contact with active TB case
- Persons with chest x-ray consistent with healed TB

10 mm or More
- Foreign-born persons from countries with high TB prevalence in Asia, Africa, and Latin America
- IV drug users
- Medically underserved low-income population groups (including Native Americans, Hispanics, and blacks)
- Residents of long-term care facilities (nursing homes, mental institutions)
- Medical conditions that increase risk for TB (silicosis, gastrectomy, undernourishment, diabetes mellitus, high-dose corticosteroids or immunosuppression Rx, leukemia or lymphoma, other malignancies)
- Employees of long-term care facilities, schools, child-care facilities, health care facilities

15 mm or More
- All others not already listed

TB, Tuberculosis; *TU,* tuberculin units.

BOX 4-4 Factors Associated with False-Negative Tuberculin Tests

Technical Errors
- Improper administration
- Inaccurate reading
- Loss of potency of antigen

Patient-Related Factors (Anergy)
- Age (elderly)
- Nutritional status
- Medications: corticosteroids, immunosuppressive agents
- Severe tuberculosis
- Coexisting diseases
  - HIV infection
  - Viral illness or vaccination
  - Lymphoreticular malignancies
  - Sarcoidosis
  - Solid tumors
  - Lepromatous leprosy
  - Sjögren's syndrome
  - Ataxia telangiectasia
  - Uremia
  - Primary biliary cirrhosis
  - Systemic lupus erythematosus
- Severe systemic disease of any etiology

Reprinted from Stein JH (ed): *Internal medicine,* ed 4, St Louis, 1994, Mosby.

UNCONJUGATED BILIRUBIN

See BILIRUBIN, DIRECT

UREA NITROGEN, BLOOD (BUN)

Normal range: 8-18 mg/dl (3-6.5 mmol/L [CF: 0.357; SMI: 0.5 mmol/L])

Box 4-5 describes factors affecting BUN level independent of renal function.

Elevated in: Drugs (aminoglycosides and other antibiotics, diuretics, lithium, corticosteroids), dehydration, gastrointestinal bleeding, decreased renal blood flow (shock, congestive heart failure, myocardial infarction), renal disease (glomerulonephritis, pyelonephritis, diabetic nephropathy), urinary tract obstruction (prostatic hypertrophy)

Decreased in: Liver disease, malnutrition, third trimester of pregnancy, overhydration, acromegaly, celiac disease

URIC ACID (serum)

Normal range: 2-7 mg/dl

Elevated in: Renal failure, gout, excessive cell lysis (chemotherapeutic agents, radiation therapy, leukemia, lymphoma, hemolytic anemia), hereditary enzyme deficiency (hypoxanthine-guanine-phosphoribosyl transferase), acidosis, myeloproliferative disorders, diet high in purines or protein, drugs (diuretics, low doses of ASA, ethambutol, nicotinic acid), lead poisoning, hypothyroidism, Addison's disease, nephrogenic diabetes insipidus, active psoriasis, polycystic kidneys

Decreased in: Drugs (allopurinol, high doses of ASA, probenecid, warfarin, corticosteroid), deficiency of xanthine oxidase, syndrome of inappropriate antidiuretic hormone secretion, renal tubular deficits (Fanconi's syndrome), alcoholism, liver disease, diet deficient in protein or purines, Wilson's disease, hemochromatosis

BOX 4-5 Factors Affecting Blood Urea Nitrogen Level Independent of Renal Function

Disproportionate Increase in Blood Urea Nitrogen
- Volume depletion ("prerenal azotemia")
- Gastrointestinal hemorrhage
- Corticosteroid or cytotoxic agents
- High-protein diet
- Obstructive uropathy
- Sepsis
- Catabolic states tissue breakdown

Disproportionate Decrease in Blood Urea Nitrogen
- Low-protein diet
- Liver disease

Reprinted from Andreoli TE (ed): *Cecil essentials of medicine,* ed 5, Philadelphia, 2001, WB Saunders.

URINALYSIS

Normal range:

Color: light straw
Appearance: clear
Ketones: absent
pH: 4.5-8 (average, 6)
Protein: absent
Glucose: absent
Specific gravity: 1.005-1.030
Occult blood absent
Microscopic examination:
 Red blood cells: 0-5 (high-power field)
 White blood cells: 0-5 (high-power field)
 Bacteria (spun specimen): absent
 Casts: 0-4 hyaline (low-power field)

Abnormalities in the microscopic examination of urine are described in Table 4-25.

URINE AMYLASE

Normal range: 35-260 U Somogyi/hr (6.5-48.1 U/hr [CF: 0.185; SMI: 1 U/hr])

Elevated in: Pancreatitis, carcinoma of the pancreas

URINE BILE

Normal: Absent

Abnormal:

Urine bilirubin: hepatitis (viral, toxic, drug-induced), biliary obstruction
Urine urobilinogen: hepatitis (viral, toxic, drug-induced), hemolytic jaundice, liver cell dysfunction (cirrhosis, infection, metastases)

TABLE 4-25 Microscopic Examination of the Urine

Finding	Associations
Casts	
Red blood cell	Glomerulonephritis, vasculitis
White blood cell	Interstitial nephritis, pyelonephritis
Epithelial cell	Acute tubular necrosis, interstitial nephritis, glomerulonephritis
Granular	Renal parenchymal disease (nonspecific)
Waxy, broad	Advanced renal failure
Hyaline	Normal finding in concentrated urine
Fatty	Heavy proteinuria
Cells	
Red blood cell	Urinary tract infection, urinary tract inflammation
White blood cell	Urinary tract infection, urinary tract inflammation
Eosinophil	Acute interstitial nephritis
(Squamous) epithelial cell	Contaminants
Crystals	
Uric acid	Acid urine, acute uric acid nephropathy, hyperuricosuria
Calcium phosphate	Alkaline urine
Calcium oxalate	Acid urine, hyperoxaluria, ethylene glycol poisoning
Cystine	Cystinuria
Sulfur	Sulfa-containing antibiotics

From Andreoli TE (ed): *Cecil essentials of medicine,* ed 5, Philadelphia, 2001, WB Saunders.

URINE CALCIUM

Normal range: <250 mg/24 hr (<6.2 mmol/dl [CF: 0.02495; SMI: 0.1 mmol/dl])
Elevated in: Primary hyperparathyroidism, hypervitaminosis D, bone metastases, multiple myeloma, increased calcium intake, steroids, prolonged immobilization, sarcoidosis, Paget's disease, idiopathic hypercalciuria, renal tubular acidosis
Decreased in: Hypoparathyroidism, pseudohypoparathyroidism, vitamin D deficiency, vitamin D–resistant rickets, diet low in calcium, drugs (thiazide diuretics, oral contraceptives), familial hypocalciuric hypercalcemia, renal osteodystrophy, potassium citrate therapy

URINE cAMP

Elevated in: Hypercalciuria, familial hypocalciuric hypercalcemia, primary hyperparathyroidism, pseudohypoparathyroidism, rickets
Decreased in: Vitamin D intoxication, sarcoidosis

URINE CATECHOLAMINES

Normal range:
Norepinephrine: <100 μg/24 hr (<590 nmol/day [CF: 5.911; SMI: 10 nmol/day])
Epinephrine: <10 μg/24 hr (55 nmol/day [CF: 5.458; SMI: 5 nmol/day])
Elevated in: Pheochromocytoma, neuroblastoma, severe stress

URINE CHLORIDE

Normal range: 110-250 mEq/day (110-250 mmol/day [CF: 1; SMI: 1 mmol/day])
Elevated in: Corticosteroids, Bartter's syndrome, diuretics, metabolic acidosis, severe hypokalemia
Decreased in: Chloride depletion (vomiting), colonic villous adenoma, chronic renal failure, renal tubular acidosis

URINE COPPER

Normal range: <40 μg/24 hr (<0.6 μmol/day [CF: 0.01574; SMI: 0.2 μmol/day])

URINE CORTISOL, FREE

Normal range: 10-110 μg/24 hr (30-300 nmol/day [CF: 2.759; SMI: 10 nmol/day])
Elevated: See CORTISOL, PLASMA

URINE CREATININE (24 hr)

Normal range:
Male: 0.8-1.8 g/day (7-16 mmol/day [CF: 8.840; SMI: 0.1 mmol/day])
Female: 0.6-1.6 g/day (5.3-14 mmol/day)
NOTE: Useful test as an indicator of completeness of 24-hr urine collection.

URINE CRYSTALS

Uric acid: acid urine, hyperuricosuria, uric acid nephropathy
Sulfur: antibiotics containing sulfa
Calcium oxalate: ethylene glycol poisoning, acid urine, hyperoxaluria
Calcium phosphate: alkaline urine
Cystine: cystinuria

URINE EOSINOPHILS

Normal: Absent
Present in: Interstitial nephritis, acute tubular necrosis, urinary tract infection, kidney transplant rejection, hepatorenal syndrome

URINE GLUCOSE (QUALITATIVE)

Normal: Absent
Present in: Diabetes mellitus, renal glycosuria (decreased renal threshold for glucose), glucose intolerance

URINE HEMOGLOBIN, FREE

Normal: Absent
Present in: Hemolysis (with saturation of serum haptoglobin binding capacity and renal threshold for tubular absorption of hemoglobin)

URINE HEMOSIDERIN

Normal: Absent
Present in: Paroxysmal nocturnal hemoglobinuria, chronic hemolytic anemia, hemochromatosis, blood transfusion, thalassemias

URINE 5-HYDROXYINDOLE-ACETIC ACID (URINE 5-HIAA)

Normal range: 2-8 mg/24 hr (10-40 μmol/day [CF: 5.23; SMI: 5 μmol/day])
Elevated in: Carcinoid tumors, after ingestion of certain foods (bananas, plums, tomatoes, avocados, pineapples, eggplant, walnuts), drugs (monoamine oxidase inhibitors, phenacetin, methyldopa, glycerol guaiacolate, acetaminophen, salicylates, phenothiazines, imipramine, methocarbamol, reserpine, methamphetamine)

URINE INDICAN

Normal: Absent
Present in: Malabsorption secondary to intestinal bacterial overgrowth

URINE KETONES (semiquantitative)

Normal: Absent
Present in: Diabetic ketoacidosis, alcoholic ketoacidosis, starvation, isopropanol ingestion

URINE METANEPHRINES

Normal range: 0-2.0 mg/24 hr (0-11.0 μmol/day [CF: 5.458; SMI: 0.5 μmol/day])
Elevated in: Pheochromocytoma, neuroblastoma, drugs (caffeine, phenothiazines, monoamine oxidase inhibitors), stress

URINE MYOGLOBIN

Normal: Absent
Present in: Severe trauma, hyperthermia, polymyositis/dermatomyositis, carbon monoxide poisoning, drugs (narcotic and amphetamine toxicity), hypothyroidism, muscle ischemia

URINE NITRITE

Normal: Absent
Present in: Urinary tract infections

URINE OCCULT BLOOD

Normal: Negative
Positive in: Trauma to urinary tract, renal disease (glomerulonephritis, pyelonephritis), renal or ureteral calculi, bladder lesions (carcinoma, cystitis), prostatitis, prostatic carcinoma, menstrual contamination, hematopoietic disorders (hemophilia, thrombocytopenia), anticoagulants, ASA

URINE OSMOLALITY

Normal range: 50-1200 mOsm/kg (50-1200 mmol/kg [CF: 1; SMI: 1 mmol/kg])
Elevated in: Syndrome of inappropriate antidiuretic hormone secretion, dehydration, glycosuria, adrenal insufficiency, high-protein diet
Decreased in: Diabetes insipidus, excessive water intake, IV hydration with D_5W, acute renal insufficiency, glomerulonephritis

URINE pH

Normal range: 4.6-8 (average, 6)
Elevated in: Bacteriuria, vegetarian diet, renal failure with inability to form ammonia, drugs (antibiotics, sodium bicarbonate, acetazolamide)
Decreased in: Acidosis (metabolic, respiratory), drugs (ammonium chloride, methenamine mandelate), diabetes mellitus, starvation, diarrhea

URINE PHOSPHATE

Normal range: 0.8-2.0 g/24 hr
Elevated in: Acute tubular necrosis (diuretic phase), chronic renal disease, uncontrolled diabetes mellitus, hyperparathyroidism, hypomagnesemia, metabolic acidosis, metabolic alkalosis, neurofibromatosis, adult-onset vitamin D–resistant hypophosphatemic osteomalacia
Decreased in: Acromegaly, acute renal failure, decreased dietary intake, hypoparathyroidism, respiratory acidosis

URINE POTASSIUM

Normal range: 25-100 mEq/24 hr (25-100 mmol/day [CF: 1; SMI: 1 mmol/day])
Elevated in: Aldosteronism (primary, secondary), glucocorticoids, alkalosis, renal tubular acidosis, excessive dietary potassium intake
Decreased in: Acute renal failure, potassium-sparing diuretics, diarrhea, hypokalemia

URINE PROTEIN (quantitative)

Normal range: <150 mg/24 hr (<0.15 g/day [CF: 0.001; SMI: 0.01 g/day])
Elevated in:
Nephrotic syndrome as a result of primary renal diseases
Malignant hypertension
Malignancies: multiple myeloma, leukemias, Hodgkin's disease
Congestive heart failure
Diabetes mellitus
Systemic lupus erythematosus, rheumatoid arthritis
Sickle cell disease
Goodpasture's syndrome
Malaria
Amyloidosis, sarcoidosis
Tubular lesions: cystinosis
Functional (after heavy exercise)
Pyelonephritis
Pregnancy
Constrictive pericarditis
Renal vein thrombosis
Toxic nephropathies: heavy metals, drugs
Radiation nephritis
Orthostatic (postural) proteinuria
Benign proteinuria: fever, heat or cold exposure

URINE SEDIMENT

See Fig. 4-14 for evaluation of common abnormalities.

URINE SODIUM (quantitative)

Normal range: 40-220 mEq/day (40-220 mmol/day [CF: 1; SMI: 1 mmol/day])
Elevated in: Diuretic administration, high sodium intake, salt-losing nephritis, acute tubular necrosis, vomiting, Addison's disease, syndrome of inappropriate antidiuretic hormone secretion, hypothyroidism, congestive heart failure, hepatic failure, chronic renal failure, Bartter's syndrome, glucocorticoid deficiency, interstitial nephritis caused by analgesic abuse, mannitol, dextran, or glycerol therapy, milk-alkali syndrome, decreased renin secretion, postobstructive diuresis
Decreased in: Increased aldosterone, glucocorticoid excess, hyponatremia, prerenal azotemia, decreased salt intake

URINE SPECIFIC GRAVITY

Normal range: 1.005-1.03
Elevated in: Dehydration, excessive fluid losses (vomiting, diarrhea, fever), x-ray contrast media, diabetes mellitus, congestive heart failure, syndrome of inappropriate antidiuretic hormone secretion, adrenal insufficiency, decreased fluid intake
Decreased in: Diabetes insipidus, renal disease (glomerulonephritis, pyelonephritis), excessive fluid intake or IV hydration

URINE VANILLYIMANDELIC ACID (VMA)

Normal range: <6.8 mg/24 hr (<35 μmol/day [CF: 5.046; SMI: 1 μmol/day])
Elevated in: Pheochromocytoma, neuroblastoma, ganglioblastoma, drugs (isoproterenol, methocarbamol, levodopa, sulfonamides, chlorpromazine), severe stress, after ingestion of bananas, chocolate, vanilla, tea, coffee
Decreased in: Drugs (monoamine oxidase inhibitors, reserpine, guanethidine, methyldopa)

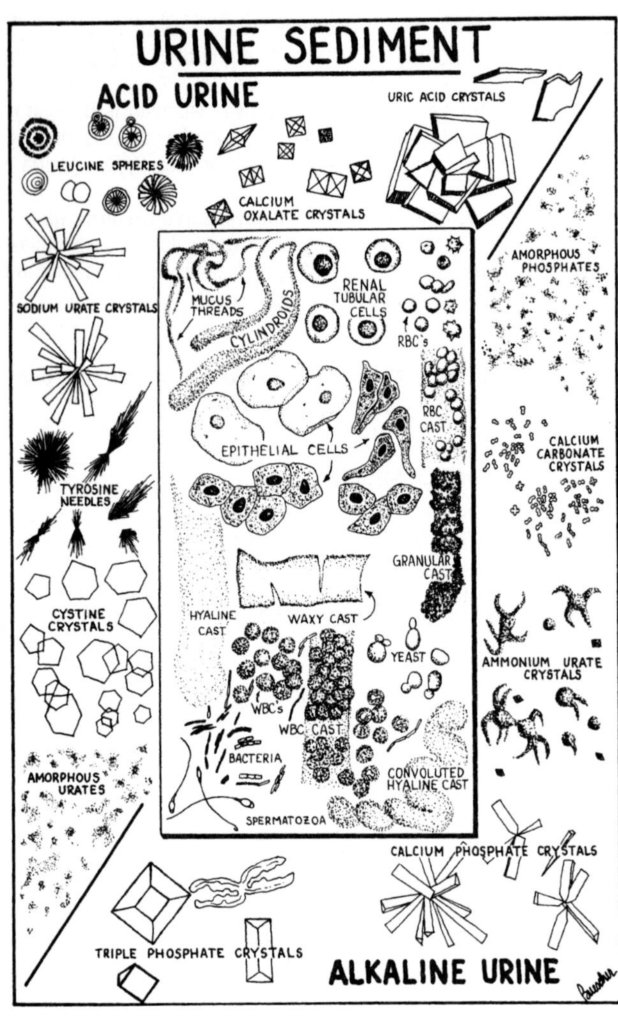

FIGURE 4-14 Microscopic examination of urinary sediment. (Reprinted from Grigorian Greene M: *The Harriet Lane handbook: a manual for pediatric house officers*, ed 17, St Louis, 2007, Mosby.)

VARICELLA-ZOSTER VIRUS (VZV) SEROLOGY

Test description: Test can be performed on whole blood, tissue, skin lesions, and CSF

VASOACTIVE INTESTINAL PEPTIDE (VIP)

Normal: <50 pg/ml
Elevated in: Pancreatic VIP-omas, neuroblastoma, pancreatic islet call hyperplasia, liver disease, MEN I, ganglioneuroma, ganglioneuroblastoma

VDRL

Normal range: Negative
Positive test: Syphilis, other treponemal diseases (yaws, pinta, bejel)

NOTE: A false-positive test may be seen in patients with systemic lupus erythematosus and other autoimmune diseases, infectious mononucleosis, HIV, atypical pneumonia, malaria, leprosy, typhus fever, rat-bite fever, relapsing fever.

NOTE: See Table 4-26 for interpretation of serologic tests for syphilis.

VISCOSITY (serum)

Normal range: 1.4-1.8 relative to water (1.10-1.22 centipoise)
Elevated in: Monoclonal gammopathies (Waldenström's macroglobulinemia, multiple myeloma), hyperfibrinogenemia, systemic lupus erythematosus, rheumatoid arthritis, polycythemia, leukemia

TABLE 4-26 Interpretation of Serologic Tests for Syphilis*

Nontreponemal Tests	Treponemal Tests	Interpretation of Finding: Is Syphilis Present?*
Nonreactive	Nonreactive	Early primary syphilis is not ruled out by negative serologic tests. Early syphilis is present in 13%-30% of patients who have a negative microhemagglutination *Treponema pallidum* test; in about 30% of patients who present with chancre but have a nonreactive reagin test; and in about 10% of patients who have a negative FTA-ABS test. Late syphilis is present in a very small fraction of patients. Adequately treated syphilis in remote past may produce these results, but treponemal tests usually remain reactive.
	Reactive	Observed in about 10% of patients with chancre. The treponemal tests may turn positive shortly before the reagin tests. Reagin tests repeated after several days are generally positive. In adequately treated early syphilis, the reagin test may return to nonreactive within 1-2 yr, whereas the treponemal tests generally do not. Late syphilis is not ruled out by a negative reagin test. The sensitivity of the reagin tests is lower than that of treponemal tests in untreated late syphilis. In secondary syphilis, rarely, a highly reactive serum appears negative when tested undiluted with a regain test because flocculation is inhibited by relative antibody excess. Not reported to occur with treponemal tests. Quantitative reagin tests are positive. False-positive treponemal tests occur in 40% of patients with Lyme disease.
Reactive	Nonreactive borderline (FTA-ABS)	Finding is not diagnostic of syphilis but constitutes a classic biologic false-positive reaction. Not diagnostic of syphilis; most patients (90%) with this pattern do not develop clinical or serologic evidence of syphilis. Repeat test is indicated. Chronic borderline results are associated with a variety of conditions other than syphilis.
	Beaded (FTA-ABS)	Not diagnostic of syphilis. Seen with collagen vascular disease.
	Reactive	Findings diagnostic of syphilis or other treponemal disease. In adequately treated syphilis, one would expect (1) a sustained fourfold drop in titer of reagin test, although reagin test may remain positive after adequate therapy; (2) treponemal tests remain positive after adequate therapy. Concurrent false-positive results on both nontreponemal and treponemal tests could occur in rare instances. It may be impossible to rule out syphilis in an individual with this test profile.

Reprinted from Stein JH (ed): *Internal medicine,* ed 4, St Louis, 1994, Mosby.
FTA-ABS, Fluorescent treponemal antibody, absorbed.
*Serologic data must always be interpreted in the light of a total clinical evaluation. Diagnosis based on serologic criteria alone is fraught with error. Serologic tests apparently in conflict with clinical diagnosis should be confirmed by repetition or possibly referral to a reference laboratory.

VITAMIN B_{12}

Normal:
190-900 ng/ml
Causes of vitamin B_{12} deficiency:
1. Pernicious anemia (antibodies against intrinsic factor and gastric parietal cells)
2. Dietary (strict lacto-ovovegetarians, food faddists)
3. Malabsorption (achlorhydria, gastrectomy, ileal resection, pancreatic insufficiency, drugs [omeprazole, cholestyramine])

Falsely low levels occur in patients with severe folate deficiency, in patients using high doses of ascorbic acid, and when cobalamin levels are measured after nuclear medicine studies (radioactivity interferes with cobalamin radioimmunoassay).

Falsely high or normal levels in patients with cobalamin deficiency can occur in severe liver disease and chronic granulocytic leukemia.

The absence of anemia or macrocytosis does not exclude the diagnosis of cobalamin deficiency.

VITAMIN D, 1,25 DIHYDROXY CALCIFEROL

Normal: 16-65 pg/ml
Elevated in: Tumor calcinosis, primary hyperparathyroidism, sarcoidosis, tuberculosis, idiopathic hypercalciuria
Decreased in: Postmenopausal osteoporosis, chronic renal failure, hypoparathyroidism, tumor-induced osteomalacia, rickets, tumor-induced osteomalacia, elevated blood lead levels

VITAMIN K

Normal: 0.10-2.20 ng/ml
Decreased in: Primary biliary cirrhosis, anticoagulants, antibiotics, choelstyramine, GI disease, pancreatic disease, cystic fibrosis, obstructive jaundice, hypoprothrombinemia, hemorrhagic disease of the newborn

VON WILLEBRAND FACTOR

Normal: Levels vary according to blood type; blood type O: 50-150 U/dl; blood type non-O: 90-200 U/dl
Decreased in: von Willebrand's disease (however, in type II von Willebrand's disease the antigen may be normal but the function is impaired)

WWBC

See COMPLETE BLOOD COUNT

WESTERGREN

See ERYTHROCYTE SEDIMENTATION RATE

WHITE BLOOD COUNT

See COMPLETE BLOOD COUNT

SECTION V

Clinical Practice Guidelines

PART A
THE PERIODIC HEALTH EXAMINATION*

Age-Specific Charts, 1468

PART B
IMMUNIZATIONS AND CHEMOPROPHYLAXIS

*Data modified from U.S. Preventive Services Task Force: *Guide to clinical preventive services: report of the U.S. Preventive Services Task Force,* ed 2, Washington, DC, 1996 (revised 2001), U.S. Department of Health and Human Services. Text downloaded from http://text.nlm.nih.gov

PART A • THE PERIODIC HEALTH EXAMINATION

Age-Specific Charts

TABLE 5-1 Birth to 10 Years

Interventions considered and recommended for the Periodic Health Examination	Leading causes of death Conditions originating in perinatal period Congenital anomalies Sudden infant death syndrome Unintentional injuries (non–motor vehicle) Motor vehicle injuries
INTERVENTIONS FOR THE GENERAL POPULATION	
Screening	**Substance use**
Height and weight	Effects of passive smoking*
Blood pressure	Antitobacco message*
Vision screen (age 3-4 yr)	**Dental health**
Hemoglobinopathy screen (birth)[1]	Regular visits to dental care provider*
Phenylalanine level (birth)[2]	Floss, brush with fluoride toothpaste daily*
Thyroxine and/or thyroid-stimulating hormone (birth)[3]	Advice about baby bottle tooth decay*
Counseling	***Immunizations***
Injury prevention	Diphtheria-tetanus-pertussis (DTaP)[4]
Child safety car seats (age <5 yr)	Inactivated poliovirus vaccine (IPV)[5]
Lap/shoulder belts (age ≥5 yr)	Measles-mumps-rubella (MMR)[6]
Bicycle helmet; avoid bicycling near traffic	*H. influenzae* type b (Hib) conjugate[7]
Smoke detector, flame-retardant sleepwear	Hepatitis A vaccine (HR4)
Hot water heater temperature <120°-130° F	Hepatitis B[8]
Window/stair guards, pool fence	Varicella[9]
Safe storage of drugs, toxic substances, firearms, and matches	Pneumococcal vaccine[10]
Syrup of ipecac, poison control phone number	Influenza[11]
CPR training for parents/caretakers	Meningococcal conjugate vaccine (MCV)[12]
Diet and exercise	Rotavirus (RV)[13]
Breastfeeding, iron-enriched formula and foods (infants and toddlers)	Human papillomavirus vaccine (HPV)[14]
Limit fat and cholesterol; maintain caloric balance; emphasize grains, fruits, vegetables (age ≥2 yr)	***Chemoprophylaxis***
Regular physical activity*	Ocular prophylaxis (birth)
INTERVENTIONS FOR HIGH-RISK POPULATIONS	
Population	***Potential Interventions (see detailed high-risk definitions)***
Preterm or low birth weight	Hemoglobin/hematocrit (HR1)
Infants of mothers at risk for HIV	HIV testing (HR2)
Low income; immigrants	Hemoglobin/hematocrit (HR1); PPD (HR3)
TB contacts	PPD (HR3)
Native American/Alaska Native	Hemoglobin/hematocrit (HR1); PPD (HR3); pneumococcal vaccine (HR5)
Residents of long-term care facilities	PPD (HR3); hepatitis A vaccine (HR4); influenza vaccine (HR6)
Certain chronic medical conditions	PPD (HR3); pneumococcal vaccine (HR5); influenza vaccine (HR6)
Increased individual or community lead exposure	Blood lead level (HR7)
Inadequate water fluoridation	Daily fluoride supplement (HR8)
Family history of skin cancer; nevi; fair skin, eyes, hair	Avoid excess/midday sun, use protective clothing* (HR9)

HR, High risk; *PPD,* purified protein derivative; *TB,* tuberculosis.

[1]Whether screening should be universal or targeted to high-risk groups depends on the proportion of high-risk individuals in the screening area and other considerations. [2]If done during first 24 hr of life, repeat by age 2 wk. [3]Optimally between day 2 and 6, but in all cases before newborn nursery discharge. [4]2, 4, 6, and 12-18 mo; once between age 4-6 yr. [5]2, 4, 6-18 mo; once between age 4-6 yr. [6]12-15 mo and 4-6 yr. [7]2, 4, 6 and 12-15 mo; no dose needed at 6 mo if PRP-OMP vaccine is used for first 2 doses. [8]Birth, 1 mo, 6 mo; or, 0-2 mo, 1-2 mo later, and 6-18 mo. If not done in infancy: current visit, and 1 and 6 mo later. [9]12-18 mo; or any child without history of chickenpox or previous immunization. Include information on risk in adulthood, duration of immunity, and potential need for booster doses. Administer a second dose of varicella vaccine at age 4-6 yr. [10]Pneumococcal polysaccharide vaccine (PPSV) can be administered at the same time as the other childhood vaccines at a separate site. [11]Influenza vaccine is recommended in children 6 mo-18 yr of age. [12]Administer meningococcal conjugate vaccine (MCV) to children aged 2 through 10 yr with terminal complement component deficiency, anatomic or functional asplenia, and certain other high risk groups (see *MMWR* 54(RR-7), 2005). Persons who received MPSV 3 or more years previously and who remain at increased risk for meningococcal disease should be revaccinated with MCV. [13]Administer first dose at 2 mo. If Rotarix® is administered at ages 2 and 4 mo, a dose at 6 mo is not indicated. [14]HPV4 may be administered in a 3-dose series to males aged 9 through 18 years to reduce the likelihood of acquiring genital warts.

*The ability of clinician counseling to influence this behavior is unproven.

HR1: Infants age 6-12 mo who are living in poverty, black, Native American or Alaska Native, immigrants from developing countries, preterm and low-birth-weight infants, infants whose principal dietary intake is unfortified cow's milk.

HR2: Infants born to high-risk mothers whose HIV status is unknown. Women at high risk include past or present injection drug users; persons who exchange sex for money or drugs and their sex partners; injection drug–using, bisexual, or HIV-positive sex partners currently or in past; persons seeking treatment for STDs; persons who received a blood transfusion between 1978 and 1985.

HR3: Persons infected with HIV, close contacts of persons with known or suspected TB, persons with medical risk factors associated with TB, immigrants from countries with high TB prevalence, medically underserved low-income populations (including homeless), residents of long-term care facilities.

HR4: Hepatitis A vaccine (Hep A) is recommended for all children at 1 yr of age (i.e., 12-23 mo). The two doses in the series should be administered at least 6 mo apart. Children who are not vaccinated by 2 yr of age can be vaccinated at subsequent visits.

HR5: Immunocompetent persons ≥2 yr with certain medical conditions, including chronic cardiac or pulmonary disease, diabetes mellitus, and anatomic asplenia, as well as cochlear implant candidates and recipients. Immunocompetent persons ≥2 yr living in high-risk environments or social settings (e.g., certain Native American and Alaska Native populations).

HR6: Annual vaccinations of children ≥6 mo who are residents of chronic care facilities or who have chronic cardiopulmonary disorders, metabolic diseases (including diabetes mellitus), hemoglobinopathies, immunosuppression, or renal dysfunction.

HR7: Children approximately age 12 mo who (1) live in communities in which the prevalence of lead levels requiring individual intervention, including residential lead hazard control or chelation, is high or undefined; (2) live in or frequently visit a home built before 1950 with dilapidated paint or with recent or ongoing renovation or remodeling; (3) have close contact with a person who has an elevated lead level; (4) live near lead industry or heavy traffic; (5) live with someone whose job or hobby involves lead exposure; (6) use lead-based pottery; or (7) take traditional ethnic remedies that contain lead.

HR8: Children living in areas with inadequate water fluoridation (<0.6 ppm).

HR9: Persons with a family history of skin cancer; a large number of moles; atypical moles; poor tanning ability; or light skin, hair, and eye color.

TABLE 5-2 Ages 11 to 24 Years

Interventions considered and recommended for the Periodic Health Examination	Leading causes of death Motor vehicle accidents/other unintentional injuries Homicide Suicide Malignant neoplasms Heart diseases
INTERVENTIONS FOR THE GENERAL POPULATION	
Screening	**Diet and exercise**
Height and weight	Limit fat and cholesterol; maintain caloric balance; emphasize grains, fruits, vegetables
Blood pressure[1]	Adequate calcium intake (females)
Papanicolaou (Pap) test[2] (females)	Regular physical activity*
Chlamydia screen[3] (females <25 yr)	**Dental health**
HIV screening	Regular visits to dental care provider*
Lipid panel (in high-risk young adults only)	Floss, brush with fluoride toothpaste daily
Rubella serology or vaccination history[4] (females >12 yr)	***Immunizations***
Assess for problem drinking	Tetanus, diphtheria, pertussis†
Counseling	Hepatitis B[5]
Injury prevention	Measles-mumps-rubella (MMR) (11-12 yr)[6]
Lap/shoulder belts	Varicella (11-12 yr)[7]
Bicycle/motorcycle/ATV helmets*	Rubella (females >12 yr)[4]
Smoke detector*	Meningococcal[8]
Safe storage/removal of firearms*	Human papilloma virus (females 11-12 yr, males 9-18 yr)[9]
Substance use	Influenza[10]
Avoid tobacco use	Pneumococcal polysaccharide vaccine (PPSV)[11]
Avoid underage drinking and illicit drug use*	***Chemoprophylaxis***
Avoid alcohol/drug use while driving, swimming, boating, etc.*	Multivitamin with folic acid (females)
Sexual behavior	
STD prevention: abstinence*; avoid high-risk behavior*; condoms/female barrier with spermicide*	
Unintended pregnancy: contraception	
INTERVENTIONS FOR HIGH-RISK POPULATIONS	
Population	***Potential Interventions (see detailed high-risk definitions)***
High-risk sexual behavior	RPR/VDRL (HR1); screen for gonorrhea (female) (HR2), HIV (HR3), chlamydia (female) (HR4); hepatitis A vaccine (HR5)
Injection or street drug use	RPR/VDRL (HR1); HIV screen (HR3); hepatitis A vaccine (HR5); PPD (HR6); advice to reduce infection risk (HR7)
TB contacts; immigrants; low income	PPD (HR6)
Native Americans/Alaska Natives	Hepatitis A vaccine (HR5); PPD (HR6); pneumococcal vaccine (HR8)
Travelers to developing countries	Hepatitis A vaccine (HR5)
Certain chronic medical conditions	PPD (HR6); pneumococcal vaccine (HR8); influenza vaccine (HR9)
Settings where adolescents and young adults congregate	Second MMR (HR10)
Susceptible to varicella, measles, mumps	Varicella vaccine (HR11); MMR (HR12)
Blood transfusion between 1975 and 1985	HIV screen (HR3)
Institutionalized persons; health care/lab workers	Hepatitis A vaccine (HR5); PPD (HR6); influenza vaccine (HR9)
Family history of skin cancer; nevi; fair skin, eyes, hair	Avoid excess/midday sun, use protective clothing* (HR13)
Prior pregnancy with neural tube defect	Folic acid 4.0 mg (HR14)
Inadequate water fluoridation	Daily fluoride supplement (HR15)
Pregnancy	HIV screen

ATV, All-terrain vehicle; *HR,* high risk; *PPD,* purified protein derivative; *RPR,* rapid plasmin reagin; *STD,* sexually transmitted disease; *TB,* tuberculosis; *VDRL,* Venereal Disease Research Laboratory.
[1]Periodic blood pressure for persons aged ≥21 yr. [2]If sexually active at present or in the past: q ≤3 yr. If sexual history is unreliable, begin Pap tests at age 18 yr. [3]If sexually active. [4]Serologic testing, documented vaccination history, and routine vaccination against rubella (preferably with MMR) are equally acceptable alternatives. [5]If not previously immunized: current visit and 1 and 6 mo later. [6]If no previous second dose of MMR. [7]If susceptible to chickenpox. [8]Meningococcal conjugate vaccine (MCV) can be administered at 11-12 yr visit, at high school entry, or at beginning of college (especially indicated in students living in college dormitories). [9]Quadrivalent human papillomavirus (types 6, 11, 16, 18) recombinant vaccine (Gardasil) should be given to all females aged 11-26 yr who have not been previously vaccinated. The vaccine is indicated for the prevention of cervical cancer and genital warts caused by the human papilloma virus (HPV) 6, 11, 16, or 18. Gardasil is an intramuscular injection for administration to the thigh or upper arm. The schedule consists of three 0.5-ml doses, with the second dose given 2 mo after the first, and the final dose administered 6 mo after the initial dose. HPV4 may also be administered in a 3-dose series to males aged 9 through 18 years to reduce their likelihood of acquiring genital warts. [10]Influenza vaccine is recommended for children 6 mo to 18 yr of age. [11]Administer to children with certain underlying medical conditions (see *MMWR* 46(RR-8), 1997), including a cochlear implant. A single revaccination should be administered to children with functional or anatomic asplenia or other immunocompromising condition after 5 yr.
*The ability of clinician counseling to influence this behavior is unproven.
†Tdap vaccine is recommended for adolescents aged 11-12 yr who have completed the recommended childhood DTP/DTaP vaccination series and have not received a Td booster dose. Adolescents aged 13-18 yr who missed the 11- 12-yr Td/Tdap booster dose should also receive a single dose of Tdap if they have completed the recommended childhood DTP/DTaP vaccination series. A 5 yr interval from the last Td dose is encouraged when Tdap is used as a booster drug; however, a shorter interval may be used if pertussis immunity is needed.

HR1: Persons who exchange sex for money or drugs and their sex partners, persons with other STDs (including HIV), and sexual contacts of persons with active syphilis. Clinicians should also consider local epidemiology.

HR2: Females who have had two or more sex partners in the last year or a sex partner with multiple sexual contacts; exchanged sex for money or drugs; or have a history of repeated episodes of gonorrhea. Clinicians should also consider local epidemiology.

HR3: Males who had sex with males after 1975; past or present injection drug users; persons who exchange sex for money or drugs and their sex partners; injection drug–using, bisexual, or HIV-positive sex partner currently or in the past; recipients of a blood transfusion between 1978 and 1985; persons seeking treatment for STDs. Clinicians should also consider local epidemiology and screening for HIV in general population.

HR4: Sexually active females with multiple risk factors, including history of prior STD, new or multiple sex partners, age $<$25 yr, nonuse or inconsistent use of barrier contraceptives, or cervical ectopy. Clinicians should consider local epidemiology of the disease in identifying other high-risk groups.

HR5: Persons living in, traveling to, or working in areas where the disease is endemic and where periodic outbreaks occur (e.g., countries with high or intermediate endemicity; certain Alaska Native, Pacific Island, Native American, and religious communities); men who have sex with men; injection or street drug users; persons with clotting factor disorders or chronic liver disease. Vaccine may be considered for institutionalized persons and workers in these institutions; military personnel; and day-care, hospital, and laboratory workers. Clinicians should also consider local epidemiology.

HR6: HIV-positive, close contacts of persons with known or suspected TB, health care workers, persons with medical risk factors associated with TB, immigrants from countries with high TB prevalence, medically underserved low-income populations (including homeless), alcoholics, injection drug users, and residents of long-term care facilities.

HR7: Persons who continue to inject drugs.

HR8: Immunocompetent persons with certain medical conditions, including chronic cardiac or pulmonary disease, diabetes mellitus, cochlear implants candidates and recipients, and anatomic asplenia. Immunocompetent persons who live in high-risk environments or social settings (e.g., certain Native American and Alaska Native populations).

HR9: Annual vaccination of residents of chronic care facilities; persons with chronic cardiopulmonary disorders, metabolic diseases (including diabetes mellitus), hemoglobinopathies, immunosuppression, or renal dysfunction; and health care providers for high-risk patients.

HR10: Adolescents and young adults in settings where such individuals congregate (e.g., high schools and colleges) if they have not previously received a second dose.

HR11: Healthy persons aged $\geq$13 yr without a history of chickenpox or previous immunization. Consider serologic testing for presumed susceptible persons aged $\geq$13 yr.

HR12: Persons born after 1956 who lack evidence of immunity to measles or mumps (e.g., documented receipt of live vaccine on or after the first birthday, laboratory evidence of immunity, or a history of physician-diagnosed measles or mumps).

HR13: Persons with a family or personal history of skin cancer; a large number of moles; atypical moles; poor tanning ability; or light skin, hair, and eye color.

HR14: Women with prior pregnancy affected by neural tube defect who are planning pregnancy.

HR15: Persons aged $<$17 yr living in areas with inadequate water fluoridation ($<$0.6 ppm).

TABLE 5-3 Ages 25 to 64 Years

Interventions considered and recommended for the Periodic Health Examination	Leading causes of death
	Malignant neoplasms Heart diseases Motor vehicle and other unintentional injuries HIV infection Suicide and homicide

INTERVENTIONS FOR THE GENERAL POPULATION

Screening	**Injury prevention**
Blood pressure	Lap/shoulder belts
Height and weight	Motorcycle/bicycle/ATV helmets*
Lipid panel (men age 35-64 yr, women age 45-64 yr)	Smoke detector*
HIV screening	Safe storage/removal of firearms*
Papanicolaou (Pap) test (women)[1]	**Sexual behavior**
Fecal occult blood test[2] and/or colonoscopy (≥50 yr)	STD prevention: avoid high-risk behavior*; condoms/female barrier with spermicide*
Mammogram ± clinical breast examination[3] (women 40-69 yr)	Unintended pregnancy: contraception
Bone density scan in postmenopausal women	**Dental health**
Assess for problem drinking	Regular visits to dental care provider*
Rubella serology or vaccination history[4] (women of childbearing age)	Floss, brush with fluoride toothpaste daily*
Counseling	***Immunizations***
Substance use	Tetanus-diphtheria (Td) boosters
Tobacco cessation	Rubella[4] (women of childbearing age)
Avoid alcohol/drug use while driving, swimming, boating, etc.*	Influenza vaccine†
Diet and exercise	Human papilloma virus[5]
Limit fat and cholesterol; maintain caloric balance; emphasize grains, fruits, vegetables	Herpes zoster (≥60 yr)[6]
Adequate calcium intake (women)	***Chemoprophylaxis***
Regular physical activity*	Multivitamin with folic acid (women planning or capable of pregnancy)

INTERVENTIONS FOR HIGH-RISK POPULATIONS

Population	***Potential Interventions (see detailed high-risk definitions)***
High-risk sexual behavior	RPR/VDRL (HR1); screen for gonorrhea (female) (HR2), HIV (HR3), Chlamydia (female) (HR4); hepatitis B vaccine (HR5); hepatitis A vaccine (HR6)
Injection or street drug use	RPR/VDRL (HR1); HIV screen (HR3); hepatitis B vaccine (HR5); hepatitis A vaccine (HR6); PPD (HR7); advice to reduce infection risk (HR8)
Low income; TB contacts; immigrants; alcoholics	PPD (HR7)
Native Americans/Alaska Natives	Hepatitis A vaccine (HR6); PPD (HR7); pneumococcal vaccine (HR9)
Travelers to developing countries	Hepatitis B vaccine (HR5); hepatitis A vaccine (HR6)
Certain chronic medical conditions	PPD (HR7); pneumococcal vaccine (HR9); influenza vaccine (HR10)
Blood product recipients	HIV screen (HR3); hepatitis B vaccine (HR5); hepatitis C screen
Susceptible to measles, mumps, or varicella	MMR (HR11); varicella vaccine (HR12)
Institutionalized persons	Hepatitis A vaccine (HR6); PPD (HR7); pneumococcal vaccine (HR9); influenza vaccine (HR10)
Health care/lab workers	Hepatitis B vaccine (HR5); hepatitis A vaccine (HR6); PPD (HR7); influenza vaccine (HR10)
Family history of skin cancer; fair skin, eyes, hair	Avoid excess/midday sun, use protective clothing* (HR13)
Previous pregnancy with neural tube defect	Folic acid 4.0 mg (HR14)
Cardiovascular risk factors	Lipid panel (HR 15)
Pregnancy	HIV screen

ATV, All-terrain vehicle; *HR,* high risk; *MMR,* measles-mumps-rubella; *PPD,* purified protein derivative; *RPR,* rapid plasma reagin; *STD,* sexually transmitted disease; *TB,* tuberculosis; *VDRL,* Venereal Disease Research Laboratory.

[1]Women who are or have been sexually active and who have a cervix: q ≤3 yr. Routine pap smear screening is unnecessary for women who have undergone a complete hysterectomy for benign disease. [2]Annually. [3]Mammogram q1-2 yr, or mammogram q1-2 yr with annual clinical breast examination. [4]Serologic testing, documented vaccination history, and routine vaccination (preferably with MMR) are equally acceptable. [5]Quadrivalent human papillomavirus (types 6, 11, 16, 18) recombinant vaccine (Gardasil) should be given to all females aged 14-26 yr who have not been previously vaccinated. The vaccine is indicated for the prevention of cervical cancer and genital warts caused by the human papilloma virus (HPV) 6, 11, 16, or 18. Gardasil is an intramuscular injection for administration to the thigh or upper arm. The schedule consists of three 0.5 ml doses, with the second dose given 2 mo after the first, and the final dose administered 6 mo after the initial dose. [6]Herpes zoster vaccine (Zostavax) is indicated for prevention of herpes zoster (shingles) in individuals 60 yr or older. Zostavax is administered as a single dose subcutaneously. It is a lyophilic preparation of the Oka/Merck strain of live, attenuated varicella zoster virus (VZV). It should not be administered to individuals with a history of primary or acquired immunodeficiency states, persons on immunosuppressive therapy (including high-dose corticosteroids), those with active untreated tuberculosis, and those who may be pregnant.

*The ability of clinician counseling to influence this behavior is unproven.

†A live attenuated influenza vaccine (LAIV, Flumist) administered intranasally is available for healthy persons aged 2 to 49 yr.

HR1: Persons who exchange sex for money or drugs and their sex partners, persons with other STDs (including HIV), and sexual contacts of persons with active syphilis. Clinicians should also consider local epidemiology.

HR2: Women who exchange sex for money or drugs or who have had repeated episodes of gonorrhea. Clinicians should also consider local epidemiology.

HR3: Men who had sex with men after 1975; past or present injection drug users; persons who exchange sex for money or drugs and their sex partners; persons with current or past injection drug–using, bisexual, or HIV-positive sex partners; recipients of a blood transfusion between 1978 and 1985; persons seeking treatment for STDs. Clinicians should also consider local epidemiology and HIV screening in the general population.

HR4: Sexually active women with multiple risk factors, including history of STD, new or multiple sex partners, nonuse or inconsistent use of barrier contraceptives, or cervical ectopy. Clinicians should also consider local epidemiology.

HR5: Blood product recipients (including hemodialysis patients), persons with frequent occupational exposure to blood or blood products, men who have sex with men, injection drug users and their sex partners, persons with multiple recent sex partners, persons with other STDs (including HIV), travelers to countries with endemic hepatitis B.

HR6: Persons living in, traveling to, or working in areas where the disease is endemic and where periodic outbreaks occur (e.g., countries with high or intermediate endemicity; certain Alaska Native, Pacific Island, Native American, and religious communities); men who have sex with men; injection or street drug users; patients with clotting factor disorders or chronic liver disease. Consider for institutionalized persons and workers in these institutions; military personnel; and day-care, hospital, and laboratory workers. Clinicians should also consider local epidemiology.

HR7: HIV-positive, close contacts of persons with known or suspected TB, health care workers, persons with medical risk factors associated with TB, immigrants from countries with high TB prevalence, medically underserved low-income populations (including homeless), alcoholics, injection drug users, and residents of long-term care facilities.

HR8: Persons who continue to inject drugs.

HR9: Immunocompetent institutionalized persons aged $\geq$50 yr and immunocompetent persons with certain medical conditions, including chronic cardiac or pulmonary disease, anatomic asplenia, or diabetes mellitus; cochlear implant candidates and recipients. Immunocompetent persons who live in high-risk environments or social settings (e.g., certain Native American and Alaska Native populations).

HR10: Annual vaccination of residents of long-term care facilities; persons with chronic cardiopulmonary disorders, metabolic diseases (including diabetes mellitus), hemoglobinopathies, immunosuppression, or renal dysfunction; and health care providers of high-risk patients.

HR11: Persons born after 1956 who lack evidence of immunity to measles or mumps (e.g., documented receipt of live vaccine on or after the first birthday, laboratory evidence of immunity, or a history of physician-diagnosed measles or mumps).

HR12: Healthy adults without a history of chickenpox or previous immunization. Consider serologic testing for presumed susceptible adults.

HR13: Persons with a family or personal history of skin cancer; a large number of moles; atypical moles; poor tanning ability; or light skin, hair, and eye color.

HR14: Women with previous pregnancy affected by neural tube disorder who are planning pregnancy.

HR15: Clinicians should consider a fasting serum lipid panel on a case-by-case basis.

TABLE 5-4 Ages 65 and Older

Interventions considered and recommended for the Periodic Health Examination	Leading causes of death Heart diseases Malignant neoplasms (lung, colorectal, breast) Cerebrovascular disease Chronic obstructive pulmonary disease Pneumonia and influenza

INTERVENTIONS FOR THE GENERAL POPULATION

Screening	**Injury prevention**
Blood pressure	Lap/shoulder belts
Height and weight	Motorcycle and bicycle helmets*
Fecal occult blood test[1] and/or colonoscopy	Fall prevention*
Mammogram ± clinical breast examination[2] (women ≤69 yr)	Safe storage/removal of firearms*
Papanicolaou (Pap) test (women)[3]	Smoke detector*
Bone density scan in postmenopausal patients	Set hot water heater to <120°-130° F
Vision screening	CPR training for household members
Assess for hearing impairment	**Dental health**
Assess for problem drinking	Regular visits to dental care provider*
Counseling	Floss, brush with fluoride toothpaste daily*
Substance use	**Sexual behavior**
Tobacco cessation	STD prevention: avoid high-risk sexual behavior*; use condoms
Avoid alcohol/drug use while driving, swimming, boating, etc.*	***Immunizations***
Diet and exercise	Pneumococcal vaccine
Limit fat and cholesterol; maintain caloric balance; emphasize grains, fruits, vegetables	Influenza[1]
Adequate calcium intake (women)	Tetanus-diphtheria (Td) boosters
Regular physical activity*	Herpes zoster[4]

INTERVENTIONS FOR HIGH-RISK POPULATIONS

Population	***Potential Interventions (see detailed high-risk definitions)***
Institutionalized persons	PPD (HR1); hepatitis A vaccine (HR2); amantadine/rimantadine (HR4)
Chronic medical conditions; TB contacts; low income; immigrants; alcoholics	PPD (HR1)
Persons ≥75 yr or ≥70 yr with risk factors for falls	Fall prevention intervention (HR5)
Cardiovascular disease risk factors	Consider lipid screening (HR6)
Family history of skin cancer; nevi; fair skin, eyes, hair	Avoid excess/midday sun, use protective clothing* (HR7)
Native Americans/Alaska Natives	PPD (HR1); hepatitis A vaccine (HR2)
Travelers to developing countries	Hepatitis A vaccine (HR2); hepatitis B vaccine (HR8)
Blood product recipients	HIV screen (HR3); hepatitis B vaccine (HR8)
High-risk sexual behavior	Hepatitis A vaccine (HR2); HIV screen (HR3); hepatitis B vaccine (HR8); RPR/VDRL (HR9)
Injection or street drug use	PPD (HR1); hepatitis A vaccine (HR2); HIV screen (HR3); hepatitis B vaccine (HR8); RPR/VDRL (HR9); advice to reduce infection risk (HR10)
Health care/lab workers	PPD (HR1); hepatitis A vaccine (HR2); amantadine/rimantadine (HR4); hepatitis B vaccine (HR8)
Persons susceptible to varicella	Varicella vaccine (HR11)
Men aged 65 to 75 who have ever smoked	Ultrasound of abdominal aorta (HR12)

HR, High risk; *PPD,* purified protein derivative; *RPR,* rapid plasma reagin; *STD,* sexually transmitted disease; *TB,* tuberculosis; *VDRL,* Venereal Disease Research Laboratory.

[1]Annually. [2]Mammogram q1-2 yr, or mammogram q1-2 yr with annual clinical breast exam. [3]All women who are or have been sexually active and who have a cervix. Consider discontinuation of testing after age 65 yr if previous regular screening with consistently normal results. [4]Herpes zoster vaccine (Zostavax) is indicated for prevention of herpes zoster (shingles) in individuals age ≥60 yr. Zostavax is administered as a single dose subcutaneously. It is a lyophilic preparation of the Oka/Merck strain of live, attenuated varicella zoster virus (VZV). It should not be administered to individuals with a history of primary or acquired immunodeficiency states, persons on immunosuppressive therapy (including high-dose corticosteroids), those with active untreated tuberculosis, and those who may be pregnant.

*The ability of clinician counseling to influence this behavior is unproven.

HR1: HIV-positive, close contacts of persons with known or suspected TB, health care workers, persons with medical risk factors associated with TB, immigrants from countries with high TB prevalence, medically underserved low-income populations (including homeless), alcoholics, injection drug users, and residents of long-term care facilities.

HR2: Persons living in, traveling to, or working in areas where the disease is endemic and where periodic outbreaks occur (e.g., countries with high or intermediate endemicity; certain Alaska Native, Pacific Island, Native American, and religious communities); men who have sex with men; injection or street drug users; persons with clotting factor disorders or chronic liver disease. Consider for institutionalized persons and workers in these institutions and day-care, hospital, and laboratory workers. Clinicians should also consider local epidemiology and HIV screening in the general population.

HR3: Men who had sex with men after 1975; past or present injection drug users; persons who exchange sex for money or drugs and their sex partners; persons with current or past injection drug–using, bisexual, or HIV-positive sex partners; recipients of a blood transfusion between 1978 and 1985; persons seeking treatment for STDs. Clinicians should also consider local epidemiology.

HR4: Consider for persons who have not received influenza vaccine or are vaccinated late, when the vaccine may be ineffective because of major antigenic changes in the virus; for unvaccinated persons who provide home care for high-risk persons; as supplemental protection in persons who are expected to have a poor antibody response; and for high-risk persons in whom the vaccine is contraindicated.

HR5: Persons aged ≥75 yr or 70-74 yr with one or more additional risk factors, including use of certain psychoactive and cardiac medications (e.g., benzodiazepines, antihypertensives); use of four or more prescription medications; impaired cognition, strength, balance, or gait. Intensive individualized, home-based multifactorial fall prevention intervention is recommended in settings where adequate resources are available to deliver such services.

HR6: Clinicians should consider fasting lipid panel screening on a case-by-case basis for persons aged 65 to 75 yr, especially in those with additional risk factors (e.g., smoking, diabetes, or hypertension).

HR7: Persons with a family or personal history of skin cancer; a large number of moles; atypical moles; poor tanning ability; or light skin, hair, and eye color.

HR8: Blood product recipients (including hemodialysis patients), persons with frequent occupational exposure to blood or blood products, men who have sex with men, injection drug users and their sex partners, persons with multiple recent sex partners, persons with other STDs (including HIV), travelers to countries with endemic hepatitis B.

HR9: Persons who exchange sex for money or drugs and their sex partners, persons with other STDs (including HIV), and sexual contacts of persons with active syphilis. Clinicians should also consider local epidemiology.

HR10: Persons who continue to inject drugs.

HR11: Healthy adults without a history of chickenpox or previous immunization. Consider serologic testing for presumed susceptible adults.

HR12: Consider ultrasound of abdominal aorta to screen for abdominal aortic aneurysm in all men aged 65 to 75 yr who have ever smoked.

TABLE 5-5 Pregnant Women*

Interventions considered and recommended for the Periodic Health Examination

INTERVENTIONS FOR THE GENERAL POPULATION	
Screening	Offer amniocentesis (15-18 wk)[1] (age ≥35 yr)
First visit	Offer multiple marker testing[1] (15-18 wk)
Blood pressure	Offer serum α-fetoprotein[1] (16-18 wk)
Hemoglobin/hematocrit	***Counseling***
Hepatitis B surface antigen (HBsAg)	Tobacco cessation; effects of passive smoking
RPR/VDRL	Alcohol/other drug use
Chlamydia screen (<25 yr)	Nutrition, including adequate calcium intake
Rubella serology or vaccination history	Encourage breastfeeding
D(Rh) typing, antibody screen	Lap/shoulder belts
Offer CVS (<13 wk)[1] or amniocentesis (15-18 wk)[1] (age ≥35 yr)	Infant safety car seats
Offer hemoglobinopathy screening	STD prevention: avoid high-risk sexual behavior[†]; use condoms[†]
Assess for problem or risk drinking	***Chemoprophylaxis***
Offer HIV screening[2]	Multivitamin with folic acid[3]
Follow-up visits	
Blood pressure	
Urine culture (12-16 wk)	

INTERVENTIONS FOR HIGH-RISK POPULATIONS	
Population	***Potential Interventions (see detailed high-risk definitions)***
High-risk sexual behavior	Screen for chlamydia (first visit) (HR1), gonorrhea (first visit) (HR2), HIV (first visit) (HR3); HBsAg (third trimester) (HR4); RPR/VDRL (third trimester) (HR5)
Blood transfusion between 1978 and 1985	HIV screen (first visit) (HR3)
Injection drug use	HIV screen (HR3); HBsAg (third trimester) (HR4); advice to reduce infection risk (HR6)
Unsensitized D-negative women	D(Rh) antibody testing (24-28 wk) (HR7)
Risk factors for Down syndrome	Offer CVS (first trimester), amniocentesis (15-18 wk)[1] (HR8)
Prior pregnancy with neural tube defect	Offer amniocentesis (15-18 wk),[1] folic acid 4.0 mg[3] (HR9)

CVS, Chorionic villus sampling; *HR,* high risk; *RPR,* rapid plasma reagin; *VDRL,* Venereal Disease Research Laboratory.

[1]Women with access to counseling and follow-up services, reliable standardized laboratories, skilled high-resolution ultrasound and, for those receiving serum marker testing, amniocentesis capabilities. [2]Universal screening is recommended. [3]Beginning at least 1 mo before conception and continuing through the first trimester.

*See Tables 5-2 and 5-3 for other preventive services recommended for women of this age group.

[†]The ability of clinician counseling to influence this behavior is unproven.

HR1: Women with history of STD or new or multiple sex partners. Clinicians should also consider local epidemiology. Chlamydia screen should be repeated in third trimester if at continued risk.

HR2: Women younger than 25 yr with two or more sex partners in the last year or whose sex partner has multiple sexual contacts, women who exchange sex for money or drugs, and women with a history of repeated episodes of gonorrhea. Clinicians should also consider local epidemiology. Gonorrhea screen should be repeated in the third trimester if at continued risk.

HR3: In areas where universal screening is not performed because of low prevalence of HIV infection, pregnant women with the following individual risk factors should be screened: past or present injection drug use; history of exchanging sex for money or drugs; injection drug–using, bisexual, or HIV-positive sex partner currently or in the past; recipients of a blood transfusion between 1978 and 1985; persons seeking treatment for STDs.

HR4: Women who are initially HBsAg negative who are at high risk because of injection drug use, who have suspected exposure to hepatitis B during pregnancy, and who have had multiple sex partners.

HR5: Women who exchange sex for money or drugs, women with other STDs (including HIV), and sexual contacts of persons with active syphilis. Clinicians should also consider local epidemiology.

HR6: Women who continue to inject drugs.

HR7: Unsensitized D-negative women.

HR8: Prior pregnancy affected by Down syndrome, advanced maternal age (≥35 yr), known carriage of chromosome rearrangement.

HR9: Women with previous pregnancy affected by neural tube defect.

PART B • IMMUNIZATIONS AND CHEMOPROPHYLAXIS

Childhood and Adolescent Immunizations

TABLE 5-6 Recommended Immunization Schedule for Persons Aged 0-6 Years—United States, 2010 (For those who fall behind or start late, see the catch-up schedule)

Vaccine ▼ Age ▶	Birth	1 Month	2 Months	4 Months	6 Months	12 Months	15 Months	18 Months	19-23 Months	2-3 Years	4-6 Years
Hepatitis B[1]	HepB	HepB		*See footnote 1*	HepB						
Rotavirus[2]			RV	RV	RV[2]						
Diphtheria, tetanus, pertussis[3]			DTaP	DTaP	DTaP	*See footnote 3*	DTaP				DTaP
Haemophilus influenzae type b[4]			Hib	Hib	Hib[4]	Hib					
Pneumococcal[5]			PCV	PCV	PCV	PCV				PPSV	
Inactivated poliovirus			IPV	IPV	IPV						IPV
Influenza[6]					Influenza (yearly)						
Measles, mumps, rubella[7]						MMR		*See footnote 7*			MMR
Varicella[8]						Varicella		*See footnote 8*			Varicella
Hepatitis A[9]						HepA (2 doses)				HepA Series	
Meningococcal[10]										MCV	

Range of recommended ages

Certain high-risk groups

This schedule indicates the recommended ages for routine administration of currently licensed vaccines, as of December 15, 2009, for children aged 0-6 years. Any dose not administered at the recommended age should be administered at any subsequent visit, when indicated and feasible. Licensed combination vaccines may be used whenever any components of the combination are indicated and other components of the vaccine are not contraindicated and if approved by the Food and Drug Administration for that dose of the series. Providers should consult the relevant Advisory Committee on Immunization Practices statement for detailed recommendations, including high-risk conditions: http://www.cdc.gov/vaccines/pubs/acip-list.htm. Clinically significant adverse events that follow immunization should be reported to the Vaccine Adverse Event Reporting System (VAERS). Guidance about how to obtain and complete a VAERS form is available at http://www.vaers.hhs.gov or by telephone, 800-822-7967.

1. **Hepatitis B vaccine (HepB).** *(Minimum age: birth)*
   At birth:
   - Administer monovalent HepB to all newborns before hospital discharge.
   - If mother is hepatitis B surface antigen (HBsAg)-positive, administer HepB and 0.5 mL of hepatitis B immune globulin (HBIG) within 12 hours of birth.
   - If mother's HBsAg status is unknown, administer HepB within 12 hours of birth. Determine mother's HBsAg status as soon as possible and, if HBsAg-positive, administer HBIG (no later than age 1 week).

   After the birth dose:
   - The HepB series should be completed with either monovalent HepB or a combination vaccine containing HepB. The second dose should be administered at age 1 or 2 months. Monovalent HepB vaccine should be used for doses administered before age 6 weeks. The final dose should be administered no earlier than age 24 weeks.
   - Infants born to HBsAg-positive mothers should be tested for HBsAg and antibody to HBsAg (anti-HBs) after completion of at least 3 doses of the HepB series, at age 9 through 18 months (generally at the next well-child visit).

   4-month dose:
   - Administration of 4 doses of HepB to infants is permissible when combination vaccines containing HepB are administered after the birth dose. The fourth dose should be administered no earlier than age 24 weeks.
2. **Rotavirus vaccine (RV).** *(Minimum age: 6 weeks)*
   - Administer the first dose at age 6 through 14 weeks *(maximum age: 14 weeks 6 days)*. Vaccination should not be initiated for infants aged 15 weeks or older (i.e., 15 weeks, 0 days or older).
   - Administer the final dose in the series by age 8 months 0 days.
   - If Rotarix® is administered at ages 2 and 4 months, a dose at 6 months is not indicated.
3. **Diphtheria and tetanus toxoids and acellular pertussis vaccine (DTaP).** *(Minimum age: 6 weeks)*
   - The fourth dose may be administered as early as age 12 months, provided at least 6 months have elapsed since the third dose.
   - Administer the final dose in the series at age 4 through 6 years.
4. **Haemophilus influenzae type b conjugate vaccine (Hib).** *(Minimum age: 6 weeks)*
   - If PRP-OMP (PedvaxHIB® or Comvax® [HepB-Hib]) is administered at ages 2 and 4 months, a dose at age 6 months is not indicated.
   - TriHiBit® (DTaP/Hib) should not be used for doses at ages 2, 4, or 6 months but can be used as the final dose in children aged 12 months or older.
5. **Pneumococcal vaccine.** *(Minimum age: 6 weeks for pneumococcal conjugate vaccine [PCV]; 2 years for pneumococcal polysaccharide vaccine [PPSV])*
   - PCV is recommended for all children aged younger than 5 years. Administer 1 dose of PCV to all healthy children aged 24 through 59 months who are not completely vaccinated for their age.
   - Administer PPSV to children aged 2 years or older with certain underlying medical conditions (see *MMWR* 2000;49[No. RR-9]), including a cochlear implant.
6. **Influenza vaccine.** *(Minimum age: 6 months for trivalent inactivated influenza vaccine [TIV]; 2 years for live, attenuated influenza vaccine [LAIV])*
   - Administer annually to children aged 6 months through 18 years
   - For healthy nonpregnant persons (i.e., those who do not have underlying medical conditions that predispose them to influenza complications) aged 2 through 49 years, either LAIV or TIV may be used.
   - Children receiving TIV should receive 0.25 mL if aged 6 through 35 months or 0.5 mL if aged 3 years or older.
   - Administer 2 doses (separated by at least 4 weeks) to children aged younger than 9 years who are receiving influenza vaccine for the first time or who were vaccinated for the first time during the previous influenza season but only received 1 dose.
7. **Measles, mumps, and rubella vaccine (MMR).** *(Minimum age: 12 months)*
   - Administer the second dose at age 4-6 years. However, the second dose may be administered before age 4, provided at least 28 days have elapsed since the first dose.
8. **Varicella vaccine.** *(Minimum age: 12 months)*
   - Administer the second dose at age 4 through 6 years. However, the second dose may be administered before age 4, provided at least 3 months have elapsed since the first dose.
   - For children aged 12 months through 12 years the minimum interval between doses is 3 months. However, if the second dose was administered at least 28 days after the first dose, it can be accepted as valid.
9. **Hepatitis A vaccine (HepA).** *(Minimum age: 12 months)*
   - Administer to all children aged 1 year (i.e., aged 12 through 23 months). Administer 2 doses at least 6 months apart.
   - Children not fully vaccinated by age 2 years can be vaccinated at subsequent visits.
   - HepA also is recommended for children older than 1 year who live in areas where vaccination programs target older children or who are at increased risk of infection. See *MMWR* 2006;55(No. RR-7).
10. **Meningococcal vaccine.** *(Minimum age: 2 years for meningococcal conjugate vaccine [MCV] and for meningococcal polysaccharide vaccine [MPSV])*
    - Administer MCV to children aged 2 through 10 years with terminal complement component deficiency, anatomic or functional asplenia, and certain other high-risk groups. See *MMWR* 2005;54(No. RR-7).
    - Persons who received MPSV 3 or more years previously and who remain at increased risk for meningococcal disease should be revaccinated with MCV.

Note: The National Childhood Vaccine Injury Act requires that health-care providers provide parents or patients with copies of vaccine information statements before administering each dose of the vaccines listed in the schedules.

The recommended immunization schedules for persons aged 0 to 18 yr are approved by the Advisory Committee on Immunization Practices (http://www.cdc.gov/vaccines/recs/acip), the American Academy of Pediatrics (http://www.aap.org), and the American Academy of Family Physicians (http://www.aafp.org).

TABLE 5-7 Recommended Immunization Schedule for Persons Aged 7-18 Years—United States, 2010 (For those who fall behind or start late, see the schedule below and the catch-up schedule)

Vaccine ▼ Age ▶	7-10 years	11-12 years	13-18 years
Tetanus, diphtheria, pertussis[1]	*See footnote 1*	Tdap	Tdap
Human papillomavirus[2]	*See footnote 2*	HPV (3 doses)	HPV Series
Meningococcal[3]	MCV	MCV	MCV
Influenza[4]	Influenza (yearly)		
Pneumococcal[5]	PPSV		
Hepatitis A[6]	HepA Series		
Hepatitis B[7]	HepB Series		
Inactivated poliovirus[8]	IPV Series		
Measles, mumps, rubella[9]	MMR Series		
Varicella[10]	Varicella Series		

Range of recommended ages

Catch-up immunization

Certain high-risk groups

This schedule indicates the recommended ages for routine administration of currently licensed vaccines, as of December 15, 2009, for children aged 7-18 years. Any dose not administered at the recommended age should be administered at any subsequent visit, when indicated and feasible. Licensed combination vaccines may be used whenever any components of the combination are indicated and other components of the vaccine are not contraindicated and if approved by the Food and Drug Administration for that dose of the series. Providers should consult the respective Advisory Committee on Immunization Practices statement for detailed recommendations, including high-risk conditions: http://www.cdc.gov/vaccines/pubs/acip-list.htm. Clinically significant adverse events that follow immunization should be reported to the Vaccine Adverse Event Reporting System (VAERS). Guidance about how to obtain and complete a VAERS form is available at http://www.vaers.hhs.gov or by telephone, 800-822-7967.

1. **Tetanus and diphtheria toxoids and acellular pertussis vaccine (Tdap).** *(Minimum age: 10 years for BOOSTRIX® and 11 years for ADACEL®)*
   - Administer at age 11 or 12 years for those who have completed the recommended childhood DTP/DTaP vaccination series and have not received a tetanus and diphtheria toxoid (Td) booster dose.
   - Persons aged 13 to 18 years who have not received Tdap should receive a dose.
   - A 5-year interval from the last Td dose is encouraged when Tdap is used as a booster dose; however, a shorter interval may be used if pertussis immunity is needed.
2. **Human papillomavirus vaccine (HPV).** *(Minimum age: 9 years)*
   - Two HPV vaccines are licensed: A quadrivalent vaccine (HPV4) for the prevention of cervical, vaginal, and vulvar cancer (in females) and genital warts (in females and males) and a bivalent vaccine (HPV2) for the prevention of cervical cancers in females.
   - HPV4 is recommended for the prevention of cervical, vaginal, and vulvar precancers and cancers and genital warts in females.
   - Administer the first dose to females at age 11 or 12 years.
   - Administer the second dose 2 months after the first dose and the third dose 6 months after the first dose (at least 24 weeks after the first dose).
   - Administer the series to females at age 13 to 18 years if not previously vaccinated.
   - HPV4 may be administered in a 3-dose series to males aged 9 through 18 years to reduce the likelihood of acquiring genital warts.
3. **Meningococcal conjugate vaccine (MCV).**
   - Administer at age 11 or 12 years, or at age 13 to 18 years if not previously vaccinated.
   - Administer to previously unvaccinated college freshmen living in a dormitory.
   - Administer MCV4 to children aged 2 through 10 years with complement component deficiency, anatomic or functional asplenia, or certain other conditions placing them at high risk.
   - Administer to children previously vaccinated with MCV4 or MPSV4 who remain at increased risk after 3 years (if first dose administered at age 7 years or older). Persons whose only risk factor is living in on-campus housing are not recommended to receive an additional dose. See *MMWR* 2009;58:1042-1043.
4. **Influenza vaccine.**
   - Administer annually to children aged 6 months to 18 years.
   - For healthy nonpregnant persons (i.e., those who do not have underlying medical conditions that predispose them to influenza complications) aged 2 to 49 years, either LAIV or TIV may be used.
   - Administer 2 doses (separated by at least 4 weeks) to children aged younger than 9 years who are receiving influenza vaccine for the first time or who were vaccinated for the first time during the previous influenza season but only received 1 dose.
5. **Pneumococcal polysaccharide vaccine (PPSV).**
   - Administer to children with certain underlying medical conditions (see *MMWR* 1997;46[No. RR-8]), including a cochlear implant. A single revaccination should be administered to children with functional or anatomic asplenia or other immunocompromising condition after 5 years.
6. **Hepatitis A vaccine (HepA).**
   - Administer 2 doses at least 6 months apart.
   - HepA is recommended for children older than 23 months who live in areas where vaccination programs target older children, who are at increased risk for infection, or for whom immunity against hepatitis A is desired.
7. **Hepatitis B vaccine (HepB).**
   - Administer the 3-dose series to those not previously vaccinated.
   - A 2-dose series (separated by at least 4 months) of adult formulation Recombivax HB® is licensed for children aged 11 to 15 years.
8. **Inactivated poliovirus vaccine (IPV).**
   - For children who received an all-IPV or all-oral poliovirus (OPV) series, a fourth dose is not necessary if the third dose was administered at age 4 years or older.
   - If both OPV and IPV were administered as part of a series, a total of 4 doses should be administered, regardless of the child's current age.
9. **Measles, mumps, and rubella vaccine (MMR).**
   - If not previously vaccinated, administer 2 doses or the second dose for those who have received only 1 dose, with at least 28 days between doses.
10. **Varicella vaccine.**
    - For persons aged 7 to 18 years without evidence of immunity (see *MMWR* 2007;56[No. RR-4]), administer 2 doses if not previously vaccinated or the second dose if they have received only 1 dose.
    - For persons aged 7 to 12 years, the minimum interval between doses is 3 months. However, if the second dose was administered at least 28 days after the first dose, it can be accepted as valid.
    - For persons aged 13 years and older, the minimum interval between doses is 28 days.

The recommended immunization schedules for persons aged 0 to 18 yr are approved by the Advisory Committee on Immunization Practices (http://www.cdc.gov.vaccines.recs.acip), the American Academy of Pediatrics (http://www.aap.org), and the American Academy of Family Physicians (http://www.aafp.org).

TABLE 5-8 Catch-Up Immunization Schedule for Persons Aged 4 Months to 18 Years Who Start Late or Who Are More than 1 Month Behind—United States

This table provides catch-up schedules and minimum intervals between doses for children whose vaccinations have been delayed. A vaccine series does not need to be restarted regardless of the time that has elapsed between doses. Use the section appropriate for the child's age.

Vaccine	Minimum Age for Dose 1	Minimum Interval Between Doses			
		Dose 1 to Dose 2	Dose 2 to Dose 3	Dose 3 to Dose 4	Dose 4 to Dose 5
CATCH-UP SCHEDULE FOR PERSONS AGED 4 MONTHS TO 6 YEARS					
Hepatitis B[1]	Birth	4 weeks	8 weeks (and at least 16 weeks after first dose)		
Rotavirus[2]	6 weeks	4 weeks	4 weeks[2]		
Diphtheria,tetanus, pertussis[3]	6 weeks	4 weeks	4 weeks	6 months	6 months[3]
Haemophilus influenzae type b[4]	6 weeks	4 weeks if first dose administered at younger than 12 months of age 8 weeks (as final dose) if first dose administered at age 12-14 months No further doses needed if first dose administered at age 15 months or older	4 weeks[4] if current age is younger than 12 months 8 weeks (as final dose)[4] if current age is 12 months or older and second dose administered at younger than 15 months of age No further doses needed if previous dose administered at age 15 months or older	8 weeks (as final dose) This dose only necessary for children aged 12 months through 59 months who received 3 doses before age 12 months	
Pneumococcal[5]	6 weeks	4 weeks if first dose administered at younger than 12 months of age 8 weeks (as final dose for healthy children) if first dose administered at age 12 months or older or current age 24 to 59 months No further doses needed for healthy children if first dose administered at age 24 months or older	4 weeks if current age is younger than 12 months 8 weeks (as final dose for healthy children) if current age is 12 months or older No further doses needed for healthy children if previous dose administered at age 24 months or older	8 weeks (as final dose) This dose only necessary for children aged 12 months to 59 months who received 3 doses before age 12 months or for high-risk children who received 3 doses at any age	
Inactivated poliovirus[6]	6 weeks	4 weeks	4 weeks	4 weeks[6]	
Measles, mumps, rubella[7]	12 months	4 weeks			
Varicella[8]	12 months	3 months			
Hepatitis A[9]	12 months	6 months			
CATCH-UP SCHEDULE FOR PERSONS AGED 7 TO 18 YEARS					
Tetanus, diphtheria/ tetanus, diphtheria, pertussis[10]	7 years[10]	4 weeks	4 weeks if first dose administered at younger than 12 months of age 6 months if first dose administered at age 12 months or older	6 months if first dose administered at younger than 12 months of age	
Human papillomavirus[11]	9 years	Routine dosing intervals are recommended[11]			
Hepatitis A[9]	12 months	6 months			
Hepatitis B[1]	Birth	4 weeks	8 weeks (and at least 16 weeks after first dose)		
Inactivated poliovirus[6]	6 weeks	4 weeks	4 weeks	6 months	
Measles, mumps, rubella[7]	12 months	4 weeks			
Varicella[8]	12 months	3 months if the person is younger than age 13 years of age 4 weeks if the person is aged 13 years or older			

1. **Hepatitis B vaccine (HepB).**
   - Administer the 3-dose series to those not previously vaccinated.
   - A 2-dose series (separated by at least 4 mo) of adult formulation Recombivax HB is licensed for children aged 11 to 15 yr.
2. **Rotavirus vaccine (RV).**
   - The maximum age for the first dose is 14 wk 6 days. Vaccination should not be initiated for infants aged 15 wk or older (i.e., 15 wk 0 days or older).
   - Administer the final dose in the series by age 8 mo 0 days.
   - If Rotarix was administered for the first and second doses, a third dose is not indicated.
3. **Diphtheria and tetanus toxoids and acellular pertussis vaccine (DTaP).**
   - The fifth dose is not necessary if the fourth dose was administered at age 4 yr or older.
4. ***Haemophilus influenzae* type b conjugate vaccine (Hib).**
   - Hib vaccine is not generally recommended for persons aged 5 yr or older. No efficacy data are available on which to base a recommendation concerning use of Hib vaccine for older children and adults. However, studies suggest good immunogenicity in persons who have sickle cell disease, leukemia, or HIV infection, or who have had a splenectomy; administering 1 dose of Hib vaccine to these persons is not contraindicated.
   - If the first 2 doses were PRP-OMP (PedvaxHIB or Comvax), and administered at age 11 mo or younger, the third (and final) dose should be administered at age 12 to 15 mo and at least 8 wk after the second dose.
   - If the first dose was administered at age 7 to 11 mo, administer 2 doses separated by 4 wk and a final dose at age 12 to 15 mo.
5. **Pneumococcal vaccine.**
   - Administer 1 dose of pneumococcal conjugate vaccine (PCV) to all healthy children aged 24 to 59 mo who have not received at least 1 dose of PCV on or after age 12 mo.
   - For children aged 24 to 59 mo with underlying medical conditions, administer 1 dose of PCV if 3 doses were received previously or administer 2 doses of PCV at least 8 wk apart if fewer than 3 doses were received previously.
   - Administer pneumococcal polysaccharide vaccine (PPSV) to children aged 2 yr or older with certain underlying medical conditions (see *MMWR* 49(RR-9), 2000), including a cochlear implant, at least 8 wk after the last dose of PCV.
6. **Inactivated poliovirus vaccine (IPV).**
   - The final dose in the series should be administered on or after the fourth birthday and at least 6 months following the previous dose.
   - A fourth dose is not necessary if the third dose was administered at age 4 or older and at least 6 months following the previous dose.
   - In the first 6 months of life, minimum age and minimum intervals are only recommended if the person is at risk for imminent exposure to circulating poliovirus (i.e., travel to a polio-endemic region or during an outbreak).
7. **Measles, mumps, and rubella vaccine (MMR).**
   - Administer the second dose at age 4 to 6 yr. However, the second dose may be administered before age 4, provided at least 28 days have elapsed since the first dose.
   - If not previously vaccinated, administer 2 doses with at least 28 days between doses.
8. **Varicella vaccine.**
   - Administer the second dose at age 4 to 6 yr. However, the second dose may be administered before age 4, provided at least 3 mo have elapsed since the first dose.
   - For persons aged 12 mo to 12 yr, the minimum interval between doses is 3 mo. However, if the second dose was administered at least 28 days after the first dose, it can be accepted as valid.
   - For persons aged 13 yr and older, the minimum interval between doses is 28 days.
9. **Hepatitis A vaccine (HepA).**
   - HepA is recommended for children older than 1 yr who live in areas where vaccination programs target older children or who are at increased risk of infection. See *MMWR* 55(RR-7), 2006.
10. **Tetanus and diphtheria toxoids vaccine (Td) and tetanus and diphtheria toxoids and acellular pertussis vaccine (Tdap).**
    - Doses of DTaP are counted as part of the Td/Tdap series.
    - dap should be substituted for a single dose of Td in the catch-up series or as a booster for children aged 10 to 18 yr; use Td for other doses.
11. **Human papillomavirus vaccine (HPV).**
    - Administer the series to females at age 13 to 18 yr if not previously vaccinated.
    - Use recommended routine dosing intervals for series catch-up (i.e., the second and third doses should be administered at 2 and 6 mo after the first dose). However, the minimum interval between the first and second doses is 4 wk. The minimum interval between the second and third doses is 12 wk, and the third dose should be given at least 24 wk after the first dose.

Information about reporting reactions after immunization is available online at http://www.vaers.hhs.gov or by telephone, 800-822-7967. Suspected cases of vaccine-preventable diseases should be reported to the state or local health department. Additional information, including precautions and contraindications for immunization, is available from the National Center for Immunization and Respiratory Diseases at http://www.cdc.gov/vaccines or by telephone at 800-CDC-INFO (800-232-4636).

QUADRIVALENT HUMAN PAPILLOMAVIRUS (HPV) VACCINE*

SUMMARY OF RATIONALE FOR QUADRIVALENT HPV VACCINE RECOMMENDATIONS*

The availability of a quadrivalent HPV vaccine offers an opportunity to decrease the burden of HPV infection and its sequelae, including cervical cancer precursors, cervical cancer, other anogenital cancers, and genital warts, in the United States. Quadrivalent HPV vaccine is licensed for use among females aged 9 to 26 years. HPV4 may also be administered in a 3-dose series to males aged 9 through 18 years to reduce their likelihood of acquiring genital warts. In this age group, clinical trials indicate that the vaccine is safe and immunogenic. Trials among females aged 16 to 26 years indicated the vaccine to be effective against HPV types 6-, 11-, 16-, and 18-related cervical, vaginal, and vulvar cancer precursors and dysplastic lesions and genital warts. HPV 16 and 18 cause approximately 70% of cervical cancers; HPV 6 and 11 cause approximately 90% of genital warts. Because HPV is sexually transmitted and often acquired soon after onset of sexual activity, vaccination should ideally occur before first sexual activity. The recommended age for vaccination is 11 to 12 years; vaccine can be administered to girls as young as age 9 years. At the beginning of a vaccination program, females older than 12 years will exist who did not have the opportunity to receive vaccine at age 11 to 12 years. Catch-up vaccination is recommended for females aged 13 to 26 years who have not yet been vaccinated.

The recommendation for routine vaccination of girls aged 11 to 12 years is based on several considerations, including studies suggesting that quadrivalent HPV vaccine among adolescents will be safe and effective, high antibody titers achieved after vaccination at age 11 to 12 years, data on HPV epidemiology and age of sexual debut in the United States, and the high probability of HPV acquisition within several years of first sexual activity. Ideally, HPV vaccine should be administered before first sexual activity, and duration of protection should extend for many years, providing protection when exposure through sexual activity might occur. The vaccine has been demonstrated to provide protection for at least 5 years without evidence of waning. Long-term follow-up studies are underway to determine duration of protection. The recommendation also considered cost-effectiveness evaluations and the established young adolescent health care visit at age 11 to 12 years recommended by several professional organizations, when other vaccines are also recommended.

Although routine vaccination is recommended at age 11 to 12 years, the majority of females aged 13 to 26 years also can benefit from vaccination. Females not yet sexually active can be expected to receive the full benefit of vaccination. Although sexually active females in this age group might have been infected with one or more vaccine HPV types, type-specific prevalence studies in the United States suggest that a small percentage of sexually active females have been infected with all four of the HPV vaccine types. These data, available from North American females aged 16 to 24 years who participated in the quadrivalent vaccine trials, are from women who were more likely to have ever had sex than similarly aged females in the general U.S. population. Among those sexually active females, the median number of lifetime sex partners (two) was similar in trial participants and females in the general U.S. population. The vaccine does not appear to protect against persistent infection, cervical cancer precursor lesions, or genital warts caused by an HPV type that females are infected with at the time of vaccination. However, females already infected with one or more vaccine HPV types before vaccination would be protected against disease caused by the other vaccine HPV types. Therefore although overall vaccine effectiveness would be lower when administered to a population of females who are sexually active and would decrease with older age and likelihood of HPV exposure with increasing number of sex partners, the majority of females in this age group will derive at least partial benefit from vaccination.

*From CDC: Quadrivalent human papillomavirus vaccine: recommendations of the Advisory Committee on Immunization Practices (ACIP), *MMWR* 56(RR-2):16-18, 2007.

RECOMMENDATIONS FOR USE OF HPV VACCINE

RECOMMENDATIONS FOR ROUTINE USE AND CATCH-UP

Routine Vaccination of Females Aged 11 to 12 Years

The Advisory Committee on Immunization Practices (ACIP) recommends routine vaccination of females aged 11 to 12 years with 3 doses of quadrivalent HPV vaccine. The vaccination series can be started as young as age 9 years.

Catch-Up Vaccination of Females Aged 13-26 Years

Vaccination also is recommended for females aged 13 to 26 years who have not been previously vaccinated or who have not completed the full series. Ideally, vaccine should be administered before potential exposure to HPV through sexual contact; however, females who might have already been exposed to HPV should be vaccinated. Sexually active females who have not been infected with any of the HPV vaccine types would receive full benefit from vaccination. Vaccination would provide less benefit to females if they have already been infected with one or more of the four vaccine HPV types. However, clinicians cannot assess the extent to which sexually active persons would benefit from vaccination, and the risk for HPV infection might continue as long as persons are sexually active. Pap testing and screening for HPV DNA or HPV antibody are not needed before vaccination at any age.

Dosage and Administration

The vaccine should be shaken well before administration. The dose of quadrivalent HPV vaccine is 0.5 ml, administered intramuscularly (IM), preferably in the deltoid muscle.

Recommended Schedule

Quadrivalent HPV vaccine is administered in a 3-dose schedule. The second and third doses should be administered 2 and 6 months after the first dose.

Minimum Dosing Intervals and Management of Persons Who Were Incorrectly Vaccinated

The minimum interval between the first and second doses of vaccine is 4 weeks. The minimum recommended interval between the second and third doses of vaccine is 12 weeks. Inadequate doses of quadrivalent HPV vaccine or vaccine doses received after a shorter-than-recommended dosing interval should be readministered.

Interrupted Vaccine Schedules

If the quadrivalent HPV vaccine schedule is interrupted, the vaccine series does not need to be restarted. If the series is interrupted after the first dose, the second dose should be administered as soon as possible and separated from the third dose by an interval of at least 12 weeks. If only the third dose is delayed, it should be administered as soon as possible.

Simultaneous Administration with Other Vaccines

Although no data exist on administration of quadrivalent HPV vaccine with vaccines other than hepatitis B vaccine, quadrivalent HPV vaccine is not a live vaccine and has no components that adversely affect safety or efficacy of other vaccinations. Quadrivalent HPV vaccine can be administered at the same visit as other age-appropriate vaccines, such as the diphtheria, tetanus, pertussis (DTP), and quadrivalent meningococcal conjugate (MCV4) vaccines. Administering all indicated vaccines together at a single visit increases the likelihood that adolescents and young adults will receive each of the vaccines on schedule. Each vaccine should be administered by a separate syringe at a different anatomic site.

Cervical Cancer Screening among Vaccinated Females

Cervical cancer screening recommendations have not changed for females who receive HPV vaccine. HPV types in the vaccine are responsible for approximately 70% of cervical cancers; females who are vaccinated could subsequently be infected with a carcinogenic HPV type for which the quadrivalent vaccine does not provide protection. Furthermore, those who were sexually active before vaccination could have been infected with a vaccine-type HPV before vaccination. Health care providers administering quadrivalent HPV vaccine should educate women about the importance of cervical cancer screening.

GROUPS FOR WHICH VACCINE IS NOT LICENSED

Vaccination of Females Aged <9 Years and >26 Years

Quadrivalent HPV vaccine is not licensed for use in girls younger than 9 years or women older than 26 years. Studies are ongoing among women older than 26 years. No studies are underway among girls younger than 9 years.

Vaccination of Males

Quadrivalent HPV vaccine is not licensed for use among males. Although data on immunogenicity and safety are available for males aged 9 to 15 years, no data exist on efficacy in males at any age. Efficacy studies in males are underway.

SPECIAL SITUATIONS AMONG FEMALES AGED 9 TO 26 YEARS

Equivocal or Abnormal Pap Test or Known HPV Infection

Females who have an equivocal or abnormal Pap test could be infected with any of approximately 40 high-risk or low-risk genital HPV types. Such females are unlikely to be infected with all four HPV vaccine types, and they might not be infected with any HPV vaccine type. Vaccination would provide protection against infection with HPV vaccine types not already acquired. With increasing severity of Pap test findings, the likelihood of infection with HPV 16 or 18 increases and the benefit of vaccination would decrease. Women should be advised that results from clinical trials do not indicate the vaccine will have any therapeutic effect on existing HPV infection or cervical lesions.

Females who have a positive HC2 high-risk test result conducted in conjunction with a Pap test could have infection with any of 13 high-risk types. This assay does not identify specific HPV types, and testing for specific HPV types is not conducted routinely in clinical practice. Women with a positive HC2 high-risk test result might not have been infected with any of the four HPV vaccine types. Vaccination would provide protection against infection with HPV vaccine types not already acquired. However, women should be advised that results from clinical trials do not indicate the vaccine will have any therapeutic effect on existing HPV infection or cervical lesions.

Genital Warts

A history of genital warts or clinically evident genital warts indicates infection with HPV, most often types 6 or 11. However, these females might not have infection with both HPV 6 and 11 or infection with HPV 16 or 18. Vaccination would provide protection against infection with HPV vaccine types not already acquired. However, females should be advised that results from clinical trials do not indicate the vaccine will have any therapeutic effect on existing HPV infection or genital warts.

Lactating Women

Lactating women can receive the HPV vaccine.

Immunocompromised Persons

Because quadrivalent HPV vaccine is a noninfectious vaccine, it can be administered to females who are immunosuppressed as a result of disease or medications. However, the immune response and vaccine efficacy might be less than that in persons who are immunocompetent.

Vaccination during Pregnancy

Quadrivalent HPV vaccine is not recommended for use in pregnancy. The vaccine has not been causally associated with adverse outcomes of pregnancy or adverse events in the developing fetus. However, data on vaccination during pregnancy are limited. Until additional information is available, initiation of the vaccine series should be delayed until after completion of the pregnancy. If a woman is found to be pregnant after initiating the vaccination series, the remainder of the 3-dose regimen should be delayed until after completion of the pregnancy. If a vaccine dose has been administered during pregnancy, no intervention is needed. A vaccine-in-pregnancy registry has been established; patients and health care providers should report any exposure to quadrivalent HPV vaccine during pregnancy by calling 800-986-8999.

PRECAUTIONS AND CONTRAINDICATIONS

Acute Illnesses

Quadrivalent HPV vaccine can be administered to persons with minor acute illnesses (e.g., diarrhea or mild upper respiratory tract infections with or without fever). Vaccination of persons with moderate or severe acute illnesses should be deferred until after the patient improves.

Hypersensitivity or Allergy to Vaccine Components

Quadrivalent HPV vaccine is contraindicated for persons with a history of immediate hypersensitivity to yeast or to any vaccine component. Data from passive surveillance in the Vaccine Adverse Event Reporting System (VAERS) indicate that recombinant yeast-derived vaccines pose a minimal risk for anaphylactic reactions in persons with a history of allergic reactions to *Saccharomyces cerevisiae* (baker's yeast).

Preventing Syncope after Vaccination

Syncope (i.e., vasovagal or vasodepressor reaction) can occur after vaccination, most commonly among adolescents and young adults. Among reports to VAERS for any vaccine that was coded as triggering syncope from 1990 to 2004, 35% of these episodes were reported among persons aged 10 to 18 years. Through January 2007, the second most common report to VAERS after receipt of HPV vaccine was syncope (Centers for Disease Control and Prevention, unpublished data, 2007). Vaccine providers should consider observing patients for 15 minutes after they receive HPV vaccine.

General Recommendations on Immunization

TABLE 5-9 Recommended and Minimum Ages and Intervals between Vaccine Doses of Routinely Recommended Vaccines[a]

Vaccine and Dose Number	Recommended Age for this Dose	Minimum Age for this Dose	Recommended Interval to Next Dose	Minimum Interval to Next Dose
Hepatitis B (HepB)-1[b]	Birth	Birth	1-4 mo	4 wk
HepB-2	1-2 mo	4 wk	2-17 mo	8 wk
HepB-3[c]	6-18 mo	24 wk	—	—
Diphtheria-tetanus-acellular pertussis (DTaP)-1[b]	2 mo	6 wk	2 mo	4 wk
DTaP-2	4 mo	10 wk	2 mo	4 wk
DTaP-3	6 mo	14 wk	6-12 mo[d]	6 mo[d,e]
DTaP-4	15-18 mo	12 mo	3 yr	6 mo[d]
DTaP-5	4-6 yr	4 yr	—	—
Haemophilus influenzae type b (Hib)-1[b,f]	2 mo	6 wk	2 mo	4 wk
Hib-2	4 mo	10 wk	2 mo	4 wk
Hib-3[g]	6 mo	14 wk	6-9 mo[d]	8 wk
Hib-4	12-15 mo	12 mo	—	—
Inactivated poliovirus (IPV)-1[b]	2 mo	6 wk	2 mo	4 wk
IPV-2	4 mo	10 wk	2-14 mo	4 wk
IPV-3	6-18 mo	14 wk	3-5 yr	4 wk
IPV-4	4-6 yr	18 wk	—	—
Pneumococcal conjugate (PCV)-1[f]	2 mo	6 wk	2 mo	4 wk
PCV-2	4 mo	10 wk	2 mo	4 wk
PCV-3	6 mo	14 wk	6 mo	8 wk
PCV-4	12-15 mo	12 mo	—	—
Measles-mumps-rubella (MMR)-1[h]	12-15 mo	12 mo	3-5 yr	4 wk
MMR-2[h]	4-6 yr	13 mo	—	—
Varicella (Var)-1[h]	12-15 mo	12 mo	3-5 yr	12 wk[i]
Var-2[h]	4-6 yr	15 mo	—	—
Hepatitis A (HepA)-1[b]	12-23 mo	12 mo	6-18 mo[d]	6 mo[d]
HepA-2	18-41 mo	18 mo	—	—
Influenza inactivated[j]	6-59 mo	6 mo[k]	1 mo	4 wk
Influenza live attenuated[j]	—	5 yr	6-10 wk	6 wk
Meningococcal conjugate[b]	11-12 yr	11 yr	—	—
Meningococcal polysaccharide (MPSV)-1	—	2 yr	5 yr[k]	5 yr[l]
MPSV-2[m]	—	7 yr	—	—
Tetanus-diphtheria	11-12 yr	7 yr	10 yr	5 yr
Tetanus-diphtheria acellular pertussis (Tdap)[n]	≥11 yr	10 yr	—	—
Pneumococcal polysaccharide (PPV)-1	—	2 yr	5 yr	5 yr
PPV-2[o]	—	7 yr	—	—
Human papillomavirus (HPV)-1[p]	11-12 yr	9 yr	2 mo	4 wk
HPV-2	11-12 yr (+2 mo)	109 mo	4 mo	12 wk
HPV-3	11-12 yr (+6 mo)	112 mo	—	—
Rotavirus (RV)-1[q]	2 mo	6 wk	2 mo	4 wk
RV-2	4 mo	10 wk	2 mo	4 wk
RV-3	6 mo	14 wk	—	—
Zoster[r]	60 yr	60 yr	—	

TABLE 5-9 Recommended and Minimum Ages and Intervals between Vaccine Doses of Routinely Recommended Vaccines—cont'd

From CDC: General recommendations on immunization: recommendations of the Advisory Committee on Immunization Practices (ACIP), *MMWR* 55:(RR-15), 2006.

[a]Combination vaccines are available. Use of licensed combination vaccines is preferred over separate injections of their equivalent component vaccines. (Source: CDC: Combination vaccines for childhood immunization: recommendations of the Advisory Committee on Immunization Practices [ACIP], the American Academy of Pediatrics [AAP], and the American Academy of Family Physicians [AAFP], *MMWR* 48:[RR-5], 1999.) When administering combination vaccines, the minimum age for administration is the oldest age for any of the individual components; the minimum interval between doses is equal to the greatest interval of any of the individual components.

[b]Combination vaccines containing the hepatitis B component are available (HepB-Hib, DTaP-HepB-IPV, and HepA-HepB). These vaccines should not be administered to infants aged <6 wk because of the other components (i.e., Hib, DTaP, HepA, and IPV).

[c]HepB-3 should be administered at least 8 wk after HepB-2 and at least 16 wk after HepB-1 and should not be administered before age 24 wk.

[d]Calendar months.

[e]The minimum recommended interval between DTaP-3 and DTaP-4 is 6 mo. However, DTaP-4 need not be repeated if administered at least 4 mo after DTaP-3.

[f]For Hib and PCV, children receiving the first dose of vaccine at age ≥7 mo require fewer doses to complete the series. (Source: Centers for Disease Control and Prevention: Recommended childhood and adolescent immunization schedule—United States, 2006, *MMWR* 54[51 & 52]:Q1-Q4, 2005.)

[g]If PRP-OMP (Pedvax-Hib, Merck) was administered at age 2 and 4 mo, a dose at age 6 mo is not required.

[h]Combination measles-mumps-rubella-varicella (MMRV) vaccine can be used for children aged 12 mo to 12 yr.

[i]The minimum interval from VAR-1 to VAR-2 for persons beginning the series at age ≥13 yr is 4 wk.

[j]Two doses of influenza vaccine are recommended for children aged <9 yr who are receiving the vaccine for the first time. Children aged <9 yr who have previously received influenza vaccine and persons aged ≥9 yr require only 1 dose per influenza season.

[k]The minimum age for inactivated influenza vaccine varies by vaccine manufacturer. Only Fluzone (Sanofi Pasteur) is approved for children aged 6-35 mo. The minimum age for Fluvirin (Novartis) is 4 yr. For Fluarix and FluLeval (GlaxoSmithKline), the minimum age is 18 yr.

[l]Certain experts recommend a second dose of MPSV 3 yr after the first dose for persons at increased risk for meningococcal disease.

[m]A second dose of meningococcal vaccine is recommended for persons previously vaccinated with MPSV who remain at high risk for meningococcal disease. MCV4 is preferred when revaccinating persons aged 11-55 yr, but a second dose of MPSV is acceptable. (Source: Centers for Disease Control and Prevention: Prevention and control of meningococcal disease: recommendations of the Advisory Committee on Immunization Practices [ACIP], *MMWR* 54:[RR-7], 2005.)

[n]Only 1 dose of Tdap is recommended. Subsequent doses should be administered as Td. If vaccination to prevent tetanus and/or diphtheria disease is required for children aged 7-9 yr, Td should be administered (minimum age for Td is 7 yr). For one brand of Tdap, the minimum age is 11 yr. The preferred interval between Tdap and a previous dose of Td is 5 yr. In persons who have received a primary series of tetanus-toxoid-containing vaccine, for management of a tetanus-prone wound, the minimum interval after a previous dose of any tetanus-containing vaccine is 5 yr.

[o]A second dose of PPV is recommended for persons at highest risk for serious pneumococcal infection and those who are likely to have a rapid decline in pneumococcal antibody concentration. Revaccination 3 yr after the previous dose can be considered for children at highest risk for severe pneumococcal infection who would be aged <10 yr at the time of revaccination. (Source: Centers for Disease Control and Prevention: Prevention of pneumococcal disease: recommendations of the Advisory Committee on Immunization Practices [ACIP], *MMWR* 46:[RR-8], 1997.)

[p]HPV is approved only for females aged 9-26 yr.

[q]The first dose of RV must be administered at age 6-12 wk. The vaccine series should not be started at age ≥13 wk. RV should not be administered to children aged ≥33 wk regardless of the number of doses received at age 6-32 wk.

[r]Herpes zoster vaccine is approved as a single dose for persons who are aged ≥60 yr with a history of varicella.

TABLE 5-10 Guidelines for Spacing of Live and Inactivated Antigens

Antigen Combination	Recommended Minimum Interval between Doses
Two or more inactivated*	Can be administered simultaneously or at any interval between doses
Inactivated and live	Can be administered simultaneously or at any interval between doses
Two or more live intranasal or injectable†	4-wk minimum interval if not administered simultaneously

From Centers for Disease Control and Prevention: General recommendations on immunization: recommendations of the Advisory Committee on Immunization Practices (ACIP), *MMWR* 55:(RR-15), 2006.

*Certain experts suggest a 1-mo interval between tetanus toxoid, reduced diphtheria toxoid, and reduced acellular pertussis vaccine and quadrivalent meningococcal conjugate vaccine if they are not administered simultaneously.

†Live oral vaccines (e.g., Ty21a typhoid vaccine and rotavirus vaccine) can be administered simultaneously or at any interval before or after inactivated or live injectable vaccines.

TABLE 5-11 Guidelines for Administering Antibody-Containing Products* and Vaccines

SIMULTANEOUS ADMINISTRATION

Combination	Recommended Minimum Interval between Doses
Antibody-containing products and inactivated antigen	Can be administered simultaneously at different sites or at any time interval between doses.
Antibody-containing products and live antigen	Should not be administered simultaneously.† If simultaneous administration of measles-containing vaccine or varicella vaccine is unavoidable, administer at different sites and revaccinate or test for seroconversion after the recommended interval.

NONSIMULTANEOUS ADMINISTRATION

PRODUCT ADMINISTERED		
First	**Second**	**Recommended Minimum Interval between Doses**
Antibody-containing products	Inactivated antigen	Not applicable
Inactivated antigen	Antibody-containing products	Not applicable
Antibody-containing products	Live antigen	Dose-related†‡§
Live antigen	Antibody-containing products	2 weeks†

From Centers for Disease Control and Prevention: General recommendations on immunization: recommendations of the Advisory Committee on Immunization Practices (ACIP), *MMWR* 55(RR-15), 2006.

*Blood products containing substantial amounts of immunoglobulin include intramuscular and intravenous immune globulin, specific hyperimmune globulin (e.g., hepatitis B immune globulin, tetanus immune globulin, varicella zoster immune globulin, and rabies immune globulin), whole blood, packed red cells, plasma, and platelet products.

†Yellow fever, oral Ty21a typhoid vaccine, and live-attenuated influenza vaccine are exceptions to these recommendations. These live-attenuated vaccines can be administered at any time before, after, or simultaneously with an antibody-containing product without substantially decreasing the antibody response.

‡Rotavirus vaccine (RV) should be deferred for 6 wk after receipt of an antibody-containing product if possible. However, if the 6-wk deferral would cause the first dose of RV to be scheduled for age >13 wk, a shorter deferral interval should be used to ensure the first dose of RV is administered no later than age 13 wk.

§The duration of interference of antibody-containing products with the immune response to the measles component of measles-containing vaccine, and possibly varicella vaccine, is dose related.

TABLE 5-12 Suggested Intervals between Administration of Antibody-Containing Products for Different Indications and Measles-Containing Vaccine and Varicella-Containing Vaccine*

Product/Indication	Dose, Including mg Immunoglobulin G (IgG)/kg Body Weight*	Recommended Interval before Measles or Varicella-Containing Vaccine Administration (mo)
Respiratory syncytial virus immune globulin (IG) monoclonal antibody (Synagis)†	15 mg/kg intramuscularly (IM)	None
Tetanus IG	250 units (10 mg IgG/kg) IM	3
Hepatitis A IG		
Contact prophylaxis	0.02 ml/kg (3.3 mg IgG/kg) IM	3
International travel	0.06 ml/kg (10 mg IgG/kg) IM	3
Hepatitis B IG	0.06 ml/kg (10 mg IgG/kg) IM	3
Rabies IG	20 international units/kg (22 mg IgG/kg) IM	4
Measles prophylaxis IG		
Standard (i.e., nonimmunocompromised) contact	0.25 ml/kg (40 mg IgG/kg) IM	5
Immunocompromised contact	0.50 ml/kg (80 mg IgG/kg) IM	6
Blood transfusion		
Red blood cells (RBCs), washed	10 ml/kg negligible IgG/kg intravenously (IV)	None
RBCs, adenine-saline added	10 ml/kg (10 mg IgG/kg) IV	3
Packed RBCs (hematocrit 65%)‡	10 ml/kg (60 mg IgG/kg) IV	6
Whole blood (hematocrit 35%-50%)‡	10 ml/kg (80-100 mg IgG/kg) IV	6
Plasma/platelet products	10 ml/kg (160 mg IgG/kg) IV	7
Cytomegalovirus intravenous immune globulin (IGIV)	150 mg/kg maximum	6
IGIV		
Replacement therapy for immune deficiencies§	300-400 mg/kg IV§	8
Immune thrombocytopenic purpura	400 mg/kg IV	8
Postexposure varicella prophylaxis¶	400 mg/kg IV	8
Immune thrombocytopenic purpura	1000 mg/kg IV	10
Kawasaki disease	2 g/kg IV	11

From Centers for Disease Control and Prevention: General recommendations on immunization: recommendations of the Advisory Committee on Immunization Practices (ACIP), *MMWR* 55:(RR-15), 2006.

*This table is not intended to provide the correct indications and dosages for using antibody-containing products. Unvaccinated persons might not be fully protected against measles during the entire recommended interval, and additional doses of immune globulin or measles vaccine might be indicated after measles exposure. Concentrations of measles antibody in an immune globulin preparation can vary by manufacturer's lot. Rates of antibody clearance after receipt of an immune globulin preparation also may vary. Recommended intervals are extrapolated from an estimated half-life of 30 days for passively acquired antibody and an observed interference with the immune response to measles vaccine for 5 mo after a dose of 80 mg IgG/kg.

†Contains antibody only to respiratory syncytial virus.

‡Assumes a serum IgG concentration of 16 mg/ml.

§Measles and varicella vaccinations are recommended for children with asymptomatic or mildly symptomatic human immunodeficiency virus (HIV) infection but are contraindicated for persons with severe immunosuppression from HIV or any other immunosuppressive disorder.

¶The investigational product VariZIG, similar to licensed VZIG, is a purified human immune globulin preparation made from plasma containing high levels of antivaricella antibodies (immunoglobulin class G [IgG]). When indicated, health care providers should make every effort to obtain and administer VariZIG. In situations in which administration of VariZIG does not appear possible within 96 hours of exposure, administration of immune globulin intravenous (IGIV) should be considered as an alternative. IGIV also should be administered within 96 hours of exposure. Although licensed IGIV preparations are known to contain antivaricella antibody titers, the titer of any specific lot of IGIV that might be available is uncertain because IGIV is not routinely tested for antivaricella antibodies. The recommended IGIV dose for postexposure prophylaxis of varicella is 400 mg/kg administered once. For pregnant women who cannot receive VariZIG within 96 hours of exposure, clinicians can choose either to administer IGIV or closely monitor the women for signs and symptoms of varicella and institute treatment with acyclovir if illness occurs. (Source: Centers for Disease Control and Prevention: A new product for postexposure prophylaxis available under an investigational new drug application expanded access protocol, *MMWR* 55 [RR-8]:209-210, 2006.)

TABLE 5-13 Contraindications to and Precautions for Commonly Used Vaccines[a]

Vaccine	True Contraindications and Precautions[a]	Untrue (Vaccines Can Be Administered)
General for all routine vaccines, including diphtheria and tetanus toxoids and acellular pertussis vaccine (DTaP); pediatric diphtheria-tetanus toxoid (DT); adult tetanus-diphtheria toxoid (Td); tetanus-reduced-diphtheria toxoid and acellular pertussis vaccine (Tdap), inactivated poliovirus vaccine (IPV); measles, mumps, and rubella vaccine (MMR); *Haemophilus influenzae* type b vaccine (Hib); hepatitis A vaccine; hepatitis B vaccine; varicella vaccine; Rotavirus vaccine; pneumococcal conjugate vaccine (PCV); inactivated influenza vaccine (TIV); live-attenuated influenza vaccine (LAIV); pneumococcal polysaccharide vaccine (PPV); meningococcal conjugate vaccine (MCV4); meningococcal polysaccharide vaccine (MPSV); human papillomavirus vaccine (HPV); and herpes zoster vaccine (HZ)	***Contraindication*** Severe allergic reaction (e.g., anaphylaxis) after a previous vaccine dose or to a vaccine component ***Precaution*** Moderate or severe acute illness with or without fever	Mild acute illness with or without fever Mild-to-moderate local reaction (e.g., swelling, redness, and soreness), low-grade or moderate fever Lack of previous physical examination in well-appearing person after current antimicrobial therapy[b] Previous convalescent preterm birth (hepatitis B vaccine is an exception in certain circumstances)[c] phase of illness dose Recent exposure to an infectious disease History of penicillin allergy, other nonvaccine allergies, relatives with allergies, receiving allergen extract immunotherapy Breastfeeding
DTaP	***Contraindications*** Severe allergic reaction (e.g., anaphylaxis) after a previous vaccine dose or to a vaccine component Encephalopathy (e.g., coma, decreased level of consciousness, prolonged seizures) not attributable to another identifiable cause within 7 days of administration of previous dose of DTP or DTaP Progressive neurologic disorder, including infantile spasms, uncontrolled epilepsy, progressive encephalopathy: defer DTaP until neurologic status clarified and stabilized ***Precautions*** Temperature of ≥105° F (≥40.5° C) ≤48 hours after vaccination with a previous dose of DTP or DTaP Collapse or shocklike state (i.e., hypotonic hyporesponsive episode) ≤48 hours after receiving a previous dose of DTP/DTaP Seizure ≤3 days after receiving a previous dose of DTP/DTaP[d] Persistent, inconsolable crying lasting ≥3 hours within 48 hr after receiving a previous dose of DTP/DTaP Guillain-Barré syndrome (GBS) <6 wk after previous dose of tetanus toxoid–containing vaccine Moderate or severe acute illness with or without fever	Temperature of ≤104° F (≤40.5° C), fussiness, or mild drowsiness after a previous dose of diphtheria toxoid-tetanus toxoid-pertussis vaccine (DTP/DTaP) Family history of seizures[d] Family history of sudden infant death syndrome Family history of an adverse event after DTP or DTaP administration Stable neurologic conditions (e.g., cerebral palsy, well-controlled seizure disorder, developmental delay)
DT, Td	***Contraindication*** Severe allergic reaction (e.g., anaphylaxis) after a previous vaccine dose or to a vaccine component ***Precautions*** GBS <6 wk after previous dose of tetanus toxoid–containing vaccine Moderate or severe acute illness with or without fever	
Tdap	***Contraindications*** Severe allergic reaction (e.g., anaphylaxis) after a previous vaccine dose or to a vaccine component Encephalopathy (e.g., coma, decreased level of consciousness, and prolonged seizures) not attributable to another identifiable cause within 7 days of administration of previous dose of DTP, DTaP, or Tdap ***Precautions*** Moderate or severe acute illness with or without fever GBS ≤6 wk after a previous dose of tetanus-toxoid-containing vaccine Progressive or unstable neurologic disorder, uncontrolled seizures or progressive encephalopathy until a treatment regimen has been established and the condition has stabilized History of arthus-type hypersensitivity reactions following a previous dose of tetanus toxoid–containing vaccine: defer vaccination until at least 10 yr have elapsed since the last tetanus toxoid–containing vaccine	Temperature of >104° F (>40.5° C) ≤48 hours after vaccination with a previous dose of DTP or DTaP Collapse or shocklike state (i.e., hypotonic hyporesponsive episode) ≤48 hours after receiving a previous dose of DTP/DTaP Seizure ≤3 days after receiving a previous dose of DTP/DTaP[d] Persistent, inconsolable crying lasting ≥3 hours within 48 hours after receiving a previous dose of DTP/DTaP History of extensive limb swelling after DTP/DTaP/Td that is not an arthus-type reaction Stable neurologic disorder Brachial neuritis Latex allergy that is not anaphylactic Breastfeeding Immunosuppression

TABLE 5-13 Contraindications to and Precautions for Commonly Used Vaccines—cont'd

Vaccine	True Contraindications and Precautions[a]	Untrue (Vaccines Can Be Administered)
IPV	***Contraindication*** Severe allergic reaction (e.g., anaphylaxis) after a previous vaccine dose or to a vaccine component ***Precautions*** Pregnancy Moderate or severe acute illness with or without fever	Previous receipt of one or more doses of oral polio vaccine
MMR[e]	***Contraindications*** Severe allergic reaction (e.g., anaphylaxis) after a previous vaccine dose or to a vaccine component Pregnancy Known severe immunodeficiency (e.g., hematologic and solid tumors, receiving chemotherapy, congenital immunodeficiency, long-term immunosuppressive therapy,[f] or patients with HIV infection who are severely immunocompromised) ***Precautions*** Recent ($\leq$11 mo) receipt of antibody-containing blood product (specific interval depends on product)[h] History of thrombocytopenia or thrombocytopenic purpura Moderate or severe acute illness with or without fever	Positive tuberculin skin test Simultaneous tuberculosis skin testing[g] Breastfeeding Pregnancy of recipient's mother or other close or household contact Recipient is female of childbearing age Immunodeficient family member or household contact Asymptomatic or mildly symptomatic HIV infection Allergy to eggs
Hib	***Contraindications*** Severe allergic reaction (e.g., anaphylaxis) after a previous vaccine dose or to a vaccine component Age <6 wk ***Precaution*** Moderate or severe acute illness with or without fever	
Hepatitis B	***Contraindication*** Severe allergic reaction (e.g., anaphylaxis) after a previous vaccine dose or to a vaccine component ***Precautions*** Infant weighing <2000 g[c] Moderate or severe acute illness with or without fever	Pregnancy Autoimmune disease (e.g., systemic lupus erythematosus or rheumatoid arthritis)
Hepatitis A	***Contraindication*** Severe allergic reaction (e.g., anaphylaxis) after a previous vaccine dose or to a vaccine component ***Precautions*** Pregnancy Moderate or severe acute illness with or without fever	
Varicella	***Contraindications*** Severe allergic reaction (e.g., anaphylaxis) after a previous vaccine dose or to a vaccine component Substantial suppression of cellular immunity Pregnancy ***Precautions*** Recent ($\leq$11 mo) receipt of antibody-containing blood product (specific interval depends on product)[h] Moderate or severe acute illness with or without fever	Pregnancy of recipient's mother or other close or household contact Immunodeficient family member or household contact[i] Asymptomatic or mildly symptomatic HIV infection Humoral immunodeficiency (e.g., a gammaglobulinemia)[j]
PCV	***Contraindication*** Severe allergic reaction (e.g., anaphylaxis) after a previous vaccine dose or to a vaccine component ***Precaution*** Moderate or severe acute illness with or without fever	
TIV	***Contraindication*** Severe allergic reaction (e.g., anaphylaxis) after a previous vaccine dose or to a vaccine component ***Precaution*** Moderate or severe acute illness with or without fever	Nonsevere (e.g., contact) allergy to latex or thimerosal Concurrent administration of warfarin or aminophylline

Continued on following page

TABLE 5-13 Contraindications to and Precautions for Commonly Used Vaccines—cont'd

Vaccine	True Contraindications and Precautions[a]	Untrue (Vaccines Can Be Administered)
LAIV	***Contraindications*** Severe allergic reaction (e.g., anaphylaxis) after a previous vaccine dose or to a vaccine component Pregnancy Known severe immunodeficiency (e.g., hematologic and solid tumors, receiving chemotherapy, congenital immunodeficiency, long-term immunosuppressive therapy,[f] or patients with HIV infection who are severely immunocompromised) Previous history of GBS Certain chronic medical conditions[k] ***Precaution*** Moderate or severe acute illness with or without fever	
PPV	***Contraindication*** Severe allergic reaction (e.g., anaphylaxis) after a previous vaccine dose or to a vaccine component ***Precaution*** Moderate or severe acute illness with or without fever	History of invasive pneumococcal disease or pneumonia
MCV4	***Contraindication*** Severe allergic reaction (e.g., anaphylaxis) after a previous vaccine dose or to a vaccine component ***Precautions*** Moderate or severe acute illness with or without fever History of GBS (if not at high risk for meningococcal disease)	
MPSV	***Contraindication*** Severe allergic reaction after a previous dose or to a vaccine component ***Precaution*** Moderate or severe acute illness with or without fever	
HPV	***Contraindication*** Severe allergic reaction after a previous dose or to a vaccine component ***Precautions*** Moderate or severe acute illness with or without fever Pregnancy	
Rotavirus	***Contraindication*** Severe allergic reaction after a previous dose or to a vaccine component ***Precautions*** Moderate or severe acute illness with or without fever Immunosuppression Receipt of an antibody-containing blood product within 6 wk[l] Preexisting gastrointestinal disease Previous history of intussusception	Preterm births Immunosuppression in household contacts Pregnant household contacts

From Centers for Disease Control and Prevention: General recommendations on immunization: recommendations of the Advisory Committee on Immunization Practices (ACIP), *MMWR* 55:(RR-15), 2006.

[a]Events or conditions listed as precautions should be reviewed carefully. Benefits of and risks for administering a specific vaccine to a person under these circumstances should be considered. If the risk from the vaccine is believed to outweigh the benefit, the vaccine should not be administered. If the benefit of vaccination is believed to outweigh the risk, the vaccine should be administered. Whether and when to administer DTaP to children with proven or suspected underlying neurologic disorders should be decided on a case-by-case basis.

[b]Antibacterial drugs and mefloquine might interfere with Ty21a oral typhoid vaccine, and certain antiviral drugs might interfere with varicella-containing and live-attenuated influenza virus vaccine.

[c]Hepatitis B vaccination should be deferred for infants weighing <2000 g if the mother is documented to be hepatitis B surface antigen (HBsAg) negative at the time of the infant's birth. Vaccination can begin at chronologic age 1 mo. For infants born to women who are HBsAg positive, hepatitis B immunoglobulin and hepatitis B vaccine should be administered at or soon after birth regardless of weight.

[d]Acetaminophen or other appropriate antipyretic can be administered to infants and children with a history of previous seizures at the time of DTaP vaccination and every 4 hours for 24 hours thereafter to reduce the possibility of postvaccination fever. (Source: American Academy of Pediatrics: Active immunization. In Pickering LK, Baker CJ, Long SS, et al (eds): *2006 red book: report of the Committee on Infectious Diseases,* ed 27, Elk Grove Village, IL, 2006, American Academy of Pediatrics.)

[e]MMR and varicella vaccines can be administered on the same day. If not administered on the same day, these vaccines should be separated by at least 28 days.

[f]Substantially immunosuppressive steroid dose is considered to be ≥2 wk of daily receipt of ≥20 mg or ≥2 mg/kg body weight of prednisone or equivalent.

[g]Measles vaccination might suppress tuberculin reactivity temporarily. Measles-containing vaccine can be administered on the same day as tuberculin skin testing. If testing cannot be performed until after the day of MMR vaccination, the test should be postponed for ≥4 wk after the vaccination. If an urgent need exists to skin test, do so with the understanding that reactivity might be reduced by the vaccine.

[h]See text for details.

[i]If a patient experiences a presumed vaccine-related rash 7-25 days after vaccination, he or she should avoid direct contact with immunocompromised persons for the duration of the rash if possible.

[j]Vaccine should be deferred for the appropriate interval if replacement immune globulin products are being administered.

[k]For details see Centers for Disease Control and Prevention: Prevention and control of influenza: recommendations of the Advisory Committee on Immunization Practices (ACIP), *MMWR* 55:(RR-10), 2006.

[l]Rotavirus vaccine (RV) should be deferred for 6 wk after receipt of an antibody-containing product if possible. However, if the 6-wk deferral would cause the first dose of RV to be scheduled for age ≥13 wk, a shorter deferral interval should be used to ensure the first dose of RV is administered no later than age 13 wk.

TABLE 5-14 Dose and Route of Administration for Selected Vaccines

Vaccines	Dose	Route
Diphtheria, tetanus, pertussis (DTaP, DT, Td, Tdap)	0.5 ml	IM
Diphtheria, tetanus, acellular pertussis, inactivated polio, hepatitis B vaccine (DTaP-IPV-HepB)	0.5 ml	IM
Diphtheria, tetanus, acellular pertussis, *Haemophilus influenzae* type b vaccine (DTaP-Hib)	0.5 ml	IM
Haemophilus influenzae type b (Hib)	0.5 ml	IM
Haemophilus influenzae type b–Hepatitis B (Hib-HepB)	0.5 ml	IM
Hepatitis A (HepA)	≤18 yr: 0.5 ml ≥19 yr: 1.0 ml	IM
HepB	≤19 yr: 0.5 ml* ≥20 yr: 1.0 ml	IM
HepA/HepB	≥18 yr: 1.0 ml	IM
Influenza, live attenuated	0.5 ml	Intranasal spray
Influenza, trivalent inactivated	6-35 mo: 0.25 ml ≥3 yr: 0.5 ml	IM
Measles, mumps, rubella	0.5 ml	SC
Measles, mumps, rubella, varicella	0.5 ml	SC
Meningococcal conjugate	0.5 ml	IM
Meningococcal polysaccharide	0.5 ml	SC
Pneumococcal conjugate	0.5 ml	IM
Pneumococcal polysaccharide	0.5 ml	IM or SC
Human papillomavirus	0.5 ml	IM
Polio, inactivated	0.5 ml	IM or SC
Rotavirus	2.0 ml	Oral
Varicella	0.5 ml	SC
Zoster	0.7 ml	SC

From CDC: General recommendations on immunization: recommendations of the Advisory Committee on Immunization Practices (ACIP), *MMWR* 55:(RR-15), 2006. Adapted from Immunization Action Coalition (http://www.immunize.org).

IM, Intramuscularly; *SC,* subcutaneously.

*Persons aged 11-15 yr can be administered Recombivax HB (Merck) 1.0 ml (adult formulation) on a 2-dose schedule.

VACCINE ADMINISTRATION*

INFECTION CONTROL AND STERILE TECHNIQUE

Persons administering vaccines should follow appropriate precautions to minimize risk for spread of disease. Hands should be cleansed with an alcohol-based, waterless antiseptic hand rub or washed with soap and water between each patient contact. Occupational Safety and Health Administration (OSHA) regulations do not require that gloves be worn when administering vaccinations unless persons administering vaccinations are likely to come into contact with potentially infectious body fluids or have open lesions on their hands. Needles used for injections must be sterile and disposable to minimize the risk for contamination. A separate needle and syringe should be used for each injection. Changing needles between drawing vaccine from a vial and injecting it into a recipient is not necessary. Different vaccines should never be mixed in the same syringe unless specifically licensed for such use, and no attempt should be made to transfer between syringes.

For all intramuscular injections, the needle should be long enough to reach the muscle mass and prevent vaccine from seeping into subcutaneous tissue but not so long as to involve underlying nerves, blood vessels, or bone. Vaccinators should be familiar with the anatomy of the area where they are injecting vaccine. Intramuscular injections are administered at a 90-degree angle to the skin, preferably into the anterolateral aspect of the thigh or the deltoid muscle of the upper arm depending on the age of the patient.

Decision on needle size and site of injection must be made for each person on the basis of the size of the muscle, the thickness of adipose tissue at the injection site, the volume of the material to be administered, injection technique, and the depth below the muscle surface into which the material is to be injected (Fig. 5-1). Aspiration before injection of vaccines or toxoids (i.e., pulling back on the syringe plunger after needle insertion before injection) is not required because no large blood vessel exists at the recommended injection sites.

INFANTS (AGED <12 MONTHS)

For the majority of infants, the anterolateral aspect of the thigh is the recommended site for injection because it provides a large muscle mass (Fig. 5-2). The muscles of the buttock have not been used for administration of vaccines in infants and children because of concern about potential injury to the sciatic nerve, which is well documented after injection of antimicrobial agents into the buttock. If the gluteal muscle must be used, care should be taken to define the anatomic landmarks.† Injection technique is the most important parameter to ensure efficient intramuscular vaccine delivery. If the subcutaneous and muscle tissue are bunched to minimize the chance of striking bone, a 1-inch needle is required to ensure intramuscular administration in infants. For the majority of infants, a 1-inch, 22- to 25-gauge needle is sufficient to penetrate muscle in an infant's thigh. For newborn (first 28 days of life) and premature infants, a ⅝-inch-long needle usually is adequate if the skin is stretched flat between thumb and forefinger and the needle inserted at a 90-degree angle to the skin.

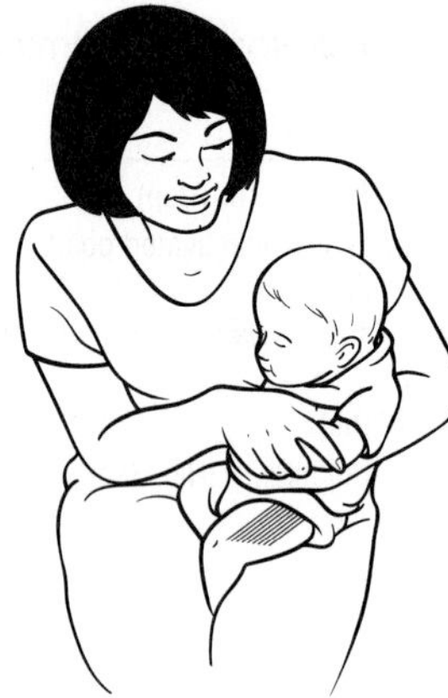

FIGURE 5-2 Intramuscular/subcutaneous site of administration: anterolateral thigh. (Adapted from Minnesota Department of Health. In Centers for Disease Control and Prevention: General recommendations on immunization: recommendations of the Advisory Committee on Immunization Practices [ACIP], *MMWR* 55[RR-15]:6, 2006.)

TODDLERS AND OLDER CHILDREN (AGED 12 MONTHS TO 10 YEARS)

The deltoid muscle should be used if the muscle mass is adequate. The needle size for deltoid site injections can range from 22 to 25 gauge and from ⅝ to 1 inch on the basis of the size of the muscle and the thickness of adipose tissue at the injection site (Fig. 5-3). A ⅝-inch needle is adequate only for the deltoid muscle and only if the skin is stretched flat between the thumb and forefinger and the needle inserted at a 90-degree

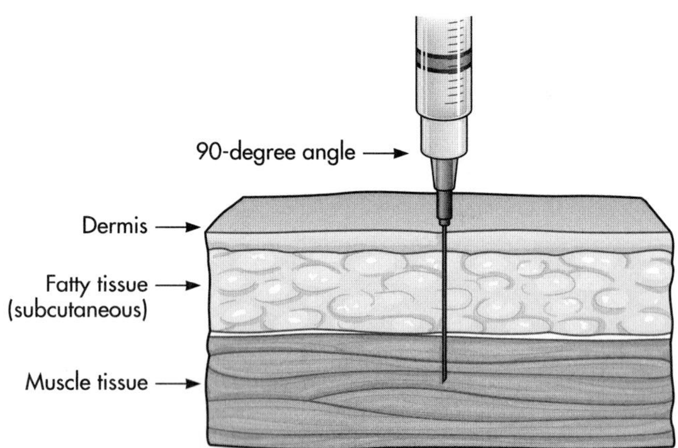

FIGURE 5-1 Intramuscular needle insertion. (Adapted from California Immunization Branch. In Centers for Disease Control and Prevention: General recommendations on immunization: recommendations of the Advisory Committee on Immunization Practices [ACIP], *MMWR* 55[RR-15]:16, 2006.)

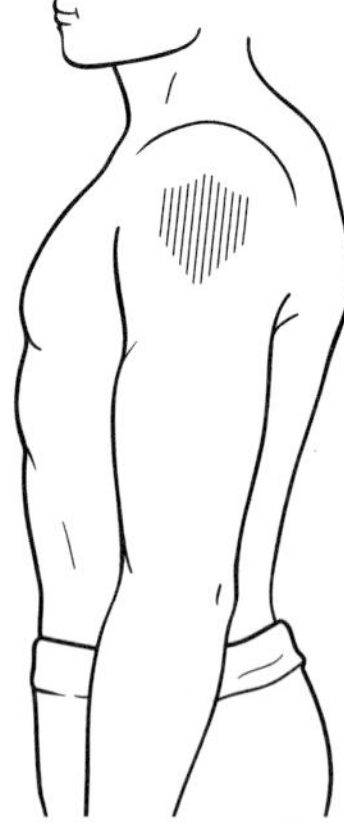

FIGURE 5-3 Intramuscular site of administration: deltoid. (Adapted from Minnesota Department of Health. In Centers for Disease Control and Prevention: General recommendations on immunization: recommendations of the Advisory Committee on Immunization Practices [ACIP], *MMWR* 55[RR-15]:17, 2006.)

*From Centers for Disease Control and Prevention: General recommendations on immunization: recommendations of the Advisory Committee on Immunization Practices (ACIP), *MMWR* 55(RR-15):14-16, 2006.

†If the gluteal muscle is chosen, injection should be administered lateral and superior to a line between the posterior superior iliac spine and the greater trochanter or in the ventrogluteal site, the center of a triangle bounded by the anterior superior iliac spine, the tubercle of the iliac crest, and the upper border of the greater trochanter.

angle to the skin. For toddlers, the anterolateral thigh can be used, but the needle should be at least 1 inch in length.

ADOLESCENTS AND ADULTS (AGED >11 YEARS)

For adults and adolescents, the deltoid muscle is recommended for routine intramuscular vaccinations. The anterolateral thigh also can be used. For men and women weighing <130 lb (<60 kg) a ⅝- to 1-inch needle is sufficient to ensure intramuscular injection. For women weighing 130 to 200 lb (60 to 90 kg) and men 130 to 260 lb (60 to 118 kg), a 1- to 1½-inch needle is needed. For women weighing >200 lb (>90 kg) or men weighing >260 lb (>118 kg), a 1½-inch needle is required.

SUBCUTANEOUS INJECTIONS

Subcutaneous injections are administered at a 45-degree angle, usually into the thigh for infants younger than 12 months and in the upper-outer triceps area of persons aged 12 months and older. Subcutaneous injections can be administered into the upper-outer triceps area of an infant if necessary. A ⅝-inch, 23- to 25-gauge needle should be inserted into the subcutaneous tissue (Figs. 5-4 and 5-5).

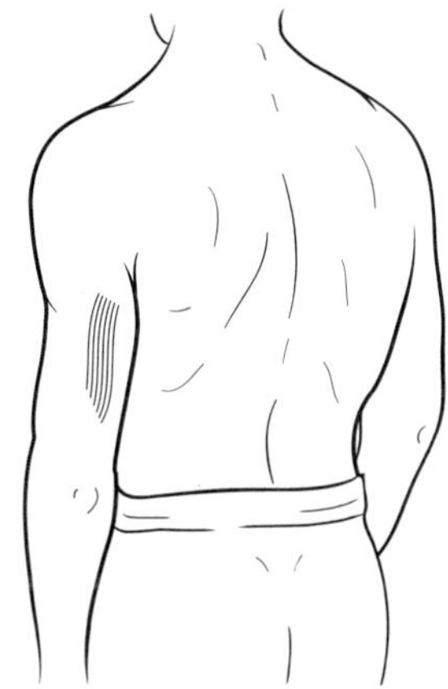

FIGURE 5-4 Subcutaneous site of administration: triceps. (Adapted from Minnesota Department of Health. In Centers for Disease Control and Prevention: General recommendations on immunization: recommendations of the Advisory Committee on Immunization Practices [ACIP], *MMWR* 55[RR-15]:17, 2006.)

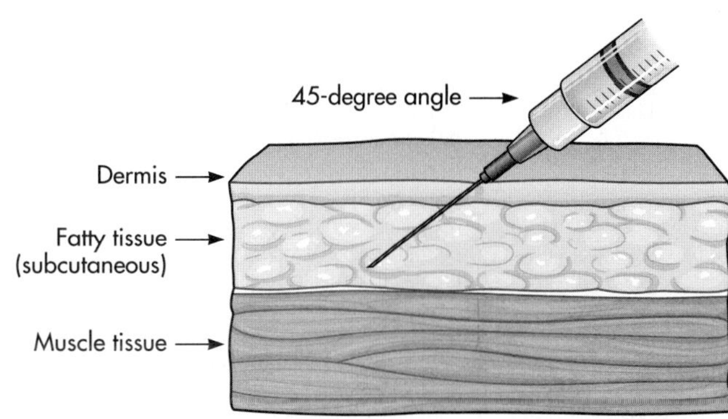

FIGURE 5-5 Subcutaneous needle insertion. (Adapted from California Administration Branch. In Centers for Disease Control and Prevention: General recommendations on immunization: recommendations of the Advisory Committee on Immunization Practices [ACIP], *MMWR* 55[RR-15]:17, 2006.)

TABLE 5-15 Treatment of Anaphylaxis with Intramuscular or Oral Pharmaceuticals

Drug	Dosage
Child	
Primary regimen	
Epinephrine 1:1000 (aqueous) (1 mg/ml)*	0.01 mg/kg up to 0.5 mg (administer 0.01 ml/kg/dose up to 0.5 ml) IM repeated every 10-20 min up to 3 doses
Secondary regimen	
Diphenhydramine	1-2 mg/kg oral, IM or IV, every 4-6 hr (maximum single dose: 100 mg)
Hydroxyzine	0.5-1 mg/kg oral, IM, every 4-6 hr (maximum single dose: 100 mg)
Prednisone	1.5-2 mg/kg oral (maximum single dose: 60 mg); use corticosteroids as long as needed
Adult	
Primary regimen	
Epinephrine 1:1000 (aqueous)*	0.01 mg/kg up to 0.5 mg (give 0.01 ml/kg/dose up to 0.5 ml) IM repeated every 10-20 min up to 3 doses
Secondary regimen	
Diphenhydramine	1-2 mg/kg up to 100 mg IM or oral every 4-6 hr

From Centers for Disease Control and Prevention: General recommendations on immunization: recommendations of the Advisory Committee on Immunization Practices (ACIP), *MMWR* 55:(RR-15), 2006. Adapted from American Academy of Pediatrics: Passive immunization. In Pickering LK, Baker CJ, Long SS, et al (eds): *Red book: 2006 report of the Committee on Infectious Diseases,* ed 27, Elk Grove, IL, 2006, American Academy of Pediatrics; and Immunization Action Coalition: Medical management of anaphylaxis in adult patients. Available at http://www.immunize.org/catg.d/p3082.pdf, and Mosby's Drug Consult 2005.

IM, Intramuscular; *IV,* intravenous.

*If agent causing anaphylactic reaction was administered by injection, epinephrine can be injected into the same site to slow absorption.

TABLE 5-16 Vaccination of Persons with Primary and Secondary Immune Deficiencies

Category	Specific Immunodeficiency	Vaccines Contraindicated*	Risk-Specific Vaccines Recommended*	Effectiveness and Comments
		PRIMARY		
B-lymphocyte (humoral)	Severe antibody deficiencies (e.g., X-linked agammaglobulinemia and common variable immunodeficiency)	Oral poliovirus (OPV)† Smallpox Live-attenuated influenza vaccine (LAIV) BCG Live oral typhoid (Ty21a)	Pneumococcal Influenza (TIV) Consider measles and varicella vaccination	The effectiveness of any vaccine will be uncertain if it depends only on the humoral response; IV immune globulin interferes with the immune response to measles vaccine and possibly varicella vaccine
	Less severe antibody deficiencies (e.g., selective IgA deficiency and IgG subclass deficiency)	OPV† Other live vaccines appear to be safe	Pneumococcal influenza (TIV)	All vaccines probably effective; immune response may be attenuated
T-lymphocyte (cell mediated and humoral)	Complete defects (e.g., severe combined immunodeficiency [SCID] disease, complete DiGeorge syndrome)	All live vaccines‡§	Pneumococcal influenza (TIV)	Vaccines may be ineffective
	Partial defects (e.g., the majority of patients with DiGeorge syndrome, Wiskott-Aldrich syndrome, ataxia-telangiectasia)	All live vaccines‡§	Pneumococcal Meningococcal *Haemophilus influenza* type b (Hib) (if not administered in infancy) Influenza (TIV)	Effectiveness of any vaccine depends on degree of immune suppression
Complement	Deficiency of early components (C1, C2, C3, and C4)	None	Pneumococcal Meningococcal Influenza (TIV)	All routine vaccines probably effective
	Deficiency of late components (C5-C9) and C3, properdin, factor B	None	Pneumococcal Meningococcal Influenza (TIV)	All routine vaccines probably effective
Phagocytic function	Chronic granulomatous disease, leukocyte adhesion defect, and myeloperoxidase deficiency	Live bacterial vaccines‡	Pneumococcal‖ Influenza (TIV) (to decrease secondary bacterial infection)	All inactivated vaccines safe and probably effective Live viral vaccines probably safe and effective
		SECONDARY		
	HIV/AIDS	OPV Smallpox BCG LAIV Withhold MMR and varicella in severely immunocompromised persons	Influenza (TIV) Pneumococcal Consider Hib (if not administered in infancy) and meningococcal vaccination	Measles, mumps, rubella (MMR); varicella; and all inactivated vaccines, including inactivated influenza, might be effective¶
	Malignant neoplasm, transplantation, immunosuppressive or radiation therapy	Live viral and bacterial, depending on immune status	Influenza (TIV) Pneumococcal	Effectiveness of any vaccine depends on degree of immune suppression
	Asplenia	None	Pneumococcal Meningococcal Hib (if not administered in infancy)	All routine vaccines probably effective
	Chronic renal disease	LAIV	Pneumococcal Influenza (TIV) Hepatitis B	All routine vaccines probably effective

From Centers for Disease Control and Prevention (CDC): General recommendations on immunization: recommendations of the Advisory Committee on Immunization Practices (ACIP), *MMWR* 55(RR-15), 2006. Modified from American Academy of Pediatrics: Passive immunization. In Pickering LK, Baker CJ, Long SS, et al (eds): *Red book: 2006 report of the Committee on Infectious Diseases,* ed 27, Elk Grove, IL, 2006, American Academy of Pediatrics; and CDC: Use of vaccines and immune globulins in persons with altered immunocompetence: recommendations of the Advisory Committee on Immunization Practices (ACIP), *MMWR* 42(RR-4):42, 1993.

BCG, Bacille Calmette-Guérin; *Ig,* immunoglobulin; *IV,* intravenous.

*Other vaccines that are universally or routinely recommended should be administered if not contraindicated.

†OPV is no longer available for routine use in the United States.

‡Live bacterial vaccines: BCG and Ty21a *Salmonella typhi* vaccine.

§Live viral vaccines: MMR, OPV, LAIV, yellow fever, and varicella, including measles-mumps-rubella-varicella (MMRV) and herpes zoster (HZ) vaccine, and vaccinia (smallpox). Smallpox vaccine is not recommended for children or the general public.

‖Pneumococcal vaccine is not indicated for children with chronic granulomatous disease.

¶Children infected with HIV should receive IG after exposure to measles and can receive varicella and measles vaccine if CD4+ lymphocyte count is >15%.

TABLE 5-17 Approaches to the Evaluation and Vaccination of Internationally Adopted Children with No or Questionable Vaccination Records

Vaccine	Recommended Approach	Alternative Approach
Measles, mumps, and rubella (MMR)	Revaccinate with MMR	Serologic testing for immunoglobulin G (IgG) antibody to measles, mumps, and rubella
Haemophilus influenzae type b (Hib)	Age-appropriate revaccination	—
Hepatitis A	Age-appropriate revaccination	Serologic testing for IgG antibody to hepatitis A virus
Hepatitis B (Hep B)	Age-appropriate revaccination and serologic testing for HBsAg*	—
Poliovirus	Revaccinate with inactivated poliovirus vaccine (IPV)	Serologic testing for neutralizing antibody to poliovirus types 1, 2, and 3 (limited availability)
Diphtheria and tetanus toxoids and acellular pertussis (DTaP)	Revaccination with DTaP, with serologic testing for specific IgG antibody to tetanus and diphtheria toxins in the event of a severe local reaction	Children whose records indicate receipt of ≥3 doses: serologic testing for specific IgG antibody to diphtheria and tetanus toxins before administering additional doses or administer a single booster dose of DTaP, followed by serologic testing after 1 mo for specific IgG antibody to diphtheria and tetanus toxins with revaccination as appropriate
Varicella	Age-appropriate vaccination of children who lack evidence of varicella immunity	—
Pneumococcal conjugate	Age-appropriate vaccination	—

From Centers for Disease Control and Prevention (CDC): General recommendations on immunization: recommendations of the Advisory Committee on Immunization Practices (ACIP), *MMWR* 55:(RR-15), 2006.

*Very rarely, Hep B vaccine can give a false-positive hepatitis B surface antigen (HBsAg) result up to 18 days after vaccination; therefore blood should be drawn to test for HBsAg before vaccinating. (Source: CDC: A comprehensive immunization strategy to eliminate transmission of hepatitis B virus infection in the United States: recommendations of the Advisory Committee on Immunization Practices [ACIP]; Part I: immunization in infants, children, and adolescents, *MMWR* 54[RR-16], 2005.)

Immunizations for Adults

TABLE 5-18 Recommended Adult Immunization Schedule, by Vaccine and Age Group—United States, 2010

Note: These recommendations *must* be read with the footnotes that follow containing number of doses, intervals between doses, and other important information.

VACCINE ▼ AGE GROUP ▶	19-26 years	27-49 years	50-59 years	60-64 years	≥65 years
Tetanus, diphtheria, pertussis (Td/Tdap)[1,*]	Substitute 1-time dose of Tdap for Td booster; then boost with Td every 10 yr				Td booster every 10 yrs
Human papillomavirus (HPV)[2,*]	3 doses (females)				
Varicella[3,*]	2 doses				
Zoster[4]				1 dose	
Measles, mumps, rubella (MMR)[5,*]	1 or 2 doses		1 dose		
Influenza[6,*]			1 dose annually		
Pneumococcal (polysaccharide)[7,8]	1 or 2 doses				1 dose
Hepatitis A[9,*]	2 doses				
Hepatitis B[10,*]	3 doses				
Meningococcal[11,*]	1 or more doses				

*Covered by the Vaccine Injury Compensation Program.

Light shading: For all persons in this category who meet the age requirements and who lack evidence of immunity (e.g., lack documentation of vaccination or have no evidence of prior infection)

Dark shading: Recommended if some other risk factor is present (e.g., on the basis of medical, occupational, lifestyle, or other indications)

No shading: No recommendation

*These schedules indicate the recommended age groups and medical indications for which administration of currently licensed vaccines is commonly indicated for adults ages 19 years and older, as of January 1, 2010. Licensed combination vaccines may be used whenever any components of the combination are indicated and when the vaccine's other components are not contraindicated. For detailed recommendations on all vaccines, including those used primarily for travelers or that are issued during the year, consult the manufacturers' package inserts and the complete statements from the Advisory Committee on Immunization Practices (http://www.cdc.gov/vaccines/pubs/acip-list.htm).

Report all clinically significant postvaccination reactions to the Vaccine Adverse Event Reporting System (VAERS). Reporting forms and instructions on filing a VAERS report are available at www.vaers.hhs.gov or by telephone, 800-822-7967.

Information on how to file a Vaccine Injury Compensation Program claim is available at www.hrsa.gov/vaccinecompensation or by telephone, 800-338-2382. To file a claim for vaccine injury, contact the U.S. Court of Federal Claims, 717 Madison Place, N.W., Washington, D.C. 20005; telephone, 202-357-6400.

Additional information about the vaccines in this schedule, extent of available data, and contraindications for vaccination is also available at www.cdc.gov/vaccines or from the CDC-INFO Contact Center at 800-CDC-INFO (800-232-4636) in English and Spanish, 24 hours a day, 7 days a week.

Use of trade names and commercial sources is for identification only and does not imply endorsement by the U.S. Department of Health and Human Services.

[1]Tetanus, diphtheria, and acellular pertussis (Td/Tdap) vaccination

Tdap should replace a single dose of Td for adults age 19 through 64 yr who have not received a dose of Tdap previously.

Adults with uncertain or incomplete history of primary vaccination series with tetanus and diphtheria toxoid–containing vaccines should begin or complete a primary vaccination series. A primary series for adults is 3 doses of tetanus and diphtheria toxoid–containing vaccines; administer the first 2 doses at least 4 wk apart and the third dose 6-12 mo after the second. However, Tdap can substitute for any one of the doses of Td in the 3-dose primary series. The booster dose of tetanus and diphtheria toxoid–containing vaccine should be administered to adults who have completed a primary series and if the last vaccination was received 10 or more yr previously. Tdap or Td vaccine may be used, as indicated.

If a woman is pregnant and received the last Td vaccination 10 or more yr previously, administer Td during the second or third trimester. If the woman received the last Td vaccination less than 10 yr previously, administer Tdap during the immediate postpartum period. A dose of Tdap is recommended for postpartum women, close contacts of infants age less than 12 mo, and all health care personnel with direct patient contact if they have not previously received Tdap. An interval as short as 2 yr from the last Td is suggested; shorter intervals can be used. Td may be deferred during pregnancy and Tdap substituted in the immediate postpartum period, or Tdap may be administered instead of Td to a pregnant woman after an informed discussion with the woman.

Consult the ACIP statement for recommendations for administering Td as prophylaxis in wound management.

[2]Human papillomavirus (HPV) vaccination

HPV vaccination is recommended for all females age 11 through 26 yr (and may begin at age 9 yr) who have not completed the vaccine series. History of genital warts, abnormal Papanicolaou test result, or positive HPV DNA test result is not evidence of prior infection with all vaccine HPV types; HPV vaccination is recommended for persons with such histories.

Ideally, vaccine should be administered before potential exposure to HPV through sexual activity; however, females who are sexually active should still be vaccinated consistent with age-based recommendations. Sexually active females who have not been infected with any of the 4 HPV vaccine types receive the full benefit of the vaccination. Vaccination is less beneficial for females who have already been infected with 1 or more of the HPV vaccine types.

A complete series consists of 3 doses. The second dose should be administered 2 mo after the first dose; the third dose should be administered 6 mo after the first dose.

HPV vaccination is not specifically recommended for females with the medical indications described in Table 5-19. Because it is not a live-virus vaccine, it can be administered to persons with the medical indications noted. However, the immune response and vaccine efficacy might be less for persons with the noted medical indications than in persons who do not have the medical indications described or who are immunocompetent. Health care personnel are not at increased risk because of occupational exposure and should be vaccinated consistent with age-based recommendations.

HPV4 may be given to males aged 9 through 26 years to reduce the likelihood of acquiring genital warts.

HPV4 would be most effective when given before exposure to HPV through sexual contact.

[3]Varicella vaccination

All adults without evidence of immunity to varicella should receive 2 doses of single-antigen varicella vaccine if not previously vaccinated or the second dose if they have received only 1 dose, unless they have a medical contraindication. Special consideration should be given to those who 1) have close contact with persons at high risk for severe disease (e.g., health care personnel and family contacts of persons with immunocompromising conditions) or 2) are at high risk for exposure or transmission (e.g., teachers; child care employees; residents and staff members of institutional settings, including correctional institutions; college students; military personnel; adolescents and adults living in households with children; nonpregnant women of childbearing age; and international travelers).

Evidence of immunity to varicella in adults includes any of the following: 1) documentation of 2 doses of varicella vaccine at least 4 wk apart; 2) U.S.-born before 1980 (although for health care personnel and pregnant women, birth before 1980 should not be considered evidence of immunity); 3) history of varicella based on diagnosis or verification of varicella by a health care provider (for a patient reporting a history of or presenting with an atypical case, a mild case, or both, health care providers should seek either an epidemiologic link to a typical varicella case or to a laboratory-confirmed case or evidence of laboratory confirmation, if it was performed at the time of acute disease); 4) history of herpes zoster based on health care provider diagnosis or verification of herpes zoster by a health care provider; or 5) laboratory evidence of immunity or laboratory confirmation of disease.

TABLE 5-18 Recommended Adult Immunization Schedule, by Vaccine and Age Group—United States, 2010—cont'd

Pregnant women should be assessed for evidence of varicella immunity. Women who do not have evidence of immunity should receive the first dose of varicella vaccine upon completion or termination of pregnancy and before discharge from the health care facility. The second dose should be administered 4-8 wk after the first dose.

[4]Herpes zoster vaccination

A single dose of zoster vaccine is recommended for adults age 60 yr and older regardless of whether they report a prior episode of herpes zoster. Persons with chronic medical conditions may be vaccinated unless their condition constitutes a contraindication.

[5]Measles, mumps, rubella (MMR) vaccination

Measles component: Adults born before 1957 generally are considered immune to measles. Adults born during or after 1957 should receive 1 or more doses of MMR unless they have a medical contraindication, documentation of 1 or more doses, history of measles based on health care provider diagnosis, or laboratory evidence of immunity.

A second dose of MMR is recommended for adults who 1) have been recently exposed to measles or are in an outbreak setting; 2) have been vaccinated previously with killed measles vaccine; 3) have been vaccinated with an unknown type of measles vaccine during 1963-1967; 4) are students in postsecondary educational institutions; 5) work in a health care facility; or 6) plan to travel internationally.

Mumps component: Adults born before 1957 generally are considered immune to mumps. Adults born during or after 1957 should receive 1 dose of MMR unless they have a medical contraindication, history of mumps based on health care provider diagnosis, or laboratory evidence of immunity.

A second dose of MMR is recommended for adults who 1) live in a community experiencing a mumps outbreak and are in an affected age group; 2) are students in postsecondary educational institutions; 3) work in a health care facility; or 4) plan to travel internationally. For unvaccinated health care personnel born before 1957 who do not have other evidence of mumps immunity, administering 1 dose on a routine basis should be considered and administering a second dose during an outbreak should also be strongly considered.

Rubella component: 1 dose of MMR vaccine is recommended for women whose rubella vaccination history is unreliable or who lack laboratory evidence of immunity. For women of childbearing age, regardless of birth yr, rubella immunity should be determined and women should be counseled regarding congenital rubella syndrome. Women who do not have evidence of immunity should receive MMR vaccine upon completion or termination of pregnancy and before discharge from the health care facility.

[6]Influenza vaccination

Medical indications: Chronic disorders of the cardiovascular or pulmonary systems, including asthma; chronic metabolic diseases, including diabetes mellitus, renal or hepatic dysfunction, hemoglobinopathies, or immunocompromising conditions (including immunocompromising conditions caused by medications or HIV); any condition that compromises respiratory function or the handling of respiratory secretions or that can increase the risk of aspiration (e.g., cognitive dysfunction, spinal cord injury, or seizure disorder or other neuromuscular disorder); and pregnancy during the influenza season. No data exist on the risk for severe or complicated influenza disease among persons with asplenia; however, influenza is a risk factor for secondary bacterial infections that can cause severe disease among persons with asplenia.

Occupational indications: All health care personnel, including those employed by long-term care and assisted-living facilities, and caregivers of children younger than 5 yr.

Other indications: Residents of nursing homes and other long-term care and assisted-living facilities; persons likely to transmit influenza to persons at high risk (e.g., in-home household contacts and caregivers of children younger than 5 yr, persons 65 yr and older, and persons of all ages with high-risk condition[s]); and anyone who would like to decrease their risk of getting influenza. Healthy, nonpregnant adults younger than 50 yr without high-risk medical conditions who are not contacts of severely immunocompromised persons in special care units can receive either intranasally administered live, attenuated influenza vaccine (FluMist) or inactivated vaccine. Other persons should receive the inactivated vaccine.

[7]Pneumococcal polysaccharide (PPSV) vaccination

Medical indications: Chronic lung disease (including asthma); chronic cardiovascular diseases; diabetes mellitus; chronic liver diseases, cirrhosis; chronic alcoholism, chronic renal failure, or nephrotic syndrome; functional or anatomic asplenia (e.g., sickle cell disease or splenectomy [if elective splenectomy is planned, vaccinate at least 2 wk before surgery]); immunocompromising conditions; and cochlear implants and cerebrospinal fluid leaks. Vaccinate as close to HIV diagnosis as possible.

Other indications: Residents of nursing homes or other long-term care facilities and persons who smoke cigarettes. Routine use of PPSV is not recommended for Alaska Native or American Indian persons younger than 65 yr unless they have underlying medical conditions that are PPSV indications. However, public health authorities may consider recommending PPSV for Alaska Natives and American Indians 50 through 64 yr of age who are living in areas in which the risk of invasive pneumococcal disease is increased.

[8]Revaccination with PPSV

One-time revaccination after 5 yr for persons with chronic renal failure or nephrotic syndrome, functional or anatomic asplenia (e.g., sickle cell disease or splenectomy), and persons with immunocompromising conditions. For persons age 65 yr or older, 1-time revaccination if they were vaccinated 5 or more yr previously and were younger than 65 yr at the time of primary vaccination.

[9]Hepatitis A vaccination

Medical indications: Persons with chronic liver disease and persons who receive clotting factor concentrates.

Behavioral indications: Men who have sex with men and persons who use illegal drugs.

Occupational indications: Persons working with hepatitis A virus (HAV)–infected primates or with HAV in a research laboratory setting.

Other indications: Persons traveling to or working in countries that have high or intermediate endemicity of hepatitis A (a list of countries is available at wwwn.cdc.gov/travel/contentdiseases.aspx) and any person seeking protection from HAV infection. Unvaccinated persons who anticipate close personal contact (e.g., household contact or regular babysitting) with an international adoptee from a country of high or intermediate endemicity during the first 60 days following arrival of the adoptee in the United States should consider vaccination. The first dose of the 2-dose HepA series should be administered as soon as adoption is planned, ideally 2 or more weeks before the arrival of the adoptee.

Single-antigen vaccine formulations should be administered in a 2-dose schedule at either 0 and 6-12 mo (Havrix) or 0 and 6-18 mo (Vaqta). If the combined hepatitis A and hepatitis B vaccine (Twinrix) is used, administer 3 doses at 0, 1, and 6 mo; alternatively, a 4-dose schedule, administered on days 0, 7, and 21 to 30 followed by a booster dose at mo 12 may be used.

[10]Hepatitis B vaccination

Medical indications: Persons with end-stage renal disease, including patients receiving hemodialysis; persons with HIV infection; and persons with chronic liver disease.

Occupational indications: Health care personnel and public-safety workers who are exposed to blood or other potentially infectious body fluids.

Behavioral indications: Sexually active persons who are not in a long-term, mutually monogamous relationship (e.g., persons with more than 1 sex partner during the previous 6 mo); persons seeking evaluation or treatment for a sexually transmitted disease (STD); current or recent injection-drug users; and men who have sex with men.

Other indications: Household contacts and sex partners of persons with chronic hepatitis B virus (HBV) infection; clients and staff members of institutions for persons with developmental disabilities; international travelers to countries with high or intermediate prevalence of chronic HBV infection (a list of countries is available at wwwn.cdc.gov/travel/contentdiseases.aspx); and any adult seeking protection from HBV infection.

Hepatitis B vaccination is recommended for all adults in the following settings: STD treatment facilities, HIV testing and treatment facilities, facilities providing drug-abuse treatment and prevention services, health care settings targeting services to injection-drug users or men who have sex with men, correctional facilities, end-stage renal disease programs and facilities for chronic hemodialysis patients, and institutions and nonresidential day care facilities for persons with developmental disabilities.

If the combined hepatitis A and hepatitis B vaccine (Twinrix) is used, administer 3 doses at 0, 1, and 6 mo; alternatively, a 4-dose schedule, administered on days 0, 7, and 21 to 30 followed by a booster dose at mo 12 may be used.

Special formulation indications: For adult patients receiving hemodialysis or with other immunocompromising conditions, 1 dose of 40 μg/mL (Recombivax HB) administered on a 3-dose schedule or 2 doses of 20 μg/mL (Engerix-B) administered simultaneously on a 4-dose schedule at 0, 1, 2, and 6 mo.

[11]Meningococcal vaccination

Medical indications: Adults with anatomic or functional asplenia or terminal complement component deficiencies.

Other indications: First-yr college students living in dormitories; microbiologists who are routinely exposed to isolates of Neisseria meningitidis; military recruits; and persons who travel to or live in countries in which meningococcal disease is hyperendemic or epidemic (e.g., the "meningitis belt" of sub-Saharan Africa during the dry season [December-June]), particularly if their contact with local populations will be prolonged. Vaccination is required by the government of Saudi Arabia for all travelers to Mecca during the annual Hajj.

Meningococcal conjugate vaccine (MCV4) is preferred for adults aged 56 years and older. Revaccination with MCV4 after 5 years is recommended for adults previously vaccinated with MCV4 or MPSV4 who remain at increased risk for infection (e.g., adults with anatomic or functional asplenia). Persons whose only risk factor is living in on-campus housing are not recommended to receive an additional dose.

[12]Selected conditions for which Haemophilus influenzae type b (Hib) vaccine may be used

Hib vaccine generally is not recommended for persons aged 5 years and older. No efficacy data are available on which to base a recommendation concerning use of Hib vaccine for older children and adults. However, studies suggest good immunogenicity in patients who have sickle cell disease, leukemia, or HIV infection or who have had a splenectomy; administering 1 dose of vaccine to these patients is not contraindicated.

[13]Immunocompromising conditions

Inactivated vaccines generally are acceptable (e.g., pneumococcal, meningococcal, and influenza [trivalent inactive influenza vaccine]) and live vaccines generally are avoided in persons with immune deficiencies or immuno-compromising conditions. Information on specific conditions is available at http://www.cdc.gov/vaccines/pubs/acip-list.htm.

TABLE 5-19 Vaccines That Might Be Indicated for Adults Based on Medical and Other Indications—United States, 2010

Note: These recommendations *must* be read with the footnotes that follow containing number of doses, intervals between doses, and other important information.

INDICATION ▶ / VACCINE ▼	Pregnancy	Immuno-compromising conditions (excluding human immunodeficiency virus [HIV])[13]	HIV infection[3,12,13] CD4+ T lymphocyte count <200 cells/μL	HIV infection[3,12,13] CD4+ T lymphocyte count ≥200 cells/μL	Diabetes, heart disease, chronic lung disease, chronic alcoholism	Asplenia[12] (including elective splenectomy and terminal complement component deficiencies)	Chronic liver disease	Kidney failure, end-stage renal disease, receipt of hemodialysis	Health-care personnel
Tetanus, diphtheria, pertussis (Td/Tdap)[1,*]	Td	Substitute 1-time dose of Tdap for Td booster; then boost with Td every 10 yrs							
Human papillomavirus (HPV)[2,*]		3 doses for females through age 26 yrs							
Varicella[3,*]	Contraindicated			2 doses					
Zoster[4]	Contraindicated				1 dose				
Measles, mumps, rubella (MMR)[5,*]	Contraindicated			1 or 2 doses					
Influenza[6,*]	1 dose TIV annually								1 dose TIV or LAIV annually
Pneumococcal (polysaccharide)[7,8]		1 or 2 doses							
Hepatitis A[9,*]					2 doses				
Hepatitis B[10,*]					3 doses				
Meningococcal[11,*]					1 or more doses				

*Covered by the Vaccine Injury Compensation Program.

For all persons in this category who meet the age requirements and who lack evidence of immunity (e.g., lack documentation of vaccination or have no evidence of prior infection)

Recommended if some other risk factor is present (e.g., on the basis of medical, occupational, lifestyle, or other indications)

No recommendation

These schedules indicate the recommended age groups and medical indications for which administration of currently licensed vaccines is commonly indicated for adults ages 19 years and older, as of January 1, 2010. Licensed combination vaccines may be used whenever any components of the combination are indicated and when the vaccine's other components are not contraindicated. For detailed recommendations on all vaccines, including those used primarily for travelers or that are issued during the year, consult the manufacturers' package inserts and the complete statements from the Advisory Committee on Immunization Practices (http://www.cdc.gov/vaccines/pubs/acip-list.htm).

[1]Tetanus, diphtheria, and acellular pertussis (Td/Tdap) vaccination

Tdap should replace a single dose of Td for adults age 19 through 64 yr who have not received a dose of Tdap previously.

Adults with uncertain or incomplete history of primary vaccination series with tetanus and diphtheria toxoid–containing vaccines should begin or complete a primary vaccination series. A primary series for adults is 3 doses of tetanus and diphtheria toxoid–containing vaccines; administer the first 2 doses at least 4 wk apart and the third dose 6-12 mo after the second. However, Tdap can substitute for any one of the doses of Td in the 3-dose primary series. The booster dose of tetanus and diphtheria toxoid–containing vaccine should be administered to adults who have completed a primary series and if the last vaccination was received 10 or more yr previously. Tdap or Td vaccine may be used, as indicated.

If a woman is pregnant and received the last Td vaccination 10 or more yr previously, administer Td during the second or third trimester. If the woman received the last Td vaccination less than 10 yr previously, administer Tdap during the immediate postpartum period. A dose of Tdap is recommended for postpartum women, close contacts of infants age less than 12 mo, and all health care personnel with direct patient contact if they have not previously received Tdap. An interval as short as 2 yr from the last Td is suggested; shorter intervals can be used. Td may be deferred during pregnancy and Tdap substituted in the immediate postpartum period, or Tdap may be administered instead of Td to a pregnant woman after an informed discussion with the woman.

Consult the ACIP statement for recommendations for administering Td as prophylaxis in wound management.

[2]Human papillomavirus (HPV) vaccination

HPV vaccination is recommended for all females age 11 through 26 yr (and may begin at age 9 yr) who have not completed the vaccine series. History of genital warts, abnormal Papanicolaou test result, or positive HPV DNA test result is not evidence of prior infection with all vaccine HPV types; HPV vaccination is recommended for persons with such histories.

Ideally, vaccine should be administered before potential exposure to HPV through sexual activity; however, females who are sexually active should still be vaccinated consistent with age-based recommendations. Sexually active females who have not been infected with any of the 4 HPV vaccine types receive the full benefit of the vaccination. Vaccination is less beneficial for females who have already been infected with 1 or more of the HPV vaccine types.

A complete series consists of 3 doses. The second dose should be administered 2 mo after the first dose; the third dose should be administered 6 mo after the first dose.

HPV vaccination is not specifically recommended for females with the medical indications described in Table 5-19. Because it is not a live-virus vaccine, it can be administered to persons with the medical indications noted. However, the immune response and vaccine efficacy might be less for persons with the noted medical indications than in persons who do not have the medical indications described or who are immunocompetent. Health care personnel are not at increased risk because of occupational exposure and should be vaccinated consistent with age-based recommendations.

[3]Varicella vaccination

All adults without evidence of immunity to varicella should receive 2 doses of single-antigen varicella vaccine if not previously vaccinated or the second dose if they have received only 1 dose, unless they have a medical contraindication. Special consideration should be given to those who 1) have close contact with persons at high risk for severe disease (e.g., health care personnel and family contacts of persons with immunocompromising conditions) or 2) are at high risk for exposure or transmission (e.g., teachers; child care employees; residents and staff members of institutional settings, including correctional institutions; college students; military personnel; adolescents and adults living in households with children; nonpregnant women of childbearing age; and international travelers).

Evidence of immunity to varicella in adults includes any of the following: 1) documentation of 2 doses of varicella vaccine at least 4 wk apart; 2) U.S.-born before 1980 (although for health care personnel and pregnant women, birth before 1980 should not be considered evidence of immunity); 3) history of varicella based on diagnosis or verification of varicella by a health care provider (for a patient reporting a history of or presenting with an atypical case, a mild case, or both, health care providers should seek either an epidemiologic link to a typical varicella case or to a laboratory-confirmed case or evidence of laboratory confirmation, if it was performed at the time of acute disease); 4) history of herpes zoster based on health care provider diagnosis or verification of herpes zoster by a health care provider; or 5) laboratory evidence of immunity or laboratory confirmation of disease.

Pregnant women should be assessed for evidence of varicella immunity. Women who do not have evidence of immunity should receive the first dose of varicella vaccine upon completion or termination of pregnancy and before discharge from the health care facility. The second dose should be administered 4-8 wk after the first dose.

TABLE 5-19 Vaccines That Might Be Indicated for Adults Based on Medical and Other Indications—United States, 2010—cont'd

[4]Herpes zoster vaccination

A single dose of zoster vaccine is recommended for adults age 60 yr and older regardless of whether they report a prior episode of herpes zoster. Persons with chronic medical conditions may be vaccinated unless their condition constitutes a contraindication.

[5]Measles, mumps, rubella (MMR) vaccination

Measles component: Adults born before 1957 generally are considered immune to measles. Adults born during or after 1957 should receive 1 or more doses of MMR unless they have a medical contraindication, documentation of 1 or more doses, history of measles based on health care provider diagnosis, or laboratory evidence of immunity.

A second dose of MMR is recommended for adults who 1) have been recently exposed to measles or are in an outbreak setting; 2) have been vaccinated previously with killed measles vaccine; 3) have been vaccinated with an unknown type of measles vaccine during 1963-1967; 4) are students in postsecondary educational institutions; 5) work in a health care facility; or 6) plan to travel internationally.

Mumps component: Adults born before 1957 generally are considered immune to mumps. Adults born during or after 1957 should receive 1 dose of MMR unless they have a medical contraindication, history of mumps based on health care provider diagnosis, or laboratory evidence of immunity.

A second dose of MMR is recommended for adults who 1) live in a community experiencing a mumps outbreak and are in an affected age group; 2) are students in postsecondary educational institutions; 3) work in a health care facility; or 4) plan to travel internationally. For unvaccinated health care personnel born before 1957 who do not have other evidence of mumps immunity, administering 1 dose on a routine basis should be considered and administering a second dose during an outbreak should also be strongly considered.

Rubella component: 1 dose of MMR vaccine is recommended for women whose rubella vaccination history is unreliable or who lack laboratory evidence of immunity. For women of childbearing age, regardless of birth yr, rubella immunity should be determined and women should be counseled regarding congenital rubella syndrome. Women who do not have evidence of immunity should receive MMR vaccine upon completion or termination of pregnancy and before discharge from the health care facility.

[6]Influenza vaccination

Medical indications: Chronic disorders of the cardiovascular or pulmonary systems, including asthma; chronic metabolic diseases, including diabetes mellitus, renal or hepatic dysfunction, hemoglobinopathies, or immunocompromising conditions (including immunocompromising conditions caused by medications or HIV); any condition that compromises respiratory function or the handling of respiratory secretions or that can increase the risk of aspiration (e.g., cognitive dysfunction, spinal cord injury, or seizure disorder or other neuromuscular disorder); and pregnancy during the influenza season. No data exist on the risk for severe or complicated influenza disease among persons with asplenia; however, influenza is a risk factor for secondary bacterial infections that can cause severe disease among persons with asplenia.

Occupational indications: All health care personnel, including those employed by long-term care and assisted-living facilities, and caregivers of children younger than 5 yr.

Other indications: Residents of nursing homes and other long-term care and assisted-living facilities; persons likely to transmit influenza to persons at high risk (e.g., in-home household contacts and caregivers of children younger than 5 yr, persons 65 yr and older, and persons of all ages with high-risk condition[s]); and anyone who would like to decrease their risk of getting influenza. Healthy, nonpregnant adults younger than 50 yr without high-risk medical conditions who are not contacts of severely immunocompromised persons in special care units can receive either intranasally administered live, attenuated influenza vaccine (FluMist) or inactivated vaccine. Other persons should receive the inactivated vaccine.

[7]Pneumococcal polysaccharide (PPSV) vaccination

Medical indications: Chronic lung disease (including asthma); chronic cardiovascular diseases; diabetes mellitus; chronic liver diseases, cirrhosis; chronic alcoholism, chronic renal failure, or nephrotic syndrome; functional or anatomic asplenia (e.g., sickle cell disease or splenectomy [if elective splenectomy is planned, vaccinate at least 2 wk before surgery]); immunocompromising conditions; and cochlear implants and cerebrospinal fluid leaks. Vaccinate as close to HIV diagnosis as possible.

Other indications: Residents of nursing homes or other long-term care facilities and persons who smoke cigarettes. Routine use of PPSV is not recommended for Alaska Native or American Indian persons younger than 65 yr unless they have underlying medical conditions that are PPSV indications. However, public health authorities may consider recommending PPSV for Alaska Natives and American Indians 50 through 64 yr of age who are living in areas in which the risk of invasive pneumococcal disease is increased.

[8]Revaccination with PPSV

One-time revaccination after 5 yr for persons with chronic renal failure or nephrotic syndrome, functional or anatomic asplenia (e.g., sickle cell disease or splenectomy), and persons with immunocompromising conditions. For persons age 65 yr or older, 1-time revaccination if they were vaccinated 5 or more yr previously and were younger than 65 yr at the time of primary vaccination.

[9]Hepatitis A vaccination

Medical indications: Persons with chronic liver disease and persons who receive clotting factor concentrates.

Behavioral indications: Men who have sex with men and persons who use illegal drugs.

Occupational indications: Persons working with hepatitis A virus (HAV)–infected primates or with HAV in a research laboratory setting.

Other indications: Persons traveling to or working in countries that have high or intermediate endemicity of hepatitis A (a list of countries is available at wwwn.cdc.gov/travel/contentdiseases.aspx) and any person seeking protection from HAV infection.

Single-antigen vaccine formulations should be administered in a 2-dose schedule at either 0 and 6-12 mo (Havrix) or 0 and 6-18 mo (Vaqta). If the combined hepatitis A and hepatitis B vaccine (Twinrix) is used, administer 3 doses at 0, 1, and 6 mo; alternatively, a 4-dose schedule, administered on days 0, 7, and 21 to 30 followed by a booster dose at mo 12 may be used.

[10]Hepatitis B vaccination

Medical indications: Persons with end-stage renal disease, including patients receiving hemodialysis; persons with HIV infection; and persons with chronic liver disease.

Occupational indications: Health care personnel and public-safety workers who are exposed to blood or other potentially infectious body fluids.

Behavioral indications: Sexually active persons who are not in a long-term, mutually monogamous relationship (e.g., persons with more than 1 sex partner during the previous 6 mo); persons seeking evaluation or treatment for a sexually transmitted disease (STD); current or recent injection-drug users; and men who have sex with men.

Other indications: Household contacts and sex partners of persons with chronic hepatitis B virus (HBV) infection; clients and staff members of institutions for persons with developmental disabilities; international travelers to countries with high or intermediate prevalence of chronic HBV infection (a list of countries is available at wwwn.cdc.gov/travel/contentdiseases.aspx); and any adult seeking protection from HBV infection.

Hepatitis B vaccination is recommended for all adults in the following settings: STD treatment facilities, HIV testing and treatment facilities, facilities providing drug-abuse treatment and prevention services, health care settings targeting services to injection-drug users or men who have sex with men, correctional facilities, end-stage renal disease programs and facilities for chronic hemodialysis patients, and institutions and nonresidential day care facilities for persons with developmental disabilities.

If the combined hepatitis A and hepatitis B vaccine (Twinrix) is used, administer 3 doses at 0, 1, and 6 mo; alternatively, a 4-dose schedule, administered on days 0, 7, and 21 to 30 followed by a booster dose at mo 12 may be used.

Special formulation indications: For adult patients receiving hemodialysis or with other immunocompromising conditions, 1 dose of 40 μg/mL (Recombivax HB) administered on a 3-dose schedule or 2 doses of 20 μg/mL (Engerix-B) administered simultaneously on a 4-dose schedule at 0, 1, 2, and 6 mo.

[11]Meningococcal vaccination

Medical indications: Adults with anatomic or functional asplenia or terminal complement component deficiencies.

Other indications: First-yr college students living in dormitories; microbiologists who are routinely exposed to isolates of Neisseria meningitidis; military recruits; and persons who travel to or live in countries in which meningococcal disease is hyperendemic or epidemic (e.g., the "meningitis belt" of sub-Saharan Africa during the dry season [December-June]), particularly if their contact with local populations will be prolonged. Vaccination is required by the government of Saudi Arabia for all travelers to Mecca during the annual Hajj.

Meningococcal conjugate vaccine (MCV) is preferred for adults with any of the preceding indications who are aged 55 years or younger, although meningococcal polysaccharide vaccine (MPSV) is an acceptable alternative. Revaccination with MCV after 5 years might be indicated for adults previously vaccinated with MPSV who remain at increased risk for infection (e.g., persons residing in areas in which disease is epidemic).

[12]Selected conditions for which Haemophilus influenzae type b (Hib) vaccine may be used

Hib vaccine generally is not recommended for persons aged 5 years and older. No efficacy data are available on which to base a recommendation concerning use of Hib vaccine for older children and adults. However, studies suggest good immunogenicity in patients who have sickle cell disease, leukemia, or HIV infection or who have had a splenectomy; administering 1 dose of vaccine to these patients is not contraindicated.

[13]Immunocompromising conditions

Inactivated vaccines generally are acceptable (e.g., pneumococcal, meningococcal, and influenza [trivalent inactive influenza vaccine]) and live vaccines generally are avoided in persons with immune deficiencies or immuno-compromising conditions. Information on specific conditions is available at http://www.cdc.gov/vaccines/pubs/acip-list.htm.

TABLE 5-20 Immunization and Pregnancy

Vaccine	Before Pregnancy	During Pregnancy	After Pregnancy	Type of Vaccine	Route
Hepatitis A	If at high risk for disease	If at high risk for disease	If at high risk for disease	Inactivated	IM
Hepatitis B	Yes, if at risk	Yes, if at risk	Yes, if at risk	Inactivated	IM
Human Papillomavirus (HPV)	Yes, if 9 to 26 years of age	No, under study	Yes, if 9 to 26 years of age	Inactivated	IM
Influenza TIV	Yes	Yes	Yes	Inactivated	IM
Influenza LAIV	Yes, if <50 years and healthy; avoid conception for 4 weeks	No	Yes, if <50 years and healthy; avoid conception for 4 weeks	Live	Nasal spray
MMR	Yes, avoid conception for 4 weeks	No	Yes, give immediately postpartum if susceptible to rubella	Live	SC
Meningococcal:	If indicated	If indicated	If indicated		
• Polysaccharide				Inactivated	SC
• Conjugate				Inactivated	IM
Pneumococcal Polysaccharide	If indicated	If indicated	If indicated	Inactivated	IM or SC
Tetanus/Diphtheria Td	Yes, Tdap preferred	If indicated	Yes, Tdap preferred	Toxoid	IM
Tdap, one dose only	Yes, preferred	If high risk of pertussis; otherwise, Td preferred	Yes, preferred	Toxoid/inactivated	IM
Varicella	Yes, avoid conception for 4 weeks	No	Yes, give immediately postpartum if susceptible	Live	SC

TABLE 5-21 Immunizing Agents and Immunization Schedules for Health Care Workers (HCWs)*

Generic Name	Primary Schedule and Booster(s)	Indications	Major Precautions and Contraindications	Special Considerations
Immunizing Agents Strongly Recommended for Health Care Workers				
Hepatitis B (HB) recombinant vaccine	Two doses IM 4 wk apart; third dose 5 mo after second; booster doses not necessary	**Preexposure:** HCWs at risk for exposure to blood or body fluids	Based on limited data no risk of adverse effects to developing fetuses is apparent. Pregnancy should *not* be considered a contraindication to vaccination of women. Previous anaphylactic reaction to common baker's yeast is a contraindication to vaccination.	The vaccine produces neither therapeutic nor adverse effects on HB-infected persons. Prevaccination serologic screening is not indicated for persons being vaccinated because of occupational risk. HCWs who have contact with patients or blood should be tested 1-2 mo after vaccination to determine serologic response.
Hepatitis B immune globulin (HBIG)	0.06 ml/kg IM as soon as possible after exposure. A second dose of HBIG should be administered 1 mo later if the HB vaccine series has not been started.	**Postexposure prophylaxis:** For persons exposed to blood or body fluids containing HBsAg and who are not immune to HBV infection—0.06 ml/kg IM as soon as possible (but no later than 7 days after exposure)		
Influenza vaccine (inactivated whole-virus and split-virus vaccines)	Annual vaccination with current vaccine Administered IM	HCWs who have contact with patients at high risk for influenza or its complications; HCWs who work in long-term care facilities, HCWs with high-risk medical conditions or who are aged ≥65 yr	History of anaphylactic hypersensitivity to egg ingestion	No evidence exists of risk to mother or fetus when the vaccine is administered to a pregnant woman with an underlying high-risk condition. Influenza vaccination is recommended during second and third trimesters of pregnancy because of increased risk for hospitalization.
Measles live-virus vaccine	One dose SC; second dose at least 1 mo later	HCWs† born during or after 1957 who do not have documentation of having received two doses of live vaccine on or after the first birthday **or** a history of physician-diagnosed measles or serologic evidence of immunity. Vaccination should be considered for all HCWs who lack proof of immunity, including those born before 1957.	Pregnancy; immunocompromised persons,‡ including HIV-infected persons who have evidence of severe immunosuppression; anaphylaxis after gelatin ingestion or administration of neomycin; recent administration of immune globulin.	MMR is the vaccine of choice if recipients are likely to be susceptible to rubella and/or mumps as well as measles. Persons vaccinated between 1963 and 1967 with a killed measles vaccine alone, killed vaccine followed by live vaccine, or with a vaccine of unknown type should be revaccinated with two doses of live measles virus vaccine.
Mumps live-virus vaccine	One dose SC; second dose at least 1 mo later	HCWs† believed to be susceptible can be vaccinated. Adults born before 1957 can be considered immune.	Pregnancy; immunocompromised persons,‡ history of anaphylactic reaction after gelatin ingestion or administration of neomycin	MMR is the vaccine of choice if recipients are likely to be susceptible to measles and rubella, as well as mumps.
Hepatitis A virus (HAV) vaccine	Two doses of vaccine either 6-12 mo apart (HAVRIX), or 6 mo apart (VAQTA)	Not routinely indicated for HCWs in the United States. Persons who work with HAV-infected primates or with HAV in a research laboratory setting should be vaccinated.	History of anaphylactic hypersensitivity to alum or, for HAVRIX, the preservative 2-phenoxyethanol. The safety of the vaccine in pregnant women has not been determined; the risk associated with vaccination should be weighed against the risk for hepatitis A in women who may be at high risk for exposure to HAV.	
Meningococcal polysaccharide vaccine (tetravalent A, C, W135, and Y)	One dose in volume and by route specified by manufacturer; need for boosters unknown	Not routinely indicated for HCWs in the United States.	The safety of the vaccine in pregnant women has not been evaluated; it should not be administered during pregnancy unless the risk for infection is high.	

Modified from *MMWR* 46(RR-18), 1998.

HBsAg, Hepatitis B surface antigen; *HBV,* hepatitis B virus; *HIV,* human immunodeficiency virus; *IM,* intramuscular; *MMR,* measles, mumps, rubella vaccine; *SC,* subcutaneous; *TB,* tuberculosis.

*Persons who provide health care to patients or work in institutions that provide patient care (e.g., physicians, nurses, emergency medical personnel, dental professionals and students, medical and nursing students, laboratory technicians, hospital volunteers, and administrative and support staff in health care institutions).

†All HCWs (i.e., medical or nonmedical, paid or volunteer, full time or part time, student or nonstudent, with or without patient-care responsibilities) who work in health care institutions (e.g., inpatient and outpatient, public and private) should be immune to measles, rubella, and varicella.

‡Persons immunocompromised because of immune deficiency diseases, HIV infection, leukemia, lymphoma or generalized malignancy, or immunosuppressed as a result of therapy with corticosteroids, alkylating drugs, antimetabolites, or radiation.

Continued on following page

TABLE 5-21 Immunizing Agents and Immunization Schedules for Health Care Workers (HCWs)—cont'd

Generic Name	Primary Schedule and Booster(s)	Indications	Major Precautions and Contraindications	Special Considerations
Typhoid vaccine, IM, SC, and oral	IM vaccine: One 0.5-ml/dose, booster 0.5 ml every 2 yr SC vaccine: Two 0.5 ml doses, ≥4 wk apart, booster 0.5 ml SC or 0.1 ID every 3 yr if exposure continues Oral vaccine: Four doses on alternate days. The manufacturer recommends revaccination with the entire 4-dose series every 5 yr	Workers in microbiology laboratories who frequently work with *Salmonella typhi*	Severe local or systemic reaction to a previous dose. Ty21a (oral) vaccine should not be administered to immunocompromised persons† or to persons receiving antimicrobial agents.	Vaccination should not be considered an alternative to the use of proper procedures when handling specimens and cultures in the laboratory.
Vaccinia vaccine (smallpox)	One dose administered with a bifurcated needle; boosters administered every 10 yr	Laboratory workers who directly handle cultures with vaccinia, recombinant vaccinia viruses, or orthopox viruses that infect human beings	The vaccine is contraindicated in pregnancy, in persons with eczema or a history of eczema, and in immunocompromised persons† and their household contacts.	Vaccination may be considered for HCWs who have direct contact with contaminated dressings or other infectious material from volunteers in clinical studies involving recombinant vaccinia virus.
Other Vaccine-Preventable Diseases				
Tetanus and diphtheria (toxoids [Td])	Two IM doses 4 wk apart; third dose 6-12 mo after second dose; booster every 10 yr	All adults	Except in the first trimester, pregnancy is not a precaution. History of a neurologic reaction or immediate hypersensitivity reaction after a previous dose. History of severe local (arthus-type) reaction after a previous dose. Such persons should not receive further routine or emergency doses of Td for 10 yr.	Tetanus prophylaxis in wound management‡
Pneumococcal polysaccharide vaccine (23 valent)	One dose, 0.5 ml, IM or SC; revaccination recommended for those at highest risk ≥5 yr after the first dose	Adults who are at increased risk of pneumococcal disease and its complications because of underlying health conditions; older adults, especially those age ≥65 who are healthy	The safety of vaccine in pregnant women has not been evaluated; it should not be administered during pregnancy unless the risk for infection is high. Previous recipients of any type of pneumococcal polysaccharide vaccine who are at highest risk for fatal infection or antibody loss may be revaccinated ≥5 yr after the first dose.	
Rubella live-virus vaccine	One dose SC; second dose at least 1 mo later	Indicated for HCWs,† both men and women, who do not have documentation of having received live vaccine on or after their first birthday **or** laboratory evidence of immunity. Adults born before 1957, **except women who can become pregnant,** can be considered immune.	Pregnancy; immunocompromised persons†; history of anaphylactic reaction after administration of neomycin	The risk for rubella vaccine–associated malformations in the offspring of women pregnant when vaccinated or who become pregnant within 3 mo after vaccination is negligible. Such women should be counseled regarding the theoretic basis of concern for the fetus. MMR is the vaccine of choice if recipients are likely to be susceptible to measles or mumps as well as rubella.
Varicella zoster live-virus vaccine	Two 0.5-ml doses SC 4-8 wk apart if ≥13 yr	Indicated for HCWs† who do not have either a reliable history of varicella or serologic evidence of immunity	Pregnancy, immunocompromised persons,‡ history of anaphylactic reaction after receipt of neomycin or gelatin. Avoid salicylate use for 6 wk after vaccination.	Vaccine is available from the manufacturer for certain patients with acute lymphocytic leukemia in remission. Because 71%-93% of persons without a history of varicella are immune, serologic testing before vaccination is likely to be cost effective.

TABLE 5-21 Immunizing Agents and Immunization Schedules for Health Care Workers (HCWs)—cont'd

Generic Name	Primary Schedule and Booster(s)	Indications	Major Precautions and Contraindications	Special Considerations
Varicella-zoster immune globulin (VZIG)	Persons <50 kg: 125 μ/10 kg IM; persons ≥50 kg: 625 μ[§]	Persons known or likely to be susceptible (particularly those at high risk for complications, e.g., pregnant women) who have close and prolonged exposure to a contact case or to an infectious hospital staff worker or patient		Serologic testing may help in assessing whether to administer VZIG. If use of VZIG prevents varicella disease, patient should be vaccinated subsequently.
BCG Vaccination				
Bacille Calmette-Guérin (BCG) vaccine (TB)	One percutaneous dose of 0.3 ml; no booster dose recommended	Should be considered only for HCWs in areas where multi-drug TB is prevalent, a strong likelihood of infection exists, and where comprehensive infection control precautions have failed to prevent TB transmission to HCWs	Should not be administered to immunocompromised persons,[‡] pregnant women	In the United States TB-control efforts are directed toward early identification, treatment of cases, and preventive therapy with isoniazid.
Other Immunobiologics that Are or May Be Indicated for HCWs				
Immune globulin (hepatitis A)	**Postexposure**—One IM dose of 0.02 ml/kg administered ≤2 wk after exposure	Indicated for HCWs exposed to feces of infectious patients	Contraindicated in persons with IgA deficiency; do not administer within 2 wk after MMR vaccine or 3 wk after varicella vaccine. Delay administration of MMR vaccine for ≥3 mo and varicella vaccine ≥5 mo after administration of immune globulin	Administer in large muscle mass (deltoid, gluteal).

Modified from *MMWR* 46(RR-18), 1998.

HBsAg, Hepatitis B surface antigen; *HBV,* hepatitis B virus; *HIV,* human immunodeficiency virus; *IM,* intramuscular; *MMR,* measles, mumps, rubella vaccine; *SC,* subcutaneous; *TB,* tuberculosis.

*Persons who provide health care to patients or work in institutions that provide patient care (e.g., physicians, nurses, emergency medical personnel, dental professionals and students, medical and nursing students, laboratory technicians, hospital volunteers, and administrative and support staff in health care institutions).

†All HCWs (i.e., medical or nonmedical, paid or volunteer, full time or part time, student or nonstudent, with or without patient-care responsibilities) who work in health care institutions (e.g., inpatient and outpatient, public and private) should be immune to measles, rubella, and varicella.

‡Persons immunocompromised because of immune deficiency diseases, HIV infection, leukemia, lymphoma or generalized malignancy, or immunosuppressed as a result of therapy with corticosteroids, alkylating drugs, antimetabolites, or radiation.

§Some experts recommend 125 μ/10 kg regardless of total body weight.

TABLE 5-22 Recommendations for Persons with Medical Conditions Requiring Special Vaccination Considerations

Condition	Td	MMR	Varicella	HBV	HAV	Pneumovax[a]	Influenza[b]	HbCV	Meningococcal	IPV	Other Live Vaccines[c]	Other Killed Vaccines[d]
HIV infection	Rou	Rou/Contr[e]	Contr[f]	Rou[g]	Rou	Rec	Rec	Cons	Rou	Rou	Contr	Rou
Severe immunocompromise[h]	Rou	Contr	Contr[f]	Rou[g]	Rou	Rec	Rec	Rou[i]	Rou	Rou	Contr	Rou
Renal failure	Rou	Rou	Rou	Rec[g]	Rou	Rec	Rec	Rou	Rou	Rou	Rou	Rou
Diabetes	Rou	Rou	Rou	Rou	Rou	Rec	Rec	Rou	Rou	Rou	Rou	Rou
Chronic liver disease	Rou	Rou	Rou	Rou	Rec	Rec	Rec	Rou	Rou	Rou	Rou	Rou
Cardiac disease	Rou	Rou	Rou	Rou	Rou	Rec	Rec	Rou	Rou	Rou	Rou	Rou
Pulmonary disease	Rou	Rou	Rou	Rou	Rou	Rec	Rec	Rou	Rou	Rou	Rou	Rou
Alcoholism	Rou	Rou	Rou	Rou	Rou	Rec	Rec	Rou	Rou	Rou	Rou	Rou
Functional/anatomic asplenia	Rou	Rou	Rou	Rou	Rou	Rec[j]	Rec	Rec[j]	Rec[j]	Rou	Rou	Rou
Terminal complement deficiency	Rou	Rou	Rou	Rou	Rou	Rou	Rou	Rou	Rec	Rou	Rou	
Clotting factor disorders	Rou	Rou	Rou	Rec	Rec	Rou	Rou	Rou	Rou	Rou	Rou	Rou

Modified and updated from *MMWR* 42(RR-4):16, 1993.

Cons, Consider vaccination; *Contr,* contraindicated; *HbCV, Haemophilus influenzae* conjugate vaccine; *HBV,* hepatitis B virus; *IPV,* inactivated poliomyelitis vaccine; *MMR,* measles-mumps-rubella; *Rec,* recommended; *Rou,* routine as outlined for all adults.

[a]Pneumovax should be repeated in 5 yr for patients in whom vaccine is recommended. Asthma without chronic obstructive pulmonary disease is not an indication for the vaccine.

[b]Influenza vaccine should also be given to caregivers and household members.

[c]Includes bacille Calmette-Guérin, vaccinia, oral typhoid, yellow fever (if exposure cannot be avoided, persons with HIV can be given yellow fever vaccine; see text).

[d]Includes rabies (check postvaccination titers in HIV or severely immunocompromised persons), Lyme disease, inactivated typhoid, cholera, plague, and anthrax.

[e]For asymptomatic, nonseverely immunocompromised persons with HIV, MMR can be used; it is contraindicated in severely immunocompromised persons. MMR can be considered in symptomatic HIV patients without severe immunocompromise.

[f]Varicella can be given to household members and caregivers, but if varicella-like rash develops after vaccination, contact should be avoided.

[g]Recommended for persons with severe chronic renal failure approaching or already receiving dialysis, and higher doses should be given. Antibody titers should be measured after vaccination in these patients and in those with HIV or severe immunocompromise (who may require higher doses) to ensure adequate response. Yearly titers should be measured in dialysis patients.

[h]Severe immunocompromise can result from congenital immunodeficiency, leukemia, lymphoma, malignancy, organ transplant, chemotherapy, radiation therapy, or high-dose corticosteroids.

[i]Only for persons with Hodgkin's disease.

[j]Give at least 2 wk in advance of elective splenectomy.

TABLE 5-23 Vaccinations for International Travel

Disease*	Areas Affected†	Prophylaxis Recommended	Ideal Time between Last Vaccine Dose and Travel
Tetanus	All	All travelers; vaccine series/booster	Probably 30 days for series Anamnestic response to booster
Measles	All	If born after 1956; ensure immunity by antibody titer, diagnosed measles, or two doses of vaccine	As MMR, 7-14 days
Rubella	All	If born after 1956 and any female of childbearing age; rubella titer or one dose of vaccine	As MMR, 7-14 days
Mumps	All	If born after 1956; ensure immunity by antibody titer, diagnosed mumps, or one dose of vaccine	As MMR, 7-14 days
Varicella	All	All travelers; antibody titer, reported illness, or vaccine series	7-14 days
Hepatitis B	5%-20% of population are carriers in Africa, Middle East except Israel, all Southeast Asia, Amazon basin, Haiti, and Dominican Republic; 1%-5% of population are carriers in south-central and southwest Asia, Israel, Japan, Americas, Russia, and eastern and southern Europe	Travelers for more than 6 mo in close contact with population or for less time but with high-risk activities (close household contact, seeking dental or medical care, sex); vaccine series	Probably 30 days
Hepatitis A	Developing countries	Travelers to rural areas; eating and drinking in settings of poor sanitation; vaccine or pooled immune globulin	Vaccine, 30 days Pooled IG, 2 days
Influenza	Tropics throughout the year; southern hemisphere from April to September	Travelers for whom vaccine is otherwise indicated; give current vaccine and revaccinate in fall as usual	7-14 days
Meningococcus*	Sub-Saharan Africa "belt" (Senegal to Ethiopia) from December to June; required for pilgrims to Saudi Arabia during Haj; epidemics reported in other African nations, India, Nepal, and Mongolia	All travelers; vaccine.	7-10 days
Rabies	Endemic dog rabies exists in Mexico, El Salvador, Guatemala, Peru, Colombia, Ecuador, India, Nepal, Philippines, Sri Lanka, Thailand, and Vietnam	Travelers staying for more than 30 days or at high risk of exposure to domestic or wild animals; vaccine series/booster	7-14 days
Poliomyelitis	Developing countries not in western hemisphere; at risk all year in tropics; in temperate zones, incidence increases in summer and fall	All travelers; vaccine series/booster	Parenteral vaccine series, 28 day (see text)
Typhoid fever	Many countries in Asia, Africa, Central America, and South America	Travelers with prolonged stay in rural areas with poor sanitation; vaccine series/booster	Oral vaccine, 7 days Parenteral vaccine, probably 14 days
Yellow fever*	North and central South America, forest-savannah zones of Africa; some countries in Africa, Asia, and Middle East require travelers from endemic areas to be vaccinated	All travelers; vaccine/booster at approved yellow fever vaccination center.	10 days
Japanese encephalitis	Seasonally in most areas of Asia, Indian subcontinent, and western Pacific islands; in temperate zones, incidence increases in summer and early fall; in tropics, year-round incidence	Travelers staying for more than 30 days in high-risk rural areas; staying outdoors during transmission season; vaccine series	10 days
Cholera*	Certain undeveloped countries	If required by local authorities, one dose usually suffices; primary series only for those living in high-risk areas under poor sanitary conditions or those with compromised gastric defense mechanisms (achlorhydria, antacid therapy, previous ulcer surgery); booster every 6 mo	Probably 30 days
Plague	Africa, Asia, and Americas in rural mountainous or upland areas	Travelers whose research or field activities bring them in contact with rodents; vaccine series/booster; consider taking tetracycline (500 mg four times a day) for chemoprophylaxis (inferred from clinical experience in treating plague)	Probably 30 days

From Noble J: *Primary care medicine,* ed 3, St Louis, 2001, Mosby.
MMR, Measles-mumps-rubella.
*Only yellow fever vaccine is required for entry by any country; cholera vaccine may be required by some local authorities. Meningococcus vaccine is required for pilgrims to Mecca, in Saudia Arabia, during Haj. However, it is important to follow Centers for Disease Control and Prevention (CDC) recommendations for all vaccines to prevent disease. If a required vaccine is contraindicated or withheld for any reason, attempts should be made to obtain a waiver from the country's consulate or embassy.
†Because areas affected can change, and for more specific details, consult the CDC's traveler's hotline.

Recommendations and Implementation Strategies for Hepatitis B Vaccination of Adults

BOX 5-1 Adults Recommended to Receive Hepatitis B Vaccination

Persons at Risk for Infection by Sexual Exposure
- Sex partners of persons who are HBsAg positive
- Sexually active persons who are not in a long-term, mutually monogamous relationship (e.g., persons who have had more than one sex partner during the previous 6 months)
- Persons seeking evaluation or treatment for a sexually transmitted disease
- Men who have sex with men

Persons at Risk for Infection by Percutaneous or Mucosal Exposure to Blood
- Current or recent users of injection drugs
- Household contacts of persons who are HBsAg positive
- Residents and staff of facilities for developmentally disabled persons
- Health care and public safety workers with reasonably anticipated risk for exposure to blood or blood-contaminated body fluids
- Persons with end-stage renal disease, including predialysis, hemodialysis, peritoneal dialysis, and home dialysis patients

Others
- International travelers to regions with high or intermediate levels (HBsAg prevalence of ≥2%) of endemic HBV infection
- Persons with chronic liver disease
- Persons with HIV infection
- All other persons seeking protection from HBV infection

From CDC: A comprehensive immunization strategy to eliminate transmission of hepatitis B virus infection in the United States: recommendations of the Advisory Committee on Immunization Practices (ACIP), *MMWR* 55(RR-16):15, 2006.

HbsAg, Hepatitis B surface antigen.

BOX 5-2 Hepatitis B Vaccine Schedules for Adults (Aged ≥20 yr)*

0, 1, and 6 months
0, 1, and 4 months
0, 2, and 4 months
0, 1, 2, and 12 months†

From CDC: A comprehensive immunization strategy to eliminate transmission of hepatitis B virus infection in the United States: recommendations of the Advisory Committee on Immunization Practices (ACIP), *MMWR* 55(RR-16):15, 2006.

*All schedules are applicable to single-antigen hepatitis B vaccines; Twinrix (combined hepatitis A and hepatitis B vaccine) may be administered at 0, 1, and 6 months.

†A 4-dose schedule of Engerix-B is licensed for all age groups.

TABLE 5-24 Recommended Doses of Currently Licensed Formulations of Adult Hepatitis B Vaccine by Group and Vaccine Type

	SINGLE-ANTIGEN VACCINE				COMBINATION VACCINE	
	Recombivax HB[a]		Engerix-B[b]		Twinrix[b,c]	
Group	Dose (μg)[d]	Vol. (ml)	Dose (μg)[d]	Vol. (ml)	Dose (μg)[d]	Vol. (ml)
Adults (aged ≥20 yr)	10	1.0	20	1.0	20	1.0
Hemodialysis patients and other immunocompromised persons aged ≥20 yr	40[e]	1.0	40[f]	2.0	—[g]	—

From Centers for Disease Control and Prevention: A comprehensive immunization strategy to eliminate transmission of hepatitis B virus infection in the United States: recommendations of the Advisory Committee on Immunization Practices (ACIP), *MMWR* 55(RR-16):10, 2006.
HB, Hepatitis B.
[a]Merck & Co., Inc., Whitehouse Station, New Jersey.
[b]GlaxoSmithKline Biologicals, Rixensart, Belgium.
[c]Combined hepatitis A and hepatitis B vaccine, recommended for persons aged >18 yr who are at increased risk for both hepatitis B virus and hepatitis A virus infections.
[d]Recombinant hepatitis B surface antigen protein dose.
[e]Dialysis formulation administered on a 3-dose schedule at 0, 1, and 6 mo.
[f]Two 1.0-ml doses administered in 1 or 2 injections on a 4-dose schedule at 0, 1, 2, and 6 mo.
[g]Not applicable.

TABLE 5-25 Recommended HIV/AIDS, Sexually Transmitted Disease (STD), and Viral Hepatitis Prevention Services by Risk Population

Risk Population[a]	Recommended Services
High-Risk Heterosexuals	
Persons seeking sexually transmitted disease evaluation or treatment	Hepatitis B vaccination Testing for HIV infection[b] Testing for syphilis, gonorrhea, and chlamydia, as clinically indicated[c]
Sexually active men not in a long-term, mutually monogamous relationship	Hepatitis B vaccination Annual testing for HIV infection[b,d]
Sexually active women not in a long-term, mutually monogamous relationship	Hepatitis B vaccination[e] Annual testing for HIV infection[b,d] Annual testing for chlamydia (NOTE: Also recommended for all sexually active females aged <25 yr)[c]
Men Who Have Sex with Men (MSM)	
All MSM	Hepatitis A vaccination Hepatitis B vaccination[e]
Sexually active MSM not in a long-term, mutually monogamous relationship	Hepatitis A vaccination Hepatitis B vaccination[e] Annual testing for HIV infection[b] Annual testing for syphilis, gonorrhea, and chlamydia[c]
Injection-Drug Users	
	Hepatitis A vaccination[f] Hepatitis B vaccination Testing for hepatitis C virus infection[g] Annual testing for HIV infection[b] Substance-abuse treatment[h]

From Centers for Disease Control and Prevention (CDC): A comprehensive immunization strategy to eliminate transmission of hepatitis B virus infection in the United States: recommendations of the Advisory Committee on Immunization Practices (ACIP), *MMWR* 55(RR-16):17, 2006.
[a]Testing for HIV infection, chlamydia, gonorrhea, syphilis, and hepatitis B surface antigen also is recommended for pregnant women. (CDC: Revised recommendations for HIV testing of adults, adolescents, and pregnant women in health care settings, *MMWR* 55[RR-14], 2006; CDC: Sexually transmitted diseases treatment guidelines, *MMWR* 55[RR-11], 2006; CDC: A comprehensive immunization strategy to eliminate transmission of hepatitis B virus infection in the United States: recommendations of the Advisory Committee on Immunization Practices [ACIP]. Part 1: immunization of infants, children, and adolescents, *MMWR* 54[RR-16], 2005.)
[b]CDC: Revised recommendations for HIV testing of adults, adolescents, and pregnant women in health care settings, *MMWR* 55(RR-14), 2006.
[c]CDC: Sexually transmitted diseases treatment guidelines 2006, *MMWR* 55(RR-11), 2006.
[d]HIV screening is recommended for all persons aged 13-64 yr. Repeat screening is recommended at least annually for persons likely to be at high risk for HIV infection, including MSM or heterosexuals who themselves or whose sex partners have had more than one partner since their most recent HIV test.
[e]Hepatitis B vaccination is recommended for persons who have had more than one sex partner during the previous 6 mo.
[f]CDC: Prevention of hepatitis A through active or passive immunization: recommendations of the Advisory Committee on Immunization Practices (ACIP), *MMWR* 55(RR-7), 2006.
[g]CDC: Recommendations for prevention and control of hepatitis C virus (HCV) infection and HCV-related chronic disease, *MMWR* 47(RR-19), 1998. Recommended frequency of testing for hepatitis C virus infection has not been determined.
[h]CDC: *Substance abuse treatment for injection drug users: a strategy with many benefits,* Atlanta, GA, 2002, U.S. Department of Health and Human Services, CDC. Available at http://www.cdc.gov/idu/facts/treatment.htm.

TABLE 5-26 Guidelines for Postexposure Prophylaxis* of Persons with Nonoccupational Exposures† to Blood or Body Fluids that Contain Blood by Exposure Type and Vaccination Status

	TREATMENT	
Exposure	**Unvaccinated Person‡**	**Previously Vaccinated Person§**
HBsAg-Positive Source		
Percutaneous (e.g., bite or needlestick) or mucosal exposure to HBsAg-positive blood or body fluids	Administer hepatitis B vaccine series and hepatitis B immune globulin (HBIG)	Administer hepatitis B vaccine booster dose
Sex or needle-sharing contact with a person who is HBsAg positive	Administer hepatitis B vaccine series and HBIG	Administer hepatitis B vaccine booster dose
Victim of sexual assault/abuse by a perpetrator who is HBsAg positive	Administer hepatitis B vaccine series and HBIG	Administer hepatitis B vaccine booster dose
Source with Unknown HBsAg Status		
Victim of sexual assault/abuse by a perpetrator with unknown HBsAg status	Administer hepatitis B vaccine series	No treatment
Percutaneous (e.g., bite or needlestick) or mucosal exposure to potentially infectious blood or body fluids from a source with unknown HBsAg status	Administer hepatitis B vaccine series	No treatment
Sexual or needle-sharing contact with person with unknown HBsAg status	Administer hepatitis B vaccine series	No treatment

From Centers for Disease Control and Prevention: A comprehensive immunization strategy to eliminate transmission of hepatitis B virus infection in the United States: recommendations of the Advisory Committee on Immunization Practices (ACIP), *MMWR* 55(RR-16):30, 2006.

HBsAg, Hepatitis B surface antigen.

*When indicated, immunoprophylaxis should be initiated as soon as possible, preferably within 24 hours. Studies are limited on the maximum interval after exposure during which postexposure prophylaxis is effective, but the interval is unlikely to exceed 7 days for percutaneous exposures or 14 days for sexual exposures. The hepatitis B vaccine series should be completed.

†These guidelines apply to nonoccupational exposures. Guidelines for management of occupational exposures have been published separately and also can be used for management of nonoccupational exposures if feasible.

‡A person who is in the process of being vaccinated but has not completed the vaccine series should complete the series and receive treatment as indicated.

§A person who has written documentation of a complete hepatitis B vaccine series and did not receive postvaccination testing.

TABLE 5-27 Typical Interpretation of Serologic Test Results for Hepatitis B Virus Infection

SEROLOGIC MARKER				
HBsAg	**Total Anti-HBc**	**IgM Anti-HBc**	**Anti-HBs**	**Interpretation**
–*	–	–	–	Never infected
+†‡	–	–	–	Early acute infection; transient (up to 18 days) after vaccination
+	+	+	–	Acute infection
–	+	+	+ or –	Acute resolving infection
–	+	–	+	Recovered from past infection and immune
+	+	–	–	Chronic infection
–	+	–	–	False-positive (i.e., susceptible), past infection, "low-level" chronic infection,§ or passive transfer of anti-HBc to infant born to mother who is HBsAg positive
–	–	–	+	Immune if concentration is >10 mIU/ml after vaccine series completion‖; passive transfer after hepatitis B immune globulin administration

From Centers for Disease Control and Prevention: A comprehensive immunization strategy to eliminate transmission of hepatitis B virus infection in the United States: recommendations of the Advisory Committee on Immunization Practices (ACIP), *MMWR* 55(RR-16):4, 2006.

HBc, Antibody to hepatitis B core antigen; *HBs,* antibody to HBsAg; *HBsAg,* hepatitis B surface antigen; *Ig,* immunoglobulin.

*Negative test result.

†Positive test result.

‡To ensure that an HBsAg-positive test result is not a false-positive, samples with reactive HBsAg results should be tested with a licensed neutralizing confirmatory test if recommended in the manufacturer's package insert.

§Persons positive only for anti-HBc are unlikely to be infectious except under unusual circumstances in which they are the source for direct percutaneous exposure of susceptible recipients to large quantities of virus (e.g., blood transfusion or organ transplant).

‖Milliinternational units per milliliter.

Hepatitis A Prophylaxis

TABLE 5-28 Recommended Dosages of Hepatitis A Immune Globulin

Setting	Duration of Coverage	Dose
Preexposure prophylaxis	Short term (<3 mo)	0.02 ml/kg
	Long term (3-5 mo)*	0.06 ml/kg
Postexposure prophylaxis	—	0.02 ml/kg

Modified from Centers for Disease Control and Prevention: Prevention of hepatitis A through active or passive immunization: recommendations of the Advisory Committee on Immunization Practices (ACIP), *MMWR* 55(RR-07):9, 2006.

NOTE Immune globulin should be administered intramuscularly into the deltoid or gluteal muscle in children younger than 24 mo; it may be administered in the anterolateral thigh muscle.

*Repeat every 5 mo if continued exposure to hepatitis A virus occurs.

TABLE 5-29 Licensed Dosages of Hepatitis A Vaccines

Vaccine	Patient's Age	Dose	Volume (ml)	Number of Doses	Schedule (mo)*
Hepatitis A vaccine, inactivated (Havrix)	12 mo to 18 yr	720 EL.U.	0.5	2	0, 6-12
	≥19 yr	1440 EL.U.	1.0	2	0, 6-12
Hepatitis A vaccine, inactivated (Vaqta)	12 mo to 18 yr	25 U	0.5	2	0, 6-18
	≥19 yr	50 U	1.0	2	0, 6-18
Combined hepatitis A and hepatitis B vaccine (Twinrix)	≥18 yr	720 EL.U. of hepatitis A antigen and 20 mcg of hepatitis B surface antigen protein	1.0	3	0, 1, and 6

Modified from Centers for Disease Control and Prevention: Prevention of hepatitis A through active or passive immunization: recommendations of the Advisory Committee on Immunization Practices (ACIP), *MMWR* 55(RR-07):10, 2006.

*Zero represents the timing of the initial dose; subsequent numbers represent months after the initial dose.

Influenza Treatment and Prophylaxis

BOX 5-3 Summary of Seasonal Influenza Vaccination Recommendations

Children

All children aged 6 months-18 years should be vaccinated annually.

Children and adolescents at higher risk for influenza complications should continue to be a focus for vaccination efforts as providers and programs transition to routinely vaccinating all children and adolescents, including those who:

- are aged 6 months-4 years (59 months)
- have chronic pulmonary (including asthma), cardiovascular (except hypertension), renal, hepatic, cognitive, neurologic/neuromuscular, hematologic, or metabolic disorders (including diabetes mellitus)
- are immunosuppressed (including immunosuppression caused by medications or by human immunodeficiency virus)
- are receiving long-term aspirin therapy and therefore might be at risk for experiencing Reye's syndrome after influenza virus infection
- are residents of long-term care facilities
- will be pregnant during the influenza season

Note: Children aged <6 months cannot receive influenza vaccination. Household and other close contacts (e.g., daycare providers) of children aged <6 months, including older children and adolescents, should be vaccinated.

Adults

Annual vaccination against influenza is recommended for any adult who wants to reduce the risk of becoming ill with influenza or of transmitting it to others. Vaccination is recommended for all adults without contraindications in the following groups, because these persons either are at higher risk for influenza complications, or are close contacts of the persons at higher risk:

- persons aged ≥50 years
- women who will be pregnant during the influenza season
- persons who have chronic pulmonary (including asthma), cardiovascular (except hypertension), renal, hepatic, cognitive, neurologic/neuromuscular, hematologic, or metabolic disorders (including diabetes mellitus)
- persons who have immunosuppression (including immunosuppression caused by medications or by human immunodeficiency virus)
- residents of nursing homes and other long-term care facilities
- health-care personnel
- household contacts and caregivers of children aged <5 years and adults aged ≥50 years, with particular emphasis on vaccinating contacts of children aged <6 months
- household contacts and caregivers of persons with medical conditions that put them at higher risk for severe complications from influenza

Modified from *MMWR* 58:(RR-8), 2009.

RECOMMENDED VACCINES FOR DIFFERENT AGE GROUPS

When vaccinating children aged 6 to 35 months with TIV, health care providers should use TIV that has been licensed by the FDA for this age group (i.e., TIV manufactured by Sanofi Pasteur [FluZone]). TIV from Novartis (Fluvirin) is FDA approved in the United States for use among persons aged 4 years and older. TIV from GlaxoSmithKline (Fluarix and FluLaval) or CSL Biotherapies (Afluria) is labeled for use in persons aged 18 years and older because data to demonstrate efficacy among younger persons have not been provided to the FDA. LAIV from MedImmune (FluMist) is licensed for use by healthy, nonpregnant persons aged 2 to 49 years. A vaccine dose does not need to be repeated if inadvertently administered to a person who does not have an age indication for the vaccine formulation given. Expanded age and risk group indications for licensed vaccines are likely over the next several years, and vaccination providers should be alert to these changes. In addition, several new vaccine formulations are being evaluated in immunogenicity and efficacy trials; when licensed, these new products will increase the influenza vaccine supply and provide additional vaccine choices for practitioners and their patients.

INFLUENZA VACCINES AND USE OF INFLUENZA ANTIVIRAL MEDICATIONS

Administration of TIV and influenza antivirals during the same medical visit is acceptable. The effect on safety and effectiveness of LAIV coadministration with influenza antiviral medications has not been studied. However, because influenza antivirals reduce replication of influenza viruses, LAIV should not be administered until 48 hours after cessation of influenza antiviral therapy, and influenza antiviral medications should not be administered for 2 weeks after receipt of LAIV. Persons receiving antivirals within the period 2 days before to 14 days after vaccination with LAIV should be revaccinated at a later date.

PERSONS WHO SHOULD NOT BE VACCINATED WITH TIV

TIV should not be administered to persons known to have anaphylactic hypersensitivity to eggs or other components of the influenza vaccine. Prophylactic use of antiviral agents is an option for preventing influenza among such persons. Information about vaccine components is located in package inserts from each manufacturer. Persons with moderate to severe acute febrile illness usually should not be vaccinated until their symptoms have abated. However, minor illnesses with or without fever do not contraindicate use of influenza vaccine. Guillaine-Barré syndrome within 6 weeks after a previous dose of TIV is considered a precaution for use of TIV.

CONSIDERATIONS WHEN USING LAIV

LAIV is an option for vaccination of healthy, nonpregnant persons aged 2 to 49 years, including health care providers and other close contacts of high-risk persons (except severely immunocompromised persons who require care in a protected environment). No preference is indicated for LAIV or TIV when considering vaccination of healthy, nonpregnant persons aged 2 to 49 years. Use of the term *healthy* in this recommendation refers to persons who do not have any of the underlying medical conditions that confer high risk for severe complications (see "Persons Who Should Not Be Vaccinated with LAIV"). However, during periods when inactivated vaccine is in short supply, use of LAIV is encouraged when feasible for eligible persons (including health care providers) because use of LAIV by these persons might increase availability of TIV for persons in groups targeted for vaccination but who cannot receive LAIV. Possible advantages of LAIV include its potential to induce a broad mucosal and systemic immune response in children, its ease of administration, and possibly increased acceptability of an intranasal rather than intramuscular route of administration.

If the vaccine recipient sneezes after administration, the dose should not be repeated. However, if nasal congestion is present that might impede delivery of the vaccine to the nasopharyngeal mucosa, deferral of administration should be considered until resolution of the illness, or TIV should be administered instead. No data exist about concomitant use of nasal corticosteroids or other intranasal medications.

Although FDA licensure of LAIV excludes children aged 2 to 4 years with a history of asthma or recurrent wheezing, the precise risk, if any, of wheezing caused by LAIV among these children is unknown because experience with LAIV among these young children is limited. Young children might not have a history of recurrent wheezing if their exposure to respiratory viruses has been limited because of their age. Certain children might have a history of wheezing with respiratory illnesses but have not had asthma diagnosed. The following screening recommendations should be used to assist persons who administer influenza vaccines in providing the appropriate vaccine for children aged 2 to 4 years.

Clinicians and vaccination programs should screen for possible reactive airways diseases when considering use of LAIV for children aged 2 to 4 years and should avoid use of this vaccine in children with asthma or a recent wheezing episode. Health care providers should consult the medical record, when available, to identify children aged 2 to 4 years with asthma or recurrent wheezing that might indicate asthma. In addition, to identify children who might be at greater risk for asthma and possibly at increased risk for wheezing after receiving LAIV, parents or caregivers of children aged 2 to 4 years should be asked, "In the past 12 months, has a health care provider ever told you that your child had wheezing or asthma?" Children whose parents or caregivers answer "yes" to this question and children who have asthma or who had a wheezing episode noted in the medical record during the preceding 12 months should not receive LAIV. TIV is available for use in children with asthma or possible reactive airways diseases.

LAIV can be administered to persons with minor acute illnesses (e.g., diarrhea or mild upper respiratory tract infection with or without fever). However, if nasal congestion is present that might impede delivery of the vaccine to the nasopharyngeal mucosa, deferral of administration should be considered until resolution of the illness.

PERSONS WHO SHOULD NOT BE VACCINATED WITH LAIV

The effectiveness or safety of LAIV is not known for the following groups, who should not be vaccinated with LAIV:

- Persons with a history of hypersensitivity, including anaphylaxis, to any of the components of LAIV or eggs
- Persons younger than 2 years or aged 50 years or older
- Persons with any of the underlying medical conditions that serve as an indication for routine influenza vaccination, including asthma, reactive airways disease, or other chronic disorders of the pulmonary or cardiovascular systems; other underlying medical conditions, including metabolic diseases such as diabetes, renal dysfunction, and hemoglobinopathies; or known or suspected immunodeficiency diseases or immunosuppressed states
- Children aged 2 to 4 years whose parents or caregivers report that a health care provider has told them during the preceding 12 months that their child had wheezing or asthma, or whose medical record indicates a wheezing episode has occurred during the preceding 12 months
- Children or adolescents receiving aspirin or other salicylates (because of the association of Reye syndrome with wild-type influenza virus infection)
- Persons with a history of Guillaine-Barré syndrome after influenza vaccination
- Pregnant women

Concurrent Administration of Influenza Vaccine with Other Vaccines

Use of LAIV concurrently with measles, mumps, rubella (MMR) alone, and MMR and varicella vaccine among children aged 12 to 15 months has been studied, and no interference with immunogenicity to antigens in any of the vaccines was observed. Among adults aged 50 years or older, the safety and immunogenicity of zoster vaccine and TIV were similar whether administered simultaneously or spaced 4 weeks apart. In the absence of specific data indicating interference, following ACIP's general recommendations for vaccination is prudent. Inactivated vaccines do not interfere with the immune response to other inactivated vaccines or to live vaccines. Inactivated or live vaccines can be administered simultaneously with LAIV. However, after administration of a live vaccine, at least 4 weeks should pass before another live vaccine is administered.

TABLE 5-30 Live Attenuated Influenza Vaccine (LAIV) Compared with Inactivated Influenza Vaccine (TIV) for Seasonal Influenza, United States Formulations

Factor	LAIV	TIV
Route of administration	Intranasal spray	Intramuscular injection
Type of vaccine	Live virus	Noninfectious virus (i.e.,inactivated)
Number of included virus strains	3 (2 influenza A, 1 influenza B)	3 (2 influenza A, 1 influenza B)
Vaccine virus strains updated	Annually	Annually
Frequency of administration	Annually*	Annually*
Approved age	Persons aged 2-49 yr	Persons aged ≥6 mo
Interval between 2 doses recommended for children aged ≥6 mo to 8 yr who are receiving influenza vaccine for the first time	4 wk	4 wk
Can be administered to persons with medical risk factors for influenza-related complications†	No	Yes
Can be administered to children with asthma or children aged 2-4 yr with wheezing during the preceding year§	No	Yes
Can be administered to family members or close contacts of immunosuppressed persons not requiring a protected environment	Yes	Yes
Can be administered to family members or close contacts of immunosuppressed persons requiring a protected environment (e.g., hematopoietic stem cell transplant recipient)	No	Yes
Can be administered to family members or close contacts of persons at high risk but not severely immunosuppressed	Yes	Yes
Can be simultaneously administered with other vaccines	Yes¶	Yes**
If not simultaneously administered, can be administered within 4 wk of another live vaccine	Prudent to space 4 wk apart	Yes
If not simultaneously administered, can be administered within 4 wk of an inactivated vaccine	Yes	Yes

Modified from *MMWR* 56(RR-6), 2007.

LAIV, Live attenuated influenza vaccine; *TIV,* inactivated influenza vaccine.

*Children aged 6 months-8 years who have never received influenza vaccine before should receive 2 doses. Those who only receive 1 dose in their first year of vaccination should receive 2 doses in the following year, spaced 4 weeks apart.

†Persons at higher risk for complications of influenza infection because of underlying medical conditions should not receive LAIV. Persons at higher risk for complications of influenza infection because of underlying medical conditions include adults and children with chronic disorders of the pulmonary or cardiovascular systems; adults and children with chronic metabolic diseases (including diabetes mellitus), renal dysfunction, hemoglobinopathies, or immunosuppression; children and adolescents receiving long-term aspirin therapy (at risk for developing Reye's syndrome after wild-type influenza infection); persons who have any condition (e.g., cognitive dysfunction, spinal cord injuries, seizure disorders, or other neuromuscular disorders) that can compromise respiratory function or the handling of respiratory secretions or that can increase the risk for aspiration; pregnant women; and residents of nursing homes and other chronic-care facilities that house persons with chronic medical conditions.

§Clinicians and immunization programs should screen for possible reactive airways diseases when considering use of LAIV for children aged 2-4 years and should avoid use of this vaccine in children with asthma or a recent wheezing episode. Health-care providers should consult the medical record, when available, to identify children aged 2-4 years with asthma or recurrent wheezing that might indicate asthma. In addition, to identify children who might be at greater risk for asthma and possibly at increased risk for wheezing after receiving LAIV, parents or caregivers of children aged 2-4 years should be asked: "In the past 12 months, has a health-care provider ever told you that your child had wheezing or asthma?" Children whose parents or caregivers answer "yes" to this question and children who have asthma or who had a wheezing episode noted in the medical record during the preceding 12 months should not receive LAIV.

¶LAIV coadministration has been evaluated systematically only among children aged 12–15 months who received measles, mumps, and rubella vaccine or varicella vaccine.

**TIV coadministration has been evaluated systematically only among adults who received pneumococcal polysaccharide or zoster vaccine.

INDICATIONS FOR USE OF ANTIVIRALS

PERSONS FOR WHOM ANTIVIRAL TREATMENT SHOULD BE CONSIDERED

If possible, antiviral treatment should be started within 48 hours of influenza illness onset. The effectiveness of initiating antiviral treatment more than 48 hours after illness onset has not been established. Persons for whom antiviral treatment should be considered include:

- Persons hospitalized with laboratory-confirmed influenza (limited data suggest benefit even for persons whose antiviral treatment is initiated more than 48 hours after illness onset)
- Persons with laboratory-confirmed influenza pneumonia
- Persons with laboratory-confirmed influenza and bacterial coinfection
- Persons with laboratory-confirmed influenza infection who are at higher risk for influenza complications
- Persons presenting to medical care with laboratory-confirmed influenza within 48 hours of influenza illness onset who want to decrease the duration or severity of their symptoms and transmission of influenza to others at higher risk for complications

PERSONS FOR WHOM ANTIVIRAL CHEMOPROPHYLAXIS SHOULD BE CONSIDERED DURING PERIODS OF INCREASED INFLUENZA ACTIVITY IN THE COMMUNITY

- Persons at high risk during the 2 weeks after influenza vaccination (after the second dose for children younger than 9 years who have not previously been vaccinated) if influenza viruses are circulating in the community
- Persons at high risk for whom influenza vaccine is contraindicated
- Family members or health care providers who are unvaccinated and are likely to have ongoing, close exposure to persons at high risk or unvaccinated persons or infants younger than 6 months
- Persons and their family members and close contacts and health care workers when circulating strains of influenza virus in the community are not matched with vaccine strains
- Persons with immune deficiencies or those who might not respond to vaccination (e.g., persons infected with HIV or other immunosuppressed conditions or who are receiving immunosuppressive medications)
- Unvaccinated staff and persons during response to an outbreak in a closed institutional setting with residents at high risk (e.g., extended-care facilities)

Modified from *MMWR* 57(RR-7), 2008.

Note: Recommended antiviral medications (neuraminidase inhibitors) are not licensed for chemoprophylaxis of children younger than 1 year (oseltamivir) or younger than 5 years (zanamivir). Updates or supplements to these recommendations (e.g., expanded age or risk group indications for licensed vaccines) might be required. Health care providers should be alert to announcements of recommendation updates and should check the CDC influenza Web site periodically for additional information (http://www.cdc.gov/flu).

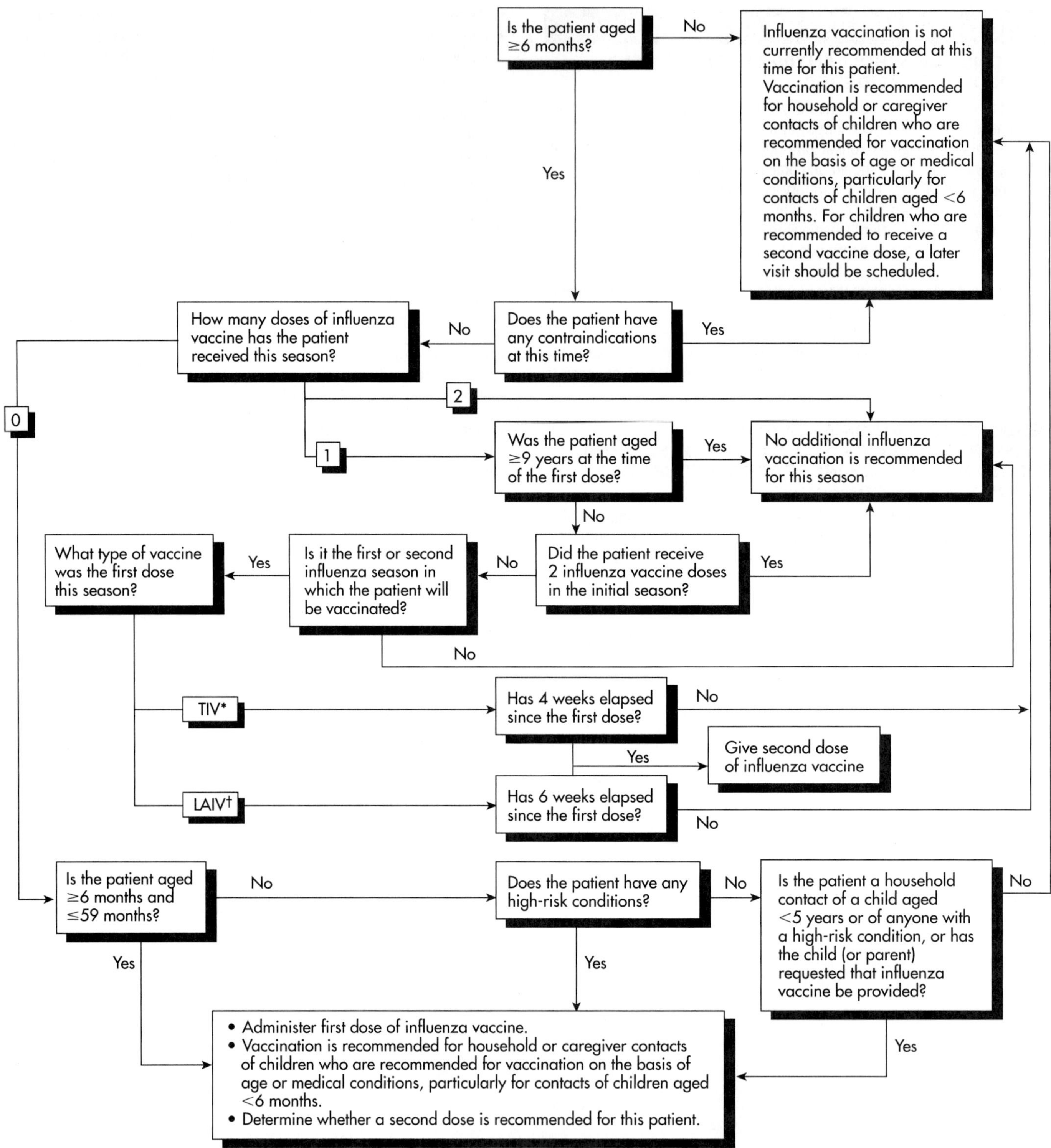

*Trivalent inactivated influenza vaccine.
†Live, attenuated influenza vaccine.

FIGURE 5-6 Algorithm for determining recommended influenza immunization actions for children. (Modified with permission from the American Academy of Pediatrics' Committee on Infectious Diseases: Prevention of influenza: recommendations for influenza immunization of children, 2006-2007, *Pediatrics* 119:846-51.315, 2007.)

HIV Testing and Postexposure Prophylaxis

RECOMMENDATIONS FOR HIV TESTING OF ADULTS, ADOLESCENTS, AND PREGNANT WOMEN

RECOMMENDATIONS FOR ADULTS AND ADOLESCENTS*

The CDC recommends that diagnostic human immunodeficiency virus (HIV) testing and opt-out HIV screening be a part of routine clinical care in all health care settings while also preserving the patient's option to decline HIV testing and ensuring a provider-patient relationship conducive to optimal clinical and preventive care. The recommendations are intended for providers in all health care settings, including hospital emergency departments, urgent-care clinics, inpatient services, sexually transmitted disease (STD) clinics or other venues offering clinical STD services, tuberculosis (TB) clinics, substance abuse treatment clinics, other public health clinics, community clinics, correctional health care facilities, and primary care settings. The guidelines address HIV testing in health care settings only; they do not modify existing guidelines concerning HIV counseling, testing, and referral for persons at high risk for HIV who seek or receive HIV testing in nonclinical settings (e.g., community-based organizations, outreach settings, or mobile vans).

SCREENING FOR HIV INFECTION

- In all health care settings, screening for HIV infection should be performed routinely for all patients aged 13 to 64 years. Health care providers should initiate screening unless prevalence of undiagnosed HIV infection in their patients has been documented to be less than 0.1%. In the absence of existing data for HIV prevalence, health care providers should initiate voluntary HIV screening until they establish that the diagnostic yield is less than 1 per 1000 patients screened, at which point such screening is no longer warranted.
- All patients initiating treatment for TB should be screened routinely for HIV infection.
- All patients seeking treatment for STDs, including all patients visiting STD clinics, should be screened routinely for HIV during each visit for a new complaint, regardless of whether the patient is known or suspected to have specific behavior risks for HIV infection.

REPEAT SCREENING

- Health care providers should subsequently test all persons likely to be at high risk for HIV at least annually. Persons likely to be at high risk include users of injection drugs and their sex partners, persons who exchange sex for money or drugs, sex partners of persons who are HIV infected, and men who have sex with men (MSM) or heterosexual persons who themselves or whose sex partners have had more than one sex partner since their most recent HIV test.
- Health care providers should encourage patients and their prospective sex partners to be tested before initiating a new sexual relationship.
- Repeat screening of persons not likely to be at high risk for HIV should be performed on the basis of clinical judgment.
- Unless recent HIV test results are immediately available, any person whose blood or body fluid is the source of an occupational exposure for a health care provider should be informed of the incident and tested for HIV infection at the time the exposure occurs.

CONSENT AND PRETEST INFORMATION

- Screening should be voluntary and undertaken only with the patient's knowledge and understanding that HIV testing is planned.
- Patients should be informed orally or in writing that HIV testing will be performed unless they decline (opt-out screening). Oral or written information should include an explanation of HIV infection and the meanings of positive and negative test results, and the patient should be offered an opportunity to ask questions and decline testing. With such notification, consent for HIV screening should be incorporated into the patient's general informed consent for medical care on the same basis as are other screening or diagnostic tests; a separate consent form for HIV testing is not recommended.
- Easily understood informational materials should be made available in the languages of the commonly encountered populations within the service area. The competence of interpreters and bilingual staff to provide language assistance to patients with limited English proficiency must be ensured.
- If a patient declines an HIV test, this decision should be documented in the medical record.

DIAGNOSTIC TESTING FOR HIV INFECTION

- All patients with signs or symptoms consistent with HIV infection or an opportunistic illness characteristic of acquired immunodeficiency syndrome (AIDS) should be tested for HIV.
- Clinicians should maintain a high level of suspicion for acute HIV infection in all patients who have a compatible clinical syndrome and who report recent high-risk behavior. When acute retroviral syndrome is a possibility, a plasma RNA test should be used in conjunction with an HIV antibody test to diagnose acute HIV infection.
- Patients or persons responsible for the patient's care should be notified orally that testing is planned, advised of the indication for testing and the implications of positive and negative test results, and offered an opportunity to ask questions and decline testing. With such notification, the patient's general consent for medical care is considered sufficient for diagnostic HIV testing.

HIV SCREENING FOR PREGNANT WOMEN AND THEIR INFANTS*

UNIVERSAL OPT-OUT SCREENING

- All pregnant women in the United States should be screened for HIV infection.
- Screening should occur after a woman is notified that HIV screening is recommended for all pregnant patients and that she will receive an HIV test as part of the routine panel of prenatal tests unless she declines (opt-out screening).
- HIV testing must be voluntary and free from coercion. No woman should be tested without her knowledge.
- Pregnant women should receive oral or written information that includes an explanation of HIV infection, a description of interventions that can reduce HIV transmission from mother to infant, and the meanings of positive and negative test results. They should be offered an opportunity to ask questions and decline testing.
- No additional process or written documentation of informed consent beyond what is required for other routine prenatal tests should be required for HIV testing.
- If a patient declines an HIV test, this decision should be documented in the medical record.

ADDRESSING REASONS FOR DECLINING TESTING

- Providers should discuss and address reasons for declining an HIV test (e.g., lack of perceived risk, fear of the disease, and concerns regarding partner violence or potential stigma or discrimination).
- Women who decline an HIV test because they have had a previous negative test result should be informed of the importance of retesting during each pregnancy.
- Logistical reasons for not testing (e.g., scheduling) should be resolved.
- Certain women who initially decline an HIV test might accept at a later date, especially if their concerns are discussed. Certain women will continue to decline testing, and their decisions should be respected and documented in the medical record.

TIMING OF HIV TESTING

- To promote informed and timely therapeutic decisions, health care providers should test women for HIV as early as possible during each pregnancy. Women who decline the test early in prenatal care should be encouraged to be tested at a subsequent visit.

**MMWR* 57(RR-10), 2008.

- A second HIV test during the third trimester, preferably less than 36 weeks of gestation, is cost effective even in areas of low HIV prevalence and may be considered for all pregnant women. A second HIV test during the third trimester is recommended for women who meet one or more of the following criteria:
  - Women who receive health care in jurisdictions with elevated incidence of HIV or AIDS among women aged 15 to 45 years. In 2004, these jurisdictions included Alabama, Connecticut, Delaware, the District of Columbia, Florida, Georgia, Illinois, Louisiana, Maryland, Massachusetts, Mississippi, Nevada, New Jersey, New York, North Carolina, Pennsylvania, Puerto Rico, Rhode Island, South Carolina, Tennessee, Texas, and Virginia.[†]
  - Women who receive health care in facilities in which prenatal screening identifies at least one pregnant woman who is infected with HIV per 1000 women screened.
  - Women who are known to be at high risk for acquiring HIV (e.g., users of injection drugs and their sex partners, women who exchange sex for money or drugs, women who are sex partners of persons who are infected with HIV, and women who have had a new or more than one sex partner during this pregnancy).
  - Women who have signs or symptoms consistent with acute HIV infection. When acute retroviral syndrome is a possibility, a plasma RNA test should be used in conjunction with an HIV antibody test to diagnose acute HIV infection.

[†]A second HIV test in the third trimester is as cost effective as other common health interventions when HIV incidence among women of childbearing age is ≥17 HIV cases per 100,000 person-years. In 2004, in jurisdictions with available data on HIV case rates, a rate of 17 new HIV diagnoses per year per 100,000 women aged 15 to 45 years was associated with an AIDS case rate of at least nine AIDS diagnoses per year per 100,000 women aged 15 to 45 years (CDC, unpublished data, 2005). As of 2004, the jurisdictions listed above exceeded these thresholds. The list of specific jurisdictions where a second test in the third trimester is recommended will be updated periodically based on surveillance data.

RAPID TESTING DURING LABOR

- Any woman with undocumented HIV status at the time of labor should be screened with a rapid HIV test unless she declines (opt-out screening).
- Reasons for declining a rapid test should be explored (see "Addressing Reasons for Declining Testing").
- Immediate initiation of appropriate antiretroviral prophylaxis should be recommended to women on the basis of a reactive rapid test result without waiting for the result of a confirmatory test.

POSTPARTUM/NEWBORN TESTING

- When a woman's HIV status is still unknown at the time of delivery, she should be screened immediately postpartum with a rapid HIV test unless she declines (opt-out screening).
- When the mother's HIV status is unknown postpartum, rapid testing of the newborn as soon as possible after birth is recommended so that antiretroviral prophylaxis can be offered to infants exposed to HIV. Women should be informed that identifying HIV antibodies in the newborn indicates that the mother is infected.
- For infants whose HIV exposure status is unknown and who are in foster care, the person legally authorized to provide consent should be informed that rapid HIV testing is recommended for infants whose biologic mothers have not been tested.
- The benefits of neonatal antiretroviral prophylaxis are best realized when it is initiated within 12 hours after birth.

CONFIRMATORY TESTING

- Whenever possible, uncertainties regarding laboratory test results indicating HIV infection status should be resolved before final decisions are made regarding reproductive options, antiretroviral therapy, cesarean delivery, or other interventions.
- If the confirmatory test result is not available before delivery, immediate initiation of appropriate antiretroviral prophylaxis should be recommended to any pregnant patient whose HIV screening test result is reactive to reduce the risk for perinatal transmission.

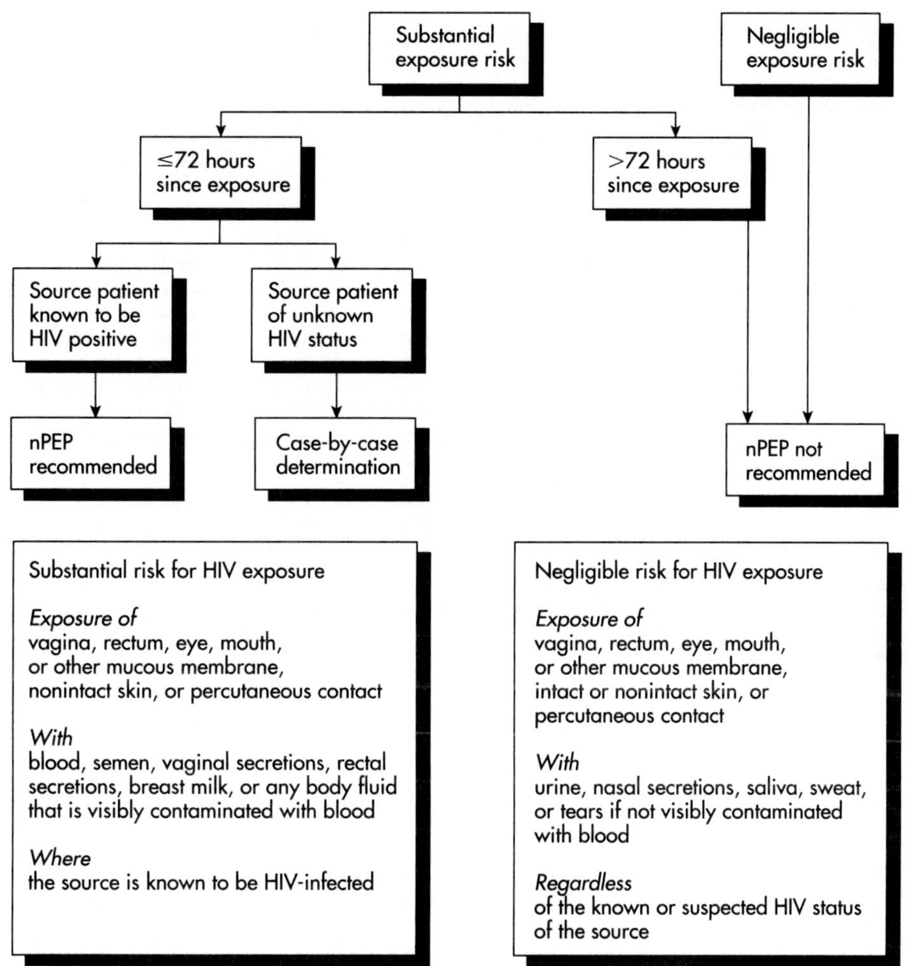

FIGURE 5-7 Algorithm for evaluation and treatment of possible nonoccupational HIV exposure. *nPEP,* Nonoccupational postexposure prophylaxis. (Modified from *MMWR* 54[RR-2], 2005.)

TABLE 5-31 HIV Exposure, Estimated Per-Act Risk

Exposure Route	Risk per 10,000 Exposures to an Infected Source
Blood transfusion	9000
Needle-sharing injection drug use	67
Receptive anal intercourse	50
Percutaneous needle stick	30
Receptive penile-vaginal intercourse	10
Insertive anal intercourse	6.5
Insertive penile-vaginal intercourse	5
Receptive oral intercourse	1
Insertive oral intercourse	0.5

Modified from *MMWR* 54(RR-2), 2005.
Estimates of risk for transmission from sexual exposures assume no condom use.
Source refers to oral intercourse performed on a man.

TABLE 5-32 Antiretroviral Regimens for Nonoccupational Postexposure Prophylaxis of HIV Infection

Preferred Regimens	
NNRTI based*	Efavirenz* plus (lamivudine or emtricitabine) plus (zidovudine or tenofovir)
PI based	Lopinavir/ritonavir (co-formulated as Kaletra) plus (lamivudine or emtricitabine) plus zidovudine
Alternative Regimens	
NNRTI based	Efavirenz plus (lamivudine or emtricitabine) plus abacavir or didanosine or stavudine†
PI based	Atazanavir plus (lamivudine or emtricitabine) plus (zidovudine or stavudine or abacavir or didanosine) or (tenofovir plus ritonavir [100 mg/day]) Fosamprenavir plus (lamivudine or emtricitabine) plus (zidovudine or stavudine) or (abacavir or tenofovir or didanosine) Fosamprenavir/ritonavir‡ plus (lamivudine or emtricitabine) plus (zidovudine or stavudine or abacavir or tenofovir or didanosine) Indinavir/ritonavir‡§ plus (lamivudine or emtricitabine) plus (zidovudine or stavudine or abacavir or tenofovir or didanosine) Lopinavir/ritonavir (co-formulated as Kaletra) plus (lamivudine or emtricitabine) plus (stavudine or abacavir or tenofovir or idanosine) Nelfinavir plus (lamivudine or emtricitabine) plus (zidovudine or stavudine or abacavir or tenofovir or didanosine) Saquinavir (hgc or sgc)/ritonavir† plus (lamivudine or emtricitabine) plus (zidovudine or stavudine or abacavir or tenofovir or didanosine)
Triple NRTI*	Abacavir plus lamivudine plus zidovudine (only when an NNRTI- or PI-based regimen cannot or should not be used)

Modified from *MMWR* 54(RR-2), 2005.

Source: U.S. Department of Health and Human Services. Guidelines for the use of antiretroviral agents in HIV-infected adults and adolescents, October 29, 2004 revision. Available at http://www.aidsinfo.nih.gov/guidelines/default_db2.asp?id=50. This document is updated periodically; refer to Web site for updated versions.

hgc, Hard-gel saquinavir capsule (Invirase); *NNRTI,* nonnucleoside reverse transcriptase inhibitor; *NRTI,* nucleoside reverse transcriptase inhibitor; *PI,* protease inhibitor; *sgc,* soft-gel saquinavir capsule (Fortovase).

*Efavirenz should be avoided in pregnant women and women of childbearing potential.

†Higher incidence of lipoatrophy, hyperlipidemia, and mitochondrial toxicities associated with stavudine than with other NRTIs.

‡Low-dose (100-400 mg) ritonavir. See Table 5-31 for doses used with specific PIs.

§Use of ritonavir with indinavir might increase risk for renal adverse events.

TABLE 5-33 Highly Active Antiretroviral Therapy Medications, Adult Dosage, and Side Effects

Medication	Adult Dosage*	Side Effects and Toxicities
Combination Tablets		
Lopinavir/ritonavir (Kaletra)‡	3 tablets twice daily 400 mg lopinavir/100 mg ritonavir	Diarrhea, nausea, vomiting; asthenia; elevated transaminases; hyperglycemia; fat redistribution; lipid abnormalities; possible increased bleeding in persons with hemophilia; pancreatitis
Zidovudine/lamivudine (Combivir)	1 tablet twice daily 300 mg zidovudine/150 mg lamivudine	See following individual medications
Zidovudine/lamivudine/abacavir (Trizivir)	1 tablet twice daily 300 mg zidovudine/150 mg lamivudine/300 mg abacavir	See following individual medications
Lamivudine/abacavir (Epzicom)	1 tablet once daily 300 mg lamivudine/600 mg abacavir	See following individual medications
Emtricitabine/tenofovir (Truvada)	1 tablet once daily 200 mg emtricitabine/300 mg tenofovir	See following individual medications
Single Agents		
Nucleoside and nucleotide reverse transcriptase inhibitors (side effects as a class: lactic acidosis, severe hepatomegaly with steatosis, including some fatal cases)		
Abacavir (Ziagen, ABC)‡	300 mg twice daily or 600 mg once daily	Severe hypersensitivity reaction (can be fatal); nausea; vomiting
Didanosine (Videx, ddl)‡	>60 kg (132 lb) body weight: 200 mg twice daily or 400 mg daily; if with tenofovir, 250 mg/daily <60 kg (132 lb): 125 mg twice daily or 250 mg daily; if with tenofovir, dose not established Do not use with stavudine (d4T, Zerit) during pregnancy; avoid ddl/d4T combination in general because of increased risk for adverse events (e.g., neuropathy, pancreatitis, and hyperlactatemia)	Pancreatitis; nausea, diarrhea; peripheral neuropathy
Emtricitabine (Emtriva, FTC)	200 mg once daily	Minimal toxicity; lactic acidosis and hepatic steatosis a rare but possibly life-threatening event
Lamivudine (Epivir, 3TC)‡	150 mg twice daily or 300 mg once daily	Minimal toxicity; lactic acidosis and hepatic steatosis a rare but possibly life-threatening event
Stavudine (Zerit, d4T)‡	>60 kg (132 lb) body weight: 40 mg twice daily <60 kg (132 lb) body weight: 30 mg twice daily Do not use with didanosine (ddl, Videx) during pregnancy; avoid ddl/d4T combination in general because of increased risk of adverse events (e.g., neuropathy, pancreatitis, and hyperlactatemia)	Pancreatitis; peripheral neuropathy; rapidly progressive ascending neuromuscular weakness (rare)
Tenofovir (Viread)	300 mg daily	Nausea, vomiting, diarrhea; headache; asthenia; flatulence; renal impairment
Zidovudine (Retrovir, AZT)‡	200 mg three times daily or 300 mg twice daily	Bone marrow suppression (anemia, neutropenia); gastrointestinal intolerance; headache; insomnia; asthenia; and myopathy
Nonnucleoside reverse transcriptase inhibitors (side effects as a class: Stevens-Johnson syndrome)		
Efavirenz (Sustiva)	600 mg daily at bedtime	Rash; central nervous system symptoms (e.g., dizziness, impaired concentration, insomnia, and abnormal dreams); transaminase elevation; false-positive cannabinoid test
Protease inhibitors (side effects as a class: gastrointestinal intolerance, hyperlipidemia, hyperglycemia, diabetes, fat redistribution, and possible increased bleeding in hemophiliacs; do not use during known or possible pregnancy)		
Atazanavir (Reyataz)	400 mg once daily; if administered with tenofovir plus ritonavir, 300 mg once daily	Indirect hyperbilirubinemia; prolonged PR interval (use caution in patients with underlying cardiac conduction defects or on concomitant medications that can cause PR prolongation)
Fosamprenavir (Lexiva)‡	1400 mg twice daily	Gastrointestinal intolerance, nausea, vomiting, diarrhea; rash; elevated transaminases; headache
Indinavir (Crixivan)	800 mg q8h With ritonavir (might increase risk for renal adverse events): 800 mg indinavir and 100 mg ritonavir q12h or 800 mg indinavir and 200 mg ritonavir every q12h	Gastrointestinal intolerance, nausea; nephrolithiasis; headache; asthenia; blurred vision; metallic taste; thrombocytopenia; hemolytic anemia; indirect hyperbilirubinemia (inconsequential)
Nelfinavir (Viracept)‡	750 mg three times daily or one 250 mg twice daily	Diarrhea; elevated transaminases
Ritonavir (Norvir)‡	See doses used in combination with other specific protease inhibitors	Gastrointestinal intolerance; nausea, vomiting, diarrhea; paresthesias; hepatitis; pancreatitis; asthenia; taste perversion; many drug interactions
Saquinavir (hard-gel capsule) (Invirase)	With ritonavir: 400 mg saquinavir and 400 mg ritonavir twice daily or 1000 mg saquinavir and 100 mg ritonavir twice daily	Gastrointestinal intolerance; nausea, diarrhea; headache; elevated transaminases
Saquinavir (soft-gel capsule) (Fortavase)	With ritonavir: 400 mg saquinavir and 400 mg ritonavir twice daily or 1000 mg saquinavir and 100 mg ritonavir twice daily	Gastrointestinal intolerance; nausea, diarrhea; abdominal pain; dyspepsia; headache; elevated transaminases

*For pediatric dosing information, see *Guidelines for Use of Antiretroviral Agents in Pediatric HIV Infection*, available at http://www.aidsinfo.nih.gov/guidelines/default_db2.asp?id=51.
‡Pediatric formulation available.

Sources: Modified from U.S. Department of Health and Human Services and the Henry J. Kaiser Family Foundation. Guidelines for the use of antiretroviral agents in HIV-infected adults and adolescents. Available at http://www.aidsinfo.nih.gov/guidelines/default_db2.asp?id=50 (refer to Web site for updated versions). Bartlett JG, Finkbeiner AK: HIV drugs: the guide to living with HIV infection, 2001, available at http://www.thebody.com/jh/bartlett/drugs.html.

TABLE 5-34 Recommended Laboratory Evaluation of Nonoccupational Prophylaxis (nPEP) of HIV Infection

Test	Baseline	During nPEP*	4-6 Wk after Exposure	3 Mo after Exposure	6 Mo after Exposure
HIV antibody testing	E, S†		E	E	E
Complete blood count with differential	E	E			
Serum liver enzymes	E	E			
Blood urea nitrogen/creatinine	E	E			
Sexually transmitted diseases screen (gonorrhea, chlamydia, syphilis)	E, S	E‡	E‡		
Hepatitis B serology	E, S		E‡	E‡	
Hepatitis C serology	E, S			E	E
Pregnancy test (for women of reproductive age)	E	E‡	E‡		
HIV viral load	S		E§	E§	E§
HIV resistance testing	S		E§	E§	E§
CD4+ T-lymphocyte count	S		E§	E§	E§

Modified from *MMWR* 54(RR-2), 2005.
E, Exposed patient; *S*, source.
*Other specific tests might be indicated depending on the antiretrovirals prescribed. Literature pertaining to individual agents should be consulted.
†HIV antibody testing of the source patient is indicated for sources of unknown serostatus.
‡Additional testing for pregnancy, sexually transmitted diseases, and hepatitis B should be performed as clinically indicated.
§If determined to be HIV infected on follow-up testing, perform as clinically indicated once diagnosed.

BOX 5-4 Situations for Which Expert Consultation for HIV Postexposure Prophylaxis Is Advised*

- Delayed (i.e., later than 24-36 hours) exposure report
  - The interval after which there is no benefit from postexposure prophylaxis (PEP) is undefined
- Unknown source (e.g., needle in sharps disposal container or laundry)
  - Decide use of PEP on a case-by-case basis
  - Consider the severity of the exposure and the epidemiologic likelihood of HIV exposure
  - Do not test needles or other sharp instruments for HIV
- Known or suspected pregnancy in the exposed person
  - Does not preclude the use of optimal PEP regimens
  - Do not deny PEP solely on the basis of pregnancy
- Resistance of the source virus to antiretroviral agents
  - Influence of drug resistance on transmission risk is unknown
  - Selection of drugs to which the source person's virus is unlikely to be resistant is recommended if the source person's virus is known or suspected to be resistant to one or more of the drugs considered for the PEP regimen
  - Resistance testing of the source person's virus at the time of the exposure is not recommended
- Toxicity of the initial PEP regimen
  - Adverse symptoms such as nausea and diarrhea are common with PEP
  - Symptoms often can be managed without changing the PEP regimen by prescribing antimotility and/or antiemetic agents
  - Modification of dose intervals (i.e., administering a lower dose of drug more frequently throughout the day, as recommended by the manufacturer) in other situations might help alleviate symptoms

*Local experts and/or the National Clinicians' Postexposure Prophylaxis Hotline (PEPline [1-888-448-4911]).

BOX 5-5 Occupational Exposure Management Resources

National Clinicians' Postexposure Prophylaxis Hotline (PEPline) Run by University of California–San Francisco/San Francisco General Hospital staff; supported by the Health Resources and Services Administration, Ryan White CARE Act, HIV/AIDS Bureau, AIDS Education and Training Centers, and CDC	Phone: 888-448-4911 Internet: http://www.ucsf.edu/hivcntr
Needlestick! A website to help clinicians manage and document occupational blood and body fluid exposures. Developed and maintained by the University of California, Los Angeles (UCLA), Emergency Medicine Center, UCLA School of Medicine, and funded in part by CDC and the Agency for Healthcare Research and Quality	Internet: http://www.needlestick.mednet.ucla.edu
Hepatitis Hotline	Phone: 888-443-7232 Internet: http://www.cdc.gov/ncidod/diseases/hepatitis/index.htm
Reporting to CDC: Occupationally acquired HIV infections and failures of PEP	Phone: 800-893-0485
HIV Antiretroviral Pregnancy Registry	Phone: 800-258-4263 Fax: 800-800-1052 Address: 1410 Commonwealth Dr., Suite 215, Wilmington, NC 28405 Internet: http://www.glaxowellcome.com/preg_reg/antiretroviral
Food and Drug Administration Report unusual or severe toxicity to antiretroviral agents	Phone: 800-332-1088 Address: MedWatch, HF-2, FDA, 5600 Fishers Lane, Rockville, MD 20857 Internet: http://www.fda.gov/medwatch
HIV/AIDS Treatment Information Service	Internet: http://www.hivatis.org

BOX 5-6 Management of Occupational Blood Exposures

Provide immediate care to the exposure site:
- Wash wounds and skin with soap and water
- Flush mucous membranes with water

Determine risk associated with exposure:
- Type of fluid (e.g., blood, visibly bloody fluid, other potentially infectious fluid or tissue, and concentrated virus)
- Type of exposure (e.g., percutaneous injury, mucous membrane or nonintact skin exposure, and bites resulting in blood exposure)

Evaluate exposure source:
- Assess the risk of infection using available information
- Test known sources for HBsAg, anti-HCV, and HIV antibodies (consider using rapid testing)
- For unknown sources, assess risk of exposure to HBV, HCV, or HIV infection
- Do not test discarded needles or syringes for virus contamination

Evaluate the exposed person:
- Assess immune status for HBV infection (i.e., by history of hepatitis B vaccination and vaccine response)

Give PEP for exposures posing risk of infection transmission:
- HBV: See Table 5-26
- HCV: PEP not recommended
- HIV: See Tables 5-34, 5-35, and 5-36 and Figure 5-7
  - Initiate PEP as soon as possible, preferably within hours of exposure
  - Offer pregnancy testing to all women of childbearing age not known to be pregnant
  - Seek expert consultation if viral resistance is suspected
  - Administer PEP for 4 weeks if tolerated

Perform follow-up testing and provide counseling:
- Advise exposed persons to seek medical evaluation for any acute illness occurring during follow-up

HBV exposures
- Perform follow-up anti-HBs testing in persons who receive hepatitis B vaccine
  - Test for anti-HBs 1 to 2 months after last dose of vaccine
  - Anti-HBs response to vaccine cannot be ascertained if HBIG was received in the previous 3 to 4 months

HCV exposures
- Perform baseline and follow-up testing for anti-HCV and alanine aminotransferase 4 to 6 months after exposures
- Perform HCV RNA at 4 to 6 weeks if earlier diagnosis of HCV infection desired
- Confirm repeatedly reactive anti-HCV enzyme immunoassays with supplemental tests

HIV exposures
- Perform HIV-antibody testing for at least 6 months after exposure (e.g., at baseline, 6 weeks, 3 months, and 6 months)
- Perform HIV-antibody testing if illness compatible with an acute retroviral syndrome occurs
- Advise exposed persons to use precautions to prevent secondary transmission during the follow-up period
- Evaluate exposed persons taking PEP within 72 hr after exposure and monitor for drug toxicity for at least 2 weeks

HBIG, Hepatitis B immune globulin; *HBsAg,* hepatitis B surface antigen; *HBV,* hepatitis B virus; *HCV,* hepatitis C virus; *HIV,* human immunodeficiency virus; *PEP,* post-exposure prophylaxis; *RNA,* ribonucleic acid.

Endocarditis Prophylaxis*

TABLE 5-35 Cardiac Conditions Associated with the Highest Risk of Adverse Outcome from Endocarditis for Which Prophylaxis with Dental Procedures Is Recommended

Prosthetic cardiac valve

Previous infective endocarditis

CHD*

Unrepaired cyanotic CHD, including palliative shunts and conduits

Completely repaired congenital heart defect with prosthetic material or device, whether placed by surgery or by catheter intervention, during the first 6 mo after the procedure[†]

Repaired CHD with residual defects at the site or adjacent to the site of a prosthetic patch or prosthetic device (that inhibit endothelialization)

Cardiac transplant recipients who develop cardiac valvulopathy

CHD, Congenital heart disease.
*Except for the conditions listed above, antibiotic prophylaxis is no longer recommended for any other form of CHD.
†Prophylaxis is recommended because endothelialization of prosthetic material occurs within 6 mo after the procedure.

TABLE 5-36 Dental Procedures for Which Endocarditis Prophylaxis Is Recommended for Patients in Table 5-35

All dental procedures that involve manipulation of gingival tissue or the periapical region of teeth or perforation of the oral mucosa*

*The following procedures and events do not need prophylaxis: routine anesthetic injections through noninfected tissue, taking dental radiographs, placement of removable prosthodontic or orthodontic appliances, adjustment of orthodontic appliances, placement of orthodontic brackets, shedding of deciduous teeth, and bleeding from trauma to the lips or oral mucosa.

TABLE 5-37 Regimens for a Dental Procedure

	REGIMEN: SINGLE DOSE 30-60 MIN BEFORE PROCEDURE		
Situation	**Agent**	**Adults**	**Children**
Oral	Amoxicillin	2 g	50 mg/kg
Unable to take oral medication	Ampicillin	2 g IM or IV	50 mg/kg IM or IV
	OR		
	Cefazolin or ceftriaxone*	1 g IM or IV	50 mg/kg IM or IV
Allergic to penicillins or ampicillin, oral	Cephalexin*[†]	2 g	50 mg/kg
	OR		
	Clindamycin	600 mg	20 mg/kg
	OR		
	Azithromycin or clarithromycin	500 mg	15 mg/kg
Allergic to penicillins or ampicillin and unable to take oral medicine	Cefazolin or ceftriaxone[†]	1 g IM or IV	50 mg/kg IM or IV
	OR		
	Clindamycin	600 mg IM or IV	20 mg/kg IM or IV

IM, Intramuscular; *IV,* intravenous.
*Or other first-generation or second-generation oral cephalosporin in equivalent adult or pediatric dosage.
†Cephalosporins should not be used in an individual with a history of anaphylaxis, angioedema, or urticaria with penicillins or ampicillin.

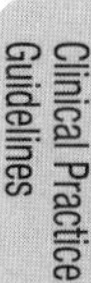

*From Prevention of infective endocarditis. A guideline from the American Heart Association Rheumatic Fever, Endocarditis, and Kawasaki Disease Committee, Council on Cardiovascular Disease in the Young, and the Council on Clinical Cardiology, Council on Cardiovascular Surgery and Anesthesia, and the Quality of Care and Outcomes Research Interdisciplinary Working Group. *Circulation* published online Apr 19, 2007, DOI: 10.1161/CIRCULATIONAHA.106.183095. Print ISSN: 0009-7322. Online ISSN: 1524-4539.

TABLE 5-38 Summary of Major Changes in Updated Recommendations

We concluded that bacteremia resulting from daily activities is much more likely to cause IE than bacteremia associated with a dental procedure.
We concluded that only an extremely small number of cases of IE might be prevented by antibiotic prophylaxis even if prophylaxis is 100% effective.
Antibiotic prophylaxis is not recommended based solely on an increased lifetime risk of acquisition of IE.
Limit recommendations for IE prophylaxis only to those conditions listed in Table 5-37.
Antibiotic prophylaxis is no longer recommended for any other form of CHD, except for the conditions listed in Table 5-37.
Antibiotic prophylaxis is recommended for all dental procedures that involve manipulation of gingival tissues or periapical region of teeth or perforation of oral mucosa only for patients with underlying cardiac conditions associated with the highest risk of adverse outcome from IE (see Table 5-37).
Antibiotic prophylaxis is recommended for procedures on respiratory tract or infected skin, skin structures, or musculoskeletal tissue only for patients with underlying cardiac conditions associated with the highest risk of adverse outcome from IE (see Table 5-37).
Antibiotic prophylaxis solely to prevent IE is not recommended for GU or GI tract procedures.
The writing group reaffirms the procedures noted in the 1997 prophylaxis guidelines for which endocarditis prophylaxis is not recommended and extends this to other common procedures, including ear and body piercing, tattooing, and vaginal delivery and hysterectomy.

A guide to the clinical preventive services described is available online at http://www.ahrq.gov/clinic/pocketgd07/.
CHD, Congenital heart disease; *GI,* gastrointestinal; *GU,* genitourinary; *IE,* infective endocarditis.

PART C • GUIDE TO CLINICAL PREVENTIVE SERVICES*

1. Cancer
   a. Screening for bladder cancer in adults
   b. Genetic risk assessment and BRCA mutation testing for breast and ovarian cancer susceptibility
   c. Screening for breast cancer
   d. Screening for cervical cancer
   e. Screening for colorectal cancer
   f. Lung cancer screening
   g. Screening for ovarian cancer
   h. Screening for pancreatic cancer
   i. Screening for prostate cancer
   j. Counseling to prevent skin cancer
   k. Screening for testicular cancer
2. Heart and vascular diseases
   a. Screening for abdominal aortic aneurysm
   b. Aspirin for the primary prevention of cardiovascular events
   c. Screening for coronary heart disease
   d. Screening for lipid disorders in adults
   e. Screening for peripheral arterial disease
3. Infectious diseases
   a. Screening for asymptomatic bacteriuria
   b. Screening for chlamydial infection
   c. Screening for genital herpes
   d. Screening for gonorrhea
   e. Screening for hepatitis B virus infection
   f. Screening for hepatitis C in adults
   g. Screening for syphilis infection
4. Injury and violence
   a. Screening for family and intimate partner violence
5. Mental health conditions and substance abuse
   a. Screening and behavioral counseling interventions in primary care to reduce alcohol misuse
   b. Screening for dementia
   c. Screening for depression
   d. Screening for suicide risk
6. Counseling to prevent tobacco use and tobacco-caused disease
7. Metabolic, nutritional, and endocrine conditions
   a. Behavioral counseling in primary care to promote a healthy diet
   b. Hormone therapy for the prevention of chronic conditions in postmenopausal women
   c. Screening for obesity in adults
   d. Behavioral counseling in primary care to promote physical activity
   e. Screening for thyroid disease
   f. Screening for type 2 diabetes mellitus in adults
8. Musculoskeletal conditions
   a. Primary care interventions to prevent low back pain in adults
   b. Screening for osteoporosis in postmenopausal women
9. Vision disorders
   a. Screening for glaucoma

*Available online.

APPENDIX

I. Complementary and Alternative Medicine

II. Primary Care Procedures (available online)

Appendix Ia

Dietary Supplements: What Every Primary Care Provider Should Know

Primary care providers must be knowledgeable regarding the safety, efficacy, and drug interactions associated with common dietary supplements because of the following:

- An estimated 38% of adults ages 18 years and older reported the use of at least one form of complementary and alternative medicine (CAM) according to the National Health Interview Survey In 2007.
- Almost 17.8% of adults specifically reported the use of dietary supplements, with fish oil, glucosamine, echinacea, flaxseed, and ginseng most frequently used.
- Although the use of dietary supplements has plateaued as a result of consumer concerns about effectiveness and potential adverse effects, usage remains common and potentially dangerous.

COMMON TERMINOLOGY

- A *dietary supplement* is defined as an oral product containing vitamins, minerals, herbs, or other botanicals; amino acids; dietary substances used to supplement the diet by increasing the total dietary intake; or a concentrate, metabolite, constituent, extract, or combination.
- *CAM* refers to the broad domain of healing practices that include diverse health systems, modalities, and practices and their accompanying theories and beliefs (see glossary of terms in Appendix Id).
- *Complementary therapies* are those that are used *in addition to* conventional therapies, whereas *alternative therapies* are those that are used *instead of* conventional therapies. Most consumers in the United States use dietary supplements as a complementary therapy.
- *Standardization* refers to the practice of producing dietary supplements with a specific amount of a given compound that may or may not include the actual active ingredient. For example, feverfew has been standardized to its parthenolide content.

LEGISLATION

The U.S. Food and Drug Administration (FDA) is frequently criticized for not closely regulating dietary supplements and monitoring their safety. However, although the agency regulates prescription drugs and over-the-counter (OTC) products, the FDA has limited regulatory authority over dietary supplements. This is because the Dietary Supplement and Health Education Act (DSHEA) of 1994 and its resulting regulations limit the FDA's authority. As a result of DSHEA, the FDA is able to act only when a dietary supplement has been documented to contain a prescription drug, as was the case with glyburide in a natural treatment for diabetes and diazepam in an osteoarthritis preparation. In addition, the FDA can act when safety issues related to a product have been clearly documented, although these cases are frequently challenged in the courts.

HEALTH CLAIMS

Dietary supplements generally are marketed under three types of health claims. The first category is the "nutrient content" claim, in which the product is identified as an excellent source of, typically, a mineral such as calcium, based on recommended daily values. The second type is the "significant scientific agreement" claim; these claims are used when some evidence of the product's efficacy exists (e.g., fish oil supplements). The third and most common type of health claim is called a "structure/function" claim; these claims state that the product has some effect on health—for example, "helps to maintain a healthy heart." However, dietary supplements are not permitted to carry claims stating that they are effective in preventing, treating, or curing diseases.

INFORMATION RESOURCES

Appendix 1b provides a brief overview of common dietary supplements. Until recently, few evidence-based resources on dietary supplements were available. Clinical studies and systematic reviews on dietary supplements are now widely available through PubMed, EMBASE, and the Cochrane Database of Systematic Reviews. Although more information is available, references on specific products vary in their interpretation of the available evidence and may exhibit an unintentional bias, either pro or con, regarding the safety and efficacy of dietary supplements.

"Gold standard" evidence-based databases on dietary supplements (subscription required) include the following:

- Natural Medicines Comprehensive Database (http://www.naturaldatabase.com): This database includes listings for many dietary supplements and is organized in a clinician-friendly manner. Monographs include the different common and scientific names; uses and likely effectiveness for different uses; chemical constituents; interactions with drugs, diseases, foods, and laboratory tests; adverse effects; and cautions. The information is extensively referenced and is updated on a daily basis. The primary limitation is that the evaluation of data on clinical effectiveness could be more rigorous.
- Natural Standard (http://www.naturalstandard.com): This database includes listings for dietary supplements and other forms of complementary and alternative medicine. The evidence supporting the assessments in this database is critically evaluated and rigorous in nature. The primary limitation is that many fewer dietary supplements are included in this database.

Evidence-based free websites on dietary supplements include the following:

- National Center for Complementary and Alternative Medicine (NCCAM) (http://nccam.nih.gov)
- Office of Dietary Supplements International Bibliographic Information on Dietary Supplements (http://dietary-supplements.info.nih.gov/Health_Information/IBIDS.aspx)
- Memorial Sloan-Kettering Cancer Center (http://www.mskcc.org/mskcc/html/11570.cfm)

DRUG INTERACTIONS

Clinically significant interactions have been documented between dietary supplements and prescription or OTC drugs. The challenge for primary care providers is to identify real, clinically relevant interactions versus potential or theoretical interactions. Data on interactions with dietary supplements are usually based on isolated case reports or on studies enrolling healthy volunteers. As with drug-drug interactions, the likelihood of an interaction and its severity are influenced especially by concomitant medical conditions, such as heart failure and presence or absence of impaired kidney and liver function.

Appendix Ic lists interactions between selected natural products and prescription and nonprescription drugs. The following two broad interactions are particularly important in primary care practice:

- St. John's wort, commonly used for depression, is a potent inducer of cytochrome P450 3A4 isoenzymes and has been documented to increase the clearance of many drugs that are metabolized through this (and other) pathways. (For a list of common drugs cleared in this manner, readers should consult http://medicine.iupui.edu/flockhart/clinlist.htm.) In addition, St. John's wort may also induce p-glycoprotein transporter systems that are important for digoxin and some chemotherapeutic agents. St. John's wort has also been associated with the development of serotonin syndrome when used with drugs that have significant serotonergic activity.
- Dietary supplements such as garlic, ginkgo, and feverfew, as well as many others, have been purported to either have antiplatelet activity or have effects on the clotting cascade. This may be important for adults also taking aspirin (and other platelet-active agents) or warfarin.

COUNSELING POINTS

The single most important counseling point related to dietary supplements is always to ask patients about their use of these products and to do so in an open, nonjudgmental manner. The approach should emphasize that many consumers have been interested in vitamins, minerals, herbs, teas, and so on, to maintain their health or to treat illness. If the clinician is unaware of the safety, efficacy, and interactions of a specific product, several websites are available to quickly scan for information. Also, access to drug information centers at colleges of pharmacy is almost always available, and some hospitals now offer programs in integrative medicine.

Patients should be asked about their goals in using the product, as well as how long they have taken it and in what dosage. Allergies to plants should be documented because cross-allergies are common. Clinicians should appreciate that an individual who uses dietary supplements may be interested in making lifestyle changes and potentially decreasing their use of prescription drugs. In addition, if an individual is also consulting an alternative medicine practitioner, clinicians should recognize that some alternative health systems discourage the use of established therapies such as vaccines.

Although problems with safety and efficacy have been identified, many dietary supplements are benign except for their cost. Some patients are at higher risk for adverse outcomes from the use of dietary supplements (e.g., those with chronic kidney and liver disease). Patients should be counseled specifically to avoid purchasing dietary supplements over the Internet.

RESEARCH ISSUES

Many clinical and observational studies of dietary supplements have been published. In the past, clinicians frequently stated that published studies of dietary supplements either did not exist or only a few were available. The reason for this finding was that until recently the National Library of Medicine did not abstract from the peer-reviewed alternative medicine literature. Fortunately, much more research is now readily available. As with all research, the more rigorous the study methodology, the less likely the dietary supplement is to demonstrate clinical benefit.

In evaluating published studies of dietary supplements, the following should be considered:

- Has the correct plant and part of the plant (root, stem, leaf) been used? This critical information may not be known to many clinicians. Consulting a resource such as the National Medicines Comprehensive Database can usually provide the needed information to judge this component of the study.
- Has the content of active ingredients been verified throughout the study? In a recent review of 81 major randomized controlled trials of herbal products, only 12 (15%) reported performing tests to quantify actual contents, and 3 (4%) provided adequate data to compare actual with expected content values of at least one chemical constituent.
- Is the severity of the disease appropriate for study? Negative studies with dietary supplements sometimes inappropriately enroll participants who have moderate-to-severe disease (e.g., those with depression or benign prostatic hyperplasia) when only mild disease would be appropriate.
- Is the duration of the study appropriate? Early studies comparing glucosamine and nonsteroidal anti-inflammatory agents (NSAIA) demonstrated greater efficacy with the NSAIA because of an inadequate study duration for glucosamine to show any benefit.
- Is a placebo group included? Recent studies with dietary supplements for menopausal symptoms and osteoarthritis have demonstrated placebo responses over 40% to 50%.
- Was the blinding maintained throughout the study? Some dietary supplements, such as saw palmetto, have distinctive odors and tastes that are not easily masked.
- Is the preparation commercially available? Most importantly, when a study with dietary supplements does show benefit, it frequently is difficult to use the product in practice because the specific formulation studied is not commercially available.

AUTHOR: **ANNE L. HUME, PHARM.D.**

Appendix Ib

Overview of Selected Natural Products

This table includes a few of the common uses and side effects of selected natural products. The evidence supporting the uses and side effects of these products varies considerably and may be based on anecdotal information or theoretical concerns with the natural products.

Natural Products	Common Use(s)	Adverse Effects/Potential Concerns
African plum (Pygeum)	Benign prostatic hyperplasia	Nausea and abdominal pain have been reported, but pygeum is generally well tolerated. Pygeum does not decrease prostate size or influence PSA concentrations.
Andrographis	Prevention and treatment of viral respiratory infections	Headache, fatigue, rash, diarrhea, and vomiting. Products are standardized to 4%-6% andrographolide; this botanical is commonly used in combination products.
Black cohosh	Menopausal symptoms (hot flashes), induction of labor in pregnant women, premenstrual syndrome	Dyspepsia, rash, weight gain, headache, and cramping have been reported. Concern exists that black cohosh causes liver toxicity. The potential development of mild estrogen-like adverse effects, especially endometrial hyperplasia, is of concern.
Butterbur	Prevention of migraine headaches; allergic rhinitis; urinary tract spasms; pain	Diarrhea, stomach upset, fatigue, belching, headache, and drowsiness may occur. Due to concern about hepatotoxicity, butterbur products should be free of pyrrolizidine alkaloids. Products should be standardized to 15% petasin and isopetasin.
Chamomile (German)	Motion sickness, anxiety, insomnia; gastrointestinal spasms; mucositis	Allergic reactions occur on rare occasion. Patients with a ragweed allergy should use chamomile with caution.
Chasteberry	Premenstrual dysphoric disorder, premenstrual syndrome, menopausal symptoms, female infertility, mastalgia	Gastrointestinal upset, headache, rash, acne, weight gain, and menstrual bleeding have been reported.
Chitosan	Weight loss, Crohn's disease, hypercholesterolemia, anemia	Gastrointestinal upset, nausea, flatulence, and constipation have been reported. Patients with a shellfish allergy should avoid the use of chitosan.
Chondroitin sulfate	Osteoarthritis, osteoporosis, hyperlipidemia	Gastrointestinal upset, nausea, diarrhea, constipation, and alopecia. Concern exists that chondroitin may have anticoagulant activity due to its structural similarity to part of heparin.
Cinnamon	Type 2 diabetes mellitus, flatulence, gastrointestinal spasms, anorexia, menopausal symptoms, impotence	Cassia cinnamon is one of three types of cinnamon in commercial food products; this is the only type that may have minor effects to improve blood glucose concentrations.
Coenzyme Q10	Congestive heart failure, angina, dilated cardiomyopathy, statin-induced myopathy, Parkinson's disease, chronic fatigue syndrome, HIV/AIDS	Nausea, vomiting, diarrhea, anorexia, heartburn, and rash have been reported. Coenzyme Q10 is structurally similar to vitamin K; concern exists about potential interaction with warfarin.
Cranberry	Prevention and treatment of urinary tract infections; type 2 diabetes mellitus; chronic fatigue syndrome; pleurisy	Gastrointestinal upset and diarrhea have been reported with large doses of cranberry. Uric acid kidney stone formation is also possible with large doses of cranberry over prolonged periods of time.
Dehydroepiandrosterone (DHEA)	Slow or reverse aging, weight loss, metabolic syndrome, erectile dysfunction, immune stimulant, osteoporosis, systemic lupus erythematosus, multiple sclerosis, depression, schizophrenia	Acne and other androgenic effects commonly occur in women. Alopecia, insulin resistance, hepatic dysfunction, and hypertension have been reported. Ingested wild yam and soy cannot be converted into DHEA by humans.
Devil's claw	Osteoarthritis, atherosclerosis, gout, myalgias, fever, migraines	Diarrhea, nausea, and vomiting, as well as allergic reactions, have been reported.

AIDS, Acquired immune deficiency syndrome; *HIV*, human immunodeficiency virus.

Continued on following page

Natural Products	Common Use(s)	Adverse Effects/Potential Concerns
Echinacea	Prevention and treatment of viral respiratory infections; urinary tract infections; chronic fatigue syndrome; attention deficit hyperactivity disorder	Nausea, vomiting, diarrhea, heartburn, headaches, dizziness, arthralgias, and allergic reactions have been reported with echinacea. Patients with a ragweed allergy should use echinacea with caution because the risk of allergic reactions may be increased.
Eleuthero (Siberian ginseng)	Maintenance of a normal blood pressure; atherosclerosis; Alzheimer's disease; chronic fatigue syndrome; diabetes; herpes simplex infections	Drowsiness, anxiety, and irritability have been reported.
Evening primrose oil (EPO)	Premenstrual syndrome, mastalgia, osteoporosis, asthma, menopausal symptoms, eczema, chronic fatigue syndrome	EPO is well tolerated.
Fenugreek	Type 2 diabetes mellitus, anorexia, atherosclerosis; also used as galactogogue	Gastrointestinal upset, flatulence, and hypoglycemia are possible side effects. Patients with a peanut allergy (and an allergy to related plants) should use fenugreek with caution. Nursing mothers who use fenugreek may notice a "maple syrup" smell in their sweat and in the urine of their infants. This may be mistaken to be "Maple Syrup Urine Disease" in the infant.
Feverfew	Prevention of migraines; fever; menstrual-related problems; arthritis; infertility; asthma	Gastrointestinal side effects are the most common with feverfew. A "post-feverfew syndrome" has been reported in individuals who have taken feverfew for prolonged periods of time and then have abruptly stopped the herbal.
Fish oil	Hypertriglyceridemia, coronary heart disease, hypertension, asthma, depression, rheumatoid arthritis, osteoporosis, psoriasis	Heartburn, nausea, rash, and a "fishy" aftertaste can occur. Contamination with pesticides (as well as with mercury and other heavy metals) is a potential concern, although this is unlikely.
Garlic	Hyperlipidemia, hypertension, peripheral arterial disease, type 2 diabetes mellitus	Nausea, vomiting, heartburn, and body odor are most common. "Deodorized" garlic products may lack the active ingredient, allicin.
Ginger	Nausea and vomiting secondary to pregnancy, chemotherapy, motion sickness, surgery	Heartburn, belching, and dermatitis have been reported. In overdoses, ginger has been associated with central nervous system depression and arrhythmias. Efficacy for hyperemesis gravidarum is unknown, and use is not recommended.
Ginkgo	Alzheimer's disease, vascular dementias, tinnitus, acute mountain sickness, intermittent claudication	Gastrointestinal side effects, headaches, dizziness, and allergic skin reactions. Seizures have been reported in several case reports. Products should contain 24% ginkgo flavone glycosides and 6% terpenoids.
Ginseng (Panax)	Increased resistance to stress and improved well-being; increased physical stamina; depression; diabetes; erectile dysfunction	Insomnia has been reported with ginseng. Vaginal bleeding, mastalgia, and amenorrhea have also been reported.
Glucosamine sulfate	Osteoarthritis	Nausea, heartburn, skin reactions, and headache have been reported. Increased glucose concentrations have been a concern but have not been well documented. Patients with a shellfish allergy should use glucosamine with caution.
Green tea	Improve cognitive performance; prevention of breast, prostate, and colon cancer; hyperlipidemia; Parkinson's disease; obesity; diabetes; cardiovascular disease	Nausea, vomiting, dyspepsia, dizziness, insomnia, and nervousness have been reported. Side effects may be a result of the large amount of caffeine in green tea products. Hepatotoxicity has been a potential concern with green tea.
Hawthorn	Mild heart failure, angina, arrhythmias, hypertension	Mild gastrointestinal effects, dizziness, rash, palpitations, and nervousness have been reported.
Hoodia	Obesity	Side effects have not been reported. Many products lack the actual ingredient.
Horse chestnut	Chronic venous insufficiency, including varicose veins; benign prostate hyperplasia; diarrhea	Mild nausea, vomiting, dizziness, headache, and itching. Products are standardized to 16%-20% aescin.
Huperzine	Alzheimer's disease, increased alertness and energy, myasthenia gravis, memory enhancement	Nausea, vomiting, diarrhea, sweating, and blurred vision as a result of the cholinergic effects of huperzine have been reported.
Kava	Anxiety, insomnia, restlessness, seizure disorders, depression, chronic fatigue syndrome	Gastrointestinal upset, headache, dizziness, "kava" dermopathy, and allergic skin reactions. Hepatotoxicity is the primary concern with kava; some countries have banned the use of kava.
Melatonin	Jet lag, insomnia, migraine, chronic fatigue syndrome, breast cancer, osteoporosis; also used for insomnia in children with ADHD	Daytime drowsiness, headache, and dizziness have been reported. Vaginal bleeding has occurred in perimenopausal women. Melatonin from animal sources should be avoided.
Melissa	Cold sores (topically), anxiety, insomnia, Alzheimer's disease, hypertension, dyspepsia	Nausea, vomiting, dizziness, and wheezing have occurred with oral melissa.
Methylsulfonylmethane (MSM)	Chronic pain, arthritis, diabetes, osteoporosis, allergies, obesity, premenstrual syndrome	Nausea, bloating, diarrhea, fatigue, and insomnia have been associated with MSM. This substance is used frequently in combination with glucosamine and chondroitin.
Milk thistle	Protective agent against liver damage due to alcohol, acetaminophen, and carbon tetrachloride; hepatitis C	Nausea, abdominal fullness, diarrhea, and allergic reactions. Patients with a ragweed allergy should use milk thistle with caution.
Peppermint	Irritable bowel syndrome, sinusitis, morning sickness, dysmenorrhea	Heartburn has been reported, as well as laryngeal and bronchial spasm in infants and children.

Natural Products	Common Use(s)	Adverse Effects/Potential Concerns
Policosanol	Hyperlipidemia, intermittent claudication, atherosclerosis	Migraines, insomnia, dizziness, skin rash, and bleeding have been reported with policosanol. The product has antiplatelet effects.
Probiotics	Treatment and prevention of diarrhea including antibiotic-associated diarrhea; irritable bowel syndrome; atopic dermatitis; Crohn's disease	Theoretically, probiotic products may increase risk of infections in immunocompromised individuals.
Red clover phytoestrogens	Menopausal symptoms, premenstrual syndrome, asthma	Rash, myalgias, headaches, and vaginal bleeding have been reported. Theoretically, endometrial hyperplasia is an adverse effect from the use of these compounds.
Red yeast rice	Hyperlipidemia, indigestion, diarrhea, circulatory conditions, HIV/AIDS	Gastrointestinal upset and dizziness may occur. Red yeast rice may contain lovastatin-like compounds and potentially cause rhabdomyolysis.
S-adenosylmethionine (SAM-e)	Depression, anxiety, dementia, osteoarthritis, heart disease	Nausea, vomiting, diarrhea, headache, and nervousness have been reported. Concern exists that SAM-e raises homocysteine levels.
St. John's wort	Depression, anxiety, chronic fatigue syndrome, HIV/AIDS	Anxiety, gastrointestinal upset, vaginal bleeding, neuropathy, and rash can occur. Hypomania has been induced by St. John's wort.
Tea tree oil	Topical use for acne, fungal infections, lice, scabies	Local inflammation and contact dermatitis may occur.
Valerian	Insomnia, depression, chronic fatigue syndrome, menstrual cramps	Headaches, gastrointestinal upset, and drowsiness can occur. Hepatotoxicity is a potential concern with valerian.

AUTHOR: **ANNE L. HUME, PHARM.D.**

Appendix Ic

Natural Products and Drug Interactions

This table lists interactions between selected natural products and prescription and nonprescription drugs. Although many of the listed interactions are theoretical in nature and have not been documented to occur in humans, those involving St. John's wort are potentially life threatening in nature, depending on the individual drug. Other interactions are based on small studies of healthy volunteers and use pharmaceutical-quality natural products that may or may not be commercially available.

Natural Products	Drugs	Interactions
Andrographis	Immune suppressants	Andrographis may stimulate immune function, potentially decreasing the effectiveness of drugs such as cyclosporine, tacrolimus, and prednisone.
	Antihypertensive agents	Andrographis may lower blood pressure, potentiating the hypotensive effects of antihypertensive agents.
	Antiplatelet and anticoagulant agents	Andrographis may have antiplatelet activity, potentially increasing the risk of bleeding.
Black cohosh	Hepatotoxic drugs	Concern exists that the risk of hepatotoxicity with black cohosh is increased in the presence of hepatotoxic drugs such as acetaminophen.
	Cisplatin	Animal studies suggest that the efficacy of cisplatin against breast cancer cells may be decreased by black cohosh.
	CYP2D6 substrates	Black cohosh may modestly inhibit CYP2D6 enzyme activity to result in higher drug concentrations.
Butterbur	CYP3A4 inducers (Rifampin, carbamazepine, etc.)	Drugs that induce the activity of CYP3A4 increase the risk of the formation of hepatotoxic metabolites from pyrrolizidine alkaloids from some butterbur products.
Chamomile	CNS depressants (benzodiazepines, opiates, barbiturates, etc.)	Chamomile may have additive CNS depressant effects.
	CYP1A2 substrates	Chamomile may inhibit CYP1A2 enzyme activity to result in higher drug concentrations.
	CYP3A4 substrates	Chamomile may inhibit CYP3A4 enzyme activity to result in higher drug concentrations.
	Estrogens	Chamomile may compete for estrogen receptors.
	Tamoxifen	Chamomile may interfere with the effects of tamoxifen because of its estrogenic effects.
Chaste tree berry	Antipsychotic agents	Chaste tree berry may antagonize the effects of antipsychotic agents through its dopaminergic activity.
	Metoclopramide	Chaste tree berry may antagonize the effects of metoclopramide through its dopaminergic activity.
	Dopamine agonists	Chaste tree berry may possess additive effects to drugs such as levodopa and ropinirole through its dopaminergic activity.
	Oral contraceptives/estrogens	Chaste tree berry may possess additive hormonal effects.
Chondroitin	Warfarin	High-dose chondroitin has structural similarity to a heparinoid and may possess weak anticoagulant effects.
Cinnamon	Hypoglycemic agents	Cinnamon may possess additive effects on blood glucose to those of hypoglycemic agents.
Coenzyme Q10	Antihypertensive agents	Coenzyme Q10 may possess additive effects on blood pressure to those of antihypertensive agents.
	Warfarin	Coenzyme Q10 may lessen the anticoagulant effects of warfarin because of its structural similarity to vitamin K.
	Chemotherapy	The antioxidant effects of coenzyme Q10 may blunt the efficacy of certain chemotherapeutic agents that depend on the formation of free radicals.
Cranberry	CYP2C9 substrates (warfarin)	Cranberry may inhibit CYP2C9 enzyme activity to result in higher drug concentrations; evidence with warfarin is contradictory.
Dehydroepiandrosterone (DHEA)	Tamoxifen and aromatase inhibitors such as anastrozole and exemestane	DHEA may interfere with the antiestrogenic effects of these drugs.
	CYP3A4 substrates	DHEA may slightly inhibit CYP3A4 enzyme activity to result in higher drug concentrations.

AChE, Acetylcholinesterase; *CCB,* calcium channel blockers; *CNS,* central nervous system; *MAOI,* monoamine oxidase inhibitor; *PPI,* proton pump inhibitors; *SSRI,* selective serotonin reuptake inhibitors.

Continued on following page

Natural Products	Drugs	Interactions
Devil's claw	Antihypertensive agents	Devil's claw may possess additive effects on blood pressure to those of antihypertensive agents.
	Hypoglycemic agents	Devil's claw may possess additive effects on blood glucose to those of hypoglycemic agents.
	H_2 antagonists and PPI	Devil's claw may raise gastric pH and blunt the efficacy of H_2 antagonists and PPI.
	CYP3A4 substrates	Devil's claw may inhibit CYP3A4 enzyme activity to result in higher drug concentrations.
	CYP2C9 substrates	Devil's claw may inhibit CYP2C9 enzyme activity to result in higher drug concentrations.
	CYP2C19 substrates	Devil's claw may inhibit CYP2C19 enzyme activity to result in higher drug concentrations.
	Warfarin	Devil's claw may inhibit CYP2C9 enzyme activity to result in higher concentrations of warfarin; purpura has been reported.
Echinacea	Immune suppressants	Echinacea may stimulate immune function, potentially decreasing the effectiveness of drugs such as cyclosporine, tacrolimus, and prednisone.
	CYP3A4 substrates	Echinacea may modestly induce hepatic CYP3A4 enzyme activity to result in lower drug concentrations.
	CYP1A2 substrates	Echinacea may inhibit CYP1A2 enzyme activity to result in higher drug concentrations.
Eleuthero (Siberian ginseng)	CNS depressants (benzodiazepines, opiates, barbiturates, etc.)	Eleuthero may have additive CNS depressant effects.
	Antiplatelet and anticoagulant agents	Eleuthero may have antiplatelet activity, potentially increasing the risk of bleeding.
	CYP3A4 substrates	Eleuthero may inhibit CYP3A4 enzyme activity to result in higher drug concentrations.
	CYP1A2 substrates	Eleuthero may modestly inhibit CYP1A2 enzyme activity to result in higher drug concentrations.
	CYP2C9 substrates	Eleuthero may modestly inhibit CYP2C9 enzyme activity to result in higher drug concentrations.
	CYP2D6 substrates	Eleuthero may inhibit CYP2D6 enzyme activity to result in higher drug concentrations.
	Digoxin	Concentration of digoxin has been reported to increase but without evidence of toxicity.
Evening primrose oil (EPO)	Antiplatelet and anticoagulant agents	EPO may have anticoagulant activity, potentially increasing the risk of bleeding.
Fenugreek	Antiplatelet and anticoagulant agents	Fenugreek may have antiplatelet activity, potentially increasing the risk of bleeding.
	Hypoglycemic agents	Fenugreek may potentially lower blood glucose concentrations and have additive effects with hypoglycemic agents.
Feverfew	Antiplatelet and anticoagulant agents	Feverfew may have antiplatelet activity, potentially increasing the risk of bleeding.
	CYP3A4 substrates	Feverfew may inhibit CYP3A4 enzyme activity to result in higher drug concentrations.
	CYP1A2 substrates	Feverfew may inhibit CYP1A2 enzyme activity to result in higher drug concentrations.
	CYP2C9 substrates	Feverfew may inhibit CYP2C9 enzyme activity to result in higher drug concentrations.
	CYP2C19 substrates	Feverfew may inhibit CYP2C19 enzyme activity to result in higher drug concentrations.
Fish oils (omega-3 fatty acids)	Antiplatelet and anticoagulant agents	Fish oils may have antiplatelet activity, potentially increasing the risk of bleeding, although this has not been documented in humans.
	Antihypertensive agents	Fish oils may possess additive effects on blood pressure to those of antihypertensive agents.
	Oral contraceptives	Oral contraceptives may potentially interfere with the triglyceride-lowering effects of fish oil.
Garlic	Antiplatelet and anticoagulant agents	Garlic may have antiplatelet activity, potentially increasing the risk of bleeding.
	CYP3A4 substrates	Garlic may potentially induce CYP3A4 enzyme activity to result in lower drug concentrations; evidence is contradictory.
	CYP2E1 substrates	Garlic may modestly inhibit CYP2E1 enzyme activity to result in higher drug concentrations.
Ginger	Antiplatelet and anticoagulant agents	Ginger may have antiplatelet activity, potentially increasing the risk of bleeding.
	Hypoglycemic agents	Ginger may potentially lower blood glucose concentrations and have additive effects with hypoglycemic agents.
Ginkgo	Antiplatelet and anticoagulant agents	Ginkgo may have antiplatelet activity, potentially increasing the risk of bleeding.
	CYP2C19 substrates	Ginkgo may induce CYP2C19 enzyme activity to result in lower drug concentrations.
	CYP1A2 substrates	Ginkgo may modestly inhibit CYP1A2 enzyme activity to result in higher drug levels.
	CYP2C9 substrates	Ginkgo may modestly inhibit CYP2C9 enzyme activity to result in higher drug concentrations.
	CYP2D6 substrates	Ginkgo may inhibit CYP2D6 enzyme activity to result in higher drug concentrations.
Ginseng (Panax)	Antiplatelet and anticoagulant agents	Panax ginseng may have antiplatelet properties; American ginseng may decrease the effectiveness (international normalized ration [INR]) of warfarin.
	CYP2D6 substrates	Panax ginseng may modestly inhibit CYP2D6 enzyme activity to result in higher drug concentrations.
	Immune suppressants	Panax ginseng may stimulate immune function, potentially decreasing the effectiveness of drugs such as cyclosporine, tacrolimus, and prednisone.
	Hypoglycemic agents	Panax ginseng may potentially lower blood glucose levels and have additive effects with hypoglycemic agents.
Glucosamine	Warfarin	High-dose glucosamine (along with high-dose chondroitin) may have additive effects to those of warfarin because of structural similarity to heparin.

AChE, Acetylcholinesterase; *CCB,* calcium channel blockers; *CNS,* central nervous system; *MAOI,* monoamine oxidase inhibitor; *PPI,* proton pump inhibitors; *SSRI,* selective serotonin reuptake inhibitors.

Natural Products	Drugs	Interactions
Green tea extract	Antiplatelet agents	Green tea possesses compounds that may have antiplatelet activity, potentially increasing the risk of bleeding.
	Amphetamines	Caffeine in green tea may increase the risk of CNS toxicity.
	Cocaine	Caffeine in green tea may increase the risk of CNS toxicity.
	Oral contraceptives	Oral contraceptives may decrease the clearance of caffeine in green tea.
	Warfarin	Small amounts of vitamin K have been reported to be present in green tea, potentially decreasing the effectiveness of warfarin.
	Theophylline	Caffeine potentially decreases theophylline clearance.
	Verapamil	Verapamil decreases caffeine clearance, resulting in increased concentrations.
	Quinolone antibiotics	Some quinolone antibiotics decrease the clearance of caffeine.
	Hepatotoxic drugs	Concern exists that the risk of hepatotoxicity with green tea is increased in the presence of hepatotoxic drugs such as acetaminophen.
Hawthorn	β-blockers	Hawthorn and β-blockers may have additive effects on blood pressure and heart rate.
	CCB, nitrates	Hawthorn and CCB (or nitrates) may have additive effects due to coronary vasodilation.
	Digoxin	Hawthorn may have additive effects to those of digoxin.
	Phosphodiesterase inhibitors	Hawthorn may have additive vasodilatory and hypotensive effects with sildenafil, tadalafil, and vardenafil.
Horse chestnut seed extract (HCSE)	Antiplatelet and anticoagulant agents	HCSE may have antiplatelet activity, potentially increasing the risk of bleeding.
	Hypoglycemic agents	HCSE may potentially lower blood glucose concentrations and have additive effects with hypoglycemic agents.
Huperzine	AChE inhibitors (donepezil, etc.)	Huperzine may have additive effects when combined with AChE inhibitors.
	Anticholinergic drugs	The effectiveness of huperzine and/or the anticholinergic drug may be decreased by their concomitant administration.
	Cholinergic drugs (bethanechol, neostigmine, etc.)	Huperzine may have additive effects when combined with cholinergic drugs.
Kava	CYP3A4 substrates	Kava may inhibit CYP3A4 enzyme activity to result in higher drug concentrations.
	CYP1A2 substrates	Kava may inhibit CYP1A2 enzyme activity to result in higher drug concentrations.
	CYP2C9 substrates, CYP2C19 substrates	Kava may inhibit CYP2C9 and CYP2C19 enzyme activity to result in higher drug concentrations.
	CYP2D6 substrates	Kava may inhibit CYP2D6 enzyme activity to result in higher drug concentrations.
	P-glycoprotein substrates (digoxin; etoposide, paclitaxel, vinblastine, vincristine; itraconazole; diltiazem, verapamil; and many other drugs)	Kava may inhibit P-glycoprotein transporter systems.
	Hepatotoxic drugs	Concern exists that the risk of hepatotoxicity from kava is increased in the presence of hepatotoxic drugs such as acetaminophen.
Melatonin	Antiplatelet and anticoagulant agents	Melatonin may potentiate the effects of antiplatelets and anticoagulants, although the mechanism is unknown.
	CNS depressants	Melatonin may have additive CNS depressant effects.
	Fluvoxamine	Fluvoxamine may increase levels of melatonin.
	Immune suppressants	Melatonin may stimulate immune function, potentially decreasing the effectiveness of drugs such as cyclosporine, tacrolimus, and prednisone.
	Hypoglycemic agents	Melatonin may impair glucose utilization and may decrease the efficacy of hypoglycemic agents.
Milk thistle	Estrogens (and other drugs that undergo glucuronidation)	Silymarin may increase the clearance of estrogens.
	CYP2C9 substrates	Milk thistle may modestly inhibit CYP2C9 enzyme activity to result in higher drug concentrations.
Peppermint oil	H_2 antagonists and proton pump inhibitors	Peppermint oil may raise gastric pH and blunt efficacy of H_2 antagonists and PPI.
	CYP3A4 substrates	Peppermint oil may modestly inhibit CYP3A4 enzyme activity to result in higher drug concentrations.
	CYP1A2 substrates	Peppermint oil may modestly inhibit CYP1A2 enzyme activity to result in higher drug concentrations.
	CYP2C9 substrates, CYP2C19 substrates	Peppermint oil may modestly inhibit CYP2C9 and CYP2C19 enzyme activity to result in higher drug concentrations.
Policosanol	Antiplatelet and anticoagulant agents	Policosanol may have antiplatelet activity, potentially increasing the risk of bleeding.
Probiotics	Antibiotics	Antibiotics may kill the live organisms in different probiotic preparations.
	Immune suppressants	Theoretically, probiotics may cause bacterial or fungal infections in patients who are taking immune suppressants chronically.

Continued on following page

Natural Products	Drugs	Interactions
Red clover phytoestrogens	Antiplatelet and anticoagulant agents Tamoxifen/aromatase inhibitors	Theoretically, red clover may possess coumarins, which increase the risk of bleeding with antiplatelet and anticoagulants.
	CYP3A4 substrates	Red clover may inhibit CYP3A4 enzyme activity to result in higher drug concentrations.
	CYP2C9 substrates, CYP2C19 substrates	Red clover may inhibit CYP2C9 and CYP2C19 enzyme activity to result in higher drug concentrations.
	CYP1A2 substrates	Red clover may inhibit CYP1A2 enzyme activity to result in higher drug concentrations.
Red yeast rice	CYP3A4 inhibitors	Drugs that inhibit CYP3A4 may decrease the metabolism of lovastatin in red yeast rice.
	Statins	Red yeast rice contains lovastatin and increases the risk of myopathy (and hepatotoxicity).
	Fibrates and niacin	Fibrates and niacin may increase concentrations of lovastatin in red yeast rice.
S-adenosylmethionine (SAM-e)	Antidepressants (including MAOIs)	Additive effects are possible, and there is potential for toxicity.
	Serotonergic drugs (triptans, SSRIs, tramadol, meperidine, dextromethorphan, etc.)	SAM-e may increase the risk of development of serotonin syndrome when used concomitantly.
Soy phytoestrogens	Antibiotics	Antibiotics may decrease the efficacy of soy because intestinal bacteria convert isoflavones into more active forms.
	Estrogens	Soy potentially may inhibit the effects of estrogen.
	Tamoxifen/aromatase inhibitors	Soy's estrogenic effects may antagonize the antitumor effects of tamoxifen/aromatase inhibitors.
	MAOIs	Fermented soy products may contain tyramine.
St. John's wort	CYP3A4 substrates	St. John's wort strongly induces CYP3A4 enzyme activity to result in lower drug concentrations.
	CYP1A2 substrates	St. John's wort modestly induces CYP1A2 enzyme activity to result in lower drug levels.
	CYP2C9 substrates	St. John's wort induces CYP2C9 enzyme activity to result in lower drug concentrations.
	P-glycoprotein substrates (digoxin; etoposide, paclitaxel, vinblastine, vincristine; itraconazole; diltiazem, verapamil; and other drugs)	St. John's wort induces P-glycoprotein transporter systems.
	Serotonergic drugs (triptans, SSRIs, tramadol, meperidine, dextromethorphan, etc.)	St. John's wort may increase the risk of development of serotonin syndrome when used concomitantly.
Valerian	CNS depressants (benzodiazepines, opiates, barbiturates, alcohol, etc.)	Valerian may increase the sedative effects of CNS depressants.
	CYP3A4 substrates	Valerian may modestly inhibit the CYP3A4 enzyme activity.

AChE, Acetylcholinesterase; *CCB,* calcium channel blockers; *CNS,* central nervous system; *MAOI,* monoamine oxidase inhibitor; *PPI,* proton pump inhibitors; *SSRI,* selective serotonin reuptake inhibitors.

EXAMPLES OF DRUGS METABOLIZED BY CYP ENZYMES

The following are example drugs that are metabolized through the different cytochrome P450 isoenzymes:

CYP1A2 substrates: theophylline, imipramine, clozapine, naproxen

CYP2C9 substrates: warfarin, tamoxifen, irbesartan, ibuprofen, glipizide

CYP2C19 substrates: omeprazole and other proton pump inhibitors, phenytoin, phenobarbital, cyclophosphamide

CYP2D6 substrates: S-metoprolol, propafenone, paroxetine, risperidone, tramadol

CYP2E1 substrates: acetaminophen, alcohol

CYP3A4 substrates: most statins, indinavir, amlodipine, verapamil, alprazolam, buspirone

(For a complete list of drugs and their respective metabolic pathways through the cytochrome P450 isoenzyme systems go to http://medicine.iupui.edu/flockhart.)

AUTHOR: **ANNE L. HUME, PHARM.D.**

Definitions of Complementary and Alternative Medicine Terms

Acupuncture Thin needles are inserted superficially on the skin at locations throughout the body. These points are located along "channels" of energy. Heat can be applied by burning (moxibustion), electric current (electroacupuncture), or pressure (acupressure). Healing is proposed by the restoration of a balance of energy flow called *Qi*. Another explanation suggests that, possibly, the stimulation activates endorphin receptors.

Alexander Technique A bodywork technique in which rebalancing of "postural sets" (i.e., physical alignment) is taught by mentally focusing on the way correct alignments should look and feel and through verbal and tactile guidance by the practitioner.

Applied Kinesiology A form of treatment that uses nutrition, physical manipulation, vitamins, diets, and exercise to restore and energize the body. Weak muscles are proposed as a source of dysfunctional health.

Aromatherapy A form of herbal medicine that uses various oils from plants. Route of administration can be through absorption in the skin or inhalation. The aromatic biochemical structures of certain herbs are thought to act in areas of the brain related to past experiences and emotions (e.g., limbic system).

Ayurveda A major health system that originated in India and incorporates the body, mind, and spirit to prevent and treat disease. Includes special types of diets, herbs, and minerals.

Biofeedback A mind-body therapy procedure in which sensors are placed on the body to measure muscle tension, heart rate, and sweat responses or neural activity. Information is provided by visual, auditory, or body-muscle cell activation so as to teach either to increase or decrease physiologic activity, which, when reconstituted, is proposed to improve health problems (e.g., pain, anxiety, or high blood pressure). In some cases, relaxation exercises complement this procedure.

Chelation Therapy Involves the removal—through intravenous infusion of a chelating agent (synthetic amino acid ethylenediamine tetraacetic acid [EDTA])—of heavy metals, including lead, nickel, and cadmium, as a way to treat certain diseases. Ancillary treatments include the use of vitamins, changes in diet, and exercise.

Cognitive Therapy Psychologic therapy in which the major focus is altering and changing irrational beliefs through a type of Socratic dialogue and self-evaluation of certain illogical thoughts. Conditioning and learning are important components of this therapy.

Craniosacral Therapy A form of gentle manual manipulation used for diagnosis and for making corrections in a system made up of cerebrospinal fluid, cranial and dural membranes, cranial bones, and sacrum. This system is proposed to be dynamic, with its own physiologic frequency. Through touch and pressure, tension is proposed to be reduced and cranial rhythms normalized, leading to improvement in health and disease.

Modified from Spencer JW: *Complementary/alternative medicine: an evidence-based approach*, St Louis, 1999, Mosby.

Diathermy The use of high-frequency electrical currents as a form of physical therapy and in surgical procedures. The term *diathermy,* derived from the Greek words *dia* and *therma,* literally means "heating through." The three forms of diathermy used by physical therapists are short wave, ultrasound, and microwave.

Eye Movement Desensitization and Reprocessing (EMDR) A technique that proposes to remove painful memories by behavioral techniques. Rhythmic, multisaccadic eye movements are produced by allowing the patient to track and follow a moving object while imagining a stressful memory or event. By using deconditioning, including verbal interaction with the therapist, the painful memory is extinguished and health improved.

Feldenkrais Method A bodywork technique that integrates physics, judo, and yoga. The practitioner directs sequences of movement using verbal or hands-on techniques or teaches a system of self-directed exercise to treat physical impairments through the learning of new movement patterns.

Hatha Yoga The branch of yoga practice that involves physical exercise, breathing practices, and movement. These exercises are designed to have a salutary effect on posture, flexibility, and strength and are intended ultimately to prepare the body to remain still for long periods of meditation.

Hellerwork A bodywork technique that treats and improves proper body alignment through the development of a more complete awareness of the physical body. The goal is to realign fascia for improvement of standing, sitting, and breathing using "body energy," verbal feedback, and changing emotions and attitudes.

Homeopathy A form of treatment in which substances (minerals, plant extracts, chemicals, or disease-producing germs), which in sufficient doses would produce a set of illness symptoms in healthy individuals, are given in microdoses to produce a "cure" of those same symptoms. The *symptom* is not thought to be part of the illness but part of a curative process.

Hyperbaric Oxygen A therapy in which 100% oxygen is given at or above atmospheric pressure. An increase in oxygen in the tissue is proposed to increase blood circulation and improve healing and health and influence the course of disease.

Jin Shin Jyutsu An ancient bodywork technique to harmonize body, mind, and spirit by gentle touch that uses specific "healing points" at the body surface. The points are proposed to overlie flowing energy (Qi). The therapist's fingers are used to "redirect, balance, and provide a more efficient energy flow" to and throughout the body.

Light Therapy Natural light or light of specified wavelengths is used to treat disease. This may include ultraviolet light, colored light, or low-intensity laser light. Generally, the eye is the initial entry point for the light because of its direct connection to the brain.

Magnetic Therapy Magnets are placed directly on the skin, theoretically stimulating living cells and increasing blood flow by ionic currents that are created from polarities on the magnets.

Mediterranean Diet A diet that is thought to provide optimal distribution of daily caloric intake of different nutrients and includes 50% to 60% carbohydrates, 30% fats, and 10% proteins. The diet is derived from the eating habits of people in the Mediterranean area, who were shown to have reduced rates of cardiovascular disease.

Mind-Body Therapies A group of therapies that emphasize using the mind or brain in conjunction with the body to assist healing. Mind-body therapies can involve varying degrees of levels of consciousness, including *hypnosis,* in which selective attention is used to induce a specific altered state (trance) for memory retrieval, relaxation, or suggestion; *visual imagery,* in which the focus is on a target visual stimulus; *yoga,* which involves integration of posture and controlled breathing, relaxation, and/or meditation; *relaxation,* which includes lighter levels of altered states of consciousness through indirect or direct focus; and *meditation,* in which there is an intentional use of posture, concentration, contemplation, and visualization.

Muscle Energy Technique A manual therapy in osteopathic medicine that includes both passive mobilization and muscle reeducation. Diagnosis of somatic dysfunction is performed by the practitioner, after which the patient is guided to provide corrective muscle contraction.

Music Therapy The use of music in an either active or passive mode. Used mainly to reduce stress, anxiety, and pain.

Naturopathy A major health system that includes practices that emphasize diet, nutrition, homeopathy, acupuncture, herbal medicine, manipulation, and various mind-body therapies. Focal points include self-healing and treatment through changes in lifestyle and emphasis on health prevention.

Ornish Diet A life-choice program based on eating a vegetarian diet containing less than 10% fat. The diet is high in complex carbohydrates and fiber. Meat and fish are generally avoided.

Oslo Diet An eating plan that emphasizes increased intake of fish and reduced total fat intake. Diet is combined with regular endurance exercise.

Pilates An educational and exercise approach using the proper body mechanics, movements, truncal and pelvic stabilization, coordinated breathing, and muscle contractions to promote strengthening. Attention is paid to the entire musculoskeletal system.

Prayer The use of prayer(s) that are offered to "some higher being" or authority to heal and/or arrest disease. May be practiced by the individual patient, by groups, or by other(s) with or without the patient's knowledge (e.g., intercessory).

Pritikin Diet A weight management plan that is based on a vegetarian framework. Meals are low in fat, high in fiber, and high in complex carbohydrates.

Qi Gong A form of Chinese exercise-stimulation therapy that proposes to improve health by redirecting mental focus, breathing, coordination, and relaxation. The goal is to "rebalance" the body's own healing capacities by activating proposed electrical or energetic currents that flow along meridians located throughout the body. These meridians, however, do not follow conventional nerve or muscle pathways. In Chinese medical training and practice this therapy includes "external Qi," which is energy transmitted from one person to another so as to heal.

Raja Yoga Yoga practice that includes all of the other forms of yoga. The practitioner is instructed to follow moral directives, physical exercises, breathing exercises, meditation, devotion, and service to others to facilitate religious awakening.

Reflexology A bodywork technique that uses reflex points on the hands and feet. Pressure is applied at points that correspond to various body parts, to eliminate blockages thought to produce pain or disease.

Reiki Comes from the Japanese word meaning "universal life force energy." The practitioner serves as a conduit for healing energy directed into the body or energy field of the recipient without physical contact with the body.

Rolfing A bodywork technique that involves the myofascia. The body is realigned by using the hands to apply deep pressure and friction that allows more sufficient posture, movement, and the "release" of emotions from the body.

Shiatsu A Japanese bodywork technique involving finger pressure at specific points on the body mainly to balance "energy" in the body. The major focus is on prevention by keeping the body healthy. The therapy uses more than 600 points on the skin that are proposed to be connected to pathways through which energy flows.

T'ai Chi A technique that uses slow, purposeful motor-physical movements of the body to control and achieve a more balanced physiologic and psychologic state.

Therapeutic Touch A body energy field technique in which hands are passed over the body without actually touching to recreate and change proposed "energy imbalances" for restoring innate healing forces. Verbal interaction between patient and therapist helps maximize effects.

Traditional Chinese Medicine An ancient form of medicine that focuses on prevention and secondarily treats disease with an emphasis on maintaining balance through the body by stimulating a constant, smooth-flowing Qi energy. Herbs, acupuncture, massage, diet, and exercise are also used.

Trager Psychophysical Integration A bodywork technique in which the practitioner enters a meditative state and guides the client through gentle, light, rhythmic, nonintrusive movements. "Mentastics" exercises using self-healing movements are taught to the clients.

AUTHOR: **ANNE L. HUME, PHARM.D.**

Appendix Ie

Relaxation Techniques

Relaxation Techniques

Relaxation Technique	Summary	Further Resources
Breathing exercise	This is the foundation of most relaxation techniques. Have patients place one hand on the chest and the other on the abdomen. Instruct them to take a slow, deep breath, as if they were sucking in all the air in the room. While doing this, the hand on the abdomen should rise higher than the hand on the chest. This promotes diaphragmatic breathing that increases alveolar expansion in the bases of the lungs. Have them hold the breath for a count of 7 and then exhale. Exhalation should take twice as long as inhalation. Repeat this for a total of five breaths, and encourage patients to do this three times a day.	*Conscious Breathing* by Gay Hendricks is one of many good resources on using breathing for relaxation and health.
Meditation		
Transcendental/The relaxation response	To prevent distracting thoughts, the subject repeats a mantra (a word or sound) over and over again while sitting in a comfortable position. If a distracting thought comes to mind, it is accepted and let go, with the mind focusing again on the mantra.	www.mindbody.harvard.edu or *The Relaxation Response* by Herbert Benson; www.tm.org for information on transcendental meditation.
Mindful meditation	This represents the philosophy of living in the present or in the moment. The *body scan* is one technique where the subject uses breathing to obtain a relaxed state while lying or sitting. The mind progressively focuses on different parts of the body, where it feels any and all sensations intentionally but nonjudgmentally before moving on to another part of the body. A patient with back pain may focus on the quality and characteristics of the pain as if to better understand it and bring it under control.	*Full Catastrophe Living* by Jon Kabat-Zinn describes this technique in full and the program for stress reduction at the University of Massachusetts Medical Center.
Centering prayer	This is a form similar to transcendental meditation that has a more religious foundation. The subject repeats a "sacred word" similar to a mantra. As thoughts come to mind, they are accepted and let go, clearing the mind to become more centered on the spirit within, as if the mind's preoccupied thoughts are the layers of an onion that are peeled away, allowing better understanding of the spirit at the core.	www.Centeringprayer.com; look under "method of centering prayer" for a nondenominational discussion.
Progressive muscle relaxation (PMR)	A form of relaxation in which the subject is attuned to the difference in feeling when the muscles are tensed and then relaxed. In a comfortable position, start by tensing the whole body from head to toe. While doing this, notice the feelings of tightness. Take a deep breath in and as you let it out, let the tension release and the muscles relax. This is then followed by progressive tension and relaxation throughout the body. One may start by clenching the fists and then tensing the arms, shoulders, chest, abdomen, hips, legs, and so on, with each step followed by relaxation.	www.uaex.edu/publications/pub/fshei28.htm is a good review of PMR as well as other relaxation exercises. It is sponsored by the University of Arkansas. *You Must Relax* is a book by the founder of this technique, Edmund Jacobson.
Visualization/Self-hypnosis	The subject uses visualization to recruit images that create a relaxed state. For example, if a person is anxious, visualizing images of a place and a time that were peaceful and comforting would help induce relaxation. This is best used in conjunction with a breathing exercise.	There are many audiocassettes that can guide people through a visualization "script" that can result in relaxation. Emmett Miller is one well-known author.
Autogenic training	This induces a physiologic response by using simple phrases. For example, "My legs are heavy and warm" is meant to increase the blood flow to this area, resulting in relaxation. This is done progressively from head to toe with the use of deep breathing and repetition of the phrase. After completing this, focus attention on any body part that may still be tense, and then focus the breath and phrase to that area until the whole body is relaxed.	The British Autogenic Society at www.autogenictherapy.org.uk is a good resource for more information.

From Rakel RE (ed): *Principles of family practice,* ed 6, Philadelphia, 2002, WB Saunders.

Continued on following page

Relaxation Techniques—cont'd

Relaxation Technique	Summary	Further Resources
Exercise/Movement		
Aerobic	While performing an aerobic exercise, focus attention on a phrase, sound, word, or prayer and passively disregard other thoughts that may enter the mind. Some may focus on their breathing, saying to themselves, "In" with inhalation and "Out" with exhalation, or repeating "one-two, one-two" with each step they take with jogging. Doing this will help the mind focus, preventing other thoughts that may cause tension.	*Beyond the Relaxation Response* by Herbert Benson includes discussion of his research on inducing the relaxation response while exercising.
Yoga	This has been practiced for thousands of years in India. In America, it has been divided into three aspects: breathing (pranayama yoga), bodily postures or asanas (hatha yoga), and meditation to maintain balance and health. Regular practice induces relaxation.	For the following therapies, it is best to encourage patients to take a class at a local community center or gym and to pick up an introductory book at a library or bookstore.
T'ai chi	An ancient Chinese martial art that uses slow, graceful movements combined with inner mindfulness and breathing techniques to help bring balance between the mind and body.	See above.
Qi gong	A traditional Chinese practice that uses movement, meditation, and controlled breathing to balance the body's vital energy force, Qi.	See above.

Index

A

Bolded page numbers indicate principal textual treatment. Page numbers followed by f indicate figures; t, tables; b, boxes.

C

D

F

H

I

J

K

L

M

O

P

U

W

OPHTHALMOLOGY

ORTHOPEDICS

OTORHINOLARYNGOLOGY (ENT)

PEDIATRICS